Length of Stay
by Diagnosis
Western Region, 2008

LOS
Length of Stay

ISBN   978-1-57372-391-6
ISSN   0895-9862

Statistics reported in the 2008 edition are drawn from individual patient discharge records for the time period October 1, 2006, through September 30, 2007 (federal fiscal year 2007). This volume is one of the books in the *Length of Stay by Diagnosis and Operation* series

Length of Stay by Diagnosis and Operation, United States
ISSN 0895-9824

Length of Stay by Diagnosis and Operation, Northeastern Region
ISSN 0895-9838

Length of Stay by Diagnosis and Operation, North Central Region
ISSN 0895-9846

Length of Stay by Diagnosis and Operation, Southern Region
ISSN 0895-9854

Length of Stay by Diagnosis and Operation, Western Region
ISSN 0895-9862

Pediatric Length of Stay by Diagnosis and Operation, United States
ISSN 0891-1223

Thomson Reuters
777 E. Eisenhower Parkway
Ann Arbor, MI 48108
+1 800 366 7526

Length of Stay by Diagnosis and Operation, Western Region, 2008

Printed and bound in the United States of America

Limitations of Thomson Reuters (The Publisher) Liability
It is understood by users of this publication that the information contained herein is intended to serve as a guide and basis for general comparisons and evaluations, but not as the sole basis upon which any specific material conduct is to be recommended or undertaken. All users of this publication agree to hold The Publisher harmless from any and all claims, losses, damages, obligations or liabilities, directly or indirectly relating to this publication, caused thereby or arising therefrom. In no event shall The Publisher have any liability for lost profits or for indirect, special, punitive, or consequential damages or any liability to any third party, even if The Publisher is advised of the possibility of such damages.

Publications Return Policy
Printed books may be returned, in good condition, for a full refund (minus a $50 handling fee) within 10 **business** days of receipt. Electronic files (i.e., CDs, tapes, diskettes) are not refundable but are guaranteed against physical defects. If your publication arrives damaged, or you need to return it for another reason, please call Customer Service immediately at (800) 568-3282.

ISSN 0895-9862
ISBN 978-1-57372-391-6

CONTENTS

INTRODUCTION

The *Length of Stay* Series: Real Patient Data for Powerful Decision Making

Today's health care professionals are challenged to reduce unnecessary stays and services without sacrificing quality of care. As a result, medical management continues to move toward a more aggressive style of managing inpatient care. This approach makes it essential to establish *Length of Stay* targets that are not only realistic, but based on real benchmark data that reflect the complexity of your patient population.

The *Length of Stay* (LOS) series is unique. It is the only resource based solely on objective, quantitative data that are consistent and complete across the United States. This methodology ensures that the focus is on statistical rather than anecdotal evidence. This series provides empirical data based on millions of discharges, enabling you to identify true utilization and achieve benchmark performance.

The *Length of Stay* series was created to help you provide quality care while reducing health care costs—by efficiently managing inpatient cases. With LOS percentiles and demographic breakdowns, this product is the industry's most powerful tool to determine stays by any sizable patient population—from the lowest realistic level to median stays, and stays at the highest outlier levels. While these percentiles are based on real data from actual inpatient records, other products' panel-determined goals are based on subjective analysis.

Each patient is unique, and the *Length of Stay* series allows you to factor in those differences. These LOS standards address the illness complexity and age of your patients by providing norms for both simple and more complex patients. Unlike some panel-determined goals, which address only the simple uncomplicated patient, our LOS provides figures for multiple diagnosis patients who have had a significant procedure performed and those who have not.

Designed for Easy Use

We designed the *Length of Stay by Diagnosis and Operation* series to be user-friendly. The front section of each book includes information on practical applications of the data, a step-by-step guide to using the tables, and a description of the data source. The LOS tables themselves include data organized by ICD-9-CM code and represent every diagnosis and procedure group. The tables examine average, median, and percentile length of stay for patients in five age groups, with single and multiple diagnoses or procedures, and according to whether the patient's stay included a significant procedure.

The appendices include counts of U.S. hospitals by bed size, region, census division, setting (rural or urban), and teaching intensity; a list of the states included in each LOS comparative region; and in the procedure volume, a table showing operative status of every procedure code included in the book. The glossary defines all of the terms used in the tables. An alphabetical index of diagnoses and procedures grouped according to classification categories can assist users who do not know the ICD-9-CM code for a particular diagnosis.

Length of Stay Data for a Variety of Needs

There are seven different editions of *Length of Stay*, making it easy to find the information you need. Each book in the series is updated annually.

Length of Stay by Diagnosis and Operation provides data representing every ICD-9-CM diagnosis and procedure group.

- National and regional (Northeastern, North Central, Southern, and Western) editions
- National Pediatric edition, with data for patients 19 years old and younger

Psychiatric Length of Stay by Diagnosis catalogs diagnoses unique to psychiatric and substance abuse treatment.

- National—available in electronic format only

Each title is available electronically for efficient analysis. The files load easily onto virtually any system, and give you the convenience to review, set LOS targets, and plan your utilization management quickly. With these files, you can generate custom reports and incorporate the data into your own decision support systems. Call at 800-568-3282 or send an email to healthcare.pubs@thomsonreuters.com for details.

About Thomson Reuters

The Healthcare business of Thomson Reuters produces insights, information, benchmarks and analysis that enable organizations to manage costs, improve performance and enhance the quality of healthcare. Thomson Reuters is the world's leading source of intelligent information for businesses and professionals. We combine industry expertise with innovative technology to deliver critical information to leading decision makers in the financial, legal, tax and accounting, scientific, healthcare and media markets, powered by the world's most trusted news organization. With headquarters in New York and major operations in London and Eagan, Minnesota, Thomson Reuters employs more than 50,000 people in 93 countries. Thomson Reuters shares are listed on the New York Stock Exchange (NYSE: TRI); Toronto Stock Exchange (TSX: TRI); London Stock Exchange (LSE: TRIL); and Nasdaq (NASDAQ: TRIN). For more information, go to www.thomsonreuters.com.

DESCRIPTION OF THE DATABASE

Thomson Reuters LOS standards are based on all-payer data gathered from more than 20 million actual inpatient records, representing more than 50 percent of discharges from U.S. hospitals annually. This detail-rich database is our Projected Inpatient Database (PIDB), which is the largest all-payer inpatient database available in the marketplace. The PIDB supports publications, products, and custom studies whose results are applicable to all short-term, general, nonfederal (STGNF) hospitals in the United States. This exclusive database combines data from both public and proprietary state data as well as individual and group hospital contracts. Updated quarterly, the PIDB is used to create the Length of Stay series and many other of our methodologies and products.

Methodology

The PIDB is created as an external, stable, consolidated database to enable users to make accurate evaluations about the entire universe of U.S. short-term, general, nonfederal (STGNF) hospitals. To make this possible, we project the data in the PIDB so that it accurately represents the universe. First, the data are standardized from all sources to create a consolidated patient record database. Then each discharge is assigned a projection factor (or weight) to indicate the number of discharges it represents. In this way, we project the data to represent the universe of all inpatient discharges.

To create the projection factors, we use the National Inpatient Sample (NIS) for creating the universe, and other sources such as the Medicare Provider Analysis and Review File (MedPAR) are used to validate the projections. NIS is a nationally representative sample produced and published by the Agency for Healthcare Research and Quality that describes the entire universe of non-federal, general (medical or surgical) or children's general, acute care hospitals in the United States. MedPAR, produced by the Centers for Medicare & Medicaid Services, contains a complete census of all Medicare inpatient discharges.

The universe of inpatients discharged from all acute care, general, non-federal U.S. hospitals is defined using NIS. The hospital characteristics are defined according to the American Hospital Association criteria:

Short-Term: The average length of stay for all patients at the facility is less than 30 days, or more than 50 percent of all patients are admitted to units in which the average length of stay is less than 30 days.

General: The primary function of the institution is to provide patient services, diagnostic and therapeutic, for a variety of medical conditions.

Nonfederal: The facility is controlled by a state, county, city, city-county, hospital district authority, or church.

U.S. hospitals include those in the 50 states and the District of Columbia. Data from long-term specialty institutions, e.g., long-term psychiatric or rehabilitation facilities, are also excluded. For the Length of Stay publications, several exclusions are applied to the average length of stay data to eliminate discharge records that do not represent a typical short-term inpatient stay. These exclusions include admission from other short-term hospital, discharge to other short-term hospital, discharge against medical advice, and death.

Data Quality and Validation

Data from all sources in the PIDB are standardized and run through a set of standard edit screens to ensure their quality. Examples of discrepancies detected by the audit include records with invalid diagnosis or procedure codes, invalid or unrecorded principal diagnosis, sex- or age-specific diagnosis or procedure inconsistencies, and incalculable age or length of stay. All records from hospitals with more than 5 percent of discharges failing any screen are deleted from the database.

The projection methodology ensures that the PIDB will be representative of the inpatient universe defined by NIS. Using data that were not used to create the projection factors, representativeness of the PIDB has been demonstrated at the ICD-9-CM diagnosis and procedure level as well as by DRG.

To perform a comparison between PIDB data and NHDS, the weighted discharges in the PIDB were grouped within ICD-9-CM diagnosis and procedure chapters, as were the discharges in NIS. PIDB patients were compared to the NIS for the same age range. The diagnosis and procedure chapter distributions of the PIDB were found to be highly representative of NIS.

Concordance between DRG-specific Medicare estimates from the PIDB and the actual Medicare counts as found in MedPAR were compared. The correlation between the PIDB and MedPAR counts is 99.9%. Because the PIDB projection methodology accounts for payer, the representativeness of the PIDB is not limited to the Medicare population, but rather is applicable across all payer types.

BENEFITS AND APPLICATIONS

The *Length of Stay* series is an invaluable standard reference for health care professionals who want to measure inpatient utilization. Using the hospital stay data found in this series, you can compare regional and national norms to an individual institution or a special population. Specifically, the *Length of Stay* series allows you to

- establish baselines (benchmarking);

- pre-authorize procedures;

- identify candidates for utilization review;

- project extended stay reviews;

- develop forecasts;

- and report lengths of stay versus benchmarks.

Patient severity, managed care market presence, and varying practice patterns all have significant impact on actual LOS statistics. As technological advances and financial pressures reduce inpatient days and increase outpatient volumes, only the most severely ill patients are left in the hospitals. Consequently, health care professionals must have detailed measurement criteria to make truly accurate, patient-focused assessments of appropriate lengths of stay.

Because the *Length of Stay* series is based on real patient data, you can tailor your LOS analyses to a particular patient age group, or compare the norms for patients with single or multiple diagnoses. You may also study regional variations, as well as specialized groups including pediatric and psychiatric patient populations. And the 10th, 25th, 50th, 75th, 95th, and 99th percentile groups enhance the average length of stay data by allowing you to pick a realistic goal for an individual patient. Our LOS data can help pinpoint whether patients are being cared for efficiently, targeting areas that may need further clinical analysis.

The proliferation of new laws regulating utilization management procedures—in part, by requiring the disclosure of criteria used—is fueling the demand for high quality data. To comply with these new legal stipulations and to track fluctuating LOS trends, utilization managers must have reliable, industry-accepted criteria sets. Because we update the *Length of Stay* series annually with millions of new patient records, it provides extremely useful trend information—including significant developments from one year to the next and over even longer periods of time. Compiled from our exclusive Projected Inpatient Database (PIDB), the largest all-payor inpatient database available in the marketplace, this series is the most comprehensive, current source for length of stay data available.

HOW TO USE THE TABLES

The data in each *Length of Stay* volume are organized numerically by the International Classification of Diseases, 9th Revision, Clinical Modification (ICD-9-CM) coding system. Each Diagnosis volume contains every diagnosis chapter (three-digit code), including both summary and valid detail codes, and the approximately 1,500 four- and five-digit codes highest in projected volume. Each Operation volume contains every procedure chapter (two-digit code) including both summary codes and valid detail codes, and the approximately 950 four-digit codes highest in projected volume.

Data are categorized by number of observed patients, average length of stay, variance, and distribution percentiles. In addition, two subtotals and a grand total are included. All data elements except the number of observed patients are calculated using the projection methodology described in the "Description of the Database" section.

Determining length of stay would be easy if all patients were identical, but they are not. Illness, complexity, age, and region of the country will cause some variation in the LOS of patients admitted with the same diagnosis or procedure. We recognize those differences and our data tables let you to do the same. The *Length of Stay* series gives you detailed length of stay breakdowns—by individual ICD-9-CM code—listed by age groups, single versus multiple diagnosis patient, and operated versus non-operated status. You can find specific length of stay norms by taking the following steps

Step 1 Find the desired ICD-9-CM code in the tables in one of the *Length of Stay* volumes. If you do not know a patient's ICD-9-CM code, refer to the index, which provides an alphabetical listing of the descriptive titles for all codes included in the book.

The **Observed Patients** column gives you the number of patients in the stratified group as reported in our projected inpatient database. "Observed" means that this data element, unlike the other elements in the LOS tables, is not projected. Patients with stays longer than 99 days (indicated as ">99") are not included.

Step 2 For each diagnosis code, patients are stratified by single or multiple diagnoses, operated or not operated status, and age. For each procedure code, patients are stratified by single or multiple diagnoses and age. Find the appropriate portion of the table for review by using the following patient information

- Number of diagnoses

- Operated status

- Age

Single or Multiple Diagnoses

More than 80 percent of all admissions are complicated (have more than one diagnosis). The data tables include rows for patients with single and multiple diagnoses. This enables you to identify stays that are realistic and on-target with the patient's unique characteristics.

Patients are classified in the multiple diagnoses category if they had at least one valid secondary diagnosis in addition to the principal one. The following codes are not considered valid secondary diagnoses for purposes of this classification

1. Manifestation codes (conditions that evolved from underlying diseases [etiology] and are in italics in ICD-9-CM, Volume 1)

2. Codes V27.0-V27.9 (outcome of delivery)

3. E Codes (external causes of injury and poisoning)

Operated or Not Operated

In the diagnosis tables, operated patients are those who had at least one procedure that is classified by CMS as an operating room procedure. CMS physician panels classify every ICD-9-CM procedure code according to whether the procedure would in most hospitals be performed in the operating room. This classification system differs slightly from that used in *Length of Stay* publications published before 1995, in which patients were categorized as "operated" if any of their procedures were labeled as Uniform Hospital Discharge Data Set (UHDDS) Class 1. Appendix C contains a list of procedure codes included in this series and their CMS-defined operative status.

Patient's Age

The data tables illustrate the impact of age by providing five age group breakouts. These ages are from the day of the patient's admission.

For diagnosis codes V30-V39, which pertain exclusively to newborns, age is replaced by birth weight in grams. Newborns with unrecorded birth weights with secondary diagnosis codes in the 764.01-764.99 and 765.01-765.19 ranges have been assigned to the appropriate birth weight category on the basis of the fifth digit of these codes. (Data for patients whose birth weights cannot be determined by using this method are included only in the Subtotal and Total rows of the table.)

Step 3 Choose from the average stay or the 10th, 25th, 50th, 75th, 95th, and 99th percentile columns to find the appropriate length of stay for your patient. Our LOS standards document the statistical range of stays for each patient group. These ranges are represented as percentiles, so that you can determine a more aggressive (benchmark) or less aggressive (norm) LOS for your patient, depending on individual variables, and are all backed by actual patient data.

Average Length of Stay

The average length of stay is calculated from the admission and discharge dates by counting the day of admission as the first day; the day of discharge is not included. The average is figured by adding the lengths of stay for each patient and then dividing by the total number of patients. Patients discharged on the day of admission are counted as staying one day. Patients with stays over 99 days (>99) are excluded from this calculation.

Median and Percentiles

A statistical range of stays are presented for each patient group. These ranges are represented as percentiles, so that you can determine a more aggressive or less aggressive LOS for your patient, depending on individual variables such as illness complications, age, etc. A length of stay percentile for a stratified group of patients is determined by arranging the individual patient stays from low to high. Counting up from the lowest stay to the point where one-half of the patients have been counted yields the value of the 50th percentile. Counting one-tenth of the total patients gives the 10th percentile, and so on.

The 10th, 25th, 50th, 75th, 90th, 95th, and 99th percentiles of stay are displayed in days. If, for example, the 10th percentile for a group of patients is four, then 10 percent of the patients stayed four days or fewer. The 50th percentile is the median. Any percentile with a value of 100 days or more is listed as >99. Patients who were hospitalized more than 99 days (>99) are not included in the total patients, average stay, and variance categories. The percentiles, however, do include these patients.

Step 4 Consult the total patient sample (**Observed Patients** column) and variance to consider the homogeneity of the data (i.e., to what extent length of stay averages are clustered or spread out within a particular patient group).

The **Total** row represents a subtotal for each of the patient age groups. The **Grand Total** row represents the total number of patients in the specified diagnosis or procedure category.

The **variance** is a measure of the spread of the data (from the lowest to the highest value) around the average. As such, it shows how much individual patient stays ranged around the average. The smallest variance is zero, indicating that all lengths of stay are equal. In tables in which there is a large variance and the patient group size is relatively small, the average stay may appear high. This sometimes occurs when one or two patients with long hospitalizations fall into the group.

FEATURES OF A DIAGNOSIS TABLE

ICD-9-CM diagnosis code and title ⎯⎯⎯

008.8 VIRAL ENTERITIS NOS

Type of Patients	Observed Patients	Avg. Stay	Vari-ance	Percentiles						
				10th	25th	50th	75th	90th	95th	99th
1. SINGLE DX										
A. Not Operated										
0–19 Years	1346	1.9	2	1	1	2	2	3	4	5
20–34	416	1.7	<1	1	1	2	2	3	3	5
35–49	213	2.3	3	1	1	2	3	3	5	10
50–64	89	2.0	3	1	1	1	3	3	4	12
65+	55	2.8	3	1	2	2	3	6	6	9
B. Operated										
0–19 Years	24	2.5	1	1	2	2	3	4	5	6
20–34	21	2.6	<1	1	2	3	3	3	3	4
35–49	6	4.2	2	2	4	5	5	5	5	6
50–64	1	2.0	0	2	2	2	2	2	2	2
65+	0									
2. MULTIPLE DX										
A. Not Operated										
0–19 Years	5020	2.3	5	1	1	2	3	4	5	8
20–34	1625	2.2	3	1	1	2	3	4	5	7
35–49	1453	2.7	3	1	1	2	3	5	6	9
50–64	1301	2.9	3	1	2	2	4	5	6	9
65+	2964	3.6	7	1	2	3	4	7	9	13
B. Operated										
0–19 Years	35	4.3	9	2	2	4	4	8	9	13
20–34	32	3.8	9	1	2	3	4	8	12	12
35–49	23	5.7	20	1	3	4	8	11	20	20
50–64	10	8.0	50	3	4	6	7	25	25	28
65+	27	14.0	92	4	7	10	18	30	31	43
SUBTOTALS										
1. SINGLE DX										
A. Not Operated	2119	1.9	2	1	1	2	2	3	4	7
B. Operated	52	2.9	1	1	2	3	3	5	5	6
2. MULTIPLE DX										
A. Not Operated	12363	2.7	5	1	1	2	3	5	6	10
B. Operated	127	6.7	46	2	3	4	8	15	20	31
1. SINGLE DX	**2171**	**2.0**	**2**	**1**	**1**	**2**	**2**	**3**	**4**	**7**
2. MULTIPLE DX	**12490**	**2.7**	**6**	**1**	**1**	**2**	**3**	**5**	**7**	**10**
A. NOT OPERATED	**14482**	**2.6**	**5**	**1**	**1**	**2**	**3**	**5**	**6**	**9**
B. OPERATED	**179**	**5.2**	**31**	**2**	**2**	**3**	**5**	**10**	**15**	**30**
TOTAL										
0–19 Years	6425	2.3	4	1	1	2	3	4	5	8
20–34	2094	2.1	3	1	1	2	3	4	4	7
35–49	1695	2.7	4	1	1	2	3	5	6	10
50–64	1401	2.8	4	1	2	2	3	5	6	9
65+	3046	3.7	8	1	2	3	5	7	9	15
GRAND TOTAL	**14661**	**2.6**	**5**	**1**	**1**	**2**	**3**	**5**	**6**	**10**

Because each patient is unique, we stratify patients by single or multiple diagnoses, operated or not operated, status, and age.

Length of stay (in days) by percentile document the statistical range of stays for each patient group, so you can determine the right length of stay for your patient.

Total number of patients

Observed Patients is the actual number of patient discharges. We derive length of stay figures from real patient data projected to represent the inpatient universe. See "Description of the Database" for further explanation.

The variance shows how much the individual patient lengths of stay ranged around the average.

Average length of stay, in days, calculated from the admission and discharge dates

LENGTH OF STAY TABLES

DIAGNOSIS CODES

Western Region, October 2006–September 2007 Data, by Diagnosis

SUMMARY OF ALL PATIENTS IN DIAGNOSIS CODES

Type of Patients	Observed Patients	Avg. Stay	Variance	Percentiles						
				10th	25th	50th	75th	90th	95th	99th
1. SINGLE DX										
A. Not Operated										
0–19 Years	320,030	1.9	1	1	1	2	2	3	3	4
20–34	170,100	1.9	3	1	1	2	2	3	3	7
35–49	22,602	2.6	13	1	1	2	2	4	7	19
50–64	8,613	3.1	25	1	1	2	3	6	9	26
65+	3,171	2.5	12	1	1	2	3	5	7	17
B. Operated										
0–19 Years	61,226	2.0	1	1	1	2	2	3	4	6
20–34	59,700	2.4	2	1	1	2	3	4	4	6
35–49	25,949	2.1	3	1	1	2	3	4	5	8
50–64	20,589	2.3	3	1	1	2	3	4	5	8
65+	8,880	2.3	2	1	1	2	3	4	5	7
2. MULTIPLE DX										
A. Not Operated										
0–19 Years	694,408	3.2	27	1	1	2	3	5	8	27
20–34	518,570	3.0	14	1	1	2	3	5	8	19
35–49	441,492	3.9	22	1	2	3	4	8	11	24
50–64	575,039	4.4	26	1	2	3	5	9	13	25
65+	1,119,795	4.6	19	1	2	3	6	9	12	22
B. Operated										
0–19 Years	135,780	4.0	54	1	2	2	4	6	12	51
20–34	275,503	3.8	19	1	2	3	4	6	8	22
35–49	272,049	4.1	28	1	2	3	4	8	12	28
50–64	361,659	4.8	38	1	2	3	5	10	15	31
65+	494,348	5.4	34	1	2	4	7	11	16	29
SUBTOTALS:										
1. SINGLE DX										
A. Not Operated	524,516	1.9	3	1	1	2	2	3	3	6
B. Operated	176,344	2.2	2	1	1	2	3	4	4	7
2. MULTIPLE DX										
A. Not Operated	3,349,304	3.9	22	1	2	3	4	8	11	23
B. Operated	1,539,339	4.6	33	1	2	3	5	9	14	29
1. SINGLE DX	700,860	2.0	3	1	1	2	2	3	4	7
2. MULTIPLE DX	4,888,643	4.1	26	1	2	3	5	8	12	25
A. NOT OPERATED	3,873,820	3.7	20	1	2	2	4	7	10	22
B. OPERATED	1,715,683	4.4	31	1	2	3	5	9	13	28
TOTAL										
0–19 Years	1,211,444	2.9	23	1	1	2	3	4	7	23
20–34	1,023,873	3.0	13	1	2	2	3	5	7	18
35–49	762,092	3.9	24	1	2	3	4	8	11	25
50–64	965,900	4.5	30	1	2	3	5	9	13	28
65+	1,626,194	4.8	23	1	2	3	6	10	13	24
GRAND TOTAL	5,589,503	3.9	23	1	2	3	4	8	11	24

SUMMARY OF ALL PATIENTS IN DIAGNOSIS CODES EXCEPT NEWBORNS

Type of Patients	Observed Patients	Avg. Stay	Variance	Percentiles						
				10th	25th	50th	75th	90th	95th	99th
1. SINGLE DX										
A. Not Operated										
0–19 Years	61,732	2.0	3	1	2	2	2	3	4	8
20–34	170,100	1.9	3	1	1	2	2	3	3	7
35–49	22,602	2.6	13	1	1	2	2	4	7	19
50–64	8,613	3.1	25	1	1	2	3	6	9	26
65+	3,171	2.5	12	1	1	2	3	5	7	17
B. Operated										
0–19 Years	23,755	2.1	3	1	2	2	3	4	5	8
20–34	59,700	2.4	2	1	1	2	3	4	4	6
35–49	25,949	2.1	3	1	1	2	3	4	5	8
50–64	20,589	2.3	3	1	1	2	3	4	5	8
65+	8,880	2.3	2	1	1	2	3	4	5	7
2. MULTIPLE DX										
A. Not Operated										
0–19 Years	205,012	3.2	16	1	2	2	3	6	9	20
20–34	518,570	3.0	14	1	1	2	3	5	8	19
35–49	441,492	3.9	22	1	2	3	4	8	11	24
50–64	575,039	4.4	26	1	2	3	5	9	13	25
65+	1,119,795	4.6	19	1	2	3	6	9	12	22
B. Operated										
0–19 Years	53,267	4.7	43	1	2	3	5	9	14	36
20–34	275,503	3.8	19	1	2	3	4	6	8	22
35–49	272,049	4.1	28	1	2	3	4	8	12	28
50–64	361,659	4.8	38	1	2	3	5	10	15	31
65+	494,348	5.4	34	1	2	4	7	11	16	29
SUBTOTALS:										
1. SINGLE DX										
A. Not Operated	266,218	2.0	5	1	2	2	2	3	4	9
B. Operated	138,873	2.3	2	1	2	2	3	4	5	7
2. MULTIPLE DX										
A. Not Operated	2,859,908	4.0	20	1	2	3	5	8	11	22
B. Operated	1,456,826	4.7	32	1	2	3	5	9	14	28
1. SINGLE DX	405,091	2.1	4	1	2	2	2	3	4	8
2. MULTIPLE DX	4,316,734	4.3	24	1	2	3	5	8	12	25
A. NOT OPERATED	3,126,126	3.9	19	1	2	3	4	8	11	22
B. OPERATED	1,595,699	4.5	30	1	2	3	5	9	13	28
TOTAL										
0–19 Years	343,766	3.1	18	1	2	2	3	6	8	20
20–34	1,023,873	3.0	13	1	2	2	3	5	7	18
35–49	762,092	3.9	24	1	2	3	4	8	11	25
50–64	965,900	4.5	30	1	2	3	5	9	13	28
65+	1,626,194	4.8	23	1	2	3	6	10	13	24
GRAND TOTAL	4,721,825	4.1	23	1	2	3	5	8	12	24

Length of Stay by Diagnosis and Operation, Western Region, 2008

Western Region, October 2006–September 2007 Data, by Diagnosis

001: CHOLERA

Type of Patients	Observed Patients	Avg. Stay	Variance	10th	25th	50th	75th	90th	95th	99th
1. SINGLE DX										
A. *Not Operated*										
0–19 Years	0									
20–34	0									
35–49	1	5.0	0	5	5	5	5	5	5	5
50–64	0									
65+	0									
B. *Operated*										
0–19 Years	0									
20–34	0									
35–49	0									
50–64	0									
65+	0									
2. MULTIPLE DX										
A. *Not Operated*										
0–19 Years	0									
20–34	0									
35–49	0									
50–64	0									
65+	0									
B. *Operated*										
0–19 Years	0									
20–34	0									
35–49	0									
50–64	0									
65+	0									
SUBTOTALS:										
1. SINGLE DX										
A. *Not Operated*	1	5.0	0	5	5	5	5	5	5	5
B. *Operated*	0									
2. MULTIPLE DX										
A. *Not Operated*	0									
B. *Operated*	0									
1. SINGLE DX	1	5.0	0	5	5	5	5	5	5	5
2. MULTIPLE DX	0									
A. NOT OPERATED	1	5.0	0	5	5	5	5	5	5	5
B. OPERATED	0									
TOTAL										
0–19 Years	0									
20–34	0									
35–49	1	5.0	0	5	5	5	5	5	5	5
50–64	0									
65+	0									
GRAND TOTAL	**1**	**5.0**	**0**	**5**	**5**	**5**	**5**	**5**	**5**	**5**

002: TYPHOID/PARATYPHOID FEV

Type of Patients	Observed Patients	Avg. Stay	Variance	10th	25th	50th	75th	90th	95th	99th
1. SINGLE DX										
A. *Not Operated*										
0–19 Years	5	4.8	<1	4	4	5	5	6	6	6
20–34	3	4.0	7	1	1	5	6	6	6	6
35–49	1	2.0	0	2	2	2	2	2	2	2
50–64	0									
65+	0									
B. *Operated*										
0–19 Years	0									
20–34	0									
35–49	0									
50–64	0									
65+	0									
2. MULTIPLE DX										
A. *Not Operated*										
0–19 Years	12	5.6	4	4	5	6	7	8	8	8
20–34	24	5.6	13	2	2	4	8	11	12	13
35–49	3	7.0	31	2	2	6	13	13	13	13
50–64	7	6.6	21	1	2	6	10	15	15	15
65+	3	8.0	31	2	2	9	13	13	13	13
B. *Operated*										
0–19 Years	0									
20–34	0									
35–49	0									
50–64	0									
65+	1	16.0	0	16	16	16	16	16	16	16
SUBTOTALS:										
1. SINGLE DX										
A. *Not Operated*	9	4.2	3	1	4	5	5	6	6	6
B. *Operated*	0									
2. MULTIPLE DX										
A. *Not Operated*	49	6.0	13	2	4	6	8	12	13	15
B. *Operated*	1	16.0	0	16	16	16	16	16	16	16
1. SINGLE DX	9	4.2	3	1	4	5	5	6	6	6
2. MULTIPLE DX	50	6.2	15	2	4	6	8	12	13	16
A. NOT OPERATED	58	5.7	12	2	4	5	8	11	13	15
B. OPERATED	1	16.0	0	16	16	16	16	16	16	16
TOTAL										
0–19 Years	17	5.4	3	4	4	5	6	8	8	8
20–34	27	5.4	12	1	2	4	8	11	12	13
35–49	4	5.8	27	2	2	6	13	13	13	13
50–64	7	6.6	21	1	4	6	10	15	15	15
65+	4	10.0	37	2	2	9	16	16	16	16
GRAND TOTAL	**59**	**5.9**	**13**	**2**	**4**	**5**	**8**	**12**	**13**	**16**

003: OTH SALMONELLA INFECTION

Type of Patients	Observed Patients	Avg. Stay	Variance	10th	25th	50th	75th	90th	95th	99th
1. SINGLE DX										
A. *Not Operated*										
0–19 Years	36	3.7	5	2	2	3	4	7	9	10
20–34	3	2.3	1	1	1	3	3	3	3	3
35–49	0									
50–64	1	5.0	0	5	5	5	5	5	5	5
65+	0									
B. *Operated*										
0–19 Years	0									
20–34	0									
35–49	0									
50–64	0									
65+	0									
2. MULTIPLE DX										
A. *Not Operated*										
0–19 Years	179	4.2	8	2	2	4	5	7	10	20
20–34	73	4.1	6	2	3	3	5	7	9	13
35–49	102	4.6	8	2	3	4	6	7	9	16
50–64	121	5.1	9	2	3	4	7	9	10	14
65+	183	5.7	11	3	3	5	6	9	12	19
B. *Operated*										
0–19 Years	4	6.0	2	5	5	6	8	8	8	8
20–34	4	7.8	16	3	6	6	10	12	12	12
35–49	4	15.5	40	7	7	18	18	22	22	22
50–64	6	9.5	11	5	8	9	11	15	15	15
65+	6	13.2	77	5	8	11	14	30	30	30
SUBTOTALS:										
1. SINGLE DX										
A. *Not Operated*	40	3.6	5	2	2	3	4	7	9	10
B. *Operated*	0									
2. MULTIPLE DX										
A. *Not Operated*	658	4.8	9	2	3	4	6	9	11	17
B. *Operated*	24	10.5	38	5	6	9	12	18	22	30
1. SINGLE DX	40	3.6	5	2	2	3	4	7	9	10
2. MULTIPLE DX	682	5.0	11	2	3	4	6	9	11	19
A. NOT OPERATED	698	4.8	9	2	3	4	6	9	10	17
B. OPERATED	24	10.5	38	5	6	9	12	18	22	30
TOTAL										
0–19 Years	219	4.1	8	2	2	3	5	7	9	13
20–34	80	4.2	7	2	3	3	5	8	10	13
35–49	106	5.0	13	2	3	4	6	8	11	19
50–64	128	5.3	10	2	3	4	7	9	11	15
65+	189	5.9	14	3	4	5	7	11	12	22
GRAND TOTAL	**722**	**4.9**	**11**	**2**	**3**	**4**	**6**	**9**	**11**	**19**

Length of Stay by Diagnosis and Operation, Western Region, 2008

Western Region, October 2006–September 2007 Data, by Diagnosis

003.0: SALMONELLA ENTERITIS

Type of Patients	Observed Patients	Avg. Stay	Vari- ance	10th	25th	50th	75th	90th	95th	99th
1. SINGLE DX										
A. Not Operated										
0–19 Years	22	3.1	4	1	2	3	3	5	7	10
20–34	3	2.3	1	1	1	3	3	3	3	3
35–49	0									
50–64	0									
65+	0									
B. Operated										
0–19 Years	0									
20–34	0									
35–49	0									
50–64	0									
65+	0									
2. MULTIPLE DX										
A. Not Operated										
0–19 Years	151	3.9	7	2	2	3	4	6	9	13
20–34	50	3.7	6	2	3	3	5	7	9	13
35–49	82	4.3	5	2	3	4	6	7	7	16
50–64	93	4.7	7	2	3	4	6	9	10	13
65+	134	5.1	9	3	3	4	6	9	12	16
B. Operated										
0–19 Years	3	5.3	<1	5	5	5	6	6	6	6
20–34	3	9.3	9	6	6	10	12	12	12	12
35–49	1	18.0	0	18	18	18	18	18	18	18
50–64	1	5.0	0	5	5	5	5	5	5	5
65+	3	10.0	21	5	5	11	14	14	14	14
SUBTOTALS:										
1. SINGLE DX										
A. Not Operated	25	3.0	4	1	2	3	3	5	7	10
B. Operated	0									
2. MULTIPLE DX										
A. Not Operated	510	4.4	7	2	3	4	5	7	10	13
B. Operated	11	8.8	20	5	5	6	12	14	18	18
1. SINGLE DX	25	3.0	4	1	2	3	3	5	7	10
2. MULTIPLE DX	521	4.5	8	2	3	4	5	8	10	14
A. NOT OPERATED	535	4.3	7	2	3	4	5	7	10	13
B. OPERATED	11	8.8	20	5	5	6	12	14	18	18
TOTAL										
0–19 Years	176	3.8	7	2	2	3	4	6	9	13
20–34	56	3.9	7	2	2	3	5	8	10	13
35–49	83	4.4	7	2	3	4	6	7	8	18
50–64	94	4.7	7	2	3	4	6	9	10	13
65+	137	5.2	10	3	3	4	6	9	12	16
GRAND TOTAL	546	4.4	8	2	3	4	5	8	10	14

004: SHIGELLOSIS

Type of Patients	Observed Patients	Avg. Stay	Vari- ance	10th	25th	50th	75th	90th	95th	99th
1. SINGLE DX										
A. Not Operated										
0–19 Years	18	2.4	1	1	2	2	2	3	5	5
20–34	2	3.0	2	2	2	4	4	4	4	4
35–49	1	1.0	0	1	1	1	1	1	1	1
50–64	1	3.0	0	3	3	3	3	3	3	3
65+	0									
B. Operated										
0–19 Years	0									
20–34	0									
35–49	0									
50–64	0									
65+	0									
2. MULTIPLE DX										
A. Not Operated										
0–19 Years	91	3.1	2	2	2	3	4	5	6	9
20–34	19	3.3	2	1	2	3	5	5	5	5
35–49	16	3.9	4	2	3	3	5	7	9	9
50–64	10	7.1	23	4	4	5	9	11	19	19
65+	14	4.1	2	2	3	4	5	6	7	7
B. Operated										
0–19 Years	0									
20–34	0									
35–49	0									
50–64	0									
65+	0									
SUBTOTALS:										
1. SINGLE DX										
A. Not Operated	22	2.5	1	1	2	2	2	3	4	5
B. Operated	0									
2. MULTIPLE DX										
A. Not Operated	150	3.6	5	2	2	3	4	5	7	11
B. Operated	0									
1. SINGLE DX	22	2.5	1	2	2	2	2	3	4	5
2. MULTIPLE DX	150	3.6	5	2	2	3	4	5	7	11
A. NOT OPERATED	172	3.4	4	2	2	3	4	5	7	11
B. OPERATED	0									
TOTAL										
0–19 Years	109	3.0	2	2	2	3	4	5	6	8
20–34	21	3.2	2	1	2	3	4	5	5	5
35–49	17	3.8	4	2	3	3	5	7	9	9
50–64	11	6.7	22	3	4	5	9	11	19	19
65+	14	4.1	2	2	3	4	5	6	7	7
GRAND TOTAL	172	3.4	4	2	2	3	4	5	7	11

005: OTHER FOOD POISONING

Type of Patients	Observed Patients	Avg. Stay	Vari- ance	10th	25th	50th	75th	90th	95th	99th
1. SINGLE DX										
A. Not Operated										
0–19 Years	15	3.2	14	1	1	1	1	4	11	13
20–34	6	1.2	<1	1	1	1	1	1	2	2
35–49	2	1.0	0	1	1	1	1	1	1	1
50–64	2	1.0	0	1	1	1	1	1	1	1
65+	0									
B. Operated										
0–19 Years	0									
20–34	0									
35–49	0									
50–64	0									
65+	0									
2. MULTIPLE DX										
A. Not Operated										
0–19 Years	46	4.3	123	1	1	1	2	12	12	74
20–34	75	2.0	10	1	1	1	2	3	4	27
35–49	86	3.3	84	1	1	2	2	4	8	75
50–64	147	2.2	3	1	1	2	3	4	6	9
65+	209	2.2	2	1	1	2	3	4	5	9
B. Operated										
0–19 Years	0									
20–34	0									
35–49	1	67.0	0	67	67	67	67	67	67	67
50–64	1	9.0	0	9	9	9	9	9	9	9
65+	1	3.0	0	3	3	3	3	3	3	3
SUBTOTALS:										
1. SINGLE DX										
A. Not Operated	25	2.4	10	1	1	1	2	2	11	13
B. Operated	0									
2. MULTIPLE DX										
A. Not Operated	563	2.5	26	1	1	2	2	4	6	12
B. Operated	3	26.4	>999	3	3	9	67	67	67	67
1. SINGLE DX	25	2.4	10	1	1	1	2	5	11	13
2. MULTIPLE DX	566	2.6	33	1	1	2	2	4	7	13
A. NOT OPERATED	588	2.5	25	1	1	2	2	4	6	13
B. OPERATED	3	26.4	>999	3	3	9	67	67	67	67
TOTAL										
0–19 Years	61	4.1	95	1	1	1	2	11	12	74
20–34	81	2.0	9	1	1	1	2	3	4	27
35–49	89	4.0	127	1	1	2	3	4	9	75
50–64	150	2.2	3	1	1	2	3	4	6	9
65+	210	2.2	2	1	1	2	3	4	5	9
GRAND TOTAL	591	2.6	32	1	1	2	2	4	7	13

Length of Stay by Diagnosis and Operation, Western Region, 2008

Western Region, October 2006–September 2007 Data, by Diagnosis

005.9: FOOD POISONING NOS

Type of Patients	Observed Patients	Avg. Stay	Variance	10th	25th	50th	75th	90th	95th	99th
1. SINGLE DX										
A. *Not Operated*										
0–19 Years	8	1.3	<1	1	1	1	2	2	2	2
20–34	6	1.2	<1	1	1	1	1	2	2	2
35–49	2	1.0	0	1	1	1	1	1	1	1
50–64	2	1.0	0	1	1	1	1	1	1	1
65+	0									
B. *Operated*										
0–19 Years	0									
20–34	0									
35–49	0									
50–64	0									
65+	0									
2. MULTIPLE DX										
A. *Not Operated*										
0–19 Years	34	1.3	<1	1	1	1	2	2	2	2
20–34	68	1.7	<1	1	1	1	2	3	4	5
35–49	71	1.7	1	1	1	1	2	3	3	8
50–64	131	2.0	2	1	1	2	2	3	5	7
65+	188	2.1	2	1	1	2	3	4	4	9
B. *Operated*										
0–19 Years	0									
20–34	0									
35–49	0									
50–64	0									
65+	1	3.0	0	3	3	3	3	3	3	3
SUBTOTALS:										
1. SINGLE DX										
A. *Not Operated*	18	1.2	<1	1	1	1	1	2	2	2
B. *Operated*	0									
2. MULTIPLE DX										
A. *Not Operated*	492	1.9	2	1	1	2	2	3	4	7
B. *Operated*	1	3.0	0	3	3	3	3	3	3	3
1. SINGLE DX	18	1.2	<1	1	1	1	1	2	2	2
2. MULTIPLE DX	493	1.9	2	1	1	2	2	3	4	7
A. NOT OPERATED	510	1.9	2	1	1	1	2	3	4	7
B. OPERATED	1	3.0	0	3	3	3	3	3	3	3
TOTAL										
0–19 Years	42	1.3	<1	1	1	1	2	2	2	2
20–34	74	1.7	<1	1	1	1	2	3	4	5
35–49	73	1.7	1	1	1	1	2	3	3	8
50–64	133	2.0	2	1	1	2	2	3	5	7
65+	189	2.1	2	1	1	2	3	4	4	9
GRAND TOTAL	511	1.9	2	1	1	1	2	3	4	7

006: AMEBIASIS

Type of Patients	Observed Patients	Avg. Stay	Variance	10th	25th	50th	75th	90th	95th	99th
1. SINGLE DX										
A. *Not Operated*										
0–19 Years	1	2.0	0	2	2	2	2	2	2	2
20–34	8	4.9	3	2	5	5	5	8	8	8
35–49	3	7.0	3	6	6	6	9	9	9	9
50–64	1	7.0	0	7	7	7	7	7	7	7
65+	0									
B. *Operated*										
0–19 Years	0									
20–34	0									
35–49	0									
50–64	0									
65+	0									
2. MULTIPLE DX										
A. *Not Operated*										
0–19 Years	5	8.2	30	2	4	9	10	16	16	16
20–34	18	6.9	23	2	3	6	9	15	20	20
35–49	31	7.4	49	2	3	6	8	11	15	41
50–64	23	7.3	35	2	3	5	9	20	20	23
65+	13	7.4	25	3	5	6	10	11	21	21
B. *Operated*										
0–19 Years	0									
20–34	0									
35–49	3	16.1	180	5	5	12	31	31	31	31
50–64	3	25.9	484	7	7	20	50	50	50	50
65+	0									
SUBTOTALS:										
1. SINGLE DX										
A. *Not Operated*	13	5.3	4	2	5	5	6	8	9	9
B. *Operated*	0									
2. MULTIPLE DX										
A. *Not Operated*	90	7.3	34	2	4	6	9	15	20	41
B. *Operated*	6	21.0	295	5	7	20	31	50	50	50
1. SINGLE DX	13	5.3	4	2	5	5	6	8	9	9
2. MULTIPLE DX	96	8.2	59	2	4	6	10	16	21	50
A. NOT OPERATED	103	7.1	31	2	4	6	8	11	16	23
B. OPERATED	6	21.0	295	5	7	20	31	50	50	50
TOTAL										
0–19 Years	6	7.1	30	2	2	4	10	16	16	16
20–34	26	6.3	18	2	4	5	8	11	15	20
35–49	37	8.1	57	2	5	6	8	12	31	41
50–64	27	9.3	103	2	3	7	10	20	23	50
65+	13	7.4	25	3	5	6	10	11	21	21
GRAND TOTAL	109	7.8	53	2	4	6	9	15	20	41

007: OTH PROTOZOAL INTEST DIS

Type of Patients	Observed Patients	Avg. Stay	Variance	10th	25th	50th	75th	90th	95th	99th
1. SINGLE DX										
A. *Not Operated*										
0–19 Years	1	3.0	0	3	3	3	3	3	3	3
20–34	1	2.0	0	2	2	2	2	2	2	2
35–49	0									
50–64	0									
65+	0									
B. *Operated*										
0–19 Years	0									
20–34	0									
35–49	0									
50–64	0									
65+	0									
2. MULTIPLE DX										
A. *Not Operated*										
0–19 Years	31	5.7	31	1	2	3	8	14	18	21
20–34	28	4.8	32	1	2	3	6	10	17	28
35–49	40	4.3	11	2	2	4	5	8	10	18
50–64	33	3.3	4	2	2	3	4	5	8	10
65+	26	4.3	12	2	2	3	5	7	10	18
B. *Operated*										
0–19 Years	0									
20–34	1	2.0	0	2	2	2	2	2	2	2
35–49	1	9.0	0	9	9	9	9	9	9	9
50–64	1	7.0	0	7	7	7	7	7	7	7
65+	1	16.0	0	16	16	16	16	16	16	16
SUBTOTALS:										
1. SINGLE DX										
A. *Not Operated*	2	2.5	<1	2	2	2	3	3	3	3
B. *Operated*	0									
2. MULTIPLE DX										
A. *Not Operated*	158	4.5	17	1	2	3	5	9	14	21
B. *Operated*	4	8.5	34	2	2	7	16	16	16	16
1. SINGLE DX	2	2.5	<1	2	2	2	3	3	3	3
2. MULTIPLE DX	162	4.6	18	1	2	3	5	9	14	21
A. NOT OPERATED	160	4.4	17	1	2	3	5	8	13	21
B. OPERATED	4	8.5	34	2	2	7	16	16	16	16
TOTAL										
0–19 Years	32	5.6	30	1	2	3	8	14	18	21
20–34	30	4.6	30	1	2	3	6	7	17	28
35–49	41	4.4	11	2	2	4	5	8	10	18
50–64	34	3.4	4	2	2	3	4	5	8	10
65+	27	4.8	17	2	2	3	6	10	16	18
GRAND TOTAL	164	4.5	18	1	2	3	5	9	14	21

Length of Stay by Diagnosis and Operation, Western Region, 2008

Western Region, October 2006–September 2007 Data, by Diagnosis

008: INTEST INF D/T ORG NEC

Type of Patients	Observed Patients	Avg. Stay	Variance	Percentiles						
				10th	25th	50th	75th	90th	95th	99th
1. SINGLE DX										
A. Not Operated										
0–19 Years	435	1.9	1	1	1	1	2	3	4	5
20–34	59	2.1	2	1	1	2	2	4	5	8
35–49	39	2.0	1	1	1	2	3	3	5	5
50–64	23	2.1	1	1	1	2	2	3	4	6
65+	11	2.6	3	1	1	2	3	5	7	7
B. Operated										
0–19 Years	2	1.5	<1	1	1	2	2	2	2	2
20–34	3	2.0	0	2	2	2	2	2	2	2
35–49	0									
50–64	0									
65+	0									
2. MULTIPLE DX										
A. Not Operated										
0–19 Years	3,958	2.4	4	1	1	2	3	4	5	11
20–34	1,489	3.3	10	1	2	2	4	6	9	18
35–49	2,449	3.9	13	1	2	3	5	7	10	20
50–64	4,077	4.7	19	1	2	3	6	9	13	21
65+	11,997	5.5	22	2	3	4	7	11	14	24
B. Operated										
0–19 Years	20	9.0	211	1	2	4	6	14	46	55
20–34	15	13.6	136	2	3	10	27	30	36	36
35–49	30	10.0	77	3	4	8	13	23	27	42
50–64	85	14.8	177	4	7	11	19	32	40	>99
65+	248	14.9	106	5	8	12	20	27	30	58
SUBTOTALS:										
1. SINGLE DX										
A. Not Operated	567	1.9	1	1	1	2	2	3	4	5
B. Operated	5	1.8	<1	1	2	2	2	2	2	2
2. MULTIPLE DX										
A. Not Operated	23,970	4.6	18	1	2	3	6	9	13	22
B. Operated	398	14.2	127	4	7	11	19	27	36	75
1. SINGLE DX	572	1.9	1	1	2	2	2	3	4	6
2. MULTIPLE DX	24,368	4.7	22	1	2	3	6	10	13	24
A. NOT OPERATED	24,537	4.5	18	1	2	3	5	9	12	22
B. OPERATED	403	14.0	128	4	7	11	19	27	36	75
TOTAL										
0–19 Years	4,415	2.3	5	1	1	2	3	4	5	10
20–34	1,566	3.4	12	1	2	2	4	6	9	19
35–49	2,518	3.9	14	1	2	3	5	7	10	21
50–64	4,185	4.8	24	1	2	3	6	10	14	25
65+	12,256	5.7	25	2	3	4	7	11	15	26
GRAND TOTAL	24,940	4.6	21	1	2	3	6	10	13	23

008.43: CAMPYLOBACTER ENTERITIS

Type of Patients	Observed Patients	Avg. Stay	Variance	Percentiles						
				10th	25th	50th	75th	90th	95th	99th
1. SINGLE DX										
A. Not Operated										
0–19 Years	9	2.2	2	1	1	2	3	3	5	5
20–34	4	3.0	<1	2	3	3	4	4	4	4
35–49	2	1.5	<1	1	1	2	2	2	2	2
50–64	0									
65+	0									
B. Operated										
0–19 Years	0									
20–34	0									
35–49	0									
50–64	0									
65+	0									
2. MULTIPLE DX										
A. Not Operated										
0–19 Years	41	2.7	3	1	2	2	3	4	7	9
20–34	45	2.8	2	2	2	3	4	5	5	7
35–49	71	3.4	3	2	2	3	4	5	7	11
50–64	77	3.6	3	2	2	3	4	6	7	11
65+	125	4.3	7	2	3	3	5	7	9	16
B. Operated										
0–19 Years	1	4.0	0	4	4	4	4	4	4	4
20–34	0									
35–49	0									
50–64	0									
65+	1	15.0	0	15	15	15	15	15	15	15
SUBTOTALS:										
1. SINGLE DX										
A. Not Operated	15	2.3	2	1	1	2	3	4	5	5
B. Operated	0									
2. MULTIPLE DX										
A. Not Operated	359	3.6	5	2	2	3	4	6	7	11
B. Operated	2	9.5	59	4	4	15	15	15	15	15
1. SINGLE DX	15	2.3	2	1	2	2	3	4	5	5
2. MULTIPLE DX	361	3.6	5	2	2	3	4	6	7	11
A. NOT OPERATED	374	3.5	5	2	2	3	4	6	7	11
B. OPERATED	2	9.5	59	4	4	15	15	15	15	15
TOTAL										
0–19 Years	51	2.7	3	1	2	2	3	4	5	9
20–34	49	2.9	2	1	2	2	4	6	5	7
35–49	73	3.3	3	2	2	3	4	5	7	11
50–64	77	3.6	3	2	2	3	4	6	7	11
65+	126	4.3	8	2	3	3	5	7	10	16
GRAND TOTAL	376	3.6	5	2	2	3	4	6	7	11

008.45: C. DIFFICILE ENTERITIS

Type of Patients	Observed Patients	Avg. Stay	Variance	Percentiles						
				10th	25th	50th	75th	90th	95th	99th
1. SINGLE DX										
A. Not Operated										
0–19 Years	21	3.2	4	2	2	3	4	5	5	10
20–34	21	2.8	3	1	2	2	3	5	6	8
35–49	20	2.3	2	1	1	2	3	5	5	5
50–64	6	3.2	3	2	2	3	4	6	6	6
65+	5	3.8	5	2	2	3	5	7	7	7
B. Operated										
0–19 Years	0									
20–34	0									
35–49	0									
50–64	0									
2. MULTIPLE DX										
A. Not Operated										
0–19 Years	253	4.6	16	1	2	3	6	9	13	17
20–34	510	4.9	18	2	2	4	6	9	13	20
35–49	1,162	5.2	21	2	3	4	6	10	13	26
50–64	2,307	6.0	25	2	3	5	7	12	16	25
65+	8,257	6.6	25	2	3	5	8	12	16	26
B. Operated										
0–19 Years	5	14.3	319	4	4	6	12	46	46	46
20–34	12	15.8	141	3	6	11	28	30	36	36
35–49	20	12.2	96	3	6	11	17	27	42	42
50–64	68	15.8	197	6	8	12	19	32	68	>99
65+	219	15.8	111	6	9	13	20	27	31	58
SUBTOTALS:										
1. SINGLE DX										
A. Not Operated	73	2.9	3	1	2	2	4	5	6	10
B. Operated	0									
2. MULTIPLE DX										
A. Not Operated	12,489	6.2	25	2	3	5	8	12	16	26
B. Operated	324	15.5	131	5	8	12	20	29	40	87
1. SINGLE DX	73	2.9	3	1	2	2	4	5	6	10
2. MULTIPLE DX	12,813	6.5	29	2	3	5	8	13	17	27
A. NOT OPERATED	12,562	6.2	25	2	3	5	8	12	16	26
B. OPERATED	324	15.5	131	5	8	12	20	29	40	87
TOTAL										
0–19 Years	279	4.6	21	1	2	3	6	10	13	23
20–34	543	5.0	23	2	3	4	6	10	13	27
35–49	1,202	5.3	22	2	3	4	6	10	13	27
50–64	2,381	6.3	32	2	3	5	7	13	17	29
65+	8,481	6.8	30	2	3	5	8	13	17	27
GRAND TOTAL	12,886	6.5	29	2	3	5	8	13	17	27

008.61: ROTAVIRUS ENTERITIS

Type of Patients	Observed Patients	Avg. Stay	Variance	Percentiles						
				10th	25th	50th	75th	90th	95th	99th
1. SINGLE DX										
A. *Not Operated*										
0–19 Years	83	2.3	1	1	1	2	3	4	4	6
20–34	0									
35–49	0									
50–64	0									
65+	0									
B. *Operated*										
0–19 Years	0									
20–34	0									
35–49	0									
50–64	0									
65+	0									
2. MULTIPLE DX										
A. *Not Operated*										
0–19 Years	1,488	2.5	3	1	2	2	3	4	5	10
20–34	2	2.5	<1	2	1	3	3	3	3	3
35–49	6	4.5	14	1	1	4	6	11	11	11
50–64	6	3.3	3	1	2	4	5	5	5	5
65+	10	3.8	6	2	3	3	4	10	10	10
B. *Operated*										
0–19 Years	2	28.3	>999	2	2	2	55	55	55	55
20–34	0									
35–49	0									
50–64	0									
65+	0									
SUBTOTALS:										
1. SINGLE DX										
A. *Not Operated*	83	2.3	1	1	1	2	3	4	4	6
B. *Operated*	0									
2. MULTIPLE DX										
A. *Not Operated*	1,512	2.5	3	1	2	2	3	4	5	10
B. *Operated*	2	28.3	>999	2	2	2	55	55	55	55
1. SINGLE DX	83	2.3	1	1	1	2	3	4	4	6
2. MULTIPLE DX	1,514	2.5	4	1	2	2	3	4	5	10
A. NOT OPERATED	1,595	2.5	3	1	2	2	3	4	5	10
B. OPERATED	2	28.3	>999	2	2	2	55	55	55	55
TOTAL										
0–19 Years	1,573	2.5	4	1	2	2	3	4	5	10
20–34	2	2.5	<1	2	2	3	3	3	3	3
35–49	6	4.5	14	1	1	4	6	11	11	11
50–64	6	3.3	3	1	2	4	5	5	5	5
65+	10	3.8	6	2	3	3	4	10	10	10
GRAND TOTAL	1,597	2.5	4	1	2	2	3	4	5	10

008.8: VIRAL ENTERITIS NOS

Type of Patients	Observed Patients	Avg. Stay	Variance	Percentiles						
				10th	25th	50th	75th	90th	95th	99th
1. SINGLE DX										
A. *Not Operated*										
0–19 Years	301	1.6	<1	1	1	1	2	3	3	5
20–34	32	1.5	<1	1	1	1	2	2	3	4
35–49	14	1.8	1	1	1	1	3	3	4	4
50–64	15	1.7	<1	1	1	2	2	3	3	3
65+	6	1.7	<1	1	1	2	2	3	3	3
B. *Operated*										
0–19 Years	2	1.5	<1	1	1	2	2	2	2	2
20–34	3	2.0	0	2	2	2	2	2	2	2
35–49	0									
50–64	0									
65+	0									
2. MULTIPLE DX										
A. *Not Operated*										
0–19 Years	2,035	1.9	2	1	1	2	2	3	4	7
20–34	856	2.4	5	1	1	2	3	4	5	9
35–49	1,109	2.5	3	1	1	2	3	6	6	9
50–64	1,532	2.7	5	1	1	2	3	5	6	11
65+	3,262	3.0	4	1	2	2	4	5	7	10
B. *Operated*										
0–19 Years	9	2.4	2	1	2	2	4	4	4	4
20–34	3	5.0	37	1	1	2	12	12	12	12
35–49	8	5.0	6	3	3	5	9	9	9	9
50–64	11	6.5	20	3	3	4	12	13	14	14
65+	22	7.7	27	3	4	7	8	14	20	23
SUBTOTALS:										
1. SINGLE DX										
A. *Not Operated*	368	1.6	<1	1	1	1	2	3	3	5
B. *Operated*	5	1.8	<1	1	2	2	2	2	2	2
2. MULTIPLE DX										
A. *Not Operated*	8,794	2.6	4	1	1	2	3	5	6	10
B. *Operated*	53	6.0	21	2	3	5	8	12	14	23
1. SINGLE DX	373	1.6	<1	1	1	1	2	3	3	5
2. MULTIPLE DX	8,847	2.6	4	1	1	2	3	5	6	10
A. NOT OPERATED	9,162	2.5	4	1	1	2	3	5	6	10
B. OPERATED	58	5.7	20	2	2	4	7	12	14	23
TOTAL										
0–19 Years	2,347	1.9	2	1	1	2	2	3	4	7
20–34	894	2.4	5	1	1	2	3	4	5	10
35–49	1,131	2.5	3	1	1	2	3	4	6	9
50–64	1,558	2.7	5	1	2	2	4	5	6	12
65+	3,290	3.0	5	1	2	2	4	5	7	11
GRAND TOTAL	9,220	2.5	4	1	1	2	3	5	6	10

009: ILL-DEFINED INTEST INF

Type of Patients	Observed Patients	Avg. Stay	Variance	Percentiles						
				10th	25th	50th	75th	90th	95th	99th
1. SINGLE DX										
A. *Not Operated*										
0–19 Years	41	2.0	<1	1	1	2	2	4	4	5
20–34	41	2.0	<1	1	1	2	2	3	4	5
35–49	17	2.1	1	1	2	2	3	5	5	5
50–64	13	2.4	<1	1	2	2	3	5	5	5
65+	3	3.3	4	1	1	4	5	5	5	5
B. *Operated*										
0–19 Years	1	2.0	0	2	2	2	2	2	2	2
20–34	2	3.0	0	3	3	3	3	3	3	3
35–49	0									
50–64	0									
65+	0									
2. MULTIPLE DX										
A. *Not Operated*										
0–19 Years	211	2.6	9	1	1	2	3	4	5	13
20–34	379	2.7	4	1	1	2	3	5	6	11
35–49	597	3.0	4	1	2	2	4	5	7	11
50–64	676	3.2	5	1	2	3	4	6	8	11
65+	845	3.5	6	1	2	3	4	6	8	14
B. *Operated*										
0–19 Years	2	10.4	141	2	2	2	19	19	19	19
20–34	4	19.4	>999	1	1	3	67	67	67	67
35–49	10	5.0	5	3	3	5	6	9	9	9
50–64	7	8.3	15	4	4	9	11	14	14	14
65+	11	7.3	37	4	4	5	7	14	23	23
SUBTOTALS:										
1. SINGLE DX										
A. *Not Operated*	115	2.1	1	1	1	2	3	4	4	5
B. *Operated*	3	2.7	<1	2	2	3	3	3	3	3
2. MULTIPLE DX										
A. *Not Operated*	2,708	3.1	5	1	2	3	4	6	7	12
B. *Operated*	34	8.4	132	2	3	6	9	14	23	67
1. SINGLE DX	118	2.1	1	1	1	2	3	4	4	5
2. MULTIPLE DX	2,742	3.2	7	1	2	3	4	6	7	12
A. NOT OPERATED	2,823	3.1	5	1	2	3	4	5	7	12
B. OPERATED	37	8.0	123	2	3	5	7	14	23	67
TOTAL										
0–19 Years	255	2.6	9	1	1	2	3	4	5	19
20–34	426	2.8	13	1	1	2	3	5	6	11
35–49	624	3.0	4	1	1	2	4	5	7	11
50–64	696	3.3	5	1	2	3	4	6	8	12
65+	859	3.6	6	1	2	3	4	6	8	14
GRAND TOTAL	2,860	3.2	7	1	2	3	4	6	7	12

Length of Stay by Diagnosis and Operation, Western Region, 2008

Western Region, October 2006–September 2007 Data, by Diagnosis

009.0: INFECTIOUS ENTERITIS NOS

Type of Patients	Observed Patients	Avg. Stay	Variance	Percentiles						
				10th	25th	50th	75th	90th	95th	99th
1. SINGLE DX										
A. Not Operated										
0–19 Years	30	1.9	1	1	1	2	2	4	4	5
20–34	32	2.0	<1	1	1	2	2	3	4	5
35–49	11	2.0	<1	1	1	2	2	3	3	3
50–64	9	2.6	2	1	2	3	3	5	5	5
65+	3	3.3	4	1	1	4	5	5	5	5
B. Operated										
0–19 Years	1	2.0	0	2	2	2	2	2	2	2
20–34	2	3.0	0	3	3	3	3	3	3	3
35–49	0									
50–64	0									
65+	0									
2. MULTIPLE DX										
A. Not Operated										
0–19 Years	127	2.4	3	1	1	2	3	4	5	8
20–34	265	2.8	3	1	2	2	3	5	6	10
35–49	394	3.0	3	1	2	3	4	5	7	11
50–64	461	3.3	5	1	2	3	4	6	8	11
65+	526	3.5	5	1	2	3	4	6	8	13
B. Operated										
0–19 Years	1	2.0	0	2	2	2	2	2	2	2
20–34	2	34.0	>999	1	1	34	67	67	67	67
35–49	8	5.3	6	2	3	6	7	9	9	9
50–64	5	8.8	14	4	4	9	10	14	14	14
65+	7	9.0	51	2	5	6	14	23	23	23
SUBTOTALS:										
1. SINGLE DX										
A. Not Operated	85	2.1	1	1	1	2	2	4	4	5
B. Operated	3	2.7	<1	2	2	3	3	3	3	3
2. MULTIPLE DX										
A. Not Operated	1,773	3.1	5	1	2	3	4	6	7	12
B. Operated	23	9.6	183	2	3	6	9	14	23	67
1. SINGLE DX	88	2.1	1	1	2	2	3	4	4	5
2. MULTIPLE DX	1,796	3.2	7	1	2	3	4	6	7	12
A. NOT OPERATED	1,858	3.1	4	1	2	3	4	5	7	11
B. OPERATED	26	8.8	166	2	3	6	9	14	23	67
TOTAL										
0–19 Years	159	2.3	2	1	1	2	2	4	5	8
20–34	301	2.9	17	1	1	2	3	5	6	10
35–49	413	3.0	3	1	2	3	3	5	7	10
50–64	475	3.3	5	1	2	3	4	6	8	13
65+	536	3.6	6	1	2	3	4	6	8	14
GRAND TOTAL	1,884	3.2	7	1	2	3	4	6	7	12

009.1: ENTERITIS PRESUM INF

Type of Patients	Observed Patients	Avg. Stay	Variance	Percentiles						
				10th	25th	50th	75th	90th	95th	99th
1. SINGLE DX										
A. Not Operated										
0–19 Years	6	2.5	<1	2	2	2	3	4	4	4
20–34	6	2.3	1	1	2	2	3	4	4	4
35–49	4	1.8	<1	1	1	2	2	2	2	2
50–64	3	2.0	<1	1	1	2	3	3	3	3
65+	0									
B. Operated										
0–19 Years	0									
20–34	0									
35–49	0									
50–64	0									
65+	0									
2. MULTIPLE DX										
A. Not Operated										
0–19 Years	50	3.6	31	1	1	2	3	7	12	33
20–34	65	2.6	2	1	2	2	3	5	6	7
35–49	114	3.2	5	1	2	2	4	6	8	10
50–64	110	3.2	5	1	2	3	4	6	8	12
65+	151	3.7	7	1	2	3	4	6	8	15
B. Operated										
0–19 Years	1	19.0	0	19	19	19	19	19	19	19
20–34	2	4.5	4	3	3	3	6	6	6	6
35–49	2	4.0	2	3	3	5	5	5	5	5
50–64	0									
65+	4	4.3	<1	4	4	4	5	5	5	5
SUBTOTALS:										
1. SINGLE DX										
A. Not Operated	19	2.2	<1	1	2	2	3	4	4	4
B. Operated	0									
2. MULTIPLE DX										
A. Not Operated	490	3.3	8	1	2	3	4	6	8	14
B. Operated	9	5.9	25	3	4	4	5	19	19	19
1. SINGLE DX	19	2.2	<1	1	2	2	3	4	4	4
2. MULTIPLE DX	499	3.4	8	1	2	3	4	6	8	15
A. NOT OPERATED	509	3.3	8	1	2	3	4	6	7	14
B. OPERATED	9	5.9	25	3	4	4	5	19	19	19
TOTAL										
0–19 Years	57	3.8	32	1	2	2	3	7	19	33
20–34	73	2.7	2	1	2	2	3	5	6	7
35–49	120	3.2	4	1	2	2	4	6	7	10
50–64	113	3.2	5	1	2	3	4	6	8	12
65+	155	3.7	6	1	2	3	4	6	8	15
GRAND TOTAL	518	3.3	8	1	2	3	4	6	8	14

009.2: INFECTIOUS DIARRHEA NOS

Type of Patients	Observed Patients	Avg. Stay	Variance	Percentiles						
				10th	25th	50th	75th	90th	95th	99th
1. SINGLE DX										
A. Not Operated										
0–19 Years	3	2.0	0	2	2	2	2	2	2	2
20–34	3	2.0	<1	1	2	2	3	3	3	3
35–49	0									
50–64	1	2.0	0	2	2	2	2	2	2	2
65+	0									
B. Operated										
0–19 Years	0									
20–34	0									
35–49	0									
50–64	0									
65+	0									
2. MULTIPLE DX										
A. Not Operated										
0–19 Years	23	2.1	1	1	1	2	3	4	4	4
20–34	30	2.6	5	1	2	3	3	5	8	11
35–49	62	2.5	1	1	2	3	3	4	4	6
50–64	74	3.0	3	1	2	3	4	5	7	8
65+	117	3.5	5	1	2	3	4	7	8	10
B. Operated										
0–19 Years	0									
20–34	0									
35–49	0									
50–64	1	11.0	0	11	11	11	11	11	11	11
65+	0									
SUBTOTALS:										
1. SINGLE DX										
A. Not Operated	7	2.0	<1	1	2	2	2	3	3	3
B. Operated	0									
2. MULTIPLE DX										
A. Not Operated	306	3.0	4	1	2	3	4	5	7	9
B. Operated	1	11.0	0	11	11	11	11	11	11	11
1. SINGLE DX	7	2.0	<1	1	2	2	2	3	3	3
2. MULTIPLE DX	307	3.0	4	1	2	3	4	6	7	10
A. NOT OPERATED	313	3.0	4	1	2	2	4	5	7	9
B. OPERATED	1	11.0	0	11	11	11	11	11	11	11
TOTAL										
0–19 Years	26	2.1	<1	1	1	2	3	4	4	4
20–34	33	2.6	5	1	2	2	3	5	8	11
35–49	62	2.5	1	2	2	2	3	4	4	6
50–64	76	3.1	4	2	3	3	4	6	7	11
65+	117	3.5	5	1	2	3	4	7	8	10
GRAND TOTAL	314	3.0	4	1	2	2	4	5	7	10

Length of Stay by Diagnosis and Operation, Western Region, 2008

Western Region, October 2006–September 2007 Data, by Diagnosis

010: PRIMARY TB INFECTION

Type of Patients	Observed Patients	Avg. Stay	Vari-ance	Percentiles 10th	25th	50th	75th	90th	95th	99th
1. SINGLE DX										
A. Not Operated										
0–19 Years	0									
20–34	1	4.0	0	4	4	4	4	4	4	4
35–49	0									
50–64	0									
65+	0									
B. Operated										
0–19 Years	0									
20–34	0									
35–49	0									
50–64	0									
65+	0									
2. MULTIPLE DX										
A. Not Operated										
0–19 Years	4	5.8	6	4	4	4	9	9	9	9
20–34	2	19.5	83	13	13	26	26	26	26	26
35–49	4	4.0	12	1	3	3	9	9	9	9
50–64	2	15.6	262	4	4	27	27	27	27	27
65+	4	8.5	62	3	4	7	20	20	20	20
B. Operated										
0–19 Years	1	47.0	0	47	47	47	47	47	47	47
20–34	0									
35–49	0									
50–64	1	30.0	0	30	30	30	30	30	30	30
65+	2	19.0	2	18	18	18	20	20	20	20
SUBTOTALS:										
1. SINGLE DX										
A. Not Operated	1	4.0	0	4	4	4	4	4	4	4
B. Operated	0									
2. MULTIPLE DX										
A. Not Operated	16	9.0	69	3	4	6	13	26	27	27
B. Operated	4	28.7	175	18	18	20	30	47	47	47
1. SINGLE DX	1	4.0	0	4	4	4	4	4	4	4
2. MULTIPLE DX	20	12.9	148	3	4	9	20	29	39	47
A. NOT OPERATED	17	8.7	66	3	4	4	9	26	27	27
B. OPERATED	4	28.7	175	18	18	20	30	47	47	47
TOTAL										
0–19 Years	5	14.0	344	4	4	6	9	47	47	47
20–34	3	14.4	121	4	4	13	26	26	26	26
35–49	4	4.0	12	1	3	3	9	9	9	9
50–64	3	20.4	200	4	4	27	30	30	30	30
65+	6	12.0	67	3	4	18	20	20	20	20
GRAND TOTAL	21	12.5	145	3	4	7	20	30	47	47

011: PULMONARY TUBERCULOSIS

Type of Patients	Observed Patients	Avg. Stay	Vari-ance	Percentiles 10th	25th	50th	75th	90th	95th	99th
1. SINGLE DX										
A. Not Operated										
0–19 Years	14	10.0	80	3	3	6	17	26	28	28
20–34	27	11.9	63	1	4	12	18	24	24	27
35–49	10	9.7	64	3	3	7	17	18	24	24
50–64	1	1.0	0	1	1	1	1	1	1	1
65+	3	7.0	28	3	3	5	13	13	13	13
B. Operated										
0–19 Years	0									
20–34	2	16.5	24	13	13	13	20	20	20	20
35–49	1	3.0	0	3	3	3	3	3	3	3
50–64	1	7.0	0	7	7	7	7	7	7	7
65+	0									
2. MULTIPLE DX										
A. Not Operated										
0–19 Years	33	11.5	86	3	5	9	16	27	32	38
20–34	154	12.6	156	3	6	8	17	31	43	>99
35–49	193	15.1	221	3	6	11	19	30	46	75
50–64	231	15.1	222	3	6	10	19	36	50	>99
65+	237	13.6	170	3	6	11	16	28	36	94
B. Operated										
0–19 Years	2	11.0	0	11	11	11	11	11	11	11
20–34	19	13.0	62	6	7	10	17	26	35	35
35–49	18	14.8	93	6	7	12	22	30	32	32
50–64	27	14.2	139	3	6	11	18	34	43	43
65+	38	14.0	70	3	8	13	18	29	31	35
SUBTOTALS:										
1. SINGLE DX										
A. Not Operated	55	10.6	65	3	3	7	18	24	26	28
B. Operated	4	10.8	54	3	7	10	13	20	20	20
2. MULTIPLE DX										
A. Not Operated	848	14.1	190	3	6	10	18	30	43	97
B. Operated	104	13.9	87	4	7	12	18	29	33	43
1. SINGLE DX	59	10.6	63	3	3	7	18	24	26	28
2. MULTIPLE DX	952	14.1	179	3	6	10	18	30	41	94
A. NOT OPERATED	903	13.9	183	3	6	10	18	29	41	94
B. OPERATED	108	13.8	86	4	7	12	18	29	33	43
TOTAL										
0–19 Years	49	11.1	79	3	4	8	16	27	29	38
20–34	202	12.6	133	3	6	9	18	28	36	>99
35–49	222	14.7	203	3	6	11	19	30	40	70
50–64	260	14.9	212	3	6	10	19	36	46	>99
65+	278	13.6	155	3	6	11	17	28	35	94
GRAND TOTAL	1,011	13.9	173	3	6	10	18	29	39	89

012: OTHER RESPIRATORY TB

Type of Patients	Observed Patients	Avg. Stay	Vari-ance	Percentiles 10th	25th	50th	75th	90th	95th	99th
1. SINGLE DX										
A. Not Operated										
0–19 Years	2	6.0	18	3	3	3	9	9	9	9
20–34	1	7.0	0	7	7	7	7	7	7	7
35–49	2	5.5	<1	5	5	5	6	6	6	6
50–64	0									
65+	0									
B. Operated										
0–19 Years	0									
20–34	0									
35–49	0									
50–64	0									
65+	0									
2. MULTIPLE DX										
A. Not Operated										
0–19 Years	1	3.0	0	3	3	3	3	3	3	3
20–34	12	10.3	16	5	7	11	13	15	18	18
35–49	10	11.4	134	4	5	8	12	18	42	42
50–64	10	9.9	44	2	6	7	15	17	24	24
65+	10	13.9	90	4	7	13	15	26	34	34
B. Operated										
0–19 Years	4	9.5	6	8	8	9	13	13	13	13
20–34	5	12.0	16	7	11	11	13	18	18	18
35–49	9	12.7	88	3	3	10	16	28	28	28
50–64	5	19.8	38	14	16	17	23	29	29	29
65+	4	13.8	38	5	14	14	17	19	19	19
SUBTOTALS:										
1. SINGLE DX										
A. Not Operated	5	6.0	5	3	5	6	7	9	9	9
B. Operated	0									
2. MULTIPLE DX										
A. Not Operated	43	11.1	65	4	5	8	13	18	26	42
B. Operated	27	13.6	51	5	8	13	17	27	28	29
1. SINGLE DX	5	6.0	5	3	5	6	7	9	9	9
2. MULTIPLE DX	70	12.1	61	4	7	11	15	23	28	42
A. NOT OPERATED	48	10.6	61	4	5	8	13	18	26	42
B. OPERATED	27	13.6	51	5	8	13	17	27	28	29
TOTAL										
0–19 Years	7	7.6	13	3	3	8	9	13	13	13
20–34	18	10.6	16	5	7	11	13	18	18	18
35–49	21	11.4	100	4	5	7	13	27	28	42
50–64	15	13.2	62	4	7	13	17	24	29	29
65+	14	13.8	71	5	7	13	17	26	34	34
GRAND TOTAL	75	11.7	59	4	7	9	15	23	28	42

Length of Stay by Diagnosis and Operation, Western Region, 2008

Western Region, October 2006–September 2007 Data, by Diagnosis

013: CNS TUBERCULOSIS

Type of Patients	Observed Patients	Avg. Stay	Vari-ance	10th	25th	50th	75th	90th	95th	99th
1. SINGLE DX										
A. Not Operated										
0–19 Years	0									
20–34	0									
35–49	2	9.0	0	9	9	9	9	9	9	9
50–64	0									
65+	0									
B. Operated										
0–19 Years	0									
20–34	0									
35–49	0									
50–64	0									
65+	0									
2. MULTIPLE DX										
A. Not Operated										
0–19 Years	3	16.0	74	6	6	21	21	21	21	21
20–34	11	12.3	62	4	7	9	18	19	29	29
35–49	19	9.1	55	2	4	8	16	27	27	>99
50–64	7	14.9	44	8	9	14	17	28	28	28
65+	10	22.9	394	6	7	20	31	72	72	72
B. Operated										
0–19 Years	0									
20–34	4	14.0	29	8	8	18	19	19	19	19
35–49	4	16.0	117	5	5	14	14	31	31	31
50–64	2	17.5	260	6	6	29	29	29	29	29
65+	5	23.2	161	12	14	22	24	44	44	44
SUBTOTALS:										
1. SINGLE DX										
A. Not Operated	2	9.0	0	9	9	9	9	9	9	9
B. Operated	0									
2. MULTIPLE DX										
A. Not Operated	50	13.8	140	4	6	10	20	28	32	>99
B. Operated	15	18.1	112	6	11	14	24	31	44	44
1. SINGLE DX	2	9.0	0	9	9	9	9	9	9	9
2. MULTIPLE DX	65	14.8	135	4	7	13	20	29	32	>99
A. NOT OPERATED	52	13.6	136	4	7	9	19	28	32	>99
B. OPERATED	15	18.1	112	6	11	14	24	31	44	44
TOTAL										
0–19 Years	3	16.0	74	6	6	21	21	21	21	21
20–34	15	12.8	51	4	8	11	18	19	29	29
35–49	25	10.2	63	2	5	9	15	27	31	>99
50–64	9	15.5	67	6	9	14	17	28	29	29
65+	15	23.0	300	7	12	20	31	44	72	72
GRAND TOTAL	67	14.6	132	4	7	13	20	29	32	>99

014: INTESTINAL TB

Type of Patients	Observed Patients	Avg. Stay	Vari-ance	10th	25th	50th	75th	90th	95th	99th
1. SINGLE DX										
A. Not Operated										
0–19 Years	0									
20–34	0									
35–49	0									
50–64	0									
65+	0									
B. Operated										
0–19 Years	0									
20–34	0									
35–49	0									
50–64	0									
65+	0									
2. MULTIPLE DX										
A. Not Operated										
0–19 Years	0									
20–34	9	10.9	50	4	6	8	12	25	25	25
35–49	10	7.2	67	1	2	3	8	24	24	24
50–64	7	7.9	33	1	4	6	13	18	18	18
65+	6	9.2	21	4	5	9	14	15	15	15
B. Operated										
0–19 Years	3	22.0	364	9	9	13	44	44	44	44
20–34	6	13.0	122	6	6	8	17	34	34	34
35–49	6	10.1	31	5	6	7	15	19	19	19
50–64	6	19.6	45	10	16	18	25	29	29	29
65+	7	9.7	53	3	3	9	17	22	22	22
SUBTOTALS:										
1. SINGLE DX										
A. Not Operated	0									
B. Operated	0									
2. MULTIPLE DX										
A. Not Operated	32	8.8	44	2	4	7	13	19	24	25
B. Operated	28	14.0	98	5	7	10	18	29	34	44
1. SINGLE DX	0									
2. MULTIPLE DX	60	11.2	75	3	5	8	17	24	25	44
A. NOT OPERATED	32	8.8	44	2	4	7	13	19	24	25
B. OPERATED	28	14.0	98	5	7	10	18	29	34	44
TOTAL										
0–19 Years	3	22.0	364	9	9	13	44	44	44	44
20–34	15	11.7	73	5	6	8	17	25	34	34
35–49	16	8.3	53	2	2	7	9	20	24	24
50–64	13	13.3	73	4	6	13	18	25	29	29
65+	13	9.5	35	3	5	9	14	17	22	22
GRAND TOTAL	60	11.2	75	3	5	8	17	24	25	44

015: BONE & JOINT TB

Type of Patients	Observed Patients	Avg. Stay	Vari-ance	10th	25th	50th	75th	90th	95th	99th
1. SINGLE DX										
A. Not Operated										
0–19 Years	1	7.0	0	7	7	7	7	7	7	7
20–34	2	1.5	<1	1	1	2	2	2	2	2
35–49	0									
50–64	0									
65+	1	14.0	0	14	14	14	14	14	14	14
B. Operated										
0–19 Years	0									
20–34	0									
35–49	0									
50–64	0									
65+	0									
2. MULTIPLE DX										
A. Not Operated										
0–19 Years	0									
20–34	3	17.0	57	9	9	18	24	24	24	24
35–49	6	8.0	27	2	3	8	11	16	16	16
50–64	6	15.7	662	2	4	5	9	68	68	68
65+	8	14.1	66	5	5	13	21	27	27	27
B. Operated										
0–19 Years	1	7.0	0	7	7	7	7	7	7	7
20–34	2	9.5	<1	9	9	10	10	10	10	10
35–49	13	9.5	24	6	6	9	10	17	19	19
50–64	6	18.4	86	6	13	19	29	>99	>99	>99
65+	11	14.5	196	4	4	10	16	32	48	48
SUBTOTALS:										
1. SINGLE DX										
A. Not Operated	4	6.0	35	1	1	2	7	14	14	14
B. Operated	0									
2. MULTIPLE DX										
A. Not Operated	23	13.3	195	3	5	9	18	24	27	68
B. Operated	33	12.7	97	4	6	10	16	29	48	>99
1. SINGLE DX	4	6.0	35	1	1	2	7	14	14	14
2. MULTIPLE DX	56	12.9	134	4	6	10	16	29	48	>99
A. NOT OPERATED	27	12.2	176	2	5	8	16	24	27	68
B. OPERATED	33	12.7	97	4	6	10	16	29	48	>99
TOTAL										
0–19 Years	2	7.0	0	7	7	7	7	7	7	7
20–34	7	10.4	67	1	2	9	18	24	24	24
35–49	19	9.0	24	2	6	9	11	17	19	19
50–64	12	17.0	343	4	6	13	29	68	>99	>99
65+	20	14.3	128	4	5	13	16	32	48	48
GRAND TOTAL	60	12.5	130	3	6	9	16	27	32	>99

Length of Stay by Diagnosis and Operation, Western Region, 2008

Western Region, October 2006–September 2007 Data, by Diagnosis

016: GENITOURINARY TB

Type of Patients	Observed Patients	Avg. Stay	Variance	10th	25th	50th	75th	90th	95th	99th
1. SINGLE DX										
A. Not Operated										
0–19 Years	0									
20–34	0									
35–49	0									
50–64	0									
65+	0									
B. Operated										
0–19 Years	0									
20–34	0									
35–49	0									
50–64	0									
65+	0									
2. MULTIPLE DX										
A. Not Operated										
0–19 Years	0									
20–34	1	1.0	0	1	1	1	1	1	1	1
35–49	2	2.5	<1	2	2	3	3	3	3	3
50–64	2	34.3	>999	2	2	67	67	67	67	67
65+	1	7.0	0	7	7	7	7	7	7	7
B. Operated										
0–19 Years	0									
20–34	3	13.3	290	2	2	5	33	33	33	33
35–49	3	7.3	14	2	3	3	10	10	10	10
50–64	2	12.5	4	11	11	14	14	14	14	14
65+	1	5.0	0	5	5	5	5	5	5	5
SUBTOTALS:										
1. SINGLE DX — A. Not Operated	0									
1. SINGLE DX — B. Operated	0									
2. MULTIPLE DX — A. Not Operated	6	13.7	689	1	2	2	7	67	67	67
2. MULTIPLE DX — B. Operated	9	10.2	88	2	5	9	11	33	33	33
1. SINGLE DX	0									
2. MULTIPLE DX	15	11.6	299	2	2	5	11	33	67	67
A. NOT OPERATED	6	13.7	689	1	2	2	7	67	67	67
B. OPERATED	9	10.2	88	2	5	9	11	33	33	33
TOTAL										
0–19 Years	0									
20–34	4	10.2	232	1	2	2	5	33	33	33
35–49	5	5.4	14	2	3	3	9	10	10	10
50–64	4	23.4	861	2	5	14	14	67	67	67
65+	2	6.0	2	5	5	5	7	7	7	7
GRAND TOTAL	15	11.6	299	2	2	5	11	33	67	67

017: OTHER TUBERCULOSIS

Type of Patients	Observed Patients	Avg. Stay	Variance	10th	25th	50th	75th	90th	95th	99th
1. SINGLE DX										
A. Not Operated										
0–19 Years	1	1.0	0	1	1	1	1	1	1	1
20–34	0									
35–49	0									
50–64	0									
65+	0									
B. Operated										
0–19 Years	0									
20–34	1	9.0	0	9	9	9	9	9	9	9
35–49	1	2.0	0	2	2	2	2	2	2	2
50–64	0									
65+	0									
2. MULTIPLE DX										
A. Not Operated										
0–19 Years	3	7.0	21	2	2	8	11	11	11	11
20–34	3	8.7	20	4	4	9	13	13	13	13
35–49	3	8.7	30	5	5	6	15	15	15	15
50–64	2	9.5	24	6	6	6	15	13	13	13
65+	2	9.0	18	6	6	12	12	12	12	12
B. Operated										
0–19 Years	2	9.5	39	5	5	10	14	14	14	14
20–34	5	3.8	11	1	1	3	5	9	9	9
35–49	2	7.0	8	5	5	7	7	9	9	9
50–64	3	14.1	56	6	8	15	21	21	21	21
65+	4	11.8	9	8	8	13	15	15	15	15
SUBTOTALS:										
1. SINGLE DX — A. Not Operated	1	1.0	0	1	1	1	1	1	1	1
1. SINGLE DX — B. Operated	2	5.5	24	2	2	2	9	9	9	9
2. MULTIPLE DX — A. Not Operated	13	8.5	16	4	6	8	12	13	15	15
2. MULTIPLE DX — B. Operated	16	8.8	32	1	5	9	14	15	21	21
1. SINGLE DX	3	4.0	19	1	1	2	9	9	9	9
2. MULTIPLE DX	29	8.7	24	2	5	8	13	15	15	21
A. NOT OPERATED	14	7.9	19	2	5	6	12	13	15	15
B. OPERATED	18	8.5	31	1	5	9	13	15	21	21
TOTAL										
0–19 Years	6	6.8	26	1	2	5	11	14	14	14
20–34	9	6.0	17	1	3	5	9	13	13	13
35–49	6	7.0	20	2	5	6	9	15	15	15
50–64	5	12.2	41	6	6	13	15	21	21	21
65+	6	10.9	11	6	8	12	13	15	15	15
GRAND TOTAL	32	8.2	25	2	5	8	13	15	15	21

018: MILIARY TUBERCULOSIS

Type of Patients	Observed Patients	Avg. Stay	Variance	10th	25th	50th	75th	90th	95th	99th
1. SINGLE DX										
A. Not Operated										
0–19 Years	0									
20–34	0									
35–49	0									
50–64	0									
65+	0									
B. Operated										
0–19 Years	0									
20–34	0									
35–49	0									
50–64	0									
65+	0									
2. MULTIPLE DX										
A. Not Operated										
0–19 Years	1	3.0	0	3	3	3	3	3	3	3
20–34	10	23.9	63	18	19	23	29	31	40	40
35–49	13	20.4	420	3	6	12	20	55	57	57
50–64	7	16.4	338	3	3	7	24	>99	>99	>99
65+	15	14.7	136	3	3	15	18	31	41	41
B. Operated										
0–19 Years	1	10.0	0	10	10	10	10	10	10	10
20–34	5	16.4	23	8	17	18	19	20	20	20
35–49	5	9.4	18	6	6	7	14	14	14	14
50–64	2	16.5	59	11	11	17	22	22	22	22
65+	4	31.2	>999	4	4	16	16	97	97	97
SUBTOTALS:										
1. SINGLE DX — A. Not Operated	0									
1. SINGLE DX — B. Operated	0									
2. MULTIPLE DX — A. Not Operated	46	18.3	231	3	7	17	24	53	55	>99
2. MULTIPLE DX — B. Operated	17	17.4	449	6	8	14	18	22	97	97
1. SINGLE DX	0									
2. MULTIPLE DX	63	18.1	284	3	7	14	22	41	55	>99
A. NOT OPERATED	46	18.3	231	3	7	17	24	53	55	>99
B. OPERATED	17	17.4	449	6	8	14	18	22	97	97
TOTAL										
0–19 Years	2	6.5	24	3	3	10	10	10	10	10
20–34	15	21.4	61	11	18	20	24	31	40	40
35–49	18	17.3	326	3	6	12	19	55	57	57
50–64	9	16.4	261	3	7	11	24	55	>99	>99
65+	19	18.2	479	3	4	15	18	41	97	97
GRAND TOTAL	63	18.1	284	3	7	14	22	41	55	>99

Length of Stay by Diagnosis and Operation, Western Region, 2008

Western Region, October 2006–September 2007 Data, by Diagnosis

020: PLAGUE

Type of Patients	Observed Patients	Avg. Stay	Variance	10th	25th	50th	75th	90th	95th	99th
1. SINGLE DX										
A. Not Operated										
0–19 Years	0									
20–34	0									
35–49	0									
50–64	0									
65+	0									
B. Operated										
0–19 Years	0									
20–34	0									
35–49	0									
50–64	0									
65+	0									
2. MULTIPLE DX										
A. Not Operated										
0–19 Years	0									
20–34	1	1.0	0	1	1	1	1	1	1	1
35–49	2	9.0	0	9	9	9	9	9	9	9
50–64	1	30.0	0	30	30	30	30	30	30	30
65+	0									
B. Operated										
0–19 Years	0									
20–34	0									
35–49	0									
50–64	0									
65+	0									
SUBTOTALS:										
1. SINGLE DX										
A. Not Operated	0									
B. Operated	0									
2. MULTIPLE DX										
A. Not Operated	4	12.3	155	1	1	9	9	30	30	30
B. Operated	0									
1. SINGLE DX	0									
2. MULTIPLE DX	4	12.3	155	1	1	9	9	30	30	30
A. NOT OPERATED	4	12.3	155	1	1	9	9	30	30	30
B. OPERATED	0									
TOTAL										
0–19 Years	0									
20–34	1	1.0	0	1	1	1	1	1	1	1
35–49	2	9.0	0	9	9	9	9	9	9	9
50–64	1	30.0	0	30	30	30	30	30	30	30
65+	0									
GRAND TOTAL	4	12.3	155	1	1	9	9	30	30	30

021: TULAREMIA

Type of Patients	Observed Patients	Avg. Stay	Variance	10th	25th	50th	75th	90th	95th	99th
1. SINGLE DX										
A. Not Operated										
0–19 Years	0									
20–34	0									
35–49	0									
50–64	0									
65+	0									
B. Operated										
0–19 Years	0									
20–34	0									
35–49	0									
50–64	0									
65+	0									
2. MULTIPLE DX										
A. Not Operated										
0–19 Years	0									
20–34	0									
35–49	0									
50–64	0									
65+	0									
B. Operated										
0–19 Years	0									
20–34	0									
35–49	0									
50–64	0									
65+	0									
SUBTOTALS:										
1. SINGLE DX										
A. Not Operated	0									
B. Operated	0									
2. MULTIPLE DX										
A. Not Operated	0									
B. Operated	0									
1. SINGLE DX	0									
2. MULTIPLE DX	0									
A. NOT OPERATED	0									
B. OPERATED	0									
TOTAL										
0–19 Years	0									
20–34	0									
35–49	0									
50–64	0									
65+	0									
GRAND TOTAL	0									

022: ANTHRAX

Type of Patients	Observed Patients	Avg. Stay	Variance	10th	25th	50th	75th	90th	95th	99th
1. SINGLE DX										
A. Not Operated										
0–19 Years	0									
20–34	0									
35–49	0									
50–64	0									
65+	0									
B. Operated										
0–19 Years	0									
20–34	0									
35–49	0									
50–64	0									
65+	0									
2. MULTIPLE DX										
A. Not Operated										
0–19 Years	0									
20–34	0									
35–49	0									
50–64	0									
65+	0									
B. Operated										
0–19 Years	0									
20–34	0									
35–49	0									
50–64	0									
65+	0									
SUBTOTALS:										
1. SINGLE DX										
A. Not Operated	0									
B. Operated	0									
2. MULTIPLE DX										
A. Not Operated	0									
B. Operated	0									
1. SINGLE DX	0									
2. MULTIPLE DX	0									
A. NOT OPERATED	0									
B. OPERATED	0									
TOTAL										
0–19 Years	0									
20–34	0									
35–49	0									
50–64	0									
65+	0									
GRAND TOTAL	0									

Length of Stay by Diagnosis and Operation, Western Region, 2008

Western Region, October 2006–September 2007 Data, by Diagnosis

023: BRUCELLOSIS

Type of Patients	Observed Patients	Avg. Stay	Variance	Percentiles						
				10th	25th	50th	75th	90th	95th	99th
1. SINGLE DX										
A. *Not Operated*										
0–19 Years	1	8.0	0	8	8	8	8	8	8	8
20–34	2	8.5	60	3	3	3	14	14	14	14
35–49	0									
50–64	0									
65+	0									
B. *Operated*										
0–19 Years	0									
20–34	0									
35–49	0									
50–64	0									
65+	0									
2. MULTIPLE DX										
A. *Not Operated*										
0–19 Years	1	7.0	0	7	7	7	7	7	7	7
20–34	6	8.5	97	1	3	4	8	28	28	28
35–49	6	5.0	15	1	2	4	9	10	10	10
50–64	6	6.2	12	1	4	8	9	10	10	10
65+	3	7.4	85	2	2	2	18	18	18	18
B. *Operated*										
0–19 Years	1	7.0	0	7	7	7	7	7	7	7
20–34	0									
35–49	1	4.0	0	4	4	4	4	4	4	4
50–64	0									
65+	0									
SUBTOTALS:										
1. SINGLE DX										
A. *Not Operated*	3	8.3	30	3	3	8	14	14	14	14
B. *Operated*	0									
2. MULTIPLE DX										
A. *Not Operated*	22	6.7	40	1	2	6	9	10	18	28
B. *Operated*	2	5.5	4	4	4	6	7	7	7	7
1. SINGLE DX	3	8.3	30	3	3	8	14	14	14	14
2. MULTIPLE DX	24	6.6	37	1	2	6	9	10	18	28
A. NOT OPERATED	25	6.9	38	1	2	6	9	14	18	28
B. OPERATED	2	5.5	4	4	4	6	7	7	7	7
TOTAL										
0–19 Years	3	7.3	<1	7	7	7	8	8	8	8
20–34	8	8.5	78	1	3	4	8	28	28	28
35–49	7	4.9	13	1	2	4	9	10	10	10
50–64	6	6.2	12	1	2	8	9	10	10	10
65+	3	7.4	85	2	2	8	18	18	18	18
GRAND TOTAL	27	6.8	35	1	2	6	9	14	18	28

024: GLANDERS

Type of Patients	Observed Patients	Avg. Stay	Variance	Percentiles						
				10th	25th	50th	75th	90th	95th	99th
1. SINGLE DX										
A. *Not Operated*										
0–19 Years	0									
20–34	0									
35–49	0									
50–64	0									
65+	0									
B. *Operated*										
0–19 Years	0									
20–34	0									
35–49	0									
50–64	0									
65+	0									
2. MULTIPLE DX										
A. *Not Operated*										
0–19 Years	0									
20–34	0									
35–49	0									
50–64	0									
65+	0									
B. *Operated*										
0–19 Years	0									
20–34	0									
35–49	0									
50–64	0									
65+	0									
SUBTOTALS:										
1. SINGLE DX A. *Not Operated*	0									
B. *Operated*	0									
2. MULTIPLE DX A. *Not Operated*	0									
B. *Operated*	0									
1. SINGLE DX	0									
2. MULTIPLE DX	0									
A. NOT OPERATED	0									
B. OPERATED	0									
TOTAL										
0–19 Years	0									
20–34	0									
35–49	0									
50–64	0									
65+	0									
GRAND TOTAL	0									

025: MELIOIDOSIS

Type of Patients	Observed Patients	Avg. Stay	Variance	Percentiles						
				10th	25th	50th	75th	90th	95th	99th
1. SINGLE DX										
A. *Not Operated*										
0–19 Years	0									
20–34	0									
35–49	0									
50–64	0									
65+	0									
B. *Operated*										
0–19 Years	0									
20–34	0									
35–49	0									
50–64	0									
65+	0									
2. MULTIPLE DX										
A. *Not Operated*										
0–19 Years	0									
20–34	0									
35–49	1	1.0	0	1	1	1	1	1	1	1
50–64	0									
65+	0									
B. *Operated*										
0–19 Years	0									
20–34	1	15.0	0	15	15	15	15	15	15	15
35–49	0									
50–64	0									
65+	0									
SUBTOTALS:										
1. SINGLE DX A. *Not Operated*	0									
B. *Operated*	0									
2. MULTIPLE DX A. *Not Operated*	1	1.0	0	1	1	1	1	1	1	1
B. *Operated*	1	15.0	0	15	15	15	15	15	15	15
1. SINGLE DX	0									
2. MULTIPLE DX	2	8.0	96	1	1	1	1	15	15	15
A. NOT OPERATED	1	1.0	0	1	1	1	1	1	1	1
B. OPERATED	1	15.0	0	15	15	15	15	15	15	15
TOTAL										
0–19 Years	0									
20–34	1	15.0	0	15	15	15	15	15	15	15
35–49	1	1.0	0	1	1	1	1	1	1	1
50–64	0									
65+	0									
GRAND TOTAL	2	8.0	96	1	1	1	1	15	15	15

Length of Stay by Diagnosis and Operation, Western Region, 2008

Western Region, October 2006–September 2007 Data, by Diagnosis

026: RAT-BITE FEVER

Type of Patients	Observed Patients	Avg. Stay	Variance	10th	25th	50th	75th	90th	95th	99th
1. SINGLE DX										
A. Not Operated										
0–19 Years	0									
20–34	0									
35–49	0									
50–64	0									
65+	0									
B. Operated										
0–19 Years	0									
20–34	0									
35–49	0									
50–64	0									
65+	0									
2. MULTIPLE DX										
A. Not Operated										
0–19 Years	4	5.0	2	3	3	6	6	6	6	6
20–34	4	8.8	34	4	4	11	16	16	16	16
35–49	2	5.0	2	4	4	5	6	6	6	6
50–64	2	5.0	8	3	3	7	7	7	7	7
65+	2	4.0	2	3	3	5	5	5	5	5
B. Operated										
0–19 Years	0									
20–34	0									
35–49	0									
50–64	0									
65+	0									
SUBTOTALS:										
1. SINGLE DX										
A. Not Operated	0									
B. Operated	0									
2. MULTIPLE DX										
A. Not Operated	14	5.9	13	3	4	5	6	11	16	16
B. Operated	0									
1. SINGLE DX	0									
2. MULTIPLE DX	14	5.9	13	3	4	5	6	11	16	16
A. NOT OPERATED	14	5.9	13	3	4	5	6	11	16	16
B. OPERATED	0									
TOTAL										
0–19 Years	4	5.0	2	3	3	6	6	6	6	6
20–34	4	8.8	34	4	4	11	16	16	16	16
35–49	2	5.0	2	4	4	5	6	6	6	6
50–64	2	5.0	8	3	3	7	7	7	7	7
65+	2	4.0	2	3	3	5	5	5	5	5
GRAND TOTAL	14	5.9	13	3	4	5	6	11	16	16

027: OTHER BACTERIAL ZOONOSES

Type of Patients	Observed Patients	Avg. Stay	Variance	10th	25th	50th	75th	90th	95th	99th
1. SINGLE DX										
A. Not Operated										
0–19 Years	0									
20–34	0									
35–49	0									
50–64	0									
65+	0									
B. Operated										
0–19 Years	0									
20–34	0									
35–49	0									
50–64	0									
65+	0									
2. MULTIPLE DX										
A. Not Operated										
0–19 Years	0									
20–34	1	2.0	0	2	2	2	2	2	2	2
35–49	4	6.7	20	3	3	4	7	13	13	13
50–64	16	7.1	10	4	5	6	10	11	14	14
65+	45	8.3	47	3	4	6	11	15	19	38
B. Operated										
0–19 Years	0									
20–34	1	6.0	0	6	6	6	6	6	6	6
35–49	2	5.0	2	4	4	5	6	6	6	6
50–64	3	6.6	40	3	3	3	14	14	14	14
65+	2	9.5	59	4	4	15	15	15	15	15
SUBTOTALS:										
1. SINGLE DX										
A. Not Operated	0									
B. Operated	0									
2. MULTIPLE DX										
A. Not Operated	66	7.8	36	3	4	6	10	14	16	38
B. Operated	8	6.9	23	3	3	4	6	15	15	15
1. SINGLE DX	0									
2. MULTIPLE DX	74	7.7	34	3	4	6	10	14	16	38
A. NOT OPERATED	66	7.8	36	3	4	6	10	14	16	38
B. OPERATED	8	6.9	23	3	3	4	6	15	15	15
TOTAL										
0–19 Years	0									
20–34	2	4.0	8	2	2	2	6	6	6	6
35–49	6	6.1	13	3	4	4	7	13	13	13
50–64	19	7.0	13	3	4	6	10	14	14	14
65+	47	8.4	47	3	4	6	11	15	19	38
GRAND TOTAL	74	7.7	34	3	4	6	10	14	16	38

030: LEPROSY

Type of Patients	Observed Patients	Avg. Stay	Variance	10th	25th	50th	75th	90th	95th	99th
1. SINGLE DX										
A. Not Operated										
0–19 Years	0									
20–34	1	2.0	0	2	2	2	2	2	2	2
35–49	0									
50–64	0									
65+	0									
B. Operated										
0–19 Years	0									
20–34	0									
35–49	0									
50–64	0									
65+	0									
2. MULTIPLE DX										
A. Not Operated										
0–19 Years	0									
20–34	7	3.9	9	1	2	3	5	10	10	10
35–49	0									
50–64	0									
65+	0									
B. Operated										
0–19 Years	0									
20–34	0									
35–49	0									
50–64	1	1.0	0	1	1	1	1	1	1	1
65+	0									
SUBTOTALS:										
1. SINGLE DX										
A. Not Operated	1	2.0	0	2	2	2	2	2	2	2
B. Operated	0									
2. MULTIPLE DX										
A. Not Operated	7	3.9	9	1	2	3	5	10	10	10
B. Operated	1	1.0	0	1	1	1	1	1	1	1
1. SINGLE DX	1	2.0	0	2	2	2	2	2	2	2
2. MULTIPLE DX	8	3.5	9	1	2	3	5	10	10	10
A. NOT OPERATED	8	3.6	8	1	2	2	4	10	10	10
B. OPERATED	1	1.0	0	1	1	1	1	1	1	1
TOTAL										
0–19 Years	0									
20–34	8	3.6	8	1	2	2	4	10	10	10
35–49	0									
50–64	1	1.0	0	1	1	1	1	1	1	1
65+	0									
GRAND TOTAL	9	3.3	8	1	2	2	4	10	10	10

Length of Stay by Diagnosis and Operation, Western Region, 2008

14

Western Region, October 2006–September 2007 Data, by Diagnosis

031: OTHER MYCOBACTERIAL DIS

Type of Patients	Observed Patients	Avg. Stay	Vari-ance	10th	25th	50th	75th	90th	95th	99th
1. SINGLE DX										
A. Not Operated										
0–19 Years	0									
20–34	1	13.0	0	13	13	13	13	13	13	13
35–49	1	1.0	0	1	1	1	1	1	1	1
50–64	0									
65+	0									
B. Operated										
0–19 Years	0									
20–34	0									
35–49	0									
50–64	2	3.5	<1	3	3	3	4	4	4	4
65+	0									
2. MULTIPLE DX										
A. Not Operated										
0–19 Years	4	9.8	55	3	3	8	20	20	20	20
20–34	8	15.1	59	4	8	21	22	24	24	24
35–49	26	10.7	58	3	5	9	14	18	25	36
50–64	67	8.4	66	2	4	7	11	15	17	58
65+	179	9.1	51	2	4	7	12	20	24	30
B. Operated										
0–19 Years	0									
20–34	5	13.0	177	2	3	8	18	34	34	34
35–49	11	10.3	120	1	1	5	18	25	25	25
50–64	38	9.7	253	1	3	5	8	24	29	94
65+	31	10.2	75	3	4	7	15	22	42	>99
SUBTOTALS:										
1. SINGLE DX										
A. Not Operated	2	7.1	71	1	1	13	13	13	13	13
B. Operated	2	3.5	<1	3	3	3	4	4	4	4
2. MULTIPLE DX										
A. Not Operated	284	9.3	56	3	4	7	13	20	24	30
B. Operated	85	10.1	162	2	3	6	14	25	34	>99
1. SINGLE DX	4	5.3	28	1	3	4	13	13	13	13
2. MULTIPLE DX	369	9.5	80	2	4	7	13	21	25	42
A. NOT OPERATED	286	9.2	56	3	4	7	13	20	24	30
B. OPERATED	87	10.0	159	2	3	6	14	25	34	>99
TOTAL										
0–19 Years	4	9.8	55	3	3	8	20	20	20	20
20–34	13	14.3	95	3	8	11	21	24	34	34
35–49	38	10.6	72	2	4	9	14	25	34	36
50–64	108	8.7	129	2	3	5	11	17	26	58
65+	210	9.2	54	3	4	7	13	21	24	30
GRAND TOTAL	373	9.4	80	2	4	7	13	21	25	42

031.0: PULMONARY MYCOBACTERIA

Type of Patients	Observed Patients	Avg. Stay	Vari-ance	10th	25th	50th	75th	90th	95th	99th
1. SINGLE DX										
A. Not Operated										
0–19 Years	0									
20–34	0									
35–49	1	13.0	0	13	13	13	13	13	13	13
50–64	0									
65+	0									
B. Operated										
0–19 Years	0									
20–34	0									
35–49	0									
50–64	2	3.5	<1	3	3	3	4	4	4	4
65+	0									
2. MULTIPLE DX										
A. Not Operated										
0–19 Years	0									
20–34	6	15.2	63	4	10	21	21	24	24	24
35–49	11	9.9	25	2	6	9	13	17	18	18
50–64	43	8.0	29	2	3	7	11	14	17	29
65+	119	8.7	44	2	3	7	12	19	22	29
B. Operated										
0–19 Years	0									
20–34	3	14.6	285	2	2	8	34	34	34	34
35–49	8	10.4	123	1	3	5	18	34	34	34
50–64	26	9.5	339	1	3	4	7	23	29	94
65+	21	11.4	88	3	4	8	15	22	42	>99
SUBTOTALS:										
1. SINGLE DX										
A. Not Operated	1	13.0	0	13	13	13	13	13	13	13
B. Operated	2	3.5	<1	3	3	3	4	4	4	4
2. MULTIPLE DX										
A. Not Operated	179	8.8	41	3	4	7	12	18	22	29
B. Operated	58	10.6	206	2	3	6	14	29	42	>99
1. SINGLE DX	3	6.7	30	3	3	4	13	13	13	13
2. MULTIPLE DX	237	9.2	81	2	4	7	12	20	24	42
A. NOT OPERATED	180	8.8	41	2	4	7	12	18	22	29
B. OPERATED	60	10.3	201	2	3	6	12	23	34	>99
TOTAL										
0–19 Years	0									
20–34	9	15.0	111	2	8	11	21	34	34	34
35–49	20	10.2	59	1	5	9	13	18	18	34
50–64	71	8.4	139	2	4	6	11	14	23	94
65+	140	9.1	51	3	4	7	13	20	22	42
GRAND TOTAL	240	9.2	80	2	4	7	12	20	24	42

032: DIPHTHERIA

Type of Patients	Observed Patients	Avg. Stay	Vari-ance	10th	25th	50th	75th	90th	95th	99th
1. SINGLE DX										
A. Not Operated										
0–19 Years	0									
20–34	0									
35–49	0									
50–64	0									
65+	0									
B. Operated										
0–19 Years	0									
20–34	0									
35–49	0									
50–64	0									
65+	0									
2. MULTIPLE DX										
A. Not Operated										
0–19 Years	1	1.0	0	1	1	1	1	1	1	1
20–34	0									
35–49	3	10.0	21	6	6	9	15	15	15	15
50–64	0									
65+	1	7.0	0	7	7	7	7	7	7	7
B. Operated										
0–19 Years	0									
20–34	0									
35–49	0									
50–64	0									
65+	1	6.0	0	6	6	6	6	6	6	6
SUBTOTALS:										
1. SINGLE DX										
A. Not Operated	0									
B. Operated	0									
2. MULTIPLE DX										
A. Not Operated	5	7.6	26	1	6	7	9	15	15	15
B. Operated	1	6.0	0	6	6	6	6	6	6	6
1. SINGLE DX	0									
2. MULTIPLE DX	6	7.3	21	1	6	6	9	15	15	15
A. NOT OPERATED	5	7.6	26	1	6	7	9	15	15	15
B. OPERATED	1	6.0	0	6	6	6	6	6	6	6
TOTAL										
0–19 Years	1	1.0	0	1	1	1	1	1	1	1
20–34	0									
35–49	3	10.0	21	6	6	9	15	15	15	15
50–64	0									
65+	2	6.5	<1	6	6	6	7	7	7	7
GRAND TOTAL	6	7.3	21	1	6	6	9	15	15	15

Length of Stay by Diagnosis and Operation, Western Region, 2008

Western Region, October 2006–September 2007 Data, by Diagnosis

033: WHOOPING COUGH

Type of Patients	Observed Patients	Avg. Stay	Vari-ance	10th	25th	50th	75th	90th	95th	99th
1. SINGLE DX										
A. Not Operated										
0–19 Years	43	3.7	11	1	1	2	5	8	11	14
20–34	0									
35–49	0									
50–64	0									
65+	0									
B. Operated										
0–19 Years	0									
20–34	0									
35–49	0									
50–64	0									
65+	0									
2. MULTIPLE DX										
A. Not Operated										
0–19 Years	93	5.3	49	1	2	3	6	12	20	44
20–34	6	3.3	6	1	2	3	4	8	8	8
35–49	4	5.0	13	1	1	3	7	9	9	9
50–64	9	5.6	4	3	5	5	6	9	9	9
65+	11	4.9	6	3	3	5	7	7	10	10
B. Operated										
0–19 Years	0									
20–34	0									
35–49	0									
50–64	0									
65+	0									
SUBTOTALS:										
1. SINGLE DX										
A. Not Operated	43	3.7	11	1	1	2	5	8	11	14
B. Operated	0									
2. MULTIPLE DX										
A. Not Operated	123	5.2	38	1	2	3	6	9	17	35
B. Operated	0									
1. SINGLE DX	43	3.7	11	1	1	2	5	8	11	14
2. MULTIPLE DX	123	5.2	38	1	2	3	6	9	17	35
A. NOT OPERATED	166	4.8	32	1	2	3	6	9	13	35
B. OPERATED	0									
TOTAL										
0–19 Years	136	4.8	37	1	2	3	6	10	17	35
20–34	6	3.3	6	1	2	3	4	8	8	8
35–49	4	5.0	13	1	1	3	7	9	9	9
50–64	9	5.6	4	3	5	5	6	7	10	10
65+	11	4.9	6	3	3	5	7	7	10	10
GRAND TOTAL	166	4.8	32	1	2	3	6	9	13	35

034: STREP THROAT/SCARLET FEV

Type of Patients	Observed Patients	Avg. Stay	Vari-ance	10th	25th	50th	75th	90th	95th	99th
1. SINGLE DX										
A. Not Operated										
0–19 Years	43	1.7	1	1	1	1	2	4	4	5
20–34	11	1.7	<1	1	1	2	2	2	3	3
35–49	4	2.0	<1	1	1	2	2	3	3	3
50–64	2	3.0	0	3	3	3	3	3	3	3
65+	0									
B. Operated										
0–19 Years	0									
20–34	1	2.0	0	2	2	2	2	2	2	2
35–49	0									
50–64	0									
65+	0									
2. MULTIPLE DX										
A. Not Operated										
0–19 Years	290	2.1	2	1	1	2	3	4	4	8
20–34	183	2.5	5	1	1	2	3	4	6	10
35–49	98	2.7	5	1	1	2	3	6	7	12
50–64	37	3.0	2	1	2	3	4	5	6	7
65+	36	2.8	7	1	1	2	3	6	11	12
B. Operated										
0–19 Years	10	3.5	5	1	2	3	5	7	7	7
20–34	7	4.6	23	1	2	3	5	15	15	15
35–49	7	5.7	16	1	2	6	8	12	12	12
50–64	0									
65+	0									
SUBTOTALS:										
1. SINGLE DX										
A. Not Operated	60	1.8	1	1	1	2	2	3	4	5
B. Operated	1	2.0	0	2	2	2	2	2	2	2
2. MULTIPLE DX										
A. Not Operated	644	2.4	4	1	1	2	3	4	6	10
B. Operated	24	4.5	13	1	2	3	6	8	12	15
1. SINGLE DX	61	1.8	1	1	1	2	2	3	4	5
2. MULTIPLE DX	668	2.5	4	1	1	2	3	4	6	11
A. NOT OPERATED	704	2.3	3	1	1	2	3	4	6	10
B. OPERATED	25	4.4	13	1	2	3	6	8	12	15
TOTAL										
0–19 Years	343	2.1	2	1	1	2	3	4	4	7
20–34	202	2.5	5	1	1	2	3	4	6	10
35–49	109	2.8	6	1	1	2	3	6	8	12
50–64	39	3.0	2	1	2	3	4	5	6	7
65+	36	2.8	7	1	1	2	3	6	11	12
GRAND TOTAL	729	2.4	4	1	1	2	3	4	6	11

034.0: STREP SORE THROAT

Type of Patients	Observed Patients	Avg. Stay	Vari-ance	10th	25th	50th	75th	90th	95th	99th
1. SINGLE DX										
A. Not Operated										
0–19 Years	38	1.7	1	1	1	2	2	4	4	5
20–34	10	1.8	<1	1	1	2	2	3	3	3
35–49	4	2.0	<1	1	1	2	2	3	3	3
50–64	2	3.0	0	3	3	3	3	3	3	3
65+	0									
B. Operated										
0–19 Years	0									
20–34	1	2.0	0	2	2	2	2	2	2	2
35–49	0									
50–64	0									
65+	0									
2. MULTIPLE DX										
A. Not Operated										
0–19 Years	261	2.0	1	1	1	2	2	3	4	6
20–34	177	2.5	5	1	1	2	3	4	6	10
35–49	97	2.7	5	1	1	2	3	6	7	12
50–64	37	3.0	2	1	2	3	4	5	6	7
65+	34	2.8	7	1	1	2	3	6	11	12
B. Operated										
0–19 Years	10	3.5	5	1	2	3	5	7	7	7
20–34	7	4.6	23	1	2	3	5	15	15	15
35–49	7	5.7	16	1	2	6	8	12	12	12
50–64	0									
65+	0									
SUBTOTALS:										
1. SINGLE DX										
A. Not Operated	54	1.8	1	1	1	2	2	3	4	5
B. Operated	1	2.0	0	2	2	2	2	2	2	2
2. MULTIPLE DX										
A. Not Operated	606	2.4	3	1	1	2	3	4	6	9
B. Operated	24	4.5	13	1	2	3	6	8	12	15
1. SINGLE DX	55	1.8	1	1	1	2	2	3	4	5
2. MULTIPLE DX	630	2.4	4	1	1	2	3	4	6	11
A. NOT OPERATED	660	2.3	3	1	1	2	3	4	6	9
B. OPERATED	25	4.4	13	1	2	3	6	8	12	15
TOTAL										
0–19 Years	309	2.0	1	1	1	2	3	4	4	6
20–34	195	2.5	5	1	1	2	3	4	6	15
35–49	108	2.9	6	1	1	2	3	6	8	12
50–64	39	3.0	2	1	2	3	4	5	6	7
65+	34	2.8	7	1	1	2	3	6	11	12
GRAND TOTAL	685	2.4	4	1	1	2	3	4	6	11

Length of Stay by Diagnosis and Operation, Western Region, 2008

Western Region, October 2006–September 2007 Data, by Diagnosis

035: ERYSIPELAS

Type of Patients	Observed Patients	Avg. Stay	Variance	10th	25th	50th	75th	90th	95th	99th
1. SINGLE DX										
A. Not Operated										
0–19 Years	4	3.0	<1	2	3	3	3	4	4	4
20–34	3	3.0	7	1	1	2	6	6	6	6
35–49	1	2.0	0	2	2	2	2	2	2	2
50–64	3	2.3	<1	2	2	2	3	3	3	3
65+	0									
B. Operated										
0–19 Years	0									
20–34	0									
35–49	0									
50–64	0									
65+	0									
2. MULTIPLE DX										
A. Not Operated										
0–19 Years	10	3.1	1	2	2	3	4	5	5	5
20–34	19	2.3	<1	1	2	3	3	3	4	4
35–49	52	3.0	2	1	2	3	4	4	5	8
50–64	79	4.3	10	2	2	3	5	9	11	18
65+	76	3.7	4	1	2	3	5	7	8	11
B. Operated										
0–19 Years	0									
20–34	1	4.0	0	4	4	4	4	4	4	4
35–49	1	9.0	0	9	9	9	9	9	9	9
50–64	1	5.0	0	5	5	5	5	5	5	5
65+	1	8.0	0	8	8	8	8	8	8	8
SUBTOTALS:										
1. SINGLE DX A. Not Operated	11	2.7	2	2	2	2	3	4	6	6
1. SINGLE DX B. Operated	0									
2. MULTIPLE DX A. Not Operated	236	3.6	6	1	2	3	4	7	9	13
2. MULTIPLE DX B. Operated	4	6.5	6	4	4	5	8	9	9	9
1. SINGLE DX	11	2.7	2	2	2	2	3	4	6	6
2. MULTIPLE DX	240	3.6	6	1	2	3	4	7	9	13
A. NOT OPERATED	247	3.6	6	1	2	3	4	6	8	13
B. OPERATED	4	6.5	6	4	4	5	8	9	9	9
TOTAL										
0–19 Years	15	3.1	1	2	2	3	4	5	5	5
20–34	22	2.4	1	1	2	2	3	3	4	6
35–49	54	3.1	3	1	2	3	4	5	6	9
50–64	83	4.2	10	2	2	3	5	9	11	18
65+	77	3.7	5	1	2	3	5	7	8	11
GRAND TOTAL	251	3.6	6	1	2	3	4	7	9	13

036: MENINGOCOCCAL INFECTION

Type of Patients	Observed Patients	Avg. Stay	Variance	10th	25th	50th	75th	90th	95th	99th
1. SINGLE DX										
A. Not Operated										
0–19 Years	7	5.0	12	2	3	3	8	10	10	10
20–34	0									
35–49	0									
50–64	1	3.0	0	3	3	3	3	3	3	3
65+	0									
B. Operated										
0–19 Years	0									
20–34	0									
35–49	0									
50–64	0									
65+	0									
2. MULTIPLE DX										
A. Not Operated										
0–19 Years	44	6.5	12	3	4	6	8	10	13	18
20–34	31	7.7	22	2	4	7	10	13	15	22
35–49	23	9.2	39	2	4	8	13	19	20	26
50–64	26	9.4	87	3	5	7	11	14	18	51
65+	18	8.6	21	3	5	8	12	14	20	20
B. Operated										
0–19 Years	1	31.0	0	31	31	31	31	31	31	31
20–34	2	30.5	142	22	22	31	39	39	39	39
35–49	0									
50–64	1	36.0	0	36	36	36	36	36	36	36
65+	1	13.0	0	13	13	13	13	13	13	13
SUBTOTALS:										
1. SINGLE DX A. Not Operated	8	4.8	11	2	3	3	10	10	10	10
1. SINGLE DX B. Operated	0									
2. MULTIPLE DX A. Not Operated	142	8.0	34	3	4	7	10	13	18	26
2. MULTIPLE DX B. Operated	5	28.2	113	13	22	31	36	39	39	39
1. SINGLE DX	8	4.8	11	2	3	3	10	10	10	10
2. MULTIPLE DX	147	8.7	49	3	5	7	10	15	20	39
A. NOT OPERATED	150	7.8	33	2	4	7	10	13	18	26
B. OPERATED	5	28.2	113	13	22	31	36	39	39	39
TOTAL										
0–19 Years	52	6.8	24	3	4	6	8	10	17	31
20–34	33	9.1	55	2	5	7	10	15	22	39
35–49	23	9.2	39	2	4	8	13	19	20	26
50–64	28	10.1	108	3	5	7	11	18	36	51
65+	19	8.9	21	3	5	8	13	14	20	20
GRAND TOTAL	155	8.5	48	3	4	7	10	14	20	39

037: TETANUS

Type of Patients	Observed Patients	Avg. Stay	Variance	10th	25th	50th	75th	90th	95th	99th
1. SINGLE DX										
A. Not Operated										
0–19 Years	0									
20–34	0									
35–49	0									
50–64	0									
65+	0									
B. Operated										
0–19 Years	0									
20–34	0									
35–49	0									
50–64	0									
65+	0									
2. MULTIPLE DX										
A. Not Operated										
0–19 Years	1	1.0	0	1	1	1	1	1	1	1
20–34	3	1.3	<1	1	1	1	2	2	2	2
35–49	5	14.2	523	2	3	4	7	55	55	55
50–64	0									
65+	1	6.0	0	6	6	6	6	6	6	6
B. Operated										
0–19 Years	0									
20–34	0									
35–49	0									
50–64	0									
65+	0									
SUBTOTALS:										
1. SINGLE DX A. Not Operated	0									
1. SINGLE DX B. Operated	0									
2. MULTIPLE DX A. Not Operated	10	8.2	274	1	1	2	6	7	55	55
2. MULTIPLE DX B. Operated	0									
1. SINGLE DX	0									
2. MULTIPLE DX	10	8.2	274	1	1	3	7	55	>99	>99
A. NOT OPERATED	10	8.2	274	1	1	2	6	7	55	55
B. OPERATED	0									
TOTAL										
0–19 Years	1	1.0	0	1	1	1	1	1	1	1
20–34	3	1.3	<1	1	1	1	2	2	2	2
35–49	5	14.2	523	2	3	4	7	55	55	55
50–64										
65+	1	6.0	0	6	6	6	6	6	6	6
GRAND TOTAL	10	8.2	274	1	1	3	7	55	>99	>99

Length of Stay by Diagnosis and Operation, Western Region, 2008

Western Region, October 2006–September 2007 Data, by Diagnosis

038: SEPTICEMIA

Type of Patients	Observed Patients	Avg. Stay	Variance	10th	25th	50th	75th	90th	95th	99th
1. SINGLE DX										
A. Not Operated										
0–19 Years	13	4.0	22	2	2	2	3	10	18	18
20–34	1	4.0	0	4	4	4	4	4	4	4
35–49	0									
50–64	8	3.9	12	1	1	4	8	10	10	10
65+	9	7.6	16	4	4	7	9	14	14	14
B. Operated										
0–19 Years	0									
20–34	0									
35–49	0									
50–64	0									
65+	0									
2. MULTIPLE DX										
A. Not Operated										
0–19 Years	1,292	6.2	38	2	3	4	8	13	16	39
20–34	2,420	7.0	59	2	3	5	8	14	20	44
35–49	5,905	8.1	62	2	4	6	10	16	22	43
50–64	13,721	8.3	58	3	4	6	10	17	22	39
65+	41,308	7.3	35	2	4	6	9	14	18	29
B. Operated										
0–19 Years	122	15.5	237	3	6	11	20	48	59	>99
20–34	451	15.2	204	4	6	11	20	33	48	>99
35–49	1,217	16.8	203	5	8	13	21	34	49	>99
50–64	2,436	17.1	201	5	8	13	21	35	48	>99
65+	4,418	15.3	121	5	8	13	19	28	36	63
SUBTOTALS:										
1. SINGLE DX										
A. Not Operated	31	5.0	19	2	2	4	7	10	14	18
B. Operated	0									
2. MULTIPLE DX										
A. Not Operated	64,646	7.5	44	2	4	6	9	15	20	33
B. Operated	8,644	16.0	162	5	8	13	20	31	43	87
1. SINGLE DX	31	5.0	19	2	2	4	7	10	14	18
2. MULTIPLE DX	73,290	8.5	65	3	4	6	10	17	23	43
A. NOT OPERATED	64,677	7.5	44	2	4	6	9	15	20	33
B. OPERATED	8,644	16.0	162	5	8	13	20	31	43	87
TOTAL										
0–19 Years	1,427	7.0	62	2	3	4	9	14	21	50
20–34	2,872	8.3	91	2	3	5	9	18	27	57
35–49	7,122	9.5	97	2	4	6	12	20	28	57
50–64	16,165	9.6	89	3	4	7	12	20	27	53
65+	45,735	8.1	49	3	4	6	10	16	21	36
GRAND TOTAL	73,321	8.5	65	3	4	6	10	17	23	43

038.0: STREPTOCOCCAL SEPTICEMIA

Type of Patients	Observed Patients	Avg. Stay	Variance	10th	25th	50th	75th	90th	95th	99th
1. SINGLE DX										
A. Not Operated										
0–19 Years	3	4.7	21	2	2	2	10	10	10	10
20–34	0									
35–49	0									
50–64	0									
65+	3	5.0	3	4	4	4	7	7	7	7
B. Operated										
0–19 Years	0									
20–34	0									
35–49	0									
50–64	0									
65+	0									
2. MULTIPLE DX										
A. Not Operated										
0–19 Years	103	8.5	26	3	5	7	10	14	17	23
20–34	121	8.0	38	3	4	5	10	15	22	28
35–49	389	8.8	60	3	5	7	10	16	22	43
50–64	867	9.2	64	3	4	7	11	17	24	48
65+	2,224	8.5	42	3	4	7	10	16	21	34
B. Operated										
0–19 Years	10	16.9	273	4	6	17	22	23	59	59
20–34	36	13.0	57	4	7	11	16	23	29	34
35–49	124	19.2	251	6	9	15	22	39	54	87
50–64	241	18.8	223	6	9	14	25	38	55	84
65+	286	16.5	133	6	9	14	21	32	40	89
SUBTOTALS:										
1. SINGLE DX										
A. Not Operated	6	4.8	10	2	2	4	7	10	10	10
B. Operated	0									
2. MULTIPLE DX										
A. Not Operated	3,704	8.7	49	3	4	7	11	16	22	36
B. Operated	697	17.6	185	6	9	14	22	33	46	86
1. SINGLE DX	6	4.8	10	2	2	4	7	10	10	10
2. MULTIPLE DX	4,401	10.1	81	3	5	7	12	20	27	49
A. NOT OPERATED	3,710	8.7	49	3	4	7	11	16	22	36
B. OPERATED	697	17.6	185	6	9	14	22	33	46	86
TOTAL										
0–19 Years	116	9.1	51	3	5	8	11	16	22	30
20–34	157	9.1	46	3	4	7	13	18	23	33
35–49	513	11.3	125	3	5	8	13	22	34	69
50–64	1,108	11.3	114	3	5	8	14	23	31	64
65+	2,513	9.4	59	3	5	7	12	18	24	39
GRAND TOTAL	4,407	10.1	81	3	5	7	12	20	27	49

038.10: STAPH SEPTICEMIA NOS

Type of Patients	Observed Patients	Avg. Stay	Variance	10th	25th	50th	75th	90th	95th	99th
1. SINGLE DX										
A. Not Operated										
0–19 Years	0									
20–34	0									
35–49	0									
50–64	0									
65+	0									
B. Operated										
0–19 Years	0									
20–34	0									
35–49	0									
50–64	0									
65+	0									
2. MULTIPLE DX										
A. Not Operated										
0–19 Years	9	6.9	27	1	3	6	10	16	16	16
20–34	26	6.6	16	3	3	5	8	13	13	17
35–49	43	9.4	87	3	5	7	12	16	25	56
50–64	130	10.4	117	3	5	7	13	18	23	59
65+	284	8.3	35	3	4	7	10	15	19	32
B. Operated										
0–19 Years	2	17.7	476	2	2	33	33	33	33	33
20–34	5	19.5	558	7	7	9	12	62	62	62
35–49	12	13.7	91	4	6	13	17	37	>99	>99
50–64	17	14.3	39	8	11	12	15	26	28	28
65+	27	19.0	170	6	9	15	25	42	47	53
SUBTOTALS:										
1. SINGLE DX										
A. Not Operated	0									
B. Operated	0									
2. MULTIPLE DX										
A. Not Operated	492	8.8	61	3	4	7	11	16	21	38
B. Operated	63	16.7	148	6	9	13	21	37	47	>99
1. SINGLE DX	0									
2. MULTIPLE DX	555	9.7	77	3	5	7	12	18	25	53
A. NOT OPERATED	492	8.8	61	3	4	7	11	16	21	38
B. OPERATED	63	16.7	148	6	9	13	21	37	47	>99
TOTAL										
0–19 Years	11	8.9	88	1	2	6	12	16	21	33
20–34	31	8.7	111	3	4	7	10	13	17	62
35–49	55	10.3	89	3	4	8	13	25	37	>99
50–64	147	10.8	110	3	5	8	14	18	26	59
65+	311	9.3	56	3	5	7	11	17	24	42
GRAND TOTAL	555	9.7	77	3	5	7	12	18	25	53

Length of Stay by Diagnosis and Operation, Western Region, 2008

Western Region, October 2006–September 2007 Data, by Diagnosis

038.11: STAPH AUREUS SEPTICEMIA

Type of Patients	Observed Patients	Avg. Stay	Vari- ance	10th	25th	50th	75th	90th	95th	99th
1. SINGLE DX										
A. *Not Operated*										
0–19 Years	1	18.0	0	18	18	18	18	18	18	18
20–34	0									
35–49	0									
50–64	2	7.0	18	4	4	4	4	10	10	10
65+	1	7.0	0	7	7	7	7	7	7	7
B. *Operated*										
0–19 Years	0									
20–34	0									
35–49	0									
50–64	0									
65+	0									
2. MULTIPLE DX										
A. *Not Operated*										
0–19 Years	63	8.3	34	3	4	6	11	16	21	26
20–34	226	11.9	123	3	5	8	14	25	39	57
35–49	586	12.0	95	4	6	10	14	23	30	59
50–64	1,187	11.9	97	4	6	8	15	20	29	56
65+	2,408	10.3	57	4	6	8	13	19	24	41
B. *Operated*										
0–19 Years	27	20.2	221	8	9	15	31	54	55	>99
20–34	80	18.5	221	5	9	15	24	45	62	>99
35–49	228	19.4	238	6	9	15	25	43	55	>99
50–64	466	20.1	285	6	10	15	24	40	63	>99
65+	551	17.5	171	7	9	14	21	31	48	76
SUBTOTALS:										
1. SINGLE DX										
A. *Not Operated*	4	9.7	36	4	4	7	10	18	18	18
B. *Operated*	0									
2. MULTIPLE DX										
A. *Not Operated*	4,470	11.0	76	4	6	8	13	21	27	48
B. *Operated*	1,352	18.8	226	6	9	15	23	38	54	>99
1. SINGLE DX	4	9.7	36	4	4	7	10	18	18	18
2. MULTIPLE DX	5,822	12.8	122	4	6	10	16	25	34	67
A. NOT OPERATED	4,474	11.0	76	4	6	8	13	21	27	48
B. OPERATED	1,352	18.8	226	6	9	15	23	38	54	>99
TOTAL										
0–19 Years	91	11.9	118	3	5	8	14	24	43	>99
20–34	306	13.6	157	3	5	10	17	30	44	68
35–49	814	14.0	146	4	7	10	17	26	40	72
50–64	1,655	14.2	163	4	7	10	17	27	39	85
65+	2,960	11.6	86	6	9	9	14	22	28	51
GRAND TOTAL	5,826	12.8	122	4	6	10	16	25	34	67

038.19: STAPH SEPTICEMIA NEC

Type of Patients	Observed Patients	Avg. Stay	Vari- ance	10th	25th	50th	75th	90th	95th	99th
1. SINGLE DX										
A. *Not Operated*										
0–19 Years	0									
20–34	0									
35–49	0									
50–64	0									
65+	0									
B. *Operated*										
0–19 Years	0									
20–34	0									
35–49	0									
50–64	0									
65+	0									
2. MULTIPLE DX										
A. *Not Operated*										
0–19 Years	28	9.4	51	3	5	7	11	14	29	34
20–34	49	10.1	70	3	5	7	13	24	31	35
35–49	133	10.9	121	3	5	8	12	24	38	66
50–64	347	9.9	62	3	5	7	11	21	28	36
65+	883	9.1	44	3	5	7	11	16	21	38
B. *Operated*										
0–19 Years	1	13.0	0	13	13	58	>99	>99	>99	>99
20–34	8	23.3	810	2	12	13	23	92	92	92
35–49	20	20.0	172	7	10	18	29	45	49	>99
50–64	61	20.8	247	7	10	18	25	44	66	>99
65+	105	17.3	140	6	9	14	22	33	39	53
SUBTOTALS:										
1. SINGLE DX										
A. *Not Operated*	0									
B. *Operated*	0									
2. MULTIPLE DX										
A. *Not Operated*	1,440	9.5	57	3	5	7	11	18	24	41
B. *Operated*	195	18.9	202	6	9	15	24	39	53	>99
1. SINGLE DX	0									
2. MULTIPLE DX	1,635	10.6	83	4	5	8	13	21	29	51
A. NOT OPERATED	1,440	9.5	57	3	5	7	11	18	24	41
B. OPERATED	195	18.9	202	6	9	15	24	39	53	>99
TOTAL										
0–19 Years	29	9.6	50	3	5	7	13	14	34	>99
20–34	57	12.0	183	3	5	7	14	24	32	92
35–49	153	12.1	136	4	5	9	14	29	46	>99
50–64	408	11.6	104	4	5	8	14	25	32	60
65+	988	9.9	61	4	5	8	12	19	25	43
GRAND TOTAL	1,635	10.6	83	4	5	8	13	21	29	51

038.2: PNEUMOCOCCAL SEPTICEMIA

Type of Patients	Observed Patients	Avg. Stay	Vari- ance	10th	25th	50th	75th	90th	95th	99th
1. SINGLE DX										
A. *Not Operated*										
0–19 Years	0									
20–34	0									
35–49	0									
50–64	0									
65+	0									
B. *Operated*										
0–19 Years	0									
20–34	0									
35–49	0									
50–64	0									
65+	0									
2. MULTIPLE DX										
A. *Not Operated*										
0–19 Years	48	6.9	63	2	3	4	6	16	20	51
20–34	64	8.1	99	2	3	5	9	15	17	75
35–49	212	8.9	67	3	4	7	11	17	24	37
50–64	366	10.1	81	3	4	7	12	20	25	47
65+	582	9.0	49	3	5	7	11	16	21	37
B. *Operated*										
0–19 Years	0									
20–34	5	30.5	639	6	11	29	37	70	70	70
35–49	17	20.4	85	9	14	18	26	36	36	36
50–64	38	21.8	352	7	11	17	23	49	94	>99
65+	41	17.3	128	8	11	15	21	28	34	66
SUBTOTALS:										
1. SINGLE DX										
A. *Not Operated*	0									
B. *Operated*	0									
2. MULTIPLE DX										
A. *Not Operated*	1,272	9.2	65	3	4	7	11	18	24	41
B. *Operated*	101	20.2	230	8	11	17	23	36	49	94
1. SINGLE DX	0									
2. MULTIPLE DX	1,373	10.0	85	3	4	7	12	20	26	51
A. NOT OPERATED	1,272	9.2	65	3	4	7	11	18	24	41
B. OPERATED	101	20.2	230	8	11	17	23	36	49	94
TOTAL										
0–19 Years	48	6.9	63	2	3	4	6	16	20	51
20–34	69	9.7	163	2	4	6	10	17	29	75
35–49	229	9.8	77	3	4	7	12	22	26	37
50–64	404	11.2	118	3	5	8	14	22	29	72
65+	623	9.6	58	4	5	7	12	19	23	41
GRAND TOTAL	1,373	10.0	85	3	4	7	12	20	26	51

Length of Stay by Diagnosis and Operation, Western Region, 2008

Western Region, October 2006–September 2007 Data, by Diagnosis

038.3: ANAEROBIC SEPTICEMIA

Type of Patients	Observed Patients	Avg. Stay	Vari-ance	10th	25th	50th	75th	90th	95th	99th
1. SINGLE DX										
A. Not Operated										
0–19 Years	0									
20–34	0									
35–49	0									
50–64	0									
65+	0									
B. Operated										
0–19 Years	0									
20–34	0									
35–49	0									
50–64	0									
65+	0									
2. MULTIPLE DX										
A. Not Operated										
0–19 Years	3	12.4	16	10	10	10	17	17	17	17
20–34	17	7.1	26	2	3	6	9	14	19	19
35–49	42	9.8	62	2	5	7	12	22	27	34
50–64	101	10.7	105	3	5	8	13	22	27	45
65+	315	8.6	33	3	5	7	11	15	20	30
B. Operated										
0–19 Years	4	11.2	57	5	5	7	11	22	22	22
20–34	8	27.6	301	7	19	25	38	64	64	64
35–49	18	18.0	192	6	7	14	23	41	56	56
50–64	28	17.6	386	5	7	13	18	28	73	91
65+	66	18.8	174	7	10	16	21	33	46	77
SUBTOTALS:										
1. SINGLE DX										
A. Not Operated	0									
B. Operated	0									
2. MULTIPLE DX										
A. Not Operated	478	9.1	51	3	5	7	11	17	23	32
B. Operated	124	18.7	229	6	9	15	22	34	55	77
1. SINGLE DX	0									
2. MULTIPLE DX	602	11.1	102	3	5	8	14	22	28	56
A. NOT OPERATED	478	9.1	51	3	5	7	11	17	23	32
B. OPERATED	124	18.7	229	6	9	15	22	34	55	77
TOTAL										
0–19 Years	7	11.7	34	5	7	10	17	22	22	22
20–34	25	13.6	200	2	3	8	19	30	38	64
35–49	60	12.2	113	3	5	8	17	25	34	56
50–64	129	12.2	172	3	5	8	15	24	28	79
65+	381	10.3	72	4	5	8	13	20	25	46
GRAND TOTAL	602	11.1	102	3	5	8	14	22	28	56

038.40: GRAM-NEG SEPTICEMIA NOS

Type of Patients	Observed Patients	Avg. Stay	Vari-ance	10th	25th	50th	75th	90th	95th	99th
1. SINGLE DX										
A. Not Operated										
0–19 Years	0									
20–34	0									
35–49	0									
50–64	0									
65+	0									
B. Operated										
0–19 Years	0									
20–34	0									
35–49	0									
50–64	0									
65+	0									
2. MULTIPLE DX										
A. Not Operated										
0–19 Years	10	6.9	29	2	3	5	10	20	20	20
20–34	25	6.6	79	2	3	5	7	10	11	47
35–49	66	5.7	28	2	2	4	7	11	18	30
50–64	175	7.6	75	2	3	5	8	18	22	46
65+	460	6.5	26	2	3	5	8	13	16	26
B. Operated										
0–19 Years	1	4.0	0	4	4	4	4	4	4	4
20–34	2	4.5	4	3	3	3	3	6	6	6
35–49	17	16.5	212	3	7	12	21	42	54	54
50–64	22	14.0	97	3	6	11	18	30	32	35
65+	63	13.3	116	5	6	11	16	28	42	>99
SUBTOTALS:										
1. SINGLE DX										
A. Not Operated	0									
B. Operated	0									
2. MULTIPLE DX										
A. Not Operated	736	6.7	40	2	3	5	8	14	18	36
B. Operated	105	13.7	126	4	6	11	17	29	42	56
1. SINGLE DX	0									
2. MULTIPLE DX	841	7.6	56	2	3	5	9	16	21	42
A. NOT OPERATED	736	6.7	40	2	3	5	8	14	18	36
B. OPERATED	105	13.7	126	4	6	11	17	29	42	56
TOTAL										
0–19 Years	11	6.7	27	3	3	5	8	10	10	20
20–34	27	6.4	73	2	3	5	7	10	11	47
35–49	83	7.9	82	2	3	5	9	18	28	54
50–64	197	8.3	81	2	3	5	10	18	30	46
65+	523	7.3	42	2	4	5	9	15	18	36
GRAND TOTAL	841	7.6	56	2	3	5	9	16	21	42

038.42: E. COLI SEPTICEMIA

Type of Patients	Observed Patients	Avg. Stay	Vari-ance	10th	25th	50th	75th	90th	95th	99th
1. SINGLE DX										
A. Not Operated										
0–19 Years	0									
20–34	1	4.0	0	4	4	4	4	4	4	4
35–49	0									
50–64	2	6.0	8	4	4	6	8	8	8	8
65+	1	4.0	0	4	4	4	4	4	4	4
B. Operated										
0–19 Years	0									
20–34	0									
35–49	0									
50–64	0									
65+	0									
2. MULTIPLE DX										
A. Not Operated										
0–19 Years	161	7.3	30	3	4	6	9	14	15	30
20–34	309	5.8	45	2	3	4	6	9	17	31
35–49	714	6.6	35	2	3	5	8	13	17	28
50–64	1,796	6.8	33	3	3	5	8	13	17	29
65+	6,270	6.3	21	3	4	5	8	11	15	24
B. Operated										
0–19 Years	8	16.1	215	4	5	15	16	50	50	50
20–34	37	12.7	261	4	4	7	13	34	83	>99
35–49	106	13.8	179	4	6	10	18	28	42	>99
50–64	210	15.9	218	4	7	11	19	25	51	79
65+	563	13.9	104	5	7	11	18	25	32	57
SUBTOTALS:										
1. SINGLE DX										
A. Not Operated	4	5.0	4	4	4	4	6	8	8	8
B. Operated	0									
2. MULTIPLE DX										
A. Not Operated	9,250	6.4	25	3	3	5	8	12	15	26
B. Operated	924	14.3	146	5	7	11	18	28	38	79
1. SINGLE DX	4	5.0	4	4	4	4	6	8	8	8
2. MULTIPLE DX	10,174	7.1	41	3	4	5	8	13	19	34
A. NOT OPERATED	9,254	6.4	25	3	3	5	8	12	15	26
B. OPERATED	924	14.3	146	5	7	11	18	28	38	79
TOTAL										
0–19 Years	169	7.7	41	3	4	6	9	14	18	42
20–34	347	6.5	72	2	3	4	7	11	22	70
35–49	820	7.5	59	3	4	5	8	15	20	44
50–64	2,008	7.7	60	3	4	5	9	20	20	43
65+	6,834	6.9	32	3	4	5	8	13	17	29
GRAND TOTAL	10,178	7.1	41	3	4	5	8	13	19	34

Length of Stay by Diagnosis and Operation, Western Region, 2008

Western Region, October 2006–September 2007 Data, by Diagnosis

038.43: PSEUDOMONAS SEPTICEMIA

Type of Patients	Observed Patients	Avg. Stay	Variance	Percentiles						
				10th	25th	50th	75th	90th	95th	99th
1. SINGLE DX										
A. Not Operated										
0–19 Years	0									
20–34	0									
35–49	0									
50–64	0									
65+	0									
B. Operated										
0–19 Years	0									
20–34	0									
35–49	0									
50–64	0									
65+	0									
2. MULTIPLE DX										
A. Not Operated										
0–19 Years	13	14.3	152	3	8	11	16	40	41	41
20–34	20	7.2	23	3	4	7	8	12	24	24
35–49	71	11.9	113	3	5	8	15	25	33	54
50–64	231	9.4	53	3	5	7	12	18	22	37
65+	608	8.9	43	3	5	7	11	16	21	34
B. Operated										
0–19 Years	2	56.0	126	48	48	56	64	64	64	64
20–34	6	35.5	257	20	31	32	67	>99	>99	>99
35–49	7	24.0	215	9	11	18	42	45	45	45
50–64	34	17.7	169	6	8	16	22	37	50	57
65+	63	15.6	219	5	7	12	17	26	36	93
SUBTOTALS:										
1. SINGLE DX										
A. Not Operated	0									
B. Operated	0									
2. MULTIPLE DX										
A. Not Operated	943	9.3	52	3	5	7	12	17	22	39
B. Operated	112	18.5	245	6	9	14	22	42	60	93
1. SINGLE DX	0									
2. MULTIPLE DX	1,055	10.3	81	3	5	8	13	19	27	53
A. NOT OPERATED	943	9.3	52	3	5	7	12	17	22	39
B. OPERATED	112	18.5	245	6	9	14	22	42	60	93
TOTAL										
0–19 Years	15	19.8	354	3	8	12	40	48	64	64
20–34	26	13.7	217	4	4	8	24	32	67	>99
35–49	78	13.0	132	3	5	9	16	28	42	54
50–64	265	10.5	75	3	5	8	13	20	27	50
65+	671	9.5	63	4	5	7	12	17	22	39
GRAND TOTAL	1,055	10.3	81	3	5	8	13	19	27	53

038.49: GRAM-NEG SEPTICEMIA NEC

Type of Patients	Observed Patients	Avg. Stay	Variance	Percentiles						
				10th	25th	50th	75th	90th	95th	99th
1. SINGLE DX										
A. Not Operated										
0–19 Years	0									
20–34	0									
35–49	0									
50–64	0									
65+	0									
B. Operated										
0–19 Years	0									
20–34	0									
35–49	0									
50–64	0									
65+	0									
2. MULTIPLE DX										
A. Not Operated										
0–19 Years	63	8.6	35	3	5	8	11	13	15	39
20–34	97	7.3	41	3	4	6	8	14	19	52
35–49	310	8.1	60	3	4	6	10	15	23	52
50–64	822	8.7	51	3	4	6	11	17	21	35
65+	2,346	7.4	33	3	4	6	9	14	18	29
B. Operated										
0–19 Years	4	18.1	710	4	4	5	58	58	58	58
20–34	29	16.1	201	6	7	10	22	47	49	53
35–49	52	16.3	311	5	6	11	20	28	91	>99
50–64	127	16.4	203	5	8	12	19	38	57	>99
65+	313	13.7	87	5	8	11	18	25	33	58
SUBTOTALS:										
1. SINGLE DX										
A. Not Operated	0									
B. Operated	0									
2. MULTIPLE DX										
A. Not Operated	3,638	7.7	40	3	4	6	9	15	19	31
B. Operated	525	14.8	147	5	7	12	18	28	43	93
1. SINGLE DX	0									
2. MULTIPLE DX	4,163	8.6	59	3	4	6	10	17	22	43
A. NOT OPERATED	3,638	7.7	40	3	4	6	9	15	19	31
B. OPERATED	525	14.8	147	5	7	12	18	28	43	93
TOTAL										
0–19 Years	67	9.2	70	3	5	8	11	14	20	58
20–34	126	9.3	91	3	4	6	10	20	26	52
35–49	362	9.3	103	3	4	6	11	18	25	91
50–64	949	9.7	78	3	4	7	12	19	26	57
65+	2,659	8.1	43	3	4	6	10	16	20	33
GRAND TOTAL	4,163	8.6	59	3	4	6	10	17	22	43

038.8: SEPTICEMIA NEC

Type of Patients	Observed Patients	Avg. Stay	Variance	Percentiles						
				10th	25th	50th	75th	90th	95th	99th
1. SINGLE DX										
A. Not Operated										
0–19 Years	0									
20–34	0									
35–49	0									
50–64	0									
65+	1	14.0	0	14	14	14	14	14	14	14
B. Operated										
0–19 Years	0									
20–34	0									
35–49	0									
50–64	0									
65+	0									
2. MULTIPLE DX										
A. Not Operated										
0–19 Years	38	6.7	44	2	3	4	9	15	21	36
20–34	47	7.5	28	3	3	5	12	16	20	>99
35–49	131	10.1	98	3	4	7	13	21	29	50
50–64	234	9.7	67	3	4	7	13	19	26	38
65+	690	7.9	48	3	4	6	10	15	20	38
B. Operated										
0–19 Years	2	5.0	2	4	4	5	6	6	6	6
20–34	12	19.4	255	5	7	12	34	44	48	48
35–49	23	20.7	265	6	8	17	27	48	50	63
50–64	56	22.6	266	7	10	20	31	60	>99	>99
65+	78	15.8	146	5	8	12	20	28	52	65
SUBTOTALS:										
1. SINGLE DX										
A. Not Operated	1	14.0	0	14	14	14	14	14	14	14
B. Operated	0									
2. MULTIPLE DX										
A. Not Operated	1,140	8.4	57	3	4	6	10	17	23	42
B. Operated	171	18.8	215	6	9	15	24	44	54	>99
1. SINGLE DX	1	14.0	0	14	14	14	14	14	14	14
2. MULTIPLE DX	1,311	9.8	90	3	4	7	12	21	29	54
A. NOT OPERATED	1,141	8.4	57	3	4	6	10	17	23	42
B. OPERATED	171	18.8	215	6	9	15	24	44	54	>99
TOTAL										
0–19 Years	40	6.6	42	2	3	4	8	10	18	36
20–34	59	9.9	94	3	4	7	13	20	35	>99
35–49	154	11.7	136	3	4	8	14	24	41	62
50–64	290	12.1	131	3	5	9	16	27	37	>99
65+	769	8.7	64	3	4	6	10	17	23	42
GRAND TOTAL	1,312	9.8	90	3	4	7	12	21	29	54

Length of Stay by Diagnosis and Operation, Western Region, 2008

Western Region, October 2006–September 2007 Data, by Diagnosis

038.9: SEPTICEMIA NOS

Type of Patients	Observed Patients	Avg. Stay	Variance	10th	25th	50th	75th	90th	95th	99th
1. SINGLE DX										
A. Not Operated										
0–19 Years	9	2.2	<1	2	2	2	2	3	3	3
20–34	0									
35–49	0									
50–64	4	1.3	<1	1	1	1	2	2	2	2
65+	3	9.3	20	5	5	9	14	14	14	14
B. Operated										
0–19 Years	0									
20–34	0									
35–49	0									
50–64	0									
65+	0									
2. MULTIPLE DX										
A. Not Operated										
0–19 Years	739	4.9	33	2	2	3	5	9	14	30
20–34	1,415	6.2	51	2	3	4	7	13	18	36
35–49	3,180	7.2	52	2	3	5	9	15	21	39
50–64	7,398	7.6	50	2	3	6	9	15	21	36
65+	24,092	6.9	34	2	3	5	8	14	18	28
B. Operated										
0–19 Years	60	12.3	187	2	4	8	14	29	48	>99
20–34	221	12.7	146	3	5	9	16	29	33	84
35–49	586	15.4	174	5	7	12	19	32	42	92
50–64	1,125	15.2	141	5	7	12	20	30	40	90
65+	2,247	14.9	108	5	8	12	19	28	35	56
SUBTOTALS:										
1. SINGLE DX										
A. Not Operated	16	3.3	12	1	2	2	3	9	14	14
B. Operated	0									
2. MULTIPLE DX										
A. Not Operated	36,824	7.0	39	2	3	5	9	14	19	31
B. Operated	4,239	14.9	129	5	7	12	19	29	37	70
1. SINGLE DX	**16**	**3.3**	**12**	**1**	**2**	**2**	**3**	**9**	**14**	**14**
2. MULTIPLE DX	**41,063**	**7.8**	**54**	**2**	**3**	**6**	**10**	**16**	**22**	**37**
A. NOT OPERATED	**36,840**	**7.0**	**39**	**2**	**3**	**5**	**9**	**14**	**19**	**31**
B. OPERATED	**4,239**	**14.9**	**129**	**5**	**7**	**12**	**19**	**29**	**37**	**70**
TOTAL										
0–19 Years	808	5.4	48	2	2	3	6	11	15	48
20–34	1,636	7.1	69	2	3	4	8	15	23	44
35–49	3,766	8.5	80	2	3	6	10	18	26	48
50–64	8,527	8.6	69	2	4	6	11	18	24	44
65+	26,342	7.6	45	2	3	6	9	15	20	33
GRAND TOTAL	**41,079**	**7.8**	**54**	**2**	**3**	**6**	**10**	**16**	**22**	**37**

039: ACTINOMYCOTIC INFECTIONS

Type of Patients	Observed Patients	Avg. Stay	Variance	10th	25th	50th	75th	90th	95th	99th
1. SINGLE DX										
A. Not Operated										
0–19 Years	1	3.0	0	3	3	3	3	3	3	3
20–34	0									
35–49	0									
50–64	0									
65+	0									
B. Operated										
0–19 Years	0									
20–34	0									
35–49	0									
50–64	0									
65+	0									
2. MULTIPLE DX										
A. Not Operated										
0–19 Years	2	4.0	8	2	2	2	6	6	6	6
20–34	5	15.1	253	2	8	11	12	43	43	43
35–49	15	8.0	63	2	3	5	11	18	31	31
50–64	27	8.1	35	2	3	6	11	18	19	22
65+	71	10.6	60	4	5	8	13	21	22	42
B. Operated										
0–19 Years	1	1.0	0	1	1	1	1	1	1	1
20–34	6	10.2	25	5	6	10	14	18	18	18
35–49	8	12.0	52	4	4	11	15	22	22	22
50–64	10	11.7	80	1	4	8	17	30	30	30
65+	18	16.0	254	5	8	11	18	31	74	74
SUBTOTALS:										
1. SINGLE DX										
A. Not Operated	1	3.0	0	3	3	3	3	3	3	3
B. Operated	0									
2. MULTIPLE DX										
A. Not Operated	120	9.8	62	2	4	8	12	20	22	42
B. Operated	43	13.1	141	4	6	11	17	21	30	74
1. SINGLE DX	**1**	**3.0**	**0**	**3**	**3**	**3**	**3**	**3**	**3**	**3**
2. MULTIPLE DX	**163**	**10.6**	**85**	**3**	**4**	**8**	**14**	**21**	**22**	**43**
A. NOT OPERATED	**121**	**9.7**	**62**	**3**	**4**	**8**	**12**	**20**	**22**	**42**
B. OPERATED	**43**	**13.1**	**141**	**4**	**6**	**11**	**17**	**21**	**30**	**74**
TOTAL										
0–19 Years	4	3.0	5	1	2	3	3	6	6	6
20–34	11	12.4	120	5	6	10	14	18	43	43
35–49	23	9.4	60	2	4	7	13	21	22	31
50–64	37	9.1	48	2	4	7	15	18	22	30
65+	89	11.7	102	4	6	9	14	22	28	74
GRAND TOTAL	**164**	**10.6**	**84**	**3**	**4**	**8**	**14**	**21**	**22**	**43**

040: OTH BACTERIAL DISEASES

Type of Patients	Observed Patients	Avg. Stay	Variance	10th	25th	50th	75th	90th	95th	99th
1. SINGLE DX										
A. Not Operated										
0–19 Years	2	2.0	0	2	2	2	2	2	2	2
20–34	0									
35–49	0									
50–64	0									
65+	0									
B. Operated										
0–19 Years	0									
20–34	0									
35–49	0									
50–64	0									
65+	0									
2. MULTIPLE DX										
A. Not Operated										
0–19 Years	38	5.1	12	2	3	4	7	11	14	15
20–34	31	5.2	13	1	3	5	7	11	13	14
35–49	28	4.8	7	2	3	4	6	9	9	13
50–64	15	11.9	149	3	6	9	11	32	48	48
65+	16	6.6	23	2	3	5	9	14	19	19
B. Operated										
0–19 Years	3	10.3	36	4	4	11	16	16	16	16
20–34	5	9.4	46	5	5	8	8	21	21	21
35–49	17	15.0	176	4	7	15	17	59	>99	>99
50–64	25	14.2	72	6	6	12	21	24	32	32
65+	11	11.1	31	5	5	12	15	15	21	21
SUBTOTALS:										
1. SINGLE DX										
A. Not Operated	2	2.0	0	2	2	2	2	2	2	2
B. Operated	0									
2. MULTIPLE DX										
A. Not Operated	128	6.0	32	2	3	5	7	12	14	32
B. Operated	61	13.3	89	5	6	11	17	23	32	>99
1. SINGLE DX	**2**	**2.0**	**0**	**2**	**2**	**2**	**2**	**2**	**2**	**2**
2. MULTIPLE DX	**189**	**8.4**	**62**	**2**	**4**	**6**	**11**	**16**	**23**	**59**
A. NOT OPERATED	**130**	**6.0**	**32**	**2**	**3**	**5**	**7**	**11**	**14**	**32**
B. OPERATED	**61**	**13.3**	**89**	**5**	**6**	**11**	**17**	**23**	**32**	**>99**
TOTAL										
0–19 Years	43	5.3	14	2	2	4	7	11	14	16
20–34	36	5.8	18	1	3	5	8	12	14	21
35–49	45	8.6	94	2	4	6	10	17	31	>99
50–64	40	13.3	99	4	6	9	18	32	32	48
65+	27	8.4	30	2	5	6	14	15	19	21
GRAND TOTAL	**191**	**8.3**	**61**	**2**	**4**	**6**	**11**	**16**	**23**	**59**

Length of Stay by Diagnosis and Operation, Western Region, 2008

Western Region, October 2006–September 2007 Data, by Diagnosis

041: BACT INF IN CCE/SITE NOS

Type of Patients	Observed Patients	Avg. Stay	Variance	10th	25th	50th	75th	90th	95th	99th
1. SINGLE DX										
A. Not Operated										
0–19 Years	1	6.0	0	6	6	6	6	6	6	6
20–34	0									
35–49	0									
50–64	0									
65+	0									
B. Operated										
0–19 Years	0									
20–34	0									
35–49	0									
50–64	0									
65+	0									
2. MULTIPLE DX										
A. Not Operated										
0–19 Years	13	4.9	8	1	2	5	7	9	10	10
20–34	10	4.3	14	1	2	3	5	14	14	14
35–49	13	4.4	18	1	2	3	5	8	16	16
50–64	14	5.0	18	1	2	4	6	10	16	16
65+	33	6.5	38	1	2	5	9	16	22	25
B. Operated										
0–19 Years	1	14.0	0	14	14	14	14	14	14	14
20–34	0									
35–49	1	22.0	0	22	22	22	22	22	22	22
50–64	3	10.4	21	5	5	13	13	13	13	13
65+	1	8.0	0	8	8	8	8	8	8	8
SUBTOTALS:										
1. SINGLE DX										
A. Not Operated	1	6.0	0	6	6	6	6	6	6	6
B. Operated	0									
2. MULTIPLE DX										
A. Not Operated	83	5.4	24	1	2	4	7	12	16	25
B. Operated	6	12.5	34	5	8	13	14	22	22	22
1. SINGLE DX	1	6.0	0	6	6	6	6	6	6	6
2. MULTIPLE DX	89	5.9	27	1	2	5	7	14	16	25
A. NOT OPERATED	84	5.4	24	1	2	4	7	12	16	25
B. OPERATED	6	12.5	34	5	8	13	14	22	22	22
TOTAL										
0–19 Years	15	5.5	13	1	2	5	7	10	14	14
20–34	10	4.3	14	1	2	3	5	14	14	14
35–49	14	5.7	38	1	2	4	7	13	22	22
50–64	17	5.9	21	1	2	5	8	13	16	16
65+	34	6.5	37	1	2	5	9	16	22	25
GRAND TOTAL	90	5.9	27	1	2	5	7	13	16	25

042: HIV DISEASE

Type of Patients	Observed Patients	Avg. Stay	Variance	10th	25th	50th	75th	90th	95th	99th
1. SINGLE DX										
A. Not Operated										
0–19 Years	0									
20–34	1	8.0	0	8	8	8	8	8	8	8
35–49	2	2.5	<1	2	2	3	3	3	3	3
50–64	0									
65+	0									
B. Operated										
0–19 Years	0									
20–34	0									
35–49	0									
50–64	0									
65+	0									
2. MULTIPLE DX										
A. Not Operated										
0–19 Years	20	7.7	84	1	2	4	8	27	27	35
20–34	991	8.0	70	2	3	5	10	16	23	46
35–49	3,224	8.0	69	2	3	5	9	17	24	42
50–64	1,349	7.7	59	2	3	5	9	16	22	43
65+	129	8.4	66	2	4	6	10	17	20	49
B. Operated										
0–19 Years	2	12.8	238	2	2	2	24	24	24	24
20–34	115	15.3	149	5	9	12	20	38	64	>99
35–49	302	12.8	111	3	3	10	17	32	32	54
50–64	137	16.1	245	3	6	11	21	37	56	83
65+	18	12.5	106	3	6	9	16	27	45	45
SUBTOTALS:										
1. SINGLE DX										
A. Not Operated	3	4.4	10	2	2	3	3	8	8	8
B. Operated	0									
2. MULTIPLE DX										
A. Not Operated	5,713	7.9	67	2	3	5	9	17	23	43
B. Operated	574	14.1	152	3	6	11	19	29	41	>99
1. SINGLE DX	3	4.4	10	2	2	3	3	8	8	8
2. MULTIPLE DX	6,287	8.5	78	2	3	6	10	18	25	49
A. NOT OPERATED	5,716	7.9	67	2	3	5	9	17	23	43
B. OPERATED	574	14.1	152	3	6	11	19	29	41	>99
TOTAL										
0–19 Years	22	8.2	90	2	2	4	9	24	27	35
20–34	1,107	8.8	83	2	3	6	11	19	26	55
35–49	3,528	8.4	75	2	3	6	10	18	25	46
50–64	1,486	8.4	82	2	3	6	10	18	25	53
65+	147	8.9	72	2	4	7	10	17	22	49
GRAND TOTAL	6,290	8.5	78	2	3	6	10	18	25	49

045: ACUTE POLIOMYELITIS

Type of Patients	Observed Patients	Avg. Stay	Variance	10th	25th	50th	75th	90th	95th	99th
1. SINGLE DX										
A. Not Operated										
0–19 Years	0									
20–34	0									
35–49	0									
50–64	0									
65+	0									
B. Operated										
0–19 Years	0									
20–34	0									
35–49	0									
50–64	0									
65+	0									
2. MULTIPLE DX										
A. Not Operated										
0–19 Years	0									
20–34	0									
35–49	0									
50–64	1	2.0	0	2	2	2	2	2	2	2
65+	0									
B. Operated										
0–19 Years	0									
20–34	0									
35–49	0									
50–64	1	3.0	0	3	3	3	3	3	3	3
65+	0									
SUBTOTALS:										
1. SINGLE DX										
A. Not Operated	0									
B. Operated	0									
2. MULTIPLE DX										
A. Not Operated	1	2.0	0	2	2	2	2	2	2	2
B. Operated	1	3.0	0	3	3	3	3	3	3	3
1. SINGLE DX	0									
2. MULTIPLE DX	2	2.5	<1	2	2	3	3	3	3	3
A. NOT OPERATED	1	2.0	0	2	2	2	2	2	2	2
B. OPERATED	1	3.0	0	3	3	3	3	3	3	3
TOTAL										
0–19 Years	0									
20–34	0									
35–49	0									
50–64	2	2.5	<1	2	2	3	3	3	3	3
65+	0									
GRAND TOTAL	2	2.5	<1	2	2	3	3	3	3	3

Length of Stay by Diagnosis and Operation, Western Region, 2008

Western Region, October 2006–September 2007 Data, by Diagnosis

046: CNS SLOW VIRUS INFECTION

Type of Patients	Observed Patients	Avg. Stay	Vari-ance	Percentiles						
				10th	25th	50th	75th	90th	95th	99th
1. SINGLE DX										
A. Not Operated										
0–19 Years	0									
20–34	0									
35–49	0									
50–64	2	4.5	12	2	2	7	7	7	7	7
65+	0									
B. Operated										
0–19 Years	0									
20–34	0									
35–49	0									
50–64	0									
65+	0									
2. MULTIPLE DX										
A. Not Operated										
0–19 Years	1	1.0	0	1	1	1	1	1	1	1
20–34	0									
35–49	5	15.4	91	4	6	21	22	24	24	24
50–64	20	7.6	66	2	2	4	9	18	18	36
65+	22	8.7	52	2	4	8	11	16	26	29
B. Operated										
0–19 Years	0									
20–34	1	16.0	0	16	16	16	16	16	16	16
35–49	1	15.0	0	15	15	15	15	15	15	15
50–64	0									
65+	0									
SUBTOTALS:										
1. SINGLE DX										
A. Not Operated	2	4.5	12	2	2	7	7	7	7	7
B. Operated	0									
2. MULTIPLE DX										
A. Not Operated	48	8.8	64	2	3	6	11	22	26	36
B. Operated	2	15.5	<1	15	15	16	16	16	16	16
1. SINGLE DX	2	4.5	12	2	2	7	7	7	7	7
2. MULTIPLE DX	50	9.1	63	2	4	8	12	22	26	36
A. NOT OPERATED	50	8.6	62	2	3	6	11	22	26	36
B. OPERATED	2	15.5	<1	15	15	16	16	16	16	16
TOTAL										
0–19 Years	1	1.0	0	1	1	1	1	1	1	1
20–34	1	16.0	0	16	16	16	16	16	16	16
35–49	5	15.4	91	4	6	21	22	24	24	24
50–64	23	7.7	61	2	2	4	9	15	18	36
65+	22	8.7	52	2	4	8	11	16	26	29
GRAND TOTAL	52	8.9	62	2	4	7	12	21	26	36

047: ENTEROVIRAL MENINGITIS

Type of Patients	Observed Patients	Avg. Stay	Vari-ance	Percentiles						
				10th	25th	50th	75th	90th	95th	99th
1. SINGLE DX										
A. Not Operated										
0–19 Years	507	2.6	2	1	2	2	3	4	5	7
20–34	261	2.4	2	1	1	2	3	4	5	6
35–49	143	2.8	7	2	2	2	3	4	6	8
50–64	35	1.9	<1	1	1	2	3	4	4	4
65+	2	2.0	0	2	2	2	2	2	2	2
B. Operated										
0–19 Years	2	2.0	2	1	1	3	3	3	3	3
20–34	1	2.0	0	2	2	2	2	2	2	2
35–49	0									
50–64	0									
65+	0									
2. MULTIPLE DX										
A. Not Operated										
0–19 Years	733	3.1	5	1	2	3	4	5	7	13
20–34	1,102	3.3	7	1	2	3	4	6	7	12
35–49	980	3.5	7	1	2	3	4	6	8	14
50–64	586	3.7	8	1	2	3	4	7	8	15
65+	262	5.0	15	2	3	4	6	10	12	19
B. Operated										
0–19 Years	4	3.5	2	2	3	4	5	5	5	5
20–34	8	5.8	14	2	3	4	10	12	12	12
35–49	13	10.2	91	2	4	6	14	25	33	33
50–64	6	4.5	9	1	2	4	7	9	9	9
65+	4	11.5	41	3	10	10	17	17	17	17
SUBTOTALS:										
1. SINGLE DX										
A. Not Operated	948	2.5	3	1	2	2	3	4	5	7
B. Operated	3	2.0	<1	1	1	2	2	3	3	3
2. MULTIPLE DX										
A. Not Operated	3,663	3.5	7	1	2	3	4	6	8	14
B. Operated	35	7.6	49	2	3	5	10	16	25	33
1. SINGLE DX	951	2.5	3	1	2	2	3	4	5	7
2. MULTIPLE DX	3,698	3.5	8	1	2	3	4	6	8	14
A. NOT OPERATED	4,611	3.3	7	1	2	3	4	6	8	13
B. OPERATED	38	7.1	47	2	3	4	10	16	25	33
TOTAL										
0–19 Years	1,246	2.9	4	1	2	2	3	5	6	11
20–34	1,372	3.1	6	1	2	3	4	5	7	11
35–49	1,136	3.5	8	1	2	3	4	6	8	14
50–64	627	3.6	8	1	2	3	4	7	8	15
65+	268	5.1	16	2	3	4	6	10	12	19
GRAND TOTAL	4,649	3.3	7	1	2	3	4	6	8	13

047.8: VIRAL MENINGITIS NEC

Type of Patients	Observed Patients	Avg. Stay	Vari-ance	Percentiles						
				10th	25th	50th	75th	90th	95th	99th
1. SINGLE DX										
A. Not Operated										
0–19 Years	60	2.7	1	1	2	2	3	4	5	7
20–34	16	2.4	1	1	3	3	3	4	4	4
35–49	10	2.5	2	1	1	2	4	5	5	5
50–64	2	1.5	<1	1	1	1	2	2	2	2
65+	0									
B. Operated										
0–19 Years	0									
20–34	0									
35–49	0									
50–64	0									
65+	0									
2. MULTIPLE DX										
A. Not Operated										
0–19 Years	80	3.3	5	1	2	3	4	6	8	13
20–34	71	2.9	2	1	2	3	4	5	6	7
35–49	71	3.5	6	1	2	3	4	6	8	14
50–64	44	4.0	15	2	2	3	4	6	13	22
65+	18	4.3	7	1	2	5	6	7	12	12
B. Operated										
0–19 Years	1	5.0	0	5	5	5	5	5	5	5
20–34	2	5.5	12	3	3	3	8	8	8	8
35–49	2	6.0	0	6	6	6	6	6	6	6
50–64	0									
65+	0									
SUBTOTALS:										
1. SINGLE DX										
A. Not Operated	88	2.6	1	1	2	2	3	4	5	7
B. Operated	0									
2. MULTIPLE DX										
A. Not Operated	284	3.4	6	1	2	3	4	6	7	14
B. Operated	5	5.6	3	3	5	6	6	8	8	8
1. SINGLE DX	88	2.6	1	1	2	2	3	4	5	7
2. MULTIPLE DX	289	3.5	6	1	2	3	4	6	8	14
A. NOT OPERATED	372	3.2	5	1	2	3	4	6	7	13
B. OPERATED	5	5.6	3	3	5	6	6	8	8	8
TOTAL										
0–19 Years	141	3.0	3	1	2	3	4	5	6	12
20–34	89	2.9	2	1	2	3	4	5	6	8
35–49	83	3.5	6	1	2	3	4	6	8	14
50–64	46	3.9	14	2	2	3	4	6	13	22
65+	18	4.3	7	1	2	5	6	7	12	12
GRAND TOTAL	377	3.3	5	1	2	3	4	6	7	13

Western Region, October 2006–September 2007 Data, by Diagnosis

047.9: VIRAL MENINGITIS NOS

Type of Patients	Observed Patients	Avg. Stay	Variance	10th	25th	50th	75th	90th	95th	99th
1. SINGLE DX										
A. Not Operated										
0–19 Years	446	2.5	2	1	2	2	3	4	5	7
20–34	245	2.4	2	1	1	2	3	4	5	6
35–49	133	2.8	7	1	2	2	3	4	5	8
50–64	33	1.9	<1	1	1	2	3	3	4	4
65+	2	2.0	0	2	2	2	2	2	2	2
B. Operated										
0–19 Years	2	2.0	0	2	2	3	3	3	3	3
20–34	1	2.0	0	2	2	2	2	2	2	2
35–49	0									
50–64	0									
65+	0									
2. MULTIPLE DX										
A. Not Operated										
0–19 Years	653	3.1	5	1	2	3	4	5	7	13
20–34	1,027	3.3	7	1	2	3	4	6	7	13
35–49	909	3.5	7	1	2	3	4	6	8	13
50–64	542	3.7	7	1	2	3	4	7	8	15
65+	244	5.1	16	2	3	4	6	10	12	19
B. Operated										
0–19 Years	3	3.0	1	2	3	4	4	4	4	4
20–34	6	5.9	17	2	3	4	10	12	12	12
35–49	11	10.9	105	2	4	6	16	25	33	33
50–64	6	4.5	9	1	2	4	7	9	9	9
65+	4	11.5	41	3	10	10	17	17	17	17
SUBTOTALS:										
1. SINGLE DX										
A. Not Operated	859	2.5	3	1	2	2	3	4	5	7
B. Operated	3	2.0	<1	1	1	2	3	3	3	3
2. MULTIPLE DX										
A. Not Operated	3,375	3.5	7	1	2	3	4	6	8	14
B. Operated	30	7.9	56	2	3	4	10	17	25	33
1. SINGLE DX	862	2.5	3	1	2	2	3	4	5	7
2. MULTIPLE DX	3,405	3.6	8	1	2	3	4	6	8	14
A. NOT OPERATED	4,234	3.3	7	1	2	3	4	6	8	13
B. OPERATED	33	7.4	54	2	3	4	10	16	25	33
TOTAL										
0–19 Years	1,104	2.8	4	1	2	2	3	5	6	11
20–34	1,279	3.2	6	1	2	3	4	6	7	12
35–49	1,053	3.5	9	1	2	3	4	6	8	16
50–64	581	3.6	7	1	2	3	4	7	8	15
65+	250	5.2	17	2	3	4	6	10	13	19
GRAND TOTAL	4,267	3.3	7	1	2	3	4	6	8	14

048: OTH ENTEROVIRAL CNS DIS

Type of Patients	Observed Patients	Avg. Stay	Variance	10th	25th	50th	75th	90th	95th	99th
1. SINGLE DX										
A. Not Operated										
0–19 Years	9	3.9	4	1	3	3	6	7	7	7
20–34	4	2.5	<1	2	2	2	3	3	3	3
35–49	0									
50–64	0									
65+	0									
B. Operated										
0–19 Years	0									
20–34	0									
35–49	0									
50–64	0									
65+	0									
2. MULTIPLE DX										
A. Not Operated										
0–19 Years	27	5.6	15	2	3	4	7	9	10	21
20–34	36	10.6	213	2	3	6	12	25	34	83
35–49	24	6.5	12	2	4	6	8	12	13	14
50–64	26	4.8	10	2	3	4	6	9	11	15
65+	35	8.7	29	4	5	7	11	15	19	27
B. Operated										
0–19 Years	0									
20–34	2	70.0	0	70	70	70	70	70	70	70
35–49	0									
50–64	0									
65+	1	46.0	0	46	46	46	46	46	46	46
SUBTOTALS:										
1. SINGLE DX										
A. Not Operated	13	3.5	3	2	2	3	4	6	7	7
B. Operated	0									
2. MULTIPLE DX										
A. Not Operated	148	7.6	69	2	4	6	9	14	19	34
B. Operated	2	57.9	286	46	46	46	70	70	70	70
1. SINGLE DX	13	3.5	3	2	2	3	4	6	7	7
2. MULTIPLE DX	150	8.2	103	2	4	6	9	14	22	70
A. NOT OPERATED	161	7.2	64	2	3	6	8	13	19	34
B. OPERATED	2	57.9	286	46	46	46	70	70	70	70
TOTAL										
0–19 Years	36	5.1	13	2	3	4	6	9	10	11
20–34	41	11.2	279	2	3	6	12	25	34	83
35–49	24	6.5	12	2	4	6	8	12	13	14
50–64	26	4.8	10	2	3	4	6	9	11	15
65+	36	9.8	66	4	5	7	11	19	27	46
GRAND TOTAL	163	7.8	96	2	3	6	8	14	21	70

049: OTH NONARTHROP CNS VIRUS

Type of Patients	Observed Patients	Avg. Stay	Variance	10th	25th	50th	75th	90th	95th	99th
1. SINGLE DX										
A. Not Operated										
0–19 Years	9	2.8	3	1	2	2	3	3	7	7
20–34	3	3.7	2	2	2	4	5	5	5	5
35–49	2	3.0	2	2	2	3	4	4	4	4
50–64	1	4.0	0	4	4	4	4	4	4	4
65+	0									
B. Operated										
0–19 Years	0									
20–34	0									
35–49	0									
50–64	0									
65+	0									
2. MULTIPLE DX										
A. Not Operated										
0–19 Years	28	6.5	43	2	3	4	6	15	22	30
20–34	52	6.7	60	3	3	5	9	11	15	55
35–49	65	5.9	14	2	3	5	8	11	13	17
50–64	69	8.1	58	2	4	5	9	21	31	>99
65+	72	8.7	28	3	5	8	12	15	21	23
B. Operated										
0–19 Years	1	3.0	0	3	3	3	3	3	3	3
20–34	2	15.0	71	9	9	21	>99	>99	>99	>99
35–49	2	5.0	31	1	1	1	9	9	9	9
50–64	2	12.5	<1	12	12	13	13	13	13	13
65+	3	5.0	13	1	1	6	8	8	8	8
SUBTOTALS:										
1. SINGLE DX										
A. Not Operated	15	3.1	2	2	2	3	4	5	7	7
B. Operated	0									
2. MULTIPLE DX										
A. Not Operated	286	7.4	40	2	3	5	9	15	21	34
B. Operated	10	8.3	37	1	3	9	13	21	>99	>99
1. SINGLE DX	15	3.1	2	2	2	3	4	5	7	7
2. MULTIPLE DX	296	7.4	40	2	3	5	9	15	21	55
A. NOT OPERATED	301	7.1	39	2	3	5	9	14	21	34
B. OPERATED	10	8.3	37	1	3	9	13	21	>99	>99
TOTAL										
0–19 Years	38	5.5	35	2	3	3	6	15	22	30
20–34	57	6.8	59	2	3	5	9	13	21	>99
35–49	69	5.8	14	2	3	5	8	11	13	17
50–64	72	8.2	57	2	4	5	9	21	31	>99
65+	75	8.6	28	3	4	7	12	15	21	23
GRAND TOTAL	311	7.2	39	2	3	5	9	14	21	34

Length of Stay by Diagnosis and Operation, Western Region, 2008

Western Region, October 2006–September 2007 Data, by Diagnosis

050: SMALLPOX

Type of Patients	Observed Patients	Avg. Stay	Variance	10th	25th	50th	75th	90th	95th	99th
1. SINGLE DX										
A. Not Operated										
0–19 Years	0									
20–34	0									
35–49	0									
50–64	0									
65+	0									
B. Operated										
0–19 Years	0									
20–34	0									
35–49	0									
50–64	0									
65+	0									
2. MULTIPLE DX										
A. Not Operated										
0–19 Years	0									
20–34	1	2.0	0	2	2	2	2	2	2	2
35–49	0									
50–64	0									
65+	0									
B. Operated										
0–19 Years	0									
20–34	0									
35–49	0									
50–64	0									
65+	0									
SUBTOTALS:										
1. SINGLE DX A. Not Operated	0									
B. Operated	0									
2. MULTIPLE DX A. Not Operated	1	2.0	0	2	2	2	2	2	2	2
B. Operated	0									
1. SINGLE DX	0									
2. MULTIPLE DX	1	2.0	0	2	2	2	2	2	2	2
A. NOT OPERATED	1	2.0	0	2	2	2	2	2	2	2
B. OPERATED	0									
TOTAL										
0–19 Years	0									
20–34	1	2.0	0	2	2	2	2	2	2	2
35–49	0									
50–64	0									
65+	0									
GRAND TOTAL	1	2.0	0	2	2	2	2	2	2	2

051: COWPOX & PARAVACCINIA

Type of Patients	Observed Patients	Avg. Stay	Variance	10th	25th	50th	75th	90th	95th	99th
1. SINGLE DX										
A. Not Operated										
0–19 Years	0									
20–34	0									
35–49	0									
50–64	0									
65+	0									
B. Operated										
0–19 Years	0									
20–34	0									
35–49	0									
50–64	0									
65+	0									
2. MULTIPLE DX										
A. Not Operated										
0–19 Years	0									
20–34	0									
35–49	0									
50–64	0									
65+	0									
B. Operated										
0–19 Years	0									
20–34	0									
35–49	0									
50–64	0									
65+	0									
SUBTOTALS:										
1. SINGLE DX A. Not Operated	0									
B. Operated	0									
2. MULTIPLE DX A. Not Operated	0									
B. Operated	0									
1. SINGLE DX	0									
2. MULTIPLE DX	0									
A. NOT OPERATED	0									
B. OPERATED	0									
TOTAL										
0–19 Years	0									
20–34	0									
35–49	0									
50–64	0									
65+	0									
GRAND TOTAL	0									

052: CHICKENPOX

Type of Patients	Observed Patients	Avg. Stay	Variance	10th	25th	50th	75th	90th	95th	99th
1. SINGLE DX										
A. Not Operated										
0–19 Years	16	3.8	17	1	1	2	4	12	15	15
20–34	9	5.4	7	2	4	5	8	10	10	10
35–49	3	1.7	1	1	1	1	3	3	3	3
50–64	0									
65+	0									
B. Operated										
0–19 Years	0									
20–34	0									
35–49	0									
50–64	0									
65+	0									
2. MULTIPLE DX										
A. Not Operated										
0–19 Years	54	3.7	6	1	2	3	5	7	8	13
20–34	33	4.5	10	2	2	4	6	8	13	15
35–49	35	4.7	11	2	2	4	6	7	11	19
50–64	18	5.5	13	1	2	5	8	10	14	14
65+	17	5.2	13	2	3	4	6	10	14	14
B. Operated										
0–19 Years	0									
20–34	0									
35–49	0									
50–64	0									
65+	0									
SUBTOTALS:										
1. SINGLE DX A. Not Operated	28	4.1	13	1	1	3	5	10	12	15
B. Operated	0									
2. MULTIPLE DX A. Not Operated	157	4.5	10	2	2	4	6	8	10	15
B. Operated	0									
1. SINGLE DX	28	4.1	13	1	1	3	5	10	12	15
2. MULTIPLE DX	157	4.5	10	2	2	4	6	8	10	15
A. NOT OPERATED	185	4.4	10	1	2	4	6	8	10	15
B. OPERATED	0									
TOTAL										
0–19 Years	70	3.8	8	1	2	3	5	7	10	15
20–34	42	4.7	10	2	2	4	6	8	10	15
35–49	38	4.4	11	2	2	3	6	7	11	19
50–64	18	5.5	13	1	2	5	8	10	14	14
65+	17	5.2	13	2	3	4	6	10	14	14
GRAND TOTAL	185	4.4	10	1	2	4	6	8	10	15

Length of Stay by Diagnosis and Operation, Western Region, 2008

26

Western Region, October 2006–September 2007 Data, by Diagnosis

053: HERPES ZOSTER

Type of Patients	Observed Patients	Avg. Stay	Variance	Percentiles						
				10th	25th	50th	75th	90th	95th	99th
1. SINGLE DX										
A. Not Operated										
0–19 Years	7	3.2	2	1	2	3	5	5	5	5
20–34	2	2.5	<1	2	2	3	3	3	3	3
35–49	12	2.8	4	1	1	2	4	5	7	7
50–64	10	2.7	2	1	2	2	4	5	5	5
65+	3	3.3	1	2	2	4	4	4	4	4
B. Operated										
0–19 Years	1	4.0	0	4	4	4	4	4	4	4
20–34	0									
35–49	0									
50–64	1	5.0	0	5	5	5	5	5	5	5
65+	0									
2. MULTIPLE DX										
A. Not Operated										
0–19 Years	69	4.7	8	2	2	4	7	8	11	15
20–34	85	4.1	9	2	2	4	5	7	10	17
35–49	205	3.9	6	2	2	3	5	7	9	12
50–64	434	4.1	10	1	2	3	5	8	10	16
65+	1,284	4.9	17	1	2	4	6	9	12	20
B. Operated										
0–19 Years	1	15.0	0	15	15	15	15	15	15	15
20–34	1	2.0	0	2	2	2	2	2	2	2
35–49	1	14.0	0	14	14	14	14	14	14	14
50–64	12	12.3	263	2	2	6	12	25	59	59
65+	19	5.4	25	1	2	3	10	14	17	17
SUBTOTALS:										
1. SINGLE DX										
A. Not Operated	34	2.9	2	1	2	3	4	5	5	7
B. Operated	2	4.5	<1	4	4	5	5	5	5	5
2. MULTIPLE DX										
A. Not Operated	2,077	4.6	14	1	2	4	6	9	11	19
B. Operated	34	8.3	116	1	2	4	12	15	25	59
1. SINGLE DX	36	3.0	2	1	2	3	4	5	5	7
2. MULTIPLE DX	2,111	4.7	16	1	2	4	6	9	12	19
A. NOT OPERATED	2,111	4.6	14	1	2	4	6	9	11	18
B. OPERATED	36	8.1	110	1	2	5	12	15	25	59
TOTAL										
0–19 Years	78	4.7	9	2	2	4	7	8	11	15
20–34	88	4.0	8	1	2	4	5	7	10	17
35–49	218	3.9	6	1	2	3	5	7	10	12
50–64	457	4.3	17	1	2	3	5	8	11	18
65+	1,306	4.9	17	1	2	4	6	9	12	20
GRAND TOTAL	2,147	4.6	15	1	2	4	6	9	11	19

053.19: HZ NERV SYST COMPS NEC

Type of Patients	Observed Patients	Avg. Stay	Variance	Percentiles						
				10th	25th	50th	75th	90th	95th	99th
1. SINGLE DX										
A. Not Operated										
0–19 Years	0									
20–34	0									
35–49	1	4.0	0	4	4	4	4	4	4	4
50–64	0									
65+	0									
B. Operated										
0–19 Years	0									
20–34	0									
35–49	0									
50–64	0									
65+	0									
2. MULTIPLE DX										
A. Not Operated										
0–19 Years	1	2.0	0	2	2	2	2	2	2	2
20–34	5	2.8	7	1	1	1	4	7	7	7
35–49	19	3.9	6	1	2	3	5	9	10	10
50–64	66	4.5	12	1	2	3	6	8	13	18
65+	299	5.0	17	1	2	4	7	10	12	19
B. Operated										
0–19 Years	0									
20–34	0									
35–49	0									
50–64	4	2.0	<1	1	2	2	2	3	3	3
65+	10	3.0	9	1	2	2	3	11	11	11
SUBTOTALS:										
1. SINGLE DX										
A. Not Operated	1	4.0	0	4	4	4	4	4	4	4
B. Operated	0									
2. MULTIPLE DX										
A. Not Operated	390	4.8	16	1	2	4	6	9	12	18
B. Operated	14	2.7	6	1	2	2	3	4	11	11
1. SINGLE DX	1	4.0	0	4	4	4	4	4	4	4
2. MULTIPLE DX	404	4.8	15	1	2	4	6	9	12	17
A. NOT OPERATED	391	4.8	16	1	2	4	6	9	12	18
B. OPERATED	14	2.7	6	1	2	2	3	4	11	11
TOTAL										
0–19 Years	1	2.0	0	2	2	2	2	2	2	2
20–34	5	2.8	7	1	1	1	4	7	7	7
35–49	20	3.9	6	1	2	3	5	7	10	10
50–64	70	4.4	12	1	2	3	5	8	13	18
65+	309	5.0	17	1	2	4	6	10	11	17
GRAND TOTAL	405	4.8	15	1	2	4	6	9	12	17

053.79: H ZOSTER COMPLICATED NEC

Type of Patients	Observed Patients	Avg. Stay	Variance	Percentiles						
				10th	25th	50th	75th	90th	95th	99th
1. SINGLE DX										
A. Not Operated										
0–19 Years	1	4.0	0	4	4	4	4	4	4	4
20–34	0									
35–49	3	2.3	2	1	1	2	4	4	4	4
50–64	1	3.0	0	3	3	3	3	3	3	3
65+	0									
B. Operated										
0–19 Years	0									
20–34	0									
35–49	0									
50–64	0									
65+	0									
2. MULTIPLE DX										
A. Not Operated										
0–19 Years	9	3.4	3	2	2	3	4	7	7	7
20–34	12	5.5	12	2	2	5	6	10	13	13
35–49	30	4.4	8	1	2	4	7	7	10	12
50–64	51	4.2	9	2	2	4	5	7	10	16
65+	155	5.2	18	2	3	4	6	11	15	24
B. Operated										
0–19 Years	0									
20–34	0									
35–49	0									
50–64	3	29.7	745	5	5	25	59	59	59	59
65+	2	8.0	49	3	3	3	13	13	13	13
SUBTOTALS:										
1. SINGLE DX										
A. Not Operated	5	2.8	2	1	2	3	4	4	4	4
B. Operated	0									
2. MULTIPLE DX										
A. Not Operated	257	4.9	14	2	2	4	6	10	12	20
B. Operated	5	20.9	525	3	5	13	25	59	59	59
1. SINGLE DX	5	2.8	2	1	2	3	4	4	4	4
2. MULTIPLE DX	262	5.2	27	2	2	4	6	10	13	24
A. NOT OPERATED	262	4.8	14	2	2	4	6	10	12	20
B. OPERATED	5	20.9	525	3	5	13	25	59	59	59
TOTAL										
0–19 Years	10	3.5	3	2	2	4	4	5	7	7
20–34	12	5.5	12	2	2	5	6	10	13	13
35–49	33	4.2	8	1	2	3	6	7	10	12
50–64	55	5.6	70	2	2	4	5	10	16	59
65+	157	5.2	18	2	3	4	6	11	15	24
GRAND TOTAL	267	5.1	27	2	2	4	6	10	13	24

Length of Stay by Diagnosis and Operation, Western Region, 2008

Western Region, October 2006–September 2007 Data, by Diagnosis

053.9: HERPES ZOSTER NOS

Type of Patients	Observed Patients	Avg. Stay	Vari-ance	10th	25th	50th	75th	90th	95th	99th
1. SINGLE DX										
A. Not Operated										
0–19 Years	1	1.0	0	1	1	1	1	1	1	1
20–34	2	2.5	<1	2	2	3	3	3	3	3
35–49	1	7.0	0	7	7	7	7	7	7	7
50–64	3	2.7	4	1	1	2	5	5	5	5
65+	1	4.0	0	4	4	4	4	4	4	4
B. Operated										
0–19 Years	1	4.0	0	4	4	4	4	4	4	4
20–34	0									
35–49	0									
50–64	0									
65+	0									
2. MULTIPLE DX										
A. Not Operated										
0–19 Years	50	5.1	10	2	3	4	7	9	11	15
20–34	33	3.7	7	1	2	3	5	7	10	12
35–49	86	3.8	5	1	2	4	5	6	9	12
50–64	211	3.8	8	1	2	3	5	7	9	15
65+	525	4.5	15	1	2	3	6	8	10	21
B. Operated										
0–19 Years	0									
20–34	0									
35–49	0									
50–64	5	10.2	12	6	7	12	12	14	14	14
65+	2	9.0	50	4	4	4	14	14	14	14
SUBTOTALS:										
1. SINGLE DX										
A. Not Operated	8	3.1	4	1	2	3	5	7	7	7
B. Operated	1	4.0	0	4	4	4	4	4	4	4
2. MULTIPLE DX										
A. Not Operated	905	4.3	12	1	2	3	5	8	10	18
B. Operated	7	9.8	17	4	6	12	14	14	14	14
1. SINGLE DX	9	3.2	4	1	2	3	4	7	7	7
2. MULTIPLE DX	912	4.3	13	1	2	3	5	8	10	18
A. NOT OPERATED	913	4.3	12	1	2	3	5	8	10	18
B. OPERATED	8	9.1	19	4	6	7	12	14	14	14
TOTAL										
0–19 Years	52	5.0	10	2	3	4	5	7	11	15
20–34	35	3.6	7	1	2	3	5	7	10	12
35–49	87	3.9	5	1	2	4	5	7	9	12
50–64	219	4.0	9	1	2	3	5	7	10	15
65+	528	4.5	15	1	2	3	6	8	10	21
GRAND TOTAL	921	4.3	12	1	2	3	5	8	10	18

054: HERPES SIMPLEX

Type of Patients	Observed Patients	Avg. Stay	Vari-ance	10th	25th	50th	75th	90th	95th	99th
1. SINGLE DX										
A. Not Operated										
0–19 Years	35	3.9	13	1	1	3	5	7	7	16
20–34	17	2.8	5	1	1	2	4	4	10	10
35–49	9	3.2	3	1	2	3	5	6	6	6
50–64	6	3.3	7	1	1	4	4	8	8	8
65+	1	3.0	0	3	3	3	3	3	3	3
B. Operated										
0–19 Years	0									
20–34	0									
35–49	0									
50–64	0									
2. MULTIPLE DX										
A. Not Operated										
0–19 Years	221	4.5	31	1	2	3	4	9	13	23
20–34	176	4.8	11	1	3	4	6	9	11	16
35–49	169	5.3	17	2	3	4	7	9	14	25
50–64	161	7.1	38	2	3	5	10	15	19	29
65+	165	10.2	66	3	5	8	12	21	26	43
B. Operated										
0–19 Years	3	7.3	10	5	5	6	11	11	11	11
20–34	6	4.8	5	3	3	4	4	9	9	9
35–49	6	19.7	197	5	12	15	28	44	44	44
50–64	8	20.6	244	4	12	17	19	57	57	57
65+	7	20.0	117	3	15	17	28	37	37	37
SUBTOTALS:										
1. SINGLE DX										
A. Not Operated	68	3.5	9	1	2	3	4	7	7	16
B. Operated	0									
2. MULTIPLE DX										
A. Not Operated	892	6.2	36	2	3	4	8	13	18	35
B. Operated	30	15.8	165	4	5	15	19	28	44	57
1. SINGLE DX	68	3.5	9	1	2	3	4	7	10	16
2. MULTIPLE DX	922	6.6	43	2	3	4	8	14	19	36
A. NOT OPERATED	960	6.0	35	2	3	4	7	13	18	29
B. OPERATED	30	15.8	165	4	5	15	19	28	44	57
TOTAL										
0–19 Years	259	4.4	28	1	2	3	5	9	14	23
20–34	199	4.6	11	1	3	4	5	9	11	16
35–49	184	5.7	28	2	3	4	7	10	16	28
50–64	175	7.6	54	2	3	5	10	17	21	37
65+	173	10.6	71	3	5	8	14	22	28	43
GRAND TOTAL	990	6.3	42	2	3	4	8	14	19	36

054.2: HS GINGIVOSTOMATITIS

Type of Patients	Observed Patients	Avg. Stay	Vari-ance	10th	25th	50th	75th	90th	95th	99th
1. SINGLE DX										
A. Not Operated										
0–19 Years	11	3.4	3	2	2	3	5	6	6	6
20–34	0									
35–49	0									
50–64	0									
65+	0									
B. Operated										
0–19 Years	0									
20–34	0									
35–49	0									
50–64	0									
2. MULTIPLE DX										
A. Not Operated										
0–19 Years	99	3.2	6	1	2	3	4	5	6	21
20–34	11	4.5	4	2	4	4	5	7	9	9
35–49	11	4.0	8	1	2	3	7	8	9	9
50–64	10	5.7	52	2	2	4	5	6	26	26
65+	7	7.6	50	2	4	5	8	23	23	23
B. Operated										
0–19 Years	1	11.0	0	11	11	11	11	11	11	11
20–34	0									
35–49	0									
50–64	0									
SUBTOTALS:										
1. SINGLE DX										
A. Not Operated	11	3.4	3	2	2	3	5	6	6	6
B. Operated	0									
2. MULTIPLE DX										
A. Not Operated	138	3.8	12	1	2	3	4	6	8	23
B. Operated	1	11.0	0	11	11	11	11	11	11	11
1. SINGLE DX	11	3.4	3	2	2	3	5	6	6	6
2. MULTIPLE DX	139	3.8	12	1	2	3	4	6	9	23
A. NOT OPERATED	149	3.7	11	1	2	3	4	6	8	23
B. OPERATED	1	11.0	0	11	11	11	11	11	11	11
TOTAL										
0–19 Years	111	3.3	6	1	2	3	4	5	6	11
20–34	11	4.5	4	2	4	4	5	7	9	9
35–49	11	4.0	8	1	2	3	7	8	9	9
50–64	10	5.7	52	2	2	4	5	6	26	26
65+	7	7.6	50	2	4	5	8	23	23	23
GRAND TOTAL	150	3.8	12	2	2	3	4	6	8	23

Length of Stay by Diagnosis and Operation, Western Region, 2008

Western Region, October 2006–September 2007 Data, by Diagnosis

054.3: HS MENINGOENCEPHALITIS

Type of Patients	Observed Patients	Avg. Stay	Vari- ance	Percentiles						
				10th	25th	50th	75th	90th	95th	99th
1. SINGLE DX										
A. *Not Operated*										
0–19 Years	1	7.0	0	7	7	7	7	7	7	7
20–34	1	2.0	0	2	2	2	2	2	2	2
35–49	1	5.0	0	5	5	5	5	5	5	5
50–64	2	4.5	24	1	1	1	8	8	8	8
65+	0									
B. *Operated*										
0–19 Years	0									
20–34	0									
35–49	0									
50–64	0									
65+	0									
2. MULTIPLE DX										
A. *Not Operated*										
0–19 Years	16	16.9	183	5	8	15	22	35	57	57
20–34	17	7.8	27	3	4	7	9	16	21	21
35–49	38	8.2	40	3	4	6	11	18	25	27
50–64	63	10.8	51	3	6	9	14	20	23	37
65+	103	12.0	72	4	6	9	16	23	29	39
B. *Operated*										
0–19 Years	0									
20–34	0									
35–49	4	24.2	224	12	13	21	28	44	44	44
50–64	1	21.0	0	21	21	21	21	21	21	21
65+	4	16.0	104	3	16	17	17	28	28	28
SUBTOTALS:										
1. SINGLE DX										
A. *Not Operated*	5	4.6	9	1	2	5	7	8	8	8
B. *Operated*	0									
2. MULTIPLE DX										
A. *Not Operated*	237	11.1	69	3	5	9	14	22	26	39
B. *Operated*	9	20.2	141	3	13	17	28	44	44	44
1. SINGLE DX	5	4.6	9	1	2	5	7	8	8	8
2. MULTIPLE DX	246	11.4	74	3	5	9	15	23	28	43
A. NOT OPERATED	242	11.0	69	3	5	8	14	21	26	39
B. OPERATED	9	20.2	141	3	13	17	28	44	44	44
TOTAL										
0–19 Years	17	16.3	177	5	8	14	21	35	57	57
20–34	18	7.5	27	2	4	6	9	16	21	21
35–49	43	9.6	74	3	4	7	13	21	27	44
50–64	66	10.8	52	3	6	9	14	21	23	37
65+	107	12.2	73	4	6	9	16	24	29	39
GRAND TOTAL	251	11.3	74	3	5	9	15	22	28	43

055: MEASLES

Type of Patients	Observed Patients	Avg. Stay	Vari- ance	Percentiles						
				10th	25th	50th	75th	90th	95th	99th
1. SINGLE DX										
A. *Not Operated*										
0–19 Years	0									
20–34	0									
35–49	0									
50–64	0									
65+	0									
B. *Operated*										
0–19 Years	0									
20–34	0									
35–49	0									
50–64	0									
65+	0									
2. MULTIPLE DX										
A. *Not Operated*										
0–19 Years	1	1.0	0	1	1	1	1	1	1	1
20–34	2	1.5	<1	1	1	1	2	2	2	2
35–49	0									
50–64	0									
65+	0									
B. *Operated*										
0–19 Years	0									
20–34	0									
35–49	0									
50–64	0									
65+	0									
SUBTOTALS:										
1. SINGLE DX										
A. *Not Operated*	0									
B. *Operated*	0									
2. MULTIPLE DX										
A. *Not Operated*	3	1.3	<1	1	1	1	2	2	2	2
B. *Operated*	0									
1. SINGLE DX	0									
2. MULTIPLE DX	3	1.3	<1	1	1	1	2	2	2	2
A. NOT OPERATED	3	1.3	<1	1	1	1	2	2	2	2
B. OPERATED	0									
TOTAL										
0–19 Years	1	1.0	0	1	1	1	1	1	1	1
20–34	2	1.5	<1	1	1	1	2	2	2	2
35–49	0									
50–64	0									
65+	0									
GRAND TOTAL	3	1.3	<1	1	1	1	2	2	2	2

056: RUBELLA

Type of Patients	Observed Patients	Avg. Stay	Vari- ance	Percentiles						
				10th	25th	50th	75th	90th	95th	99th
1. SINGLE DX										
A. *Not Operated*										
0–19 Years	0									
20–34	0									
35–49	0									
50–64	0									
65+	0									
B. *Operated*										
0–19 Years	0									
20–34	0									
35–49	0									
50–64	0									
65+	0									
2. MULTIPLE DX										
A. *Not Operated*										
0–19 Years	0									
20–34	0									
35–49	0									
50–64	1	7.0	0	7	7	7	7	7	7	7
65+	0									
B. *Operated*										
0–19 Years	0									
20–34	0									
35–49	0									
50–64	0									
65+	0									
SUBTOTALS:										
1. SINGLE DX										
A. *Not Operated*	0									
B. *Operated*	0									
2. MULTIPLE DX										
A. *Not Operated*	1	7.0	0	7	7	7	7	7	7	7
B. *Operated*	0									
1. SINGLE DX	0									
2. MULTIPLE DX	1	7.0	0	7	7	7	7	7	7	7
A. NOT OPERATED	1	7.0	0	7	7	7	7	7	7	7
B. OPERATED	0									
TOTAL										
0–19 Years	0									
20–34	0									
35–49	0									
50–64	1	7.0	0	7	7	7	7	7	7	7
65+	0									
GRAND TOTAL	1	7.0	0	7	7	7	7	7	7	7

Length of Stay by Diagnosis and Operation, Western Region, 2008

Western Region, October 2006–September 2007 Data, by Diagnosis

057: OTHER VIRAL EXANTHEMATA

Type of Patients	Observed Patients	Avg. Stay	Variance	Percentiles 10th	25th	50th	75th	90th	95th	99th
1. SINGLE DX										
A. Not Operated										
0–19 Years	38	2.1	1	1	1	2	3	4	4	4
20–34	4	1.3	<1	1	1	1	1	2	2	2
35–49	1	3.0	0	3	3	3	3	3	3	3
50–64	0									
65+	0									
B. Operated										
0–19 Years	0									
20–34	0									
35–49	0									
50–64	0									
65+	0									
2. MULTIPLE DX										
A. Not Operated										
0–19 Years	100	2.1	<1	1	1	2	3	4	4	4
20–34	24	3.4	3	1	2	3	4	5	6	9
35–49	12	3.6	7	2	2	3	3	5	11	11
50–64	11	3.6	2	2	2	3	5	5	6	6
65+	8	4.0	7	1	2	3	5	9	9	9
B. Operated										
0–19 Years	0									
20–34	0									
35–49	0									
50–64	0									
65+	0									
SUBTOTALS:										
1. SINGLE DX										
A. Not Operated	43	2.1	1	1	1	2	3	4	4	4
B. Operated	0									
2. MULTIPLE DX										
A. Not Operated	155	2.6	2	1	2	2	3	4	5	9
B. Operated	0									
1. SINGLE DX	43	2.1	1	1	1	2	3	4	4	4
2. MULTIPLE DX	155	2.6	2	1	2	2	3	4	5	9
A. NOT OPERATED	198	2.5	2	1	2	2	3	4	5	9
B. OPERATED	0									
TOTAL										
0–19 Years	138	2.1	<1	1	1	2	3	4	4	4
20–34	28	3.1	3	1	2	3	4	5	6	9
35–49	13	3.5	6	2	2	3	3	5	11	11
50–64	11	3.6	2	2	2	3	5	5	6	6
65+	8	4.0	7	1	2	3	5	9	9	9
GRAND TOTAL	198	2.5	2	1	2	2	3	4	5	9

060: YELLOW FEVER

Type of Patients	Observed Patients	Avg. Stay	Variance	Percentiles 10th	25th	50th	75th	90th	95th	99th
1. SINGLE DX										
A. Not Operated										
0–19 Years	0									
20–34	0									
35–49	0									
50–64	0									
65+	0									
B. Operated										
0–19 Years	0									
20–34	0									
35–49	0									
50–64	0									
65+	0									
2. MULTIPLE DX										
A. Not Operated										
0–19 Years	0									
20–34	0									
35–49	0									
50–64	0									
65+	0									
B. Operated										
0–19 Years	0									
20–34	0									
35–49	0									
50–64	0									
65+	0									
SUBTOTALS:										
1. SINGLE DX										
A. Not Operated	0									
B. Operated	0									
2. MULTIPLE DX										
A. Not Operated	0									
B. Operated	0									
1. SINGLE DX	0									
2. MULTIPLE DX	0									
A. NOT OPERATED	0									
B. OPERATED	0									
TOTAL										
0–19 Years	0									
20–34	0									
35–49	0									
50–64	0									
65+	0									
GRAND TOTAL	0									

061: DENGUE

Type of Patients	Observed Patients	Avg. Stay	Variance	Percentiles 10th	25th	50th	75th	90th	95th	99th
1. SINGLE DX										
A. Not Operated										
0–19 Years	0									
20–34	1	3.0	0	3	3	3	3	3	3	3
35–49	1	5.0	0	5	5	5	5	5	5	5
50–64	0									
65+	0									
B. Operated										
0–19 Years	0									
20–34	0									
35–49	0									
50–64	0									
65+	0									
2. MULTIPLE DX										
A. Not Operated										
0–19 Years	6	4.3	7	2	2	4	7	8	8	8
20–34	11	4.5	31	2	2	3	4	5	21	21
35–49	7	2.1	1	1	1	2	3	4	4	4
50–64	8	2.8	2	1	2	2	4	5	5	5
65+	1	3.0	0	3	3	3	3	3	3	3
B. Operated										
0–19 Years	0									
20–34	0									
35–49	0									
50–64	0									
65+	0									
SUBTOTALS:										
1. SINGLE DX										
A. Not Operated	2	4.0	2	3	3	4	5	5	5	5
B. Operated	0									
2. MULTIPLE DX										
A. Not Operated	33	3.5	12	2	2	2	4	5	8	21
B. Operated	0									
1. SINGLE DX	2	4.0	2	3	3	4	5	5	5	5
2. MULTIPLE DX	33	3.5	12	2	2	2	4	5	8	21
A. NOT OPERATED	35	3.5	12	2	2	3	4	5	8	21
B. OPERATED	0									
TOTAL										
0–19 Years	6	4.3	7	2	2	4	7	8	8	8
20–34	12	4.3	28	2	2	3	3	5	21	21
35–49	8	2.5	2	1	1	2	4	5	5	5
50–64	8	2.8	2	1	2	2	4	5	5	5
65+	1	3.0	0	3	3	3	3	3	3	3
GRAND TOTAL	35	3.5	12	2	2	3	4	5	8	21

Length of Stay by Diagnosis and Operation, Western Region, 2008

Western Region, October 2006–September 2007 Data, by Diagnosis

062: MOSQUITO-BORNE VE

Type of Patients	Observed Patients	Avg. Stay	Variance	Percentiles						
				10th	25th	50th	75th	90th	95th	99th
1. SINGLE DX										
A. *Not Operated*										
0–19 Years	0									
20–34	0									
35–49	0									
50–64	0									
65+	0									
B. *Operated*										
0–19 Years	0									
20–34	0									
35–49	0									
50–64	0									
65+	0									
2. MULTIPLE DX										
A. *Not Operated*										
0–19 Years	0									
20–34	0									
35–49	0									
50–64	1	4.0	0	4	4	4	4	4	4	4
65+	1	8.0	0	8	8	8	8	8	8	8
B. *Operated*										
0–19 Years	0									
20–34	0									
35–49	0									
50–64	0									
65+	0									
SUBTOTALS:										
1. SINGLE DX										
A. *Not Operated*	0									
B. *Operated*	0									
2. MULTIPLE DX										
A. *Not Operated*	2	6.0	8	4	4	8	8	8	8	8
B. *Operated*	0									
1. SINGLE DX	0									
2. MULTIPLE DX	2	6.0	8	4	4	8	8	8	8	8
A. NOT OPERATED	2	6.0	8	4	4	8	8	8	8	8
B. OPERATED	0									
TOTAL										
0–19 Years	0									
20–34	0									
35–49	0									
50–64	1	4.0	0	4	4	4	4	4	4	4
65+	1	8.0	0	8	8	8	8	8	8	8
GRAND TOTAL	2	6.0	8	4	4	8	8	8	8	8

063: TICK-BORNE VIRAL ENCEPH

Type of Patients	Observed Patients	Avg. Stay	Variance	Percentiles						
				10th	25th	50th	75th	90th	95th	99th
1. SINGLE DX										
A. *Not Operated*										
0–19 Years	0									
20–34	0									
35–49	0									
50–64	0									
65+	0									
B. *Operated*										
0–19 Years	0									
20–34	0									
35–49	0									
50–64	0									
65+	0									
2. MULTIPLE DX										
A. *Not Operated*										
0–19 Years	0									
20–34	0									
35–49	0									
50–64	1	4.0	0	4	4	4	4	4	4	4
65+	0									
B. *Operated*										
0–19 Years	0									
20–34	0									
35–49	0									
50–64	0									
65+	0									
SUBTOTALS:										
1. SINGLE DX										
A. *Not Operated*	0									
B. *Operated*	0									
2. MULTIPLE DX										
A. *Not Operated*	1	4.0	0	4	4	4	4	4	4	4
B. *Operated*	0									
1. SINGLE DX	0									
2. MULTIPLE DX	1	4.0	0	4	4	4	4	4	4	4
A. NOT OPERATED	1	4.0	0	4	4	4	4	4	4	4
B. OPERATED	0									
TOTAL										
0–19 Years	0									
20–34	0									
35–49	0									
50–64	1	4.0	0	4	4	4	4	4	4	4
65+	0									
GRAND TOTAL	1	4.0	0	4	4	4	4	4	4	4

064: ARTHROPOD-BORNE VE NEC

Type of Patients	Observed Patients	Avg. Stay	Variance	Percentiles						
				10th	25th	50th	75th	90th	95th	99th
1. SINGLE DX										
A. *Not Operated*										
0–19 Years	0									
20–34	0									
35–49	0									
50–64	0									
65+	0									
B. *Operated*										
0–19 Years	0									
20–34	0									
35–49	0									
50–64	0									
65+	0									
2. MULTIPLE DX										
A. *Not Operated*										
0–19 Years	0									
20–34	0									
35–49	0									
50–64	0									
65+	0									
B. *Operated*										
0–19 Years	0									
20–34	0									
35–49	0									
50–64	0									
65+	0									
SUBTOTALS:										
1. SINGLE DX A. *Not Operated*	0									
1. SINGLE DX B. *Operated*	0									
2. MULTIPLE DX A. *Not Operated*	0									
2. MULTIPLE DX B. *Operated*	0									
1. SINGLE DX	0									
2. MULTIPLE DX	0									
A. NOT OPERATED	0									
B. OPERATED	0									
TOTAL										
0–19 Years	0									
20–34	0									
35–49	0									
50–64	0									
65+	0									
GRAND TOTAL	0									

Length of Stay by Diagnosis and Operation, Western Region, 2008

Western Region, October 2006–September 2007 Data, by Diagnosis

065: ARTHROPOD HEMOR FEVER

Type of Patients	Observed Patients	Avg. Stay	Vari-ance	10th	25th	50th	75th	90th	95th	99th
1. SINGLE DX										
A. Not Operated										
0–19 Years	0									
20–34	0									
35–49	0									
50–64	0									
65+	0									
B. Operated										
0–19 Years	0									
20–34	0									
35–49	0									
50–64	0									
65+	0									
2. MULTIPLE DX										
A. Not Operated										
0–19 Years	0									
20–34	1	2.0	0	2	2	2	2	2	2	2
35–49	0									
50–64	0									
65+	0									
B. Operated										
0–19 Years	0									
20–34	0									
35–49	0									
50–64	0									
65+	0									
SUBTOTALS:										
1. SINGLE DX										
A. Not Operated	0									
B. Operated	0									
2. MULTIPLE DX										
A. Not Operated	1	2.0	0	2	2	2	2	2	2	2
B. Operated	0									
1. SINGLE DX	0									
2. MULTIPLE DX	1	2.0	0	2	2	2	2	2	2	2
A. NOT OPERATED	1	2.0	0	2	2	2	2	2	2	2
B. OPERATED	0									
TOTAL										
0–19 Years	0									
20–34	1	2.0	0	2	2	2	2	2	2	2
35–49	0									
50–64	0									
65+	0									
GRAND TOTAL	1	2.0	0	2	2	2	2	2	2	2

066: OTH ARTHROPOD VIRUS DIS

Type of Patients	Observed Patients	Avg. Stay	Vari-ance	10th	25th	50th	75th	90th	95th	99th
1. SINGLE DX										
A. Not Operated										
0–19 Years	1	3.0	0	3	3	3	3	3	3	3
20–34	3	5.3	1	4	4	6	6	6	6	6
35–49	2	7.0	8	5	5	7	9	9	9	9
50–64	3	4.7	16	1	1	4	9	9	9	9
65+	0									
B. Operated										
0–19 Years	0									
20–34	0									
35–49	0									
50–64	0									
65+	0									
2. MULTIPLE DX										
A. Not Operated										
0–19 Years	6	4.7	10	1	2	5	6	10	10	10
20–34	9	4.2	5	1	3	4	5	8	8	8
35–49	31	9.7	125	2	3	7	12	19	27	59
50–64	56	9.6	45	4	5	8	11	21	24	28
65+	106	11.1	54	3	6	9	14	22	27	29
B. Operated										
0–19 Years	0									
20–34	1	28.0	0	28	28	28	28	28	28	28
35–49	1	18.0	0	18	18	18	18	18	18	18
50–64	1	12.0	0	12	12	12	12	12	12	12
65+	5	23.6	41	16	18	25	28	31	31	31
SUBTOTALS:										
1. SINGLE DX										
A. Not Operated	9	5.2	7	1	4	5	6	9	9	9
B. Operated	0									
2. MULTIPLE DX										
A. Not Operated	208	10.0	61	3	4	8	12	20	25	29
B. Operated	8	22.0	47	12	16	18	28	31	31	31
1. SINGLE DX	9	5.2	7	1	4	5	6	9	9	9
2. MULTIPLE DX	216	10.4	65	3	5	8	14	22	27	31
A. NOT OPERATED	217	9.8	59	3	4	8	12	20	25	29
B. OPERATED	8	22.0	47	12	16	18	28	31	31	31
TOTAL										
0–19 Years	7	4.4	9	1	2	4	6	10	10	10
20–34	13	6.3	45	2	3	5	6	8	28	28
35–49	34	9.8	116	2	4	7	12	19	27	59
50–64	60	9.3	43	4	4	8	11	20	24	28
65+	111	11.6	60	3	6	9	16	24	28	31
GRAND TOTAL	225	10.2	64	3	4	8	13	22	27	31

070: VIRAL HEPATITIS

Type of Patients	Observed Patients	Avg. Stay	Vari-ance	10th	25th	50th	75th	90th	95th	99th
1. SINGLE DX										
A. Not Operated										
0–19 Years	14	2.0	<1	1	1	2	3	3	4	4
20–34	26	2.5	3	1	2	2	4	5	6	7
35–49	10	2.4	1	1	2	2	3	5	5	5
50–64	7	2.3	3	1	1	2	3	6	6	6
65+	0									
B. Operated										
0–19 Years	0									
20–34	0									
35–49	0									
50–64	1	6.0	0	6	6	6	6	6	6	6
65+	0									
2. MULTIPLE DX										
A. Not Operated										
0–19 Years	52	3.2	8	1	1	3	4	5	10	15
20–34	243	4.2	10	1	2	3	5	8	11	13
35–49	780	4.3	15	1	2	3	5	9	12	20
50–64	1,220	4.4	20	1	2	4	6	9	12	20
65+	356	4.7	15	1	2	4	6	9	12	18
B. Operated										
0–19 Years	0									
20–34	4	8.0	11	4	8	8	12	12	12	12
35–49	35	10.6	50	2	7	10	12	17	28	35
50–64	121	14.7	252	4	6	10	15	35	51	91
65+	14	8.4	4	6	7	8	10	11	13	13
SUBTOTALS:										
1. SINGLE DX										
A. Not Operated	57	2.3	2	1	1	2	3	4	6	7
B. Operated	1	6.0	0	6	6	6	6	6	6	6
2. MULTIPLE DX										
A. Not Operated	2,651	4.3	17	1	2	3	5	9	12	20
B. Operated	174	13.2	191	4	6	9	14	29	47	91
1. SINGLE DX	58	2.4	2	1	1	2	3	5	6	7
2. MULTIPLE DX	2,825	4.9	32	1	2	3	6	10	13	26
A. NOT OPERATED	2,708	4.3	16	1	2	3	5	9	12	19
B. OPERATED	175	13.2	190	4	6	9	14	29	47	91
TOTAL										
0–19 Years	66	2.9	7	1	1	2	3	5	9	15
20–34	273	4.1	10	1	2	3	5	8	11	13
35–49	825	4.5	18	1	2	3	6	9	12	22
50–64	1,349	5.3	49	1	2	3	6	11	15	38
65+	370	4.8	15	1	2	4	6	9	12	18
GRAND TOTAL	2,883	4.8	31	1	2	3	6	10	13	26

Western Region, October 2006–September 2007 Data, by Diagnosis

070.30: AC VH B S COMA OR DELTA

Type of Patients	Observed Patients	Avg. Stay	Variance	Percentiles						
				10th	25th	50th	75th	90th	95th	99th
1. SINGLE DX										
A. Not Operated										
0–19 Years	0									
20–34	5	3.6	7	1	2	2	5	7	7	7
35–49	4	3.0	2	2	2	3	6	5	5	5
50–64	1	2.0	0	2	2	2	2	2	2	2
65+	0									
B. Operated										
0–19 Years	0									
20–34	0									
35–49	0									
50–64	0									
65+	0									
2. MULTIPLE DX										
A. Not Operated										
0–19 Years	1	5.0	0	5	5	5	5	5	5	5
20–34	56	4.4	10	1	2	4	5	10	12	13
35–49	98	4.8	11	1	2	4	7	10	12	15
50–64	61	6.0	17	2	3	5	7	11	15	20
65+	17	6.7	24	2	3	5	9	16	18	18
B. Operated										
0–19 Years	0									
20–34	0									
35–49	3	5.7	16	1	1	8	8	8	8	8
50–64	1	8.0	0	8	8	8	8	8	8	8
65+	0									
SUBTOTALS:										
1. SINGLE DX										
A. Not Operated	10	3.2	4	1	2	2	5	6	7	7
B. Operated	0									
2. MULTIPLE DX										
A. Not Operated	233	5.2	14	1	3	4	7	10	13	17
B. Operated	4	6.2	12	1	1	8	8	8	8	8
1. SINGLE DX	10	3.2	4	1	2	2	5	6	7	7
2. MULTIPLE DX	237	5.2	14	1	3	4	7	10	13	17
A. NOT OPERATED	243	5.1	13	1	2	4	7	10	12	17
B. OPERATED	4	6.2	12	1	1	8	8	8	8	8
TOTAL										
0–19 Years	1	5.0	0	5	5	5	5	5	5	5
20–34	61	4.4	9	1	2	4	5	9	11	13
35–49	105	4.8	11	1	2	4	7	10	11	15
50–64	63	6.0	17	2	3	5	8	11	15	20
65+	17	6.7	24	2	3	5	9	16	18	18
GRAND TOTAL	247	5.1	13	1	2	4	7	10	12	17

070.44: CHR VH C W COMA

Type of Patients	Observed Patients	Avg. Stay	Variance	Percentiles						
				10th	25th	50th	75th	90th	95th	99th
1. SINGLE DX										
A. Not Operated										
0–19 Years	0									
20–34	0									
35–49	0									
50–64	0									
65+	0									
B. Operated										
0–19 Years	0									
20–34	0									
35–49	0									
50–64	0									
65+	0									
2. MULTIPLE DX										
A. Not Operated										
0–19 Years	0									
20–34	4	5.3	22	1	2	5	9	11	11	11
35–49	211	4.1	14	1	2	3	5	9	12	18
50–64	547	4.6	23	1	2	3	6	10	13	23
65+	124	4.7	17	2	2	3	6	9	12	16
B. Operated										
0–19 Years	0									
20–34	0									
35–49	13	9.2	21	3	6	10	12	16	17	17
50–64	24	24.3	532	6	9	15	38	72	91	>99
65+	4	8.3	11	6	6	8	13	13	13	13
SUBTOTALS:										
1. SINGLE DX										
A. Not Operated	0									
B. Operated	0									
2. MULTIPLE DX										
A. Not Operated	886	4.5	20	1	2	3	6	9	12	22
B. Operated	41	17.9	371	6	7	12	18	47	72	>99
1. SINGLE DX	0									
2. MULTIPLE DX	927	5.1	43	1	2	3	6	11	15	32
A. NOT OPERATED	886	4.5	20	1	2	3	6	9	12	22
B. OPERATED	41	17.9	371	6	7	12	18	47	72	>99
TOTAL										
0–19 Years	0									
20–34	4	5.3	22	1	2	5	9	11	11	11
35–49	224	4.4	16	1	2	3	6	10	13	18
50–64	571	5.5	59	1	2	3	8	11	17	47
65+	128	4.8	18	2	2	4	6	9	12	16
GRAND TOTAL	927	5.1	43	1	2	3	6	11	15	32

070.54: CHR VH C W/O COMA

Type of Patients	Observed Patients	Avg. Stay	Variance	Percentiles						
				10th	25th	50th	75th	90th	95th	99th
1. SINGLE DX										
A. Not Operated										
0–19 Years	1	1.0	0	1	1	1	1	1	1	1
20–34	0									
35–49	0									
50–64	1	6.0	0	6	6	6	6	6	6	6
65+	0									
B. Operated										
0–19 Years	0									
20–34	0									
35–49	0									
50–64	1	6.0	0	6	6	6	6	6	6	6
65+	0									
2. MULTIPLE DX										
A. Not Operated										
0–19 Years	5	2.8	16	1	1	4	6	10	10	10
20–34	8	4.4	5	1	2	4	5	8	8	8
35–49	102	3.8	10	1	2	3	5	8	10	15
50–64	155	4.0	34	1	1	3	5	8	11	16
65+	37	3.9	5	1	2	3	5	7	8	9
B. Operated										
0–19 Years	0									
20–34	0									
35–49	11	12.9	85	6	7	11	17	22	35	35
50–64	66	12.5	165	4	6	9	13	22	31	72
65+	8	8.8	2	7	8	8	10	11	11	11
SUBTOTALS:										
1. SINGLE DX										
A. Not Operated	2	3.5	12	1	1	6	6	6	6	6
B. Operated	1	6.0	0	6	6	6	6	6	6	6
2. MULTIPLE DX										
A. Not Operated	307	3.9	21	1	1	3	5	8	10	16
B. Operated	85	12.2	140	4	7	9	12	22	31	72
1. SINGLE DX	3	4.3	8	1	1	6	6	6	6	6
2. MULTIPLE DX	392	5.7	58	1	2	4	7	11	16	51
A. NOT OPERATED	309	3.9	21	1	1	3	5	8	10	16
B. OPERATED	86	12.2	138	4	6	9	12	22	31	72
TOTAL										
0–19 Years	6	2.5	14	1	1	1	6	10	10	10
20–34	8	4.4	5	1	2	4	6	8	8	8
35–49	113	4.7	24	1	2	3	6	10	14	22
50–64	223	6.5	87	2	2	4	7	13	19	64
65+	45	4.7	8	2	2	4	7	9	10	11
GRAND TOTAL	395	5.7	58	1	2	4	7	11	16	51

Length of Stay by Diagnosis and Operation, Western Region, 2008

Western Region, October 2006–September 2007 Data, by Diagnosis

070.71: VH C NOS W COMA

Type of Patients	Observed Patients	Avg. Stay	Variance	10th	25th	Percentiles 50th	75th	90th	95th	99th
1. SINGLE DX										
A. Not Operated										
0–19 Years	0									
20–34	0									
35–49	0									
50–64	0									
65+	0									
B. Operated										
0–19 Years	0									
20–34	0									
35–49	0									
50–64	0									
65+	0									
2. MULTIPLE DX										
A. Not Operated										
0–19 Years	0									
20–34	3	2.7	4	1	1	2	5	5	5	5
35–49	87	4.9	27	1	2	3	6	11	14	29
50–64	192	3.9	10	1	2	3	5	8	10	17
65+	48	3.8	10	1	2	3	4	10	12	13
B. Operated										
0–19 Years	0									
20–34	0									
35–49	1	10.0	0	10	10	10	10	10	10	10
50–64	7	13.7	188	2	4	7	32	35	35	35
65+	0									
SUBTOTALS:										
1. SINGLE DX										
A. Not Operated	0									
B. Operated	0									
2. MULTIPLE DX										
A. Not Operated	330	4.1	15	1	2	3	5	9	12	21
B. Operated	8	13.2	163	2	4	9	10	35	35	35
1. SINGLE DX	0									
2. MULTIPLE DX	338	4.3	20	1	2	3	5	9	12	24
A. NOT OPERATED	330	4.1	15	1	2	3	5	9	12	21
B. OPERATED	8	13.2	163	2	4	9	10	35	35	35
TOTAL										
0–19 Years	0									
20–34	3	2.7	4	1	1	2	5	5	5	5
35–49	88	4.9	27	1	2	3	6	11	14	29
50–64	199	4.2	19	1	2	3	5	9	11	21
65+	48	3.8	10	1	2	3	4	10	12	13
GRAND TOTAL	338	4.3	20	1	2	3	5	9	12	24

071: RABIES

Type of Patients	Observed Patients	Avg. Stay	Variance	10th	25th	Percentiles 50th	75th	90th	95th	99th
1. SINGLE DX										
A. Not Operated										
0–19 Years	0									
20–34	0									
35–49	0									
50–64	0									
65+	0									
B. Operated										
0–19 Years	0									
20–34	0									
35–49	0									
50–64	0									
65+	0									
2. MULTIPLE DX										
A. Not Operated										
0–19 Years	0									
20–34	0									
35–49	0									
50–64	0									
65+	0									
B. Operated										
0–19 Years	0									
20–34	0									
35–49	0									
50–64	0									
65+	0									
SUBTOTALS:										
1. SINGLE DX										
A. Not Operated	0									
B. Operated	0									
2. MULTIPLE DX										
A. Not Operated	0									
B. Operated	0									
1. SINGLE DX	0									
2. MULTIPLE DX	0									
A. NOT OPERATED	0									
B. OPERATED	0									
TOTAL										
0–19 Years	0									
20–34	0									
35–49	0									
50–64	0									
65+	0									
GRAND TOTAL	0									

072: MUMPS

Type of Patients	Observed Patients	Avg. Stay	Variance	10th	25th	Percentiles 50th	75th	90th	95th	99th
1. SINGLE DX										
A. Not Operated										
0–19 Years	0									
20–34	0									
35–49	0									
50–64	0									
65+	0									
B. Operated										
0–19 Years	0									
20–34	0									
35–49	0									
50–64	0									
65+	0									
2. MULTIPLE DX										
A. Not Operated										
0–19 Years	4	2.3	<1	2	2	2	3	3	3	3
20–34	3	4.7	6	2	2	5	7	7	7	7
35–49	2	3.5	5	2	2	4	5	5	5	5
50–64	2	3.0	2	2	2	3	4	4	4	4
65+	0									
B. Operated										
0–19 Years	0									
20–34	0									
35–49	0									
50–64	0									
65+	0									
SUBTOTALS:										
1. SINGLE DX										
A. Not Operated	0									
B. Operated	0									
2. MULTIPLE DX										
A. Not Operated	11	3.3	3	2	2	2	5	5	7	7
B. Operated	0									
1. SINGLE DX	0									
2. MULTIPLE DX	11	3.3	3	2	2	2	5	5	7	7
A. NOT OPERATED	11	3.3	3	2	2	2	5	5	7	7
B. OPERATED	0									
TOTAL										
0–19 Years	4	2.3	<1	2	2	2	3	3	3	3
20–34	3	4.7	6	2	2	5	7	7	7	7
35–49	2	3.5	5	2	2	4	5	5	5	5
50–64	2	3.0	2	2	2	3	4	4	4	4
65+	0									
GRAND TOTAL	11	3.3	3	2	2	2	5	5	7	7

Length of Stay by Diagnosis and Operation, Western Region, 2008

Western Region, October 2006–September 2007 Data, by Diagnosis

073: ORNITHOSIS

Type of Patients	Observed Patients	Avg. Stay	Vari- ance	Percentiles 10th	25th	50th	75th	90th	95th	99th
1. SINGLE DX										
A. Not Operated										
0–19 Years	0									
20–34	0									
35–49	0									
50–64	0									
65+	0									
B. Operated										
0–19 Years	0									
20–34	0									
35–49	0									
50–64	0									
65+	0									
2. MULTIPLE DX										
A. Not Operated										
0–19 Years	2	3.5	<1	3	3	4	4	4	4	4
20–34	2	4.5	4	3	3	6	6	6	6	6
35–49	4	6.0	18	4	4	5	11	11	11	11
50–64	1	3.0	0	3	3	3	3	3	3	3
65+	1	11.0	0	11	11	11	11	11	11	11
B. Operated										
0–19 Years	0									
20–34	0									
35–49	1	13.0	0	13	13	13	13	13	13	13
50–64	1	7.0	0	7	7	7	7	7	7	7
65+	0									
SUBTOTALS:										
1. SINGLE DX										
A. Not Operated	0									
B. Operated	0									
2. MULTIPLE DX										
A. Not Operated	10	5.4	10	3	3	4	6	11	11	11
B. Operated	2	10.0	18	7	7	13	13	13	13	13
1. SINGLE DX	0									
2. MULTIPLE DX	12	6.2	13	3	4	5	11	11	13	13
A. NOT OPERATED	10	5.4	10	3	3	4	6	11	11	11
B. OPERATED	2	10.0	18	7	7	13	13	13	13	13
TOTAL										
0–19 Years	2	3.5	<1	3	3	4	4	4	4	4
20–34	2	4.5	4	3	3	6	6	6	6	6
35–49	5	7.4	18	4	4	5	11	13	13	13
50–64	2	5.0	0	3	3	7	7	7	7	7
65+	1	11.0	0	11	11	11	11	11	11	11
GRAND TOTAL	12	6.2	13	3	4	5	11	11	13	13

074: COXSACKIE VIRAL DISEASE

Type of Patients	Observed Patients	Avg. Stay	Vari- ance	Percentiles 10th	25th	50th	75th	90th	95th	99th
1. SINGLE DX										
A. Not Operated										
0–19 Years	5	2.0	1	1	1	2	3	3	3	3
20–34	2	2.0	2	1	1	3	3	3	3	3
35–49	0									
50–64	0									
65+	0									
B. Operated										
0–19 Years	0									
20–34	0									
35–49	0									
50–64	0									
65+	0									
2. MULTIPLE DX										
A. Not Operated										
0–19 Years	53	2.4	2	1	1	2	3	4	6	8
20–34	6	3.7	2	2	3	3	5	6	6	6
35–49	4	3.8	10	1	1	4	6	7	7	7
50–64	4	8.8	121	2	2	4	16	25	25	25
65+	5	4.6	42	1	1	2	3	16	16	16
B. Operated										
0–19 Years	0									
20–34	0									
35–49	0									
50–64	0									
65+	2	19.0	197	9	9	29	29	29	29	29
SUBTOTALS:										
1. SINGLE DX										
A. Not Operated	7	2.0	1	1	1	2	3	3	3	3
B. Operated	0									
2. MULTIPLE DX										
A. Not Operated	72	3.1	12	1	1	2	3	6	7	25
B. Operated	2	19.0	197	9	9	29	29	29	29	29
1. SINGLE DX	7	2.0	1	1	1	2	3	3	3	3
2. MULTIPLE DX	74	3.5	21	1	1	2	4	6	9	29
A. NOT OPERATED	79	3.0	11	1	1	2	3	6	7	25
B. OPERATED	2	19.0	197	9	9	29	29	29	29	29
TOTAL										
0–19 Years	58	2.3	2	1	1	2	3	4	6	8
20–34	8	3.3	2	1	3	3	6	6	6	6
35–49	4	3.8	10	1	1	4	6	7	7	7
50–64	4	8.8	121	2	2	4	16	25	25	25
65+	7	8.8	110	1	1	2	16	29	29	29
GRAND TOTAL	81	3.4	20	1	1	2	3	6	8	29

075: INFECTIOUS MONONUCLEOSIS

Type of Patients	Observed Patients	Avg. Stay	Vari- ance	Percentiles 10th	25th	50th	75th	90th	95th	99th
1. SINGLE DX										
A. Not Operated										
0–19 Years	35	2.0	1	1	1	2	2	4	4	5
20–34	17	2.1	2	1	1	1	3	4	6	6
35–49	1	2.0	0	2	2	2	2	2	2	2
50–64	0									
65+	0									
B. Operated										
0–19 Years	0									
20–34	0									
35–49	0									
50–64	0									
65+	0									
2. MULTIPLE DX										
A. Not Operated										
0–19 Years	404	2.6	4	1	1	2	3	5	6	10
20–34	181	3.4	5	1	2	3	4	8	8	11
35–49	37	3.2	3	1	2	3	4	6	8	8
50–64	24	3.3	2	2	2	3	4	5	6	7
65+	11	6.2	49	2	2	3	8	8	26	26
B. Operated										
0–19 Years	15	6.6	33	1	3	4	9	10	24	24
20–34	11	3.9	5	1	2	4	5	7	8	8
35–49	3	4.0	13	1	1	3	8	8	8	8
50–64	2	21.0	629	3	3	21	39	39	39	39
65+	4	7.3	23	2	5	9	13	13	13	13
SUBTOTALS:										
1. SINGLE DX										
A. Not Operated	53	2.0	2	1	1	2	2	4	4	6
B. Operated	0									
2. MULTIPLE DX										
A. Not Operated	657	2.9	5	1	1	2	3	5	6	11
B. Operated	35	6.5	53	1	3	4	8	10	24	39
1. SINGLE DX	53	2.0	2	1	1	2	2	4	4	6
2. MULTIPLE DX	692	3.1	8	1	1	2	4	6	8	12
A. NOT OPERATED	710	2.8	5	1	1	2	3	5	7	10
B. OPERATED	35	6.5	53	1	3	4	8	10	24	39
TOTAL										
0–19 Years	454	2.7	5	1	1	2	3	5	7	11
20–34	209	3.3	5	1	2	3	4	6	8	10
35–49	41	3.3	4	1	2	3	4	6	8	8
50–64	26	4.6	52	2	2	3	4	6	7	39
65+	15	6.5	40	2	2	5	8	13	26	26
GRAND TOTAL	745	3.0	8	1	1	2	4	6	8	11

Length of Stay by Diagnosis and Operation, Western Region, 2008

Western Region, October 2006–September 2007 Data, by Diagnosis

076: TRACHOMA

Type of Patients	Observed Patients	Avg. Stay	Variance	10th	25th	50th	75th	90th	95th	99th
1. SINGLE DX										
A. Not Operated										
0–19 Years	0									
20–34	0									
35–49	0									
50–64	0									
65+	0									
B. Operated										
0–19 Years	0									
20–34	0									
35–49	0									
50–64	0									
65+	0									
2. MULTIPLE DX										
A. Not Operated										
0–19 Years	0									
20–34	0									
35–49	0									
50–64	0									
65+	0									
B. Operated										
0–19 Years	0									
20–34	0									
35–49	0									
50–64	0									
65+	0									
SUBTOTALS:										
1. SINGLE DX A. Not Operated	0									
B. Operated	0									
2. MULTIPLE DX A. Not Operated	0									
B. Operated	0									
1. SINGLE DX	0									
2. MULTIPLE DX	0									
A. NOT OPERATED	0									
B. OPERATED	0									
TOTAL										
0–19 Years	0									
20–34	0									
35–49	0									
50–64	0									
65+	0									
GRAND TOTAL	0									

077: VIRAL/CHLAM CONJUNCT NEC

Type of Patients	Observed Patients	Avg. Stay	Variance	10th	25th	50th	75th	90th	95th	99th
1. SINGLE DX										
A. Not Operated										
0–19 Years	4	1.5	<1	1	1	1	1	3	3	3
20–34	0									
35–49	0									
50–64	0									
65+	0									
B. Operated										
0–19 Years	0									
20–34	0									
35–49	0									
50–64	0									
65+	0									
2. MULTIPLE DX										
A. Not Operated										
0–19 Years	4	2.5	<1	2	2	3	3	3	3	3
20–34	5	2.6	4	1	1	2	3	6	6	6
35–49	3	2.0	<1	1	1	2	3	3	3	3
50–64	3	2.7	2	1	1	3	4	4	4	4
65+	4	6.3	37	1	1	11	12	12	12	12
B. Operated										
0–19 Years	0									
20–34	0									
35–49	0									
50–64	0									
65+	0									
SUBTOTALS:										
1. SINGLE DX A. Not Operated	4	1.5	<1	1	1	1	1	3	3	3
B. Operated	0									
2. MULTIPLE DX A. Not Operated	19	3.3	10	1	1	2	3	11	12	12
B. Operated	0									
1. SINGLE DX	4	1.5	<1	1	1	1	1	3	3	3
2. MULTIPLE DX	19	3.3	10	1	1	2	3	11	12	12
A. NOT OPERATED	23	3.0	9	1	1	2	3	6	11	12
B. OPERATED	0									
TOTAL										
0–19 Years	8	2.0	<1	1	1	2	2	3	3	3
20–34	5	2.6	4	1	1	2	3	6	6	6
35–49	3	2.0	<1	1	1	2	3	3	3	3
50–64	3	2.7	2	1	1	3	4	4	4	4
65+	4	6.3	37	1	1	11	12	12	12	12
GRAND TOTAL	23	3.0	9	1	1	2	3	6	11	12

078: OTHER VIRAL DISEASE

Type of Patients	Observed Patients	Avg. Stay	Variance	10th	25th	50th	75th	90th	95th	99th
1. SINGLE DX										
A. Not Operated										
0–19 Years	8	2.9	3	1	2	3	3	7	7	7
20–34	3	1.3	<1	1	1	1	2	2	2	2
35–49	0									
50–64	0									
65+	0									
B. Operated										
0–19 Years	8	2.0	1	1	1	1	3	4	4	4
20–34	1	1.0	0	1	1	1	1	1	1	1
35–49	0									
50–64	0									
65+	0									
2. MULTIPLE DX										
A. Not Operated										
0–19 Years	62	4.0	27	1	1	2	4	8	12	36
20–34	43	5.5	10	3	3	5	7	10	11	14
35–49	70	6.4	35	1	2	4	8	15	20	28
50–64	105	6.5	27	1	3	5	9	14	17	25
65+	74	8.0	54	1	2	6	11	19	26	29
B. Operated										
0–19 Years	7	23.9	>999	1	1	2	67	91	91	91
20–34	16	6.1	86	1	1	4	6	19	37	37
35–49	17	3.8	19	1	1	1	5	13	15	15
50–64	18	7.9	92	1	1	2	17	27	27	27
65+	15	18.1	401	1	5	15	21	33	82	82
SUBTOTALS:										
1. SINGLE DX A. Not Operated	11	2.5	3	1	1	2	3	3	7	7
B. Operated	9	1.9	1	1	1	1	3	4	4	4
2. MULTIPLE DX A. Not Operated	354	6.2	33	1	2	4	8	14	18	28
B. Operated	73	10.2	290	1	1	4	13	23	37	91
1. SINGLE DX	20	2.2	2	1	1	2	3	4	7	7
2. MULTIPLE DX	427	6.9	79	1	2	4	8	15	20	36
A. NOT OPERATED	365	6.1	33	1	2	4	8	14	18	28
B. OPERATED	82	9.3	265	1	1	2	12	21	33	91
TOTAL										
0–19 Years	77	5.7	171	1	1	2	4	9	14	91
20–34	70	5.1	27	1	2	4	7	10	12	37
35–49	88	5.9	33	1	2	4	7	15	20	28
50–64	123	6.7	36	1	2	5	10	15	18	27
65+	89	9.7	123	1	2	7	14	21	28	82
GRAND TOTAL	447	6.7	76	1	2	4	8	15	20	36

36

Length of Stay by Diagnosis and Operation, Western Region, 2008

078.5: CYTOMEGALOVIRAL DISEASE

Type of Patients	Observed Patients	Avg. Stay	Variance	10th	25th	50th	75th	90th	95th	99th
1. SINGLE DX										
A. Not Operated										
0–19 Years	2	4.5	12	2	2	7	7	7	7	7
20–34	0									
35–49	0									
50–64	0									
65+	0									
B. Operated										
0–19 Years	0									
20–34	0									
35–49	0									
50–64	0									
65+	0									
2. MULTIPLE DX										
A. Not Operated										
0–19 Years	24	7.0	53	1	3	5	9	13	14	36
20–34	33	6.3	10	3	4	6	8	10	12	14
35–49	52	7.9	39	2	4	7	11	17	20	28
50–64	90	7.3	27	3	4	5	10	14	17	27
65+	41	12.2	53	5	7	10	17	21	28	29
B. Operated										
0–19 Years	2	79.0	283	67	67	79	91	91	91	91
20–34	2	12.0	95	5	5	12	19	19	19	19
35–49	2	11.0	31	7	7	7	15	15	15	15
50–64	6	15.8	77	1	12	17	20	27	27	27
65+	11	24.0	419	11	13	20	23	33	82	82
SUBTOTALS:										
1. SINGLE DX										
A. Not Operated	2	4.5	12	2	2	7	7	7	7	7
B. Operated	0									
2. MULTIPLE DX										
A. Not Operated	240	8.1	37	2	4	7	11	17	20	28
B. Operated	23	24.4	548	7	12	18	23	67	82	91
1. SINGLE DX	2	4.5	12	2	2	7	7	7	7	7
2. MULTIPLE DX	263	9.5	102	2	4	7	12	19	23	67
A. NOT OPERATED	242	8.1	37	2	4	7	11	16	20	28
B. OPERATED	23	24.4	548	7	12	18	23	67	82	91
TOTAL										
0–19 Years	28	12.0	416	1	3	6	11	36	67	91
20–34	35	6.6	14	3	4	6	8	11	14	19
35–49	54	8.0	38	2	4	7	11	17	20	28
50–64	96	7.8	33	2	4	6	11	16	19	27
65+	52	14.7	147	5	8	12	20	26	29	82
GRAND TOTAL	265	9.5	101	2	4	7	12	19	23	67

079: VIR/CHLAMYD INF CCE/NOS

Type of Patients	Observed Patients	Avg. Stay	Variance	10th	25th	50th	75th	90th	95th	99th
1. SINGLE DX										
A. Not Operated										
0–19 Years	595	2.1	<1	1	1	2	3	3	4	5
20–34	24	1.9	1	1	1	2	3	3	4	5
35–49	14	1.7	<1	1	1	2	3	3	3	3
50–64	6	2.2	<1	1	1	2	3	3	3	3
65+	1	2.0	0	2	2	2	2	2	2	2
B. Operated										
0–19 Years	1	2.0	0	2	2	2	2	2	2	2
20–34	0									
35–49	0									
50–64	0									
65+	0									
2. MULTIPLE DX										
A. Not Operated										
0–19 Years	1,589	2.3	2	1	1	2	3	4	5	8
20–34	383	2.8	4	1	1	2	3	5	6	14
35–49	481	2.7	3	1	2	2	3	5	6	9
50–64	566	2.6	4	1	1	2	3	5	6	12
65+	914	2.7	3	1	1	2	3	5	6	8
B. Operated										
0–19 Years	2	1.5	<1	1	1	1	1	2	2	2
20–34	3	5.7	14	3	3	4	10	10	10	10
35–49	6	3.3	5	1	3	4	4	7	7	7
50–64	5	6.8	10	4	4	6	9	11	11	11
65+	6	5.2	15	1	3	3	6	12	12	12
SUBTOTALS:										
1. SINGLE DX										
A. Not Operated	640	2.1	<1	1	1	2	3	3	4	5
B. Operated	1	2.0	0	2	2	2	2	2	2	2
2. MULTIPLE DX										
A. Not Operated	3,933	2.5	3	1	1	2	3	4	5	9
B. Operated	22	4.8	11	3	4	6	11	20	82	91
1. SINGLE DX	641	2.1	<1	1	1	2	3	3	4	5
2. MULTIPLE DX	3,955	2.5	3	1	1	2	3	4	6	9
A. NOT OPERATED	4,573	2.5	3	1	1	2	3	4	5	8
B. OPERATED	23	4.7	11	1	2	4	6	10	11	12
TOTAL										
0–19 Years	2,187	2.2	2	1	1	2	3	4	4	7
20–34	410	2.7	4	1	1	2	3	5	6	12
35–49	501	2.7	3	1	1	2	3	5	6	9
50–64	577	2.7	4	1	1	2	3	5	6	12
65+	921	2.7	3	1	1	2	3	5	6	8
GRAND TOTAL	4,596	2.5	3	1	1	2	3	4	5	9

079.99: VIRAL INFECTION NOS

Type of Patients	Observed Patients	Avg. Stay	Variance	10th	25th	50th	75th	90th	95th	99th
1. SINGLE DX										
A. Not Operated										
0–19 Years	552	2.1	<1	1	1	2	3	3	4	5
20–34	24	1.9	1	1	1	2	3	3	4	5
35–49	14	1.7	<1	1	1	2	3	3	3	3
50–64	6	2.2	<1	1	1	2	3	3	3	3
65+	1	2.0	0	2	2	2	2	2	2	2
B. Operated										
0–19 Years	1	2.0	0	2	2	2	2	2	2	2
20–34	0									
35–49	0									
50–64	0									
65+	0									
2. MULTIPLE DX										
A. Not Operated										
0–19 Years	1,456	2.2	2	1	1	2	3	4	5	7
20–34	372	2.7	4	1	1	2	3	5	6	12
35–49	469	2.7	3	1	2	2	3	5	6	9
50–64	556	2.6	4	1	1	2	3	5	6	12
65+	905	2.6	3	1	1	2	3	5	6	8
B. Operated										
0–19 Years	2	1.5	<1	1	1	1	1	2	2	2
20–34	3	5.7	14	3	3	4	10	10	10	10
35–49	5	3.8	5	1	3	4	4	7	7	7
50–64	5	6.8	10	4	4	6	9	11	11	11
65+	6	5.2	15	1	3	3	6	12	12	12
SUBTOTALS:										
1. SINGLE DX										
A. Not Operated	597	2.1	<1	1	1	2	3	3	4	5
B. Operated	1	2.0	0	2	2	2	2	2	2	2
2. MULTIPLE DX										
A. Not Operated	3,758	2.5	3	1	1	2	3	4	5	9
B. Operated	21	5.0	11	3	4	6	10	11	12	12
1. SINGLE DX	598	2.1	<1	1	1	2	3	3	4	5
2. MULTIPLE DX	3,779	2.5	3	1	1	2	3	4	5	9
A. NOT OPERATED	4,355	2.4	3	1	1	2	3	4	5	8
B. OPERATED	22	4.8	10	1	3	4	6	10	11	12
TOTAL										
0–19 Years	2,011	2.2	2	1	1	2	3	4	4	6
20–34	399	2.7	4	1	1	2	3	5	6	10
35–49	488	2.7	3	1	1	2	3	5	6	9
50–64	567	2.7	4	1	1	2	3	5	6	12
65+	912	2.7	3	1	1	2	3	5	6	8
GRAND TOTAL	4,377	2.5	3	1	1	2	3	4	5	8

Length of Stay by Diagnosis and Operation, Western Region, 2008

Western Region, October 2006–September 2007 Data, by Diagnosis

080: LOUSE-BORNE TYPHUS

Type of Patients	Observed Patients	Avg. Stay	Variance	Percentiles						
				10th	25th	50th	75th	90th	95th	99th
1. SINGLE DX										
A. Not Operated										
0–19 Years	0									
20–34	0									
35–49	0									
50–64	0									
65+	0									
B. Operated										
0–19 Years	0									
20–34	0									
35–49	0									
50–64	0									
65+	0									
2. MULTIPLE DX										
A. Not Operated										
0–19 Years	0									
20–34	0									
35–49	0									
50–64	0									
65+	0									
B. Operated										
0–19 Years	0									
20–34	0									
35–49	0									
50–64	0									
65+	0									
SUBTOTALS:										
1. SINGLE DX *A. Not Operated*	0									
B. Operated	0									
2. MULTIPLE DX *A. Not Operated*	0									
B. Operated	0									
1. SINGLE DX	0									
2. MULTIPLE DX	0									
A. NOT OPERATED	0									
B. OPERATED	0									
TOTAL										
0–19 Years	0									
20–34	0									
35–49	0									
50–64	0									
65+	0									
GRAND TOTAL	0									

081: OTHER TYPHUS

Type of Patients	Observed Patients	Avg. Stay	Variance	Percentiles						
				10th	25th	50th	75th	90th	95th	99th
1. SINGLE DX										
A. Not Operated										
0–19 Years	0									
20–34	0									
35–49	0									
50–64	0									
65+	0									
B. Operated										
0–19 Years	0									
20–34	0									
35–49	0									
50–64	0									
65+	0									
2. MULTIPLE DX										
A. Not Operated										
0–19 Years	3	4.3	10	2	2	3	8	8	8	8
20–34	4	3.8	6	1	1	3	7	7	7	7
35–49	2	3.0	0	3	3	3	3	3	3	3
50–64	7	6.0	29	2	4	4	6	18	18	18
65+	4	6.0	6	3	3	5	8	8	8	8
B. Operated										
0–19 Years	0									
20–34	0									
35–49	0									
50–64	0									
65+	0									
SUBTOTALS:										
1. SINGLE DX *A. Not Operated*	0									
B. Operated	0									
2. MULTIPLE DX *A. Not Operated*	20	5.0	14	3	3	4	6	8	8	18
B. Operated	0									
1. SINGLE DX	0									
2. MULTIPLE DX	20	5.0	14	3	3	4	6	8	8	18
A. NOT OPERATED	20	5.0	14	3	3	4	6	8	8	18
B. OPERATED	0									
TOTAL										
0–19 Years	3	4.3	10	2	2	3	8	8	8	8
20–34	4	3.8	6	1	1	3	7	7	7	7
35–49	2	3.0	0	3	3	3	3	3	3	3
50–64	7	6.0	29	2	4	4	6	18	18	18
65+	4	6.0	6	3	3	5	8	8	8	8
GRAND TOTAL	20	5.0	14	2	3	4	6	8	8	18

082: TICK-BORNE RICKETTSIOSES

Type of Patients	Observed Patients	Avg. Stay	Variance	Percentiles						
				10th	25th	50th	75th	90th	95th	99th
1. SINGLE DX										
A. Not Operated										
0–19 Years	3	2.3	<1	2	2	2	2	3	3	3
20–34	0									
35–49	0									
50–64	0									
65+	0									
B. Operated										
0–19 Years	0									
20–34	0									
35–49	0									
50–64	0									
65+	0									
2. MULTIPLE DX										
A. Not Operated										
0–19 Years	2	6.5	4	5	5	8	8	8	8	8
20–34	2	4.0	18	1	1	7	7	7	7	7
35–49	5	5.6	10	1	5	6	6	10	10	10
50–64	7	4.1	14	1	2	2	8	11	11	11
65+	4	6.5	14	4	4	6	6	12	12	12
B. Operated										
0–19 Years	0									
20–34	0									
35–49	0									
50–64	0									
65+	0									
SUBTOTALS:										
1. SINGLE DX *A. Not Operated*	3	2.3	<1	2	2	2	2	3	3	3
B. Operated	0									
2. MULTIPLE DX *A. Not Operated*	20	5.2	11	1	2	5	7	10	11	12
B. Operated	0									
1. SINGLE DX	3	2.3	<1	2	2	2	3	3	3	3
2. MULTIPLE DX	20	5.2	11	1	2	5	7	10	11	12
A. NOT OPERATED	23	4.8	11	1	2	4	7	10	11	12
B. OPERATED	0									
TOTAL										
0–19 Years	5	4.0	6	2	2	3	5	8	8	8
20–34	2	4.0	18	1	1	7	7	7	7	7
35–49	5	5.6	10	1	5	6	6	10	10	10
50–64	7	4.1	14	1	2	2	8	11	11	11
65+	4	6.5	14	4	4	6	6	12	12	12
GRAND TOTAL	23	4.8	11	2	2	4	7	10	11	12

Length of Stay by Diagnosis and Operation, Western Region, 2008

38

Western Region, October 2006–September 2007 Data, by Diagnosis

083: OTHER RICKETTSIOSES

Type of Patients	Observed Patients	Avg. Stay	Variance	10th	25th	50th	75th	90th	95th	99th
						Percentiles				
1. SINGLE DX										
A. *Not Operated*										
0–19 Years	0									
20–34	0									
35–49	0									
50–64	0									
65+	0									
B. *Operated*										
0–19 Years	0									
20–34	0									
35–49	0									
50–64	0									
65+	0									
2. MULTIPLE DX										
A. *Not Operated*										
0–19 Years	0									
20–34	6	4.2	7	1	3	4	5	9	9	9
35–49	4	8.2	32	4	4	4	9	16	16	16
50–64	4	10.0	25	5	5	10	16	16	16	16
65+	4	2.8	4	1	1	4	5	5	5	5
B. *Operated*										
0–19 Years	0									
20–34	0									
35–49	2	26.8	960	5	5	5	49	49	49	49
50–64	0									
65+	0									
SUBTOTALS:										
1. SINGLE DX										
A. *Not Operated*	0									
B. *Operated*	0									
2. MULTIPLE DX										
A. *Not Operated*	18	6.1	21	1	3	5	9	16	16	16
B. *Operated*	2	26.8	960	5	5	5	49	49	49	49
1. SINGLE DX	**0**									
2. MULTIPLE DX	**20**	**8.1**	**110**	**1**	**4**	**5**	**9**	**16**	**16**	**49**
A. NOT OPERATED	**18**	**6.1**	**21**	**1**	**3**	**5**	**9**	**16**	**16**	**16**
B. OPERATED	**2**	**26.8**	**960**	**5**	**5**	**5**	**49**	**49**	**49**	**49**
TOTAL										
0–19 Years	0									
20–34	6	4.2	7	1	3	4	5	9	9	9
35–49	6	14.4	302	4	4	10	16	49	49	49
50–64	4	10.0	25	5	5	10	16	16	16	16
65+	4	2.8	4	1	1	4	5	5	5	5
GRAND TOTAL	**20**	**8.1**	**110**	**1**	**4**	**5**	**9**	**16**	**16**	**49**

084: MALARIA

Type of Patients	Observed Patients	Avg. Stay	Variance	10th	25th	50th	75th	90th	95th	99th
						Percentiles				
1. SINGLE DX										
A. *Not Operated*										
0–19 Years	0									
20–34	10	2.7	5	1	1	2	3	5	8	8
35–49	1	1.0	0	1	1	1	1	1	1	1
50–64	0									
65+	0									
B. *Operated*										
0–19 Years	0									
20–34	0									
35–49	0									
50–64	0									
65+	0									
2. MULTIPLE DX										
A. *Not Operated*										
0–19 Years	14	2.9	5	1	1	2	3	6	9	9
20–34	45	3.0	3	1	2	3	4	6	6	7
35–49	30	2.4	2	1	2	2	3	4	4	7
50–64	36	4.3	10	1	2	4	6	8	9	18
65+	6	3.7	2	2	2	4	5	5	5	5
B. *Operated*										
0–19 Years	0									
20–34	0									
35–49	0									
50–64	0									
65+	0									
SUBTOTALS:										
1. SINGLE DX										
A. *Not Operated*	11	2.5	5	1	1	2	3	5	8	8
B. *Operated*	0									
2. MULTIPLE DX										
A. *Not Operated*	131	3.2	5	2	2	3	4	6	7	9
B. *Operated*	0									
1. SINGLE DX	**11**	**2.5**	**5**	**1**	**1**	**2**	**3**	**5**	**8**	**8**
2. MULTIPLE DX	**131**	**3.2**	**5**	**1**	**2**	**3**	**4**	**6**	**7**	**9**
A. NOT OPERATED	**142**	**3.2**	**5**	**1**	**2**	**3**	**4**	**6**	**7**	**9**
B. OPERATED	**0**									
TOTAL										
0–19 Years	14	2.9	5	1	1	2	3	6	9	9
20–34	55	2.9	3	1	1	2	4	6	7	8
35–49	31	2.4	2	1	1	2	3	4	4	7
50–64	36	4.3	10	1	2	4	6	8	9	18
65+	6	3.7	2	2	2	4	5	5	5	5
GRAND TOTAL	**142**	**3.2**	**5**	**1**	**2**	**3**	**4**	**6**	**7**	**9**

085: LEISHMANIASIS

Type of Patients	Observed Patients	Avg. Stay	Variance	10th	25th	50th	75th	90th	95th	99th
						Percentiles				
1. SINGLE DX										
A. *Not Operated*										
0–19 Years	0									
20–34	0									
35–49	0									
50–64	0									
65+	0									
B. *Operated*										
0–19 Years	0									
20–34	0									
35–49	0									
50–64	0									
65+	0									
2. MULTIPLE DX										
A. *Not Operated*										
0–19 Years	0									
20–34	0									
35–49	1	2.0	0	2	2	2	2	2	2	2
50–64	1	2.0	0	2	2	2	2	2	2	2
65+	0									
B. *Operated*										
0–19 Years	0									
20–34	0									
35–49	0									
50–64	0									
65+	0									
SUBTOTALS:										
1. SINGLE DX										
A. *Not Operated*	0									
B. *Operated*	0									
2. MULTIPLE DX										
A. *Not Operated*	2	2.0	0	2	2	2	2	2	2	2
B. *Operated*	0									
1. SINGLE DX	**0**									
2. MULTIPLE DX	**2**	**2.0**	**0**	**2**	**2**	**2**	**2**	**2**	**2**	**2**
A. NOT OPERATED	**2**	**2.0**	**0**	**2**	**2**	**2**	**2**	**2**	**2**	**2**
B. OPERATED	**0**									
TOTAL										
0–19 Years	0									
20–34	0									
35–49	1	2.0	0	2	2	2	2	2	2	2
50–64	1	2.0	0	2	2	2	2	2	2	2
65+	0									
GRAND TOTAL	**2**	**2.0**	**0**	**2**	**2**	**2**	**2**	**2**	**2**	**2**

Length of Stay by Diagnosis and Operation, Western Region, 2008

Western Region, October 2006–September 2007 Data, by Diagnosis

086: TRYPANOSOMIASIS

Type of Patients	Observed Patients	Avg. Stay	Variance	10th	25th	50th	75th	90th	95th	99th
1. SINGLE DX										
A. Not Operated										
0–19 Years	0									
20–34	0									
35–49	0									
50–64	0									
65+	0									
B. Operated										
0–19 Years	0									
20–34	0									
35–49	0									
50–64	0									
65+	0									
2. MULTIPLE DX										
A. Not Operated										
0–19 Years	0									
20–34	1	5.0	0	5	5	5	5	5	5	5
35–49	0									
50–64	0									
65+	1	4.0	0	4	4	4	4	4	4	4
B. Operated										
0–19 Years	0									
20–34	1	1.0	0	1	1	1	1	1	1	1
35–49	0									
50–64	0									
65+	0									
SUBTOTALS:										
1. SINGLE DX A. Not Operated	0									
1. SINGLE DX B. Operated	0									
2. MULTIPLE DX A. Not Operated	2	4.5	<1	4	4	4	5	5	5	5
2. MULTIPLE DX B. Operated	1	1.0	0	1	1	1	1	1	1	1
1. SINGLE DX	0									
2. MULTIPLE DX	3	3.3	4	1	1	4	5	5	5	5
A. NOT OPERATED	2	4.5	<1	4	4	4	5	5	5	5
B. OPERATED	1	1.0	0	1	1	1	1	1	1	1
TOTAL										
0–19 Years	0									
20–34	1	5.0	0	5	5	5	5	5	5	5
35–49	1	1.0	0	1	1	1	1	1	1	1
50–64	0									
65+	1	4.0	0	4	4	4	4	4	4	4
GRAND TOTAL	3	3.3	4	1	1	4	5	5	5	5

087: RELAPSING FEVER

Type of Patients	Observed Patients	Avg. Stay	Variance	10th	25th	50th	75th	90th	95th	99th
1. SINGLE DX										
A. Not Operated										
0–19 Years	0									
20–34	0									
35–49	0									
50–64	0									
65+	0									
B. Operated										
0–19 Years	0									
20–34	0									
35–49	0									
50–64	0									
65+	0									
2. MULTIPLE DX										
A. Not Operated										
0–19 Years	0									
20–34	2	2.5	4	1	1	1	4	4	4	4
35–49	0									
50–64	0									
65+	2	2.5	<1	2	2	2	3	3	3	3
B. Operated										
0–19 Years	0									
20–34	0									
35–49	0									
50–64	0									
65+	0									
SUBTOTALS:										
1. SINGLE DX A. Not Operated	0									
1. SINGLE DX B. Operated	0									
2. MULTIPLE DX A. Not Operated	4	2.5	2	1	1	2	3	4	4	4
2. MULTIPLE DX B. Operated	0									
1. SINGLE DX	0									
2. MULTIPLE DX	4	2.5	2	1	1	2	3	4	4	4
A. NOT OPERATED	4	2.5	2	1	1	2	3	4	4	4
B. OPERATED	0									
TOTAL										
0–19 Years	0									
20–34	2	2.5	4	1	1	1	4	4	4	4
35–49	0									
50–64	0									
65+	2	2.5	<1	2	2	2	3	3	3	3
GRAND TOTAL	4	2.5	2	1	1	2	3	4	4	4

088: OTH ARTHROPOD-BORNE DIS

Type of Patients	Observed Patients	Avg. Stay	Variance	10th	25th	50th	75th	90th	95th	99th
1. SINGLE DX										
A. Not Operated										
0–19 Years	2	2.0	2	1	1	2	3	3	3	3
20–34	0									
35–49	1	9.0	0	9	9	9	9	9	9	9
50–64	0									
65+	1	1.0	0	1	1	1	1	1	1	1
B. Operated										
0–19 Years	0									
20–34	0									
35–49	0									
50–64	0									
2. MULTIPLE DX										
A. Not Operated										
0–19 Years	0									
20–34	11	7.6	180	1	2	4	6	7	48	48
35–49	10	2.5	<1	1	2	3	3	3	4	4
50–64	10	4.7	8	1	3	4	7	8	9	9
65+	6	3.3	1	2	3	3	4	5	5	5
B. Operated										
0–19 Years	0									
20–34	0									
35–49	0									
50–64	0									
65+	2	3.5	4	2	2	2	5	5	5	5
SUBTOTALS:										
1. SINGLE DX A. Not Operated	4	3.5	14	1	1	1	3	9	9	9
1. SINGLE DX B. Operated	0									
2. MULTIPLE DX A. Not Operated	37	4.7	57	1	2	3	5	7	9	48
2. MULTIPLE DX B. Operated	2	3.5	4	2	2	2	5	5	5	5
1. SINGLE DX	4	3.5	14	1	1	1	3	9	9	9
2. MULTIPLE DX	39	4.7	54	1	2	3	5	7	9	48
A. NOT OPERATED	41	4.6	52	1	2	3	5	7	9	48
B. OPERATED	2	3.5	4	2	2	2	5	5	5	5
TOTAL										
0–19 Years	2	2.0	2	1	1	2	3	3	3	3
20–34	11	7.6	180	1	2	4	6	7	48	48
35–49	11	3.1	5	1	2	3	3	4	9	9
50–64	10	4.7	8	1	3	4	7	8	9	9
65+	9	3.1	2	1	2	3	4	5	5	5
GRAND TOTAL	43	4.6	50	1	2	3	5	7	9	48

Length of Stay by Diagnosis and Operation, Western Region, 2008

Western Region, October 2006–September 2007 Data, by Diagnosis

088.81: LYME DISEASE

Type of Patients	Observed Patients	Avg. Stay	Variance	Percentiles 10th	25th	50th	75th	90th	95th	99th
1. SINGLE DX										
A. Not Operated										
0–19 Years	2	2.0	2	1	1	2	3	3	3	3
20–34	0									
35–49	1	9.0	0	9	9	9	9	9	9	9
50–64	0									
65+	1	1.0	0	1	1	1	1	1	1	1
B. Operated										
0–19 Years	0									
20–34	0									
35–49	0									
50–64	0									
65+	0									
2. MULTIPLE DX										
A. Not Operated										
0–19 Years	0									
20–34	10	7.7	200	1	2	4	6	7	48	48
35–49	10	2.5	<1	1	2	3	3	3	4	4
50–64	7	3.7	6	1	1	3	7	7	7	7
65+	6	3.3	1	2	3	3	4	5	5	5
B. Operated										
0–19 Years	0									
20–34	0									
35–49	0									
50–64	0									
65+	2	3.5	4	2	2	2	5	5	5	5
SUBTOTALS:										
1. SINGLE DX A. Not Operated	4	3.5	14	1	1	1	3	9	9	9
1. SINGLE DX B. Operated	0									
2. MULTIPLE DX A. Not Operated	33	4.5	63	1	2	3	4	7	7	48
2. MULTIPLE DX B. Operated	2	3.5	4	2	2	2	5	5	5	5
1. SINGLE DX	4	3.5	14	1	1	1	3	9	9	9
2. MULTIPLE DX	35	4.4	59	1	2	3	4	7	7	48
A. NOT OPERATED	37	4.4	57	1	2	3	4	7	9	48
B. OPERATED	2	3.5	4	2	2	2	5	5	5	5
TOTAL										
0–19 Years	2	2.0	2	1	1	2	3	3	3	3
20–34	10	7.7	200	1	2	4	6	7	48	48
35–49	11	3.1	5	1	2	3	3	4	9	9
50–64	7	3.7	6	1	1	3	7	7	7	7
65+	9	3.1	2	2	3	3	4	5	5	5
GRAND TOTAL	39	4.3	54	1	2	3	4	7	9	48

090: CONGENITAL SYPHILIS

Type of Patients	Observed Patients	Avg. Stay	Variance	Percentiles 10th	25th	50th	75th	90th	95th	99th
1. SINGLE DX										
A. Not Operated										
0–19 Years	7	7.7	15	1	3	10	10	10	10	10
20–34	0									
35–49	0									
50–64	0									
65+	0									
B. Operated										
0–19 Years	0									
20–34	0									
35–49	0									
50–64	0									
65+	0									
2. MULTIPLE DX										
A. Not Operated										
0–19 Years	14	9.2	8	6	9	10	10	11	14	14
20–34	0									
35–49	0									
50–64	1	4.0	0	4	4	4	4	4	4	4
65+	1	12.0	0	12	12	12	12	12	12	12
B. Operated										
0–19 Years	0									
20–34	0									
35–49	0									
50–64	0									
65+	0									
SUBTOTALS:										
1. SINGLE DX A. Not Operated	7	7.7	15	1	3	10	10	10	10	10
1. SINGLE DX B. Operated	0									
2. MULTIPLE DX A. Not Operated	16	9.1	10	4	9	10	10	12	14	14
2. MULTIPLE DX B. Operated	0									
1. SINGLE DX	7	7.7	15	1	3	10	10	10	10	10
2. MULTIPLE DX	16	9.1	10	4	9	10	10	12	14	14
A. NOT OPERATED	23	8.7	11	3	9	10	10	11	12	14
B. OPERATED	0									
TOTAL										
0–19 Years	21	8.7	11	3	9	10	10	10	11	14
20–34	0									
35–49	0									
50–64	1	4.0	0	4	4	4	4	4	4	4
65+	1	12.0	0	12	12	12	12	12	12	12
GRAND TOTAL	23	8.7	11	3	9	10	10	11	12	14

091: EARLY SYMPTOMATIC SYPH

Type of Patients	Observed Patients	Avg. Stay	Variance	Percentiles 10th	25th	50th	75th	90th	95th	99th
1. SINGLE DX										
A. Not Operated										
0–19 Years	0									
20–34	0									
35–49	0									
50–64	0									
65+	0									
B. Operated										
0–19 Years	0									
20–34	0									
35–49	0									
50–64	0									
65+	0									
2. MULTIPLE DX										
A. Not Operated										
0–19 Years	1	4.0	0	4	4	4	4	4	4	4
20–34	8	7.9	13	3	6	8	10	15	15	15
35–49	11	4.1	15	2	2	2	4	10	13	13
50–64	5	4.4	4	3	3	3	6	8	7	7
65+	1	8.0	0	8	8	8	8	8	8	8
B. Operated										
0–19 Years	0									
20–34	0									
35–49	0									
50–64	0									
65+	0									
SUBTOTALS:										
1. SINGLE DX A. Not Operated	0									
1. SINGLE DX B. Operated	0									
2. MULTIPLE DX A. Not Operated	26	5.5	14	2	3	4	8	10	13	15
2. MULTIPLE DX B. Operated	0									
1. SINGLE DX	0									
2. MULTIPLE DX	26	5.5	14	2	3	4	8	10	13	15
A. NOT OPERATED	26	5.5	14	2	3	4	8	10	13	15
B. OPERATED	0									
TOTAL										
0–19 Years	1	4.0	0	4	4	4	4	4	4	4
20–34	8	7.9	13	3	6	8	10	15	15	15
35–49	11	4.1	15	2	2	2	4	10	13	13
50–64	5	4.4	4	3	3	3	6	8	7	7
65+	1	8.0	0	8	8	8	8	8	8	8
GRAND TOTAL	26	5.5	14	2	3	4	8	10	13	15

Length of Stay by Diagnosis and Operation, Western Region, 2008

Western Region, October 2006–September 2007 Data, by Diagnosis

092: EARLY SYPHILIS LATENT

Type of Patients	Observed Patients	Avg. Stay	Variance	10th	25th	50th	75th	90th	95th	99th
1. SINGLE DX										
A. Not Operated										
0–19 Years	0									
20–34	0									
35–49	0									
50–64	0									
65+	0									
B. Operated										
0–19 Years	0									
20–34	0									
35–49	0									
50–64	0									
65+	0									
2. MULTIPLE DX										
A. Not Operated										
0–19 Years	0									
20–34	0									
35–49	0									
50–64	1	3.0	0	3	3	3	3	3	3	3
65+	0									
B. Operated										
0–19 Years	0									
20–34	0									
35–49	0									
50–64	0									
65+	0									
SUBTOTALS:										
1. SINGLE DX										
A. Not Operated	0									
B. Operated	0									
2. MULTIPLE DX										
A. Not Operated	1	3.0	0	3	3	3	3	3	3	3
B. Operated	0									
1. SINGLE DX	0									
2. MULTIPLE DX	1	3.0	0	3	3	3	3	3	3	3
A. NOT OPERATED	1	3.0	0	3	3	3	3	3	3	3
B. OPERATED	0									
TOTAL										
0–19 Years	0									
20–34	0									
35–49	0									
50–64	1	3.0	0	3	3	3	3	3	3	3
65+	0									
GRAND TOTAL	1	3.0	0	3	3	3	3	3	3	3

093: CARDIOVASCULAR SYPHILIS

Type of Patients	Observed Patients	Avg. Stay	Variance	10th	25th	50th	75th	90th	95th	99th
1. SINGLE DX										
A. Not Operated										
0–19 Years	0									
20–34	0									
35–49	0									
50–64	0									
65+	0									
B. Operated										
0–19 Years	0									
20–34	0									
35–49	0									
50–64	0									
65+	0									
2. MULTIPLE DX										
A. Not Operated										
0–19 Years	0									
20–34	0									
35–49	0									
50–64	1	4.0	0	4	4	4	4	4	4	4
65+	1	27.0	0	27	27	27	27	27	27	27
B. Operated										
0–19 Years	0									
20–34	0									
35–49	0									
50–64	0									
65+	0									
SUBTOTALS:										
1. SINGLE DX										
A. Not Operated	0									
B. Operated	0									
2. MULTIPLE DX										
A. Not Operated	2	15.4	259	4	4	4	27	27	27	27
B. Operated	0									
1. SINGLE DX	0									
2. MULTIPLE DX	2	15.4	259	4	4	4	27	27	27	27
A. NOT OPERATED	2	15.4	259	4	4	4	27	27	27	27
B. OPERATED	0									
TOTAL										
0–19 Years	0									
20–34	0									
35–49	0									
50–64	1	4.0	0	4	4	4	4	4	4	4
65+	1	27.0	0	27	27	27	27	27	27	27
GRAND TOTAL	2	15.4	259	4	4	4	27	27	27	27

094: NEUROSYPHILIS

Type of Patients	Observed Patients	Avg. Stay	Variance	10th	25th	50th	75th	90th	95th	99th
1. SINGLE DX										
A. Not Operated										
0–19 Years	0									
20–34	3	6.3	44	2	2	3	14	14	14	14
35–49	2	2.0	0	2	2	2	2	2	2	2
50–64	1	1.0	0	1	1	1	1	1	1	1
65+	0									
B. Operated										
0–19 Years	0									
20–34	0									
35–49	0									
50–64	1	8.0	0	8	8	8	8	8	8	8
65+	0									
2. MULTIPLE DX										
A. Not Operated										
0–19 Years	1	8.0	0	8	8	8	8	8	8	8
20–34	20	8.9	28	3	5	9	14	17	20	20
35–49	56	7.3	52	1	3	5	10	14	21	39
50–64	52	8.9	67	2	3	6	13	17	23	44
65+	43	7.5	50	2	3	5	10	14	18	42
B. Operated										
0–19 Years	0									
20–34	3	8.7	37	2	2	10	14	14	14	14
35–49	14	5.2	18	2	2	3	10	10	15	15
50–64	32	3.9	12	1	2	3	5	7	11	17
65+	21	9.9	443	1	2	3	5	8	58	85
SUBTOTALS:										
1. SINGLE DX										
A. Not Operated	6	4.0	24	1	2	2	3	14	14	14
B. Operated	1	8.0	0	8	8	8	8	8	8	8
2. MULTIPLE DX										
A. Not Operated	172	8.0	53	2	3	5	11	16	20	42
B. Operated	70	6.2	145	1	2	3	5	10	15	85
1. SINGLE DX	7	4.6	23	1	2	2	8	14	14	14
2. MULTIPLE DX	242	7.5	80	2	3	5	10	14	18	44
A. NOT OPERATED	178	7.9	52	2	3	5	11	16	20	42
B. OPERATED	71	6.2	143	1	2	3	6	10	15	85
TOTAL										
0–19 Years	1	8.0	0	8	8	8	8	8	8	8
20–34	26	8.6	28	2	4	9	14	15	17	20
35–49	72	6.7	45	1	2	4	10	14	17	39
50–64	86	6.9	51	1	3	4	9	16	17	44
65+	64	8.3	175	2	3	4	8	14	20	85
GRAND TOTAL	249	7.4	78	2	3	4	10	14	18	44

Length of Stay by Diagnosis and Operation, Western Region, 2008

Western Region, October 2006–September 2007 Data, by Diagnosis

095: LATE SYPHILIS NEC W SX

Type of Patients	Observed Patients	Avg. Stay	Variance	10th	25th	50th	75th	90th	95th	99th
1. SINGLE DX										
A. *Not Operated*										
0–19 Years	0									
20–34	0									
35–49	0									
50–64	0									
65+	0									
B. *Operated*										
0–19 Years	0									
20–34	0									
35–49	0									
50–64	0									
65+	0									
2. MULTIPLE DX										
A. *Not Operated*										
0–19 Years	0									
20–34	1	14.0	0	14	14	14	14	14	14	14
35–49	1	1.0	0	1	1	1	1	1	1	1
50–64	2	8.6	60	3	3	14	14	14	14	14
65+	3	3.3	2	2	2	3	5	5	5	5
B. *Operated*										
0–19 Years	0									
20–34	1	15.0	0	15	15	15	15	15	15	15
35–49	0									
50–64	0									
65+	0									
SUBTOTALS:										
1. SINGLE DX										
A. *Not Operated*	0									
B. *Operated*	0									
2. MULTIPLE DX										
A. *Not Operated*	7	6.0	31	1	2	3	14	14	14	14
B. *Operated*	1	15.0	0	15	15	15	15	15	15	15
1. SINGLE DX	0									
2. MULTIPLE DX	8	7.2	37	1	3	5	14	15	15	15
A. NOT OPERATED	7	6.0	31	1	2	3	14	14	14	14
B. OPERATED	1	15.0	0	15	15	15	15	15	15	15
TOTAL										
0–19 Years	0									
20–34	2	14.5	<1	14	14	15	15	15	15	15
35–49	1	1.0	0	1	1	1	1	1	1	1
50–64	2	8.6	60	3	3	14	14	14	14	14
65+	3	3.3	2	2	2	3	5	5	5	5
GRAND TOTAL	8	7.2	37	1	3	5	14	15	15	15

096: LATENT LATE SYPHILIS

Type of Patients	Observed Patients	Avg. Stay	Variance	10th	25th	50th	75th	90th	95th	99th
1. SINGLE DX										
A. *Not Operated*										
0–19 Years	0									
20–34	0									
35–49	0									
50–64	0									
65+	0									
B. *Operated*										
0–19 Years	0									
20–34	0									
35–49	0									
50–64	0									
65+	0									
2. MULTIPLE DX										
A. *Not Operated*										
0–19 Years	0									
20–34	2	6.0	2	5	5	6	7	7	7	7
35–49	0									
50–64	0									
65+	3	9.3	12	6	6	9	13	13	13	13
B. *Operated*										
0–19 Years	0									
20–34	0									
35–49	0									
50–64	0									
65+	0									
SUBTOTALS:										
1. SINGLE DX										
A. *Not Operated*	0									
B. *Operated*	0									
2. MULTIPLE DX										
A. *Not Operated*	5	8.0	10	5	6	7	9	13	13	13
B. *Operated*	0									
1. SINGLE DX	0									
2. MULTIPLE DX	5	8.0	10	5	6	7	9	13	13	13
A. NOT OPERATED	5	8.0	10	5	6	7	9	13	13	13
B. OPERATED	0									
TOTAL										
0–19 Years	0									
20–34	2	6.0	2	5	5	6	7	7	7	7
35–49	0									
50–64	0									
65+	3	9.3	12	6	6	9	13	13	13	13
GRAND TOTAL	5	8.0	10	5	6	7	9	13	13	13

097: SYPHILIS NEC & NOS

Type of Patients	Observed Patients	Avg. Stay	Variance	10th	25th	50th	75th	90th	95th	99th
1. SINGLE DX										
A. *Not Operated*										
0–19 Years	0									
20–34	0									
35–49	0									
50–64	0									
65+	1	1.0	0	1	1	1	1	1	1	1
B. *Operated*										
0–19 Years	0									
20–34	0									
35–49	0									
50–64	0									
65+	0									
2. MULTIPLE DX										
A. *Not Operated*										
0–19 Years	1	3.0	0	3	3	3	3	3	3	3
20–34	3	4.7	2	3	3	5	6	6	6	6
35–49	11	5.7	26	2	3	3	7	15	16	16
50–64	4	4.5	3	3	4	4	7	7	7	7
65+	7	7.0	23	1	3	8	10	14	14	14
B. *Operated*										
0–19 Years	0									
20–34	0									
35–49	0									
50–64	1	3.0	0	3	3	3	3	3	3	3
65+	0									
SUBTOTALS:										
1. SINGLE DX										
A. *Not Operated*	1	1.0	0	1	1	1	1	1	1	1
B. *Operated*	0									
2. MULTIPLE DX										
A. *Not Operated*	26	5.6	18	2	3	4	7	14	15	16
B. *Operated*	1	3.0	0	3	3	3	3	3	3	3
1. SINGLE DX	1	1.0	0	1	1	1	1	1	1	1
2. MULTIPLE DX	27	5.5	17	2	3	4	7	14	15	16
A. NOT OPERATED	27	5.4	18	1	3	4	7	14	15	16
B. OPERATED	1	3.0	0	3	3	3	3	3	3	3
TOTAL										
0–19 Years	1	3.0	0	3	3	3	3	3	3	3
20–34	3	4.7	2	3	3	5	6	6	6	6
35–49	11	5.7	26	2	3	3	7	15	16	16
50–64	5	4.2	3	3	3	3	4	7	7	7
65+	7	6.2	24	1	3	8	10	14	14	14
GRAND TOTAL	28	5.4	17	1	3	4	7	14	15	16

Length of Stay by Diagnosis and Operation, Western Region, 2008

Western Region, October 2006–September 2007 Data, by Diagnosis

098: GONOCOCCAL INFECTIONS

Type of Patients	Observed Patients	Avg. Stay	Variance	Percentiles						
				10th	25th	50th	75th	90th	95th	99th
1. SINGLE DX										
A. Not Operated										
0–19 Years	5	2.8	<1	2	2	3	3	4	4	4
20–34	8	3.4	1	2	3	3	5	5	5	5
35–49	3	1.7	<1	1	1	2	2	2	2	2
50–64	0									
65+	0									
B. Operated										
0–19 Years	0									
20–34	2	2.5	<1	2	2	2	3	3	3	3
35–49	0									
50–64	0									
65+	0									
2. MULTIPLE DX										
A. Not Operated										
0–19 Years	26	3.1	2	2	2	3	4	5	5	7
20–34	62	4.2	15	1	2	3	5	6	8	30
35–49	22	4.4	28	2	2	3	5	6	6	27
50–64	10	4.8	15	2	3	3	5	15	15	15
65+	0									
B. Operated										
0–19 Years	5	4.4	3	2	4	4	5	5	7	7
20–34	11	5.5	2	4	5	6	6	7	8	8
35–49	9	4.0	8	1	3	5	5	10	10	10
50–64	2	5.0	8	3	8	8	7	7	7	7
65+	1	8.0	0	8	8	8	8	8	8	8
SUBTOTALS:										
1. SINGLE DX										
A. Not Operated	16	2.9	1	2	2	3	4	5	5	5
B. Operated	2	2.5	<1	2	2	2	3	3	3	3
2. MULTIPLE DX										
A. Not Operated	120	4.0	15	2	2	3	5	6	8	27
B. Operated	28	4.9	5	2	3	5	6	8	8	10
1. SINGLE DX	18	2.8	1	2	2	3	3	5	5	5
2. MULTIPLE DX	148	4.2	13	2	2	3	5	6	8	27
A. NOT OPERATED	136	3.9	13	2	2	3	4	6	7	27
B. OPERATED	30	4.7	5	3	3	5	6	8	8	10
TOTAL										
0–19 Years	36	3.3	2	1	2	3	4	5	7	7
20–34	83	4.2	12	2	2	3	5	6	8	30
35–49	34	4.1	20	1	2	3	5	6	10	27
50–64	12	4.8	13	2	3	3	5	7	15	15
65+	1	8.0	0	8	8	8	8	8	8	8
GRAND TOTAL	166	4.0	12	2	2	3	5	6	8	27

099: OTHER VENEREAL DISEASE

Type of Patients	Observed Patients	Avg. Stay	Variance	Percentiles						
				10th	25th	50th	75th	90th	95th	99th
1. SINGLE DX										
A. Not Operated										
0–19 Years	2	2.0	0	2	2	2	2	2	2	2
20–34	2	4.5	12	2	2	2	7	7	7	7
35–49	0									
50–64	0									
65+										
B. Operated										
0–19 Years	0									
20–34	0									
35–49	0									
50–64	0									
65+	0									
2. MULTIPLE DX										
A. Not Operated										
0–19 Years	30	2.8	4	1	2	2	4	5	7	8
20–34	53	3.0	4	1	2	3	5	5	7	10
35–49	12	4.4	11	1	2	4	8	9	10	10
50–64	10	4.5	12	2	2	3	4	13	13	13
65+	1	7.0	0	7	7	7	7	7	7	7
B. Operated										
0–19 Years	3	5.7	1	5	5	5	7	7	7	7
20–34	15	3.9	3	2	2	5	5	6	6	6
35–49	3	3.3	4	1	1	4	5	5	5	5
50–64	1	4.0	0	4	4	4	4	4	4	4
65+	0									
SUBTOTALS:										
1. SINGLE DX										
A. Not Operated	4	3.2	6	2	2	2	2	7	7	7
B. Operated	0									
2. MULTIPLE DX										
A. Not Operated	106	3.3	5	1	2	3	4	7	8	10
B. Operated	22	4.1	3	2	3	5	5	6	6	7
1. SINGLE DX	4	3.2	6	2	2	2	2	7	7	7
2. MULTIPLE DX	128	3.4	5	1	2	3	4	7	8	10
A. NOT OPERATED	110	3.3	5	1	2	3	4	7	8	10
B. OPERATED	22	4.1	3	2	3	5	5	6	6	7
TOTAL										
0–19 Years	35	3.0	4	1	2	3	4	5	7	8
20–34	70	3.3	4	1	2	3	4	6	7	10
35–49	15	4.2	9	1	1	4	7	9	10	10
50–64	11	4.5	11	2	2	3	4	8	13	13
65+	1	7.0	0	7	7	7	7	7	7	7
GRAND TOTAL	132	3.4	5	1	2	3	4	7	8	10

100: LEPTOSPIROSIS

Type of Patients	Observed Patients	Avg. Stay	Variance	Percentiles						
				10th	25th	50th	75th	90th	95th	99th
1. SINGLE DX										
A. Not Operated										
0–19 Years	0									
20–34	0									
35–49	0									
50–64	0									
65+										
B. Operated										
0–19 Years	0									
20–34	0									
35–49	0									
50–64	0									
65+	0									
2. MULTIPLE DX										
A. Not Operated										
0–19 Years	1	2.0	0	2	2	2	2	2	2	2
20–34	6	4.8	5	3	3	5	5	5	9	9
35–49	2	3.5	<1	3	3	3	4	4	4	4
50–64	2	3.0	2	2	2	4	4	4	4	4
65+	0									
B. Operated										
0–19 Years	0									
20–34	0									
35–49	0									
50–64	0									
65+	0									
SUBTOTALS:										
1. SINGLE DX										
A. Not Operated	0									
B. Operated	0									
2. MULTIPLE DX										
A. Not Operated	11	4.0	4	2	3	4	5	5	5	9
B. Operated	0									
1. SINGLE DX	0									
2. MULTIPLE DX	11	4.0	4	2	3	4	5	5	5	9
A. NOT OPERATED	11	4.0	4	2	3	4	5	5	5	9
B. OPERATED	0									
TOTAL										
0–19 Years	1	2.0	0	2	2	2	2	2	2	2
20–34	6	4.8	5	3	3	5	5	5	9	9
35–49	2	3.5	<1	3	3	3	4	4	4	4
50–64	2	3.0	2	2	2	4	4	4	4	4
65+										
GRAND TOTAL	11	4.0	4	2	3	4	5	5	5	9

Length of Stay by Diagnosis and Operation, Western Region, 2008

Western Region, October 2006–September 2007 Data, by Diagnosis

101: VINCENT'S ANGINA

Type of Patients	Observed Patients	Avg. Stay	Variance	Percentiles						
				10th	25th	50th	75th	90th	95th	99th
1. SINGLE DX										
A. *Not Operated*										
0–19 Years	0									
20–34	0									
35–49	0									
50–64	0									
65+	0									
B. *Operated*										
0–19 Years	0									
20–34	0									
35–49	0									
50–64	0									
65+	0									
2. MULTIPLE DX										
A. *Not Operated*										
0–19 Years	1	3.0	0	3	3	3	3	3	3	3
20–34	3	2.0	0	2	2	2	2	2	2	2
35–49	0									
50–64	1	4.0	0	4	4	4	4	4	4	4
65+	0									
B. *Operated*										
0–19 Years	0									
20–34	0									
35–49	1	15.0	0	15	15	15	15	15	15	15
50–64	0									
65+	0									
SUBTOTALS:										
1. SINGLE DX										
A. *Not Operated*	0									
B. *Operated*	0									
2. MULTIPLE DX										
A. *Not Operated*	5	2.6	<1	2	2	2	3	4	4	4
B. *Operated*	1	15.0	0	15	15	15	15	15	15	15
1. SINGLE DX	0									
2. MULTIPLE DX	6	4.7	26	2	2	2	4	15	15	15
A. NOT OPERATED	5	2.6	<1	2	2	2	3	4	4	4
B. OPERATED	1	15.0	0	15	15	15	15	15	15	15
TOTAL										
0–19 Years	1	3.0	0	3	3	3	3	3	3	3
20–34	3	2.0	0	2	2	2	2	2	2	2
35–49	1	15.0	0	15	15	15	15	15	15	15
50–64	1	4.0	0	4	4	4	4	4	4	4
65+	0									
GRAND TOTAL	6	4.7	26	2	2	2	4	15	15	15

102: YAWS

Type of Patients	Observed Patients	Avg. Stay	Variance	Percentiles						
				10th	25th	50th	75th	90th	95th	99th
1. SINGLE DX — A. Not Operated — 0–19 Years	0									
20–34	0									
35–49	0									
50–64	0									
65+	0									
B. Operated — 0–19 Years	0									
20–34	0									
35–49	0									
50–64	0									
65+	0									
2. MULTIPLE DX — A. Not Operated — 0–19 Years	0									
20–34	0									
35–49	0									
50–64	0									
65+	0									
B. Operated — 0–19 Years	0									
20–34	0									
35–49	0									
50–64	0									
65+	0									
SUBTOTALS 1A Not Operated	0									
1B Operated	0									
2A Not Operated	0									
2B Operated	0									
1. SINGLE DX	0									
2. MULTIPLE DX	0									
A. NOT OPERATED	0									
B. OPERATED	0									
TOTAL 0–19 Years	0									
20–34	0									
35–49	0									
50–64	0									
65+	0									
GRAND TOTAL	0									

103: PINTA

Type of Patients	Observed Patients	Avg. Stay	Variance	Percentiles						
				10th	25th	50th	75th	90th	95th	99th
1. SINGLE DX — A. Not Operated — 0–19 Years	0									
20–34	0									
35–49	0									
50–64	0									
65+	0									
B. Operated — 0–19 Years	0									
20–34	0									
35–49	0									
50–64	0									
65+	0									
2. MULTIPLE DX — A. Not Operated — 0–19 Years	0									
20–34	0									
35–49	0									
50–64	0									
65+	0									
B. Operated — 0–19 Years	0									
20–34	0									
35–49	0									
50–64	0									
65+	0									
SUBTOTALS 1A Not Operated	0									
1B Operated	0									
2A Not Operated	0									
2B Operated	0									
1. SINGLE DX	0									
2. MULTIPLE DX	0									
A. NOT OPERATED	0									
B. OPERATED	0									
TOTAL 0–19 Years	0									
20–34	0									
35–49	0									
50–64	0									
65+	0									
GRAND TOTAL	0									

Length of Stay by Diagnosis and Operation, Western Region, 2008

45

Western Region, October 2006–September 2007 Data, by Diagnosis

104: OTHER SPIROCHETAL INFECT

Type of Patients	Observed Patients	Avg. Stay	Variance	10th	25th	50th	75th	90th	95th	99th
1. SINGLE DX										
A. Not Operated										
0–19 Years	0									
20–34	0									
35–49	0									
50–64	0									
65+	0									
B. Operated										
0–19 Years	0									
20–34	0									
35–49	0									
50–64	0									
65+	0									
2. MULTIPLE DX										
A. Not Operated										
0–19 Years	1	1.0	0	1	1	1	1	1	1	1
20–34	1	4.0	0	4	4	4	4	4	4	4
35–49	1	1.0	0	1	1	1	1	1	1	1
50–64	0									
65+	0									
B. Operated										
0–19 Years	0									
20–34	0									
35–49	0									
50–64	0									
65+	0									
SUBTOTALS:										
1. SINGLE DX										
A. Not Operated	0									
B. Operated	0									
2. MULTIPLE DX										
A. Not Operated	3	2.0	3	1	1	1	1	4	4	4
B. Operated	0									
1. SINGLE DX	0									
2. MULTIPLE DX	3	2.0	3	1	1	1	1	4	4	4
A. NOT OPERATED	3	2.0	3	1	1	1	1	4	4	4
B. OPERATED	0									
TOTAL										
0–19 Years	1	1.0	0	1	1	1	1	1	1	1
20–34	1	4.0	0	4	4	4	4	4	4	4
35–49	1	1.0	0	1	1	1	1	1	1	1
50–64	0									
65+	0									
GRAND TOTAL	3	2.0	3	1	1	1	1	4	4	4

110: DERMATOPHYTOSIS

Type of Patients	Observed Patients	Avg. Stay	Variance	10th	25th	50th	75th	90th	95th	99th
1. SINGLE DX										
A. Not Operated										
0–19 Years	5	2.4	10	1	1	1	1	8	8	8
20–34	0									
35–49	0									
50–64	1	2.0	0	2	2	2	2	2	2	2
65+	1	2.0	0	2	2	2	2	2	2	2
B. Operated										
0–19 Years	0									
20–34	0									
35–49	0									
50–64	0									
65+	0									
2. MULTIPLE DX										
A. Not Operated										
0–19 Years	7	2.1	<1	1	1	2	3	3	3	3
20–34	17	2.4	1	1	1	2	3	4	4	4
35–49	11	3.5	15	1	2	3	4	6	14	14
50–64	25	3.9	10	1	2	3	5	7	8	16
65+	30	3.5	10	1	1	2	4	7	10	15
B. Operated										
0–19 Years	0									
20–34	0									
35–49	1	15.0	0	15	15	15	15	15	15	15
50–64	0									
65+	0									
SUBTOTALS:										
1. SINGLE DX										
A. Not Operated	7	2.3	7	1	1	1	2	8	8	8
B. Operated	0									
2. MULTIPLE DX										
A. Not Operated	90	3.3	8	1	1	3	4	7	8	16
B. Operated	1	15.0	0	15	15	15	15	15	15	15
1. SINGLE DX	7	2.3	7	1	1	1	2	8	8	8
2. MULTIPLE DX	91	3.4	10	1	1	3	4	7	10	16
A. NOT OPERATED	97	3.2	8	1	1	2	4	7	8	16
B. OPERATED	1	15.0	0	15	15	15	15	15	15	15
TOTAL										
0–19 Years	12	2.3	4	1	1	1	3	3	8	8
20–34	17	2.4	1	1	1	2	3	4	4	4
35–49	12	4.4	25	1	1	2	4	14	15	15
50–64	26	3.8	10	1	2	3	5	7	8	16
65+	31	3.5	10	1	1	2	4	7	10	15
GRAND TOTAL	98	3.3	10	1	1	2	4	7	10	16

111: DERMATOMYCOSIS NEC & NOS

Type of Patients	Observed Patients	Avg. Stay	Variance	10th	25th	50th	75th	90th	95th	99th
1. SINGLE DX										
A. Not Operated										
0–19 Years	0									
20–34	0									
35–49	0									
50–64	0									
65+	0									
B. Operated										
0–19 Years	0									
20–34	0									
35–49	0									
50–64	0									
65+	0									
2. MULTIPLE DX										
A. Not Operated										
0–19 Years	1	3.0	0	3	3	3	3	3	3	3
20–34	0									
35–49	4	2.5	9	1	1	1	1	7	7	7
50–64	2	3.5	4	2	2	4	5	5	5	5
65+	2	7.0	18	4	4	10	10	10	10	10
B. Operated										
0–19 Years	0									
20–34	1	7.0	0	7	7	7	7	7	7	7
35–49	0									
50–64	2	4.5	12	2	2	2	7	7	7	7
65+	1	7.0	0	7	7	7	7	7	7	7
SUBTOTALS:										
1. SINGLE DX										
A. Not Operated	0									
B. Operated	0									
2. MULTIPLE DX										
A. Not Operated	9	3.8	10	1	1	3	5	10	10	10
B. Operated	4	5.7	6	2	2	7	7	7	7	7
1. SINGLE DX	0									
2. MULTIPLE DX	13	4.4	9	1	2	4	7	7	10	10
A. NOT OPERATED	9	3.8	10	1	1	3	5	10	10	10
B. OPERATED	4	5.7	6	2	2	7	7	7	7	7
TOTAL										
0–19 Years	1	3.0	0	3	3	3	3	3	3	3
20–34	1	7.0	0	7	7	7	7	7	7	7
35–49	4	2.5	9	1	1	1	1	7	7	7
50–64	4	4.0	6	2	2	2	5	7	7	7
65+	3	7.0	9	4	4	7	10	10	10	10
GRAND TOTAL	13	4.4	9	1	2	4	7	7	10	10

Length of Stay by Diagnosis and Operation, Western Region, 2008

Western Region, October 2006–September 2007 Data, by Diagnosis

112: CANDIDIASIS

Type of Patients	Observed Patients	Avg. Stay	Vari- ance	Percentiles						
				10th	25th	50th	75th	90th	95th	99th
1. SINGLE DX										
A. Not Operated										
0–19 Years	3	5.0	13	2	2	4	9	9	9	9
20–34	1	2.0	0	2	2	2	2	2	2	2
35–49	0									
50–64	1	8.0	0	8	8	8	8	8	8	8
65+	0									
B. Operated										
0–19 Years	0									
20–34	0									
35–49	0									
50–64	0									
65+	0									
2. MULTIPLE DX										
A. Not Operated										
0–19 Years	49	6.0	45	1	2	3	6	17	22	30
20–34	119	5.6	36	1	2	4	7	11	16	28
35–49	254	6.3	67	2	2	4	7	13	19	57
50–64	458	6.5	35	2	3	5	8	13	17	29
65+	1,220	6.7	31	2	3	5	8	14	18	26
B. Operated										
0–19 Years	3	10.9	72	3	7	10	20	20	20	20
20–34	9	18.2	506	7	7	9	12	70	70	70
35–49	9	20.9	22	16	18	22	27	>99	>99	>99
50–64	25	15.9	123	6	9	12	26	41	>99	>99
65+	65	17.4	242	6	8	11	20	35	52	90
SUBTOTALS:										
1. SINGLE DX										
A. Not Operated	5	5.0	11	2	2	4	8	9	9	9
B. Operated	0									
2. MULTIPLE DX										
A. Not Operated	2,100	6.6	37	2	3	5	8	13	17	29
B. Operated	111	17.2	210	6	8	12	22	41	60	>99
1. SINGLE DX	5	5.0	11	2	2	4	8	9	9	9
2. MULTIPLE DX	2,211	7.1	51	2	3	5	8	15	20	39
A. NOT OPERATED	2,105	6.5	37	2	3	5	8	13	17	29
B. OPERATED	111	17.2	210	6	8	12	22	60	60	>99
TOTAL										
0–19 Years	55	6.2	45	1	2	3	7	17	22	30
20–34	129	6.4	75	1	2	4	7	11	17	51
35–49	263	6.8	72	2	2	4	7	14	21	64
50–64	484	7.0	44	2	3	5	9	14	20	42
65+	1,285	7.3	47	2	3	5	9	15	19	35
GRAND TOTAL	2,216	7.1	51	2	3	5	8	15	20	39

112.0: THRUSH

Type of Patients	Observed Patients	Avg. Stay	Vari- ance	Percentiles						
				10th	25th	50th	75th	90th	95th	99th
1. SINGLE DX										
A. Not Operated										
0–19 Years	0									
20–34	0									
35–49	0									
50–64	0									
65+	0									
B. Operated										
0–19 Years	0									
20–34	0									
35–49	0									
50–64	0									
65+	0									
2. MULTIPLE DX										
A. Not Operated										
0–19 Years	17	2.4	2	1	1	2	3	5	6	6
20–34	15	7.7	39	1	2	7	11	17	21	21
35–49	29	3.0	6	1	2	2	4	7	8	11
50–64	42	5.0	17	1	2	4	7	9	14	18
65+	77	4.4	13	1	2	4	6	8	14	20
B. Operated										
0–19 Years	0									
20–34	0									
35–49	0									
50–64	0									
65+	2	25.1	198	15	15	35	35	35	35	35
SUBTOTALS:										
1. SINGLE DX										
A. Not Operated	0									
B. Operated	0									
2. MULTIPLE DX										
A. Not Operated	180	4.4	15	1	2	3	6	8	14	20
B. Operated	2	25.1	198	15	15	35	35	35	35	35
1. SINGLE DX	0									
2. MULTIPLE DX	182	4.6	21	1	2	3	6	9	15	21
A. NOT OPERATED	180	4.4	15	1	2	3	6	8	14	20
B. OPERATED	2	25.1	198	15	15	35	35	35	35	35
TOTAL										
0–19 Years	17	2.4	2	1	1	2	3	5	6	6
20–34	15	7.7	39	1	2	7	11	17	21	21
35–49	29	3.0	6	1	2	2	4	7	8	11
50–64	42	5.0	17	1	2	4	7	9	14	18
65+	79	4.9	26	1	2	4	6	9	16	35
GRAND TOTAL	182	4.6	21	1	2	3	6	9	15	21

112.2: GU CANDIDIASIS NEC

Type of Patients	Observed Patients	Avg. Stay	Vari- ance	Percentiles						
				10th	25th	50th	75th	90th	95th	99th
1. SINGLE DX										
A. Not Operated										
0–19 Years	1	2.0	0	2	2	2	2	2	2	2
20–34	0									
35–49	0									
50–64	0									
65+	0									
B. Operated										
0–19 Years	0									
20–34	0									
35–49	0									
50–64	0									
65+	0									
2. MULTIPLE DX										
A. Not Operated										
0–19 Years	15	4.7	15	1	2	4	5	7	17	17
20–34	26	5.4	14	2	3	4	6	11	14	16
35–49	50	6.2	14	2	3	6	7	13	14	20
50–64	106	5.9	23	2	3	5	8	10	12	29
65+	528	6.5	25	2	3	5	8	13	17	23
B. Operated										
0–19 Years	1	3.0	0	3	3	3	3	3	3	3
20–34	2	4.0	18	1	1	4	7	7	7	7
35–49	1	27.0	0	27	27	27	27	27	27	27
50–64	4	9.5	3	8	8	9	9	12	12	12
65+	19	12.9	115	4	6	10	17	20	52	52
SUBTOTALS:										
1. SINGLE DX										
A. Not Operated	1	2.0	0	2	2	2	2	2	2	2
B. Operated	0									
2. MULTIPLE DX										
A. Not Operated	725	6.3	23	2	3	5	8	12	16	23
B. Operated	27	11.9	99	3	6	10	14	20	27	52
1. SINGLE DX	1	2.0	0	2	2	2	2	2	2	2
2. MULTIPLE DX	752	6.5	27	2	3	5	8	13	17	27
A. NOT OPERATED	726	6.3	23	2	3	5	8	12	16	23
B. OPERATED	27	11.9	99	3	6	10	14	20	27	52
TOTAL										
0–19 Years	17	4.4	14	1	2	4	5	7	16	17
20–34	28	5.3	14	1	3	4	6	11	14	16
35–49	51	6.6	22	2	3	6	8	13	14	27
50–64	110	6.0	23	2	3	5	8	11	12	29
65+	547	6.7	29	2	3	5	8	13	17	24
GRAND TOTAL	753	6.5	27	2	3	5	8	13	17	27

Length of Stay by Diagnosis and Operation, Western Region, 2008

Western Region, October 2006–September 2007 Data, by Diagnosis

112.4: LUNG CANDIDIASIS

Type of Patients	Observed Patients	Avg. Stay	Variance	Percentiles						
				10th	25th	50th	75th	90th	95th	99th
1. SINGLE DX										
A. Not Operated										
0–19 Years	0									
20–34	0									
35–49	0									
50–64	0									
65+	0									
B. Operated										
0–19 Years	0									
20–34	0									
35–49	0									
50–64	0									
65+	0									
2. MULTIPLE DX										
A. Not Operated										
0–19 Years	2	21.5	<1	21	21	21	22	22	22	22
20–34	5	7.0	10	4	5	6	8	12	12	12
35–49	16	6.1	19	3	3	5	6	11	20	20
50–64	46	10.2	29	6	7	8	12	18	24	26
65+	124	8.3	22	4	5	7	10	15	17	23
B. Operated										
0–19 Years	0									
20–34	4	9.0	9	5	9	10	12	12	12	12
35–49	2	19.0	18	16	16	19	22	22	22	22
50–64	2	12.0	32	8	8	16	>99	>99	>99	>99
65+	9	15.3	117	6	9	10	18	41	41	41
SUBTOTALS:										
1. SINGLE DX										
A. Not Operated	0									
B. Operated	0									
2. MULTIPLE DX										
A. Not Operated	193	8.7	26	4	5	7	11	16	20	26
B. Operated	17	13.9	74	6	9	10	18	41	>99	>99
1. SINGLE DX	0									
2. MULTIPLE DX	210	9.1	31	4	5	8	11	17	21	26
A. NOT OPERATED	193	8.7	26	4	5	7	11	16	20	26
B. OPERATED	17	13.9	74	6	9	10	18	41	>99	>99
TOTAL										
0–19 Years	2	21.5	<1	21	21	21	22	22	22	22
20–34	9	7.9	9	4	5	8	10	12	12	12
35–49	18	7.5	35	3	4	5	10	20	22	22
50–64	48	10.3	28	6	7	8	13	19	25	26
65+	133	8.8	31	4	5	7	11	17	19	23
GRAND TOTAL	210	9.1	31	4	5	8	11	17	21	26

112.5: DISSEMINATED CANDIDIASIS

Type of Patients	Observed Patients	Avg. Stay	Variance	Percentiles						
				10th	25th	50th	75th	90th	95th	99th
1. SINGLE DX										
A. Not Operated										
0–19 Years	0									
20–34	0									
35–49	0									
50–64	0									
65+	0									
B. Operated										
0–19 Years	0									
20–34	0									
35–49	0									
50–64	0									
65+	0									
2. MULTIPLE DX										
A. Not Operated										
0–19 Years	4	20.3	62	12	16	23	30	30	30	30
20–34	12	11.7	200	3	4	6	10	28	51	51
35–49	30	17.7	311	6	7	10	20	38	64	68
50–64	47	13.1	113	4	7	10	16	27	29	57
65+	119	12.2	79	4	6	10	16	24	28	49
B. Operated										
0–19 Years	0									
20–34	3	39.8	923	9	9	41	70	70	70	70
35–49	4	21.5	32	15	19	24	28	>99	>99	>99
50–64	11	20.8	141	8	12	26	37	39	>99	>99
65+	27	23.1	390	7	9	19	29	58	60	90
SUBTOTALS:										
1. SINGLE DX										
A. Not Operated	0									
B. Operated	0									
2. MULTIPLE DX										
A. Not Operated	212	13.3	127	4	6	10	17	27	35	57
B. Operated	45	23.5	327	8	9	20	33	60	90	>99
1. SINGLE DX	0									
2. MULTIPLE DX	257	15.1	176	4	7	11	19	30	49	90
A. NOT OPERATED	212	13.3	127	4	6	10	17	27	35	57
B. OPERATED	45	23.5	327	8	9	20	33	60	90	>99
TOTAL										
0–19 Years	4	20.3	62	12	16	23	30	30	30	30
20–34	15	17.3	423	3	4	9	9	51	70	70
35–49	34	18.2	278	6	8	12	24	57	68	>99
50–64	58	14.5	125	4	7	11	19	30	42	>99
65+	146	14.2	152	4	6	11	19	27	33	60
GRAND TOTAL	257	15.1	176	4	7	11	19	30	49	90

112.84: ESOPHAGEAL CANDIDIASIS

Type of Patients	Observed Patients	Avg. Stay	Variance	Percentiles						
				10th	25th	50th	75th	90th	95th	99th
1. SINGLE DX										
A. Not Operated										
0–19 Years	0									
20–34	1	2.0	0	2	2	2	2	2	2	2
35–49	0									
50–64	0									
65+	0									
B. Operated										
0–19 Years	0									
20–34	0									
35–49	0									
50–64	0									
65+	0									
2. MULTIPLE DX										
A. Not Operated										
0–19 Years	8	6.1	21	1	1	6	11	13	13	13
20–34	45	3.9	5	1	2	3	5	7	8	9
35–49	109	4.3	16	1	2	3	5	8	9	24
50–64	184	4.8	14	1	2	4	6	10	12	26
65+	310	5.2	14	2	3	4	6	9	12	21
B. Operated										
0–19 Years	1	10.0	0	10	10	10	10	10	10	10
20–34	0									
35–49	1	18.0	0	18	18	18	18	18	18	18
50–64	5	11.2	15	9	9	10	10	18	18	18
65+	5	7.0	7	3	6	8	9	9	9	9
SUBTOTALS:										
1. SINGLE DX										
A. Not Operated	1	2.0	0	2	2	2	2	2	2	2
B. Operated	0									
2. MULTIPLE DX										
A. Not Operated	656	4.9	14	2	3	4	6	9	12	21
B. Operated	12	9.9	18	6	8	9	10	18	18	18
1. SINGLE DX	1	2.0	0	2	2	2	2	2	2	2
2. MULTIPLE DX	668	5.0	14	2	3	4	6	9	12	21
A. NOT OPERATED	657	4.9	14	2	3	4	6	9	12	21
B. OPERATED	12	9.9	18	6	8	9	10	18	18	18
TOTAL										
0–19 Years	9	6.6	20	1	2	6	10	13	13	13
20–34	46	3.8	5	1	2	3	5	7	8	9
35–49	110	4.5	17	1	2	3	5	8	11	24
50–64	189	5.0	15	2	2	4	6	10	13	26
65+	315	5.3	14	2	3	4	7	9	12	21
GRAND TOTAL	669	5.0	14	2	3	4	6	9	12	21

Length of Stay by Diagnosis and Operation, Western Region, 2008

Western Region, October 2006–September 2007 Data, by Diagnosis

114: COCCIDIOIDOMYCOSIS

Type of Patients	Observed Patients	Avg. Stay	Variance	Percentiles 10th	25th	50th	75th	90th	95th	99th
1. SINGLE DX										
A. Not Operated										
0–19 Years	4	3.5	6	1	1	5	6	6	6	6
20–34	20	5.2	7	1	2	6	8	8	9	9
35–49	21	7.2	38	3	4	6	8	10	18	29
50–64	4	4.0	16	2	2	2	2	10	10	10
65+	1	7.0	0	7	7	7	7	7	7	7
B. Operated										
0–19 Years	2	4.5	24	1	1	8	8	8	8	8
20–34	2	4.5	24	1	1	8	8	8	8	8
35–49	1	2.0	0	2	2	2	2	2	2	2
50–64	1	7.0	0	7	7	7	7	7	7	7
65+	1	2.0	0	2	2	2	2	2	2	2
2. MULTIPLE DX										
A. Not Operated										
0–19 Years	53	7.6	64	2	3	5	9	15	21	41
20–34	251	6.6	48	2	3	5	8	12	15	60
35–49	403	7.7	85	2	3	6	9	15	23	85
50–64	414	8.2	85	2	4	6	9	16	22	62
65+	325	7.8	34	3	4	6	10	14	20	31
B. Operated										
0–19 Years	7	17.7	323	3	4	35	35	48	48	48
20–34	92	13.1	172	4	6	9	17	36	41	>99
35–49	145	12.2	225	3	5	8	14	25	45	>99
50–64	178	10.5	146	3	4	6	12	21	35	74
65+	110	10.0	86	3	5	7	13	20	28	44
SUBTOTALS:										
1. SINGLE DX										
A. Not Operated	50	5.8	21	2	3	5	8	9	10	29
B. Operated	7	4.2	11	1	1	2	8	8	8	8
2. MULTIPLE DX										
A. Not Operated	1,446	7.7	66	2	4	6	9	14	21	50
B. Operated	532	11.4	162	3	4	7	14	23	39	94
1. SINGLE DX	57	5.6	20	1	2	5	8	9	10	29
2. MULTIPLE DX	1,978	8.7	95	2	4	6	10	17	24	69
A. NOT OPERATED	1,496	7.6	65	2	4	6	9	14	20	50
B. OPERATED	539	11.3	161	3	4	7	13	23	39	94
TOTAL										
0–19 Years	66	8.3	94	2	3	5	9	21	35	48
20–34	365	8.1	85	2	4	6	9	15	22	93
35–49	570	8.8	122	2	4	6	10	17	25	98
50–64	597	8.9	104	2	4	6	10	16	27	68
65+	437	8.4	48	3	4	6	10	17	22	35
GRAND TOTAL	2,035	8.6	93	2	4	6	10	17	24	68

114.0: PRIMARY COCCIDIOIDOMYCOS

Type of Patients	Observed Patients	Avg. Stay	Variance	Percentiles 10th	25th	50th	75th	90th	95th	99th
1. SINGLE DX										
A. Not Operated										
0–19 Years	3	4.4	4	2	2	5	6	6	6	6
20–34	16	5.4	6	2	3	6	8	9	9	9
35–49	17	7.8	44	3	4	6	9	18	29	29
50–64	4	4.0	16	2	2	2	2	10	10	10
65+	1	7.0	0	7	7	7	7	7	7	7
B. Operated										
0–19 Years	2	4.5	24	1	1	8	8	8	8	8
20–34	0									
35–49	0									
50–64	1	7.0	0	7	7	7	7	7	7	7
65+	1	2.0	0	2	2	2	2	2	2	2
2. MULTIPLE DX										
A. Not Operated										
0–19 Years	36	6.6	28	2	3	5	9	14	21	21
20–34	148	6.2	46	2	3	5	7	10	12	21
35–49	260	7.9	86	2	3	6	9	17	23	36
50–64	286	7.5	64	2	4	6	9	13	19	50
65+	259	7.8	36	3	4	6	10	14	21	32
B. Operated										
0–19 Years	1	35.0	0	35	35	35	35	35	35	35
20–34	35	14.5	276	5	7	9	17	36	39	93
35–49	67	11.2	72	5	5	9	15	20	25	54
50–64	83	12.2	180	3	5	8	14	22	29	81
65+	64	10.6	57	4	5	7	13	20	23	44
SUBTOTALS:										
1. SINGLE DX										
A. Not Operated	41	6.2	23	2	3	6	8	9	10	29
B. Operated	4	4.5	12	1	2	7	8	8	8	8
2. MULTIPLE DX										
A. Not Operated	989	7.5	58	2	4	6	9	14	19	38
B. Operated	250	11.9	134	4	5	9	14	22	32	74
1. SINGLE DX	45	6.1	22	2	3	6	8	9	10	29
2. MULTIPLE DX	1,239	8.4	77	2	4	6	10	16	22	44
A. NOT OPERATED	1,030	7.4	57	2	4	6	9	14	19	37
B. OPERATED	254	11.8	133	4	5	9	14	22	32	74
TOTAL										
0–19 Years	42	7.0	45	2	3	5	9	14	21	35
20–34	199	7.6	92	2	4	6	8	12	18	76
35–49	344	8.5	82	2	4	6	10	18	23	36
50–64	374	8.5	92	2	4	6	10	16	22	56
65+	325	8.3	41	3	4	6	10	16	22	32
GRAND TOTAL	1,284	8.3	75	2	4	6	10	16	22	44

115: HISTOPLASMOSIS

Type of Patients	Observed Patients	Avg. Stay	Variance	Percentiles 10th	25th	50th	75th	90th	95th	99th
1. SINGLE DX										
A. Not Operated										
0–19 Years	0									
20–34	0									
35–49	0									
50–64	0									
65+	0									
B. Operated										
0–19 Years	0									
20–34	0									
35–49	0									
50–64	0									
65+	0									
2. MULTIPLE DX										
A. Not Operated										
0–19 Years	1	25.0	0	25	25	25	25	25	25	25
20–34	6	11.8	99	4	6	7	19	29	29	29
35–49	3	7.0	75	1	1	3	17	17	17	17
50–64	4	15.2	71	5	5	18	25	25	25	25
65+	4	9.2	29	4	4	6	11	16	16	16
B. Operated										
0–19 Years	1	7.0	0	7	7	7	7	7	7	7
20–34	3	15.3	24	12	12	13	21	21	21	21
35–49	3	8.0	43	2	2	7	15	15	15	15
50–64	3	29.0	>999	4	4	13	70	70	70	70
65+	0									
SUBTOTALS:										
1. SINGLE DX										
A. Not Operated	0									
B. Operated	0									
2. MULTIPLE DX										
A. Not Operated	18	11.9	75	3	5	7	18	25	29	29
B. Operated	10	16.4	386	2	7	12	15	70	70	70
1. SINGLE DX	0									
2. MULTIPLE DX	28	13.5	180	3	5	11	17	25	29	70
A. NOT OPERATED	18	11.9	75	3	5	7	18	25	29	29
B. OPERATED	10	16.4	386	2	7	12	15	70	70	70
TOTAL										
0–19 Years	2	16.1	158	7	7	25	25	25	25	25
20–34	9	13.0	71	4	6	12	19	29	29	29
35–49	6	7.5	48	1	2	3	15	17	17	17
50–64	7	21.1	516	4	5	13	25	70	70	70
65+	4	9.2	29	4	4	6	11	16	16	16
GRAND TOTAL	28	13.5	180	3	5	11	17	25	29	70

Length of Stay by Diagnosis and Operation, Western Region, 2008

Western Region, October 2006–September 2007 Data, by Diagnosis

116: BLASTOMYCOTIC INFECTION

Type of Patients	Observed Patients	Avg. Stay	Variance	10th	25th	50th	75th	90th	95th	99th
1. SINGLE DX										
A. Not Operated										
0–19 Years	0									
20–34	1	1.0	0		1		1	1	1	1
35–49	0									
50–64	0									
65+	0									
B. Operated										
0–19 Years	0									
20–34	0									
35–49	0									
50–64	0									
65+	0									
2. MULTIPLE DX										
A. Not Operated										
0–19 Years	0									
20–34	0									
35–49	0									
50–64	2	10.6	60	5	5	16	16	16	16	16
65+	1	6.0	0	6	6	6	6	6	6	6
B. Operated										
0–19 Years	0									
20–34	1	16.0	0	16	16	16	16	16	16	16
35–49	1	2.0	0	2	2	2	2	2	2	2
50–64	0									
65+	1	4.0	0	4	4	4	4	4	4	4
SUBTOTALS:										
1. SINGLE DX										
A. Not Operated	1	1.0	0	1	1	1	1	1	1	1
B. Operated	0									
2. MULTIPLE DX										
A. Not Operated	3	9.1	37	5	5	6	16	16	16	16
B. Operated	3	7.3	57	2	2	4	16	16	16	16
1. SINGLE DX	1	1.0	0	1	1	1	1	1	1	1
2. MULTIPLE DX	6	8.2	39	2	4	6	16	16	16	16
A. NOT OPERATED	4	7.1	41	1	5	6	16	16	16	16
B. OPERATED	3	7.3	57	2	2	4	16	16	16	16
TOTAL										
0–19 Years	0									
20–34	2	8.6	111	1	1	16	16	16	16	16
35–49	1	2.0	0	2	2	2	2	2	2	2
50–64	2	10.6	60	5	5	16	16	16	16	16
65+	2	5.0	2	4	4	4	6	6	6	6
GRAND TOTAL	7	7.2	40	1	2	5	16	16	16	16

117: OTHER MYCOSES

Type of Patients	Observed Patients	Avg. Stay	Variance	10th	25th	50th	75th	90th	95th	99th
1. SINGLE DX										
A. Not Operated										
0–19 Years	1	1.0	0	1	1	1	1	1	1	1
20–34	2	1.5	<1	1	1	1	2	2	2	2
35–49	1	10.0	0	10	10	10	10	10	10	10
50–64	2	2.0	2	1	1	3	3	3	3	3
65+	0									
B. Operated										
0–19 Years	0									
20–34	1	2.0	0	2	2	2	2	2	2	2
35–49	1	6.0	0	6	6	6	6	6	6	6
50–64	0									
65+	0									
2. MULTIPLE DX										
A. Not Operated										
0–19 Years	10	9.6	60	3	3	9	13	16	27	27
20–34	66	8.8	58	2	3	7	12	20	22	45
35–49	99	9.7	82	2	3	7	13	21	29	44
50–64	192	8.5	45	2	4	7	11	16	20	53
65+	239	10.4	67	3	5	9	13	21	23	37
B. Operated										
0–19 Years	5	18.4	539	2	2	12	18	58	58	58
20–34	19	8.8	37	1	4	9	13	19	22	22
35–49	39	13.8	183	3	5	9	17	32	55	>99
50–64	74	13.5	196	3	4	10	16	30	51	>99
65+	80	13.2	96	3	7	11	17	24	29	50
SUBTOTALS:										
1. SINGLE DX										
A. Not Operated	6	3.0	12	1	1	2	3	10	10	10
B. Operated	2	4.0	8	2	2	4	6	6	6	6
2. MULTIPLE DX										
A. Not Operated	606	9.5	61	2	4	7	13	19	23	40
B. Operated	217	13.2	149	3	5	10	17	28	46	89
1. SINGLE DX	8	3.3	10	1	1	2	6	10	10	10
2. MULTIPLE DX	823	10.5	87	2	4	8	14	21	27	53
A. NOT OPERATED	612	9.4	61	2	4	7	13	19	23	40
B. OPERATED	219	13.1	149	3	5	10	17	27	42	89
TOTAL										
0–19 Years	16	11.8	205	2	2	9	13	27	58	58
20–34	88	8.6	53	2	3	7	12	19	22	45
35–49	140	10.8	111	2	4	7	15	26	32	55
50–64	268	9.8	91	2	4	7	14	19	27	89
65+	319	11.1	75	3	5	9	15	22	25	40
GRAND TOTAL	831	10.4	87	2	4	8	14	21	27	53

117.3: ASPERGILLOSIS

Type of Patients	Observed Patients	Avg. Stay	Variance	10th	25th	50th	75th	90th	95th	99th
1. SINGLE DX										
A. Not Operated										
0–19 Years	0									
20–34	1	1.0	0	1	1	1	1	1	1	1
35–49	0									
50–64	1	3.0	0	3	3	3	3	3	3	3
65+	0									
B. Operated										
0–19 Years	0									
20–34	0									
35–49	0									
50–64	0									
65+	0									
2. MULTIPLE DX										
A. Not Operated										
0–19 Years	3	2.7	<1	2	2	3	3	3	3	3
20–34	28	7.8	68	2	4	6	9	12	19	45
35–49	47	9.1	69	1	4	5	12	21	26	37
50–64	94	8.8	58	2	4	7	11	18	23	53
65+	150	10.2	74	3	4	9	13	19	23	40
B. Operated										
0–19 Years	0									
20–34	7	11.5	52	4	5	11	19	22	22	22
35–49	24	12.4	140	3	5	8	17	21	30	55
50–64	45	10.3	71	3	4	7	14	23	26	37
65+	53	14.8	104	5	8	13	17	28	34	50
SUBTOTALS:										
1. SINGLE DX										
A. Not Operated	2	2.0	2	1	1	3	3	3	3	3
B. Operated	0									
2. MULTIPLE DX										
A. Not Operated	322	9.3	68	2	4	7	12	19	23	40
B. Operated	129	12.6	98	3	5	10	17	24	31	50
1. SINGLE DX	2	2.0	2	1	1	3	3	3	3	3
2. MULTIPLE DX	451	10.3	79	3	4	8	14	21	25	50
A. NOT OPERATED	324	9.3	68	2	4	7	12	19	23	40
B. OPERATED	129	12.6	98	3	5	10	17	24	31	50
TOTAL										
0–19 Years	3	2.7	<1	2	2	3	3	3	3	3
20–34	36	8.3	65	2	4	6	11	19	22	45
35–49	71	10.2	94	2	4	6	17	21	28	55
50–64	140	9.2	62	2	4	7	11	19	24	37
65+	203	11.4	86	3	5	9	15	22	25	50
GRAND TOTAL	453	10.2	79	3	4	8	14	21	25	50

Length of Stay by Diagnosis and Operation, Western Region, 2008

50

Western Region, October 2006–September 2007 Data, by Diagnosis

118: OPPORTUNISTIC MYCOSES

Type of Patients	Observed Patients	Avg. Stay	Vari-ance	10th	25th	50th	75th	90th	95th	99th
1. SINGLE DX										
A. *Not Operated*										
0–19 Years	0									
20–34	0									
35–49	0									
50–64	0									
65+	0									
B. *Operated*										
0–19 Years	0									
20–34	0									
35–49	0									
50–64	0									
65+	0									
2. MULTIPLE DX										
A. *Not Operated*										
0–19 Years	0									
20–34	0									
35–49	0									
50–64	0									
65+	0									
B. *Operated*										
0–19 Years	0									
20–34	0									
35–49	0									
50–64	0									
65+	0									
SUBTOTALS:										
1. SINGLE DX A. *Not Operated*	0									
B. *Operated*	0									
2. MULTIPLE DX A. *Not Operated*	0									
B. *Operated*	0									
1. SINGLE DX	0									
2. MULTIPLE DX	0									
A. NOT OPERATED	0									
B. OPERATED	0									
TOTAL										
0–19 Years	0									
20–34	0									
35–49	0									
50–64	0									
65+	0									
GRAND TOTAL	0									

120: SCHISTOSOMIASIS

Type of Patients	Observed Patients	Avg. Stay	Vari-ance	10th	25th	50th	75th	90th	95th	99th
1. SINGLE DX										
A. *Not Operated*										
0–19 Years	0									
20–34	0									
35–49	0									
50–64	0									
65+	0									
B. *Operated*										
0–19 Years	0									
20–34	0									
35–49	0									
50–64	0									
65+	0									
2. MULTIPLE DX										
A. *Not Operated*										
0–19 Years	1	2.0	0	2	2	2	2	2	2	2
20–34	0									
35–49	0									
50–64	2	5.5	25	2	2	6	9	9	9	9
65+	0									
B. *Operated*										
0–19 Years	0									
20–34	0									
35–49	0									
50–64	0									
65+	1	13.0	0	13	13	13	13	13	13	13
SUBTOTALS:										
1. SINGLE DX A. *Not Operated*	0									
B. *Operated*	0									
2. MULTIPLE DX A. *Not Operated*	3	4.3	16	2	2	2	9	9	13	9
B. *Operated*	1	13.0	0	13	13	13	13	13	13	13
1. SINGLE DX	0									
2. MULTIPLE DX	4	6.5	30	2	2	2	9	13	13	13
A. NOT OPERATED	3	4.3	16	2	2	2	9	9	13	9
B. OPERATED	1	13.0	0	13	13	13	13	13	13	13
TOTAL										
0–19 Years	1	2.0	0	2	2	2	2	2	2	2
20–34	0									
35–49	0									
50–64	2	5.5	25	2	2	6	9	9	9	9
65+	1	13.0	0	13	13	13	13	13	13	13
GRAND TOTAL	4	6.5	30	2	2	2	9	13	13	13

121: OTH TREMATODE INFECTION

Type of Patients	Observed Patients	Avg. Stay	Vari-ance	10th	25th	50th	75th	90th	95th	99th
1. SINGLE DX										
A. *Not Operated*										
0–19 Years	0									
20–34	1	17.0	0	17	17	17	17	17	17	17
35–49	0									
50–64	0									
65+	0									
B. *Operated*										
0–19 Years	0									
20–34	0									
35–49	0									
50–64	0									
65+	0									
2. MULTIPLE DX										
A. *Not Operated*										
0–19 Years	0									
20–34	1	12.0	0	12	12	12	12	12	12	12
35–49	3	2.0	3	1	1	1	4	4	4	4
50–64	0									
65+	0									
B. *Operated*										
0–19 Years	0									
20–34	0									
35–49	1	3.0	0	3	3	3	3	3	3	3
50–64	0									
65+	0									
SUBTOTALS:										
1. SINGLE DX A. *Not Operated*	1	17.0	0	17	17	17	17	17	17	17
B. *Operated*	0									
2. MULTIPLE DX A. *Not Operated*	4	4.5	27	1	1	4	4	12	12	12
B. *Operated*	1	3.0	0	3	3	3	3	3	3	3
1. SINGLE DX	1	17.0	0	17	17	17	17	17	17	17
2. MULTIPLE DX	5	4.2	20	1	1	3	4	12	12	12
A. NOT OPERATED	5	7.0	51	1	1	4	12	17	17	17
B. OPERATED	1	3.0	0	3	3	3	3	3	3	3
TOTAL										
0–19 Years	0									
20–34	2	14.5	12	12	12	17	17	17	17	17
35–49	4	2.3	2	1	1	3	4	4	4	4
50–64	0									
65+	0									
GRAND TOTAL	6	6.3	44	1	1	3	12	17	17	17

Length of Stay by Diagnosis and Operation, Western Region, 2008

51

Western Region, October 2006–September 2007 Data, by Diagnosis

122: ECHINOCOCCOSIS

Type of Patients	Observed Patients	Avg. Stay	Vari-ance	Percentiles 10th	25th	50th	75th	90th	95th	99th
1. SINGLE DX										
A. Not Operated										
0–19 Years	0									
20–34	2	1.0	0	1	1	1	1	1	1	1
35–49	1	2.0	0	2	2	2	2	2	2	2
50–64	0									
65+	0									
B. Operated										
0–19 Years	1	2.0	0	2	2	2	2	2	2	2
20–34	1	1.0	0	1	1	1	1	1	1	1
35–49	1	7.0	0	7	7	7	7	7	7	7
50–64	0									
65+	0									
2. MULTIPLE DX										
A. Not Operated										
0–19 Years	0									
20–34	1	1.0	0	1	1	1	1	1	1	1
35–49	0									
50–64	0									
65+	2	2.0	2	1	1	2	3	3	3	3
B. Operated										
0–19 Years	0									
20–34	1	6.0	0	6	6	6	6	6	6	6
35–49	0									
50–64	3	4.0	9	1	1	4	7	7	7	7
65+	2	9.0	8	7	7	11	11	11	11	11
SUBTOTALS:										
1. SINGLE DX — A. Not Operated	3	1.3	<1	1	1	1	2	2	2	2
1. SINGLE DX — B. Operated	3	3.3	10	1	1	2	2	7	7	7
2. MULTIPLE DX — A. Not Operated	3	1.7	1	1	1	1	3	3	3	3
2. MULTIPLE DX — B. Operated	6	6.0	11	1	4	6	7	11	11	11
1. SINGLE DX	6	2.3	5	1	1	2	2	7	7	7
2. MULTIPLE DX	9	4.5	12	1	1	4	7	11	11	11
A. NOT OPERATED	6	1.5	<1	1	1	1	2	3	3	3
B. OPERATED	9	5.1	11	1	2	6	7	11	11	11
TOTAL										
0–19 Years	1	2.0	0	2	2	2	2	2	2	2
20–34	5	2.0	5	1	1	1	1	6	6	6
35–49	2	4.5	12	2	2	4	7	7	7	7
50–64	3	4.0	9	1	1	4	7	7	7	7
65+	4	5.5	20	1	1	5	7	11	11	11
GRAND TOTAL	**15**	**3.7**	**10**	**1**	**1**	**2**	**7**	**7**	**11**	**11**

123: OTHER CESTODE INFECTION

Type of Patients	Observed Patients	Avg. Stay	Vari-ance	Percentiles 10th	25th	50th	75th	90th	95th	99th
1. SINGLE DX										
A. Not Operated										
0–19 Years	0									
20–34	8	2.1	4	1	1	1	2	7	7	7
35–49	6	2.7	2	1	2	2	3	5	5	5
50–64	1	3.0	0	3	3	3	3	3	3	3
65+	0									
B. Operated										
0–19 Years	0									
20–34	0									
35–49	0									
50–64	0									
65+	0									
2. MULTIPLE DX										
A. Not Operated										
0–19 Years	14	1.7	<1	1	1	2	2	3	3	3
20–34	90	4.2	12	1	2	3	5	9	13	17
35–49	75	4.6	14	1	2	4	6	8	11	24
50–64	40	5.6	38	1	2	4	6	13	20	27
65+	19	5.4	18	1	2	4	9	11	16	16
B. Operated										
0–19 Years	2	5.5	4	4	4	4	7	7	7	7
20–34	15	12.7	486	2	3	6	10	28	88	88
35–49	11	14.1	70	4	8	12	19	34	>99	>99
50–64	6	7.2	6	4	5	7	8	11	11	11
65+	1	12.0	0	12	12	12	12	12	12	12
SUBTOTALS:										
1. SINGLE DX — A. Not Operated	15	2.4	3	1	1	2	3	5	7	7
1. SINGLE DX — B. Operated	0									
2. MULTIPLE DX — A. Not Operated	238	4.5	17	1	2	3	5	9	13	24
2. MULTIPLE DX — B. Operated	35	11.7	230	3	5	8	14	28	88	>99
1. SINGLE DX	15	2.4	3	1	1	2	3	5	7	7
2. MULTIPLE DX	273	5.4	50	1	2	4	6	11	16	34
A. NOT OPERATED	253	4.4	17	1	2	3	5	9	13	24
B. OPERATED	35	11.7	230	3	5	8	14	28	88	>99
TOTAL										
0–19 Years	16	2.2	2	1	1	1	3	4	7	7
20–34	113	5.2	79	1	2	3	5	9	14	28
35–49	92	5.6	30	1	3	4	7	12	19	>99
50–64	47	5.7	33	1	2	5	7	13	20	27
65+	20	5.8	19	1	3	5	10	12	16	16
GRAND TOTAL	**288**	**5.3**	**48**	**2**	**2**	**3**	**6**	**10**	**16**	**34**

124: TRICHINOSIS

Type of Patients	Observed Patients	Avg. Stay	Vari-ance	Percentiles 10th	25th	50th	75th	90th	95th	99th
1. SINGLE DX										
A. Not Operated										
0–19 Years	0									
20–34	0									
35–49	0									
50–64	0									
65+	0									
B. Operated										
0–19 Years	0									
20–34	0									
35–49	0									
50–64	0									
65+	0									
2. MULTIPLE DX										
A. Not Operated										
0–19 Years	0									
20–34	1	5.0	0	5	5	5	5	5	5	5
35–49	1	3.0	0	3	3	3	3	3	3	3
50–64	0									
65+	0									
B. Operated										
0–19 Years	0									
20–34	0									
35–49	0									
50–64	0									
65+	0									
SUBTOTALS:										
1. SINGLE DX — A. Not Operated	0									
1. SINGLE DX — B. Operated	0									
2. MULTIPLE DX — A. Not Operated	2	4.0	2	3	3	4	5	5	5	5
2. MULTIPLE DX — B. Operated	0									
1. SINGLE DX	0									
2. MULTIPLE DX	2	4.0	2	3	3	4	5	5	5	5
A. NOT OPERATED	2	4.0	2	3	3	4	5	5	5	5
B. OPERATED	0									
TOTAL										
0–19 Years	0									
20–34	1	5.0	0	5	5	5	5	5	5	5
35–49	1	3.0	0	3	3	3	3	3	3	3
50–64	0									
65+	0									
GRAND TOTAL	**2**	**4.0**	**2**	**3**	**3**	**4**	**5**	**5**	**5**	**5**

Length of Stay by Diagnosis and Operation, Western Region, 2008

Western Region, October 2006–September 2007 Data, by Diagnosis

125: FILARIAL INFECTION

Type of Patients	Observed Patients	Avg. Stay	Variance	10th	25th	50th	75th	90th	95th	99th
1. SINGLE DX										
A. *Not Operated*										
0–19 Years	0									
20–34	0									
35–49	0									
50–64	0									
65+	0									
B. *Operated*										
0–19 Years	0									
20–34	0									
35–49	0									
50–64	0									
65+	0									
2. MULTIPLE DX										
A. *Not Operated*										
0–19 Years	0									
20–34	0									
35–49	0									
50–64	1	5.0	0	5	5	5	5	5	5	5
65+	0									
B. *Operated*										
0–19 Years	0									
20–34	0									
35–49	0									
50–64	0									
65+	1	31.0	0	31	31	31	31	31	31	31
SUBTOTALS:										
1. SINGLE DX										
A. Not Operated	0									
B. Operated	0									
2. MULTIPLE DX										
A. Not Operated	1	5.0	0	5	5	5	5	5	5	5
B. Operated	1	31.0	0	31	31	31	31	31	31	31
1. SINGLE DX	0									
2. MULTIPLE DX	2	18.0	333	5	5	18	31	31	31	31
A. NOT OPERATED	1	5.0	0	5	5	5	5	5	5	5
B. OPERATED	1	31.0	0	31	31	31	31	31	31	31
TOTAL										
0–19 Years	0									
20–34	0									
35–49	0									
50–64	1	5.0	0	5	5	5	5	5	5	5
65+	1	31.0	0	31	31	31	31	31	31	31
GRAND TOTAL	2	18.0	333	5	5	18	31	31	31	31

126: ANCYLOSTOMIASIS

Type of Patients	Observed Patients	Avg. Stay	Variance	10th	25th	50th	75th	90th	95th	99th
1. SINGLE DX										
A. *Not Operated*										
0–19 Years	0									
20–34	0									
35–49	0									
50–64	0									
65+	0									
B. *Operated*										
0–19 Years	0									
20–34	0									
35–49	0									
50–64	0									
65+	0									
2. MULTIPLE DX										
A. *Not Operated*										
0–19 Years	0									
20–34	1	2.0	0	2	2	2	2	2	2	2
35–49	0									
50–64	1	2.0	0	2	2	2	2	2	2	2
65+	0									
B. *Operated*										
0–19 Years	0									
20–34	0									
35–49	0									
50–64	0									
65+	0									
SUBTOTALS:										
1. SINGLE DX										
A. Not Operated	0									
B. Operated	0									
2. MULTIPLE DX										
A. Not Operated	2	2.0	0	2	2	2	2	2	2	2
B. Operated	0									
1. SINGLE DX	0									
2. MULTIPLE DX	2	2.0	0	2	2	2	2	2	2	2
A. NOT OPERATED	2	2.0	0	2	2	2	2	2	2	2
B. OPERATED	0									
TOTAL										
0–19 Years	0									
20–34	1	2.0	0	2	2	2	2	2	2	2
35–49	0									
50–64	1	2.0	0	2	2	2	2	2	2	2
65+	0									
GRAND TOTAL	2	2.0	0	2	2	2	2	2	2	2

127: OTH INTEST HELMINTHIASES

Type of Patients	Observed Patients	Avg. Stay	Variance	10th	25th	50th	75th	90th	95th	99th
1. SINGLE DX										
A. *Not Operated*										
0–19 Years	0									
20–34	0									
35–49	0									
50–64	0									
65+	0									
B. *Operated*										
0–19 Years	2	1.5	<1	1	1	2	2	2	2	2
20–34	0									
35–49	0									
50–64	0									
65+	0									
2. MULTIPLE DX										
A. *Not Operated*										
0–19 Years	2	5.0	2	4	4	6	6	6	6	6
20–34	4	2.7	3	1	1	3	3	5	5	5
35–49	4	2.7	<1	1	1	3	3	4	4	4
50–64	3	5.7	<1	5	5	6	6	6	6	6
65+	10	7.6	32	4	4	5	10	21	21	21
B. *Operated*										
0–19 Years	2	3.0	2	2	2	4	4	4	4	4
20–34	0									
35–49	1	5.0	0	5	5	5	5	5	5	5
50–64	0									
65+	0									
SUBTOTALS:										
1. SINGLE DX										
A. Not Operated	0									
B. Operated	2	1.5	<1	1	1	2	2	2	2	2
2. MULTIPLE DX										
A. Not Operated	23	5.5	19	2	3	5	6	10	13	21
B. Operated	3	3.7	2	2	2	4	5	5	5	5
1. SINGLE DX	2	1.5	<1	1	1	2	2	2	2	2
2. MULTIPLE DX	26	5.2	17	2	3	5	6	10	13	21
A. NOT OPERATED	23	5.5	19	2	3	5	6	10	13	21
B. OPERATED	5	2.8	3	1	2	2	4	5	5	5
TOTAL										
0–19 Years	6	3.2	3	1	2	4	4	6	6	6
20–34	4	2.7	3	1	1	3	3	5	5	5
35–49	5	3.2	2	1	3	3	4	4	5	5
50–64	3	5.7	<1	5	5	6	6	6	6	6
65+	10	7.6	32	4	4	5	10	21	21	21
GRAND TOTAL	28	5.0	17	1	3	4	6	10	13	21

Length of Stay by Diagnosis and Operation, Western Region, 2008

Western Region, October 2006–September 2007 Data, by Diagnosis

128: HELMINTHIASES NEC & NOS

Type of Patients	Observed Patients	Avg. Stay	Vari-ance	10th	25th	50th	75th	90th	95th	99th
1. SINGLE DX										
A. Not Operated										
0–19 Years	0									
20–34	0									
35–49	0									
50–64	0									
65+	0									
B. Operated										
0–19 Years	0									
20–34	0									
35–49	0									
50–64	0									
65+	0									
2. MULTIPLE DX										
A. Not Operated										
0–19 Years	0									
20–34	0									
35–49	0									
50–64	0									
65+	0									
B. Operated										
0–19 Years	0									
20–34	0									
35–49	0									
50–64	0									
65+	0									
SUBTOTALS:										
1. SINGLE DX A. Not Operated	0									
1. SINGLE DX B. Operated	0									
2. MULTIPLE DX A. Not Operated	0									
2. MULTIPLE DX B. Operated	0									
1. SINGLE DX	0									
2. MULTIPLE DX	0									
A. NOT OPERATED	0									
B. OPERATED	0									
TOTAL										
0–19 Years	0									
20–34	0									
35–49	0									
50–64	0									
65+	0									
GRAND TOTAL	0									

129: INTEST PARASITISM NOS

Type of Patients	Observed Patients	Avg. Stay	Vari-ance	10th	25th	50th	75th	90th	95th	99th
1. SINGLE DX										
A. Not Operated										
0–19 Years	0									
20–34	0									
35–49	0									
50–64	0									
65+	0									
B. Operated										
0–19 Years	0									
20–34	0									
35–49	0									
50–64	0									
65+	0									
2. MULTIPLE DX										
A. Not Operated										
0–19 Years	0									
20–34	2	4.5	<1	4	4	5	5	5	5	5
35–49	0									
50–64	0									
65+	2	3.5	<1	3	3	4	4	4	4	4
B. Operated										
0–19 Years	0									
20–34	0									
35–49	0									
50–64	0									
65+	0									
SUBTOTALS:										
1. SINGLE DX A. Not Operated	0									
1. SINGLE DX B. Operated	0									
2. MULTIPLE DX A. Not Operated	4	4.0	<1	3	4	4	5	5	5	5
2. MULTIPLE DX B. Operated	0									
1. SINGLE DX	0									
2. MULTIPLE DX	4	4.0	<1	3	4	4	5	5	5	5
A. NOT OPERATED	4	4.0	<1	3	4	4	5	5	5	5
B. OPERATED	0									
TOTAL										
0–19 Years	0									
20–34	2	4.5	<1	4	4	5	5	5	5	5
35–49	0									
50–64	0									
65+	2	3.5	<1	3	3	4	4	4	4	4
GRAND TOTAL	4	4.0	<1	3	4	4	5	5	5	5

130: TOXOPLASMOSIS

Type of Patients	Observed Patients	Avg. Stay	Vari-ance	10th	25th	50th	75th	90th	95th	99th
1. SINGLE DX										
A. Not Operated										
0–19 Years	0									
20–34	0									
35–49	0									
50–64	0									
65+	0									
B. Operated										
0–19 Years	0									
20–34	0									
35–49	0									
50–64	0									
65+	0									
2. MULTIPLE DX										
A. Not Operated										
0–19 Years	0									
20–34	2	10.9	160	2	2	2	20	20	20	20
35–49	9	11.6	69	1	6	10	13	26	26	26
50–64	3	6.0	3	4	4	7	7	7	7	7
65+	0									
B. Operated										
0–19 Years	0									
20–34	0									
35–49	1	6.0	0	6	6	6	6	6	6	6
50–64	1	3.0	0	3	3	3	3	3	3	3
65+	0									
SUBTOTALS:										
1. SINGLE DX A. Not Operated	0									
1. SINGLE DX B. Operated	0									
2. MULTIPLE DX A. Not Operated	14	10.3	61	2	5	7	13	24	26	26
2. MULTIPLE DX B. Operated	2	4.5	4	3	3	3	6	6	6	6
1. SINGLE DX	0									
2. MULTIPLE DX	16	9.6	57	2	4	7	10	24	26	26
A. NOT OPERATED	14	10.3	61	2	5	7	13	24	26	26
B. OPERATED	2	4.5	4	3	3	3	6	6	6	6
TOTAL										
0–19 Years	0									
20–34	2	10.9	160	2	2	2	20	20	20	20
35–49	10	11.1	65	1	6	10	13	24	26	26
50–64	4	5.3	4	3	4	4	7	7	7	7
65+	0									
GRAND TOTAL	16	9.6	57	2	4	7	10	24	26	26

Length of Stay by Diagnosis and Operation, Western Region, 2008

Western Region, October 2006–September 2007 Data, by Diagnosis

131: TRICHOMONIASIS

Type of Patients	Observed Patients	Avg. Stay	Vari-ance	10th	25th	50th	75th	90th	95th	99th
1. SINGLE DX										
A. Not Operated										
0–19 Years	0									
20–34	0									
35–49	0									
50–64	0									
65+	0									
B. Operated										
0–19 Years	0									
20–34	0									
35–49	0									
50–64	0									
65+	0									
2. MULTIPLE DX										
A. Not Operated										
0–19 Years	3	3.0	4	1	1	3	5	5	5	5
20–34	8	2.4	<1	1	2	2	3	3	4	4
35–49	9	3.0	6	1	1	2	5	4	8	8
50–64	4	4.5	4	3	3	4	5	8	7	7
65+	5	2.2	1	1	1	3	3	3	3	3
B. Operated										
0–19 Years	0									
20–34	0									
35–49	1	2.0	0	2	2	2	2	2	2	2
50–64	0									
65+	0									
SUBTOTALS:										
1. SINGLE DX										
A. Not Operated	0									
B. Operated	0									
2. MULTIPLE DX										
A. Not Operated	29	2.9	3	1	2	3	3	5	7	8
B. Operated	1	2.0	0	2	2	2	2	2	2	2
1. SINGLE DX	0									
2. MULTIPLE DX	30	2.9	3	1	2	2	3	5	7	8
A. NOT OPERATED	29	2.9	3	1	2	3	3	5	7	8
B. OPERATED	1	2.0	0	2	2	2	2	2	2	2
TOTAL										
0–19 Years	3	3.0	4	1	1	3	5	5	5	5
20–34	8	2.4	<1	1	2	2	3	4	4	4
35–49	10	2.9	5	1	1	2	5	5	8	8
50–64	4	4.5	4	3	3	4	5	8	7	7
65+	5	2.2	1	1	1	3	3	3	3	3
GRAND TOTAL	30	2.9	3	1	2	2	3	5	7	8

132: PEDICULOSIS & PHTHIRUS

Type of Patients	Observed Patients	Avg. Stay	Vari-ance	10th	25th	50th	75th	90th	95th	99th
1. SINGLE DX										
A. Not Operated										
0–19 Years	0									
20–34	0									
35–49	0									
50–64	0									
65+	0									
B. Operated										
0–19 Years	0									
20–34	0									
35–49	0									
50–64	0									
65+	0									
2. MULTIPLE DX										
A. Not Operated										
0–19 Years	1	2.0	0	2	2	2	2	2	2	2
20–34	0									
35–49	1	7.0	0	7	7	7	7	7	7	7
50–64	0									
65+	0									
B. Operated										
0–19 Years	0									
20–34	0									
35–49	0									
50–64	0									
65+	0									
SUBTOTALS:										
1. SINGLE DX										
A. Not Operated	0									
B. Operated	0									
2. MULTIPLE DX										
A. Not Operated	2	4.5	12	2	2	7	7	7	7	7
B. Operated	0									
1. SINGLE DX	0									
2. MULTIPLE DX	2	4.5	12	2	2	7	7	7	7	7
A. NOT OPERATED	2	4.5	12	2	2	7	7	7	7	7
B. OPERATED	0									
TOTAL										
0–19 Years	1	2.0	0	2	2	2	2	2	2	2
20–34	0									
35–49	1	7.0	0	7	7	7	7	7	7	7
50–64	0									
65+	0									
GRAND TOTAL	2	4.5	12	2	2	7	7	7	7	7

133: ACARIASIS

Type of Patients	Observed Patients	Avg. Stay	Vari-ance	10th	25th	50th	75th	90th	95th	99th
1. SINGLE DX										
A. Not Operated										
0–19 Years	4	3.5	10	1	1	2	3	8	8	8
20–34	0									
35–49	0									
50–64	0									
65+	0									
B. Operated										
0–19 Years	0									
20–34	0									
35–49	0									
50–64	0									
65+	0									
2. MULTIPLE DX										
A. Not Operated										
0–19 Years	6	2.2	1	1	1	2	3	4	4	4
20–34	3	2.3	1	1	1	3	3	3	3	3
35–49	17	2.6	3	1	1	2	3	5	7	7
50–64	19	4.1	14	1	2	3	5	8	17	17
65+	38	4.8	24	1	2	4	5	11	15	26
B. Operated										
0–19 Years	0									
20–34	0									
35–49	0									
50–64	0									
65+	0									
SUBTOTALS:										
1. SINGLE DX										
A. Not Operated	4	3.5	10	1	1	2	3	8	8	8
B. Operated	0									
2. MULTIPLE DX										
A. Not Operated	83	3.9	15	1	2	3	5	7	11	26
B. Operated	0									
1. SINGLE DX	4	3.5	10	1	1	2	3	8	8	8
2. MULTIPLE DX	83	3.9	15	1	2	3	5	7	11	26
A. NOT OPERATED	87	3.9	15	1	2	3	5	7	11	26
B. OPERATED	0									
TOTAL										
0–19 Years	10	2.7	4	1	1	2	3	4	8	8
20–34	3	2.3	1	1	1	3	3	3	3	3
35–49	17	2.6	3	1	2	2	3	5	7	7
50–64	19	4.1	14	1	2	4	5	8	17	17
65+	38	4.8	24	1	2	4	5	11	15	26
GRAND TOTAL	87	3.9	15	1	2	3	5	7	11	26

55

Length of Stay by Diagnosis and Operation, Western Region, 2008

Western Region, October 2006–September 2007 Data, by Diagnosis

134: OTHER INFESTATION

Type of Patients	Observed Patients	Avg. Stay	Variance	10th	25th	50th	75th	90th	95th	99th
1. SINGLE DX										
A. Not Operated										
0–19 Years	0									
20–34	0									
35–49	0									
50–64	0									
65+	0									
B. Operated										
0–19 Years	0									
20–34	0									
35–49	0									
50–64	0									
65+	0									
2. MULTIPLE DX										
A. Not Operated										
0–19 Years	0									
20–34	0									
35–49	0									
50–64	0									
65+	0									
B. Operated										
0–19 Years	0									
20–34	0									
35–49	0									
50–64	0									
65+	1	10.0	0	10	10	10	10	10	10	10
SUBTOTALS:										
1. SINGLE DX A. Not Operated	0									
B. Operated	0									
2. MULTIPLE DX A. Not Operated	0									
B. Operated	1	10.0	0	10	10	10	10	10	10	10
1. SINGLE DX	0									
2. MULTIPLE DX	1	10.0	0	10	10	10	10	10	10	10
A. NOT OPERATED	0									
B. OPERATED	1	10.0	0	10	10	10	10	10	10	10
TOTAL										
0–19 Years	0									
20–34	0									
35–49	0									
50–64	0									
65+	1	10.0	0	10	10	10	10	10	10	10
GRAND TOTAL	1	10.0	0	10	10	10	10	10	10	10

135: SARCOIDOSIS

Type of Patients	Observed Patients	Avg. Stay	Variance	10th	25th	50th	75th	90th	95th	99th
1. SINGLE DX										
A. Not Operated										
0–19 Years	1	6.0	0	6	6	6	6	6	6	6
20–34	0									
35–49	1	2.0	0	2	2	2	2	2	2	2
50–64	1	5.0	0	5	5	5	5	5	5	5
65+	0									
B. Operated										
0–19 Years	0									
20–34	2	4.0	2	3	3	3	5	5	5	5
35–49	4	1.0	0	1	1	1	1	1	1	1
50–64	2	2.5	4	1	1	1	1	4	4	4
65+	0									
2. MULTIPLE DX										
A. Not Operated										
0–19 Years	3	13.0	102	4	4	11	24	24	24	24
20–34	24	4.3	10	1	2	4	5	6	13	13
35–49	93	4.3	10	1	2	4	5	8	9	24
50–64	120	5.4	51	1	2	4	6	10	15	25
65+	76	4.9	13	1	3	4	7	10	13	17
B. Operated										
0–19 Years	2	2.5	4	1	1	1	4	4	4	4
20–34	18	6.6	61	1	2	4	7	16	33	33
35–49	64	5.7	39	1	2	4	7	14	19	33
50–64	58	6.1	30	1	2	4	8	16	18	21
65+	32	5.4	28	1	1	4	8	11	18	23
SUBTOTALS:										
1. SINGLE DX A. Not Operated	3	4.3	4	2	3	5	6	6	6	6
B. Operated	8	2.1	3	1	1	1	3	5	5	5
2. MULTIPLE DX A. Not Operated	316	4.9	27	1	2	4	6	9	13	24
B. Operated	174	5.8	35	1	2	4	7	14	18	33
1. SINGLE DX	11	2.7	4	1	2	2	5	5	6	6
2. MULTIPLE DX	490	5.3	30	1	2	4	6	11	15	25
A. NOT OPERATED	319	4.9	27	1	2	4	6	9	13	24
B. OPERATED	182	5.7	34	1	1	4	7	14	18	33
TOTAL										
0–19 Years	6	8.4	70	1	4	6	11	24	24	24
20–34	44	5.2	31	1	2	4	6	12	13	33
35–49	162	4.7	22	1	2	4	6	9	13	27
50–64	181	5.6	43	1	2	4	7	12	17	25
65+	108	5.1	17	1	2	4	8	10	13	18
GRAND TOTAL	501	5.2	30	1	2	4	6	11	15	24

136: INF/PARASIT DIS NEC&NOS

Type of Patients	Observed Patients	Avg. Stay	Variance	10th	25th	50th	75th	90th	95th	99th
1. SINGLE DX										
A. Not Operated										
0–19 Years	6	3.8	7	2	2	3	6	8	8	8
20–34	3	5.3	<1	5	5	5	6	6	6	6
35–49	3	2.0	<1	2	2	2	2	2	2	2
50–64	3	3.0	0	2	2	3	4	4	4	4
65+	1	1.0	0	1	1	1	1	1	1	1
B. Operated										
0–19 Years	0									
20–34	0									
35–49	0									
50–64	0									
65+	0									
2. MULTIPLE DX										
A. Not Operated										
0–19 Years	29	7.8	65	2	3	5	8	22	31	33
20–34	53	8.4	67	2	3	6	11	18	24	50
35–49	85	6.2	25	2	3	5	8	12	18	25
50–64	104	8.3	45	2	4	7	10	15	19	24
65+	119	7.9	62	2	3	6	9	15	24	40
B. Operated										
0–19 Years	0									
20–34	3	7.0	13	4	4	6	11	11	11	11
35–49	11	13.5	70	4	7	13	18	24	30	30
50–64	20	11.3	46	4	7	9	15	25	26	26
65+	16	15.0	178	2	4	13	23	34	49	49
SUBTOTALS:										
1. SINGLE DX A. Not Operated	16	3.4	4	2	2	3	5	6	8	8
B. Operated	0									
2. MULTIPLE DX A. Not Operated	390	7.7	50	2	3	6	9	15	21	40
B. Operated	50	12.7	92	4	6	10	15	25	31	49
1. SINGLE DX	16	3.4	4	2	2	3	5	6	8	8
2. MULTIPLE DX	440	8.3	58	2	3	6	10	17	24	40
A. NOT OPERATED	406	7.5	49	2	3	6	9	15	21	37
B. OPERATED	50	12.7	92	4	6	10	15	25	31	49
TOTAL										
0–19 Years	35	7.1	57	2	3	5	8	13	21	33
20–34	59	8.2	61	2	3	6	11	18	24	50
35–49	99	6.9	34	2	3	5	9	17	20	25
50–64	127	8.7	45	2	4	7	11	16	23	26
65+	136	8.6	80	2	3	6	10	18	31	49
GRAND TOTAL	456	8.1	56	2	3	6	10	17	24	40

Length of Stay by Diagnosis and Operation, Western Region, 2008

Western Region, October 2006–September 2007 Data, by Diagnosis

136.3: PNEUMOCYSTOSIS

Type of Patients	Observed Patients	Avg. Stay	Variance	10th	25th	50th	75th	90th	95th	99th
1. SINGLE DX										
A. Not Operated										
0–19 Years	0									
20–34	1	6.0	0	6	6	6	6	6	6	6
35–49	1	2.0	0	2	2	2	2	2	2	2
50–64	2	3.0	2	2	2	4	4	4	4	4
65+	0									
B. Operated										
0–19 Years	0									
20–34	0									
35–49	0									
50–64	0									
65+	0									
2. MULTIPLE DX										
A. Not Operated										
0–19 Years	4	13.1	197	2	2	12	33	33	33	33
20–34	24	6.7	13	3	4	6	10	12	13	13
35–49	44	6.7	27	2	3	6	8	17	18	21
50–64	67	9.3	54	3	5	8	11	16	23	52
65+	52	12.4	101	4	6	10	15	24	37	50
B. Operated										
0–19 Years	0									
20–34	1	11.0	0	11	11	11	11	11	11	11
35–49	8	15.2	81	3	9	13	18	30	30	30
50–64	19	11.6	46	4	7	9	15	25	26	26
65+	14	15.9	195	2	4	14	23	34	49	49
SUBTOTALS:										
1. SINGLE DX										
A. Not Operated	4	3.5	4	2	2	4	6	6	6	6
B. Operated	0									
2. MULTIPLE DX										
A. Not Operated	191	9.3	62	3	4	8	11	17	24	50
B. Operated	42	13.7	100	4	7	11	18	26	31	49
1. SINGLE DX	4	3.5	4	2	2	4	6	6	6	6
2. MULTIPLE DX	233	10.1	71	3	5	8	12	20	26	49
A. NOT OPERATED	195	9.2	61	2	4	8	11	17	24	50
B. OPERATED	42	13.7	100	4	7	11	18	26	31	49
TOTAL										
0–19 Years	4	13.1	197	2	2	12	33	33	33	33
20–34	26	6.8	12	3	4	6	10	12	13	13
35–49	53	7.9	43	2	3	6	10	18	21	30
50–64	88	9.7	53	3	5	8	11	17	24	52
65+	66	13.1	120	4	6	10	15	31	37	50
GRAND TOTAL	237	10.0	71	2	5	8	12	20	26	49

137: LATE EFFECT TUBERCULOSIS

Type of Patients	Observed Patients	Avg. Stay	Variance	10th	25th	50th	75th	90th	95th	99th
1. SINGLE DX										
A. Not Operated										
0–19 Years	0									
20–34	0									
35–49	0									
50–64	0									
65+	0									
B. Operated										
0–19 Years	0									
20–34	0									
35–49	0									
50–64	0									
65+	0									
2. MULTIPLE DX										
A. Not Operated										
0–19 Years	0									
20–34	0									
35–49	0									
50–64	1	8.0	0	8	8	8	8	8	8	8
65+	0									
B. Operated										
0–19 Years	0									
20–34	0									
35–49	0									
50–64	0									
65+	0									
SUBTOTALS:										
1. SINGLE DX										
A. Not Operated	0									
B. Operated	0									
2. MULTIPLE DX										
A. Not Operated	1	8.0	0	8	8	8	8	8	8	8
B. Operated	0									
1. SINGLE DX	0									
2. MULTIPLE DX	1	8.0	0	8	8	8	8	8	8	8
A. NOT OPERATED	1	8.0	0	8	8	8	8	8	8	8
B. OPERATED	0									
TOTAL										
0–19 Years	0									
20–34	0									
35–49	0									
50–64	1	8.0	0	8	8	8	8	8	8	8
65+	0									
GRAND TOTAL	1	8.0	0	8	8	8	8	8	8	8

138: LATE EFFECT ACUTE POLIO

Type of Patients	Observed Patients	Avg. Stay	Variance	10th	25th	50th	75th	90th	95th	99th
1. SINGLE DX										
A. Not Operated										
0–19 Years	0									
20–34	0									
35–49	0									
50–64	0									
65+	0									
B. Operated										
0–19 Years	0									
20–34	0									
35–49	0									
50–64	0									
65+	0									
2. MULTIPLE DX										
A. Not Operated										
0–19 Years	0									
20–34	0									
35–49	0									
50–64	5	4.0	7	1	3	3	5	8	8	8
65+	8	6.4	21	1	2	5	11	13	13	13
B. Operated										
0–19 Years	1	8.0	0	8	8	8	8	8	8	8
20–34	1	1.0	0	1	1	1	1	1	1	1
35–49	0									
50–64	1	1.0	0	1	1	1	1	1	1	1
65+	0									
SUBTOTALS:										
1. SINGLE DX										
A. Not Operated	0									
B. Operated	0									
2. MULTIPLE DX										
A. Not Operated	13	5.5	16	1	3	5	8	11	13	13
B. Operated	3	3.3	16	1	1	1	3	8	8	8
1. SINGLE DX	0									
2. MULTIPLE DX	16	5.1	16	1	3	5	8	11	13	13
A. NOT OPERATED	13	5.5	16	1	3	5	8	11	13	13
B. OPERATED	3	3.3	16	1	1	1	3	8	8	8
TOTAL										
0–19 Years	1	8.0	0	8	8	8	8	8	8	8
20–34	1	1.0	0	1	1	1	1	1	1	1
35–49	0									
50–64	6	3.5	7	1	1	3	5	8	8	8
65+	8	6.4	21	1	2	5	11	13	13	13
GRAND TOTAL	16	5.1	16	1	1	3	8	11	13	13

Length of Stay by Diagnosis and Operation, Western Region, 2008

Western Region, October 2006–September 2007 Data, by Diagnosis

139: LATE EFFECT INFECT NEC

Type of Patients	Observed Patients	Avg. Stay	Vari-ance	10th	25th	50th	75th	90th	95th	99th
1. SINGLE DX										
A. Not Operated										
0–19 Years	0									
20–34	0									
35–49	0									
50–64	0									
65+	0									
B. Operated										
0–19 Years	0									
20–34	0									
35–49	0									
50–64	0									
65+	0									
2. MULTIPLE DX										
A. Not Operated										
0–19 Years	0									
20–34	0									
35–49	0									
50–64	0									
65+	1	1.0	0	1	1	1	1	1	1	1
B. Operated										
0–19 Years	0									
20–34	1	7.0	0	7	7	7	7	7	7	7
35–49	0									
50–64	1	6.0	0	6	6	6	6	6	6	6
65+	0									
SUBTOTALS:										
1. SINGLE DX										
A. Not Operated	0									
B. Operated	0									
2. MULTIPLE DX										
A. Not Operated	1	1.0	0	1	1	1	1	1	1	1
B. Operated	2	6.5	<1	6	6	6	6	7	7	7
1. SINGLE DX	0									
2. MULTIPLE DX	3	4.7	10	1	1	6	7	7	7	7
A. NOT OPERATED	1	1.0	0	1	1	1	1	1	1	1
B. OPERATED	2	6.5	<1	6	6	6	7	7	7	7
TOTAL										
0–19 Years	0									
20–34	1	7.0	0	7	7	7	7	7	7	7
35–49	0									
50–64	1	6.0	0	6	6	6	6	6	6	6
65+	1	1.0	0	1	1	1	1	1	1	1
GRAND TOTAL	3	4.7	10	1	1	6	7	7	7	7

140: LIP CA

Type of Patients	Observed Patients	Avg. Stay	Vari-ance	10th	25th	50th	75th	90th	95th	99th
1. SINGLE DX										
A. Not Operated										
0–19 Years	0									
20–34	0									
35–49	0									
50–64	0									
65+	0									
B. Operated										
0–19 Years	1	1.0	0	1	1	1	1	1	1	1
20–34	0									
35–49	1	1.0	0	1	1	1	1	1	1	1
50–64	2	5.5	40	1	1	1	10	10	10	10
65+	0									
2. MULTIPLE DX										
A. Not Operated										
0–19 Years	1	5.0	0	5	5	5	5	5	5	5
20–34	0									
35–49	1	17.0	0	17	17	17	17	17	17	17
50–64	1	5.0	0	5	5	5	5	5	5	5
65+	2	6.5	4	5	5	7	8	8	8	8
B. Operated										
0–19 Years	0									
20–34	2	3.0	8	1	1	3	5	5	5	5
35–49	15	4.4	26	1	1	2	6	14	15	15
50–64	19	4.9	26	1	1	2	8	13	17	17
65+	22	4.2	20	1	1	3	6	8	10	20
SUBTOTALS:										
1. SINGLE DX										
A. Not Operated	0									
B. Operated	4	3.3	20	1	1	1	1	10	10	10
2. MULTIPLE DX										
A. Not Operated	5	8.0	27	5	5	5	8	17	17	17
B. Operated	58	4.5	22	1	1	2	6	13	15	20
1. SINGLE DX	4	3.3	20	1	1	1	1	10	10	10
2. MULTIPLE DX	63	4.7	23	1	1	3	6	13	15	20
A. NOT OPERATED	5	8.0	27	5	5	5	8	17	17	17
B. OPERATED	62	4.4	22	1	1	2	6	12	14	20
TOTAL										
0–19 Years	2	3.0	8	1	1	1	5	5	5	5
20–34	2	3.0	8	1	1	3	5	5	5	5
35–49	17	4.9	33	1	1	2	6	15	17	17
50–64	22	5.0	25	1	1	3	10	12	13	17
65+	24	4.4	19	1	1	4	6	8	10	20
GRAND TOTAL	67	4.6	23	1	1	2	6	13	15	20

141: TONGUE CA

Type of Patients	Observed Patients	Avg. Stay	Vari-ance	10th	25th	50th	75th	90th	95th	99th
1. SINGLE DX										
A. Not Operated										
0–19 Years	0									
20–34	0									
35–49	2	8.1	97	1	1	15	15	15	15	15
50–64	0									
65+	3	1.0	0	1	1	1	1	1	1	1
B. Operated										
0–19 Years	1	3.0	0	3	3	3	3	3	3	3
20–34	8	4.4	12	1	1	3	7	10	10	10
35–49	16	3.2	7	1	1	2	4	7	11	11
50–64	16	2.7	5	1	1	2	2	7	9	9
65+	8	2.4	3	1	1	2	3	6	6	6
2. MULTIPLE DX										
A. Not Operated										
0–19 Years	1	1.0	0	1	1	1	1	1	1	1
20–34	8	5.1	11	1	3	5	8	11	11	11
35–49	36	6.9	63	1	2	4	9	17	20	43
50–64	107	7.0	99	1	2	4	9	17	21	88
65+	87	5.6	34	1	2	4	7	11	19	32
B. Operated										
0–19 Years	1	4.0	0	4	4	4	4	4	4	4
20–34	10	7.7	33	2	2	9	12	18	18	18
35–49	88	6.2	45	1	1	5	8	12	16	48
50–64	281	6.0	66	1	2	4	7	11	18	37
65+	280	6.0	62	1	2	4	8	13	18	29
SUBTOTALS:										
1. SINGLE DX										
A. Not Operated	5	3.8	39	1	1	1	1	15	15	15
B. Operated	49	3.1	6	1	1	2	4	7	9	11
2. MULTIPLE DX										
A. Not Operated	239	6.4	67	1	2	4	8	16	20	43
B. Operated	660	6.1	61	1	2	4	7	13	18	31
1. SINGLE DX	54	3.2	9	1	1	2	4	7	10	15
2. MULTIPLE DX	899	6.2	62	1	2	4	8	13	18	35
A. NOT OPERATED	244	6.3	66	1	2	4	8	16	20	43
B. OPERATED	709	5.9	58	1	2	4	7	12	17	29
TOTAL										
0–19 Years	3	2.7	2	1	1	3	4	4	4	4
20–34	26	5.9	21	1	2	5	9	12	13	18
35–49	142	6.1	46	1	2	4	8	12	17	43
50–64	404	6.2	73	1	2	4	7	12	19	37
65+	378	5.8	55	1	2	3	7	13	18	29
GRAND TOTAL	953	6.0	60	1	2	4	7	13	18	32

Length of Stay by Diagnosis and Operation, Western Region, 2008

Western Region, October 2006–September 2007 Data, by Diagnosis

141.0: TONGUE BASE CA

Type of Patients	Observed Patients	Avg. Stay	Variance	Percentiles						
				10th	25th	50th	75th	90th	95th	99th
1. SINGLE DX										
A. *Not Operated*										
0–19 Years	0									
20–34	0									
35–49	2	8.1	97	1	1	15	15	15	15	15
50–64	0									
65+	2	1.0	0	1	1	1	1	1	1	1
B. *Operated*										
0–19 Years	0									
20–34	2	3.0	8	1	1	1	5	5	5	5
35–49	4	3.3	8	1	1	4	4	7	7	7
50–64	4	4.7	15	1	1	2	7	9	9	9
65+	1	6.0	0	6	6	6	6	6	6	6
2. MULTIPLE DX										
A. *Not Operated*										
0–19 Years	0									
20–34	3	7.7	12	4	4	8	11	11	11	11
35–49	20	8.5	93	1	2	6	11	17	17	43
50–64	68	8.5	142	1	2	5	10	21	26	>99
65+	49	5.5	30	1	2	4	7	10	17	32
B. *Operated*										
0–19 Years	0									
20–34	1	12.0	0	12	12	12	12	12	12	12
35–49	32	6.5	39	1	2	6	8	12	26	26
50–64	117	6.1	50	1	3	4	7	11	18	26
65+	95	8.0	120	1	2	6	10	16	24	95
SUBTOTALS:										
1. SINGLE DX										
A. *Not Operated*	4	4.5	49	1	1	1	15	15	15	15
B. *Operated*	11	4.0	9	1	1	4	7	7	9	9
2. MULTIPLE DX										
A. *Not Operated*	140	7.4	94	1	2	5	9	17	21	88
B. *Operated*	245	6.9	76	1	2	5	8	13	21	31
1. SINGLE DX	15	4.1	17	1	1	2	7	9	15	15
2. MULTIPLE DX	385	7.1	82	1	2	5	9	16	21	60
A. NOT OPERATED	144	7.3	92	1	2	5	9	17	21	88
B. OPERATED	256	6.8	73	1	2	5	8	13	21	31
TOTAL										
0–19 Years	0									
20–34	6	6.8	18	1	1	5	11	12	12	12
35–49	58	7.0	57	1	2	5	8	16	26	43
50–64	189	6.9	83	1	2	4	9	16	21	88
65+	147	7.0	89	1	2	5	8	15	20	32
GRAND TOTAL	400	7.0	80	1	2	5	9	15	21	43

142: MAJOR SALIVARY GLAND CA

Type of Patients	Observed Patients	Avg. Stay	Variance	Percentiles						
				10th	25th	50th	75th	90th	95th	99th
1. SINGLE DX										
A. *Not Operated*										
0–19 Years	0									
20–34	0									
35–49	0									
50–64	0									
65+	0									
B. *Operated*										
0–19 Years	3	1.0	0	1	1	1	1	1	1	1
20–34	6	2.5	<1	2	2	3	3	3	3	3
35–49	7	1.9	<1	1	1	2	2	3	3	3
50–64	14	1.9	<1	1	1	2	2	4	5	5
65+	10	1.6	<1	1	1	1	2	2	4	4
2. MULTIPLE DX										
A. *Not Operated*										
0–19 Years	1	3.0	0	3	3	3	3	3	3	3
20–34	3	2.7	1	1	2	2	3	4	4	4
35–49	4	2.7	3	1	1	2	3	5	5	5
50–64	7	2.9	8	1	1	2	3	9	9	9
65+	18	7.2	60	2	3	4	7	27	28	28
B. *Operated*										
0–19 Years	4	4.0	13	1	1	2	4	9	9	9
20–34	8	3.1	16	1	1	2	2	13	13	13
35–49	32	2.8	8	1	1	2	3	6	7	14
50–64	89	3.2	10	1	1	2	4	7	10	19
65+	195	3.4	12	1	1	2	4	7	9	18
SUBTOTALS:										
1. SINGLE DX										
A. *Not Operated*	0									
B. *Operated*	40	1.9	<1	1	1	2	2	3	4	5
2. MULTIPLE DX										
A. *Not Operated*	33	5.2	39	1	2	3	6	9	27	28
B. *Operated*	328	3.3	11	1	1	2	4	7	9	17
1. SINGLE DX	40	1.9	<1	1	1	2	2	3	4	5
2. MULTIPLE DX	361	3.4	14	1	1	2	4	7	10	19
A. NOT OPERATED	33	5.2	39	1	2	3	6	9	27	28
B. OPERATED	368	3.1	10	1	1	2	4	6	9	17
TOTAL										
0–19 Years	8	2.7	8	1	1	2	3	9	9	9
20–34	17	2.8	8	1	1	2	3	4	13	13
35–49	43	2.7	6	1	1	2	3	6	7	14
50–64	110	3.0	9	1	1	2	3	6	9	13
65+	223	3.6	17	1	1	2	4	7	10	27
GRAND TOTAL	401	3.3	13	1	2	2	4	7	9	18

142.0: PAROTID GLAND CA

Type of Patients	Observed Patients	Avg. Stay	Variance	Percentiles						
				10th	25th	50th	75th	90th	95th	99th
1. SINGLE DX										
A. *Not Operated*										
0–19 Years	0									
20–34	0									
35–49	0									
50–64	0									
65+	0									
B. *Operated*										
0–19 Years	3	1.0	0	1	1	1	1	1	1	1
20–34	4	2.5	<1	2	2	3	3	3	3	3
35–49	5	2.2	<1	2	2	2	2	3	3	3
50–64	12	1.9	<1	1	1	1	2	4	5	5
65+	10	1.6	<1	1	1	1	2	2	4	4
2. MULTIPLE DX										
A. *Not Operated*										
0–19 Years	1	3.0	0	3	3	3	3	3	3	3
20–34	2	2.0	0	1	2	2	2	2	2	2
35–49	4	2.7	3	1	1	2	3	5	5	5
50–64	4	2.0	<1	1	1	2	2	3	3	3
65+	13	8.4	77	3	3	5	7	27	28	28
B. *Operated*										
0–19 Years	4	4.0	13	1	1	2	4	9	9	9
20–34	9	3.1	16	1	1	2	2	13	13	13
35–49	28	2.7	9	1	1	2	3	7	9	9
50–64	79	3.1	10	1	1	2	4	7	10	19
65+	176	3.3	11	1	1	2	4	7	9	17
SUBTOTALS:										
1. SINGLE DX										
A. *Not Operated*	0									
B. *Operated*	34	1.9	1	1	1	2	2	3	4	5
2. MULTIPLE DX										
A. *Not Operated*	24	5.6	50	2	2	3	6	10	27	28
B. *Operated*	295	3.2	11	1	1	2	4	7	9	17
1. SINGLE DX	34	1.9	1	1	1	2	2	3	4	5
2. MULTIPLE DX	319	3.4	14	1	1	2	4	7	10	19
A. NOT OPERATED	24	5.6	50	2	2	3	6	10	27	28
B. OPERATED	329	3.0	10	1	1	2	4	6	9	15
TOTAL										
0–19 Years	8	2.7	8	1	1	2	3	9	9	9
20–34	14	2.8	9	1	1	2	3	4	13	13
35–49	37	2.7	7	1	1	2	3	6	9	14
50–64	95	2.9	8	1	1	2	4	6	9	19
65+	199	3.5	16	1	1	2	4	7	10	28
GRAND TOTAL	353	3.2	13	1	2	2	4	7	9	19

Length of Stay by Diagnosis and Operation, Western Region, 2008

Western Region, October 2006–September 2007 Data, by Diagnosis

143: GUM CA

Type of Patients	Observed Patients	Avg. Stay	Vari-ance	10th	25th	50th	75th	90th	95th	99th
1. SINGLE DX										
A. Not Operated										
0–19 Years	0									
20–34	0									
35–49	0									
50–64	1	2.0	0	2	2	2	2	2	2	2
65+	0									
B. Operated										
0–19 Years	0									
20–34	0									
35–49	1	4.0	0	4	4	4	4	4	4	4
50–64	2	3.5	12	1	1	6	6	6	6	6
65+	4	3.0	11	1	1	1	2	8	8	8
2. MULTIPLE DX										
A. Not Operated										
0–19 Years	1	1.0	0	1	1	1	1	1	1	1
20–34	1	4.0	0	4	4	4	4	4	4	4
35–49	2	8.9	71	3	3	3	15	15	15	15
50–64	1	5.0	0	5	5	5	5	5	5	5
65+	8	3.6	22	1	1	2	3	15	15	15
B. Operated										
0–19 Years	3	12.7	30	9	9	10	19	19	19	19
20–34	3	3.0	0	3	3	3	3	3	3	3
35–49	2	12.5	4	11	11	13	14	14	14	14
50–64	19	9.0	107	2	2	7	10	18	48	48
65+	71	5.8	23	1	2	5	8	10	15	25
SUBTOTALS:										
1. SINGLE DX										
A. Not Operated	1	2.0	0	2	2	2	2	2	2	2
B. Operated	7	3.3	8	1	1	2	6	8	8	8
2. MULTIPLE DX										
A. Not Operated	13	4.4	24	1	1	3	4	15	15	15
B. Operated	96	6.7	42	1	2	6	9	13	18	48
1. SINGLE DX	8	3.1	7	1	1	2	4	8	8	8
2. MULTIPLE DX	109	6.5	40	1	2	5	9	14	17	25
A. NOT OPERATED	14	4.2	22	1	1	2	4	15	15	15
B. OPERATED	103	6.5	40	1	2	6	9	12	17	25
TOTAL										
0–19 Years	4	9.7	54	1	1	9	10	19	19	19
20–34	3	3.7	<1	3	3	4	4	4	4	4
35–49	4	10.7	30	3	3	11	14	15	15	15
50–64	23	8.0	93	2	2	6	8	13	18	48
65+	83	5.5	23	1	2	4	8	10	15	25
GRAND TOTAL	117	6.2	38	1	2	5	8	13	17	25

144: MOUTH FLOOR CA

Type of Patients	Observed Patients	Avg. Stay	Vari-ance	10th	25th	50th	75th	90th	95th	99th
1. SINGLE DX										
A. Not Operated										
0–19 Years	0									
20–34	0									
35–49	0									
50–64	1	1.0	0	1	1	1	1	1	1	1
65+	1	1.0	0	1	1	1	1	1	1	1
B. Operated										
0–19 Years	0									
20–34	0									
35–49	0									
50–64	1	2.0	0	2	2	2	2	2	2	2
65+	1	3.0	0	3	3	3	3	3	3	3
2. MULTIPLE DX										
A. Not Operated										
0–19 Years	0									
20–34	1	5.0	0	5	5	5	5	5	5	5
35–49	2	6.5	40	2	2	7	11	11	11	11
50–64	10	10.2	110	2	2	6	13	17	36	36
65+	13	3.5	4	2	2	3	5	7	7	7
B. Operated										
0–19 Years	0									
20–34	0									
35–49	16	10.3	118	2	4	7	14	18	46	46
50–64	84	10.5	95	1	4	9	12	18	33	49
65+	74	8.7	102	1	3	6	11	15	24	65
SUBTOTALS:										
1. SINGLE DX										
A. Not Operated	2	1.0	0	1	1	1	1	1	1	1
B. Operated	2	2.5	<1	2	2	3	3	3	3	3
2. MULTIPLE DX										
A. Not Operated	26	6.4	53	2	2	3	7	13	17	36
B. Operated	174	9.7	100	1	3	8	12	16	33	49
1. SINGLE DX	4	1.7	<1	1	1	2	2	3	3	3
2. MULTIPLE DX	200	9.3	95	2	3	7	12	16	33	49
A. NOT OPERATED	28	6.0	51	1	2	3	7	13	17	36
B. OPERATED	176	9.6	99	1	3	8	12	16	33	49
TOTAL										
0–19 Years	0									
20–34	1	5.0	0	5	5	5	5	5	5	5
35–49	18	9.9	108	2	3	7	14	18	46	46
50–64	96	10.3	96	1	3	9	12	18	36	49
65+	89	7.8	89	1	3	5	9	15	18	65
GRAND TOTAL	204	9.1	94	1	3	7	11	16	31	49

145: MOUTH CA NEC & NOS

Type of Patients	Observed Patients	Avg. Stay	Vari-ance	10th	25th	50th	75th	90th	95th	99th
1. SINGLE DX										
A. Not Operated										
0–19 Years	0									
20–34	0									
35–49	0									
50–64	1	1.0	0	1	1	1	1	1	1	1
65+	0									
B. Operated										
0–19 Years	0									
20–34	0									
35–49	2	3.0	8	1	1	5	5	5	5	5
50–64	5	2.8	3	1	1	3	4	5	5	5
65+	4	2.3	2	1	1	3	4	4	4	4
2. MULTIPLE DX										
A. Not Operated										
0–19 Years	0									
20–34	1	1.0	0	1	1	1	1	1	1	1
35–49	3	1.7	1	1	1	1	3	3	3	3
50–64	10	4.7	39	1	2	3	4	22	22	22
65+	28	4.8	23	1	1	3	5	11	15	21
B. Operated										
0–19 Years	0									
20–34	5	3.0	6	1	2	2	3	7	7	7
35–49	25	6.0	23	1	3	5	8	11	16	20
50–64	83	6.9	37	1	2	6	9	15	18	36
65+	111	7.9	48	1	3	6	11	17	22	30
SUBTOTALS:										
1. SINGLE DX										
A. Not Operated	1	1.0	0	1	1	1	1	1	1	1
B. Operated	11	2.7	3	1	1	3	4	5	5	5
2. MULTIPLE DX										
A. Not Operated	42	4.5	24	1	1	3	5	10	15	22
B. Operated	224	7.2	41	1	2	6	9	16	21	30
1. SINGLE DX	12	2.5	3	1	1	3	4	5	5	5
2. MULTIPLE DX	266	6.8	39	1	2	5	9	15	21	30
A. NOT OPERATED	43	4.4	24	1	1	3	5	10	15	22
B. OPERATED	235	7.0	40	1	2	5	9	15	21	30
TOTAL										
0–19 Years	0									
20–34	6	2.7	5	1	1	2	3	7	7	7
35–49	30	5.4	22	1	1	3	8	10	16	20
50–64	99	6.4	36	1	2	4	9	15	18	36
65+	143	7.2	43	1	2	5	9	15	22	30
GRAND TOTAL	278	6.6	38	1	2	4	9	15	21	30

Length of Stay by Diagnosis and Operation, Western Region, 2008

Western Region, October 2006–September 2007 Data, by Diagnosis

146: OROPHARYNX CA

Type of Patients	Observed Patients	Avg. Stay	Variance	10th	25th	50th	75th	90th	95th	99th
1. SINGLE DX										
A. *Not Operated*										
0–19 Years	0									
20–34	0									
35–49	2	4.5	4	3	3	5	6	6	6	6
50–64	3	1.0	0	1	1	1	1	1	1	1
65+	0									
B. *Operated*										
0–19 Years	0									
20–34	0									
35–49	4	3.0	5	1	1	5	5	5	5	5
50–64	12	4.6	8	1	2	4	6	8	11	11
65+	0									
2. MULTIPLE DX										
A. *Not Operated*										
0–19 Years	1	7.0	0	7	7	7	7	7	7	7
20–34	1	2.0	0	2	2	2	2	2	2	2
35–49	27	6.8	32	2	3	5	9	12	21	25
50–64	76	6.2	43	1	2	4	7	16	23	32
65+	45	5.1	63	1	2	3	6	9	13	53
B. *Operated*										
0–19 Years	0									
20–34	1	3.0	0	3	3	3	3	3	3	3
35–49	58	5.3	43	1	2	3	6	10	24	35
50–64	140	5.4	27	1	2	4	7	11	15	27
65+	69	6.9	81	1	2	4	8	14	17	57
SUBTOTALS:										
1. SINGLE DX A. *Not Operated*	5	2.4	5	1	1	1	3	6	6	6
B. *Operated*	16	4.2	8	1	2	4	6	8	11	11
2. MULTIPLE DX A. *Not Operated*	150	5.9	47	1	2	4	7	11	21	32
B. *Operated*	268	5.8	44	1	2	3	7	13	15	36
1. SINGLE DX	21	3.8	7	1	1	4	5	6	8	11
2. MULTIPLE DX	418	5.8	45	1	2	4	7	12	17	35
A. NOT OPERATED	155	5.8	46	1	2	4	7	11	21	32
B. OPERATED	284	5.7	42	1	2	4	7	11	15	36
TOTAL										
0–19 Years	1	7.0	0	7	7	7	7	7	7	7
20–34	2	2.5	<1	2	2	3	3	3	3	3
35–49	91	5.6	37	1	2	4	7	10	21	35
50–64	231	5.5	32	1	2	4	7	11	17	27
65+	114	6.2	74	1	2	4	7	13	15	53
GRAND TOTAL	439	5.7	43	1	2	4	7	11	16	35

146.0: TONSIL CA

Type of Patients	Observed Patients	Avg. Stay	Variance	10th	25th	50th	75th	90th	95th	99th
1. SINGLE DX										
A. *Not Operated*										
0–19 Years	0									
20–34	0									
35–49	2	4.5	4	3	3	5	6	6	6	6
50–64	1	1.0	0	1	1	1	1	1	1	1
65+	0									
B. *Operated*										
0–19 Years	0									
20–34	0									
35–49	3	2.3	5	1	1	1	5	5	5	5
50–64	9	4.1	4	1	3	4	5	8	8	8
65+	0									
2. MULTIPLE DX										
A. *Not Operated*										
0–19 Years	0									
20–34	1	2.0	0	2	2	2	2	2	2	2
35–49	13	6.8	39	2	3	5	9	11	25	25
50–64	43	5.8	52	1	1	3	7	16	25	32
65+	16	4.0	10	1	2	2	7	8	11	11
B. *Operated*										
0–19 Years	0									
20–34	1	3.0	0	3	3	3	3	3	3	3
35–49	44	4.2	23	1	2	3	5	8	8	30
50–64	98	4.2	10	1	2	3	6	8	11	15
65+	42	6.2	77	2	3	4	7	10	15	57
SUBTOTALS:										
1. SINGLE DX A. *Not Operated*	3	3.3	6	1	1	3	6	6	6	6
B. *Operated*	12	3.7	5	1	2	4	5	6	8	8
2. MULTIPLE DX A. *Not Operated*	73	5.5	40	1	2	3	7	11	25	32
B. *Operated*	185	4.6	29	1	2	3	6	8	13	30
1. SINGLE DX	15	3.6	5	1	1	4	5	6	8	8
2. MULTIPLE DX	258	4.9	32	1	2	3	6	9	14	30
A. NOT OPERATED	76	5.5	39	1	2	3	7	11	25	32
B. OPERATED	197	4.6	27	1	2	3	6	8	13	30
TOTAL										
0–19 Years	0									
20–34	2	2.5	<1	2	2	3	3	3	3	3
35–49	62	4.7	26	1	2	3	6	8	11	30
50–64	151	4.6	22	1	2	3	6	8	13	25
65+	58	5.6	59	1	2	4	7	10	15	57
GRAND TOTAL	273	4.8	30	1	2	3	6	9	13	30

147: NASOPHARYNX CA

Type of Patients	Observed Patients	Avg. Stay	Variance	10th	25th	50th	75th	90th	95th	99th
1. SINGLE DX										
A. *Not Operated*										
0–19 Years	2	8.5	83	2	2	2	2	15	15	15
20–34	1	6.0	0	6	6	6	6	6	6	6
35–49	0									
50–64	1	1.0	0	1	1	1	1	1	1	1
65+	2	1.0	0	1	1	1	1	1	1	1
B. *Operated*										
0–19 Years	0									
20–34	0									
35–49	1	1.0	0	1	1	1	1	1	1	1
50–64	0									
65+	0									
2. MULTIPLE DX										
A. *Not Operated*										
0–19 Years	0									
20–34	10	10.8	430	1	1	3	7	18	68	68
35–49	23	4.7	7	2	2	4	6	8	10	12
50–64	49	5.8	35	1	2	4	8	11	13	38
65+	24	6.6	52	2	2	4	8	14	23	30
B. *Operated*										
0–19 Years	1	15.0	0	15	15	15	15	15	15	15
20–34	7	5.3	23	2	2	3	8	15	15	15
35–49	16	8.1	113	1	2	6	8	21	43	43
50–64	16	6.9	28	2	2	7	12	15	16	16
65+	0									
SUBTOTALS:										
1. SINGLE DX A. *Not Operated*	6	4.3	31	1	1	2	6	15	15	15
B. *Operated*	1	1.0	0	1	1	1	1	1	1	1
2. MULTIPLE DX A. *Not Operated*	106	6.2	68	1	2	4	7	12	14	38
B. *Operated*	40	7.3	61	1	2	5	12	15	16	43
1. SINGLE DX	7	3.9	27	1	1	1	6	15	15	15
2. MULTIPLE DX	146	6.5	66	1	2	4	8	13	16	43
A. NOT OPERATED	112	6.1	66	1	2	4	7	12	15	38
B. OPERATED	41	7.1	60	1	2	5	9	15	16	43
TOTAL										
0–19 Years	3	10.7	56	2	2	15	15	15	15	15
20–34	18	8.4	355	1	1	4	7	18	68	68
35–49	40	6.0	55	1	2	4	7	11	14	38
50–64	66	6.0	53	1	2	4	8	11	16	38
65+	26	6.2	41	2	2	4	8	14	16	30
GRAND TOTAL	153	6.4	64	1	2	4	8	13	16	43

Length of Stay by Diagnosis and Operation, Western Region, 2008

Western Region, October 2006–September 2007 Data, by Diagnosis

148: HYPOPHARYNX CA

Type of Patients	Observed Patients	Avg. Stay	Vari-ance	Percentiles 10th	25th	50th	75th	90th	95th	99th
1. SINGLE DX										
A. Not Operated										
0–19 Years	0									
20–34	0									
35–49	1	1.0	0	1	1	1	1	1	1	1
50–64	1	4.0	0	4	4	4	4	4	4	4
65+	1	1.0	0	1	1	1	1	1	1	1
B. Operated										
0–19 Years	0									
20–34	0									
35–49	0									
50–64	1	7.0	0	7	7	7	7	7	7	7
65+	0									
2. MULTIPLE DX										
A. Not Operated										
0–19 Years	0									
20–34	11	18.8	590	3	3	12	21	52	78	78
35–49	24	5.3	23	1	1	4	7	13	14	20
50–64	35	7.5	58	1	2	6	10	14	26	39
B. Operated										
0–19 Years	0									
20–34	9	14.0	0	14	14	14	14	14	14	14
35–49	9	11.0	81	2	3	9	17	28	28	28
50–64	34	7.3	41	1	3	5	10	15	21	29
65+	31	9.3	46	2	5	8	13	18	22	30
SUBTOTALS:										
1. SINGLE DX — A. Not Operated	3	2.0	3	1	1	1	4	4	4	4
1. SINGLE DX — B. Operated	1	7.0	0	7	7	7	7	7	7	7
2. MULTIPLE DX — A. Not Operated	70	8.5	143	1	2	5	10	17	26	78
2. MULTIPLE DX — B. Operated	75	8.6	48	2	3	7	13	18	22	30
1. SINGLE DX	4	3.2	8	1	1	1	7	7	7	7
2. MULTIPLE DX	145	8.6	93	1	3	6	11	18	22	52
A. NOT OPERATED	73	8.2	139	1	2	5	9	15	26	78
B. OPERATED	76	8.6	47	2	3	7	12	18	22	30
TOTAL										
0–19 Years	0									
20–34	1	14.0	0	14	14	14	14	14	14	14
35–49	21	14.6	352	2	3	9	17	28	52	78
50–64	60	6.4	33	1	3	5	7	14	18	29
65+	67	8.2	52	1	2	7	11	18	22	39
GRAND TOTAL	149	8.4	91	1	3	6	11	18	22	52

149: OTHER OROPHARYNX CA

Type of Patients	Observed Patients	Avg. Stay	Vari-ance	Percentiles 10th	25th	50th	75th	90th	95th	99th
1. SINGLE DX										
A. Not Operated										
0–19 Years	0									
20–34	0									
35–49	1	1.0	0	1	1	1	1	1	1	1
50–64	5	3.6	23	1	1	1	3	12	12	12
65+	0									
B. Operated										
0–19 Years	0									
20–34	0									
35–49	1	13.0	0	13	13	13	13	13	13	13
50–64	1	2.0	0	2	2	2	2	2	2	2
65+	0									
2. MULTIPLE DX										
A. Not Operated										
0–19 Years	0									
20–34	6	3.3	12	1	1	1	4	10	10	10
35–49	26	6.7	101	1	2	4	7	15	21	50
50–64	30	5.7	27	1	2	5	7	13	14	25
B. Operated										
0–19 Years	0									
20–34	3	15.0	0	15	15	15	15	15	15	15
35–49	3	3.4	10	1	1	2	5	7	7	7
50–64	14	9.3	62	1	2	9	14	20	27	27
65+	12	13.1	111	5	5	10	13	32	33	33
SUBTOTALS:										
1. SINGLE DX — A. Not Operated	6	3.2	19	1	1	1	3	12	12	12
1. SINGLE DX — B. Operated	2	7.5	60	2	2	2	13	13	13	13
2. MULTIPLE DX — A. Not Operated	62	5.9	56	1	2	4	7	12	15	50
2. MULTIPLE DX — B. Operated	30	10.4	80	1	5	9	14	23	32	33
1. SINGLE DX	8	4.2	26	1	1	1	3	13	13	13
2. MULTIPLE DX	92	7.4	67	1	2	5	10	15	25	50
A. NOT OPERATED	68	5.7	53	1	1	4	7	12	15	50
B. OPERATED	32	10.2	77	1	5	9	13	23	32	33
TOTAL										
0–19 Years	0									
20–34	1	15.0	0	15	15	15	15	15	15	15
35–49	11	4.0	18	1	1	2	7	10	13	13
50–64	46	7.1	79	1	2	4	9	17	21	50
65+	42	7.8	60	1	2	6	10	14	25	33
GRAND TOTAL	100	7.1	65	1	2	5	10	15	25	33

150: ESOPHAGUS CA

Type of Patients	Observed Patients	Avg. Stay	Vari-ance	Percentiles 10th	25th	50th	75th	90th	95th	99th
1. SINGLE DX										
A. Not Operated										
0–19 Years	0									
20–34	0									
35–49	1	3.0	0	3	3	3	3	3	3	3
50–64	8	4.1	23	1	1	2	6	15	15	15
65+	1	7.0	0	7	7	7	7	7	7	7
B. Operated										
0–19 Years	0									
20–34	0									
35–49	0									
50–64	3	9.0	4	7	7	9	11	11	11	11
65+	2	7.5	4	6	6	9	9	9	9	9
2. MULTIPLE DX										
A. Not Operated										
0–19 Years	0									
20–34	5	11.0	152	1	3	4	17	30	30	30
35–49	80	5.5	31	1	2	4	7	7	15	29
50–64	321	6.1	44	1	2	4	7	12	17	27
65+	577	5.9	38	2	2	4	7	12	14	29
B. Operated										
0–19 Years	0									
20–34	3	9.0	19	4	4	11	12	12	12	12
35–49	42	12.2	119	4	5	10	16	24	29	56
50–64	213	13.3	89	5	8	11	16	23	29	52
65+	259	13.1	83	5	8	10	16	24	34	49
SUBTOTALS:										
1. SINGLE DX — A. Not Operated	10	4.3	19	1	1	3	6	15	15	15
1. SINGLE DX — B. Operated	5	8.4	4	6	7	9	9	11	11	11
2. MULTIPLE DX — A. Not Operated	983	5.9	40	1	2	4	7	12	15	29
2. MULTIPLE DX — B. Operated	517	13.1	88	5	8	11	16	24	32	51
1. SINGLE DX	15	5.7	17	1	2	6	9	11	15	15
2. MULTIPLE DX	1,500	8.4	68	2	3	6	11	18	23	43
A. NOT OPERATED	993	5.9	40	1	2	4	7	12	15	29
B. OPERATED	522	13.0	87	5	8	10	16	24	31	51
TOTAL										
0–19 Years	0									
20–34	8	10.2	93	1	3	4	12	30	30	30
35–49	123	7.8	70	2	3	5	10	18	24	39
50–64	545	8.9	73	2	3	7	11	19	23	42
65+	839	8.1	63	2	3	6	10	16	23	43
GRAND TOTAL	1,515	8.4	68	2	3	6	11	18	23	42

Western Region, October 2006–September 2007 Data, by Diagnosis

150.5: LOWER 3RD ESOPHAGUS CA

Type of Patients	Observed Patients	Avg. Stay	Variance	10th	25th	50th	75th	90th	95th	99th
1. SINGLE DX										
A. Not Operated										
0–19 Years	0									
20–34	0									
35–49	0									
50–64	0									
65+	0									
B. Operated										
0–19 Years	0									
20–34	0									
35–49	0									
50–64	2	8.0	2	7	7	9	9	9	9	9
65+	2	7.5	4	6	6	9	9	9	9	9
2. MULTIPLE DX										
A. Not Operated										
0–19 Years	0									
20–34	3	17.0	169	4	4	17	30	30	30	30
35–49	29	5.2	25	1	2	5	7	15	15	22
50–64	103	6.6	35	2	3	5	8	12	17	25
65+	185	6.0	25	1	2	5	7	13	16	25
B. Operated										
0–19 Years	0									
20–34	1	4.0	0	4	4	4	4	4	4	4
35–49	24	13.5	137	3	6	11	20	24	29	56
50–64	124	12.7	69	7	8	11	15	22	24	33
65+	159	13.5	88	6	8	10	16	24	34	49
SUBTOTALS:										
1. SINGLE DX										
A. Not Operated	0									
B. Operated	4	7.8	2	6	7	9	9	9	9	9
2. MULTIPLE DX										
A. Not Operated	320	6.2	30	2	3	5	8	13	16	25
B. Operated	308	13.1	83	6	6	10	16	23	30	49
1. SINGLE DX	4	7.8	2	6	7	9	9	9	9	9
2. MULTIPLE DX	628	9.6	68	2	4	8	12	20	24	43
A. NOT OPERATED	320	6.2	30	2	3	5	8	13	16	25
B. OPERATED	312	13.1	83	6	8	10	16	23	30	49
TOTAL										
0–19 Years	0									
20–34	4	13.7	155	4	4	4	30	30	30	30
35–49	53	9.0	91	2	3	6	11	21	24	56
50–64	229	9.9	62	3	5	8	12	20	23	33
65+	346	9.4	67	2	4	8	11	20	24	46
GRAND TOTAL	632	9.6	68	2	4	8	12	20	24	43

150.8: ESOPHAGUS CA NEC

Type of Patients	Observed Patients	Avg. Stay	Variance	10th	25th	50th	75th	90th	95th	99th
1. SINGLE DX										
A. Not Operated										
0–19 Years	0									
20–34	0									
35–49	1	3.0	0	3	3	3	3	3	3	3
50–64	2	9.0	70	3	3	15	15	15	15	15
65+	0									
B. Operated										
0–19 Years	0									
20–34	0									
35–49	0									
50–64	0									
65+	0									
2. MULTIPLE DX										
A. Not Operated										
0–19 Years	0									
20–34	1	3.0	0	3	3	3	3	3	3	3
35–49	13	4.0	7	1	2	3	7	7	8	8
50–64	81	7.1	96	1	2	5	8	12	23	78
65+	123	6.1	91	2	2	4	7	9	13	64
B. Operated										
0–19 Years	0									
20–34	1	11.0	0	11	11	11	11	11	11	11
35–49	6	13.5	159	5	8	9	10	39	39	39
50–64	22	20.7	226	7	10	17	27	41	44	62
65+	29	11.7	41	4	8	12	16	22	29	>99
SUBTOTALS:										
1. SINGLE DX										
A. Not Operated	3	7.0	48	3	3	3	15	15	15	15
B. Operated	0									
2. MULTIPLE DX										
A. Not Operated	218	6.3	87	2	2	4	7	10	16	64
B. Operated	58	15.3	136	5	8	11	21	37	44	>99
1. SINGLE DX	3	7.0	48	3	3	3	15	15	15	15
2. MULTIPLE DX	276	8.2	110	2	3	5	9	17	29	78
A. NOT OPERATED	221	6.3	87	2	2	4	7	10	15	64
B. OPERATED	58	15.3	136	5	8	11	21	37	44	>99
TOTAL										
0–19 Years	0									
20–34	2	7.0	31	3	3	3	11	11	11	11
35–49	20	6.7	65	1	2	3	5	8	10	39
50–64	105	10.0	150	1	3	6	10	24	32	62
65+	152	7.2	86	2	3	5	8	14	22	79
GRAND TOTAL	279	8.2	110	2	3	5	9	17	27	78

150.9: ESOPHAGUS CA NOS

Type of Patients	Observed Patients	Avg. Stay	Variance	10th	25th	50th	75th	90th	95th	99th
1. SINGLE DX										
A. Not Operated										
0–19 Years	0									
20–34	0									
35–49	0									
50–64	5	1.8	2	1	1	1	2	4	4	4
65+	0									
B. Operated										
0–19 Years	0									
20–34	0									
35–49	0									
50–64	0									
65+	0									
2. MULTIPLE DX										
A. Not Operated										
0–19 Years	0									
20–34	1	1.0	0	1	1	1	1	1	1	1
35–49	26	4.8	29	2	3	3	4	8	9	29
50–64	85	4.3	14	1	2	3	5	8	13	18
65+	162	5.4	25	1	2	4	7	11	13	29
B. Operated										
0–19 Years	0									
20–34	1	12.0	0	12	12	12	12	12	12	12
35–49	4	9.3	144	1	3	6	27	27	27	27
50–64	32	12.1	84	2	7	12	14	19	22	52
65+	31	11.8	87	3	6	10	14	21	30	46
SUBTOTALS:										
1. SINGLE DX										
A. Not Operated	5	1.8	2	1	1	1	2	4	4	4
B. Operated	0									
2. MULTIPLE DX										
A. Not Operated	274	5.0	22	1	2	4	6	9	13	29
B. Operated	68	11.8	85	2	6	11	13	22	29	52
1. SINGLE DX	5	1.8	2	1	1	1	2	4	4	4
2. MULTIPLE DX	342	6.4	42	1	2	4	8	13	18	30
A. NOT OPERATED	279	5.0	22	1	2	4	6	9	13	29
B. OPERATED	68	11.8	85	2	6	11	13	22	29	52
TOTAL										
0–19 Years	0									
20–34	2	6.5	59	1	1	3	12	12	12	12
35–49	30	5.4	42	1	3	3	6	8	27	29
50–64	122	6.2	44	2	3	4	8	13	18	22
65+	193	6.5	40	2	3	4	8	12	18	33
GRAND TOTAL	347	6.3	42	1	2	4	8	13	18	30

63

Length of Stay by Diagnosis and Operation, Western Region, 2008

Western Region, October 2006–September 2007 Data, by Diagnosis

151: STOMACH CA

Type of Patients	Observed Patients	Avg. Stay	Vari-ance	Percentiles 10th	25th	50th	75th	90th	95th	99th
1. SINGLE DX										
A. Not Operated										
0–19 Years	0									
20–34	2	1.0	0	1	1	1	1	1	1	1
35–49	0									
50–64	7	4.7	27	1	2	3	6	16	16	16
65+	1	1.0	0	1	1	1	1	1	1	1
B. Operated										
0–19 Years	0									
20–34	1	5.0	0	5	5	5	5	5	5	5
35–49	7	6.7	13	1	5	7	8	13	13	13
50–64	14	6.9	5	4	5	6	9	9	11	11
65+	7	6.1	6	4	4	6	8	10	10	10
2. MULTIPLE DX										
A. Not Operated										
0–19 Years	1	13.0	0	13	13	13	13	13	13	13
20–34	46	8.4	127	1	2	6	12	17	18	73
35–49	204	6.1	32	1	2	4	8	14	19	25
50–64	455	6.4	41	2	2	4	8	14	18	36
65+	889	5.5	22	2	3	4	7	11	14	22
B. Operated										
0–19 Years	2	11.5	<1	11	11	12	12	12	12	12
20–34	35	11.4	35	5	7	10	15	19	22	26
35–49	187	12.0	69	5	7	10	14	24	31	57
50–64	557	12.2	72	5	7	10	15	23	29	49
65+	1,064	12.3	75	5	7	10	15	22	28	56
SUBTOTALS:										
1. SINGLE DX										
A. Not Operated	10	3.6	22	1	1	2	3	16	16	16
B. Operated	29	6.6	6	4	5	6	8	10	11	13
2. MULTIPLE DX										
A. Not Operated	1,595	5.9	32	2	2	4	7	13	17	25
B. Operated	1,845	12.2	72	5	7	10	15	23	28	49
1. SINGLE DX	39	5.9	12	1	4	6	8	10	13	16
2. MULTIPLE DX	3,440	9.3	63	2	4	7	12	18	24	43
A. NOT OPERATED	1,605	5.9	32	2	2	4	7	13	17	25
B. OPERATED	1,874	12.2	72	5	7	10	15	22	28	49
TOTAL										
0–19 Years	3	12.0	<1	11	11	12	13	13	13	13
20–34	84	9.4	87	2	3	8	13	18	19	73
35–49	398	8.9	58	2	3	7	12	20	26	36
50–64	1,033	9.5	65	2	4	8	12	19	26	46
65+	1,961	9.2	62	2	4	7	12	18	23	42
GRAND TOTAL	3,479	9.3	63	2	4	7	12	18	24	43

151.0: STOMACH CARDIA CA

Type of Patients	Observed Patients	Avg. Stay	Vari-ance	Percentiles 10th	25th	50th	75th	90th	95th	99th
1. SINGLE DX										
A. Not Operated										
0–19 Years	0									
20–34	0									
35–49	0									
50–64	3	7.0	60	2	2	3	16	16	16	16
65+	0									
B. Operated										
0–19 Years	0									
20–34	1	1.0	0	1	1	1	1	1	1	1
35–49	3	8.0	3	6	6	9	9	9	9	9
50–64										
65+	2	9.0	2	8	8	10	10	10	10	10
2. MULTIPLE DX										
A. Not Operated										
0–19 Years	0									
20–34	5	7.8	43	2	2	6	12	17	17	17
35–49	53	5.5	25	2	2	3	7	11	17	25
50–64	165	5.5	19	2	3	4	7	11	14	23
65+	293	5.7	27	2	2	4	7	11	16	26
B. Operated										
0–19 Years	0									
20–34	4	13.2	45	6	6	9	19	19	19	19
35–49	42	13.7	73	7	8	10	17	24	32	38
50–64	191	12.7	81	6	8	10	15	22	29	54
65+	271	13.4	86	6	8	11	15	24	29	57
SUBTOTALS:										
1. SINGLE DX										
A. Not Operated	3	7.0	60	2	2	3	16	16	16	16
B. Operated	6	7.2	11	1	6	9	9	10	10	10
2. MULTIPLE DX										
A. Not Operated	516	5.6	24	2	2	4	7	12	15	23
B. Operated	508	13.1	82	6	8	11	15	24	29	54
1. SINGLE DX	9	7.1	22	1	3	8	9	16	16	16
2. MULTIPLE DX	1,024	9.4	67	2	4	8	12	18	24	45
A. NOT OPERATED	519	5.6	24	2	2	4	7	12	15	23
B. OPERATED	514	13.1	82	6	8	11	15	24	29	54
TOTAL										
0–19 Years	0									
20–34	9	10.2	47	2	6	9	17	19	19	19
35–49	96	9.0	63	2	3	7	13	20	25	38
50–64	362	9.4	64	2	4	8	12	18	24	49
65+	566	9.4	70	2	4	8	12	18	24	45
GRAND TOTAL	1,033	9.3	67	2	4	8	12	18	24	45

151.2: PYLORIC ANTRUM CA

Type of Patients	Observed Patients	Avg. Stay	Vari-ance	Percentiles 10th	25th	50th	75th	90th	95th	99th
1. SINGLE DX										
A. Not Operated										
0–19 Years	0									
20–34	0									
35–49	0									
50–64	1	6.0	0	6	6	6	6	6	6	6
65+	0									
B. Operated										
0–19 Years	0									
20–34	0									
35–49	1	8.0	0	8	8	8	8	8	8	8
50–64	1	4.0	0	4	4	4	4	4	4	4
65+	0									
2. MULTIPLE DX										
A. Not Operated										
0–19 Years	1	13.0	0	13	13	13	13	13	13	13
20–34	5	10.8	47	3	7	8	17	19	19	19
35–49	10	5.7	47	1	2	4	9	14	22	22
50–64	29	10.2	187	2	3	7	17	17	54	60
65+	122	5.2	15	2	2	4	6	11	13	18
B. Operated										
0–19 Years	0									
20–34	10	12.0	20	12	8	12	12	12	12	12
35–49	33	12.6	31	6	8	10	15	17	20	31
50–64	86	12.1	64	5	7	9	15	23	26	44
65+	237	12.5	55	6	7	10	15	22	27	39
SUBTOTALS:										
1. SINGLE DX										
A. Not Operated	1	6.0	0	6	6	6	6	6	6	6
B. Operated	2	6.0	8	4	4	4	8	8	8	8
2. MULTIPLE DX										
A. Not Operated	167	6.3	51	2	2	4	7	13	17	54
B. Operated	367	12.2	54	6	7	10	15	22	26	42
1. SINGLE DX	3	6.0	4	4	4	6	8	8	8	8
2. MULTIPLE DX	534	10.4	60	3	6	8	14	20	24	42
A. NOT OPERATED	168	6.3	51	2	2	4	7	13	17	54
B. OPERATED	369	12.2	54	6	7	10	15	22	26	42
TOTAL										
0–19 Years	2	12.5	<1	12	12	13	13	13	13	13
20–34	15	12.0	27	7	8	11	16	19	22	22
35–49	44	9.4	38	2	5	8	13	17	20	31
50–64	117	11.5	93	4	6	8	14	23	27	54
65+	359	10.0	53	3	5	8	13	20	23	38
GRAND TOTAL	537	10.4	60	3	6	8	14	20	24	42

Length of Stay by Diagnosis and Operation, Western Region, 2008

Western Region, October 2006–September 2007 Data, by Diagnosis

151.4: STOMACH BODY CA

Type of Patients	Observed Patients	Avg. Stay	Variance	Percentiles						
				10th	25th	50th	75th	90th	95th	99th
1. SINGLE DX										
A. *Not Operated*										
0–19 Years	0									
20–34	1	1.0	0			1	1	1	1	1
35–49	0									
50–64	1	2.0	0	2	2	2	2	2	2	2
65+	0									
B. *Operated*										
0–19 Years	0									
20–34	0									
35–49	0									
50–64	3	7.0	12	5	5	5	11	11	11	11
65+	0									
2. MULTIPLE DX										
A. *Not Operated*										
0–19 Years	0									
20–34	6	6.6	17	2	3	4	10	12	12	12
35–49	18	6.3	54	1	3	3	7	24	27	27
50–64	40	7.7	51	2	2	4	11	17	23	29
65+	82	4.4	9	1	3	4	5	8	9	17
B. *Operated*										
0–19 Years	0									
20–34	6	10.5	36	5	6	10	10	22	22	22
35–49	24	10.8	57	3	6	10	14	22	26	31
50–64	55	10.7	46	4	6	9	13	22	26	32
65+	106	10.5	37	5	7	9	12	20	25	28
SUBTOTALS:										
1. SINGLE DX										
A. *Not Operated*	2	1.5	<1	1	1	1	2	2	2	2
B. *Operated*	3	7.0	12	5	5	5	11	11	11	11
2. MULTIPLE DX										
A. *Not Operated*	146	5.6	28	2	2	4	7	11	17	27
B. *Operated*	191	10.6	41	5	6	9	13	21	26	32
1. SINGLE DX	5	4.8	15	1	2	5	5	11	11	11
2. MULTIPLE DX	337	8.5	41	2	4	7	11	17	23	30
A. NOT OPERATED	148	5.6	27	1	2	4	7	11	17	27
B. OPERATED	194	10.6	41	5	6	9	13	21	26	32
TOTAL										
0–19 Years	0									
20–34	13	8.0	30	2	4	9	10	12	22	22
35–49	42	8.9	60	2	3	3	11	22	26	31
50–64	99	9.3	49	4	4	8	12	17	24	30
65+	188	7.9	34	2	4	7	10	15	21	28
GRAND TOTAL	342	8.4	41	2	4	7	11	17	23	30

151.8: STOMACH CA NEC

Type of Patients	Observed Patients	Avg. Stay	Variance	Percentiles						
				10th	25th	50th	75th	90th	95th	99th
1. SINGLE DX										
A. *Not Operated*										
0–19 Years	0									
20–34	0									
35–49	0									
50–64	1	3.0	0	3	3	3	3	3	3	3
65+	1	1.0	0	1	1	1	1	1	1	1
B. *Operated*										
0–19 Years	0									
20–34	1	5.0	0	5	5	5	5	5	5	5
35–49	2	10.0	18	7	7	13	13	13	13	13
50–64	2	8.5	<1	8	8	8	9	9	9	9
65+	3	5.0	3	4	4	4	7	7	7	7
2. MULTIPLE DX										
A. *Not Operated*										
0–19 Years	0									
20–34	15	11.2	326	1	2	6	13	18	73	73
35–49	50	7.9	40	2	4	6	9	18	21	32
50–64	93	6.9	53	2	3	4	8	15	19	46
65+	149	5.7	25	2	2	4	7	11	16	18
B. *Operated*										
0–19 Years	0									
20–34	8	11.0	0	11	11	11	11	11	11	11
35–49	41	12.4	124	4	6	9	14	32	35	>99
50–64	100	12.3	62	5	7	10	16	26	29	33
65+	188	13.7	133	5	7	10	16	27	39	83
SUBTOTALS:										
1. SINGLE DX										
A. *Not Operated*	2	2.0	2	1	1	1	3	3	3	3
B. *Operated*	8	7.1	9	4	4	7	8	13	13	13
2. MULTIPLE DX										
A. *Not Operated*	307	6.7	51	2	3	5	8	15	18	36
B. *Operated*	338	13.0	108	5	7	10	16	27	33	67
1. SINGLE DX	10	6.1	12	1	4	5	8	13	13	13
2. MULTIPLE DX	645	10.0	91	2	4	7	12	21	28	58
A. NOT OPERATED	309	6.7	51	2	3	5	8	15	18	36
B. OPERATED	346	12.9	107	5	7	10	15	27	33	67
TOTAL										
0–19 Years	1	11.0	0	11	11	11	11	11	11	11
20–34	24	10.6	211	1	2	7	15	17	18	73
35–49	93	9.9	80	2	5	8	12	23	32	>99
50–64	196	9.6	64	2	4	7	12	21	28	36
65+	341	10.1	100	2	4	7	12	20	28	59
GRAND TOTAL	655	10.0	90	2	4	7	12	21	28	58

151.9: STOMACH CA NOS

Type of Patients	Observed Patients	Avg. Stay	Variance	Percentiles						
				10th	25th	50th	75th	90th	95th	99th
1. SINGLE DX										
A. *Not Operated*										
0–19 Years	0									
20–34	1	1.0	0	1	1	1	1	1	1	1
35–49	0									
50–64	1	1.0	0	1	1	1	1	1	1	1
65+	0									
B. *Operated*										
0–19 Years	0									
20–34	0									
35–49	2	6.5	<1	6	6	6	7	7	7	7
50–64	4	6.2	5	4	4	5	7	9	9	9
65+	0									
2. MULTIPLE DX										
A. *Not Operated*										
0–19 Years	0									
20–34	12	4.7	21	1	2	3	5	9	17	17
35–49	56	4.7	18	2	4	3	6	13	15	20
50–64	104	5.7	22	1	2	3	8	15	15	25
65+	170	5.8	23	1	2	4	7	12	15	24
B. *Operated*										
0–19 Years	0									
20–34	17	21.5	40	17	17	17	26	26	26	26
35–49	17	14.3	58	7	9	12	17	27	31	31
50–64	53	12.4	104	4	6	9	15	24	30	60
65+	79	10.7	54	5	6	9	13	20	25	43
SUBTOTALS:										
1. SINGLE DX										
A. *Not Operated*	2	1.0	0	1	1	1	1	1	1	1
B. *Operated*	6	6.3	3	4	5	6	7	9	9	9
2. MULTIPLE DX										
A. *Not Operated*	342	5.5	22	1	2	4	7	12	15	24
B. *Operated*	151	11.9	73	5	6	9	15	23	29	43
1. SINGLE DX	8	5.0	8	1	4	5	7	9	9	9
2. MULTIPLE DX	493	7.5	46	2	3	6	10	15	21	37
A. NOT OPERATED	344	5.5	22	1	2	4	7	12	15	24
B. OPERATED	157	11.6	72	5	6	9	14	23	29	43
TOTAL										
0–19 Years	0									
20–34	15	6.7	56	1	2	3	9	17	26	26
35–49	75	6.9	42	1	3	5	9	15	23	31
50–64	162	7.8	58	1	3	6	10	16	22	60
65+	249	7.4	38	2	3	6	10	14	20	27
GRAND TOTAL	501	7.4	45	2	3	6	10	15	20	37

Length of Stay by Diagnosis and Operation, Western Region, 2008

Western Region, October 2006–September 2007 Data, by Diagnosis

152: SMALL INTESTINE CA

Type of Patients	Observed Patients	Avg. Stay	Variance	10th	25th	50th	75th	90th	95th	99th
1. SINGLE DX										
A. Not Operated										
0–19 Years	0									
20–34	0									
35–49	0									
50–64	0									
65+	0									
B. Operated										
0–19 Years	0									
20–34	1	6.0	0	6	6	6	6	6	6	6
35–49	2	10.6	83	4	4	17	17	17	17	17
50–64	0									
65+	0									
2. MULTIPLE DX										
A. Not Operated										
0–19 Years	0									
20–34	1	27.0	0	27	27	27	27	27	27	27
35–49	11	8.7	212	2	3	4	7	7	52	52
50–64	29	7.3	58	1	3	4	8	19	21	35
65+	98	6.7	43	2	3	5	8	13	17	51
B. Operated										
0–19 Years	0									
20–34	7	10.9	49	6	7	8	11	26	26	26
35–49	67	9.3	50	4	5	7	10	21	23	33
50–64	179	10.2	79	4	5	7	12	19	26	63
65+	270	12.3	72	4	7	10	15	22	32	56
SUBTOTALS:										
1. SINGLE DX										
A. Not Operated	0									
B. Operated	3	9.0	49	4	4	6	17	17	17	17
2. MULTIPLE DX										
A. Not Operated	139	7.1	61	2	3	5	8	15	21	51
B. Operated	523	11.2	72	4	6	9	14	22	29	46
1. SINGLE DX	3	9.0	49	4	4	6	17	17	17	17
2. MULTIPLE DX	662	10.3	72	3	5	8	13	20	28	51
A. NOT OPERATED	139	7.1	61	2	3	5	8	15	21	51
B. OPERATED	526	11.1	72	4	6	9	14	22	29	46
TOTAL										
0–19 Years	0									
20–34	8	12.9	74	6	7	8	26	27	27	27
35–49	79	9.2	69	3	4	6	10	21	29	52
50–64	210	9.8	77	3	5	7	11	18	26	36
65+	368	10.8	70	3	5	9	14	20	29	51
GRAND TOTAL	665	10.3	72	3	5	8	13	20	28	51

152.0: DUODENUM CA

Type of Patients	Observed Patients	Avg. Stay	Variance	10th	25th	50th	75th	90th	95th	99th
1. SINGLE DX										
A. Not Operated										
0–19 Years	0									
20–34	0									
35–49	0									
50–64	0									
65+	0									
B. Operated										
0–19 Years	0									
20–34	0									
35–49	0									
50–64	1	17.0	0	17	17	17	17	17	17	17
65+	0									
2. MULTIPLE DX										
A. Not Operated										
0–19 Years	0									
20–34	0									
35–49	11	8.7	212	2	3	4	7	7	52	52
50–64	15	6.1	33	1	2	4	8	18	19	19
65+	75	6.5	47	2	3	4	8	11	14	51
B. Operated										
0–19 Years	0									
20–34	13	16.5	177	7	7	17	26	26	26	26
35–49	13	17.0	97	8	8	13	23	30	33	33
50–64	51	14.2	136	4	6	11	16	28	35	69
65+	82	16.2	101	7	9	14	20	30	41	>99
SUBTOTALS:										
1. SINGLE DX										
A. Not Operated	0									
B. Operated	1	17.0	0	17	17	17	17	17	17	17
2. MULTIPLE DX										
A. Not Operated	101	6.6	61	2	3	4	8	11	18	51
B. Operated	148	15.6	112	6	8	13	19	30	37	69
1. SINGLE DX	1	17.0	0	17	17	17	17	17	17	17
2. MULTIPLE DX	249	12.0	111	3	5	9	15	26	34	56
A. NOT OPERATED	101	6.6	61	2	3	4	8	11	18	51
B. OPERATED	149	15.6	111	6	8	13	19	30	37	69
TOTAL										
0–19 Years	0									
20–34	2	16.5	177	7	7	17	26	26	26	26
35–49	24	13.2	161	3	5	8	23	30	33	52
50–64	67	12.4	122	3	5	10	16	26	33	69
65+	157	11.5	99	3	5	9	15	23	37	56
GRAND TOTAL	250	12.0	110	3	5	9	15	26	34	56

153: COLON CA

Type of Patients	Observed Patients	Avg. Stay	Variance	10th	25th	50th	75th	90th	95th	99th
1. SINGLE DX										
A. Not Operated										
0–19 Years	1	1.0	0	1	1	1	1	1	1	1
20–34	0									
35–49	1	3.0	0	3	3	3	3	3	3	3
50–64	2	1.5	<1	1	1	2	2	2	2	2
65+	2	2.5	4	1	1	4	4	4	4	4
B. Operated										
0–19 Years	3	3.0	4	1	4	3	5	5	5	5
20–34	11	4.7	2	4	4	5	5	6	7	7
35–49	59	4.7	11	3	3	5	5	7	8	27
50–64	140	4.1	3	2	3	4	5	6	7	9
65+	67	4.8	5	2	3	5	6	7	8	14
2. MULTIPLE DX										
A. Not Operated										
0–19 Years	0									
20–34	20	7.5	81	2	3	5	6	12	21	41
35–49	150	4.6	16	1	2	4	6	10	11	27
50–64	449	5.1	23	1	2	4	6	9	15	21
65+	1,199	4.9	16	1	2	4	6	9	13	19
B. Operated										
0–19 Years	6	3.2	6	1	3	3	3	8	8	8
20–34	125	7.7	27	3	5	7	10	13	14	24
35–49	901	8.2	40	4	6	7	10	14	18	39
50–64	3,280	7.6	34	3	4	6	9	14	18	32
65+	8,271	8.8	38	4	5	7	10	16	21	33
SUBTOTALS:										
1. SINGLE DX										
A. Not Operated	6	2.0	2	1	1	3	3	4	4	4
B. Operated	280	4.4	5	2	3	5	5	7	7	12
2. MULTIPLE DX										
A. Not Operated	1,818	5.0	18	1	2	4	6	10	13	20
B. Operated	12,583	8.4	37	4	5	7	10	15	20	33
1. SINGLE DX	286	4.4	5	2	3	4	5	7	7	12
2. MULTIPLE DX	14,401	8.0	36	3	4	6	9	15	19	32
A. NOT OPERATED	1,824	5.0	18	1	2	4	6	10	13	20
B. OPERATED	12,863	8.3	37	4	5	7	10	15	20	33
TOTAL										
0–19 Years	10	2.9	5	1	1	3	3	5	8	8
20–34	156	7.5	32	3	4	6	9	13	15	41
35–49	1,111	7.5	37	3	4	6	9	13	17	35
50–64	3,871	7.2	32	3	4	6	8	13	18	31
65+	9,539	8.3	37	3	5	7	10	15	20	31
GRAND TOTAL	14,687	7.9	36	3	4	6	9	14	19	31

Length of Stay by Diagnosis and Operation, Western Region, 2008

Western Region, October 2006–September 2007 Data, by Diagnosis

153.0: HEPATIC FLEXURE CA

Type of Patients	Observed Patients	Avg. Stay	Variance	Percentiles 10th	25th	50th	75th	90th	95th	99th
1. SINGLE DX										
A. *Not Operated*										
0–19 Years	0									
20–34	0									
35–49	0									
50–64	0									
65+	0									
B. *Operated*										
0–19 Years	0									
20–34	0									
35–49	0									
50–64	7	3.9	1	2	3		5	5	5	5
65+	6	3.8	3	1	3		5	6	6	6
2. MULTIPLE DX										
A. *Not Operated*										
0–19 Years	0									
20–34	1	2.0	0	2	2	2	2	2	2	2
35–49	4	7.5	43	1	1	3	11	15	15	15
50–64	13	5.4	44	1	2	3	4	19	21	21
65+	62	5.1	12	2	3	4	6	9	13	16
B. *Operated*										
0–19 Years	0									
20–34	6	8.5	16	3	5	10	11	14	14	14
35–49	41	7.9	19	4	5	7	10	14	15	23
50–64	161	8.1	35	4	5	7	9	13	17	42
65+	490	9.4	49	4	5	7	11	17	23	43
SUBTOTALS:										
1. SINGLE DX										
A. *Not Operated*	0									
B. *Operated*	13	3.9	2	2	3	4	5	5	5	6
2. MULTIPLE DX										
A. *Not Operated*	80	5.3	18	1	3	4	6	11	15	21
B. *Operated*	698	9.0	44	4	5	7	11	16	22	38
1. SINGLE DX	13	3.9	2	2	3	4	5	5	5	6
2. MULTIPLE DX	778	8.6	43	3	5	7	10	15	21	38
A. NOT OPERATED	80	5.3	18	1	3	4	6	11	15	21
B. OPERATED	711	8.9	44	4	5	7	10	16	22	38
TOTAL										
0–19 Years	0									
20–34	7	7.6	20	2	3	8	11	14	14	14
35–49	45	7.8	21	3	5	7	11	14	15	23
50–64	181	7.8	35	3	4	7	9	13	18	42
65+	558	8.9	47	3	5	7	10	16	22	38
GRAND TOTAL	791	8.6	42	3	5	7	10	15	21	38

153.1: TRANSVERSE COLON CA

Type of Patients	Observed Patients	Avg. Stay	Variance	Percentiles 10th	25th	50th	75th	90th	95th	99th
1. SINGLE DX										
A. *Not Operated*										
0–19 Years	0									
20–34	0									
35–49	0									
50–64	0									
65+	0									
B. *Operated*										
0–19 Years	0									
20–34	0									
35–49	2	15.0	280	3	3	15	27	27	27	27
50–64	12	5.0	1	4	4	5	6	6	7	7
65+	8	4.4	5	2	2	4	5	9	9	9
2. MULTIPLE DX										
A. *Not Operated*										
0–19 Years	0									
20–34	0									
35–49	6	4.0	5	1	3	3	6	7	7	7
50–64	20	4.4	11	1	2	3	7	10	12	12
65+	73	4.7	12	2	2	4	6	8	9	22
B. *Operated*										
0–19 Years	0									
20–34	17	9.8	18	5	7	10	11	14	21	21
35–49	74	9.5	30	4	6	8	12	18	23	>99
50–64	292	8.6	46	4	5	7	10	16	20	28
65+	944	9.0	35	4	5	7	11	16	21	33
SUBTOTALS:										
1. SINGLE DX										
A. *Not Operated*	0									
B. *Operated*	22	5.7	26	3	4	4	6	7	9	27
2. MULTIPLE DX										
A. *Not Operated*	99	4.6	11	1	2	4	6	9	10	22
B. *Operated*	1,327	8.9	37	4	5	7	11	16	21	32
1. SINGLE DX	22	5.7	26	3	4	4	6	7	9	27
2. MULTIPLE DX	1,426	8.6	36	4	5	7	10	15	21	31
A. NOT OPERATED	99	4.6	11	1	2	4	6	9	10	22
B. OPERATED	1,349	8.9	37	4	5	7	10	16	21	32
TOTAL										
0–19 Years	0									
20–34	17	9.8	18	5	7	10	11	14	21	21
35–49	82	9.2	34	4	5	8	11	18	23	>99
50–64	324	8.2	44	3	5	6	9	15	20	28
65+	1,025	8.6	34	4	5	7	10	15	20	32
GRAND TOTAL	1,448	8.6	36	4	5	7	10	15	21	31

153.2: DESCENDING COLON CA

Type of Patients	Observed Patients	Avg. Stay	Variance	Percentiles 10th	25th	50th	75th	90th	95th	99th
1. SINGLE DX										
A. *Not Operated*										
0–19 Years	0									
20–34	0									
35–49	1	3.0	0	3	3	3	3	3	3	3
50–64	0									
65+	0									
B. *Operated*										
0–19 Years	0									
20–34	1	5.0	0	5	5	5	5	5	5	5
35–49	9	4.2	2	2	3	5	5	6	6	6
50–64	9	5.1	3	2	4	5	6	7	7	7
65+	0									
2. MULTIPLE DX										
A. *Not Operated*										
0–19 Years	0									
20–34	0									
35–49	4	3.7	9	1	1	3	3	8	8	8
50–64	17	4.1	10	1	2	4	5	8	13	13
65+	51	5.7	16	2	3	4	8	11	14	18
B. *Operated*										
0–19 Years	0									
20–34	9	6.7	21	3	4	5	6	6	18	18
35–49	70	8.2	43	4	5	7	9	14	15	54
50–64	213	7.7	21	4	5	6	9	14	17	23
65+	468	9.1	52	4	5	7	11	17	22	31
SUBTOTALS:										
1. SINGLE DX										
A. *Not Operated*	1	3.0	0	3	3	3	3	3	3	3
B. *Operated*	19	4.7	2	2	4	5	5	6	7	7
2. MULTIPLE DX										
A. *Not Operated*	72	5.2	15	1	2	4	4	10	14	18
B. *Operated*	760	8.6	42	4	5	7	10	16	20	29
1. SINGLE DX	20	4.6	2	2	4	5	6	6	7	7
2. MULTIPLE DX	832	8.3	41	3	5	7	10	16	20	29
A. NOT OPERATED	73	5.2	15	1	2	4	4	10	14	18
B. OPERATED	779	8.5	41	4	5	7	10	16	20	29
TOTAL										
0–19 Years	0									
20–34	10	6.5	19	3	4	5	6	9	18	18
35–49	84	7.5	38	3	4	6	8	13	14	54
50–64	239	7.3	20	3	4	5	7	13	16	23
65+	519	8.7	49	4	5	7	10	17	22	30
GRAND TOTAL	852	8.2	40	3	5	6	10	16	20	29

Length of Stay by Diagnosis and Operation, Western Region, 2008

Western Region, October 2006–September 2007 Data, by Diagnosis

153.3: SIGMOID COLON CA

Type of Patients	Observed Patients	Avg. Stay	Variance	10th	25th	50th	75th	90th	95th	99th
1. SINGLE DX										
A. Not Operated										
0–19 Years	0									
20–34	0									
35–49	0									
50–64	1	1.0	0	1	1	1	1	1	1	1
65+	0									
B. Operated										
0–19 Years	0									
20–34	4	4.8	<1	4	4	4	6	6	6	6
35–49	31	4.4	3	3	3	4	5	7	8	10
50–64	51	4.1	3	3	3	4	5	6	6	9
65+	16	4.1	2	2	4	4	5	5	7	7
2. MULTIPLE DX										
A. Not Operated										
0–19 Years	0									
20–34	2	4.5	<1	4	4	5	5	5	5	5
35–49	28	5.5	29	1	2	4	6	12	15	27
50–64	74	5.7	43	1	2	3	6	13	16	38
65+	176	5.3	30	1	2	4	6	11	15	34
B. Operated										
0–19 Years	0									
20–34	30	7.3	8	5	5	7	9	11	12	15
35–49	337	7.8	35	3	4	6	10	13	19	32
50–64	1,104	7.4	38	3	4	6	8	13	19	36
65+	1,738	8.7	39	4	5	7	10	15	20	35
SUBTOTALS:										
1. SINGLE DX										
A. Not Operated	1	1.0	0	1	1	1	1	1	1	1
B. Operated	102	4.2	3	2	3	4	5	6	7	9
2. MULTIPLE DX										
A. Not Operated	280	5.4	33	1	2	4	6	12	15	34
B. Operated	3,209	8.1	38	3	5	6	10	15	19	35
1. SINGLE DX	103	4.2	3	2	3	4	5	6	7	9
2. MULTIPLE DX	3,489	7.9	39	3	4	6	9	14	19	35
A. NOT OPERATED	281	5.4	33	1	2	4	6	12	15	34
B. OPERATED	3,311	8.0	38	3	4	6	9	14	19	34
TOTAL										
0–19 Years	0									
20–34	36	6.8	8	4	5	6	9	11	12	15
35–49	396	7.4	33	3	4	6	9	13	19	32
50–64	1,230	7.2	37	3	4	5	8	13	19	36
65+	1,930	8.3	39	3	5	7	10	15	19	34
GRAND TOTAL	3,592	7.8	38	3	4	6	9	14	19	34

153.4: CECUM CA

Type of Patients	Observed Patients	Avg. Stay	Variance	10th	25th	50th	75th	90th	95th	99th
1. SINGLE DX										
A. Not Operated										
0–19 Years	0									
20–34	0									
35–49	0									
50–64	0									
65+	0									
B. Operated										
0–19 Years	0									
20–34	1	4.0	0	4	4	4	4	4	4	4
35–49	9	3.8	<1	2	3	4	4	5	5	5
50–64	18	3.4	1	2	3	4	4	5	5	5
65+	12	4.6	4	2	3	4	6	7	7	7
2. MULTIPLE DX										
A. Not Operated										
0–19 Years	0									
20–34	4	7.0	5	5	5	7	10	10	10	10
35–49	18	6.2	38	1	3	4	8	13	27	27
50–64	66	4.7	14	1	2	4	6	8	11	21
65+	231	4.7	11	1	2	4	6	9	12	17
B. Operated										
0–19 Years	1	3.0	0	3	3	3	3	3	3	3
20–34	15	7.2	10	3	5	6	9	13	13	13
35–49	128	7.5	13	3	5	7	10	13	15	17
50–64	566	7.3	23	3	4	6	8	13	17	29
65+	1,891	8.6	34	4	5	7	10	16	20	29
SUBTOTALS:										
1. SINGLE DX										
A. Not Operated	0									
B. Operated	40	3.9	2	2	3	4	4	6	7	7
2. MULTIPLE DX										
A. Not Operated	319	4.8	13	1	2	4	6	9	12	19
B. Operated	2,601	8.2	31	4	5	7	10	15	19	28
1. SINGLE DX	40	3.9	2	2	3	4	5	6	7	7
2. MULTIPLE DX	2,920	7.9	30	3	4	6	9	14	18	28
A. NOT OPERATED	319	4.8	13	1	2	4	6	9	12	19
B. OPERATED	2,641	8.2	31	3	5	7	10	14	19	28
TOTAL										
0–19 Years	1	3.0	0	3	3	3	3	3	3	3
20–34	20	7.0	9	4	5	6	9	10	13	13
35–49	155	7.2	16	3	4	6	9	13	15	18
50–64	650	6.9	23	3	4	6	8	12	16	27
65+	2,134	8.1	33	3	5	7	10	15	19	28
GRAND TOTAL	2,960	7.8	30	3	4	6	9	14	18	28

153.5: APPENDIX CA

Type of Patients	Observed Patients	Avg. Stay	Variance	10th	25th	50th	75th	90th	95th	99th
1. SINGLE DX										
A. Not Operated										
0–19 Years	0									
20–34	0									
35–49	0									
50–64	0									
65+	0									
B. Operated										
0–19 Years	2	2.0	2	1	1	1	3	3	3	3
20–34	2	3.5	4	2	2	5	5	5	5	5
35–49	3	5.0	8	3	3	3	7	7	7	7
50–64	4	2.3	2	1	1	3	3	4	4	4
65+	0									
2. MULTIPLE DX										
A. Not Operated										
0–19 Years	0									
20–34	1	3.0	0	3	3	3	3	3	3	3
35–49	5	6.6	60	1	2	4	6	20	20	20
50–64	4	3.8	3	2	3	4	6	6	6	6
65+	0									
B. Operated										
0–19 Years	4	2.0	1	1	1	2	3	3	3	3
20–34	18	4.0	10	3	3	3	5	9	13	13
35–49	35	8.5	83	2	4	5	9	17	35	44
50–64	97	6.5	20	2	4	5	8	12	15	27
65+	78	8.4	32	3	5	7	10	15	22	30
SUBTOTALS:										
1. SINGLE DX										
A. Not Operated	0									
B. Operated	10	3.0	4	1	1	3	4	5	7	7
2. MULTIPLE DX										
A. Not Operated	10	5.1	30	1	2	4	6	20	20	20
B. Operated	232	7.2	34	2	4	6	9	14	17	30
1. SINGLE DX	10	3.0	4	1	1	3	4	5	7	7
2. MULTIPLE DX	242	7.1	34	2	4	6	9	14	17	30
A. NOT OPERATED	10	5.1	30	1	2	4	6	20	20	20
B. OPERATED	242	7.0	34	2	4	6	9	13	17	30
TOTAL										
0–19 Years	6	2.0	1	1	1	1	3	3	3	3
20–34	20	4.0	9	1	2	4	5	9	13	13
35–49	38	8.2	78	3	4	5	9	17	35	44
50–64	106	6.4	22	2	4	5	7	12	15	21
65+	82	8.2	31	3	5	7	10	14	18	30
GRAND TOTAL	252	6.9	33	2	3	5	8	13	17	30

Length of Stay by Diagnosis and Operation, Western Region, 2008

Western Region, October 2006–September 2007 Data, by Diagnosis

153.6: ASCENDING COLON CA

Type of Patients	Observed Patients	Avg. Stay	Variance	10th	25th	50th	75th	90th	95th	99th
1. SINGLE DX										
A. *Not Operated*										
0–19 Years	0									
20–34	0									
35–49	0									
50–64	1	2.0	0	2	2	2	2	2	2	2
65+	0									
B. *Operated*										
0–19 Years	1	5.0	0	5	5	5	5	5	5	5
20–34	2	6.0	2	5	5	7	7	7	7	7
35–49	5	4.8	4	3	4	4	5	8	8	8
50–64	24	4.2	5	2	3	4	5	6	8	12
65+	21	5.8	6	4	4	6	6	7	10	14
2. MULTIPLE DX										
A. *Not Operated*										
0–19 Years	0									
20–34	0									
35–49	9	3.4	7	1	2	3	4	10	10	10
50–64	30	4.9	14	2	3	4	6	12	12	18
65+	213	4.8	14	2	2	4	6	9	12	19
B. *Operated*										
0–19 Years	1	8.0	0	8	8	8	8	8	8	8
20–34	15	8.6	9	6	6	8	12	13	15	15
35–49	124	7.6	20	4	5	6	9	12	14	22
50–64	562	7.0	23	3	4	6	8	13	16	26
65+	2,122	8.5	39	4	5	7	10	15	20	35
SUBTOTALS:										
1. SINGLE DX										
A. *Not Operated*	1	2.0	0	2	2	2	2	2	2	2
B. *Operated*	53	5.0	6	2	4	5	7	7	10	14
2. MULTIPLE DX										
A. *Not Operated*	252	4.8	13	2	2	4	6	9	12	19
B. *Operated*	2,824	8.2	35	4	5	6	10	14	20	32
1. SINGLE DX	54	4.9	6	2	3	5	6	7	10	14
2. MULTIPLE DX	3,076	7.9	34	3	4	6	9	14	19	32
A. NOT OPERATED	253	4.8	13	2	2	4	6	9	12	19
B. OPERATED	2,877	8.1	35	3	5	6	10	14	19	32
TOTAL										
0–19 Years	2	6.5	5	5	5	7	8	8	8	8
20–34	17	8.3	9	5	5	6	9	13	15	15
35–49	138	7.2	20	3	4	6	9	12	14	22
50–64	617	6.8	22	3	4	5	8	12	15	24
65+	2,356	8.2	37	3	5	6	10	15	20	33
GRAND TOTAL	3,130	7.9	34	3	4	6	9	14	18	31

153.7: SPLENIC FLEXURE CA

Type of Patients	Observed Patients	Avg. Stay	Variance	10th	25th	50th	75th	90th	95th	99th
1. SINGLE DX										
A. *Not Operated*										
0–19 Years	0									
20–34	0									
35–49	0									
50–64	0									
65+	0									
B. *Operated*										
0–19 Years	0									
20–34	0									
35–49	0									
50–64	5	3.8	<1	3	4	4	4	4	4	4
65+	2	5.0	8	3	3	5	7	7	7	7
2. MULTIPLE DX										
A. *Not Operated*										
0–19 Years	0									
20–34	0									
35–49	4	7.5	6	4	8	8	10	10	10	10
50–64	15	3.7	11	1	1	3	5	6	14	14
65+	18	5.0	16	1	2	4	6	14	16	16
B. *Operated*										
0–19 Years	0									
20–34	7	14.6	213	4	5	8	24	44	44	44
35–49	36	10.6	69	4	5	8	14	16	39	40
50–64	119	9.4	69	4	5	7	11	15	26	46
65+	247	9.5	31	4	6	8	11	18	21	28
SUBTOTALS:										
1. SINGLE DX										
A. *Not Operated*	0									
B. *Operated*	7	4.1	2	3	3	4	4	7	7	7
2. MULTIPLE DX										
A. *Not Operated*	37	4.8	14	1	2	4	6	10	14	16
B. *Operated*	409	9.6	48	4	6	8	11	18	23	39
1. SINGLE DX	7	4.1	2	3	3	4	4	7	7	7
2. MULTIPLE DX	446	9.2	47	4	5	7	11	16	22	39
A. NOT OPERATED	37	4.8	14	1	2	4	6	10	14	16
B. OPERATED	416	9.5	48	4	6	8	11	17	23	39
TOTAL										
0–19 Years	0									
20–34	7	14.6	213	4	5	8	24	44	44	44
35–49	40	10.2	63	4	5	8	13	16	39	40
50–64	139	8.6	64	3	4	6	10	14	24	46
65+	267	9.1	31	4	6	8	11	17	21	28
GRAND TOTAL	453	9.1	47	4	5	7	11	16	22	39

153.8: LARGE INTESTINE CA NEC

Type of Patients	Observed Patients	Avg. Stay	Variance	10th	25th	50th	75th	90th	95th	99th
1. SINGLE DX										
A. *Not Operated*										
0–19 Years	1	1.0	0	1	1	1	1	1	1	1
20–34	0									
35–49	0									
50–64	0									
65+	0									
B. *Operated*										
0–19 Years	0									
20–34	1	5.0	0	5	5	5	5	5	5	5
35–49	1	4.0	0	4	4	4	4	4	4	4
50–64	3	3.7	2	2	2	4	5	5	5	5
65+	2	5.5	12	3	3	6	8	8	8	8
2. MULTIPLE DX										
A. *Not Operated*										
0–19 Years	0									
20–34	5	16.8	226	4	6	12	21	41	41	41
35–49	22	5.0	12	1	3	5	6	11	11	14
50–64	51	5.0	19	1	2	3	7	11	13	20
65+	86	5.1	11	2	3	5	6	9	11	17
B. *Operated*										
0–19 Years	0									
20–34	5	7.2	19	3	5	5	9	14	14	14
35–49	25	14.8	268	3	5	9	14	40	54	66
50–64	97	9.8	62	4	5	7	11	21	22	55
65+	161	10.1	34	4	6	8	13	19	22	28
SUBTOTALS:										
1. SINGLE DX										
A. *Not Operated*	1	1.0	0	1	1	1	1	1	1	1
B. *Operated*	7	4.4	4	2	3	4	5	8	8	8
2. MULTIPLE DX										
A. *Not Operated*	164	5.4	23	1	2	4	7	11	13	21
B. *Operated*	288	10.3	64	4	5	8	13	20	24	54
1. SINGLE DX	8	4.0	5	1	2	4	5	8	8	8
2. MULTIPLE DX	452	8.6	55	2	4	7	11	17	22	40
A. NOT OPERATED	165	5.4	23	1	2	4	7	11	13	21
B. OPERATED	295	10.2	64	4	5	8	13	20	24	54
TOTAL										
0–19 Years	1	1.0	0	1	1	1	1	1	1	1
20–34	11	11.3	125	4	5	6	14	21	41	41
35–49	48	10.1	167	2	3	6	11	18	40	66
50–64	151	8.1	52	2	4	6	10	17	22	37
65+	249	8.3	31	3	4	7	11	16	20	28
GRAND TOTAL	460	8.5	54	2	4	6	11	17	21	40

Western Region, October 2006–September 2007 Data, by Diagnosis

153.9: COLON CA NOS

Type of Patients	Observed Patients	Avg. Stay	Vari-ance	Percentiles						
				10th	25th	50th	75th	90th	95th	99th
1. SINGLE DX										
A. *Not Operated*										
0–19 Years	0									
20–34	0									
35–49	0									
50–64	0									
65+	2	2.5	4	1	1	4	4	4	4	4
B. *Operated*										
0–19 Years	0									
20–34	0									
35–49	0									
50–64	7	5.0	5	3	4	4	7	9	9	9
65+	0									
2. MULTIPLE DX										
A. *Not Operated*										
0–19 Years	0									
20–34	8	3.5	3	2	2	3	5	6	6	6
35–49	54	3.5	5	1	2	3	5	6	7	10
50–64	158	5.2	21	1	2	4	7	11	15	20
65+	285	4.9	15	1	2	4	6	10	13	18
B. *Operated*										
0–19 Years	0									
20–34	3	8.4	17	5	5	7	13	13	13	13
35–49	31	7.8	19	4	4	7	10	13	18	21
50–64	69	7.1	20	3	4	6	8	15	18	23
65+	132	8.8	33	4	5	8	10	17	22	28
SUBTOTALS:										
1. SINGLE DX										
A. *Not Operated*	2	2.5	4	1	1	4	4	4	4	4
B. *Operated*	7	5.0	5	3	4	4	7	9	9	9
2. MULTIPLE DX										
A. *Not Operated*	505	4.8	16	1	2	4	6	10	13	19
B. *Operated*	235	8.1	27	4	5	7	9	16	20	28
1. SINGLE DX	9	4.4	5	1	4	4	4	9	9	9
2. MULTIPLE DX	740	5.9	22	1	3	5	8	12	15	23
A. NOT OPERATED	507	4.8	16	1	2	4	6	10	13	19
B. OPERATED	242	8.1	27	4	4	7	9	15	20	28
TOTAL										
0–19 Years	0									
20–34	11	4.8	10	2	2	5	6	7	10	13
35–49	85	5.0	14	2	3	4	6	10	11	21
50–64	234	5.8	21	2	3	4	7	11	15	20
65+	419	6.1	24	1	3	5	8	12	16	23
GRAND TOTAL	749	5.9	22	1	3	5	8	12	15	23

154: RECTUM & ANUS CA

Type of Patients	Observed Patients	Avg. Stay	Vari-ance	Percentiles						
				10th	25th	50th	75th	90th	95th	99th
1. SINGLE DX										
A. *Not Operated*										
0–19 Years	0									
20–34	1	2.0	0	2	2	2	2	2	2	2
35–49	8	3.5	8	1	2	2	3	10	10	10
50–64	7	2.9	3	1	1	3	3	6	6	6
65+	5	1.8	2	1	1	1	2	4	4	4
B. *Operated*										
0–19 Years	0									
20–34	8	4.9	2	3	4	5	7	7	7	7
35–49	39	5.1	7	3	3	5	6	9	10	15
50–64	109	5.2	6	2	4	5	6	8	9	13
65+	32	5.0	6	2	3	5	7	8	9	11
2. MULTIPLE DX										
A. *Not Operated*										
0–19 Years	0									
20–34	25	5.5	20	2	2	4	6	15	16	16
35–49	201	5.8	60	1	1	4	7	11	13	50
50–64	432	5.4	24	1	2	4	7	11	14	26
65+	650	5.5	37	1	2	4	7	10	15	35
B. *Operated*										
0–19 Years	2	6.5	24	3	3	3	10	10	10	10
20–34	65	9.9	56	4	6	7	12	20	24	40
35–49	637	8.8	65	3	5	7	10	16	23	40
50–64	1,846	7.9	38	3	5	6	9	14	19	31
65+	2,711	9.0	46	4	5	7	11	16	22	35
SUBTOTALS:										
1. SINGLE DX										
A. *Not Operated*	21	2.8	5	1	1	2	3	5	6	10
B. *Operated*	188	5.1	6	2	4	5	6	8	9	15
2. MULTIPLE DX										
A. *Not Operated*	1,308	5.5	36	1	2	4	7	11	14	28
B. *Operated*	5,261	8.6	46	4	4	7	10	15	21	35
1. SINGLE DX	209	4.9	6	2	3	5	6	8	9	13
2. MULTIPLE DX	6,569	8.0	45	3	4	6	9	15	20	35
A. NOT OPERATED	1,329	5.5	35	1	2	4	7	11	14	28
B. OPERATED	5,449	8.5	45	4	5	7	10	15	21	35
TOTAL										
0–19 Years	2	6.5	24	3	3	3	10	10	10	10
20–34	99	8.3	46	3	4	6	10	16	23	40
35–49	885	7.9	63	2	4	6	9	14	20	43
50–64	2,394	7.3	35	3	3	6	9	13	17	30
65+	3,398	8.3	46	3	5	7	10	15	21	35
GRAND TOTAL	6,778	7.9	44	3	4	6	9	14	20	35

154.0: RECTOSIGMOID JUNCTION CA

Type of Patients	Observed Patients	Avg. Stay	Vari-ance	Percentiles						
				10th	25th	50th	75th	90th	95th	99th
1. SINGLE DX										
A. *Not Operated*										
0–19 Years	0									
20–34	0									
35–49	2	6.0	32	2	2	6	10	10	10	10
50–64	2	3.0	0	3	3	3	3	3	3	3
65+	1	1.0	0	1	1	1	1	1	1	1
B. *Operated*										
0–19 Years	0									
20–34	2	3.5	<1	3	3	4	4	4	4	4
35–49	12	4.1	4	3	3	4	5	6	9	9
50–64	42	4.9	2	3	4	5	6	7	7	7
65+	12	5.3	6	3	4	5	5	9	11	11
2. MULTIPLE DX										
A. *Not Operated*										
0–19 Years	0									
20–34	10	6.0	18	2	3	4	9	10	15	15
35–49	52	7.2	136	1	2	4	7	13	15	71
50–64	118	5.4	47	1	2	4	7	11	14	21
65+	189	5.8	47	2	2	4	6	11	15	48
B. *Operated*										
0–19 Years	2	6.5	24	3	3	3	10	10	10	10
20–34	18	8.5	55	3	5	6	8	16	35	35
35–49	205	8.6	48	3	5	7	8	15	20	34
50–64	645	7.9	29	4	5	6	9	14	19	30
65+	1,048	9.5	49	4	5	7	11	18	22	38
SUBTOTALS:										
1. SINGLE DX										
A. *Not Operated*	5	3.8	13	1	2	3	3	10	10	10
B. *Operated*	68	4.8	3	3	3	5	6	7	7	11
2. MULTIPLE DX										
A. *Not Operated*	369	5.8	49	2	2	4	7	12	15	48
B. *Operated*	1,918	8.9	43	4	5	7	10	16	21	34
1. SINGLE DX	73	4.7	3	3	3	4	6	7	9	11
2. MULTIPLE DX	2,287	8.4	45	3	5	7	10	15	20	35
A. NOT OPERATED	374	5.8	49	2	2	4	7	12	15	48
B. OPERATED	1,986	8.7	42	4	5	7	10	16	21	34
TOTAL										
0–19 Years	2	6.5	24	3	3	3	10	10	10	10
20–34	30	7.3	40	3	4	6	8	13	16	35
35–49	271	8.1	63	3	4	6	10	14	19	50
50–64	807	7.3	27	4	4	6	9	14	18	28
65+	1,250	8.9	50	3	5	7	11	17	21	38
GRAND TOTAL	2,360	8.3	44	3	5	6	10	15	20	34

Western Region, October 2006–September 2007 Data, by Diagnosis

154.1: RECTUM CA

Type of Patients	Observed Patients	Avg. Stay	Variance	10th	25th	50th	75th	90th	95th	99th
1. SINGLE DX										
A. Not Operated										
0–19 Years	0									
20–34	1	2.0	0	2	2	2	2	2	2	2
35–49	3	2.0	<1	1	1	2	3	3	3	3
50–64	5	2.8	4	1	1	3	3	6	6	6
65+	4	2.0	2	1	1	2	4	4	4	4
B. Operated										
0–19 Years	0									
20–34	6	5.3	2	4	4	5	7	7	7	7
35–49	24	5.3	5	3	4	5	7	8	9	10
50–64	55	5.3	8	2	4	5	7	8	10	16
65+	18	4.8	6	1	3	5	7	8	9	9
2. MULTIPLE DX										
A. Not Operated										
0–19 Years	0									
20–34	14	5.1	24	1	2	3	6	16	16	16
35–49	109	4.9	17	1	2	4	7	10	13	17
50–64	249	5.2	27	1	2	4	6	10	14	28
65+	403	5.3	30	1	2	4	7	10	13	23
B. Operated										
0–19 Years	0									
20–34	44	10.3	59	4	6	7	12	23	24	40
35–49	365	8.8	55	4	5	7	9	16	24	40
50–64	1,041	7.7	30	3	5	6	9	13	17	29
65+	1,468	8.6	41	3	5	7	10	15	21	34
SUBTOTALS:										
1. SINGLE DX										
A. Not Operated	13	2.3	2	1	1	2	3	4	6	6
B. Operated	103	5.2	6	2	4	5	7	8	9	13
2. MULTIPLE DX										
A. Not Operated	775	5.2	27	1	2	4	6	10	13	27
B. Operated	2,918	8.3	40	4	5	7	10	15	20	34
1. SINGLE DX	116	4.9	7	2	3	5	6	8	9	13
2. MULTIPLE DX	3,693	7.7	39	2	4	6	9	14	19	32
A. NOT OPERATED	788	5.2	27	1	2	4	6	10	13	27
B. OPERATED	3,021	8.2	39	3	5	7	9	14	20	34
TOTAL										
0–19 Years	0									
20–34	65	8.6	51	3	4	7	9	19	23	40
35–49	501	7.7	47	2	4	6	9	14	20	36
50–64	1,350	7.1	30	2	4	6	8	12	16	29
65+	1,893	7.9	40	2	4	6	9	14	19	34
GRAND TOTAL	3,809	7.6	38	2	4	6	9	14	18	32

154.8: RECTUM & ANUS CA NEC

Type of Patients	Observed Patients	Avg. Stay	Variance	10th	25th	50th	75th	90th	95th	99th
1. SINGLE DX										
A. Not Operated										
0–19 Years	0									
20–34	0									
35–49	1	3.0	0	3	3	3	3	3	3	3
50–64	0									
65+	0									
B. Operated										
0–19 Years	0									
20–34	0									
35–49	3	8.4	34	4	4	6	6	15	15	15
50–64	8	6.5	12	2	4	8	8	11	11	11
65+	2	4.5	24	1	1	8	8	8	8	8
2. MULTIPLE DX										
A. Not Operated										
0–19 Years	0									
20–34	0									
35–49	20	8.1	151	2	2	5	6	13	54	54
50–64	41	5.7	20	1	3	4	7	12	13	19
65+	37	5.1	17	2	3	4	6	10	13	22
B. Operated										
0–19 Years	0									
20–34	0									
35–49	44	11.8	247	4	6	7	13	16	29	98
50–64	118	9.8	133	3	5	7	9	13	28	51
65+	151	10.1	55	3	5	8	12	20	26	36
SUBTOTALS:										
1. SINGLE DX										
A. Not Operated	1	3.0	0	3	3	3	3	3	3	3
B. Operated	13	6.6	16	2	4	6	8	11	15	15
2. MULTIPLE DX										
A. Not Operated	98	5.9	45	1	3	4	7	12	17	54
B. Operated	315	10.2	110	3	5	7	11	19	28	50
1. SINGLE DX	14	6.4	16	2	3	6	8	11	15	15
2. MULTIPLE DX	413	9.2	98	3	4	7	10	17	24	50
A. NOT OPERATED	99	5.9	45	1	3	4	7	12	17	54
B. OPERATED	328	10.1	107	3	5	7	11	19	26	50
TOTAL										
0–19 Years	0									
20–34	2	10.0	0	10	10	10	10	10	10	10
35–49	68	10.4	206	3	5	6	11	20	29	98
50–64	167	8.6	102	3	4	6	10	15	19	51
65+	190	9.1	51	4	4	7	11	19	23	36
GRAND TOTAL	427	9.1	95	3	4	7	10	17	23	50

155: LIVER & INTRAHEP DUCT CA

Type of Patients	Observed Patients	Avg. Stay	Variance	10th	25th	50th	75th	90th	95th	99th
1. SINGLE DX										
A. Not Operated										
0–19 Years	3	5.0	7	3	3	4	8	8	8	8
20–34	0									
35–49	3	2.0	<1	1	1	2	3	3	3	3
50–64	15	2.1	2	1	1	1	4	4	5	5
65+	12	2.0	5	1	1	1	3	4	8	8
B. Operated										
0–19 Years	1	7.0	0	7	7	7	7	7	7	7
20–34	0									
35–49	1	1.0	0	1	1	1	1	1	1	1
50–64	3	1.3	<1	1	1	1	2	2	2	2
65+	5	1.2	<1	1	1	1	1	2	2	2
2. MULTIPLE DX										
A. Not Operated										
0–19 Years	17	5.1	13	1	3	4	8	9	14	14
20–34	29	7.5	81	1	2	3	8	18	30	38
35–49	196	4.9	16	1	2	4	7	10	12	32
50–64	931	5.1	20	1	2	4	7	11	14	21
65+	1,026	5.5	20	1	2	4	7	12	15	20
B. Operated										
0–19 Years	23	13.4	146	5	6	9	15	33	38	51
20–34	10	10.3	81	4	5	6	11	26	28	28
35–49	76	7.3	27	2	3	5	11	15	18	23
50–64	350	7.4	47	1	3	6	9	15	20	34
65+	329	7.0	32	1	4	6	9	14	17	26
SUBTOTALS:										
1. SINGLE DX										
A. Not Operated	33	2.3	4	1	1	1	3	4	8	8
B. Operated	10	1.8	4	1	1	1	2	7	7	7
2. MULTIPLE DX										
A. Not Operated	2,199	5.3	20	1	2	4	7	11	14	22
B. Operated	788	7.4	43	1	3	6	9	15	19	34
1. SINGLE DX	43	2.2	4	1	1	1	3	4	7	8
2. MULTIPLE DX	2,987	5.9	27	1	2	4	8	12	15	26
A. NOT OPERATED	2,232	5.3	20	1	2	4	7	11	14	21
B. OPERATED	798	7.4	43	1	3	6	9	15	19	34
TOTAL										
0–19 Years	44	9.4	97	2	4	7	11	17	33	51
20–34	39	8.2	81	1	3	5	11	26	30	38
35–49	276	5.5	20	2	2	4	7	12	15	23
50–64	1,299	5.7	28	2	4	4	8	11	15	26
65+	1,372	5.8	23	1	2	5	8	12	15	24
GRAND TOTAL	3,030	5.8	27	1	2	4	8	12	15	26

Length of Stay by Diagnosis and Operation, Western Region, 2008

Western Region, October 2006–September 2007 Data, by Diagnosis

155.0: PRIMARY LIVER CA

Type of Patients	Observed Patients	Avg. Stay	Vari-ance	10th	25th	50th	75th	90th	95th	99th
1. SINGLE DX										
A. Not Operated										
0–19 Years	3	5.0	7	3	3	4	8	8	8	8
20–34	0									
35–49	2	2.0	2	1	1	1	3	3	3	3
50–64	11	2.2	2	1	1	1	4	4	5	5
65+	7	1.3	<1	1	1	1	1	3	3	3
B. Operated										
0–19 Years	1	7.0	0	7	7	7	7	7	7	7
20–34	0									
35–49	1	1.0	0	1	1	1	1	1	1	1
50–64	3	1.3	<1	1	1	1	2	2	2	2
65+	3	1.0	0	1	1	1	1	1	1	1
2. MULTIPLE DX										
A. Not Operated										
0–19 Years	17	5.1	13	1	3	4	8	9	14	14
20–34	23	6.4	51	1	2	3	8	16	18	30
35–49	152	5.0	16	2	2	4	7	10	12	32
50–64	760	5.1	20	1	2	4	7	10	13	23
65+	707	5.1	16	1	2	4	7	10	13	17
B. Operated										
0–19 Years	22	13.7	150	5	7	9	15	33	38	51
20–34	6	9.6	72	4	5	6	11	26	26	26
35–49	62	7.0	24	2	4	5	11	14	16	23
50–64	283	7.3	51	1	3	6	9	15	22	38
65+	256	6.4	23	1	3	5	8	13	15	24
SUBTOTALS:										
1. SINGLE DX										
A. Not Operated	23	2.3	3	1	1	1	3	4	5	8
B. Operated	8	1.9	4	1	1	1	1	7	7	7
2. MULTIPLE DX										
A. Not Operated	1,659	5.1	18	1	2	4	7	10	13	19
B. Operated	629	7.2	42	1	3	6	9	14	19	34
1. SINGLE DX	31	2.2	3	1	1	1	3	4	7	8
2. MULTIPLE DX	2,288	5.7	25	1	2	4	7	11	15	26
A. NOT OPERATED	1,682	5.0	18	1	2	4	7	10	13	19
B. OPERATED	637	7.1	42	1	3	6	9	14	19	34
TOTAL										
0–19 Years	43	9.5	99	2	4	7	12	17	33	51
20–34	29	7.1	55	1	2	4	8	18	26	30
35–49	217	5.6	19	1	2	4	7	11	15	23
50–64	1,057	5.6	29	1	2	4	7	11	15	29
65+	973	5.4	18	1	2	4	7	11	14	20
GRAND TOTAL	2,319	5.6	25	1	2	4	7	11	14	25

155.1: INTRAHEPATIC DUCT CA

Type of Patients	Observed Patients	Avg. Stay	Vari-ance	10th	25th	50th	75th	90th	95th	99th
1. SINGLE DX										
A. Not Operated										
0–19 Years	0									
20–34	0									
35–49	1	2.0	0	2	2	2	2	2	2	2
50–64	3	2.3	2	1	1	2	4	4	4	4
65+	3	4.3	12	1	1	4	8	8	8	8
B. Operated										
0–19 Years	0									
20–34	0									
35–49	0									
50–64	0									
65+	1	2.0	0	2	2	2	2	2	2	2
2. MULTIPLE DX										
A. Not Operated										
0–19 Years	0									
20–34	6	11.7	203	1	3	7	18	38	38	38
35–49	29	5.4	21	1	1	4	8	12	16	17
50–64	122	6.3	25	1	3	5	9	14	16	21
65+	230	6.9	33	2	3	5	9	15	18	28
B. Operated										
0–19 Years	0									
20–34	3	13.6	153	6	6	7	28	28	28	28
35–49	10	10.2	44	4	5	8	14	23	23	23
50–64	52	8.4	34	2	5	7	11	16	20	29
65+	56	10.2	68	2	6	8	13	17	24	52
SUBTOTALS:										
1. SINGLE DX										
A. Not Operated	7	3.2	6	1	1	2	4	8	8	8
B. Operated	1	2.0	0	2	2	2	2	2	2	2
2. MULTIPLE DX										
A. Not Operated	387	6.6	32	1	3	5	9	14	17	28
B. Operated	121	9.5	53	2	5	8	13	17	22	33
1. SINGLE DX	8	3.0	5	1	1	2	4	8	8	8
2. MULTIPLE DX	508	7.3	38	2	3	6	10	15	18	29
A. NOT OPERATED	394	6.6	32	1	2	5	9	14	17	28
B. OPERATED	122	9.5	53	2	5	8	13	17	22	33
TOTAL										
0–19 Years	0									
20–34	9	12.3	167	1	3	7	18	38	38	38
35–49	40	6.5	30	1	2	5	9	16	18	23
50–64	177	6.8	28	2	3	5	9	14	17	26
65+	290	7.5	41	2	3	6	10	15	18	33
GRAND TOTAL	516	7.3	38	2	3	6	10	15	18	29

156: GALLBLADDER & DUCT CA

Type of Patients	Observed Patients	Avg. Stay	Vari-ance	10th	25th	50th	75th	90th	95th	99th
1. SINGLE DX										
A. Not Operated										
0–19 Years	0									
20–34	0									
35–49	2	3.5	5	2	2	4	5	5	5	5
50–64	4	5.0	15	2	2	2	10	10	10	10
65+	2	2.5	<1	2	2	3	3	3	3	3
B. Operated										
0–19 Years	0									
20–34	4	6.0	0	6	6	6	6	6	6	6
35–49	4	12.8	124	5	5	6	29	29	29	29
50–64	4	5.5	11	3	3	6	10	10	10	10
65+	2	1.0	0	1	1	1	1	1	1	1
2. MULTIPLE DX										
A. Not Operated										
0–19 Years	0									
20–34	2	8.5	4	7	7	7	10	10	10	10
35–49	36	7.7	78	2	3	6	8	15	18	52
50–64	133	5.7	15	2	3	4	8	11	13	19
65+	408	6.4	21	2	3	5	8	13	15	22
B. Operated										
0–19 Years	1	3.0	0	3	3	3	3	3	3	3
20–34	3	10.0	42	4	4	9	17	17	17	17
35–49	44	9.9	40	4	6	8	13	19	22	33
50–64	173	10.7	93	4	5	8	12	21	27	59
65+	348	11.4	110	4	6	8	13	21	28	50
SUBTOTALS:										
1. SINGLE DX										
A. Not Operated	8	4.0	8	2	2	3	6	10	10	10
B. Operated	11	7.4	62	1	3	6	10	11	29	29
2. MULTIPLE DX										
A. Not Operated	579	6.3	23	2	3	5	8	12	15	22
B. Operated	569	11.1	99	4	6	8	13	21	27	50
1. SINGLE DX	19	6.0	41	1	2	5	6	11	29	29
2. MULTIPLE DX	1,148	8.7	66	2	4	7	11	16	21	43
A. NOT OPERATED	587	6.3	23	2	3	5	8	12	15	22
B. OPERATED	580	11.0	98	4	6	8	13	21	28	50
TOTAL										
0–19 Years	1	3.0	0	3	3	3	3	3	3	3
20–34	6	8.8	20	4	6	9	10	17	17	17
35–49	86	9.0	60	2	4	8	11	18	22	52
50–64	314	8.4	64	2	4	7	10	16	21	41
65+	760	8.7	68	2	4	7	11	16	21	43
GRAND TOTAL	1,167	8.6	66	2	4	7	10	16	21	43

Western Region, October 2006–September 2007 Data, by Diagnosis

156.0: GALLBLADDER CA

Type of Patients	Observed Patients	Avg. Stay	Variance	10th	25th	50th	75th	90th	95th	99th
1. SINGLE DX										
A. Not Operated										
0–19 Years	0									
20–34	0									
35–49	1	2.0	0	2	2	2	2	2	2	2
50–64	1	6.0	0	6	6	6	6	6	6	6
65+	0									
B. Operated										
0–19 Years	0									
20–34	0									
35–49	2	5.5	<1	5	5	5	6	6	6	6
50–64	1	3.0	0	3	3	3	3	3	3	3
65+	1	1.0	0	1	1	1	1	1	1	1
2. MULTIPLE DX										
A. Not Operated										
0–19 Years	0									
20–34	1	7.0	0	7	7	7	7	7	7	7
35–49	12	4.9	8	1	2	6	8	8	9	9
50–64	53	5.8	18	1	3	5	8	10	16	20
65+	70	6.3	26	2	3	4	8	14	16	27
B. Operated										
0–19 Years	0									
20–34	2	10.6	84	4	4	17	17	17	17	17
35–49	17	7.7	64	2	4	6	8	22	33	33
50–64	67	6.7	54	2	4	6	7	11	13	59
65+	169	8.2	34	3	5	7	10	15	19	36
SUBTOTALS:										
1. SINGLE DX										
A. Not Operated	2	4.0	8	2	2	4	6	6	6	6
B. Operated	4	3.8	5	1	3	5	5	6	6	6
2. MULTIPLE DX										
A. Not Operated	136	6.0	21	1	3	5	8	11	16	23
B. Operated	255	7.8	42	3	4	6	9	14	19	36
1. SINGLE DX	6	3.8	5	1	2	5	6	6	6	6
2. MULTIPLE DX	391	7.2	35	2	4	6	8	13	18	33
A. NOT OPERATED	138	6.0	21	1	3	5	8	11	16	23
B. OPERATED	259	7.7	41	3	4	6	9	14	18	36
TOTAL										
0–19 Years	0									
20–34	3	9.4	46	4	4	7	17	17	17	17
35–49	32	6.3	38	2	3	6	7	8	22	33
50–64	122	6.3	38	2	3	5	7	10	13	20
65+	240	7.6	32	3	4	6	9	14	18	28
GRAND TOTAL	397	7.1	35	2	4	6	8	13	18	33

156.1: EXTRAHEPATIC DUCT CA

Type of Patients	Observed Patients	Avg. Stay	Variance	10th	25th	50th	75th	90th	95th	99th
1. SINGLE DX										
A. Not Operated										
0–19 Years	0									
20–34	0									
35–49	0									
50–64	2	2.0	0	2	2	2	2	2	2	2
65+	1	2.0	0	2	2	2	2	2	2	2
B. Operated										
0–19 Years	0									
20–34	1	6.0	0	6	6	6	6	6	6	6
35–49	0									
50–64	1	6.0	0	6	6	6	6	6	6	6
65+	1	1.0	0	1	1	1	1	1	1	1
2. MULTIPLE DX										
A. Not Operated										
0–19 Years	0									
20–34	0									
35–49	9	9.6	29	3	5	8	15	17	17	17
50–64	47	5.9	12	2	3	4	9	11	11	16
65+	185	6.7	21	2	3	6	9	13	15	22
B. Operated										
0–19 Years	0									
20–34	1	9.0	0	9	9	9	9	9	9	9
35–49	8	9.1	18	5	6	8	10	19	19	19
50–64	41	13.5	133	6	8	10	15	21	27	75
65+	73	13.1	121	5	7	10	16	22	33	80
SUBTOTALS:										
1. SINGLE DX										
A. Not Operated	3	2.0	0	2	2	2	2	2	2	2
B. Operated	3	4.3	8	1	1	6	6	6	6	6
2. MULTIPLE DX										
A. Not Operated	241	6.7	20	2	3	6	9	13	15	20
B. Operated	123	13.0	117	5	7	10	15	22	28	75
1. SINGLE DX	6	3.2	5	1	2	2	6	6	6	6
2. MULTIPLE DX	364	8.8	62	2	4	7	11	16	20	37
A. NOT OPERATED	244	6.6	20	2	3	6	9	13	15	20
B. OPERATED	126	12.8	116	5	7	10	15	22	28	75
TOTAL										
0–19 Years	0									
20–34	2	7.5	4	6	6	8	9	9	9	9
35–49	17	9.4	23	3	6	8	12	17	19	33
50–64	91	9.3	81	2	4	8	11	18	21	75
65+	260	8.5	58	2	4	7	11	16	21	37
GRAND TOTAL	370	8.7	61	2	4	7	11	16	20	37

156.2: AMPULLA OF VATER CA

Type of Patients	Observed Patients	Avg. Stay	Variance	10th	25th	50th	75th	90th	95th	99th
1. SINGLE DX										
A. Not Operated										
0–19 Years	0									
20–34	0									
35–49	1	5.0	0	5	5	5	5	5	5	5
50–64	1	10.0	0	10	10	10	10	10	10	10
65+	0									
B. Operated										
0–19 Years	0									
20–34	0									
35–49	2	20.1	158	11	11	29	29	29	29	29
50–64	1	10.0	0	10	10	10	10	10	10	10
65+	0									
2. MULTIPLE DX										
A. Not Operated										
0–19 Years	0									
20–34	0									
35–49	4	3.5	3	2	3	3	3	6	6	6
50–64	13	4.9	12	2	2	4	5	11	12	12
65+	84	5.6	15	2	3	4	7	11	12	19
B. Operated										
0–19 Years	0									
20–34	1	3.0	0	3	3	3	3	3	3	3
35–49	12	11.8	26	8	8	11	14	17	25	25
50–64	40	13.6	76	6	8	11	18	25	36	41
65+	73	17.4	203	8	9	14	20	35	47	94
SUBTOTALS:										
1. SINGLE DX										
A. Not Operated	2	7.5	12	5	5	10	10	10	10	10
B. Operated	3	16.7	113	10	10	11	29	29	29	29
2. MULTIPLE DX										
A. Not Operated	101	5.5	14	2	3	4	7	11	12	19
B. Operated	126	15.5	149	7	8	12	18	28	41	50
1. SINGLE DX	5	13.1	85	5	10	10	11	29	29	29
2. MULTIPLE DX	227	11.1	114	2	4	8	13	22	29	49
A. NOT OPERATED	103	5.5	14	2	3	4	7	11	12	17
B. OPERATED	129	15.6	148	7	8	12	18	29	41	50
TOTAL										
0–19 Years	1	3.0	0	3	3	3	3	3	3	3
20–34	0									
35–49	19	10.6	50	3	6	9	13	25	29	29
50–64	55	11.4	71	3	6	9	12	23	31	41
65+	157	11.1	136	2	4	8	14	25	35	50
GRAND TOTAL	232	11.1	113	2	4	8	13	22	29	49

Length of Stay by Diagnosis and Operation, Western Region, 2008

Western Region, October 2006–September 2007 Data, by Diagnosis

157: PANCREAS CA

Type of Patients	Observed Patients	Avg. Stay	Variance	10th	25th	50th	75th	90th	95th	99th
1. SINGLE DX										
A. Not Operated										
0–19 Years	0									
20–34	0									
35–49	1	10.0	0	10	10	10	10	10	10	10
50–64	6	3.3	23	1	1	2	2	13	13	13
65+	1	3.0	0	3	3	3	3	3	3	3
B. Operated										
0–19 Years	1	8.0	0	8	8	8	8	8	8	8
20–34	0									
35–49	2	9.0	0	9	9	9	9	9	9	9
50–64	13	7.5	33	2	4	6	8	17	21	21
65+	6	6.3	1	5	5	6	7	8	8	8
2. MULTIPLE DX										
A. Not Operated										
0–19 Years	2	7.0	8	5	5	7	9	9	9	9
20–34	8	3.3	2	1	3	3	4	6	6	6
35–49	178	5.4	25	2	3	4	7	10	13	31
50–64	814	6.0	36	2	3	5	7	12	15	26
65+	1,809	5.6	17	2	3	5	7	11	13	21
B. Operated										
0–19 Years	2	11.5	4	10	10	12	13	13	13	13
20–34	14	14.4	171	5	6	8	15	41	43	43
35–49	148	12.0	79	4	7	10	14	24	28	43
50–64	601	12.8	98	5	7	10	16	24	31	49
65+	868	12.2	71	5	7	10	15	22	27	45
SUBTOTALS:										
1. SINGLE DX — A. Not Operated	8	4.1	22	1	1	2	3	13	13	13
1. SINGLE DX — B. Operated	22	7.3	20	3	5	7	8	11	17	21
2. MULTIPLE DX — A. Not Operated	2,811	5.7	23	2	3	4	7	11	14	23
2. MULTIPLE DX — B. Operated	1,633	12.4	82	5	7	10	15	23	29	47
1. SINGLE DX	30	6.5	22	2	3	6	8	13	17	21
2. MULTIPLE DX	4,444	8.2	56	2	3	6	10	16	21	38
A. NOT OPERATED	2,819	5.7	23	2	3	4	7	11	14	23
B. OPERATED	1,655	12.4	82	5	7	10	15	23	29	47
TOTAL										
0–19 Years	5	9.0	8	5	8	9	10	13	13	13
20–34	22	10.4	137	3	3	6	11	28	41	43
35–49	329	8.4	60	2	3	7	11	17	24	38
50–64	1,434	8.9	74	2	3	7	11	18	24	43
65+	2,684	7.8	44	2	3	6	10	15	20	32
GRAND TOTAL	4,474	8.2	55	2	3	6	10	16	21	38

157.0: PANCREAS HEAD CA

Type of Patients	Observed Patients	Avg. Stay	Variance	10th	25th	50th	75th	90th	95th	99th
1. SINGLE DX										
A. Not Operated										
0–19 Years	0									
20–34	0									
35–49	1	10.0	0	10	10	10	10	10	10	10
50–64	2	1.5	<1	1	1	2	2	2	2	2
65+	0									
B. Operated										
0–19 Years	0									
20–34	0									
35–49	2	9.0	0	9	9	9	9	9	9	9
50–64	4	10.3	25	6	7	11	17	17	17	17
65+	2	6.0	2	5	5	5	7	7	7	7
2. MULTIPLE DX										
A. Not Operated										
0–19 Years	0									
20–34	2	3.0	0	3	3	3	3	3	3	3
35–49	58	5.4	27	2	3	4	7	9	19	31
50–64	312	6.2	47	2	3	5	7	12	15	26
65+	832	5.8	17	2	3	5	8	11	14	21
B. Operated										
0–19 Years	0									
20–34	3	16.3	101	10	10	11	28	28	28	28
35–49	85	13.2	77	8	8	11	16	26	33	43
50–64	364	14.0	103	8	8	11	17	26	35	50
65+	495	13.1	70	8	8	11	16	24	29	39
SUBTOTALS:										
1. SINGLE DX — A. Not Operated	3	4.3	24	1	1	2	10	10	10	10
1. SINGLE DX — B. Operated	8	8.9	15	5	7	9	11	17	17	17
2. MULTIPLE DX — A. Not Operated	1,204	5.9	25	2	3	5	8	11	14	23
2. MULTIPLE DX — B. Operated	947	13.5	83	6	8	11	17	25	31	45
1. SINGLE DX	11	7.7	20	2	5	7	10	11	17	17
2. MULTIPLE DX	2,151	9.2	65	2	4	7	12	18	24	40
A. NOT OPERATED	1,207	5.9	25	2	3	5	8	11	14	23
B. OPERATED	955	13.5	83	6	8	11	17	25	31	45
TOTAL										
0–19 Years	0									
20–34	5	11.0	104	3	3	10	11	28	28	28
35–49	146	10.0	69	2	4	8	13	20	27	39
50–64	682	10.4	92	2	4	8	13	20	27	48
65+	1,329	8.5	49	2	4	7	11	17	22	33
GRAND TOTAL	2,162	9.2	65	2	4	7	12	18	24	40

157.1: PANCREAS BODY CA

Type of Patients	Observed Patients	Avg. Stay	Variance	10th	25th	50th	75th	90th	95th	99th
1. SINGLE DX										
A. Not Operated										
0–19 Years	0									
20–34	0									
35–49	0									
50–64	0									
65+	0									
B. Operated										
0–19 Years	1	8.0	0	8	8	8	8	8	8	8
20–34	0									
35–49	0									
50–64	3	3.3	1	2	2	4	4	4	4	4
65+	0									
2. MULTIPLE DX										
A. Not Operated										
0–19 Years	0									
20–34	2	3.5	<1	3	3	4	4	4	4	4
35–49	11	5.1	11	1	3	5	5	7	9	12
50–64	44	7.3	49	2	3	5	10	14	18	41
65+	115	5.5	12	2	3	5	8	11	12	14
B. Operated										
0–19 Years	0									
20–34	1	6.0	0	6	6	6	6	6	6	6
35–49	19	10.4	18	5	8	11	13	16	21	21
50–64	47	9.8	29	5	7	8	12	18	23	24
65+	78	9.8	60	4	6	8	11	17	23	59
SUBTOTALS:										
1. SINGLE DX — A. Not Operated	0									
1. SINGLE DX — B. Operated	4	4.5	6	2	2	4	8	8	8	8
2. MULTIPLE DX — A. Not Operated	172	5.9	21	2	3	5	8	11	13	20
2. MULTIPLE DX — B. Operated	145	9.8	44	4	6	8	12	17	21	27
1. SINGLE DX	4	4.5	6	2	2	4	8	8	8	8
2. MULTIPLE DX	317	7.7	35	2	4	7	10	13	18	27
A. NOT OPERATED	172	5.9	21	2	3	5	8	11	13	20
B. OPERATED	149	9.7	43	4	6	8	12	17	21	27
TOTAL										
0–19 Years	1	8.0	0	8	8	8	8	8	8	8
20–34	3	4.3	2	3	3	4	6	6	6	6
35–49	30	8.4	22	2	5	8	12	13	16	21
50–64	94	8.4	39	2	4	8	11	17	20	41
65+	193	7.2	35	2	4	6	9	13	15	27
GRAND TOTAL	321	7.7	35	2	4	6	10	13	18	27

Length of Stay by Diagnosis and Operation, Western Region, 2008

Western Region, October 2006–September 2007 Data, by Diagnosis

75

157.2: PANCREAS TAIL CA

Type of Patients	Observed Patients	Avg. Stay	Variance	10th	25th	50th	75th	90th	95th	99th
1. SINGLE DX										
A. *Not Operated*										
0–19 Years	0									
20–34	0									
35–49	0									
50–64	0									
65+	0									
B. *Operated*										
0–19 Years	0									
20–34	0									
35–49	0									
50–64	1	2.0	0	2	2	2	2	2	2	2
65+	1	7.0	0	7	7	7	7	7	7	7
2. MULTIPLE DX										
A. *Not Operated*										
0–19 Years	0									
20–34	1	1.0	0	1	1	1	1	1	1	1
35–49	15	6.9	65	2	2	4	11	12	33	33
50–64	75	6.0	22	2	3	5	8	12	15	26
65+	113	5.3	13	2	3	4	7	9	12	16
B. *Operated*										
0–19 Years	1	10.0	0	10	10	10	10	10	10	10
20–34	3	17.8	464	4	4	7	43	43	43	43
35–49	17	6.7	7	4	5	7	8	10	11	11
50–64	55	10.9	179	4	5	7	11	20	38	76
65+	77	8.8	37	3	6	7	10	17	22	36
SUBTOTALS:										
1. SINGLE DX										
A. *Not Operated*	0									
B. *Operated*	2	4.5	12	2	2	2	7	7	7	7
2. MULTIPLE DX										
A. *Not Operated*	204	5.6	20	2	3	4	7	11	13	24
B. *Operated*	153	9.5	92	4	5	7	10	17	23	66
1. SINGLE DX	2	4.5	12	2	2	2	7	7	7	7
2. MULTIPLE DX	357	7.3	55	2	3	6	9	13	18	38
A. NOT OPERATED	204	5.6	20	2	3	4	7	11	13	24
B. OPERATED	155	9.5	92	4	5	7	10	17	23	66
TOTAL										
0–19 Years	1	10.0	0	10	10	10	10	10	10	10
20–34	4	13.7	381	1	4	6	7	43	43	43
35–49	32	6.8	33	2	4	6	10	11	12	33
50–64	131	8.0	93	2	3	6	9	14	20	66
65+	191	6.7	26	2	3	6	8	13	16	27
GRAND TOTAL	359	7.3	54	2	3	6	9	13	18	38

157.8: PANCREAS CA NEC

Type of Patients	Observed Patients	Avg. Stay	Variance	10th	25th	50th	75th	90th	95th	99th
1. SINGLE DX										
A. *Not Operated*										
0–19 Years	0									
20–34	0									
35–49	0									
50–64	2	7.5	60	2	2	8	13	13	13	13
65+	0									
B. *Operated*										
0–19 Years	0									
20–34	0									
35–49	0									
50–64	2	5.0	8	3	3	3	7	7	7	7
65+	2	7.0	2	6	6	6	8	8	8	8
2. MULTIPLE DX										
A. *Not Operated*										
0–19 Years	1	9.0	0	9	9	9	9	9	9	9
20–34	2	4.5	4	3	3	5	6	6	6	6
35–49	28	5.1	16	1	2	4	7	10	12	19
50–64	125	5.8	22	1	2	4	8	13	15	20
65+	220	6.1	24	2	3	4	8	13	16	24
B. *Operated*										
0–19 Years	1	13.0	0	13	13	13	13	13	13	13
20–34	3	21.0	312	7	7	15	41	41	41	41
35–49	11	10.9	48	5	5	8	17	19	24	41
50–64	71	11.1	57	4	6	8	15	23	26	36
65+	105	12.9	81	4	7	11	17	23	29	45
SUBTOTALS:										
1. SINGLE DX										
A. *Not Operated*	2	7.5	60	2	2	8	8	13	13	13
B. *Operated*	4	6.0	5	3	6	6	6	8	8	8
2. MULTIPLE DX										
A. *Not Operated*	376	5.9	23	3	3	4	8	13	15	23
B. *Operated*	191	12.3	73	4	6	10	17	23	28	45
1. SINGLE DX	6	6.5	15	2	3	6	8	13	13	13
2. MULTIPLE DX	567	8.1	49	2	3	6	11	18	22	36
A. NOT OPERATED	378	5.9	23	1	3	4	8	13	15	23
B. OPERATED	195	12.1	73	4	6	10	17	23	28	45
TOTAL										
0–19 Years	2	11.0	8	9	9	11	13	13	13	13
20–34	5	14.4	239	3	6	7	15	41	41	41
35–49	39	6.7	31	1	3	5	11	17	19	24
50–64	200	7.7	40	1	3	6	11	17	21	28
65+	327	8.3	52	2	3	6	12	19	22	37
GRAND TOTAL	573	8.0	48	2	3	6	11	18	22	36

157.9: PANCREAS CA NOS

Type of Patients	Observed Patients	Avg. Stay	Variance	10th	25th	50th	75th	90th	95th	99th
1. SINGLE DX										
A. *Not Operated*										
0–19 Years	0									
20–34	0									
35–49	0									
50–64	2	1.0	0	1	1	1	1	1	1	1
65+	1	3.0	0	3	3	3	3	3	3	3
B. *Operated*										
0–19 Years	0									
20–34	0									
35–49	0									
50–64	1	8.0	0	8	8	8	8	8	8	8
65+	1	5.0	0	5	5	5	5	5	5	5
2. MULTIPLE DX										
A. *Not Operated*										
0–19 Years	1	5.0	0	5	5	5	5	5	5	5
20–34	1	3.0	0	3	3	3	3	3	3	3
35–49	62	5.3	24	2	2	4	7	9	11	29
50–64	244	5.6	32	1	2	4	7	12	14	33
65+	500	5.3	17	1	2	4	7	10	13	22
B. *Operated*										
0–19 Years	0									
20–34	1	11.0	0	11	11	11	11	11	11	11
35–49	8	10.2	59	1	4	11	14	24	24	24
50–64	41	10.4	51	4	6	9	14	19	22	32
65+	77	10.4	61	3	6	9	13	18	21	60
SUBTOTALS:										
1. SINGLE DX										
A. *Not Operated*	3	1.7	1	1	1	1	3	3	3	3
B. *Operated*	2	6.5	4	5	5	5	8	8	8	8
2. MULTIPLE DX										
A. *Not Operated*	808	5.4	22	1	2	4	7	10	13	24
B. *Operated*	127	10.4	56	3	6	9	13	18	22	32
1. SINGLE DX	5	3.6	9	1	1	3	5	8	8	8
2. MULTIPLE DX	935	6.1	30	1	3	5	8	12	16	27
A. NOT OPERATED	811	5.4	22	1	2	4	7	10	13	24
B. OPERATED	129	10.3	56	3	6	9	13	18	22	32
TOTAL										
0–19 Years	1	5.0	0	5	5	5	5	5	5	5
20–34	2	7.0	31	3	3	11	11	11	11	11
35–49	70	5.9	29	2	2	4	7	11	17	29
50–64	288	6.3	38	1	2	5	8	12	18	33
65+	579	5.9	26	2	3	5	8	12	14	26
GRAND TOTAL	940	6.0	30	1	3	5	8	12	16	27

Western Region, October 2006–September 2007 Data, by Diagnosis

158: PERITONEUM CA

Type of Patients	Observed Patients	Avg. Stay	Variance	10th	25th	50th	75th	90th	95th	99th
1. SINGLE DX										
A. Not Operated										
0–19 Years	0									
20–34	1	2.0	0	2	2	2	2	2	2	2
35–49	2	4.0	2	3	3	5	5	5	5	5
50–64	0									
65+	1	1.0	0	1	1	1	1	1	1	1
B. Operated										
0–19 Years	4	2.5	2	1	2	3	3	4	4	4
20–34	2	2.0	0	2	3	2	2	4	4	4
35–49	5	3.6	1	2	3	4	4	5	5	5
50–64	9	3.9	5	1	3	4	5	8	8	8
65+	3	4.7	4	3	3	4	7	7	7	7
2. MULTIPLE DX										
A. Not Operated										
0–19 Years	3	10.1	170	1	1	4	25	25	25	25
20–34	8	9.0	64	2	3	7	8	24	24	24
35–49	27	5.9	28	2	2	4	8	14	18	21
50–64	53	5.5	22	1	2	4	7	13	16	18
65+	83	5.8	22	1	2	4	9	13	14	24
B. Operated										
0–19 Years	11	13.3	220	3	5	12	17	55	>99	>99
20–34	18	9.1	51	3	3	7	10	21	29	29
35–49	83	7.1	28	3	4	6	8	14	15	38
50–64	239	8.7	86	3	5	7	9	15	21	45
65+	286	8.9	48	4	5	7	10	17	22	38
SUBTOTALS:										
1. SINGLE DX										
A. Not Operated	4	2.8	3	1	1	2	2	5	5	5
B. Operated	23	3.5	3	1	2	3	5	5	5	5
2. MULTIPLE DX										
A. Not Operated	174	5.9	27	1	2	4	8	13	18	24
B. Operated	637	8.7	63	3	5	7	10	16	21	42
1. SINGLE DX	27	3.4	3	1	2	3	5	5	7	8
2. MULTIPLE DX	811	8.1	56	3	4	6	9	16	20	38
A. NOT OPERATED	178	5.9	26	1	2	4	8	13	18	24
B. OPERATED	660	8.5	61	3	5	6	10	16	21	42
TOTAL										
0–19 Years	18	10.4	170	1	3	5	15	55	>99	>99
20–34	29	8.3	52	2	3	7	8	21	24	29
35–49	117	6.6	27	2	3	5	8	14	16	26
50–64	301	8.0	74	3	4	6	8	14	20	40
65+	373	8.2	43	3	4	7	10	16	20	35
GRAND TOTAL	838	7.9	55	2	4	6	9	16	20	38

158.0: RETROPERITONEUM CA

Type of Patients	Observed Patients	Avg. Stay	Variance	10th	25th	50th	75th	90th	95th	99th
1. SINGLE DX										
A. Not Operated										
0–19 Years	0									
20–34	1	2.0	0	2	2	2	2	2	2	2
35–49	2	4.0	2	3	3	5	5	5	5	5
50–64	0									
65+	0									
B. Operated										
0–19 Years	3	3.0	<1	2	2	3	4	4	4	4
20–34	0									
35–49	3	4.0	<1	3	3	4	5	5	5	5
50–64	8	3.8	5	1	1	3	5	8	8	8
65+	3	4.7	4	3	3	4	7	7	7	7
2. MULTIPLE DX										
A. Not Operated										
0–19 Years	1	25.0	0	25	25	25	25	25	25	25
20–34	3	9.6	58	3	3	8	18	18	18	18
35–49	14	5.5	18	2	2	4	5	12	14	14
50–64	20	3.8	8	1	2	3	5	8	10	10
65+	22	3.8	7	1	1	3	5	7	9	9
B. Operated										
0–19 Years	10	13.2	244	3	4	12	15	55	55	55
20–34	11	9.1	39	5	5	7	12	20	21	21
35–49	46	6.4	31	2	4	5	7	9	14	38
50–64	109	9.0	75	4	5	7	10	16	21	40
65+	120	9.1	59	4	5	7	10	18	27	42
SUBTOTALS:										
1. SINGLE DX										
A. Not Operated	3	3.3	2	2	2	3	5	5	5	5
B. Operated	17	3.8	3	1	3	4	5	7	8	8
2. MULTIPLE DX										
A. Not Operated	60	4.8	20	1	2	4	7	10	14	25
B. Operated	296	8.8	67	3	5	7	10	16	21	53
1. SINGLE DX	20	3.8	3	2	3	3	5	5	7	8
2. MULTIPLE DX	356	8.1	61	2	4	6	9	15	21	42
A. NOT OPERATED	63	4.8	19	1	2	3	7	9	12	25
B. OPERATED	313	8.5	64	3	5	6	9	16	21	42
TOTAL										
0–19 Years	14	11.9	202	2	3	8	15	55	55	55
20–34	15	8.7	40	2	4	7	12	20	21	21
35–49	65	6.0	26	2	3	5	7	10	14	38
50–64	137	7.9	65	3	5	6	8	14	21	40
65+	145	8.2	54	2	4	6	9	16	22	42
GRAND TOTAL	376	7.9	59	2	4	6	9	14	21	42

158.8: PERITONEUM CA NEC

Type of Patients	Observed Patients	Avg. Stay	Variance	10th	25th	50th	75th	90th	95th	99th
1. SINGLE DX										
A. Not Operated										
0–19 Years	0									
20–34	0									
35–49	0									
50–64	0									
65+	1	1.0	0	1	1	1	1	1	1	1
B. Operated										
0–19 Years	1	1.0	0	1	1	1	1	1	1	1
20–34	2	2.0	0	2	2	2	2	2	2	2
35–49	2	3.0	2	2	2	2	4	4	4	4
50–64	0									
65+	0									
2. MULTIPLE DX										
A. Not Operated										
0–19 Years	2	2.5	4	1	1	4	4	4	4	4
20–34	3	5.7	10	2	2	7	8	8	8	8
35–49	9	6.7	56	1	2	3	5	21	21	21
50–64	17	7.7	30	2	3	7	13	16	18	18
65+	37	7.3	29	2	3	7	10	14	18	24
B. Operated										
0–19 Years	5	14.0	0	14	14	14	>99	>99	>99	>99
20–34	5	5.8	5	3	4	6	6	8	8	8
35–49	26	7.0	15	3	4	6	10	14	15	16
50–64	106	8.8	114	3	4	6	8	16	20	45
65+	134	9.0	44	4	4	7	11	18	22	35
SUBTOTALS:										
1. SINGLE DX										
A. Not Operated	1	1.0	0	1	1	1	1	1	1	1
B. Operated	5	2.2	1	1	2	2	2	4	4	4
2. MULTIPLE DX										
A. Not Operated	68	7.1	31	2	3	5	7	10	14	24
B. Operated	272	8.7	68	3	4	6	10	16	21	45
1. SINGLE DX	6	2.0	1	1	1	2	2	4	4	4
2. MULTIPLE DX	340	8.4	61	3	4	6	10	16	20	38
A. NOT OPERATED	69	7.0	31	2	3	5	7	9	15	24
B. OPERATED	277	8.6	67	3	4	6	10	16	21	45
TOTAL										
0–19 Years	4	5.0	38	1	1	4	4	>99	>99	>99
20–34	10	5.0	7	2	3	6	8	8	8	8
35–49	37	6.7	24	2	3	5	8	15	18	21
50–64	123	8.6	102	3	4	6	9	16	20	45
65+	172	8.6	41	3	4	7	11	17	21	35
GRAND TOTAL	346	8.2	60	3	4	6	10	16	20	38

Length of Stay by Diagnosis and Operation, Western Region, 2008

Western Region, October 2006–September 2007 Data, by Diagnosis

159: OTH DIGESTIVE ORGAN CA

Type of Patients	Observed Patients	Avg. Stay	Vari-ance	10th	25th	50th	75th	90th	95th	99th
1. SINGLE DX										
A. Not Operated										
0–19 Years	0									
20–34	0									
35–49	0									
50–64	0									
65+	0									
B. Operated										
0–19 Years	0									
20–34	0									
35–49	0									
50–64	0									
65+	0									
2. MULTIPLE DX										
A. Not Operated										
0–19 Years	1	2.0	0	2	2	2	2	2	2	2
20–34	1	10.0	0	10	10	10	10	10	10	10
35–49	0									
50–64	5	6.6	44	1	4	4	6	18	18	18
65+	16	8.7	56	3	3	6	9	20	30	30
B. Operated										
0–19 Years	1	14.0	0	14	14	14	14	14	14	14
20–34	3	13.0	37	9	9	10	20	20	20	20
35–49	3	8.3	30	3	3	8	14	14	14	14
50–64	7	11.0	69	4	5	8	14	28	28	28
65+	14	10.0	29	4	6	8	13	17	22	22
SUBTOTALS:										
1. SINGLE DX										
A. Not Operated	0									
B. Operated	0									
2. MULTIPLE DX										
A. Not Operated	23	8.0	49	2	3	6	10	18	20	30
B. Operated	28	10.5	36	4	6	9	14	20	22	28
1. SINGLE DX	0									
2. MULTIPLE DX	51	9.4	43	3	4	8	13	18	22	30
A. NOT OPERATED	23	8.0	49	2	3	6	10	18	20	30
B. OPERATED	28	10.5	36	4	6	9	14	20	22	28
TOTAL										
0–19 Years	2	8.0	70	2	2	8	14	14	14	14
20–34	4	12.3	27	9	10	10	20	20	20	20
35–49	3	8.3	30	3	3	8	14	14	14	14
50–64	12	9.2	59	4	4	6	12	18	28	28
65+	30	9.3	43	3	5	8	12	20	22	30
GRAND TOTAL	51	9.4	43	3	4	8	13	18	22	30

160: NASAL/ME/SINUS CA

Type of Patients	Observed Patients	Avg. Stay	Vari-ance	10th	25th	50th	75th	90th	95th	99th
1. SINGLE DX										
A. Not Operated										
0–19 Years	0									
20–34	1	1.0	0	1	1	1	1	1	1	1
35–49	0									
50–64	1	7.0	0	7	7	7	7	7	7	7
65+	0									
B. Operated										
0–19 Years	0									
20–34	5	3.8	5	2	2	3	5	7	7	7
35–49	1	2.0	0	2	2	2	2	2	2	2
50–64	8	2.9	2	1	2	2	4	5	5	5
65+	5	1.4	<1	1	1	1	2	2	2	2
2. MULTIPLE DX										
A. Not Operated										
0–19 Years	1	3.0	0	3	3	3	3	3	3	3
20–34	5	4.8	13	2	2	3	7	10	10	10
35–49	10	5.2	8	3	4	5	5	8	12	12
50–64	9	5.3	14	1	2	4	9	12	12	12
65+	24	4.0	8	1	2	3	5	8	9	11
B. Operated										
0–19 Years	2	5.0	0	5	5	5	5	5	5	5
20–34	6	6.9	23	1	4	8	10	14	14	14
35–49	29	7.0	28	1	3	6	10	17	17	19
50–64	57	5.9	45	1	2	3	7	14	22	35
65+	78	4.8	33	1	1	3	6	9	15	40
SUBTOTALS:										
1. SINGLE DX										
A. Not Operated	2	4.0	18	1	1	7	7	7	7	7
B. Operated	19	2.7	3	1	2	2	4	5	7	7
2. MULTIPLE DX										
A. Not Operated	49	4.5	9	1	2	4	6	9	11	12
B. Operated	172	5.6	35	1	2	4	7	12	17	35
1. SINGLE DX	21	2.8	3	1	2	2	4	5	7	7
2. MULTIPLE DX	221	5.4	30	1	2	4	7	12	15	28
A. NOT OPERATED	51	4.5	9	1	2	4	6	9	11	12
B. OPERATED	191	5.3	33	1	2	4	7	12	16	35
TOTAL										
0–19 Years	3	4.3	1	3	3	5	5	5	5	5
20–34	17	5.0	14	2	2	4	6	10	14	14
35–49	40	6.4	23	3	3	5	8	15	17	19
50–64	75	5.5	37	1	3	4	7	12	16	35
65+	107	4.5	26	1	1	3	5	8	12	21
GRAND TOTAL	242	5.2	28	1	2	4	6	11	15	28

161: LARYNX CA

Type of Patients	Observed Patients	Avg. Stay	Vari-ance	10th	25th	50th	75th	90th	95th	99th
1. SINGLE DX										
A. Not Operated										
0–19 Years	0									
20–34	0									
35–49	0									
50–64	8	2.0	1	1	1	2	2	4	4	4
65+	4	4.8	7	1	1	6	7	7	7	7
B. Operated										
0–19 Years	0									
20–34	0									
35–49	0									
50–64	20	5.5	13	1	1	5	9	10	10	11
65+	4	4.8	32	1	1	4	13	13	13	13
2. MULTIPLE DX										
A. Not Operated										
0–19 Years	0									
20–34	0									
35–49	22	7.9	52	2	4	5	10	18	24	30
50–64	147	8.1	101	1	3	6	9	15	21	48
65+	173	6.9	52	1	2	5	9	14	18	35
B. Operated										
0–19 Years	0									
20–34	2	13.5	<1	13	13	14	14	14	14	14
35–49	38	10.5	77	2	6	9	12	17	30	49
50–64	201	9.7	90	2	4	7	12	18	24	44
65+	219	10.2	102	2	5	8	12	18	28	51
SUBTOTALS:										
1. SINGLE DX										
A. Not Operated	12	2.9	4	1	1	2	4	6	7	7
B. Operated	24	5.4	15	1	1	4	9	10	11	13
2. MULTIPLE DX										
A. Not Operated	342	7.5	73	1	3	5	9	14	20	44
B. Operated	460	10.0	94	2	5	8	12	18	26	49
1. SINGLE DX	36	4.6	12	1	3	4	7	10	11	13
2. MULTIPLE DX	802	8.9	87	2	4	7	11	17	24	48
A. NOT OPERATED	354	7.3	72	1	3	5	9	14	20	44
B. OPERATED	484	9.8	91	2	5	7	12	18	26	49
TOTAL										
0–19 Years	0									
20–34	2	13.5	<1	13	13	14	14	14	14	14
35–49	60	9.5	69	2	5	7	10	17	25	49
50–64	376	8.7	90	2	4	6	10	18	24	46
65+	400	8.7	81	2	4	7	10	16	26	48
GRAND TOTAL	838	8.7	84	2	4	7	10	17	24	48

Length of Stay by Diagnosis and Operation, Western Region, 2008

Western Region, October 2006–September 2007 Data, by Diagnosis

161.0: GLOTTIS CA

Type of Patients	Observed Patients	Avg. Stay	Variance	10th	25th	50th	75th	90th	95th	99th
1. SINGLE DX										
A. Not Operated										
0–19 Years	0									
20–34	0									
35–49	0									
50–64	2	1.5	<1	1	1	2	2	2	2	2
65+	0									
B. Operated										
0–19 Years	0									
20–34	0									
35–49	0									
50–64	5	3.2	12	1	1	1	4	9	9	9
65+	2	7.0	71	1	1	7	13	13	13	13
2. MULTIPLE DX										
A. Not Operated										
0–19 Years	0									
20–34	0									
35–49	2	17.9	282	6	6	6	30	30	30	30
50–64	27	8.1	77	2	3	6	9	20	20	44
65+	33	6.6	38	2	3	5	7	17	19	27
B. Operated										
0–19 Years	0									
20–34	0									
35–49	7	11.6	55	2	6	10	16	25	25	25
50–64	52	11.0	179	3	5	7	11	20	30	89
65+	69	10.3	161	1	4	7	12	21	26	94
SUBTOTALS:										
1. SINGLE DX A. Not Operated	2	1.5	<1	1	1	2	2	2	2	2
1. SINGLE DX B. Operated	7	4.3	24	1	1	1	9	13	13	13
2. MULTIPLE DX A. Not Operated	62	7.6	62	2	3	5	9	18	20	44
2. MULTIPLE DX B. Operated	128	10.7	161	2	5	7	13	21	26	89
1. SINGLE DX	9	3.6	19	1	1	1	4	13	13	13
2. MULTIPLE DX	190	9.7	130	2	4	7	12	20	26	89
A. NOT OPERATED	64	7.4	61	2	3	5	9	18	20	44
B. OPERATED	135	10.3	155	1	4	7	12	21	26	89
TOTAL										
0–19 Years	0									
20–34	0									
35–49	9	13.0	85	6	6	10	16	30	30	30
50–64	86	9.4	137	2	4	7	10	20	22	89
65+	104	9.1	122	1	3	7	12	18	24	40
GRAND TOTAL	199	9.4	126	1	3	7	11	20	26	44

161.1: SUPRAGLOTTIS CA

Type of Patients	Observed Patients	Avg. Stay	Variance	10th	25th	50th	75th	90th	95th	99th
1. SINGLE DX										
A. Not Operated										
0–19 Years	0									
20–34	0									
35–49	0									
50–64	1	4.0	0	4	4	4	4	4	4	4
65+	2	5.5	<1	5	5	6	6	6	6	6
B. Operated										
0–19 Years	0									
20–34	0									
35–49	0									
50–64	7	6.0	8	1	4	6	8	10	10	10
65+	1	1.0	0	1	1	1	1	1	1	1
2. MULTIPLE DX										
A. Not Operated										
0–19 Years	0									
20–34	0									
35–49	8	5.3	13	2	2	3	10	11	11	11
50–64	55	8.5	62	2	4	7	12	19	21	48
65+	61	7.4	88	1	2	5	9	14	16	60
B. Operated										
0–19 Years	0									
20–34	1	13.0	0	13	13	13	13	13	13	13
35–49	15	8.5	46	2	5	7	11	12	30	30
50–64	65	8.4	66	2	3	7	10	14	20	46
65+	62	9.3	50	2	5	8	12	16	26	35
SUBTOTALS:										
1. SINGLE DX A. Not Operated	3	5.0	<1	4	4	5	6	6	6	6
1. SINGLE DX B. Operated	8	5.4	10	1	4	6	8	10	10	10
2. MULTIPLE DX A. Not Operated	124	7.8	72	1	2	6	10	14	20	44
2. MULTIPLE DX B. Operated	143	8.8	56	2	4	7	11	15	26	41
1. SINGLE DX	11	5.3	7	1	4	6	7	8	10	10
2. MULTIPLE DX	267	8.3	63	2	3	7	10	15	21	46
A. NOT OPERATED	127	7.7	70	1	2	6	9	14	20	48
B. OPERATED	151	8.7	54	2	4	7	11	15	26	41
TOTAL										
0–19 Years	0									
20–34	1	13.0	0	13	13	13	13	13	13	13
35–49	23	7.4	36	2	3	6	10	12	12	30
50–64	128	8.3	61	2	4	6	10	15	20	46
65+	126	8.2	68	1	3	7	10	15	26	35
GRAND TOTAL	278	8.2	61	2	3	7	10	15	21	46

161.8: LARYNX CA NEC

Type of Patients	Observed Patients	Avg. Stay	Variance	10th	25th	50th	75th	90th	95th	99th
1. SINGLE DX										
A. Not Operated										
0–19 Years	0									
20–34	0									
35–49	0									
50–64	4	2.0	<1	1	2	2	2	3	3	3
65+	1	1.0	0	1	1	1	1	1	1	1
B. Operated										
0–19 Years	0									
20–34	0									
35–49	0									
50–64	5	7.0	18	1	4	9	10	11	11	11
65+	0									
2. MULTIPLE DX										
A. Not Operated										
0–19 Years	0									
20–34	0									
35–49	2	4.5	<1	4	4	5	5	5	5	5
50–64	28	10.0	295	1	4	6	9	15	31	91
65+	24	7.5	18	2	4	8	10	12	12	19
B. Operated										
0–19 Years	0									
20–34	1	14.0	0	14	14	14	14	14	14	14
35–49	8	13.7	226	2	7	9	17	49	49	49
50–64	50	10.0	60	2	5	8	14	18	24	44
65+	44	10.0	36	4	6	10	12	15	18	35
SUBTOTALS:										
1. SINGLE DX A. Not Operated	5	1.8	<1	1	1	2	2	3	3	3
1. SINGLE DX B. Operated	5	7.0	18	1	4	9	10	11	11	11
2. MULTIPLE DX A. Not Operated	54	8.7	160	1	4	6	10	14	19	91
2. MULTIPLE DX B. Operated	103	10.3	61	3	6	8	13	17	24	44
1. SINGLE DX	10	4.4	16	1	1	2	9	10	11	11
2. MULTIPLE DX	157	9.8	95	2	5	8	12	17	24	49
A. NOT OPERATED	59	8.1	150	1	3	6	9	14	19	91
B. OPERATED	108	10.2	59	3	6	9	13	17	24	44
TOTAL										
0–19 Years	0									
20–34	1	14.0	0	14	14	14	14	14	14	14
35–49	10	11.8	191	4	5	8	13	17	49	49
50–64	87	9.5	131	2	4	6	13	17	24	91
65+	69	9.0	31	3	6	8	11	15	18	35
GRAND TOTAL	167	9.4	92	2	4	8	12	16	22	49

Length of Stay by Diagnosis and Operation, Western Region, 2008

Western Region, October 2006–September 2007 Data, by Diagnosis

162: TRACHEA/BRONCHUS/LUNG CA

Type of Patients	Observed Patients	Avg. Stay	Variance	10th	25th	50th	75th	90th	95th	99th
1. SINGLE DX										
A. *Not Operated*										
0–19 Years	0									
20–34	0									
35–49	5	1.6	<1	1	1	1	2	3	3	3
50–64	17	1.9	2	1	1	1	3	4	4	4
65+	10	3.1	3	2	2	3	4	7	7	7
B. *Operated*										
0–19 Years	2	5.5	4	4	4	7	7	7	7	7
20–34	4	5.2	4	4	3	5	7	8	8	8
35–49	15	4.7	5	2	3	4	5	7	8	8
50–64	38	4.0	4	1	2	4	5	6	8	9
65+	35	3.9	4	1	2	4	5	6	8	8
2. MULTIPLE DX										
A. *Not Operated*										
0–19 Years	3	2.3	<1	2	2	2	3	3	3	3
20–34	30	5.4	30	2	2	3	9	13	14	24
35–49	414	6.5	43	1	2	4	8	14	20	28
50–64	2,286	6.1	31	1	2	5	8	13	16	27
65+	5,105	6.0	22	2	3	5	8	12	15	24
B. *Operated*										
0–19 Years	6	7.3	7	3	6	8	9	11	11	11
20–34	28	9.8	95	4	5	5	12	22	23	50
35–49	418	7.9	66	3	4	5	7	14	21	39
50–64	2,371	7.4	34	3	4	6	9	16	18	29
65+	5,197	7.8	36	3	4	6	9	14	19	29
SUBTOTALS:										
1. SINGLE DX										
A. *Not Operated*	32	2.3	2	1	1	2	4	4		7
B. *Operated*	94	4.2	4	2	2	4	6	7		9
2. MULTIPLE DX										
A. *Not Operated*	7,838	6.0	26	2	3	5	8	12	16	25
B. *Operated*	8,020	7.7	37	3	4	6	9	14	19	30
1. SINGLE DX	126	3.7	4	1	2	4	5	7	8	9
2. MULTIPLE DX	15,858	6.9	32	2	3	6	8	13	17	27
A. NOT OPERATED	7,870	6.0	26	2	3	5	8	12	16	25
B. OPERATED	8,114	7.6	37	3	4	6	9	14	19	30
TOTAL										
0–19 Years	11	5.6	9	2	3	6	8	9	11	11
20–34	62	7.4	61	1	2	5	9	14	22	50
35–49	852	7.1	54	2	3	5	8	15	20	36
50–64	4,712	6.7	33	3	3	6	8	13	17	28
65+	10,347	6.9	30	2	3	6	9	13	17	27
GRAND TOTAL	15,984	6.8	32	2	3	5	8	13	17	27

162.2: MAIN BRONCHUS CA

Type of Patients	Observed Patients	Avg. Stay	Variance	10th	25th	50th	75th	90th	95th	99th
1. SINGLE DX										
A. *Not Operated*										
0–19 Years	0									
20–34	0									
35–49	2	1.5	<1	1	1	2	2	2	2	2
50–64	3	2.0	<1	1	1	2	3	3	3	3
65+	0									
B. *Operated*										
0–19 Years	0									
20–34	2	4.0	2	3	3	4	5	5	5	5
35–49	2	6.5	<1	6	6	6	7	7	7	7
50–64	0									
65+	0									
2. MULTIPLE DX										
A. *Not Operated*										
0–19 Years	1	2.0	0	2	2	2	2	2	2	2
20–34	3	5.0	13	2	2	4	9	9	9	9
35–49	38	6.0	26	1	2	5	7	13	21	22
50–64	224	6.4	38	1	3	5	9	12	14	28
65+	427	6.3	23	2	3	5	8	13	15	24
B. *Operated*										
0–19 Years	2	6.5	<1	6	6	7	7	7	7	7
20–34	2	8.4	40	4	4	4	13	13	13	13
35–49	22	6.6	26	1	3	6	8	10	19	21
50–64	131	8.5	70	2	4	7	11	16	22	47
65+	170	7.5	21	3	4	7	10	14	16	22
SUBTOTALS:										
1. SINGLE DX										
A. *Not Operated*	5	1.8	<1	1	1	2	2	3	3	3
B. *Operated*	4	5.3	3	3	3	5	6	7	7	7
2. MULTIPLE DX										
A. *Not Operated*	693	6.3	28	2	3	5	8	12	15	24
B. *Operated*	327	7.8	41	2	4	6	10	14	19	24
1. SINGLE DX	9	3.3	5	1	2	3	5	7	7	7
2. MULTIPLE DX	1,020	6.8	32	2	3	6	9	13	16	24
A. NOT OPERATED	698	6.3	28	2	3	5	8	12	15	24
B. OPERATED	331	7.8	41	2	4	6	10	14	19	24
TOTAL										
0–19 Years	3	5.0	7	2	2	6	7	7	7	7
20–34	7	5.7	15	3	3	4	9	13	13	13
35–49	64	6.1	25	1	3	5	7	12	19	22
50–64	358	7.1	51	1	3	6	9	14	18	30
65+	597	6.6	22	3	4	6	9	13	15	24
GRAND TOTAL	1,029	6.8	32	2	3	6	9	13	16	24

162.3: UP LOBE BRONCHUS/LUNG CA

Type of Patients	Observed Patients	Avg. Stay	Variance	10th	25th	50th	75th	90th	95th	99th
1. SINGLE DX										
A. *Not Operated*										
0–19 Years	0									
20–34	0									
35–49	1	3.0	0	3	3	3	3	3	3	3
50–64	6	1.7	1	1	1	1	2	3	4	4
65+	3	2.3	2	1	1	2	4	4	4	4
B. *Operated*										
0–19 Years	1	4.0	0	4	4	4	4	4	4	4
20–34	0									
35–49	3	3.7	2	2	2	4	5	5	5	5
50–64	15	3.7	2	2	2	4	5	5	6	6
65+	20	3.7	5	1	2	4	5	6	9	9
2. MULTIPLE DX										
A. *Not Operated*										
0–19 Years	0									
20–34	3	9.4	52	1	1	13	14	14	14	14
35–49	109	6.9	37	1	3	5	9	15	20	27
50–64	671	6.5	35	2	3	5	8	13	17	27
65+	1,551	6.1	25	2	3	5	8	12	15	24
B. *Operated*										
0–19 Years	1	11.0	0	11	11	11	11	11	11	11
20–34	8	7.3	34	3	5	5	13	19	19	19
35–49	210	7.8	85	3	4	6	9	13	20	38
50–64	1,231	7.4	30	3	4	6	9	13	18	27
65+	2,686	7.9	35	4	4	6	9	14	19	31
SUBTOTALS:										
1. SINGLE DX										
A. *Not Operated*	10	2.0	2	1	1	2	3	4	4	4
B. *Operated*	39	3.7	3	1	2	4	5	6	6	9
2. MULTIPLE DX										
A. *Not Operated*	2,334	6.3	28	2	3	5	8	12	16	25
B. *Operated*	4,136	7.7	36	3	4	6	9	14	19	30
1. SINGLE DX	49	3.3	3	1	2	3	5	6	6	9
2. MULTIPLE DX	6,470	7.2	33	2	4	6	9	13	18	29
A. NOT OPERATED	2,344	6.2	28	2	3	5	8	12	16	25
B. OPERATED	4,175	7.7	36	3	4	6	9	14	19	30
TOTAL										
0–19 Years	2	7.5	24	4	4	11	11	11	11	11
20–34	11	7.9	35	1	5	5	13	14	19	19
35–49	323	7.5	68	2	4	5	9	13	20	36
50–64	1,923	7.0	32	2	4	6	9	13	18	27
65+	4,260	7.2	32	2	4	6	9	13	18	29
GRAND TOTAL	6,519	7.2	33	2	4	6	9	13	18	28

Length of Stay by Diagnosis and Operation, Western Region, 2008

Western Region, October 2006–September 2007 Data, by Diagnosis

162.4: MID LOBE BRONCH/LUNG CA

Type of Patients	Observed Patients	Avg. Stay	Variance	10th	25th	50th	75th	90th	95th	99th
1. SINGLE DX										
A. Not Operated										
0–19 Years	0									
20–34	0									
35–49	0									
50–64	0									
65+	2	4.0	0	4	4	4	4	4	4	4
B. Operated										
0–19 Years	0									
20–34	0									
35–49	2	5.5	4	4	4	6	7	7	7	7
50–64	2	3.0	2	2	2	2	4	4	4	4
65+	2	2.0	2	1	1	1	3	3	3	3
2. MULTIPLE DX										
A. Not Operated										
0–19 Years	0									
20–34	0									
35–49	13	9.0	43	3	4	7	11	17	25	25
50–64	45	5.7	21	1	2	6	7	11	13	27
65+	158	6.2	18	2	3	5	7	11	15	24
B. Operated										
0–19 Years	0									
20–34	3	13.1	72	5	5	12	22	22	22	22
35–49	21	9.1	90	2	4	5	8	22	23	39
50–64	140	6.6	23	2	4	5	8	13	16	25
65+	270	6.4	35	3	4	5	7	10	15	28
SUBTOTALS:										
1. SINGLE DX										
A. Not Operated	2	4.0	0	4	4	4	4	4	4	4
B. Operated	6	3.5	4	1	2	4	4	7	7	7
2. MULTIPLE DX										
A. Not Operated	216	6.2	20	2	3	5	8	11	15	25
B. Operated	434	6.6	34	2	4	5	7	12	16	27
1. SINGLE DX	8	3.6	3	1	2	4	4	7	7	7
2. MULTIPLE DX	650	6.5	29	2	4	5	7	11	16	27
A. NOT OPERATED	218	6.2	20	2	3	5	8	11	15	25
B. OPERATED	440	6.6	34	2	4	5	7	12	16	27
TOTAL										
0–19 Years	0									
20–34	3	13.1	72	5	5	12	22	22	22	22
35–49	36	8.8	67	2	4	6	10	22	25	39
50–64	187	6.3	22	2	3	5	8	12	16	27
65+	432	6.3	28	2	4	5	7	10	15	24
GRAND TOTAL	658	6.5	29	2	4	5	7	11	16	27

162.5: LOW LOBE BRONCH/LUNG CA

Type of Patients	Observed Patients	Avg. Stay	Variance	10th	25th	50th	75th	90th	95th	99th
1. SINGLE DX										
A. Not Operated										
0–19 Years	0									
20–34	0									
35–49	0									
50–64	0									
65+	1	3.0	0	3	3	3	3	3	3	3
B. Operated										
0–19 Years	0									
20–34	1	8.0	0	8	8	8	8	8	8	8
35–49	6	4.7	5	2	3	4	7	7	8	8
50–64	15	4.4	5	1	3	4	6	8	9	9
65+	10	4.2	3	3	3	4	5	8	8	8
2. MULTIPLE DX										
A. Not Operated										
0–19 Years	1	3.0	0	3	3	3	3	3	3	3
20–34	3	4.7	30	1	1	2	11	11	15	15
35–49	50	5.8	18	2	3	4	8	12	15	18
50–64	294	6.8	35	2	3	5	8	13	18	30
65+	874	6.8	28	2	3	6	8	13	17	26
B. Operated										
0–19 Years	2	5.5	12	3	3	3	8	8	8	8
20–34	8	6.5	14	3	4	6	7	14	14	14
35–49	94	7.3	27	4	4	6	8	17	20	25
50–64	599	7.1	28	3	4	6	8	13	18	30
65+	1,579	7.7	38	3	4	6	9	14	19	28
SUBTOTALS:										
1. SINGLE DX										
A. Not Operated	1	3.0	0	3	3	3	3	3	3	3
B. Operated	32	4.5	5	2	3	4	6	8	8	9
2. MULTIPLE DX										
A. Not Operated	1,222	6.7	29	2	3	5	8	13	17	27
B. Operated	2,282	7.5	35	3	4	6	9	14	18	28
1. SINGLE DX	33	4.5	5	2	3	4	6	8	8	9
2. MULTIPLE DX	3,504	7.2	33	2	4	6	9	14	18	28
A. NOT OPERATED	1,223	6.7	29	2	3	5	8	13	17	27
B. OPERATED	2,314	7.4	34	3	4	6	9	14	18	28
TOTAL										
0–19 Years	3	4.7	8	3	3	3	8	8	8	8
20–34	12	6.2	15	2	4	5	8	11	14	14
35–49	150	6.7	24	2	4	5	8	15	18	23
50–64	908	6.9	30	2	4	5	8	13	18	30
65+	2,464	7.3	34	2	4	6	9	14	18	27
GRAND TOTAL	3,537	7.2	33	2	4	6	9	14	18	28

162.8: BRONCHUS/LUNG CA NEC

Type of Patients	Observed Patients	Avg. Stay	Variance	10th	25th	50th	75th	90th	95th	99th
1. SINGLE DX										
A. Not Operated										
0–19 Years	0									
20–34	0									
35–49	2	1.0	0	1	1	1	1	1	1	1
50–64	3	2.0	3	1	1	1	4	4	4	4
65+	0									
B. Operated										
0–19 Years	0									
20–34	1	1.0	0	1	1	1	1	1	1	1
35–49	4	5.0	6	2	2	5	8	8	8	8
50–64	3	5.3	4	3	3	6	7	7	7	7
2. MULTIPLE DX										
A. Not Operated										
0–19 Years	0									
20–34	3	2.3	2	1	1	2	4	4	4	4
35–49	66	7.2	73	1	2	4	7	21	25	45
50–64	346	6.5	30	1	3	5	9	14	15	23
65+	613	5.7	21	1	2	4	7	11	15	24
B. Operated										
0–19 Years	0									
20–34	6	17.2	300	5	7	7	23	50	50	50
35–49	33	9.7	62	4	4	7	12	20	23	41
50–64	125	8.4	68	2	4	6	10	16	20	39
65+	252	8.1	38	3	4	6	10	17	23	28
SUBTOTALS:										
1. SINGLE DX										
A. Not Operated	5	1.6	2	1	1	1	1	1	4	4
B. Operated	8	4.6	6	1	2	5	7	8	8	8
2. MULTIPLE DX										
A. Not Operated	1,028	6.0	28	1	2	5	8	13	16	25
B. Operated	416	8.5	53	3	4	6	10	17	23	35
1. SINGLE DX	13	3.5	6	1	1	3	5	7	8	8
2. MULTIPLE DX	1,444	6.7	36	2	3	5	9	14	18	27
A. NOT OPERATED	1,033	6.0	28	1	2	5	8	13	16	25
B. OPERATED	424	8.4	52	3	4	6	10	17	23	35
TOTAL										
0–19 Years	0									
20–34	9	12.2	243	1	4	7	11	50	50	50
35–49	102	7.8	70	1	3	5	9	20	24	41
50–64	478	6.9	40	2	3	5	8	14	17	35
65+	868	6.4	27	2	3	5	8	13	17	26
GRAND TOTAL	1,457	6.7	36	2	3	5	8	14	18	27

Length of Stay by Diagnosis and Operation, Western Region, 2008

Western Region, October 2006–September 2007 Data, by Diagnosis

162.9: BRONCHUS/LUNG CA NOS

Type of Patients	Observed Patients	Avg. Stay	Variance	Percentiles 10th	25th	50th	75th	90th	95th	99th
1. SINGLE DX										
A. Not Operated										
0–19 Years	0									
20–34	0									
35–49	0									
50–64	5	2.2	3	1	1	1	4	4	4	4
65+	4	3.3	6	2	2	2	7	7	7	7
B. Operated										
0–19 Years	0									
20–34	1	5.0	0	5	5	5	5	5	5	5
35–49	0									
50–64	2	2.5	4	1	1	1	4	4	5	5
65+	0									
2. MULTIPLE DX										
A. Not Operated										
0–19 Years	1	2.0	0	2	2	2	2	2	2	2
20–34	18	5.5	34	1	2	3	7	14	24	24
35–49	134	6.2	47	1	2	4	8	14	18	28
50–64	702	5.3	24	1	2	4	7	12	16	24
65+	1,474	5.3	18	2	3	4	7	10	14	20
B. Operated										
0–19 Years	1	9.0	0	9	9	9	9	9	9	9
20–34	1	4.0	0	4	4	4	4	4	4	4
35–49	37	8.2	71	1	4	7	10	15	17	51
50–64	138	7.8	35	2	4	6	10	16	19	30
65+	231	8.8	45	3	4	7	11	18	23	28
SUBTOTALS:										
1. SINGLE DX A. Not Operated	9	2.7	4	1	1	2	4	7	7	7
B. Operated	3	3.3	4	1	1	4	5	5	5	5
2. MULTIPLE DX A. Not Operated	2,329	5.4	21	2	2	4	7	11	15	23
B. Operated	408	8.4	44	2	4	7	11	16	21	29
1. SINGLE DX	12	2.8	4	1	1	2	4	5	7	7
2. MULTIPLE DX	2,737	5.8	26	1	2	4	7	12	16	25
A. NOT OPERATED	2,338	5.3	21	1	2	4	7	11	15	23
B. OPERATED	411	8.4	44	2	4	7	11	16	21	29
TOTAL										
0–19 Years	2	5.5	24	2	2	6	9	9	9	9
20–34	20	5.4	31	1	2	4	6	10	14	24
35–49	171	6.6	53	1	2	4	9	14	18	51
50–64	847	5.7	27	1	2	4	7	12	16	26
65+	1,709	5.8	23	2	3	4	7	11	15	24
GRAND TOTAL	2,749	5.8	26	1	2	4	7	12	16	25

163: PLEURA CA

Type of Patients	Observed Patients	Avg. Stay	Variance	Percentiles 10th	25th	50th	75th	90th	95th	99th
1. SINGLE DX										
A. Not Operated										
0–19 Years	1	1.0	0	1	1	1	1	1	1	1
20–34	1	1.0	0	1	1	1	1	1	1	1
35–49	1	5.0	0	5	5	5	5	5	5	5
50–64	0									
65+	0									
B. Operated										
0–19 Years	0									
20–34	0									
35–49	0									
50–64	2	3.0	2	2	2	3	4	4	4	4
65+	1	3.0	0	3	3	3	3	3	3	3
2. MULTIPLE DX										
A. Not Operated										
0–19 Years	1	11.0	0	11	11	11	11	11	11	11
20–34	1	3.0	0	3	3	3	3	3	3	3
35–49	2	5.0	8	3	3	7	7	7	7	7
50–64	25	4.3	9	1	2	3	6	9	10	10
65+	108	5.5	20	1	2	4	7	10	14	22
B. Operated										
0–19 Years	1	12.0	0	12	12	12	12	12	12	12
20–34	3	5.6	17	1	1	7	9	9	9	9
35–49	3	6.7	6	4	4	7	9	9	9	9
50–64	39	7.0	22	1	4	6	10	15	16	21
65+	118	7.4	26	2	4	6	10	14	18	24
SUBTOTALS:										
1. SINGLE DX A. Not Operated	3	2.3	5	1	1	1	5	5	5	5
B. Operated	3	3.0	<1	2	2	3	4	4	4	4
2. MULTIPLE DX A. Not Operated	137	5.3	18	1	2	4	7	11	13	22
B. Operated	164	7.3	24	2	4	6	10	14	16	24
1. SINGLE DX	6	2.7	3	1	1	2	4	5	5	5
2. MULTIPLE DX	301	6.4	22	2	3	5	9	13	15	23
A. NOT OPERATED	140	5.2	18	2	2	4	7	11	13	22
B. OPERATED	167	7.2	24	2	4	6	10	14	16	24
TOTAL										
0–19 Years	3	8.0	36	1	1	11	12	12	12	12
20–34	5	4.2	13	1	1	3	7	9	9	9
35–49	6	5.9	5	3	4	7	7	9	9	9
50–64	66	5.9	18	1	2	5	9	11	15	21
65+	227	6.5	24	2	3	5	9	13	15	24
GRAND TOTAL	307	6.3	22	2	3	5	9	13	15	23

164: THYMUS/HEART/MEDIAST CA

Type of Patients	Observed Patients	Avg. Stay	Variance	Percentiles 10th	25th	50th	75th	90th	95th	99th
1. SINGLE DX										
A. Not Operated										
0–19 Years	1	6.0	0	6	6	6	6	6	6	6
20–34	0									
35–49	1	1.0	0	1	1	1	1	1	1	1
50–64	0									
65+	0									
B. Operated										
0–19 Years	2	5.0	32	1	1	·	9	9	9	9
20–34	4	5.7	27	2	2	4	6	13	13	13
35–49	1	5.0	0	5	5	5	5	5	5	5
50–64	4	3.8	<1	3	3	3	5	5	5	5
65+	0									
2. MULTIPLE DX										
A. Not Operated										
0–19 Years	5	5.8	17	1	3	5	9	11	11	11
20–34	17	6.9	27	1	3	6	9	15	21	21
35–49	20	5.9	26	1	2	5	6	11	15	22
50–64	51	6.0	44	1	2	4	7	12	18	36
65+	40	6.1	20	1	3	5	9	13	14	20
B. Operated										
0–19 Years	7	11.7	32	5	6	11	22	>99	>99	>99
20–34	27	8.5	62	3	6	8	8	20	21	40
35–49	34	9.7	45	4	4	8	14	20	22	29
50–64	54	7.2	32	2	4	5	9	14	20	29
65+	61	7.6	40	2	4	6	9	16	19	38
SUBTOTALS:										
1. SINGLE DX A. Not Operated	2	3.5	12	1	1	6	6	6	6	6
B. Operated	11	4.8	12	2	2	4	6	9	13	13
2. MULTIPLE DX A. Not Operated	133	6.1	30	1	2	5	8	12	15	29
B. Operated	183	8.2	42	2	4	6	10	17	21	40
1. SINGLE DX	13	4.6	12	1	2	4	6	9	13	13
2. MULTIPLE DX	316	7.3	38	2	3	5	9	15	21	36
A. NOT OPERATED	135	6.1	30	1	2	5	8	12	15	29
B. OPERATED	194	8.0	41	2	4	6	10	16	21	40
TOTAL										
0–19 Years	15	8.5	31	1	5	9	11	22	15	29
20–34	48	7.7	47	2	4	6	8	15	21	40
35–49	56	8.1	41	2	4	6	11	18	22	29
50–64	109	6.5	37	1	3	5	9	14	18	29
65+	101	7.0	33	1	4	6	9	14	17	22
GRAND TOTAL	329	7.2	37	2	3	5	9	15	20	36

Length of Stay by Diagnosis and Operation, Western Region, 2008

Western Region, October 2006–September 2007 Data, by Diagnosis

165: OTHER RESP/INTRATHOR CA

Type of Patients	Observed Patients	Avg. Stay	Variance	10th	25th	50th	75th	90th	95th	99th
1. SINGLE DX										
A. *Not Operated*										
0–19 Years	0									
20–34	0									
35–49	0									
50–64	0									
65+	0									
B. *Operated*										
0–19 Years	0									
20–34	1	4.0	0	4	4	4	4	4	4	4
35–49	0									
50–64	0									
65+	0									
2. MULTIPLE DX										
A. *Not Operated*										
0–19 Years	0									
20–34	0									
35–49	0									
50–64	0									
65+	0									
B. *Operated*										
0–19 Years	0									
20–34	0									
35–49	0									
50–64	0									
65+	0									
SUBTOTALS:										
1. SINGLE DX										
A. *Not Operated*	0									
B. *Operated*	1	4.0	0	4	4	4	4	4	4	4
2. MULTIPLE DX										
A. *Not Operated*	0									
B. *Operated*	0									
1. SINGLE DX	1	4.0	0	4	4	4	4	4	4	4
2. MULTIPLE DX	0									
A. NOT OPERATED	0									
B. OPERATED	1	4.0	0	4	4	4	4	4	4	4
TOTAL										
0–19 Years	0									
20–34	1	4.0	0	4	4	4	4	4	4	4
35–49	0									
50–64	0									
65+	0									
GRAND TOTAL	1	4.0	0	4	4	4	4	4	4	4

170: BONE & ARTICULAR CART CA

Type of Patients	Observed Patients	Avg. Stay	Variance	10th	25th	50th	75th	90th	95th	99th
1. SINGLE DX										
A. *Not Operated*										
0–19 Years	11	4.1	5	2	2	3	5	7	9	9
20–34	3	3.7	6	1	1	4	6	6	6	6
35–49	1	8.0	0	8	8	8	8	8	8	8
50–64	0									
65+	0									
B. *Operated*										
0–19 Years	26	4.2	17	1	2	3	7	9	14	17
20–34	37	4.0	9	1	2	3	6	7	9	16
35–49	26	3.7	10	1	2	3	4	7	12	13
50–64	12	3.0	4	1	1	3	4	6	7	7
65+	7	5.1	10	1	3	4	9	9	9	9
2. MULTIPLE DX										
A. *Not Operated*										
0–19 Years	55	4.6	27	1	1	3	6	10	12	27
20–34	31	6.3	21	2	2	6	8	12	16	20
35–49	29	5.6	25	1	2	4	7	12	14	23
50–64	19	5.4	15	2	4	4	5	9	19	19
65+	21	4.3	10	1	2	4	6	7	8	14
B. *Operated*										
0–19 Years	40	10.1	195	3	4	7	10	17	24	85
20–34	68	7.7	40	2	4	6	10	19	22	>99
35–49	78	7.1	51	2	3	6	10	13	17	42
50–64	122	6.7	42	1	2	5	8	12	22	34
65+	123	8.2	86	2	3	6	10	17	22	55
SUBTOTALS:										
1. SINGLE DX										
A. *Not Operated*	15	4.3	6	2	2	4	6	8	9	9
B. *Operated*	108	4.0	10	1	2	3	5	7	9	16
2. MULTIPLE DX										
A. *Not Operated*	155	5.2	21	1	2	4	7	11	14	25
B. *Operated*	431	7.7	70	2	3	6	9	16	22	42
1. SINGLE DX	123	4.0	10	1	2	3	6	7	9	16
2. MULTIPLE DX	586	7.0	59	1	3	5	8	14	21	38
A. NOT OPERATED	170	5.1	20	1	2	4	7	11	13	25
B. OPERATED	539	6.9	61	1	3	5	8	14	21	38
TOTAL										
0–19 Years	132	6.2	79	1	2	4	7	12	17	38
20–34	139	6.3	29	1	3	5	8	13	19	30
35–49	134	6.2	39	2	2	4	8	12	15	36
50–64	153	6.2	37	1	2	4	8	12	19	34
65+	151	7.5	74	1	3	5	9	16	21	55
GRAND TOTAL	709	6.5	51	1	2	4	8	13	18	36

171: SOFT TISSUE CA

Type of Patients	Observed Patients	Avg. Stay	Variance	10th	25th	50th	75th	90th	95th	99th
1. SINGLE DX										
A. *Not Operated*										
0–19 Years	8	2.5	6	1	1	1	3	8	8	8
20–34	3	4.0	7	1	1	5	6	6	6	6
35–49	7	3.7	5	1	2	3	6	7	7	7
50–64	2	1.5	<1	1	1	2	2	2	2	2
65+	2	5.5	24	2	2	2	9	9	9	9
B. *Operated*										
0–19 Years	13	2.9	6	1	1	2	2	2	8	8
20–34	33	3.9	19	1	2	2	5	6	10	25
35–49	48	2.9	4	1	2	2	5	6	6	7
50–64	49	3.0	5	1	1	2	4	7	9	10
65+	24	3.3	5	1	1	3	4	6	7	9
2. MULTIPLE DX										
A. *Not Operated*										
0–19 Years	28	8.7	162	1	2	5	7	25	28	64
20–34	28	4.4	10	1	2	4	6	9	10	14
35–49	51	6.7	26	2	3	4	10	15	16	23
50–64	78	6.9	34	2	3	4	7	18	20	24
65+	111	5.7	41	1	2	4	7	12	16	22
B. *Operated*										
0–19 Years	35	10.9	235	2	5	7	10	17	46	84
20–34	65	8.6	85	2	3	6	10	21	28	43
35–49	165	6.2	38	1	2	4	8	11	15	36
50–64	362	6.6	56	1	2	4	8	14	21	46
65+	502	6.3	39	1	2	5	8	13	16	29
SUBTOTALS:										
1. SINGLE DX										
A. *Not Operated*	22	3.3	6	1	1	2	5	7	8	9
B. *Operated*	167	3.2	8	1	1	2	4	6	8	10
2. MULTIPLE DX										
A. *Not Operated*	296	6.4	45	2	3	4	8	14	18	28
B. *Operated*	1,129	6.6	54	1	2	5	8	13	21	42
1. SINGLE DX	189	3.2	7	1	1	2	4	6	8	10
2. MULTIPLE DX	1,425	6.6	52	1	2	4	8	14	20	41
A. NOT OPERATED	318	6.1	43	1	2	4	8	13	18	25
B. OPERATED	1,296	6.2	49	1	2	4	8	13	19	41
TOTAL										
0–19 Years	84	8.1	161	1	2	5	8	14	28	84
20–34	129	6.4	55	1	2	4	7	14	25	41
35–49	271	5.7	30	1	2	4	8	11	15	29
50–64	491	6.2	48	1	2	4	8	14	21	45
65+	639	6.1	39	1	2	4	8	13	16	29
GRAND TOTAL	1,614	6.2	48	1	2	4	8	13	18	36

Length of Stay by Diagnosis and Operation, Western Region, 2008

Western Region, October 2006–September 2007 Data, by Diagnosis

171.3: LOW LIMB SOFT TISSUE CA

Type of Patients	Observed Patients	Avg. Stay	Vari-ance	10th	25th	50th	75th	90th	95th	99th
1. SINGLE DX										
A. Not Operated										
0–19 Years	0									
20–34	0									
35–49	2	2.5	<1	2	2	2	3	3		3
50–64	0									
65+	1	9.0	0	9	9	9	9	9		9
B. Operated										
0–19 Years	8	3.1	8	1	1	2	2	8	8	8
20–34	13	5.1	42	1	2	2	5	10	25	25
35–49	19	3.7	4	1	2	3	6	7	7	7
50–64	25	2.6	4	1	2	2	3	5	5	10
65+	18	2.9	4	1	1	3	4	5	7	7
2. MULTIPLE DX										
A. Not Operated										
0–19 Years	2	4.0	2	3	3	3	5	5	5	5
20–34	2	2.0	2	1	1	2	3	3	3	3
35–49	4	7.3	110	1	1	3	23	23	23	23
50–64	9	9.6	67	1	3	6	13	23	23	23
65+	12	7.4	31	3	4	5	9	12	22	22
B. Operated										
0–19 Years	5	4.0	6	2	3	3	4	8	8	8
20–34	25	7.1	44	1	3	4	9	21	21	26
35–49	62	5.3	33	2	2	4	7	9	11	42
50–64	109	4.8	38	1	2	3	5	10	14	30
65+	161	5.0	15	2	2	4	6	10	13	21
SUBTOTALS:										
1. SINGLE DX										
A. Not Operated	3	4.7	14	2	2	3	3	9	9	9
B. Operated	83	3.4	10	1	2	2	4	6	7	25
2. MULTIPLE DX										
A. Not Operated	29	7.5	48	1	3	5	11	22	23	23
B. Operated	362	5.1	27	1	2	4	6	10	13	26
1. SINGLE DX	86	3.4	10	1	2	2	4	7	8	25
2. MULTIPLE DX	391	5.3	29	1	2	4	7	10	14	26
A. NOT OPERATED	32	7.2	45	2	3	4	9	21	23	23
B. OPERATED	445	4.8	24	1	2	3	6	10	12	25
TOTAL										
0–19 Years	15	3.5	6	1	2	3	3	8	8	8
20–34	40	6.2	42	1	2	2	8	21	25	26
35–49	87	4.9	29	1	2	3	6	11	11	42
50–64	143	4.7	36	1	2	3	5	10	14	30
65+	192	5.0	16	2	2	4	6	10	13	22
GRAND TOTAL	477	4.9	26	1	2	3	6	10	13	25

171.5: ABDOMEN SOFT TISSUE CA

Type of Patients	Observed Patients	Avg. Stay	Vari-ance	10th	25th	50th	75th	90th	95th	99th
1. SINGLE DX										
A. Not Operated										
0–19 Years	0									
20–34	2	3.0	8	1	1	1	5	5	5	5
35–49	2	4.0	18	1	1	4	7	7	7	7
50–64	1	2.0	0	2	2	2	2	2	2	2
65+	0									
B. Operated										
0–19 Years	0									
20–34	0									
35–49	2	5.0	2	4	4	6	6	6	6	6
50–64	5	6.0	12	1	4	7	8	10	10	10
65+	1	6.0	0	6	6	6	6	6	6	6
2. MULTIPLE DX										
A. Not Operated										
0–19 Years	6	8.7	65	3	5	6	7	25	25	25
20–34	11	4.6	18	1	1	4	8	9	14	14
35–49	21	8.5	28	3	4	8	13	15	16	18
50–64	36	7.1	31	2	3	4	8	18	19	24
65+	45	5.2	16	1	2	4	8	10	13	16
B. Operated										
0–19 Years	8	10.2	90	5	6	6	8	33	33	33
20–34	12	14.2	151	4	7	11	15	34	43	43
35–49	43	7.5	32	2	3	6	10	14	16	29
50–64	90	10.3	80	2	5	7	13	22	31	>99
65+	118	10.0	66	4	5	7	12	19	29	42
SUBTOTALS:										
1. SINGLE DX										
A. Not Operated	5	3.2	7	1	1	2	5	7	7	7
B. Operated	8	5.8	8	1	4	6	8	10	10	10
2. MULTIPLE DX										
A. Not Operated	119	6.5	26	2	3	4	9	15	18	24
B. Operated	271	9.9	70	3	5	7	12	21	29	47
1. SINGLE DX	13	4.8	9	1	2	5	7	8	10	10
2. MULTIPLE DX	390	8.9	59	2	4	7	11	18	26	43
A. NOT OPERATED	124	6.3	26	2	3	4	8	15	16	24
B. OPERATED	279	9.8	69	3	5	7	12	21	29	47
TOTAL										
0–19 Years	14	9.6	74	5	5	6	8	25	33	33
20–34	25	9.1	102	1	4	7	11	19	34	43
35–49	68	7.6	30	2	4	6	11	15	16	29
50–64	132	9.2	66	2	4	7	11	21	28	47
65+	164	8.7	57	2	4	7	10	16	22	42
GRAND TOTAL	403	8.7	58	2	4	7	11	18	25	42

172: SKIN MALIGNANT MELANOMA

Type of Patients	Observed Patients	Avg. Stay	Vari-ance	10th	25th	50th	75th	90th	95th	99th
1. SINGLE DX										
A. Not Operated										
0–19 Years	0									
20–34	0									
35–49	2	4.5	12	2	2	2	7	7	7	7
50–64	2	2.5	4	1	1	3	4	4	4	4
65+	1	1.0	0	1	1	1	1	1	1	1
B. Operated										
0–19 Years	0									
20–34	6	3.0	12	1	1	2	3	10	10	10
35–49	12	2.5	4	1	1	2	3	5	7	7
50–64	25	1.8	2	1	1	1	2	5	5	6
65+	16	2.2	1	1	1	2	3	4	4	4
2. MULTIPLE DX										
A. Not Operated										
0–19 Years	0									
20–34	8	4.4	17	1	3	3	6	14	14	14
35–49	17	5.3	16	2	2	4	7	11	16	16
50–64	35	4.5	19	1	2	3	5	7	18	20
65+	44	5.0	19	1	2	4	8	11	12	21
B. Operated										
0–19 Years	1	1.0	0	1	1	1	1	1	1	1
20–34	22	2.2	2	1	1	2	3	5	5	6
35–49	46	3.0	7	1	1	2	4	8	8	9
50–64	140	2.8	10	1	1	2	3	6	8	17
65+	255	2.6	7	1	1	2	3	6	8	15
SUBTOTALS:										
1. SINGLE DX										
A. Not Operated	5	3.0	6	1	1	2	4	7	7	7
B. Operated	59	2.2	3	1	1	1	3	5	6	10
2. MULTIPLE DX										
A. Not Operated	104	4.8	18	1	2	3	6	11	13	20
B. Operated	464	2.7	8	1	1	2	3	6	8	15
1. SINGLE DX	64	2.3	3	1	1	1	3	5	6	10
2. MULTIPLE DX	568	3.1	10	1	1	2	4	7	9	17
A. NOT OPERATED	109	4.7	17	1	2	3	6	11	13	20
B. OPERATED	523	2.6	7	1	1	2	3	6	8	13
TOTAL										
0–19 Years	1	1.0	0	1	1	1	1	1	1	1
20–34	36	2.8	7	1	1	2	3	6	10	14
35–49	77	3.4	9	1	1	2	5	8	9	16
50–64	202	2.9	11	1	1	2	3	6	8	18
65+	316	2.9	9	1	1	2	4	7	9	15
GRAND TOTAL	632	3.0	10	1	1	2	4	7	9	16

Western Region, October 2006–September 2007 Data, by Diagnosis

173: OTHER SKIN CA

Type of Patients	Observed Patients	Avg. Stay	Vari-ance	10th	25th	50th	75th	90th	95th	99th
1. SINGLE DX										
A. Not Operated										
0–19 Years	2	1.0	0	1	1	1	1	1	1	1
20–34	0									
35–49	3	4.0	7	1	1	5	6	6	6	6
50–64	4	5.8	8	4	4	5	8	10	10	10
65+	2	5.5	40	1	1	10	10	10	10	10
B. Operated										
0–19 Years	3	1.3	<1	1	1	1	2	2	2	2
20–34	7	1.9	1	1	1	1	3	4	4	4
35–49	15	3.3	7	1	1	2	5	7	10	10
50–64	20	2.6	3	1	1	2	3	5	6	6
65+	30	2.0	2	1	1	1	2	5	6	7
2. MULTIPLE DX										
A. Not Operated										
0–19 Years	1	6.0	0	6	6	6	6	6	6	6
20–34	4	2.5	2	1	2	3	3	4	4	4
35–49	10	5.7	34	1	2	3	12	16	16	16
50–64	56	5.2	27	1	2	3	7	14	18	22
65+	103	4.8	22	1	2	3	7	10	12	22
B. Operated										
0–19 Years	4	1.8	2	1	1	1	4	4	4	4
20–34	12	4.6	18	1	1	3	9	9	13	13
35–49	62	4.3	14	1	2	3	6	6	8	23
50–64	160	4.8	28	1	1	3	6	8	14	27
65+	500	4.2	22	1	1	3	5	8	13	24
SUBTOTALS:										
1. SINGLE DX										
A. Not Operated	11	4.4	11	1	1	4	7	10	10	10
B. Operated	75	2.4	3	1	1	2	3	5	6	10
2. MULTIPLE DX										
A. Not Operated	174	4.9	23	1	2	3	7	11	15	22
B. Operated	738	4.3	22	1	2	3	6	8	13	24
1. SINGLE DX	86	2.6	5	1	1	2	3	6	7	10
2. MULTIPLE DX	912	4.4	23	1	1	3	6	9	13	24
A. NOT OPERATED	185	4.9	23	1	2	3	6	11	15	22
B. OPERATED	813	4.1	21	1	1	3	5	8	13	24
TOTAL										
0–19 Years	10	1.9	3	1	1	1	2	4	6	6
20–34	23	3.4	11	1	1	2	4	9	9	13
35–49	90	4.2	15	1	2	3	6	8	12	23
50–64	240	4.7	25	1	2	3	6	9	14	25
65+	635	4.2	21	1	1	3	5	9	13	24
GRAND TOTAL	998	4.3	21	1	1	3	6	9	13	24

173.3: OTHER FACE SKIN CA NEC

Type of Patients	Observed Patients	Avg. Stay	Vari-ance	10th	25th	50th	75th	90th	95th	99th
1. SINGLE DX										
A. Not Operated										
0–19 Years	0									
20–34	0									
35–49	0									
50–64	0									
65+	2	5.5	40	1	1	10	10	10	10	10
B. Operated										
0–19 Years	0									
20–34	2	1.5	<1	1	1	2	2	2	2	2
35–49	5	2.0	3	1	1	1	2	5	5	5
50–64	1	1.0	0	1	1	1	1	1	1	1
65+	6	1.2	<1	1	1	1	1	2	2	2
2. MULTIPLE DX										
A. Not Operated										
0–19 Years	0									
20–34	4	7.8	55	1	1	2	16	16	16	16
35–49	12	4.9	34	1	2	3	6	8	22	22
50–64	18	6.0	55	1	1	3	9	15	31	31
B. Operated										
0–19 Years	0									
20–34	2	4.0	18	1	1	7	7	7	7	7
35–49	8	3.3	5	1	2	3	3	8	8	8
50–64	38	4.2	23	1	1	3	5	7	22	23
65+	139	3.9	27	1	1	2	5	8	10	31
SUBTOTALS:										
1. SINGLE DX										
A. Not Operated	2	5.5	40	1	1	10	10	10	10	10
B. Operated	14	1.5	1	1	1	1	2	2	5	5
2. MULTIPLE DX										
A. Not Operated	34	5.8	46	1	2	3	8	15	22	31
B. Operated	187	3.9	25	1	1	2	5	7	10	31
1. SINGLE DX	16	2.0	6	1	1	1	2	5	10	10
2. MULTIPLE DX	221	4.2	28	1	1	2	5	8	12	31
A. NOT OPERATED	36	5.8	44	1	2	3	9	15	22	31
B. OPERATED	201	3.7	24	1	1	2	5	7	10	23
TOTAL										
0–19 Years	0									
20–34	4	2.8	8	1	1	2	7	7	7	7
35–49	17	3.9	18	1	1	2	5	12	16	16
50–64	51	4.3	25	1	2	3	5	7	22	23
65+	165	4.0	29	1	1	2	5	8	10	31
GRAND TOTAL	237	4.1	27	1	1	2	5	8	12	31

174: FEMALE BREAST CA

Type of Patients	Observed Patients	Avg. Stay	Vari-ance	10th	25th	50th	75th	90th	95th	99th
1. SINGLE DX										
A. Not Operated										
0–19 Years	0									
20–34	0									
35–49	3	1.0	0	1	1	1	1	1	1	1
50–64	10	3.4	17	1	2	2	3	3	15	15
65+	3	2.7	2	1	1	3	4	4	4	4
B. Operated										
0–19 Years	0									
20–34	55	1.5	<1	1	1	1	2	2	3	5
35–49	422	1.6	1	1	1	1	2	3	4	5
50–64	517	1.6	1	1	1	1	2	3	4	5
65+	225	1.4	<1	1	1	1	2	2	3	4
2. MULTIPLE DX										
A. Not Operated										
0–19 Years	1	3.0	0	3	3	3	3	3	3	3
20–34	16	4.6	26	1	2	3	6	11	21	21
35–49	175	5.5	28	1	2	4	8	12	16	23
50–64	318	5.5	34	1	2	3	8	11	18	29
65+	253	5.1	20	1	2	4	7	11	15	22
B. Operated										
0–19 Years	0									
20–34	193	2.3	8	1	1	2	3	4	5	18
35–49	2,121	2.1	6	1	1	2	2	3	5	11
50–64	4,012	1.9	4	1	1	1	2	3	4	9
65+	4,264	1.9	4	1	1	1	2	3	5	10
SUBTOTALS:										
1. SINGLE DX										
A. Not Operated	16	2.8	11	1	1	2	3	4	15	15
B. Operated	1,219	1.6	1	1	1	1	2	3	4	5
2. MULTIPLE DX										
A. Not Operated	763	5.3	28	1	2	4	7	11	16	24
B. Operated	10,590	2.0	4	1	1	1	2	3	5	10
1. SINGLE DX	1,235	1.6	1	1	1	1	2	3	4	5
2. MULTIPLE DX	11,353	2.2	6	1	1	1	2	4	6	13
A. NOT OPERATED	779	5.3	27	1	2	3	7	11	15	24
B. OPERATED	11,809	1.9	4	1	1	1	2	3	5	9
TOTAL										
0–19 Years	1	3.0	0	3	3	3	3	3	3	3
20–34	264	2.3	8	1	1	2	3	4	5	18
35–49	2,721	2.3	7	1	1	2	3	4	6	13
50–64	4,857	2.1	6	1	1	2	3	4	6	12
65+	4,745	2.1	5	1	1	2	3	4	6	12
GRAND TOTAL	12,588	2.1	6	1	1	1	2	4	6	12

Length of Stay by Diagnosis and Operation, Western Region, 2008

Western Region, October 2006–September 2007 Data, by Diagnosis

174.0: FEMALE NIPPLE/AREOLA CA

Type of Patients	Observed Patients	Avg. Stay	Variance	10th	25th	50th	75th	90th	95th	99th
1. SINGLE DX										
A. Not Operated										
0–19 Years	0									
20–34	0									
35–49	0									
50–64	0									
65+	0									
B. Operated										
0–19 Years	0									
20–34	3	1.0	0	1	1	1	1	1	1	1
35–49	8	1.5	<1	1	1	1	2	3	3	3
50–64	14	1.1	<1	1	1	1	1	2	2	2
65+	5	1.6	<1	1	1	1	2	3	3	3
2. MULTIPLE DX										
A. Not Operated										
0–19 Years	0									
20–34	0									
35–49	0									
50–64	3	15.2	138	8	8	9	29	29	29	29
65+	4	5.5	10	2	2	7	9	9	9	9
B. Operated										
0–19 Years	0									
20–34	5	2.0	2	1	1	2	2	4	4	4
35–49	42	1.8	<1	1	1	2	2	3	4	5
50–64	106	1.8	4	1	1	1	2	3	4	7
65+	164	1.8	3	1	1	1	2	3	4	10
SUBTOTALS:										
1. SINGLE DX										
A. Not Operated	0									
B. Operated	30	1.3	<1	1	1	1	1	2	3	3
2. MULTIPLE DX										
A. Not Operated	7	9.7	78	1	1	1	8	29	29	29
B. Operated	317	1.8	3	1	1	1	2	3	4	9
1. SINGLE DX	30	1.3	<1	1	1	1	1	2	3	3
2. MULTIPLE DX	324	2.0	6	1	1	1	2	3	5	10
A. NOT OPERATED	7	9.7	78	1	2	8	9	29	29	29
B. OPERATED	347	1.8	3	1	1	1	2	3	4	9
TOTAL										
0–19 Years	0									
20–34	8	1.6	1	1	1	1	2	4	4	4
35–49	50	1.8	<1	1	1	2	2	3	4	5
50–64	123	2.1	10	1	1	1	2	3	5	20
65+	173	1.9	3	1	1	1	2	3	5	10
GRAND TOTAL	354	1.9	5	1	1	1	2	3	4	10

174.1: FEMALE CENTRAL BREAST CA

Type of Patients	Observed Patients	Avg. Stay	Variance	10th	25th	50th	75th	90th	95th	99th
1. SINGLE DX										
A. Not Operated										
0–19 Years	0									
20–34	0									
35–49	1	1.0	0	1	1	1	1	1	1	1
50–64	0									
65+	1	1.0	0	1	1	1	1	1	1	1
B. Operated										
0–19 Years	0									
20–34	1	1.0	0	1	1	1	1	1	1	1
35–49	14	1.6	1	1	1	1	2	3	5	5
50–64	21	1.5	<1	1	1	1	2	2	2	4
65+	15	1.5	<1	1	1	1	2	3	3	3
2. MULTIPLE DX										
A. Not Operated										
0–19 Years	0									
20–34	0									
35–49	1	6.0	0	6	6	6	6	6	6	6
50–64	6	7.0	50	2	3	4	7	21	21	21
65+	3	4.3	5	3	3	3	7	7	7	7
B. Operated										
0–19 Years	0									
20–34	10	5.4	83	1	2	2	4	31	31	31
35–49	84	2.4	9	1	1	2	3	3	5	22
50–64	171	1.8	3	1	1	1	2	3	4	7
65+	233	1.8	2	1	1	1	2	3	5	7
SUBTOTALS:										
1. SINGLE DX										
A. Not Operated	2	1.0	0	1	1	1	1	1	1	1
B. Operated	51	1.5	<1	1	1	1	2	2	3	5
2. MULTIPLE DX										
A. Not Operated	10	6.1	30	3	3	4	7	7	21	21
B. Operated	498	2.0	5	1	1	1	2	3	5	12
1. SINGLE DX	53	1.5	<1	1	1	1	2	2	3	5
2. MULTIPLE DX	508	2.1	6	1	1	1	2	3	5	12
A. NOT OPERATED	12	5.2	29	1	2	3	6	7	21	21
B. OPERATED	549	1.9	5	1	1	1	2	3	4	11
TOTAL										
0–19 Years	0									
20–34	11	5.0	76	1	1	1	4	6	31	31
35–49	100	2.3	8	1	1	2	3	4	6	13
50–64	198	1.9	5	1	1	1	2	3	4	21
65+	252	1.8	2	1	1	1	2	3	5	7
GRAND TOTAL	561	2.0	6	1	1	1	2	3	5	12

174.2: FEMALE UIQ BREAST CA

Type of Patients	Observed Patients	Avg. Stay	Variance	10th	25th	50th	75th	90th	95th	99th
1. SINGLE DX										
A. Not Operated										
0–19 Years	0									
20–34	0									
35–49	0									
50–64	1	2.0	0	2	2	2	2	2	2	2
65+	0									
B. Operated										
0–19 Years	0									
20–34	3	1.3	<1	1	1	1	2	2	2	2
35–49	15	1.3	<1	1	1	1	1	2	2	2
50–64	20	1.3	<1	1	1	1	1	2	2	3
65+	5	1.0	0	1	1	1	1	1	1	1
2. MULTIPLE DX										
A. Not Operated										
0–19 Years	0									
20–34	0									
35–49	2	3.5	4	2	2	5	5	5	5	5
50–64	2	9.5	142	1	1	10	18	18	18	18
65+	3	6.0	<1	5	5	6	7	7	7	7
B. Operated										
0–19 Years	0									
20–34	12	3.2	23	1	1	2	3	3	18	18
35–49	98	2.0	5	1	1	1	3	4	5	19
50–64	240	1.7	1	1	1	1	2	3	4	7
65+	265	1.7	2	1	1	1	2	3	4	7
SUBTOTALS:										
1. SINGLE DX										
A. Not Operated	1	2.0	0	2	2	2	2	2	2	2
B. Operated	43	1.3	<1	1	1	1	1	2	2	3
2. MULTIPLE DX										
A. Not Operated	7	6.3	31	1	2	5	7	18	18	18
B. Operated	615	1.8	2	1	1	1	2	3	4	7
1. SINGLE DX	44	1.3	<1	1	1	1	1	2	2	3
2. MULTIPLE DX	622	1.8	3	1	1	1	2	3	5	8
A. NOT OPERATED	8	5.8	29	1	2	5	7	18	18	18
B. OPERATED	658	1.7	2	1	1	1	2	3	4	7
TOTAL										
0–19 Years	0									
20–34	15	2.8	18	1	1	1	3	3	3	3
35–49	115	2.0	4	1	1	1	2	3	5	5
50–64	263	1.7	2	1	1	1	2	3	4	7
65+	273	1.7	2	1	1	1	2	3	4	7
GRAND TOTAL	666	1.8	3	1	1	1	2	3	4	8

Length of Stay by Diagnosis and Operation, Western Region, 2008

174.3: FEMALE LIQ BREAST CA

Type of Patients	Observed Patients	Avg. Stay	Vari- ance	Percentiles						
				10th	25th	50th	75th	90th	95th	99th
1. SINGLE DX										
A. Not Operated										
0–19 Years	0									
20–34	0									
35–49	0									
50–64	0									
65+	0									
B. Operated										
0–19 Years	0									
20–34	0									
35–49	8	1.8	<1	1	1	2	2	3	3	3
50–64	9	1.7	<1	1	1	2	2	2	2	2
65+	6	1.2	<1	1	1	1	1	2	2	2
2. MULTIPLE DX										
A. Not Operated										
0–19 Years	0									
20–34	0									
35–49	1	2.0	0	2	2	2	2	2	2	2
50–64	0									
65+	4	4.7	14	1	1	2	8	8	8	8
B. Operated										
0–19 Years	0									
20–34	4	2.0	2	1	1	2	2	4	4	4
35–49	58	2.2	4	1	1	2	2	4	6	14
50–64	119	1.9	3	1	1	1	2	3	4	12
65+	153	1.7	2	1	1	1	1	3	5	9
SUBTOTALS:										
1. SINGLE DX										
A. Not Operated	0									
B. Operated	23	1.6	<1	1	1	2	2	2	2	3
2. MULTIPLE DX										
A. Not Operated	5	4.2	12	2	2	2	8	8	8	8
B. Operated	334	1.9	3	1	1	1	2	2	5	11
1. SINGLE DX	23	1.6	<1	1	1	2	2	2	2	3
2. MULTIPLE DX	339	1.9	3	1	1	1	2	4	5	11
A. NOT OPERATED	5	4.2	12	2	2	2	8	8	8	8
B. OPERATED	357	1.8	3	1	1	1	2	3	5	11
TOTAL										
0–19 Years	0									
20–34	4	2.0	2	1	1	2	4	4	4	4
35–49	67	2.1	4	1	1	2	2	4	5	14
50–64	128	1.8	3	1	1	1	2	3	4	12
65+	163	1.8	3	1	1	1	2	3	5	9
GRAND TOTAL	362	1.9	3	1	1	1	2	3	5	11

174.4: FEMALE UOQ BREAST CA

Type of Patients	Observed Patients	Avg. Stay	Vari- ance	Percentiles						
				10th	25th	50th	75th	90th	95th	99th
1. SINGLE DX										
A. Not Operated										
0–19 Years	0									
20–34	0									
35–49	0									
50–64	1	3.0	0	3	3	3	3	3	3	3
65+	0									
B. Operated										
0–19 Years	0									
20–34	10	1.2	<1	1	1	1	1	2	3	3
35–49	83	1.5	<1	1	1	1	2	2	3	5
50–64	65	1.6	1	1	1	1	2	3	3	6
65+	35	1.3	<1	1	1	1	1	2	2	3
2. MULTIPLE DX										
A. Not Operated										
0–19 Years	0									
20–34	1	4.0	0	4	4	4	4	4	4	4
35–49	5	4.2	16	1	1	2	8	9	9	9
50–64	18	3.0	7	1	1	2	4	8	10	10
65+	18	4.4	8	1	2	5	7	8	10	10
B. Operated										
0–19 Years	0									
20–34	50	2.3	2	1	1	1	2	3	4	7
35–49	467	1.9	2	1	1	1	1	2	3	10
50–64	796	1.9	3	1	1	1	2	3	4	8
65+	936	1.8	2	1	1	1	2	3	4	7
SUBTOTALS:										
1. SINGLE DX										
A. Not Operated	1	3.0	0	3	3	3	3	3	3	3
B. Operated	193	1.5	<1	1	1	1	2	2	3	6
2. MULTIPLE DX										
A. Not Operated	42	3.8	8	1	1	3	6	8	9	10
B. Operated	2,249	1.8	2	1	1	1	2	3	4	8
1. SINGLE DX	194	1.5	<1	1	1	1	2	2	3	6
2. MULTIPLE DX	2,291	1.9	2	1	1	1	2	4	5	8
A. NOT OPERATED	43	3.8	8	1	1	3	6	8	9	10
B. OPERATED	2,442	1.8	2	1	1	1	2	3	4	8
TOTAL										
0–19 Years	0									
20–34	61	2.2	2	1	1	2	3	4	5	7
35–49	555	1.9	2	1	1	1	2	3	5	9
50–64	880	1.9	3	1	1	1	2	3	5	8
65+	989	1.8	2	1	1	1	2	3	4	8
GRAND TOTAL	2,485	1.9	2	1	1	1	2	3	4	8

174.5: FEMALE LOQ BREAST CA

Type of Patients	Observed Patients	Avg. Stay	Vari- ance	Percentiles						
				10th	25th	50th	75th	90th	95th	99th
1. SINGLE DX										
A. Not Operated										
0–19 Years	0									
20–34	0									
35–49	0									
50–64	0									
65+	0									
B. Operated										
0–19 Years	0									
20–34	2	1.5	<1	1	1	2	2	2	2	2
35–49	19	1.9	24	1	1	2	2	4	5	5
50–64	19	1.5	<1	1	1	2	2	3	3	3
65+	7	1.6	2	1	1	1	1	5	5	5
2. MULTIPLE DX										
A. Not Operated										
0–19 Years	0									
20–34	0									
35–49	2	4.5	24	1	1	8	8	8	8	8
50–64	3	6.0	16	2	2	6	10	10	10	10
65+	1	1.0	0	1	1	1	1	1	1	1
B. Operated										
0–19 Years	0									
20–34	7	2.6	4	1	1	2	3	7	7	7
35–49	101	1.8	1	1	1	1	1	3	4	8
50–64	166	2.2	5	1	1	2	2	4	5	15
65+	174	2.0	6	1	1	1	2	3	5	18
SUBTOTALS:										
1. SINGLE DX										
A. Not Operated	0									
B. Operated	47	1.7	1	1	1	1	2	3	4	5
2. MULTIPLE DX										
A. Not Operated	6	4.7	15	1	1	6	6	8	10	10
B. Operated	448	2.0	5	1	1	1	2	4	5	15
1. SINGLE DX	47	1.7	1	1	1	1	2	3	4	5
2. MULTIPLE DX	454	2.1	5	1	1	1	2	4	5	15
A. NOT OPERATED	6	4.7	15	1	1	6	6	8	10	10
B. OPERATED	495	2.0	4	1	1	1	2	4	5	15
TOTAL										
0–19 Years	0									
20–34	9	2.3	3	1	1	2	2	7	7	7
35–49	122	1.8	2	1	1	1	1	3	4	8
50–64	188	2.2	5	1	1	2	2	4	6	15
65+	182	2.0	6	1	1	1	2	3	5	18
GRAND TOTAL	501	2.0	5	1	1	1	2	4	5	12

Length of Stay by Diagnosis and Operation, Western Region, 2008

Western Region, October 2006–September 2007 Data, by Diagnosis

174.8: FEMALE BREAST CA NEC

Type of Patients	Observed Patients	Avg. Stay	Variance	10th	25th	50th	75th	90th	95th	99th
1. SINGLE DX										
A. *Not Operated*										
0–19 Years	0									
20–34	0									
35–49	1	1.0	0	1	1	1	1	1	1	1
50–64	5	5.0	31	2	2	3	3	15	15	15
65+	1	3.0	0	3	3	3	3	3	3	3
B. *Operated*										
0–19 Years	0									
20–34	18	1.7	1	1	1	2	2	2	3	5
35–49	130	1.7	1	1	1	1	2	3	4	6
50–64	186	1.7	2	1	1	1	2	3	4	6
65+	81	1.4	<1	1	1	1	2	2	3	3
2. MULTIPLE DX										
A. *Not Operated*										
0–19 Years	1	3.0	0	3	3	3	3	3	3	3
20–34	8	3.4	4	1	1	3	6	6	6	6
35–49	75	5.5	34	2	2	3	7	12	15	38
50–64	139	6.0	38	1	2	4	8	12	22	28
65+	88	5.3	26	1	2	4	7	11	19	23
B. *Operated*										
0–19 Years	0									
20–34	62	2.0	2	1	1	2	2	3	4	8
35–49	685	2.3	9	1	1	2	2	4	5	19
50–64	1,334	2.0	3	1	1	1	2	4	5	10
65+	1,333	2.0	5	1	1	1	2	4	6	13
SUBTOTALS:										
1. SINGLE DX										
A. *Not Operated*	7	4.1	23	1	2	3	3	15	15	15
B. *Operated*	415	1.6	1	1	1	1	2	3	4	6
2. MULTIPLE DX										
A. *Not Operated*	311	5.6	33	2	2	4	7	12	19	28
B. *Operated*	3,414	2.1	5	1	1	1	2	4	5	12
1. SINGLE DX	422	1.7	2	1	1	1	2	3	4	6
2. MULTIPLE DX	3,725	2.4	8	1	1	1	2	4	7	16
A. NOT OPERATED	318	5.6	32	2	2	4	7	12	18	28
B. OPERATED	3,829	2.0	5	1	1	1	2	4	5	11
TOTAL										
0–19 Years	1	3.0	0	3	3	3	3	3	3	3
20–34	88	2.0	2	1	1	2	3	4	5	8
35–49	891	2.5	11	1	1	2	2	4	5	19
50–64	1,664	2.3	8	1	1	1	2	4	6	14
65+	1,503	2.2	7	1	1	1	2	4	6	16
GRAND TOTAL	4,147	2.3	8	1	1	1	2	4	6	15

174.9: FEMALE BREAST CA NOS

Type of Patients	Observed Patients	Avg. Stay	Variance	10th	25th	50th	75th	90th	95th	99th
1. SINGLE DX										
A. *Not Operated*										
0–19 Years	0									
20–34	0									
35–49	1	1.0	0	1	1	1	1	1	1	1
50–64	3	1.3	<1	1	1	1	2	2	2	2
65+	1	4.0	0	4	4	4	4	4	4	4
B. *Operated*										
0–19 Years	0									
20–34	18	1.6	<1	1	1	2	2	2	4	4
35–49	140	1.6	1	1	1	1	2	3	4	6
50–64	178	1.7	<1	1	1	2	2	3	4	5
65+	70	1.4	<1	1	1	1	2	2	3	4
2. MULTIPLE DX										
A. *Not Operated*										
0–19 Years	0									
20–34	7	6.2	55	1	1	3	11	21	21	21
35–49	89	5.7	26	1	2	4	8	13	19	22
50–64	146	4.9	29	1	2	3	7	11	15	30
65+	131	5.1	19	1	2	4	6	11	15	20
B. *Operated*										
0–19 Years	0									
20–34	41	1.8	2	1	1	1	2	3	4	7
35–49	567	2.1	5	1	1	2	2	4	5	8
50–64	1,047	2.0	5	1	1	1	2	4	5	8
65+	981	2.0	4	1	1	1	2	4	5	10
SUBTOTALS:										
1. SINGLE DX										
A. *Not Operated*	5	1.8	2	1	1	1	2	4	4	4
B. *Operated*	406	1.6	1	1	1	1	2	3	4	5
2. MULTIPLE DX										
A. *Not Operated*	373	5.2	25	1	2	3	7	11	15	24
B. *Operated*	2,636	2.0	5	1	1	1	2	4	5	9
1. SINGLE DX	411	1.6	1	1	1	1	2	3	4	5
2. MULTIPLE DX	3,009	2.4	8	1	1	2	3	5	7	15
A. NOT OPERATED	378	5.2	25	1	2	3	7	11	15	24
B. OPERATED	3,042	2.0	4	1	1	1	2	4	5	9
TOTAL										
0–19 Years	0									
20–34	66	2.2	8	1	1	2	3	4	5	21
35–49	797	2.4	8	1	1	2	3	5	7	16
50–64	1,374	2.3	8	1	1	2	2	4	6	12
65+	1,183	2.3	6	1	1	1	2	4	7	15
GRAND TOTAL	3,420	2.3	7	1	1	1	2	4	7	15

175: MALE BREAST CA

Type of Patients	Observed Patients	Avg. Stay	Variance	10th	25th	50th	75th	90th	95th	99th
1. SINGLE DX										
A. *Not Operated*										
0–19 Years	0									
20–34	0									
35–49	0									
50–64	0									
65+	0									
B. *Operated*										
0–19 Years	0									
20–34	0									
35–49	0									
50–64	3	1.0	0	1	1	1	1	1	1	1
65+	2	1.5	<1	1	1	2	2	2	2	2
2. MULTIPLE DX										
A. *Not Operated*										
0–19 Years	0									
20–34	2	4.0	18	1	1	1	7	7	7	7
35–49	1	4.0	0	4	4	4	4	4	4	4
50–64	3	15.3	56	8	8	15	23	23	23	23
B. *Operated*										
0–19 Years	0									
20–34	3	1.3	<1	1	1	1	1	2	2	2
35–49	18	2.8	13	1	1	2	3	6	16	16
50–64	54	1.7	2	1	1	1	2	2	4	10
SUBTOTALS:										
1. SINGLE DX										
A. *Not Operated*	0									
B. *Operated*	5	1.2	<1	1	1	1	1	2	2	2
2. MULTIPLE DX										
A. *Not Operated*	6	9.7	64	1	4	8	15	23	23	23
B. *Operated*	75	1.9	5	1	1	1	2	3	6	16
1. SINGLE DX	5	1.2	<1	1	1	1	1	2	2	2
2. MULTIPLE DX	81	2.5	13	1	1	1	2	4	8	23
A. NOT OPERATED	6	9.7	64	1	4	8	15	23	23	23
B. OPERATED	80	1.9	5	1	1	1	2	3	4	16
TOTAL										
0–19 Years	0									
20–34	5	2.4	7	1	1	1	2	7	7	7
35–49	22	2.6	11	1	1	1	3	4	6	16
50–64	59	2.4	13	1	1	1	2	4	10	23
GRAND TOTAL	86	2.4	12	1	1	1	2	4	8	23

Western Region, October 2006–September 2007 Data, by Diagnosis

176: KAPOSI'S SARCOMA

Type of Patients	Observed Patients	Avg. Stay	Variance	10th	25th	50th	75th	90th	95th	99th
1. SINGLE DX										
A. *Not Operated*										
0–19 Years	0									
20–34	0									
35–49	0									
50–64	0									
65+	0									
B. *Operated*										
0–19 Years	0									
20–34	0									
35–49	0									
50–64	0									
65+	0									
2. MULTIPLE DX										
A. *Not Operated*										
0–19 Years	0									
20–34	1	3.0	0	3	3	3	3	3	3	3
35–49	2	8.6	83	2	2	15	15	15	15	15
50–64	3	10.0	28	6	6	8	16	16	16	16
65+	2	8.0	8	6	6	6	10	10	10	10
B. *Operated*										
0–19 Years	0									
20–34	1	14.0	0	14	14	14	14	14	14	14
35–49	1	6.0	0	6	6	6	6	6	6	6
50–64	0									
65+	2	4.5	<1	4	4	4	5	5	5	5
SUBTOTALS:										
1. SINGLE DX										
A. *Not Operated*	0									
B. *Operated*	0									
2. MULTIPLE DX										
A. *Not Operated*	8	8.3	26	2	6	8	15	16	16	16
B. *Operated*	4	7.3	21	4	5	6	14	15	16	14
1. SINGLE DX	0									
2. MULTIPLE DX	12	7.9	23	3	5	6	14	15	16	16
A. NOT OPERATED	8	8.3	26	2	6	8	15	16	16	16
B. OPERATED	4	7.3	21	4	5	6	14	15	16	14
TOTAL										
0–19 Years	0									
20–34	2	8.6	60	3	3	14	14	14	14	14
35–49	3	7.7	44	2	2	6	15	15	15	15
50–64	3	10.0	28	6	6	8	16	16	16	16
65+	4	6.2	7	4	4	6	6	10	10	10
GRAND TOTAL	12	7.9	23	3	5	6	14	15	16	16

179: UTERUS CA NOS

Type of Patients	Observed Patients	Avg. Stay	Variance	10th	25th	50th	75th	90th	95th	99th
1. SINGLE DX										
A. *Not Operated*										
0–19 Years	0									
20–34	0									
35–49	0									
50–64	0									
65+	0									
B. *Operated*										
0–19 Years	0									
20–34	0									
35–49	3	2.0	<1	1	1	2	3	3	3	3
50–64	5	2.4	4	1	1	2	2	6	6	6
65+	4	2.8	2	1	1	4	4	4	4	4
2. MULTIPLE DX										
A. *Not Operated*										
0–19 Years	0									
20–34	1	2.0	0	2	2	2	2	2	2	2
35–49	8	5.1	21	2	2	5	7	15	15	15
50–64	24	5.2	61	1	1	3	6	11	16	38
65+	26	3.3	3	2	2	3	5	5	6	7
B. *Operated*										
0–19 Years	0									
20–34	2	2.0	2	1	1	1	3	3	3	3
35–49	34	3.9	6	2	2	3	5	6	11	11
50–64	102	5.4	81	2	3	3	5	9	13	26
65+	80	5.6	15	3	3	4	7	12	14	22
SUBTOTALS:										
1. SINGLE DX										
A. *Not Operated*	0									
B. *Operated*	12	2.4	2	1	1	2	3	4	6	6
2. MULTIPLE DX										
A. *Not Operated*	59	4.3	29	2	2	3	5	7	13	38
B. *Operated*	218	5.2	45	2	3	4	6	9	13	22
1. SINGLE DX	12	2.4	2	1	2	2	3	4	5	6
2. MULTIPLE DX	277	5.0	41	2	2	3	6	9	13	26
A. NOT OPERATED	59	4.3	29	1	2	3	5	7	15	38
B. OPERATED	230	5.1	43	2	3	4	6	9	13	22
TOTAL										
0–19 Years	0									
20–34	3	2.0	1	1	1	2	3	3	3	3
35–49	45	4.0	8	1	2	3	5	7	11	15
50–64	131	5.2	75	2	3	3	5	9	14	38
65+	110	4.9	13	2	3	4	6	10	13	17
GRAND TOTAL	289	4.9	40	2	2	3	6	9	13	26

180: CERVIX UTERI CA

Type of Patients	Observed Patients	Avg. Stay	Variance	10th	25th	50th	75th	90th	95th	99th
1. SINGLE DX										
A. *Not Operated*										
0–19 Years	0									
20–34	2	1.5	<1	1	1	2	2	2	2	2
35–49	6	1.3	<1	1	1	1	2	2	2	2
50–64	7	1.3	<1	1	1	1	2	2	2	2
65+	1	1.0	0	1	1	1	1	1	1	1
B. *Operated*										
0–19 Years	0									
20–34	35	2.5	2	1	2	3	3	4	4	6
35–49	107	2.6	2	1	2	2	3	5	5	5
50–64	65	2.6	2	1	2	3	3	5	5	6
65+	11	2.0	1	1	1	2	3	3	4	4
2. MULTIPLE DX										
A. *Not Operated*										
0–19 Years	0									
20–34	40	4.1	11	2	2	3	7	10	11	13
35–49	147	4.8	23	1	2	3	6	11	15	24
50–64	123	4.0	19	1	1	3	5	9	13	21
65+	59	4.4	14	2	2	3	6	9	11	23
B. *Operated*										
0–19 Years	0									
20–34	167	4.6	50	1	2	3	4	6	10	44
35–49	607	4.2	17	1	2	3	5	7	10	23
50–64	491	4.9	53	1	2	3	5	8	13	43
65+	235	5.2	36	2	2	3	5	10	15	31
SUBTOTALS:										
1. SINGLE DX										
A. *Not Operated*	16	1.3	<1	1	1	1	2	2	2	2
B. *Operated*	218	2.6	2	1	2	3	3	4	5	6
2. MULTIPLE DX										
A. *Not Operated*	369	4.4	19	1	2	3	5	10	13	23
B. *Operated*	1,501	4.6	36	1	2	3	5	8	12	30
1. SINGLE DX	234	2.5	2	1	2	2	3	4	5	6
2. MULTIPLE DX	1,870	4.6	32	1	2	3	5	8	12	29
A. NOT OPERATED	385	4.3	18	1	2	3	5	9	13	23
B. OPERATED	1,719	4.3	32	1	2	3	4	7	11	29
TOTAL										
0–19 Years	1	1.0	0	1	1	1	1	1	1	1
20–34	244	4.2	36	1	2	3	4	7	10	42
35–49	867	4.1	17	1	2	3	4	7	10	23
50–64	686	4.5	42	1	2	3	5	8	12	28
65+	306	4.9	31	2	2	3	5	10	14	30
GRAND TOTAL	2,104	4.3	29	1	2	3	5	8	11	28

Western Region, October 2006–September 2007 Data, by Diagnosis

180.0: ENDOCERVIX CA

Type of Patients	Observed Patients	Avg. Stay	Variance	Percentiles						
				10th	25th	50th	75th	90th	95th	99th
1. SINGLE DX										
A. Not Operated										
0–19 Years	0									
20–34	0									
35–49	0									
50–64	0									
65+	0									
B. Operated										
0–19 Years	0									
20–34	10	2.8	2	1	2	3	4	4	6	6
35–49	14	2.6	<1	1	2	3	3	3	4	4
50–64	9	2.6	2	1	1	3	3	4	4	4
65+	0									
2. MULTIPLE DX										
A. Not Operated										
0–19 Years	0									
20–34	4	2.0	4	1	1	1	1	5	5	5
35–49	11	7.4	61	1	2	6	10	13	28	28
50–64	6	2.3	<1	1	2	3	3	3	3	3
65+	0									
B. Operated										
0–19 Years	0									
20–34	34	2.9	2	1	2	3	4	4	5	6
35–49	136	3.8	9	2	2	3	4	5	7	12
50–64	112	4.5	21	2	3	4	5	7	9	16
65+	61	4.5	7	2	3	4	5	9	10	15
SUBTOTALS:										
1. SINGLE DX										
A. Not Operated	0									
B. Operated	33	2.6	1	1	2	3	3	4	4	4
2. MULTIPLE DX										
A. Not Operated	21	4.9	38	1	1	3	6	10	13	28
B. Operated	343	4.0	12	2	3	3	4	6	8	15
1. SINGLE DX	33	2.6	1	1	2	3	3	4	4	4
2. MULTIPLE DX	364	4.1	14	1	2	3	5	7	9	16
A. NOT OPERATED	21	4.9	38	1	1	3	6	10	13	28
B. OPERATED	376	3.9	11	1	2	3	4	6	8	15
TOTAL										
0–19 Years	0									
20–34	48	2.8	2	1	2	3	4	4	5	6
35–49	161	3.9	12	1	2	3	4	6	7	28
50–64	127	4.2	19	1	2	3	5	7	8	16
65+	61	4.5	7	2	3	4	5	9	10	15
GRAND TOTAL	397	4.0	13	1	2	3	4	6	8	16

180.8: CERVIX CA NEC

Type of Patients	Observed Patients	Avg. Stay	Variance	Percentiles						
				10th	25th	50th	75th	90th	95th	99th
1. SINGLE DX										
A. Not Operated										
0–19 Years	0									
20–34	1	2.0	0	2	2	2	2	2	2	2
35–49	1	1.0	0	1	1	1	1	1	1	1
50–64	3	1.0	0	1	1	1	1	1	1	1
65+	0									
B. Operated										
0–19 Years	0									
20–34	11	2.6	1	1	1	3	4	4	4	4
35–49	37	3.0	3	1	2	3	4	5	5	8
50–64	24	2.7	2	1	1	2	3	5	5	5
65+	6	2.3	1	1	1	2	3	4	4	4
2. MULTIPLE DX										
A. Not Operated										
0–19 Years	0									
20–34	13	3.8	8	1	2	2	2	7	10	10
35–49	53	4.5	18	1	2	3	5	10	15	20
50–64	37	4.2	22	1	2	3	4	9	21	21
65+	25	3.4	6	1	2	3	4	7	9	11
B. Operated										
0–19 Years	0									
20–34	44	6.2	135	1	2	3	4	5	42	55
35–49	177	5.1	32	2	3	4	5	9	15	35
50–64	163	5.3	88	1	2	3	5	10	13	72
65+	82	5.8	45	1	2	4	6	14	17	39
SUBTOTALS:										
1. SINGLE DX										
A. Not Operated	5	1.2	<1	1	1	1	1	2	2	2
B. Operated	78	2.8	2	1	2	3	4	5	5	8
2. MULTIPLE DX										
A. Not Operated	128	4.1	16	1	2	3	5	9	11	21
B. Operated	466	5.4	63	1	2	3	5	10	17	44
1. SINGLE DX	83	2.7	2	1	1	3	4	5	5	8
2. MULTIPLE DX	594	5.1	53	1	2	3	5	10	15	43
A. NOT OPERATED	133	4.0	15	1	2	3	5	8	11	21
B. OPERATED	544	5.0	55	1	2	3	5	9	15	43
TOTAL										
0–19 Years	0									
20–34	69	5.1	89	1	2	3	4	7	19	55
35–49	268	4.6	25	1	2	3	5	9	14	25
50–64	227	4.8	68	1	2	3	5	9	11	43
65+	113	5.1	35	1	2	3	5	11	17	31
GRAND TOTAL	677	4.8	48	1	2	3	5	9	14	42

180.9: CERVIX UTERI CA NOS

Type of Patients	Observed Patients	Avg. Stay	Variance	Percentiles						
				10th	25th	50th	75th	90th	95th	99th
1. SINGLE DX										
A. Not Operated										
0–19 Years	0									
20–34	1	1.0	0	1	1	1	1	1	1	1
35–49	5	1.4	<1	1	1	1	2	2	2	2
50–64	3	1.3	<1	1	1	1	2	2	2	2
65+	1	1.0	0	1	1	1	1	1	1	1
B. Operated										
0–19 Years	0									
20–34	13	2.2	<1	1	1	2	3	3	4	4
35–49	55	2.4	1	1	2	2	3	4	5	5
50–64	31	2.5	1	1	2	2	3	4	5	6
65+	4	1.8	<1	1	1	2	3	3	3	3
2. MULTIPLE DX										
A. Not Operated										
0–19 Years	0									
20–34	22	4.4	12	1	2	3	7	10	11	13
35–49	83	4.7	21	1	2	3	5	10	13	24
50–64	80	4.1	20	1	1	3	5	9	13	29
65+	33	5.1	19	1	2	4	7	9	12	23
B. Operated										
0–19 Years	1	1.0	0	1	1	1	1	1	1	1
20–34	79	4.2	25	1	2	3	4	7	8	33
35–49	279	3.8	13	1	2	3	4	7	10	23
50–64	205	4.8	45	1	2	3	5	9	13	27
65+	88	4.9	43	1	2	3	5	10	13	51
SUBTOTALS:										
1. SINGLE DX										
A. Not Operated	10	1.3	<1	1	1	1	2	2	2	2
B. Operated	103	2.4	1	1	2	2	3	4	5	5
2. MULTIPLE DX										
A. Not Operated	218	4.5	19	1	2	3	5	6	13	23
B. Operated	652	4.3	28	1	2	3	5	8	11	28
1. SINGLE DX	113	2.3	1	1	1	2	3	4	5	5
2. MULTIPLE DX	870	4.4	26	1	2	3	5	8	12	27
A. NOT OPERATED	228	4.3	19	1	2	3	5	7	10	23
B. OPERATED	755	4.0	25	1	2	3	4	7	10	27
TOTAL										
0–19 Years	1	1.0	0	1	1	1	1	1	1	1
20–34	115	4.0	20	1	2	3	4	7	10	29
35–49	422	3.8	13	1	2	3	4	7	10	20
50–64	319	4.3	34	1	2	3	5	8	13	27
65+	126	4.8	35	1	2	3	5	10	13	29
GRAND TOTAL	983	4.1	24	1	2	3	5	8	11	26

Length of Stay by Diagnosis and Operation, Western Region, 2008

Western Region, October 2006–September 2007 Data, by Diagnosis

181: PLACENTA CA

Type of Patients	Observed Patients	Avg. Stay	Variance	Percentiles						
				10th	25th	50th	75th	90th	95th	99th
1. SINGLE DX										
A. Not Operated										
0–19 Years	0									
20–34	0									
35–49	1	2.0	0	2	2	2	2	2	2	2
50–64	1	1.0	0	1	1	1	1	1	1	1
65+	0									
B. Operated										
0–19 Years	0									
20–34	0									
35–49	0									
50–64	0									
65+	0									
2. MULTIPLE DX										
A. Not Operated										
0–19 Years	1	3.0	0	3	3	3	3	3	3	3
20–34	3	10.4	74	1	1	12	18	18	18	18
35–49	0									
50–64	0									
65+	0									
B. Operated										
0–19 Years	0									
20–34	1	5.0	0	5	5	5	5	5	5	5
35–49	1	4.0	0	4	4	4	4	4	4	4
50–64	0									
65+	0									
SUBTOTALS:										
1. SINGLE DX										
A. Not Operated	2	1.5	<1	1	1	1	2	2	2	2
B. Operated	0									
2. MULTIPLE DX										
A. Not Operated	4	8.5	63	1	3	3	18	18	18	18
B. Operated	2	4.5	<1	4	4	4	5	5	5	5
1. SINGLE DX	2	1.5	<1	1	1	1	2	2	2	2
2. MULTIPLE DX	6	7.2	42	1	3	4	12	18	18	18
A. NOT OPERATED	6	6.2	51	1	1	2	12	18	18	18
B. OPERATED	2	4.5	<1	4	4	4	5	5	5	5
TOTAL										
0–19 Years	1	3.0	0	3	3	3	3	3	3	3
20–34	4	9.0	57	1	5	9	18	18	18	18
35–49	2	3.0	2	2	2	4	4	4	4	4
50–64	1	1.0	0	1	1	1	1	1	1	1
65+	0									
GRAND TOTAL	8	5.7	37	1	2	3	5	18	18	18

182: UTERUS BODY CA

Type of Patients	Observed Patients	Avg. Stay	Variance	Percentiles						
				10th	25th	50th	75th	90th	95th	99th
1. SINGLE DX										
A. Not Operated										
0–19 Years	0									
20–34	2	2.5	<1	2	2	3	3	3	3	3
35–49	2	3.5	<1	3	3	4	4	4	4	4
50–64	2	2.0	2	1	1	2	3	3	3	3
65+	2	1.0	0	1	1	1	1	1	1	1
B. Operated										
0–19 Years	0									
20–34	6	2.8	<1	2	2	3	3	4	4	4
35–49	50	2.5	1	1	2	3	3	4	4	5
50–64	182	2.5	1	1	2	2	3	4	4	6
65+	50	2.7	1	1	2	3	3	4	5	5
2. MULTIPLE DX										
A. Not Operated										
0–19 Years	0									
20–34	10	3.9	5	2	2	4	6	8	8	8
35–49	29	2.8	6	1	1	2	3	6	6	12
50–64	80	4.9	25	1	2	3	7	10	19	25
65+	72	4.5	24	1	1	2	5	11	14	30
B. Operated										
0–19 Years	1	5.0	0	5	5	5	5	5	5	5
20–34	61	3.2	2	2	2	3	4	5	6	7
35–49	656	3.4	4	2	2	3	4	5	7	11
50–64	2,563	3.6	8	2	2	3	4	6	8	16
65+	2,099	4.5	16	2	3	3	5	8	12	21
SUBTOTALS:										
1. SINGLE DX										
A. Not Operated	8	2.2	1	1	1	2	3	4	4	4
B. Operated	288	2.5	1	1	2	3	3	4	4	5
2. MULTIPLE DX										
A. Not Operated	191	4.4	21	1	1	3	5	10	13	25
B. Operated	5,380	3.9	11	2	2	3	4	6	9	19
1. SINGLE DX	296	2.5	1	1	2	3	3	4	4	5
2. MULTIPLE DX	5,571	3.9	11	2	2	3	4	7	9	19
A. NOT OPERATED	199	4.3	20	1	1	3	5	10	13	24
B. OPERATED	5,668	3.9	10	2	2	3	4	6	9	18
TOTAL										
0–19 Years	1	5.0	0	5	5	5	5	5	5	5
20–34	79	3.3	2	2	2	3	4	5	6	8
35–49	737	3.3	4	1	2	3	4	5	7	11
50–64	2,827	3.6	8	2	2	3	4	6	8	16
65+	2,223	4.5	16	2	2	3	5	8	12	21
GRAND TOTAL	5,867	3.9	11	2	2	3	4	6	9	19

182.0: CORPUS UTERI CA NEC

Type of Patients	Observed Patients	Avg. Stay	Variance	Percentiles						
				10th	25th	50th	75th	90th	95th	99th
1. SINGLE DX										
A. Not Operated										
0–19 Years	0									
20–34	2	2.5	<1	2	2	3	3	3	3	3
35–49	2	3.5	<1	3	3	4	4	4	4	4
50–64	2	2.0	2	1	1	2	3	3	3	3
65+	2	1.0	0	1	1	1	1	1	1	1
B. Operated										
0–19 Years	0									
20–34	6	2.8	<1	2	2	3	3	4	4	4
35–49	50	2.5	1	1	2	3	3	4	4	5
50–64	179	2.5	1	1	2	2	3	4	4	6
65+	49	2.7	1	1	2	3	3	4	5	5
2. MULTIPLE DX										
A. Not Operated										
0–19 Years	0									
20–34	10	3.9	5	2	2	4	6	8	8	8
35–49	29	2.8	6	1	1	2	3	6	6	12
50–64	75	5.0	26	1	1	4	7	10	19	25
65+	71	4.5	24	1	1	2	5	11	14	30
B. Operated										
0–19 Years	0									
20–34	60	3.2	2	2	2	3	4	5	6	7
35–49	646	3.4	4	2	2	3	4	5	7	11
50–64	2,535	3.6	7	2	2	3	4	6	7	15
65+	2,078	4.5	16	2	3	3	5	8	12	21
SUBTOTALS:										
1. SINGLE DX										
A. Not Operated	8	2.2	1	1	1	2	3	4	4	4
B. Operated	284	2.5	1	2	2	3	3	4	4	5
2. MULTIPLE DX										
A. Not Operated	185	4.4	21	1	1	3	5	10	13	25
B. Operated	5,320	3.9	10	2	2	3	4	6	9	18
1. SINGLE DX	292	2.5	1	2	2	3	3	4	4	5
2. MULTIPLE DX	5,505	3.9	11	2	2	3	4	7	9	19
A. NOT OPERATED	193	4.3	21	1	1	3	5	10	13	25
B. OPERATED	5,604	3.8	10	2	2	3	4	6	9	18
TOTAL										
0–19 Years	1	5.0	0	5	5	5	5	5	5	5
20–34	78	3.3	2	2	2	3	4	5	6	8
35–49	727	3.3	4	1	2	3	4	5	7	11
50–64	2,791	3.6	7	2	2	3	4	6	7	15
65+	2,200	4.4	16	2	2	3	5	8	12	21
GRAND TOTAL	5,797	3.9	10	2	2	3	4	6	9	18

Length of Stay by Diagnosis and Operation, Western Region, 2008

Western Region, October 2006–September 2007 Data, by Diagnosis

183: OVARY/UTER ADNEXA CA NEC

Type of Patients	Observed Patients	Avg. Stay	Variance	10th	25th	50th	75th	90th	95th	99th
1. SINGLE DX										
A. Not Operated										
0–19 Years	0									
20–34	2	1.5	<1	1	1	2	2	2	2	2
35–49	6	2.5	12	1	1	3	3	4	4	4
50–64	12	1.7	3	1	1	1	2	2	7	7
65+	5	1.8	1	1	1	1	3	3	3	3
B. Operated										
0–19 Years	6	3.0	1	1	3	3	4	4	4	4
20–34	18	2.9	3	1	2	3	3	5	9	9
35–49	33	3.4	2	2	3	3	4	5	6	9
50–64	44	3.4	2	1	3	4	4	5	6	7
65+	6	2.5	1	1	2	3	3	4	4	4
2. MULTIPLE DX										
A. Not Operated										
0–19 Years	4	2.5	9	1	1	1	7	7	7	7
20–34	28	4.3	12	1	1	3	7	9	10	14
35–49	117	4.4	23	1	2	3	5	10	13	24
50–64	306	5.7	42	1	2	4	7	11	19	28
65+	420	5.5	18	2	3	4	7	12	15	19
B. Operated										
0–19 Years	27	5.2	13	2	2	5	7	9	15	15
20–34	126	4.8	14	2	3	4	5	8	12	21
35–49	560	5.6	21	2	3	4	7	10	13	26
50–64	1,346	6.9	38	3	4	5	8	13	18	32
65+	1,083	7.6	39	3	4	6	9	14	19	34
SUBTOTALS:										
1. SINGLE DX										
A. Not Operated	25	1.9	2	1	1	1	3	3	4	7
B. Operated	107	3.2	2	1	2	3	4	5	6	9
2. MULTIPLE DX										
A. Not Operated	875	5.4	27	1	2	4	7	12	15	24
B. Operated	3,142	6.8	35	3	4	5	8	13	17	32
1. SINGLE DX	132	3.0	2	1	2	3	4	4	6	9
2. MULTIPLE DX	4,017	6.5	33	2	3	5	8	12	17	28
A. NOT OPERATED	900	5.3	27	1	2	4	7	11	15	24
B. OPERATED	3,249	6.7	34	3	3	5	8	12	17	31
TOTAL										
0–19 Years	37	4.6	12	1	2	4	6	8	15	15
20–34	174	4.5	13	1	2	3	5	9	12	21
35–49	716	5.2	21	2	3	4	6	10	13	24
50–64	1,708	6.6	38	2	3	5	8	12	18	32
65+	1,514	7.0	34	2	4	5	8	13	17	28
GRAND TOTAL	4,149	6.4	33	2	3	5	8	12	16	28

183.0: OVARY CA

Type of Patients	Observed Patients	Avg. Stay	Variance	10th	25th	50th	75th	90th	95th	99th
1. SINGLE DX										
A. Not Operated										
0–19 Years	0									
20–34	2	1.5	<1	1	1	2	2	2	2	2
35–49	6	2.5	3	1	1	3	3	4	4	4
50–64	11	1.7	3	1	1	1	2	2	7	7
65+	5	1.8	1	1	1	1	3	3	3	3
B. Operated										
0–19 Years	6	3.0	1	1	3	3	4	4	4	4
20–34	17	2.9	4	1	2	3	3	5	9	9
35–49	30	3.4	2	2	3	4	4	5	6	9
50–64	42	3.4	2	1	3	4	4	5	6	7
65+	6	2.5	1	1	2	3	3	4	4	4
2. MULTIPLE DX										
A. Not Operated										
0–19 Years	4	2.5	9	1	1	1	7	7	7	7
20–34	26	4.5	12	1	1	4	7	9	10	14
35–49	112	4.4	23	1	2	3	5	10	13	24
50–64	301	5.6	42	1	2	4	7	11	19	28
65+	419	5.5	18	2	3	4	7	12	15	19
B. Operated										
0–19 Years	27	5.2	13	2	2	5	7	9	15	15
20–34	125	4.8	14	2	3	4	5	8	12	21
35–49	536	5.6	22	2	3	4	7	10	13	26
50–64	1,259	7.0	39	3	4	5	8	13	18	33
65+	1,028	7.7	40	3	4	6	9	14	19	34
SUBTOTALS:										
1. SINGLE DX										
A. Not Operated	24	1.9	2	1	1	1	3	3	4	7
B. Operated	101	3.2	2	1	2	3	4	5	6	9
2. MULTIPLE DX										
A. Not Operated	862	5.4	27	1	2	4	7	12	15	24
B. Operated	2,975	6.9	36	3	4	5	8	13	17	32
1. SINGLE DX	125	3.0	2	1	2	3	4	4	6	9
2. MULTIPLE DX	3,837	6.5	34	2	3	5	8	12	17	28
A. NOT OPERATED	886	5.3	27	1	2	4	7	11	15	24
B. OPERATED	3,076	6.8	35	3	3	5	8	13	17	32
TOTAL										
0–19 Years	37	4.6	12	1	2	4	6	8	15	15
20–34	170	4.5	13	1	3	4	6	9	12	21
35–49	684	5.3	21	2	3	4	6	10	13	26
50–64	1,613	6.6	39	2	3	5	8	12	18	32
65+	1,458	7.0	35	2	4	5	8	13	17	28
GRAND TOTAL	3,962	6.4	34	2	3	5	8	12	16	28

184: OTHER FEMALE GENITAL CA

Type of Patients	Observed Patients	Avg. Stay	Variance	10th	25th	50th	75th	90th	95th	99th
1. SINGLE DX										
A. Not Operated										
0–19 Years	1	10.0	0	10	10	10	10	10	10	10
20–34	0									
35–49	0									
50–64	0									
65+	0									
B. Operated										
0–19 Years	1	2.0	0	2	2	2	2	2	2	2
20–34	1	1.0	0	1	1	1	1	1	1	1
35–49	10	2.4	1	1	2	2	3	4	4	4
50–64	10	2.3	2	1	1	2	3	5	5	5
65+	12	2.5	2	1	1	2	4	5	5	5
2. MULTIPLE DX										
A. Not Operated										
0–19 Years	2	4.0	8	2	2	4	6	6	6	6
20–34	1	4.0	0	4	4	4	4	4	4	4
35–49	6	7.7	66	1	3	5	10	23	23	23
50–64	20	10.4	446	1	2	4	7	19	97	97
65+	29	5.1	19	2	2	4	7	10	11	21
B. Operated										
0–19 Years	3	12.6	133	5	5	7	26	26	26	26
20–34	8	2.8	3	1	2	3	4	4	6	6
35–49	56	3.7	13	1	2	3	4	6	11	22
50–64	139	5.0	43	1	2	3	5	13	18	32
65+	326	4.8	42	1	2	3	5	9	15	35
SUBTOTALS:										
1. SINGLE DX										
A. Not Operated	1	10.0	0	10	10	10	10	10	10	10
B. Operated	34	2.4	1	1	1	2	3	4	5	5
2. MULTIPLE DX										
A. Not Operated	58	7.1	170	1	2	4	7	14	21	97
B. Operated	532	4.7	39	1	2	3	5	10	16	33
1. SINGLE DX	35	2.6	3	1	1	2	3	4	5	10
2. MULTIPLE DX	590	5.0	52	1	2	3	5	10	17	35
A. NOT OPERATED	59	7.2	168	1	2	4	9	14	21	97
B. OPERATED	566	4.6	37	1	2	3	5	9	16	33
TOTAL										
0–19 Years	7	8.3	68	2	2	6	10	26	26	26
20–34	10	2.7	3	1	1	3	4	4	6	6
35–49	72	3.8	16	1	2	3	4	6	11	23
50–64	169	5.5	90	1	2	3	5	14	18	43
65+	367	4.7	39	1	2	3	5	9	15	35
GRAND TOTAL	625	4.8	50	1	2	3	5	10	16	33

Length of Stay by Diagnosis and Operation, Western Region, 2008

Western Region, October 2006–September 2007 Data, by Diagnosis

184.4: VULVA CA NOS

Type of Patients	Observed Patients	Avg. Stay	Variance	10th	25th	50th	75th	90th	95th	99th
1. SINGLE DX										
A. Not Operated										
0–19 Years	0									
20–34	0									
35–49	0									
50–64	0									
65+	0									
B. Operated										
0–19 Years	0									
20–34	1	1.0	0	1	1	1	1	1	1	1
35–49	6	2.5	2	1	1	3	4	4	4	4
50–64	9	2.1	2	1	1	2	2	5	5	5
65+	8	2.8	2	2	2	2	3	5	5	5
2. MULTIPLE DX										
A. Not Operated										
0–19 Years	0									
20–34	1	4.0	0	4	4	4	4	4	4	4
35–49	2	12.0	238	1	1	1	23	23	23	23
50–64	11	14.0	780	1	3	4	11	14	97	97
65+	19	5.4	25	1	2	4	5	9	11	21
B. Operated										
0–19 Years	1	26.0	0	26	26	26	26	26	26	26
20–34	6	2.8	3	1	2	3	3	6	6	6
35–49	36	3.5	14	1	2	3	4	6	11	22
50–64	102	4.8	45	1	2	3	4	10	18	30
65+	254	4.4	25	1	2	3	5	9	13	33
SUBTOTALS:										
1. SINGLE DX A. Not Operated	0									
1. SINGLE DX B. Operated	24	2.4	2	1	1	2	3	4	5	5
2. MULTIPLE DX A. Not Operated	33	8.6	282	1	2	4	9	14	23	97
2. MULTIPLE DX B. Operated	399	4.4	30	1	2	3	4	9	16	30
1. SINGLE DX	24	2.4	2	1	1	2	3	4	5	5
2. MULTIPLE DX	432	4.7	50	1	2	3	5	9	17	33
A. NOT OPERATED	33	8.6	282	1	2	4	9	14	23	97
B. OPERATED	423	4.3	29	1	2	3	4	9	15	30
TOTAL										
0–19 Years	1	26.0	0	26	26	26	26	26	26	26
20–34	8	2.8	3	1	2	3	4	6	6	6
35–49	44	3.7	20	1	2	3	4	6	11	23
50–64	122	5.4	110	1	2	3	5	11	18	43
65+	281	4.4	25	1	2	3	5	9	13	33
GRAND TOTAL	456	4.6	48	1	2	3	5	9	16	33

185: PROSTATE CA

Type of Patients	Observed Patients	Avg. Stay	Variance	10th	25th	50th	75th	90th	95th	99th
1. SINGLE DX										
A. Not Operated										
0–19 Years	0									
20–34	0									
35–49	0									
50–64	4	1.5	1	1	1	1	3	3	3	3
65+	1	1.0	0	1	1	1	1	1	1	1
B. Operated										
0–19 Years	0									
20–34	0									
35–49	140	1.7	<1	1	1	2	2	3	3	3
50–64	1,183	1.9	<1	1	1	2	2	3	3	5
65+	548	1.8	<1	1	2	2	3	3	3	5
2. MULTIPLE DX										
A. Not Operated										
0–19 Years	3	6.0	49	1	1	3	14	14	14	14
20–34	0									
35–49	12	4.3	18	2	2	3	5	9	16	16
50–64	167	4.3	29	1	1	3	5	9	13	28
65+	574	4.5	14	1	2	4	6	9	12	18
B. Operated										
0–19 Years	1	7.0	0	7	7	7	7	7	7	7
20–34	0									
35–49	429	2.4	3	1	1	2	3	4	5	10
50–64	6,769	2.3	3	1	1	2	3	4	5	9
65+	6,339	2.5	6	1	1	2	3	4	6	12
SUBTOTALS:										
1. SINGLE DX A. Not Operated	5	1.4	<1	1	1	1	1	3	3	3
1. SINGLE DX B. Operated	1,871	1.9	<1	1	2	2	2	3	3	5
2. MULTIPLE DX A. Not Operated	756	4.4	18	1	2	3	6	9	13	19
2. MULTIPLE DX B. Operated	13,538	2.4	4	1	1	2	3	4	5	10
1. SINGLE DX	1,876	1.9	<1	1	1	2	2	3	3	3
2. MULTIPLE DX	14,294	2.5	5	1	1	2	3	4	6	12
A. NOT OPERATED	761	4.4	18	1	2	3	6	9	13	19
B. OPERATED	15,409	2.3	4	1	1	2	3	4	5	10
TOTAL										
0–19 Years	4	6.3	33	1	1	3	14	14	14	14
20–34	0									
35–49	581	2.3	3	1	1	2	3	4	5	10
50–64	8,123	2.3	3	1	1	2	3	4	5	9
65+	7,462	2.6	6	1	1	2	3	5	7	13
GRAND TOTAL	16,170	2.4	5	1	1	2	3	4	5	11

186: TESTIS CA

Type of Patients	Observed Patients	Avg. Stay	Variance	10th	25th	50th	75th	90th	95th	99th
1. SINGLE DX										
A. Not Operated										
0–19 Years	0									
20–34	3	3.6	14	1	1	2	8	8	8	8
35–49	1	4.0	0	4	4	4	4	4	4	4
50–64	0									
65+	0									
B. Operated										
0–19 Years	8	3.1	5	1	1	2	4	6	6	6
20–34	43	2.8	4	1	2	3	4	6	6	8
35–49	13	2.5	7	1	1	3	5	5	10	10
50–64	1	1.0	0	1	1	1	1	1	1	1
65+	1	2.0	0	2	2	2	2	2	2	2
2. MULTIPLE DX										
A. Not Operated										
0–19 Years	4	3.8	7	1	1	2	6	6	6	6
20–34	41	6.4	34	3	3	5	9	13	17	29
35–49	21	6.1	10	3	4	6	8	11	12	13
50–64	3	3.7	2	3	3	3	5	5	5	5
65+	5	4.2	2	2	4	5	5	5	5	5
B. Operated										
0–19 Years	10	13.0	355	1	2	5	16	62	62	62
20–34	140	7.8	94	2	2	5	10	18	22	34
35–49	60	7.7	125	1	2	4	8	16	28	60
50–64	20	5.1	14	1	2	4	7	13	13	13
65+	3	6.3	30	1	1	6	12	12	12	12
SUBTOTALS:										
1. SINGLE DX A. Not Operated	4	3.7	10	1	1	2	4	8	8	8
1. SINGLE DX B. Operated	66	2.7	4	1	2	3	4	6	6	10
2. MULTIPLE DX A. Not Operated	74	5.9	23	2	3	6	9	13	17	29
2. MULTIPLE DX B. Operated	233	7.7	105	2	5	9	17	22	28	60
1. SINGLE DX	70	2.8	5	1	2	3	4	6	6	10
2. MULTIPLE DX	307	7.3	86	2	5	9	14	20	22	58
A. NOT OPERATED	78	5.8	22	3	5	8	11	13	20	29
B. OPERATED	299	6.6	87	4	8	11	14	20	28	60
TOTAL										
0–19 Years	22	7.7	179	1	2	4	16	16	24	62
20–34	227	6.5	68	1	2	4	8	14	19	33
35–49	95	6.6	85	1	2	4	8	12	18	60
50–64	24	4.7	13	1	2	3	7	9	13	13
65+	9	4.7	10	2	2	5	5	12	12	12
GRAND TOTAL	377	6.4	74	1	2	4	8	13	19	58

Western Region, October 2006–September 2007 Data, by Diagnosis

186.9: TESTIS CA NEC & NOS

Type of Patients	Observed Patients	Avg. Stay	Variance	10th	25th	50th	75th	90th	95th	99th
1. SINGLE DX										
A. Not Operated										
0–19 Years	0									
20–34	2	5.0	18	2	2	2	8	8	8	8
35–49	1	4.0	0	4	4	4	4	4	4	4
50–64	0									
65+	0									
B. Operated										
0–19 Years	8	3.1	5	1	1	2	4	6	6	6
20–34	43	2.8	4	1	1	2	4	6	6	8
35–49	12	2.7	7	1	1	1	3	5	10	10
50–64	1	1.0	0	1	1	1	1	1	1	1
65+	1	2.0	0	2	2	2	2	2	2	2
2. MULTIPLE DX										
A. Not Operated										
0–19 Years	4	3.8	7	1	1	2	6	6	6	6
20–34	41	6.4	34	1	3	5	9	13	17	29
35–49	21	6.1	10	3	4	6	8	11	12	13
50–64	3	3.7	1	3	3	3	5	5	5	5
65+	5	4.2	2	2	4	5	5	5	5	5
B. Operated										
0–19 Years	10	13.0	355	1	2	5	16	62	62	62
20–34	138	7.8	95	1	2	5	10	18	22	34
35–49	59	7.7	127	1	2	4	9	16	28	60
50–64	18	5.4	15	1	2	5	8	13	13	13
65+	3	6.3	30	1	1	6	12	12	12	12
SUBTOTALS:										
1. SINGLE DX *A. Not Operated*	3	4.7	9	2	2	4	8	8	8	8
1. SINGLE DX *B. Operated*	65	2.8	4	1	1	2	4	6	6	10
2. MULTIPLE DX *A. Not Operated*	74	5.9	23	1	3	5	8	11	13	29
2. MULTIPLE DX *B. Operated*	228	7.8	107	1	2	5	9	18	22	60
1. SINGLE DX	68	2.8	5	1	1	2	4	6	6	10
2. MULTIPLE DX	302	7.3	87	1	2	5	9	14	20	58
A. NOT OPERATED	77	5.9	22	1	3	5	8	11	13	29
B. OPERATED	293	6.7	88	1	2	4	8	14	20	60
TOTAL										
0–19 Years	22	7.7	179	1	2	4	6	16	24	62
20–34	224	6.6	69	1	2	4	8	14	19	33
35–49	93	6.7	86	1	2	4	8	11	18	60
50–64	22	5.0	13	1	2	4	7	9	13	13
65+	9	4.7	10	2	2	5	5	12	12	12
GRAND TOTAL	370	6.5	75	1	2	4	8	13	19	58

187: PENIS/MALE GENITAL CA

Type of Patients	Observed Patients	Avg. Stay	Variance	10th	25th	50th	75th	90th	95th	99th
1. SINGLE DX										
A. Not Operated										
0–19 Years	0									
20–34	0									
35–49	0									
50–64	0									
65+	0									
B. Operated										
0–19 Years	0									
20–34	2	1.5	<1	1	1	2	2	2	2	2
35–49	2	5.0	18	2	2	8	8	8	8	8
50–64	7	1.7	1	1	1	1	2	4	4	4
65+	3	2.7	8	1	1	1	6	6	6	6
2. MULTIPLE DX										
A. Not Operated										
0–19 Years	0									
20–34	1	2.0	0	2	2	2	2	2	2	2
35–49	1	4.0	0	4	4	4	4	4	4	4
50–64	2	6.0	32	2	2	10	10	10	10	10
65+	6	7.4	81	1	1	5	13	23	23	23
B. Operated										
0–19 Years	1	3.0	0	3	3	3	3	3	3	3
20–34	1	3.0	0	3	3	3	3	3	3	3
35–49	12	3.6	8	1	1	2	5	6	10	10
50–64	32	3.9	6	1	2	3	5	7	9	11
65+	57	4.0	23	1	1	2	5	9	13	26
SUBTOTALS:										
1. SINGLE DX *A. Not Operated*	0									
1. SINGLE DX *B. Operated*	14	2.4	5	1	1	1	2	6	8	8
2. MULTIPLE DX *A. Not Operated*	10	6.2	52	2	4	4	10	23	23	23
2. MULTIPLE DX *B. Operated*	103	3.9	16	1	1	3	5	9	10	22
1. SINGLE DX	14	2.4	5	1	1	1	2	6	8	8
2. MULTIPLE DX	113	4.1	19	1	1	3	5	9	11	23
A. NOT OPERATED	10	6.2	52	2	4	4	10	23	23	23
B. OPERATED	117	3.7	15	1	1	3	5	8	10	22
TOTAL										
0–19 Years	1	3.0	0	3	3	3	3	3	3	3
20–34	4	2.0	<1	1	2	2	3	3	3	3
35–49	15	3.8	8	1	1	3	6	8	10	10
50–64	41	3.6	7	1	2	4	5	7	9	11
65+	66	4.3	28	1	1	4	5	10	13	26
GRAND TOTAL	127	3.9	18	1	1	3	5	8	11	23

188: BLADDER CA

Type of Patients	Observed Patients	Avg. Stay	Variance	10th	25th	50th	75th	90th	95th	99th
1. SINGLE DX										
A. Not Operated										
0–19 Years	0									
20–34	0									
35–49	0									
50–64	2	1.5	<1	1	1	2	2	2	2	2
65+	2	1.0	0	1	1	1	1	1	1	1
B. Operated										
0–19 Years	1	2.0	0	2	2	2	2	2	2	2
20–34	2	2.0	2	1	1	2	2	3	3	3
35–49	14	2.5	6	1	1	1	3	7	9	9
50–64	41	2.9	8	1	1	1	4	7	10	10
65+	53	2.1	4	1	1	1	3	5	7	8
2. MULTIPLE DX										
A. Not Operated										
0–19 Years	1	1.0	0	1	1	1	1	1	1	1
20–34	0									
35–49	16	3.9	9	1	2	3	7	9	9	9
50–64	88	4.6	26	1	2	4	5	9	17	31
65+	290	4.7	20	2	2	4	6	9	14	22
B. Operated										
0–19 Years	2	6.5	12	4	4	9	9	9	9	9
20–34	7	9.5	123	1	1	10	10	33	33	33
35–49	131	8.3	116	1	2	6	6	18	23	67
50–64	930	6.3	39	1	1	5	9	13	17	29
65+	3,482	5.4	33	1	1	3	8	12	16	28
SUBTOTALS:										
1. SINGLE DX *A. Not Operated*	4	1.3	<1	1	1	1	2	2	2	2
1. SINGLE DX *B. Operated*	111	2.5	5	1	1	1	3	7	8	10
2. MULTIPLE DX *A. Not Operated*	395	4.6	20	1	2	3	6	9	14	22
2. MULTIPLE DX *B. Operated*	4,552	5.7	37	1	1	4	8	12	16	29
1. SINGLE DX	115	2.4	5	1	1	1	3	7	8	10
2. MULTIPLE DX	4,947	5.6	36	1	1	4	8	12	16	29
A. NOT OPERATED	399	4.6	20	1	2	3	6	9	14	22
B. OPERATED	4,663	5.6	36	1	1	4	8	12	16	29
TOTAL										
0–19 Years	4	4.0	13	1	1	4	4	9	9	9
20–34	9	7.8	103	1	2	3	9	33	33	33
35–49	161	7.4	99	1	2	5	8	15	22	67
50–64	1,061	6.0	37	1	1	4	8	12	17	29
65+	3,827	5.3	32	1	1	3	7	11	15	27
GRAND TOTAL	5,062	5.5	35	1	1	4	8	12	16	28

Length of Stay by Diagnosis and Operation, Western Region, 2008

Western Region, October 2006–September 2007 Data, by Diagnosis

188.0: BLADDER TRIGONE CA

Type of Patients	Observed Patients	Avg. Stay	Vari-ance	Percentiles 10th	25th	50th	75th	90th	95th	99th
1. SINGLE DX										
A. *Not Operated*										
0–19 Years	0									
20–34	0									
35–49	0									
50–64	0									
65+	0									
B. *Operated*										
0–19 Years	1	1.0	0	1	1	1	1	1	1	1
20–34	0									
35–49	1									
50–64	4	2.8	12	1	1	1	8	8	8	8
65+	3	1.0	0	1	1	1	1	1	1	1
2. MULTIPLE DX										
A. *Not Operated*										
0–19 Years	0									
20–34	0									
35–49	0									
50–64	2	3.5	<1	3	3	4	4	4	4	4
65+	4	3.0	7	1	2	2	2	7	7	7
B. *Operated*										
0–19 Years	0									
20–34	0									
35–49	14	10.0	289	1	2	5	10	12	68	68
50–64	51	6.9	75	1	1	5	9	15	21	54
65+	210	4.7	23	1	1	3	7	11	14	21
SUBTOTALS:										
1. SINGLE DX										
A. *Not Operated*	0									
B. *Operated*	8	1.9	6	1	1	1	1	8	8	8
2. MULTIPLE DX										
A. *Not Operated*	6	3.2	5	1	2	2	4	7	7	7
B. *Operated*	275	5.4	47	1	1	3	7	12	15	30
1. SINGLE DX	8	1.9	6	1	1	1	1	8	8	8
2. MULTIPLE DX	281	5.3	46	1	1	3	7	12	15	30
A. NOT OPERATED	6	3.2	5	1	2	2	4	7	7	7
B. OPERATED	283	5.3	46	1	1	3	7	12	15	30
TOTAL										
0–19 Years	0									
20–34	1	1.0	0	1	1	1	1	1	1	1
35–49	14	10.0	289	1	2	5	10	12	68	68
50–64	57	6.5	69	1	1	4	8	15	21	54
65+	217	4.6	23	1	1	3	7	11	14	21
GRAND TOTAL	289	5.2	45	1	1	3	7	12	15	30

188.1: BLADDER DOME CA

Type of Patients	Observed Patients	Avg. Stay	Vari-ance	Percentiles 10th	25th	50th	75th	90th	95th	99th
1. SINGLE DX										
A. *Not Operated*										
0–19 Years	0									
20–34	0									
35–49	0									
50–64	0									
65+	0									
B. *Operated*										
0–19 Years	1	2.0	0	2	2	2	2	2	2	2
20–34	0									
35–49	1	1.0	0	1	1	1	1	1	1	1
50–64	2	2.5	<1	2	2	3	3	3	3	3
65+	4	2.5	<1	1	1	3	3	3	3	3
2. MULTIPLE DX										
A. *Not Operated*										
0–19 Years	0									
20–34	0									
35–49	0									
50–64	4	12.6	192	1	1	15	31	31	31	31
65+	8	2.8	2	1	1	2	4	5	5	5
B. *Operated*										
0–19 Years	1	4.0	0	4	4	4	4	4	4	4
20–34	2	6.0	32	2	2	2	10	10	10	10
35–49	5	9.8	28	6	7	8	9	19	19	19
50–64	38	6.2	64	1	1	2	9	16	25	36
65+	209	4.7	21	1	1	3	7	11	12	22
SUBTOTALS:										
1. SINGLE DX										
A. *Not Operated*	0									
B. *Operated*	8	2.3	<1	1	1	2	3	3	3	3
2. MULTIPLE DX										
A. *Not Operated*	12	6.0	77	1	1	3	4	15	31	31
B. *Operated*	255	5.1	28	1	1	3	7	11	15	25
1. SINGLE DX	8	2.3	<1	1	1	3	3	3	3	3
2. MULTIPLE DX	267	5.1	30	1	1	3	7	11	15	27
A. NOT OPERATED	12	6.0	77	1	1	3	4	15	31	31
B. OPERATED	263	5.0	27	1	1	3	7	11	14	25
TOTAL										
0–19 Years	2	3.0	2	2	2	2	4	4	4	4
20–34	2	6.0	32	2	2	2	10	10	10	10
35–49	6	8.3	35	1	6	7	9	19	19	19
50–64	44	6.6	73	1	1	3	9	16	25	36
65+	221	4.6	20	1	1	3	7	11	12	22
GRAND TOTAL	275	5.0	29	1	1	3	7	11	15	27

188.2: BLADDER LATERAL WALL CA

Type of Patients	Observed Patients	Avg. Stay	Vari-ance	Percentiles 10th	25th	50th	75th	90th	95th	99th
1. SINGLE DX										
A. *Not Operated*										
0–19 Years	0									
20–34	0									
35–49	0									
50–64	0									
65+	0									
B. *Operated*										
0–19 Years	0									
20–34	1	3.0	0	3	3	3	3	3	3	3
35–49	3	4.3	17	1	1	3	9	9	9	9
50–64	5	4.2	12	1	2	4	4	10	10	10
65+	10	1.3	<1	1	1	1	1	2	3	3
2. MULTIPLE DX										
A. *Not Operated*										
0–19 Years	0									
20–34	0									
35–49	0									
50–64	3	5.0	13	1	1	6	8	8	8	8
65+	13	9.0	38	1	4	8	14	18	20	20
B. *Operated*										
0–19 Years	0									
20–34	0									
35–49	12	7.2	49	1	1	5	9	15	25	25
50–64	130	4.6	25	1	1	2	8	11	15	24
65+	471	4.6	29	1	1	3	6	10	14	27
SUBTOTALS:										
1. SINGLE DX										
A. *Not Operated*	0									
B. *Operated*	19	2.6	7	1	1	1	3	9	10	10
2. MULTIPLE DX										
A. *Not Operated*	16	8.2	35	1	4	8	10	18	20	20
B. *Operated*	613	4.6	29	1	1	3	6	10	14	25
1. SINGLE DX	19	2.6	7	1	1	1	3	9	10	10
2. MULTIPLE DX	629	4.7	29	1	1	3	7	10	15	25
A. NOT OPERATED	16	8.2	35	1	4	8	10	18	20	20
B. OPERATED	632	4.6	28	1	1	3	6	10	14	25
TOTAL										
0–19 Years	0									
20–34	1	3.0	0	3	3	3	3	3	3	3
35–49	15	6.7	42	1	1	5	9	15	25	25
50–64	138	4.6	25	1	1	2	8	11	15	24
65+	494	4.6	29	1	1	3	6	10	14	27
GRAND TOTAL	648	4.7	29	1	1	3	6	10	15	25

Length of Stay by Diagnosis and Operation, Western Region, 2008

Western Region, October 2006–September 2007 Data, by Diagnosis

188.4: BLADDER POST WALL CA

Type of Patients	Observed Patients	Avg. Stay	Variance	10th	25th	50th	75th	90th	95th	99th
1. SINGLE DX										
A. Not Operated										
0–19 Years	0									
20–34	0									
35–49	0									
50–64	0									
65+	0									
B. Operated										
0–19 Years	0									
20–34	0									
35–49	0									
50–64	1	3.0	0	3	3	3	3	3	3	3
65+	2	1.5	<1	1	1	2	2	2	2	2
2. MULTIPLE DX										
A. Not Operated										
0–19 Years	0									
20–34	0									
35–49	0									
50–64	0									
65+	10	4.5	5	2	3	4	6	8	8	8
B. Operated										
0–19 Years	0									
20–34	0									
35–49	12	6.5	16	1	3	8	10	11	13	13
50–64	76	6.0	45	1	1	4	8	13	18	37
65+	303	4.3	31	1	1	3	6	9	11	23
SUBTOTALS:										
1. SINGLE DX										
A. Not Operated	0									
B. Operated	3	2.0	<1	1	1	2	3	3	3	3
2. MULTIPLE DX										
A. Not Operated	10	4.5	5	2	3	4	6	8	8	8
B. Operated	391	4.7	34	1	1	3	7	10	13	35
1. SINGLE DX	3	2.0	<1	1	1	2	3	3	3	3
2. MULTIPLE DX	401	4.7	33	1	1	3	7	10	13	35
A. NOT OPERATED	10	4.5	5	2	3	4	6	8	8	8
B. OPERATED	394	4.7	34	1	1	3	7	10	13	35
TOTAL										
0–19 Years	0									
20–34	0									
35–49	12	6.5	16	3	3	8	10	11	13	13
50–64	77	6.0	45	1	1	4	8	13	18	37
65+	315	4.3	30	1	1	3	6	9	11	23
GRAND TOTAL	404	4.7	33	1	1	3	7	10	13	29

188.5: BLADDER NECK CA

Type of Patients	Observed Patients	Avg. Stay	Variance	10th	25th	50th	75th	90th	95th	99th
1. SINGLE DX										
A. Not Operated										
0–19 Years	0									
20–34	0									
35–49	0									
50–64	0									
65+	0									
B. Operated										
0–19 Years	0									
20–34	0									
35–49	0									
50–64	4	1.3	<1	1	1	1	1	2	2	2
65+	4	2.5	9	1	1	1	1	7	7	7
2. MULTIPLE DX										
A. Not Operated										
0–19 Years	0									
20–34	0									
35–49	2	4.9	32	1	1	1	9	9	9	9
50–64	2	4.0	2	3	3	4	5	5	5	5
65+	3	2.7	<1	2	2	3	3	3	3	3
B. Operated										
0–19 Years	0									
20–34	0									
35–49	5	3.8	21	1	1	2	3	12	12	12
50–64	52	5.3	29	1	1	2	7	13	16	26
65+	213	3.6	18	1	1	2	4	9	11	23
SUBTOTALS:										
1. SINGLE DX										
A. Not Operated	0									
B. Operated	8	1.9	4	1	1	1	1	7	7	7
2. MULTIPLE DX										
A. Not Operated	7	3.7	7	1	2	3	5	9	9	9
B. Operated	270	3.9	20	1	1	2	6	9	13	25
1. SINGLE DX	8	1.9	4	1	1	1	3	7	7	7
2. MULTIPLE DX	277	3.9	20	1	1	2	6	9	13	25
A. NOT OPERATED	7	3.7	7	1	2	3	5	9	9	9
B. OPERATED	278	3.9	20	1	1	2	6	9	13	25
TOTAL										
0–19 Years	0									
20–34	0									
35–49	7	4.1	20	1	1	2	9	12	12	12
50–64	58	4.9	27	1	1	2	7	13	16	26
65+	220	3.6	17	1	1	2	4	9	11	23
GRAND TOTAL	285	3.9	19	1	1	2	6	9	13	25

188.8: BLADDER CA NEC

Type of Patients	Observed Patients	Avg. Stay	Variance	10th	25th	50th	75th	90th	95th	99th
1. SINGLE DX										
A. Not Operated										
0–19 Years	0									
20–34	0									
35–49	0									
50–64	2	1.5	<1	1	1	2	2	2	2	2
65+	0									
B. Operated										
0–19 Years	0									
20–34	0									
35–49	2	2.0	2	1	1	1	3	3	3	3
50–64	16	3.1	9	1	1	2	6	7	10	10
65+	17	2.6	5	1	1	1	3	7	8	8
2. MULTIPLE DX										
A. Not Operated										
0–19 Years	0									
20–34	0									
35–49	6	4.0	10	1	1	4	6	9	9	9
50–64	34	3.6	12	1	1	3	5	7	12	18
65+	93	5.0	18	1	2	4	6	9	15	22
B. Operated										
0–19 Years	1	9.0	0	9	9	9	9	9	9	9
20–34	4	11.3	222	1	2	9	33	33	33	33
35–49	48	8.5	127	1	1	7	9	22	23	67
50–64	369	7.0	42	1	2	6	9	13	18	35
65+	1,247	6.2	40	1	2	5	8	13	18	34
SUBTOTALS:										
1. SINGLE DX										
A. Not Operated	2	1.5	<1	1	1	2	2	2	2	2
B. Operated	35	2.8	6	1	1	1	4	7	8	10
2. MULTIPLE DX										
A. Not Operated	133	4.6	16	1	2	3	6	9	14	22
B. Operated	1,669	6.4	43	1	2	5	9	13	18	35
1. SINGLE DX	37	2.7	6	1	1	1	3	7	8	10
2. MULTIPLE DX	1,802	6.3	42	1	2	5	8	13	18	34
A. NOT OPERATED	135	4.5	16	1	2	3	6	9	14	22
B. OPERATED	1,704	6.4	43	1	2	5	9	13	18	35
TOTAL										
0–19 Years	1	9.0	0	9	9	9	9	9	9	9
20–34	4	11.3	222	1	2	9	33	33	33	33
35–49	56	7.8	113	1	2	5	9	19	23	67
50–64	421	6.5	39	1	2	6	9	13	17	33
65+	1,357	6.1	38	1	2	4	8	13	17	33
GRAND TOTAL	1,839	6.2	41	1	2	5	8	13	18	34

Length of Stay by Diagnosis and Operation, Western Region, 2008

Western Region, October 2006–September 2007 Data, by Diagnosis

188.9: BLADDER CA NOS

Type of Patients	Observed Patients	Avg. Stay	Variance	10th	25th	50th	75th	90th	95th	99th
1. SINGLE DX										
A. Not Operated										
0–19 Years	0									
20–34	0									
35–49	0									
50–64	0									
65+	2	1.0	0		1		1	1	1	1
B. Operated										
0–19 Years	0									
20–34										
35–49	5	2.4	7	1	1	1			7	7
50–64	6	3.3	15	1	1	1	6	7	10	10
65+	9	2.4	4	1	1	2	3	7	7	7
2. MULTIPLE DX										
A. Not Operated										
0–19 Years	1	1.0	0	1	1	1	1	1	1	1
20–34	8	3.5	7	2	2	3	5	7	8	8
35–49	42	4.6	22	1	2	3	5	8	17	22
50–64	151	4.4	19	1	2	3	5	8	12	26
B. Operated										
0–19 Years	0									
20–34	1	9.0	0	9	9	9	9	9	9	9
35–49	24	8.6	160	2	4	5	7	20	23	63
50–64	167	6.6	27	1	2	6	8	13	14	28
65+	567	6.6	35	1	2	6	9	14	18	26
SUBTOTALS:										
1. SINGLE DX										
A. Not Operated	2	1.0	0	1	1	1	1	1	1	1
B. Operated	20	2.7	7	1	1	1	3	7	7	10
2. MULTIPLE DX										
A. Not Operated	202	4.4	19	1	2	3	5	8	12	22
B. Operated	759	6.7	37	1	2	6	9	14	18	29
1. SINGLE DX	22	2.6	7	1	1	1	3	7	7	10
2. MULTIPLE DX	961	6.2	34	2	2	5	8	13	17	29
A. NOT OPERATED	204	4.3	19	1	2	3	5	8	12	22
B. OPERATED	779	6.6	37	1	2	6	9	14	18	29
TOTAL										
0–19 Years	1	1.0	0	1	1	1	1	1	1	1
20–34	1	9.0	0	9	9	9	9	9	9	9
35–49	37	6.7	112	1	2	4	7	9	23	63
50–64	215	6.1	26	1	2	6	8	12	15	26
65+	729	6.1	33	1	2	5	8	13	17	29
GRAND TOTAL	983	6.1	34	1	2	5	8	13	17	29

189: KIDNEY/URINARY CA NEC

Type of Patients	Observed Patients	Avg. Stay	Variance	10th	25th	50th	75th	90th	95th	99th
1. SINGLE DX										
A. Not Operated										
0–19 Years	4	3.2	7	1	1		5	6	6	6
20–34	0									
35–49	0									
50–64	3	3.0	4	1	1	3	5	5	5	5
65+	1	1.0	0	1	1		1	1	1	1
B. Operated										
0–19 Years	12	5.6	5	3	4	6	7	8	10	10
20–34	11	3.9	2	2	3	4	5	6	6	6
35–49	76	3.3	2	2	2	3	4	5	5	7
50–64	127	3.2	2	2	2	3	4	5	5	7
65+	47	3.9	6	1	2	4	5	7	10	11
2. MULTIPLE DX										
A. Not Operated										
0–19 Years	17	3.1	3	1	2	3	4	5	7	7
20–34	6	6.9	18	2	4	8	8	14	14	14
35–49	76	4.3	21	1	2	3	5	8	14	31
50–64	251	5.2	30	1	2	4	6	10	15	28
65+	435	5.1	20	1	2	4	6	10	13	22
B. Operated										
0–19 Years	44	10.6	125	4	5	7	10	22	33	53
20–34	78	4.4	9	2	3	4	5	7	10	23
35–49	670	4.5	11	2	3	4	5	7	10	19
50–64	2,178	4.7	14	2	3	4	5	7	10	21
65+	3,042	5.4	21	2	3	4	6	9	13	24
SUBTOTALS:										
1. SINGLE DX										
A. Not Operated	8	2.9	5	1	1	3	5	6	6	6
B. Operated	273	3.4	3	2	2	3	4	5	6	10
2. MULTIPLE DX										
A. Not Operated	785	5.0	23	1	2	4	6	10	13	27
B. Operated	6,012	5.1	18	2	3	4	6	8	11	23
1. SINGLE DX	281	3.4	3	2	2	3	4	5	6	10
2. MULTIPLE DX	6,797	5.1	19	2	3	4	6	9	12	24
A. NOT OPERATED	793	5.0	23	1	2	4	6	10	13	27
B. OPERATED	6,285	5.0	18	2	3	4	6	8	11	23
TOTAL										
0–19 Years	77	7.8	84	2	4	5	8	14	33	53
20–34	95	4.5	9	2	3	4	5	8	10	23
35–49	822	4.4	11	2	3	4	5	7	9	18
50–64	2,559	4.6	15	2	3	4	5	8	10	22
65+	3,525	5.3	21	2	3	4	6	9	13	23
GRAND TOTAL	7,078	5.0	18	2	3	4	6	8	12	23

189.0: KIDNEY CA NEC

Type of Patients	Observed Patients	Avg. Stay	Variance	10th	25th	50th	75th	90th	95th	99th
1. SINGLE DX										
A. Not Operated										
0–19 Years	4	3.2	7	1	1		5	6	6	6
20–34	0									
35–49	0									
50–64	3	3.0	4	1	1	3	5	5	5	5
65+	0									
B. Operated										
0–19 Years	12	5.6	5	3	4	6	7	8	10	10
20–34	11	3.9	2	2	3	4	5	6	6	6
35–49	73	3.3	2	2	2	3	4	5	5	7
50–64	119	3.2	2	2	2	3	4	5	5	7
65+	39	3.6	5	1	2	4	5	6	10	11
2. MULTIPLE DX										
A. Not Operated										
0–19 Years	17	3.1	3	1	2	3	4	5	7	7
20–34	6	6.9	18	2	4	8	8	14	14	14
35–49	71	4.4	22	1	2	3	5	8	14	31
50–64	236	5.1	29	1	2	4	6	10	15	27
65+	351	5.1	17	1	2	4	7	10	13	21
B. Operated										
0–19 Years	44	10.6	125	4	5	7	10	22	33	53
20–34	75	4.4	9	2	3	4	5	7	10	23
35–49	630	4.5	11	2	3	4	5	7	9	19
50–64	2,014	4.7	14	2	3	4	5	7	10	21
65+	2,404	5.2	20	2	3	4	6	9	12	23
SUBTOTALS:										
1. SINGLE DX										
A. Not Operated	7	3.1	5	1	1	3	5	6	6	6
B. Operated	254	3.4	3	2	2	3	4	5	6	10
2. MULTIPLE DX										
A. Not Operated	681	5.0	22	1	2	4	6	10	13	25
B. Operated	5,167	4.9	18	2	3	4	6	8	11	22
1. SINGLE DX	261	3.4	3	2	2	3	4	5	6	10
2. MULTIPLE DX	5,848	4.9	18	2	3	4	6	8	11	23
A. NOT OPERATED	688	5.0	22	1	2	4	6	10	13	25
B. OPERATED	5,421	4.9	17	2	3	4	6	8	11	22
TOTAL										
0–19 Years	77	7.8	84	2	4	5	8	14	33	53
20–34	92	4.5	9	2	3	4	5	8	10	23
35–49	774	4.4	12	2	3	4	5	7	9	19
50–64	2,372	4.6	15	2	3	4	5	8	10	22
65+	2,794	5.2	20	2	3	4	6	9	12	22
GRAND TOTAL	6,109	4.9	18	2	3	4	6	8	11	22

Length of Stay by Diagnosis and Operation, Western Region, 2008

Western Region, October 2006–September 2007 Data, by Diagnosis

189.1: RENAL PELVIS CA

Type of Patients	Observed Patients	Avg. Stay	Variance	10th	25th	50th	75th	90th	95th	99th
1. SINGLE DX										
A. Not Operated										
0–19 Years	0									
20–34	0									
35–49	0									
50–64	0									
65+	1	1.0	0						1	1
B. Operated										
0–19 Years	0									
20–34	0									
35–49	3	2.7	<1	2	2	3	3	3	3	3
50–64	5	2.6	<1	2	2	3	3	3	3	3
65+	4	5.7	8	4	4	4	5	10	10	10
2. MULTIPLE DX										
A. Not Operated										
0–19 Years	0									
20–34	0									
35–49	1	1.0	0	1	1	1	1	1	1	1
50–64	6	6.9	12	3	4	8	9	12	12	12
65+	39	5.1	29	1	2	4	6	9	16	31
B. Operated										
0–19 Years	0									
20–34	3	3.3	<1	3	3	3	4	4	4	4
35–49	33	4.6	5	2	3	4	6	7	9	10
50–64	101	4.8	26	2	3	4	6	7	9	13
65+	341	5.7	15	2	3	5	7	10	12	25
SUBTOTALS:										
1. SINGLE DX										
A. Not Operated	1	1.0	0	1	1	1	1	1	1	1
B. Operated	12	3.7	5	2	3	3	4	5	10	10
2. MULTIPLE DX										
A. Not Operated	46	5.2	27	1	2	4	6	9	12	31
B. Operated	478	5.4	17	2	3	4	6	9	12	25
1. SINGLE DX	13	3.5	5	2	2	3	4	5	10	10
2. MULTIPLE DX	524	5.4	18	2	3	4	6	9	12	25
A. NOT OPERATED	47	5.1	27	1	2	4	6	9	12	31
B. OPERATED	490	5.4	17	2	3	4	6	9	11	25
TOTAL										
0–19 Years	0									
20–34	3	3.3	<1	3	3	3	4	4	4	4
35–49	37	4.3	5	2	3	4	6	7	9	10
50–64	112	4.8	24	2	3	4	6	8	9	13
65+	385	5.6	17	2	3	5	7	10	12	27
GRAND TOTAL	537	5.4	18	2	3	4	6	9	12	25

189.2: URETER CA

Type of Patients	Observed Patients	Avg. Stay	Variance	10th	25th	50th	75th	90th	95th	99th
1. SINGLE DX										
A. Not Operated										
0–19 Years	0									
20–34	0									
35–49	0									
50–64	0									
65+	0									
B. Operated										
0–19 Years	0									
20–34	0									
35–49	0									
50–64	3	3.0	<1	2	3	3	4	4	4	4
65+	3	5.3	10	3	3	4	9	9	9	9
2. MULTIPLE DX										
A. Not Operated										
0–19 Years	0									
20–34	0									
35–49	2	3.0	8	1	1	3	5	5	5	5
50–64	6	5.6	28	1	3	3	8	15	15	15
65+	31	4.6	16	1	3	3	7	9	13	17
B. Operated										
0–19 Years	0									
20–34	0									
35–49	4	3.5	2	3	3	4	5	5	5	5
50–64	52	4.2	5	2	3	4	5	7	8	14
65+	262	6.5	24	2	4	5	8	13	16	26
SUBTOTALS:										
1. SINGLE DX										
A. Not Operated	0									
B. Operated	6	4.2	6	2	3	4	4	9	9	9
2. MULTIPLE DX										
A. Not Operated	39	4.7	17	1	3	3	7	12	15	17
B. Operated	318	6.1	22	2	3	5	7	12	16	25
1. SINGLE DX	6	4.2	6	2	3	4	4	9	9	9
2. MULTIPLE DX	357	5.9	21	2	3	5	7	12	15	25
A. NOT OPERATED	39	4.7	17	1	3	3	7	12	15	17
B. OPERATED	324	6.1	21	2	3	5	7	11	15	25
TOTAL										
0–19 Years	0									
20–34	0									
35–49	6	3.3	3	1	2	4	5	5	5	5
50–64	61	4.3	7	1	3	4	5	7	8	15
65+	296	6.3	23	2	3	5	8	13	16	26
GRAND TOTAL	363	5.9	21	2	3	5	7	11	15	25

190: EYE CA

Type of Patients	Observed Patients	Avg. Stay	Variance	10th	25th	50th	75th	90th	95th	99th
1. SINGLE DX										
A. Not Operated										
0–19 Years	1	5.0	0	5	5	5	5	5	5	5
20–34	1	1.0	0	1	1	1	1	1	1	1
35–49	0									
50–64	0									
65+	0									
B. Operated										
0–19 Years	13	1.7	1	1	1	1	2	3	4	4
20–34	0									
35–49	1	2.0	0	2	2	2	2	2	2	2
50–64	2	1.0	0	1	1	1	1	1	1	1
65+	0									
2. MULTIPLE DX										
A. Not Operated										
0–19 Years	3	4.0	<1	3	3	4	5	5	5	5
20–34	5	5.2	11	3	3	4	5	11	11	11
35–49	1	3.0	0	3	3	3	3	3	3	3
50–64	0									
65+	4	2.8	<1	2	3	3	3	3	3	3
B. Operated										
0–19 Years	2	11.5	216	1	1	12	22	22	22	22
20–34	2	2.0	0	2	2	2	2	2	2	2
35–49	4	1.8	<1	1	1	2	2	2	2	2
50–64	6	6.0	12	2	4	6	7	12	12	12
65+	21	5.3	80	1	2	2	4	10	16	41
SUBTOTALS:										
1. SINGLE DX										
A. Not Operated	2	3.0	8	1	1	3	5	5	5	5
B. Operated	16	1.6	<1	1	1	1	2	3	4	4
2. MULTIPLE DX										
A. Not Operated	13	4.0	5	3	3	3	4	5	11	11
B. Operated	34	5.2	61	1	2	2	5	12	22	41
1. SINGLE DX	18	1.8	1	1	1	1	2	4	5	5
2. MULTIPLE DX	47	4.9	45	1	2	3	5	11	16	41
A. NOT OPERATED	15	3.9	5	1	3	3	5	5	11	11
B. OPERATED	50	4.1	44	1	2	2	4	10	16	41
TOTAL										
0–19 Years	19	3.3	23	1	1	2	4	5	22	22
20–34	7	4.2	11	1	2	3	5	11	11	11
35–49	6	2.0	<1	1	2	2	3	3	3	3
50–64	8	4.8	14	1	3	5	7	12	12	12
65+	25	4.9	67	1	2	3	3	10	16	41
GRAND TOTAL	65	4.0	35	1	1	2	4	7	12	41

Length of Stay by Diagnosis and Operation, Western Region, 2008

Western Region, October 2006–September 2007 Data, by Diagnosis

191: BRAIN CA

Type of Patients	Observed Patients	Avg. Stay	Variance	Percentiles						
				10th	25th	50th	75th	90th	95th	99th
1. SINGLE DX										
A. Not Operated										
0–19 Years	13	3.0	8	1	2	2	3	4	12	12
20–34	14	2.1	1	1	1	2	2	3	5	5
35–49	17	2.1	2	1	1	2	3	4	5	5
50–64	23	2.4	4	1	1	1	4	4	5	9
65+	9	2.6	4	1	1	2	3	7	7	7
B. Operated										
0–19 Years	29	3.8	4	2	2	4	4	6	7	11
20–34	35	3.5	3	2	2	3	4	6	8	8
35–49	48	4.0	10	2	2	3	5	8	10	16
50–64	61	3.6	5	2	2	3	4	7	8	11
65+	14	3.5	6	2	2	3	4	9	9	9
2. MULTIPLE DX										
A. Not Operated										
0–19 Years	118	5.8	49	1	2	3	7	15	18	33
20–34	136	4.6	29	1	2	3	5	9	20	26
35–49	317	4.5	19	1	2	3	6	9	14	23
50–64	636	4.7	29	1	1	3	6	10	14	28
65+	648	4.9	18	1	2	4	6	10	12	23
B. Operated										
0–19 Years	159	10.5	129	2	3	7	13	23	33	63
20–34	266	6.8	52	2	3	5	8	13	19	43
35–49	518	6.6	56	2	3	5	8	12	18	36
50–64	856	7.2	55	2	3	5	8	14	20	42
65+	650	7.9	39	2	3	6	10	15	20	29
SUBTOTALS:										
1. SINGLE DX										
A. Not Operated	76	2.4	4	1	1	2	3	4	5	12
B. Operated	187	3.7	6	2	2	3	4	7	9	12
2. MULTIPLE DX										
A. Not Operated	1,855	4.8	25	1	2	3	6	10	14	26
B. Operated	2,449	7.4	56	2	3	5	9	15	20	39
1. SINGLE DX	263	3.3	5	1	2	3	4	6	8	12
2. MULTIPLE DX	4,304	6.3	45	2	3	4	8	13	18	33
A. NOT OPERATED	1,931	4.7	24	1	2	3	6	10	13	24
B. OPERATED	2,636	7.2	54	2	3	5	9	14	20	37
TOTAL										
0–19 Years	319	7.8	90	2	3	5	9	18	24	49
20–34	451	5.7	41	2	2	4	7	11	16	31
35–49	900	5.6	41	1	2	4	7	11	16	28
50–64	1,576	6.0	44	1	3	4	7	12	17	35
65+	1,321	6.3	31	2	3	5	8	12	17	27
GRAND TOTAL	4,567	6.1	43	1	2	4	7	12	17	32

191.1: FRONTAL LOBE CA

Type of Patients	Observed Patients	Avg. Stay	Variance	Percentiles						
				10th	25th	50th	75th	90th	95th	99th
1. SINGLE DX										
A. Not Operated										
0–19 Years	0									
20–34	3	2.3	<1	2	2	2	3	3	3	3
35–49	4	2.5	2	1	2	2	3	4	4	4
50–64	3	1.7	<1	1	1	2	2	2	2	2
65+	3	3.0	12	1	1	1	7	7	7	7
B. Operated										
0–19 Years	1	2.0	0	2	2	2	2	2	2	2
20–34	12	3.2	3	2	2	4	4	6	7	7
35–49	21	2.6	3	1	2	2	2	5	7	7
50–64	17	3.7	7	2	2	3	4	8	10	16
65+	5	2.4	1	1	2	2	3	4	4	4
2. MULTIPLE DX										
A. Not Operated										
0–19 Years	11	2.3	1	1	1	3	3	3	4	4
20–34	38	4.3	20	1	2	3	4	9	16	24
35–49	90	3.6	10	1	1	3	4	8	9	20
50–64	149	4.2	21	1	1	3	4	9	13	24
65+	160	5.0	20	1	2	3	6	10	12	26
B. Operated										
0–19 Years	26	9.4	73	3	3	7	13	20	23	40
20–34	106	5.6	26	2	3	4	8	11	13	19
35–49	220	6.1	33	2	3	4	8	11	16	33
50–64	313	7.1	47	2	3	5	8	13	20	32
65+	211	8.2	38	3	4	7	10	16	21	34
SUBTOTALS:										
1. SINGLE DX										
A. Not Operated	13	2.4	3	1	1	2	3	4	7	7
B. Operated	56	3.0	4	1	2	2	4	7	7	10
2. MULTIPLE DX										
A. Not Operated	448	4.3	18	1	2	3	5	9	12	24
B. Operated	876	7.0	40	2	3	5	9	13	19	35
1. SINGLE DX	69	2.9	4	1	2	2	3	7	7	12
2. MULTIPLE DX	1,324	6.1	35	2	3	4	8	12	17	29
A. NOT OPERATED	461	4.3	18	1	2	3	5	9	12	24
B. OPERATED	932	6.8	39	2	3	5	8	13	18	34
TOTAL										
0–19 Years	38	7.1	61	1	3	4	9	18	23	40
20–34	159	5.1	23	2	2	4	6	10	13	24
35–49	335	5.2	26	1	2	4	7	10	13	28
50–64	482	6.0	39	2	3	5	7	12	17	30
65+	379	6.7	33	2	3	5	9	13	20	28
GRAND TOTAL	1,393	5.9	33	2	3	4	7	12	17	29

191.2: TEMPORAL LOBE CA

Type of Patients	Observed Patients	Avg. Stay	Variance	Percentiles						
				10th	25th	50th	75th	90th	95th	99th
1. SINGLE DX										
A. Not Operated										
0–19 Years	0									
20–34	3	1.7	<1	1	1	2	2	2	2	2
35–49	3	1.0	0	1	1	1	1	1	1	1
50–64	5	1.8	2	1	1	2	2	4	4	4
65+	1	2.0	0	2	2	2	2	2	2	2
B. Operated										
0–19 Years	10	3.5	8	2	2	3	4	11	11	11
20–34	6	2.7	<1	2	2	3	3	3	3	3
35–49	13	5.5	12	2	2	5	8	10	12	12
50–64	19	3.5	5	2	2	3	4	5	11	11
65+	3	4.6	14	2	2	3	9	9	9	9
2. MULTIPLE DX										
A. Not Operated										
0–19 Years	6	6.6	37	1	1	2	11	15	15	15
20–34	17	4.0	13	1	1	3	5	10	12	12
35–49	29	3.8	11	2	2	3	4	8	11	16
50–64	80	3.8	23	1	1	2	5	8	12	35
65+	113	4.9	20	1	2	4	6	9	13	22
B. Operated										
0–19 Years	20	6.1	16	2	4	6	8	14	16	16
20–34	44	7.0	82	2	3	4	8	14	20	57
35–49	118	6.1	26	2	3	5	8	12	17	25
50–64	215	6.0	32	2	3	4	7	11	16	30
65+	188	7.8	44	2	3	6	9	14	21	29
SUBTOTALS:										
1. SINGLE DX										
A. Not Operated	12	1.6	<1	1	1	2	2	2	4	4
B. Operated	51	4.0	7	2	2	3	5	9	11	12
2. MULTIPLE DX										
A. Not Operated	245	4.4	20	1	1	3	5	9	12	22
B. Operated	585	6.7	38	2	3	5	8	13	17	29
1. SINGLE DX	63	3.5	7	1	2	3	4	8	10	12
2. MULTIPLE DX	830	6.0	34	2	2	4	7	12	16	29
A. NOT OPERATED	257	4.3	19	1	1	3	5	9	12	22
B. OPERATED	636	6.5	36	2	3	5	8	12	17	29
TOTAL										
0–19 Years	36	5.5	18	2	2	4	8	12	15	16
20–34	70	5.7	58	2	2	3	7	12	15	57
35–49	163	5.5	23	2	2	4	8	11	16	25
50–64	319	5.2	29	1	2	5	6	11	14	30
65+	305	6.7	37	2	3	5	8	13	18	29
GRAND TOTAL	893	5.8	32	2	2	4	7	12	16	29

Length of Stay by Diagnosis and Operation, Western Region, 2008

Western Region, October 2006–September 2007 Data, by Diagnosis

191.3: PARIETAL LOBE CA

Type of Patients	Observed Patients	Avg. Stay	Variance	10th	25th	50th	75th	90th	95th	99th
1. SINGLE DX										
A. Not Operated										
0–19 Years	0									
20–34	0									
35–49	3	1.7	1	1	1	1	3	3	3	3
50–64	4	3.3	2	1	1	4	4	4	4	4
65+	3	2.0	<1	1	1	2	3	3	3	3
B. Operated										
0–19 Years	1	3.0	0	3	3	3	3	3	3	3
20–34	5	4.6	4	3	4	4	4	8	8	8
35–49	3	3.7	8	2	2	2	7	7	7	7
50–64	13	3.2	3	2	2	3	3	7	7	7
65+	0									
2. MULTIPLE DX										
A. Not Operated										
0–19 Years	6	5.7	45	1	2	2	9	18	18	18
20–34	13	2.0	2	1	1	1	2	4	6	6
35–49	42	4.5	15	1	2	3	6	9	10	20
50–64	102	4.9	24	1	1	3	7	10	13	23
65+	86	4.3	10	1	2	4	6	9	11	16
B. Operated										
0–19 Years	11	3.4	4	2	2	3	3	4	9	9
20–34	20	4.5	8	2	2	4	5	10	10	11
35–49	63	6.4	75	2	3	4	7	11	16	66
50–64	152	8.5	118	2	3	6	9	15	30	81
65+	121	7.2	28	2	3	6	10	14	18	22
SUBTOTALS:										
1. SINGLE DX										
A. Not Operated	10	2.4	2	1	1	3	4	4	4	4
B. Operated	22	3.6	4	2	2	3	4	7	7	8
2. MULTIPLE DX										
A. Not Operated	249	4.5	17	1	1	3	6	10	12	20
B. Operated	367	7.3	72	2	3	5	9	14	19	66
1. SINGLE DX	32	3.2	3	1	2	3	4	7	7	8
2. MULTIPLE DX	616	6.2	52	2	2	4	8	12	17	37
A. NOT OPERATED	259	4.4	17	1	1	3	6	9	12	20
B. OPERATED	389	7.1	69	2	3	5	8	14	19	66
TOTAL										
0–19 Years	18	4.1	17	2	2	3	3	9	18	18
20–34	38	3.6	7	1	1	3	5	8	10	11
35–49	111	5.5	49	2	2	4	6	8	15	20
50–64	271	6.8	79	3	3	5	8	13	20	76
65+	210	5.9	22	2	3	5	8	13	16	20
GRAND TOTAL	648	6.0	50	1	2	4	7	12	16	37

191.8: BRAIN CA NEC

Type of Patients	Observed Patients	Avg. Stay	Variance	10th	25th	50th	75th	90th	95th	99th
1. SINGLE DX										
A. Not Operated										
0–19 Years	2	1.5	<1	1	1	2	2	2	2	2
20–34	1	1.0	0	1	1	1	1	1	1	1
35–49	0									
50–64	3	4.3	17	1	1	3	3	9	9	9
65+	0									
B. Operated										
0–19 Years	0									
20–34	3	5.7	6	3	3	6	6	8	8	8
35–49	1	3.0	0	3	3	3	3	3	3	3
50–64	3	4.4	16	2	2	2	3	9	9	9
65+	2	6.0	18	3	3	9	9	9	9	9
2. MULTIPLE DX										
A. Not Operated										
0–19 Years	17	3.6	10	1	1	3	3	5	10	11
20–34	13	9.5	117	1	3	5	9	26	35	35
35–49	64	5.4	31	1	2	3	7	10	15	27
50–64	86	5.4	33	1	2	4	7	12	14	35
65+	80	5.1	21	1	3	4	7	10	12	28
B. Operated										
0–19 Years	25	13.9	235	3	5	9	17	23	26	78
20–34	21	6.1	17	3	3	4	4	10	13	19
35–49	45	7.2	46	2	3	5	8	14	22	36
50–64	62	6.3	20	2	3	5	9	12	15	20
65+	37	7.4	38	3	3	5	10	15	24	26
SUBTOTALS:										
1. SINGLE DX										
A. Not Operated	6	2.8	10	1	1	2	3	4	4	4
B. Operated	9	5.0	9	2	3	3	8	9	9	9
2. MULTIPLE DX										
A. Not Operated	260	5.4	32	2	3	4	7	11	15	31
B. Operated	190	7.7	62	2	3	6	10	16	22	36
1. SINGLE DX	15	4.1	10	1	2	3	8	9	9	9
2. MULTIPLE DX	450	6.4	46	1	2	4	8	13	20	31
A. NOT OPERATED	266	5.3	31	1	2	4	7	10	15	31
B. OPERATED	199	7.6	60	2	3	5	10	15	22	36
TOTAL										
0–19 Years	44	9.3	162	1	2	3	5	22	23	78
20–34	38	7.1	52	1	3	5	8	19	26	35
35–49	110	6.1	37	1	2	4	6	14	22	27
50–64	154	5.7	27	1	2	4	8	12	15	31
65+	119	5.9	27	1	3	4	7	12	16	26
GRAND TOTAL	465	6.3	45	1	2	4	8	13	20	31

191.9: BRAIN CA NOS

Type of Patients	Observed Patients	Avg. Stay	Variance	10th	25th	50th	75th	90th	95th	99th
1. SINGLE DX										
A. Not Operated										
0–19 Years	0									
20–34	3	1.7	<1	1	1	2	2	2	2	2
35–49	3	3.4	4	1	1	4	5	5	5	5
50–64	1	1.0	0	1	1	1	1	1	1	1
65+	1	3.0	0	3	3	3	3	3	3	3
B. Operated										
0–19 Years	2	4.5	<1	4	4	4	5	5	5	5
20–34	0									
35–49	1	3.0	0	3	3	3	3	3	3	3
50–64	2	5.5	<1	5	5	6	6	6	6	6
65+	2	3.5	<1	3	3	3	4	4	4	4
2. MULTIPLE DX										
A. Not Operated										
0–19 Years	20	5.2	19	1	2	4	5	11	15	15
20–34	22	4.1	20	1	1	3	4	10	11	20
35–49	54	4.5	19	1	1	3	6	12	14	22
50–64	136	5.3	35	1	2	4	6	12	14	24
65+	123	5.1	22	1	2	4	6	10	13	23
B. Operated										
0–19 Years	11	9.9	82	2	2	4	19	22	23	23
20–34	10	8.4	98	2	2	6	6	6	28	28
35–49	13	7.4	73	2	3	5	6	17	33	33
50–64	34	8.1	57	2	3	6	9	17	26	35
65+	15	9.7	54	1	5	9	12	20	28	28
SUBTOTALS:										
1. SINGLE DX										
A. Not Operated	8	2.4	2	1	1	2	4	5	5	5
B. Operated	7	4.3	1	3	3	4	5	6	6	6
2. MULTIPLE DX										
A. Not Operated	355	5.0	26	1	2	4	6	11	14	23
B. Operated	83	8.5	64	2	3	6	12	20	26	35
1. SINGLE DX	15	3.3	3	1	2	3	5	5	6	6
2. MULTIPLE DX	438	5.7	35	1	2	4	7	12	17	28
A. NOT OPERATED	363	4.9	26	1	2	3	6	11	14	23
B. OPERATED	90	8.2	61	2	3	5	10	20	26	35
TOTAL										
0–19 Years	33	6.8	42	1	2	4	10	18	22	23
20–34	35	5.1	43	1	2	3	5	11	26	28
35–49	71	4.9	29	1	2	4	6	9	17	33
50–64	173	5.8	39	1	2	4	7	12	17	35
65+	141	5.5	27	1	2	4	7	11	14	28
GRAND TOTAL	453	5.6	34	1	2	4	7	12	17	28

Length of Stay by Diagnosis and Operation, Western Region, 2008

Western Region, October 2006–September 2007 Data, by Diagnosis

192: OTHER NERVOUS SYSTEM CA

Type of Patients	Observed Patients	Avg. Stay	Variance	10th	25th	50th	75th	90th	95th	99th
1. SINGLE DX										
A. Not Operated										
0–19 Years	0									
20–34	0									
35–49	1	5.0	0	5	5	5	5	5	5	5
50–64	0									
65+	0									
B. Operated										
0–19 Years	0									
20–34	4	6.0	24	2	3	6	6	13	13	13
35–49	4	9.5	86	2	2	7	8	23	23	23
50–64	5	4.4	3	2	4	5	5	6	6	6
65+	2	6.0	18	3	3	9	9	9	9	9
2. MULTIPLE DX										
A. Not Operated										
0–19 Years	4	4.0	16	2	2	2	10	10	10	10
20–34	4	7.0	40	1	1	12	12	13	13	13
35–49	4	2.5	<1	2	2	3	3	3	3	3
50–64	12	7.5	45	2	3	7	8	20	22	22
65+	27	5.5	14	1	3	5	7	10	12	18
B. Operated										
0–19 Years	9	11.7	95	1	4	7	18	30	30	30
20–34	20	7.3	32	3	3	7	10	13	27	27
35–49	38	6.4	19	2	3	7	8	14	17	21
50–64	77	7.7	49	3	4	6	9	14	23	48
65+	52	9.6	93	3	4	7	11	22	30	55
SUBTOTALS:										
1. SINGLE DX										
A. Not Operated	1	5.0	0	5	5	5	5	5	5	5
B. Operated	15	6.4	30	2	3	5	8	13	23	23
2. MULTIPLE DX										
A. Not Operated	51	5.8	23	2	2	4	7	12	18	22
B. Operated	196	8.1	56	3	4	6	9	17	23	48
1. SINGLE DX	16	6.3	28	2	3	5	8	13	22	23
2. MULTIPLE DX	247	7.6	50	2	3	6	9	15	22	30
A. NOT OPERATED	52	5.7	22	2	3	4	7	12	18	22
B. OPERATED	211	8.0	54	2	4	6	9	16	23	30
TOTAL										
0–19 Years	13	9.3	81	2	2	5	16	20	30	30
20–34	28	7.1	30	2	3	6	11	13	13	27
35–49	47	6.3	23	2	3	5	8	14	17	23
50–64	94	7.5	46	2	4	6	9	14	22	48
65+	81	8.2	68	3	3	6	9	18	23	55
GRAND TOTAL	263	7.5	49	2	3	6	9	15	22	30

193: THYROID CA

Type of Patients	Observed Patients	Avg. Stay	Variance	10th	25th	50th	75th	90th	95th	99th
1. SINGLE DX										
A. Not Operated										
0–19 Years	8	1.9	<1	1	1	2	2	3	3	3
20–34	96	1.8	<1	1	1	2	2	3	3	3
35–49	166	1.8	<1	1	1	2	2	3	3	3
50–64	131	1.9	<1	1	1	2	2	3	3	3
65+	36	1.8	<1	1	1	2	2	3	3	4
B. Operated										
0–19 Years	33	1.5	<1	1	1	1	2	3	3	4
20–34	186	1.4	<1	1	1	1	2	2	3	4
35–49	291	1.4	<1	1	1	1	2	2	3	4
50–64	194	1.4	<1	1	1	1	2	2	3	5
65+	42	1.3	<1	1	1	1	2	2	2	3
2. MULTIPLE DX										
A. Not Operated										
0–19 Years	16	1.8	<1	1	1	2	2	2	3	3
20–34	145	2.0	<1	1	1	2	2	3	3	5
35–49	320	2.1	4	1	1	2	2	3	4	10
50–64	307	2.2	4	1	1	2	3	3	4	12
65+	247	2.8	7	2	2	2	3	5	7	17
B. Operated										
0–19 Years	27	2.7	3	1	1	2	4	6	7	7
20–34	465	2.1	7	1	1	1	2	4	5	12
35–49	923	1.8	2	1	1	1	2	3	5	8
50–64	1,170	2.1	12	1	1	1	2	3	5	15
65+	769	2.5	10	1	2	2	2	5	7	16
SUBTOTALS:										
1. SINGLE DX										
A. Not Operated	437	1.8	<1	1	1	2	2	3	3	3
B. Operated	746	1.4	<1	1	1	1	2	2	3	4
2. MULTIPLE DX										
A. Not Operated	1,035	2.3	4	1	1	2	2	3	5	11
B. Operated	3,354	2.1	8	1	1	1	2	4	6	13
1. SINGLE DX	1,183	1.6	<1	1	1	1	2	3	3	4
2. MULTIPLE DX	4,389	2.2	7	1	1	1	2	4	5	13
A. NOT OPERATED	1,472	2.2	3	1	1	2	2	3	4	10
B. OPERATED	4,100	2.0	7	1	1	1	2	3	5	12
TOTAL										
0–19 Years	84	2.0	2	1	1	1	2	4	4	7
20–34	892	1.9	4	1	1	1	2	3	4	9
35–49	1,700	1.8	2	1	1	1	2	3	4	8
50–64	1,802	2.1	9	1	1	1	2	3	5	13
65+	1,094	2.5	9	1	2	2	3	4	7	16
GRAND TOTAL	5,572	2.0	6	1	1	1	2	3	5	11

194: OTH ENDOCRINE GLAND CA

Type of Patients	Observed Patients	Avg. Stay	Variance	10th	25th	50th	75th	90th	95th	99th
1. SINGLE DX										
A. Not Operated										
0–19 Years	3	4.3	17	1	1	3	9	9	9	9
20–34	0									
35–49	0									
50–64	0									
65+	1	1.0	0	1	1	1	1	1	1	1
B. Operated										
0–19 Years	4	7.2	6	4	4	7	8	10	10	10
20–34	4	3.5	4	2	2	5	5	5	5	5
35–49	4	3.0	2	2	1	3	5	5	5	5
50–64	3	2.7	4	1	1	2	5	5	5	5
65+	0									
2. MULTIPLE DX										
A. Not Operated										
0–19 Years	25	7.3	84	1	2	3	7	23	31	36
20–34	10	3.6	8	1	2	3	4	10	10	10
35–49	5	3.2	4	1	3	3	4	6	6	6
50–64	17	5.5	15	2	3	4	7	10	18	18
65+	16	6.2	22	1	3	4	10	13	16	16
B. Operated										
0–19 Years	28	13.4	209	3	4	7	21	28	30	72
20–34	12	7.3	29	2	4	6	13	13	20	20
35–49	22	6.0	22	1	3	4	10	14	15	15
50–64	36	5.5	34	1	2	4	7	7	17	33
65+	25	4.1	9	1	2	3	6	8	10	11
SUBTOTALS:										
1. SINGLE DX										
A. Not Operated	4	3.5	14	1	1	3	9	9	9	9
B. Operated	13	4.3	7	2	2	4	5	8	10	10
2. MULTIPLE DX										
A. Not Operated	73	5.8	39	1	2	4	7	11	18	36
B. Operated	123	7.3	76	1	3	5	8	15	23	33
1. SINGLE DX	17	4.1	8	1	2	3	5	9	10	10
2. MULTIPLE DX	196	6.7	62	1	2	4	7	14	23	36
A. NOT OPERATED	77	5.7	38	1	2	4	7	11	18	36
B. OPERATED	136	7.0	70	1	2	5	8	14	23	33
TOTAL										
0–19 Years	60	10.0	141	2	3	6	11	27	31	72
20–34	24	5.4	21	2	2	4	7	13	13	20
35–49	31	5.2	18	1	2	4	6	11	15	15
50–64	56	5.3	27	2	2	4	7	9	17	33
65+	42	4.8	15	1	2	3	7	11	12	16
GRAND TOTAL	213	6.5	59	1	2	4	7	13	21	33

Length of Stay by Diagnosis and Operation, Western Region, 2008

Western Region, October 2006—September 2007 Data, by Diagnosis

195: OTHER & ILL-DEFINED CA

Type of Patients	Observed Patients	Avg. Stay	Variance	10th	25th	50th	75th	90th	95th	99th
						Percentiles				
1. SINGLE DX										
A. Not Operated										
0–19 Years	2	3.5	<1	3	3	4	4	4	4	4
20–34	1	4.0	0	4	4	4	4	4	4	4
35–49	2	1.0	0	1	1	1	1	1	1	1
50–64	2	2.5	4	1	1	3	4	4	4	4
65+	3	2.3	2	1	1	2	4	4	4	4
B. Operated										
0–19 Years	1	4.0	0	4	4	4	4	4	4	4
20–34	3	2.7	2	1	1	3	4	4	4	4
35–49	1	2.0	0	2	2	2	2	2	2	2
50–64	3	3.7	4	2	2	3	6	6	6	6
65+	3	2.3	<1	2	2	2	3	3	3	3
2. MULTIPLE DX										
A. Not Operated										
0–19 Years	4	7.8	105	1	1	4	23	23	23	23
20–34	4	8.2	37	4	4	8	8	17	17	17
35–49	19	5.8	24	1	2	4	8	11	21	21
50–64	80	7.1	115	1	2	4	8	15	22	85
65+	105	5.0	16	1	2	4	6	11	13	18
B. Operated										
0–19 Years	9	10.9	67	5	6	8	9	30	30	30
20–34	5	10.7	98	2	5	7	12	27	27	27
35–49	18	9.5	64	2	3	5	17	20	27	27
50–64	60	6.2	51	1	2	4	8	12	18	42
65+	74	7.1	59	1	3	5	9	15	21	55
SUBTOTALS:										
1. SINGLE DX										
A. Not Operated	10	2.5	2	1	1	3	4	4	4	4
B. Operated	11	2.9	2	2	2	3	4	4	6	6
2. MULTIPLE DX										
A. Not Operated	212	6.0	56	1	2	4	8	12	17	26
B. Operated	166	7.4	58	1	2	5	9	17	21	42
1. SINGLE DX	21	2.7	2	1	2	3	4	4	4	6
2. MULTIPLE DX	378	6.6	57	1	2	4	8	15	19	32
A. NOT OPERATED	222	5.8	54	1	2	4	7	12	17	26
B. OPERATED	177	7.1	56	1	2	5	9	17	21	42
TOTAL										
0–19 Years	16	8.8	65	3	4	5	9	23	30	30
20–34	13	7.6	54	2	4	4	8	17	27	27
35–49	40	7.1	45	1	2	4	10	18	20	27
50–64	145	6.6	85	1	2	4	8	15	19	42
65+	185	5.8	34	1	2	4	8	13	15	22
GRAND TOTAL	399	6.4	55	1	2	4	8	15	19	32

196: 2ND & NOS LYMPH NODE CA

Type of Patients	Observed Patients	Avg. Stay	Variance	10th	25th	50th	75th	90th	95th	99th
						Percentiles				
1. SINGLE DX										
A. Not Operated										
0–19 Years	0									
20–34	0									
35–49	0									
50–64	0									
65+	0									
B. Operated										
0–19 Years	0									
20–34	0									
35–49	0									
50–64	2	1.5	<1	1	1	1	2	2	2	2
65+	0									
2. MULTIPLE DX										
A. Not Operated										
0–19 Years	0									
20–34	16	4.2	9	1	2	4	6	9	11	11
35–49	67	4.9	13	1	2	4	7	10	13	15
50–64	137	6.5	71	1	2	4	7	14	20	38
65+	210	6.0	22	2	3	5	8	11	14	25
B. Operated										
0–19 Years	19	5.6	69	1	2	3	7	11	38	38
20–34	139	3.6	7	1	1	3	5	8	9	12
35–49	309	3.1	17	1	1	2	3	6	9	20
50–64	670	3.4	13	1	1	2	4	7	10	19
65+	733	3.8	15	1	1	3	5	8	10	19
SUBTOTALS:										
1. SINGLE DX										
A. Not Operated	0									
B. Operated	2	1.5	<1	1	1	1	2	2	2	2
2. MULTIPLE DX										
A. Not Operated	430	5.9	36	1	2	5	7	11	15	30
B. Operated	1,870	3.5	14	1	1	2	4	7	10	19
1. SINGLE DX	2	1.5	<1	1	1	1	2	2	2	2
2. MULTIPLE DX	2,300	4.0	19	1	1	3	5	8	11	20
A. NOT OPERATED	430	5.9	36	1	2	5	7	11	15	30
B. OPERATED	1,872	3.5	14	1	1	2	4	7	10	19
TOTAL										
0–19 Years	19	5.6	69	1	2	3	7	11	38	38
20–34	155	3.6	7	1	1	3	5	8	9	12
35–49	376	3.4	17	1	1	2	4	7	10	20
50–64	809	3.9	24	1	1	3	5	8	12	21
65+	943	4.3	17	1	1	3	6	9	12	19
GRAND TOTAL	2,302	4.0	19	1	1	3	5	8	11	20

196.0: 2ND/NOS HEAD/NECK LN CA

Type of Patients	Observed Patients	Avg. Stay	Variance	10th	25th	50th	75th	90th	95th	99th
						Percentiles				
1. SINGLE DX										
A. Not Operated										
0–19 Years	0									
20–34	0									
35–49	0									
50–64	0									
65+	0									
B. Operated										
0–19 Years	0									
20–34	0									
35–49	0									
50–64	2	1.5	<1	1	1	1	2	2	2	2
65+	0									
2. MULTIPLE DX										
A. Not Operated										
0–19 Years	0									
20–34	7	2.9	9	1	1	2	4	9	9	9
35–49	23	4.7	16	1	2	3	7	10	14	15
50–64	33	8.7	191	2	2	4	9	21	21	77
65+	30	6.2	18	2	3	4	8	12	16	18
B. Operated										
0–19 Years	10	7.2	124	1	2	3	7	11	38	38
20–34	66	2.5	5	1	1	2	3	5	7	13
35–49	152	2.7	16	1	1	2	3	4	7	13
50–64	326	3.1	12	1	2	2	3	6	9	18
65+	301	3.3	10	1	2	2	4	7	9	15
SUBTOTALS:										
1. SINGLE DX										
A. Not Operated	0									
B. Operated	2	1.5	<1	1	1	1	2	2	2	2
2. MULTIPLE DX										
A. Not Operated	93	6.5	80	1	2	4	7	14	18	77
B. Operated	855	3.1	13	1	1	2	4	6	8	16
1. SINGLE DX	2	1.5	<1	1	1	1	2	2	2	2
2. MULTIPLE DX	948	3.4	20	1	1	2	4	7	10	21
A. NOT OPERATED	93	6.5	80	1	2	4	7	14	18	77
B. OPERATED	857	3.1	13	1	1	2	4	6	8	16
TOTAL										
0–19 Years	10	7.2	124	1	2	3	7	11	38	38
20–34	73	2.5	5	1	1	2	3	5	8	13
35–49	175	2.9	16	1	1	2	3	5	8	15
50–64	361	3.6	31	1	1	3	4	6	13	21
65+	331	3.6	11	1	1	3	4	7	10	16
GRAND TOTAL	950	3.4	20	1	1	2	4	7	10	21

Length of Stay by Diagnosis and Operation, Western Region, 2008

Western Region, October 2006–September 2007 Data, by Diagnosis

196.1: 2ND/NOS INTRATHOR LN CA

Type of Patients	Observed Patients	Avg. Stay	Variance	Percentiles						
				10th	25th	50th	75th	90th	95th	99th
1. SINGLE DX										
A. Not Operated										
0–19 Years	0									
20–34	0									
35–49	0									
50–64	0									
65+	0									
B. Operated										
0–19 Years	0									
20–34	0									
35–49	0									
50–64	0									
65+	0									
2. MULTIPLE DX										
A. Not Operated										
0–19 Years	0									
20–34	1	3.0	0	3	3	3	3	3	3	3
35–49	10	3.7	11	1	1	3	4	10	10	10
50–64	17	4.7	18	1	2	4	5	10	16	16
65+	36	5.0	9	1	2	5	7	9	12	12
B. Operated										
0–19 Years	1	2.0	0	2	2	2	2	2	2	2
20–34	6	2.2	3	1	1	2	3	5	5	5
35–49	17	2.9	3	1	1	3	4	6	7	7
50–64	54	3.7	11	1	1	2	5	8	12	15
65+	98	4.0	19	1	1	2	5	10	15	19
SUBTOTALS:										
1. SINGLE DX A. Not Operated	0									
B. Operated	0									
2. MULTIPLE DX A. Not Operated	64	4.7	11	1	2	4	7	10	10	16
B. Operated	176	3.7	14	1	1	2	5	9	10	18
1. SINGLE DX	0									
2. MULTIPLE DX	240	4.0	14	1	2	3	5	9	12	17
A. NOT OPERATED	64	4.7	11	1	2	4	7	10	10	16
B. OPERATED	176	3.7	14	1	1	2	5	9	12	18
TOTAL										
0–19 Years	1	2.0	0	2	2	2	2	2	2	2
20–34	7	2.3	2	1	1	2	3	5	5	5
35–49	27	3.2	6	1	1	3	4	7	9	10
50–64	71	3.9	13	1	1	2	5	9	12	16
65+	134	4.3	16	1	1	3	6	10	13	18
GRAND TOTAL	240	4.0	14	1	1	3	5	9	12	17

196.2: 2ND/NOS INTRA-ABD LN CA

Type of Patients	Observed Patients	Avg. Stay	Variance	Percentiles						
				10th	25th	50th	75th	90th	95th	99th
1. SINGLE DX										
A. Not Operated										
0–19 Years	0									
20–34	0									
35–49	0									
50–64	0									
65+	0									
B. Operated										
0–19 Years	0									
20–34	0									
35–49	0									
50–64	0									
65+	0									
2. MULTIPLE DX										
A. Not Operated										
0–19 Years	0									
20–34	3	7.0	16	3	3	7	11	11	11	11
35–49	19	4.6	12	1	1	5	5	10	14	14
50–64	51	6.0	34	1	3	5	8	10	15	38
65+	84	6.4	33	2	3	5	8	11	13	35
B. Operated										
0–19 Years	5	5.6	9	2	4	5	7	10	10	10
20–34	37	6.0	6	3	4	6	8	9	11	12
35–49	41	5.5	19	2	4	4	6	9	13	22
50–64	65	5.8	12	3	4	5	7	9	12	21
65+	85	6.2	15	2	3	5	8	13	15	19
SUBTOTALS:										
1. SINGLE DX A. Not Operated	0									
B. Operated	0									
2. MULTIPLE DX A. Not Operated	157	6.1	30	1	3	5	8	11	14	35
B. Operated	233	5.9	13	2	3	5	7	10	13	20
1. SINGLE DX	0									
2. MULTIPLE DX	390	6.0	20	2	3	5	8	10	13	22
A. NOT OPERATED	157	6.1	30	1	3	5	8	11	14	35
B. OPERATED	233	5.9	13	2	3	5	7	10	13	20
TOTAL										
0–19 Years	5	5.6	9	2	4	5	7	10	10	10
20–34	40	6.1	7	3	4	6	8	10	11	12
35–49	60	5.2	17	1	3	4	6	9	14	22
50–64	116	5.9	21	2	3	5	7	10	15	21
65+	169	6.3	24	2	3	5	8	11	15	33
GRAND TOTAL	390	6.0	20	2	3	5	8	10	13	22

196.3: 2ND/NOS AXILLA/UL LN CA

Type of Patients	Observed Patients	Avg. Stay	Variance	Percentiles						
				10th	25th	50th	75th	90th	95th	99th
1. SINGLE DX										
A. Not Operated										
0–19 Years	0									
20–34	0									
35–49	0									
50–64	0									
65+	0									
B. Operated										
0–19 Years	0									
20–34	0									
35–49	0									
50–64	0									
65+	0									
2. MULTIPLE DX										
A. Not Operated										
0–19 Years	0									
20–34	1	6.0	0	6	6	6	6	6	6	6
35–49	6	6.0	15	2	3	6	7	13	13	13
50–64	14	6.5	45	1	2	4	12	18	20	20
65+	21	6.9	33	2	3	5	7	13	17	25
B. Operated										
0–19 Years	7	1.0	0	1	1	1	1	1	1	1
20–34	7	1.0	0	1	1	1	1	1	1	1
35–49	56	1.9	6	1	1	1	2	3	7	16
50–64	120	1.9	9	1	1	1	2	3	5	11
65+	115	2.4	9	1	1	1	2	6	9	18
SUBTOTALS:										
1. SINGLE DX A. Not Operated	0									
B. Operated	0									
2. MULTIPLE DX A. Not Operated	42	6.6	32	2	3	5	7	15	18	25
B. Operated	299	2.0	7	1	1	1	2	4	7	18
1. SINGLE DX	0									
2. MULTIPLE DX	341	2.6	12	1	1	1	2	6	10	19
A. NOT OPERATED	42	6.6	32	2	3	5	7	15	18	25
B. OPERATED	299	2.0	7	1	1	1	2	4	7	18
TOTAL										
0–19 Years	1	1.0	0	1	1	1	1	1	1	1
20–34	8	1.6	3	1	1	1	1	6	6	6
35–49	62	2.3	8	1	1	1	2	5	7	16
50–64	134	2.4	12	1	1	1	2	4	10	20
65+	136	3.1	15	1	1	3	3	7	11	19
GRAND TOTAL	341	2.6	12	1	1	1	2	6	10	19

Length of Stay by Diagnosis and Operation, Western Region, 2008

Western Region, October 2006–September 2007 Data, by Diagnosis

197: SECONDARY RESP/DIGEST CA

Type of Patients	Observed Patients	Avg. Stay	Variance	10th	25th	50th	75th	90th	95th	99th
1. SINGLE DX										
A. Not Operated										
0–19 Years	0									
20–34	0									
35–49	1	1.0	0	1	1	1	1	1	1	1
50–64	1	3.0	0	3	3	3	3	3	3	3
65+	2	2.5	4	1	1	4	4	4	4	4
B. Operated										
0–19 Years	0									
20–34	0									
35–49	2	6.5	4	5	5	7	8	8	8	8
50–64	1	8.0	0	8	8	8	8	8	8	8
65+	1	5.0	0	5	5	5	5	5	5	5
2. MULTIPLE DX										
A. Not Operated										
0–19 Years	38	5.9	42	1	2	4	7	17	20	30
20–34	213	5.6	31	1	2	4	7	11	16	32
35–49	1,237	5.8	34	1	2	4	7	13	17	27
50–64	3,446	5.7	24	1	2	4	7	12	15	25
65+	5,904	5.7	22	1	3	4	7	11	14	22
B. Operated										
0–19 Years	59	6.3	48	2	3	7	7	11	22	43
20–34	152	7.5	64	2	3	5	9	15	21	48
35–49	675	8.3	57	2	4	6	10	18	23	40
50–64	1,941	8.3	60	2	4	6	10	17	23	42
65+	2,337	8.6	47	2	4	7	11	17	22	31
SUBTOTALS:										
1. SINGLE DX										
A. Not Operated	4	2.3	2	1	1	3	3	4	4	4
B. Operated	4	6.5	3	5	5	8	8	8	8	8
2. MULTIPLE DX										
A. Not Operated	10,838	5.7	24	1	2	4	7	12	15	24
B. Operated	5,164	8.4	54	2	4	6	11	17	22	36
1. SINGLE DX	8	4.4	7	1	3	5	8	8	8	8
2. MULTIPLE DX	16,002	6.6	35	2	3	5	8	13	18	29
A. NOT OPERATED	10,842	5.7	24	1	2	4	7	12	15	24
B. OPERATED	5,168	8.4	54	2	4	6	11	17	22	36
TOTAL										
0–19 Years	97	6.1	46	1	2	4	7	14	20	43
20–34	365	6.4	46	1	3	5	8	12	19	36
35–49	1,915	6.7	43	1	3	5	8	15	19	32
50–64	5,389	6.6	39	2	3	5	8	13	18	30
65+	8,244	6.5	31	2	3	5	8	13	17	27
GRAND TOTAL	16,010	6.6	35	2	3	5	8	13	18	29

197.0: SECONDARY LUNG CA

Type of Patients	Observed Patients	Avg. Stay	Variance	10th	25th	50th	75th	90th	95th	99th
1. SINGLE DX										
A. Not Operated										
0–19 Years	0									
20–34	0									
35–49	0									
50–64	0									
65+	0									
B. Operated										
0–19 Years	0									
20–34	0									
35–49	0									
50–64	0									
65+	0									
2. MULTIPLE DX										
A. Not Operated										
0–19 Years	23	4.1	15	1	1	3	6	7	12	17
20–34	52	5.3	42	1	2	3	6	11	17	34
35–49	205	5.6	51	1	2	3	6	11	16	34
50–64	511	5.0	22	1	2	3	6	10	14	24
65+	877	5.4	18	1	3	4	7	11	13	22
B. Operated										
0–19 Years	37	5.2	23	2	3	4	6	9	10	30
20–34	68	4.7	10	1	3	4	6	9	10	17
35–49	188	4.9	24	1	3	4	6	9	13	20
50–64	471	5.2	24	1	2	4	6	10	13	28
65+	470	6.0	34	2	3	4	7	11	16	29
SUBTOTALS:										
1. SINGLE DX										
A. Not Operated	0									
B. Operated	0									
2. MULTIPLE DX										
A. Not Operated	1,668	5.3	24	1	2	4	7	11	14	24
B. Operated	1,234	5.4	27	1	2	4	6	10	14	28
1. SINGLE DX	0									
2. MULTIPLE DX	2,902	5.3	25	1	2	4	7	11	14	25
A. NOT OPERATED	1,668	5.3	24	1	2	4	7	11	14	24
B. OPERATED	1,234	5.4	27	1	2	4	6	10	14	28
TOTAL										
0–19 Years	60	4.8	20	1	2	4	6	9	10	30
20–34	120	4.9	24	1	2	4	6	9	11	32
35–49	393	5.3	38	1	2	4	6	11	16	34
50–64	982	5.1	23	1	2	4	6	10	13	25
65+	1,347	5.6	24	1	3	4	7	11	14	23
GRAND TOTAL	2,902	5.3	25	1	2	4	7	11	14	25

197.2: SECONDARY PLEURA CA

Type of Patients	Observed Patients	Avg. Stay	Variance	10th	25th	50th	75th	90th	95th	99th
1. SINGLE DX										
A. Not Operated										
0–19 Years	0									
20–34	0									
35–49	0									
50–64	0									
65+	1	4.0	0	4	4	4	4	4	4	4
B. Operated										
0–19 Years	0									
20–34	0									
35–49	0									
50–64	0									
65+	1	5.0	0	5	5	5	5	5	5	5
2. MULTIPLE DX										
A. Not Operated										
0–19 Years	3	10.7	16	7	7	10	15	15	15	15
20–34	30	3.6	10	1	2	5	5	7	11	13
35–49	303	6.3	36	1	2	5	8	14	17	29
50–64	978	6.0	26	1	3	5	8	12	16	25
65+	2,073	6.0	24	2	3	5	8	12	15	24
B. Operated										
0–19 Years	8	7.5	24	4	4	7	11	11	11	11
20–34	8	8.4	27	3	6	7	9	20	20	20
35–49	78	10.4	54	3	6	9	11	21	28	43
50–64	248	10.1	57	3	5	9	13	19	23	32
65+	440	9.1	34	3	5	8	12	17	19	28
SUBTOTALS:										
1. SINGLE DX										
A. Not Operated	1	4.0	0	4	4	4	4	4	4	4
B. Operated	1	5.0	0	5	5	5	5	5	5	5
2. MULTIPLE DX										
A. Not Operated	3,387	6.0	25	1	3	5	8	12	15	25
B. Operated	776	9.5	44	3	5	8	12	18	22	29
1. SINGLE DX	2	4.5	<1	4	4	4	5	5	5	5
2. MULTIPLE DX	4,163	6.7	31	2	3	5	9	14	17	27
A. NOT OPERATED	3,388	6.0	25	1	3	5	8	12	15	25
B. OPERATED	777	9.5	44	3	5	8	12	18	22	29
TOTAL										
0–19 Years	5	9.4	17	4	7	10	11	15	15	15
20–34	38	4.6	16	1	2	3	7	10	13	20
35–49	381	7.1	42	1	3	5	9	15	20	34
50–64	1,226	6.9	35	2	3	5	9	13	18	27
65+	2,515	6.5	27	2	3	5	9	13	17	26
GRAND TOTAL	4,165	6.7	31	2	3	5	9	14	17	27

Length of Stay by Diagnosis and Operation, Western Region, 2008

Western Region, October 2006–September 2007 Data, by Diagnosis

197.4: SECONDARY SM INTEST CA

Type of Patients	Observed Patients	Avg. Stay	Variance	10th	25th	50th	75th	90th	95th	99th
1. SINGLE DX										
A. Not Operated										
0–19 Years	0									
20–34	0									
35–49	0									
50–64	0									
65+	0									
B. Operated										
0–19 Years	0									
20–34	0									
35–49	0									
50–64	0									
65+	0									
2. MULTIPLE DX										
A. Not Operated										
0–19 Years	1	5.0	0	5	5	5	5	5	5	5
20–34	7	8.7	43	2	4	8	13	21	21	21
35–49	21	5.3	15	2	3	4	7	10	11	16
50–64	75	6.9	26	2	3	5	9	16	19	21
65+	95	6.3	25	2	3	5	7	12	18	26
B. Operated										
0–19 Years	2	14.5	110	7	7	22	22	22	22	22
20–34	4	15.0	199	6	7	9	23	36	36	36
35–49	40	12.6	48	6	8	11	14	26	27	32
50–64	165	13.3	120	5	6	10	17	24	33	71
65+	189	12.6	55	4	7	11	16	23	26	30
SUBTOTALS:										
1. SINGLE DX										
A. Not Operated	0									
B. Operated	0									
2. MULTIPLE DX										
A. Not Operated	199	6.5	25	2	3	5	8	14	18	25
B. Operated	400	12.9	82	5	7	10	16	24	28	53
1. SINGLE DX	0									
2. MULTIPLE DX	599	10.8	72	3	5	9	14	21	26	42
A. NOT OPERATED	199	6.5	25	2	3	5	8	14	18	25
B. OPERATED	400	12.9	82	5	7	10	16	24	28	53
TOTAL										
0–19 Years	3	11.4	85	5	5	7	22	22	22	22
20–34	11	11.0	95	4	4	8	13	21	36	36
35–49	61	10.1	48	3	5	9	12	20	26	32
50–64	240	11.3	99	3	5	8	14	21	28	53
65+	284	10.5	54	3	5	9	15	21	24	30
GRAND TOTAL	599	10.8	72	3	5	9	14	21	26	42

197.5: SECONDARY LG INTEST CA

Type of Patients	Observed Patients	Avg. Stay	Variance	10th	25th	50th	75th	90th	95th	99th
1. SINGLE DX										
A. Not Operated										
0–19 Years	0									
20–34	0									
35–49	0									
50–64	0									
65+	0									
B. Operated										
0–19 Years	0									
20–34	0									
35–49	0									
50–64	0									
65+	0									
2. MULTIPLE DX										
A. Not Operated										
0–19 Years	0									
20–34	3	8.3	72	2	2	5	18	18	18	18
35–49	32	6.8	55	1	2	4	9	12	25	36
50–64	60	6.8	29	2	3	6	8	16	17	26
65+	120	6.2	31	1	2	4	8	14	17	25
B. Operated										
0–19 Years	0									
20–34	4	8.0	11	3	9	10	10	10	10	10
35–49	44	11.8	54	5	7	9	17	22	25	32
50–64	122	10.6	60	5	8	8	12	19	23	47
65+	209	11.9	63	5	7	10	15	20	28	34
SUBTOTALS:										
1. SINGLE DX										
A. Not Operated	0									
B. Operated	0									
2. MULTIPLE DX										
A. Not Operated	215	6.5	34	1	3	5	8	14	18	26
B. Operated	379	11.4	61	5	6	9	15	20	25	47
1. SINGLE DX	0									
2. MULTIPLE DX	594	9.6	57	3	5	8	12	19	23	35
A. NOT OPERATED	215	6.5	34	1	3	5	8	14	18	26
B. OPERATED	379	11.4	61	5	6	9	15	20	25	47
TOTAL										
0–19 Years	0									
20–34	7	8.1	30	2	3	3	9	18	18	18
35–49	76	9.7	60	2	4	8	13	21	25	36
50–64	182	9.3	52	4	5	7	11	17	22	47
65+	329	9.8	59	2	5	8	13	18	23	34
GRAND TOTAL	594	9.6	57	3	5	8	12	19	23	35

197.6: SECONDARY PERITONEUM CA

Type of Patients	Observed Patients	Avg. Stay	Variance	10th	25th	50th	75th	90th	95th	99th
1. SINGLE DX										
A. Not Operated										
0–19 Years	0									
20–34	0									
35–49	0									
50–64	0									
65+	1	1.0	0	1	1	1	1	1	1	1
B. Operated										
0–19 Years	0									
20–34	1	8.0	0	8	8	8	8	8	8	8
35–49	1	8.0	0	8	8	8	8	8	8	8
50–64	0									
65+										
2. MULTIPLE DX										
A. Not Operated										
0–19 Years	9	9.9	110	1	2	4	19	30	30	30
20–34	61	6.6	42	2	3	5	7	12	22	35
35–49	281	6.4	37	1	2	4	9	15	18	26
50–64	711	5.7	27	1	2	4	7	12	17	28
65+	1,030	5.9	26	2	3	5	7	11	15	27
B. Operated										
0–19 Years	10	6.6	24	1	4	5	9	14	16	16
20–34	40	12.3	155	3	4	9	18	23	40	55
35–49	144	10.0	86	3	4	7	12	22	29	44
50–64	397	10.0	87	3	4	7	12	21	29	52
65+	495	9.5	49	3	5	8	12	17	23	35
SUBTOTALS:										
1. SINGLE DX										
A. Not Operated	1	1.0	0	1	1	1	1	1	1	1
B. Operated	2	8.0	0	8	8	8	8	8	8	8
2. MULTIPLE DX										
A. Not Operated	2,092	5.9	29	1	3	4	7	12	16	28
B. Operated	1,086	9.8	72	3	4	7	12	20	26	45
1. SINGLE DX	3	5.7	16	1	1	8	8	8	8	8
2. MULTIPLE DX	3,178	7.3	47	2	3	5	9	15	20	33
A. NOT OPERATED	2,093	5.9	29	1	3	4	7	12	16	28
B. OPERATED	1,088	9.8	72	3	4	7	12	20	26	45
TOTAL										
0–19 Years	19	8.1	64	1	3	5	14	20	30	30
20–34	101	8.9	94	2	3	5	10	21	22	48
35–49	426	7.7	56	2	3	5	10	17	18	35
50–64	1,109	7.2	53	2	3	5	9	16	21	36
65+	1,526	7.1	36	2	3	5	9	14	17	31
GRAND TOTAL	3,181	7.3	47	2	3	5	9	15	20	33

Length of Stay by Diagnosis and Operation, Western Region, 2008

Western Region, October 2006–September 2007 Data, by Diagnosis

197.7: SECONDARY LIVER CA

Type of Patients	Observed Patients	Avg. Stay	Variance	10th	25th	50th	75th	90th	95th	99th
1. SINGLE DX										
A. Not Operated										
0-19 Years	0									
20-34	0									
35-49	1	1.0	0	1	1	1	1	1	1	1
50-64	1	3.0	0	3	3	3	3	3	3	3
65+	0									
B. Operated										
0-19 Years	0									
20-34	0									
35-49	1	5.0	0	5	5	5	5	5	5	5
50-64	0									
65+	0									
2. MULTIPLE DX										
A. Not Operated										
0-19 Years	1	1.0	0	1	1	1	1	1	1	1
20-34	55	5.4	17	1	2	4	7	10	16	18
35-49	327	4.8	16	1	2	4	6	10	13	21
50-64	914	5.4	22	1	2	4	7	11	13	23
65+	1,420	5.3	18	1	2	4	7	10	13	20
B. Operated										
0-19 Years	4	13.9	383	3	4	5	43	43	43	43
20-34	16	6.9	17	1	5	6	8	10	19	19
35-49	143	7.1	37	2	4	5	7	13	19	40
50-64	432	6.2	25	1	4	5	7	10	15	26
65+	426	6.6	37	1	3	5	8	12	19	36
SUBTOTALS:										
1. SINGLE DX										
A. Not Operated	2	2.0	2	1	1	2	2	3	3	3
B. Operated	1	5.0	0	5	5	5	5	5	5	5
2. MULTIPLE DX										
A. Not Operated	2,717	5.2	19	1	2	4	7	10	13	21
B. Operated	1,021	6.6	33	1	4	5	8	12	17	33
1. SINGLE DX	3	3.0	4	1	1	3	5	5	5	5
2. MULTIPLE DX	3,738	5.6	23	1	3	5	7	11	14	24
A. NOT OPERATED	2,719	5.2	19	1	2	4	7	10	13	21
B. OPERATED	1,022	6.6	32	1	4	5	8	12	17	33
TOTAL										
0-19 Years	5	11.3	320	1	3	4	5	43	43	43
20-34	71	5.8	17	1	3	5	7	10	16	19
35-49	472	5.5	24	1	3	4	7	11	14	25
50-64	1,347	5.7	23	1	3	5	7	11	14	24
65+	1,846	5.6	22	1	3	4	7	11	14	23
GRAND TOTAL	3,741	5.6	23	1	3	5	7	11	14	24

197.8: 2ND DIGEST/SPLEEN CA

Type of Patients	Observed Patients	Avg. Stay	Variance	10th	25th	50th	75th	90th	95th	99th
1. SINGLE DX										
A. Not Operated										
0-19 Years	0									
20-34	0									
35-49	0									
50-64	0									
65+	0									
B. Operated										
0-19 Years	0									
20-34	0									
35-49	0									
50-64	0									
65+	0									
2. MULTIPLE DX										
A. Not Operated										
0-19 Years	0									
20-34	3	3.0	3	1	3	4	4	4	4	4
35-49	56	7.0	33	2	3	5	9	17	22	24
50-64	153	6.6	24	2	3	5	9	12	18	22
65+	225	5.8	22	1	3	5	7	11	13	20
B. Operated										
0-19 Years	0									
20-34	2	5.5	<1	5	5	6	6	6	6	6
35-49	23	10.5	83	3	5	8	12	20	31	39
50-64	65	8.8	39	3	5	7	12	19	21	30
65+	64	10.0	42	2	6	9	14	18	19	30
SUBTOTALS:										
1. SINGLE DX										
A. Not Operated	0									
B. Operated	0									
2. MULTIPLE DX										
A. Not Operated	437	6.2	24	2	3	5	8	12	16	23
B. Operated	154	9.5	46	3	5	8	13	19	21	31
1. SINGLE DX	0									
2. MULTIPLE DX	591	7.0	32	2	3	5	9	14	19	29
A. NOT OPERATED	437	6.2	24	2	3	5	8	12	16	23
B. OPERATED	154	9.5	46	3	5	8	13	19	21	31
TOTAL										
0-19 Years	0									
20-34	5	4.0	4	1	4	6	5	6	6	6
35-49	79	8.0	50	2	3	6	10	17	23	39
50-64	218	7.2	30	2	3	6	10	14	20	27
65+	289	6.7	30	1	3	5	9	13	17	29
GRAND TOTAL	591	7.0	32	2	3	5	9	14	19	29

198: OTHER SECONDARY CA

Type of Patients	Observed Patients	Avg. Stay	Variance	10th	25th	50th	75th	90th	95th	99th
1. SINGLE DX										
A. Not Operated										
0-19 Years	0									
20-34	0									
35-49	0									
50-64	0									
65+	3	2.7	1	2	2	2	2	4	4	4
B. Operated										
0-19 Years	0									
20-34	0									
35-49	2	1.0	0	1	1	1	1	1	1	1
50-64	4	1.8	<1	1	1	2	2	3	3	3
65+	1	2.0	0	2	2	2	2	2	2	2
2. MULTIPLE DX										
A. Not Operated										
0-19 Years	40	6.0	35	1	2	4	9	12	13	33
20-34	150	6.4	60	1	2	5	8	12	17	33
35-49	899	5.4	27	1	2	4	7	11	15	27
50-64	2,484	5.3	26	1	2	4	7	11	15	25
65+	3,753	5.4	22	2	3	4	7	10	14	23
B. Operated										
0-19 Years	43	12.5	265	2	3	6	16	29	50	80
20-34	121	7.5	90	1	3	5	10	14	21	42
35-49	680	7.2	50	2	3	5	10	16	21	37
50-64	1,970	7.5	52	2	3	5	10	16	21	34
65+	2,235	7.0	41	2	3	5	9	14	19	32
SUBTOTALS:										
1. SINGLE DX										
A. Not Operated	3	2.7	1	2	2	2	4	4	4	4
B. Operated	7	1.6	<1	1	1	1	2	3	3	3
2. MULTIPLE DX										
A. Not Operated	7,326	5.4	25	1	2	4	7	11	15	25
B. Operated	5,049	7.3	50	2	3	5	9	15	20	35
1. SINGLE DX	10	1.9	<1	1	1	2	2	4	4	4
2. MULTIPLE DX	12,375	6.2	36	1	3	4	8	13	17	29
A. NOT OPERATED	7,329	5.4	25	1	2	4	7	11	15	25
B. OPERATED	5,056	7.3	50	2	3	5	9	15	20	35
TOTAL										
0-19 Years	83	9.3	163	1	2	6	10	24	30	80
20-34	271	6.9	74	1	2	5	9	12	20	42
35-49	1,581	6.2	38	1	2	4	8	13	18	32
50-64	4,458	6.3	39	1	2	4	8	12	18	29
65+	5,992	6.0	30	2	3	4	8	12	16	28
GRAND TOTAL	12,385	6.2	36	1	3	4	8	13	17	29

Length of Stay by Diagnosis and Operation, Western Region, 2008

Western Region, October 2006–September 2007 Data, by Diagnosis

198.1: SECONDARY URINARY CA NEC

Type of Patients	Observed Patients	Avg. Stay	Vari-ance	10th	25th	50th	75th	90th	95th	99th
1. SINGLE DX										
A. Not Operated										
0–19 Years	0									
20–34	0									
35–49	0									
50–64	0									
65+	0									
B. Operated										
0–19 Years	0									
20–34	0									
35–49	0									
50–64	0									
65+	0									
2. MULTIPLE DX										
A. Not Operated										
0–19 Years	0									
20–34	1	12.0	0	12	12	12	12	12	12	12
35–49	6	7.3	15	3	3	7	12	12	12	12
50–64	14	4.9	33	1	2	4	5	5	7	24
65+	68	5.8	22	1	3	4	7	11	17	25
B. Operated										
0–19 Years	0									
20–34	2	5.5	<1	5	5	6	6	6	6	6
35–49	16	7.9	23	3	4	8	9	13	22	22
50–64	61	8.8	57	2	4	6	11	20	23	39
65+	154	6.5	49	1	2	4	8	14	18	28
SUBTOTALS:										
1. SINGLE DX										
A. Not Operated	0									
B. Operated	0									
2. MULTIPLE DX										
A. Not Operated	89	5.8	23	1	3	4	7	12	17	25
B. Operated	233	7.2	50	1	3	5	9	15	21	29
1. SINGLE DX	0									
2. MULTIPLE DX	322	6.8	43	1	3	5	9	14	19	28
A. NOT OPERATED	89	5.8	23	1	3	4	7	12	17	25
B. OPERATED	233	7.2	50	1	3	5	9	15	21	29
TOTAL										
0–19 Years	0									
20–34	3	7.7	14	5	5	6	12	12	12	12
35–49	22	7.8	20	3	4	7	10	12	13	22
50–64	75	8.1	54	2	4	5	10	20	24	39
65+	222	6.2	41	1	2	4	8	13	17	28
GRAND TOTAL	322	6.8	43	1	3	5	9	14	19	28

198.3: SECONDARY BRAIN/SPINE CA

Type of Patients	Observed Patients	Avg. Stay	Vari-ance	10th	25th	50th	75th	90th	95th	99th
1. SINGLE DX										
A. Not Operated										
0–19 Years	0									
20–34	0									
35–49	0									
50–64	0									
65+	3	2.7	1	2	2	2	4	4	4	4
B. Operated										
0–19 Years	0									
20–34	0									
35–49	0									
50–64	1	3.0	0	3	3	3	3	3	3	3
65+	0									
2. MULTIPLE DX										
A. Not Operated										
0–19 Years	11	3.4	15	1	1	2	4	8	13	13
20–34	62	5.2	27	1	2	4	5	10	14	29
35–49	413	4.8	25	1	2	3	6	9	15	25
50–64	1,309	4.9	25	1	2	3	6	10	14	25
65+	1,714	4.9	17	1	2	4	6	9	13	20
B. Operated										
0–19 Years	5	10.6	64	5	5	7	12	24	24	24
20–34	33	7.2	58	1	3	5	8	11	20	42
35–49	239	6.3	25	2	3	5	8	12	16	29
50–64	731	7.3	46	2	3	5	9	15	20	29
65+	625	7.4	34	2	3	6	10	14	18	30
SUBTOTALS:										
1. SINGLE DX										
A. Not Operated	3	2.7	1	2	2	2	4	4	4	4
B. Operated	1	3.0	0	3	3	3	3	3	3	3
2. MULTIPLE DX										
A. Not Operated	3,509	4.9	21	1	2	4	6	10	14	24
B. Operated	1,633	7.2	39	2	3	6	9	14	19	30
1. SINGLE DX	4	2.8	<1	2	2	3	4	4	4	4
2. MULTIPLE DX	5,142	5.6	28	1	2	4	7	11	15	25
A. NOT OPERATED	3,512	4.9	21	1	2	4	6	10	14	24
B. OPERATED	1,634	7.2	39	2	3	6	9	14	19	30
TOTAL										
0–19 Years	16	5.6	39	1	1	3	8	13	24	24
20–34	95	5.9	38	1	2	4	8	11	18	42
35–49	652	5.3	26	1	2	4	7	11	15	27
50–64	2,041	5.7	34	1	2	4	7	12	16	27
65+	2,342	5.5	23	2	2	4	7	11	14	22
GRAND TOTAL	5,146	5.6	28	1	2	4	7	11	15	25

198.4: 2ND NERV SYST CA NEC

Type of Patients	Observed Patients	Avg. Stay	Vari-ance	10th	25th	50th	75th	90th	95th	99th
1. SINGLE DX										
A. Not Operated										
0–19 Years	0									
20–34	0									
35–49	0									
50–64	0									
65+	0									
B. Operated										
0–19 Years	0									
20–34	1	1.0	0	1	1	1	1	1	1	1
35–49	0									
50–64	0									
2. MULTIPLE DX										
A. Not Operated										
0–19 Years	1	9.0	0	9	9	9	9	9	9	9
20–34	7	4.6	7	2	3	4	6	10	10	10
35–49	56	5.5	18	1	3	4	8	11	14	20
50–64	98	6.1	19	2	3	5	8	12	16	20
65+	76	6.8	27	2	4	5	8	13	16	30
B. Operated										
0–19 Years	0									
20–34	7	5.7	19	1	2	4	5	12	12	12
35–49	32	8.6	119	2	3	6	9	16	37	56
50–64	80	7.8	45	1	3	7	10	16	23	29
65+	77	8.5	61	2	4	6	10	16	28	>99
SUBTOTALS:										
1. SINGLE DX										
A. Not Operated	0									
B. Operated	1	1.0	0	1	1	1	1	1	1	1
2. MULTIPLE DX										
A. Not Operated	238	6.1	21	2	3	5	8	12	16	20
B. Operated	196	8.1	62	2	3	6	10	16	27	56
1. SINGLE DX	1	1.0	0	1	1	1	1	1	1	1
2. MULTIPLE DX	434	7.0	40	2	3	5	9	14	18	30
A. NOT OPERATED	238	6.1	21	2	3	5	8	12	16	20
B. OPERATED	197	8.1	62	2	3	6	10	16	27	56
TOTAL										
0–19 Years	1	9.0	0	9	9	9	9	9	9	9
20–34	14	5.2	13	2	3	4	7	11	12	12
35–49	89	6.5	56	1	3	4	9	12	17	56
50–64	178	6.9	31	1	3	6	10	15	18	28
65+	153	7.6	44	2	4	6	10	15	22	53
GRAND TOTAL	435	7.0	40	2	3	5	9	14	18	30

Length of Stay by Diagnosis and Operation, Western Region, 2008

Western Region, October 2006–September 2007 Data, by Diagnosis

198.5: SECONDARY BONE CA

Type of Patients	Observed Patients	Avg. Stay	Variance	Percentiles						
				10th	25th	50th	75th	90th	95th	99th
1. SINGLE DX										
A. *Not Operated*										
0–19 Years	0									
20–34	0									
35–49	0									
50–64	0									
65+	0									
B. *Operated*										
0–19 Years	0									
20–34	0									
35–49	0									
50–64	1	2.0	0	2	2	2	2	2	2	2
65+	0									
2. MULTIPLE DX										
A. *Not Operated*										
0–19 Years	21	5.7	16	1	2	5	8	12	12	13
20–34	47	7.9	138	2	3	5	7	16	21	76
35–49	280	6.1	35	2	2	4	8	16	17	34
50–64	749	5.8	30	1	3	4	7	12	16	28
65+	1,478	5.9	25	2	3	5	7	11	15	28
B. *Operated*										
0–19 Years	27	16.3	370	2	3	8	25	50	56	80
20–34	20	11.8	289	2	3	11	11	18	80	80
35–49	154	9.6	75	2	4	7	13	18	28	57
50–64	531	9.0	59	2	4	7	12	18	24	38
65+	717	8.1	45	2	4	6	10	17	20	34
SUBTOTALS:										
1. SINGLE DX										
A. *Not Operated*	0									
B. *Operated*	1	2.0	0	2	2	2	2	2	2	2
2. MULTIPLE DX										
A. *Not Operated*	2,575	6.0	30	2	3	4	7	12	15	28
B. *Operated*	1,449	8.8	64	2	4	7	11	18	23	42
1. SINGLE DX	1	2.0	0	2	2	2	2	2	2	2
2. MULTIPLE DX	4,024	7.0	44	2	3	5	9	14	19	32
A. NOT OPERATED	2,575	6.0	30	2	3	4	7	12	15	28
B. OPERATED	1,450	8.8	64	2	4	7	11	18	23	42
TOTAL										
0–19 Years	48	11.7	240	1	3	6	12	29	50	80
20–34	67	9.0	182	2	3	5	10	16	27	80
35–49	434	7.4	52	2	3	5	10	16	20	39
50–64	1,281	7.2	44	2	3	5	9	15	18	34
65+	2,195	6.6	33	2	2	5	8	13	18	29
GRAND TOTAL	4,025	7.0	44	2	3	5	9	14	19	32

198.89: SECONDARY CA NEC

Type of Patients	Observed Patients	Avg. Stay	Variance	Percentiles						
				10th	25th	50th	75th	90th	95th	99th
1. SINGLE DX										
A. *Not Operated*										
0–19 Years	0									
20–34	0									
35–49	0									
50–64	0									
65+	0									
B. *Operated*										
0–19 Years	0									
20–34	0									
35–49	0									
50–64	1	1.0	0	1	1	1	1	1	1	1
65+	1	1.0	0	1	1	1	1	1	1	1
2. MULTIPLE DX										
A. *Not Operated*										
0–19 Years	5	13.9	118	7	8	10	11	33	33	33
20–34	24	6.4	20	2	3	6	8	11	11	22
35–49	109	6.1	17	1	3	5	8	11	15	18
50–64	235	5.9	27	1	2	4	7	12	19	25
65+	308	5.3	21	2	3	4	7	10	14	25
B. *Operated*										
0–19 Years	9	4.1	6	1	2	4	6	7	7	7
20–34	43	6.7	58	1	2	4	9	14	21	40
35–49	148	7.2	51	1	2	4	9	19	23	35
50–64	377	6.5	63	1	2	4	8	14	21	42
65+	461	5.7	34	1	2	4	7	13	17	29
SUBTOTALS:										
1. SINGLE DX										
A. *Not Operated*	0									
B. *Operated*	2	1.0	0	1	1	1	1	1	1	1
2. MULTIPLE DX										
A. *Not Operated*	681	5.8	24	1	3	4	7	11	15	25
B. *Operated*	1,038	6.2	48	1	2	4	7	14	20	34
1. SINGLE DX	2	1.0	0	1	1	1	1	1	1	1
2. MULTIPLE DX	1,719	6.0	38	1	2	4	7	13	18	29
A. NOT OPERATED	681	5.8	24	1	3	4	7	11	15	25
B. OPERATED	1,040	6.2	48	1	2	4	7	14	20	34
TOTAL										
0–19 Years	14	7.6	64	1	3	7	8	11	33	33
20–34	67	6.6	44	1	2	4	9	14	21	40
35–49	258	6.7	37	1	3	5	10	16	20	28
50–64	613	6.2	49	1	2	4	8	13	19	30
65+	769	5.5	29	1	2	4	7	11	16	28
GRAND TOTAL	1,721	6.0	38	1	2	4	7	13	18	29

199: CA SITE NOS

Type of Patients	Observed Patients	Avg. Stay	Variance	Percentiles						
				10th	25th	50th	75th	90th	95th	99th
1. SINGLE DX										
A. *Not Operated*										
0–19 Years	0									
20–34	0									
35–49	0									
50–64	0									
65+	2	5.5	40	1	1	1	1	10	10	10
B. *Operated*										
0–19 Years	0									
20–34	0									
35–49	0									
50–64	1	5.0	0	5	5	5	5	5	5	5
65+	0									
2. MULTIPLE DX										
A. *Not Operated*										
0–19 Years	4	3.5	6	2	2	3	7	7	7	7
20–34	13	6.5	59	1	2	4	7	11	30	30
35–49	45	6.1	24	1	2	6	8	10	13	29
50–64	133	6.4	31	1	3	5	8	15	19	25
65+	203	5.1	15	1	2	4	7	9	12	22
B. *Operated*										
0–19 Years	1	2.0	0	2	2	2	2	2	2	2
20–34	6	8.3	83	1	1	3	14	24	24	24
35–49	26	15.3	147	5	8	12	19	35	41	52
50–64	65	11.2	104	2	4	9	15	24	29	53
65+	63	8.6	32	3	4	8	11	18	20	25
SUBTOTALS:										
1. SINGLE DX										
A. *Not Operated*	2	5.5	40	1	1	1	1	10	10	10
B. *Operated*	1	5.0	0	5	5	5	5	5	5	5
2. MULTIPLE DX										
A. *Not Operated*	398	5.7	23	1	2	4	7	10	15	28
B. *Operated*	161	10.7	86	2	4	8	15	21	26	52
1. SINGLE DX	3	5.3	20	1	1	5	10	10	10	10
2. MULTIPLE DX	559	7.1	46	1	3	5	9	15	21	34
A. NOT OPERATED	400	5.7	23	1	2	4	7	10	15	28
B. OPERATED	162	10.6	85	2	4	8	15	21	26	52
TOTAL										
0–19 Years	5	3.2	5	2	2	2	3	7	7	7
20–34	19	7.1	64	1	2	4	9	24	30	30
35–49	71	9.5	88	2	3	7	10	19	29	52
50–64	199	8.0	59	2	4	5	10	17	24	45
65+	268	5.9	21	1	3	5	8	11	15	22
GRAND TOTAL	562	7.1	46	1	3	5	9	15	20	34

Length of Stay by Diagnosis and Operation, Western Region, 2008

Western Region, October 2006–September 2007 Data, by Diagnosis

199.1: MALIGNANT NEOPLASM NEC

Type of Patients	Observed Patients	Avg. Stay	Vari-ance	10th	25th	50th	75th	90th	95th	99th
1. SINGLE DX										
A. Not Operated										
0–19 Years	0									
20–34	0									
35–49	0									
50–64	0									
65+	2	5.5	40	1	1	1	10	10	10	10
B. Operated										
0–19 Years	0									
20–34	0									
35–49	0									
50–64	0									
65+	0									
2. MULTIPLE DX										
A. Not Operated										
0–19 Years	3	4.0	7	2	2	3	7	7	7	7
20–34	5	8.9	151	1	2	2	9	30	30	30
35–49	24	5.2	13	1	2	4	7	7	10	15
50–64	78	6.0	34	1	2	4	7	13	22	30
65+	123	5.1	15	3	3	4	7	9	12	22
B. Operated										
0–19 Years	0									
20–34	2	1.0	0	1	1	1	1	1	1	1
35–49	12	13.0	101	2	5	10	17	25	35	35
50–64	35	8.0	79	2	2	5	11	15	29	45
65+	37	7.1	24	2	4	6	9	15	19	20
SUBTOTALS:										
1. SINGLE DX										
A. Not Operated	2	5.5	40	1	1	1	10	10	10	10
B. Operated	0									
2. MULTIPLE DX										
A. Not Operated	233	5.5	23	1	2	4	7	10	15	25
B. Operated	86	8.1	60	1	3	6	11	18	20	45
1. SINGLE DX	2	5.5	40	1	1	1	10	10	10	10
2. MULTIPLE DX	319	6.2	34	1	2	5	8	13	18	30
A. NOT OPERATED	235	5.5	23	1	2	4	7	10	15	25
B. OPERATED	86	8.1	60	1	3	6	11	18	20	45
TOTAL										
0–19 Years	3	4.0	7	2	2	3	7	7	7	7
20–34	7	6.6	115	1	1	2	9	30	30	30
35–49	36	7.8	54	1	3	6	10	17	25	35
50–64	113	6.6	48	1	2	5	8	14	22	30
65+	162	5.6	17	1	3	4	7	10	14	22
GRAND TOTAL	321	6.2	34	1	2	5	8	13	18	30

200: LYMPHOSARC/RETICULOSARC

Type of Patients	Observed Patients	Avg. Stay	Vari-ance	10th	25th	50th	75th	90th	95th	99th
1. SINGLE DX										
A. Not Operated										
0–19 Years	5	6.0	21	2	4	5	5	14	14	14
20–34	7	3.2	1	2	2	4	4	4	4	4
35–49	3	8.4	57	3	3	5	17	17	17	17
50–64	5	4.6	3	2	4	5	6	6	6	6
65+	5	1.6	<1	1	1	1	2	3	3	3
B. Operated										
0–19 Years	4	6.2	96	1	1	1	8	21	21	21
20–34	2	4.5	24	1	1	1	8	8	8	8
35–49	7	3.4	3	1	1	1	5	5	5	5
50–64	4	8.2	44	1	1	6	9	17	17	17
65+	3	3.0	12	1	1	1	7	7	7	7
2. MULTIPLE DX										
A. Not Operated										
0–19 Years	21	10.8	92	4	4	6	13	27	28	35
20–34	41	12.0	133	3	5	7	20	24	28	58
35–49	89	9.0	76	3	6	6	12	20	23	60
50–64	147	8.0	64	2	3	5	10	16	23	42
65+	252	8.2	53	2	3	6	11	19	23	33
B. Operated										
0–19 Years	27	11.7	96	3	5	9	14	26	29	45
20–34	30	17.7	139	4	7	15	29	32	34	46
35–49	63	13.5	132	5	5	10	21	33	47	>99
50–64	128	13.8	179	2	5	9	21	29	31	72
65+	184	11.1	77	3	5	9	15	22	27	63
SUBTOTALS:										
1. SINGLE DX										
A. Not Operated	25	4.3	14	1	2	4	5	6	14	17
B. Operated	20	5.0	30	1	1	4	6	9	21	21
2. MULTIPLE DX										
A. Not Operated	550	8.7	68	2	3	6	11	20	25	37
B. Operated	432	12.7	123	3	5	9	18	28	33	72
1. SINGLE DX	45	4.6	21	1	1	4	5	9	17	21
2. MULTIPLE DX	982	10.5	96	2	4	7	14	23	29	58
A. NOT OPERATED	575	8.5	66	2	3	6	11	20	24	37
B. OPERATED	452	12.4	121	2	5	9	18	27	32	72
TOTAL										
0–19 Years	57	10.5	88	2	4	7	13	26	29	45
20–34	80	13.2	138	2	4	8	21	29	34	58
35–49	162	10.5	101	2	4	7	15	25	31	>99
50–64	284	10.6	123	2	3	6	13	24	30	70
65+	444	9.3	65	2	4	7	13	21	25	38
GRAND TOTAL	1,027	10.2	94	2	4	7	14	23	29	51

200.00: RETICULOSARC XNODAL/NOS

Type of Patients	Observed Patients	Avg. Stay	Vari-ance	10th	25th	50th	75th	90th	95th	99th
1. SINGLE DX										
A. Not Operated										
0–19 Years	1	2.0	0	2	2	2	2	2	2	2
20–34	1	1.0	0	1	1	1	1	1	1	1
35–49	0									
50–64	0									
65+	1	1.0	0	1	1	1	1	1	1	1
B. Operated										
0–19 Years	0									
20–34	0									
35–49	0									
50–64	1	6.0	0	6	6	6	6	6	6	6
65+	0									
2. MULTIPLE DX										
A. Not Operated										
0–19 Years	3	4.7	9	2	2	4	8	8	8	8
20–34	5	6.8	22	3	5	5	6	15	15	15
35–49	22	7.1	36	1	3	4	8	11	20	20
50–64	52	6.5	50	2	3	6	8	11	22	42
65+	89	8.2	54	2	4	6	10	19	23	35
B. Operated										
0–19 Years	4	11.1	76	6	6	8	8	24	24	24
20–34	7	14.1	88	4	5	13	24	25	25	25
35–49	11	13.0	87	5	7	12	25	>99	>99	>99
50–64	32	17.8	336	2	7	11	24	>99	70	72
65+	40	9.9	68	1	4	9	14	18	24	38
SUBTOTALS:										
1. SINGLE DX										
A. Not Operated	3	1.3	<1	1	1	1	1	2	2	2
B. Operated	1	6.0	0	6	6	6	6	6	6	6
2. MULTIPLE DX										
A. Not Operated	171	7.4	49	2	3	5	9	16	22	35
B. Operated	94	13.3	170	2	5	10	21	27	60	>99
1. SINGLE DX	4	2.5	6	1	1	2	6	6	6	6
2. MULTIPLE DX	265	9.5	99	2	4	6	12	23	27	72
A. NOT OPERATED	174	7.3	49	2	3	5	9	16	22	35
B. OPERATED	95	13.2	169	2	5	10	21	27	60	>99
TOTAL										
0–19 Years	8	7.5	50	2	4	6	8	24	24	24
20–34	13	10.3	72	3	5	6	15	24	25	25
35–49	33	9.0	59	1	3	8	14	25	>99	>99
50–64	85	10.7	184	2	3	6	11	24	27	72
65+	130	8.6	59	2	4	6	12	19	24	35
GRAND TOTAL	269	9.4	99	2	3	6	12	22	27	72

Length of Stay by Diagnosis and Operation, Western Region, 2008

Western Region, October 2006–September 2007 Data, by Diagnosis

201: HODGKIN'S DISEASE

Type of Patients	Observed Patients	Avg. Stay	Vari-ance	10th	25th	50th	75th	90th	95th	99th
1. SINGLE DX										
A. Not Operated										
0–19 Years	18	3.8	8	1	1	3	5	8	8	10
20–34	10	2.8	4	1	2	2	4	6	6	6
35–49	4	3.0	3	1	2	4	5	5	5	5
50–64	2	2.5	<1	2	2	3	3	3	3	3
65+	1	1.0	0	1	1	1	1	1	1	1
B. Operated										
0–19 Years	7	6.0	21	1	2	4	11	12	12	12
20–34	12	2.0	1	1	1	2	3	3	5	5
35–49	9	3.3	5	1	2	3	5	7	7	7
50–64	2	1.0	0	1	1	1	1	1	1	1
65+	0									
2. MULTIPLE DX										
A. Not Operated										
0–19 Years	34	4.2	10	2	2	3	5	8	12	15
20–34	73	7.2	143	2	3	4	7	11	18	79
35–49	59	5.7	22	2	3	4	7	13	20	21
50–64	61	7.2	49	1	3	5	8	18	21	34
65+	48	7.2	38	2	3	6	9	15	19	34
B. Operated										
0–19 Years	26	10.8	52	3	6	10	13	19	20	36
20–34	134	12.2	114	2	4	10	19	23	26	86
35–49	66	9.9	58	1	3	7	19	21	25	25
50–64	80	10.9	56	2	4	9	18	21	24	31
65+	61	13.1	94	4	6	10	17	26	30	50
SUBTOTALS:										
1. SINGLE DX										
A. Not Operated	35	3.3	6	1	1	2	5	6	7	10
B. Operated	30	3.3	9	1	1	2	4	9	11	12
2. MULTIPLE DX										
A. Not Operated	275	6.5	62	2	3	4	7	14	19	34
B. Operated	367	11.6	84	2	4	9	18	22	25	41
1. SINGLE DX	65	3.3	7	1	1	2	5	7	9	12
2. MULTIPLE DX	642	9.4	80	2	3	6	14	21	24	36
A. NOT OPERATED	310	6.2	56	2	2	4	7	12	18	34
B. OPERATED	397	10.9	83	2	4	8	18	21	25	41
TOTAL										
0–19 Years	85	6.3	32	1	2	4	10	13	17	36
20–34	229	9.7	123	2	3	6	16	21	25	79
35–49	138	7.5	43	1	3	6	10	20	21	24
50–64	145	9.1	56	1	3	6	15	21	21	31
65+	110	10.4	77	2	5	7	14	21	28	41
GRAND TOTAL	707	8.8	77	2	3	6	13	20	22	35

202: OTH MAL LYMPH/HIST NEOPL

Type of Patients	Observed Patients	Avg. Stay	Vari-ance	10th	25th	50th	75th	90th	95th	99th
1. SINGLE DX										
A. Not Operated										
0–19 Years	6	3.3	2	2	2	4	5	5	5	5
20–34	7	3.6	11	1	2	2	7	7	9	9
35–49	13	2.3	1	1	2	2	3	4	4	4
50–64	13	2.8	3	1	1	2	3	6	6	6
65+	20	2.5	5	1	1	2	3	4	11	11
B. Operated										
0–19 Years	8	9.0	252	1	1	1	10	47	47	47
20–34	8	2.3	<1	2	2	2	2	4	4	4
35–49	19	2.6	3	1	1	2	4	7	7	7
50–64	31	3.1	7	1	1	2	6	7	7	10
65+	15	2.7	5	1	1	2	4	7	7	7
2. MULTIPLE DX										
A. Not Operated										
0–19 Years	51	9.2	96	2	4	6	10	26	33	49
20–34	112	8.0	55	2	3	5	10	18	23	38
35–49	326	7.0	56	1	3	5	9	17	22	28
50–64	778	7.5	61	2	3	5	9	16	21	41
65+	1,510	7.2	42	2	3	5	9	15	20	33
B. Operated										
0–19 Years	10	8.6	166	1	1	4	7	13	44	44
20–34	99	10.8	79	2	4	8	17	21	27	52
35–49	249	9.8	69	1	4	7	14	22	24	33
50–64	661	11.9	131	2	4	8	18	26	34	54
65+	923	9.3	65	2	4	7	12	20	25	34
SUBTOTALS:										
1. SINGLE DX										
A. Not Operated	59	2.7	4	1	1	2	3	5	7	11
B. Operated	81	3.4	30	1	1	2	4	7	7	47
2. MULTIPLE DX										
A. Not Operated	2,777	7.3	50	2	3	5	9	16	21	37
B. Operated	1,942	10.3	90	2	4	7	14	22	28	42
1. SINGLE DX	140	3.1	19	1	1	2	4	7	7	11
2. MULTIPLE DX	4,719	8.5	69	2	3	6	11	20	24	39
A. NOT OPERATED	2,836	7.2	50	2	3	5	9	15	21	37
B. OPERATED	2,023	10.0	90	2	4	7	13	22	27	42
TOTAL										
0–19 Years	75	8.6	111	1	2	4	9	26	33	49
20–34	226	8.9	66	2	3	6	12	21	23	38
35–49	607	7.9	62	1	3	5	10	20	23	32
50–64	1,483	9.3	96	2	3	6	12	21	29	46
65+	2,468	7.9	51	2	3	6	10	17	22	33
GRAND TOTAL	4,859	8.4	68	2	3	6	10	19	24	39

202.80: XNODAL/NOS LYMPHOMA NEC

Type of Patients	Observed Patients	Avg. Stay	Vari-ance	10th	25th	50th	75th	90th	95th	99th
1. SINGLE DX										
A. Not Operated										
0–19 Years	1	2.0	0	2	2	2	2	2	2	2
20–34	2	5.0	32	1	1	1	9	9	9	9
35–49	6	2.0	1	1	1	1	2	4	4	4
50–64	8	3.1	4	1	2	3	6	6	6	6
65+	12	1.9	<1	1	1	2	3	3	4	4
B. Operated										
0–19 Years	0									
20–34	1	2.0	0	2	2	2	2	2	2	2
35–49	3	2.0	3	1	1	1	4	4	4	4
50–64	13	1.9	3	1	1	1	2	3	7	7
65+	6	2.7	6	1	1	2	4	7	7	7
2. MULTIPLE DX										
A. Not Operated										
0–19 Years	8	6.0	33	1	3	6	7	19	19	19
20–34	35	6.8	36	3	3	5	7	14	23	25
35–49	115	6.4	39	1	2	4	8	13	23	28
50–64	314	7.1	45	2	3	5	9	15	19	35
65+	634	7.1	43	2	3	5	8	15	20	33
B. Operated										
0–19 Years	0									
20–34	20	12.9	83	1	6	12	21	21	26	27
35–49	65	10.6	69	1	4	8	17	23	24	32
50–64	191	13.4	122	2	5	10	20	28	37	49
65+	264	9.8	59	2	5	8	13	21	26	34
SUBTOTALS:										
1. SINGLE DX										
A. Not Operated	29	2.5	3	1	1	2	3	3	6	9
B. Operated	23	2.1	3	1	1	1	3	4	7	7
2. MULTIPLE DX										
A. Not Operated	1,106	7.0	43	2	3	5	8	15	20	33
B. Operated	540	11.3	86	2	5	8	17	24	29	40
1. SINGLE DX	52	2.3	3	1	1	2	3	4	7	9
2. MULTIPLE DX	1,646	8.4	61	2	3	6	11	20	25	37
A. NOT OPERATED	1,135	6.9	43	2	3	5	8	15	20	33
B. OPERATED	563	10.9	85	2	4	8	17	24	28	40
TOTAL										
0–19 Years	9	5.6	31	1	2	5	6	19	19	19
20–34	58	8.7	59	1	3	5	14	21	25	27
35–49	189	7.6	53	1	2	5	10	20	24	32
50–64	526	9.2	82	2	3	6	12	21	28	40
65+	916	7.8	49	2	3	6	9	17	24	33
GRAND TOTAL	1,698	8.2	60	2	3	6	10	19	24	37

Length of Stay by Diagnosis and Operation, Western Region, 2008

Western Region, October 2006–September 2007 Data, by Diagnosis

202.81: HEAD MAL LYMPHOMA NEC

Type of Patients	Observed Patients	Avg. Stay	Variance	10th	25th	50th	75th	90th	95th	99th
1. SINGLE DX										
A. Not Operated										
0–19 Years	0									
20–34	1	1.0	0	1	1	1	1	1	1	1
35–49	2	3.0	0	3	3	3	3	3	3	3
50–64	1	5.0	0	5	5	5	5	5	5	5
65+	3	5.0	28	1	1	3	11	11	11	11
B. Operated										
0–19 Years	1	47.0	0	47	47	47	47	47	47	47
20–34	2	2.0	0	2	2	2	2	2	2	2
35–49	8	2.5	5	1	1	2	3	7	7	7
50–64	3	6.0	16	2	2	6	10	10	10	10
65+	3	1.7	1	1	1	1	3	3	3	3
2. MULTIPLE DX										
A. Not Operated										
0–19 Years	3	6.7	2	5	5	7	8	8	8	8
20–34	10	8.6	132	1	1	5	8	38	38	38
35–49	25	7.6	53	1	3	5	9	21	22	24
50–64	74	6.4	58	1	2	4	7	17	22	40
65+	133	6.0	25	2	3	5	7	11	17	22
B. Operated										
0–19 Years	0									
20–34	16	11.9	206	2	3	7	10	41	52	52
35–49	32	10.0	57	1	5	8	14	21	22	28
50–64	79	9.4	125	1	2	6	13	20	31	75
65+	124	8.5	74	1	3	7	10	19	22	42
SUBTOTALS:										
1. SINGLE DX										
A. Not Operated	7	3.9	12	1	1	3	5	11	11	11
B. Operated	17	5.5	120	1	1	2	4	10	47	47
2. MULTIPLE DX										
A. Not Operated	245	6.4	42	1	3	5	7	14	20	37
B. Operated	251	9.2	96	1	3	7	12	20	27	52
1. SINGLE DX	24	5.0	87	1	1	2	4	10	11	47
2. MULTIPLE DX	496	7.8	71	1	3	5	9	19	22	41
A. NOT OPERATED	252	6.3	41	1	3	5	7	14	20	37
B. OPERATED	268	8.9	97	1	2	6	11	20	27	52
TOTAL										
0–19 Years	4	16.7	405	5	5	8	8	47	47	47
20–34	29	9.7	163	1	2	6	10	38	41	52
35–49	67	8.0	53	1	2	5	12	21	22	28
50–64	157	7.9	92	1	2	5	9	20	26	40
65+	263	7.1	49	1	3	5	8	16	20	36
GRAND TOTAL	520	7.7	72	1	3	5	9	19	22	41

202.82: THOR MAL LYMPHOMA NEC

Type of Patients	Observed Patients	Avg. Stay	Variance	10th	25th	50th	75th	90th	95th	99th
1. SINGLE DX										
A. Not Operated										
0–19 Years	1	4.0	0	4	4	4	4	4	4	4
20–34	2	4.0	18	1	1	7	7	7	7	7
35–49	0									
50–64	1	1.0	0	1	1	1	1	1	1	1
65+	0									
B. Operated										
0–19 Years	2	5.5	40	1	1	10	10	10	10	10
20–34	4	2.0	<1	1	2	2	3	3	3	3
35–49	1	3.0	0	3	3	3	3	3	3	3
50–64	1	1.0	0	1	1	1	1	1	1	1
65+	3	2.3	5	1	1	1	5	5	5	5
2. MULTIPLE DX										
A. Not Operated										
0–19 Years	14	6.2	11	3	4	5	10	11	12	12
20–34	21	6.9	23	2	4	5	11	12	15	18
35–49	15	7.8	27	1	3	7	11	13	21	21
50–64	31	5.7	32	2	3	4	7	10	18	30
65+	86	7.0	48	2	3	5	9	14	17	50
B. Operated										
0–19 Years	1	13.0	0	13	13	13	13	13	13	13
20–34	21	8.1	26	3	4	7	12	13	17	22
35–49	19	8.7	138	1	3	6	11	22	52	52
50–64	28	7.5	36	2	3	7	11	14	14	23
65+	51	8.9	38	2	4	8	12	16	20	28
SUBTOTALS:										
1. SINGLE DX										
A. Not Operated	4	3.3	8	1	1	4	7	7	7	7
B. Operated	11	2.7	7	1	1	2	3	5	10	10
2. MULTIPLE DX										
A. Not Operated	167	6.8	37	2	3	5	9	13	17	30
B. Operated	120	8.4	47	2	4	7	11	15	20	28
1. SINGLE DX	15	2.9	7	1	1	2	4	7	10	10
2. MULTIPLE DX	287	7.5	42	2	3	6	10	14	18	30
A. NOT OPERATED	171	6.7	36	2	2	5	9	13	17	30
B. OPERATED	131	8.0	46	1	3	7	11	14	20	28
TOTAL										
0–19 Years	18	6.4	14	2	4	5	10	12	13	13
20–34	48	6.9	24	2	3	6	10	13	17	22
35–49	35	8.2	85	1	3	7	11	14	22	52
50–64	61	6.3	29	2	3	5	8	11	14	30
65+	140	7.6	44	2	3	6	10	15	18	28
GRAND TOTAL	302	7.2	41	2	3	5	10	14	18	28

202.83: ABD MAL LYMPHOMAS NEC

Type of Patients	Observed Patients	Avg. Stay	Variance	10th	25th	50th	75th	90th	95th	99th
1. SINGLE DX										
A. Not Operated										
0–19 Years	0									
20–34	0									
35–49	2	1.5	<1	1	1	2	2	2	2	2
50–64	1	1.0	0	1	1	1	1	1	1	1
65+	3	1.7	1	1	1	1	3	3	3	3
B. Operated										
0–19 Years	1	10.0	0	10	10	10	10	10	10	10
20–34	1	4.0	0	4	4	4	4	4	4	4
35–49	4	4.5	4	2	2	4	7	7	7	7
50–64	2	3.5	12	1	1	6	6	6	6	6
65+	3	4.3	6	2	2	4	7	7	7	7
2. MULTIPLE DX										
A. Not Operated										
0–19 Years	1	5.0	0	5	5	5	5	5	5	5
20–34	14	12.0	114	3	5	8	16	31	38	38
35–49	63	8.0	116	2	3	5	11	13	20	81
50–64	150	7.5	45	2	3	5	10	17	21	34
65+	300	7.3	34	2	3	6	10	15	19	31
B. Operated										
0–19 Years	2	22.2	911	1	6	8	8	44	44	44
20–34	9	9.2	65	1	6	8	8	16	19	29
35–49	28	6.9	23	1	4	6	11	13	20	20
50–64	108	10.1	95	3	4	7	11	25	29	42
65+	143	9.3	52	2	4	7	12	21	23	32
SUBTOTALS:										
1. SINGLE DX										
A. Not Operated	6	1.5	<1	1	1	1	2	2	3	3
B. Operated	11	4.7	7	2	2	4	7	7	10	10
2. MULTIPLE DX										
A. Not Operated	528	7.6	49	2	3	5	10	15	21	34
B. Operated	290	9.5	70	2	4	7	11	21	26	42
1. SINGLE DX	17	3.6	7	1	1	3	5	7	10	10
2. MULTIPLE DX	818	8.2	57	2	3	6	10	17	22	38
A. NOT OPERATED	534	7.5	49	2	3	5	10	15	21	34
B. OPERATED	301	9.3	68	2	4	7	11	21	25	40
TOTAL										
0–19 Years	4	14.8	380	1	1	5	10	44	44	44
20–34	24	10.6	91	3	4	8	15	29	31	38
35–49	97	7.4	83	2	3	5	9	13	20	81
50–64	261	8.6	67	2	3	6	10	18	25	42
65+	449	7.9	40	2	3	6	10	16	22	31
GRAND TOTAL	835	8.2	56	2	3	6	10	17	22	38

Western Region, October 2006–September 2007 Data, by Diagnosis

202.88: MULT LN MAL LYMPHOMA NEC

Type of Patients	Observed Patients	Avg. Stay	Variance	Percentiles						
				10th	25th	50th	75th	90th	95th	99th
1. SINGLE DX										
A. Not Operated										
0–19 Years	0									
20–34	0									
35–49	1	2.0	0	2	2	2	2	2	2	2
50–64	2	2.0	2	1	1	1	3	3	3	3
65+	2	3.0	2	2	2	2	4	4	4	4
B. Operated										
0–19 Years	0									
20–34	0									
35–49	0									
50–64	1	1.0	0	1	1	1	1	1	1	1
65+	1	1.0	0	1	1	1	1	1	1	1
2. MULTIPLE DX										
A. Not Operated										
0–19 Years	2	14.6	361	1	1	28	28	28	28	28
20–34	8	9.3	35	2	5	8	8	20	20	20
35–49	34	9.2	71	2	4	5	13	23	26	32
50–64	69	11.0	170	2	4	7	12	22	45	63
65+	171	7.4	50	2	3	6	9	16	20	44
B. Operated										
0–19 Years	0									
20–34	10	9.0	47	2	5	6	10	21	21	21
35–49	29	13.5	85	3	5	15	19	29	31	32
50–64	68	18.7	225	3	8	21	24	34	40	90
65+	75	12.7	83	3	6	11	18	25	28	52
SUBTOTALS:										
1. SINGLE DX										
A. Not Operated	5	2.4	1	2	2	2	3	4	4	4
B. Operated	2	1.0	0	1	1	1	1	1	1	1
2. MULTIPLE DX										
A. Not Operated	284	8.6	84	2	3	6	10	19	22	58
B. Operated	182	14.9	142	3	6	12	22	28	33	65
1. SINGLE DX	7	2.0	1	1	1	2	3	4	4	4
2. MULTIPLE DX	466	11.0	116	2	4	7	16	23	29	58
A. NOT OPERATED	289	8.5	84	2	3	6	9	19	22	58
B. OPERATED	184	14.7	143	3	6	12	22	28	33	65
TOTAL										
0–19 Years	2	14.6	361	1	1	28	28	28	28	28
20–34	18	9.1	39	2	5	8	11	21	21	21
35–49	65	10.9	81	2	4	7	18	24	29	32
50–64	140	14.6	210	2	4	9	22	34	42	65
65+	248	9.0	66	2	3	6	12	20	23	44
GRAND TOTAL	473	10.9	116	2	4	7	16	23	29	58

203: MULTIPLE MYELOMA ET AL

Type of Patients	Observed Patients	Avg. Stay	Variance	Percentiles						
				10th	25th	50th	75th	90th	95th	99th
1. SINGLE DX										
A. Not Operated										
0–19 Years	0									
20–34	0									
35–49	3	3.0	12	1	1	1	7	7	7	7
50–64	8	1.5	<1	1	1	1	2	3	3	3
65+	4	2.5	6	1	1	2	6	6	6	6
B. Operated										
0–19 Years	0									
20–34	0									
35–49	0									
50–64	5	6.0	47	1	1	1	13	14	14	14
65+	2	3.0	8	1	1	3	5	5	5	5
2. MULTIPLE DX										
A. Not Operated										
0–19 Years	1	1.0	0	1	1	1	1	1	1	1
20–34	8	6.5	12	3	4	6	8	14	14	14
35–49	113	8.0	50	2	3	6	11	19	24	30
50–64	495	7.2	41	2	3	5	9	14	18	31
65+	811	7.5	46	2	3	6	9	15	19	29
B. Operated										
0–19 Years	0									
20–34	1	1.0	0	1	1	1	1	1	1	1
35–49	74	14.8	141	2	8	15	17	21	31	87
50–64	298	14.5	66	4	9	15	18	24	29	42
65+	224	13.2	81	3	7	13	18	23	28	38
SUBTOTALS:										
1. SINGLE DX										
A. Not Operated	15	2.1	4	1	1	1	2	6	7	7
B. Operated	7	5.1	35	1	1	1	13	14	14	14
2. MULTIPLE DX										
A. Not Operated	1,428	7.4	44	2	3	6	9	15	19	30
B. Operated	597	14.0	81	3	8	14	18	23	29	42
1. SINGLE DX	22	3.1	14	1	1	1	3	7	13	14
2. MULTIPLE DX	2,025	9.4	64	2	4	7	14	19	23	37
A. NOT OPERATED	1,443	7.4	44	2	3	6	9	15	19	30
B. OPERATED	604	13.9	81	3	8	14	18	23	29	42
TOTAL										
0–19 Years	1	1.0	0	1	1	1	1	1	1	1
20–34	9	5.9	14	1	4	5	8	14	14	14
35–49	190	10.6	96	2	3	8	15	21	25	46
50–64	806	9.8	63	2	4	8	15	19	23	37
65+	1,041	8.7	59	2	4	7	11	18	21	34
GRAND TOTAL	2,047	9.3	64	2	4	7	14	19	23	37

203.00: MULT MYELOMA W/O REMISS

Type of Patients	Observed Patients	Avg. Stay	Variance	Percentiles						
				10th	25th	50th	75th	90th	95th	99th
1. SINGLE DX										
A. Not Operated										
0–19 Years	0									
20–34	0									
35–49	3	3.0	12	1	1	1	7	7	7	7
50–64	8	1.5	<1	1	1	1	2	3	3	3
65+	4	2.5	6	1	1	2	6	6	6	6
B. Operated										
0–19 Years	0									
20–34	0									
35–49	0									
50–64	4	7.3	52	1	1	13	13	14	14	14
65+	2	3.0	8	1	1	3	5	5	5	5
2. MULTIPLE DX										
A. Not Operated										
0–19 Years	1	1.0	0	1	1	1	1	1	1	1
20–34	8	6.5	12	3	4	6	8	14	14	14
35–49	108	7.9	48	2	3	6	11	18	24	30
50–64	481	7.1	41	2	3	5	9	14	18	31
65+	788	7.4	46	2	3	6	9	15	19	33
B. Operated										
0–19 Years	0									
20–34	1	1.0	0	1	1	1	1	1	1	1
35–49	62	15.8	155	3	11	15	17	22	31	87
50–64	260	15.0	64	4	11	15	18	24	29	42
65+	194	13.1	87	3	7	13	18	23	29	42
SUBTOTALS:										
1. SINGLE DX										
A. Not Operated	15	2.1	4	1	1	1	2	6	7	7
B. Operated	6	5.8	37	1	1	5	13	14	14	14
2. MULTIPLE DX										
A. Not Operated	1,386	7.4	44	2	3	6	9	15	19	31
B. Operated	517	14.4	84	3	8	14	18	24	29	42
1. SINGLE DX	21	3.2	15	1	1	1	3	7	13	14
2. MULTIPLE DX	1,903	9.3	65	2	4	7	13	18	23	37
A. NOT OPERATED	1,401	7.3	44	2	3	6	9	15	19	30
B. OPERATED	523	14.3	85	3	8	14	18	24	29	42
TOTAL										
0–19 Years	1	1.0	0	1	1	1	1	1	1	1
20–34	9	5.9	14	1	4	5	8	14	14	14
35–49	173	10.7	100	2	4	8	15	21	26	46
50–64	753	9.8	63	2	4	8	15	19	23	37
65+	988	8.5	59	2	3	6	11	18	21	35
GRAND TOTAL	1,924	9.2	65	2	4	7	13	18	23	37

Length of Stay by Diagnosis and Operation, Western Region, 2008

Western Region, October 2006–September 2007 Data, by Diagnosis

204: LYMPHOID LEUKEMIA

Type of Patients	Observed Patients	Avg. Stay	Variance	Percentiles 10th	25th	50th	75th	90th	95th	99th
1. SINGLE DX										
A. Not Operated										
0–19 Years	65	4.5	17	1	1	3	7	9	11	23
20–34	6	8.0	61	1	1	8	17	18	18	18
35–49	7	3.9	4	1	2	4	5	7	7	7
50–64	5	3.6	4	1	2	5	5	5	5	5
65+	5	1.6	<1	1	1	1	2	3	3	3
B. Operated										
0–19 Years	3	8.7	14	6	6	7	13	13	13	13
20–34	2	2.5	4	1	1	4	4	4	4	4
35–49	1	1.0	0	1	1	1	1	1	1	1
50–64	5	1.0	0	1	1	1	1	1	1	1
65+	0									
2. MULTIPLE DX										
A. Not Operated										
0–19 Years	449	9.3	104	2	3	6	11	22	27	56
20–34	183	17.9	265	2	5	15	26	37	54	>99
35–49	147	14.1	221	2	3	8	23	36	44	59
50–64	228	10.6	127	2	3	6	14	26	34	49
65+	442	7.0	47	1	3	5	9	14	22	36
B. Operated										
0–19 Years	47	32.4	491	6	12	30	41	72	82	84
20–34	44	25.0	222	5	15	25	33	49	50	>99
35–49	47	23.7	228	3	9	24	35	45	51	54
50–64	80	17.8	295	2	5	14	26	40	54	85
65+	45	15.0	252	1	5	10	18	33	44	83
SUBTOTALS:										
1. SINGLE DX										
A. Not Operated	88	4.5	18	1	1	3	7	9	11	23
B. Operated	11	3.4	15	1	1	1	6	7	13	13
2. MULTIPLE DX										
A. Not Operated	1,449	10.4	134	2	3	6	13	25	32	61
B. Operated	263	22.2	329	3	6	21	31	47	56	84
1. SINGLE DX	99	4.3	17	1	1	3	6	9	13	18
2. MULTIPLE DX	1,712	12.2	182	2	3	7	18	29	40	72
A. NOT OPERATED	1,537	10.0	130	1	3	6	12	25	32	59
B. OPERATED	274	21.4	330	2	6	21	30	46	56	84
TOTAL										
0–19 Years	564	10.6	170	1	3	6	11	26	32	73
20–34	235	18.8	261	2	5	17	27	42	54	>99
35–49	202	15.9	236	2	3	8	26	39	46	54
50–64	318	12.1	178	1	3	6	19	29	37	63
65+	492	7.7	71	1	3	5	9	16	25	44
GRAND TOTAL	1,811	11.8	176	1	3	7	16	29	39	70

204.00: ALL W/O REMISSION

Type of Patients	Observed Patients	Avg. Stay	Variance	Percentiles 10th	25th	50th	75th	90th	95th	99th
1. SINGLE DX										
A. Not Operated										
0–19 Years	60	4.7	17	1	1	4	7	9	11	23
20–34	6	8.0	61	1	1	8	17	18	18	18
35–49	7	3.9	4	1	2	4	5	7	7	7
50–64	2	3.5	4	2	2	2	5	5	5	5
65+	2	1.0	0	1	1	1	1	1	1	1
B. Operated										
0–19 Years	3	8.7	14	6	6	7	13	13	13	13
20–34	2	2.5	4	1	1	4	4	4	4	4
35–49	0									
50–64	2	1.0	0	1	1	1	1	1	1	1
65+	0									
2. MULTIPLE DX										
A. Not Operated										
0–19 Years	398	9.5	105	2	3	7	11	22	27	56
20–34	172	18.2	272	2	5	16	26	39	57	>99
35–49	117	15.7	247	2	3	8	25	40	47	59
50–64	100	16.0	189	2	4	13	26	35	38	63
65+	78	12.0	116	2	4	8	18	28	36	50
B. Operated										
0–19 Years	33	29.7	623	5	10	26	38	72	82	84
20–34	30	23.2	208	5	13	26	31	37	63	>99
35–49	27	26.4	214	5	17	25	36	50	51	54
50–64	26	24.6	383	1	9	25	30	49	54	85
65+	4	38.1	>999	1	1	29	83	83	83	83
SUBTOTALS:										
1. SINGLE DX										
A. Not Operated	77	4.8	19	1	1	4	7	9	17	23
B. Operated	7	4.7	20	1	1	4	7	13	13	13
2. MULTIPLE DX										
A. Not Operated	865	13.1	180	2	4	8	20	30	39	70
B. Operated	120	26.5	385	4	10	26	35	54	72	85
1. SINGLE DX	84	4.8	19	1	2	4	7	9	13	23
2. MULTIPLE DX	985	14.7	224	2	4	9	22	34	45	82
A. NOT OPERATED	942	12.4	172	2	3	8	19	29	38	70
B. OPERATED	127	25.3	390	2	9	25	35	54	72	85
TOTAL										
0–19 Years	494	10.3	156	1	3	7	11	23	35	72
20–34	210	18.5	262	2	5	17	27	37	57	>99
35–49	151	17.0	254	2	4	8	27	40	49	59
50–64	130	17.3	239	2	4	14	25	36	46	72
65+	84	13.0	185	2	3	8	19	31	38	83
GRAND TOTAL	1,069	13.9	215	2	4	8	21	32	42	81

204.10: CLL W/O REMISSION

Type of Patients	Observed Patients	Avg. Stay	Variance	Percentiles 10th	25th	50th	75th	90th	95th	99th
1. SINGLE DX										
A. Not Operated										
0–19 Years	0									
20–34	0									
35–49	0									
50–64	3	3.7	5	1	1	5	5	5	5	5
65+	3	2.0	<1	1	1	2	3	3	3	3
B. Operated										
0–19 Years	0									
20–34	0									
35–49	1	1.0	0	1	1	1	1	1	1	1
50–64	1	1.0	0	1	1	1	1	1	1	1
65+	0									
2. MULTIPLE DX										
A. Not Operated										
0–19 Years	0									
20–34	4	5.3	16	2	2	7	10	10	10	10
35–49	23	5.5	25	2	3	3	7	10	18	21
50–64	122	6.0	25	1	3	5	7	11	17	26
65+	359	5.9	24	2	3	5	8	11	14	26
B. Operated										
0–19 Years	0									
20–34	0									
35–49	9	12.4	81	1	5	10	21	26	26	26
50–64	44	13.6	208	2	5	7	22	26	35	80
65+	39	12.9	133	1	5	10	17	27	44	51
SUBTOTALS:										
1. SINGLE DX										
A. Not Operated	6	2.8	3	1	1	2	5	5	5	5
B. Operated	2	1.0	0	1	1	1	1	1	1	1
2. MULTIPLE DX										
A. Not Operated	508	5.9	24	1	3	5	7	11	15	26
B. Operated	94	13.0	159	2	5	8	18	26	35	80
1. SINGLE DX	8	2.4	3	1	1	3	3	5	5	5
2. MULTIPLE DX	602	7.0	52	1	3	5	8	14	21	33
A. NOT OPERATED	514	5.8	24	1	3	5	7	11	15	26
B. OPERATED	96	12.8	159	2	5	8	18	26	35	80
TOTAL										
0–19 Years	0									
20–34	6	5.3	10	2	2	5	7	10	10	10
35–49	33	7.2	49	2	2	5	8	21	21	26
50–64	170	7.9	83	1	3	5	8	18	25	40
65+	401	6.5	39	2	3	5	8	13	17	31
GRAND TOTAL	610	6.9	51	1	3	5	8	14	21	33

Length of Stay by Diagnosis and Operation, Western Region, 2008

112

205: MYELOID LEUKEMIA

Type of Patients	Observed Patients	Avg. Stay	Vari-ance	10th	25th	50th	75th	90th	95th	99th
1. SINGLE DX										
A. Not Operated										
0–19 Years	6	2.4	4	1	1	2	3	6	6	6
20–34	11	3.3	8	1	1	2	4	8	9	9
35–49	8	3.4	4	1	1	4	5	6	6	6
50–64	7	2.6	3	1	1	2	5	5	5	5
65+	9	2.0	5	1	1	1	2	8	8	8
B. Operated										
0–19 Years	0									
20–34	2	15.0	159	6	6	6	24	24	24	24
35–49	0									
50–64	1	1.0	0	1	1	1	1	1	1	1
65+	4	1.0	0	1	1	1	1	1	1	1
2. MULTIPLE DX										
A. Not Operated										
0–19 Years	74	16.9	329	1	3	11	29	38	61	>99
20–34	198	17.1	272	2	4	11	29	38	52	94
35–49	303	16.8	212	2	5	12	27	36	48	59
50–64	496	18.2	260	2	5	13	29	38	44	77
65+	958	10.2	132	2	3	6	12	27	34	50
B. Operated										
0–19 Years	29	38.1	395	24	26	33	48	93	>99	>99
20–34	65	27.7	269	8	20	27	33	48	53	86
35–49	69	25.1	191	5	21	25	30	37	42	97
50–64	122	26.1	233	6	20	25	33	47	52	72
65+	76	22.4	334	1	7	22	30	55	70	>99
SUBTOTALS:										
1. SINGLE DX										
A. Not Operated	41	2.8	5	1	1	2	4	6	8	9
B. Operated	7	5.0	73	1	6	6	6	24	24	24
2. MULTIPLE DX										
A. Not Operated	2,029	14.1	209	2	4	7	24	33	42	63
B. Operated	361	26.4	277	5	19	25	33	48	63	>99
1. SINGLE DX	48	3.1	14	1	1	2	4	6	8	24
2. MULTIPLE DX	2,390	15.9	239	2	4	9	26	36	45	75
A. NOT OPERATED	2,070	13.8	208	2	3	7	24	33	41	63
B. OPERATED	368	26.0	282	4	17	25	33	47	63	>99
TOTAL										
0–19 Years	109	21.7	433	1	3	22	31	52	87	>99
20–34	276	19.0	289	2	5	15	30	42	52	86
35–49	380	18.0	218	2	5	15	28	36	42	63
50–64	626	19.5	265	2	5	18	29	41	47	75
65+	1,047	11.0	156	2	3	6	14	29	37	63
GRAND TOTAL	2,438	15.7	238	2	4	9	26	36	44	73

205.00: AML W/O REMISSION

Type of Patients	Observed Patients	Avg. Stay	Vari-ance	10th	25th	50th	75th	90th	95th	99th
1. SINGLE DX										
A. Not Operated										
0–19 Years	4	1.5	1	1	1	1	3	3	3	3
20–34	7	3.7	11	1	1	2	8	9	9	9
35–49	6	3.5	4	1	1	4	5	6	6	6
50–64	5	2.8	4	1	1	2	5	5	5	5
65+	7	2.3	7	1	1	1	2	8	8	8
B. Operated										
0–19 Years	0									
20–34	1	6.0	0	6	6	6	6	6	6	6
35–49	0									
50–64	1	1.0	0	1	1	1	1	1	1	1
65+	1	1.0	0	1	1	1	1	1	1	1
2. MULTIPLE DX										
A. Not Operated										
0–19 Years	64	18.2	354	1	3	16	29	41	61	>99
20–34	144	20.8	261	2	7	20	31	42	52	82
35–49	210	21.1	228	3	6	23	31	39	48	63
50–64	375	21.3	276	3	6	23	31	42	46	79
65+	781	10.8	148	2	3	6	13	28	35	53
B. Operated										
0–19 Years	17	40.6	359	24	26	38	54	>99	>99	>99
20–34	42	30.6	323	8	21	30	37	53	68	86
35–49	32	28.8	260	10	23	28	34	39	46	97
50–64	81	27.5	268	6	21	25	34	47	55	83
65+	42	24.4	430	1	7	24	37	68	72	>99
SUBTOTALS:										
1. SINGLE DX										
A. Not Operated	29	2.9	6	1	1	2	4	8	8	9
B. Operated	3	2.7	8	1	1	1	6	6	6	6
2. MULTIPLE DX										
A. Not Operated	1,574	15.9	233	2	4	9	27	36	43	66
B. Operated	214	28.7	327	6	21	27	36	54	71	>99
1. SINGLE DX	32	2.9	6	1	1	2	5	6	8	9
2. MULTIPLE DX	1,788	17.4	262	2	4	11	28	38	47	79
A. NOT OPERATED	1,603	15.7	232	2	4	9	27	36	43	66
B. OPERATED	217	28.4	332	6	20	27	35	53	69	>99
TOTAL										
0–19 Years	85	21.9	435	1	3	22	31	54	87	>99
20–34	194	22.2	293	2	7	22	31	46	53	86
35–49	248	21.7	240	3	6	24	31	39	47	66
50–64	462	22.1	281	3	6	23	32	42	50	79
65+	831	11.4	170	2	3	6	15	30	39	63
GRAND TOTAL	1,820	17.2	261	2	4	11	28	38	47	79

205.10: CML W/O REMISSION

Type of Patients	Observed Patients	Avg. Stay	Vari-ance	10th	25th	50th	75th	90th	95th	99th
1. SINGLE DX										
A. Not Operated										
0–19 Years	2	4.0	8	2	2	6	6	6	6	6
20–34	4	2.5	2	1	2	3	4	4	4	4
35–49	1	1.0	0	1	1	1	1	1	1	1
50–64	2	2.0	2	1	1	2	3	3	3	3
65+	2	1.0	0	1	1	1	1	1	1	1
B. Operated										
0–19 Years	0									
20–34	0									
35–49	0									
50–64	0									
2. MULTIPLE DX										
A. Not Operated										
0–19 Years	5	7.2	45	1	2	5	11	17	17	17
20–34	38	4.1	9	1	2	4	6	8	8	16
35–49	75	6.8	38	2	3	5	8	15	22	34
50–64	94	7.4	69	1	2	5	8	15	26	47
65+	155	6.9	46	2	3	4	8	15	24	33
B. Operated										
0–19 Years	2	10.5	59	5	5	16	16	16	16	16
20–34	8	26.2	226	6	12	28	43	48	48	48
35–49	5	23.4	37	16	18	26	27	30	30	30
50–64	11	28.1	150	13	20	26	36	44	49	49
65+	12	14.3	87	4	6	13	24	25	27	27
SUBTOTALS:										
1. SINGLE DX										
A. Not Operated	11	2.3	3	1	1	2	3	4	6	6
B. Operated	0									
2. MULTIPLE DX										
A. Not Operated	367	6.7	47	1	2	5	8	15	21	34
B. Operated	38	21.8	156	5	12	24	28	43	48	49
1. SINGLE DX	11	2.3	3	1	1	2	3	4	6	6
2. MULTIPLE DX	405	8.1	76	2	3	5	10	20	27	43
A. NOT OPERATED	378	6.6	46	1	2	5	8	15	21	34
B. OPERATED	38	21.8	156	5	12	24	28	43	48	49
TOTAL										
0–19 Years	9	7.2	36	1	2	5	11	17	17	17
20–34	50	7.5	107	1	3	4	7	21	35	48
35–49	81	7.7	54	2	3	5	10	19	24	34
50–64	107	9.5	116	1	3	6	11	26	34	47
65+	169	7.4	52	2	3	5	9	18	24	33
GRAND TOTAL	416	8.0	75	1	3	5	9	20	27	43

Percentiles

113

Length of Stay by Diagnosis and Operation, Western Region, 2008

Western Region, October 2006–September 2007 Data, by Diagnosis

206: MONOCYTIC LEUKEMIA

Type of Patients	Observed Patients	Avg. Stay	Variance	10th	25th	50th	75th	90th	95th	99th
1. SINGLE DX										
A. Not Operated										
0–19 Years	0									
20–34	0									
35–49	0									
50–64	0									
65+	0									
B. Operated										
0–19 Years	0									
20–34	0									
35–49	0									
50–64	0									
65+	0									
2. MULTIPLE DX										
A. Not Operated										
0–19 Years	1	5.0	0	5	5	5	5	5	5	5
20–34	1	45.0	0	45	45	45	45	45	45	45
35–49	4	15.1	222	1	4	23	32	32	32	32
50–64	4	14.2	188	1	1	4	28	28	28	28
65+	20	8.1	56	3	4	5	8	13	25	31
B. Operated										
0–19 Years	2	21.0	504	5	5	21	37	37	37	37
20–34	0									
35–49	0									
50–64	0									
65+	0									
SUBTOTALS:										
1. SINGLE DX										
A. Not Operated	0									
B. Operated	0									
2. MULTIPLE DX										
A. Not Operated	30	11.0	130	1	4	5	13	31	32	45
B. Operated	2	21.0	504	5	5	21	37	37	37	37
1. SINGLE DX	0									
2. MULTIPLE DX	32	11.6	144	3	4	5	13	31	37	45
A. NOT OPERATED	30	11.0	130	1	4	5	13	31	32	45
B. OPERATED	2	21.0	504	5	5	21	37	37	37	37
TOTAL										
0–19 Years	3	15.6	337	5	5	5	37	37	37	37
20–34	1	45.0	0	45	45	45	45	45	45	45
35–49	4	15.1	222	1	4	23	32	32	32	32
50–64	4	14.2	188	1	1	4	28	28	28	28
65+	20	8.1	56	3	4	5	8	13	25	31
GRAND TOTAL	32	11.6	144	3	4	5	13	31	37	45

207: OTHER SPECIFIED LEUKEMIA

Type of Patients	Observed Patients	Avg. Stay	Variance	10th	25th	50th	75th	90th	95th	99th
1. SINGLE DX										
A. Not Operated										
0–19 Years	0									
20–34	0									
35–49	0									
50–64	0									
65+	0									
B. Operated										
0–19 Years	0									
20–34	0									
35–49	0									
50–64	0									
65+	0									
2. MULTIPLE DX										
A. Not Operated										
0–19 Years	0									
20–34	0									
35–49	2	16.0	332	3	3	3	29	29	29	29
50–64	0									
65+	1	2.0	0	2	2	2	2	2	2	2
B. Operated										
0–19 Years	1	29.0	0	29	29	29	29	29	29	29
20–34	0									
35–49	0									
50–64	2	15.0	197	5	5	15	25	25	25	25
65+	1	6.0	0	6	6	6	6	6	6	6
SUBTOTALS:										
1. SINGLE DX										
A. Not Operated	0									
B. Operated	0									
2. MULTIPLE DX										
A. Not Operated	3	11.3	232	2	2	3	29	29	29	29
B. Operated	4	16.2	156	5	6	6	25	29	29	29
1. SINGLE DX	0									
2. MULTIPLE DX	7	14.1	163	2	3	6	29	29	29	29
A. NOT OPERATED	3	11.3	232	2	2	3	29	29	29	29
B. OPERATED	4	16.2	156	5	6	6	25	29	29	29
TOTAL										
0–19 Years	1	29.0	0	29	29	29	29	29	29	29
20–34	0									
35–49	2	16.0	332	3	3	3	29	29	29	29
50–64	2	15.0	197	5	5	15	25	25	25	25
65+	2	4.0	8	2	2	6	6	6	6	6
GRAND TOTAL	7	14.1	163	2	3	6	29	29	29	29

208: LEUKEMIA NOS CELL TYPE

Type of Patients	Observed Patients	Avg. Stay	Variance	10th	25th	50th	75th	90th	95th	99th
1. SINGLE DX										
A. Not Operated										
0–19 Years	0									
20–34	1	5.0	0	5	5	5	5	5	5	5
35–49	1	30.0	0	30	30	30	30	30	30	30
50–64	2	2.0	2	1	1	1	1	3	3	3
65+	3	1.3	<1	1	1	1	2	2	2	2
B. Operated										
0–19 Years	1	1.0	0	1	1	1	1	1	1	1
20–34	0									
35–49	0									
50–64	0									
65+	0									
2. MULTIPLE DX										
A. Not Operated										
0–19 Years	9	13.9	176	1	5	7	30	32	32	32
20–34	7	4.4	10	1	2	4	6	10	10	10
35–49	9	11.9	170	1	7	7	13	39	39	39
50–64	27	4.3	25	1	1	2	6	8	17	22
65+	116	5.3	48	1	2	3	6	11	18	41
B. Operated										
0–19 Years	0									
20–34	1	3.0	0	3	3	3	3	3	3	3
35–49	1	3.0	0	3	3	3	3	3	3	3
50–64	2	7.6	24	4	4	11	11	11	11	11
65+	2	5.5	12	3	3	3	8	8	8	8
SUBTOTALS:										
1. SINGLE DX										
A. Not Operated	7	6.1	112	1	1	2	5	30	30	30
B. Operated	1	1.0	0	1	1	1	1	1	1	1
2. MULTIPLE DX										
A. Not Operated	168	5.9	60	1	2	3	6	14	22	41
B. Operated	6	5.4	12	3	3	4	8	11	11	11
1. SINGLE DX	8	5.5	99	1	1	2	3	30	30	30
2. MULTIPLE DX	174	5.9	58	1	2	3	6	13	22	41
A. NOT OPERATED	175	5.9	61	1	2	3	6	14	27	41
B. OPERATED	7	4.7	12	1	3	3	8	11	11	11
TOTAL										
0–19 Years	10	12.6	173	1	1	7	30	32	32	32
20–34	9	4.3	8	1	2	4	6	10	10	10
35–49	11	12.7	176	1	2	7	27	30	39	39
50–64	31	4.3	24	1	1	3	6	8	17	22
65+	121	5.2	46	1	2	3	6	10	17	41
GRAND TOTAL	182	5.9	59	1	2	3	6	13	22	41

Length of Stay by Diagnosis and Operation, Western Region, 2008

Western Region, October 2006–September 2007 Data, by Diagnosis

210: BEN MOUTH/PHARYNX NEOPL

Type of Patients	Observed Patients	Avg. Stay	Vari-ance	10th	25th	50th	75th	90th	95th	99th
1. SINGLE DX										
A. Not Operated										
0–19 Years	1	8.0	0	8	8	8	8	8	8	8
20–34	0									
35–49	0									
50–64	2	2.0	2	1	1	1	3	3	3	3
65+	0									
B. Operated										
0–19 Years	12	2.8	5	1	1	1	5	6	7	7
20–34	67	1.3	<1	1	1	1	1	2	3	4
35–49	73	1.5	<1	1	1	1	2	2	3	7
50–64	75	1.3	<1	1	1	1	1	2	3	3
65+	20	1.5	<1	1	1	1	2	3	4	4
2. MULTIPLE DX										
A. Not Operated										
0–19 Years	7	3.3	6	1	1	1	6	7	7	7
20–34	2	4.0	0	4	4	4	4	4	4	4
35–49	3	3.3	10	1	1	2	7	7	7	7
50–64	7	4.3	22	1	1	3	6	14	14	14
65+	8	3.5	11	1	1	2	8	9	9	9
B. Operated										
0–19 Years	20	7.6	44	1	3	4	8	16	25	25
20–34	53	1.8	2	1	1	1	2	3	5	6
35–49	135	1.6	2	1	1	1	2	3	3	7
50–64	289	1.5	1	1	1	1	1	2	3	7
65+	245	1.5	1	1	1	1	2	2	3	6
SUBTOTALS:										
1. SINGLE DX										
A. Not Operated	3	4.0	13	1	1	3	3	8	8	8
B. Operated	247	1.4	<1	1	1	1	2	2	3	6
2. MULTIPLE DX										
A. Not Operated	27	3.7	10	1	1	3	3	8	9	14
B. Operated	742	1.7	4	1	1	1	2	3	4	9
1. SINGLE DX	250	1.5	1	1	1	1	2	3	3	7
2. MULTIPLE DX	769	1.8	4	1	1	1	2	3	5	11
A. NOT OPERATED	30	3.7	10	1	1	3	6	8	9	14
B. OPERATED	989	1.6	3	1	1	1	2	3	4	8
TOTAL										
0–19 Years	40	5.4	29	1	1	3	7	15	20	25
20–34	122	1.6	1	1	1	1	2	2	4	6
35–49	211	1.6	2	1	1	1	2	2	3	7
50–64	373	1.5	2	1	1	1	2	2	3	7
65+	273	1.5	2	1	1	1	2	3	3	9
GRAND TOTAL	1,019	1.7	3	1	1	1	2	3	4	9

210.2: BENIGN MAJOR SG NEOPLASM

Type of Patients	Observed Patients	Avg. Stay	Vari-ance	10th	25th	50th	75th	90th	95th	99th
1. SINGLE DX										
A. Not Operated										
0–19 Years	0									
20–34	0									
35–49	0									
50–64	2	2.0	2	1	1	1	3	3	3	3
65+	0									
B. Operated										
0–19 Years	5	1.0	0	1	1	1	1	1	1	1
20–34	63	1.3	<1	1	1	1	1	2	3	3
35–49	70	1.4	<1	1	1	1	2	2	2	7
50–64	72	1.2	<1	1	1	1	1	2	2	2
65+	20	1.5	<1	1	1	1	2	3	4	4
2. MULTIPLE DX										
A. Not Operated										
0–19 Years	0									
20–34	0									
35–49	0									
50–64	2	2.0	2	1	1	1	3	3	3	3
65+	5	3.2	9	1	1	2	4	8	8	8
B. Operated										
0–19 Years	2	1.0	0	1	1	1	1	1	1	1
20–34	41	1.7	1	1	1	1	1	2	3	6
35–49	120	1.4	<1	1	1	1	2	2	3	7
50–64	270	1.5	<1	1	1	1	2	2	3	6
65+	234	1.5	1	1	1	1	2	2	3	6
SUBTOTALS:										
1. SINGLE DX										
A. Not Operated	2	2.0	2	1	1	1	3	3	3	3
B. Operated	230	1.3	<1	1	1	1	2	2	3	4
2. MULTIPLE DX										
A. Not Operated	7	2.9	7	1	1	2	4	8	8	8
B. Operated	667	1.5	1	1	1	1	2	2	3	6
1. SINGLE DX	232	1.3	<1	1	1	1	1	2	3	4
2. MULTIPLE DX	674	1.5	1	1	1	1	2	2	3	7
A. NOT OPERATED	9	2.7	5	1	1	2	3	8	8	8
B. OPERATED	897	1.4	<1	1	1	1	2	2	3	6
TOTAL										
0–19 Years	7	1.0	0	1	1	1	1	1	1	1
20–34	104	1.4	<1	1	1	1	2	3	3	5
35–49	190	1.4	<1	1	1	1	2	2	3	7
50–64	346	1.4	<1	1	1	1	2	2	3	6
65+	259	1.5	1	1	1	1	2	2	3	8
GRAND TOTAL	906	1.4	<1	1	1	1	2	2	3	6

211: BENIGN DIGESTIVE NEOPL

Type of Patients	Observed Patients	Avg. Stay	Vari-ance	10th	25th	50th	75th	90th	95th	99th
1. SINGLE DX										
A. Not Operated										
0–19 Years	8	1.3	<1	1	1	1	1	3	3	3
20–34	1	5.0	0	5	5	5	5	5	5	5
35–49	4	1.8	<1	1	1	2	3	3	3	3
50–64	4	3.0	16	1	1	1	9	9	9	9
65+	6	1.0	0	1	1	1	1	1	1	1
B. Operated										
0–19 Years	5	4.2	2	1	4	4	5	6	6	6
20–34	15	3.9	8	1	1	3	7	7	9	9
35–49	34	4.0	9	2	2	3	5	6	7	18
50–64	128	4.0	5	1	3	4	5	6	7	12
65+	82	3.8	3	2	3	4	5	6	6	8
2. MULTIPLE DX										
A. Not Operated										
0–19 Years	15	2.1	4	1	1	1	2	4	8	8
20–34	38	3.8	10	1	2	3	4	7	14	15
35–49	137	2.9	4	1	2	2	4	6	7	9
50–64	339	3.7	19	1	2	3	4	7	9	21
65+	852	4.0	11	1	2	3	5	8	9	14
B. Operated										
0–19 Years	25	8.3	42	3	5	7	9	16	17	33
20–34	139	6.6	12	3	4	6	8	11	12	17
35–49	366	6.2	26	2	4	5	7	11	16	28
50–64	1,518	5.3	15	3	3	4	6	9	12	22
65+	2,398	6.3	24	3	4	5	7	11	15	27
SUBTOTALS:										
1. SINGLE DX										
A. Not Operated	23	1.7	3	1	1	1	1	3	5	9
B. Operated	264	3.9	5	1	3	4	5	6	7	12
2. MULTIPLE DX										
A. Not Operated	1,381	3.8	12	1	2	3	5	7	9	15
B. Operated	4,446	6.0	21	2	4	5	7	10	14	25
1. SINGLE DX	287	3.8	5	1	2	4	5	6	7	12
2. MULTIPLE DX	5,827	5.5	20	2	3	4	6	9	13	24
A. NOT OPERATED	1,404	3.8	12	2	2	3	5	7	9	14
B. OPERATED	4,710	5.9	20	2	3	5	7	10	14	25
TOTAL										
0–19 Years	53	5.1	31	1	1	4	7	10	16	33
20–34	193	5.8	12	2	3	5	7	11	12	17
35–49	541	5.2	21	2	3	4	6	8	14	27
50–64	1,989	5.0	15	2	3	4	6	8	11	22
65+	3,338	5.6	21	2	3	5	7	10	13	24
GRAND TOTAL	6,114	5.4	19	2	3	4	6	9	13	24

Length of Stay by Diagnosis and Operation, Western Region, 2008

Western Region, October 2006–September 2007 Data, by Diagnosis

211.1: BENIGN STOMACH NEOPLASM

Type of Patients	Observed Patients	Avg. Stay	Vari-ance	10th	25th	50th	75th	90th	95th	99th
1. SINGLE DX										
A. Not Operated										
0–19 Years	0									
20–34	0									
35–49	1	2.0	0	2	2	2	2	2	2	2
50–64	0									
65+	0									
B. Operated										
0–19 Years	1	5.0	0	5	5	5	5	5	5	5
20–34	0									
35–49	2	1.5	<1	1	1	1	1	2	2	2
50–64	4	4.0	<1	3	3	4	4	5	5	5
65+	1	5.0	0	5	5	5	5	5	5	5
2. MULTIPLE DX										
A. Not Operated										
0–19 Years	0									
20–34	6	2.2	1	1	1	2	3	4	4	4
35–49	18	2.5	1	1	2	2	3	4	5	5
50–64	46	4.1	11	2	2	3	5	7	8	21
65+	145	3.8	6	1	2	3	4	7	9	12
B. Operated										
0–19 Years	1	7.0	0	7	7	7	7	7	7	7
20–34	1	5.0	0	5	5	5	7	7	7	7
35–49	25	7.5	34	2	4	6	9	17	19	22
50–64	44	6.6	19	2	4	6	8	11	14	24
65+	60	7.7	16	4	5	7	10	14	15	22
SUBTOTALS:										
1. SINGLE DX										
A. Not Operated	1	2.0	0	2	2	2	2	2	2	2
B. Operated	8	3.6	2	1	2	4	5	5	5	5
2. MULTIPLE DX										
A. Not Operated	215	3.7	6	1	2	3	4	7	8	12
B. Operated	131	7.3	20	2	4	7	9	14	16	22
1. SINGLE DX	9	3.4	2	1	2	4	5	5	5	5
2. MULTIPLE DX	346	5.0	15	2	2	4	7	10	12	21
A. NOT OPERATED	216	3.7	6	1	2	3	4	7	8	12
B. OPERATED	139	7.1	20	2	4	6	9	14	16	22
TOTAL										
0–19 Years	2	6.0	2	5	5	7	7	7	7	7
20–34	7	2.6	2	1	1	2	4	5	5	5
35–49	46	5.2	26	1	2	4	6	15	17	22
50–64	94	5.2	16	2	3	4	7	9	14	24
65+	206	4.9	12	2	2	4	7	10	12	15
GRAND TOTAL	355	5.0	14	2	2	4	7	9	12	21

211.3: BENIGN LG INTEST NEOPL

Type of Patients	Observed Patients	Avg. Stay	Vari-ance	10th	25th	50th	75th	90th	95th	99th
1. SINGLE DX										
A. Not Operated										
0–19 Years	7	1.3	<1	1	1	1	1	3	3	3
20–34	0									
35–49	2	2.0	2	1	1	3	3	3	3	3
50–64	1	9.0	0	9	9	9	9	9	9	9
65+	2	1.0	0	1	1	1	1	1	1	1
B. Operated										
0–19 Years	3	4.0	4	2	2	4	6	6	6	6
20–34	4	3.8	10	2	1	6	6	7	7	7
35–49	15	3.5	2	2	2	3	5	6	6	6
50–64	91	3.9	3	2	3	4	4	6	7	12
65+	69	3.9	2	2	3	4	5	6	6	7
2. MULTIPLE DX										
A. Not Operated										
0–19 Years	11	1.5	<1	1	1	1	2	2	3	3
20–34	11	2.7	2	1	2	2	4	6	6	6
35–49	79	2.9	4	1	1	2	4	6	7	9
50–64	218	3.6	24	1	2	3	5	8	8	27
65+	521	4.1	13	1	2	3	5	8	9	19
B. Operated										
0–19 Years	12	6.8	10	5	5	5	7	9	15	15
20–34	46	6.6	8	3	4	6	9	11	12	13
35–49	149	6.0	16	3	4	5	9	12	15	18
50–64	1,132	5.0	11	3	4	4	6	8	11	20
65+	1,929	6.0	19	3	4	5	7	10	13	26
SUBTOTALS:										
1. SINGLE DX										
A. Not Operated	12	2.0	5	1	1	1	3	3	9	9
B. Operated	182	3.9	3	2	3	4	5	6	6	10
2. MULTIPLE DX										
A. Not Operated	840	3.8	15	1	2	3	5	7	9	20
B. Operated	3,268	5.6	16	3	4	5	6	9	12	24
1. SINGLE DX	194	3.8	3	2	3	4	5	6	7	10
2. MULTIPLE DX	4,108	5.3	16	2	3	4	6	9	12	23
A. NOT OPERATED	852	3.8	15	1	2	3	5	7	9	20
B. OPERATED	3,450	5.6	15	3	3	5	6	9	12	23
TOTAL										
0–19 Years	33	3.6	11	1	1	2	5	7	9	15
20–34	61	5.7	10	2	4	5	7	10	11	13
35–49	245	4.8	13	1	3	4	6	9	13	17
50–64	1,442	4.7	12	2	3	4	5	8	10	20
65+	2,521	5.5	18	2	3	5	6	9	12	24
GRAND TOTAL	4,302	5.2	16	2	3	4	6	9	11	22

211.4: BENIGN RECTUM/ANUS NEOPL

Type of Patients	Observed Patients	Avg. Stay	Vari-ance	10th	25th	50th	75th	90th	95th	99th
1. SINGLE DX										
A. Not Operated										
0–19 Years	1	1.0	0	1	1	1	1	1	1	1
20–34	0									
35–49	0									
50–64	3	1.0	0	1	1	1	1	1	1	1
65+	4	1.0	0	1	1	1	1	1	1	1
B. Operated										
0–19 Years	0									
20–34	1	1.0	0	1	1	1	1	1	1	1
35–49	6	4.0	4	1	3	3	6	6	6	6
50–64	16	2.7	4	1	1	2	4	6	7	7
65+	10	3.2	4	1	1	2	5	6	6	6
2. MULTIPLE DX										
A. Not Operated										
0–19 Years	0									
20–34	12	4.0	14	1	2	3	4	6	15	15
35–49	17	3.2	5	1	1	2	4	7	7	7
50–64	31	2.5	2	1	1	3	3	5	6	6
65+	103	3.1	5	1	1	3	4	6	8	11
B. Operated										
0–19 Years	0									
20–34	7	5.0	11	4	4	5	7	10	10	10
35–49	33	5.3	19	1	2	4	6	11	16	18
50–64	96	5.9	37	1	3	5	6	10	17	41
65+	192	6.3	58	2	2	5	7	12	16	53
SUBTOTALS:										
1. SINGLE DX										
A. Not Operated	8	1.0	0	1	1	1	1	1	1	1
B. Operated	33	3.1	4	1	1	3	5	6	6	7
2. MULTIPLE DX										
A. Not Operated	163	3.1	5	1	1	2	4	6	7	11
B. Operated	329	6.0	46	1	2	5	7	11	16	37
1. SINGLE DX	41	2.7	4	1	1	2	4	6	6	7
2. MULTIPLE DX	492	5.1	35	1	2	4	6	9	14	31
A. NOT OPERATED	171	3.0	5	1	1	2	4	6	7	11
B. OPERATED	362	5.8	43	1	2	5	7	10	16	37
TOTAL										
0–19 Years	2	2.5	4	1	1	4	4	4	4	4
20–34	20	4.2	13	1	1	3	5	7	10	15
35–49	56	4.5	13	1	2	4	6	9	14	18
50–64	146	4.7	28	1	1	4	6	8	11	31
65+	309	5.1	40	1	2	4	6	10	14	23
GRAND TOTAL	533	4.9	33	1	2	4	6	9	14	25

Length of Stay by Diagnosis and Operation, Western Region, 2008

Western Region, October 2006–September 2007 Data, by Diagnosis

211.6: BEN PANCREAS NEOPL NEC

Type of Patients	Observed Patients	Avg. Stay	Vari-ance	10th	25th	50th	75th	90th	95th	99th
1. SINGLE DX										
A. Not Operated										
0–19 Years	0									
20–34	0									
35–49	0									
50–64	0									
65+	0									
B. Operated										
0–19 Years	0									
20–34	3	7.0	4	5	5	7	9	9	9	9
35–49	3	5.0	4	3	3	5	7	7	7	7
50–64	5	7.6	6	5	6	7	9	11	11	11
65+	1	1.0	0	1	1	1	1	1	1	1
2. MULTIPLE DX										
A. Not Operated										
0–19 Years	1	4.0	0	4	4	4	4	4	4	4
20–34	0									
35–49	1	2.0	0	2	2	2	2	2	2	2
50–64	7	3.6	9	1	2	2	5	10	10	10
65+	13	4.8	14	1	2	3	7	11	12	12
B. Operated										
0–19 Years	3	20.3	129	11	11	17	33	33	33	33
20–34	20	7.4	10	4	5	7	8	16	16	16
35–49	38	8.2	47	4	5	6	8	11	27	36
50–64	81	8.6	36	4	5	7	9	15	22	41
65+	86	10.4	50	5	6	8	13	20	21	46
SUBTOTALS:										
1. SINGLE DX A. Not Operated	0									
1. SINGLE DX B. Operated	12	6.3	7	3	5	7	7	9	11	11
2. MULTIPLE DX A. Not Operated	22	4.2	11	1	2	3	6	10	11	12
2. MULTIPLE DX B. Operated	228	9.3	44	4	5	7	10	17	22	37
1. SINGLE DX	12	6.3	7	3	5	7	7	9	11	11
2. MULTIPLE DX	250	8.8	43	4	5	7	10	16	21	37
A. NOT OPERATED	22	4.2	11	1	2	3	6	10	11	12
B. OPERATED	240	9.1	42	4	5	7	10	17	22	37
TOTAL										
0–19 Years	4	16.3	152	4	11	11	33	33	33	33
20–34	23	7.3	9	5	5	8	8	11	15	16
35–49	42	7.9	44	4	5	6	8	11	27	36
50–64	93	8.1	34	3	5	7	9	13	22	41
65+	100	9.6	49	5	5	8	12	17	20	46
GRAND TOTAL	262	8.7	42	4	5	7	10	16	21	37

212: BENIGN INTRATHOR NEOPL

Type of Patients	Observed Patients	Avg. Stay	Vari-ance	10th	25th	50th	75th	90th	95th	99th
1. SINGLE DX										
A. Not Operated										
0–19 Years	0									
20–34	1	2.0	0	2	2	2	2	2	2	2
35–49	0									
50–64	0									
65+	0									
B. Operated										
0–19 Years	6	3.5	3	1	2	3	5	6	6	6
20–34	6	3.7	2	2	3	4	4	6	6	6
35–49	10	3.2	4	1	2	3	3	6	7	7
50–64	14	2.1	1	1	1	1	3	4	4	4
65+	3	5.0	4	3	3	5	7	7	7	7
2. MULTIPLE DX										
A. Not Operated										
0–19 Years	5	2.4	3	1	1	2	3	5	5	5
20–34	15	4.7	24	2	2	3	6	11	20	20
35–49	12	5.0	22	1	2	4	8	10	17	17
50–64	23	3.6	8	1	1	3	5	7	8	12
65+	36	5.1	23	2	2	3	7	15	18	18
B. Operated										
0–19 Years	28	4.6	18	2	2	3	5	9	16	19
20–34	39	6.2	33	2	3	4	8	10	26	29
35–49	96	4.5	10	1	3	4	6	8	10	22
50–64	217	4.6	22	1	2	4	5	8	11	28
65+	219	5.6	26	1	3	4	7	10	12	22
SUBTOTALS:										
1. SINGLE DX A. Not Operated	1	2.0	0	2	2	2	2	2	2	2
1. SINGLE DX B. Operated	39	3.1	3	1	1	3	4	6	7	7
2. MULTIPLE DX A. Not Operated	91	4.5	18	2	2	3	5	10	15	20
2. MULTIPLE DX B. Operated	599	5.1	23	1	3	4	6	9	12	26
1. SINGLE DX	40	3.0	3	1	1	3	4	6	6	7
2. MULTIPLE DX	690	5.0	22	1	2	4	6	9	12	26
A. NOT OPERATED	92	4.5	18	1	2	3	5	10	15	20
B. OPERATED	638	4.9	22	1	3	4	6	9	11	26
TOTAL										
0–19 Years	39	4.1	14	1	2	3	5	8	16	19
20–34	61	5.5	28	2	3	4	7	10	11	29
35–49	118	4.5	11	1	3	4	6	8	10	17
50–64	254	4.4	20	1	3	3	5	8	11	28
65+	258	5.5	26	1	3	4	7	10	14	22
GRAND TOTAL	730	4.9	21	1	2	4	6	9	12	22

213: BENIGN BONE/CART NEOPL

Type of Patients	Observed Patients	Avg. Stay	Vari-ance	10th	25th	50th	75th	90th	95th	99th
1. SINGLE DX										
A. Not Operated										
0–19 Years	2	1.5	<1	1	1	2	2	2	2	2
20–34	1	1.0	0	1	1	1	1	1	1	1
35–49	1	14.0	0	14	14	14	14	14	14	14
50–64	0									
65+	0									
B. Operated										
0–19 Years	77	1.5	1	1	1	1	1	3	4	6
20–34	53	1.8	1	1	1	1	2	4	4	5
35–49	32	2.9	11	1	1	2	3	5	7	18
50–64	18	1.8	<1	1	1	2	3	3	3	3
65+	2	1.5	<1	1	1	1	2	2	2	2
2. MULTIPLE DX										
A. Not Operated										
0–19 Years	2	8.5	24	5	5	12	12	12	12	12
20–34	5	3.0	5	2	2	3	3	7	7	7
35–49	4	3.0	2	1	2	3	4	4	4	4
50–64	5	2.8	3	2	2	3	4	6	6	6
65+	6	3.5	12	1	1	3	4	10	10	10
B. Operated										
0–19 Years	46	2.9	8	1	1	1	3	7	9	12
20–34	75	2.9	10	1	1	2	3	6	11	19
35–49	77	2.9	6	1	1	2	3	6	8	12
50–64	98	3.5	22	1	2	3	3	7	9	36
65+	43	4.6	34	1	3	6	6	8	11	30
SUBTOTALS:										
1. SINGLE DX A. Not Operated	4	4.5	40	1	1	2	2	14	14	14
1. SINGLE DX B. Operated	182	1.9	3	1	1	1	2	4	4	7
2. MULTIPLE DX A. Not Operated	22	3.6	9	2	2	3	4	7	10	12
2. MULTIPLE DX B. Operated	339	3.3	15	1	1	2	4	7	9	26
1. SINGLE DX	186	1.9	4	1	1	1	2	4	4	14
2. MULTIPLE DX	361	3.3	15	1	1	2	4	7	9	26
A. NOT OPERATED	26	3.7	12	1	2	2	4	10	12	14
B. OPERATED	521	2.8	11	1	1	2	3	6	8	18
TOTAL										
0–19 Years	127	2.1	5	1	1	1	2	4	6	12
20–34	134	2.5	6	1	1	2	3	4	6	16
35–49	114	3.0	8	1	1	2	4	6	8	14
50–64	121	3.2	18	1	1	3	3	6	9	26
65+	51	4.4	30	1	1	3	6	8	11	30
GRAND TOTAL	547	2.8	11	1	1	2	3	6	8	18

Length of Stay by Diagnosis and Operation, Western Region, 2008

Western Region, October 2006–September 2007 Data, by Diagnosis

214: LIPOMA

Type of Patients	Observed Patients	Avg. Stay	Vari-ance	Percentiles						
				10th	25th	50th	75th	90th	95th	99th
1. SINGLE DX										
A. Not Operated										
0–19 Years	0									
20–34	6	1.8	<1	1	1	2	2	3	3	3
35–49	8	2.5	10	1	1	1	1	10	10	10
50–64	11	1.0	0	1	1	1	1	1	1	1
65+	2	1.0	0	1	1	1	1	1	1	1
B. Operated										
0–19 Years	7	1.4	1	1	1	1	1	4	4	4
20–34	9	1.2	<1	1	1	1	1	2	2	2
35–49	20	2.2	3	1	1	1	2	6	6	6
50–64	25	1.6	1	1	1	1	2	4	4	5
65+	13	2.2	3	1	1	2	2	6	6	6
2. MULTIPLE DX										
A. Not Operated										
0–19 Years	5	1.6	<1	1	1	1	2	3	3	3
20–34	9	1.3	<1	1	1	1	1	3	3	3
35–49	29	2.4	3	1	1	2	3	6	6	6
50–64	25	2.4	8	1	1	1	3	4	4	15
65+	25	2.4	4	1	1	2	3	6	7	7
B. Operated										
0–19 Years	7	2.6	3	1	1	2	4	5	5	5
20–34	25	3.3	10	1	1	2	4	8	12	12
35–49	69	3.3	10	1	1	3	4	6	7	23
50–64	173	3.7	17	1	1	3	5	7	9	28
65+	119	4.7	20	2	2	4	6	10	14	22
SUBTOTALS:										
1. SINGLE DX										
A. Not Operated	27	1.6	3	1	1	1	2	3	3	10
B. Operated	74	1.8	2	1	1	1	2	4	6	6
2. MULTIPLE DX										
A. Not Operated	93	2.3	4	1	1	1	3	5	6	15
B. Operated	393	3.9	16	1	1	3	5	7	10	25
1. SINGLE DX	101	1.7	2	1	1	1	2	4	5	6
2. MULTIPLE DX	486	3.6	14	1	1	3	5	7	9	23
A. NOT OPERATED	120	2.1	4	1	1	1	3	4	6	10
B. OPERATED	467	3.6	15	1	1	2	5	7	9	23
TOTAL										
0–19 Years	19	1.9	2	1	1	1	3	4	5	5
20–34	49	2.4	6	1	1	1	3	5	8	12
35–49	126	2.8	7	1	1	2	4	6	6	10
50–64	234	3.2	14	1	1	3	6	6	9	25
65+	159	4.1	17	1	1	3	6	7	12	22
GRAND TOTAL	587	3.3	13	1	1	2	4	6	9	22

214.8: LIPOMA NEC

Type of Patients	Observed Patients	Avg. Stay	Vari-ance	Percentiles						
				10th	25th	50th	75th	90th	95th	99th
1. SINGLE DX										
A. Not Operated										
0–19 Years	0									
20–34	3	2.0	<1	1	1	2	3	3	3	3
35–49	2	2.0	2	1	1	1	1	3	3	3
50–64	2	1.0	0	1	1	1	1	1	1	1
65+	0									
B. Operated										
0–19 Years	4	1.0	0	1	1	1	1	1	1	1
20–34	5	1.4	<1	1	1	1	2	2	2	2
35–49	10	1.2	<1	1	1	1	1	2	2	2
50–64	17	1.3	<1	1	1	1	1	2	2	4
65+	7	1.4	<1	1	1	2	2	2	2	2
2. MULTIPLE DX										
A. Not Operated										
0–19 Years	2	2.5	<1	2	2	3	3	3	3	3
20–34	4	1.0	0	1	1	1	1	1	1	1
35–49	3	2.7	<1	2	2	3	3	3	3	3
50–64	5	4.2	36	1	1	1	2	15	15	15
65+	3	1.3	<1	1	1	2	2	2	2	2
B. Operated										
0–19 Years	6	2.2	2	1	1	1	4	4	4	4
20–34	16	2.8	9	1	1	2	5	5	12	12
35–49	34	3.2	17	1	1	3	3	7	9	23
50–64	84	2.5	5	1	1	2	3	5	6	11
65+	52	2.9	4	2	2	2	4	5	7	9
SUBTOTALS:										
1. SINGLE DX										
A. Not Operated	7	1.7	<1	1	1	1	3	3	3	3
B. Operated	43	1.3	<1	1	1	1	1	2	2	4
2. MULTIPLE DX										
A. Not Operated	17	2.5	11	1	1	2	2	3	15	15
B. Operated	192	2.7	7	1	1	2	3	5	8	12
1. SINGLE DX	50	1.3	<1	1	1	1	2	2	3	4
2. MULTIPLE DX	209	2.7	7	1	1	2	3	5	8	12
A. NOT OPERATED	24	2.3	8	1	1	1	2	3	3	15
B. OPERATED	235	2.5	6	1	1	2	3	5	7	11
TOTAL										
0–19 Years	12	1.8	1	1	1	1	3	4	4	4
20–34	28	2.2	5	1	1	1	3	5	5	12
35–49	49	2.7	13	1	1	1	3	6	9	23
50–64	108	2.3	5	1	1	2	3	5	6	11
65+	62	2.6	3	1	2	2	3	5	6	9
GRAND TOTAL	259	2.4	6	1	1	2	3	5	7	12

215: BENIGN SOFT TISSUE NEOPL

Type of Patients	Observed Patients	Avg. Stay	Vari-ance	Percentiles						
				10th	25th	50th	75th	90th	95th	99th
1. SINGLE DX										
A. Not Operated										
0–19 Years	1	4.0	0	4	4	4	4	4	4	4
20–34	1	4.0	0	4	4	4	4	4	4	4
35–49	1	2.0	0	2	2	2	2	2	2	2
50–64	0									
65+	0									
B. Operated										
0–19 Years	14	2.9	13	1	1	2	3	6	14	14
20–34	21	2.2	5	1	1	1	1	2	6	10
35–49	24	2.6	3	1	1	3	4	5	6	6
50–64	32	2.2	2	1	1	2	3	4	5	7
65+	7	3.7	4	1	2	3	5	7	7	7
2. MULTIPLE DX										
A. Not Operated										
0–19 Years	2	1.0	0	1	1	1	1	1	1	1
20–34	5	2.6	1	1	2	3	3	4	4	4
35–49	3	2.0	0	2	2	2	2	2	2	2
50–64	19	4.9	23	1	2	3	7	14	19	19
65+	14	4.6	12	2	2	4	5	9	15	15
B. Operated										
0–19 Years	26	4.3	31	1	1	3	5	8	9	29
20–34	60	3.5	8	1	2	3	4	8	9	19
35–49	112	3.6	8	1	1	3	5	8	10	12
50–64	168	3.5	9	1	1	3	5	7	9	17
65+	115	4.9	17	2	2	3	7	10	14	16
SUBTOTALS:										
1. SINGLE DX										
A. Not Operated	3	3.3	1	2	2	4	4	4	4	4
B. Operated	98	2.5	5	1	1	2	3	5	6	14
2. MULTIPLE DX										
A. Not Operated	43	4.1	15	1	2	3	5	8	14	19
B. Operated	481	3.9	12	1	2	3	5	8	10	17
1. SINGLE DX	101	2.5	4	1	1	2	3	5	6	14
2. MULTIPLE DX	524	3.9	12	1	2	3	5	8	10	17
A. NOT OPERATED	46	4.1	14	1	2	3	4	8	14	19
B. OPERATED	579	3.7	11	1	1	3	5	8	10	16
TOTAL										
0–19 Years	43	3.7	23	1	1	2	4	7	9	29
20–34	87	3.2	7	1	1	2	4	6	8	19
35–49	140	3.4	7	1	1	2	4	7	10	12
50–64	219	3.4	10	1	2	2	6	7	9	17
65+	136	4.8	16	2	2	3	5	9	14	16
GRAND TOTAL	625	3.7	11	1	1	3	5	8	10	16

Length of Stay by Diagnosis and Operation, Western Region, 2008

216: BENIGN SKIN NEOPLASM

Type of Patients	Observed Patients	Avg. Stay	Variance	10th	25th	50th	75th	90th	95th	99th
1. SINGLE DX										
A. Not Operated										
0–19 Years	9	1.2	<1	1	1	1	1			
20–34	1	3.0	0	3	3	3	3	3	3	3
35–49	1	1.0	0	1	1	1	1	1	1	1
50–64	0									
65+	0									
B. Operated										
0–19 Years	8	1.4	<1	1	1	1	2	3	3	3
20–34	3	2.3	5	1	1	1	5	5	5	5
35–49	0									
50–64	0									
65+	0									
2. MULTIPLE DX										
A. Not Operated										
0–19 Years	3	1.0	0	1	1	1	1	1	1	1
20–34	2	1.0	0	1	1	1	1	1	1	1
35–49	3	1.3	<1	1	1	1	2	2	2	2
50–64	4	2.8	12	1	1	1	8	8	8	8
65+	0									
B. Operated										
0–19 Years	6	1.3	<1	1	1	1	1	3	3	3
20–34	5	2.0	5	1	1	1	1	6	6	6
35–49	9	2.2	1	1	1	2	3	4	4	4
50–64	6	3.3	7	1	1	2	5	8	8	8
65+	4	12.7	379	3	3	3	5	42	42	42
SUBTOTALS:										
1. SINGLE DX										
A. Not Operated	11	1.4	<1	1	1	1	1	3	3	3
B. Operated	11	1.6	2	1	1	1	2	3	3	3
2. MULTIPLE DX										
A. Not Operated	12	1.7	4	1	1	1	3	2	8	8
B. Operated	30	3.6	55	1	1	1	3	6	8	42
1. SINGLE DX	22	1.5	1	1	1	1	1	3	3	3
2. MULTIPLE DX	42	3.1	41	1	1	1	3	5	8	42
A. NOT OPERATED	23	1.5	2	1	1	1	1	3	3	3
B. OPERATED	41	3.1	41	1	1	1	3	5	6	42
TOTAL										
0–19 Years	26	1.3	<1	1	1	1	1	3	3	3
20–34	11	2.0	3	1	1	1	3	5	6	6
35–49	13	1.9	1	1	1	2	2	4	4	4
50–64	10	3.1	8	1	1	2	5	8	8	8
65+	4	12.7	379	3	3	3	5	42	42	42
GRAND TOTAL	64	2.5	28	1	1	1	2	5	6	42

217: BENIGN BREAST NEOPLASM

Type of Patients	Observed Patients	Avg. Stay	Variance	10th	25th	50th	75th	90th	95th	99th
1. SINGLE DX										
A. Not Operated										
0–19 Years	0									
20–34	0									
35–49	1	1.0	0	1	1	1	1	1	1	1
50–64	0									
65+	0									
B. Operated										
0–19 Years	2	2.0	2	1	1	3	3	3	3	3
20–34	1	1.0	0	1	1	1	1	1	1	1
35–49	9	1.1	<1	1	1	1	1	2	2	2
50–64	3	1.3	<1	1	1	1	2	2	2	2
65+	0									
2. MULTIPLE DX										
A. Not Operated										
0–19 Years	0									
20–34	0									
35–49	0									
50–64	0									
65+	1	6.0	0	6	6	6	6	6	6	6
B. Operated										
0–19 Years	0									
20–34	7	2.0	2	1	1	1	4	4	4	4
35–49	14	2.0	1	1	1	2	2	3	5	5
50–64	18	2.3	3	1	1	2	3	6	6	6
65+	11	1.3	<1	1	1	1	2	2	2	2
SUBTOTALS:										
1. SINGLE DX										
A. Not Operated	1	1.0	0	1	1	1	1	1	1	1
B. Operated	15	1.3	<1	1	1	1	2	2	3	3
2. MULTIPLE DX										
A. Not Operated	1	6.0	0	6	6	6	6	6	6	6
B. Operated	50	1.9	2	1	1	1	2	4	5	42
1. SINGLE DX	16	1.3	<1	1	1	1	1	2	3	3
2. MULTIPLE DX	51	2.0	2	1	1	1	2	4	6	6
A. NOT OPERATED	2	3.5	12	1	1	6	6	6	6	6
B. OPERATED	65	1.8	2	1	1	1	2	4	5	6
TOTAL										
0–19 Years	2	2.0	2	1	1	3	3	3	3	3
20–34	8	1.9	2	1	1	1	2	4	4	4
35–49	24	1.6	<1	1	1	2	2	4	3	3
50–64	21	2.1	3	1	1	2	2	5	6	6
65+	12	1.7	2	1	1	1	2	2	6	6
GRAND TOTAL	67	1.8	2	1	1	1	2	4	5	6

218: UTERINE LEIOMYOMA

Type of Patients	Observed Patients	Avg. Stay	Variance	10th	25th	50th	75th	90th	95th	99th
1. SINGLE DX										
A. Not Operated										
0–19 Years	0									
20–34	8	1.9	2	1	1	1	2	4	4	4
35–49	101	1.3	<1	1	1	1	1	2	2	3
50–64	36	1.1	<1	1	1	1	1	2	2	3
65+	0									
B. Operated										
0–19 Years	2	1.5	<1	1	1	2	2	2	2	2
20–34	267	2.2	<1	1	2	2	3	3	3	4
35–49	1,165	2.2	<1	1	2	2	3	3	3	4
50–64	378	2.2	<1	1	2	2	3	3	3	4
65+	8	2.8	<1	2	3	3	3	3	3	3
2. MULTIPLE DX										
A. Not Operated										
0–19 Years	0									
20–34	65	2.0	3	1	1	2	2	3	6	11
35–49	645	1.6	2	1	1	1	2	3	4	7
50–64	199	1.7	2	1	1	2	2	3	4	9
65+	19	3.5	10	1	1	2	5	9	12	12
B. Operated										
0–19 Years	3	2.0	<1	1	1	2	3	3	3	3
20–34	1,899	2.5	2	1	2	2	3	3	3	7
35–49	21,406	2.4	2	1	2	2	3	3	4	7
50–64	8,111	2.4	2	1	2	2	3	4	4	7
65+	434	2.8	5	1	2	2	3	4	6	12
SUBTOTALS:										
1. SINGLE DX										
A. Not Operated	145	1.3	<1	1	1	1	1	2	3	3
B. Operated	1,820	2.2	<1	1	1	2	3	3	3	4
2. MULTIPLE DX										
A. Not Operated	928	1.7	2	1	1	1	2	3	4	8
B. Operated	31,853	2.4	2	1	1	2	3	3	4	7
1. SINGLE DX	1,965	2.1	<1	1	2	2	3	3	3	4
2. MULTIPLE DX	32,781	2.4	2	1	2	2	3	3	4	7
A. NOT OPERATED	1,073	1.7	2	1	1	1	2	3	4	8
B. OPERATED	33,673	2.4	2	1	2	2	3	3	4	7
TOTAL										
0–19 Years	5	1.8	<1	1	2	2	2	3	3	3
20–34	2,239	2.4	1	1	1	2	3	3	4	6
35–49	23,317	2.4	2	1	2	2	3	3	4	7
50–64	8,724	2.4	2	1	2	2	3	3	4	7
65+	461	2.9	5	1	2	2	3	4	6	12
GRAND TOTAL	34,746	2.4	2	1	2	2	3	3	4	7

Length of Stay by Diagnosis and Operation, Western Region, 2008

Western Region, October 2006–September 2007 Data, by Diagnosis

218.0: UTER SUBMUCOUS LEIOMYOMA

Type of Patients	Observed Patients	Avg. Stay	Vari-ance	10th	25th	50th	75th	90th	95th	99th
1. SINGLE DX										
A. Not Operated										
0–19 Years	0									
20–34	0									
35–49	1	1.0	0	1	1	1	1	1	1	1
50–64	0									
65+	0									
B. Operated										
0–19 Years	0									
20–34	11	2.2	<1	1	2	2	3	3	3	3
35–49	77	2.0	<1	1	1	2	3	3	4	4
50–64	25	2.4	<1	1	2	3	3	3	3	4
65+	1	3.0	0	3	3	3	3	3	3	3
2. MULTIPLE DX										
A. Not Operated										
0–19 Years	0									
20–34	5	3.8	18	1	1	1	4	11	11	11
35–49	50	1.7	2	1	1	1	2	2	3	8
50–64	10	1.4	<1	1	1	1	2	2	2	2
65+	2	6.5	12	4	4	9	9	9	9	9
B. Operated										
0–19 Years	1	1.0	0	1	1	1	1	1	1	1
20–34	248	2.4	1	1	2	2	3	4	5	7
35–49	3,096	2.4	2	1	2	2	3	4	4	7
50–64	1,142	2.4	4	1	2	2	3	4	4	7
65+	65	2.9	3	3	2	2	3	4	6	10
SUBTOTALS:										
1. SINGLE DX										
A. Not Operated	1	1.0	0	1	1	1	1	1	1	1
B. Operated	114	2.1	<1	1	1	2	3	3	3	3
2. MULTIPLE DX										
A. Not Operated	67	1.9	4	1	1	1	2	4	6	11
B. Operated	4,552	2.4	2	1	2	2	3	4	4	7
1. SINGLE DX	115	2.1	<1	1	1	2	3	3	3	3
2. MULTIPLE DX	4,619	2.4	2	1	2	2	3	4	4	7
A. NOT OPERATED	68	1.9	4	1	1	1	2	4	6	11
B. OPERATED	4,666	2.4	2	1	2	2	3	4	4	7
TOTAL										
0–19 Years	1	1.0	0	1	1	1	1	1	1	1
20–34	264	2.4	2	1	2	2	3	3	5	9
35–49	3,224	2.4	2	1	2	2	3	3	4	7
50–64	1,177	2.4	3	1	2	2	3	3	4	7
65+	68	3.0	3	3	3	3	3	5	6	10
GRAND TOTAL	4,734	2.4	2	1	2	2	3	4	4	7

218.1: UTER INTRAMUR LEIOMYOMA

Type of Patients	Observed Patients	Avg. Stay	Vari-ance	10th	25th	50th	75th	90th	95th	99th
1. SINGLE DX										
A. Not Operated										
0–19 Years	0									
20–34	0									
35–49	2	2.0	2	1	1	2	3	3	3	3
50–64	0									
65+	0									
B. Operated										
0–19 Years	0									
20–34	53	2.1	<1	1	2	2	2	3	3	5
35–49	270	2.2	<1	1	2	2	3	3	3	4
50–64	77	2.2	<1	1	2	2	3	3	3	5
65+	1	2.0	0	2	2	2	2	2	2	2
2. MULTIPLE DX										
A. Not Operated										
0–19 Years	0									
20–34	3	2.3	1	1	1	2	3	3	3	3
35–49	44	1.8	<1	1	1	2	2	3	3	4
50–64	11	2.1	1	1	1	2	3	3	4	4
65+	0									
B. Operated										
0–19 Years	2	3.0	0	3	3	3	3	3	3	3
20–34	525	2.4	1	1	2	2	3	3	4	6
35–49	7,183	2.4	2	1	2	2	3	3	4	6
50–64	2,689	2.5	2	1	2	2	3	3	4	7
65+	155	2.8	5	2	2	2	3	4	6	16
SUBTOTALS:										
1. SINGLE DX										
A. Not Operated	2	2.0	2	1	1	2	3	3	3	3
B. Operated	401	2.2	<1	1	2	2	3	3	3	4
2. MULTIPLE DX										
A. Not Operated	58	1.9	<1	1	1	2	2	3	3	4
B. Operated	10,553	2.4	2	1	2	2	3	3	4	7
1. SINGLE DX	403	2.2	<1	1	2	2	3	3	3	4
2. MULTIPLE DX	10,611	2.4	2	1	2	2	3	3	4	7
A. NOT OPERATED	60	1.9	<1	1	1	2	2	3	3	4
B. OPERATED	10,954	2.4	2	1	2	2	3	3	4	6
TOTAL										
0–19 Years	1	3.0	0	3	3	3	3	3	3	3
20–34	581	2.4	1	1	2	2	3	3	3	6
35–49	7,499	2.4	2	1	2	2	3	3	4	6
50–64	2,777	2.5	2	1	2	2	3	3	4	6
65+	156	2.8	5	2	2	2	3	4	6	16
GRAND TOTAL	11,014	2.4	2	1	2	2	3	3	4	6

218.2: UTER SUBSEROUS LEIOMYOMA

Type of Patients	Observed Patients	Avg. Stay	Vari-ance	10th	25th	50th	75th	90th	95th	99th
1. SINGLE DX										
A. Not Operated										
0–19 Years	0									
20–34	1	4.0	0	4	4	4	4	4	4	4
35–49	1	2.0	0	2	2	2	2	2	2	2
50–64	0									
65+	0									
B. Operated										
0–19 Years	0									
20–34	52	2.1	<1	1	2	2	3	3	3	4
35–49	136	2.3	<1	1	2	2	3	3	3	4
50–64	38	2.1	<1	1	2	2	3	3	3	4
65+	0									
2. MULTIPLE DX										
A. Not Operated										
0–19 Years	0									
20–34	6	1.7	<1	1	1	2	2	2	2	2
35–49	25	1.9	3	1	1	1	3	3	4	8
50–64	3	2.7	4	1	1	2	5	5	5	5
65+	0									
B. Operated										
0–19 Years	0									
20–34	284	2.4	<1	1	2	2	3	3	4	6
35–49	2,392	2.4	2	1	2	2	3	3	4	7
50–64	937	2.5	2	1	2	2	3	4	4	7
65+	65	2.6	2	1	2	2	3	3	6	10
SUBTOTALS:										
1. SINGLE DX										
A. Not Operated	2	3.0	2	2	2	4	4	4	4	4
B. Operated	226	2.2	<1	1	2	2	3	3	3	4
2. MULTIPLE DX										
A. Not Operated	34	1.9	2	1	1	1	3	3	5	8
B. Operated	3,678	2.4	2	1	2	2	3	3	4	7
1. SINGLE DX	228	2.2	<1	1	2	2	3	3	3	4
2. MULTIPLE DX	3,712	2.4	2	1	2	2	3	3	4	7
A. NOT OPERATED	36	2.0	2	1	1	1	3	4	5	8
B. OPERATED	3,904	2.4	2	1	2	2	3	3	4	7
TOTAL										
0–19 Years	0									
20–34	343	2.4	<1	1	2	2	3	3	4	6
35–49	2,554	2.4	2	1	2	2	3	3	4	7
50–64	978	2.5	1	1	2	2	3	3	4	7
65+	65	2.6	2	1	2	2	3	3	6	10
GRAND TOTAL	3,940	2.4	2	1	2	2	3	3	4	7

Western Region, October 2006–September 2007 Data, by Diagnosis

218.9: UTERINE LEIOMYOMA NOS

Type of Patients	Observed Patients	Avg. Stay	Variance	10th	25th	50th	75th	90th	95th	99th
1. SINGLE DX										
A. Not Operated										
0–19 Years	0									
20–34	7	1.6	<1	1	1	1	3	3	3	3
35–49	97	1.3	<1	1	1	1	1	2	2	3
50–64	36	1.1	<1	1	1	1	1	2	2	3
65+	0									
B. Operated										
0–19 Years	2	1.5	<1	1	1	2	2	2	2	2
20–34	151	2.2	<1	1	2	2	3	3	3	4
35–49	682	2.2	<1	1	2	2	3	3	3	4
50–64	238	2.2	<1	1	2	2	3	3	3	4
65+	6	2.8	<1	2	3	3	3	3	3	3
2. MULTIPLE DX										
A. Not Operated										
0–19 Years	0									
20–34	51	1.9	2	1	1	1	2	3	3	6
35–49	526	1.6	2	1	1	1	2	3	4	7
50–64	175	1.7	2	1	1	1	2	3	4	9
65+	17	3.2	9	1	1	2	4	8	12	12
B. Operated										
0–19 Years	1	2.0	0	2	2	2	2	2	2	2
20–34	842	2.5	2	1	2	2	3	4	4	7
35–49	8,735	2.4	2	1	2	2	3	3	4	7
50–64	3,343	2.4	2	1	2	2	3	4	4	7
65+	149	2.9	8	1	2	2	3	5	8	20
SUBTOTALS:										
1. SINGLE DX A. Not Operated	140	1.2	<1	1	1	1	1	2	2	3
B. Operated	1,079	2.2	<1	1	2	2	3	3	3	4
2. MULTIPLE DX A. Not Operated	769	1.7	2	1	1	1	2	3	4	8
B. Operated	13,070	2.4	2	1	2	2	3	3	4	7
1. SINGLE DX	1,219	2.1	<1	1	2	2	3	3	3	4
2. MULTIPLE DX	13,839	2.4	2	1	2	2	3	3	4	7
A. NOT OPERATED	909	1.6	2	1	1	1	2	3	4	7
B. OPERATED	14,149	2.4	2	1	2	2	3	3	4	7
TOTAL										
0–19 Years	3	1.7	<1	1	1	2	2	2	2	2
20–34	1,051	2.4	2	1	2	2	3	3	4	7
35–49	10,040	2.3	2	1	2	2	3	3	4	7
50–64	3,792	2.4	2	1	2	2	3	3	4	7
65+	172	3.0	8	2	3	3	3	5	8	20
GRAND TOTAL	15,058	2.3	2	1	2	2	3	3	4	7

219: OTH BENIGN UTERUS NEOPL

Type of Patients	Observed Patients	Avg. Stay	Variance	10th	25th	50th	75th	90th	95th	99th
1. SINGLE DX										
A. Not Operated										
0–19 Years	0									
20–34	0									
35–49	1	2.0	0	2	2	2	2	2	2	2
50–64	0									
65+	0									
B. Operated										
0–19 Years	1	3.0	0	3	3	3	3	3	3	3
20–34	2	3.0	0	3	3	3	3	3	3	3
35–49	5	1.4	<1	1	1	1	2	2	2	2
50–64	2	2.5	<1	2	2	3	3	3	3	3
65+	1	3.0	0	3	3	3	3	3	3	3
2. MULTIPLE DX										
A. Not Operated										
0–19 Years	0									
20–34	0									
35–49	1	1.0	0	1	1	1	1	1	1	1
50–64	3	1.0	0	1	1	1	1	1	1	1
65+	0									
B. Operated										
0–19 Years	1	5.0	0	5	5	5	5	5	5	5
20–34	14	2.1	<1	1	1	2	2	3	4	4
35–49	99	2.5	3	1	2	2	3	3	4	18
50–64	60	3.0	11	1	2	2	3	4	5	23
65+	9	3.2	2	1	3	3	4	5	5	5
SUBTOTALS:										
1. SINGLE DX A. Not Operated	1	2.0	0	2	2	2	2	2	2	2
B. Operated	11	2.2	<1	1	1	2	3	3	3	3
2. MULTIPLE DX A. Not Operated	4	1.0	0	1	1	1	1	1	1	1
B. Operated	183	2.7	6	1	2	2	3	4	5	18
1. SINGLE DX	12	2.2	<1	1	1	2	3	3	3	3
2. MULTIPLE DX	187	2.6	6	1	2	2	3	4	5	18
A. NOT OPERATED	5	1.2	<1	1	1	1	1	2	2	2
B. OPERATED	194	2.6	5	1	2	2	3	4	5	18
TOTAL										
0–19 Years	2	4.0	2	3	3	3	3	5	5	5
20–34	16	2.3	<1	1	2	2	3	3	4	4
35–49	106	2.4	3	1	2	2	3	3	4	7
50–64	65	2.9	10	1	2	2	3	4	5	23
65+	10	3.2	2	2	3	3	4	5	5	5
GRAND TOTAL	199	2.6	5	1	2	2	3	4	5	17

220: BENIGN OVARY NEOPLASM

Type of Patients	Observed Patients	Avg. Stay	Variance	10th	25th	50th	75th	90th	95th	99th
1. SINGLE DX										
A. Not Operated										
0–19 Years	0									
20–34	2	1.5	<1	1	1	2	2	2	2	2
35–49	0									
50–64	0									
65+	0									
B. Operated										
0–19 Years	83	2.3	2	1	1	2	3	3	3	10
20–34	342	2.0	<1	1	1	2	3	3	3	4
35–49	176	2.0	<1	1	1	2	3	3	3	5
50–64	97	2.3	<1	1	2	2	3	3	4	6
65+	23	2.6	2	1	1	3	3	4	5	6
2. MULTIPLE DX										
A. Not Operated										
0–19 Years	4	1.5	<1	1	1	1	2	3	3	3
20–34	7	1.4	<1	1	1	1	2	3	3	3
35–49	17	2.4	4	1	1	2	3	6	8	8
50–64	14	2.4	<1	1	2	2	3	4	4	4
65+	3	1.7	1	1	1	1	3	3	3	3
B. Operated										
0–19 Years	190	2.8	2	1	2	2	4	5	5	8
20–34	939	2.4	1	1	2	2	3	3	5	7
35–49	1,547	2.7	4	1	2	2	3	4	5	10
50–64	1,629	3.0	4	1	2	3	3	5	6	11
65+	1,063	3.8	12	2	2	3	4	7	9	17
SUBTOTALS:										
1. SINGLE DX A. Not Operated	2	1.5	<1	1	1	2	2	2	2	2
B. Operated	721	2.1	<1	1	1	2	3	3	3	5
2. MULTIPLE DX A. Not Operated	45	2.1	2	1	1	2	3	4	4	8
B. Operated	5,368	3.0	6	1	2	3	3	5	6	12
1. SINGLE DX	723	2.1	<1	1	1	2	3	3	3	5
2. MULTIPLE DX	5,413	3.0	6	1	2	3	3	5	6	12
A. NOT OPERATED	47	2.1	2	1	1	2	3	4	4	8
B. OPERATED	6,089	2.9	5	1	2	2	3	4	6	11
TOTAL										
0–19 Years	277	2.6	2	1	2	2	3	4	5	8
20–34	1,290	2.3	2	1	1	2	3	3	4	7
35–49	1,740	2.7	4	1	2	2	3	4	5	10
50–64	1,740	2.9	4	1	2	3	3	4	6	10
65+	1,089	3.7	12	1	2	3	4	6	9	17
GRAND TOTAL	6,136	2.8	5	1	2	2	3	4	6	11

Length of Stay by Diagnosis and Operation, Western Region, 2008

Western Region, October 2006–September 2007 Data, by Diagnosis

221: BEN NEOPL OTH FE GENITAL

Type of Patients	Observed Patients	Avg. Stay	Variance	10th	25th	50th	75th	90th	95th	99th
1. SINGLE DX										
A. Not Operated										
0–19 Years	0									
20–34	0									
35–49	0									
50–64	0									
65+	0									
B. Operated										
0–19 Years	3	1.7	<1	1	1	2	2	2	2	2
20–34	10	1.8	<1	1	1	2	2	2	4	4
35–49	9	1.8	<1	1	1	2	2	2	3	3
50–64	8	1.8	<1	1	1	2	2	3	3	3
65+	0									
2. MULTIPLE DX										
A. Not Operated										
0–19 Years	0									
20–34	1	4.0	0	4	4	4	4	4	4	4
35–49	0									
50–64	5	6.4	23	1	2	7	10	12	12	12
65+	0									
B. Operated										
0–19 Years	8	3.4	7	1	1	2	2	4	9	9
20–34	29	2.5	2	1	2	2	3	3	4	8
35–49	80	3.0	3	1	2	3	4	5	6	10
50–64	90	2.5	2	1	2	2	3	4	5	9
65+	26	3.0	3	1	1	3	3	6	7	7
SUBTOTALS:										
1. SINGLE DX										
A. Not Operated	0									
B. Operated	30	1.8	<1	1	1	2	2	2	3	4
2. MULTIPLE DX										
A. Not Operated	6	6.0	20	4	4	4	10	12	12	12
B. Operated	233	2.8	3	1	2	2	3	4	6	9
1. SINGLE DX	30	1.8	<1	1	1	2	2	2	3	4
2. MULTIPLE DX	239	2.8	3	1	2	2	3	5	7	10
A. NOT OPERATED	6	6.0	20	4	4	4	10	12	12	12
B. OPERATED	263	2.7	2	1	2	2	3	4	5	9
TOTAL										
0–19 Years	11	2.9	5	1	1	2	2	4	4	4
20–34	40	2.4	2	1	1	2	3	4	4	8
35–49	89	2.9	3	1	2	3	4	4	5	10
50–64	103	2.6	3	1	1	2	3	4	6	10
65+	26	3.0	3	1	1	3	3	6	7	7
GRAND TOTAL	269	2.7	3	1	2	2	3	4	6	10

222: BENIGN MALE GENIT NEOPL

Type of Patients	Observed Patients	Avg. Stay	Variance	10th	25th	50th	75th	90th	95th	99th
1. SINGLE DX										
A. Not Operated										
0–19 Years	0									
20–34	0									
35–49	0									
50–64	0									
65+	0									
B. Operated										
0–19 Years	0									
20–34	1	4.0	0	4	4	4	4	4	4	4
35–49	1	1.0	0	1	1	1	1	1	1	1
50–64	0									
65+	0									
2. MULTIPLE DX										
A. Not Operated										
0–19 Years	0									
20–34	0									
35–49	0									
50–64	1	1.0	0	1	1	1	1	1	1	1
65+	0									
B. Operated										
0–19 Years	0									
20–34	1	7.0	0	7	7	7	7	7	7	7
35–49	3	1.0	0	1	1	1	1	1	1	1
50–64	1	1.0	0	1	1	1	1	1	1	1
65+	3	1.0	0	1	1	1	1	1	1	1
SUBTOTALS:										
1. SINGLE DX										
A. Not Operated	0									
B. Operated	2	2.5	4	1	1	2	4	4	4	4
2. MULTIPLE DX										
A. Not Operated	1	1.0	0	1	1	1	1	1	1	1
B. Operated	8	1.8	5	1	1	1	1	7	7	7
1. SINGLE DX	2	2.5	4	1	1	2	4	4	4	4
2. MULTIPLE DX	9	1.7	4	1	1	1	1	7	7	7
A. NOT OPERATED	1	1.0	0	1	1	1	1	1	1	1
B. OPERATED	10	1.9	4	1	1	1	1	4	7	7
TOTAL										
0–19 Years	0									
20–34	2	5.5	4	4	4	6	7	7	7	7
35–49	4	1.0	0	1	1	1	1	1	1	1
50–64	2	1.0	0	1	1	1	1	1	1	1
65+	3	1.0	0	1	1	1	1	1	1	1
GRAND TOTAL	11	1.8	4	1	1	1	1	4	7	7

223: BENIGN KIDNEY/URIN NEOPL

Type of Patients	Observed Patients	Avg. Stay	Variance	10th	25th	50th	75th	90th	95th	99th
1. SINGLE DX										
A. Not Operated										
0–19 Years	0									
20–34	0									
35–49	2	1.5	<1	1	1	2	2	2	2	2
50–64	0									
65+	0									
B. Operated										
0–19 Years	1	4.0	0	4	4	4	4	4	4	4
20–34	2	3.5	<1	3	3	4	4	4	5	5
35–49	14	2.9	1	2	2	3	3	4	4	5
50–64	12	2.5	1	2	2	3	3	5	5	5
65+	10	2.9	2	2	2	3	3	7	7	7
2. MULTIPLE DX										
A. Not Operated										
0–19 Years	3	3.3	<1	3	3	3	4	4	4	4
20–34	4	22.7	>999	6	6	7	7	71	71	71
35–49	11	1.9	1	1	1	2	2	3	3	4
50–64	9	3.3	7	1	2	2	5	9	9	9
65+	9	3.0	5	1	1	2	2	6	6	6
B. Operated										
0–19 Years	8	3.6	3	2	2	4	5	5	6	6
20–34	25	5.5	25	2	3	4	6	11	12	25
35–49	90	4.6	25	2	2	4	5	7	9	39
50–64	227	4.0	14	1	2	3	4	7	9	18
65+	307	3.9	6	1	2	4	5	7	9	15
SUBTOTALS:										
1. SINGLE DX										
A. Not Operated	2	1.5	<1	1	1	2	2	2	2	2
B. Operated	39	2.9	2	2	2	3	3	5	5	7
2. MULTIPLE DX										
A. Not Operated	36	5.0	135	1	1	2	5	6	9	71
B. Operated	657	4.1	12	1	2	4	5	7	9	18
1. SINGLE DX	41	2.8	2	1	2	3	3	4	5	7
2. MULTIPLE DX	693	4.1	18	1	2	4	5	7	9	20
A. NOT OPERATED	38	4.8	128	1	1	3	5	6	9	71
B. OPERATED	696	4.0	12	1	2	3	5	7	9	18
TOTAL										
0–19 Years	12	3.6	2	2	2	4	4	5	6	6
20–34	31	7.6	161	2	3	4	7	11	25	71
35–49	117	4.1	21	1	2	3	4	6	8	28
50–64	248	3.9	13	1	2	3	4	7	9	18
65+	326	3.8	6	1	2	3	5	7	8	15
GRAND TOTAL	734	4.1	17	1	2	3	5	7	9	18

Length of Stay by Diagnosis and Operation, Western Region, 2008

Western Region, October 2006–September 2007 Data, by Diagnosis

223.0: BENIGN KIDNEY NEOPL NEC

Type of Patients	Observed Patients	Avg. Stay	Vari-ance	10th	25th	50th	75th	90th	95th	99th
1. SINGLE DX										
A. Not Operated										
0–19 Years	0									
20–34	0									
35–49	2	1.5	<1		1	2	2	2	2	2
50–64	0									
65+	0									
B. Operated										
0–19 Years	1	4.0	0	4	4	4	4	4	4	4
20–34	2	3.5	<1	3	3	4	4	4	4	4
35–49	12	2.9	1	2	2	3	4	4	5	5
50–64	11	2.5	2	1	1	2	3	5	5	5
65+	9	3.0	3	2	2	3	3	7	7	7
2. MULTIPLE DX										
A. Not Operated										
0–19 Years	3	3.3	<1	3	3	3	4	4	4	4
20–34	4	22.7	>999	6	6	7	71	71	71	71
35–49	11	1.9	1	1	1	2	3	3	4	4
50–64	9	3.3	7	1	2	2	5	9	9	9
65+	8	3.1	6	1	1	1	5	6	6	6
B. Operated										
0–19 Years	2	4.5	<1	4	4	5	5	5	5	5
20–34	16	6.4	33	2	3	5	7	12	25	25
35–49	80	4.8	27	2	3	4	5	7	8	39
50–64	205	4.0	13	1	2	3	4	6	9	15
65+	239	4.3	6	2	3	4	5	7	9	15
SUBTOTALS:										
1. SINGLE DX										
A. Not Operated	2	1.5	<1	1	1	2	2	2	2	2
B. Operated	35	2.9	2	1	2	3	4	5	5	7
2. MULTIPLE DX										
A. Not Operated	35	5.1	138	1	1	3	5	6	9	71
B. Operated	542	4.3	13	1	3	4	5	7	9	18
1. SINGLE DX	37	2.8	2	1	2	3	3	5	5	7
2. MULTIPLE DX	577	4.4	20	2	2	4	5	7	9	25
A. NOT OPERATED	37	4.9	131	1	1	2	5	6	9	71
B. OPERATED	577	4.2	12	2	2	4	5	7	9	18
TOTAL										
0–19 Years	6	3.8	<1	3	3	4	4	5	5	5
20–34	22	9.1	219	3	3	5	7	12	25	71
35–49	105	4.3	22	2	2	3	5	6	8	28
50–64	225	3.9	12	1	2	3	4	6	9	15
65+	256	4.2	6	2	3	4	5	7	9	15
GRAND TOTAL	614	4.3	19	2	2	4	5	7	9	18

224: BENIGN EYE NEOPLASM

Type of Patients	Observed Patients	Avg. Stay	Vari-ance	10th	25th	50th	75th	90th	95th	99th
1. SINGLE DX										
A. Not Operated										
0–19 Years	0									
20–34	0									
35–49	0									
50–64	0									
65+	0									
B. Operated										
0–19 Years	0									
20–34	0									
35–49	0									
50–64	0									
65+	1	1.0	0	1	1	1	1	1	1	1
2. MULTIPLE DX										
A. Not Operated										
0–19 Years	0									
20–34	0									
35–49	0									
50–64	0									
65+	1	1.0	0	1	1	1	1	1	1	1
B. Operated										
0–19 Years	1	1.0	0	1	1	1	1	1	1	1
20–34	1	2.0	0	2	2	2	2	2	2	2
35–49	4	4.5	11	1	4	4	9	9	9	9
50–64	3	3.0	12	1	1	1	7	7	7	7
65+	2	2.5	4	1	1	4	4	4	4	4
SUBTOTALS:										
1. SINGLE DX										
A. Not Operated	0									
B. Operated	1	1.0	0	1	1	1	1	1	1	1
2. MULTIPLE DX										
A. Not Operated	1	1.0	0	1	1	1	1	1	1	1
B. Operated	11	3.2	8	1	1	2	4	7	9	9
1. SINGLE DX	1	1.0	0	1	1	1	1	1	1	1
2. MULTIPLE DX	12	3.0	7	1	1	2	4	7	9	9
A. NOT OPERATED	1	1.0	0	1	1	1	1	1	1	1
B. OPERATED	12	3.0	7	1	1	2	4	7	9	9
TOTAL										
0–19 Years	1	1.0	0	1	1	1	1	1	1	1
20–34	1	2.0	0	2	2	2	2	2	2	2
35–49	4	4.5	11	1	4	4	9	9	9	9
50–64	3	3.0	12	1	1	1	7	7	7	7
65+	4	1.8	2	1	1	1	4	4	4	4
GRAND TOTAL	13	2.9	7	1	1	1	4	7	9	9

225: BENIGN NERV SYST NEOPL

Type of Patients	Observed Patients	Avg. Stay	Vari-ance	10th	25th	50th	75th	90th	95th	99th
1. SINGLE DX										
A. Not Operated										
0–19 Years	2	4.0	2	3	3	4	5	5	5	5
20–34	2	1.0	0	1	1	1	1	1	1	1
35–49	7	1.9	<1	1	1	2	3	3	3	3
50–64	12	2.1	3	1	1	1	2	5	6	6
65+	2	2.5	<1	2	2	3	3	3	3	3
B. Operated										
0–19 Years	9	4.0	14	2	1	4	5	13	13	13
20–34	49	3.2	4	1	2	3	4	5	6	10
35–49	95	3.8	4	2	2	3	5	6	8	11
50–64	115	4.0	6	2	2	3	5	6	10	14
65+	27	3.2	2	2	2	3	4	5	5	6
2. MULTIPLE DX										
A. Not Operated										
0–19 Years	5	4.2	2	2	4	4	5	6	6	6
20–34	36	3.0	7	1	1	2	4	9	9	10
35–49	73	2.6	5	1	1	2	3	5	6	15
50–64	164	4.3	64	1	1	2	4	8	13	35
65+	376	4.1	17	1	2	3	3	8	10	17
B. Operated										
0–19 Years	43	7.9	53	2	3	5	12	20	22	33
20–34	211	5.6	22	2	3	4	7	11	15	29
35–49	629	5.5	24	2	3	4	6	11	14	34
50–64	1,200	5.7	34	2	3	4	6	11	15	34
65+	829	7.0	39	2	3	5	8	14	19	34
SUBTOTALS:										
1. SINGLE DX										
A. Not Operated	25	2.1	2	1	1	3	3	5	5	6
B. Operated	295	3.7	5	2	2	4	4	6	8	13
2. MULTIPLE DX										
A. Not Operated	654	3.9	27	1	1	3	5	8	10	20
B. Operated	2,912	6.0	33	2	3	4	7	12	16	33
1. SINGLE DX	320	3.6	5	1	2	3	4	6	8	12
2. MULTIPLE DX	3,566	5.6	32	2	3	4	7	11	15	32
A. NOT OPERATED	679	3.9	26	1	1	3	5	8	10	20
B. OPERATED	3,207	5.8	31	2	3	4	7	11	16	31
TOTAL										
0–19 Years	59	6.9	44	2	3	4	8	20	22	33
20–34	298	4.9	18	2	2	4	6	9	13	29
35–49	804	5.0	20	2	3	4	6	10	13	23
50–64	1,491	5.3	35	2	3	4	6	10	14	33
65+	1,234	6.0	33	2	3	4	7	12	16	33
GRAND TOTAL	3,886	5.5	30	2	3	4	6	10	15	30

Length of Stay by Diagnosis and Operation, Western Region, 2008

Western Region, October 2006–September 2007 Data, by Diagnosis

225.0: BENIGN BRAIN NEOPLASM

Type of Patients	Observed Patients	Avg. Stay	Vari-ance	10th	25th	50th	75th	90th	95th	99th
1. SINGLE DX										
A. Not Operated										
0–19 Years	2	4.0	2	3	3	4	5	5	5	5
20–34	0									
35–49	0									
50–64	0									
65+	0									
B. Operated										
0–19 Years	4	2.0	2	1	1	2	4	4	4	4
20–34	12	2.7	2	2	2	2	3	4	6	6
35–49	7	3.7	4	2	2	3	5	7	7	7
50–64	6	4.3	10	2	2	4	6	10	10	10
65+	1	4.0	0	4	4	4	4	4	4	4
2. MULTIPLE DX										
A. Not Operated										
0–19 Years	4	4.7	<1	4	4	5	5	6	6	6
20–34	13	4.1	10	1	1	3	6	9	10	10
35–49	7	3.1	10	1	1	3	3	10	10	10
50–64	11	5.4	10	1	4	5	9	10	10	10
65+	14	4.7	17	1	2	4	6	8	17	17
B. Operated										
0–19 Years	20	7.6	71	2	3	4	8	20	33	33
20–34	46	7.0	34	2	3	6	8	13	17	29
35–49	53	7.5	41	3	4	6	8	15	23	34
50–64	71	6.6	53	2	3	4	7	17	24	>99
65+	32	7.9	91	2	3	5	8	17	24	50
SUBTOTALS:										
1. SINGLE DX										
A. Not Operated	2	4.0	2	3	3	4	5	5	5	5
B. Operated	30	3.2	4	2	2	2	4	6	7	10
2. MULTIPLE DX										
A. Not Operated	49	4.5	11	1	2	4	6	10	10	17
B. Operated	222	7.2	53	2	3	5	8	15	23	49
1. SINGLE DX	32	3.3	4	2	2	3	4	6	7	10
2. MULTIPLE DX	271	6.7	46	2	3	4	7	13	22	49
A. NOT OPERATED	51	4.5	11	1	2	4	6	9	10	17
B. OPERATED	252	6.7	48	2	3	4	7	13	22	49
TOTAL										
0–19 Years	30	6.2	51	2	3	4	5	20	22	33
20–34	71	5.7	27	2	3	4	7	11	13	29
35–49	67	6.6	37	2	3	5	7	14	20	34
50–64	88	6.3	45	2	3	4	7	12	21	>99
65+	47	6.9	68	2	3	4	7	17	22	50
GRAND TOTAL	303	6.3	43	2	3	4	7	12	20	34

225.1: BENIGN CRAN NERVE NEOPL

Type of Patients	Observed Patients	Avg. Stay	Vari-ance	10th	25th	50th	75th	90th	95th	99th
1. SINGLE DX										
A. Not Operated										
0–19 Years	0									
20–34	0									
35–49	0									
50–64	1	1.0	0	1	1	1	1	1	1	1
65+	0									
B. Operated										
0–19 Years	1	5.0	0	5	5	5	5	5	5	5
20–34	11	4.6	4	3	3	4	5	6	10	10
35–49	22	4.0	4	2	3	4	5	5	6	11
50–64	22	4.4	4	2	3	4	5	8	8	10
65+	1	4.0	0	4	4	4	4	4	4	4
2. MULTIPLE DX										
A. Not Operated										
0–19 Years	0									
20–34	5	1.6	<1	1	1	2	2	3	3	3
35–49	10	2.5	2	1	2	3	4	5	5	5
50–64	11	4.0	7	1	2	3	6	6	10	10
65+	25	2.6	8	1	1	2	3	4	4	15
B. Operated										
0–19 Years	5	4.6	3	2	4	5	6	6	6	6
20–34	34	5.4	16	2	3	4	6	12	17	19
35–49	104	4.6	8	2	3	4	6	8	8	14
50–64	198	5.1	23	2	3	4	5	8	14	33
65+	56	6.0	18	3	4	5	7	12	17	22
SUBTOTALS:										
1. SINGLE DX										
A. Not Operated	1	1.0	0	1	1	1	1	1	1	1
B. Operated	57	4.3	4	2	3	4	5	6	10	11
2. MULTIPLE DX										
A. Not Operated	51	2.8	6	1	1	2	4	5	6	15
B. Operated	397	5.1	18	2	3	4	6	8	13	22
1. SINGLE DX	58	4.2	4	2	3	4	5	6	10	11
2. MULTIPLE DX	448	4.9	17	2	3	4	5	8	13	22
A. NOT OPERATED	52	2.8	6	1	1	2	3	5	6	15
B. OPERATED	454	5.0	16	2	3	4	6	8	12	22
TOTAL										
0–19 Years	6	4.7	2	2	4	5	6	6	6	6
20–34	50	4.8	13	2	3	4	5	8	12	19
35–49	136	4.4	7	2	3	4	5	8	10	14
50–64	232	5.0	21	2	3	4	5	8	11	26
65+	82	5.0	17	1	3	4	6	10	13	22
GRAND TOTAL	506	4.8	15	2	3	4	5	8	12	21

225.2: BEN CEREB MENINGES NEOPL

Type of Patients	Observed Patients	Avg. Stay	Vari-ance	10th	25th	50th	75th	90th	95th	99th
1. SINGLE DX										
A. Not Operated										
0–19 Years	0									
20–34	2	1.0	0	1	1	1	1	1	1	1
35–49	7	1.9	<1	1	1	2	3	3	3	3
50–64	11	2.2	3	1	1	2	3	5	6	6
65+	2	2.5	<1	2	2	3	3	3	3	3
B. Operated										
0–19 Years	0									
20–34	16	3.1	3	1	2	3	3	4	8	8
35–49	45	3.7	4	2	2	3	4	7	8	9
50–64	62	3.9	7	2	2	3	4	6	8	16
65+	20	2.8	1	1	2	2	4	4	5	5
2. MULTIPLE DX										
A. Not Operated										
0–19 Years	1	2.0	0	2	2	2	2	2	2	2
20–34	18	2.6	6	1	1	2	2	9	9	9
35–49	54	2.5	6	1	1	2	3	5	6	15
50–64	142	4.2	73	1	1	2	4	8	14	35
65+	329	4.2	17	1	2	3	5	9	10	17
B. Operated										
0–19 Years	8	9.3	69	1	3	4	13	23	23	23
20–34	100	4.9	14	2	3	4	6	6	15	22
35–49	386	5.4	24	2	3	4	6	11	14	26
50–64	759	5.8	37	2	3	5	7	11	16	34
65+	570	7.3	41	3	3	5	9	15	20	35
SUBTOTALS:										
1. SINGLE DX										
A. Not Operated	22	2.0	2	1	1	2	3	3	5	6
B. Operated	143	3.6	5	2	2	3	4	6	8	12
2. MULTIPLE DX										
A. Not Operated	544	4.0	30	1	1	3	5	8	10	22
B. Operated	1,823	6.2	35	2	3	4	7	12	16	34
1. SINGLE DX	165	3.4	5	1	2	3	4	6	8	12
2. MULTIPLE DX	2,367	5.7	35	2	3	4	7	11	15	33
A. NOT OPERATED	566	3.9	29	1	1	3	5	8	10	22
B. OPERATED	1,966	6.0	34	2	3	4	7	12	16	33
TOTAL										
0–19 Years	9	8.5	66	1	3	4	13	23	23	23
20–34	136	4.3	13	2	2	3	5	8	12	21
35–49	492	4.9	21	2	2	3	6	10	13	23
50–64	974	5.4	41	2	2	4	6	11	15	34
65+	921	6.1	34	2	2	4	8	12	17	34
GRAND TOTAL	2,532	5.5	33	2	2	4	6	11	15	32

Length of Stay by Diagnosis and Operation, Western Region, 2008

225.4: BEN SPIN MENINGES NEOPL

Type of Patients	Observed Patients	Avg. Stay	Vari-ance	10th	25th	50th	75th	90th	95th	99th
1. SINGLE DX										
A. Not Operated										
0–19 Years	0									
20–34	0									
35–49	0									
50–64	0									
65+	0									
B. Operated										
0–19 Years	1	4.0	0	4	4	4	4	4	4	4
20–34	8	2.4	1	1	2	2	2	4	4	4
35–49	11	3.6	2	2	3	4	4	5	6	6
50–64	16	3.2	3	1	2	3	4	6	7	7
65+	4	4.5	3	2	5	5	5	6	6	6
2. MULTIPLE DX										
A. Not Operated										
0–19 Years	0									
20–34	0									
35–49	1	2.0	0	2	2	2	2	2	2	2
50–64	0									
65+	8	3.8	19	1	1	2	3	14	14	14
B. Operated										
0–19 Years	5	7.6	20	1	6	8	10	13	13	13
20–34	18	7.1	55	1	3	5	8	21	30	30
35–49	54	5.6	34	2	3	4	5	10	16	34
50–64	107	4.6	8	2	3	4	6	8	10	14
65+	128	5.8	19	2	3	5	7	10	15	22
SUBTOTALS:										
1. SINGLE DX — A. Not Operated	0									
B. Operated	40	3.3	2	1	2	3	4	5	6	7
2. MULTIPLE DX — A. Not Operated	9	3.6	17	1	2	3	4	5	6	7
B. Operated	312	5.5	20	2	3	4	7	10	14	28
1. SINGLE DX	40	3.3	2	1	2	3	4	5	6	7
2. MULTIPLE DX	321	5.4	20	2	3	4	7	10	14	28
A. NOT OPERATED	9	3.6	17	1	2	3	4	5	6	7
B. OPERATED	352	5.2	18	2	3	4	6	9	13	28
TOTAL										
0–19 Years	6	7.0	18	1	4	6	10	13	13	13
20–34	26	5.7	43	1	3	4	7	11	21	30
35–49	66	5.2	29	2	3	4	5	9	15	34
50–64	123	4.4	18	2	2	4	6	7	9	14
65+	140	5.7	18	2	3	5	7	10	14	22
GRAND TOTAL	361	5.2	18	2	3	4	6	9	13	28

226: BENIGN THYROID NEOPLASM

Type of Patients	Observed Patients	Avg. Stay	Vari-ance	10th	25th	50th	75th	90th	95th	99th
1. SINGLE DX										
A. Not Operated										
0–19 Years	0									
20–34	0									
35–49	0									
50–64	0									
65+	0									
B. Operated										
0–19 Years	19	1.3	<1	1	1	1	1	2	2	4
20–34	93	1.1	<1	1	1	1	1	1	2	2
35–49	146	1.1	<1	1	1	1	1	1	2	2
50–64	154	1.1	<1	1	1	1	1	2	2	2
65+	32	1.1	<1	1	1	1	1	1	2	3
2. MULTIPLE DX										
A. Not Operated										
0–19 Years	0									
20–34	0									
35–49	5	4.8	30	1	1	3	8	13	13	13
50–64	4	3.3	4	1	1	3	6	6	6	6
65+	6	5.9	11	2	3	7	7	11	11	11
B. Operated										
0–19 Years	5	1.2	<1	1	1	1	1	2	2	2
20–34	131	1.3	<1	1	1	1	1	2	2	2
35–49	335	1.3	<1	1	1	1	1	2	3	4
50–64	591	1.4	2	1	1	1	1	2	3	6
65+	430	1.6	3	1	1	1	2	2	3	8
SUBTOTALS:										
1. SINGLE DX — A. Not Operated	0									
B. Operated	444	1.1	<1	1	1	1	1	2	2	2
2. MULTIPLE DX — A. Not Operated	15	4.8	14	1	1	3	7	11	13	13
B. Operated	1,492	1.4	2	1	1	1	1	2	3	6
1. SINGLE DX	444	1.1	<1	1	1	1	1	2	2	2
2. MULTIPLE DX	1,507	1.5	2	1	1	1	2	2	3	7
A. NOT OPERATED	15	4.8	14	1	1	3	7	11	13	13
B. OPERATED	1,936	1.4	1	1	1	1	1	2	3	5
TOTAL										
0–19 Years	24	1.3	<1	1	1	1	1	2	2	4
20–34	224	1.2	<1	1	1	1	1	2	2	3
35–49	486	1.3	<1	1	1	1	1	2	2	4
50–64	749	1.4	<1	1	1	1	2	2	2	6
65+	468	1.6	3	1	1	1	2	2	3	8
GRAND TOTAL	1,951	1.4	2	1	1	1	1	2	3	6

227: BEN NEOPL OTH ENDOCRINE

Type of Patients	Observed Patients	Avg. Stay	Vari-ance	10th	25th	50th	75th	90th	95th	99th
1. SINGLE DX										
A. Not Operated										
0–19 Years	0									
20–34	1	6.0	0	6	6	6	6	6	6	6
35–49	1	2.0	0	2	2	2	2	2	2	2
50–64	0									
65+	0									
B. Operated										
0–19 Years	10	2.7	3	1	2	2	3	6	6	6
20–34	43	2.6	3	1	1	2	3	5	5	10
35–49	73	2.2	2	1	1	2	3	4	4	7
50–64	61	2.1	2	1	1	2	3	4	5	6
65+	19	1.7	1	1	1	1	3	3	4	4
2. MULTIPLE DX										
A. Not Operated										
0–19 Years	8	5.5	11	1	3	7	7	11	11	11
20–34	29	3.4	7	1	1	3	4	10	10	10
35–49	47	3.2	10	1	1	3	4	7	9	17
50–64	81	4.2	16	1	1	3	5	9	12	21
65+	97	5.0	16	1	3	4	6	10	14	23
B. Operated										
0–19 Years	28	3.5	11	1	2	3	5	7	7	17
20–34	232	3.7	12	1	2	3	4	7	10	20
35–49	589	3.2	16	1	1	2	4	6	9	18
50–64	1,239	2.9	11	1	1	2	3	6	8	19
65+	985	2.9	16	1	2	2	3	6	8	18
SUBTOTALS:										
1. SINGLE DX — A. Not Operated	2	4.0	8	2	2	2	6	6	6	6
B. Operated	206	2.2	2	1	1	2	3	4	5	6
2. MULTIPLE DX — A. Not Operated	262	4.3	14	1	2	3	5	9	11	21
B. Operated	3,073	3.0	14	1	1	2	3	6	9	18
1. SINGLE DX	208	2.3	2	1	1	2	3	4	5	6
2. MULTIPLE DX	3,335	3.1	14	1	1	2	4	6	9	19
A. NOT OPERATED	264	4.3	14	1	2	3	5	9	11	21
B. OPERATED	3,279	3.0	13	1	1	2	3	6	8	18
TOTAL										
0–19 Years	46	3.7	9	1	1	3	5	7	8	17
20–34	305	3.5	10	2	2	3	4	7	10	16
35–49	710	3.1	14	1	1	2	4	6	8	17
50–64	1,381	2.9	11	1	1	2	3	6	9	19
65+	1,101	3.0	16	1	1	2	3	6	9	20
GRAND TOTAL	3,543	3.1	13	1	1	2	3	6	9	18

Length of Stay by Diagnosis and Operation, Western Region, 2008

Western Region, October 2006–September 2007 Data, by Diagnosis

227.0: BENIGN ADRENAL NEOPLASM

Type of Patients	Observed Patients	Avg. Stay	Vari-ance	10th	25th	50th	75th	90th	95th	99th
1. SINGLE DX										
A. *Not Operated*										
0–19 Years	0									
20–34	0									
35–49	0									
50–64	0									
65+	0									
B. *Operated*										
0–19 Years	1	1.0	0	1	1	1	1	1	1	1
20–34	2	2.5	4	1	1	1	4	4	4	4
35–49	9	2.3	3	1	1	2	3	6	6	6
50–64	8	3.1	3	1	2	3	4	6	6	6
65+	2	1.5	<1	1	1	1	2	2	2	2
2. MULTIPLE DX										
A. *Not Operated*										
0–19 Years	4	7.3	8	4	7	7	7	11	11	11
20–34	7	4.7	14	1	2	3	10	10	10	10
35–49	12	3.5	9	1	2	3	5	12	12	12
50–64	16	5.4	32	1	1	3	7	16	21	21
65+	17	7.4	37	2	4	4	9	20	21	21
B. *Operated*										
0–19 Years	9	4.7	24	1	2	4	5	17	17	17
20–34	39	3.4	12	1	1	2	4	7	7	21
35–49	137	3.2	6	1	2	3	4	5	7	15
50–64	205	3.7	10	1	2	3	5	7	10	17
65+	89	4.2	10	2	2	4	5	7	13	15
SUBTOTALS:										
1. SINGLE DX										
A. *Not Operated*	0									
B. *Operated*	22	2.5	3	1	1	2	3	5	6	6
2. MULTIPLE DX										
A. *Not Operated*	56	5.7	26	1	2	4	7	14	20	21
B. *Operated*	479	3.6	9	1	2	3	5	6	9	17
1. SINGLE DX	22	2.5	3	1	1	2	3	5	6	6
2. MULTIPLE DX	535	3.8	11	1	2	3	5	7	11	17
A. NOT OPERATED	56	5.7	26	1	2	4	7	14	20	21
B. OPERATED	501	3.6	9	1	2	3	5	6	9	17
TOTAL										
0–19 Years	14	5.2	19	1	2	4	4	11	17	17
20–34	48	3.5	12	1	2	3	3	7	10	21
35–49	158	3.1	6	1	2	3	4	5	7	15
50–64	229	3.8	12	1	2	3	5	7	11	17
65+	108	4.7	15	1	2	4	6	10	14	20
GRAND TOTAL	557	3.8	11	1	2	3	5	7	11	17

227.1: BENIGN PARATHYROID NEOPL

Type of Patients	Observed Patients	Avg. Stay	Vari-ance	10th	25th	50th	75th	90th	95th	99th
1. SINGLE DX										
A. *Not Operated*										
0–19 Years	0									
20–34	0									
35–49	0									
50–64	0									
65+	0									
B. *Operated*										
0–19 Years	0									
20–34	0									
35–49	14	1.0	0	1	1	1	1	1	1	1
50–64	16	1.1	<1	1	1	1	1	1	2	2
65+	6	1.0	0	1	1	1	1	1	1	1
2. MULTIPLE DX										
A. *Not Operated*										
0–19 Years	1	3.0	0	3	3	3	3	3	3	3
20–34	2	2.5	<1	2	2	2	3	3	3	3
35–49	5	1.2	<1	1	1	1	1	2	2	2
50–64	17	4.1	9	1	1	4	6	9	10	10
65+	14	6.5	30	2	4	5	7	11	23	23
B. *Operated*										
0–19 Years	5	1.0	0	1	1	1	1	1	1	1
20–34	38	2.2	5	1	1	1	2	6	8	8
35–49	194	1.7	3	1	1	1	2	3	4	13
50–64	561	1.6	4	1	1	1	1	2	4	9
65+	571	1.9	7	1	2	1	2	3	5	16
SUBTOTALS:										
1. SINGLE DX										
A. *Not Operated*	0									
B. *Operated*	36	1.0	<1	1	1	1	1	1	1	2
2. MULTIPLE DX										
A. *Not Operated*	39	4.5	17	1	1	1	4	10	11	23
B. *Operated*	1,369	1.7	5	1	1	1	1	3	5	14
1. SINGLE DX	36	1.0	<1	1	1	1	1	1	1	2
2. MULTIPLE DX	1,408	1.8	6	1	1	1	2	3	5	14
A. NOT OPERATED	39	4.5	17	1	1	1	4	10	11	23
B. OPERATED	1,405	1.7	5	1	1	1	1	3	4	14
TOTAL										
0–19 Years	6	1.3	<1	1	1	1	1	3	3	3
20–34	40	2.2	4	1	2	1	2	6	8	8
35–49	213	1.6	3	1	1	1	2	3	4	11
50–64	594	1.6	4	1	1	1	1	3	4	10
65+	591	2.0	8	1	2	1	2	3	7	17
GRAND TOTAL	1,444	1.8	6	1	1	1	2	3	5	14

227.3: BENIGN PITUITARY NEOPL

Type of Patients	Observed Patients	Avg. Stay	Vari-ance	10th	25th	50th	75th	90th	95th	99th
1. SINGLE DX										
A. *Not Operated*										
0–19 Years	0									
20–34	1	6.0	0	6	6	6	6	6	6	6
35–49	1	2.0	0	2	2	2	2	2	2	2
50–64	0									
65+	0									
B. *Operated*										
0–19 Years	9	2.9	3	1	2	2	3	6	6	6
20–34	40	2.6	3	1	2	2	3	5	5	10
35–49	49	2.5	1	1	2	2	3	4	4	7
50–64	36	2.4	1	1	2	2	3	4	5	5
65+	10	2.2	1	1	1	3	3	4	4	4
2. MULTIPLE DX										
A. *Not Operated*										
0–19 Years	3	4.0	13	1	1	3	8	8	8	8
20–34	20	3.1	5	1	2	2	4	5	6	10
35–49	30	3.5	11	1	2	3	4	7	9	17
50–64	48	3.9	13	1	1	3	5	9	12	19
65+	66	4.1	6	1	2	4	5	7	8	12
B. *Operated*										
0–19 Years	14	3.7	4	1	2	4	5	5	7	7
20–34	154	4.1	13	2	2	3	4	7	13	20
35–49	257	4.4	27	2	2	3	5	8	11	23
50–64	469	4.0	16	2	2	3	4	7	11	23
65+	318	4.3	30	2	2	3	5	7	11	30
SUBTOTALS:										
1. SINGLE DX										
A. *Not Operated*	2	4.0	8	2	2	2	6	6	6	6
B. *Operated*	144	2.5	2	1	2	3	3	4	5	7
2. MULTIPLE DX										
A. *Not Operated*	167	3.8	9	1	1	3	5	7	9	17
B. *Operated*	1,212	4.2	22	2	2	3	5	8	11	23
1. SINGLE DX	146	2.5	2	1	2	3	3	4	5	7
2. MULTIPLE DX	1,379	4.1	20	1	2	3	5	8	11	23
A. NOT OPERATED	169	3.8	9	1	2	3	5	7	9	17
B. OPERATED	1,356	4.0	20	2	2	3	4	7	10	23
TOTAL										
0–19 Years	26	3.5	4	1	2	3	5	7	7	8
20–34	215	3.8	11	1	2	3	4	7	10	16
35–49	337	4.1	23	1	2	3	5	8	10	22
50–64	553	3.9	15	2	2	3	4	7	11	23
65+	394	4.2	25	2	2	3	5	7	10	30
GRAND TOTAL	1,525	4.0	19	1	2	3	4	7	10	22

Length of Stay by Diagnosis and Operation, Western Region, 2008

Western Region, October 2006–September 2007 Data, by Diagnosis

228: HEMANGIOMA/LYMPHANGIOMA

Type of Patients	Observed Patients	Avg. Stay	Variance	10th	25th	50th	75th	90th	95th	99th
1. SINGLE DX										
A. Not Operated										
0–19 Years	26	1.9	4	1	1	1	2	4	4	10
20–34	9	1.5	<1	1	1	1	2	3	3	3
35–49	7	2.1	2	1	1	2	3	5	5	5
50–64	1	2.0	0	2	2	2	2	2	2	2
65+	0									
B. Operated										
0–19 Years	44	2.3	5	1	1	1	3	5	6	12
20–34	23	2.4	2	1	1	2	3	5	5	6
35–49	23	3.2	5	1	1	3	4	7	7	9
50–64	16	2.5	2	1	1	2	3	4	6	6
65+	3	2.7	2	1	1	3	4	4	4	4
2. MULTIPLE DX										
A. Not Operated										
0–19 Years	50	4.8	51	1	2	3	5	8	10	50
20–34	36	3.9	12	1	1	3	6	8	12	15
35–49	45	2.9	6	1	1	2	4	6	8	11
50–64	58	3.6	15	1	1	3	4	7	11	21
65+	53	4.3	11	2	2	3	5	7	10	21
B. Operated										
0–19 Years	35	5.8	62	1	1	3	8	12	31	37
20–34	61	4.8	38	2	2	3	5	8	15	44
35–49	106	4.5	10	2	2	4	6	8	10	15
50–64	107	4.8	15	1	2	4	6	9	13	21
65+	53	4.4	10	1	1	4	7	9	10	12
SUBTOTALS:										
1. SINGLE DX										
A. Not Operated	43	1.8	3	1	1	1	2	3	4	10
B. Operated	109	2.6	4	1	1	2	3	5	6	9
2. MULTIPLE DX										
A. Not Operated	242	3.9	19	1	1	3	5	7	10	21
B. Operated	362	4.7	21	1	2	4	6	9	12	21
1. SINGLE DX	152	2.4	3	1	2	2	3	5	6	10
2. MULTIPLE DX	604	4.4	21	1	2	3	6	8	11	21
A. NOT OPERATED	285	3.6	17	1	1	3	4	7	10	21
B. OPERATED	471	4.2	18	1	2	3	5	8	11	21
TOTAL										
0–19 Years	155	3.8	34	1	1	2	4	8	12	37
20–34	129	3.9	23	1	1	3	4	7	11	17
35–49	181	3.8	8	1	2	3	5	7	9	15
50–64	182	4.2	14	1	2	3	6	8	11	21
65+	109	4.3	10	1	2	4	6	9	10	13
GRAND TOTAL	756	4.0	18	1	2	3	5	8	10	21

228.02: INTRACRANIAL HEMANGIOMA

Type of Patients	Observed Patients	Avg. Stay	Variance	10th	25th	50th	75th	90th	95th	99th
1. SINGLE DX										
A. Not Operated										
0–19 Years	1	1.0	0	1	1	1	1	1	1	1
20–34	2	1.0	0	1	1	1	1	1	1	1
35–49	4	2.0	<1	1	1	2	2	3	3	3
50–64	0									
65+	0									
B. Operated										
0–19 Years	2	2.5	<1	2	2	3	3	3	3	3
20–34	7	2.9	1	2	2	3	3	5	5	5
35–49	5	3.2	3	2	2	3	3	6	6	6
50–64	1	1.0	0	1	1	1	1	1	1	1
65+	0									
2. MULTIPLE DX										
A. Not Operated										
0–19 Years	3	4.3	2	3	3	4	6	6	6	6
20–34	17	3.8	13	1	1	2	5	11	12	12
35–49	22	3.0	5	1	1	2	5	6	6	9
50–64	32	3.3	14	1	2	3	4	7	8	21
65+	22	4.4	19	1	2	3	6	8	10	21
B. Operated										
0–19 Years	8	3.8	8	1	2	2	8	8	8	8
20–34	21	4.0	12	1	2	3	5	8	7	17
35–49	47	4.7	12	2	2	3	6	9	12	18
50–64	27	4.8	18	1	2	3	7	10	11	21
65+	14	5.6	18	2	3	6	10	11	12	12
SUBTOTALS:										
1. SINGLE DX										
A. Not Operated	7	1.6	<1	1	1	1	2	3	3	3
B. Operated	15	2.8	2	2	2	3	3	5	6	6
2. MULTIPLE DX										
A. Not Operated	96	3.6	12	2	1	2	4	7	10	21
B. Operated	117	4.6	14	2	2	3	6	10	12	18
1. SINGLE DX	22	2.4	2	1	2	2	3	3	5	6
2. MULTIPLE DX	213	4.2	13	1	2	3	6	8	11	21
A. NOT OPERATED	103	3.5	12	1	1	2	4	7	9	21
B. OPERATED	132	4.4	13	2	2	3	6	9	11	18
TOTAL										
0–19 Years	14	3.5	5	1	2	3	4	8	8	8
20–34	47	3.6	10	1	2	2	5	7	11	17
35–49	78	4.0	10	1	2	3	5	7	10	18
50–64	60	3.9	16	1	2	3	5	8	10	21
65+	36	4.8	19	1	2	3	8	10	12	21
GRAND TOTAL	235	4.0	12	1	2	3	5	8	11	21

229: BENIGN NEOPLASM NEC&NOS

Type of Patients	Observed Patients	Avg. Stay	Variance	10th	25th	50th	75th	90th	95th	99th
1. SINGLE DX										
A. Not Operated										
0–19 Years	1	1.0	0	1	1	1	1	1	1	1
20–34	0									
35–49	0									
50–64	2	3.5	<1	3	3	4	4	4	4	4
65+	0									
B. Operated										
0–19 Years	2	7.0	8	5	5	7	9	9	9	9
20–34	1	1.0	0	1	1	1	1	1	1	1
35–49	2	2.0	0	1	1	3	3	3	3	3
50–64	2	2.0	0	1	1	2	3	3	3	3
65+	1	2.0	0	2	2	2	2	2	2	2
2. MULTIPLE DX										
A. Not Operated										
0–19 Years	1	1.0	0	1	1	1	1	1	1	1
20–34	2	2.5	<1	1	2	3	3	3	3	3
35–49	5	2.4	1	1	1	2	3	4	4	4
50–64	4	4.8	20	1	1	7	10	10	10	10
65+	2	3.0	8	1	1	5	5	5	5	5
B. Operated										
0–19 Years	2	4.5	<1	4	4	5	5	5	5	5
20–34	12	6.0	31	2	3	4	6	11	21	21
35–49	25	4.5	18	1	1	4	5	6	14	20
50–64	26	3.7	7	1	3	3	5	6	7	7
65+	18	4.3	12	2	3	3	6	8	15	15
SUBTOTALS:										
1. SINGLE DX										
A. Not Operated	3	2.7	2	1	1	3	4	4	4	4
B. Operated	8	3.1	8	1	1	3	5	9	9	9
2. MULTIPLE DX										
A. Not Operated	14	3.1	7	1	1	2	4	7	10	10
B. Operated	83	4.4	14	1	2	4	5	7	11	21
1. SINGLE DX	11	3.0	6	1	1	3	4	5	9	9
2. MULTIPLE DX	97	4.2	13	1	2	3	5	7	11	21
A. NOT OPERATED	17	3.0	6	1	1	2	4	7	10	10
B. OPERATED	91	4.3	13	1	2	3	5	7	11	21
TOTAL										
0–19 Years	6	4.2	9	1	1	5	5	9	9	9
20–34	15	5.2	27	1	2	4	6	11	21	21
35–49	32	4.0	15	1	2	3	4	6	14	20
50–64	34	3.7	4	1	3	3	5	6	7	10
65+	21	4.1	11	1	2	3	6	8	15	15
GRAND TOTAL	108	4.1	12	1	2	3	5	7	10	20

Length of Stay by Diagnosis and Operation, Western Region, 2008

127

Western Region, October 2006–September 2007 Data, by Diagnosis

230: DIGESTIVE CA IN SITU

Type of Patients	Observed Patients	Avg. Stay	Variance	10th	25th	50th	75th	90th	95th	99th
1. SINGLE DX										
A. Not Operated										
0–19 Years	0									
20–34	0									
35–49	0									
50–64	0									
65+	1	2.0	0	2	2	2	2	2	2	2
B. Operated										
0–19 Years	0									
20–34	0									
35–49	2	3.5	4	2	2	2	5	5	5	5
50–64	6	3.2	6	1	1	1	6	6	6	6
65+	5	4.4	3	2	4	4	6	6	6	6
2. MULTIPLE DX										
A. Not Operated										
0–19 Years	0									
20–34	0									
35–49	4	4.8	4	2	5	5	7	7	7	7
50–64	10	5.8	31	2	2	3	8	19	19	19
65+	34	5.5	29	2	2	3	6	13	22	22
B. Operated										
0–19 Years	0									
20–34	0									
35–49	8	7.1	20	1	1	8	10	12	12	12
50–64	109	6.0	71	2	3	5	6	9	13	26
65+	162	8.2	79	2	4	6	9	15	23	55
SUBTOTALS:										
1. SINGLE DX										
A. Not Operated	1	2.0	0	2	2	2	2	2	2	2
B. Operated	13	3.7	4	1	2	4	6	6	6	6
2. MULTIPLE DX										
A. Not Operated	48	5.5	27	2	2	3	6	13	19	22
B. Operated	279	7.3	75	2	3	5	8	13	20	55
1. SINGLE DX	14	3.6	4	1	2	4	6	6	6	6
2. MULTIPLE DX	327	7.0	68	2	3	5	8	13	19	42
A. NOT OPERATED	49	5.4	26	2	2	3	6	13	19	22
B. OPERATED	292	7.1	72	2	3	5	8	12	19	55
TOTAL										
0–19 Years	0									
20–34	0									
35–49	14	5.9	14	1	2	5	10	11	12	12
50–64	125	5.9	65	2	3	5	6	9	13	26
65+	202	7.6	70	2	3	5	8	14	22	42
GRAND TOTAL	341	6.9	66	2	3	5	8	12	19	42

230.3: COLON CA IN SITU

Type of Patients	Observed Patients	Avg. Stay	Variance	10th	25th	50th	75th	90th	95th	99th
1. SINGLE DX										
A. Not Operated										
0–19 Years	0									
20–34	0									
35–49	0									
50–64	0									
65+	0									
B. Operated										
0–19 Years	0									
20–34	0									
35–49	1	2.0	0	2	2	2	2	2	2	2
50–64	3	5.3	1	4	4	6	6	6	6	6
65+	2	5.0	2	4	4	6	6	6	6	6
2. MULTIPLE DX										
A. Not Operated										
0–19 Years	0									
20–34	0									
35–49	1	7.0	0	7	7	7	7	7	7	7
50–64	2	10.6	143	2	2	19	19	19	19	19
65+	14	5.2	29	2	2	3	6	9	22	22
B. Operated										
0–19 Years	0									
20–34	0									
35–49	3	8.3	14	4	4	10	11	11	11	11
50–64	67	5.1	7	3	3	5	6	8	11	16
65+	99	7.9	60	3	4	6	8	15	21	42
SUBTOTALS:										
1. SINGLE DX										
A. Not Operated	0									
B. Operated	6	4.7	3	2	4	4	6	6	6	6
2. MULTIPLE DX										
A. Not Operated	17	5.9	35	2	2	4	7	19	22	22
B. Operated	169	6.8	40	3	4	5	7	12	18	42
1. SINGLE DX	6	4.7	3	2	4	4	6	6	6	6
2. MULTIPLE DX	186	6.7	40	3	4	5	7	12	19	42
A. NOT OPERATED	17	5.9	35	2	2	4	7	19	22	22
B. OPERATED	175	6.8	39	3	4	5	7	11	18	42
TOTAL										
0–19 Years	0									
20–34	0									
35–49	5	6.8	15	3	4	7	10	11	11	11
50–64	72	5.3	10	3	3	5	6	8	13	19
65+	115	7.5	56	3	4	5	8	14	21	42
GRAND TOTAL	192	6.7	39	3	4	5	7	11	19	42

231: RESPIRATORY CA IN SITU

Type of Patients	Observed Patients	Avg. Stay	Variance	10th	25th	50th	75th	90th	95th	99th
1. SINGLE DX										
A. Not Operated										
0–19 Years	0									
20–34	0									
35–49	0									
50–64	1	1.0	0	1	1	1	1	1	1	1
65+	0									
B. Operated										
0–19 Years	0									
20–34	0									
35–49	0									
50–64	0									
65+	0									
2. MULTIPLE DX										
A. Not Operated										
0–19 Years	0									
20–34	0									
35–49	1	3.0	0	3	3	3	3	3	3	3
50–64	9	5.6	21	1	3	4	6	14	14	14
B. Operated										
0–19 Years	0									
20–34	0									
35–49	0									
50–64	3	6.7	30	1	1	7	12	12	12	12
65+	4	10.5	116	1	1	8	26	26	26	26
SUBTOTALS:										
1. SINGLE DX										
A. Not Operated	1	1.0	0	1	1	1	1	1	1	1
B. Operated	0									
2. MULTIPLE DX										
A. Not Operated	10	5.3	20	1	3	4	6	14	14	14
B. Operated	7	8.9	73	1	1	7	12	26	26	26
1. SINGLE DX	1	1.0	0	1	1	1	1	1	1	1
2. MULTIPLE DX	17	6.8	41	1	3	6	8	14	26	26
A. NOT OPERATED	11	4.9	19	1	1	3	6	12	14	14
B. OPERATED	7	8.9	73	1	1	7	12	26	26	26
TOTAL										
0–19 Years	0									
20–34	0									
35–49	0									
50–64	5	4.8	22	1	1	3	7	12	12	12
65+	13	7.1	49	1	3	6	8	14	26	26
GRAND TOTAL	18	6.5	41	1	1	5	8	14	26	26

Length of Stay by Diagnosis and Operation, Western Region, 2008

Western Region, October 2006—September 2007 Data, by Diagnosis

232: SKIN CA IN SITU

Type of Patients	Observed Patients	Avg. Stay	Variance	Percentiles 10th	25th	50th	75th	90th	95th	99th
1. SINGLE DX										
A. Not Operated										
0–19 Years	0									
20–34	1	1.0	0							
35–49	0									
50–64	0									
65+	0									
B. Operated										
0–19 Years	0									
20–34	0									
35–49	1	1.0	0		1	1	1	1	1	1
50–64	0									
65+	1	1.0	0	1	1	1	1	1	1	1
2. MULTIPLE DX										
A. Not Operated										
0–19 Years	0									
20–34	0									
35–49	1	1.0	0	1	1	1	1	1	1	1
50–64	1	1.0	0	1	1	1	1	1	1	1
65+	2	2.0	2	1	1	3	3	3	3	3
B. Operated										
0–19 Years	0									
20–34	0									
35–49	3	3.0	3	2	2	2	5	5	5	5
50–64	9	1.9	2	1	1	1	3	4	4	4
65+	15	3.8	9	1	2	2	6	7	11	11
SUBTOTALS:										
1. SINGLE DX										
A. Not Operated	1	1.0	0	1	1	1	1	1	1	1
B. Operated	2	1.0	0	1	1	1	1	1	1	1
2. MULTIPLE DX										
A. Not Operated	4	1.5	<1	1	1	1	1	3	3	3
B. Operated	27	3.1	6	1	1	2	5	7	7	11
1. SINGLE DX	3	1.0	0	1	1	1	1	1	1	1
2. MULTIPLE DX	31	2.9	6	1	1	2	4	6	7	11
A. NOT OPERATED	5	1.4	<1	1	1	1	1	3	3	3
B. OPERATED	29	2.9	6	1	1	2	4	7	7	11
TOTAL										
0–19 Years	0									
20–34	1	1.0	0	1	1	1	1	1	1	1
35–49	5	2.2	3	1	1	2	2	5	5	5
50–64	10	1.8	2	1	1	1	3	4	4	4
65+	18	3.4	8	1	1	2	5	7	11	11
GRAND TOTAL	34	2.7	6	1	1	2	4	6	7	11

233: BREAST/GU CA IN SITU

Type of Patients	Observed Patients	Avg. Stay	Variance	Percentiles 10th	25th	50th	75th	90th	95th	99th
1. SINGLE DX										
A. Not Operated										
0–19 Years	0									
20–34	1	2.0	0	2	2	2	2	2	2	2
35–49	0									
50–64	1	1.0	0	1	1	1	1	1	1	1
65+	0									
B. Operated										
0–19 Years	1	1.0	0	1	1	1	1	1	1	1
20–34	88	1.8	<1	1	1	2	2	3	3	4
35–49	224	1.8	<1	1	1	2	2	3	4	5
50–64	178	1.8	1	1	1	1	2	3	4	5
65+	59	1.5	1	1	1	1	2	2	3	9
2. MULTIPLE DX										
A. Not Operated										
0–19 Years	0									
20–34	2	3.0	8	1	1	3	5	5	5	5
35–49	3	2.7	4	1	1	1	5	5	5	5
50–64	9	1.8	2	1	1	1	2	5	5	5
65+	19	1.7	3	1	1	1	2	3	8	8
B. Operated										
0–19 Years	0									
20–34	313	1.9	1	1	1	2	2	3	3	5
35–49	1,067	2.1	2	1	1	2	3	4	4	7
50–64	1,079	2.2	3	1	1	2	3	4	5	8
65+	895	2.4	9	1	1	2	3	4	7	15
SUBTOTALS:										
1. SINGLE DX										
A. Not Operated	2	1.5	<1	1	1	2	2	2	2	2
B. Operated	550	1.8	1	1	1	2	2	3	4	5
2. MULTIPLE DX										
A. Not Operated	33	1.9	3	1	1	2	3	5	5	8
B. Operated	3,354	2.2	4	1	1	2	3	4	5	9
1. SINGLE DX	552	1.8	1	1	1	1	2	3	4	5
2. MULTIPLE DX	3,387	2.2	4	1	1	2	3	4	5	9
A. NOT OPERATED	35	1.9	2	1	1	1	2	5	5	8
B. OPERATED	3,904	2.1	4	1	1	2	3	4	5	9
TOTAL										
0–19 Years	1	1.0	0	1	1	1	1	1	1	1
20–34	404	1.9	<1	1	1	2	2	3	3	5
35–49	1,294	2.1	2	1	1	2	3	4	4	7
50–64	1,267	2.1	2	1	1	2	3	4	5	8
65+	973	2.3	9	1	1	1	2	4	7	14
GRAND TOTAL	3,939	2.1	4	1	1	2	2	4	5	9

233.0: BREAST CA IN SITU

Type of Patients	Observed Patients	Avg. Stay	Variance	Percentiles 10th	25th	50th	75th	90th	95th	99th
1. SINGLE DX										
A. Not Operated										
0–19 Years	0									
20–34	0									
35–49	0									
50–64	1	1.0	0	1	1	1	1	1	1	1
65+	0									
B. Operated										
0–19 Years	0									
20–34	7	1.3	<1	1	1	1	2	2	2	2
35–49	117	1.7	1	1	1	1	2	3	4	5
50–64	136	1.8	1	1	1	1	2	4	4	5
65+	46	1.2	<1	1	1	1	1	2	2	2
2. MULTIPLE DX										
A. Not Operated										
0–19 Years	0									
20–34	0									
35–49	1	2.0	0	2	2	2	2	2	2	2
50–64	4	2.0	4	1	1	1	1	5	5	5
65+	7	2.1	7	1	1	2	2	8	8	8
B. Operated										
0–19 Years	0									
20–34	24	2.2	1	1	1	2	3	3	4	5
35–49	396	2.1	2	1	1	2	2	4	5	8
50–64	689	2.1	3	1	1	2	2	4	5	7
65+	612	1.7	1	1	1	1	2	3	4	7
SUBTOTALS:										
1. SINGLE DX										
A. Not Operated		1.0	0	1	1	1	1	1	1	1
B. Operated	306	1.7	1	1	1	1	2	3	4	5
2. MULTIPLE DX										
A. Not Operated	12	2.1	5	1	1	2	2	5	8	8
B. Operated	1,721	1.9	2	1	1	1	2	4	5	7
1. SINGLE DX	307	1.6	1	1	1	1	2	3	4	5
2. MULTIPLE DX	1,733	1.9	2	1	1	1	2	4	5	7
A. NOT OPERATED	13	2.0	4	1	1	1	2	5	8	8
B. OPERATED	2,027	1.9	2	1	1	1	2	4	4	7
TOTAL										
0–19 Years	0									
20–34	31	2.0	2	1	1	2	2	3	3	5
35–49	514	2.0	2	1	1	1	2	4	5	7
50–64	830	2.0	2	1	1	1	2	4	5	7
65+	665	1.6	1	1	1	1	2	3	4	7
GRAND TOTAL	2,040	1.9	2	1	1	1	2	4	4	7

Length of Stay by Diagnosis and Operation, Western Region, 2008

Western Region, October 2006–September 2007 Data, by Diagnosis

233.1: CERVIX UTERI CA IN SITU

Type of Patients	Observed Patients	Avg. Stay	Variance	Percentiles 10th	25th	50th	75th	90th	95th	99th
1. SINGLE DX										
A. Not Operated										
0–19 Years	0									
20–34	1	2.0	0	2	2	2	2	2	2	2
35–49	0									
50–64	0									
65+	0									
B. Operated										
0–19 Years	1	1.0	0	1	1	1	1	1	1	1
20–34	79	1.8	<1	1	1	2	2	3	3	4
35–49	102	1.9	<1	1	1	2	2	3	3	4
50–64	40	2.0	<1	1	1	2	2	3	3	3
65+	8	1.8	<1	1	1	2	2	3	3	3
2. MULTIPLE DX										
A. Not Operated										
0–19 Years	0									
20–34	2	3.0	8	1	1	3	5	5	5	5
35–49	2	3.0	8	1	1	3	5	5	5	5
50–64	3	1.7	<1	1	1	2	2	2	2	2
65+	3	1.3	<1	1	1	1	2	2	2	2
B. Operated										
0–19 Years	0									
20–34	284	1.9	1	1	1	2	2	3	3	6
35–49	634	2.2	2	1	1	2	3	3	4	6
50–64	293	2.3	2	1	2	2	3	3	5	8
65+	108	3.0	7	1	2	3	3	5	6	10
SUBTOTALS:										
1. SINGLE DX										
A. Not Operated	1	2.0	0	2	2	2	2	2	2	2
B. Operated	230	1.9	<1	1	1	2	2	3	3	4
2. MULTIPLE DX										
A. Not Operated	10	2.1	3	1	1	1	2	2	2	5
B. Operated	1,319	2.2	2	1	1	2	3	3	4	7
1. SINGLE DX	231	1.9	<1	1	1	2	2	3	3	4
2. MULTIPLE DX	1,329	2.2	2	1	1	2	3	3	4	7
A. NOT OPERATED	11	2.1	2	1	1	2	2	3	5	5
B. OPERATED	1,549	2.2	2	1	1	2	3	3	4	6
TOTAL										
0–19 Years	1	1.0	0	1	1	1	1	1	1	1
20–34	366	1.9	<1	1	1	2	2	3	3	5
35–49	738	2.1	2	1	1	2	3	3	4	6
50–64	336	2.3	2	1	2	2	3	3	5	7
65+	119	2.8	6	1	2	2	3	4	6	10
GRAND TOTAL	1,560	2.2	2	1	1	2	3	3	4	6

234: CA IN SITU NEC & NOS

Type of Patients	Observed Patients	Avg. Stay	Variance	Percentiles 10th	25th	50th	75th	90th	95th	99th
1. SINGLE DX										
A. Not Operated										
0–19 Years	0									
20–34	0									
35–49	0									
50–64	0									
65+	0									
B. Operated										
0–19 Years	0									
20–34	1	1.0	0	1	1	1	1	1	1	1
35–49	0									
50–64	0									
65+	0									
2. MULTIPLE DX										
A. Not Operated										
0–19 Years	0									
20–34	0									
35–49	0									
50–64	0									
65+	1	5.0	0	5	5	5	5	5	5	5
B. Operated										
0–19 Years	0									
20–34	0									
35–49	1	1.0	0	1	1	1	1	1	1	1
50–64	3	5.7	40	2	2	2	13	13	13	13
65+	0									
SUBTOTALS:										
1. SINGLE DX										
A. Not Operated	0									
B. Operated	1	1.0	0	1	1	1	1	1	1	1
2. MULTIPLE DX										
A. Not Operated	1	5.0	0	5	5	5	5	5	5	5
B. Operated	4	4.5	32	1	2	2	2	13	13	13
1. SINGLE DX	1	1.0	0	1	1	1	1	1	1	1
2. MULTIPLE DX	5	4.6	24	1	2	2	5	13	13	13
A. NOT OPERATED	1	5.0	0	5	5	5	5	5	5	5
B. OPERATED	5	3.8	27	1	1	2	2	13	13	13
TOTAL										
0–19 Years	0									
20–34	1	1.0	0	1	1	1	1	1	1	1
35–49	1	1.0	0	1	1	1	1	1	1	1
50–64	3	5.7	40	2	2	2	13	13	13	13
65+	1	5.0	0	5	5	5	5	5	5	5
GRAND TOTAL	6	4.0	22	1	1	2	5	13	13	13

235: GI/RESP UNC BEHAV NEOPL

Type of Patients	Observed Patients	Avg. Stay	Variance	Percentiles 10th	25th	50th	75th	90th	95th	99th
1. SINGLE DX										
A. Not Operated										
0–19 Years	1	2.0	0	2	2	2	2	2	2	2
20–34	3	1.3	<1	1	1	1	2	2	2	2
35–49	4	2.5	2	1	1	3	4	4	4	4
50–64	5	2.2	7	1	1	1	1	7	7	7
65+	1	1.0	0	1	1	1	1	1	1	1
B. Operated										
0–19 Years	4	2.5	2	1	1	3	3	4	4	4
20–34	10	3.0	4	1	2	2	5	5	7	7
35–49	15	3.5	3	1	2	4	4	5	7	7
50–64	34	3.9	9	1	2	3	5	6	9	17
65+	15	2.9	3	1	1	3	5	5	5	5
2. MULTIPLE DX										
A. Not Operated										
0–19 Years	8	6.5	14	2	4	5	7	14	14	14
20–34	12	3.8	5	1	3	4	5	6	8	8
35–49	35	4.6	8	1	2	4	5	9	10	12
50–64	84	4.0	10	1	2	3	5	7	9	18
65+	184	4.4	12	1	2	3	6	9	10	18
B. Operated										
0–19 Years	9	3.8	8	1	1	4	5	5	8	8
20–34	54	6.5	24	1	3	5	7	14	20	21
35–49	128	5.5	16	1	3	5	7	11	15	19
50–64	334	5.6	21	2	3	4	7	10	15	24
65+	514	6.4	34	2	3	5	8	10	18	30
SUBTOTALS:										
1. SINGLE DX										
A. Not Operated	14	2.0	3	1	1	1	2	4	7	7
B. Operated	78	3.4	6	1	2	3	5	5	7	17
2. MULTIPLE DX										
A. Not Operated	323	4.3	11	1	2	3	6	8	10	17
B. Operated	1,039	6.0	27	2	3	5	7	10	15	26
1. SINGLE DX	92	3.2	6	1	1	3	4	5	7	17
2. MULTIPLE DX	1,362	5.6	23	2	3	4	7	10	14	24
A. NOT OPERATED	337	4.2	11	1	2	3	5	8	10	17
B. OPERATED	1,117	5.8	26	2	3	5	7	10	15	25
TOTAL										
0–19 Years	22	4.5	11	1	2	4	7	8	9	14
20–34	79	5.4	20	1	3	5	7	12	17	21
35–49	182	5.1	13	1	3	4	6	10	12	19
50–64	457	5.2	18	2	3	4	6	9	14	23
65+	714	5.8	28	2	3	5	7	10	15	26
GRAND TOTAL	1,454	5.5	23	1	3	4	7	10	14	23

Western Region, October 2006–September 2007 Data, by Diagnosis

235.2: GI UNC BEHAV NEOPL

Type of Patients	Observed Patients	Avg. Stay	Variance	10th	25th	50th	75th	90th	95th	99th
1. SINGLE DX										
A. Not Operated										
0–19 Years	0									
20–34	0									
35–49	2	1.5	<1	1	1	2	2	2	2	2
50–64	0									
65+	0									
B. Operated										
0–19 Years	3	3.0	<1	2	2	3	4	4	4	4
20–34	6	3.8	5	1	2	3	5	7	7	7
35–49	8	3.6	4	1	1	4	4	7	7	7
50–64	26	3.7	4	1	2	4	5	6	8	9
65+	9	3.6	3	1	3	4	5	5	5	5
2. MULTIPLE DX										
A. Not Operated										
0–19 Years	0									
20–34	1	8.0	0	8	8	8	8	8	8	8
35–49	10	5.4	9	3	3	4	7	12	12	12
50–64	21	2.9	3	1	1	3	4	5	6	6
65+	77	4.0	7	1	2	3	5	8	10	16
B. Operated										
0–19 Years	5	1.8	2	1	1	1	1	4	4	4
20–34	20	6.7	40	1	2	5	10	21	21	21
35–49	58	5.3	10	2	3	5	6	9	11	18
50–64	233	5.5	17	2	3	4	7	9	14	23
65+	407	6.4	34	2	3	5	8	10	15	30
SUBTOTALS:										
1. SINGLE DX										
A. Not Operated	2	1.5	<1	1	1	2	2	2	2	2
B. Operated	52	3.7	4	1	2	4	5	5	7	9
2. MULTIPLE DX										
A. Not Operated	109	4.0	7	1	2	3	5	8	9	12
B. Operated	723	6.0	27	2	3	5	7	10	15	26
1. SINGLE DX	54	3.6	4	1	2	4	5	5	7	9
2. MULTIPLE DX	832	5.8	25	2	3	5	7	10	14	25
A. NOT OPERATED	111	3.9	7	1	2	3	5	7	9	12
B. OPERATED	775	5.9	26	2	3	5	7	10	14	26
TOTAL										
0–19 Years	8	2.3	2	1	1	2	3	4	4	4
20–34	27	6.1	32	1	2	5	7	14	21	21
35–49	78	5.0	10	2	3	4	6	9	11	18
50–64	280	5.2	16	2	3	4	6	9	13	23
65+	493	6.0	30	2	3	5	7	10	14	30
GRAND TOTAL	886	5.6	24	2	3	4	7	10	14	25

235.7: TRACH/LUNG UNC BEHAV NEO

Type of Patients	Observed Patients	Avg. Stay	Variance	10th	25th	50th	75th	90th	95th	99th
1. SINGLE DX										
A. Not Operated										
0–19 Years	0									
20–34	0									
35–49	0									
50–64	2	1.0	0	1	1	1	1	1	1	1
65+	0									
B. Operated										
0–19 Years	0									
20–34	0									
35–49	5	4.0	<1	3	4	4	4	5	5	5
50–64	2	3.0	8	1	1	1	5	5	5	5
65+	1	2.0	0	2	2	2	2	2	2	2
2. MULTIPLE DX										
A. Not Operated										
0–19 Years	2	5.5	4	4	4	4	7	7	7	7
20–34	4	2.8	3	1	1	3	5	5	5	5
35–49	10	5.4	9	1	3	4	8	10	10	10
50–64	19	4.7	15	1	2	4	6	9	18	18
65+	37	4.2	14	1	2	3	5	8	17	18
B. Operated										
0–19 Years	0									
20–34	13	6.0	7	4	4	5	7	9	13	13
35–49	26	5.7	15	2	3	5	7	12	13	16
50–64	42	4.9	26	2	3	4	5	7	10	34
65+	52	4.8	15	1	2	4	5	9	12	20
SUBTOTALS:										
1. SINGLE DX										
A. Not Operated	2	1.0	0	1	1	1	1	1	1	1
B. Operated	8	3.5	2	1	2	4	4	5	5	5
2. MULTIPLE DX										
A. Not Operated	72	4.5	13	1	2	3	6	8	10	18
B. Operated	133	5.1	18	2	3	4	6	9	13	20
1. SINGLE DX	10	3.0	3	1	1	3	4	5	5	5
2. MULTIPLE DX	205	4.9	16	2	3	4	6	9	12	18
A. NOT OPERATED	74	4.4	13	1	2	3	6	8	10	18
B. OPERATED	141	5.0	17	2	3	4	6	9	12	20
TOTAL										
0–19 Years	2	5.5	4	4	4	4	7	7	7	7
20–34	17	5.2	8	2	4	5	5	9	13	13
35–49	41	5.4	12	2	3	4	7	10	12	16
50–64	65	4.7	22	2	3	5	5	7	10	34
65+	90	4.5	14	1	2	3	5	8	12	20
GRAND TOTAL	215	4.8	15	1	3	4	6	9	12	18

236: GU UNC BEHAV NEOPL

Type of Patients	Observed Patients	Avg. Stay	Variance	10th	25th	50th	75th	90th	95th	99th
1. SINGLE DX										
A. Not Operated										
0–19 Years	0									
20–34	1	1.0	0	1	1	1	1	1	1	1
35–49	1	1.0	0	1	1	1	1	1	1	1
50–64	0									
65+	2	1.5	<1	1	1	2	2	2	2	2
B. Operated										
0–19 Years	3	3.0	4	1	1	3	5	5	5	5
20–34	24	2.3	1	1	1	2	3	4	4	5
35–49	17	2.4	2	1	2	2	3	4	5	5
50–64	14	2.4	2	1	2	2	3	5	5	5
65+	6	2.3	4	1	1	1	3	6	6	6
2. MULTIPLE DX										
A. Not Operated										
0–19 Years	0									
20–34	5	2.4	2	1	1	3	3	4	4	4
35–49	11	3.0	10	1	1	2	4	4	12	12
50–64	15	3.9	17	1	1	2	5	10	15	15
65+	24	2.9	5	1	1	2	4	6	7	8
B. Operated										
0–19 Years	11	4.2	5	2	2	4	5	6	9	9
20–34	76	3.1	5	1	2	3	4	6	6	10
35–49	191	3.5	5	2	2	3	4	6	7	12
50–64	184	3.5	5	2	2	3	4	6	7	10
65+	144	3.9	46	1	2	3	4	7	8	14
SUBTOTALS:										
1. SINGLE DX										
A. Not Operated	4	1.3	<1	1	1	1	2	2	2	2
B. Operated	64	2.4	2	1	1	2	3	4	5	6
2. MULTIPLE DX										
A. Not Operated	55	3.1	8	1	1	2	4	7	10	15
B. Operated	606	3.6	14	1	2	3	4	6	8	12
1. SINGLE DX	68	2.3	2	1	1	2	3	4	5	6
2. MULTIPLE DX	661	3.5	14	1	2	3	4	6	8	12
A. NOT OPERATED	59	3.0	8	1	1	2	4	7	10	15
B. OPERATED	670	3.5	13	1	2	3	4	6	7	12
TOTAL										
0–19 Years	14	3.9	4	2	2	4	5	6	9	9
20–34	106	2.9	3	1	2	3	4	5	6	9
35–49	220	3.4	5	1	2	3	4	6	7	12
50–64	213	3.5	5	2	2	3	4	6	8	10
65+	176	3.7	38	1	1	3	4	7	8	14
GRAND TOTAL	729	3.4	13	1	2	3	4	6	8	12

Length of Stay by Diagnosis and Operation, Western Region, 2008

Western Region, October 2006–September 2007 Data, by Diagnosis

236.2: OVARY UNC BEHAV NEOPL

Type of Patients	Observed Patients	Avg. Stay	Vari-ance	10th	25th	50th	75th	90th	95th	99th
1. SINGLE DX										
A. Not Operated										
0–19 Years	0									
20–34	0									
35–49	0									
50–64	0									
65+	1	1.0	0		1	1		1	1	1
B. Operated										
0–19 Years	0									
20–34	20	2.3	2	1	1	2	3	4	5	5
35–49	11	2.7	2	1	2	3	4	4	5	5
50–64	9	2.9	2	2	2	3	3	5	5	5
65+	2	4.5	4	3	3	3	6	6	6	6
2. MULTIPLE DX										
A. Not Operated										
0–19 Years	0									
20–34	1	1.0	0	1	1	1	1	1	1	1
35–49	3	1.7	<1	1	1	1	2	2	2	2
50–64	3	6.0	13	3	3	5	10	10	10	10
65+	7	1.7	<1	1	1	2	2	2	2	2
B. Operated										
0–19 Years	8	4.1	6	2	2	4	5	9	9	9
20–34	61	3.2	4	1	2	3	4	6	6	10
35–49	133	3.7	6	2	2	3	4	6	8	12
50–64	147	3.7	5	2	2	3	4	6	8	10
65+	61	5.8	98	2	3	4	6	8	12	79
SUBTOTALS:										
1. SINGLE DX										
A. Not Operated	1	1.0	0	1	1	1	1	1	1	1
B. Operated	42	2.6	2	1	2	2	3	5	5	6
2. MULTIPLE DX										
A. Not Operated	14	2.6	6	1	1	1	2	5	10	10
B. Operated	410	3.9	20	2	2	3	4	7	8	12
1. SINGLE DX	43	2.6	2	1	2	2	3	5	5	6
2. MULTIPLE DX	424	3.9	19	2	2	3	4	7	8	12
A. NOT OPERATED	15	2.5	5	1	1	2	2	5	10	10
B. OPERATED	452	3.8	18	2	2	3	4	6	8	12
TOTAL										
0–19 Years	8	4.1	6	2	2	4	5	9	9	9
20–34	82	3.0	3	1	2	3	4	5	6	10
35–49	147	3.6	6	2	2	3	4	6	7	12
50–64	159	3.7	5	2	2	3	4	6	8	10
65+	71	5.3	86	2	3	3	5	8	12	79
GRAND TOTAL	467	3.8	18	2	2	3	4	6	8	12

237: UNC NEOPL ENDOCR/NERV

Type of Patients	Observed Patients	Avg. Stay	Vari-ance	10th	25th	50th	75th	90th	95th	99th
1. SINGLE DX										
A. Not Operated										
0–19 Years	2	1.0	0	1	1	1	1	1	1	1
20–34	2	1.0	0	1	1	1	1	1	1	1
35–49	4	4.0	6	1	1	3	6	6	6	6
50–64	4	2.0	4	1	1	1	1	5	5	5
65+	2	2.0	2	1	1	2	3	3	3	3
B. Operated										
0–19 Years	9	3.8	9	1	2	3	5	10	10	10
20–34	15	3.9	14	1	2	3	4	7	7	16
35–49	25	4.0	35	1	1	3	4	6	8	30
50–64	16	2.6	2	1	1	3	3	5	5	6
65+	1	2.0	0	2	2	2	2	2	2	2
2. MULTIPLE DX										
A. Not Operated										
0–19 Years	21	3.3	8	1	1	2	5	6	7	12
20–34	27	3.9	15	1	1	2	5	9	13	16
35–49	46	4.3	24	1	2	3	5	8	10	32
50–64	71	3.7	12	1	1	3	5	8	11	21
65+	81	4.3	14	1	2	3	6	7	10	27
B. Operated										
0–19 Years	58	7.4	48	2	3	6	9	18	23	33
20–34	111	6.1	28	2	3	4	8	12	18	26
35–49	142	6.5	49	2	2	5	8	14	20	31
50–64	192	5.2	26	1	2	3	7	11	15	26
65+	111	4.9	28	1	2	3	6	11	17	22
SUBTOTALS:										
1. SINGLE DX										
A. Not Operated	14	2.3	4	1	1	1	3	6	6	6
B. Operated	66	3.6	18	1	1	3	3	6	10	30
2. MULTIPLE DX										
A. Not Operated	246	4.0	15	1	2	3	5	8	11	21
B. Operated	614	5.8	35	2	2	4	7	12	18	30
1. SINGLE DX	80	3.3	16	1	1	3	3	6	7	30
2. MULTIPLE DX	860	5.3	30	2	2	3	7	11	15	29
A. NOT OPERATED	260	3.9	14	1	2	3	5	8	10	21
B. OPERATED	680	5.6	33	1	2	4	7	12	17	30
TOTAL										
0–19 Years	90	6.0	37	2	2	4	7	12	19	33
20–34	155	5.5	25	1	2	4	7	12	16	26
35–49	217	5.7	42	1	2	4	7	11	19	31
50–64	283	4.6	21	1	2	3	6	10	13	26
65+	195	4.6	22	1	2	3	6	10	14	27
GRAND TOTAL	940	5.1	29	1	2	3	6	11	15	29

237.5: CNS UNC BEHAV NEOPL

Type of Patients	Observed Patients	Avg. Stay	Vari-ance	10th	25th	50th	75th	90th	95th	99th
1. SINGLE DX										
A. Not Operated										
0–19 Years	2	1.0	0	1	1	1	1	1	1	1
20–34	2	1.0	0	1	1	1	1	1	1	1
35–49	3	3.3	6	1	1	1	6	6	6	6
50–64	2	1.0	0	1	1	1	1	1	1	1
65+	2	2.0	2	1	1	2	3	3	3	3
B. Operated										
0–19 Years	4	5.5	14	2	2	3	7	10	10	10
20–34	7	5.6	23	3	3	3	7	16	16	16
35–49	9	7.7	78	3	3	4	6	30	30	30
50–64	4	3.8	2	3	3	3	3	6	6	6
65+	0									
2. MULTIPLE DX										
A. Not Operated										
0–19 Years	9	3.1	5	1	1	3	5	7	7	7
20–34	13	5.2	25	1	2	3	8	13	16	16
35–49	31	4.7	33	1	1	3	6	6	7	32
50–64	44	3.2	6	1	1	3	4	6	7	13
65+	60	4.1	9	1	2	3	5	8	10	14
B. Operated										
0–19 Years	26	5.9	20	2	2	6	7	12	15	19
20–34	48	6.6	30	2	2	5	8	13	19	29
35–49	59	6.9	28	2	3	6	8	14	16	30
50–64	72	7.3	32	3	4	6	8	14	17	31
65+	30	6.1	23	2	2	5	9	11	17	22
SUBTOTALS:										
1. SINGLE DX										
A. Not Operated	10	1.9	3	1	1	1	3	3	6	6
B. Operated	24	6.0	38	3	3	3	6	12	16	30
2. MULTIPLE DX										
A. Not Operated	157	4.0	14	1	2	3	5	8	11	16
B. Operated	235	6.7	28	2	3	5	8	13	17	29
1. SINGLE DX	34	4.8	31	1	3	3	6	10	16	30
2. MULTIPLE DX	392	5.6	24	1	2	4	7	11	15	29
A. NOT OPERATED	167	3.9	14	1	1	3	5	8	10	16
B. OPERATED	259	6.7	29	2	3	5	8	13	17	30
TOTAL										
0–19 Years	41	5.0	17	1	2	4	7	10	12	19
20–34	69	6.2	28	2	3	4	8	13	16	29
35–49	102	6.2	34	2	3	5	7	12	15	30
50–64	122	5.6	25	2	3	4	7	11	15	26
65+	92	4.7	14	1	2	3	6	9	11	22
GRAND TOTAL	426	5.6	25	1	2	4	7	11	15	29

Western Region, October 2006–September 2007 Data, by Diagnosis

238: UNC BEHAV NEOPL NEC&NOS

Type of Patients	Observed Patients	Avg. Stay	Variance	10th	25th	50th	75th	90th	95th	99th
1. SINGLE DX										
A. Not Operated										
0–19 Years	1	1.0	0	1	1	1	1	1	1	1
20–34	4	3.5	4	1	1	3	6	6	6	6
35–49	2	2.0	2	1	1	1	3	3	3	3
50–64	8	2.4	6	1	1	1	4	8	8	8
65+	15	1.4	1	1	1	1	1	2	5	5
B. Operated										
0–19 Years	6	1.2	<1	1	1	1	1	1	2	2
20–34	26	2.8	8	1	2	3	4	4	5	6
35–49	15	4.5	9	1	2	4	7	7	12	12
50–64	27	2.9	4	1	2	2	4	6	7	7
65+	2	6.5	<1	6	6	6	7	7	7	7
2. MULTIPLE DX										
A. Not Operated										
0–19 Years	35	2.7	10	1	1	2	3	5	11	17
20–34	35	3.1	5	1	2	2	4	7	8	9
35–49	105	4.5	18	1	1	3	6	9	12	20
50–64	289	5.2	29	1	2	4	7	11	14	32
65+	1,255	4.5	17	1	2	3	6	9	12	20
B. Operated										
0–19 Years	21	11.0	193	1	2	4	12	35	39	42
20–34	61	5.9	51	1	2	3	6	15	26	35
35–49	105	8.6	120	1	3	5	9	22	38	47
50–64	193	8.8	95	1	3	5	10	26	30	43
65+	195	7.9	51	2	3	6	10	16	22	44
SUBTOTALS:										
1. SINGLE DX										
A. Not Operated	30	2.0	3	1	1	1	2	5	6	8
B. Operated	76	3.1	5	1	1	3	4	6	7	12
2. MULTIPLE DX										
A. Not Operated	1,719	4.5	19	1	2	3	6	9	12	21
B. Operated	575	8.2	84	1	3	5	9	21	29	43
1. SINGLE DX	106	2.8	4	1	1	2	4	6	7	8
2. MULTIPLE DX	2,294	5.4	38	1	2	4	7	11	16	35
A. NOT OPERATED	1,749	4.5	18	1	2	3	6	9	12	21
B. OPERATED	651	7.6	77	1	2	5	9	18	28	42
TOTAL										
0–19 Years	63	5.3	84	1	1	2	4	12	35	42
20–34	126	4.4	28	1	2	3	5	8	15	28
35–49	227	6.4	69	1	2	4	7	12	25	42
50–64	517	6.4	56	1	2	4	7	14	25	36
65+	1,467	4.9	23	1	2	3	6	10	13	23
GRAND TOTAL	2,400	5.3	36	1	2	4	6	11	16	34

238.1: SFT TISS UNC BEHAV NEOPL

Type of Patients	Observed Patients	Avg. Stay	Variance	10th	25th	50th	75th	90th	95th	99th
1. SINGLE DX										
A. Not Operated										
0–19 Years	0									
20–34	1	4.0	0	4	4	4	4	4	4	4
35–49	1	3.0	0	3	3	3	3	3	3	3
50–64	1	2.0	0	2	2	2	2	2	2	2
65+	0									
B. Operated										
0–19 Years	2	1.0	0	1	1	1	1	1	1	1
20–34	12	2.5	1	2	2	3	3	4	4	4
35–49	10	4.5	5	2	2	5	7	7	7	7
50–64	16	3.4	4	1	2	3	5	7	7	7
65+	1	6.0	0	6	6	6	6	6	6	6
2. MULTIPLE DX										
A. Not Operated										
0–19 Years	1	3.0	0	3	3	3	3	3	3	3
20–34	4	1.8	<1	1	2	2	2	2	2	2
35–49	14	4.7	10	2	2	4	5	8	13	13
50–64	12	5.5	10	2	2	5	9	9	10	10
65+	30	4.4	12	2	2	3	6	9	13	14
B. Operated										
0–19 Years	4	4.8	7	2	3	7	7	7	7	7
20–34	29	4.7	11	2	3	4	6	11	11	15
35–49	49	5.9	28	1	3	5	7	11	12	30
50–64	95	5.9	14	3	3	5	9	11	14	17
65+	102	5.9	15	3	3	5	8	12	13	14
SUBTOTALS:										
1. SINGLE DX										
A. Not Operated	3	3.0	1	2	2	3	4	4	4	4
B. Operated	41	3.3	4	1	2	3	5	7	7	7
2. MULTIPLE DX										
A. Not Operated	61	4.5	10	2	2	3	6	9	10	14
B. Operated	279	5.8	16	2	3	5	7	11	13	22
1. SINGLE DX	44	3.3	4	1	2	3	5	7	7	7
2. MULTIPLE DX	340	5.5	15	2	3	5	7	11	13	17
A. NOT OPERATED	64	4.4	10	1	2	3	6	9	10	14
B. OPERATED	320	5.4	15	2	3	5	7	11	13	17
TOTAL										
0–19 Years	7	3.4	7	1	1	3	5	7	7	7
20–34	46	3.8	9	1	2	3	5	8	11	15
35–49	74	5.4	21	1	2	5	7	10	12	30
50–64	124	5.5	13	2	3	4	7	10	13	16
65+	133	5.6	14	2	2	5	7	11	13	14
GRAND TOTAL	384	5.3	15	1	2	4	7	10	13	17

238.75: MDS NOS

Type of Patients	Observed Patients	Avg. Stay	Variance	10th	25th	50th	75th	90th	95th	99th
1. SINGLE DX										
A. Not Operated										
0–19 Years	0									
20–34	0									
35–49	0									
50–64	0									
65+	0									
B. Operated										
0–19 Years	0									
20–34	0									
35–49	0									
50–64	5	1.6	2	1	1	1	1	4	4	4
65+	11	1.2	<1	1	1	1	1	2	2	2
2. MULTIPLE DX										
A. Not Operated										
0–19 Years	7	2.0	2	1	1	1	3	5	5	5
20–34	3	4.7	9	2	2	4	8	8	8	8
35–49	16	6.9	49	1	2	5	9	16	27	27
50–64	100	5.2	35	1	2	4	6	11	14	43
65+	749	4.2	15	1	2	3	6	9	12	19
B. Operated										
0–19 Years	2	37.0	8	35	35	37	39	39	39	39
20–34	2	26.0	0	26	26	26	26	26	26	26
35–49	7	33.1	179	17	21	36	42	53	53	53
50–64	19	20.5	150	7	7	23	28	35	41	41
65+	15	11.1	81	2	5	7	20	24	30	30
SUBTOTALS:										
1. SINGLE DX										
A. Not Operated	16	1.3	<1	1	1	1	1	2	4	4
B. Operated	0									
2. MULTIPLE DX										
A. Not Operated	875	4.4	18	1	2	3	6	9	12	22
B. Operated	45	20.3	181	2	7	22	28	39	41	53
1. SINGLE DX	16	1.3	<1	1	1	1	1	2	4	4
2. MULTIPLE DX	920	5.1	37	1	2	3	6	11	16	35
A. NOT OPERATED	891	4.3	17	1	2	3	6	9	12	22
B. OPERATED	45	20.3	181	2	7	22	28	39	41	53
TOTAL										
0–19 Years	9	9.8	240	1	1	2	5	39	39	39
20–34	5	13.1	140	2	4	8	26	26	26	26
35–49	23	14.9	234	1	2	9	22	41	42	53
50–64	124	7.4	82	1	2	4	7	22	28	41
65+	775	4.3	17	1	2	3	6	9	12	22
GRAND TOTAL	936	5.1	37	1	2	3	6	11	16	35

Length of Stay by Diagnosis and Operation, Western Region, 2008

Western Region, October 2006–September 2007 Data, by Diagnosis

238.79: LN UNC BEHAV NEOPL NEC

Type of Patients	Observed Patients	Avg. Stay	Variance	10th	25th	50th	75th	90th	95th	99th
1. SINGLE DX										
A. Not Operated										
0–19 Years	0									
20–34	0									
35–49	0									
50–64	0									
65+	1	5.0	0	5	5	5	5	5	5	5
B. Operated										
0–19 Years	0									
20–34	0									
35–49	0									
50–64	1	1.0	0	1	1	1	1	1	1	1
65+	0									
2. MULTIPLE DX										
A. Not Operated										
0–19 Years	12	3.8	26	1	1	1	5	11	17	17
20–34	5	3.4	4	2	2	3	3	5	7	7
35–49	12	3.3	3	1	1	3	5	5	6	6
50–64	64	5.9	37	1	2	4	7	13	20	29
65+	154	4.9	23	1	2	4	6	10	12	20
B. Operated										
0–19 Years	3	20.8	326	9	9	12	42	42	42	42
20–34	3	17.3	109	7	7	17	17	28	28	28
35–49	7	15.2	296	3	3	7	31	47	47	47
50–64	12	9.4	51	2	2	8	9	19	26	26
65+	16	14.8	182	5	5	14	26	34	50	50
SUBTOTALS:										
1. SINGLE DX										
A. Not Operated	1	5.0	0	5	5	5	5	5	5	5
B. Operated	1	1.0	0	1	1	1	1	1	1	1
2. MULTIPLE DX										
A. Not Operated	247	5.0	25	1	2	4	6	11	13	28
B. Operated	41	13.9	160	2	6	9	17	31	42	50
1. SINGLE DX	2	3.0	8	1	1	3	5	5	5	5
2. MULTIPLE DX	288	6.3	54	1	2	4	7	13	20	42
A. NOT OPERATED	248	5.0	25	1	2	4	6	11	13	28
B. OPERATED	42	13.6	160	2	5	9	17	31	42	50
TOTAL										
0–19 Years	15	7.2	116	1	1	3	11	17	17	42
20–34	8	8.6	86	2	2	5	7	28	28	28
35–49	19	7.7	134	1	2	4	6	31	47	47
50–64	77	6.4	40	1	2	4	8	15	21	29
65+	171	5.9	45	1	2	4	7	12	17	42
GRAND TOTAL	290	6.3	53	1	2	4	7	13	20	42

239: UNSPECIFIED NEOPLASM

Type of Patients	Observed Patients	Avg. Stay	Variance	10th	25th	50th	75th	90th	95th	99th
1. SINGLE DX										
A. Not Operated										
0–19 Years	2	2.0	2	1	1	2	3	3	3	3
20–34	8	2.0	4	1	1	1	2	4	6	6
35–49	5	1.8	1	1	1	1	3	3	3	3
50–64	10	1.5	<1	1	1	1	2	3	3	3
65+	2	1.5	<1	1	1	2	2	2	2	2
B. Operated										
0–19 Years	5	2.2	1	1	2	2	2	4	4	4
20–34	20	1.9	1	1	1	2	2	3	4	4
35–49	28	2.6	3	1	1	2	4	4	7	8
50–64	12	2.4	4	1	1	2	4	4	8	8
65+	9	1.6	2	1	1	1	1	5	5	5
2. MULTIPLE DX										
A. Not Operated										
0–19 Years	10	2.1	2	1	1	1	3	5	5	5
20–34	34	2.9	6	1	1	2	3	6	9	11
35–49	65	2.9	6	1	1	2	4	6	7	13
50–64	158	3.6	9	1	2	3	5	7	9	15
65+	329	4.2	11	1	2	3	6	9	11	14
B. Operated										
0–19 Years	13	4.2	21	1	1	3	3	6	18	18
20–34	37	3.2	6	1	1	3	5	6	7	13
35–49	104	4.1	9	1	2	3	5	7	10	15
50–64	194	4.2	17	1	1	3	5	8	14	20
65+	224	4.7	25	1	2	3	6	10	13	22
SUBTOTALS:										
1. SINGLE DX										
A. Not Operated	27	1.7	2	1	1	2	2	3	4	6
B. Operated	74	2.2	2	1	1	2	3	4	5	8
2. MULTIPLE DX										
A. Not Operated	596	3.8	10	1	2	3	5	8	10	14
B. Operated	572	4.3	18	1	2	3	5	9	13	21
1. SINGLE DX	101	2.1	2	1	1	2	3	4	5	8
2. MULTIPLE DX	1,168	4.0	14	1	2	3	5	8	11	19
A. NOT OPERATED	623	3.7	10	1	2	3	5	8	10	14
B. OPERATED	646	4.1	16	1	1	3	5	8	12	20
TOTAL										
0–19 Years	30	3.0	11	1	1	2	4	5	6	18
20–34	99	2.8	5	1	1	2	3	6	7	13
35–49	202	3.4	7	2	2	3	5	6	8	15
50–64	374	3.8	13	1	2	3	6	8	11	20
65+	564	4.3	16	1	2	3	6	9	12	21
GRAND TOTAL	1,269	3.9	13	1	2	3	5	8	11	18

239.0: DIGESTIVE NEOPLASM NOS

Type of Patients	Observed Patients	Avg. Stay	Variance	10th	25th	50th	75th	90th	95th	99th
1. SINGLE DX										
A. Not Operated										
0–19 Years	0									
20–34	0									
35–49	0									
50–64	2	1.5	<1	1	1	2	2	2	2	2
65+	1	2.0	0	2	2	2	2	2	2	2
B. Operated										
0–19 Years	0									
20–34	1	3.0	0	3	3	3	3	3	3	3
35–49	4	3.2	7	1	1	3	3	7	7	7
50–64	3	2.0	<1	1	1	2	3	3	3	3
65+	4	2.0	4	1	1	1	5	5	5	5
2. MULTIPLE DX										
A. Not Operated										
0–19 Years	1	2.0	0	2	2	2	2	2	2	2
20–34	3	3.0	<1	2	2	3	4	4	4	4
35–49	13	2.1	2	1	1	1	3	5	5	5
50–64	35	4.7	13	1	2	4	7	9	14	14
65+	83	4.7	15	1	2	3	7	10	13	19
B. Operated										
0–19 Years	3	4.3	4	2	2	5	6	6	6	6
20–34	3	3.7	6	1	1	4	6	6	6	6
35–49	19	5.8	9	2	4	5	7	10	15	15
50–64	58	6.3	28	1	3	5	8	15	20	22
65+	60	6.5	32	2	3	5	8	12	22	35
SUBTOTALS:										
1. SINGLE DX										
A. Not Operated	3	1.7	<1	1	1	2	2	2	2	2
B. Operated	12	2.5	4	1	1	3	3	5	7	7
2. MULTIPLE DX										
A. Not Operated	135	4.4	13	1	2	3	6	10	13	14
B. Operated	143	6.3	26	2	3	5	7	12	16	22
1. SINGLE DX	15	2.3	3	1	1	2	3	5	7	7
2. MULTIPLE DX	278	5.4	21	1	2	4	7	11	14	22
A. NOT OPERATED	138	4.4	13	1	2	3	6	10	13	14
B. OPERATED	155	6.0	25	1	3	5	7	11	16	22
TOTAL										
0–19 Years	4	3.8	4	2	2	5	5	6	6	6
20–34	7	3.3	3	1	1	3	4	6	6	6
35–49	36	4.2	9	1	1	4	6	7	10	15
50–64	98	5.5	22	2	2	4	7	14	16	22
65+	148	5.4	22	2	2	4	7	11	13	22
GRAND TOTAL	293	5.2	20	1	2	4	7	11	14	22

Length of Stay by Diagnosis and Operation, Western Region, 2008

Western Region, October 2006–September 2007 Data, by Diagnosis

239.6: BRAIN NEOPLASM NOS

Type of Patients	Observed Patients	Avg. Stay	Variance	Percentiles 10th	25th	50th	75th	90th	95th	99th
1. SINGLE DX										
A. Not Operated										
0–19 Years	1	1.0	0	1	1	1	1	1	1	1
20–34	3	1.0	0	1	1	1	1	1	1	1
35–49	4	1.5	1	1	1	1	3	3	3	3
50–64	6	1.5	<1	1	1	1	2	3	3	3
65+	0									
B. Operated										
0–19 Years	0									
20–34	5	2.6	3	1	1	2	4	5	5	5
35–49	2	2.5	4	1	1	4	4	4	4	4
50–64	1	3.0	0	3	3	3	3	3	3	3
65+	0									
2. MULTIPLE DX										
A. Not Operated										
0–19 Years	3	2.7	2	1	1	3	4	4	4	4
20–34	19	2.4	5	1	1	2	3	6	9	9
35–49	36	3.0	8	1	1	2	4	6	10	13
50–64	72	3.0	5	1	1	2	4	6	7	14
65+	115	3.9	10	1	2	3	5	7	10	12
B. Operated										
0–19 Years	2	3.5	<1	3	3	4	4	4	4	4
20–34	13	3.5	5	1	1	3	5	6	7	7
35–49	23	4.6	14	2	2	3	6	7	15	15
50–64	12	3.9	9	1	2	3	8	8	10	10
65+	15	4.7	7	3	3	4	6	9	10	10
SUBTOTALS:										
1. SINGLE DX										
A. Not Operated	14	1.4	<1	1	1	1	1	3	3	3
B. Operated	8	2.6	3	1	1	3	4	5	5	5
2. MULTIPLE DX										
A. Not Operated	245	3.4	8	1	2	2	4	7	9	13
B. Operated	65	4.2	9	1	2	3	6	8	10	15
1. SINGLE DX	22	1.8	2	1	1	1	3	4	4	5
2. MULTIPLE DX	310	3.6	8	1	2	3	5	7	9	14
A. NOT OPERATED	259	3.3	8	1	1	2	4	7	9	13
B. OPERATED	73	4.1	8	1	2	3	6	7	10	15
TOTAL										
0–19 Years	6	2.7	2	1	1	3	4	4	4	4
20–34	40	2.7	4	1	1	2	3	6	7	9
35–49	65	3.5	10	1	1	2	5	6	10	15
50–64	91	3.0	6	1	1	2	4	6	8	14
65+	130	4.0	10	1	2	3	6	7	10	12
GRAND TOTAL	332	3.5	8	1	1	3	4	7	9	14

240: SIMPLE & NOS GOITER

Type of Patients	Observed Patients	Avg. Stay	Variance	Percentiles 10th	25th	50th	75th	90th	95th	99th
1. SINGLE DX										
A. Not Operated										
0–19 Years	0									
20–34	0									
35–49	0									
50–64	1	7.0	0	7	7	7	7	7	7	7
65+	0									
B. Operated										
0–19 Years	2	1.0	0	1	1	1	1	1	1	1
20–34	14	1.6	<1	1	1	1	2	3	4	4
35–49	33	1.3	<1	1	1	1	2	2	2	3
50–64	30	1.2	<1	1	1	1	1	1	2	5
65+	6	1.5	<1	1	1	1	2	3	3	3
2. MULTIPLE DX										
A. Not Operated										
0–19 Years	0									
20–34	4	1.8	<1	1	1	1	2	3	3	3
35–49	3	1.0	0	1	1	1	1	1	1	1
50–64	13	2.3	6	1	1	1	2	4	10	10
65+	16	4.6	19	1	2	3	6	12	15	15
B. Operated										
0–19 Years	2	2.0	2	1	1	1	3	3	3	3
20–34	23	1.6	<1	1	1	1	2	2	3	4
35–49	55	1.7	<1	1	1	1	2	3	4	4
50–64	127	2.1	12	1	1	1	2	3	5	13
65+	75	2.0	3	1	1	1	2	4	5	10
SUBTOTALS:										
1. SINGLE DX										
A. Not Operated	1	7.0	0	7	7	7	7	7	7	7
B. Operated	85	1.3	<1	1	1	1	1	2	3	5
2. MULTIPLE DX										
A. Not Operated	36	3.1	12	1	1	1	4	9	12	15
B. Operated	282	2.0	7	1	1	1	2	3	4	11
1. SINGLE DX	86	1.4	<1	1	1	1	1	2	3	7
2. MULTIPLE DX	318	2.1	7	1	1	1	2	4	5	12
A. NOT OPERATED	37	3.2	12	1	1	1	4	9	12	15
B. OPERATED	367	1.8	5	1	1	1	2	3	4	10
TOTAL										
0–19 Years	4	1.5	<1	1	1	1	1	3	3	3
20–34	41	1.6	<1	1	1	1	2	3	3	4
35–49	91	1.5	<1	1	1	1	2	3	3	4
50–64	171	2.0	10	1	1	1	2	3	5	13
65+	97	2.4	6	1	1	1	3	5	9	15
GRAND TOTAL	404	1.9	6	1	1	1	2	3	5	11

240.9: GOITER NOS

Type of Patients	Observed Patients	Avg. Stay	Variance	Percentiles 10th	25th	50th	75th	90th	95th	99th
1. SINGLE DX										
A. Not Operated										
0–19 Years	0									
20–34	0									
35–49	0									
50–64	1	7.0	0	7	7	7	7	7	7	7
65+	0									
B. Operated										
0–19 Years	2	1.0	0	1	1	1	1	1	1	1
20–34	14	1.6	<1	1	1	1	2	3	4	4
35–49	33	1.3	<1	1	1	1	2	2	2	3
50–64	29	1.2	<1	1	1	1	1	1	2	5
65+	6	1.5	<1	1	1	1	2	3	3	3
2. MULTIPLE DX										
A. Not Operated										
0–19 Years	0									
20–34	4	1.8	<1	1	1	1	2	3	3	3
35–49	3	1.0	0	1	1	1	1	1	1	1
50–64	13	2.3	6	1	1	1	2	4	10	10
65+	16	4.6	19	1	2	3	6	12	15	15
B. Operated										
0–19 Years	2	2.0	2	1	1	1	3	3	3	3
20–34	23	1.6	<1	1	1	1	2	2	3	4
35–49	55	1.7	<1	1	1	1	2	3	4	4
50–64	126	2.1	12	1	1	1	2	3	5	13
65+	74	2.0	3	1	1	1	2	4	5	10
SUBTOTALS:										
1. SINGLE DX										
A. Not Operated	1	7.0	0	7	7	7	7	7	7	7
B. Operated	84	1.3	<1	1	1	1	1	2	3	5
2. MULTIPLE DX										
A. Not Operated	36	3.1	12	1	1	1	4	9	12	15
B. Operated	280	2.0	7	1	1	1	2	3	4	11
1. SINGLE DX	85	1.4	<1	1	1	1	1	2	3	7
2. MULTIPLE DX	316	2.1	7	1	1	1	2	4	5	12
A. NOT OPERATED	37	3.2	12	1	1	1	4	9	12	15
B. OPERATED	364	1.8	5	1	1	1	2	3	4	10
TOTAL										
0–19 Years	4	1.5	<1	1	1	1	1	3	3	3
20–34	41	1.6	<1	1	1	1	2	3	3	4
35–49	91	1.5	<1	1	1	1	2	3	3	4
50–64	169	2.0	10	1	1	1	2	3	5	13
65+	96	2.4	6	1	1	1	3	5	9	15
GRAND TOTAL	401	1.9	6	1	1	1	2	3	5	11

Length of Stay by Diagnosis and Operation, Western Region, 2008

Western Region, October 2006–September 2007 Data, by Diagnosis

241: NONTOXIC NODULAR GOITER

Type of Patients	Observed Patients	Avg. Stay	Vari- ance	Percentiles 10th	25th	50th	75th	90th	95th	99th
1. SINGLE DX										
A. Not Operated										
0–19 Years	0									
20–34	1	2.0	0	2	2	2	2	2	2	2
35–49	0									
50–64	1	1.0	0	1	1	1	1	1	1	1
65+	1	2.0	0	2	2	2	2	2	2	2
B. Operated										
0–19 Years	16	1.1	<1	1	1	1	1	2	2	2
20–34	152	1.1	<1	1	1	1	1	2	2	2
35–49	273	1.2	<1	1	1	1	1	2	2	3
50–64	270	1.3	<1	1	1	1	2	2	2	3
65+	53	1.2	<1	1	1	1	1	2	2	4
2. MULTIPLE DX										
A. Not Operated										
0–19 Years	3	1.7	1	1	1	1	3	3	3	3
20–34	12	3.2	7	1	1	2	6	7	7	7
35–49	22	2.4	4	1	1	1	4	6	7	7
50–64	39	3.0	5	1	1	3	4	6	8	10
B. Operated										
0–19 Years	13	1.7	<1	1	1	1	2	3	4	4
20–34	207	1.6	<1	1	1	1	2	3	3	5
35–49	662	1.6	2	1	1	1	2	3	3	6
50–64	1,192	1.6	8	1	1	1	2	2	3	7
65+	745	1.9	5	1	1	1	2	3	4	12
SUBTOTALS:										
1. SINGLE DX										
A. Not Operated	3	1.7	<1	1	1	2	1	2	2	2
B. Operated	764	1.2	<1	1	1	1	1	2	2	3
2. MULTIPLE DX										
A. Not Operated	76	2.8	5	1	1	2	4	6	7	10
B. Operated	2,819	1.7	5	1	1	1	2	3	4	8
1. SINGLE DX	767	1.2	<1	1	1	1	1	2	2	3
2. MULTIPLE DX	2,895	1.7	5	1	1	1	2	3	4	8
A. NOT OPERATED	79	2.8	5	1	1	2	4	6	7	10
B. OPERATED	3,583	1.6	4	1	1	1	2	2	3	7
TOTAL										
0–19 Years	29	1.3	<1	1	1	1	1	2	3	4
20–34	363	1.4	<1	1	1	1	2	2	3	5
35–49	947	1.5	2	1	1	1	2	2	3	6
50–64	1,485	1.6	6	1	1	1	2	2	3	6
65+	838	1.9	5	1	1	1	2	3	4	10
GRAND TOTAL	3,662	1.6	4	1	1	1	2	2	3	7

241.0: NONTOXIC UNINOD GOITER

Type of Patients	Observed Patients	Avg. Stay	Vari- ance	Percentiles 10th	25th	50th	75th	90th	95th	99th
1. SINGLE DX										
A. Not Operated										
0–19 Years	0									
20–34	1	2.0	0	2	2	2	2	2	2	2
35–49	0									
50–64	0									
65+	0									
B. Operated										
0–19 Years	12	1.0	0	1	1	1	1	1	1	1
20–34	83	1.1	<1	1	1	1	1	1	2	2
35–49	118	1.1	<1	1	1	1	1	2	2	2
50–64	97	1.2	<1	1	1	1	1	2	2	4
65+	17	1.1	<1	1	1	1	1	2	2	2
2. MULTIPLE DX										
A. Not Operated										
0–19 Years	0									
20–34	3	1.7	1	1	1	1	3	3	3	3
35–49	2	2.5	4	1	1	2	4	4	4	4
50–64	7	2.4	5	1	1	1	4	7	7	7
65+	16	3.4	6	1	1	3	4	7	10	10
B. Operated										
0–19 Years	5	1.2	<1	1	1	1	1	2	2	2
20–34	76	1.2	<1	1	1	1	1	2	2	3
35–49	203	1.3	<1	1	1	1	1	2	3	5
50–64	348	1.3	<1	1	1	1	1	2	2	5
65+	189	1.5	2	1	1	1	2	2	3	9
SUBTOTALS:										
1. SINGLE DX										
A. Not Operated	1	2.0	0	2	2	2	2	2	2	2
B. Operated	327	1.1	<1	1	1	1	1	2	2	2
2. MULTIPLE DX										
A. Not Operated	28	2.9	5	1	1	3	4	7	7	10
B. Operated	821	1.3	<1	1	1	1	1	2	3	5
1. SINGLE DX	328	1.1	<1	1	1	1	1	2	2	2
2. MULTIPLE DX	849	1.4	<1	1	1	1	1	2	3	5
A. NOT OPERATED	29	2.9	5	1	1	3	4	7	7	10
B. OPERATED	1,148	1.3	<1	1	1	1	1	2	2	4
TOTAL										
0–19 Years	17	1.1	<1	1	1	1	1	1	2	2
20–34	163	1.2	<1	1	1	1	1	2	2	3
35–49	323	1.2	<1	1	1	1	2	2	2	4
50–64	452	1.3	<1	1	1	1	1	2	2	5
65+	222	1.6	2	1	1	1	2	3	4	9
GRAND TOTAL	1,177	1.3	<1	1	1	1	1	2	3	5

241.1: NONTOXIC MULTINOD GOITER

Type of Patients	Observed Patients	Avg. Stay	Vari- ance	Percentiles 10th	25th	50th	75th	90th	95th	99th
1. SINGLE DX										
A. Not Operated										
0–19 Years	0									
20–34	0									
35–49	0									
50–64	1	1.0	0	1	1	1	1	1	1	1
65+	1	2.0	0	2	2	2	2	2	2	2
B. Operated										
0–19 Years	3	1.3	<1	1	1	1	2	2	2	2
20–34	58	1.2	<1	1	1	1	1	2	2	3
35–49	138	1.3	<1	1	1	1	2	2	2	3
50–64	153	1.3	<1	1	1	1	2	2	2	3
65+	32	1.3	<1	1	1	1	1	2	2	4
2. MULTIPLE DX										
A. Not Operated										
0–19 Years	0									
20–34	0									
35–49	10	3.3	8	1	1	2	6	7	7	7
50–64	12	2.2	4	1	1	1	2	5	7	7
65+	21	2.5	4	1	1	2	3	5	6	8
B. Operated										
0–19 Years	8	2.0	1	1	1	2	2	4	4	4
20–34	120	1.8	1	1	1	1	2	3	5	6
35–49	423	1.8	3	1	1	1	2	3	4	8
50–64	779	1.8	12	1	1	1	2	3	3	7
65+	505	2.0	7	1	1	1	2	3	5	14
SUBTOTALS:										
1. SINGLE DX										
A. Not Operated	2	1.5	<1	1	1	2	2	2	2	2
B. Operated	384	1.3	1	1	1	1	1	2	2	3
2. MULTIPLE DX										
A. Not Operated	43	2.6	5	1	1	2	4	6	7	8
B. Operated	1,835	1.8	8	1	1	1	2	3	4	9
1. SINGLE DX	386	1.3	<1	1	1	1	1	2	2	3
2. MULTIPLE DX	1,878	1.9	7	1	1	1	2	3	4	9
A. NOT OPERATED	45	2.5	4	1	1	2	3	6	7	8
B. OPERATED	2,219	1.7	6	1	1	1	2	3	4	8
TOTAL										
0–19 Years	11	1.8	<1	1	1	1	2	3	4	4
20–34	178	1.6	1	1	1	1	2	3	4	6
35–49	571	1.7	3	1	1	1	2	3	4	7
50–64	945	1.7	10	1	1	1	2	3	3	7
65+	559	2.0	6	1	1	1	2	3	5	14
GRAND TOTAL	2,264	1.8	6	1	1	1	2	3	4	8

Length of Stay by Diagnosis and Operation, Western Region, 2008

Western Region, October 2006–September 2007 Data, by Diagnosis

241.9: NONTOXIC NOD GOITER NOS

Type of Patients	Observed Patients	Avg. Stay	Variance	Percentiles 10th	25th	50th	75th	90th	95th	99th
1. SINGLE DX										
A. Not Operated										
0–19 Years	0									
20–34	0									
35–49	0									
50–64	0									
65+	0									
B. Operated										
0–19 Years	1	1.0	0						1	1
20–34	11	1.1	<1	1	1	1	1	1	2	2
35–49	17	1.1	<1	1	1	1	1	1	2	2
50–64	20	1.2	<1	1	1	1	1	2	3	3
65+	4	1.5	<1	1	1	2	2	2	2	2
2. MULTIPLE DX										
A. Not Operated										
0–19 Years	0									
20–34	0									
35–49	0									
50–64	3	3.3	6	1	1	3	6	6	6	6
65+	2	5.0	2	4	4	6	6	6	6	6
B. Operated										
0–19 Years	0									
20–34	11	1.7	<1	1	1	2	2	3	3	3
35–49	36	1.2	<1	1	1	1	1	1	3	6
50–64	65	1.5	1	1	1	1	2	2	3	8
65+	51	1.9	6	1	1	1	2	2	3	16
SUBTOTALS:										
1. SINGLE DX										
A. Not Operated	0									
B. Operated	53	1.1	<1	1	1	1	1	2	2	3
2. MULTIPLE DX										
A. Not Operated	5	4.0	5	1	3	4	6	6	6	6
B. Operated	163	1.6	3	1	1	1	2	2	3	10
1. SINGLE DX	53	1.1	<1	1	1	1	1	2	2	3
2. MULTIPLE DX	168	1.7	3	1	1	1	2	3	4	10
A. NOT OPERATED	5	4.0	5	1	3	4	6	6	6	6
B. OPERATED	216	1.5	2	1	1	1	2	2	3	8
TOTAL										
0–19 Years	1	1.0	0	1	1	1	1	1	1	1
20–34	22	1.4	<1	1	1	1	2	2	3	3
35–49	53	1.2	<1	1	1	1	1	1	2	6
50–64	88	1.5	1	1	1	1	2	2	3	8
65+	57	2.0	6	1	1	1	2	3	6	16
GRAND TOTAL	221	1.5	2	1	1	1	2	2	3	8

242: THYROTOXICOSIS

Type of Patients	Observed Patients	Avg. Stay	Variance	Percentiles 10th	25th	50th	75th	90th	95th	99th
1. SINGLE DX										
A. Not Operated										
0–19 Years	6	1.2	<1	1	1	1	1	2	2	2
20–34	9	2.1	3	1	1	1	3	6	6	6
35–49	13	2.2	2	1	1	2	3	4	6	6
50–64	4	1.8	<1	1	2	2	2	2	2	2
65+	0									
B. Operated										
0–19 Years	7	1.6	<1	1	1	1	2	3	3	3
20–34	39	1.5	<1	1	1	1	2	2	3	3
35–49	40	1.6	<1	1	1	1	2	3	4	4
50–64	30	1.3	<1	1	1	1	1	2	3	3
65+	7	1.7	1	1	1	1	2	4	4	4
2. MULTIPLE DX										
A. Not Operated										
0–19 Years	30	2.3	3	1	1	2	3	4	5	8
20–34	282	2.7	6	1	1	2	3	5	7	13
35–49	287	3.3	7	1	1	3	4	7	9	13
50–64	249	3.6	10	1	2	3	5	6	8	21
65+	205	3.9	8	1	2	3	5	7	9	13
B. Operated										
0–19 Years	11	2.3	2	1	1	2	3	4	5	5
20–34	105	2.6	6	1	1	2	3	5	9	12
35–49	155	2.0	5	1	1	1	2	3	5	13
50–64	199	2.2	37	1	1	1	2	3	5	14
65+	95	2.2	9	1	1	1	2	3	9	19
SUBTOTALS:										
1. SINGLE DX										
A. Not Operated	32	1.9	2	1	1	2	2	3	6	6
B. Operated	123	1.5	<1	1	1	1	2	2	3	4
2. MULTIPLE DX										
A. Not Operated	1,053	3.3	8	1	1	2	4	6	8	13
B. Operated	565	2.2	17	1	1	1	2	4	5	15
1. SINGLE DX	155	1.6	<1	1	1	1	2	3	3	6
2. MULTIPLE DX	1,618	2.9	11	1	1	2	4	6	8	13
A. NOT OPERATED	1,085	3.3	8	1	1	2	4	6	8	13
B. OPERATED	688	2.1	14	1	1	1	2	3	5	14
TOTAL										
0–19 Years	54	2.1	2	1	1	2	3	4	5	8
20–34	435	2.6	6	1	1	2	3	5	7	12
35–49	495	2.7	6	1	1	2	3	6	8	13
50–64	482	2.9	21	1	1	2	3	5	7	21
65+	307	3.3	9	1	1	2	4	7	9	14
GRAND TOTAL	1,773	2.8	11	1	1	2	3	6	8	13

242.00: TOX DIF GOITER W/O CRIS

Type of Patients	Observed Patients	Avg. Stay	Variance	Percentiles 10th	25th	50th	75th	90th	95th	99th
1. SINGLE DX										
A. Not Operated										
0–19 Years	5	1.2	<1	1	1	1	1	2	2	2
20–34	4	1.5	1	1	1	1	3	3	3	3
35–49	6	2.7	<1	2	2	2	3	4	4	4
50–64	1	2.0	0	2	2	2	2	2	2	2
65+	0									
B. Operated										
0–19 Years	5	1.6	<1	1	1	1	2	3	3	3
20–34	22	1.6	<1	1	1	2	2	2	3	3
35–49	23	1.6	<1	1	1	1	2	2	3	4
50–64	16	1.3	<1	1	1	1	1	2	3	3
65+	2	2.5	4					4	4	4
2. MULTIPLE DX										
A. Not Operated										
0–19 Years	9	2.3	2	1	1	2	4	5	5	5
20–34	81	2.9	4	1	1	2	4	5	8	10
35–49	81	3.2	6	1	1	2	4	6	8	13
50–64	60	4.2	22	1	2	3	5	8	12	28
65+	22	4.3	6	2	3	4	5	5	9	13
B. Operated										
0–19 Years	9	2.1	1	1	1	2	3	4	4	4
20–34	63	2.5	4	1	1	2	3	5	7	9
35–49	71	2.0	7	1	1	1	2	4	5	21
50–64	78	1.6	1	1	1	1	2	3	4	7
65+	23	1.5	<1	1	1	1	2	2	4	3
SUBTOTALS:										
1. SINGLE DX										
A. Not Operated	16	1.9	<1	1	1	2	2	3	4	4
B. Operated	68	1.6	<1	1	1	1	2	3	3	4
2. MULTIPLE DX										
A. Not Operated	253	3.4	9	1	2	3	4	6	8	13
B. Operated	244	2.0	4	1	1	1	2	4	5	9
1. SINGLE DX	84	1.6	<1	1	1	1	2	3	3	4
2. MULTIPLE DX	497	2.7	7	1	1	2	3	5	7	13
A. NOT OPERATED	269	3.3	9	1	1	2	4	6	8	13
B. OPERATED	312	1.9	3	1	1	1	2	3	5	8
TOTAL										
0–19 Years	28	1.9	1	1	1	2	2	3	4	5
20–34	170	2.5	4	1	1	2	3	5	7	10
35–49	181	2.5	6	1	1	2	3	5	6	13
50–64	155	2.6	11	1	1	2	3	5	7	23
65+	47	2.9	5	1	1	2	4	5	5	13
GRAND TOTAL	581	2.5	6	1	1	2	3	5	7	12

Length of Stay by Diagnosis and Operation, Western Region, 2008

Western Region, October 2006–September 2007 Data, by Diagnosis

242.20: TOX MULTINOD GOIT S CRIS

Type of Patients	Observed Patients	Avg. Stay	Vari-ance	10th	25th	50th	75th	90th	95th	99th
1. SINGLE DX										
A. Not Operated										
0–19 Years	0									
20–34	0									
35–49	0									
50–64	0									
65+	0									
B. Operated										
0–19 Years	0									
20–34	9	1.3	<1	1	1	1	1	3	3	3
35–49	7	1.6	1	1	1	1	2	4	4	4
50–64	9	1.3	<1	1	1	1	1	3	3	3
65+	3	1.3	<1	1	1	1	2	2	2	2
2. MULTIPLE DX										
A. Not Operated										
0–19 Years	0									
20–34	3	3.7	14	1	1	2	8	8	8	8
35–49	7	3.7	15	1	1	3	4	12	12	12
50–64	6	4.2	3	1	3	5	5	6	6	6
65+	16	4.3	7	1	2	5	6	8	10	10
B. Operated										
0–19 Years	0	1.0	0	1	1	1	1	1	1	1
20–34	17	1.8	1	1	1	1	2	4	5	5
35–49	43	1.6	<1	1	1	1	2	3	3	3
50–64	76	1.6	<1	1	1	1	2	2	3	3
65+	49	1.9	7	1	1	1	2	3	4	19
SUBTOTALS:										
1. SINGLE DX										
A. Not Operated	0									
B. Operated	28	1.4	<1	1	1	1	1	3	3	4
2. MULTIPLE DX										
A. Not Operated	32	4.1	8	1	2	3	6	8	10	12
B. Operated	186	1.7	2	1	1	1	2	3	4	6
1. SINGLE DX	28	1.4	<1	1	1	1	1	3	3	4
2. MULTIPLE DX	218	2.0	4	1	1	1	2	4	5	10
A. NOT OPERATED	32	4.1	8	1	2	3	6	8	10	12
B. OPERATED	214	1.6	2	1	1	1	2	3	4	5
TOTAL										
0–19 Years	1	1.0	0	1	1	1	1	1	1	1
20–34	29	1.8	2	1	1	1	2	4	5	8
35–49	57	1.9	3	1	1	1	2	3	4	12
50–64	91	1.7	1	1	1	1	2	3	5	6
65+	68	2.4	8	1	1	1	2	5	7	19
GRAND TOTAL	246	2.0	4	1	1	1	2	4	5	10

242.90: THYROTOX NOS W/O CRISIS

Type of Patients	Observed Patients	Avg. Stay	Vari-ance	10th	25th	50th	75th	90th	95th	99th
1. SINGLE DX										
A. Not Operated										
0–19 Years	1	1.0	0	1	1	1	1	1	1	1
20–34	2	1.0	0	1	1	1	1	1	1	1
35–49	5	1.2	<1	1	1	1	1	2	2	2
50–64	2	1.5	<1	1	1	2	2	2	2	2
65+	0									
B. Operated										
0–19 Years	1	1.0	0	1	1	1	1	1	1	1
20–34	3	1.7	<1	1	1	2	2	2	2	2
35–49	5	1.4	<1	1	1	1	1	3	3	3
50–64	2	1.0	0	1	1	1	1	1	1	1
65+	1	2.0	0	2	2	2	2	2	2	2
2. MULTIPLE DX										
A. Not Operated										
0–19 Years	12	2.3	5	1	1	2	3	5	8	8
20–34	90	2.3	3	1	1	2	3	4	6	12
35–49	116	2.7	4	1	1	2	4	6	7	9
50–64	115	3.1	5	1	2	2	4	6	7	11
65+	103	3.8	7	1	2	3	5	7	9	13
B. Operated										
0–19 Years	1	5.0	0	5	5	5	5	5	5	5
20–34	8	2.6	7	1	1	2	3	9	9	9
35–49	14	3.0	14	1	1	1	2	10	13	13
50–64	17	2.0	10	1	1	1	1	2	14	14
65+	4	9.0	14	4	4	9	13	13	13	13
SUBTOTALS:										
1. SINGLE DX										
A. Not Operated	10	1.2	<1	1	1	1	1	2	2	2
B. Operated	12	1.4	<1	1	1	1	2	2	3	3
2. MULTIPLE DX										
A. Not Operated	436	3.0	5	1	1	2	4	6	7	11
B. Operated	44	3.1	14	1	1	1	3	10	13	14
1. SINGLE DX	22	1.3	<1	1	1	1	2	2	2	3
2. MULTIPLE DX	480	3.0	6	1	1	2	4	6	8	13
A. NOT OPERATED	446	2.9	5	1	1	2	4	6	7	11
B. OPERATED	56	2.8	12	1	1	1	2	9	13	14
TOTAL										
0–19 Years	15	2.3	4	1	1	2	3	5	8	8
20–34	103	2.3	3	1	1	2	2	4	6	10
35–49	140	2.7	5	1	1	2	4	6	7	10
50–64	136	2.9	5	1	1	2	4	5	7	12
65+	108	3.9	9	1	2	3	5	8	11	13
GRAND TOTAL	502	2.9	6	1	1	2	4	6	8	13

243: CONG HYPOTHYROIDISM

Type of Patients	Observed Patients	Avg. Stay	Vari-ance	10th	25th	50th	75th	90th	95th	99th
1. SINGLE DX										
A. Not Operated										
0–19 Years	3	1.3	<1	1	1	1	2	2	2	2
20–34	0									
35–49	0									
50–64	0									
65+	0									
B. Operated										
0–19 Years	0									
20–34	0									
35–49	0									
50–64	0									
65+	0									
2. MULTIPLE DX										
A. Not Operated										
0–19 Years	8	4.1	9	1	2	2	5	9	9	9
20–34	1	1.0	0	1	1	1	1	1	1	1
35–49	0									
50–64	0									
65+	0									
B. Operated										
0–19 Years	0									
20–34	0									
35–49	0									
50–64	0									
65+	0									
SUBTOTALS:										
1. SINGLE DX										
A. Not Operated	3	1.3	<1	1	1	1	2	2	2	2
B. Operated	0									
2. MULTIPLE DX										
A. Not Operated	9	3.8	9	1	2	2	5	9	9	9
B. Operated	0									
1. SINGLE DX	3	1.3	<1	1	1	1	2	2	2	2
2. MULTIPLE DX	9	3.8	9	1	2	2	5	9	9	9
A. NOT OPERATED	12	3.2	8	1	1	2	4	8	9	9
B. OPERATED	0									
TOTAL										
0–19 Years	11	3.4	8	1	1	2	5	8	9	9
20–34	1	1.0	0	1	1	1	1	1	1	1
35–49	0									
50–64	0									
65+	0									
GRAND TOTAL	12	3.2	8	1	1	2	4	8	9	9

Length of Stay by Diagnosis and Operation, Western Region, 2008

Western Region, October 2006–September 2007 Data, by Diagnosis

244: ACQUIRED HYPOTHYROIDISM

Type of Patients	Observed Patients	Avg. Stay	Vari-ance	10th	25th	50th	75th	90th	95th	99th
1. SINGLE DX										
A. *Not Operated*										
0–19 Years	0									
20–34	3	1.3	<1	1	1	1	2	2	2	2
35–49	2	2.0	2	1	1	1	3	3	3	3
50–64	0									
65+	0									
B. *Operated*										
0–19 Years	0									
20–34	2	4.5	12	2	2	2	7	7	7	7
35–49	0									
50–64	0									
65+	0									
2. MULTIPLE DX										
A. *Not Operated*										
0–19 Years	3	3.7	21	1	1	1	9	9	9	9
20–34	43	3.7	9	1	2	3	4	7	9	16
35–49	129	2.6	5	1	1	2	3	5	6	13
50–64	210	4.4	32	1	2	3	5	8	13	30
65+	436	4.5	12	1	2	4	6	8	11	19
B. *Operated*										
0–19 Years	0									
20–34	3	13.4	65	4	4	17	19	19	19	19
35–49	6	3.3	23	1	1	3	3	13	13	13
50–64	6	6.5	54	1	1	2	12	19	19	19
65+	6	7.4	35	1	3	8	11	17	17	17
SUBTOTALS:										
1. SINGLE DX										
A. *Not Operated*	5	1.6	<1	1	1	1	2	2	2	3
B. *Operated*	2	4.5	12	2	2	2	7	7	7	7
2. MULTIPLE DX										
A. *Not Operated*	821	4.1	16	1	2	3	5	8	11	22
B. *Operated*	21	6.8	45	2	1	4	12	17	19	19
1. SINGLE DX	7	2.4	5	1	1	2	3	7	7	7
2. MULTIPLE DX	842	4.2	17	1	2	3	5	8	12	22
A. NOT OPERATED	826	4.1	16	1	2	3	5	8	11	22
B. OPERATED	23	6.6	42	1	1	4	12	17	19	19
TOTAL										
0–19 Years	3	3.7	21	1	1	1	9	9	9	9
20–34	51	4.2	16	1	2	3	6	8	16	19
35–49	137	2.6	6	1	1	2	3	5	7	13
50–64	216	4.4	33	1	2	3	5	8	13	30
65+	442	4.5	13	1	2	4	6	8	11	19
GRAND TOTAL	849	4.2	17	1	2	3	5	8	12	22

244.9: HYPOTHYROIDISM NOS

Type of Patients	Observed Patients	Avg. Stay	Vari-ance	10th	25th	50th	75th	90th	95th	99th
1. SINGLE DX										
A. *Not Operated*										
0–19 Years	0									
20–34	3	1.3	<1	1	1	1	1	2	2	2
35–49	2	2.0	2	1	1	1	3	3	3	3
50–64	0									
65+	0									
B. *Operated*										
0–19 Years	0									
20–34	1	7.0	0	7	7	7	7	7	7	7
35–49	0									
50–64	0									
65+	0									
2. MULTIPLE DX										
A. *Not Operated*										
0–19 Years	3	3.7	21	1	1	1	9	9	9	9
20–34	29	3.8	11	1	2	3	4	7	9	16
35–49	83	2.5	4	1	1	2	3	5	6	13
50–64	162	4.2	22	1	2	3	5	8	13	30
65+	369	4.4	11	1	2	3	6	8	11	17
B. *Operated*										
0–19 Years	0									
20–34	2	10.5	83	4	4	17	17	17	17	17
35–49	4	4.0	36	1	1	1	3	13	13	13
50–64	5	4.0	21	1	1	2	12	19	19	19
65+	6	7.4	35	1	3	8	11	17	17	17
SUBTOTALS:										
1. SINGLE DX										
A. *Not Operated*	5	1.6	<1	1	1	1	2	3	3	3
B. *Operated*	1	7.0	0	7	7	7	7	7	7	7
2. MULTIPLE DX										
A. *Not Operated*	646	4.1	13	1	2	3	5	8	11	19
B. *Operated*	17	6.0	34	1	1	4	11	17	17	17
1. SINGLE DX	6	2.5	5	1	1	1	3	3	7	7
2. MULTIPLE DX	663	4.1	14	1	2	3	5	8	11	19
A. NOT OPERATED	651	4.1	13	1	2	3	5	8	11	19
B. OPERATED	18	6.0	32	1	2	4	11	17	11	17
TOTAL										
0–19 Years	3	3.7	21	1	1	1	9	9	9	9
20–34	35	4.1	15	1	2	3	4	9	16	17
35–49	89	2.5	5	1	1	2	3	5	7	13
50–64	167	4.2	22	1	2	3	5	8	13	30
65+	375	4.4	11	1	2	3	6	8	11	17
GRAND TOTAL	669	4.1	14	1	2	3	5	8	11	19

245: THYROIDITIS

Type of Patients	Observed Patients	Avg. Stay	Vari-ance	10th	25th	50th	75th	90th	95th	99th
1. SINGLE DX										
A. *Not Operated*										
0–19 Years	0									
20–34	0									
35–49	0									
50–64	0									
65+	0									
B. *Operated*										
0–19 Years	2	2.0	0	2	2	2	2	2	2	2
20–34	13	1.1	<1	1	1	1	1	1	2	2
35–49	31	1.3	<1	1	1	1	1	2	3	3
50–64	29	1.2	<1	1	1	1	1	2	2	3
65+	7	1.3	<1	1	1	1	2	2	2	2
2. MULTIPLE DX										
A. *Not Operated*										
0–19 Years	4	5.3	17	1	4	4	5	11	11	11
20–34	15	3.7	9	1	2	3	4	9	13	13
35–49	12	3.2	9	1	2	3	4	5	9	9
50–64	14	6.6	72	3	3	4	5	11	35	35
65+	9	4.6	9	3	3	4	6	10	10	10
B. *Operated*										
0–19 Years	6	2.5	3	1	1	2	3	6	6	6
20–34	45	2.4	5	1	1	2	2	2	6	10
35–49	144	1.7	1	1	1	1	2	2	4	11
50–64	160	1.6	2	1	1	1	2	3	4	8
65+	65	2.0	7	1	1	1	2	4	6	16
SUBTOTALS:										
1. SINGLE DX										
A. *Not Operated*	0									
B. *Operated*	82	1.2	<1	1	1	1	1	2	2	3
2. MULTIPLE DX										
A. *Not Operated*	54	4.6	25	1	2	3	5	9	11	35
B. *Operated*	420	1.8	3	1	1	1	2	3	5	11
1. SINGLE DX	82	1.2	<1	1	1	1	1	2	2	3
2. MULTIPLE DX	474	2.1	7	1	1	1	3	4	6	11
A. NOT OPERATED	54	4.6	25	1	2	3	5	9	11	35
B. OPERATED	502	1.7	3	1	1	1	2	3	4	10
TOTAL										
0–19 Years	12	3.3	8	1	2	2	4	6	11	11
20–34	73	2.4	5	1	1	2	3	5	8	13
35–49	187	1.7	3	1	1	1	2	3	4	11
50–64	203	1.9	8	1	1	1	2	3	4	11
65+	81	2.3	7	1	2	1	2	5	8	16
GRAND TOTAL	556	2.0	6	1	1	1	2	4	6	11

Length of Stay by Diagnosis and Operation, Western Region, 2008

Western Region, October 2006–September 2007 Data, by Diagnosis

245.2: CHR LYMPHOCYT THYROIDIT

Type of Patients	Observed Patients	Avg. Stay	Vari-ance	Percentiles						
				10th	25th	50th	75th	90th	95th	99th
1. SINGLE DX										
A. Not Operated										
0–19 Years	0									
20–34	0									
35–49	0									
50–64	0									
65+	0									
B. Operated										
0–19 Years	2	2.0	0	2	2	2	2	2	2	2
20–34	10	1.1	<1	1	1	1	1	2	2	2
35–49	26	1.2	<1	1	1	1	1	2	2	3
50–64	28	1.2	<1	1	1	1	1	2	3	3
65+	6	1.3	<1	1	1	1	2	2	2	2
2. MULTIPLE DX										
A. Not Operated										
0–19 Years	2	7.5	24	4	4	4	11	11	11	11
20–34	9	4.0	15	1	2	3	4	13	13	13
35–49	4	3.0	2	1	3	4	4	4	4	4
50–64	6	10.0	159	3	3	4	11	35	35	35
65+	2	9.0	2	8	8	10	10	10	10	10
B. Operated										
0–19 Years	5	1.8	<1	1	1	2	2	3	3	3
20–34	42	2.2	4	1	1	2	2	5	7	9
35–49	128	1.7	3	1	1	1	2	2	4	6
50–64	138	1.7	2	1	1	1	2	3	4	8
65+	56	2.2	7	1	1	1	2	4	10	16
SUBTOTALS:										
1. SINGLE DX										
A. Not Operated	0									
B. Operated	72	1.2	<1	1	1	1	1	2	2	3
2. MULTIPLE DX										
A. Not Operated	23	6.1	52	1	3	4	8	11	13	35
B. Operated	369	1.8	3	1	1	1	2	3	5	11
1. SINGLE DX	72	1.2	<1	1	1	1	1	2	2	3
2. MULTIPLE DX	392	2.1	7	1	1	1	2	4	6	13
A. NOT OPERATED	23	6.1	52	1	3	4	8	11	13	35
B. OPERATED	441	1.7	3	1	1	1	2	3	4	10
TOTAL										
0–19 Years	9	3.1	10	1	2	2	2	11	11	11
20–34	61	2.3	5	1	1	2	2	5	7	13
35–49	158	1.7	3	1	1	1	2	3	4	6
50–64	172	1.9	9	1	1	1	2	3	4	11
65+	64	2.3	8	1	1	2	2	5	10	16
GRAND TOTAL	464	2.0	6	1	1	1	2	3	5	11

246: OTH DISORDERS OF THYROID

Type of Patients	Observed Patients	Avg. Stay	Vari-ance	Percentiles						
				10th	25th	50th	75th	90th	95th	99th
1. SINGLE DX										
A. Not Operated										
0–19 Years	0									
20–34	1	1.0	0	1	1	1	1	1	1	1
35–49	0									
50–64	0									
65+	0									
B. Operated										
0–19 Years	3	1.3	<1	1	1	2	2	2	2	2
20–34	16	1.3	<1	1	1	1	1	2	2	3
35–49	29	1.2	<1	1	1	1	1	2	2	3
50–64	26	1.2	<1	1	1	1	1	2	2	3
65+	8	1.1	<1	1	1	1	2	2	2	2
2. MULTIPLE DX										
A. Not Operated										
0–19 Years	0									
20–34	3	1.3	<1	1	1	1	2	2	2	2
35–49	8	3.8	24	1	1	2	4	14	14	14
50–64	13	3.0	5	1	2	3	5	5	9	9
65+	10	3.3	10	1	2	3	5	11	11	11
B. Operated										
0–19 Years	5	1.4	<1	1	1	1	2	2	2	2
20–34	21	1.4	<1	1	1	1	2	2	2	5
35–49	50	1.6	3	1	1	1	1	2	3	13
50–64	76	1.3	<1	1	1	1	1	2	2	5
65+	35	1.6	2	1	1	1	2	2	6	7
SUBTOTALS:										
1. SINGLE DX										
A. Not Operated	1	1.0	0	1	1	1	1	1	1	1
B. Operated	82	1.2	<1	1	1	1	1	2	2	3
2. MULTIPLE DX										
A. Not Operated	34	3.1	10	1	1	2	4	9	11	14
B. Operated	187	1.5	2	1	1	1	2	2	3	7
1. SINGLE DX	83	1.2	<1	1	1	1	1	2	2	3
2. MULTIPLE DX	221	1.7	3	1	1	1	2	3	5	11
A. NOT OPERATED	35	3.1	10	1	1	2	4	9	11	14
B. OPERATED	269	1.4	1	1	1	1	1	2	3	6
TOTAL										
0–19 Years	8	1.4	<1	1	1	1	2	2	2	2
20–34	41	1.4	<1	1	1	1	2	2	2	5
35–49	87	1.7	4	1	1	1	2	3	3	14
50–64	115	1.5	1	1	1	1	2	2	4	5
65+	53	1.9	3	1	1	1	2	3	6	11
GRAND TOTAL	304	1.6	2	1	1	1	2	2	4	9

250: DIABETES MELLITUS

Type of Patients	Observed Patients	Avg. Stay	Vari-ance	Percentiles						
				10th	25th	50th	75th	90th	95th	99th
1. SINGLE DX										
A. Not Operated										
0–19 Years	587	2.6	2	1	2	2	3	4	5	8
20–34	150	2.0	1	1	1	2	3	3	4	5
35–49	89	1.8	<1	1	1	2	2	3	4	5
50–64	56	2.1	1	1	1	2	3	4	5	5
65+	32	2.0	3	1	1	2	2	4	5	10
B. Operated										
0–19 Years	0									
20–34	0									
35–49	2	1.0	0	1	1	1	1	1	1	1
50–64	2	6.0	32	2	2	6	10	10	10	10
65+	1	2.0	0	2	2	2	2	2	2	2
2. MULTIPLE DX										
A. Not Operated										
0–19 Years	3,530	2.6	4	1	1	2	3	4	5	9
20–34	9,156	3.2	10	1	2	2	4	6	8	15
35–49	12,671	3.7	12	1	2	3	4	7	9	19
50–64	14,520	4.0	15	1	2	3	5	8	10	19
65+	16,120	3.9	13	1	2	3	5	8	10	17
B. Operated										
0–19 Years	23	6.9	65	2	2	5	8	11	11	41
20–34	466	8.7	51	3	4	7	11	17	24	39
35–49	2,672	9.0	67	3	4	7	11	17	23	47
50–64	5,886	9.0	63	2	4	7	11	17	24	41
65+	5,457	8.7	52	2	4	7	11	17	22	36
SUBTOTALS:										
1. SINGLE DX										
A. Not Operated	914	2.4	2	1	1	2	3	4	5	7
B. Operated	4	3.7	17	1	2	2	2	10	10	10
2. MULTIPLE DX										
A. Not Operated	55,997	3.7	12	1	2	3	4	7	9	17
B. Operated	14,504	8.9	59	2	4	7	11	17	23	40
1. SINGLE DX	918	2.4	2	1	1	2	3	4	5	7
2. MULTIPLE DX	70,501	4.7	26	1	2	3	6	10	14	26
A. NOT OPERATED	56,911	3.7	12	1	2	3	4	7	9	17
B. OPERATED	14,508	8.9	59	2	4	7	11	17	23	40
TOTAL										
0–19 Years	4,140	2.6	4	1	1	2	3	4	5	10
20–34	9,772	3.4	13	1	2	2	4	6	9	19
35–49	15,433	4.6	25	1	2	3	5	9	13	25
50–64	20,464	5.4	33	1	2	4	7	11	15	29
65+	21,610	5.1	27	1	2	4	6	11	15	26
GRAND TOTAL	71,419	4.7	26	1	2	3	6	10	14	26

Length of Stay by Diagnosis and Operation, Western Region, 2008

Western Region, October 2006–September 2007 Data, by Diagnosis

250.00: DM2/NOS UNCOMP NSU

Type of Patients	Observed Patients	Avg. Stay	Variance	Percentiles						
				10th	25th	50th	75th	90th	95th	99th
1. SINGLE DX										
A. Not Operated										
0–19 Years	33	2.4	2	1	2	2	3	4	5	7
20–34	10	1.5	<1	1	1	1	2	3	3	3
35–49	12	1.9	1	1	1	2	2	3	5	5
50–64	4	1.5	<1	1	1	2	2	2	2	2
65+	1	1.0	0	1	1	1	1	1	1	1
B. Operated										
0–19 Years	0									
20–34	0									
35–49	0									
50–64	0									
65+	0									
2. MULTIPLE DX										
A. Not Operated										
0–19 Years	100	2.9	2	1	2	3	4	5	6	8
20–34	201	2.2	2	1	1	2	3	4	5	7
35–49	422	2.3	2	1	1	2	3	4	5	7
50–64	444	2.5	3	1	1	2	3	4	6	8
65+	312	3.1	10	1	2	2	4	6	8	13
B. Operated										
0–19 Years	1	5.0	0	5	5	5	5	5	5	5
20–34	2	4.0	2	3	3	4	5	5	5	5
35–49	11	3.3	9	1	1	2	6	7	9	9
50–64	28	5.4	95	1	1	2	5	12	17	51
65+	10	3.8	8	1	1	3	5	9	9	9
SUBTOTALS:										
1. SINGLE DX — A. Not Operated	60	2.1	1	1	1	2	2	3	4	7
1. SINGLE DX — B. Operated	0									
2. MULTIPLE DX — A. Not Operated	1,479	2.6	4	1	1	2	3	4	6	9
2. MULTIPLE DX — B. Operated	52	4.6	54	1	1	2	5	9	12	51
1. SINGLE DX	60	2.1	1	1	1	2	3	3	4	7
2. MULTIPLE DX	1,531	2.6	6	1	1	2	3	5	6	9
A. NOT OPERATED	1,539	2.5	4	1	1	2	3	4	6	9
B. OPERATED	52	4.6	54	1	1	2	5	9	12	51
TOTAL										
0–19 Years	134	2.8	2	1	2	3	4	4	5	8
20–34	213	2.2	2	1	1	2	3	4	5	7
35–49	445	2.3	2	1	1	2	3	4	5	8
50–64	476	2.6	9	1	1	2	3	5	6	12
65+	323	3.1	10	1	2	2	4	6	8	13
GRAND TOTAL	1,591	2.6	6	1	1	2	3	5	6	9

250.01: DM1 UNCOMP NSU

Type of Patients	Observed Patients	Avg. Stay	Variance	Percentiles						
				10th	25th	50th	75th	90th	95th	99th
1. SINGLE DX										
A. Not Operated										
0–19 Years	173	2.5	2	1	2	2	3	4	5	7
20–34	5	1.6	<1	1	1	1	2	3	3	3
35–49	0									
50–64	1	2.0	0	2	2	2	2	2	2	2
65+	1	2.0	0	2	2	2	2	2	2	2
B. Operated										
0–19 Years	0									
20–34	0									
35–49	0									
50–64	1	2.0	0	2	2	2	2	2	2	2
65+	0									
2. MULTIPLE DX										
A. Not Operated										
0–19 Years	285	2.6	2	1	2	2	3	4	5	7
20–34	58	2.0	3	1	1	1	2	4	5	10
35–49	41	2.0	1	1	1	2	2	4	4	7
50–64	21	3.3	5	1	2	3	4	8	9	>99
65+	8	2.8	3	1	2	2	5	>99	>99	>99
B. Operated										
0–19 Years	0									
20–34	0									
35–49	3	10.0	13	6	6	11	13	13	13	13
50–64	0									
65+	0									
SUBTOTALS:										
1. SINGLE DX — A. Not Operated	180	2.5	2	1	2	2	3	4	4	7
1. SINGLE DX — B. Operated	1	2.0	0	2	2	2	2	2	2	2
2. MULTIPLE DX — A. Not Operated	413	2.5	2	1	1	2	3	4	5	9
2. MULTIPLE DX — B. Operated	3	10.0	13	6	6	11	13	13	13	13
1. SINGLE DX	181	2.5	2	1	2	2	3	4	4	7
2. MULTIPLE DX	416	2.6	3	1	1	2	3	5	5	11
A. NOT OPERATED	593	2.5	2	1	2	2	3	4	5	9
B. OPERATED	4	8.0	25	2	6	11	13	13	13	13
TOTAL										
0–19 Years	458	2.6	2	1	2	2	3	4	5	7
20–34	63	2.0	3	1	1	1	2	4	5	10
35–49	44	2.5	6	1	1	2	3	4	6	13
50–64	23	3.2	5	1	2	3	4	8	9	>99
65+	9	2.7	3	1	2	2	5	>99	>99	>99
GRAND TOTAL	597	2.5	3	1	2	2	3	4	5	11

250.02: DM2/NOS UNCOMP UNC

Type of Patients	Observed Patients	Avg. Stay	Variance	Percentiles						
				10th	25th	50th	75th	90th	95th	99th
1. SINGLE DX										
A. Not Operated										
0–19 Years	6	4.3	15	1	2	3	7	11	11	11
20–34	15	1.9	<1	1	1	2	3	3	3	3
35–49	14	1.7	<1	1	1	2	2	3	4	4
50–64	14	1.8	1	1	1	2	2	4	4	4
65+	5	2.2	3	1	1	2	2	5	5	5
B. Operated										
0–19 Years	0									
20–34	0									
35–49	0									
50–64	0									
65+	0									
2. MULTIPLE DX										
A. Not Operated										
0–19 Years	41	2.3	2	1	1	2	3	4	5	6
20–34	294	2.5	2	1	1	2	3	5	6	8
35–49	912	2.7	4	1	1	2	3	5	6	10
50–64	1,370	3.0	7	1	2	2	4	5	7	12
65+	1,257	3.7	7	1	2	3	4	7	8	15
B. Operated										
0–19 Years	0									
20–34	2	4.0	0	4	4	4	4	4	4	4
35–49	7	4.6	11	1	2	4	7	>99	>99	>99
50–64	25	6.4	33	1	2	5	8	16	18	24
65+	24	8.9	55	2	4	7	13	18	27	29
SUBTOTALS:										
1. SINGLE DX — A. Not Operated	54	2.1	3	1	2	2	2	4	5	11
1. SINGLE DX — B. Operated	0									
2. MULTIPLE DX — A. Not Operated	3,874	3.1	6	1	2	2	4	6	7	12
2. MULTIPLE DX — B. Operated	58	7.1	40	1	3	6	9	18	27	>99
1. SINGLE DX	54	2.1	3	1	1	2	2	4	5	11
2. MULTIPLE DX	3,932	3.2	7	1	2	3	4	6	7	14
A. NOT OPERATED	3,928	3.1	6	1	2	2	4	6	7	12
B. OPERATED	58	7.1	40	1	3	6	9	18	27	>99
TOTAL										
0–19 Years	47	2.6	4	1	1	2	3	5	6	11
20–34	311	2.5	2	1	1	2	3	5	6	8
35–49	933	2.7	4	1	1	2	3	5	6	10
50–64	1,409	3.0	7	1	1	2	4	5	7	13
65+	1,286	3.8	9	1	2	3	5	7	9	16
GRAND TOTAL	3,986	3.1	7	1	2	2	4	6	7	14

141

Length of Stay by Diagnosis and Operation, Western Region, 2008

Western Region, October 2006–September 2007 Data, by Diagnosis

250.03: DM1 UNCOMP UNC

Type of Patients	Observed Patients	Avg. Stay	Vari-ance	10th	25th	50th	75th	90th	95th	99th
1. SINGLE DX										
A. Not Operated										
0–19 Years	34	2.5	2	1	1	2	3	5	5	6
20–34	3	2.0	<1	1	1	2	3	3	3	3
35–49	0									
50–64	1	1.0	0	1	1	1	1	1	1	1
65+	0									
B. Operated										
0–19 Years	0									
20–34	0									
35–49	0									
50–64	0									
65+	0									
2. MULTIPLE DX										
A. Not Operated										
0–19 Years	99	2.8	9	1	1	2	3	5	6	12
20–34	137	2.3	3	1	1	2	3	4	5	11
35–49	122	3.2	7	1	1	2	4	6	7	14
50–64	66	3.4	12	1	2	2	4	7	8	25
65+	53	4.1	5	2	3	4	5	7	9	12
B. Operated										
0–19 Years	2	2.0	0	2	2	2	2	2	2	2
20–34	3	4.3	6	2	2	4	7	7	7	7
35–49	2	8.0	6	7	7	7	9	9	9	9
50–64	3	4.7	6	2	2	5	7	7	7	7
65+	2	7.0	18	4	4	4	10	10	10	10
SUBTOTALS:										
1. SINGLE DX – A. Not Operated	38	2.4	2	1	1	2	3	5	5	6
1. SINGLE DX – B. Operated	0									
2. MULTIPLE DX – A. Not Operated	477	3.0	7	1	1	2	4	5	7	13
2. MULTIPLE DX – B. Operated	12	5.1	8	2	2	5	7	9	10	10
1. SINGLE DX	38	2.4	2	1	1	2	3	5	5	6
2. MULTIPLE DX	489	3.0	7	1	1	2	4	6	7	13
A. NOT OPERATED	515	2.9	7	1	1	2	4	5	7	12
B. OPERATED	12	5.1	8	2	2	5	7	9	10	10
TOTAL										
0–19 Years	135	2.7	7	1	1	2	3	5	5	12
20–34	143	2.4	3	1	1	2	3	4	5	11
35–49	124	3.3	8	1	2	3	4	6	8	14
50–64	70	3.4	12	1	2	4	5	7	8	25
65+	55	4.2	6	2	3	4	5	7	10	12
GRAND TOTAL	527	3.0	7	1	1	2	4	5	7	12

250.10: DM2/NOS W KETOACID NSU

Type of Patients	Observed Patients	Avg. Stay	Vari-ance	10th	25th	50th	75th	90th	95th	99th
1. SINGLE DX										
A. Not Operated										
0–19 Years	3	2.4	5	1	1	1		5	5	5
20–34	4	2.5	3	1	2	2		5	5	5
35–49	4	1.8	<1	1	1	1		2	3	3
50–64	2	2.5	5	1	1	3		4	4	4
65+	0									
B. Operated										
0–19 Years	0									
20–34	0									
35–49	0									
50–64	0									
65+	0									
2. MULTIPLE DX										
A. Not Operated										
0–19 Years	33	2.9	5	1	2	2	3	5	7	13
20–34	169	2.9	4	1	2	2	4	5	7	14
35–49	312	3.6	7	1	2	3	4	6	8	15
50–64	210	3.7	6	1	2	3	5	7	8	11
65+	82	4.5	7	2	3	4	6	8	10	14
B. Operated										
0–19 Years	0									
20–34	3	6.7	2	5	5	7	8	8	8	8
35–49	5	6.4	11	2	5	6	8	11	11	11
50–64	6	8.7	6	5	7	10	10	12	12	12
65+	1	8.0	0	8	8	8	8	8	8	8
SUBTOTALS:										
1. SINGLE DX – A. Not Operated	13	2.2	2	1	1	2	3	5	5	5
1. SINGLE DX – B. Operated	0									
2. MULTIPLE DX – A. Not Operated	806	3.6	6	1	2	3	5	6	8	13
2. MULTIPLE DX – B. Operated	15	7.5	7	5	5	8	10	11	12	10
1. SINGLE DX	13	2.2	2	1	1	2	3	5	5	6
2. MULTIPLE DX	821	3.6	7	1	2	3	5	7	8	14
A. NOT OPERATED	819	3.5	6	1	2	3	5	6	8	14
B. OPERATED	15	7.5	7	5	5	8	10	11	12	12
TOTAL										
0–19 Years	36	2.8	5	1	2	2	3	5	7	13
20–34	176	3.0	4	1	2	2	4	6	7	14
35–49	321	3.6	7	1	2	3	4	6	8	15
50–64	218	3.8	7	1	3	3	6	7	9	12
65+	83	4.6	7	2	3	4	6	8	10	14
GRAND TOTAL	834	3.6	7	1	2	3	5	7	8	14

250.11: DM1 W KETOACIDOSIS NSU

Type of Patients	Observed Patients	Avg. Stay	Vari-ance	10th	25th	50th	75th	90th	95th	99th
1. SINGLE DX										
A. Not Operated										
0–19 Years	72	2.5	2	1	2	2	3	4	5	7
20–34	7	2.0	1	1	2	2	3	4	4	4
35–49	4	1.8	<1	1	2	2	2	2	2	2
50–64	1	2.0	0	2	2	2	2	2	2	2
65+	0									
B. Operated										
0–19 Years	0									
20–34	0									
35–49	0									
50–64	0									
65+	0									
2. MULTIPLE DX										
A. Not Operated										
0–19 Years	315	2.7	4	1	2	2	3	5	6	11
20–34	477	2.9	8	1	2	2	3	5	7	13
35–49	295	3.4	13	1	2	3	4	6	7	14
50–64	96	3.9	9	2	2	3	5	6	11	18
65+	20	4.8	9	2	3	3	6	10	12	12
B. Operated										
0–19 Years	0									
20–34	6	9.7	19	5	5	8	14	15	15	15
35–49	5	11.8	29	5	11	11	12	20	20	20
50–64	2	15.5	24	12	12	12	19	19	19	19
65+	0									
SUBTOTALS:										
1. SINGLE DX – A. Not Operated	84	2.5	2	1	2	2	3	4	5	7
1. SINGLE DX – B. Operated	0									
2. MULTIPLE DX – A. Not Operated	1,203	3.1	8	1	2	2	4	5	7	13
2. MULTIPLE DX – B. Operated	13	11.4	24	5	8	11	14	19	20	20
1. SINGLE DX	84	2.5	2	1	2	2	3	4	5	7
2. MULTIPLE DX	1,216	3.2	9	1	2	2	4	5	8	14
A. NOT OPERATED	1,287	3.0	8	1	2	2	3	5	7	13
B. OPERATED	13	11.4	24	5	8	11	14	19	20	20
TOTAL										
0–19 Years	387	2.6	3	1	2	2	3	5	6	11
20–34	490	3.0	9	1	2	2	3	5	8	15
35–49	304	3.5	14	1	2	3	4	6	8	14
50–64	99	4.1	12	2	2	3	5	7	13	18
65+	20	4.8	9	2	3	3	6	10	12	12
GRAND TOTAL	1,300	3.1	9	1	2	2	4	5	7	14

Western Region, October 2006–September 2007 Data, by Diagnosis

250.12: DM2/NOS W KETOACID UNC

Type of Patients	Observed Patients	Avg. Stay	Variance	Percentiles 10th	25th	50th	75th	90th	95th	99th
1. SINGLE DX										
A. *Not Operated*										
0–19 Years	14	3.0	4	2	2	2	3	4	9	9
20–34	21	2.1	<1	1	2	2	3	3	3	4
35–49	22	2.1	1	1	1	2	3	4	4	5
50–64	9	2.3	2	1	1	2	3	5	5	5
65+	0									
B. *Operated*										
0–19 Years	0									
20–34	0									
35–49	0									
50–64	0									
65+	0									
2. MULTIPLE DX										
A. *Not Operated*										
0–19 Years	112	3.2	6	1	2	3	4	6	8	11
20–34	989	3.3	9	1	2	3	4	6	7	15
35–49	1,854	3.5	7	1	2	3	4	6	8	15
50–64	1,703	4.1	16	1	2	3	5	7	9	17
65+	650	4.6	11	2	2	4	6	9	11	18
B. *Operated*										
0–19 Years	2	23.6	598	6	6	41	41	41	41	41
20–34	18	10.4	97	2	5	7	11	34	37	37
35–49	47	12.0	201	3	5	7	14	25	36	72
50–64	50	13.1	91	4	5	10	18	26	30	47
65+	27	10.8	31	5	7	10	13	19	20	27
SUBTOTALS:										
1. SINGLE DX										
A. *Not Operated*	66	2.3	2	1	2	2	3	4	4	9
B. *Operated*	0									
2. MULTIPLE DX										
A. *Not Operated*	5,308	3.8	11	1	2	3	5	7	9	16
B. *Operated*	144	12.1	120	4	5	8	16	25	33	63
1. SINGLE DX	66	2.3	2	1	2	2	3	4	4	9
2. MULTIPLE DX	5,452	4.0	16	1	2	3	5	7	10	19
A. NOT OPERATED	5,374	3.8	11	1	2	3	5	7	9	16
B. OPERATED	144	12.1	120	4	5	8	16	25	33	63
TOTAL										
0–19 Years	128	3.5	17	1	2	3	4	6	8	18
20–34	1,028	3.4	11	1	2	3	4	6	8	17
35–49	1,923	3.7	14	1	2	3	4	7	8	18
50–64	1,762	4.3	21	1	2	3	5	8	10	24
65+	677	4.9	14	2	3	4	6	9	13	20
GRAND TOTAL	5,518	4.0	16	1	2	3	5	7	10	19

250.13: DM1 W KETOACIDOSIS UNC

Type of Patients	Observed Patients	Avg. Stay	Variance	Percentiles 10th	25th	50th	75th	90th	95th	99th
1. SINGLE DX										
A. *Not Operated*										
0–19 Years	229	2.6	3	1	1	2	3	5	5	8
20–34	73	2.2	1	1	1	2	3	4	4	6
35–49	21	1.8	<1	1	1	2	2	3	3	3
50–64	5	2.6	1	1	2	3	3	4	4	4
65+	0									
B. *Operated*										
0–19 Years	0									
20–34	0									
35–49	0									
50–64	0									
65+	0									
2. MULTIPLE DX										
A. *Not Operated*										
0–19 Years	2,328	2.5	3	1	1	2	3	4	5	8
20–34	4,680	2.9	8	1	2	2	3	5	6	12
35–49	2,878	3.4	8	1	2	3	4	6	8	15
50–64	1,238	4.0	11	1	2	3	5	7	9	18
65+	319	4.9	31	1	3	4	6	8	11	28
B. *Operated*										
0–19 Years	13	5.5	12	2	2	5	7	11	11	11
20–34	52	9.3	87	2	4	6	10	18	27	48
35–49	57	14.8	258	3	7	11	17	20	60	85
50–64	39	13.2	155	4	6	10	14	31	48	65
65+	14	14.7	321	3	4	9	17	25	72	72
SUBTOTALS:										
1. SINGLE DX										
A. *Not Operated*	328	2.5	2	1	1	2	3	4	5	8
B. *Operated*	0									
2. MULTIPLE DX										
A. *Not Operated*	11,443	3.1	8	1	2	2	4	5	7	13
B. *Operated*	175	12.1	176	3	5	8	15	20	42	76
1. SINGLE DX	328	2.5	2	1	1	2	3	4	5	8
2. MULTIPLE DX	11,618	3.2	12	1	2	2	4	6	8	16
A. NOT OPERATED	11,771	3.1	8	1	2	2	4	5	7	13
B. OPERATED	175	12.1	176	3	5	8	15	20	42	76
TOTAL										
0–19 Years	2,570	2.5	3	1	1	2	3	4	5	9
20–34	4,805	2.9	9	1	2	2	3	5	6	13
35–49	2,956	3.6	15	1	2	3	4	6	8	18
50–64	1,282	4.3	18	1	2	3	5	8	10	22
65+	333	5.3	46	1	3	4	6	9	13	28
GRAND TOTAL	11,946	3.2	12	1	2	2	4	6	8	15

250.20: DM2/NOS W HYPEROSMOL NSU

Type of Patients	Observed Patients	Avg. Stay	Variance	Percentiles 10th	25th	50th	75th	90th	95th	99th
1. SINGLE DX										
A. *Not Operated*										
0–19 Years	0									
20–34	2	2.5	<1	2	2	2	3	3	3	3
35–49	0									
50–64	1	2.0	0	2	2	2	2	2	2	2
65+	0									
B. *Operated*										
0–19 Years	0									
20–34	0									
35–49	0									
50–64	0									
65+	0									
2. MULTIPLE DX										
A. *Not Operated*										
0–19 Years	8	4.1	14	1	2	2	4	13	13	13
20–34	44	2.7	3	1	2	2	3	3	5	10
35–49	168	3.3	5	1	2	3	4	6	8	11
50–64	245	3.5	6	1	2	3	4	6	8	13
65+	215	4.5	9	2	2	3	5	9	11	14
B. *Operated*										
0–19 Years	0									
20–34	1	18.0	0	18	18	18	18	18	18	18
35–49	3	6.7	10	3	3	8	9	9	9	9
50–64	8	9.0	17	5	5	7	14	16	16	16
65+	3	15.4	68	6	6	18	22	22	22	22
SUBTOTALS:										
1. SINGLE DX										
A. *Not Operated*	3	2.3	<1	2	2	2	3	3	3	3
B. *Operated*	0									
2. MULTIPLE DX										
A. *Not Operated*	680	3.7	7	1	2	3	5	7	9	13
B. *Operated*	15	10.4	33	5	6	9	16	18	22	22
1. SINGLE DX	3	2.3	<1	2	2	2	3	3	3	3
2. MULTIPLE DX	695	3.9	8	1	2	3	5	8	10	15
A. NOT OPERATED	683	3.7	7	1	2	3	5	7	9	13
B. OPERATED	15	10.4	33	5	6	9	16	18	22	22
TOTAL										
0–19 Years	8	4.1	14	1	2	2	4	13	13	13
20–34	47	3.0	8	1	2	2	3	5	8	18
35–49	171	3.4	5	1	2	3	4	7	9	11
50–64	254	3.7	7	1	2	3	5	7	9	14
65+	218	4.6	11	2	2	4	6	9	11	16
GRAND TOTAL	698	3.8	8	1	2	3	5	8	10	15

Length of Stay by Diagnosis and Operation, Western Region, 2008

Western Region, October 2006–September 2007 Data, by Diagnosis

250.22: DM2/NOS W HYPEROSMOL UNC

Type of Patients	Observed Patients	Avg. Stay	Variance	10th	25th	50th	75th	90th	95th	99th
1. SINGLE DX										
A. Not Operated										
0–19 Years	0									
20–34	0									
35–49	2	1.5	<1	1	1	1	2	2	2	2
50–64	2	2.0	2	1	1	2	3	3	3	3
65+	0									
B. Operated										
0–19 Years	0									
20–34	0									
35–49	0									
50–64	0									
65+	0									
2. MULTIPLE DX										
A. Not Operated										
0–19 Years	2	1.5	<1	1	1	2	2	2	2	2
20–34	55	3.4	7	1	2	3	4	6	10	14
35–49	191	4.0	14	1	2	3	5	7	11	24
50–64	309	4.1	11	1	2	3	5	8	10	16
65+	288	5.1	20	2	3	4	6	10	13	23
B. Operated										
0–19 Years	0									
20–34	5	10.8	9	6	10	12	13	13	13	13
35–49	7	13.8	93	4	6	13	18	32	32	32
50–64	7	11.1	30	4	7	10	14	21	21	21
65+										
SUBTOTALS:										
1. SINGLE DX										
A. Not Operated	4	1.7	<1	1	1	1	2	3	3	3
B. Operated	0									
2. MULTIPLE DX										
A. Not Operated	845	4.4	15	1	2	3	5	8	11	21
B. Operated	19	12.0	45	4	7	12	14	21	32	32
1. SINGLE DX	4	1.7	<1	1	1	2	2	3	3	3
2. MULTIPLE DX	864	4.5	17	1	2	3	5	9	12	22
A. NOT OPERATED	849	4.4	15	1	2	3	5	8	11	21
B. OPERATED	19	12.0	45	4	7	12	14	21	32	32
TOTAL										
0–19 Years	2	1.5	<1	1	1	2	2	2	2	2
20–34	55	3.4	7	1	2	3	4	6	10	14
35–49	198	4.1	15	1	2	3	5	8	12	24
50–64	318	4.3	15	1	2	3	5	8	11	19
65+	295	5.3	21	2	3	4	6	11	14	23
GRAND TOTAL	868	4.5	17	1	2	3	5	9	12	22

250.30: DM2/NOS W COMA NEC NSU

Type of Patients	Observed Patients	Avg. Stay	Variance	10th	25th	50th	75th	90th	95th	99th
1. SINGLE DX										
A. Not Operated										
0–19 Years	0									
20–34	0									
35–49	0									
50–64	0									
65+	0									
B. Operated										
0–19 Years	0									
20–34	0									
35–49	0									
50–64	0									
65+	0									
2. MULTIPLE DX										
A. Not Operated										
0–19 Years	1	3.0	0	3	3	3	3	3	3	3
20–34	5	4.2	11	1	2	3	6	9	9	9
35–49	19	5.7	90	1	1	2	6	15	42	42
50–64	59	7.3	123	1	2	3	8	20	38	>99
65+	180	3.7	9	1	2	3	5	8	10	15
B. Operated										
0–19 Years	0									
20–34	2	6.0	2	5	5	6	7	7	7	7
35–49	2	14.0	70	8	8	8	20	20	20	20
50–64	4	10.3	23	5	8	12	12	16	16	16
65+										
SUBTOTALS:										
1. SINGLE DX										
A. Not Operated	0									
B. Operated	0									
2. MULTIPLE DX										
A. Not Operated	264	4.6	42	1	2	3	5	9	13	44
B. Operated	8	10.1	29	5	6	8	12	20	20	20
1. SINGLE DX	0									
2. MULTIPLE DX	272	4.8	42	1	2	3	5	10	15	44
A. NOT OPERATED	264	4.6	42	1	2	3	5	9	13	44
B. OPERATED	8	10.1	29	5	6	8	12	20	20	20
TOTAL										
0–19 Years	1	3.0	0	3	3	3	3	3	3	3
20–34	5	4.2	11	1	2	3	6	9	9	9
35–49	21	5.7	81	1	1	3	6	8	15	42
50–64	61	7.5	121	1	2	3	8	20	38	>99
65+	184	3.8	10	1	2	3	5	9	11	16
GRAND TOTAL	272	4.8	42	1	2	3	5	10	15	44

250.40: DM2/NOS W REN MANIF NSU

Type of Patients	Observed Patients	Avg. Stay	Variance	10th	25th	50th	75th	90th	95th	99th
1. SINGLE DX										
A. Not Operated										
0–19 Years	0									
20–34	0									
35–49	1	1.0	0	1	1	1	1	1	1	1
50–64	0									
65+	2	5.5	39	1	1	6	10	10	10	10
B. Operated										
0–19 Years	0									
20–34	0									
35–49	0									
50–64	0									
65+	0									
2. MULTIPLE DX										
A. Not Operated										
0–19 Years	1	6.0	0	6	6	6	6	6	6	6
20–34	53	4.9	17	1	2	4	6	10	13	22
35–49	359	5.0	23	1	2	4	6	11	14	26
50–64	956	4.9	22	1	2	4	6	11	14	21
65+	950	4.9	17	1	2	4	6	10	13	20
B. Operated										
0–19 Years	0									
20–34	9	4.3	5	1	4	5	6	>99	>99	>99
35–49	152	7.1	28	2	4	5	9	13	17	26
50–64	464	7.0	31	2	4	6	9	13	17	31
65+	322	6.4	23	1	3	5	9	13	16	24
SUBTOTALS:										
1. SINGLE DX										
A. Not Operated	3	4.0	27	1	1	1	1	10	10	10
B. Operated	0									
2. MULTIPLE DX										
A. Not Operated	2,319	4.9	20	1	2	4	6	10	13	21
B. Operated	947	6.8	28	1	3	5	9	13	17	27
1. SINGLE DX	3	4.0	27	1	1	1	1	10	10	10
2. MULTIPLE DX	3,266	5.5	23	1	2	4	7	11	14	24
A. NOT OPERATED	2,322	4.9	20	1	2	4	6	10	13	21
B. OPERATED	947	6.8	28	1	3	5	9	13	17	27
TOTAL										
0–19 Years	1	6.0	0	6	6	6	6	6	6	6
20–34	62	4.8	15	1	2	4	6	10	13	>99
35–49	512	5.6	25	1	2	4	7	12	16	26
50–64	1,420	5.6	26	1	2	4	7	12	15	24
65+	1,274	5.3	19	1	2	4	7	11	14	21
GRAND TOTAL	3,269	5.5	23	1	2	4	7	11	14	24

Length of Stay by Diagnosis and Operation, Western Region, 2008

Western Region, October 2006–September 2007 Data, by Diagnosis

250.41: DM1 W RENAL MANIFEST NSU

Type of Patients	Observed Patients	Avg. Stay	Vari-ance	Percentiles 10th	25th	50th	75th	90th	95th	99th
1. SINGLE DX										
A. Not Operated										
0–19 Years	0									
20–34	0									
35–49	0									
50–64	0									
65+	0									
B. Operated										
0–19 Years	0									
20–34	0									
35–49	0									
50–64	0									
65+	0									
2. MULTIPLE DX										
A. Not Operated										
0–19 Years	1	1.0	0	1	1	1	1	1	1	1
20–34	68	4.2	13	1	2	3	5	9	11	20
35–49	98	3.9	13	1	1	3	5	8	10	21
50–64	70	4.8	24	1	2	3	5	11	18	24
65+	23	6.7	36	1	2	5	10	18	20	21
B. Operated										
0–19 Years	0									
20–34	34	9.2	28	4	5	8	13	17	21	21
35–49	121	9.4	57	4	6	8	10	15	22	47
50–64	66	8.4	33	3	5	7	9	16	19	30
65+	13	9.3	79	2	3	6	10	22	31	31
SUBTOTALS:										
1. SINGLE DX										
A. Not Operated	0									
B. Operated	0									
2. MULTIPLE DX										
A. Not Operated	260	4.4	18	1	2	3	5	10	13	21
B. Operated	234	9.1	47	3	5	8	10	16	22	35
1. SINGLE DX	0									
2. MULTIPLE DX	494	6.6	37	1	2	5	9	14	19	30
A. NOT OPERATED	260	4.4	18	1	2	3	5	10	13	21
B. OPERATED	234	9.1	47	3	5	8	10	16	22	35
TOTAL										
0–19 Years	1	1.0	0	1	1	1	1	1	1	1
20–34	102	5.8	23	1	2	5	8	13	16	21
35–49	219	6.9	45	1	3	6	9	14	19	35
50–64	136	6.6	31	1	3	5	9	15	19	26
65+	36	7.6	51	1	2	6	10	20	22	31
GRAND TOTAL	494	6.6	37	1	2	5	9	14	19	30

250.42: DM2/NOS W REN MANIF UNC

Type of Patients	Observed Patients	Avg. Stay	Vari-ance	Percentiles 10th	25th	50th	75th	90th	95th	99th
1. SINGLE DX										
A. Not Operated										
0–19 Years	0									
20–34	0									
35–49	0									
50–64	0									
65+	0									
B. Operated										
0–19 Years	0									
20–34	0									
35–49	0									
50–64	0									
65+	0									
2. MULTIPLE DX										
A. Not Operated										
0–19 Years	0									
20–34	32	5.5	31	1	2	4	7	10	18	28
35–49	148	4.9	17	1	2	3	6	10	12	22
50–64	336	5.3	19	2	2	4	6	11	14	21
65+	339	4.8	21	1	2	4	6	9	12	20
B. Operated										
0–19 Years	0									
20–34	0									
35–49	32	6.6	21	2	4	6	8	13	17	23
50–64	66	8.2	22	4	5	7	11	14	15	26
65+	33	11.6	62	4	6	11	14	22	30	35
SUBTOTALS:										
1. SINGLE DX										
A. Not Operated	0									
B. Operated	0									
2. MULTIPLE DX										
A. Not Operated	855	5.0	20	2	3	4	6	10	13	22
B. Operated	131	8.7	35	3	4	7	12	14	22	30
1. SINGLE DX	0									
2. MULTIPLE DX	986	5.5	23	2	3	4	7	11	14	24
A. NOT OPERATED	855	5.0	20	2	3	4	6	10	13	22
B. OPERATED	131	8.7	35	3	4	7	12	14	22	30
TOTAL										
0–19 Years	0									
20–34	32	5.5	31	1	2	4	7	10	18	28
35–49	180	5.2	18	2	2	4	6	10	14	23
50–64	402	5.8	21	2	3	4	7	11	14	21
65+	372	5.4	28	1	2	4	7	11	14	26
GRAND TOTAL	986	5.5	23	2	3	4	7	11	14	24

250.43: DM1 W RENAL MANIFEST UNC

Type of Patients	Observed Patients	Avg. Stay	Vari-ance	Percentiles 10th	25th	50th	75th	90th	95th	99th
1. SINGLE DX										
A. Not Operated										
0–19 Years	0									
20–34	0									
35–49	0									
50–64	0									
65+	0									
B. Operated										
0–19 Years	0									
20–34	0									
35–49	0									
50–64	0									
65+	0									
2. MULTIPLE DX										
A. Not Operated										
0–19 Years	2	3.0	2		2	4	4	4	4	4
20–34	78	5.2	23	2	2	4	7	11	13	32
35–49	74	5.8	47	1	2	4	7	12	19	43
50–64	41	5.5	31	1	2	4	6	11	18	24
65+	19	6.5	30	3	4	5	7	10	27	27
B. Operated										
0–19 Years	0									
20–34	8	12.1	212	1	2	7	16	46	46	46
35–49	11	8.9	165	2	3	6	8	10	47	47
50–64	5	6.8	8	3	5	8	8	10	10	10
65+	1	4.0	0	4	4	4	4	4	4	4
SUBTOTALS:										
1. SINGLE DX										
A. Not Operated	0									
B. Operated	0									
2. MULTIPLE DX										
A. Not Operated	214	5.6	33	1	2	4	7	11	16	29
B. Operated	25	9.3	137	2	4	6	8	16	46	47
1. SINGLE DX	0									
2. MULTIPLE DX	239	6.0	44	1	2	4	7	11	17	43
A. NOT OPERATED	214	5.6	33	1	2	4	7	11	16	29
B. OPERATED	25	9.3	137	2	4	6	8	16	46	47
TOTAL										
0–19 Years	2	3.0	2		2	4	4	4	4	4
20–34	86	5.9	42	2	2	4	7	12	15	46
35–49	85	6.2	61	1	2	4	7	12	19	47
50–64	46	5.6	29	1	3	4	7	11	18	24
65+	20	6.4	28	3	4	5	7	10	27	27
GRAND TOTAL	239	6.0	44	1	2	4	7	11	17	43

Length of Stay by Diagnosis and Operation, Western Region, 2008

Western Region, October 2006–September 2007 Data, by Diagnosis

250.60: DM2/NOS W NEUR MANIF NSU

Type of Patients	Observed Patients	Avg. Stay	Variance	10th	25th	50th	75th	90th	95th	99th
1. SINGLE DX										
A. Not Operated										
0–19 Years	0									
20–34	0									
35–49	1	1.0	0	1	1	1	1	1	1	1
50–64	1	2.0	0	2	2	2	2	2	2	2
65+	2	2.5	<1	2	2	3	3	3	3	3
B. Operated										
0–19 Years	0									
20–34	0									
35–49	0									
50–64	0									
65+	0									
2. MULTIPLE DX										
A. Not Operated										
0–19 Years	3	12.0	215	3	3	4	29	29	29	29
20–34	260	4.1	19	1	2	3	4	8	10	24
35–49	1,037	4.2	14	1	2	3	5	8	11	22
50–64	1,468	4.3	14	1	2	3	5	8	11	19
65+	1,305	4.5	14	2	2	4	6	8	11	17
B. Operated										
0–19 Years	1	3.0	0	3	3	3	3	3	3	3
20–34	13	5.5	7	2	4	6	6	9	11	11
35–49	204	8.4	64	2	4	6	10	17	23	47
50–64	573	7.5	35	2	4	6	9	15	19	32
65+	421	6.9	38	1	3	5	9	15	19	29
SUBTOTALS:										
1. SINGLE DX — A. Not Operated	4	2.0	<1	1	1	2	2	2	3	3
1. SINGLE DX — B. Operated	0									
2. MULTIPLE DX — A. Not Operated	4,073	4.3	14	1	2	3	5	8	11	20
2. MULTIPLE DX — B. Operated	1,212	7.4	41	2	4	6	9	15	19	33
1. SINGLE DX	4	2.0	<1	1	2	2	2	3	3	3
2. MULTIPLE DX	5,285	5.0	22	1	2	4	6	10	13	24
A. NOT OPERATED	4,077	4.3	14	1	2	3	5	8	11	20
B. OPERATED	1,212	7.4	41	2	4	6	9	15	19	33
TOTAL										
0–19 Years	4	9.8	165	3	3	4	29	29	29	29
20–34	273	4.1	19	1	2	3	5	8	10	24
35–49	1,242	4.9	24	1	2	4	6	10	13	24
50–64	2,042	5.2	22	1	2	4	6	10	14	24
65+	1,728	5.1	21	1	2	4	6	10	13	22
GRAND TOTAL	5,289	5.0	22	1	2	4	6	10	13	24

250.61: DM1 W NEURO MANIFEST NSU

Type of Patients	Observed Patients	Avg. Stay	Variance	10th	25th	50th	75th	90th	95th	99th
1. SINGLE DX										
A. Not Operated										
0–19 Years	0									
20–34	0									
35–49	0									
50–64	0									
65+	0									
B. Operated										
0–19 Years	0									
20–34	0									
35–49	0									
50–64	0									
65+	0									
2. MULTIPLE DX										
A. Not Operated										
0–19 Years	15	3.0	5	1	1	2	4	6	9	9
20–34	443	3.8	10	1	2	3	5	7	10	15
35–49	456	4.3	14	1	2	3	5	8	12	20
50–64	152	4.6	13	1	2	4	6	8	12	19
65+	36	5.1	31	1	2	4	6	11	20	29
B. Operated										
20–34	27	7.3	47	1	3	5	9	16	25	30
35–49	67	8.4	96	2	3	5	9	24	26	59
50–64	49	8.1	71	1	3	7	10	15	21	51
65+	11	5.6	17	1	2	6	8	12	12	12
SUBTOTALS:										
1. SINGLE DX — A. Not Operated	0									
1. SINGLE DX — B. Operated	0									
2. MULTIPLE DX — A. Not Operated	1,102	4.2	13	1	2	3	5	8	11	20
2. MULTIPLE DX — B. Operated	154	7.9	74	2	3	5	9	16	25	51
1. SINGLE DX	0									
2. MULTIPLE DX	1,256	4.6	22	1	2	3	5	9	12	25
A. NOT OPERATED	1,102	4.2	13	1	2	3	5	8	11	20
B. OPERATED	154	7.9	74	2	3	5	9	16	25	51
TOTAL										
0–19 Years	15	3.0	5	1	1	2	4	6	9	9
20–34	470	4.0	13	1	2	3	5	8	11	22
35–49	523	4.8	26	1	2	3	5	9	14	26
50–64	201	5.4	29	1	2	4	7	11	13	26
65+	47	5.2	27	1	2	4	6	11	12	29
GRAND TOTAL	1,256	4.6	22	1	2	3	5	9	12	25

250.62: DM2/NOS W NEUR MANIF UNC

Type of Patients	Observed Patients	Avg. Stay	Variance	10th	25th	50th	75th	90th	95th	99th
1. SINGLE DX										
A. Not Operated										
0–19 Years	0									
20–34	0									
35–49	0									
50–64	0									
65+	0									
B. Operated										
0–19 Years	0									
20–34	0									
35–49	0									
50–64	0									
65+	0									
2. MULTIPLE DX										
A. Not Operated										
0–19 Years	2	2.0	0	2	2	2	2	2	2	2
20–34	124	5.5	26	2	2	4	6	10	16	28
35–49	636	4.2	13	1	2	3	5	8	10	21
50–64	732	4.4	13	1	2	3	6	8	11	19
65+	392	4.5	12	1	2	4	6	9	11	19
B. Operated										
20–34	15	7.2	10	3	4	7	9	11	13	13
35–49	142	9.6	91	3	4	7	11	17	23	61
50–64	210	8.9	59	3	5	7	11	16	20	53
65+	85	8.4	60	3	5	7	9	14	17	54
SUBTOTALS:										
1. SINGLE DX — A. Not Operated	0									
1. SINGLE DX — B. Operated	0									
2. MULTIPLE DX — A. Not Operated	1,886	4.4	14	1	2	3	5	8	11	20
2. MULTIPLE DX — B. Operated	452	9.0	68	3	5	7	11	15	22	54
1. SINGLE DX	0									
2. MULTIPLE DX	2,338	5.3	27	1	2	4	6	10	14	26
A. NOT OPERATED	1,886	4.4	14	1	2	3	5	8	11	20
B. OPERATED	452	9.0	68	3	5	7	11	15	22	54
TOTAL										
0–19 Years	2	2.0	0	2	2	2	2	2	2	2
20–34	139	5.6	25	2	2	4	7	11	16	28
35–49	778	5.2	32	1	2	4	6	10	14	27
50–64	942	5.4	27	2	2	4	7	10	14	26
65+	477	5.2	22	2	2	4	7	10	13	20
GRAND TOTAL	2,338	5.3	27	2	2	4	6	10	14	26

Length of Stay by Diagnosis and Operation, Western Region, 2008

Western Region, October 2006–September 2007 Data, by Diagnosis

250.63: DM1 W NEURO MANIFEST UNC

Type of Patients	Observed Patients	Avg. Stay	Vari-ance	Percentiles						
				10th	25th	50th	75th	90th	95th	99th
1. SINGLE DX										
A. Not Operated										
0–19 Years	0									
20–34	0									
35–49	0									
50–64	0									
65+	1	2.0	0	2	2	2	2	2	2	2
B. Operated										
0–19 Years	0									
20–34	0									
35–49	0									
50–64	0									
65+	0									
2. MULTIPLE DX										
A. Not Operated										
0–19 Years	6	4.9	61	1	1	1	3	21	21	21
20–34	322	4.7	19	1	2	3	5	10	14	22
35–49	298	4.2	10	1	2	3	5	8	11	15
50–64	84	5.0	30	2	2	4	6	8	11	45
65+	28	5.0	29	2	3	4	5	7	10	31
B. Operated										
0–19 Years	0									
20–34	11	15.3	112	6	7	12	24	26	39	39
35–49	44	11.8	182	3	5	7	10	30	38	72
50–64	14	7.9	16	4	4	8	10	13	15	15
65+	4	14.5	2	13	13	14	15	16	16	16
SUBTOTALS:										
1. SINGLE DX										
A. Not Operated	1	2.0	0	2	2	2	2	2	2	2
B. Operated	0									
2. MULTIPLE DX										
A. Not Operated	738	4.6	18	1	2	3	5	9	12	21
B. Operated	73	11.8	132	3	6	9	13	24	38	72
1. SINGLE DX	1	2.0	0	2	2	2	2	2	2	2
2. MULTIPLE DX	811	5.2	32	1	2	4	6	10	14	30
A. NOT OPERATED	739	4.5	17	1	2	3	5	9	12	21
B. OPERATED	73	11.8	132	3	6	9	13	24	38	72
TOTAL										
0–19 Years	6	4.9	61	1	1	1	3	21	21	21
20–34	333	5.1	26	1	2	3	6	11	15	26
35–49	342	5.2	38	1	2	4	6	9	13	36
50–64	98	5.4	29	2	2	4	7	10	13	45
65+	33	6.1	36	2	3	4	5	14	16	31
GRAND TOTAL	812	5.2	32	1	2	4	6	10	14	30

250.70: DM2/NOS W CIRC DIS NSU

Type of Patients	Observed Patients	Avg. Stay	Vari-ance	Percentiles						
				10th	25th	50th	75th	90th	95th	99th
1. SINGLE DX										
A. Not Operated										
0–19 Years	0									
20–34	0									
35–49	0									
50–64	0									
65+	1	2.0	0	2	2	2	2	2	2	2
B. Operated										
0–19 Years	0									
20–34	0									
35–49	0									
50–64	0									
65+	1	2.0	0	2	2	2	2	2	2	2
2. MULTIPLE DX										
A. Not Operated										
0–19 Years	0									
20–34	6	5.3	23	2	2	3	7	14	14	14
35–49	76	5.9	17	2	3	4	8	12	16	19
50–64	330	5.0	14	1	2	4	7	10	12	16
65+	620	5.9	23	2	3	5	7	12	15	23
B. Operated										
0–19 Years	0									
20–34	22	6.8	28	2	3	5	9	12	14	24
35–49	295	10.1	68	3	5	8	13	21	29	43
50–64	1,350	9.9	82	2	4	8	12	20	26	40
65+	2,333	9.1	56	4	4	7	12	18	23	34
SUBTOTALS:										
1. SINGLE DX										
A. Not Operated	0									
B. Operated	1	2.0	0	2	2	2	2	2	2	2
2. MULTIPLE DX										
A. Not Operated	1,032	5.6	20	1	3	4	7	11	14	22
B. Operated	4,000	9.4	66	2	4	7	12	19	25	37
1. SINGLE DX	1	2.0	0	2	2	2	2	2	2	2
2. MULTIPLE DX	5,032	8.7	59	2	4	7	11	17	23	36
A. NOT OPERATED	1,032	5.6	20	1	3	4	7	11	14	22
B. OPERATED	4,001	9.4	66	2	4	7	12	19	25	37
TOTAL										
0–19 Years	0									
20–34	28	6.5	26	1	3	5	9	14	14	24
35–49	371	9.2	60	2	4	7	12	18	27	42
50–64	1,680	8.9	72	2	4	7	11	18	24	39
65+	2,954	8.4	51	2	4	7	11	17	22	33
GRAND TOTAL	5,033	8.7	59	2	4	7	11	17	23	36

250.71: DM1 W CIRC DISORD NSU

Type of Patients	Observed Patients	Avg. Stay	Vari-ance	Percentiles						
				10th	25th	50th	75th	90th	95th	99th
1. SINGLE DX										
A. Not Operated										
0–19 Years	0									
20–34	0									
35–49	0									
50–64	0									
65+	0									
B. Operated										
0–19 Years	0									
20–34	0									
35–49	0									
50–64	0									
65+	0									
2. MULTIPLE DX										
A. Not Operated										
0–19 Years	0									
20–34	4	7.3	47	2	3	7	17	17	17	17
35–49	23	4.9	5	2	3	5	7	7	8	8
50–64	29	6.0	10	2	3	5	9	10	12	12
65+	13	8.9	160	2	4	6	7	11	50	50
B. Operated										
0–19 Years	0									
20–34	11	11.5	93	4	5	7	19	29	29	29
35–49	76	9.6	59	3	4	7	13	21	28	36
50–64	118	9.7	70	3	4	7	13	20	33	41
65+	49	8.6	31	3	5	7	10	18	21	26
SUBTOTALS:										
1. SINGLE DX										
A. Not Operated	0									
B. Operated	0									
2. MULTIPLE DX										
A. Not Operated	69	6.2	38	2	3	5	7	10	12	50
B. Operated	254	9.5	60	3	5	7	12	20	27	41
1. SINGLE DX	0									
2. MULTIPLE DX	323	8.8	57	3	4	7	10	18	25	41
A. NOT OPERATED	69	6.2	38	2	3	5	7	10	12	50
B. OPERATED	254	9.5	60	3	5	7	12	20	27	41
TOTAL										
0–19 Years	0									
20–34	15	10.3	80	3	4	7	17	29	29	29
35–49	99	8.5	50	3	4	6	10	21	27	29
50–64	147	9.0	60	2	4	7	11	17	22	41
65+	62	8.6	56	3	5	7	10	15	21	50
GRAND TOTAL	323	8.8	57	3	4	7	10	18	25	41

Length of Stay by Diagnosis and Operation, Western Region, 2008

Western Region, October 2006–September 2007 Data, by Diagnosis

250.72: DM2/NOS W CIRC DIS UNC

Type of Patients	Observed Patients	Avg. Stay	Vari-ance	10th	25th	50th	75th	90th	95th	99th
1. SINGLE DX										
A. Not Operated										
0–19 Years	0									
20–34	0									
35–49	0									
50–64	0									
65+	0									
B. Operated										
0–19 Years	0									
20–34	0									
35–49	0									
50–64	0									
65+	0									
2. MULTIPLE DX										
A. Not Operated										
0–19 Years	0									
20–34	7	7.6	41	1	3	6	11	20	20	20
35–49	36	5.6	15	1	3	4	8	13	14	14
50–64	122	6.0	20	2	3	5	8	11	14	22
65+	114	7.3	52	2	4	6	8	12	16	30
B. Operated										
0–19 Years	0									
20–34	17	11.7	111	4	5	7	17	31	39	39
35–49	143	10.8	96	3	5	8	12	20	34	54
50–64	402	12.0	98	4	6	9	15	25	30	49
65+	342	11.8	79	5	6	9	14	21	32	45
SUBTOTALS:										
1. SINGLE DX										
A. Not Operated	0									
B. Operated	0									
2. MULTIPLE DX										
A. Not Operated	279	6.5	33	2	3	5	8	12	15	25
B. Operated	904	11.7	91	4	6	9	14	22	31	49
1. SINGLE DX	0									
2. MULTIPLE DX	1,183	10.5	82	3	5	8	13	21	29	49
A. NOT OPERATED	279	6.5	33	2	3	5	8	12	15	25
B. OPERATED	904	11.7	91	4	6	9	14	22	31	49
TOTAL										
0–19 Years	0									
20–34	24	10.5	91	3	4	7	17	22	31	39
35–49	179	9.8	84	3	5	8	11	18	28	54
50–64	524	10.6	87	3	5	8	13	22	29	48
65+	456	10.6	76	4	6	8	13	20	30	45
GRAND TOTAL	1,183	10.5	82	3	5	8	13	21	29	49

250.80: DM2/NOS W MANIF NEC NSU

Type of Patients	Observed Patients	Avg. Stay	Vari-ance	10th	25th	50th	75th	90th	95th	99th
1. SINGLE DX										
A. Not Operated										
0–19 Years	2	4.0	0	4	4	4	4	4	4	4
20–34	3	1.0	0	1	1	1	1	1	1	1
35–49	3	1.0	0	1	1	1	1	1	1	1
50–64	10	2.1	2	1	1	2	3	3	5	5
65+	18	1.6	<1	1	1	1	2	3	4	4
B. Operated										
0–19 Years	0									
20–34	0									
35–49	0									
50–64	0									
65+	0									
2. MULTIPLE DX										
A. Not Operated										
0–19 Years	29	2.1	<1	1	1	2	2	3	4	5
20–34	163	3.2	15	1	1	2	4	6	10	21
35–49	1,100	3.8	17	1	2	3	5	7	11	19
50–64	3,065	3.5	12	1	1	2	4	7	9	19
65+	7,478	3.2	9	1	1	2	4	6	8	14
B. Operated										
0–19 Years	1	5.0	0	5	5	5	5	5	5	5
20–34	61	7.8	37	3	4	6	10	16	22	27
35–49	677	7.5	34	3	4	6	10	14	18	31
50–64	1,589	8.2	46	2	4	7	10	16	20	35
65+	1,408	8.1	42	2	4	7	10	15	19	32
SUBTOTALS:										
1. SINGLE DX										
A. Not Operated	36	1.8	1	1	1	1	2	4	4	5
B. Operated	0									
2. MULTIPLE DX										
A. Not Operated	11,835	3.3	10	1	1	2	4	6	9	16
B. Operated	3,736	8.0	42	2	4	6	10	15	20	34
1. SINGLE DX	36	1.8	1	1	1	1	2	4	4	5
2. MULTIPLE DX	15,571	4.4	22	1	2	3	6	9	13	23
A. NOT OPERATED	11,871	3.3	10	1	1	2	4	6	9	16
B. OPERATED	3,736	8.0	42	2	4	6	10	15	20	34
TOTAL										
0–19 Years	32	2.3	1	1	1	2	3	4	5	5
20–34	227	4.4	25	1	1	3	5	10	14	26
35–49	1,780	5.2	27	1	2	4	7	11	15	25
50–64	4,664	5.1	28	2	2	3	6	11	15	27
65+	8,904	3.9	17	1	2	3	5	8	11	20
GRAND TOTAL	15,607	4.4	22	2	2	3	6	9	13	23

250.81: DM1 W MANIFEST NEC NSU

Type of Patients	Observed Patients	Avg. Stay	Vari-ance	10th	25th	50th	75th	90th	95th	99th
1. SINGLE DX										
A. Not Operated										
0–19 Years	14	2.4	1	1	2	2	3	4	4	4
20–34	0									
35–49	0									
50–64	0									
65+	0									
B. Operated										
0–19 Years	0									
20–34	0									
35–49	0									
50–64	0									
65+	0									
2. MULTIPLE DX										
A. Not Operated										
0–19 Years	60	2.1	2	1	1	2	3	3	5	10
20–34	159	3.3	24	1	1	2	3	6	8	29
35–49	231	3.2	10	1	1	2	4	6	8	16
50–64	179	3.8	18	1	1	3	5	7	10	30
65+	142	3.3	8	1	1	2	4	7	9	15
B. Operated										
0–19 Years	2	7.5	<1	7	7	7	8	8	8	8
20–34	49	9.0	50	3	4	6	12	20	23	32
35–49	108	8.5	32	3	5	7	10	16	19	29
50–64	109	9.0	107	3	4	6	10	16	26	59
65+	28	8.8	96	2	4	6	9	17	18	53
SUBTOTALS:										
1. SINGLE DX										
A. Not Operated	14	2.4	1	1	2	2	3	4	4	4
B. Operated	0									
2. MULTIPLE DX										
A. Not Operated	771	3.3	14	1	1	2	4	7	8	17
B. Operated	296	8.8	68	3	4	7	10	16	21	53
1. SINGLE DX	14	2.4	1	1	2	2	3	4	4	4
2. MULTIPLE DX	1,067	4.8	35	1	2	3	6	10	14	30
A. NOT OPERATED	785	3.3	14	1	2	2	4	7	8	17
B. OPERATED	296	8.8	68	3	4	7	10	16	21	53
TOTAL										
0–19 Years	76	2.3	3	1	1	2	3	4	6	10
20–34	208	4.6	36	1	1	3	5	10	16	30
35–49	339	4.9	23	1	2	3	7	10	15	24
50–64	288	5.8	57	1	2	4	7	11	15	53
65+	170	4.2	26	2	2	3	5	9	12	18
GRAND TOTAL	1,081	4.8	34	1	2	3	6	10	14	30

Western Region, October 2006–September 2007 Data, by Diagnosis

250.82: DM2/NOS W MANIF NEC UNC

Type of Patients	Observed Patients	Avg. Stay	Vari-ance	Percentiles 10th	25th	50th	75th	90th	95th	99th
1. SINGLE DX										
A. Not Operated										
0–19 Years	0									
20–34	1	2.0	0	2	2	2	2	2	2	2
35–49	1	1.0	0	1	1	1	1	1	1	1
50–64	3	3.7	1	3	3	3	5	5	5	5
65+	0									
B. Operated										
0–19 Years	0									
20–34	0									
35–49	0									
50–64	1	10.0	0	10	10	10	10	10	10	10
65+	0									
2. MULTIPLE DX										
A. Not Operated										
0–19 Years	5	2.6	<1	2	2	2	3	4	4	4
20–34	72	4.2	22	1	2	3	4	9	15	27
35–49	398	4.9	25	1	2	4	6	10	13	25
50–64	721	5.1	28	1	2	4	6	10	13	23
65+	933	4.5	18	1	2	3	6	8	12	22
B. Operated										
0–19 Years	0									
20–34	37	7.5	23	3	4	6	9	16	19	20
35–49	344	9.2	55	3	5	7	12	17	21	42
50–64	586	9.7	58	4	5	7	12	17	24	46
65+	260	9.4	43	4	5	7	11	17	22	34
SUBTOTALS:										
1. SINGLE DX										
A. Not Operated	5	2.8	2	1	2	3	3	5	5	5
B. Operated	1	10.0	0	10	10	10	10	10	10	10
2. MULTIPLE DX										
A. Not Operated	2,129	4.8	23	1	2	3	6	9	12	23
B. Operated	1,227	9.4	53	4	5	7	12	17	23	42
1. SINGLE DX	6	4.0	10	1	2	3	5	10	10	10
2. MULTIPLE DX	3,356	6.5	39	2	3	5	8	13	17	34
A. NOT OPERATED	2,134	4.8	23	1	2	3	6	9	12	23
B. OPERATED	1,228	9.4	53	4	5	7	12	17	23	42
TOTAL										
0–19 Years	5	2.6	<1	2	2	2	3	4	4	4
20–34	110	5.3	24	1	2	4	7	12	17	20
35–49	743	6.9	43	2	3	5	8	14	18	38
50–64	1,311	7.2	47	2	3	5	9	14	19	36
65+	1,193	5.6	27	1	2	4	7	11	15	28
GRAND TOTAL	3,362	6.5	39	2	3	5	8	13	17	34

250.83: DM1 W MANIFEST NEC UNC

Type of Patients	Observed Patients	Avg. Stay	Vari-ance	Percentiles 10th	25th	50th	75th	90th	95th	99th
1. SINGLE DX										
A. Not Operated										
0–19 Years	1	2.0	0	2	2	2	2	2	2	2
20–34	1	2.0	0	2	2	2	2	2	2	2
35–49	0									
50–64	0									
65+	0									
B. Operated										
0–19 Years	0									
20–34	0									
35–49	0									
50–64	0									
65+	0									
2. MULTIPLE DX										
A. Not Operated										
0–19 Years	12	4.1	37	1	1	2	3	10	22	22
20–34	78	4.4	30	1	2	3	5	8	9	45
35–49	106	4.7	27	1	2	3	5	8	13	25
50–64	65	4.7	16	1	2	4	6	9	14	23
65+	37	5.7	60	1	2	4	6	12	16	46
B. Operated										
0–19 Years	0									
20–34	48	9.4	32	4	6	8	12	17	21	29
35–49	50	9.3	50	4	5	7	10	16	22	45
50–64	46	9.7	95	3	4	7	10	20	22	58
65+	10	13.8	48	5	7	14	20	22	22	22
SUBTOTALS:										
1. SINGLE DX										
A. Not Operated	2	2.0	0	2	2	2	2	2	2	2
B. Operated	0									
2. MULTIPLE DX										
A. Not Operated	298	4.7	30	1	2	3	5	9	14	42
B. Operated	154	9.7	58	4	5	8	11	18	22	45
1. SINGLE DX	2	2.0	0	2	2	2	2	2	2	2
2. MULTIPLE DX	452	6.4	45	1	2	5	8	13	18	42
A. NOT OPERATED	300	4.7	30	1	2	3	5	9	14	42
B. OPERATED	154	9.7	58	4	5	8	11	18	22	45
TOTAL										
0–19 Years	13	3.9	35	1	1	2	2	10	22	22
20–34	127	6.3	36	1	3	5	7	13	17	29
35–49	156	6.1	39	1	3	5	7	11	17	42
50–64	111	6.8	55	2	3	5	8	13	20	39
65+	47	7.4	68	1	2	4	10	17	22	46
GRAND TOTAL	454	6.4	45	1	2	5	8	13	18	42

250.92: DM2/NOS W COMP NOS UNC

Type of Patients	Observed Patients	Avg. Stay	Vari-ance	Percentiles 10th	25th	50th	75th	90th	95th	99th
1. SINGLE DX										
A. Not Operated										
0–19 Years	0									
20–34	1	2.0	0	2	2	2	2	2	2	2
35–49	0									
50–64	1	1.0	0	1	1	1	1	1	1	1
65+	0									
B. Operated										
0–19 Years	0									
20–34	0									
35–49	0									
50–64	0									
65+	0									
2. MULTIPLE DX										
A. Not Operated										
0–19 Years	6	2.2	2	1	1	2	2	5	5	5
20–34	29	2.7	8	1	1	2	3	6	6	15
35–49	156	2.8	8	1	1	2	3	5	6	12
50–64	171	3.0	5	2	2	2	4	6	7	13
65+	135	3.2	6	2	2	3	4	6	7	10
B. Operated										
0–19 Years	0									
20–34	0									
35–49	2	8.0	2	7	7	7	9	9	9	9
50–64	0									
65+	2	5.0	2	4	4	5	6	6	6	6
SUBTOTALS:										
1. SINGLE DX										
A. Not Operated	2	1.5	<1	1	1	2	2	2	2	2
B. Operated	0									
2. MULTIPLE DX										
A. Not Operated	497	3.0	6	1	1	2	4	5	7	13
B. Operated	4	6.5	4	4	4	6	7	9	9	9
1. SINGLE DX	2	1.5	<1	1	1	2	2	2	2	2
2. MULTIPLE DX	501	3.0	6	1	1	2	4	6	7	13
A. NOT OPERATED	499	3.0	6	1	1	2	4	5	7	13
B. OPERATED	4	6.5	4	4	4	6	7	9	9	9
TOTAL										
0–19 Years	6	2.2	2	1	1	2	2	5	5	5
20–34	30	2.7	8	1	1	2	3	6	6	15
35–49	158	2.9	8	1	1	2	3	5	6	12
50–64	172	3.0	5	2	2	2	4	6	7	13
65+	137	3.2	6	2	2	3	4	6	7	10
GRAND TOTAL	503	3.0	6	1	1	2	4	6	7	12

149

Length of Stay by Diagnosis and Operation, Western Region, 2008

Western Region, October 2006–September 2007 Data, by Diagnosis

251: OTH PANCREATIC DISORDER

Type of Patients	Observed Patients	Avg. Stay	Variance	10th	25th	50th	75th	90th	95th	99th
1. SINGLE DX										
A. Not Operated										
0–19 Years	27	1.4	<1	1	1	1	2	2	2	2
20–34	4	2.8	3	1	1	3	5	5	5	5
35–49	4	2.0	2	1	1	1	4	4	4	4
50–64	2	4.5	5	3	3	5	6	6	6	6
65+	3	1.3	<1	1	1	1	2	2	2	2
B. Operated										
0–19 Years	0									
20–34	0									
35–49	0									
50–64	0									
65+	0									
2. MULTIPLE DX										
A. Not Operated										
0–19 Years	120	3.6	40	1	1	2	3	7	11	39
20–34	67	2.5	5	1	1	2	3	4	6	16
35–49	189	3.3	12	1	1	2	4	7	11	24
50–64	238	3.3	11	1	1	2	4	7	10	16
65+	536	3.3	7	1	2	3	4	6	8	13
B. Operated										
0–19 Years	0									
20–34	1	5.0	0	5	5	5	5	5	5	5
35–49	6	11.0	27	6	7	12	13	20	20	20
50–64	5	13.6	71	6	10	11	13	28	28	28
65+	5	13.6	66	1	11	15	20	21	21	21
SUBTOTALS:										
1. SINGLE DX										
A. Not Operated	40	1.8	1	1	1	1	2	3	4	6
B. Operated	0									
2. MULTIPLE DX										
A. Not Operated	1,150	3.3	12	1	1	2	4	7	9	18
B. Operated	17	12.2	48	5	7	11	15	21	28	28
1. SINGLE DX	40	1.8	1	1	1	1	2	3	4	6
2. MULTIPLE DX	1,167	3.4	14	1	1	2	4	7	10	20
A. NOT OPERATED	1,190	3.2	12	1	1	2	4	6	9	18
B. OPERATED	17	12.2	48	5	7	11	15	21	28	28
TOTAL										
0–19 Years	147	3.2	33	1	1	2	3	7	8	39
20–34	72	2.6	5	1	1	2	3	4	6	16
35–49	199	3.5	14	1	1	2	4	7	12	24
50–64	245	3.6	14	1	1	2	4	7	11	20
65+	544	3.4	9	1	2	3	4	7	9	17
GRAND TOTAL	1,207	3.4	13	1	1	2	4	7	10	20

251.1: HYPOGLYCEMIA NEC

Type of Patients	Observed Patients	Avg. Stay	Variance	10th	25th	50th	75th	90th	95th	99th
1. SINGLE DX										
A. Not Operated										
0–19 Years	9	1.6	<1	1	1	2	2	2	2	2
20–34	1	5.0	0	5	5	5	5	5	5	5
35–49	1	2.0	0	2	2	2	2	2	2	2
50–64	1	6.0	0	6	6	6	6	6	6	6
65+	1	1.0	0	1	1	1	1	1	1	1
B. Operated										
0–19 Years	0									
20–34	0									
35–49	0									
50–64	0									
65+	0									
2. MULTIPLE DX										
A. Not Operated										
0–19 Years	56	3.2	10	1	1	2	4	7	12	14
20–34	14	2.9	4	1	1	2	3	5	8	8
35–49	61	3.3	16	1	1	2	3	6	11	24
50–64	74	3.7	17	1	1	2	4	8	11	26
65+	177	3.7	12	1	2	3	5	8	10	20
B. Operated										
0–19 Years	0									
20–34	0									
35–49	1	8.0	0	8	8	8	8	8	8	8
50–64	0									
65+	0									
SUBTOTALS:										
1. SINGLE DX										
A. Not Operated	13	2.2	2	1	1	2	2	5	6	6
B. Operated	0									
2. MULTIPLE DX										
A. Not Operated	382	3.5	13	1	1	2	4	7	11	20
B. Operated	1	8.0	0	8	8	8	8	8	8	8
1. SINGLE DX	13	2.2	2	1	1	2	2	5	6	6
2. MULTIPLE DX	383	3.5	13	1	1	2	4	7	11	20
A. NOT OPERATED	395	3.5	13	1	1	2	4	7	11	20
B. OPERATED	1	8.0	0	8	8	8	8	8	8	8
TOTAL										
0–19 Years	65	2.9	9	1	1	2	3	7	11	14
20–34	15	3.1	4	1	1	3	4	5	8	8
35–49	63	3.3	16	1	1	2	3	6	11	24
50–64	75	3.7	17	1	1	2	4	8	11	26
65+	178	3.7	12	1	2	3	5	8	10	20
GRAND TOTAL	396	3.5	13	1	1	2	4	7	11	20

251.2: HYPOGLYCEMIA NOS

Type of Patients	Observed Patients	Avg. Stay	Variance	10th	25th	50th	75th	90th	95th	99th
1. SINGLE DX										
A. Not Operated										
0–19 Years	18	1.3	<1	1	1	1	2	2	2	2
20–34	3	2.0	<1	1	1	2	3	3	3	3
35–49	3	2.0	3	1	1	1	4	4	4	4
50–64	1	3.0	0	3	3	3	3	3	3	3
65+	1	2.0	0	2	2	2	2	2	2	2
B. Operated										
0–19 Years	0									
20–34	0									
35–49	0									
50–64	0									
65+	0									
2. MULTIPLE DX										
A. Not Operated										
0–19 Years	62	3.9	68	1	1	2	3	5	8	52
20–34	46	2.0	1	1	1	2	3	4	4	6
35–49	83	2.8	8	1	1	2	3	5	8	>99
50–64	106	3.0	8	1	1	2	3	6	9	13
65+	285	3.0	5	1	2	2	4	5	8	10
B. Operated										
0–19 Years	0									
20–34	0									
35–49	3	15.0	19	12	12	13	20	20	20	20
50–64	1	11.0	0	11	11	11	11	11	11	11
65+	3	9.0	52	11	11	11	15	15	15	15
SUBTOTALS:										
1. SINGLE DX										
A. Not Operated	26	1.6	<1	1	1	1	2	3	3	4
B. Operated	0									
2. MULTIPLE DX										
A. Not Operated	582	3.0	12	1	1	2	3	5	8	16
B. Operated	7	11.8	33	1	11	12	15	20	20	20
1. SINGLE DX	26	1.6	<1	1	1	1	2	3	3	4
2. MULTIPLE DX	589	3.1	13	1	1	2	3	6	8	20
A. NOT OPERATED	608	2.9	12	1	1	2	3	5	8	16
B. OPERATED	7	11.8	33	1	11	12	15	20	20	20
TOTAL										
0–19 Years	80	3.3	54	1	1	2	2	4	8	52
20–34	49	2.0	1	1	1	2	3	4	4	6
35–49	89	3.2	13	1	1	2	3	6	12	>99
50–64	108	3.1	8	1	1	2	3	7	11	13
65+	289	3.0	5	1	2	2	4	6	8	13
GRAND TOTAL	615	3.0	13	1	1	2	3	6	8	16

Length of Stay by Diagnosis and Operation, Western Region, 2008

252: PARATHYROID DISORDER

Type of Patients	Observed Patients	Avg. Stay	Vari- ance	Percentiles						
				10th	25th	50th	75th	90th	95th	99th
1. SINGLE DX										
A. *Not Operated*										
0–19 Years	2	4.0	2	3	3	4	5	5	5	5
20–34	1	2.0	0	2	2	2	2	2	2	2
35–49	0									
50–64	2	4.5	4	3	3	3	6	6	6	6
65+	0									
B. *Operated*										
0–19 Years	1	1.0	0	1	1	1	1	1	1	1
20–34	4	1.0	0	1	1	1	1	1	1	1
35–49	20	1.1	<1	1	1	1	1	1	1	1
50–64	38	1.2	<1	1	1	1	1	2	2	2
65+	16	1.3	<1	1	1	1	1	3	3	3
2. MULTIPLE DX										
A. *Not Operated*										
0–19 Years	13	6.8	54	1	1	4	9	20	23	23
20–34	35	3.9	9	1	2	3	6	8	10	13
35–49	73	3.8	13	1	2	3	4	6	12	23
50–64	105	4.3	11	1	2	3	6	9	10	16
65+	208	4.9	24	1	2	4	6	10	13	27
B. *Operated*										
0–19 Years	4	4.3	11	1	1	6	8	8	8	8
20–34	53	3.3	15	1	1	2	4	8	12	22
35–49	123	2.4	6	1	1	1	3	5	7	12
50–64	373	1.9	5	1	1	1	2	3	6	12
65+	394	2.0	7	1	1	1	2	4	8	16
SUBTOTALS:										
1. SINGLE DX										
A. *Not Operated*	5	3.8	3	2	3	3	3	5	6	6
B. *Operated*	79	1.1	<1	1	1	1	1	2	2	3
2. MULTIPLE DX										
A. *Not Operated*	434	4.6	19	1	2	3	6	9	12	23
B. *Operated*	947	2.1	6	1	1	1	2	4	7	13
1. SINGLE DX	84	1.3	<1	1	1	1	1	2	3	6
2. MULTIPLE DX	1,381	2.9	12	1	1	2	3	6	9	17
A. NOT OPERATED	439	4.6	18	1	2	3	6	9	11	23
B. OPERATED	1,026	2.0	6	1	1	1	2	4	7	13
TOTAL										
0–19 Years	20	5.8	39	1	1	3	8	20	23	23
20–34	93	3.4	12	1	1	2	5	6	8	22
35–49	216	2.7	8	1	1	2	3	6	8	15
50–64	518	2.3	7	1	1	1	2	5	8	13
65+	618	3.0	14	1	1	1	3	6	10	17
GRAND TOTAL	1,465	2.8	11	1	1	1	3	6	9	16

252.00: HYPERPARATHYROIDISM NOS

Type of Patients	Observed Patients	Avg. Stay	Vari- ance	Percentiles						
				10th	25th	50th	75th	90th	95th	99th
1. SINGLE DX										
A. *Not Operated*										
0–19 Years	0									
20–34	0									
35–49	0									
50–64	0									
65+	0									
B. *Operated*										
0–19 Years	0									
20–34	1	1.0	0	1	1	1	1	1	1	1
35–49	2	1.0	0	1	1	1	1	1	1	1
50–64	11	1.2	<1	1	1	1	1	2	2	2
65+	5	1.0	0	1	1	1	1	1	1	1
2. MULTIPLE DX										
A. *Not Operated*										
0–19 Years	2	16.5	83	10	10	23	23	23	23	23
20–34	4	2.5	2	1	1	3	3	4	4	4
35–49	12	2.6	2	1	2	2	4	4	5	5
50–64	21	3.2	6	1	2	2	5	5	9	10
65+	39	3.9	18	1	2	3	5	6	14	24
B. *Operated*										
0–19 Years	1	1.0	0	1	1	1	1	1	1	1
20–34	8	2.5	5	1	1	2	3	8	8	8
35–49	28	2.3	5	1	1	2	3	4	4	12
50–64	53	1.9	3	1	1	1	2	3	5	10
65+	59	1.8	2	1	1	1	2	4	5	8
SUBTOTALS:										
1. SINGLE DX										
A. *Not Operated*	0									
B. *Operated*	19	1.1	<1	1	1	1	1	2	2	2
2. MULTIPLE DX										
A. *Not Operated*	78	3.8	17	1	2	3	4	6	10	24
B. *Operated*	149	1.9	3	1	1	1	2	3	5	10
1. SINGLE DX	19	1.1	<1	1	1	1	1	2	2	2
2. MULTIPLE DX	227	2.6	8	1	1	2	3	5	7	14
A. NOT OPERATED	78	3.8	17	1	2	3	4	6	10	24
B. OPERATED	168	1.8	3	1	1	1	2	3	5	10
TOTAL										
0–19 Years	3	11.4	121	1	1	10	23	23	23	23
20–34	13	2.4	4	1	1	2	3	4	8	8
35–49	42	2.3	4	1	1	2	3	4	4	12
50–64	85	2.1	4	1	1	1	2	5	5	10
65+	103	2.5	9	1	1	1	3	5	6	14
GRAND TOTAL	246	2.5	8	1	1	2	3	5	6	14

252.01: PRIM HYPERPARATHYROIDISM

Type of Patients	Observed Patients	Avg. Stay	Vari- ance	Percentiles						
				10th	25th	50th	75th	90th	95th	99th
1. SINGLE DX										
A. *Not Operated*										
0–19 Years	0									
20–34	0									
35–49	0									
50–64	0									
65+	0									
B. *Operated*										
0–19 Years	1	1.0	0	1	1	1	1	1	1	1
20–34	3	1.0	0	1	1	1	1	1	1	1
35–49	16	1.0	0	1	1	1	1	1	1	1
50–64	26	1.2	<1	1	1	1	1	2	2	3
65+	11	1.4	<1	1	1	1	1	3	3	3
2. MULTIPLE DX										
A. *Not Operated*										
0–19 Years	1	3.0	0	3	3	3	3	3	3	3
20–34	4	3.7	8	2	2	2	3	8	8	8
35–49	14	6.3	36	2	3	4	8	15	23	23
50–64	20	5.0	13	2	2	3	8	10	11	13
65+	93	5.6	22	1	3	5	7	10	13	29
B. *Operated*										
0–19 Years	1	2.0	0	2	2	2	2	2	2	2
20–34	27	2.2	4	1	1	1	3	6	6	8
35–49	73	1.8	3	1	1	1	2	4	5	12
50–64	266	1.5	3	1	1	1	1	2	4	9
65+	302	1.9	7	1	1	1	2	3	6	15
SUBTOTALS:										
1. SINGLE DX										
A. *Not Operated*	0									
B. *Operated*	57	1.1	<1	1	1	1	1	1	1	3
2. MULTIPLE DX										
A. *Not Operated*	132	5.5	21	2	3	4	7	10	13	27
B. *Operated*	669	1.8	4	1	1	1	2	3	5	11
1. SINGLE DX	57	1.1	<1	1	1	1	1	1	1	3
2. MULTIPLE DX	801	2.4	9	1	1	1	2	6	8	15
A. NOT OPERATED	132	5.5	21	2	3	4	7	10	13	27
B. OPERATED	726	1.7	4	1	1	1	2	3	5	11
TOTAL										
0–19 Years	3	2.0	1	1	1	1	3	3	3	3
20–34	34	2.2	4	1	1	1	3	6	8	8
35–49	103	2.3	9	1	1	1	2	4	7	15
50–64	312	1.7	4	1	1	1	2	3	5	10
65+	406	2.8	12	1	1	1	3	7	10	16
GRAND TOTAL	858	2.3	9	1	1	1	2	5	8	15

Length of Stay by Diagnosis and Operation, Western Region, 2008

151

Western Region, October 2006–September 2007 Data, by Diagnosis

253: PITUITARY GLAND DISORD

Type of Patients	Observed Patients	Avg. Stay	Vari-ance	10th	25th	50th	75th	90th	95th	99th
1. SINGLE DX										
A. Not Operated										
0–19 Years	2	1.0	0	1	1	1	1	1	1	1
20–34	0									
35–49	4	1.8	<1	1	1	2	2	2	2	2
50–64	3	2.0	<1	1	1	2	3	3	3	3
65+	2	5.5	4	4	4	7	7	7	7	7
B. Operated										
0–19 Years	2	2.5	<1	2	2	2	3	3	3	3
20–34	3	1.7	<1	1	1	2	2	2	2	2
35–49	6	2.2	<1	1	1	2	3	3	3	3
50–64	6	2.2	<1	2	2	2	2	3	3	3
65+	0									
2. MULTIPLE DX										
A. Not Operated										
0–19 Years	57	6.5	88	1	2	3	7	12	23	56
20–34	54	4.6	12	1	2	3	6	9	13	15
35–49	169	4.7	24	1	2	3	5	9	15	32
50–64	524	4.5	15	1	2	3	6	9	12	22
65+	2,208	5.3	18	2	3	4	7	10	12	18
B. Operated										
0–19 Years	3	6.0	37	2	2	3	13	13	13	13
20–34	26	4.4	28	2	2	3	4	8	19	24
35–49	20	4.1	11	1	1	3	5	8	15	15
50–64	29	5.7	48	1	2	4	6	11	22	34
65+	55	8.6	44	2	3	7	12	15	22	38
SUBTOTALS:										
1. SINGLE DX										
A. Not Operated	11	2.4	3	1	1	2	3	4	7	7
B. Operated	17	2.1	<1	1	2	2	2	3	3	3
2. MULTIPLE DX										
A. Not Operated	3,012	5.1	19	2	3	4	6	10	12	20
B. Operated	133	6.4	39	2	2	4	8	14	19	34
1. SINGLE DX	28	2.2	1	1	2	2	3	3	4	7
2. MULTIPLE DX	3,145	5.2	20	2	3	4	7	10	12	22
A. NOT OPERATED	3,023	5.1	19	2	3	4	6	10	12	20
B. OPERATED	150	5.9	37	2	2	3	7	13	18	34
TOTAL										
0–19 Years	64	6.2	81	1	2	3	7	12	15	56
20–34	83	4.4	16	1	2	3	5	9	13	24
35–49	199	4.5	22	1	2	3	5	9	14	27
50–64	562	4.5	17	1	2	3	6	9	12	23
65+	2,265	5.4	19	2	3	4	7	10	12	19
GRAND TOTAL	3,173	5.2	20	2	3	4	6	10	12	22

253.6: NEUROHYPOPH DISORD NEC

Type of Patients	Observed Patients	Avg. Stay	Vari-ance	10th	25th	50th	75th	90th	95th	99th
1. SINGLE DX										
A. Not Operated										
0–19 Years	0									
20–34	0									
35–49	1	2.0	0	2	2	2	2	2	2	2
50–64	2	2.5	<1	2	2	3	3	3	3	3
65+	2	5.5	4	4	4	7	7	7	7	7
B. Operated										
0–19 Years	0									
20–34	0									
35–49	0									
50–64	0									
65+	0									
2. MULTIPLE DX										
A. Not Operated										
0–19 Years	11	5.6	16	2	2	4	11	11	11	11
20–34	23	4.4	7	1	3	4	6	9	9	10
35–49	109	4.2	12	1	2	3	5	8	11	16
50–64	461	4.4	14	1	2	3	6	8	10	22
65+	2,142	5.3	17	2	3	4	7	10	12	18
B. Operated										
0–19 Years	0									
20–34	1	9.0	0	9	9	9	9	9	9	9
35–49	1	2.0	0	2	2	2	2	2	2	2
50–64	8	11.8	115	4	5	7	22	34	34	34
65+	37	10.0	47	5	6	8	12	17	26	38
SUBTOTALS:										
1. SINGLE DX										
A. Not Operated	5	3.6	4	2	2	3	4	7	7	7
B. Operated	0									
2. MULTIPLE DX										
A. Not Operated	2,746	5.1	17	2	3	4	6	10	12	18
B. Operated	47	10.1	56	4	6	8	12	22	26	38
1. SINGLE DX	5	3.6	4	2	2	3	4	7	7	7
2. MULTIPLE DX	2,793	5.2	18	2	3	4	7	10	12	19
A. NOT OPERATED	2,751	5.1	17	2	3	4	6	10	12	18
B. OPERATED	47	10.1	56	4	6	8	12	22	26	38
TOTAL										
0–19 Years	11	5.6	16	2	2	4	11	11	11	11
20–34	24	4.5	8	1	3	4	6	9	9	10
35–49	111	4.2	12	1	2	3	5	9	11	16
50–64	471	4.5	16	1	2	3	6	8	11	24
65+	2,181	5.4	18	2	3	4	7	10	12	18
GRAND TOTAL	2,798	5.2	18	2	3	4	7	10	12	19

254: DISEASES OF THYMUS GLAND

Type of Patients	Observed Patients	Avg. Stay	Vari-ance	10th	25th	50th	75th	90th	95th	99th
1. SINGLE DX										
A. Not Operated										
0–19 Years	0									
20–34	0									
35–49	0									
50–64	0									
65+	0									
B. Operated										
0–19 Years	0									
20–34	2	2.5	<1	2	2	3	3	3	3	3
35–49	4	3.0	5	1	1	2	3	6	6	6
50–64	4	1.8	<1	1	1	1	2	3	3	3
65+	0									
2. MULTIPLE DX										
A. Not Operated										
0–19 Years	3	1.7	1	1	1	1	3	3	3	3
20–34	0									
35–49	2	4.0	18	1	1	1	7	7	7	7
50–64	1	15.0	0	15	15	15	15	15	15	15
65+	0									
B. Operated										
0–19 Years	3	2.3	<1	2	2	2	3	3	3	3
20–34	19	3.6	3	2	3	3	4	6	6	9
35–49	22	3.7	4	2	3	3	4	5	7	11
50–64	14	3.5	3	2	2	3	4	6	7	7
65+	4	2.8	2	1	1	3	4	4	4	4
SUBTOTALS:										
1. SINGLE DX										
A. Not Operated	0									
B. Operated	10	2.4	2	1	1	2	3	6	6	6
2. MULTIPLE DX										
A. Not Operated	6	4.7	31	1	1	1	4	15	15	15
B. Operated	62	3.5	3	2	3	3	4	5	7	11
1. SINGLE DX	10	2.4	2	1	1	2	3	6	6	6
2. MULTIPLE DX	68	3.6	5	1	2	3	4	6	7	15
A. NOT OPERATED	6	4.7	31	1	1	1	4	15	15	15
B. OPERATED	72	3.4	3	2	2	3	4	5	7	11
TOTAL										
0–19 Years	6	2.0	<1	1	1	2	3	3	3	3
20–34	21	3.5	2	2	3	3	4	4	6	6
35–49	28	3.6	5	1	3	3	4	7	7	11
50–64	19	3.7	10	2	2	3	4	7	15	15
65+	4	2.8	2	1	1	3	4	4	4	4
GRAND TOTAL	78	3.5	5	1	2	3	4	6	7	15

Length of Stay by Diagnosis and Operation, Western Region. 2008

Western Region, October 2006–September 2007 Data, by Diagnosis

255: ADRENAL GLAND DISORDERS

Type of Patients	Observed Patients	Avg. Stay	Variance	10th	25th	50th	75th	90th	95th	99th
1. SINGLE DX										
A. Not Operated										
0–19 Years	4	1.3	<1	1	1	1	1	2	2	2
20–34	2	1.5	<1	1	1	2	2	2	2	2
35–49	1	1.0	0	1	1	1	1	1	1	1
50–64	0									
65+	0									
B. Operated										
0–19 Years	2	2.0	2	1	1	3	3	3	3	3
20–34	3	2.3	1	1	1	3	3	3	3	3
35–49	4	2.5	2	1	2	3	3	4	4	4
50–64	8	2.2	2	1	1	2	3	5	5	5
65+	0									
2. MULTIPLE DX										
A. Not Operated										
0–19 Years	52	3.0	6	1	1	2	4	7	9	11
20–34	139	3.5	6	1	2	3	4	6	9	14
35–49	234	4.1	9	1	2	3	5	8	10	15
50–64	332	4.4	14	1	2	3	5	9	11	19
65+	413	4.3	10	1	2	4	5	8	11	18
B. Operated										
0–19 Years	2	2.5	4	1	1	1	1	4	4	4
20–34	20	3.9	8	1	2	3	4	10	10	12
35–49	57	4.7	28	1	2	3	5	9	14	36
50–64	81	3.5	8	1	2	3	5	7	9	15
65+	37	4.6	14	1	2	4	6	10	14	15
SUBTOTALS:										
1. SINGLE DX										
A. Not Operated	7	1.3	<1	1	1	1	1	2	2	2
B. Operated	17	2.3	1	1	1	2	2	4	5	5
2. MULTIPLE DX										
A. Not Operated	1,170	4.1	11	1	2	3	5	8	11	18
B. Operated	197	4.1	15	1	2	3	5	8	11	17
1. SINGLE DX	24	2.0	1	1	1	2	3	3	4	5
2. MULTIPLE DX	1,367	4.1	11	1	2	3	5	8	11	17
A. NOT OPERATED	1,177	4.1	10	1	2	3	5	8	11	18
B. OPERATED	214	3.9	14	1	2	3	5	8	11	15
TOTAL										
0–19 Years	60	2.8	6	1	1	2	3	7	9	11
20–34	164	3.5	6	1	2	3	4	6	10	14
35–49	296	4.2	12	1	2	3	5	8	11	16
50–64	421	4.2	13	1	2	3	5	8	11	19
65+	450	4.3	11	1	2	4	5	8	11	18
GRAND TOTAL	1,391	4.1	11	2	2	3	5	8	11	17

255.4: CORTICOADR INSUFFICIENCY

Type of Patients	Observed Patients	Avg. Stay	Variance	10th	25th	50th	75th	90th	95th	99th
1. SINGLE DX										
A. Not Operated										
0–19 Years	1	1.0	0	1	1	1	1	1	1	1
20–34	2	1.5	<1	1	1	2	2	2	2	2
35–49	1	1.0	0	1	1	1	1	1	1	1
50–64	0									
65+	0									
B. Operated										
0–19 Years	0									
20–34	0									
35–49	0									
50–64	1	2.0	0	2	2	2	2	2	2	2
65+	0									
2. MULTIPLE DX										
A. Not Operated										
0–19 Years	28	2.8	5	1	1	2	4	7	9	9
20–34	116	3.4	5	1	2	3	4	5	9	14
35–49	173	4.2	10	1	2	3	5	8	11	15
50–64	275	4.4	14	1	2	3	5	9	11	19
65+	360	4.2	10	1	2	3	5	8	11	19
B. Operated										
0–19 Years	0									
20–34	0									
35–49	2	6.0	2	5	5	7	7	7	7	7
50–64	4	7.3	8	5	5	8	8	11	11	11
65+	6	8.3	9	5	6	7	10	13	13	13
SUBTOTALS:										
1. SINGLE DX										
A. Not Operated	4	1.3	<1	1	1	1	1	2	2	2
B. Operated	1	2.0	0	2	2	2	2	2	2	2
2. MULTIPLE DX										
A. Not Operated	952	4.1	11	1	2	3	5	8	11	18
B. Operated	12	7.6	7	5	5	7	9	11	13	13
1. SINGLE DX	5	1.4	<1	1	1	1	2	2	2	2
2. MULTIPLE DX	964	4.2	11	1	2	3	5	8	11	18
A. NOT OPERATED	956	4.1	11	1	2	3	5	8	11	18
B. OPERATED	13	7.1	9	5	5	7	9	11	13	13
TOTAL										
0–19 Years	29	2.7	5	1	1	2	3	7	7	9
20–34	118	3.4	5	1	2	3	4	5	9	14
35–49	176	4.2	10	1	2	3	5	8	11	15
50–64	280	4.4	14	1	2	3	5	8	11	19
65+	366	4.3	11	1	2	4	5	8	11	19
GRAND TOTAL	969	4.2	11	1	2	3	5	8	11	18

256: OVARIAN DYSFUNCTION

Type of Patients	Observed Patients	Avg. Stay	Variance	10th	25th	50th	75th	90th	95th	99th
1. SINGLE DX										
A. Not Operated										
0–19 Years	0									
20–34	5	2.0	1	1	1	2	2	4	4	4
35–49	1	2.0	0	2	2	2	2	2	2	2
50–64	0									
65+	0									
B. Operated										
0–19 Years	0									
20–34	3	2.7	<1	2	2	3	3	3	3	3
35–49	0									
50–64	0									
65+	0									
2. MULTIPLE DX										
A. Not Operated										
0–19 Years	3	1.0	0	1	1	1	1	1	1	1
20–34	77	3.2	10	1	1	3	4	6	7	25
35–49	12	2.7	5	1	1	1	4	6	7	7
50–64	2	3.5	<1	3	3	3	4	4	4	4
65+	0									
B. Operated										
0–19 Years	4	1.8	<1	1	1	2	2	3	3	3
20–34	49	2.3	1	1	2	2	2	4	4	7
35–49	37	2.1	<1	1	2	2	3	3	4	5
50–64	10	1.9	1	1	1	2	3	4	4	4
65+	0									
SUBTOTALS:										
1. SINGLE DX										
A. Not Operated	6	2.0	1	1	1	2	2	4	4	4
B. Operated	3	2.7	<1	2	2	3	3	3	3	3
2. MULTIPLE DX										
A. Not Operated	94	3.1	9	1	1	2	4	6	7	25
B. Operated	100	2.1	1	1	1	2	3	3	4	7
1. SINGLE DX	9	2.2	<1	1	2	2	3	4	4	4
2. MULTIPLE DX	194	2.6	5	1	1	2	3	5	6	10
A. NOT OPERATED	100	3.0	9	1	1	2	4	6	7	25
B. OPERATED	103	2.2	1	1	2	2	3	3	4	5
TOTAL										
0–19 Years	7	1.4	<1	1	1	1	2	2	3	3
20–34	134	2.8	7	1	1	2	3	5	6	10
35–49	50	2.3	2	1	1	2	3	4	6	7
50–64	12	2.2	1	1	1	2	3	4	4	4
65+	0									
GRAND TOTAL	203	2.6	5	1	1	2	3	5	6	8

Length of Stay by Diagnosis and Operation, Western Region, 2008

Western Region, October 2006–September 2007 Data, by Diagnosis

257: TESTICULAR DYSFUNCTION

Type of Patients	Observed Patients	Avg. Stay	Variance	10th	25th	50th	75th	90th	95th	99th
1. SINGLE DX										
A. Not Operated										
0–19 Years	0									
20–34	0									
35–49	0									
50–64	0									
65+	0									
B. Operated										
0–19 Years	0									
20–34	0									
35–49	0									
50–64	0									
65+	0									
2. MULTIPLE DX										
A. Not Operated										
0–19 Years	0									
20–34	5	1.6	<1	1	1	2	2	2	2	2
35–49	4	1.3	<1	1	1	1	2	2	2	2
50–64	17	1.7	<1	1	1	2	2	2	3	3
65+	5	4.2	30	1	2	2	2	14	14	14
B. Operated										
0–19 Years	1	1.0	0	1	1	1	1	1	1	1
20–34	0									
35–49	0									
50–64	1	2.0	0	2	2	2	2	2	2	2
65+	0									
SUBTOTALS:										
1. SINGLE DX										
A. Not Operated	0									
B. Operated	0									
2. MULTIPLE DX										
A. Not Operated	31	2.0	5	1	1	2	2	2	3	14
B. Operated	2	1.5	<1	1	1	2	2	2	2	2
1. SINGLE DX	0									
2. MULTIPLE DX	33	2.0	5	1	1	2	2	2	3	14
A. NOT OPERATED	31	2.0	5	1	1	2	2	2	3	14
B. OPERATED	2	1.5	<1	1	1	2	2	2	2	2
TOTAL										
0–19 Years	0									
20–34	6	1.5	<1	1	1	2	2	2	2	2
35–49	4	1.3	<1	1	1	1	2	2	2	2
50–64	18	1.7	<1	1	1	2	2	2	3	3
65+	5	4.2	30	1	2	2	2	14	14	14
GRAND TOTAL	33	2.0	5	1	1	2	2	2	3	14

258: POLYGLANDULAR DYSFUNCT

Type of Patients	Observed Patients	Avg. Stay	Variance	10th	25th	50th	75th	90th	95th	99th
1. SINGLE DX										
A. Not Operated										
0–19 Years	0									
20–34	0									
35–49	0									
50–64	0									
65+	0									
B. Operated										
0–19 Years	1	2.0	0	2	2	2	2	2	2	2
20–34	0									
35–49	0									
50–64	0									
65+	0									
2. MULTIPLE DX										
A. Not Operated										
0–19 Years	0									
20–34	5	3.0	1	2	2	3	4	4	4	4
35–49	2	3.0	8	1	1	5	5	5	5	5
50–64	2	4.0	18	1	1	1	7	7	7	7
65+	3	4.3	2	3	3	4	6	6	6	6
B. Operated										
0–19 Years	1	2.0	0	2	2	2	2	2	2	2
20–34	1	23.0	0	23	23	23	23	23	23	23
35–49	1	2.0	0	2	2	2	2	2	2	2
50–64	4	3.0	5	1	2	2	6	6	6	6
65+	1	8.0	0	8	8	8	8	8	8	8
SUBTOTALS:										
1. SINGLE DX										
A. Not Operated	0									
B. Operated	1	2.0	0	2	2	2	2	2	2	2
2. MULTIPLE DX										
A. Not Operated	12	3.5	4	2	2	4	5	6	7	7
B. Operated	8	5.9	54	1	2	3	8	23	23	23
1. SINGLE DX	1	2.0	0	2	2	2	2	2	2	2
2. MULTIPLE DX	20	4.5	23	1	2	3	6	8	23	23
A. NOT OPERATED	12	3.5	4	1	2	4	5	6	7	7
B. OPERATED	9	5.5	49	1	2	2	6	23	23	23
TOTAL										
0–19 Years	2	2.0	0	2	2	2	2	2	2	2
20–34	6	6.4	67	2	2	4	4	23	23	23
35–49	3	2.7	4	1	1	2	5	5	5	5
50–64	6	3.3	7	1	1	2	6	7	7	7
65+	4	5.3	5	3	3	6	6	8	8	8
GRAND TOTAL	21	4.4	22	1	2	3	5	7	8	23

259: OTH ENDOCRINE DISORDERS

Type of Patients	Observed Patients	Avg. Stay	Variance	10th	25th	50th	75th	90th	95th	99th
1. SINGLE DX										
A. Not Operated										
0–19 Years	0									
20–34	0									
35–49	0									
50–64	0									
65+	0									
B. Operated										
0–19 Years	1	1.0	0	1	1	1	1	1	1	1
20–34	0									
35–49	0									
50–64	0									
65+	0									
2. MULTIPLE DX										
A. Not Operated										
0–19 Years	2	1.5	<1	1	1	1	2	2	2	2
20–34	2	3.5	<1	3	3	3	4	4	4	4
35–49	6	3.0	4	1	1	3	4	6	6	6
50–64	14	4.1	8	2	2	3	5	9	10	10
65+	27	5.3	18	1	3	4	7	9	18	18
B. Operated										
0–19 Years	1	6.0	0	6	6	6	6	6	6	6
20–34	0									
35–49	0									
50–64	2	2.0	2	1	1	1	3	3	3	3
65+	1	7.0	0	7	7	7	7	7	7	7
SUBTOTALS:										
1. SINGLE DX										
A. Not Operated	0									
B. Operated	1	1.0	0	1	1	1	1	1	1	1
2. MULTIPLE DX										
A. Not Operated	51	4.5	13	1	2	3	6	8	10	18
B. Operated	4	4.3	8	1	1	6	7	7	7	7
1. SINGLE DX	1	1.0	0	1	1	1	1	1	1	1
2. MULTIPLE DX	55	4.5	12	1	2	3	6	8	10	18
A. NOT OPERATED	51	4.5	13	1	2	3	6	8	10	18
B. OPERATED	5	3.6	8	1	1	3	6	7	7	7
TOTAL										
0–19 Years	4	2.5	6	1	1	1	6	6	6	6
20–34	2	3.5	<1	3	3	3	4	4	4	4
35–49	6	3.0	4	1	1	3	4	6	6	6
50–64	16	3.9	7	1	2	3	5	9	10	10
65+	28	5.3	18	1	3	4	7	9	18	18
GRAND TOTAL	56	4.4	12	1	2	3	6	8	10	18

Length of Stay by Diagnosis and Operation, Western Region. 2008

Western Region, October 2006–September 2007 Data, by Diagnosis

260: KWASHIORKOR

Type of Patients	Observed Patients	Avg. Stay	Variance	Percentiles 10th	25th	50th	75th	90th	95th	99th
1. SINGLE DX										
A. Not Operated										
0–19 Years	0									
20–34	0									
35–49	0									
50–64	0									
65+	0									
B. Operated										
0–19 Years	0									
20–34	0									
35–49	0									
50–64	0									
65+	0									
2. MULTIPLE DX										
A. Not Operated										
0–19 Years	3	13.0	12	11	11	11	17	17	17	17
20–34	1	10.0	0	10	10	10	10	10	10	10
35–49	3	7.3	4	5	5	8	9	9	9	9
50–64	8	7.7	18	1	7	8	9	14	14	14
65+	11	5.5	6	3	3	5	8	8	10	10
B. Operated										
0–19 Years	0									
20–34	0									
35–49	0									
50–64	0									
65+	1	2.0	0	2	2	2	2	2	2	2
SUBTOTALS:										
1. SINGLE DX										
A. Not Operated	0									
B. Operated	0									
2. MULTIPLE DX										
A. Not Operated	26	7.4	15	3	4	8	10	12	14	17
B. Operated	1	2.0	0	2	2	2	2	2	2	2
1. SINGLE DX	0									
2. MULTIPLE DX	27	7.2	15	2	4	8	10	12	14	17
A. NOT OPERATED	26	7.4	15	3	4	8	10	12	14	17
B. OPERATED	1	2.0	0	2	2	2	2	2	2	2
TOTAL										
0–19 Years	3	13.0	12	11	11	11	17	17	17	17
20–34	1	10.0	0	10	10	10	10	10	10	10
35–49	3	7.3	4	5	5	8	9	9	9	9
50–64	8	7.7	18	1	7	8	9	14	14	14
65+	12	5.2	7	2	3	5	8	8	10	10
GRAND TOTAL	27	7.2	15	2	4	8	10	12	14	17

261: NUTRITIONAL MARASMUS

Type of Patients	Observed Patients	Avg. Stay	Variance	Percentiles 10th	25th	50th	75th	90th	95th	99th
1. SINGLE DX										
A. Not Operated										
0–19 Years	0									
20–34	0									
35–49	0									
50–64	0									
65+	0									
B. Operated										
0–19 Years	0									
20–34	0									
35–49	0									
50–64	0									
65+	0									
2. MULTIPLE DX										
A. Not Operated										
0–19 Years	10	11.4	62	2	7	7	16	25	25	25
20–34	9	13.2	169	3	5	11	12	45	45	45
35–49	17	6.7	27	2	4	6	8	11	24	24
50–64	44	6.2	18	2	4	5	9	14	15	19
65+	76	7.7	29	3	4	6	9	14	20	27
B. Operated										
0–19 Years	1	36.0	0	36	36	36	36	36	36	36
20–34	0									
35–49	2	11.5	40	7	7	12	16	16	16	16
50–64	3	5.7	9	3	3	5	9	9	9	9
65+	4	29.2	407	5	5	32	54	54	54	54
SUBTOTALS:										
1. SINGLE DX										
A. Not Operated	0									
B. Operated	0									
2. MULTIPLE DX										
A. Not Operated	156	7.7	37	3	4	6	10	14	20	27
B. Operated	10	19.3	293	5	5	16	32	54	54	54
1. SINGLE DX	0									
2. MULTIPLE DX	166	8.4	59	3	4	6	10	16	24	45
A. NOT OPERATED	156	7.7	37	3	4	6	10	14	20	27
B. OPERATED	10	19.3	293	5	5	16	32	54	54	54
TOTAL										
0–19 Years	11	13.6	110	5	7	10	24	25	36	36
20–34	9	13.2	169	3	5	11	12	45	45	45
35–49	19	7.2	28	2	4	6	9	16	24	24
50–64	47	6.2	17	2	4	5	9	14	15	19
65+	80	8.7	65	3	4	6	10	15	24	54
GRAND TOTAL	166	8.4	59	3	4	6	10	16	24	45

262: OTH SEVERE MALNUTRITION

Type of Patients	Observed Patients	Avg. Stay	Variance	Percentiles 10th	25th	50th	75th	90th	95th	99th
1. SINGLE DX										
A. Not Operated										
0–19 Years	0									
20–34	0									
35–49	0									
50–64	0									
65+	0									
B. Operated										
0–19 Years	0									
20–34	0									
35–49	0									
50–64	0									
65+	0									
2. MULTIPLE DX										
A. Not Operated										
0–19 Years	2	8.5	12	6	6	11	11	11	11	11
20–34	8	11.4	114	1	4	7	20	31	31	31
35–49	13	9.3	48	2	4	7	14	16	25	25
50–64	17	8.2	27	3	5	6	9	19	19	19
65+	21	8.9	70	3	4	6	7	21	22	34
B. Operated										
0–19 Years	1	23.0	0	23	23	23	23	23	23	23
20–34	0									
35–49	0									
50–64	2	16.0	288	4	4	16	28	28	28	28
65+	2	11.5	12	9	9	14	14	14	14	14
SUBTOTALS:										
1. SINGLE DX										
A. Not Operated	0									
B. Operated	0									
2. MULTIPLE DX										
A. Not Operated	61	9.1	54	3	4	6	13	19	22	34
B. Operated	5	15.6	96	4	9	14	23	28	28	28
1. SINGLE DX	0									
2. MULTIPLE DX	66	9.6	59	3	4	6	14	21	25	34
A. NOT OPERATED	61	9.1	54	3	4	6	13	19	22	34
B. OPERATED	5	15.6	96	4	9	14	23	28	28	28
TOTAL										
0–19 Years	3	13.4	76	6	6	11	23	23	23	23
20–34	8	11.4	114	1	4	7	20	31	31	31
35–49	13	9.3	48	2	4	7	14	16	25	25
50–64	19	9.0	45	3	4	6	12	19	28	28
65+	23	9.1	65	3	4	6	14	21	22	34
GRAND TOTAL	66	9.6	59	3	4	6	14	21	25	34

Length of Stay by Diagnosis and Operation, Western Region, 2008

Western Region, October 2006–September 2007 Data, by Diagnosis

263: PROT-CAL MALNUT NEC&NOS

Type of Patients	Observed Patients	Avg. Stay	Vari-ance	10th	25th	50th	75th	90th	95th	99th
1. SINGLE DX										
A. Not Operated										
0–19 Years	0									
20–34	0									
35–49	1	4.0	0	4	4	4	4	4	4	4
50–64	0									
65+	1	3.0	0	3	3	3	3	3	3	3
B. Operated										
0–19 Years	0									
20–34	0									
35–49	0									
50–64	0									
65+	0									
2. MULTIPLE DX										
A. Not Operated										
0–19 Years	55	7.0	52	1	2	5	9	16	21	43
20–34	27	7.1	83	2	3	4	7	12	34	40
35–49	70	6.4	29	2	3	5	8	14	18	29
50–64	182	5.7	18	2	3	4	7	12	14	21
65+	517	5.9	28	2	3	4	7	12	15	28
B. Operated										
0–19 Years	2	7.5	12	5	5	8	10	10	10	10
20–34	3	17.6	209	3	3	18	32	32	32	32
35–49	6	9.1	49	1	4	10	20	>99	>99	>99
50–64	16	7.4	39	2	4	6	9	15	27	27
65+	22	9.5	58	2	4	7	12	23	24	25
SUBTOTALS:										
1. SINGLE DX										
A. Not Operated	2	3.5	<1	3	3	3	4	4	4	4
B. Operated	0									
2. MULTIPLE DX										
A. Not Operated	851	6.0	29	2	3	4	7	12	16	29
B. Operated	49	9.2	57	2	4	7	12	24	27	>99
1. SINGLE DX	2	3.5	<1	3	3	3	4	4	4	4
2. MULTIPLE DX	900	6.2	31	2	3	5	7	12	16	29
A. NOT OPERATED	853	6.0	29	2	3	4	7	12	16	29
B. OPERATED	49	9.2	57	2	4	7	12	24	27	>99
TOTAL										
0–19 Years	57	7.0	50	1	2	5	9	16	21	43
20–34	30	8.2	99	2	3	4	8	18	34	40
35–49	77	6.6	30	2	3	5	9	15	20	>99
50–64	198	5.8	20	2	3	4	8	12	15	27
65+	540	6.1	30	2	3	5	7	12	16	28
GRAND TOTAL	902	6.2	31	2	3	5	7	12	16	29

263.9: PROTEIN-CAL MALNUT NOS

Type of Patients	Observed Patients	Avg. Stay	Vari-ance	10th	25th	50th	75th	90th	95th	99th
1. SINGLE DX										
A. Not Operated										
0–19 Years	0									
20–34	0									
35–49	1	4.0	0	4	4	4	4	4	4	4
50–64	0									
65+	1	3.0	0	3	3	3	3	3	3	3
B. Operated										
0–19 Years	0									
20–34	0									
35–49	0									
50–64	0									
65+	0									
2. MULTIPLE DX										
A. Not Operated										
0–19 Years	40	5.4	23	1	2	4	7	11	15	21
20–34	24	6.2	61	2	3	4	5	11	12	40
35–49	62	6.6	31	2	3	5	9	14	18	29
50–64	152	5.6	19	2	3	4	7	11	14	21
65+	436	5.8	25	2	3	4	7	11	14	27
B. Operated										
0–19 Years	2	7.5	12	5	5	8	10	10	10	10
20–34	3	17.6	209	3	3	18	32	32	32	32
35–49	4	11.2	64	1	10	14	20	>99	>99	>99
50–64	13	7.9	48	2	4	6	9	15	27	27
65+	16	11.4	65	3	7	9	21	24	25	25
SUBTOTALS:										
1. SINGLE DX										
A. Not Operated	2	3.5	<1	3	3	3	4	4	4	4
B. Operated	0									
2. MULTIPLE DX										
A. Not Operated	714	5.8	25	2	3	4	7	11	15	27
B. Operated	38	10.5	66	2	4	9	18	25	32	>99
1. SINGLE DX	2	3.5	<1	3	3	3	4	4	4	4
2. MULTIPLE DX	752	6.0	28	2	3	4	7	12	16	28
A. NOT OPERATED	716	5.8	25	2	3	4	7	11	15	27
B. OPERATED	38	10.5	66	2	4	9	18	25	32	>99
TOTAL										
0–19 Years	42	5.5	23	2	3	4	9	11	15	21
20–34	27	7.4	84	2	3	4	8	18	32	40
35–49	67	6.8	33	2	3	5	10	16	20	>99
50–64	165	5.8	21	2	3	4	7	12	15	27
65+	453	6.0	27	2	3	4	7	12	15	27
GRAND TOTAL	754	6.0	28	2	3	4	7	12	16	28

264: VITAMIN A DEFICIENCY

Type of Patients	Observed Patients	Avg. Stay	Vari-ance	10th	25th	50th	75th	90th	95th	99th
1. SINGLE DX										
A. Not Operated										
0–19 Years	0									
20–34	0									
35–49	0									
50–64	0									
65+										
B. Operated										
0–19 Years	0									
20–34	0									
35–49	0									
50–64	0									
65+	0									
2. MULTIPLE DX										
A. Not Operated										
0–19 Years	0									
20–34	0									
35–49	0									
50–64	1	2.0	0	2	2	2	2	2	2	2
65+	0									
B. Operated										
0–19 Years	0									
20–34	0									
35–49	0									
50–64	0									
65+	0									
SUBTOTALS:										
1. SINGLE DX										
A. Not Operated	0									
B. Operated	0									
2. MULTIPLE DX										
A. Not Operated	1	2.0	0	2	2	2	2	2	2	2
B. Operated	0									
1. SINGLE DX	0									
2. MULTIPLE DX	1	2.0	0	2	2	2	2	2	2	2
A. NOT OPERATED	1	2.0	0	2	2	2	2	2	2	2
B. OPERATED	0									
TOTAL										
0–19 Years	0									
20–34	0									
35–49	0									
50–64	1	2.0	0	2	2	2	2	2	2	2
65+	0									
GRAND TOTAL	1	2.0	0	2	2	2	2	2	2	2

Western Region, October 2006–September 2007 Data, by Diagnosis

265: THIAMINE & NIACIN DEF

Type of Patients	Observed Patients	Avg. Stay	Variance	Percentiles 10th	25th	50th	75th	90th	95th	99th
1. SINGLE DX										
A. Not Operated										
0–19 Years	0									
20–34	0									
35–49	0									
50–64	0									
65+	0									
B. Operated										
0–19 Years	0									
20–34	0									
35–49	0									
50–64	0									
65+	0									
2. MULTIPLE DX										
A. Not Operated										
0–19 Years	1	3.0	0	3	3	3	3	3	3	3
20–34	4	10.2	84	5	5	5	7	24	24	24
35–49	17	5.9	18	2	3	4	9	13	15	15
50–64	45	12.1	273	2	4	6	12	30	47	89
65+	35	5.5	29	1	2	4	6	13	18	25
B. Operated										
0–19 Years	0									
20–34	0									
35–49	0									
50–64	1	22.0	0	22	22	22	22	22	22	22
65+	0									
SUBTOTALS:										
1. SINGLE DX										
A. Not Operated	0									
B. Operated	0									
2. MULTIPLE DX										
A. Not Operated	102	8.7	144	2	3	4	10	15	30	49
B. Operated	1	22.0	0	22	22	22	22	22	22	22
1. SINGLE DX	0									
2. MULTIPLE DX	103	8.8	145	2	3	4	10	18	30	49
A. NOT OPERATED	102	8.7	144	2	3	4	10	15	30	49
B. OPERATED	1	22.0	0	22	22	22	22	22	22	22
TOTAL										
0–19 Years	1	3.0	0	3	3	3	3	3	3	3
20–34	4	10.2	84	5	5	5	7	24	24	24
35–49	17	5.9	18	2	3	4	9	13	15	15
50–64	46	12.3	269	2	4	7	12	30	47	89
65+	35	5.5	29	1	2	4	6	13	18	25
GRAND TOTAL	103	8.8	145	2	3	4	10	18	30	49

266: B-COMPLEX DEFICIENCIES

Type of Patients	Observed Patients	Avg. Stay	Variance	Percentiles 10th	25th	50th	75th	90th	95th	99th
1. SINGLE DX										
A. Not Operated										
0–19 Years	0									
20–34	0									
35–49	0									
50–64	0									
65+	0									
B. Operated										
0–19 Years	0									
20–34	0									
35–49	0									
50–64	0									
65+	0									
2. MULTIPLE DX										
A. Not Operated										
0–19 Years	0									
20–34	12	2.8	2	1	2	3	4	4	6	6
35–49	12	5.9	23	2	2	5	8	10	18	18
50–64	24	6.1	71	2	2	4	6	13	15	42
65+	71	4.4	7	2	2	4	6	8	9	12
B. Operated										
0–19 Years	0									
20–34	0									
35–49	0									
50–64	0									
65+	2	9.0	8	7	7	7	11	11	11	11
SUBTOTALS:										
1. SINGLE DX										
A. Not Operated	0									
B. Operated	0									
2. MULTIPLE DX										
A. Not Operated	119	4.7	21	2	2	4	6	9	11	18
B. Operated	2	9.0	8	7	7	7	11	11	11	11
1. SINGLE DX	0									
2. MULTIPLE DX	121	4.8	21	2	2	4	6	9	11	18
A. NOT OPERATED	119	4.7	21	2	2	4	6	9	11	18
B. OPERATED	2	9.0	8	7	7	7	11	11	11	11
TOTAL										
0–19 Years	0									
20–34	12	2.8	2	1	2	3	4	4	6	6
35–49	12	5.9	23	2	2	5	8	10	18	18
50–64	24	6.1	71	2	2	4	6	13	15	42
65+	73	4.5	7	2	2	4	6	8	10	12
GRAND TOTAL	121	4.8	21	2	2	4	6	9	11	18

267: ASCORBIC ACID DEFICIENCY

Type of Patients	Observed Patients	Avg. Stay	Variance	Percentiles 10th	25th	50th	75th	90th	95th	99th
1. SINGLE DX										
A. Not Operated										
0–19 Years	0									
20–34	0									
35–49	0									
50–64	0									
65+	0									
B. Operated										
0–19 Years	0									
20–34	0									
35–49	0									
50–64	0									
65+	0									
2. MULTIPLE DX										
A. Not Operated										
0–19 Years	0									
20–34	0									
35–49	0									
50–64	0									
65+	0									
B. Operated										
0–19 Years	0									
20–34	0									
35–49	0									
50–64	0									
65+	0									
SUBTOTALS:										
1. SINGLE DX										
A. Not Operated	0									
B. Operated	0									
2. MULTIPLE DX										
A. Not Operated	0									
B. Operated	0									
1. SINGLE DX	0									
2. MULTIPLE DX	0									
A. NOT OPERATED	0									
B. OPERATED	0									
TOTAL										
0–19 Years	0									
20–34	0									
35–49	0									
50–64	0									
65+	0									
GRAND TOTAL	0									

Length of Stay by Diagnosis and Operation, Western Region, 2008

Western Region, October 2006–September 2007 Data, by Diagnosis

268: VITAMIN D DEFICIENCY

Type of Patients	Observed Patients	Avg. Stay	Variance	10th	25th	50th	75th	90th	95th	99th
1. SINGLE DX										
A. Not Operated										
0–19 Years	0									
20–34	0									
35–49	0									
50–64	0									
65+	0									
B. Operated										
0–19 Years	0									
20–34	0									
35–49	1	3.0	0	3	3	3	3	3	3	3
50–64	0									
65+	0									
2. MULTIPLE DX										
A. Not Operated										
0–19 Years	4	3.3	2	2	2	3	5	5	5	5
20–34	1	2.0	0	2	2	2	2	2	2	2
35–49	6	6.3	8	3	4	7	7	11	11	11
50–64	4	6.8	3	5	6	7	9	9	9	9
65+	6	3.8	7	1	2	3	6	8	8	8
B. Operated										
0–19 Years	2	13.5	59	8	8	14	19	19	19	19
20–34	1	1.0	0	1	1	1	1	1	1	1
35–49	0									
50–64	0									
65+	0									
SUBTOTALS:										
1. SINGLE DX										
A. Not Operated	0									
B. Operated	1	3.0	0	3	3	3	3	3	3	3
2. MULTIPLE DX										
A. Not Operated	21	4.9	7	2	3	5	7	8	9	11
B. Operated	3	9.4	81	1	1	8	19	19	19	19
1. SINGLE DX	1	3.0	0	3	3	3	3	3	3	3
2. MULTIPLE DX	24	5.5	16	2	3	5	7	9	11	19
A. NOT OPERATED	21	4.9	7	2	3	5	7	8	9	11
B. OPERATED	4	7.8	65	1	3	8	19	19	19	19
TOTAL										
0–19 Years	6	6.7	41	2	3	5	8	19	19	19
20–34	2	1.5	<1	1	1	1	2	2	2	2
35–49	7	5.9	8	3	3	6	7	11	11	11
50–64	4	6.8	3	5	6	7	9	9	9	9
65+	6	3.8	7	1	2	3	6	8	8	8
GRAND TOTAL	25	5.4	15	2	3	5	7	9	11	19

269: OTH NUTRITION DEFICIENCY

Type of Patients	Observed Patients	Avg. Stay	Variance	10th	25th	50th	75th	90th	95th	99th
1. SINGLE DX										
A. Not Operated										
0–19 Years	0									
20–34	0									
35–49	0									
50–64	0									
65+	0									
B. Operated										
0–19 Years	0									
20–34	0									
35–49	0									
50–64	0									
65+	0									
2. MULTIPLE DX										
A. Not Operated										
0–19 Years	3	7.7	44	2	2	6	15	15	15	15
20–34	3	12.3	142	4	4	7	26	26	26	26
35–49	1	6.0		6	6	6	6	6	6	6
50–64	7	3.0	5	1	1	2	6	6	6	6
65+	17	3.3	2	1	2	3	4	5	6	6
B. Operated										
0–19 Years	2	2.5	<1	2	2	3	3	3	3	3
20–34	0									
35–49	0									
50–64	0									
65+	0									
SUBTOTALS:										
1. SINGLE DX										
A. Not Operated	0									
B. Operated	0									
2. MULTIPLE DX										
A. Not Operated	31	4.6	23	1	2	4	6	6	15	26
B. Operated	2	2.5	<1	2	2	3	3	3	3	3
1. SINGLE DX	0									
2. MULTIPLE DX	33	4.5	22	1	2	4	5	6	15	26
A. NOT OPERATED	31	4.6	23	1	2	4	6	6	15	26
B. OPERATED	2	2.5	<1	2	2	3	3	3	3	3
TOTAL										
0–19 Years	5	5.6	30	2	2	3	6	15	15	15
20–34	3	12.3	142	4	4	7	26	26	26	26
35–49	1	6.0	0	6	6	6	6	6	6	6
50–64	7	3.0	5	1	1	2	6	6	6	6
65+	17	3.3	2	1	2	3	4	5	6	6
GRAND TOTAL	33	4.5	22	1	2	4	5	6	15	26

270: AA METABOLISM DISORDER

Type of Patients	Observed Patients	Avg. Stay	Variance	10th	25th	50th	75th	90th	95th	99th
1. SINGLE DX										
A. Not Operated										
0–19 Years	11	2.5	3	1	1	2	4	5	6	6
20–34	0									
35–49	0									
50–64	0									
65+	0									
B. Operated										
0–19 Years	0									
20–34	0									
35–49	0									
50–64	0									
65+	0									
2. MULTIPLE DX										
A. Not Operated										
0–19 Years	59	4.7	18	1	2	3	6	11	14	20
20–34	13	3.5	2	2	3	3	4	5	7	7
35–49	22	2.5	6	1	1	2	2	5	8	11
50–64	20	6.3	40	1	3	4	7	12	13	29
65+	17	4.5	22	2	2	3	4	14	19	19
B. Operated										
0–19 Years	3	26.3	856	2	2	18	59	59	59	59
20–34	1	7.0	0	7	7	7	7	7	7	7
35–49	0									
50–64	2	7.5	59	2	2	13	13	13	13	13
65+	0									
SUBTOTALS:										
1. SINGLE DX										
A. Not Operated	11	2.5	3	1	1	2	4	5	6	6
B. Operated	0									
2. MULTIPLE DX										
A. Not Operated	131	4.4	19	1	2	3	5	10	13	20
B. Operated	6	16.8	466	2	2	13	18	59	59	59
1. SINGLE DX	11	2.5	3	1	1	2	4	5	6	6
2. MULTIPLE DX	137	5.0	42	1	2	3	5	11	14	29
A. NOT OPERATED	142	4.3	18	1	2	3	4	10	12	20
B. OPERATED	6	16.8	466	2	2	13	18	59	59	59
TOTAL										
0–19 Years	73	5.3	59	1	2	3	5	11	18	59
20–34	14	3.7	3	2	2	4	5	7	7	7
35–49	22	2.5	6	1	1	2	2	5	8	11
50–64	22	6.4	39	2	3	4	8	13	13	29
65+	17	4.5	22	2	2	3	4	14	19	19
GRAND TOTAL	148	4.8	39	1	2	3	5	11	14	29

Length of Stay by Diagnosis and Operation, Western Region, 2008

Western Region, October 2006–September 2007 Data, by Diagnosis

271: DISORD COH & METABOLISM

Type of Patients	Observed Patients	Avg. Stay	Vari-ance	Percentiles 10th	25th	50th	75th	90th	95th	99th
1. SINGLE DX										
A. Not Operated										
0–19 Years	9	1.2	<1	1	1	1	1		2	2
20–34	0									
35–49	0									
50–64	0									
65+	0									
B. Operated										
0–19 Years	0									
20–34	0									
35–49	0									
50–64	0									
65+	0									
2. MULTIPLE DX										
A. Not Operated										
0–19 Years	46	2.5	6	1	1	2	3	4	7	13
20–34	6	5.7	41	1	1	4	7	18	18	18
35–49	6	1.7	1	1	1	1	2	4	4	4
50–64	4	8.1	24	2	7	9	14	14	14	14
65+	18	3.5	7	1	2	2	5	8	11	11
B. Operated										
0–19 Years	1	47.0	0	47	47	>99	>99	>99	>99	>99
20–34	1	12.0	0	12	12	12	12	12	12	12
35–49	2	8.0	8	6	6	6	10	10	10	10
50–64	1	14.0	0	14	14	14	14	14	14	14
65+	0									
SUBTOTALS:										
1. SINGLE DX										
A. Not Operated	9	1.2	<1	1	1	1	1	2	2	2
B. Operated	0									
2. MULTIPLE DX										
A. Not Operated	80	3.2	10	1	1	2	4	7	11	18
B. Operated	5	17.7	272	6	10	14	>99	>99	>99	>99
1. SINGLE DX	9	1.2	<1	1	1	1	1	2	2	2
2. MULTIPLE DX	85	4.0	35	1	1	2	4	11	14	>99
A. NOT OPERATED	89	3.0	10	1	1	2	3	7	10	18
B. OPERATED	5	17.7	272	6	10	14	>99	>99	>99	>99
TOTAL										
0–19 Years	56	3.1	40	1	1	2	3	7	47	>99
20–34	7	6.6	40	1	1	4	12	18	18	18
35–49	8	3.3	11	1	1	2	6	10	10	10
50–64	5	9.2	25	2	7	9	14	14	14	14
65+	18	3.5	7	1	2	2	5	8	11	11
GRAND TOTAL	94	3.8	32	1	1	2	4	10	14	>99

272: DISORD LIPOID METABOL

Type of Patients	Observed Patients	Avg. Stay	Vari-ance	Percentiles 10th	25th	50th	75th	90th	95th	99th
1. SINGLE DX										
A. Not Operated										
0–19 Years	0									
20–34	0									
35–49	1	1.0	0	1	1	1	1	1	1	1
50–64	0									
65+	0									
B. Operated										
0–19 Years	2	3.0	8	1	1	1	5	5	5	5
20–34	0									
35–49	1	1.0	0	1	1	1	1	1	1	1
50–64	3	1.0	0	1	1	1	1	1	1	1
65+	0									
2. MULTIPLE DX										
A. Not Operated										
0–19 Years	5	3.8	13	1	1	2	6	9	9	9
20–34	8	2.9	3	1	2	2	3	7	7	7
35–49	39	3.4	11	1	1	2	4	7	13	14
50–64	26	2.8	8	1	1	2	3	5	7	14
65+	27	4.2	21	1	2	3	5	6	18	20
B. Operated										
0–19 Years	2	23.7	678	5	5	42	42	42	42	42
20–34	6	2.3	1	1	1	3	3	4	4	4
35–49	27	2.2	3	1	1	2	3	5	5	8
50–64	30	2.0	1	1	1	2	3	4	4	>99
65+	4	3.8	10	1	1	3	6	7	7	7
SUBTOTALS:										
1. SINGLE DX										
A. Not Operated	1	1.0	0	1	1	1	1	1	1	1
B. Operated	6	1.7	3	1	1	1	1	5	5	5
2. MULTIPLE DX										
A. Not Operated	105	3.4	12	1	1	2	4	7	12	18
B. Operated	69	2.9	25	1	1	2	3	5	7	>99
1. SINGLE DX	7	1.6	2	1	1	1	1	5	5	5
2. MULTIPLE DX	174	3.2	17	1	1	2	4	6	9	42
A. NOT OPERATED	106	3.4	12	1	1	2	4	7	12	18
B. OPERATED	75	2.8	24	1	1	2	3	5	7	>99
TOTAL										
0–19 Years	9	8.0	171	1	1	2	5	7	42	42
20–34	14	2.6	3	1	2	2	3	4	7	7
35–49	68	2.9	8	1	1	2	4	6	8	14
50–64	59	2.3	4	1	1	2	3	4	5	>99
65+	31	4.1	19	1	1	3	5	6	18	20
GRAND TOTAL	181	3.1	17	1	1	2	4	6	8	42

273: PLASMA PROT METABOL PBX

Type of Patients	Observed Patients	Avg. Stay	Vari-ance	Percentiles 10th	25th	50th	75th	90th	95th	99th
1. SINGLE DX										
A. Not Operated										
0–19 Years	1	1.0	0	1	1	1	1	1	1	1
20–34	0									
35–49	1	1.0	0	1	1	1	1	1	1	1
50–64	1	1.0	0	1	1	1	1	1	1	1
65+	1	2.0	0	2	2	2	2	2	2	2
B. Operated										
0–19 Years	0									
20–34	0									
35–49	0									
50–64	0									
65+	0									
2. MULTIPLE DX										
A. Not Operated										
0–19 Years	16	4.8	15	1	1	3	9	11	12	12
20–34	8	4.5	12	1	2	4	8	11	11	11
35–49	38	5.0	21	1	2	3	6	9	17	24
50–64	99	7.3	79	2	3	5	9	15	21	74
65+	142	5.6	22	1	2	4	8	10	14	24
B. Operated										
0–19 Years	0									
20–34	2	15.5	24	12	12	16	19	19	19	19
35–49	5	19.3	176	7	8	15	29	37	37	37
50–64	6	12.0	87	1	2	14	15	26	26	26
65+	11	6.5	32	1	1	6	11	15	15	15
SUBTOTALS:										
1. SINGLE DX										
A. Not Operated	4	1.3	<1	1	1	1	1	2	2	2
B. Operated	0									
2. MULTIPLE DX										
A. Not Operated	303	6.0	41	1	2	4	8	11	16	26
B. Operated	24	11.3	91	1	2	11	15	26	29	37
1. SINGLE DX	4	1.3	<1	1	1	1	1	2	2	2
2. MULTIPLE DX	327	6.4	46	1	2	4	8	14	17	30
A. NOT OPERATED	307	6.0	40	1	2	4	8	11	16	26
B. OPERATED	24	11.3	91	1	2	11	15	26	29	37
TOTAL										
0–19 Years	17	4.5	15	1	1	3	7	11	12	12
20–34	10	6.7	33	2	2	5	11	12	19	19
35–49	44	6.5	57	1	2	5	8	15	24	37
50–64	106	7.5	80	1	3	5	9	15	21	30
65+	154	5.7	23	1	2	4	8	11	15	24
GRAND TOTAL	331	6.3	46	1	2	4	8	14	17	30

Length of Stay by Diagnosis and Operation, Western Region, 2008

Western Region, October 2006–September 2007 Data, by Diagnosis

274: GOUT

Type of Patients	Observed Patients	Avg. Stay	Vari-ance	10th	25th	50th	75th	90th	95th	99th
1. SINGLE DX										
A. Not Operated										
0–19 Years	0									
20–34	4	2.3	4	1	1	2	5	5	5	5
35–49	10	1.5	<1	1	1	1	2	4	2	4
50–64	4	1.8	<1	1	1	1	3	3	3	3
65+	2	1.0	0	1	1	1	1	1	1	1
B. Operated										
0–19 Years	0									
20–34	0									
35–49	4	4.5	10	2	2	3	9	9	9	9
50–64	2	1.0	0	1	1	1	1	1	1	1
65+	1	2.0	0	2	2	2	2	2	2	2
2. MULTIPLE DX										
A. Not Operated										
0–19 Years	0									
20–34	53	2.8	4	1	2	2	3	5	6	11
35–49	251	3.5	8	1	2	3	4	7	8	14
50–64	464	3.6	8	1	2	3	5	7	8	15
65+	1,112	4.0	9	1	2	3	5	7	9	16
B. Operated										
0–19 Years	0									
20–34	5	4.4	14	2	2	3	4	11	11	11
35–49	27	3.4	6	1	1	3	5	5	7	8
50–64	56	4.7	32	1	2	3	5	8	10	37
65+	122	5.6	26	2	3	4	7	10	12	33
SUBTOTALS:										
1. SINGLE DX										
A. Not Operated	20	1.7	1	1	1	1	2	4	5	5
B. Operated	7	3.1	8	1	1	2	4	9	9	9
2. MULTIPLE DX										
A. Not Operated	1,880	3.8	9	1	2	3	5	7	9	16
B. Operated	210	5.0	25	1	2	4	6	9	12	33
1. SINGLE DX	27	2.0	3	1	1	1	2	4	5	9
2. MULTIPLE DX	2,090	3.9	11	1	2	3	5	7	9	16
A. NOT OPERATED	1,900	3.8	9	1	2	3	5	7	9	16
B. OPERATED	217	5.0	25	1	2	4	6	9	12	33
TOTAL										
0–19 Years	0									
20–34	62	2.9	5	1	2	2	4	5	6	11
35–49	292	3.4	7	1	2	3	4	7	8	14
50–64	526	3.7	10	1	2	3	5	7	8	16
65+	1,237	4.2	11	1	2	3	5	8	10	17
GRAND TOTAL	2,117	3.9	10	1	2	3	5	7	9	16

274.0: GOUTY ARTHROPATHY

Type of Patients	Observed Patients	Avg. Stay	Vari-ance	10th	25th	50th	75th	90th	95th	99th
1. SINGLE DX										
A. Not Operated										
0–19 Years	0									
20–34	3	2.7	4	1	1	2	5	5	5	5
35–49	7	1.3	<1	1	1	1	2	2	2	2
50–64	4	1.8	<1	1	1	1	3	3	3	3
65+	2	1.0	0	1	1	1	1	1	1	1
B. Operated										
0–19 Years	0									
20–34	0									
35–49	3	3.0	1	2	2	3	4	4	4	4
50–64	2	1.0	0	1	1	1	1	1	1	1
65+	0									
2. MULTIPLE DX										
A. Not Operated										
0–19 Years	0									
20–34	42	2.7	4	1	2	2	3	5	6	11
35–49	190	3.7	9	1	2	3	4	7	8	20
50–64	330	3.8	8	1	2	3	5	7	10	15
65+	824	4.1	9	1	2	3	5	8	10	16
B. Operated										
0–19 Years	0									
20–34	4	5.0	17	2	2	3	4	11	11	11
35–49	22	3.3	4	1	2	3	4	5	7	8
50–64	34	5.3	49	1	2	4	5	8	26	37
65+	87	5.2	17	2	3	4	7	9	12	33
SUBTOTALS:										
1. SINGLE DX										
A. Not Operated	16	1.6	1	1	1	1	2	3	5	5
B. Operated	5	2.2	2	1	1	2	3	4	4	4
2. MULTIPLE DX										
A. Not Operated	1,386	3.9	9	1	2	3	5	7	9	16
B. Operated	147	4.9	23	2	3	4	5	8	11	33
1. SINGLE DX	21	1.8	1	1	1	1	2	3	4	5
2. MULTIPLE DX	1,533	4.0	10	1	2	3	5	8	10	16
A. NOT OPERATED	1,402	3.9	9	1	2	3	5	7	9	16
B. OPERATED	152	4.8	22	2	2	4	5	8	11	33
TOTAL										
0–19 Years	0									
20–34	49	2.9	5	1	2	2	4	5	6	11
35–49	222	3.6	8	1	2	3	4	7	8	14
50–64	370	3.9	12	1	2	3	5	7	10	17
65+	913	4.2	10	1	2	3	5	8	10	16
GRAND TOTAL	1,554	4.0	10	1	2	3	5	8	10	16

274.9: GOUT NOS

Type of Patients	Observed Patients	Avg. Stay	Vari-ance	10th	25th	50th	75th	90th	95th	99th
1. SINGLE DX										
A. Not Operated										
0–19 Years	0									
20–34	1	1.0	0	1	1	1	1	1	1	1
35–49	3	2.0	3	1	1	1	4	4	4	4
50–64	0									
65+	0									
B. Operated										
0–19 Years	0									
20–34	0									
35–49	1	9.0	0	9	9	9	9	9	9	9
50–64	0									
65+	0									
2. MULTIPLE DX										
A. Not Operated										
0–19 Years	0									
20–34	10	2.7	2	1	1	3	3	5	5	5
35–49	52	2.8	3	1	1	2	4	5	6	8
50–64	110	3.0	4	2	2	2	4	6	8	8
65+	253	3.7	9	1	2	3	5	6	8	13
B. Operated										
0–19 Years	0									
20–34	1	2.0	0	2	2	2	2	2	2	2
35–49	1	8.0	0	8	8	8	8	8	8	8
50–64	1	10.0	0	10	10	10	10	10	10	10
65+	10	4.0	5	2	2	4	5	9	9	9
SUBTOTALS:										
1. SINGLE DX										
A. Not Operated	4	1.8	2	1	1	1	4	4	4	4
B. Operated	1	9.0	0	9	9	9	9	9	9	9
2. MULTIPLE DX										
A. Not Operated	425	3.4	7	1	2	3	4	6	8	11
B. Operated	13	4.6	8	2	2	4	6	9	10	10
1. SINGLE DX	5	3.2	12	1	1	1	4	9	9	9
2. MULTIPLE DX	438	3.4	7	1	2	3	4	6	8	11
A. NOT OPERATED	429	3.4	7	1	2	3	4	6	8	11
B. OPERATED	14	4.9	9	2	2	5	8	9	10	10
TOTAL										
0–19 Years	0									
20–34	12	2.5	2	1	1	3	3	4	5	5
35–49	57	3.0	4	1	1	3	4	5	8	9
50–64	111	3.1	4	2	2	2	4	6	8	8
65+	263	3.7	9	1	2	3	5	6	8	13
GRAND TOTAL	443	3.4	7	1	2	3	4	6	8	11

Length of Stay by Diagnosis and Operation, Western Region, 2008

275: DISORD MINERAL METABOL

Type of Patients	Observed Patients	Avg. Stay	Vari-ance	10th	25th	50th	75th	90th	95th	99th
1. SINGLE DX										
A. Not Operated										
0–19 Years	0									
20–34	2	2.5	<1	2	2	3	3	3	3	3
35–49	5	1.0	0	1	1	1	1	1	1	1
50–64	4	4.0	0	4	4	4	4	4	4	4
65+	4	2.2	<1	1	1	2	3	3	3	3
B. Operated										
0–19 Years	0									
20–34	0									
35–49	0									
50–64	1	4.0	0	4	4	4	4	4	4	4
65+	0									
2. MULTIPLE DX										
A. Not Operated										
0–19 Years	54	3.8	8	1	1	3	5	8	9	13
20–34	126	3.2	8	1	1	2	4	6	8	16
35–49	277	3.5	7	1	2	3	5	6	9	13
50–64	568	4.3	17	1	2	3	5	8	11	20
65+	1,115	4.4	12	1	2	4	5	8	10	19
B. Operated										
0–19 Years	3	10.6	95	5	5	5	22	22	22	22
20–34	8	8.0	61	1	4	6	9	26	26	26
35–49	12	5.8	15	1	4	5	8	11	13	13
50–64	29	9.3	184	1	2	3	11	23	42	62
65+	50	8.7	53	2	4	7	12	17	20	43
SUBTOTALS:										
1. SINGLE DX										
A. Not Operated	12	1.9	1	1	1	2	3	3	4	4
B. Operated	1	4.0	0	4	4	4	4	4	4	4
2. MULTIPLE DX										
A. Not Operated	2,140	4.2	13	1	2	3	5	8	10	18
B. Operated	102	8.5	86	1	3	5	11	17	22	43
1. SINGLE DX	13	2.1	1	1	1	2	3	4	4	4
2. MULTIPLE DX	2,242	4.4	17	1	2	3	5	8	11	20
A. NOT OPERATED	2,152	4.1	12	1	2	3	5	8	10	18
B. OPERATED	103	8.5	85	1	3	5	11	17	22	43
TOTAL										
0–19 Years	57	4.1	14	1	1	3	5	9	10	22
20–34	136	3.5	12	1	1	3	4	7	9	19
35–49	294	3.6	7	1	2	3	5	7	9	13
50–64	599	4.5	26	1	2	3	5	9	12	26
65+	1,169	4.6	15	1	2	4	6	8	11	20
GRAND TOTAL	2,255	4.3	17	1	2	3	5	8	11	20

275.41: HYPOCALCEMIA

Type of Patients	Observed Patients	Avg. Stay	Vari-ance	10th	25th	50th	75th	90th	95th	99th
1. SINGLE DX										
A. Not Operated										
0–19 Years	0									
20–34	1	2.0	0	2	2	2	2	2	2	2
35–49	3	1.0	0	1	1	1	1	1	1	1
50–64	0									
65+	2	2.5	<1	2	2	2	2	3	3	3
B. Operated										
0–19 Years	0									
20–34	0									
35–49	0									
50–64	0									
65+	0									
2. MULTIPLE DX										
A. Not Operated										
0–19 Years	19	4.3	11	1	1	3	8	9	10	10
20–34	63	3.3	8	1	1	2	4	7	9	16
35–49	133	3.0	4	1	2	3	4	6	7	10
50–64	164	3.4	11	1	2	3	4	7	9	18
65+	147	3.9	9	1	2	3	5	7	7	19
B. Operated										
0–19 Years	2	5.0	0	5	5	5	5	5	5	5
20–34	4	10.0	125	1	1	6	26	26	26	26
35–49	5	5.6	35	1	1	2	11	13	13	13
50–64	2	4.9	32	1	2	3	9	9	9	9
65+	3	5.0	9	2	2	5	8	8	8	8
SUBTOTALS:										
1. SINGLE DX										
A. Not Operated	6	1.7	<1	1	1	2	2	3	3	3
B. Operated	0									
2. MULTIPLE DX										
A. Not Operated	526	3.5	8	1	2	3	5	7	8	15
B. Operated	16	6.4	42	1	1	5	9	13	26	26
1. SINGLE DX	6	1.7	<1	1	1	2	2	3	3	3
2. MULTIPLE DX	542	3.6	9	1	2	3	5	7	9	16
A. NOT OPERATED	532	3.4	8	1	2	3	5	7	8	15
B. OPERATED	16	6.4	42	1	1	5	9	13	26	26
TOTAL										
0–19 Years	21	4.3	10	1	1	3	4	9	9	10
20–34	68	3.7	15	1	1	2	4	7	10	26
35–49	141	3.0	6	1	1	3	4	6	8	13
50–64	166	3.5	11	1	2	3	4	7	9	18
65+	152	3.9	8	1	2	3	5	7	8	19
GRAND TOTAL	548	3.5	9	1	2	3	5	7	9	16

275.42: HYPERCALCEMIA

Type of Patients	Observed Patients	Avg. Stay	Vari-ance	10th	25th	50th	75th	90th	95th	99th
1. SINGLE DX										
A. Not Operated										
0–19 Years	0									
20–34	0									
35–49	1	1.0	0	1	1	1	1	1	1	1
50–64	1	4.0	0	4	4	4	4	4	4	4
65+	0									
B. Operated										
0–19 Years	0									
20–34	0									
35–49	0									
50–64	0									
65+	0									
2. MULTIPLE DX										
A. Not Operated										
0–19 Years	7	3.6	6	1	1	4	5	8	8	8
20–34	20	2.6	3	1	1	2	3	5	5	7
35–49	96	4.4	10	1	2	4	5	9	11	18
50–64	295	4.8	20	2	3	4	6	9	11	21
65+	625	4.8	14	2	3	4	6	8	11	19
B. Operated										
0–19 Years	0									
20–34	1	6.0	0	6	6	6	6	6	6	6
35–49	4	7.3	5	5	5	6	10	10	10	10
50–64	9	10.4	62	1	5	11	17	23	23	23
65+	24	9.3	38	3	4	7	14	20	20	22
SUBTOTALS:										
1. SINGLE DX										
A. Not Operated	2	2.5	4	1	1	4	4	4	4	4
B. Operated	0									
2. MULTIPLE DX										
A. Not Operated	1,043	4.7	15	1	2	4	6	9	11	19
B. Operated	38	9.3	38	3	5	7	14	20	22	23
1. SINGLE DX	2	2.5	4	1	1	4	4	4	4	4
2. MULTIPLE DX	1,081	4.9	17	1	3	4	6	9	11	20
A. NOT OPERATED	1,045	4.7	15	1	2	4	6	9	11	19
B. OPERATED	38	9.3	38	3	5	7	14	20	22	23
TOTAL										
0–19 Years	7	3.6	6	1	1	4	5	8	8	8
20–34	21	2.7	3	1	1	2	3	5	6	7
35–49	101	4.5	10	1	2	4	6	9	10	13
50–64	305	5.0	22	2	3	4	6	10	13	21
65+	649	4.9	16	2	3	4	6	9	11	20
GRAND TOTAL	1,083	4.9	17	1	3	4	6	9	11	20

Length of Stay by Diagnosis and Operation, Western Region, 2008

Western Region, October 2006–September 2007 Data, by Diagnosis

275.49: CA METABOL DISORDER NEC

Type of Patients	Observed Patients	Avg. Stay	Variance	10th	25th	50th	75th	90th	95th	99th
1. SINGLE DX										
A. Not Operated										
0–19 Years	0									
20–34	1	3.0	0	3	3	3	3	3	3	3
35–49	1	1.0	0	1	1	1	1	1	1	1
50–64	0									
65+	2	2.0	2	1	1	1	3	3	3	3
B. Operated										
0–19 Years	0									
20–34	0									
35–49	0									
50–64	1	4.0	0	4	4	4	4	4	4	4
65+	0									
2. MULTIPLE DX										
A. Not Operated										
0–19 Years	5	3.4	3	1	2	4	5	5	5	5
20–34	12	3.5	11	1	1	2	4	5	13	13
35–49	17	3.7	6	1	2	2	5	8	10	10
50–64	35	4.0	7	1	2	3	5	9	10	11
65+	241	4.0	10	1	2	3	5	7	8	21
B. Operated										
0–19 Years	0									
20–34	3	6.0	0	6	6	6	6	6	6	6
35–49	3	4.3	<1	4	4	4	5	5	5	5
50–64	16	10.1	296	1	2	3	6	42	62	62
65+	21	8.1	81	2	4	5	10	12	17	43
SUBTOTALS:										
1. SINGLE DX										
A. Not Operated	4	2.0	1	1	1	3	3	3	3	3
B. Operated	1	4.0	0	4	4	4	4	4	4	4
2. MULTIPLE DX										
A. Not Operated	310	4.0	10	1	2	3	5	7	9	15
B. Operated	41	8.6	154	2	3	5	8	17	42	62
1. SINGLE DX	5	2.4	2	1	1	3	3	4	4	4
2. MULTIPLE DX	351	4.5	28	1	2	3	5	8	11	27
A. NOT OPERATED	314	3.9	9	1	2	3	5	7	9	15
B. OPERATED	42	8.5	151	2	3	5	8	17	42	62
TOTAL										
0–19 Years	5	3.4	3	1	2	4	5	5	5	5
20–34	14	3.7	10	1	2	3	4	6	13	13
35–49	21	3.7	6	1	2	4	5	6	8	10
50–64	52	5.9	100	1	2	3	5	10	17	62
65+	264	4.3	17	1	2	3	5	8	11	22
GRAND TOTAL	356	4.5	28	1	2	3	5	8	11	27

276: FLUID/ELECTROLYTE DISORD

Type of Patients	Observed Patients	Avg. Stay	Variance	10th	25th	50th	75th	90th	95th	99th
1. SINGLE DX										
A. Not Operated										
0–19 Years	87	1.4	<1	1	1	1	2	2	3	4
20–34	6	1.5	<1	1	1	1	2	3	3	3
35–49	10	2.1	<1	1	1	2	3	3	4	4
50–64	9	2.3	<1	1	2	2	3	4	4	4
65+	9	2.7	5	1	1	2	4	7	7	7
B. Operated										
0–19 Years	0									
20–34	0									
35–49	0									
50–64	0									
65+	0									
2. MULTIPLE DX										
A. Not Operated										
0–19 Years	8,774	2.0	2	1	1	2	2	3	4	7
20–34	2,479	2.7	10	1	1	2	3	5	7	14
35–49	5,585	3.0	9	1	1	2	3	6	8	15
50–64	11,467	3.3	12	1	1	2	4	6	8	16
65+	33,339	3.6	9	1	2	3	4	7	9	15
B. Operated										
0–19 Years	21	9.1	68	1	2	8	15	18	34	>99
20–34	45	7.3	35	1	3	5	11	16	18	26
35–49	139	7.7	68	1	3	5	10	17	21	54
50–64	314	7.7	100	2	3	5	9	16	23	44
65+	601	8.7	58	2	4	7	11	17	22	37
SUBTOTALS:										
1. SINGLE DX										
A. Not Operated	121	1.7	<1	1	1	1	2	3	3	5
B. Operated	0									
2. MULTIPLE DX										
A. Not Operated	61,644	3.2	9	1	1	2	4	6	8	14
B. Operated	1,120	8.2	70	2	3	6	10	17	22	48
1. SINGLE DX	121	1.7	<1	1	1	2	2	3	3	5
2. MULTIPLE DX	62,764	3.3	10	1	2	3	4	6	8	16
A. NOT OPERATED	61,765	3.2	9	1	1	2	4	6	8	14
B. OPERATED	1,120	8.2	70	2	3	6	10	17	22	48
TOTAL										
0–19 Years	8,882	2.0	2	1	1	2	2	3	4	8
20–34	2,530	2.8	11	1	1	2	3	5	7	14
35–49	5,734	3.1	10	1	1	2	4	6	8	16
50–64	11,790	3.4	14	1	1	2	4	7	9	18
65+	33,949	3.6	10	1	2	3	4	7	9	16
GRAND TOTAL	62,885	3.3	10	1	1	2	4	6	8	16

276.0: HYPEROSMOLALITY

Type of Patients	Observed Patients	Avg. Stay	Variance	10th	25th	50th	75th	90th	95th	99th
1. SINGLE DX										
A. Not Operated										
0–19 Years	3	1.3	<1	1	1	1	2	2	2	2
20–34	0									
35–49	0									
50–64	0									
65+	0									
B. Operated										
0–19 Years	0									
20–34	0									
35–49	0									
50–64	0									
65+	0									
2. MULTIPLE DX										
A. Not Operated										
0–19 Years	97	3.9	15	1	2	3	4	8	12	22
20–34	39	4.4	17	1	2	4	5	8	17	18
35–49	62	5.4	28	2	2	3	6	12	14	31
50–64	135	5.0	16	2	3	3	6	10	16	21
65+	938	5.3	16	2	3	4	6	10	13	21
B. Operated										
0–19 Years	1	15.0	0	15	15	78	>99	>99	>99	>99
20–34	1	21.0	0	21	21	21	21	21	21	21
35–49	2	29.8	>999	6	6	6	54	54	54	54
50–64	1	8.0	0	8	8	8	8	8	8	8
65+	22	12.1	72	5	6	9	15	21	32	36
SUBTOTALS:										
1. SINGLE DX										
A. Not Operated	3	1.3	<1	1	1	1	2	2	2	2
B. Operated	0									
2. MULTIPLE DX										
A. Not Operated	1,271	5.1	16	2	3	4	6	10	14	22
B. Operated	27	13.7	129	5	6	11	17	36	54	>99
1. SINGLE DX	3	1.3	<1	1	1	1	2	2	2	2
2. MULTIPLE DX	1,298	5.3	20	2	3	4	6	10	14	22
A. NOT OPERATED	1,274	5.1	16	2	3	4	6	10	14	22
B. OPERATED	27	13.7	129	5	6	11	17	36	54	>99
TOTAL										
0–19 Years	101	3.9	16	1	2	3	4	9	15	22
20–34	40	4.9	23	1	2	4	5	8	17	21
35–49	64	6.2	64	2	2	3	7	12	15	54
50–64	136	5.0	16	2	3	4	6	10	16	21
65+	960	5.5	18	2	3	4	6	10	14	22
GRAND TOTAL	1,301	5.3	20	2	3	4	6	10	14	22

276.1: HYPOSMOLALITY

Type of Patients	Observed Patients	Avg. Stay	Variance	Percentiles						
				10th	25th	50th	75th	90th	95th	99th
1. SINGLE DX										
A. Not Operated										
0–19 Years	2	1.0	0	1	1	1	1	1	1	1
20–34	0									
35–49	2	2.5	<1	2	2	3	3	3	3	3
50–64	0									
65+	1	2.0	0	2	2	2	2	2	2	2
B. Operated										
0–19 Years	0									
20–34	0									
35–49	0									
50–64	0									
65+	0									
2. MULTIPLE DX										
A. Not Operated										
0–19 Years	236	2.9	9	1	1	2	3	5	8	18
20–34	181	2.8	5	1	1	2	4	5	7	11
35–49	866	3.4	14	1	2	2	4	6	9	18
50–64	2,448	3.3	12	1	2	2	4	6	9	17
65+	8,722	3.5	8	1	2	3	4	6	8	14
B. Operated										
0–19 Years	1	13.0	0	13	13	13	13	13	13	13
20–34	2	7.6	83	1	1	14	14	14	14	14
35–49	9	6.7	52	1	1	4	9	22	22	22
50–64	30	13.1	128	3	4	10	20	31	37	44
65+	117	8.8	62	3	4	7	10	16	23	50
SUBTOTALS:										
1. SINGLE DX										
A. Not Operated	5	1.8	<1	1	1	2	2	2	3	3
B. Operated	0									
2. MULTIPLE DX										
A. Not Operated	12,453	3.4	9	1	2	3	4	6	8	14
B. Operated	159	9.5	75	2	4	7	11	19	25	50
1. SINGLE DX	5	1.8	<1	1	1	2	2	2	3	3
2. MULTIPLE DX	12,612	3.5	10	1	2	3	4	6	9	15
A. NOT OPERATED	12,458	3.4	9	1	2	3	4	6	8	14
B. OPERATED	159	9.5	75	2	4	7	11	19	25	50
TOTAL										
0–19 Years	239	2.9	9	1	1	2	3	5	8	18
20–34	183	2.8	5	1	1	2	4	6	7	11
35–49	877	3.4	14	1	2	2	4	6	9	18
50–64	2,478	3.4	15	1	2	3	4	6	9	19
65+	8,840	3.6	9	1	2	3	4	7	8	14
GRAND TOTAL	12,617	3.5	10	1	2	3	4	6	9	15

276.2: ACIDOSIS

Type of Patients	Observed Patients	Avg. Stay	Variance	Percentiles						
				10th	25th	50th	75th	90th	95th	99th
1. SINGLE DX										
A. Not Operated										
0–19 Years	0									
20–34	0									
35–49	0									
50–64	0									
65+	0									
B. Operated										
0–19 Years	0									
20–34	0									
35–49	0									
50–64	0									
65+	0									
2. MULTIPLE DX										
A. Not Operated										
0–19 Years	51	2.9	10	1	1	2	3	5	7	22
20–34	62	3.0	7	1	1	2	4	8	9	12
35–49	176	3.2	6	1	1	2	4	7	8	14
50–64	195	3.7	9	1	2	3	4	7	9	13
65+	178	4.1	11	1	2	3	5	7	9	17
B. Operated										
0–19 Years	0									
20–34	0									
35–49	3	8.0	37	4	4	5	15	15	15	15
50–64	4	11.2	110	1	1	8	10	26	26	26
65+	7	9.8	43	4	4	7	15	21	21	21
SUBTOTALS:										
1. SINGLE DX										
A. Not Operated	0									
B. Operated	0									
2. MULTIPLE DX										
A. Not Operated	662	3.5	9	1	2	3	4	7	9	14
B. Operated	14	9.8	53	4	4	7	15	21	26	26
1. SINGLE DX	0									
2. MULTIPLE DX	676	3.7	10	1	2	3	5	7	9	17
A. NOT OPERATED	662	3.5	9	1	2	3	4	7	9	14
B. OPERATED	14	9.8	53	4	4	7	15	21	26	26
TOTAL										
0–19 Years	51	2.9	10	1	1	2	3	5	7	22
20–34	62	3.0	7	1	1	2	4	8	9	12
35–49	179	3.2	7	1	1	3	4	7	8	14
50–64	199	3.8	11	1	2	3	5	7	10	26
65+	185	4.3	13	1	2	3	5	8	11	21
GRAND TOTAL	676	3.7	10	1	2	3	5	7	9	17

276.50: VOLUME DEPLETION NOS

Type of Patients	Observed Patients	Avg. Stay	Variance	Percentiles						
				10th	25th	50th	75th	90th	95th	99th
1. SINGLE DX										
A. Not Operated										
0–19 Years	0									
20–34	0									
35–49	0									
50–64	1	1.0	0	1	1	1	1	1	1	1
65+	0									
B. Operated										
0–19 Years	0									
20–34	0									
35–49	0									
50–64	0									
65+	0									
2. MULTIPLE DX										
A. Not Operated										
0–19 Years	37	1.7	<1	1	1	2	2	3	3	4
20–34	25	2.7	3	1	2	2	3	5	7	8
35–49	44	2.4	4	1	1	2	3	4	6	13
50–64	119	2.7	4	1	1	2	3	5	6	9
65+	422	3.1	5	1	2	3	4	6	8	11
B. Operated										
0–19 Years	0									
20–34	0									
35–49	1	8.0	0	8	8	8	8	8	8	8
50–64	1	5.0	0	5	5	5	5	5	5	5
65+	4	7.5	51	3	3	5	12	18	18	18
SUBTOTALS:										
1. SINGLE DX										
A. Not Operated	1	1.0	0	1	1	1	1	1	1	1
B. Operated	0									
2. MULTIPLE DX										
A. Not Operated	647	2.9	5	1	2	2	3	5	7	11
B. Operated	6	7.2	32	3	3	5	8	18	18	18
1. SINGLE DX	1	1.0	0	1	1	1	1	1	1	1
2. MULTIPLE DX	653	2.9	5	1	2	2	4	5	7	13
A. NOT OPERATED	648	2.9	5	1	1	2	3	5	7	11
B. OPERATED	6	7.2	32	3	3	5	8	18	18	18
TOTAL										
0–19 Years	37	1.7	<1	1	1	2	2	3	3	4
20–34	25	2.7	3	1	1	2	3	5	7	8
35–49	45	2.6	5	1	1	2	3	4	6	13
50–64	121	2.7	4	1	1	2	3	5	6	9
65+	426	3.2	6	1	2	3	4	6	8	13
GRAND TOTAL	654	2.9	5	1	2	2	4	5	7	13

Length of Stay by Diagnosis and Operation, Western Region, 2008

Western Region, October 2006–September 2007 Data, by Diagnosis

276.51: DEHYDRATION

Type of Patients	Observed Patients	Avg. Stay	Variance	Percentiles 10th	25th	50th	75th	90th	95th	99th
1. SINGLE DX										
A. Not Operated										
0–19 Years	78	1.4	<1	1	1	1	2	2	3	3
20–34	5	1.6	<1	1	1	1	2	3	3	3
35–49	5	2.2	2	1	1	2	3	4	4	4
50–64	2	2.0	0	2	2	2	2	2	2	2
65+	6	3.2	7	1	1	4	5	7	7	7
B. Operated										
0–19 Years	0									
20–34	0									
35–49	0									
50–64	0									
65+	0									
2. MULTIPLE DX										
A. Not Operated										
0–19 Years	8,169	1.9	2	1	1	2	2	3	4	7
20–34	1,442	2.7	12	1	1	2	3	5	7	14
35–49	2,600	3.0	7	1	1	2	3	5	7	14
50–64	5,388	3.4	12	1	2	2	4	7	9	17
65+	18,068	3.6	9	1	2	3	4	7	9	15
B. Operated										
0–19 Years	16	9.3	82	1	2	8	17	18	34	34
20–34	8	9.5	28	4	5	6	12	18	18	18
35–49	28	9.5	42	3	4	6	12	18	21	28
50–64	64	8.7	69	2	4	6	10	18	30	39
65+	199	10.2	68	3	5	8	14	18	23	50
SUBTOTALS:										
1. SINGLE DX A. Not Operated	96	1.6	<1	1	1	1	2	3	3	7
B. Operated	0									
2. MULTIPLE DX A. Not Operated	35,667	3.1	8	1	1	2	4	6	8	14
B. Operated	315	9.8	65	2	5	7	13	18	23	39
1. SINGLE DX	96	1.6	<1	1	1	1	2	3	3	7
2. MULTIPLE DX	35,982	3.1	9	1	1	2	4	6	8	15
A. NOT OPERATED	35,763	3.1	8	1	1	2	4	6	8	14
B. OPERATED	315	9.8	65	2	5	7	13	18	23	39
TOTAL										
0–19 Years	8,263	1.9	2	1	1	2	2	3	4	7
20–34	1,455	2.8	12	1	1	2	3	5	7	14
35–49	2,633	3.0	7	1	2	2	4	6	8	14
50–64	5,454	3.4	13	1	2	2	4	7	9	18
65+	18,273	3.7	10	1	2	3	4	7	9	16
GRAND TOTAL	36,078	3.1	9	1	1	2	4	6	8	15

276.52: HYPOVOLEMIA

Type of Patients	Observed Patients	Avg. Stay	Variance	Percentiles 10th	25th	50th	75th	90th	95th	99th
1. SINGLE DX										
A. Not Operated										
0–19 Years	0									
20–34	0									
35–49	0									
50–64	0									
65+	1	1.0	0	1	1	1	1	1	1	1
B. Operated										
0–19 Years	0									
20–34	0									
35–49	0									
50–64	0									
65+	0									
2. MULTIPLE DX										
A. Not Operated										
0–19 Years	16	1.8	1	1	1	2	2	3	5	5
20–34	17	2.8	5	1	1	2	3	6	9	9
35–49	60	2.8	4	1	1	2	4	5	7	11
50–64	168	3.5	59	1	1	2	4	5	7	21
65+	515	3.4	10	2	2	3	4	6	8	14
B. Operated										
0–19 Years	0									
20–34	0									
35–49	2	9.5	24	6	6	13	13	13	13	13
50–64	2	10.0	50	5	5	5	15	15	15	15
65+	18	8.8	32	2	3	9	14	16	17	17
SUBTOTALS:										
1. SINGLE DX A. Not Operated	1	1.0	0	1	1	1	1	1	1	1
B. Operated	0									
2. MULTIPLE DX A. Not Operated	776	3.3	20	1	1	2	4	6	8	15
B. Operated	22	8.9	30	2	4	9	14	16	16	17
1. SINGLE DX	1	1.0	0	1	1	1	1	1	1	1
2. MULTIPLE DX	798	3.5	21	1	2	3	4	6	9	17
A. NOT OPERATED	777	3.3	20	1	1	2	4	6	8	15
B. OPERATED	22	8.9	30	2	4	9	14	16	16	17
TOTAL										
0–19 Years	16	1.8	1	1	1	2	2	3	5	5
20–34	17	2.8	5	1	1	2	3	6	9	9
35–49	62	3.0	6	1	1	2	4	6	7	13
50–64	170	3.6	59	1	2	2	4	5	8	21
65+	534	3.6	11	2	2	3	4	7	9	17
GRAND TOTAL	799	3.5	21	1	1	3	4	6	9	17

276.6: FLUID OVERLOAD

Type of Patients	Observed Patients	Avg. Stay	Variance	Percentiles 10th	25th	50th	75th	90th	95th	99th
1. SINGLE DX										
A. Not Operated										
0–19 Years	0									
20–34	0									
35–49	0									
50–64	0									
65+	0									
B. Operated										
0–19 Years	0									
20–34	0									
35–49	0									
50–64	0									
65+	0									
2. MULTIPLE DX										
A. Not Operated										
0–19 Years	16	2.9	3	1	2	2	4	6	7	7
20–34	92	2.6	9	1	1	2	3	4	6	27
35–49	303	3.2	9	1	2	2	4	7	8	17
50–64	422	3.4	9	1	2	3	4	7	9	15
65+	449	3.3	7	1	2	3	4	6	8	12
B. Operated										
0–19 Years	0									
20–34	6	7.4	32	2	4	4	11	17	17	17
35–49	17	5.8	11	2	3	5	7	12	12	12
50–64	23	7.1	17	3	3	6	10	12	14	17
65+	21	5.7	14	3	3	4	8	10	11	15
SUBTOTALS:										
1. SINGLE DX A. Not Operated	0									
B. Operated	0									
2. MULTIPLE DX A. Not Operated	1,282	3.2	8	1	1	2	4	6	8	16
B. Operated	67	6.3	16	2	3	6	9	12	14	17
1. SINGLE DX	0									
2. MULTIPLE DX	1,349	3.4	9	1	2	2	4	7	9	16
A. NOT OPERATED	1,282	3.2	8	1	1	2	4	6	8	16
B. OPERATED	67	6.3	16	2	3	6	9	12	14	17
TOTAL										
0–19 Years	16	2.9	3	1	2	2	4	6	7	7
20–34	98	2.9	12	1	1	2	3	5	8	27
35–49	320	3.4	10	1	2	2	4	7	9	17
50–64	445	3.6	10	1	2	3	4	7	9	16
65+	470	3.4	8	2	3	3	4	7	8	13
GRAND TOTAL	1,349	3.4	9	1	2	2	4	7	9	16

Western Region, October 2006–September 2007 Data, by Diagnosis

276.7: HYPERPOTASSEMIA

Type of Patients	Observed Patients	Avg. Stay	Variance	Percentiles 10th	25th	50th	75th	90th	95th	99th
1. SINGLE DX										
A. Not Operated										
0–19 Years	3	1.0	0	1	1	1	1	1	1	1
20–34	0									
35–49	0									
50–64	0									
65+	0									
B. Operated										
0–19 Years	0									
20–34	0									
35–49	0									
50–64	0									
65+	0									
2. MULTIPLE DX										
A. Not Operated										
0–19 Years	45	2.7	6	1	1	2	3	5	7	14
20–34	286	2.5	6	1	1	2	3	5	7	14
35–49	803	2.4	6	1	1	2	3	4	7	14
50–64	1,542	2.7	7	1	1	2	3	5	7	14
65+	2,274	3.1	7	1	1	2	4	6	8	14
B. Operated										
0–19 Years	2	3.0	0	3	3	3	3	3	3	3
20–34	25	6.1	33	1	3	4	10	12	13	26
35–49	63	6.5	76	1	2	3	6	17	20	57
50–64	169	6.0	90	1	2	3	7	13	16	61
65+	179	6.8	46	1	2	5	9	13	22	35
SUBTOTALS:										
1. SINGLE DX										
A. Not Operated	3	1.0	0	1	1	1	1	1	1	1
B. Operated	0									
2. MULTIPLE DX										
A. Not Operated	4,950	2.8	7	1	1	2	3	5	7	14
B. Operated	438	6.4	66	1	2	4	8	13	18	35
1. SINGLE DX	3	1.0	0	1	1	1	1	1	1	1
2. MULTIPLE DX	5,388	3.1	13	1	1	2	4	6	9	17
A. NOT OPERATED	4,953	2.8	7	1	1	2	3	5	7	14
B. OPERATED	438	6.4	66	1	2	4	8	13	18	35
TOTAL										
0–19 Years	50	2.6	5	1	1	2	3	5	7	14
20–34	311	2.8	9	1	1	2	3	6	9	14
35–49	866	2.7	12	1	1	2	3	5	9	17
50–64	1,711	3.0	16	1	1	2	3	6	8	16
65+	2,453	3.3	11	1	1	2	4	7	9	17
GRAND TOTAL	5,391	3.1	13	1	1	2	4	6	9	17

276.8: HYPOPOTASSEMIA

Type of Patients	Observed Patients	Avg. Stay	Variance	Percentiles 10th	25th	50th	75th	90th	95th	99th
1. SINGLE DX										
A. Not Operated										
0–19 Years	1	4.0	0	4	4	4	4	4	4	4
20–34	1	1.0	0	1	1	1	1	1	1	1
35–49	3	1.7	<1	1	1	2	2	2	2	2
50–64	6	2.7	<1	2	2	2	3	4	4	4
65+	1	2.0	0	2	2	3	2	2	2	2
B. Operated										
0–19 Years	0									
20–34	0									
35–49	0									
50–64	0									
65+	0									
2. MULTIPLE DX										
A. Not Operated										
0–19 Years	94	2.4	5	1	1	2	3	5	6	14
20–34	316	2.5	6	1	1	2	3	5	7	13
35–49	619	3.0	11	1	1	2	3	6	8	16
50–64	946	3.2	10	1	1	2	4	6	8	15
65+	1,587	3.2	7	2	2	3	4	6	8	13
B. Operated										
0–19 Years	1	2.0	0	2	2	2	2	2	2	2
20–34	0									
35–49	13	8.7	32	2	4	9	11	12	23	23
50–64	18	9.9	344	2	2	3	9	26	81	81
65+	31	8.2	59	2	4	6	10	14	28	37
SUBTOTALS:										
1. SINGLE DX										
A. Not Operated	12	2.3	<1	1	2	2	2	3	4	4
B. Operated	0									
2. MULTIPLE DX										
A. Not Operated	3,562	3.1	8	1	1	2	4	6	8	14
B. Operated	63	8.7	131	2	3	6	10	14	26	81
1. SINGLE DX	12	2.3	<1	1	2	2	3	4	4	4
2. MULTIPLE DX	3,625	3.2	11	1	1	2	4	6	8	15
A. NOT OPERATED	3,574	3.1	8	1	1	2	4	6	8	14
B. OPERATED	63	8.7	131	2	3	6	10	14	26	81
TOTAL										
0–19 Years	95	2.4	5	1	1	2	3	5	6	14
20–34	318	2.5	6	1	1	2	3	5	7	13
35–49	635	3.1	12	1	1	2	3	5	9	17
50–64	970	3.3	16	1	1	2	4	6	8	16
65+	1,619	3.3	8	2	2	3	4	6	8	14
GRAND TOTAL	3,637	3.2	11	1	1	2	4	6	8	15

276.9: ELECT/FLUID DISORD NEC

Type of Patients	Observed Patients	Avg. Stay	Variance	Percentiles 10th	25th	50th	75th	90th	95th	99th
1. SINGLE DX										
A. Not Operated										
0–19 Years	0									
20–34	0									
35–49	0									
50–64	0									
65+	0									
B. Operated										
0–19 Years	0									
20–34	0									
35–49	0									
50–64	0									
65+	0									
2. MULTIPLE DX										
A. Not Operated										
0–19 Years	6	1.5	<1	1	1	1	2	3	3	3
20–34	7	1.9	2	1	1	1	2	5	5	5
35–49	33	2.7	3	1	1	2	4	5	6	8
50–64	76	3.6	7	1	2	3	5	7	8	13
65+	137	3.9	14	1	2	3	4	7	10	22
B. Operated										
0–19 Years	1	8.0	0	8	8	8	8	8	8	8
20–34	0									
35–49	0									
50–64	2	10.0	8	8	8	8	12	12	12	12
65+	3	12.0	16	8	8	12	16	16	16	16
SUBTOTALS:										
1. SINGLE DX										
A. Not Operated	0									
B. Operated	0									
2. MULTIPLE DX										
A. Not Operated	259	3.6	10	1	2	3	4	7	8	20
B. Operated	6	10.6	11	8	8	8	12	16	16	16
1. SINGLE DX	0									
2. MULTIPLE DX	265	3.7	11	1	2	3	5	7	9	20
A. NOT OPERATED	259	3.6	10	1	2	3	4	7	8	20
B. OPERATED	6	10.6	11	8	8	8	12	16	16	16
TOTAL										
0–19 Years	7	2.4	7	1	1	3	3	5	8	8
20–34	7	1.9	2	1	1	2	2	5	5	5
35–49	33	2.7	3	1	1	2	4	5	6	8
50–64	78	3.8	8	1	2	3	6	8	9	13
65+	140	4.1	15	1	2	3	4	8	12	22
GRAND TOTAL	265	3.7	11	1	2	3	5	7	9	20

Length of Stay by Diagnosis and Operation, Western Region, 2008

Western Region, October 2006–September 2007 Data, by Diagnosis

277: METABOL DISORD NEC & NOS

Type of Patients	Observed Patients	Avg. Stay	Variance	10th	25th	50th	75th	90th	95th	99th
1. SINGLE DX										
A. Not Operated										
0–19 Years	38	4.8	21	1	1	2	9	11	15	16
20–34	18	3.3	9	1	1	3	4	11	11	11
35–49	8	7.5	16	2	3	6	9	13	13	13
50–64	14	2.3	1	1	1	2	3	4	5	5
65+	0									
B. Operated										
0–19 Years	11	2.2	5	1	1	1	2	4	8	8
20–34	3	1.0	0	1	1	1	1	1	1	1
35–49	0									
50–64	0									
65+	0									
2. MULTIPLE DX										
A. Not Operated										
0–19 Years	425	8.3	35	2	3	7	13	17	20	24
20–34	626	8.3	39	2	4	7	12	15	19	29
35–49	235	7.6	48	1	3	5	11	20	21	30
50–64	199	6.3	43	1	2	4	8	14	17	39
65+	155	5.7	34	1	2	4	7	12	15	34
B. Operated										
0–19 Years	27	16.3	205	3	5	12	27	43	43	51
20–34	44	15.5	190	2	5	13	18	27	36	82
35–49	29	14.5	156	2	4	13	20	34	46	49
50–64	32	15.6	144	3	8	16	18	25	62	>99
65+	29	13.7	89	2	6	12	21	26	29	38
SUBTOTALS:										
1. SINGLE DX										
A. Not Operated	78	4.3	16	1	1	2	7	11	12	16
B. Operated	14	1.9	4	1	1	1	2	4	8	8
2. MULTIPLE DX										
A. Not Operated	1,640	7.7	40	2	3	6	11	15	19	29
B. Operated	161	15.1	156	2	6	13	19	29	43	82
1. SINGLE DX	92	3.9	15	1	1	2	5	10	11	16
2. MULTIPLE DX	1,801	8.4	55	2	3	6	13	17	21	36
A. NOT OPERATED	1,718	7.6	40	1	3	6	11	15	19	28
B. OPERATED	175	14.1	157	2	4	12	19	29	43	82
TOTAL										
0–19 Years	501	8.3	47	1	3	7	13	17	21	30
20–34	691	8.6	52	2	3	7	13	16	20	34
35–49	272	8.3	63	1	3	5	10	19	22	45
50–64	245	7.3	65	1	2	4	9	17	20	48
65+	184	7.0	51	1	2	4	9	15	22	38
GRAND TOTAL	1,893	8.2	54	1	3	6	12	16	21	36

277.02: CF W PULMON MANIFEST

Type of Patients	Observed Patients	Avg. Stay	Variance	10th	25th	50th	75th	90th	95th	99th
1. SINGLE DX										
A. Not Operated										
0–19 Years	18	7.4	22	1	3	7	11	15	16	16
20–34	2	7.0	31	3	3	11	11	11	11	11
35–49	0									
50–64	1	5.0	0	5	5	5	5	5	5	5
65+	0									
B. Operated										
0–19 Years	0									
20–34	0									
35–49	0									
50–64	0									
65+	0									
2. MULTIPLE DX										
A. Not Operated										
0–19 Years	289	10.0	34	3	5	9	14	18	21	25
20–34	427	9.8	36	3	5	9	14	16	20	29
35–49	77	10.9	36	4	6	10	15	20	21	27
50–64	34	11.6	73	3	6	10	15	18	22	48
65+	5	7.4	29	4	5	5	6	17	17	17
B. Operated										
0–19 Years	13	18.9	154	6	11	15	27	38	43	43
20–34	23	18.8	262	7	9	16	25	30	36	82
35–49	6	23.7	175	13	15	20	26	49	49	49
50–64	3	29.4	140	22	22	23	43	43	43	43
65+	0									
SUBTOTALS:										
1. SINGLE DX										
A. Not Operated	21	7.2	20	2	3	7	11	11	15	16
B. Operated	0									
2. MULTIPLE DX										
A. Not Operated	832	10.0	37	3	5	9	14	17	21	27
B. Operated	45	20.2	208	6	12	17	26	38	43	82
1. SINGLE DX	21	7.2	20	2	3	7	11	11	15	16
2. MULTIPLE DX	877	10.5	50	3	5	10	14	18	22	35
A. NOT OPERATED	853	9.9	37	3	5	9	14	17	21	27
B. OPERATED	45	20.2	208	6	12	17	26	38	43	82
TOTAL										
0–19 Years	320	10.2	41	3	5	9	14	18	21	27
20–34	452	10.2	51	3	5	9	14	17	21	34
35–49	83	11.8	56	4	6	11	15	21	22	49
50–64	38	12.8	97	3	6	10	16	22	43	48
65+	5	7.4	29	4	5	5	6	17	17	17
GRAND TOTAL	898	10.5	50	3	5	9	14	18	22	35

277.1: DISORD PORPHYRIN METABOL

Type of Patients	Observed Patients	Avg. Stay	Variance	10th	25th	50th	75th	90th	95th	99th
1. SINGLE DX										
A. Not Operated										
0–19 Years	0									
20–34	4	3.3	2	1	4	4	4	4	4	4
35–49	7	8.3	13	3	6	9	12	13	13	13
50–64	8	2.1	2	1	1	1	3	4	4	4
65+	0									
B. Operated										
0–19 Years	0									
20–34	0									
35–49	0									
50–64	0									
65+	0									
2. MULTIPLE DX										
A. Not Operated										
0–19 Years	11	5.7	33	2	2	5	6	11	21	21
20–34	50	5.8	60	2	2	4	6	6	13	52
35–49	77	5.4	22	1	2	4	6	13	19	21
50–64	55	5.5	28	2	3	4	6	10	15	35
65+	4	4.8	27	1	1	5	12	12	12	12
B. Operated										
0–19 Years	0									
20–34	0									
35–49	3	8.3	22	3	3	10	12	12	12	12
50–64	0									
65+	1	7.0	0	7	7	7	7	7	7	7
SUBTOTALS:										
1. SINGLE DX										
A. Not Operated	19	4.6	14	1	1	4	6	12	13	13
B. Operated	0									
2. MULTIPLE DX										
A. Not Operated	197	5.5	34	2	3	4	6	12	15	35
B. Operated	4	8.0	15	3	7	10	12	>99	>99	>99
1. SINGLE DX	19	4.6	14	1	1	4	6	12	13	13
2. MULTIPLE DX	201	5.6	33	2	3	4	6	12	15	35
A. NOT OPERATED	216	5.5	32	1	3	4	6	12	15	26
B. OPERATED	4	8.0	15	3	7	10	12	>99	>99	>99
TOTAL										
0–19 Years	11	5.7	33	2	2	5	6	11	21	21
20–34	54	5.6	56	2	2	4	6	9	13	52
35–49	87	5.7	22	1	3	4	7	13	15	21
50–64	63	5.1	26	1	3	4	6	10	15	>99
65+	5	5.2	21	1	1	5	7	12	12	12
GRAND TOTAL	220	5.5	32	1	3	4	6	12	15	35

Length of Stay by Diagnosis and Operation. Western Region. 2008

166

277.39: AMYLOIDOSIS NEC

Type of Patients	Observed Patients	Avg. Stay	Variance	10th	25th	50th	75th	90th	95th	99th
1. SINGLE DX										
A. Not Operated										
0–19 Years	0									
20–34	0									
35–49	0									
50–64	0									
65+	0									
B. Operated										
0–19 Years	0									
20–34	0									
35–49	0									
50–64	0									
65+	0									
2. MULTIPLE DX										
A. Not Operated										
0–19 Years	0									
20–34	4	11.8	140	4	4	10	29	29	29	29
35–49	26	11.3	133	1	3	6	16	30	33	45
50–64	40	7.8	57	2	4	5	9	14	29	39
65+	102	6.7	44	2	3	5	8	14	15	34
B. Operated										
0–19 Years	0									
20–34	3	8.4	12	5	5	8	12	12	12	12
35–49	10	18.0	143	4	11	18	20	46	46	46
50–64	20	16.4	149	4	13	16	18	25	62	62
65+	21	15.8	96	4	6	16	22	26	29	38
SUBTOTALS:										
1. SINGLE DX										
A. Not Operated	0									
B. Operated	0									
2. MULTIPLE DX										
A. Not Operated	172	7.8	64	2	3	5	10	15	29	40
B. Operated	54	16.0	119	4	8	16	20	26	38	62
1. SINGLE DX	0									
2. MULTIPLE DX	226	9.7	89	3	3	6	14	21	29	45
A. NOT OPERATED	172	7.8	64	2	3	5	10	15	29	40
B. OPERATED	54	16.0	119	4	8	16	20	26	38	62
TOTAL										
0–19 Years	0									
20–34	7	10.3	78	4	4	8	12	29	29	29
35–49	36	13.2	141	1	3	9	20	30	45	46
50–64	60	10.7	102	2	4	8	15	19	29	62
65+	123	8.2	64	2	3	6	11	19	26	38
GRAND TOTAL	226	9.7	89	2	3	6	14	21	29	45

278: OVERWEIGHT/OBESE/HYPERAL

Type of Patients	Observed Patients	Avg. Stay	Variance	10th	25th	50th	75th	90th	95th	99th
1. SINGLE DX										
A. Not Operated										
0–19 Years	0									
20–34	2	1.5	<1	1	1	1	2	2	2	2
35–49	1	1.0	0	1	1	1	1	1	1	1
50–64	1	1.0	0	1	1	1	1	1	1	1
65+	0									
B. Operated										
0–19 Years	12	1.7	<1	1	1	2	2	3	3	3
20–34	61	1.8	<1	1	1	2	2	3	3	4
35–49	61	1.9	<1	1	2	2	2	3	3	5
50–64	51	1.7	<1	1	2	2	2	3	3	4
65+	1	3.0	0	3	3	3	3	3	3	3
2. MULTIPLE DX										
A. Not Operated										
0–19 Years	24	1.2	<1	1	1	1	1	1	3	3
20–34	22	2.8	21	1	1	1	3	5	7	22
35–49	70	4.3	43	1	1	2	5	9	12	41
50–64	116	5.2	54	1	1	3	6	13	18	38
65+	42	4.5	12	2	2	4	7	8	8	20
B. Operated										
0–19 Years	69	1.9	<1	1	1	2	2	3	3	4
20–34	2,845	2.2	3	1	1	2	3	3	4	7
35–49	5,432	2.3	4	1	1	2	3	3	4	8
50–64	6,725	2.4	9	1	1	2	3	4	5	10
65+	546	2.3	4	1	1	2	3	4	6	13
SUBTOTALS:										
1. SINGLE DX										
A. Not Operated	4	1.3	<1	1	1	1	1	2	2	2
B. Operated	186	1.8	<1	1	1	2	2	3	3	4
2. MULTIPLE DX										
A. Not Operated	274	4.3	38	1	1	2	5	9	14	38
B. Operated	15,617	2.3	6	1	1	2	3	4	5	9
1. SINGLE DX	190	1.8	<1	1	1	2	2	3	3	4
2. MULTIPLE DX	15,891	2.4	7	1	1	2	3	4	5	9
A. NOT OPERATED	278	4.3	38	1	1	2	5	9	14	38
B. OPERATED	15,803	2.3	6	1	1	2	3	4	5	9
TOTAL										
0–19 Years	105	1.7	<1	1	1	2	2	3	3	4
20–34	2,930	2.2	3	1	1	2	3	3	4	7
35–49	5,564	2.3	4	1	1	2	3	3	5	9
50–64	6,893	2.5	10	1	1	2	3	4	5	11
65+	589	2.5	5	1	1	2	3	5	6	15
GRAND TOTAL	16,081	2.4	7	1	1	2	3	4	5	9

278.01: MORBID OBESITY

Type of Patients	Observed Patients	Avg. Stay	Variance	10th	25th	50th	75th	90th	95th	99th
1. SINGLE DX										
A. Not Operated										
0–19 Years	0									
20–34	2	1.5	<1	1	1	1	2	2	2	2
35–49	1	1.0	0	1	1	1	1	1	1	1
50–64	0									
65+	0									
B. Operated										
0–19 Years	12	1.7	<1	1	1	2	2	3	3	3
20–34	49	1.9	<1	1	1	2	2	3	3	4
35–49	52	2.0	<1	1	2	2	2	3	3	5
50–64	33	1.9	<1	1	1	2	2	3	3	4
65+	1	3.0	0	3	3	3	3	3	3	3
2. MULTIPLE DX										
A. Not Operated										
0–19 Years	1	1.0	0	1	1	1	1	1	1	1
20–34	12	2.2	4	1	1	1	3	5	7	7
35–49	44	3.6	30	1	1	2	3	7	12	35
50–64	70	4.7	39	1	1	3	5	13	17	38
65+	19	3.6	5	1	2	3	5	7	8	8
B. Operated										
0–19 Years	69	1.9	<1	1	1	2	2	3	3	4
20–34	2,771	2.2	3	1	1	2	3	3	4	7
35–49	5,179	2.3	4	1	1	2	3	3	4	8
50–64	6,370	2.4	10	1	1	2	3	4	5	10
65+	497	2.1	3	1	1	2	3	4	5	7
SUBTOTALS:										
1. SINGLE DX										
A. Not Operated	3	1.3	<1	1	1	1	1	2	2	2
B. Operated	147	1.9	<1	1	1	2	2	3	3	4
2. MULTIPLE DX										
A. Not Operated	146	4.0	29	1	1	2	4	10	13	35
B. Operated	14,886	2.3	6	1	1	2	3	4	4	9
1. SINGLE DX	150	1.9	<1	1	1	2	2	3	3	4
2. MULTIPLE DX	15,032	2.3	6	1	1	2	3	4	5	9
A. NOT OPERATED	149	4.0	29	1	1	2	4	10	13	35
B. OPERATED	15,033	2.3	6	1	1	2	3	4	4	9
TOTAL										
0–19 Years	82	1.8	<1	1	1	2	2	3	3	4
20–34	2,834	2.2	3	1	1	2	3	3	4	7
35–49	5,276	2.3	4	1	1	2	3	3	5	8
50–64	6,473	2.5	10	1	1	2	3	4	5	11
65+	517	2.2	3	1	1	2	3	4	5	7
GRAND TOTAL	15,182	2.3	6	1	1	2	3	4	5	9

Length of Stay by Diagnosis and Operation, Western Region, 2008

Western Region, October 2006–September 2007 Data, by Diagnosis

278.1: LOCALIZED ADIPOSITY

Type of Patients	Observed Patients	Avg. Stay	Variance	10th	25th	50th	75th	90th	95th	99th
1. SINGLE DX										
A. Not Operated										
0–19 Years	0									
20–34	0									
35–49	0									
50–64	1	1.0								
65+	0									
B. Operated										
0–19 Years	0									
20–34	10	1.5	<1	1	1	1	2	3	3	3
35–49	9	1.3	<1	1	1	1	1	3	3	3
50–64	17	1.2	<1	1	1	1	1	2	3	3
65+	0									
2. MULTIPLE DX										
A. Not Operated										
0–19 Years	0									
20–34	2	1.0	0	1	1	1	1	1	1	1
35–49	3	1.0	0	1	1	1	1	1	1	1
50–64	5	1.2	<1	1	1	1	1	2	2	2
65+	1	4.0	0	4	4	4	4	4	4	4
B. Operated										
0–19 Years	0									
20–34	67	2.1	2	1	1	2	2	4	5	7
35–49	235	2.3	3	1	1	2	3	4	5	9
50–64	328	2.4	4	1	1	2	3	4	6	11
65+	47	3.6	12	1	1	3	5	6	13	17
SUBTOTALS:										
1. SINGLE DX A. Not Operated	1	1.0	0	1	1	1	1	1	1	1
* B. Operated*	36	1.3	<1	1	1	1	2	3	3	3
2. MULTIPLE DX A. Not Operated	11	1.4	<1	1	1	1	1	2	4	4
* B. Operated*	677	2.4	4	1	1	2	3	4	6	12
1. SINGLE DX	37	1.3	<1	1	1	1	2	3	3	3
2. MULTIPLE DX	688	2.4	4	1	1	2	3	4	6	12
A. NOT OPERATED	12	1.3	<1	1	1	1	2	2	4	4
B. OPERATED	713	2.4	4	1	1	2	3	4	6	11
TOTAL										
0–19 Years	0									
20–34	79	2.0	2	1	2	2	2	4	5	7
35–49	247	2.3	3	1	2	2	3	4	5	9
50–64	351	2.3	4	1	1	2	3	4	6	11
65+	48	3.7	12	1	3	3	5	6	13	17
GRAND TOTAL	725	2.3	4	1	1	2	3	4	6	11

279: DISORD IMMUNE MECHANISM

Type of Patients	Observed Patients	Avg. Stay	Variance	10th	25th	50th	75th	90th	95th	99th
1. SINGLE DX										
A. Not Operated										
0–19 Years	23	1.0	0	1	1	1	1	1	1	1
20–34	0									
35–49	0									
50–64	1	1.0	0	1	1	1	1	1	1	1
65+	1	1.0	0	1	1	1	1	1	1	1
B. Operated										
0–19 Years	0									
20–34	0									
35–49	0									
50–64	0									
65+	0									
2. MULTIPLE DX										
A. Not Operated										
0–19 Years	61	5.1	82	1	1	1	5	14	21	60
20–34	15	5.7	28	1	2	3	11	15	17	17
35–49	38	3.4	8	1	1	2	5	7	11	12
50–64	18	4.2	11	1	2	3	4	9	14	14
65+	25	6.6	48	1	2	4	9	15	19	28
B. Operated										
0–19 Years	3	6.0	74	1	1	3	16	16	16	16
20–34	3	12.4	99	1	2	13	22	22	22	22
35–49	3	7.0	74	2	2	2	17	17	17	17
50–64	2	15.0	18	12	12	15	18	18	18	18
65+	1	19.0	0	19	19	19	19	19	19	19
SUBTOTALS:										
1. SINGLE DX A. Not Operated	25	1.0	0	1	1	1	1	1	1	1
* B. Operated*	0									
2. MULTIPLE DX A. Not Operated	157	4.9	46	1	1	3	6	12	16	28
* B. Operated*	12	10.4	67	1	2	13	17	19	22	22
1. SINGLE DX	25	1.0	0	1	1	1	1	1	1	1
2. MULTIPLE DX	169	5.3	49	1	1	3	6	14	18	28
A. NOT OPERATED	182	4.4	41	1	1	2	5	11	15	28
B. OPERATED	12	10.4	67	1	2	13	17	19	22	22
TOTAL										
0–19 Years	87	4.1	63	1	1	2	4	12	16	60
20–34	18	6.8	41	1	2	4	11	17	22	22
35–49	41	3.7	12	1	1	2	5	7	11	17
50–64	21	5.1	21	1	2	3	6	12	14	18
65+	27	6.8	51	1	2	4	10	19	19	28
GRAND TOTAL	194	4.7	45	1	1	2	6	14	17	28

280: IRON DEFICIENCY ANEMIAS

Type of Patients	Observed Patients	Avg. Stay	Variance	10th	25th	50th	75th	90th	95th	99th
1. SINGLE DX										
A. Not Operated										
0–19 Years	38	1.6	<1	1	1	1	2	2	4	5
20–34	18	1.7	2	1	1	1	2	4	7	7
35–49	39	1.4	<1	1	1	1	2	2	3	5
50–64	25	1.5	<1	1	1	1	2	3	3	3
65+	22	1.5	<1	1	1	2	2	3	3	4
B. Operated										
0–19 Years	0									
20–34	1	1.0	0	1	1	1	1	1	1	1
35–49	1	1.0	0	1	1	1	1	1	1	1
50–64	1	1.0	0	1	1	1	1	1	1	1
65+	0									
2. MULTIPLE DX										
A. Not Operated										
0–19 Years	188	2.1	3	1	1	2	2	4	6	8
20–34	564	2.2	3	1	1	2	3	4	5	8
35–49	2,100	2.3	4	1	1	2	3	4	5	10
50–64	1,897	2.9	7	1	2	3	3	5	7	14
65+	4,847	3.2	7	1	2	3	4	6	7	13
B. Operated										
0–19 Years	1	19.0	0	19	19	19	19	19	19	19
20–34	15	3.3	5	1	2	2	4	7	9	9
35–49	75	3.5	14	1	2	2	4	8	15	23
50–64	55	5.6	23	2	2	4	8	13	15	19
65+	85	10.8	89	2	5	9	14	22	28	65
SUBTOTALS:										
1. SINGLE DX A. Not Operated	142	1.6	<1	1	1	1	2	3	3	5
* B. Operated*	3	1.0	0	1	1	1	1	1	1	1
2. MULTIPLE DX A. Not Operated	9,596	2.8	6	1	1	2	3	5	7	12
* B. Operated*	231	6.8	54	2	4	13	17	21	21	30
1. SINGLE DX	145	1.5	<1	1	1	1	2	3	3	5
2. MULTIPLE DX	9,827	2.9	7	1	1	2	3	6	7	14
A. NOT OPERATED	9,738	2.8	6	1	1	2	3	5	7	12
B. OPERATED	234	6.7	54	2	4	9	9	15	21	30
TOTAL										
0–19 Years	227	2.1	3	1	1	2	2	4	5	8
20–34	598	2.2	3	1	1	2	3	4	6	9
35–49	2,215	2.3	4	1	1	2	3	4	6	10
50–64	1,978	2.9	8	1	2	3	3	5	8	14
65+	4,954	3.3	9	1	2	3	4	6	8	15
GRAND TOTAL	9,972	2.9	7	1	2	2	4	6	7	14

Length of Stay by Diagnosis and Operation, Western Region, 2008

280.0: CHR BLOOD LOSS ANEMIA

Type of Patients	Observed Patients	Avg. Stay	Variance	Percentiles						
				10th	25th	50th	75th	90th	95th	99th
1. SINGLE DX										
A. Not Operated										
0–19 Years	2	1.5	<1	1	1	1	2	2	2	2
20–34	4	1.3	<1	1	1	1	1	2	2	2
35–49	11	1.3	<1	1	1	1	1	2	3	3
50–64	3	2.0	<1	1	1	2	3	3	3	3
65+	7	1.6	<1	1	1	2	2	3	3	3
B. Operated										
0–19 Years	0									
20–34	1	1.0	0	1	1	1	1	1	1	1
35–49	1	1.0	0	1	1	1	1	1	1	1
50–64	1	1.0	0	1	1	1	1	1	1	1
65+	0									
2. MULTIPLE DX										
A. Not Operated										
0–19 Years	72	1.9	2	1	1	1	2	3	4	7
20–34	302	1.9	2	1	1	1	2	3	4	7
35–49	1,120	2.1	3	1	1	2	2	4	5	10
50–64	820	2.6	6	1	1	2	3	5	7	11
65+	2,191	3.1	8	1	1	2	4	6	8	14
B. Operated										
0–19 Years	0									
20–34	13	3.0	5	1	2	2	4	5	9	9
35–49	63	3.5	15	1	1	2	4	8	9	23
50–64	37	5.1	22	1	2	3	7	12	14	19
65+	48	11.3	114	2	4	9	15	22	28	65
SUBTOTALS:										
1. SINGLE DX										
A. Not Operated	27	1.4	<1	1	1	1	2	2	3	3
B. Operated	3	1.0	0	1	1	1	1	1	1	1
2. MULTIPLE DX										
A. Not Operated	4,505	2.7	6	1	1	2	3	5	7	12
B. Operated	161	6.1	57	1	2	3	8	14	20	30
1. SINGLE DX	30	1.4	<1	1	1	1	2	2	3	3
2. MULTIPLE DX	4,666	2.8	8	1	1	2	3	5	7	14
A. NOT OPERATED	4,532	2.7	6	1	1	2	3	5	7	12
B. OPERATED	164	6.0	56	1	2	3	8	14	20	30
TOTAL										
0–19 Years	74	1.9	2	1	1	1	2	3	4	7
20–34	320	1.9	2	1	1	1	2	4	4	7
35–49	1,195	2.2	4	1	1	2	3	4	6	11
50–64	861	2.7	7	1	1	2	3	5	8	13
65+	2,246	3.3	12	1	1	2	4	6	8	17
GRAND TOTAL	4,696	2.8	8	1	1	2	3	5	7	14

280.8: IRON DEF ANEMIA NEC

Type of Patients	Observed Patients	Avg. Stay	Variance	Percentiles						
				10th	25th	50th	75th	90th	95th	99th
1. SINGLE DX										
A. Not Operated										
0–19 Years	3	1.3	<1	1	1	1	2	2	2	2
20–34	1	1.0	0	1	1	1	1	1	1	1
35–49	0									
50–64	0									
65+	0									
B. Operated										
0–19 Years	0									
20–34	0									
35–49	0									
50–64	0									
65+	0									
2. MULTIPLE DX										
A. Not Operated										
0–19 Years	7	1.7	<1	1	1	1	2	3	3	3
20–34	22	2.8	7	1	1	1	4	6	7	11
35–49	81	2.3	2	1	1	2	3	4	5	8
50–64	59	2.7	3	1	2	2	4	5	7	9
65+	104	3.0	3	1	2	3	4	5	6	7
B. Operated										
0–19 Years	0									
20–34	0									
35–49	1	3.0	0	3	3	3	3	3	3	3
50–64	1	5.0	0	5	5	5	5	5	5	5
65+	0									
SUBTOTALS:										
1. SINGLE DX										
A. Not Operated	4	1.3	<1	1	1	1	1	2	2	2
B. Operated	0									
2. MULTIPLE DX										
A. Not Operated	273	2.7	3	1	1	2	3	5	6	8
B. Operated	2	4.0	2	3	3	4	5	5	5	5
1. SINGLE DX	4	1.3	<1	1	1	1	1	2	2	2
2. MULTIPLE DX	275	2.7	3	1	1	2	3	5	6	8
A. NOT OPERATED	277	2.7	3	1	1	2	3	5	6	8
B. OPERATED	2	4.0	2	3	3	4	5	5	5	5
TOTAL										
0–19 Years	10	1.6	<1	1	1	1	2	3	3	3
20–34	23	2.7	7	1	1	1	4	6	7	11
35–49	82	2.3	2	1	1	2	3	4	5	8
50–64	60	2.8	3	1	1	2	4	5	7	9
65+	104	3.0	3	1	2	3	4	5	6	7
GRAND TOTAL	279	2.7	3	1	1	2	3	5	6	8

280.9: IRON DEF ANEMIA NOS

Type of Patients	Observed Patients	Avg. Stay	Variance	Percentiles						
				10th	25th	50th	75th	90th	95th	99th
1. SINGLE DX										
A. Not Operated										
0–19 Years	28	1.8	<1	1	1	2	2	3	4	5
20–34	13	1.9	3	1	1	1	2	4	7	7
35–49	27	1.5	<1	1	1	1	2	2	3	5
50–64	22	1.5	<1	1	1	1	2	3	3	3
65+	13	1.5	<1	1	1	1	1	3	4	4
B. Operated										
0–19 Years	0									
20–34	0									
35–49	0									
50–64	0									
65+	0									
2. MULTIPLE DX										
A. Not Operated										
0–19 Years	100	2.3	3	1	1	2	3	5	6	10
20–34	237	2.5	5	1	1	2	3	5	6	12
35–49	882	2.4	4	1	1	2	3	4	6	9
50–64	1,006	3.1	8	1	2	2	4	6	8	14
65+	2,532	3.2	5	1	2	3	4	6	7	12
B. Operated										
0–19 Years	1	19.0	0	19	19	19	19	19	19	19
20–34	2	5.0	8	3	3	5	7	7	7	7
35–49	11	3.8	11	1	1	3	5	7	12	12
50–64	17	6.8	25	3	3	5	9	15	17	17
65+	36	9.9	55	2	5	8	13	21	29	31
SUBTOTALS:										
1. SINGLE DX										
A. Not Operated	103	1.6	1	1	1	1	2	3	4	5
B. Operated	0									
2. MULTIPLE DX										
A. Not Operated	4,757	3.0	6	1	1	2	4	6	7	12
B. Operated	67	8.1	45	2	3	6	11	17	21	31
1. SINGLE DX	103	1.6	1	1	1	1	2	3	4	5
2. MULTIPLE DX	4,824	3.0	7	1	1	2	4	6	7	13
A. NOT OPERATED	4,860	2.9	6	1	1	2	4	6	7	12
B. OPERATED	67	8.1	45	2	3	6	11	17	21	31
TOTAL										
0–19 Years	129	2.3	5	1	1	2	3	5	6	10
20–34	252	2.5	5	1	1	2	3	5	7	12
35–49	920	2.4	4	1	1	2	3	4	6	9
50–64	1,045	3.1	8	1	2	2	4	6	8	14
65+	2,581	3.3	7	1	2	3	4	6	8	13
GRAND TOTAL	4,927	3.0	7	1	1	2	4	6	7	13

Length of Stay by Diagnosis and Operation, Western Region, 2008

Western Region, October 2006–September 2007 Data, by Diagnosis

281: OTHER DEFICIENCY ANEMIA

Type of Patients	Observed Patients	Avg. Stay	Variance	Percentiles						
				10th	25th	50th	75th	90th	95th	99th
1. SINGLE DX										
A. Not Operated										
0–19 Years	3	1.3	<1	1	1	1	2	2	2	2
20–34	0									
35–49	4	5.2	25	1	2	2	6	12	12	12
50–64	2	1.5	<1	1	1	1	2	2	2	2
65+	5	1.2	<1	1	1	1	1	2	2	2
B. Operated										
0–19 Years	0									
20–34	0									
35–49	0									
50–64	0									
65+	0									
2. MULTIPLE DX										
A. Not Operated										
0–19 Years	8	2.1	<1	1	2	2	3	4	4	4
20–34	24	3.4	6	1	2	3	4	7	9	11
35–49	97	3.2	7	1	1	3	4	6	8	14
50–64	137	3.3	11	1	1	2	4	6	9	14
65+	453	3.4	8	1	1	3	4	7	8	14
B. Operated										
0–19 Years	0									
20–34	0									
35–49	1	2.0	0	2	2	2	2	2	2	2
50–64	3	10.4	164	1	1	5	25	25	25	25
65+	8	6.2	12	3	3	5	6	13	13	13
SUBTOTALS:										
1. SINGLE DX										
A. Not Operated	14	2.4	9	1	1	1	2	2	2	2
B. Operated	0									
2. MULTIPLE DX										
A. Not Operated	719	3.3	8	1	1	3	4	6	8	14
B. Operated	12	6.9	44	2	3	5	6	13	25	25
1. SINGLE DX	14	2.4	9	1	1	1	2	2	12	12
2. MULTIPLE DX	731	3.4	9	1	1	3	4	6	9	14
A. NOT OPERATED	733	3.3	8	1	1	3	4	6	8	14
B. OPERATED	12	6.9	44	2	3	5	6	13	25	25
TOTAL										
0–19 Years	11	1.9	<1	1	1	2	3	4	4	4
20–34	24	3.4	6	1	2	3	4	7	9	11
35–49	102	3.3	8	1	1	3	4	6	8	13
50–64	142	3.4	14	1	1	2	4	6	9	25
65+	466	3.4	8	1	1	3	4	7	8	14
GRAND TOTAL	745	3.4	9	1	1	3	4	6	9	14

281.9: DEFICIENCY ANEMIA NOS

Type of Patients	Observed Patients	Avg. Stay	Variance	Percentiles						
				10th	25th	50th	75th	90th	95th	99th
1. SINGLE DX										
A. Not Operated										
0–19 Years	2	1.5	<1	1	1	2	2	2	2	2
20–34	0									
35–49	2	1.5	<1	1	1	2	2	2	2	2
50–64	0									
65+	3	1.3	<1	1	1	1	2	2	2	2
B. Operated										
0–19 Years	0									
20–34	0									
35–49	0									
50–64	0									
65+	0									
2. MULTIPLE DX										
A. Not Operated										
0–19 Years	6	1.8	<1	1	1	2	2	3	3	3
20–34	9	2.8	6	1	1	2	3	9	9	9
35–49	47	2.3	2	1	1	2	3	4	5	7
50–64	77	2.4	3	1	1	2	3	5	7	9
65+	303	3.0	6	1	1	2	4	6	7	14
B. Operated										
0–19 Years	0									
20–34	0									
35–49	1	2.0	0	2	2	2	2	2	2	2
50–64	3	10.4	164	1	1	5	25	25	25	25
65+	5	5.4	8	3	3	5	6	10	10	10
SUBTOTALS:										
1. SINGLE DX										
A. Not Operated	7	1.4	<1	1	1	1	2	2	2	2
B. Operated	0									
2. MULTIPLE DX										
A. Not Operated	442	2.8	5	1	1	2	4	5	7	13
B. Operated	9	6.7	54	3	3	5	6	25	25	25
1. SINGLE DX	7	1.4	<1	1	1	1	2	2	2	2
2. MULTIPLE DX	451	2.9	6	1	1	2	4	6	7	14
A. NOT OPERATED	449	2.8	5	1	1	2	4	5	7	13
B. OPERATED	9	6.7	54	3	3	5	6	25	25	25
TOTAL										
0–19 Years	8	1.8	<1	1	1	2	2	3	3	3
20–34	9	2.8	6	1	1	2	3	9	9	9
35–49	50	2.3	2	1	1	2	3	4	5	7
50–64	80	2.7	10	1	1	2	4	5	8	25
65+	311	3.0	6	1	1	2	4	6	7	14
GRAND TOTAL	458	2.9	6	1	1	2	4	6	7	14

282: HERED HEMOLYTIC ANEMIA

Type of Patients	Observed Patients	Avg. Stay	Variance	Percentiles						
				10th	25th	50th	75th	90th	95th	99th
1. SINGLE DX										
A. Not Operated										
0–19 Years	224	3.3	9	1	1	2	4	6	9	14
20–34	224	4.1	18	1	2	2	5	8	11	22
35–49	92	3.9	14	1	1	3	5	8	9	24
50–64	6	5.5	10	2	2	7	7	10	10	10
65+	0									
B. Operated										
0–19 Years	8	3.4	10	1	1	3	3	11	11	11
20–34	4	3.5	3	2	2	3	3	6	6	6
35–49	0									
50–64	0									
65+	0									
2. MULTIPLE DX										
A. Not Operated										
0–19 Years	731	4.7	17	1	2	3	6	10	13	19
20–34	2,081	6.4	35	2	3	5	8	13	16	32
35–49	1,204	5.7	26	2	3	4	7	11	14	25
50–64	337	5.4	21	1	2	4	7	11	14	24
65+	50	3.4	16	1	2	2	4	6	8	27
B. Operated										
0–19 Years	38	4.7	35	1	2	3	5	12	13	34
20–34	42	11.1	229	2	4	7	11	23	27	95
35–49	19	16.2	262	4	5	8	28	51	54	54
50–64	7	9.2	101	1	2	8	8	31	31	31
65+	4	13.4	152	3	3	4	18	29	29	29
SUBTOTALS:										
1. SINGLE DX										
A. Not Operated	546	3.8	13	1	1	3	5	7	10	19
B. Operated	12	3.4	7	1	2	3	3	6	11	11
2. MULTIPLE DX										
A. Not Operated	4,403	5.8	29	1	2	4	7	12	15	27
B. Operated	110	9.7	168	2	3	6	11	25	34	54
1. SINGLE DX	558	3.8	13	1	1	3	5	7	10	19
2. MULTIPLE DX	4,513	5.9	33	1	2	4	7	12	15	29
A. NOT OPERATED	4,949	5.6	28	1	2	4	7	11	15	26
B. OPERATED	122	9.1	156	2	3	5	10	23	34	54
TOTAL										
0–19 Years	1,001	4.4	16	1	2	3	6	9	12	18
20–34	2,351	6.2	38	2	3	5	8	12	16	32
35–49	1,315	5.7	30	1	3	4	7	11	14	28
50–64	350	5.5	23	1	2	4	7	11	14	25
65+	54	4.1	31	1	2	4	7	6	18	29
GRAND TOTAL	5,071	5.7	31	1	2	4	7	11	15	28

Western Region, October 2006–September 2007 Data, by Diagnosis

282.42: THAL HB-S DIS W CRISIS

Type of Patients	Observed Patients	Avg. Stay	Vari-ance	10th	25th	50th	75th	90th	95th	99th
1. SINGLE DX										
A. Not Operated										
0–19 Years	8	3.3	6	1	1	3	6	6	6	6
20–34	7	2.9	4	1	1	3	3	7	7	7
35–49	2	2.5	<1	2	2	3	3	3	3	3
50–64	0									
65+	0									
B. Operated										
0–19 Years	0									
20–34	0									
35–49	0									
50–64	0									
65+	0									
2. MULTIPLE DX										
A. Not Operated										
0–19 Years	38	5.7	26	1	2	4	8	11	19	25
20–34	85	7.0	73	1	3	5	8	15	17	70
35–49	31	6.7	42	1	2	4	10	14	20	28
50–64	11	9.2	104	2	3	5	11	16	37	37
65+	0									
B. Operated										
0–19 Years	1	13.0	0	13	13	13	13	13	13	13
20–34	1	10.0	0	10	10	10	10	10	10	10
35–49	1	20.0	0	20	20	20	20	20	20	20
50–64	1	6.0	0	6	6	6	6	6	6	6
65+	0									
SUBTOTALS:										
1. SINGLE DX										
A. Not Operated	17	3.0	4	1	1	3	3	6	7	7
B. Operated	0									
2. MULTIPLE DX										
A. Not Operated	165	6.8	58	1	3	4	8	15	18	37
B. Operated	4	12.3	35	6	10	13	20	20	20	20
1. SINGLE DX	17	3.0	4	1	1	3	3	6	7	7
2. MULTIPLE DX	169	6.9	58	1	3	4	9	15	19	37
A. NOT OPERATED	182	6.4	54	1	2	4	8	13	18	37
B. OPERATED	4	12.3	35	6	10	13	20	20	20	20
TOTAL										
0–19 Years	47	5.4	24	1	2	4	7	11	15	25
20–34	93	6.7	69	1	3	4	8	12	17	70
35–49	34	6.8	44	1	2	4	10	14	20	28
50–64	12	8.9	95	2	3	6	11	16	37	37
65+	0									
GRAND TOTAL	186	6.5	54	1	2	4	8	14	18	37

282.60: SICKLE-CELL DISEASE NOS

Type of Patients	Observed Patients	Avg. Stay	Vari-ance	10th	25th	50th	75th	90th	95th	99th
1. SINGLE DX										
A. Not Operated										
0–19 Years	10	1.7	<1	1	1	1	3	3	3	3
20–34	7	1.9	2	1	1	1	3	5	5	5
35–49	2	1.0	0	1	1	1	1	1	1	1
50–64	0									
65+	0									
B. Operated										
0–19 Years	1	3.0	0	3	3	3	3	3	3	3
20–34	0									
35–49	0									
50–64	0									
65+	0									
2. MULTIPLE DX										
A. Not Operated										
0–19 Years	37	2.7	4	1	2	2	3	5	8	10
20–34	48	4.2	17	1	1	2	6	9	12	22
35–49	35	2.6	6	1	1	2	3	6	6	13
50–64	16	2.7	5	1	2	2	4	7	8	8
65+	1	2.0	0	2	2	2	2	2	2	2
B. Operated										
0–19 Years	0									
20–34	0									
35–49	0									
50–64	0									
65+	1	29.0	0	29	29	29	29	29	29	29
SUBTOTALS:										
1. SINGLE DX										
A. Not Operated	19	1.7	1	1	1	1	3	3	5	5
B. Operated	1	3.0	0	3	3	3	3	3	3	3
2. MULTIPLE DX										
A. Not Operated	137	3.2	9	1	1	2	4	7	9	13
B. Operated	1	29.0	0	29	29	29	29	29	29	29
1. SINGLE DX	20	1.8	1	1	1	1	3	3	5	5
2. MULTIPLE DX	138	3.4	14	1	1	2	4	8	10	22
A. NOT OPERATED	156	3.0	8	1	1	2	3	6	9	13
B. OPERATED	2	16.0	338	3	3	16	29	29	29	29
TOTAL										
0–19 Years	48	2.5	3	1	1	2	3	5	5	10
20–34	55	3.9	16	1	1	2	5	8	12	22
35–49	37	2.5	5	1	1	2	3	6	6	13
50–64	16	2.7	5	1	2	2	4	7	8	8
65+	2	15.3	359	2	2	2	29	29	29	29
GRAND TOTAL	158	3.2	13	1	1	2	3	6	9	22

282.62: HB-SS DISEASE W CRISIS

Type of Patients	Observed Patients	Avg. Stay	Vari-ance	10th	25th	50th	75th	90th	95th	99th
1. SINGLE DX										
A. Not Operated										
0–19 Years	150	4.0	11	1	2	3	5	8	11	17
20–34	186	4.4	20	1	2	3	5	8	13	27
35–49	82	3.8	12	1	2	3	5	7	9	24
50–64	6	5.5	10	2	2	7	7	10	10	10
65+	0									
B. Operated										
0–19 Years	1	11.0	0	11	11	11	11	11	11	11
20–34	1	6.0	0	6	6	6	6	6	6	6
35–49	0									
50–64	0									
65+	0									
2. MULTIPLE DX										
A. Not Operated										
0–19 Years	514	5.2	18	1	2	4	7	10	14	19
20–34	1,761	6.5	36	2	3	5	8	13	17	34
35–49	1,021	5.9	28	2	3	5	7	11	14	25
50–64	253	5.5	19	1	2	4	7	11	14	24
65+	6	7.2	95	2	3	3	5	27	27	27
B. Operated										
0–19 Years	6	5.8	21	2	2	3	10	13	13	13
20–34	23	16.9	343	6	8	11	19	27	34	95
35–49	15	18.5	294	5	6	11	34	51	54	54
50–64	4	13.8	131	8	8	8	20	31	31	31
65+	1	18.0	0	18	18	18	18	18	18	18
SUBTOTALS:										
1. SINGLE DX										
A. Not Operated	424	4.2	15	1	2	3	5	8	11	20
B. Operated	2	8.5	12	6	6	6	11	11	11	11
2. MULTIPLE DX										
A. Not Operated	3,555	6.0	30	2	3	5	8	12	15	29
B. Operated	49	15.8	269	5	7	10	18	34	51	95
1. SINGLE DX	426	4.2	15	1	2	3	5	8	11	20
2. MULTIPLE DX	3,604	6.2	34	2	3	5	8	12	16	31
A. NOT OPERATED	3,979	5.8	29	2	3	4	7	11	15	28
B. OPERATED	51	15.5	261	5	6	10	18	34	51	95
TOTAL										
0–19 Years	671	4.9	17	1	2	4	6	10	13	19
20–34	1,971	6.4	39	2	3	5	8	13	17	34
35–49	1,118	5.9	32	2	3	4	7	11	14	33
50–64	263	5.6	21	1	2	5	7	11	14	25
65+	7	8.7	96	2	3	3	18	27	27	27
GRAND TOTAL	4,030	6.0	33	2	3	4	7	12	15	30

Length of Stay by Diagnosis and Operation, Western Region, 2008

Western Region, October 2006–September 2007 Data, by Diagnosis

282.64: HB-S/HB-C DIS W CRISIS

Type of Patients	Observed Patients	Avg. Stay	Variance	10th	25th	50th	75th	90th	95th	99th
1. SINGLE DX										
A. Not Operated										
0–19 Years	4	2.5	2	1	2	3	4	4	4	4
20–34	3	4.0	4	2	2	4	6	6	6	6
35–49	3	10.7	54	5	5	8	19	19	19	19
50–64	0									
65+	0									
B. Operated										
0–19 Years	0									
20–34	0									
35–49	0									
50–64	0									
65+	0									
2. MULTIPLE DX										
A. Not Operated										
0–19 Years	16	5.7	22	1	2	4	11	13	14	14
20–34	35	6.5	19	3	3	5	9	12	18	21
35–49	19	4.9	5	3	3	4	6	9	10	10
50–64	9	4.1	7	1	2	3	6	9	9	9
65+	0									
B. Operated										
0–19 Years	0									
20–34	0									
35–49	0									
50–64	0									
65+	0									
SUBTOTALS:										
1. SINGLE DX										
A. Not Operated	10	5.4	27	2	2	4	6	6	6	19
B. Operated	0									
2. MULTIPLE DX										
A. Not Operated	79	5.7	15	2	3	5	8	11	14	21
B. Operated	0									
1. SINGLE DX	10	5.4	27	2	2	4	6	19	19	19
2. MULTIPLE DX	79	5.7	15	2	3	5	8	11	13	21
A. NOT OPERATED	89	5.7	16	2	3	4	8	11	13	21
B. OPERATED	0									
TOTAL										
0–19 Years	20	5.1	19	1	2	3	9	13	14	14
20–34	38	6.3	18	3	3	5	8	12	18	21
35–49	22	5.7	14	3	4	4	7	9	10	19
50–64	9	4.1	7	1	2	3	6	9	9	9
65+	0									
GRAND TOTAL	89	5.7	16	2	3	4	8	11	13	21

282.69: HB-S DIS NEC W CRISIS

Type of Patients	Observed Patients	Avg. Stay	Variance	10th	25th	50th	75th	90th	95th	99th
1. SINGLE DX										
A. Not Operated										
0–19 Years	15	3.3	2	2	3	3	4	5	6	6
20–34	15	3.2	6	1	1	2	5	6	9	9
35–49	1	2.0	0	2	2	2	2	2	2	2
50–64	0									
65+	0									
B. Operated										
0–19 Years	0									
20–34	0									
35–49	0									
50–64	0									
65+	0									
2. MULTIPLE DX										
A. Not Operated										
0–19 Years	46	4.0	6	2	2	4	5	8	8	11
20–34	112	5.7	17	2	3	5	7	11	15	16
35–49	63	5.8	15	2	3	5	7	11	14	20
50–64	30	6.1	22	2	2	5	8	13	14	20
65+	0									
B. Operated										
0–19 Years	1	12.0	0	12	12	12	12	12	12	12
20–34	0									
35–49	0									
50–64	0									
65+	0									
SUBTOTALS:										
1. SINGLE DX										
A. Not Operated	31	3.2	3	1	2	3	4	6	6	9
B. Operated	0									
2. MULTIPLE DX										
A. Not Operated	251	5.5	15	2	3	4	7	11	14	20
B. Operated	1	12.0	0	12	12	12	12	12	12	12
1. SINGLE DX	31	3.2	3	1	2	3	4	6	6	9
2. MULTIPLE DX	252	5.5	15	2	3	5	7	11	14	20
A. NOT OPERATED	282	5.2	14	2	2	4	7	10	13	20
B. OPERATED	1	12.0	0	12	12	12	12	12	12	12
TOTAL										
0–19 Years	62	4.0	6	2	2	3	5	7	8	12
20–34	127	5.4	16	2	2	4	7	11	14	16
35–49	64	5.8	15	2	3	5	7	11	14	20
50–64	30	6.1	22	2	2	5	8	13	14	20
65+	0									
GRAND TOTAL	283	5.3	15	2	2	4	7	11	13	20

283: ACQ HEMOLYTIC ANEMIA

Type of Patients	Observed Patients	Avg. Stay	Variance	10th	25th	50th	75th	90th	95th	99th
1. SINGLE DX										
A. Not Operated										
0–19 Years	17	3.0	7	1	1	2	3	8	10	10
20–34	5	1.8	<1	1	1	2	2	2	3	3
35–49	6	2.2	<1	1	2	2	2	4	4	4
50–64	6	3.3	4	2	2	4	4	7	7	7
65+	3	1.7	<1	1	1	2	2	2	2	2
B. Operated										
0–19 Years	0									
20–34	2	4.0	0	4	4	4	4	4	4	4
35–49	2	1.0	0	1	1	1	1	1	1	1
50–64	1	6.0	0	6	6	6	6	6	6	6
65+	1	2.0	0	2	2	2	2	2	2	2
2. MULTIPLE DX										
A. Not Operated										
0–19 Years	85	5.3	34	1	2	3	6	11	16	34
20–34	100	4.7	22	1	2	3	5	9	14	29
35–49	116	4.8	20	1	2	4	7	10	11	22
50–64	231	4.9	14	1	2	4	6	10	12	18
65+	478	5.1	21	1	2	4	6	10	13	22
B. Operated										
0–19 Years	3	18.7	80	10	10	18	28	28	28	28
20–34	14	9.4	113	10	5	5	10	26	36	36
35–49	19	11.2	138	3	5	6	15	25	53	53
50–64	25	5.7	35	1	3	3	8	14	18	23
65+	34	7.7	47	2	3	5	8	17	27	28
SUBTOTALS:										
1. SINGLE DX										
A. Not Operated	37	2.7	4	1	1	2	3	5	8	10
B. Operated	6	3.0	4	1	1	4	4	6	6	6
2. MULTIPLE DX										
A. Not Operated	1,010	5.0	20	1	2	4	6	10	13	24
B. Operated	95	8.5	76	2	3	5	12	19	27	53
1. SINGLE DX	43	2.7	4	1	1	2	3	5	7	10
2. MULTIPLE DX	1,105	5.3	26	1	2	4	6	11	14	27
A. NOT OPERATED	1,047	4.9	20	1	2	4	6	10	13	24
B. OPERATED	101	8.1	74	2	3	5	10	18	26	36
TOTAL										
0–19 Years	105	5.3	36	1	2	3	6	11	16	28
20–34	121	5.1	33	1	2	3	5	11	14	29
35–49	143	5.5	39	1	2	4	7	11	14	33
50–64	263	4.9	16	1	2	4	6	10	12	23
65+	516	5.3	23	1	2	4	6	10	13	27
GRAND TOTAL	1,148	5.2	25	1	2	4	6	10	14	27

Length of Stay by Diagnosis and Operation, Western Region, 2008

Western Region, October 2006–September 2007 Data, by Diagnosis

283.0: AUTOIMMUNE HEMOLY ANEMIA

Type of Patients	Observed Patients	Avg. Stay	Vari-ance	Percentiles						
				10th	25th	50th	75th	90th	95th	99th
1. SINGLE DX										
A. Not Operated										
0–19 Years	8	3.9	12	1	1	2	8	10	10	10
20–34	4	1.5	<1	1	1	2	2	2	2	2
35–49	2	3.0	2	2	2	2	4	4	4	4
50–64	2	3.0	2	2	2	4	4	4	4	4
65+	1	1.0	0	1	1	1	1	1	1	1
B. Operated										
0–19 Years	0									
20–34	2	4.0	0	4	4	4	4	4	4	4
35–49	1	1.0	0	1	1	1	1	1	1	1
50–64	1	6.0	0	6	6	6	6	6	6	6
65+	0									
2. MULTIPLE DX										
A. Not Operated										
0–19 Years	48	4.2	22	1	2	3	5	7	10	26
20–34	43	5.3	21	2	3	4	6	9	18	22
35–49	52	5.2	10	2	3	5	7	10	11	14
50–64	129	5.1	13	2	3	4	7	9	12	18
65+	274	5.5	18	2	3	4	7	11	13	27
B. Operated										
0–19 Years	0									
20–34	7	14.6	170	1	5	9	26	36	36	36
35–49	13	9.0	26	3	5	8	14	16	17	17
50–64	17	5.1	31	2	2	3	6	14	23	23
65+	27	7.5	42	2	3	5	12	17	19	27
SUBTOTALS:										
1. SINGLE DX										
A. Not Operated	17	3.0	7	1	1	2	4	8	10	10
B. Operated	4	3.7	4	1	1	4	4	6	6	6
2. MULTIPLE DX										
A. Not Operated	546	5.3	17	2	3	4	7	10	13	22
B. Operated	64	8.0	54	2	3	5	11	17	23	36
1. SINGLE DX	21	3.1	6	1	1	2	4	6	8	10
2. MULTIPLE DX	610	5.5	21	2	3	4	7	11	14	26
A. NOT OPERATED	563	5.2	17	2	2	4	7	10	13	22
B. OPERATED	68	7.7	52	2	3	5	10	17	23	36
TOTAL										
0–19 Years	56	4.2	20	1	1	3	5	8	10	26
20–34	56	6.2	46	1	3	3	6	18	22	36
35–49	68	5.8	15	2	3	5	8	11	14	17
50–64	149	5.1	15	2	2	4	7	9	12	23
65+	302	5.7	21	2	3	4	7	11	14	27
GRAND TOTAL	631	5.5	21	2	3	4	7	11	14	26

283.9: ACQ HEMOLYTIC ANEMIA NOS

Type of Patients	Observed Patients	Avg. Stay	Vari-ance	Percentiles						
				10th	25th	50th	75th	90th	95th	99th
1. SINGLE DX										
A. Not Operated										
0–19 Years	5	2.6	2	1	2	2	3	5	5	5
20–34	1	3.0	0	3	3	3	3	3	3	3
35–49	3	1.7	<1	1	1	2	2	2	2	2
50–64	4	3.5	6	2	2	2	3	7	7	7
65+	2	2.0	0	2	2	2	2	2	2	2
B. Operated										
0–19 Years	0									
20–34	0									
35–49	1	1.0	0	1	1	1	1	1	1	1
50–64	0									
65+	1	2.0	0	2	2	2	2	2	2	2
2. MULTIPLE DX										
A. Not Operated										
0–19 Years	8	3.4	6	1	2	3	4	9	9	9
20–34	33	3.3	5	1	2	3	4	6	7	12
35–49	40	3.8	9	1	2	3	4	9	10	14
50–64	67	4.5	10	1	2	4	6	8	11	17
65+	172	4.6	23	1	2	4	6	9	11	18
B. Operated										
0–19 Years	0									
20–34	5	2.4	3	1	1	2	3	5	5	5
35–49	2	3.5	4	2	2	5	5	5	5	5
50–64	7	6.2	48	1	1	3	14	18	18	18
65+	6	8.7	91	3	3	6	12	28	28	28
SUBTOTALS:										
1. SINGLE DX										
A. Not Operated	15	2.6	2	1	2	2	3	5	7	7
B. Operated	2	1.5	<1	1	1	2	2	2	2	2
2. MULTIPLE DX										
A. Not Operated	320	4.3	16	1	2	3	5	9	11	16
B. Operated	20	5.7	46	1	2	3	6	18	18	28
1. SINGLE DX	17	2.5	2	1	2	2	3	5	7	7
2. MULTIPLE DX	340	4.4	18	1	2	3	5	9	11	18
A. NOT OPERATED	335	4.3	16	1	2	3	5	8	11	16
B. OPERATED	22	5.3	43	1	2	3	6	14	18	28
TOTAL										
0–19 Years	13	3.1	4	1	2	3	3	5	9	9
20–34	39	3.2	5	1	2	3	4	6	7	12
35–49	46	3.6	8	1	2	3	4	6	10	14
50–64	78	4.6	13	1	2	4	6	10	11	18
65+	181	4.7	25	1	2	4	6	9	11	28
GRAND TOTAL	357	4.3	18	1	2	3	5	8	11	18

284: APLAST ANEM&OTH BM FAIL

Type of Patients	Observed Patients	Avg. Stay	Vari-ance	Percentiles						
				10th	25th	50th	75th	90th	95th	99th
1. SINGLE DX										
A. Not Operated										
0–19 Years	34	1.8	3	1	1	1	2	3	5	9
20–34	15	3.7	7	1	1	3	6	6	11	11
35–49	15	1.6	2	1	1	1	2	4	5	5
50–64	11	1.4	<1	1	1	1	2	2	2	2
65+	9	2.6	11	1	1	1	2	11	11	11
B. Operated										
0–19 Years	0									
20–34	0									
35–49	0									
50–64	0									
65+	0									
2. MULTIPLE DX										
A. Not Operated										
0–19 Years	249	4.5	20	1	2	3	6	10	13	21
20–34	231	5.0	22	1	2	3	7	11	14	23
35–49	495	4.9	28	1	2	3	6	10	13	31
50–64	1,059	4.9	25	1	2	3	6	10	14	23
65+	1,610	4.8	21	1	2	4	6	10	13	23
B. Operated										
0–19 Years	13	26.0	275	9	10	30	32	46	62	62
20–34	14	15.2	90	5	6	11	26	27	28	28
35–49	15	16.6	90	3	11	16	21	28	40	40
50–64	21	14.8	89	5	9	12	18	35	41	>99
65+	27	12.2	49	6	7	11	17	22	27	30
SUBTOTALS:										
1. SINGLE DX										
A. Not Operated	84	2.1	4	1	1	1	2	4	6	11
B. Operated	0									
2. MULTIPLE DX										
A. Not Operated	3,644	4.8	23	1	2	3	6	10	13	23
B. Operated	90	16.0	118	5	8	13	22	31	40	>99
1. SINGLE DX	84	2.1	4	1	1	1	2	4	6	11
2. MULTIPLE DX	3,734	5.1	28	1	2	4	6	11	14	27
A. NOT OPERATED	3,728	4.8	23	1	2	3	6	10	13	23
B. OPERATED	90	16.0	118	5	8	13	22	31	40	>99
TOTAL										
0–19 Years	296	5.2	49	1	1	3	6	11	16	37
20–34	260	5.5	30	1	2	4	7	12	16	28
35–49	525	5.1	33	1	2	3	6	11	16	31
50–64	1,091	5.1	28	1	2	3	7	10	15	27
65+	1,646	4.9	23	1	2	4	6	10	13	24
GRAND TOTAL	3,818	5.0	28	1	2	3	6	11	14	27

Length of Stay by Diagnosis and Operation, Western Region, 2008

Western Region, October 2006–September 2007 Data, by Diagnosis

284.1: PANCYTOPENIA

Type of Patients	Observed Patients	Avg. Stay	Variance	Percentiles						
				10th	25th	50th	75th	90th	95th	99th
1. SINGLE DX										
A. Not Operated										
0–19 Years	6	1.3	<1	1	1		1	3	3	3
20–34	6	3.7	4	1	3	3	6	6	6	6
35–49	7	1.7	1	1	1	1	2	4	4	4
50–64	4	1.8	<1	1	2	2	2	2	2	2
65+	2	1.0	0	1	1	1	1	1	1	1
B. Operated										
0–19 Years	0									
20–34	0									
35–49	0									
50–64	0									
65+	0									
2. MULTIPLE DX										
A. Not Operated										
0–19 Years	106	4.5	23	1	2	3	5	9	13	20
20–34	91	4.8	21	1	2	4	6	10	12	28
35–49	294	5.0	31	1	2	4	6	10	12	34
50–64	578	4.5	17	1	2	3	6	9	12	22
65+	877	4.3	15	1	2	3	6	8	11	22
B. Operated										
0–19 Years	3	21.3	478	4	4	14	46	46	46	46
20–34	4	6.5	10	4	4	5	6	11	11	11
35–49	7	12.1	27	3	10	11	18	18	18	18
50–64	13	14.0	69	5	8	12	18	22	35	35
65+	12	10.3	21	6	7	9	13	15	22	22
SUBTOTALS:										
1. SINGLE DX A. Not Operated	25	2.1	2	1	1	1	3	4	6	6
B. Operated	0									
2. MULTIPLE DX A. Not Operated	1,946	4.5	19	1	2	3	6	9	12	23
B. Operated	39	12.3	70	5	6	11	15	22	35	46
1. SINGLE DX	25	2.1	2	1	1	1	3	4	6	6
2. MULTIPLE DX	1,985	4.7	21	1	2	3	6	9	12	23
A. NOT OPERATED	1,971	4.5	19	1	2	3	6	9	12	23
B. OPERATED	39	12.3	70	5	6	11	15	22	35	46
TOTAL										
0–19 Years	115	4.8	38	1	2	3	5	10	14	37
20–34	101	4.8	19	1	2	4	6	10	11	22
35–49	308	5.1	31	1	2	4	6	10	13	31
50–64	595	4.7	20	1	2	3	6	9	14	23
65+	891	4.4	16	1	2	3	6	9	11	22
GRAND TOTAL	2,010	4.6	21	1	2	3	6	9	12	23

284.8: APLASTIC ANEMIAS NEC

Type of Patients	Observed Patients	Avg. Stay	Variance	Percentiles						
				10th	25th	50th	75th	90th	95th	99th
1. SINGLE DX										
A. Not Operated										
0–19 Years	9	1.3	<1	1	1	1	1	3	3	3
20–34	2	2.0	2	1	1	3	3	3	3	3
35–49	5	1.8	3	1	1	1	1	5	5	5
50–64	1	1.0	0	1	1	1	1	1	1	1
65+	4	4.0	22	1	2	2	11	11	11	11
B. Operated										
0–19 Years	0									
20–34	0									
35–49	0									
50–64	0									
65+	0									
2. MULTIPLE DX										
A. Not Operated										
0–19 Years	106	5.0	18	1	2	3	6	11	14	21
20–34	95	5.2	25	1	2	3	6	12	16	28
35–49	166	5.1	26	1	2	3	6	11	15	24
50–64	425	5.5	37	1	2	4	7	11	16	31
65+	649	5.5	30	1	2	4	7	11	14	25
B. Operated										
0–19 Years	6	28.3	380	9	9	31	32	62	62	62
20–34	6	14.5	83	9	6	10	23	28	28	28
35–49	7	19.4	129	3	12	21	23	40	40	40
50–64	5	13.8	52	3	11	16	17	22	22	22
65+	14	14.4	65	6	7	14	19	27	30	30
SUBTOTALS:										
1. SINGLE DX A. Not Operated	21	2.0	5	1	1	1	2	3	5	11
B. Operated	0									
2. MULTIPLE DX A. Not Operated	1,441	5.4	30	1	2	4	7	11	15	25
B. Operated	38	17.5	139	6	9	16	23	31	40	62
1. SINGLE DX	21	2.0	5	1	1	1	2	3	5	11
2. MULTIPLE DX	1,479	5.7	36	1	2	4	7	12	16	30
A. NOT OPERATED	1,462	5.3	30	1	2	4	7	11	15	25
B. OPERATED	38	17.5	139	6	9	16	23	31	40	62
TOTAL										
0–19 Years	121	5.9	59	1	2	3	7	12	16	32
20–34	103	5.7	32	1	2	3	7	14	16	28
35–49	178	5.5	36	1	2	3	7	13	20	33
50–64	431	5.6	38	1	2	4	7	12	16	31
65+	667	5.6	32	1	2	4	7	11	15	27
GRAND TOTAL	1,500	5.6	36	1	2	4	7	12	16	28

284.9: APLASTIC ANEMIA NOS

Type of Patients	Observed Patients	Avg. Stay	Variance	Percentiles						
				10th	25th	50th	75th	90th	95th	99th
1. SINGLE DX										
A. Not Operated										
0–19 Years	10	2.8	7	1	1	2	4	9	9	9
20–34	7	4.2	12	1	1	4	6	11	11	11
35–49	2	1.0	0	1	1	1	1	1	1	1
50–64	6	1.2	<1	1	1	1	1	2	2	2
65+	3	1.7	1	1	1	1	3	3	3	3
B. Operated										
0–19 Years	0									
20–34	0									
35–49	0									
50–64	0									
65+	0									
2. MULTIPLE DX										
A. Not Operated										
0–19 Years	27	3.6	15	1	1	2	4	9	11	17
20–34	38	5.8	21	1	2	4	9	12	16	18
35–49	28	3.3	15	1	1	3	5	10	11	17
50–64	50	4.5	14	1	2	3	7	10	12	17
65+	80	4.1	16	1	1	3	6	10	11	24
B. Operated										
0–19 Years	4	26.1	113	10	30	31	33	33	33	33
20–34	3	24.3	14	20	20	26	27	27	27	27
35–49	1	28.0	0	28	28	28	28	28	28	28
50–64	3	20.2	316	9	11	11	>99	>99	>99	>99
65+	1	4.0	0	4	4	4	4	4	4	4
SUBTOTALS:										
1. SINGLE DX A. Not Operated	28	2.5	6	1	1	1	3	6	9	11
B. Operated	0									
2. MULTIPLE DX A. Not Operated	223	4.3	17	1	1	3	6	11	12	17
B. Operated	12	22.5	133	9	11	27	31	41	>99	>99
1. SINGLE DX	28	2.5	6	1	1	1	3	6	9	11
2. MULTIPLE DX	235	5.3	38	1	1	3	7	12	17	33
A. NOT OPERATED	251	4.1	16	1	1	3	6	11	12	17
B. OPERATED	12	22.5	133	9	11	27	31	41	>99	>99
TOTAL										
0–19 Years	41	5.6	66	1	1	2	6	11	30	33
20–34	48	6.7	40	1	2	4	11	16	20	27
35–49	31	4.0	34	1	1	1	5	10	17	28
50–64	59	5.0	37	1	1	3	7	11	13	>99
65+	84	4.0	16	1	1	3	5	10	11	24
GRAND TOTAL	263	5.0	35	1	1	3	7	11	17	33

Length of Stay by Diagnosis and Operation, Western Region, 2008

Western Region, October 2006–September 2007 Data, by Diagnosis

285: ANEMIA NEC & NOS

Type of Patients	Observed Patients	Avg. Stay	Variance	10th	25th	50th	75th	90th	95th	99th
1. SINGLE DX										
A. Not Operated										
0–19 Years	11	1.3	<1	1	1	1	1	2	2	2
20–34	15	1.4	<1	1	1	1	2	2	3	3
35–49	36	1.3	<1	1	1	1	1	2	3	3
50–64	35	1.1	<1	1	1	1	1	2	2	2
65+	80	1.1	<1	1	1	1	1	1	2	3
B. Operated										
0–19 Years	0									
20–34	0									
35–49	0									
50–64	0									
65+	1	5.0	0	5	5	5	5	5	5	5
2. MULTIPLE DX										
A. Not Operated										
0–19 Years	149	1.8	3	1	1	1	2	3	4	11
20–34	404	2.1	4	1	1	1	2	4	5	10
35–49	1,389	2.4	5	1	1	2	3	5	6	11
50–64	2,388	2.7	8	1	1	2	3	5	7	14
65+	7,164	3.0	7	1	2	2	4	6	8	13
B. Operated										
0–19 Years	3	10.3	163	1	1	5	25	25	25	25
20–34	23	4.4	37	1	1	2	6	9	20	24
35–49	59	4.9	46	1	1	2	5	10	20	37
50–64	70	7.3	46	1	2	5	9	18	22	29
65+	142	8.5	48	2	4	7	11	17	20	35
SUBTOTALS:										
1. SINGLE DX A. Not Operated	177	1.2	<1	1	1	1	1	2	2	3
B. Operated	1	5.0	0	5	5	5	5	5	5	5
2. MULTIPLE DX A. Not Operated	11,494	2.8	7	1	1	2	3	6	7	13
B. Operated	297	7.2	49	1	2	5	10	17	21	35
1. SINGLE DX	178	1.2	<1	1	1	1	2	2	2	3
2. MULTIPLE DX	11,791	2.9	8	1	1	2	4	6	8	15
A. NOT OPERATED	11,671	2.8	7	1	1	2	3	6	7	13
B. OPERATED	298	7.2	49	1	2	5	10	17	21	35
TOTAL										
0–19 Years	163	1.9	6	1	1	1	2	3	4	16
20–34	442	2.2	6	1	1	1	2	4	6	15
35–49	1,484	2.5	7	1	1	2	3	5	6	13
50–64	2,493	2.8	9	1	1	2	3	6	7	17
65+	7,387	3.1	8	1	1	2	4	6	8	14
GRAND TOTAL	11,969	2.9	8	1	1	2	4	6	8	15

285.1: ACUTE POSTHEMOR ANEMIA

Type of Patients	Observed Patients	Avg. Stay	Variance	10th	25th	50th	75th	90th	95th	99th
1. SINGLE DX										
A. Not Operated										
0–19 Years	0									
20–34	3	1.3	<1	1	1	1	2	2	2	2
35–49	3	2.3	1	1	1	3	3	3	3	3
50–64	0									
65+	2	2.0	2	1	1	2	3	3	3	3
B. Operated										
0–19 Years	0									
20–34	0									
35–49	0									
50–64	0									
65+	0									
2. MULTIPLE DX										
A. Not Operated										
0–19 Years	29	2.0	8	1	1	1	2	3	4	16
20–34	116	1.7	1	1	1	1	2	3	4	5
35–49	340	2.3	4	1	1	2	3	5	6	10
50–64	322	2.9	6	1	1	2	4	5	7	13
65+	858	3.3	8	2	2	3	4	6	8	14
B. Operated										
0–19 Years	3	10.3	163	1	1	5	25	25	25	25
20–34	16	2.8	7	1	1	1	2	5	9	9
35–49	26	4.8	50	1	2	3	5	10	11	37
50–64	19	5.4	37	1	1	3	6	19	24	24
65+	47	7.6	43	1	3	5	11	17	20	32
SUBTOTALS:										
1. SINGLE DX A. Not Operated	8	1.9	<1	1	1	2	3	3	3	3
B. Operated	0									
2. MULTIPLE DX A. Not Operated	1,665	2.9	6	1	1	2	4	6	7	13
B. Operated	111	5.9	43	1	2	4	7	14	20	32
1. SINGLE DX	8	1.9	<1	1	1	2	3	3	3	3
2. MULTIPLE DX	1,776	3.1	9	1	1	2	4	6	8	15
A. NOT OPERATED	1,673	2.9	6	1	1	2	4	6	7	13
B. OPERATED	111	5.9	43	1	2	4	7	14	20	32
TOTAL										
0–19 Years	32	2.8	24	1	1	1	2	4	16	25
20–34	135	1.9	2	1	1	1	3	5	5	8
35–49	369	2.5	7	1	1	2	3	5	6	11
50–64	341	3.0	8	1	1	2	4	6	8	13
65+	907	3.5	10	2	2	3	4	7	9	15
GRAND TOTAL	1,784	3.1	9	1	1	2	4	6	8	15

285.21: ANEMIA IN CKD

Type of Patients	Observed Patients	Avg. Stay	Variance	10th	25th	50th	75th	90th	95th	99th
1. SINGLE DX										
A. Not Operated										
0–19 Years	0									
20–34	0									
35–49	0									
50–64	0									
65+	0									
B. Operated										
0–19 Years	0									
20–34	0									
35–49	0									
50–64	0									
65+	0									
2. MULTIPLE DX										
A. Not Operated										
0–19 Years	5	1.4	<1	1	1	1	1	3	3	3
20–34	19	2.3	4	1	1	2	3	4	10	10
35–49	94	2.8	5	1	1	2	4	6	7	14
50–64	244	3.1	9	1	1	2	4	6	8	17
65+	733	3.1	8	1	1	2	4	6	8	16
B. Operated										
0–19 Years	0									
20–34	1	20.0	0	20	20	20	20	20	20	20
35–49	3	9.0	93	2	2	5	5	20	20	20
50–64	10	10.2	73	2	4	8	15	29	29	29
65+	17	9.7	82	2	5	7	10	22	39	39
SUBTOTALS:										
1. SINGLE DX A. Not Operated	0									
B. Operated	0									
2. MULTIPLE DX A. Not Operated	1,095	3.1	8	1	1	2	4	6	8	17
B. Operated	31	10.1	75	2	5	7	15	20	29	39
1. SINGLE DX	0									
2. MULTIPLE DX	1,126	3.3	11	1	1	2	4	7	9	19
A. NOT OPERATED	1,095	3.1	8	1	1	2	4	6	8	17
B. OPERATED	31	10.1	75	2	5	7	15	20	29	39
TOTAL										
0–19 Years	5	1.4	<1	1	1	1	1	3	3	3
20–34	20	3.2	20	1	1	2	3	10	20	20
35–49	97	3.0	8	1	1	2	4	7	8	20
50–64	254	3.4	13	1	1	2	4	7	10	19
65+	750	3.3	11	1	1	2	4	7	8	18
GRAND TOTAL	1,126	3.3	11	1	1	2	4	7	9	19

Length of Stay by Diagnosis and Operation, Western Region, 2008

Western Region, October 2006–September 2007 Data, by Diagnosis

285.22: ANEMIA IN NEOPL DISEASE

Type of Patients	Observed Patients	Avg. Stay	Vari-ance	10th	25th	50th	75th	90th	95th	99th
1. SINGLE DX										
A. Not Operated										
0–19 Years	0									
20–34	0									
35–49	2	2.0	0	1	1	1	2	3	3	3
50–64	1	1.0	0	1	1	1	1	1	1	1
65+	1	1.0	0	1	1	1	1	1	1	1
B. Operated										
0–19 Years	0									
20–34	0									
35–49	0									
50–64	0									
65+	0									
2. MULTIPLE DX										
A. Not Operated										
0–19 Years	18	1.3	<1	1	1	1	1	3	4	4
20–34	16	1.8	3	1	1	1	2	6	6	6
35–49	113	2.5	8	1	1	1	3	5	8	16
50–64	348	2.5	7	1	1	2	3	5	7	14
65+	869	2.6	6	1	1	2	3	5	7	12
B. Operated										
0–19 Years	0									
20–34	2	9.1	127	1	1	17	17	17	17	17
35–49	7	9.0	64	1	3	6	18	22	22	22
50–64										
65+	16	9.1	12	3	9	10	12	13	13	13
SUBTOTALS:										
1. SINGLE DX — A. Not Operated	4	1.5	<1	1	1	1	1	3	3	3
B. Operated	0									
2. MULTIPLE DX — A. Not Operated	1,364	2.5	6	1	1	2	3	5	7	13
B. Operated	25	9.1	29	2	4	9	12	17	18	22
1. SINGLE DX	4	1.5	<1	1	1	1	1	3	3	3
2. MULTIPLE DX	1,389	2.7	8	1	1	2	3	6	8	14
A. NOT OPERATED	1,368	2.5	6	1	1	2	3	5	7	13
B. OPERATED	25	9.1	29	2	4	9	12	17	18	22
TOTAL										
0–19 Years	18	1.3	<1	1	1	1	1	3	4	4
20–34	16	1.8	3	1	1	1	2	6	6	6
35–49	117	2.6	10	1	1	1	3	5	10	17
50–64	356	2.6	9	1	1	2	3	5	7	16
65+	886	2.7	7	1	1	2	3	6	8	13
GRAND TOTAL	1,393	2.7	8	1	1	2	3	6	8	14

285.29: ANEMIA CHR DISEASE NEC

Type of Patients	Observed Patients	Avg. Stay	Vari-ance	10th	25th	50th	75th	90th	95th	99th
1. SINGLE DX										
A. Not Operated										
0–19 Years	0									
20–34	0									
35–49	0									
50–64	1	2.0	0	2	2	2	2	2	2	2
65+	2	1.0	0	1	1	1	1	1	1	1
B. Operated										
0–19 Years	0									
20–34	0									
35–49	0									
50–64	0									
65+	0									
2. MULTIPLE DX										
A. Not Operated										
0–19 Years	8	1.4	<1	1	1	1	2	3	3	3
20–34	32	3.1	8	1	1	2	4	6	9	15
35–49	129	3.2	8	1	1	2	3	7	8	14
50–64	272	3.0	9	1	1	2	4	6	7	17
65+	859	3.3	9	1	1	2	4	6	8	15
B. Operated										
0–19 Years	0									
20–34	2	4.5	12	2	2	5	7	7	7	7
35–49	9	10.0	53	2	5	7	18	21	21	21
50–64										
65+	10	11.0	45	3	5	8	17	19	20	20
SUBTOTALS:										
1. SINGLE DX — A. Not Operated	3	1.3	<1	1	1	1	2	2	2	2
B. Operated	0									
2. MULTIPLE DX — A. Not Operated	1,300	3.2	9	1	1	2	4	6	8	15
B. Operated	21	10.0	45	3	5	7	17	19	21	21
1. SINGLE DX	3	1.3	<1	1	1	1	2	2	2	2
2. MULTIPLE DX	1,321	3.3	10	1	1	2	4	7	9	18
A. NOT OPERATED	1,303	3.2	9	1	1	2	4	6	8	15
B. OPERATED	21	10.0	45	3	5	7	17	19	20	21
TOTAL										
0–19 Years	8	1.4	<1	1	1	1	2	3	3	3
20–34	32	3.1	8	1	1	2	4	6	9	15
35–49	131	3.2	8	1	1	2	4	7	8	14
50–64	282	3.2	12	1	1	2	4	6	9	21
65+	871	3.4	10	1	1	2	4	7	9	17
GRAND TOTAL	1,324	3.3	10	1	1	2	4	7	9	18

285.8: ANEMIA NEC

Type of Patients	Observed Patients	Avg. Stay	Vari-ance	10th	25th	50th	75th	90th	95th	99th
1. SINGLE DX										
A. Not Operated										
0–19 Years	1	2.0	0	2	2	2	2	2	2	2
20–34	1	3.0	0	3	3	3	3	3	3	3
35–49	1	2.0	0	2	2	2	2	2	2	2
50–64	2	1.0	0	1	1	1	1	1	1	1
65+	1	1.0	0	1	1	1	1	1	1	1
B. Operated										
0–19 Years	0									
20–34	0									
35–49	0									
50–64	0									
65+	0									
2. MULTIPLE DX										
A. Not Operated										
0–19 Years	6	1.8	2	1	1	1	3	4	4	4
20–34	26	2.2	2	1	1	2	3	4	5	8
35–49	58	2.1	3	1	1	1	3	4	6	10
50–64	103	2.7	3	1	1	2	4	5	7	7
65+	285	3.2	6	1	2	2	4	6	8	14
B. Operated										
0–19 Years	0									
20–34	3	13.6	219	3	3	24	24	24	24	24
35–49	3	2.3	5	1	1	1	5	5	5	5
50–64	4	3.8	10	1	1	6	7	7	7	7
65+	5	5.6	13	1	3	6	8	10	10	10
SUBTOTALS:										
1. SINGLE DX — A. Not Operated	6	1.7	<1	1	1	2	2	3	3	3
B. Operated	0									
2. MULTIPLE DX — A. Not Operated	478	2.9	5	1	1	2	4	6	7	10
B. Operated	14	5.5	37	1	5	5	7	10	24	24
1. SINGLE DX	6	1.7	<1	1	1	2	2	3	3	3
2. MULTIPLE DX	492	2.9	6	1	1	2	4	6	7	10
A. NOT OPERATED	484	2.9	5	1	1	2	4	6	7	10
B. OPERATED	14	5.5	37	1	5	5	7	10	24	24
TOTAL										
0–19 Years	7	1.9	1	1	1	1	3	4	4	4
20–34	29	3.0	18	1	1	2	3	5	8	24
35–49	62	2.1	3	1	1	1	3	4	5	10
50–64	109	2.7	4	1	1	2	4	6	7	7
65+	291	3.2	6	1	1	2	4	6	8	14
GRAND TOTAL	498	2.9	6	1	2	2	4	6	7	10

Length of Stay by Diagnosis and Operation, Western Region, 2008

Western Region, October 2006–September 2007 Data, by Diagnosis

285.9: ANEMIA NOS

Type of Patients	Observed Patients	Avg. Stay	Variance	Percentiles						
				10th	25th	50th	75th	90th	95th	99th
1. SINGLE DX										
A. Not Operated										
0–19 Years	10	1.2	<1	1	1	1	1	2	2	2
20–34	11	1.3	<1	1	1	1	2	2	2	2
35–49	30	1.1	<1	1	1	1	1	1	2	2
50–64	31	1.1	<1	1	1	1	1	2	2	2
65+	74	1.1	<1	1	1	1	1	1	2	3
B. Operated										
0–19 Years	0									
20–34	0									
35–49	0									
50–64	0									
65+	1	5.0	0	5	5	5	5	5	5	5
2. MULTIPLE DX										
A. Not Operated										
0–19 Years	77	1.9	3	1	1	1	2	3	4	11
20–34	195	2.1	5	1	1	1	2	4	6	15
35–49	652	2.3	4	1	1	2	3	5	6	9
50–64	1,097	2.6	8	1	1	2	3	5	7	13
65+	3,548	2.9	6	1	1	2	4	6	7	13
B. Operated										
0–19 Years	0									
20–34	4	2.3	<1	1	1	2	3	3	3	3
35–49	23	4.6	45	1	1	2	6	8	10	33
50–64	21	6.5	36	1	2	6	7	14	17	23
65+	47	8.5	59	2	4	5	12	17	23	35
SUBTOTALS:										
1. SINGLE DX										
A. Not Operated	156	1.1	<1	1	1	1	1	2	2	2
B. Operated	1	5.0	0	5	5	5	5	5	5	5
2. MULTIPLE DX										
A. Not Operated	5,569	2.7	6	1	1	2	3	5	7	12
B. Operated	95	6.8	51	1	2	5	9	15	23	35
1. SINGLE DX	157	1.2	<1	1	1	1	1	2	2	3
2. MULTIPLE DX	5,664	2.8	7	1	1	2	3	5	7	13
A. NOT OPERATED	5,725	2.7	6	1	1	2	3	5	7	12
B. OPERATED	96	6.8	50	1	2	5	8	15	23	35
TOTAL										
0–19 Years	87	1.8	2	1	1	1	2	3	4	11
20–34	210	2.1	5	1	1	1	2	4	5	11
35–49	705	2.3	6	1	1	2	3	5	6	9
50–64	1,149	2.6	8	1	1	2	3	5	7	14
65+	3,670	2.9	7	1	1	2	4	6	8	13
GRAND TOTAL	5,821	2.7	7	1	1	2	3	5	7	13

286: COAGULATION DEFECTS

Type of Patients	Observed Patients	Avg. Stay	Variance	Percentiles						
				10th	25th	50th	75th	90th	95th	99th
1. SINGLE DX										
A. Not Operated										
0–19 Years	23	2.2	3	1	1	2	3	4	4	8
20–34	1	3.0	0	3	3	3	3	3	3	3
35–49	0									
50–64	0									
65+	0									
B. Operated										
0–19 Years	0									
20–34	0									
35–49	1	1.0	0	1	1	1	1	1	1	1
50–64	0									
65+	0									
2. MULTIPLE DX										
A. Not Operated										
0–19 Years	70	3.5	9	1	1	2	4	9	9	15
20–34	78	4.6	14	1	2	3	7	9	13	20
35–49	113	4.3	13	1	2	3	6	9	14	16
50–64	206	4.8	18	1	2	3	6	10	15	20
65+	527	5.0	24	1	2	3	6	11	14	26
B. Operated										
0–19 Years	6	5.3	36	1	1	2	12	14	14	14
20–34	8	6.3	38	1	2	6	11	19	19	19
35–49	8	4.0	6	1	2	4	5	9	9	9
50–64	11	9.1	56	2	3	6	13	17	26	26
65+	23	10.4	258	2	3	5	9	17	52	67
SUBTOTALS:										
1. SINGLE DX										
A. Not Operated	24	2.3	2	1	1	2	3	4	4	8
B. Operated	1	1.0	0	1	1	1	1	1	1	1
2. MULTIPLE DX										
A. Not Operated	994	4.7	20	1	2	3	6	10	14	22
B. Operated	56	8.1	129	1	2	5	9	17	26	67
1. SINGLE DX	25	2.2	2	1	1	2	3	4	4	8
2. MULTIPLE DX	1,050	4.9	26	1	2	3	6	10	14	25
A. NOT OPERATED	1,018	4.7	20	1	2	3	6	10	14	22
B. OPERATED	57	8.0	127	1	2	5	9	17	26	67
TOTAL										
0–19 Years	99	3.3	9	1	1	2	4	8	10	15
20–34	87	4.8	16	1	2	3	7	10	13	20
35–49	122	4.3	13	1	2	3	6	11	11	16
50–64	217	5.0	21	1	2	3	6	11	15	24
65+	550	5.2	35	1	2	3	6	11	15	27
GRAND TOTAL	1,075	4.9	26	1	2	3	6	10	14	25

286.7: ACQ COAG FACTOR DEF

Type of Patients	Observed Patients	Avg. Stay	Variance	Percentiles						
				10th	25th	50th	75th	90th	95th	99th
1. SINGLE DX										
A. Not Operated										
0–19 Years	1	1.0	0	1	1	1	1	1	1	1
20–34	0									
35–49	0									
50–64	0									
65+	0									
B. Operated										
0–19 Years	0									
20–34	0									
35–49	0									
50–64	0									
65+	0									
2. MULTIPLE DX										
A. Not Operated										
0–19 Years	2	1.0	0	1	1	1	1	1	1	1
20–34	5	7.0	26	1	3	8	9	14	14	14
35–49	32	4.6	16	1	2	3	6	11	15	16
50–64	49	5.3	21	1	2	4	6	15	16	19
65+	103	4.6	21	1	2	3	6	10	13	21
B. Operated										
0–19 Years	0									
20–34	0									
35–49	3	2.3	2	1	1	2	4	4	4	4
50–64	3	16.3	99	6	6	17	26	26	26	26
65+	3	7.4	8	4	4	9	9	9	9	9
SUBTOTALS:										
1. SINGLE DX										
A. Not Operated	1	1.0	0	1	1	1	1	1	1	1
B. Operated	0									
2. MULTIPLE DX										
A. Not Operated	191	4.8	20	1	2	3	6	11	15	21
B. Operated	9	8.7	65	1	4	6	9	26	26	26
1. SINGLE DX	1	1.0	0	1	1	1	1	1	1	1
2. MULTIPLE DX	200	5.0	23	1	2	3	6	11	16	26
A. NOT OPERATED	192	4.8	20	1	2	3	6	11	15	21
B. OPERATED	9	8.7	65	1	4	6	9	26	26	26
TOTAL										
0–19 Years	3	1.0	0	1	1	1	1	1	1	1
20–34	5	7.0	26	1	3	8	9	14	14	14
35–49	35	4.4	16	1	2	3	6	11	15	16
50–64	52	6.0	31	1	3	4	7	16	18	26
65+	106	4.7	20	1	2	3	6	10	13	21
GRAND TOTAL	201	5.0	22	1	2	3	6	11	16	26

Length of Stay by Diagnosis and Operation, Western Region, 2008

Western Region, October 2006–September 2007 Data, by Diagnosis

286.9: COAG DEFECT NEC & NOS

Type of Patients	Observed Patients	Avg. Stay	Variance	10th	25th	50th	75th	90th	95th	99th
1. SINGLE DX										
A. Not Operated										
0–19 Years	0									
20–34	0									
35–49	0									
50–64	0									
65+	0									
B. Operated										
0–19 Years	0									
20–34	0									
35–49	0									
50–64	0									
65+	0									
2. MULTIPLE DX										
A. Not Operated										
0–19 Years	4	2.5	2	1	1	2	3	4	4	4
20–34	10	2.8	5	1	1	2	4	4	5	8
35–49	34	4.1	13	1	2	2	5	8	14	15
50–64	72	4.3	16	1	2	3	5	8	15	24
65+	157	4.4	14	1	2	3	5	10	13	20
B. Operated										
0–19 Years	0									
20–34	0									
35–49	2	4.5	<1	4	4	5	5	5	5	5
50–64	1	10.0	0	10	10	10	10	10	10	10
65+	9	4.8	10	1	2	4	7	10	10	10
SUBTOTALS:										
1. SINGLE DX										
A. Not Operated	0									
B. Operated	0									
2. MULTIPLE DX										
A. Not Operated	277	4.3	14	1	2	3	5	9	13	20
B. Operated	12	5.2	10	2	3	4	7	10	10	10
1. SINGLE DX	0									
2. MULTIPLE DX	289	4.3	14	1	2	3	5	9	12	20
A. NOT OPERATED	277	4.3	14	1	2	3	5	9	13	20
B. OPERATED	12	5.2	10	2	3	4	7	10	13	20
TOTAL										
0–19 Years	4	2.5	2	1	1	2	3	4	4	4
20–34	10	2.8	5	1	1	2	4	4	8	8
35–49	36	4.1	12	1	1	2	5	8	14	15
50–64	73	4.4	16	1	2	3	5	10	15	24
65+	166	4.4	14	1	2	3	5	10	12	20
GRAND TOTAL	289	4.3	14	1	2	3	5	9	12	20

287: PURPURA & OTH HEMOR COND

Type of Patients	Observed Patients	Avg. Stay	Variance	10th	25th	50th	75th	90th	95th	99th
1. SINGLE DX										
A. Not Operated										
0–19 Years	261	1.7	1	1	1	1	2	3	4	6
20–34	54	2.5	2	1	1	2	3	4	5	7
35–49	38	2.2	1	1	1	2	3	4	5	5
50–64	29	2.3	3	1	1	2	3	5	5	8
65+	15	1.7	<1	1	1	1	2	3	3	3
B. Operated										
0–19 Years	11	3.2	3	1	1	3	5	5	5	5
20–34	25	2.5	3	1	1	2	4	5	5	7
35–49	11	2.8	3	1	2	2	4	5	6	6
50–64	4	2.0	<1	1	1	2	3	3	3	3
65+	3	2.3	1	1	1	3	3	3	3	3
2. MULTIPLE DX										
A. Not Operated										
0–19 Years	509	2.5	5	1	2	2	3	5	7	10
20–34	392	3.9	22	1	2	3	4	7	10	22
35–49	528	4.1	17	1	2	3	5	8	12	21
50–64	855	3.9	14	1	2	3	5	8	11	19
65+	1,271	4.8	21	1	2	4	6	9	13	24
B. Operated										
0–19 Years	17	6.5	52	2	3	4	9	10	32	32
20–34	64	6.0	54	1	2	3	8	12	16	48
35–49	83	6.7	135	2	2	3	6	14	20	95
50–64	106	7.1	119	1	2	4	7	14	28	33
65+	129	8.1	67	2	3	5	10	19	23	41
SUBTOTALS:										
1. SINGLE DX										
A. Not Operated	397	1.9	2	1	1	1	2	3	5	6
B. Operated	54	2.7	2	1	1	2	4	5	5	7
2. MULTIPLE DX										
A. Not Operated	3,555	4.1	17	1	2	3	5	8	11	21
B. Operated	399	7.1	92	1	2	4	8	16	23	48
1. SINGLE DX	451	2.0	2	1	1	2	2	4	5	6
2. MULTIPLE DX	3,954	4.4	26	1	2	3	5	9	12	24
A. NOT OPERATED	3,952	3.8	16	1	2	3	5	8	11	20
B. OPERATED	453	6.6	84	1	2	4	7	15	22	41
TOTAL										
0–19 Years	798	2.4	6	1	1	2	3	4	6	10
20–34	535	4.0	24	1	2	3	4	7	11	22
35–49	660	4.3	32	1	2	3	5	8	13	24
50–64	994	4.2	26	1	2	3	5	8	12	27
65+	1,418	5.1	26	1	2	4	6	10	14	25
GRAND TOTAL	4,405	4.1	24	1	2	3	5	8	12	23

287.0: ALLERGIC PURPURA

Type of Patients	Observed Patients	Avg. Stay	Variance	10th	25th	50th	75th	90th	95th	99th
1. SINGLE DX										
A. Not Operated										
0–19 Years	51	1.3	<1	1	1	1	1	2	3	5
20–34	1	7.0	0	7	7	7	7	7	7	7
35–49	0									
50–64	0									
65+	0									
B. Operated										
0–19 Years	0									
20–34	0									
35–49	0									
50–64	0									
65+	0									
2. MULTIPLE DX										
A. Not Operated										
0–19 Years	138	2.4	3	1	1	2	3	4	7	9
20–34	13	4.4	20	1	2	3	4	10	17	17
35–49	18	4.4	9	2	2	4	6	10	13	13
50–64	15	5.3	14	1	3	4	7	10	15	15
65+	24	4.8	10	2	2	4	7	11	11	12
B. Operated										
0–19 Years	1	3.0	0	3	3	3	3	3	3	3
20–34	1	1.0	0	1	1	1	1	1	1	1
35–49	0									
50–64	0									
65+	0									
SUBTOTALS:										
1. SINGLE DX										
A. Not Operated	52	1.4	1	1	1	1	1	2	3	7
B. Operated	0									
2. MULTIPLE DX										
A. Not Operated	208	3.2	7	1	1	2	4	7	9	13
B. Operated	2	2.0	2	1	1	3	3	3	3	3
1. SINGLE DX	52	1.4	1	1	1	1	1	2	3	7
2. MULTIPLE DX	210	3.2	7	1	1	2	4	7	9	13
A. NOT OPERATED	260	2.8	6	1	1	2	3	6	8	13
B. OPERATED	2	2.0	2	1	1	3	3	3	3	3
TOTAL										
0–19 Years	190	2.1	3	1	1	2	3	4	5	9
20–34	15	4.3	19	1	1	3	6	10	17	17
35–49	18	4.4	9	2	2	4	6	8	13	13
50–64	15	5.3	14	1	3	4	7	10	15	15
65+	24	4.8	10	2	2	4	7	11	11	12
GRAND TOTAL	262	2.8	6	1	1	2	3	6	7	13

Length of Stay by Diagnosis and Operation, Western Region, 2008

Western Region, October 2006–September 2007 Data, by Diagnosis

287.31: IMMUN THROMBOCYT PURPURA

Type of Patients	Observed Patients	Avg. Stay	Variance	Percentiles						
				10th	25th	50th	75th	90th	95th	99th
1. SINGLE DX										
A. *Not Operated*										
0–19 Years	190	1.8	2	1	1	1	2	3	4	6
20–34	48	2.4	2	1	1	2	3	4	5	6
35–49	29	2.4	1	1	2	2	3	4	5	5
50–64	25	2.4	3	1	1	2	3	5	5	8
65+	10	1.8	<1	1	1	1	3	3	3	3
B. *Operated*										
0–19 Years	11	3.2	3	1	1	3	5	5	5	5
20–34	25	2.5	3	1	1	2	4	5	5	7
35–49	11	2.8	3	1	2	2	4	5	6	6
50–64	3	2.0	1	1	1	2	3	3	3	3
65+	3	2.3	1	1	1	3	3	3	3	3
2. MULTIPLE DX										
A. *Not Operated*										
0–19 Years	243	2.5	5	1	1	2	3	4	6	11
20–34	255	3.9	18	1	2	3	4	7	11	20
35–49	290	4.0	12	1	2	3	4	7	12	18
50–64	392	4.2	16	1	2	3	5	8	12	19
65+	557	5.4	24	2	2	4	6	11	15	26
B. *Operated*										
0–19 Years	12	4.7	10	2	3	4	9	10	10	10
20–34	59	5.5	47	1	2	3	8	12	16	48
35–49	77	6.9	145	2	2	4	6	16	24	95
50–64	95	6.3	52	1	2	4	7	14	28	33
65+	113	7.8	68	2	3	5	9	18	22	41
SUBTOTALS:										
1. SINGLE DX										
A. *Not Operated*	302	2.0	2	1	1	2	2	4	5	6
B. *Operated*	53	2.7	2	1	1	2	4	5	5	7
2. MULTIPLE DX										
A. *Not Operated*	1,737	4.3	17	1	2	3	5	8	12	22
B. *Operated*	356	6.7	75	1	2	4	8	16	21	41
1. SINGLE DX	355	2.1	2	1	1	2	3	4	5	6
2. MULTIPLE DX	2,093	4.7	28	1	2	3	5	9	14	27
A. NOT OPERATED	2,039	3.9	16	1	2	3	5	8	11	20
B. OPERATED	409	6.2	67	1	2	4	7	14	20	35
TOTAL										
0–19 Years	456	2.3	4	1	1	2	3	4	6	10
20–34	387	3.9	20	1	2	3	4	8	11	20
35–49	407	4.4	37	1	2	3	5	8	13	24
50–64	515	4.5	22	1	2	3	5	8	13	29
65+	683	5.7	32	2	2	4	7	12	17	29
GRAND TOTAL	2,448	4.3	25	1	2	3	5	8	13	24

287.4: 2ND THROMBOCYTOPENIA

Type of Patients	Observed Patients	Avg. Stay	Variance	Percentiles						
				10th	25th	50th	75th	90th	95th	99th
1. SINGLE DX										
A. *Not Operated*										
0–19 Years	0									
20–34	1	1.0	0	1	1	1	1	1	1	1
35–49	1	2.0	0	2	2	2	2	2	2	2
50–64	0									
65+	0									
B. *Operated*										
0–19 Years	0									
20–34	0									
35–49	0									
50–64	0									
65+	0									
2. MULTIPLE DX										
A. *Not Operated*										
0–19 Years	20	1.9	1	1	1	2	3	4	4	4
20–34	43	4.2	49	1	1	3	4	7	8	47
35–49	99	4.3	17	1	2	3	5	9	15	21
50–64	200	3.6	11	1	1	3	4	8	10	14
65+	285	4.4	21	1	2	3	6	8	13	21
B. *Operated*										
0–19 Years	0									
20–34	1	9.0	0	9	9	9	9	9	9	9
35–49	0									
50–64	5	3.6	4	1	2	4	5	6	6	6
65+	6	12.9	85	2	3	14	22	24	24	24
SUBTOTALS:										
1. SINGLE DX										
A. *Not Operated*	2	1.5	<1	1	1	1	2	2	2	2
B. *Operated*	0									
2. MULTIPLE DX										
A. *Not Operated*	647	4.0	19	1	1	3	5	8	11	20
B. *Operated*	12	8.7	62	2	3	6	14	22	24	24
1. SINGLE DX	2	1.5	<1	1	1	1	2	2	2	2
2. MULTIPLE DX	659	4.1	20	1	1	3	5	8	12	21
A. NOT OPERATED	649	4.0	19	1	1	3	5	8	11	20
B. OPERATED	12	8.7	62	2	3	6	14	22	24	24
TOTAL										
0–19 Years	20	1.9	1	1	1	2	3	4	4	4
20–34	45	4.2	48	1	1	3	4	7	9	47
35–49	100	4.3	17	1	2	3	5	8	15	20
50–64	205	3.6	11	1	1	3	5	8	10	14
65+	291	4.6	23	1	2	3	6	9	13	24
GRAND TOTAL	661	4.1	20	1	1	3	5	8	12	21

287.5: THROMBOCYTOPENIA NOS

Type of Patients	Observed Patients	Avg. Stay	Variance	Percentiles						
				10th	25th	50th	75th	90th	95th	99th
1. SINGLE DX										
A. *Not Operated*										
0–19 Years	6	1.5	<1	1	1	1	2	2	2	2
20–34	3	2.3	5	1	1	3	3	3	3	3
35–49	6	1.3	<1	1	1	1	1	3	3	3
50–64	3	1.7	1	1	1	1	3	3	3	3
65+	2	1.0	0	1	1	1	1	1	1	1
B. *Operated*										
0–19 Years	0									
20–34	0									
35–49	0									
50–64	0									
65+	0									
2. MULTIPLE DX										
A. *Not Operated*										
0–19 Years	59	3.1	16	1	1	2	3	7	9	25
20–34	62	3.0	5	1	2	2	4	6	7	11
35–49	88	3.1	5	1	1	2	4	6	9	11
50–64	213	3.5	13	1	1	3	4	7	9	18
65+	318	4.1	13	1	2	3	5	8	11	20
B. *Operated*										
0–19 Years	1	6.0	0	6	6	6	6	6	6	6
20–34	1	3.0	0	3	3	3	3	3	3	3
35–49	2	1.5	<1	1	1	2	2	2	2	2
50–64	2	8.5	24	5	5	5	12	12	12	12
65+	4	7.7	16	2	2	8	10	11	11	11
SUBTOTALS:										
1. SINGLE DX										
A. *Not Operated*	20	1.6	<1	1	1	1	2	3	3	3
B. *Operated*	0									
2. MULTIPLE DX										
A. *Not Operated*	740	3.6	12	1	1	3	4	7	10	18
B. *Operated*	10	6.0	16	1	2	5	10	11	12	12
1. SINGLE DX	20	1.6	<1	1	1	1	2	3	3	3
2. MULTIPLE DX	750	3.6	12	1	1	3	4	8	10	18
A. NOT OPERATED	760	3.6	11	1	1	3	4	7	9	18
B. OPERATED	10	6.0	16	1	2	5	10	11	12	12
TOTAL										
0–19 Years	66	3.0	15	1	1	2	3	6	8	25
20–34	66	3.0	5	1	2	2	4	6	7	11
35–49	96	2.9	5	1	1	2	4	6	9	11
50–64	218	3.5	13	1	1	3	4	7	10	18
65+	324	4.1	13	1	2	3	5	8	11	20
GRAND TOTAL	770	3.6	12	1	1	3	4	7	10	18

Length of Stay by Diagnosis and Operation, Western Region, 2008

Western Region, October 2006–September 2007 Data, by Diagnosis

288: WBC DISORDERS

Type of Patients	Observed Patients	Avg. Stay	Variance	10th	25th	50th	75th	90th	95th	99th
1. SINGLE DX										
A. Not Operated										
0–19 Years	9	2.8	6	1	2	2	3	9	9	9
20–34	3	2.3	2	1	1	2	4	4	4	4
35–49	0									
50–64	0									
65+	0									
B. Operated										
0–19 Years	0									
20–34	0									
35–49	0									
50–64	0									
65+	0									
2. MULTIPLE DX										
A. Not Operated										
0–19 Years	981	5.0	28	2	2	4	6	10	13	26
20–34	584	4.7	15	2	2	3	6	10	13	20
35–49	1,109	4.7	15	2	2	4	6	9	11	21
50–64	2,098	5.1	18	2	3	4	6	9	13	23
65+	2,523	5.5	21	2	3	4	7	10	14	23
B. Operated										
0–19 Years	11	9.3	56	4	4	5	17	18	22	22
20–34	9	13.2	353	3	5	7	10	63	63	63
35–49	17	16.2	487	2	6	9	14	39	95	95
50–64	24	15.5	185	6	6	13	22	29	30	67
65+	31	12.4	109	3	5	9	17	25	30	48
SUBTOTALS:										
1. SINGLE DX										
A. Not Operated	12	2.7	5	1	2	2	3	4	9	9
B. Operated	0									
2. MULTIPLE DX										
A. Not Operated	7,295	5.1	20	2	3	4	6	10	13	23
B. Operated	92	13.6	211	3	6	9	17	26	39	95
1. SINGLE DX	12	2.7	5	1	2	2	3	4	9	9
2. MULTIPLE DX	7,387	5.2	23	2	3	4	6	10	14	24
A. NOT OPERATED	7,307	5.1	20	2	3	4	6	10	13	23
B. OPERATED	92	13.6	211	3	6	9	17	26	39	95
TOTAL										
0–19 Years	1,001	5.1	28	2	2	4	6	10	14	25
20–34	596	4.8	21	2	2	3	6	10	13	20
35–49	1,126	4.9	23	2	2	4	6	9	12	23
50–64	2,122	5.2	21	2	3	4	6	10	14	24
65+	2,554	5.6	23	2	3	4	7	11	14	25
GRAND TOTAL	7,399	5.2	23	2	3	4	6	10	14	24

288.00: NEUTROPENIA NOS

Type of Patients	Observed Patients	Avg. Stay	Variance	10th	25th	50th	75th	90th	95th	99th
1. SINGLE DX										
A. Not Operated										
0–19 Years	4	2.0	<1	1	2	2	2	3	3	3
20–34	0									
35–49	0									
50–64	0									
65+	0									
B. Operated										
0–19 Years	0									
20–34	0									
35–49	0									
50–64	0									
65+	0									
2. MULTIPLE DX										
A. Not Operated										
0–19 Years	517	4.8	17	2	2	4	6	10	12	24
20–34	267	5.0	19	2	3	4	6	10	13	21
35–49	543	4.8	14	2	3	4	6	9	12	20
50–64	995	5.2	17	2	3	4	6	9	13	22
65+	1,107	5.5	22	2	3	4	7	10	14	25
B. Operated										
0–19 Years	4	7.3	42	4	4	4	17	18	17	17
20–34	2	34.0	>999	4	5	34	63	63	63	63
35–49	6	17.3	154	6	8	14	25	39	39	39
50–64	12	15.1	303	6	5	7	17	26	67	67
65+	10	12.1	117	3	5	6	21	25	30	30
SUBTOTALS:										
1. SINGLE DX										
A. Not Operated	4	2.0	<1	1	2	2	2	3	3	3
B. Operated	0									
2. MULTIPLE DX										
A. Not Operated	3,429	5.1	18	2	3	4	6	10	13	23
B. Operated	34	14.8	243	4	6	8	17	26	39	67
1. SINGLE DX	4	2.0	<1	1	2	2	2	3	3	3
2. MULTIPLE DX	3,463	5.2	21	2	3	4	6	10	13	24
A. NOT OPERATED	3,433	5.1	18	2	3	4	6	10	13	23
B. OPERATED	34	14.8	243	4	6	8	17	26	39	67
TOTAL										
0–19 Years	525	4.8	18	2	2	4	6	10	14	24
20–34	269	5.3	31	2	3	4	6	10	13	24
35–49	549	4.9	17	2	3	4	6	9	12	21
50–64	1,007	5.3	21	2	3	4	6	10	13	22
65+	1,117	5.6	24	2	3	4	7	11	14	29
GRAND TOTAL	3,467	5.2	21	2	3	4	6	10	13	24

288.03: DRUG-IND NEUTROPENIA

Type of Patients	Observed Patients	Avg. Stay	Variance	10th	25th	50th	75th	90th	95th	99th
1. SINGLE DX										
A. Not Operated										
0–19 Years	0									
20–34	0									
35–49	0									
50–64	0									
65+	0									
B. Operated										
0–19 Years	0									
20–34	0									
35–49	0									
50–64	0									
65+	0									
2. MULTIPLE DX										
A. Not Operated										
0–19 Years	304	5.2	31	2	2	4	6	11	14	22
20–34	192	5.0	14	2	3	4	6	10	14	18
35–49	376	4.7	13	2	3	4	6	9	11	17
50–64	760	5.2	20	2	3	4	6	10	14	24
65+	850	5.7	22	2	3	4	7	11	15	23
B. Operated										
0–19 Years	4	12.5	78	4	5	5	22	22	22	22
20–34	2	10.0	0	10	10	10	10	10	10	10
35–49	6	23.0	>999	4	8	9	14	95	95	95
50–64	6	18.1	55	9	13	15	22	25	30	30
65+	11	16.4	155	6	8	15	22	25	48	48
SUBTOTALS:										
1. SINGLE DX										
A. Not Operated	0									
B. Operated	0									
2. MULTIPLE DX										
A. Not Operated	2,482	5.3	21	2	3	4	6	10	14	22
B. Operated	28	17.4	318	5	8	13	20	30	48	95
1. SINGLE DX	0									
2. MULTIPLE DX	2,510	5.4	25	2	3	4	7	10	14	23
A. NOT OPERATED	2,482	5.3	21	2	3	4	6	10	14	22
B. OPERATED	28	17.4	318	5	8	13	20	30	48	95
TOTAL										
0–19 Years	308	5.3	32	2	2	4	6	11	15	22
20–34	193	5.1	14	2	3	4	6	10	14	18
35–49	382	5.0	34	2	3	4	6	9	11	23
50–64	766	5.3	22	2	3	4	7	10	14	24
65+	861	5.9	24	2	3	4	7	11	15	25
GRAND TOTAL	2,510	5.4	25	2	3	4	7	10	14	23

Length of Stay by Diagnosis and Operation, Western Region 2008

288.09: NEUTROPENIA NEC

Type of Patients	Observed Patients	Avg. Stay	Variance	10th	25th	50th	75th	90th	95th	99th
1. SINGLE DX										
A. Not Operated										
0–19 Years	1	2.0	0	2	2	2	2	2	2	2
20–34	0									
35–49	0									
50–64	0									
65+	0									
B. Operated										
0–19 Years	0									
20–34	0									
35–49	0									
50–64	0									
65+	0									
2. MULTIPLE DX										
A. Not Operated										
0–19 Years	61	6.3	23	2	3	5	8	12	15	23
20–34	23	3.8	3	2	3	3	5	6	7	7
35–49	37	6.3	31	2	3	5	7	11	21	27
50–64	92	5.4	21	2	3	4	6	12	15	25
65+	114	5.6	27	2	3	4	6	9	12	32
B. Operated										
0–19 Years	2	10.5	83	4	4	4	17	17	17	17
20–34	0									
35–49	0									
50–64	0									
65+	2	11.6	111	4	4	19	19	19	19	19
SUBTOTALS:										
1. SINGLE DX										
A. Not Operated	1	2.0	0	2	2	2	2	2	2	2
B. Operated	0									
2. MULTIPLE DX										
A. Not Operated	327	5.6	23	2	3	4	7	11	15	27
B. Operated	4	11.0	66	4	4	17	19	19	19	19
1. SINGLE DX	1	2.0	0	2	2	2	2	2	2	2
2. MULTIPLE DX	331	5.7	24	2	3	4	7	11	15	27
A. NOT OPERATED	328	5.6	23	2	3	4	7	11	15	27
B. OPERATED	4	11.0	66	4	4	17	19	19	19	19
TOTAL										
0–19 Years	64	6.3	24	2	3	5	8	14	17	23
20–34	23	3.8	3	2	3	3	5	6	7	7
35–49	37	6.3	31	2	3	5	7	11	21	27
50–64	92	5.4	21	2	3	4	6	12	15	25
65+	116	5.7	28	2	3	4	6	9	13	32
GRAND TOTAL	332	5.7	24	2	3	4	7	11	15	27

288.60: LEUKOCYTOSIS NOS

Type of Patients	Observed Patients	Avg. Stay	Variance	10th	25th	50th	75th	90th	95th	99th
1. SINGLE DX										
A. Not Operated										
0–19 Years	2	2.0	2	1	1	3	3	3	3	3
20–34	2	1.5	<1	1	1	2	2	2	2	2
35–49	0									
50–64	0									
65+	0									
B. Operated										
0–19 Years	0									
20–34	0									
35–49	0									
50–64	0									
65+	0									
2. MULTIPLE DX										
A. Not Operated										
0–19 Years	28	1.9	1	1	1	2	2	3	3	6
20–34	45	3.0	10	1	1	2	3	6	8	20
35–49	77	3.2	5	1	2	2	4	6	8	12
50–64	123	3.7	9	1	2	3	4	7	10	16
65+	284	4.5	12	1	2	4	6	9	11	18
B. Operated										
0–19 Years	0									
20–34	0									
35–49	0									
50–64	1	24.0	0	24	24	24	24	24	24	24
65+	8	7.7	29	2	3	9	13	16	16	16
SUBTOTALS:										
1. SINGLE DX										
A. Not Operated	4	1.8	<1	1	1	2	3	3	3	3
B. Operated	0									
2. MULTIPLE DX										
A. Not Operated	557	3.9	10	1	2	3	5	8	10	16
B. Operated	9	9.5	55	2	3	9	13	24	24	24
1. SINGLE DX	4	1.8	<1	1	1	2	3	3	3	3
2. MULTIPLE DX	566	4.0	12	1	2	3	5	9	10	18
A. NOT OPERATED	561	3.9	10	1	2	3	5	8	10	16
B. OPERATED	9	9.5	55	2	3	9	13	24	24	24
TOTAL										
0–19 Years	30	1.9	1	1	1	2	2	3	3	6
20–34	47	3.0	10	1	1	2	3	6	8	20
35–49	77	3.2	5	1	1	2	4	6	8	12
50–64	124	3.8	13	1	2	3	4	7	10	20
65+	292	4.6	13	1	2	4	6	9	11	18
GRAND TOTAL	570	4.0	11	1	2	3	5	9	10	18

289: OTHER BLOOD DISEASE

Type of Patients	Observed Patients	Avg. Stay	Variance	10th	25th	50th	75th	90th	95th	99th
1. SINGLE DX										
A. Not Operated										
0–19 Years	197	1.9	1	1	1	1	2	4	4	6
20–34	21	1.9	6	1	1	1	2	2	2	12
35–49	10	2.1	2	1	1	2	3	4	4	4
50–64	2	2.0	2	1	1	3	3	3	3	3
65+	0									
B. Operated										
0–19 Years	59	1.9	1	1	1	2	2	3	5	7
20–34	17	2.5	4	1	1	2	3	5	9	9
35–49	8	2.1	4	1	1	1	5	6	6	6
50–64	5	2.2	2	1	1	2	3	4	4	4
65+	0									
2. MULTIPLE DX										
A. Not Operated										
0–19 Years	431	2.5	3	1	1	3	3	5	6	10
20–34	165	3.8	12	1	2	3	5	8	9	19
35–49	156	4.1	14	1	2	3	5	8	12	16
50–64	197	4.3	20	1	2	3	5	9	12	20
65+	231	4.5	12	1	2	3	6	9	11	17
B. Operated										
0–19 Years	85	3.0	5	1	1	2	4	6	7	14
20–34	100	4.8	16	1	2	4	6	10	13	17
35–49	114	6.3	37	1	3	5	8	13	15	35
50–64	109	7.4	62	1	3	5	9	17	20	41
65+	82	8.0	61	1	3	6	9	17	26	40
SUBTOTALS:										
1. SINGLE DX										
A. Not Operated	230	1.9	2	1	1	1	2	4	4	6
B. Operated	89	2.0	2	1	1	2	2	4	5	9
2. MULTIPLE DX										
A. Not Operated	1,180	3.6	11	1	2	3	5	7	10	16
B. Operated	490	5.9	39	1	2	4	7	12	17	35
1. SINGLE DX	319	1.9	2	1	1	1	2	4	5	6
2. MULTIPLE DX	1,670	4.3	20	1	2	3	5	9	12	22
A. NOT OPERATED	1,410	3.3	10	1	1	2	4	7	9	15
B. OPERATED	579	5.3	36	1	2	4	7	11	16	35
TOTAL										
0–19 Years	772	2.4	3	1	1	2	3	4	5	9
20–34	303	3.9	13	1	2	3	5	9	10	17
35–49	288	4.8	24	1	2	4	6	10	14	29
50–64	313	5.3	36	1	2	4	6	11	17	34
65+	313	5.4	27	1	2	4	7	10	15	28
GRAND TOTAL	1,989	3.9	18	1	1	3	5	8	11	20

Length of Stay by Diagnosis and Operation, Western Region, 2008

Western Region, October 2006–September 2007 Data, by Diagnosis

289.2: MESENTERIC LYMPHADENITIS

Type of Patients	Observed Patients	Avg. Stay	Vari-ance	10th	25th	50th	75th	90th	95th	99th
1. SINGLE DX										
A. *Not Operated*										
0–19 Years	118	1.5	<1	1	1	1	2	2	3	5
20–34	19	1.9	6	1	1	1	2	2	12	12
35–49	6	2.0	2	1	1	2	3	4	4	4
50–64	0									
65+	0									
B. *Operated*										
0–19 Years	46	1.6	<1	1	1	1	2	2	3	3
20–34	9	1.6	<1	1	1	1	2	3	3	3
35–49	2	1.0	0	1	1	1	1	1	1	1
50–64	2	1.0	0	1	1	1	1	1	1	1
65+	0									
2. MULTIPLE DX										
A. *Not Operated*										
0–19 Years	238	1.9	2	1	1	2	2	4	4	9
20–34	58	2.4	4	1	1	2	3	4	8	10
35–49	20	2.1	<1	1	1	2	3	3	4	4
50–64	20	2.3	5	1	1	1	3	6	10	10
65+	11	3.5	5	1	2	3	6	7	7	7
B. *Operated*										
0–19 Years	60	2.3	2	1	1	2	3	3	7	8
20–34	32	3.4	11	1	1	2	3	4	11	15
35–49	19	3.4	8	1	1	2	4	8	11	11
50–64	10	5.2	20	2	2	4	6	17	17	17
65+	0									
SUBTOTALS:										
1. SINGLE DX										
A. *Not Operated*	143	1.5	1	1	1	1	2	2	3	5
B. *Operated*	59	1.5	<1	1	1	1	2	2	3	3
2. MULTIPLE DX										
A. *Not Operated*	347	2.1	3	1	1	2	2	4	5	9
B. *Operated*	121	3.0	7	1	1	2	3	6	8	15
1. SINGLE DX	202	1.5	1	1	1	1	2	2	3	5
2. MULTIPLE DX	468	2.3	4	1	1	2	3	4	7	10
A. NOT OPERATED	490	1.9	2	1	1	1	2	3	4	9
B. OPERATED	180	2.5	6	1	1	2	3	5	7	15
TOTAL										
0–19 Years	462	1.8	2	1	1	1	2	3	4	8
20–34	118	2.5	6	1	1	2	3	5	9	12
35–49	47	2.6	4	1	1	2	3	4	8	11
50–64	32	3.1	11	1	1	2	4	6	10	17
65+	11	3.5	5	1	2	3	6	7	7	7
GRAND TOTAL	670	2.1	3	1	1	2	3	4	5	10

289.3: LYMPHADENITIS NOS

Type of Patients	Observed Patients	Avg. Stay	Vari-ance	10th	25th	50th	75th	90th	95th	99th
1. SINGLE DX										
A. *Not Operated*										
0–19 Years	73	2.7	2	1	2	2	2	4	5	6
20–34	1	2.0	0	2	2	2	2	2	2	2
35–49	2	2.0	2	1	1	2	3	3	3	3
50–64	0									
65+	0									
B. *Operated*										
0–19 Years	6	3.2	6	1	2	3	5	7	7	7
20–34	2	3.5	4	2	2	5	5	5	5	5
35–49	1	1.0	0	1	1	1	1	1	1	1
50–64	0									
65+	0									
2. MULTIPLE DX										
A. *Not Operated*										
0–19 Years	161	3.1	3	1	2	3	4	5	6	10
20–34	23	2.8	2	1	2	2	4	5	5	6
35–49	25	2.6	3	1	2	2	4	5	6	7
50–64	22	3.5	10	1	2	2	4	9	11	12
65+	15	2.3	1	1	2	2	3	4	5	5
B. *Operated*										
0–19 Years	8	5.1	4	2	4	5	7	9	9	9
20–34	16	4.3	13	1	2	3	6	11	12	12
35–49	9	5.9	17	1	3	6	8	14	14	14
50–64	14	3.0	6	1	1	4	4	5	9	9
65+	7	3.0	12	1	1	1	8	8	8	8
SUBTOTALS:										
1. SINGLE DX										
A. *Not Operated*	76	2.6	2	1	2	2	4	4	5	6
B. *Operated*	9	3.0	5	1	1	2	5	7	7	7
2. MULTIPLE DX										
A. *Not Operated*	246	3.0	4	1	2	3	4	5	6	11
B. *Operated*	54	4.2	11	1	1	4	6	8	11	14
1. SINGLE DX	85	2.7	2	1	2	2	4	5	5	7
2. MULTIPLE DX	300	3.2	5	1	2	3	4	6	8	11
A. NOT OPERATED	322	2.9	3	1	2	3	4	5	6	10
B. OPERATED	63	4.0	10	1	1	4	6	8	9	14
TOTAL										
0–19 Years	248	3.1	3	1	2	3	4	5	6	10
20–34	42	3.4	6	1	2	2	5	6	8	12
35–49	37	3.3	8	1	1	3	4	7	8	14
50–64	36	3.3	8	1	1	2	4	9	11	12
65+	22	2.5	4	1	1	2	3	5	8	8
GRAND TOTAL	385	3.1	4	1	2	3	4	5	7	11

289.59: SPLEEN DISEASE NEC

Type of Patients	Observed Patients	Avg. Stay	Vari-ance	10th	25th	50th	75th	90th	95th	99th
1. SINGLE DX										
A. *Not Operated*										
0–19 Years	5	1.6	<1	1	1	1	2	3	3	3
20–34	1	2.0	0	2	2	2	2	2	2	2
35–49	1	4.0	0	4	4	4	4	4	4	4
50–64	0									
65+	0									
B. *Operated*										
0–19 Years	5	2.2	<1	1	2	2	3	3	3	3
20–34	5	2.6	1	1	2	3	3	4	4	4
35–49	4	3.3	7	1	1	5	6	6	6	6
50–64	3	3.0	<1	2	2	3	4	4	4	4
65+	0									
2. MULTIPLE DX										
A. *Not Operated*										
0–19 Years	16	3.9	7	1	2	3	6	8	9	9
20–34	33	4.6	6	2	3	4	6	8	9	11
35–49	53	5.3	20	1	3	4	7	9	12	29
50–64	65	4.1	8	2	2	3	5	7	19	19
65+	86	5.3	13	2	3	5	7	10	13	19
B. *Operated*										
0–19 Years	15	4.6	11	2	2	4	5	9	14	14
20–34	42	5.8	16	2	4	5	7	11	13	22
35–49	63	7.2	41	2	4	6	9	14	16	44
50–64	50	9.5	66	3	4	6	13	19	24	41
65+	44	11.1	80	4	6	8	12	26	31	40
SUBTOTALS:										
1. SINGLE DX										
A. *Not Operated*	7	2.0	1	1	1	2	3	4	4	4
B. *Operated*	17	2.7	2	1	2	3	3	5	6	6
2. MULTIPLE DX										
A. *Not Operated*	253	4.8	12	2	2	4	6	9	11	19
B. *Operated*	214	8.1	52	2	4	6	9	17	22	40
1. SINGLE DX	24	2.5	2	1	1	2	3	4	5	6
2. MULTIPLE DX	467	6.3	33	2	3	5	7	12	17	34
A. NOT OPERATED	260	4.7	12	1	2	4	6	9	11	19
B. OPERATED	231	7.7	50	2	4	6	9	16	22	40
TOTAL										
0–19 Years	41	3.7	8	1	2	3	5	7	9	14
20–34	81	5.1	11	2	3	4	6	9	10	22
35–49	121	6.2	31	1	3	5	7	11	15	29
50–64	118	6.4	40	2	3	4	9	15	19	34
65+	130	7.3	43	2	3	6	9	15	20	35
GRAND TOTAL	491	6.1	32	2	3	5	7	12	17	34

Western Region, October 2006–September 2007 Data, by Diagnosis

290: DEMENTIAS

Type of Patients	Observed Patients	Avg. Stay	Vari-ance	Percentiles 10th	25th	50th	75th	90th	95th	99th
1. SINGLE DX										
A. Not Operated										
0–19 Years	0									
20–34	0									
35–49	0									
50–64	0									
65+	7	9.9	79	1	1	8	21	21	21	21
B. Operated										
0–19 Years	0									
20–34	0									
35–49	0									
50–64	0									
65+	0									
2. MULTIPLE DX										
A. Not Operated										
0–19 Years	0									
20–34	2	8.5	109	1	1	9	16	16	16	16
35–49	6	8.3	29	2	3	8	14	15	15	15
50–64	98	13.5	180	2	4	11	16	29	38	77
65+	1,616	9.4	71	2	3	7	13	20	25	40
B. Operated										
0–19 Years	0									
20–34	0									
35–49	0									
50–64	2	30.5	<1	30	30	30	31	31	31	31
65+	15	15.0	109	5	10	12	18	26	47	47
SUBTOTALS:										
1. SINGLE DX										
A. Not Operated	7	9.9	79	1	1	8	21	21	21	21
B. Operated	0									
2. MULTIPLE DX										
A. Not Operated	1,722	9.7	78	2	3	7	14	20	26	41
B. Operated	17	16.8	122	5	10	13	20	31	47	47
1. SINGLE DX	7	9.9	79	1	1	8	21	21	21	21
2. MULTIPLE DX	1,739	9.7	79	2	3	7	14	20	26	42
A. NOT OPERATED	1,729	9.7	78	2	3	7	14	20	26	41
B. OPERATED	17	16.8	122	5	10	13	20	31	47	47
TOTAL										
0–19 Years	0									
20–34	2	8.5	109	1	1	9	16	16	16	16
35–49	6	8.3	29	2	3	8	14	15	15	15
50–64	100	13.8	182	2	4	11	18	30	38	77
65+	1,638	9.5	72	2	3	7	13	20	25	41
GRAND TOTAL	1,746	9.7	79	2	3	7	14	20	26	42

290.0: SENILE DEMENTIA UNCOMP

Type of Patients	Observed Patients	Avg. Stay	Vari-ance	Percentiles 10th	25th	50th	75th	90th	95th	99th
1. SINGLE DX										
A. Not Operated										
0–19 Years	0									
20–34	0									
35–49	0									
50–64	0									
65+	1	3.0	0	3	3	3	3	3	3	3
B. Operated										
0–19 Years	0									
20–34	0									
35–49	0									
50–64	0									
65+	0									
2. MULTIPLE DX										
A. Not Operated										
0–19 Years	0									
20–34	0									
35–49	1	8.0	0	8	8	8	8	8	8	8
50–64	3	2.7	2	1	1	3	4	4	4	4
65+	177	6.7	51	1	3	4	8	14	20	30
B. Operated										
0–19 Years	0									
20–34	0									
35–49	0									
50–64	0									
65+	2	18.6	111	11	11	26	26	26	26	26
SUBTOTALS:										
1. SINGLE DX										
A. Not Operated	1	3.0	0	3	3	3	3	3	3	3
B. Operated	0									
2. MULTIPLE DX										
A. Not Operated	181	6.6	50	1	3	4	8	14	20	30
B. Operated	2	18.6	111	11	11	26	26	26	26	26
1. SINGLE DX	1	3.0	0	3	3	3	3	3	3	3
2. MULTIPLE DX	183	6.7	51	1	3	4	8	14	20	30
A. NOT OPERATED	182	6.6	50	1	3	4	8	14	20	30
B. OPERATED	2	18.6	111	11	11	26	26	26	26	26
TOTAL										
0–19 Years	0									
20–34	0									
35–49	1	8.0	0	8	8	8	8	8	8	8
50–64	3	2.7	2	1	1	3	4	4	4	4
65+	180	6.8	52	1	3	4	8	14	21	30
GRAND TOTAL	184	6.7	51	1	3	4	8	14	20	30

290.20: SENILE DELUSION

Type of Patients	Observed Patients	Avg. Stay	Vari-ance	Percentiles 10th	25th	50th	75th	90th	95th	99th
1. SINGLE DX										
A. Not Operated										
0–19 Years	0									
20–34	0									
35–49	0									
50–64	0									
65+	1	14.0	0	14	14	14	14	14	14	14
B. Operated										
0–19 Years	0									
20–34	0									
35–49	0									
50–64	0									
65+	0									
2. MULTIPLE DX										
A. Not Operated										
0–19 Years	0									
20–34	0									
35–49	0									
50–64	9	16.5	74	2	14	16	21	30	30	30
65+	241	14.2	91	4	7	13	18	28	32	44
B. Operated										
0–19 Years	0									
20–34	0									
35–49	0									
50–64	1	30.0	0	30	30	30	30	30	30	30
65+	2	16.0	32	12	12	16	20	20	20	20
SUBTOTALS:										
1. SINGLE DX										
A. Not Operated	1	14.0	0	14	14	14	14	14	14	14
B. Operated	0									
2. MULTIPLE DX										
A. Not Operated	250	14.2	90	4	7	13	18	28	32	44
B. Operated	3	20.7	81	12	12	20	30	30	30	30
1. SINGLE DX	1	14.0	0	14	14	14	14	14	14	14
2. MULTIPLE DX	253	14.3	90	4	7	13	18	28	32	44
A. NOT OPERATED	251	14.2	89	4	7	13	18	28	32	44
B. OPERATED	3	20.7	81	12	12	20	30	30	30	30
TOTAL										
0–19 Years	0									
20–34	0									
35–49	0									
50–64	10	17.9	84	7	14	16	25	30	30	30
65+	244	14.2	90	4	7	13	18	28	32	44
GRAND TOTAL	254	14.3	90	4	7	13	18	28	32	44

Length of Stay by Diagnosis and Operation, Western Region, 2008

Western Region, October 2006–September 2007 Data, by Diagnosis

Type of Patients	290.3: SENILE DELIRIUM										290.40: VASCULAR DEMENTIA UNCOMP										290.41: VASC DEMENTIA W DELIRIUM									
	Obs. Patients	Avg. Stay	Vari-ance	10th	25th	50th	75th	90th	95th	99th	Obs. Patients	Avg. Stay	Vari-ance	10th	25th	50th	75th	90th	95th	99th	Obs. Patients	Avg. Stay	Vari-ance	10th	25th	50th	75th	90th	95th	99th
1. SINGLE DX																														
A. Not Operated																														
0–19 Years	0										0										0									
20–34	0										0										0									
35–49	0										0										0									
50–64	0										0										0									
65+	3	14.4	133	1	1	21	21	21	21	21	0										0									
B. Operated																														
0–19 Years	0										0										0									
20–34	0										0										0									
35–49	0										0										0									
50–64	0										0										0									
65+	0										0										0									
2. MULTIPLE DX																														
A. Not Operated																														
0–19 Years	0										0										0									
20–34	0										0										0									
35–49	0										1	3.0	0	3	3	3	3	3	3	3	2	11.0	18	8	8	14	14	14	14	14
50–64	5	7.0	41	2	3	6	6	18	18	18	33	14.0	270	3	4	10	15	37	51	77	20	9.8	76	2	3	8	14	27	33	33
65+	272	7.1	46	2	3	5	9	15	22	33	301	7.3	55	2	3	5	9	16	24	41	246	7.2	42	2	3	5	9	15	21	29
B. Operated																														
0–19 Years	0										0										0									
20–34	0										0										0									
35–49	0										0										0									
50–64	0										0										0									
65+	4	7.2	7	5	5	5	9	10	10	10	3	12.3	4	10	10	13	14	14	14	14	1	10.0	0	10	10	10	10	10	10	10
SUBTOTALS:																														
1. SINGLE DX																														
A. Not Operated	3	14.4	133	1	1	21	21	21	21	21	0										0									
B. Operated	0										0										0									
2. MULTIPLE DX																														
A. Not Operated	277	7.1	46	2	3	5	9	16	22	33	335	7.9	80	2	3	5	10	17	25	48	268	7.4	44	2	3	5	10	16	22	33
B. Operated	4	7.2	7	5	5	5	9	10	10	10	3	12.3	4	10	10	13	14	14	14	14	1	10.0	0	10	10	10	10	10	10	10
1. SINGLE DX	3	14.4	133	1	1	21	21	21	21	21	0										0									
2. MULTIPLE DX	281	7.1	46	2	3	5	9	15	21	33	338	8.0	79	2	3	5	10	17	25	48	269	7.5	44	2	3	5	10	16	22	33
A. NOT OPERATED	280	7.2	47	2	3	5	9	16	21	33	335	7.9	80	2	3	5	10	17	25	48	268	7.4	44	2	3	5	10	16	22	33
B. OPERATED	4	7.2	7	5	5	5	9	10	10	10	3	12.3	4	10	10	13	14	14	14	14	1	10.0	0	10	10	10	10	10	10	10
TOTAL																														
0–19 Years	0										0										0									
20–34	0										0										0									
35–49	0										1	3.0	0	3	3	3	3	3	3	3	2	11.0	18	8	8	14	14	14	14	14
50–64	5	7.0	41	2	3	6	6	18	18	18	33	14.0	270	3	4	10	15	37	51	77	20	9.8	76	2	3	8	14	27	33	33
65+	279	7.2	47	2	3	5	9	16	22	33	304	7.3	55	2	3	5	9	16	22	33	247	7.2	42	2	3	5	9	15	21	29
GRAND TOTAL	284	7.2	47	2	3	5	9	16	21	33	338	8.0	79	2	3	5	10	17	25	48	269	7.5	44	2	3	5	10	16	22	33

291: ALC-INDUCED MENTAL DIS

Type of Patients	Observed Patients	Avg. Stay	Vari-ance	Percentiles						
				10th	25th	50th	75th	90th	95th	99th
1. SINGLE DX										
A. Not Operated										
0–19 Years	0									
20–34	5	2.8	<1	2	2	3	3	4	4	4
35–49	9	1.7	<1	1	1	1	1	3	3	3
50–64	1	1.0	0	1	1	1	1	1	1	1
65+	0									
B. Operated										
0–19 Years	0									
20–34	0									
35–49	0									
50–64	0									
65+	0									
2. MULTIPLE DX										
A. Not Operated										
0–19 Years	42	3.5	11	1	1	2	4	10	10	14
20–34	1,781	3.5	10	1	2	3	4	6	9	16
35–49	7,479	4.2	15	1	2	3	5	8	11	20
50–64	6,121	5.1	33	1	2	4	6	10	14	27
65+	1,367	5.7	27	2	3	4	7	11	15	25
B. Operated										
0–19 Years	0									
20–34	5	9.8	16	5	6	12	13	13	13	13
35–49	28	10.1	52	4	6	8	11	18	28	33
50–64	50	11.4	52	4	7	10	13	19	29	36
65+	18	10.2	19	6	7	10	13	15	21	21
SUBTOTALS:										
1. SINGLE DX										
A. Not Operated	15	2.0	1	1	1	2	2	3	4	4
B. Operated	0									
2. MULTIPLE DX										
A. Not Operated	16,790	4.6	22	1	2	3	5	9	12	23
B. Operated	101	10.8	44	4	7	10	13	18	28	33
1. SINGLE DX	15	2.0	1	1	1	2	2	3	4	4
2. MULTIPLE DX	16,891	4.6	23	1	2	3	5	9	12	23
A. NOT OPERATED	16,805	4.6	22	1	2	3	5	9	12	23
B. OPERATED	101	10.8	44	4	7	10	13	18	28	33
TOTAL										
0–19 Years	42	3.5	11	1	1	2	4	10	10	14
20–34	1,791	3.5	10	1	2	3	4	6	9	16
35–49	7,516	4.2	16	1	2	3	5	8	11	20
50–64	6,172	5.2	33	1	2	4	6	10	14	28
65+	1,385	5.7	27	2	3	4	7	11	15	25
GRAND TOTAL	16,906	4.6	23	1	2	3	5	9	12	23

291.0: DELIRIUM TREMENS

Type of Patients	Observed Patients	Avg. Stay	Vari-ance	Percentiles						
				10th	25th	50th	75th	90th	95th	99th
1. SINGLE DX										
A. Not Operated										
0–19 Years	0									
20–34	0									
35–49	1	3.0	0	3	3	3	3	3	3	3
50–64	0									
65+	0									
B. Operated										
0–19 Years	0									
20–34	0									
35–49	0									
50–64	0									
65+	0									
2. MULTIPLE DX										
A. Not Operated										
0–19 Years	2	3.0	2	2	2	2	4	4	4	4
20–34	378	3.9	9	1	2	3	5	8	10	17
35–49	1,786	4.9	19	1	2	4	6	9	12	21
50–64	1,599	6.2	37	2	3	5	7	12	17	29
65+	365	6.8	48	2	3	5	8	13	17	36
B. Operated										
0–19 Years	0									
20–34	0									
35–49	10	11.6	82	4	7	12	16	33	33	33
50–64	21	11.6	67	4	7	10	13	18	29	36
65+	7	12.2	25	6	7	12	15	21	21	21
SUBTOTALS:										
1. SINGLE DX										
A. Not Operated	1	3.0	0	3	3	3	3	3	3	3
B. Operated	0									
2. MULTIPLE DX										
A. Not Operated	4,130	5.5	28	1	2	4	7	9	12	25
B. Operated	38	11.7	60	4	7	10	15	18	33	36
1. SINGLE DX	1	3.0	0	3	3	3	3	3	3	3
2. MULTIPLE DX	4,168	5.5	29	1	2	4	7	9	15	26
A. NOT OPERATED	4,131	5.5	28	1	2	4	7	9	12	25
B. OPERATED	38	11.7	60	4	7	10	15	18	33	36
TOTAL										
0–19 Years	2	3.0	2	2	2	2	4	4	4	4
20–34	378	3.9	9	1	2	3	5	8	10	17
35–49	1,797	4.9	20	1	2	4	6	9	12	22
50–64	1,620	6.2	37	2	3	5	7	12	17	29
65+	372	6.9	48	2	3	5	9	14	18	36
GRAND TOTAL	4,169	5.5	29	1	2	4	7	11	15	26

291.2: ALC-IND PERSIST DEMENTIA

Type of Patients	Observed Patients	Avg. Stay	Vari-ance	Percentiles						
				10th	25th	50th	75th	90th	95th	99th
1. SINGLE DX										
A. Not Operated										
0–19 Years	0									
20–34	0									
35–49	0									
50–64	0									
65+	0									
B. Operated										
0–19 Years	0									
20–34	0									
35–49	0									
50–64	0									
65+	0									
2. MULTIPLE DX										
A. Not Operated										
0–19 Years	0									
20–34	6	4.2	9	1	3	4	4	10	10	10
35–49	40	8.6	105	1	2	5	11	27	41	>99
50–64	108	13.1	367	2	3	6	14	50	70	>99
65+	107	8.1	40	2	4	6	10	15	24	31
B. Operated										
0–19 Years	0									
20–34	0									
35–49	0									
50–64	1	15.0	0	15	15	15	15	15	15	15
65+	0									
SUBTOTALS:										
1. SINGLE DX										
A. Not Operated	0									
B. Operated	0									
2. MULTIPLE DX										
A. Not Operated	261	10.1	190	2	3	6	11	24	43	>99
B. Operated	1	15.0	0	15	15	15	15	15	15	15
1. SINGLE DX	0									
2. MULTIPLE DX	262	10.1	189	2	3	6	11	24	43	>99
A. NOT OPERATED	261	10.1	190	2	3	6	11	24	43	>99
B. OPERATED	1	15.0	0	15	15	15	15	15	15	15
TOTAL										
0–19 Years	0									
20–34	6	4.2	9	1	3	4	4	10	10	10
35–49	40	8.6	105	1	2	5	11	27	41	>99
50–64	109	13.1	364	2	3	6	14	47	70	>99
65+	107	8.1	40	2	4	6	10	15	24	31
GRAND TOTAL	262	10.1	189	2	3	6	11	24	43	>99

Length of Stay by Diagnosis and Operation, Western Region, 2008

Western Region, October 2006–September 2007 Data, by Diagnosis

291.3: ALC-IND PSYCH W HALLUCIN

Type of Patients	Observed Patients	Avg. Stay	Variance	10th	25th	50th	75th	90th	95th	99th
1. SINGLE DX										
A. Not Operated										
0–19 Years	0									
20–34	0									
35–49	0									
50–64	1	1.0	0	1	1	1	1	1	1	1
65+	0									
B. Operated										
0–19 Years	0									
20–34	0									
35–49	0									
50–64	0									
65+	0									
2. MULTIPLE DX										
A. Not Operated										
0–19 Years	1	1.0	0	1	1	1	1	1	1	1
20–34	46	3.3	7	1	1	2	4	7	9	12
35–49	144	3.7	7	1	2	3	5	7	9	12
50–64	95	4.9	12	1	2	4	7	10	12	19
65+	26	5.0	16	2	2	3	6	13	14	16
B. Operated										
0–19 Years	0									
20–34	0									
35–49	1	11.0	0	11	11	11	11	11	11	11
50–64	2	11.5	4	10	10	12	13	13	13	13
65+	0									
SUBTOTALS:										
1. SINGLE DX										
A. Not Operated	1	1.0	0	1	1	1	1	1	1	1
B. Operated	0									
2. MULTIPLE DX										
A. Not Operated	312	4.1	10	1	2	3	6	8	11	14
B. Operated	3	11.3	2	10	10	11	13	13	13	13
1. SINGLE DX	1	1.0	0	1	1	1	1	1	1	1
2. MULTIPLE DX	315	4.2	10	1	2	3	6	9	11	14
A. NOT OPERATED	313	4.1	10	1	2	3	6	8	11	14
B. OPERATED	3	11.3	2	10	10	11	13	13	13	13
TOTAL										
0–19 Years	1	1.0	0	1	1	1	1	1	1	1
20–34	46	3.3	7	1	2	2	4	7	9	12
35–49	145	3.8	8	1	2	3	5	7	9	12
50–64	98	5.0	12	1	2	4	7	11	12	19
65+	26	5.0	16	2	2	3	6	13	14	16
GRAND TOTAL	316	4.2	10	1	2	3	6	9	11	14

291.81: ALCOHOL WITHDRAWAL

Type of Patients	Observed Patients	Avg. Stay	Variance	10th	25th	50th	75th	90th	95th	99th
1. SINGLE DX										
A. Not Operated										
0–19 Years	0									
20–34	2	3.0	2	2	2	4	4	4	4	4
35–49	8	1.5	<1	1	1	1	1	2	3	3
50–64	0									
65+	0									
B. Operated										
0–19 Years	0									
20–34	0									
35–49	0									
50–64	0									
65+	0									
2. MULTIPLE DX										
A. Not Operated										
0–19 Years	25	4.1	14	1	2	3	5	10	13	14
20–34	1,221	3.4	10	1	2	3	5	6	8	16
35–49	5,262	3.9	13	1	2	3	5	7	10	18
50–64	4,146	4.4	18	1	2	3	5	8	11	20
65+	830	4.8	14	1	3	4	6	9	13	19
B. Operated										
0–19 Years	0									
20–34	5	9.8	16	5	6	12	13	13	13	13
35–49	17	9.2	39	4	6	7	11	17	28	28
50–64	23	10.4	37	4	6	9	13	19	20	28
65+	10	9.0	14	6	6	10	13	14	14	14
SUBTOTALS:										
1. SINGLE DX										
A. Not Operated	10	1.8	1	1	1	2	2	4	4	4
B. Operated	0									
2. MULTIPLE DX										
A. Not Operated	11,484	4.1	15	1	2	3	5	7	10	19
B. Operated	55	9.7	30	4	6	9	13	16	20	28
1. SINGLE DX	10	1.8	1	1	1	2	2	4	4	4
2. MULTIPLE DX	11,539	4.1	15	1	2	3	5	8	11	19
A. NOT OPERATED	11,494	4.1	15	1	2	3	5	7	10	19
B. OPERATED	55	9.7	30	4	6	9	13	16	20	28
TOTAL										
0–19 Years	25	4.1	14	1	2	3	5	10	13	14
20–34	1,228	3.4	10	1	2	3	4	6	9	16
35–49	5,287	4.0	13	1	2	3	5	7	10	19
50–64	4,169	4.5	18	1	2	3	5	8	12	20
65+	840	4.9	14	1	3	4	6	9	13	19
GRAND TOTAL	11,549	4.1	15	1	2	3	5	8	11	19

291.89: ALC-IND MENTAL DIS NEC

Type of Patients	Observed Patients	Avg. Stay	Variance	10th	25th	50th	75th	90th	95th	99th
1. SINGLE DX										
A. Not Operated										
0–19 Years	0									
20–34	3	2.7	<1	2	2	3	3	3	3	3
35–49	0									
50–64	0									
65+	0									
B. Operated										
0–19 Years	0									
20–34	0									
35–49	0									
50–64	0									
65+	0									
2. MULTIPLE DX										
A. Not Operated										
0–19 Years	13	2.7	6	1	1	2	3	4	10	10
20–34	112	3.1	5	1	1	2	3	6	8	9
35–49	203	3.3	8	1	2	3	4	6	8	13
50–64	99	3.7	14	1	2	3	5	7	9	33
65+	7	4.8	22	1	2	3	5	15	15	15
B. Operated										
0–19 Years	0									
20–34	0									
35–49	0									
50–64	1	10.0	0	10	10	10	10	10	10	10
65+	0									
SUBTOTALS:										
1. SINGLE DX										
A. Not Operated	3	2.7	<1	2	2	3	3	3	3	3
B. Operated	0									
2. MULTIPLE DX										
A. Not Operated	434	3.4	9	1	2	3	4	6	9	13
B. Operated	1	10.0	0	10	10	10	10	10	10	10
1. SINGLE DX	3	2.7	<1	2	2	3	3	3	3	3
2. MULTIPLE DX	435	3.4	9	1	2	3	4	6	9	13
A. NOT OPERATED	437	3.3	9	1	2	3	4	6	9	13
B. OPERATED	1	10.0	0	10	10	10	10	10	10	10
TOTAL										
0–19 Years	13	2.7	6	1	1	2	3	4	10	10
20–34	115	3.1	5	1	1	2	4	6	8	9
35–49	203	3.3	8	1	2	3	4	6	8	13
50–64	100	3.8	14	1	2	3	4	7	9	12
65+	7	4.8	22	1	2	3	5	15	15	15
GRAND TOTAL	438	3.4	9	1	2	3	4	6	9	13

Length of Stay by Diagnosis and Operation, Western Region, 2008

Western Region, October 2006–September 2007 Data, by Diagnosis

292: DRUG-INDUCED MENTAL DIS

Type of Patients	Observed Patients	Avg. Stay	Vari-ance	Percentiles						
				10th	25th	50th	75th	90th	95th	99th
1. SINGLE DX										
A. *Not Operated*										
0–19 Years	5	1.4	<1	1	1	1	1	3	3	3
20–34	16	4.0	14	1	2	3	5	9	15	15
35–49	5	1.6	<1	1	1	1	2	3	3	3
50–64	4	3.5	6	1	2	3	5	7	7	7
65+	1	6.0	0	6	6	6	6	6	6	6
B. *Operated*										
0–19 Years	0									
20–34	0									
35–49	0									
50–64	0									
65+	0									
2. MULTIPLE DX										
A. *Not Operated*										
0–19 Years	291	4.6	26	1	2	4	5	8	8	23
20–34	2,223	4.3	13	1	2	3	5	8	11	18
35–49	2,505	4.2	11	1	2	3	5	8	10	18
50–64	2,019	4.5	15	1	2	4	6	8	11	20
65+	1,523	4.3	14	1	2	3	5	8	11	17
B. *Operated*										
0–19 Years	2	3.0	8	1	1	1	5	5	5	5
20–34	6	6.4	16	1	2	8	9	11	11	11
35–49	12	9.2	25	1	5	11	13	15	16	16
50–64	9	13.3	66	5	8	9	17	31	31	31
65+	29	8.5	23	2	5	8	10	18	18	19
SUBTOTALS:										
1. SINGLE DX										
A. *Not Operated*	31	3.2	9	1	1	2	4	6	9	15
B. *Operated*	0									
2. MULTIPLE DX										
A. *Not Operated*	8,561	4.3	13	1	2	3	5	8	10	18
B. *Operated*	58	9.0	32	2	5	9	11	17	18	31
1. SINGLE DX	31	3.2	9	1	1	2	4	6	9	15
2. MULTIPLE DX	8,619	4.4	14	1	2	3	5	8	11	18
A. NOT OPERATED	8,592	4.3	13	1	2	3	5	8	10	18
B. OPERATED	58	9.0	32	2	5	9	11	17	18	31
TOTAL										
0–19 Years	298	4.5	25	1	2	4	5	8	13	23
20–34	2,245	4.3	13	1	2	3	5	8	11	18
35–49	2,522	4.2	11	1	2	3	5	8	10	17
50–64	2,032	4.5	15	1	2	4	6	8	11	21
65+	1,553	4.4	14	1	2	3	6	9	11	18
GRAND TOTAL	8,650	4.4	14	1	2	3	5	8	11	18

292.0: DRUG WITHDRAWAL

Type of Patients	Observed Patients	Avg. Stay	Vari-ance	Percentiles						
				10th	25th	50th	75th	90th	95th	99th
1. SINGLE DX										
A. *Not Operated*										
0–19 Years	0									
20–34	0									
35–49	0									
50–64	0									
65+	0									
B. *Operated*										
0–19 Years	0									
20–34	0									
35–49	0									
50–64	0									
65+	0									
2. MULTIPLE DX										
A. *Not Operated*										
0–19 Years	154	4.3	8	2	3	4	5	6	8	18
20–34	1,285	4.4	9	2	3	4	5	7	10	15
35–49	1,512	4.5	10	2	3	4	6	8	10	18
50–64	1,209	4.7	14	1	3	4	6	8	11	19
65+	288	4.7	14	1	2	4	6	9	12	22
B. *Operated*										
0–19 Years	1	5.0	0	5	5	5	5	5	5	5
20–34	4	7.3	15	2	7	9	9	11	11	11
35–49	6	10.4	6	6	9	11	12	13	13	13
50–64	3	14.0	19	9	9	16	17	17	17	17
65+	3	7.7	30	2	2	8	13	13	13	13
SUBTOTALS:										
1. SINGLE DX										
A. *Not Operated*	0									
B. *Operated*	0									
2. MULTIPLE DX										
A. *Not Operated*	4,448	4.5	11	1	3	4	6	8	10	18
B. *Operated*	17	9.5	18	2	7	9	12	16	17	17
1. SINGLE DX	0									
2. MULTIPLE DX	4,465	4.5	11	1	3	4	6	8	10	18
A. NOT OPERATED	4,448	4.5	11	1	3	4	6	8	10	18
B. OPERATED	17	9.5	18	2	7	9	12	16	17	17
TOTAL										
0–19 Years	155	4.3	8	2	3	4	5	6	8	18
20–34	1,289	4.4	9	2	3	4	5	7	10	15
35–49	1,518	4.5	10	2	3	4	6	8	10	18
50–64	1,212	4.7	14	1	3	4	6	8	11	19
65+	291	4.8	14	1	2	4	6	9	12	22
GRAND TOTAL	4,465	4.5	11	1	3	4	6	8	10	18

292.12: DRG-IND PSYCH W HALLUCIN

Type of Patients	Observed Patients	Avg. Stay	Vari-ance	Percentiles						
				10th	25th	50th	75th	90th	95th	99th
1. SINGLE DX										
A. *Not Operated*										
0–19 Years	0									
20–34	1	15.0	0	15	15	15	15	15	15	15
35–49	0									
50–64	0									
65+	0									
B. *Operated*										
0–19 Years	0									
20–34	0									
35–49	0									
50–64	0									
65+	0									
2. MULTIPLE DX										
A. *Not Operated*										
0–19 Years	24	5.4	159	1	1	2	5	10	10	63
20–34	93	4.1	13	1	2	3	5	9	12	20
35–49	102	3.9	17	1	2	3	5	7	10	22
50–64	73	3.6	17	1	1	2	4	8	12	25
65+	161	3.7	7	1	2	3	5	7	10	12
B. *Operated*										
0–19 Years	1	1.0	0	1	1	1	1	1	1	1
20–34	0									
35–49	2	15.5	<1	15	15	15	16	16	16	16
50–64	2	6.5	4	5	5	8	8	8	8	8
65+	2	13.5	40	9	9	18	18	18	18	18
SUBTOTALS:										
1. SINGLE DX										
A. *Not Operated*	1	15.0	0	15	15	15	15	15	15	15
B. *Operated*	0									
2. MULTIPLE DX										
A. *Not Operated*	453	3.9	20	1	2	3	5	8	11	20
B. *Operated*	7	10.3	39	1	5	9	16	18	18	18
1. SINGLE DX	1	15.0	0	15	15	15	15	15	15	15
2. MULTIPLE DX	460	4.0	21	1	2	3	5	8	11	20
A. NOT OPERATED	454	3.9	20	1	2	3	5	8	11	20
B. OPERATED	7	10.3	39	1	5	9	16	18	18	18
TOTAL										
0–19 Years	25	5.2	153	1	1	1	5	10	10	63
20–34	94	4.2	14	1	2	3	5	10	12	20
35–49	104	4.2	20	1	2	3	5	8	13	22
50–64	75	3.7	17	1	1	2	5	8	12	25
65+	163	3.8	9	1	2	3	5	8	10	17
GRAND TOTAL	461	4.0	21	1	2	3	5	8	11	20

Length of Stay by Diagnosis and Operation, Western Region, 2008

Western Region, October 2006–September 2007 Data, by Diagnosis

292.81: DRUG-INDUCED DELIRIUM

Type of Patients	Observed Patients	Avg. Stay	Variance	10th	25th	50th	75th	90th	95th	99th
1. SINGLE DX										
A. Not Operated										
0–19 Years	1	1.0	0	1	1	1	1	1	1	1
20–34	2	1.5	<1	1	1	2	2	2	2	2
35–49	1	1.0	0	1	1	1	1	1	1	1
50–64	0									
65+	1	6.0	0	6	6	6	6	6	6	6
B. Operated										
0–19 Years	0									
20–34	0									
35–49	0									
50–64	0									
65+	0									
2. MULTIPLE DX										
A. Not Operated										
0–19 Years	20	3.1	15	1	1	2	3	8	17	17
20–34	68	3.5	16	1	1	2	4	8	11	23
35–49	163	3.5	9	1	2	3	4	7	10	13
50–64	448	4.0	16	1	2	3	5	8	11	21
65+	949	4.2	13	1	2	3	5	8	10	15
B. Operated										
0–19 Years	0									
20–34	1	8.0	0	8	8	8	8	8	8	8
35–49	3	2.3	5	1	1	1	5	5	5	5
50–64	4	16.2	119	8	8	8	18	31	31	31
65+	24	8.2	22	3	5	8	10	14	18	19
SUBTOTALS:										
1. SINGLE DX A. Not Operated	5	2.2	5	1	1	1	2	6	6	6
1. SINGLE DX B. Operated	0									
2. MULTIPLE DX A. Not Operated	1,648	4.0	14	1	2	3	5	8	11	19
2. MULTIPLE DX B. Operated	32	8.6	39	2	5	8	10	18	19	31
1. SINGLE DX	5	2.2	5	1	1	1	2	6	6	6
2. MULTIPLE DX	1,680	4.1	14	1	2	3	5	8	11	19
A. NOT OPERATED	1,653	4.0	14	1	2	3	5	8	11	19
B. OPERATED	32	8.6	39	2	5	8	10	18	19	31
TOTAL										
0–19 Years	21	3.0	14	1	1	2	3	7	8	17
20–34	71	3.5	16	1	1	2	4	8	11	23
35–49	167	3.5	9	1	2	3	4	7	10	13
50–64	452	4.1	17	1	2	3	5	8	11	22
65+	974	4.3	14	1	2	3	5	8	11	16
GRAND TOTAL	1,685	4.1	14	1	2	3	5	8	11	19

292.84: DRUG-IND MOOD DISORDER

Type of Patients	Observed Patients	Avg. Stay	Variance	10th	25th	50th	75th	90th	95th	99th
1. SINGLE DX										
A. Not Operated										
0–19 Years	0									
20–34	3	2.7	4	1	1	2	5	5	5	5
35–49	0									
50–64	1	7.0	0	7	7	7	7	7	7	7
65+	0									
B. Operated										
0–19 Years	0									
20–34	0									
35–49	0									
50–64	0									
65+	0									
2. MULTIPLE DX										
A. Not Operated										
0–19 Years	43	4.4	14	2	2	3	5	7	13	19
20–34	365	4.0	12	2	2	3	5	9	11	18
35–49	364	4.1	11	1	2	3	5	8	9	14
50–64	120	4.7	9	2	3	4	6	9	10	14
65+	18	9.5	76	2	4	5	10	22	35	35
B. Operated										
0–19 Years	0									
20–34	1	1.0	0	1	1	1	1	1	1	1
35–49	1	10.0	0	10	10	10	10	10	10	10
50–64	0									
65+	0									
SUBTOTALS:										
1. SINGLE DX A. Not Operated	4	3.8	8	1	1	5	7	7	7	7
1. SINGLE DX B. Operated	0									
2. MULTIPLE DX A. Not Operated	910	4.2	13	1	2	3	5	8	10	18
2. MULTIPLE DX B. Operated	2	5.5	41	1	1	6	10	10	10	10
1. SINGLE DX	4	3.8	8	1	1	5	7	7	7	7
2. MULTIPLE DX	912	4.3	13	1	2	3	5	8	10	18
A. NOT OPERATED	914	4.2	13	1	2	3	5	8	10	18
B. OPERATED	2	5.5	41	1	2	6	10	10	10	10
TOTAL										
0–19 Years	43	4.4	14	2	2	3	5	7	13	19
20–34	369	4.0	12	2	2	3	5	9	11	18
35–49	365	4.1	11	1	2	3	5	8	9	14
50–64	121	4.7	9	2	3	4	6	9	10	14
65+	18	9.5	76	2	4	5	10	22	35	35
GRAND TOTAL	916	4.2	13	1	2	3	5	8	10	18

292.9: DRUG MENTAL DISORDER NOS

Type of Patients	Observed Patients	Avg. Stay	Variance	10th	25th	50th	75th	90th	95th	99th
1. SINGLE DX										
A. Not Operated										
0–19 Years	1	1.0	0	1	1	1	1	1	1	1
20–34	5	3.6	4	1	3	3	5	6	6	6
35–49	2	1.0	0	1	1	1	1	1	1	1
50–64	2	3.0	0	3	3	3	3	3	3	3
65+	0									
B. Operated										
0–19 Years	0									
20–34	0									
35–49	0									
50–64	0									
65+	0									
2. MULTIPLE DX										
A. Not Operated										
0–19 Years	31	5.2	17	1	2	4	6	11	15	16
20–34	232	4.4	27	1	2	3	5	10	12	26
35–49	202	3.7	11	1	2	3	5	7	10	16
50–64	90	4.2	19	1	2	3	5	8	12	30
65+	41	4.4	6	1	3	4	6	7	8	11
B. Operated										
0–19 Years	0									
20–34	0									
35–49	0									
50–64	0									
65+	0									
SUBTOTALS:										
1. SINGLE DX A. Not Operated	10	2.7	3	1	1	3	3	5	6	6
1. SINGLE DX B. Operated	0									
2. MULTIPLE DX A. Not Operated	596	4.2	19	1	2	3	5	8	11	22
2. MULTIPLE DX B. Operated	0									
1. SINGLE DX	10	2.7	3	1	1	3	3	5	6	6
2. MULTIPLE DX	596	4.2	19	1	2	3	5	8	11	22
A. NOT OPERATED	606	4.2	18	1	2	3	5	8	11	22
B. OPERATED	0									
TOTAL										
0–19 Years	32	5.1	17	1	2	4	6	11	15	16
20–34	237	4.4	27	1	2	3	5	10	12	26
35–49	204	3.7	11	1	2	3	5	7	10	16
50–64	92	4.2	19	1	2	3	5	8	12	30
65+	41	4.4	6	1	3	4	6	7	8	11
GRAND TOTAL	606	4.2	18	1	2	3	5	8	11	22

Western Region, October 2006–September 2007 Data, by Diagnosis

293: TRANS MENTAL DIS D/T CCE

Type of Patients	Observed Patients	Avg. Stay	Vari-ance	10th	25th	50th	75th	90th	95th	99th
1. SINGLE DX										
A. Not Operated										
0–19 Years	1	1.0	0	1	1	1	1	1	1	1
20–34	1	1.0	0	1	1	1	1	1	1	1
35–49	1	2.0		2	2	2	2	2	2	2
50–64	0									
65+	0									
B. Operated										
0–19 Years	0									
20–34	0									
35–49	0									
50–64	0									
65+	0									
2. MULTIPLE DX										
A. Not Operated										
0–19 Years	9	2.8	3	1	2	2	4	6	6	6
20–34	16	6.4	64	2	2	4	7	11	34	34
35–49	52	4.3	17	1	2	3	5	11	15	20
50–64	120	5.3	33	1	2	3	7	14	17	28
65+	418	5.7	40	1	2	4	7	12	16	34
B. Operated										
0–19 Years	0									
20–34	0									
35–49	0									
50–64	3	7.3	1	6	6	8	8	8	8	8
65+	10	5.5	14	1	2	7	9	12	12	12
SUBTOTALS:										
1. SINGLE DX										
A. Not Operated	3	1.3	<1	1	1	1	1	2	2	2
B. Operated	0									
2. MULTIPLE DX										
A. Not Operated	615	5.4	37	1	2	3	7	12	16	29
B. Operated	13	5.9	12	2	3	7	8	9	12	12
1. SINGLE DX	3	1.3	<1	1	1	1	2	2	2	2
2. MULTIPLE DX	628	5.5	36	1	2	3	7	12	16	29
A. NOT OPERATED	618	5.4	37	1	2	3	7	12	16	29
B. OPERATED	13	5.9	12	2	3	7	8	9	12	12
TOTAL										
0–19 Years	10	2.6	3	1	1	2	4	6	6	6
20–34	17	6.1	62	1	2	3	6	11	34	34
35–49	53	4.3	17	1	2	3	5	11	15	20
50–64	123	5.3	32	1	2	3	7	14	17	28
65+	428	5.7	39	1	2	4	7	12	16	34
GRAND TOTAL	631	5.4	36	1	2	3	7	12	16	29

293.0: DELIRIUM D/T CCE

Type of Patients	Observed Patients	Avg. Stay	Vari-ance	10th	25th	50th	75th	90th	95th	99th
1. SINGLE DX										
A. Not Operated										
0–19 Years	1	1.0	0	1	1	1	1	1	1	1
20–34	1	1.0	0	1	1	1	1	1	1	1
35–49	0									
50–64	0									
65+	0									
B. Operated										
0–19 Years	0									
20–34	0									
35–49	0									
50–64	0									
65+	0									
2. MULTIPLE DX										
A. Not Operated										
0–19 Years	5	2.2	2	1	1	2	3	4	4	4
20–34	8	3.4	4	1	2	2	5	6	6	6
35–49	33	3.6	12	1	1	2	4	6	13	15
50–64	95	4.6	27	1	1	3	5	12	17	29
65+	365	5.1	31	1	2	3	7	10	13	24
B. Operated										
0–19 Years	0									
20–34	0									
35–49	0									
50–64	3	7.3	1	6	6	8	8	8	8	8
65+	6	6.0	16	2	3	7	9	12	12	12
SUBTOTALS:										
1. SINGLE DX										
A. Not Operated	2	1.0	0	1	1	1	1	1	1	1
B. Operated	0									
2. MULTIPLE DX										
A. Not Operated	506	4.9	29	1	2	3	6	10	14	22
B. Operated	9	6.5	11	2	3	7	8	12	12	12
1. SINGLE DX	2	1.0	0	1	1	1	1	1	1	1
2. MULTIPLE DX	515	4.9	28	1	2	3	6	10	14	22
A. NOT OPERATED	508	4.9	28	1	2	3	6	10	14	22
B. OPERATED	9	6.5	11	2	3	7	8	12	12	12
TOTAL										
0–19 Years	6	2.0	2	1	1	2	3	4	4	4
20–34	9	3.1	4	1	2	2	4	6	6	6
35–49	33	3.6	12	1	1	2	4	6	13	15
50–64	98	4.7	26	1	2	3	5	12	17	29
65+	371	5.2	31	1	2	3	7	10	13	24
GRAND TOTAL	517	4.9	28	1	2	3	6	10	14	22

293.83: MOOD DISORDER IN CCE

Type of Patients	Observed Patients	Avg. Stay	Vari-ance	10th	25th	50th	75th	90th	95th	99th
1. SINGLE DX										
A. Not Operated										
0–19 Years	0									
20–34	0									
35–49	1	2.0		2	2	2	2	2	2	2
50–64	0									
65+	0									
B. Operated										
0–19 Years	0									
20–34	0									
35–49	0									
50–64	0									
65+	0									
2. MULTIPLE DX										
A. Not Operated										
0–19 Years	3	4.0	4	2	2	4	6	6	6	6
20–34	5	13.2	146	3	7	11	11	34	34	34
35–49	11	6.2	37	1	2	6	6	15	20	20
50–64	14	10.0	63	3	3	8	14	24	28	28
65+	13	8.7	73	1	5	7	8	16	34	34
B. Operated										
0–19 Years	0									
20–34	0									
35–49	0									
50–64	0									
65+	0									
SUBTOTALS:										
1. SINGLE DX										
A. Not Operated	1	2.0	0	2	2	2	2	2	2	2
B. Operated	0									
2. MULTIPLE DX										
A. Not Operated	46	8.7	65	2	3	7	11	20	28	34
B. Operated	0									
1. SINGLE DX	1	2.0	0	2	2	2	2	2	2	2
2. MULTIPLE DX	46	8.7	65	2	3	7	11	20	28	34
A. NOT OPERATED	47	8.6	65	2	3	6	11	20	28	34
B. OPERATED	0									
TOTAL										
0–19 Years	3	4.0	4	2	2	4	6	6	6	6
20–34	5	13.2	146	3	7	11	11	34	34	34
35–49	12	5.8	35	1	3	3	6	15	20	20
50–64	14	10.0	63	3	3	8	14	24	28	28
65+	13	8.7	73	1	5	7	8	16	34	34
GRAND TOTAL	47	8.6	65	2	3	6	11	20	28	34

Length of Stay by Diagnosis and Operation, Western Region, 2008

Western Region, October 2006–September 2007 Data, by Diagnosis

294: PERSIST MENT DIS D/T CCE

Type of Patients	Observed Patients	Avg. Stay	Vari-ance	Percentiles						
				10th	25th	50th	75th	90th	95th	99th
1. SINGLE DX										
A. *Not Operated*										
0–19 Years	0									
20–34	0									
35–49	0									
50–64	3	5.0	28	1	1	3	11	11	11	11
65+	12	5.0	44	1	2	3	4	14	23	23
B. *Operated*										
0–19 Years	0									
20–34	0									
35–49	0									
50–64	0									
65+	0									
2. MULTIPLE DX										
A. *Not Operated*										
0–19 Years	1	5.0	0	5	5	5	5	5	5	5
20–34	16	14.1	331	2	4	7	16	30	74	74
35–49	31	10.3	89	2	2	8	18	21	34	36
50–64	133	10.1	149	2	3	6	11	27	32	64
65+	2,015	7.7	61	2	3	5	10	17	23	40
B. *Operated*										
0–19 Years	0									
20–34	0									
35–49	0									
50–64	0									
65+	12	12.3	29	6	6	14	16	18	21	21
SUBTOTALS:										
1. SINGLE DX										
A. *Not Operated*	15	5.0	39	1	1	3	4	14	23	23
B. *Operated*	0									
2. MULTIPLE DX										
A. *Not Operated*	2,196	8.0	69	2	3	5	10	18	24	44
B. *Operated*	12	12.3	29	6	6	14	16	18	21	21
1. SINGLE DX	15	5.0	39	1	1	3	4	14	23	23
2. MULTIPLE DX	2,208	8.0	69	2	3	5	10	18	24	44
A. NOT OPERATED	2,211	8.0	69	2	3	5	10	18	24	44
B. OPERATED	12	12.3	29	6	6	14	16	18	21	21
TOTAL										
0–19 Years	1	5.0	0	5	5	5	5	5	5	5
20–34	16	14.1	331	2	4	7	16	30	74	74
35–49	31	10.3	89	1	2	8	18	21	34	36
50–64	136	10.0	147	2	3	6	11	27	32	64
65+	2,039	7.8	61	2	3	5	10	18	23	40
GRAND TOTAL	2,223	8.0	69	2	3	5	10	18	24	44

294.8: OTH PERSIST MENT DIS CCE

Type of Patients	Observed Patients	Avg. Stay	Vari-ance	Percentiles						
				10th	25th	50th	75th	90th	95th	99th
1. SINGLE DX										
A. *Not Operated*										
0–19 Years	0									
20–34	0									
35–49	0									
50–64	2	7.0	31	3	3	3	11	11	11	11
65+	10	3.5	15	1	1	3	3	14	14	14
B. *Operated*										
0–19 Years	0									
20–34	0									
35–49	0									
50–64	0									
65+	0									
2. MULTIPLE DX										
A. *Not Operated*										
0–19 Years	0									
20–34	3	11.7	20	7	7	12	16	16	16	16
35–49	19	13.3	104	2	4	10	20	34	36	36
50–64	111	10.6	146	2	4	6	13	27	32	64
65+	1,979	7.7	62	2	3	5	10	17	23	40
B. *Operated*										
0–19 Years	0									
20–34	0									
35–49	0									
50–64	0									
65+	12	12.3	29	6	6	14	16	18	21	21
SUBTOTALS:										
1. SINGLE DX										
A. *Not Operated*	12	4.1	17	1	2	3	4	11	14	14
B. *Operated*	0									
2. MULTIPLE DX										
A. *Not Operated*	2,112	7.9	67	2	3	5	10	18	24	42
B. *Operated*	12	12.3	29	6	6	14	16	18	21	21
1. SINGLE DX	12	4.1	17	1	2	3	4	11	14	14
2. MULTIPLE DX	2,124	8.0	67	2	3	5	10	18	24	42
A. NOT OPERATED	2,124	7.9	67	2	3	5	10	18	24	42
B. OPERATED	12	12.3	29	6	6	14	16	18	21	21
TOTAL										
0–19 Years	0									
20–34	3	11.7	20	7	7	12	16	16	16	16
35–49	19	13.3	104	2	4	10	20	34	36	36
50–64	113	10.5	144	2	4	6	13	27	32	64
65+	2,001	7.7	61	2	3	5	10	17	23	40
GRAND TOTAL	2,136	7.9	67	2	3	5	10	18	24	42

295: SCHIZOPHRENIC DISORDERS

Type of Patients	Observed Patients	Avg. Stay	Vari-ance	Percentiles						
				10th	25th	50th	75th	90th	95th	99th
1. SINGLE DX										
A. *Not Operated*										
0–19 Years	97	12.5	190	2	5	8	14	25	44	86
20–34	1,134	10.6	128	2	4	7	13	22	31	70
35–49	899	10.3	114	2	4	7	13	21	31	60
50–64	532	11.4	163	2	4	7	14	25	39	71
65+	28	12.7	95	2	6	10	20	30	36	>99
B. *Operated*										
0–19 Years	0									
20–34	0									
35–49	0									
50–64	0									
65+	0									
2. MULTIPLE DX										
A. *Not Operated*										
0–19 Years	656	11.7	162	3	4	8	15	24	34	85
20–34	9,002	10.0	115	3	4	7	12	21	30	65
35–49	11,911	9.7	96	3	4	7	12	20	28	57
50–64	9,609	11.6	126	3	5	8	14	24	35	70
65+	1,628	14.2	128	4	7	12	18	27	38	64
B. *Operated*										
0–19 Years	8	11.5	59	6	6	6	17	17	17	17
20–34	8	28.1	>999	5	6	16	63	92	92	92
35–49	14	15.8	204	3	5	8	18	41	45	45
50–64	20	16.2	171	4	8	16	18	31	61	>99
65+	8	18.7	112	7	11	19	20	40	40	40
SUBTOTALS:										
1. SINGLE DX										
A. *Not Operated*	2,690	10.7	132	2	4	7	13	23	33	69
B. *Operated*	0									
2. MULTIPLE DX										
A. *Not Operated*	32,806	10.6	114	3	4	7	13	22	31	65
B. *Operated*	52	18.1	294	4	7	16	19	41	63	>99
1. SINGLE DX	2,690	10.7	132	2	4	7	13	23	33	69
2. MULTIPLE DX	32,858	10.6	115	3	4	7	13	22	31	65
A. NOT OPERATED	35,496	10.6	116	3	4	7	13	22	31	65
B. OPERATED	52	18.1	294	4	7	16	19	41	63	>99
TOTAL										
0–19 Years	755	11.8	165	3	4	8	15	24	34	85
20–34	10,144	10.1	118	2	4	7	12	21	31	66
35–49	12,824	9.8	97	3	4	7	12	20	28	57
50–64	10,161	11.6	128	3	5	8	14	24	36	70
65+	1,664	14.2	128	4	7	12	18	27	38	64
GRAND TOTAL	35,548	10.6	116	3	4	7	13	22	31	65

Western Region, October 2006–September 2007 Data, by Diagnosis

295.10: HEBEPHRENIA-UNSPEC

Type of Patients	Observed Patients	Avg. Stay	Vari-ance	Percentiles						
				10th	25th	50th	75th	90th	95th	99th
1. SINGLE DX										
A. Not Operated										
0–19 Years	1	7.0	0	7	7	7	7	7	7	7
20–34	13	13.3	164	2	8	10	14	22	41	51
35–49	7	9.7	88	1	1	8	19	26	32	26
50–64	7	21.5	662	4	5	15	21	78	78	78
65+	1	26.0	0	26	26	26	>99	>99	>99	>99
B. Operated										
0–19 Years	0									
20–34	0									
35–49	0									
50–64	0									
65+	0									
2. MULTIPLE DX										
A. Not Operated										
0–19 Years	12	14.3	91	4	8	12	19	29	34	34
20–34	60	15.8	251	3	6	10	17	39	41	88
35–49	52	15.5	243	4	6	9	17	41	53	71
50–64	53	20.1	203	5	9	17	28	45	56	>99
65+	3	6.7	14	4	4	5	11	11	11	11
B. Operated										
0–19 Years	1	6.0	0	6	6	6	6	6	6	6
20–34	0									
35–49	0									
50–64	0									
65+	0									
SUBTOTALS:										
1. SINGLE DX										
A. Not Operated	29	14.6	257	2	5	10	20	26	35	>99
B. Operated	0									
2. MULTIPLE DX										
A. Not Operated	180	16.7	223	4	6	13	21	38	49	88
B. Operated	1	6.0	0	6	6	6	6	6	6	6
1. SINGLE DX	29	14.6	257	2	5	10	20	26	35	>99
2. MULTIPLE DX	181	16.7	222	4	6	13	21	38	49	88
A. NOT OPERATED	209	16.4	227	3	6	12	21	38	53	88
B. OPERATED	1	6.0	0	6	6	6	6	6	6	6
TOTAL										
0–19 Years	14	13.1	85	4	6	12	17	29	34	34
20–34	73	15.3	234	3	6	10	17	35	46	88
35–49	59	14.8	226	3	5	9	18	41	53	71
50–64	60	20.3	247	5	9	17	26	45	56	>99
65+	4	11.5	102	4	5	11	26	>99	>99	>99
GRAND TOTAL	210	16.4	226	3	6	12	21	38	53	88

295.30: PARANOID SCHIZ-UNSPEC

Type of Patients	Observed Patients	Avg. Stay	Vari-ance	Percentiles						
				10th	25th	50th	75th	90th	95th	99th
1. SINGLE DX										
A. Not Operated										
0–19 Years	19	12.3	154	4	7	9	13	22	59	59
20–34	271	11.9	186	2	4	8	15	25	41	89
35–49	223	11.5	128	2	4	8	15	25	32	60
50–64	126	11.2	147	2	4	7	14	27	43	55
65+	7	18.8	104	5	6	20	28	30	30	30
B. Operated										
0–19 Years	0									
20–34	0									
35–49	0									
50–64	0									
65+	0									
2. MULTIPLE DX										
A. Not Operated										
0–19 Years	99	14.6	192	3	5	12	19	31	42	64
20–34	1,328	11.0	144	2	4	7	13	23	34	73
35–49	1,518	10.0	106	2	4	7	12	21	29	54
50–64	1,251	11.7	133	3	5	8	15	24	38	71
65+	270	13.7	122	4	7	11	17	27	39	61
B. Operated										
0–19 Years	1	17.0	0	17	17	17	17	17	17	17
20–34	0									
35–49	0									
50–64	0									
65+	1	11.0	0	11	11	11	11	11	11	11
SUBTOTALS:										
1. SINGLE DX										
A. Not Operated	646	11.7	156	2	4	8	15	25	35	73
B. Operated	0									
2. MULTIPLE DX										
A. Not Operated	4,466	11.1	129	3	4	7	14	23	34	67
B. Operated	2	14.0	18	11	11	17	17	17	17	17
1. SINGLE DX	646	11.7	156	2	4	8	15	25	35	73
2. MULTIPLE DX	4,468	11.1	129	3	4	7	14	23	34	67
A. NOT OPERATED	5,112	11.2	133	2	4	7	14	23	34	68
B. OPERATED	2	14.0	18	11	11	17	17	17	17	17
TOTAL										
0–19 Years	119	14.2	184	3	5	11	17	29	42	64
20–34	1,599	11.2	151	2	4	7	13	24	34	78
35–49	1,741	10.2	109	2	4	7	13	22	31	55
50–64	1,377	11.6	134	3	5	8	15	24	38	71
65+	278	13.8	121	4	7	11	17	27	39	61
GRAND TOTAL	5,114	11.2	132	2	4	7	14	23	34	68

295.32: PARANOID SCHIZ-CHRONIC

Type of Patients	Observed Patients	Avg. Stay	Vari-ance	Percentiles						
				10th	25th	50th	75th	90th	95th	99th
1. SINGLE DX										
A. Not Operated										
0–19 Years	12	14.0	139	6	8	10	15	24	48	48
20–34	132	10.8	111	2	4	8	13	24	29	54
35–49	105	10.4	159	2	4	7	12	23	36	82
50–64	79	13.4	162	3	6	10	17	23	53	70
65+	4	16.2	184	6	9	9	14	36	36	36
B. Operated										
0–19 Years	0									
20–34	0									
35–49	0									
50–64	0									
65+	0									
2. MULTIPLE DX										
A. Not Operated										
0–19 Years	37	9.8	47	3	5	7	13	21	24	29
20–34	806	10.2	107	3	4	7	13	23	30	72
35–49	965	10.7	116	3	4	7	13	23	32	77
50–64	902	12.1	139	3	5	8	16	27	42	>99
65+	134	15.3	150	4	7	13	20	28	48	60
B. Operated										
0–19 Years	0									
20–34	1	92.0	0	92	92	92	92	92	92	92
35–49	3	20.9	480	2	2	16	45	45	45	45
50–64	2	23.5	111	16	16	24	31	31	31	31
65+	1	20.0	0	20	20	20	20	20	20	20
SUBTOTALS:										
1. SINGLE DX										
A. Not Operated	332	11.5	140	3	5	8	14	24	33	70
B. Operated	0									
2. MULTIPLE DX										
A. Not Operated	2,844	11.2	123	3	4	8	14	24	34	85
B. Operated	7	31.8	895	2	16	20	45	92	92	92
1. SINGLE DX	332	11.5	140	3	5	8	14	24	33	70
2. MULTIPLE DX	2,851	11.3	125	3	4	8	14	24	35	91
A. NOT OPERATED	3,176	11.3	125	3	4	8	14	24	34	77
B. OPERATED	7	31.8	895	2	16	20	45	92	92	92
TOTAL										
0–19 Years	49	10.8	70	4	6	8	13	22	24	48
20–34	939	10.4	115	3	4	7	13	23	30	74
35–49	1,073	10.7	120	3	4	7	13	23	33	77
50–64	983	12.3	141	3	5	9	16	27	42	>99
65+	139	15.4	149	4	7	13	20	28	48	60
GRAND TOTAL	3,183	11.3	127	3	4	8	14	24	34	77

Length of Stay by Diagnosis and Operation, Western Region, 2008

Western Region, October 2006–September 2007 Data, by Diagnosis

295.34: PARANOID-CHR/EXACER

Type of Patients	Observed Patients	Avg. Stay	Variance	Percentiles						
				10th	25th	50th	75th	90th	95th	99th
1. SINGLE DX										
A. Not Operated										
0–19 Years	5	9.2	95	1	5	6	8	26	26	26
20–34	83	10.4	88	2	4	8	15	21	31	>99
35–49	72	9.8	97	3	4	7	11	19	28	52
50–64	40	10.1	102	3	4	7	10	21	25	55
65+	4	10.0	83	2	2	6	23	23	23	23
B. Operated										
0–19 Years	0									
20–34	0									
35–49	0									
50–64	0									
65+	0									
2. MULTIPLE DX										
A. Not Operated										
0–19 Years	52	12.0	104	4	6	9	15	23	25	66
20–34	1,099	10.1	105	3	4	7	12	21	29	53
35–49	1,624	9.6	86	3	4	7	11	18	25	51
50–64	1,537	11.7	112	3	5	9	14	23	32	66
65+	323	14.3	121	4	7	12	18	27	35	50
B. Operated										
0–19 Years	0									
20–34	1	7.0	0	7	7	7	7	7	7	7
35–49	2	7.5	<1	7	7	8	8	8	8	8
50–64	3	13.3	30	7	7	16	17	17	17	17
65+	1	15.0	0	15	15	15	15	15	15	15
SUBTOTALS:										
1. SINGLE DX										
A. Not Operated	204	10.1	92	3	4	7	12	21	28	54
B. Operated	0									
2. MULTIPLE DX										
A. Not Operated	4,635	10.8	103	3	5	8	13	21	28	59
B. Operated	7	11.0	22	7	7	8	16	17	17	17
1. SINGLE DX	204	10.1	92	3	4	7	12	21	28	54
2. MULTIPLE DX	4,642	10.8	103	3	5	8	13	21	28	59
A. NOT OPERATED	4,839	10.7	103	3	5	8	13	21	28	58
B. OPERATED	7	11.0	22	7	7	8	16	17	17	17
TOTAL										
0–19 Years	57	11.7	102	4	6	8	15	24	26	66
20–34	1,183	10.1	103	3	4	7	12	21	30	57
35–49	1,698	9.6	86	3	4	7	11	18	25	51
50–64	1,580	11.7	111	3	5	9	14	23	32	66
65+	328	14.2	120	4	7	12	18	27	35	50
GRAND TOTAL	4,846	10.7	102	3	5	8	13	21	28	58

295.60: RESID TYPE SCHIZ DIS NOS

Type of Patients	Observed Patients	Avg. Stay	Variance	Percentiles						
				10th	25th	50th	75th	90th	95th	99th
1. SINGLE DX										
A. Not Operated										
0–19 Years	0									
20–34	7	6.9	10	3	4	6	10	11	11	11
35–49	6	20.9	506	2	5	20	22	64	64	64
50–64	3	44.6	>999	2	2	61	71	71	71	71
65+	0									
B. Operated										
0–19 Years	0									
20–34	0									
35–49	0									
50–64	0									
65+	0									
2. MULTIPLE DX										
A. Not Operated										
0–19 Years	4	17.6	386	4	4	5	46	46	46	46
20–34	49	9.7	90	2	4	7	12	22	38	>99
35–49	57	11.8	194	2	3	8	15	29	34	86
50–64	66	10.3	85	3	4	7	12	25	31	37
65+	7	14.2	79	4	5	13	20	30	30	30
B. Operated										
0–19 Years	0									
20–34	0									
35–49	1	6.0	0	6	6	6	6	6	6	6
50–64	0									
65+	0									
SUBTOTALS:										
1. SINGLE DX										
A. Not Operated	16	19.2	560	3	5	10	22	64	71	71
B. Operated	0									
2. MULTIPLE DX										
A. Not Operated	183	10.9	125	2	4	7	14	26	33	86
B. Operated	1	6.0	0	6	6	6	6	6	6	6
1. SINGLE DX	16	19.2	560	3	5	10	22	64	71	71
2. MULTIPLE DX	184	10.9	125	2	4	7	14	26	33	86
A. NOT OPERATED	199	11.6	163	2	4	7	15	27	37	71
B. OPERATED	1	6.0	0	6	6	6	6	6	6	6
TOTAL										
0–19 Years	4	17.6	386	4	4	5	46	46	46	46
20–34	56	9.4	81	2	4	7	11	22	38	>99
35–49	64	12.5	221	2	3	8	16	29	34	86
50–64	69	11.8	172	2	4	7	13	25	37	71
65+	7	14.2	79	4	5	13	20	30	30	30
GRAND TOTAL	200	11.5	162	2	4	7	14	27	37	71

295.62: RESID TYPE SCHIZ-CHRONIC

Type of Patients	Observed Patients	Avg. Stay	Variance	Percentiles						
				10th	25th	50th	75th	90th	95th	99th
1. SINGLE DX										
A. Not Operated										
0–19 Years	1	12.0	0	12	12	12	12	12	12	12
20–34	14	13.1	47	5	8	15	18	22	24	24
35–49	16	10.1	78	3	5	8	11	17	39	39
50–64	12	15.1	115	4	5	12	17	27	40	40
65+	1	2.0	0	2	2	2	2	2	2	2
B. Operated										
0–19 Years	0									
20–34	0									
35–49	0									
50–64	0									
65+	0									
2. MULTIPLE DX										
A. Not Operated										
0–19 Years	6	10.2	129	3	4	7	8	33	33	33
20–34	111	8.9	83	2	3	6	12	19	27	49
35–49	150	10.1	90	2	4	7	13	22	32	51
50–64	155	12.0	143	3	4	8	16	23	38	58
65+	25	14.3	169	4	6	9	15	29	40	56
B. Operated										
0–19 Years	0									
20–34	0									
35–49	0									
50–64	0									
65+	0									
SUBTOTALS:										
1. SINGLE DX										
A. Not Operated	44	12.3	78	3	5	10	17	23	27	40
B. Operated	0									
2. MULTIPLE DX										
A. Not Operated	447	10.7	112	2	4	7	14	22	32	56
B. Operated	0									
1. SINGLE DX	44	12.3	78	3	5	10	17	23	27	40
2. MULTIPLE DX	447	10.7	112	2	4	7	14	22	32	56
A. NOT OPERATED	491	10.8	109	3	4	7	14	22	32	56
B. OPERATED	0									
TOTAL										
0–19 Years	7	10.5	108	3	4	7	12	33	33	33
20–34	125	9.4	80	2	3	6	12	21	25	49
35–49	166	10.1	88	3	4	7	12	22	32	51
50–64	167	12.2	141	3	4	8	16	24	38	58
65+	26	13.8	168	3	6	8	15	29	40	56
GRAND TOTAL	491	10.8	109	3	4	7	14	22	32	56

Length of Stay by Diagnosis and Operation, Western Region, 2008

295.64: RESID SCHIZ-CHR/EXACER

Type of Patients	Observed Patients	Avg. Stay	Variance	10th	25th	50th	75th	90th	95th	99th
1. SINGLE DX										
A. Not Operated										
0–19 Years	1	15.0	0	15	15	15	15	15	15	15
20–34	5	6.4	5	3	3	6	7	7	7	9
35–49	4	7.5	20	4	4	5	7	14	14	14
50–64	2	3.5	<1	3	3	3	4	4	4	4
65+	0									
B. Operated										
0–19 Years	0									
20–34	0									
35–49	0									
50–64	0									
65+	0									
2. MULTIPLE DX										
A. Not Operated										
0–19 Years	5	5.2	11	3	3	4	5	11	11	11
20–34	102	9.6	125	2	4	6	12	22	42	>99
35–49	147	10.3	91	3	4	7	13	22	32	46
50–64	158	11.8	152	3	5	8	15	23	32	69
65+	23	13.6	59	6	7	13	18	23	26	34
B. Operated										
0–19 Years	0									
20–34	0									
35–49	0									
50–64	0									
65+	0									
SUBTOTALS:										
1. SINGLE DX										
A. Not Operated	12	7.0	16	3	4	6	7	14	15	15
B. Operated	0									
2. MULTIPLE DX										
A. Not Operated	435	10.8	120	3	4	7	14	23	34	69
B. Operated	0									
1. SINGLE DX	12	7.0	16	3	4	6	7	14	15	15
2. MULTIPLE DX	435	10.8	120	3	4	7	14	23	34	69
A. NOT OPERATED	447	10.7	117	3	4	7	13	23	32	69
B. OPERATED	0									
TOTAL										
0–19 Years	6	6.8	25	3	3	5	11	15	15	15
20–34	107	9.4	120	2	4	6	11	22	42	>99
35–49	151	10.2	90	3	4	7	13	21	32	46
50–64	160	11.7	151	3	4	8	14	23	30	69
65+	23	13.6	59	6	7	13	18	23	26	34
GRAND TOTAL	447	10.7	117	3	4	7	13	23	32	69

295.70: SCHIZOAFF DISORDER NOS

Type of Patients	Observed Patients	Avg. Stay	Variance	10th	25th	50th	75th	90th	95th	99th
1. SINGLE DX										
A. Not Operated										
0–19 Years	32	13.7	342	1	4	8	15	24	62	86
20–34	322	9.7	110	2	3	6	13	21	28	58
35–49	289	9.5	92	2	3	6	12	20	29	54
50–64	163	9.4	124	2	3	6	13	21	29	94
65+	6	8.2	34	1	2	8	12	16	16	16
B. Operated										
0–19 Years	0									
20–34	0									
35–49	0									
50–64	0									
65+	0									
2. MULTIPLE DX										
A. Not Operated										
0–19 Years	241	11.5	216	3	4	7	13	22	37	96
20–34	3,305	9.6	125	2	4	6	11	20	31	75
35–49	4,533	9.3	94	2	4	6	11	19	28	60
50–64	3,086	11.2	125	3	4	8	14	24	35	81
65+	400	15.1	151	4	8	13	18	28	42	82
B. Operated										
0–19 Years	0									
20–34	3	29.0	899	6	6	18	63	63	63	63
35–49	2	4.5	<1	4	4	5	5	5	5	5
50–64	5	10.2	32	4	8	12	19	>99	>99	>99
65+	2	18.9	127	11	11	11	27	27	27	27
SUBTOTALS:										
1. SINGLE DX										
A. Not Operated	812	9.7	115	2	3	6	13	21	29	58
B. Operated	0									
2. MULTIPLE DX										
A. Not Operated	11,565	10.2	117	2	4	7	12	21	31	71
B. Operated	12	15.4	274	4	6	11	19	63	>99	>99
1. SINGLE DX	812	9.7	115	2	3	6	13	21	29	58
2. MULTIPLE DX	11,577	10.2	117	2	4	7	12	21	31	71
A. NOT OPERATED	12,377	10.1	117	2	4	7	12	21	31	70
B. OPERATED	12	15.4	274	4	6	11	19	63	>99	>99
TOTAL										
0–19 Years	273	11.8	231	2	4	7	13	23	37	96
20–34	3,630	9.6	124	2	4	6	11	21	31	75
35–49	4,824	9.3	94	2	4	6	11	19	28	59
50–64	3,254	11.1	125	3	4	7	14	24	35	83
65+	408	15.1	149	4	8	13	18	28	42	73
GRAND TOTAL	12,389	10.1	117	2	4	7	12	21	31	70

295.72: SCHIZOAFF DISORD-CHRONIC

Type of Patients	Observed Patients	Avg. Stay	Variance	10th	25th	50th	75th	90th	95th	99th
1. SINGLE DX										
A. Not Operated										
0–19 Years	0									
20–34	7	6.6	12	1	5	7	9	12	12	12
35–49	2	7.5	12	5	5	8	10	10	10	10
50–64	2	2.5	4	1	1	1	4	4	4	4
65+	0									
B. Operated										
0–19 Years	0									
20–34	0									
35–49	0									
50–64	0									
65+	0									
2. MULTIPLE DX										
A. Not Operated										
0–19 Years	2	5.0	18	2	2	8	8	8	8	8
20–34	78	8.9	109	2	3	6	10	19	40	>99
35–49	116	11.0	145	2	5	7	16	22	31	63
50–64	92	12.6	92	3	5	11	17	25	29	54
65+	40	15.0	108	7	8	14	17	20	35	50
B. Operated										
0–19 Years	0									
20–34	0									
35–49	0									
50–64	1	30.0	0	30	30	30	30	30	30	30
65+	0									
SUBTOTALS:										
1. SINGLE DX										
A. Not Operated	11	6.0	12	1	4	5	9	10	12	12
B. Operated	0									
2. MULTIPLE DX										
A. Not Operated	328	11.4	119	3	4	8	16	22	31	61
B. Operated	1	30.0	0	30	30	30	30	30	30	30
1. SINGLE DX	11	6.0	12	1	4	5	9	10	12	12
2. MULTIPLE DX	329	11.5	120	3	4	8	16	22	31	61
A. NOT OPERATED	339	11.2	117	3	4	7	16	22	31	61
B. OPERATED	1	30.0	0	30	30	30	30	30	30	30
TOTAL										
0–19 Years	2	5.0	18	2	2	8	8	8	8	8
20–34	85	8.7	101	2	4	6	9	16	27	>99
35–49	118	10.9	143	2	3	7	15	22	31	63
50–64	95	12.6	95	3	5	11	17	26	29	54
65+	40	15.0	108	7	8	14	17	20	35	50
GRAND TOTAL	340	11.3	117	3	4	8	16	22	30	61

Length of Stay by Diagnosis and Operation, Western Region, 2008

Western Region, October 2006–September 2007 Data, by Diagnosis

295.74: SCHIZOAFF DIS-CHR/EXACER

Type of Patients	Observed Patients	Avg. Stay	Variance	10th	25th	50th	75th	90th	95th	99th
1. SINGLE DX										
A. Not Operated										
0–19 Years	1	7.0	0	7	7	7	7	7	7	7
20–34	54	11.9	131	2	4	9	14	33	39	45
35–49	45	13.4	207	3	4	9	18	27	30	69
50–64	17	15.9	241	1	3	12	28	42	45	45
65+	2	10.5	12	8	8	13	13	13	13	13
B. Operated										
0–19 Years	0									
20–34	0									
35–49	0									
50–64	0									
65+	0									
2. MULTIPLE DX										
A. Not Operated										
0–19 Years	43	8.2	54	3	4	6	10	17	21	42
20–34	1,006	8.5	49	3	4	7	11	17	22	38
35–49	1,744	9.2	63	3	4	7	11	17	25	42
50–64	1,496	11.3	107	3	5	8	14	22	29	60
65+	233	15.2	131	5	8	14	19	28	34	92
B. Operated										
0–19 Years	0									
20–34	0									
35–49	4	27.2	150	15	15	19	34	41	41	41
50–64	6	13.0	26	4	11	13	16	18	18	18
65+	1	7.0	0	7	7	7	7	7	7	7
SUBTOTALS:										
1. SINGLE DX										
A. Not Operated	119	13.0	171	2	4	9	17	33	42	67
B. Operated	0									
2. MULTIPLE DX										
A. Not Operated	4,522	10.0	81	3	5	7	12	20	27	51
B. Operated	11	17.6	119	7	11	16	19	34	41	41
1. SINGLE DX	119	13.0	171	2	4	9	17	33	42	67
2. MULTIPLE DX	4,533	10.1	81	3	5	7	12	20	27	51
A. NOT OPERATED	4,641	10.1	83	3	5	7	13	20	27	51
B. OPERATED	11	17.6	119	7	11	16	19	34	41	41
TOTAL										
0–19 Years	44	8.2	53	3	4	6	10	17	21	42
20–34	1,060	8.7	54	3	4	7	11	17	23	39
35–49	1,793	9.3	68	3	4	7	11	18	26	42
50–64	1,519	11.4	108	3	5	8	14	22	29	56
65+	236	15.2	130	5	8	14	19	28	34	92
GRAND TOTAL	4,652	10.1	83	3	5	7	13	20	27	51

295.90: SCHIZOPHRENIA NOS-UNSPEC

Type of Patients	Observed Patients	Avg. Stay	Variance	10th	25th	50th	75th	90th	95th	99th
1. SINGLE DX										
A. Not Operated										
0–19 Years	15	10.4	135	1	2	6	11	34	36	36
20–34	143	9.1	83	2	3	6	13	19	23	45
35–49	91	8.0	44	2	3	6	10	17	21	37
50–64	59	11.2	199	2	3	6	14	21	38	97
65+	2	3.0	0	3	3	3	3	3	3	3
B. Operated										
0–19 Years	0									
20–34	0									
35–49	0									
50–64	0									
65+	0									
2. MULTIPLE DX										
A. Not Operated										
0–19 Years	72	11.6	164	2	3	8	15	22	32	77
20–34	596	10.1	82	2	4	7	13	23	27	52
35–49	580	10.4	123	2	4	7	15	22	34	57
50–64	423	11.6	154	2	4	7	15	26	38	60
65+	84	9.4	65	1	4	7	13	18	24	>99
B. Operated										
0–19 Years	0									
20–34	2	11.0	70	5	5	17	17	17	17	17
35–49	2	10.0	96	3	3	3	17	17	17	17
50–64	2	30.8	>999	1	1	1	61	61	61	61
65+	0									
SUBTOTALS:										
1. SINGLE DX										
A. Not Operated	310	9.2	96	2	3	6	12	19	25	39
B. Operated	0									
2. MULTIPLE DX										
A. Not Operated	1,755	10.6	116	2	4	7	14	23	32	57
B. Operated	6	17.3	502	1	3	5	17	61	61	61
1. SINGLE DX	310	9.2	96	2	3	6	12	19	25	39
2. MULTIPLE DX	1,761	10.6	117	2	4	7	14	23	32	57
A. NOT OPERATED	2,065	10.4	113	2	4	7	14	22	31	56
B. OPERATED	6	17.3	502	1	3	5	17	61	61	61
TOTAL										
0–19 Years	87	11.4	158	1	3	8	15	24	34	77
20–34	741	9.9	82	2	4	7	13	21	27	47
35–49	673	10.1	112	2	4	7	14	22	31	55
50–64	484	11.6	164	2	4	7	15	26	38	63
65+	86	9.2	64	1	3	7	13	18	24	>99
GRAND TOTAL	2,071	10.4	114	2	4	7	14	22	31	57

295.92: SCHIZOPHRENIA NOS-CHR

Type of Patients	Observed Patients	Avg. Stay	Variance	10th	25th	50th	75th	90th	95th	99th
1. SINGLE DX										
A. Not Operated										
0–19 Years	0									
20–34	9	7.4	45	1	3	6	9	21	21	21
35–49	6	14.0	127	3	6	11	15	35	35	35
50–64	4	4.5	16	1	1	4	5	10	10	10
65+	0									
B. Operated										
0–19 Years	0									
20–34	0									
35–49	0									
50–64	0									
65+	0									
2. MULTIPLE DX										
A. Not Operated										
0–19 Years	2	9.0	18	6	6	12	12	12	12	12
20–34	54	11.3	128	3	4	6	16	31	39	>99
35–49	61	9.0	53	2	3	6	13	13	27	>99
50–64	63	16.4	225	3	7	13	22	36	91	>99
65+	6	10.8	156	3	4	7	9	36	36	36
B. Operated										
0–19 Years	0									
20–34	0									
35–49	0									
50–64	0									
65+	0									
SUBTOTALS:										
1. SINGLE DX										
A. Not Operated	19	8.9	73	1	3	6	14	21	35	35
B. Operated	0									
2. MULTIPLE DX										
A. Not Operated	186	12.2	144	2	4	9	18	31	39	>99
B. Operated	0									
1. SINGLE DX	19	8.9	73	1	3	6	14	21	35	35
2. MULTIPLE DX	186	12.2	144	2	4	9	18	31	39	>99
A. NOT OPERATED	205	11.9	138	2	4	9	17	31	37	>99
B. OPERATED	0									
TOTAL										
0–19 Years	2	9.0	18	6	6	12	12	12	12	12
20–34	63	10.7	117	2	4	6	15	31	36	>99
35–49	67	9.4	60	2	3	6	14	21	28	>99
50–64	67	15.7	220	3	7	12	22	37	91	>99
65+	6	10.8	156	3	4	7	9	36	36	36
GRAND TOTAL	205	11.9	138	2	4	9	17	31	37	>99

Western Region, October 2006–September 2007 Data, by Diagnosis

295.94: SCHIZ NOS-CHR/EXACER

Type of Patients	Observed Patients	Avg. Stay	Variance	10th	25th	50th	75th	90th	95th	99th
1. SINGLE DX										
A. Not Operated										
0–19 Years	0									
20–34	8	15.6	202		8	12	30	44	44	44
35–49	8	8.6	55	1	1	4	13	22	22	22
50–64	1	6.0	0	6	6	6	6	6	6	6
65+	0									
B. Operated										
0–19 Years	0									
20–34	0									
35–49	0									
50–64	0									
65+	0									
2. MULTIPLE DX										
A. Not Operated										
0–19 Years	2	9.5	40	5	5	5	14	14	14	14
20–34	60	10.2	87	2	4	6	15	24	34	36
35–49	80	11.7	170	2	5	8	13	26	31	78
50–64	53	10.2	53	4	4	8	14	21	24	33
65+	5	9.2	36	2	6	9	11	18	18	18
B. Operated										
0–19 Years	0									
20–34	0									
35–49	0									
50–64	0									
65+	0									
SUBTOTALS:										
1. SINGLE DX										
A. Not Operated	17	11.7	127	1	4	9	13	30	44	44
B. Operated	0									
2. MULTIPLE DX										
A. Not Operated	200	10.8	109	2	4	7	14	24	30	38
B. Operated	0									
1. SINGLE DX	17	11.7	127	1	4	9	13	30	44	44
2. MULTIPLE DX	200	10.8	109	2	4	7	14	24	30	38
A. NOT OPERATED	217	10.8	110	2	4	8	14	24	31	44
B. OPERATED	0									
TOTAL										
0–19 Years	2	9.5	40	5	5	5	14	14	14	14
20–34	68	10.8	101	2	4	6	15	27	34	44
35–49	88	11.4	160	1	4	8	13	26	31	78
50–64	54	10.1	52	4	4	8	14	21	24	33
65+	5	9.2	36	2	6	9	11	18	18	18
GRAND TOTAL	217	10.8	110	2	4	8	14	24	31	44

296: EPISODIC MOOD DISORDER

Type of Patients	Observed Patients	Avg. Stay	Variance	10th	25th	50th	75th	90th	95th	99th
1. SINGLE DX										
A. Not Operated										
0–19 Years	390	6.0	32	1	3	4	7	12	17	28
20–34	1,001	6.1	50	1	2	4	7	13	19	34
35–49	773	5.9	31	1	2	4	7	13	16	27
50–64	407	6.8	55	1	2	4	8	15	19	32
65+	49	10.0	134	1	3	7	13	23	46	>99
B. Operated										
0–19 Years	1	1.0	0	1	1	1	1	1	1	1
20–34	0									
35–49	0									
50–64	0									
65+	0									
2. MULTIPLE DX										
A. Not Operated										
0–19 Years	4,376	6.9	55	2	3	5	8	13	18	45
20–34	13,487	6.0	38	2	3	4	7	12	16	31
35–49	17,362	6.6	40	2	3	5	8	13	17	32
50–64	13,047	7.9	59	2	3	6	10	16	21	40
65+	5,203	11.6	82	3	5	10	15	22	28	48
B. Operated										
0–19 Years	1	5.0	0	5	5	5	5	5	5	5
20–34	15	9.0	78	2	3	7	10	24	33	33
35–49	17	17.8	330	1	6	11	22	52	66	66
50–64	31	16.0	160	3	6	14	21	34	42	56
65+	33	19.6	137	8	11	15	26	36	48	51
SUBTOTALS:										
1. SINGLE DX										
A. Not Operated	2,620	6.2	44	1	2	4	7	13	18	34
B. Operated	1	1.0	0	1	1	1	1	1	1	1
2. MULTIPLE DX										
A. Not Operated	53,475	7.3	52	2	3	5	9	15	20	37
B. Operated	97	16.4	176	3	7	14	22	34	48	66
1. SINGLE DX	2,621	6.2	44	1	2	4	7	13	18	34
2. MULTIPLE DX	53,572	7.3	52	2	3	5	9	15	20	37
A. NOT OPERATED	56,095	7.2	52	2	3	5	9	15	20	37
B. OPERATED	98	16.2	177	3	7	13	22	34	48	66
TOTAL										
0–19 Years	4,768	6.8	53	2	3	5	8	13	18	43
20–34	14,503	6.0	38	2	3	4	7	12	16	31
35–49	18,152	6.6	40	2	3	5	8	13	17	32
50–64	13,485	7.9	60	2	3	6	10	16	21	40
65+	5,285	11.7	83	3	5	10	15	22	28	48
GRAND TOTAL	56,193	7.2	52	2	3	5	9	15	20	37

296.20: MDD ONE EPIS-NOS

Type of Patients	Observed Patients	Avg. Stay	Variance	10th	25th	50th	75th	90th	95th	99th
1. SINGLE DX										
A. Not Operated										
0–19 Years	45	4.9	14	1	3	5	6	6	8	24
20–34	74	3.4	6	1	1	3	4	7	9	10
35–49	38	5.4	39	1	2	3	7	13	15	36
50–64	22	3.0	4	1	2	3	4	5	6	9
65+	4	4.5	20	1		2	4	11	11	11
B. Operated										
0–19 Years	0									
20–34	0									
35–49	0									
50–64	0									
65+	0									
2. MULTIPLE DX										
A. Not Operated										
0–19 Years	385	6.3	43	2	3	5	7	12	17	24
20–34	1,135	4.2	12	1	2	3	5	8	11	18
35–49	1,352	5.0	20	1	2	4	6	10	12	20
50–64	1,060	5.9	36	1	3	4	7	12	16	33
65+	532	9.3	55	2	4	7	13	19	23	31
B. Operated										
0–19 Years	0									
20–34	2	1.5	<1	1	1	2	2	2	2	2
35–49	3	4.7	30	1	1	2	11	11	11	11
50–64	2	11.5	111	4	4	12	19	19	19	19
65+	4	10.7	13	6	6	10	13	14	14	14
SUBTOTALS:										
1. SINGLE DX										
A. Not Operated	183	4.1	15	1	2	3	5	8	9	24
B. Operated	0									
2. MULTIPLE DX										
A. Not Operated	4,464	5.6	30	1	2	4	7	12	16	26
B. Operated	11	7.5	38	1	2	6	13	14	19	19
1. SINGLE DX	183	4.1	15	1	2	3	5	8	9	24
2. MULTIPLE DX	4,475	5.6	30	1	2	4	7	12	16	26
A. NOT OPERATED	4,647	5.6	30	1	2	4	7	11	15	26
B. OPERATED	11	7.5	38	1	2	6	13	14	19	19
TOTAL										
0–19 Years	430	6.1	40	1	3	5	7	12	16	24
20–34	1,211	4.2	12	1	2	3	5	8	11	18
35–49	1,393	5.0	21	1	2	4	6	10	12	20
50–64	1,084	5.9	36	1	3	4	7	12	16	33
65+	540	9.2	55	2	4	7	13	19	23	31
GRAND TOTAL	4,658	5.6	30	1	2	4	7	11	15	26

Length of Stay by Diagnosis and Operation, Western Region, 2008

Western Region, October 2006–September 2007 Data, by Diagnosis

296.22: MDD ONE EPIS-MODERATE

Type of Patients	Observed Patients	Avg. Stay	Variance	10th	25th	50th	75th	90th	95th	99th
1. SINGLE DX										
A. Not Operated										
0–19 Years	8	4.1	14	1	1	3	4	13	13	13
20–34	9	2.9	2	1	2	2	4	6	6	6
35–49	7	3.7	4	1	3	3	5	7	7	7
50–64	1	1.0	0	1	1	1	1	1	1	1
65+	0									
B. Operated										
0–19 Years	0									
20–34	0									
35–49	0									
50–64	0									
65+	0									
2. MULTIPLE DX										
A. Not Operated										
0–19 Years	68	5.0	11	2	3	5	6	9	10	21
20–34	111	3.0	7	1	1	2	4	6	7	12
35–49	104	4.2	7	1	2	4	5	8	10	11
50–64	71	5.8	36	1	2	4	8	13	17	32
65+	63	8.0	30	2	3	7	13	15	18	22
B. Operated										
0–19 Years	0									
20–34	0									
35–49	0									
50–64	0									
65+	1	14.0	0	14	14	14	14	14	14	14
SUBTOTALS:										
1. SINGLE DX										
A. Not Operated	25	3.4	6	1	2	3	4	6	7	13
B. Operated	0									
2. MULTIPLE DX										
A. Not Operated	417	4.9	18	1	2	4	6	10	14	19
B. Operated	1	14.0	0	14	14	14	14	14	14	14
1. SINGLE DX	25	3.4	6	1	2	3	4	6	7	13
2. MULTIPLE DX	418	4.9	18	1	2	4	6	11	14	19
A. NOT OPERATED	442	4.8	18	1	2	4	6	10	14	19
B. OPERATED	1	14.0	0	14	14	14	14	14	14	14
TOTAL										
0–19 Years	76	4.9	11	1	3	4	6	9	11	21
20–34	120	3.0	6	1	1	2	4	6	7	12
35–49	111	4.2	7	1	2	4	5	7	10	11
50–64	72	5.7	35	1	2	3	7	13	17	32
65+	64	8.1	30	2	3	7	13	15	18	22
GRAND TOTAL	443	4.8	18	1	2	4	6	10	14	19

296.23: MDD ONE EPIS-SEVERE

Type of Patients	Observed Patients	Avg. Stay	Variance	10th	25th	50th	75th	90th	95th	99th
1. SINGLE DX										
A. Not Operated										
0–19 Years	45	4.8	14	2	3	4	6	7	10	23
20–34	57	3.2	6	1	2	3	4	6	8	14
35–49	30	4.3	17	1	2	3	4	9	15	17
50–64	21	5.5	30	1	2	3	6	15	16	21
65+	1	5.0	0	5	5	5	5	5	5	5
B. Operated										
0–19 Years	0									
20–34	0									
35–49	0									
50–64	0									
65+	0									
2. MULTIPLE DX										
A. Not Operated										
0–19 Years	318	5.8	17	2	3	5	7	10	13	21
20–34	591	4.1	11	1	2	3	5	8	11	16
35–49	621	5.4	21	2	2	4	7	11	14	22
50–64	483	6.3	39	2	2	5	8	12	17	36
65+	283	9.2	49	2	4	7	12	19	22	38
B. Operated										
0–19 Years	0									
20–34	0									
35–49	0									
50–64	4	8.9	93	2	2	3	8	23	23	23
65+	2	25.5	5	24	24	26	27	27	27	27
SUBTOTALS:										
1. SINGLE DX										
A. Not Operated	154	4.2	14	1	2	3	5	8	14	21
B. Operated	0									
2. MULTIPLE DX										
A. Not Operated	2,296	5.8	28	2	2	4	7	12	15	26
B. Operated	6	14.4	130	2	3	8	24	27	27	27
1. SINGLE DX	154	4.2	14	1	2	3	5	8	14	21
2. MULTIPLE DX	2,302	5.8	28	2	2	4	7	12	15	27
A. NOT OPERATED	2,450	5.7	27	2	2	4	7	12	15	26
B. OPERATED	6	14.4	130	2	3	8	24	27	27	27
TOTAL										
0–19 Years	363	5.7	17	2	3	5	7	10	12	23
20–34	648	4.0	11	1	2	3	5	8	11	16
35–49	651	5.4	21	2	2	4	7	11	15	22
50–64	508	6.3	39	2	2	5	8	13	17	28
65+	286	9.3	51	2	4	7	12	19	24	38
GRAND TOTAL	2,456	5.7	27	2	2	4	7	12	15	26

296.24: MDD ONE EPIS-SEV W PSYCH

Type of Patients	Observed Patients	Avg. Stay	Variance	10th	25th	50th	75th	90th	95th	99th
1. SINGLE DX										
A. Not Operated										
0–19 Years	18	8.4	28	2	4	8	8	16	20	20
20–34	42	7.6	67	2	3	5	9	12	27	41
35–49	28	6.2	34	1	2	5	9	16	18	25
50–64	16	6.8	29	2	2	6	8	16	19	19
65+	4	9.1	72	1	3	13	19	19	19	19
B. Operated										
0–19 Years	0									
20–34	0									
35–49	0									
50–64	0									
2. MULTIPLE DX										
A. Not Operated										
0–19 Years	138	7.8	40	3	4	6	9	16	21	33
20–34	312	6.7	30	2	3	5	9	14	17	26
35–49	422	7.1	36	2	4	5	9	14	18	30
50–64	400	9.2	73	2	4	6	12	18	28	41
65+	297	11.5	53	3	6	10	15	21	25	37
B. Operated										
0–19 Years	0									
20–34	1	4.0	2	3	3	5	5	5	5	5
35–49	1	14.0	0	14	14	14	14	14	14	14
50–64	2	13.0	49	8	8	8	18	18	18	18
65+	7	27.6	285	10	13	22	48	51	51	51
SUBTOTALS:										
1. SINGLE DX										
A. Not Operated	108	7.3	46	2	3	5	10	16	19	34
B. Operated	0									
2. MULTIPLE DX										
A. Not Operated	1,569	8.4	51	2	4	6	11	17	22	36
B. Operated	12	20.2	256	5	10	15	34	48	51	51
1. SINGLE DX	108	7.3	46	2	3	5	10	16	19	34
2. MULTIPLE DX	1,581	8.5	53	2	4	6	11	17	22	37
A. NOT OPERATED	1,677	8.4	50	2	4	6	11	17	22	36
B. OPERATED	12	20.2	256	5	10	15	34	48	51	51
TOTAL										
0–19 Years	156	7.9	38	3	4	6	9	16	21	33
20–34	356	6.8	34	2	3	5	9	14	18	29
35–49	451	7.1	35	2	3	5	9	14	18	30
50–64	418	9.1	71	2	4	6	12	18	28	40
65+	308	11.9	63	3	6	11	15	22	25	40
GRAND TOTAL	1,689	8.5	53	2	4	6	11	17	22	37

Length of Stay by Diagnosis and Operation, Western Region, 2008

Western Region, October 2006–September 2007 Data, by Diagnosis

296.30: RECURRENT MDD-UNSPEC

Type of Patients	Observed Patients	Avg. Stay	Variance	10th	25th	50th	75th	90th	95th	99th
1. SINGLE DX										
A. Not Operated										
0–19 Years	9	5.3	9	1	3	6	6	11	11	11
20–34	36	3.2	5	1	1	2	4	7	9	9
35–49	38	4.4	9	1	2	4	5	9	11	15
50–64	22	6.2	33	1	2	4	8	15	16	23
65+	2	2.5	<1	2	2	3	3	3	3	3
B. Operated										
0–19 Years	0									
20–34	0									
35–49	0									
50–64	0									
65+	0									
2. MULTIPLE DX										
A. Not Operated										
0–19 Years	163	5.8	22	2	2	5	7	11	15	26
20–34	707	5.0	24	1	2	4	6	9	13	27
35–49	1,221	5.5	23	2	3	4	7	11	14	23
50–64	877	6.7	46	2	3	5	8	14	18	28
65+	355	10.4	66	3	4	8	14	20	24	41
B. Operated										
0–19 Years	0									
20–34	0									
35–49	0									
50–64	3	10.6	72	1	1	14	17	17	17	17
65+	2	9.5	40	5	5	10	14	14	14	14
SUBTOTALS:										
1. SINGLE DX										
A. Not Operated	107	4.4	13	1	2	4	5	9	11	16
B. Operated	0									
2. MULTIPLE DX										
A. Not Operated	3,323	6.3	36	2	3	5	7	13	17	27
B. Operated	5	10.2	47	1	5	14	14	17	17	17
1. SINGLE DX	107	4.4	13	1	2	4	5	9	11	16
2. MULTIPLE DX	3,328	6.3	36	2	3	5	7	13	17	27
A. NOT OPERATED	3,430	6.2	36	2	3	5	7	13	17	27
B. OPERATED	5	10.2	47	1	5	14	14	17	17	17
TOTAL										
0–19 Years	172	5.8	22	2	2	5	7	11	15	26
20–34	743	4.9	23	1	2	4	6	9	13	25
35–49	1,259	5.5	23	2	3	4	7	11	14	23
50–64	902	6.7	45	2	3	5	8	14	18	27
65+	359	10.3	66	3	4	8	14	20	24	41
GRAND TOTAL	3,435	6.2	36	2	3	5	7	13	17	27

296.32: RECURRENT MDD-MOD

Type of Patients	Observed Patients	Avg. Stay	Variance	10th	25th	50th	75th	90th	95th	99th
1. SINGLE DX										
A. Not Operated										
0–19 Years	11	4.3	17	1	2	3	4	9	15	15
20–34	14	2.4	3	1	2	2	2	4	8	8
35–49	8	6.5	20	1	3	5	10	13	13	13
50–64	8	7.4	76	1	3	4	5	27	27	27
65+	1	1.0	0	1	1	1	1	1	1	1
B. Operated										
0–19 Years	0									
20–34	0									
35–49	0									
50–64	0									
65+	0									
2. MULTIPLE DX										
A. Not Operated										
0–19 Years	130	5.6	27	2	3	5	7	9	11	21
20–34	240	4.4	29	1	2	3	5	8	10	31
35–49	409	4.8	17	1	2	4	6	9	11	20
50–64	279	5.7	29	1	3	5	7	11	15	26
65+	125	9.1	64	2	4	7	13	17	22	63
B. Operated										
0–19 Years	0									
20–34	1	7.0	0	7	7	7	7	7	7	7
35–49	1	4.0	0	4	4	4	4	4	4	4
50–64	0									
65+	1	23.0	0	23	23	23	23	23	23	23
SUBTOTALS:										
1. SINGLE DX										
A. Not Operated	42	4.6	26	1	2	3	5	12	13	27
B. Operated	0									
2. MULTIPLE DX										
A. Not Operated	1,183	5.5	30	1	2	4	7	11	14	30
B. Operated	3	11.3	103	4	4	7	23	23	23	23
1. SINGLE DX	42	4.6	26	1	2	3	5	12	13	27
2. MULTIPLE DX	1,186	5.5	30	1	2	4	7	11	14	30
A. NOT OPERATED	1,225	5.4	30	1	2	4	7	11	14	29
B. OPERATED	3	11.3	103	4	4	7	23	23	23	23
TOTAL										
0–19 Years	141	5.5	27	2	3	5	7	9	11	21
20–34	255	4.3	28	1	2	3	5	8	10	31
35–49	418	4.8	17	1	2	4	6	9	12	20
50–64	287	5.7	30	1	3	5	7	11	15	27
65+	127	9.2	65	2	4	7	13	18	23	63
GRAND TOTAL	1,228	5.5	30	1	2	4	7	11	14	29

296.33: RECURRENT MDD-SEVERE

Type of Patients	Observed Patients	Avg. Stay	Variance	10th	25th	50th	75th	90th	95th	99th
1. SINGLE DX										
A. Not Operated										
0–19 Years	38	7.6	59	2	3	6	8	14	28	42
20–34	83	3.9	12	1	2	3	5	8	9	25
35–49	58	4.1	13	1	2	3	5	7	8	20
50–64	43	4.9	35	1	2	3	5	10	12	35
65+	7	7.8	38	3	4	6	8	21	21	21
B. Operated										
0–19 Years	0									
20–34	0									
35–49	0									
50–64	0									
65+	0									
2. MULTIPLE DX										
A. Not Operated										
0–19 Years	478	5.6	16	2	3	5	7	10	12	19
20–34	1,597	5.3	26	2	2	4	6	10	14	25
35–49	2,412	6.4	42	2	3	5	8	12	18	32
50–64	2,146	6.9	35	2	3	5	9	14	18	30
65+	946	10.9	66	3	5	9	14	21	26	44
B. Operated										
0–19 Years	1	5.0	0	5	5	5	5	5	5	5
20–34	3	5.3	10	3	3	4	9	9	9	9
35–49	4	21.0	125	7	7	19	24	34	34	34
50–64	4	35.4	370	10	10	34	42	56	56	56
65+	3	17.4	164	8	8	12	32	32	32	32
SUBTOTALS:										
1. SINGLE DX										
A. Not Operated	229	4.9	27	1	2	3	6	9	13	28
B. Operated	0									
2. MULTIPLE DX										
A. Not Operated	7,579	6.8	41	2	3	5	8	14	18	30
B. Operated	15	19.9	264	4	7	12	34	42	56	56
1. SINGLE DX	229	4.9	27	1	2	3	6	9	13	28
2. MULTIPLE DX	7,594	6.8	41	2	3	5	8	14	18	31
A. NOT OPERATED	7,808	6.8	40	2	3	5	8	14	18	30
B. OPERATED	15	19.9	264	4	7	12	34	42	56	56
TOTAL										
0–19 Years	517	5.8	19	2	3	5	7	10	13	24
20–34	1,683	5.2	26	2	2	4	6	10	14	25
35–49	2,474	6.4	42	2	3	5	8	12	18	32
50–64	2,193	6.9	37	2	3	5	9	14	18	30
65+	956	10.9	66	3	5	9	14	21	26	44
GRAND TOTAL	7,823	6.8	41	2	3	5	8	14	18	31

Length of Stay by Diagnosis and Operation, Western Region, 2008

©2009 Thomson Reuters. All rights reserved.

Western Region, October 2006–September 2007 Data, by Diagnosis

296.34: RECURRENT MDD-SEV PSYCH

Type of Patients	Observed Patients	Avg. Stay	Variance	10th	25th	50th	75th	90th	95th	99th
1. SINGLE DX										
A. Not Operated										
0–19 Years	15	4.9	5	3	3	4	7	8	9	9
20–34	48	5.4	17	1	2	4	7	13	14	17
35–49	65	6.0	17	2	3	6	8	13	14	21
50–64	32	8.3	81	1	3	5	9	19	27	41
65+	5	13.8	176	4	6	7	16	36	36	36
B. Operated										
0–19 Years	0									
20–34	0									
35–49	0									
50–64	0									
65+	0									
2. MULTIPLE DX										
A. Not Operated										
0–19 Years	150	7.8	42	2	4	6	9	13	23	35
20–34	572	6.9	44	2	3	5	8	14	20	36
35–49	1,086	7.8	50	2	4	6	10	15	19	42
50–64	1,021	9.2	77	2	4	7	11	18	25	49
65+	613	14.0	105	4	7	12	17	25	33	53
B. Operated										
0–19 Years	0									
20–34	1	33.0	0	33	33	33	33	33	33	33
35–49	0									
50–64	4	7.5	14	5	6	6	13	13	13	13
65+	5	13.6	54	7	10	11	14	26	26	26
SUBTOTALS:										
1. SINGLE DX										
A. Not Operated	165	6.4	35	2	3	5	8	14	16	36
B. Operated	0									
2. MULTIPLE DX										
A. Not Operated	3,442	9.2	72	2	4	7	12	18	25	46
B. Operated	10	13.1	86	6	6	11	14	26	33	33
1. SINGLE DX	165	6.4	35	2	3	5	8	14	16	36
2. MULTIPLE DX	3,452	9.2	72	2	4	7	12	18	25	46
A. NOT OPERATED	3,607	9.0	71	2	4	7	11	18	24	45
B. OPERATED	10	13.1	86	6	6	11	14	26	33	33
TOTAL										
0–19 Years	165	7.5	39	2	4	6	9	13	20	35
20–34	621	6.8	43	2	3	5	8	14	19	33
35–49	1,151	7.7	48	2	4	6	9	15	19	40
50–64	1,057	9.2	77	2	4	7	11	19	25	49
65+	623	14.0	105	4	7	12	17	25	33	53
GRAND TOTAL	3,617	9.1	71	2	4	7	11	18	25	45

296.40: BPI-RECENT MANIC NOS

Type of Patients	Observed Patients	Avg. Stay	Variance	10th	25th	50th	75th	90th	95th	99th
1. SINGLE DX										
A. Not Operated										
0–19 Years	13	8.2	37	2	4	7	9	19	19	19
20–34	68	7.9	42	2	3	5	10	20	23	28
35–49	59	7.2	66	1	2	5	8	17	20	52
50–64	31	10.1	60	2	5	9	14	21	22	37
65+	6	9.3	68	2	3	4	15	23	23	23
B. Operated										
0–19 Years	0									
20–34	0									
35–49	0									
50–64	0									
65+	0									
2. MULTIPLE DX										
A. Not Operated										
0–19 Years	72	10.3	82	2	4	7	15	23	28	42
20–34	474	8.2	54	2	3	6	11	17	20	32
35–49	529	8.1	61	2	3	6	10	17	22	46
50–64	531	9.8	81	2	4	7	13	20	27	48
65+	212	11.6	80	3	6	10	15	21	28	50
B. Operated										
0–19 Years	0									
20–34	0									
35–49	1	66.0	0	66	66	66	66	66	66	66
50–64	1	14.0	0	14	14	14	14	14	14	14
65+	0									
SUBTOTALS:										
1. SINGLE DX										
A. Not Operated	177	8.1	54	2	3	6	10	19	22	37
B. Operated	0									
2. MULTIPLE DX										
A. Not Operated	1,818	9.1	69	2	4	7	12	19	24	46
B. Operated	2	40.1	>999	14	14	66	66	66	66	66
1. SINGLE DX	177	8.1	54	2	3	6	10	19	22	37
2. MULTIPLE DX	1,820	9.2	71	2	4	7	12	19	24	46
A. NOT OPERATED	1,995	9.0	68	2	4	7	12	19	23	46
B. OPERATED	2	40.1	>999	14	14	66	66	66	66	66
TOTAL										
0–19 Years	85	10.0	75	2	4	7	15	22	27	42
20–34	542	8.2	52	2	3	6	11	17	21	31
35–49	589	8.2	67	2	3	6	10	17	22	48
50–64	563	9.8	79	2	4	7	13	20	26	48
65+	218	11.5	80	2	6	10	15	21	28	50
GRAND TOTAL	1,997	9.1	70	2	4	7	12	19	24	46

296.43: BPI-RECENT MANIC SEVERE

Type of Patients	Observed Patients	Avg. Stay	Variance	10th	25th	50th	75th	90th	95th	99th
1. SINGLE DX										
A. Not Operated										
0–19 Years	3	20.0	327	9	9	10	41	41	41	41
20–34	12	7.5	54	2	5	5	11	12	27	27
35–49	10	6.1	7	4	5	6	7	7	11	11
50–64	4	3.5	7	1	2	3	7	7	7	7
65+	0									
B. Operated										
0–19 Years	0									
20–34	0									
35–49	0									
50–64	0									
65+	0									
2. MULTIPLE DX										
A. Not Operated										
0–19 Years	25	11.8	47	3	7	11	15	19	27	29
20–34	101	8.3	65	3	3	6	11	19	24	30
35–49	122	7.8	40	2	3	5	10	18	20	29
50–64	138	9.6	68	2	4	7	12	20	28	37
65+	59	12.6	62	4	6	12	17	24	28	37
B. Operated										
0–19 Years	0									
20–34	0									
35–49	1	6.0	0	6	6	6	6	6	6	6
50–64	0									
65+	0									
SUBTOTALS:										
1. SINGLE DX										
A. Not Operated	29	7.8	68	1	3	6	9	12	27	41
B. Operated	0									
2. MULTIPLE DX										
A. Not Operated	445	9.3	60	3	4	7	12	20	25	36
B. Operated	1	6.0	0	6	6	6	6	6	6	6
1. SINGLE DX	29	7.8	68	1	3	6	9	12	27	41
2. MULTIPLE DX	446	9.3	59	3	4	7	12	20	25	36
A. NOT OPERATED	474	9.2	60	2	4	7	12	20	25	37
B. OPERATED	1	6.0	0	6	6	6	6	6	6	6
TOTAL										
0–19 Years	28	12.7	73	3	8	11	17	27	29	41
20–34	113	8.2	63	2	3	6	9	19	25	30
35–49	133	7.7	37	2	3	6	10	17	20	29
50–64	142	9.4	67	2	4	7	12	19	26	37
65+	59	12.6	62	4	6	12	17	24	28	37
GRAND TOTAL	475	9.2	60	2	4	7	12	20	25	37

Length of Stay by Diagnosis and Operation, Western Region, 2008

Western Region, October 2006–September 2007 Data, by Diagnosis

296.44: BPI-RECENT MANIC PSYCH

Type of Patients	Observed Patients	Avg. Stay	Vari-ance	10th	25th	50th	75th	90th	95th	99th
1. SINGLE DX										
A. Not Operated										
0–19 Years	18	12.0	127	2	3	7	20	23	46	46
20–34	106	12.0	174	3	4	7	14	30	34	66
35–49	82	8.3	42	1	3	7	13	16	20	37
50–64	52	11.4	165	3	4	8	15	19	27	88
65+	8	21.4	393	6	9	12	19	59	59	59
B. Operated										
0–19 Years	0									
20–34	0									
35–49	0									
50–64	0									
65+	0									
2. MULTIPLE DX										
A. Not Operated										
0–19 Years	88	10.4	57	3	6	9	11	19	28	41
20–34	744	12.0	116	3	5	9	15	25	34	58
35–49	751	11.7	108	3	5	8	16	24	32	56
50–64	750	12.9	149	3	5	9	16	25	37	66
65+	293	15.3	123	5	8	12	20	30	35	67
B. Operated										
0–19 Years	0									
20–34	1	10.0	0	10	10	10	10	10	10	10
35–49	2	16.0	72	10	10	16	22	22	22	22
50–64	1	16.0	0	16	16	16	16	16	16	16
65+	2	21.5	40	17	17	26	26	26	26	26
SUBTOTALS:										
1. SINGLE DX										
A. Not Operated	266	11.0	138	2	4	8	13	21	31	66
B. Operated	0									
2. MULTIPLE DX										
A. Not Operated	2,626	12.5	123	3	5	9	16	25	35	58
B. Operated	6	16.8	41	10	10	16	22	26	26	26
1. SINGLE DX	266	11.0	138	2	4	8	13	21	31	66
2. MULTIPLE DX	2,632	12.5	123	3	5	9	16	25	35	58
A. NOT OPERATED	2,892	12.3	125	3	5	9	16	25	34	59
B. OPERATED	6	16.8	41	10	10	16	22	26	26	26
TOTAL										
0–19 Years	106	10.7	69	3	6	9	11	21	28	41
20–34	851	12.0	123	3	5	9	15	25	34	62
35–49	835	11.4	102	3	5	8	15	23	31	55
50–64	803	12.8	150	3	5	9	16	25	35	66
65+	303	15.5	129	5	8	12	21	30	38	67
GRAND TOTAL	2,898	12.4	125	3	5	9	16	25	34	59

296.50: BPI-RECENT DEPR NOS

Type of Patients	Observed Patients	Avg. Stay	Vari-ance	10th	25th	50th	75th	90th	95th	99th
1. SINGLE DX										
A. Not Operated										
0–19 Years	14	4.6	5	2	3	4	7	8	8	8
20–34	48	4.1	12	1	3	3	5	7	7	23
35–49	36	6.1	22	1	3	5	7	14	17	18
50–64	19	5.2	36	1	2	4	5	13	27	27
65+	4	9.4	117	1	1	3	9	25	25	25
B. Operated										
0–19 Years	0									
20–34	0									
35–49	0									
50–64	0									
65+	0									
2. MULTIPLE DX										
A. Not Operated										
0–19 Years	154	6.4	25	2	3	5	8	12	14	29
20–34	912	5.4	20	2	3	4	7	10	14	22
35–49	1,401	6.0	21	2	3	5	7	11	14	26
50–64	845	7.1	35	2	4	6	9	14	19	28
65+	182	11.8	74	3	6	10	15	21	23	42
B. Operated										
0–19 Years	0									
20–34	1	7.0	0	7	7	7	7	7	7	7
35–49	1	1.0	0	1	1	1	1	1	1	1
50–64	2	12.4	179	3	3	3	22	22	22	22
65+	2	26.0	197	16	16	36	36	36	36	36
SUBTOTALS:										
1. SINGLE DX										
A. Not Operated	121	5.1	21	1	2	4	6	11	14	25
B. Operated	0									
2. MULTIPLE DX										
A. Not Operated	3,494	6.4	29	2	3	5	8	12	16	27
B. Operated	6	14.2	178	1	3	12	22	36	36	36
1. SINGLE DX	121	5.1	21	1	2	4	6	11	14	25
2. MULTIPLE DX	3,500	6.4	29	2	3	5	8	12	16	27
A. NOT OPERATED	3,615	6.4	29	2	3	5	8	12	16	27
B. OPERATED	6	14.2	178	1	3	12	22	36	36	36
TOTAL										
0–19 Years	168	6.3	23	2	3	5	8	12	14	29
20–34	961	5.4	19	2	3	4	7	10	13	22
35–49	1,438	6.0	21	2	3	5	7	11	14	26
50–64	866	7.1	35	2	4	6	9	14	19	28
65+	188	11.9	77	3	6	10	15	21	23	42
GRAND TOTAL	3,621	6.4	29	2	3	5	8	12	16	27

296.52: BPI-RECENT DEPR MOD

Type of Patients	Observed Patients	Avg. Stay	Vari-ance	10th	25th	50th	75th	90th	95th	99th
1. SINGLE DX										
A. Not Operated										
0–19 Years	2	6.5	<1	6	6	7	7	7	7	7
20–34	5	4.4	7	2	2	4	6	8	8	8
35–49	3	3.7	4	2	2	3	6	6	6	6
50–64	1	2.0	0	2	2	2	2	2	2	2
65+	0									
B. Operated										
0–19 Years	0									
20–34	0									
35–49	0									
50–64	0									
65+	0									
2. MULTIPLE DX										
A. Not Operated										
0–19 Years	11	9.4	138	2	3	6	11	12	43	43
20–34	59	5.2	28	2	3	4	6	8	16	33
35–49	77	6.8	27	2	3	5	9	15	17	24
50–64	63	7.5	47	2	4	6	8	14	16	51
65+	10	9.1	41	1	6	7	10	15	24	24
B. Operated										
0–19 Years	0									
20–34	0									
35–49	0									
50–64	0									
65+	0									
SUBTOTALS:										
1. SINGLE DX										
A. Not Operated	11	4.4	5	2	2	4	6	7	8	8
B. Operated	0									
2. MULTIPLE DX										
A. Not Operated	220	6.8	40	2	3	5	8	14	17	33
B. Operated	0									
1. SINGLE DX	11	4.4	5	2	2	4	6	7	8	8
2. MULTIPLE DX	220	6.8	40	2	3	5	8	14	17	33
A. NOT OPERATED	231	6.7	38	2	3	5	7	13	17	33
B. OPERATED	0									
TOTAL										
0–19 Years	13	9.0	116	2	4	6	9	12	43	43
20–34	64	5.2	26	2	3	4	6	8	10	33
35–49	80	6.7	27	2	3	5	9	15	17	24
50–64	64	7.4	47	2	4	6	8	14	16	51
65+	10	9.1	41	1	6	7	10	15	24	24
GRAND TOTAL	231	6.7	38	2	3	5	7	13	17	33

Length of Stay by Diagnosis and Operation, Western Region, 2008

Western Region, October 2006–September 2007 Data, by Diagnosis

296.53: BPI-RECENT DEPR SEVERE

Type of Patients	Observed Patients	Avg. Stay	Variance	Percentiles						
				10th	25th	50th	75th	90th	95th	99th
1. SINGLE DX										
A. Not Operated										
0–19 Years	7	4.4	5	2	2	4	6	8	8	8
20–34	22	4.0	8	2	2	3	4	7	9	12
35–49	16	4.3	9	2	2	3	7	7	12	12
50–64	4	7.0	16	4	4	5	6	13	13	13
65+	1	9.0	0	9	9	9	9	9	9	9
B. Operated										
0–19 Years	0									
20–34	0									
35–49	0									
50–64	0									
65+	0									
2. MULTIPLE DX										
A. Not Operated										
0–19 Years	71	6.2	42	2	3	5	7	10	13	40
20–34	413	5.8	40	2	3	4	7	11	14	25
35–49	671	7.2	41	2	3	5	9	16	19	33
50–64	440	7.9	36	2	3	6	10	16	21	29
65+	106	12.0	69	4	6	10	15	21	27	48
B. Operated										
0–19 Years	0									
20–34	0									
35–49	0									
50–64	2	17.5	5	16	16	18	19	19	19	19
65+	0									
SUBTOTALS:										
1. SINGLE DX										
A. Not Operated	50	4.5	8	2	2	4	6	8	12	13
B. Operated	0									
2. MULTIPLE DX										
A. Not Operated	1,701	7.3	43	2	3	5	9	14	19	31
B. Operated	2	17.5	5	16	16	18	19	19	19	19
1. SINGLE DX	50	4.5	8	2	2	4	6	8	12	13
2. MULTIPLE DX	1,703	7.3	43	2	3	5	9	14	19	30
A. NOT OPERATED	1,751	7.2	43	2	3	5	9	14	19	30
B. OPERATED	2	17.5	5	16	16	18	19	19	19	19
TOTAL										
0–19 Years	78	6.0	39	2	3	4	7	10	13	40
20–34	435	5.7	38	2	3	4	7	11	14	25
35–49	687	7.1	40	2	3	5	9	14	19	33
50–64	446	7.9	36	2	4	6	10	16	20	29
65+	107	12.0	68	4	6	10	15	21	27	48
GRAND TOTAL	1,753	7.2	43	2	3	5	9	14	19	30

296.54: BPI-RECENT DEPR PSYCH

Type of Patients	Observed Patients	Avg. Stay	Variance	10th	25th	50th	75th	90th	95th	99th
1. SINGLE DX										
A. Not Operated										
0–19 Years	6	7.5	26	3	4	8	8	8	17	17
20–34	23	8.4	30	2	5	6	12	17	18	19
35–49	15	5.6	14	2	3	5	7	10	16	16
50–64	6	9.0	48	2	6	6	10	22	22	22
65+	0									
B. Operated										
0–19 Years	0									
20–34	0									
35–49	0									
50–64	0									
65+	0									
2. MULTIPLE DX										
A. Not Operated										
0–19 Years	54	8.0	31	3	4	7	10	13	16	31
20–34	429	6.9	29	2	4	5	9	13	17	29
35–49	613	7.8	51	3	4	6	10	15	20	36
50–64	482	9.7	89	3	4	7	12	20	24	51
65+	115	16.6	161	4	7	15	22	29	36	61
B. Operated										
0–19 Years	0									
20–34	0									
35–49	1	52.0	0	52	52	52	52	52	52	52
50–64	2	23.0	332	10	10	10	36	36	36	36
65+	0									
SUBTOTALS:										
1. SINGLE DX										
A. Not Operated	50	7.5	27	2	4	6	10	17	18	22
B. Operated	0									
2. MULTIPLE DX										
A. Not Operated	1,693	8.7	68	3	4	6	10	17	23	42
B. Operated	3	32.7	445	10	10	36	52	52	52	52
1. SINGLE DX	50	7.5	27	2	4	6	10	17	18	22
2. MULTIPLE DX	1,696	8.8	70	3	4	6	10	18	24	44
A. NOT OPERATED	1,743	8.7	67	3	4	6	10	17	22	42
B. OPERATED	3	32.7	445	10	10	36	52	52	52	52
TOTAL										
0–19 Years	60	8.0	30	3	4	7	10	14	16	31
20–34	452	6.9	30	2	4	5	8	13	17	29
35–49	629	7.9	53	3	4	6	9	15	20	38
50–64	490	9.7	89	3	4	7	12	20	25	51
65+	115	16.6	161	4	7	15	22	29	36	61
GRAND TOTAL	1,746	8.7	69	3	4	6	10	17	23	42

296.60: BPI-RECENT MIXED NOS

Type of Patients	Observed Patients	Avg. Stay	Variance	10th	25th	50th	75th	90th	95th	99th
1. SINGLE DX										
A. Not Operated										
0–19 Years	9	8.7	61	2	2	5	12	24	24	24
20–34	31	6.1	16	2	3	5	9	12	13	19
35–49	26	5.2	27	2	3	4	6	9	12	27
50–64	9	4.1	4	1	3	4	5	8	8	8
65+	0									
B. Operated										
0–19 Years	0									
20–34	0									
35–49	0									
50–64	0									
65+	0									
2. MULTIPLE DX										
A. Not Operated										
0–19 Years	128	7.1	44	2	3	6	9	12	15	43
20–34	432	5.5	19	2	3	4	7	11	14	23
35–49	560	6.4	31	2	4	5	8	12	16	27
50–64	340	7.9	70	2	4	6	9	14	22	42
65+	73	11.0	94	3	5	8	15	22	27	67
B. Operated										
0–19 Years	0									
20–34	0									
35–49	0									
50–64	0									
65+	0									
SUBTOTALS:										
1. SINGLE DX										
A. Not Operated	75	5.8	24	2	3	4	7	12	17	27
B. Operated	0									
2. MULTIPLE DX										
A. Not Operated	1,533	6.8	42	2	3	5	8	13	17	34
B. Operated	0									
1. SINGLE DX	75	5.8	24	2	3	4	7	12	17	27
2. MULTIPLE DX	1,533	6.8	42	2	3	5	8	13	17	34
A. NOT OPERATED	1,608	6.7	41	2	3	5	8	13	17	34
B. OPERATED	0									
TOTAL										
0–19 Years	137	7.2	45	2	3	6	9	12	17	43
20–34	463	5.6	18	2	3	4	7	11	14	23
35–49	586	6.3	31	2	3	5	7	12	16	27
50–64	349	7.8	69	2	4	6	8	14	22	42
65+	73	11.0	94	3	5	8	15	22	27	67
GRAND TOTAL	1,608	6.7	41	2	3	5	8	13	17	34

Length of Stay by Diagnosis and Operation, Western Region, 2008

Western Region, October 2006–September 2007 Data, by Diagnosis

296.63: BPI-RECENT MIXED SEVERE

Type of Patients	Observed Patients	Avg. Stay	Variance	Percentiles						
				10th	25th	50th	75th	90th	95th	99th
1. SINGLE DX										
A. Not Operated										
0–19 Years	3	4.3	5	3	3	3	7	7	7	7
20–34	15	3.0	3	2	2	3	3	4	8	8
35–49	9	8.6	108	1	2	5	7	33	33	33
50–64	8	8.1	61	1	4	6	10	26	26	26
65+	1	14.0	0	14	14	14	14	14	14	14
B. Operated										
0–19 Years	0									
20–34	0									
35–49	0									
50–64	0									
65+	0									
2. MULTIPLE DX										
A. Not Operated										
0–19 Years	57	7.7	79	2	3	5	7	16	30	54
20–34	268	4.9	11	2	3	4	6	10	11	17
35–49	291	6.1	34	2	3	5	7	12	15	29
50–64	247	6.8	47	2	3	5	8	12	17	42
65+	27	7.4	17	2	5	6	12	14	14	15
B. Operated										
0–19 Years	0									
20–34	1	16.0	0	16	16	16	16	16	16	16
35–49	0									
50–64	0									
65+	0									
SUBTOTALS:										
1. SINGLE DX										
A. Not Operated	36	6.0	47	1	2	3	7	14	26	33
B. Operated	0									
2. MULTIPLE DX										
A. Not Operated	890	6.1	34	2	3	5	7	11	15	30
B. Operated	1	16.0	0	16	16	16	16	16	16	16
1. SINGLE DX	36	6.0	47	1	2	3	7	14	26	33
2. MULTIPLE DX	891	6.1	34	2	3	5	7	12	15	30
A. NOT OPERATED	926	6.1	35	2	3	5	7	11	15	30
B. OPERATED	1	16.0	0	16	16	16	16	16	16	16
TOTAL										
0–19 Years	60	7.6	76	2	3	5	7	16	30	54
20–34	284	4.9	12	2	3	4	6	9	11	17
35–49	300	6.1	36	2	3	5	7	12	15	33
50–64	255	6.9	48	2	3	5	9	12	18	42
65+	28	7.7	18	2	5	6	12	14	14	15
GRAND TOTAL	927	6.1	35	2	3	5	7	12	15	30

296.64: BPI-RECENT MIXED PSYCH

Type of Patients	Observed Patients	Avg. Stay	Variance	Percentiles						
				10th	25th	50th	75th	90th	95th	99th
1. SINGLE DX										
A. Not Operated										
0–19 Years	9	6.8	14	3	3	7	9	12	12	12
20–34	25	9.6	135	1	3	6	9	31	42	42
35–49	33	7.9	68	2	3	6	9	14	24	44
50–64	10	5.1	10	3	3	4	6	13	13	13
65+	0									
B. Operated										
0–19 Years	0									
20–34	0									
35–49	0									
50–64	0									
65+	0									
2. MULTIPLE DX										
A. Not Operated										
0–19 Years	84	9.3	92	3	5	6	10	16	26	63
20–34	495	7.6	74	2	4	6	8	13	18	49
35–49	711	7.7	43	3	4	6	9	15	18	36
50–64	512	8.6	49	3	4	6	10	16	21	35
65+	102	13.9	99	6	7	11	16	25	32	56
B. Operated										
0–19 Years	0									
20–34	0									
35–49	0									
50–64	0									
65+	1	37.0	0	37	37	37	37	37	37	37
SUBTOTALS:										
1. SINGLE DX										
A. Not Operated	77	8.0	76	2	3	6	9	14	31	44
B. Operated	0									
2. MULTIPLE DX										
A. Not Operated	1,904	8.3	60	3	4	6	10	15	21	43
B. Operated	1	37.0	0	37	37	37	37	37	37	37
1. SINGLE DX	77	8.0	76	2	3	6	9	14	31	44
2. MULTIPLE DX	1,905	8.3	60	3	4	6	10	15	21	43
A. NOT OPERATED	1,981	8.3	60	3	4	6	10	15	21	44
B. OPERATED	1	37.0	0	37	37	37	37	37	37	37
TOTAL										
0–19 Years	93	9.0	85	3	5	6	10	16	26	63
20–34	520	7.7	77	2	4	6	8	13	19	44
35–49	744	7.7	44	3	4	6	9	15	18	37
50–64	522	8.5	49	3	4	6	10	16	21	35
65+	103	14.1	103	6	7	11	16	25	32	56
GRAND TOTAL	1,982	8.3	61	3	4	6	10	15	21	44

296.7: BIPOLAR I-RECENT NOS

Type of Patients	Observed Patients	Avg. Stay	Variance	Percentiles						
				10th	25th	50th	75th	90th	95th	99th
1. SINGLE DX										
A. Not Operated										
0–19 Years	15	7.2	40	2	2	5	12	19	21	21
20–34	32	5.7	29	1	2	3	8	14	19	20
35–49	13	7.5	38	2	3	5	10	13	24	24
50–64	12	6.1	18	2	2	6	11	13	13	13
65+	1	8.0	0	8	8	8	8	8	8	8
B. Operated										
0–19 Years	0									
20–34	0									
35–49	0									
50–64	0									
65+	0									
2. MULTIPLE DX										
A. Not Operated										
0–19 Years	105	7.3	49	2	3	6	8	14	18	43
20–34	307	5.7	24	1	3	4	7	12	14	26
35–49	352	6.8	47	2	3	5	8	14	20	44
50–64	286	9.6	54	2	4	7	13	20	25	37
65+	90	13.4	90	2	6	11	19	25	32	42
B. Operated										
0–19 Years	0									
20–34	0									
35–49	0									
50–64	0									
65+	1	8.0	0	8	8	8	8	8	8	8
SUBTOTALS:										
1. SINGLE DX										
A. Not Operated	73	6.4	30	1	2	5	8	13	19	24
B. Operated	0									
2. MULTIPLE DX										
A. Not Operated	1,140	7.8	51	2	3	6	10	16	22	38
B. Operated	1	8.0	0	8	8	8	8	8	8	8
1. SINGLE DX	73	6.4	30	1	2	5	8	13	19	24
2. MULTIPLE DX	1,141	7.8	51	2	3	6	10	16	22	38
A. NOT OPERATED	1,213	7.7	50	2	3	6	10	16	22	37
B. OPERATED	1	8.0	0	8	8	8	8	8	8	8
TOTAL										
0–19 Years	120	7.3	48	2	3	6	8	14	19	43
20–34	339	5.7	25	1	3	4	7	12	14	26
35–49	365	6.8	46	2	3	5	8	14	20	44
50–64	298	9.5	53	2	4	7	13	20	25	37
65+	92	13.3	89	2	6	11	18	25	32	42
GRAND TOTAL	1,214	7.7	49	2	3	6	10	16	22	37

Length of Stay by Diagnosis and Operation, Western Region, 2008

Western Region, October 2006–September 2007 Data, by Diagnosis

296.80: BIPOLAR DISORDER NOS

Type of Patients	Observed Patients	Avg. Stay	Variance	10th	25th	50th	75th	90th	95th	99th
1. SINGLE DX										
A. Not Operated										
0–19 Years	38	5.4	20	1	2	4	7	12	15	16
20–34	126	6.1	30	1	2	4	7	14	18	22
35–49	97	5.0	29	1	2	3	5	11	18	31
50–64	49	5.2	21	1	2	4	6	14	15	23
65+	0									
B. Operated										
0–19 Years	1	1.0	0	1	1	1	1	1	1	1
20–34	0									
35–49	0									
50–64	0									
65+	0									
2. MULTIPLE DX										
A. Not Operated										
0–19 Years	401	7.9	98	2	3	6	9	15	22	96
20–34	1,334	6.1	37	2	3	4	7	13	18	31
35–49	1,399	6.3	35	2	3	5	8	13	17	29
50–64	839	7.5	59	3	3	5	9	15	19	36
65+	228	12.2	100	3	4	10	17	25	29	41
B. Operated										
0–19 Years	0									
20–34	3	11.9	111	4	4	8	24	24	24	24
35–49	2	14.5	24	11	11	11	18	18	18	18
50–64	0									
65+	0									
SUBTOTALS:										
1. SINGLE DX										
A. Not Operated	310	5.5	27	1	2	4	7	13	17	25
B. Operated	1	1.0	0	1	1	1	1	1	1	1
2. MULTIPLE DX										
A. Not Operated	4,201	6.9	52	2	3	5	9	14	20	36
B. Operated	5	12.9	63	4	8	11	18	24	24	24
1. SINGLE DX	311	5.5	27	1	2	4	7	13	17	25
2. MULTIPLE DX	4,206	6.9	52	2	3	5	9	14	20	36
A. NOT OPERATED	4,511	6.8	50	2	3	5	8	14	19	36
B. OPERATED	6	11.0	74	1	4	8	18	24	24	24
TOTAL										
0–19 Years	440	7.7	92	2	3	6	9	15	21	96
20–34	1,463	6.1	37	1	2	4	7	13	18	31
35–49	1,498	6.2	35	2	3	4	8	13	17	29
50–64	888	7.3	57	2	3	5	9	15	19	36
65+	228	12.2	100	3	4	10	17	26	31	56
GRAND TOTAL	4,517	6.8	51	2	3	5	8	14	19	36

296.89: BIPOLAR DISORDER NEC

Type of Patients	Observed Patients	Avg. Stay	Variance	10th	25th	50th	75th	90th	95th	99th
1. SINGLE DX										
A. Not Operated										
0–19 Years	8	6.0	21	1	2	5	7	14	14	14
20–34	30	7.0	44	2	2	4	12	19	20	25
35–49	24	4.3	10	1	2	4	5	7	8	16
50–64	13	5.8	24	1	2	5	7	14	15	15
65+	2	1.0	0	1	1	1	1	1	1	1
B. Operated										
0–19 Years	0									
20–34	0									
35–49	0									
50–64	0									
65+	0									
2. MULTIPLE DX										
A. Not Operated										
0–19 Years	178	8.3	80	2	4	6	9	14	20	55
20–34	728	5.4	23	2	3	4	7	11	15	26
35–49	748	6.3	34	2	3	5	8	12	16	28
50–64	471	8.0	57	2	3	6	9	17	22	44
65+	157	14.0	126	3	6	11	17	32	39	48
B. Operated										
0–19 Years	0									
20–34	0									
35–49	0									
50–64	1	16.0	0	16	16	16	16	16	16	16
65+	1	21.0	0	21	21	21	21	21	21	21
SUBTOTALS:										
1. SINGLE DX										
A. Not Operated	77	5.7	28	1	2	4	7	15	16	25
B. Operated	0									
2. MULTIPLE DX										
A. Not Operated	2,282	7.1	50	2	3	5	8	14	20	39
B. Operated	2	18.5	12	16	16	16	21	21	21	21
1. SINGLE DX	77	5.7	28	1	2	4	7	15	16	25
2. MULTIPLE DX	2,284	7.1	50	2	3	5	8	14	20	39
A. NOT OPERATED	2,359	7.0	49	2	3	5	8	14	20	39
B. OPERATED	2	18.5	12	16	16	16	21	21	21	21
TOTAL										
0–19 Years	186	8.2	78	2	4	6	9	14	19	55
20–34	758	5.5	24	1	3	4	7	11	15	26
35–49	772	6.2	33	2	3	5	7	12	16	28
50–64	485	7.9	56	2	3	6	10	16	21	44
65+	160	13.9	126	3	6	11	17	30	39	48
GRAND TOTAL	2,361	7.0	49	2	3	5	8	14	20	39

296.90: EPISODIC MOOD DISORD NOS

Type of Patients	Observed Patients	Avg. Stay	Variance	10th	25th	50th	75th	90th	95th	99th
1. SINGLE DX										
A. Not Operated										
0–19 Years	44	4.0	9	1	2	3	6	7	9	17
20–34	57	4.2	16	1	2	3	5	7	18	21
35–49	31	4.5	15	1	2	3	5	9	15	16
50–64	9	4.2	11	2	2	3	4	11	11	11
65+	1	2.0	0	2	2	2	2	2	2	2
B. Operated										
0–19 Years	0									
20–34	0									
35–49	0									
50–64	0									
65+	0									
2. MULTIPLE DX										
A. Not Operated										
0–19 Years	995	6.7	84	2	3	5	8	13	19	>99
20–34	1,227	5.2	31	1	2	4	6	11	14	27
35–49	1,163	5.6	27	1	2	4	7	12	15	26
50–64	517	6.5	39	2	3	5	8	13	18	38
65+	192	11.5	78	3	5	9	15	24	26	55
B. Operated										
0–19 Years	0									
20–34	0									
35–49	0									
50–64	2	14.0	98	7	7	14	21	21	21	21
65+	1	21.0	0	21	21	21	21	21	21	21
SUBTOTALS:										
1. SINGLE DX										
A. Not Operated	142	4.2	13	1	2	3	5	9	10	18
B. Operated	0									
2. MULTIPLE DX										
A. Not Operated	4,094	6.1	48	1	3	4	7	13	17	41
B. Operated	3	16.4	65	7	7	21	21	21	21	21
1. SINGLE DX	142	4.2	13	1	2	3	5	9	10	18
2. MULTIPLE DX	4,097	6.1	48	1	3	4	7	13	17	41
A. NOT OPERATED	4,236	6.1	47	1	3	4	7	12	17	39
B. OPERATED	3	16.4	65	7	7	21	21	21	21	21
TOTAL										
0–19 Years	1,039	6.6	81	2	3	5	7	12	18	>99
20–34	1,284	5.1	30	1	2	3	6	10	14	27
35–49	1,194	5.5	27	1	2	4	7	12	15	26
50–64	528	6.5	39	2	3	5	8	13	19	38
65+	194	11.5	78	3	5	9	15	24	26	55
GRAND TOTAL	4,239	6.1	47	1	3	4	7	12	17	39

Western Region, October 2006–September 2007 Data, by Diagnosis

296.99: EPISODIC MOOD DISORD NEC

Type of Patients	Observed Patients	Avg. Stay	Vari-ance	10th	25th	50th	75th	90th	95th	99th
1. SINGLE DX										
A. Not Operated										
0–19 Years	2	1.0	0	1	1	1	1	1	1	1
20–34	1	4.0	0	4	4	4	4	4	4	4
35–49	2	3.5	12	1	1	4	6	6	6	6
50–64	1	2.0	0	2	2	2	2	2	2	2
65+	0									
B. Operated										
0–19 Years	0									
20–34	0									
35–49	0									
50–64	0									
65+	0									
2. MULTIPLE DX										
A. Not Operated										
0–19 Years	45	7.8	53	2	4	7	10	14	15	47
20–34	69	4.3	12	1	2	3	5	8	12	20
35–49	48	4.8	11	1	3	4	7	10	12	16
50–64	44	9.0	48	2	4	7	16	18	20	28
65+	16	9.6	72	1	3	10	14	16	33	33
B. Operated										
0–19 Years	0									
20–34	0									
35–49	0									
50–64	0									
65+	0									
SUBTOTALS:										
1. SINGLE DX										
A. Not Operated	6	2.5	4	1	1	2	4	6	6	6
B. Operated	0									
2. MULTIPLE DX										
A. Not Operated	222	6.4	35	1	3	5	8	14	17	28
B. Operated	0									
1. SINGLE DX	6	2.5	4	1	1	2	4	6	6	6
2. MULTIPLE DX	222	6.4	35	1	3	5	8	14	17	28
A. NOT OPERATED	228	6.3	35	1	3	4	8	14	17	28
B. OPERATED	0									
TOTAL										
0–19 Years	47	7.5	53	1	3	7	10	14	15	47
20–34	70	4.3	12	1	2	3	5	8	12	20
35–49	50	4.8	11	1	3	4	7	9	12	16
50–64	45	8.9	48	2	4	6	12	18	20	28
65+	16	9.6	72	1	3	10	14	16	33	33
GRAND TOTAL	228	6.3	35	1	3	4	8	14	17	28

297: DELUSIONAL DISORDERS

Type of Patients	Observed Patients	Avg. Stay	Vari-ance	10th	25th	50th	75th	90th	95th	99th
1. SINGLE DX										
A. Not Operated										
0–19 Years	1	6.0	0	6	6	6	6	6	6	6
20–34	8	7.6	148	1	2	3	4	37	37	37
35–49	8	10.3	147	1	1	4	13	29	29	29
50–64	9	7.4	45	1	3	5	9	23	23	23
65+	0									
B. Operated										
0–19 Years	0									
20–34	0									
35–49	0									
50–64	0									
65+	0									
2. MULTIPLE DX										
A. Not Operated										
0–19 Years	6	9.0	93	1	1	9	17	24	24	24
20–34	57	5.5	28	1	2	4	7	14	15	28
35–49	128	7.5	54	1	3	5	9	16	22	37
50–64	120	8.6	67	1	3	6	12	21	25	35
65+	255	10.3	102	2	3	7	14	21	31	55
B. Operated										
0–19 Years	0									
20–34	0									
35–49	0									
50–64	0									
65+	1	15.0	0	15	15	15	15	15	15	15
SUBTOTALS:										
1. SINGLE DX										
A. Not Operated	26	8.3	99	1	2	4	10	29	29	37
B. Operated	0									
2. MULTIPLE DX										
A. Not Operated	566	8.8	78	1	3	6	12	20	25	43
B. Operated	1	15.0	0	15	15	15	15	15	15	15
1. SINGLE DX	26	8.3	99	1	2	4	10	29	29	37
2. MULTIPLE DX	567	8.8	78	1	3	6	12	20	25	43
A. NOT OPERATED	592	8.8	79	1	3	6	12	20	26	43
B. OPERATED	1	15.0	0	15	15	15	15	15	15	15
TOTAL										
0–19 Years	7	8.6	79	1	1	7	10	14	15	47
20–34	65	5.7	41	1	2	4	7	14	15	37
35–49	136	7.7	59	1	3	5	9	16	26	37
50–64	129	8.5	65	1	3	6	12	21	25	35
65+	256	10.4	102	2	3	7	14	21	31	55
GRAND TOTAL	593	8.8	79	1	3	6	12	20	26	43

297.1: DELUSIONAL DISORDER

Type of Patients	Observed Patients	Avg. Stay	Vari-ance	10th	25th	50th	75th	90th	95th	99th
1. SINGLE DX										
A. Not Operated										
0–19 Years	1	6.0	0	6	6	6	6	6	6	6
20–34	7	8.4	167	1	1	3	10	37	37	37
35–49	6	12.2	186	1	1	1	29	29	29	42
50–64	7	8.3	54	1	3	7	11	23	23	23
65+	0									
B. Operated										
0–19 Years	0									
20–34	0									
35–49	0									
50–64	0									
65+	0									
2. MULTIPLE DX										
A. Not Operated										
0–19 Years	3	11.3	135	1	1	9	24	24	24	24
20–34	34	5.5	29	1	2	4	7	11	15	28
35–49	91	7.6	62	1	3	5	10	15	25	42
50–64	87	9.2	79	2	3	6	13	22	25	39
65+	198	11.3	114	2	4	8	16	22	34	55
B. Operated										
0–19 Years	0									
20–34	0									
35–49	0									
50–64	0									
65+	0									
SUBTOTALS:										
1. SINGLE DX										
A. Not Operated	21	9.4	117	1	1	4	11	29	29	37
B. Operated	0									
2. MULTIPLE DX										
A. Not Operated	413	9.6	91	2	3	6	13	21	29	43
B. Operated	0									
1. SINGLE DX	21	9.4	117	1	1	4	11	29	29	37
2. MULTIPLE DX	413	9.6	91	2	3	6	13	21	29	43
A. NOT OPERATED	434	9.6	92	1	3	6	13	22	29	43
B. OPERATED	0									
TOTAL										
0–19 Years	4	10.0	98	1	1	9	9	24	24	24
20–34	41	6.0	50	1	2	4	7	11	15	37
35–49	97	7.9	69	1	3	5	10	15	29	42
50–64	94	9.1	76	2	3	6	13	22	25	39
65+	198	11.3	114	2	4	8	16	22	34	55
GRAND TOTAL	434	9.6	92	1	3	6	13	22	29	43

Length of Stay by Diagnosis and Operation, Western Region, 2008

Western Region, October 2006–September 2007 Data, by Diagnosis

298: OTH NONORGANIC PSYCHOSES

Type of Patients	Observed Patients	Avg. Stay	Vari-ance	Percentiles						
				10th	25th	50th	75th	90th	95th	99th
1. SINGLE DX										
A. Not Operated										
0–19 Years	76	7.1	38	2	3	5	9	17	21	29
20–34	439	5.8	38	1	2	4	7	12	17	29
35–49	266	5.8	44	1	2	4	7	12	18	32
50–64	156	6.7	38	1	2	5	8	17	20	27
65+	13	4.0	10	1	2	3	7	7	11	11
B. Operated										
0–19 Years	0									
20–34	0									
35–49	0									
50–64	0									
65+	0									
2. MULTIPLE DX										
A. Not Operated										
0–19 Years	528	8.1	58	2	4	6	10	16	21	34
20–34	2,793	6.9	55	2	3	5	8	14	19	42
35–49	2,305	6.8	49	2	3	5	8	14	19	34
50–64	1,710	8.2	78	2	3	5	11	18	25	52
65+	1,814	9.9	83	2	3	7	14	20	27	44
B. Operated										
0–19 Years	1	1.0	0	1	1	1	1	1	1	1
20–34	0									
35–49	5	8.4	17	2	7	9	12	12	12	12
50–64	3	34.4	>999	9	9	20	75	75	75	75
65+	11	7.7	35	3	3	6	10	12	22	22
SUBTOTALS:										
1. SINGLE DX										
A. Not Operated	950	6.0	39	1	2	4	7	13	18	29
B. Operated	0									
2. MULTIPLE DX										
A. Not Operated	9,150	7.8	65	2	3	5	10	16	22	42
B. Operated	20	11.5	252	1	3	9	12	22	22	75
1. SINGLE DX	950	6.0	39	1	2	4	7	13	18	29
2. MULTIPLE DX	9,170	7.8	65	2	3	5	10	16	22	42
A. NOT OPERATED	10,100	7.6	63	2	3	5	10	16	21	41
B. OPERATED	20	11.5	252	1	3	9	12	22	22	75
TOTAL										
0–19 Years	605	8.0	56	2	3	6	10	16	21	34
20–34	3,232	6.8	53	2	3	5	8	14	19	39
35–49	2,576	6.7	48	2	3	5	8	14	19	32
50–64	1,869	8.1	77	2	3	5	10	18	25	52
65+	1,838	9.8	83	2	3	7	14	20	27	44
GRAND TOTAL	10,120	7.6	63	2	3	5	10	16	21	41

298.9: PSYCHOSIS NOS

Type of Patients	Observed Patients	Avg. Stay	Vari-ance	Percentiles						
				10th	25th	50th	75th	90th	95th	99th
1. SINGLE DX										
A. Not Operated										
0–19 Years	74	7.1	39	2	3	5	9	17	21	29
20–34	430	5.8	38	1	2	4	7	12	17	29
35–49	263	5.8	44	1	2	4	7	12	18	32
50–64	151	6.7	39	1	2	5	8	17	20	27
65+	12	4.3	10	1	2	3	7	7	11	11
B. Operated										
0–19 Years	0									
20–34	0									
35–49	0									
50–64	0									
65+	0									
2. MULTIPLE DX										
A. Not Operated										
0–19 Years	515	8.0	55	2	4	6	10	16	21	34
20–34	2,736	6.9	54	2	3	5	8	14	19	42
35–49	2,251	6.8	49	2	3	5	8	14	19	34
50–64	1,668	8.3	79	2	3	6	11	18	26	52
65+	1,759	9.9	84	2	3	8	14	20	27	45
B. Operated										
0–19 Years	1	1.0	0	1	1	1	1	1	1	1
20–34	0									
35–49	4	8.3	23	1	2	12	12	12	12	12
50–64	3	34.4	>999	9	9	20	75	75	75	75
65+	10	7.8	38	3	3	6	10	22	22	22
SUBTOTALS:										
1. SINGLE DX										
A. Not Operated	930	6.1	40	1	2	4	7	14	19	29
B. Operated	0									
2. MULTIPLE DX										
A. Not Operated	8,929	7.8	65	2	3	5	10	16	22	42
B. Operated	18	12.0	279	1	3	9	12	22	75	75
1. SINGLE DX	930	6.1	40	1	2	4	7	14	19	29
2. MULTIPLE DX	8,947	7.8	65	2	3	5	10	16	22	42
A. NOT OPERATED	9,859	7.6	63	2	3	5	10	16	21	41
B. OPERATED	18	12.0	279	1	3	9	12	22	75	75
TOTAL										
0–19 Years	590	7.9	53	2	3	6	10	16	21	34
20–34	3,166	6.8	52	2	3	5	8	14	19	38
35–49	2,518	6.7	49	2	3	5	8	14	19	32
50–64	1,822	8.2	78	2	3	6	10	18	25	52
65+	1,781	9.9	83	2	3	7	14	20	27	45
GRAND TOTAL	9,877	7.6	63	2	3	5	10	16	21	41

299: PERVASIVE DEVEL DISORDER

Type of Patients	Observed Patients	Avg. Stay	Vari-ance	Percentiles						
				10th	25th	50th	75th	90th	95th	99th
1. SINGLE DX										
A. Not Operated										
0–19 Years	6	2.2	2	1	1	2	2	5	5	5
20–34	1	7.0	0	7	7	7	7	7	7	7
35–49	1	8.0	0	8	8	8	8	8	8	8
50–64	0									
65+	0									
B. Operated										
0–19 Years	0									
20–34	0									
35–49	0									
50–64	0									
65+	0									
2. MULTIPLE DX										
A. Not Operated										
0–19 Years	96	7.3	55	1	2	6	10	17	29	>99
20–34	37	10.8	146	2	3	4	14	27	47	48
35–49	8	11.0	329	2	3	6	7	56	56	56
50–64	2	9.5	142	1	1	10	18	18	18	18
65+	1	4.0	0	4	4	4	4	4	4	4
B. Operated										
0–19 Years	1	2.0	0	2	2	2	2	2	2	2
20–34	0									
35–49	0									
50–64	0									
65+	0									
SUBTOTALS:										
1. SINGLE DX										
A. Not Operated	8	3.5	8	1	1	2	5	8	8	8
B. Operated	0									
2. MULTIPLE DX										
A. Not Operated	144	8.4	93	1	2	6	10	21	29	56
B. Operated	1	2.0	0	2	2	2	2	2	2	2
1. SINGLE DX	8	3.5	8	1	1	2	5	8	8	8
2. MULTIPLE DX	145	8.4	93	1	2	6	10	21	29	56
A. NOT OPERATED	152	8.2	90	1	2	6	10	20	29	56
B. OPERATED	1	2.0	0	2	2	2	2	2	2	2
TOTAL										
0–19 Years	103	7.0	53	1	2	5	9	15	21	47
20–34	38	10.7	143	2	3	6	14	27	47	48
35–49	9	10.7	290	2	3	6	8	56	56	56
50–64	2	9.5	142	1	1	10	18	18	18	18
65+	1	4.0	0	4	4	4	4	4	4	4
GRAND TOTAL	153	8.1	90	1	2	5	10	20	29	56

Western Region, October 2006–September 2007 Data, by Diagnosis

300: ANX/DISSOC/SOMAT DISORD

Type of Patients	Observed Patients	Avg. Stay	Vari-ance	Percentiles						
				10th	25th	50th	75th	90th	95th	99th
1. SINGLE DX										
A. Not Operated										
0–19 Years	33	2.9	9	1	1	2	3	6	8	17
20–34	38	4.5	32	1	1	2	6	8	25	26
35–49	19	1.6	1	1	1	1	2	4	4	4
50–64	11	2.5	3	1	1	2	4	5	6	6
65+	4	1.3	<1	1	1	1	2	2	2	2
B. Operated										
0–19 Years	0									
20–34	0									
35–49	0									
50–64	0									
65+	0									
2. MULTIPLE DX										
A. Not Operated										
0–19 Years	330	4.1	38	1	1	3	5	8	10	28
20–34	814	3.5	19	1	1	2	4	7	10	19
35–49	1,212	3.2	13	1	1	2	4	7	9	19
50–64	1,129	2.9	8	1	1	2	3	6	8	15
65+	877	3.7	20	1	1	2	4	9	13	22
B. Operated										
0–19 Years	0									
20–34	2	1.0	0	1	1	1	1	1	1	1
35–49	10	3.1	6	1	1	2	5	8	8	8
50–64	7	3.8	21	1	1	2	7	13	13	13
65+	7	7.3	71	1	1	4	9	25	25	25
SUBTOTALS:										
1. SINGLE DX										
A. Not Operated	105	3.2	16	1	1	2	3	7	8	25
B. Operated	0									
2. MULTIPLE DX										
A. Not Operated	4,362	3.3	16	1	1	2	4	7	10	20
B. Operated	26	4.3	28	1	1	2	5	9	13	25
1. SINGLE DX	105	3.2	16	1	1	2	3	7	8	25
2. MULTIPLE DX	4,388	3.4	16	1	1	2	4	7	8	20
A. NOT OPERATED	4,467	3.3	16	1	1	2	4	7	10	20
B. OPERATED	26	4.3	28	1	1	2	5	9	13	25
TOTAL										
0–19 Years	363	4.0	36	1	1	3	5	8	10	28
20–34	854	3.6	20	1	1	2	4	7	10	21
35–49	1,241	3.1	13	1	1	2	4	7	9	19
50–64	1,147	2.9	8	1	1	2	3	6	8	15
65+	888	3.8	20	1	1	2	4	9	13	22
GRAND TOTAL	4,493	3.3	16	1	1	2	4	7	10	20

300.00: ANXIETY STATE NOS

Type of Patients	Observed Patients	Avg. Stay	Vari-ance	Percentiles						
				10th	25th	50th	75th	90th	95th	99th
1. SINGLE DX										
A. Not Operated										
0–19 Years	2	2.5	<1	2	2	3	3	3	3	3
20–34	7	3.4	8	1	1	2	6	7	8	8
35–49	3	1.0	0	1	1	1	1	1	1	1
50–64	2	1.5	<1	1	1	1	2	2	2	2
65+	2	1.0	0	1	1	1	1	1	1	1
B. Operated										
0–19 Years	0									
20–34	0									
35–49	0									
50–64	0									
65+	0									
2. MULTIPLE DX										
A. Not Operated										
0–19 Years	51	5.6	151	1	2	3	6	10	10	>99
20–34	120	3.1	16	1	1	2	3	7	10	17
35–49	301	2.0	5	1	1	1	2	4	5	13
50–64	392	2.1	5	1	1	1	2	4	6	12
65+	362	2.7	10	1	1	2	3	5	9	16
B. Operated										
0–19 Years	0									
20–34	0									
35–49	2	1.0	0	1	1	1	1	1	1	1
50–64	5	3.8	26	1	1	2	2	13	13	13
65+	3	2.0	3	1	1	4	4	4	4	4
SUBTOTALS:										
1. SINGLE DX										
A. Not Operated	16	2.3	5	1	1	2	3	7	8	8
B. Operated	0									
2. MULTIPLE DX										
A. Not Operated	1,226	2.5	14	1	1	2	3	5	8	15
B. Operated	10	2.7	14	1	1	2	2	4	13	13
1. SINGLE DX	16	2.3	5	1	1	2	3	7	8	8
2. MULTIPLE DX	1,236	2.5	14	1	1	2	3	5	8	15
A. NOT OPERATED	1,242	2.5	14	1	1	2	3	5	8	15
B. OPERATED	10	2.7	14	1	1	2	2	4	13	13
TOTAL										
0–19 Years	53	5.5	146	1	2	3	6	10	10	>99
20–34	127	3.1	16	1	1	2	3	7	9	17
35–49	306	2.0	5	1	1	2	2	4	5	13
50–64	399	2.1	5	1	1	2	2	4	6	13
65+	367	2.7	9	1	1	2	3	5	9	16
GRAND TOTAL	1,252	2.5	14	1	1	2	3	5	8	15

300.01: PANIC DIS W/O AGORAPHOB

Type of Patients	Observed Patients	Avg. Stay	Vari-ance	Percentiles						
				10th	25th	50th	75th	90th	95th	99th
1. SINGLE DX										
A. Not Operated										
0–19 Years	1	2.0	0	2	2	2	2	2	2	2
20–34	4	1.8	<1	1	1	1	3	3	3	3
35–49	3	2.0	3	1	1	1	4	4	4	4
50–64	2	1.0	0	1	1	1	1	1	1	1
65+	0									
B. Operated										
0–19 Years	0									
20–34	0									
35–49	0									
50–64	0									
65+	0									
2. MULTIPLE DX										
A. Not Operated										
0–19 Years	25	2.7	5	1	1	2	4	5	6	10
20–34	104	2.5	6	1	1	2	3	5	9	11
35–49	167	2.0	3	1	1	1	2	4	5	11
50–64	178	2.0	4	1	1	1	2	4	5	11
65+	185	2.5	7	1	1	2	3	5	7	13
B. Operated										
0–19 Years	0									
20–34	1	1.0	0	1	1	1	1	1	1	1
35–49	0									
50–64	0									
65+	0									
SUBTOTALS:										
1. SINGLE DX										
A. Not Operated	10	1.7	1	1	1	1	2	3	4	4
B. Operated	0									
2. MULTIPLE DX										
A. Not Operated	659	2.3	5	1	1	1	3	5	6	11
B. Operated	1	1.0	0	1	1	1	1	1	1	1
1. SINGLE DX	10	1.7	1	1	1	1	2	3	4	4
2. MULTIPLE DX	660	2.3	5	1	1	1	3	5	6	11
A. NOT OPERATED	669	2.3	5	1	1	1	3	5	6	11
B. OPERATED	1	1.0	0	1	1	1	1	1	1	1
TOTAL										
0–19 Years	26	2.6	5	1	1	2	4	5	6	10
20–34	109	2.5	6	1	1	2	3	5	9	11
35–49	170	2.0	3	1	1	1	2	4	5	11
50–64	180	2.0	4	1	1	1	2	4	5	11
65+	185	2.5	7	1	1	2	3	5	7	13
GRAND TOTAL	670	2.3	5	1	1	1	3	5	6	11

Length of Stay by Diagnosis and Operation, Western Region, 2008

Western Region, October 2006–September 2007 Data, by Diagnosis

300.02: GENERAL ANXIETY DISORD

Type of Patients	Observed Patients	Avg. Stay	Vari-ance	Percentiles 10th	25th	50th	75th	90th	95th	99th
1. SINGLE DX										
A. Not Operated										
0–19 Years	2	9.9	97	3	3	3	17	17	17	17
20–34	0									
35–49	0									
50–64	0									
65+	1	1.0	0	1	1	1	1	1	1	1
B. Operated										
0–19 Years	0									
20–34	0									
35–49	0									
50–64	0									
65+	0									
2. MULTIPLE DX										
A. Not Operated										
0–19 Years	21	5.3	14	1	3	5	6	10	13	14
20–34	46	3.2	5	1	2	3	4	5	7	12
35–49	56	4.2	11	1	2	3	6	8	12	13
50–64	56	4.4	14	1	2	3	7	8	11	22
65+	51	6.9	35	1	2	6	10	13	17	29
B. Operated										
0–19 Years	0									
20–34	0									
35–49	0									
50–64	0									
65+	1	25.0	0	25	25	25	25	25	25	25
SUBTOTALS:										
1. SINGLE DX										
A. Not Operated	3	6.9	75	1	1	3	17	17	17	17
B. Operated	0									
2. MULTIPLE DX										
A. Not Operated	230	4.8	18	1	2	3	7	10	12	22
B. Operated	1	25.0	0	25	25	25	25	25	25	25
1. SINGLE DX	3	6.9	75	1	1	3	17	17	17	17
2. MULTIPLE DX	231	4.8	19	1	2	3	7	10	13	25
A. NOT OPERATED	233	4.8	18	1	2	3	7	10	13	22
B. OPERATED	1	25.0	0	25	25	25	25	25	25	25
TOTAL										
0–19 Years	23	5.7	19	1	3	5	8	13	14	17
20–34	46	3.2	5	1	2	3	4	5	7	12
35–49	56	4.2	11	1	2	3	6	10	12	13
50–64	56	4.4	14	1	2	3	7	8	11	22
65+	53	7.2	40	1	2	6	10	14	25	29
GRAND TOTAL	234	4.9	20	1	2	3	7	10	13	25

300.11: CONVERSION DISORDER

Type of Patients	Observed Patients	Avg. Stay	Vari-ance	Percentiles 10th	25th	50th	75th	90th	95th	99th
1. SINGLE DX										
A. Not Operated										
0–19 Years	8	1.9	<1	1	1	2	2	3	3	3
20–34	12	4.4	10	1	1	3	3	7	11	11
35–49	2	1.5	<1	1	1	2	2	2	2	2
50–64	2	4.5	<1	4	4	5	5	5	5	5
65+	0									
B. Operated										
0–19 Years	0									
20–34	0									
35–49	0									
50–64	0									
65+	0									
2. MULTIPLE DX										
A. Not Operated										
0–19 Years	65	3.1	9	1	1	2	4	5	8	21
20–34	154	3.2	6	1	2	3	4	6	7	17
35–49	222	3.2	6	1	2	3	4	6	8	10
50–64	157	3.5	8	1	2	3	4	6	10	15
65+	44	4.7	13	1	2	4	6	9	11	20
B. Operated										
0–19 Years	0									
20–34	0									
35–49	4	3.8	2	2	2	4	5	5	5	5
50–64	0									
65+	2	5.5	12	3	3	8	8	8	8	8
SUBTOTALS:										
1. SINGLE DX										
A. Not Operated	24	3.3	7	1	1	2	5	7	7	11
B. Operated	0									
2. MULTIPLE DX										
A. Not Operated	642	3.3	7	1	2	3	4	6	8	15
B. Operated	6	4.3	5	2	3	5	5	8	8	8
1. SINGLE DX	24	3.3	7	1	1	2	5	7	7	11
2. MULTIPLE DX	648	3.4	7	1	2	3	4	6	8	15
A. NOT OPERATED	666	3.3	7	1	2	3	4	6	8	15
B. OPERATED	6	4.3	5	2	3	5	5	8	8	8
TOTAL										
0–19 Years	73	2.9	8	1	1	2	3	5	8	21
20–34	166	3.3	7	1	2	3	4	6	7	17
35–49	228	3.2	6	1	2	3	4	6	8	10
50–64	159	3.5	8	1	2	3	4	6	10	15
65+	46	4.7	13	1	2	4	6	9	11	20
GRAND TOTAL	672	3.4	7	1	2	3	4	6	8	15

300.4: DYSTHYMIC DISORDER

Type of Patients	Observed Patients	Avg. Stay	Vari-ance	Percentiles 10th	25th	50th	75th	90th	95th	99th
1. SINGLE DX										
A. Not Operated										
0–19 Years	8	4.0	5	1	3	3	5	8	8	8
20–34	6	1.5	<1	1	1	2	2	3	3	2
35–49	3	2.0	<1	1	2	2	3	3	3	3
50–64	5	2.8	4	1	2	3	3	6	6	6
65+	0									
B. Operated										
0–19 Years	0									
20–34	0									
35–49	0									
50–64	0									
65+	0									
2. MULTIPLE DX										
A. Not Operated										
0–19 Years	79	4.0	6	1	2	4	5	7	9	11
20–34	170	3.4	9	1	1	3	4	6	8	17
35–49	229	4.2	15	1	1	3	5	8	12	19
50–64	182	3.7	11	1	1	3	5	7	11	17
65+	152	5.6	36	1	2	3	7	14	20	23
B. Operated										
0–19 Years	0									
20–34	0									
35–49	3	2.0	3	1	1	1	4	4	4	4
50–64	2	4.0	18	1	1	7	7	7	7	7
65+	1	9.0	0	9	9	9	9	9	9	9
SUBTOTALS:										
1. SINGLE DX										
A. Not Operated	22	2.8	4	1	1	2	3	6	6	8
B. Operated	0									
2. MULTIPLE DX										
A. Not Operated	812	4.2	16	1	2	3	5	8	12	20
B. Operated	6	3.8	12	1	1	1	7	9	9	9
1. SINGLE DX	22	2.8	4	1	1	2	3	6	6	8
2. MULTIPLE DX	818	4.2	16	1	2	3	5	8	12	20
A. NOT OPERATED	834	4.1	16	1	2	3	5	8	12	20
B. OPERATED	6	3.8	12	1	1	1	7	9	9	9
TOTAL										
0–19 Years	87	4.0	6	1	2	4	5	7	9	11
20–34	176	3.3	9	1	1	3	4	6	8	17
35–49	235	4.2	15	1	2	3	5	8	12	19
50–64	189	3.6	10	1	1	3	5	7	11	17
65+	153	5.6	36	1	2	3	7	14	20	23
GRAND TOTAL	840	4.1	16	1	2	3	5	8	12	20

Length of Stay by Diagnosis and Operation, Western Region, 2008

Western Region, October 2006–September 2007 Data, by Diagnosis

300.9: NONPSYCH MENTAL DIS NOS

Type of Patients	Observed Patients	Avg. Stay	Vari-ance	Percentiles						
				10th	25th	50th	75th	90th	95th	99th
1. SINGLE DX										
A. *Not Operated*										
0–19 Years	10	1.4	<1	1	1	1	1	4	4	4
20–34	3	18.2	154	4	4	25	26	26	26	26
35–49	6	1.3	<1	1	1	1	2	2	2	2
50–64	0									
65+	1	2.0	0	2	2	2	2	2	2	2
B. *Operated*										
0–19 Years	0									
20–34	0									
35–49	0									
50–64	0									
65+	0									
2. MULTIPLE DX										
A. *Not Operated*										
0–19 Years	50	2.1	3	1	1	1	3	4	5	8
20–34	106	3.1	10	1	1	2	4	7	10	16
35–49	119	3.5	26	1	1	2	4	6	9	32
50–64	69	3.0	12	1	1	2	4	7	9	20
65+	28	5.9	31	1	2	3	9	15	17	19
B. *Operated*										
0–19 Years	0									
20–34	0									
35–49	1	8.0	0	8	8	8	8	8	8	8
50–64	0									
65+	0									
SUBTOTALS:										
1. SINGLE DX										
A. *Not Operated*	20	3.9	55	1	1	1	2	4	25	26
B. *Operated*	0									
2. MULTIPLE DX										
A. *Not Operated*	372	3.3	17	1	1	2	4	7	10	23
B. *Operated*	1	8.0	0	8	8	8	8	8	8	8
1. SINGLE DX	20	3.9	55	1	1	1	2	4	25	26
2. MULTIPLE DX	373	3.3	17	1	1	2	4	7	10	23
A. NOT OPERATED	392	3.3	18	1	1	2	4	7	11	25
B. OPERATED	1	8.0	0	8	8	8	8	8	8	8
TOTAL										
0–19 Years	60	2.0	2	1	1	1	3	4	5	8
20–34	109	3.5	19	1	1	1	4	8	11	25
35–49	126	3.4	25	1	1	2	4	6	9	32
50–64	69	3.0	12	1	1	2	4	7	9	20
65+	29	5.7	31	1	2	3	9	15	17	19
GRAND TOTAL	393	3.3	18	1	1	2	4	7	11	25

301: PERSONALITY DISORDERS

Type of Patients	Observed Patients	Avg. Stay	Vari-ance	Percentiles						
				10th	25th	50th	75th	90th	95th	99th
1. SINGLE DX										
A. *Not Operated*										
0–19 Years	2	1.0	0	1	1	1	1	1	1	1
20–34	4	4.5	8	1	4	5	8	8	8	8
35–49	3	11.6	94	1	1	14	20	20	20	20
50–64	3	1.0	0	1	1	1	1	1	1	1
65+	0									
B. *Operated*										
0–19 Years	0									
20–34	0									
35–49	0									
50–64	0									
65+	0									
2. MULTIPLE DX										
A. *Not Operated*										
0–19 Years	36	6.5	72	1	2	4	7	11	36	41
20–34	98	4.6	22	1	1	4	6	9	13	36
35–49	78	4.2	12	1	2	3	6	8	11	20
50–64	68	4.1	12	1	2	3	5	9	11	16
65+	37	7.1	62	1	3	5	10	13	32	39
B. *Operated*										
0–19 Years	0									
20–34	1	3.0	0	3	3	3	3	3	3	3
35–49	0									
50–64	0									
65+	0									
SUBTOTALS:										
1. SINGLE DX										
A. *Not Operated*	12	4.8	39	1	1	1	8	14	20	20
B. *Operated*	0									
2. MULTIPLE DX										
A. *Not Operated*	317	4.9	28	1	2	3	6	10	13	36
B. *Operated*	1	3.0	0	3	3	3	3	3	3	3
1. SINGLE DX	12	4.8	39	1	1	1	8	14	20	20
2. MULTIPLE DX	318	4.9	28	1	2	3	6	10	13	36
A. NOT OPERATED	329	4.9	28	1	2	3	6	10	13	36
B. OPERATED	1	3.0	0	3	3	3	3	3	3	3
TOTAL										
0–19 Years	38	6.2	70	1	2	4	7	11	36	41
20–34	103	4.5	21	1	1	4	6	9	11	17
35–49	81	4.5	16	1	2	3	6	8	13	20
50–64	71	4.0	12	1	1	3	5	9	11	16
65+	37	7.1	62	1	3	5	10	13	32	39
GRAND TOTAL	330	4.9	28	1	2	3	6	10	13	36

302: SEX/GENDER ID DISORDERS

Type of Patients	Observed Patients	Avg. Stay	Vari-ance	Percentiles						
				10th	25th	50th	75th	90th	95th	99th
1. SINGLE DX										
A. *Not Operated*										
0–19 Years	0									
20–34	0									
35–49	0									
50–64	0									
65+	0									
B. *Operated*										
0–19 Years	0									
20–34	1	1.0	0	1	1	1	1	1	1	1
35–49	1	1.0	0	1	1	1	1	1	1	1
50–64	0									
65+	0									
2. MULTIPLE DX										
A. *Not Operated*										
0–19 Years	2	4.0	0	4	4	4	4	4	4	4
20–34	2	1.5	<1	1	1	1	1	2	2	2
35–49	1	3.0	0	3	3	3	3	3	3	3
50–64	1	1.0	0	1	1	1	1	1	1	1
65+	0									
B. *Operated*										
0–19 Years	0									
20–34	7	1.0	0	1	1	1	1	1	1	1
35–49	1	2.0	0	2	2	2	2	2	2	2
50–64	1	1.0	0	1	1	1	1	1	1	1
65+	1	1.0	0	1	1	1	1	1	1	1
SUBTOTALS:										
1. SINGLE DX										
A. *Not Operated*	0									
B. *Operated*	2	1.0	0	1	1	1	1	1	1	1
2. MULTIPLE DX										
A. *Not Operated*	6	2.5	2	1	1	3	4	4	4	4
B. *Operated*	10	1.1	<1	1	1	1	1	1	2	2
1. SINGLE DX	2	1.0	0	1	1	1	1	1	1	1
2. MULTIPLE DX	16	1.6	1	1	1	1	2	4	4	4
A. NOT OPERATED	6	2.5	2	1	1	3	4	4	4	4
B. OPERATED	12	1.1	<1	1	1	1	1	1	2	2
TOTAL										
0–19 Years	2	4.0	0	4	4	4	4	4	4	4
20–34	10	1.1	<1	1	1	1	1	1	2	2
35–49	3	2.0	1	1	1	1	3	3	3	3
50–64	2	1.0	0	1	1	1	1	1	1	1
65+	1	1.0	0	1	1	1	1	1	1	1
GRAND TOTAL	18	1.6	1	1	1	1	2	4	4	4

Length of Stay by Diagnosis and Operation, Western Region, 2008

Western Region, October 2006–September 2007 Data, by Diagnosis

303: ALCOHOL DEPENDENCE SYND

Type of Patients	Observed Patients	Avg. Stay	Vari-ance	10th	25th	50th	75th	90th	95th	99th
1. SINGLE DX										
A. Not Operated										
0–19 Years	3	12.3	232	3	3	4	30	30	30	30
20–34	54	14.6	394	1	3	4	29	30	58	90
35–49	119	13.0	205	1	3	5	28	30	30	>99
50–64	67	11.0	248	1	2	4	14	30	30	89
65+	9	21.6	148	2	8	29	30	31	31	31
B. Operated										
0–19 Years	0									
20–34	0									
35–49	0									
50–64	0									
65+	0									
2. MULTIPLE DX										
A. Not Operated										
0–19 Years	74	10.1	117	1	1	5	16	30	30	42
20–34	954	6.8	66	1	2	4	8	19	28	30
35–49	2,814	5.7	40	1	2	4	7	14	19	30
50–64	2,323	5.7	34	1	2	4	7	13	18	29
65+	662	5.8	34	1	2	4	7	14	17	30
B. Operated										
0–19 Years	0									
20–34	0									
35–49	5	13.5	214	1	4	6	21	36	36	36
50–64	9	8.1	21	3	4	8	12	15	15	15
65+	4	12.2	76	3	3	8	23	23	23	23
SUBTOTALS:										
1. SINGLE DX										
A. Not Operated	252	13.1	255	1	2	5	28	30	30	90
B. Operated	0									
2. MULTIPLE DX										
A. Not Operated	6,827	5.9	42	1	2	4	7	14	20	30
B. Operated	18	10.5	80	3	4	8	15	23	36	36
1. SINGLE DX	252	13.1	255	1	2	5	28	30	30	90
2. MULTIPLE DX	6,845	5.9	42	1	2	4	7	14	20	30
A. NOT OPERATED	7,079	6.2	51	1	2	4	7	14	21	30
B. OPERATED	18	10.5	80	3	4	8	15	23	36	36
TOTAL										
0–19 Years	77	10.2	119	1	1	5	16	30	30	42
20–34	1,008	7.2	86	1	2	4	8	20	29	30
35–49	2,938	6.0	49	1	2	4	7	14	20	30
50–64	2,399	5.9	41	1	2	4	7	14	19	30
65+	675	6.1	39	1	2	4	7	14	18	30
GRAND TOTAL	7,097	6.2	51	1	2	4	7	14	21	30

303.00: AC ALCOHOL INTOX-UNSPEC

Type of Patients	Observed Patients	Avg. Stay	Vari-ance	10th	25th	50th	75th	90th	95th	99th
1. SINGLE DX										
A. Not Operated										
0–19 Years	0									
20–34	6	1.7	<1	1	1	1	2	2	3	3
35–49	7	1.3	<1	1	1	1	2	2	2	2
50–64	5	1.0	0	1	1	1	1	1	1	1
65+	0									
B. Operated										
0–19 Years	0									
20–34	0									
35–49	0									
50–64	0									
65+	0									
2. MULTIPLE DX										
A. Not Operated										
0–19 Years	12	1.4	<1	1	1	1	2	2	4	4
20–34	120	2.2	2	1	1	2	3	4	5	7
35–49	377	2.7	5	1	1	2	3	6	7	11
50–64	291	2.7	4	1	1	2	4	5	6	10
65+	109	4.4	32	1	1	3	5	10	13	20
B. Operated										
0–19 Years	0									
20–34	0									
35–49	1	6.0	0	6	6	6	6	6	6	6
50–64	3	5.3	16	3	3	3	10	10	10	10
65+	1	23.0	0	23	23	23	23	23	23	23
SUBTOTALS:										
1. SINGLE DX										
A. Not Operated	18	1.3	<1	1	1	1	2	2	3	3
B. Operated	0									
2. MULTIPLE DX										
A. Not Operated	909	2.8	8	1	1	2	3	6	7	12
B. Operated	5	9.0	69	3	3	6	10	23	23	23
1. SINGLE DX	18	1.3	<1	1	1	2	2	2	3	3
2. MULTIPLE DX	914	2.9	9	1	1	2	3	6	7	12
A. NOT OPERATED	927	2.8	8	1	1	2	3	6	7	12
B. OPERATED	5	9.0	69	3	3	6	10	23	23	23
TOTAL										
0–19 Years	12	1.4	<1	1	1	1	2	2	4	4
20–34	126	2.1	2	1	1	2	3	4	5	7
35–49	385	2.7	5	1	1	2	3	6	7	11
50–64	299	2.7	4	1	1	2	4	5	7	10
65+	110	4.6	35	1	1	3	5	10	18	23
GRAND TOTAL	932	2.8	8	1	1	2	3	6	7	12

303.01: AC ALCOHOL INTOX-CONT

Type of Patients	Observed Patients	Avg. Stay	Vari-ance	10th	25th	50th	75th	90th	95th	99th
1. SINGLE DX										
A. Not Operated										
0–19 Years	0									
20–34	2	2.0	2	1	1	1	3	3	3	3
35–49	14	4.4	54	1	1	3	3	8	29	29
50–64	11	4.1	64	1	1	1	3	4	28	28
65+	0									
B. Operated										
0–19 Years	0									
20–34	0									
35–49	0									
50–64	0									
65+	0									
2. MULTIPLE DX										
A. Not Operated										
0–19 Years	8	1.8	1	1	1	1	2	4	4	4
20–34	171	2.9	5	1	1	2	4	5	7	12
35–49	670	3.3	9	1	1	3	4	7	9	15
50–64	605	4.2	20	1	2	3	5	8	12	24
65+	218	4.4	20	1	2	3	6	8	11	27
B. Operated										
0–19 Years	0									
20–34	0									
35–49	2	2.5	4	1	1	3	4	4	4	4
50–64	2	10.0	8	8	8	12	12	12	12	12
65+	1	15.0	0	15	15	15	15	15	15	15
SUBTOTALS:										
1. SINGLE DX										
A. Not Operated	27	4.1	52	1	1	2	3	8	28	29
B. Operated	0									
2. MULTIPLE DX										
A. Not Operated	1,672	3.7	14	1	2	3	5	7	10	21
B. Operated	5	8.0	32	1	4	8	12	15	15	15
1. SINGLE DX	27	4.1	52	1	1	2	3	8	28	29
2. MULTIPLE DX	1,677	3.7	15	1	2	3	5	7	10	21
A. NOT OPERATED	1,699	3.7	15	1	1	3	5	7	10	23
B. OPERATED	5	8.0	32	1	4	8	12	15	15	15
TOTAL										
0–19 Years	8	1.8	1	1	1	1	2	4	4	4
20–34	173	2.9	4	1	1	2	4	5	7	12
35–49	686	3.4	10	1	1	3	4	7	9	15
50–64	618	4.2	21	1	2	3	5	8	12	26
65+	219	4.5	21	1	2	3	6	8	11	27
GRAND TOTAL	1,704	3.7	15	1	1	3	5	7	10	23

Western Region, October 2006–September 2007 Data, by Diagnosis

303.90: ALC DEP NEC & NOS-UNSPEC

Type of Patients	Observed Patients	Avg. Stay	Variance	Percentiles						
				10th	25th	50th	75th	90th	95th	99th
1. SINGLE DX										
A. Not Operated										
0–19 Years	0									
20–34	8	17.7	939	1	1	4	30	90	90	90
35–49	15	14.1	242	1	2	14	21	30	57	57
50–64	9	6.2	61	1	2	3	6	24	24	24
65+	1	30.0	0	30	30	30	30	30	30	30
B. Operated										
0–19 Years	0									
20–34	0									
35–49	0									
50–64	0									
65+	0									
2. MULTIPLE DX										
A. Not Operated										
0–19 Years	15	9.5	70	2	3	5	16	20	30	30
20–34	178	6.4	46	1	2	3	7	16	21	30
35–49	496	6.4	60	1	2	4	8	14	19	30
50–64	356	6.4	41	2	3	4	7	14	19	27
65+	73	5.6	38	2	2	4	6	14	15	33
B. Operated										
0–19 Years	0									
20–34	0									
35–49	0									
50–64	2	8.5	40	4	4	13	13	13	13	13
65+	0									
SUBTOTALS:										
1. SINGLE DX										
A. Not Operated	33	13.3	354	1	2	4	18	30	57	90
B. Operated	0									
2. MULTIPLE DX										
A. Not Operated	1,118	6.4	51	1	2	4	8	15	20	30
B. Operated	2	8.5	40	4	4	13	13	13	13	13
1. SINGLE DX	33	13.3	354	1	2	4	18	30	57	90
2. MULTIPLE DX	1,120	6.4	51	1	2	4	8	15	20	30
A. NOT OPERATED	1,151	6.6	60	1	2	4	8	15	21	30
B. OPERATED	2	8.5	40	4	4	13	13	13	13	13
TOTAL										
0–19 Years	15	9.5	70	2	3	5	16	20	30	30
20–34	186	6.9	84	1	2	3	8	16	21	30
35–49	511	6.6	67	1	2	4	8	14	20	30
50–64	367	6.4	41	2	2	4	7	14	19	27
65+	74	5.9	46	2	2	4	6	14	28	33
GRAND TOTAL	1,153	6.6	60	1	2	4	8	15	21	30

303.91: ALC DEP NEC & NOS-CONT

Type of Patients	Observed Patients	Avg. Stay	Variance	Percentiles						
				10th	25th	50th	75th	90th	95th	99th
1. SINGLE DX										
A. Not Operated										
0–19 Years	3	12.3	232	3	3	4	30	30	30	30
20–34	36	17.4	352	1	3	9	29	30	58	89
35–49	81	15.4	218	2	4	10	29	30	30	>99
50–64	41	13.9	282	3	4	5	30	30	30	89
65+	8	20.6	157	2	7	28	30	31	31	31
B. Operated										
0–19 Years	0									
20–34	0									
35–49	0									
50–64	0									
65+	0									
2. MULTIPLE DX										
A. Not Operated										
0–19 Years	32	14.2	102	3	6	11	21	30	30	31
20–34	402	9.3	101	1	3	5	11	28	30	30
35–49	1,104	7.3	47	2	3	5	9	14	21	30
50–64	942	7.1	40	2	3	5	8	14	21	30
65+	219	7.1	36	2	3	5	10	14	21	30
B. Operated										
0–19 Years	0									
20–34	0									
35–49	2	28.4	112	21	21	21	36	36	36	36
50–64	2	10.0	50	5	5	5	15	15	15	15
65+	1	8.0	0	8	8	8	8	8	8	8
SUBTOTALS:										
1. SINGLE DX										
A. Not Operated	169	15.6	257	2	4	8	29	30	31	>99
B. Operated	0									
2. MULTIPLE DX										
A. Not Operated	2,699	7.6	53	2	3	5	9	15	26	30
B. Operated	5	17.0	151	5	8	15	21	36	36	36
1. SINGLE DX	169	15.6	257	2	4	8	29	30	31	>99
2. MULTIPLE DX	2,704	7.6	54	2	3	5	9	15	26	30
A. NOT OPERATED	2,868	8.1	69	2	3	5	10	20	29	30
B. OPERATED	5	17.0	151	5	8	15	21	36	36	36
TOTAL										
0–19 Years	35	14.0	107	3	4	11	23	30	30	31
20–34	438	10.0	126	1	3	5	12	29	30	37
35–49	1,187	7.9	64	2	3	5	9	15	21	30
50–64	985	7.4	51	2	3	5	9	14	23	30
65+	228	7.6	46	2	3	5	10	14	23	30
GRAND TOTAL	2,873	8.1	69	2	3	5	10	20	29	30

304: DRUG DEPENDENCE

Type of Patients	Observed Patients	Avg. Stay	Variance	Percentiles						
				10th	25th	50th	75th	90th	95th	99th
1. SINGLE DX										
A. Not Operated										
0–19 Years	5	7.7	159	1	1	2	4	30	30	30
20–34	58	10.2	153	1	2	4	15	30	30	57
35–49	47	8.6	134	2	3	4	7	30	30	>99
50–64	23	3.2	3	1	2	3	4	6	6	6
65+	1	5.0	0	5	5	5	5	5	5	5
B. Operated										
0–19 Years	0									
20–34	0									
35–49	0									
50–64	0									
65+	0									
2. MULTIPLE DX										
A. Not Operated										
0–19 Years	223	17.0	244	1	4	10	29	42	42	42
20–34	974	7.7	72	2	3	5	9	18	24	31
35–49	1,020	6.7	40	1	3	4	8	14	20	30
50–64	680	6.6	27	2	3	5	8	14	17	27
65+	82	7.3	28	2	3	6	10	14	18	28
B. Operated										
0–19 Years	1	42.0	0	42	42	42	42	42	42	42
20–34	0									
35–49	3	9.0	7	6	6	10	11	11	11	11
50–64	1	5.0	0	5	5	5	5	5	5	5
65+	0									
SUBTOTALS:										
1. SINGLE DX										
A. Not Operated	134	8.3	123	1	2	4	6	30	30	59
B. Operated	0									
2. MULTIPLE DX										
A. Not Operated	2,979	7.8	69	2	3	5	9	17	25	42
B. Operated	5	14.8	236	5	6	10	11	42	42	42
1. SINGLE DX	134	8.3	123	1	2	4	6	30	30	59
2. MULTIPLE DX	2,984	7.8	70	2	3	5	9	17	25	42
A. NOT OPERATED	3,113	7.8	72	2	3	5	9	18	27	42
B. OPERATED	5	14.8	236	5	6	10	11	42	42	42
TOTAL										
0–19 Years	229	16.9	245	1	3	10	29	42	42	42
20–34	1,032	7.8	77	2	3	5	9	18	26	31
35–49	1,070	6.7	44	1	3	4	8	15	21	30
50–64	704	6.5	26	2	3	5	8	14	17	27
65+	83	7.3	28	2	3	6	10	14	18	28
GRAND TOTAL	3,118	7.8	72	2	3	5	9	18	27	42

Length of Stay by Diagnosis and Operation, Western Region, 2008

Western Region, October 2006–September 2007 Data, by Diagnosis

304.00: OPIOID DEPENDENCE-UNSPEC

Type of Patients	Observed Patients	Avg. Stay	Vari-ance	10th	25th	50th	75th	90th	95th	99th
1. SINGLE DX										
A. Not Operated										
0–19 Years	0									
20–34	4	12.3	151	2	2	14	29	29	29	29
35–49	1	2.0	0	2	2	2	2	2	2	2
50–64	0									
65+	0									
B. Operated										
0–19 Years	0									
20–34	0									
35–49	0									
50–64	0									
65+	0									
2. MULTIPLE DX										
A. Not Operated										
0–19 Years	17	5.9	30	2	2	5	6	14	23	23
20–34	113	5.5	22	1	3	4	6	13	14	21
35–49	97	5.9	36	2	3	4	6	15	21	>99
50–64	82	6.2	33	2	3	4	8	14	19	27
65+	12	7.4	72	1	1	4	8	20	28	28
B. Operated										
0–19 Years	0									
20–34	0									
35–49	1	11.0	0	11	11	11	11	11	11	11
50–64	0									
65+	0									
SUBTOTALS:										
1. SINGLE DX										
A. Not Operated	5	10.2	135	2	2	4	14	29	29	29
B. Operated	0									
2. MULTIPLE DX										
A. Not Operated	321	5.9	31	2	3	4	7	14	19	28
B. Operated	1	11.0	0	11	11	11	11	11	11	11
1. SINGLE DX	5	10.2	135	2	2	4	14	29	29	29
2. MULTIPLE DX	322	5.9	31	2	3	4	7	14	19	28
A. NOT OPERATED	326	6.0	32	2	3	4	7	14	20	29
B. OPERATED	1	11.0	0	11	11	11	11	11	11	11
TOTAL										
0–19 Years	17	5.9	30	2	2	5	6	14	23	23
20–34	117	5.7	27	1	3	4	7	14	14	28
35–49	99	5.9	35	2	3	4	6	15	21	>99
50–64	82	6.2	33	2	3	4	8	14	19	27
65+	12	7.4	72	1	1	4	8	20	28	28
GRAND TOTAL	327	6.0	32	2	3	4	7	14	20	29

304.01: OPIOID DEPENDENCE-CONT

Type of Patients	Observed Patients	Avg. Stay	Vari-ance	10th	25th	50th	75th	90th	95th	99th
1. SINGLE DX										
A. Not Operated										
0–19 Years	4	9.3	193	1	2	4	30	30	30	30
20–34	32	6.7	80	2	2	3	5	22	30	30
35–49	26	5.0	28	3	3	4	5	7	7	30
50–64	16	3.5	2	2	3	3	4	6	6	6
65+	1	5.0	0	5	5	5	5	5	5	5
B. Operated										
0–19 Years	0									
20–34	0									
35–49	0									
50–64	0									
65+	0									
2. MULTIPLE DX										
A. Not Operated										
0–19 Years	30	6.4	48	2	2	5	6	18	27	30
20–34	334	6.1	39	2	3	4	7	11	21	30
35–49	373	5.6	23	2	3	4	7	10	14	29
50–64	324	5.7	13	2	4	5	7	9	12	19
65+	37	6.1	16	2	4	6	7	10	16	21
B. Operated										
0–19 Years	0									
20–34	0									
35–49	1	10.0	0	10	10	10	10	10	10	10
50–64	1	5.0	0	5	5	5	5	5	5	5
65+	0									
SUBTOTALS:										
1. SINGLE DX										
A. Not Operated	79	5.6	51	2	2	3	5	29	30	30
B. Operated	0									
2. MULTIPLE DX										
A. Not Operated	1,098	5.8	25	2	3	5	7	10	14	30
B. Operated	2	7.5	12	5	5	11	10	10	10	10
1. SINGLE DX	79	5.6	51	2	2	3	5	29	30	30
2. MULTIPLE DX	1,100	5.8	25	2	3	5	7	10	14	30
A. NOT OPERATED	1,177	5.8	27	2	3	5	7	10	14	30
B. OPERATED	2	7.5	12	5	5	5	10	10	10	10
TOTAL										
0–19 Years	34	6.7	61	2	2	4	6	18	30	30
20–34	366	6.1	42	2	3	4	7	12	21	30
35–49	400	5.5	23	2	3	4	6	10	14	30
50–64	341	5.6	13	2	3	5	7	9	12	19
65+	38	6.1	15	2	4	6	7	10	16	21
GRAND TOTAL	1,179	5.8	27	2	3	5	7	10	14	30

304.11: SEDATIVE DEPENDENCE-CONT

Type of Patients	Observed Patients	Avg. Stay	Vari-ance	10th	25th	50th	75th	90th	95th	99th
1. SINGLE DX										
A. Not Operated										
0–19 Years	0									
20–34	2	4.5	12	2	2	5	7	7	7	7
35–49	0									
50–64	1	6.0	0	6	6	6	6	6	6	6
65+	0									
B. Operated										
0–19 Years	0									
20–34	0									
35–49	0									
50–64	0									
65+	0									
2. MULTIPLE DX										
A. Not Operated										
0–19 Years	2	7.0	8	5	5	9	9	9	9	9
20–34	17	7.1	27	1	4	5	9	14	21	21
35–49	29	6.2	36	1	3	4	7	13	14	31
50–64	36	6.7	30	2	4	6	8	10	21	30
65+	8	9.1	10	5	6	8	11	14	14	14
B. Operated										
0–19 Years	0									
20–34	0									
35–49	0									
50–64	0									
65+	0									
SUBTOTALS:										
1. SINGLE DX										
A. Not Operated	3	5.0	7	2	2	6	7	7	7	7
B. Operated	0									
2. MULTIPLE DX										
A. Not Operated	92	6.8	29	2	4	5	9	12	14	31
B. Operated	0									
1. SINGLE DX	3	5.0	7	2	2	6	7	7	7	7
2. MULTIPLE DX	92	6.8	29	2	4	5	9	12	14	31
A. NOT OPERATED	95	6.8	28	2	4	5	8	12	14	31
B. OPERATED	0									
TOTAL										
0–19 Years	2	7.0	8	5	5	9	9	9	9	9
20–34	17	7.1	27	1	4	5	9	14	21	21
35–49	31	6.1	34	2	2	4	7	13	14	31
50–64	37	6.7	29	2	4	6	8	10	21	30
65+	8	9.1	10	5	6	8	11	14	14	14
GRAND TOTAL	95	6.8	28	2	4	5	8	12	14	31

Length of Stay by Diagnosis and Operation, Western Region, 2008

Western Region, October 2006–September 2007 Data, by Diagnosis

304.20: COCAINE DEP-UNSPEC

Type of Patients	Observed Patients	Avg. Stay	Variance	10th	25th	50th	75th	90th	95th	99th
1. SINGLE DX										
A. Not Operated										
0–19 Years	0									
20–34	0									
35–49	1	9.0	0	9	9	9	9	9	9	9
50–64	0									
65+	0									
B. Operated										
0–19 Years	0									
20–34	0									
35–49	0									
50–64	0									
65+	0									
2. MULTIPLE DX										
A. Not Operated										
0–19 Years	10	5.4	34	1	1	2	8	19	19	19
20–34	30	6.3	52	2	2	4	7	14	30	30
35–49	56	5.4	22	1	2	4	7	13	15	23
50–64	18	5.7	34	1	2	3	8	14	23	23
65+	0									
B. Operated										
0–19 Years	0									
20–34	0									
35–49	0									
50–64	0									
65+	0									
SUBTOTALS:										
1. SINGLE DX										
A. Not Operated	1	9.0	0	9	9	9	9	9	9	9
B. Operated	0									
2. MULTIPLE DX										
A. Not Operated	114	5.7	32	1	2	4	7	14	15	30
B. Operated	0									
1. SINGLE DX	1	9.0	0	9	9	9	9	9	9	9
2. MULTIPLE DX	114	5.7	32	1	2	4	7	14	15	30
A. NOT OPERATED	115	5.7	32	1	2	4	8	14	15	30
B. OPERATED	0									
TOTAL										
0–19 Years	10	5.4	34	1	1	2	8	19	19	19
20–34	30	6.3	52	2	2	4	7	14	30	30
35–49	57	5.4	21	1	2	4	7	13	15	23
50–64	18	5.7	34	1	2	3	8	14	23	23
65+	0									
GRAND TOTAL	115	5.7	32	1	2	4	8	14	15	30

304.21: COCAINE DEP-CONT

Type of Patients	Observed Patients	Avg. Stay	Variance	10th	25th	50th	75th	90th	95th	99th
1. SINGLE DX										
A. Not Operated										
0–19 Years	0									
20–34	2	16.0	442	1	1	31	31	31	31	31
35–49	7	21.2	434	1	3	21	30	59	59	59
50–64	1	1.0	0	1	1	1	1	1	1	1
65+	0									
B. Operated										
0–19 Years	0									
20–34	0									
35–49	0									
50–64	0									
65+	0									
2. MULTIPLE DX										
A. Not Operated										
0–19 Years	8	18.2	104	2	18	18	24	30	30	30
20–34	54	11.8	244	1	2	5	17	29	39	91
35–49	123	7.6	47	1	3	5	9	16	21	30
50–64	51	7.7	35	2	3	6	14	14	14	29
65+	2	6.0	31	2	2	2	10	10	10	10
B. Operated										
0–19 Years	0									
20–34	0									
35–49	0									
50–64	0									
65+	0									
SUBTOTALS:										
1. SINGLE DX										
A. Not Operated	10	18.1	380	1	1	21	30	31	59	59
B. Operated	0									
2. MULTIPLE DX										
A. Not Operated	238	8.9	96	1	3	5	13	21	29	39
B. Operated	0									
1. SINGLE DX	10	18.1	380	1	1	21	30	31	59	59
2. MULTIPLE DX	238	8.9	96	1	3	5	13	21	29	39
A. NOT OPERATED	248	9.3	109	1	3	5	14	21	30	50
B. OPERATED	0									
TOTAL										
0–19 Years	8	18.2	104	2	18	18	24	30	30	30
20–34	56	11.9	244	1	2	5	19	30	39	91
35–49	130	8.3	75	1	3	5	10	21	30	30
50–64	52	7.6	35	2	3	5	14	14	14	29
65+	2	6.0	31	2	2	2	10	10	10	10
GRAND TOTAL	248	9.3	109	1	3	5	14	21	30	50

304.31: CANNABIS DEP-CONT

Type of Patients	Observed Patients	Avg. Stay	Variance	10th	25th	50th	75th	90th	95th	99th
1. SINGLE DX										
A. Not Operated										
0–19 Years	0									
20–34	0									
35–49	2	30.0	0	30	30	30	30	30	30	30
50–64	0									
65+	0									
B. Operated										
0–19 Years	0									
20–34	0									
35–49	0									
50–64	0									
65+	0									
2. MULTIPLE DX										
A. Not Operated										
0–19 Years	22	18.2	80	7	12	18	27	29	30	34
20–34	10	5.8	68	1	1	2	8	28	28	28
35–49	2	7.4	83	1	1	1	14	14	14	14
50–64	2	12.9	125	5	5	5	21	21	21	21
65+	0									
B. Operated										
0–19 Years	0									
20–34	0									
35–49	0									
50–64	0									
65+	0									
SUBTOTALS:										
1. SINGLE DX										
A. Not Operated	2	30.0	0	30	30	30	30	30	30	30
B. Operated	0									
2. MULTIPLE DX										
A. Not Operated	36	13.9	105	1	5	13	22	28	30	34
B. Operated	0									
1. SINGLE DX	2	30.0	0	30	30	30	30	30	30	30
2. MULTIPLE DX	36	13.9	105	1	5	13	22	28	30	34
A. NOT OPERATED	38	14.7	112	1	5	14	25	30	30	34
B. OPERATED	0									
TOTAL										
0–19 Years	22	18.2	80	7	12	18	27	29	30	34
20–34	10	5.8	68	1	1	2	8	28	28	28
35–49	4	18.7	197	1	1	30	30	30	30	30
50–64	2	12.9	125	5	5	5	21	21	21	21
65+	0									
GRAND TOTAL	38	14.7	112	1	5	14	25	30	30	34

211

Length of Stay by Diagnosis and Operation, Western Region, 2008

Western Region, October 2006–September 2007 Data, by Diagnosis

304.70: OPIOID/OTHER DEP-UNSPEC

Type of Patients	Observed Patients	Avg. Stay	Variance	10th	25th	50th	75th	90th	95th	99th
1. SINGLE DX										
A. Not Operated										
0–19 Years	0									
20–34	1	14.0	0	14	14	14	14	14	14	14
35–49	0									
50–64	0									
65+	0									
B. Operated										
0–19 Years	0									
20–34	0									
35–49	0									
50–64	0									
65+	0									
2. MULTIPLE DX										
A. Not Operated										
0–19 Years	6	9.2	79	3	3	3	14	25	25	25
20–34	46	11.3	187	2	2	6	17	21	30	84
35–49	27	6.8	50	1	1	3	10	18	21	28
50–64	15	6.8	52	1	2	4	12	14	27	27
65+	2	8.5	59	3	3	14	14	14	14	14
B. Operated										
0–19 Years	0									
20–34	1	6.0	0	6	6	6	6	6	6	6
35–49	0									
50–64	0									
65+	0									
SUBTOTALS:										
1. SINGLE DX										
A. Not Operated	1	14.0	0	14	14	14	14	14	14	14
B. Operated	0									
2. MULTIPLE DX										
A. Not Operated	96	9.1	119	1	2	5	14	21	21	84
B. Operated	1	6.0	0	6	6	6	6	6	6	6
1. SINGLE DX	1	14.0	0	14	14	14	14	14	14	14
2. MULTIPLE DX	97	9.1	118	1	2	5	14	21	27	84
A. NOT OPERATED	97	9.2	118	1	2	5	14	21	27	84
B. OPERATED	1	6.0	0	6	6	6	6	6	6	6
TOTAL										
0–19 Years	6	9.2	79	3	3	3	14	25	25	25
20–34	47	11.3	183	2	2	7	17	21	29	84
35–49	28	6.8	48	1	2	3	9	18	27	28
50–64	15	6.8	52	1	2	4	12	14	27	27
65+	2	8.5	59	3	3	14	14	14	14	14
GRAND TOTAL	98	9.2	117	1	2	5	14	21	27	84

304.71: OPIOID/OTHER DEP-CONT

Type of Patients	Observed Patients	Avg. Stay	Variance	10th	25th	50th	75th	90th	95th	99th
1. SINGLE DX										
A. Not Operated										
0–19 Years	0									
20–34	6	23.0	414	2	5	29	30	57	57	57
35–49	2	4.5	4	3	3	6	6	6	6	6
50–64	1	1.0	0	1	1	1	1	1	1	1
65+	0									
B. Operated										
0–19 Years	0									
20–34	0									
35–49	0									
50–64	0									
65+	0									
2. MULTIPLE DX										
A. Not Operated										
0–19 Years	10	4.6	14	1	1	4	7	10	11	11
20–34	81	8.6	46	2	4	7	10	15	26	30
35–49	52	8.6	49	2	4	7	11	16	27	30
50–64	57	7.8	29	2	4	7	14	17	21	24
65+	6	8.3	31	1	4	6	14	15	15	15
B. Operated										
0–19 Years	0									
20–34	0									
35–49	0									
50–64	0									
65+	0									
SUBTOTALS:										
1. SINGLE DX										
A. Not Operated	9	16.5	357	1	3	6	29	57	57	57
B. Operated	0									
2. MULTIPLE DX										
A. Not Operated	206	8.1	40	2	4	7	10	16	24	30
B. Operated	0									
1. SINGLE DX	9	16.5	357	1	3	6	29	57	57	57
2. MULTIPLE DX	206	8.1	40	2	4	7	10	16	24	30
A. NOT OPERATED	215	8.5	55	2	4	7	10	17	26	30
B. OPERATED	0									
TOTAL										
0–19 Years	10	4.6	14	1	1	4	7	10	11	11
20–34	87	9.6	81	2	4	7	10	26	29	57
35–49	54	8.4	48	2	4	7	11	16	27	30
50–64	58	7.7	29	2	4	7	10	17	21	24
65+	6	8.3	31	1	4	6	14	15	15	15
GRAND TOTAL	215	8.5	55	2	4	7	10	17	26	30

305: NONDEPENDENT DRUG ABUSE

Type of Patients	Observed Patients	Avg. Stay	Variance	10th	25th	50th	75th	90th	95th	99th
1. SINGLE DX										
A. Not Operated										
0–19 Years	50	1.2	<1	1	1	1	1	1	2	4
20–34	31	2.7	30	1	1	1	2	3	13	30
35–49	34	1.8	6	1	1	1	2	2	4	15
50–64	17	1.2	<1	1	1	1	1	2	2	2
65+	4	1.3	<1	1	1	2	2	2	2	2
B. Operated										
0–19 Years	0									
20–34	0									
35–49	0									
50–64	0									
65+	0									
2. MULTIPLE DX										
A. Not Operated										
0–19 Years	321	2.2	9	1	1	1	2	4	8	19
20–34	728	2.1	6	1	1	1	2	4	5	13
35–49	1,029	2.4	9	1	1	2	3	5	7	14
50–64	654	2.5	5	1	1	2	3	5	7	11
65+	240	2.8	11	1	1	2	3	5	6	21
B. Operated										
0–19 Years	0									
20–34	7	3.3	8	1	2	2	5	9	9	9
35–49	4	3.0	2	1	3	4	4	4	4	4
50–64	4	7.0	30	1	4	7	13	13	13	13
65+	4	6.5	23	1	4	10	11	11	11	11
SUBTOTALS:										
1. SINGLE DX										
A. Not Operated	136	1.7	9	1	1	1	1	2	3	15
B. Operated	0									
2. MULTIPLE DX										
A. Not Operated	2,972	2.4	8	1	1	2	3	5	6	13
B. Operated	19	4.7	15	1	2	4	9	11	13	13
1. SINGLE DX	136	1.7	9	1	1	1	1	2	3	15
2. MULTIPLE DX	2,991	2.4	8	1	1	2	3	5	6	13
A. NOT OPERATED	3,108	2.3	8	1	1	1	3	4	6	13
B. OPERATED	19	4.7	15	1	2	4	9	11	13	13
TOTAL										
0–19 Years	371	2.1	8	1	1	1	2	3	6	19
20–34	766	2.1	7	1	1	1	2	4	5	13
35–49	1,067	2.4	9	1	1	2	3	5	7	14
50–64	675	2.4	6	1	1	2	3	5	7	11
65+	248	2.8	11	1	1	2	3	5	7	21
GRAND TOTAL	3,127	2.3	8	1	1	1	3	5	6	13

Length of Stay by Diagnosis and Operation, Western Region, 2008

Western Region, October 2006–September 2007 Data, by Diagnosis

305.00: ALCOHOL ABUSE-UNSPEC

Type of Patients	Observed Patients	Avg. Stay	Vari-ance	10th	25th	50th	75th	90th	95th	99th
1. SINGLE DX										
A. Not Operated										
0–19 Years	43	1.1	<1	1	1	1	1	1	2	2
20–34	18	1.2	<1	1	1	1	1	2	2	2
35–49	19	1.2	<1	1	1	1	1	2	2	2
50–64	9	1.2	<1	1	1	1	1	2	2	2
65+	2	1.0	0	1	1	1	1	1	1	1
B. Operated										
0–19 Years	0									
20–34	0									
35–49	0									
50–64	0									
65+	0									
2. MULTIPLE DX										
A. Not Operated										
0–19 Years	206	1.7	4	1	1	1	2	3	3	13
20–34	301	1.7	5	1	1	1	2	3	3	10
35–49	383	2.0	5	1	1	1	2	4	5	9
50–64	292	2.1	4	1	1	1	2	4	6	8
65+	143	2.6	13	1	1	2	3	5	6	22
B. Operated										
0–19 Years	0									
20–34	0									
35–49	1	3.0	0	3	3	3	3	3	3	3
50–64	0									
65+	2	7.0	18	4	4	7	10	10	10	10
SUBTOTALS:										
1. SINGLE DX										
A. Not Operated	91	1.1	<1	1	1	1	1	2	2	2
B. Operated	0									
2. MULTIPLE DX										
A. Not Operated	1,325	2.0	6	1	1	1	2	4	5	11
B. Operated	3	5.7	14	3	3	4	10	10	10	10
1. SINGLE DX	91	1.1	<1	1	1	1	1	2	2	2
2. MULTIPLE DX	1,328	2.0	6	1	1	1	2	4	5	11
A. NOT OPERATED	1,416	1.9	5	1	1	1	2	3	5	10
B. OPERATED	3	5.7	14	3	3	4	10	10	10	10
TOTAL										
0–19 Years	249	1.6	4	1	1	1	1	2	3	13
20–34	319	1.6	4	1	1	1	2	3	3	10
35–49	403	2.0	5	1	1	1	2	4	5	9
50–64	301	2.0	4	1	1	1	2	4	6	8
65+	147	2.7	13	1	1	2	3	5	6	22
GRAND TOTAL	1,419	1.9	5	1	1	1	2	3	5	10

305.01: ALCOHOL ABUSE-CONTINUOUS

Type of Patients	Observed Patients	Avg. Stay	Vari-ance	10th	25th	50th	75th	90th	95th	99th
1. SINGLE DX										
A. Not Operated										
0–19 Years	1	3.0	0	3	3	3	3	3	3	3
20–34	1	1.0	0	1	1	1	1	1	1	1
35–49	4	1.5	<1	1	1	1	2	2	2	2
50–64	2	1.0	0	1	1	1	1	1	1	1
65+	2	1.5	<1	1	1	2	2	2	2	2
B. Operated										
0–19 Years	0									
20–34	0									
35–49	0									
50–64	0									
65+	0									
2. MULTIPLE DX										
A. Not Operated										
0–19 Years	16	1.6	3	1	1	1	2	2	8	8
20–34	55	2.2	6	1	1	1	2	4	8	14
35–49	133	2.5	11	1	1	2	2	5	6	23
50–64	105	2.6	5	1	1	2	3	6	7	11
65+	60	2.5	3	1	1	2	4	5	5	9
B. Operated										
0–19 Years	0									
20–34	1	2.0	0	2	2	2	2	2	2	2
35–49	0									
50–64	2	7.0	70	1	1	13	13	13	13	13
65+	2	6.1	49	1	1	11	11	11	11	11
SUBTOTALS:										
1. SINGLE DX										
A. Not Operated	10	1.5	<1	1	1	1	2	3	3	3
B. Operated	0									
2. MULTIPLE DX										
A. Not Operated	369	2.4	7	1	1	2	3	5	6	12
B. Operated	5	5.7	35	1	1	2	11	13	13	13
1. SINGLE DX	10	1.5	<1	1	1	1	2	3	3	3
2. MULTIPLE DX	374	2.5	7	1	1	2	3	5	7	13
A. NOT OPERATED	379	2.4	6	1	1	2	3	5	6	12
B. OPERATED	5	5.7	35	1	1	2	11	13	13	13
TOTAL										
0–19 Years	17	1.7	3	1	1	1	2	2	3	8
20–34	57	2.2	6	1	1	1	2	4	8	14
35–49	137	2.5	10	1	1	2	2	5	6	23
50–64	109	2.6	6	1	1	2	3	6	7	12
65+	64	2.6	4	1	1	2	4	5	6	11
GRAND TOTAL	384	2.4	7	1	1	2	3	5	6	13

305.51: OPIOID ABUSE-CONTINUOUS

Type of Patients	Observed Patients	Avg. Stay	Vari-ance	10th	25th	50th	75th	90th	95th	99th
1. SINGLE DX										
A. Not Operated										
0–19 Years	0									
20–34	2	2.5	4	1	1	4	4	4	4	4
35–49	2	3.5	<1	3	3	4	4	4	4	4
50–64	0									
65+	0									
B. Operated										
0–19 Years	0									
20–34	0									
35–49	0									
50–64	0									
65+	0									
2. MULTIPLE DX										
A. Not Operated										
0–19 Years	0									
20–34	7	2.7	1	2	2	2	3	5	5	5
35–49	9	3.6	10	1	1	2	7	9	9	9
50–64	14	5.4	49	1	2	3	5	11	27	27
65+	1	6.0	0	6	6	6	6	6	6	6
B. Operated										
0–19 Years	0									
20–34	0									
35–49	0									
50–64	0									
65+	0									
SUBTOTALS:										
1. SINGLE DX										
A. Not Operated	4	3.0	2	1	3	4	4	4	4	4
B. Operated	0									
2. MULTIPLE DX										
A. Not Operated	31	4.3	25	1	2	2	5	9	11	27
B. Operated	0									
1. SINGLE DX	4	3.0	2	1	3	4	4	4	4	4
2. MULTIPLE DX	31	4.3	25	1	2	2	5	9	11	27
A. NOT OPERATED	35	4.2	23	1	2	3	5	9	11	27
B. OPERATED	0									
TOTAL										
0–19 Years	0									
20–34	9	2.7	2	2	2	3	3	5	5	5
35–49	11	3.6	8	1	1	3	7	7	9	9
50–64	14	5.4	49	1	2	3	5	11	27	27
65+	1	6.0	0	6	6	6	6	6	6	6
GRAND TOTAL	35	4.2	23	1	2	3	5	9	11	27

Length of Stay by Diagnosis and Operation, Western Region, 2008

213

Western Region, October 2006–September 2007 Data, by Diagnosis

305.60: COCAINE ABUSE-UNSPEC

Type of Patients	Observed Patients	Avg. Stay	Vari-ance	10th	25th	50th	75th	90th	95th	99th
1. SINGLE DX										
A. Not Operated										
0–19 Years	1	1.0	0	1	1	1	1	1	1	1
20–34	0									
35–49	1	3.0	0	3	3	3	3	3	3	3
50–64	1	2.0	0	2	2	2	2	2	2	2
65+	0									
B. Operated										
0–19 Years	0									
20–34	0									
35–49	0									
50–64	0									
65+	0									
2. MULTIPLE DX										
A. Not Operated										
0–19 Years	16	4.0	23	1	1	2	6	13	13	13
20–34	74	2.2	4	1	1	2	2	4	7	13
35–49	136	2.8	6	1	1	2	3	6	8	12
50–64	52	2.5	3	1	1	2	3	5	6	9
65+	4	7.0	89	1	1	2	21	21	21	21
B. Operated										
0–19 Years	0									
20–34	0									
35–49	0									
50–64	0									
65+	0									
SUBTOTALS:										
1. SINGLE DX										
A. Not Operated	3	2.0	<1	1	1	2	3	3	3	3
B. Operated	0									
2. MULTIPLE DX										
A. Not Operated	282	2.7	7	1	1	2	3	6	8	13
B. Operated	0									
1. SINGLE DX	3	2.0	<1	1	1	2	3	3	3	3
2. MULTIPLE DX	282	2.7	7	1	1	2	3	6	8	13
A. NOT OPERATED	285	2.7	7	1	1	2	3	6	8	13
B. OPERATED	0									
TOTAL										
0–19 Years	17	3.8	22	1	1	1	6	13	13	13
20–34	74	2.2	4	1	1	2	2	4	7	13
35–49	137	2.8	6	1	1	2	3	6	8	12
50–64	53	2.4	3	1	1	2	3	5	6	9
65+	4	7.0	89	1	1	2	21	21	21	21
GRAND TOTAL	285	2.7	7	1	1	2	3	6	8	13

305.90: DRUG ABUSE NEC-UNSPEC

Type of Patients	Observed Patients	Avg. Stay	Vari-ance	10th	25th	50th	75th	90th	95th	99th
1. SINGLE DX										
A. Not Operated										
0–19 Years	2	2.5	4	1	1	4	4	4	4	4
20–34	1	13.0	0	13	13	13	13	13	13	13
35–49	2	1.0	0	1	1	1	1	1	1	1
50–64	1	1.0	0	1	1	1	1	1	1	1
65+	0									
B. Operated										
0–19 Years	0									
20–34	0									
35–49	0									
50–64	0									
65+	0									
2. MULTIPLE DX										
A. Not Operated										
0–19 Years	16	3.0	8	1	1	2	5	6	12	12
20–34	56	2.8	7	1	1	2	3	6	11	13
35–49	58	2.8	12	1	1	2	3	6	8	21
50–64	36	3.2	4	1	2	3	4	5	8	8
65+	4	2.5	2	1	2	3	4	4	4	4
B. Operated										
0–19 Years	0									
20–34	1	2.0	0	2	2	2	2	2	2	2
35–49	0									
50–64	1	4.0	0	4	4	4	4	4	4	4
65+	0									
SUBTOTALS:										
1. SINGLE DX										
A. Not Operated	6	3.5	23	1	1	2	4	13	13	13
B. Operated	0									
2. MULTIPLE DX										
A. Not Operated	170	2.9	8	1	1	2	4	5	8	15
B. Operated	2	3.0	2	2	2	4	4	4	4	4
1. SINGLE DX	6	3.5	23	1	1	2	4	13	13	13
2. MULTIPLE DX	172	2.9	8	1	1	2	4	5	8	15
A. NOT OPERATED	176	2.9	8	1	1	2	4	6	8	15
B. OPERATED	2	3.0	2	2	2	4	4	4	4	4
TOTAL										
0–19 Years	18	3.0	8	1	1	2	4	6	12	12
20–34	58	2.9	9	1	1	2	3	6	11	13
35–49	60	2.8	11	1	1	2	3	5	7	21
50–64	38	3.2	4	1	2	3	4	5	8	8
65+	4	2.5	2	1	2	3	4	4	4	4
GRAND TOTAL	178	2.9	8	1	1	2	4	6	8	15

306: PSYCHOPHYSIOLOGIC PBX

Type of Patients	Observed Patients	Avg. Stay	Vari-ance	10th	25th	50th	75th	90th	95th	99th
1. SINGLE DX										
A. Not Operated										
0–19 Years	3	1.7	1	1	1	2	3	3	3	3
20–34	1	2.0	0	2	2	2	2	2	2	2
35–49	1	1.0	0	1	1	1	1	1	1	1
50–64	1	1.0	0	1	1	1	1	1	1	1
65+	0									
B. Operated										
0–19 Years	0									
20–34	0									
35–49	0									
50–64	0									
65+	0									
2. MULTIPLE DX										
A. Not Operated										
0–19 Years	36	3.9	11	1	1	3	5	10	12	12
20–34	63	2.9	10	1	1	2	3	6	8	18
35–49	80	2.9	11	1	1	2	3	6	7	27
50–64	106	2.9	7	1	1	2	4	6	8	10
65+	89	2.8	6	1	1	2	4	6	8	14
B. Operated										
0–19 Years	1	2.0	0	2	2	2	2	2	2	2
20–34	1	3.0	2	2	2	3	4	4	4	4
35–49	1	13.0	0	13	13	13	13	13	13	13
50–64	0									
65+	0									
SUBTOTALS:										
1. SINGLE DX										
A. Not Operated	6	1.5	<1	1	1	1	2	3	3	3
B. Operated	0									
2. MULTIPLE DX										
A. Not Operated	374	3.0	8	1	1	2	4	5	8	14
B. Operated	4	5.3	27	2	2	4	4	13	13	13
1. SINGLE DX	6	1.5	<1	1	1	1	2	3	3	3
2. MULTIPLE DX	378	3.0	8	1	1	2	4	6	9	14
A. NOT OPERATED	380	2.9	8	1	1	2	4	6	8	14
B. OPERATED	4	5.3	27	2	2	4	13	13	13	13
TOTAL										
0–19 Years	40	3.7	10	1	1	3	5	10	12	12
20–34	66	2.9	9	1	1	2	3	6	8	18
35–49	82	3.0	12	1	1	2	3	6	7	27
50–64	107	2.9	7	1	1	2	4	6	8	10
65+	89	2.8	6	1	1	2	4	6	8	14
GRAND TOTAL	384	3.0	8	1	1	2	4	6	8	14

Length of Stay by Diagnosis and Operation, Western Region, 2008

Western Region, October 2006–September 2007 Data, by Diagnosis

307: SPECIAL SYMPTOM NEC

Type of Patients	Observed Patients	Avg. Stay	Vari-ance	Percentiles						
				10th	25th	50th	75th	90th	95th	99th
1. SINGLE DX										
A. Not Operated										
0–19 Years	16	2.6	7	1	1	1	3	6	11	11
20–34	3	1.7	1	1	1	1	3	3	3	3
35–49	4	2.0	<1	1	1	2	2	3	3	3
50–64	3	1.0	0	1	1	1	1	1	1	1
65+	0									
B. Operated										
0–19 Years	0									
20–34	0									
35–49	0									
50–64	0									
65+	0									
2. MULTIPLE DX										
A. Not Operated										
0–19 Years	224	8.1	80	1	2	4	11	21	28	44
20–34	214	5.2	66	1	1	3	5	9	25	62
35–49	209	3.3	9	1	1	2	4	7	11	14
50–64	193	4.6	66	1	1	2	4	7	15	49
65+	248	4.0	12	1	2	3	5	8	10	15
B. Operated										
0–19 Years	3	7.4	42	1	1	7	14	14	14	14
20–34	1	1.0		1	1	1	1	1	1	1
35–49	3	16.4	180	3	3	16	30	30	30	30
50–64	2	7.5	24	4	4	4	11	11	11	11
65+	7	6.4	12	2	3	7	10	11	11	11
SUBTOTALS:										
1. SINGLE DX										
A. Not Operated	26	2.2	5	1	1	1	3	4	6	11
B. Operated	0									
2. MULTIPLE DX										
A. Not Operated	1,088	5.0	48	1	2	3	5	11	16	42
B. Operated	16	8.3	55	1	3	7	11	16	30	30
1. SINGLE DX	26	2.2	5	1	1	1	3	4	6	11
2. MULTIPLE DX	1,104	5.1	48	1	2	3	6	11	16	37
A. NOT OPERATED	1,114	5.0	47	1	1	3	5	11	16	37
B. OPERATED	16	8.3	55	1	3	7	11	16	30	30
TOTAL										
0–19 Years	243	7.7	77	1	2	4	10	19	27	44
20–34	218	5.1	66	1	1	3	5	9	25	62
35–49	216	3.5	13	1	1	2	4	8	11	16
50–64	198	4.6	64	1	1	2	4	7	15	49
65+	255	4.1	12	1	2	3	5	8	10	15
GRAND TOTAL	1,130	5.0	48	1	1	3	6	11	16	37

307.1: ANOREXIA NERVOSA

Type of Patients	Observed Patients	Avg. Stay	Vari-ance	Percentiles						
				10th	25th	50th	75th	90th	95th	99th
1. SINGLE DX										
A. Not Operated										
0–19 Years	3	7.0	13	4	4	6	11	11	11	11
20–34	0									
35–49	0									
50–64	0									
65+	0									
B. Operated										
0–19 Years	0									
20–34	0									
35–49	0									
50–64	0									
65+	0									
2. MULTIPLE DX										
A. Not Operated										
0–19 Years	121	11.5	101	2	4	9	15	27	31	45
20–34	75	8.9	153	1	2	5	9	27	37	>99
35–49	38	6.3	22	1	3	5	9	14	15	19
50–64	25	12.2	220	2	3	7	15	31	45	64
65+	2	6.5	4	5	5	7	8	8	8	8
B. Operated										
0–19 Years	1	14.0	0	14	14	14	14	14	14	14
20–34	0									
35–49	1	30.0	0	30	30	30	30	30	30	30
50–64	0									
65+	1	7.0	0	7	7	7	7	7	7	7
SUBTOTALS:										
1. SINGLE DX										
A. Not Operated	3	7.0	13	4	4	6	11	11	11	11
B. Operated	0									
2. MULTIPLE DX										
A. Not Operated	261	10.0	118	1	3	6	13	25	32	64
B. Operated	3	17.0	137	7	7	14	30	30	30	30
1. SINGLE DX	3	7.0	13	4	4	6	11	11	11	11
2. MULTIPLE DX	264	10.1	118	1	3	6	13	26	32	64
A. NOT OPERATED	264	10.0	117	1	3	6	13	25	32	64
B. OPERATED	3	17.0	137	7	7	14	30	30	30	30
TOTAL										
0–19 Years	125	11.4	99	2	4	9	15	27	31	45
20–34	75	8.9	153	1	2	5	9	27	37	>99
35–49	39	6.9	35	1	3	5	11	14	19	30
50–64	25	12.2	220	2	3	7	15	31	45	64
65+	3	6.7	2	5	5	7	8	8	8	8
GRAND TOTAL	267	10.1	117	1	3	6	13	26	32	64

307.81: TENSION HEADACHE

Type of Patients	Observed Patients	Avg. Stay	Vari-ance	Percentiles						
				10th	25th	50th	75th	90th	95th	99th
1. SINGLE DX										
A. Not Operated										
0–19 Years	3	2.3	1	1	1	3	3	3	3	3
20–34	2	2.0	2	1	1	3	3	3	3	3
35–49	2	1.5	<1	1	1	2	2	2	2	2
50–64	3	1.0	0	1	1	1	1	1	1	1
65+	0									
B. Operated										
0–19 Years	0									
20–34	0									
35–49	0									
50–64	0									
65+	0									
2. MULTIPLE DX										
A. Not Operated										
0–19 Years	12	2.3	2	1	1	2	4	4	4	4
20–34	58	2.5	3	1	1	2	4	5	5	6
35–49	93	2.2	2	1	1	2	3	4	5	8
50–64	93	2.2	2	1	1	2	3	4	6	7
65+	64	2.8	3	1	2	2	3	5	6	11
B. Operated										
0–19 Years	0									
20–34	0									
35–49	0									
50–64	2	7.5	24	4	4	4	11	11	11	11
65+	4	7.0	17	3	3	7	10	11	11	11
SUBTOTALS:										
1. SINGLE DX										
A. Not Operated	10	1.7	<1	1	1	1	3	3	3	3
B. Operated	0									
2. MULTIPLE DX										
A. Not Operated	320	2.4	2	1	1	2	3	4	5	7
B. Operated	6	7.2	15	3	4	4	11	11	11	11
1. SINGLE DX	10	1.7	<1	1	1	1	3	3	3	3
2. MULTIPLE DX	326	2.5	3	1	1	2	3	5	6	10
A. NOT OPERATED	330	2.4	2	1	1	2	3	4	5	7
B. OPERATED	6	7.2	15	3	4	4	11	11	11	11
TOTAL										
0–19 Years	15	2.3	2	1	1	2	4	4	4	4
20–34	60	2.5	2	1	1	2	4	5	5	6
35–49	95	2.2	2	1	1	2	3	4	5	8
50–64	98	2.3	3	1	1	2	3	5	6	11
65+	68	3.0	5	1	2	2	4	6	7	11
GRAND TOTAL	336	2.4	3	1	1	2	3	5	6	10

Length of Stay by Diagnosis and Operation, Western Region, 2008

Western Region, October 2006–September 2007 Data, by Diagnosis

307.9: SPECIAL SYMPTOM NEC&NOS

Type of Patients	Observed Patients	Avg. Stay	Variance	10th	25th	50th	75th	90th	95th	99th
1. SINGLE DX										
A. Not Operated										
0–19 Years	1	1.0	0	1	1	1	1	1	1	1
20–34	1	1.0	0	1	1	1	1	1	1	1
35–49	0									
50–64	0									
65+	0									
B. Operated										
0–19 Years	0									
20–34	0									
35–49	0									
50–64	0									
65+	0									
2. MULTIPLE DX										
A. Not Operated										
0–19 Years	11	3.0	20	1	1	1	3	5	16	16
20–34	18	1.9	2	1	1	1	3	4	6	6
35–49	28	2.7	5	1	1	2	4	6	6	10
50–64	30	5.0	35	2	2	3	6	8	11	34
65+	145	4.8	16	1	2	4	6	9	12	19
B. Operated										
0–19 Years	0									
20–34	0									
35–49	0									
50–64	0									
65+	2	5.0	18	2	2	2	8	8	8	8
SUBTOTALS:										
1. SINGLE DX										
A. Not Operated	2	1.0	0	1	1	1	1	1	1	1
B. Operated	0									
2. MULTIPLE DX										
A. Not Operated	232	4.2	17	1	2	3	5	8	11	19
B. Operated	2	5.0	18	2	2	2	8	8	8	8
1. SINGLE DX	2	1.0	0	1	1	1	1	1	1	1
2. MULTIPLE DX	234	4.2	17	1	2	3	5	8	11	19
A. NOT OPERATED	234	4.2	17	1	2	3	5	8	11	19
B. OPERATED	2	5.0	18	2	2	2	8	8	8	8
TOTAL										
0–19 Years	12	2.8	19	1	1	1	2	5	16	16
20–34	19	1.9	2	1	1	1	3	4	6	6
35–49	28	2.7	5	1	1	2	4	6	6	10
50–64	30	5.0	35	2	2	3	6	8	11	34
65+	147	4.8	16	1	2	4	6	9	12	19
GRAND TOTAL	236	4.2	17	1	2	3	5	8	11	19

308: ACUTE REACTION TO STRESS

Type of Patients	Observed Patients	Avg. Stay	Variance	10th	25th	50th	75th	90th	95th	99th
1. SINGLE DX										
A. Not Operated										
0–19 Years	2	1.0	0	1	1	1	1	1	1	1
20–34	2	1.0	0	1	1	1	1	1	1	1
35–49	4	1.5	<1	1	1	2	2	2	2	2
50–64	1	1.0	0	1	1	1	1	1	1	1
65+	0									
B. Operated										
0–19 Years	0									
20–34	0									
35–49	0									
50–64	0									
65+	0									
2. MULTIPLE DX										
A. Not Operated										
0–19 Years	15	2.7	4	1	1	2	4	6	7	7
20–34	47	2.2	6	1	1	1	2	4	6	13
35–49	113	1.7	2	1	1	1	2	3	5	8
50–64	125	1.5	1	1	1	1	2	3	3	5
65+	78	1.7	1	1	1	1	2	3	4	7
B. Operated										
0–19 Years	0									
20–34	2	3.0	2	2	2	3	4	4	4	4
35–49	1	1.0	0	1	1	1	1	1	1	1
50–64	0									
65+	1	14.0	0	14	14	14	14	14	14	14
SUBTOTALS:										
1. SINGLE DX										
A. Not Operated	9	1.2	<1	1	1	1	1	2	2	2
B. Operated	0									
2. MULTIPLE DX										
A. Not Operated	378	1.7	2	1	1	1	2	3	4	8
B. Operated	4	5.2	35	1	1	3	4	14	14	14
1. SINGLE DX	9	1.2	<1	1	1	1	1	2	2	2
2. MULTIPLE DX	382	1.8	3	1	1	1	2	3	4	10
A. NOT OPERATED	387	1.7	2	1	1	1	2	3	4	8
B. OPERATED	4	5.2	35	1	1	3	4	14	14	14
TOTAL										
0–19 Years	17	2.5	4	1	1	1	2	3	6	7
20–34	49	2.1	5	1	1	1	2	4	6	13
35–49	119	1.7	2	1	1	1	2	3	5	8
50–64	127	1.5	1	1	1	1	2	3	3	5
65+	79	1.9	3	1	1	1	2	3	4	14
GRAND TOTAL	391	1.8	3	1	1	1	2	3	4	10

309: ADJUSTMENT REACTION

Type of Patients	Observed Patients	Avg. Stay	Variance	10th	25th	50th	75th	90th	95th	99th
1. SINGLE DX										
A. Not Operated										
0–19 Years	67	3.1	9	1	1	2	4	7	9	17
20–34	113	2.0	4	1	1	1	2	3	5	12
35–49	62	1.8	3	1	1	1	2	3	4	8
50–64	33	2.1	3	1	1	2	3	4	7	8
65+	3	1.7	1	1	1	1	3	3	3	3
B. Operated										
0–19 Years	0									
20–34	0									
35–49	0									
50–64	0									
65+	0									
2. MULTIPLE DX										
A. Not Operated										
0–19 Years	578	4.3	25	1	2	3	5	9	12	23
20–34	1,266	3.3	23	1	1	3	4	6	9	19
35–49	1,058	3.8	16	1	1	3	5	8	11	18
50–64	565	3.9	14	1	1	3	5	9	12	19
65+	174	4.3	22	1	2	3	5	10	13	26
B. Operated										
0–19 Years	2	1.0	0	1	1	1	1	1	1	1
20–34	1	1.0	0	1	1	1	1	1	1	1
35–49	0									
50–64	2	3.0	2	2	2	2	4	4	4	4
65+	0									
SUBTOTALS:										
1. SINGLE DX										
A. Not Operated	278	2.2	5	1	1	2	3	4	6	13
B. Operated	0									
2. MULTIPLE DX										
A. Not Operated	3,641	3.7	20	1	1	2	4	8	11	21
B. Operated	5	1.8	2	1	1	1	2	4	4	4
1. SINGLE DX	278	2.2	5	1	1	2	3	4	6	13
2. MULTIPLE DX	3,646	3.7	20	1	1	2	4	8	11	21
A. NOT OPERATED	3,919	3.6	19	1	1	2	4	7	11	20
B. OPERATED	5	1.8	2	1	1	1	2	4	4	4
TOTAL										
0–19 Years	645	4.2	23	1	1	3	5	9	12	22
20–34	1,381	3.2	21	1	1	2	4	6	8	19
35–49	1,121	3.6	15	1	1	2	4	8	11	18
50–64	600	3.8	14	1	1	2	5	8	12	19
65+	177	4.3	21	1	1	3	5	10	13	26
GRAND TOTAL	3,924	3.6	19	1	1	2	4	7	11	20

Length of Stay by Diagnosis and Operation, Western Region, 2008

Western Region, October 2006–September 2007 Data, by Diagnosis

309.0: ADJUSTMENT DIS-DEPRESSED

Type of Patients	Observed Patients	Avg. Stay	Vari-ance	Percentiles 10th	25th	50th	75th	90th	95th	99th
1. SINGLE DX										
A. Not Operated										
0–19 Years	20	3.0	7	1	1	2	3	8	11	11
20–34	47	1.6	<1	1	1	1	2	3	4	5
35–49	24	1.7	<1	1	1	1	2	3	3	4
50–64	13	2.2	1	1	1	2	3	3	4	4
65+	0									
B. Operated										
0–19 Years	0									
20–34	0									
35–49	0									
50–64	0									
65+	0									
2. MULTIPLE DX										
A. Not Operated										
0–19 Years	153	2.9	6	1	1	2	3	5	7	13
20–34	385	2.4	4	1	1	2	3	4	6	11
35–49	271	2.9	7	1	1	2	4	6	8	16
50–64	154	3.5	11	1	1	2	4	7	12	15
65+	71	4.7	33	1	1	2	5	10	24	26
B. Operated										
0–19 Years	0									
20–34	0									
35–49	0									
50–64	2	3.0	2	2	2	2	4	4	4	4
65+	0									
SUBTOTALS:										
1. SINGLE DX										
A. Not Operated	104	2.0	2	1	1	2	2	3	4	8
B. Operated	0									
2. MULTIPLE DX										
A. Not Operated	1,034	2.9	8	1	1	2	3	6	8	14
B. Operated	2	3.0	2	2	2	2	4	4	4	4
1. SINGLE DX	104	2.0	2	1	1	2	2	3	4	8
2. MULTIPLE DX	1,036	2.9	8	1	1	2	3	6	8	14
A. NOT OPERATED	1,138	2.8	8	1	1	2	3	5	8	14
B. OPERATED	2	3.0	2	2	2	2	4	4	4	4
TOTAL										
0–19 Years	173	2.9	6	1	1	2	3	6	7	13
20–34	432	2.3	4	1	1	2	3	4	6	11
35–49	295	2.8	7	1	1	2	3	5	8	16
50–64	169	3.4	10	1	1	2	4	7	12	15
65+	71	4.7	33	1	1	2	5	10	24	26
GRAND TOTAL	1,140	2.8	8	1	1	2	3	5	8	14

309.28: ADJUST DIS-ANXIETY/DEPR

Type of Patients	Observed Patients	Avg. Stay	Vari-ance	Percentiles 10th	25th	50th	75th	90th	95th	99th
1. SINGLE DX										
A. Not Operated										
0–19 Years	9	1.8	3	1	1	1	2	6	6	6
20–34	15	2.1	2	1	1	1	3	4	6	6
35–49	6	3.0	2	2	2	3	4	5	5	5
50–64	5	1.6	<1	1	1	2	2	2	2	2
65+	1	3.0	0	3	3	3	3	3	3	3
B. Operated										
0–19 Years	0									
20–34	0									
35–49	0									
50–64	0									
65+	0									
2. MULTIPLE DX										
A. Not Operated										
0–19 Years	36	3.3	12	1	1	2	3	4	7	19
20–34	150	2.5	4	1	1	2	3	4	6	13
35–49	132	3.0	7	1	1	2	4	6	7	15
50–64	78	3.5	8	1	2	2	4	8	9	15
65+	44	4.1	9	1	2	3	6	9	10	12
B. Operated										
0–19 Years	0									
20–34	0									
35–49	0									
50–64	0									
65+	0									
SUBTOTALS:										
1. SINGLE DX										
A. Not Operated	36	2.1	2	1	1	2	2	3	4	6
B. Operated	0									
2. MULTIPLE DX										
A. Not Operated	440	3.1	7	1	1	2	3	4	6	14
B. Operated	0									
1. SINGLE DX	36	2.1	2	1	1	2	2	3	4	6
2. MULTIPLE DX	440	3.1	7	1	1	2	3	4	6	14
A. NOT OPERATED	476	3.0	7	1	1	2	3	5	8	14
B. OPERATED	0									
TOTAL										
0–19 Years	45	3.0	11	1	1	2	3	6	8	19
20–34	165	2.4	4	1	1	2	3	4	6	13
35–49	138	3.0	6	1	1	2	3	5	7	15
50–64	83	3.4	8	1	2	2	4	8	9	15
65+	45	4.1	9	1	2	3	6	9	10	12
GRAND TOTAL	476	3.0	7	1	1	2	3	5	8	14

309.4: ADJUST DIS-EMOT/CONDUCT

Type of Patients	Observed Patients	Avg. Stay	Vari-ance	Percentiles 10th	25th	50th	75th	90th	95th	99th
1. SINGLE DX										
A. Not Operated										
0–19 Years	19	3.7	10	1	1	3	5	9	13	13
20–34	26	2.2	5	1	1	1	2	5	5	12
35–49	10	1.7	1	1	1	1	2	4	4	4
50–64	4	1.3	<1	1	1	1	1	2	2	2
65+	1	1.0	0	1	1	1	1	1	1	1
B. Operated										
0–19 Years	0									
20–34	0									
35–49	0									
50–64	0									
65+	0									
2. MULTIPLE DX										
A. Not Operated										
0–19 Years	141	3.5	11	1	1	2	4	7	12	16
20–34	260	2.7	6	1	1	2	3	6	7	11
35–49	186	3.3	17	1	1	2	3	6	10	18
50–64	82	3.5	15	1	1	2	3	7	14	18
65+	27	4.4	22	1	1	3	5	10	16	20
B. Operated										
0–19 Years	0									
20–34	2	1.0	0	1	1	1	1	1	1	1
35–49	1	1.0	0	1	1	1	1	1	1	1
50–64	0									
65+	0									
SUBTOTALS:										
1. SINGLE DX										
A. Not Operated	60	2.5	6	1	1	2	3	5	9	13
B. Operated	0									
2. MULTIPLE DX										
A. Not Operated	696	3.2	11	1	1	2	4	6	9	17
B. Operated	3	1.0	0	1	1	1	1	1	1	1
1. SINGLE DX	60	2.5	6	1	1	2	3	5	9	13
2. MULTIPLE DX	699	3.2	11	1	1	2	4	6	9	17
A. NOT OPERATED	756	3.1	11	1	1	2	4	6	9	17
B. OPERATED	3	1.0	0	1	1	1	1	1	1	1
TOTAL										
0–19 Years	160	3.5	11	1	1	2	4	7	12	16
20–34	288	2.7	6	1	1	2	3	6	7	12
35–49	197	3.2	16	1	1	2	3	6	10	18
50–64	86	3.4	15	1	1	2	3	7	14	18
65+	28	4.3	21	1	1	3	5	10	16	20
GRAND TOTAL	759	3.1	11	1	1	2	4	6	9	17

Length of Stay by Diagnosis and Operation, Western Region, 2008

Western Region, October 2006–September 2007 Data, by Diagnosis

309.81: POSTTRAUMATIC STRESS DIS

Type of Patients	Observed Patients	Avg. Stay	Variance	10th	25th	50th	75th	90th	95th	99th
1. SINGLE DX										
A. Not Operated										
0–19 Years	6	6.2	32	1	3	4	7	17	17	17
20–34	7	4.6	31	1	1	3	4	17	17	17
35–49	3	1.0	0	1	1	1	1	1	1	1
50–64	3	3.7	14	1	1	2	8	8	8	8
65+	0									
B. Operated										
0–19 Years	0									
20–34	0									
35–49	0									
50–64	0									
65+	0									
2. MULTIPLE DX										
A. Not Operated										
0–19 Years	164	7.2	52	2	3	6	9	13	18	45
20–34	271	6.1	68	1	2	4	7	13	18	38
35–49	313	5.5	19	1	2	4	7	11	14	20
50–64	140	5.8	18	1	3	5	8	11	14	20
65+	9	6.6	32	1	3	5	8	18	18	18
B. Operated										
0–19 Years	0									
20–34	0									
35–49	0									
50–64	0									
65+	0									
SUBTOTALS:										
1. SINGLE DX										
A. Not Operated	19	4.4	24	1	1	3	5	17	17	17
B. Operated	0									
2. MULTIPLE DX										
A. Not Operated	897	6.1	40	1	3	4	7	12	16	31
B. Operated	0									
1. SINGLE DX	19	4.4	24	1	1	3	5	17	17	17
2. MULTIPLE DX	897	6.1	40	1	3	4	7	12	16	31
A. NOT OPERATED	916	6.0	40	1	3	4	7	12	16	31
B. OPERATED	0									
TOTAL										
0–19 Years	170	7.1	51	2	3	6	9	13	18	45
20–34	278	6.1	67	1	2	4	7	13	18	38
35–49	316	5.5	19	1	3	4	7	11	14	20
50–64	143	5.7	18	1	2	5	8	11	14	20
65+	9	6.6	32	1	3	5	8	18	18	18
GRAND TOTAL	916	6.0	40	1	3	4	7	12	16	31

309.9: ADJUSTMENT REACTION NOS

Type of Patients	Observed Patients	Avg. Stay	Variance	10th	25th	50th	75th	90th	95th	99th
1. SINGLE DX										
A. Not Operated										
0–19 Years	8	2.5	2	1	1	2	3	5	5	5
20–34	11	1.3	<1	1	1	1	1	2	2	2
35–49	13	1.5	1	1	1	1	1	3	5	5
50–64	6	2.7	6	1	1	2	4	7	7	7
65+	0									
B. Operated										
0–19 Years	0									
20–34	0									
35–49	0									
50–64	0									
65+	0									
2. MULTIPLE DX										
A. Not Operated										
0–19 Years	37	2.9	6	1	1	2	3	7	8	11
20–34	115	2.3	31	1	1	1	2	3	4	6
35–49	81	2.2	4	1	1	2	2	4	7	12
50–64	60	3.1	16	1	1	2	4	6	7	29
65+	10	2.6	2	1	1	2	5	5	>99	>99
B. Operated										
0–19 Years	0									
20–34	0									
35–49	0									
50–64	0									
65+	0									
SUBTOTALS:										
1. SINGLE DX										
A. Not Operated	38	1.8	2	1	1	1	2	4	5	7
B. Operated	0									
2. MULTIPLE DX										
A. Not Operated	303	2.5	17	1	1	2	3	5	6	12
B. Operated	0									
1. SINGLE DX	38	1.8	2	1	1	1	2	4	5	7
2. MULTIPLE DX	303	2.5	17	1	1	2	3	5	6	12
A. NOT OPERATED	341	2.5	15	1	1	2	3	5	6	12
B. OPERATED	0									
TOTAL										
0–19 Years	45	2.8	5	1	1	2	3	6	8	11
20–34	126	2.2	28	1	1	1	2	3	4	6
35–49	94	2.2	4	1	1	2	2	4	7	12
50–64	66	3.1	15	1	1	2	4	6	>99	29
65+	10	2.6	2	1	1	2	5	5	>99	>99
GRAND TOTAL	341	2.5	15	1	1	2	3	5	6	12

310: NONPSYCHOTIC OBS

Type of Patients	Observed Patients	Avg. Stay	Variance	10th	25th	50th	75th	90th	95th	99th
1. SINGLE DX										
A. Not Operated										
0–19 Years	16	1.6	1	1	1	1	2	3	5	5
20–34	5	2.2	5	1	1	1	2	6	6	6
35–49	5	1.4	<1	1	1	1	1	1	2	2
50–64	3	1.0	0	1	1	1	1	1	1	1
65+	1	7.0	0	7	7	7	7	7	7	7
B. Operated										
0–19 Years	0									
20–34	0									
35–49	0									
50–64	0									
65+	0									
2. MULTIPLE DX										
A. Not Operated										
0–19 Years	68	2.1	6	1	1	1	2	4	5	18
20–34	88	4.5	81	1	1	2	4	9	14	78
35–49	115	4.8	51	1	2	2	6	11	13	39
50–64	120	5.7	65	1	2	3	6	14	23	49
65+	220	4.9	30	1	2	3	5	10	14	27
B. Operated										
0–19 Years	0									
20–34	1	6.0	0	6	6	6	6	6	6	6
35–49	1	23.0	0	23	23	23	23	23	23	23
50–64	0									
65+	0									
SUBTOTALS:										
1. SINGLE DX										
A. Not Operated	30	1.8	2	1	1	1	2	3	6	7
B. Operated	0									
2. MULTIPLE DX										
A. Not Operated	611	4.7	46	1	1	3	5	10	15	39
B. Operated	2	14.5	142	6	6	6	23	23	23	23
1. SINGLE DX	30	1.8	2	1	1	1	2	3	6	7
2. MULTIPLE DX	613	4.7	47	1	1	3	5	10	15	39
A. NOT OPERATED	641	4.5	44	1	1	3	5	10	14	39
B. OPERATED	2	14.5	142	6	6	6	23	23	23	23
TOTAL										
0–19 Years	84	2.0	5	1	1	1	2	4	5	18
20–34	94	4.4	76	1	1	2	4	9	14	78
35–49	121	4.8	51	1	2	2	6	11	13	39
50–64	123	5.6	64	1	2	3	6	14	23	49
65+	221	4.9	30	1	1	3	5	10	14	27
GRAND TOTAL	643	4.6	45	1	1	3	5	10	15	39

Western Region, October 2006–September 2007 Data, by Diagnosis

310.2: POSTCONCUSSION SYNDROME

Type of Patients	Observed Patients	Avg. Stay	Vari- ance	Percentiles						
				10th	25th	50th	75th	90th	95th	99th
1. SINGLE DX										
A. Not Operated										
0–19 Years	16	1.6	1	1	1	1	2	3	5	5
20–34	5	2.2	5	1	1	1	2	6	6	6
35–49	5	1.4	<1	1	1	1	2	2	2	2
50–64	3	1.0	0	1	1	1	1	1	1	1
65+	0									
B. Operated										
0–19 Years	0									
20–34	0									
35–49	0									
50–64	0									
65+	0									
2. MULTIPLE DX										
A. Not Operated										
0–19 Years	65	2.0	5	1	1	1	2	3	4	18
20–34	69	2.4	4	1	1	2	3	5	8	11
35–49	88	2.9	6	1	1	2	4	6	8	13
50–64	82	3.4	18	1	1	3	4	6	8	34
65+	145	3.9	22	1	2	3	4	8	11	27
B. Operated										
0–19 Years	0									
20–34	1	6.0	0	6	6	6	6	6	6	6
35–49	1	23.0	0	23	23	23	23	23	23	23
50–64	0									
65+	0									
SUBTOTALS:										
1. SINGLE DX										
A. Not Operated	29	1.6	2	1	1	1	2	3	5	6
B. Operated	0									
2. MULTIPLE DX										
A. Not Operated	449	3.1	14	1	1	2	3	7	9	17
B. Operated	2	14.5	142	6	6	6	23	23	23	23
1. SINGLE DX	**29**	**1.6**	**2**	**1**	**1**	**1**	**2**	**3**	**5**	**6**
2. MULTIPLE DX	**451**	**3.2**	**14**	**1**	**1**	**2**	**3**	**7**	**9**	**18**
A. NOT OPERATED	**478**	**3.0**	**13**	**1**	**1**	**2**	**3**	**6**	**8**	**17**
B. OPERATED	**2**	**14.5**	**142**	**6**	**6**	**6**	**23**	**23**	**23**	**23**
TOTAL										
0–19 Years	81	1.9	5	1	1	1	2	3	4	18
20–34	75	2.4	4	1	1	1	3	5	6	11
35–49	94	3.1	10	1	1	2	4	6	9	23
50–64	85	3.4	17	1	1	3	4	6	8	34
65+	145	3.9	22	1	2	3	4	8	11	27
GRAND TOTAL	**480**	**3.1**	**14**	**1**	**1**	**2**	**3**	**6**	**8**	**18**

311: DEPRESSIVE DISORDER NEC

Type of Patients	Observed Patients	Avg. Stay	Vari- ance	Percentiles						
				10th	25th	50th	75th	90th	95th	99th
1. SINGLE DX										
A. Not Operated										
0–19 Years	116	3.9	8	1	2	3	5	7	9	16
20–34	149	2.5	5	1	1	2	3	5	6	13
35–49	93	3.1	6	1	1	2	4	7	8	13
50–64	41	2.7	3	1	1	2	3	5	6	9
65+	5	3.6	10	1	2	3	3	9	9	9
B. Operated										
0–19 Years	0									
20–34	0									
35–49	0									
50–64	1	1.0	0	1	1	1	1	1	1	1
65+	0									
2. MULTIPLE DX										
A. Not Operated										
0–19 Years	993	4.4	17	1	2	3	6	8	10	18
20–34	1,925	3.6	15	1	2	3	4	7	9	18
35–49	2,063	4.2	16	1	2	3	5	8	11	21
50–64	1,143	4.7	25	1	2	3	6	10	13	25
65+	345	6.5	38	1	2	4	8	15	19	33
B. Operated										
0–19 Years	0									
20–34	3	4.0	9	1	1	4	7	7	7	7
35–49	8	7.1	30	1	3	6	9	19	19	19
50–64	6	7.7	28	1	3	6	13	14	14	14
65+	2	11.0	8	9	9	11	13	13	13	13
SUBTOTALS:										
1. SINGLE DX										
A. Not Operated	404	3.1	6	1	1	2	4	6	8	13
B. Operated	1	1.0	0	1	1	1	1	1	1	1
2. MULTIPLE DX										
A. Not Operated	6,469	4.3	19	1	2	3	5	8	12	21
B. Operated	19	7.2	24	1	3	6	9	14	19	19
1. SINGLE DX	**405**	**3.1**	**6**	**1**	**1**	**2**	**4**	**6**	**8**	**13**
2. MULTIPLE DX	**6,488**	**4.3**	**19**	**1**	**2**	**3**	**5**	**8**	**12**	**21**
A. NOT OPERATED	**6,873**	**4.2**	**18**	**1**	**2**	**3**	**5**	**8**	**12**	**21**
B. OPERATED	**20**	**6.9**	**25**	**1**	**3**	**6**	**9**	**14**	**19**	**19**
TOTAL										
0–19 Years	1,109	4.3	16	1	2	3	5	8	10	18
20–34	2,077	3.5	14	1	2	3	4	7	9	18
35–49	2,164	4.2	16	1	2	3	5	8	11	20
50–64	1,191	4.7	25	1	2	3	6	10	13	25
65+	352	6.5	38	1	2	4	8	14	19	33
GRAND TOTAL	**6,893**	**4.2**	**18**	**1**	**2**	**3**	**5**	**8**	**12**	**20**

312: CONDUCT DISTURBANCE NEC

Type of Patients	Observed Patients	Avg. Stay	Vari- ance	Percentiles						
				10th	25th	50th	75th	90th	95th	99th
1. SINGLE DX										
A. Not Operated										
0–19 Years	30	4.6	10	1	2	4	6	9	10	14
20–34	8	3.2	5	1	1	3	4	8	8	8
35–49	4	4.5	49	1	1	1	1	15	15	15
50–64	2	8.5	5	7	7	9	10	10	10	10
65+	0									
B. Operated										
0–19 Years	0									
20–34	0									
35–49	0									
50–64	0									
65+	0									
2. MULTIPLE DX										
A. Not Operated										
0–19 Years	399	6.1	35	1	2	5	7	12	17	41
20–34	166	6.0	102	1	2	3	6	11	25	41
35–49	87	8.5	112	1	2	5	10	23	38	>99
50–64	41	7.7	89	1	2	4	9	16	32	44
65+	53	9.4	63	1	3	8	13	22	27	32
B. Operated										
0–19 Years	1	2.0	0	2	2	2	2	2	2	2
20–34	0									
35–49	0									
50–64	1	72.0	0	72	72	72	72	72	72	72
65+	1	32.0	0	32	32	32	32	32	32	32
SUBTOTALS:										
1. SINGLE DX										
A. Not Operated	44	4.5	12	1	1	4	6	10	10	15
B. Operated	0									
2. MULTIPLE DX										
A. Not Operated	746	6.7	65	1	2	4	8	15	22	44
B. Operated	3	35.2	>999	2	32	32	72	72	72	72
1. SINGLE DX	**44**	**4.5**	**12**	**1**	**1**	**4**	**6**	**10**	**10**	**15**
2. MULTIPLE DX	**749**	**6.8**	**71**	**1**	**2**	**4**	**8**	**15**	**22**	**50**
A. NOT OPERATED	**790**	**6.5**	**62**	**1**	**2**	**4**	**8**	**14**	**21**	**44**
B. OPERATED	**3**	**35.2**	**>999**	**2**	**32**	**32**	**72**	**72**	**72**	**72**
TOTAL										
0–19 Years	430	6.0	33	1	2	5	7	12	17	34
20–34	174	5.8	98	1	2	3	6	10	25	41
35–49	91	8.3	110	1	2	5	10	22	38	>99
50–64	44	9.2	177	1	2	4	10	17	34	72
65+	54	9.8	71	1	3	8	13	24	27	32
GRAND TOTAL	**793**	**6.7**	**68**	**1**	**2**	**4**	**8**	**14**	**22**	**50**

Length of Stay by Diagnosis and Operation, Western Region, 2008

Western Region, October 2006–September 2007 Data, by Diagnosis

312.30: IMPULSE CONTROL PBX NOS

Type of Patients	Observed Patients	Avg. Stay	Vari-ance	10th	25th	50th	75th	90th	95th	99th
1. SINGLE DX										
A. Not Operated										
0–19 Years	8	4.4	9	1	1	4	6	10	10	10
20–34	6	3.7	6	1	2	4	4	8	8	8
35–49	2	8.0	96	1	1	8	15	15	15	15
50–64	1	7.0	0	7	7	7	7	7	7	7
65+	0									
B. Operated										
0–19 Years	0									
20–34	0									
35–49	0									
50–64	0									
65+	0									
2. MULTIPLE DX										
A. Not Operated										
0–19 Years	89	6.7	37	1	3	6	7	13	17	41
20–34	76	5.0	47	1	2	3	5	9	21	41
35–49	48	8.4	107	1	2	5	10	23	38	>99
50–64	19	8.7	132	1	3	4	11	34	44	44
65+	16	14.1	56	5	6	13	22	25	27	27
B. Operated										
0–19 Years	0									
20–34	0									
35–49	0									
50–64	0									
65+	1	32.0	0	32	32	32	32	32	32	32
SUBTOTALS:										
1. SINGLE DX										
A. Not Operated	17	4.7	14	1	2	4	6	10	15	15
B. Operated	0									
2. MULTIPLE DX										
A. Not Operated	248	7.2	66	1	2	5	8	17	25	44
B. Operated	1	32.0	0	32	32	32	32	32	32	32
1. SINGLE DX	17	4.7	14	1	2	4	6	10	15	15
2. MULTIPLE DX	249	7.3	68	1	2	5	8	18	26	44
A. NOT OPERATED	265	7.0	63	1	2	5	8	17	23	44
B. OPERATED	1	32.0	0	32	32	32	32	32	32	32
TOTAL										
0–19 Years	97	6.5	35	1	3	6	7	13	17	41
20–34	82	4.9	44	1	2	3	5	9	11	41
35–49	50	8.4	104	1	2	5	13	23	38	>99
50–64	20	8.7	125	1	3	4	9	15	34	44
65+	17	15.2	71	5	7	15	22	27	32	32
GRAND TOTAL	266	7.1	65	1	2	5	8	17	25	44

312.34: INTERMITT EXPLOS DISORD

Type of Patients	Observed Patients	Avg. Stay	Vari-ance	10th	25th	50th	75th	90th	95th	99th
1. SINGLE DX										
A. Not Operated										
0–19 Years	5	5.2	<1	4	5	5	6	6	6	6
20–34	2	2.0	2	1	1	2	3	3	3	3
35–49	0									
50–64	1	10.0	0	10	10	10	10	10	10	10
65+	0									
B. Operated										
0–19 Years	0									
20–34	0									
35–49	0									
50–64	0									
65+	0									
2. MULTIPLE DX										
A. Not Operated										
0–19 Years	117	6.2	53	1	3	5	7	12	19	66
20–34	67	5.6	55	1	2	3	6	12	23	40
35–49	28	7.5	113	1	2	4	9	17	18	56
50–64	10	5.3	15	1	2	5	7	8	14	14
65+	5	6.2	13	3	4	4	9	11	11	11
B. Operated										
0–19 Years	0									
20–34	0									
35–49	0									
50–64	0									
65+	0									
SUBTOTALS:										
1. SINGLE DX										
A. Not Operated	8	5.0	7	1	3	5	6	10	10	10
B. Operated	0									
2. MULTIPLE DX										
A. Not Operated	227	6.1	58	1	2	4	7	12	18	56
B. Operated	0									
1. SINGLE DX	8	5.0	7	1	3	5	6	10	10	10
2. MULTIPLE DX	227	6.1	58	1	2	4	7	12	18	56
A. NOT OPERATED	235	6.1	56	1	2	4	7	12	18	56
B. OPERATED	0									
TOTAL										
0–19 Years	122	6.2	51	1	3	5	7	11	17	66
20–34	69	5.5	54	1	2	3	6	12	23	40
35–49	28	7.5	113	1	2	4	9	17	18	56
50–64	11	5.7	16	2	2	6	8	10	14	14
65+	5	6.2	13	3	4	4	9	11	11	11
GRAND TOTAL	235	6.1	56	1	2	4	7	12	18	56

312.9: CONDUCT DISTURBANCE NOS

Type of Patients	Observed Patients	Avg. Stay	Vari-ance	10th	25th	50th	75th	90th	95th	99th
1. SINGLE DX										
A. Not Operated										
0–19 Years	6	8.2	15	3	5	8	10	14	14	14
20–34	1	1.0	0	1	1	1	1	1	1	1
35–49	0									
50–64	0									
65+										
B. Operated										
0–19 Years	0									
20–34	0									
35–49	0									
50–64	0									
65+	0									
2. MULTIPLE DX										
A. Not Operated										
0–19 Years	107	5.9	19	2	3	5	7	12	16	20
20–34	5	25.9	>999	1	1	6	26	96	96	96
35–49	2	17.7	261	6	6	29	29	29	29	29
50–64	4	10.0	216	2	2	4	32	32	32	32
65+	12	5.4	13	1	3	4	8	10	11	11
B. Operated										
0–19 Years	0									
20–34	0									
35–49	0									
50–64	0									
65+	0									
SUBTOTALS:										
1. SINGLE DX										
A. Not Operated	7	7.1	20	1	3	8	10	14	14	14
B. Operated	0									
2. MULTIPLE DX										
A. Not Operated	130	6.9	91	2	3	5	8	13	17	32
B. Operated	0									
1. SINGLE DX	7	7.1	20	1	3	8	10	14	14	14
2. MULTIPLE DX	130	6.9	91	2	3	5	8	13	17	32
A. NOT OPERATED	137	6.9	87	2	3	5	8	13	17	32
B. OPERATED	0									
TOTAL										
0–19 Years	113	6.0	19	2	3	5	8	12	16	20
20–34	5	25.9	>999	1	1	6	26	96	96	96
35–49	3	12.1	222	1	1	6	29	29	29	29
50–64	4	10.0	216	2	2	2	2	32	32	32
65+	12	5.4	13	1	3	4	8	10	11	11
GRAND TOTAL	137	6.9	87	2	3	5	8	13	17	32

Length of Stay by Diagnosis and Operation, Western Region, 2008

313: EMOTIONAL DIS CHILD/ADOL

Type of Patients	Observed Patients	Avg. Stay	Variance	Percentiles 10th	25th	50th	75th	90th	95th	99th
1. SINGLE DX										
A. Not Operated										
0–19 Years	11	4.3	7	1	2	5	5	6	10	10
20–34	0									
35–49	0									
50–64	0									
65+	0									
B. Operated										
0–19 Years	0									
20–34	0									
35–49	0									
50–64	0									
65+	0									
2. MULTIPLE DX										
A. Not Operated										
0–19 Years	182	6.1	24	2	3	5	7	12	15	26
20–34	0									
35–49	0									
50–64	0									
65+	0									
B. Operated										
0–19 Years	0									
20–34	0									
35–49	0									
50–64	0									
65+	0									
SUBTOTALS:										
1. SINGLE DX										
A. Not Operated	11	4.3	7	1	2	5	5	6	10	10
B. Operated	0									
2. MULTIPLE DX										
A. Not Operated	182	6.1	24	2	3	5	7	12	15	26
B. Operated	0									
1. SINGLE DX	11	4.3	7	1	2	5	5	6	10	10
2. MULTIPLE DX	182	6.1	24	2	3	5	7	12	15	26
A. NOT OPERATED	193	6.0	23	1	3	5	7	12	15	26
B. OPERATED	0									
TOTAL										
0–19 Years	193	6.0	23	1	3	5	7	12	15	26
20–34	0									
35–49	0									
50–64	0									
65+	0									
GRAND TOTAL	193	6.0	23	1	3	5	7	12	15	26

313.81: OPPOSITIONAL DEFIANT DIS

Type of Patients	Observed Patients	Avg. Stay	Variance	Percentiles 10th	25th	50th	75th	90th	95th	99th
1. SINGLE DX										
A. Not Operated										
0–19 Years	10	4.5	7	1	2	5	5	10	10	10
20–34	0									
35–49	0									
50–64	0									
65+	0									
B. Operated										
0–19 Years	0									
20–34	0									
35–49	0									
50–64	0									
65+	0									
2. MULTIPLE DX										
A. Not Operated										
0–19 Years	158	5.8	23	2	3	4	7	11	15	26
20–34	0									
35–49	0									
50–64	0									
65+	0									
B. Operated										
0–19 Years	0									
20–34	0									
35–49	0									
50–64	0									
65+	0									
SUBTOTALS:										
1. SINGLE DX										
A. Not Operated	10	4.5	7	1	2	5	5	10	10	10
B. Operated	0									
2. MULTIPLE DX										
A. Not Operated	158	5.8	23	2	3	4	7	11	15	26
B. Operated	0									
1. SINGLE DX	10	4.5	7	1	2	5	5	10	10	10
2. MULTIPLE DX	158	5.8	23	2	3	4	7	11	15	26
A. NOT OPERATED	168	5.7	22	1	3	4	7	11	15	26
B. OPERATED	0									
TOTAL										
0–19 Years	168	5.7	22	1	3	4	7	11	15	26
20–34	0									
35–49	0									
50–64	0									
65+	0									
GRAND TOTAL	168	5.7	22	1	3	4	7	11	15	26

314: HYPERKINETIC SYNDROME

Type of Patients	Observed Patients	Avg. Stay	Variance	Percentiles 10th	25th	50th	75th	90th	95th	99th
1. SINGLE DX										
A. Not Operated										
0–19 Years	3	12.7	284	1	1	5	32	32	32	32
20–34	0									
35–49	0									
50–64	0									
65+	0									
B. Operated										
0–19 Years	0									
20–34	0									
35–49	0									
50–64	0									
65+	0									
2. MULTIPLE DX										
A. Not Operated										
0–19 Years	156	7.5	43	2	4	7	9	12	17	29
20–34	15	2.9	4	1	2	3	3	6	9	9
35–49	4	2.5	<1	2	2	2	3	3	3	3
50–64	1	3.0	0	3	3	3	3	3	3	3
65+	0									
B. Operated										
0–19 Years	0									
20–34	0									
35–49	1	7.0	0	7	7	7	7	7	7	7
50–64	0									
65+	0									
SUBTOTALS:										
1. SINGLE DX										
A. Not Operated	3	12.7	284	1	1	5	32	32	32	32
B. Operated	0									
2. MULTIPLE DX										
A. Not Operated	176	7.0	41	2	3	6	9	12	16	29
B. Operated	1	7.0	0	7	7	7	7	7	7	7
1. SINGLE DX	3	12.7	284	1	1	5	32	32	32	32
2. MULTIPLE DX	177	7.0	41	2	3	6	9	12	16	29
A. NOT OPERATED	179	7.1	44	2	3	6	9	12	17	32
B. OPERATED	1	7.0	0	7	7	7	7	7	7	7
TOTAL										
0–19 Years	159	7.6	47	2	4	7	9	13	18	32
20–34	15	2.9	4	1	2	3	3	6	9	9
35–49	5	3.4	4	2	3	3	3	3	7	7
50–64	1	3.0	0	3	3	3	3	3	3	3
65+	0									
GRAND TOTAL	180	7.1	44	2	3	6	9	12	17	32

Length of Stay by Diagnosis and Operation, Western Region, 2008

Western Region, October 2006–September 2007 Data, by Diagnosis

314.01: ADD CHILD W HYPERACT

Type of Patients	Observed Patients	Avg. Stay	Variance	10th	25th	50th	75th	90th	95th	99th
1. SINGLE DX										
A. Not Operated										
0–19 Years	3	12.7	284	1	1	5	32	32	32	32
20–34	0									
35–49	0									
50–64	0									
65+	0									
B. Operated										
0–19 Years	0									
20–34	0									
35–49	0									
50–64	0									
65+	0									
2. MULTIPLE DX										
A. Not Operated										
0–19 Years	148	7.7	44	2	4	7	10	13	17	29
20–34	9	3.4	6	1	2	3	3	9	9	9
35–49	4	2.5	<1	2	2	2	3	3	3	3
50–64	0									
65+	0									
B. Operated										
0–19 Years	0									
20–34	0									
35–49	0									
50–64	0									
65+	0									
SUBTOTALS:										
1. SINGLE DX										
A. Not Operated	3	12.7	284	1	1	5	32	32	32	32
B. Operated	0									
2. MULTIPLE DX										
A. Not Operated	161	7.4	43	2	3	6	9	12	16	29
B. Operated	0									
1. SINGLE DX	3	12.7	284	1	1	5	32	32	32	32
2. MULTIPLE DX	161	7.4	43	2	3	6	9	12	16	29
A. NOT OPERATED	164	7.5	46	2	3	6	9	12	17	32
B. OPERATED	0									
TOTAL										
0–19 Years	151	7.8	48	2	4	7	10	13	18	32
20–34	9	3.4	6	1	2	3	3	9	9	9
35–49	4	2.5	<1	2	2	2	3	3	3	3
50–64	0									
65+	0									
GRAND TOTAL	164	7.5	46	2	3	6	9	12	17	32

315: SPECIFIC DEVELOP DELAYS

Type of Patients	Observed Patients	Avg. Stay	Variance	10th	25th	50th	75th	90th	95th	99th
1. SINGLE DX										
A. Not Operated										
0–19 Years	1	1.0	0	1	1	1	1	1	1	1
20–34	0									
35–49	0									
50–64	0									
65+	0									
B. Operated										
0–19 Years	0									
20–34	0									
35–49	0									
50–64	0									
65+	0									
2. MULTIPLE DX										
A. Not Operated										
0–19 Years	14	4.3	30	1	1	2	6	16	17	17
20–34	4	5.9	39	1	1	1	8	14	14	14
35–49	2	39.2	>999	4	4	4	75	75	75	75
50–64	0									
65+	0									
B. Operated										
0–19 Years	0									
20–34	0									
35–49	0									
50–64	1	2.0	0	2	2	2	2	2	2	2
65+	0									
SUBTOTALS:										
1. SINGLE DX										
A. Not Operated	1	1.0	0	1	1	1	1	1	1	1
B. Operated	0									
2. MULTIPLE DX										
A. Not Operated	20	8.1	271	1	1	2	6	17	17	75
B. Operated	1	2.0	0	2	2	2	2	2	2	2
1. SINGLE DX	1	1.0	0	1	1	1	1	1	1	1
2. MULTIPLE DX	21	7.8	259	1	1	2	6	16	17	75
A. NOT OPERATED	21	7.8	260	1	1	2	6	16	17	75
B. OPERATED	1	2.0	0	2	2	2	2	2	2	2
TOTAL										
0–19 Years	15	4.1	28	1	1	2	6	16	17	17
20–34	4	5.9	39	1	1	1	8	14	14	14
35–49	2	39.2	>999	4	4	4	75	75	75	75
50–64	1	2.0	0	2	2	2	2	2	2	2
65+	0									
GRAND TOTAL	22	7.5	249	1	1	2	6	16	17	75

316: PSYCHIC FACTOR W DCE

Type of Patients	Observed Patients	Avg. Stay	Variance	10th	25th	50th	75th	90th	95th	99th
1. SINGLE DX										
A. Not Operated										
0–19 Years	0									
20–34	0									
35–49	0									
50–64	0									
65+	0									
B. Operated										
0–19 Years	0									
20–34	0									
35–49	0									
50–64	0									
65+	0									
2. MULTIPLE DX										
A. Not Operated										
0–19 Years	4	2.5	3	1	1	3	4	4	4	4
20–34	6	3.0	2	1	2	4	4	5	5	5
35–49	14	3.1	6	1	2	2	3	5	11	11
50–64	12	2.8	2	1	1	3	3	4	6	6
65+	9	2.7	2	1	1	2	4	5	5	5
B. Operated										
0–19 Years	0									
20–34	0									
35–49	0									
50–64	0									
65+	0									
SUBTOTALS:										
1. SINGLE DX										
A. Not Operated	0									
B. Operated	0									
2. MULTIPLE DX										
A. Not Operated	45	2.9	3	1	2	3	4	5	5	11
B. Operated	0									
1. SINGLE DX	0									
2. MULTIPLE DX	45	2.9	3	1	2	3	4	5	5	11
A. NOT OPERATED	45	2.9	3	1	2	3	4	5	5	11
B. OPERATED	0									
TOTAL										
0–19 Years	4	2.5	3	1	1	3	4	4	4	4
20–34	6	3.0	2	1	2	4	4	5	5	5
35–49	14	3.1	6	1	2	2	3	5	11	11
50–64	12	2.8	2	1	1	3	3	4	6	6
65+	9	2.7	2	1	1	2	4	5	5	5
GRAND TOTAL	45	2.9	3	1	2	3	4	5	5	11

317: MILD MENTAL RETARDATION

Type of Patients	Observed Patients	Avg. Stay	Variance	10th	25th	50th	75th	90th	95th	99th
1. SINGLE DX										
A. *Not Operated*										
0–19 Years	0									
20–34	0									
35–49	0									
50–64	0									
65+	0									
B. *Operated*										
0–19 Years	0									
20–34	0									
35–49	0									
50–64	0									
65+	0									
2. MULTIPLE DX										
A. *Not Operated*										
0–19 Years	1	6.0	0	6	6	6	6	6	6	6
20–34	5	5.2	17	2	3	3	6	12	12	12
35–49	2	5.5	4	4	4	6	7	7	7	7
50–64	3	9.7	16	5	5	12	12	12	12	12
65+	1	19.0	0	19	19	19	19	19	19	19
B. *Operated*										
0–19 Years	0									
20–34	0									
35–49	0									
50–64	0									
65+	0									
SUBTOTALS:										
1. SINGLE DX										
A. *Not Operated*	0									
B. *Operated*	0									
2. MULTIPLE DX										
A. *Not Operated*	12	7.6	26	3	3	6	12	12	19	19
B. *Operated*	0									
1. SINGLE DX	0									
2. MULTIPLE DX	12	7.6	26	3	3	6	12	12	19	19
A. NOT OPERATED	12	7.6	26	3	3	6	12	12	19	19
B. OPERATED	0									
TOTAL										
0–19 Years	1	6.0	0	6	6	6	6	6	6	6
20–34	5	5.2	17	2	3	3	6	12	12	12
35–49	2	5.5	4	4	4	6	7	7	7	7
50–64	3	9.7	16	5	5	12	12	12	12	12
65+	1	19.0	0	19	19	19	19	19	19	19
GRAND TOTAL	12	7.6	26	3	3	6	12	12	19	19

318: OTHER MENTAL RETARDATION

Type of Patients	Observed Patients	Avg. Stay	Variance	10th	25th	50th	75th	90th	95th	99th
1. SINGLE DX										
A. *Not Operated*										
0–19 Years	0									
20–34	0									
35–49	0									
50–64	0									
65+	0									
B. *Operated*										
0–19 Years	0									
20–34	0									
35–49	0									
50–64	0									
65+	0									
2. MULTIPLE DX										
A. *Not Operated*										
0–19 Years	4	10.8	130	1	1	13	26	26	26	26
20–34	3	31.7	>999	2	2	10	83	83	83	83
35–49	2	3.5	12	1	1	4	6	6	6	6
50–64	3	11.7	141	2	2	8	25	25	25	25
65+	1	2.0	0	2	2	2	2	2	2	2
B. *Operated*										
0–19 Years	0									
20–34	0									
35–49	0									
50–64	0									
65+	0									
SUBTOTALS:										
1. SINGLE DX										
A. *Not Operated*	0									
B. *Operated*	0									
2. MULTIPLE DX										
A. *Not Operated*	13	14.0	500	1	2	6	13	26	83	83
B. *Operated*	0									
1. SINGLE DX	0									
2. MULTIPLE DX	13	14.0	500	1	2	6	13	26	83	83
A. NOT OPERATED	13	14.0	500	1	2	6	13	26	83	83
B. OPERATED	0									
TOTAL										
0–19 Years	4	10.8	130	1	1	13	26	26	26	26
20–34	3	31.7	>999	2	2	10	83	83	83	83
35–49	2	3.5	12	1	1	4	6	6	6	6
50–64	3	11.7	141	2	2	8	25	25	25	25
65+	1	2.0	0	2	2	2	2	2	2	2
GRAND TOTAL	13	14.0	500	1	2	6	13	26	83	83

319: MENTAL RETARDATION NOS

Type of Patients	Observed Patients	Avg. Stay	Variance	10th	25th	50th	75th	90th	95th	99th
1. SINGLE DX										
A. *Not Operated*										
0–19 Years	0									
20–34	0									
35–49	0									
50–64	0									
65+	0									
B. *Operated*										
0–19 Years	0									
20–34	0									
35–49	0									
50–64	0									
65+	0									
2. MULTIPLE DX										
A. *Not Operated*										
0–19 Years	4	13.3	97	5	5	6	26	26	26	26
20–34	8	13.8	199	1	4	11	14	37	37	37
35–49	5	5.4	9	1	4	6	7	9	9	9
50–64	8	6.7	39	1	2	6	15	17	17	17
65+	1	22.0	0	22	22	22	22	22	22	22
B. *Operated*										
0–19 Years	0									
20–34	0									
35–49	0									
50–64	0									
65+	0									
SUBTOTALS:										
1. SINGLE DX										
A. *Not Operated*	0									
B. *Operated*	0									
2. MULTIPLE DX										
A. *Not Operated*	26	10.2	100	1	4	7	15	26	34	37
B. *Operated*	0									
1. SINGLE DX	0									
2. MULTIPLE DX	26	10.2	100	1	4	7	15	26	34	37
A. NOT OPERATED	26	10.2	100	1	4	7	15	26	34	37
B. OPERATED	0									
TOTAL										
0–19 Years	4	13.3	97	5	5	6	26	26	26	26
20–34	8	13.8	199	1	4	11	14	37	37	37
35–49	5	5.4	9	1	4	6	7	9	9	9
50–64	8	6.7	39	1	2	6	15	17	17	17
65+	1	22.0	0	22	22	22	22	22	22	22
GRAND TOTAL	26	10.2	100	1	4	7	15	26	34	37

Length of Stay by Diagnosis and Operation, Western Region, 2008

Western Region, October 2006–September 2007 Data, by Diagnosis

Type of Patients	320: BACTERIAL MENINGITIS										320.9: BACTERIAL MENINGITIS NOS										321: OTH ORGANISM MENINGITIS									
	Observed Patients	Avg. Stay	Vari-ance	10th	25th	50th	75th	90th	95th	99th	Observed Patients	Avg. Stay	Vari-ance	10th	25th	50th	75th	90th	95th	99th	Observed Patients	Avg. Stay	Vari-ance	10th	25th	50th	75th	90th	95th	99th
1. SINGLE DX																														
A. Not Operated																														
0–19 Years	28	8.9	25	3	5	10	13	14	17	21	17	8.8	19	3	5	9	13	14	14	14	0									
20–34	9	3.9	3	1	3	4	6	6	6	6	6	3.7	4	1	2	4	6	6	6	6	0									
35–49	3	3.7	9	1	1	3	7	7	7	7	3	3.7	9	1	1	3	7	7	7	7	0									
50–64	4	8.0	21	4	5	9	14	14	14	14	3	7.7	30	4	4	5	14	14	14	14	0									
65+	0										0										0									
B. Operated																														
0–19 Years	0										0										0									
20–34	0										0										0									
35–49	0										0										0									
50–64	0										0										0									
65+	0										0																				
2. MULTIPLE DX																														
A. Not Operated																														
0–19 Years	139	10.5	41	3	6	10	14	19	24	32	47	8.3	18	3	5	9	11	14	15	19	0									
20–34	110	7.6	40	2	4	6	9	18	20	30	57	6.0	25	2	3	5	7	11	18	30	0									
35–49	140	9.0	65	3	5	7	10	15	24	54	55	7.3	30	3	4	6	8	13	19	31	0									
50–64	188	9.3	56	3	4	7	13	16	18	44	65	8.1	44	3	4	6	10	16	18	44	0									
65+	143	10.0	92	4	5	7	11	19	22	49	58	9.4	38	3	5	7	13	20	24	25	0									
B. Operated																														
0–19 Years	12	22.4	236	11	11	17	28	50	51	51	0										0									
20–34	9	14.5	32	8	10	13	18	26	26	26	0										0									
35–49	18	18.7	416	4	8	13	25	29	94	94	4	12.7	128	4	4	6	12	29	29	29	0									
50–64	27	17.4	197	6	8	14	20	26	46	72	3	24.0	409	6	6	20	46	46	46	46	0									
65+	16	15.7	97	5	9	15	21	27	43	43	4	16.3	86	8	9	21	27	27	27	27	0									
SUBTOTALS:																														
1. SINGLE DX																														
A. Not Operated	44	7.4	23	2	4	6	10	14	14	21	29	7.1	20	1	3	6	10	14	14	14	0									
B. Operated	0										0										0									
2. MULTIPLE DX																														
A. Not Operated	720	9.4	60	3	5	8	12	17	21	39	282	7.8	33	3	4	7	10	15	19	30	0									
B. Operated	82	17.8	209	6	9	14	21	28	46	94	11	17.1	168	6	6	12	27	29	46	46	0									
1. SINGLE DX	44	7.4	23	2	4	6	10	14	14	21	29	7.1	20	1	3	6	10	14	14	14	**0**									
2. MULTIPLE DX	802	10.2	82	3	5	8	13	19	25	49	293	8.2	40	3	4	7	10	16	20	31	**0**									
A. NOT OPERATED	764	9.2	58	3	4	8	12	16	21	39	311	7.8	31	3	4	7	10	14	19	25	**0**									
B. OPERATED	82	17.8	209	6	9	14	21	28	46	94	11	17.1	168	6	6	12	27	29	46	46	**0**									
TOTAL																														
0–19 Years	179	11.0	60	3	6	10	14	20	25	50	64	8.5	18	3	5	9	12	14	14	19	0									
20–34	128	7.8	41	2	4	6	9	18	20	30	63	5.8	23	2	3	4	7	11	13	30	0									
35–49	161	10.0	111	3	5	8	11	17	27	61	62	7.5	35	3	4	6	8	13	19	31	0									
50–64	219	10.2	79	3	5	8	14	18	22	46	71	8.7	64	3	4	6	11	16	20	46	0									
65+	159	10.6	95	4	5	8	13	20	25	49	62	9.9	42	4	5	8	13	21	24	27	0									
GRAND TOTAL	**846**	**10.1**	**79**	**3**	**5**	**8**	**13**	**19**	**24**	**49**	**322**	**8.1**	**38**	**3**	**4**	**7**	**10**	**15**	**19**	**30**	**0**									

Length of Stay by Diagnosis and Operation, Western Region, 2008

322: MENINGITIS CAUSE NOS

Type of Patients	Observed Patients	Avg. Stay	Vari-ance	10th	25th	50th	75th	90th	95th	99th
1. SINGLE DX										
A. Not Operated										
0–19 Years	28	4.9	12	1	2	3	9	10	10	12
20–34	10	2.3	2	1	1	2	3	4	5	5
35–49	7	4.0	4	1	2	4	5	7	7	7
50–64	1	3.0	0	3	3	3	3	3	3	3
65+	0									
B. Operated										
0–19 Years	0									
20–34	0									
35–49	0									
50–64	1	1.0	0	1	1	1	1	1	1	1
65+	1	1.0	0	1	1	1	1	1	1	1
2. MULTIPLE DX										
A. Not Operated										
0–19 Years	65	6.3	24	2	2	4	9	14	15	20
20–34	75	4.6	15	1	2	3	6	9	10	26
35–49	81	6.2	28	2	3	5	7	11	16	30
50–64	103	5.3	11	2	3	5	7	10	12	13
65+	88	8.2	47	3	4	6	11	16	20	44
B. Operated										
0–19 Years	0									
20–34	5	8.2	14	4	6	8	9	14	14	14
35–49	9	9.0	21	1	8	10	10	16	16	16
50–64	12	10.4	92	2	3	5	18	21	31	31
65+	15	5.8	50	1	2	4	7	11	29	29
SUBTOTALS:										
1. SINGLE DX										
A. Not Operated	46	4.2	9	1	2	3	5	10	10	12
B. Operated	2	1.0	0	1	1	1	1	1	1	1
2. MULTIPLE DX										
A. Not Operated	412	6.1	26	2	3	5	8	12	15	26
B. Operated	41	8.2	52	1	3	6	10	18	21	31
1. SINGLE DX	48	4.0	9	1	2	3	5	10	10	12
2. MULTIPLE DX	453	6.3	29	2	3	5	8	13	16	29
A. NOT OPERATED	458	5.9	25	2	3	5	8	12	15	26
B. OPERATED	43	7.8	52	1	2	6	10	18	21	31
TOTAL										
0–19 Years	93	5.9	21	2	2	4	9	13	15	20
20–34	90	4.6	15	1	2	3	6	9	10	26
35–49	97	6.3	26	2	3	5	8	11	16	30
50–64	117	5.8	21	2	3	5	7	12	13	21
65+	104	7.8	47	2	4	6	10	16	20	31
GRAND TOTAL	501	6.1	27	2	3	5	8	12	16	28

322.9: MENINGITIS NOS

Type of Patients	Observed Patients	Avg. Stay	Vari-ance	10th	25th	50th	75th	90th	95th	99th
1. SINGLE DX										
A. Not Operated										
0–19 Years	28	4.9	12	1	2	3	9	10	10	12
20–34	9	2.3	2	1	1	2	3	5	5	5
35–49	7	4.0	4	1	2	4	5	7	7	7
50–64	1	3.0	0	3	3	3	3	3	3	3
65+	0									
B. Operated										
0–19 Years	0									
20–34	0									
35–49	0									
50–64	1	1.0	0	1	1	1	1	1	1	1
65+	1	1.0	0	1	1	1	1	1	1	1
2. MULTIPLE DX										
A. Not Operated										
0–19 Years	60	6.3	23	2	2	4	9	14	15	20
20–34	65	4.5	9	1	2	3	6	9	10	14
35–49	72	6.1	23	2	3	5	7	11	16	30
50–64	84	5.3	11	2	3	5	7	10	12	18
65+	79	7.7	27	3	4	6	11	16	20	26
B. Operated										
0–19 Years	0									
20–34	4	8.0	19	4	4	6	9	14	14	14
35–49	7	9.6	23	1	8	10	10	16	16	16
50–64	11	10.4	101	2	3	5	19	21	31	31
65+	13	5.9	58	1	2	3	7	11	29	29
SUBTOTALS:										
1. SINGLE DX										
A. Not Operated	45	4.2	9	1	2	3	5	10	10	12
B. Operated	2	1.0	0	1	1	1	1	1	1	1
2. MULTIPLE DX										
A. Not Operated	360	6.0	20	2	3	5	8	12	14	22
B. Operated	35	8.3	60	1	2	6	11	19	29	31
1. SINGLE DX	47	4.1	9	1	2	3	5	10	10	12
2. MULTIPLE DX	395	6.2	23	2	3	5	8	13	16	26
A. NOT OPERATED	405	5.8	19	2	3	5	8	12	14	20
B. OPERATED	37	7.9	60	1	2	5	10	18	29	31
TOTAL										
0–19 Years	88	5.8	20	2	2	4	9	13	15	20
20–34	78	4.4	10	1	2	3	6	9	10	14
35–49	86	6.2	23	2	3	5	8	11	16	30
50–64	97	5.8	23	2	3	5	7	12	18	31
65+	93	7.4	31	2	4	6	10	14	20	29
GRAND TOTAL	442	6.0	22	2	3	5	8	12	15	22

323: ENCEPHALOMYELITIS

Type of Patients	Observed Patients	Avg. Stay	Vari-ance	10th	25th	50th	75th	90th	95th	99th
1. SINGLE DX										
A. Not Operated										
0–19 Years	5	3.2	5	1	2	2	5	6	6	6
20–34	5	4.6	2	2	5	5	5	6	6	6
35–49	5	3.2	4	1	2	3	4	6	6	6
50–64	1	5.0	0	5	5	5	5	5	5	5
65+	0									
B. Operated										
0–19 Years	0									
20–34	0									
35–49	0									
50–64	2	3.0	8	1	1	5	5	5	5	5
65+	1	1.0	0	1	1	1	1	1	1	1
2. MULTIPLE DX										
A. Not Operated										
0–19 Years	50	8.0	109	1	2	5	10	22	23	66
20–34	60	7.2	39	2	3	4	10	16	21	27
35–49	98	8.2	84	2	4	6	9	14	18	63
50–64	107	8.3	41	2	4	7	11	15	17	31
65+	119	8.7	41	2	5	7	11	18	24	29
B. Operated										
0–19 Years	4	7.5	108	1	2	2	4	23	23	23
20–34	5	17.3	124	4	11	14	29	29	29	29
35–49	5	16.7	926	2	3	3	4	71	71	71
50–64	15	20.3	445	2	4	9	39	44	70	70
65+	4	8.9	37	2	2	6	13	15	15	15
SUBTOTALS:										
1. SINGLE DX										
A. Not Operated	16	3.8	3	1	2	4	5	6	6	6
B. Operated	3	2.3	5	1	1	1	1	5	5	5
2. MULTIPLE DX										
A. Not Operated	434	8.2	58	2	4	6	10	16	22	31
B. Operated	33	16.4	364	2	3	8	23	44	70	71
1. SINGLE DX	19	3.5	4	1	2	4	5	6	6	6
2. MULTIPLE DX	467	8.8	83	2	4	6	10	17	24	61
A. NOT OPERATED	450	8.1	57	2	4	6	10	16	22	31
B. OPERATED	36	15.2	349	2	3	6	23	44	70	71
TOTAL										
0–19 Years	59	7.6	100	1	2	5	9	22	23	66
20–34	70	7.8	48	2	3	5	10	18	26	29
35–49	108	8.4	115	2	3	6	9	14	18	63
50–64	125	9.6	101	2	4	7	11	17	31	45
65+	124	8.7	40	2	5	7	11	17	29	29
GRAND TOTAL	486	8.6	81	2	4	6	10	17	24	61

Length of Stay by Diagnosis and Operation, Western Region, 2008

Western Region, October 2006–September 2007 Data, by Diagnosis

324: CNS ABSCESS

Type of Patients	Observed Patients	Avg. Stay	Variance	10th	25th	50th	75th	90th	95th	99th
1. SINGLE DX										
A. Not Operated										
0–19 Years	1	5.0	0	5	5	5	5	5	5	5
20–34	0									
35–49	1	6.0	0	6	6	6	6	6	6	6
50–64	3	2.3	2	1	1	2	4	4	4	4
65+	0									
B. Operated										
0–19 Years	1	9.0	0	9	9	9	9	9	9	9
20–34	0									
35–49	1	2.0	0	2	2	2	2	2	2	2
50–64	1	2.0	0	2	2	2	2	2	2	2
65+	1	1.0	0	1	1	1	1	1	1	1
2. MULTIPLE DX										
A. Not Operated										
0–19 Years	10	6.3	68	1	2	3	5	8	28	28
20–34	18	6.7	14	1	4	6	6	8	14	14
35–49	77	11.1	107	3	5	8	13	25	41	54
50–64	125	10.3	77	3	5	7	13	19	28	45
65+	113	10.2	89	3	5	8	12	18	29	56
B. Operated										
0–19 Years	26	16.5	367	5	6	9	16	53	62	77
20–34	51	14.7	176	4	6	10	18	30	42	62
35–49	139	15.4	215	4	7	11	19	36	44	90
50–64	263	15.6	189	5	7	11	20	34	46	73
65+	135	13.5	150	4	6	10	18	29	35	56
SUBTOTALS:										
1. SINGLE DX										
A. Not Operated	5	3.6	4	1	2	4	5	5	5	6
B. Operated	4	3.5	13	1	2	2	2	9	9	9
2. MULTIPLE DX										
A. Not Operated	343	10.2	85	3	5	7	12	21	29	54
B. Operated	614	15.1	192	4	7	11	19	31	43	77
1. SINGLE DX	9	3.5	7	1	2	2	5	9	9	9
2. MULTIPLE DX	957	13.3	159	4	6	9	16	28	40	69
A. NOT OPERATED	348	10.1	84	3	5	7	12	21	29	54
B. OPERATED	618	15.0	192	4	7	11	19	31	43	77
TOTAL										
0–19 Years	38	13.3	287	2	5	8	12	33	62	77
20–34	69	12.6	145	3	5	8	15	29	37	62
35–49	218	13.8	180	4	6	10	16	29	43	88
50–64	392	13.8	159	4	6	10	16	28	38	69
65+	249	12.0	125	4	5	9	14	26	31	56
GRAND TOTAL	966	13.2	159	4	6	9	15	28	38	69

324.0: INTRACRANIAL ABSCESS

Type of Patients	Observed Patients	Avg. Stay	Variance	10th	25th	50th	75th	90th	95th	99th
1. SINGLE DX										
A. Not Operated										
0–19 Years	1	5.0	0	5	5	5	5	5	5	5
20–34	0									
35–49	0									
50–64	3	2.3	2	1	1	2	4	4	4	4
65+	0									
B. Operated										
0–19 Years	0									
20–34	0									
35–49	0									
50–64	1	2.0	0	2	2	2	2	2	2	2
65+	1	1.0	0	1	1	1	1	1	1	1
2. MULTIPLE DX										
A. Not Operated										
0–19 Years	8	6.3	83	1	2	2	5	28	28	28
20–34	8	6.5	15	3	6	6	8	14	14	14
35–49	14	11.9	119	4	5	6	15	22	43	43
50–64	32	9.8	96	2	5	7	12	16	23	54
65+	27	8.2	26	3	4	7	11	17	17	22
B. Operated										
0–19 Years	23	17.9	399	5	7	10	18	53	62	77
20–34	25	11.2	60	3	6	9	15	21	29	30
35–49	51	15.0	217	3	7	11	18	28	42	90
50–64	78	14.8	120	4	6	12	21	34	42	>99
65+	40	14.1	118	5	7	11	19	27	35	56
SUBTOTALS:										
1. SINGLE DX										
A. Not Operated	4	3.0	3	1	1	2	4	5	5	5
B. Operated	2	1.5	<1	1	1	1	2	2	2	2
2. MULTIPLE DX										
A. Not Operated	89	9.0	70	2	4	7	11	17	22	54
B. Operated	217	14.6	164	4	6	11	19	31	42	77
1. SINGLE DX	6	2.5	3	1	1	2	4	5	5	5
2. MULTIPLE DX	306	13.0	143	3	5	9	16	28	37	62
A. NOT OPERATED	93	8.8	68	2	4	6	11	17	22	54
B. OPERATED	219	14.5	164	3	6	11	19	30	41	77
TOTAL										
0–19 Years	32	14.6	331	2	5	8	12	33	62	77
20–34	33	10.0	53	3	5	8	15	21	29	30
35–49	65	14.3	195	3	6	11	18	28	42	90
50–64	114	13.0	118	3	6	9	16	29	37	54
65+	68	11.6	89	3	5	9	14	22	28	56
GRAND TOTAL	312	12.8	142	3	5	9	16	28	37	62

324.1: INTRASPINAL ABSCESS

Type of Patients	Observed Patients	Avg. Stay	Variance	10th	25th	50th	75th	90th	95th	99th
1. SINGLE DX										
A. Not Operated										
0–19 Years	0									
20–34	0									
35–49	1	6.0	0	6	6	6	6	6	6	6
50–64	0									
65+	0									
B. Operated										
0–19 Years	1	9.0	0	9	9	9	9	9	9	9
20–34	0									
35–49	1	2.0	0	2	2	2	2	2	2	2
50–64	0									
65+	0									
2. MULTIPLE DX										
A. Not Operated										
0–19 Years	2	6.5	25	3	3	7	10	10	10	10
20–34	10	6.8	16	1	5	6	10	11	14	14
35–49	61	11.1	109	3	5	8	12	25	31	54
50–64	90	10.3	70	3	5	7	13	20	29	45
65+	85	10.6	104	3	5	8	12	20	29	67
B. Operated										
0–19 Years	3	5.7	<1	5	5	6	6	6	6	6
20–34	25	18.6	272	5	7	12	24	42	58	62
35–49	87	15.7	219	4	7	11	19	40	50	>99
50–64	182	16.0	222	5	7	11	19	34	51	73
65+	91	13.4	171	4	6	10	15	29	35	97
SUBTOTALS:										
1. SINGLE DX										
A. Not Operated	1	6.0	0	6	6	6	6	6	6	6
B. Operated	2	5.5	24	2	2	2	2	9	9	9
2. MULTIPLE DX										
A. Not Operated	248	10.4	89	3	5	7	12	21	29	54
B. Operated	388	15.4	212	4	7	11	19	34	48	88
1. SINGLE DX	3	5.6	12	2	2	6	9	9	9	9
2. MULTIPLE DX	636	13.5	169	4	6	10	15	28	41	69
A. NOT OPERATED	249	10.4	88	3	5	7	12	21	29	54
B. OPERATED	390	15.4	211	4	7	11	19	34	48	88
TOTAL										
0–19 Years	6	6.5	7	3	5	6	9	10	10	10
20–34	35	15.2	225	4	6	10	17	37	58	62
35–49	150	13.7	177	4	6	10	15	29	43	88
50–64	272	14.2	178	4	6	10	17	28	42	69
65+	176	12.0	140	4	5	9	14	27	31	67
GRAND TOTAL	639	13.4	169	4	6	10	15	28	41	69

325: PHLEBITIS IC VEN SINUS

Type of Patients	Observed Patients	Avg. Stay	Variance	10th	25th	50th	75th	90th	95th	99th
1. SINGLE DX										
A. *Not Operated*										
0–19 Years	1	4.0	0	4	4	4	4	4	4	4
20–34	1	12.0	0	12	12	12	12	12	12	12
35–49	4	3.2	7	1	2	3	3	7	7	7
50–64	1	6.0	0	6	6	6	6	6	6	6
65+	0									
B. *Operated*										
0–19 Years	0									
20–34	0									
35–49	0									
50–64	0									
65+	0									
2. MULTIPLE DX										
A. *Not Operated*										
0–19 Years	7	5.0	5	1	4	5	7	8	8	8
20–34	47	5.3	9	2	3	5	8	9	10	14
35–49	45	5.2	9	1	3	5	7	9	9	13
50–64	24	4.6	13	1	2	4	6	8	9	18
65+	10	8.6	106	1	2	6	12	14	35	35
B. *Operated*										
0–19 Years	3	14.2	123	6	6	10	27	27	27	27
20–34	3	15.0	21	11	11	14	20	20	20	20
35–49	3	14.3	120	7	7	9	27	27	27	27
50–64	1	13.0	0	13	13	13	13	13	13	13
65+	0									
SUBTOTALS:										
1. SINGLE DX										
A. *Not Operated*	7	5.0	14	1	2	4	7	12	12	12
B. *Operated*	0									
2. MULTIPLE DX										
A. *Not Operated*	133	5.3	17	1	3	5	7	9	12	18
B. *Operated*	10	14.4	59	6	9	13	20	27	27	27
1. SINGLE DX	7	5.0	14	1	2	4	7	12	12	12
2. MULTIPLE DX	143	6.0	25	2	3	5	8	10	14	27
A. NOT OPERATED	140	5.3	16	1	3	5	7	9	12	18
B. OPERATED	10	14.4	59	6	9	13	20	27	27	27
TOTAL										
0–19 Years	11	7.4	47	4	4	5	8	10	27	27
20–34	51	6.0	15	2	3	5	8	11	14	20
35–49	52	5.5	18	1	3	5	7	9	12	27
50–64	26	5.0	15	1	2	4	6	9	13	18
65+	10	8.6	106	1	2	6	12	14	35	35
GRAND TOTAL	150	5.9	24	1	3	5	8	11	14	27

326: LATE EFF IC ABSCESS

Type of Patients	Observed Patients	Avg. Stay	Variance	10th	25th	50th	75th	90th	95th	99th
1. SINGLE DX										
A. *Not Operated*										
0–19 Years	0									
20–34	0									
35–49	0									
50–64	0									
65+	0									
B. *Operated*										
0–19 Years	0									
20–34	0									
35–49	0									
50–64	0									
65+	0									
2. MULTIPLE DX										
A. *Not Operated*										
0–19 Years	0									
20–34	0									
35–49	1	1.0	0	1	1	1	1	1	1	1
50–64	0									
65+	0									
B. *Operated*										
0–19 Years	0									
20–34	0									
35–49	1	7.0	0	7	7	7	7	7	7	7
50–64	0									
65+	0									
SUBTOTALS:										
1. SINGLE DX										
A. *Not Operated*	0									
B. *Operated*	0									
2. MULTIPLE DX										
A. *Not Operated*	1	1.0	0	1	1	1	1	1	1	1
B. *Operated*	1	7.0	0	7	7	7	7	7	7	7
1. SINGLE DX	0									
2. MULTIPLE DX	2	4.0	17	1	1	4	7	7	7	7
A. NOT OPERATED	1	1.0	0	1	1	1	1	1	1	1
B. OPERATED	1	7.0	0	7	7	7	7	7	7	7
TOTAL										
0–19 Years	0									
20–34	0									
35–49	2	4.0	17	1	1	4	7	7	7	7
50–64	0									
65+	0									
GRAND TOTAL	2	4.0	17	1	1	4	7	7	7	7

327: ORGANIC SLEEP DISORDERS

Type of Patients	Observed Patients	Avg. Stay	Variance	10th	25th	50th	75th	90th	95th	99th
1. SINGLE DX										
A. *Not Operated*										
0–19 Years	0									
20–34	0									
35–49	1	3.0	0	3	3	3	3	3	3	3
50–64	3	2.7	2	1	1	3	4	4	4	4
65+	1	3.0	0	3	3	3	3	3	3	3
B. *Operated*										
0–19 Years	22	1.1	<1	1	1	1	1	1	1	2
20–34	20	1.5	<1	1	1	1	2	3	3	4
35–49	50	1.5	<1	1	1	1	2	3	3	4
50–64	35	1.6	<1	1	1	1	2	3	3	3
65+	4	1.0	0	1	1	1	1	1	1	1
2. MULTIPLE DX										
A. *Not Operated*										
0–19 Years	66	3.1	15	1	1	2	3	6	9	23
20–34	53	4.2	21	1	2	3	5	8	13	28
35–49	201	3.5	9	1	2	3	4	8	9	17
50–64	228	3.5	8	1	2	3	4	6	9	13
65+	161	3.6	6	1	2	3	5	7	8	12
B. *Operated*										
0–19 Years	296	1.6	3	1	1	2	2	3	5	11
20–34	239	1.8	15	1	1	1	2	3	4	7
35–49	559	1.7	3	1	1	1	2	3	4	8
50–64	512	1.7	3	1	1	1	2	3	4	7
65+	90	1.8	4	1	1	1	2	3	4	17
SUBTOTALS:										
1. SINGLE DX										
A. *Not Operated*	5	2.8	<1	1	1	3	3	4	4	4
B. *Operated*	131	1.4	<1	1	1	1	2	3	3	4
2. MULTIPLE DX										
A. *Not Operated*	709	3.5	10	1	1	3	4	7	9	16
B. *Operated*	1,696	1.7	4	1	1	1	2	3	4	8
1. SINGLE DX	136	1.5	<1	1	1	1	2	3	3	4
2. MULTIPLE DX	2,405	2.3	6	1	1	1	3	4	6	12
A. NOT OPERATED	714	3.5	9	1	1	3	4	7	9	16
B. OPERATED	1,827	1.7	4	1	1	1	2	3	4	7
TOTAL										
0–19 Years	384	1.9	5	1	1	1	2	4	5	14
20–34	312	2.2	16	1	1	1	2	4	5	13
35–49	811	2.1	4	1	1	1	2	4	6	12
50–64	778	2.2	5	1	1	2	3	4	6	12
65+	256	2.9	6	1	2	2	4	6	8	12
GRAND TOTAL	2,541	2.2	6	1	1	1	2	4	6	12

Length of Stay by Diagnosis and Operation, Western Region, 2008

Western Region, October 2006–September 2007 Data, by Diagnosis

327.23: OBSTRUCTIVE SLEEP APNEA

Type of Patients	Observed Patients	Avg. Stay	Variance	10th	25th	50th	75th	90th	95th	99th
1. SINGLE DX										
A. Not Operated										
0–19 Years	0									
20–34	0									
35–49	1	3.0	0	3	3	3	3	3	3	3
50–64	2	2.5	4	1	1	3	4	4	4	4
65+	1	3.0	0	3	3	3	3	3	3	3
B. Operated										
0–19 Years	22	1.1	<1	1	1	1	1	1	1	2
20–34	20	1.5	<1	1	1	1	2	3	3	4
35–49	50	1.5	<1	1	1	1	2	3	3	4
50–64	35	1.6	<1	1	1	1	2	3	3	3
65+	4	1.0	0	1	1	1	1	1	1	1
2. MULTIPLE DX										
A. Not Operated										
0–19 Years	51	3.0	16	1	1	2	3	6	9	23
20–34	51	4.2	22	1	1	3	5	8	13	28
35–49	194	3.5	10	1	2	3	4	6	10	17
50–64	215	3.5	8	1	2	3	4	6	9	13
65+	148	3.6	6	1	2	3	5	7	8	12
B. Operated										
0–19 Years	296	1.6	3	1	1	1	1	3	5	11
20–34	238	1.5	1	1	1	1	2	3	3	6
35–49	559	1.7	2	1	1	1	2	3	4	8
50–64	511	1.7	3	1	1	1	2	3	4	7
65+	90	1.8	4	1	1	1	2	3	4	17
SUBTOTALS:										
1. SINGLE DX										
A. Not Operated	4	2.8	2	1	1	3	3	4	4	4
B. Operated	131	1.4	<1	1	1	1	2	3	3	4
2. MULTIPLE DX										
A. Not Operated	659	3.5	10	1	1	3	4	7	9	17
B. Operated	1,694	1.7	2	1	1	1	2	3	4	8
1. SINGLE DX	135	1.5	<1	1	1	1	2	3	3	4
2. MULTIPLE DX	2,353	2.2	5	1	1	1	2	4	6	12
A. NOT OPERATED	663	3.5	10	1	1	3	4	7	9	17
B. OPERATED	1,825	1.7	2	1	1	1	2	3	4	7
TOTAL										
0–19 Years	369	1.8	5	1	1	1	2	3	5	14
20–34	309	2.0	6	1	1	1	2	4	5	11
35–49	804	2.1	4	1	1	1	2	4	6	12
50–64	763	2.2	5	1	1	1	3	4	6	11
65+	243	2.9	6	1	1	2	4	6	7	12
GRAND TOTAL	2,488	2.2	5	1	1	1	2	4	6	12

330: CEREB DEGEN IN CHILD

Type of Patients	Observed Patients	Avg. Stay	Variance	10th	25th	50th	75th	90th	95th	99th
1. SINGLE DX										
A. Not Operated										
0–19 Years	0									
20–34	1	4.0	0	4	4	4	4	4	4	4
35–49	0									
50–64	0									
65+	0									
B. Operated										
0–19 Years	0									
20–34	0									
35–49	0									
50–64	0									
65+	0									
2. MULTIPLE DX										
A. Not Operated										
0–19 Years	18	5.4	27	1	2	4	6	16	18	18
20–34	3	13.7	121	3	3	13	25	25	25	25
35–49	3	8.8	154	1	1	2	23	23	23	23
50–64	2	5.5	<1	5	5	6	6	6	6	6
65+	2	30.2	716	11	11	49	49	49	49	49
B. Operated										
0–19 Years	9	10.3	265	2	3	5	7	53	53	53
20–34	0									
35–49	0									
50–64	0									
65+	0									
SUBTOTALS:										
1. SINGLE DX										
A. Not Operated	1	4.0	0	4	4	4	4	4	4	4
B. Operated	0									
2. MULTIPLE DX										
A. Not Operated	28	8.4	108	1	3	5	13	23	25	49
B. Operated	9	10.3	265	2	3	5	7	53	53	53
1. SINGLE DX	1	4.0	0	4	4	4	4	4	4	4
2. MULTIPLE DX	37	8.9	141	1	3	5	11	23	49	53
A. NOT OPERATED	29	8.3	105	1	3	4	11	23	25	49
B. OPERATED	9	10.3	265	2	3	5	7	53	53	53
TOTAL										
0–19 Years	27	7.1	105	1	2	4	6	16	18	53
20–34	4	11.2	104	3	3	4	25	25	25	25
35–49	3	8.8	154	1	1	2	23	23	23	23
50–64	2	5.5	<1	5	5	6	6	6	6	6
65+	2	30.2	716	11	11	49	49	49	49	49
GRAND TOTAL	38	8.8	138	1	3	5	11	23	49	53

331: CEREBRAL DEGENERATION

Type of Patients	Observed Patients	Avg. Stay	Variance	10th	25th	50th	75th	90th	95th	99th
1. SINGLE DX										
A. Not Operated										
0–19 Years	1	2.0	0	2	2	2	2	2	2	2
20–34	2	5.5	24	2	2	9	9	9	9	9
35–49	0									
50–64	8	11.6	180	1	4	7	14	43	43	43
65+	38	5.0	24	1	2	3	9	11	15	23
B. Operated										
0–19 Years	16	2.7	5	1	1	2	3	8	8	8
20–34	6	2.2	2	1	1	1	4	4	4	4
35–49	23	4.0	14	1	2	3	5	7	10	18
50–64	22	2.0	<1	1	1	2	3	3	3	3
65+	23	2.2	2	1	1	2	3	4	4	6
2. MULTIPLE DX										
A. Not Operated										
0–19 Years	18	3.1	5	1	1	3	3	7	9	9
20–34	27	3.3	4	1	2	3	4	7	8	9
35–49	46	8.7	279	1	2	4	8	17	32	88
50–64	372	9.7	138	1	3	5	11	23	33	59
65+	5,967	8.3	58	2	3	6	11	18	23	37
B. Operated										
0–19 Years	99	6.1	124	1	2	3	6	12	27	91
20–34	104	7.3	90	1	2	4	8	16	18	49
35–49	170	7.4	152	1	2	4	7	16	32	>99
50–64	327	6.0	47	1	2	3	7	15	22	37
65+	971	4.7	27	1	2	3	5	11	15	30
SUBTOTALS:										
1. SINGLE DX										
A. Not Operated	49	6.0	52	1	2	3	9	13	15	43
B. Operated	90	2.7	6	1	1	2	3	4	7	18
2. MULTIPLE DX										
A. Not Operated	6,430	8.3	64	2	3	6	11	18	24	40
B. Operated	1,671	5.5	54	1	2	3	6	12	18	46
1. SINGLE DX	139	3.9	24	1	1	2	4	9	11	23
2. MULTIPLE DX	8,101	7.7	63	1	3	5	10	17	23	41
A. NOT OPERATED	6,479	8.3	64	2	3	6	11	18	24	41
B. OPERATED	1,761	5.3	52	1	2	3	6	12	17	44
TOTAL										
0–19 Years	134	5.3	95	1	2	3	5	9	14	48
20–34	139	6.3	72	1	2	4	7	15	18	49
35–49	239	7.3	164	1	2	4	7	16	30	96
50–64	729	7.8	98	1	2	4	10	19	28	54
65+	6,999	7.8	55	2	3	5	11	17	22	36
GRAND TOTAL	8,240	7.7	63	1	3	5	10	17	23	41

Length of Stay by Diagnosis and Operation, Western Region, 2008

331.0: ALZHEIMER'S DISEASE

Type of Patients	Observed Patients	Avg. Stay	Variance	10th	25th	50th	75th	90th	95th	99th
1. SINGLE DX										
A. Not Operated										
0–19 Years	0									
20–34	0									
35–49	0									
50–64	6	8.2	19	4	4	7	13	14	14	14
65+	31	5.5	27	1	2	3	10	11	15	23
B. Operated										
0–19 Years	0									
20–34	0									
35–49	0									
50–64	0									
65+	0									
2. MULTIPLE DX										
A. Not Operated										
0–19 Years	0									
20–34	1	9.0	0	9	9	9	9	9	9	9
35–49	6	22.3	772	3	4	9	32	75	75	75
50–64	182	10.6	116	2	3	7	13	22	32	54
65+	4,566	8.9	63	2	3	6	12	19	24	40
B. Operated										
0–19 Years	0									
20–34	0									
35–49	0									
50–64	1	11.0	0	11	11	11	11	11	11	11
65+	23	12.2	117	3	4	9	19	33	46	>99
SUBTOTALS:										
1. SINGLE DX										
A. Not Operated	37	6.0	26	1	2	4	10	13	15	23
B. Operated	0									
2. MULTIPLE DX										
A. Not Operated	4,755	8.9	66	2	3	6	12	19	24	42
B. Operated	24	12.2	112	3	5	9	18	33	46	>99
1. SINGLE DX	37	6.0	26	1	2	4	10	13	15	23
2. MULTIPLE DX	4,779	9.0	67	2	3	6	12	19	24	42
A. NOT OPERATED	4,792	8.9	66	2	3	6	12	19	24	42
B. OPERATED	24	12.2	112	3	5	9	18	33	46	>99
TOTAL										
0–19 Years	0									
20–34	1	9.0	0	9	9	9	9	9	9	9
35–49	6	22.3	772	3	4	9	32	75	75	75
50–64	189	10.5	112	2	3	7	13	22	32	54
65+	4,620	8.8	63	2	3	6	12	19	24	40
GRAND TOTAL	4,816	8.9	66	2	3	6	12	19	24	42

331.3: COMMUNIC HYDROCEPHALUS

Type of Patients	Observed Patients	Avg. Stay	Variance	10th	25th	50th	75th	90th	95th	99th
1. SINGLE DX										
A. Not Operated										
0–19 Years	0									
20–34	1	9.0	0	9	9	9	9	9	9	9
35–49	0									
50–64	0									
65+	3	2.7	8	1	1	1	6	6	6	6
B. Operated										
0–19 Years	3	2.3	1	1	1	3	3	3	3	3
20–34	0									
35–49	7	2.9	2	1	2	2	4	5	5	5
50–64	7	1.7	<1	1	1	1	3	3	3	3
65+	19	2.2	2	1	1	2	3	4	6	6
2. MULTIPLE DX										
A. Not Operated										
0–19 Years	2	3.0	0	3	3	3	3	3	3	3
20–34	3	5.7	10	2	2	7	8	8	8	8
35–49	4	8.0	44	2	2	9	17	17	17	17
50–64	37	4.8	17	1	2	4	5	11	11	21
65+	290	5.2	19	1	2	4	7	10	12	22
B. Operated										
0–19 Years	17	4.2	13	1	2	3	6	12	12	12
20–34	16	9.9	227	2	4	5	11	16	64	64
35–49	30	10.5	334	1	2	4	13	30	96	>99
50–64	129	5.8	40	1	2	3	8	15	19	43
65+	728	4.3	21	1	2	3	5	9	14	22
SUBTOTALS:										
1. SINGLE DX										
A. Not Operated	4	4.3	16	1	1	4	9	9	9	9
B. Operated	36	2.2	2	1	1	2	3	4	5	6
2. MULTIPLE DX										
A. Not Operated	336	5.2	19	1	2	4	7	10	12	21
B. Operated	920	4.8	39	1	2	3	5	10	15	30
1. SINGLE DX	40	2.4	3	1	1	2	3	5	6	9
2. MULTIPLE DX	1,256	4.9	33	1	2	3	6	10	15	30
A. NOT OPERATED	340	5.2	19	1	2	4	7	10	12	21
B. OPERATED	956	4.7	38	1	2	3	5	10	15	30
TOTAL										
0–19 Years	22	3.9	11	1	2	3	4	9	12	12
20–34	20	9.3	183	2	4	6	9	16	64	64
35–49	41	8.9	254	1	2	4	9	22	32	>99
50–64	173	5.4	34	1	2	3	6	13	17	43
65+	1,040	4.5	21	1	2	3	6	9	13	22
GRAND TOTAL	1,296	4.8	33	1	2	3	6	10	15	30

331.4: OBSTR HYDROCEPHALUS

Type of Patients	Observed Patients	Avg. Stay	Variance	10th	25th	50th	75th	90th	95th	99th
1. SINGLE DX										
A. Not Operated										
0–19 Years	0									
20–34	1	2.0	0	2	2	2	2	2	2	2
35–49	0									
50–64	1	1.0	0	1	1	1	1	1	1	1
65+	0									
B. Operated										
0–19 Years	13	2.8	6	1	1	2	3	8	8	8
20–34	6	2.2	2	1	1	1	4	4	4	4
35–49	16	4.5	19	1	2	3	5	10	18	18
50–64	15	2.2	<1	1	2	2	3	3	4	4
65+	4	2.3	<1	1	1	2	3	3	3	3
2. MULTIPLE DX										
A. Not Operated										
0–19 Years	15	2.9	5	1	1	3	3	7	9	9
20–34	22	2.8	1	1	2	3	4	4	4	5
35–49	23	2.8	3	1	1	3	4	5	5	8
50–64	49	4.8	26	1	2	3	5	11	15	24
65+	73	4.6	13	1	2	3	6	9	12	18
B. Operated										
0–19 Years	81	6.5	149	1	2	3	5	13	27	91
20–34	88	6.8	66	1	2	4	8	17	18	49
35–49	140	6.8	113	1	2	3	6	15	24	66
50–64	195	6.1	52	1	2	4	7	13	23	37
65+	206	4.8	25	1	2	3	6	12	15	23
SUBTOTALS:										
1. SINGLE DX										
A. Not Operated	2	1.5	<1	1	1	2	2	2	2	2
B. Operated	54	3.0	8	1	1	2	3	7	8	18
2. MULTIPLE DX										
A. Not Operated	182	4.1	14	1	2	3	5	8	11	24
B. Operated	710	6.0	69	1	2	3	6	14	19	49
1. SINGLE DX	56	3.0	8	1	1	2	3	7	8	18
2. MULTIPLE DX	892	5.6	58	1	2	3	6	12	17	48
A. NOT OPERATED	184	4.0	14	1	2	3	5	8	11	24
B. OPERATED	764	5.8	65	1	2	3	6	13	18	49
TOTAL										
0–19 Years	109	5.6	114	1	2	3	5	9	15	48
20–34	117	5.8	53	1	2	3	6	14	18	38
35–49	179	6.1	92	1	2	3	6	11	22	66
50–64	260	5.6	45	1	2	3	7	12	23	30
65+	283	4.7	22	1	2	3	6	11	15	23
GRAND TOTAL	948	5.4	56	1	2	3	6	12	17	44

Length of Stay by Diagnosis and Operation, Western Region, 2008

Western Region, October 2006–September 2007 Data, by Diagnosis

331.82: DEMENTIA W LEWY BODIES

Type of Patients	Observed Patients	Avg. Stay	Variance	Percentiles						
				10th	25th	50th	75th	90th	95th	99th
1. SINGLE DX										
A. Not Operated										
0–19 Years	0									
20–34	0									
35–49	0									
50–64	0									
65+	3	2.3	<1	2	2	2	3	3	3	3
B. Operated										
0–19 Years	0									
20–34	0									
35–49	0									
50–64	0									
65+	0									
2. MULTIPLE DX										
A. Not Operated										
0–19 Years	0									
20–34	0									
35–49	2	4.5	4	3	3	3	6	6	6	6
50–64	46	9.9	138	1	3	6	12	27	47	>99
65+	886	7.0	38	2	3	5	9	16	20	30
B. Operated										
0–19 Years	0									
20–34	0									
35–49	0									
50–64	1	1.0	0	1	1	1	1	1	1	1
65+	13	9.7	53	3	6	8	12	25	>99	>99
SUBTOTALS:										
1. SINGLE DX										
A. Not Operated	3	2.3	<1	2	2	2	3	3	3	3
B. Operated	0									
2. MULTIPLE DX										
A. Not Operated	934	7.1	44	2	3	5	9	16	21	30
B. Operated	14	9.1	54	1	4	8	12	25	>99	>99
1. SINGLE DX	3	2.3	<1	2	2	2	3	3	3	3
2. MULTIPLE DX	948	7.2	44	2	3	5	9	16	21	31
A. NOT OPERATED	937	7.1	43	2	3	5	9	16	21	30
B. OPERATED	14	9.1	54	1	4	8	12	25	>99	>99
TOTAL										
0–19 Years	0									
20–34	0									
35–49	2	4.5	4	3	3	3	6	6	6	6
50–64	47	9.7	137	3	3	6	11	27	47	>99
65+	902	7.0	39	2	3	5	9	16	20	30
GRAND TOTAL	951	7.2	44	2	3	5	9	16	21	31

332: PARKINSON'S DISEASE

Type of Patients	Observed Patients	Avg. Stay	Variance	Percentiles						
				10th	25th	50th	75th	90th	95th	99th
1. SINGLE DX										
A. Not Operated										
0–19 Years	0									
20–34	0									
35–49	1	2.0	0	2	2	2	2	2	2	2
50–64	3	1.3	<1	1	1	1	2	2	2	2
65+	4	2.0	<1	1	1	2	2	3	3	3
B. Operated										
0–19 Years	0									
20–34	0									
35–49	9	1.2	<1	1	1	1	1	2	2	2
50–64	48	1.7	1	1	1	1	2	3	4	6
65+	45	1.5	1	1	1	1	2	3	3	7
2. MULTIPLE DX										
A. Not Operated										
0–19 Years	0									
20–34	1	5.0	0	5	5	5	5	5	5	5
35–49	22	7.0	64	1	3	5	7	12	15	39
50–64	233	5.0	28	1	3	4	6	8	11	29
65+	1,088	4.4	14	1	3	3	5	8	11	21
B. Operated										
0–19 Years	2	18.5	535	2	2	2	35	35	35	35
20–34	2	1.5	<1	1	1	1	2	2	2	2
35–49	20	1.8	3	1	1	1	2	4	4	8
50–64	153	1.9	6	1	1	1	2	4	5	12
65+	252	2.6	23	1	1	2	2	5	9	26
SUBTOTALS:										
1. SINGLE DX										
A. Not Operated	8	1.8	<1	1	1	2	2	3	3	3
B. Operated	102	1.6	1	1	1	1	2	3	3	6
2. MULTIPLE DX										
A. Not Operated	1,344	4.6	17	1	2	3	5	8	11	21
B. Operated	429	2.4	18	1	1	1	2	5	8	24
1. SINGLE DX	110	1.6	1	1	1	1	2	3	3	6
2. MULTIPLE DX	1,773	4.0	18	1	2	3	5	8	11	21
A. NOT OPERATED	1,352	4.5	17	1	2	3	5	8	11	21
B. OPERATED	531	2.2	15	1	1	1	2	4	7	14
TOTAL										
0–19 Years	2	18.5	535	2	2	2	35	35	35	35
20–34	3	2.7	4	1	1	2	5	5	5	5
35–49	52	3.9	35	1	1	2	5	8	12	39
50–64	437	3.5	19	1	1	2	4	7	10	20
65+	1,389	4.0	16	1	2	3	5	8	10	21
GRAND TOTAL	1,883	3.9	18	1	1	3	5	7	10	21

332.0: PARALYSIS AGITANS

Type of Patients	Observed Patients	Avg. Stay	Variance	Percentiles						
				10th	25th	50th	75th	90th	95th	99th
1. SINGLE DX										
A. Not Operated										
0–19 Years	0									
20–34	0									
35–49	1	2.0	0	2	2	2	2	2	2	2
50–64	3	1.3	<1	1	1	1	2	2	2	2
65+	4	2.0	<1	1	1	2	2	3	3	3
B. Operated										
0–19 Years	0									
20–34	0									
35–49	9	1.2	<1	1	1	1	1	2	2	2
50–64	48	1.7	1	1	1	1	2	3	4	6
65+	45	1.5	1	1	1	1	2	3	3	7
2. MULTIPLE DX										
A. Not Operated										
0–19 Years	0									
20–34	0									
35–49	14	7.3	96	1	2	5	7	15	39	39
50–64	207	4.9	27	1	2	4	6	8	11	20
65+	1,054	4.4	14	1	2	3	5	8	11	21
B. Operated										
0–19 Years	2	18.5	535	2	2	2	35	35	35	35
20–34	2	1.5	<1	1	1	1	2	2	2	2
35–49	20	1.8	3	1	1	1	2	4	4	8
50–64	153	1.9	6	1	1	1	2	4	5	12
65+	251	2.7	23	1	1	2	2	5	9	26
SUBTOTALS:										
1. SINGLE DX										
A. Not Operated	8	1.8	<1	1	1	2	2	3	3	3
B. Operated	102	1.6	1	1	1	1	2	3	3	6
2. MULTIPLE DX										
A. Not Operated	1,275	4.5	17	1	2	3	5	8	11	21
B. Operated	428	2.4	18	1	1	1	2	5	8	24
1. SINGLE DX	110	1.6	1	1	1	1	2	3	3	6
2. MULTIPLE DX	1,703	4.0	18	1	2	3	5	7	10	21
A. NOT OPERATED	1,283	4.5	17	1	2	3	5	8	11	21
B. OPERATED	530	2.2	15	1	1	1	2	4	7	14
TOTAL										
0–19 Years	2	18.5	535	2	2	2	35	35	35	35
20–34	2	1.5	<1	1	1	1	2	2	2	2
35–49	44	3.4	37	1	1	1	4	7	8	39
50–64	411	3.4	18	1	2	2	4	7	9	19
65+	1,354	4.0	16	1	2	3	5	8	10	21
GRAND TOTAL	1,813	3.8	18	1	1	3	5	7	10	21

Length of Stay by Diagnosis and Operation, Western Region, 2008

333: EXTRAPYRAMID DISORD NEC

Type of Patients	Observed Patients	Avg. Stay	Vari-ance	Percentiles						
				10th	25th	50th	75th	90th	95th	99th
1. SINGLE DX										
A. Not Operated										
0–19 Years	31	1.8	1	1	1	1	2	4	4	5
20–34	5	1.2	<1	1	1	1	1	2	2	2
35–49	4	2.5	<1	2	2	2	3	3	3	3
50–64	3	21.6	>999	1	1	5	59	59	59	59
65+	1	2.0	0	2	2	2	2	2	2	2
B. Operated										
0–19 Years	1	1.0	0	1	1	1	1	1	1	1
20–34	4	1.3	<1	1	1	1	2	2	2	2
35–49	3	2.7	2	1	1	3	4	4	4	4
50–64	6	1.2	<1	1	1	1	1	2	2	2
65+	8	1.1	<1	1	1	1	1	2	2	2
2. MULTIPLE DX										
A. Not Operated										
0–19 Years	124	3.3	18	1	1	2	3	6	9	26
20–34	153	6.1	103	1	2	3	5	13	22	61
35–49	245	4.8	28	1	2	3	6	10	18	29
50–64	389	5.0	44	1	2	3	6	10	14	24
65+	900	4.3	16	1	2	3	5	8	11	19
B. Operated										
0–19 Years	2	15.0	385	1	1	29	29	29	29	29
20–34	3	11.3	232	2	2	3	29	29	29	29
35–49	17	1.9	4	1	1	1	2	3	3	9
50–64	44	3.2	77	1	1	1	2	3	7	59
65+	92	2.3	6	1	1	1	2	6	7	13
SUBTOTALS:										
1. SINGLE DX										
A. Not Operated	44	3.2	75	1	1	2	3	4	5	59
B. Operated	22	1.4	<1	1	1	1	1	2	3	4
2. MULTIPLE DX										
A. Not Operated	1,811	4.6	31	1	2	3	5	9	13	27
B. Operated	158	2.8	34	1	1	1	2	6	9	29
1. SINGLE DX	66	2.6	51	1	1	1	2	4	4	59
2. MULTIPLE DX	1,969	4.5	32	1	2	3	5	9	13	29
A. NOT OPERATED	1,855	4.6	32	1	2	3	5	9	13	29
B. OPERATED	180	2.7	30	1	1	1	2	4	8	29
TOTAL										
0–19 Years	158	3.2	19	1	1	2	3	5	9	29
20–34	165	6.0	100	1	2	3	5	13	22	61
35–49	269	4.6	26	1	2	3	6	10	18	29
50–64	442	4.9	53	1	2	3	6	9	14	30
65+	1,001	4.1	15	1	2	3	5	8	11	19
GRAND TOTAL	2,035	4.4	32	1	2	3	5	9	12	29

333.0: DEGEN BASAL GANGLIA NEC

Type of Patients	Observed Patients	Avg. Stay	Vari-ance	Percentiles						
				10th	25th	50th	75th	90th	95th	99th
1. SINGLE DX										
A. Not Operated										
0–19 Years	0									
20–34	0									
35–49	0									
50–64	0									
65+	1	2.0	0	2	2	2	2	2	2	2
B. Operated										
0–19 Years	0									
20–34	1	1.0	0	1	1	1	1	1	1	1
35–49	0									
50–64	0									
65+	0									
2. MULTIPLE DX										
A. Not Operated										
0–19 Years	0									
20–34	3	3.3	5	2	2	2	6	6	6	6
35–49	7	7.1	69	1	2	2	14	23	23	23
50–64	41	7.7	119	2	3	4	8	14	18	67
65+	378	4.8	19	2	2	4	6	9	12	21
B. Operated										
0–19 Years	0									
20–34	0									
35–49	0									
50–64	2	2.5	<1	2	2	3	3	3	3	3
65+	9	6.8	10	2	5	7	8	13	13	13
SUBTOTALS:										
1. SINGLE DX										
A. Not Operated	1	2.0	0	2	2	2	2	2	2	2
B. Operated	1	1.0	0	1	1	1	1	1	1	1
2. MULTIPLE DX										
A. Not Operated	429	5.1	30	2	2	4	6	9	13	23
B. Operated	11	6.0	11	2	3	6	8	9	13	13
1. SINGLE DX	2	1.5	<1	1	1	2	2	2	2	2
2. MULTIPLE DX	440	5.1	29	2	2	4	6	9	13	23
A. NOT OPERATED	430	5.1	30	2	2	4	6	9	13	23
B. OPERATED	12	5.6	12	2	3	5	8	9	13	13
TOTAL										
0–19 Years	0									
20–34	4	2.7	5	1	2	2	2	6	6	6
35–49	7	7.1	69	1	2	2	14	23	23	23
50–64	43	7.4	115	2	3	4	8	14	18	67
65+	388	4.9	19	2	2	4	6	9	12	21
GRAND TOTAL	442	5.1	29	2	2	4	6	9	13	23

333.1: TREMOR NEC

Type of Patients	Observed Patients	Avg. Stay	Vari-ance	Percentiles						
				10th	25th	50th	75th	90th	95th	99th
1. SINGLE DX										
A. Not Operated										
0–19 Years	1	1.0	0	1	1	1	1	1	1	1
20–34	1	1.0	0	1	1	1	1	1	1	1
35–49	0									
50–64	0									
65+	0									
B. Operated										
0–19 Years	0									
20–34	1	1.0	0	1	1	1	1	1	1	1
35–49	1	1.0	0	1	1	1	1	1	1	1
50–64	4	1.0	0	1	1	1	1	1	1	1
65+	7	1.0	0	1	1	1	1	1	1	1
2. MULTIPLE DX										
A. Not Operated										
0–19 Years	6	2.2	1	1	1	2	3	4	4	4
20–34	5	4.0	6	1	2	5	5	7	7	7
35–49	36	2.6	2	1	1	3	3	5	5	6
50–64	81	3.4	7	1	2	3	4	6	8	14
65+	158	2.7	4	1	1	2	4	6	7	9
B. Operated										
0–19 Years	0									
20–34	1	2.0	0	2	2	2	2	2	2	2
35–49	6	1.3	<1	2	1	1	2	3	3	3
50–64	27	1.5	<1	1	1	1	2	3	3	3
65+	76	1.5	<1	1	1	1	2	3	4	6
SUBTOTALS:										
1. SINGLE DX										
A. Not Operated	2	1.0	0	1	1	1	1	1	1	1
B. Operated	13	1.0	0	1	1	1	1	1	1	1
2. MULTIPLE DX										
A. Not Operated	286	2.9	5	1	1	2	4	6	7	10
B. Operated	110	1.5	<1	1	1	1	2	3	4	4
1. SINGLE DX	15	1.0	0	1	1	1	1	1	1	1
2. MULTIPLE DX	396	2.5	4	1	1	2	3	5	7	10
A. NOT OPERATED	288	2.9	5	1	1	2	4	6	7	10
B. OPERATED	123	1.5	<1	1	1	1	2	3	4	4
TOTAL										
0–19 Years	7	2.0	1	1	1	2	3	4	4	4
20–34	8	3.0	5	1	1	2	5	7	7	7
35–49	43	2.4	2	1	1	2	3	5	5	6
50–64	112	2.8	6	1	1	2	4	6	8	12
65+	241	2.3	3	1	1	1	3	5	6	8
GRAND TOTAL	411	2.5	4	1	1	2	3	5	6	9

231

Length of Stay by Diagnosis and Operation, Western Region, 2008

Western Region, October 2006–September 2007 Data, by Diagnosis

333.2: MYOCLONUS

Type of Patients	Observed Patients	Avg. Stay	Vari-ance	10th	25th	50th	75th	90th	95th	99th
1. SINGLE DX										
A. Not Operated										
0–19 Years	22	1.9	1	1	1	2	2	2	4	5
20–34	1	2.0	0	2	2	2	2	2	2	2
35–49	3	2.3	<1	2	2	2	3	3	3	3
50–64	0									
65+	0									
B. Operated										
0–19 Years	0									
20–34	0									
35–49	0									
50–64	0									
65+	0									
2. MULTIPLE DX										
A. Not Operated										
0–19 Years	45	2.4	3	1	1	2	2	4	5	10
20–34	27	4.1	22	1	2	2	4	9	14	22
35–49	35	5.2	20	2	2	4	6	11	18	21
50–64	59	3.9	9	1	2	3	5	8	11	17
65+	123	3.7	7	1	2	3	5	7	9	12
B. Operated										
0–19 Years	1	29.0	0	29	29	29	29	29	29	29
20–34	1	29.0	0	29	29	29	29	29	29	29
35–49	2	5.5	24	2	2	9	9	9	9	9
50–64	0									
65+	2	4.5	4	3	3	6	6	6	6	6
SUBTOTALS:										
1. SINGLE DX										
A. Not Operated	26	2.0	1	1	1	2	2	2	4	5
B. Operated	0									
2. MULTIPLE DX										
A. Not Operated	289	3.8	10	1	2	3	5	8	10	18
B. Operated	6	13.0	159	2	3	9	29	29	29	29
1. SINGLE DX	26	2.0	1	1	2	2	2	4	4	5
2. MULTIPLE DX	295	3.9	14	1	2	3	5	8	10	22
A. NOT OPERATED	315	3.6	10	1	2	3	4	7	10	17
B. OPERATED	6	13.0	159	2	3	9	29	29	29	29
TOTAL										
0–19 Years	68	2.6	13	1	1	2	3	4	5	29
20–34	29	4.9	42	2	2	2	4	14	22	29
35–49	40	5.0	19	2	2	3	6	11	18	21
50–64	59	3.9	9	1	2	3	5	8	11	17
65+	125	3.7	7	1	2	3	5	7	9	12
GRAND TOTAL	321	3.8	14	1	2	3	4	7	10	21

334: SPINOCEREBELLAR DISEASE

Type of Patients	Observed Patients	Avg. Stay	Vari-ance	10th	25th	50th	75th	90th	95th	99th
1. SINGLE DX										
A. Not Operated										
0–19 Years	7	1.3	<1	1	1	1	2	2	2	2
20–34	0									
35–49	0									
50–64	1	3.0	0	3	3	3	3	3	3	3
65+	0									
B. Operated										
0–19 Years	1	2.0	0	2	2	2	2	2	2	2
20–34	0									
35–49	0									
50–64	0									
65+	0									
2. MULTIPLE DX										
A. Not Operated										
0–19 Years	19	3.1	10	1	1	2	3	11	12	12
20–34	8	5.1	8	1	2	5	6	10	10	10
35–49	9	4.8	20	2	2	3	5	16	16	16
50–64	23	7.7	127	2	2	4	7	20	21	53
65+	52	4.4	9	1	2	4	6	8	11	14
B. Operated										
0–19 Years	4	7.5	121	1	1	2	3	24	24	24
20–34	0									
35–49	3	23.7	513	5	5	17	49	49	49	49
50–64	2	4.0	18	1	1	1	7	7	7	7
65+	0									
SUBTOTALS:										
1. SINGLE DX										
A. Not Operated	8	1.5	<1	1	1	1	2	3	3	3
B. Operated	1	2.0	0	2	2	2	2	2	2	2
2. MULTIPLE DX										
A. Not Operated	111	4.9	35	1	2	3	6	10	14	21
B. Operated	9	12.1	255	1	2	5	17	49	49	49
1. SINGLE DX	9	1.6	<1	1	1	1	2	3	3	3
2. MULTIPLE DX	120	5.5	53	1	2	3	6	11	16	49
A. NOT OPERATED	119	4.7	34	1	2	3	5	10	14	21
B. OPERATED	10	11.1	237	1	2	5	17	49	49	49
TOTAL										
0–19 Years	31	3.2	21	1	1	2	3	5	12	24
20–34	8	5.1	8	1	2	5	6	10	10	10
35–49	12	9.5	181	2	2	5	16	17	49	49
50–64	26	7.3	114	1	2	4	7	20	21	53
65+	52	4.4	9	1	2	4	6	8	11	14
GRAND TOTAL	129	5.2	51	1	2	3	5	11	16	49

335: ANT HORN CELL DISEASE

Type of Patients	Observed Patients	Avg. Stay	Vari-ance	10th	25th	50th	75th	90th	95th	99th
1. SINGLE DX										
A. Not Operated										
0–19 Years	3	1.0	0	1	1	1	1	1	1	1
20–34	0									
35–49	2	3.0	8	1	1	1	5	5	5	5
50–64	2	1.5	<1	1	1	2	2	2	2	2
65+	0									
B. Operated										
0–19 Years	2	7.0	8	5	5	5	9	9	9	9
20–34	0									
35–49	0									
50–64	0									
65+	0									
2. MULTIPLE DX										
A. Not Operated										
0–19 Years	17	7.9	193	1	1	3	5	43	46	46
20–34	5	9.8	146	1	3	7	7	31	31	31
35–49	32	3.7	10	1	1	3	5	7	13	14
50–64	103	5.6	39	1	2	3	6	15	24	29
65+	142	5.3	29	1	2	4	6	10	15	28
B. Operated										
0–19 Years	7	7.0	24	1	3	5	12	13	13	13
20–34	0									
35–49	3	7.0	75	1	1	3	17	17	17	17
50–64	11	8.9	101	1	1	5	16	25	29	29
65+	8	12.4	45	5	6	11	15	26	26	26
SUBTOTALS:										
1. SINGLE DX										
A. Not Operated	7	1.7	2	1	1	1	2	3	5	5
B. Operated	2	7.0	8	5	5	5	9	9	9	9
2. MULTIPLE DX										
A. Not Operated	299	5.5	42	1	2	4	6	13	18	41
B. Operated	29	9.2	63	1	3	6	13	25	26	29
1. SINGLE DX	9	2.9	8	1	1	1	5	9	9	9
2. MULTIPLE DX	328	5.8	45	1	2	4	7	14	20	41
A. NOT OPERATED	306	5.4	41	1	2	4	6	11	18	41
B. OPERATED	31	9.0	59	1	3	6	13	17	26	29
TOTAL										
0–19 Years	29	6.9	120	1	1	4	7	13	43	46
20–34	5	9.8	146	1	3	7	7	31	31	31
35–49	37	3.9	14	1	1	3	5	7	14	17
50–64	116	5.9	45	1	2	3	7	15	27	29
65+	150	5.7	32	1	2	4	7	11	16	28
GRAND TOTAL	337	5.7	44	1	2	4	7	14	20	41

Western Region, October 2006–September 2007 Data, by Diagnosis

335.20: AMYOTROPHIC SCLEROSIS

Type of Patients	Observed Patients	Avg. Stay	Variance	10th	25th	50th	75th	90th	95th	99th
1. SINGLE DX										
A. Not Operated										
0–19 Years	0									
20–34	0									
35–49	2	3.0	8							
50–64	1	1.0	0	1	1	1	1	1	1	1
65+	0									
B. Operated										
0–19 Years	0									
20–34	0									
35–49	0									
50–64	0									
65+	0									
2. MULTIPLE DX										
A. Not Operated										
0–19 Years	0									
20–34	1	3.0	0	3	3	3	3	3	3	3
35–49	28	3.4	7	1	1	3	5	7	7	13
50–64	98	5.8	41	1	2	3	7	15	27	29
65+	120	4.9	19	1	2	4	6	10	13	24
B. Operated										
0–19 Years	0									
20–34	0									
35–49	3	7.0	75	1	5	3	17	17	17	17
50–64	6	11.1	101	1	5	6	16	29	29	29
65+	7	13.0	49	5	6	13	15	26	26	26
SUBTOTALS:										
1. SINGLE DX — A. Not Operated	3	2.3	5	1	1	1	5	5	5	5
1. SINGLE DX — B. Operated	0									
2. MULTIPLE DX — A. Not Operated	247	5.1	27	1	2	4	6	10	15	28
2. MULTIPLE DX — B. Operated	16	11.2	69	1	5	10	15	26	29	29
1. SINGLE DX	3	2.3	5	1	1	1	5	5	5	5
2. MULTIPLE DX	263	5.5	31	1	2	4	6	13	17	29
A. NOT OPERATED	250	5.1	27	1	2	4	6	10	15	28
B. OPERATED	16	11.2	69	1	5	10	15	26	29	29
TOTAL										
0–19 Years	0									
20–34	1	3.0	0	3	3	3	3	3	3	3
35–49	33	3.7	12	1	1	3	5	7	13	17
50–64	105	6.0	45	1	2	4	7	15	27	29
65+	127	5.4	24	1	2	4	7	11	15	26
GRAND TOTAL	266	5.4	31	1	2	4	6	13	17	29

336: SPINAL CORD DISEASE NEC

Type of Patients	Observed Patients	Avg. Stay	Variance	10th	25th	50th	75th	90th	95th	99th
1. SINGLE DX										
A. Not Operated										
0–19 Years	1	5.0	0	5	5	5	5	5	5	5
20–34	2	1.0	0	1	1	1	1	1	1	1
35–49	3	6.7	41	2	2	4	14	14	14	14
50–64	2	2.0	0	2	2	2	2	2	2	2
65+	0									
B. Operated										
0–19 Years	2	2.5	<1	2	2	3	3	3	3	3
20–34	1	4.0	0	4	4	4	4	4	4	4
35–49	2	6.0	18	3	3	3	9	9	9	9
50–64	5	5.0	2	4	4	5	5	7	7	7
65+	0									
2. MULTIPLE DX										
A. Not Operated										
0–19 Years	7	1.7	2	1	1	1	3	4	4	4
20–34	20	4.0	16	1	1	3	5	7	17	17
35–49	39	7.6	60	2	3	5	10	15	29	37
50–64	59	5.1	22	2	2	3	6	13	17	21
65+	68	6.5	24	3	3	5	8	11	13	30
B. Operated										
0–19 Years	15	7.8	129	2	2	4	6	25	43	43
20–34	21	6.9	111	2	2	3	4	16	22	47
35–49	27	6.1	34	2	3	4	6	13	23	25
50–64	73	7.5	66	3	3	5	8	17	30	46
65+	51	8.3	126	2	2	6	9	16	21	74
SUBTOTALS:										
1. SINGLE DX — A. Not Operated	7	4.2	21	1	1	2	5	14	14	14
1. SINGLE DX — B. Operated	10	4.6	4	3	3	4	5	7	9	9
2. MULTIPLE DX — A. Not Operated	193	5.8	31	1	2	4	7	13	17	30
2. MULTIPLE DX — B. Operated	187	7.5	86	1	3	4	7	17	25	47
1. SINGLE DX	17	4.4	10	1	2	4	5	9	14	14
2. MULTIPLE DX	380	6.6	58	1	3	4	7	14	21	43
A. NOT OPERATED	200	5.8	30	1	2	4	7	13	17	30
B. OPERATED	197	7.3	82	2	3	4	7	16	25	47
TOTAL										
0–19 Years	25	5.6	84	1	1	3	5	8	25	43
20–34	44	5.2	62	1	3	4	4	11	17	47
35–49	71	6.9	47	2	3	4	8	15	23	37
50–64	138	6.3	46	1	3	4	7	15	19	32
65+	119	7.3	68	2	3	6	9	13	21	32
GRAND TOTAL	397	6.5	57	1	3	4	7	14	21	43

337: AUTONOMIC NERVE DISORDER

Type of Patients	Observed Patients	Avg. Stay	Variance	10th	25th	50th	75th	90th	95th	99th
1. SINGLE DX										
A. Not Operated										
0–19 Years	1	13.0	0	13	13	13	13	13	13	13
20–34	0									
35–49	3	1.7	<1	1	1	2	2	2	2	2
50–64	1	2.0	0	2	2	2	2	2	2	2
65+	2	1.0	0	1	1	1	1	1	1	1
B. Operated										
0–19 Years	1	3.0	0	3	3	3	3	3	3	3
20–34	2	1.5	<1	1	1	2	2	2	2	2
35–49	6	1.7	1	1	1	1	2	4	4	4
50–64	3	1.0	0	1	1	1	1	1	1	1
65+	0									
2. MULTIPLE DX										
A. Not Operated										
0–19 Years	22	7.7	55	2	3	4	11	16	25	28
20–34	66	6.6	36	1	2	4	9	14	23	27
35–49	90	4.4	37	1	2	3	4	8	9	55
50–64	103	4.7	19	1	2	3	6	11	14	16
65+	165	4.2	14	1	2	3	6	8	11	20
B. Operated										
0–19 Years	3	7.0	52	1	1	5	15	15	15	15
20–34	18	2.8	4	1	1	2	3	5	9	9
35–49	46	2.8	6	1	1	2	4	5	7	12
50–64	23	4.5	16	1	1	3	7	9	12	16
65+	12	4.9	37	1	1	2	3	15	19	19
SUBTOTALS:										
1. SINGLE DX — A. Not Operated	7	3.2	19	1	1	2	2	13	13	13
1. SINGLE DX — B. Operated	12	1.6	<1	1	1	1	2	3	4	4
2. MULTIPLE DX — A. Not Operated	446	4.9	26	1	2	3	6	11	14	24
2. MULTIPLE DX — B. Operated	102	3.6	13	1	1	2	5	8	12	16
1. SINGLE DX	19	2.2	8	1	1	1	2	4	13	13
2. MULTIPLE DX	548	4.6	23	1	2	3	6	10	14	23
A. NOT OPERATED	453	4.9	25	1	2	3	6	11	14	24
B. OPERATED	114	3.4	12	1	1	2	4	7	12	16
TOTAL										
0–19 Years	27	7.7	50	1	3	4	11	16	25	28
20–34	86	5.7	31	1	2	3	7	14	14	27
35–49	145	3.7	25	1	2	3	4	7	9	15
50–64	130	4.5	18	1	1	3	6	11	14	16
65+	179	4.2	15	1	2	3	6	8	12	20
GRAND TOTAL	567	4.6	23	1	2	3	5	10	14	23

Length of Stay by Diagnosis and Operation, Western Region, 2008

Western Region, October 2006–September 2007 Data, by Diagnosis

338: PAIN NEC

Type of Patients	Observed Patients	Avg. Stay	Variance	10th	25th	50th	75th	90th	95th	99th
1. SINGLE DX										
A. Not Operated										
0–19 Years	13	1.8	1	1	1	1	2	3	5	5
20–34	42	1.7	1	1	1	1	2	3	4	6
35–49	30	1.8	<1	1	1	2	2	3	3	3
50–64	19	2.2	4	1	1	2	2	7	7	7
65+	5	1.4	<1	1	1	1	2	2	2	2
B. Operated										
0–19 Years	2	3.5	5	2	2	4	5	5	5	5
20–34	1	1.0	0	1	1	1	1	1	1	1
35–49	1	1.0	0	1	1	1	1	1	1	1
50–64	0									
65+	0									
2. MULTIPLE DX										
A. Not Operated										
0–19 Years	132	2.6	4	1	1	2	3	6	7	9
20–34	620	3.0	10	1	1	2	4	6	8	15
35–49	1,169	3.4	13	1	1	2	4	7	9	17
50–64	1,349	3.7	10	1	2	3	5	7	9	17
65+	1,306	3.9	10	1	2	3	5	7	10	17
B. Operated										
0–19 Years	32	2.4	6	1	1	1	3	5	9	10
20–34	123	2.6	9	1	1	2	3	5	8	15
35–49	238	2.7	11	1	1	2	3	5	8	19
50–64	284	2.7	7	1	1	2	3	6	9	14
65+	235	3.0	11	1	2	3	5	7	10	19
SUBTOTALS:										
1. SINGLE DX										
A. Not Operated	109	1.8	1	1	1	2	2	3	4	7
B. Operated	5	2.0	3	1	1	1	2	5	5	5
2. MULTIPLE DX										
A. Not Operated	4,576	3.6	11	1	2	3	4	7	9	17
B. Operated	912	2.7	9	1	1	2	3	6	9	17
1. SINGLE DX	114	1.8	1	1	1	1	2	3	4	7
2. MULTIPLE DX	5,488	3.4	11	1	1	2	4	7	9	17
A. NOT OPERATED	4,685	3.5	11	1	2	3	4	7	9	17
B. OPERATED	917	2.7	9	1	1	2	3	6	9	17
TOTAL										
0–19 Years	179	2.5	4	1	1	2	3	5	7	10
20–34	787	2.9	10	1	1	2	3	5	8	15
35–49	1,438	3.3	12	1	1	2	4	6	9	17
50–64	1,652	3.5	10	1	2	3	4	7	9	17
65+	1,546	3.8	10	1	2	3	5	7	10	18
GRAND TOTAL	5,602	3.4	11	1	1	2	4	7	9	17

338.11: ACUTE PAIN D/T TRAUMA

Type of Patients	Observed Patients	Avg. Stay	Variance	10th	25th	50th	75th	90th	95th	99th
1. SINGLE DX										
A. Not Operated										
0–19 Years	0									
20–34	2	2.0	2	1	1	1	3	3	3	3
35–49	0									
50–64	0									
65+	0									
B. Operated										
0–19 Years	0									
20–34	0									
35–49	0									
50–64	0									
65+	0									
2. MULTIPLE DX										
A. Not Operated										
0–19 Years	5	2.8	5	1	1	2	4	6	6	6
20–34	24	3.7	19	1	1	2	4	8	14	19
35–49	49	3.0	6	1	1	3	3	7	7	14
50–64	52	3.1	5	1	2	2	3	6	8	12
65+	176	3.7	5	2	2	3	5	6	8	11
B. Operated										
0–19 Years	0									
20–34	0									
35–49	0									
50–64	0									
65+	0									
SUBTOTALS:										
1. SINGLE DX										
A. Not Operated	2	2.0	2	1	1	1	3	3	3	3
B. Operated	0									
2. MULTIPLE DX										
A. Not Operated	306	3.4	6	1	2	3	4	6	8	14
B. Operated	0									
1. SINGLE DX	2	2.0	2	1	1	1	3	3	3	3
2. MULTIPLE DX	306	3.4	6	1	2	3	4	6	8	14
A. NOT OPERATED	308	3.4	6	1	2	3	4	6	8	14
B. OPERATED	0									
TOTAL										
0–19 Years	5	2.8	5	1	1	2	4	6	6	6
20–34	26	3.6	18	1	1	2	4	8	14	19
35–49	49	3.0	6	1	1	3	3	7	7	14
50–64	52	3.1	5	1	2	2	3	6	8	12
65+	176	3.7	5	2	2	3	5	6	8	11
GRAND TOTAL	308	3.4	6	1	2	3	4	6	8	14

338.18: ACUTE POSTOP PAIN NEC

Type of Patients	Observed Patients	Avg. Stay	Variance	10th	25th	50th	75th	90th	95th	99th
1. SINGLE DX										
A. Not Operated										
0–19 Years	12	1.8	1	1	1	1	2	3	5	5
20–34	39	1.7	1	1	1	1	2	3	4	6
35–49	28	1.8	<1	1	1	2	2	3	3	3
50–64	17	2.0	2	1	1	2	2	4	7	7
65+	4	1.3	<1	1	1	1	2	2	2	2
B. Operated										
0–19 Years	1	5.0	0	5	5	5	5	5	5	5
20–34	1	1.0	0	1	1	1	1	1	1	1
35–49	1	1.0	0	1	1	1	1	1	1	1
50–64	0									
65+	0									
2. MULTIPLE DX										
A. Not Operated										
0–19 Years	83	2.2	3	1	1	2	3	3	5	15
20–34	340	2.4	5	1	1	2	3	4	5	10
35–49	480	2.4	4	1	1	2	3	4	6	9
50–64	425	2.6	4	1	1	2	3	5	7	9
65+	270	2.9	5	1	1	2	4	5	7	11
B. Operated										
0–19 Years	26	1.9	3	1	1	1	2	4	5	9
20–34	84	1.9	3	1	1	1	2	3	5	13
35–49	145	1.8	2	1	1	1	2	3	4	6
50–64	172	1.9	2	1	1	1	2	3	4	7
65+	161	2.1	2	1	1	2	3	4	5	9
SUBTOTALS:										
1. SINGLE DX										
A. Not Operated	100	1.8	1	1	1	1	2	3	3	7
B. Operated	3	2.3	5	1	1	1	5	5	5	5
2. MULTIPLE DX										
A. Not Operated	1,598	2.5	4	1	1	2	3	5	6	10
B. Operated	588	1.9	2	1	1	1	2	4	5	9
1. SINGLE DX	103	1.8	1	1	1	1	2	3	4	6
2. MULTIPLE DX	2,186	2.4	4	1	1	2	3	4	6	10
A. NOT OPERATED	1,698	2.5	4	1	1	2	3	5	6	10
B. OPERATED	591	1.9	2	1	1	1	2	4	5	9
TOTAL										
0–19 Years	122	2.1	3	1	1	2	3	4	5	9
20–34	464	2.3	5	1	1	2	3	4	5	10
35–49	654	2.3	3	1	1	2	3	4	6	9
50–64	614	2.4	3	1	1	2	3	5	6	9
65+	435	2.6	4	1	1	2	3	5	6	10
GRAND TOTAL	2,289	2.4	4	1	1	2	3	4	6	9

234

Length of Stay by Diagnosis and Operation, Western Region, 2008

Western Region, October 2006–September 2007 Data, by Diagnosis

338.19: ACUTE PAIN NEC

Type of Patients	Observed Patients	Avg. Stay	Vari-ance	10th	25th	50th	75th	90th	95th	99th
1. SINGLE DX										
A. Not Operated										
0–19 Years	0									
20–34	0									
35–49	1	3.0	0			3	3	3	3	3
50–64	0									
65+	0									
B. Operated										
0–19 Years	0									
20–34	0									
35–49	0									
50–64	0									
65+	0									
2. MULTIPLE DX										
A. Not Operated										
0–19 Years	8	3.1	6	1	1	2	3	8	8	8
20–34	38	3.1	4	1	2	3	4	7	8	8
35–49	78	3.2	7	1	1	3	4	7	9	17
50–64	103	3.7	8	1	2	3	5	8	9	14
65+	119	3.5	4	1	2	3	4	6	7	8
B. Operated										
0–19 Years	1	3.0	0	3	3	3	3	3	3	3
20–34	0									
35–49	2	4.5	24	1	1	1	8	8	8	8
50–64	0									
65+	2	6.5	59	1	1	1	12	12	12	12
SUBTOTALS:										
1. SINGLE DX										
A. Not Operated	1	3.0	0	3	3	3	3	3	3	3
B. Operated	0									
2. MULTIPLE DX										
A. Not Operated	346	3.4	6	1	2	3	4	7	8	12
B. Operated	5	5.0	23	1	1	3	8	12	12	12
1. SINGLE DX	1	3.0	0	3	3	3	3	3	3	3
2. MULTIPLE DX	351	3.4	6	1	2	3	4	7	8	12
A. NOT OPERATED	347	3.4	6	1	2	3	4	7	8	12
B. OPERATED	5	5.0	23	1	1	3	8	12	12	12
TOTAL										
0–19 Years	9	3.1	6	1	2	2	3	8	8	8
20–34	38	3.1	4	1	2	3	4	7	8	8
35–49	81	3.2	7	1	1	3	4	7	8	17
50–64	103	3.7	8	1	2	3	5	8	9	14
65+	121	3.5	4	1	2	3	4	6	7	12
GRAND TOTAL	352	3.4	6	1	2	3	4	7	8	12

338.29: CHRONIC PAIN NEC

Type of Patients	Observed Patients	Avg. Stay	Vari-ance	10th	25th	50th	75th	90th	95th	99th
1. SINGLE DX										
A. Not Operated										
0–19 Years	0									
20–34	1	4.0	0	4	4	4	4	4	4	4
35–49	0									
50–64	1	7.0	0	7	7	7	7	7	7	7
65+	0									
B. Operated										
0–19 Years	0									
20–34	0									
35–49	0									
50–64	0									
65+	0									
2. MULTIPLE DX										
A. Not Operated										
0–19 Years	8	4.2	6	2	2	3	4	9	9	9
20–34	73	4.0	32	1	1	2	4	7	14	40
35–49	149	4.0	8	1	2	3	5	8	11	12
50–64	139	4.2	12	1	2	3	6	8	11	14
65+	160	4.1	11	1	2	3	5	7	10	17
B. Operated										
0–19 Years	3	6.0	21	1	1	7	10	10	10	10
20–34	20	2.9	9	1	2	3	3	5	15	15
35–49	37	3.3	14	1	1	2	3	8	12	19
50–64	21	2.8	7	1	1	2	3	7	9	10
65+	12	7.1	46	1	1	6	13	14	23	23
SUBTOTALS:										
1. SINGLE DX										
A. Not Operated	2	5.5	4	4	4	4	7	7	7	7
B. Operated	0									
2. MULTIPLE DX										
A. Not Operated	529	4.1	13	1	2	3	5	8	11	16
B. Operated	93	3.7	17	1	1	2	4	10	13	23
1. SINGLE DX	2	5.5	4	4	4	4	7	7	7	7
2. MULTIPLE DX	622	4.0	14	1	2	3	5	8	11	17
A. NOT OPERATED	531	4.1	13	1	2	3	5	8	11	16
B. OPERATED	93	3.7	17	1	1	2	4	10	13	23
TOTAL										
0–19 Years	11	4.7	9	2	2	4	7	9	10	10
20–34	94	3.8	27	1	1	2	4	7	14	40
35–49	186	3.8	9	1	2	3	5	8	11	16
50–64	161	4.0	11	1	2	3	5	8	11	14
65+	172	4.3	14	1	2	3	5	7	13	23
GRAND TOTAL	624	4.0	14	1	2	3	5	8	11	17

338.3: NEOPLASM RELATED PAIN

Type of Patients	Observed Patients	Avg. Stay	Vari-ance	10th	25th	50th	75th	90th	95th	99th
1. SINGLE DX										
A. Not Operated										
0–19 Years	0									
20–34	0									
35–49	0									
50–64	0									
65+	0									
B. Operated										
0–19 Years	0									
20–34	0									
35–49	0									
50–64	0									
65+	0									
2. MULTIPLE DX										
A. Not Operated										
0–19 Years	9	3.7	6	1	2	3	5	8	8	8
20–34	64	4.1	10	1	2	3	5	8	11	15
35–49	210	5.0	29	1	2	3	6	10	15	27
50–64	419	4.6	17	1	2	3	6	9	13	19
65+	439	4.4	15	1	2	3	5	9	11	20
B. Operated										
0–19 Years	0									
20–34	4	9.5	43	2	6	15	15	15	15	15
35–49	21	5.7	45	1	2	3	7	11	17	29
50–64	58	4.7	18	1	2	3	6	12	14	18
65+	40	5.4	22	1	2	4	7	11	15	19
SUBTOTALS:										
1. SINGLE DX										
A. Not Operated	0									
B. Operated	0									
2. MULTIPLE DX										
A. Not Operated	1,141	4.6	18	1	2	3	6	9	12	20
B. Operated	123	5.3	25	1	2	3	7	12	15	19
1. SINGLE DX	0									
2. MULTIPLE DX	1,264	4.6	18	1	2	3	6	9	13	20
A. NOT OPERATED	1,141	4.6	18	1	2	3	6	9	12	20
B. OPERATED	123	5.3	25	1	2	3	7	12	15	19
TOTAL										
0–19 Years	9	3.7	6	1	2	3	5	8	8	8
20–34	68	4.4	13	1	2	3	6	10	13	15
35–49	231	5.1	31	1	2	3	6	10	15	29
50–64	477	4.6	17	1	2	3	6	9	13	19
65+	479	4.5	15	1	2	3	5	9	12	20
GRAND TOTAL	1,264	4.6	18	1	2	3	6	9	13	20

Length of Stay by Diagnosis and Operation, Western Region, 2008

Western Region, October 2006–September 2007 Data, by Diagnosis

338.4: CHRONIC PAIN SYNDROME

Type of Patients	Observed Patients	Avg. Stay	Variance	10th	25th	50th	75th	90th	95th	99th
1. SINGLE DX										
A. Not Operated										
0–19 Years	1	2.0	0	2	2	2	2	2	2	2
20–34	0									
35–49	1	2.0	0	2	2	2	2	2	2	2
50–64	0									
65+	0									
B. Operated										
0–19 Years	1	2.0	0	2	2	2	2	2	2	2
20–34	1	1.0	0	1	1	1	1	1	1	1
35–49	0									
50–64	0									
65+	0									
2. MULTIPLE DX										
A. Not Operated										
0–19 Years	9	4.4	7	1	3	5	6	8	8	8
20–34	49	4.0	13	1	2	3	5	7	13	17
35–49	118	4.1	18	1	2	3	5	9	11	25
50–64	132	4.3	9	1	2	3	6	8	10	12
65+	79	4.8	17	1	3	4	6	10	14	29
B. Operated										
0–19 Years	1	4.0	0	4	4	4	4	4	4	4
20–34	10	2.9	7	1	1	2	4	7	8	8
35–49	16	3.3	19	1	1	1	2	10	17	17
50–64	17	3.1	6	1	1	1	4	7	9	9
65+	13	2.7	8	1	1	1	3	7	10	10
SUBTOTALS:										
1. SINGLE DX										
A. Not Operated	2	2.0	0	2	2	2	2	2	2	2
B. Operated	2	1.5	<1	1	1	1	2	2	2	2
2. MULTIPLE DX										
A. Not Operated	387	4.3	14	1	2	3	5	9	11	24
B. Operated	57	3.0	10	1	1	2	4	7	10	17
1. SINGLE DX	4	1.8	<1	1	2	2	2	2	2	2
2. MULTIPLE DX	444	4.1	13	1	2	3	5	8	10	19
A. NOT OPERATED	389	4.3	14	1	2	3	5	9	11	24
B. OPERATED	59	3.0	9	1	1	2	4	7	10	17
TOTAL										
0–19 Years	12	4.0	6	1	2	3	6	7	8	8
20–34	60	3.7	12	1	1	2	5	7	13	17
35–49	135	4.0	18	1	2	3	5	9	11	25
50–64	149	4.1	9	1	2	3	6	8	10	12
65+	92	4.5	17	1	2	3	6	10	11	29
GRAND TOTAL	448	4.1	13	1	2	3	5	8	10	19

340: MULTIPLE SCLEROSIS

Type of Patients	Observed Patients	Avg. Stay	Variance	10th	25th	50th	75th	90th	95th	99th
1. SINGLE DX										
A. Not Operated										
0–19 Years	13	3.8	12	1	2	3	4	10	12	12
20–34	72	3.5	11	1	2	3	4	5	6	23
35–49	44	3.5	5	1	2	3	5	6	7	11
50–64	27	2.6	2	1	1	2	3	4	5	6
65+	4	2.3	<1	1	1	2	3	3	3	3
B. Operated										
0–19 Years	0									
20–34	3	3.0	12	1	1	1	7	7	7	7
35–49	0									
50–64	1	2.0	0	2	2	2	2	2	2	2
65+	0									
2. MULTIPLE DX										
A. Not Operated										
0–19 Years	28	3.4	4	1	2	3	4	6	8	10
20–34	488	4.4	14	1	2	3	5	9	12	20
35–49	893	4.2	12	1	2	4	5	7	10	21
50–64	824	4.7	23	1	2	4	5	8	11	24
65+	160	4.2	10	2	2	4	5	7	9	21
B. Operated										
0–19 Years	3	19.5	223	10	10	12	37	37	37	37
20–34	5	14.6	61	5	9	16	18	25	25	25
35–49	24	4.6	24	1	2	3	3	10	16	21
50–64	43	5.4	34	1	2	3	8	13	20	22
65+	7	10.6	56	2	6	8	14	25	25	25
SUBTOTALS:										
1. SINGLE DX										
A. Not Operated	160	3.4	7	1	2	3	4	5	7	17
B. Operated	4	2.7	8	1	1	1	2	7	7	7
2. MULTIPLE DX										
A. Not Operated	2,393	4.4	16	1	2	4	5	8	10	22
B. Operated	82	6.7	50	1	2	4	8	18	22	37
1. SINGLE DX	164	3.3	7	1	2	3	4	5	7	17
2. MULTIPLE DX	2,475	4.5	17	1	2	4	5	8	11	24
A. NOT OPERATED	2,553	4.4	16	1	2	4	5	8	10	21
B. OPERATED	86	6.5	49	1	2	3	8	18	22	37
TOTAL										
0–19 Years	44	4.6	33	1	2	3	4	10	12	37
20–34	568	4.4	14	1	2	3	5	8	13	23
35–49	961	4.2	12	1	2	4	5	7	10	21
50–64	895	4.7	23	1	2	4	5	8	11	24
65+	171	4.5	13	2	2	4	5	8	11	25
GRAND TOTAL	2,639	4.4	17	1	2	4	5	8	11	23

341: OTHER CNS DEMYELINATION

Type of Patients	Observed Patients	Avg. Stay	Variance	10th	25th	50th	75th	90th	95th	99th
1. SINGLE DX										
A. Not Operated										
0–19 Years	3	2.7	4	1	1	2	5	5	5	5
20–34	9	4.4	8	1	2	4	5	5	10	10
35–49	7	3.0	5	1	1	3	4	7	7	7
50–64	3	1.3	<1	1	1	1	2	2	2	2
65+	1	4.0	0	4	4	4	4	4	4	4
B. Operated										
0–19 Years	0									
20–34	0									
35–49	0									
50–64	0									
65+	0									
2. MULTIPLE DX										
A. Not Operated										
0–19 Years	18	3.1	3	1	2	3	4	6	6	6
20–34	86	6.3	32	2	3	5	8	13	15	40
35–49	92	8.1	114	1	3	5	10	15	38	>99
50–64	88	7.3	94	2	3	5	7	15	17	83
65+	40	8.0	51	2	4	6	11	15	15	43
B. Operated										
0–19 Years	0									
20–34	1	7.0	0	7	7	7	7	7	7	7
35–49	4	11.9	168	3	3	4	10	31	31	31
50–64	4	19.9	>999	1	1	3	72	72	72	72
65+	6	11.2	28	11	11	11	15	15	15	15
SUBTOTALS:										
1. SINGLE DX										
A. Not Operated	23	3.4	6	1	1	3	5	7	7	10
B. Operated	0									
2. MULTIPLE DX										
A. Not Operated	324	7.1	73	2	3	5	8	14	17	52
B. Operated	15	13.4	324	1	3	10	15	31	72	72
1. SINGLE DX	23	3.4	6	1	1	3	5	7	7	10
2. MULTIPLE DX	339	7.4	85	2	3	5	9	14	20	67
A. NOT OPERATED	347	6.9	70	1	3	5	8	13	16	52
B. OPERATED	15	13.4	324	1	3	10	15	31	72	72
TOTAL										
0–19 Years	21	3.1	3	1	2	3	4	6	6	6
20–34	96	6.1	30	2	3	5	7	12	15	40
35–49	103	7.9	109	1	3	4	10	15	31	67
50–64	95	7.7	133	2	3	5	7	13	24	83
65+	47	8.3	48	2	4	7	12	15	15	43
GRAND TOTAL	362	7.1	81	1	3	5	8	14	17	67

Length of Stay by Diagnosis and Operation, Western Region, 2008

Western Region, October 2006–September 2007 Data, by Diagnosis

342: HEMIPLEGIA

Type of Patients	Observed Patients	Avg. Stay	Variance	Percentiles						
				10th	25th	50th	75th	90th	95th	99th
1. SINGLE DX										
A. Not Operated										
0–19 Years	0									
20–34	0									
35–49	0									
50–64	0									
65+	0									
B. Operated										
0–19 Years	1	1.0	0	1	1	1	1	1	1	1
20–34	0									
35–49	0									
50–64	0									
65+	0									
2. MULTIPLE DX										
A. Not Operated										
0–19 Years	5	2.8	6	1	1	2	3	7	7	7
20–34	58	3.1	6	1	1	3	4	6	9	11
35–49	101	3.6	8	1	2	3	4	8	9	18
50–64	118	3.7	8	1	2	3	5	7	8	11
65+	72	3.3	4	1	2	3	4	6	7	10
B. Operated										
0–19 Years	2	2.0	2	1	1	1	3	3	3	3
20–34	2	3.0	0	3	3	3	3	3	3	3
35–49	0									
50–64	2	11.1	50	6	6	16	16	16	16	16
65+	2	3.0	0	3	3	3	3	3	3	3
SUBTOTALS:										
1. SINGLE DX										
A. Not Operated	0									
B. Operated	1	1.0	0	1	1	1	1	1	1	1
2. MULTIPLE DX										
A. Not Operated	354	3.5	7	1	2	3	4	7	8	11
B. Operated	8	4.7	23	1	3	3	4	16	16	16
1. SINGLE DX	1	1.0	0	1	1	1	1	1	1	1
2. MULTIPLE DX	362	3.5	7	1	2	3	4	7	8	13
A. NOT OPERATED	354	3.5	7	1	2	3	4	7	8	11
B. OPERATED	9	4.3	21	1	3	3	3	16	16	16
TOTAL										
0–19 Years	8	2.4	4	1	1	1	3	7	7	7
20–34	60	3.1	5	1	1	3	4	6	8	11
35–49	101	3.6	8	1	2	3	4	8	9	18
50–64	120	3.8	9	1	2	3	5	7	9	16
65+	74	3.3	4	1	2	3	4	6	7	10
GRAND TOTAL	363	3.5	7	1	2	3	4	7	8	13

342.90: UNSPEC HEMIPLEG-SIDE NOS

Type of Patients	Observed Patients	Avg. Stay	Variance	Percentiles						
				10th	25th	50th	75th	90th	95th	99th
1. SINGLE DX										
A. Not Operated										
0–19 Years	0									
20–34	0									
35–49	0									
50–64	0									
65+	0									
B. Operated										
0–19 Years	1	1.0	0	1	1	1	1	1	1	1
20–34	0									
35–49	0									
50–64	0									
65+	0									
2. MULTIPLE DX										
A. Not Operated										
0–19 Years	4	2.7	8	1	1	2	3	7	7	7
20–34	45	3.4	6	1	2	3	4	7	9	11
35–49	70	3.2	6	1	2	3	4	7	8	11
50–64	93	3.6	9	1	2	3	4	6	9	24
65+	49	3.5	4	1	2	3	5	6	7	10
B. Operated										
0–19 Years	2	2.0	2	1	1	1	3	3	3	3
20–34	0									
35–49	0									
50–64	0									
65+	1	3.0	0	3	3	3	3	3	3	3
SUBTOTALS:										
1. SINGLE DX										
A. Not Operated	0									
B. Operated	1	1.0	0	1	1	1	1	1	1	1
2. MULTIPLE DX										
A. Not Operated	261	3.4	7	1	2	3	4	6	8	11
B. Operated	3	2.3	1	1	1	3	3	3	3	3
1. SINGLE DX	1	1.0	0	1	1	1	1	1	1	1
2. MULTIPLE DX	264	3.4	7	1	2	3	4	6	8	11
A. NOT OPERATED	261	3.4	7	1	2	3	4	6	8	11
B. OPERATED	4	2.0	1	1	1	1	3	3	3	3
TOTAL										
0–19 Years	7	2.3	5	1	1	1	3	7	7	7
20–34	45	3.4	6	1	2	3	4	6	9	11
35–49	70	3.2	6	1	2	3	4	7	8	11
50–64	93	3.6	9	1	2	3	4	6	9	24
65+	50	3.4	4	1	2	3	5	6	7	10
GRAND TOTAL	265	3.4	7	1	2	3	4	6	8	11

343: INFANTILE CEREBRAL PALSY

Type of Patients	Observed Patients	Avg. Stay	Variance	Percentiles						
				10th	25th	50th	75th	90th	95th	99th
1. SINGLE DX										
A. Not Operated										
0–19 Years	0									
20–34	0									
35–49	0									
50–64	0									
65+	0									
B. Operated										
0–19 Years	11	2.6	4	1	1	2	4	4	7	7
20–34	0									
35–49	0									
50–64	0									
65+	0									
2. MULTIPLE DX										
A. Not Operated										
0–19 Years	33	3.9	28	1	1	2	4	8	11	30
20–34	13	4.7	16	1	2	4	6	10	14	14
35–49	14	3.9	6	2	2	3	5	8	9	9
50–64	11	6.7	54	1	2	3	7	19	23	23
65+	4	3.0	2	1	1	3	4	4	4	4
B. Operated										
0–19 Years	81	3.1	7	1	2	2	4	6	6	18
20–34	8	2.0	<1	1	2	2	3	3	3	3
35–49	4	2.3		1	1	1	4	4	4	4
50–64	2	4.5	5	3	3	5	6	6	6	6
65+	0									
SUBTOTALS:										
1. SINGLE DX										
A. Not Operated	0									
B. Operated	11	2.6	4	1	1	2	4	4	7	7
2. MULTIPLE DX										
A. Not Operated	75	4.4	24	1	2	3	6	8	14	30
B. Operated	95	3.0	6	1	2	2	4	6	6	18
1. SINGLE DX	11	2.6	4	1	2	2	4	4	7	7
2. MULTIPLE DX	170	3.6	15	1	2	3	4	7	9	23
A. NOT OPERATED	75	4.4	24	1	2	3	6	8	14	30
B. OPERATED	106	3.0	6	1	2	2	4	6	6	13
TOTAL										
0–19 Years	125	3.3	12	1	2	2	4	6	8	18
20–34	21	3.7	11	1	2	3	5	10	14	14
35–49	18	3.5	5	1	2	3	4	8	9	9
50–64	13	6.4	47	1	3	3	6	19	23	23
65+	4	3.0	2	1	1	3	4	4	4	4
GRAND TOTAL	181	3.6	14	1	2	2	4	7	9	23

Length of Stay by Diagnosis and Operation, Western Region, 2008

Western Region, October 2006–September 2007 Data, by Diagnosis

344: OTH PARALYTIC SYNDROMES

Type of Patients	Observed Patients	Avg. Stay	Variance	Percentiles 10th	25th	50th	75th	90th	95th	99th
1. SINGLE DX										
A. Not Operated										
0–19 Years	1	1.0	0	1	1	1	1	1	1	1
20–34	0									
35–49	0									
50–64	1	2.0	0	2	2	2	2	2	2	2
65+	0									
B. Operated										
0–19 Years	1	3.0	0	3	3	3	3	3	3	3
20–34	1	1.0	0	1	1	1	1	1	1	1
35–49	1	3.0	0	3	3	3	3	3	3	3
50–64	1	2.0	0	2	2	2	2	2	2	2
65+	1	1.0	0	1	1	1	1	1	1	1
2. MULTIPLE DX										
A. Not Operated										
0–19 Years	11	4.6	28	1	1	3	9	9	16	18
20–34	56	6.1	48	2	2	4	7	17	21	35
35–49	69	6.4	44	2	2	4	8	15	18	38
50–64	90	6.7	77	2	2	3	7	21	30	>99
65+	110	5.1	23	2	2	4	6	9	17	27
B. Operated										
0–19 Years	12	3.4	3	2	2	3	4	6	6	6
20–34	24	5.0	18	2	2	3	8	10	11	18
35–49	31	8.0	100	3	5	5	9	19	45	>99
50–64	57	5.3	26	2	4	4	7	15	17	>99
65+	44	6.9	99	2	2	4	8	11	21	58
SUBTOTALS:										
1. SINGLE DX A. Not Operated	2	1.5	<1	1	1	2	2	2	2	2
1. SINGLE DX B. Operated	5	2.0	1	1	2	3	3	3	3	3
2. MULTIPLE DX A. Not Operated	336	5.9	46	2	2	4	7	15	21	38
2. MULTIPLE DX B. Operated	168	6.1	57	2	2	4	7	12	19	>99
1. SINGLE DX	7	1.9	<1	1	1	2	3	3	3	3
2. MULTIPLE DX	504	6.0	50	2	2	4	7	14	21	44
A. NOT OPERATED	338	5.9	46	2	2	3	7	15	21	38
B. OPERATED	173	5.9	56	2	2	4	7	12	19	>99
TOTAL										
0–19 Years	25	3.8	14	1	1	3	4	9	9	18
20–34	81	5.7	38	2	2	4	7	12	19	35
35–49	101	6.9	61	2	2	4	8	15	23	45
50–64	149	6.1	57	2	2	3	7	17	26	>99
65+	155	5.6	45	1	2	4	6	10	17	35
GRAND TOTAL	511	5.9	49	2	2	4	7	14	21	44

345: EPIL & RECUR SEIZURES

Type of Patients	Observed Patients	Avg. Stay	Variance	Percentiles 10th	25th	50th	75th	90th	95th	99th
1. SINGLE DX										
A. Not Operated										
0–19 Years	534	2.2	4	1	1	2	3	4	6	9
20–34	304	3.7	6	1	2	3	5	7	8	11
35–49	159	3.6	5	1	2	3	5	7	8	12
50–64	98	3.6	5	1	2	3	5	7	8	11
65+	14	2.3	3	1	1	1	3	4		7
B. Operated										
0–19 Years	19	4.6	15	1	1	4	7	11	11	11
20–34	36	7.2	22	2	3	6	10	12	16	23
35–49	19	6.6	22	2	3	4	10	16	17	17
50–64	14	5.1	14	1	3	4	6	10	14	14
65+	0									
2. MULTIPLE DX										
A. Not Operated										
0–19 Years	1,891	2.9	9	1	1	2	3	6	8	16
20–34	1,986	3.7	20	1	2	3	4	7	9	21
35–49	2,841	3.7	16	1	2	3	5	7	10	20
50–64	2,857	4.1	16	1	2	3	5	8	11	21
65+	2,718	4.3	19	2	2	3	5	8	11	21
B. Operated										
0–19 Years	65	8.4	144	1	2	4	12	19	26	76
20–34	114	7.8	72	1	3	5	10	15	25	33
35–49	125	7.3	49	2	3	5	10	15	20	28
50–64	106	9.3	127	2	3	6	10	20	28	44
65+	39	11.3	151	2	5	8	13	18	36	75
SUBTOTALS:										
1. SINGLE DX A. Not Operated	1,109	2.9	5	1	1	2	4	6	7	11
1. SINGLE DX B. Operated	88	6.2	20	1	3	5	9	11	15	23
2. MULTIPLE DX A. Not Operated	12,293	3.8	16	1	2	3	5	7	10	20
2. MULTIPLE DX B. Operated	449	8.4	96	1	3	5	11	17	25	49
1. SINGLE DX	1,197	3.2	7	1	1	2	4	7	8	13
2. MULTIPLE DX	12,742	4.0	20	2	2	3	5	8	11	21
A. NOT OPERATED	13,402	3.7	15	1	2	3	4	7	10	20
B. OPERATED	537	8.1	84	1	3	5	10	16	24	44
TOTAL										
0–19 Years	2,509	2.9	13	1	1	2	3	6	8	17
20–34	2,440	3.9	21	1	2	3	5	7	10	22
35–49	3,144	3.8	17	1	2	3	4	7	10	20
50–64	3,075	4.3	20	1	2	3	5	8	11	22
65+	2,771	4.4	21	1	2	3	5	8	12	22
GRAND TOTAL	13,939	3.9	19	2	2	3	5	8	11	21

345.10: GRAND MAL W/O INTRACT

Type of Patients	Observed Patients	Avg. Stay	Variance	Percentiles 10th	25th	50th	75th	90th	95th	99th
1. SINGLE DX										
A. Not Operated										
0–19 Years	54	1.9	1	1	1	2	2	3	5	6
20–34	26	1.9	<1	1	1	2	2	4	4	4
35–49	13	2.9	7	1	1	2	4	4	11	11
50–64	11	2.3	1	1	1	2	3	3	5	5
65+	2	1.5	<1	1	1	2	2	2	2	2
B. Operated										
0–19 Years	0									
20–34	0									
35–49	0									
50–64	0									
65+	0									
2. MULTIPLE DX										
A. Not Operated										
0–19 Years	173	2.6	17	1	1	2	3	4	7	25
20–34	270	3.1	12	1	1	3	3	6	8	23
35–49	351	3.3	14	1	1	4	4	6	9	21
50–64	379	3.6	11	2	2	3	4	7	10	20
65+	377	3.8	8	2	2	3	5	7	9	12
B. Operated										
0–19 Years	1	9.0	0	9	9	9	9	9	9	9
20–34	3	2.7	8	1	1	1	6	6	6	6
35–49	5	3.4	3	1	2	4	4	5	5	5
50–64	7	5.3	16	1	2	5	7	13	13	13
65+	5	11.6	10	7	10	13	15	15	15	15
SUBTOTALS:										
1. SINGLE DX A. Not Operated	106	2.1	2	1	1	2	2	4	4	6
1. SINGLE DX B. Operated	0									
2. MULTIPLE DX A. Not Operated	1,550	3.4	12	1	1	3	5	7	9	18
2. MULTIPLE DX B. Operated	21	6.1	20	1	2	5	11	13	13	15
1. SINGLE DX	106	2.1	2	1	1	2	2	4	4	6
2. MULTIPLE DX	1,571	3.4	12	1	1	3	4	7	9	18
A. NOT OPERATED	1,656	3.3	11	1	1	3	4	6	9	18
B. OPERATED	21	6.1	20	1	2	5	9	13	13	15
TOTAL										
0–19 Years	228	2.5	13	1	1	2	3	4	6	16
20–34	299	2.9	11	1	1	2	3	6	7	23
35–49	369	3.3	14	1	2	3	4	6	9	21
50–64	397	3.6	11	2	2	3	5	7	10	20
65+	384	3.9	8	2	2	3	5	8	9	13
GRAND TOTAL	1,677	3.3	12	1	1	2	4	6	9	18

345.11: GRAND MAL W INTRACT EPIL

Type of Patients	Observed Patients	Avg. Stay	Variance	10th	25th	50th	75th	90th	95th	99th
1. SINGLE DX										
A. Not Operated										
0–19 Years	14	2.6	7	1	1	1	3	8	9	9
20–34	11	3.5	6	1	2	3	6	7	8	8
35–49	5	3.0	<1	2	3	3	3	5	4	4
50–64	2	5.0	8	3	3	7	7	7	7	7
65+	0									
B. Operated										
0–19 Years	0									
20–34	1	16.0	0	16	16	16	16	16	16	16
35–49	0									
50–64	0									
65+	0									
2. MULTIPLE DX										
A. Not Operated										
0–19 Years	60	3.6	15	1	1	2	4	10	14	19
20–34	72	5.2	94	1	2	4	6	9	11	83
35–49	43	4.7	20	1	2	3	6	11	13	21
50–64	26	4.8	28	1	2	4	6	8	29	>99
65+	10	3.4	4	1	2	3	5	7	7	7
B. Operated										
0–19 Years	6	3.2	6	1	1	3	5	7	7	7
20–34	7	8.4	91	1	2	3	15	27	27	27
35–49	4	2.0	2	1	1	1	2	4	4	4
50–64	1	10.0	0	10	10	10	10	10	10	10
65+	0									
SUBTOTALS:										
1. SINGLE DX										
A. Not Operated	32	3.1	6	1	1	3	3	7	8	9
B. Operated	1	16.0	0	16	16	16	16	16	16	16
2. MULTIPLE DX										
A. Not Operated	211	4.5	44	1	1	2	5	9	12	29
B. Operated	18	5.3	44	1	1	3	7	15	27	27
1. SINGLE DX	33	3.5	10	1	1	3	4	8	9	16
2. MULTIPLE DX	229	4.6	44	1	2	3	5	10	13	29
A. NOT OPERATED	243	4.3	39	1	2	3	5	9	12	29
B. OPERATED	19	5.9	47	1	1	3	8	16	27	27
TOTAL										
0–19 Years	80	3.4	13	1	1	2	4	9	11	19
20–34	91	5.4	84	1	2	3	6	9	13	83
35–49	52	4.3	17	1	2	3	5	11	13	21
50–64	29	5.0	26	2	2	4	7	8	29	>99
65+	10	3.4	4	1	2	3	5	7	7	7
GRAND TOTAL	262	4.4	40	1	2	3	5	9	12	29

345.3: GRAND MAL STATUS

Type of Patients	Observed Patients	Avg. Stay	Variance	10th	25th	50th	75th	90th	95th	99th
1. SINGLE DX										
A. Not Operated										
0–19 Years	81	1.5	<1	1	1	1	2	3	3	4
20–34	20	2.1	1	1	1	2	3	4	4	4
35–49	10	3.0	5	1	1	2	5	5	8	8
50–64	2	1.5	<1	1	1	2	2	2	2	2
65+	3	2.7	2	1	1	3	4	4	4	4
B. Operated										
0–19 Years	0									
20–34	0									
35–49	1	10.0	0	10	10	10	10	10	10	10
50–64	0									
65+	0									
2. MULTIPLE DX										
A. Not Operated										
0–19 Years	513	3.1	11	1	1	2	4	6	9	17
20–34	368	4.6	34	1	2	3	5	9	12	33
35–49	560	4.7	35	1	2	3	5	9	15	28
50–64	478	5.5	28	1	2	4	7	12	18	31
65+	393	6.4	36	3	3	5	8	14	19	30
B. Operated										
0–19 Years	9	17.7	534	2	4	12	19	76	76	76
20–34	4	7.7	118	1	1	7	24	24	24	24
35–49	7	14.3	106	3	5	9	24	28	28	28
50–64	12	25.6	583	5	14	19	39	44	91	91
65+	11	19.3	414	5	8	14	20	36	75	75
SUBTOTALS:										
1. SINGLE DX										
A. Not Operated	116	1.8	1	1	1	1	2	3	4	5
B. Operated	1	10.0	0	10	10	10	10	10	10	10
2. MULTIPLE DX										
A. Not Operated	2,312	4.8	29	1	2	3	6	10	15	27
B. Operated	43	18.9	406	3	5	14	24	39	75	91
1. SINGLE DX	117	1.8	2	1	1	1	2	4	4	8
2. MULTIPLE DX	2,355	5.0	40	1	2	3	6	10	16	30
A. NOT OPERATED	2,428	4.6	29	1	2	3	5	9	15	27
B. OPERATED	44	18.6	398	3	5	14	24	39	75	91
TOTAL										
0–19 Years	603	3.1	20	1	1	2	3	6	9	19
20–34	392	4.5	33	1	2	3	5	9	12	33
35–49	578	4.8	37	1	2	3	5	9	15	28
50–64	492	6.0	50	1	2	4	7	13	19	39
65+	407	6.7	50	2	3	5	8	14	20	30
GRAND TOTAL	2,472	4.9	38	1	2	3	6	10	16	29

345.40: LRE W CPS W/O INTRACT

Type of Patients	Observed Patients	Avg. Stay	Variance	10th	25th	50th	75th	90th	95th	99th
1. SINGLE DX										
A. Not Operated										
0–19 Years	24	3.5	12	1	1	2	4	6	7	17
20–34	31	4.3	8	1	2	4	6	9	10	10
35–49	15	3.3	5	1	1	3	5	6	8	10
50–64	8	4.9	2	3	4	4	7	7	7	8
65+	0									
B. Operated										
0–19 Years	0									
20–34	3	3.3	2	2	2	3	5	5	5	5
35–49	0									
50–64	1	14.0	0	14	14	14	14	14	14	14
65+	0									
2. MULTIPLE DX										
A. Not Operated										
0–19 Years	67	3.1	14	1	1	2	4	7	7	24
20–34	87	3.8	7	1	2	3	5	7	8	16
35–49	110	3.5	8	1	2	3	4	7	9	10
50–64	104	4.0	26	1	2	3	5	6	8	18
65+	131	3.9	9	1	2	3	5	8	10	16
B. Operated										
0–19 Years	0									
20–34	4	4.5	14	2	2	3	10	10	10	10
35–49	4	8.0	34	2	4	8	12	14	14	14
50–64	2	4.5	12	2	2	5	7	7	7	7
65+	2	7.0	49	2	2	12	12	12	12	12
SUBTOTALS:										
1. SINGLE DX										
A. Not Operated	78	3.9	8	1	2	3	5	7	10	17
B. Operated	4	6.0	30	2	3	4	5	14	14	14
2. MULTIPLE DX										
A. Not Operated	499	3.7	13	1	2	3	5	7	9	18
B. Operated	12	6.1	22	2	2	4	12	12	14	14
1. SINGLE DX	82	4.0	9	1	2	3	5	7	10	17
2. MULTIPLE DX	511	3.8	13	1	2	3	5	7	9	17
A. NOT OPERATED	577	3.7	12	1	2	3	5	7	9	17
B. OPERATED	16	6.1	22	2	2	4	10	14	14	14
TOTAL										
0–19 Years	91	3.2	13	1	1	2	4	6	7	24
20–34	125	3.9	7	1	2	4	5	8	10	11
35–49	129	3.6	9	1	2	3	4	7	9	14
50–64	115	4.2	25	1	2	3	5	7	9	18
65+	133	4.0	9	1	2	3	5	8	11	16
GRAND TOTAL	593	3.8	12	1	2	3	5	7	9	17

Length of Stay by Diagnosis and Operation, Western Region, 2008

Western Region, October 2006–September 2007 Data, by Diagnosis

345.41: LRE W CPS W INTRACT

Type of Patients	Observed Patients	Avg. Stay	Variance	Percentiles						
				10th	25th	50th	75th	90th	95th	99th
1. SINGLE DX										
A. Not Operated										
0–19 Years	21	3.7	5	1	2	4	5	6	6	10
20–34	52	4.2	3	2	3	4	5	7	7	11
35–49	36	4.3	5	2	3	4	6	7	8	12
50–64	15	4.7	7	1	3	4	6	8	11	11
65+	0									
B. Operated										
0–19 Years	4	8.0	12	5	5	5	11	11	11	11
20–34	15	6.9	11	3	4	7	10	11	12	12
35–49	6	8.9	29	2	4	11	11	17	17	17
50–64	7	4.4	3	2	3	4	6	6	6	6
65+	0									
2. MULTIPLE DX										
A. Not Operated										
0–19 Years	43	3.7	12	1	1	3	4	7	10	18
20–34	100	4.6	9	2	3	4	6	7	10	20
35–49	85	4.9	7	2	3	4	7	8	10	12
50–64	77	5.0	9	2	3	4	6	8	11	18
65+	21	4.6	10	2	2	4	5	8	9	14
B. Operated										
0–19 Years	13	6.4	20	3	3	4	8	14	15	15
20–34	44	8.4	36	2	4	7	13	17	18	25
35–49	30	6.9	26	1	3	5	10	13	18	20
50–64	20	7.3	36	3	4	6	9	11	11	30
65+	1	13.0	0	13	13	13	13	13	13	13
SUBTOTALS:										
1. SINGLE DX										
A. Not Operated	124	4.2	4	2	3	4	5	7	8	11
B. Operated	32	6.9	14	3	4	6	10	11	12	17
2. MULTIPLE DX										
A. Not Operated	326	4.7	9	2	3	4	6	8	10	15
B. Operated	108	7.6	31	2	3	6	11	14	18	25
1. SINGLE DX	156	4.8	7	2	3	4	6	8	11	12
2. MULTIPLE DX	434	5.4	16	2	3	4	7	10	13	20
A. NOT OPERATED	450	4.5	8	2	3	4	6	8	10	14
B. OPERATED	140	7.4	27	2	3	6	10	14	17	25
TOTAL										
0–19 Years	81	4.3	12	1	2	3	5	7	10	18
20–34	211	5.5	16	2	3	4	7	10	13	20
35–49	157	5.3	12	2	3	4	7	10	12	18
50–64	119	5.3	13	2	3	4	7	9	11	18
65+	22	5.0	13	2	2	4	8	9	13	14
GRAND TOTAL	590	5.2	14	2	3	4	7	10	12	18

345.50: LRE W SPS W/O INTRACT

Type of Patients	Observed Patients	Avg. Stay	Variance	Percentiles						
				10th	25th	50th	75th	90th	95th	99th
1. SINGLE DX										
A. Not Operated										
0–19 Years	44	2.1	<1	1	1	2	3	3	4	4
20–34	26	4.4	8	1	2	4	7	8	9	11
35–49	12	4.6	6	2	4	4	7	8	9	9
50–64	10	3.5	8	1	3	3	4	5	11	11
65+	4	3.2	8	1	1	1	4	7	7	7
B. Operated										
0–19 Years	0									
20–34	1	4.0	0	4	4	4	4	4	4	4
35–49	0									
50–64	0									
65+	0									
2. MULTIPLE DX										
A. Not Operated										
0–19 Years	100	2.9	5	1	1	2	4	5	7	11
20–34	79	3.4	11	1	1	2	4	6	10	20
35–49	106	3.2	5	1	2	2	4	6	8	11
50–64	149	3.7	7	1	2	3	5	8	10	11
65+	208	3.9	10	1	2	3	5	8	9	17
B. Operated										
0–19 Years	0									
20–34	1	2.0	0	2	2	2	2	2	2	2
35–49	2	7.0	2	6	6	8	8	8	8	8
50–64	1	7.0	0	7	7	7	7	7	7	7
65+	5	9.6	33	5	5	7	13	18	18	18
SUBTOTALS:										
1. SINGLE DX										
A. Not Operated	96	3.2	6	1	2	3	4	7	8	11
B. Operated	1	4.0	0	4	4	4	4	4	4	4
2. MULTIPLE DX										
A. Not Operated	642	3.5	8	1	2	3	4	7	9	14
B. Operated	9	7.9	23	2	5	7	8	18	18	25
1. SINGLE DX	97	3.2	6	1	2	3	4	7	8	11
2. MULTIPLE DX	651	3.6	8	1	2	3	5	7	9	15
A. NOT OPERATED	738	3.5	7	1	2	3	4	7	9	12
B. OPERATED	10	7.5	22	2	5	7	8	18	18	25
TOTAL										
0–19 Years	144	2.6	4	1	1	2	3	5	6	11
20–34	107	3.6	10	1	2	3	4	7	9	18
35–49	120	3.4	5	1	2	3	4	7	8	11
50–64	160	3.7	7	1	2	3	5	8	10	11
65+	217	4.1	11	1	2	3	5	8	10	17
GRAND TOTAL	748	3.5	8	1	2	3	4	7	9	14

345.51: LRE W SPS W INTRACT

Type of Patients	Observed Patients	Avg. Stay	Variance	Percentiles						
				10th	25th	50th	75th	90th	95th	99th
1. SINGLE DX										
A. Not Operated										
0–19 Years	25	2.7	3	1	2	3	3	4	7	8
20–34	15	4.1	2	2	3	4	5	6	7	7
35–49	8	3.5	3	1	3	3	4	7	7	7
50–64	8	4.4	3	2	3	5	5	7	7	7
65+	0									
B. Operated										
0–19 Years	2	2.5	4	1	1	1	4	4	4	4
20–34	6	11.5	49	2	9	10	15	23	23	23
35–49	3	8.3	44	4	4	5	16	16	16	16
50–64	0									
65+	0									
2. MULTIPLE DX										
A. Not Operated										
0–19 Years	40	3.6	9	1	1	3	5	7	9	16
20–34	42	4.1	16	1	3	3	5	8	9	24
35–49	38	5.1	13	1	3	4	7	9	12	20
50–64	27	5.6	31	2	3	5	7	12	16	27
65+	17	6.7	22	3	3	5	9	12	20	20
B. Operated										
0–19 Years	3	15.3	9	12	12	16	18	18	18	18
20–34	5	3.0	0	3	3	3	3	3	3	3
35–49	11	7.2	19	3	3	7	10	14	15	15
50–64	4	12.0	56	3	3	12	14	21	21	21
65+	0									
SUBTOTALS:										
1. SINGLE DX										
A. Not Operated	56	3.4	3	1	2	3	4	6	7	8
B. Operated	11	9.0	46	2	4	9	15	16	23	23
2. MULTIPLE DX										
A. Not Operated	164	4.7	17	1	2	4	6	9	12	24
B. Operated	23	8.2	33	3	3	7	14	16	18	21
1. SINGLE DX	67	4.4	14	1	2	3	5	8	11	23
2. MULTIPLE DX	187	5.2	20	1	2	4	7	10	15	24
A. NOT OPERATED	220	4.4	14	1	2	4	5	8	10	20
B. OPERATED	34	8.4	37	3	3	8	14	16	21	23
TOTAL										
0–19 Years	70	3.8	13	1	1	3	4	8	12	18
20–34	68	4.7	18	1	3	3	6	9	11	24
35–49	60	5.4	15	2	3	4	7	10	14	20
50–64	39	6.0	30	2	3	4	7	14	21	27
65+	17	6.7	22	3	3	5	9	12	20	20
GRAND TOTAL	254	5.0	19	1	2	4	6	10	15	23

Western Region, October 2006–September 2007 Data, by Diagnosis

345.80: EPILEPSY NEC W/O INTRACT

Type of Patients	Observed Patients	Avg. Stay	Vari-ance	Percentiles						
				10th	25th	50th	75th	90th	95th	99th
1. SINGLE DX										
A. *Not Operated*										
0–19 Years	40	2.2	9	1	1	2	2	3	4	20
20–34	10	5.2	10	2	3	4	7	12	12	12
35–49	8	3.3	8	1	1	3	4	8	8	8
50–64	6	3.7	10	1	2	3	4	10	10	10
65+	0									
B. *Operated*										
0–19 Years	0									
20–34	1	5.0	0	5	5	5	5	5	5	5
35–49	2	5.5	4	4	4	7	7	7	7	7
50–64	0									
65+	0									
2. MULTIPLE DX										
A. *Not Operated*										
0–19 Years	73	2.5	4	1	1	2	3	5	7	11
20–34	65	3.2	8	1	1	3	4	6	7	17
35–49	107	3.3	10	1	1	2	4	7	9	15
50–64	109	4.7	14	2	2	4	6	8	12	20
65+	90	4.2	16	1	2	3	5	7	10	27
B. *Operated*										
0–19 Years	2	21.0	32	17	17	17	25	25	25	25
20–34	3	8.4	42	2	2	3	15	15	15	15
35–49	1	7.0	0	7	7	7	7	7	7	7
50–64	0									
65+	2	6.0	8	4	4	6	8	8	8	8
SUBTOTALS:										
1. SINGLE DX										
A. *Not Operated*	64	3.0	10	1	1	2	3	7	8	20
B. *Operated*	3	5.3	2	4	4	5	7	7	7	7
2. MULTIPLE DX										
A. *Not Operated*	444	3.7	11	1	2	3	5	7	9	17
B. *Operated*	8	10.7	58	2	7	8	15	25	25	25
1. SINGLE DX	67	3.1	10	1	1	2	4	7	8	20
2. MULTIPLE DX	452	3.8	13	1	2	3	5	7	10	20
A. NOT OPERATED	508	3.6	11	1	1	3	5	7	9	17
B. OPERATED	11	9.3	48	4	4	7	15	17	25	25
TOTAL										
0–19 Years	115	2.7	12	1	1	2	3	5	9	20
20–34	79	3.7	10	1	2	3	4	7	12	17
35–49	118	3.4	9	1	1	2	4	7	8	15
50–64	115	4.7	13	2	2	4	6	8	12	20
65+	92	4.2	16	1	2	3	5	7	10	27
GRAND TOTAL	519	3.7	13	1	2	3	5	7	10	20

345.90: EPILEPSY NOS W/O INTRACT

Type of Patients	Observed Patients	Avg. Stay	Vari-ance	Percentiles						
				10th	25th	50th	75th	90th	95th	99th
1. SINGLE DX										
A. *Not Operated*										
0–19 Years	143	1.9	2	1	1	1	2	3	4	8
20–34	77	3.2	5	1	2	3	4	6	7	11
35–49	33	3.2	7	1	1	2	4	7	10	12
50–64	21	2.8	3	1	1	2	4	4	7	7
65+	5	1.6	<1	1	1	1	2	3	3	3
B. *Operated*										
0–19 Years	2	1.0	0	1	1	1	1	1	1	1
20–34	1	3.0	0	3	3	3	3	3	3	3
35–49	0									
50–64	1	3.0	0	3	3	3	3	3	3	3
65+	0									
2. MULTIPLE DX										
A. *Not Operated*										
0–19 Years	526	2.5	6	1	1	2	3	5	7	14
20–34	729	3.0	10	1	1	3	4	6	7	13
35–49	1,231	3.1	8	1	1	2	4	6	8	16
50–64	1,337	3.5	9	1	2	3	4	7	9	16
65+	1,358	3.8	13	2	2	3	5	7	9	16
B. *Operated*										
0–19 Years	6	2.5	2	1	1	2	4	4	4	4
20–34	9	7.7	83	1	3	3	7	27	27	27
35–49	18	11.7	136	1	3	8	16	26	49	49
50–64	28	7.1	21	2	3	7	10	12	15	22
65+	11	6.9	21	2	5	5	9	11	18	18
SUBTOTALS:										
1. SINGLE DX										
A. *Not Operated*	279	2.5	4	1	1	2	3	5	7	11
B. *Operated*	4	2.0	1	1	1	3	3	3	3	3
2. MULTIPLE DX										
A. *Not Operated*	5,181	3.3	10	1	1	2	4	6	8	16
B. *Operated*	72	7.9	60	2	3	6	10	17	22	49
1. SINGLE DX	283	2.5	4	1	1	2	3	5	7	11
2. MULTIPLE DX	5,253	3.4	11	1	2	3	4	7	9	16
A. NOT OPERATED	5,460	3.3	10	1	1	3	5	7	8	15
B. OPERATED	76	7.6	58	3	5	5	10	17	22	49
TOTAL										
0–19 Years	677	2.4	5	1	1	2	3	4	7	14
20–34	816	3.1	11	1	1	2	4	6	7	14
35–49	1,282	3.2	11	1	1	2	4	6	8	17
50–64	1,387	3.6	9	1	2	3	4	7	9	16
65+	1,374	3.8	14	2	2	3	5	7	9	17
GRAND TOTAL	5,536	3.3	11	1	2	2	4	6	8	16

345.91: INTRACTABLE EPILEPSY NOS

Type of Patients	Observed Patients	Avg. Stay	Vari-ance	Percentiles						
				10th	25th	50th	75th	90th	95th	99th
1. SINGLE DX										
A. *Not Operated*										
0–19 Years	34	3.1	16	1	1	2	4	6	8	23
20–34	21	5.3	15	1	3	4	8	10	13	14
35–49	12	3.4	5	1	2	4	4	5	9	9
50–64	11	3.1	1	2	2	3	4	5	5	5
65+	0									
B. *Operated*										
0–19 Years	9	5.2	15	1	2	5	7	11	11	11
20–34	4	3.7	3	2	2	3	4	6	6	6
35–49	5	4.0	12	1	3	3	3	10	10	10
50–64	4	3.5	14	1	1	3	3	9	9	9
65+	0									
2. MULTIPLE DX										
A. *Not Operated*										
0–19 Years	95	3.1	10	1	1	2	4	6	9	26
20–34	107	4.0	10	1	2	3	5	7	9	16
35–49	104	4.0	6	1	2	4	5	7	8	11
50–64	81	4.9	17	1	2	4	7	8	10	28
65+	21	6.1	17	3	4	4	7	11	13	18
B. *Operated*										
0–19 Years	16	6.0	130	1	1	2	5	26	42	42
20–34	28	9.2	167	1	3	5	10	33	33	66
35–49	25	4.8	22	1	2	3	7	11	12	20
50–64	23	6.5	29	3	3	4	9	13	13	24
65+	1	1.0	0	1	1	1	1	1	1	1
SUBTOTALS:										
1. SINGLE DX										
A. *Not Operated*	78	3.8	13	1	1	3	4	8	10	23
B. *Operated*	22	4.4	11	1	2	3	6	10	11	11
2. MULTIPLE DX										
A. *Not Operated*	408	4.1	11	1	2	3	5	7	10	18
B. *Operated*	93	6.7	86	2	3	4	9	13	24	66
1. SINGLE DX	100	3.9	12	1	1	3	5	8	10	14
2. MULTIPLE DX	501	4.6	26	1	2	3	5	9	12	26
A. NOT OPERATED	486	4.0	11	1	2	3	5	7	10	18
B. OPERATED	115	6.3	72	1	2	3	8	13	20	42
TOTAL										
0–19 Years	154	3.5	24	1	1	2	4	7	10	26
20–34	160	5.1	40	1	2	4	6	10	13	33
35–49	146	4.1	9	1	2	4	5	6	10	15
50–64	119	5.0	18	1	2	4	7	9	13	24
65+	22	5.8	17	2	4	4	7	11	13	18
GRAND TOTAL	601	4.5	24	1	2	3	5	9	11	24

Length of Stay by Diagnosis and Operation, Western Region, 2008

Western Region, October 2006–September 2007 Data, by Diagnosis

346: MIGRAINE

Type of Patients	Observed Patients	Avg. Stay	Variance	10th	25th	50th	75th	90th	95th	99th
1. SINGLE DX										
A. Not Operated										
0–19 Years	99	1.7	1	1	1	1	2	3	4	6
20–34	128	2.2	3	1	1	2	3	4	5	9
35–49	132	2.1	2	1	1	2	3	3	5	7
50–64	37	1.7	<1	1	1	2	2	3	3	3
65+	7	2.0	1	1	1	2	3	3	3	3
B. Operated										
0–19 Years	0									
20–34	0									
35–49	0									
50–64	0									
65+	0									
2. MULTIPLE DX										
A. Not Operated										
0–19 Years	346	2.6	4	1	1	2	3	5	7	12
20–34	1,224	2.8	4	1	1	2	3	5	7	10
35–49	1,915	2.8	5	1	1	2	3	5	6	12
50–64	1,258	2.7	5	1	1	2	3	5	6	11
65+	446	2.5	4	1	1	2	3	4	6	9
B. Operated										
0–19 Years	1	3.0	0	3	3	3	3	3	3	3
20–34	6	4.3	11	1	2	3	8	9	9	9
35–49	16	6.5	20	1	2	7	11	12	15	15
50–64	13	7.3	40	3	3	5	8	20	21	21
65+	6	6.7	25	3	4	6	10	15	15	15
SUBTOTALS:										
1. SINGLE DX										
A. Not Operated	403	2.0	2	1	1	2	2	3	4	7
B. Operated	0									
2. MULTIPLE DX										
A. Not Operated	5,189	2.7	5	1	1	2	3	5	7	11
B. Operated	42	6.4	25	1	3	5	9	12	15	21
1. SINGLE DX	403	2.0	2	1	1	2	2	3	4	7
2. MULTIPLE DX	5,231	2.8	5	1	1	2	3	5	7	11
A. NOT OPERATED	5,592	2.7	4	1	1	2	3	5	7	11
B. OPERATED	42	6.4	25	1	3	5	9	12	15	21
TOTAL										
0–19 Years	446	2.4	4	1	1	2	3	5	6	11
20–34	1,358	2.7	4	1	1	2	3	5	7	10
35–49	2,063	2.8	5	1	1	2	3	5	7	12
50–64	1,308	2.7	6	1	1	2	3	5	7	11
65+	459	2.5	4	1	1	2	3	4	6	11
GRAND TOTAL	5,634	2.7	5	1	1	2	3	5	7	11

346.00: CLASS MIGRAINE S INTRACT

Type of Patients	Observed Patients	Avg. Stay	Variance	10th	25th	50th	75th	90th	95th	99th
1. SINGLE DX										
A. Not Operated										
0–19 Years	2	1.0	0	1	1	1	1	1	1	1
20–34	3	1.7	1	1	1	1	1	3	3	3
35–49	5	1.0	0	1	1	1	1	1	1	1
50–64	5	1.2	<1	1	1	1	1	2	2	2
65+	0									
B. Operated										
0–19 Years	0									
20–34	0									
35–49	0									
50–64	0									
65+	0									
2. MULTIPLE DX										
A. Not Operated										
0–19 Years	3	2.0	0	2	2	2	2	2	2	2
20–34	35	2.2	4	1	1	2	3	4	5	11
35–49	70	2.4	3	1	1	2	3	5	6	10
50–64	36	1.9	1	1	1	2	3	3	4	6
65+	18	2.4	6	1	1	2	3	3	4	12
B. Operated										
0–19 Years	0									
20–34	1	3.0	0	3	3	3	3	3	3	3
35–49	0									
50–64	0									
65+	0									
SUBTOTALS:										
1. SINGLE DX										
A. Not Operated	15	1.2	<1	1	1	1	1	2	3	3
B. Operated	0									
2. MULTIPLE DX										
A. Not Operated	162	2.2	3	1	1	2	3	4	5	11
B. Operated	1	3.0	0	3	3	3	3	3	3	3
1. SINGLE DX	15	1.2	<1	1	1	1	1	2	3	3
2. MULTIPLE DX	163	2.3	3	1	1	2	3	4	5	11
A. NOT OPERATED	177	2.2	3	1	1	2	3	4	5	11
B. OPERATED	1	3.0	0	3	3	3	3	3	3	3
TOTAL										
0–19 Years	5	1.6	<1	1	1	1	2	2	2	2
20–34	39	2.2	3	1	1	2	3	4	5	11
35–49	75	2.4	3	1	1	2	3	4	6	10
50–64	41	1.8	1	1	1	2	3	3	3	6
65+	18	2.4	6	1	1	2	3	3	4	12
GRAND TOTAL	178	2.2	3	1	1	2	3	4	5	11

346.10: COMN MIGRAINE S INTRACT

Type of Patients	Observed Patients	Avg. Stay	Variance	10th	25th	50th	75th	90th	95th	99th
1. SINGLE DX										
A. Not Operated										
0–19 Years	5	1.4	<1	1	1	1	2	2	2	2
20–34	3	1.3	<1	1	1	1	2	2	2	2
35–49	4	1.0	0	1	1	1	1	1	1	1
50–64	1	1.0	0	1	1	1	1	1	1	1
65+	0									
B. Operated										
0–19 Years	0									
20–34	0									
35–49	0									
50–64	0									
65+	0									
2. MULTIPLE DX										
A. Not Operated										
0–19 Years	19	2.0	6	1	1	2	2	3	3	12
20–34	50	2.1	2	1	2	2	3	4	4	7
35–49	80	2.3	3	1	2	2	3	4	5	11
50–64	59	2.8	7	1	2	2	3	6	10	14
65+	22	2.5	1	1	2	2	3	4	4	5
B. Operated										
0–19 Years	0									
20–34	0									
35–49	1	5.0	0	5	5	5	5	5	5	5
50–64	1	4.0	0	4	4	4	4	4	4	4
65+	0									
SUBTOTALS:										
1. SINGLE DX										
A. Not Operated	13	1.2	<1	1	1	1	1	2	2	2
B. Operated	0									
2. MULTIPLE DX										
A. Not Operated	230	2.4	4	1	1	2	3	4	6	11
B. Operated	2	4.5	<1	4	4	4	5	5	5	5
1. SINGLE DX	13	1.2	<1	1	1	1	1	2	2	2
2. MULTIPLE DX	232	2.4	4	1	1	2	3	4	6	11
A. NOT OPERATED	243	2.3	4	1	1	2	3	4	5	11
B. OPERATED	2	4.5	<1	4	4	4	5	5	5	5
TOTAL										
0–19 Years	24	1.9	5	1	1	1	2	3	3	12
20–34	53	2.1	2	1	1	2	3	4	4	7
35–49	85	2.2	3	1	1	2	3	4	5	11
50–64	61	2.8	7	1	2	2	3	6	8	14
65+	22	2.5	1	1	2	2	3	4	4	5
GRAND TOTAL	245	2.3	4	1	1	2	3	4	5	11

Length of Stay by Diagnosis and Operation, Western Region 2008

Western Region, October 2006–September 2007 Data, by Diagnosis

346.20: MIGRAINE VRNT S INTRACT

Type of Patients	Observed Patients	Avg. Stay	Vari-ance	10th	25th	50th	75th	90th	95th	99th
1. SINGLE DX										
A. Not Operated										
0–19 Years	7	1.4	<1	1	1	1	2	2	2	2
20–34	4	1.3	<1	1	1	1	2	2	2	2
35–49	7	1.6	<1	1	1	2	2	2	2	2
50–64	0									
65+	1	1.0	0	1	1	1	1	1	1	1
B. Operated										
0–19 Years	0									
20–34	0									
35–49	0									
50–64	0									
65+	0									
2. MULTIPLE DX										
A. Not Operated										
0–19 Years	20	2.8	5	1	1	2	3	6	7	10
20–34	40	2.5	2	1	1	2	3	4	5	7
35–49	82	2.7	6	1	1	2	3	5	8	13
50–64	74	2.7	5	1	1	2	4	5	8	13
65+	36	2.3	3	1	1	2	3	4	6	8
B. Operated										
0–19 Years	0									
20–34	0									
35–49	0									
50–64	1	3.0	0	3	3	3	3	3	3	3
65+	1	10.0	0	10	10	10	10	10	10	10
SUBTOTALS:										
1. SINGLE DX										
A. Not Operated	19	1.4	<1	1	1	1	2	2	2	2
B. Operated	0									
2. MULTIPLE DX										
A. Not Operated	252	2.6	5	1	1	2	3	5	8	12
B. Operated	2	6.5	24	3	3	7	10	10	10	10
1. SINGLE DX	19	1.4	<1	1	1	1	2	2	2	2
2. MULTIPLE DX	254	2.7	5	1	1	2	3	5	8	12
A. NOT OPERATED	271	2.5	4	1	1	2	3	5	8	12
B. OPERATED	2	6.5	24	3	3	7	10	10	10	10
TOTAL										
0–19 Years	27	2.5	4	1	1	2	3	6	7	10
20–34	44	2.3	2	1	1	2	3	4	5	7
35–49	89	2.6	6	1	1	2	3	5	8	13
50–64	75	2.7	5	1	1	2	4	5	8	13
65+	38	2.5	4	1	1	2	3	5	8	10
GRAND TOTAL	273	2.6	5	1	1	2	3	5	8	12

346.80: MIGRAINE NEC W/O INTRACT

Type of Patients	Observed Patients	Avg. Stay	Vari-ance	10th	25th	50th	75th	90th	95th	99th
1. SINGLE DX										
A. Not Operated										
0–19 Years	25	1.3	<1	1	1	1	2	2	2	3
20–34	26	2.6	3	1	1	2	3	5	6	7
35–49	34	2.4	5	1	1	2	3	4	7	12
50–64	8	1.7	<1	1	1	1	2	3	3	3
65+	2	1.5	<1	1	1	2	2	2	2	2
B. Operated										
0–19 Years	0									
20–34	0									
35–49	0									
50–64	0									
65+	0									
2. MULTIPLE DX										
A. Not Operated										
0–19 Years	72	2.7	5	1	1	2	3	6	8	12
20–34	268	2.6	3	1	1	2	3	5	6	9
35–49	489	2.5	4	1	1	2	3	5	6	12
50–64	335	2.5	5	1	1	2	3	5	6	12
65+	119	2.3	2	1	1	2	3	4	6	7
B. Operated										
0–19 Years	0									
20–34	1	1.0	0	1	1	1	1	1	1	1
35–49	3	7.4	12	4	4	7	11	11	11	11
50–64	3	4.7	2	3	3	5	6	6	6	6
65+	2	5.0	2	4	4	6	6	6	6	6
SUBTOTALS:										
1. SINGLE DX										
A. Not Operated	95	2.1	3	1	1	2	3	4	6	12
B. Operated	0									
2. MULTIPLE DX										
A. Not Operated	1,283	2.5	4	1	1	2	3	5	6	11
B. Operated	9	5.2	8	1	4	5	6	11	11	11
1. SINGLE DX	95	2.1	3	1	1	2	3	4	6	12
2. MULTIPLE DX	1,292	2.5	4	1	1	2	3	5	6	11
A. NOT OPERATED	1,378	2.5	4	1	1	2	3	5	6	11
B. OPERATED	9	5.2	8	1	4	5	6	11	11	11
TOTAL										
0–19 Years	97	2.3	4	1	1	2	3	5	8	12
20–34	295	2.6	3	1	1	2	3	5	6	9
35–49	526	2.6	4	1	1	2	3	5	6	12
50–64	346	2.5	5	1	1	2	3	5	6	12
65+	123	2.3	2	1	1	2	3	4	6	7
GRAND TOTAL	1,387	2.5	4	1	1	2	3	5	6	11

346.81: INTRACTABLE MIGRAINE NEC

Type of Patients	Observed Patients	Avg. Stay	Vari-ance	10th	25th	50th	75th	90th	95th	99th
1. SINGLE DX										
A. Not Operated										
0–19 Years	6	2.5	4	1	1	2	4	6	6	6
20–34	10	2.1	2	1	1	2	3	3	5	5
35–49	10	2.7	3	1	2	2	3	7	7	7
50–64	0									
65+	0									
B. Operated										
0–19 Years	0									
20–34	0									
35–49	0									
50–64	0									
65+	0									
2. MULTIPLE DX										
A. Not Operated										
0–19 Years	16	3.4	9	1	2	2	4	9	12	12
20–34	82	3.7	9	1	2	3	5	7	10	20
35–49	122	4.0	8	1	2	3	5	7	10	13
50–64	57	3.5	4	1	2	3	4	7	8	9
65+	15	3.5	10	1	2	3	4	6	14	14
B. Operated										
0–19 Years	0									
20–34	2	2.5	<1	2	2	2	3	3	3	3
35–49	1	11.0	0	11	11	11	11	11	11	11
50–64	1	8.0	0	8	8	8	8	8	8	8
65+	0									
SUBTOTALS:										
1. SINGLE DX										
A. Not Operated	26	2.4	3	1	1	2	3	5	6	7
B. Operated	0									
2. MULTIPLE DX										
A. Not Operated	292	3.7	7	1	2	3	5	7	10	13
B. Operated	4	6.0	18	2	2	6	8	11	11	11
1. SINGLE DX	26	2.4	3	1	1	2	3	5	6	7
2. MULTIPLE DX	296	3.8	8	1	2	3	5	7	10	13
A. NOT OPERATED	318	3.6	7	1	2	3	5	7	9	13
B. OPERATED	4	6.0	18	2	2	6	8	11	11	11
TOTAL										
0–19 Years	22	3.2	8	1	1	2	4	6	9	12
20–34	94	3.5	8	1	2	3	4	6	10	20
35–49	133	3.9	8	1	2	3	5	7	10	13
50–64	58	3.5	4	1	2	3	4	8	8	9
65+	15	3.5	10	1	2	3	4	6	14	14
GRAND TOTAL	322	3.7	7	1	2	3	5	7	9	13

Length of Stay by Diagnosis and Operation, Western Region, 2008

Western Region, October 2006–September 2007 Data, by Diagnosis

346.90: MIGRAINE NOS W/O INTRACT

Type of Patients	Observed Patients	Avg. Stay	Variance	Percentiles 10th	25th	50th	75th	90th	95th	99th
1. SINGLE DX										
A. Not Operated										
0–19 Years	34	1.7	<1	1	1	2	2	3	4	4
20–34	50	1.9	2	1	1	2	2	3	3	9
35–49	39	2.0	1	1	1	2	3	3	5	5
50–64	10	1.9	<1	1	1	1	3	3	3	3
65+	3	2.3	1	1	1	3	3	3	3	3
B. Operated										
0–19 Years	0									
20–34	0									
35–49	0									
50–64	0									
65+	0									
2. MULTIPLE DX										
A. Not Operated										
0–19 Years	153	2.3	3	1	1	2	3	4	5	11
20–34	490	2.6	3	1	1	2	3	4	6	9
35–49	725	2.5	3	1	1	2	3	4	6	9
50–64	492	2.5	4	1	1	2	3	5	6	9
65+	195	2.4	4	1	1	2	3	4	6	11
B. Operated										
0–19 Years	0									
20–34	2	8.5	<1	8	8	8	9	9	9	9
35–49	4	5.3	19	1	2	8	10	10	10	10
50–64	3	2.7	2	1	1	3	3	4	4	4
65+	2	2.5	4	1	1	3	4	4	4	4
SUBTOTALS:										
1. SINGLE DX										
A. Not Operated	136	1.9	1	1	1	2	2	3	3	5
B. Operated	0									
2. MULTIPLE DX										
A. Not Operated	2,055	2.5	4	1	1	2	3	5	6	9
B. Operated	11	4.6	12	1	1	4	8	9	10	10
1. SINGLE DX	136	1.9	1	1	1	2	2	3	4	5
2. MULTIPLE DX	2,066	2.5	4	1	1	2	3	5	6	9
A. NOT OPERATED	2,191	2.5	3	1	1	2	3	4	6	9
B. OPERATED	11	4.6	12	1	1	4	8	9	10	10
TOTAL										
0–19 Years	187	2.2	3	1	1	2	3	4	4	11
20–34	542	2.5	3	1	1	2	3	5	6	9
35–49	768	2.5	3	1	1	2	3	4	6	10
50–64	505	2.5	4	1	1	2	3	5	6	8
65+	200	2.4	4	1	1	2	3	4	5	11
GRAND TOTAL	2,202	2.5	4	1	1	2	3	4	6	9

346.91: INTRACTABLE MIGRAINE NOS

Type of Patients	Observed Patients	Avg. Stay	Variance	Percentiles 10th	25th	50th	75th	90th	95th	99th
1. SINGLE DX										
A. Not Operated										
0–19 Years	17	2.0	1	1	1	2	2	3	6	6
20–34	29	2.6	6	1	1	2	3	4	4	14
35–49	28	2.2	1	1	1	2	3	3	4	5
50–64	11	1.8	<1	1	1	2	2	2	3	3
65+	1	3.0	0	3	3	3	3	3	3	3
B. Operated										
0–19 Years	0									
20–34	0									
35–49	0									
50–64	0									
2. MULTIPLE DX										
A. Not Operated										
0–19 Years	52	3.2	4	1	2	3	4	6	7	9
20–34	205	3.3	4	1	2	3	4	6	8	10
35–49	286	3.6	7	1	2	3	4	7	8	14
50–64	171	3.4	6	1	2	3	4	6	7	17
65+	30	2.8	5	1	1	2	4	8	8	8
B. Operated										
0–19 Years	0									
20–34	0									
35–49	5	7.0	40	1	1	6	12	15	15	15
50–64	3	12.7	54	7	7	10	21	21	21	21
65+	0									
SUBTOTALS:										
1. SINGLE DX										
A. Not Operated	86	2.2	3	1	1	2	3	3	4	14
B. Operated	0									
2. MULTIPLE DX										
A. Not Operated	744	3.4	6	1	2	3	4	6	8	13
B. Operated	8	9.1	47	1	1	7	12	21	21	21
1. SINGLE DX	86	2.2	3	1	1	2	3	3	4	14
2. MULTIPLE DX	752	3.5	7	1	2	3	4	6	8	14
A. NOT OPERATED	830	3.3	6	1	2	3	4	6	8	13
B. OPERATED	8	9.1	47	1	1	7	12	21	21	21
TOTAL										
0–19 Years	69	2.9	4	1	1	2	4	6	7	9
20–34	234	3.2	5	1	2	3	4	6	8	11
35–49	319	3.6	7	1	2	3	4	6	9	14
50–64	185	3.4	8	1	2	3	4	6	8	18
65+	31	2.8	5	1	1	2	4	7	8	8
GRAND TOTAL	838	3.4	6	1	2	3	4	6	8	14

347: CATAPLEXY & NARCOLEPSY

Type of Patients	Observed Patients	Avg. Stay	Variance	Percentiles 10th	25th	50th	75th	90th	95th	99th
1. SINGLE DX										
A. Not Operated										
0–19 Years	1	1.0	0	1	1	1	1	1	1	1
20–34	0									
35–49	0									
50–64	0									
65+	0									
B. Operated										
0–19 Years	0									
20–34	0									
35–49	0									
50–64	0									
2. MULTIPLE DX										
A. Not Operated										
0–19 Years	1	1.0	0	1	1	1	1	1	1	1
20–34	2	4.5	<1	4	4	4	5	5	5	5
35–49	3	4.0	7	1	1	5	6	6	6	6
50–64	3	4.0	<1	3	3	3	5	5	5	5
65+	11	3.2	3	1	2	3	5	5	5	6
B. Operated										
0–19 Years	0									
20–34	0									
35–49	0									
50–64	0									
SUBTOTALS:										
1. SINGLE DX										
A. Not Operated	1	1.0	0	1	1	1	1	1	1	1
B. Operated	0									
2. MULTIPLE DX										
A. Not Operated	20	3.5	3	1	2	4	5	5	6	6
B. Operated	0									
1. SINGLE DX	1	1.0	0	1	1	1	1	1	1	1
2. MULTIPLE DX	20	3.5	3	1	2	4	5	5	6	6
A. NOT OPERATED	21	3.3	3	1	2	4	5	5	6	6
B. OPERATED	0									
TOTAL										
0–19 Years	2	1.0	0	1	1	1	1	1	1	1
20–34	2	4.5	<1	4	4	4	5	5	5	5
35–49	3	4.0	7	1	1	5	6	6	6	6
50–64	3	4.0	<1	3	3	3	5	5	5	5
65+	11	3.2	3	1	2	3	4	5	6	6
GRAND TOTAL	21	3.3	3	1	2	4	5	5	6	6

348: OTHER BRAIN CONDITIONS

Type of Patients	Observed Patients	Avg. Stay	Variance	10th	25th	50th	75th	90th	95th	99th
1. SINGLE DX										
A. Not Operated										
0–19 Years	19	2.8	19	1	1	1	2	6	20	20
20–34	13	2.7	4	1	1	2	4	5	7	7
35–49	13	1.8	<1	1	1	2	2	3	3	3
50–64	7	1.7	<1	1	1	1	3	3	3	3
65+	1	6.0	0	6	6	6	6	6	6	6
B. Operated										
0–19 Years	25	2.7	5	1	2	2	3	4	6	12
20–34	33	2.6	3	1	2	2	3	4	5	9
35–49	31	3.1	4	1	2	3	4	5	6	10
50–64	15	3.5	<1	3	3	3	4	6	6	6
65+	1	3.0	0	3	3	3	3	3	3	3
2. MULTIPLE DX										
A. Not Operated										
0–19 Years	144	4.5	38	1	1	3	5	11	15	29
20–34	302	4.8	57	1	2	3	5	8	13	42
35–49	502	5.3	28	1	2	4	7	11	15	30
50–64	983	6.0	40	1	2	4	7	12	18	31
65+	2,229	6.0	31	2	3	4	7	11	15	29
B. Operated										
0–19 Years	191	5.2	51	2	2	3	5	10	15	60
20–34	271	5.0	27	2	2	3	6	10	14	32
35–49	288	4.4	20	1	2	3	5	9	12	20
50–64	200	5.9	81	1	2	3	5	11	17	64
65+	128	10.3	107	1	3	7	15	22	29	39
SUBTOTALS:										
1. SINGLE DX										
A. Not Operated	53	2.4	8	1	1	2	3	4	6	20
B. Operated	105	2.9	3	1	2	3	4	5	6	10
2. MULTIPLE DX										
A. Not Operated	4,160	5.8	35	1	2	4	7	11	15	31
B. Operated	1,078	5.7	52	1	2	3	6	12	18	39
1. SINGLE DX	158	2.8	5	1	1	2	3	5	6	12
2. MULTIPLE DX	5,238	5.8	38	1	2	4	7	11	16	33
A. NOT OPERATED	4,213	5.7	35	1	2	4	7	11	15	30
B. OPERATED	1,183	5.4	48	1	2	3	6	11	17	39
TOTAL										
0–19 Years	379	4.6	42	1	2	3	5	10	14	55
20–34	619	4.7	41	1	2	3	5	9	13	35
35–49	834	4.9	24	1	2	3	6	10	14	28
50–64	1,205	5.9	46	1	2	4	7	12	17	33
65+	2,359	6.3	36	2	3	5	8	12	16	33
GRAND TOTAL	5,396	5.7	38	1	2	4	7	11	16	33

348.0: CEREBRAL CYSTS

Type of Patients	Observed Patients	Avg. Stay	Variance	10th	25th	50th	75th	90th	95th	99th
1. SINGLE DX										
A. Not Operated										
0–19 Years	1	1.0	0	1	1	1	1	1	1	1
20–34	2	4.0	18	1	1	2	7	7	7	7
35–49	5	1.8	1	1	1	1	3	3	3	3
50–64	0									
65+	0									
B. Operated										
0–19 Years	8	3.5	15	1	1	2	6	12	12	12
20–34	7	2.4	<1	1	2	3	3	3	3	3
35–49	7	2.6	3	1	2	2	3	6	6	6
50–64	5	3.6	<1	3	3	4	4	4	4	4
65+	0									
2. MULTIPLE DX										
A. Not Operated										
0–19 Years	11	2.2	2	1	1	2	3	4	5	5
20–34	26	1.7	2	1	1	1	2	2	6	6
35–49	22	3.7	7	1	2	3	5	7	9	10
50–64	26	4.3	26	1	2	2	4	14	18	20
65+	21	3.3	6	1	2	2	4	8	8	8
B. Operated										
0–19 Years	63	4.9	16	1	2	3	7	11	13	21
20–34	39	4.6	15	1	2	3	6	8	14	19
35–49	82	4.4	27	2	2	3	5	7	11	42
50–64	51	4.2	12	2	2	3	5	7	9	21
65+	39	5.3	21	1	2	3	7	12	14	23
SUBTOTALS:										
1. SINGLE DX										
A. Not Operated	8	2.2	4	1	1	1	3	7	7	7
B. Operated	27	3.0	5	1	2	3	3	6	6	12
2. MULTIPLE DX										
A. Not Operated	106	3.1	10	1	1	2	4	6	8	18
B. Operated	274	4.6	19	1	2	3	6	9	13	21
1. SINGLE DX	35	2.8	5	1	1	2	3	6	7	12
2. MULTIPLE DX	380	4.2	17	1	2	3	5	8	12	21
A. NOT OPERATED	114	3.1	10	1	1	2	4	6	8	18
B. OPERATED	301	4.5	18	1	2	3	6	8	12	21
TOTAL										
0–19 Years	83	4.4	15	1	2	3	4	6	9	12
20–34	74	3.4	11	1	1	2	4	6	8	19
35–49	116	4.1	21	1	2	3	5	7	11	19
50–64	82	4.2	15	1	2	3	5	7	14	21
65+	60	4.6	16	1	2	3	6	9	12	23
GRAND TOTAL	415	4.1	16	1	2	3	5	8	12	20

348.1: ANOXIC BRAIN DAMAGE

Type of Patients	Observed Patients	Avg. Stay	Variance	10th	25th	50th	75th	90th	95th	99th
1. SINGLE DX										
A. Not Operated										
0–19 Years	0									
20–34	0									
35–49	0									
50–64	0									
65+	0									
B. Operated										
0–19 Years	0									
20–34	0									
35–49	0									
50–64	0									
65+	0									
2. MULTIPLE DX										
A. Not Operated										
0–19 Years	16	11.8	172	2	4	8	15	23	55	55
20–34	30	15.8	257	2	4	8	23	42	57	58
35–49	41	12.5	100	3	6	10	17	30	35	>99
50–64	58	13.5	144	2	4	11	18	29	33	70
65+	89	11.0	126	2	3	7	14	25	32	59
B. Operated										
0–19 Years	2	46.9	127	39	39	39	55	55	55	55
20–34	5	22.2	150	20	20	20	32	35	35	35
35–49	2	12.0	125	4	4	4	20	20	20	20
50–64	4	22.0	131	14	16	16	19	39	39	39
65+	4	24.4	162	8	8	21	33	36	36	36
SUBTOTALS:										
1. SINGLE DX										
A. Not Operated	0									
B. Operated	0									
2. MULTIPLE DX										
A. Not Operated	234	12.5	146	2	4	8	17	29	37	59
B. Operated	17	24.3	194	4	16	20	35	39	55	55
1. SINGLE DX	0									
2. MULTIPLE DX	251	13.3	157	2	4	9	19	31	39	59
A. NOT OPERATED	234	12.5	146	2	4	8	17	29	37	59
B. OPERATED	17	24.3	194	4	16	20	35	39	55	55
TOTAL										
0–19 Years	18	15.7	288	2	4	8	18	55	55	55
20–34	35	16.7	242	2	4	13	26	37	57	58
35–49	43	12.5	98	3	5	10	17	30	35	>99
50–64	62	14.1	146	3	5	12	19	29	33	70
65+	93	11.6	134	2	3	8	15	27	36	59
GRAND TOTAL	251	13.3	157	2	4	9	19	31	39	59

Length of Stay by Diagnosis and Operation, Western Region, 2008

Western Region, October 2006–September 2007 Data, by Diagnosis

348.2: BENIGN INTRACRANIAL HTN

Type of Patients	Observed Patients	Avg. Stay	Vari-ance	10th	25th	50th	75th	90th	95th	99th
1. SINGLE DX										
A. Not Operated										
0–19 Years	9	2.0	3	1	1	1	2	6	6	6
20–34	5	2.6	2	1	1	3	4	4	4	4
35–49	6	1.8	<1	2	2	2	2	2	2	2
50–64	0									
65+	0									
B. Operated										
0–19 Years	0									
20–34	9	1.8	<1	1	1	2	2	3	3	3
35–49	8	2.0	2	1	1	2	2	4	4	4
50–64	0									
65+	0									
2. MULTIPLE DX										
A. Not Operated										
0–19 Years	45	3.3	8	1	1	2	4	8	10	13
20–34	119	3.4	5	1	2	3	5	7	8	11
35–49	60	3.6	7	1	2	3	4	7	11	14
50–64	21	4.0	15	1	1	3	5	7	9	18
65+	1	1.0	0	1	1	1	1	1	1	1
B. Operated										
0–19 Years	19	6.0	27	1	1	5	10	15	17	17
20–34	78	4.8	25	1	1	4	6	10	12	29
35–49	48	3.9	16	1	1	3	5	10	12	17
50–64	20	4.1	35	1	1	2	3	17	17	24
65+	1	2.0	0	2	2	2	2	2	2	2
SUBTOTALS:										
1. SINGLE DX										
A. Not Operated	20	2.1	2	1	1	2	2	4	6	6
B. Operated	17	1.9	1	1	1	2	2	4	4	4
2. MULTIPLE DX										
A. Not Operated	246	3.5	7	1	2	3	4	7	9	13
B. Operated	166	4.6	24	1	1	3	6	10	15	27
1. SINGLE DX	37	2.0	1	1	1	2	2	4	4	6
2. MULTIPLE DX	412	3.9	14	1	2	3	5	8	11	18
A. NOT OPERATED	266	3.4	7	1	2	3	4	7	9	13
B. OPERATED	183	4.3	22	1	1	2	5	10	13	27
TOTAL										
0–19 Years	73	3.8	14	1	1	2	5	10	13	17
20–34	211	3.8	13	1	2	3	5	7	10	19
35–49	122	3.5	10	1	2	2	4	9	11	16
50–64	41	4.0	24	1	2	2	5	7	17	24
65+	2	1.5	<1	1	1	2	2	2	2	2
GRAND TOTAL	449	3.7	13	1	1	3	5	8	10	18

348.30: ENCEPHALOPATHY NOS

Type of Patients	Observed Patients	Avg. Stay	Vari-ance	10th	25th	50th	75th	90th	95th	99th
1. SINGLE DX										
A. Not Operated										
0–19 Years	3	8.3	103	1	1	4	4	6	20	20
20–34	1	4.0	0	4	4	4	4	4	4	4
35–49	0									
50–64	0									
65+	1	6.0	0	6	6	6	6	6	6	6
B. Operated										
0–19 Years	0									
20–34	0									
35–49	0									
50–64	0									
65+	0									
2. MULTIPLE DX										
A. Not Operated										
0–19 Years	21	4.7	21	1	1	3	5	8	13	15
20–34	23	4.0	7	1	2	4	5	7	11	11
35–49	100	5.1	19	2	2	4	6	10	14	19
50–64	237	5.5	26	1	2	4	7	12	16	21
65+	660	5.6	23	2	3	4	7	11	14	27
B. Operated										
0–19 Years	0									
20–34	0									
35–49	4	8.5	43	2	2	5	17	17	17	17
50–64	5	22.9	>999	4	6	9	14	81	81	81
65+	13	9.7	39	4	5	7	17	18	21	21
SUBTOTALS:										
1. SINGLE DX										
A. Not Operated	5	7.0	56	1	4	4	6	20	20	20
B. Operated	0									
2. MULTIPLE DX										
A. Not Operated	1,041	5.5	23	2	3	4	7	11	14	25
B. Operated	22	12.5	266	4	5	8	17	18	21	81
1. SINGLE DX	5	7.0	56	1	4	4	6	20	20	20
2. MULTIPLE DX	1,063	5.6	29	2	3	4	7	11	15	27
A. NOT OPERATED	1,046	5.5	23	2	3	4	7	11	14	25
B. OPERATED	22	12.5	266	4	5	8	17	18	21	81
TOTAL										
0–19 Years	24	5.1	29	1	1	3	5	10	13	17
20–34	24	4.0	7	1	2	4	5	6	11	19
35–49	104	5.2	20	2	2	4	7	10	15	19
50–64	242	5.9	49	1	2	4	7	12	16	27
65+	674	5.7	23	2	3	4	7	11	14	27
GRAND TOTAL	1,068	5.7	29	2	3	4	7	11	15	27

348.31: METABOLIC ENCEPHALOPATHY

Type of Patients	Observed Patients	Avg. Stay	Vari-ance	10th	25th	50th	75th	90th	95th	99th
1. SINGLE DX										
A. Not Operated										
0–19 Years	0									
20–34	1	1.0	0	1	1	1	1	1	1	1
35–49	0									
50–64	0									
65+	0									
B. Operated										
0–19 Years	0									
20–34	0									
35–49	0									
50–64	0									
65+	0									
2. MULTIPLE DX										
A. Not Operated										
0–19 Years	4	6.3	63	1	2	4	18	18	18	18
20–34	15	3.5	4	1	2	3	5	6	8	8
35–49	84	5.9	32	1	2	5	7	11	16	33
50–64	292	5.6	18	2	3	4	8	12	13	23
65+	864	6.3	31	2	3	5	7	12	15	25
B. Operated										
0–19 Years	0									
20–34	0									
35–49	3	16.4	251	3	3	12	12	34	34	34
50–64	7	19.1	247	5	6	9	38	42	42	42
65+	28	14.8	95	3	7	12	20	29	34	39
SUBTOTALS:										
1. SINGLE DX										
A. Not Operated	1	1.0	0	1	1	1	1	1	1	1
B. Operated	0									
2. MULTIPLE DX										
A. Not Operated	1,259	6.1	28	2	3	5	7	11	14	25
B. Operated	38	15.7	126	3	7	12	22	34	39	42
1. SINGLE DX	1	1.0	0	1	1	1	1	1	1	1
2. MULTIPLE DX	1,297	6.4	33	2	3	5	8	12	16	29
A. NOT OPERATED	1,260	6.1	28	2	3	5	7	11	14	25
B. OPERATED	38	15.7	126	3	7	12	22	34	39	42
TOTAL										
0–19 Years	4	6.3	63	1	2	4	18	18	18	18
20–34	16	3.3	4	1	2	2	5	6	8	8
35–49	87	6.3	40	1	2	5	7	12	20	34
50–64	299	6.0	26	2	3	5	8	11	14	27
65+	892	6.5	36	2	3	5	8	12	16	33
GRAND TOTAL	1,298	6.3	33	2	3	5	8	12	16	29

Length of Stay by Diagnosis and Operation, Western Region, 2008

Western Region, October 2006–September 2007 Data, by Diagnosis

348.39: ENCEPHALOPATHY NEC

Type of Patients	Observed Patients	Avg. Stay	Vari-ance	10th	25th	50th	75th	90th	95th	99th
1. SINGLE DX										
A. Not Operated										
0–19 Years	2	2.0	0		2	2	2	2	2	2
20–34	1	2.0	0		2	2	2	2	2	2
35–49	0									
50–64	0									
65+	0									
B. Operated										
0–19 Years	0									
20–34	0									
35–49	0									
50–64	0									
65+	1	3.0	0	3	3	3	3	3	3	3
2. MULTIPLE DX										
A. Not Operated										
0–19 Years	24	4.0	34	1	1	3	4	6	11	29
20–34	16	7.8	260	1	2	3	6	10	68	68
35–49	78	5.0	11	1	2	4	7	10	11	15
50–64	173	6.6	52	2	3	5	8	14	19	40
65+	388	6.3	24	2	3	5	8	11	15	25
B. Operated										
0–19 Years	1	14.0	0	14	14	14	14	14	14	14
20–34	1	15.0	0	15	15	15	15	15	15	15
35–49	1	8.0	0	8	8	8	8	8	8	8
50–64	3	27.2	>999	5	5	13	64	64	64	64
65+	10	22.1	354	3	14	16	23	72	72	72
SUBTOTALS:										
1. SINGLE DX										
A. Not Operated	3	2.0	0	2	2	2	2	2	2	2
B. Operated	1	3.0	0	3	3	3	3	3	3	3
2. MULTIPLE DX										
A. Not Operated	679	6.2	36	2	3	5	8	11	15	32
B. Operated	16	21.2	375	5	13	14	20	64	72	72
1. SINGLE DX	4	2.3	<1	2	2	2	3	3	3	3
2. MULTIPLE DX	695	6.6	48	2	3	5	8	12	17	40
A. NOT OPERATED	682	6.2	36	2	3	5	8	11	15	32
B. OPERATED	17	20.1	371	3	13	14	20	64	72	72
TOTAL										
0–19 Years	27	4.2	34	1	1	2	5	11	14	29
20–34	18	7.9	235	1	2	3	6	15	68	68
35–49	79	5.1	11	1	2	4	8	10	11	15
50–64	176	7.0	70	2	3	5	8	14	20	63
65+	399	6.7	38	2	3	5	8	12	17	29
GRAND TOTAL	699	6.5	48	2	3	5	8	12	17	33

348.4: BRAIN COMPRESSION

Type of Patients	Observed Patients	Avg. Stay	Vari-ance	10th	25th	50th	75th	90th	95th	99th
1. SINGLE DX										
A. Not Operated										
0–19 Years	0									
20–34	0									
35–49	0									
50–64	0									
65+	0									
B. Operated										
0–19 Years	17	2.2	<1	1	2	2	3	4	4	4
20–34	15	2.9	1	2	2	3	4	5	5	5
35–49	15	3.5	2	2	2	3	5	5	6	6
50–64	10	3.5	1	2	3	3	4	5	6	6
65+	0									
2. MULTIPLE DX										
A. Not Operated										
0–19 Years	7	3.3	3	1	2	3	5	6	6	6
20–34	9	2.7	3	1	2	2	3	6	6	6
35–49	5	3.0	6	1	2	2	3	7	7	7
50–64	7	1.9	1	1	1	2	2	4	4	4
65+	3	3.0	3	2	2	2	5	5	5	5
B. Operated										
0–19 Years	101	4.2	39	2	2	3	4	6	7	60
20–34	130	4.4	9	2	3	3	5	9	11	14
35–49	119	3.9	7	2	2	3	4	7	9	15
50–64	78	4.1	6	2	3	3	4	8	10	15
65+	9	7.8	29	3	5	7	8	21	21	21
SUBTOTALS:										
1. SINGLE DX										
A. Not Operated	0									
B. Operated	57	3.0	2	2	2	3	4	5	5	6
2. MULTIPLE DX										
A. Not Operated	31	2.7	3	1	2	2	4	5	6	7
B. Operated	437	4.2	15	2	3	3	5	7	10	17
1. SINGLE DX	57	3.0	2	2	2	3	4	5	5	6
2. MULTIPLE DX	468	4.1	15	2	2	3	5	7	10	17
A. NOT OPERATED	31	2.7	3	1	2	3	4	5	6	7
B. OPERATED	494	4.1	14	2	2	3	4	7	9	17
TOTAL										
0–19 Years	125	3.9	33	2	2	3	4	6	7	60
20–34	154	4.2	8	2	2	3	5	8	11	14
35–49	139	3.8	6	2	2	3	4	7	9	15
50–64	95	3.9	5	2	3	3	4	7	9	15
65+	12	6.6	26	2	3	7	8	9	21	21
GRAND TOTAL	525	4.0	13	2	2	3	4	7	9	16

348.8: BRAIN CONDITIONS NEC

Type of Patients	Observed Patients	Avg. Stay	Vari-ance	10th	25th	50th	75th	90th	95th	99th
1. SINGLE DX										
A. Not Operated										
0–19 Years	0									
20–34	1	1.0	0	1	1	1	1	1	1	1
35–49	1	1.0	0	1	1	1	1	1	1	1
50–64	5	2.0	1		1	2	3		3	3
65+	0									
B. Operated										
0–19 Years	0									
20–34	1	1.0	0	1	1	1	1	1	1	1
35–49	1	10.0	0	10	10	10	10	10	10	10
50–64	0									
65+	0									
2. MULTIPLE DX										
A. Not Operated										
0–19 Years	11	2.7	5	1	1	2	4	5	8	8
20–34	49	3.6	11	1	1	2	4	9	9	16
35–49	73	4.3	13	1	2	3	6	8	10	24
50–64	99	5.0	42	1	2	3	6	11	19	27
65+	118	4.0	15	1	2	3	5	9	11	28
B. Operated										
0–19 Years	3	10.4	161	2	2	4	25	25	25	25
20–34	13	6.8	117	1	3	4	5	9	42	42
35–49	26	4.7	16	1	2	3	7	11	12	16
50–64	23	4.9	22	1	2	4	7	8	13	22
65+	17	6.5	89	1	1	3	7	20	38	38
SUBTOTALS:										
1. SINGLE DX										
A. Not Operated	7	1.7	<1	1	1	1	3	3	3	3
B. Operated	2	5.5	41	1	1	6	10	10	10	10
2. MULTIPLE DX										
A. Not Operated	350	4.2	21	1	2	3	5	9	11	27
B. Operated	82	5.7	52	1	2	4	7	11	20	42
1. SINGLE DX	9	2.6	8	1	1	1	3	10	10	10
2. MULTIPLE DX	432	4.5	27	1	2	3	6	9	12	28
A. NOT OPERATED	357	4.2	21	1	2	3	5	9	11	27
B. OPERATED	84	5.7	51	1	2	4	7	11	20	42
TOTAL										
0–19 Years	14	4.4	40	1	1	2	4	8	25	25
20–34	64	4.2	33	1	1	3	4	9	9	42
35–49	101	4.4	14	1	2	3	6	9	10	24
50–64	127	4.8	37	1	2	3	6	10	14	27
65+	135	4.3	24	1	1	3	5	9	12	38
GRAND TOTAL	441	4.5	27	1	2	3	6	9	12	28

Length of Stay by Diagnosis and Operation, Western Region, 2008

Western Region, October 2006–September 2007 Data, by Diagnosis

349: NERV SYST DISORD NEC&NOS

Type of Patients	Observed Patients	Avg. Stay	Variance	Percentiles 10th	25th	50th	75th	90th	95th	99th
1. SINGLE DX										
A. Not Operated										
0–19 Years	9	2.6	2	1	1	3	3	5	5	5
20–34	19	2.0	1	1	1	2	2	4	4	4
35–49	17	2.5	3	1	1	2	4	5	7	7
50–64	7	4.0	15	1	1	2	8	11	11	11
65+	1	3.0	0	3	3	3	3	3	3	3
B. Operated										
0–19 Years	0									
20–34	8	5.0	19	1	1	3	6	13	13	13
35–49	13	3.1	6	1	1	3	4	5	10	10
50–64	8	4.5	18	1	1	4	6	14	14	14
65+	1	2.0	0	2	2	2	2	2	2	2
2. MULTIPLE DX										
A. Not Operated										
0–19 Years	75	2.9	9	1	1	2	3	5	8	17
20–34	217	2.9	4	1	2	2	4	5	8	10
35–49	283	3.7	16	1	2	2	4	7	9	26
50–64	343	4.8	25	1	2	4	6	8	12	26
65+	640	6.1	24	2	3	5	7	11	15	27
B. Operated										
0–19 Years	19	4.0	11	1	1	4	5	9	14	14
20–34	37	6.8	28	1	3	6	11	14	18	23
35–49	88	5.2	18	2	3	4	6	10	17	22
50–64	146	5.2	38	1	2	4	5	10	15	36
65+	86	7.1	48	1	2	6	10	14	15	43
SUBTOTALS:										
1. SINGLE DX										
A. Not Operated	53	2.5	4	1	1	2	3	4	7	11
B. Operated	30	3.9	13	1	1	3	5	10	13	14
2. MULTIPLE DX										
A. Not Operated	1,558	4.8	21	1	2	4	6	9	13	25
B. Operated	376	5.7	34	1	2	4	7	12	15	36
1. SINGLE DX	83	3.0	7	1	1	2	4	6	10	14
2. MULTIPLE DX	1,934	5.0	23	1	2	4	6	10	14	25
A. NOT OPERATED	1,611	4.7	20	1	2	4	6	9	12	25
B. OPERATED	406	5.6	33	1	2	4	7	12	15	25
TOTAL										
0–19 Years	103	3.0	9	1	1	2	4	5	8	15
20–34	281	3.4	9	1	2	2	4	8	10	14
35–49	401	3.9	16	1	2	3	5	8	10	22
50–64	504	4.9	29	1	2	4	6	9	14	26
65+	728	6.2	26	2	3	5	8	12	15	28
GRAND TOTAL	2,017	4.9	23	1	2	4	6	10	14	25

349.0: LUMBAR PUNCTURE REACTION

Type of Patients	Observed Patients	Avg. Stay	Variance	Percentiles 10th	25th	50th	75th	90th	95th	99th
1. SINGLE DX										
A. Not Operated										
0–19 Years	8	2.8	2	1	2	3	4	5	5	5
20–34	19	2.0	1	1	1	2	3	4	4	4
35–49	14	2.4	3	1	1	2	3	4	7	7
50–64	6	3.4	15	1	1	2	3	11	11	11
65+	0									
B. Operated										
0–19 Years	0									
20–34	0									
35–49	0									
50–64	1	2.0	0	2	2	2	2	2	2	2
65+	0									
2. MULTIPLE DX										
A. Not Operated										
0–19 Years	53	2.6	5	1	1	2	3	4	6	15
20–34	177	2.9	3	1	2	2	4	5	6	10
35–49	163	2.9	4	1	2	2	4	5	6	10
50–64	60	3.6	9	1	2	3	4	7	8	20
65+	18	3.9	8	1	2	2	6	7	12	12
B. Operated										
0–19 Years	0									
20–34	3	7.6	26	2	2	9	12	12	12	12
35–49	6	3.3	4	2	2	2	4	7	7	7
50–64	3	4.0	12	2	2	2	8	8	8	8
65+	0									
SUBTOTALS:										
1. SINGLE DX										
A. Not Operated	47	2.4	3	1	1	2	3	4	5	11
B. Operated	1	2.0	0	2	2	2	2	2	2	2
2. MULTIPLE DX										
A. Not Operated	471	3.0	5	1	2	2	4	6	7	10
B. Operated	12	4.6	12	2	2	2	7	9	12	12
1. SINGLE DX	48	2.4	3	1	1	2	3	4	5	11
2. MULTIPLE DX	483	3.0	5	1	2	2	4	6	7	11
A. NOT OPERATED	518	3.0	5	1	2	2	4	6	7	10
B. OPERATED	13	4.4	12	2	2	2	7	9	12	12
TOTAL										
0–19 Years	61	2.6	5	1	1	2	3	5	6	15
20–34	199	2.9	4	1	2	2	4	5	6	10
35–49	183	2.9	4	1	2	2	4	5	6	10
50–64	70	3.6	9	1	2	3	4	7	9	20
65+	18	3.9	8	1	2	2	6	7	12	12
GRAND TOTAL	531	3.0	5	1	2	2	4	6	7	11

349.82: TOXIC ENCEPHALOPATHY

Type of Patients	Observed Patients	Avg. Stay	Variance	Percentiles 10th	25th	50th	75th	90th	95th	99th
1. SINGLE DX										
A. Not Operated										
0–19 Years	0									
20–34	0									
35–49	0									
50–64	0									
65+	1	3.0	0	3	3	3	3	3	3	3
B. Operated										
0–19 Years	0									
20–34	0									
35–49	0									
50–64	0									
65+	0									
2. MULTIPLE DX										
A. Not Operated										
0–19 Years	9	1.4	<1	1	1	1	2	3	3	3
20–34	29	2.6	4	1	1	2	3	5	5	10
35–49	83	5.2	43	1	3	3	6	12	18	35
50–64	243	5.1	28	1	2	4	6	9	12	26
65+	573	6.2	24	2	3	5	8	12	16	28
B. Operated										
0–19 Years	0									
20–34	0									
35–49	2	19.0	2	18	18	20	20	20	20	20
50–64	6	16.2	150	4	6	13	25	36	36	36
65+	21	11.6	52	7	8	9	13	15	16	40
SUBTOTALS:										
1. SINGLE DX										
A. Not Operated	1	3.0	0	3	3	3	3	3	3	3
B. Operated	0									
2. MULTIPLE DX										
A. Not Operated	937	5.7	27	2	3	4	7	11	15	28
B. Operated	29	13.1	70	6	8	11	15	25	36	40
1. SINGLE DX	1	3.0	0	3	3	3	3	3	3	3
2. MULTIPLE DX	966	5.9	30	2	3	4	7	11	16	30
A. NOT OPERATED	938	5.7	27	2	3	4	7	11	15	28
B. OPERATED	29	13.1	70	6	8	11	15	25	36	40
TOTAL										
0–19 Years	9	1.4	<1	1	1	1	2	3	3	3
20–34	29	2.6	4	1	1	2	3	5	5	10
35–49	85	5.5	46	1	2	3	6	14	20	35
50–64	249	5.4	34	2	2	4	6	10	15	36
65+	595	6.4	26	2	3	5	8	12	16	29
GRAND TOTAL	967	5.9	30	2	3	4	7	11	16	30

Western Region, October 2006–September 2007 Data, by Diagnosis

350: TRIGEM NERVE DISORDER

Type of Patients	Observed Patients	Avg. Stay	Vari-ance	10th	25th	50th	75th	90th	95th	99th
1. SINGLE DX										
A. *Not Operated*										
0–19 Years	0									
20–34	3	2.3		1	1	2	4	4	4	4
35–49	2	1.5	2	1	1	2	2	2	2	2
50–64	3	4.7	<1	4	4	5	5	5	5	5
65+	2	4.0	18	1	1	7	7	7	7	7
B. *Operated*										
0–19 Years	0									
20–34	3	3.3	5	2	2	2	6	6	6	6
35–49	16	3.6	3	2	2	3	4	6	8	8
50–64	41	2.4	<1	1	1	2	3	3	4	5
65+	5	1.8	<1	1	1	2	2	3	3	3
2. MULTIPLE DX										
A. *Not Operated*										
0–19 Years	1	7.0	0	7	7	7	7	7	7	7
20–34	4	3.5	6	1	1	5	6	6	6	6
35–49	46	2.9	9	1	1	2	4	9	10	13
50–64	73	3.0	10	1	1	2	4	7	8	22
65+	150	4.0	14	1	1	3	6	9	12	17
B. *Operated*										
0–19 Years	1	3.0	0	3	3	3	3	3	3	3
20–34	12	4.2	8	2	2	3	4	8	10	10
35–49	61	3.1	2	1	2	3	4	5	6	8
50–64	156	3.3	8	2	2	3	3	5	7	21
65+	136	3.4	6	2	2	3	4	6	8	12
SUBTOTALS:										
1. SINGLE DX										
A. *Not Operated*	10	3.2	4	1	1	4	5	5	7	7
B. *Operated*	65	2.7	2	1	2	2	3	4	5	8
2. MULTIPLE DX										
A. *Not Operated*	274	3.6	12	1	1	2	5	8	10	17
B. *Operated*	366	3.3	6	2	2	3	4	5	7	13
1. SINGLE DX	75	2.7	2	1	2	2	3	5	6	8
2. MULTIPLE DX	640	3.4	9	1	2	3	4	7	9	15
A. NOT OPERATED	284	3.6	12	1	1	2	5	8	10	17
B. OPERATED	431	3.2	6	2	2	3	4	5	7	12
TOTAL										
0–19 Years	2	5.0	8	3	3	7	7	7	7	7
20–34	22	3.7	6	1	2	3	5	8	8	10
35–49	125	3.1	5	1	2	3	4	6	8	10
50–64	273	3.1	7	1	2	3	3	5	7	21
65+	293	3.7	10	1	2	3	5	7	10	17
GRAND TOTAL	715	3.4	8	1	2	3	4	6	9	15

350.1: TRIGEMINAL NEURALGIA

Type of Patients	Observed Patients	Avg. Stay	Vari-ance	10th	25th	50th	75th	90th	95th	99th
1. SINGLE DX										
A. *Not Operated*										
0–19 Years	0									
20–34	2	2.5	4	1	1	2	4	4	4	4
35–49	2	1.5	<1	1	1	2	2	2	2	2
50–64	3	4.7	<1	4	4	5	5	5	5	5
65+	2	4.0	18	1	1	7	7	7	7	7
B. *Operated*										
0–19 Years	0									
20–34	3	3.3	5	2	2	2	6	6	6	6
35–49	15	3.5	3	2	2	3	4	6	8	8
50–64	41	2.4	<1	1	1	2	3	3	4	5
65+	5	1.8	<1	1	1	2	2	3	3	3
2. MULTIPLE DX										
A. *Not Operated*										
0–19 Years	1	7.0	0	7	7	7	7	7	7	7
20–34	3	3.0	7	1	1	5	6	6	6	6
35–49	35	3.0	10	1	1	2	4	9	10	13
50–64	68	3.2	11	1	1	2	4	7	8	22
65+	144	4.0	14	1	1	3	6	9	12	17
B. *Operated*										
0–19 Years	1	3.0	0	3	3	3	3	3	3	3
20–34	11	4.2	9	2	2	3	4	8	10	10
35–49	60	3.2	2	2	2	3	4	5	6	8
50–64	155	3.3	8	2	2	3	3	5	7	21
65+	134	3.4	6	2	2	3	4	6	8	12
SUBTOTALS:										
1. SINGLE DX										
A. *Not Operated*	9	3.3	5	1	1	4	5	5	7	7
B. *Operated*	64	2.6	2	1	2	2	3	4	5	8
2. MULTIPLE DX										
A. *Not Operated*	251	3.6	13	1	1	2	5	8	10	17
B. *Operated*	361	3.3	6	2	2	3	4	5	7	13
1. SINGLE DX	73	2.7	2	1	2	2	3	5	6	8
2. MULTIPLE DX	612	3.5	9	1	2	3	4	7	9	15
A. NOT OPERATED	260	3.6	12	1	1	2	5	8	10	17
B. OPERATED	425	3.2	6	2	2	3	4	5	7	12
TOTAL										
0–19 Years	2	5.0	8	3	3	7	7	7	7	7
20–34	19	3.7	7	2	2	3	5	6	8	10
35–49	112	3.1	5	1	2	3	4	6	8	10
50–64	267	3.1	8	1	2	3	3	5	7	21
65+	285	3.7	10	1	2	3	5	7	10	17
GRAND TOTAL	685	3.4	8	2	2	3	4	6	8	15

351: FACIAL NERVE DISORDERS

Type of Patients	Observed Patients	Avg. Stay	Vari-ance	10th	25th	50th	75th	90th	95th	99th
1. SINGLE DX										
A. *Not Operated*										
0–19 Years	8	1.4	<1	1	1	1	1	1	3	3
20–34	12	1.4	<1	1	1	1	2	2	3	3
35–49	12	1.3	<1	1	1	1	1	2	3	3
50–64	7	1.6	<1	1	1	1	2	3	3	3
65+	1	1.0	0	1	1	1	1	1	1	1
B. *Operated*										
0–19 Years	0									
20–34	0									
35–49	8	2.3	<1	1	2	2	3	3	3	3
50–64	6	2.7	1	1	2	3	3	4	4	4
65+	2	1.0	0	1	1	1	1	1	1	1
2. MULTIPLE DX										
A. *Not Operated*										
0–19 Years	14	1.8	1	1	1	1	2	2	4	4
20–34	78	2.3	4	1	1	2	3	5	7	9
35–49	240	2.2	5	1	1	2	2	4	5	13
50–64	314	2.1	3	1	1	2	2	4	5	10
65+	291	2.3	3	1	1	2	3	4	5	10
B. *Operated*										
0–19 Years	3	1.7	<1	1	1	2	2	2	2	2
20–34	3	2.0	1	1	1	2	2	3	3	3
35–49	22	3.6	4	1	2	2	4	6	7	9
50–64	46	2.8	2	1	2	3	3	4	6	7
65+	31	3.4	4	1	2	3	5	6	7	8
SUBTOTALS:										
1. SINGLE DX										
A. *Not Operated*	40	1.4	<1	1	1	1	2	2	3	3
B. *Operated*	16	2.3	<1	1	1	2	3	3	4	4
2. MULTIPLE DX										
A. *Not Operated*	937	2.2	4	1	1	2	3	4	5	10
B. *Operated*	105	3.1	3	1	2	3	4	6	6	8
1. SINGLE DX	56	1.6	<1	1	1	1	2	3	3	4
2. MULTIPLE DX	1,042	2.3	4	1	1	2	3	4	6	9
A. NOT OPERATED	977	2.2	3	1	1	2	3	4	5	10
B. OPERATED	121	2.9	3	1	2	3	4	5	6	8
TOTAL										
0–19 Years	25	1.6	<1	1	1	1	2	3	4	4
20–34	93	2.2	3	1	1	2	3	4	6	9
35–49	282	2.3	5	1	1	2	3	4	6	13
50–64	373	2.2	3	1	1	2	3	4	5	10
65+	325	2.4	3	1	1	2	3	5	6	9
GRAND TOTAL	1,098	2.3	3	1	1	2	3	4	6	9

Length of Stay by Diagnosis and Operation, Western Region, 2008

Western Region, October 2006–September 2007 Data, by Diagnosis

351.0: BELL'S PALSY

Type of Patients	Observed Patients	Avg. Stay	Variance	10th	25th	50th	75th	90th	95th	99th
1. SINGLE DX										
A. Not Operated										
0–19 Years	8	1.4	<1	1	1	1	1	3	3	3
20–34	12	1.4	<1	1	1	1	2	2	3	3
35–49	12	1.3	<1	1	1	1	1	2	3	3
50–64	7	1.6	<1	1	1	1	2	3	3	3
65+	1	1.0	0	1	1	1	1	1	1	1
B. Operated										
0–19 Years	0									
20–34	0									
35–49	0									
50–64	0									
65+	1	1.0	0	1	1	1	1	1	1	1
2. MULTIPLE DX										
A. Not Operated										
0–19 Years	14	1.8	1	1	1	1	2	4	4	4
20–34	70	2.1	2	1	1	1	3	4	5	8
35–49	232	2.2	5	1	1	2	2	4	5	13
50–64	304	2.0	3	1	1	2	2	4	5	9
65+	279	2.3	3	1	1	2	3	4	5	10
B. Operated										
0–19 Years	3	1.7	<1	1	1	2	2	2	2	2
20–34	2	2.5	<1	1	1	2	2	2	2	2
35–49	8	3.4	5	2	2	3	6	7	7	7
50–64	7	1.4	<1	1	1	1	2	2	2	2
65+	14	3.3	4	1	1	3	5	6	7	7
SUBTOTALS:										
1. SINGLE DX										
A. Not Operated	40	1.4	<1	1	1	1	2	2	3	3
B. Operated	1	1.0	0	1	1	1	1	1	1	1
2. MULTIPLE DX										
A. Not Operated	899	2.2	3	1	1	2	3	4	5	9
B. Operated	34	2.7	4	1	1	2	4	6	7	7
1. SINGLE DX	41	1.4	<1	1	1	1	2	2	3	3
2. MULTIPLE DX	933	2.2	3	1	1	2	3	4	5	9
A. NOT OPERATED	939	2.1	3	1	1	2	3	4	5	9
B. OPERATED	35	2.6	3	1	1	2	4	6	7	7
TOTAL										
0–19 Years	25	1.6	<1	1	1	1	2	3	4	4
20–34	84	2.0	2	1	1	1	2	4	5	8
35–49	252	2.2	5	1	1	2	2	4	6	13
50–64	318	2.0	3	1	1	2	2	4	5	9
65+	295	2.4	3	1	1	3	3	5	6	10
GRAND TOTAL	974	2.2	3	1	1	2	3	4	5	9

352: DISORDER CRAN NERVE NEC

Type of Patients	Observed Patients	Avg. Stay	Variance	10th	25th	50th	75th	90th	95th	99th
1. SINGLE DX										
A. Not Operated										
0–19 Years	0									
20–34	1	1.0	0	1	1	1	1	1	1	1
35–49	1	1.0	0	1	1	1	1	1	1	1
50–64	0									
65+	0									
B. Operated										
0–19 Years	0									
20–34	1	5.0	0	5	5	5	5	5	5	5
35–49	0									
50–64	1	4.0	0	4	4	4	4	4	4	4
65+	0									
2. MULTIPLE DX										
A. Not Operated										
0–19 Years	2	2.5	4	1	2	3	4	4	4	4
20–34	5	2.8	4	1	2	2	3	6	6	6
35–49	10	4.9	11	2	2	4	6	11	11	11
50–64	16	4.3	15	1	2	2	7	10	14	14
65+	23	5.6	19	1	3	4	7	13	14	16
B. Operated										
0–19 Years	1	4.0	0	4	4	4	4	4	4	4
20–34	2	5.5	<1	5	5	6	6	6	6	6
35–49	4	2.3	<1	1	1	2	3	3	3	3
50–64	6	9.4	82	1	4	10	11	26	26	26
65+	4	6.0	30	2	3	5	14	14	14	14
SUBTOTALS:										
1. SINGLE DX										
A. Not Operated	2	1.0	0	1	1	1	1	1	1	1
B. Operated	2	4.5	<1	4	4	5	5	5	5	5
2. MULTIPLE DX										
A. Not Operated	56	4.7	15	1	2	4	6	11	14	16
B. Operated	17	6.2	40	1	3	4	6	14	26	26
1. SINGLE DX	4	2.8	4	1	1	4	5	5	5	5
2. MULTIPLE DX	73	5.1	20	1	2	4	6	11	14	26
A. NOT OPERATED	58	4.6	15	1	2	3	6	11	14	16
B. OPERATED	19	6.0	35	1	3	4	6	14	26	26
TOTAL										
0–19 Years	3	3.0	3	1	1	2	4	4	4	4
20–34	9	3.4	4	1	2	3	5	6	6	6
35–49	15	3.9	10	1	2	3	6	10	11	11
50–64	23	5.6	34	1	2	4	8	11	14	26
65+	27	5.6	19	1	3	4	7	14	14	16
GRAND TOTAL	77	4.9	20	1	2	4	6	11	14	26

353: NERVE ROOT/PLEXUS DISORD

Type of Patients	Observed Patients	Avg. Stay	Variance	10th	25th	50th	75th	90th	95th	99th
1. SINGLE DX										
A. Not Operated										
0–19 Years	1	1.0	0	1	1	1	1	1	1	1
20–34	0									
35–49	2	1.5	<1	1	1	1	2	2	2	2
50–64	0									
65+	0									
B. Operated										
0–19 Years	10	1.0	0	1	1	1	1	1	1	1
20–34	37	1.8	2	1	1	1	2	3	3	9
35–49	41	1.9	2	1	1	1	2	3	4	7
50–64	23	1.7	1	1	1	1	2	3	4	4
65+	1	1.0	0	1	1	1	1	1	1	1
2. MULTIPLE DX										
A. Not Operated										
0–19 Years	3	3.3	2	2	2	3	5	5	5	5
20–34	14	3.1	2	2	2	3	4	4	6	6
35–49	38	3.4	7	1	1	2	5	8	9	10
50–64	48	3.9	11	1	2	3	6	8	11	15
65+	57	4.4	12	1	2	3	6	9	14	15
B. Operated										
0–19 Years	21	3.3	7	1	1	2	5	7	8	10
20–34	100	2.5	3	1	1	2	3	5	7	11
35–49	140	2.8	5	1	1	2	3	5	9	12
50–64	95	2.9	31	1	1	1	3	5	9	50
65+	13	4.7	30	1	1	2	6	9	21	21
SUBTOTALS:										
1. SINGLE DX										
A. Not Operated	3	1.3	<1	1	1	1	2	2	2	2
B. Operated	112	1.7	2	1	1	1	2	3	4	7
2. MULTIPLE DX										
A. Not Operated	160	3.9	9	1	2	3	5	8	10	15
B. Operated	369	2.8	12	1	1	2	3	5	8	14
1. SINGLE DX	115	1.7	2	1	1	1	2	3	4	7
2. MULTIPLE DX	529	3.2	12	1	1	2	4	7	9	15
A. NOT OPERATED	163	3.8	9	1	2	3	5	8	10	15
B. OPERATED	481	2.6	10	1	1	2	3	5	7	14
TOTAL										
0–19 Years	35	2.6	5	1	1	2	3	6	8	10
20–34	151	2.4	3	1	1	2	3	4	6	9
35–49	221	2.7	5	1	1	2	3	5	8	12
50–64	166	3.0	21	1	2	2	3	6	9	15
65+	71	4.4	15	2	3	3	6	9	14	21
GRAND TOTAL	644	2.9	10	1	1	2	3	6	8	14

250

Western Region, October 2006–September 2007 Data, by Diagnosis

353.0: BRACHIAL PLEXUS LESIONS

Type of Patients	Observed Patients	Avg. Stay	Variance	10th	25th	50th	75th	90th	95th	99th
1. SINGLE DX										
A. Not Operated										
0–19 Years	1	1.0	0			1			1	1
20–34	0									
35–49	1	2.0	0	2	2	2	2	2	2	2
50–64	0									
65+	0									
B. Operated										
0–19 Years	10	1.0	0	1	1	1	1	1	1	1
20–34	37	1.8	2	1	1	1	2	3	3	9
35–49	41	1.9	2	1	1	1	2	3	4	7
50–64	22	1.6	1	1	1	1	2	3	4	4
65+	1	1.0	0					1	1	1
2. MULTIPLE DX										
A. Not Operated										
0–19 Years	2	2.5	<1	2	2	2	3	3	3	3
20–34	10	3.0	6	1	2	3	4	6	6	6
35–49	24	3.1	6	1	1	2	5	5	9	10
50–64	19	3.4	9	1	1	2	4	9	11	11
65+	23	4.2	4	2	3	4	6	7	7	10
B. Operated										
0–19 Years	19	2.7	4	1	1	2	4	6	8	8
20–34	97	2.5	3	1	1	2	3	5	7	11
35–49	138	2.8	5	1	1	2	3	5	9	12
50–64	90	2.8	32	1	1	1	3	5	8	50
65+	9	3.1	8	1	2	2	5	9	9	9
SUBTOTALS:										
1. SINGLE DX										
A. Not Operated	2	1.5	<1	1	1	2	2	2	2	2
B. Operated	111	1.7	2	1	1	2	3	4	4	7
2. MULTIPLE DX										
A. Not Operated	78	3.5	6	1	2	3	4	7	9	11
B. Operated	353	2.7	11	1	1	2	3	5	8	14
1. SINGLE DX	113	1.7	2	1	1	1	2	3	4	7
2. MULTIPLE DX	431	2.9	10	1	1	2	3	5	8	12
A. NOT OPERATED	80	3.4	6	1	2	3	4	7	9	11
B. OPERATED	464	2.5	9	1	1	2	3	4	7	12
TOTAL										
0–19 Years	32	2.1	3	1	1	1	3	5	6	8
20–34	144	2.4	3	1	1	1	3	4	6	9
35–49	204	2.7	5	1	1	2	3	5	7	12
50–64	131	2.7	23	1	1	1	3	4	8	15
65+	33	3.8	6	2	2	3	5	7	9	10
GRAND TOTAL	544	2.6	9	1	1	2	3	5	7	12

354: MONONEURITIS UPPER LIMB

Type of Patients	Observed Patients	Avg. Stay	Variance	10th	25th	50th	75th	90th	95th	99th
1. SINGLE DX										
A. Not Operated										
0–19 Years	0									
20–34	1	1.0	0	1	1	1	1	1	1	1
35–49	2	2.5	4	1	1	2	4	4	4	4
50–64	2	1.0	0	1	1	1	1	1	1	1
65+	0									
B. Operated										
0–19 Years	1	1.0	0	1	1	1	1	1	1	1
20–34	5	1.2	<1	1	1	1	1	2	2	2
35–49	6	1.5	2	1	1	1	2	4	4	4
50–64	9	1.2	<1	1	1	1	2	2	2	2
65+	4	1.0	0	1	1	1	1	1	1	1
2. MULTIPLE DX										
A. Not Operated										
0–19 Years	3	4.3	12	2	1	4	8	8	8	8
20–34	14	2.1	3	1	1	2	2	5	7	7
35–49	78	2.2	3	1	1	2	2	4	6	12
50–64	128	2.4	5	1	1	2	3	5	5	10
65+	113	2.7	4	2	1	2	3	5	7	9
B. Operated										
0–19 Years	3	1.0	0	1	1	1	1	1	1	1
20–34	33	3.9	165	1	1	2	2	4	5	75
35–49	71	2.4	7	1	1	2	3	5	7	14
50–64	83	1.7	2	1	1	1	2	4	4	9
65+	53	2.0	6	1	1	2	2	4	6	17
SUBTOTALS:										
1. SINGLE DX										
A. Not Operated	5	1.6	2	1	1	2	2	4	4	4
B. Operated	25	1.2	<1	1	1	1	1	2	2	4
2. MULTIPLE DX										
A. Not Operated	336	2.4	4	1	1	2	3	5	6	10
B. Operated	243	2.3	26	1	1	2	2	4	6	14
1. SINGLE DX	30	1.3	<1	1	1	1	1	2	4	4
2. MULTIPLE DX	579	2.4	14	1	1	2	3	4	6	13
A. NOT OPERATED	341	2.4	4	1	1	2	3	5	6	10
B. OPERATED	268	2.2	24	1	1	2	2	4	5	14
TOTAL										
0–19 Years	7	2.4	7	1	1	1	4	5	6	8
20–34	53	3.1	103	1	1	1	3	4	5	75
35–49	157	2.3	5	1	1	2	2	5	6	13
50–64	222	2.1	4	1	1	1	3	4	5	10
65+	170	2.4	5	1	1	2	3	4	7	15
GRAND TOTAL	609	2.3	13	1	1	2	3	4	6	12

355: MONONEURITIS LEG & NOS

Type of Patients	Observed Patients	Avg. Stay	Variance	10th	25th	50th	75th	90th	95th	99th
1. SINGLE DX										
A. Not Operated										
0–19 Years	1	1.0	0	1	1	1	1	1	1	1
20–34	4	2.5	<1	1	1	3	3	3	3	3
35–49	2	1.0	0	1	1	1	1	1	1	1
50–64	2	1.0	0	1	1	1	1	1	1	1
65+	0									
B. Operated										
0–19 Years	1	1.0	0	1	1	1	1	1	1	1
20–34	2	1.0	0	1	1	1	1	1	1	1
35–49	8	1.3	<1	1	1	1	1	2	2	2
50–64	7	1.6	<1	1	1	1	2	3	3	3
65+	0									
2. MULTIPLE DX										
A. Not Operated										
0–19 Years	8	3.1	11	1	1	3	3	11	11	11
20–34	43	2.9	6	1	1	2	4	6	9	9
35–49	107	4.0	13	1	2	3	5	9	11	18
50–64	139	4.4	70	1	2	3	5	8	11	97
65+	240	3.9	7	1	2	3	5	8	9	13
B. Operated										
0–19 Years	0									
20–34	14	2.7	15	1	1	1	2	6	15	15
35–49	41	2.0	2	1	1	1	2	5	6	6
50–64	68	2.1	3	1	1	2	3	4	5	11
65+	55	3.7	32	1	1	3	3	8	18	27
SUBTOTALS:										
1. SINGLE DX										
A. Not Operated	9	1.7	1	1	1	1	3	3	3	3
B. Operated	18	1.3	<1	1	1	1	2	2	3	3
2. MULTIPLE DX										
A. Not Operated	537	4.0	25	1	2	3	5	8	10	15
B. Operated	178	2.6	13	1	1	1	3	6	7	26
1. SINGLE DX	27	1.4	<1	1	1	1	2	3	3	3
2. MULTIPLE DX	715	3.6	22	1	1	3	4	7	9	18
A. NOT OPERATED	546	3.9	24	1	2	3	5	8	9	15
B. OPERATED	196	2.5	12	1	1	1	3	5	6	26
TOTAL										
0–19 Years	10	2.7	9	1	1	2	3	3	11	11
20–34	63	2.8	7	1	1	2	3	6	9	15
35–49	158	3.3	10	1	1	2	4	7	9	18
50–64	216	3.6	47	1	1	2	4	7	10	15
65+	295	3.9	12	1	2	3	5	8	9	18
GRAND TOTAL	742	3.6	21	1	1	3	4	7	9	18

Length of Stay by Diagnosis and Operation, Western Region, 2008

Western Region, October 2006–September 2007 Data, by Diagnosis

355.8: MONONEURITIS LEG NOS

Type of Patients	Observed Patients	Avg. Stay	Variance	10th	25th	50th	75th	90th	95th	99th
1. SINGLE DX										
A. Not Operated										
0–19 Years	1	1.0	0	1	1		1	1	1	1
20–34	3	2.3	1	1	1		3	3	3	3
35–49	0									
50–64	1	1.0	0	1	1		1	1	1	1
65+	0									
B. Operated										
0–19 Years	0									
20–34	0									
35–49	2	1.0	0	1	1		1	1	1	1
50–64	2	1.5	<1	1	1		1	2	2	2
65+	0									
2. MULTIPLE DX										
A. Not Operated										
0–19 Years	3	2.3	1	1	1	3	3	3	3	3
20–34	22	2.9	5	1	1	2	4	6	7	9
35–49	73	4.1	12	1	2	3	6	8	11	20
50–64	83	3.6	7	1	2	3	5	8	11	>99
65+	170	3.9	6	1	2	3	5	8	9	11
B. Operated										
0–19 Years	0									
20–34	4	5.3	43	1	1	3	15	15	15	15
35–49	5	1.6	<1	1	1	1	2	3	3	3
50–64	14	2.2	2	1	1	2	4	4	5	5
65+	20	6.8	70	1	1	3	6	18	27	27
SUBTOTALS:										
1. SINGLE DX										
A. Not Operated	5	1.8	1	1	1	1	3	3	3	3
B. Operated	4	1.3	<1	1	1	1	2	2	2	2
2. MULTIPLE DX										
A. Not Operated	351	3.8	8	1	2	3	5	8	9	14
B. Operated	43	4.5	41	1	1	2	4	15	18	27
1. SINGLE DX	9	1.6	<1	1	1	1	2	3	3	3
2. MULTIPLE DX	394	3.9	11	1	2	3	5	8	9	20
A. NOT OPERATED	356	3.8	8	1	2	3	5	8	9	14
B. OPERATED	47	4.3	38	1	1	2	4	15	18	27
TOTAL										
0–19 Years	4	2.0	1	1	1	3	3	3	3	3
20–34	29	3.2	10	1	1	2	5	7	9	15
35–49	80	3.9	12	1	2	3	6	8	11	20
50–64	100	3.3	7	1	2	2	4	7	9	13
65+	190	4.2	13	1	2	3	5	8	9	26
GRAND TOTAL	403	3.8	11	1	2	3	5	8	9	18

356: HERED PERIPH NEUROPAT

Type of Patients	Observed Patients	Avg. Stay	Variance	10th	25th	50th	75th	90th	95th	99th
1. SINGLE DX										
A. Not Operated										
0–19 Years	1	3.0	0	3	3	3	3	3	3	3
20–34	0									
35–49	1	3.0	0	3	3	3	3	3	3	3
50–64	5	2.4	4	1	1	1	4	5	5	5
65+	0									
B. Operated										
0–19 Years	1	6.0	0	6	6	6	6	6	6	6
20–34	0									
35–49	0									
50–64	1	1.0	0	1	1	1	1	1	1	1
65+	0									
2. MULTIPLE DX										
A. Not Operated										
0–19 Years	5	7.0	17	2	3	9	10	11	11	11
20–34	22	5.7	67	1	2	3	5	14	16	38
35–49	54	5.7	71	1	2	3	6	8	21	57
50–64	82	4.5	10	2	2	4	6	9	10	18
65+	203	4.9	23	2	2	4	6	8	11	28
B. Operated										
0–19 Years	3	10.0	49	2	2	13	15	15	15	15
20–34	6	2.3	1	1	2	2	2	4	4	4
35–49	8	5.2	45	1	2	2	10	20	20	20
50–64	23	5.5	67	1	1	3	5	18	28	29
65+	32	2.8	14	1	1	1	3	8	12	17
SUBTOTALS:										
1. SINGLE DX										
A. Not Operated	7	2.6	3	1	1	3	4	5	5	5
B. Operated	2	3.5	12	1	1	1	6	6	6	6
2. MULTIPLE DX										
A. Not Operated	366	5.0	30	2	2	4	6	9	12	30
B. Operated	72	4.2	36	1	1	2	4	12	18	29
1. SINGLE DX	9	2.8	4	1	1	3	4	6	6	6
2. MULTIPLE DX	438	4.9	31	2	2	3	5	9	14	29
A. NOT OPERATED	373	4.9	29	2	2	4	6	9	12	30
B. OPERATED	74	4.2	35	1	1	2	4	12	18	27
TOTAL										
0–19 Years	10	7.4	23	2	3	6	11	13	15	15
20–34	28	5.0	54	1	2	3	5	14	16	38
35–49	63	5.6	66	1	2	3	6	10	20	57
50–64	111	4.6	21	1	2	3	5	7	9	28
65+	235	4.6	22	1	2	3	5	8	12	28
GRAND TOTAL	447	4.8	30	1	2	3	5	9	14	29

356.9: IDIO PERIPH NEUROPAT NOS

Type of Patients	Observed Patients	Avg. Stay	Variance	10th	25th	50th	75th	90th	95th	99th
1. SINGLE DX										
A. Not Operated										
0–19 Years	0									
20–34	0									
35–49	1	3.0	0	3	3	3	3	3	3	3
50–64	4	1.8	2	1	1	1	1	4	4	4
65+	0									
B. Operated										
0–19 Years	0									
20–34	0									
35–49	0									
50–64	1	1.0	0	1	1	1	1	1	1	1
65+	0									
2. MULTIPLE DX										
A. Not Operated										
0–19 Years	1	10.0	0	10	10	10	10	10	10	10
20–34	15	6.6	96	1	1	3	5	16	38	38
35–49	40	4.0	12	1	2	3	5	8	12	19
50–64	62	4.6	12	2	2	3	7	9	11	18
65+	160	4.7	24	1	2	3	5	9	11	30
B. Operated										
0–19 Years	1	13.0	0	13	13	13	13	13	13	13
20–34	1	4.0	0	4	4	4	4	4	4	4
35–49	2	11.1	160	2	2	20	20	20	20	20
50–64	8	9.6	143	1	1	5	9	29	29	29
65+	4	7.5	17	4	4	10	10	12	12	12
SUBTOTALS:										
1. SINGLE DX										
A. Not Operated	5	2.0	2	1	1	1	3	4	4	4
B. Operated	1	1.0	0	1	1	1	1	1	1	1
2. MULTIPLE DX										
A. Not Operated	278	4.7	23	1	2	3	5	9	12	30
B. Operated	16	9.1	85	1	3	5	13	28	29	29
1. SINGLE DX	6	1.8	2	1	1	1	3	4	4	4
2. MULTIPLE DX	294	4.9	27	1	2	3	6	9	14	30
A. NOT OPERATED	283	4.6	23	1	2	3	5	9	12	30
B. OPERATED	17	8.7	84	1	2	4	12	28	29	29
TOTAL										
0–19 Years	2	11.5	4	10	10	13	13	13	13	13
20–34	16	6.4	90	1	2	3	5	16	38	38
35–49	43	4.3	17	1	2	3	5	8	12	20
50–64	75	5.0	27	1	2	3	7	9	14	29
65+	164	4.8	23	1	2	3	5	9	11	30
GRAND TOTAL	300	4.9	27	1	2	3	6	9	14	30

Length of Stay by Diagnosis and Operation, Western Region, 2008

Western Region, October 2006–September 2007 Data, by Diagnosis

357: INFLAM/TOXIC NEUROPATHY

Type of Patients	Observed Patients	Avg. Stay	Variance	10th	25th	50th	75th	90th	95th	99th
1. SINGLE DX										
A. Not Operated										
0–19 Years	25	3.7	7	2	2	3	4	7	7	14
20–34	19	4.9	4	2	3	5	6	8	9	9
35–49	20	5.6	11	3	4	5	7	9	11	16
50–64	37	1.7	3	1	1	1	1	4	5	10
65+	1	3.0	0	3	3	3	3	3	3	3
B. Operated										
0–19 Years	0									
20–34	0									
35–49	0									
50–64	0									
65+	0									
2. MULTIPLE DX										
A. Not Operated										
0–19 Years	58	8.3	57	2	4	6	10	18	24	46
20–34	139	8.5	45	3	5	6	10	19	22	36
35–49	238	9.1	106	2	4	6	10	18	28	49
50–64	416	8.4	89	2	3	6	9	19	25	64
65+	412	7.7	54	2	3	6	10	15	20	39
B. Operated										
0–19 Years	2	36.3	>999	6	6	6	67	67	67	67
20–34	7	22.9	634	6	6	13	28	78	78	78
35–49	9	14.6	157	2	4	15	31	34	>99	>99
50–64	18	23.8	690	2	6	12	39	69	94	94
65+	18	24.1	384	4	8	18	40	58	68	68
SUBTOTALS:										
1. SINGLE DX										
A. Not Operated	102	3.6	8	1	1	3	5	7	9	14
B. Operated	0									
2. MULTIPLE DX										
A. Not Operated	1,263	8.3	75	2	4	6	10	17	23	48
B. Operated	54	22.7	495	3	6	15	34	67	78	>99
1. SINGLE DX	102	3.6	8	1	1	3	5	7	9	14
2. MULTIPLE DX	1,317	8.9	100	2	4	6	10	18	27	58
A. NOT OPERATED	1,365	7.9	71	2	3	6	9	16	23	48
B. OPERATED	54	22.7	495	3	6	15	34	67	78	>99
TOTAL										
0–19 Years	85	7.6	88	2	3	5	8	14	22	67
20–34	165	8.7	72	3	5	6	9	17	22	37
35–49	267	9.0	102	2	4	6	10	20	31	52
50–64	471	8.4	117	1	3	5	9	19	26	69
65+	431	8.3	78	2	3	6	10	17	24	50
GRAND TOTAL	1,419	8.5	95	2	3	6	10	18	25	58

357.0: AC INFECT POLYNEURITIS

Type of Patients	Observed Patients	Avg. Stay	Variance	10th	25th	50th	75th	90th	95th	99th
1. SINGLE DX										
A. Not Operated										
0–19 Years	18	4.2	9	1	2	3	6	7	14	14
20–34	18	5.1	4	3	4	5	6	8	9	9
35–49	17	5.7	12	2	4	5	6	11	16	16
50–64	5	5.2	8	3	3	5	5	10	10	10
65+	0									
B. Operated										
0–19 Years	0									
20–34	0									
35–49	0									
50–64	0									
65+	0									
2. MULTIPLE DX										
A. Not Operated										
0–19 Years	52	8.8	61	3	4	7	10	18	24	46
20–34	109	8.9	45	4	5	7	10	19	22	36
35–49	155	10.4	114	3	5	7	12	21	31	48
50–64	237	10.7	126	3	5	7	12	23	30	74
65+	176	10.2	82	3	5	8	12	18	25	58
B. Operated										
0–19 Years	2	36.3	>999	6	6	6	67	67	67	67
20–34	3	32.2	>999	6	6	13	78	78	78	78
35–49	3	22.4	103	15	18	18	34	>99	>99	>99
50–64	7	36.8	>999	8	10	16	69	94	>99	>99
65+	10	33.5	450	3	18	31	45	63	68	68
SUBTOTALS:										
1. SINGLE DX										
A. Not Operated	58	5.0	8	2	3	5	6	8	11	16
B. Operated	0									
2. MULTIPLE DX										
A. Not Operated	729	10.1	96	3	5	7	12	21	28	58
B. Operated	25	33.2	692	6	13	26	58	78	94	>99
1. SINGLE DX	58	5.0	8	2	3	5	6	8	11	16
2. MULTIPLE DX	754	10.9	132	3	5	7	12	22	31	69
A. NOT OPERATED	787	9.7	91	3	5	7	11	20	26	58
B. OPERATED	25	33.2	692	6	13	26	58	78	94	>99
TOTAL										
0–19 Years	72	8.4	99	2	3	6	9	14	24	67
20–34	130	8.9	76	3	5	6	10	15	22	37
35–49	175	10.2	108	3	5	7	12	21	31	95
50–64	249	11.3	167	3	5	7	12	25	31	87
65+	186	11.4	127	3	5	8	13	24	39	61
GRAND TOTAL	812	10.5	125	3	5	7	12	21	30	68

357.81: CHR INFL DEMYEL POLYNEUR

Type of Patients	Observed Patients	Avg. Stay	Variance	10th	25th	50th	75th	90th	95th	99th
1. SINGLE DX										
A. Not Operated										
0–19 Years	7	2.4	<1	2	2	2	3	3	3	3
20–34	0									
35–49	2	3.5	<1	3	3	4	4	4	4	4
50–64	30	1.1	<1	1	1	1	1	1	2	2
65+	1	3.0	0	3	3	3	3	3	3	3
B. Operated										
0–19 Years	0									
20–34	0									
35–49	0									
50–64	0									
65+	0									
2. MULTIPLE DX										
A. Not Operated										
0–19 Years	5	3.0	<1	2	3	3	3	4	4	4
20–34	11	6.2	27	3	3	5	6	9	21	21
35–49	45	7.9	130	1	2	5	7	13	37	52
50–64	93	5.2	30	2	2	3	6	12	19	32
65+	134	5.3	17	2	2	5	7	11	13	18
B. Operated										
0–19 Years	0									
20–34	2	9.5	24	6	6	13	13	13	13	13
35–49	4	14.7	198	2	2	4	22	31	31	31
50–64	8	14.4	302	2	2	8	30	51	51	51
65+	3	17.3	130	6	6	17	29	29	29	29
SUBTOTALS:										
1. SINGLE DX										
A. Not Operated	40	1.5	<1	1	1	2	2	3	3	4
B. Operated	0									
2. MULTIPLE DX										
A. Not Operated	288	5.7	39	2	2	4	7	11	18	37
B. Operated	17	14.4	192	2	4	8	22	31	51	51
1. SINGLE DX	40	1.5	<1	1	1	1	2	3	3	4
2. MULTIPLE DX	305	6.2	51	2	2	4	7	12	19	37
A. NOT OPERATED	328	5.2	37	1	2	3	6	10	14	32
B. OPERATED	17	14.4	192	2	4	8	22	31	51	51
TOTAL										
0–19 Years	12	2.7	<1	2	2	3	3	3	4	4
20–34	13	6.7	26	3	4	5	6	13	21	21
35–49	51	8.3	130	1	2	5	8	22	37	52
50–64	131	4.9	46	1	1	2	5	11	19	32
65+	138	5.6	22	2	2	5	7	11	14	28
GRAND TOTAL	345	5.6	48	1	2	4	6	12	19	37

Length of Stay by Diagnosis and Operation, Western Region, 2008

Western Region, October 2006–September 2007 Data, by Diagnosis

358: MYONEURAL DISORDERS

Type of Patients	Observed Patients	Avg. Stay	Vari-ance	10th	25th	50th	75th	90th	95th	99th
1. SINGLE DX										
A. Not Operated										
0–19 Years	8	3.8	4	1	2	3	6	7	7	7
20–34	10	3.4	9	1	2	3	5	11	11	11
35–49	4	3.3	5	1	1	4	6	6	6	6
50–64	5	3.4	11	1	1	3	3	9	9	9
65+	5	4.6	4	2	3	5	6	7	7	7
B. Operated										
0–19 Years	3	2.7	4	1	1	2	5	5	5	5
20–34	3	3.0	4	1	1	3	5	5	5	5
35–49	3	3.0	<1	2	2	3	4	4	4	4
50–64	2	4.0	0	4	4	4	4	4	4	4
65+	0									
2. MULTIPLE DX										
A. Not Operated										
0–19 Years	17	10.3	426	1	2	5	8	13	89	89
20–34	84	4.7	14	1	2	3	6	10	11	21
35–49	139	7.0	84	2	3	5	8	14	19	28
50–64	194	6.3	34	2	3	5	8	13	16	33
65+	273	7.2	59	2	3	5	9	14	21	36
B. Operated										
0–19 Years	14	8.9	175	3	3	4	9	11	54	54
20–34	31	5.4	22	2	3	4	6	11	15	23
35–49	32	5.8	25	2	2	3	8	15	18	19
50–64	29	9.4	93	2	3	5	12	25	32	39
65+	16	17.2	260	3	5	9	33	43	49	49
SUBTOTALS:										
1. SINGLE DX										
A. Not Operated	32	3.7	6	1	2	3	5	7	7	11
B. Operated	11	3.1	2	1	2	3	4	5	5	5
2. MULTIPLE DX										
A. Not Operated	707	6.7	61	2	3	5	8	13	18	33
B. Operated	122	8.4	99	2	3	4	9	19	32	49
1. SINGLE DX	43	3.5	5	1	2	3	5	6	7	11
2. MULTIPLE DX	829	6.9	67	2	3	5	8	14	19	40
A. NOT OPERATED	739	6.5	59	2	3	5	8	13	18	33
B. OPERATED	133	8.0	93	2	3	4	9	18	32	49
TOTAL										
0–19 Years	42	8.0	231	1	3	4	7	11	13	89
20–34	128	4.7	15	1	2	3	6	10	11	21
35–49	178	6.6	70	2	3	4	8	14	18	28
50–64	230	6.6	42	2	3	5	8	14	19	33
65+	294	7.7	74	2	3	5	9	16	25	43
GRAND TOTAL	872	6.8	64	2	3	5	8	13	19	40

358.00: MG W/O EXACERBATION

Type of Patients	Observed Patients	Avg. Stay	Vari-ance	10th	25th	50th	75th	90th	95th	99th
1. SINGLE DX										
A. Not Operated										
0–19 Years	8	3.8	4	1	2	3	6	7	7	7
20–34	6	3.0	3	1	2	2	5	5	5	5
35–49	0									
50–64	3	1.7	1	1	1	1	3	3	3	3
65+	2	4.0	8	2	2	4	6	6	6	6
B. Operated										
0–19 Years	3	2.7	4	1	1	2	5	5	5	5
20–34	3	3.0	4	1	1	2	5	5	5	5
35–49	3	3.0	<1	2	2	3	4	4	4	4
50–64	2	4.0	0	4	4	4	4	4	4	4
65+	0									
2. MULTIPLE DX										
A. Not Operated										
0–19 Years	4	3.5	11	1	1	2	4	8	8	8
20–34	16	3.8	10	1	2	2	4	8	11	11
35–49	27	6.6	38	1	2	4	10	19	20	22
50–64	56	5.5	44	2	2	3	6	11	16	46
65+	91	6.1	23	2	3	4	9	13	17	22
B. Operated										
0–19 Years	7	5.0	10	3	3	3	9	10	10	10
20–34	27	4.0	5	2	3	3	5	7	8	11
35–49	24	4.9	24	2	2	3	4	15	16	19
50–64	20	7.0	53	2	3	3	6	23	25	25
65+	6	3.8	2	2	3	3	5	6	6	6
SUBTOTALS:										
1. SINGLE DX										
A. Not Operated	19	3.2	4	1	2	3	5	6	7	7
B. Operated	11	3.1	2	1	2	3	4	5	5	5
2. MULTIPLE DX										
A. Not Operated	194	5.7	30	1	2	4	8	13	17	33
B. Operated	84	5.0	23	2	3	3	5	10	16	25
1. SINGLE DX	30	3.2	3	1	2	3	5	6	6	7
2. MULTIPLE DX	278	5.5	28	2	2	4	7	12	17	23
A. NOT OPERATED	213	5.5	28	1	2	4	7	11	16	22
B. OPERATED	95	4.8	21	2	3	3	5	10	16	25
TOTAL										
0–19 Years	22	3.9	7	1	2	3	5	8	9	10
20–34	52	3.8	6	1	2	3	5	8	8	11
35–49	54	5.6	30	2	3	3	7	15	19	22
50–64	81	5.7	44	2	3	3	8	14	18	46
65+	99	5.9	22	2	3	4	8	13	17	22
GRAND TOTAL	308	5.3	26	2	2	3	6	11	16	22

358.01: MG W EXACERBATION

Type of Patients	Observed Patients	Avg. Stay	Vari-ance	10th	25th	50th	75th	90th	95th	99th
1. SINGLE DX										
A. Not Operated										
0–19 Years	0									
20–34	4	4.0	23	1	1	3	11	11	11	11
35–49	4	3.3	5	1	1	4	6	6	6	6
50–64	2	6.0	18	3	3	3	9	9	9	9
65+	3	5.0	4	3	3	5	7	7	7	7
B. Operated										
0–19 Years	0									
20–34	0									
35–49	0									
50–64	0									
65+	0									
2. MULTIPLE DX										
A. Not Operated										
0–19 Years	10	5.4	14	2	2	5	7	11	12	12
20–34	67	5.0	15	1	2	4	6	10	11	21
35–49	110	7.1	97	2	3	5	8	13	14	28
50–64	127	6.7	31	2	3	5	8	13	16	27
65+	171	7.9	80	2	3	5	9	17	27	43
B. Operated										
0–19 Years	0									
20–34	4	15.0	35	9	9	15	23	23	23	23
35–49	8	8.4	22	2	6	8	10	18	18	18
50–64	7	11.5	93	4	5	9	12	32	32	32
65+	9	27.0	236	9	14	30	40	49	49	49
SUBTOTALS:										
1. SINGLE DX										
A. Not Operated	13	4.3	10	1	2	3	6	9	11	11
B. Operated	0									
2. MULTIPLE DX										
A. Not Operated	485	6.9	61	2	3	5	8	13	19	33
B. Operated	28	16.1	164	5	8	12	23	40	43	49
1. SINGLE DX	13	4.3	10	1	2	3	6	9	11	11
2. MULTIPLE DX	513	7.4	71	2	3	5	9	14	21	40
A. NOT OPERATED	498	6.9	60	2	3	5	8	13	19	33
B. OPERATED	28	16.1	164	5	8	12	23	40	43	49
TOTAL										
0–19 Years	10	5.4	14	2	2	5	7	11	12	12
20–34	75	5.4	21	1	2	4	7	11	15	23
35–49	122	7.1	89	2	3	5	9	13	14	28
50–64	136	6.9	34	2	3	5	9	13	20	32
65+	183	8.8	103	2	3	5	10	19	30	49
GRAND TOTAL	526	7.4	70	2	3	5	9	14	21	40

Length of Stay by Diagnosis and Operation, Western Region 2008

359: MUSCULAR DYSTROPHIES

Type of Patients	Observed Patients	Avg. Stay	Vari-ance	Percentiles						
				10th	25th	50th	75th	90th	95th	99th
1. SINGLE DX										
A. *Not Operated*										
0–19 Years	4	2.0	-1	1	1	1	3	3	3	3
20–34	0									
35–49	2	2.0	2	1	1	1	3	3	3	3
50–64	0									
65+	0									
B. *Operated*										
0–19 Years	0									
20–34	0									
35–49	1	3.0	0	3	3	3	3	3	3	3
50–64	0									
65+	0									
2. MULTIPLE DX										
A. *Not Operated*										
0–19 Years	26	6.7	195	1	1	3	5	10	26	70
20–34	64	3.4	11	1	1	2	4	6	9	21
35–49	71	4.8	72	1	1	3	5	8	14	70
50–64	84	5.6	34	1	2	4	7	14	17	32
65+	185	5.4	21	2	3	4	6	11	12	26
B. *Operated*										
0–19 Years	18	7.3	66	1	4	6	7	11	38	38
20–34	5	13.1	188	1	4	5	25	31	31	31
35–49	7	12.6	88	4	5	7	20	28	28	28
50–64	12	10.0	64	3	4	6	17	20	27	27
65+	18	7.3	13	2	5	7	9	13	15	15
SUBTOTALS:										
1. SINGLE DX										
A. *Not Operated*	6	2.0	1	1	1	1	3	3	3	3
B. *Operated*	1	3.0	0	3	3	3	3	3	3	3
2. MULTIPLE DX										
A. *Not Operated*	430	5.1	41	1	2	4	6	10	14	26
B. *Operated*	60	8.9	61	2	4	6	11	20	28	38
1. SINGLE DX	7	2.1	1	1	1	3	3	3	3	3
2. MULTIPLE DX	490	5.6	45	1	2	4	6	11	16	32
A. NOT OPERATED	436	5.1	41	1	2	4	6	9	14	26
B. OPERATED	61	8.8	61	3	4	6	10	20	27	38
TOTAL										
0–19 Years	48	6.6	129	1	1	4	6	10	26	70
20–34	69	4.1	28	1	1	3	4	8	13	31
35–49	81	5.4	75	1	1	3	5	9	15	70
50–64	96	6.2	39	1	2	4	7	15	20	32
65+	203	5.5	20	2	3	4	7	11	13	23
GRAND TOTAL	497	5.5	45	1	2	4	6	11	16	32

359.4: TOXIC MYOPATHY

Type of Patients	Observed Patients	Avg. Stay	Vari-ance	Percentiles						
				10th	25th	50th	75th	90th	95th	99th
1. SINGLE DX										
A. *Not Operated*										
0–19 Years	0									
20–34	0									
35–49	0									
50–64	0									
65+	0									
B. *Operated*										
0–19 Years	0									
20–34	0									
35–49	0									
50–64	0									
65+	0									
2. MULTIPLE DX										
A. *Not Operated*										
0–19 Years	1	9.0	0	9	9	9	9	9	9	9
20–34	1	3.0	0	3	3	3	3	3	3	3
35–49	16	3.8	5	1	2	4	5	7	8	8
50–64	42	5.8	31	1	2	4	7	14	15	24
65+	123	5.0	16	2	3	4	6	9	12	22
B. *Operated*										
0–19 Years	0									
20–34	0									
35–49	0									
50–64	0									
65+	4	9.5	19	6	6	11	15	15	15	15
SUBTOTALS:										
1. SINGLE DX										
A. *Not Operated*	0									
B. *Operated*	0									
2. MULTIPLE DX										
A. *Not Operated*	183	5.1	19	2	3	4	6	9	14	23
B. *Operated*	4	9.5	19	6	6	11	15	15	15	15
1. SINGLE DX	0									
2. MULTIPLE DX	187	5.1	19	2	3	4	7	9	15	23
A. NOT OPERATED	183	5.1	19	2	3	4	6	9	14	23
B. OPERATED	4	9.5	19	6	6	11	15	15	15	15
TOTAL										
0–19 Years	1	9.0	0	9	9	9	9	9	9	9
20–34	1	3.0	0	3	3	3	3	3	3	3
35–49	16	3.8	5	1	2	4	5	7	8	8
50–64	42	5.8	31	1	2	4	7	14	15	24
65+	127	5.1	17	2	3	4	6	9	12	22
GRAND TOTAL	187	5.1	19	2	3	4	7	9	15	23

360: DISORDERS OF THE GLOBE

Type of Patients	Observed Patients	Avg. Stay	Vari-ance	Percentiles						
				10th	25th	50th	75th	90th	95th	99th
1. SINGLE DX										
A. *Not Operated*										
0–19 Years	3	1.7	<1	1	1	2	2	2	2	2
20–34	1	4.0	0	4	4	4	4	4	4	4
35–49	0									
50–64	0									
65+	0									
B. *Operated*										
0–19 Years	0									
20–34	2	2.5	4	1	1	4	4	4	4	4
35–49	0									
50–64	0									
65+	4	3.2	2	2	2	2	4	5	5	5
2. MULTIPLE DX										
A. *Not Operated*										
0–19 Years	7	4.4	7	2	2	4	7	8	8	8
20–34	7	3.4	12	1	1	2	6	10	10	10
35–49	10	3.9	9	1	1	3	5	11	11	11
50–64	22	6.0	43	2	3	4	6	13	13	32
65+	23	5.2	13	1	2	5	8	9	9	17
B. *Operated*										
0–19 Years	10	3.8	18	1	1	2	4	8	14	14
20–34	7	7.3	43	1	2	6	13	19	19	19
35–49	16	3.5	16	1	1	1	4	9	15	15
50–64	15	6.0	27	2	3	4	7	11	22	22
65+	43	3.8	9	1	1	3	6	7	10	14
SUBTOTALS:										
1. SINGLE DX										
A. *Not Operated*	4	2.3	2	1	1	2	4	4	4	4
B. *Operated*	6	3.0	2	1	2	2	4	5	5	5
2. MULTIPLE DX										
A. *Not Operated*	69	5.0	21	1	2	4	6	9	13	32
B. *Operated*	91	4.4	17	1	1	3	6	9	14	22
1. SINGLE DX	10	2.7	2	1	2	2	4	4	5	5
2. MULTIPLE DX	160	4.7	19	1	2	4	6	9	13	22
A. NOT OPERATED	73	4.8	21	1	2	4	6	9	13	32
B. OPERATED	97	4.3	17	1	1	3	6	9	14	22
TOTAL										
0–19 Years	20	3.7	11	1	2	2	4	8	8	14
20–34	17	5.0	25	1	1	3	6	13	19	19
35–49	26	3.7	13	1	1	3	5	7	11	15
50–64	37	6.0	36	2	3	4	7	13	22	32
65+	70	4.2	10	1	2	3	6	8	10	17
GRAND TOTAL	170	4.5	18	1	2	3	6	9	13	22

Length of Stay by Diagnosis and Operation, Western Region, 2008

Western Region, October 2006–September 2007 Data, by Diagnosis

361: RETINAL DETACHMENT

Type of Patients	Observed Patients	Avg. Stay	Variance	10th	25th	50th	75th	90th	95th	99th
1. SINGLE DX										
A. Not Operated										
0–19 Years	0									
20–34	0									
35–49	0									
50–64	0									
65+	0									
B. Operated										
0–19 Years	3	1.3	<1	1	1	1	2	2	2	2
20–34	9	1.7	<1	1	1	1	2	2	3	3
35–49	17	1.6	1	1	1	1	2	3	3	5
50–64	42	1.1	<1	1	1	1	1	1	2	4
65+	6	1.0	0	1	1	1	1	1	1	1
2. MULTIPLE DX										
A. Not Operated										
0–19 Years	0									
20–34	0									
35–49	2	1.0	0	1	1	1	1	1	1	1
50–64	15	2.2	4	1	1	1	3	7	7	7
65+	6	2.5	1	2	2	3	3	4	4	4
B. Operated										
0–19 Years	11	7.3	296	1	1	2	4	5	59	59
20–34	17	1.8	1	1	1	1	2	4	5	5
35–49	32	1.7	2	1	1	1	2	3	4	7
50–64	123	1.7	2	1	1	1	2	3	5	8
65+	62	1.5	<1	1	1	1	2	2	3	5
SUBTOTALS:										
1. SINGLE DX — A. Not Operated	0									
1. SINGLE DX — B. Operated	77	1.3	<1	1	1	1	2	2	4	4
2. MULTIPLE DX — A. Not Operated	23	2.2	3	1	1	1	3	4	7	7
2. MULTIPLE DX — B. Operated	245	1.9	15	1	1	1	2	3	5	8
1. SINGLE DX	77	1.3	<1	1	1	1	2	2	4	4
2. MULTIPLE DX	268	1.9	14	1	1	1	2	3	5	8
A. NOT OPERATED	23	2.2	3	1	1	1	3	4	7	7
B. OPERATED	322	1.7	12	1	1	1	2	3	4	7
TOTAL										
0–19 Years	14	6.0	234	1	1	1	3	5	59	59
20–34	26	1.8	1	1	1	1	2	3	4	5
35–49	51	1.6	1	1	1	1	2	3	4	7
50–64	180	1.6	2	1	1	1	2	3	4	8
65+	74	1.5	<1	1	1	1	2	3	4	5
GRAND TOTAL	345	1.8	11	1	1	1	2	3	4	7

362: RETINAL DISORDERS NEC

Type of Patients	Observed Patients	Avg. Stay	Variance	10th	25th	50th	75th	90th	95th	99th
1. SINGLE DX										
A. Not Operated										
0–19 Years	9	1.5	1	1	1	1	1	4	4	4
20–34	2	1.5	<1	1	1	1	2	2	2	2
35–49	0									
50–64	2	3.5	<1	3	3	4	4	4	4	4
65+	0									
B. Operated										
0–19 Years	6	1.0	0	1	1	1	1	1	1	1
20–34	0									
35–49	2	3.5	12	1	1	4	6	6	6	6
50–64	1	1.0	0	1	1	1	1	1	1	1
65+	2	1.0	0	1	1	1	1	1	1	1
2. MULTIPLE DX										
A. Not Operated										
0–19 Years	25	5.1	89	1	1	2	4	14	22	44
20–34	11	4.5	25	1	2	3	4	6	19	19
35–49	30	2.7	4	1	1	2	4	5	6	10
50–64	84	2.7	7	1	1	2	3	5	7	16
65+	140	2.5	3	1	1	2	3	5	6	7
B. Operated										
0–19 Years	19	2.7	10	1	1	1	3	11	11	11
20–34	2	4.5	5	3	3	5	6	6	6	6
35–49	4	1.0	0	1	1	1	1	1	1	1
50–64	11	2.4	9	1	1	1	2	3	11	11
65+	26	2.2	5	1	1	1	2	5	7	10
SUBTOTALS:										
1. SINGLE DX — A. Not Operated	13	1.8	1	1	1	1	2	4	4	4
1. SINGLE DX — B. Operated	11	1.5	2	1	1	1	1	1	6	6
2. MULTIPLE DX — A. Not Operated	290	2.9	12	1	1	2	3	5	7	19
2. MULTIPLE DX — B. Operated	62	2.4	7	1	1	1	2	5	10	11
1. SINGLE DX	24	1.6	2	1	1	1	1	4	4	6
2. MULTIPLE DX	352	2.8	11	1	1	2	3	5	7	16
A. NOT OPERATED	303	2.8	12	1	1	2	3	5	6	16
B. OPERATED	73	2.3	6	1	1	1	2	5	10	11
TOTAL										
0–19 Years	59	3.4	43	1	1	1	3	8	14	44
20–34	15	4.1	20	1	2	3	4	6	19	19
35–49	36	2.6	4	1	1	2	4	6	6	10
50–64	98	2.6	7	1	1	2	3	5	8	16
65+	168	2.5	3	1	1	2	3	5	6	9
GRAND TOTAL	376	2.7	11	1	1	2	3	5	7	16

363: CHOROIDAL DISORDERS

Type of Patients	Observed Patients	Avg. Stay	Variance	10th	25th	50th	75th	90th	95th	99th
1. SINGLE DX										
A. Not Operated										
0–19 Years	0									
20–34	0									
35–49	0									
50–64	0									
65+	0									
B. Operated										
0–19 Years	1	4.0	0	4	4	4	4	4	4	4
20–34	0									
35–49	1	1.0	0	1	1	1	1	1	1	1
50–64	0									
65+	0									
2. MULTIPLE DX										
A. Not Operated										
0–19 Years	1	3.0	0	3	3	3	3	3	3	3
20–34	2	4.5	<1	4	4	5	5	5	5	5
35–49	2	4.5	24	1	1	1	4	8	8	8
50–64	2	4.5	4	3	3	6	6	6	6	6
65+	3	4.3	1	3	3	5	5	5	5	5
B. Operated										
0–19 Years	0									
20–34	2	11.5	59	6	6	12	17	17	17	17
35–49	0									
50–64	0									
65+	7	2.9	3	1	1	3	3	6	6	6
SUBTOTALS:										
1. SINGLE DX — A. Not Operated	0									
1. SINGLE DX — B. Operated	2	2.5	4	1	1	4	4	4	4	4
2. MULTIPLE DX — A. Not Operated	10	4.3	4	1	3	5	5	5	8	8
2. MULTIPLE DX — B. Operated	9	4.8	24	1	3	3	6	17	17	17
1. SINGLE DX	2	2.5	4	1	1	4	4	4	4	4
2. MULTIPLE DX	19	4.5	13	1	3	3	6	8	17	17
A. NOT OPERATED	10	4.3	4	1	3	5	5	6	8	8
B. OPERATED	11	4.4	21	1	1	3	6	17	17	17
TOTAL										
0–19 Years	2	3.5	<1	3	3	4	4	4	4	4
20–34	4	8.0	36	4	5	6	12	17	17	17
35–49	2	4.5	24	1	1	1	4	8	8	8
50–64	3	3.4	6	1	1	3	3	6	6	6
65+	10	3.3	3	1	3	3	5	6	6	6
GRAND TOTAL	21	4.3	12	1	3	3	5	6	8	17

Length of Stay by Diagnosis and Operation, Western Region 2008

364: IRIS/CILIARY BODY DISORD

Type of Patients	Observed Patients	Avg. Stay	Variance	10th	25th	50th	75th	90th	95th	99th
1. SINGLE DX										
A. *Not Operated*										
0–19 Years	0									
20–34	2	2.0	2		1	3	3	3	3	3
35–49	0									
50–64	2	1.0	0		1	1	1	1	1	1
65+	0									
B. *Operated*										
0–19 Years	0									
20–34	0									
35–49	0									
50–64	0									
65+	0									
2. MULTIPLE DX										
A. *Not Operated*										
0–19 Years	2	2.0	2	1	1	3	3	3	3	3
20–34	5	3.0	4	1	1	3	5	5	5	5
35–49	16	2.9	3	1	2	2	5	6	6	6
50–64	5	5.2	45	1	1	3	4	17	17	17
65+	7	2.4	2	1	1	2	4	5	5	5
B. *Operated*										
0–19 Years	2	3.5	12	1	1	1	6	6	6	6
20–34	0									
35–49	1	4.0	0	4	4	4	4	4	4	4
50–64	4	2.0	1	1	1	1	3	3	3	3
65+	2	1.5	<1	1	1	2	2	2	2	2
SUBTOTALS:										
1. SINGLE DX										
A. *Not Operated*	4	1.5	1	1	1	1	3	3	3	3
B. *Operated*	0									
2. MULTIPLE DX										
A. *Not Operated*	35	3.1	8	1	1	2	4	5	6	17
B. *Operated*	9	2.4	3	1	1	2	3	6	6	6
1. SINGLE DX	4	1.5	1	1	1	1	3	3	3	3
2. MULTIPLE DX	44	3.0	7	1	1	2	4	5	6	17
A. NOT OPERATED	39	2.9	8	1	1	2	4	5	6	17
B. OPERATED	9	2.4	3	1	1	2	3	6	6	6
TOTAL										
0–19 Years	4	2.7	6	1	1	1	3	6	6	6
20–34	7	2.7	3	1	1	3	5	6	6	6
35–49	17	2.9	3	1	2	2	4	6	6	6
50–64	11	3.3	22	1	1	1	3	4	17	17
65+	9	2.2	2	1	1	2	2	5	5	5
GRAND TOTAL	48	2.8	7	1	1	2	3	5	6	17

365: GLAUCOMA

Type of Patients	Observed Patients	Avg. Stay	Variance	10th	25th	50th	75th	90th	95th	99th
1. SINGLE DX										
A. *Not Operated*										
0–19 Years	0									
20–34	0									
35–49	2	1.0	0	1	1	1	1	1	1	1
50–64	1	1.0	0	1	1	1	1	1	1	1
65+	3	1.0	0	1	1	1	1	1	1	1
B. *Operated*										
0–19 Years	0									
20–34	1	1.0	0	1	1	1	1	1	1	1
35–49	2	4.6	24	1	1	8	8	8	8	8
50–64	5	1.6	<1	1	1	2	2	2	2	2
65+	2	1.0	0	1	1	1	1	1	1	1
2. MULTIPLE DX										
A. *Not Operated*										
0–19 Years	1	1.0	0	1	1	1	1	1	1	1
20–34	5	3.0	4	1	1	3	5	5	5	5
35–49	8	2.5	1	1	2	2	3	4	4	4
50–64	10	1.4	<1	1	1	1	1	3	3	3
65+	36	2.8	6	1	1	2	3	6	8	13
B. *Operated*										
0–19 Years	1	1.0	0	1	1	1	1	1	1	1
20–34	0									
35–49	8	2.3	6	1	1	1	5	7	7	7
50–64	29	3.7	25	1	1	3	3	10	12	24
65+	21	2.9	4	1	1	2	5	5	5	8
SUBTOTALS:										
1. SINGLE DX										
A. *Not Operated*	6	1.0	0	1	1	1	1	1	1	1
B. *Operated*	10	2.0	5	1	1	2	2	8	8	8
2. MULTIPLE DX										
A. *Not Operated*	60	2.5	5	1	1	2	3	5	6	13
B. *Operated*	59	3.2	14	1	1	2	5	7	10	24
1. SINGLE DX	16	1.6	3	1	1	1	1	2	8	8
2. MULTIPLE DX	119	2.8	9	1	1	2	4	6	8	13
A. NOT OPERATED	66	2.4	4	1	1	2	3	5	6	13
B. OPERATED	69	3.0	13	1	1	2	4	7	9	24
TOTAL										
0–19 Years	2	1.0	0	1	1	1	1	1	1	1
20–34	6	2.7	4	1	1	3	5	5	5	5
35–49	20	2.5	4	1	1	2	4	6	8	8
50–64	45	2.9	17	1	1	1	3	7	10	24
65+	62	2.7	5	1	1	2	4	5	6	13
GRAND TOTAL	135	2.7	9	1	1	2	3	6	8	13

366: CATARACT

Type of Patients	Observed Patients	Avg. Stay	Variance	10th	25th	50th	75th	90th	95th	99th
1. SINGLE DX										
A. *Not Operated*										
0–19 Years	0									
20–34	0									
35–49	0									
50–64	0									
65+	0									
B. *Operated*										
0–19 Years	0									
20–34	0									
35–49	1	2.0	0	2	2	2	2	2	2	2
50–64	1	1.0	0	1	1	1	1	1	1	1
65+	2	1.0	0	1	1	1	1	1	1	1
2. MULTIPLE DX										
A. *Not Operated*										
0–19 Years	0									
20–34	0									
35–49	1	1.0	0	1	1	1	1	1	1	1
50–64	3	1.3	<1	1	1	1	2	2	2	2
65+	10	2.1	2	1	1	2	3	4	5	5
B. *Operated*										
0–19 Years	3	1.3	<1	1	1	1	2	2	2	2
20–34	1	2.0	0	2	2	2	2	2	2	2
35–49	3	1.3	<1	1	1	1	2	2	2	2
50–64	15	2.7	22	1	1	2	2	5	19	19
65+	15	3.1	13	1	1	2	3	10	13	13
SUBTOTALS:										
1. SINGLE DX										
A. *Not Operated*	0									
B. *Operated*	4	1.3	<1	1	1	1	1	2	2	2
2. MULTIPLE DX										
A. *Not Operated*	14	1.9	2	1	1	1	3	4	5	5
B. *Operated*	37	2.6	14	1	1	2	2	5	13	19
1. SINGLE DX	4	1.3	<1	1	1	1	1	2	2	2
2. MULTIPLE DX	51	2.4	11	1	1	1	2	5	10	19
A. NOT OPERATED	14	1.9	2	1	1	1	3	4	5	5
B. OPERATED	41	2.5	13	1	1	1	2	5	10	19
TOTAL										
0–19 Years	3	1.3	<1	1	1	1	2	2	2	2
20–34	1	2.0	0	2	2	2	2	2	2	2
35–49	5	1.4	<1	1	1	1	2	2	2	2
50–64	19	2.4	17	1	1	2	2	5	19	19
65+	27	2.6	8	1	1	2	3	5	10	13
GRAND TOTAL	55	2.3	10	1	1	1	2	5	10	19

Length of Stay by Diagnosis and Operation, Western Region, 2008

Western Region, October 2006–September 2007 Data, by Diagnosis

367: DISORDERS OF REFRACTION

Type of Patients	Observed Patients	Avg. Stay	Variance	10th	25th	50th	75th	90th	95th	99th
1. SINGLE DX										
A. Not Operated										
0–19 Years	0									
20–34	0									
35–49	0									
50–64	0									
65+	0									
B. Operated										
0–19 Years	0									
20–34	0									
35–49	0									
50–64	0									
65+	0									
2. MULTIPLE DX										
A. Not Operated										
0–19 Years	0									
20–34	0									
35–49	0									
50–64	0									
65+	0									
B. Operated										
0–19 Years	0									
20–34	0									
35–49	0									
50–64	0									
65+	0									
SUBTOTALS:										
1. SINGLE DX										
A. Not Operated	0									
B. Operated	0									
2. MULTIPLE DX										
A. Not Operated	0									
B. Operated	0									
1. SINGLE DX	0									
2. MULTIPLE DX	0									
A. NOT OPERATED	0									
B. OPERATED	0									
TOTAL										
0–19 Years	0									
20–34	0									
35–49	0									
50–64	0									
65+	0									
GRAND TOTAL	**0**									

368: VISUAL DISTURBANCES

Type of Patients	Observed Patients	Avg. Stay	Variance	10th	25th	50th	75th	90th	95th	99th
1. SINGLE DX										
A. Not Operated										
0–19 Years	0									
20–34	2	2.0	0	2	2	2	2	2	2	2
35–49	1	1.0	0	1	1	1	1	1	1	1
50–64	1	2.0	0	2	2	2	2	2	2	2
65+	1	1.0	0	1	1	1	1	1	1	1
B. Operated										
0–19 Years	0									
20–34	0									
35–49	0									
50–64	0									
65+	0									
2. MULTIPLE DX										
A. Not Operated										
0–19 Years	8	3.1	6	1	1	4	6	7	7	7
20–34	48	2.2	4	1	1	2	3	3	4	12
35–49	82	2.3	5	1	1	2	3	4	5	13
50–64	168	1.9	2	1	1	2	2	4	4	7
65+	231	2.6	4	1	1	2	3	5	7	11
B. Operated										
0–19 Years	1	3.0	0	3	3	3	3	3	3	3
20–34	0									
35–49	3	3.3	4	1	1	4	5	5	5	5
50–64	4	4.3	7	2	3	4	8	8	8	8
65+	10	11.5	743	1	1	4	5	6	89	89
SUBTOTALS:										
1. SINGLE DX										
A. Not Operated	5	1.6	<1	1	1	2	2	2	2	2
B. Operated	0									
2. MULTIPLE DX										
A. Not Operated	537	2.3	4	1	1	2	3	4	6	11
B. Operated	18	8.1	411	1	2	4	5	8	89	89
1. SINGLE DX	5	1.6	<1	1	1	2	2	2	2	2
2. MULTIPLE DX	555	2.5	17	1	1	2	3	4	6	12
A. NOT OPERATED	542	2.3	3	1	1	2	3	4	5	11
B. OPERATED	18	8.1	411	2	2	4	5	8	89	89
TOTAL										
0–19 Years	9	3.1	5	1	1	3	4	7	7	7
20–34	50	2.2	4	1	1	2	3	3	4	12
35–49	86	2.4	5	1	1	2	3	4	5	13
50–64	173	2.0	2	1	1	2	2	4	4	8
65+	242	2.9	35	1	1	2	3	5	7	13
GRAND TOTAL	**560**	**2.5**	**17**	**1**	**1**	**2**	**3**	**4**	**6**	**12**

368.2: DIPLOPIA

Type of Patients	Observed Patients	Avg. Stay	Variance	10th	25th	50th	75th	90th	95th	99th
1. SINGLE DX										
A. Not Operated										
0–19 Years	0									
20–34	1	2.0	0	2	2	2	2	2	2	2
35–49	0									
50–64	0									
65+	1	1.0	0	1	1	1	1	1	1	1
B. Operated										
0–19 Years	0									
20–34	0									
35–49	0									
50–64	0									
65+	0									
2. MULTIPLE DX										
A. Not Operated										
0–19 Years	2	2.5	4	1	1	1	4	4	4	4
20–34	16	2.4	7	1	1	2	3	3	12	12
35–49	39	2.4	5	1	1	2	3	4	6	13
50–64	82	1.8	1	1	1	2	2	3	4	5
65+	80	2.2	2	1	1	2	3	4	6	8
B. Operated										
0–19 Years	0									
20–34	0									
35–49	1	1.0	0	1	1	1	1	1	1	1
50–64	1	2.0	0	2	2	2	2	2	2	2
65+	1	1.0	0	1	1	1	1	1	1	1
SUBTOTALS:										
1. SINGLE DX										
A. Not Operated	2	1.5	<1	1	1	2	2	2	2	2
B. Operated	0									
2. MULTIPLE DX										
A. Not Operated	219	2.1	3	1	1	2	3	4	5	11
B. Operated	3	1.3	<1	1	1	1	2	2	2	2
1. SINGLE DX	2	1.5	<1	1	1	2	2	2	2	2
2. MULTIPLE DX	222	2.1	3	1	1	2	3	4	4	8
A. NOT OPERATED	221	2.1	3	1	1	2	3	4	4	8
B. OPERATED	3	1.3	<1	1	1	1	2	2	2	2
TOTAL										
0–19 Years	2	2.5	4	1	1	1	4	4	4	4
20–34	17	2.4	7	1	1	2	3	3	12	12
35–49	40	2.4	4	1	1	2	3	4	6	13
50–64	83	1.8	1	1	1	2	2	3	4	5
65+	82	2.2	2	1	1	2	3	4	6	8
GRAND TOTAL	**224**	**2.1**	**3**	**1**	**1**	**2**	**3**	**4**	**4**	**8**

Length of Stay by Diagnosis and Operation, Western Region, 2008

369: BLINDNESS & LOW VISION

Type of Patients	Observed Patients	Avg. Stay	Vari-ance	10th	25th	50th	75th	90th	95th	99th
1. SINGLE DX										
A. *Not Operated*										
0–19 Years	0									
20–34	0									
35–49	0									
50–64	0									
65+	0									
B. *Operated*										
0–19 Years	0									
20–34	0									
35–49	0									
50–64	0									
65+	0									
2. MULTIPLE DX										
A. *Not Operated*										
0–19 Years	1	1.0	0				1	1	1	1
20–34	7	4.2	20	1	1	3	4	14	14	14
35–49	11	4.8	29	2	2	3	5	7	20	20
50–64	13	1.9	1	1	1	1	2	4	4	4
65+	19	2.6	9	1	1	1	3	8	13	13
B. *Operated*										
0–19 Years	0									
20–34	1	1.0	0	1	1	1	1	1	1	1
35–49	2	9.0	0	9	9	9	9	9	9	9
50–64	4	3.8	14	1	1	4	9	9	9	9
65+	2	1.0	0	1	1	1	1	1	1	1
SUBTOTALS:										
1. SINGLE DX										
A. *Not Operated*	0									
B. *Operated*	0									
2. MULTIPLE DX										
A. *Not Operated*	51	3.1	13	1	1	2	3	5	13	20
B. *Operated*	9	4.0	15	1	1	4	9	9	9	9
1. SINGLE DX	0									
2. MULTIPLE DX	60	3.2	13	1	1	2	4	9	13	20
A. NOT OPERATED	51	3.1	13	1	1	2	3	5	13	20
B. OPERATED	9	4.0	15	1	1	4	9	9	9	9
TOTAL										
0–19 Years	1	1.0	0	1	1	1	1	1	1	1
20–34	8	3.8	19	1	1	3	4	14	14	14
35–49	13	5.5	26	2	2	3	7	7	20	20
50–64	17	2.3	4	1	1	1	3	4	9	9
65+	21	2.4	8	1	1	1	2	4	8	13
GRAND TOTAL	60	3.2	13	1	1	2	4	9	13	20

370: KERATITIS

Type of Patients	Observed Patients	Avg. Stay	Vari-ance	10th	25th	50th	75th	90th	95th	99th
1. SINGLE DX										
A. *Not Operated*										
0–19 Years	2	8.0	31	4	4	4	12	12	12	12
20–34	2	2.5	<1	2	2	3	3	3	3	3
35–49	5	11.0	54	3	8	10	11	23	23	23
50–64	0									
65+	1	6.0	0	6	6	6	6	6	6	6
B. *Operated*										
0–19 Years	0									
20–34	0									
35–49	1	10.0	0	10	10	10	10	10	10	10
50–64	3	12.7	339	2	2	2	34	34	34	34
65+	1	1.0	0	1	1	1	1	1	1	1
2. MULTIPLE DX										
A. *Not Operated*										
0–19 Years	9	9.5	296	1	2	5	5	55	55	55
20–34	10	4.5	10	1	2	3	8	8	9	9
35–49	39	7.0	42	1	3	6	9	19	26	28
50–64	22	4.9	20	2	2	3	7	9	12	20
65+	22	3.7	7	1	2	3	5	7	8	11
B. *Operated*										
0–19 Years	1	13.0	0	13	13	13	13	13	13	13
20–34	4	7.3	68	1	1	2	19	19	19	19
35–49	11	6.9	23	2	3	5	13	14	14	14
50–64	10	6.3	31	1	1	7	8	16	16	16
65+	20	6.9	63	1	1	5	9	22	32	32
SUBTOTALS:										
1. SINGLE DX										
A. *Not Operated*	10	8.2	40	2	3	6	11	23	23	23
B. *Operated*	5	9.8	195	1	2	2	10	34	34	34
2. MULTIPLE DX										
A. *Not Operated*	102	5.8	49	1	2	4	7	11	19	28
B. *Operated*	46	6.9	43	1	2	5	9	15	19	32
1. SINGLE DX	15	8.7	82	2	2	6	11	23	34	34
2. MULTIPLE DX	148	6.2	47	1	2	4	8	13	19	32
A. NOT OPERATED	112	6.0	48	1	2	5	8	11	20	28
B. OPERATED	51	7.2	55	1	2	5	9	15	22	34
TOTAL										
0–19 Years	12	9.5	220	1	2	5	6	13	55	55
20–34	16	4.9	22	1	3	3	7	11	19	19
35–49	56	7.4	39	2	3	6	10	14	23	28
50–64	35	6.0	45	1	2	3	8	15	20	34
65+	44	5.2	34	1	1	3	7	9	12	32
GRAND TOTAL	163	6.4	50	1	2	4	8	13	20	34

371: CORNEAL OPACITY & NEC

Type of Patients	Observed Patients	Avg. Stay	Vari-ance	10th	25th	50th	75th	90th	95th	99th
1. SINGLE DX										
A. *Not Operated*										
0–19 Years	0									
20–34	0									
35–49	0									
50–64	0									
65+	0									
B. *Operated*										
0–19 Years	0									
20–34	2	1.5	<1	1	1	2	2	2	2	2
35–49	0									
50–64	0									
65+	0									
2. MULTIPLE DX										
A. *Not Operated*										
0–19 Years	0									
20–34	1	1.0	0	1	1	1	1	1	1	1
35–49	1	8.0	0	8	8	8	8	8	8	8
50–64	1	1.0	0	1	1	1	1	1	1	1
65+	3	1.3	<1	1	1	1	2	2	2	2
B. *Operated*										
0–19 Years	1	1.0	0	1	1	1	1	1	1	1
20–34	1	3.0	0	3	3	3	3	3	3	3
35–49	5	1.2	<1	1	1	1	1	2	2	2
50–64	5	1.2	<1	1	1	1	1	2	2	2
65+	5	1.0	0	1	1	1	1	1	1	1
SUBTOTALS:										
1. SINGLE DX										
A. *Not Operated*	0									
B. *Operated*	2	1.5	<1	1	1	2	2	2	2	2
2. MULTIPLE DX										
A. *Not Operated*	6	2.3	8	1	1	1	2	8	8	8
B. *Operated*	17	1.2	<1	1	1	1	1	2	3	3
1. SINGLE DX	2	1.5	<1	1	1	2	2	2	2	2
2. MULTIPLE DX	23	1.5	2	1	1	1	1	2	3	8
A. NOT OPERATED	6	2.3	8	1	1	1	2	8	8	8
B. OPERATED	19	1.3	<1	1	1	1	1	2	3	3
TOTAL										
0–19 Years	1	1.0	0	1	1	1	1	1	1	1
20–34	4	1.8	<1	1	1	2	3	3	3	3
35–49	6	2.3	8	1	1	1	2	8	8	8
50–64	6	1.2	<1	1	1	1	1	2	2	2
65+	8	1.1	<1	1	1	1	1	2	2	2
GRAND TOTAL	25	1.5	2	1	1	1	1	2	3	8

Length of Stay by Diagnosis and Operation, Western Region, 2008

Western Region, October 2006–September 2007 Data, by Diagnosis

372: DISORDERS OF CONJUNCTIVA

Type of Patients	Observed Patients	Avg. Stay	Variance	10th	25th	50th	75th	90th	95th	99th
1. SINGLE DX										
A. Not Operated										
0–19 Years	13	1.5	<1	1	1	1	1	1	3	4
20–34	0									
35–49	0									
50–64	0									
65+	0									
B. Operated										
0–19 Years	0									
20–34	1	1.0	0	1	1	1	1	1	1	1
35–49	1	4.0	0	4	4	4	4	4	4	4
50–64	0									
65+	0									
2. MULTIPLE DX										
A. Not Operated										
0–19 Years	23	2.5	3	1	1	2	3	5	6	8
20–34	7	2.2	1	1	1	2	3	4	4	4
35–49	9	3.0	5	1	1	2	5	5	7	7
50–64	25	3.6	10	1	2	3	4	6	10	15
65+	41	3.3	7	1	1	2	5	7	9	13
B. Operated										
0–19 Years	1	2.0	0	2	2	2	2	2	2	2
20–34	1	2.0	0	2	2	2	2	2	2	2
35–49	1	1.0	0	1	1	1	1	1	1	1
50–64	2	6.5	24	3	3	7	10	10	10	10
65+	3	3.3	16	1	1	1	1	8	8	8
SUBTOTALS:										
1. SINGLE DX										
A. Not Operated	13	1.5	<1	1	1	1	1	1	3	4
B. Operated	2	2.5	4	1	1	1	4	4	4	4
2. MULTIPLE DX										
A. Not Operated	105	3.1	6	1	1	2	4	4	6	13
B. Operated	8	3.5	12	1	1	2	2	8	10	10
1. SINGLE DX	15	1.6	1	1	1	1	2	4	4	4
2. MULTIPLE DX	113	3.1	7	1	1	2	4	6	9	13
A. NOT OPERATED	118	2.9	6	1	1	2	4	6	8	13
B. OPERATED	10	3.3	10	1	1	2	4	10	10	10
TOTAL										
0–19 Years	37	2.1	3	1	1	2	3	4	6	8
20–34	9	2.0	1	1	1	2	2	4	4	4
35–49	11	2.9	4	1	1	2	5	5	7	7
50–64	27	3.8	11	1	2	3	4	10	10	15
65+	44	3.3	8	1	1	2	5	8	9	13
GRAND TOTAL	128	2.9	6	1	1	2	4	6	8	13

373: INFLAMMATION OF EYELIDS

Type of Patients	Observed Patients	Avg. Stay	Variance	10th	25th	50th	75th	90th	95th	99th
1. SINGLE DX										
A. Not Operated										
0–19 Years	51	2.3	3	1	1	2	3	3	5	12
20–34	6	3.2	3	1	2	3	5	5	5	5
35–49	3	2.7	1	2	2	2	4	4	4	4
50–64	2	2.0	0	2	2	2	2	2	2	2
65+	0									
B. Operated										
0–19 Years	0									
20–34	0									
35–49	0									
50–64	0									
65+	0									
2. MULTIPLE DX										
A. Not Operated										
0–19 Years	140	2.9	2	1	2	2	4	5	6	6
20–34	74	3.3	4	1	2	3	5	5	6	15
35–49	83	3.8	5	2	2	3	5	7	9	12
50–64	47	3.7	8	1	2	3	5	7	10	15
65+	27	4.8	7	2	3	4	7	9	10	11
B. Operated										
0–19 Years	5	4.6	7	3	3	3	5	9	9	9
20–34	2	4.0	0	4	4	4	4	4	4	4
35–49	4	6.5	7	4	4	7	10	10	10	10
50–64	1	4.0	0	4	4	4	4	4	4	4
65+	3	10.0	13	7	7	9	14	14	14	14
SUBTOTALS:										
1. SINGLE DX										
A. Not Operated	62	2.4	3	1	2	2	3	4	5	12
B. Operated	0									
2. MULTIPLE DX										
A. Not Operated	371	3.4	5	1	2	3	4	6	8	11
B. Operated	15	6.1	10	3	4	5	9	10	14	14
1. SINGLE DX	62	2.4	3	1	2	2	3	4	5	12
2. MULTIPLE DX	386	3.5	5	1	2	3	4	6	9	12
A. NOT OPERATED	433	3.3	4	1	2	3	4	6	7	11
B. OPERATED	15	6.1	10	3	4	5	9	10	14	14
TOTAL										
0–19 Years	196	2.8	3	1	2	2	3	5	6	11
20–34	82	3.3	4	1	2	3	4	5	5	15
35–49	90	3.9	6	2	2	3	5	8	9	12
50–64	50	3.6	7	1	2	3	4	7	10	15
65+	30	5.3	10	2	3	4	7	10	11	14
GRAND TOTAL	448	3.4	5	1	2	3	4	6	8	12

373.13: EYELID ABSCESS

Type of Patients	Observed Patients	Avg. Stay	Variance	10th	25th	50th	75th	90th	95th	99th
1. SINGLE DX										
A. Not Operated										
0–19 Years	51	2.3	3	1	1	2	3	3	5	12
20–34	6	3.2	3	1	2	3	5	5	5	5
35–49	3	2.7	1	2	2	2	4	4	4	4
50–64	2	2.0	0	2	2	2	2	2	2	2
65+	0									
B. Operated										
0–19 Years	0									
20–34	0									
35–49	0									
50–64	0									
65+	0									
2. MULTIPLE DX										
A. Not Operated										
0–19 Years	134	2.8	2	1	2	2	3	5	6	6
20–34	70	3.2	3	1	2	3	4	5	5	9
35–49	79	3.8	5	1	2	3	5	7	9	12
50–64	44	3.8	8	2	2	3	5	7	10	15
65+	25	4.9	7	2	3	4	7	9	10	11
B. Operated										
0–19 Years	5	4.6	7	3	3	3	5	9	9	9
20–34	2	4.0	0	4	4	4	4	4	4	4
35–49	4	6.5	7	4	4	7	10	10	10	10
50–64	1	4.0	0	4	4	4	4	4	4	4
65+	3	10.0	13	7	7	9	14	14	14	14
SUBTOTALS:										
1. SINGLE DX										
A. Not Operated	62	2.4	3	1	2	2	3	4	5	12
B. Operated	0									
2. MULTIPLE DX										
A. Not Operated	352	3.4	4	1	2	3	4	6	8	11
B. Operated	15	6.1	10	3	4	5	9	10	14	14
1. SINGLE DX	62	2.4	3	1	2	2	3	4	5	12
2. MULTIPLE DX	367	3.5	5	1	2	3	4	6	8	11
A. NOT OPERATED	414	3.2	4	1	2	3	4	6	7	11
B. OPERATED	15	6.1	10	3	4	5	9	10	14	14
TOTAL										
0–19 Years	190	2.7	3	1	2	2	3	5	6	11
20–34	78	3.3	2	1	2	3	4	5	5	9
35–49	86	3.9	6	2	2	3	5	7	9	12
50–64	47	3.7	8	1	3	3	5	7	10	15
65+	28	5.4	10	2	3	4	7	10	11	14
GRAND TOTAL	429	3.3	5	1	2	3	4	6	8	11

Length of Stay by Diagnosis and Operation, Western Region, 2008

374: DISORDERS OF EYELIDS NEC

Type of Patients	Observed Patients	Avg. Stay	Vari- ance	Percentiles						
				10th	25th	50th	75th	90th	95th	99th
1. SINGLE DX										
A. Not Operated										
0–19 Years	2	1.0	0		1	1	1	1	1	1
20–34	0									
35–49	0									
50–64	0									
65+	0									
B. Operated										
0–19 Years	0									
20–34	1	1.0	0	1	1	1	1	1	1	1
35–49	1	1.0	0	1	1	1	1	1	1	1
50–64	3	1.0	0	1	1	1	1	1	1	1
65+	0									
2. MULTIPLE DX										
A. Not Operated										
0–19 Years	1	1.0	0	1	1	1	1	1	1	1
20–34	1	1.0	0	1	1	1	1	1	1	1
35–49	7	3.9	39	1	1	1	3	18	18	18
50–64	10	2.9	3	1	2	3	4	6	6	6
65+	7	2.3	3	1	1	2	4	5	5	5
B. Operated										
0–19 Years	2	1.0	0	1	1	1	1	1	1	1
20–34	2	1.0	0	1	1	1	1	1	1	1
35–49	9	2.8	9	1	1	1	3	10	10	10
50–64	23	1.3	1	1	1	1	1	2	2	2
65+	14	2.2	10	1	1	2	4	8	11	11
SUBTOTALS:										
1. SINGLE DX										
A. Not Operated	2	1.0	0	1	1	1	1	1	1	1
B. Operated	5	1.0	0	1	1	1	1	1	1	1
2. MULTIPLE DX										
A. Not Operated	26	2.9	12	1	1	2	4	5	6	18
B. Operated	50	1.8	5	1	1	1	1	3	8	11
1. SINGLE DX	7	1.0	0	1	1	1	1	1	1	1
2. MULTIPLE DX	76	2.1	7	1	1	1	2	4	8	18
A. NOT OPERATED	28	2.7	11	1	1	2	4	5	6	18
B. OPERATED	55	1.7	5	1	1	1	1	3	8	11
TOTAL										
0–19 Years	5	1.0	0	1	1	1	1	1	1	1
20–34	4	1.0	0	1	1	1	1	1	1	1
35–49	17	3.1	20	1	1	1	3	10	18	18
50–64	36	1.7	2	1	1	1	2	4	6	6
65+	21	2.2	7	1	1	2	2	5	8	11
GRAND TOTAL	83	2.1	7	1	1	1	2	4	6	18

375: LACRIMAL SYSTEM DISORDER

Type of Patients	Observed Patients	Avg. Stay	Vari- ance	Percentiles						
				10th	25th	50th	75th	90th	95th	99th
1. SINGLE DX										
A. Not Operated										
0–19 Years	5	2.6	<1	2	2	2	3	4	4	4
20–34	2	2.0	2	1	1	2	3	3	3	3
35–49	0									
50–64	0									
65+	0									
B. Operated										
0–19 Years	2	3.5	12	1	1	4	6	6	6	6
20–34	0									
35–49	0									
50–64	0									
65+	0									
2. MULTIPLE DX										
A. Not Operated										
0–19 Years	20	3.6	9	1	2	3	3	8	9	13
20–34	7	3.6	11	1	2	3	3	11	11	11
35–49	10	2.7	3	1	2	2	4	6	6	6
50–64	11	2.5	1	1	2	2	3	4	5	5
65+	17	4.5	5	3	3	3	6	8	9	9
B. Operated										
0–19 Years	12	4.8	11	1	2	4	6	10	10	10
20–34	3	3.7	14	1	1	2	8	8	8	8
35–49	4	3.8	<1	3	3	4	4	5	5	5
50–64	9	3.3	3	1	3	3	4	6	6	6
65+	10	3.3	4	2	2	3	4	8	8	8
SUBTOTALS:										
1. SINGLE DX										
A. Not Operated	7	2.4	<1	1	1	2	3	4	4	4
B. Operated	2	3.5	12	1	1	4	6	6	6	6
2. MULTIPLE DX										
A. Not Operated	65	3.5	6	1	2	3	4	8	9	13
B. Operated	38	3.9	6	1	2	3	5	8	10	10
1. SINGLE DX	9	2.7	2	1	2	2	3	6	6	6
2. MULTIPLE DX	103	3.6	6	1	2	3	4	8	9	11
A. NOT OPERATED	72	3.4	6	1	2	3	4	7	9	13
B. OPERATED	40	3.8	6	1	2	3	5	8	8	10
TOTAL										
0–19 Years	39	3.8	8	1	2	3	5	9	10	13
20–34	12	3.3	9	1	1	3	3	8	11	11
35–49	14	3.0	2	1	2	2	4	5	6	6
50–64	20	2.9	2	1	2	3	4	5	6	6
65+	27	4.0	5	2	3	3	5	8	8	9
GRAND TOTAL	112	3.6	6	1	2	3	4	8	9	11

376: DISORDERS OF THE ORBIT

Type of Patients	Observed Patients	Avg. Stay	Vari- ance	Percentiles						
				10th	25th	50th	75th	90th	95th	99th
1. SINGLE DX										
A. Not Operated										
0–19 Years	82	2.5	2	1	1	2	3	4	6	10
20–34	16	2.4	2	1	1	3	3	4	5	5
35–49	7	2.3	2	1	1	2	4	4	4	4
50–64	8	1.9	<1	1	1	2	2	3	4	4
65+	2	2.5	<1	2	2	3	3	3	3	3
B. Operated										
0–19 Years	5	1.6	<1	1	1	1	2	3	3	3
20–34	1	6.0	0	6	6	6	6	6	6	6
35–49	0									
50–64	1	1.0	0	1	1	1	1	1	1	1
65+	0									
2. MULTIPLE DX										
A. Not Operated										
0–19 Years	267	3.2	6	1	2	3	4	6	7	12
20–34	136	3.5	4	2	2	3	4	5	7	13
35–49	164	3.4	4	1	2	3	4	6	7	12
50–64	150	3.7	8	2	2	3	4	6	8	15
65+	114	4.8	14	2	2	4	6	10	13	18
B. Operated										
0–19 Years	33	6.0	20	2	3	5	7	11	18	20
20–34	23	2.7	2	1	1	3	4	5	5	6
35–49	45	6.2	19	1	3	5	8	14	15	18
50–64	40	4.4	14	1	1	4	6	10	12	14
65+	18	6.1	21	4	4	5	8	11	21	21
SUBTOTALS:										
1. SINGLE DX										
A. Not Operated	115	2.4	2	1	1	2	3	4	5	7
B. Operated	7	2.1	3	1	1	1	3	6	6	6
2. MULTIPLE DX										
A. Not Operated	831	3.6	7	1	2	3	4	6	8	15
B. Operated	159	5.2	17	1	2	4	7	10	14	20
1. SINGLE DX	122	2.4	2	1	1	2	3	4	5	7
2. MULTIPLE DX	990	3.9	9	1	2	3	5	7	9	17
A. NOT OPERATED	946	3.5	7	1	2	3	4	6	8	14
B. OPERATED	166	5.0	17	1	2	4	7	10	14	20
TOTAL										
0–19 Years	387	3.3	7	1	2	3	4	6	7	15
20–34	176	3.3	4	1	2	3	4	5	6	13
35–49	216	4.0	9	1	2	3	5	7	10	15
50–64	199	3.7	9	1	2	3	4	7	10	14
65+	134	4.9	14	2	2	4	6	10	13	20
GRAND TOTAL	1,112	3.7	8	1	2	3	4	7	9	15

Length of Stay by Diagnosis and Operation, Western Region, 2008

Western Region, October 2006–September 2007 Data, by Diagnosis

376.01: ORBITAL CELLULITIS

Type of Patients	Observed Patients	Avg. Stay	Variance	10th	25th	50th	75th	90th	95th	99th
1. SINGLE DX										
A. Not Operated										
0–19 Years	77	2.5	3	1	2	2	3	4	6	10
20–34	16	2.4	2	1	1	3	3	4	5	5
35–49	6	2.5	2	1	1	3	4	4	5	5
50–64	7	1.9	1	1	1	2	2	4	4	4
65+	2	2.5	<1	2	2	3	3	3	3	3
B. Operated										
0–19 Years	2	2.5	<1	2	2	2	3	3	3	3
20–34	1	6.0	0	6	6	6	6	6	6	6
35–49	0									
50–64	0									
65+	0									
2. MULTIPLE DX										
A. Not Operated										
0–19 Years	262	3.2	6	1	2	3	4	5	6	12
20–34	122	3.5	4	2	2	3	4	5	6	13
35–49	158	3.4	4	1	2	3	4	6	7	12
50–64	136	3.7	8	1	2	3	4	6	8	13
65+	100	4.7	14	2	2	3	6	10	14	18
B. Operated										
0–19 Years	28	6.6	20	3	3	6	7	14	18	20
20–34	12	3.2	1	2	2	3	4	4	6	6
35–49	34	7.1	17	3	4	6	9	14	17	18
50–64	21	6.2	16	2	3	5	10	12	13	14
65+	13	6.5	26	2	4	5	8	11	21	21
SUBTOTALS:										
1. SINGLE DX										
A. Not Operated	108	2.5	2	1	1	2	3	4	5	7
B. Operated	3	3.7	4	2	2	3	6	6	6	6
2. MULTIPLE DX										
A. Not Operated	778	3.6	7	1	2	3	4	6	8	15
B. Operated	108	6.3	18	2	3	5	8	12	15	20
1. SINGLE DX	111	2.5	2	1	1	2	3	4	6	7
2. MULTIPLE DX	886	3.9	9	2	2	3	5	7	9	17
A. NOT OPERATED	886	3.4	6	1	2	3	4	6	7	14
B. OPERATED	111	6.2	18	2	3	5	8	11	15	20
TOTAL										
0–19 Years	369	3.3	7	1	2	3	4	6	7	15
20–34	151	3.4	4	2	2	3	4	5	6	13
35–49	198	4.0	8	1	2	3	5	7	10	17
50–64	164	3.9	9	2	2	3	4	6	10	14
65+	115	4.9	15	2	2	4	6	10	14	20
GRAND TOTAL	997	3.8	8	1	2	3	4	7	9	15

377: DISORDERS OF OPTIC NERVE

Type of Patients	Observed Patients	Avg. Stay	Variance	10th	25th	50th	75th	90th	95th	99th
1. SINGLE DX										
A. Not Operated										
0–19 Years	19	2.8	2	1	2	3	3	3	6	6
20–34	20	2.8	1	1	2	3	4	4	4	4
35–49	11	2.6	2	1	2	3	4	5	5	5
50–64	4	4.8	<1	4	4	5	6	6	6	6
65+	0									
B. Operated										
0–19 Years	0									
20–34	1	2.0	0	2	2	2	2	2	2	2
35–49	1	9.0	0	9	9	9	9	9	9	9
50–64	0									
65+	1	3.0	0	3	3	3	3	3	3	3
2. MULTIPLE DX										
A. Not Operated										
0–19 Years	28	3.4	3	1	3	3	4	5	6	9
20–34	72	3.1	3	1	2	3	4	5	6	9
35–49	93	3.7	6	2	2	3	5	6	9	18
50–64	61	3.2	4	1	2	3	4	5	6	11
65+	44	3.6	5	2	2	3	4	8	8	10
B. Operated										
0–19 Years	3	1.3	<1	1	1	1	2	2	2	2
20–34	2	7.0	2	6	6	8	8	8	8	8
35–49	6	3.8	8	1	1	2	6	7	7	7
50–64	5	2.4	2	1	1	3	3	4	4	4
65+	10	7.3	100	1	2	4	7	35	35	35
SUBTOTALS:										
1. SINGLE DX										
A. Not Operated	54	2.9	2	1	2	3	4	4	6	6
B. Operated	3	4.7	14	2	2	3	9	9	9	9
2. MULTIPLE DX										
A. Not Operated	298	3.4	4	1	2	3	4	6	8	10
B. Operated	26	4.8	44	1	1	3	6	8	8	35
1. SINGLE DX	57	3.0	2	1	2	3	4	5	6	7
2. MULTIPLE DX	324	3.5	7	1	2	3	4	6	8	10
A. NOT OPERATED	352	3.3	4	1	2	3	4	5	7	10
B. OPERATED	29	4.8	40	1	2	3	6	8	9	35
TOTAL										
0–19 Years	50	3.1	3	1	2	3	4	5	6	9
20–34	95	3.1	3	1	2	3	4	5	6	9
35–49	111	3.6	6	1	2	3	5	6	9	18
50–64	70	3.2	4	1	2	3	4	6	6	11
65+	55	4.3	23	2	2	3	4	8	10	35
GRAND TOTAL	381	3.4	7	1	2	3	4	6	7	10

377.30: OPTIC NEURITIS NOS

Type of Patients	Observed Patients	Avg. Stay	Variance	10th	25th	50th	75th	90th	95th	99th
1. SINGLE DX										
A. Not Operated										
0–19 Years	13	2.8	2	1	2	3	3	4	6	6
20–34	17	2.7	<1	1	2	3	3	4	4	4
35–49	9	3.0	1	1	2	3	4	5	5	5
50–64	0									
65+	0									
B. Operated										
0–19 Years	0									
20–34	0									
35–49	0									
50–64	0									
65+	0									
2. MULTIPLE DX										
A. Not Operated										
0–19 Years	15	3.5	2	1	2	4	5	5	6	6
20–34	56	3.1	3	1	2	3	4	5	7	9
35–49	60	4.0	7	2	3	3	5	6	9	18
50–64	36	3.5	5	1	2	3	5	6	7	11
65+	18	3.9	6	2	2	3	5	8	10	10
B. Operated										
0–19 Years	0									
20–34	0									
35–49	2	6.0	0	6	6	6	6	6	6	6
50–64	0									
65+	0									
SUBTOTALS:										
1. SINGLE DX										
A. Not Operated	39	2.8	1	1	2	3	3	4	5	6
B. Operated	0									
2. MULTIPLE DX										
A. Not Operated	185	3.6	5	1	2	3	4	6	8	11
B. Operated	3	6.3	<1	6	6	6	7	7	7	7
1. SINGLE DX	39	2.8	1	1	2	3	3	4	5	6
2. MULTIPLE DX	188	3.6	5	1	2	3	4	6	8	11
A. NOT OPERATED	224	3.5	4	1	2	3	4	6	7	10
B. OPERATED	3	6.3	<1	6	6	6	7	7	7	7
TOTAL										
0–19 Years	28	3.1	2	1	2	3	3	5	6	6
20–34	74	3.0	2	1	2	3	4	5	6	9
35–49	71	4.0	6	2	3	3	5	6	9	18
50–64	36	3.5	5	1	2	3	5	6	7	11
65+	18	3.9	6	2	2	3	5	8	10	10
GRAND TOTAL	227	3.5	4	1	2	3	4	6	7	10

378: STRABISMUS

Type of Patients	Observed Patients	Avg. Stay	Vari-ance	Percentiles						
				10th	25th	50th	75th	90th	95th	99th
1. SINGLE DX										
A. *Not Operated*										
0–19 Years	7	2.0	2	1	1	1	3	5	5	5
20–34	2	2.5	4	1	1	4	4	4	4	4
35–49	5	2.8	2	1	2	3	4	4	4	4
50–64	1	3.0	0	3	3	3	3	3	3	3
65+	1	1.0	0	1	1	1	1	1	1	1
B. *Operated*										
0–19 Years	1	1.0	0	1	1	1	1	1	1	1
20–34	1	2.0	0	2	2	2	2	2	2	2
35–49	0									
50–64	0									
65+	0									
2. MULTIPLE DX										
A. *Not Operated*										
0–19 Years	14	2.4	5	1	1	2	3	5	9	9
20–34	21	2.5	6	1	1	2	2	5	7	10
35–49	55	3.3	7	1	2	3	4	6	9	15
50–64	134	2.8	4	1	1	2	3	6	7	10
65+	149	2.8	5	1	1	2	4	6	7	8
B. *Operated*										
0–19 Years	8	3.9	55	1	1	1	3	22	22	22
20–34	0									
35–49	4	2.8	2	1	1	3	4	4	4	4
50–64	3	7.0	13	4	4	6	11	11	11	11
65+	6	6.5	19	1	4	6	8	14	14	14
SUBTOTALS:										
1. SINGLE DX										
A. *Not Operated*	16	2.3	2	1	1	2	4	4	5	5
B. *Operated*	2	1.5	<1	1	1	2	2	2	2	2
2. MULTIPLE DX										
A. *Not Operated*	373	2.8	5	1	1	2	4	6	7	10
B. *Operated*	21	4.9	28	1	1	3	6	11	14	22
1. SINGLE DX	18	2.2	2	1	1	2	3	4	5	5
2. MULTIPLE DX	394	2.9	6	1	1	2	4	6	7	14
A. NOT OPERATED	389	2.8	5	1	1	2	4	6	7	10
B. OPERATED	23	4.6	27	1	1	3	6	11	14	22
TOTAL										
0–19 Years	30	2.7	17	1	1	1	3	5	9	22
20–34	24	2.5	5	1	1	2	4	5	7	10
35–49	64	3.2	6	2	2	3	4	6	7	15
50–64	138	2.9	5	1	1	2	3	6	7	11
65+	156	2.9	6	1	1	2	4	6	7	14
GRAND TOTAL	412	2.9	6	1	1	2	4	6	7	14

379: EYE DISORDERS NEC

Type of Patients	Observed Patients	Avg. Stay	Vari-ance	Percentiles						
				10th	25th	50th	75th	90th	95th	99th
1. SINGLE DX										
A. *Not Operated*										
0–19 Years	8	1.5	<1	1	1	1	2	2	2	2
20–34	2	2.0	2	1	1	2	3	3	3	3
35–49	4	1.8	<1	1	1	1	2	3	3	3
50–64	2	1.0	0	1	1	1	1	1	1	1
65+	0									
B. *Operated*										
0–19 Years	0									
20–34	0									
35–49	3	2.0	<1	1	1	2	3	3	3	3
50–64	1	1.0	0	1	1	1	1	1	1	1
65+	1	1.0	0	1	1	1	1	1	1	1
2. MULTIPLE DX										
A. *Not Operated*										
0–19 Years	19	1.7	1	1	1	1	2	3	5	5
20–34	22	2.6	8	1	1	1	3	5	7	13
35–49	30	2.4	4	1	1	2	3	5	6	9
50–64	32	2.6	6	1	1	2	3	5	10	11
65+	35	2.7	3	1	2	2	4	5	7	7
B. *Operated*										
0–19 Years	4	2.5	2	1	1	1	3	4	4	4
20–34	1	2.0	0	2	2	2	2	2	2	2
35–49	10	1.0	0	1	1	1	1	1	1	1
50–64	22	1.9	4	1	1	1	1	5	6	9
65+	22	5.7	37	1	1	3	11	16	16	17
SUBTOTALS:										
1. SINGLE DX										
A. *Not Operated*	16	1.6	<1	1	1	1	2	3	3	3
B. *Operated*	5	1.6	<1	1	1	1	2	3	3	3
2. MULTIPLE DX										
A. *Not Operated*	138	2.5	4	1	1	2	3	5	7	11
B. *Operated*	59	3.2	19	1	1	3	6	11	14	17
1. SINGLE DX	21	1.6	<1	1	1	1	2	3	3	3
2. MULTIPLE DX	197	2.7	9	1	1	2	3	5	9	16
A. NOT OPERATED	154	2.4	4	1	1	2	3	5	6	11
B. OPERATED	64	3.1	18	1	1	3	6	11	15	17
TOTAL										
0–19 Years	31	1.8	1	1	1	1	3	3	4	5
20–34	25	2.5	7	1	1	2	4	5	7	13
35–49	47	2.0	3	1	1	2	3	4	5	9
50–64	57	2.2	5	1	1	2	3	5	9	11
65+	58	3.8	17	1	2	2	5	11	16	17
GRAND TOTAL	218	2.6	8	1	1	2	3	5	9	16

380: DISORDER OF EXTERNAL EAR

Type of Patients	Observed Patients	Avg. Stay	Vari-ance	Percentiles						
				10th	25th	50th	75th	90th	95th	99th
1. SINGLE DX										
A. *Not Operated*										
0–19 Years	42	2.5	2	1	1	2	3	4	5	7
20–34	15	2.3	<1	1	1	2	3	3	4	4
35–49	11	2.0	1	1	1	2	3	3	4	4
50–64	7	2.7	9	1	1	2	3	9	9	9
65+	1	2.0	0	2	2	2	2	2	2	2
B. *Operated*										
0–19 Years	0									
20–34	0									
35–49	2	1.0	0	1	1	1	1	1	1	1
50–64	0									
65+	0									
2. MULTIPLE DX										
A. *Not Operated*										
0–19 Years	134	2.7	3	1	1	2	3	5	6	10
20–34	92	3.0	3	1	2	3	4	5	6	8
35–49	169	2.9	3	1	2	3	4	5	5	10
50–64	166	3.2	4	1	2	3	4	6	7	11
65+	125	3.6	6	1	2	3	4	7	8	12
B. *Operated*										
0–19 Years	13	3.6	16	1	1	3	4	5	16	16
20–34	6	2.7	3	1	2	3	3	4	6	8
35–49	7	5.0	24	1	1	3	9	14	14	14
50–64	8	2.0	3	1	1	1	1	5	5	5
65+	8	5.8	93	1	1	1	7	29	29	29
SUBTOTALS:										
1. SINGLE DX										
A. *Not Operated*	76	2.4	2	1	1	2	3	4	5	9
B. *Operated*	2	1.0	0	1	1	1	1	1	1	1
2. MULTIPLE DX										
A. *Not Operated*	686	3.1	4	1	2	3	4	5	7	11
B. *Operated*	42	3.8	27	1	1	2	4	7	14	29
1. SINGLE DX	78	2.3	2	1	1	2	3	4	5	9
2. MULTIPLE DX	728	3.1	5	1	2	3	4	5	7	11
A. NOT OPERATED	762	3.0	4	1	2	3	4	5	7	10
B. OPERATED	44	3.7	26	1	1	2	4	7	14	29
TOTAL										
0–19 Years	189	2.7	4	1	1	2	3	5	6	11
20–34	113	2.9	2	1	2	3	4	5	6	7
35–49	189	2.9	4	1	2	3	4	5	6	11
50–64	181	3.1	4	1	2	3	4	5	7	11
65+	134	3.7	11	1	2	3	4	7	8	14
GRAND TOTAL	806	3.0	5	1	2	3	4	5	7	11

Length of Stay by Diagnosis and Operation, Western Region, 2008

Western Region, October 2006–September 2007 Data, by Diagnosis

380.10: INF OTITIS EXTERNA NOS

Type of Patients	Observed Patients	Avg. Stay	Vari-ance	10th	25th	50th	75th	90th	95th	99th
1. SINGLE DX										
A. Not Operated										
0–19 Years	37	2.6	2	1	2	2	3	4	5	7
20–34	10	2.5	<1	1	2	3	3	3	4	4
35–49	9	2.2	<1	1	2	2	3	3	4	4
50–64	2	2.0	2	1	1	2	3	3	3	3
65+	0									
B. Operated										
0–19 Years	0									
20–34	0									
35–49	0									
50–64	0									
65+	0									
2. MULTIPLE DX										
A. Not Operated										
0–19 Years	103	2.5	2	1	1	2	3	4	5	7
20–34	68	2.8	2	1	2	3	4	5	6	7
35–49	125	2.9	3	1	2	3	4	5	6	10
50–64	111	2.8	3	1	2	3	3	4	5	8
65+	86	3.7	5	1	2	3	5	7	8	12
B. Operated										
0–19 Years	8	4.8	22	1	2	4	5	16	16	16
20–34	2	3.0	2	2	3	3	4	4	4	4
35–49	5	2.4	3	1	1	3	3	5	5	5
50–64	2	5.0	0	5	5	5	5	5	5	5
65+	0									
SUBTOTALS:										
1. SINGLE DX										
A. Not Operated	58	2.5	1	1	2	2	3	4	5	7
B. Operated	0									
2. MULTIPLE DX										
A. Not Operated	493	2.9	3	1	2	3	4	5	6	10
B. Operated	17	3.9	12	1	2	3	5	5	16	16
1. SINGLE DX	58	2.5	1	1	2	2	3	4	5	7
2. MULTIPLE DX	510	2.9	3	1	2	3	4	5	6	10
A. NOT OPERATED	551	2.9	3	1	2	3	4	5	6	9
B. OPERATED	17	3.9	12	1	2	3	5	5	16	16
TOTAL										
0–19 Years	148	2.6	3	1	1	2	3	4	5	8
20–34	80	2.8	2	1	2	3	4	4	6	7
35–49	139	2.8	3	1	2	3	4	4	5	10
50–64	115	2.8	3	1	2	3	3	4	5	8
65+	86	3.7	5	1	2	3	5	7	8	12
GRAND TOTAL	568	2.9	3	1	2	3	4	5	6	10

381: NOM & ET DISORDERS

Type of Patients	Observed Patients	Avg. Stay	Vari-ance	10th	25th	50th	75th	90th	95th	99th
1. SINGLE DX										
A. Not Operated										
0–19 Years	4	2.8	<1	2	3	3	3	3	3	3
20–34	0									
35–49	1	2.0	0	2	2	2	2	2	2	2
50–64	1	4.0	0	4	4	4	4	4	4	4
65+	0									
B. Operated										
0–19 Years	6	1.7	1	1	1	1	2	4	4	4
20–34	0									
35–49	2	1.5	<1	1	1	1	2	2	2	2
50–64	1	1.0	0	1	1	1	1	1	1	1
65+	0									
2. MULTIPLE DX										
A. Not Operated										
0–19 Years	26	1.8	<1	1	1	2	2	3	4	4
20–34	6	2.2	1	1	1	2	3	4	4	4
35–49	8	2.3	3	1	1	2	2	6	6	6
50–64	9	4.6	60	1	1	2	3	25	25	25
65+	15	2.8	3	2	2	2	3	6	7	7
B. Operated										
0–19 Years	135	1.5	2	1	1	1	1	2	4	8
20–34	2	2.0	2	1	1	3	3	3	3	3
35–49	6	4.5	8	2	3	3	5	10	10	10
50–64	3	2.3	1	1	1	3	3	3	3	3
65+	6	1.3	<1	1	1	1	2	2	2	2
SUBTOTALS:										
1. SINGLE DX										
A. Not Operated	6	2.8	<1	2	2	3	3	4	4	4
B. Operated	9	1.6	1	1	1	1	2	4	4	4
2. MULTIPLE DX										
A. Not Operated	64	2.5	10	1	1	2	3	4	6	25
B. Operated	152	1.7	2	1	1	1	2	3	4	8
1. SINGLE DX	15	2.1	1	1	1	2	3	4	4	7
2. MULTIPLE DX	216	1.9	5	1	1	2	2	3	5	8
A. NOT OPERATED	70	2.6	9	1	1	2	3	4	6	25
B. OPERATED	161	1.6	2	1	1	1	2	3	4	8
TOTAL										
0–19 Years	171	1.6	2	1	1	1	2	3	4	8
20–34	8	2.1	1	1	2	2	3	4	4	4
35–49	17	2.9	5	1	2	2	3	6	10	10
50–64	14	3.8	39	1	1	2	3	4	25	25
65+	21	2.4	3	1	2	2	3	5	6	7
GRAND TOTAL	231	1.9	4	1	1	2	2	3	5	8

382: SUPPURATIVE/NOS OMED

Type of Patients	Observed Patients	Avg. Stay	Vari-ance	10th	25th	50th	75th	90th	95th	99th
1. SINGLE DX										
A. Not Operated										
0–19 Years	47	1.7	<1	1	1	1	2	3	3	5
20–34	0									
35–49	1	1.0	0	1	1	1	1	1	1	1
50–64	0									
65+	0									
B. Operated										
0–19 Years	5	1.4	<1	1	1	1	1	3	3	3
20–34	1	1.0	0	1	1	1	1	1	1	1
35–49	1	1.0	0	1	1	1	1	1	1	1
50–64	0									
65+	0									
2. MULTIPLE DX										
A. Not Operated										
0–19 Years	280	2.1	2	1	1	2	3	3	4	7
20–34	20	2.6	2	1	1	3	4	5	5	5
35–49	29	2.1	<1	1	1	2	2	4	5	5
50–64	44	2.6	3	1	1	2	4	5	6	8
65+	37	3.6	6	1	3	3	5	7	9	12
B. Operated										
0–19 Years	58	2.3	4	1	1	2	3	6	8	9
20–34	18	2.0	3	1	1	2	2	3	5	7
35–49	7	2.3	2	1	1	2	3	5	5	5
50–64	9	3.3	8	1	1	3	4	8	8	8
65+	11	4.1	28	1	1	2	5	10	18	18
SUBTOTALS:										
1. SINGLE DX										
A. Not Operated	48	1.7	<1	1	1	1	2	3	3	5
B. Operated	7	1.3	<1	1	1	1	1	3	3	3
2. MULTIPLE DX										
A. Not Operated	410	2.3	2	1	1	2	3	4	5	8
B. Operated	103	2.5	7	1	1	2	3	6	8	10
1. SINGLE DX	55	1.7	<1	1	1	1	2	3	3	5
2. MULTIPLE DX	513	2.3	3	1	1	2	3	4	6	9
A. NOT OPERATED	458	2.2	2	1	1	2	3	4	5	8
B. OPERATED	110	2.4	7	1	1	2	3	6	8	10
TOTAL										
0–19 Years	390	2.1	2	1	1	2	3	4	5	8
20–34	39	2.3	2	1	1	2	3	5	6	7
35–49	38	2.1	1	1	1	2	2	4	5	5
50–64	53	2.8	4	1	1	2	4	6	8	8
65+	48	3.7	11	1	3	3	5	8	10	18
GRAND TOTAL	568	2.3	3	1	1	2	3	4	6	9

382.9: OTITIS MEDIA NOS

Type of Patients	Observed Patients	Avg. Stay	Variance	Percentiles						
				10th	25th	50th	75th	90th	95th	99th
1. SINGLE DX										
A. Not Operated										
0–19 Years	42	1.6	<1	1	1	1	2	3	3	3
20–34	0									
35–49	0									
50–64	0									
65+	0									
B. Operated										
0–19 Years	3	1.0	0	1	1	1	1	1	1	1
20–34	1	1.0	0	1	1	1	1	1	1	1
35–49	1	1.0	0	1	1	1	1	1	1	1
50–64	0									
65+	0									
2. MULTIPLE DX										
A. Not Operated										
0–19 Years	247	2.0	1	1	1	2	3	3	4	6
20–34	12	2.7	2	1	1	3	4	5	5	5
35–49	24	2.1	<1	1	1	2	2	3	4	5
50–64	40	2.5	3	1	1	2	3	5	6	8
65+	34	3.6	7	1	1	3	5	7	9	12
B. Operated										
0–19 Years	46	2.1	3	1	1	1	3	4	6	8
20–34	13	2.2	4	1	1	2	2	6	7	7
35–49	5	2.8	2	1	2	3	3	5	5	5
50–64	8	3.6	9	1	1	3	8	8	8	8
65+	8	3.0	10	1	1	1	3	10	10	10
SUBTOTALS:										
1. SINGLE DX										
A. Not Operated	42	1.6	<1	1	1	1	2	3	3	3
B. Operated	5	1.0	0	1	1	1	1	1	1	1
2. MULTIPLE DX										
A. Not Operated	357	2.2	2	1	1	2	3	4	5	8
B. Operated	80	2.4	5	1	1	1	3	6	8	10
1. SINGLE DX	47	1.5	<1	1	1	1	2	3	3	3
2. MULTIPLE DX	437	2.3	3	1	1	2	3	4	5	8
A. NOT OPERATED	399	2.2	2	1	1	2	3	4	5	8
B. OPERATED	85	2.3	4	1	1	1	3	6	8	10
TOTAL										
0–19 Years	338	2.0	1	1	1	2	2	3	4	7
20–34	26	2.4	3	1	1	2	3	5	6	7
35–49	30	2.2	1	1	1	2	3	3	5	5
50–64	48	2.7	4	1	1	2	3	6	8	8
65+	42	3.5	7	1	1	3	5	7	9	12
GRAND TOTAL	484	2.2	2	1	1	2	3	4	5	8

383: MASTOIDITIS ET AL

Type of Patients	Observed Patients	Avg. Stay	Variance	Percentiles						
				10th	25th	50th	75th	90th	95th	99th
1. SINGLE DX										
A. Not Operated										
0–19 Years	13	1.8	<1	1	1	2	2	3	4	4
20–34	1	4.0	0	4	4	4	4	4	4	4
35–49	4	2.3	2	1	1	3	4	4	4	4
50–64	1	2.0	0	2	2	2	2	2	2	2
65+	2	1.5	<1	1	1	2	2	2	2	2
B. Operated										
0–19 Years	11	3.0	1	2	2	3	4	5	5	5
20–34	0									
35–49	1	6.0	0	6	6	6	6	6	6	6
50–64	2	3.0	8	1	1	5	5	5	5	5
65+	0									
2. MULTIPLE DX										
A. Not Operated										
0–19 Years	117	2.9	4	1	2	2	3	5	7	10
20–34	36	3.1	4	1	2	3	4	7	7	9
35–49	69	3.1	4	1	2	3	4	6	7	11
50–64	56	3.5	12	1	2	3	4	7	9	20
65+	76	3.5	9	2	2	3	4	8	10	17
B. Operated										
0–19 Years	86	5.5	35	2	3	4	5	11	15	40
20–34	21	3.9	6	2	2	3	5	7	7	10
35–49	37	4.1	14	1	2	3	5	10	12	17
50–64	31	9.7	214	1	2	6	9	18	42	75
65+	30	5.0	31	1	1	3	6	13	15	26
SUBTOTALS:										
1. SINGLE DX										
A. Not Operated	21	2.0	1	1	1	2	2	4	4	4
B. Operated	14	3.2	2	2	2	3	5	5	6	6
2. MULTIPLE DX										
A. Not Operated	354	3.2	6	1	2	2	4	6	8	14
B. Operated	205	5.7	57	2	2	4	6	11	15	40
1. SINGLE DX	35	2.5	2	1	1	2	3	5	5	6
2. MULTIPLE DX	559	4.1	26	1	2	3	5	8	11	25
A. NOT OPERATED	375	3.1	6	1	2	2	4	6	8	14
B. OPERATED	219	5.5	54	2	2	4	6	11	15	40
TOTAL										
0–19 Years	227	3.8	17	1	2	3	4	7	10	25
20–34	58	3.4	5	1	2	3	4	6	8	10
35–49	111	3.4	7	1	2	3	4	6	9	12
50–64	90	5.6	88	1	2	3	6	10	18	75
65+	108	3.9	15	2	2	3	4	9	12	17
GRAND TOTAL	594	4.0	25	1	2	3	4	7	11	25

383.00: AC MASTOIDITIS W/O COMP

Type of Patients	Observed Patients	Avg. Stay	Variance	Percentiles						
				10th	25th	50th	75th	90th	95th	99th
1. SINGLE DX										
A. Not Operated										
0–19 Years	10	1.7	<1	1	1	2	2	3	3	3
20–34	0									
35–49	2	1.0	0	1	1	1	1	1	1	1
50–64	1	2.0	0	2	2	2	2	2	2	2
65+	1	2.0	0	2	2	2	2	2	2	2
B. Operated										
0–19 Years	3	2.7	1	2	2	2	4	4	4	4
20–34	0									
35–49	1	6.0	0	6	6	6	6	6	6	6
50–64	0									
65+	0									
2. MULTIPLE DX										
A. Not Operated										
0–19 Years	67	2.6	2	1	2	2	3	4	6	7
20–34	25	3.4	5	1	2	3	5	7	7	9
35–49	46	3.0	5	1	2	2	4	5	8	11
50–64	23	3.3	10	1	2	3	4	5	6	16
65+	32	3.3	6	1	2	3	4	6	10	10
B. Operated										
0–19 Years	44	5.4	44	2	2	4	5	9	11	40
20–34	9	4.0	5	1	3	3	5	8	8	8
35–49	16	4.4	10	1	3	3	5	10	12	12
50–64	11	5.7	13	2	3	5	7	10	13	13
65+	9	7.3	22	1	5	6	11	15	15	15
SUBTOTALS:										
1. SINGLE DX										
A. Not Operated	14	1.6	<1	1	1	2	2	2	3	3
B. Operated	4	3.5	4	2	2	3	5	6	6	6
2. MULTIPLE DX										
A. Not Operated	193	3.0	5	1	2	2	3	6	7	11
B. Operated	89	5.3	28	2	3	4	6	10	13	40
1. SINGLE DX	18	2.1	2	1	1	2	2	4	6	6
2. MULTIPLE DX	282	3.7	13	1	2	3	4	7	10	16
A. NOT OPERATED	207	2.9	4	1	2	2	3	6	7	10
B. OPERATED	93	5.2	27	2	3	4	6	10	13	40
TOTAL										
0–19 Years	124	3.5	19	1	2	3	4	6	7	25
20–34	34	3.5	5	1	2	3	5	7	8	9
35–49	65	3.4	7	1	2	3	4	7	9	12
50–64	35	4.0	11	1	2	3	5	7	13	16
65+	42	4.2	12	1	2	3	5	10	11	15
GRAND TOTAL	300	3.6	12	1	2	3	4	7	9	16

Length of Stay by Diagnosis and Operation, Western Region, 2008

Western Region, October 2006–September 2007 Data, by Diagnosis

384: OTH DISORD TYMPANIC MEMB

Type of Patients	Observed Patients	Avg. Stay	Variance	10th	25th	50th	75th	90th	95th	99th
1. SINGLE DX										
A. Not Operated										
0–19 Years	0									
20–34	0									
35–49	0									
50–64	1	1.0	0	1	1	1	1	1	1	1
65+	0									
B. Operated										
0–19 Years	0									
20–34	3	1.0	0	1	1	1	1	1	1	1
35–49	0									
50–64	1	1.0	0	1	1	1	1	1	1	1
65+	0									
2. MULTIPLE DX										
A. Not Operated										
0–19 Years	2	4.0	0	4	4	4	4	4	4	4
20–34	0									
35–49	0									
50–64	0									
65+	6	3.7	6	1	2	3	5	8	8	8
B. Operated										
0–19 Years	6	1.2	<1	1	1	1	1	2	2	2
20–34	2	1.0	0	1	1	1	1	1	1	1
35–49	2	1.0	0	1	1	1	1	1	1	1
50–64	8	1.3	<1	1	1	1	1	3	3	3
65+	5	2.0	1	1	1	2	2	4	4	4
SUBTOTALS:										
1. SINGLE DX — A. Not Operated	1	1.0	0	1	1	1	1	1	1	1
1. SINGLE DX — B. Operated	4	1.0	0	1	1	1	1	1	1	1
2. MULTIPLE DX — A. Not Operated	8	3.8	5	1	2	3	4	8	8	8
2. MULTIPLE DX — B. Operated	23	1.3	<1	1	1	1	1	2	3	4
1. SINGLE DX	5	1.0	0	1	1	1	1	1	1	1
2. MULTIPLE DX	31	2.0	3	1	1	1	3	4	5	8
A. NOT OPERATED	9	3.4	5	1	2	3	4	8	8	8
B. OPERATED	27	1.3	<1	1	1	1	1	2	3	4
TOTAL										
0–19 Years	8	1.9	2	1	1	1	2	4	4	4
20–34	5	1.0	0	1	1	1	1	1	1	1
35–49	2	1.0	0	1	1	1	1	1	1	1
50–64	10	1.2	<1	1	1	1	2	4	5	8
65+	11	2.9	4	1	1	2	2	5	8	8
GRAND TOTAL	36	1.8	2	1	1	1	2	4	5	8

385: MID EAR/MASTOID PBX NEC

Type of Patients	Observed Patients	Avg. Stay	Variance	10th	25th	50th	75th	90th	95th	99th
1. SINGLE DX										
A. Not Operated										
0–19 Years	0									
20–34	0									
35–49	0									
50–64	1	1.0	0	1	1	1	1	1	1	1
65+	0									
B. Operated										
0–19 Years	3	1.0	0	1	1	1	1	1	1	1
20–34	5	1.2	<1	1	1	1	1	2	2	2
35–49	3	1.0	0	1	1	1	1	1	1	1
50–64	1	1.0	0	1	1	1	1	1	1	1
65+	0									
2. MULTIPLE DX										
A. Not Operated										
0–19 Years	3	2.3	5	1	1	2	5	5	5	5
20–34	4	2.3	4	1	1	2	5	5	5	5
35–49	0									
50–64	4	4.2	7	2	3	3	4	8	8	8
65+	8	1.9	<1	1	1	2	2	4	4	4
B. Operated										
0–19 Years	6	1.8	3	1	1	1	1	5	5	5
20–34	13	3.9	38	1	1	1	1	16	19	19
35–49	27	2.2	3	1	1	2	3	5	6	8
50–64	25	3.7	80	1	1	1	3	5	7	46
65+	13	2.2	3	1	1	2	3	4	7	7
SUBTOTALS:										
1. SINGLE DX — A. Not Operated	1	1.0	0	1	1	1	1	1	1	1
1. SINGLE DX — B. Operated	12	1.1	<1	1	1	1	1	2	2	2
2. MULTIPLE DX — A. Not Operated	19	2.5	4	1	1	2	4	5	8	8
2. MULTIPLE DX — B. Operated	84	2.9	31	1	1	2	3	5	7	46
1. SINGLE DX	13	1.1	<1	1	1	1	1	1	2	2
2. MULTIPLE DX	103	2.8	26	1	1	1	3	5	7	19
A. NOT OPERATED	20	2.5	4	1	1	2	3	5	5	8
B. OPERATED	96	2.7	27	1	1	1	2	5	7	46
TOTAL										
0–19 Years	12	1.8	2	1	1	1	1	5	5	5
20–34	22	3.0	23	1	1	1	2	5	16	19
35–49	30	2.1	3	1	1	2	3	4	6	8
50–64	31	3.6	65	1	1	1	3	5	8	46
65+	21	2.0	2	1	1	2	2	4	4	7
GRAND TOTAL	116	2.6	23	1	1	1	3	5	7	19

386: VERTIGINOUS SYNDROMES

Type of Patients	Observed Patients	Avg. Stay	Variance	10th	25th	50th	75th	90th	95th	99th
1. SINGLE DX										
A. Not Operated										
0–19 Years	2	1.0	0	1	1	1	1	1	1	1
20–34	12	1.8	2	1	1	1	2	2	6	6
35–49	24	1.5	<1	1	1	2	2	3	3	4
50–64	28	1.4	<1	1	1	1	2	3	3	3
65+	16	1.4	<1	1	1	1	2	2	3	3
B. Operated										
0–19 Years	0									
20–34	0									
35–49	4	2.0	2	1	1	2	2	4	4	4
50–64	7	2.6	<1	1	2	3	3	4	4	4
65+	0									
2. MULTIPLE DX										
A. Not Operated										
0–19 Years	16	1.6	<1	1	1	2	2	3	4	4
20–34	79	2.1	2	1	1	2	3	4	5	9
35–49	431	2.2	3	1	1	2	3	4	5	10
50–64	1,145	2.1	2	1	1	2	3	4	5	7
65+	2,854	2.5	3	1	1	2	3	4	6	9
B. Operated										
0–19 Years	1	2.0	0	2	2	2	2	2	2	2
20–34	5	2.2	2	1	2	3	3	4	4	4
35–49	17	3.2	3	1	2	3	4	6	7	7
50–64	47	2.9	2	1	2	3	4	5	6	7
65+	35	6.3	105	1	2	3	6	10	27	59
SUBTOTALS:										
1. SINGLE DX — A. Not Operated	82	1.5	<1	1	1	1	2	2	3	6
1. SINGLE DX — B. Operated	11	2.4	1	1	2	2	3	4	4	4
2. MULTIPLE DX — A. Not Operated	4,525	2.4	3	1	1	2	3	4	5	9
2. MULTIPLE DX — B. Operated	105	4.0	38	1	2	3	4	6	7	27
1. SINGLE DX	93	1.6	<1	1	1	1	2	3	3	6
2. MULTIPLE DX	4,630	2.4	4	1	1	2	3	4	5	9
A. NOT OPERATED	4,607	2.3	3	1	1	2	3	4	5	8
B. OPERATED	116	3.9	35	1	2	3	4	6	7	27
TOTAL										
0–19 Years	19	1.5	<1	1	1	2	2	3	4	4
20–34	96	2.1	2	1	1	2	3	4	5	9
35–49	476	2.2	3	1	1	2	3	4	5	10
50–64	1,227	2.1	2	1	1	2	3	4	5	7
65+	2,905	2.5	5	1	1	3	3	4	6	9
GRAND TOTAL	4,723	2.4	4	1	1	2	3	4	5	9

Length of Stay by Diagnosis and Operation, Western Region, 2008

Western Region, October 2006–September 2007 Data, by Diagnosis

386.00: MENIERE'S DISEASE NOS

Type of Patients	Observed Patients	Avg. Stay	Vari- ance	10th	25th	50th	75th	90th	95th	99th
1. SINGLE DX										
A. Not Operated										
0–19 Years	0									
20–34	1	2.0	0	2	2	2	2	2	2	2
35–49	1	1.0	0	1	1	1	1	1	1	1
50–64	2	1.0	0	1	1	1	1	1	1	1
65+	2	2.0	2	1	1	1	3	3	3	3
B. Operated										
0–19 Years	0									
20–34	0									
35–49	3	2.0	3	1	1	1	4	4	4	4
50–64	4	2.5	2	1	1	2	4	4	4	4
65+	0									
2. MULTIPLE DX										
A. Not Operated										
0–19 Years	2	1.0	0	1	1	1	1	1	1	1
20–34	3	3.7	21	1	1	1	9	9	9	9
35–49	20	2.1	<1	1	1	2	3	3	3	4
50–64	50	2.4	2	1	1	2	3	5	6	7
65+	128	2.4	3	1	1	2	3	5	7	9
B. Operated										
0–19 Years	1	2.0	0	2	2	2	2	2	2	2
20–34	0									
35–49	2	3.0	2	2	2	2	4	4	4	4
50–64	20	2.8	<1	2	2	3	4	4	4	4
65+	15	2.9	3	1	2	3	4	5	7	7
SUBTOTALS:										
1. SINGLE DX										
A. Not Operated	6	1.5	<1	1	1	1	2	3	3	3
B. Operated	7	2.3	2	1	1	2	4	4	4	4
2. MULTIPLE DX										
A. Not Operated	203	2.4	3	1	1	2	3	5	6	9
B. Operated	38	2.8	1	1	2	3	3	4	5	7
1. SINGLE DX	13	1.9	1	1	1	1	3	4	4	4
2. MULTIPLE DX	241	2.5	3	1	1	2	3	4	6	9
A. NOT OPERATED	209	2.4	3	1	1	2	3	5	6	9
B. OPERATED	45	2.8	1	1	2	3	3	4	4	7
TOTAL										
0–19 Years	3	1.3	<1	1	1	1	2	2	2	2
20–34	4	3.3	15	1	1	1	9	9	9	9
35–49	26	2.1	1	1	1	2	3	4	4	4
50–64	76	2.5	2	1	1	2	3	4	5	7
65+	145	2.5	3	1	1	2	3	5	7	9
GRAND TOTAL	254	2.4	3	1	1	2	3	4	6	9

386.10: PERIPHERAL VERTIGO NOS

Type of Patients	Observed Patients	Avg. Stay	Vari- ance	10th	25th	50th	75th	90th	95th	99th
1. SINGLE DX										
A. Not Operated										
0–19 Years	0									
20–34	0									
35–49	0									
50–64	1	1.0	0	1	1	1	1	1	1	1
65+	0									
B. Operated										
0–19 Years	0									
20–34	0									
35–49	0									
50–64	0									
65+	0									
2. MULTIPLE DX										
A. Not Operated										
0–19 Years	1	4.0	0	4	4	4	4	4	4	4
20–34	9	1.9	1	1	1	1	3	4	4	4
35–49	21	2.0	1	1	1	2	2	3	3	5
50–64	73	2.0	1	1	1	2	2	4	4	5
65+	188	2.5	3	1	1	2	3	4	5	9
B. Operated										
0–19 Years	0									
20–34	1	4.0	0	4	4	4	4	4	4	4
35–49	0									
50–64	0									
65+	2	3.5	<1	3	3	4	4	4	4	4
SUBTOTALS:										
1. SINGLE DX										
A. Not Operated	1	1.0	0	1	1	1	1	1	1	1
B. Operated	0									
2. MULTIPLE DX										
A. Not Operated	292	2.3	2	1	1	2	3	4	5	8
B. Operated	3	3.7	<1	3	3	4	4	4	4	4
1. SINGLE DX	1	1.0	0	1	1	1	1	1	1	1
2. MULTIPLE DX	295	2.3	2	1	1	2	3	4	5	8
A. NOT OPERATED	293	2.3	2	1	1	2	3	4	5	8
B. OPERATED	3	3.7	<1	3	3	4	4	4	4	4
TOTAL										
0–19 Years	1	4.0	0	4	4	4	4	4	4	4
20–34	10	2.1	2	1	1	2	2	4	4	4
35–49	21	2.0	1	1	1	2	3	4	4	5
50–64	74	2.0	1	1	1	2	2	4	4	5
65+	190	2.5	3	1	1	2	3	4	5	9
GRAND TOTAL	296	2.3	2	1	1	2	3	4	5	8

386.11: BEN PAROXYSMAL VERTIGO

Type of Patients	Observed Patients	Avg. Stay	Vari- ance	10th	25th	50th	75th	90th	95th	99th
1. SINGLE DX										
A. Not Operated										
0–19 Years	1	1.0	0	1	1	1	1	1	1	1
20–34	2	2.0	0	2	2	2	2	2	2	2
35–49	9	1.6	1	1	1	1	2	3	4	4
50–64	11	1.3	<1	1	1	1	1	2	3	3
65+	6	1.5	<1	1	1	2	2	2	2	2
B. Operated										
0–19 Years	0									
20–34	0									
35–49	0									
50–64	1	2.0	0	2	2	2	2	2	2	2
65+	0									
2. MULTIPLE DX										
A. Not Operated										
0–19 Years	7	1.4	<1	1	1	1	2	2	2	3
20–34	22	1.9	1	1	1	2	2	3	4	5
35–49	148	2.0	2	1	1	2	2	3	5	7
50–64	466	2.0	2	1	1	2	2	4	5	8
65+	1,286	2.5	4	1	1	2	3	4	6	10
B. Operated										
0–19 Years	0									
20–34	1	3.0	0	3	3	3	3	3	3	3
35–49	1	4.0	0	4	4	4	4	4	4	4
50–64	2	2.0	0	2	2	2	2	2	2	2
65+	6	4.8	6	2	3	5	6	9	9	9
SUBTOTALS:										
1. SINGLE DX										
A. Not Operated	29	1.5	<1	1	1	1	2	2	3	4
B. Operated	1	2.0	0	2	2	2	2	2	2	2
2. MULTIPLE DX										
A. Not Operated	1,929	2.3	4	1	1	2	3	4	5	9
B. Operated	10	4.0	5	2	2	4	4	6	9	9
1. SINGLE DX	30	1.5	<1	1	1	1	1	2	3	4
2. MULTIPLE DX	1,939	2.3	4	1	1	2	3	4	5	9
A. NOT OPERATED	1,958	2.3	3	1	1	2	3	4	5	9
B. OPERATED	11	3.8	5	2	2	3	4	6	9	9
TOTAL										
0–19 Years	8	1.4	<1	1	1	2	2	2	3	3
20–34	25	1.9	1	1	1	2	2	3	4	5
35–49	158	2.0	2	1	1	2	2	3	5	7
50–64	480	1.9	2	1	1	2	2	4	5	8
65+	1,298	2.5	4	1	1	2	3	4	6	9
GRAND TOTAL	1,969	2.3	4	1	1	2	3	4	5	9

Length of Stay by Diagnosis and Operation, Western Region, 2008

Western Region, October 2006–September 2007 Data, by Diagnosis

386.12: VESTIBULAR NEURONITIS

Type of Patients	Observed Patients	Avg. Stay	Variance	10th	25th	50th	75th	90th	95th	99th
1. SINGLE DX										
A. Not Operated										
0–19 Years	0									
20–34	5	2.2	5	1	1	1	2	6	6	6
35–49	5	1.0	0	1	1	1	1	1	2	1
50–64	2	1.5	<1	1	1	2	2	2	2	2
65+	1	1.0	0	1	1	1	1	1	1	1
B. Operated										
0–19 Years	0									
20–34	0									
35–49	0									
50–64	1	3.0		3	3	3	3	3	3	3
65+	0									
2. MULTIPLE DX										
A. Not Operated										
0–19 Years	0									
20–34	17	2.2	3	1	1	2	2	2	8	8
35–49	52	2.6	4	1	1	2	3	4	5	11
50–64	111	2.1	<1	1	1	2	3	3	4	5
65+	291	2.7	2	1	2	2	3	5	6	8
B. Operated										
0–19 Years	0									
20–34	1	1.0	0	1	1	1	1	1	1	1
35–49	1	4.0	0	4	4	4	4	4	4	4
50–64	0									
65+	3	10.0	16	6	6	10	14	14	14	14
SUBTOTALS:										
1. SINGLE DX										
A. Not Operated	13	1.5	2	1	1	1	1	2	6	6
B. Operated	1	3.0	0	3	3	3	3	3	3	3
2. MULTIPLE DX										
A. Not Operated	471	2.5	2	1	2	2	3	4	5	8
B. Operated	5	7.0	26	1	4	6	10	14	14	14
1. SINGLE DX	14	1.6	2	1	1	1	2	3	6	6
2. MULTIPLE DX	476	2.6	3	1	2	2	3	4	6	9
A. NOT OPERATED	484	2.5	2	1	1	2	3	4	5	8
B. OPERATED	6	6.3	23	1	3	4	10	14	14	14
TOTAL										
0–19 Years	0									
20–34	23	2.2	3	1	1	2	2	4	6	8
35–49	58	2.5	4	1	1	2	3	4	5	11
50–64	114	2.1	1	1	1	2	3	3	4	5
65+	295	2.8	3	1	2	2	3	5	6	9
GRAND TOTAL	490	2.6	3	1	1	2	3	4	6	9

386.30: LABYRINTHITIS NOS

Type of Patients	Observed Patients	Avg. Stay	Variance	10th	25th	50th	75th	90th	95th	99th
1. SINGLE DX										
A. Not Operated										
0–19 Years	0									
20–34	4	1.3	<1	1	1	1	1	2	2	2
35–49	6	1.5	<1	1	1	1	2	3	3	3
50–64	8	1.3	<1	1	1	2	2	2	2	2
65+	3	1.3	<1	1	1	1	2	2	2	2
B. Operated										
0–19 Years	0									
20–34	0									
35–49	0									
50–64	0									
65+	0									
2. MULTIPLE DX										
A. Not Operated										
0–19 Years	4	1.3	<1	1	1	2	2	2	2	2
20–34	13	2.5	3	1	2	2	3	5	5	5
35–49	133	2.3	3	1	2	2	3	4	6	10
50–64	296	2.2	2	1	2	2	3	4	5	8
65+	613	2.4	3	1	2	2	3	4	5	8
B. Operated										
0–19 Years	0									
20–34	0									
35–49	0									
50–64	1	4.0	0	4	4	4	4	4	4	4
65+	4	23.6	662	2	2	7	27	59	59	59
SUBTOTALS:										
1. SINGLE DX										
A. Not Operated	21	1.3	<1	1	1	1	2	2	2	3
B. Operated	0									
2. MULTIPLE DX										
A. Not Operated	1,059	2.3	3	1	2	2	3	4	5	8
B. Operated	5	19.6	573	2	4	7	27	59	59	59
1. SINGLE DX	21	1.3	<1	1	1	1	2	2	2	3
2. MULTIPLE DX	1,064	2.4	6	1	2	2	3	4	6	9
A. NOT OPERATED	1,080	2.3	3	1	2	2	3	4	5	8
B. OPERATED	5	19.6	573	2	4	7	27	59	59	59
TOTAL										
0–19 Years	4	1.3	<1	1	1	2	2	2	2	2
20–34	17	2.2	2	1	1	2	3	5	5	5
35–49	139	2.3	3	1	1	2	3	4	6	10
50–64	305	2.2	2	1	1	2	3	4	5	7
65+	620	2.5	9	1	2	2	3	4	6	11
GRAND TOTAL	1,085	2.4	6	1	1	2	3	4	5	9

386.35: VIRAL LABYRINTHITIS

Type of Patients	Observed Patients	Avg. Stay	Variance	10th	25th	50th	75th	90th	95th	99th
1. SINGLE DX										
A. Not Operated										
0–19 Years	1	1.0	0	1	1	1	1	1	1	1
20–34	0									
35–49	1	3.0	0	3	3	3	3	3	3	3
50–64	4	2.5	<1	2	2	2	3	3	3	3
65+	2	1.5	<1	1	1	1	2	2	2	2
B. Operated										
0–19 Years	0									
20–34	0									
35–49	0									
50–64	0									
65+	0									
2. MULTIPLE DX										
A. Not Operated										
0–19 Years	0									
20–34	11	2.1	2	1	1	2	3	3	5	5
35–49	30	2.1	10	1	1	1	2	3	4	18
50–64	83	2.0	1	1	1	2	2	4	5	5
65+	146	2.4	3	1	1	2	3	5	5	8
B. Operated										
0–19 Years	0									
20–34	0									
35–49	0									
50–64	1	6.0	0	6	6	6	6	6	6	6
65+	0									
SUBTOTALS:										
1. SINGLE DX										
A. Not Operated	8	2.1	<1	1	1	2	3	3	3	3
B. Operated	0									
2. MULTIPLE DX										
A. Not Operated	270	2.3	3	1	1	2	3	4	5	8
B. Operated	1	6.0	0	6	6	6	6	6	6	6
1. SINGLE DX	8	2.1	<1	1	1	2	3	3	3	3
2. MULTIPLE DX	271	2.3	3	1	1	2	3	4	5	8
A. NOT OPERATED	278	2.2	3	1	1	2	3	4	5	8
B. OPERATED	1	6.0	0	6	6	6	6	6	6	6
TOTAL										
0–19 Years	1	1.0	0	1	1	1	1	1	1	1
20–34	11	2.1	2	1	1	2	3	3	5	5
35–49	31	2.2	9	1	1	1	2	3	4	18
50–64	88	2.1	1	1	1	2	3	4	5	6
65+	148	2.4	3	1	1	2	3	5	5	8
GRAND TOTAL	279	2.3	3	1	1	2	3	4	5	8

Length of Stay by Diagnosis and Operation, Western Region, 2008

387: OTOSCLEROSIS

Type of Patients	Observed Patients	Avg. Stay	Variance	10th	25th	50th	75th	90th	95th	99th
1. SINGLE DX										
A. Not Operated										
0–19 Years	0									
20–34	0									
35–49	0									
50–64	0									
65+	0									
B. Operated										
0–19 Years	0									
20–34	1	2.0	0	2	2	2	2	2	2	2
35–49	1	1.0	0	1	1	1	1	1	1	1
50–64	3	1.0	0	1	1	1	1	1	1	1
65+	0									
2. MULTIPLE DX										
A. Not Operated										
0–19 Years	0									
20–34	0									
35–49	1	1.0	0	1	1	1	1	1	1	1
50–64	0									
65+	0									
B. Operated										
0–19 Years	0									
20–34	1	1.0	<1	1	1	1	1	1	1	1
35–49	7	1.4	<1	1	1	1	2	2	3	3
50–64	10	1.5	<1	1	1	1	2	3	3	3
65+	5	1.8	2	1	1	1	2	4	4	4
SUBTOTALS:										
1. SINGLE DX										
A. Not Operated	0									
B. Operated	5	1.2	<1	1	1	1	1	2	2	2
2. MULTIPLE DX										
A. Not Operated	1	1.0	0	1	1	1	1	1	1	1
B. Operated	23	1.5	<1	1	1	1	2	3	3	4
1. SINGLE DX	5	1.2	<1	1	1	1	1	2	2	2
2. MULTIPLE DX	24	1.5	<1	1	1	1	2	3	3	4
A. NOT OPERATED	1	1.0	0	1	1	1	1	1	1	1
B. OPERATED	28	1.5	<1	1	1	1	2	3	3	4
TOTAL										
0–19 Years	0									
20–34	2	1.5	<1	1	1	1	2	2	2	2
35–49	9	1.3	<1	1	1	1	1	3	3	3
50–64	13	1.4	<1	1	1	1	2	3	3	3
65+	5	1.8	2	1	1	1	2	4	4	4
GRAND TOTAL	29	1.5	<1	1	1	1	2	3	3	4

388: DISORDERS OF EAR NEC

Type of Patients	Observed Patients	Avg. Stay	Variance	10th	25th	50th	75th	90th	95th	99th
1. SINGLE DX										
A. Not Operated										
0–19 Years	3	1.0	0	1	1	1	1	1	1	1
20–34	1	1.0	0	1	1	1	1	1	1	1
35–49	1	1.0	0	1	1	1	1	1	1	1
50–64	0									
65+	0									
B. Operated										
0–19 Years	0									
20–34	2	3.5	<1	3	3	4	4	4	4	4
35–49	1	2.0	0	2	2	2	2	2	2	2
50–64	1	4.0	0	4	4	4	4	4	4	4
65+	0									
2. MULTIPLE DX										
A. Not Operated										
0–19 Years	7	2.3	2	1	1	2	4	4	4	4
20–34	4	2.5	2	1	1	2	3	4	4	4
35–49	19	2.2	3	1	1	2	3	5	8	8
50–64	31	3.1	23	1	1	2	3	4	6	28
65+	44	2.6	5	1	1	2	3	5	7	10
B. Operated										
0–19 Years	1	1.0	0	1	1	1	1	1	1	1
20–34	4	3.7	10	1	1	1	6	7	7	7
35–49	13	4.0	6	2	2	3	5	7	10	10
50–64	14	6.1	79	1	2	3	7	12	35	35
65+	6	4.2	7	2	2	3	5	9	9	9
SUBTOTALS:										
1. SINGLE DX										
A. Not Operated	5	1.0	0	1	1	1	1	1	1	1
B. Operated	4	3.3	<1	2	3	4	4	4	4	4
2. MULTIPLE DX										
A. Not Operated	105	2.6	9	1	1	2	3	4	7	10
B. Operated	38	4.7	33	1	2	3	6	9	12	35
1. SINGLE DX	9	2.0	2	1	1	1	3	4	4	4
2. MULTIPLE DX	143	3.2	16	1	1	2	4	6	8	28
A. NOT OPERATED	110	2.6	9	1	1	2	3	4	7	10
B. OPERATED	42	4.6	30	1	2	3	5	7	10	35
TOTAL										
0–19 Years	11	1.8	2	1	1	1	3	4	4	4
20–34	11	3.0	4	1	1	3	4	6	7	7
35–49	34	2.9	5	1	1	2	3	6	8	10
50–64	46	4.0	40	1	1	2	4	7	12	35
65+	50	2.7	5	1	2	2	4	5	9	10
GRAND TOTAL	152	3.1	15	1	1	2	4	6	8	28

389: HEARING LOSS

Type of Patients	Observed Patients	Avg. Stay	Variance	10th	25th	50th	75th	90th	95th	99th
1. SINGLE DX										
A. Not Operated										
0–19 Years	1	1.0	0	1	1	1	1	1	1	1
20–34	0									
35–49	0									
50–64	0									
65+	0									
B. Operated										
0–19 Years	5	1.0	0	1	1	1	1	1	1	1
20–34	0									
35–49	1	1.0	0	1	1	1	1	1	1	1
50–64	1	3.0	0	3	3	3	3	3	3	3
65+	2	1.0	0	1	1	1	1	1	1	1
2. MULTIPLE DX										
A. Not Operated										
0–19 Years	2	1.0	0	1	1	1	1	1	1	1
20–34	2	3.0	8	1	1	3	5	5	5	5
35–49	9	3.6	7	1	2	3	4	10	10	10
50–64	12	3.1	5	1	1	2	6	6	7	7
65+	14	3.5	5	1	2	3	6	6	7	7
B. Operated										
0–19 Years	6	1.0	0	1	1	1	1	1	1	1
20–34	3	2.0	3	1	1	1	4	4	4	4
35–49	5	1.6	<1	1	1	1	2	3	3	3
50–64	9	1.9	2	1	1	1	2	5	5	5
65+	18	1.3	<1	1	1	1	1	3	3	3
SUBTOTALS:										
1. SINGLE DX										
A. Not Operated	1	1.0	0	1	1	1	1	1	1	1
B. Operated	9	1.2	<1	1	1	1	1	3	3	3
2. MULTIPLE DX										
A. Not Operated	39	3.2	5	1	1	2	5	6	7	10
B. Operated	41	1.5	<1	1	1	1	2	3	3	5
1. SINGLE DX	10	1.2	<1	1	1	1	1	3	3	3
2. MULTIPLE DX	80	2.3	4	1	1	1	3	5	6	10
A. NOT OPERATED	40	3.2	5	1	1	2	5	6	7	10
B. OPERATED	50	1.4	<1	1	1	1	1	3	3	5
TOTAL										
0–19 Years	14	1.0	0	1	1	1	1	1	1	1
20–34	5	2.4	4	1	1	1	4	5	5	5
35–49	15	2.7	5	1	1	2	3	5	10	10
50–64	22	2.6	3	1	1	2	3	6	6	7
65+	34	2.2	3	1	1	1	3	6	6	7
GRAND TOTAL	90	2.2	3	1	1	1	3	5	6	10

Length of Stay by Diagnosis and Operation, Western Region, 2008

Western Region, October 2006–September 2007 Data, by Diagnosis

390: RHF W/O HEART INVOLV

Type of Patients	Observed Patients	Avg. Stay	Vari-ance	Percentiles 10th	25th	50th	75th	90th	95th	99th
1. SINGLE DX										
A. Not Operated										
0–19 Years	6	2.3	1	1	1	3	3	4	4	4
20–34	2	3.0	0	3	3	3	3	3	3	3
35–49	0									
50–64	0									
65+	0									
B. Operated										
0–19 Years	0									
20–34	0									
35–49	0									
50–64	0									
65+	0									
2. MULTIPLE DX										
A. Not Operated										
0–19 Years	6	4.8	5	1	4	5	7	7	7	7
20–34	15	3.7	6	1	2	3	5	7	8	8
35–49	6	2.7	3	1	1	3	4	5	5	5
50–64	8	3.4	5	1	2	3	6	7	7	7
65+	6	5.3	22	1	2	3	6	14	14	14
B. Operated										
0–19 Years	0									
20–34	0									
35–49	2	6.0	8	4	4	4	8	8	8	8
50–64	1	13.0	0	13	13	13	13	13	13	13
65+	0									
SUBTOTALS:										
1. SINGLE DX										
A. Not Operated	8	2.5	1	1	2	3	3	4	4	4
B. Operated	0									
2. MULTIPLE DX										
A. Not Operated	41	3.9	7	1	2	3	6	7	7	14
B. Operated	3	8.3	20	4	4	8	13	13	13	13
1. SINGLE DX	8	2.5	1	1	2	3	3	4	4	4
2. MULTIPLE DX	44	4.2	9	1	2	4	6	7	8	14
A. NOT OPERATED	49	3.7	7	1	2	3	5	7	7	14
B. OPERATED	3	8.3	20	4	4	8	13	13	13	13
TOTAL										
0–19 Years	12	3.6	5	1	2	4	6	7	7	7
20–34	17	3.6	5	1	2	3	5	7	8	8
35–49	8	3.5	5	1	2	4	5	8	8	8
50–64	9	4.4	15	1	2	3	6	13	13	13
65+	6	5.3	22	1	2	3	6	14	14	14
GRAND TOTAL	52	3.9	8	1	2	3	5	7	8	14

391: RHF W HEART INVOLVEMENT

Type of Patients	Observed Patients	Avg. Stay	Vari-ance	Percentiles 10th	25th	50th	75th	90th	95th	99th
1. SINGLE DX										
A. Not Operated										
0–19 Years	0									
20–34	1	2.0	0	2	2	2	2	2	2	2
35–49	0									
50–64	0									
65+	0									
B. Operated										
0–19 Years	0									
20–34	0									
35–49	0									
50–64	1	11.0	0	11	11	11	11	11	11	11
65+	0									
2. MULTIPLE DX										
A. Not Operated										
0–19 Years	3	4.3	6	2	2	4	7	7	7	7
20–34	8	4.1	7	1	2	3	4	8	8	8
35–49	13	6.8	48	1	3	4	8	17	25	25
50–64	15	5.3	20	1	2	5	7	11	18	18
65+	25	5.5	17	1	2	5	7	11	14	17
B. Operated										
0–19 Years	1	9.0	0	9	9	9	9	9	9	9
20–34	0									
35–49	8	9.7	25	5	6	8	11	19	19	19
50–64	11	20.3	154	9	11	14	30	34	48	48
65+	9	11.8	28	4	9	12	14	21	21	21
SUBTOTALS:										
1. SINGLE DX										
A. Not Operated	1	2.0	0	2	2	2	2	2	2	2
B. Operated	1	11.0	0	11	11	11	11	11	11	11
2. MULTIPLE DX										
A. Not Operated	64	5.5	22	1	2	4	7	11	17	25
B. Operated	29	14.4	92	5	9	12	16	30	34	48
1. SINGLE DX	2	6.5	40	2	2	2	11	11	11	11
2. MULTIPLE DX	93	8.3	60	2	3	6	11	17	23	48
A. NOT OPERATED	65	5.4	22	1	2	4	7	11	17	25
B. OPERATED	30	14.2	89	5	9	12	16	30	34	48
TOTAL										
0–19 Years	4	5.5	10	2	2	4	7	9	9	9
20–34	9	3.9	6	1	2	3	4	8	8	8
35–49	22	8.1	38	3	3	6	11	17	19	25
50–64	26	11.7	130	2	3	7	14	30	34	48
65+	34	7.2	27	1	3	6	11	14	17	21
GRAND TOTAL	95	8.2	59	2	3	6	11	17	23	48

392: RHEUMATIC CHOREA

Type of Patients	Observed Patients	Avg. Stay	Vari-ance	Percentiles 10th	25th	50th	75th	90th	95th	99th
1. SINGLE DX										
A. Not Operated										
0–19 Years	0									
20–34	0									
35–49	0									
50–64	0									
65+	0									
B. Operated										
0–19 Years	0									
20–34	0									
35–49	0									
50–64	0									
65+	0									
2. MULTIPLE DX										
A. Not Operated										
0–19 Years	3	3.0	1	2	2	3	4	4	4	4
20–34	0									
35–49	0									
50–64	0									
65+	1	5.0	0	5	5	5	5	5	5	5
B. Operated										
0–19 Years	0									
20–34	0									
35–49	0									
50–64	0									
65+	0									
SUBTOTALS:										
1. SINGLE DX										
A. Not Operated	0									
B. Operated	0									
2. MULTIPLE DX										
A. Not Operated	4	3.5	2	2	2	4	5	5	5	5
B. Operated	0									
1. SINGLE DX	0									
2. MULTIPLE DX	4	3.5	2	2	2	4	5	5	5	5
A. NOT OPERATED	4	3.5	2	2	2	4	5	5	5	5
B. OPERATED	0									
TOTAL										
0–19 Years	3	3.0	1	2	2	3	4	4	4	4
20–34	0									
35–49	0									
50–64	0									
65+	1	5.0	0	5	5	5	5	5	5	5
GRAND TOTAL	4	3.5	2	2	2	4	5	5	5	5

Length of Stay by Diagnosis and Operation, Western Region, 2008

393: CHR RHEUMATIC PERICARD

Type of Patients	Observed Patients	Avg. Stay	Vari-ance	10th	25th	50th	75th	90th	95th	99th
1. SINGLE DX										
A. Not Operated										
0–19 Years	0									
20–34	0									
35–49	0									
50–64	0									
65+	0									
B. Operated										
0–19 Years	0									
20–34	0									
35–49	0									
50–64	0									
65+	0									
2. MULTIPLE DX										
A. Not Operated										
0–19 Years	0									
20–34	0									
35–49	0									
50–64	1	3.0	0	3	3	3	3	3	3	3
65+	3	7.0	28	3	3	5	13	13	13	13
B. Operated										
0–19 Years	0									
20–34	0									
35–49	2	5.0	2	4	4	5	6	6	6	6
50–64	3	11.6	36	6	6	11	18	18	18	18
65+	2	19.0	8	17	17	17	21	21	21	21
SUBTOTALS:										
1. SINGLE DX										
A. Not Operated	0									
B. Operated	0									
2. MULTIPLE DX										
A. Not Operated	4	6.0	22	3	3	5	5	13	13	13
B. Operated	7	11.8	46	4	6	11	18	21	21	21
1. SINGLE DX	0									
2. MULTIPLE DX	11	9.7	43	3	4	6	17	18	21	21
A. NOT OPERATED	4	6.0	22	3	3	5	5	13	13	13
B. OPERATED	7	11.8	46	4	6	11	18	21	21	21
TOTAL										
0–19 Years	0									
20–34	0									
35–49	2	5.0	2	4	4	5	6	6	6	6
50–64	4	9.5	43	3	3	6	18	18	18	18
65+	5	11.8	59	3	5	13	17	21	21	21
GRAND TOTAL	11	9.7	43	3	4	6	17	18	21	21

394: DISEASES OF MITRAL VALVE

Type of Patients	Observed Patients	Avg. Stay	Vari-ance	10th	25th	50th	75th	90th	95th	99th
1. SINGLE DX										
A. Not Operated										
0–19 Years	0									
20–34	0									
35–49	0									
50–64	0									
65+	0									
B. Operated										
0–19 Years	0									
20–34	1	1.0	0	1	1	1	1	1	1	1
35–49	1	1.0	0	1	1	1	1	1	1	1
50–64	1	1.0	0	1	1	1	1	1	1	1
65+	1	1.0	0	1	1	1	1	1	1	1
2. MULTIPLE DX										
A. Not Operated										
0–19 Years	0									
20–34	4	10.0	30	6	6	7	9	18	18	18
35–49	22	4.6	33	1	1	2	5	10	20	21
50–64	36	5.5	36	1	2	3	7	15	22	25
65+	38	4.1	11	1	1	3	6	9	11	12
B. Operated										
0–19 Years	1	11.0	0	11	11	11	11	11	11	11
20–34	19	8.8	54	1	3	6	14	23	24	24
35–49	66	7.8	28	1	4	7	9	15	19	25
50–64	144	8.5	32	3	5	7	10	15	20	30
65+	167	10.3	52	4	6	8	13	18	23	41
SUBTOTALS:										
1. SINGLE DX										
A. Not Operated	0									
B. Operated	4	1.0	0	1	1	1	1	1	1	1
2. MULTIPLE DX										
A. Not Operated	100	4.9	26	1	1	3	7	11	18	25
B. Operated	397	9.1	42	2	5	8	11	17	21	33
1. SINGLE DX	4	1.0	0	1	1	1	1	1	1	1
2. MULTIPLE DX	497	8.3	41	1	4	7	10	17	21	30
A. NOT OPERATED	100	4.9	26	1	1	3	7	11	18	25
B. OPERATED	401	9.0	42	2	5	8	11	17	21	30
TOTAL										
0–19 Years	1	11.0	0	11	11	11	11	11	11	11
20–34	24	8.7	49	1	4	6	12	19	23	24
35–49	89	6.9	31	1	2	6	9	15	19	25
50–64	181	7.8	34	1	5	7	9	15	20	30
65+	206	9.1	50	1	5	8	11	17	22	33
GRAND TOTAL	501	8.2	41	1	4	7	10	16	21	28

395: DISEASES OF AORTIC VALVE

Type of Patients	Observed Patients	Avg. Stay	Vari-ance	10th	25th	50th	75th	90th	95th	99th
1. SINGLE DX										
A. Not Operated										
0–19 Years	0									
20–34	0									
35–49	0									
50–64	0									
65+	0									
B. Operated										
0–19 Years	0									
20–34	0									
35–49	0									
50–64	0									
65+	0									
2. MULTIPLE DX										
A. Not Operated										
0–19 Years	1	4.0	0	4	4	4	4	4	4	4
20–34	0									
35–49	1	1.0	0	1	1	1	1	1	1	1
50–64	7	4.3	14	1	1	3	7	10	10	10
65+	6	2.7	2	1	1	3	3	5	5	5
B. Operated										
0–19 Years	1	5.0	0	5	5	5	5	5	5	5
20–34	3	7.7	21	5	5	5	13	13	13	13
35–49	7	7.4	13	4	4	7	10	14	14	14
50–64	27	7.0	7	4	5	6	10	11	12	12
65+	49	8.5	37	4	5	7	10	16	19	39
SUBTOTALS:										
1. SINGLE DX										
A. Not Operated	0									
B. Operated	0									
2. MULTIPLE DX										
A. Not Operated	15	3.4	8	1	1	3	5	7	10	10
B. Operated	87	7.9	25	4	5	6	10	13	16	39
1. SINGLE DX	0									
2. MULTIPLE DX	102	7.2	24	3	5	6	9	12	16	20
A. NOT OPERATED	15	3.4	8	1	1	3	5	7	10	10
B. OPERATED	87	7.9	25	4	5	6	10	13	16	39
TOTAL										
0–19 Years	2	4.5	<1	4	4	4	5	5	5	5
20–34	3	7.7	21	5	5	5	13	13	13	13
35–49	8	6.6	16	1	4	6	10	14	14	14
50–64	34	6.4	16	3	5	6	9	11	12	12
65+	55	7.9	36	3	5	7	10	16	19	39
GRAND TOTAL	102	7.2	24	3	5	6	9	12	16	20

Length of Stay by Diagnosis and Operation, Western Region, 2008

Western Region, October 2006–September 2007 Data, by Diagnosis

396: MITRAL/AORTIC VALVE DIS

Type of Patients	Observed Patients	Avg. Stay	Variance	10th	25th	50th	75th	90th	95th	99th
1. SINGLE DX										
A. Not Operated										
0–19 Years	0									
20–34	0									
35–49	1	5.0	0	5	5	5	5	5	5	5
50–64	0									
65+	0									
B. Operated										
0–19 Years	0									
20–34	1	3.0	0	3	3	3	3	3	3	3
35–49	3	1.0	0	1	1	1	1	1	1	1
50–64	3	5.0	7	3	3	4	8	8	8	8
65+	1	7.0	0	7	7	7	7	7	7	7
2. MULTIPLE DX										
A. Not Operated										
0–19 Years	0									
20–34	9	5.1	20	1	2	3	8	13	13	13
35–49	20	4.5	11	2	2	3	6	8	8	14
50–64	48	3.3	5	1	2	3	5	6	8	11
65+	295	3.6	8	1	2	3	5	7	10	15
B. Operated										
0–19 Years	2	13.0	49	8	8	8	18	18	18	18
20–34	18	13.7	216	4	5	8	18	26	65	65
35–49	70	12.0	95	4	5	8	16	25	28	62
50–64	260	9.6	46	4	5	7	11	19	22	30
65+	967	11.3	74	5	6	9	13	20	27	50
SUBTOTALS:										
1. SINGLE DX A. Not Operated	1	5.0	0	5	5	5	5	5	5	5
1. SINGLE DX B. Operated	8	3.5	7	1	1	3	7	8	8	8
2. MULTIPLE DX A. Not Operated	372	3.6	8	1	2	3	5	7	10	14
2. MULTIPLE DX B. Operated	1,317	11.0	72	5	6	8	13	20	26	50
1. SINGLE DX	9	3.7	7	1	1	3	5	8	8	8
2. MULTIPLE DX	1,689	9.4	67	2	5	7	11	18	24	47
A. NOT OPERATED	373	3.6	8	1	2	3	5	7	10	14
B. OPERATED	1,325	11.0	72	5	6	8	13	20	26	50
TOTAL										
0–19 Years	2	13.0	49	8	8	8	18	18	18	18
20–34	28	10.6	161	2	4	7	13	23	26	65
35–49	94	10.0	85	3	4	7	13	21	25	62
50–64	311	8.6	45	3	5	7	10	17	21	28
65+	1,263	9.5	69	2	5	7	12	18	25	48
GRAND TOTAL	1,698	9.4	67	2	5	7	11	18	24	46

396.2: MVI & AORTIC STENOSIS

Type of Patients	Observed Patients	Avg. Stay	Variance	10th	25th	50th	75th	90th	95th	99th
1. SINGLE DX										
A. Not Operated										
0–19 Years	0									
20–34	0									
35–49	0									
50–64	0									
65+	0									
B. Operated										
0–19 Years	0									
20–34	0									
35–49	0									
50–64	0									
65+	0									
2. MULTIPLE DX										
A. Not Operated										
0–19 Years	0									
20–34	0									
35–49	5	4.8	7	2	3	4	7	8	8	8
50–64	11	3.5	5	2	2	2	6	6	8	8
65+	148	3.6	7	1	2	3	4	7	10	13
B. Operated										
0–19 Years	0									
20–34	1	5.0	0	5	5	5	5	5	5	5
35–49	7	9.0	37	4	4	6	14	20	20	20
50–64	82	9.8	42	4	5	7	13	21	23	30
65+	514	11.1	57	5	6	9	14	20	26	36
SUBTOTALS:										
1. SINGLE DX A. Not Operated	0									
1. SINGLE DX B. Operated	0									
2. MULTIPLE DX A. Not Operated	164	3.6	7	1	2	3	5	7	10	13
2. MULTIPLE DX B. Operated	604	10.9	55	5	6	9	14	20	25	35
1. SINGLE DX	0									
2. MULTIPLE DX	768	9.4	54	3	5	7	12	18	23	34
A. NOT OPERATED	164	3.6	7	1	2	3	5	7	10	13
B. OPERATED	604	10.9	55	5	6	9	14	20	25	35
TOTAL										
0–19 Years	0									
20–34	1	5.0	0	5	5	5	5	5	5	5
35–49	12	7.2	27	3	4	5	8	14	20	20
50–64	93	9.1	42	3	5	7	11	20	23	30
65+	662	9.4	56	3	5	8	12	18	24	35
GRAND TOTAL	768	9.4	54	3	5	7	12	18	23	34

396.3: MVI & AVI

Type of Patients	Observed Patients	Avg. Stay	Variance	10th	25th	50th	75th	90th	95th	99th
1. SINGLE DX										
A. Not Operated										
0–19 Years	0									
20–34	0									
35–49	0									
50–64	0									
65+	0									
B. Operated										
0–19 Years	0									
20–34	1	3.0	0	3	3	3	3	3	3	3
35–49	0									
50–64	1	3.0	0	3	3	3	3	3	3	3
65+	0									
2. MULTIPLE DX										
A. Not Operated										
0–19 Years	0									
20–34	4	3.7	8	2	2	2	3	8	8	8
35–49	4	4.2	21	1	1	2	3	11	11	11
50–64	18	2.1	9	1	1	3	3	6	6	6
65+	59	3.6	9	1	1	3	5	7	10	17
B. Operated										
0–19 Years	6	13.0	49	8	8	8	18	18	18	18
20–34	6	20.9	522	4	5	12	26	65	65	65
35–49	34	13.1	147	4	4	9	16	28	36	62
50–64	90	9.9	74	4	5	8	11	18	24	72
65+	220	11.1	86	5	6	8	13	19	31	51
SUBTOTALS:										
1. SINGLE DX A. Not Operated	0									
1. SINGLE DX B. Operated	2	3.0	0	3	3	3	3	3	3	3
2. MULTIPLE DX A. Not Operated	85	3.3	8	1	2	2	4	7	9	17
2. MULTIPLE DX B. Operated	352	11.2	96	5	6	8	13	20	28	62
1. SINGLE DX	2	3.0	0	3	3	3	3	3	3	3
2. MULTIPLE DX	437	9.7	89	2	5	7	11	18	26	60
A. NOT OPERATED	85	3.3	8	1	2	2	4	7	9	17
B. OPERATED	354	11.1	96	5	6	8	13	20	28	62
TOTAL										
0–19 Years	2	13.0	49	8	8	8	18	18	18	18
20–34	11	13.1	347	2	3	8	12	26	65	65
35–49	38	12.1	140	3	4	9	15	28	36	62
50–64	109	8.6	70	2	4	7	10	16	21	28
65+	279	9.5	79	2	5	7	11	18	25	51
GRAND TOTAL	439	9.6	89	2	5	7	11	18	26	60

396.8: MITRAL/AO MULT INVOLV

Type of Patients	Observed Patients	Avg. Stay	Variance	10th	25th	Percentiles 50th	75th	90th	95th	99th
1. SINGLE DX										
A. *Not Operated*										
0–19 Years	0									
20–34	0									
35–49	1	5.0	0	5	5	5	5	5	5	5
50–64	0									
65+	0									
B. *Operated*										
0–19 Years	0									
20–34	0									
35–49	0									
50–64	1	8.0	0	8	8	8	8	8	8	8
65+	0									
2. MULTIPLE DX										
A. *Not Operated*										
0–19 Years	0									
20–34	3	7.7	32	3	3	6	14	14	14	14
35–49	9	4.7	9	1	2	5	6	11	11	11
50–64	49	3.3	8	1	1	3	4	6	7	16
65+										
B. *Operated*										
0–19 Years	0									
20–34	6	9.5	32	4	5	8	15	18	18	18
35–49	16	11.3	50	4	6	8	14	24	25	25
50–64	45	8.6	19	4	5	8	9	16	17	21
65+	138	11.9	107	5	6	9	14	24	33	55
SUBTOTALS:										
1. SINGLE DX										
A. *Not Operated*	1	5.0	0	5	5	5	5	5	5	5
B. *Operated*	1	8.0	0	8	8	8	8	8	8	8
2. MULTIPLE DX										
A. *Not Operated*	61	3.7	10	1	2	3	5	6	11	16
B. *Operated*	205	11.1	82	5	6	8	13	21	27	50
1. SINGLE DX	2	6.5	4	5	5	7	8	8	8	8
2. MULTIPLE DX	266	9.4	75	2	5	7	11	18	25	50
A. NOT OPERATED	62	3.7	10	1	2	3	5	6	11	16
B. OPERATED	206	11.1	82	5	6	8	13	21	27	50
TOTAL										
0–19 Years	0									
20–34	6	9.5	32	4	5	8	15	18	18	18
35–49	20	10.4	46	4	5	8	14	21	24	25
50–64	55	7.9	19	4	5	7	9	15	17	21
65+	187	9.7	95	2	4	7	11	20	27	55
GRAND TOTAL	268	9.4	75	2	5	7	11	18	25	50

397: ENDOCARDIAL DISEASE NEC

Type of Patients	Observed Patients	Avg. Stay	Variance	10th	25th	Percentiles 50th	75th	90th	95th	99th
1. SINGLE DX										
A. *Not Operated*										
0–19 Years	0									
20–34	0									
35–49	0									
50–64	0									
65+	0									
B. *Operated*										
0–19 Years	0									
20–34	0									
35–49	0									
50–64	0									
65+	0									
2. MULTIPLE DX										
A. *Not Operated*										
0–19 Years	0									
20–34	0									
35–49	8	9.5	173	1	1	2	7	36	36	36
50–64	10	8.6	176	1	1	4	8	45	45	45
65+	15	3.8	5	1	2	3	5	8	9	9
B. *Operated*										
0–19 Years	1	8.0	0	8	8	8	8	8	8	8
20–34	3	5.7	14	3	3	4	10	10	10	10
35–49	6	7.0	21	4	4	6	7	16	16	16
50–64	16	15.6	263	3	6	8	20	41	63	63
65+	29	12.0	308	5	6	7	10	23	35	97
SUBTOTALS:										
1. SINGLE DX										
A. *Not Operated*	0									
B. *Operated*	0									
2. MULTIPLE DX										
A. *Not Operated*	33	6.6	97	1	2	4	6	12	36	45
B. *Operated*	55	12.1	245	4	6	7	10	23	41	97
1. SINGLE DX	0									
2. MULTIPLE DX	88	10.0	194	1	4	6	9	23	36	97
A. NOT OPERATED	33	6.6	97	1	2	4	6	12	36	45
B. OPERATED	55	12.1	245	4	6	7	10	23	41	97
TOTAL										
0–19 Years	1	8.0	0	8	8	8	8	8	8	8
20–34	3	5.7	14	3	3	4	10	10	10	10
35–49	14	8.4	103	1	1	5	7	24	36	36
50–64	26	12.9	233	1	4	7	18	41	45	63
65+	44	9.2	218	2	4	6	8	12	23	97
GRAND TOTAL	88	10.0	194	1	4	6	9	23	36	97

398: OTH RHEUMATIC HEART DIS

Type of Patients	Observed Patients	Avg. Stay	Variance	10th	25th	Percentiles 50th	75th	90th	95th	99th
1. SINGLE DX										
A. *Not Operated*										
0–19 Years	0									
20–34	0									
35–49	0									
50–64	0									
65+	0									
B. *Operated*										
0–19 Years	0									
20–34	0									
35–49	0									
50–64	0									
65+	0									
2. MULTIPLE DX										
A. *Not Operated*										
0–19 Years	0									
20–34	22	5.6	17	1	3	5	7	12	13	17
35–49	120	4.3	9	1	2	4	6	8	9	17
50–64	445	5.4	27	2	2	4	6	11	14	22
65+	3,485	5.0	15	2	3	4	6	9	12	20
B. *Operated*										
0–19 Years	0									
20–34	4	10.2	15	5	5	10	12	14	14	14
35–49	25	18.7	165	6	10	17	21	46	47	54
50–64	80	12.9	102	4	7	10	18	23	24	73
65+	255	12.4	98	2	6	10	17	24	31	49
SUBTOTALS:										
1. SINGLE DX										
A. *Not Operated*	0									
B. *Operated*	0									
2. MULTIPLE DX										
A. *Not Operated*	4,072	5.0	16	2	3	4	6	9	12	20
B. *Operated*	364	12.9	105	3	6	10	18	24	31	53
1. SINGLE DX	0									
2. MULTIPLE DX	4,436	5.7	28	2	3	4	7	11	15	26
A. NOT OPERATED	4,072	5.0	16	2	3	4	6	9	12	20
B. OPERATED	364	12.9	105	3	6	10	18	24	31	53
TOTAL										
0–19 Years	0									
20–34	26	6.3	19	3	3	5	9	13	14	17
35–49	145	6.8	64	2	3	4	7	17	20	47
50–64	525	6.5	45	3	3	4	8	14	19	31
65+	3,740	5.5	24	2	3	4	7	10	14	25
GRAND TOTAL	4,436	5.7	28	2	3	4	7	11	15	26

Length of Stay by Diagnosis and Operation, Western Region, 2008

Western Region, October 2006–September 2007 Data, by Diagnosis

398.91: RHEUMATIC HEART FAILURE

Type of Patients	Observed Patients	Avg. Stay	Variance	10th	25th	50th	75th	90th	95th	99th
1. SINGLE DX										
A. Not Operated										
0–19 Years	0									
20–34	0									
35–49	0									
50–64	0									
65+	0									
B. Operated										
0–19 Years	0									
20–34	0									
35–49	0									
50–64	0									
65+	0									
2. MULTIPLE DX										
A. Not Operated										
0–19 Years	0									
20–34	20	5.7	17	2	3	5	7	13	17	17
35–49	118	4.3	8	1	3	4	6	8	9	17
50–64	438	5.4	27	2	3	4	6	11	14	22
65+	3,481	5.0	15	2	3	4	6	9	12	20
B. Operated										
0–19 Years	0									
20–34	4	10.2	15	5	5	10	12	14	14	14
35–49	24	19.2	166	6	13	17	21	46	47	54
50–64	79	12.9	103	4	7	10	18	23	31	73
65+	255	12.4	98	2	6	10	17	24	31	49
SUBTOTALS:										
1. SINGLE DX										
A. Not Operated	0									
B. Operated	0									
2. MULTIPLE DX										
A. Not Operated	4,057	5.0	16	2	3	4	6	9	12	20
B. Operated	362	12.9	105	3	6	10	18	24	31	53
1. SINGLE DX	0									
2. MULTIPLE DX	4,419	5.7	28	2	3	4	7	11	15	26
A. NOT OPERATED	4,057	5.0	16	2	3	4	6	9	12	20
B. OPERATED	362	12.9	105	3	6	10	18	24	31	53
TOTAL										
0–19 Years	0									
20–34	24	6.5	19	2	3	5	10	13	14	17
35–49	142	6.8	66	2	2	4	7	17	20	47
50–64	517	6.6	46	2	3	4	8	14	20	31
65+	3,736	5.5	24	2	3	4	7	11	14	25
GRAND TOTAL	4,419	5.7	28	2	3	4	7	11	15	26

401: ESSENTIAL HYPERTENSION

Type of Patients	Observed Patients	Avg. Stay	Variance	10th	25th	50th	75th	90th	95th	99th
1. SINGLE DX										
A. Not Operated										
0–19 Years	6	3.3	1	1	3	4	4	4	4	4
20–34	17	2.2	2	1	1	2	3	4	5	5
35–49	30	1.9	2	1	1	1	2	4	5	7
50–64	47	1.5	<1	1	1	1	2	2	3	5
65+	25	1.6	<1	1	1	1	2	3	3	4
B. Operated										
0–19 Years	0									
20–34	0									
35–49	1	1.0	0	1	1	1	1	1	1	1
50–64	0									
65+	0									
2. MULTIPLE DX										
A. Not Operated										
0–19 Years	61	3.5	9	1	2	3	4	8	10	15
20–34	361	2.4	4	1	1	2	3	5	6	9
35–49	1,997	2.4	4	1	1	2	3	4	6	9
50–64	3,082	2.4	5	1	1	2	3	5	6	11
65+	4,290	2.6	4	1	2	2	3	5	6	11
B. Operated										
0–19 Years	1	2.0	0	2	2	2	2	2	2	2
20–34	5	4.0	9	2	3	3	4	9	9	9
35–49	36	5.2	43	1	2	3	5	15	22	31
50–64	86	4.3	43	1	2	2	4	9	10	46
65+	115	4.7	19	1	1	3	7	11	13	20
SUBTOTALS:										
1. SINGLE DX										
A. Not Operated	125	1.8	1	1	1	1	2	3	4	5
B. Operated	1	1.0	0	1	1	1	1	1	1	1
2. MULTIPLE DX										
A. Not Operated	9,791	2.5	4	1	1	2	3	5	6	10
B. Operated	243	4.6	31	1	1	3	6	10	13	31
1. SINGLE DX	126	1.8	1	1	1	1	2	3	4	5
2. MULTIPLE DX	10,034	2.6	5	1	1	2	3	5	6	11
A. NOT OPERATED	9,916	2.5	4	1	1	2	3	5	6	10
B. OPERATED	244	4.6	31	1	1	3	6	10	13	31
TOTAL										
0–19 Years	68	3.5	8	1	2	3	4	8	10	15
20–34	383	2.4	4	1	1	2	3	5	6	9
35–49	2,064	2.4	4	1	1	2	3	4	6	10
50–64	3,215	2.4	6	1	1	2	3	5	6	12
65+	4,430	2.7	5	1	1	2	3	5	7	11
GRAND TOTAL	10,160	2.5	5	1	1	2	3	5	6	11

401.0: MALIGNANT HYPERTENSION

Type of Patients	Observed Patients	Avg. Stay	Variance	10th	25th	50th	75th	90th	95th	99th
1. SINGLE DX										
A. Not Operated										
0–19 Years	0									
20–34	2	3.5	4	2	2	5	5	5	5	5
35–49	5	1.8	<1	1	1	2	2	3	3	3
50–64	13	1.5	<1	1	1	2	2	3	3	3
65+	7	1.7	<1	1	1	1	3	3	3	3
B. Operated										
0–19 Years	0									
20–34	0									
35–49	0									
50–64	0									
65+	0									
2. MULTIPLE DX										
A. Not Operated										
0–19 Years	11	4.7	6	3	3	3	7	9	9	9
20–34	94	3.0	6	1	1	2	3	7	8	13
35–49	473	2.7	4	1	1	2	3	5	7	10
50–64	655	2.9	7	1	1	2	3	5	8	15
65+	1,001	3.1	7	1	2	2	4	6	8	15
B. Operated										
0–19 Years	1	2.0	0	2	2	2	2	2	2	2
20–34										
35–49	9	10.7	113	2	3	3	15	31	31	31
50–64	13	7.2	95	1	2	4	8	10	38	38
65+	23	5.7	23	1	2	5	8	11	13	20
SUBTOTALS:										
1. SINGLE DX										
A. Not Operated	27	1.9	<1	1	1	2	2	3	3	5
B. Operated	0									
2. MULTIPLE DX										
A. Not Operated	2,234	3.0	6	1	1	2	4	6	8	13
B. Operated	46	7.0	61	1	2	4	9	15	22	38
1. SINGLE DX	27	1.9	<1	1	1	2	2	3	3	5
2. MULTIPLE DX	2,280	3.1	8	1	1	2	4	6	8	15
A. NOT OPERATED	2,261	3.0	6	1	1	2	4	6	8	13
B. OPERATED	46	7.0	61	1	2	4	9	15	22	38
TOTAL										
0–19 Years	12	4.4	6	2	3	3	4	7	9	9
20–34	96	3.0	6	1	1	2	4	7	8	13
35–49	487	2.9	7	1	1	2	3	6	7	15
50–64	681	3.0	9	1	1	2	3	5	8	15
65+	1,031	3.2	7	1	1	2	4	6	8	15
GRAND TOTAL	2,307	3.0	8	1	1	2	4	6	8	15

Length of Stay by Diagnosis and Operation, Western Region, 2008

Western Region, October 2006–September 2007 Data, by Diagnosis

401.9: HYPERTENSION NOS

Type of Patients	Observed Patients	Avg. Stay	Vari-ance	10th	25th	50th	75th	90th	95th	99th
1. SINGLE DX										
A. Not Operated										
0–19 Years	6	3.3	1	1	3	4	4	4	4	4
20–34	14	2.0	1	1	1	1	3	4	4	4
35–49	25	1.9	2	1	1	1	2	4	5	7
50–64	34	1.4	<1	1	1	1	1	2	3	5
65+	18	1.6	<1	1	1	1	2	3	4	4
B. Operated										
0–19 Years	0									
20–34	0									
35–49	1	1.0	0		1	1	1	1	1	1
50–64	0									
65+	0									
2. MULTIPLE DX										
A. Not Operated										
0–19 Years	50	3.3	10	1	1	2	4	6	11	15
20–34	267	2.1	2	1	1	2	3	4	5	8
35–49	1,518	2.2	3	1	1	2	3	4	5	9
50–64	2,421	2.3	4	1	1	2	3	4	6	10
65+	3,279	2.5	4	1	1	2	3	5	6	9
B. Operated										
0–19 Years	0									
20–34	5	4.0	9	1	3	3	4	9	9	9
35–49	27	3.3	8	1	2	2	5	6	7	15
50–64	73	3.8	33	1	2	2	4	8	9	46
65+	92	4.4	18	1	1	3	6	10	12	25
SUBTOTALS:										
1. SINGLE DX										
A. Not Operated	97	1.7	1	1	1	1	2	2	4	7
B. Operated	1	1.0	0	1	1	1	1	1	1	1
2. MULTIPLE DX										
A. Not Operated	7,535	2.4	4	1	1	2	3	5	6	9
B. Operated	197	4.0	22	1	1	2	5	9	12	25
1. SINGLE DX	98	1.7	1	1	1	1	2	4	4	7
2. MULTIPLE DX	7,732	2.4	4	1	1	2	3	5	6	10
A. NOT OPERATED	7,632	2.4	4	1	1	2	3	4	6	9
B. OPERATED	198	4.0	22	1	1	2	5	9	12	25
TOTAL										
0–19 Years	56	3.3	9	1	2	2	4	6	11	15
20–34	286	2.2	2	1	1	2	3	4	5	9
35–49	1,571	2.3	3	1	1	2	3	4	5	9
50–64	2,528	2.3	5	1	1	2	3	4	6	10
65+	3,389	2.5	4	1	1	2	3	5	6	10
GRAND TOTAL	7,830	2.4	4	1	1	2	3	5	6	10

402: HYPERTENSIVE HEART DIS

Type of Patients	Observed Patients	Avg. Stay	Vari-ance	10th	25th	50th	75th	90th	95th	99th
1. SINGLE DX										
A. Not Operated										
0–19 Years	0									
20–34	0									
35–49	4	1.3	<1	1	1	1	2	2	2	2
50–64	1	1.0	0	1	1	1	1	1	1	1
65+	3	1.3	<1	1	1	1	2	2	2	2
B. Operated										
0–19 Years	0									
20–34	0									
35–49	0									
50–64	0									
65+	0									
2. MULTIPLE DX										
A. Not Operated										
0–19 Years	2	2.0	0	2	2	2	2	2	2	2
20–34	72	3.4	4	1	2	3	4	6	7	11
35–49	609	3.5	7	1	2	3	4	6	8	14
50–64	1,196	4.0	13	1	2	3	5	7	9	16
65+	3,337	4.4	11	2	2	4	5	8	10	16
B. Operated										
0–19 Years	0									
20–34	3	6.3	<1	6	6	6	7	7	7	7
35–49	15	7.5	59	1	1	5	8	16	30	30
50–64	72	7.4	45	1	2	5	11	16	23	29
65+	164	7.2	32	3	3	6	9	13	20	28
SUBTOTALS:										
1. SINGLE DX										
A. Not Operated	8	1.3	<1	1	1	1	2	2	2	2
B. Operated	0									
2. MULTIPLE DX										
A. Not Operated	5,216	4.2	11	1	2	3	5	8	10	16
B. Operated	254	7.3	36	1	3	6	9	14	21	29
1. SINGLE DX	8	1.3	<1	1	1	1	2	2	2	2
2. MULTIPLE DX	5,470	4.3	13	1	2	3	5	8	10	18
A. NOT OPERATED	5,224	4.1	11	1	2	3	5	8	10	16
B. OPERATED	254	7.3	36	3	3	6	9	14	21	29
TOTAL										
0–19 Years	2	2.0	0	2	2	2	2	2	2	2
20–34	75	3.5	4	1	2	3	4	6	7	11
35–49	628	3.6	8	1	2	3	4	6	8	15
50–64	1,269	4.2	16	1	2	3	5	8	10	20
65+	3,504	4.5	12	2	2	4	6	8	10	19
GRAND TOTAL	5,478	4.3	13	1	2	3	5	8	10	18

402.00: MAL HTN HRT DIS W/O HF

Type of Patients	Observed Patients	Avg. Stay	Vari-ance	10th	25th	50th	75th	90th	95th	99th
1. SINGLE DX										
A. Not Operated										
0–19 Years	0									
20–34	0									
35–49	1	1.0	0	1	1	1	1	1	1	1
50–64	0									
65+	0									
B. Operated										
0–19 Years	0									
20–34	0									
35–49	0									
50–64	0									
65+	0									
2. MULTIPLE DX										
A. Not Operated										
0–19 Years	1	2.0	0	2	2	2	2	2	2	2
20–34	3	2.0	3	1	1	1	4	4	4	4
35–49	29	2.9	5	1	1	2	4	5	5	11
50–64	43	3.2	4	1	2	3	4	6	8	9
65+	59	3.2	4	1	2	3	4	6	7	11
B. Operated										
0–19 Years	0									
20–34	0									
35–49	0									
50–64	0									
65+	4	11.5	36	6	8	10	16	20	20	20
SUBTOTALS:										
1. SINGLE DX										
A. Not Operated	1	1.0	0	1	1	1	1	1	1	1
B. Operated	0									
2. MULTIPLE DX										
A. Not Operated	135	3.1	4	1	2	3	4	6	7	11
B. Operated	4	11.5	36	6	8	10	16	20	20	20
1. SINGLE DX	1	1.0	0	1	1	1	1	1	1	1
2. MULTIPLE DX	139	3.4	7	1	2	3	4	6	9	11
A. NOT OPERATED	136	3.1	4	1	2	3	4	6	7	11
B. OPERATED	4	11.5	36	6	8	10	16	20	20	20
TOTAL										
0–19 Years	1	2.0	0	2	2	2	2	2	2	2
20–34	3	2.0	3	1	1	1	4	4	4	4
35–49	30	2.8	5	1	1	2	4	5	5	11
50–64	43	3.2	4	1	2	3	4	6	8	9
65+	63	3.8	10	1	2	3	5	7	9	20
GRAND TOTAL	140	3.3	7	1	2	3	4	6	9	11

Length of Stay by Diagnosis and Operation, Western Region, 2008

Western Region, October 2006–September 2007 Data, by Diagnosis

402.01: MAL HTN HEART DIS W HF

Type of Patients	Observed Patients	Avg. Stay	Variance	Percentiles 10th	25th	50th	75th	90th	95th	99th
1. SINGLE DX										
A. Not Operated										
0–19 Years	0									
20–34	0									
35–49	0									
50–64	0									
65+	0									
B. Operated										
0–19 Years	0									
20–34	0									
35–49	0									
50–64	0									
65+	0									
2. MULTIPLE DX										
A. Not Operated										
0–19 Years	1	2.0	0	2	2	2	2	2	2	2
20–34	12	4.8	5	2	3	5	6	6	10	10
35–49	58	3.5	3	2	2	3	5	6	7	8
50–64	63	5.1	51	2	2	4	6	7	9	58
65+	119	4.1	9	1	2	3	5	8	9	13
B. Operated										
0–19 Years	0									
20–34	1	6.0	0	6	6	6	6	6	6	6
35–49	0									
50–64	3	10.6	79	5	5	6	21	21	21	21
65+	5	10.0	26	6	6	10	11	18	18	18
SUBTOTALS:										
1. SINGLE DX A. Not Operated	0									
B. Operated	0									
2. MULTIPLE DX A. Not Operated	253	4.2	18	2	2	3	5	7	9	15
B. Operated	9	9.8	35	5	6	6	11	21	21	21
1. SINGLE DX	0									
2. MULTIPLE DX	262	4.4	19	2	2	3	5	8	9	20
A. NOT OPERATED	253	4.2	18	2	2	3	5	7	9	15
B. OPERATED	9	9.8	35	5	6	6	11	21	21	21
TOTAL										
0–19 Years	1	2.0	0	2	2	2	2	2	2	2
20–34	13	4.9	5	2	2	4	6	6	10	10
35–49	58	3.5	3	2	2	3	5	6	7	8
50–64	66	5.3	53	2	3	4	6	8	11	58
65+	124	4.3	10	1	2	3	6	8	10	18
GRAND TOTAL	262	4.4	19	2	2	3	5	8	9	20

402.90: HTN HRT DIS NOS W/O HF

Type of Patients	Observed Patients	Avg. Stay	Variance	Percentiles 10th	25th	50th	75th	90th	95th	99th
1. SINGLE DX										
A. Not Operated										
0–19 Years	0									
20–34	0									
35–49	3	1.3	<1	1	1	1	2	2	2	2
50–64	1	1.0	0	1	1	1	1	1	1	1
65+	2	1.0	0	1	1	1	1	1	1	1
B. Operated										
0–19 Years	0									
20–34	0									
35–49	0									
50–64	0									
65+	0									
2. MULTIPLE DX										
A. Not Operated										
0–19 Years	0									
20–34	12	2.2	<1	1	1	2	3	3	4	4
35–49	113	2.7	4	1	1	2	3	5	6	11
50–64	206	2.5	3	1	2	2	3	5	6	9
65+	294	3.1	5	1	2	3	4	6	7	12
B. Operated										
0–19 Years	0									
20–34	0									
35–49	2	1.0	0	1	1	1	1	1	1	1
50–64	8	2.5	4	1	1	2	4	7	7	7
65+	19	4.8	17	2	3	3	8	10	16	16
SUBTOTALS:										
1. SINGLE DX A. Not Operated	6	1.2	<1	1	1	1	1	2	2	2
B. Operated	0									
2. MULTIPLE DX A. Not Operated	625	2.8	4	1	1	2	3	5	7	11
B. Operated	29	3.9	14	1	2	2	6	10	10	16
1. SINGLE DX	6	1.2	<1	1	1	1	1	2	2	2
2. MULTIPLE DX	654	2.9	5	1	1	2	4	5	7	11
A. NOT OPERATED	631	2.8	4	1	1	2	3	5	7	11
B. OPERATED	29	3.9	14	1	2	2	6	10	10	16
TOTAL										
0–19 Years	0									
20–34	12	2.2	<1	1	1	2	3	3	4	4
35–49	118	2.6	3	1	1	2	3	5	6	11
50–64	215	2.5	3	1	2	2	3	5	6	9
65+	315	3.2	6	1	2	3	4	6	9	12
GRAND TOTAL	660	2.8	5	1	1	2	4	5	7	11

402.91: HTN HEART DIS NOS W HF

Type of Patients	Observed Patients	Avg. Stay	Variance	Percentiles 10th	25th	50th	75th	90th	95th	99th
1. SINGLE DX										
A. Not Operated										
0–19 Years	0									
20–34	0									
35–49	0									
50–64	0									
65+	0									
B. Operated										
0–19 Years	0									
20–34	0									
35–49	0									
50–64	0									
65+	0									
2. MULTIPLE DX										
A. Not Operated										
0–19 Years	0									
20–34	45	3.3	4	2	2	3	4	5	7	11
35–49	408	3.8	8	1	2	3	5	7	9	15
50–64	880	4.3	13	1	2	4	5	8	9	17
65+	2,849	4.5	12	2	2	4	6	8	10	18
B. Operated										
0–19 Years	0									
20–34	2	6.5	<1	6	6	6	7	7	7	7
35–49	13	8.5	61	1	5	6	8	16	30	30
50–64	61	7.9	47	1	6	6	12	16	23	29
65+	134	7.3	33	2	4	6	9	13	23	28
SUBTOTALS:										
1. SINGLE DX A. Not Operated	0									
B. Operated	0									
2. MULTIPLE DX A. Not Operated	4,182	4.4	12	2	2	4	5	8	10	17
B. Operated	210	7.6	38	1	4	6	10	14	23	29
1. SINGLE DX	0									
2. MULTIPLE DX	4,392	4.5	13	2	2	4	6	8	10	19
A. NOT OPERATED	4,182	4.4	12	2	2	4	5	8	10	17
B. OPERATED	210	7.6	38	1	4	6	10	14	23	29
TOTAL										
0–19 Years	0									
20–34	47	3.5	4	2	2	3	4	6	7	11
35–49	421	3.9	10	1	2	3	5	8	9	17
50–64	941	4.5	16	1	2	4	5	8	11	22
65+	2,983	4.7	13	2	2	4	6	9	11	19
GRAND TOTAL	4,392	4.5	13	2	2	4	6	8	10	19

403: HYPERTENSIVE CKD

Type of Patients	Observed Patients	Avg. Stay	Vari- ance	Percentiles						
				10th	25th	50th	75th	90th	95th	99th
1. SINGLE DX										
A. Not Operated										
0–19 Years	0									
20–34	1	2.0	0	2	2	2	2	2	2	2
35–49	2	1.0	0	1	1	1	1	1	1	1
50–64	0									
65+	2	1.0	0	1	1	1	1	1	1	1
B. Operated										
0–19 Years	0									
20–34	0									
35–49	1	4.0	0	4	4	4	4	4	4	4
50–64	0									
65+	1	2.0	0	2	2	2	2	2	2	2
2. MULTIPLE DX										
A. Not Operated										
0–19 Years	102	4.0	18	1	1	3	5	8	11	20
20–34	950	4.0	14	1	2	3	5	8	12	19
35–49	2,029	4.0	19	1	2	3	5	8	11	21
50–64	3,043	4.5	28	1	2	3	6	9	13	24
65+	3,965	4.7	19	1	2	3	6	9	12	21
B. Operated										
0–19 Years	74	10.0	54	4	6	7	12	19	26	37
20–34	334	6.6	35	2	4	5	8	12	16	36
35–49	636	6.2	27	1	3	5	7	12	17	27
50–64	1,201	6.2	37	1	3	5	8	12	15	33
65+	978	5.9	39	2	4	6	9	13	17	28
SUBTOTALS:										
1. SINGLE DX										
A. Not Operated	5	1.2	<1	1	1	1	2	2	2	2
B. Operated	2	3.0	2	2	2	3	4	4	4	4
2. MULTIPLE DX										
A. Not Operated	10,089	4.4	21	1	2	3	6	9	12	22
B. Operated	3,223	6.3	36	1	3	5	8	12	17	33
1. SINGLE DX	7	1.7	1	1	1	1	2	4	4	4
2. MULTIPLE DX	13,312	4.9	26	1	2	4	6	10	13	24
A. NOT OPERATED	10,094	4.4	21	1	2	3	6	9	12	22
B. OPERATED	3,225	6.3	36	1	3	5	8	12	17	33
TOTAL										
0–19 Years	176	6.5	42	2	2	5	8	14	20	33
20–34	1,285	4.7	20	1	2	3	6	9	13	22
35–49	2,668	4.6	22	1	2	3	6	9	13	22
50–64	4,244	5.0	31	1	2	4	6	10	14	26
65+	4,946	4.9	23	1	2	4	6	10	13	22
GRAND TOTAL	13,319	4.9	26	1	2	4	6	10	13	24

403.00: MAL HTN CKD I-IV/NOS

Type of Patients	Observed Patients	Avg. Stay	Vari- ance	Percentiles						
				10th	25th	50th	75th	90th	95th	99th
1. SINGLE DX										
A. Not Operated										
0–19 Years	0									
20–34	0									
35–49	0									
50–64	0									
65+	0									
B. Operated										
0–19 Years	0									
20–34	0									
35–49	0									
50–64	0									
65+	0									
2. MULTIPLE DX										
A. Not Operated										
0–19 Years	3	5.3	6	3	3	5	8	8	8	8
20–34	69	4.2	5	2	3	4	6	8	8	13
35–49	161	5.2	61	2	2	4	6	9	13	22
50–64	175	5.5	46	2	3	5	7	8	10	27
65+	268	4.7	12	2	2	4	6	10	11	19
B. Operated										
0–19 Years	1	7.0	0	7	7	7	7	7	7	7
20–34	4	9.8	14	5	10	10	14	14	14	14
35–49	8	9.6	50	1	3	10	13	21	21	21
50–64	14	7.4	11	4	5	7	9	12	14	14
65+	26	8.6	31	1	3	10	12	16	17	20
SUBTOTALS:										
1. SINGLE DX										
A. Not Operated	0									
B. Operated	0									
2. MULTIPLE DX										
A. Not Operated	676	5.0	32	2	2	4	6	9	11	20
B. Operated	53	8.5	26	2	5	9	12	15	17	21
1. SINGLE DX	0									
2. MULTIPLE DX	729	5.3	32	2	2	4	6	10	13	20
A. NOT OPERATED	676	5.0	32	2	2	4	6	9	11	20
B. OPERATED	53	8.5	26	2	5	9	12	15	17	21
TOTAL										
0–19 Years	4	5.8	5	3	3	5	7	8	8	8
20–34	73	4.5	7	2	3	4	6	8	10	14
35–49	169	5.4	61	1	2	4	6	10	13	22
50–64	189	5.6	44	2	3	5	7	9	12	27
65+	294	5.1	15	2	2	4	6	11	14	19
GRAND TOTAL	729	5.3	32	2	2	4	6	10	13	20

403.01: MAL HTN CKD V-ESRD

Type of Patients	Observed Patients	Avg. Stay	Vari- ance	Percentiles						
				10th	25th	50th	75th	90th	95th	99th
1. SINGLE DX										
A. Not Operated										
0–19 Years	0									
20–34	0									
35–49	0									
50–64	0									
65+	0									
B. Operated										
0–19 Years	0									
20–34	0									
35–49	0									
50–64	0									
65+	0									
2. MULTIPLE DX										
A. Not Operated										
0–19 Years	8	2.8	3	1	2	2	4	6	6	6
20–34	162	4.1	12	1	2	3	5	9	11	15
35–49	193	4.7	15	1	2	4	6	9	12	22
50–64	206	5.0	18	2	2	3	7	10	13	20
65+	131	5.5	24	2	3	4	7	12	16	23
B. Operated										
0–19 Years	5	13.0	25	6	10	14	17	18	18	18
20–34	18	6.3	18	2	5	5	8	15	16	16
35–49	20	9.2	30	4	5	9	12	16	23	23
50–64	28	8.7	62	2	5	7	11	16	20	42
65+	23	7.5	27	1	4	6	8	16	17	20
SUBTOTALS:										
1. SINGLE DX										
A. Not Operated	0									
B. Operated	0									
2. MULTIPLE DX										
A. Not Operated	700	4.8	17	1	2	4	6	9	13	22
B. Operated	94	8.3	37	2	4	7	11	16	18	42
1. SINGLE DX	0									
2. MULTIPLE DX	794	5.2	20	1	2	4	7	10	15	22
A. NOT OPERATED	700	4.8	17	1	2	4	6	9	13	22
B. OPERATED	94	8.3	37	2	4	7	11	16	18	42
TOTAL										
0–19 Years	13	6.7	37	1	2	4	10	17	18	18
20–34	180	4.3	12	1	2	3	5	9	12	16
35–49	213	5.1	18	1	2	4	7	10	15	22
50–64	234	5.4	24	1	2	4	7	10	14	23
65+	154	5.8	25	1	3	4	7	13	17	23
GRAND TOTAL	794	5.2	20	1	2	4	7	10	15	22

Length of Stay by Diagnosis and Operation, Western Region, 2008

Western Region, October 2006–September 2007 Data, by Diagnosis

403.90: HTN CKD NOS I-IV/NOS

Type of Patients	Observed Patients	Avg. Stay	Vari-ance	10th	25th	50th	75th	90th	95th	99th
1. SINGLE DX										
A. Not Operated										
0–19 Years	0									
20–34	0									
35–49	2	1.0	0	1	1	1	1	1	1	1
50–64	0									
65+	0									
B. Operated										
0–19 Years	0									
20–34	0									
35–49	0									
50–64	0									
65+	0									
2. MULTIPLE DX										
A. Not Operated										
0–19 Years	22	3.0	6	1	1	3	3	6	6	11
20–34	103	3.6	11	1	1	3	4	8	11	15
35–49	388	3.3	6	1	2	3	4	6	8	14
50–64	698	4.1	17	1	2	3	5	8	11	20
65+	1,388	4.3	15	1	2	3	5	8	11	21
B. Operated										
0–19 Years	3	11.3	1	10	10	12	12	12	12	12
20–34	16	7.7	35	2	4	6	11	17	21	21
35–49	27	4.8	13	1	1	4	7	9	10	17
50–64	64	4.8	29	1	1	4	6	10	14	34
65+	118	5.0	23	1	1	3	7	11	15	22
SUBTOTALS:										
1. SINGLE DX										
A. Not Operated	2	1.0	0	1	1	1	1	1	1	1
B. Operated	0									
2. MULTIPLE DX										
A. Not Operated	2,599	4.1	14	1	2	3	5	8	11	20
B. Operated	228	5.2	25	1	1	4	7	11	16	22
1. SINGLE DX	2	1.0	0	1	1	1	1	1	1	1
2. MULTIPLE DX	2,827	4.2	15	1	2	3	5	8	11	20
A. NOT OPERATED	2,601	4.1	14	1	2	3	5	8	11	20
B. OPERATED	228	5.2	25	1	1	4	7	11	16	22
TOTAL										
0–19 Years	25	4.0	13	2	2	3	3	6	12	12
20–34	119	4.1	16	1	1	3	5	10	12	21
35–49	417	3.3	6	2	2	3	4	7	8	14
50–64	762	4.1	18	1	2	3	5	9	11	20
65+	1,506	4.4	15	1	2	3	5	9	11	21
GRAND TOTAL	2,829	4.2	15	1	2	3	5	8	11	20

403.91: HTN CKD NOS V-ESRD

Type of Patients	Observed Patients	Avg. Stay	Vari-ance	10th	25th	50th	75th	90th	95th	99th
1. SINGLE DX										
A. Not Operated										
0–19 Years	0									
20–34	1	2.0	0	2	2	2	2	2	2	2
35–49	0									
50–64	0									
65+	2	1.0	0	1	1	1	1	1	1	1
B. Operated										
0–19 Years	0									
20–34	0									
35–49	1	4.0	0	4	4	4	4	4	4	4
50–64	0									
65+	1	2.0	0	2	2	2	2	2	2	2
2. MULTIPLE DX										
A. Not Operated										
0–19 Years	69	4.4	24	1	1	3	5	9	15	30
20–34	612	4.0	16	1	1	3	5	9	12	19
35–49	1,284	4.0	18	1	1	3	6	9	12	22
50–64	1,958	4.6	32	1	2	3	6	9	14	27
65+	2,166	4.8	22	1	2	4	6	10	13	22
B. Operated										
0–19 Years	65	9.8	59	4	5	7	11	20	26	37
20–34	296	6.5	36	2	4	5	7	11	16	49
35–49	581	6.1	27	1	3	5	8	12	16	34
50–64	1,093	6.3	37	1	3	5	8	12	15	33
65+	810	6.0	42	1	2	5	8	12	18	28
SUBTOTALS:										
1. SINGLE DX										
A. Not Operated	3	1.3	<1	1	1	2	2	2	2	2
B. Operated	2	3.0	2	2	2	3	4	4	4	4
2. MULTIPLE DX										
A. Not Operated	6,089	4.5	24	1	2	3	6	9	13	23
B. Operated	2,845	6.2	37	1	3	5	8	12	17	34
1. SINGLE DX	5	2.0	1	1	1	2	2	4	4	4
2. MULTIPLE DX	8,934	5.1	29	1	2	4	6	10	14	25
A. NOT OPERATED	6,092	4.5	24	1	2	3	6	9	13	23
B. OPERATED	2,847	6.2	37	1	3	5	8	12	17	34
TOTAL										
0–19 Years	134	7.0	48	1	3	5	8	15	25	33
20–34	909	4.8	24	1	2	4	6	10	13	23
35–49	1,866	4.7	22	1	2	3	6	10	14	24
50–64	3,051	5.2	35	1	2	4	6	10	15	29
65+	2,979	5.1	28	1	2	4	7	10	14	24
GRAND TOTAL	8,939	5.1	29	1	2	4	6	10	14	25

404: HTN HEART & CKD

Type of Patients	Observed Patients	Avg. Stay	Vari-ance	10th	25th	50th	75th	90th	95th	99th
1. SINGLE DX										
A. Not Operated										
0–19 Years	0									
20–34	0									
35–49	0									
50–64	0									
65+	0									
B. Operated										
0–19 Years	0									
20–34	0									
35–49	0									
50–64	0									
65+	0									
2. MULTIPLE DX										
A. Not Operated										
0–19 Years	14	3.6	4	1	2	3	6	6	6	6
20–34	111	5.0	26	1	2	4	6	8	17	28
35–49	468	4.9	22	1	2	4	6	9	14	22
50–64	1,069	5.3	20	2	2	4	7	10	13	25
65+	2,899	5.8	22	2	3	5	7	11	15	26
B. Operated										
0–19 Years	16	16.0	0	16	16	16	16	16	16	16
20–34	16	7.0	15	2	4	6	9	12	16	16
35–49	50	10.4	107	2	5	7	13	20	33	54
50–64	134	10.8	74	3	5	8	15	20	30	40
65+	284	10.7	57	3	6	9	14	20	27	41
SUBTOTALS:										
1. SINGLE DX										
A. Not Operated	0									
B. Operated	0									
2. MULTIPLE DX										
A. Not Operated	4,561	5.6	22	2	3	4	7	11	14	25
B. Operated	485	10.6	66	3	5	9	14	20	29	41
1. SINGLE DX	0									
2. MULTIPLE DX	5,046	6.1	28	2	3	5	8	12	16	28
A. NOT OPERATED	4,561	5.6	22	2	3	4	7	11	14	25
B. OPERATED	485	10.6	66	3	5	9	14	20	29	41
TOTAL										
0–19 Years	15	4.4	14	1	2	3	6	6	6	16
20–34	127	5.2	25	1	2	4	6	10	16	28
35–49	518	5.4	33	1	2	4	6	10	16	32
50–64	1,203	5.9	29	2	3	4	7	12	16	27
65+	3,183	6.3	27	2	3	5	8	12	16	28
GRAND TOTAL	5,046	6.1	28	2	3	5	8	12	16	28

Length of Stay by Diagnosis and Operation, Western Region, 2008

404.01: MH HRT&CKD I-IV/NOS W HF

Type of Patients	Observed Patients	Avg. Stay	Vari- ance	10th	25th	50th	75th	90th	95th	99th
1. SINGLE DX										
A. Not Operated										
0–19 Years	0									
20–34	0									
35–49	0									
50–64	0									
65+	0									
B. Operated										
0–19 Years	0									
20–34	0									
35–49	0									
50–64	0									
65+	0									
2. MULTIPLE DX										
A. Not Operated										
0–19 Years	2	2.0	2	1	1	1	3	3	3	3
20–34	9	3.8	4	1	3	3	4	8	8	8
35–49	28	5.0	10	1	3	5	7	8	9	16
50–64	55	4.8	6	2	3	5	7	8	9	12
65+	113	5.2	14	2	3	4	6	10	13	19
B. Operated										
0–19 Years	0									
20–34	1	4.0	0	4	4	4	4	4	4	4
35–49	1	6.0	0	6	6	6	6	6	6	6
50–64	6	5.3	3	3	4	5	7	8	8	8
65+	9	8.9	38	2	5	7	12	22	22	22
SUBTOTALS:										
1. SINGLE DX										
A. Not Operated	0									
B. Operated	0									
2. MULTIPLE DX										
A. Not Operated	207	5.0	11	2	3	4	6	9	11	17
B. Operated	17	7.2	24	3	4	5	8	13	22	22
1. SINGLE DX	0									
2. MULTIPLE DX	224	5.2	12	2	3	4	7	9	12	19
A. NOT OPERATED	207	5.0	11	2	3	4	6	9	11	17
B. OPERATED	17	7.2	24	3	4	5	8	13	22	22
TOTAL										
0–19 Years	2	2.0	2	1	1	1	3	3	3	3
20–34	10	3.8	4	1	3	3	4	8	8	8
35–49	29	5.0	10	1	3	5	6	8	9	16
50–64	61	4.9	6	2	3	5	7	8	9	12
65+	122	5.5	17	2	3	5	7	11	13	20
GRAND TOTAL	224	5.2	12	2	3	4	7	9	12	19

404.03: MH HRT&CKD V-ESRD W HF

Type of Patients	Observed Patients	Avg. Stay	Vari- ance	10th	25th	50th	75th	90th	95th	99th
1. SINGLE DX										
A. Not Operated										
0–19 Years	0									
20–34	0									
35–49	0									
50–64	0									
65+	0									
B. Operated										
0–19 Years	0									
20–34	0									
35–49	0									
50–64	0									
65+	0									
2. MULTIPLE DX										
A. Not Operated										
0–19 Years	1	3.0	0	3	3	3	3	3	3	3
20–34	14	6.3	38	1	2	5	7	15	23	23
35–49	26	6.9	86	2	2	4	8	14	16	48
50–64	53	4.6	29	1	2	3	5	8	11	38
65+	54	5.9	36	2	2	4	6	11	22	31
B. Operated										
0–19 Years	0									
20–34	6	8.8	5	6	7	9	10	12	12	12
35–49	7	12.0	111	3	6	7	15	34	34	34
50–64	4	14.5	290	4	6	8	40	40	40	40
65+	6	6.7	5	4	5	7	9	9	9	9
SUBTOTALS:										
1. SINGLE DX										
A. Not Operated	0									
B. Operated	0									
2. MULTIPLE DX										
A. Not Operated	148	5.6	42	1	2	4	7	11	15	38
B. Operated	23	10.2	80	4	6	8	10	15	34	40
1. SINGLE DX	0									
2. MULTIPLE DX	171	6.2	49	2	2	4	7	11	16	40
A. NOT OPERATED	148	5.6	42	1	2	4	7	11	15	38
B. OPERATED	23	10.2	80	4	6	8	10	15	34	40
TOTAL										
0–19 Years	1	3.0	0	3	3	3	3	3	3	3
20–34	20	7.0	28	2	3	6	9	12	23	23
35–49	33	8.0	93	2	3	5	10	15	34	48
50–64	57	5.3	49	1	2	3	6	8	11	40
65+	60	6.0	33	2	3	4	7	11	13	31
GRAND TOTAL	171	6.2	49	2	2	4	7	11	16	40

404.91: HTN HRT&CKD I-IV W HF

Type of Patients	Observed Patients	Avg. Stay	Vari- ance	10th	25th	50th	75th	90th	95th	99th
1. SINGLE DX										
A. Not Operated										
0–19 Years	0									
20–34	0									
35–49	0									
50–64	0									
65+	0									
B. Operated										
0–19 Years	0									
20–34	0									
35–49	0									
50–64	0									
65+	0									
2. MULTIPLE DX										
A. Not Operated										
0–19 Years	1	6.0	0	6	6	6	6	6	6	6
20–34	23	5.9	33	2	3	4	6	8	17	28
35–49	182	4.9	20	2	2	4	6	8	11	28
50–64	477	5.8	23	2	3	4	8	11	14	26
65+	1,902	5.9	20	2	3	5	7	11	15	24
B. Operated										
0–19 Years	0									
20–34	1	16.0	0	16	16	16	16	16	16	16
35–49	15	10.5	93	2	5	9	11	32	33	33
50–64	34	12.6	72	3	6	12	16	26	29	32
65+	126	11.3	56	4	6	10	15	24	27	41
SUBTOTALS:										
1. SINGLE DX										
A. Not Operated	0									
B. Operated	0									
2. MULTIPLE DX										
A. Not Operated	2,585	5.8	20	2	3	5	7	11	14	24
B. Operated	176	11.5	61	4	6	10	15	25	29	41
1. SINGLE DX	0									
2. MULTIPLE DX	2,761	6.2	25	2	3	5	8	12	16	26
A. NOT OPERATED	2,585	5.8	20	2	3	5	7	11	14	24
B. OPERATED	176	11.5	61	4	6	10	15	25	29	41
TOTAL										
0–19 Years	1	6.0	0	6	6	6	6	6	6	6
20–34	24	6.3	36	2	3	4	6	16	17	28
35–49	197	5.3	27	2	3	4	6	10	14	33
50–64	511	6.2	29	2	3	4	8	12	17	27
65+	2,028	6.2	24	2	3	5	8	12	16	26
GRAND TOTAL	2,761	6.2	25	2	3	5	8	12	16	26

Percentiles

Length of Stay by Diagnosis and Operation, Western Region, 2008

Western Region, October 2006–September 2007 Data, by Diagnosis

404.92: HTN HRT&CKD V-ESRD S HF

Type of Patients	Observed Patients	Avg. Stay	Variance	10th	25th	50th	75th	90th	95th	99th
1. SINGLE DX										
A. Not Operated										
0–19 Years	0									
20–34	0									
35–49	0									
50–64	0									
65+	0									
B. Operated										
0–19 Years	0									
20–34	0									
35–49	0									
50–64	0									
65+	0									
2. MULTIPLE DX										
A. Not Operated										
0–19 Years	3	2.0	1	1	1	2	3	3	3	3
20–34	13	4.7	37	1	1	3	4	10	23	23
35–49	32	4.2	18	1	2	3	4	10	15	20
50–64	53	4.8	12	1	2	4	7	10	12	16
65+	61	5.2	21	2	2	4	7	10	14	23
B. Operated										
0–19 Years	1	16.0	0	16	16	16	16	16	16	16
20–34	4	4.2	6	1	1	4	6	6	6	6
35–49	7	14.4	347	1	2	7	20	54	54	54
50–64	18	8.7	48	3	4	6	10	17	31	31
65+	19	8.7	47	1	3	7	13	16	29	29
SUBTOTALS:										
1. SINGLE DX										
A. Not Operated	0									
B. Operated	0									
2. MULTIPLE DX										
A. Not Operated	162	4.8	18	1	2	4	6	10	12	23
B. Operated	49	9.3	85	1	4	7	12	17	29	54
1. SINGLE DX	0									
2. MULTIPLE DX	211	5.8	37	1	2	4	8	12	16	29
A. NOT OPERATED	162	4.8	18	1	2	4	6	10	12	23
B. OPERATED	49	9.3	85	1	4	7	12	17	29	54
TOTAL										
0–19 Years	4	5.5	50	1	1	3	16	16	16	16
20–34	17	4.6	29	1	1	3	6	10	23	23
35–49	39	6.0	85	1	2	3	6	15	20	54
50–64	71	5.8	24	1	3	4	8	11	12	31
65+	80	6.0	29	2	2	4	8	14	15	29
GRAND TOTAL	211	5.8	37	1	2	4	8	12	16	29

404.93: HTN HRT&CKD V-ESRD W HF

Type of Patients	Observed Patients	Avg. Stay	Variance	10th	25th	50th	75th	90th	95th	99th
1. SINGLE DX										
A. Not Operated										
0–19 Years	0									
20–34	0									
35–49	0									
50–64	0									
65+	0									
B. Operated										
0–19 Years	0									
20–34	0									
35–49	0									
50–64	0									
65+	0									
2. MULTIPLE DX										
A. Not Operated										
0–19 Years	6	4.2	5	1	2	6	6	6	6	6
20–34	45	4.8	25	2	2	3	5	7	11	30
35–49	141	4.9	19	1	2	3	6	10	14	18
50–64	377	5.1	18	1	2	4	6	11	15	20
65+	668	6.2	31	2	3	5	8	12	16	29
B. Operated										
0–19 Years	0									
20–34	3	5.7	17	1	1	7	9	9	9	9
35–49	17	9.2	58	1	5	7	12	19	30	30
50–64	61	11.0	82	3	5	8	15	20	30	47
65+	113	10.9	57	3	6	9	14	20	29	39
SUBTOTALS:										
1. SINGLE DX										
A. Not Operated	0									
B. Operated	0									
2. MULTIPLE DX										
A. Not Operated	1,237	5.6	26	1	2	4	7	11	15	27
B. Operated	194	10.7	64	2	6	9	14	20	30	39
1. SINGLE DX	0									
2. MULTIPLE DX	1,431	6.3	34	2	3	4	8	13	17	30
A. NOT OPERATED	1,237	5.6	26	1	2	4	7	11	15	27
B. OPERATED	194	10.7	64	2	6	9	14	20	30	39
TOTAL										
0–19 Years	6	4.2	5	1	2	6	6	6	6	6
20–34	48	4.9	24	1	2	3	6	9	11	30
35–49	158	5.3	25	1	2	4	7	12	16	29
50–64	438	5.9	31	1	2	4	8	13	17	26
65+	781	6.9	37	2	3	5	9	14	18	31
GRAND TOTAL	1,431	6.3	34	2	3	4	8	13	17	30

405: SECONDARY HYPERTENSION

Type of Patients	Observed Patients	Avg. Stay	Variance	10th	25th	50th	75th	90th	95th	99th
1. SINGLE DX										
A. Not Operated										
0–19 Years	0									
20–34	1	2.0	0	2	2	2	2	2	2	2
35–49	1	3.0	0	3	3	3	3	3	3	3
50–64	1	2.0	0	2	2	2	2	2	2	2
65+	1	1.0	0	1	1	1	1	1	1	1
B. Operated										
0–19 Years	0									
20–34	0									
35–49	0									
50–64	1	1.0	0	1	1	1	1	1	1	1
65+	0									
2. MULTIPLE DX										
A. Not Operated										
0–19 Years	7	2.6	4	1	1	2	4	6	6	6
20–34	10	2.6	3	1	2	2	4	6	6	6
35–49	9	2.3	1	1	2	2	3	4	4	4
50–64	19	3.4	6	1	2	3	4	7	11	11
65+	42	3.1	4	1	2	3	5	6	7	8
B. Operated										
0–19 Years	3	2.0	<1	1	1	2	2	3	3	3
20–34	4	4.0	0	4	4	4	4	4	4	4
35–49	3	3.0	7	1	1	2	6	6	6	6
50–64	15	2.8	5	1	1	2	5	5	9	9
65+	35	4.2	40	1	1	2	4	12	14	34
SUBTOTALS:										
1. SINGLE DX										
A. Not Operated	4	2.0	<1	1	2	2	3	3	3	3
B. Operated	1	1.0	0	1	1	1	1	1	1	1
2. MULTIPLE DX										
A. Not Operated	87	3.0	4	1	2	2	4	6	7	11
B. Operated	57	3.6	27	1	1	2	4	9	12	34
1. SINGLE DX	5	1.8	<1	1	1	2	2	3	3	3
2. MULTIPLE DX	144	3.3	13	1	1	2	4	6	8	14
A. NOT OPERATED	91	3.0	4	1	2	2	4	6	7	11
B. OPERATED	58	3.6	26	1	1	2	4	9	12	34
TOTAL										
0–19 Years	10	2.4	3	1	1	2	3	4	6	6
20–34	12	2.7	2	1	1	2	4	4	6	6
35–49	13	2.5	2	2	2	2	3	4	6	6
50–64	36	3.1	6	1	2	3	4	6	9	11
65+	78	3.6	20	1	2	3	4	7	12	34
GRAND TOTAL	149	3.2	13	1	1	2	4	6	8	14

Length of Stay by Diagnosis and Operation, Western Region, 2008

410: AMI

Type of Patients	Observed Patients	Avg. Stay	Variance	10th	25th	50th	75th	90th	95th	99th
1. SINGLE DX										
A. *Not Operated*										
0–19 Years	2	1.5	<1	1	1	2	2	2	2	2
20–34	7	1.7	<1	1	1	2	2	3	3	3
35–49	18	2.0	2	1	1	1	2	5	6	6
50–64	29	2.7	3	1	1	2	4	5	6	7
65+	14	2.4	3	1	1	2	4	4	6	6
B. *Operated*										
0–19 Years	0									
20–34	1	4.0	0	4	4	4	4	4	4	4
35–49	17	2.8	3	2	2	2	3	5	8	8
50–64	36	2.5	2	1	2	2	3	4	4	9
65+	14	2.4	2	1	2	2	3	3	6	6
2. MULTIPLE DX										
A. *Not Operated*										
0–19 Years	22	3.5	23	1	1	2	3	4	17	19
20–34	206	3.2	9	1	2	2	4	5	8	17
35–49	1,531	3.4	8	1	2	3	4	6	8	13
50–64	4,904	4.2	18	1	2	3	5	8	11	21
65+	19,561	5.0	14	2	3	4	6	9	12	19
B. *Operated*										
0–19 Years	2	3.0	2	2	2	4	4	4	4	4
20–34	237	3.6	7	2	2	3	4	6	8	18
35–49	4,483	3.8	16	2	2	3	4	7	10	21
50–64	13,840	4.6	25	2	2	3	5	9	13	26
65+	15,546	6.0	34	2	2	4	8	13	17	29
SUBTOTALS:										
1. SINGLE DX										
A. *Not Operated*	70	2.3	2	1	1	2	3	5	6	7
B. *Operated*	68	2.6	2	1	2	2	3	4	6	9
2. MULTIPLE DX										
A. *Not Operated*	26,224	4.7	15	2	2	4	6	9	12	20
B. *Operated*	34,108	5.2	29	2	2	3	6	11	15	27
1. SINGLE DX	138	2.4	2	1	1	2	3	5	6	8
2. MULTIPLE DX	60,332	5.0	23	2	2	3	6	10	13	24
A. NOT OPERATED	26,294	4.7	15	2	2	4	6	9	12	20
B. OPERATED	34,176	5.1	29	2	2	3	6	11	15	27
TOTAL										
0–19 Years	26	3.3	20	1	1	2	3	4	17	19
20–34	451	3.4	8	1	2	3	4	6	8	18
35–49	6,049	3.7	14	1	2	3	4	7	10	20
50–64	18,809	4.5	23	2	2	3	5	9	13	25
65+	35,135	5.5	23	2	3	4	7	11	14	25
GRAND TOTAL	60,470	5.0	23	2	2	3	6	10	13	24

410.01: ANTEROLAT AMI-INITIAL

Type of Patients	Observed Patients	Avg. Stay	Variance	10th	25th	50th	75th	90th	95th	99th
1. SINGLE DX										
A. *Not Operated*										
0–19 Years	0									
20–34	0									
35–49	1	2.0	0	2	2	2	2	2	2	2
50–64	0									
65+	0									
B. *Operated*										
0–19 Years	0									
20–34	0									
35–49	0									
50–64	2	2.5	<1	2	2	2	3	3	3	3
65+	0									
2. MULTIPLE DX										
A. *Not Operated*										
0–19 Years	0									
20–34	4	2.5	<1	2	2	3	3	3	3	3
35–49	40	3.1	2	1	2	3	4	5	6	7
50–64	74	5.1	62	2	2	3	5	8	15	66
65+	250	5.5	17	3	3	4	6	9	13	23
B. *Operated*										
0–19 Years	1	4.0	0	4	4	4	4	4	4	4
20–34	19	3.7	3	2	2	3	4	6	8	8
35–49	216	4.7	35	2	2	3	4	7	14	25
50–64	546	5.1	47	2	2	3	5	9	14	26
65+	497	6.5	43	2	3	4	8	13	19	43
SUBTOTALS:										
1. SINGLE DX										
A. *Not Operated*	1	2.0	0	2	2	2	2	2	2	2
B. *Operated*	2	2.5	<1	2	2	2	3	3	3	3
2. MULTIPLE DX										
A. *Not Operated*	368	5.1	25	2	3	4	6	9	13	23
B. *Operated*	1,279	5.5	43	2	3	4	6	11	15	37
1. SINGLE DX	3	2.3	<1	2	2	2	3	3	3	3
2. MULTIPLE DX	1,647	5.5	39	2	3	4	6	10	13	30
A. NOT OPERATED	369	5.1	25	2	3	4	6	9	13	23
B. OPERATED	1,281	5.5	43	2	3	4	6	11	15	37
TOTAL										
0–19 Years	1	4.0	0	4	4	4	4	4	4	4
20–34	23	3.5	3	2	2	3	4	5	6	8
35–49	257	4.5	30	2	2	3	4	7	10	25
50–64	622	5.1	48	2	2	3	5	9	14	26
65+	747	6.2	35	2	3	4	7	12	16	33
GRAND TOTAL	1,650	5.4	39	2	3	4	6	10	15	30

410.11: ANT AMI NEC-INITIAL

Type of Patients	Observed Patients	Avg. Stay	Variance	10th	25th	50th	75th	90th	95th	99th
1. SINGLE DX										
A. *Not Operated*										
0–19 Years	0									
20–34	2	2.0	2	1	1	1	3	3	3	3
35–49	1	1.0	0	1	1	1	1	1	1	1
50–64	4	4.0	<1	3	3	4	4	5	5	5
65+	0									
B. *Operated*										
0–19 Years	0									
20–34	0									
35–49	7	3.6	5	2	2	3	5	8	8	8
50–64	8	2.6	<1	2	2	3	3	4	4	4
65+	9	2.8	2	1	2	3	3	6	6	6
2. MULTIPLE DX										
A. *Not Operated*										
0–19 Years	2	11.0	128	3	3	11	19	19	19	19
20–34	5	3.0	7	2	2	3	3	5	5	5
35–49	111	3.6	7	1	2	3	4	8	9	12
50–64	322	4.6	14	1	2	3	6	9	12	19
65+	994	5.4	14	2	3	4	7	10	12	20
B. *Operated*										
0–19 Years	0									
20–34	58	4.2	10	2	2	3	5	8	9	20
35–49	899	4.3	19	2	2	3	4	8	11	23
50–64	2,434	4.7	25	2	2	3	5	9	12	27
65+	2,230	6.0	31	2	3	4	7	12	17	28
SUBTOTALS:										
1. SINGLE DX										
A. *Not Operated*	7	3.0	2	1	1	3	4	5	5	5
B. *Operated*	24	3.0	2	2	2	3	3	5	6	8
2. MULTIPLE DX										
A. *Not Operated*	1,434	5.1	14	2	3	4	7	9	12	19
B. *Operated*	5,621	5.1	27	2	2	3	6	10	14	27
1. SINGLE DX	31	3.0	2	2	2	3	3	5	6	8
2. MULTIPLE DX	7,055	5.1	24	2	2	4	6	10	14	25
A. NOT OPERATED	1,441	5.1	13	2	3	4	6	9	12	19
B. OPERATED	5,645	5.1	27	2	2	3	6	10	14	27
TOTAL										
0–19 Years	2	11.0	128	3	3	11	19	19	19	19
20–34	65	4.0	9	2	2	3	5	8	8	20
35–49	1,018	4.2	17	2	2	3	4	8	11	22
50–64	2,768	4.7	24	2	2	3	5	9	12	25
65+	3,233	5.8	26	2	3	4	7	11	15	26
GRAND TOTAL	7,086	5.1	24	2	2	4	6	10	14	25

Length of Stay by Diagnosis and Operation, Western Region, 2008

Western Region, October 2006–September 2007 Data, by Diagnosis

410.21: INFEROLAT AMI-INITIAL

Type of Patients	Observed Patients	Avg. Stay	Variance	10th	25th	50th	75th	90th	95th	99th
1. SINGLE DX										
A. Not Operated										
0–19 Years	0									
20–34	0									
35–49	0									
50–64	1	3.0	0	3	3	3	3	3	3	3
65+	0									
B. Operated										
0–19 Years	0									
20–34	0									
35–49	0									
50–64	2	3.0	2	2	2	2	4	4	4	4
65+	1	2.0	0	2	2	2	2	2	2	2
2. MULTIPLE DX										
A. Not Operated										
0–19 Years	2	9.0	125	1	1	17	17	17	17	17
20–34	9	2.2	2	1	2	2	3	3	5	5
35–49	31	4.8	21	2	2	3	6	11	16	21
50–64	75	4.5	21	2	2	3	5	10	13	27
65+	184	4.7	14	2	3	4	5	8	10	26
B. Operated										
0–19 Years	0									
20–34	7	3.4	7	1	2	2	6	8	8	8
35–49	191	4.0	24	2	2	3	4	7	9	30
50–64	503	4.2	20	2	2	3	4	8	11	19
65+	477	5.0	24	2	2	3	6	10	14	27
SUBTOTALS:										
1. SINGLE DX										
A. Not Operated	1	3.0	0	3	3	3	3	3	3	3
B. Operated	3	2.7	1	2	2	2	2	4	4	4
2. MULTIPLE DX										
A. Not Operated	301	4.6	16	2	2	3	5	9	12	24
B. Operated	1,178	4.5	22	2	2	3	5	9	12	25
1. SINGLE DX	4	2.8	<1	2	2	2	3	4	4	4
2. MULTIPLE DX	1,479	4.5	21	2	2	3	5	9	12	25
A. NOT OPERATED	302	4.6	16	2	2	3	5	9	12	24
B. OPERATED	1,181	4.5	22	2	2	3	5	9	12	25
TOTAL										
0–19 Years	2	9.0	125	1	1	17	17	17	17	17
20–34	16	2.8	4	1	2	2	3	6	8	8
35–49	222	4.1	23	2	2	3	4	7	10	21
50–64	581	4.2	20	2	2	3	5	9	12	24
65+	662	5.0	21	2	2	3	6	10	13	27
GRAND TOTAL	1,483	4.5	21	2	2	3	5	9	12	25

410.31: INFEROPOST AMI-INITIAL

Type of Patients	Observed Patients	Avg. Stay	Variance	10th	25th	50th	75th	90th	95th	99th
1. SINGLE DX										
A. Not Operated										
0–19 Years	0									
20–34	0									
35–49	0									
50–64	1	3.0	0	3	3	3	3	3	3	3
65+	0									
B. Operated										
0–19 Years	0									
20–34	0									
35–49	0									
50–64	1	1.0	0	1	1	1	1	1	1	1
65+	0									
2. MULTIPLE DX										
A. Not Operated										
0–19 Years	0									
20–34	0									
35–49	15	3.9	8	2	2	3	5	8	12	12
50–64	43	4.7	20	1	2	3	5	11	14	21
65+	87	5.6	10	3	3	5	7	10	13	17
B. Operated										
0–19 Years	0									
20–34	5	4.2	5	2	3	3	6	7	7	7
35–49	133	3.9	16	2	2	3	4	7	11	26
50–64	394	4.5	28	2	2	3	4	9	13	30
65+	328	5.7	44	2	3	4	6	11	16	30
SUBTOTALS:										
1. SINGLE DX										
A. Not Operated	1	3.0	0	3	3	3	3	3	3	3
B. Operated	1	1.0	0	1	1	1	1	1	1	1
2. MULTIPLE DX										
A. Not Operated	145	5.2	13	2	3	4	6	10	13	18
B. Operated	860	4.9	32	2	2	3	5	10	14	30
1. SINGLE DX	2	2.0	2	1	1	2	3	3	3	3
2. MULTIPLE DX	1,005	4.9	30	2	2	3	5	10	14	26
A. NOT OPERATED	146	5.1	13	2	3	4	6	10	13	18
B. OPERATED	861	4.9	32	2	2	3	5	10	14	30
TOTAL										
0–19 Years	0									
20–34	5	4.2	5	2	2	3	6	7	7	7
35–49	148	3.9	15	2	2	3	4	7	11	26
50–64	439	4.5	27	2	2	3	4	9	13	27
65+	415	5.7	37	2	3	4	7	11	15	26
GRAND TOTAL	1,007	4.9	29	2	2	3	5	10	14	26

410.41: INF AMI NEC-INITIAL

Type of Patients	Observed Patients	Avg. Stay	Variance	10th	25th	50th	75th	90th	95th	99th
1. SINGLE DX										
A. Not Operated										
0–19 Years	1	2.0	0	2	2	2	2	2	2	2
20–34	1	2.0	0	2	2	2	2	2	2	2
35–49	4	3.3	7	1	1	3	6	6	6	6
50–64	3	3.3	2	2	2	3	3	5	5	5
65+	0									
B. Operated										
0–19 Years	0									
20–34	0									
35–49	5	1.8	<1	1	2	2	2	2	2	2
50–64	9	2.1	<1	1	2	2	3	3	3	3
65+	2	1.5	<1	1	1	1	2	2	2	2
2. MULTIPLE DX										
A. Not Operated										
0–19 Years	4	1.5	1	1	1	1	3	3	3	3
20–34	19	3.6	15	1	1	3	4	10	17	17
35–49	151	3.4	6	1	2	3	4	6	8	13
50–64	387	3.8	15	1	2	3	4	7	10	22
65+	890	4.8	12	2	3	4	6	9	11	18
B. Operated										
0–19 Years	0									
20–34	60	3.1	2	2	2	3	3	5	7	8
35–49	1,118	3.2	8	2	2	3	3	5	7	14
50–64	3,384	4.0	18	2	2	3	4	7	11	22
65+	2,932	5.1	24	2	2	3	6	10	15	26
SUBTOTALS:										
1. SINGLE DX										
A. Not Operated	9	3.0	4	1	2	2	5	6	6	6
B. Operated	16	1.9	<1	1	1	2	2	3	3	3
2. MULTIPLE DX										
A. Not Operated	1,451	4.4	12	2	2	3	5	8	11	19
B. Operated	7,494	4.3	19	2	2	3	5	8	12	23
1. SINGLE DX	25	2.3	2	1	2	2	3	5	5	6
2. MULTIPLE DX	8,945	4.3	18	2	2	3	5	8	12	22
A. NOT OPERATED	1,460	4.4	12	2	2	3	5	8	11	19
B. OPERATED	7,510	4.3	19	2	2	3	5	8	12	23
TOTAL										
0–19 Years	5	1.6	<1	1	1	1	2	3	3	3
20–34	80	3.2	5	1	2	3	3	5	7	17
35–49	1,278	3.2	8	2	2	3	3	5	8	14
50–64	3,783	3.9	17	2	2	3	4	7	11	22
65+	3,824	5.0	21	2	2	3	6	10	14	24
GRAND TOTAL	8,970	4.3	18	2	2	3	5	8	12	22

410.51: LAT AMI NEC-INITIAL

Type of Patients	Observed Patients	Avg. Stay	Vari-ance	Percentiles 10th	25th	50th	75th	90th	95th	99th
1. SINGLE DX										
A. Not Operated										
0–19 Years	0									
20–34	0									
35–49	0									
50–64	1	5.0	0	5	5	5	5	5	5	5
65+	0									
B. Operated										
0–19 Years	0									
20–34	0									
35–49	0									
50–64	0									
65+	0									
2. MULTIPLE DX										
A. Not Operated										
0–19 Years	0									
20–34	5	2.0	<1	1	2	2	2	3	3	3
35–49	17	2.7	2	1	2	2	4	5	6	6
50–64	62	3.5	5	2	2	3	4	5	8	12
65+	166	5.0	16	2	3	4	6	10	13	19
B. Operated										
0–19 Years	0									
20–34	7	3.4	4	1	2	3	4	7	7	7
35–49	123	3.1	6	2	2	2	3	5	7	11
50–64	275	4.2	25	2	2	3	4	8	12	42
65+	324	5.4	22	2	2	4	6	11	14	23
SUBTOTALS:										
1. SINGLE DX										
A. Not Operated	1	5.0	0	5	5	5	5	5	5	5
B. Operated	0									
2. MULTIPLE DX										
A. Not Operated	250	4.4	13	2	2	4	5	8	11	17
B. Operated	729	4.6	21	2	2	3	5	9	13	23
1. SINGLE DX	**1**	**5.0**	**0**	**5**	**5**	**5**	**5**	**5**	**5**	**5**
2. MULTIPLE DX	**979**	**4.5**	**19**	**2**	**2**	**3**	**5**	**9**	**12**	**23**
A. NOT OPERATED	**251**	**4.4**	**13**	**2**	**2**	**4**	**5**	**8**	**11**	**17**
B. OPERATED	**729**	**4.6**	**21**	**2**	**2**	**3**	**5**	**9**	**13**	**23**
TOTAL										
0–19 Years	0									
20–34	12	2.8	3	1	2	3	3	4	7	7
35–49	140	3.1	5	2	2	2	3	5	6	11
50–64	338	4.1	21	2	2	3	4	8	11	37
65+	490	5.3	20	2	3	4	6	11	14	23
GRAND TOTAL	**980**	**4.5**	**19**	**2**	**2**	**3**	**5**	**9**	**12**	**23**

410.61: POSTERIOR AMI-INITIAL

Type of Patients	Observed Patients	Avg. Stay	Vari-ance	Percentiles 10th	25th	50th	75th	90th	95th	99th
1. SINGLE DX										
A. Not Operated										
0–19 Years	0									
20–34	1	2.0	0	2	2	2	2	2	2	2
35–49	0									
50–64	1	6.0	0	6	6	6	6	6	6	6
65+	0									
B. Operated										
0–19 Years	0									
20–34	0									
35–49	1	5.0	0	5	5	5	5	5	5	5
50–64	1	2.0	0	2	2	2	2	2	2	2
65+	0									
2. MULTIPLE DX										
A. Not Operated										
0–19 Years	0									
20–34	0									
35–49	1	7.0	0	7	7	7	7	7	7	7
50–64	9	3.7	13	1	2	2	3	12	12	12
65+	38	5.6	10	3	3	5	8	9	14	16
B. Operated										
0–19 Years	0									
20–34	1	3.0	0	3	3	3	3	3	3	3
35–49	31	3.0	9	1	2	2	3	4	11	15
50–64	75	4.5	16	2	2	3	5	10	14	21
65+	86	5.8	42	2	2	4	7	10	18	45
SUBTOTALS:										
1. SINGLE DX										
A. Not Operated	2	4.0	8	2	2	6	6	6	6	6
B. Operated	2	3.5	4	2	2	5	5	5	5	5
2. MULTIPLE DX										
A. Not Operated	48	5.3	11	2	3	4	7	9	12	16
B. Operated	193	4.8	27	2	2	3	6	10	15	29
1. SINGLE DX	**4**	**3.8**	**4**	**2**	**2**	**5**	**6**	**6**	**6**	**6**
2. MULTIPLE DX	**241**	**4.9**	**24**	**2**	**2**	**3**	**6**	**10**	**14**	**23**
A. NOT OPERATED	**50**	**5.2**	**11**	**2**	**3**	**4**	**7**	**9**	**12**	**16**
B. OPERATED	**195**	**4.8**	**27**	**2**	**2**	**3**	**6**	**10**	**15**	**29**
TOTAL										
0–19 Years	0									
20–34	2	2.5	<1	2	2	3	3	3	3	3
35–49	33	3.2	9	1	2	2	3	7	11	15
50–64	86	4.4	16	2	2	3	5	10	12	21
65+	124	5.7	32	2	3	4	7	10	15	29
GRAND TOTAL	**245**	**4.9**	**24**	**2**	**2**	**3**	**6**	**10**	**14**	**23**

410.71: SUBEND INFARCT-INITIAL

Type of Patients	Observed Patients	Avg. Stay	Vari-ance	Percentiles 10th	25th	50th	75th	90th	95th	99th
1. SINGLE DX										
A. Not Operated										
0–19 Years	0									
20–34	1	2.0	0	2	2	2	2	2	2	2
35–49	8	1.8	1	1	1	2	2	4	4	4
50–64	14	1.8	3	1	1	1	2	4	7	7
65+	10	2.6	3	1	1	2	4	6	6	6
B. Operated										
0–19 Years	0									
20–34	1	4.0	0	4	4	4	4	4	4	4
35–49	3	2.3	<1	2	2	2	3	3	3	3
50–64	7	3.3	9	1	1	2	6	9	9	9
65+	2	2.0	0	2	2	2	2	2	2	2
2. MULTIPLE DX										
A. Not Operated										
0–19 Years	8	2.0	<1	1	2	2	2	3	3	3
20–34	131	3.1	5	1	2	2	4	5	7	13
35–49	1,021	3.3	9	1	2	3	4	6	8	13
50–64	3,495	4.3	18	1	2	3	5	8	11	21
65+	14,974	5.0	15	2	3	4	6	9	12	20
B. Operated										
0–19 Years	0									
20–34	66	3.5	9	2	2	3	4	6	8	19
35–49	1,561	3.9	17	1	2	3	4	8	11	22
50–64	5,539	5.0	28	1	2	3	6	10	14	27
65+	7,834	6.5	38	2	2	4	9	14	18	30
SUBTOTALS:										
1. SINGLE DX										
A. Not Operated	33	2.0	2	1	1	1	2	4	6	7
B. Operated	13	2.9	5	1	2	2	3	6	9	9
2. MULTIPLE DX										
A. Not Operated	19,629	4.8	15	2	2	4	6	9	12	20
B. Operated	15,000	5.6	33	2	2	3	7	12	16	28
1. SINGLE DX	**46**	**2.3**	**3**	**1**	**1**	**2**	**2**	**4**	**6**	**9**
2. MULTIPLE DX	**34,629**	**5.1**	**23**	**2**	**2**	**4**	**6**	**10**	**14**	**24**
A. NOT OPERATED	**19,662**	**4.8**	**15**	**2**	**2**	**4**	**6**	**9**	**12**	**20**
B. OPERATED	**15,013**	**5.6**	**33**	**2**	**2**	**3**	**7**	**12**	**16**	**28**
TOTAL										
0–19 Years	8	2.0	<1	1	2	2	2	3	3	3
20–34	199	3.3	6	1	2	3	4	6	8	14
35–49	2,593	3.7	14	1	2	3	4	7	10	21
50–64	9,055	4.7	24	1	2	3	6	10	13	25
65+	22,820	5.5	23	2	3	4	7	11	14	24
GRAND TOTAL	**34,675**	**5.1**	**23**	**2**	**2**	**4**	**6**	**10**	**14**	**24**

Western Region, October 2006–September 2007 Data, by Diagnosis

410.72: SUBEND INFARCT-SUBSQ

Type of Patients	Observed Patients	Avg. Stay	Variance	10th	25th	50th	75th	90th	95th	99th
1. SINGLE DX										
A. Not Operated										
0–19 Years	0									
20–34	0									
35–49	0									
50–64	0									
65+	1	1.0	0	1	1	1	1	1	1	1
B. Operated										
0–19 Years	0									
20–34	0									
35–49	0									
50–64	0									
65+	0									
2. MULTIPLE DX										
A. Not Operated										
0–19 Years	1	1.0	0	1	1	1	1	1	1	1
20–34	2	2.0	0	1	1	1	1	1	1	1
35–49	14	3.3	9	1	2	2	4	5	13	13
50–64	47	2.5	2	1	1	2	3	5	5	7
65+	97	4.1	17	1	2	3	5	8	11	30
B. Operated										
0–19 Years	0									
20–34	2									
35–49	6	13.9	395	2	2	3	18	53	53	53
50–64	39	4.3	18	1	1	3	6	9	15	20
65+	57	4.2	46	1	1	2	5	11	12	48
SUBTOTALS:										
1. SINGLE DX										
A. Not Operated	1	1.0	0	1	1	1	1	1	1	1
B. Operated	0									
2. MULTIPLE DX										
A. Not Operated	161	3.5	12	1	2	3	4	7	9	20
B. Operated	102	4.8	57	1	1	2	6	11	13	48
1. SINGLE DX	1	1.0	0	1	1	1	1	1	1	1
2. MULTIPLE DX	263	4.0	30	1	1	3	5	8	12	30
A. NOT OPERATED	162	3.5	12	1	2	3	4	7	9	20
B. OPERATED	102	4.8	57	1	1	2	6	11	13	48
TOTAL										
0–19 Years	1	1.0	0	1	1	1	1	1	1	1
20–34	2	2.0	0	1	1	1	1	1	1	1
35–49	20	6.5	136	2	2	3	5	13	18	53
50–64	86	3.3	10	1	1	2	4	7	9	20
65+	155	4.1	27	1	2	3	5	8	12	30
GRAND TOTAL	264	4.0	30	1	1	3	5	8	12	30

410.81: AMI NEC-INITIAL EPISODE

Type of Patients	Observed Patients	Avg. Stay	Variance	10th	25th	50th	75th	90th	95th	99th
1. SINGLE DX										
A. Not Operated										
0–19 Years	0									
20–34	0									
35–49	0									
50–64	2	2.0	0	2	2	2	2	2	2	2
65+	0									
B. Operated										
0–19 Years	0									
20–34	0									
35–49	0									
50–64	3	1.7	<1	1	1	2	2	2	2	2
65+	0									
2. MULTIPLE DX										
A. Not Operated										
0–19 Years	1	3.0	0	3	3	3	3	3	3	3
20–34	10	2.4	<1	1	2	2	3	4	4	4
35–49	34	3.1	7	1	2	2	3	7	10	13
50–64	80	4.7	35	1	2	3	5	8	15	40
65+	383	4.7	9	2	3	4	6	8	11	16
B. Operated										
0–19 Years	1	2.0	0	2	2	2	2	2	2	2
20–34	2	7.0	31	3	3	7	11	11	11	11
35–49	55	4.8	18	2	2	3	6	10	15	23
50–64	166	5.0	22	1	2	3	7	12	15	26
65+	210	6.8	34	2	3	5	9	15	18	30
SUBTOTALS:										
1. SINGLE DX										
A. Not Operated	2	2.0	0	2	2	2	2	2	2	2
B. Operated	3	1.7	<1	1	1	2	2	2	2	2
2. MULTIPLE DX										
A. Not Operated	508	4.6	13	2	2	4	6	8	11	17
B. Operated	434	5.8	28	2	2	4	8	13	17	27
1. SINGLE DX	5	1.8	<1	1	2	2	2	2	2	2
2. MULTIPLE DX	942	5.2	20	2	2	4	7	11	14	24
A. NOT OPERATED	510	4.5	13	2	2	4	6	8	11	17
B. OPERATED	437	5.8	28	2	2	4	8	13	17	27
TOTAL										
0–19 Years	2	2.5	<1	2	2	3	3	3	3	3
20–34	12	3.2	7	1	2	3	3	4	11	11
35–49	89	4.2	15	1	2	3	5	7	13	23
50–64	251	4.9	26	1	2	3	6	12	15	29
65+	593	5.4	19	2	3	4	7	10	13	24
GRAND TOTAL	947	5.1	20	2	2	4	7	11	14	24

410.91: AMI NOS-INITIAL EPISODE

Type of Patients	Observed Patients	Avg. Stay	Variance	10th	25th	50th	75th	90th	95th	99th
1. SINGLE DX										
A. Not Operated										
0–19 Years	0									
20–34	2	1.0	0	1	1	1	1	1	1	1
35–49	3	1.7	<1	1	2	2	2	2	2	2
50–64	1	2.0	0	2	2	2	2	2	2	2
65+	1	4.0	0	4	4	4	4	4	4	4
B. Operated										
0–19 Years	0									
20–34	0									
35–49	0									
50–64	3	2.7	<1	2	2	3	3	3	3	3
65+	0									
2. MULTIPLE DX										
A. Not Operated										
0–19 Years	4	2.5	2	1	1	2	4	4	4	4
20–34	21	4.5	35	1	1	2	4	9	19	23
35–49	76	3.2	7	1	2	3	4	6	7	16
50–64	223	4.6	20	1	2	3	6	9	14	24
65+	1,370	4.6	11	2	2	4	6	8	10	16
B. Operated										
0–19 Years	0									
20–34	8	5.0	29	1	3	4	4	18	18	18
35–49	129	3.7	7	2	2	3	5	8	9	12
50–64	402	5.2	27	2	2	3	7	10	14	26
65+	510	6.8	46	2	3	5	9	14	19	28
SUBTOTALS:										
1. SINGLE DX										
A. Not Operated	7	1.9	1	1	1	2	2	4	4	4
B. Operated	3	2.7	<1	2	2	3	3	3	3	3
2. MULTIPLE DX										
A. Not Operated	1,694	4.6	12	1	2	4	6	8	10	18
B. Operated	1,049	5.8	35	2	2	4	7	12	16	27
1. SINGLE DX	10	2.1	<1	1	1	2	3	4	4	4
2. MULTIPLE DX	2,743	5.0	21	2	2	4	6	10	13	23
A. NOT OPERATED	1,701	4.6	12	1	2	4	6	8	10	18
B. OPERATED	1,052	5.8	35	2	2	4	7	12	16	27
TOTAL										
0–19 Years	4	2.5	2	1	1	2	4	4	4	4
20–34	31	4.4	31	1	1	3	4	9	19	23
35–49	208	3.5	7	1	2	3	4	7	9	12
50–64	629	5.0	24	1	2	3	6	10	14	26
65+	1,881	5.2	21	2	2	4	7	10	13	22
GRAND TOTAL	2,753	5.0	21	2	2	4	6	10	13	23

Length of Stay by Diagnosis and Operation, Western Region 2008

Western Region, October 2006–September 2007 Data, by Diagnosis

411: OTH AC ISCHEMIC HRT DIS

Type of Patients	Observed Patients	Avg. Stay	Vari-ance	10th	25th	50th	75th	90th	95th	99th
1. SINGLE DX										
A. Not Operated										
0–19 Years	0									
20–34	2	1.0	0	1	1	1	1	1	1	1
35–49	18	1.6	<1	1	1	1	2	3	3	3
50–64	15	1.5	<1	1	1	1	2	2	3	3
65+	13	1.6	<1	1	1	2	2	2	3	3
B. Operated										
0–19 Years	0									
20–34	0									
35–49	0									
50–64	1	1.0	0	1	1	1	1	1	1	1
65+	0									
2. MULTIPLE DX										
A. Not Operated										
0–19 Years	3	3.7	14	1	1	2	8	8	8	8
20–34	66	1.8	3	1	1	1	2	3	4	8
35–49	722	2.1	3	1	1	2	2	4	5	9
50–64	1,779	2.2	6	1	1	2	3	4	5	10
65+	2,028	2.4	4	1	1	2	3	5	6	9
B. Operated										
0–19 Years	0									
20–34	1	19.0	0	19	19	19	19	19	19	19
35–49	31	2.7	3	1	2	2	3	5	7	7
50–64	119	3.2	11	1	1	2	4	8	10	17
65+	134	3.8	13	1	1	2	5	9	11	16
SUBTOTALS:										
1. SINGLE DX										
A. Not Operated	48	1.5	<1	1	1	1	2	2	3	3
B. Operated	1	1.0	0	1	1	1	1	1	1	1
2. MULTIPLE DX										
A. Not Operated	4,598	2.3	5	1	1	2	3	4	5	9
B. Operated	285	3.5	12	1	1	2	4	8	10	19
1. SINGLE DX	49	1.5	<1	1	1	1	2	2	3	3
2. MULTIPLE DX	4,883	2.3	5	1	1	2	3	4	6	10
A. NOT OPERATED	4,646	2.3	4	1	1	2	3	4	5	9
B. OPERATED	286	3.5	12	1	1	2	4	8	10	19
TOTAL										
0–19 Years	3	3.7	14	1	1	2	8	8	8	8
20–34	69	2.0	6	1	1	1	2	3	4	19
35–49	771	2.1	3	1	1	2	2	4	5	9
50–64	1,914	2.2	7	1	1	2	3	4	6	10
65+	2,175	2.5	4	1	1	2	3	5	6	11
GRAND TOTAL	4,932	2.3	5	1	1	2	3	4	6	10

411.1: INTERMED CORONARY SYND

Type of Patients	Observed Patients	Avg. Stay	Vari-ance	10th	25th	50th	75th	90th	95th	99th
1. SINGLE DX										
A. Not Operated										
0–19 Years	0									
20–34	2	1.0	0	1	1	1	1	1	1	1
35–49	17	1.6	<1	1	1	1	1	3	3	3
50–64	15	1.5	<1	1	1	1	2	2	3	3
65+	13	1.6	<1	1	1	2	2	2	3	3
B. Operated										
0–19 Years	0									
20–34	0									
35–49	0									
50–64	1	1.0	0	1	1	1	1	1	1	1
65+	0									
2. MULTIPLE DX										
A. Not Operated										
0–19 Years	1	1.0	0	1	1	1	1	1	1	1
20–34	60	1.7	1	1	1	1	2	3	4	8
35–49	663	2.0	3	1	1	2	2	3	4	9
50–64	1,641	2.1	6	1	1	2	3	4	5	9
65+	1,825	2.3	3	1	1	2	3	4	5	8
B. Operated										
0–19 Years	0									
20–34	0									
35–49	22	2.7	2	1	2	2	3	5	6	7
50–64	90	3.2	10	1	1	2	4	7	10	19
65+	88	3.9	13	1	1	2	5	9	10	22
SUBTOTALS:										
1. SINGLE DX										
A. Not Operated	47	1.5	<1	1	1	1	2	2	3	3
B. Operated	1	1.0	0	1	1	1	1	1	1	1
2. MULTIPLE DX										
A. Not Operated	4,190	2.2	4	1	1	2	3	4	5	8
B. Operated	200	3.4	11	1	1	2	4	8	10	19
1. SINGLE DX	48	1.5	<1	1	1	1	2	2	3	3
2. MULTIPLE DX	4,390	2.2	4	1	1	2	3	4	5	9
A. NOT OPERATED	4,237	2.2	4	1	1	2	3	4	5	8
B. OPERATED	201	3.4	11	1	1	2	4	8	10	16
TOTAL										
0–19 Years	1	1.0	0	1	1	1	1	1	1	1
20–34	62	1.7	1	1	1	1	2	3	3	8
35–49	702	2.0	3	1	1	2	2	3	4	9
50–64	1,747	2.2	6	1	1	2	3	4	5	10
65+	1,926	2.4	3	1	1	2	3	4	6	9
GRAND TOTAL	4,438	2.2	4	1	1	2	3	4	5	9

411.89: AC ISCHEMIC HRT DIS-NEC

Type of Patients	Observed Patients	Avg. Stay	Vari-ance	10th	25th	50th	75th	90th	95th	99th
1. SINGLE DX										
A. Not Operated										
0–19 Years	0									
20–34	0									
35–49	1	1.0	0	1	1	1	1	1	1	1
50–64	0									
65+	0									
B. Operated										
0–19 Years	0									
20–34	0									
35–49	0									
50–64	0									
65+	0									
2. MULTIPLE DX										
A. Not Operated										
0–19 Years	2	5.0	18	2	2	2	8	8	8	8
20–34	4	2.3	2	1	2	2	2	4	4	4
35–49	32	3.1	14	1	1	3	4	4	6	22
50–64	62	3.2	23	1	1	2	4	7	8	36
65+	119	2.8	4	1	1	2	3	5	7	10
B. Operated										
0–19 Years	0									
20–34	0									
35–49	0									
50–64	7	1.1	<1	1	1	1	1	2	2	2
65+	14	3.1	7	1	1	2	5	7	9	9
SUBTOTALS:										
1. SINGLE DX										
A. Not Operated	1	1.0	0	1	1	1	1	1	1	1
B. Operated	0									
2. MULTIPLE DX										
A. Not Operated	219	2.9	11	1	1	2	4	5	8	10
B. Operated	21	2.4	5	1	1	1	2	6	7	9
1. SINGLE DX	1	1.0	0	1	1	1	1	1	1	1
2. MULTIPLE DX	240	2.9	10	1	1	2	4	5	7	10
A. NOT OPERATED	220	2.9	11	1	1	2	4	5	7	10
B. OPERATED	21	2.4	5	1	1	1	2	6	7	9
TOTAL										
0–19 Years	2	5.0	18	2	2	2	8	8	8	8
20–34	4	2.3	2	1	2	2	2	4	4	4
35–49	33	3.1	13	1	1	2	3	4	6	22
50–64	69	3.0	21	1	1	2	3	4	8	36
65+	133	2.8	4	1	1	2	3	5	7	10
GRAND TOTAL	241	2.9	10	1	1	2	3	5	7	10

Length of Stay by Diagnosis and Operation, Western Region, 2008

Western Region, October 2006–September 2007 Data, by Diagnosis

412: OLD MYOCARDIAL INFARCT

Type of Patients	Observed Patients	Avg. Stay	Vari-ance	Percentiles						
				10th	25th	50th	75th	90th	95th	99th
1. SINGLE DX										
A. Not Operated										
0–19 Years	0									
20–34	0									
35–49	0									
50–64	0									
65+	0									
B. Operated										
0–19 Years	0									
20–34	0									
35–49	0									
50–64	0									
65+	0									
2. MULTIPLE DX										
A. Not Operated										
0–19 Years	0									
20–34	0									
35–49	2	2.5	4	1	1	4	4	4	4	4
50–64	2	8.0	8	6	6	10	10	10	10	10
65+	1	5.0	0	5	5	5	5	5	5	5
B. Operated										
0–19 Years	0									
20–34	0									
35–49	0									
50–64	0									
65+	0									
SUBTOTALS:										
1. SINGLE DX A. Not Operated	0									
B. Operated	0									
2. MULTIPLE DX A. Not Operated	5	5.2	11	1	4	5	6	10	10	10
B. Operated	0									
1. SINGLE DX	0									
2. MULTIPLE DX	5	5.2	11	1	4	5	6	10	10	10
A. NOT OPERATED	5	5.2	11	1	4	5	6	10	10	10
B. OPERATED	0									
TOTAL										
0–19 Years	0									
20–34	0									
35–49	2	2.5	4	1	1	4	4	4	4	4
50–64	2	8.0	8	6	6	10	10	10	10	10
65+	1	5.0	0	5	5	5	5	5	5	5
GRAND TOTAL	5	5.2	11	1	4	5	6	10	10	10

413: ANGINA PECTORIS

Type of Patients	Observed Patients	Avg. Stay	Vari-ance	Percentiles						
				10th	25th	50th	75th	90th	95th	99th
1. SINGLE DX										
A. Not Operated										
0–19 Years	0									
20–34	1	1.0	0	1	1	1	1	1	1	1
35–49	10	1.7	<1	1	1	1	3	3	3	3
50–64	20	1.3	<1	1	1	1	1	2	2	3
65+	8	1.3	<1	1	1	1	2	2	2	2
B. Operated										
0–19 Years	0									
20–34	0									
35–49	0									
50–64	0									
65+	0									
2. MULTIPLE DX										
A. Not Operated										
0–19 Years	6	2.2	3	1	1	2	3	5	5	5
20–34	42	2.0	1	1	1	2	3	3	4	6
35–49	566	2.0	2	1	1	1	3	4	5	8
50–64	1,150	1.9	2	1	1	2	2	3	4	7
65+	1,379	2.1	2	1	1	2	3	4	5	8
B. Operated										
0–19 Years	0									
20–34	1	2.0	0	2	2	2	2	2	2	2
35–49	10	4.2	21	2	2	3	4	17	17	17
50–64	16	2.5	7	1	1	1	3	5	11	11
65+	27	2.9	14	1	1	2	3	7	8	18
SUBTOTALS:										
1. SINGLE DX A. Not Operated	39	1.4	<1	1	1	1	2	3	3	3
B. Operated	0									
2. MULTIPLE DX A. Not Operated	3,143	2.0	2	1	1	2	2	4	5	7
B. Operated	54	3.0	13	1	1	2	4	7	11	18
1. SINGLE DX	39	1.4	<1	1	1	1	2	3	3	3
2. MULTIPLE DX	3,197	2.0	2	1	1	2	2	4	5	8
A. NOT OPERATED	3,182	2.0	2	1	1	2	2	4	5	7
B. OPERATED	54	3.0	13	1	1	2	4	7	11	18
TOTAL										
0–19 Years	6	2.2	3	1	1	2	3	5	5	5
20–34	44	2.0	1	1	1	2	3	3	4	6
35–49	586	2.0	3	1	1	2	2	4	5	8
50–64	1,186	1.9	2	1	1	1	2	3	4	7
65+	1,414	2.1	2	1	1	2	3	4	5	8
GRAND TOTAL	3,236	2.0	2	1	1	2	2	4	5	8

413.1: PRINZMETAL ANGINA

Type of Patients	Observed Patients	Avg. Stay	Vari-ance	Percentiles						
				10th	25th	50th	75th	90th	95th	99th
1. SINGLE DX										
A. Not Operated										
0–19 Years	0									
20–34	0									
35–49	1	1.0	0	1	1	1	1	1	1	1
50–64	1	2.0	0	2	2	2	2	2	2	2
65+	0									
B. Operated										
0–19 Years	0									
20–34	0									
35–49	0									
50–64	0									
65+	0									
2. MULTIPLE DX										
A. Not Operated										
0–19 Years	5	2.4	3	1	1	2	3	5	5	5
20–34	21	1.9	2	1	1	1	2	3	3	6
35–49	119	2.3	3	1	1	2	3	4	6	8
50–64	146	1.9	2	1	1	2	2	4	4	7
65+	75	2.0	2	1	1	2	2	4	5	7
B. Operated										
0–19 Years	0									
20–34	0									
35–49	2	3.5	<1	3	3	4	4	4	4	4
50–64	1	4.0	0	4	4	4	4	4	4	4
65+	1	7.0	0	7	7	7	7	7	7	7
SUBTOTALS:										
1. SINGLE DX A. Not Operated	2	1.5	<1	1	1	1	2	2	2	2
B. Operated	0									
2. MULTIPLE DX A. Not Operated	366	2.1	2	1	1	2	2	4	5	7
B. Operated	4	4.5	3	3	3	4	4	7	7	7
1. SINGLE DX	2	1.5	<1	1	1	1	2	2	2	2
2. MULTIPLE DX	370	2.1	2	1	1	2	2	4	5	7
A. NOT OPERATED	368	2.1	2	1	1	2	2	4	5	7
B. OPERATED	4	4.5	3	3	3	4	4	7	7	7
TOTAL										
0–19 Years	5	2.4	3	1	1	2	3	5	5	5
20–34	21	1.9	2	1	1	1	2	3	3	6
35–49	122	2.3	3	1	1	2	3	4	6	8
50–64	148	2.0	2	1	1	2	2	4	4	7
65+	76	2.1	2	1	1	2	2	4	6	7
GRAND TOTAL	372	2.1	2	1	1	2	2	4	5	7

413.9: ANGINA PECTORIS NEC&NOS

Type of Patients	Observed Patients	Avg. Stay	Vari-ance	Percentiles 10th	25th	50th	75th	90th	95th	99th
1. SINGLE DX										
A. *Not Operated*										
0–19 Years	0									
20–34	1	1.0	0			1				1
35–49	9	1.8	<1	1	1	1	3	3	3	3
50–64	19	1.3	<1	1	1	1	1	2	3	3
65+	8	1.3	<1	1	1	1	2	2	2	2
B. *Operated*										
0–19 Years	0									
20–34	0									
35–49	0									
50–64	0									
65+	0									
2. MULTIPLE DX										
A. *Not Operated*										
0–19 Years	1	1.0	0			1				1
20–34	21	2.1	1	1	1	2	3	4	4	5
35–49	446	1.9	2	1	1	1	2	4	5	7
50–64	1,004	1.9	2	1	1	1	2	3	4	6
65+	1,303	2.1	2	1	1	2	3	4	5	8
B. *Operated*										
0–19 Years	0									
20–34	1	2.0	0	2	2	2	2	2	2	2
35–49	8	4.4	27	1	2	3	4	17	17	17
50–64	15	2.4	7	1	1	1	3	5	11	11
65+	26	2.7	14	1	1	1	3	7	8	18
SUBTOTALS:										
1. SINGLE DX										
A. *Not Operated*	37	1.4	<1	1	1	1	2		3	3
B. *Operated*	0									
2. MULTIPLE DX										
A. *Not Operated*	2,775	2.0	2	1	1	2	2	4	5	7
B. *Operated*	50	2.9	14	1	1	1	3	7	11	18
1. SINGLE DX	37	1.4	<1	1	1	1	2		3	3
2. MULTIPLE DX	2,825	2.0	2	1	1	2	2	4	5	8
A. NOT OPERATED	2,812	2.0	2	1	1	1	2	4	5	7
B. OPERATED	50	2.9	14	1	1	1	3	7	11	18
TOTAL										
0–19 Years	1	1.0	0	1	1	1	1	1	1	1
20–34	23	2.0	1	1	1	2	3	4	4	5
35–49	463	1.9	2	1	1	1	2	4	5	7
50–64	1,038	1.9	2	1	1	1	2	3	4	6
65+	1,337	2.1	2	1	1	2	3	4	5	8
GRAND TOTAL	2,862	2.0	2	1	1	1	2	4	5	8

414: OTH CHR ISCHEMIC HRT DIS

Type of Patients	Observed Patients	Avg. Stay	Vari-ance	Percentiles 10th	25th	50th	75th	90th	95th	99th
1. SINGLE DX										
A. *Not Operated*										
0–19 Years	0									
20–34	1	1.0	0	1	1	1	1	1	1	1
35–49	10	1.2	<1	1	1	1	1	2	2	2
50–64	36	1.1	<1	1	1	1	1	2	2	3
65+	36	1.4	<1	1	1	1	3	3	3	5
B. *Operated*										
0–19 Years	0									
20–34	2	3.5	12	1	1	1	6	6	6	6
35–49	68	1.2	<1	1	1	1	1	2	3	4
50–64	277	1.2	<1	1	1	1	1	1	2	5
65+	389	1.3	2	1	1	1	2	2	3	7
2. MULTIPLE DX										
A. *Not Operated*										
0–19 Years	2	3.0	2	2	2	2	4	4	4	4
20–34	116	2.2	3	1	1	2	3	4	6	8
35–49	2,669	2.4	4	1	1	2	3	4	6	10
50–64	9,740	2.5	5	1	1	2	3	5	6	11
65+	17,489	2.7	5	1	1	2	3	5	6	11
B. *Operated*										
0–19 Years	1	4.0	0	4	4	4	4	4	4	4
20–34	110	3.5	15	1	1	2	5	9	12	18
35–49	4,690	3.0	10	1	1	2	4	7	9	14
50–64	25,559	3.4	16	1	1	2	5	8	10	18
65+	39,812	3.7	21	1	1	2	5	9	12	21
SUBTOTALS:										
1. SINGLE DX										
A. *Not Operated*	83	1.3	<1	1	1	1	1	2	3	5
B. *Operated*	736	1.2	1	1	1	1	1	2	2	6
2. MULTIPLE DX										
A. *Not Operated*	30,016	2.6	5	1	1	2	3	5	6	11
B. *Operated*	70,172	3.6	18	1	1	2	5	8	11	20
1. SINGLE DX	819	1.2	<1	1	1	1	1	2	2	6
2. MULTIPLE DX	100,188	3.3	15	1	1	2	4	7	10	18
A. NOT OPERATED	30,099	2.6	5	1	1	2	3	5	6	11
B. OPERATED	70,908	3.5	18	1	1	2	5	8	11	20
TOTAL										
0–19 Years	3	3.3	1	2	2	4	4	4	4	4
20–34	229	2.8	9	1	1	2	3	6	9	16
35–49	7,437	2.8	8	1	1	2	3	6	8	13
50–64	35,612	3.1	13	1	1	2	4	7	9	17
65+	57,726	3.4	16	1	1	2	4	8	10	19
GRAND TOTAL	101,007	3.2	15	1	1	2	4	7	10	18

414.00: COR AS-GRAFT TYPE NOS

Type of Patients	Observed Patients	Avg. Stay	Vari-ance	Percentiles 10th	25th	50th	75th	90th	95th	99th
1. SINGLE DX										
A. *Not Operated*										
0–19 Years	0									
20–34	0									
35–49	0									
50–64	3	1.0	0	1	1	1	3	3	3	3
65+	3	1.7	1	1	1	1	3	3	3	3
B. *Operated*										
0–19 Years	0									
20–34	1	1.0	0	1	1	1	1	1	1	1
35–49	1	4.0	0	4	4	4	4	4	4	4
50–64	1	1.0	0	1	1	1	1	1	1	1
65+	1	1.0	0	1	1	1	1	1	1	1
2. MULTIPLE DX										
A. *Not Operated*										
0–19 Years	0									
20–34	8	2.5	2	1	1	3	3	5	5	5
35–49	307	2.2	4	1	1	2	3	4	5	11
50–64	1,238	2.3	3	1	1	2	3	4	5	9
65+	2,859	2.4	3	1	1	2	3	4	6	10
B. *Operated*										
0–19 Years	0									
20–34	1	1.0	0	1	1	1	1	1	1	1
35–49	58	2.9	8	1	1	2	4	7	8	13
50–64	306	3.2	15	1	1	2	4	7	11	20
65+	496	3.7	29	1	1	2	4	8	11	24
SUBTOTALS:										
1. SINGLE DX										
A. *Not Operated*	4	1.5	1	1	1	1	3	3	3	3
B. *Operated*	4	1.8	2	1	1	1	1	4	4	4
2. MULTIPLE DX										
A. *Not Operated*	4,412	2.4	3	1	1	2	3	4	6	10
B. *Operated*	861	3.4	22	1	1	2	4	7	11	22
1. SINGLE DX	8	1.6	1	1	1	1	3	4	4	4
2. MULTIPLE DX	5,273	2.5	7	1	1	2	3	5	6	12
A. NOT OPERATED	4,416	2.4	3	1	1	2	3	4	6	10
B. OPERATED	865	3.4	22	1	1	2	4	7	11	22
TOTAL										
0–19 Years	0									
20–34	10	2.2	2	1	1	2	3	5	5	5
35–49	366	2.3	4	1	1	2	3	4	7	12
50–64	1,546	2.5	6	1	1	2	3	5	6	13
65+	3,359	2.6	7	1	1	2	3	5	6	12
GRAND TOTAL	5,281	2.5	7	1	1	2	3	5	6	12

Length of Stay by Diagnosis and Operation, Western Region, 2008

Western Region, October 2006–September 2007 Data, by Diagnosis

414.01: COR AS-NATIVE VESSEL

Type of Patients	Observed Patients	Avg. Stay	Variance	10th	25th	50th	75th	90th	95th	99th
1. SINGLE DX										
A. Not Operated										
0–19 Years	0									
20–34	1	1.0	0	1	1	1	1	1	1	1
35–49	9	1.2	<1	1	1	1	1	2	2	2
50–64	33	1.2	<1	1	1	1	1	2	2	3
65+	32	1.4	<1	1	1	1	1	2	3	5
B. Operated										
0–19 Years	0									
20–34	1	6.0	0	6	6	6	6	6	6	6
35–49	65	1.2	<1	1	1	1	1	1	2	3
50–64	261	1.2	<1	1	1	1	1	1	2	5
65+	368	1.3	2	1	1	1	1	1	2	7
2. MULTIPLE DX										
A. Not Operated										
0–19 Years	1	4.0	0	4	4	4	4	4	4	4
20–34	95	2.2	3	1	1	2	3	4	7	9
35–49	2,207	2.3	4	1	1	2	3	4	6	9
50–64	7,950	2.5	5	1	1	2	3	5	6	11
65+	13,436	2.7	5	1	1	2	3	5	7	11
B. Operated										
0–19 Years	0	4.0	0	4	4	4	4	4	4	4
20–34	95	3.5	14	1	1	2	5	7	12	18
35–49	4,432	3.0	9	1	1	2	4	7	9	14
50–64	23,577	3.4	15	1	1	2	5	8	10	18
65+	35,615	3.8	21	1	1	2	5	9	12	21
SUBTOTALS:										
1. SINGLE DX A. Not Operated	75	1.3	<1	1	1	1	1	2	3	5
1. SINGLE DX B. Operated	695	1.2	1	1	1	1	1	1	2	6
2. MULTIPLE DX A. Not Operated	23,689	2.6	5	1	1	2	3	5	6	11
2. MULTIPLE DX B. Operated	63,720	3.6	18	1	1	2	5	8	11	20
1. SINGLE DX	770	1.2	<1	1	1	1	1	2	2	6
2. MULTIPLE DX	87,409	3.3	15	1	1	2	4	8	10	18
A. NOT OPERATED	23,764	2.6	5	1	1	2	3	5	6	11
B. OPERATED	64,415	3.6	18	1	1	2	5	8	11	20
TOTAL										
0–19 Years	2	4.0	0	4	4	4	4	4	4	4
20–34	192	2.9	9	1	1	2	3	6	9	16
35–49	6,713	2.8	8	1	1	2	3	6	8	13
50–64	31,821	3.1	13	1	1	2	4	7	9	16
65+	49,451	3.5	17	1	1	2	5	8	11	19
GRAND TOTAL	88,179	3.3	15	1	1	2	4	8	10	18

414.02: COR AS-AUTOLOG GRAFT

Type of Patients	Observed Patients	Avg. Stay	Variance	10th	25th	50th	75th	90th	95th	99th
1. SINGLE DX										
A. Not Operated										
0–19 Years	0									
20–34	0									
35–49	0									
50–64	0									
65+	1	1.0	0	1	1	1	1	1	1	1
B. Operated										
0–19 Years	0									
20–34	0									
35–49	0									
50–64	3	2.0	3	1	1	1	4	4	4	4
65+	7	1.7	2	1	1	1	2	5	5	5
2. MULTIPLE DX										
A. Not Operated										
0–19 Years	0									
20–34	1	1.0	0	1	1	1	1	1	1	1
35–49	44	3.4	10	1	1	3	4	7	10	17
50–64	187	2.8	5	1	1	2	3	5	7	13
65+	508	3.0	14	1	1	2	4	5	7	12
B. Operated										
0–19 Years	0									
20–34	2	1.5	<1	1	1	1	2	2	2	2
35–49	79	3.1	11	1	1	2	4	7	11	22
50–64	891	2.6	12	1	1	1	3	6	8	18
65+	2,209	2.8	15	1	1	2	3	6	9	17
SUBTOTALS:										
1. SINGLE DX A. Not Operated	1	1.0	0	1	1	1	1	1	1	1
1. SINGLE DX B. Operated	10	1.8	2	1	1	1	2	5	5	6
2. MULTIPLE DX A. Not Operated	740	3.0	12	1	1	2	3	5	7	13
2. MULTIPLE DX B. Operated	3,181	2.8	14	1	1	2	3	6	9	18
1. SINGLE DX	11	1.7	2	1	1	1	2	4	5	5
2. MULTIPLE DX	3,921	2.8	13	1	1	2	3	6	9	17
A. NOT OPERATED	741	3.0	12	1	1	2	3	5	7	13
B. OPERATED	3,191	2.8	14	1	1	2	3	6	9	18
TOTAL										
0–19 Years	0									
20–34	3	1.3	<1	1	1	1	2	2	2	2
35–49	123	3.2	11	1	1	2	4	7	10	17
50–64	1,081	2.6	11	1	1	1	3	5	8	17
65+	2,725	2.9	14	1	1	2	3	6	9	17
GRAND TOTAL	3,932	2.8	13	1	1	2	3	6	9	17

414.04: COR AS-ART BYPASS GRAFT

Type of Patients	Observed Patients	Avg. Stay	Variance	10th	25th	50th	75th	90th	95th	99th
1. SINGLE DX										
A. Not Operated										
0–19 Years	0									
20–34	0									
35–49	0									
50–64	0									
65+	0									
B. Operated										
0–19 Years	0									
20–34	0									
35–49	0									
50–64	1	1.0	0	1	1	1	1	1	1	1
65+	1	1.0	0	1	1	1	1	1	1	1
2. MULTIPLE DX										
A. Not Operated										
0–19 Years	0									
20–34	0									
35–49	9	2.6	2	1	2	2	3	6	6	6
50–64	40	2.2	2	1	1	2	3	4	4	7
65+	94	2.5	2	1	1	2	3	4	6	8
B. Operated										
0–19 Years	0									
20–34	1	1.0	0	1	1	1	1	1	1	1
35–49	14	2.3	8	1	1	1	1	9	9	9
50–64	96	3.5	30	1	1	2	4	7	12	47
65+	183	3.6	30	1	1	1	3	9	13	38
SUBTOTALS:										
1. SINGLE DX A. Not Operated	0									
1. SINGLE DX B. Operated	2	1.0	0	1	1	1	1	1	1	1
2. MULTIPLE DX A. Not Operated	143	2.4	2	1	1	2	3	4	6	7
2. MULTIPLE DX B. Operated	294	3.5	29	1	1	1	4	9	13	38
1. SINGLE DX	2	1.0	0	1	1	1	1	1	1	1
2. MULTIPLE DX	437	3.2	20	1	1	2	3	7	11	21
A. NOT OPERATED	143	2.4	2	1	1	2	3	4	6	7
B. OPERATED	296	3.5	28	1	1	1	4	9	13	38
TOTAL										
0–19 Years	0									
20–34	1	1.0	0	1	1	1	1	1	1	1
35–49	23	2.4	6	1	1	1	3	6	9	9
50–64	137	3.1	22	1	1	2	4	6	11	15
65+	278	3.2	21	1	1	2	3	7	12	26
GRAND TOTAL	439	3.1	20	1	1	2	3	7	11	21

Length of Stay by Diagnosis and Operation, Western Region, 2008

Western Region, October 2006–September 2007 Data, by Diagnosis

414.05: COR AS-BYPASS GRAFT NOS

Type of Patients	Observed Patients	Avg. Stay	Variance	10th	25th	50th	75th	90th	95th	99th
1. SINGLE DX										
A. Not Operated										
0–19 Years	0									
20–34	0									
35–49	0									
50–64	0									
65+	0									
B. Operated										
0–19 Years	0									
20–34	0									
35–49	1	1.0	0	1	1	1	1	1	1	1
50–64	0									
65+	0									
2. MULTIPLE DX										
A. Not Operated										
0–19 Years	0									
20–34	0									
35–49	11	3.6	10	1	1	3	6	7	11	11
50–64	35	2.8	7	1	1	2	3	5	9	14
65+	73	3.0	7	1	1	2	4	6	8	16
B. Operated										
0–19 Years	0									
20–34	1	5.0	0	5	5	5	5	5	5	5
35–49	4	1.5	1	1	1	1	3	3	3	3
50–64	50	4.0	35	1	1	2	5	10	10	40
65+	83	4.0	24	1	1	2	5	9	12	25
SUBTOTALS:										
1. SINGLE DX										
A. Not Operated	0									
B. Operated	1	1.0	0	1	1	1	1	1	1	1
2. MULTIPLE DX										
A. Not Operated	119	3.0	7	1	1	2	3	6	9	14
B. Operated	138	3.9	27	1	1	2	5	9	12	25
1. SINGLE DX	1	1.0	0	1	1	1	1	1	1	1
2. MULTIPLE DX	257	3.5	18	1	1	2	4	7	11	21
A. NOT OPERATED	119	3.0	7	1	1	2	3	6	9	14
B. OPERATED	139	3.9	27	1	1	2	5	9	12	25
TOTAL										
0–19 Years	0									
20–34	1	5.0	0	5	5	5	5	5	5	5
35–49	16	2.9	8	1	1	2	3	7	11	11
50–64	85	3.5	24	1	1	2	4	7	10	40
65+	156	3.5	16	1	1	2	5	7	12	21
GRAND TOTAL	258	3.5	18	1	1	2	4	7	11	21

414.8: CHR ISCHEMIC HRT DIS NEC

Type of Patients	Observed Patients	Avg. Stay	Variance	10th	25th	50th	75th	90th	95th	99th
1. SINGLE DX										
A. Not Operated										
0–19 Years	0									
20–34	0									
35–49	1	1.0	0	1	1	1	1	1	1	1
50–64	1	1.0	0	1	1	1	1	1	1	1
65+	0									
B. Operated										
0–19 Years	0									
20–34	0									
35–49	1	1.0	0	1	1	1	1	1	1	1
50–64	9	1.0	0	1	1	1	1	1	1	1
65+	12	1.5	<1	1	1	1	3	3	3	3
2. MULTIPLE DX										
A. Not Operated										
0–19 Years	1	2.0	0	2	2	2	2	2	2	2
20–34	10	2.6	3	1	1	2	4	6	6	6
35–49	57	3.1	7	1	1	2	4	6	7	14
50–64	233	3.3	12	1	1	2	4	6	8	14
65+	439	3.3	6	1	1	3	4	6	8	15
B. Operated										
0–19 Years	0									
20–34	5	5.7	56	1	1	4	4	19	19	19
35–49	86	3.2	45	1	1	1	2	6	12	53
50–64	597	3.2	52	1	1	2	2	7	14	42
65+	1,174	2.3	19	1	1	2	2	5	8	19
SUBTOTALS:										
1. SINGLE DX										
A. Not Operated	2	1.0	0	1	1	1	1	1	1	1
B. Operated	22	1.3	<1	1	1	1	1	3	3	3
2. MULTIPLE DX										
A. Not Operated	740	3.3	8	1	1	3	4	6	8	14
B. Operated	1,862	2.7	31	1	1	1	2	5	10	22
1. SINGLE DX	24	1.3	<1	1	1	1	1	3	3	3
2. MULTIPLE DX	2,602	2.8	25	1	1	2	3	6	9	21
A. NOT OPERATED	742	3.3	8	1	1	3	4	6	8	14
B. OPERATED	1,884	2.7	31	1	1	2	2	5	10	22
TOTAL										
0–19 Years	1	2.0	0	2	2	2	2	2	2	2
20–34	15	3.7	21	2	1	2	4	6	19	19
35–49	145	3.2	29	1	1	2	3	6	11	24
50–64	840	3.2	40	1	1	2	3	7	12	31
65+	1,625	2.6	16	1	1	2	3	6	8	17
GRAND TOTAL	2,626	2.8	24	1	1	1	3	6	9	21

415: ACUTE PULMONARY HRT DIS

Type of Patients	Observed Patients	Avg. Stay	Variance	10th	25th	50th	75th	90th	95th	99th
1. SINGLE DX										
A. Not Operated										
0–19 Years	8	3.5	3	2	2	3	5	7	7	7
20–34	57	2.6	2	1	2	2	3	4	5	8
35–49	73	2.8	3	1	2	2	4	5	6	7
50–64	54	2.5	3	2	1	2	3	5	6	7
65+	27	3.2	2	2	2	3	4	5	6	6
B. Operated										
0–19 Years	0									
20–34	2	3.0	8	1	1	1	5	5	5	5
35–49	1	8.0	0	8	8	8	8	8	8	8
50–64	1	3.0	0	3	3	3	3	3	3	3
65+	0									
2. MULTIPLE DX										
A. Not Operated										
0–19 Years	95	4.2	6	1	2	4	6	8	9	11
20–34	1,260	4.3	12	1	2	4	6	8	10	14
35–49	3,332	4.6	12	2	2	4	6	8	10	17
50–64	5,125	4.9	13	2	3	4	6	9	10	17
65+	9,231	5.2	11	2	3	5	6	9	11	17
B. Operated										
0–19 Years	5	15.0	173	3	4	10	26	32	32	32
20–34	111	8.7	54	2	4	6	11	18	23	35
35–49	315	8.1	49	2	4	6	10	15	20	32
50–64	674	8.3	48	3	4	7	10	15	21	42
65+	1,348	8.0	33	3	4	6	10	15	20	29
SUBTOTALS:										
1. SINGLE DX										
A. Not Operated	219	2.7	2	2	2	2	4	5	6	7
B. Operated	4	4.3	9	1	1	3	8	8	8	8
2. MULTIPLE DX										
A. Not Operated	19,043	4.9	12	1	3	4	6	9	11	17
B. Operated	2,453	8.1	40	3	4	6	10	15	20	34
1. SINGLE DX	223	2.8	3	1	2	2	4	5	6	7
2. MULTIPLE DX	21,496	5.3	16	2	3	5	7	9	12	20
A. NOT OPERATED	19,262	4.9	12	2	3	4	6	9	11	17
B. OPERATED	2,457	8.1	40	3	4	6	10	15	20	34
TOTAL										
0–19 Years	108	4.6	17	1	2	4	6	8	9	26
20–34	1,430	4.6	16	1	2	4	6	8	11	19
35–49	3,721	4.9	16	2	2	4	6	8	11	19
50–64	5,854	5.3	18	2	3	5	6	9	12	21
65+	10,606	5.5	15	2	3	5	7	10	12	20
GRAND TOTAL	21,719	5.3	16	2	3	5	7	9	12	20

Length of Stay by Diagnosis and Operation, Western Region, 2008

Western Region, October 2006–September 2007 Data, by Diagnosis

415.11: IATRO PULM EMBOL/INFARCT

Type of Patients	Observed Patients	Avg. Stay	Vari-ance	10th	25th	50th	75th	90th	95th	99th
1. SINGLE DX										
A. Not Operated										
0–19 Years	4	4.0	6	2	2	5	7	7	7	7
20–34	8	2.1	<1	1	2	2	3	4	4	4
35–49	11	3.0	3	1	1	2	5	5	6	6
50–64	13	2.6	1	1	2	2	3	4	5	5
65+	4	3.5	1	2	4	4	4	4	4	4
B. Operated										
0–19 Years	0									
20–34	0									
35–49	0									
50–64	0									
65+	0									
2. MULTIPLE DX										
A. Not Operated										
0–19 Years	4	5.5	10	3	4	4	5	10	10	10
20–34	101	4.0	6	1	3	3	5	7	9	11
35–49	282	4.5	9	2	2	4	6	8	10	16
50–64	386	4.3	7	2	2	4	6	8	9	13
65+	455	5.0	9	2	3	4	6	8	11	17
B. Operated										
0–19 Years	0									
20–34	6	6.7	16	1	3	6	10	11	11	11
35–49	26	5.7	5	4	4	5	7	7	8	14
50–64	50	7.2	23	3	4	6	9	13	18	25
65+	65	8.2	45	3	4	6	11	15	20	41
SUBTOTALS:										
1. SINGLE DX										
A. Not Operated	40	2.9	2	1	2	2	4	5	6	7
B. Operated	0									
2. MULTIPLE DX										
A. Not Operated	1,228	4.6	8	2	3	4	6	8	10	14
B. Operated	147	7.3	30	3	4	6	9	13	16	29
1. SINGLE DX	40	2.9	2	1	2	2	4	5	6	7
2. MULTIPLE DX	1,375	4.9	11	2	3	4	6	8	11	17
A. NOT OPERATED	1,268	4.5	8	2	3	4	6	8	10	14
B. OPERATED	147	7.3	30	3	4	6	9	13	16	29
TOTAL										
0–19 Years	8	4.8	7	2	3	5	5	10	10	10
20–34	115	4.0	7	1	2	3	5	8	10	11
35–49	319	4.6	8	2	3	4	6	8	10	15
50–64	449	4.6	10	2	2	4	6	8	10	15
65+	524	5.3	15	2	3	5	6	9	13	20
GRAND TOTAL	1,415	4.8	11	2	3	4	6	8	11	17

415.19: PULMON EMBOL/INFARCT NEC

Type of Patients	Observed Patients	Avg. Stay	Vari-ance	10th	25th	50th	75th	90th	95th	99th
1. SINGLE DX										
A. Not Operated										
0–19 Years	4	3.0	0	3	3	3	3	3	3	3
20–34	49	2.7	2	1	2	3	3	4	5	8
35–49	62	2.7	3	1	2	2	4	5	6	7
50–64	41	2.4	3	1	2	2	3	6	6	7
65+	23	3.2	2	2	2	3	5	5	6	6
B. Operated										
0–19 Years	0									
20–34	2	3.0	8	1	1	1	5	5	5	5
35–49	1	8.0	0	8	8	8	8	8	8	8
50–64	1	3.0	0	3	3	3	3	3	3	3
65+	0									
2. MULTIPLE DX										
A. Not Operated										
0–19 Years	90	4.1	6	1	2	4	6	7	9	11
20–34	1,156	4.4	12	1	2	4	6	8	10	14
35–49	3,028	4.7	12	2	2	4	6	8	10	17
50–64	4,690	4.9	14	2	3	4	6	9	11	18
65+	8,669	5.2	11	2	3	5	6	9	11	17
B. Operated										
0–19 Years	5	15.0	173	3	4	10	26	32	32	32
20–34	105	8.8	56	2	4	6	11	19	23	35
35–49	289	8.3	53	2	4	6	11	15	20	33
50–64	624	8.3	50	3	4	7	10	15	21	42
65+	1,283	7.9	33	3	4	6	10	15	19	29
SUBTOTALS:										
1. SINGLE DX										
A. Not Operated	179	2.7	3	1	1	2	4	5	6	7
B. Operated	4	4.3	9	1	1	3	8	8	8	8
2. MULTIPLE DX										
A. Not Operated	17,633	5.0	12	2	3	4	6	9	11	17
B. Operated	2,306	8.1	41	3	4	7	10	15	20	34
1. SINGLE DX	183	2.7	3	1	2	2	4	5	6	8
2. MULTIPLE DX	19,939	5.3	16	2	3	5	7	9	12	20
A. NOT OPERATED	17,812	4.9	12	2	3	4	6	9	11	17
B. OPERATED	2,310	8.1	41	3	4	7	10	15	20	34
TOTAL										
0–19 Years	99	4.6	18	1	2	4	6	8	9	26
20–34	1,312	4.6	17	1	2	4	6	9	11	20
35–49	3,380	4.9	17	2	2	4	6	9	11	20
50–64	5,356	5.3	19	2	3	4	7	10	12	22
65+	9,975	5.5	15	2	3	5	7	10	12	20
GRAND TOTAL	20,122	5.3	16	2	3	5	7	9	12	20

416: CHR PULMONARY HEART DIS

Type of Patients	Observed Patients	Avg. Stay	Vari-ance	10th	25th	50th	75th	90th	95th	99th
1. SINGLE DX										
A. Not Operated										
0–19 Years	2	1.5	<1	1	1	1	2	2	2	2
20–34	6	2.2	<1	1	2	2	3	3	3	3
35–49	4	1.3	<1	1	1	1	1	2	2	2
50–64	0									
65+	1	1.0	0	1	1	1	1	1	1	1
B. Operated										
0–19 Years	0									
20–34	0									
35–49	0									
50–64	0									
65+	0									
2. MULTIPLE DX										
A. Not Operated										
0–19 Years	28	9.5	243	1	2	5	8	28	54	68
20–34	134	4.1	13	1	2	3	6	8	10	18
35–49	419	4.8	23	1	2	3	6	10	14	27
50–64	656	5.3	27	1	2	4	7	11	15	26
65+	991	5.0	19	1	2	4	6	9	13	20
B. Operated										
0–19 Years	2	8.0	31	4	4	8	12	12	12	12
20–34	9	18.3	148	5	8	17	22	40	40	40
35–49	17	10.7	49	3	8	10	13	15	33	33
50–64	14	10.7	62	1	6	9	14	22	31	31
65+	21	9.8	73	3	4	8	11	22	28	34
SUBTOTALS:										
1. SINGLE DX										
A. Not Operated	13	1.7	<1	1	1	2	2	3	3	3
B. Operated	0									
2. MULTIPLE DX										
A. Not Operated	2,228	5.1	25	1	2	4	6	10	14	23
B. Operated	63	11.4	77	3	5	9	14	22	33	40
1. SINGLE DX	13	1.7	<1	1	1	2	2	3	3	3
2. MULTIPLE DX	2,291	5.2	27	1	2	4	6	10	14	28
A. NOT OPERATED	2,241	5.0	25	1	2	4	6	10	14	23
B. OPERATED	63	11.4	77	3	5	9	14	22	33	40
TOTAL										
0–19 Years	32	8.9	216	1	2	4	8	12	54	68
20–34	149	4.9	32	1	2	3	6	10	14	33
35–49	440	5.0	25	1	2	3	6	10	15	28
50–64	670	5.4	28	1	2	4	7	11	15	26
65+	1,013	5.1	20	1	2	4	6	9	14	21
GRAND TOTAL	2,304	5.2	27	1	2	4	6	10	14	27

Length of Stay by Diagnosis and Operation, Western Region 2008

Western Region, October 2006–September 2007 Data, by Diagnosis

416.0: PRIMARY PULMONARY HTN

Type of Patients	Observed Patients	Avg. Stay	Variance	10th	25th	50th	75th	90th	95th	99th
1. SINGLE DX										
A. Not Operated										
0–19 Years	2	1.5	<1	1	1	1	2	2	2	2
20–34	2	2.5	<1	2	2	3	3	3	3	3
35–49	1	1.0	0	1	1	1	1	1	1	1
50–64	0									
65+	0									
B. Operated										
0–19 Years	0									
20–34	0									
35–49	0									
50–64	0									
65+	0									
2. MULTIPLE DX										
A. Not Operated										
0–19 Years	6	15.7	455	1	3	4	28	54	54	54
20–34	36	4.3	8	1	2	3	6	8	10	10
35–49	93	4.8	30	1	2	3	6	10	15	40
50–64	91	5.5	22	1	2	4	9	12	15	22
65+	94	5.4	20	1	2	4	7	12	17	21
B. Operated										
0–19 Years	1	12.0	0	12	12	12	12	12	12	12
20–34	1	33.0	0	33	33	33	33	33	33	33
35–49	6	9.9	23	1	8	12	13	14	14	14
50–64	3	13.7	227	3	3	7	31	31	31	31
65+	2	10.0	18	7	7	10	13	13	13	13
SUBTOTALS:										
1. SINGLE DX										
A. Not Operated	5	1.8	<1	1	1	2	2	3	3	3
B. Operated	0									
2. MULTIPLE DX										
A. Not Operated	320	5.3	31	1	2	4	7	11	15	22
B. Operated	13	12.7	89	3	7	12	13	31	33	33
1. SINGLE DX	5	1.8	<1	1	2	2	2	3	3	3
2. MULTIPLE DX	333	5.6	35	1	2	4	7	12	16	31
A. NOT OPERATED	325	5.3	30	1	2	4	7	11	15	22
B. OPERATED	13	12.7	89	3	7	12	13	31	33	33
TOTAL										
0–19 Years	9	12.2	322	1	2	4	12	54	54	54
20–34	39	4.9	28	1	2	3	6	9	10	33
35–49	100	5.1	30	1	2	4	6	12	15	22
50–64	94	5.7	28	1	2	4	9	12	17	31
65+	96	5.5	20	1	2	5	7	12	17	21
GRAND TOTAL	338	5.6	34	1	2	4	7	12	16	31

416.8: CHR PULMON HEART DIS NEC

Type of Patients	Observed Patients	Avg. Stay	Variance	10th	25th	50th	75th	90th	95th	99th
1. SINGLE DX										
A. Not Operated										
0–19 Years	0									
20–34	4	2.0	<1	1	1	2	2	3	3	3
35–49	3	1.3	<1	1	1	1	2	2	2	2
50–64	0									
65+	1	1.0	0	1	1	1	1	1	1	1
B. Operated										
0–19 Years	0									
20–34	0									
35–49	0									
50–64	0									
65+	0									
2. MULTIPLE DX										
A. Not Operated										
0–19 Years	22	7.8	189	2	2	6	8	9	10	68
20–34	91	4.0	16	1	2	3	5	8	12	27
35–49	296	4.7	19	1	2	3	6	9	14	27
50–64	481	5.2	29	1	2	4	6	10	14	29
65+	742	4.8	18	1	2	4	6	9	12	20
B. Operated										
0–19 Years	1	4.0	0	4	4	4	4	4	4	4
20–34	8	16.4	134	5	8	17	22	40	40	40
35–49	11	11.2	66	5	6	10	15	15	33	33
50–64	11	9.9	32	1	6	12	14	15	18	18
65+	18	9.1	75	2	4	6	9	28	34	34
SUBTOTALS:										
1. SINGLE DX										
A. Not Operated	8	1.6	<1	1	1	2	2	2	3	3
B. Operated	0									
2. MULTIPLE DX										
A. Not Operated	1,632	4.9	24	1	2	4	6	9	13	23
B. Operated	49	10.8	74	3	5	9	14	22	33	40
1. SINGLE DX	8	1.6	<1	1	1	2	2	2	3	3
2. MULTIPLE DX	1,681	5.1	26	1	2	4	6	10	14	27
A. NOT OPERATED	1,640	4.9	24	1	2	4	6	9	13	23
B. OPERATED	49	10.8	74	3	5	9	14	22	33	40
TOTAL										
0–19 Years	23	7.7	181	2	2	5	8	9	10	68
20–34	103	4.9	35	1	2	3	5	10	17	27
35–49	310	4.9	22	1	2	4	6	10	14	27
50–64	492	5.3	29	1	2	4	7	11	15	29
65+	761	4.9	19	1	2	4	6	9	12	20
GRAND TOTAL	1,689	5.1	26	1	2	4	6	10	14	27

416.9: CHR PULMON HEART DIS NOS

Type of Patients	Observed Patients	Avg. Stay	Variance	10th	25th	50th	75th	90th	95th	99th
1. SINGLE DX										
A. Not Operated										
0–19 Years	0									
20–34	0									
35–49	0									
50–64	0									
65+	0									
B. Operated										
0–19 Years	0									
20–34	0									
35–49	0									
50–64	0									
65+	0									
2. MULTIPLE DX										
A. Not Operated										
0–19 Years	0									
20–34	7	3.4	5	1	2	2	6	6	6	6
35–49	30	6.1	32	2	3	4	7	12	18	28
50–64	84	5.6	22	2	3	4	7	12	17	23
65+	155	5.7	24	2	3	5	7	10	16	25
B. Operated										
0–19 Years	0									
20–34	0									
35–49	0									
50–64	0									
65+	1	22.0	0	22	22	22	22	22	22	22
SUBTOTALS:										
1. SINGLE DX										
A. Not Operated	0									
B. Operated	0									
2. MULTIPLE DX										
A. Not Operated	276	5.7	23	2	3	4	7	11	16	25
B. Operated	1	22.0	0	22	22	22	22	22	22	22
1. SINGLE DX	0									
2. MULTIPLE DX	277	5.7	24	2	3	4	7	11	17	25
A. NOT OPERATED	276	5.7	23	2	3	4	7	11	16	25
B. OPERATED	1	22.0	0	22	22	22	22	22	22	22
TOTAL										
0–19 Years	0									
20–34	7	3.4	5	1	2	2	6	6	6	6
35–49	30	6.1	32	2	3	4	7	12	18	28
50–64	84	5.6	25	2	3	4	7	11	17	23
65+	156	5.8	25	2	3	5	7	11	16	25
GRAND TOTAL	277	5.7	24	2	3	4	7	11	17	25

Length of Stay by Diagnosis and Operation, Western Region, 2008

Western Region, October 2006–September 2007 Data, by Diagnosis

417: OTH PULMON CIRC DISEASE

Type of Patients	Observed Patients	Avg. Stay	Variance	10th	25th	50th	75th	90th	95th	99th
1. SINGLE DX										
A. *Not Operated*										
0–19 Years	0									
20–34	0									
35–49	0									
50–64	0									
65+	0									
B. *Operated*										
0–19 Years	1	1.0	0			1	1	1	1	1
20–34	0									
35–49	1	2.0	0	2	2	2	2	2	2	2
50–64	0									
65+	0									
2. MULTIPLE DX										
A. *Not Operated*										
0–19 Years	3	1.3	<1	1	1	1	2	2	2	2
20–34	2	10.0	31	6	6	6	14	14	14	14
35–49	8	2.8	1	1	2	2	4	4	4	4
50–64	10	8.5	73	2	2	5	12	28	28	28
65+	13	6.2	30	2	3	4	7	16	18	18
B. *Operated*										
0–19 Years	12	7.5	114	1	1	4	8	14	39	39
20–34	1	28.0	0	28	28	28	28	28	28	28
35–49	6	8.2	41	1	5	5	14	18	18	18
50–64	6	4.5	17	1	1	5	9	10	10	10
65+	6	5.5	23	1	2	4	11	12	12	12
SUBTOTALS:										
1. SINGLE DX										
A. *Not Operated*	0									
B. *Operated*	2	1.5	<1	1	1	2	2	2	2	2
2. MULTIPLE DX										
A. *Not Operated*	36	5.9	37	1	2	3	7	16	18	28
B. *Operated*	31	7.3	72	1	1	5	10	14	28	39
1. SINGLE DX	2	1.5	<1	1	1	2	2	2	2	2
2. MULTIPLE DX	67	6.6	53	1	2	4	9	16	18	39
A. NOT OPERATED	36	5.9	37	1	2	3	7	16	18	28
B. OPERATED	33	7.0	70	1	1	5	10	14	28	39
TOTAL										
0–19 Years	16	5.9	92	1	1	1	8	14	39	39
20–34	3	16.1	123	6	6	14	28	28	28	28
35–49	15	4.9	23	1	2	4	5	14	18	18
50–64	16	7.0	54	2	2	5	9	16	28	28
65+	19	6.0	26	1	2	4	11	16	18	18
GRAND TOTAL	69	6.4	52	1	2	4	8	16	18	39

420: ACUTE PERICARDITIS

Type of Patients	Observed Patients	Avg. Stay	Variance	10th	25th	50th	75th	90th	95th	99th
1. SINGLE DX										
A. *Not Operated*										
0–19 Years	10	2.2	1	1	1	2	3	4	4	4
20–34	20	1.8	1	1	1	1	2	4	4	4
35–49	18	1.6	<1	1	1	1	2	3	4	4
50–64	11	1.5	<1	1	1	1	2	2	3	3
65+	3	1.7	<1	1	1	2	2	2	2	2
B. *Operated*										
0–19 Years	0									
20–34	0									
35–49	0									
50–64	0									
65+	0									
2. MULTIPLE DX										
A. *Not Operated*										
0–19 Years	50	2.3	3	1	1	1	3	4	5	9
20–34	261	2.6	4	1	1	2	3	5	7	11
35–49	346	2.6	6	1	1	2	3	5	7	11
50–64	492	3.2	13	1	2	2	4	6	8	24
65+	479	3.9	13	1	2	3	5	9	11	18
B. *Operated*										
0–19 Years	6	13.1	102	4	9	12	12	33	33	33
20–34	27	13.6	248	4	5	10	13	27	35	82
35–49	64	9.4	113	3	5	6	10	20	23	74
50–64	117	9.9	45	3	6	9	13	18	21	36
65+	115	9.2	35	4	5	8	12	17	24	29
SUBTOTALS:										
1. SINGLE DX										
A. *Not Operated*	62	1.7	<1	1	1	1	2	3	4	4
B. *Operated*	0									
2. MULTIPLE DX										
A. *Not Operated*	1,628	3.2	10	1	1	2	4	7	9	16
B. *Operated*	329	9.9	72	3	5	8	12	18	24	36
1. SINGLE DX	62	1.7	<1	1	1	1	2	3	4	4
2. MULTIPLE DX	1,957	4.3	27	1	1	3	5	9	13	24
A. NOT OPERATED	1,690	3.1	10	1	1	2	4	6	9	16
B. OPERATED	329	9.9	72	3	5	8	12	18	24	36
TOTAL										
0–19 Years	66	3.3	20	1	1	2	4	7	9	33
20–34	308	3.5	35	1	1	2	4	7	10	24
35–49	428	3.6	28	1	1	2	4	7	10	23
50–64	620	4.4	26	1	2	3	5	10	13	27
65+	597	4.9	21	1	2	3	7	11	14	24
GRAND TOTAL	2,019	4.2	26	1	1	3	5	9	13	24

420.90: ACUTE PERICARDITIS NOS

Type of Patients	Observed Patients	Avg. Stay	Variance	10th	25th	50th	75th	90th	95th	99th
1. SINGLE DX										
A. *Not Operated*										
0–19 Years	2	2.5	<1	2	2	3	3	3	3	3
20–34	9	1.7	<1	1	1	1	2	4	4	4
35–49	12	1.5	<1	1	1	1	2	2	4	4
50–64	4	1.5	<1	1	1	1	2	2	2	2
65+	2	2.0	0	2	2	2	2	2	2	2
B. *Operated*										
0–19 Years	0									
20–34	0									
35–49	0									
50–64	0									
65+	0									
2. MULTIPLE DX										
A. *Not Operated*										
0–19 Years	17	2.2	2	1	1	2	2	4	5	5
20–34	119	2.3	3	1	1	2	3	4	5	8
35–49	181	2.6	8	1	1	2	3	5	7	16
50–64	235	3.3	18	1	1	2	4	7	8	27
65+	271	3.9	15	1	1	2	5	9	12	19
B. *Operated*										
0–19 Years	2	22.4	216	12	12	12	33	33	33	33
20–34	10	21.3	537	3	10	11	24	82	82	82
35–49	24	9.2	199	3	5	6	9	12	12	74
50–64	65	10.5	56	3	6	9	13	19	23	41
65+	53	10.0	48	4	6	8	11	18	26	35
SUBTOTALS:										
1. SINGLE DX										
A. *Not Operated*	29	1.7	<1	1	1	1	2	3	4	4
B. *Operated*	0									
2. MULTIPLE DX										
A. *Not Operated*	823	3.2	13	1	1	2	4	7	9	18
B. *Operated*	154	11.0	113	4	6	8	12	19	32	74
1. SINGLE DX	29	1.7	<1	1	1	1	2	3	4	4
2. MULTIPLE DX	977	4.4	36	1	1	2	5	10	13	29
A. NOT OPERATED	852	3.1	12	1	1	2	3	7	9	18
B. OPERATED	154	11.0	113	4	6	8	12	19	32	74
TOTAL										
0–19 Years	21	4.1	50	1	1	2	4	5	12	33
20–34	138	3.7	62	1	1	2	3	6	10	35
35–49	217	3.2	32	1	1	2	3	5	9	16
50–64	304	4.8	35	1	1	3	6	11	15	32
65+	326	4.9	25	1	2	3	6	11	14	25
GRAND TOTAL	1,006	4.3	36	1	1	2	5	10	13	28

Length of Stay by Diagnosis and Operation, Western Region, 2008

Western Region, October 2006–September 2007 Data, by Diagnosis

420.91: AC IDIOPATHIC PERICARD

Type of Patients	Observed Patients	Avg. Stay	Variance	10th	25th	50th	75th	90th	95th	99th
1. SINGLE DX										
A. Not Operated										
0–19 Years	6	2.0	2	1	1	2	3	4	4	4
20–34	11	1.8	1	1	1	1	2	4	4	4
35–49	4	2.0	<1	1	1	2	2	3	3	3
50–64	7	1.4	<1	1	1	1	2	3	3	3
65+	1	1.0	0	1	1	1	1	1	1	1
B. Operated										
0–19 Years	0									
20–34	0									
35–49	0									
50–64	0									
65+	0									
2. MULTIPLE DX										
A. Not Operated										
0–19 Years	28	2.5	4	1	1	2	3	5	7	9
20–34	117	2.5	3	1	1	2	3	5	6	8
35–49	132	2.6	3	1	1	2	3	5	6	11
50–64	216	2.9	6	1	1	2	4	5	7	11
65+	158	3.7	9	1	2	3	5	8	11	16
B. Operated										
0–19 Years	4	8.5	11	4	4	9	12	12	12	12
20–34	12	7.1	24	4	4	5	8	11	21	21
35–49	23	8.4	72	3	4	6	8	20	29	36
50–64	25	9.3	35	3	4	9	13	16	18	27
65+	40	9.1	25	3	5	8	12	16	17	24
SUBTOTALS:										
1. SINGLE DX										
A. Not Operated	29	1.8	1	1	1	1	2	4	4	4
B. Operated	0									
2. MULTIPLE DX										
A. Not Operated	651	2.9	6	1	1	2	4	5	7	11
B. Operated	104	8.7	36	3	4	7	11	16	20	29
1. SINGLE DX	29	1.8	1	1	1	1	2	4	4	4
2. MULTIPLE DX	755	3.7	14	1	1	3	4	8	11	18
A. NOT OPERATED	680	2.9	6	1	1	2	4	5	7	11
B. OPERATED	104	8.7	36	3	4	7	11	16	20	29
TOTAL										
0–19 Years	38	3.1	7	1	1	2	4	9	9	12
20–34	140	2.8	6	1	1	2	4	5	7	11
35–49	159	3.4	17	1	1	2	4	6	9	29
50–64	248	3.5	13	1	1	2	4	7	10	18
65+	199	4.8	17	1	2	3	7	11	14	18
GRAND TOTAL	784	3.7	14	1	1	3	4	8	11	18

421: AC/SUBAC ENDOCARDITIS

Type of Patients	Observed Patients	Avg. Stay	Variance	10th	25th	50th	75th	90th	95th	99th
1. SINGLE DX										
A. Not Operated										
0–19 Years	0									
20–34	0									
35–49	1	4.0	0	4	4	4	4	4	4	4
50–64	0									
65+	0									
B. Operated										
0–19 Years	0									
20–34	0									
35–49	0									
50–64	0									
65+	0									
2. MULTIPLE DX										
A. Not Operated										
0–19 Years	29	9.6	47	2	4	8	13	17	25	29
20–34	128	11.4	112	3	5	8	15	26	41	46
35–49	261	12.5	141	3	5	8	15	29	40	64
50–64	384	9.5	69	3	4	7	11	19	25	47
65+	663	9.3	47	3	5	7	12	17	21	36
B. Operated										
0–19 Years	4	31.5	>999	5	5	15	97	97	97	97
20–34	21	21.1	186	6	10	21	31	45	48	>99
35–49	77	17.7	177	6	8	14	22	37	46	66
50–64	107	18.9	127	9	12	16	23	32	44	56
65+	83	19.2	125	8	12	16	24	37	38	63
SUBTOTALS:										
1. SINGLE DX										
A. Not Operated	1	4.0	0	4	4	4	4	4	4	4
B. Operated	0									
2. MULTIPLE DX										
A. Not Operated	1,465	10.1	76	3	5	7	12	19	27	46
B. Operated	292	19.0	164	7	10	16	24	37	45	70
1. SINGLE DX	1	4.0	0	4	4	4	4	4	4	4
2. MULTIPLE DX	1,757	11.6	102	3	5	8	14	23	31	53
A. NOT OPERATED	1,466	10.1	76	3	5	7	12	19	27	46
B. OPERATED	292	19.0	164	7	10	16	24	37	45	70
TOTAL										
0–19 Years	33	12.2	276	2	5	8	14	17	29	97
20–34	149	12.8	133	3	5	9	16	31	42	57
35–49	339	13.6	154	3	6	9	17	30	42	64
50–64	491	11.5	96	3	5	8	15	23	30	53
65+	746	10.4	65	4	5	8	13	20	26	41
GRAND TOTAL	1,758	11.6	102	3	5	8	14	23	31	53

421.0: AC/SUBAC BACT ENDOCARD

Type of Patients	Observed Patients	Avg. Stay	Variance	10th	25th	50th	75th	90th	95th	99th
1. SINGLE DX										
A. Not Operated										
0–19 Years	0									
20–34	0									
35–49	1	4.0	0	4	4	4	4	4	4	4
50–64	0									
65+	0									
B. Operated										
0–19 Years	0									
20–34	0									
35–49	0									
50–64	0									
65+	0									
2. MULTIPLE DX										
A. Not Operated										
0–19 Years	28	9.7	48	2	4	8	13	17	25	29
20–34	121	11.6	116	3	5	8	14	26	41	46
35–49	251	12.5	142	3	5	8	15	29	38	64
50–64	363	9.4	64	3	4	7	11	19	25	47
65+	645	9.3	45	3	5	8	12	17	21	35
B. Operated										
0–19 Years	4	31.5	>999	5	5	15	97	97	97	97
20–34	21	21.1	186	6	10	21	31	45	48	>99
35–49	76	17.8	178	6	8	14	22	37	46	66
50–64	106	18.7	123	9	12	16	22	32	44	56
65+	79	19.2	129	8	12	16	24	37	39	63
SUBTOTALS:										
1. SINGLE DX										
A. Not Operated	1	4.0	0	4	4	4	4	4	4	4
B. Operated	0									
2. MULTIPLE DX										
A. Not Operated	1,408	10.1	75	3	5	7	12	19	27	44
B. Operated	286	19.0	164	7	10	16	24	37	45	70
1. SINGLE DX	1	4.0	0	4	4	4	4	4	4	4
2. MULTIPLE DX	1,694	11.6	101	3	5	8	14	23	31	53
A. NOT OPERATED	1,409	10.1	75	3	5	7	12	19	27	44
B. OPERATED	286	19.0	164	7	10	16	24	37	45	70
TOTAL										
0–19 Years	32	12.4	283	2	4	8	15	17	29	97
20–34	142	13.0	137	3	5	9	17	31	42	57
35–49	328	13.7	155	3	6	9	17	30	42	64
50–64	469	11.5	92	3	5	8	15	23	30	47
65+	724	10.4	64	4	5	8	13	20	25	39
GRAND TOTAL	1,695	11.6	101	3	5	8	14	23	31	53

293

Length of Stay by Diagnosis and Operation, Western Region, 2008

Western Region, October 2006–September 2007 Data, by Diagnosis

422: ACUTE MYOCARDITIS

Type of Patients	Observed Patients	Avg. Stay	Variance	10th	25th	50th	75th	90th	95th	99th
1. SINGLE DX										
A. Not Operated										
0–19 Years	3	2.7	1	2	2	2	4	4	4	4
20–34	11	2.0	1	1	1	2	3	4	4	4
35–49	6	1.2	<1	1	1	1	1	1	2	2
50–64	1	1.0	0	1	1	1	1	1	1	1
65+	0									
B. Operated										
0–19 Years	0									
20–34	0									
35–49	0									
50–64	0									
65+	0									
2. MULTIPLE DX										
A. Not Operated										
0–19 Years	28	3.2	5	1	2	3	5	5	8	10
20–34	81	3.0	6	1	2	2	3	6	6	17
35–49	63	2.6	3	1	1	2	3	4	5	10
50–64	47	3.7	12	1	1	3	5	7	10	17
65+	19	4.6	7	2	2	4	6	8	12	12
B. Operated										
0–19 Years	1	54.0	0	54	54	54	54	54	54	54
20–34	2	9.4	142	1	6	1	18	18	18	18
35–49	3	8.3	4	6	6	9	10	10	10	10
50–64	2	24.1	388	10	10	38	38	38	38	38
65+	1	14.0	0	14	14	14	14	14	14	14
SUBTOTALS:										
1. SINGLE DX										
A. Not Operated	21	1.8	<1	1	1	2	2	3	4	4
B. Operated	0									
2. MULTIPLE DX										
A. Not Operated	238	3.2	7	1	2	2	4	6	8	15
B. Operated	9	17.8	295	1	9	10	18	54	54	54
1. SINGLE DX	21	1.8	<1	1	1	2	2	3	4	4
2. MULTIPLE DX	247	3.7	24	1	2	2	4	6	10	18
A. NOT OPERATED	259	3.1	6	1	2	2	4	6	8	15
B. OPERATED	9	17.8	295	1	9	10	18	54	54	54
TOTAL										
0–19 Years	32	4.7	85	1	2	3	5	5	10	54
20–34	94	3.0	8	1	2	2	3	6	7	18
35–49	72	2.7	5	1	1	2	3	5	9	10
50–64	50	4.5	35	1	2	3	5	10	15	38
65+	20	5.0	11	2	2	4	6	8	12	14
GRAND TOTAL	268	3.5	22	1	2	2	4	6	10	18

423: OTH PERICARDIAL DISEASE

Type of Patients	Observed Patients	Avg. Stay	Variance	10th	25th	50th	75th	90th	95th	99th
1. SINGLE DX										
A. Not Operated										
0–19 Years	4	1.7	<1	1	1	1	2	3	3	3
20–34	12	1.6	<1	1	1	1	2	2	4	4
35–49	14	1.6	<1	1	1	1	2	2	4	4
50–64	10	1.4	<1	1	1	1	2	2	3	3
65+	1	1.0	0	1	1	1	1	1	1	1
B. Operated										
0–19 Years	0									
20–34	1	3.0	0	3	3	3	3	3	3	3
35–49	3	3.3	4	1	1	4	5	5	5	5
50–64	4	2.0	1	1	1	3	3	3	3	3
65+	1	4.0	0	4	4	4	4	4	4	4
2. MULTIPLE DX										
A. Not Operated										
0–19 Years	48	2.5	3	1	1	2	3	5	7	10
20–34	183	3.0	8	1	1	2	4	6	7	13
35–49	371	3.0	11	1	1	2	4	6	8	15
50–64	571	3.2	8	1	1	3	4	6	9	14
65+	681	4.2	17	2	2	3	6	8	11	18
B. Operated										
0–19 Years	8	8.0	159	3	3	5	5	39	39	39
20–34	35	9.2	57	3	5	7	11	17	27	41
35–49	129	8.5	48	3	4	6	10	17	21	32
50–64	241	7.9	36	2	4	6	11	15	19	35
65+	330	8.6	62	3	4	7	10	17	21	34
SUBTOTALS:										
1. SINGLE DX										
A. Not Operated	41	1.5	<1	1	1	1	2	2	3	4
B. Operated	9	2.8	2	1	1	3	4	5	5	5
2. MULTIPLE DX										
A. Not Operated	1,854	3.5	12	1	1	2	4	7	9	16
B. Operated	743	8.3	52	3	4	6	10	16	21	35
1. SINGLE DX	50	1.8	1	1	1	2	2	3	4	5
2. MULTIPLE DX	2,597	4.9	28	1	2	3	6	10	14	25
A. NOT OPERATED	1,895	3.5	12	1	1	3	4	7	9	16
B. OPERATED	752	8.3	52	3	4	6	10	16	21	35
TOTAL										
0–19 Years	60	3.2	25	1	1	3	5	5	7	39
20–34	231	3.9	20	1	1	3	5	8	12	24
35–49	517	4.3	25	1	1	3	5	10	14	25
50–64	826	4.5	21	1	2	3	6	10	13	23
65+	1,013	5.6	36	1	2	4	7	11	15	27
GRAND TOTAL	2,647	4.8	28	1	2	3	6	10	14	25

423.8: PERICARDIAL DISEASE NEC

Type of Patients	Observed Patients	Avg. Stay	Variance	10th	25th	50th	75th	90th	95th	99th
1. SINGLE DX										
A. Not Operated										
0–19 Years	1	3.0	0	3	3	3	3	3	3	3
20–34	1	1.0	0	1	1	1	1	1	1	1
35–49	1	2.0	0	2	2	2	2	2	2	2
50–64	1	1.0	0	1	1	1	1	1	1	1
65+	0									
B. Operated										
0–19 Years	0									
20–34	0									
35–49	1	1.0	0	1	1	1	1	1	1	1
50–64	3	2.3	1	1	1	3	3	3	3	3
65+	1	4.0	0	4	4	4	4	4	4	4
2. MULTIPLE DX										
A. Not Operated										
0–19 Years	4	2.8	2	1	3	3	3	4	4	4
20–34	10	2.4	2	1	1	2	3	4	4	4
35–49	42	2.9	5	1	2	2	4	6	7	9
50–64	39	4.7	18	1	2	3	5	11	15	20
65+	46	3.8	5	1	2	4	5	7	8	8
B. Operated										
0–19 Years	4	2.0	2	1	1	3	3	3	3	3
20–34	6	7.2	24	2	2	6	12	12	12	12
35–49	35	9.3	88	2	4	6	12	18	28	51
50–64	65	7.1	35	2	3	5	10	14	16	37
65+	63	8.1	27	3	5	7	11	14	16	33
SUBTOTALS:										
1. SINGLE DX										
A. Not Operated	4	1.8	<1	1	1	2	2	3	3	3
B. Operated	5	2.4	2	1	1	3	3	4	4	4
2. MULTIPLE DX										
A. Not Operated	141	3.7	8	1	2	3	5	7	8	15
B. Operated	171	7.9	42	2	4	6	10	14	18	37
1. SINGLE DX	9	2.1	1	1	1	2	3	4	4	4
2. MULTIPLE DX	312	6.0	31	1	2	4	7	12	15	28
A. NOT OPERATED	145	3.6	8	1	2	3	5	7	8	15
B. OPERATED	176	7.7	42	2	4	6	10	14	18	37
TOTAL										
0–19 Years	7	2.6	1	1	1	3	3	4	4	4
20–34	17	4.0	14	1	1	3	4	12	12	12
35–49	79	5.7	51	2	2	4	7	12	18	51
50–64	108	6.0	29	2	3	5	8	13	16	20
65+	110	6.3	22	2	3	5	8	12	14	19
GRAND TOTAL	321	5.9	31	1	2	4	7	12	15	28

423.9: PERICARDIAL DISEASE NOS

Type of Patients	Observed Patients	Avg. Stay	Variance	10th	25th	50th	75th	90th	95th	99th
1. SINGLE DX										
A. Not Operated										
0–19 Years	3	1.3	<1	1	1	1	2	2	2	2
20–34	11	1.6	<1	1	1	1	2	2	4	4
35–49	13	1.5	<1	1	1	1	2	2	4	4
50–64	9	1.4	<1	1	1	1	2	3	3	3
65+	1	1.0	0	1	1	1	1	1	1	1
B. Operated										
0–19 Years	0									
20–34	0									
35–49	1	4.0	0	4	4	4	4	4	4	4
50–64	1	1.0	0	1	1	1	1	1	1	1
65+	0									
2. MULTIPLE DX										
A. Not Operated										
0–19 Years	44	2.5	4	1	1	2	3	5	7	10
20–34	158	3.0	9	1	1	2	3	6	8	13
35–49	313	3.0	12	1	1	2	3	6	8	15
50–64	488	3.0	7	1	2	3	4	6	8	13
65+	561	3.9	17	1	2	3	5	7	9	18
B. Operated										
0–19 Years	5	11.0	245	2	4	5	5	39	39	39
20–34	19	8.3	21	3	5	7	11	17	18	18
35–49	62	7.3	24	3	4	6	10	12	14	29
50–64	121	7.3	27	2	4	6	9	13	16	28
65+	197	8.2	44	3	4	6	9	18	21	34
SUBTOTALS:										
1. SINGLE DX										
A. Not Operated	37	1.5	<1	1	1	1	2	2	3	4
B. Operated	2	2.5	4	1	1	1	4	4	4	4
2. MULTIPLE DX										
A. Not Operated	1,564	3.3	12	1	1	2	4	7	9	15
B. Operated	404	7.8	37	3	4	6	10	15	19	34
1. SINGLE DX	39	1.6	<1	1	1	1	2	3	4	4
2. MULTIPLE DX	1,968	4.2	20	1	2	3	5	9	12	23
A. NOT OPERATED	1,601	3.3	12	1	1	2	4	6	9	15
B. OPERATED	406	7.8	37	3	4	6	10	15	19	34
TOTAL										
0–19 Years	52	3.3	29	1	1	2	3	5	7	39
20–34	188	3.5	12	1	1	2	4	7	11	18
35–49	389	3.6	16	1	1	2	4	8	11	23
50–64	619	3.8	14	1	1	2	5	8	11	17
65+	759	5.0	27	1	2	4	6	9	15	27
GRAND TOTAL	2,007	4.2	20	1	2	3	5	9	12	22

424: OTH ENDOCARDIAL DISEASE

Type of Patients	Observed Patients	Avg. Stay	Variance	10th	25th	50th	75th	90th	95th	99th
1. SINGLE DX										
A. Not Operated										
0–19 Years	1	3.0	0	3	3	3	3	3	3	3
20–34	3	3.3	6	1	1	3	6	6	6	6
35–49	5	1.4	<1	1	1	1	3	3	3	3
50–64	4	1.0	0	1	1	1	1	1	1	1
65+	4	1.3	<1	1	1	1	2	2	2	2
B. Operated										
0–19 Years	4	2.7	4	1	1	1	4	5	5	5
20–34	1	4.0	0	4	4	4	4	4	4	4
35–49	21	3.6	2	2	3	4	4	5	5	6
50–64	22	4.1	2	2	3	4	5	6	7	7
65+	8	6.4	14	1	5	5	8	14	14	14
2. MULTIPLE DX										
A. Not Operated										
0–19 Years	11	6.6	207	1	1	2	3	4	50	50
20–34	42	4.7	57	1	1	2	3	11	18	43
35–49	128	3.3	15	1	1	2	3	7	9	21
50–64	312	3.8	23	1	1	3	4	8	11	24
65+	1,481	3.4	10	1	1	3	4	7	8	16
B. Operated										
0–19 Years	30	5.3	20	2	3	4	6	10	11	24
20–34	133	6.6	21	3	4	5	8	11	16	17
35–49	529	7.2	23	4	4	6	8	12	15	26
50–64	2,083	7.8	30	4	5	6	9	14	18	30
65+	5,030	9.4	45	4	6	7	11	16	21	36
SUBTOTALS:										
1. SINGLE DX										
A. Not Operated	17	1.7	2	1	1	1	2	3	6	6
B. Operated	56	4.2	5	1	3	4	5	7	7	14
2. MULTIPLE DX										
A. Not Operated	1,974	3.5	14	1	1	2	4	7	9	21
B. Operated	7,805	8.8	40	4	5	7	10	15	20	34
1. SINGLE DX	73	3.6	5	1	2	4	5	6	7	14
2. MULTIPLE DX	9,779	7.7	39	2	4	6	9	14	19	33
A. NOT OPERATED	1,991	3.5	14	1	1	2	4	7	9	21
B. OPERATED	7,861	8.7	40	4	5	7	10	15	20	34
TOTAL										
0–19 Years	46	5.3	60	1	2	4	5	10	11	50
20–34	179	6.1	29	1	3	5	7	11	16	41
35–49	683	6.3	24	2	4	5	7	11	14	26
50–64	2,421	7.2	31	3	4	6	8	13	17	29
65+	6,523	8.0	43	4	7	7	10	15	20	34
GRAND TOTAL	9,852	7.7	39	2	4	6	9	14	19	32

424.0: MITRAL VALVE DISORDER

Type of Patients	Observed Patients	Avg. Stay	Variance	10th	25th	50th	75th	90th	95th	99th
1. SINGLE DX										
A. Not Operated										
0–19 Years	1	3.0	0	3	3	3	3	3	3	3
20–34	1	3.0	0	3	3	3	3	3	3	3
35–49	3	1.0	0	1	1	1	1	1	1	1
50–64	3	1.0	0	1	1	1	1	1	1	1
65+	1	1.0	0	1	1	1	1	1	1	1
B. Operated										
0–19 Years	1	5.0	0	5	5	5	5	5	5	5
20–34	0									
35–49	13	3.4	2	1	3	4	4	5	5	5
50–64	16	4.1	2	2	3	4	4	6	7	7
65+	4	5.2	2	4	5	5	5	7	7	7
2. MULTIPLE DX										
A. Not Operated										
0–19 Years	5	2.6	2	1	2	2	2	4	4	4
20–34	16	3.6	21	1	1	2	4	9	19	19
35–49	50	3.1	12	1	1	2	4	7	7	21
50–64	124	3.3	18	1	1	2	4	7	9	24
65+	203	3.3	8	1	1	3	4	7	8	15
B. Operated										
0–19 Years	10	8.0	42	3	3	6	6	11	24	24
20–34	61	7.2	32	3	4	6	8	13	16	41
35–49	280	7.1	23	3	4	6	8	12	15	24
50–64	848	8.0	37	4	5	6	9	14	19	32
65+	1,164	9.7	43	4	6	8	11	17	22	35
SUBTOTALS:										
1. SINGLE DX										
A. Not Operated	9	1.5	<1	1	1	1	2	3	3	3
B. Operated	34	4.0	2	2	3	4	5	6	7	7
2. MULTIPLE DX										
A. Not Operated	398	3.3	12	1	1	2	4	7	8	21
B. Operated	2,363	8.7	39	4	7	7	10	15	20	34
1. SINGLE DX	43	3.4	3	1	2	4	5	5	6	7
2. MULTIPLE DX	2,761	7.9	39	3	4	6	10	15	19	32
A. NOT OPERATED	407	3.2	12	1	1	2	4	7	8	21
B. OPERATED	2,397	8.6	39	4	5	7	10	15	20	34
TOTAL										
0–19 Years	17	5.9	31	2	3	4	6	11	24	24
20–34	78	6.4	32	1	4	5	8	13	16	41
35–49	346	6.3	23	2	4	5	8	12	14	23
50–64	991	7.3	37	3	4	6	8	14	18	31
65+	1,372	8.7	43	3	5	7	10	16	21	33
GRAND TOTAL	2,804	7.9	39	2	4	6	9	14	19	32

Length of Stay by Diagnosis and Operation, Western Region, 2008

Western Region, October 2006–September 2007 Data, by Diagnosis

424.1: AORTIC VALVE DISORDER

Type of Patients	Observed Patients	Avg. Stay	Vari-ance	10th	25th	50th	75th	90th	95th	99th
1. SINGLE DX										
A. Not Operated										
0–19 Years	0									
20–34	2	3.5	12	1	1	1	6	6	6	6
35–49	2	2.0	0	1	1	2	3	3	3	3
50–64	1	1.0	0	1	1	1	1	1	1	1
65+	3	1.3	<1	1	1	1	2	2	2	2
B. Operated										
0–19 Years	2	2.5	4	1	1	4	4	4	4	4
20–34	1	4.0	0	4	4	4	4	4	4	4
35–49	8	4.0	1	3	3	4	5	6	6	6
50–64	6	4.3	3	2	3	4	5	7	7	7
65+	3	9.7	14	7	7	8	14	14	14	14
2. MULTIPLE DX										
A. Not Operated										
0–19 Years	3	1.3	<1	1	1	1	2	2	2	2
20–34	17	1.8	1	1	1	1	2	3	5	5
35–49	56	2.9	16	1	1	2	3	7	8	28
50–64	169	3.3	10	1	1	2	4	8	9	17
65+	1,243	3.4	10	1	1	3	4	7	9	15
B. Operated										
0–19 Years	10	4.5	7	1	3	5	6	9	9	9
20–34	53	6.5	11	4	5	5	6	11	17	17
35–49	230	7.2	22	4	5	6	8	12	15	26
50–64	1,220	7.6	25	4	5	6	9	13	16	27
65+	3,856	9.3	45	4	6	7	11	16	21	36
SUBTOTALS:										
1. SINGLE DX A. Not Operated	8	2.0	3	1	1	1	2	6	6	6
1. SINGLE DX B. Operated	20	4.8	8	3	3	4	6	8	14	14
2. MULTIPLE DX A. Not Operated	1,488	3.3	10	1	1	2	4	7	9	16
2. MULTIPLE DX B. Operated	5,369	8.8	40	4	5	7	10	15	20	35
1. SINGLE DX	28	4.0	8	1	2	4	5	7	8	14
2. MULTIPLE DX	6,857	7.6	39	2	4	6	9	14	18	33
A. NOT OPERATED	1,496	3.3	10	1	1	2	4	7	9	16
B. OPERATED	5,389	8.8	40	4	5	7	10	15	20	35
TOTAL										
0–19 Years	15	3.6	7	1	1	3	6	7	9	9
20–34	73	5.3	12	1	4	5	6	9	13	17
35–49	296	6.3	23	2	4	5	7	11	14	28
50–64	1,396	7.1	25	3	4	6	8	12	15	26
65+	5,105	7.8	43	4	4	6	9	15	19	34
GRAND TOTAL	6,885	7.6	39	2	4	6	9	14	18	33

425: CARDIOMYOPATHY

Type of Patients	Observed Patients	Avg. Stay	Vari-ance	10th	25th	50th	75th	90th	95th	99th
1. SINGLE DX										
A. Not Operated										
0–19 Years	1	1.0	0	1	1	1	1	1	1	1
20–34	4	1.0	0	1	1	1	1	1	1	1
35–49	2	3.5	12	1	1	1	6	6	6	6
50–64	2	3.0	8	1	1	3	5	5	5	5
65+	2	1.0	0	1	1	1	1	1	1	1
B. Operated										
0–19 Years	2	5.0	31	1	1	5	9	9	9	9
20–34	4	1.5	<1	1	1	1	1	3	3	3
35–49	12	1.3	<1	1	1	1	1	2	3	3
50–64	20	1.2	<1	1	1	1	1	1	2	3
65+	10	1.4	2	1	1	1	1	5	5	5
2. MULTIPLE DX										
A. Not Operated										
0–19 Years	25	8.7	161	1	2	3	9	31	33	53
20–34	152	5.0	52	1	2	3	6	10	13	51
35–49	468	3.5	11	1	2	2	4	7	10	18
50–64	656	3.8	18	1	2	3	4	7	10	24
65+	577	3.9	12	1	2	3	5	8	11	19
B. Operated										
0–19 Years	17	10.0	211	1	4	4	9	35	53	53
20–34	61	5.2	54	1	2	2	6	12	16	44
35–49	214	4.3	77	1	1	1	4	9	17	48
50–64	462	3.4	24	1	1	1	4	8	14	29
65+	524	2.9	30	1	1	1	2	7	9	29
SUBTOTALS:										
1. SINGLE DX A. Not Operated	11	1.8	3	1	1	1	1	5	6	6
1. SINGLE DX B. Operated	48	1.4	2	1	1	1	1	3	3	9
2. MULTIPLE DX A. Not Operated	1,878	3.9	19	2	2	3	4	8	11	22
2. MULTIPLE DX B. Operated	1,278	3.5	40	1	1	3	4	8	12	31
1. SINGLE DX	59	1.5	2	1	1	1	1	3	5	9
2. MULTIPLE DX	3,156	3.8	28	1	1	2	4	8	12	26
A. NOT OPERATED	1,889	3.9	19	2	2	3	4	8	11	22
B. OPERATED	1,326	3.4	39	1	1	2	4	8	12	30
TOTAL										
0–19 Years	45	8.9	168	1	1	3	9	31	35	53
20–34	221	5.0	51	1	1	3	6	11	14	44
35–49	696	3.7	31	1	1	2	4	8	12	23
50–64	1,140	3.6	20	1	1	2	4	7	11	25
65+	1,113	3.4	21	1	1	2	4	7	10	20
GRAND TOTAL	3,215	3.7	27	1	1	2	4	8	11	26

425.1: HYPERTR OBSTR CARDIOMYOP

Type of Patients	Observed Patients	Avg. Stay	Vari-ance	10th	25th	50th	75th	90th	95th	99th
1. SINGLE DX										
A. Not Operated										
0–19 Years	0									
20–34	4	1.0	0	1	1	1	1	1	1	1
35–49	0									
50–64	1	6.0	0	6	6	6	6	6	6	6
65+	1	1.0	0	1	1	1	1	1	1	1
B. Operated										
0–19 Years	0									
20–34	2	2.0	2	1	1	1	3	3	3	3
35–49	4	1.8	<1	1	1	2	3	3	3	3
50–64	7	1.3	<1	1	1	1	1	3	3	3
65+	0									
2. MULTIPLE DX										
A. Not Operated										
0–19 Years	0									
20–34	11	3.9	11	1	1	2	8	9	9	9
35–49	28	2.3	6	1	1	2	2	5	6	13
50–64	61	2.6	4	1	1	2	4	5	6	11
65+	110	3.9	16	1	2	3	5	7	11	24
B. Operated										
0–19 Years	5	1.8	2	1	1	2	2	4	4	4
20–34	14	5.4	24	1	1	5	6	14	16	16
35–49	28	3.6	12	1	1	2	4	8	12	15
50–64	54	5.0	37	1	1	3	6	14	20	30
65+	48	5.9	75	2	2	3	7	12	21	52
SUBTOTALS:										
1. SINGLE DX A. Not Operated	6	1.8	4	1	1	1	1	6	6	6
1. SINGLE DX B. Operated	13	1.5	<1	1	1	2	2	3	3	3
2. MULTIPLE DX A. Not Operated	210	3.3	11	1	1	2	4	6	9	14
2. MULTIPLE DX B. Operated	149	4.9	42	1	1	3	6	12	15	30
1. SINGLE DX	19	1.6	2	1	1	1	2	3	6	6
2. MULTIPLE DX	359	4.0	25	1	1	2	5	8	12	26
A. NOT OPERATED	216	3.3	11	1	1	2	4	6	9	14
B. OPERATED	162	4.7	40	1	1	2	5	11	15	30
TOTAL										
0–19 Years	5	1.8	2	1	1	2	2	4	4	4
20–34	31	4.1	17	1	1	2	6	9	14	16
35–49	61	2.9	9	1	1	2	3	6	8	15
50–64	122	3.6	20	1	1	2	4	7	11	25
65+	159	4.5	34	2	2	3	5	10	12	29
GRAND TOTAL	378	3.9	24	1	1	2	5	8	12	26

Length of Stay by Diagnosis and Operation, Western Region, 2008

Western Region, October 2006–September 2007 Data, by Diagnosis

425.4: PRIM CARDIOMYOPATHY NEC

Type of Patients	Observed Patients	Avg. Stay	Variance	Percentiles 10th	25th	50th	75th	90th	95th	99th
1. SINGLE DX										
A. Not Operated										
0–19 Years	1	1.0	0	1	1	1	1	1	1	1
20–34	0									
35–49	1	1.0	0	1	1	1	1	1	1	1
50–64	2	3.0	8	1	1	3	5	5	5	5
65+	0									
B. Operated										
0–19 Years	2	5.0	31	1	1	5	9	9	9	9
20–34	2	1.0	0	1	1	1	1	1	1	1
35–49	8	1.0	0	1	1	1	1	1	1	1
50–64	13	1.1	<1	1	1	1	1	1	2	2
65+	10	1.4	2	1	1	1	1	5	5	5
2. MULTIPLE DX										
A. Not Operated										
0–19 Years	22	6.7	85	1	2	3	7	16	31	33
20–34	124	5.4	61	1	2	3	6	11	14	51
35–49	344	3.3	9	1	1	2	4	7	10	15
50–64	501	3.6	17	1	2	3	4	7	9	21
65+	431	3.8	11	1	2	3	4	8	10	19
B. Operated										
0–19 Years	11	11.5	238	1	1	9	10	25	53	53
20–34	44	3.8	22	1	1	1	5	12	8	20
35–49	177	4.4	89	1	1	1	4	9	10	63
50–64	387	3.0	20	1	1	1	3	8	12	27
65+	470	2.5	24	1	1	1	2	5	9	28
SUBTOTALS:										
1. SINGLE DX										
A. Not Operated	4	2.0	4	1	1	1	1	5	5	5
B. Operated	35	1.4	2	1	1	1	1	1	5	9
2. MULTIPLE DX										
A. Not Operated	1,422	3.8	19	1	2	3	4	7	11	20
B. Operated	1,089	3.1	36	1	1	1	3	8	11	29
1. SINGLE DX	39	1.4	2	1	1	1	1	2	5	9
2. MULTIPLE DX	2,511	3.5	26	1	2	2	4	7	11	25
A. NOT OPERATED	1,426	3.8	18	1	2	2	4	7	10	20
B. OPERATED	1,124	3.1	35	1	1	1	3	7	10	28
TOTAL										
0–19 Years	36	7.9	127	1	1	3	9	25	33	53
20–34	170	4.9	51	1	1	3	6	11	14	51
35–49	530	3.6	36	1	1	2	4	7	11	23
50–64	903	3.3	18	1	1	2	4	7	10	22
65+	911	3.1	18	1	1	2	4	7	10	19
GRAND TOTAL	2,550	3.5	26	1	1	2	4	7	10	25

426: CONDUCTION DISORDERS

Type of Patients	Observed Patients	Avg. Stay	Variance	Percentiles 10th	25th	50th	75th	90th	95th	99th
1. SINGLE DX										
A. Not Operated										
0–19 Years	13	1.8	2	1	1	1	2	3	3	6
20–34	12	1.3	<1	1	1	1	1	3	6	6
35–49	7	1.6	<1	1	1	1	2	2	3	3
50–64	16	1.6	<1	1	1	1	2	3	3	3
65+	46	1.2	<1	1	1	1	1	2	2	4
B. Operated										
0–19 Years	24	1.0	<1	1	1	1	1	1	1	2
20–34	38	1.1	<1	1	1	1	1	1	2	3
35–49	16	1.1	<1	1	1	1	1	1	3	3
50–64	7	1.1	<1	1	1	1	1	2	2	2
65+	3	1.3	<1	1	2	1	2	2	2	2
2. MULTIPLE DX										
A. Not Operated										
0–19 Years	39	2.6	7	1	1	2	3	6	10	13
20–34	94	1.9	2	1	1	1	2	4	6	7
35–49	217	2.6	5	1	1	2	3	5	6	10
50–64	853	2.8	6	1	1	2	3	5	7	12
65+	5,503	3.2	8	1	1	2	4	6	8	13
B. Operated										
0–19 Years	42	2.1	5	1	1	1	2	6	6	10
20–34	64	2.7	9	1	1	1	4	7	8	17
35–49	99	3.2	20	1	1	2	4	8	10	35
50–64	167	3.6	17	1	1	2	5	9	12	23
65+	597	5.0	21	2	2	4	6	10	15	25
SUBTOTALS:										
1. SINGLE DX										
A. Not Operated	94	1.4	<1	1	1	1	2	2	3	6
B. Operated	88	1.1	<1	1	1	1	1	1	2	3
2. MULTIPLE DX										
A. Not Operated	6,706	3.1	8	1	1	2	4	6	8	13
B. Operated	969	4.3	20	1	1	3	5	10	13	24
1. SINGLE DX	182	1.3	<1	1	1	1	1	2	3	4
2. MULTIPLE DX	7,675	3.2	9	1	1	2	4	6	8	15
A. NOT OPERATED	6,800	3.1	7	1	1	2	4	6	7	13
B. OPERATED	1,057	4.0	19	1	1	2	5	10	12	23
TOTAL										
0–19 Years	118	2.0	5	1	1	1	2	5	6	10
20–34	208	2.0	4	1	1	1	2	4	6	10
35–49	339	2.7	9	1	1	1	3	5	8	14
50–64	1,043	2.9	8	1	1	2	3	6	8	16
65+	6,149	3.3	9	1	1	2	4	6	8	15
GRAND TOTAL	7,857	3.2	9	1	1	2	4	6	8	15

426.0: COMPLETE A/V BLOCK

Type of Patients	Observed Patients	Avg. Stay	Variance	Percentiles 10th	25th	50th	75th	90th	95th	99th
1. SINGLE DX										
A. Not Operated										
0–19 Years	2	1.0	0	1	1	1	1	1	1	1
20–34	4	2.0	1	1	1	3	3	3	3	3
35–49	3	1.3	<1	1	1	2	2	2	2	2
50–64	8	1.8	<1	1	1	2	2	3	3	3
65+	23	1.3	<1	1	1	1	1	2	2	4
B. Operated										
0–19 Years	2	1.5	<1	1	1	2	2	2	2	2
20–34	0									
35–49	0									
50–64	0									
65+	2	1.5	<1	1	1	2	2	2	2	2
2. MULTIPLE DX										
A. Not Operated										
0–19 Years	10	3.6	15	1	1	2	6	13	13	13
20–34	21	2.1	3	1	1	1	2	5	6	6
35–49	81	3.1	8	1	1	2	3	6	8	17
50–64	486	2.9	7	1	1	2	4	5	7	14
65+	3,356	3.3	8	1	2	2	4	6	8	15
B. Operated										
0–19 Years	5	4.8	11	2	2	4	6	10	10	10
20–34	4	2.3	4	1	1	2	4	4	4	4
35–49	23	6.3	52	1	2	4	8	11	14	35
50–64	66	4.1	18	1	1	2	5	11	12	24
65+	408	5.4	24	2	2	4	7	11	15	25
SUBTOTALS:										
1. SINGLE DX										
A. Not Operated	40	1.5	<1	1	1	2	2	2	3	4
B. Operated	4	1.5	<1	1	1	2	2	2	2	2
2. MULTIPLE DX										
A. Not Operated	3,954	3.2	8	1	2	2	4	6	8	14
B. Operated	506	5.2	25	1	2	4	7	11	15	25
1. SINGLE DX	44	1.5	<1	1	1	1	2	2	3	4
2. MULTIPLE DX	4,460	3.5	11	1	2	3	4	7	9	16
A. NOT OPERATED	3,994	3.2	8	1	2	2	4	6	8	14
B. OPERATED	510	5.2	24	1	2	4	7	11	15	25
TOTAL										
0–19 Years	19	3.4	12	1	1	2	6	10	13	13
20–34	29	2.1	2	1	1	1	3	3	6	6
35–49	107	3.7	19	1	1	2	4	8	10	17
50–64	560	3.1	9	1	1	2	4	6	8	14
65+	3,789	3.5	11	2	2	3	4	7	9	17
GRAND TOTAL	4,504	3.4	10	2	2	2	4	7	9	16

Length of Stay by Diagnosis and Operation, Western Region, 2008

Western Region, October 2006–September 2007 Data, by Diagnosis

426.11: 1ST DEGREE A/V BLOCK

Type of Patients	Observed Patients	Avg. Stay	Vari-ance	10th	25th	50th	75th	90th	95th	99th
1. SINGLE DX										
A. Not Operated										
0–19 Years	1	1.0	0	1	1	1	1	1	1	1
20–34	0									
35–49	1	1.0	0	1	1	1	1	1	1	1
50–64	0									
65+	1	1.0	0	1	1	1	1	1	1	1
B. Operated										
0–19 Years	0									
20–34	0									
35–49	0									
50–64	0									
65+	0									
2. MULTIPLE DX										
A. Not Operated										
0–19 Years	0									
20–34	8	1.4	<1	1	1	1	2	2	2	2
35–49	8	1.9	1	1	1	2	3	4	4	4
50–64	23	2.7	4	1	1	2	4	5	6	8
65+	159	3.0	4	1	1	2	4	6	7	12
B. Operated										
0–19 Years	0									
20–34	0									
35–49	2	2.0	0	2	2	2	2	2	2	2
50–64	3	5.4	44	1	1	2	13	13	13	13
65+	20	3.5	11	1	1	2	4	10	11	11
SUBTOTALS:										
1. SINGLE DX										
A. Not Operated	3	1.0	0	1	1	1	1	1	1	1
B. Operated	0									
2. MULTIPLE DX										
A. Not Operated	198	2.8	4	1	1	2	4	5	7	12
B. Operated	25	3.6	13	1	1	2	4	10	11	13
1. SINGLE DX	3	1.0	0	1	1	1	1	1	1	1
2. MULTIPLE DX	223	2.9	5	1	1	2	4	6	7	12
A. NOT OPERATED	201	2.8	4	1	1	2	4	5	6	10
B. OPERATED	25	3.6	13	1	1	2	4	10	11	13
TOTAL										
0–19 Years	1	1.0	0	1	1	1	1	1	1	1
20–34	8	1.4	<1	1	1	1	2	2	2	2
35–49	11	1.8	<1	1	1	2	2	3	4	4
50–64	26	3.0	8	1	1	2	4	6	8	13
65+	180	3.0	5	1	1	2	4	6	7	12
GRAND TOTAL	226	2.9	5	1	1	2	4	6	7	12

426.12: MOBITZ II A/V BLOCK

Type of Patients	Observed Patients	Avg. Stay	Vari-ance	10th	25th	50th	75th	90th	95th	99th
1. SINGLE DX										
A. Not Operated										
0–19 Years	1	1.0	0	1	1	1	1	1	1	1
20–34	1	1.0	0	1	1	1	1	1	1	1
35–49	0									
50–64	2	2.0	2	1	1	1	3	3	3	3
65+	2	1.5	<1	1	1	1	2	2	2	2
B. Operated										
0–19 Years	0									
20–34	0									
35–49	0									
50–64	0									
65+	0									
2. MULTIPLE DX										
A. Not Operated										
0–19 Years	0									
20–34	3	2.3	2	1	1	2	4	4	4	4
35–49	9	2.5	1	2	2	3	3	3	4	4
50–64	57	2.7	3	1	1	2	3	5	6	8
65+	467	3.0	5	1	1	2	4	6	8	13
B. Operated										
0–19 Years	0									
20–34	1	7.0	0	7	7	7	7	7	7	7
35–49	1	3.0	0	3	3	3	3	3	3	3
50–64	5	8.0	91	1	1	3	12	23	23	23
65+	32	4.1	7	2	2	3	5	8	10	10
SUBTOTALS:										
1. SINGLE DX										
A. Not Operated	6	1.5	<1	1	1	1	2	3	3	3
B. Operated	0									
2. MULTIPLE DX										
A. Not Operated	536	3.0	5	1	1	2	4	6	8	12
B. Operated	39	4.6	17	2	2	3	6	10	12	23
1. SINGLE DX	6	1.5	<1	1	1	1	2	3	3	3
2. MULTIPLE DX	575	3.1	6	1	1	2	4	6	8	13
A. NOT OPERATED	542	3.0	5	1	1	2	4	6	8	12
B. OPERATED	39	4.6	17	2	2	3	6	10	12	23
TOTAL										
0–19 Years	1	1.0	0	1	1	1	1	1	1	1
20–34	5	3.0	7	1	1	2	4	7	7	7
35–49	10	2.5	<1	2	2	3	3	4	4	4
50–64	64	3.1	10	1	1	2	3	5	7	23
65+	501	3.1	6	1	2	2	4	6	8	13
GRAND TOTAL	581	3.1	6	1	2	2	4	6	8	13

426.13: 2ND DEGREE A/V BLOCK NEC

Type of Patients	Observed Patients	Avg. Stay	Vari-ance	10th	25th	50th	75th	90th	95th	99th
1. SINGLE DX										
A. Not Operated										
0–19 Years	0									
20–34	2	1.0	0	1	1	1	1	1	1	1
35–49	1	2.0	0	2	2	2	2	2	2	2
50–64	1	1.0	0	1	1	1	1	1	1	1
65+	13	1.0	0	1	1	1	1	1	1	1
B. Operated										
0–19 Years	0									
20–34	1	1.0	0	1	1	1	1	1	1	1
35–49	0									
50–64	0									
65+	0									
2. MULTIPLE DX										
A. Not Operated										
0–19 Years	2	1.5	<1	1	1	1	2	2	2	2
20–34	10	2.0	3	1	1	1	2	3	7	7
35–49	29	2.6	5	1	1	2	3	5	8	10
50–64	136	2.7	4	1	1	2	4	5	7	9
65+	998	3.0	7	1	1	2	4	5	7	12
B. Operated										
0–19 Years	1	2.0	0	2	2	2	2	2	2	2
20–34	1	1.0	0	1	1	1	1	1	1	1
35–49	2	1.5	<1	1	1	2	2	2	2	2
50–64	12	5.7	34	1	2	3	8	17	17	17
65+	63	4.1	11	1	1	3	6	10	10	15
SUBTOTALS:										
1. SINGLE DX										
A. Not Operated	17	1.1	<1	1	1	1	1	2	2	2
B. Operated	1	1.0	0	1	1	1	1	1	1	1
2. MULTIPLE DX										
A. Not Operated	1,175	2.9	6	1	1	2	4	5	7	11
B. Operated	79	4.2	14	2	2	3	6	10	13	17
1. SINGLE DX	18	1.1	<1	1	1	1	1	2	2	2
2. MULTIPLE DX	1,254	3.0	7	1	1	2	4	6	7	13
A. NOT OPERATED	1,192	2.9	6	1	1	2	4	5	7	11
B. OPERATED	80	4.2	14	1	1	3	6	10	13	17
TOTAL										
0–19 Years	3	1.7	<1	1	1	2	2	2	2	2
20–34	14	1.8	3	1	1	2	3	3	7	7
35–49	32	2.4	4	1	1	3	3	5	8	10
50–64	149	2.9	7	1	1	2	4	6	7	17
65+	1,074	3.0	7	1	1	2	4	6	7	13
GRAND TOTAL	1,272	3.0	7	1	1	2	4	6	7	13

Length of Stay by Diagnosis and Operation, Western Region 2008

Western Region, October 2006–September 2007 Data, by Diagnosis

426.7: ANOMALOUS A/V EXCITATION

Type of Patients	Observed Patients	Avg. Stay	Variance	10th	25th	50th	75th	90th	95th	99th
1. SINGLE DX										
A. *Not Operated*										
0–19 Years	7	1.7	<1	1	1	2	2	3	3	3
20–34	5	1.0	0	1	1	1	1	1	1	1
35–49	1	2.0	0	2	2	2	2	2	2	2
50–64	1	1.0	0	1	1	1	1	1	1	1
65+	0									
B. *Operated*										
0–19 Years	19	1.0	0	1	1	1	1	1	1	1
20–34	36	1.1	<1	1	1	1	1	1	1	3
35–49	14	1.1	<1	1	1	1	1	2	3	3
50–64	7	1.1	<1	1	1	1	1	2	2	2
65+	1	1.0	0	1	1	1	1	1	1	1
2. MULTIPLE DX										
A. *Not Operated*										
0–19 Years	16	2.3	2	1	1	2	2	5	5	5
20–34	37	1.8	2	1	1	1	2	4	6	7
35–49	49	2.0	2	1	1	1	3	4	5	6
50–64	34	1.8	2	1	1	2	2	3	5	7
65+	13	1.9	<1	1	1	2	2	3	4	4
B. *Operated*										
0–19 Years	31	1.3	<1	1	1	1	1	1	3	6
20–34	47	1.7	2	1	1	1	2	4	5	7
35–49	54	1.8	3	1	1	1	2	4	7	8
50–64	50	2.0	8	1	1	2	2	3	6	19
65+	17	3.9	13	1	1	2	5	10	11	11
SUBTOTALS:										
1. SINGLE DX										
A. *Not Operated*	14	1.4	<1	1	1	1	2	2	3	3
B. *Operated*	77	1.1	<1	1	1	1	1	1	1	1
2. MULTIPLE DX										
A. *Not Operated*	149	1.9	2	1	1	1	2	4	5	7
B. *Operated*	199	1.9	5	1	1	1	2	4	7	11
1. SINGLE DX	91	1.1	<1	1	1	1	1	1	2	3
2. MULTIPLE DX	348	1.9	3	1	1	1	2	4	6	10
A. NOT OPERATED	163	1.9	2	1	1	1	2	4	5	7
B. OPERATED	276	1.7	4	1	1	1	1	3	5	10
TOTAL										
0–19 Years	73	1.5	1	1	1	1	1	2	2	5
20–34	125	1.5	1	1	1	1	1	3	4	7
35–49	118	1.8	2	1	1	1	2	4	5	7
50–64	92	1.8	5	1	1	1	2	3	5	19
65+	31	3.0	8	1	1	2	4	7	10	11
GRAND TOTAL	439	1.8	3	1	1	1	2	3	5	8

427: CARDIAC DYSRHYTHMIAS

Type of Patients	Observed Patients	Avg. Stay	Variance	10th	25th	50th	75th	90th	95th	99th
1. SINGLE DX										
A. *Not Operated*										
0–19 Years	41	1.7	<1	1	1	1	2	3	3	4
20–34	107	1.3	<1	1	1	1	1	2	3	3
35–49	199	1.4	<1	1	1	1	2	2	3	4
50–64	291	1.5	<1	1	1	1	2	3	3	6
65+	281	1.5	2	1	1	1	2	3	3	6
B. *Operated*										
0–19 Years	53	1.1	<1	1	1	1	1	1	1	3
20–34	131	1.1	<1	1	1	1	1	1	2	3
35–49	176	1.2	<1	1	1	1	1	2	3	3
50–64	310	1.2	<1	1	1	1	1	2	2	4
65+	139	1.1	<1	1	1	1	1	2	2	2
2. MULTIPLE DX										
A. *Not Operated*										
0–19 Years	310	3.9	29	1	1	2	4	9	15	25
20–34	1,315	2.3	6	1	1	1	3	4	6	11
35–49	4,730	2.5	8	1	1	2	3	5	7	12
50–64	14,838	2.7	9	1	1	2	3	5	7	13
65+	50,939	3.2	8	1	1	2	4	6	8	14
B. *Operated*										
0–19 Years	66	4.7	52	1	1	2	5	9	18	45
20–34	328	3.3	21	1	1	1	4	8	10	26
35–49	1,069	3.1	15	1	1	1	4	7	10	22
50–64	3,535	3.3	19	1	1	1	4	8	11	21
65+	6,233	4.4	30	1	1	2	6	10	14	25
SUBTOTALS:										
1. SINGLE DX										
A. *Not Operated*	919	1.5	1	1	1	1	2	2	3	5
B. *Operated*	809	1.1	<1	1	1	1	1	1	2	3
2. MULTIPLE DX										
A. *Not Operated*	72,132	3.0	8	1	1	2	4	6	8	14
B. *Operated*	11,231	3.9	26	1	1	2	5	9	12	24
1. SINGLE DX	1,728	1.3	<1	1	1	1	1	2	3	4
2. MULTIPLE DX	83,363	3.1	10	1	1	2	4	6	8	15
A. NOT OPERATED	73,051	3.0	8	1	1	2	4	6	8	13
B. OPERATED	12,040	3.7	24	1	1	2	5	9	12	23
TOTAL										
0–19 Years	470	3.5	28	1	1	2	3	8	12	26
20–34	1,881	2.3	8	1	1	1	3	5	7	15
35–49	6,174	2.6	9	1	1	2	3	5	7	13
50–64	18,974	2.8	10	1	1	2	3	6	8	15
65+	57,592	3.3	10	1	1	2	4	7	9	15
GRAND TOTAL	85,091	3.1	10	1	1	2	4	6	8	15

427.0: PSVT

Type of Patients	Observed Patients	Avg. Stay	Variance	10th	25th	50th	75th	90th	95th	99th
1. SINGLE DX										
A. *Not Operated*										
0–19 Years	9	1.9	1	1	1	2	2	4	4	4
20–34	11	1.4	<1	1	1	1	2	2	3	3
35–49	25	1.6	<1	1	1	1	2	2	3	4
50–64	14	1.3	<1	1	1	1	1	2	3	3
65+	3	1.3	<1	1	1	1	2	2	2	2
B. *Operated*										
0–19 Years	18	1.1	<1	1	1	1	1	1	2	2
20–34	62	1.1	<1	1	1	1	2	1	2	3
35–49	45	1.1	<1	1	1	1	1	1	2	3
50–64	55	1.1	<1	1	1	1	1	1	1	5
65+	15	1.0	0	1	1	1	1	1	1	1
2. MULTIPLE DX										
A. *Not Operated*										
0–19 Years	32	2.0	3	1	1	2	2	4	5	9
20–34	98	2.0	7	1	1	1	2	4	4	23
35–49	288	2.1	3	1	1	2	2	4	6	9
50–64	648	2.2	4	1	1	2	3	4	6	12
65+	1,409	2.8	6	1	1	2	3	5	7	12
B. *Operated*										
0–19 Years	16	1.9	6	1	1	1	2	3	11	11
20–34	68	1.6	2	1	1	1	2	3	4	6
35–49	158	1.6	2	1	1	1	1	3	5	10
50–64	250	2.1	11	1	1	2	2	5	6	14
65+	308	3.1	13	1	1	4	4	7	9	16
SUBTOTALS:										
1. SINGLE DX										
A. *Not Operated*	62	1.5	<1	1	1	1	2	2	3	4
B. *Operated*	195	1.1	<1	1	1	1	1	1	2	3
2. MULTIPLE DX										
A. *Not Operated*	2,475	2.5	5	1	1	2	3	5	7	12
B. *Operated*	800	2.3	10	1	1	1	3	5	7	15
1. SINGLE DX	257	1.2	<1	1	1	1	1	2	2	4
2. MULTIPLE DX	3,275	2.5	7	1	1	2	3	5	7	13
A. NOT OPERATED	2,537	2.5	5	1	1	2	3	5	7	11
B. OPERATED	995	2.1	8	1	1	2	2	5	7	15
TOTAL										
0–19 Years	75	1.8	3	1	1	2	2	3	4	11
20–34	239	1.6	3	1	1	2	2	4	4	7
35–49	516	1.8	2	1	1	1	2	4	5	8
50–64	967	2.1	6	1	1	1	2	4	6	12
65+	1,735	2.9	8	1	1	2	3	6	7	14
GRAND TOTAL	3,532	2.4	6	1	1	2	3	5	7	12

Length of Stay by Diagnosis and Operation, Western Region, 2008

Western Region, October 2006–September 2007 Data, by Diagnosis

427.1: PVT

Type of Patients	Observed Patients	Avg. Stay	Vari-ance	10th	25th	50th	75th	90th	95th	99th
1. SINGLE DX										
A. Not Operated										
0–19 Years	2	1.0	0	1	1	1	1	1	1	1
20–34	11	1.3	<1	1	1	1	2	2	2	2
35–49	7	1.0	0	1	1	1	1	1	1	1
50–64	8	1.4	<1	1	1	1	2	2	2	2
65+	3	1.0	0	1	1	1	1	1	1	1
B. Operated										
0–19 Years	0									
20–34	18	1.2	<1	1	1	1	1	2	3	3
35–49	17	1.3	<1	1	1	1	1	3	3	3
50–64	14	2.1	1	1	1	2	3	4	4	4
65+	9	1.2	<1	1	1	1	1	2	2	2
2. MULTIPLE DX										
A. Not Operated										
0–19 Years	20	3.9	13	1	2	3	4	10	15	15
20–34	73	2.3	4	1	1	2	3	3	7	10
35–49	298	3.3	35	1	1	2	3	5	8	14
50–64	814	3.2	8	1	1	2	4	6	8	15
65+	1,831	3.6	9	1	2	3	5	7	9	14
B. Operated										
0–19 Years	10	4.5	7	2	2	4	7	9	9	9
20–34	57	4.2	23	1	1	3	6	8	10	26
35–49	184	4.0	14	1	1	3	5	8	11	20
50–64	645	4.4	21	1	1	3	6	10	13	22
65+	1,191	4.7	21	1	1	4	6	10	13	22
SUBTOTALS:										
1. SINGLE DX										
A. Not Operated	31	1.2	<1	1	1	1	1	2	2	2
B. Operated	58	1.5	<1	1	1	1	2	3	3	4
2. MULTIPLE DX										
A. Not Operated	3,036	3.4	11	1	2	3	4	7	9	15
B. Operated	2,087	4.5	20	1	1	3	6	10	13	22
1. SINGLE DX	89	1.4	<1	1	1	1	2	2	3	4
2. MULTIPLE DX	5,123	3.9	15	1	1	3	5	8	11	18
A. NOT OPERATED	3,067	3.4	11	1	2	3	4	7	9	15
B. OPERATED	2,145	4.4	20	1	1	3	6	10	13	22
TOTAL										
0–19 Years	32	3.9	11	1	2	3	5	9	10	15
20–34	159	2.8	11	1	1	2	3	6	8	24
35–49	506	3.4	26	1	1	2	4	7	10	14
50–64	1,481	3.7	14	1	2	3	5	8	11	20
65+	3,034	4.0	14	1	2	3	5	8	11	18
GRAND TOTAL	5,212	3.8	15	1	1	3	5	8	11	18

427.31: ATRIAL FIBRILLATION

Type of Patients	Observed Patients	Avg. Stay	Vari-ance	10th	25th	50th	75th	90th	95th	99th
1. SINGLE DX										
A. Not Operated										
0–19 Years	5	1.2	<1	1	1	1	1	1	2	2
20–34	55	1.2	<1	1	1	1	1	2	2	3
35–49	112	1.4	<1	1	1	1	2	2	3	4
50–64	187	1.6	1	1	1	1	2	3	3	6
65+	127	1.9	4	1	1	1	2	3	4	7
B. Operated										
0–19 Years	0									
20–34	11	1.0	0	1	1	1	1	1	1	1
35–49	45	1.3	<1	1	1	1	1	2	3	3
50–64	137	1.1	<1	1	1	1	1	2	2	3
65+	57	1.1	<1	1	1	1	1	2	2	2
2. MULTIPLE DX										
A. Not Operated										
0–19 Years	24	1.9	3	1	1	1	2	5	6	6
20–34	534	1.9	3	1	1	1	2	3	5	10
35–49	2,455	2.5	6	1	1	2	3	5	7	11
50–64	8,389	2.7	7	1	1	2	3	5	7	12
65+	26,293	3.2	8	1	1	2	4	6	8	13
B. Operated										
0–19 Years	3	2.0	3	1	1	1	3	4	4	4
20–34	41	2.7	13	1	1	1	3	4	7	22
35–49	328	2.8	13	1	1	2	3	6	8	18
50–64	1,476	2.8	15	1	1	2	3	6	9	22
65+	2,197	4.7	44	1	1	2	6	11	15	32
SUBTOTALS:										
1. SINGLE DX										
A. Not Operated	486	1.6	2	1	1	1	2	3	3	6
B. Operated	250	1.2	<1	1	1	1	1	2	2	3
2. MULTIPLE DX										
A. Not Operated	37,695	3.0	7	1	1	2	4	6	8	13
B. Operated	4,045	3.8	32	1	1	3	5	9	13	27
1. SINGLE DX	736	1.4	1	1	1	1	2	2	3	5
2. MULTIPLE DX	41,740	3.1	10	1	1	2	4	6	8	15
A. NOT OPERATED	38,181	3.0	7	1	1	2	4	6	8	13
B. OPERATED	4,295	3.6	30	1	1	3	4	9	13	26
TOTAL										
0–19 Years	32	1.8	2	1	1	1	2	4	6	6
20–34	641	1.9	3	1	1	1	2	3	5	10
35–49	2,940	2.4	7	1	1	2	3	5	7	11
50–64	10,189	2.6	8	1	1	2	3	5	7	13
65+	28,674	3.3	11	1	1	2	4	6	8	15
GRAND TOTAL	42,476	3.1	10	1	1	2	4	6	8	14

427.32: ATRIAL FLUTTER

Type of Patients	Observed Patients	Avg. Stay	Vari-ance	10th	25th	50th	75th	90th	95th	99th
1. SINGLE DX										
A. Not Operated										
0–19 Years	0									
20–34	3	2.0	1	1	1	3	3	3	3	3
35–49	5	1.0	0	1	1	1	1	1	1	1
50–64	21	1.3	<1	1	1	1	1	2	2	4
65+	11	1.3	<1	1	1	1	1	2	3	3
B. Operated										
0–19 Years	2	1.0	0	1	1	1	1	1	1	1
20–34	12	1.1	<1	1	1	1	1	1	2	2
35–49	30	1.0	<1	1	1	1	1	1	1	2
65+	33	1.1	<1	1	1	1	1	1	2	2
2. MULTIPLE DX										
A. Not Operated										
0–19 Years	11	3.1	6	1	1	2	5	5	8	8
20–34	70	2.8	6	1	1	2	3	3	6	17
35–49	310	2.9	7	1	1	2	3	6	8	13
50–64	1,175	2.9	10	1	1	2	4	6	7	14
65+	2,559	3.1	6	1	1	2	4	6	8	13
B. Operated										
0–19 Years	5	4.2	13	1	1	3	7	9	9	9
20–34	29	2.8	5	1	1	2	4	7	8	8
35–49	107	2.5	5	1	1	1	3	5	7	10
50–64	492	2.5	12	1	1	1	3	6	8	15
65+	922	2.8	11	1	1	2	3	6	9	17
SUBTOTALS:										
1. SINGLE DX										
A. Not Operated	40	1.3	<1	1	1	1	1	2	3	4
B. Operated	77	1.1	<1	1	1	1	1	1	2	2
2. MULTIPLE DX										
A. Not Operated	4,125	3.0	7	1	1	2	4	6	8	13
B. Operated	1,555	2.7	11	1	1	1	3	6	8	15
1. SINGLE DX	117	1.1	<1	1	1	1	1	2	2	3
2. MULTIPLE DX	5,680	2.9	8	1	1	2	4	6	8	14
A. NOT OPERATED	4,165	3.0	7	1	1	2	4	6	8	13
B. OPERATED	1,632	2.6	10	1	1	1	3	6	8	15
TOTAL										
0–19 Years	16	3.4	8	1	1	3	5	8	9	9
20–34	104	2.7	6	1	1	2	3	6	7	9
35–49	434	2.7	6	1	1	2	3	6	8	13
50–64	1,718	2.7	10	1	1	2	3	6	7	14
65+	3,525	3.0	8	1	1	2	4	6	8	13
GRAND TOTAL	5,797	2.9	8	1	1	2	4	6	8	14

Length of Stay by Diagnosis and Operation, Western Region, 2008

427.41: VENTRICULAR FIBRILLATION

Type of Patients	Observed Patients	Avg. Stay	Variance	10th	25th	50th	75th	90th	95th	99th
1. SINGLE DX										
A. Not Operated										
0–19 Years	0									
20–34	0									
35–49	0									
50–64	0									
65+	0									
B. Operated										
0–19 Years	0									
20–34	0									
35–49	0									
50–64	0									
65+	0									
2. MULTIPLE DX										
A. Not Operated										
0–19 Years	2	4.0	18	1	1	7	7	7	7	7
20–34	12	10.3	103	2	2	5	11	25	32	32
35–49	47	8.0	98	1	2	4	11	18	30	53
50–64	104	8.0	172	1	2	4	8	16	32	76
65+	188	5.8	32	1	2	4	7	14	19	25
B. Operated										
0–19 Years	4	8.5	65	2	2	8	20	20	20	20
20–34	39	9.4	55	1	5	7	10	18	32	32
35–49	67	8.4	50	2	4	7	9	19	24	38
50–64	163	7.7	42	2	4	6	10	15	19	38
65+	180	8.4	51	1	3	6	11	17	22	38
SUBTOTALS:										
1. SINGLE DX										
A. Not Operated	0									
B. Operated	0									
2. MULTIPLE DX										
A. Not Operated	353	6.9	85	1	2	4	8	16	22	48
B. Operated	453	8.2	48	1	4	6	10	17	22	38
1. SINGLE DX	0									
2. MULTIPLE DX	806	7.6	64	1	3	5	10	16	22	38
A. NOT OPERATED	353	6.9	85	1	2	4	8	16	22	48
B. OPERATED	453	8.2	48	1	4	6	10	17	22	38
TOTAL										
0–19 Years	6	7.0	48	1	2	7	8	20	20	20
20–34	51	9.6	65	2	4	7	11	21	32	32
35–49	114	8.3	69	1	3	6	10	18	26	38
50–64	267	7.8	92	1	3	5	9	16	21	48
65+	368	7.1	43	1	2	5	9	15	21	35
GRAND TOTAL	806	7.6	64	1	3	5	10	16	22	38

427.61: ATRIAL PREMATURE BEATS

Type of Patients	Observed Patients	Avg. Stay	Variance	10th	25th	50th	75th	90th	95th	99th
1. SINGLE DX										
A. Not Operated										
0–19 Years	0									
20–34	0									
35–49	0									
50–64	0									
65+	0									
B. Operated										
0–19 Years	0									
20–34	0									
35–49	2	1.0	0	1	1	1	1	1	1	1
50–64	0									
65+	0									
2. MULTIPLE DX										
A. Not Operated										
0–19 Years	4	3.0	4	2	2	2	6	6	6	6
20–34	2	1.0	0	1	1	1	1	1	1	1
35–49	22	1.4	<1	1	1	1	2	2	2	4
50–64	40	2.0	8	1	1	1	2	4	7	18
65+	119	2.0	2	1	1	2	3	4	5	7
B. Operated										
0–19 Years	0									
20–34	0									
35–49	3	1.0	0	1	1	1	1	1	1	1
50–64	3	1.0	0	1	1	1	1	1	1	1
65+	4	1.8	2	1	1	1	4	4	4	4
SUBTOTALS:										
1. SINGLE DX										
A. Not Operated	0									
B. Operated	2	1.0	0	1	1	1	1	1	1	1
2. MULTIPLE DX										
A. Not Operated	187	1.9	3	1	1	1	2	3	5	8
B. Operated	10	1.3	<1	1	1	1	1	4	4	4
1. SINGLE DX	2	1.0	0	1	1	1	1	1	1	1
2. MULTIPLE DX	197	1.9	3	1	1	1	2	3	5	8
A. NOT OPERATED	187	1.9	3	1	1	1	2	3	5	8
B. OPERATED	12	1.3	<1	1	1	1	1	1	1	4
TOTAL										
0–19 Years	4	3.0	4	2	2	2	6	6	6	6
20–34	2	1.0	0	1	1	1	1	1	1	1
35–49	27	1.3	<1	1	1	1	2	2	2	4
50–64	43	1.9	8	1	1	1	2	3	4	18
65+	123	2.0	2	1	1	2	3	4	5	7
GRAND TOTAL	199	1.9	3	1	1	1	2	3	5	7

427.69: PREMATURE BEATS NEC

Type of Patients	Observed Patients	Avg. Stay	Variance	10th	25th	50th	75th	90th	95th	99th
1. SINGLE DX										
A. Not Operated										
0–19 Years	2	2.0	0	2	2	2	2	2	2	2
20–34	2	1.0	0	1	1	1	1	1	1	1
35–49	6	1.2	<1	1	1	1	1	2	2	2
50–64	4	1.3	<1	1	1	1	1	2	2	2
65+	0									
B. Operated										
0–19 Years	1	1.0	0	1	1	1	1	1	1	1
20–34	1	1.0	0	1	1	1	1	1	1	1
35–49	2	1.0	0	1	1	1	1	1	1	1
50–64	3	1.0	0	1	1	1	1	1	1	1
65+	1	1.0	0	1	1	1	1	1	1	1
2. MULTIPLE DX										
A. Not Operated										
0–19 Years	9	2.1	1	1	1	2	3	4	4	4
20–34	29	2.0	<1	1	1	2	3	3	3	4
35–49	93	1.7	<1	1	1	1	2	3	3	6
50–64	169	1.9	3	1	1	1	2	3	4	7
65+	296	2.2	3	1	1	2	3	4	5	10
B. Operated										
0–19 Years	1	1.0	0	1	1	1	1	1	1	1
20–34	12	1.0	0	1	1	1	1	1	1	1
35–49	22	1.8	2	1	1	1	2	3	5	6
50–64	37	1.8	2	1	1	1	2	4	6	7
65+	30	2.4	4	1	1	2	3	6	7	8
SUBTOTALS:										
1. SINGLE DX										
A. Not Operated	14	1.3	<1	1	1	1	2	2	2	2
B. Operated	8	1.0	0	1	1	1	1	1	1	1
2. MULTIPLE DX										
A. Not Operated	596	2.0	2	1	1	2	2	4	5	7
B. Operated	102	1.9	3	1	1	1	2	4	6	7
1. SINGLE DX	22	1.2	<1	1	1	1	1	2	2	2
2. MULTIPLE DX	698	2.0	2	1	1	1	2	4	5	7
A. NOT OPERATED	610	2.0	2	1	1	2	2	4	5	7
B. OPERATED	110	1.8	3	1	1	1	2	4	6	7
TOTAL										
0–19 Years	13	1.9	<1	1	1	2	2	3	4	4
20–34	44	1.6	<1	1	1	1	1	3	3	4
35–49	123	1.7	<1	1	1	1	2	3	3	6
50–64	213	1.8	3	1	1	2	2	3	4	7
65+	327	2.3	3	1	1	2	3	4	6	9
GRAND TOTAL	720	2.0	2	1	1	1	2	4	5	7

Length of Stay by Diagnosis and Operation, Western Region, 2008

301

427.81: SINOATRIAL NODE DYSFUNCT

Type of Patients	Observed Patients	Avg. Stay	Vari-ance	10th	25th	50th	75th	90th	95th	99th
1. SINGLE DX										
A. Not Operated										
0–19 Years	0									
20–34	4	1.5	<1	1	1	1	2	3	3	3
35–49	10	1.4	<1	1	1	1	2	3	3	3
50–64	23	1.2	<1	1	1	1	1	2	2	3
65+	108	1.2	<1	1	1	1	1	2	3	5
B. Operated										
0–19 Years	0									
20–34	0									
35–49	1	1.0	0	1	1	1	1	1	1	1
50–64	0									
65+	2	1.0	0	1	1	1	1	1	1	1
2. MULTIPLE DX										
A. Not Operated										
0–19 Years	6	2.0	4	1	1	1	2	6	6	6
20–34	49	2.8	6	1	1	2	3	5	7	15
35–49	214	3.0	5	1	1	2	4	6	8	10
50–64	1,011	3.1	8	1	1	2	4	6	8	13
65+	9,257	3.4	9	1	1	3	5	7	9	15
B. Operated										
0–19 Years	0									
20–34	4	4.3	22	1	1	1	11	11	11	11
35–49	18	4.8	26	1	1	3	6	13	20	20
50–64	93	5.4	29	1	1	3	7	13	18	24
65+	754	4.8	25	1	1	3	7	10	13	22
SUBTOTALS:										
1. SINGLE DX										
A. Not Operated	145	1.3	<1	1	1	1	1	2	3	5
B. Operated	3	1.0	0	1	1	1	1	1	1	1
2. MULTIPLE DX										
A. Not Operated	10,537	3.4	9	1	1	3	4	7	9	15
B. Operated	869	4.9	25	1	1	3	7	10	14	22
1. SINGLE DX	148	1.2	<1	1	1	1	1	2	3	5
2. MULTIPLE DX	11,406	3.5	10	1	1	3	5	7	9	15
A. NOT OPERATED	10,682	3.3	9	1	1	3	4	7	9	15
B. OPERATED	872	4.9	25	1	1	3	7	10	14	22
TOTAL										
0–19 Years	6	2.0	4	1	1	1	2	6	6	6
20–34	57	2.8	7	1	1	2	3	5	9	15
35–49	243	3.0	7	1	1	2	4	6	8	13
50–64	1,127	3.3	10	1	1	2	4	7	9	16
65+	10,121	3.5	10	1	1	3	5	7	9	15
GRAND TOTAL	11,554	3.5	10	1	1	3	5	7	9	15

427.89: OTH CARDIAC DYSRHYTHMIAS

Type of Patients	Observed Patients	Avg. Stay	Vari-ance	10th	25th	50th	75th	90th	95th	99th
1. SINGLE DX										
A. Not Operated										
0–19 Years	22	1.7	<1	1	1	1	3	3	3	4
20–34	21	1.3	<1	1	1	1	2	2	2	3
35–49	34	1.5	<1	1	1	1	2	2	3	4
50–64	34	1.4	<1	1	1	1	2	3	3	3
65+	29	1.2	<1	1	1	1	1	2	2	3
B. Operated										
0–19 Years	34	1.1	<1	1	1	1	1	1	1	3
20–34	37	1.0	0	1	1	1	1	1	1	1
35–49	52	1.1	<1	1	1	1	1	1	2	3
50–64	70	1.2	<1	1	1	1	1	2	3	4
65+	22	1.1	<1	1	1	1	1	1	1	4
2. MULTIPLE DX										
A. Not Operated										
0–19 Years	198	4.7	41	1	1	2	5	12	19	39
20–34	425	2.2	4	1	1	2	3	5	5	10
35–49	975	2.2	4	1	1	2	3	4	6	10
50–64	2,385	2.4	4	1	1	2	3	5	6	10
65+	8,781	2.8	5	1	1	2	3	5	7	11
B. Operated										
0–19 Years	24	3.7	21	1	1	1	4	6	17	18
20–34	77	2.1	9	1	1	1	2	4	6	19
35–49	179	2.2	8	1	1	1	2	5	6	20
50–64	357	2.7	9	1	1	1	3	6	9	14
65+	622	4.2	31	1	1	3	5	9	14	24
SUBTOTALS:										
1. SINGLE DX										
A. Not Operated	140	1.4	<1	1	1	1	2	3	3	4
B. Operated	215	1.1	<1	1	1	1	1	1	2	3
2. MULTIPLE DX										
A. Not Operated	12,764	2.7	6	1	1	2	3	5	7	12
B. Operated	1,259	3.4	21	1	1	2	4	7	11	21
1. SINGLE DX	355	1.2	<1	1	1	1	1	2	3	4
2. MULTIPLE DX	14,023	2.8	7	1	1	2	3	5	7	13
A. NOT OPERATED	12,904	2.7	6	1	1	2	3	5	7	12
B. OPERATED	1,474	3.0	19	1	1	1	4	7	10	20
TOTAL										
0–19 Years	278	3.9	33	1	1	2	4	11	17	26
20–34	560	2.1	4	1	1	1	2	4	5	11
35–49	1,240	2.2	4	1	1	1	3	4	6	10
50–64	2,846	2.4	5	1	1	2	3	5	6	11
65+	9,454	2.9	7	1	1	2	4	5	7	13
GRAND TOTAL	14,378	2.7	7	1	1	2	3	5	7	13

427.9: CARDIAC DYSRHYTHMIA NOS

Type of Patients	Observed Patients	Avg. Stay	Vari-ance	10th	25th	50th	75th	90th	95th	99th
1. SINGLE DX										
A. Not Operated										
0–19 Years	1	2.0	0	2	2	2	2	2	2	2
20–34	0									
35–49	0									
50–64	0									
65+	0									
B. Operated										
0–19 Years	0									
20–34	0									
35–49	0									
50–64	0									
65+	0									
2. MULTIPLE DX										
A. Not Operated										
0–19 Years	3	2.0	1	1	1	2	3	3	3	3
20–34	14	2.4	2	1	1	2	3	3	5	6
35–49	14	1.6	<1	1	1	1	2	2	3	3
50–64	46	2.1	3	1	1	2	3	4	4	10
65+	109	2.7	8	1	1	2	3	5	6	16
B. Operated										
0–19 Years	0									
20–34	0									
35–49	0									
50–64	5	4.4	20	1	1	2	7	11	11	11
65+	6	4.0	7	3	3	4	4	9	9	9
SUBTOTALS:										
1. SINGLE DX										
A. Not Operated	1	2.0	0	2	2	2	2	2	2	2
B. Operated	0									
2. MULTIPLE DX										
A. Not Operated	186	2.4	5	1	1	2	3	4	5	16
B. Operated	12	3.9	11	1	1	3	4	9	11	11
1. SINGLE DX	1	2.0	0	2	2	2	2	2	2	2
2. MULTIPLE DX	198	2.5	6	1	1	2	3	4	6	16
A. NOT OPERATED	187	2.4	5	1	1	2	3	4	5	16
B. OPERATED	12	3.9	11	1	1	3	4	9	11	11
TOTAL										
0–19 Years	4	2.0	<1	1	1	2	3	3	3	3
20–34	15	2.3	2	1	1	2	3	3	6	6
35–49	14	1.6	<1	1	1	1	2	3	3	3
50–64	51	2.3	5	1	1	2	3	4	7	11
65+	115	2.7	8	1	1	2	3	5	6	16
GRAND TOTAL	199	2.5	6	1	1	2	3	4	6	16

302

428: HEART FAILURE

Type of Patients	Observed Patients	Avg. Stay	Variance	Percentiles						
				10th	25th	50th	75th	90th	95th	99th
1. SINGLE DX										
A. Not Operated										
0–19 Years	1	6.0	0	6	6	6	6	6	6	6
20–34	2	1.0	0	1	1	1	1	1	1	1
35–49	11	3.2	12	1	1	2	3	9	11	11
50–64	14	2.9	10	1	1	2	3	4	13	13
65+	26	2.9	3	1	2	3	4	6	6	6
B. Operated										
0–19 Years	0									
20–34	0									
35–49	0									
50–64	6	1.0	0	1	1	1	1	1	1	1
65+	4	1.8	<1	1	1	1	2	3	3	3
2. MULTIPLE DX										
A. Not Operated										
0–19 Years	118	6.0	49	1	2	4	7	13	18	40
20–34	1,422	4.3	15	1	2	3	5	9	11	19
35–49	7,261	4.0	12	1	2	3	5	7	10	17
50–64	20,588	4.4	17	1	2	3	5	8	11	20
65+	75,347	4.5	12	1	2	4	6	8	11	18
B. Operated										
0–19 Years	16	21.9	486	7	8	14	24	89	>99	>99
20–34	134	10.6	155	1	4	7	14	23	35	87
35–49	593	7.3	62	1	1	5	10	16	24	45
50–64	2,196	7.9	87	1	1	5	10	18	26	48
65+	5,526	7.3	61	1	1	5	10	16	22	38
SUBTOTALS:										
1. SINGLE DX										
A. Not Operated	54	2.9	6	1	1	2	4	6	9	13
B. Operated	10	1.3	<1	1	1	1	1	2	3	3
2. MULTIPLE DX										
A. Not Operated	104,736	4.4	13	1	2	3	6	8	11	18
B. Operated	8,465	7.5	71	1	1	5	10	17	23	42
1. SINGLE DX	**64**	**2.7**	**6**	**1**	**1**	**2**	**3**	**6**	**6**	**13**
2. MULTIPLE DX	**113,201**	**4.7**	**18**	**1**	**2**	**4**	**6**	**9**	**12**	**21**
A. NOT OPERATED	**104,790**	**4.4**	**13**	**1**	**2**	**3**	**6**	**8**	**11**	**18**
B. OPERATED	**8,475**	**7.5**	**71**	**1**	**2**	**5**	**10**	**17**	**23**	**42**
TOTAL										
0–19 Years	135	7.9	123	1	2	4	9	17	37	89
20–34	1,558	4.8	30	1	2	3	6	10	14	27
35–49	7,865	4.3	17	1	2	3	5	8	11	21
50–64	22,804	4.8	25	1	2	3	6	9	13	25
65+	80,903	4.7	16	1	2	4	6	9	12	20
GRAND TOTAL	**113,265**	**4.7**	**18**	**2**	**2**	**4**	**6**	**9**	**12**	**21**

428.0: CHF NOS

Type of Patients	Observed Patients	Avg. Stay	Variance	Percentiles						
				10th	25th	50th	75th	90th	95th	99th
1. SINGLE DX										
A. Not Operated										
0–19 Years	1	6.0	0	6	6	6	6	6	6	6
20–34	2	1.0	0	1	1	1	1	1	1	1
35–49	11	3.2	12	1	1	2	3	9	11	11
50–64	14	2.9	10	1	1	2	3	4	13	13
65+	26	2.9	3	1	2	3	4	6	6	6
B. Operated										
0–19 Years	0									
20–34	0									
35–49	0									
50–64	6	1.0	0	1	1	1	1	1	1	1
65+	4	1.8	<1	1	1	1	2	3	3	3
2. MULTIPLE DX										
A. Not Operated										
0–19 Years	107	5.4	39	1	2	4	7	11	15	37
20–34	1,302	4.2	13	1	2	3	5	8	11	19
35–49	6,647	4.0	12	1	2	3	5	7	10	17
50–64	18,365	4.4	17	1	2	3	5	8	11	20
65+	65,998	4.5	12	1	2	4	6	8	11	17
B. Operated										
0–19 Years	13	17.3	209	7	8	13	21	53	>99	>99
20–34	123	10.4	149	1	3	7	14	23	35	87
35–49	533	7.5	65	1	1	5	10	17	24	40
50–64	2,004	7.8	83	1	1	5	10	19	26	48
65+	5,002	7.1	61	1	1	5	10	16	22	37
SUBTOTALS:										
1. SINGLE DX										
A. Not Operated	54	2.9	6	1	1	2	4	6	9	13
B. Operated	10	1.3	<1	1	1	1	1	2	3	3
2. MULTIPLE DX										
A. Not Operated	92,419	4.4	13	1	2	3	5	8	11	18
B. Operated	7,675	7.4	69	1	1	5	10	17	23	42
1. SINGLE DX	**64**	**2.7**	**6**	**1**	**1**	**2**	**3**	**6**	**6**	**13**
2. MULTIPLE DX	**100,094**	**4.6**	**18**	**1**	**2**	**4**	**6**	**9**	**12**	**21**
A. NOT OPERATED	**92,473**	**4.4**	**13**	**1**	**2**	**3**	**5**	**8**	**11**	**18**
B. OPERATED	**7,685**	**7.4**	**69**	**1**	**2**	**5**	**10**	**17**	**23**	**42**
TOTAL										
0–19 Years	121	6.7	69	1	2	4	8	14	21	53
20–34	1,427	4.8	28	1	2	3	6	9	14	26
35–49	7,191	4.2	17	1	2	3	5	8	11	20
50–64	20,389	4.7	24	1	2	3	6	9	13	25
65+	71,030	4.6	16	1	2	4	6	9	12	20
GRAND TOTAL	**100,158**	**4.6**	**18**	**2**	**2**	**4**	**6**	**9**	**12**	**21**

428.1: LEFT HEART FAILURE

Type of Patients	Observed Patients	Avg. Stay	Variance	Percentiles						
				10th	25th	50th	75th	90th	95th	99th
1. SINGLE DX										
A. Not Operated										
0–19 Years	0									
20–34	0									
35–49	0									
50–64	0									
65+	0									
B. Operated										
0–19 Years	0									
20–34	0									
35–49	0									
50–64	0									
65+	0									
2. MULTIPLE DX										
A. Not Operated										
0–19 Years	1	4.0	0	4	4	4	4	4	4	4
20–34	8	3.5	4	1	2	4	6	6	6	6
35–49	13	3.1	10	1	2	2	3	5	13	13
50–64	25	4.3	10	1	2	4	5	7	11	15
65+	103	4.0	8	1	2	3	5	8	8	14
B. Operated										
0–19 Years	0									
20–34	1	2.0	0	2	2	2	2	2	2	2
35–49	5	5.1	39	1	1	1	8	15	15	15
50–64	8	6.9	34	1	1	9	11	15	15	15
65+	10	8.9	103	1	1	2	11	28	28	28
SUBTOTALS:										
1. SINGLE DX										
A. Not Operated	0									
B. Operated	0									
2. MULTIPLE DX										
A. Not Operated	150	3.9	8	1	2	3	5	7	11	15
B. Operated	24	7.2	61	1	1	2	11	15	25	28
1. SINGLE DX	**0**									
2. MULTIPLE DX	**174**	**4.4**	**17**	**1**	**2**	**3**	**5**	**9**	**13**	**25**
A. NOT OPERATED	**150**	**3.9**	**8**	**1**	**2**	**3**	**5**	**7**	**11**	**15**
B. OPERATED	**24**	**7.2**	**61**	**1**	**2**	**3**	**11**	**15**	**25**	**28**
TOTAL										
0–19 Years	1	4.0	0	4	4	4	4	4	4	4
20–34	9	3.3	4	1	2	3	5	6	6	6
35–49	18	3.7	17	1	2	2	4	13	15	15
50–64	33	5.0	16	1	2	4	6	8	15	15
65+	113	4.4	18	1	2	3	6	8	11	25
GRAND TOTAL	**174**	**4.4**	**17**	**2**	**2**	**3**	**5**	**9**	**13**	**25**

Length of Stay by Diagnosis and Operation, Western Region, 2008

Western Region, October 2006–September 2007 Data, by Diagnosis

428.20: SYSTOLIC HF NOS

Type of Patients	Observed Patients	Avg. Stay	Vari-ance	Percentiles 10th	25th	50th	75th	90th	95th	99th
1. SINGLE DX										
A. Not Operated										
0–19 Years	0									
20–34	0									
35–49	0									
50–64	0									
65+	0									
B. Operated										
0–19 Years	0									
20–34	0									
35–49	0									
50–64	0									
65+	0									
2. MULTIPLE DX										
A. Not Operated										
0–19 Years	3	7.7	113	1	1	2	20	20	20	20
20–34	20	4.6	9	1	2	3	7	10	11	11
35–49	79	4.7	26	1	2	3	5	10	15	30
50–64	235	4.9	17	1	2	4	6	9	13	22
65+	684	4.5	11	2	2	4	6	9	10	15
B. Operated										
0–19 Years	0									
20–34	1	4.0	0	4	4	4	4	4	4	4
35–49	7	5.1	16	1	1	6	7	12	12	12
50–64	39	6.2	28	1	1	5	9	15	17	20
65+	92	6.6	33	1	2	5	10	14	19	25
SUBTOTALS:										
1. SINGLE DX										
A. Not Operated	0									
B. Operated	0									
2. MULTIPLE DX										
A. Not Operated	1,021	4.6	13	2	2	4	6	9	11	19
B. Operated	139	6.4	31	1	1	5	9	14	17	23
1. SINGLE DX	0									
2. MULTIPLE DX	1,160	4.8	16	1	2	4	6	9	12	21
A. NOT OPERATED	1,021	4.6	13	2	2	4	6	9	11	19
B. OPERATED	139	6.4	31	1	1	5	9	14	17	23
TOTAL										
0–19 Years	3	7.7	113	1	1	2	20	20	20	20
20–34	21	4.5	9	1	2	4	6	9	10	11
35–49	86	4.8	25	1	2	3	5	10	13	30
50–64	274	5.0	19	1	2	4	6	10	15	22
65+	776	4.7	14	1	2	4	6	9	11	19
GRAND TOTAL	1,160	4.8	16	1	2	4	6	9	12	21

428.21: ACUTE SYSTOLIC HF

Type of Patients	Observed Patients	Avg. Stay	Vari-ance	Percentiles 10th	25th	50th	75th	90th	95th	99th
1. SINGLE DX										
A. Not Operated										
0–19 Years	0									
20–34	0									
35–49	0									
50–64	0									
65+	0									
B. Operated										
0–19 Years	0									
20–34	0									
35–49	0									
50–64	0									
65+	0									
2. MULTIPLE DX										
A. Not Operated										
0–19 Years	1	13.0	0	13	13	13	13	13	13	13
20–34	17	3.9	11	1	2	3	4	9	15	15
35–49	80	4.1	7	1	2	3	5	8	10	12
50–64	170	4.7	11	2	2	4	6	8	11	18
65+	467	4.9	31	2	2	4	6	8	12	20
B. Operated										
0–19 Years	0									
20–34	0									
35–49	5	7.6	4	5	6	8	9	10	10	10
50–64	15	9.5	32	2	5	10	12	16	22	22
65+	33	8.5	22	3	5	8	11	13	16	22
SUBTOTALS:										
1. SINGLE DX										
A. Not Operated	0									
B. Operated	0									
2. MULTIPLE DX										
A. Not Operated	735	4.7	24	2	2	4	6	9	11	19
B. Operated	53	8.7	23	3	5	8	11	15	16	22
1. SINGLE DX	0									
2. MULTIPLE DX	788	5.0	25	2	2	4	6	10	12	20
A. NOT OPERATED	735	4.7	24	2	2	4	6	9	11	19
B. OPERATED	53	8.7	23	3	5	8	11	15	16	22
TOTAL										
0–19 Years	1	13.0	0	13	13	13	13	13	13	13
20–34	17	3.9	11	1	2	3	4	9	15	15
35–49	85	4.3	8	1	2	4	5	9	10	12
50–64	185	5.1	14	2	2	4	6	10	12	20
65+	500	5.1	32	2	2	4	6	9	12	20
GRAND TOTAL	788	5.0	25	2	2	4	6	10	12	20

428.22: CHRONIC SYSTOLIC HF

Type of Patients	Observed Patients	Avg. Stay	Vari-ance	Percentiles 10th	25th	50th	75th	90th	95th	99th
1. SINGLE DX										
A. Not Operated										
0–19 Years	0									
20–34	0									
35–49	0									
50–64	0									
65+	0									
B. Operated										
0–19 Years	0									
20–34	0									
35–49	0									
50–64	0									
65+	0									
2. MULTIPLE DX										
A. Not Operated										
0–19 Years	0									
20–34	7	5.4	12	2	3	4	9	11	11	11
35–49	22	5.0	25	2	2	3	5	12	14	21
50–64	55	4.2	7	1	2	4	6	8	10	11
65+	190	4.7	19	1	2	3	5	10	14	25
B. Operated										
0–19 Years	0									
20–34	2	28.3	>999	1	1	55	55	55	55	55
35–49	19	4.9	39	1	1	2	6	14	26	26
50–64	42	7.7	239	1	1	7	7	18	30	87
65+	95	4.1	50	1	1	1	5	10	14	58
SUBTOTALS:										
1. SINGLE DX										
A. Not Operated	0									
B. Operated	0									
2. MULTIPLE DX										
A. Not Operated	274	4.6	17	1	2	3	5	10	13	23
B. Operated	158	5.4	115	1	1	1	5	13	23	58
1. SINGLE DX	0									
2. MULTIPLE DX	432	4.9	53	1	1	3	5	10	14	30
A. NOT OPERATED	274	4.6	17	1	2	3	5	10	13	23
B. OPERATED	158	5.4	115	1	1	1	5	13	23	58
TOTAL										
0–19 Years	0									
20–34	9	10.5	291	1	3	4	9	55	55	55
35–49	41	4.9	31	1	2	3	5	12	14	26
50–64	97	5.7	109	1	1	3	6	10	18	87
65+	285	4.5	29	1	1	3	5	10	14	25
GRAND TOTAL	432	4.9	53	1	1	3	5	10	14	30

Length of Stay by Diagnosis and Operation, Western Region, 2008

428.23: AC & CHR SYSTOLIC HF

Type of Patients	Observed Patients	Avg. Stay	Variance	Percentiles 10th	25th	50th	75th	90th	95th	99th
1. SINGLE DX										
A. Not Operated										
0–19 Years	0									
20–34	0									
35–49	0									
50–64	0									
65+	0									
B. Operated										
0–19 Years	0									
20–34	0									
35–49	0									
50–64	0									
65+	0									
2. MULTIPLE DX										
A. Not Operated										
0–19 Years	1	14.0	0	14	14	14	14	14	14	14
20–34	18	7.9	126	1	2	4	8	30	44	44
35–49	83	4.3	10	1	2	3	5	8	9	22
50–64	284	4.9	15	1	2	4	6	10	13	20
65+	880	4.6	14	1	2	4	6	9	11	19
B. Operated										
0–19 Years	1	89.0	0	89	89	89	89	89	89	89
20–34	1	10.0	0	10	10	10	10	10	10	10
35–49	7	10.0	15	4	8	9	14	15	15	15
50–64	22	9.5	100	1	4	6	11	15	23	47
65+	58	10.0	48	3	5	9	14	20	27	29
SUBTOTALS:										
1. SINGLE DX										
A. Not Operated	0									
B. Operated	0									
2. MULTIPLE DX										
A. Not Operated	1,266	4.7	16	1	2	4	6	9	12	19
B. Operated	89	10.7	125	2	5	9	14	20	27	89
1. SINGLE DX	0									
2. MULTIPLE DX	1,355	5.1	25	1	2	4	6	10	13	22
A. NOT OPERATED	1,266	4.7	16	1	2	4	6	9	12	19
B. OPERATED	89	10.7	125	2	5	9	14	20	27	89
TOTAL										
0–19 Years	2	51.5	>999	14	14	52	89	89	89	89
20–34	19	8.0	119	1	2	4	8	30	44	44
35–49	90	4.7	13	1	2	3	6	8	12	22
50–64	306	5.2	22	1	2	4	6	11	14	22
65+	938	4.9	18	2	2	4	6	10	12	20
GRAND TOTAL	1,355	5.1	25	1	2	4	6	10	13	22

428.30: DIASTOLIC HF NOS

Type of Patients	Observed Patients	Avg. Stay	Variance	Percentiles 10th	25th	50th	75th	90th	95th	99th
1. SINGLE DX										
A. Not Operated										
0–19 Years	0									
20–34	0									
35–49	0									
50–64	0									
65+	0									
B. Operated										
0–19 Years	0									
20–34	0									
35–49	0									
50–64	0									
65+	0									
2. MULTIPLE DX										
A. Not Operated										
0–19 Years	2	11.0	8	9	9	13	13	13	13	13
20–34	20	3.7	4	2	2	3	5	6	9	9
35–49	145	3.9	7	1	2	3	5	7	9	15
50–64	601	4.7	19	1	2	3	6	9	12	23
65+	3,035	4.7	14	2	2	4	6	9	11	19
B. Operated										
0–19 Years	0									
20–34	4	7.3	10	4	4	8	10	10	10	10
35–49	3	4.7	12	1	1	5	8	8	8	8
50–64	17	10.2	191	3	4	6	11	14	62	62
65+	102	11.3	71	3	6	10	14	24	29	40
SUBTOTALS:										
1. SINGLE DX										
A. Not Operated	0									
B. Operated	0									
2. MULTIPLE DX										
A. Not Operated	3,803	4.7	14	2	2	4	6	9	11	20
B. Operated	126	10.9	84	3	5	9	13	23	29	42
1. SINGLE DX	0									
2. MULTIPLE DX	3,929	4.9	18	2	2	4	6	9	12	22
A. NOT OPERATED	3,803	4.7	14	2	2	4	6	9	11	20
B. OPERATED	126	10.9	84	3	5	9	13	23	29	42
TOTAL										
0–19 Years	2	11.0	8	9	9	13	13	13	13	13
20–34	24	4.3	6	2	3	4	5	9	10	10
35–49	148	3.9	7	1	2	3	5	7	9	15
50–64	618	4.9	24	1	2	4	6	9	12	23
65+	3,137	4.9	17	2	2	4	6	9	12	22
GRAND TOTAL	3,929	4.9	18	2	2	4	6	9	12	22

428.31: ACUTE DIASTOLIC HF

Type of Patients	Observed Patients	Avg. Stay	Variance	Percentiles 10th	25th	50th	75th	90th	95th	99th
1. SINGLE DX										
A. Not Operated										
0–19 Years	0									
20–34	0									
35–49	0									
50–64	0									
65+	0									
B. Operated										
0–19 Years	0									
20–34	0									
35–49	0									
50–64	0									
65+	0									
2. MULTIPLE DX										
A. Not Operated										
0–19 Years	0									
20–34	5	3.4	<1	3	3	3	4	4	4	4
35–49	48	5.1	25	1	3	4	6	8	9	35
50–64	223	4.7	15	2	2	4	5	10	12	19
65+	1,110	4.6	11	2	2	4	6	9	11	17
B. Operated										
0–19 Years	0									
20–34	0									
35–49	4	11.2	129	4	4	4	9	28	28	28
50–64	10	15.1	140	6	7	10	16	36	37	37
65+	38	11.9	50	5	7	9	17	25	25	33
SUBTOTALS:										
1. SINGLE DX										
A. Not Operated	0									
B. Operated	0									
2. MULTIPLE DX										
A. Not Operated	1,386	4.6	12	2	2	4	6	9	11	18
B. Operated	52	12.5	70	5	7	9	17	25	33	37
1. SINGLE DX	0									
2. MULTIPLE DX	1,438	4.9	16	2	2	4	6	9	12	20
A. NOT OPERATED	1,386	4.6	12	2	2	4	6	9	11	18
B. OPERATED	52	12.5	70	5	7	9	17	25	33	37
TOTAL										
0–19 Years	0									
20–34	5	3.4	<1	3	3	3	4	4	4	4
35–49	52	5.6	33	2	3	4	6	9	12	35
50–64	233	5.2	24	2	2	4	6	11	14	29
65+	1,148	4.8	14	2	2	4	6	9	11	20
GRAND TOTAL	1,438	4.9	16	2	2	4	6	9	12	20

Length of Stay by Diagnosis and Operation, Western Region, 2008

Western Region, October 2006–September 2007 Data, by Diagnosis

428.32: CHRONIC DIASTOLIC HF

Type of Patients	Observed Patients	Avg. Stay	Vari-ance	10th	25th	50th	75th	90th	95th	99th
1. SINGLE DX										
A. Not Operated										
0–19 Years	0									
20–34	0									
35–49	0									
50–64	0									
65+	0									
B. Operated										
0–19 Years	0									
20–34	0									
35–49	0									
50–64	0									
65+	0									
2. MULTIPLE DX										
A. Not Operated										
0–19 Years	0									
20–34	4	3.3	5	1	1	4	4	6	6	6
35–49	14	5.3	29	2	3	3	5	9	23	23
50–64	88	5.3	52	1	2	3	6	10	13	61
65+	491	4.4	10	1	2	4	6	8	10	17
B. Operated										
0–19 Years	0									
20–34	1	20.0	0	20	20	20	20	20	20	20
35–49	1	3.0	0	3	3	3	3	3	3	3
50–64	2	15.1	160	6	6	24	24	24	24	24
65+	19	8.5	73	1	2	7	11	17	38	38
SUBTOTALS:										
1. SINGLE DX										
A. Not Operated	0									
B. Operated	0									
2. MULTIPLE DX										
A. Not Operated	597	4.6	17	1	2	4	6	8	11	19
B. Operated	23	9.3	78	1	3	7	12	20	24	38
1. SINGLE DX	0									
2. MULTIPLE DX	620	4.8	20	1	2	4	6	9	12	20
A. NOT OPERATED	597	4.6	17	1	2	4	6	8	11	19
B. OPERATED	23	9.3	78	1	3	7	12	20	24	38
TOTAL										
0–19 Years	0									
20–34	5	6.6	59	1	2	4	6	20	20	20
35–49	15	5.1	28	2	3	3	5	9	23	23
50–64	90	5.5	55	2	2	3	6	10	14	61
65+	510	4.6	13	1	2	4	6	9	11	17
GRAND TOTAL	620	4.8	20	1	2	4	6	9	12	20

428.33: AC & CHR DIASTOLIC HF

Type of Patients	Observed Patients	Avg. Stay	Vari-ance	10th	25th	50th	75th	90th	95th	99th
1. SINGLE DX										
A. Not Operated										
0–19 Years	0									
20–34	0									
35–49	0									
50–64	0									
65+	0									
B. Operated										
0–19 Years	0									
20–34	0									
35–49	0									
50–64	0									
65+	0									
2. MULTIPLE DX										
A. Not Operated										
0–19 Years	0									
20–34	8	4.1	6	1	2	3	5	9	9	9
35–49	65	4.7	17	2	2	3	5	9	12	21
50–64	341	4.7	21	1	2	3	5	9	12	20
65+	1,702	4.6	13	1	2	4	6	9	12	19
B. Operated										
0–19 Years	0									
20–34	0									
35–49	1	3.0	0	3	3	3	3	3	3	3
50–64	12	13.4	250	3	5	11	16	16	61	61
65+	38	11.9	78	4	6	10	16	24	33	40
SUBTOTALS:										
1. SINGLE DX										
A. Not Operated	0									
B. Operated	0									
2. MULTIPLE DX										
A. Not Operated	2,116	4.6	14	1	2	4	6	9	12	20
B. Operated	51	12.1	115	3	5	9	16	21	33	61
1. SINGLE DX	0									
2. MULTIPLE DX	2,167	4.8	18	1	2	4	6	9	12	20
A. NOT OPERATED	2,116	4.6	14	1	2	4	6	9	12	20
B. OPERATED	51	12.1	115	3	5	9	16	21	33	61
TOTAL										
0–19 Years	0									
20–34	8	4.1	6	1	2	3	5	9	9	9
35–49	66	4.7	17	2	2	3	5	9	12	21
50–64	353	5.0	31	2	2	4	6	10	13	33
65+	1,740	4.8	16	1	2	4	6	9	12	20
GRAND TOTAL	2,167	4.8	18	1	2	4	6	9	12	20

428.40: SYS & DIASTOLIC HF NOS

Type of Patients	Observed Patients	Avg. Stay	Vari-ance	10th	25th	50th	75th	90th	95th	99th
1. SINGLE DX										
A. Not Operated										
0–19 Years	0									
20–34	0									
35–49	0									
50–64	0									
65+	0									
B. Operated										
0–19 Years	0									
20–34	0									
35–49	0									
50–64	0									
65+	0									
2. MULTIPLE DX										
A. Not Operated										
0–19 Years	1	40.0	0	40	40	40	40	40	40	40
20–34	2	4.5	12	2	2	7	7	7	7	7
35–49	16	3.8	2	1	2	4	5	6	6	6
50–64	59	4.3	27	2	2	3	5	8	11	38
65+	239	4.8	16	2	2	4	6	9	12	19
B. Operated										
0–19 Years	1	13.0	0	13	13	13	13	13	13	13
20–34	0									
35–49	0									
50–64	1	12.0	0	12	12	12	12	12	12	12
65+	13	10.1	60	1	4	9	14	18	28	28
SUBTOTALS:										
1. SINGLE DX										
A. Not Operated	0									
B. Operated	0									
2. MULTIPLE DX										
A. Not Operated	317	4.8	21	2	2	4	6	9	11	26
B. Operated	15	10.4	52	1	4	11	14	18	28	28
1. SINGLE DX	0									
2. MULTIPLE DX	332	5.0	24	2	2	4	6	10	12	28
A. NOT OPERATED	317	4.8	21	2	2	4	6	9	11	26
B. OPERATED	15	10.4	52	1	4	11	14	18	28	28
TOTAL										
0–19 Years	2	26.4	356	13	13	13	40	40	40	40
20–34	2	4.5	12	2	2	7	7	7	7	7
35–49	16	3.8	2	1	3	4	5	6	6	6
50–64	60	4.4	27	2	2	3	5	8	11	38
65+	252	5.1	20	2	2	4	6	10	12	26
GRAND TOTAL	332	5.0	24	2	2	4	6	10	12	28

Length of Stay by Diagnosis and Operation, Western Region, 2008

428.43: ACCHR SYS & DIASTOLIC HF

Type of Patients	Observed Patients	Avg. Stay	Vari-ance	Percentiles						
				10th	25th	50th	75th	90th	95th	99th
1. SINGLE DX										
A. Not Operated										
0–19 Years	0									
20–34	0									
35–49	0									
50–64	0									
65+	0									
B. Operated										
0–19 Years	0									
20–34	0									
35–49	0									
50–64	0									
65+	0									
2. MULTIPLE DX										
A. Not Operated										
0–19 Years	0									
20–34	8	7.9	39	1	2	7	12	20	20	20
35–49	19	4.9	30	1	2	3	5	10	25	25
50–64	74	5.2	19	2	3	4	6	9	14	25
65+	261	5.3	16	2	3	4	6	10	13	22
B. Operated										
0–19 Years	0									
20–34	0									
35–49	5	8.0	17	2	6	10	13	>99	>99	>99
50–64	6	20.2	192	7	7	24	30	41	41	41
65+	14	11.3	46	2	7	11	13	23	25	25
SUBTOTALS:										
1. SINGLE DX										
A. Not Operated	0									
B. Operated	0									
2. MULTIPLE DX										
A. Not Operated	362	5.3	18	2	3	4	6	10	13	25
B. Operated	25	12.8	87	2	7	11	17	30	41	>99
1. SINGLE DX	0									
2. MULTIPLE DX	387	5.8	25	2	3	5	7	12	16	28
A. NOT OPERATED	362	5.3	18	2	3	4	6	10	13	25
B. OPERATED	25	12.8	87	2	7	11	17	30	41	>99
TOTAL										
0–19 Years	0									
20–34	8	7.9	39	1	2	7	12	20	20	20
35–49	24	5.5	28	1	2	4	9	13	25	>99
50–64	80	6.3	46	2	3	4	6	12	24	41
65+	275	5.6	19	2	3	5	7	11	14	25
GRAND TOTAL	387	5.8	25	2	3	5	7	12	16	28

429: ILL-DEFINED HEART DIS

Type of Patients	Observed Patients	Avg. Stay	Vari-ance	Percentiles						
				10th	25th	50th	75th	90th	95th	99th
1. SINGLE DX										
A. Not Operated										
0–19 Years	0									
20–34	8	1.6	<1	1	1	1	3	3	3	3
35–49	3	1.3	<1	1	1	1	2	2	2	2
50–64	1	1.0	0	1	1	1	1	1	1	1
65+	1	1.0	0	1	1	1	1	1	1	1
B. Operated										
0–19 Years	0									
20–34	1	1.0	0	1	1	1	1	1	1	1
35–49	1	1.0	0	1	1	1	1	1	1	1
50–64	0									
65+	0									
2. MULTIPLE DX										
A. Not Operated										
0–19 Years	31	3.5	15	1	1	3	4	6	10	21
20–34	55	2.6	2	1	1	2	4	5	5	8
35–49	109	2.8	5	1	1	2	3	6	8	12
50–64	270	3.2	7	1	1	2	4	6	8	15
65+	379	4.3	14	2	2	3	5	8	11	22
B. Operated										
0–19 Years	11	6.7	14	4	4	7	9	10	15	15
20–34	12	6.0	8	2	5	6	9	9	11	11
35–49	19	5.5	8	1	3	5	8	9	10	10
50–64	49	6.6	85	1	1	4	8	14	26	53
65+	83	7.5	131	1	1	3	8	17	27	76
SUBTOTALS:										
1. SINGLE DX										
A. Not Operated	13	1.5	<1	1	1	1	2	3	3	3
B. Operated	2	1.0	0	1	1	1	1	1	1	1
2. MULTIPLE DX										
A. Not Operated	844	3.6	10	1	2	3	4	7	9	18
B. Operated	174	6.9	88	1	1	5	8	14	22	53
1. SINGLE DX	15	1.4	<1	1	1	1	2	3	3	3
2. MULTIPLE DX	1,018	4.2	25	1	2	3	5	8	12	23
A. NOT OPERATED	857	3.6	10	1	2	3	4	7	9	18
B. OPERATED	176	6.8	88	1	1	4	8	14	22	53
TOTAL										
0–19 Years	42	4.4	17	1	1	3	5	9	10	21
20–34	76	3.0	5	1	1	2	4	6	8	11
35–49	132	3.1	7	1	1	2	4	7	9	12
50–64	320	3.7	20	1	2	2	4	8	9	18
65+	463	4.8	36	2	2	3	6	9	14	33
GRAND TOTAL	1,033	4.1	25	1	2	3	5	8	11	23

429.4: HRT DIS POSTCARDIAC SURG

Type of Patients	Observed Patients	Avg. Stay	Vari-ance	Percentiles						
				10th	25th	50th	75th	90th	95th	99th
1. SINGLE DX										
A. Not Operated										
0–19 Years	0									
20–34	0									
35–49	0									
50–64	0									
65+	0									
B. Operated										
0–19 Years	0									
20–34	0									
35–49	0									
50–64	0									
65+	0									
2. MULTIPLE DX										
A. Not Operated										
0–19 Years	18	3.8	21	1	1	3	4	6	21	21
20–34	6	4.5	5	1	3	5	5	8	8	8
35–49	28	4.3	10	1	2	3	7	9	10	12
50–64	82	4.4	12	1	2	4	6	9	10	16
65+	145	5.3	18	2	3	4	7	10	14	23
B. Operated										
0–19 Years	9	7.4	13	4	5	7	9	15	15	15
20–34	4	7.0	7	5	6	6	11	11	11	11
35–49	3	8.0	<1	7	7	8	9	9	9	9
50–64	11	6.7	79	1	1	3	8	14	31	31
65+	35	7.6	221	1	1	7	7	22	37	76
SUBTOTALS:										
1. SINGLE DX										
A. Not Operated	0									
B. Operated	0									
2. MULTIPLE DX										
A. Not Operated	279	4.8	15	1	2	4	6	9	12	21
B. Operated	62	7.4	138	1	1	4	8	15	31	76
1. SINGLE DX	0									
2. MULTIPLE DX	341	5.3	38	1	2	4	7	10	15	31
A. NOT OPERATED	279	4.8	15	1	2	4	6	9	12	21
B. OPERATED	62	7.4	138	1	1	4	8	15	31	76
TOTAL										
0–19 Years	27	5.0	20	1	2	4	6	10	15	21
20–34	10	5.5	7	3	5	5	6	11	11	11
35–49	31	4.6	10	1	2	5	8	9	10	12
50–64	93	4.6	19	1	2	4	6	9	14	31
65+	180	5.8	57	2	3	4	7	11	17	37
GRAND TOTAL	341	5.3	38	1	2	4	7	10	15	31

Length of Stay by Diagnosis and Operation, Western Region, 2008

Western Region, October 2006–September 2007 Data, by Diagnosis

Type of Patients	430: SUBARACHNOID HEMORRHAGE										431: INTRACEREBRAL HEMORRHAGE										432: ICH NEC & NOS									
	Observed Patients	Avg. Stay	Vari-ance	10th	25th	50th	75th	90th	95th	99th	Observed Patients	Avg. Stay	Vari-ance	10th	25th	50th	75th	90th	95th	99th	Observed Patients	Avg. Stay	Vari-ance	10th	25th	50th	75th	90th	95th	99th
1. SINGLE DX																														
A. *Not Operated*																														
0–19 Years	2	1.0	0	1	1	1	1	1	1	1	2	2.0	0	2	2	2	2	2	2	2	4	4.0	3	2	2	3	5	6	6	6
20–34	5	2.0	<1	1	1	2	3	3	3	3	10	2.3	3	1	1	1	3	4	6	6	2	2.0	2	2	1	3	3	3	3	3
35–49	20	4.6	12	1	2	4	7	9	9	13	5	2.8	2	2	2	2	3	5	5	5	5	1.6	<1	1	1	2	2	2	2	2
50–64	17	4.2	9	1	2	6	7	9	10	13	3	4.7	22	1	1	3	10	10	10	10	9	3.1	6	1	1	2	5	7	7	7
65+	3	3.3	4	1	1	4	5	5	5	5	5	3.2	<1	3	3	3	3	4	4	4	4	1.5	<1	1	1	1	1	3	3	3
B. *Operated*																														
0–19 Years	6	8.5	30	3	4	5	12	17	17	17	1	3.0	0	3	3	3	3	3	3	3	1	3.4	16	1	2	2	5	12	12	12
20–34	5	9.0	29	1	8	8	13	15	15	15	3	8.0	12	3	6	6	12	12	12	12	3	2.5	<1	2	2	3	3	3	3	3
35–49	14	11.1	22	5	8	11	14	16	22	22	3	8.4	16	6	6	6	13	13	13	13	12	3.4	3	2	2	3	5	5	7	7
50–64	11	8.7	32	2	6	8	10	17	20	20	2	5.5	4	4	4	4	7	7	7	7	23	4.1	16	2	3	3	5	7	8	20
65+	2	16.0	49	11	11	21	21	21	21	21	0										9	4.3	4	3	4	4	6	7	7	7
2. MULTIPLE DX																														
A. *Not Operated*																														
0–19 Years	17	6.0	41	1	2	4	8	14	26	26	18	4.5	14	1	2	3	7	11	12	12	15	6.4	31	2	3	4	10	12	22	22
20–34	46	6.0	39	1	3	4	9	12	13	37	102	6.2	30	2	3	5	10	14	18	26	45	6.4	68	2	2	4	7	15	19	48
35–49	182	6.9	38	2	3	5	9	14	19	34	479	8.5	88	2	3	6	10	19	25	51	137	6.1	69	1	2	4	7	13	18	30
50–64	299	7.1	32	2	3	6	9	14	16	38	1,345	7.9	69	2	3	6	8	16	24	45	346	6.5	73	1	2	4	7	11	21	55
65+	367	5.9	21	2	2	4	8	13	15	20	3,630	6.2	32	2	3	5	8	12	16	29	1,159	4.9	19	1	2	4	6	10	12	20
B. *Operated*																														
0–19 Years	12	12.2	30	8	8	11	14	19	21	21	14	16.5	109	7	10	12	19	32	40	40	24	8.0	37	2	3	6	12	15	18	23
20–34	90	19.6	177	7	12	16	23	35	47	82	35	12.8	59	5	7	11	18	28	31	>99	40	10.5	86	2	5	7	16	22	24	48
35–49	275	18.4	155	7	11	16	22	33	41	83	152	21.8	249	11	11	18	28	39	59	75	142	10.0	101	3	4	7	13	21	28	68
50–64	522	20.6	185	9	13	18	25	35	48	92	328	20.7	222	7	10	17	26	43	55	81	442	8.3	58	2	4	6	10	15	25	37
65+	259	19.5	124	9	13	18	24	31	41	63	421	15.9	119	6	8	13	21	29	36	55	1,232	8.1	41	3	4	6	9	15	20	33
SUBTOTALS:																														
1. SINGLE DX																														
A. *Not Operated*	47	3.9	9	1	1	3	6	9	9	13	25	2.8	4	1	2	3	3	5	6	10	24	2.6	4	1	1	2	3	6	6	7
B. *Operated*	38	10.0	29	3	6	9	13	17	21	22	9	7.0	11	3	6	6	7	13	13	13	55	3.8	10	1	2	3	5	7	8	20
2. MULTIPLE DX																														
A. *Not Operated*	911	6.5	29	1	3	5	9	13	16	25	5,574	6.8	46	2	3	5	8	13	19	36	1,702	5.4	35	1	2	4	6	10	15	26
B. *Operated*	1,158	19.7	163	8	12	17	24	34	43	83	950	18.4	180	6	9	15	24	35	47	72	1,880	8.3	50	3	4	6	10	16	22	37
1. SINGLE DX	85	6.6	27	1	2	6	9	14	17	22	34	3.9	9	1	2	3	6	7	12	13	79	3.4	8	1	2	3	5	7	7	20
2. MULTIPLE DX	2,069	13.9	147	2	5	11	19	28	35	65	6,524	8.5	82	2	3	6	10	18	26	49	3,582	6.9	45	2	3	5	8	14	19	33
A. NOT OPERATED	958	6.4	29	2	3	5	9	13	16	25	5,599	6.8	46	2	3	5	8	13	18	36	1,726	5.3	35	1	2	4	6	10	14	26
B. OPERATED	1,196	19.4	162	7	12	17	23	33	43	82	959	18.3	179	6	9	15	24	35	47	72	1,935	8.2	50	3	4	6	10	16	21	37
TOTAL																														
0–19 Years	37	8.2	42	1	3	7	12	17	21	26	35	9.1	87	1	2	5	12	19	32	40	50	6.5	31	2	2	4	11	14	18	23
20–34	146	14.3	166	2	5	12	20	28	40	69	150	7.5	44	2	3	5	10	18	23	31	91	7.9	77	1	3	5	10	19	24	48
35–49	491	13.4	135	2	5	11	18	28	35	63	639	11.6	157	2	4	7	15	27	36	64	296	7.8	85	1	3	5	10	18	23	68
50–64	849	15.4	170	3	7	13	20	29	39	83	1,678	10.4	124	2	4	7	13	23	34	63	820	7.4	64	2	3	5	8	16	23	38
65+	631	11.5	108	2	4	9	16	24	29	49	4,056	7.2	50	2	3	5	9	15	20	36	2,404	6.5	32	2	3	5	8	13	16	28
GRAND TOTAL	2,154	13.6	144	2	5	11	19	27	35	65	6,558	8.5	82	2	3	6	10	18	26	49	3,661	6.8	45	2	3	5	8	14	19	33

432.1: SUBDURAL HEMORRHAGE

Type of Patients	Observed Patients	Avg. Stay	Vari-ance	10th	25th	50th	75th	90th	95th	99th
1. SINGLE DX										
A. Not Operated										
0–19 Years	4	4.0	3	2	2	3	5	6	6	6
20–34	1	3.0	0	3	3	3	3	3	3	3
35–49	5	1.6	<1	1	1	2	2	2	2	2
50–64	6	2.5	6	1	1	1	5	6	6	6
65+	2	1.0	0	1	1	1	1	1	1	1
B. Operated										
0–19 Years	7	3.4	16	1	1	2	5	12	12	12
20–34	4	2.5	<1	2	2	3	3	3	3	3
35–49	12	3.4	3	2	2	3	5	5	7	7
50–64	22	4.2	16	2	2	3	5	7	8	20
65+	9	4.3	4	1	3	4	6	7	7	7
2. MULTIPLE DX										
A. Not Operated										
0–19 Years	12	6.6	34	2	3	5	8	12	22	22
20–34	28	5.7	32	1	2	4	6	15	17	26
35–49	80	4.7	18	1	2	3	7	10	13	21
50–64	210	6.1	81	1	2	4	6	12	19	55
65+	852	4.8	20	1	2	3	6	10	12	20
B. Operated										
0–19 Years	24	8.0	37	2	3	6	12	15	18	23
20–34	33	9.1	48	2	4	6	12	21	24	28
35–49	126	8.9	73	3	4	6	12	19	27	57
50–64	417	8.1	56	2	4	6	9	18	24	37
65+	1,200	8.0	39	3	4	6	10	15	20	31
SUBTOTALS:										
1. SINGLE DX										
A. Not Operated	18	2.5	3	1	1	2	3	6	6	6
B. Operated	54	3.8	10	1	2	3	5	7	8	20
2. MULTIPLE DX										
A. Not Operated	1,182	5.0	31	2	2	4	6	10	14	25
B. Operated	1,800	8.1	46	3	4	6	10	16	21	35
1. SINGLE DX	72	3.5	9	1	2	3	5	7	7	20
2. MULTIPLE DX	2,982	6.9	42	2	3	5	8	14	18	31
A. NOT OPERATED	1,200	5.0	31	1	2	4	6	10	14	23
B. OPERATED	1,854	8.0	45	2	4	6	10	15	21	35
TOTAL										
0–19 Years	47	6.6	32	1	2	5	11	14	18	23
20–34	66	7.1	41	2	3	5	10	17	21	28
35–49	223	6.9	53	1	3	5	10	15	21	44
50–64	655	7.3	63	2	3	5	8	15	22	40
65+	2,063	6.6	34	2	3	5	8	13	16	28
GRAND TOTAL	3,054	6.8	41	2	3	5	8	14	18	31

432.9: INTRACRANIAL HEMOR NOS

Type of Patients	Observed Patients	Avg. Stay	Vari-ance	10th	25th	50th	75th	90th	95th	99th
1. SINGLE DX										
A. Not Operated										
0–19 Years	0									
20–34	1	1.0	0	1	1	1	1	1	1	1
35–49	0									
50–64	2	5.5	4	4	4	7	7	7	7	7
65+	1	1.0	0	1	1	1	1	1	1	1
B. Operated										
0–19 Years	0									
20–34	0									
35–49	0									
50–64	0									
65+	0									
2. MULTIPLE DX										
A. Not Operated										
0–19 Years	3	5.6	32	1	1	4	12	12	12	12
20–34	16	7.4	139	1	1	3	5	19	48	48
35–49	57	8.1	135	2	4	5	8	18	20	83
50–64	132	7.2	61	2	3	5	8	15	22	35
65+	302	5.3	15	2	3	4	7	10	12	20
B. Operated										
0–19 Years	0									
20–34	4	26.3	214	17	17	22	22	48	48	48
35–49	13	22.3	240	9	13	20	23	34	68	68
50–64	14	17.7	72	7	8	15	26	28	29	29
65+	20	14.3	100	2	6	15	19	27	34	35
SUBTOTALS:										
1. SINGLE DX										
A. Not Operated	4	3.2	8	1	1	1	4	7	7	7
B. Operated	0									
2. MULTIPLE DX										
A. Not Operated	510	6.2	45	2	3	5	7	11	17	30
B. Operated	51	18.2	143	6	9	16	25	29	35	68
1. SINGLE DX	4	3.2	8	1	1	1	4	7	7	7
2. MULTIPLE DX	561	7.3	66	2	3	5	8	15	22	35
A. NOT OPERATED	514	6.2	45	2	3	5	7	11	17	30
B. OPERATED	51	18.2	143	6	9	16	25	29	35	68
TOTAL										
0–19 Years	3	5.6	32	1	1	4	12	12	12	12
20–34	21	10.7	198	1	2	5	17	22	48	48
35–49	70	10.8	182	2	4	6	13	21	30	83
50–64	148	8.2	70	2	4	6	15	21	24	35
65+	323	5.9	25	2	3	5	7	11	15	28
GRAND TOTAL	565	7.3	65	2	3	5	8	15	22	35

433: PRECEREBRAL OCCLUSION

Type of Patients	Observed Patients	Avg. Stay	Vari-ance	10th	25th	50th	75th	90th	95th	99th
1. SINGLE DX										
A. Not Operated										
0–19 Years	0									
20–34	0									
35–49	0									
50–64	8	3.0	7	1	1	2	7	7	7	7
65+	9	1.8	3	1	1	1	2	6	6	6
B. Operated										
0–19 Years	0									
20–34	0									
35–49	6	2.0	<1	1	1	2	3	3	3	3
50–64	58	1.2	<1	1	1	1	1	2	2	3
65+	228	1.2	<1	1	1	1	1	2	3	3
2. MULTIPLE DX										
A. Not Operated										
0–19 Years	5	4.4	8	1	4	4	4	9	9	9
20–34	23	5.0	16	3	3	4	5	7	9	22
35–49	222	5.8	42	2	2	4	7	11	13	47
50–64	1,106	4.9	31	1	2	3	6	10	13	24
65+	3,503	4.4	14	1	2	3	5	8	11	19
B. Operated										
0–19 Years	2	3.0	8	1	1	1	5	5	5	5
20–34	11	3.6	14	1	1	2	8	9	11	11
35–49	200	3.9	25	1	1	2	4	9	13	19
50–64	3,146	2.5	16	1	1	1	2	5	8	19
65+	12,114	2.3	9	1	1	1	2	5	7	14
SUBTOTALS:										
1. SINGLE DX										
A. Not Operated	17	2.4	5	1	1	1	2	7	7	7
B. Operated	292	1.2	<1	1	1	1	1	2	3	3
2. MULTIPLE DX										
A. Not Operated	4,859	4.5	19	1	2	3	6	9	12	22
B. Operated	15,473	2.4	11	1	1	1	2	5	8	15
1. SINGLE DX	309	1.3	<1	1	1	1	1	2	3	5
2. MULTIPLE DX	20,332	2.9	14	1	1	2	3	6	9	17
A. NOT OPERATED	4,876	4.5	19	1	2	3	6	9	12	22
B. OPERATED	15,765	2.4	10	1	1	1	2	5	8	15
TOTAL										
0–19 Years	7	4.0	7	1	1	4	5	9	9	9
20–34	34	4.5	16	1	2	4	5	5	11	22
35–49	428	4.8	35	1	2	3	6	10	13	40
50–64	4,318	3.1	21	1	1	2	3	6	10	15
65+	15,854	2.8	11	1	1	2	3	6	8	15
GRAND TOTAL	20,641	2.9	13	1	1	2	3	6	9	17

Length of Stay by Diagnosis and Operation, Western Region, 2008

Western Region, October 2006–September 2007 Data, by Diagnosis

433.10: CAROTID OCCL S INFARCT

Type of Patients	Observed Patients	Avg. Stay	Vari-ance	10th	25th	50th	75th	90th	95th	99th
1. SINGLE DX										
A. Not Operated										
0–19 Years	0									
20–34	0									
35–49	0									
50–64	6	2.5	6	1	1	1	3	7	7	7
65+	5	1.0	0	1	1	1	1	1	1	1
B. Operated										
0–19 Years	0									
20–34	0									
35–49	3	1.3	<1	1	1	1	2	2	2	2
50–64	57	1.2	<1	1	1	1	1	2	2	2
65+	221	1.2	<1	1	1	1	1	2	3	3
2. MULTIPLE DX										
A. Not Operated										
0–19 Years	0									
20–34	6	3.3	2	1	3	4	4	5	5	5
35–49	40	3.1	5	1	2	3	4	8	8	9
50–64	296	3.1	7	1	1	2	4	6	8	15
65+	1,143	3.3	8	1	1	3	4	6	8	13
B. Operated										
0–19 Years	0									
20–34	7	1.4	<1	1	1	1	2	3	3	3
35–49	147	2.6	8	1	1	2	3	6	8	14
50–64	2,771	2.1	8	1	1	1	2	4	6	13
65+	11,051	2.1	6	1	1	1	2	4	6	12
SUBTOTALS:										
1. SINGLE DX										
A. Not Operated	11	1.8	3	1	1	1	2	3	7	7
B. Operated	281	1.2	<1	1	1	1	1	2	2	3
2. MULTIPLE DX										
A. Not Operated	1,485	3.2	7	1	1	2	4	6	8	13
B. Operated	13,976	2.1	7	1	1	1	2	4	6	12
1. SINGLE DX	292	1.3	<1	1	1	1	1	2	2	4
2. MULTIPLE DX	15,461	2.2	7	1	1	1	2	4	7	12
A. NOT OPERATED	1,496	3.2	7	1	1	2	4	6	8	13
B. OPERATED	14,257	2.1	7	1	1	1	2	4	6	12
TOTAL										
0–19 Years	0									
20–34	13	2.3	2	1	1	2	3	4	5	5
35–49	190	2.7	7	1	1	2	3	6	8	14
50–64	3,130	2.1	8	1	1	1	2	4	6	13
65+	12,420	2.2	7	1	1	1	2	4	7	12
GRAND TOTAL	15,753	2.2	7	1	1	1	2	4	7	12

433.11: CAROTID OCCL W INFARCT

Type of Patients	Observed Patients	Avg. Stay	Vari-ance	10th	25th	50th	75th	90th	95th	99th
1. SINGLE DX										
A. Not Operated										
0–19 Years	0									
20–34	0									
35–49	0									
50–64	1	2.0	0	2	2	2	2	2	2	2
65+	2	4.0	8	2	2	6	6	6	6	6
B. Operated										
0–19 Years	0									
20–34	0									
35–49	3	2.7	<1	2	3	3	3	3	3	3
50–64	1	3.0	0	3	3	3	3	3	3	3
65+	2	1.0	0	1	1	1	1	1	1	1
2. MULTIPLE DX										
A. Not Operated										
0–19 Years	3	5.7	8	4	4	4	9	9	9	9
20–34	2	4.0	2	3	3	5	5	5	5	5
35–49	117	6.1	48	2	3	4	7	11	21	47
50–64	523	5.6	38	2	3	4	7	11	16	32
65+	1,579	5.0	16	2	3	4	6	9	12	21
B. Operated										
0–19 Years	0									
20–34	3	7.4	22	2	2	9	11	11	11	11
35–49	31	5.8	20	1	2	5	7	11	17	19
50–64	192	7.5	60	1	3	6	9	16	24	56
65+	479	6.9	33	1	3	6	9	13	18	27
SUBTOTALS:										
1. SINGLE DX										
A. Not Operated	3	3.4	5	2	2	2	6	6	6	6
B. Operated	6	2.2	<1	1	1	2	3	3	3	3
2. MULTIPLE DX										
A. Not Operated	2,224	5.2	23	2	3	4	6	10	13	25
B. Operated	705	7.0	40	1	3	6	9	14	19	29
1. SINGLE DX	9	2.6	2	1	2	2	3	6	6	6
2. MULTIPLE DX	2,929	5.6	27	2	3	4	7	11	14	26
A. NOT OPERATED	2,227	5.2	23	2	3	4	6	10	13	25
B. OPERATED	711	6.9	39	1	3	6	9	14	19	29
TOTAL										
0–19 Years	3	5.7	8	4	4	4	9	9	9	9
20–34	5	6.0	15	2	3	5	9	11	11	11
35–49	151	6.0	41	2	2	4	7	11	17	47
50–64	717	6.1	44	2	3	4	7	12	18	41
65+	2,062	5.4	20	2	3	4	7	11	13	24
GRAND TOTAL	2,938	5.6	27	2	3	4	7	11	14	26

433.21: VERT ART OCCL W INFARCT

Type of Patients	Observed Patients	Avg. Stay	Vari-ance	10th	25th	50th	75th	90th	95th	99th
1. SINGLE DX										
A. Not Operated										
0–19 Years	0									
20–34	0									
35–49	0									
50–64	1	7.0	0	7	7	7	7	7	7	7
65+	0									
B. Operated										
0–19 Years	0									
20–34	0									
35–49	0									
50–64	0									
65+	0									
2. MULTIPLE DX										
A. Not Operated										
0–19 Years	0									
20–34	8	5.3	4	4	4	4	6	9	9	9
35–49	23	6.7	14	3	4	6	8	13	14	15
50–64	79	5.7	23	2	3	4	7	12	17	27
65+	125	4.9	15	2	2	4	6	8	11	19
B. Operated										
0–19 Years	0									
20–34	1	8.0	0	8	8	8	8	8	8	8
35–49	4	21.6	338	2	12	28	44	44	44	44
50–64	7	10.7	24	3	6	13	15	16	16	16
65+	10	11.2	86	3	4	6	14	30	30	30
SUBTOTALS:										
1. SINGLE DX										
A. Not Operated	1	7.0	0	7	7	7	7	7	7	7
B. Operated	0									
2. MULTIPLE DX										
A. Not Operated	235	5.4	17	2	3	4	7	10	14	20
B. Operated	22	12.8	111	3	6	12	15	28	30	44
1. SINGLE DX	1	7.0	0	7	7	7	7	7	7	7
2. MULTIPLE DX	257	6.0	29	2	3	4	7	12	16	30
A. NOT OPERATED	236	5.4	17	2	3	4	7	10	14	20
B. OPERATED	22	12.8	111	3	6	12	15	28	30	44
TOTAL										
0–19 Years	0									
20–34	9	5.6	4	2	4	4	7	9	9	9
35–49	27	8.9	80	2	4	6	12	15	28	44
50–64	87	6.2	24	2	3	5	7	13	17	27
65+	135	5.3	22	2	3	4	6	9	14	30
GRAND TOTAL	258	6.0	29	2	3	4	7	12	16	30

Length of Stay by Diagnosis and Operation, Western Region 2008

Western Region, October 2006–September 2007 Data, by Diagnosis

434: CEREBRAL ARTERY OCCLUS

Type of Patients	Observed Patients	Avg. Stay	Variance	10th	25th	50th	75th	90th	95th	99th
1. SINGLE DX										
A. Not Operated										
0–19 Years	1	6.0	0	6	6	6	6	6	6	6
20–34	5	2.2	<1	1	2	2	3	3	3	3
35–49	27	2.8	3	1	2	2	4	5	6	7
50–64	19	2.4	6	1	1	2	2	6	11	11
65+	34	2.2	2	1	1	2	3	4	5	6
B. Operated										
0–19 Years	0									
20–34	0									
35–49	0									
50–64	0									
65+	0									
2. MULTIPLE DX										
A. Not Operated										
0–19 Years	53	5.4	25	1	2	4	8	10	15	29
20–34	471	5.1	40	1	2	3	5	10	15	28
35–49	3,056	4.7	23	1	2	3	6	9	13	23
50–64	10,532	4.7	25	1	2	3	5	9	13	25
65+	34,581	4.5	15	2	2	4	5	8	11	20
B. Operated										
0–19 Years	3	11.4	26	7	10	17	17	>99	>99	>99
20–34	24	14.6	185	4	6	10	19	30	67	>99
35–49	114	15.6	164	4	7	11	20	31	45	56
50–64	315	14.6	193	4	6	10	19	30	44	93
65+	646	11.6	89	4	6	9	14	23	30	49
SUBTOTALS:										
1. SINGLE DX										
A. Not Operated	86	2.5	3	1	1	2	3	5	6	11
B. Operated	0									
2. MULTIPLE DX										
A. Not Operated	48,693	4.6	18	1	2	3	5	9	12	21
B. Operated	1,102	12.9	131	4	6	9	16	27	35	72
1. SINGLE DX	86	2.5	3	1	1	2	3	5	6	11
2. MULTIPLE DX	49,795	4.8	22	1	2	3	6	9	12	24
A. NOT OPERATED	48,779	4.6	18	1	2	3	5	9	12	21
B. OPERATED	1,102	12.9	131	4	6	9	16	27	35	72
TOTAL										
0–19 Years	57	5.8	26	1	2	4	8	13	17	>99
20–34	500	5.5	51	1	2	4	6	11	18	30
35–49	3,197	5.0	32	1	2	3	6	9	14	30
50–64	10,866	4.9	32	1	2	3	6	10	14	29
65+	35,261	4.7	18	2	2	4	6	9	12	21
GRAND TOTAL	49,881	4.8	22	1	2	3	6	9	12	24

433.31: MULT PREC OCCL W INFARCT

Type of Patients	Observed Patients	Avg. Stay	Variance	10th	25th	50th	75th	90th	95th	99th
1. SINGLE DX										
A. Not Operated										
0–19 Years	0									
20–34	0									
35–49	0									
50–64	0									
65+	0									
B. Operated										
0–19 Years	0									
20–34	0									
35–49	0									
50–64	0									
65+	0									
2. MULTIPLE DX										
A. Not Operated										
0–19 Years	0									
20–34	0									
35–49	9	6.7	12	2	5	6	9	13	13	13
50–64	49	5.2	24	1	2	4	7	11	14	28
65+	146	5.1	26	2	3	4	6	9	12	28
B. Operated										
0–19 Years	0									
20–34	0									
35–49	3	13.0	9	10	10	13	16	16	16	16
50–64	14	13.0	634	1	2	4	10	27	97	97
65+	23	6.1	17	2	3	6	8	11	14	17
SUBTOTALS:										
1. SINGLE DX										
A. Not Operated	0									
B. Operated	0									
2. MULTIPLE DX										
A. Not Operated	204	5.2	25	2	3	4	6	9	13	28
B. Operated	40	9.0	234	1	3	6	10	16	27	97
1. SINGLE DX	0									
2. MULTIPLE DX	244	5.9	61	2	3	4	7	10	14	28
A. NOT OPERATED	204	5.2	25	2	3	4	6	9	13	28
B. OPERATED	40	9.0	234	1	3	6	10	16	27	97
TOTAL										
0–19 Years	0									
20–34	0									
35–49	12	8.3	18	3	5	9	13	13	16	16
50–64	63	7.0	163	1	2	4	7	11	19	97
65+	169	5.3	25	2	3	4	6	10	13	28
GRAND TOTAL	244	5.9	61	2	3	4	7	10	14	28

433.30: MULT PREC OCCL S INFARCT

Type of Patients	Observed Patients	Avg. Stay	Variance	10th	25th	50th	75th	90th	95th	99th
1. SINGLE DX										
A. Not Operated										
0–19 Years	0									
20–34	0									
35–49	0									
50–64	0									
65+	0									
B. Operated										
0–19 Years	0									
20–34	0									
35–49	0									
50–64	0									
65+	4	1.3	<1	1	1	1	1	2	2	2
2. MULTIPLE DX										
A. Not Operated										
0–19 Years	0									
20–34	0									
35–49	2	1.5	<1	1	1	1	2	2	2	2
50–64	30	3.8	6	1	2	3	6	7	8	10
65+	188	3.5	8	1	2	3	4	7	9	12
B. Operated										
0–19 Years	0									
20–34	0									
35–49	8	3.6	6	1	2	3	5	9	9	9
50–64	120	2.6	12	1	1	1	3	5	7	18
65+	471	2.5	14	1	1	1	3	5	8	14
SUBTOTALS:										
1. SINGLE DX										
A. Not Operated	0									
B. Operated	4	1.3	<1	1	1	1	1	2	2	2
2. MULTIPLE DX										
A. Not Operated	220	3.5	7	1	2	3	4	7	9	12
B. Operated	599	2.6	13	1	1	1	3	5	8	17
1. SINGLE DX	4	1.3	<1	1	1	1	1	2	2	2
2. MULTIPLE DX	819	2.8	12	1	1	2	3	6	8	14
A. NOT OPERATED	220	3.5	7	1	2	3	4	7	9	12
B. OPERATED	603	2.6	13	1	1	1	3	5	8	14
TOTAL										
0–19 Years	0									
20–34	0									
35–49	10	3.2	6	1	2	2	4	6	9	9
50–64	150	2.9	11	1	1	2	3	6	8	18
65+	663	2.8	12	1	1	2	3	6	8	14
GRAND TOTAL	823	2.8	12	1	1	2	3	6	8	14

Length of Stay by Diagnosis and Operation, Western Region, 2008

Western Region, October 2006–September 2007 Data, by Diagnosis

434.01: CEREB THROMB W INFARCT

Type of Patients	Observed Patients	Avg. Stay	Variance	Percentiles						
				10th	25th	50th	75th	90th	95th	99th
1. SINGLE DX										
A. Not Operated										
0–19 Years	0									
20–34	0									
35–49	0									
50–64	0									
65+	0									
B. Operated										
0–19 Years	0									
20–34	0									
35–49	0									
50–64	0									
65+	0									
2. MULTIPLE DX										
A. Not Operated										
0–19 Years	5	7.4	28	2	3	7	10	15	15	15
20–34	25	7.5	52	3	3	5	8	19	23	32
35–49	91	5.3	25	1	2	4	6	10	16	34
50–64	290	5.7	33	2	2	4	6	13	16	29
65+	804	5.2	26	2	3	4	6	9	12	22
B. Operated										
0–19 Years	0									
20–34	2	42.3	>999	18	18	67	>99	>99	>99	>99
35–49	13	14.3	237	4	7	9	11	38	56	56
50–64	24	16.3	352	4	6	11	15	28	72	75
65+	33	10.7	76	4	6	8	13	19	29	46
SUBTOTALS:										
1. SINGLE DX										
A. Not Operated	0									
B. Operated	0									
2. MULTIPLE DX										
A. Not Operated	1,215	5.4	28	2	3	4	6	10	14	23
B. Operated	72	14.1	235	4	6	9	15	29	67	>99
1. SINGLE DX	0									
2. MULTIPLE DX	1,287	5.9	44	2	3	4	7	11	16	31
A. NOT OPERATED	1,215	5.4	28	2	3	4	6	10	14	23
B. OPERATED	72	14.1	235	4	6	9	15	29	67	>99
TOTAL										
0–19 Years	5	7.4	28	2	3	7	10	15	15	15
20–34	27	10.1	181	3	3	6	10	32	67	>99
35–49	104	6.4	59	2	3	5	7	11	18	38
50–64	314	6.5	64	2	2	4	7	14	18	31
65+	837	5.5	29	2	3	4	7	10	13	23
GRAND TOTAL	1,287	5.9	44	2	3	4	7	11	16	31

434.11: CEREBRAL EMBOL W INFARCT

Type of Patients	Observed Patients	Avg. Stay	Variance	Percentiles						
				10th	25th	50th	75th	90th	95th	99th
1. SINGLE DX										
A. Not Operated										
0–19 Years	0									
20–34	1	2.0	0	2	2	2	2	2	2	2
35–49	2	2.0	0	2	2	2	2	2	2	2
50–64	1	1.0	0	1	1	1	1	1	1	1
65+	1	3.0	0	3	3	3	3	3	3	3
B. Operated										
0–19 Years	0									
20–34	0									
35–49	0									
50–64	0									
65+	0									
2. MULTIPLE DX										
A. Not Operated										
0–19 Years	9	8.0	74	1	2	5	9	29	29	29
20–34	78	5.3	19	2	2	4	6	12	15	26
35–49	376	6.1	37	2	3	4	8	11	16	33
50–64	1,102	6.0	35	2	3	4	7	11	16	32
65+	4,836	5.6	22	2	3	4	7	10	13	25
B. Operated										
0–19 Years	0									
20–34	8	13.9	48	4	8	11	22	23	23	23
35–49	36	16.0	194	5	8	11	19	30	50	74
50–64	75	16.5	262	4	6	11	22	35	54	93
65+	173	12.2	107	4	6	9	14	22	32	53
SUBTOTALS:										
1. SINGLE DX										
A. Not Operated	5	2.0	<1	2	2	2	2	3	3	3
B. Operated	0									
2. MULTIPLE DX										
A. Not Operated	6,401	5.7	25	2	3	4	7	11	14	26
B. Operated	292	13.8	158	4	6	10	17	29	39	74
1. SINGLE DX	5	2.0	<1	2	2	2	2	3	3	3
2. MULTIPLE DX	6,693	6.1	33	2	3	5	7	11	15	29
A. NOT OPERATED	6,406	5.7	25	2	3	4	7	11	14	26
B. OPERATED	292	13.8	158	4	6	10	17	29	39	74
TOTAL										
0–19 Years	9	8.0	74	1	2	5	9	29	29	29
20–34	87	6.1	27	2	2	4	8	14	16	26
35–49	414	6.9	58	2	3	5	9	13	19	35
50–64	1,178	6.7	56	2	3	5	8	12	19	39
65+	5,010	5.9	26	2	3	5	7	11	14	26
GRAND TOTAL	6,698	6.1	33	2	3	5	7	11	15	29

434.91: CEREB ART OCCL W INFARCT

Type of Patients	Observed Patients	Avg. Stay	Variance	Percentiles						
				10th	25th	50th	75th	90th	95th	99th
1. SINGLE DX										
A. Not Operated										
0–19 Years	1	6.0	0	6	6	6	6	6	6	6
20–34	4	2.3	<1	1	1	3	3	3	3	3
35–49	23	2.7	3	1	2	2	4	5	5	7
50–64	18	2.5	6	1	1	2	2	6	11	11
65+	32	2.2	2	1	1	2	3	4	5	6
B. Operated										
0–19 Years	0									
20–34	0									
35–49	0									
50–64	0									
65+	0									
2. MULTIPLE DX										
A. Not Operated										
0–19 Years	35	4.6	12	1	2	4	7	9	10	16
20–34	363	4.9	44	1	2	3	5	10	14	28
35–49	2,570	4.5	20	1	2	3	5	9	12	23
50–64	9,099	4.5	23	1	2	3	5	9	12	24
65+	28,780	4.3	14	1	2	3	5	8	11	19
B. Operated										
0–19 Years	2	12.0	49	7	7	17	>99	>99	>99	>99
20–34	14	11.1	76	5	6	7	17	27	30	30
35–49	64	15.8	138	5	8	13	21	31	42	55
50–64	210	14.1	153	4	6	10	18	29	40	98
65+	436	11.5	84	4	6	9	14	23	29	47
SUBTOTALS:										
1. SINGLE DX										
A. Not Operated	78	2.5	3	1	1	2	3	5	6	11
B. Operated	0									
2. MULTIPLE DX										
A. Not Operated	40,847	4.4	16	1	2	3	5	8	11	20
B. Operated	726	12.6	110	4	6	9	16	26	33	55
1. SINGLE DX	78	2.5	3	1	1	2	3	5	6	11
2. MULTIPLE DX	41,573	4.5	19	1	2	3	5	8	12	22
A. NOT OPERATED	40,925	4.4	16	1	2	3	5	8	11	20
B. OPERATED	726	12.6	110	4	6	9	16	26	33	55
TOTAL										
0–19 Years	38	5.0	15	1	2	4	7	10	17	>99
20–34	381	5.1	46	1	2	3	5	10	16	29
35–49	2,657	4.7	26	1	2	3	5	9	13	27
50–64	9,327	4.7	28	1	2	3	5	9	13	28
65+	29,248	4.5	15	1	2	3	5	8	11	20
GRAND TOTAL	41,651	4.5	19	1	2	3	5	8	12	22

Length of Stay by Diagnosis and Operation, Western Region, 2008

Western Region, October 2006–September 2007 Data, by Diagnosis

435: TRANSIENT CEREB ISCHEMIA

Type of Patients	Observed Patients	Avg. Stay	Vari-ance	Percentiles						
				10th	25th	50th	75th	90th	95th	99th
1. SINGLE DX										
A. Not Operated										
0–19 Years	0									
20–34	6	2.0	2	1	1	2	3	4	4	4
35–49	42	1.8	1	1	1	1	2	3	5	5
50–64	67	1.6	<1	1	1	1	2	3	3	5
65+	40	1.5	<1	1	1	1	2	3	3	5
B. Operated										
0–19 Years	0									
20–34	0									
35–49	0									
50–64	0									
65+	1	1.0	0	1	1	1	1	1	1	1
2. MULTIPLE DX										
A. Not Operated										
0–19 Years	21	2.6	4	1	1	2	3	6	7	8
20–34	234	2.0	2	1	1	2	2	3	4	7
35–49	1,668	2.1	2	1	1	2	3	4	5	8
50–64	5,331	2.2	3	1	1	2	3	4	5	8
65+	15,571	2.5	4	1	1	2	3	5	6	9
B. Operated										
0–19 Years	0									
20–34	0									
35–49	19	5.7	30	1	2	4	9	11	24	24
50–64	69	4.4	23	1	1	3	5	12	16	25
65+	273	5.9	24	1	1	5	8	12	15	26
SUBTOTALS:										
1. SINGLE DX										
A. Not Operated	155	1.7	<1	1	1	1	2	3	4	5
B. Operated	1	1.0	0	1	1	1	1	1	1	1
2. MULTIPLE DX										
A. Not Operated	22,825	2.4	3	1	1	2	3	4	6	9
B. Operated	361	5.6	24	1	2	4	8	12	15	25
1. SINGLE DX	156	1.6	<1	1	1	1	2	3	4	5
2. MULTIPLE DX	23,186	2.4	4	1	1	2	3	4	6	10
A. NOT OPERATED	22,980	2.4	3	1	1	2	3	4	5	9
B. OPERATED	362	5.6	24	1	2	4	8	12	15	25
TOTAL										
0–19 Years	21	2.6	4	1	1	2	3	6	7	8
20–34	240	2.0	2	1	1	2	2	3	4	7
35–49	1,729	2.1	3	1	1	2	3	4	5	9
50–64	5,467	2.2	3	1	1	2	3	4	5	9
65+	15,885	2.5	4	1	1	2	3	5	6	10
GRAND TOTAL	23,342	2.4	4	1	1	2	3	4	6	10

435.3: VERTBASILAR ART SYNDROME

Type of Patients	Observed Patients	Avg. Stay	Vari-ance	Percentiles						
				10th	25th	50th	75th	90th	95th	99th
1. SINGLE DX										
A. Not Operated										
0–19 Years	0									
20–34	0									
35–49	0									
50–64	1	1.0	0							
65+	1	5.0	0	5	5	5	5	5	5	5
B. Operated										
0–19 Years	0									
20–34	0									
35–49	0									
50–64	0									
65+	0									
2. MULTIPLE DX										
A. Not Operated										
0–19 Years	0									
20–34	1	1.0	0	1	1	2	1	1	1	1
35–49	5	2.4	1	1	2	2	3	4	4	4
50–64	45	2.4	3	1	1	2	3	5	6	8
65+	202	3.2	4	1	2	3	4	6	7	10
B. Operated										
0–19 Years	0									
20–34	0									
35–49	0									
50–64	3	1.7	<1	1	1	2	2	2	2	2
65+	9	9.4	85	1	4	4	11	28	28	28
SUBTOTALS:										
1. SINGLE DX										
A. Not Operated	2	3.0	8	1	1	1	5	5	5	5
B. Operated	0									
2. MULTIPLE DX										
A. Not Operated	253	3.0	4	1	2	2	4	5	7	10
B. Operated	12	7.4	74	1	2	4	9	21	28	28
1. SINGLE DX	2	3.0	8	1	1	1	5	5	5	5
2. MULTIPLE DX	265	3.2	8	1	2	2	4	6	8	15
A. NOT OPERATED	255	3.0	4	1	2	2	4	5	7	10
B. OPERATED	12	7.4	74	1	2	4	9	21	28	28
TOTAL										
0–19 Years	0									
20–34	1	1.0	0	1	1	2	1	1	1	1
35–49	5	2.4	1	1	2	2	3	4	4	4
50–64	49	2.3	3	1	2	2	3	5	6	8
65+	212	3.5	9	2	3	3	4	6	8	15
GRAND TOTAL	267	3.2	8	1	2	2	4	6	8	15

435.8: TRANS CEREB ISCHEMIA NEC

Type of Patients	Observed Patients	Avg. Stay	Vari-ance	Percentiles						
				10th	25th	50th	75th	90th	95th	99th
1. SINGLE DX										
A. Not Operated										
0–19 Years	0									
20–34	0									
35–49	0									
50–64	4	1.8	<1	1	1	2	2	2	2	2
65+	0									
B. Operated										
0–19 Years	0									
20–34	0									
35–49	0									
50–64	0									
65+	0									
2. MULTIPLE DX										
A. Not Operated										
0–19 Years	2	4.0	8	2	2	6	6	6	6	6
20–34	12	1.8	1	1	1	1	2	3	5	5
35–49	98	2.3	2	1	1	2	3	4	5	9
50–64	306	2.5	7	1	1	2	3	5	6	10
65+	868	2.7	4	1	1	2	3	5	6	10
B. Operated										
0–19 Years	0									
20–34	0									
35–49	1	11.0	0	11	11	11	11	11	11	11
50–64	1	13.0	0	13	13	13	13	13	13	13
65+	10	4.4	6	2	3	5	6	7	9	9
SUBTOTALS:										
1. SINGLE DX										
A. Not Operated	4	1.8	<1	1	1	2	2	2	2	2
B. Operated	0									
2. MULTIPLE DX										
A. Not Operated	1,286	2.6	5	1	1	2	3	5	6	10
B. Operated	12	5.7	14	1	3	5	9	11	13	13
1. SINGLE DX	4	1.8	<1	1	1	2	2	2	2	2
2. MULTIPLE DX	1,298	2.6	5	1	1	2	3	5	6	10
A. NOT OPERATED	1,290	2.6	5	1	1	2	3	5	6	10
B. OPERATED	12	5.7	14	2	3	5	9	11	13	13
TOTAL										
0–19 Years	2	4.0	8	2	2	6	6	6	6	6
20–34	12	1.8	1	1	1	1	2	3	5	5
35–49	99	2.4	3	1	1	2	3	4	5	11
50–64	311	2.5	7	1	1	2	3	5	6	10
65+	878	2.7	4	1	1	2	3	5	6	10
GRAND TOTAL	1,302	2.6	5	1	1	2	3	5	6	10

Length of Stay by Diagnosis and Operation, Western Region, 2008

Western Region, October 2006–September 2007 Data, by Diagnosis

435.9: TRANS CEREB ISCHEMIA NOS

Type of Patients	Observed Patients	Avg. Stay	Variance	10th	25th	50th	75th	90th	95th	99th
1. SINGLE DX										
A. Not Operated										
0–19 Years	0									
20–34	6	2.0	2	1	1	2	3	4	4	4
35–49	42	1.8	1	1	1	1	2	3	5	5
50–64	62	1.6	<1	1	1	1	2	3	3	5
65+	39	1.4	<1	1	1	1	2	2	3	3
B. Operated										
0–19 Years	0									
20–34	0									
35–49	0									
50–64	0									
65+	0									
2. MULTIPLE DX										
A. Not Operated										
0–19 Years	18	2.5	4	1	1	2	3	7	8	8
20–34	220	2.0	2	1	1	2	2	3	4	7
35–49	1,563	2.1	2	1	1	2	3	3	4	8
50–64	4,962	2.1	3	1	1	2	3	4	5	8
65+	14,424	2.5	4	1	1	2	3	4	6	9
B. Operated										
0–19 Years	0									
20–34	0									
35–49	11	6.9	37	3	3	5	9	9	24	24
50–64	35	6.4	32	1	3	4	7	16	18	25
65+	179	7.1	23	2	3	6	9	13	15	26
SUBTOTALS:										
1. SINGLE DX										
A. Not Operated	149	1.6	<1	1	1	1	2	3	3	5
B. Operated	0									
2. MULTIPLE DX										
A. Not Operated	21,187	2.4	3	1	1	2	3	4	5	9
B. Operated	225	7.0	25	2	3	6	9	13	16	25
1. SINGLE DX	149	1.6	<1	1	1	1	2	3	3	5
2. MULTIPLE DX	21,412	2.4	4	1	1	2	3	4	6	10
A. NOT OPERATED	21,336	2.4	3	1	1	2	3	4	5	9
B. OPERATED	225	7.0	25	2	3	6	9	13	16	25
TOTAL										
0–19 Years	18	2.5	4	1	1	2	3	7	8	8
20–34	226	2.0	2	1	1	2	2	3	4	7
35–49	1,616	2.1	3	1	1	2	3	3	4	9
50–64	5,059	2.2	3	1	1	2	3	4	5	9
65+	14,642	2.5	4	1	1	2	3	5	6	10
GRAND TOTAL	21,561	2.4	4	1	1	2	3	4	6	10

436: ACUTE ILL-DEFINED CVD

Type of Patients	Observed Patients	Avg. Stay	Variance	10th	25th	50th	75th	90th	95th	99th
1. SINGLE DX										
A. Not Operated										
0–19 Years	0									
20–34	0									
35–49	0									
50–64	0									
65+	1	2.0	0	2	2	2	2	2	2	2
B. Operated										
0–19 Years	0									
20–34	0									
35–49	0									
50–64	0									
65+	0									
2. MULTIPLE DX										
A. Not Operated										
0–19 Years	0									
20–34	2	4.0	2	3	3	5	5	5	5	5
35–49	13	3.8	4	2	2	4	5	7	7	7
50–64	38	3.4	8	1	1	2	6	8	11	11
65+	93	3.2	5	1	2	3	4	7	8	10
B. Operated										
0–19 Years	0									
20–34	0									
35–49	0									
50–64	0									
65+	0									
SUBTOTALS:										
1. SINGLE DX										
A. Not Operated	1	2.0	0	2	2	2	2	2	2	2
B. Operated	0									
2. MULTIPLE DX										
A. Not Operated	146	3.3	6	1	2	3	4	7	8	11
B. Operated	0									
1. SINGLE DX	1	2.0	0	2	2	2	2	2	2	2
2. MULTIPLE DX	146	3.3	6	1	2	3	4	7	8	11
A. NOT OPERATED	147	3.3	5	1	2	3	4	7	8	11
B. OPERATED	0									
TOTAL										
0–19 Years	0									
20–34	2	4.0	2	3	3	5	5	5	5	5
35–49	13	3.8	4	2	2	4	5	7	7	7
50–64	38	3.4	8	1	1	2	6	8	11	11
65+	94	3.2	5	1	2	3	4	7	8	10
GRAND TOTAL	147	3.3	5	1	2	3	4	7	8	11

437: OTH CEREBROVASC DISEASE

Type of Patients	Observed Patients	Avg. Stay	Variance	10th	25th	50th	75th	90th	95th	99th
1. SINGLE DX										
A. Not Operated										
0–19 Years	3	1.7	1	1	1	3	3	3	3	3
20–34	5	3.8	5	1	2	5	5	6	6	6
35–49	5	1.2	<1	1	1	1	1	1	2	2
50–64	30	1.6	<1	1	1	1	2	2	4	4
65+	6	1.3	<1	1	1	1	2	2	2	2
B. Operated										
0–19 Years	6	4.5	12	2	2	3	6	11	11	11
20–34	18	3.2	6	1	1	2	5	7	9	9
35–49	35	2.3	3	1	1	1	4	5	6	7
50–64	54	2.2	3	1	1	1	4	6	6	7
65+	10	2.4	5	1	1	1	4	4	8	8
2. MULTIPLE DX										
A. Not Operated										
0–19 Years	25	8.7	115	1	2	4	12	24	24	46
20–34	91	3.7	6	2	2	3	5	7	8	13
35–49	260	3.9	19	1	2	3	5	7	10	17
50–64	831	3.6	23	1	1	2	4	7	10	20
65+	1,349	4.1	24	1	2	3	5	9	12	24
B. Operated										
0–19 Years	27	6.4	65	2	2	3	6	14	27	36
20–34	87	5.6	40	2	2	3	6	13	16	46
35–49	323	4.0	16	1	1	3	5	8	12	21
50–64	748	4.5	32	1	1	3	6	9	14	24
65+	424	4.7	39	1	1	3	6	10	17	24
SUBTOTALS:										
1. SINGLE DX										
A. Not Operated	49	1.8	2	1	1	2	2	4	5	6
B. Operated	123	2.5	4	1	1	4	4	5	6	9
2. MULTIPLE DX										
A. Not Operated	2,556	4.0	24	1	1	3	5	8	11	23
B. Operated	1,609	4.6	32	1	1	3	6	10	14	24
1. SINGLE DX	172	2.3	3	1	1	3	3	5	6	9
2. MULTIPLE DX	4,165	4.2	27	1	1	3	5	9	13	24
A. NOT OPERATED	2,605	3.9	23	1	1	2	5	8	11	21
B. OPERATED	1,732	4.4	30	1	1	3	5	9	14	24
TOTAL										
0–19 Years	61	6.9	79	1	2	3	6	16	24	46
20–34	201	4.5	21	1	2	3	5	9	12	19
35–49	623	3.9	17	1	1	3	5	8	11	20
50–64	1,663	3.9	26	1	2	2	5	8	12	21
65+	1,789	4.3	28	1	1	3	5	9	13	24
GRAND TOTAL	4,337	4.1	26	1	1	3	5	8	12	24

Western Region, October 2006–September 2007 Data, by Diagnosis

437.0: CEREBRAL ATHEROSCLEROSIS

Type of Patients	Observed Patients	Avg. Stay	Vari-ance	Percentiles						
				10th	25th	50th	75th	90th	95th	99th
1. SINGLE DX										
A. Not Operated										
0–19 Years	0									
20–34	0									
35–49	1	1.0	0	1	1	1	1	1	1	1
50–64	0									
65+	0									
B. Operated										
0–19 Years	0									
20–34	0									
35–49	0									
50–64	0									
65+	0									
2. MULTIPLE DX										
A. Not Operated										
0–19 Years	1	3.0	0	3	3	3	3	3	3	3
20–34	1	4.0	0	4	4	4	4	4	4	4
35–49	3	2.3	2	1	1	2	4	4	4	4
50–64	39	4.4	10	1	2	4	6	9	13	14
65+	311	7.0	64	2	3	4	9	15	20	70
B. Operated										
0–19 Years	0									
20–34	2	2.0	2	1	1	3	3	3	3	3
35–49	6	4.0	21	1	1	3	4	13	13	13
50–64	9	1.9	3	1	1	1	2	6	6	6
65+	22	2.1	2	1	1	2	3	4	4	4
SUBTOTALS:										
1. SINGLE DX										
A. Not Operated	1	1.0	0	1	1	1	1	1	1	1
B. Operated	0									
2. MULTIPLE DX										
A. Not Operated	355	6.7	58	2	3	4	8	14	19	70
B. Operated	39	2.4	5	1	1	2	3	6	6	13
1. SINGLE DX	1	1.0	0	1	1	1	1	1	1	1
2. MULTIPLE DX	394	6.2	54	1	2	4	8	14	19	70
A. NOT OPERATED	356	6.7	58	2	3	4	8	14	19	70
B. OPERATED	39	2.4	5	1	1	2	3	4	6	13
TOTAL										
0–19 Years	1	3.0	0	3	3	3	3	3	3	3
20–34	3	2.7	2	1	1	3	4	4	4	4
35–49	10	3.2	13	1	1	3	4	13	13	13
50–64	48	4.0	9	1	1	3	6	7	10	14
65+	333	6.7	61	2	2	4	9	14	20	70
GRAND TOTAL	395	6.2	54	1	2	4	8	14	19	70

437.1: AC CEREBROVASC INSUF NOS

Type of Patients	Observed Patients	Avg. Stay	Vari-ance	Percentiles						
				10th	25th	50th	75th	90th	95th	99th
1. SINGLE DX										
A. Not Operated										
0–19 Years	0									
20–34	0									
35–49	1	2.0	0	2	2	2	2	2	2	2
50–64	0									
65+	0									
B. Operated										
0–19 Years	0									
20–34	0									
35–49	0									
50–64	0									
65+	0									
2. MULTIPLE DX										
A. Not Operated										
0–19 Years	0									
20–34	2	2.5	4	1	1	3	4	4	4	4
35–49	9	2.9	2	1	2	3	3	6	6	6
50–64	37	3.7	22	1	2	2	4	7	17	26
65+	110	3.4	8	1	2	3	4	7	10	14
B. Operated										
0–19 Years	0									
20–34	0									
35–49	0									
50–64	2	3.5	12	1	1	1	6	6	6	6
65+	3	11.3	44	7	7	8	19	19	19	19
SUBTOTALS:										
1. SINGLE DX										
A. Not Operated	1	2.0	0	2	2	2	2	2	2	2
B. Operated	0									
2. MULTIPLE DX										
A. Not Operated	158	3.5	11	1	2	3	4	6	10	17
B. Operated	5	8.2	43	1	6	7	8	19	19	19
1. SINGLE DX	1	2.0	0	2	2	2	2	2	2	2
2. MULTIPLE DX	163	3.6	12	1	2	3	4	7	10	19
A. NOT OPERATED	159	3.5	11	1	2	3	4	6	10	17
B. OPERATED	5	8.2	43	1	6	7	8	19	19	19
TOTAL										
0–19 Years	0									
20–34	2	2.5	4	1	1	3	4	4	4	4
35–49	10	2.8	2	2	2	3	3	4	6	6
50–64	39	3.7	22	1	2	2	4	7	17	26
65+	113	3.7	10	1	2	3	5	8	10	15
GRAND TOTAL	164	3.6	12	1	2	3	4	7	10	19

437.2: HTN ENCEPHALOPATHY

Type of Patients	Observed Patients	Avg. Stay	Vari-ance	Percentiles						
				10th	25th	50th	75th	90th	95th	99th
1. SINGLE DX										
A. Not Operated										
0–19 Years	0									
20–34	0									
35–49	0									
50–64	0									
65+	0									
B. Operated										
0–19 Years	0									
20–34	0									
35–49	0									
50–64	0									
65+	0									
2. MULTIPLE DX										
A. Not Operated										
0–19 Years	8	13.0	238	2	3	5	24	46	46	46
20–34	38	4.1	6	2	2	4	5	8	10	11
35–49	125	4.0	7	1	2	3	6	8	9	12
50–64	324	5.2	43	1	2	4	6	10	14	25
65+	460	3.9	9	1	2	3	5	8	10	16
B. Operated										
0–19 Years	0									
20–34	3	12.3	20	8	8	12	17	17	17	17
35–49	5	9.8	46	4	5	6	15	19	19	19
50–64	11	8.8	18	5	5	8	14	14	16	16
65+	7	9.3	56	2	3	8	12	24	24	24
SUBTOTALS:										
1. SINGLE DX										
A. Not Operated	0									
B. Operated	0									
2. MULTIPLE DX										
A. Not Operated	955	4.4	23	1	2	3	5	8	11	20
B. Operated	26	9.6	31	3	5	8	14	17	19	24
1. SINGLE DX	0									
2. MULTIPLE DX	981	4.6	24	1	2	3	6	9	12	20
A. NOT OPERATED	955	4.4	23	1	2	3	5	8	11	20
B. OPERATED	26	9.6	31	3	5	8	14	17	19	24
TOTAL										
0–19 Years	8	13.0	238	2	3	5	24	46	46	46
20–34	41	4.7	11	2	2	4	6	9	11	17
35–49	130	4.3	10	1	2	3	6	8	10	15
50–64	335	5.3	43	1	2	4	6	10	14	25
65+	467	4.0	10	1	2	3	5	8	10	16
GRAND TOTAL	981	4.6	24	1	2	3	6	9	12	20

Length of Stay by Diagnosis and Operation, Western Region, 2008

Western Region, October 2006–September 2007 Data, by Diagnosis

437.3: NONRUPT CEREBRAL ANRYSM

Type of Patients	Observed Patients	Avg. Stay	Variance	10th	25th	50th	75th	90th	95th	99th
1. SINGLE DX										
A. Not Operated										
0–19 Years	2	2.0	2	1	1	2	3	3	3	3
20–34	2	5.5	<1	5	5	6	6	6	6	6
35–49	1	1.0	0	1	1	1	1	1	1	1
50–64	11	1.8	2	1	1	1	3	4	4	4
65+	0									
B. Operated										
0–19 Years	2	7.0	32	3	3	3	11	11	11	11
20–34	13	2.9	5	1	1	2	5	5	7	7
35–49	32	2.3	3	1	1	1	4	5	6	7
50–64	54	2.2	3	1	1	1	4	4	6	7
65+	10	2.4	5	1	1	1	4	4	8	8
2. MULTIPLE DX										
A. Not Operated										
0–19 Years	0									
20–34	11	3.8	10	1	1	2	2	8	8	8
35–49	50	2.6	7	1	1	2	3	5	6	17
50–64	91	2.8	4	1	1	2	4	6	7	9
65+	109	2.8	5	1	1	2	4	6	7	9
B. Operated										
0–19 Years	11	4.6	17	1	2	3	5	11	14	14
20–34	44	5.0	22	1	2	3	7	12	13	22
35–49	265	3.7	13	1	1	3	5	8	10	18
50–64	691	4.3	27	1	1	3	5	9	14	23
65+	381	4.6	36	1	1	3	6	10	16	24
SUBTOTALS:										
1. SINGLE DX										
A. Not Operated	17	2.2	3	1	1	1	1	5	6	6
B. Operated	111	2.4	4	1	1	1	4	5	6	8
2. MULTIPLE DX										
A. Not Operated	261	2.8	5	1	1	2	4	6	7	9
B. Operated	1,392	4.3	27	1	1	3	5	9	13	23
1. SINGLE DX	128	2.4	4	1	1	1	4	5	6	8
2. MULTIPLE DX	1,653	4.1	24	1	1	3	5	8	12	22
A. NOT OPERATED	278	2.8	5	1	1	2	4	6	7	9
B. OPERATED	1,503	4.2	25	1	1	3	5	9	13	23
TOTAL										
0–19 Years	15	4.5	17	1	2	3	5	11	14	14
20–34	70	4.4	17	1	2	3	6	10	13	22
35–49	349	3.4	11	1	1	2	4	7	10	17
50–64	847	4.0	23	1	1	3	5	8	13	20
65+	500	4.1	29	1	1	2	5	9	13	24
GRAND TOTAL	1,781	3.9	22	1	1	3	5	8	12	22

437.7: TRANSIENT GLOBAL AMNESIA

Type of Patients	Observed Patients	Avg. Stay	Variance	10th	25th	50th	75th	90th	95th	99th
1. SINGLE DX										
A. Not Operated										
0–19 Years	0									
20–34	2	1.5	<1	1	1	2	2	2	2	2
35–49	1	1.0	0	1	1	1	1	1	1	1
50–64	15	1.5	<1	1	1	1	2	2	4	4
65+	6	1.3	<1	1	1	1	2	2	2	2
B. Operated										
0–19 Years	0									
20–34	0									
35–49	0									
50–64	0									
65+	0									
2. MULTIPLE DX										
A. Not Operated										
0–19 Years	1	3.0	0	3	3	3	3	3	3	3
20–34	8	2.4	5	1	1	1	5	7	7	7
35–49	33	1.5	<1	1	1	1	2	2	3	4
50–64	296	1.6	1	1	1	1	2	3	3	7
65+	275	1.7	1	1	1	1	2	3	4	5
B. Operated										
0–19 Years	0									
20–34	0									
35–49	0									
50–64	2	2.5	<1	2	2	3	3	3	3	3
65+	1	10.0	0	10	10	10	10	10	10	10
SUBTOTALS:										
1. SINGLE DX										
A. Not Operated	24	1.4	<1	1	1	1	2	2	2	4
B. Operated	0									
2. MULTIPLE DX										
A. Not Operated	613	1.7	1	1	1	1	2	3	3	6
B. Operated	3	5.0	19	2	2	3	10	10	10	10
1. SINGLE DX	24	1.4	<1	1	1	1	2	2	2	4
2. MULTIPLE DX	616	1.7	1	1	1	1	2	3	3	7
A. NOT OPERATED	637	1.6	1	1	1	1	2	3	3	6
B. OPERATED	3	5.0	19	2	2	3	10	10	10	10
TOTAL										
0–19 Years	1	3.0	0	3	3	3	3	3	3	3
20–34	10	2.2	4	1	1	1	2	7	7	7
35–49	34	1.5	<1	1	1	1	2	2	3	4
50–64	313	1.6	<1	1	1	1	2	2	3	6
65+	282	1.7	1	1	1	1	2	3	4	8
GRAND TOTAL	640	1.7	1	1	1	1	2	3	3	7

438: LATE EFF CEREBROVASC DIS

Type of Patients	Observed Patients	Avg. Stay	Variance	10th	25th	50th	75th	90th	95th	99th
1. SINGLE DX										
A. Not Operated										
0–19 Years	0									
20–34	0									
35–49	0									
50–64	0									
65+	0									
B. Operated										
0–19 Years	0									
20–34	0									
35–49	0									
50–64	0									
65+	0									
2. MULTIPLE DX										
A. Not Operated										
0–19 Years	6	3.2	16	1	1	4	4	11	11	11
20–34	26	4.9	25	1	2	4	6	11	14	24
35–49	150	6.3	76	1	2	4	6	13	22	61
50–64	430	4.5	41	1	2	3	5	9	14	43
65+	1,251	4.5	20	1	2	3	5	9	13	28
B. Operated										
0–19 Years	2	18.6	356	5	5	32	32	32	32	32
20–34	1	6.0	0	6	6	6	6	6	6	6
35–49	9	7.6	80	1	3	4	6	27	27	27
50–64	38	5.5	91	1	1	3	6	11	28	54
65+	36	6.9	29	1	3	6	9	15	17	24
SUBTOTALS:										
1. SINGLE DX										
A. Not Operated	0									
B. Operated	0									
2. MULTIPLE DX										
A. Not Operated	1,863	4.6	30	1	2	3	5	9	14	30
B. Operated	86	6.6	67	1	2	4	8	15	24	54
1. SINGLE DX	0									
2. MULTIPLE DX	1,949	4.7	31	1	2	3	5	9	14	30
A. NOT OPERATED	1,863	4.6	30	1	2	3	5	9	14	30
B. OPERATED	86	6.6	67	1	2	4	8	15	24	54
TOTAL										
0–19 Years	8	7.1	115	1	1	4	11	32	32	32
20–34	27	4.9	24	1	2	4	6	11	14	24
35–49	159	6.4	76	1	2	4	6	14	22	61
50–64	468	4.5	45	1	2	3	5	9	14	48
65+	1,287	4.6	20	1	2	3	5	9	13	28
GRAND TOTAL	1,949	4.7	31	1	2	3	5	9	14	30

Western Region, October 2006–September 2007 Data, by Diagnosis

438.20: LATE EFF CVD-HEMI NOS

Type of Patients	Observed Patients	Avg. Stay	Vari-ance	10th	25th	50th	75th	90th	95th	99th
1. SINGLE DX										
A. Not Operated										
0–19 Years	0									
20–34	0									
35–49	0									
50–64	0									
65+	0									
B. Operated										
0–19 Years	0									
20–34	0									
35–49	0									
50–64	0									
65+	0									
2. MULTIPLE DX										
A. Not Operated										
0–19 Years	0									
20–34	5	7.2	92	1	2	3	6	24	24	24
35–49	32	5.0	16	2	3	4	6	11	21	>99
50–64	62	7.8	196	1	2	3	7	21	43	>99
65+	138	4.9	26	1	2	3	5	11	17	32
B. Operated										
0–19 Years	0									
20–34	0									
35–49	3	3.4	6	1	1	3	6	6	6	6
50–64	11	7.1	248	1	1	2	3	9	54	54
65+	3	4.0	4	2	2	4	6	6	6	6
SUBTOTALS:										
1. SINGLE DX										
A. Not Operated	0									
B. Operated	0									
2. MULTIPLE DX										
A. Not Operated	237	5.7	71	1	2	3	6	13	22	>99
B. Operated	17	5.9	158	1	1	2	4	9	54	54
1. SINGLE DX	0									
2. MULTIPLE DX	254	5.7	77	1	2	3	6	13	23	>99
A. NOT OPERATED	237	5.7	71	1	2	3	6	13	22	>99
B. OPERATED	17	5.9	158	1	1	2	4	9	54	54
TOTAL										
0–19 Years	0									
20–34	5	7.2	92	1	2	3	6	24	24	24
35–49	35	4.8	15	1	3	4	6	11	21	>99
50–64	73	7.7	201	1	2	3	7	21	48	>99
65+	141	4.8	26	1	2	3	5	11	15	32
GRAND TOTAL	254	5.7	77	1	2	3	6	13	23	>99

438.82: LATE EFF CVD-DYSPHAGIA

Type of Patients	Observed Patients	Avg. Stay	Vari-ance	10th	25th	50th	75th	90th	95th	99th
1. SINGLE DX										
A. Not Operated										
0–19 Years	0									
20–34	0									
35–49	0									
50–64	0									
65+	0									
B. Operated										
0–19 Years	0									
20–34	0									
35–49	0									
50–64	0									
65+	0									
2. MULTIPLE DX										
A. Not Operated										
0–19 Years	0									
20–34	0									
35–49	3	19.7	641	5	5	5	49	49	49	49
50–64	9	4.3	11	1	2	3	6	10	10	10
65+	199	5.6	22	2	3	4	7	11	15	22
B. Operated										
0–19 Years	0									
20–34	0									
35–49	1	27.0	0	27	27	27	27	27	27	27
50–64	0									
65+	4	7.8	11	4	7	8	12	12	12	12
SUBTOTALS:										
1. SINGLE DX										
A. Not Operated	0									
B. Operated	0									
2. MULTIPLE DX										
A. Not Operated	211	5.8	30	2	3	4	7	11	15	27
B. Operated	5	11.6	82	4	7	8	12	27	27	27
1. SINGLE DX	0									
2. MULTIPLE DX	216	5.9	31	2	3	4	7	11	16	27
A. NOT OPERATED	211	5.8	30	2	3	4	7	11	15	27
B. OPERATED	5	11.6	82	4	7	8	12	27	27	27
TOTAL										
0–19 Years	0									
20–34	0									
35–49	4	21.6	440	5	5	27	27	49	49	49
50–64	9	4.3	11	1	2	3	6	10	10	10
65+	203	5.7	21	2	3	4	7	11	14	22
GRAND TOTAL	216	5.9	31	2	3	4	7	11	16	27

438.89: OTH LATE EFFECT CVD

Type of Patients	Observed Patients	Avg. Stay	Vari-ance	10th	25th	50th	75th	90th	95th	99th
1. SINGLE DX										
A. Not Operated										
0–19 Years	0									
20–34	0									
35–49	0									
50–64	0									
65+	0									
B. Operated										
0–19 Years	0									
20–34	0									
35–49	0									
50–64	0									
65+	0									
2. MULTIPLE DX										
A. Not Operated										
0–19 Years	6	3.2	16	1	1	1	4	11	11	11
20–34	21	4.3	12	1	2	4	5	7	11	14
35–49	80	5.4	37	1	2	4	6	10	16	38
50–64	275	3.7	12	1	2	3	4	7	10	21
65+	692	4.2	15	1	2	3	5	8	11	22
B. Operated										
0–19 Years	1	32.0	0	32	32	32	32	32	32	32
20–34	1	6.0	0	6	6	6	6	6	6	6
35–49	4	7.5	49	3	4	5	5	18	18	18
50–64	25	4.5	33	1	1	3	6	10	11	28
65+	25	7.4	33	3	3	8	10	15	17	24
SUBTOTALS:										
1. SINGLE DX										
A. Not Operated	0									
B. Operated	0									
2. MULTIPLE DX										
A. Not Operated	1,074	4.1	16	1	2	3	5	8	11	22
B. Operated	56	6.5	46	1	2	4	8	15	24	32
1. SINGLE DX	0									
2. MULTIPLE DX	1,130	4.3	17	1	2	3	5	8	11	23
A. NOT OPERATED	1,074	4.1	16	1	2	3	5	8	11	22
B. OPERATED	56	6.5	46	1	2	4	8	15	24	32
TOTAL										
0–19 Years	7	7.4	133	1	1	1	11	32	32	32
20–34	22	4.4	11	1	2	4	6	7	11	14
35–49	84	5.5	37	1	2	4	6	10	18	38
50–64	300	3.8	14	1	2	3	4	7	10	22
65+	717	4.3	16	1	2	3	5	8	11	22
GRAND TOTAL	1,130	4.3	17	1	2	3	5	8	11	23

317

Length of Stay by Diagnosis and Operation, Western Region, 2008

Western Region, October 2006–September 2007 Data, by Diagnosis

440: ATHEROSCLEROSIS

Type of Patients	Observed Patients	Avg. Stay	Variance	Percentiles 10th	25th	50th	75th	90th	95th	99th
1. SINGLE DX										
A. Not Operated										
0–19 Years	0									
20–34	1	1.0	0		1	1		1		1
35–49	0									
50–64	4	1.3	<1	1	1	1	2	2	2	2
65+	11	2.3	15	1	1	1	1	2	14	14
B. Operated										
0–19 Years	0									
20–34	0									
35–49	9	2.4	5	1	1	2	3	8	8	8
50–64	55	1.5	<1	1	1	1	2	3	4	5
65+	123	1.7	4	1	1	1	2	3	5	10
2. MULTIPLE DX										
A. Not Operated										
0–19 Years	0									
20–34	5	4.4	15	2	2	2	5	11	11	11
35–49	63	4.1	14	1	2	3	5	7	9	20
50–64	363	4.7	45	1	1	3	5	9	13	28
65+	1,404	4.3	15	1	1	3	6	9	11	20
B. Operated										
0–19 Years	4	5.7	13	1	1	6	6	10	10	10
20–34	24	4.9	20	1	2	3	7	11	13	18
35–49	460	6.4	52	1	1	4	8	16	21	34
50–64	3,902	5.1	39	1	1	3	6	12	16	30
65+	11,494	5.1	35	1	1	3	7	12	16	29
SUBTOTALS:										
1. SINGLE DX										
A. Not Operated	16	1.9	10	1	1	1	1	2	14	14
B. Operated	188	1.7	3	1	1	1	2	3	5	10
2. MULTIPLE DX										
A. Not Operated	1,835	4.3	21	1	1	3	6	9	11	22
B. Operated	15,884	5.2	37	1	1	3	7	12	16	29
1. SINGLE DX	204	1.7	4	1	1	1	2	3	5	10
2. MULTIPLE DX	17,719	5.1	35	1	1	3	7	12	16	29
A. NOT OPERATED	1,851	4.3	21	1	1	3	6	9	11	22
B. OPERATED	16,072	5.1	36	1	1	3	7	12	16	29
TOTAL										
0–19 Years	4	5.7	13	1	1	6	6	10	10	10
20–34	31	4.6	18	1	2	3	7	11	13	18
35–49	532	6.0	47	1	2	4	8	14	19	32
50–64	4,324	5.1	39	1	1	3	6	12	16	30
65+	13,032	5.0	33	1	1	3	7	12	16	28
GRAND TOTAL	17,923	5.0	35	1	1	3	6	12	16	29

440.1: RENAL ARTERY AS

Type of Patients	Observed Patients	Avg. Stay	Variance	Percentiles 10th	25th	50th	75th	90th	95th	99th
1. SINGLE DX										
A. Not Operated										
0–19 Years	0									
20–34	0									
35–49	0									
50–64	0									
65+	0									
B. Operated										
0–19 Years	0									
20–34	0									
35–49	0									
50–64	5	1.0	0	1	1	1	1	1	1	1
65+	10	1.0	0	1	1	1	1	1	1	1
2. MULTIPLE DX										
A. Not Operated										
0–19 Years	0									
20–34	3	5.0	27	2	2	2	11	11	11	11
35–49	4	6.0	7	3	3	5	7	9	9	9
50–64	29	4.0	13	1	1	3	5	9	14	15
65+	82	2.5	5	1	1	3	4	6	7	10
B. Operated										
0–19 Years	4	5.7	13	1	1	6	6	10	10	10
20–34	7	2.1	1	1	1	2	3	4	4	4
35–49	21	3.0	19	1	1	2	3	5	13	18
50–64	196	2.0	7	1	1	1	2	4	8	15
65+	968	1.9	5	1	1	1	2	4	7	12
SUBTOTALS:										
1. SINGLE DX										
A. Not Operated	0									
B. Operated	15	1.0	0	1	1	1	1	1	1	1
2. MULTIPLE DX										
A. Not Operated	118	3.1	8	1	1	3	5	7	9	14
B. Operated	1,196	2.0	5	1	1	1	2	4	7	13
1. SINGLE DX	15	1.0	0	1	1	1	1	1	1	1
2. MULTIPLE DX	1,314	2.1	6	1	1	1	2	5	7	13
A. NOT OPERATED	118	3.1	8	1	1	3	5	7	9	14
B. OPERATED	1,211	1.9	5	1	1	1	2	4	7	13
TOTAL										
0–19 Years	4	5.7	13	1	1	6	6	10	10	10
20–34	10	3.0	9	1	1	2	3	11	11	11
35–49	25	3.5	18	1	1	2	4	9	13	18
50–64	230	2.3	8	1	1	1	2	5	8	15
65+	1,060	1.9	5	1	1	1	2	4	7	11
GRAND TOTAL	1,329	2.0	6	1	1	1	2	5	7	13

440.20: AS NATIVE ARTERY EXT NOS

Type of Patients	Observed Patients	Avg. Stay	Variance	Percentiles 10th	25th	50th	75th	90th	95th	99th
1. SINGLE DX										
A. Not Operated										
0–19 Years	0									
20–34	0									
35–49	0									
50–64	0									
65+	3	5.3	55	1	1	1	14	14	14	14
B. Operated										
0–19 Years	0									
20–34	0									
35–49	0									
50–64	4	1.3	<1	1	1	1	2	2	2	2
65+	19	1.2	<1	1	1	1	1	2	4	4
2. MULTIPLE DX										
A. Not Operated										
0–19 Years	0									
20–34	0									
35–49	4	1.8	<1	1	1	2	2	2	2	2
50–64	47	3.5	9	1	1	3	5	7	8	17
65+	123	3.7	8	1	2	3	4	8	10	12
B. Operated										
0–19 Years	0									
20–34	2	6.0	31	2	2	2	10	10	10	10
35–49	26	4.2	8	1	1	4	5	5	9	11
50–64	217	3.7	13	1	1	3	5	7	11	19
65+	531	3.9	17	1	1	2	5	8	12	20
SUBTOTALS:										
1. SINGLE DX										
A. Not Operated	3	5.3	55	1	1	1	14	14	14	14
B. Operated	23	1.2	<1	1	1	1	1	2	2	4
2. MULTIPLE DX										
A. Not Operated	174	3.6	8	1	2	3	4	7	10	13
B. Operated	776	3.9	16	1	1	3	5	8	11	20
1. SINGLE DX	26	1.7	7	1	1	1	1	2	4	14
2. MULTIPLE DX	950	3.8	14	1	1	3	5	8	11	19
A. NOT OPERATED	177	3.6	9	1	1	3	4	8	10	14
B. OPERATED	799	3.8	16	1	1	2	5	8	11	20
TOTAL										
0–19 Years	0									
20–34	2	6.0	31	2	2	2	10	10	10	10
35–49	30	3.9	8	1	1	3	5	7	9	11
50–64	268	3.6	12	1	1	3	5	7	11	19
65+	676	3.8	15	1	1	2	5	8	11	20
GRAND TOTAL	976	3.8	14	1	1	3	5	8	11	19

Length of Stay by Diagnosis and Operation, Western Region, 2008

440.21: AS EXT W INTERMITT CLAUD

Type of Patients	Observed Patients	Avg. Stay	Variance	10th	25th	50th	75th	90th	95th	99th
1. SINGLE DX										
A. Not Operated										
0–19 Years	0									
20–34	0									
35–49	0									
50–64	4	1.3	<1	1	1	1	2	2	2	2
65+	7	1.0	0	1	1	1	1	1	1	1
B. Operated										
0–19 Years	0									
20–34	1	1.0	0	1	1	1	1	1	1	1
35–49	2	1.5	<1	1	1	2	2	2	2	2
50–64	29	1.5	<1	1	1	1	2	3	3	4
65+	66	1.8	6	1	1	1	2	4	5	19
2. MULTIPLE DX										
A. Not Operated										
0–19 Years	0									
20–34	0									
35–49	16	3.5	23	1	1	2	5	7	20	20
50–64	79	1.8	2	1	1	1	2	4	5	7
65+	251	2.2	5	1	1	1	2	5	6	13
B. Operated										
0–19 Years	0									
20–34	3	2.7	<1	2	2	3	3	3	3	3
35–49	167	3.2	17	1	1	2	4	6	8	25
50–64	1,571	2.9	10	1	1	2	4	6	8	17
65+	3,730	2.7	11	1	1	2	3	6	8	15
SUBTOTALS:										
1. SINGLE DX										
A. Not Operated	11	1.1	<1	1	1	1	1	2	2	2
B. Operated	98	1.7	4	1	1	1	2	3	4	19
2. MULTIPLE DX										
A. Not Operated	346	2.1	5	1	1	1	2	5	6	13
B. Operated	5,471	2.8	11	1	1	2	3	6	8	16
1. SINGLE DX	**109**	**1.6**	**4**	**1**	**1**	**1**	**1**	**3**	**4**	**6**
2. MULTIPLE DX	**5,817**	**2.7**	**11**	**1**	**1**	**2**	**3**	**6**	**8**	**16**
A. NOT OPERATED	**357**	**2.1**	**5**	**1**	**1**	**1**	**2**	**5**	**6**	**13**
B. OPERATED	**5,569**	**2.7**	**11**	**1**	**1**	**2**	**3**	**6**	**8**	**16**
TOTAL										
0–19 Years	0									
20–34	4	2.3	<1	1	1	3	3	3	3	3
35–49	185	3.2	17	1	1	2	4	6	8	25
50–64	1,683	2.8	9	1	1	2	3	6	8	17
65+	4,054	2.6	11	1	1	1	3	5	8	15
GRAND TOTAL	**5,926**	**2.7**	**10**	**1**	**1**	**2**	**3**	**6**	**8**	**16**

440.22: AS EXT ART W REST PAIN

Type of Patients	Observed Patients	Avg. Stay	Variance	10th	25th	50th	75th	90th	95th	99th
1. SINGLE DX										
A. Not Operated										
0–19 Years	0									
20–34	0									
35–49	0									
50–64	0									
65+	1	2.0	0	2	2	2	2	2	2	2
B. Operated										
0–19 Years	0									
20–34	0									
35–49	2	2.5	<1	2	2	2	3	3	3	3
50–64	7	1.3	<1	1	1	1	2	2	2	2
65+	15	2.5	6	1	1	1	3	5	10	10
2. MULTIPLE DX										
A. Not Operated										
0–19 Years	0									
20–34	0									
35–49	5	3.6	4	1	2	4	5	6	6	6
50–64	34	4.4	34	1	2	3	4	7	25	27
65+	135	3.8	12	1	1	3	5	9	10	15
B. Operated										
0–19 Years	0									
20–34	0									
35–49	47	5.8	24	2	2	4	8	12	14	26
50–64	416	5.0	33	1	2	4	6	10	13	21
65+	1,260	4.7	20	1	2	3	6	10	13	23
SUBTOTALS:										
1. SINGLE DX										
A. Not Operated	1	2.0	0	2	2	2	2	2	2	2
B. Operated	24	2.1	4	1	1	1	3	4	5	10
2. MULTIPLE DX										
A. Not Operated	174	3.9	16	1	1	3	4	9	11	25
B. Operated	1,723	4.8	23	1	2	4	6	10	13	23
1. SINGLE DX	**25**	**2.1**	**4**	**1**	**1**	**1**	**2**	**4**	**5**	**10**
2. MULTIPLE DX	**1,897**	**4.8**	**22**	**1**	**2**	**3**	**6**	**10**	**13**	**25**
A. NOT OPERATED	**175**	**3.9**	**16**	**1**	**1**	**3**	**4**	**9**	**11**	**25**
B. OPERATED	**1,747**	**4.8**	**23**	**1**	**2**	**3**	**6**	**10**	**13**	**23**
TOTAL										
0–19 Years	0									
20–34	0									
35–49	54	5.5	22	1	2	4	7	11	14	26
50–64	457	4.9	33	1	2	3	6	10	13	25
65+	1,411	4.6	19	1	2	3	6	9	13	23
GRAND TOTAL	**1,922**	**4.7**	**22**	**1**	**2**	**3**	**6**	**10**	**13**	**23**

440.23: AS EXT W ULCER

Type of Patients	Observed Patients	Avg. Stay	Variance	10th	25th	50th	75th	90th	95th	99th
1. SINGLE DX										
A. Not Operated										
0–19 Years	0									
20–34	0									
35–49	0									
50–64	0									
65+	0									
B. Operated										
0–19 Years	0									
20–34	0									
35–49	0									
50–64	1	5.0	0	5	5	5	5	5	5	5
65+	3	1.3	<1	1	1	1	1	2	2	2
2. MULTIPLE DX										
A. Not Operated										
0–19 Years	0									
20–34	1	5.0	0	5	5	5	5	5	5	5
35–49	7	3.9	5	1	2	4	5	8	8	8
50–64	57	6.8	131	1	2	4	7	13	22	79
65+	309	5.4	20	1	2	4	7	10	14	24
B. Operated										
0–19 Years	0									
20–34	0									
35–49	31	6.1	29	1	2	5	7	14	17	23
50–64	359	6.3	42	1	2	4	8	14	20	30
65+	1,646	6.2	38	1	2	4	8	14	17	33
SUBTOTALS:										
1. SINGLE DX										
A. Not Operated	0									
B. Operated	4	2.2	4	1	1	1	2	5	5	5
2. MULTIPLE DX										
A. Not Operated	374	5.5	36	1	2	4	7	10	15	25
B. Operated	2,036	6.2	39	1	2	4	8	14	18	32
1. SINGLE DX	**4**	**2.2**	**4**	**1**	**1**	**1**	**2**	**5**	**5**	**5**
2. MULTIPLE DX	**2,410**	**6.1**	**38**	**1**	**2**	**4**	**8**	**14**	**17**	**30**
A. NOT OPERATED	**374**	**5.5**	**36**	**1**	**2**	**4**	**7**	**10**	**15**	**25**
B. OPERATED	**2,040**	**6.2**	**39**	**1**	**2**	**4**	**8**	**14**	**17**	**32**
TOTAL										
0–19 Years	0									
20–34	1	5.0	0	5	5	5	5	5	5	5
35–49	38	5.6	25	1	2	4	7	14	17	23
50–64	417	6.4	54	1	2	4	8	14	20	32
65+	1,958	6.1	36	1	2	4	8	13	17	30
GRAND TOTAL	**2,414**	**6.1**	**38**	**1**	**2**	**4**	**8**	**14**	**17**	**30**

Length of Stay by Diagnosis and Operation, Western Region, 2008

Western Region, October 2006–September 2007 Data, by Diagnosis

440.24: AS EXT W GANGRENE

Type of Patients	Observed Patients	Avg. Stay	Vari-ance	10th	25th	50th	75th	90th	95th	99th
1. SINGLE DX										
A. Not Operated										
0–19 Years	0									
20–34	0									
35–49	0									
50–64	0									
65+	0									
B. Operated										
0–19 Years	0									
20–34	0									
35–49	4	3.3	11	1	1	3	8	8	8	8
50–64	2	3.5	4	2	2	5	5	5	5	5
65+	2	3.5	12	1	1	1	6	6	6	6
2. MULTIPLE DX										
A. Not Operated										
0–19 Years	0									
20–34	15	4.4	17	2	2	3	5	9	17	17
35–49	68	8.1	71	2	3	6	9	15	27	53
50–64	333	5.8	18	1	3	5	7	11	13	20
B. Operated										
0–19 Years	0									
20–34	8	9.0	24	2	7	8	13	18	18	18
35–49	111	12.2	98	3	5	10	16	25	30	35
50–64	720	10.7	79	3	5	8	14	22	28	45
65+	2,437	9.7	59	3	5	8	13	19	24	39
SUBTOTALS:										
1. SINGLE DX — A. Not Operated	0									
1. SINGLE DX — B. Operated	8	3.4	7	1	1	3	5	8	8	8
2. MULTIPLE DX — A. Not Operated	416	6.1	28	1	3	5	8	11	15	27
2. MULTIPLE DX — B. Operated	3,276	10.0	65	3	5	8	13	20	25	42
1. SINGLE DX	8	3.4	7	1	1	3	5	8	8	8
2. MULTIPLE DX	3,692	9.5	62	2	4	7	12	19	24	40
A. NOT OPERATED	416	6.1	28	1	3	5	8	11	15	27
B. OPERATED	3,284	10.0	65	3	5	8	13	20	25	42
TOTAL										
0–19 Years	0									
20–34	8	9.0	24	2	2	8	13	18	18	18
35–49	130	11.1	94	2	4	9	16	24	29	35
50–64	790	10.5	79	3	5	8	14	22	28	49
65+	2,772	9.2	55	2	4	7	12	18	23	37
GRAND TOTAL	3,700	9.5	62	2	4	7	12	19	24	39

440.29: ATHEROSCLEROSIS-LIMB NEC

Type of Patients	Observed Patients	Avg. Stay	Vari-ance	10th	25th	50th	75th	90th	95th	99th
1. SINGLE DX										
A. Not Operated										
0–19 Years	0									
20–34	1	1.0	0	1	1	1	1	1	1	1
35–49	0									
50–64	0									
65+	0									
B. Operated										
0–19 Years	0									
20–34	0									
35–49	1	1.0	0	1	1	1	1	1	1	1
50–64	3	1.0	0	1	1	1	1	1	1	1
65+	6	1.3	<1	1	1	1	1	3	3	3
2. MULTIPLE DX										
A. Not Operated										
0–19 Years	0									
20–34	1	2.0	0	2	2	2	2	2	2	2
35–49	2	4.5	<1	4	4	5	5	5	5	5
50–64	18	4.1	11	1	2	3	5	10	14	14
65+	73	4.2	13	1	1	3	6	8	11	20
B. Operated										
0–19 Years	0									
20–34	1	1.0	0	1	1	1	1	1	1	1
35–49	9	10.8	71	1	7	9	12	29	29	29
50–64	86	5.4	68	1	2	4	7	9	12	73
65+	197	5.5	31	1	2	4	8	11	14	23
SUBTOTALS:										
1. SINGLE DX — A. Not Operated	1	1.0	0	1	1	1	1	1	1	1
1. SINGLE DX — B. Operated	10	1.2	<1	1	1	1	1	3	3	3
2. MULTIPLE DX — A. Not Operated	94	4.1	12	1	2	3	6	8	11	20
2. MULTIPLE DX — B. Operated	293	5.6	44	1	2	4	8	11	14	29
1. SINGLE DX	11	1.2	<1	1	1	1	1	3	3	3
2. MULTIPLE DX	387	5.3	36	1	2	4	7	10	14	23
A. NOT OPERATED	95	4.1	12	1	2	3	6	8	11	20
B. OPERATED	303	5.5	43	1	2	4	7	11	14	23
TOTAL										
0–19 Years	0									
20–34	3	1.3	<1	1	1	1	2	2	2	2
35–49	12	8.9	64	1	3	8	12	18	29	29
50–64	107	5.1	57	1	2	4	6	9	12	19
65+	276	5.1	27	1	2	3	7	10	14	23
GRAND TOTAL	398	5.1	36	1	2	4	7	10	14	23

440.30: AS BYPASS GRAFT EXT NOS

Type of Patients	Observed Patients	Avg. Stay	Vari-ance	10th	25th	50th	75th	90th	95th	99th
1. SINGLE DX										
A. Not Operated										
0–19 Years	0									
20–34	0									
35–49	0									
50–64	0									
65+	0									
B. Operated										
0–19 Years	0									
20–34	0									
35–49	0									
50–64	1	2.0	0	2	2	2	2	2	2	2
65+	1	2.0	0	2	2	2	2	2	2	2
2. MULTIPLE DX										
A. Not Operated										
0–19 Years	0									
20–34	2	11.1	32	7	7	15	15	15	15	15
35–49	12	3.9	11	1	2	3	5	6	13	13
50–64	26	4.2	6	1	2	3	7	8	8	8
B. Operated										
0–19 Years	0									
20–34	1	2.0	0	2	2	2	2	2	2	2
35–49	14	7.5	48	1	1	7	13	18	22	22
50–64	59	5.8	20	1	2	5	8	14	15	16
65+	158	5.7	38	1	2	4	8	12	16	34
SUBTOTALS:										
1. SINGLE DX — A. Not Operated	0									
1. SINGLE DX — B. Operated	2	2.0	0	2	2	2	2	2	2	2
2. MULTIPLE DX — A. Not Operated	40	4.4	10	1	2	4	7	8	13	15
2. MULTIPLE DX — B. Operated	232	5.8	33	1	2	4	8	13	16	27
1. SINGLE DX	2	2.0	0	2	2	2	2	2	2	2
2. MULTIPLE DX	272	5.6	30	1	2	4	8	13	15	27
A. NOT OPERATED	40	4.4	10	1	2	4	7	8	13	15
B. OPERATED	234	5.8	33	1	2	4	8	13	16	27
TOTAL										
0–19 Years	0									
20–34	1	2.0	0	2	2	2	2	2	2	2
35–49	16	8.0	45	1	2	7	13	18	22	22
50–64	72	5.4	18	1	2	5	7	13	15	16
65+	185	5.5	33	1	2	4	8	12	15	34
GRAND TOTAL	274	5.6	30	1	2	4	8	13	15	27

Western Region, October 2006–September 2007 Data, by Diagnosis

440.31: AS AUTOLOG BYP GRAFT EXT

Type of Patients	Observed Patients	Avg. Stay	Vari-ance	10th	25th	50th	75th	90th	95th	99th
1. SINGLE DX										
A. *Not Operated*										
0–19 Years	0									
20–34	0									
35–49	0									
50–64	0									
65+	0									
B. *Operated*										
0–19 Years	0									
20–34	0									
35–49	0									
50–64	2	1.5	<1	1	1	2	2	2	2	2
65+	0									
2. MULTIPLE DX										
A. *Not Operated*										
0–19 Years	0									
20–34	0									
35–49	4	2.5	6	1	1	1	6	6	6	6
50–64	8	3.5	4	1	2	3	5	6	6	6
65+	33	4.8	27	1	2	3	5	8	10	30
B. *Operated*										
0–19 Years	0									
20–34	0									
35–49	13	8.1	19	4	5	8	9	14	19	19
50–64	129	5.2	29	1	2	3	6	12	17	24
65+	317	5.6	39	1	2	4	6	12	18	34
SUBTOTALS:										
1. SINGLE DX										
A. *Not Operated*	0									
B. *Operated*	2	1.5	<1	1	1	2	2	2	2	2
2. MULTIPLE DX										
A. *Not Operated*	45	4.3	21	1	2	3	5	8	10	30
B. *Operated*	459	5.5	36	1	2	4	7	12	17	34
1. SINGLE DX	2	1.5	<1	1	1	2	2	2	2	2
2. MULTIPLE DX	504	5.4	35	1	2	4	6	11	17	33
A. NOT OPERATED	45	4.3	21	1	2	3	5	8	10	30
B. OPERATED	461	5.5	36	1	2	4	7	12	17	34
TOTAL										
0–19 Years	0									
20–34	0									
35–49	17	6.8	21	1	4	6	9	14	19	19
50–64	139	5.0	27	1	2	3	6	11	17	24
65+	350	5.5	38	1	2	4	6	12	17	34
GRAND TOTAL	506	5.4	35	1	2	4	6	11	17	33

441: AORTIC ANEURYSM

Type of Patients	Observed Patients	Avg. Stay	Vari-ance	10th	25th	50th	75th	90th	95th	99th
1. SINGLE DX										
A. *Not Operated*										
0–19 Years	0									
20–34	0									
35–49	1	1.0	0	1	1	1	1	1	1	1
50–64	0									
65+	5	2.4	3	1	3	3	5	5	5	5
B. *Operated*										
0–19 Years	0									
20–34	2	4.0	2	3	3	5	5	5	5	5
35–49	0									
50–64	11	2.6	4	1	1	1	5	5	6	6
65+	36	2.0	3	1	1	1	2	5	7	7
2. MULTIPLE DX										
A. *Not Operated*										
0–19 Years	1	14.0	0	14	14	14	14	14	14	14
20–34	23	3.5	7	1	1	3	6	7	8	9
35–49	108	6.0	54	1	2	4	7	12	16	35
50–64	255	5.5	30	1	2	4	7	11	16	27
65+	899	4.1	13	1	2	3	5	8	10	17
B. *Operated*										
0–19 Years	8	6.8	18	3	4	5	13	14	14	14
20–34	40	10.4	177	4	5	6	9	13	44	77
35–49	158	11.8	216	3	5	7	11	20	41	79
50–64	1,189	7.4	65	1	2	5	9	15	22	42
65+	5,167	6.2	54	1	2	4	8	13	19	38
SUBTOTALS:										
1. SINGLE DX										
A. *Not Operated*	6	2.2	3	1	1	2	3	5	5	5
B. *Operated*	49	2.2	3	1	1	1	3	5	6	7
2. MULTIPLE DX										
A. *Not Operated*	1,286	4.5	21	1	2	3	6	9	12	23
B. *Operated*	6,562	6.6	62	1	2	5	8	14	20	40
1. SINGLE DX	55	2.2	3	1	1	1	3	5	6	7
2. MULTIPLE DX	7,848	6.2	55	1	2	4	8	13	19	38
A. NOT OPERATED	1,292	4.5	20	1	2	3	6	9	12	23
B. OPERATED	6,611	6.5	61	1	2	5	8	14	20	39
TOTAL										
0–19 Years	9	7.6	22	3	4	5	13	14	14	14
20–34	65	7.8	121	1	4	6	8	12	17	77
35–49	267	9.4	158	2	4	6	10	17	31	79
50–64	1,455	7.0	59	1	2	5	8	15	21	39
65+	6,107	5.8	48	1	2	4	7	13	18	35
GRAND TOTAL	7,903	6.2	55	1	2	4	8	13	19	38

441.01: THOR AORTA DISSECTION

Type of Patients	Observed Patients	Avg. Stay	Vari-ance	10th	25th	50th	75th	90th	95th	99th
1. SINGLE DX										
A. *Not Operated*										
0–19 Years	0									
20–34	0									
35–49	0									
50–64	0									
65+	0									
B. *Operated*										
0–19 Years	0									
20–34	0									
35–49	0									
50–64	0									
65+	0									
2. MULTIPLE DX										
A. *Not Operated*										
0–19 Years	1	14.0	0	14	14	14	14	14	14	14
20–34	6	2.5	3	1	1	4	4	4	4	4
35–49	34	6.2	26	1	3	5	7	14	17	25
50–64	84	6.2	22	2	3	5	8	12	13	29
65+	170	5.6	13	2	3	4	7	10	14	17
B. *Operated*										
0–19 Years	1	14.0	0	14	14	14	14	14	14	14
20–34	6	8.1	17	1	6	9	10	13	13	13
35–49	50	12.2	110	6	7	9	13	19	34	63
50–64	131	12.6	90	5	7	10	15	25	32	42
65+	143	13.6	80	5	7	11	17	27	33	39
SUBTOTALS:										
1. SINGLE DX										
A. *Not Operated*	0									
B. *Operated*	0									
2. MULTIPLE DX										
A. *Not Operated*	295	5.8	17	2	3	5	7	11	14	23
B. *Operated*	331	12.9	87	5	7	10	16	26	33	42
1. SINGLE DX	0									
2. MULTIPLE DX	626	9.6	67	2	4	7	12	19	26	39
A. NOT OPERATED	295	5.8	17	2	3	5	7	11	14	23
B. OPERATED	331	12.9	87	5	7	10	16	26	33	42
TOTAL										
0–19 Years	2	14.0	0	14	14	14	14	14	14	14
20–34	12	5.3	18	1	1	4	9	10	13	13
35–49	84	9.7	84	3	5	8	11	17	25	63
50–64	215	10.1	73	2	5	8	12	21	29	41
65+	313	9.3	59	3	4	7	12	18	26	38
GRAND TOTAL	626	9.6	67	2	4	7	12	19	26	39

Length of Stay by Diagnosis and Operation, Western Region, 2008

Western Region, October 2006–September 2007 Data, by Diagnosis

441.02: ABD AORTA DISSECTION

Type of Patients	Observed Patients	Avg. Stay	Vari-ance	10th	25th	50th	75th	90th	95th	99th
1. SINGLE DX										
A. Not Operated										
0–19 Years	0									
20–34	0									
35–49	0									
50–64	0									
65+	0									
B. Operated										
0–19 Years	0									
20–34	0									
35–49	0									
50–64	0									
65+	0									
2. MULTIPLE DX										
A. Not Operated										
0–19 Years	0									
20–34	6	3.0	8	1	1	3	4	8	8	8
35–49	15	5.3	10	2	3	4	8	9	12	12
50–64	44	7.0	40	1	3	5	10	17	23	27
65+	76	4.8	14	1	2	4	6	9	16	19
B. Operated										
0–19 Years	0									
20–34	3	6.0	9	3	3	6	9	9	9	9
35–49	3	3.3	2	2	2	3	5	5	5	5
50–64	30	13.8	135	3	6	11	17	35	42	47
65+	50	9.1	45	1	4	8	13	18	20	35
SUBTOTALS:										
1. SINGLE DX — A. Not Operated	0									
1. SINGLE DX — B. Operated	0									
2. MULTIPLE DX — A. Not Operated	141	5.5	22	1	2	4	7	10	16	23
2. MULTIPLE DX — B. Operated	86	10.4	80	2	4	8	14	20	30	47
1. SINGLE DX	0									
2. MULTIPLE DX	227	7.3	50	1	3	5	9	16	20	35
A. NOT OPERATED	141	5.5	22	1	2	4	7	10	16	23
B. OPERATED	86	10.4	80	2	4	8	14	20	30	47
TOTAL										
0–19 Years	0									
20–34	9	4.0	9	1	1	3	6	9	9	9
35–49	18	4.9	9	2	3	4	8	9	12	12
50–64	74	9.7	89	2	3	7	11	23	30	47
65+	126	6.5	31	1	3	5	9	15	18	20
GRAND TOTAL	227	7.3	50	1	3	5	9	16	20	35

441.03: THORACOABD AORTA DISSECT

Type of Patients	Observed Patients	Avg. Stay	Vari-ance	10th	25th	50th	75th	90th	95th	99th
1. SINGLE DX										
A. Not Operated										
0–19 Years	0									
20–34	0									
35–49	0									
50–64	0									
65+	0									
B. Operated										
0–19 Years	0									
20–34	0									
35–49	0									
50–64	0									
65+	0									
2. MULTIPLE DX										
A. Not Operated										
0–19 Years	0									
20–34	2	7.0	0	7	7	7	7	7	7	7
35–49	20	8.9	54	2	4	8	10	16	23	35
50–64	33	7.0	39	1	2	6	16	16	23	27
65+	54	6.5	54	1	2	5	7	12	25	43
B. Operated										
0–19 Years	0									
20–34	1	8.0	0	8	8	8	8	8	8	8
35–49	17	22.1	496	8	10	14	17	73	79	79
50–64	39	14.8	111	6	7	13	21	33	54	>99
65+	28	14.0	112	6	7	10	19	27	34	52
SUBTOTALS:										
1. SINGLE DX — A. Not Operated	0									
1. SINGLE DX — B. Operated	0									
2. MULTIPLE DX — A. Not Operated	109	7.1	48	1	3	5	8	13	23	35
2. MULTIPLE DX — B. Operated	85	15.9	192	6	8	12	19	34	52	>99
1. SINGLE DX	0									
2. MULTIPLE DX	194	11.0	130	2	5	8	14	23	34	79
A. NOT OPERATED	109	7.1	48	1	3	5	8	13	23	35
B. OPERATED	85	15.9	192	6	8	12	19	34	52	>99
TOTAL										
0–19 Years	0									
20–34	3	7.3	<1	7	7	7	8	8	8	8
35–49	37	15.0	294	4	7	10	14	37	73	79
50–64	72	11.2	92	2	5	8	16	26	33	>99
65+	82	9.0	85	2	3	6	11	20	27	52
GRAND TOTAL	194	11.0	130	2	5	8	14	23	34	79

441.2: THORACIC AORTIC ANEURYSM

Type of Patients	Observed Patients	Avg. Stay	Vari-ance	10th	25th	50th	75th	90th	95th	99th
1. SINGLE DX										
A. Not Operated										
0–19 Years	0									
20–34	0									
35–49	1	1.0	0	1	1	1	1	1	1	1
50–64	0									
65+	0									
B. Operated										
0–19 Years	0									
20–34	2	4.0	2	3	3	5	5	5	5	5
35–49	0									
50–64	0									
65+	0									
2. MULTIPLE DX										
A. Not Operated										
0–19 Years	0									
20–34	2	3.0	2	2	2	3	4	4	4	4
35–49	20	2.2	1	1	1	2	3	4	4	4
50–64	21	2.7	3	1	1	2	4	5	6	7
65+	113	3.5	8	1	2	3	5	7	8	12
B. Operated										
0–19 Years	6	5.7	14	3	4	5	5	13	13	13
20–34	23	7.2	37	4	5	6	7	9	9	34
35–49	51	6.0	6	3	4	6	8	9	10	16
50–64	155	7.0	19	3	4	6	8	13	15	22
65+	264	7.8	50	2	4	6	9	15	20	56
SUBTOTALS:										
1. SINGLE DX — A. Not Operated	1	1.0	0	1	1	1	1	1	1	1
1. SINGLE DX — B. Operated	2	4.0	2	3	3	5	5	5	5	5
2. MULTIPLE DX — A. Not Operated	156	3.2	6	1	2	2	4	6	8	12
2. MULTIPLE DX — B. Operated	499	7.3	35	2	4	6	8	13	17	34
1. SINGLE DX	3	3.0	4	1	1	3	5	5	5	5
2. MULTIPLE DX	655	6.3	31	2	3	5	8	12	15	30
A. NOT OPERATED	157	3.2	6	1	2	2	4	6	8	12
B. OPERATED	501	7.3	35	3	4	6	8	13	17	34
TOTAL										
0–19 Years	6	5.7	14	3	4	5	5	13	13	13
20–34	27	6.6	33	3	5	6	6	9	9	34
35–49	72	4.9	8	1	3	4	7	9	9	16
50–64	176	6.5	19	2	4	5	8	12	15	22
65+	377	6.5	41	2	3	5	8	12	17	39
GRAND TOTAL	658	6.3	31	2	3	5	8	12	15	30

Length of Stay by Diagnosis and Operation, Western Region, 2008

Western Region, October 2006–September 2007 Data, by Diagnosis

441.3: RUPT ABD AORTIC ANEURYSM

Type of Patients	Observed Patients	Avg. Stay	Vari-ance	Percentiles 10th	25th	50th	75th	90th	95th	99th
1. SINGLE DX										
A. Not Operated										
0–19 Years	0									
20–34	0									
35–49	0									
50–64	0									
65+	0									
B. Operated										
0–19 Years	0									
20–34	0									
35–49	0									
50–64	0									
65+	0									
2. MULTIPLE DX										
A. Not Operated										
0–19 Years	0									
20–34	0									
35–49	0									
50–64	1	3.0	0		3	3	3	3		3
65+	25	3.8	14	1	1	3	4	10	12	14
B. Operated										
0–19 Years	0									
20–34	0									
35–49	5	34.6	>999	6	11	13	56	87	87	87
50–64	78	15.0	236	4	6	10	20	32	50	>99
65+	278	14.4	128	5	7	11	18	29	40	74
SUBTOTALS:										
1. SINGLE DX										
A. Not Operated	0									
B. Operated	0									
2. MULTIPLE DX										
A. Not Operated	26	3.8	14	1	1	3	4	10	12	14
B. Operated	361	14.8	168	5	7	11	18	30	40	87
1. SINGLE DX	0									
2. MULTIPLE DX	387	14.1	165	4	7	11	17	29	40	87
A. NOT OPERATED	26	3.8	14	1	1	3	4	10	12	14
B. OPERATED	361	14.8	168	5	7	11	18	30	40	87
TOTAL										
0–19 Years	0									
20–34	0									
35–49	5	34.6	>999	6	11	13	56	87	87	87
50–64	79	14.9	235	3	6	10	20	32	50	>99
65+	303	13.6	127	4	7	11	17	27	38	60
GRAND TOTAL	387	14.1	165	4	7	11	17	29	40	87

441.4: ABD AORTIC ANEURYSM

Type of Patients	Observed Patients	Avg. Stay	Vari-ance	Percentiles 10th	25th	50th	75th	90th	95th	99th
1. SINGLE DX										
A. Not Operated										
0–19 Years	0									
20–34	0									
35–49	0									
50–64	0									
65+	5	2.4	3	1	1	2	3	5	5	5
B. Operated										
0–19 Years	0									
20–34	0									
35–49	0									
50–64	11	2.6	4	1	1	1	5	5	6	6
65+	35	2.0	3	1	1	1	2	5	7	7
2. MULTIPLE DX										
A. Not Operated										
0–19 Years	0									
20–34	2	5.5	25	2	2	6	9	9	9	9
35–49	9	9.3	332	1	3	3	4	58	58	58
50–64	54	3.2	7	1	1	3	4	7	8	12
65+	387	3.2	8	1	1	2	4	7	9	12
B. Operated										
0–19 Years	1	6.0	0	6	6	6	6	6	6	6
20–34	1	5.0	0	5	5	5	5	5	5	5
35–49	22	8.0	44	1	4	7	10	19	22	25
50–64	719	4.8	23	1	2	4	6	10	12	22
65+	4,293	5.1	38	1	1	3	7	11	15	28
SUBTOTALS:										
1. SINGLE DX										
A. Not Operated	5	2.4	3	1	1	2	3	5	5	5
B. Operated	46	2.1	3	1	1	1	3	5	6	7
2. MULTIPLE DX										
A. Not Operated	452	3.4	14	1	1	2	4	7	9	12
B. Operated	5,036	5.1	36	1	1	3	7	10	15	27
1. SINGLE DX	51	2.1	3	1	1	1	3	5	6	7
2. MULTIPLE DX	5,488	4.9	34	1	1	3	6	10	14	27
A. NOT OPERATED	457	3.3	14	1	1	2	4	7	9	12
B. OPERATED	5,082	5.0	35	1	1	3	7	10	15	27
TOTAL										
0–19 Years	1	6.0	0	6	6	6	6	6	6	6
20–34	3	5.3	12	2	2	5	9	9	9	9
35–49	31	8.4	120	1	3	5	9	19	25	58
50–64	784	4.7	22	1	2	4	6	9	12	22
65+	4,720	4.9	35	1	1	3	6	10	14	27
GRAND TOTAL	5,539	4.9	34	1	1	3	6	10	14	26

441.7: THORACOABD ANEURYSM

Type of Patients	Observed Patients	Avg. Stay	Vari-ance	Percentiles 10th	25th	50th	75th	90th	95th	99th
1. SINGLE DX										
A. Not Operated										
0–19 Years	0									
20–34	0									
35–49	0									
50–64	0									
65+	0									
B. Operated										
0–19 Years	0									
20–34	0									
35–49	0									
50–64	0									
65+	1	2.0	0	2	2	2	2	2	2	2
2. MULTIPLE DX										
A. Not Operated										
0–19 Years	0									
20–34	1	6.0	0	6	6	6	6	6	6	6
35–49	3	4.6	22	1	1	3	10	10	10	10
50–64	9	9.1	181	1	1	4	8	42	42	42
65+	42	4.3	13	1	2	3	5	8	12	19
B. Operated										
0–19 Years	0									
20–34	3	32.3	>999	7	7	13	77	77	77	77
35–49	4	27.8	674	5	5	14	64	64	64	64
50–64	31	11.1	96	2	4	8	15	25	34	39
65+	83	10.1	109	2	3	7	13	23	33	50
SUBTOTALS:										
1. SINGLE DX										
A. Not Operated	0									
B. Operated	1	2.0	0	2	2	2	2	2	2	2
2. MULTIPLE DX										
A. Not Operated	55	5.1	41	1	2	3	6	10	18	42
B. Operated	121	11.5	162	2	4	7	14	27	36	64
1. SINGLE DX	1	2.0	0	2	2	2	2	2	2	2
2. MULTIPLE DX	176	9.5	132	1	3	6	12	22	34	64
A. NOT OPERATED	55	5.1	41	1	2	3	6	10	18	42
B. OPERATED	122	11.4	161	2	4	7	14	27	36	64
TOTAL										
0–19 Years	0									
20–34	4	25.7	>999	6	7	13	13	77	77	77
35–49	7	17.8	497	1	3	10	28	64	64	64
50–64	40	10.6	112	2	3	7	15	25	34	42
65+	126	8.1	84	1	2	5	9	17	30	48
GRAND TOTAL	177	9.5	132	1	3	6	12	22	34	64

Length of Stay by Diagnosis and Operation, Western Region, 2008

Western Region, October 2006–September 2007 Data, by Diagnosis

442: OTHER ANEURYSM

Type of Patients	Observed Patients	Avg. Stay	Vari-ance	Percentiles						
				10th	25th	50th	75th	90th	95th	99th
1. SINGLE DX										
A. Not Operated										
0–19 Years	0									
20–34	2	3.5	12	1	1	1	6	6	6	6
35–49	0									
50–64	1	3.0	0	3	3	3	3	3	3	3
65+	2	1.5	<1	1	1	2	2	2	2	2
B. Operated										
0–19 Years	1	3.0	0	3	3	3	3	3	3	3
20–34	5	2.8	3	1	1	3	4	5	5	5
35–49	7	4.3	17	1	2	3	5	13	13	13
50–64	12	1.9	<1	1	1	2	2	3	4	4
65+	10	1.5	<1	1	1	1	2	2	4	4
2. MULTIPLE DX										
A. Not Operated										
0–19 Years	3	4.3	17	1	1	3	9	9	9	9
20–34	9	8.9	280	2	2	3	4	53	53	53
35–49	21	3.4	10	1	1	2	4	8	8	13
50–64	42	3.4	7	1	1	3	5	7	7	11
65+	113	3.0	5	1	1	2	4	6	7	11
B. Operated										
0–19 Years	8	4.1	6	2	2	4	8	9	9	9
20–34	32	7.0	71	2	2	5	8	18	24	39
35–49	90	5.6	43	1	1	3	6	14	19	44
50–64	346	5.4	45	1	2	3	6	11	17	37
65+	830	4.6	24	1	2	3	6	9	14	26
SUBTOTALS:										
1. SINGLE DX										
A. Not Operated	5	2.6	4	1	1	2	3	6	6	6
B. Operated	35	2.4	5	1	1	2	3	4	5	13
2. MULTIPLE DX										
A. Not Operated	188	3.4	19	1	1	2	4	7	8	13
B. Operated	1,306	5.0	32	1	2	3	6	10	16	30
1. SINGLE DX	40	2.5	5	1	1	2	3	5	5	13
2. MULTIPLE DX	1,494	4.8	31	1	2	3	6	9	15	30
A. NOT OPERATED	193	3.4	19	1	1	2	4	7	8	13
B. OPERATED	1,341	4.9	32	1	2	3	6	10	15	30
TOTAL										
0–19 Years	12	4.1	7	2	2	3	4	9	9	9
20–34	48	6.8	98	1	2	4	6	18	24	53
35–49	118	5.2	36	1	2	3	6	12	18	29
50–64	401	5.1	41	1	2	3	6	10	16	30
65+	955	4.4	22	1	2	3	6	9	13	24
GRAND TOTAL	1,534	4.7	30	1	2	3	6	9	15	30

442.2: ILIAC ARTERY ANEURYSM

Type of Patients	Observed Patients	Avg. Stay	Vari-ance	Percentiles						
				10th	25th	50th	75th	90th	95th	99th
1. SINGLE DX										
A. Not Operated										
0–19 Years	0									
20–34	0									
35–49	0									
50–64	0									
65+	0									
B. Operated										
0–19 Years	0									
20–34	0									
35–49	0									
50–64	4	1.5	<1	1	1	1	2	2	2	2
65+	7	1.6	1	1	1	1	2	4	4	4
2. MULTIPLE DX										
A. Not Operated										
0–19 Years	0									
20–34	0									
35–49	1	2.0	0	2	2	2	2	2	2	2
50–64	3	3.3	10	1	1	2	7	7	7	7
65+	22	3.0	5	1	1	3	4	7	7	8
B. Operated										
0–19 Years	0									
20–34	1	6.0	0	6	6	6	6	6	6	6
35–49	11	7.9	83	6	6	6	10	21	29	29
50–64	68	4.6	42	1	1	3	5	9	13	37
65+	252	4.4	36	1	1	2	6	9	14	30
SUBTOTALS:										
1. SINGLE DX										
A. Not Operated	0									
B. Operated	11	1.5	<1	1	1	1	2	2	2	4
2. MULTIPLE DX										
A. Not Operated	26	3.0	5	1	1	2	4	7	7	8
B. Operated	332	4.6	38	1	2	2	6	9	17	30
1. SINGLE DX	11	1.5	<1	1	1	1	2	2	2	4
2. MULTIPLE DX	358	4.5	36	1	2	2	6	9	15	30
A. NOT OPERATED	26	3.0	5	1	1	2	4	7	7	8
B. OPERATED	343	4.5	37	1	2	2	6	9	15	30
TOTAL										
0–19 Years	0									
20–34	1	6.0	0	6	6	6	6	6	6	6
35–49	12	7.4	78	1	2	4	10	21	29	29
50–64	75	4.4	39	1	1	2	5	7	13	37
65+	281	4.2	33	1	1	2	5	9	14	30
GRAND TOTAL	369	4.4	35	1	1	2	5	9	14	30

442.3: LOWER EXTREMITY ANEURYSM

Type of Patients	Observed Patients	Avg. Stay	Vari-ance	Percentiles						
				10th	25th	50th	75th	90th	95th	99th
1. SINGLE DX										
A. Not Operated										
0–19 Years	0									
20–34	0									
35–49	0									
50–64	1	3.0	0	3	3	3	3	3	3	3
65+	1	1.0	0	1	1	1	1	1	1	1
B. Operated										
0–19 Years	0									
20–34	2	4.5	<1	4	4	5	5	5	5	5
35–49	2	7.6	60	2	2	13	13	13	13	13
50–64	4	2.8	<1	2	2	3	3	4	4	4
65+	1	2.0	0	2	2	2	2	2	2	2
2. MULTIPLE DX										
A. Not Operated										
0–19 Years	0									
20–34	4	3.5	4	2	2	4	6	6	6	6
35–49	7	3.7	18	1	1	2	4	13	13	13
50–64	16	3.1	8	1	1	2	4	7	11	11
65+	56	2.4	4	1	1	2	3	5	6	11
B. Operated										
0–19 Years	0									
20–34	13	5.0	2	4	4	5	5	6	6	6
35–49	27	10.9	137	1	3	5	18	24	39	39
50–64	165	5.1	17	1	2	4	8	9	12	19
65+	456	4.3	13	1	2	3	5	8	11	19
SUBTOTALS:										
1. SINGLE DX										
A. Not Operated	2	2.0	2	1	1	1	3	3	3	3
B. Operated	9	4.1	12	2	2	3	4	13	13	13
2. MULTIPLE DX										
A. Not Operated	83	2.7	6	1	1	2	3	6	7	13
B. Operated	663	4.7	24	1	2	3	6	9	14	28
1. SINGLE DX	11	3.7	11	2	2	3	4	5	13	13
2. MULTIPLE DX	746	4.5	22	1	2	3	5	9	12	25
A. NOT OPERATED	85	2.7	5	1	1	2	3	6	7	13
B. OPERATED	672	4.7	24	1	2	3	5	9	14	28
TOTAL										
0–19 Years	2	5.0	2	4	4	5	6	6	6	6
20–34	19	8.7	103	1	2	5	10	24	39	39
35–49	36	5.0	18	1	2	4	8	12	13	19
50–64	186	5.0	39	1	2	3	5	10	17	44
65+	514	4.1	13	1	2	3	5	8	10	18
GRAND TOTAL	757	4.5	22	1	2	3	5	9	12	25

Length of Stay by Diagnosis and Operation, Western Region, 2008

Western Region, October 2006–September 2007 Data, by Diagnosis

443: OTH PERIPH VASC DISEASE

Type of Patients	Observed Patients	Avg. Stay	Variance	10th	25th	50th	75th	90th	95th	99th
1. SINGLE DX										
A. *Not Operated*										
0–19 Years	0									
20–34	4	3.0	5	1	1	3	6	6	6	6
35–49	5	2.0	2	1	1	1	3	4	4	4
50–64	6	1.3	<1	1	1	1	2	2	2	2
65+	1	1.0	0	1	1	1	1	1	1	1
B. *Operated*										
0–19 Years	0									
20–34	1	4.0	0	4	4	4	4	4	4	4
35–49	2	1.0	0	1	1	1	1	1	1	1
50–64	9	1.4	<1	1	1	1	1	3	3	3
65+	18	1.5	<1	1	1	1	2	3	4	4
2. MULTIPLE DX										
A. *Not Operated*										
0–19 Years	5	2.0	1	1	1	2	3	3	3	3
20–34	56	5.2	40	1	2	4	7	9	12	46
35–49	139	3.8	7	1	2	3	5	8	9	11
50–64	200	3.6	6	1	2	3	5	7	9	12
65+	393	4.0	12	1	3	3	5	8	11	16
B. *Operated*										
0–19 Years	3	8.3	2	7	7	8	10	10	10	10
20–34	7	10.7	561	7	1	2	4	65	65	65
35–49	78	5.7	27	1	2	4	8	11	16	29
50–64	355	5.3	40	1	1	3	6	12	17	37
65+	870	4.8	24	1	1	3	7	11	15	25
SUBTOTALS:										
1. SINGLE DX										
A. *Not Operated*	16	1.9	2	1	1	1	3	4	6	6
B. *Operated*	30	1.5	<1	1	1	1	2	3	4	4
2. MULTIPLE DX										
A. *Not Operated*	793	3.9	11	1	2	3	5	8	10	15
B. *Operated*	1,313	5.0	31	1	1	3	7	12	15	26
1. SINGLE DX	46	1.7	1	1	1	1	2	3	4	6
2. MULTIPLE DX	2,106	4.6	24	1	1	3	6	10	13	23
A. NOT OPERATED	809	3.9	11	1	2	3	5	8	10	15
B. OPERATED	1,343	4.9	31	1	1	3	7	11	15	26
TOTAL										
0–19 Years	8	4.4	12	1	2	3	8	10	10	10
20–34	68	5.6	87	1	2	3	6	9	12	65
35–49	224	4.4	14	1	2	3	6	9	11	18
50–64	570	4.6	28	1	1	3	6	9	14	25
65+	1,282	4.5	20	1	1	3	6	10	14	22
GRAND TOTAL	2,152	4.5	24	1	1	3	6	10	13	23

443.89: PERIPH VASCULAR DIS NEC

Type of Patients	Observed Patients	Avg. Stay	Variance	10th	25th	50th	75th	90th	95th	99th
1. SINGLE DX										
A. *Not Operated*										
0–19 Years	0									
20–34	0									
35–49	0									
50–64	0									
65+	0									
B. *Operated*										
0–19 Years	0									
20–34	0									
35–49	0									
50–64	1	3.0	0	3	3	3	3	3	3	3
65+	2	1.0	0	1	1	1	1	1	1	1
2. MULTIPLE DX										
A. *Not Operated*										
0–19 Years	1	3.0	0	3	3	3	3	3	3	3
20–34	4	2.5	2	1	2	3	4	4	4	4
35–49	12	3.1	3	1	2	3	5	6	6	6
50–64	29	3.6	6	1	2	3	5	7	7	12
65+	82	4.7	14	1	2	4	6	9	11	22
B. *Operated*										
0–19 Years	0									
20–34	0									
35–49	9	3.2	4	1	2	2	4	7	7	7
50–64	68	7.2	96	1	1	4	7	16	29	50
65+	179	5.8	28	1	2	4	8	14	16	26
SUBTOTALS:										
1. SINGLE DX										
A. *Not Operated*	0									
B. *Operated*	3	1.7	1	1	1	1	3	3	3	3
2. MULTIPLE DX										
A. *Not Operated*	128	4.2	11	1	2	3	5	8	11	16
B. *Operated*	256	6.1	46	1	2	4	7	14	17	37
1. SINGLE DX	3	1.7	1	1	1	1	3	3	3	3
2. MULTIPLE DX	384	5.5	35	1	2	4	7	12	16	35
A. NOT OPERATED	128	4.2	11	1	2	3	5	8	11	16
B. OPERATED	259	6.0	46	1	2	4	7	14	17	37
TOTAL										
0–19 Years	1	3.0	0	3	3	3	3	3	3	3
20–34	4	2.5	2	1	2	3	4	4	4	4
35–49	21	3.2	3	1	2	2	4	6	6	7
50–64	98	6.1	71	1	2	3	6	15	25	50
65+	263	5.4	24	1	2	4	7	12	15	23
GRAND TOTAL	387	5.4	35	1	2	4	7	12	16	35

443.9: PERIPH VASCULAR DIS NOS

Type of Patients	Observed Patients	Avg. Stay	Variance	10th	25th	50th	75th	90th	95th	99th
1. SINGLE DX										
A. *Not Operated*										
0–19 Years	0									
20–34	0									
35–49	1	1.0	0	1	1	1	1	1	1	1
50–64	3	1.0	0	1	1	1	1	1	1	1
65+	1	1.0	0	1	1	1	1	1	1	1
B. *Operated*										
0–19 Years	0									
20–34	0									
35–49	2	1.0	0	1	1	1	1	1	1	1
50–64	7	1.3	<1	1	1	1	1	1	3	3
65+	16	1.6	<1	1	1	1	2	3	4	4
2. MULTIPLE DX										
A. *Not Operated*										
0–19 Years	1	1.0	0	1	1	1	1	1	1	1
20–34	5	2.8	6	1	2	2	2	7	7	7
35–49	31	3.0	5	1	1	2	4	6	8	10
50–64	93	3.3	7	1	2	3	4	6	8	15
65+	263	3.7	11	1	1	3	5	8	10	15
B. *Operated*										
0–19 Years	0									
20–34	0									
35–49	37	5.4	25	1	1	5	8	11	18	22
50–64	259	4.6	25	1	1	3	6	10	15	23
65+	667	4.5	23	1	1	3	6	11	14	25
SUBTOTALS:										
1. SINGLE DX										
A. *Not Operated*	5	1.0	0	1	1	1	1	1	1	1
B. *Operated*	25	1.4	<1	1	1	1	2	3	3	4
2. MULTIPLE DX										
A. *Not Operated*	393	3.5	9	1	1	3	4	7	10	15
B. *Operated*	963	4.6	24	1	1	3	6	11	14	23
1. SINGLE DX	30	1.4	<1	1	1	1	1	2	3	4
2. MULTIPLE DX	1,356	4.3	20	1	1	3	6	10	13	22
A. NOT OPERATED	398	3.5	9	1	1	3	4	7	10	15
B. OPERATED	988	4.5	23	1	1	3	6	11	14	23
TOTAL										
0–19 Years	1	1.0	0	1	1	1	1	1	1	1
20–34	5	2.8	6	1	2	2	2	7	7	7
35–49	71	4.2	17	1	1	3	6	10	11	22
50–64	362	4.2	20	1	1	3	5	9	12	22
65+	947	4.3	20	1	1	3	6	10	13	22
GRAND TOTAL	1,386	4.2	20	1	1	3	5	10	13	22

Length of Stay by Diagnosis and Operation, Western Region, 2008

Western Region, October 2006–September 2007 Data, by Diagnosis

444: ARTERIAL EMBOLISM

Type of Patients	Observed Patients	Avg. Stay	Variance	10th	25th	50th	75th	90th	95th	99th
1. SINGLE DX										
A. Not Operated										
0–19 Years	0									
20–34	2	1.5	<1	1	1	2	2	2	2	2
35–49	3	1.3	<1	1	2	1	2	2	2	2
50–64	3	2.7	1	2	2	2	4	4	4	4
65+	4	1.8	<1	1	1	2	3	3	3	3
B. Operated										
0–19 Years	0									
20–34	5	4.2	3	3	3	3	5	7	7	7
35–49	5	4.0	17	1	1	3	4	11	11	11
50–64	11	2.7	7	1	1	2	3	4	10	10
65+	10	1.7	2	1	1	1	2	5	5	5
2. MULTIPLE DX										
A. Not Operated										
0–19 Years	6	4.2	20	1	2	2	4	13	13	13
20–34	32	4.7	13	1	2	4	7	8	10	19
35–49	93	4.2	9	1	2	4	6	8	10	17
50–64	198	5.0	19	1	2	3	6	10	12	23
65+	576	5.0	15	1	2	4	7	9	12	18
B. Operated										
0–19 Years	0	2.0	0	2	2	2	2	2	2	2
20–34	36	9.3	54	2	4	7	15	22	25	28
35–49	243	8.6	58	2	4	6	11	18	23	37
50–64	895	6.8	64	1	2	5	8	14	19	41
65+	1,913	6.3	36	1	3	5	8	13	16	28
SUBTOTALS:										
1. SINGLE DX										
A. Not Operated	12	1.8	<1	1	1	2	2	3	4	4
B. Operated	31	2.8	6	1	1	2	3	5	10	11
2. MULTIPLE DX										
A. Not Operated	905	4.9	15	1	2	4	6	9	12	18
B. Operated	3,088	6.6	46	1	3	5	8	14	19	34
1. SINGLE DX	43	2.6	5	1	1	2	3	5	7	11
2. MULTIPLE DX	3,993	6.2	40	1	3	5	8	13	17	32
A. NOT OPERATED	917	4.8	15	1	2	4	6	9	12	18
B. OPERATED	3,119	6.6	46	1	3	5	8	14	19	34
TOTAL										
0–19 Years	7	3.9	17	1	2	2	4	13	13	13
20–34	75	6.8	37	1	3	4	8	16	22	28
35–49	344	7.3	48	1	3	5	9	15	21	36
50–64	1,107	6.4	56	1	2	4	7	13	19	41
65+	2,503	6.0	31	1	2	5	8	12	15	28
GRAND TOTAL	4,036	6.2	40	1	2	5	8	12	17	32

444.0: ABD AORTIC EMBOLISM

Type of Patients	Observed Patients	Avg. Stay	Variance	10th	25th	50th	75th	90th	95th	99th
1. SINGLE DX										
A. Not Operated										
0–19 Years	0									
20–34	0									
35–49	1	2.0	0	2	2	2	2	2	2	2
50–64	0									
65+	0									
B. Operated										
0–19 Years	0									
20–34	0									
35–49	0									
50–64	0									
65+	0									
2. MULTIPLE DX										
A. Not Operated										
0–19 Years	0									
20–34	0									
35–49	4	5.7	8	4	4	4	5	10	10	10
50–64	21	3.9	6	1	2	3	5	7	8	10
65+	19	6.6	32	2	2	5	9	18	20	20
B. Operated										
0–19 Years	0									
20–34	1	16.0	0	16	16	16	16	16	16	16
35–49	31	9.4	76	4	4	6	11	22	33	37
50–64	156	8.8	77	4	5	6	15	22	24	46
65+	138	8.5	60	2	5	7	10	14	19	48
SUBTOTALS:										
1. SINGLE DX										
A. Not Operated	1	2.0	0	2	2	2	2	2	2	2
B. Operated	0									
2. MULTIPLE DX										
A. Not Operated	44	5.2	19	2	2	4	6	10	14	20
B. Operated	326	8.7	69	3	5	6	10	15	23	47
1. SINGLE DX	1	2.0	0	2	2	2	2	2	2	2
2. MULTIPLE DX	370	8.3	64	2	4	6	9	15	22	47
A. NOT OPERATED	45	5.2	19	2	2	4	6	10	14	20
B. OPERATED	326	8.7	69	3	5	6	10	15	23	47
TOTAL										
0–19 Years	0									
20–34	1	16.0	0	16	16	16	16	16	16	16
35–49	36	8.8	69	2	4	6	10	22	33	37
50–64	177	8.2	71	3	5	6	9	15	23	46
65+	157	8.2	57	2	4	7	10	14	19	48
GRAND TOTAL	371	8.3	64	2	4	6	9	15	22	47

444.21: UPPER EXTREMITY EMBOLISM

Type of Patients	Observed Patients	Avg. Stay	Variance	10th	25th	50th	75th	90th	95th	99th
1. SINGLE DX										
A. Not Operated										
0–19 Years	0									
20–34	0									
35–49	0									
50–64	3	2.7	1	2	2	2	4	4	4	4
65+	1	2.0	0	2	2	2	2	2	2	2
B. Operated										
0–19 Years	0									
20–34	0									
35–49	0									
50–64	2	3.0	0	3	3	3	3	3	3	3
65+	2	6.0	32	2	2	2	10	10	10	10
2. MULTIPLE DX										
A. Not Operated										
0–19 Years	2	2.0	2	1	1	1	3	3	3	3
20–34	8	4.8	5	1	1	4	7	8	8	8
35–49	29	4.8	12	1	2	4	6	9	13	16
50–64	42	5.5	33	1	2	4	7	10	10	37
65+	107	4.7	19	1	2	3	6	8	10	22
B. Operated										
0–19 Years	0									
20–34	6	6.8	48	1	2	4	13	18	18	18
35–49	25	6.8	21	2	4	7	8	12	17	19
50–64	73	5.2	23	1	2	4	7	11	13	29
65+	216	4.8	14	2	2	4	6	9	13	18
SUBTOTALS:										
1. SINGLE DX										
A. Not Operated	4	2.5	1	2	2	2	4	4	4	4
B. Operated	4	4.5	14	2	2	3	3	10	10	10
2. MULTIPLE DX										
A. Not Operated	188	4.9	20	1	3	4	7	8	10	34
B. Operated	320	5.1	17	1	2	4	7	10	13	19
1. SINGLE DX	8	3.5	7	2	2	2	3	10	10	10
2. MULTIPLE DX	508	5.0	18	1	2	4	7	9	12	21
A. NOT OPERATED	192	4.8	20	1	2	4	6	8	10	34
B. OPERATED	324	5.1	17	1	2	4	7	10	13	19
TOTAL										
0–19 Years	2	2.0	2	1	1	1	3	3	3	3
20–34	16	5.3	20	1	3	4	7	13	18	18
35–49	54	5.7	17	1	3	5	8	11	16	19
50–64	120	5.3	26	1	2	4	7	10	12	29
65+	324	4.8	15	1	2	4	6	8	10	21
GRAND TOTAL	516	5.0	18	1	2	4	7	9	12	21

Length of Stay by Diagnosis and Operation, Western Region, 2008

444.22: LOWER EXTREMITY EMBOLISM

Type of Patients	Observed Patients	Avg. Stay	Variance	10th	25th	50th	75th	90th	95th	99th
1. SINGLE DX										
A. Not Operated										
0–19 Years	0									
20–34	0									
35–49	2	1.0	0		1	1	1	1	1	1
50–64	0									
65+	2	2.0	2	1	1	3	3	3	3	3
B. Operated										
0–19 Years	0									
20–34	2	4.0	2	3	3	3	5	5	5	5
35–49	4	4.8	19	1	1	4	11	11	11	11
50–64	6	2.0	2	1	1	1	3	4	4	4
65+	9	1.8	2	1	1	1	2	5	5	5
2. MULTIPLE DX										
A. Not Operated										
0–19 Years	2	7.5	60	2	2	13	13	13	13	13
20–34	13	5.9	24	1	2	5	8	10	19	19
35–49	36	4.2	10	1	2	4	6	7	10	17
50–64	98	4.8	18	1	2	3	5	9	14	23
65+	357	5.2	13	1	2	4	7	10	12	16
B. Operated										
0–19 Years	1	2.0	0	2	2	2	2	2	2	2
20–34	17	9.0	38	3	4	7	12	16	25	25
35–49	143	8.9	52	2	4	7	12	19	23	34
50–64	512	6.5	52	1	2	4	7	14	19	41
65+	1,289	6.4	38	1	3	5	8	13	17	29
SUBTOTALS:										
1. SINGLE DX										
A. Not Operated	4	1.5	1	1	1	1	1	3	3	3
B. Operated	21	2.6	6	1	1	2	3	5	5	11
2. MULTIPLE DX										
A. Not Operated	506	5.0	14	1	2	4	7	10	12	18
B. Operated	1,962	6.6	43	1	3	5	8	14	19	32
1. SINGLE DX	25	2.4	5	1	1	2	3	5	5	11
2. MULTIPLE DX	2,468	6.3	37	1	3	5	8	13	17	30
A. NOT OPERATED	510	5.0	14	1	2	4	7	10	12	18
B. OPERATED	1,983	6.6	43	1	3	5	8	14	19	32
TOTAL										
0–19 Years	3	5.7	40	2	2	2	13	13	13	13
20–34	32	7.4	32	2	4	6	8	16	19	25
35–49	185	7.8	46	1	3	6	10	17	22	34
50–64	616	6.1	47	1	2	4	7	13	16	38
65+	1,657	6.1	32	1	2	5	8	12	16	28
GRAND TOTAL	2,493	6.3	37	1	2	5	8	13	17	30

444.81: ILIAC ARTERY EMBOLISM

Type of Patients	Observed Patients	Avg. Stay	Variance	10th	25th	50th	75th	90th	95th	99th
1. SINGLE DX										
A. Not Operated										
0–19 Years	0									
20–34	0									
35–49	0									
50–64	0									
65+	1	1.0	0	1	1	1	1	1	1	1
B. Operated										
0–19 Years	0									
20–34	0									
35–49	0									
50–64	3	2.0	<1	1	1	2	3	3	3	3
65+	1	1.0	0	1	1	1	1	1	1	1
2. MULTIPLE DX										
A. Not Operated										
0–19 Years	0									
20–34	2	3.5	<1	3	3	3	4	4	4	4
35–49	6	3.3	2	2	2	3	4	6	6	6
50–64	11	5.7	27	1	1	5	10	10	18	18
65+	29	3.9	14	1	1	2	6	9	9	16
B. Operated										
0–19 Years	0									
20–34	4	9.1	79	2	5	7	22	22	22	22
35–49	38	7.4	66	1	3	5	9	17	32	40
50–64	135	6.3	112	1	2	3	6	11	22	67
65+	227	5.7	26	1	2	5	8	12	15	25
SUBTOTALS:										
1. SINGLE DX										
A. Not Operated	1	1.0	0	1	1	1	1	1	1	1
B. Operated	4	1.8	<1	1	1	2	2	3	3	3
2. MULTIPLE DX										
A. Not Operated	48	4.2	15	1	1	3	6	9	10	18
B. Operated	404	6.1	59	1	2	4	7	12	16	35
1. SINGLE DX	5	1.6	<1	1	1	1	2	3	3	3
2. MULTIPLE DX	452	5.9	54	1	2	4	7	11	16	35
A. NOT OPERATED	49	4.1	15	1	1	3	6	9	10	18
B. OPERATED	408	6.1	58	1	2	4	7	12	16	35
TOTAL										
0–19 Years	0									
20–34	6	7.2	56	2	3	5	7	22	22	22
35–49	44	6.8	59	2	3	4	9	13	18	40
50–64	149	6.1	103	1	2	3	6	11	18	67
65+	258	5.5	25	1	2	4	7	11	15	25
GRAND TOTAL	457	5.9	54	1	2	4	7	11	16	35

445: ATHEROEMBOLISM

Type of Patients	Observed Patients	Avg. Stay	Variance	10th	25th	50th	75th	90th	95th	99th
1. SINGLE DX										
A. Not Operated										
0–19 Years	0									
20–34	0									
35–49	0									
50–64	0									
65+	1	1.0	0	1	1	1	1	1	1	1
B. Operated										
0–19 Years	0									
20–34	0									
35–49	0									
50–64	0									
65+	0									
2. MULTIPLE DX										
A. Not Operated										
0–19 Years	0									
20–34	5	4.0	2	2	3	4	5	6	6	6
35–49	6	4.3	3	2	3	4	6	6	6	6
50–64	20	4.8	18	1	2	3	6	10	10	18
65+	39	5.6	23	1	2	4	7	10	16	26
B. Operated										
0–19 Years	0									
20–34	0									
35–49	9	4.7	8	2	2	4	6	10	10	10
50–64	18	5.9	27	1	1	5	8	16	18	18
65+	42	6.3	19	2	3	5	8	12	14	20
SUBTOTALS:										
1. SINGLE DX										
A. Not Operated	1	1.0	0	1	1	1	1	1	1	1
B. Operated	0									
2. MULTIPLE DX										
A. Not Operated	70	5.1	19	1	2	4	6	10	14	26
B. Operated	69	6.0	19	1	2	5	8	12	16	20
1. SINGLE DX	1	1.0	0	1	1	1	1	1	1	1
2. MULTIPLE DX	139	5.5	19	1	2	5	8	11	16	20
A. NOT OPERATED	71	5.1	18	1	2	4	6	9	14	26
B. OPERATED	69	6.0	19	1	2	5	8	12	16	20
TOTAL										
0–19 Years	0									
20–34	5	4.0	2	2	3	4	5	6	6	6
35–49	15	4.5	6	2	3	4	6	8	10	10
50–64	38	5.3	22	1	1	4	8	12	18	18
65+	82	5.9	21	2	2	5	8	11	14	26
GRAND TOTAL	140	5.5	19	1	2	5	8	10	14	20

Length of Stay by Diagnosis and Operation, Western Region, 2008

Western Region, October 2006–September 2007 Data, by Diagnosis

446: POLYARTERIT NODOSA ET AL

Type of Patients	Observed Patients	Avg. Stay	Vari-ance	10th	25th	50th	75th	90th	95th	99th
1. SINGLE DX										
A. Not Operated										
0–19 Years	176	2.3	2	1	1	2	3	4	5	9
20–34	3	3.7	6	1	1	4	6	6	6	6
35–49	2	1.0	0	1	1	1	1	1	1	1
50–64	3	4.7	40	1	1	1	12	12	12	12
65+	1	1.0	0	1	1	1	1	1	1	1
B. Operated										
0–19 Years	0									
20–34	1	1.0	0	1	1	1	1	1	1	1
35–49	0									
50–64	1	4.0	0	4	4	4	4	4	4	4
65+	1	5.0	0	5	5	5	5	5	5	5
2. MULTIPLE DX										
A. Not Operated										
0–19 Years	327	3.9	14	1	2	3	4	7	9	23
20–34	110	9.0	121	2	3	6	10	19	27	56
35–49	125	9.0	86	2	3	6	11	20	26	49
50–64	236	8.2	72	2	3	6	10	16	24	41
65+	299	7.3	63	1	2	5	9	16	22	42
B. Operated										
0–19 Years	6	13.1	114	1	4	11	25	27	27	27
20–34	18	8.5	36	2	4	8	9	20	23	23
35–49	16	15.2	492	2	6	8	15	43	90	90
50–64	82	9.7	93	2	3	6	12	27	27	49
65+	155	5.9	27	2	3	4	7	11	17	29
SUBTOTALS:										
1. SINGLE DX										
A. Not Operated	185	2.3	2	1	1	2	3	4	5	10
B. Operated	3	3.3	4	1	1	4	5	5	5	5
2. MULTIPLE DX										
A. Not Operated	1,097	6.9	62	1	2	4	8	15	21	36
B. Operated	277	7.9	80	2	3	5	9	17	26	44
1. SINGLE DX	188	2.4	2	1	1	2	3	4	5	10
2. MULTIPLE DX	1,374	7.1	66	2	3	4	8	15	22	42
A. NOT OPERATED	1,282	6.2	56	1	2	4	7	14	19	34
B. OPERATED	280	7.8	79	2	3	5	9	17	26	44
TOTAL										
0–19 Years	509	3.5	12	1	2	3	4	6	8	23
20–34	132	8.8	106	2	3	6	10	19	27	56
35–49	143	9.6	132	2	3	6	12	20	27	56
50–64	322	8.5	77	2	3	6	11	18	26	44
65+	456	6.8	51	2	3	4	8	15	19	34
GRAND TOTAL	1,562	6.5	61	1	2	4	8	14	20	39

446.1: MUCOCUTAN LN SYNDROME

Type of Patients	Observed Patients	Avg. Stay	Vari-ance	10th	25th	50th	75th	90th	95th	99th
1. SINGLE DX										
A. Not Operated										
0–19 Years	173	2.3	2	1	1	2	3	4	5	9
20–34	0									
35–49	0									
50–64	0									
65+	0									
B. Operated										
0–19 Years	0									
20–34	0									
35–49	0									
50–64	0									
65+	0									
2. MULTIPLE DX										
A. Not Operated										
0–19 Years	297	3.4	4	1	2	3	4	6	8	10
20–34	0									
35–49	1	11.0	0	11	11	11	11	11	11	11
50–64	0									
65+	0									
B. Operated										
0–19 Years	0									
20–34	0									
35–49	0									
50–64	0									
65+	0									
SUBTOTALS:										
1. SINGLE DX										
A. Not Operated	174	2.3	2	1	1	2	3	4	5	9
B. Operated	0									
2. MULTIPLE DX										
A. Not Operated	298	3.4	4	1	2	3	4	6	8	11
B. Operated	0									
1. SINGLE DX	174	2.3	2	1	1	2	3	4	5	9
2. MULTIPLE DX	298	3.4	4	1	2	3	4	6	8	11
A. NOT OPERATED	472	3.0	4	1	2	3	4	5	7	10
B. OPERATED	0									
TOTAL										
0–19 Years	470	3.0	4	1	2	3	4	5	7	10
20–34	0									
35–49	2	6.0	49	1	1	11	11	11	11	11
50–64	0									
65+	0									
GRAND TOTAL	472	3.0	4	1	2	3	4	5	7	10

446.4: WEGENER'S GRANULOMATOSIS

Type of Patients	Observed Patients	Avg. Stay	Vari-ance	10th	25th	50th	75th	90th	95th	99th
1. SINGLE DX										
A. Not Operated										
0–19 Years	0									
20–34	0									
35–49	0									
50–64	2	1.0	0	1	1	1	1	1	1	1
65+	0									
B. Operated										
0–19 Years	0									
20–34	0									
35–49	0									
50–64	1	1.0	0	1	1	1	1	1	1	1
65+	1	4.0	0	4	4	4	4	4	4	4
2. MULTIPLE DX										
A. Not Operated										
0–19 Years	11	6.6	77	1	1	3	7	23	25	25
20–34	22	7.2	42	2	3	4	10	15	20	27
35–49	25	6.8	23	2	3	6	8	11	18	21
50–64	37	7.6	51	2	3	6	9	19	26	27
65+	43	11.6	68	3	6	9	15	19	28	42
B. Operated										
0–19 Years	4	6.8	25	1	4	11	11	11	11	11
20–34	8	6.4	9	2	3	8	8	10	10	10
35–49	4	8.2	28	1	1	10	13	13	13	13
50–64	30	12.2	147	2	3	8	16	27	44	49
65+	8	8.5	25	3	6	7	14	17	17	17
SUBTOTALS:										
1. SINGLE DX										
A. Not Operated	2	1.0	0	1	1	1	1	1	1	1
B. Operated	2	2.5	5	1	1	3	4	4	4	4
2. MULTIPLE DX										
A. Not Operated	138	8.6	55	2	3	6	12	19	26	29
B. Operated	54	10.1	94	2	3	8	11	19	27	49
1. SINGLE DX	4	1.8	2	1	1	1	3	4	4	4
2. MULTIPLE DX	192	9.0	66	2	3	7	11	19	27	44
A. NOT OPERATED	140	8.4	55	1	3	6	11	19	26	29
B. OPERATED	56	9.8	93	1	3	8	11	19	27	49
TOTAL										
0–19 Years	15	6.7	61	1	1	4	11	23	25	25
20–34	31	6.8	33	2	3	5	8	12	20	27
35–49	29	7.0	23	1	3	6	9	13	18	21
50–64	70	9.3	96	3	3	6	11	24	27	49
65+	51	11.1	62	3	6	9	14	19	28	42
GRAND TOTAL	196	8.8	65	1	3	6	11	19	27	44

446.5: GIANT CELL ARTERITIS

Type of Patients	Observed Patients	Avg. Stay	Vari-ance	10th	25th	50th	75th	90th	95th	99th
1. SINGLE DX										
A. Not Operated										
0–19 Years	0									
20–34	0									
35–49	1	1.0	0	1	1	1	1	1	1	1
50–64	0									
65+	0									
B. Operated										
0–19 Years	0									
20–34	0									
35–49	0									
50–64	0									
65+	1	5.0	0	5	5	5	5	5	5	5
2. MULTIPLE DX										
A. Not Operated										
0–19 Years	0									
20–34	0									
35–49	5	6.0	23	2	2	4	9	13	13	13
50–64	34	4.4	18	2	2	3	5	9	12	23
65+	121	3.5	8	1	2	3	4	6	9	16
B. Operated										
0–19 Years	0									
20–34	0									
35–49	2	4.5	4	3	3	6	6	6	6	6
50–64	34	5.7	21	2	2	4	7	12	17	20
65+	135	5.1	15	2	3	4	6	10	11	25
SUBTOTALS:										
1. SINGLE DX										
A. Not Operated	1	1.0	0	1	1	1	1	1	1	1
B. Operated	1	5.0	0	5	5	5	5	5	5	5
2. MULTIPLE DX										
A. Not Operated	160	3.8	11	1	2	3	4	7	10	21
B. Operated	171	5.2	16	2	3	4	6	10	12	25
1. SINGLE DX	2	3.0	8	1	1	5	5	5	5	5
2. MULTIPLE DX	331	4.5	14	2	2	3	5	9	11	21
A. NOT OPERATED	161	3.8	11	1	2	3	4	7	10	21
B. OPERATED	172	5.2	16	2	3	4	6	10	12	25
TOTAL										
0–19 Years	0									
20–34	0									
35–49	8	5.0	17	2	2	4	9	13	13	13
50–64	68	5.0	20	2	2	3	5	12	15	23
65+	257	4.4	12	1	2	3	5	8	10	21
GRAND TOTAL	333	4.5	14	2	2	3	5	9	11	21

446.6: THROMB MICROANGIOPATHY

Type of Patients	Observed Patients	Avg. Stay	Vari-ance	10th	25th	50th	75th	90th	95th	99th
1. SINGLE DX										
A. Not Operated										
0–19 Years	3	1.0	0	1	1	1	1	1	1	1
20–34	2	5.0	2	4	4	5	6	6	6	6
35–49	0									
50–64	1	12.0	0	12	12	12	12	12	12	12
65+	0									
B. Operated										
0–19 Years	0									
20–34	0									
35–49	0									
50–64	0									
65+	0									
2. MULTIPLE DX										
A. Not Operated										
0–19 Years	9	13.8	85	2	6	13	19	32	32	32
20–34	43	10.2	91	4	6	7	10	22	27	56
35–49	43	13.7	140	4	5	11	19	27	32	56
50–64	56	12.5	148	3	6	9	15	28	32	77
65+	21	16.2	156	5	8	13	21	29	34	54
B. Operated										
0–19 Years	1	27.0	0	27	27	27	27	27	27	27
20–34	2	4.0	0	4	4	4	4	4	4	4
35–49	3	19.2	433	6	6	8	43	43	43	43
50–64	4	21.8	248	2	2	28	39	39	39	39
65+	1	3.0	0	3	3	3	3	3	3	3
SUBTOTALS:										
1. SINGLE DX										
A. Not Operated	6	4.2	19	1	1	4	6	12	12	12
B. Operated	0									
2. MULTIPLE DX										
A. Not Operated	172	12.8	130	3	6	9	16	27	32	56
B. Operated	11	16.6	236	3	4	8	28	39	43	43
1. SINGLE DX	6	4.2	19	1	1	4	6	12	12	12
2. MULTIPLE DX	183	13.0	136	3	6	9	17	28	32	56
A. NOT OPERATED	178	12.5	129	3	6	9	16	27	32	56
B. OPERATED	11	16.6	236	3	4	8	28	39	43	43
TOTAL										
0–19 Years	13	11.9	108	2	4	13	19	27	32	32
20–34	47	9.7	85	4	5	7	10	22	27	56
35–49	46	14.1	152	4	5	9	19	29	43	56
50–64	61	13.1	154	3	6	9	16	28	32	77
65+	22	15.6	156	3	8	13	21	29	34	54
GRAND TOTAL	189	12.7	134	3	5	9	16	28	32	56

447: OTHER ARTERIAL DISEASE

Type of Patients	Observed Patients	Avg. Stay	Vari-ance	10th	25th	50th	75th	90th	95th	99th
1. SINGLE DX										
A. Not Operated										
0–19 Years	3	1.7	<1	1	1	2	2	2	2	2
20–34	1	3.0	0	3	3	3	3	3	3	3
35–49	2	1.0	0	1	1	1	1	1	1	1
50–64	1	1.0	0	1	1	1	1	1	1	1
65+	0									
B. Operated										
0–19 Years	0									
20–34	5	1.2	<1	1	1	1	1	2	2	2
35–49	1	1.0	0	1	1	1	1	1	1	1
50–64	5	1.4	<1	1	1	1	1	3	3	3
65+	19	1.6	2	1	1	2	2	3	6	6
2. MULTIPLE DX										
A. Not Operated										
0–19 Years	19	3.9	12	1	2	3	5	12	13	13
20–34	29	4.8	16	1	2	3	7	12	12	15
35–49	73	4.5	19	1	2	3	6	8	11	32
50–64	133	5.4	41	1	2	3	7	12	16	31
65+	179	5.4	30	1	2	4	7	11	16	29
B. Operated										
0–19 Years	7	7.9	45	1	1	8	11	20	20	20
20–34	13	11.0	326	3	3	9	9	19	69	69
35–49	70	4.7	24	1	1	3	6	12	16	24
50–64	339	3.2	20	1	1	1	4	7	11	23
65+	795	3.2	15	1	1	1	4	7	11	21
SUBTOTALS:										
1. SINGLE DX										
A. Not Operated	7	1.6	<1	1	1	1	2	2	3	3
B. Operated	30	1.5	1	1	1	1	2	3	3	6
2. MULTIPLE DX										
A. Not Operated	433	5.1	30	1	2	3	6	11	14	29
B. Operated	1,224	3.4	21	1	1	2	4	8	12	22
1. SINGLE DX	37	1.5	1	1	1	1	2	3	3	6
2. MULTIPLE DX	1,657	3.8	24	1	1	2	5	9	12	23
A. NOT OPERATED	440	5.1	30	1	2	3	6	11	14	29
B. OPERATED	1,254	3.3	20	1	1	2	4	8	12	22
TOTAL										
0–19 Years	29	4.6	21	1	2	3	6	12	13	20
20–34	48	6.1	103	1	2	3	7	12	15	69
35–49	146	4.5	21	1	1	3	6	10	12	24
50–64	478	3.8	27	1	1	2	4	8	13	25
65+	993	3.5	18	1	1	2	4	8	12	23
GRAND TOTAL	1,694	3.8	23	1	1	2	4	9	12	23

Length of Stay by Diagnosis and Operation, Western Region, 2008

Western Region, October 2006–September 2007 Data, by Diagnosis

447.1: ARTERIAL STRICTURE

Type of Patients	Observed Patients	Avg. Stay	Variance	Percentiles						
				10th	25th	50th	75th	90th	95th	99th
1. SINGLE DX										
A. Not Operated										
0–19 Years	1	2.0	0	2	2	2	2	2	2	2
20–34	0									
35–49	0									
50–64	0									
65+	0									
B. Operated										
0–19 Years	0									
20–34	0									
35–49	1	1.0	0	1	1	1	1	1	1	1
50–64	4	1.0	0	1	1	1	1	1	1	1
65+	19	1.6	2	1	1	1	2	3	6	6
2. MULTIPLE DX										
A. Not Operated										
0–19 Years	0									
20–34	3	3.0	4	1	1	3	5	5	5	5
35–49	11	2.6	4	1	1	2	3	4	8	8
50–64	35	3.2	14	1	1	2	3	7	14	19
65+	73	3.1	6	2	2	2	4	7	8	12
B. Operated										
0–19 Years	5	20.0	0	20	20	20	20	20	20	20
20–34	5	5.4	10	3	4	4	5	5	11	11
35–49	40	3.6	13	1	1	2	4	6	10	14
50–64	273	2.7	11	1	1	1	3	8	11	20
65+	710	2.8	11	1	1	1	3	6	10	16
SUBTOTALS:										
1. SINGLE DX										
A. Not Operated	1	2.0	0	2	2	2	2	2	2	2
B. Operated	24	1.5	1	1	1	1	2	3	3	6
2. MULTIPLE DX										
A. Not Operated	122	3.1	8	1	1	2	4	7	8	14
B. Operated	1,029	2.9	11	1	1	1	3	6	10	18
1. SINGLE DX	25	1.5	1	1	1	1	2	3	3	6
2. MULTIPLE DX	1,151	2.9	11	1	1	2	3	7	9	18
A. NOT OPERATED	123	3.1	8	1	1	2	4	7	8	14
B. OPERATED	1,053	2.8	11	1	1	1	3	6	9	18
TOTAL										
0–19 Years	2	11.0	162	2	2	11	20	20	20	20
20–34	8	4.5	9	1	3	4	5	11	11	11
35–49	52	3.3	11	1	1	2	4	9	12	14
50–64	312	2.8	11	1	1	1	3	6	8	19
65+	802	2.8	10	1	1	1	3	6	9	16
GRAND TOTAL	1,176	2.9	11	1	1	2	3	7	9	18

447.6: ARTERITIS NOS

Type of Patients	Observed Patients	Avg. Stay	Variance	Percentiles						
				10th	25th	50th	75th	90th	95th	99th
1. SINGLE DX										
A. Not Operated										
0–19 Years	2	1.5	<1	1	1	2	2	2	2	2
20–34	0									
35–49	1	1.0	0	1	1	1	1	1	1	1
50–64	1	1.0	0	1	1	1	1	1	1	1
65+	0									
B. Operated										
0–19 Years	0									
20–34	0									
35–49	0									
50–64	0									
65+	0									
2. MULTIPLE DX										
A. Not Operated										
0–19 Years	18	3.9	12	1	2	3	5	12	13	13
20–34	21	5.3	19	1	2	4	6	12	12	15
35–49	57	4.9	23	1	2	4	6	9	11	32
50–64	75	6.1	48	1	2	4	8	12	16	52
65+	83	7.5	48	2	3	5	10	16	23	34
B. Operated										
0–19 Years	1	10.0	0	10	10	10	10	10	10	10
20–34	2	6.5	12	4	4	4	9	9	9	9
35–49	8	9.1	16	5	6	7	11	17	17	17
50–64	10	13.7	186	6	7	8	11	36	50	50
65+	11	10.6	72	3	4	8	15	24	28	28
SUBTOTALS:										
1. SINGLE DX										
A. Not Operated	4	1.3	<1	1	1	1	2	2	2	2
B. Operated	0									
2. MULTIPLE DX										
A. Not Operated	254	6.1	38	1	2	4	8	12	16	32
B. Operated	32	10.9	86	4	6	8	11	22	28	50
1. SINGLE DX	4	1.3	<1	1	1	1	2	2	2	2
2. MULTIPLE DX	286	6.6	46	1	2	5	8	13	20	34
A. NOT OPERATED	258	6.0	38	1	2	4	8	12	16	32
B. OPERATED	32	10.9	86	4	6	8	11	22	28	50
TOTAL										
0–19 Years	21	4.0	13	1	2	3	5	10	12	13
20–34	23	5.4	18	1	2	4	9	12	12	15
35–49	66	5.3	23	1	2	4	7	11	11	32
50–64	86	6.9	68	2	3	4	9	14	20	52
65+	94	7.9	51	2	3	5	10	18	24	34
GRAND TOTAL	290	6.5	46	1	2	4	8	13	20	34

448: DISEASE OF CAPILLARIES

Type of Patients	Observed Patients	Avg. Stay	Variance	Percentiles						
				10th	25th	50th	75th	90th	95th	99th
1. SINGLE DX										
A. Not Operated										
0–19 Years	0									
20–34	0									
35–49	1	4.0	0	4	4	4	4	4	4	4
50–64	0									
65+	0									
B. Operated										
0–19 Years	0									
20–34	0									
35–49	0									
50–64	1	5.0	0	5	5	5	5	5	5	5
65+	0									
2. MULTIPLE DX										
A. Not Operated										
0–19 Years	1	7.0	0	7	7	7	7	7	7	7
20–34	1	2.0	0	2	2	2	2	2	2	2
35–49	24	5.8	29	2	3	4	7	11	14	26
50–64	33	4.1	66	1	1	3	3	6	13	47
65+	60	2.8	4	1	1	2	3	5	6	13
B. Operated										
0–19 Years	1	1.0	0	1	1	1	1	1	1	1
20–34	2	13.0	0	13	13	13	13	13	13	13
35–49	4	4.7	19	1	1	4	4	11	11	11
50–64	7	7.2	46	1	1	3	15	15	15	15
65+	7	3.0	10	1	1	2	3	10	10	10
SUBTOTALS:										
1. SINGLE DX										
A. Not Operated	1	4.0	0	4	4	4	4	4	4	4
B. Operated	1	5.0	0	5	5	5	5	5	5	5
2. MULTIPLE DX										
A. Not Operated	119	3.8	27	1	1	2	4	7	11	26
B. Operated	20	5.2	28	1	1	2	11	13	15	15
1. SINGLE DX	2	4.5	<1	4	4	5	5	5	5	5
2. MULTIPLE DX	139	4.0	27	1	1	2	4	9	13	26
A. NOT OPERATED	120	3.8	27	1	2	3	4	7	11	26
B. OPERATED	21	5.2	27	1	1	3	10	13	15	15
TOTAL										
0–19 Years	2	4.0	18	1	1	7	7	7	7	7
20–34	2	7.5	59	2	2	2	13	13	13	13
35–49	29	5.6	26	1	3	4	7	11	14	26
50–64	41	4.6	61	1	1	3	3	13	15	47
65+	67	2.8	5	1	1	2	3	5	6	13
GRAND TOTAL	141	4.0	27	1	1	3	4	8	13	26

451: THROMBOPHLEBITIS

Type of Patients	Observed Patients	Avg. Stay	Variance	Percentiles						
				10th	25th	50th	75th	90th	95th	99th
1. SINGLE DX										
A. Not Operated										
0–19 Years	0									
20–34	8	2.5	3	1	1	2	4	6	6	6
35–49	9	2.6	4	1	1	2	3	7	7	7
50–64	4	2.8	2	1	2	4	4	4	4	4
65+	1	2.0	0	2	2	2	2	2	2	2
B. Operated										
0–19 Years	0									
20–34	0									
35–49	2	4.0	18	1	1	7	7	7	7	7
50–64	2	1.5	<1	1	1	2	2	2	2	2
65+	1	9.0	0	9	9	9	9	9	9	9
2. MULTIPLE DX										
A. Not Operated										
0–19 Years	10	6.3	26	1	4	4	9	16	16	16
20–34	85	5.1	33	1	2	3	6	10	15	41
35–49	205	4.0	12	1	2	3	5	7	10	18
50–64	237	4.4	10	1	2	4	6	8	11	15
65+	388	4.4	9	1	2	4	6	8	10	15
B. Operated										
0–19 Years	0									
20–34	18	9.6	43	1	6	9	11	18	29	29
35–49	26	6.7	26	2	4	5	7	13	21	21
50–64	32	7.3	28	2	4	5	9	14	17	25
65+	64	8.3	47	3	4	6	11	15	19	47
SUBTOTALS:										
1. SINGLE DX										
A. Not Operated	22	2.6	3	1	1	2	4	4	6	7
B. Operated	5	4.0	14	1	1	2	7	9	9	9
2. MULTIPLE DX										
A. Not Operated	925	4.4	12	1	2	4	6	8	10	18
B. Operated	140	7.9	38	2	4	6	10	15	20	29
1. SINGLE DX	27	2.8	5	1	1	2	4	7	7	9
2. MULTIPLE DX	1,065	4.8	17	1	2	4	6	9	12	21
A. NOT OPERATED	947	4.3	12	1	2	4	6	8	10	18
B. OPERATED	145	7.8	38	2	4	6	10	15	19	29
TOTAL										
0–19 Years	10	6.3	26	1	4	4	9	16	16	16
20–34	111	5.7	36	1	2	4	7	11	17	29
35–49	242	4.2	14	1	2	3	5	8	10	21
50–64	275	4.7	12	1	2	4	6	9	11	18
65+	454	4.9	16	2	3	4	6	9	11	20
GRAND TOTAL	1,092	4.8	17	1	2	4	6	9	12	21

451.0: SUPERF PHLEBITIS LEG

Type of Patients	Observed Patients	Avg. Stay	Variance	Percentiles						
				10th	25th	50th	75th	90th	95th	99th
1. SINGLE DX										
A. Not Operated										
0–19 Years	0									
20–34	4	1.8	<1	1	1	2	2	3	3	3
35–49	3	1.0	0	1	1	1	1	1	1	1
50–64	3	3.0	3	1	1	4	4	4	4	4
65+	0									
B. Operated										
0–19 Years	0									
20–34	0									
35–49	0									
50–64	0									
65+	0									
2. MULTIPLE DX										
A. Not Operated										
0–19 Years	1	4.0	0	4	4	4	4	4	4	4
20–34	18	3.8	16	1	1	3	6	10	17	17
35–49	55	3.0	5	1	1	2	4	6	8	11
50–64	64	3.3	4	1	2	3	5	6	7	9
65+	80	3.7	6	1	2	3	5	7	8	14
B. Operated										
0–19 Years	0									
20–34	0									
35–49	1	5.0	0	5	5	5	5	5	5	5
50–64	5	6.2	24	1	2	7	8	13	13	13
65+	11	5.2	7	2	4	5	8	9	9	9
SUBTOTALS:										
1. SINGLE DX										
A. Not Operated	10	1.9	2	1	1	2	3	4	4	4
B. Operated	0									
2. MULTIPLE DX										
A. Not Operated	218	3.4	6	1	2	3	4	7	8	11
B. Operated	17	5.5	10	1	4	5	8	9	13	13
1. SINGLE DX	10	1.9	2	1	1	2	3	4	4	4
2. MULTIPLE DX	235	3.6	7	1	2	3	5	7	8	13
A. NOT OPERATED	228	3.4	6	1	2	3	4	7	8	11
B. OPERATED	17	5.5	10	1	4	5	8	9	13	13
TOTAL										
0–19 Years	1	4.0	0	4	4	4	4	4	4	4
20–34	22	3.5	14	1	1	3	3	6	10	17
35–49	59	3.0	5	1	1	2	4	6	8	11
50–64	72	3.5	6	1	2	3	5	7	8	13
65+	91	3.9	6	1	2	3	5	7	9	14
GRAND TOTAL	245	3.5	6	1	2	3	5	7	8	13

451.11: FEMORAL VEIN PHLEBITIS

Type of Patients	Observed Patients	Avg. Stay	Variance	Percentiles						
				10th	25th	50th	75th	90th	95th	99th
1. SINGLE DX										
A. Not Operated										
0–19 Years	0									
20–34	0									
35–49	0									
50–64	0									
65+	0									
B. Operated										
0–19 Years	0									
20–34	0									
35–49	1	7.0	0	7	7	7	7	7	7	7
50–64	0									
65+	0									
2. MULTIPLE DX										
A. Not Operated										
0–19 Years	0									
20–34	6	9.2	66	3	4	6	13	24	24	24
35–49	19	6.6	56	1	2	4	7	25	28	28
50–64	24	5.8	16	1	2	6	8	11	11	18
65+	71	4.5	6	2	3	4	6	8	9	10
B. Operated										
0–19 Years	0									
20–34	4	6.5	4	4	6	6	7	9	9	9
35–49	4	6.3	3	4	4	7	8	8	8	8
50–64	4	7.5	31	2	5	7	15	15	15	15
65+	18	7.6	30	2	4	6	10	15	23	23
SUBTOTALS:										
1. SINGLE DX										
A. Not Operated	0									
B. Operated	1	7.0	0	7	7	7	7	7	7	7
2. MULTIPLE DX										
A. Not Operated	120	5.3	19	1	3	4	7	10	11	25
B. Operated	30	7.2	22	3	4	6	8	15	15	23
1. SINGLE DX	1	7.0	0	7	7	7	7	7	7	7
2. MULTIPLE DX	150	5.7	20	2	3	5	7	10	15	25
A. NOT OPERATED	120	5.3	19	1	3	4	7	10	11	25
B. OPERATED	31	7.2	21	3	4	6	8	15	15	23
TOTAL										
0–19 Years	0									
20–34	10	8.1	40	2	4	6	9	24	24	24
35–49	24	6.6	45	1	3	4	7	11	25	28
50–64	28	6.0	17	1	3	6	8	11	15	18
65+	89	5.1	12	2	3	4	6	9	10	23
GRAND TOTAL	151	5.7	20	2	3	5	7	10	15	25

Length of Stay by Diagnosis and Operation, Western Region, 2008

Western Region, October 2006–September 2007 Data, by Diagnosis

451.19: DEEP PHLEBITIS LEG NEC

Type of Patients	Observed Patients	Avg. Stay	Variance	10th	25th	50th	75th	90th	95th	99th
1. SINGLE DX										
A. Not Operated										
0–19 Years	0									
20–34	1	4.0	0	4	4	4	4	4	4	4
35–49	4	4.2	4	3	3	3	4	7	7	7
50–64	1	2.0	0	2	2	2	2	2	2	2
65+	1	2.0	0	2	2	2	2	2	2	2
B. Operated										
0–19 Years	0									
20–34	0									
35–49	0									
50–64	0									
65+	1	9.0	0	9	9	9	9	9	9	9
2. MULTIPLE DX										
A. Not Operated										
0–19 Years	1	5.0	0	5	5	5	5	5	5	5
20–34	10	4.3	5	1	5	5	6	7	7	7
35–49	42	4.4	6	2	3	4	6	8	10	10
50–64	51	4.9	11	1	2	4	7	8	11	18
65+	116	4.5	7	2	3	4	6	8	10	13
B. Operated										
0–19 Years	0									
20–34	4	14.5	93	9	9	10	29	29	29	29
35–49	11	7.7	32	4	5	6	13	13	21	21
50–64	12	9.4	46	2	4	8	12	14	17	25
65+	23	9.2	87	3	4	7	11	15	19	47
SUBTOTALS:										
1. SINGLE DX										
A. Not Operated	7	3.6	3	2	2	3	4	7	7	7
B. Operated	1	9.0	0	9	9	9	9	9	9	9
2. MULTIPLE DX										
A. Not Operated	220	4.6	7	1	3	4	6	8	10	13
B. Operated	50	9.3	65	3	4	7	12	19	25	47
1. SINGLE DX	8	4.2	6	2	3	3	4	9	9	9
2. MULTIPLE DX	270	5.5	21	1	3	4	7	10	13	25
A. NOT OPERATED	227	4.6	7	1	3	4	6	8	10	13
B. OPERATED	51	9.3	63	3	4	7	12	17	25	47
TOTAL										
0–19 Years	1	5.0	0	5	5	5	5	5	5	5
20–34	15	7.0	46	2	3	6	9	10	29	29
35–49	57	5.1	12	2	3	4	6	10	13	21
50–64	64	5.7	20	1	2	5	7	11	14	25
65+	141	5.3	22	2	3	4	6	10	12	19
GRAND TOTAL	278	5.4	21	2	3	4	7	10	13	25

452: PORTAL VEIN THROMBOSIS

Type of Patients	Observed Patients	Avg. Stay	Variance	10th	25th	50th	75th	90th	95th	99th
1. SINGLE DX										
A. Not Operated										
0–19 Years	0									
20–34	0									
35–49	0									
50–64	0									
65+	0									
B. Operated										
0–19 Years	0									
20–34	0									
35–49	0									
50–64	0									
65+	0									
2. MULTIPLE DX										
A. Not Operated										
0–19 Years	9	6.7	29	1	4	6	6	19	19	19
20–34	20	7.0	26	3	4	6	9	12	24	24
35–49	50	4.5	6	1	2	4	7	7	9	10
50–64	61	5.8	44	2	3	5	6	10	13	50
65+	53	5.3	12	2	3	5	7	10	13	15
B. Operated										
0–19 Years	2	9.5	12	7	7	12	12	12	12	12
20–34	1	31.0	0	31	31	31	31	31	31	31
35–49	8	7.0	21	1	4	9	9	12	12	12
50–64	12	16.5	529	1	1	2	27	34	78	78
65+	2	21.9	383	8	8	8	36	36	36	36
SUBTOTALS:										
1. SINGLE DX										
A. Not Operated	0									
B. Operated	0									
2. MULTIPLE DX										
A. Not Operated	193	5.5	23	2	3	5	7	10	12	24
B. Operated	25	13.9	304	1	2	8	20	34	36	78
1. SINGLE DX	0									
2. MULTIPLE DX	218	6.5	61	2	3	5	7	11	16	36
A. NOT OPERATED	193	5.5	23	2	3	5	7	10	12	24
B. OPERATED	25	13.9	304	1	2	8	20	34	36	78
TOTAL										
0–19 Years	11	7.2	26	3	4	6	11	12	19	19
20–34	21	8.1	52	3	4	6	9	12	24	31
35–49	58	4.9	8	1	2	5	7	9	11	12
50–64	73	7.6	133	2	3	5	7	15	27	78
65+	55	6.0	28	2	3	5	7	11	14	36
GRAND TOTAL	218	6.5	61	2	3	5	7	11	16	36

453: OTH VENOUS THROMBOSIS

Type of Patients	Observed Patients	Avg. Stay	Variance	10th	25th	50th	75th	90th	95th	99th
1. SINGLE DX										
A. Not Operated										
0–19 Years	9	2.2	3	1	1	1	4	5	5	5
20–34	66	2.6	3	1	1	2	4	5	6	9
35–49	105	2.9	4	1	1	3	4	5	6	9
50–64	82	3.1	6	1	1	3	4	6	6	18
65+	36	3.8	4	1	3	4	5	7	8	8
B. Operated										
0–19 Years	4	4.2	11	1	2	2	6	8	8	8
20–34	17	2.7	2	1	1	3	4	4	6	6
35–49	10	2.1	2	1	1	2	3	3	4	4
50–64	7	1.3	<1	1	1	1	2	2	2	2
65+	6	1.3	<1	1	1	1	2	2	2	2
2. MULTIPLE DX										
A. Not Operated										
0–19 Years	80	4.2	11	1	2	4	5	7	12	18
20–34	790	3.9	11	1	2	3	5	7	9	17
35–49	2,174	4.0	13	1	2	3	5	7	9	16
50–64	3,098	4.2	11	1	2	4	5	8	10	17
65+	6,154	4.4	9	1	2	4	6	8	9	15
B. Operated										
0–19 Years	40	6.2	29	1	3	5	6	13	22	23
20–34	154	6.7	59	1	3	5	8	12	16	47
35–49	350	6.8	34	2	3	5	8	14	20	29
50–64	617	6.7	35	2	3	5	8	14	18	28
65+	1,519	6.3	28	2	3	5	8	13	17	26
SUBTOTALS:										
1. SINGLE DX										
A. Not Operated	298	3.0	4	1	1	3	4	5	7	9
B. Operated	44	2.3	3	1	1	2	3	4	6	8
2. MULTIPLE DX										
A. Not Operated	12,296	4.3	10	1	2	4	5	8	10	16
B. Operated	2,680	6.5	32	2	3	5	8	13	17	28
1. SINGLE DX	342	2.9	4	1	1	3	4	5	6	9
2. MULTIPLE DX	14,976	4.7	15	1	2	4	6	8	11	20
A. NOT OPERATED	12,594	4.2	10	1	2	4	5	8	10	16
B. OPERATED	2,724	6.4	32	2	3	5	8	13	17	28
TOTAL										
0–19 Years	133	4.6	17	1	2	4	6	9	13	22
20–34	1,027	4.2	19	1	2	3	5	8	10	20
35–49	2,639	4.3	17	1	2	3	5	8	11	20
50–64	3,804	4.6	16	1	2	4	6	9	12	20
65+	7,715	4.8	13	1	3	4	6	8	11	19
GRAND TOTAL	15,318	4.6	15	1	2	4	6	8	11	19

Length of Stay by Diagnosis and Operation, Western Region, 2008

Western Region, October 2006–September 2007 Data, by Diagnosis

453.40: DVT LEG NOS

Type of Patients	Observed Patients	Avg. Stay	Variance	Percentiles						
				10th	25th	50th	75th	90th	95th	99th
1. SINGLE DX										
A. Not Operated										
0–19 Years	1	4.0	0	4	4	4	4	4	4	4
20–34	5	3.0	3	1	1	4	4	5	5	5
35–49	14	3.6	4	1	2	3	5	5	8	8
50–64	14	4.0	18	1	2	3	4	6	18	18
65+	7	4.0	8	1	1	3	7	8	8	8
B. Operated										
0–19 Years	0									
20–34	1	3.0	0	3	3	3	3	3	3	3
35–49	1	3.0	0	3	3	3	3	3	3	3
50–64	0									
65+	0									
2. MULTIPLE DX										
A. Not Operated										
0–19 Years	6	2.3	3	1	1	1	4	5	5	5
20–34	80	3.5	6	1	2	3	5	7	7	11
35–49	228	4.0	13	1	2	3	5	8	9	25
50–64	349	4.1	11	1	2	3	5	8	10	19
65+	753	4.7	8	2	3	4	6	8	10	14
B. Operated										
0–19 Years	1	5.0	0	5	5	5	5	5	5	5
20–34	8	6.1	23	1	2	6	9	16	16	16
35–49	26	7.0	29	1	3	6	10	16	18	19
50–64	50	5.3	25	1	2	4	7	9	14	28
65+	175	5.6	24	2	2	4	7	11	14	28
SUBTOTALS:										
1. SINGLE DX										
A. Not Operated	41	3.7	9	1	2	3	5	6	8	18
B. Operated	2	3.0	0	3	3	3	3	3	3	3
2. MULTIPLE DX										
A. Not Operated	1,416	4.3	10	1	2	4	6	8	10	16
B. Operated	260	5.7	25	1	2	4	7	12	16	28
1. SINGLE DX	43	3.7	8	1	2	3	5	6	8	18
2. MULTIPLE DX	1,676	4.6	12	1	2	4	6	8	10	19
A. NOT OPERATED	1,457	4.3	10	1	2	4	5	8	10	16
B. OPERATED	262	5.7	25	1	2	4	7	11	16	28
TOTAL										
0–19 Years	8	2.9	3	1	1	2	4	5	5	5
20–34	94	3.7	7	1	2	3	5	7	9	16
35–49	269	4.3	15	1	2	3	5	9	11	25
50–64	413	4.3	13	1	2	3	5	8	10	19
65+	935	4.8	11	1	3	4	6	9	11	16
GRAND TOTAL	**1,719**	**4.5**	**12**	**1**	**2**	**4**	**6**	**8**	**10**	**19**

453.41: DVT PROXIMAL LEG

Type of Patients	Observed Patients	Avg. Stay	Variance	Percentiles						
				10th	25th	50th	75th	90th	95th	99th
1. SINGLE DX										
A. Not Operated										
0–19 Years	2	1.0	0	1	1	1	1	1	1	1
20–34	28	3.0	5	1	1	2	4	7	7	9
35–49	47	3.0	3	1	2	3	4	5	6	9
50–64	35	2.8	3	1	1	2	4	6	6	8
65+	17	3.6	3	3	3	3	4	6	8	8
B. Operated										
0–19 Years	1	2.0	0	2	2	2	2	2	2	2
20–34	6	2.2	<1	1	1	2	3	3	3	3
35–49	6	2.2	1	1	1	2	3	4	4	4
50–64	5	1.4	<1	1	1	1	2	2	2	2
65+	4	1.5	<1	1	1	2	2	2	2	2
2. MULTIPLE DX										
A. Not Operated										
0–19 Years	43	4.5	14	2	2	4	6	7	13	18
20–34	361	3.8	8	1	2	3	5	7	8	13
35–49	947	4.1	11	1	2	3	5	7	10	17
50–64	1,479	4.4	12	1	2	4	6	8	10	18
65+	3,278	4.4	9	1	2	4	6	8	9	16
B. Operated										
0–19 Years	19	8.2	44	2	4	5	11	22	23	23
20–34	78	7.7	94	2	3	5	8	14	25	65
35–49	196	7.1	39	2	3	5	8	14	21	32
50–64	324	7.0	42	2	3	5	8	13	19	31
65+	906	6.5	30	2	3	5	8	13	16	26
SUBTOTALS:										
1. SINGLE DX										
A. Not Operated	129	3.0	3	1	1	3	4	5	6	9
B. Operated	22	1.9	<1	1	1	2	2	3	3	4
2. MULTIPLE DX										
A. Not Operated	6,108	4.3	10	1	2	4	6	8	10	16
B. Operated	1,523	6.7	37	2	3	5	8	13	18	30
1. SINGLE DX	151	2.8	3	1	1	3	4	5	6	9
2. MULTIPLE DX	7,631	4.8	16	1	2	4	6	9	11	21
A. NOT OPERATED	6,237	4.3	10	1	2	4	6	8	9	16
B. OPERATED	1,545	6.7	37	2	3	5	8	13	18	30
TOTAL										
0–19 Years	65	5.4	25	2	2	4	6	13	18	23
20–34	473	4.4	24	1	2	3	5	8	10	22
35–49	1,196	4.5	17	1	2	4	6	8	11	22
50–64	1,843	4.8	18	2	2	4	6	9	12	23
65+	4,205	4.9	14	1	3	4	6	9	11	19
GRAND TOTAL	**7,782**	**4.8**	**16**	**1**	**2**	**4**	**6**	**8**	**11**	**21**

453.42: DVT DISTAL LEG

Type of Patients	Observed Patients	Avg. Stay	Variance	Percentiles						
				10th	25th	50th	75th	90th	95th	99th
1. SINGLE DX										
A. Not Operated										
0–19 Years	0									
20–34	17	2.4	3	1	1	1	3	3	6	6
35–49	29	2.2	2	1	1	2	3	5	5	6
50–64	26	3.1	4	1	1	3	4	6	7	8
65+	6	4.0	3	3	3	5	5	6	6	6
B. Operated										
0–19 Years	0									
20–34	1	1.0	0	1	1	1	1	1	1	1
35–49	1	3.0	0	3	3	3	3	3	3	3
50–64	0									
65+	0									
2. MULTIPLE DX										
A. Not Operated										
0–19 Years	10	3.8	3	1	3	3	5	5	6	6
20–34	162	3.6	6	1	2	3	5	7	8	11
35–49	565	3.9	20	1	2	3	5	7	9	13
50–64	779	4.1	11	1	2	3	5	8	10	17
65+	1,440	4.3	9	1	2	4	6	8	9	14
B. Operated										
0–19 Years	3	4.3	8	1	1	6	6	6	6	6
20–34	13	5.5	16	2	3	4	7	11	16	16
35–49	57	6.4	24	1	3	5	9	13	16	25
50–64	138	7.1	32	2	3	5	9	15	19	23
65+	324	6.2	23	2	3	5	8	12	17	22
SUBTOTALS:										
1. SINGLE DX										
A. Not Operated	78	2.7	3	1	1	2	4	5	6	8
B. Operated	2	2.0	2	1	1	3	3	3	3	3
2. MULTIPLE DX										
A. Not Operated	2,956	4.2	12	1	2	4	5	7	9	14
B. Operated	535	6.4	25	2	3	5	8	13	17	23
1. SINGLE DX	80	2.6	3	1	1	2	4	5	6	8
2. MULTIPLE DX	3,491	4.5	14	1	2	4	6	8	11	18
A. NOT OPERATED	3,034	4.1	11	1	2	3	5	7	9	14
B. OPERATED	537	6.4	25	2	3	5	8	13	17	23
TOTAL										
0–19 Years	13	3.9	4	1	3	4	6	6	6	6
20–34	193	3.6	7	1	2	3	5	7	9	13
35–49	652	4.1	20	1	2	3	5	7	10	15
50–64	943	4.5	15	1	2	4	6	9	12	20
65+	1,770	4.7	12	1	2	4	6	8	10	18
GRAND TOTAL	**3,571**	**4.5**	**14**	**1**	**2**	**4**	**6**	**8**	**11**	**18**

333

Length of Stay by Diagnosis and Operation, Western Region, 2008

Western Region, October 2006–September 2007 Data, by Diagnosis

453.8: VENOUS THROMBOSIS NEC

Type of Patients	Observed Patients	Avg. Stay	Variance	10th	25th	50th	75th	90th	95th	99th
1. SINGLE DX										
A. Not Operated										
0–19 Years	5	1.8	2	1	1	1	2	4	4	4
20–34	16	2.1	1	1	1	2	3	4	4	4
35–49	14	3.8	10	1	1	3	5	9	10	10
50–64	7	2.7	4	1	1	2	5	5	5	5
65+	6	3.8	4	1	3	4	5	7	7	7
B. Operated										
0–19 Years	3	5.0	13	1	1	6	8	8	8	8
20–34	9	3.1	3	1	2	4	4	6	6	6
35–49	2	1.0	0	1	1	1	1	1	1	1
50–64	2	1.0	0	1	1	1	1	1	1	1
65+	2	1.0	0	1	1	1	1	1	1	1
2. MULTIPLE DX										
A. Not Operated										
0–19 Years	15	3.1	4	1	2	2	4	5	8	8
20–34	163	4.3	15	1	2	3	5	8	11	21
35–49	398	3.7	8	1	2	3	5	7	9	12
50–64	453	4.0	8	1	2	3	5	8	10	14
65+	637	4.4	9	1	2	4	6	8	10	15
B. Operated										
0–19 Years	12	4.0	10	1	1	3	6	6	12	12
20–34	45	5.4	24	1	2	3	8	10	15	25
35–49	57	5.5	23	2	2	4	7	11	16	27
50–64	78	5.5	19	1	2	4	7	12	16	20
65+	97	7.2	35	2	3	5	9	15	21	28
SUBTOTALS:										
1. SINGLE DX										
A. Not Operated	48	2.9	5	1	1	2	4	5	8	10
B. Operated	18	2.7	5	1	1	1	4	6	8	8
2. MULTIPLE DX										
A. Not Operated	1,666	4.1	9	1	2	3	5	8	10	15
B. Operated	289	6.0	26	1	3	4	8	13	17	27
1. SINGLE DX	66	2.8	5	1	1	2	4	6	8	10
2. MULTIPLE DX	1,955	4.4	12	1	2	4	6	8	10	19
A. NOT OPERATED	1,714	4.1	9	1	2	3	5	8	10	15
B. OPERATED	307	5.8	26	1	2	4	8	12	16	26
TOTAL										
0–19 Years	35	3.4	6	1	1	3	5	6	8	12
20–34	233	4.3	16	1	2	3	5	9	11	21
35–49	471	3.9	10	1	2	3	5	7	9	15
50–64	540	4.2	10	1	2	3	5	8	10	16
65+	742	4.8	14	1	2	4	6	9	11	20
GRAND TOTAL	2,021	4.3	12	1	2	3	6	8	10	19

454: LEG VARICOSE VEINS

Type of Patients	Observed Patients	Avg. Stay	Variance	10th	25th	50th	75th	90th	95th	99th
1. SINGLE DX										
A. Not Operated										
0–19 Years	0									
20–34	0									
35–49	0									
50–64	0									
65+	0									
B. Operated										
0–19 Years	0									
20–34	5	2.2	7	1	1	1	1	7	7	7
35–49	10	2.8	28	1	1	1	1	2	18	18
50–64	7	2.3	9	1	1	1	2	9	9	9
65+	2	1.5	<1	1	1	2	2	2	2	2
2. MULTIPLE DX										
A. Not Operated										
0–19 Years	0									
20–34	3	2.0	<1	1	1	2	3	3	3	3
35–49	40	5.1	21	1	2	4	6	12	19	19
50–64	75	5.5	19	1	3	4	7	10	13	27
65+	147	5.5	23	2	3	4	6	9	15	26
B. Operated										
0–19 Years	1	1.0	0	1	1	1	1	1	1	1
20–34	7	7.7	108	1	1	5	9	30	30	30
35–49	49	3.0	24	1	1	4	7	7	12	27
50–64	50	5.2	36	1	1	3	7	15	18	26
65+	81	4.4	28	1	1	5	6	12	14	30
SUBTOTALS:										
1. SINGLE DX										
A. Not Operated	0									
B. Operated	24	2.4	15	1	1	1	1	7	9	18
2. MULTIPLE DX										
A. Not Operated	265	5.4	21	1	3	4	6	11	15	26
B. Operated	188	4.4	32	1	1	4	5	12	16	30
1. SINGLE DX	24	2.4	15	1	1	1	1	7	9	18
2. MULTIPLE DX	453	5.0	26	1	3	4	6	11	15	27
A. NOT OPERATED	265	5.4	21	1	3	4	6	11	15	26
B. OPERATED	212	4.1	31	1	1	4	5	11	16	27
TOTAL										
0–19 Years	1	1.0	0	1	1	1	1	1	1	1
20–34	15	4.7	57	1	1	1	6	9	30	30
35–49	99	3.8	24	1	2	2	4	11	18	27
50–64	132	5.2	25	1	2	4	7	11	16	26
65+	230	5.1	25	1	2	4	6	12	15	26
GRAND TOTAL	477	4.8	26	1	3	3	6	11	15	27

454.2: LEG VV W ULCER & INFLAM

Type of Patients	Observed Patients	Avg. Stay	Variance	10th	25th	50th	75th	90th	95th	99th
1. SINGLE DX										
A. Not Operated										
0–19 Years	0									
20–34	0									
35–49	0									
50–64	0									
65+	0									
B. Operated										
0–19 Years	0									
20–34	0									
35–49	1	18.0	0	18	18	18	18	18	18	18
50–64	1	9.0	0	9	9	9	9	9	9	9
65+	0									
2. MULTIPLE DX										
A. Not Operated										
0–19 Years	0									
20–34	1	3.0	0	3	3	3	3	3	3	3
35–49	14	4.0	7	1	3	3	4	6	12	12
50–64	43	5.7	20	2	3	5	7	9	13	27
65+	58	6.1	26	2	3	5	7	13	16	28
B. Operated										
0–19 Years	0									
20–34	1	30.0	0	30	30	30	30	30	30	30
35–49	6	9.4	88	4	5	5	12	27	27	27
50–64	11	8.9	38	6	6	7	10	13	26	26
65+	21	6.7	56	1	1	4	4	9	20	30
SUBTOTALS:										
1. SINGLE DX										
A. Not Operated	0									
B. Operated	2	13.4	40	9	9	9	18	18	18	18
2. MULTIPLE DX										
A. Not Operated	116	5.7	21	2	3	4	7	11	14	27
B. Operated	39	8.3	65	1	3	6	10	26	30	30
1. SINGLE DX	2	13.4	40	9	9	9	18	18	18	18
2. MULTIPLE DX	155	6.3	33	2	3	5	7	13	20	30
A. NOT OPERATED	116	5.7	21	2	3	4	7	11	14	27
B. OPERATED	41	8.6	64	1	4	6	10	20	27	30
TOTAL										
0–19 Years	0									
20–34	2	16.5	354	3	3	17	30	30	30	30
35–49	21	6.2	40	1	3	4	6	12	18	27
50–64	55	6.4	24	2	3	6	7	11	14	27
65+	79	6.3	33	1	3	4	7	14	20	30
GRAND TOTAL	157	6.4	34	2	3	5	7	13	18	30

455: HEMORRHOIDS

Type of Patients	Observed Patients	Avg. Stay	Vari-ance	10th	25th	50th	75th	90th	95th	99th
1. SINGLE DX										
A. Not Operated										
0–19 Years	0									
20–34	12	1.4	<1	1	1	1	2	2	3	3
35–49	11	1.2	<1	1	1	1	1	2	2	2
50–64	5	1.2	<1	1	1	1	1	2	2	2
65+	2	1.5	<1	1	1	2	2	2	2	2
B. Operated										
0–19 Years	0									
20–34	15	1.5	<1	1	1	1	2	2	3	3
35–49	23	1.4	<1	1	1	1	2	2	3	3
50–64	10	1.4	<1	1	1	1	1	4	4	4
65+	3	1.3	<1	1	1	1	2	2	2	2
2. MULTIPLE DX										
A. Not Operated										
0–19 Years	9	2.1	1	1	2	2	2	5	5	5
20–34	204	2.5	5	1	1	2	3	4	6	10
35–49	728	2.5	4	1	1	2	3	4	6	11
50–64	890	2.7	6	1	1	2	3	5	7	12
65+	1,991	3.0	6	1	2	2	4	6	8	13
B. Operated										
0–19 Years	1	3.0	0	3	3	3	3	3	3	3
20–34	112	2.9	5	1	1	2	4	6	8	9
35–49	324	3.0	6	1	1	2	3	6	8	11
50–64	347	3.3	11	1	1	2	4	7	10	15
65+	327	4.2	17	1	2	3	5	9	11	23
SUBTOTALS:										
1. SINGLE DX										
A. Not Operated	30	1.3	<1	1	1	1	2	2	2	3
B. Operated	51	1.4	<1	1	1	1	2	2	3	4
2. MULTIPLE DX										
A. Not Operated	3,822	2.8	6	1	1	2	3	5	7	12
B. Operated	1,111	3.4	11	1	1	2	4	7	10	17
1. SINGLE DX	81	1.4	<1	1	1	1	2	2	3	4
2. MULTIPLE DX	4,933	3.0	7	1	1	2	3	6	8	13
A. NOT OPERATED	3,852	2.8	6	1	1	2	3	5	7	12
B. OPERATED	1,162	3.3	11	1	1	2	4	7	9	17
TOTAL										
0–19 Years	10	2.2	1	1	2	2	2	5	5	5
20–34	343	2.5	5	1	1	2	3	5	7	10
35–49	1,086	2.6	5	1	1	2	3	5	6	11
50–64	1,252	2.9	8	1	1	2	3	5	7	12
65+	2,323	3.2	8	1	2	2	4	6	8	15
GRAND TOTAL	5,014	2.9	7	1	1	2	3	6	8	13

455.2: INT HEMORRHOID-COMP NEC

Type of Patients	Observed Patients	Avg. Stay	Vari-ance	10th	25th	50th	75th	90th	95th	99th
1. SINGLE DX										
A. Not Operated										
0–19 Years	0									
20–34	6	1.2	<1	1	1	1	1	2	2	2
35–49	4	1.3	<1	1	1	1	2	2	2	2
50–64	3	1.3	<1	1	1	1	2	2	2	2
65+	2	1.5	<1	1	1	2	2	2	2	2
B. Operated										
0–19 Years	0									
20–34	2	1.0	0	1	1	1	1	1	1	1
35–49	6	1.3	<1	1	1	1	1	3	3	3
50–64	3	1.3	<1	1	1	1	2	2	2	2
65+	0									
2. MULTIPLE DX										
A. Not Operated										
0–19 Years	6	1.7	<1	1	1	1	2	2	2	2
20–34	142	2.5	6	1	1	2	3	4	6	17
35–49	519	2.5	5	1	1	2	3	4	6	11
50–64	620	2.7	4	1	1	2	3	5	6	11
65+	1,402	3.1	7	2	2	2	4	6	7	13
B. Operated										
0–19 Years	1	3.0	0	3	3	3	3	3	3	3
20–34	63	3.4	6	1	2	2	4	8	8	12
35–49	193	3.0	5	1	2	2	4	6	9	11
50–64	221	3.6	14	1	1	2	4	7	11	15
65+	220	4.5	19	1	2	3	6	9	11	23
SUBTOTALS:										
1. SINGLE DX										
A. Not Operated	15	1.3	<1	1	1	1	2	2	2	2
B. Operated	11	1.3	<1	1	1	1	1	2	3	3
2. MULTIPLE DX										
A. Not Operated	2,689	2.9	6	1	1	2	3	5	7	12
B. Operated	698	3.7	13	1	2	3	4	8	10	20
1. SINGLE DX	26	1.3	<1	1	1	1	1	2	2	3
2. MULTIPLE DX	3,387	3.0	7	1	1	2	4	6	8	14
A. NOT OPERATED	2,704	2.9	6	1	1	2	3	5	7	12
B. OPERATED	709	3.7	12	1	2	3	4	8	10	20
TOTAL										
0–19 Years	7	1.9	<1	1	1	1	2	3	3	3
20–34	213	2.7	6	1	1	2	3	5	8	12
35–49	722	2.6	5	1	1	2	3	5	6	11
50–64	847	2.9	7	1	1	2	4	6	8	12
65+	1,624	3.3	9	2	2	3	4	6	8	16
GRAND TOTAL	3,413	3.0	7	1	1	2	4	6	8	14

455.5: EXT HEMORRHOID-COMP NEC

Type of Patients	Observed Patients	Avg. Stay	Vari-ance	10th	25th	50th	75th	90th	95th	99th
1. SINGLE DX										
A. Not Operated										
0–19 Years	0									
20–34	1	1.0	0	1	1	1	1	1	1	1
35–49	0									
50–64	0									
65+	0									
B. Operated										
0–19 Years	0									
20–34	2	2.0	0	2	2	2	2	2	2	2
35–49	2	1.5	<1	1	1	1	2	2	2	2
50–64	1	1.0	0	1	1	1	1	1	1	1
65+	0									
2. MULTIPLE DX										
A. Not Operated										
0–19 Years	1	5.0	0	5	5	5	5	5	5	5
20–34	19	2.3	1	1	1	2	3	4	4	4
35–49	87	2.4	2	1	1	2	3	4	4	11
50–64	85	2.9	7	1	2	2	4	5	6	22
65+	175	3.1	6	1	2	2	4	6	8	12
B. Operated										
0–19 Years	0									
20–34	11	2.5	2	1	1	3	3	4	5	5
35–49	24	3.4	5	2	2	3	4	7	7	10
50–64	28	3.5	10	1	1	2	5	10	11	12
65+	29	3.7	8	1	1	3	5	8	10	11
SUBTOTALS:										
1. SINGLE DX										
A. Not Operated	1	1.0	0	1	1	1	1	1	1	1
B. Operated	5	1.6	<1	1	1	2	2	2	2	2
2. MULTIPLE DX										
A. Not Operated	367	2.8	5	1	2	2	3	5	6	11
B. Operated	92	3.4	7	1	1	3	4	7	10	12
1. SINGLE DX	6	1.5	<1	1	1	1	2	2	2	2
2. MULTIPLE DX	459	2.9	5	1	1	2	4	5	7	11
A. NOT OPERATED	368	2.8	5	1	2	2	3	5	6	11
B. OPERATED	97	3.3	7	1	1	2	4	7	10	12
TOTAL										
0–19 Years	1	5.0	0	5	5	5	5	5	5	5
20–34	33	2.3	1	1	1	2	3	4	4	5
35–49	113	2.6	3	1	1	2	3	4	7	10
50–64	114	3.0	8	1	2	2	4	6	7	12
65+	204	3.2	6	1	2	2	4	6	8	11
GRAND TOTAL	465	2.9	5	1	1	2	4	5	7	11

Length of Stay by Diagnosis and Operation, Western Region, 2008

Western Region, October 2006–September 2007 Data, by Diagnosis

455.8: HEMORRHOID NOS-COMP NEC

Type of Patients	Observed Patients	Avg. Stay	Variance	10th	25th	50th	75th	90th	95th	99th
1. SINGLE DX										
A. Not Operated										
0–19 Years	0									
20–34	0									
35–49	1	1.0	0	1	1	1	1	1	1	1
50–64	1	1.0	0	1	1	1	1	1	1	1
65+	0									
B. Operated										
0–19 Years	0									
20–34	2	1.0	0	1	1	1	1	1	1	1
35–49	5	1.2	<1	1	1	1	1	2	2	2
50–64	1	1.0	0	1	1	1	1	1	1	1
65+	1	1.0	0	1	1	1	1	1	1	1
2. MULTIPLE DX										
A. Not Operated										
0–19 Years	2	2.0	0	2	2	2	2	2	2	2
20–34	26	2.1	<1	1	1	2	3	3	4	4
35–49	69	2.4	3	1	1	2	3	5	6	10
50–64	127	2.7	20	1	1	2	3	5	7	14
65+	338	2.8	5	1	1	2	3	6	7	10
B. Operated										
0–19 Years	0									
20–34	11	1.0	0	1	1	1	1	1	1	1
35–49	12	2.7	8	1	1	2	2	7	10	10
50–64	10	4.1	26	1	1	2	4	6	18	18
65+	18	5.3	45	1	1	3	4	16	27	27
SUBTOTALS:										
1. SINGLE DX										
A. Not Operated	2	1.0	0	1	1	1	1	1	1	1
B. Operated	9	1.1	<1	1	1	1	1	2	2	2
2. MULTIPLE DX										
A. Not Operated	562	2.7	8	1	1	2	3	6	7	11
B. Operated	41	4.1	29	1	1	2	4	10	16	27
1. SINGLE DX	11	1.1	<1	1	1	1	1	1	2	2
2. MULTIPLE DX	603	2.8	9	1	1	2	3	6	7	12
A. NOT OPERATED	564	2.7	8	1	1	2	3	6	7	11
B. OPERATED	50	3.6	25	1	1	2	3	9	16	27
TOTAL										
0–19 Years	2	2.0	0	2	2	2	2	2	2	2
20–34	29	2.0	<1	1	1	2	2	3	3	4
35–49	87	2.4	4	1	1	2	3	5	6	10
50–64	139	2.8	20	1	1	2	3	6	8	18
65+	357	3.0	7	1	1	2	3	6	8	12
GRAND TOTAL	614	2.8	9	1	1	2	3	6	7	12

456: VARICOSE VEINS NEC

Type of Patients	Observed Patients	Avg. Stay	Variance	10th	25th	50th	75th	90th	95th	99th
1. SINGLE DX										
A. Not Operated										
0–19 Years	0									
20–34	0									
35–49	0									
50–64	2	3.0	8	1	1	5	5	5	5	5
65+	0									
B. Operated										
0–19 Years	0									
20–34	1	2.0	0	2	2	2	2	2	2	2
35–49	1	1.0	0	1	1	1	1	1	1	1
50–64	1	1.0	0	1	1	1	1	1	1	1
65+	0									
2. MULTIPLE DX										
A. Not Operated										
0–19 Years	6	4.7	11	1	2	5	8	9	9	9
20–34	36	3.9	6	1	3	3	5	7	10	11
35–49	308	4.5	13	2	3	4	5	7	10	19
50–64	487	4.6	32	2	2	3	5	7	11	34
65+	269	4.4	11	2	3	4	5	8	10	19
B. Operated										
0–19 Years	2	1.5	<1	1	1	1	2	2	2	2
20–34	11	3.9	9	1	2	3	5	9	10	10
35–49	35	7.2	40	1	3	5	10	14	18	32
50–64	51	7.7	32	2	3	6	11	16	20	21
65+	58	6.7	25	1	3	5	9	15	17	21
SUBTOTALS:										
1. SINGLE DX										
A. Not Operated	2	3.0	8	1	1	5	5	5	5	5
B. Operated	3	1.3	<1	1	1	1	2	2	2	2
2. MULTIPLE DX										
A. Not Operated	1,106	4.5	21	2	2	4	5	7	10	21
B. Operated	157	6.9	30	2	3	5	9	15	18	21
1. SINGLE DX	5	2.0	3	1	1	1	2	5	5	5
2. MULTIPLE DX	1,263	4.8	22	2	3	4	5	9	12	21
A. NOT OPERATED	1,108	4.5	21	2	2	4	5	7	10	21
B. OPERATED	160	6.8	30	1	3	5	9	15	18	21
TOTAL										
0–19 Years	8	3.9	10	1	1	3	5	9	9	9
20–34	48	3.9	6	1	2	3	5	9	10	11
35–49	344	4.7	17	2	3	4	5	8	12	21
50–64	541	4.9	32	2	2	3	6	9	13	21
65+	327	4.8	14	2	3	4	6	9	13	19
GRAND TOTAL	1,268	4.8	22	2	2	4	5	9	12	21

456.0: ESOPH VARICES W BLEEDING

Type of Patients	Observed Patients	Avg. Stay	Variance	10th	25th	50th	75th	90th	95th	99th
1. SINGLE DX										
A. Not Operated										
0–19 Years	0									
20–34	0									
35–49	0									
50–64	2	3.0	8	1	1	5	5	5	5	5
65+	0									
B. Operated										
0–19 Years	0									
20–34	0									
35–49	0									
50–64	0									
65+	0									
2. MULTIPLE DX										
A. Not Operated										
0–19 Years	3	6.4	14	2	2	8	9	9	9	9
20–34	24	3.9	5	2	2	3	5	7	9	10
35–49	197	4.0	7	2	2	3	5	6	8	17
50–64	303	4.8	42	2	2	3	5	8	10	36
65+	159	4.4	8	2	3	4	5	8	9	15
B. Operated										
0–19 Years	1	2.0	0	2	2	2	2	2	2	2
20–34	1	9.0	0	9	9	9	9	9	9	9
35–49	4	5.7	31	2	3	3	4	14	14	14
50–64	7	6.6	21	2	3	6	7	16	16	16
65+	6	11.0	24	5	6	15	15	16	16	16
SUBTOTALS:										
1. SINGLE DX										
A. Not Operated	2	3.0	8	1	1	5	5	5	5	5
B. Operated	0									
2. MULTIPLE DX										
A. Not Operated	686	4.4	23	2	2	4	5	7	9	21
B. Operated	19	7.7	26	2	3	6	14	16	16	16
1. SINGLE DX	2	3.0	8	1	1	5	5	5	5	5
2. MULTIPLE DX	705	4.5	23	2	2	4	5	8	9	21
A. NOT OPERATED	688	4.4	23	2	2	4	5	7	9	21
B. OPERATED	19	7.7	26	2	3	6	14	16	16	16
TOTAL										
0–19 Years	4	5.3	14	2	2	8	9	9	9	9
20–34	25	4.1	6	2	3	3	5	9	9	10
35–49	201	4.0	7	2	2	3	5	6	8	16
50–64	312	4.8	41	2	3	3	5	8	10	36
65+	165	4.6	10	2	3	4	5	9	11	16
GRAND TOTAL	707	4.5	23	2	2	4	5	8	9	21

Length of Stay by Diagnosis and Operation, Western Region, 2008

Western Region, October 2006–September 2007 Data, by Diagnosis

456.8: VARICES NEC

Type of Patients	Observed Patients	Avg. Stay	Variance	10th	25th	50th	75th	90th	95th	99th
1. SINGLE DX										
A. Not Operated										
0–19 Years	0									
20–34	0									
35–49	0									
50–64	0									
65+	0									
B. Operated										
0–19 Years	0									
20–34	0									
35–49	1	1.0	0	1	1	1		1	1	1
50–64	0									
65+	0									
2. MULTIPLE DX										
A. Not Operated										
0–19 Years	0									
20–34	9	4.6	8	1	3	3	6	11	11	11
35–49	96	5.4	26	2	3	4	6	10	13	38
50–64	157	4.4	14	2	3	4	5	7	11	21
65+	94	4.6	17	2	3	4	5	7	15	29
B. Operated										
0–19 Years	0									
20–34	2	7.5	12	5	5	5	10	10	10	10
35–49	25	8.8	41	3	5	8	10	16	18	32
50–64	40	8.5	34	2	4	7	13	19	21	21
65+	50	6.3	23	1	3	5	9	13	17	29
SUBTOTALS:										
1. SINGLE DX										
A. Not Operated	0									
B. Operated	1	1.0	0	1	1	1	1	1	1	1
2. MULTIPLE DX										
A. Not Operated	356	4.8	18	2	3	4	5	8	12	27
B. Operated	117	7.6	31	2	4	6	10	15	19	21
1. SINGLE DX	1	1.0	0	1	1	1	1	1	1	1
2. MULTIPLE DX	473	5.5	23	2	3	4	6	11	15	27
A. NOT OPERATED	356	4.8	18	2	3	4	5	8	12	27
B. OPERATED	118	7.5	31	2	4	6	10	15	19	21
TOTAL										
0–19 Years	0									
20–34	11	5.1	9	3	3	5	6	10	11	11
35–49	122	6.1	31	2	3	5	6	12	16	32
50–64	197	5.2	21	2	3	4	6	11	15	21
65+	144	5.2	19	2	3	4	6	10	15	21
GRAND TOTAL	474	5.5	23	2	3	4	6	11	15	27

457: NONINF LYMPHATIC DISORD

Type of Patients	Observed Patients	Avg. Stay	Variance	10th	25th	50th	75th	90th	95th	99th
1. SINGLE DX										
A. Not Operated										
0–19 Years	1	2.0	0	2	2	2	2	2	2	2
20–34	1	3.0	0	3	3	3	3	3	3	3
35–49	1	3.0	0	3	3	3	3	3	3	3
50–64	0									
65+	1	1.0	0	1	1	1	1	1	1	1
B. Operated										
0–19 Years	1	1.0	0	1	1	1	1	1	1	1
20–34	0									
35–49	2	1.0	0	1	1	1	1	1	1	1
50–64	1	1.0	0	1	1	1	1	1	1	1
65+	0									
2. MULTIPLE DX										
A. Not Operated										
0–19 Years	10	7.3	118	1	1	2	7	19	34	34
20–34	23	3.7	12	1	2	3	3	7	11	16
35–49	53	3.4	5	1	2	3	5	6	7	14
50–64	100	4.2	12	1	2	3	6	8	10	23
65+	104	4.8	17	3	3	4	6	9	14	19
B. Operated										
0–19 Years	2	10.5	<1	10	10	10	11	11	11	11
20–34	7	8.5	150	3	3	5	5	36	36	36
35–49	20	8.9	104	2	4	5	6	21	26	41
50–64	29	5.4	37	1	2	3	6	13	13	30
65+	37	6.1	26	1	3	5	8	15	18	20
SUBTOTALS:										
1. SINGLE DX										
A. Not Operated	4	2.3	<1	1	1	3	3	3	3	3
B. Operated	4	1.0	0	1	1	1	1	1	1	1
2. MULTIPLE DX										
A. Not Operated	290	4.3	17	1	2	3	5	8	11	23
B. Operated	95	6.7	54	1	3	4	8	15	21	41
1. SINGLE DX	8	1.6	<1	1	1	1	3	3	3	3
2. MULTIPLE DX	385	4.9	27	1	2	3	6	10	14	30
A. NOT OPERATED	294	4.3	16	1	2	3	5	8	11	23
B. OPERATED	99	6.5	53	1	2	4	7	15	21	41
TOTAL										
0–19 Years	14	6.9	88	1	1	3	10	19	34	34
20–34	31	4.7	44	1	2	3	5	7	16	36
35–49	76	4.8	36	1	2	3	5	9	20	41
50–64	130	4.4	18	1	2	4	6	9	12	23
65+	142	5.1	20	1	3	4	6	10	14	20
GRAND TOTAL	393	4.9	26	1	2	3	6	10	14	30

457.1: OTHER LYMPHEDEMA

Type of Patients	Observed Patients	Avg. Stay	Variance	10th	25th	50th	75th	90th	95th	99th
1. SINGLE DX										
A. Not Operated										
0–19 Years	0									
20–34	1	3.0	0	3	3	3	3	3	3	3
35–49	0									
50–64	0									
65+	0									
B. Operated										
0–19 Years	1	1.0	0	1	1	1	1	1	1	1
20–34	0									
35–49	0									
50–64	0									
65+	0									
2. MULTIPLE DX										
A. Not Operated										
0–19 Years	4	10.2	250	1	1	2	4	34	34	34
20–34	11	4.3	8	3	3	3	6	7	11	11
35–49	28	3.1	3	1	2	2	4	6	7	7
50–64	56	4.9	16	2	2	4	6	9	12	23
65+	70	4.3	8	1	3	4	5	8	9	14
B. Operated										
0–19 Years	0									
20–34	1	5.0	0	5	5	5	5	5	5	5
35–49	5	12.2	110	3	5	6	21	26	26	26
50–64	6	2.8	1	1	2	3	4	4	4	4
65+	4	12.3	61	5	6	18	20	20	20	20
SUBTOTALS:										
1. SINGLE DX										
A. Not Operated	1	3.0	0	3	3	3	3	3	3	3
B. Operated	1	1.0	0	1	1	1	1	1	1	1
2. MULTIPLE DX										
A. Not Operated	169	4.5	15	1	2	3	6	8	10	23
B. Operated	16	8.3	64	2	3	5	18	21	26	26
1. SINGLE DX	2	2.0	2	1	1	1	3	3	3	3
2. MULTIPLE DX	185	4.8	20	1	2	3	6	8	12	26
A. NOT OPERATED	170	4.5	15	1	2	3	6	8	10	23
B. OPERATED	17	7.8	63	1	3	5	6	21	26	26
TOTAL										
0–19 Years	5	8.4	206	1	1	2	4	34	34	34
20–34	13	4.2	7	3	3	3	5	7	11	11
35–49	33	4.5	28	1	2	3	5	7	21	26
50–64	62	4.7	15	2	2	4	6	9	10	23
65+	74	4.7	13	3	3	4	6	8	14	20
GRAND TOTAL	187	4.8	20	1	2	3	6	8	12	26

Length of Stay by Diagnosis and Operation, Western Region, 2008

Western Region, October 2006–September 2007 Data, by Diagnosis

458: HYPOTENSION

Type of Patients	Observed Patients	Avg. Stay	Vari-ance	Percentiles 10th	25th	50th	75th	90th	95th	99th
1. SINGLE DX										
A. Not Operated										
0–19 Years	4	1.0	0	1	1	1	1	1	1	1
20–34	1	1.0	0		1	1	1	1	1	1
35–49	2	3.5	<1	3	3	3	4	4	4	4
50–64	4	2.7	6	1	1	2	3	6	6	6
65+	6	1.3	<1	1	1	1	1	3	3	3
B. Operated										
0–19 Years	0									
20–34	0									
35–49	0									
50–64	0									
65+	0									
2. MULTIPLE DX										
A. Not Operated										
0–19 Years	79	5.6	32	1	2	3	7	15	18	25
20–34	183	2.9	11	1	1	2	3	5	8	18
35–49	726	3.0	7	1	1	2	4	6	8	15
50–64	2,403	3.2	9	1	1	2	4	6	8	15
65+	8,237	3.2	7	1	2	2	4	6	8	13
B. Operated										
0–19 Years	2	11.0	196	1	1	11	21	21	21	21
20–34	5	1.8	<1	1	1	2	2	2	3	3
35–49	32	4.4	9	1	2	4	6	8	10	12
50–64	89	5.6	40	1	1	3	7	17	22	28
65+	226	7.1	50	1	3	5	9	16	22	39
SUBTOTALS:										
1. SINGLE DX										
A. Not Operated	17	1.8	2	1	1	1	3	4	6	6
B. Operated	0									
2. MULTIPLE DX										
A. Not Operated	11,628	3.2	8	1	1	2	4	6	8	14
B. Operated	354	6.5	45	1	2	4	8	15	21	34
1. SINGLE DX	17	1.8	2	1	1	1	3	4	6	6
2. MULTIPLE DX	11,982	3.3	9	1	1	2	4	6	8	15
A. NOT OPERATED	11,645	3.2	8	1	1	2	4	6	8	14
B. OPERATED	354	6.5	45	1	2	4	8	15	21	34
TOTAL										
0–19 Years	85	5.5	34	1	1	3	7	15	18	25
20–34	189	2.8	11	1	1	2	3	5	8	18
35–49	760	3.0	7	1	1	2	4	6	8	15
50–64	2,496	3.2	10	1	1	2	4	6	9	18
65+	8,469	3.3	9	1	2	3	4	6	8	14
GRAND TOTAL	11,999	3.3	9	1	1	2	4	6	8	15

458.0: ORTHOSTATIC HYPOTENSION

Type of Patients	Observed Patients	Avg. Stay	Vari-ance	Percentiles 10th	25th	50th	75th	90th	95th	99th
1. SINGLE DX										
A. Not Operated										
0–19 Years	4	1.0	0	1	1	1	1	1	1	1
20–34	0									
35–49	1	3.0	0	3	3	3	3	3	3	3
50–64	4	2.7	6	1	1	2	3	6	6	6
65+	3	1.7	1	1	1	1	1	3	3	3
B. Operated										
0–19 Years	0									
20–34	0									
35–49	0									
50–64	0									
65+	0									
2. MULTIPLE DX										
A. Not Operated										
0–19 Years	55	6.8	37	2	2	5	9	17	20	25
20–34	84	3.6	21	1	1	2	4	7	10	35
35–49	243	3.0	9	1	1	2	4	6	8	15
50–64	859	2.9	6	1	1	2	4	6	7	11
65+	3,894	3.2	7	1	2	3	4	6	8	12
B. Operated										
0–19 Years	1	21.0	0	21	21	21	21	21	21	21
20–34	2	1.5	<1	1	1	2	2	2	2	2
35–49	8	4.1	8	1	2	3	4	8	10	10
50–64	15	8.5	38	3	5	6	10	21	23	23
65+	85	7.5	28	3	4	6	10	15	18	>99
SUBTOTALS:										
1. SINGLE DX										
A. Not Operated	12	1.9	2	1	1	1	3	3	6	6
B. Operated	0									
2. MULTIPLE DX										
A. Not Operated	5,135	3.2	8	1	2	2	4	6	8	14
B. Operated	111	7.4	30	2	4	6	10	15	21	29
1. SINGLE DX	12	1.9	2	1	1	1	3	4	6	6
2. MULTIPLE DX	5,246	3.3	9	1	2	2	4	6	8	15
A. NOT OPERATED	5,147	3.2	8	1	2	2	4	6	8	14
B. OPERATED	111	7.4	30	2	4	6	10	15	21	29
TOTAL										
0–19 Years	60	6.7	40	1	2	5	9	18	20	25
20–34	86	3.6	20	1	1	2	4	7	10	35
35–49	252	3.0	9	1	1	2	4	6	8	15
50–64	878	3.0	7	1	2	2	4	6	8	12
65+	3,982	3.3	8	1	2	3	4	6	8	14
GRAND TOTAL	5,258	3.3	9	1	2	2	4	6	8	15

458.21: HEMODIALYSIS HYPOTENSION

Type of Patients	Observed Patients	Avg. Stay	Vari-ance	Percentiles 10th	25th	50th	75th	90th	95th	99th
1. SINGLE DX										
A. Not Operated										
0–19 Years	0									
20–34	0									
35–49	0									
50–64	0									
65+	0									
B. Operated										
0–19 Years	0									
20–34	0									
35–49	0									
50–64	0									
65+	0									
2. MULTIPLE DX										
A. Not Operated										
0–19 Years	0									
20–34	6	2.5	4	1	1	2	5	5	5	5
35–49	18	3.7	16	1	2	2	4	7	18	18
50–64	66	3.7	7	1	2	3	5	7	10	12
65+	160	3.2	7	1	1	2	4	7	10	13
B. Operated										
0–19 Years	0									
20–34	0									
35–49	2	9.0	18	6	6	12	12	12	12	12
50–64	6	7.0	69	1	2	4	9	23	23	23
65+	13	13.8	170	3	4	7	22	27	45	45
SUBTOTALS:										
1. SINGLE DX										
A. Not Operated	0									
B. Operated	0									
2. MULTIPLE DX										
A. Not Operated	250	3.3	8	1	1	2	4	7	10	13
B. Operated	21	11.4	130	2	4	6	16	26	27	45
1. SINGLE DX	0									
2. MULTIPLE DX	271	4.0	21	1	2	3	5	8	11	26
A. NOT OPERATED	250	3.3	8	1	1	2	4	7	10	13
B. OPERATED	21	11.4	130	2	4	6	16	26	27	45
TOTAL										
0–19 Years	0									
20–34	6	2.5	4	1	1	2	5	5	5	5
35–49	20	4.3	18	1	2	3	4	12	18	18
50–64	72	4.0	12	1	2	3	5	8	10	23
65+	173	4.0	26	1	2	4	8	11	11	27
GRAND TOTAL	271	4.0	21	1	2	3	5	8	11	26

Length of Stay by Diagnosis and Operation, Western Region, 2008

458.29: IATROGEN HYPOTENSION NEC

Type of Patients	Observed Patients	Avg. Stay	Variance	10th	25th	50th	75th	90th	95th	99th
1. SINGLE DX										
A. Not Operated										
0–19 Years	0									
20–34	0									
35–49	0									
50–64	0									
65+	2	1.0	0	1	1	1	1	1	1	1
B. Operated										
0–19 Years	0									
20–34	0									
35–49	0									
50–64	0									
65+	0									
2. MULTIPLE DX										
A. Not Operated										
0–19 Years	4	2.5	6	1	1	2	6	6	6	6
20–34	20	1.8	1	1	1	1	2	3	5	5
35–49	147	2.4	2	1	1	2	3	4	5	8
50–64	467	2.7	5	1	1	2	3	5	7	11
65+	1,354	2.7	4	1	1	2	3	5	7	11
B. Operated										
0–19 Years	1	1.0	0	1	1	1	1	1	1	1
20–34	3	2.0	<1	1	1	2	3	3	3	3
35–49	18	3.8	8	1	1	3	6	8	10	10
50–64	53	3.4	15	1	1	2	4	7	11	20
65+	85	4.7	36	1	1	3	5	13	14	39
SUBTOTALS:										
1. SINGLE DX										
A. Not Operated	2	1.0	0	1	1	1	1	1	1	1
B. Operated	0									
2. MULTIPLE DX										
A. Not Operated	1,992	2.7	4	1	1	2	3	5	7	11
B. Operated	160	4.1	25	1	1	3	5	9	14	30
1. SINGLE DX	2	1.0	0	1	1	1	1	1	1	1
2. MULTIPLE DX	2,152	2.8	6	1	1	2	3	5	7	12
A. NOT OPERATED	1,994	2.7	4	1	1	2	3	5	7	11
B. OPERATED	160	4.1	25	1	1	3	5	9	14	30
TOTAL										
0–19 Years	5	2.2	5	1	1	1	2	6	6	6
20–34	23	1.8	1	1	1	1	2	3	3	5
35–49	165	2.5	3	1	1	2	3	5	6	10
50–64	520	2.7	6	1	1	2	3	5	8	12
65+	1,441	2.8	6	1	1	2	3	5	7	13
GRAND TOTAL	2,154	2.8	6	1	1	2	3	5	7	12

458.8: HYPOTENSION NEC

Type of Patients	Observed Patients	Avg. Stay	Variance	10th	25th	50th	75th	90th	95th	99th
1. SINGLE DX										
A. Not Operated										
0–19 Years	0									
20–34	0									
35–49	1	4.0	0	4	4	4	4	4	4	4
50–64	0									
65+	0									
B. Operated										
0–19 Years	0									
20–34	0									
35–49	0									
50–64	0									
65+	0									
2. MULTIPLE DX										
A. Not Operated										
0–19 Years	6	4.2	29	1	1	3	3	15	15	15
20–34	15	2.2	2	1	1	3	3	4	5	5
35–49	56	3.2	6	1	1	2	4	8	9	10
50–64	170	4.1	18	1	2	3	5	9	11	20
65+	419	3.7	8	1	2	3	5	7	9	15
B. Operated										
0–19 Years	0									
20–34	0									
35–49	0									
50–64	1	1.0	0	1	1	1	1	1	1	1
65+	7	12.8	83	2	6	10	20	28	28	28
SUBTOTALS:										
1. SINGLE DX										
A. Not Operated	1	4.0	0	4	4	4	4	4	4	4
B. Operated	0									
2. MULTIPLE DX										
A. Not Operated	666	3.7	11	1	2	3	5	7	9	16
B. Operated	8	11.3	88	1	6	10	20	28	28	28
1. SINGLE DX	1	4.0	0	4	4	4	4	4	4	4
2. MULTIPLE DX	674	3.8	12	1	2	3	5	7	10	19
A. NOT OPERATED	667	3.7	11	1	2	3	5	7	9	16
B. OPERATED	8	11.3	88	1	6	10	20	28	28	28
TOTAL										
0–19 Years	6	4.2	29	1	1	3	3	15	15	15
20–34	15	2.2	2	1	1	3	3	4	5	5
35–49	57	3.3	6	1	1	2	4	8	9	10
50–64	171	4.0	18	1	2	3	5	9	11	20
65+	426	3.8	11	1	2	3	5	7	9	19
GRAND TOTAL	675	3.8	12	1	2	3	5	7	10	19

458.9: HYPOTENSION NOS

Type of Patients	Observed Patients	Avg. Stay	Variance	10th	25th	50th	75th	90th	95th	99th
1. SINGLE DX										
A. Not Operated										
0–19 Years	0									
20–34	1	1.0	0	1	1	1	1	1	1	1
35–49	0									
50–64	0									
65+	1	1.0	0	1	1	1	1	1	1	1
B. Operated										
0–19 Years	0									
20–34	0									
35–49	0									
50–64	0									
65+	0									
2. MULTIPLE DX										
A. Not Operated										
0–19 Years	14	2.0	2	1	1	2	2	4	6	6
20–34	57	2.4	3	1	1	2	3	4	6	8
35–49	257	3.0	6	1	1	2	4	6	8	14
50–64	832	3.5	12	1	1	2	4	7	9	18
65+	2,394	3.4	8	1	2	3	4	7	8	14
B. Operated										
0–19 Years	0									
20–34	0									
35–49	4	5.5	4	4	4	6	6	8	8	8
50–64	13	9.7	84	1	2	7	16	22	28	28
65+	36	8.5	59	2	4	6	11	18	29	34
SUBTOTALS:										
1. SINGLE DX										
A. Not Operated	2	1.0	0	1	1	1	1	1	1	1
B. Operated	0									
2. MULTIPLE DX										
A. Not Operated	3,554	3.3	9	1	2	3	4	7	8	15
B. Operated	53	8.6	60	2	3	6	12	20	28	34
1. SINGLE DX	2	1.0	0	1	1	1	1	1	1	1
2. MULTIPLE DX	3,607	3.4	10	1	2	3	4	7	9	16
A. NOT OPERATED	3,556	3.3	9	1	2	3	4	7	8	15
B. OPERATED	53	8.6	60	2	3	6	12	20	28	34
TOTAL										
0–19 Years	14	2.0	2	1	1	2	2	4	6	6
20–34	58	2.3	3	1	1	2	3	4	6	8
35–49	261	3.1	6	1	1	2	4	6	8	14
50–64	845	3.6	13	1	2	3	4	7	9	20
65+	2,431	3.4	9	1	2	3	4	7	9	15
GRAND TOTAL	3,609	3.4	10	1	2	3	4	7	9	16

Length of Stay by Diagnosis and Operation, Western Region, 2008

Western Region, October 2006–September 2007 Data, by Diagnosis

459: OTH CIRCULATORY DISORDER

Type of Patients	Observed Patients	Avg. Stay	Variance	10th	25th	50th	75th	90th	95th	99th
1. SINGLE DX										
A. Not Operated										
0–19 Years	1	1.0	0	1	1	1	1	1	1	1
20–34	3	2.7	1	2	2	2	4	4	4	4
35–49	1	1.0	1	1	1	1	1	1	1	1
50–64	4	1.5	1	1	1	1	3	3	3	3
65+	1	2.0	0	2	2	2	2	2	2	2
B. Operated										
0–19 Years	1	4.0	0	4	4	4	4	4	4	4
20–34	2	3.5	<1	3	3	3	4	4	4	4
35–49	3	2.3	1	2	3	3	4	4	4	4
50–64	4	1.3	<1	1	1	1	1	2	2	2
65+	1	1.0	0	1	1	1	1	1	1	1
2. MULTIPLE DX										
A. Not Operated										
0–19 Years	8	6.3	42	1	2	3	7	21	21	21
20–34	65	4.7	23	1	2	3	5	11	15	27
35–49	274	4.7	20	1	2	3	6	10	14	28
50–64	575	4.7	16	1	2	4	6	10	13	21
65+	1,214	4.9	17	2	2	4	6	9	12	20
B. Operated										
0–19 Years	2	1.0	0	1	1	1	1	1	1	1
20–34	34	5.9	30	2	2	4	7	12	19	24
35–49	103	6.4	41	1	2	5	8	15	17	33
50–64	183	7.7	63	1	3	5	9	17	23	42
65+	336	7.3	48	2	3	5	9	15	19	33
SUBTOTALS:										
1. SINGLE DX										
A. Not Operated	10	1.8	1	1	1	2	2	3	4	4
B. Operated	11	2.2	2	1	1	2	4	4	4	4
2. MULTIPLE DX										
A. Not Operated	2,136	4.8	18	1	2	4	6	9	12	21
B. Operated	658	7.2	50	1	3	5	9	15	21	35
1. SINGLE DX	21	2.0	1	1	1	2	3	4	4	4
2. MULTIPLE DX	2,794	5.4	26	1	2	4	7	10	15	28
A. NOT OPERATED	2,146	4.8	18	1	2	4	6	9	12	21
B. OPERATED	669	7.1	50	1	3	5	9	15	21	35
TOTAL										
0–19 Years	12	4.8	32	1	1	3	5	9	21	21
20–34	104	5.0	25	1	2	4	5	12	18	24
35–49	381	5.1	26	2	2	3	6	11	15	31
50–64	766	5.4	29	1	3	4	7	11	15	28
65+	1,552	5.4	25	3	3	4	7	10	14	29
GRAND TOTAL	2,815	5.4	26	1	2	4	7	10	15	28

459.0: HEMORRHAGE NOS

Type of Patients	Observed Patients	Avg. Stay	Variance	10th	25th	50th	75th	90th	95th	99th
1. SINGLE DX										
A. Not Operated										
0–19 Years	1	1.0	0	1	1	1	1	1	1	1
20–34	1	2.0	0	2	2	2	2	2	2	2
35–49	0									
50–64	1	1.0	0	1	1	1	1	1	1	1
65+	1	2.0	0	2	2	2	2	2	2	2
B. Operated										
0–19 Years	0									
20–34	2	3.5	<1	3	3	3	4	4	4	4
35–49	1	2.0	0	2	2	2	2	2	2	2
50–64	0									
65+	0									
2. MULTIPLE DX										
A. Not Operated										
0–19 Years	5	3.2	5	1	2	3	3	7	7	7
20–34	25	6.9	42	1	4	5	7	18	20	27
35–49	47	5.7	36	1	2	3	6	15	17	31
50–64	153	4.9	16	1	2	4	6	10	13	20
65+	443	5.3	19	2	3	4	7	9	12	25
B. Operated										
0–19 Years	0									
20–34	3	5.0	3	4	4	4	7	7	7	7
35–49	23	9.3	98	2	3	6	9	31	33	35
50–64	29	7.9	48	2	4	6	9	17	28	29
65+	78	8.8	67	2	5	7	10	17	29	51
SUBTOTALS:										
1. SINGLE DX										
A. Not Operated	4	1.5	<1	1	1	2	2	2	2	2
B. Operated	3	3.0	<1	2	2	3	4	4	4	4
2. MULTIPLE DX										
A. Not Operated	673	5.3	20	2	2	4	7	10	13	25
B. Operated	133	8.6	66	2	4	6	10	17	29	35
1. SINGLE DX	7	2.1	1	1	1	2	3	4	4	4
2. MULTIPLE DX	806	5.8	29	2	3	4	7	11	16	31
A. NOT OPERATED	677	5.2	20	2	2	4	6	10	13	25
B. OPERATED	136	8.5	66	2	4	6	9	17	29	35
TOTAL										
0–19 Years	6	2.8	5	1	1	3	3	7	7	7
20–34	31	6.3	36	1	3	4	7	15	20	27
35–49	71	6.8	57	1	2	3	8	16	31	35
50–64	183	5.4	22	2	2	4	7	11	14	28
65+	522	5.8	28	2	3	5	7	10	15	32
GRAND TOTAL	813	5.8	29	2	3	4	7	11	16	31

459.2: VEIN COMPRESSION

Type of Patients	Observed Patients	Avg. Stay	Variance	10th	25th	50th	75th	90th	95th	99th
1. SINGLE DX										
A. Not Operated										
0–19 Years	0									
20–34	0									
35–49	0									
50–64	0									
65+	0									
B. Operated										
0–19 Years	1	4.0	0	4	4	4	4	4	4	4
20–34	0									
35–49	1	1.0	0	1	1	1	1	1	1	1
50–64	2	1.0	0	1	1	1	1	1	1	1
65+	0									
2. MULTIPLE DX										
A. Not Operated										
0–19 Years	2	15.0	72	9	9	15	21	21	21	21
20–34	4	3.8	<1	3	4	4	4	4	4	4
35–49	28	3.8	15	1	2	2	5	11	12	18
50–64	42	5.4	20	2	2	4	6	13	14	20
65+	39	5.1	11	1	2	5	8	10	12	13
B. Operated										
0–19 Years	1	1.0	0	1	1	1	1	1	1	1
20–34	16	6.6	45	2	2	3	9	18	24	24
35–49	43	4.3	11	1	2	4	6	8	10	17
50–64	46	7.2	103	1	2	3	7	19	28	48
65+	43	4.2	17	1	2	3	5	8	11	24
SUBTOTALS:										
1. SINGLE DX										
A. Not Operated	0									
B. Operated	4	1.7	2	1	1	1	1	4	4	4
2. MULTIPLE DX										
A. Not Operated	115	5.0	17	1	2	4	7	11	13	20
B. Operated	149	5.4	46	1	2	3	6	11	18	42
1. SINGLE DX	4	1.7	2	1	1	1	1	4	4	4
2. MULTIPLE DX	264	5.2	33	1	2	3	6	11	14	28
A. NOT OPERATED	115	5.0	17	1	2	4	7	11	13	20
B. OPERATED	153	5.3	45	1	2	3	6	11	18	42
TOTAL										
0–19 Years	4	8.8	78	1	3	7	15	21	21	21
20–34	20	6.1	37	2	2	3	9	18	24	24
35–49	72	4.1	12	1	2	3	5	8	11	18
50–64	90	6.2	63	2	2	3	6	13	20	48
65+	82	4.7	14	2	2	4	7	9	11	24
GRAND TOTAL	268	5.2	33	1	2	3	6	11	14	28

459.81: VENOUS INSUFFICIENCY NOS

Type of Patients	Observed Patients	Avg. Stay	Variance	10th	25th	50th	75th	90th	95th	99th
1. SINGLE DX										
A. Not Operated										
0–19 Years	0									
20–34	2	3.0	2	2	2	2	4	4	4	4
35–49	1	1.0	0	1	1	1	1	1	1	1
50–64	3	1.7	1	1	1	1	3	3	3	3
65+	0									
B. Operated										
0–19 Years	0									
20–34	0									
35–49	0									
50–64	2	1.5	<1	1	1	1	2	2	2	2
65+	0									
2. MULTIPLE DX										
A. Not Operated										
0–19 Years	1	5.0	0	5	5	5	5	5	5	5
20–34	25	3.5	10	1	2	3	4	8	12	13
35–49	175	4.8	19	1	2	4	6	10	14	28
50–64	334	4.6	13	1	2	4	6	8	11	17
65+	658	4.7	17	2	2	4	6	8	11	22
B. Operated										
0–19 Years	0									
20–34	10	6.2	29	1	4	5	5	19	19	19
35–49	29	7.7	33	2	3	5	13	16	17	21
50–64	96	7.6	51	1	3	6	9	19	23	38
65+	167	7.8	52	1	4	6	10	15	21	33
SUBTOTALS:										
1. SINGLE DX										
A. Not Operated	6	2.0	2	1	1	2	3	4	4	4
B. Operated	2	1.5	<1	1	1	1	2	2	2	2
2. MULTIPLE DX										
A. Not Operated	1,193	4.7	16	1	2	4	6	9	11	21
B. Operated	302	7.7	48	1	3	6	10	16	21	32
1. SINGLE DX	8	1.9	1	1	1	2	3	4	4	4
2. MULTIPLE DX	1,495	5.3	24	1	2	4	6	10	14	28
A. NOT OPERATED	1,199	4.6	16	1	2	4	6	9	11	20
B. OPERATED	304	7.7	48	1	3	5	10	16	21	32
TOTAL										
0–19 Years	1	5.0	0	5	5	5	5	5	5	5
20–34	37	4.2	15	1	2	3	5	12	13	19
35–49	205	5.2	22	1	2	4	7	11	15	23
50–64	435	5.2	22	1	2	4	7	10	15	23
65+	825	5.3	26	1	3	4	8	10	14	29
GRAND TOTAL	1,503	5.3	24	1	2	4	6	10	14	28

460: ACUTE NASOPHARYNGITIS

Type of Patients	Observed Patients	Avg. Stay	Variance	10th	25th	50th	75th	90th	95th	99th
1. SINGLE DX										
A. Not Operated										
0–19 Years	0									
20–34	0									
35–49	0									
50–64	0									
65+	0									
B. Operated										
0–19 Years	0									
20–34	0									
35–49	0									
50–64	0									
65+	0									
2. MULTIPLE DX										
A. Not Operated										
0–19 Years	20	2.0	<1	1	1	2	3	3	3	3
20–34	1	3.0	0	3	3	3	3	3	3	3
35–49	1	4.0	0	4	4	4	4	4	4	4
50–64	6	1.8	<1	1	1	2	2	3	3	3
65+	2	5.0	32	1	1	5	9	9	9	9
B. Operated										
0–19 Years	0									
20–34	0									
35–49	0									
50–64	0									
65+	0									
SUBTOTALS:										
1. SINGLE DX										
A. Not Operated	0									
B. Operated	0									
2. MULTIPLE DX										
A. Not Operated	30	2.3	2	1	1	2	3	3	4	9
B. Operated	0									
1. SINGLE DX	0									
2. MULTIPLE DX	30	2.3	2	1	1	2	3	3	4	9
A. NOT OPERATED	30	2.3	2	1	1	2	3	3	4	9
B. OPERATED	0									
TOTAL										
0–19 Years	20	2.0	<1	1	1	2	3	3	3	3
20–34	1	3.0	0	3	3	3	3	3	3	3
35–49	1	4.0	0	4	4	4	4	4	4	4
50–64	6	1.8	<1	1	1	2	2	3	3	3
65+	2	5.0	32	1	1	5	9	9	9	9
GRAND TOTAL	30	2.3	2	1	1	2	3	3	4	9

461: ACUTE SINUSITIS

Type of Patients	Observed Patients	Avg. Stay	Variance	10th	25th	50th	75th	90th	95th	99th
1. SINGLE DX										
A. Not Operated										
0–19 Years	9	1.9	<1	1	1	2	2	3	3	3
20–34	5	3.2	2	2	2	3	4	5	5	5
35–49	2	1.5	<1	1	1	2	2	2	2	2
50–64	0									
65+	0									
B. Operated										
0–19 Years	0									
20–34	1	2.0	0	2	2	2	2	2	2	2
35–49	0									
50–64	0									
65+	0									
2. MULTIPLE DX										
A. Not Operated										
0–19 Years	94	2.9	3	1	2	3	4	5	6	9
20–34	95	3.2	8	1	2	3	4	5	7	20
35–49	109	2.9	4	1	2	2	4	5	7	9
50–64	124	3.2	6	1	2	2	4	7	7	11
65+	183	3.2	4	1	2	3	4	6	7	10
B. Operated										
0–19 Years	31	5.5	8	2	4	5	7	9	10	15
20–34	17	6.6	18	2	4	5	7	15	16	16
35–49	28	4.6	8	1	3	4	6	8	8	14
50–64	22	6.7	47	2	2	5	8	12	21	30
65+	16	6.4	22	1	3	6	7	15	16	16
SUBTOTALS:										
1. SINGLE DX										
A. Not Operated	16	2.3	1	1	2	2	3	4	5	5
B. Operated	1	2.0	0	2	2	2	2	2	2	2
2. MULTIPLE DX										
A. Not Operated	605	3.1	5	1	2	2	4	6	7	11
B. Operated	114	5.8	19	2	3	5	7	10	15	21
1. SINGLE DX	17	2.2	1	1	2	2	3	4	5	5
2. MULTIPLE DX	719	3.5	8	1	2	3	4	7	8	15
A. NOT OPERATED	621	3.1	5	1	2	2	4	6	7	11
B. OPERATED	115	5.8	19	2	3	5	7	10	15	21
TOTAL										
0–19 Years	134	3.4	5	1	2	3	4	6	8	10
20–34	118	3.7	11	2	2	3	4	6	12	17
35–49	139	3.3	6	1	2	3	4	6	8	14
50–64	146	3.7	13	1	2	3	5	7	9	21
65+	199	3.4	6	1	2	3	4	6	8	16
GRAND TOTAL	736	3.5	8	1	2	3	4	7	8	15

Length of Stay by Diagnosis and Operation, Western Region, 2008

Western Region, October 2006–September 2007 Data, by Diagnosis

461.0: AC MAXILLARY SINUSITIS

Type of Patients	Observed Patients	Avg. Stay	Vari-ance	Percentiles						
				10th	25th	50th	75th	90th	95th	99th
1. SINGLE DX										
A. *Not Operated*										
0–19 Years	1	3.0	0	3	3	3	3	3	3	3
20–34	1	4.0	0	4	4	4	4	4	4	4
35–49	1	2.0	0	2	2	2	2	2	2	2
50–64	0									
65+	0									
B. *Operated*										
0–19 Years	0									
20–34	1	2.0	0	2	2	2	2	2	2	2
35–49	0									
50–64	0									
65+	0									
2. MULTIPLE DX										
A. *Not Operated*										
0–19 Years	26	2.7	1	1	2	3	3	4	5	6
20–34	21	3.1	4	2	2	3	3	4	7	10
35–49	34	3.1	3	1	2	3	5	6	7	7
50–64	45	3.0	5	1	2	2	4	7	7	10
65+	63	3.7	6	2	2	3	5	6	7	17
B. *Operated*										
0–19 Years	3	4.7	<1	4	4	5	5	5	5	5
20–34	1	5.0	0	5	5	5	5	5	5	5
35–49	6	5.8	3	4	4	5	7	8	8	8
50–64	6	3.7	7	2	2	2	6	8	8	8
65+	6	8.8	43	1	3	13	15	16	16	16
SUBTOTALS:										
1. SINGLE DX										
A. *Not Operated*	3	3.0	<1	2	2	3	3	3	4	4
B. *Operated*	1	2.0	0	2	2	2	2	2	2	2
2. MULTIPLE DX										
A. *Not Operated*	189	3.2	4	1	2	3	4	6	7	10
B. *Operated*	22	5.9	17	2	3	5	7	13	15	16
1. SINGLE DX	4	2.8	<1	2	2	2	4	4	4	4
2. MULTIPLE DX	211	3.5	6	1	2	3	5	7	7	15
A. NOT OPERATED	192	3.2	4	1	2	3	4	6	7	10
B. OPERATED	23	5.7	17	2	2	5	7	13	15	16
TOTAL										
0–19 Years	30	2.9	2	1	2	3	3	5	5	6
20–34	24	3.2	4	2	2	3	4	5	7	10
35–49	41	3.5	4	1	2	3	5	7	7	7
50–64	51	3.1	5	1	2	2	5	7	7	10
65+	69	4.2	11	2	3	3	5	7	13	17
GRAND TOTAL	215	3.5	6	1	2	3	5	7	7	15

461.8: OTHER ACUTE SINUSITIS

Type of Patients	Observed Patients	Avg. Stay	Vari-ance	Percentiles						
				10th	25th	50th	75th	90th	95th	99th
1. SINGLE DX										
A. *Not Operated*										
0–19 Years	2	2.0	0	2	2	2	2	2	2	2
20–34	2	3.5	4	2	2	5	5	5	5	5
35–49	1	1.0	0	1	1	1	1	1	1	1
50–64	0									
65+	0									
B. *Operated*										
0–19 Years	0									
20–34	0									
35–49	0									
50–64	0									
65+	0									
2. MULTIPLE DX										
A. *Not Operated*										
0–19 Years	23	3.2	4	1	2	3	4	5	7	9
20–34	27	4.8	20	2	2	3	5	12	17	20
35–49	21	3.8	9	1	2	3	6	6	7	15
50–64	19	4.2	6	2	2	3	6	7	11	11
65+	34	2.8	2	1	2	2	4	5	5	6
B. *Operated*										
0–19 Years	16	5.6	12	3	3	5	6	10	15	15
20–34	2	5.0	2	4	4	4	6	6	6	6
35–49	10	5.2	14	1	2	5	6	14	14	14
50–64	4	8.0	75	3	3	5	5	21	21	21
65+	4	4.5	14	1	1	2	6	9	9	9
SUBTOTALS:										
1. SINGLE DX										
A. *Not Operated*	5	2.4	2	1	2	2	2	5	5	5
B. *Operated*	0									
2. MULTIPLE DX										
A. *Not Operated*	124	3.7	8	1	2	3	4	6	7	17
B. *Operated*	36	5.6	17	2	3	5	6	10	15	21
1. SINGLE DX	5	2.4	2	1	2	2	2	5	5	5
2. MULTIPLE DX	160	4.1	11	2	2	3	5	7	11	20
A. NOT OPERATED	129	3.6	8	1	2	3	4	6	7	17
B. OPERATED	36	5.6	17	2	3	5	6	10	15	21
TOTAL										
0–19 Years	41	4.1	8	2	2	3	5	7	9	15
20–34	31	4.7	18	2	2	4	5	7	17	20
35–49	32	4.1	11	1	2	3	5	7	14	15
50–64	23	4.8	17	2	3	4	6	7	11	21
65+	38	3.0	3	1	2	2	4	5	6	9
GRAND TOTAL	165	4.0	11	2	2	3	5	7	10	20

461.9: ACUTE SINUSITIS NOS

Type of Patients	Observed Patients	Avg. Stay	Vari-ance	Percentiles						
				10th	25th	50th	75th	90th	95th	99th
1. SINGLE DX										
A. *Not Operated*										
0–19 Years	4	1.8	<1	1	1	2	3	3	3	3
20–34	3	3.0	0	3	3	3	3	3	3	3
35–49	0									
50–64	0									
65+	0									
B. *Operated*										
0–19 Years	0									
20–34	0									
35–49	0									
50–64	0									
65+	0									
2. MULTIPLE DX										
A. *Not Operated*										
0–19 Years	20	2.8	3	1	2	2	4	5	8	8
20–34	24	2.1	3	1	1	2	3	3	3	5
35–49	32	2.6	3	1	1	2	3	5	7	8
50–64	36	2.7	7	1	1	2	3	6	11	13
65+	56	2.6	3	1	2	2	3	4	7	9
B. *Operated*										
0–19 Years	1	5.0	0	5	5	5	5	5	5	5
20–34	4	10.3	37	5	5	15	15	16	16	16
35–49	2	4.5	<1	4	4	4	5	5	5	5
50–64	2	5.0	18	2	2	5	8	8	8	8
65+	1	5.0	0	5	5	5	5	5	5	5
SUBTOTALS:										
1. SINGLE DX										
A. *Not Operated*	5	2.0	1	1	1	2	3	3	3	3
B. *Operated*	0									
2. MULTIPLE DX										
A. *Not Operated*	168	2.6	4	1	1	2	3	5	6	11
B. *Operated*	10	7.0	22	4	5	5	8	10	16	16
1. SINGLE DX	5	2.0	1	1	1	2	3	3	3	3
2. MULTIPLE DX	178	2.8	6	1	1	2	3	5	8	15
A. NOT OPERATED	173	2.5	4	1	1	2	3	5	6	11
B. OPERATED	10	7.0	22	4	5	5	8	15	16	16
TOTAL										
0–19 Years	25	2.7	3	1	1	2	4	5	5	8
20–34	29	3.2	13	1	1	2	3	5	15	16
35–49	34	2.7	3	1	1	2	4	5	7	8
50–64	38	2.8	8	1	1	2	3	6	11	13
65+	57	2.6	3	2	2	3	3	5	7	9
GRAND TOTAL	183	2.8	5	1	1	2	3	5	7	15

Western Region, October 2006–September 2007 Data, by Diagnosis

462: ACUTE PHARYNGITIS

Type of Patients	Observed Patients	Avg. Stay	Variance	10th	25th	50th	75th	90th	95th	99th
1. SINGLE DX										
A. Not Operated										
0–19 Years	33	1.8	<1	1	1	2	2	3	3	4
20–34	18	1.7	<1	1	1	1	2	3	4	4
35–49	3	1.3	<1	1	1	1	2	2	2	2
50–64	0									
65+	0									
B. Operated										
0–19 Years	0									
20–34	0									
35–49	0									
50–64	0									
65+	0									
2. MULTIPLE DX										
A. Not Operated										
0–19 Years	191	2.1	2	1	1	2	2	4	4	12
20–34	144	2.3	6	1	1	2	3	3	5	13
35–49	90	2.5	3	1	1	2	3	4	6	9
50–64	84	2.3	2	1	1	2	3	5	6	7
65+	86	3.3	20	1	1	2	4	6	8	40
B. Operated										
0–19 Years	2	3.5	<1	3	3	4	4	4	4	4
20–34	2	2.0	0	2	2	2	2	2	2	2
35–49	2	4.5	24	1	1	1	8	8	8	8
50–64	0									
65+	1	5.0	0	5	5	5	5	5	5	5
SUBTOTALS:										
1. SINGLE DX										
A. Not Operated	54	1.7	<1	1	1	2	2	3	3	4
B. Operated	0									
2. MULTIPLE DX										
A. Not Operated	595	2.4	6	1	1	2	3	4	6	10
B. Operated	7	3.6	6	1	2	3	5	8	8	8
1. SINGLE DX	54	1.7	<1	1	1	2	2	3	3	4
2. MULTIPLE DX	602	2.4	6	1	1	2	3	4	6	10
A. NOT OPERATED	649	2.4	6	1	1	2	3	4	5	10
B. OPERATED	7	3.6	6	2	2	3	5	8	8	8
TOTAL										
0–19 Years	226	2.1	2	1	1	2	2	3	4	7
20–34	164	2.3	6	1	1	2	3	4	5	13
35–49	95	2.5	3	1	1	2	3	5	6	9
50–64	84	2.3	2	1	1	2	3	5	6	7
65+	87	3.3	20	1	1	2	4	6	8	40
GRAND TOTAL	656	2.4	6	1	1	2	3	4	6	10

463: ACUTE TONSILLITIS

Type of Patients	Observed Patients	Avg. Stay	Variance	10th	25th	50th	75th	90th	95th	99th
1. SINGLE DX										
A. Not Operated										
0–19 Years	54	1.7	<1	1	1	2	2	3	3	5
20–34	34	1.4	<1	1	1	1	2	2	3	4
35–49	9	1.8	<1	1	1	2	2	3	3	3
50–64	3	1.7	<1	1	1	2	2	2	2	2
65+	0									
B. Operated										
0–19 Years	9	1.9	2	1	1	2	2	5	5	5
20–34	8	2.9	2	1	2	3	4	5	5	5
35–49	1	6.0	0	6	6	6	6	6	6	6
50–64	0									
65+	0									
2. MULTIPLE DX										
A. Not Operated										
0–19 Years	227	2.0	1	1	1	2	3	3	4	6
20–34	216	2.2	2	1	1	2	3	4	6	7
35–49	88	2.3	3	1	1	2	3	4	5	15
50–64	36	2.3	3	1	1	2	3	4	5	11
65+	6	3.0	<1	2	2	3	4	4	4	4
B. Operated										
0–19 Years	52	2.2	2	1	1	2	3	4	6	8
20–34	26	2.6	4	1	1	2	3	6	6	9
35–49	13	2.0	2	1	1	2	2	4	6	6
50–64	3	2.0	0	2	2	2	2	2	2	2
65+	2	2.0	0	2	2	2	2	2	2	2
SUBTOTALS:										
1. SINGLE DX										
A. Not Operated	100	1.6	<1	1	1	2	2	3	3	4
B. Operated	18	2.6	3	1	1	3	3	5	6	6
2. MULTIPLE DX										
A. Not Operated	573	2.2	2	1	1	2	3	4	5	7
B. Operated	96	2.3	3	1	1	2	3	5	6	9
1. SINGLE DX	118	1.7	<1	1	1	2	2	3	4	5
2. MULTIPLE DX	669	2.2	2	1	1	2	3	4	5	7
A. NOT OPERATED	673	2.1	2	1	1	2	3	4	4	7
B. OPERATED	114	2.3	3	1	1	2	3	5	6	8
TOTAL										
0–19 Years	342	2.0	1	1	1	2	2	3	4	6
20–34	284	2.2	2	1	1	2	3	4	5	7
35–49	111	2.3	3	1	1	2	3	5	5	9
50–64	42	2.3	3	1	1	2	3	3	4	11
65+	8	2.8	<1	2	2	2	3	4	4	4
GRAND TOTAL	787	2.1	2	1	1	2	3	4	5	7

464: AC LARYNGITIS/TRACHEITIS

Type of Patients	Observed Patients	Avg. Stay	Variance	10th	25th	50th	75th	90th	95th	99th
1. SINGLE DX										
A. Not Operated										
0–19 Years	831	1.3	<1	1	1	1	2	2	3	4
20–34	22	1.9	<1	1	1	2	2	3	3	6
35–49	28	2.0	<1	1	1	2	2	3	3	5
50–64	10	1.8	<1	1	1	2	2	3	3	3
65+	2	1.5	<1	1	1	2	2	2	2	2
B. Operated										
0–19 Years	0									
20–34	0									
35–49	0									
50–64	0									
65+	0									
2. MULTIPLE DX										
A. Not Operated										
0–19 Years	1,406	1.9	3	1	1	1	2	3	4	10
20–34	87	2.9	9	1	1	2	3	6	10	20
35–49	151	3.0	5	1	1	2	4	5	7	9
50–64	147	3.4	13	1	2	2	4	7	9	16
65+	116	3.5	11	1	2	2	4	6	10	20
B. Operated										
0–19 Years	4	5.7	25	1	1	2	9	11	11	11
20–34	3	10.3	185	1	1	4	26	26	26	26
35–49	7	10.6	50	3	6	9	15	24	24	24
50–64	8	15.8	186	4	5	9	19	45	45	45
65+	3	4.0	0	4	4	4	4	4	4	4
SUBTOTALS:										
1. SINGLE DX										
A. Not Operated	893	1.4	<1	1	1	1	2	2	3	4
B. Operated	0									
2. MULTIPLE DX										
A. Not Operated	1,907	2.2	5	1	1	2	2	4	6	12
B. Operated	25	10.6	104	2	4	7	14	24	26	45
1. SINGLE DX	893	1.4	<1	1	1	1	2	2	3	4
2. MULTIPLE DX	1,932	2.3	7	1	1	2	3	4	6	14
A. NOT OPERATED	2,800	2.0	4	1	1	1	2	3	5	10
B. OPERATED	25	10.6	104	2	4	7	14	24	26	45
TOTAL										
0–19 Years	2,241	1.7	2	1	1	1	2	3	4	8
20–34	112	2.9	12	1	1	2	3	5	10	20
35–49	186	3.1	8	1	1	2	4	6	8	16
50–64	165	3.9	26	2	2	3	4	8	12	31
65+	121	3.5	11	2	2	4	6	7	7	20
GRAND TOTAL	2,825	2.0	5	1	1	1	2	4	5	12

Length of Stay by Diagnosis and Operation, Western Region, 2008

Western Region, October 2006–September 2007 Data, by Diagnosis

464.30: AC EPIGLOTTITIS S OBSTR

Type of Patients	Observed Patients	Avg. Stay	Vari-ance	10th	25th	50th	75th	90th	95th	99th
1. SINGLE DX										
A. Not Operated										
0–19 Years	3	1.3	<1	1	1	1	2	2	2	2
20–34	15	1.9	2	1	1	2	2	2	6	6
35–49	25	1.9	<1	1	1	2	2	3	3	5
50–64	7	1.7	<1	1	1	2	2	3	3	3
65+	1	2.0	0	2	2	2	2	2	2	2
B. Operated										
0–19 Years	0									
20–34	0									
35–49	0									
50–64	0									
65+	0									
2. MULTIPLE DX										
A. Not Operated										
0–19 Years	16	1.9	<1	1	1	2	2	3	4	4
20–34	55	2.2	2	1	1	2	3	3	4	10
35–49	83	2.4	2	1	1	2	3	4	5	6
50–64	65	2.7	2	1	2	2	3	5	5	9
65+	40	2.8	4	1	2	2	4	5	7	11
B. Operated										
0–19 Years	3	10.3	185	1	1	4	26	26	26	26
20–34	1	6.0	0	6	6	6	6	6	6	6
35–49	1	7.0	0	7	7	7	7	7	7	7
50–64	1	4.0	0	4	4	4	4	4	4	4
65+										
SUBTOTALS:										
1. SINGLE DX										
A. Not Operated	51	1.9	1	1	1	2	2	3	3	
B. Operated	0									
2. MULTIPLE DX										
A. Not Operated	259	2.5	2	1	1	2	3	4	5	9
B. Operated	6	8.0	82	1	4	4	7	26	26	26
1. SINGLE DX	51	1.9	1	1	1	2	2	3	3	
2. MULTIPLE DX	265	2.6	5	1	1	2	3	4	5	10
A. NOT OPERATED	310	2.4	2	1	1	2	3	4	5	7
B. OPERATED	6	8.0	82	1	4	4	7	26	26	26
TOTAL										
0–19 Years	19	1.8	<1	1	1	2	2	3	4	4
20–34	73	2.5	10	1	1	2	3	3	6	26
35–49	109	2.3	2	1	1	2	3	4	5	6
50–64	73	2.7	2	1	2	2	3	5	6	9
65+	42	2.8	4	1	2	2	4	5	6	11
GRAND TOTAL	316	2.5	4	1	1	2	3	4	5	9

464.4: CROUP

Type of Patients	Observed Patients	Avg. Stay	Vari-ance	10th	25th	50th	75th	90th	95th	99th
1. SINGLE DX										
A. Not Operated										
0–19 Years	803	1.3	<1	1	1	1	2	2	3	4
20–34	0									
35–49	0									
50–64	0									
65+	0									
B. Operated										
0–19 Years	0									
20–34	0									
35–49	0									
50–64	0									
65+	0									
2. MULTIPLE DX										
A. Not Operated										
0–19 Years	1,296	1.7	1	1	1	1	2	3	4	6
20–34	2	2.0	2	1	1	3	3	3	3	3
35–49	1	1.0	0	1	1	1	1	1	1	1
50–64	0									
65+	0									
B. Operated										
0–19 Years	2	6.5	40	2	2	2	11	11	11	11
20–34	0									
35–49	0									
50–64	0									
65+	0									
SUBTOTALS:										
1. SINGLE DX										
A. Not Operated	803	1.3	<1	1	1	1	2	2	3	4
B. Operated	0									
2. MULTIPLE DX										
A. Not Operated	1,299	1.7	1	1	1	1	2	3	4	6
B. Operated	2	6.5	40	2	2	2	11	11	11	11
1. SINGLE DX	803	1.3	<1	1	1	1	2	2	3	4
2. MULTIPLE DX	1,301	1.7	1	1	1	1	2	3	4	6
A. NOT OPERATED	2,102	1.6	1	1	1	1	2	3	3	5
B. OPERATED	2	6.5	40	2	2	2	11	11	11	11
TOTAL										
0–19 Years	2,101	1.6	1	1	1	2	2	3	3	6
20–34	2	2.0	2	1	1	3	3	3	3	3
35–49	1	1.0	0	1	1	1	1	1	1	1
50–64	0									
65+	0									
GRAND TOTAL	2,104	1.6	1	1	1	2	2	3	3	6

465: AC URI MULT SITES/NOS

Type of Patients	Observed Patients	Avg. Stay	Vari-ance	10th	25th	50th	75th	90th	95th	99th
1. SINGLE DX										
A. Not Operated										
0–19 Years	323	1.7	<1	1	1	2	2	3	3	5
20–34	8	2.1	2	1	1	2	2	5	5	5
35–49	4	1.8	<1	1	1	2	3	3	3	3
50–64	1	1.0	0	1	1	1	1	1	1	1
65+	2	1.5	<1	1	1	1	2	2	2	2
B. Operated										
0–19 Years	2	1.5	<1	1	1	2	2	2	2	2
20–34	0									
35–49	0									
50–64	0									
65+	0									
2. MULTIPLE DX										
A. Not Operated										
0–19 Years	1,414	2.2	4	1	1	2	3	4	5	8
20–34	150	2.4	3	1	1	2	3	5	6	10
35–49	242	2.2	9	1	1	2	3	4	4	8
50–64	308	2.2	2	1	1	2	3	4	5	7
65+	541	2.6	3	1	1	2	3	5	6	8
B. Operated										
0–19 Years	3	10.1	193	2	2	2	26	26	26	26
20–34	5	2.6	1	1	2	3	3	4	4	4
35–49	2	5.5	24	2	2	6	9	9	9	9
50–64	2	4.0	0	4	4	4	4	4	4	4
65+	2	4.0	8	2	2	4	6	6	6	6
SUBTOTALS:										
1. SINGLE DX										
A. Not Operated	338	1.7	<1	1	1	2	2	3	3	5
B. Operated	2	1.5	<1	1	1	2	2	2	2	2
2. MULTIPLE DX										
A. Not Operated	2,655	2.3	4	1	1	2	3	4	5	8
B. Operated	14	5.0	41	2	2	3	4	9	26	26
1. SINGLE DX	340	1.7	<1	1	1	2	2	3	3	5
2. MULTIPLE DX	2,669	2.3	4	1	1	2	3	4	5	8
A. NOT OPERATED	2,993	2.2	4	1	1	2	3	4	5	8
B. OPERATED	16	4.6	37	1	2	3	4	9	26	26
TOTAL										
0–19 Years	1,742	2.1	4	1	1	2	2	4	4	8
20–34	163	2.4	3	1	1	2	3	4	6	10
35–49	248	2.2	9	1	1	2	3	4	5	8
50–64	311	2.3	2	1	1	2	3	4	5	7
65+	545	2.6	3	1	1	2	3	5	6	8
GRAND TOTAL	3,009	2.2	4	1	1	2	3	4	5	8

Length of Stay by Diagnosis and Operation, Western Region, 2008

Western Region, October 2006–September 2007 Data, by Diagnosis

465.8: ACUTE URI MULT SITES NEC

Type of Patients	Observed Patients	Avg. Stay	Vari-ance	10th	25th	50th	75th	90th	95th	99th
1. SINGLE DX										
A. Not Operated										
0–19 Years	10	1.8	2	1	1	2	2	2	5	5
20–34	4	2.8	3	1	2	3	3	5	5	5
35–49	2	2.5	<1	2	2	3	3	3	3	3
50–64	1	1.0	0	1	1	1	1	1	1	1
65+	0									
B. Operated										
0–19 Years	1	1.0	0	1	1	1	1	1	1	1
20–34	0									
35–49	0									
50–64	0									
65+	0									
2. MULTIPLE DX										
A. Not Operated										
0–19 Years	33	2.1	1	1	1	2	3	4	4	5
20–34	18	2.4	1	1	2	2	3	4	5	5
35–49	15	1.9	<1	1	1	2	2	3	3	3
50–64	10	2.9	5	1	1	2	4	7	7	7
65+	1	3.0	0	3	3	3	3	3	3	3
B. Operated										
0–19 Years	0									
20–34	5	2.6	1	1	2	3	3	4	4	4
35–49	1	2.0	0	2	2	2	2	2	2	2
50–64	0									
65+	1	2.0	0	2	2	2	2	2	2	2
SUBTOTALS:										
1. SINGLE DX										
A. Not Operated	17	2.1	2	1	1	2	2	5	5	5
B. Operated	1	1.0	0	1	1	1	1	1	1	1
2. MULTIPLE DX										
A. Not Operated	77	2.2	1	1	1	2	3	4	5	7
B. Operated	7	2.4	<1	1	2	3	3	4	4	4
1. SINGLE DX	18	2.0	2	1	1	2	2	5	5	5
2. MULTIPLE DX	84	2.3	1	1	1	2	3	4	4	7
A. NOT OPERATED	94	2.2	2	1	1	2	3	4	5	7
B. OPERATED	8	2.3	1	1	2	3	3	4	4	4
TOTAL										
0–19 Years	44	2.0	1	1	1	2	2	4	4	5
20–34	27	2.5	1	1	2	2	3	4	5	5
35–49	18	1.9	<1	1	1	2	2	3	3	3
50–64	11	2.7	4	1	1	2	4	6	7	7
65+	2	2.5	<1	2	2	3	3	3	3	3
GRAND TOTAL	102	2.2	1	1	1	2	3	4	5	6

465.9: ACUTE URI NOS

Type of Patients	Observed Patients	Avg. Stay	Vari-ance	10th	25th	50th	75th	90th	95th	99th
1. SINGLE DX										
A. Not Operated										
0–19 Years	313	1.7	<1	1	1	2	2	3	3	4
20–34	3	1.3	<1	1	1	2	2	2	2	2
35–49	2	1.0	0	1	1	1	1	1	1	1
50–64	0									
65+	2	1.5	<1	1	1	1	2	2	2	2
B. Operated										
0–19 Years	1	2.0	0	2	2	2	2	2	2	2
20–34	0									
35–49	0									
50–64	0									
65+	0									
2. MULTIPLE DX										
A. Not Operated										
0–19 Years	1,380	2.2	4	1	1	2	3	4	5	9
20–34	131	2.4	3	1	1	2	3	5	6	10
35–49	221	2.2	10	1	1	2	3	4	4	8
50–64	295	2.2	2	1	1	2	3	4	5	7
65+	539	2.6	3	1	1	3	3	5	6	8
B. Operated										
0–19 Years	3	10.1	193	2	2	2	26	26	26	26
20–34	0									
35–49	1	9.0	0	9	9	9	9	9	9	9
50–64	2	4.0	0	4	4	4	4	4	4	4
65+	1	6.0	0	6	6	6	6	6	6	6
SUBTOTALS:										
1. SINGLE DX										
A. Not Operated	320	1.7	<1	1	1	2	2	3	3	4
B. Operated	1	2.0	0	2	2	2	2	2	2	2
2. MULTIPLE DX										
A. Not Operated	2,566	2.3	4	1	1	2	3	4	5	8
B. Operated	7	7.6	72	2	2	4	9	26	26	26
1. SINGLE DX	321	1.7	<1	1	1	2	2	3	3	4
2. MULTIPLE DX	2,573	2.3	4	1	1	2	3	4	5	8
A. NOT OPERATED	2,886	2.2	4	1	1	2	3	4	5	8
B. OPERATED	8	6.9	66	2	2	4	9	26	26	26
TOTAL										
0–19 Years	1,697	2.1	4	1	1	2	3	4	4	8
20–34	134	2.4	3	1	1	2	3	5	6	10
35–49	224	2.2	10	1	1	2	3	4	4	8
50–64	297	2.2	2	1	1	2	3	4	5	7
65+	542	2.6	3	1	1	3	3	5	6	8
GRAND TOTAL	2,894	2.2	4	1	1	2	3	4	5	8

466: AC BRONCHITIS/BRONCHIOL

Type of Patients	Observed Patients	Avg. Stay	Vari-ance	10th	25th	50th	75th	90th	95th	99th
1. SINGLE DX										
A. Not Operated										
0–19 Years	4,354	2.5	2	1	1	2	3	4	5	7
20–34	5	1.8	2	1	1	1	2	4	4	4
35–49	8	2.1	2	1	1	2	3	5	5	5
50–64	10	2.0	2	1	1	1	3	3	5	5
65+	8	1.9	2	1	1	1	2	4	4	4
B. Operated										
0–19 Years	3	1.7	<1	1	1	2	2	2	2	2
20–34	0									
35–49	0									
50–64	0									
65+	0									
2. MULTIPLE DX										
A. Not Operated										
0–19 Years	12,267	3.1	6	1	2	3	4	6	7	11
20–34	300	3.9	19	1	2	3	4	9	14	23
35–49	696	3.0	5	1	1	2	4	5	7	13
50–64	1,015	2.9	5	1	1	2	4	5	7	11
65+	2,893	3.3	7	1	2	3	4	6	7	12
B. Operated										
0–19 Years	13	14.0	401	2	3	4	16	28	75	75
20–34	5	9.4	33	4	5	8	12	18	18	18
35–49	13	6.6	44	1	3	4	7	14	25	25
50–64	15	6.9	18	2	3	7	9	14	15	15
65+	27	6.5	17	3	4	5	8	11	11	22
SUBTOTALS:										
1. SINGLE DX										
A. Not Operated	4,385	2.5	2	1	1	2	3	4	5	7
B. Operated	3	1.7	<1	1	1	2	2	2	2	2
2. MULTIPLE DX										
A. Not Operated	17,171	3.2	6	1	2	3	4	6	7	12
B. Operated	73	8.1	93	2	4	5	9	15	22	75
1. SINGLE DX	4,388	2.5	2	1	1	2	3	4	5	7
2. MULTIPLE DX	17,244	3.2	7	1	2	3	4	6	7	12
A. NOT OPERATED	21,556	3.0	5	1	2	2	4	5	7	11
B. OPERATED	76	7.9	91	2	3	5	9	15	22	75
TOTAL										
0–19 Years	16,637	3.0	5	1	2	2	4	5	7	11
20–34	310	4.0	19	1	2	3	4	9	14	22
35–49	717	3.0	6	1	1	2	4	5	7	14
50–64	1,040	3.0	5	1	1	2	4	6	7	12
65+	2,928	3.4	7	1	2	3	4	6	8	12
GRAND TOTAL	21,632	3.0	6	1	2	2	4	5	7	12

Length of Stay by Diagnosis and Operation, Western Region, 2008

Western Region, October 2006–September 2007 Data, by Diagnosis

466.0: ACUTE BRONCHITIS

Type of Patients	Observed Patients	Avg. Stay	Variance	10th	25th	50th	75th	90th	95th	99th
1. SINGLE DX										
A. Not Operated										
0–19 Years	130	2.1	1	1	1	2	3	4	4	5
20–34	5	1.8	2	1	1	1	2	4	4	4
35–49	8	2.1	2	1	1	2	3	5	5	5
50–64	9	1.9	2	1	1	2	2	5	5	5
65+	7	1.6	1	1	1	1	2	4	4	4
B. Operated										
0–19 Years	0									
20–34	0									
35–49	0									
50–64	0									
65+	0									
2. MULTIPLE DX										
A. Not Operated										
0–19 Years	384	3.1	16	1	1	2	3	4	7	25
20–34	292	4.0	19	1	2	3	4	9	14	23
35–49	670	2.9	5	1	1	2	4	5	7	13
50–64	993	2.9	4	1	1	2	4	5	7	11
65+	2,842	3.3	7	1	2	3	4	6	7	12
B. Operated										
0–19 Years	1	3.0	0	3	3	3	3	3	3	3
20–34	4	10.8	32	5	8	10	18	18	18	18
35–49	5	12.0	66	4	7	10	14	25	25	25
50–64	10	6.0	20	2	5	7	9	11	15	15
65+	21	7.0	19	3	4	7	8	11	11	22
SUBTOTALS:										
1. SINGLE DX										
A. Not Operated	159	2.0	1	1	1	2	3	4	4	5
B. Operated	0									
2. MULTIPLE DX										
A. Not Operated	5,181	3.2	7	1	2	3	4	6	7	14
B. Operated	41	7.6	28	3	4	7	10	14	18	25
1. SINGLE DX	159	2.0	1	1	1	2	3	4	4	5
2. MULTIPLE DX	5,222	3.3	8	1	2	3	4	6	8	14
A. NOT OPERATED	5,340	3.2	7	1	2	3	4	6	7	14
B. OPERATED	41	7.6	28	3	4	7	10	14	18	25
TOTAL										
0–19 Years	515	2.8	12	1	1	2	3	4	5	18
20–34	301	4.0	19	1	2	3	4	9	14	23
35–49	683	3.0	6	1	1	2	4	5	7	14
50–64	1,012	2.9	5	1	1	2	4	5	7	11
65+	2,870	3.4	7	1	2	3	4	6	8	12
GRAND TOTAL	5,381	3.2	8	1	2	3	4	6	8	14

466.11: AC BRONCHIOLITIS D/T RSV

Type of Patients	Observed Patients	Avg. Stay	Variance	10th	25th	50th	75th	90th	95th	99th
1. SINGLE DX										
A. Not Operated										
0–19 Years	2,533	2.6	3	1	1	2	3	5	6	8
20–34	0									
35–49	0									
50–64	0									
65+	1	4.0	0	4	4	4	4	4	4	4
B. Operated										
0–19 Years	3	1.7	<1	1	1	2	2	2	2	2
20–34	0									
35–49	0									
50–64	0									
65+	0									
2. MULTIPLE DX										
A. Not Operated										
0–19 Years	6,390	3.4	7	1	2	3	4	6	8	12
20–34	0									
35–49	0									
50–64	1	11.0	0	11	11	11	11	11	11	11
65+	4	4.8	31	1	2	3	13	13	13	13
B. Operated										
0–19 Years	9	17.8	533	3	4	10	17	75	75	75
20–34	0									
35–49	0									
50–64	0									
65+	0									
SUBTOTALS:										
1. SINGLE DX										
A. Not Operated	2,534	2.6	3	1	1	2	3	5	6	8
B. Operated	3	1.7	<1	1	1	2	2	2	2	2
2. MULTIPLE DX										
A. Not Operated	6,395	3.4	7	1	2	3	4	6	8	12
B. Operated	9	17.8	533	3	4	10	17	75	75	75
1. SINGLE DX	2,537	2.6	3	1	1	2	3	5	6	8
2. MULTIPLE DX	6,404	3.4	8	1	2	3	4	6	8	12
A. NOT OPERATED	8,929	3.2	6	1	2	3	4	6	7	11
B. OPERATED	12	13.8	442	2	3	4	17	28	75	75
TOTAL										
0–19 Years	8,935	3.2	6	1	2	3	4	6	7	11
20–34	0									
35–49	0									
50–64	1	11.0	0	11	11	11	11	11	11	11
65+	5	4.6	23	1	2	3	4	13	13	13
GRAND TOTAL	8,941	3.2	6	1	2	3	4	6	7	11

466.19: AC BRONCHIOL D/T ORG NEC

Type of Patients	Observed Patients	Avg. Stay	Variance	10th	25th	50th	75th	90th	95th	99th
1. SINGLE DX										
A. Not Operated										
0–19 Years	1,691	2.3	2	1	1	2	3	4	5	6
20–34	0									
35–49	0									
50–64	1	3.0	0	3	3	3	3	3	3	3
65+	0									
B. Operated										
0–19 Years	0									
20–34	0									
35–49	0									
50–64	0									
65+	0									
2. MULTIPLE DX										
A. Not Operated										
0–19 Years	5,493	2.8	4	1	1	2	3	5	6	10
20–34	8	2.5	3	1	1	3	3	6	6	6
35–49	26	3.8	8	1	2	3	4	8	10	13
50–64	21	3.3	7	1	2	3	4	5	7	13
65+	47	4.4	8	2	2	4	6	7	11	14
B. Operated										
0–19 Years	3	6.0	48	2	2	2	2	14	14	14
20–34	0	4.0	0	4	4	4	4	4	4	4
35–49	8	3.2	3	1	1	3	4	6	6	6
50–64	5	8.8	11	5	7	9	9	14	14	14
65+	6	4.5	6	2	3	4	5	9	9	9
SUBTOTALS:										
1. SINGLE DX										
A. Not Operated	1,692	2.3	2	1	1	2	3	4	5	6
B. Operated	0									
2. MULTIPLE DX										
A. Not Operated	5,595	2.8	4	1	2	2	3	5	6	10
B. Operated	23	5.2	13	2	2	4	7	9	14	14
1. SINGLE DX	1,692	2.3	2	1	1	2	3	4	5	6
2. MULTIPLE DX	5,618	2.8	4	1	2	2	3	5	6	10
A. NOT OPERATED	7,287	2.7	4	1	1	2	3	5	6	9
B. OPERATED	23	5.2	13	2	2	4	7	9	14	14
TOTAL										
0–19 Years	7,187	2.6	4	1	1	2	3	5	6	9
20–34	9	2.7	3	1	1	3	3	6	6	6
35–49	34	3.7	7	1	2	3	4	7	10	13
50–64	27	4.3	12	2	2	3	5	9	13	14
65+	53	4.4	7	2	2	4	5	7	11	14
GRAND TOTAL	7,310	2.7	4	1	1	2	3	5	6	9

Length of Stay by Diagnosis and Operation, Western Region, 2008

Western Region, October 2006–September 2007 Data, by Diagnosis

470: DEVIATED NASAL SEPTUM

Type of Patients	Observed Patients	Avg. Stay	Vari-ance	10th	25th	50th	75th	90th	95th	99th
1. SINGLE DX										
A. Not Operated										
0–19 Years	0									
20–34	0									
35–49	0									
50–64	0									
65+	0									
B. Operated										
0–19 Years	0									
20–34	0									
35–49	0									
50–64	0									
65+	0									
2. MULTIPLE DX										
A. Not Operated										
0–19 Years	0									
20–34	2	1.0	0	1	1	1	1	1	1	1
35–49	2	1.0	0	1	1	1	1	1	1	1
50–64	0									
65+	0									
B. Operated										
0–19 Years	8	1.8	1	1	1	1	3	3	3	3
20–34	54	1.4	<1	1	1	1	1	2	4	6
35–49	122	1.3	<1	1	1	1	1	2	3	3
50–64	109	1.3	<1	1	1	1	1	2	3	3
65+	47	1.6	2	1	1	1	2	3	5	8
SUBTOTALS:										
1. SINGLE DX										
A. Not Operated	0									
B. Operated	0									
2. MULTIPLE DX										
A. Not Operated	4	1.0	0	1	1	1	1	1	1	1
B. Operated	340	1.3	<1	1	1	1	1	2	3	5
1. SINGLE DX	0									
2. MULTIPLE DX	344	1.3	<1	1	1	1	2	3	5	
A. NOT OPERATED	4	1.0	0	1	1	1	1	1	1	1
B. OPERATED	340	1.3	<1	1	1	1	2	3	5	
TOTAL										
0–19 Years	8	1.8	1	1	1	1	3	3	3	3
20–34	56	1.4	1	1	1	1	1	2	4	6
35–49	124	1.2	<1	1	1	1	1	2	3	3
50–64	109	1.3	<1	1	1	1	1	2	3	3
65+	47	1.6	2	1	1	1	2	3	5	8
GRAND TOTAL	344	1.3	<1	1	1	1	2	3	5	

471: NASAL POLYPS

Type of Patients	Observed Patients	Avg. Stay	Vari-ance	10th	25th	50th	75th	90th	95th	99th
1. SINGLE DX										
A. Not Operated										
0–19 Years	0									
20–34	0									
35–49	1	4.0	0	4	4	4	4	4	4	4
50–64	0									
65+	0									
B. Operated										
0–19 Years	0									
20–34	0									
35–49	1	1.0	0	1	1	1	1	1	1	1
50–64	1	2.0	0	2	2	2	2	2	2	2
65+	0									
2. MULTIPLE DX										
A. Not Operated										
0–19 Years	0									
20–34	2	1.0	0	1	1	1	1	1	1	1
35–49	3	2.0	3	1	1	1	4	4	4	4
50–64	2	1.0	0	1	1	1	1	1	1	1
65+	6	2.5	3	1	1	1	4	5	5	5
B. Operated										
0–19 Years	4	2.5	6	1	1	2	6	6	6	6
20–34	11	2.4	4	1	1	1	4	6	6	6
35–49	16	2.3	3	1	1	2	4	6	6	6
50–64	17	2.3	8	1	1	1	2	7	12	12
65+	15	1.9	2	1	1	1	2	5	6	6
SUBTOTALS:										
1. SINGLE DX										
A. Not Operated	1	4.0	0	4	4	4	4	4	4	4
B. Operated	2	1.5	<1	1	1	1	2	2	2	2
2. MULTIPLE DX										
A. Not Operated	13	1.9	2	1	1	1	3	4	5	5
B. Operated	63	2.2	4	1	1	1	2	6	6	12
1. SINGLE DX	3	2.3	2	1	1	2	4	4	4	4
2. MULTIPLE DX	76	2.2	4	1	1	1	3	6	6	12
A. NOT OPERATED	14	2.1	4	1	1	1	4	4	5	5
B. OPERATED	65	2.2	4	1	1	1	2	6	6	12
TOTAL										
0–19 Years	4	2.5	6	1	1	2	6	6	6	6
20–34	13	2.2	4	1	1	1	4	6	6	6
35–49	21	2.3	3	1	1	1	4	4	6	6
50–64	20	2.2	7	1	1	2	2	7	12	12
65+	21	2.1	5	1	1	1	3	5	5	6
GRAND TOTAL	79	2.2	4	1	1	1	3	6	6	12

472: CHR PHARYN/NASOPHARYNG

Type of Patients	Observed Patients	Avg. Stay	Vari-ance	10th	25th	50th	75th	90th	95th	99th
1. SINGLE DX										
A. Not Operated										
0–19 Years	1	2.0	0	2	2	2	2	2	2	2
20–34	0									
35–49	0									
50–64	0									
65+	0									
B. Operated										
0–19 Years	0									
20–34	0									
35–49	0									
50–64	0									
65+	0									
2. MULTIPLE DX										
A. Not Operated										
0–19 Years	5	2.8	2	1	2	3	4	4	4	4
20–34	0									
35–49	0									
50–64	2	4.0	8	2	2	4	6	6	6	6
65+	5	2.6	2	1	2	2	4	4	4	4
B. Operated										
0–19 Years	1	2.0	0	2	2	2	2	2	2	2
20–34	1	1.0	0	1	1	1	1	1	1	1
35–49	1	3.0	0	3	3	3	3	3	3	3
50–64	0									
65+	0									
SUBTOTALS:										
1. SINGLE DX										
A. Not Operated	1	2.0	0	2	2	2	2	2	2	2
B. Operated	0									
2. MULTIPLE DX										
A. Not Operated	12	2.9	2	1	2	2	4	4	6	6
B. Operated	3	2.0	<1	1	2	2	3	3	3	3
1. SINGLE DX	1	2.0	0	2	2	2	2	2	2	2
2. MULTIPLE DX	15	2.7	2	1	2	2	4	4	6	6
A. NOT OPERATED	13	2.9	2	1	2	2	4	4	6	6
B. OPERATED	3	2.0	<1	1	2	2	3	3	3	3
TOTAL										
0–19 Years	7	2.6	1	1	2	2	4	4	4	4
20–34	1	1.0	0	1	1	1	1	1	1	1
35–49	1	3.0	0	3	3	3	3	3	3	3
50–64	2	4.0	8	2	2	4	6	6	6	6
65+	5	2.6	2	1	2	2	4	4	4	4
GRAND TOTAL	16	2.7	2	1	2	2	4	4	6	6

Length of Stay by Diagnosis and Operation, Western Region, 2008

Western Region, October 2006–September 2007 Data, by Diagnosis

473: CHRONIC SINUSITIS

Type of Patients	Observed Patients	Avg. Stay	Variance	Percentiles 10th	25th	50th	75th	90th	95th	99th
1. SINGLE DX										
A. Not Operated										
0–19 Years	14	2.0	<1	1	1	2	3	3	3	3
20–34	3	2.0	<1	1	1	2	3	3	3	3
35–49	0									
50–64	2	3.0	8	1	1	3	5	5	5	5
65+	4	1.0	0	1	1	1	1	1	1	1
B. Operated										
0–19 Years	1	1.0	0	1	1	1	1	1	1	1
20–34	2	2.0	2	1	1	3	3	3	3	3
35–49	4	1.5	<1	1	1	1	1	3	3	3
50–64	5	1.4	<1	1	1	1	1	3	3	3
65+	0									
2. MULTIPLE DX										
A. Not Operated										
0–19 Years	127	2.6	2	1	2	2	3	4	5	7
20–34	82	2.7	3	1	2	2	4	5	6	7
35–49	103	2.7	2	1	2	2	4	4	5	7
50–64	150	2.6	2	1	1	2	3	4	5	9
65+	157	3.2	7	1	2	2	4	6	8	14
B. Operated										
0–19 Years	30	4.4	32	1	1	2	6	13	21	22
20–34	78	3.7	17	1	1	2	4	10	13	22
35–49	92	2.3	6	1	1	1	2	5	9	11
50–64	130	2.6	9	1	1	1	3	5	9	17
65+	105	2.8	15	1	1	1	3	6	9	20
SUBTOTALS:										
1. SINGLE DX										
A. Not Operated	23	1.9	1	1	1	2	3	3	3	5
B. Operated	12	1.5	<1	1	1	1	3	3	3	3
2. MULTIPLE DX										
A. Not Operated	619	2.8	4	1	1	2	3	5	6	10
B. Operated	435	2.9	13	1	1	1	3	7	11	20
1. SINGLE DX	35	1.8	1	1	1	1	3	3	3	5
2. MULTIPLE DX	1,054	2.8	7	1	1	2	3	5	7	16
A. NOT OPERATED	642	2.7	3	1	1	2	3	5	6	10
B. OPERATED	447	2.9	13	1	1	1	3	6	11	20
TOTAL										
0–19 Years	172	2.8	7	1	1	2	3	5	6	21
20–34	165	3.1	10	1	1	2	4	6	8	17
35–49	199	2.5	4	1	1	2	3	5	7	10
50–64	287	2.6	5	1	1	2	3	6	6	14
65+	266	3.0	10	1	1	2	3	6	8	17
GRAND TOTAL	1,089	2.8	7	1	1	2	3	5	7	16

473.0: CHR MAXILLARY SINUSITIS

Type of Patients	Observed Patients	Avg. Stay	Variance	Percentiles 10th	25th	50th	75th	90th	95th	99th
1. SINGLE DX										
A. Not Operated										
0–19 Years	1	2.0	0	2	2	2	2	2	2	2
20–34	1	2.0	0	2	2	2	2	2	2	2
35–49	0									
50–64	0									
65+	1	1.0	0	1	1	1	1	1	1	1
B. Operated										
0–19 Years	0									
20–34	1	1.0	0	1	1	1	1	1	1	1
35–49	0									
50–64	0									
65+	0									
2. MULTIPLE DX										
A. Not Operated										
0–19 Years	23	2.5	2	1	2	2	3	5	5	6
20–34	18	2.6	2	1	2	2	3	4	7	7
35–49	23	2.6	2	1	2	2	4	5	5	6
50–64	31	2.8	3	1	2	2	4	4	5	9
65+	35	3.0	8	1	2	2	3	5	7	17
B. Operated										
0–19 Years	8	5.5	58	1	1	2	12	22	22	22
20–34	8	4.6	22	1	2	3	11	13	13	13
35–49	19	2.2	3	1	1	1	2	5	8	8
50–64	25	1.7	2	1	1	1	2	4	4	6
65+	29	2.5	4	1	1	2	4	7	7	7
SUBTOTALS:										
1. SINGLE DX										
A. Not Operated	3	1.7	<1	1	1	2	2	2	2	2
B. Operated	1	1.0	0	1	1	1	1	1	1	1
2. MULTIPLE DX										
A. Not Operated	130	2.8	4	1	2	2	3	5	6	9
B. Operated	89	2.7	10	1	1	1	3	6	8	22
1. SINGLE DX	4	1.5	<1	1	1	2	2	2	2	2
2. MULTIPLE DX	219	2.7	6	1	1	2	3	5	7	13
A. NOT OPERATED	133	2.7	4	1	1	2	3	5	6	9
B. OPERATED	90	2.6	10	1	1	1	3	5	8	22
TOTAL										
0–19 Years	32	3.3	16	1	1	2	3	5	12	22
20–34	28	3.1	8	1	2	2	3	7	11	13
35–49	42	2.4	3	1	1	2	3	4	5	8
50–64	56	2.3	3	1	1	2	3	4	5	9
65+	65	2.8	6	1	1	2	3	5	7	17
GRAND TOTAL	223	2.7	6	1	1	2	3	5	7	13

473.8: CHRONIC SINUSITIS NEC

Type of Patients	Observed Patients	Avg. Stay	Variance	Percentiles 10th	25th	50th	75th	90th	95th	99th
1. SINGLE DX										
A. Not Operated										
0–19 Years	1	2.0	0	2	2	2	2	2	2	2
20–34	1	3.0	0	3	3	3	3	3	3	3
35–49	0									
50–64	0									
65+	1	1.0	0	1	1	1	1	1	1	1
B. Operated										
0–19 Years	0									
20–34	0									
35–49	1	3.0	0	3	3	3	3	3	3	3
50–64	1	1.0	0	1	1	1	1	1	1	1
65+	0									
2. MULTIPLE DX										
A. Not Operated										
0–19 Years	25	2.7	2	1	2	3	3	5	5	7
20–34	16	3.1	2	1	2	3	4	5	7	7
35–49	16	3.0	1	1	2	3	4	5	5	5
50–64	17	3.0	2	1	2	3	3	5	6	6
65+	25	4.4	10	2	2	3	6	11	11	12
B. Operated										
0–19 Years	9	5.5	50	1	1	2	6	21	21	21
20–34	24	5.2	35	1	1	2	6	16	17	22
35–49	22	2.8	10	1	1	1	3	9	10	11
50–64	27	3.0	16	1	1	1	3	9	14	17
65+	21	3.8	32	1	1	1	3	14	16	20
SUBTOTALS:										
1. SINGLE DX										
A. Not Operated	3	2.0	<1	1	1	2	3	3	3	3
B. Operated	2	2.0	2	1	1	2	3	3	3	3
2. MULTIPLE DX										
A. Not Operated	99	3.3	4	1	2	3	4	6	7	12
B. Operated	103	3.8	25	1	1	1	4	12	16	21
1. SINGLE DX	5	2.0	1	1	1	2	3	3	3	3
2. MULTIPLE DX	202	3.6	15	1	1	2	4	7	12	20
A. NOT OPERATED	102	3.2	4	1	2	3	4	5	7	11
B. OPERATED	105	3.8	25	1	1	1	4	12	16	21
TOTAL										
0–19 Years	35	3.4	15	1	1	2	3	6	13	21
20–34	42	4.3	22	1	2	3	5	10	16	22
35–49	38	2.9	7	1	1	2	4	6	10	11
50–64	45	2.9	10	1	1	2	3	5	9	17
65+	47	4.1	19	1	1	2	5	11	14	20
GRAND TOTAL	207	3.5	15	1	1	2	4	7	12	20

Length of Stay by Diagnosis and Operation, Western Region, 2008

Western Region, October 2006–September 2007 Data, by Diagnosis

473.9: CHRONIC SINUSITIS NOS

Type of Patients	Observed Patients	Avg. Stay	Vari-ance	10th	25th	50th	75th	90th	95th	99th
1. SINGLE DX										
A. Not Operated										
0–19 Years	11	2.0	<1	1	1	2	3	3	3	3
20–34	1	1.0	0	1	1	1	1	1	1	1
35–49	0									
50–64	2	3.0	8	1	1	3	5	5	5	5
65+	2	1.0	0	1	1	1	1	1	1	1
B. Operated										
0–19 Years	0									
20–34	0									
35–49	1	1.0	0	1	1	1	1	1	1	1
50–64	1	1.0	0	1	1	1	1	1	1	1
65+	0									
2. MULTIPLE DX										
A. Not Operated										
0–19 Years	52	2.4	2	1	1	2	3	4	5	6
20–34	36	2.5	3	1	1	2	3	5	6	7
35–49	47	2.7	3	1	1	2	3	5	7	8
50–64	75	2.4	2	1	1	2	4	4	5	6
65+	72	3.0	6	1	1	2	4	6	8	14
B. Operated										
0–19 Years	5	3.4	8	1	1	2	6	7	7	7
20–34	14	3.0	8	1	1	1	5	5	11	11
35–49	19	2.1	5	1	1	1	2	8	9	9
50–64	19	2.6	11	1	1	1	2	11	12	12
65+	15	1.3	<1	1	1	1	1	2	3	3
SUBTOTALS:										
1. SINGLE DX										
A. Not Operated	16	1.9	1	1	1	2	3	3	5	5
B. Operated	2	1.0	0	1	1	1	1	1	1	1
2. MULTIPLE DX										
A. Not Operated	282	2.6	3	1	1	2	3	5	6	8
B. Operated	72	2.3	7	1	1	1	2	5	9	12
1. SINGLE DX	18	1.8	1	1	1	1	3	3	5	5
2. MULTIPLE DX	354	2.6	4	1	1	2	3	5	6	11
A. NOT OPERATED	298	2.6	3	1	1	2	3	5	6	8
B. OPERATED	74	2.3	6	1	1	1	2	5	9	12
TOTAL										
0–19 Years	68	2.4	2	1	1	2	3	4	5	7
20–34	51	2.6	4	1	1	2	3	5	6	11
35–49	67	2.5	4	1	1	2	3	5	7	9
50–64	97	2.5	4	1	1	2	4	4	5	12
65+	89	2.7	5	1	1	2	3	6	7	14
GRAND TOTAL	372	2.5	4	1	1	2	3	5	6	11

474: CHR T & A DISEASE

Type of Patients	Observed Patients	Avg. Stay	Vari-ance	10th	25th	50th	75th	90th	95th	99th
1. SINGLE DX										
A. Not Operated										
0–19 Years	6	2.0	1	1	1	2	2	4	4	4
20–34	1	1.0	0	1	1	1	1	1	1	1
35–49	0									
50–64	0									
65+	0									
B. Operated										
0–19 Years	121	1.2	<1	1	1	1	1	2	2	3
20–34	13	1.2	<1	1	1	1	1	1	4	4
35–49	2	2.5	<1	2	2	3	3	3	3	3
50–64	0									
65+	0									
2. MULTIPLE DX										
A. Not Operated										
0–19 Years	29	1.8	1	1	1	2	2	4	4	4
20–34	10	2.2	2	1	1	2	4	4	5	5
35–49	6	2.8	9	1	1	2	2	9	9	9
50–64	2	1.0	0	1	1	1	1	1	1	1
65+	3	1.7	<1	1	2	2	2	2	2	2
B. Operated										
0–19 Years	883	1.5	2	1	1	1	2	3	4	7
20–34	98	1.7	2	1	1	1	2	3	5	11
35–49	84	1.5	1	1	1	1	2	3	3	8
50–64	41	1.3	<1	1	1	1	1	2	3	4
65+	2	2.0	2	1	2	2	3	3	3	3
SUBTOTALS:										
1. SINGLE DX										
A. Not Operated	7	1.9	1	1	1	2	2	4	4	4
B. Operated	136	1.2	<1	1	1	1	1	2	2	4
2. MULTIPLE DX										
A. Not Operated	50	2.0	2	1	1	2	2	4	4	9
B. Operated	1,108	1.6	2	1	1	1	2	3	4	7
1. SINGLE DX	143	1.2	<1	1	1	1	1	2	2	4
2. MULTIPLE DX	1,158	1.6	2	1	1	1	2	3	4	7
A. NOT OPERATED	57	2.0	2	1	1	1	2	4	4	9
B. OPERATED	1,244	1.5	2	1	1	1	2	3	4	7
TOTAL										
0–19 Years	1,039	1.5	2	1	1	1	2	4	4	7
20–34	122	1.7	2	1	1	1	2	3	5	7
35–49	92	1.6	1	1	1	1	2	3	3	9
50–64	43	1.3	<1	1	1	1	2	3	3	4
65+	5	1.8	<1	1	1	2	2	3	3	3
GRAND TOTAL	1,301	1.5	2	1	1	1	2	3	4	7

474.00: CHRONIC TONSILLITIS

Type of Patients	Observed Patients	Avg. Stay	Vari-ance	10th	25th	50th	75th	90th	95th	99th
1. SINGLE DX										
A. Not Operated										
0–19 Years	2	1.5	<1	1	1	2	2	2	2	2
20–34	1	1.0	0	1	1	1	1	1	1	1
35–49	0									
50–64	0									
65+	0									
B. Operated										
0–19 Years	23	1.3	<1	1	1	1	1	2	2	4
20–34	11	1.3	<1	1	1	1	1	1	4	4
35–49	0									
50–64	0									
65+	0									
2. MULTIPLE DX										
A. Not Operated										
0–19 Years	10	1.8	1	1	1	2	2	4	4	4
20–34	6	2.3	3	1	1	2	4	5	5	5
35–49	2	1.5	<1	1	1	2	2	2	2	2
50–64	0									
65+	0									
B. Operated										
0–19 Years	109	1.5	1	1	1	1	1	3	4	6
20–34	60	1.8	3	1	1	1	2	3	5	11
35–49	36	1.5	2	1	1	1	2	2	3	8
50–64	18	1.4	<1	1	1	1	1	3	4	4
65+	0									
SUBTOTALS:										
1. SINGLE DX										
A. Not Operated	3	1.3	<1	1	1	1	2	2	2	2
B. Operated	34	1.3	<1	1	1	1	1	2	4	4
2. MULTIPLE DX										
A. Not Operated	18	2.0	2	1	1	2	2	4	5	5
B. Operated	223	1.6	2	1	1	1	2	3	4	6
1. SINGLE DX	37	1.3	<1	1	1	1	1	2	4	4
2. MULTIPLE DX	241	1.6	2	1	1	1	2	3	4	6
A. NOT OPERATED	21	1.9	1	1	1	1	2	4	4	5
B. OPERATED	257	1.5	2	1	1	1	2	3	4	6
TOTAL										
0–19 Years	144	1.5	1	1	1	1	2	3	4	6
20–34	78	1.7	3	1	1	1	2	3	5	11
35–49	38	1.5	2	1	1	1	2	2	3	8
50–64	18	1.4	<1	1	1	1	1	3	4	4
65+	0									
GRAND TOTAL	278	1.6	2	1	1	1	2	3	4	6

Length of Stay by Diagnosis and Operation, Western Region, 2008

Western Region, October 2006–September 2007 Data, by Diagnosis

474.10: HYPERTR TONSIL W ADENOID

Type of Patients	Observed Patients	Avg. Stay	Variance	10th	25th	50th	75th	90th	95th	99th
1. SINGLE DX										
A. Not Operated										
0–19 Years	0									
20–34	0									
35–49	0									
50–64	0									
65+	0									
B. Operated										
0–19 Years	66	1.2	<1	1	1	1	1	2	2	3
20–34	0									
35–49	0									
50–64	0									
65+	0									
2. MULTIPLE DX										
A. Not Operated										
0–19 Years	6	2.3	2	1	1	2	4	4	4	4
20–34	0									
35–49	0									
50–64	0									
65+	0									
B. Operated										
0–19 Years	585	1.5	3	1	1	1	1	2	4	7
20–34	13	1.9	2	1	1	1	2	5	5	5
35–49	6	2.2	4	1	1	1	2	6	6	6
50–64	3	1.0	0	1	1	1	1	1	1	1
65+	0									
SUBTOTALS:										
1. SINGLE DX										
A. Not Operated	0									
B. Operated	66	1.2	<1	1	1	1	1	2	2	3
2. MULTIPLE DX										
A. Not Operated	6	2.3	2	1	1	2	4	4	4	4
B. Operated	607	1.5	3	1	1	1	1	2	4	7
1. SINGLE DX	66	1.2	<1	1	1	1	1	2	2	3
2. MULTIPLE DX	613	1.5	3	1	1	1	1	2	4	7
A. NOT OPERATED	6	2.3	2	1	1	2	4	4	4	4
B. OPERATED	673	1.5	2	1	1	1	1	2	4	7
TOTAL										
0–19 Years	657	1.5	2	1	1	1	1	2	4	7
20–34	13	1.9	2	1	1	1	2	4	5	5
35–49	6	2.2	4	1	1	1	2	6	6	6
50–64	3	1.0	0	1	1	1	1	1	1	1
65+	0									
GRAND TOTAL	679	1.5	2	1	1	1	1	2	4	7

475: PERITONSILLAR ABSCESS

Type of Patients	Observed Patients	Avg. Stay	Variance	10th	25th	50th	75th	90th	95th	99th
1. SINGLE DX										
A. Not Operated										
0–19 Years	102	1.7	<1	1	1	2	2	3	3	4
20–34	85	1.7	<1	1	1	2	2	3	3	4
35–49	22	1.6	<1	1	1	1	2	2	2	4
50–64	10	1.6	<1	1	1	1	2	3	3	3
65+	0									
B. Operated										
0–19 Years	127	1.5	<1	1	1	1	1	2	3	4
20–34	114	1.6	<1	1	1	1	2	3	3	4
35–49	36	1.4	<1	1	1	1	2	2	2	3
50–64	11	2.0	3	1	1	2	2	3	7	7
65+	3	1.7	<1	1	1	2	2	2	2	2
2. MULTIPLE DX										
A. Not Operated										
0–19 Years	174	1.9	<1	1	1	2	2	3	3	4
20–34	172	2.1	3	1	1	2	2	4	5	7
35–49	110	2.1	2	1	1	2	3	4	4	6
50–64	49	2.5	2	1	2	2	3	4	6	8
65+	17	2.8	3	1	2	2	3	6	6	6
B. Operated										
0–19 Years	257	2.0	2	1	1	2	2	3	5	8
20–34	278	2.2	3	1	1	2	3	3	6	9
35–49	160	2.8	6	1	1	2	3	7	9	12
50–64	57	4.5	45	1	2	3	4	9	17	43
65+	21	5.7	60	1	2	3	6	11	16	35
SUBTOTALS:										
1. SINGLE DX										
A. Not Operated	219	1.7	<1	1	1	2	2	3	3	4
B. Operated	291	1.6	<1	1	1	1	2	3	3	4
2. MULTIPLE DX										
A. Not Operated	522	2.1	2	1	1	2	3	3	4	7
B. Operated	773	2.5	8	1	1	2	3	5	7	12
1. SINGLE DX	510	1.6	<1	1	1	1	2	3	3	4
2. MULTIPLE DX	1,295	2.4	6	1	1	2	3	4	6	11
A. NOT OPERATED	741	2.0	2	1	1	2	2	3	4	6
B. OPERATED	1,064	2.3	6	1	1	2	2	4	6	11
TOTAL										
0–19 Years	660	1.9	1	1	1	2	2	3	4	6
20–34	649	2.0	2	1	1	2	2	4	4	9
35–49	328	2.3	4	1	1	2	3	4	7	11
50–64	127	3.3	22	1	1	2	3	6	8	25
65+	41	4.2	34	1	2	2	5	8	11	35
GRAND TOTAL	1,805	2.1	4	1	1	2	2	4	5	10

476: CHR LARYNG/LARYNGOTRACH

Type of Patients	Observed Patients	Avg. Stay	Variance	10th	25th	50th	75th	90th	95th	99th
1. SINGLE DX										
A. Not Operated										
0–19 Years	0									
20–34	0									
35–49	0									
50–64	0									
65+	0									
B. Operated										
0–19 Years	0									
20–34	0									
35–49	0									
50–64	0									
65+	0									
2. MULTIPLE DX										
A. Not Operated										
0–19 Years	0									
20–34	0									
35–49	0									
50–64	1	2.0	0	2	2	2	2	2	2	2
65+	1	1.0	0	1	1	1	1	1	1	1
B. Operated										
0–19 Years	0									
20–34	0									
35–49	0									
50–64	0									
65+	1	1.0	0	1	1	1	1	1	1	1
SUBTOTALS:										
1. SINGLE DX										
A. Not Operated	0									
B. Operated	0									
2. MULTIPLE DX										
A. Not Operated	2	1.5	<1	1	1	1	2	2	2	2
B. Operated	1	1.0	0	1	1	1	1	1	1	1
1. SINGLE DX	0									
2. MULTIPLE DX	3	1.3	<1	1	1	1	2	2	2	2
A. NOT OPERATED	2	1.5	<1	1	1	1	2	2	2	2
B. OPERATED	1	1.0	0	1	1	1	1	1	1	1
TOTAL										
0–19 Years	0									
20–34	0									
35–49	0									
50–64	1	2.0	0	2	2	2	2	2	2	2
65+	2	1.0	0	1	1	1	1	1	1	1
GRAND TOTAL	3	1.3	<1	1	1	1	2	2	2	2

Western Region, October 2006–September 2007 Data, by Diagnosis

477: ALLERGIC RHINITIS

Type of Patients	Observed Patients	Avg. Stay	Vari-ance	10th	25th	50th	75th	90th	95th	99th
1. SINGLE DX										
A. Not Operated										
0–19 Years	0									
20–34	1	8.0	0	8	8	8	8	8	8	8
35–49	0									
50–64	0									
65+	0									
B. Operated										
0–19 Years	0									
20–34	0									
35–49	0									
50–64	0									
65+	0									
2. MULTIPLE DX										
A. Not Operated										
0–19 Years	2	3.0	2	2	2	4	4	4	4	4
20–34	0									
35–49	8	1.3	<1	1	1	1	1	2	2	2
50–64	6	1.3	<1	1	1	1	2	2	2	2
65+	11	1.5	<1	1	1	1	2	2	2	2
B. Operated										
0–19 Years	0									
20–34	1	2.0	0	2	2	2	2	2	2	2
35–49	0									
50–64	1	1.0	0	1	1	1	1	1	1	1
65+	0									
SUBTOTALS:										
1. SINGLE DX										
A. Not Operated	1	8.0	0	8	8	8	8	8	8	8
B. Operated	0									
2. MULTIPLE DX										
A. Not Operated	27	1.5	<1	1	1	1	2	2	2	4
B. Operated	2	1.5	<1	1	1	1	2	2	2	2
1. SINGLE DX	1	8.0	0	8	8	8	8	8	8	8
2. MULTIPLE DX	29	1.5	<1	1	1	1	2	2	2	4
A. NOT OPERATED	28	1.7	2	1	1	1	2	2	4	8
B. OPERATED	2	1.5	<1	1	1	1	2	2	2	2
TOTAL										
0–19 Years	2	3.0	2	2	2	4	4	4	4	4
20–34	2	5.0	18	2	2	5	8	8	8	8
35–49	8	1.3	<1	1	1	1	1	2	2	2
50–64	7	1.3	<1	1	1	1	2	2	2	2
65+	11	1.5	<1	1	1	1	2	2	2	2
GRAND TOTAL	30	1.7	2	1	1	1	2	2	4	8

478: OTH UP RESPIRATORY DIS

Type of Patients	Observed Patients	Avg. Stay	Vari-ance	10th	25th	50th	75th	90th	95th	99th
1. SINGLE DX										
A. Not Operated										
0–19 Years	44	2.5	5	1	1	2	3	4	6	14
20–34	22	2.6	9	1	1	2	3	4	4	15
35–49	22	2.0	1	1	1	2	3	4	4	5
50–64	16	3.1	4	1	2	2	4	6	9	9
65+	3	2.0	1	1	1	2	3	3	3	3
B. Operated										
0–19 Years	56	2.8	4	1	1	2	4	5	6	12
20–34	16	2.4	3	1	1	2	3	6	6	6
35–49	19	2.1	2	1	1	2	3	4	6	6
50–64	16	2.4	3	1	1	2	2	5	7	7
65+	4	1.8	<1	1	1	1	2	3	3	3
2. MULTIPLE DX										
A. Not Operated										
0–19 Years	181	3.1	8	1	1	2	4	5	7	17
20–34	131	3.1	9	1	2	3	4	5	7	19
35–49	250	3.2	7	1	1	3	4	6	8	15
50–64	293	3.6	9	1	2	3	4	6	10	15
65+	277	4.4	21	1	1	3	6	10	13	25
B. Operated										
0–19 Years	149	4.4	22	1	2	3	5	9	16	23
20–34	117	3.6	12	1	1	2	5	6	12	14
35–49	158	3.6	16	1	1	2	5	8	10	23
50–64	221	4.3	55	1	1	2	5	9	11	34
65+	188	5.0	62	1	1	2	6	11	18	42
SUBTOTALS:										
1. SINGLE DX										
A. Not Operated	107	2.5	5	1	1	2	3	4	6	14
B. Operated	111	2.5	3	1	1	2	3	5	6	7
2. MULTIPLE DX										
A. Not Operated	1,132	3.6	12	1	1	3	4	7	10	19
B. Operated	833	4.2	37	1	1	2	5	9	13	26
1. SINGLE DX	218	2.5	4	1	1	2	3	5	6	12
2. MULTIPLE DX	1,965	3.8	23	1	1	3	5	8	11	23
A. NOT OPERATED	1,239	3.5	11	1	1	3	4	7	10	19
B. OPERATED	944	4.0	34	1	1	2	5	8	12	26
TOTAL										
0–19 Years	430	3.4	12	1	1	3	4	6	9	20
20–34	286	3.2	10	1	1	2	4	6	10	18
35–49	449	3.2	10	1	1	3	4	7	8	17
50–64	546	3.8	28	1	1	3	5	8	10	20
65+	472	4.6	37	1	1	3	6	10	14	26
GRAND TOTAL	2,183	3.7	21	1	1	2	4	7	10	22

478.19: NASAL & SINUS DIS NEC

Type of Patients	Observed Patients	Avg. Stay	Vari-ance	10th	25th	50th	75th	90th	95th	99th
1. SINGLE DX										
A. Not Operated										
0–19 Years	12	1.8	3	1	1	1	2	2	2	7
20–34	6	4.0	30	1	1	2	4	15	15	15
35–49	6	1.7	1	1	1	1	2	4	4	4
50–64	4	2.8	<1	2	2	3	3	4	4	4
65+	1	1.0	0	1	1	1	1	1	1	1
B. Operated										
0–19 Years	2	1.5	<1	1	1	2	2	2	2	2
20–34	0									
35–49	0									
50–64	2	1.5	<1	1	1	1	2	2	2	2
65+	0									
2. MULTIPLE DX										
A. Not Operated										
0–19 Years	36	2.5	2	1	1	2	4	5	5	7
20–34	34	3.0	3	1	2	3	4	4	5	10
35–49	66	3.3	4	1	2	3	4	6	7	10
50–64	67	3.4	4	1	2	3	4	6	7	11
65+	51	3.6	9	1	2	3	4	7	9	15
B. Operated										
0–19 Years	7	4.6	47	1	1	2	5	20	20	20
20–34	19	2.5	7	1	1	3	5	5	10	10
35–49	31	2.3	4	1	1	1	3	5	7	8
50–64	45	2.6	6	1	1	2	3	7	8	10
65+	25	2.6	6	1	2	2	3	6	7	10
SUBTOTALS:										
1. SINGLE DX										
A. Not Operated	29	2.3	8	1	1	1	2	4	7	15
B. Operated	4	1.5	<1	1	1	1	2	2	2	2
2. MULTIPLE DX										
A. Not Operated	254	3.2	5	1	1	3	4	6	7	11
B. Operated	127	2.6	8	1	1	2	3	7	8	10
1. SINGLE DX	33	2.2	7	1	1	1	2	4	7	15
2. MULTIPLE DX	381	3.0	6	1	1	2	4	6	7	11
A. NOT OPERATED	283	3.1	5	1	1	3	4	6	7	14
B. OPERATED	131	2.6	7	1	1	1	3	6	8	10
TOTAL										
0–19 Years	57	2.6	8	1	1	2	3	5	7	20
20–34	59	2.9	7	1	1	2	4	5	10	15
35–49	103	2.9	4	1	1	2	4	5	7	10
50–64	118	3.0	5	1	1	2	4	6	7	10
65+	77	3.3	8	1	1	2	4	7	9	15
GRAND TOTAL	414	3.0	6	1	1	2	4	6	7	11

Length of Stay by Diagnosis and Operation, Western Region, 2008

Western Region, October 2006–September 2007 Data, by Diagnosis

478.24: RETROPHARYNGEAL ABSCESS

Type of Patients	Observed Patients	Avg. Stay	Variance	Percentiles						
				10th	25th	50th	75th	90th	95th	99th
1. SINGLE DX										
A. *Not Operated*										
0–19 Years	15	3.3	2	2	2	3	4	6	6	6
20–34	3	2.0	0	2	2	2	2	2	2	2
35–49	3	3.0	<1	2	2	3	4	4	4	4
50–64	3	4.3	16	2	2	3	9	9	9	9
65+	2	2.5	<1	2	2	3	3	3	3	3
B. *Operated*										
0–19 Years	23	3.1	6	1	1	2	4	5	7	12
20–34	3	4.0	8	2	2	6	6	6	6	6
35–49	5	2.4	<1	2	2	2	3	3	3	3
50–64	2	4.5	12	2	2	7	7	7	7	7
65+	0									
2. MULTIPLE DX										
A. *Not Operated*										
0–19 Years	43	3.7	6	1	2	3	4	6	8	15
20–34	12	2.8	2	1	2	3	3	4	6	6
35–49	33	3.8	13	1	2	3	4	7	15	15
50–64	20	4.7	11	1	3	4	5	8	11	15
65+	11	5.8	50	2	2	3	6	9	26	26
B. *Operated*										
0–19 Years	56	3.8	3	2	3	4	4	7	8	9
20–34	12	3.3	7	1	1	3	5	8	9	9
35–49	18	7.4	38	3	3	6	8	19	26	26
50–64	22	11.7	339	3	5	6	10	16	35	88
65+	11	10.4	107	2	3	7	12	26	34	34
SUBTOTALS:										
1. SINGLE DX										
A. *Not Operated*	26	3.2	3	2	2	3	4	6	6	9
B. *Operated*	32	3.1	6	1	2	2	4	6	7	12
2. MULTIPLE DX										
A. *Not Operated*	119	4.0	12	1	2	3	5	7	10	15
B. *Operated*	119	6.4	88	2	3	4	7	10	19	35
1. SINGLE DX	58	3.1	4	1	2	3	4	6	7	12
2. MULTIPLE DX	238	5.2	52	2	2	4	5	9	15	34
A. NOT OPERATED	145	3.8	11	1	2	3	4	7	9	15
B. OPERATED	151	5.7	72	2	2	4	6	9	14	35
TOTAL										
0–19 Years	137	3.6	5	1	2	3	4	6	8	12
20–34	29	3.0	4	1	2	2	4	6	8	9
35–49	59	4.7	21	1	2	3	6	10	15	26
50–64	47	8.0	173	2	3	5	8	14	16	88
65+	24	7.7	76	2	3	4	9	26	26	34
GRAND TOTAL	296	4.8	43	1	2	3	5	8	12	34

478.29: PHARYNGEAL DISEASE NEC

Type of Patients	Observed Patients	Avg. Stay	Variance	Percentiles						
				10th	25th	50th	75th	90th	95th	99th
1. SINGLE DX										
A. *Not Operated*										
0–19 Years	3	2.0	<1	1	1	2	3	3	3	3
20–34	2	2.0	2	1	1	3	3	3	3	3
35–49	0									
50–64	1	3.0	0	3	3	3	3	3	3	3
65+	0									
B. *Operated*										
0–19 Years	6	2.3	1	1	1	2	3	4	4	4
20–34	3	2.3	2	1	1	2	4	4	4	4
35–49	2	1.5	<1	1	1	2	2	2	2	2
50–64	2	2.0	0	2	2	2	2	2	2	2
65+	0									
2. MULTIPLE DX										
A. *Not Operated*										
0–19 Years	13	2.3	2	1	1	2	4	4	5	5
20–34	19	2.5	3	1	1	2	3	4	8	8
35–49	31	3.3	18	1	2	2	4	5	8	24
50–64	32	3.5	6	1	3	3	5	5	8	14
65+	42	4.9	42	1	2	3	5	10	19	32
B. *Operated*										
0–19 Years	9	2.4	4	1	1	1	4	6	6	6
20–34	14	3.6	6	1	2	3	5	5	11	11
35–49	20	3.4	8	1	2	3	4	10	12	12
50–64	20	5.4	51	1	2	4	6	9	34	34
65+	25	6.5	49	1	2	3	10	18	19	25
SUBTOTALS:										
1. SINGLE DX										
A. *Not Operated*	6	2.2	<1	1	1	2	3	3	3	3
B. *Operated*	13	2.2	1	1	1	2	3	4	4	4
2. MULTIPLE DX										
A. *Not Operated*	137	3.6	19	1	1	2	4	6	10	15
B. *Operated*	88	4.7	30	1	2	3	5	11	18	34
1. SINGLE DX	19	2.2	1	1	1	2	3	4	4	4
2. MULTIPLE DX	225	4.0	24	1	1	3	4	8	12	25
A. NOT OPERATED	143	3.6	19	1	1	2	4	6	10	15
B. OPERATED	101	4.4	27	1	2	3	5	10	15	35
TOTAL										
0–19 Years	31	2.3	2	1	1	2	4	4	5	6
20–34	38	2.9	4	1	1	2	4	5	8	11
35–49	53	3.3	14	1	2	2	4	5	10	24
50–64	55	4.1	23	1	2	3	5	7	9	34
65+	67	5.5	44	1	2	3	6	18	19	32
GRAND TOTAL	244	3.9	22	1	1	3	4	7	11	25

478.74: LARYNGEAL STENOSIS

Type of Patients	Observed Patients	Avg. Stay	Variance	Percentiles						
				10th	25th	50th	75th	90th	95th	99th
1. SINGLE DX										
A. *Not Operated*										
0–19 Years	1	1.0	0	1	1	1	1	1	1	1
20–34	3	1.0	0	1	1	1	1	1	1	1
35–49	4	1.5	<1	1	1	1	2	2	2	2
50–64	1	2.0	0	2	2	2	2	2	2	2
65+	0									
B. *Operated*										
0–19 Years	6	1.8	<1	1	1	2	2	3	3	3
20–34	2	1.5	<1	1	1	1	1	2	2	2
35–49	3	2.7	8	1	1	1	6	6	6	6
50–64	0									
65+	0									
2. MULTIPLE DX										
A. *Not Operated*										
0–19 Years	14	5.3	46	1	1	2	4	17	22	22
20–34	5	10.8	101	1	5	5	19	24	24	24
35–49	10	4.4	8	2	3	4	5	10	10	10
50–64	16	3.4	6	1	2	3	5	6	6	6
65+	14	6.7	39	1	1	4	8	14	22	22
B. *Operated*										
0–19 Years	36	6.4	51	1	1	3	8	19	21	26
20–34	18	4.4	18	1	1	2	8	12	14	14
35–49	14	2.9	3	1	2	3	3	5	7	7
50–64	28	5.9	50	1	1	3	9	14	23	31
65+	25	4.7	18	1	1	4	6	13	14	16
SUBTOTALS:										
1. SINGLE DX										
A. *Not Operated*	9	1.3	<1	1	1	2	2	2	2	2
B. *Operated*	11	2.0	2	1	1	2	2	3	6	6
2. MULTIPLE DX										
A. *Not Operated*	59	5.4	32	1	2	3	6	14	22	24
B. *Operated*	121	5.2	34	1	1	3	7	14	18	26
1. SINGLE DX	20	1.7	1	1	1	1	2	3	6	6
2. MULTIPLE DX	180	5.3	33	1	1	3	7	14	19	26
A. NOT OPERATED	68	4.9	30	1	1	3	5	14	19	24
B. OPERATED	132	5.0	32	1	1	3	7	13	18	26
TOTAL										
0–19 Years	57	5.6	45	1	1	2	7	18	21	26
20–34	28	5.0	36	1	1	3	8	14	19	24
35–49	31	3.2	5	1	3	3	4	6	8	10
50–64	45	4.9	33	1	2	3	5	10	14	31
65+	39	5.4	26	1	1	4	7	14	16	22
GRAND TOTAL	200	4.9	31	1	1	3	6	13	18	24

Length of Stay by Diagnosis and Operation, Western Region, 2008

Western Region, October 2006–September 2007 Data, by Diagnosis

480: VIRAL PNEUMONIA

Type of Patients	Observed Patients	Avg. Stay	Vari-ance	10th	25th	50th	Percentiles 75th	90th	95th	99th
1. SINGLE DX										
A. Not Operated										
0–19 Years	352	2.7	3	1	1	2	3	5	6	9
20–34	1	7.0	0	7	7	7	7	7	7	7
35–49	1	1.0	0	1	1	1	1	1	1	1
50–64	0									
65+	0									
B. Operated										
0–19 Years	0									
20–34	0									
35–49	0									
50–64	0									
65+	0									
2. MULTIPLE DX										
A. Not Operated										
0–19 Years	1,776	3.4	8	1	2	3	4	6	8	15
20–34	61	5.8	80	1	2	4	6	11	14	68
35–49	121	4.7	19	1	2	3	5	10	14	19
50–64	201	5.4	52	1	2	3	6	10	16	48
65+	396	4.9	13	2	3	4	6	10	11	20
B. Operated										
0–19 Years	4	27.1	172	15	15	34	42	42	42	42
20–34	3	11.0	63	3	3	11	19	19	19	19
35–49	7	11.0	40	3	6	10	15	22	22	22
50–64	12	16.3	80	7	7	18	21	22	36	36
65+	6	7.5	11	3	6	7	9	13	13	13
SUBTOTALS:										
1. SINGLE DX										
A. Not Operated	354	2.7	3	1	1	2	3	5	6	9
B. Operated	0									
2. MULTIPLE DX										
A. Not Operated	2,555	3.9	15	1	2	3	5	7	10	18
B. Operated	32	14.3	94	3	7	13	19	22	36	42
1. SINGLE DX	354	2.7	3	1	2	2	3	5	6	9
2. MULTIPLE DX	2,587	4.1	17	1	2	3	5	7	11	21
A. NOT OPERATED	2,909	3.8	14	1	2	3	5	7	9	18
B. OPERATED	32	14.3	94	3	7	13	19	22	36	42
TOTAL										
0–19 Years	2,132	3.3	9	1	2	2	4	6	8	15
20–34	65	6.1	78	1	2	4	7	13	14	68
35–49	129	5.0	22	1	2	3	6	12	15	22
50–64	213	6.1	59	1	2	3	7	12	20	41
65+	402	5.0	13	2	3	4	6	10	11	18
GRAND TOTAL	2,941	3.9	16	1	2	3	5	7	10	19

480.1: RSV PNEUMONIA

Type of Patients	Observed Patients	Avg. Stay	Vari-ance	10th	25th	50th	Percentiles 75th	90th	95th	99th
1. SINGLE DX										
A. Not Operated										
0–19 Years	216	3.1	3	1	2	3	4	6	7	9
20–34	0									
35–49	0									
50–64	0									
65+	0									
B. Operated										
0–19 Years	0									
20–34	0									
35–49	0									
50–64	0									
65+	0									
2. MULTIPLE DX										
A. Not Operated										
0–19 Years	852	3.9	9	1	2	3	5	7	9	15
20–34	1	7.0	0	7	7	7	7	7	7	7
35–49	5	6.6	49	3	3	3	5	19	19	19
50–64	18	10.1	77	2	4	7	14	26	32	32
65+	14	5.4	8	3	3	5	7	10	11	11
B. Operated										
0–19 Years	1	42.0	0	42	42	42	42	42	42	42
20–34	0									
35–49	0									
50–64	1	19.0	0	19	19	19	19	19	19	19
65+	0									
SUBTOTALS:										
1. SINGLE DX										
A. Not Operated	216	3.1	3	1	2	3	4	6	7	9
B. Operated	0									
2. MULTIPLE DX										
A. Not Operated	890	4.1	11	1	2	3	5	7	9	20
B. Operated	2	30.5	260	19	19	31	42	42	42	42
1. SINGLE DX	216	3.1	3	1	2	3	4	6	7	9
2. MULTIPLE DX	892	4.1	13	1	2	3	5	7	9	21
A. NOT OPERATED	1,106	3.9	10	1	2	3	5	7	9	17
B. OPERATED	2	30.5	260	19	19	31	42	42	42	42
TOTAL										
0–19 Years	1,069	3.8	9	1	2	3	5	7	8	15
20–34	1	7.0	0	7	7	7	7	7	7	7
35–49	5	6.6	49	3	3	3	5	19	19	19
50–64	19	10.5	77	2	4	7	16	26	32	32
65+	14	5.4	8	3	3	5	7	10	11	11
GRAND TOTAL	1,108	3.9	11	1	2	3	5	7	9	19

480.9: VIRAL PNEUMONIA NOS

Type of Patients	Observed Patients	Avg. Stay	Vari-ance	10th	25th	50th	Percentiles 75th	90th	95th	99th
1. SINGLE DX										
A. Not Operated										
0–19 Years	131	2.0	<1	1	1	2	3	3	4	4
20–34	1	7.0	0	7	7	7	7	7	7	7
35–49	1	1.0	0	1	1	1	1	1	1	1
50–64	0									
65+	0									
B. Operated										
0–19 Years	0									
20–34	0									
35–49	0									
50–64	0									
65+	0									
2. MULTIPLE DX										
A. Not Operated										
0–19 Years	858	2.8	5	1	1	2	3	5	6	10
20–34	56	4.6	13	1	2	4	6	11	14	14
35–49	104	4.3	13	1	2	3	5	8	12	17
50–64	165	4.6	32	1	2	3	6	8	11	41
65+	359	4.8	11	2	3	4	6	9	11	18
B. Operated										
0–19 Years	2	16.0	2	15	15	15	17	17	17	17
20–34	3	11.0	63	3	3	11	19	19	19	19
35–49	7	11.0	40	3	6	10	15	22	22	22
50–64	7	13.4	63	2	7	17	21	22	22	22
65+	5	7.6	14	3	6	7	9	13	13	13
SUBTOTALS:										
1. SINGLE DX										
A. Not Operated	133	2.0	1	1	1	2	3	3	4	5
B. Operated	0									
2. MULTIPLE DX										
A. Not Operated	1,542	3.6	11	1	2	3	4	7	9	16
B. Operated	24	11.4	41	3	6	10	17	21	22	22
1. SINGLE DX	133	2.0	1	1	1	2	3	3	4	5
2. MULTIPLE DX	1,566	3.7	12	1	2	3	5	7	10	18
A. NOT OPERATED	1,675	3.5	10	1	2	3	4	7	9	16
B. OPERATED	24	11.4	41	3	6	10	17	21	22	22
TOTAL										
0–19 Years	991	2.7	5	1	1	2	3	5	6	10
20–34	60	4.9	16	1	2	4	7	11	14	19
35–49	112	4.7	17	1	2	3	6	10	15	18
50–64	172	4.9	36	1	2	3	6	9	13	41
65+	364	4.8	11	2	3	4	6	9	11	18
GRAND TOTAL	1,699	3.6	12	1	2	3	4	7	9	17

Length of Stay by Diagnosis and Operation, Western Region, 2008

Western Region, October 2006–September 2007 Data, by Diagnosis

481: PNEUMOCOCCAL PNEUMONIA

Type of Patients	Observed Patients	Avg. Stay	Variance	10th	25th	50th	75th	90th	95th	99th
1. SINGLE DX										
A. Not Operated										
0–19 Years	20	3.1	4	1	2	3	3	7	8	8
20–34	3	2.7	<1	2	2	3	3	3	3	3
35–49	2	2.5	<1	2	2	3	3	3	3	3
50–64	5	2.2	<1	1	2	2	3	3	3	3
65+	0									
B. Operated										
0–19 Years	0									
20–34	0									
35–49	0									
50–64	0									
65+	0									
2. MULTIPLE DX										
A. Not Operated										
0–19 Years	166	4.4	12	1	2	3	6	9	11	19
20–34	143	4.4	8	2	3	4	5	7	8	17
35–49	407	5.2	18	2	3	4	7	10	12	23
50–64	744	5.6	19	2	3	4	7	11	13	23
65+	1,512	5.6	21	2	3	5	7	10	14	20
B. Operated										
0–19 Years	16	9.6	14	5	7	10	14	14	15	15
20–34	10	8.7	18	3	6	10	12	17	>99	>99
35–49	25	17.9	125	8	9	15	22	38	39	44
50–64	42	14.3	171	4	6	9	18	25	34	69
65+	55	13.4	51	6	8	12	16	24	27	33
SUBTOTALS:										
1. SINGLE DX										
A. Not Operated	30	2.9	3	1	2	3	3	5	7	8
B. Operated	0									
2. MULTIPLE DX										
A. Not Operated	2,972	5.4	19	2	3	4	7	10	13	21
B. Operated	148	13.7	96	5	7	11	17	27	34	69
1. SINGLE DX	30	2.9	3	1	2	3	3	5	7	8
2. MULTIPLE DX	3,120	5.8	26	2	3	4	7	11	15	25
A. NOT OPERATED	3,002	5.4	19	2	3	4	7	10	13	21
B. OPERATED	148	13.7	96	5	7	11	17	27	34	69
TOTAL										
0–19 Years	202	4.6	14	1	2	3	6	10	12	15
20–34	156	4.7	10	2	3	4	6	8	11	21
35–49	434	6.0	33	2	3	4	7	11	16	32
50–64	791	6.0	30	2	3	4	7	11	16	29
65+	1,567	5.9	24	2	3	5	7	11	14	24
GRAND TOTAL	3,150	5.8	26	2	3	4	7	11	15	25

482: OTHER BACT PNEUMONIA

Type of Patients	Observed Patients	Avg. Stay	Variance	10th	25th	50th	75th	90th	95th	99th
1. SINGLE DX										
A. Not Operated										
0–19 Years	49	2.5	4	1	1	2	3	3	6	10
20–34	4	3.0	4	2	2	2	6	6	6	6
35–49	3	3.3	1	2	2	4	4	4	4	4
50–64	3	3.0	7	1	2	2	6	6	6	6
65+	1	4.0	0	4	4	4	4	4	4	4
B. Operated										
0–19 Years	0									
20–34	1	3.0	0	3	3	3	3	3	3	3
35–49	0									
50–64	0									
2. MULTIPLE DX										
A. Not Operated										
0–19 Years	676	6.7	46	1	2	4	9	14	18	37
20–34	575	9.5	79	2	4	7	13	20	25	39
35–49	997	8.0	59	2	3	6	10	17	23	34
50–64	2,395	8.1	51	3	4	6	10	16	21	37
65+	7,461	8.0	38	3	4	6	10	15	19	31
B. Operated										
0–19 Years	19	17.3	161	3	10	13	24	36	51	51
20–34	35	24.7	347	6	10	19	40	52	63	74
35–49	76	16.0	151	6	8	13	20	30	36	81
50–64	129	15.1	133	5	7	12	20	30	33	63
65+	291	15.5	114	6	9	13	19	27	35	91
SUBTOTALS:										
1. SINGLE DX										
A. Not Operated	60	2.6	4	1	1	2	4	6	7	10
B. Operated	1	3.0	0	3	3	3	3	3	3	3
2. MULTIPLE DX										
A. Not Operated	12,104	8.0	45	2	4	6	10	15	20	33
B. Operated	550	16.1	144	6	9	13	20	30	36	74
1. SINGLE DX	61	2.6	4	1	1	2	3	6	7	8
2. MULTIPLE DX	12,654	8.4	52	3	4	6	10	16	21	36
A. NOT OPERATED	12,164	8.0	45	2	4	6	10	15	20	33
B. OPERATED	551	16.1	144	6	9	13	20	30	36	74
TOTAL										
0–19 Years	744	6.7	50	1	2	4	9	14	19	37
20–34	614	10.4	106	2	4	7	14	21	28	55
35–49	1,077	8.5	69	2	3	6	11	19	24	37
50–64	2,527	8.5	58	3	4	6	10	17	22	38
65+	7,753	8.3	43	3	4	7	10	16	20	33
GRAND TOTAL	12,715	8.3	52	3	4	6	10	16	21	36

482.0: K. PNEUMONIAE PNEUMONIA

Type of Patients	Observed Patients	Avg. Stay	Variance	10th	25th	50th	75th	90th	95th	99th
1. SINGLE DX										
A. Not Operated										
0–19 Years	0									
20–34	0									
35–49	0									
50–64	0									
65+	0									
B. Operated										
0–19 Years	0									
20–34	0									
35–49	0									
50–64	0									
2. MULTIPLE DX										
A. Not Operated										
0–19 Years	10	15.9	171	4	4	15	26	40	40	40
20–34	15	7.3	20	3	3	7	9	13	18	18
35–49	32	6.4	19	3	4	5	9	11	13	22
50–64	139	8.1	43	3	4	6	9	19	21	38
65+	396	7.3	29	3	4	6	9	14	17	29
B. Operated										
0–19 Years	0									
20–34	0									
35–49	4	20.0	84	11	14	24	24	31	31	31
50–64	6	11.2	6	8	10	10	14	14	14	14
65+	17	14.0	45	5	9	12	19	25	26	26
SUBTOTALS:										
1. SINGLE DX										
A. Not Operated	0									
B. Operated	0									
2. MULTIPLE DX										
A. Not Operated	592	7.6	35	3	4	6	9	14	19	30
B. Operated	27	14.3	46	8	10	12	19	25	26	31
1. SINGLE DX	0									
2. MULTIPLE DX	619	7.9	37	3	4	6	10	15	21	30
A. NOT OPERATED	592	7.6	35	3	4	6	9	14	19	30
B. OPERATED	27	14.3	46	8	10	12	19	25	26	31
TOTAL										
0–19 Years	10	15.9	171	4	4	15	26	40	40	40
20–34	15	7.3	20	3	3	7	9	13	18	18
35–49	36	8.0	43	3	3	6	11	14	13	31
50–64	145	8.2	42	3	4	6	9	18	21	38
65+	413	7.6	31	3	4	6	9	14	19	28
GRAND TOTAL	619	7.9	37	3	4	6	10	15	21	30

Western Region, October 2006–September 2007 Data, by Diagnosis

482.1: PSEUDOMONAL PNEUMONIA

Type of Patients	Observed Patients	Avg. Stay	Variance	10th	25th	50th	75th	90th	95th	99th
1. SINGLE DX										
A. Not Operated										
0–19 Years	1	8.0	0	8	8	8	8	8	8	8
20–34	0									
35–49	0									
50–64	1	6.0	0	6	6	6	6	6	6	6
65+	1	4.0	0	4	4	4	4	4	4	4
B. Operated										
0–19 Years	0									
20–34	0									
35–49	1	3.0	0	3	3	3	3	3	3	3
50–64	0									
65+	0									
2. MULTIPLE DX										
A. Not Operated										
0–19 Years	165	11.1	65	4	6	10	14	18	22	51
20–34	205	12.1	52	3	6	11	16	21	24	31
35–49	162	10.4	103	3	5	8	13	22	26	46
50–64	389	8.8	38	3	5	7	11	16	21	33
65+	1,316	8.7	44	3	5	7	11	16	21	34
B. Operated										
0–19 Years	1	10.0	0	10	10	10	10	10	10	10
20–34	13	31.7	473	9	10	27	49	55	74	74
35–49	11	20.2	486	7	7	14	18	36	81	81
50–64	20	14.9	277	5	7	9	17	22	81	81
65+	44	19.4	250	7	10	16	21	40	44	91
SUBTOTALS:										
1. SINGLE DX										
A. Not Operated	3	6.0	4	4	4	6	8	8	8	8
B. Operated	1	3.0	0	3	3	3	3	3	3	3
2. MULTIPLE DX										
A. Not Operated	2,237	9.3	51	3	5	7	11	18	22	35
B. Operated	89	20.2	329	6	9	15	21	48	60	91
1. SINGLE DX	4	5.3	5	3	3	6	8	8	8	8
2. MULTIPLE DX	2,326	9.8	66	3	5	8	12	18	23	41
A. NOT OPERATED	2,240	9.3	51	3	5	7	11	18	22	35
B. OPERATED	90	20.0	329	6	9	14	21	48	60	91
TOTAL										
0–19 Years	167	11.1	65	4	6	10	14	18	22	51
20–34	218	13.2	97	4	6	12	18	23	29	52
35–49	174	11.0	130	3	5	8	13	22	29	81
50–64	410	9.1	51	3	5	7	11	17	21	33
65+	1,361	9.1	54	3	5	7	11	17	22	39
GRAND TOTAL	2,330	9.8	66	3	5	8	12	18	23	41

482.2: H. INFLUENZAE PNEUMONIA

Type of Patients	Observed Patients	Avg. Stay	Variance	10th	25th	50th	75th	90th	95th	99th
1. SINGLE DX										
A. Not Operated										
0–19 Years	2	5.5	40	1	1	10	10	10	10	10
20–34	1	2.0	0	2	2	2	2	2	2	2
35–49	0									
50–64	0									
65+	0									
B. Operated										
0–19 Years	0									
20–34	0									
35–49	0									
50–64	0									
65+	0									
2. MULTIPLE DX										
A. Not Operated										
0–19 Years	22	7.4	35	2	3	5	11	15	18	24
20–34	17	5.0	21	1	2	5	6	10	20	20
35–49	51	6.8	59	3	3	5	7	10	22	43
50–64	134	5.6	17	2	3	5	7	10	13	23
65+	366	6.1	16	3	3	5	8	11	13	18
B. Operated										
0–19 Years	0									
20–34	0									
35–49	2	17.4	178	8	8	8	27	27	27	27
50–64	4	11.8	55	4	8	11	21	21	21	21
65+	5	12.2	49	4	8	11	16	22	22	22
SUBTOTALS:										
1. SINGLE DX										
A. Not Operated	3	4.4	24	1	1	2	10	10	10	10
B. Operated	0									
2. MULTIPLE DX										
A. Not Operated	590	6.1	21	2	3	5	7	11	14	24
B. Operated	11	13.0	59	4	8	11	21	22	27	27
1. SINGLE DX	3	4.4	24	1	1	2	10	10	10	10
2. MULTIPLE DX	601	6.2	22	2	3	5	7	11	14	24
A. NOT OPERATED	593	6.0	21	2	3	5	7	11	14	24
B. OPERATED	11	13.0	59	4	8	11	21	22	27	27
TOTAL										
0–19 Years	24	7.3	34	2	3	6	11	15	18	24
20–34	18	4.8	20	1	2	5	6	10	20	20
35–49	53	7.2	64	3	3	5	7	10	27	43
50–64	138	5.8	19	2	3	5	7	11	14	23
65+	371	6.2	17	3	3	5	8	11	14	22
GRAND TOTAL	604	6.2	22	2	3	5	8	11	14	24

482.30: STREP PNEUMONIA NOS

Type of Patients	Observed Patients	Avg. Stay	Variance	10th	25th	50th	75th	90th	95th	99th
1. SINGLE DX										
A. Not Operated										
0–19 Years	1	1.0	0	1	1	1	1	1	1	1
20–34	0									
35–49	1	2.0	0	2	2	2	2	2	2	2
50–64	1	1.0	0	1	1	1	1	1	1	1
65+	0									
B. Operated										
0–19 Years	0									
20–34	0									
35–49	0									
50–64	0									
65+	0									
2. MULTIPLE DX										
A. Not Operated										
0–19 Years	20	4.9	34	1	1	3	6	10	25	25
20–34	23	7.0	148	2	2	4	5	15	16	60
35–49	55	4.5	11	2	2	4	5	9	11	19
50–64	112	5.9	20	2	3	4	7	13	16	18
65+	171	5.5	20	2	3	4	7	11	14	23
B. Operated										
0–19 Years	1	8.0	0	8	8	8	8	8	8	8
20–34	2	8.0	49	3	3	8	13	13	13	13
35–49	4	15.0	57	10	10	12	26	26	26	26
50–64	6	9.0	17	3	5	10	11	14	14	14
65+	9	14.0	90	4	7	12	19	30	30	30
SUBTOTALS:										
1. SINGLE DX										
A. Not Operated	3	1.3	<1	1	1	1	2	2	2	2
B. Operated	0									
2. MULTIPLE DX										
A. Not Operated	381	5.6	27	2	3	4	6	11	16	23
B. Operated	22	12.0	57	4	7	10	14	26	27	30
1. SINGLE DX	3	1.3	<1	1	1	1	2	2	2	2
2. MULTIPLE DX	403	5.9	31	2	3	4	7	12	16	26
A. NOT OPERATED	384	5.5	27	2	3	4	6	11	16	23
B. OPERATED	22	12.0	57	4	7	10	14	26	27	30
TOTAL										
0–19 Years	22	4.9	32	1	1	2	6	10	13	25
20–34	25	7.0	138	2	2	4	5	15	16	60
35–49	60	5.2	20	2	2	4	6	10	14	26
50–64	119	6.1	20	2	3	4	8	13	16	18
65+	180	5.9	27	2	3	4	7	12	19	27
GRAND TOTAL	406	5.9	31	2	3	4	7	12	16	26

Length of Stay by Diagnosis and Operation, Western Region, 2008

Western Region, October 2006–September 2007 Data, by Diagnosis

482.41: STAPH AUREUS PNEUMONIA

Type of Patients	Observed Patients	Avg. Stay	Variance	10th	25th	50th	75th	90th	95th	99th
1. SINGLE DX										
A. Not Operated										
0–19 Years	1	4.0	0	4	4	4	4	4	4	4
20–34	0									
35–49	0									
50–64	0									
65+	0									
B. Operated										
0–19 Years	0									
20–34	0									
35–49	0									
50–64	0									
65+	0									
2. MULTIPLE DX										
A. Not Operated										
0–19 Years	73	9.5	63	4	5	7	12	15	21	55
20–34	160	10.4	113	3	5	8	11	18	29	76
35–49	341	10.2	67	3	5	8	13	21	25	37
50–64	793	10.4	71	3	5	8	13	19	25	47
65+	2,754	9.7	42	4	5	8	12	17	21	34
B. Operated										
0–19 Years	6	20.3	256	8	10	13	24	51	51	51
20–34	14	24.8	244	8	13	21	35	42	63	63
35–49	32	16.2	131	6	9	13	20	30	51	52
50–64	53	19.1	142	7	10	18	24	33	35	63
65+	143	15.3	66	7	9	14	18	28	35	44
SUBTOTALS:										
1. SINGLE DX										
A. Not Operated	1	4.0	0	4	4	4	4	4	4	4
B. Operated	0									
2. MULTIPLE DX										
A. Not Operated	4,121	9.9	53	4	5	8	12	18	23	39
B. Operated	248	16.9	109	7	10	14	21	32	36	63
1. SINGLE DX	1	4.0	0	4	4	4	4	4	4	4
2. MULTIPLE DX	4,369	10.3	59	4	5	8	13	19	24	41
A. NOT OPERATED	4,122	9.9	53	4	5	8	12	18	23	39
B. OPERATED	248	16.9	109	7	10	14	21	32	36	63
TOTAL										
0–19 Years	80	10.3	82	4	5	8	12	16	27	55
20–34	174	11.5	138	3	5	8	14	25	35	76
35–49	373	10.7	75	3	5	8	14	21	25	51
50–64	846	11.0	80	4	6	9	14	21	27	52
65+	2,897	10.0	45	4	6	8	13	18	22	35
GRAND TOTAL	4,370	10.3	59	4	5	8	13	19	24	41

482.82: E. COLI PNEUMONIA

Type of Patients	Observed Patients	Avg. Stay	Variance	10th	25th	50th	75th	90th	95th	99th
1. SINGLE DX										
A. Not Operated										
0–19 Years	0									
20–34	0									
35–49	0									
50–64	0									
65+	0									
B. Operated										
0–19 Years	0									
20–34	0									
35–49	0									
50–64	0									
65+	0									
2. MULTIPLE DX										
A. Not Operated										
0–19 Years	3	7.7	41	3	3	5	15	15	15	15
20–34	4	8.0	21	4	5	7	12	14	14	14
35–49	12	8.1	29	3	5	5	11	16	18	18
50–64	63	9.2	62	3	5	7	12	20	25	47
65+	212	8.0	34	3	4	7	10	14	17	28
B. Operated										
0–19 Years	0									
20–34	0									
35–49	3	17.6	46	10	10	20	23	23	23	23
50–64	2	13.5	110	6	6	14	21	21	21	21
65+	7	26.4	947	4	11	15	27	94	94	94
SUBTOTALS:										
1. SINGLE DX										
A. Not Operated	0									
B. Operated	0									
2. MULTIPLE DX										
A. Not Operated	294	8.3	40	3	4	7	10	15	20	28
B. Operated	12	22.0	565	6	10	20	21	27	94	94
1. SINGLE DX	0									
2. MULTIPLE DX	306	8.8	66	3	5	7	11	16	21	28
A. NOT OPERATED	294	8.3	40	3	4	7	10	15	20	28
B. OPERATED	12	22.0	565	6	10	20	21	27	94	94
TOTAL										
0–19 Years	3	7.7	41	3	3	5	15	15	15	15
20–34	4	8.0	21	4	5	7	12	14	14	14
35–49	15	10.0	45	3	4	8	16	20	23	23
50–64	65	9.3	63	3	5	7	12	21	25	47
65+	219	8.6	70	3	4	7	11	15	20	28
GRAND TOTAL	306	8.8	66	3	5	7	11	16	21	28

482.83: GRAM-NEG PNEUMONIA NEC

Type of Patients	Observed Patients	Avg. Stay	Variance	10th	25th	50th	75th	90th	95th	99th
1. SINGLE DX										
A. Not Operated										
0–19 Years	2	2.0	2	1	1	3	3	3	3	3
20–34	0									
35–49	0									
50–64	0									
65+	0									
B. Operated										
0–19 Years	0									
20–34	0									
35–49	0									
50–64	0									
65+	0									
2. MULTIPLE DX										
A. Not Operated										
0–19 Years	39	7.3	31	2	3	6	8	17	18	27
20–34	27	9.9	96	3	3	5	14	27	31	40
35–49	57	6.7	27	2	3	6	8	13	15	33
50–64	175	7.6	66	3	4	6	8	14	19	32
65+	625	7.5	39	3	4	6	9	16	19	33
B. Operated										
0–19 Years	2	25.4	215	15	15	15	36	36	36	36
20–34	1	14.0	0	14	14	14	14	14	14	14
35–49	5	14.3	127	5	7	10	17	33	33	33
50–64	12	11.6	79	4	9	14	14	14	20	35
65+	18	16.1	81	6	9	15	22	31	35	36
SUBTOTALS:										
1. SINGLE DX										
A. Not Operated	2	2.0	2	1	1	3	3	3	3	3
B. Operated	0									
2. MULTIPLE DX										
A. Not Operated	923	7.5	45	3	4	6	8	15	19	33
B. Operated	38	14.9	91	4	7	13	19	33	36	36
1. SINGLE DX	2	2.0	2	1	1	3	3	3	3	3
2. MULTIPLE DX	961	7.8	49	3	4	6	9	16	20	35
A. NOT OPERATED	925	7.5	45	3	4	6	8	15	19	33
B. OPERATED	38	14.9	91	4	7	13	19	33	36	36
TOTAL										
0–19 Years	43	7.9	50	2	3	6	9	17	18	36
20–34	28	10.0	93	3	5	5	14	27	31	40
35–49	62	7.3	37	2	3	6	9	14	15	33
50–64	187	7.9	68	3	4	6	9	14	19	35
65+	643	7.7	42	3	4	6	9	16	20	34
GRAND TOTAL	963	7.8	49	3	4	6	9	16	20	35

Length of Stay by Diagnosis and Operation, Western Region, 2008

Western Region, October 2006–September 2007 Data, by Diagnosis

482.84: LEGIONNAIRES' DISEASE

Type of Patients	Observed Patients	Avg. Stay	Vari-ance	10th	25th	50th	75th	90th	95th	99th
1. SINGLE DX										
A. Not Operated										
0–19 Years	0									
20–34	0									
35–49	0									
50–64	0									
65+	0									
B. Operated										
0–19 Years	0									
20–34	0									
35–49	0									
50–64	0									
65+	0									
2. MULTIPLE DX										
A. Not Operated										
0–19 Years	2	6.5	<1	6	6	6	7	7	7	7
20–34	3	5.3	2	4	4	5	7	7	7	7
35–49	21	10.0	49	3	5	8	13	20	23	27
50–64	40	8.1	25	3	5	6	10	16	20	22
65+	59	8.3	27	3	5	7	10	15	20	27
B. Operated										
0–19 Years	0									
20–34	1	13.0	0	13	13	13	13	13		13
35–49	0									
50–64	3	18.0	209	4	4	17	33	33	33	33
65+	2	9.5	<1	9	9	10	10	10	10	10
SUBTOTALS:										
1. SINGLE DX										
A. Not Operated	0									
B. Operated	0									
2. MULTIPLE DX										
A. Not Operated	125	8.4	30	3	5	7	10	16	20	27
B. Operated	6	14.4	103	4	9	10	17	33	33	33
1. SINGLE DX	0									
2. MULTIPLE DX	131	8.7	34	3	5	7	11	17	20	27
A. NOT OPERATED	125	8.4	30	3	5	7	10	16	20	27
B. OPERATED	6	14.4	103	4	9	10	17	33	33	33
TOTAL										
0–19 Years	2	6.5	<1	6	6	6	7	7	7	7
20–34	4	7.2	16	4	4	5	7	13	13	13
35–49	21	10.0	49	3	5	8	13	20	23	27
50–64	43	8.8	40	3	5	6	11	17	20	33
65+	61	8.3	27	3	5	7	10	15	17	27
GRAND TOTAL	131	8.7	34	3	5	7	11	17	20	27

482.9: BACTERIAL PNEUMONIA NOS

Type of Patients	Observed Patients	Avg. Stay	Vari-ance	10th	25th	50th	75th	90th	95th	99th
1. SINGLE DX										
A. Not Operated										
0–19 Years	38	2.0	1	1	1	2	2	4	4	6
20–34	1	2.0	0	2	2	2	2	2	2	2
35–49	2	4.0	0	4	4	4	4	4	4	4
50–64	1	2.0	0	2	2	2	2	2	2	2
65+	0									
B. Operated										
0–19 Years	0									
20–34	0									
35–49	0									
50–64	0									
65+	0									
2. MULTIPLE DX										
A. Not Operated										
0–19 Years	297	3.2	7	1	2	3	4	6	7	13
20–34	77	4.3	16	2	2	3	5	9	10	27
35–49	190	4.0	12	1	2	3	5	7	9	22
50–64	398	4.5	15	1	2	4	5	8	12	21
65+	1,209	4.7	13	2	3	4	6	9	11	18
B. Operated										
0–19 Years	5	11.0	32	3	10	11	12	19	19	19
20–34	2	6.0	8	4	4	4	6	8	8	8
35–49	5	5.0	6	3	3	4	6	9	9	9
50–64	14	10.7	57	5	6	7	14	22	30	30
65+	25	10.0	15	5	7	10	12	15	17	20
SUBTOTALS:										
1. SINGLE DX										
A. Not Operated	42	2.1	2	1	1	2	3	4	4	6
B. Operated	0									
2. MULTIPLE DX										
A. Not Operated	2,171	4.4	13	1	2	3	5	8	11	18
B. Operated	51	9.6	29	4	6	9	12	15	20	30
1. SINGLE DX	42	2.1	2	1	2	3	3	4	4	6
2. MULTIPLE DX	2,222	4.5	14	1	2	4	5	9	11	19
A. NOT OPERATED	2,213	4.4	13	1	2	3	5	8	11	18
B. OPERATED	51	9.6	29	4	6	9	12	15	20	30
TOTAL										
0–19 Years	340	3.1	8	1	2	2	4	6	8	14
20–34	80	4.3	15	2	2	3	5	9	10	27
35–49	197	4.0	12	1	2	3	5	7	9	22
50–64	413	4.7	18	1	2	4	6	9	13	22
65+	1,234	4.8	13	2	3	4	6	9	12	18
GRAND TOTAL	2,264	4.5	14	2	3	3	5	9	11	19

483: PNEUMONIA ORGANISM NEC

Type of Patients	Observed Patients	Avg. Stay	Vari-ance	10th	25th	50th	75th	90th	95th	99th
1. SINGLE DX										
A. Not Operated										
0–19 Years	17	4.3	20	1	2	2	5	10	18	18
20–34	2	2.0	0	2	2	2	2	2	2	2
35–49	2	1.5	<1	1	1	2	2	2	2	2
50–64	0									
65+	0									
B. Operated										
0–19 Years	0									
20–34	0									
35–49	0									
50–64	0									
65+	0									
2. MULTIPLE DX										
A. Not Operated										
0–19 Years	168	3.3	5	1	2	3	4	6	8	15
20–34	39	6.0	43	1	3	4	6	13	23	35
35–49	58	5.7	18	2	3	5	7	11	14	23
50–64	68	7.2	29	2	4	6	10	14	21	30
65+	115	7.4	22	3	4	6	10	13	16	23
B. Operated										
0–19 Years	3	16.3	25	11	11	21	>99	>99	>99	>99
20–34	3	11.7	9	9	11	11	15	15	15	15
35–49	2	5.5	4	4	4	7	7	7	7	7
50–64	3	11.7	41	7	7	9	19	19	19	19
65+	6	10.0	36	6	7	8	9	22	22	22
SUBTOTALS:										
1. SINGLE DX										
A. Not Operated	21	3.9	17	1	2	2	5	9	10	18
B. Operated	0									
2. MULTIPLE DX										
A. Not Operated	448	5.5	21	2	3	4	7	11	14	23
B. Operated	17	11.2	31	6	7	9	17	22	>99	>99
1. SINGLE DX	21	3.9	17	1	2	2	5	9	10	18
2. MULTIPLE DX	465	5.7	23	2	3	4	7	11	15	23
A. NOT OPERATED	469	5.4	21	2	3	4	7	11	14	23
B. OPERATED	17	11.2	31	6	7	9	17	22	>99	>99
TOTAL										
0–19 Years	188	3.6	10	1	2	3	4	7	10	21
20–34	44	6.2	41	2	3	4	6	13	16	35
35–49	62	5.5	18	2	3	5	7	11	14	23
50–64	71	7.4	30	2	4	6	10	13	21	30
65+	121	7.5	22	3	5	6	9	13	16	23
GRAND TOTAL	486	5.6	22	2	4	4	7	11	15	23

Length of Stay by Diagnosis and Operation, Western Region, 2008

Western Region, October 2006–September 2007 Data, by Diagnosis

483.0: M. PNEUMONIAE PNEUMONIA

Type of Patients	Observed Patients	Avg. Stay	Variance	10th	25th	50th	75th	90th	95th	99th
1. SINGLE DX										
A. Not Operated										
0–19 Years	14	3.1	5	1	2	2	5	6	9	9
20–34	1	2.0	0	2	2	2	2	2	2	2
35–49	2	1.5	<1	1	1	2	2	2	2	2
50–64	0									
65+	0									
B. Operated										
0–19 Years	0									
20–34	0									
35–49	0									
50–64	0									
65+	0									
2. MULTIPLE DX										
A. Not Operated										
0–19 Years	150	3.2	5	1	2	3	4	6	7	11
20–34	29	4.8	22	1	3	4	5	9	16	23
35–49	48	5.1	13	2	3	5	7	11	12	18
50–64	49	6.2	14	2	3	6	8	12	14	15
65+	57	6.6	10	3	5	6	8	11	12	19
B. Operated										
0–19 Years	3	16.3	25	11	11	21	>99	>99	>99	>99
20–34	2	12.0	18	9	9	15	15	15	15	15
35–49	2	5.5	4	4	4	7	7	7	7	7
50–64	1	7.0	0	7	7	7	7	7	7	7
65+	3	8.3	1	7	7	9	9	9	9	9
SUBTOTALS:										
1. SINGLE DX										
A. Not Operated	17	2.9	5	1	2	2	3	6	9	9
B. Operated	0									
2. MULTIPLE DX										
A. Not Operated	333	4.7	12	1	2	4	6	9	11	16
B. Operated	11	10.6	26	7	7	9	15	21	>99	>99
1. SINGLE DX	17	2.9	5	1	2	2	3	6	9	9
2. MULTIPLE DX	344	4.8	13	1	2	4	6	10	12	19
A. NOT OPERATED	350	4.6	11	1	2	4	6	9	11	16
B. OPERATED	11	10.6	26	7	7	9	15	21	>99	>99
TOTAL										
0–19 Years	167	3.4	8	1	2	3	4	6	8	21
20–34	32	5.2	24	1	3	4	6	9	16	23
35–49	52	5.0	12	2	3	4	7	10	12	18
50–64	50	6.2	14	2	3	6	8	12	14	15
65+	60	6.7	10	3	5	6	9	11	12	19
GRAND TOTAL	361	4.7	13	1	2	4	6	10	12	19

484: PNEUM IN OTH INF DIS

Type of Patients	Observed Patients	Avg. Stay	Variance	10th	25th	50th	75th	90th	95th	99th
1. SINGLE DX										
A. Not Operated										
0–19 Years	0									
20–34	0									
35–49	0									
50–64	0									
65+	0									
B. Operated										
0–19 Years	0									
20–34	0									
35–49	0									
50–64	0									
65+	0									
2. MULTIPLE DX										
A. Not Operated										
0–19 Years	0									
20–34	0									
35–49	0									
50–64	0									
65+	0									
B. Operated										
0–19 Years	0									
20–34	0									
35–49	0									
50–64	0									
65+	0									
SUBTOTALS:										
1. SINGLE DX										
A. Not Operated	0									
B. Operated	0									
2. MULTIPLE DX										
A. Not Operated	0									
B. Operated	0									
1. SINGLE DX	0									
2. MULTIPLE DX	0									
A. NOT OPERATED	0									
B. OPERATED	0									
TOTAL										
0–19 Years	0									
20–34	0									
35–49	0									
50–64	0									
65+	0									
GRAND TOTAL	0									

485: BRONCHOPNEUMONIA ORG NOS

Type of Patients	Observed Patients	Avg. Stay	Variance	10th	25th	50th	75th	90th	95th	99th
1. SINGLE DX										
A. Not Operated										
0–19 Years	43	2.4	2	1	1	2	3	4	5	7
20–34	0									
35–49	1	4.0	0	4	4	4	4	4	4	4
50–64	1	3.0	0	3	3	3	3	3	3	3
65+	0									
B. Operated										
0–19 Years	0									
20–34	0									
35–49	0									
50–64	0									
65+	0									
2. MULTIPLE DX										
A. Not Operated										
0–19 Years	242	2.9	4	1	2	2	3	5	7	10
20–34	40	5.9	80	1	2	4	5	13	36	47
35–49	123	4.6	14	2	2	4	6	9	11	17
50–64	252	4.2	9	2	2	3	5	8	11	15
65+	794	5.0	11	2	3	4	6	9	11	16
B. Operated										
0–19 Years	1	32.0	0	32	32	32	32	32	32	32
20–34	1	4.0	0	4	4	4	4	4	4	4
35–49	4	6.5	35	2	3	5	6	15	15	15
50–64	8	13.3	109	3	5	11	19	34	34	34
65+	19	15.1	141	4	7	10	22	37	49	49
SUBTOTALS:										
1. SINGLE DX										
A. Not Operated	45	2.5	2	1	2	2	3	4	5	7
B. Operated	0									
2. MULTIPLE DX										
A. Not Operated	1,451	4.5	12	2	2	4	6	8	10	16
B. Operated	33	13.8	128	3	5	10	18	32	37	49
1. SINGLE DX	45	2.5	2	1	2	2	3	4	5	7
2. MULTIPLE DX	1,484	4.7	16	2	2	4	6	9	11	21
A. NOT OPERATED	1,496	4.5	12	2	2	4	6	8	10	16
B. OPERATED	33	13.8	128	3	5	10	18	32	37	49
TOTAL										
0–19 Years	286	3.0	7	1	2	2	3	5	7	10
20–34	41	5.8	78	1	2	4	5	10	15	47
35–49	128	4.7	15	2	2	4	6	9	11	17
50–64	261	4.5	14	2	3	3	5	8	11	18
65+	813	5.3	16	2	3	4	7	9	11	22
GRAND TOTAL	1,529	4.7	16	2	2	4	6	9	11	19

Length of Stay by Diagnosis and Operation, Western Region, 2008

Western Region, October 2006–September 2007 Data, by Diagnosis

486: PNEUMONIA ORGANISM NOS

Type of Patients	Observed Patients	Avg. Stay	Vari-ance	Percentiles						
				10th	25th	50th	75th	90th	95th	99th
1. SINGLE DX										
A. Not Operated										
0–19 Years	1,502	2.5	2	1	1	2	3	4	5	9
20–34	105	2.3	2	1	1	2	3	4	5	6
35–49	92	2.4	2	1	1	2	3	4	5	9
50–64	66	2.3	1	1	2	2	3	4	4	5
65+	63	2.8	5	1	1	2	3	5	8	11
B. Operated										
0–19 Years	0									
20–34	0									
35–49	2	6.5	24	3	3	3	10	10	10	10
50–64	1	1.0	0	1	1	1	1	1	1	1
65+	2	3.0	8	1	1	3	5	5	5	5
2. MULTIPLE DX										
A. Not Operated										
0–19 Years	9,085	3.0	5	1	2	2	4	5	7	11
20–34	3,543	3.8	11	1	2	3	5	7	10	17
35–49	9,621	4.0	12	1	2	3	5	7	10	18
50–64	20,551	4.4	14	1	2	4	5	8	11	18
65+	67,523	4.7	12	2	3	4	6	8	11	17
B. Operated										
0–19 Years	77	10.8	80	3	6	8	13	19	23	67
20–34	109	11.3	59	4	6	10	15	21	27	40
35–49	298	9.6	43	3	5	8	13	17	23	31
50–64	658	10.9	68	4	5	9	14	20	27	41
65+	1,315	10.7	58	4	6	9	14	19	24	39
SUBTOTALS:										
1. SINGLE DX										
A. Not Operated	1,828	2.5	2	1	1	2	3	4	5	9
B. Operated	5	4.0	14	1	1	3	5	10	10	10
2. MULTIPLE DX										
A. Not Operated	110,323	4.4	12	2	2	4	5	8	10	17
B. Operated	2,457	10.7	59	4	6	9	14	19	24	39
1. SINGLE DX	1,833	2.5	2	1	1	2	3	4	5	9
2. MULTIPLE DX	112,780	4.6	14	2	2	4	6	8	11	19
A. NOT OPERATED	112,151	4.4	12	1	2	4	5	8	10	17
B. OPERATED	2,462	10.7	59	4	6	9	14	19	24	39
TOTAL										
0–19 Years	10,664	3.0	6	1	2	2	4	5	7	12
20–34	3,757	4.0	14	1	2	3	5	7	10	20
35–49	10,013	4.2	13	1	2	3	5	8	11	19
50–64	21,276	4.6	17	1	2	4	6	9	11	20
65+	68,903	4.8	13	2	3	4	6	9	11	19
GRAND TOTAL	114,613	4.5	14	2	2	4	6	8	11	19

487: INFLUENZA

Type of Patients	Observed Patients	Avg. Stay	Vari-ance	Percentiles						
				10th	25th	50th	75th	90th	95th	99th
1. SINGLE DX										
A. Not Operated										
0–19 Years	123	2.0	<1	1	1	2	3	3	3	5
20–34	3	1.3	<1	1	1	1	2	2	2	2
35–49	3	3.0	7	1	1	2	6	6	6	6
50–64	2	1.0	0	1	2	2	1	1	1	1
65+	1	2.0	0	2	2	2	2	2	2	2
B. Operated										
0–19 Years	0									
20–34	0									
35–49	0									
50–64	0									
65+	0									
2. MULTIPLE DX										
A. Not Operated										
0–19 Years	520	3.4	14	1	1	2	4	5	7	18
20–34	100	4.0	58	1	1	2	4	7	11	71
35–49	159	3.0	5	1	2	3	4	6	7	12
50–64	199	4.5	28	1	2	4	5	8	15	30
65+	572	4.1	9	1	2	3	5	8	10	16
B. Operated										
0–19 Years	2	26.5	4	25	25	25	28	28	28	28
20–34	0									
35–49	3	7.3	5	6	6	6	10	10	10	10
50–64	2	34.0	568	17	17	51	51	51	51	51
65+	6	13.2	26	7	9	13	14	19	19	19
SUBTOTALS:										
1. SINGLE DX										
A. Not Operated	132	2.0	<1	1	1	2	2	3	3	5
B. Operated	0									
2. MULTIPLE DX										
A. Not Operated	1,550	3.8	16	1	2	3	4	7	10	18
B. Operated	13	17.1	154	6	9	14	19	28	51	51
1. SINGLE DX	132	2.0	<1	1	1	2	2	3	3	5
2. MULTIPLE DX	1,563	3.9	19	1	2	3	5	7	11	22
A. NOT OPERATED	1,682	3.7	15	1	2	3	4	7	10	18
B. OPERATED	13	17.1	154	6	9	14	19	28	51	51
TOTAL										
0–19 Years	645	3.2	14	1	1	2	3	5	9	18
20–34	103	3.9	57	1	1	2	5	7	10	25
35–49	165	3.1	5	1	2	3	4	6	7	12
50–64	203	4.7	39	1	2	3	5	8	16	30
65+	579	4.2	10	1	2	3	5	8	11	17
GRAND TOTAL	1,695	3.8	18	1	2	3	4	7	10	21

487.0: INFLUENZA W PNEUMONIA

Type of Patients	Observed Patients	Avg. Stay	Vari-ance	Percentiles						
				10th	25th	50th	75th	90th	95th	99th
1. SINGLE DX										
A. Not Operated										
0–19 Years	20	2.5	<1	2	2	2	3	4	5	5
20–34	2	1.5	<1	1	1	2	2	2	2	2
35–49	0									
50–64	0									
65+	0									
B. Operated										
0–19 Years	0									
20–34	0									
35–49	0									
50–64	0									
65+	0									
2. MULTIPLE DX										
A. Not Operated										
0–19 Years	177	4.8	29	1	2	3	5	10	15	35
20–34	28	4.7	13	1	2	3	6	10	11	16
35–49	48	4.0	8	1	2	3	5	8	11	13
50–64	89	6.2	51	2	2	4	6	16	28	34
65+	245	5.0	14	2	3	4	6	9	13	18
B. Operated										
0–19 Years	0									
20–34	0									
35–49	2	8.0	8	6	6	6	10	10	10	10
50–64	0									
65+	4	15.8	16	11	14	19	19	19	19	19
SUBTOTALS:										
1. SINGLE DX										
A. Not Operated	22	2.4	<1	1	2	2	3	3	4	5
B. Operated	0									
2. MULTIPLE DX										
A. Not Operated	587	5.0	24	1	2	4	6	10	14	29
B. Operated	6	13.2	27	6	10	13	19	19	19	19
1. SINGLE DX	22	2.4	<1	1	1	2	3	3	4	5
2. MULTIPLE DX	593	5.1	24	1	2	4	6	10	14	29
A. NOT OPERATED	609	4.9	23	1	2	4	6	10	14	28
B. OPERATED	6	13.2	27	6	10	13	19	19	19	19
TOTAL										
0–19 Years	197	4.5	27	1	2	3	5	9	14	35
20–34	30	4.5	13	2	2	3	6	10	11	16
35–49	50	4.2	8	1	2	3	6	8	11	13
50–64	89	6.2	51	2	2	4	6	16	28	34
65+	249	5.2	15	2	3	4	6	10	13	19
GRAND TOTAL	615	5.0	24	1	2	4	6	10	14	28

Length of Stay by Diagnosis and Operation, Western Region, 2008

Western Region, October 2006–September 2007 Data, by Diagnosis

487.1: FLU W RESP MANIFEST NEC

Type of Patients	Observed Patients	Avg. Stay	Variance	10th	25th	50th	75th	90th	95th	99th
1. SINGLE DX										
A. Not Operated										
0–19 Years	95	1.9	<1	1	1	2	2	3	3	5
20–34	0									
35–49	2	1.5	<1	1	1	2	2	2	2	2
50–64	2	1.0	0	1	1	1	1	1	1	1
65+	1	2.0	0	2	2	2	2	2	2	2
B. Operated										
0–19 Years	0									
20–34	0									
35–49	0									
50–64	0									
65+	0									
2. MULTIPLE DX										
A. Not Operated										
0–19 Years	310	2.7	5	1	1	2	3	5	8	11
20–34	54	2.9	14	1	1	2	3	6	9	25
35–49	102	2.6	3	1	1	2	3	5	5	7
50–64	93	3.1	5	1	2	2	3	6	7	14
65+	304	3.5	5	1	2	3	4	6	8	11
B. Operated										
0–19 Years	2	26.5	4	25	25	25	28	28	28	28
20–34	0									
35–49	1	6.0	0	6	6	6	6	6	6	6
50–64	2	34.0	568	17	17	51	51	51	51	51
65+	2	8.0	2	7	7	7	9	9	9	9
SUBTOTALS:										
1. SINGLE DX A. Not Operated	100	1.8	<1	1	1	2	2	3	3	5
1. SINGLE DX B. Operated	0									
2. MULTIPLE DX A. Not Operated	863	3.0	6	1	2	2	3	5	6	12
2. MULTIPLE DX B. Operated	7	20.4	257	6	7	17	28	51	51	51
1. SINGLE DX	100	1.8	<1	1	1	2	2	3	3	5
2. MULTIPLE DX	870	3.2	10	1	2	2	4	6	8	14
A. NOT OPERATED	963	2.9	5	1	1	2	3	6	7	12
B. OPERATED	7	20.4	257	6	7	17	28	51	51	51
TOTAL										
0–19 Years	407	2.6	7	1	1	2	3	5	7	12
20–34	54	2.9	14	1	1	2	3	6	9	25
35–49	105	2.6	3	1	1	2	3	5	6	7
50–64	97	3.7	31	1	2	3	4	6	9	51
65+	307	3.5	6	1	2	3	4	7	8	11
GRAND TOTAL	970	3.0	9	1	2	2	4	6	7	13

490: BRONCHITIS NOS

Type of Patients	Observed Patients	Avg. Stay	Variance	10th	25th	50th	75th	90th	95th	99th
1. SINGLE DX										
A. Not Operated										
0–19 Years	45	2.5	2	1	1	2	3	4	5	7
20–34	3	2.0	3	1	1	1	3	4	4	4
35–49	4	1.5	1	1	1	2	3	3	3	3
50–64	4	1.3	<1	1	1	2	2	2	2	2
65+	2	2.5	4	1	2	3	4	4	4	4
B. Operated										
0–19 Years	0									
20–34	0									
35–49	0									
50–64	0									
65+	0									
2. MULTIPLE DX										
A. Not Operated										
0–19 Years	171	2.4	3	1	1	2	3	4	6	10
20–34	117	2.7	4	1	1	2	3	6	7	9
35–49	283	2.5	4	1	1	2	3	5	5	12
50–64	488	2.5	2	1	1	2	3	4	5	7
65+	1,118	3.0	5	2	2	2	4	5	7	10
B. Operated										
0–19 Years	2	7.6	83	1	1	14	14	14	14	14
20–34	1	22.0	0	22	22	22	22	22	22	22
35–49	1	22.0	0	22	22	22	22	22	22	22
50–64	5	6.4	24	3	4	4	6	6	6	6
65+	9	8.4	22	3	5	9	12	9	16	9
SUBTOTALS:										
1. SINGLE DX A. Not Operated	58	2.3	2	1	1	2	3	4	5	5
1. SINGLE DX B. Operated	0									
2. MULTIPLE DX A. Not Operated	2,177	2.8	4	1	1	2	3	5	6	9
2. MULTIPLE DX B. Operated	18	8.2	36	3	5	6	13	16	22	22
1. SINGLE DX	58	2.3	2	1	1	2	3	4	5	5
2. MULTIPLE DX	2,195	2.8	4	1	1	2	4	5	6	14
A. NOT OPERATED	2,235	2.7	4	1	1	2	3	5	6	12
B. OPERATED	18	8.2	36	3	5	6	13	16	22	22
TOTAL										
0–19 Years	218	2.4	4	1	1	2	3	4	6	10
20–34	121	2.9	7	1	1	2	3	6	7	11
35–49	288	2.5	4	1	1	2	3	5	6	7
50–64	497	2.5	3	1	2	2	3	4	5	8
65+	1,129	3.0	5	2	2	2	4	6	7	11
GRAND TOTAL	2,253	2.8	4	1	2	2	3	5	6	10

491: CHRONIC BRONCHITIS

Type of Patients	Observed Patients	Avg. Stay	Variance	10th	25th	50th	75th	90th	95th	99th
1. SINGLE DX										
A. Not Operated										
0–19 Years	3	1.7	<1	1	1	2	2	2	2	2
20–34	1	2.0	0	2	2	2	2	2	2	2
35–49	27	2.4	5	1	1	2	3	5	5	12
50–64	55	2.5	3	1	1	2	3	5	7	8
65+	105	2.4	2	1	1	2	3	5	5	6
B. Operated										
0–19 Years	0									
20–34	0									
35–49	0									
50–64	0									
65+	1	2.0	0	2	2	2	2	2	2	2
2. MULTIPLE DX										
A. Not Operated										
0–19 Years	26	3.0	4	1	1	3	4	6	7	8
20–34	125	3.3	8	1	2	3	4	6	7	14
35–49	2,604	3.7	11	1	2	3	4	7	9	16
50–64	13,754	4.1	12	1	2	3	5	8	10	17
65+	33,464	4.3	12	2	2	3	5	8	10	17
B. Operated										
0–19 Years	2	13.0	0	13	13	13	13	13	13	13
20–34	1	16.0	31	12	12	16	16	20	20	20
35–49	28	12.9	137	3	6	8	14	28	43	50
50–64	164	11.2	86	3	5	9	15	23	31	>99
65+	449	11.0	67	3	5	9	14	22	26	42
SUBTOTALS:										
1. SINGLE DX A. Not Operated	191	2.4	3	1	1	2	3	5	5	9
1. SINGLE DX B. Operated	1	2.0	0	2	2	2	2	2	2	2
2. MULTIPLE DX A. Not Operated	49,973	4.2	12	3	3	3	5	8	10	17
2. MULTIPLE DX B. Operated	644	11.1	74	3	5	9	14	22	27	51
1. SINGLE DX	192	2.4	3	1	1	2	3	5	5	9
2. MULTIPLE DX	50,617	4.3	13	2	2	3	5	8	10	18
A. NOT OPERATED	50,164	4.2	12	2	2	3	5	8	10	17
B. OPERATED	645	11.1	74	3	5	9	14	22	27	51
TOTAL										
0–19 Years	30	3.2	7	1	1	2	4	7	8	13
20–34	128	3.5	10	1	2	3	4	7	9	20
35–49	2,659	3.8	13	1	2	3	5	7	9	18
50–64	13,973	4.2	14	2	2	3	5	8	10	19
65+	34,019	4.4	13	1	2	4	5	8	11	18
GRAND TOTAL	50,809	4.3	13	1	2	3	5	8	10	18

Length of Stay by Diagnosis and Operation, Western Region, 2008

Western Region, October 2006–September 2007 Data, by Diagnosis

491.20: OCB W/O EXACERBATION

Type of Patients	Observed Patients	Avg. Stay	Variance	10th	25th	50th	75th	90th	95th	99th
1. SINGLE DX										
A. Not Operated										
0–19 Years	1	1.0	0	1	1	1	1	1	1	1
20–34	0									
35–49	0									
50–64	1	5.0	0	5	5	5	5	5	5	5
65+	0									
B. Operated										
0–19 Years	0									
20–34	0									
35–49	0									
50–64	0									
65+	1	2.0	0	2	2	2	2	2	2	2
2. MULTIPLE DX										
A. Not Operated										
0–19 Years	1	1.0	0	1	1	1	1	1	1	1
20–34	2	5.0	18	2	2	8	8	8	8	8
35–49	32	3.0	5	1	2	2	4	6	8	10
50–64	122	3.7	7	1	2	3	5	8	10	12
65+	339	3.7	8	1	2	3	5	7	8	18
B. Operated										
0–19 Years	0									
20–34	0									
35–49	0									
50–64	5	7.6	71	1	3	4	8	22	22	22
65+	5	8.6	102	2	3	3	9	26	26	26
SUBTOTALS:										
1. SINGLE DX										
A. Not Operated	2	3.0	8	1	1	5	5	5	5	5
B. Operated	1	2.0	0	2	2	2	2	2	2	2
2. MULTIPLE DX										
A. Not Operated	496	3.7	8	1	2	3	5	7	9	15
B. Operated	10	8.1	78	1	3	3	9	26	26	26
1. SINGLE DX	3	2.7	4	1	1	2	5	5	5	5
2. MULTIPLE DX	506	3.7	9	1	2	3	5	8	9	18
A. NOT OPERATED	498	3.7	8	1	2	3	5	7	9	15
B. OPERATED	11	7.6	73	2	2	3	9	22	26	26
TOTAL										
0–19 Years	2	1.0	0	1	1	1	1	1	1	1
20–34	2	5.0	18	2	2	8	8	8	8	8
35–49	32	3.0	5	1	2	2	4	6	8	10
50–64	128	3.9	10	1	2	3	5	8	10	12
65+	345	3.8	10	1	2	3	5	7	8	18
GRAND TOTAL	509	3.7	9	1	2	3	5	8	9	18

491.21: OCB W EXACERBATION

Type of Patients	Observed Patients	Avg. Stay	Variance	10th	25th	50th	75th	90th	95th	99th
1. SINGLE DX										
A. Not Operated										
0–19 Years	1	2.0	0	2	2	2	2	2	2	2
20–34	1	2.0	0	2	2	2	2	2	2	2
35–49	18	2.7	7	1	1	2	3	5	12	12
50–64	45	2.5	3	1	1	2	3	5	6	7
65+	87	2.4	2	1	1	2	3	5	5	9
B. Operated										
0–19 Years	0									
20–34	0									
35–49	0									
50–64	0									
65+	0									
2. MULTIPLE DX										
A. Not Operated										
0–19 Years	16	2.3	2	1	1	2	4	5	5	5
20–34	65	3.9	11	1	2	3	4	7	9	21
35–49	1,998	3.8	12	1	2	3	5	7	9	18
50–64	11,202	4.2	13	1	2	3	5	8	10	18
65+	27,035	4.3	12	1	2	3	5	8	10	17
B. Operated										
0–19 Years	0									
20–34	1	20.0	0	20	20	20	20	20	20	20
35–49	20	12.0	115	5	6	8	13	22	27	50
50–64	137	11.2	90	3	5	8	15	24	31	>99
65+	376	11.0	73	3	5	9	14	22	27	46
SUBTOTALS:										
1. SINGLE DX										
A. Not Operated	152	2.4	3	1	1	2	3	5	6	9
B. Operated	0									
2. MULTIPLE DX										
A. Not Operated	40,316	4.2	12	1	2	3	5	8	10	17
B. Operated	534	11.1	79	3	5	9	14	22	28	51
1. SINGLE DX	152	2.4	3	1	1	2	3	5	6	9
2. MULTIPLE DX	40,850	4.3	14	1	2	3	5	8	10	18
A. NOT OPERATED	40,468	4.2	12	1	2	3	5	8	10	17
B. OPERATED	534	11.1	79	3	5	9	14	22	28	51
TOTAL										
0–19 Years	17	2.2	2	1	1	2	3	5	5	5
20–34	67	4.1	15	1	2	3	5	7	13	21
35–49	2,036	3.9	13	1	1	3	5	7	10	18
50–64	11,384	4.2	15	1	2	3	5	8	10	19
65+	27,498	4.4	13	2	2	3	5	8	10	18
GRAND TOTAL	41,002	4.3	14	1	2	3	5	8	10	18

491.22: OCB W ACUTE BRONCHITIS

Type of Patients	Observed Patients	Avg. Stay	Variance	10th	25th	50th	75th	90th	95th	99th
1. SINGLE DX										
A. Not Operated										
0–19 Years	1	2.0	0	2	2	2	2	2	2	2
20–34	0									
35–49	9	1.8	2	1	1	1	2	5	5	5
50–64	9	2.8	5	1	1	3	3	8	8	8
65+	18	2.8	2	1	2	2	4	5	5	5
B. Operated										
0–19 Years	0									
20–34	0									
35–49	0									
50–64	0									
65+	0									
2. MULTIPLE DX										
A. Not Operated										
0–19 Years	2	2.5	4	1	1	1	4	4	4	4
20–34	48	2.4	3	1	1	2	3	5	6	7
35–49	556	3.3	7	1	2	3	4	6	8	12
50–64	2,401	4.1	10	1	2	3	5	8	10	16
65+	6,015	4.5	12	2	2	4	6	8	10	17
B. Operated										
0–19 Years	0									
20–34	0									
35–49	4	22.0	279	7	10	28	28	43	43	43
50–64	17	13.5	75	3	5	14	17	23	35	35
65+	64	11.4	30	5	7	11	15	18	22	26
SUBTOTALS:										
1. SINGLE DX										
A. Not Operated	37	2.5	3	1	1	2	3	5	5	8
B. Operated	0									
2. MULTIPLE DX										
A. Not Operated	9,022	4.3	12	1	2	4	5	8	10	17
B. Operated	85	12.3	52	4	7	12	16	21	24	43
1. SINGLE DX	37	2.5	3	1	1	2	3	5	5	8
2. MULTIPLE DX	9,107	4.4	12	1	2	4	5	8	10	17
A. NOT OPERATED	9,059	4.3	12	1	2	4	5	8	10	17
B. OPERATED	85	12.3	52	4	7	12	16	21	24	43
TOTAL										
0–19 Years	3	2.3	2	1	1	2	4	4	4	4
20–34	48	2.4	3	1	1	3	3	5	6	7
35–49	569	3.4	10	1	2	3	4	6	8	13
50–64	2,427	4.1	11	1	2	3	5	8	10	17
65+	6,097	4.6	13	2	2	4	6	8	11	18
GRAND TOTAL	9,144	4.4	12	1	2	4	5	8	10	17

Western Region, October 2006–September 2007 Data, by Diagnosis

492: EMPHYSEMA

Type of Patients	Observed Patients	Avg. Stay	Variance	Percentiles 10th	25th	50th	75th	90th	95th	99th
1. SINGLE DX										
A. Not Operated										
0–19 Years	1	2.0	0	2	2	2	2	2	2	2
20–34	0									
35–49	0									
50–64	2	2.0	0	2	2	2	2	2	2	2
65+	1	1.0	0	1	1	1	1	1	1	1
B. Operated										
0–19 Years	0									
20–34	2	3.0	2	2	2	4	4	4	4	4
35–49	3	9.3	120	3	3	3	22	22	22	22
50–64	0									
65+	1	5.0	0	5	5	5	5	5	5	5
2. MULTIPLE DX										
A. Not Operated										
0–19 Years	4	3.7	13	1	1	2	3	9	9	9
20–34	12	3.4	3	2	2	5	5	5	7	7
35–49	60	3.1	3	1	2	3	4	5	6	8
50–64	269	4.3	20	1	2	3	5	9	12	21
65+	656	4.2	11	1	2	3	5	8	11	17
B. Operated										
0–19 Years	13	9.2	112	2	4	7	10	16	42	42
20–34	29	5.8	33	1	3	5	6	10	13	32
35–49	46	7.0	27	2	3	5	10	15	19	19
50–64	138	12.0	93	3	6	10	16	22	31	66
65+	75	9.8	79	2	4	8	12	17	22	61
SUBTOTALS:										
1. SINGLE DX										
A. Not Operated	4	1.8	<1	1	2	2	2	2	2	2
B. Operated	6	6.5	58	2	3	4	5	22	22	22
2. MULTIPLE DX										
A. Not Operated	1,001	4.1	13	1	2	3	5	8	10	17
B. Operated	301	10.0	79	2	4	7	14	19	24	55
1. SINGLE DX	10	4.6	38	2	2	3	4	5	22	22
2. MULTIPLE DX	1,302	5.5	34	1	2	4	7	12	16	31
A. NOT OPERATED	1,005	4.1	13	1	2	3	5	8	10	17
B. OPERATED	307	9.9	78	2	4	7	13	20	24	55
TOTAL										
0–19 Years	18	7.6	89	2	2	5	9	16	42	42
20–34	43	5.0	24	2	2	4	6	8	10	32
35–49	109	5.0	19	2	2	4	6	12	15	21
50–64	409	6.9	58	1	2	4	9	16	21	42
65+	733	4.8	21	1	2	4	6	13	13	20
GRAND TOTAL	1,312	5.5	34	2	2	4	7	12	16	31

492.0: EMPHYSEMATOUS BLEB

Type of Patients	Observed Patients	Avg. Stay	Variance	Percentiles 10th	25th	50th	75th	90th	95th	99th
1. SINGLE DX										
A. Not Operated										
0–19 Years	0									
20–34	0									
35–49	0									
50–64	0									
65+	0									
B. Operated										
0–19 Years	0									
20–34	2	3.0	2	2	2	4	4	4	4	4
35–49	3	9.3	120	3	3	3	22	22	22	22
50–64	0									
65+	1	5.0	0	5	5	5	5	5	5	5
2. MULTIPLE DX										
A. Not Operated										
0–19 Years	4	3.7	13	1	1	2	3	9	9	9
20–34	7	2.9	2	2	2	2	5	5	5	7
35–49	21	3.5	3	1	2	3	4	5	5	8
50–64	58	4.7	15	1	2	4	7	10	14	17
65+	50	5.1	15	2	2	4	6	9	14	21
B. Operated										
0–19 Years	13	9.2	112	2	4	7	10	16	42	42
20–34	26	4.9	8	1	3	4	6	8	10	13
35–49	34	7.0	30	2	3	5	9	16	19	21
50–64	65	10.0	37	3	5	8	15	19	22	25
65+	30	9.6	25	4	6	9	14	16	17	22
SUBTOTALS:										
1. SINGLE DX										
A. Not Operated	0									
B. Operated	6	6.5	58	2	3	4	5	22	22	22
2. MULTIPLE DX										
A. Not Operated	140	4.5	13	1	2	4	6	8	13	17
B. Operated	168	8.5	37	3	4	7	12	17	20	25
1. SINGLE DX	6	6.5	58	2	3	4	5	22	22	22
2. MULTIPLE DX	308	6.7	30	2	3	5	8	15	17	22
A. NOT OPERATED	140	4.5	13	1	2	4	6	8	13	17
B. OPERATED	174	8.4	38	3	4	7	12	17	21	25
TOTAL										
0–19 Years	17	8.0	92	2	3	5	9	16	42	42
20–34	35	4.4	7	2	2	4	6	8	10	13
35–49	58	5.9	26	2	3	4	7	15	19	22
50–64	123	7.5	34	2	3	6	11	16	19	23
65+	81	6.8	23	2	3	6	8	14	16	22
GRAND TOTAL	314	6.7	30	2	3	5	8	15	17	22

492.8: EMPHYSEMA NEC

Type of Patients	Observed Patients	Avg. Stay	Variance	Percentiles 10th	25th	50th	75th	90th	95th	99th
1. SINGLE DX										
A. Not Operated										
0–19 Years	1	2.0	0	2	2	2	2	2	2	2
20–34	0									
35–49	0									
50–64	2	2.0	0	2	2	2	2	2	2	2
65+	1	1.0	0	1	1	1	1	1	1	1
B. Operated										
0–19 Years	0									
20–34	0									
35–49	0									
50–64	0									
65+	0									
2. MULTIPLE DX										
A. Not Operated										
0–19 Years	0									
20–34	5	4.2	4	2	3	4	5	7	7	7
35–49	39	3.0	3	1	1	3	4	6	6	7
50–64	211	4.2	21	1	2	3	5	8	10	21
65+	606	4.1	11	1	2	3	5	8	10	16
B. Operated										
0–19 Years	0									
20–34	3	13.0	270	2	2	5	32	32	32	32
35–49	12	7.1	20	1	4	7	9	12	15	15
50–64	73	13.8	137	2	6	11	18	29	42	>99
65+	45	9.9	117	3	3	7	12	20	27	61
SUBTOTALS:										
1. SINGLE DX										
A. Not Operated	4	1.8	<1	1	2	2	2	2	2	2
B. Operated	0									
2. MULTIPLE DX										
A. Not Operated	861	4.1	13	1	2	3	5	8	10	17
B. Operated	133	11.8	125	2	5	10	16	24	34	66
1. SINGLE DX	4	1.8	<1	1	2	2	2	2	2	2
2. MULTIPLE DX	994	5.1	35	1	2	3	6	10	15	33
A. NOT OPERATED	865	4.1	13	1	2	3	5	8	10	17
B. OPERATED	133	11.8	125	2	5	10	16	24	34	66
TOTAL										
0–19 Years	1	2.0	0	2	2	2	2	2	2	2
20–34	8	7.5	102	2	2	5	5	32	32	32
35–49	51	3.9	10	1	1	3	5	7	12	15
50–64	286	6.6	68	1	2	4	8	16	22	55
65+	652	4.5	20	1	2	3	6	8	12	20
GRAND TOTAL	998	5.1	35	1	2	3	6	10	15	32

Western Region, October 2006–September 2007 Data, by Diagnosis

493: ASTHMA

Type of Patients	Observed Patients	Avg. Stay	Variance	Percentiles						
				10th	25th	50th	75th	90th	95th	99th
1. SINGLE DX										
A. *Not Operated*										
0–19 Years	3,322	1.9	1	1	1	2	2	3	4	5
20–34	375	1.8	1	1	1	2	2	3	4	5
35–49	296	2.0	2	1	1	2	2	4	4	7
50–64	138	2.1	1	1	1	2	3	4	4	5
65+	55	2.2	2	1	1	2	2	4	5	9
B. *Operated*										
0–19 Years	0									
20–34	0									
35–49	0									
50–64	0									
65+	0									
2. MULTIPLE DX										
A. *Not Operated*										
0–19 Years	9,344	2.4	2	1	1	2	3	4	5	8
20–34	3,225	2.8	4	1	1	2	3	5	7	11
35–49	7,063	3.4	8	1	2	3	4	6	8	13
50–64	8,943	3.8	9	1	2	3	5	7	9	15
65+	10,454	4.4	12	1	2	4	6	8	10	17
B. *Operated*										
0–19 Years	15	8.8	141	1	1	5	11	16	48	48
20–34	12	10.6	49	3	3	11	16	20	24	24
35–49	48	10.1	72	3	4	7	13	24	26	35
50–64	86	11.8	152	2	4	8	14	22	32	62
65+	131	12.6	125	3	5	10	16	25	32	59
SUBTOTALS:										
1. SINGLE DX										
A. *Not Operated*	4,186	1.9	1	1	1	2	2	3	4	5
B. *Operated*	0									
2. MULTIPLE DX										
A. *Not Operated*	39,029	3.5	8	1	2	3	4	5	7	14
B. *Operated*	292	11.7	122	2	4	8	15	24	32	60
1. SINGLE DX	4,186	1.9	1	1	1	2	2	3	4	5
2. MULTIPLE DX	39,321	3.5	10	1	2	3	4	5	7	15
A. NOT OPERATED	43,215	3.3	8	1	2	3	4	6	8	14
B. OPERATED	292	11.7	122	2	4	8	15	24	32	60
TOTAL										
0–19 Years	12,681	2.3	2	1	1	2	3	4	5	7
20–34	3,612	2.7	5	1	1	2	3	5	6	11
35–49	7,407	3.3	8	1	2	3	4	6	6	14
50–64	9,167	3.9	11	1	2	3	5	7	9	16
65+	10,640	4.5	14	1	2	4	6	8	11	18
GRAND TOTAL	43,507	3.4	9	1	2	3	4	6	8	15

493.01: EXTR ASTH W STATUS ASTH

Type of Patients	Observed Patients	Avg. Stay	Variance	Percentiles						
				10th	25th	50th	75th	90th	95th	99th
1. SINGLE DX										
A. *Not Operated*										
0–19 Years	128	2.0	1	1	1	2	3	3	4	6
20–34	2	1.5	<1	1	1	2	2	2	2	2
35–49	2	2.0	2	1	1	1	3	3	3	3
50–64	0									
65+	0									
B. *Operated*										
0–19 Years	0									
20–34	0									
35–49	0									
50–64	0									
65+	0									
2. MULTIPLE DX										
A. *Not Operated*										
0–19 Years	360	2.8	5	1	2	2	3	5	6	10
20–34	62	3.6	13	1	1	3	4	6	9	22
35–49	41	3.7	15	1	2	3	4	6	6	22
50–64	27	3.3	10	1	2	3	4	8	8	16
65+	10	4.4	4	1	3	4	6	7	7	7
B. *Operated*										
0–19 Years	0									
20–34	0									
35–49	0									
50–64	1	7.0	0	7	7	7	7	7	7	7
65+	0									
SUBTOTALS:										
1. SINGLE DX										
A. *Not Operated*	132	2.0	1	1	1	2	3	3	4	6
B. *Operated*	0									
2. MULTIPLE DX										
A. *Not Operated*	500	3.0	7	1	2	3	4	5	7	16
B. *Operated*	1	7.0	0	7	7	7	7	7	7	7
1. SINGLE DX	132	2.0	1	1	1	2	3	3	4	6
2. MULTIPLE DX	501	3.0	7	1	2	3	4	5	7	16
A. NOT OPERATED	632	2.8	6	1	1	3	3	5	6	15
B. OPERATED	1	7.0	0	7	7	7	7	7	7	7
TOTAL										
0–19 Years	488	2.6	4	1	1	2	3	4	6	9
20–34	64	3.6	12	1	1	3	3	5	9	22
35–49	43	3.6	14	1	2	3	4	6	6	22
50–64	28	3.5	10	1	2	3	4	7	8	16
65+	10	4.4	4	1	3	4	6	7	7	7
GRAND TOTAL	633	2.8	6	1	1	2	3	5	6	15

493.02: EXTR ASTHMA W EXACER

Type of Patients	Observed Patients	Avg. Stay	Variance	Percentiles						
				10th	25th	50th	75th	90th	95th	99th
1. SINGLE DX										
A. *Not Operated*										
0–19 Years	307	1.8	<1	1	1	2	2	3	4	5
20–34	19	1.8	<1	1	1	2	3	3	4	4
35–49	11	2.2	<1	2	2	2	3	3	3	3
50–64	2	2.5	4	1	1	1	4	4	4	4
65+	0									
B. *Operated*										
0–19 Years	0									
20–34	0									
35–49	0									
50–64	0									
65+	0									
2. MULTIPLE DX										
A. *Not Operated*										
0–19 Years	835	2.3	2	1	1	2	3	4	5	8
20–34	153	2.8	5	1	1	2	3	5	7	14
35–49	206	3.0	5	1	1	2	3	6	7	9
50–64	137	3.2	5	1	2	3	3	7	8	9
65+	76	4.4	14	1	2	3	5	7	11	24
B. *Operated*										
0–19 Years	0									
20–34	0									
35–49	0									
50–64	0									
65+	1	4.0	0	4	4	4	4	4	4	4
SUBTOTALS:										
1. SINGLE DX										
A. *Not Operated*	339	1.8	<1	1	1	2	2	3	4	5
B. *Operated*	0									
2. MULTIPLE DX										
A. *Not Operated*	1,407	2.7	4	1	1	2	3	5	7	10
B. *Operated*	1	4.0	0	4	4	4	4	4	4	4
1. SINGLE DX	339	1.8	<1	1	1	2	2	3	4	5
2. MULTIPLE DX	1,408	2.7	4	1	1	2	3	5	7	10
A. NOT OPERATED	1,746	2.5	4	1	1	2	3	5	6	9
B. OPERATED	1	4.0	0	4	4	4	4	4	4	4
TOTAL										
0–19 Years	1,142	2.2	2	1	1	2	3	4	5	7
20–34	172	2.7	5	1	1	3	3	5	7	14
35–49	217	3.0	4	1	1	2	4	6	7	9
50–64	139	3.2	5	2	2	3	4	7	8	9
65+	77	4.4	14	1	2	4	5	7	11	24
GRAND TOTAL	1,747	2.5	4	1	1	2	3	5	6	9

Length of Stay by Diagnosis and Operation, Western Region, 2008

Western Region, October 2006–September 2007 Data, by Diagnosis

493.20: CHR OBSTR ASTHMA NOS

Type of Patients	Observed Patients	Avg. Stay	Variance	10th	25th	50th	75th	90th	95th	99th
1. SINGLE DX										
A. Not Operated										
0–19 Years	0									
20–34	2	3.0	8	1	1	5	5	5	5	5
35–49	0									
50–64	5	3.2	<1	2	3	3	4	4	4	4
65+	0									
B. Operated										
0–19 Years	0									
20–34	0									
35–49	0									
50–64	0									
65+	0									
2. MULTIPLE DX										
A. Not Operated										
0–19 Years	4	3.0	2	2	2	3	4	5	5	5
20–34	11	3.2	8	1	2	2	3	5	11	11
35–49	89	3.6	21	1	2	3	4	6	8	42
50–64	181	3.3	7	1	2	3	4	6	8	18
65+	374	4.0	9	1	2	3	5	8	10	16
B. Operated										
0–19 Years	0									
20–34	0									
35–49	3	7.3	24	4	4	5	13	13	13	13
50–64	7	9.7	123	2	2	4	15	32	32	32
65+	12	13.4	431	1	1	7	11	19	77	77
SUBTOTALS:										
1. SINGLE DX										
A. Not Operated	7	3.2	2	1	2	3	3	4	5	5
B. Operated	0									
2. MULTIPLE DX										
A. Not Operated	659	3.7	10	1	2	3	5	7	9	16
B. Operated	22	11.4	269	2	2	6	13	19	32	77
1. SINGLE DX	7	3.2	2	1	2	3	4	5	5	5
2. MULTIPLE DX	681	4.0	20	1	2	3	5	7	10	19
A. NOT OPERATED	666	3.7	10	1	2	3	5	7	9	16
B. OPERATED	22	11.4	269	2	2	6	13	19	32	77
TOTAL										
0–19 Years	4	3.0	2	2	2	3	4	5	5	5
20–34	13	3.2	7	1	2	2	3	5	11	11
35–49	92	3.7	21	1	2	3	4	6	9	42
50–64	193	3.5	12	1	2	3	4	6	9	19
65+	386	4.3	24	1	2	3	5	8	10	19
GRAND TOTAL	688	4.0	20	1	2	3	5	7	10	19

493.21: CHR OBSTR ASTH W STATUS

Type of Patients	Observed Patients	Avg. Stay	Variance	10th	25th	50th	75th	90th	95th	99th
1. SINGLE DX										
A. Not Operated										
0–19 Years	1	2.0	0	2	2	2	2	2	2	2
20–34	2	1.5	<1	1	1	2	2	2	2	2
35–49	0									
50–64	2	3.0	2	2	2	4	4	4	4	4
65+	1	1.0	0	1	1	1	1	1	1	1
B. Operated										
0–19 Years	0									
20–34	0									
35–49	0									
50–64	0									
65+	0									
2. MULTIPLE DX										
A. Not Operated										
0–19 Years	5	3.6	17	2	2	2	2	11	11	11
20–34	31	3.8	5	2	2	3	5	6	9	12
35–49	170	4.2	12	1	2	3	5	8	9	25
50–64	267	5.6	18	2	3	5	7	11	13	21
65+	252	5.8	20	2	3	5	7	10	13	25
B. Operated										
0–19 Years	0									
20–34	0									
35–49	2	14.4	178	5	5	5	24	24	24	24
50–64	3	9.3	122	1	1	5	22	22	22	22
65+	1	16.0	0	16	16	16	16	16	16	16
SUBTOTALS:										
1. SINGLE DX										
A. Not Operated	6	2.0	1	1	1	2	2	4	4	4
B. Operated	0									
2. MULTIPLE DX										
A. Not Operated	725	5.2	17	2	3	4	7	10	12	21
B. Operated	6	12.1	95	1	5	5	22	24	24	24
1. SINGLE DX	6	2.0	1	1	1	2	2	4	4	4
2. MULTIPLE DX	731	5.3	18	2	3	4	7	10	13	24
A. NOT OPERATED	731	5.2	17	2	3	4	6	10	12	21
B. OPERATED	6	12.1	95	1	5	5	22	24	24	24
TOTAL										
0–19 Years	6	3.4	14	2	2	2	2	11	11	11
20–34	33	3.7	5	2	2	3	4	6	9	12
35–49	172	4.3	14	1	2	3	5	8	10	25
50–64	272	5.6	18	2	3	5	7	11	14	22
65+	254	5.8	21	2	3	5	7	11	13	25
GRAND TOTAL	737	5.3	18	2	3	4	7	10	13	24

493.22: CHR OBSTR ASTH W EXACER

Type of Patients	Observed Patients	Avg. Stay	Variance	10th	25th	50th	75th	90th	95th	99th
1. SINGLE DX										
A. Not Operated										
0–19 Years	11	2.2	1	1	2	2	2	3	5	5
20–34	8	2.1	<1	1	2	2	3	3	3	3
35–49	22	2.5	2	1	1	2	4	4	5	5
50–64	30	2.1	2	1	1	2	3	4	5	5
65+	29	2.3	3	1	1	2	3	4	5	9
B. Operated										
0–19 Years	0									
20–34	0									
35–49	0									
50–64	0									
65+	0									
2. MULTIPLE DX										
A. Not Operated										
0–19 Years	36	2.8	4	1	1	2	4	5	7	11
20–34	214	3.4	6	1	2	3	5	6	8	11
35–49	2,162	4.0	11	1	2	3	5	7	10	17
50–64	4,667	4.2	10	1	2	3	5	8	10	17
65+	6,783	4.7	14	2	2	4	6	9	11	18
B. Operated										
0–19 Years	0									
20–34	1	3.0	0	3	3	3	3	3	3	3
35–49	18	13.7	108	3	5	11	21	34	35	35
50–64	54	14.7	194	4	7	11	15	27	58	62
65+	90	13.9	105	4	7	11	19	26	32	59
SUBTOTALS:										
1. SINGLE DX										
A. Not Operated	100	2.3	2	1	1	2	3	4	5	5
B. Operated	0									
2. MULTIPLE DX										
A. Not Operated	13,862	4.4	12	1	2	4	5	8	10	17
B. Operated	163	14.1	134	4	7	11	17	27	35	60
1. SINGLE DX	100	2.3	2	1	1	2	3	4	5	5
2. MULTIPLE DX	14,025	4.5	15	1	2	4	6	8	11	19
A. NOT OPERATED	13,962	4.4	12	1	2	4	5	8	10	17
B. OPERATED	163	14.1	134	4	7	11	17	27	35	60
TOTAL										
0–19 Years	47	2.6	3	1	1	2	3	5	5	11
20–34	223	3.4	6	1	2	3	4	6	7	11
35–49	2,202	4.0	12	1	2	3	5	7	10	18
50–64	4,751	4.3	14	2	2	3	5	8	10	18
65+	6,902	4.8	16	2	2	4	6	9	11	19
GRAND TOTAL	14,125	4.5	15	1	2	4	6	8	11	19

Western Region, October 2006–September 2007 Data, by Diagnosis

493.90: ASTHMA NOS

Type of Patients	Observed Patients	Avg. Stay	Vari- ance	Percentiles 10th	25th	50th	75th	90th	95th	99th
1. SINGLE DX										
A. Not Operated										
0–19 Years	384	2.0	1	1	1	2	3	3	4	6
20–34	13	1.6	<1	1	1	1	2	3	3	3
35–49	9	2.1	<1	1	1	2	2	4	4	4
50–64	2	1.5	<1	1	1	2	2	2	2	2
65+	3	3.7	4	2	2	3	6	6	6	6
B. Operated										
0–19 Years	0									
20–34	0									
35–49	0									
50–64	0									
65+	0									
2. MULTIPLE DX										
A. Not Operated										
0–19 Years	1,171	2.2	2	1	1	2	3	4	4	6
20–34	127	2.7	4	1	1	2	3	5	6	7
35–49	253	2.5	5	1	1	2	3	5	6	10
50–64	281	2.9	3	1	2	2	4	5	7	9
65+	528	3.4	5	1	2	3	4	6	7	10
B. Operated										
0–19 Years	5	2.6	5	1	1	1	5	5	5	5
20–34	1	5.0	0	5	5	5	5	5	5	5
35–49	2	2.0	2	1	1	3	3	3	3	3
50–64	4	3.5	6	1	3	3	5	7	7	7
65+	8	4.6	16	1	2	2	7	13	13	13
SUBTOTALS:										
1. SINGLE DX										
A. Not Operated	411	2.0	1	1	1	2	3	3	4	6
B. Operated	0									
2. MULTIPLE DX										
A. Not Operated	2,360	2.6	3	1	1	2	3	5	6	9
B. Operated	20	3.7	9	1	1	3	5	7	13	13
1. SINGLE DX	411	2.0	1	1	1	2	3	3	4	6
2. MULTIPLE DX	2,380	2.6	3	1	1	2	3	5	6	9
A. NOT OPERATED	2,771	2.5	3	1	1	2	3	4	6	9
B. OPERATED	20	3.7	9	1	1	3	5	7	13	13
TOTAL										
0–19 Years	1,560	2.2	2	1	1	2	3	4	4	6
20–34	141	2.6	4	1	1	2	3	5	6	7
35–49	264	2.5	4	1	1	2	3	5	6	10
50–64	287	2.9	3	1	2	2	4	5	7	9
65+	539	3.4	5	1	2	3	4	6	7	11
GRAND TOTAL	2,791	2.5	3	1	1	2	3	5	6	9

493.91: ASTHMA W STATUS ASTH

Type of Patients	Observed Patients	Avg. Stay	Vari- ance	Percentiles 10th	25th	50th	75th	90th	95th	99th
1. SINGLE DX										
A. Not Operated										
0–19 Years	574	2.1	2	1	1	2	3	4	5	6
20–34	44	1.9	1	1	1	1	3	3	4	6
35–49	38	2.3	2	1	2	2	2	5	6	7
50–64	6	2.2	<1	1	2	2	2	4	4	4
65+	2	3.0	2	2	2	3	4	4	4	4
B. Operated										
0–19 Years	0									
20–34	0									
35–49	0									
50–64	0									
65+	0									
2. MULTIPLE DX										
A. Not Operated										
0–19 Years	1,560	2.8	3	1	2	2	3	5	6	9
20–34	439	3.1	5	1	2	2	4	6	8	12
35–49	543	3.7	10	1	2	3	5	7	8	15
50–64	329	4.6	16	1	2	4	6	9	12	20
65+	160	4.6	13	2	2	4	6	8	10	15
B. Operated										
0–19 Years	2	6.0	49	1	1	6	11	11	11	11
20–34	3	17.0	7	15	15	16	20	20	20	20
35–49	1	20.0	0	20	20	20	20	20	20	20
50–64	1	15.0	0	15	15	15	15	15	15	15
65+	2	11.5	40	7	7	16	16	16	16	16
SUBTOTALS:										
1. SINGLE DX										
A. Not Operated	664	2.1	2	1	1	2	3	4	5	6
B. Operated	0									
2. MULTIPLE DX										
A. Not Operated	3,031	3.3	7	1	2	3	4	6	8	13
B. Operated	9	13.5	38	1	11	15	16	20	20	20
1. SINGLE DX	664	2.1	2	1	1	2	3	4	5	6
2. MULTIPLE DX	3,040	3.3	7	1	2	3	4	6	8	13
A. NOT OPERATED	3,695	3.1	6	1	2	3	4	6	7	12
B. OPERATED	9	13.5	38	1	11	15	16	20	20	20
TOTAL										
0–19 Years	2,136	2.6	3	1	1	2	3	5	6	8
20–34	486	3.1	6	1	2	2	4	6	8	14
35–49	582	3.7	10	1	2	3	5	7	8	15
50–64	336	4.6	16	1	2	4	6	9	12	20
65+	164	4.7	13	2	2	4	6	8	11	16
GRAND TOTAL	3,704	3.1	7	1	2	2	4	6	7	13

493.92: ASTHMA NOS W EXACER

Type of Patients	Observed Patients	Avg. Stay	Vari- ance	Percentiles 10th	25th	50th	75th	90th	95th	99th
1. SINGLE DX										
A. Not Operated										
0–19 Years	1,880	1.8	<1	1	1	2	2	3	4	5
20–34	284	1.8	1	1	1	2	2	3	4	5
35–49	213	1.9	2	1	1	2	2	4	4	7
50–64	90	2.0	1	1	1	2	2	4	4	5
65+	19	1.7	<1	1	1	2	2	3	3	3
B. Operated										
0–19 Years	0									
20–34	0									
35–49	0									
50–64	0									
65+	0									
2. MULTIPLE DX										
A. Not Operated										
0–19 Years	5,208	2.3	2	1	1	2	3	4	5	7
20–34	2,172	2.6	4	1	1	2	3	5	6	10
35–49	3,569	3.0	4	1	2	2	4	6	7	10
50–64	3,021	3.2	5	1	2	3	4	6	7	11
65+	2,248	3.7	7	2	2	3	5	7	9	14
B. Operated										
0–19 Years	7	14.6	240	1	6	10	16	48	48	48
20–34	7	9.7	51	3	3	9	11	24	24	24
35–49	21	7.5	29	3	4	7	11	16	19	19
50–64	15	6.0	11	2	4	6	8	10	14	14
65+	16	9.9	68	3	5	7	10	22	33	33
SUBTOTALS:										
1. SINGLE DX										
A. Not Operated	2,486	1.8	1	1	1	2	2	3	4	5
B. Operated	0									
2. MULTIPLE DX										
A. Not Operated	16,218	2.8	4	1	1	2	4	5	7	11
B. Operated	66	8.7	60	3	4	7	11	17	22	48
1. SINGLE DX	2,486	1.8	1	1	1	2	2	3	4	5
2. MULTIPLE DX	16,284	2.9	5	1	1	2	4	5	7	11
A. NOT OPERATED	18,704	2.7	4	1	1	2	3	5	6	10
B. OPERATED	66	8.7	60	3	4	7	11	17	22	48
TOTAL										
0–19 Years	7,095	2.2	2	1	1	2	3	4	5	7
20–34	2,463	2.6	4	1	1	3	3	5	6	10
35–49	3,803	2.9	5	1	2	3	4	5	7	10
50–64	3,126	3.2	5	1	2	3	4	6	7	11
65+	2,283	3.7	8	1	2	3	5	7	9	14
GRAND TOTAL	18,770	2.7	4	1	1	2	3	5	6	10

Length of Stay by Diagnosis and Operation, Western Region, 2008

Western Region, October 2006–September 2007 Data, by Diagnosis

494: BRONCHIECTASIS

Type of Patients	Observed Patients	Avg. Stay	Variance	10th	25th	50th	75th	90th	95th	99th
1. SINGLE DX										
A. Not Operated										
0–19 Years	2	2.5	<1	2	2	2	3	3	3	3
20–34	2	4.5	12	2	2	7	7	7	7	7
35–49	2	3.0	2	2	2	3	4	4	4	4
50–64	1	4.0	0	4	4	4	4	4	4	4
65+	0									
B. Operated										
0–19 Years	0									
20–34	1	5.0	0	5	5	5	5	5	5	5
35–49	0									
50–64	2	4.5	<1	4	4	5	5	5	5	5
65+	0									
2. MULTIPLE DX										
A. Not Operated										
0–19 Years	37	8.8	32	3	4	7	12	15	24	24
20–34	61	5.7	17	2	3	4	7	11	15	19
35–49	80	4.3	12	1	2	3	6	9	9	25
50–64	210	5.7	64	2	2	4	6	10	13	33
65+	834	4.8	12	2	3	4	6	9	11	20
B. Operated										
0–19 Years	2	6.5	12	4	4	4	9	9	9	9
20–34	13	7.3	29	2	5	5	9	13	21	21
35–49	6	15.3	91	6	9	13	18	33	33	33
50–64	33	9.0	91	2	4	6	11	16	21	53
65+	40	6.8	19	2	3	6	8	12	16	22
SUBTOTALS:										
1. SINGLE DX										
A. Not Operated	7	3.4	3	2	2	3	4	7	7	7
B. Operated	3	4.7	<1	4	4	5	5	5	5	5
2. MULTIPLE DX										
A. Not Operated	1,222	5.1	23	2	3	4	6	9	12	22
B. Operated	94	8.2	52	2	4	6	10	15	21	53
1. SINGLE DX	10	3.8	3	2	2	4	5	7	7	7
2. MULTIPLE DX	1,316	5.3	25	2	3	4	7	10	13	22
A. NOT OPERATED	1,229	5.1	23	2	3	4	6	9	12	22
B. OPERATED	97	8.1	51	2	4	6	10	15	21	53
TOTAL										
0–19 Years	41	8.4	31	3	4	7	11	14	21	24
20–34	77	5.9	19	2	3	5	7	13	16	21
35–49	88	5.1	24	1	2	4	6	9	13	33
50–64	246	6.1	68	2	3	4	7	11	15	46
65+	874	4.9	13	2	3	4	6	9	11	20
GRAND TOTAL	1,326	5.3	25	2	3	4	7	10	13	22

494.0: BRONCHIECT W/O AC EXACER

Type of Patients	Observed Patients	Avg. Stay	Variance	10th	25th	50th	75th	90th	95th	99th
1. SINGLE DX										
A. Not Operated										
0–19 Years	2	2.5	<1	2	2	2	3	3	3	3
20–34	0									
35–49	1	2.0	0	2	2	2	2	2	2	2
50–64	0									
65+	0									
B. Operated										
0–19 Years	0									
20–34	0									
35–49	0									
50–64	2	4.5	<1	4	4	5	5	5	5	5
65+	0									
2. MULTIPLE DX										
A. Not Operated										
0–19 Years	13	10.8	62	3	4	7	14	24	24	24
20–34	18	4.5	13	1	2	3	6	10	15	15
35–49	41	3.8	6	1	2	3	5	7	8	11
50–64	89	3.8	7	1	2	3	5	7	8	14
65+	276	4.0	8	1	2	3	5	7	10	11
B. Operated										
0–19 Years	2	6.5	12	4	4	4	9	9	9	9
20–34	7	5.6	14	1	2	5	8	12	12	12
35–49	2	7.5	4	6	6	9	9	9	9	9
50–64	28	9.1	104	2	6	6	11	20	21	53
65+	25	6.3	21	2	3	5	8	12	13	22
SUBTOTALS:										
1. SINGLE DX										
A. Not Operated	3	2.3	<1	2	2	2	3	3	3	3
B. Operated	2	4.5	<1	4	4	5	5	5	5	5
2. MULTIPLE DX										
A. Not Operated	437	4.2	10	1	2	3	5	8	10	15
B. Operated	64	7.5	56	2	3	5	9	13	20	53
1. SINGLE DX	5	3.2	2	2	2	3	4	5	5	5
2. MULTIPLE DX	501	4.6	17	1	2	4	6	9	11	21
A. NOT OPERATED	440	4.2	10	1	2	3	5	7	10	15
B. OPERATED	66	7.4	55	2	3	5	9	13	20	53
TOTAL										
0–19 Years	17	9.3	56	3	4	7	11	14	24	24
20–34	25	4.8	13	1	2	4	6	10	12	15
35–49	44	3.9	6	1	2	3	6	8	9	11
50–64	119	5.1	34	1	2	4	7	11	14	21
65+	301	4.2	9	1	2	3	5	8	10	12
GRAND TOTAL	506	4.6	17	2	2	4	6	9	11	21

494.1: BRONCHIECT W AC EXACER

Type of Patients	Observed Patients	Avg. Stay	Variance	10th	25th	50th	75th	90th	95th	99th
1. SINGLE DX										
A. Not Operated										
0–19 Years	0									
20–34	2	4.5	12	2	2	7	7	7	7	7
35–49	1	4.0	0	4	4	4	4	4	4	4
50–64	1	4.0	0	4	4	4	4	4	4	4
65+	0									
B. Operated										
0–19 Years	0									
20–34	1	5.0	0	5	5	5	5	5	5	5
35–49	0									
50–64	0									
65+	0									
2. MULTIPLE DX										
A. Not Operated										
0–19 Years	24	7.7	15	2	5	8	10	13	14	15
20–34	43	6.2	19	1	3	5	6	13	16	19
35–49	39	4.9	18	1	2	4	6	8	13	25
50–64	121	7.0	103	2	3	4	8	12	17	46
65+	558	5.2	14	2	3	4	7	9	13	21
B. Operated										
0–19 Years	0									
20–34	6	9.3	45	3	5	5	13	21	21	21
35–49	4	19.2	89	13	13	13	33	33	33	33
50–64	5	8.2	21	4	4	8	10	15	15	15
65+	15	7.7	14	3	5	7	10	14	16	16
SUBTOTALS:										
1. SINGLE DX										
A. Not Operated	4	4.3	4	2	4	4	7	7	7	7
B. Operated	1	5.0	0	5	5	5	5	5	5	5
2. MULTIPLE DX										
A. Not Operated	785	5.6	29	2	3	4	7	10	13	23
B. Operated	30	9.6	42	3	5	8	13	16	21	33
1. SINGLE DX	5	4.4	3	2	4	4	5	7	7	7
2. MULTIPLE DX	815	5.8	30	2	3	5	7	10	14	23
A. NOT OPERATED	789	5.6	29	2	3	4	7	10	13	23
B. OPERATED	31	9.5	41	4	5	8	13	16	21	33
TOTAL										
0–19 Years	24	7.7	15	2	5	8	10	13	14	15
20–34	52	6.5	21	2	3	5	8	13	17	21
35–49	44	6.2	40	2	2	4	7	13	18	33
50–64	127	7.1	99	2	3	4	8	13	17	46
65+	573	5.3	15	2	3	4	7	9	13	21
GRAND TOTAL	820	5.7	30	2	3	5	7	10	14	23

Length of Stay by Diagnosis and Operation, Western Region, 2008

495: EXTR ALLERGIC ALVEOLITIS

Type of Patients	Observed Patients	Avg. Stay	Variance	Percentiles						
				10th	25th	50th	75th	90th	95th	99th
1. SINGLE DX										
A. *Not Operated*										
0–19 Years	1	2.0	0	2	2	2	2	2	2	2
20–34	0									
35–49	0									
50–64	0									
65+	0									
B. *Operated*										
0–19 Years	0									
20–34	1	1.0	0	1	1	1	1	1	1	1
35–49	0									
50–64	1	3.0	0	3	3	3	3	3	3	3
65+	0									
2. MULTIPLE DX										
A. *Not Operated*										
0–19 Years	3	3.3	<1	3	3	3	4	4	4	4
20–34	11	3.8	7	2	2	3	6	7	10	10
35–49	38	4.2	8	2	2	3	6	8	10	14
50–64	56	6.1	42	1	2	4	7	13	14	42
65+	47	5.6	17	2	3	5	7	12	15	17
B. *Operated*										
0–19 Years	0									
20–34	6	8.0	10	4	5	8	9	13	13	13
35–49	19	6.3	22	1	3	6	9	10	22	22
50–64	23	7.7	37	2	4	6	10	16	19	26
65+	11	10.5	56	4	6	9	12	18	29	29
SUBTOTALS:										
1. SINGLE DX										
A. *Not Operated*	1	2.0	0	2	2	2	2	2	2	2
B. *Operated*	2	2.0	2	1	1	2	3	3	3	3
2. MULTIPLE DX										
A. *Not Operated*	155	5.2	23	2	2	4	6	10	14	24
B. *Operated*	59	7.8	33	2	4	6	9	16	22	29
1. SINGLE DX	3	2.0	1	1	1	2	3	3	3	3
2. MULTIPLE DX	214	5.9	27	2	3	5	8	12	15	26
A. NOT OPERATED	156	5.2	23	2	2	4	6	10	14	24
B. OPERATED	61	7.6	33	2	4	6	9	14	19	29
TOTAL										
0–19 Years	4	3.0	<1	2	3	3	4	4	4	4
20–34	18	5.1	12	1	2	3	8	10	13	13
35–49	57	4.9	13	2	2	4	6	9	10	22
50–64	80	6.5	40	2	3	5	8	14	16	42
65+	58	6.5	27	2	3	5	9	13	17	29
GRAND TOTAL	217	5.9	27	2	3	5	7	12	15	26

496: CHRONIC AIRWAY OBSTR NEC

Type of Patients	Observed Patients	Avg. Stay	Variance	Percentiles						
				10th	25th	50th	75th	90th	95th	99th
1. SINGLE DX										
A. *Not Operated*										
0–19 Years	1	2.0	0	2	2	2	2	2	2	2
20–34	0									
35–49	2	1.0	0	1	1	1	1	1	1	1
50–64	4	2.0	<1	1	1	2	3	3	3	3
65+	3	4.3	16	2	2	2	9	9	9	9
B. *Operated*										
0–19 Years	0									
20–34	0									
35–49	0									
50–64	1	7.0	0	7	7	7	7	7	7	7
65+	0									
2. MULTIPLE DX										
A. *Not Operated*										
0–19 Years	7	3.9	4	2	2	3	6	7	7	7
20–34	6	1.8	1	1	1	1	2	4	4	4
35–49	80	3.1	8	1	1	2	4	6	8	18
50–64	412	3.4	9	1	2	3	4	7	9	17
65+	1,157	3.6	10	1	2	3	4	7	9	17
B. *Operated*										
0–19 Years	1	29.0	0	29	29	29	29	29	29	29
20–34	0									
35–49	2	18.0	18	15	15	21	21	21	21	21
50–64	21	9.0	57	2	4	8	12	14	22	33
65+	42	5.4	81	1	1	2	6	15	41	>99
SUBTOTALS:										
1. SINGLE DX										
A. *Not Operated*	10	2.5	6	1	1	2	2	9	9	9
B. *Operated*	1	7.0	0	7	7	7	7	7	7	7
2. MULTIPLE DX										
A. *Not Operated*	1,662	3.5	10	1	2	3	4	7	9	17
B. *Operated*	66	7.3	83	1	1	4	10	21	33	>99
1. SINGLE DX	11	2.9	7	1	1	2	3	3	9	9
2. MULTIPLE DX	1,728	3.7	13	1	2	3	4	7	10	19
A. NOT OPERATED	1,672	3.5	10	1	2	3	4	7	9	17
B. OPERATED	67	7.3	82	1	1	4	10	21	33	>99
TOTAL										
0–19 Years	9	6.5	75	2	2	3	6	29	29	29
20–34	6	1.8	1	1	1	1	2	4	4	4
35–49	84	3.4	13	1	1	2	4	7	8	21
50–64	438	3.6	13	1	1	3	4	8	11	22
65+	1,202	3.7	13	1	2	3	4	7	9	18
GRAND TOTAL	1,739	3.7	13	1	2	3	4	7	10	19

500: COAL WORKERS' PNEUMOCON

Type of Patients	Observed Patients	Avg. Stay	Variance	Percentiles						
				10th	25th	50th	75th	90th	95th	99th
1. SINGLE DX										
A. *Not Operated*										
0–19 Years	0									
20–34	0									
35–49	0									
50–64	0									
65+	0									
B. *Operated*										
0–19 Years	0									
20–34	0									
35–49	0									
50–64	0									
65+	0									
2. MULTIPLE DX										
A. *Not Operated*										
0–19 Years	0									
20–34	0									
35–49	0									
50–64	0									
65+	2	3.0	2	2	2	4	4	4	4	4
B. *Operated*										
0–19 Years	0									
20–34	0									
35–49	0									
50–64	4	5.5	10	3	4	5	10	10	10	10
65+	6	11.1	60	5	5	8	17	24	24	24
SUBTOTALS:										
1. SINGLE DX										
A. *Not Operated*	0									
B. *Operated*	0									
2. MULTIPLE DX										
A. *Not Operated*	2	3.0	2	2	2	4	4	4	4	4
B. *Operated*	10	8.9	45	4	5	5	10	17	24	24
1. SINGLE DX	0									
2. MULTIPLE DX	12	7.9	42	3	4	5	10	17	24	24
A. NOT OPERATED	2	3.0	2	2	2	4	4	4	4	4
B. OPERATED	10	8.9	45	4	5	5	10	17	24	24
TOTAL										
0–19 Years	0									
20–34	0									
35–49	0									
50–64	4	5.5	10	3	4	5	10	10	10	10
65+	8	9.1	57	2	5	5	10	24	24	24
GRAND TOTAL	12	7.9	42	3	4	5	10	17	24	24

Length of Stay by Diagnosis and Operation, Western Region, 2008

Western Region, October 2006–September 2007 Data, by Diagnosis

501: ASBESTOSIS

Type of Patients	Observed Patients	Avg. Stay	Variance	10th	25th	50th	75th	90th	95th	99th
1. SINGLE DX										
A. Not Operated										
0–19 Years	0									
20–34	0									
35–49	0									
50–64	0									
65+	0									
B. Operated										
0–19 Years	0									
20–34	0									
35–49	0									
50–64	0									
65+	0									
2. MULTIPLE DX										
A. Not Operated										
0–19 Years	0									
20–34	0									
35–49	0									
50–64	3	5.7	9	3	3	5	9	9	9	9
65+	33	5.2	27	2	2	3	6	12	14	27
B. Operated										
0–19 Years	0									
20–34	0									
35–49	0									
50–64	2	8.0	2	7	7	7	9	9	9	9
65+	7	9.0	37	3	4	8	12	21	21	21
SUBTOTALS:										
1. SINGLE DX A. Not Operated	0									
B. Operated	0									
2. MULTIPLE DX A. Not Operated	36	5.3	26	2	2	3	6	12	14	27
B. Operated	9	8.8	29	3	6	8	9	21	21	21
1. SINGLE DX	0									
2. MULTIPLE DX	45	6.0	28	2	3	4	9	12	14	27
A. NOT OPERATED	36	5.3	26	2	2	3	6	12	14	27
B. OPERATED	9	8.8	29	3	6	8	9	21	21	21
TOTAL										
0–19 Years	0									
20–34	0									
35–49	0									
50–64	5	6.6	7	3	5	7	9	9	9	9
65+	40	5.9	30	2	3	4	9	12	21	27
GRAND TOTAL	45	6.0	28	2	3	4	9	12	14	27

502: SILICA PNEUMOCON NEC

Type of Patients	Observed Patients	Avg. Stay	Variance	10th	25th	50th	75th	90th	95th	99th
1. SINGLE DX										
A. Not Operated										
0–19 Years	0									
20–34	0									
35–49	0									
50–64	0									
65+	0									
B. Operated										
0–19 Years	0									
20–34	0									
35–49	0									
50–64	0									
65+	0									
2. MULTIPLE DX										
A. Not Operated										
0–19 Years	0									
20–34	0									
35–49	1	3.0	0	3	3	3	3	3	3	3
50–64	1	3.0	0	3	3	3	3	3	3	3
65+	9	5.6	19	2	4	4	6	17	17	17
B. Operated										
0–19 Years	0									
20–34	0									
35–49	1	2.0	0	2	2	2	2	2	2	2
50–64	1	4.0	0	4	4	4	4	4	4	4
65+	4	6.7	18	1	1	7	7	11	11	11
SUBTOTALS:										
1. SINGLE DX A. Not Operated	0									
B. Operated	0									
2. MULTIPLE DX A. Not Operated	11	5.2	17	3	3	4	6	6	17	17
B. Operated	6	5.5	15	1	2	7	8	11	11	11
1. SINGLE DX	0									
2. MULTIPLE DX	17	5.3	15	2	3	4	6	11	17	17
A. NOT OPERATED	11	5.2	17	3	3	4	6	6	17	17
B. OPERATED	6	5.5	15	1	2	7	8	11	11	11
TOTAL										
0–19 Years	0									
20–34	0									
35–49	2	2.5	<1	2	2	3	3	3	3	3
50–64	2	3.5	<1	3	3	3	3	4	4	4
65+	13	6.0	18	2	4	5	7	11	17	17
GRAND TOTAL	17	5.3	15	2	3	4	6	11	17	17

503: INORG DUST PNEUMOCON NEC

Type of Patients	Observed Patients	Avg. Stay	Variance	10th	25th	50th	75th	90th	95th	99th
1. SINGLE DX										
A. Not Operated										
0–19 Years	0									
20–34	0									
35–49	0									
50–64	0									
65+	0									
B. Operated										
0–19 Years	0									
20–34	0									
35–49	0									
50–64	0									
65+	0									
2. MULTIPLE DX										
A. Not Operated										
0–19 Years	0									
20–34	0									
35–49	0									
50–64	1	4.0	0	4	4	4	4	4	4	4
65+	0									
B. Operated										
0–19 Years	0									
20–34	0									
35–49	0									
50–64	0									
65+	0									
SUBTOTALS:										
1. SINGLE DX A. Not Operated	0									
B. Operated	0									
2. MULTIPLE DX A. Not Operated	1	4.0	0	4	4	4	4	4	4	4
B. Operated	0									
1. SINGLE DX	0									
2. MULTIPLE DX	1	4.0	0	4	4	4	4	4	4	4
A. NOT OPERATED	1	4.0	0	4	4	4	4	4	4	4
B. OPERATED	0									
TOTAL										
0–19 Years	0									
20–34	0									
35–49	0									
50–64	1	4.0	0	4	4	4	4	4	4	4
65+	0									
GRAND TOTAL	1	4.0	0	4	4	4	4	4	4	4

Western Region, October 2006–September 2007 Data, by Diagnosis

504: DUST PNEUMONOPATHY NEC

Type of Patients	Observed Patients	Avg. Stay	Vari-ance	10th	25th	50th	75th	90th	95th	99th
1. SINGLE DX										
A. *Not Operated*										
0–19 Years	0									
20–34	0									
35–49	0									
50–64	0									
65+	0									
B. *Operated*										
0–19 Years	0									
20–34	0									
35–49	0									
50–64	0									
65+	0									
2. MULTIPLE DX										
A. *Not Operated*										
0–19 Years	0									
20–34	0									
35–49	0									
50–64	0									
65+	1	4.0	0	4	4	4	4	4	4	4
B. *Operated*										
0–19 Years	0									
20–34	0									
35–49	0									
50–64	0									
65+	0									
SUBTOTALS:										
1. SINGLE DX										
A. *Not Operated*	0									
B. *Operated*	0									
2. MULTIPLE DX										
A. *Not Operated*	1	4.0	0	4	4	4	4	4	4	4
B. *Operated*	0									
1. SINGLE DX	0									
2. MULTIPLE DX	1	4.0	0	4	4	4	4	4	4	4
A. NOT OPERATED	1	4.0	0	4	4	4	4	4	4	4
B. OPERATED	0									
TOTAL										
0–19 Years	0									
20–34	0									
35–49	0									
50–64	0									
65+	1	4.0	0	4	4	4	4	4	4	4
GRAND TOTAL	1	4.0	0	4	4	4	4	4	4	4

505: PNEUMOCONIOSIS NOS

Type of Patients	Observed Patients	Avg. Stay	Vari-ance	10th	25th	50th	75th	90th	95th	99th
1. SINGLE DX										
A. *Not Operated*										
0–19 Years	0									
20–34	0									
35–49	1	1.0	0	1	1	1	1	1	1	1
50–64	0									
65+	0									
B. *Operated*										
0–19 Years	0									
20–34	0									
35–49	0									
50–64	0									
65+	0									
2. MULTIPLE DX										
A. *Not Operated*										
0–19 Years	0									
20–34	0									
35–49	0									
50–64	0									
65+	2	3.5	12	1	1	4	6	6	6	6
B. *Operated*										
0–19 Years	0									
20–34	0									
35–49	0									
50–64	0									
65+	1	10.0	0	10	10	10	10	10	10	10
SUBTOTALS:										
1. SINGLE DX										
A. *Not Operated*	1	1.0	0	1	1	1	1	1	1	1
B. *Operated*	0									
2. MULTIPLE DX										
A. *Not Operated*	2	3.5	12	1	1	4	6	6	6	6
B. *Operated*	1	10.0	0	10	10	10	10	10	10	10
1. SINGLE DX	1	1.0	0	1	1	1	1	1	1	1
2. MULTIPLE DX	3	5.6	20	1	1	6	10	10	10	10
A. NOT OPERATED	3	2.7	8	1	1	1	6	6	6	6
B. OPERATED	1	10.0	0	10	10	10	10	10	10	10
TOTAL										
0–19 Years	0									
20–34	0									
35–49	1	1.0	0	1	1	1	1	1	1	1
50–64	0									
65+	3	5.6	20	1	1	6	10	10	10	10
GRAND TOTAL	4	4.5	19	1	1	1	6	10	10	10

506: FUME/VAPOR RESP DISEASES

Type of Patients	Observed Patients	Avg. Stay	Vari-ance	10th	25th	50th	75th	90th	95th	99th
1. SINGLE DX										
A. *Not Operated*										
0–19 Years	5	1.2	<1	1	1	1	1	2	2	2
20–34	1	1.0	0	1	1	1	1	1	1	1
35–49	1	2.0	0	2	2	2	2	2	2	2
50–64	1	6.0	0	6	6	6	6	6	6	6
65+	0									
B. *Operated*										
0–19 Years	0									
20–34	0									
35–49	0									
50–64	0									
65+	0									
2. MULTIPLE DX										
A. *Not Operated*										
0–19 Years	11	3.2	6	1	2	2	4	5	10	10
20–34	28	2.8	7	1	1	2	4	6	7	13
35–49	60	4.0	32	1	1	2	5	7	11	36
50–64	47	4.6	72	1	1	2	3	8	20	42
65+	33	4.9	18	1	2	4	6	8	18	18
B. *Operated*										
0–19 Years	0									
20–34	1	14.0	0	14	14	14	14	14	14	14
35–49	0									
50–64	2	40.5	59	35	35	41	46	46	46	46
65+	0									
SUBTOTALS:										
1. SINGLE DX										
A. *Not Operated*	8	1.9	3	1	1	1	2	6	6	6
B. *Operated*	0									
2. MULTIPLE DX										
A. *Not Operated*	179	4.1	34	1	1	2	5	8	11	41
B. *Operated*	3	31.7	262	14	14	35	46	46	46	46
1. SINGLE DX	8	1.9	3	1	1	1	2	6	6	6
2. MULTIPLE DX	182	4.5	49	1	1	2	5	8	14	42
A. NOT OPERATED	187	4.0	33	1	1	2	5	8	11	41
B. OPERATED	3	31.7	262	14	14	35	46	46	46	46
TOTAL										
0–19 Years	16	2.6	5	1	1	2	3	5	10	10
20–34	30	3.1	11	1	1	2	4	6	13	14
35–49	61	4.0	32	1	1	2	5	7	11	36
50–64	50	6.0	119	1	2	2	4	10	41	46
65+	33	4.9	18	1	2	4	6	8	18	18
GRAND TOTAL	190	4.4	48	1	1	2	5	8	14	42

Length of Stay by Diagnosis and Operation, Western Region, 2008

369

Western Region, October 2006–September 2007 Data, by Diagnosis

507: SOLID/LIQ PNEUMONITIS

Type of Patients	Observed Patients	Avg. Stay	Vari-ance	10th	25th	50th	75th	90th	95th	99th
1. SINGLE DX										
A. Not Operated										
0–19 Years	30	3.0	5	1	1	2	3	7	8	9
20–34	3	1.0	0	1	1	1	1	1	1	1
35–49	1	1.0	0	1	1	1	1	1	1	1
50–64	1	7.0	0	7	7	7	7	7	7	7
65+	3	2.7	4	1	1	2	5	5	5	5
B. Operated										
0–19 Years	0									
20–34	0									
35–49	0									
50–64	0									
65+	0									
2. MULTIPLE DX										
A. Not Operated										
0–19 Years	558	6.1	45	1	2	4	7	13	19	28
20–34	632	6.6	39	2	3	5	8	14	19	36
35–49	1,294	7.0	45	2	3	5	8	14	20	33
50–64	2,869	7.1	44	2	3	5	9	14	19	33
65+	16,773	7.0	30	2	4	6	9	13	17	28
B. Operated										
0–19 Years	48	20.6	204	7	10	18	26	38	45	77
20–34	16	16.6	299	3	7	9	18	53	61	61
35–49	44	19.2	224	2	8	16	28	37	40	74
50–64	116	16.9	159	5	9	13	21	35	49	54
65+	424	14.9	127	5	7	12	19	28	35	71
SUBTOTALS:										
1. SINGLE DX										
A. Not Operated	38	2.8	5	1	1	2	3	7	8	9
B. Operated	0									
2. MULTIPLE DX										
A. Not Operated	22,126	7.0	33	2	3	5	9	14	18	28
B. Operated	648	16.0	151	5	8	13	21	31	38	71
1. SINGLE DX	38	2.8	5	1	1	2	3	7	8	9
2. MULTIPLE DX	22,774	7.3	39	2	3	6	9	14	19	30
A. NOT OPERATED	22,164	7.0	33	2	3	5	9	14	18	28
B. OPERATED	648	16.0	151	5	8	13	21	31	38	71
TOTAL										
0–19 Years	636	7.0	70	1	2	5	8	17	23	41
20–34	651	6.8	47	2	3	5	8	14	20	36
35–49	1,339	7.4	56	2	3	5	9	15	22	37
50–64	2,986	7.5	52	2	3	5	9	15	20	36
65+	17,200	7.2	34	2	4	6	9	14	18	29
GRAND TOTAL	22,812	7.3	39	2	3	6	9	14	19	30

507.0: FOOD/VOMIT PNEUMONITIS

Type of Patients	Observed Patients	Avg. Stay	Vari-ance	10th	25th	50th	75th	90th	95th	99th
1. SINGLE DX										
A. Not Operated										
0–19 Years	25	3.0	5	1	1	3	3	7	8	9
20–34	3	1.0	0	1	1	1	1	1	1	1
35–49	1	1.0	0	1	1	1	1	1	1	1
50–64	1	7.0	0	7	7	7	7	7	7	7
65+	2	3.5	4	2	2	5	5	5	5	5
B. Operated										
0–19 Years	0									
20–34	0									
35–49	0									
50–64	0									
65+	0									
2. MULTIPLE DX										
A. Not Operated										
0–19 Years	543	6.2	46	1	2	4	7	13	19	28
20–34	621	6.7	39	2	3	5	8	14	19	36
35–49	1,283	7.0	45	2	3	5	8	14	20	34
50–64	2,844	7.1	44	2	3	5	9	14	19	33
65+	16,721	7.0	30	2	4	6	9	13	17	28
B. Operated										
0–19 Years	48	20.6	204	7	10	18	26	38	45	77
20–34	16	16.6	299	3	7	9	18	53	61	61
35–49	43	19.5	226	2	8	16	28	37	40	74
50–64	115	17.0	159	5	9	13	22	35	49	54
65+	421	14.9	128	5	7	12	19	28	35	71
SUBTOTALS:										
1. SINGLE DX										
A. Not Operated	32	2.9	5	1	1	2	4	6	8	9
B. Operated	0									
2. MULTIPLE DX										
A. Not Operated	22,012	7.0	34	2	3	5	9	14	18	28
B. Operated	643	16.0	152	5	8	13	21	31	38	71
1. SINGLE DX	32	2.9	5	1	1	2	4	6	8	9
2. MULTIPLE DX	22,655	7.3	39	2	3	6	9	14	19	31
A. NOT OPERATED	22,044	7.0	33	2	3	5	9	14	18	28
B. OPERATED	643	16.0	152	5	8	13	21	31	38	71
TOTAL										
0–19 Years	616	7.2	72	1	2	5	8	17	23	41
20–34	640	6.9	47	2	3	5	8	14	20	36
35–49	1,327	7.4	56	2	3	5	9	15	22	37
50–64	2,960	7.5	52	2	3	5	9	15	20	36
65+	17,144	7.2	34	2	4	6	9	14	18	29
GRAND TOTAL	22,687	7.3	39	2	3	6	9	14	19	31

508: RESP COND D/T EXT AGENT

Type of Patients	Observed Patients	Avg. Stay	Vari-ance	10th	25th	50th	75th	90th	95th	99th
1. SINGLE DX										
A. Not Operated										
0–19 Years	0									
20–34	0									
35–49	0									
50–64	0									
65+	0									
B. Operated										
0–19 Years	0									
20–34	0									
35–49	0									
50–64	0									
65+	0									
2. MULTIPLE DX										
A. Not Operated										
0–19 Years	3	4.7	6	2	2	5	7	7	7	7
20–34	8	2.7	3	1	1	2	4	6	6	6
35–49	17	4.8	29	1	2	3	5	14	22	22
50–64	49	3.8	7	1	2	3	6	7	8	11
65+	107	5.3	18	2	3	4	7	13	14	20
B. Operated										
0–19 Years	0									
20–34	0									
35–49	1	2.0	0	2	2	2	2	2	2	2
50–64	1	36.0	0	36	36	36	36	36	36	36
65+	6	10.6	56	1	4	9	16	21	21	21
SUBTOTALS:										
1. SINGLE DX										
A. Not Operated	0									
B. Operated	0									
2. MULTIPLE DX										
A. Not Operated	184	4.7	16	1	2	3	6	10	14	20
B. Operated	8	12.7	136	1	2	9	16	36	36	36
1. SINGLE DX	0									
2. MULTIPLE DX	192	5.1	23	1	2	3	6	11	14	22
A. NOT OPERATED	184	4.7	16	1	2	3	6	10	14	20
B. OPERATED	8	12.7	136	1	2	9	16	36	36	36
TOTAL										
0–19 Years	3	4.7	6	2	2	5	7	7	7	7
20–34	8	2.7	3	1	1	2	4	6	6	6
35–49	18	4.7	28	1	2	3	5	14	22	22
50–64	50	4.5	27	1	2	3	6	8	11	36
65+	113	5.6	21	2	3	4	7	13	15	20
GRAND TOTAL	192	5.1	23	1	2	3	6	11	14	22

Length of Stay by Diagnosis and Operation, Western Region, 2008

510: EMPYEMA

Type of Patients	Observed Patients	Avg. Stay	Variance	Percentiles						
				10th	25th	50th	75th	90th	95th	99th
1. SINGLE DX										
A. Not Operated										
0–19 Years	3	7.0	7	5	5	6	10	10	10	10
20–34	2	3.5	4	2	2	5	5	5	5	5
35–49	1	4.0	0	4	4	4	4	4	4	4
50–64	0									
65+	0									
B. Operated										
0–19 Years	0									
20–34	0									
35–49	4	8.5	34	1	1	7	14	14	14	14
50–64	3	5.0	13	2	2	4	9	9	9	9
65+	0									
2. MULTIPLE DX										
A. Not Operated										
0–19 Years	23	8.5	19	4	6	8	10	14	14	22
20–34	48	10.4	71	1	4	9	13	27	28	36
35–49	146	10.1	67	3	5	8	13	17	23	47
50–64	269	10.0	51	3	6	8	12	18	23	42
65+	279	9.9	47	3	5	8	13	19	22	36
B. Operated										
0–19 Years	66	11.2	69	5	7	9	13	16	21	68
20–34	126	11.9	42	5	8	11	15	19	21	36
35–49	291	12.8	67	6	8	11	15	22	28	49
50–64	401	14.1	81	6	9	12	17	25	29	50
65+	307	14.4	68	6	9	12	19	25	31	46
SUBTOTALS:										
1. SINGLE DX										
A. Not Operated	6	5.3	7	2	4	5	6	10	10	10
B. Operated	7	7.0	25	1	2	7	12	14	14	14
2. MULTIPLE DX										
A. Not Operated	765	10.0	53	3	5	8	13	19	23	38
B. Operated	1,191	13.5	70	6	8	12	17	23	29	49
1. SINGLE DX	**13**	**6.2**	**16**	**2**	**4**	**5**	**9**	**12**	**14**	**14**
2. MULTIPLE DX	**1,956**	**12.1**	**66**	**4**	**7**	**10**	**15**	**21**	**27**	**47**
A. NOT OPERATED	**771**	**9.9**	**53**	**3**	**5**	**8**	**13**	**19**	**23**	**38**
B. OPERATED	**1,198**	**13.4**	**70**	**6**	**8**	**12**	**16**	**23**	**29**	**48**
TOTAL										
0–19 Years	92	10.4	56	5	7	9	12	16	21	68
20–34	176	11.4	50	4	7	10	15	19	26	36
35–49	442	11.8	68	4	7	10	14	20	27	47
50–64	673	12.4	73	4	7	11	16	22	28	48
65+	586	12.3	63	4	7	10	16	22	28	45
GRAND TOTAL	**1,969**	**12.0**	**66**	**4**	**7**	**10**	**15**	**21**	**27**	**47**

510.9: EMPYEMA W/O FISTULA

Type of Patients	Observed Patients	Avg. Stay	Variance	Percentiles						
				10th	25th	50th	75th	90th	95th	99th
1. SINGLE DX										
A. Not Operated										
0–19 Years	3	7.0	7	5	5	6	10	10	10	10
20–34	1	5.0	0	5	5	5	5	5	5	5
35–49	1	4.0	0	4	4	4	4	4	4	4
50–64	0									
65+	0									
B. Operated										
0–19 Years	0									
20–34	0									
35–49	3	11.0	13	7	7	12	14	14	14	14
50–64	2	3.0	2	2	2	4	4	4	4	4
65+	0									
2. MULTIPLE DX										
A. Not Operated										
0–19 Years	22	8.5	20	4	6	8	10	14	14	22
20–34	41	9.9	51	2	5	9	12	19	27	29
35–49	126	9.8	52	3	5	8	13	17	21	37
50–64	239	9.8	46	3	6	8	12	18	21	34
65+	247	10.2	42	3	6	9	13	19	22	32
B. Operated										
0–19 Years	59	11.7	74	5	7	10	13	19	22	68
20–34	107	11.2	22	5	8	11	15	18	20	24
35–49	261	12.4	50	6	8	11	15	20	25	46
50–64	357	13.8	74	6	9	12	17	24	28	47
65+	268	14.1	61	6	9	12	19	24	29	45
SUBTOTALS:										
1. SINGLE DX										
A. Not Operated	5	6.0	6	4	5	6	6	10	10	10
B. Operated	5	7.8	26	2	4	7	12	14	14	14
2. MULTIPLE DX										
A. Not Operated	675	9.9	45	3	6	8	13	18	22	34
B. Operated	1,052	13.2	60	6	8	11	16	22	27	45
1. SINGLE DX	**10**	**6.9**	**15**	**4**	**4**	**5**	**10**	**14**	**14**	**14**
2. MULTIPLE DX	**1,727**	**11.9**	**57**	**5**	**7**	**10**	**15**	**21**	**25**	**40**
A. NOT OPERATED	**680**	**9.9**	**45**	**3**	**6**	**8**	**13**	**18**	**21**	**34**
B. OPERATED	**1,057**	**13.2**	**60**	**6**	**8**	**11**	**16**	**22**	**27**	**45**
TOTAL										
0–19 Years	84	10.7	59	5	7	9	12	16	21	68
20–34	149	10.8	30	5	7	10	15	19	20	28
35–49	391	11.5	52	5	7	10	14	19	25	46
50–64	598	12.2	67	5	7	10	15	21	27	47
65+	515	12.2	56	4	7	11	16	22	26	38
GRAND TOTAL	**1,737**	**11.9**	**57**	**5**	**7**	**10**	**15**	**21**	**25**	**40**

511: PLEURISY

Type of Patients	Observed Patients	Avg. Stay	Variance	Percentiles						
				10th	25th	50th	75th	90th	95th	99th
1. SINGLE DX										
A. Not Operated										
0–19 Years	0									
20–34	5	4.4	4	3	3	4	4	8	8	8
35–49	14	2.4	5	1	1	1	3	7	7	7
50–64	7	2.6	1	1	2	2	4	4	4	4
65+	7	2.4	4	1	1	2	4	6	6	6
B. Operated										
0–19 Years	0									
20–34	1	3.0	0	3	3	3	3	3	3	3
35–49	0									
50–64	2	4.5	4	3	3	3	6	6	6	6
65+	3	4.3	<1	4	4	4	5	5	5	5
2. MULTIPLE DX										
A. Not Operated										
0–19 Years	75	5.2	20	1	2	4	6	10	17	23
20–34	258	4.4	17	1	2	3	5	10	13	25
35–49	800	4.4	18	1	2	3	6	9	13	23
50–64	1,786	4.9	25	1	2	3	6	11	14	25
65+	3,914	5.0	18	1	2	4	6	10	13	21
B. Operated										
0–19 Years	11	10.9	71	5	5	8	15	15	33	33
20–34	38	11.3	37	4	8	11	13	20	26	27
35–49	111	11.3	95	3	5	9	14	22	30	49
50–64	280	11.4	106	3	5	9	14	23	28	51
65+	575	10.4	71	3	5	8	13	21	26	39
SUBTOTALS:										
1. SINGLE DX										
A. Not Operated	33	2.8	4	1	1	2	4	6	7	8
B. Operated	6	4.2	1	3	3	4	5	6	6	6
2. MULTIPLE DX										
A. Not Operated	6,833	4.9	20	1	2	4	6	10	13	22
B. Operated	1,015	10.8	82	3	5	8	14	21	28	44
1. SINGLE DX	**39**	**3.0**	**4**	**1**	**1**	**3**	**4**	**6**	**7**	**8**
2. MULTIPLE DX	**7,848**	**5.7**	**32**	**1**	**2**	**4**	**7**	**12**	**16**	**28**
A. NOT OPERATED	**6,866**	**4.9**	**20**	**1**	**2**	**4**	**6**	**10**	**13**	**22**
B. OPERATED	**1,021**	**10.8**	**82**	**3**	**5**	**8**	**14**	**21**	**28**	**44**
TOTAL										
0–19 Years	86	5.9	29	1	2	5	7	14	17	33
20–34	302	5.3	25	1	2	3	7	13	14	26
35–49	925	5.2	32	1	2	3	6	12	16	29
50–64	2,075	5.8	41	1	2	4	7	12	18	30
65+	4,499	5.7	28	1	2	4	7	11	15	27
GRAND TOTAL	**7,887**	**5.7**	**32**	**1**	**2**	**4**	**7**	**12**	**16**	**28**

371

Length of Stay by Diagnosis and Operation, Western Region, 2008

Western Region, October 2006–September 2007 Data, by Diagnosis

511.0: PLEURISY W/O EFFUS OR TB

Type of Patients	Observed Patients	Avg. Stay	Variance	10th	25th	50th	75th	90th	95th	99th
1. SINGLE DX										
A. Not Operated										
0–19 Years	0									
20–34	0									
35–49	6	1.0	0	1	1	1	1	1	1	1
50–64	2	2.0	0	2	2	2	2	2	2	2
65+	0									
B. Operated										
0–19 Years	0									
20–34	0									
35–49	0									
50–64	0									
65+	0									
2. MULTIPLE DX										
A. Not Operated										
0–19 Years	4	2.5	3	1	1	2	2	5	5	5
20–34	66	2.8	13	1	1	2	3	5	7	26
35–49	140	2.2	5	1	1	2	2	4	6	10
50–64	200	2.2	2	1	1	2	3	4	5	8
65+	235	2.4	3	1	1	2	3	5	6	9
B. Operated										
0–19 Years	0									
20–34	2	8.0	50	3	3	3	13	13	13	13
35–49	7	5.6	12	1	3	6	7	12	12	12
50–64	19	8.0	36	1	3	7	11	21	21	21
65+	32	8.1	137	1	3	5	7	15	22	65
SUBTOTALS:										
1. SINGLE DX										
A. Not Operated	8	1.3	<1	1	1	1	1	2	2	2
B. Operated	0									
2. MULTIPLE DX										
A. Not Operated	645	2.4	4	1	1	2	3	4	6	10
B. Operated	60	7.7	86	3	3	5	9	15	21	65
1. SINGLE DX	8	1.3	<1	1	1	1	1	2	2	2
2. MULTIPLE DX	705	2.8	13	1	1	2	3	5	7	15
A. NOT OPERATED	653	2.3	4	1	1	2	3	4	6	10
B. OPERATED	60	7.7	86	3	3	5	9	15	21	65
TOTAL										
0–19 Years	4	2.5	3	1	1	2	2	5	5	5
20–34	68	2.9	14	1	1	2	3	6	10	26
35–49	153	2.3	5	1	1	2	2	4	7	12
50–64	221	2.7	8	1	1	2	4	5	7	15
65+	267	3.1	22	1	1	2	4	6	7	19
GRAND TOTAL	713	2.8	13	1	1	2	3	5	7	15

511.8: PLEURAL EFFUS NEC NOT TB

Type of Patients	Observed Patients	Avg. Stay	Variance	10th	25th	50th	75th	90th	95th	99th
1. SINGLE DX										
A. Not Operated										
0–19 Years	0									
20–34	3	4.7	8	3	3	3	8	8	8	8
35–49	2	3.0	2	2	2	4	4	4	4	4
50–64	3	2.0	1	1	1	2	3	3	3	3
65+	1	4.0	0	4	4	4	4	4	4	4
B. Operated										
0–19 Years	0									
20–34	1	3.0	0	3	3	3	3	3	3	3
35–49	0									
50–64	1	3.0	0	3	3	3	3	3	3	3
65+	0									
2. MULTIPLE DX										
A. Not Operated										
0–19 Years	13	6.8	11	3	5	6	8	11	14	14
20–34	51	5.4	13	2	3	5	7	10	13	18
35–49	141	5.4	17	2	3	4	7	11	14	21
50–64	345	6.4	34	2	3	4	8	14	18	30
65+	591	6.0	24	2	3	5	8	12	15	27
B. Operated										
0–19 Years	9	12.4	73	5	8	11	15	33	33	33
20–34	15	13.0	45	5	10	12	17	24	27	27
35–49	35	13.2	115	5	6	9	17	29	39	49
50–64	84	12.1	55	5	7	10	17	22	28	37
65+	161	12.6	84	4	6	10	16	26	31	44
SUBTOTALS:										
1. SINGLE DX										
A. Not Operated	9	3.3	4	1	2	3	4	8	8	8
B. Operated	2	3.0	0	3	3	3	3	3	3	3
2. MULTIPLE DX										
A. Not Operated	1,141	6.1	26	2	3	5	8	12	16	26
B. Operated	304	12.5	77	4	7	10	16	25	31	39
1. SINGLE DX	11	3.3	3	2	2	3	4	4	8	8
2. MULTIPLE DX	1,445	7.4	43	2	3	5	10	15	21	32
A. NOT OPERATED	1,150	6.0	25	2	3	4	8	12	16	26
B. OPERATED	306	12.5	77	4	6	10	16	25	31	39
TOTAL										
0–19 Years	22	9.1	42	5	5	7	11	15	15	33
20–34	70	7.0	29	2	3	5	10	14	17	27
35–49	178	6.9	45	2	3	5	8	14	19	39
50–64	433	7.5	43	2	3	5	10	17	21	30
65+	753	7.4	44	2	3	5	10	15	21	32
GRAND TOTAL	1,456	7.4	43	2	3	5	10	15	21	32

511.9: PLEURAL EFFUSION NOS

Type of Patients	Observed Patients	Avg. Stay	Variance	10th	25th	50th	75th	90th	95th	99th
1. SINGLE DX										
A. Not Operated										
0–19 Years	0									
20–34	2	4.0	0	4	4	4	4	4	4	4
35–49	6	3.7	7	1	2	3	7	7	7	7
50–64	2	4.0	0	4	4	4	4	4	4	4
65+	6	2.2	4	1	1	1	2	6	6	6
B. Operated										
0–19 Years	0									
20–34	0									
35–49	0									
50–64	1	6.0	0	6	6	6	6	6	6	6
65+	3	4.3	<1	4	4	4	5	5	5	5
2. MULTIPLE DX										
A. Not Operated										
0–19 Years	56	5.1	23	1	2	4	6	10	17	23
20–34	139	4.6	15	1	2	3	7	10	13	17
35–49	510	4.7	19	1	2	3	6	9	13	23
50–64	1,228	4.9	24	1	2	3	6	10	13	22
65+	3,064	5.0	17	1	2	4	6	10	13	20
B. Operated										
0–19 Years	2	4.0	2	3	3	5	5	5	5	5
20–34	20	10.4	31	3	7	9	13	14	20	26
35–49	66	10.6	90	3	5	9	13	18	29	61
50–64	171	11.3	139	3	4	8	14	24	28	79
65+	377	9.7	57	3	5	8	12	20	25	39
SUBTOTALS:										
1. SINGLE DX										
A. Not Operated	16	3.2	4	1	2	4	4	7	7	7
B. Operated	4	4.8	<1	4	4	4	5	6	6	6
2. MULTIPLE DX										
A. Not Operated	4,997	4.9	19	1	2	4	6	10	13	21
B. Operated	636	10.2	82	3	5	8	12	21	26	47
1. SINGLE DX	20	3.5	4	1	2	4	5	7	7	7
2. MULTIPLE DX	5,633	5.5	29	1	2	4	7	11	15	26
A. NOT OPERATED	5,013	4.9	19	1	2	4	6	10	13	21
B. OPERATED	640	10.2	81	3	5	8	12	21	26	47
TOTAL										
0–19 Years	58	5.0	22	1	2	4	6	10	17	23
20–34	161	5.3	21	1	2	4	7	12	14	25
35–49	582	5.3	30	1	2	4	7	11	15	29
50–64	1,402	5.7	42	1	2	4	7	12	16	30
65+	3,450	5.5	23	1	2	4	7	11	14	25
GRAND TOTAL	5,653	5.5	29	1	2	4	7	11	15	26

Length of Stay by Diagnosis and Operation, Western Region, 2008

Western Region, October 2006–September 2007 Data, by Diagnosis

512: PNEUMOTHORAX

Type of Patients	Observed Patients	Avg. Stay	Variance	10th	25th	50th	75th	90th	95th	99th
1. SINGLE DX										
A. Not Operated										
0–19 Years	154	3.0	4	1	1	3	4	6	7	9
20–34	167	3.2	4	1	2	3	4	6	7	10
35–49	57	3.2	4	1	2	3	4	7	8	9
50–64	20	2.2	3	1	1	2	3	4	8	8
65+	12	1.8	1	1	1	2	2	3	4	4
B. Operated										
0–19 Years	40	5.3	9	2	3	5	6	9	10	16
20–34	45	5.7	11	2	3	5	7	10	11	17
35–49	17	4.2	4	2	3	4	5	7	8	8
50–64	4	7.0	11	3	3	6	8	11	11	11
65+	0									
2. MULTIPLE DX										
A. Not Operated										
0–19 Years	197	3.9	13	1	2	2	5	9	13	17
20–34	434	4.1	10	1	2	3	5	8	10	17
35–49	485	4.3	14	1	2	3	5	8	11	20
50–64	805	4.8	26	1	2	3	6	10	14	28
65+	1,552	5.2	30	1	2	4	7	10	14	25
B. Operated										
0–19 Years	152	6.8	22	2	4	6	9	11	15	27
20–34	281	7.3	23	3	4	6	9	13	17	24
35–49	193	8.5	47	3	5	6	10	16	20	44
50–64	224	10.5	87	3	5	8	12	21	28	38
65+	259	10.6	74	2	5	8	14	23	29	41
SUBTOTALS:										
1. SINGLE DX										
A. Not Operated	410	3.0	4	1	1	3	4	6	7	9
B. Operated	106	5.4	9	2	3	5	7	9	11	16
2. MULTIPLE DX										
A. Not Operated	3,473	4.8	24	1	2	3	6	9	13	22
B. Operated	1,109	8.9	54	3	4	7	11	18	23	37
1. SINGLE DX	516	3.5	6	1	2	3	5	7	8	11
2. MULTIPLE DX	4,582	5.8	34	1	2	4	7	12	16	29
A. NOT OPERATED	3,883	4.6	22	1	2	3	6	9	12	22
B. OPERATED	1,215	8.6	52	3	4	7	10	17	22	37
TOTAL										
0–19 Years	543	4.6	15	1	2	3	6	9	13	20
20–34	927	5.0	15	1	2	4	6	10	12	20
35–49	752	5.3	25	1	2	4	6	10	15	27
50–64	1,053	6.0	44	1	2	4	7	12	19	33
65+	1,823	5.9	40	1	2	4	7	12	18	31
GRAND TOTAL	5,098	5.5	32	1	2	4	7	11	16	28

512.0: SPONT TENS PNEUMOTHORAX

Type of Patients	Observed Patients	Avg. Stay	Vari-ance	10th	25th	50th	75th	90th	95th	99th
1. SINGLE DX										
A. Not Operated										
0–19 Years	8	3.1	3	1	2	3	4	7	7	7
20–34	6	2.7	1	1	2	3	3	4	4	4
35–49	2	2.0	2	1	1	2	3	3	3	3
50–64	0									
65+	1	4.0	0	4	4	4	4	4	4	4
B. Operated										
0–19 Years	0									
20–34	5	7.2	36	1	5	6	7	17	17	17
35–49	0									
50–64	0									
65+	0									
2. MULTIPLE DX										
A. Not Operated										
0–19 Years	5	8.2	17	2	6	10	11	12	12	12
20–34	33	6.2	17	2	3	5	9	12	15	17
35–49	19	7.4	19	2	5	6	9	16	18	18
50–64	35	7.0	35	2	3	5	8	15	22	26
65+	60	7.2	21	2	4	7	9	13	16	27
B. Operated										
0–19 Years	4	8.0	28	5	5	6	6	16	16	16
20–34	25	8.3	28	3	4	7	12	17	18	22
35–49	14	9.8	83	5	6	7	10	15	40	40
50–64	11	15.4	89	6	7	13	26	28	29	29
65+	14	16.7	139	6	8	16	24	50	>99	>99
SUBTOTALS:										
1. SINGLE DX										
A. Not Operated	17	2.9	2	1	2	3	3	4	7	7
B. Operated	5	7.2	36	1	5	6	7	17	17	17
2. MULTIPLE DX										
A. Not Operated	152	7.0	23	2	4	6	9	13	16	26
B. Operated	68	11.5	81	4	5	8	16	26	29	>99
1. SINGLE DX	22	3.9	12	1	2	3	4	7	7	17
2. MULTIPLE DX	220	8.4	45	2	4	7	10	17	22	40
A. NOT OPERATED	169	6.6	22	2	3	5	9	12	16	26
B. OPERATED	73	11.2	78	4	5	8	16	24	29	>99
TOTAL										
0–19 Years	17	5.8	18	2	3	5	7	12	16	16
20–34	69	6.7	23	2	3	5	9	14	17	22
35–49	35	8.1	46	3	5	6	9	15	18	40
50–64	46	9.0	59	2	3	7	11	22	26	29
65+	75	8.9	55	3	5	7	11	19	26	>99
GRAND TOTAL	242	8.0	43	2	4	6	10	16	21	40

512.1: IATROGENIC PNEUMOTHORAX

Type of Patients	Observed Patients	Avg. Stay	Vari-ance	10th	25th	50th	75th	90th	95th	99th
1. SINGLE DX										
A. Not Operated										
0–19 Years	1	3.0	0	3	3	3	3	3	3	3
20–34	3	1.3	<1	1	1	1	2	2	2	2
35–49	6	2.7	3	1	1	3	4	5	5	5
50–64	5	2.2	<1	1	2	2	3	3	3	3
65+	3	1.0	0	1	1	1	1	1	1	1
B. Operated										
0–19 Years	0									
20–34	0									
35–49	0									
50–64	0									
65+	0									
2. MULTIPLE DX										
A. Not Operated										
0–19 Years	7	3.4	13	1	1	1	8	9	9	9
20–34	33	4.5	9	1	2	4	6	8	12	12
35–49	122	3.8	9	1	2	3	5	8	9	12
50–64	340	3.9	14	1	2	3	5	8	11	19
65+	759	4.0	23	1	1	3	5	8	10	19
B. Operated										
0–19 Years	3	4.3	2	3	3	4	6	6	6	6
20–34	6	7.1	63	1	1	3	14	20	20	20
35–49	16	7.2	42	2	3	5	7	19	21	21
50–64	44	7.8	54	1	3	5	12	13	21	38
65+	102	7.8	59	1	2	6	11	18	22	35
SUBTOTALS:										
1. SINGLE DX										
A. Not Operated	18	2.1	1	1	1	2	3	4	5	5
B. Operated	0									
2. MULTIPLE DX										
A. Not Operated	1,261	3.9	19	1	2	3	5	8	10	19
B. Operated	171	7.7	55	1	2	5	11	18	22	37
1. SINGLE DX	18	2.1	1	1	1	2	3	4	5	5
2. MULTIPLE DX	1,432	4.4	25	1	2	3	6	9	12	22
A. NOT OPERATED	1,279	3.9	19	1	2	3	5	8	10	19
B. OPERATED	171	7.7	55	1	2	5	11	18	22	37
TOTAL										
0–19 Years	11	3.6	8	1	1	3	6	8	9	9
20–34	42	4.6	16	1	2	4	6	8	12	20
35–49	144	4.1	13	1	2	3	5	8	11	19
50–64	389	4.3	20	1	2	3	5	10	13	26
65+	864	4.4	29	1	2	3	6	9	12	23
GRAND TOTAL	1,450	4.4	24	1	2	3	6	9	12	22

Length of Stay by Diagnosis and Operation, Western Region, 2008

Western Region, October 2006–September 2007 Data, by Diagnosis

512.8: SPONT PNEUMOTHORAX NEC

Type of Patients	Observed Patients	Avg. Stay	Variance	10th	25th	50th	75th	90th	95th	99th
1. SINGLE DX										
A. Not Operated										
0–19 Years	145	3.0	4	1	1	3	4	6	7	9
20–34	158	3.2	5	1	2	3	4	6	8	10
35–49	49	3.3	4	1	2	3	4	6	8	9
50–64	15	2.2	3	1	1	2	3	4	8	8
65+	8	1.9	<1	1	1	2	2	3	3	3
B. Operated										
0–19 Years	40	5.3	9	2	3	5	6	9	10	16
20–34	40	5.5	9	2	3	5	7	10	11	14
35–49	17	4.2	4	2	3	4	5	7	8	8
50–64	4	7.0	11	3	3	6	8	11	11	11
65+	0									
2. MULTIPLE DX										
A. Not Operated										
0–19 Years	185	3.8	13	1	2	2	5	8	13	17
20–34	368	3.8	8	1	2	3	5	8	10	17
35–49	344	4.3	16	1	2	3	5	8	11	25
50–64	430	5.4	34	1	2	4	6	10	16	33
65+	733	6.3	34	2	3	5	8	13	17	26
B. Operated										
0–19 Years	145	6.8	23	2	4	6	9	11	15	27
20–34	250	7.2	22	3	4	6	9	13	17	24
35–49	163	8.5	45	3	5	7	10	16	19	44
50–64	169	10.9	93	4	6	9	12	21	28	44
65+	143	12.0	69	4	6	9	16	25	29	40
SUBTOTALS:										
1. SINGLE DX										
A. Not Operated	375	3.1	4	1	1	3	3	6	7	9
B. Operated	101	5.3	8	2	3	5	7	9	10	14
2. MULTIPLE DX										
A. Not Operated	2,060	5.1	26	1	2	4	6	10	14	26
B. Operated	870	8.9	52	3	5	7	11	17	22	36
1. SINGLE DX	476	3.5	6	1	2	3	5	7	8	11
2. MULTIPLE DX	2,930	6.2	36	2	3	5	8	13	17	31
A. NOT OPERATED	2,435	4.8	23	1	2	3	6	9	13	25
B. OPERATED	971	8.5	48	3	4	7	10	16	22	36
TOTAL										
0–19 Years	515	4.5	15	1	2	3	6	9	13	20
20–34	816	4.8	14	1	2	4	6	9	12	20
35–49	573	5.4	27	2	2	4	6	11	15	28
50–64	618	6.8	56	1	3	5	8	14	21	36
65+	884	7.2	44	2	3	5	9	15	19	35
GRAND TOTAL	3,406	5.8	33	1	2	4	7	12	16	29

513: LUNG/MEDIASTINUM ABSCESS

Type of Patients	Observed Patients	Avg. Stay	Variance	10th	25th	50th	75th	90th	95th	99th
1. SINGLE DX										
A. Not Operated										
0–19 Years	2	2.0	2	1	1	1	3	3	3	3
20–34	2	3.0	0	3	3	3	3	3	3	3
35–49	2	7.5	12	5	5	5	10	10	10	10
50–64	1	7.0	0	7	7	7	7	7	7	7
65+	0									
B. Operated										
0–19 Years	0									
20–34	0									
35–49	1	4.0	0	4	4	4	4	4	4	4
50–64	1	1.0	0	1	1	1	1	1	1	1
65+	1	5.0	0	5	5	5	5	5	5	5
2. MULTIPLE DX										
A. Not Operated										
0–19 Years	40	7.6	21	3	4	7	10	15	17	21
20–34	53	7.7	32	2	3	6	11	15	21	24
35–49	156	8.6	101	2	4	6	10	16	24	63
50–64	208	9.4	54	3	5	7	11	19	23	37
65+	237	9.0	41	3	5	8	11	16	19	31
B. Operated										
0–19 Years	12	11.9	60	5	6	9	21	22	24	24
20–34	27	12.8	270	5	5	7	16	19	46	82
35–49	66	12.7	64	6	8	11	16	20	25	42
50–64	88	11.6	74	4	5	9	16	21	31	51
65+	79	10.4	54	3	5	8	14	22	26	38
SUBTOTALS:										
1. SINGLE DX										
A. Not Operated	7	4.6	9	1	3	3	7	10	10	10
B. Operated	3	3.3	4	1	1	4	5	5	5	5
2. MULTIPLE DX										
A. Not Operated	694	8.9	56	3	4	7	11	16	21	37
B. Operated	272	11.6	84	4	6	9	16	21	26	46
1. SINGLE DX	10	4.2	8	1	3	4	5	10	10	10
2. MULTIPLE DX	966	9.6	66	3	5	8	12	18	23	42
A. NOT OPERATED	701	8.8	56	3	4	7	11	16	21	36
B. OPERATED	275	11.5	84	4	6	9	16	21	26	46
TOTAL										
0–19 Years	54	8.3	33	3	4	7	10	17	21	24
20–34	82	9.3	114	2	3	6	12	17	21	82
35–49	225	9.8	92	3	4	7	12	19	24	42
50–64	298	10.0	61	4	5	8	13	19	23	38
65+	317	9.4	44	3	5	8	12	17	22	31
GRAND TOTAL	976	9.6	65	3	5	7	12	18	23	42

513.0: LUNG ABSCESS

Type of Patients	Observed Patients	Avg. Stay	Variance	10th	25th	50th	75th	90th	95th	99th
1. SINGLE DX										
A. Not Operated										
0–19 Years	2	2.0	2	1	1	1	3	3	3	3
20–34	2	3.0	0	3	3	3	3	3	3	3
35–49	2	7.5	12	5	5	5	10	10	10	10
50–64	1	7.0	0	7	7	7	7	7	7	7
65+	0									
B. Operated										
0–19 Years	0									
20–34	0									
35–49	1	4.0	0	4	4	4	4	4	4	4
50–64	1	1.0	0	1	1	1	1	1	1	1
65+	1	5.0	0	5	5	5	5	5	5	5
2. MULTIPLE DX										
A. Not Operated										
0–19 Years	40	7.6	21	3	4	7	10	15	17	21
20–34	53	7.7	32	2	3	6	11	15	21	24
35–49	155	8.7	101	2	4	6	10	16	24	63
50–64	205	9.3	54	3	5	7	11	19	23	37
65+	236	9.0	41	3	5	8	11	16	19	31
B. Operated										
0–19 Years	12	11.9	60	5	6	9	21	22	24	24
20–34	22	10.1	92	5	5	7	14	18	19	46
35–49	62	12.8	68	6	7	11	16	20	25	42
50–64	79	11.5	81	4	5	8	16	21	31	51
65+	74	10.0	53	3	5	8	14	21	26	38
SUBTOTALS:										
1. SINGLE DX										
A. Not Operated	7	4.6	9	1	3	3	7	10	10	10
B. Operated	3	3.3	4	1	1	4	5	5	5	5
2. MULTIPLE DX										
A. Not Operated	689	8.8	56	3	4	7	11	16	21	37
B. Operated	249	11.3	69	4	6	9	16	21	26	42
1. SINGLE DX	10	4.2	8	1	3	4	5	10	10	10
2. MULTIPLE DX	938	9.5	61	3	5	8	12	18	22	40
A. NOT OPERATED	696	8.8	56	3	4	7	11	16	21	37
B. OPERATED	252	11.2	69	4	5	9	15	21	26	42
TOTAL										
0–19 Years	54	8.3	33	3	4	7	10	17	21	24
20–34	77	8.2	49	2	3	6	11	17	21	46
35–49	220	9.8	94	3	4	7	12	19	25	42
50–64	286	9.9	62	4	5	7	12	19	23	44
65+	311	9.2	44	3	5	8	11	16	21	31
GRAND TOTAL	948	9.4	61	3	5	7	12	18	22	40

Length of Stay by Diagnosis and Operation, Western Region, 2008

514: PULMONARY CONGESTION

Type of Patients	Observed Patients	Avg. Stay	Vari-ance	Percentiles						
				10th	25th	50th	75th	90th	95th	99th
1. SINGLE DX										
A. Not Operated										
0–19 Years	0									
20–34	0									
35–49	0									
50–64	0									
65+	0									
B. Operated										
0–19 Years	0									
20–34	0									
35–49	0									
50–64	0									
65+	0									
2. MULTIPLE DX										
A. Not Operated										
0–19 Years	15	4.4	11	1	2	4	5	9	13	13
20–34	27	2.2	2	1	1	2	3	3	4	7
35–49	72	3.3	10	1	1	2	4	8	11	15
50–64	144	3.5	10	1	1	3	4	8	10	15
65+	292	3.7	8	1	2	3	5	7	9	16
B. Operated										
0–19 Years	1	1.0	0	1	1	1	1	1	1	1
20–34	4	6.5	26	2	3	6	11	13	13	13
35–49	4	6.3	21	2	3	8	8	12	12	12
50–64	3	3.0	4	1	1	3	5	5	5	5
65+	11	7.3	35	3	3	6	8	11	23	23
SUBTOTALS:										
1. SINGLE DX										
A. Not Operated	0									
B. Operated	0									
2. MULTIPLE DX										
A. Not Operated	550	3.6	9	1	2	3	4	8	9	15
B. Operated	23	6.1	26	1	3	5	8	12	13	23
1. SINGLE DX	0									
2. MULTIPLE DX	573	3.7	10	1	2	3	5	8	10	15
A. NOT OPERATED	550	3.6	9	1	2	3	4	8	9	15
B. OPERATED	23	6.1	26	1	3	5	8	12	13	23
TOTAL										
0–19 Years	16	4.2	11	1	2	3	4	9	13	13
20–34	31	2.8	6	1	1	2	3	4	8	13
35–49	76	3.5	11	1	1	2	4	9	12	15
50–64	147	3.5	10	1	1	3	4	8	10	15
65+	303	3.9	10	1	2	3	5	8	10	16
GRAND TOTAL	573	3.7	10	1	2	3	5	8	10	15

515: POSTINFLAM PULM FIBROSIS

Type of Patients	Observed Patients	Avg. Stay	Vari-ance	Percentiles						
				10th	25th	50th	75th	90th	95th	99th
1. SINGLE DX										
A. Not Operated										
0–19 Years	0									
20–34	3	5.7	21	3	3	3	11	11	11	11
35–49	4	2.0	4	1	1	1	5	5	5	5
50–64	3	1.3	<1	1	1	1	2	2	2	2
65+	3	2.0	3	1	1	1	4	4	4	4
B. Operated										
0–19 Years	2	3.0	2	2	2	2	4	4	4	4
20–34	5	3.6	1	2	3	4	4	5	5	5
35–49	13	2.5	3	1	1	2	3	4	7	7
50–64	34	1.9	1	1	1	2	2	4	4	5
65+	14	1.9	1	1	1	2	3	3	4	4
2. MULTIPLE DX										
A. Not Operated										
0–19 Years	12	6.3	40	1	2	5	13	16	19	19
20–34	43	4.7	16	2	2	4	5	9	12	23
35–49	126	5.0	21	1	2	4	6	9	12	25
50–64	426	5.2	30	1	2	4	7	11	13	23
65+	1,616	5.0	16	1	2	4	6	9	13	19
B. Operated										
0–19 Years	8	4.9	26	1	1	3	12	13	13	13
20–34	32	4.9	34	1	2	4	4	10	20	27
35–49	189	5.5	62	1	2	3	6	10	14	51
50–64	556	4.8	24	1	2	3	6	11	14	26
65+	564	5.6	32	2	2	4	7	12	16	26
SUBTOTALS:										
1. SINGLE DX										
A. Not Operated	13	2.7	8	1	1	1	3	5	11	11
B. Operated	68	2.2	2	1	1	2	3	4	4	7
2. MULTIPLE DX										
A. Not Operated	2,223	5.0	19	1	2	4	6	10	13	21
B. Operated	1,349	5.2	33	1	2	3	6	11	15	27
1. SINGLE DX	81	2.3	3	1	1	2	3	4	5	11
2. MULTIPLE DX	3,572	5.1	24	1	2	4	6	10	14	24
A. NOT OPERATED	2,236	5.0	19	1	2	4	6	10	13	21
B. OPERATED	1,417	5.1	32	1	2	3	6	11	15	27
TOTAL										
0–19 Years	22	5.5	31	1	1	3	7	13	16	19
20–34	83	4.7	22	1	2	4	5	10	13	27
35–49	332	5.2	44	1	2	3	6	9	13	43
50–64	1,019	4.9	26	1	2	3	6	11	14	25
65+	2,197	5.1	20	1	2	4	6	10	14	22
GRAND TOTAL	3,653	5.0	24	1	2	4	6	10	14	24

516: OTH ALVEO PNEUMONOPATHY

Type of Patients	Observed Patients	Avg. Stay	Vari-ance	Percentiles						
				10th	25th	50th	75th	90th	95th	99th
1. SINGLE DX										
A. Not Operated										
0–19 Years	4	3.3	<1	2	2	4	4	4	4	4
20–34	2	1.0	0	1	1	1	1	1	1	1
35–49	1	1.0	0	1	1	1	1	1	1	1
50–64	3	4.3	33	1	1	1	11	11	11	11
65+	1	4.0	0	4	4	4	4	4	4	4
B. Operated										
0–19 Years	0									
20–34	1	1.0	0	1	1	1	1	1	1	1
35–49	4	2.0	1	1	1	1	3	3	3	3
50–64	4	1.5	<1	1	1	1	1	3	3	3
65+	4	2.8	<1	2	2	3	3	3	3	3
2. MULTIPLE DX										
A. Not Operated										
0–19 Years	41	5.3	103	1	2	3	4	8	30	>99
20–34	25	4.9	28	1	2	3	5	11	12	26
35–49	97	8.0	73	2	3	5	9	18	26	47
50–64	196	6.3	36	2	3	4	8	13	18	32
65+	496	6.3	27	2	3	5	8	13	16	26
B. Operated										
0–19 Years	5	10.2	70	2	6	6	14	23	23	23
20–34	18	5.4	20	2	2	5	7	12	17	17
35–49	78	10.2	94	2	3	8	12	25	29	49
50–64	166	10.0	95	2	3	7	13	23	30	54
65+	220	10.1	83	2	4	7	15	20	27	48
SUBTOTALS:										
1. SINGLE DX										
A. Not Operated	11	3.0	9	1	1	2	4	4	11	11
B. Operated	13	2.0	1	1	1	2	3	3	3	3
2. MULTIPLE DX										
A. Not Operated	855	6.4	38	2	3	5	8	13	18	32
B. Operated	487	9.9	87	2	3	7	13	22	29	49
1. SINGLE DX	24	2.5	5	1	1	2	3	3	4	11
2. MULTIPLE DX	1,342	7.7	58	2	3	5	9	16	23	43
A. NOT OPERATED	866	6.4	38	2	3	5	8	13	18	32
B. OPERATED	500	9.7	86	2	3	7	13	22	28	48
TOTAL										
0–19 Years	50	5.7	92	1	2	3	4	14	30	>99
20–34	46	4.8	24	1	2	3	6	11	12	26
35–49	180	8.8	82	2	3	6	10	17	26	47
50–64	369	7.9	66	2	3	5	10	16	24	44
65+	721	7.4	47	2	3	5	10	16	19	37
GRAND TOTAL	1,366	7.6	58	2	3	5	9	16	23	43

Length of Stay by Diagnosis and Operation, Western Region, 2008

375

Western Region, October 2006–September 2007 Data, by Diagnosis

516.3: IDIO FIBROSIS ALVEOLITIS

Type of Patients	Observed Patients	Avg. Stay	Variance	10th	25th	50th	75th	90th	95th	99th
1. SINGLE DX										
A. Not Operated										
0–19 Years	0									
20–34	0									
35–49	0									
50–64	0									
65+	1	4.0	0	4	4	4	4	4	4	4
B. Operated										
0–19 Years	0									
20–34	0									
35–49	2	3.0	0	3	3	3	3	3	3	3
50–64	2	2.0	2	1	1	2	3	3	3	3
65+	0									
2. MULTIPLE DX										
A. Not Operated										
0–19 Years	2	10.0	70	4	4	4	16	16	16	16
20–34	4	4.0	9	1	3	4	4	4	8	8
35–49	17	7.6	55	2	3	5	7	23	26	26
50–64	62	4.6	9	2	3	4	6	8	9	19
65+	211	5.4	18	2	3	4	7	11	14	23
B. Operated										
0–19 Years	2	23.0	0	23	23	23	23	23	23	23
20–34	2	9.0	18	6	6	6	12	12	12	12
35–49	23	9.4	160	2	2	6	10	29	40	49
50–64	48	10.5	112	2	3	8	13	24	30	56
65+	63	8.8	75	2	3	5	12	22	32	>99
SUBTOTALS:										
1. SINGLE DX — A. Not Operated	1	4.0	0	4	4	4	4	4	4	4
1. SINGLE DX — B. Operated	4	2.5	<1	1	3	3	3	3	3	3
2. MULTIPLE DX — A. Not Operated	296	5.4	19	2	3	4	7	11	14	24
2. MULTIPLE DX — B. Operated	137	9.6	101	2	3	6	12	24	32	56
1. SINGLE DX	5	2.8	1	1	3	3	3	4	4	4
2. MULTIPLE DX	433	6.7	48	2	3	4	8	14	22	40
A. NOT OPERATED	297	5.4	19	2	3	4	7	11	14	24
B. OPERATED	141	9.4	99	2	3	5	12	23	32	56
TOTAL										
0–19 Years	3	14.3	92	4	4	16	23	23	23	23
20–34	6	5.7	15	1	3	4	8	12	12	12
35–49	42	8.3	110	2	3	4	9	23	29	49
50–64	112	7.0	61	2	3	4	8	13	24	32
65+	275	6.2	33	2	3	4	7	13	18	35
GRAND TOTAL	438	6.7	48	3	3	4	8	14	22	40

516.8: ALVEO PNEUMONOPATHY NEC

Type of Patients	Observed Patients	Avg. Stay	Variance	10th	25th	50th	75th	90th	95th	99th
1. SINGLE DX										
A. Not Operated										
0–19 Years	4	3.3	<1	2	2	4	4	4	4	4
20–34	0									
35–49	0									
50–64	1	11.0	0	11	11	11	11	11	11	11
65+	0									
B. Operated										
0–19 Years	0									
20–34	0									
35–49	0									
50–64	2	1.0	0	1	1	1	1	1	1	1
65+	4	2.8	<1	2	2	3	3	3	3	3
2. MULTIPLE DX										
A. Not Operated										
0–19 Years	38	3.6	22	1	2	3	4	7	30	>99
20–34	18	4.5	33	1	3	3	4	8	26	26
35–49	76	7.8	60	2	3	5	9	17	23	39
50–64	126	7.3	48	2	3	5	9	16	23	32
65+	284	7.0	32	2	3	6	9	14	18	27
B. Operated										
0–19 Years	4	7.0	25	2	6	6	6	14	14	14
20–34	11	5.9	23	2	2	5	9	11	17	17
35–49	53	10.9	67	3	5	9	14	23	26	42
50–64	116	9.9	90	2	3	7	14	23	30	44
65+	156	10.5	86	2	4	8	15	19	27	48
SUBTOTALS:										
1. SINGLE DX — A. Not Operated	5	4.8	13	2	3	4	4	11	11	11
1. SINGLE DX — B. Operated	6	2.2	<1	1	1	2	3	3	3	3
2. MULTIPLE DX — A. Not Operated	542	6.9	40	2	3	5	9	14	18	32
2. MULTIPLE DX — B. Operated	340	10.2	82	2	4	8	14	21	27	44
1. SINGLE DX	11	3.4	7	1	2	3	4	4	11	11
2. MULTIPLE DX	882	8.2	59	2	3	6	11	17	23	42
A. NOT OPERATED	547	6.9	40	2	3	5	8	14	18	32
B. OPERATED	346	10.1	82	2	4	8	14	21	27	44
TOTAL										
0–19 Years	46	3.9	21	1	2	3	4	7	14	>99
20–34	29	5.0	29	1	2	3	6	11	17	26
35–49	129	9.1	65	2	4	7	11	20	26	39
50–64	245	8.5	69	2	3	6	11	18	25	44
65+	444	8.2	54	2	3	6	11	17	20	42
GRAND TOTAL	893	8.1	58	2	3	6	11	17	23	42

517: LUNG INVOLV IN DCE

Type of Patients	Observed Patients	Avg. Stay	Variance	10th	25th	50th	75th	90th	95th	99th
1. SINGLE DX										
A. Not Operated										
0–19 Years	0									
20–34	0									
35–49	0									
50–64	0									
65+	0									
B. Operated										
0–19 Years	0									
20–34	0									
35–49	0									
50–64	0									
65+	0									
2. MULTIPLE DX										
A. Not Operated										
0–19 Years	0									
20–34	0									
35–49	0									
50–64	0									
65+	0									
B. Operated										
0–19 Years	0									
20–34	0									
35–49	0									
50–64	0									
65+	0									
SUBTOTALS:										
1. SINGLE DX — A. Not Operated	0									
1. SINGLE DX — B. Operated	0									
2. MULTIPLE DX — A. Not Operated	0									
2. MULTIPLE DX — B. Operated	0									
1. SINGLE DX	0									
2. MULTIPLE DX	0									
A. NOT OPERATED	0									
B. OPERATED	0									
TOTAL										
0–19 Years	0									
20–34	0									
35–49	0									
50–64	0									
65+	0									
GRAND TOTAL	0									

Length of Stay by Diagnosis and Operation, Western Region, 2008

518: OTHER LUNG DISEASES

Type of Patients	Observed Patients	Avg. Stay	Vari-ance	Percentiles						
				10th	25th	50th	75th	90th	95th	99th
1. SINGLE DX										
A. Not Operated										
0–19 Years	26	1.7	1	1	1	1	2	4	4	5
20–34	10	1.9	3	1	1	1	2	6	6	6
35–49	9	2.3	2	1	1	2	3	5	5	5
50–64	3	1.7	1	1	1	1	3	3	3	3
65+	5	4.0	11	1	2	2	7	8	8	8
B. Operated										
0–19 Years	2	2.0	2	1	1	3	3	3	3	3
20–34	6	3.8	4	1	3	4	5	7	7	7
35–49	4	2.0	<1	1	2	2	3	3	3	3
50–64	14	3.8	8	1	2	3	4	8	11	11
65+	3	2.7	<1	2	2	3	3	3	3	3
2. MULTIPLE DX										
A. Not Operated										
0–19 Years	906	7.3	81	1	2	4	9	17	25	44
20–34	1,507	6.0	43	1	2	4	7	13	18	37
35–49	3,622	7.2	60	2	3	5	9	15	20	39
50–64	9,755	7.9	56	2	3	6	10	16	21	38
65+	21,092	7.5	41	2	4	6	9	15	19	31
B. Operated										
0–19 Years	76	15.5	303	2	3	8	20	36	56	75
20–34	133	12.9	181	2	3	8	17	34	43	58
35–49	334	12.4	184	2	3	8	17	30	40	79
50–64	785	12.6	176	2	4	8	17	29	42	80
65+	1,190	13.0	143	2	5	10	17	27	37	72
SUBTOTALS:										
1. SINGLE DX										
A. Not Operated	53	2.1	3	1	1	1	2	4	6	8
B. Operated	29	3.3	5	1	2	3	4	7	8	11
2. MULTIPLE DX										
A. Not Operated	36,882	7.5	48	2	3	6	9	15	20	34
B. Operated	2,518	12.9	166	2	4	9	17	29	39	74
1. SINGLE DX	82	2.5	4	1	1	2	3	5	7	11
2. MULTIPLE DX	39,400	7.8	57	2	3	6	10	16	21	39
A. NOT OPERATED	36,935	7.5	48	2	3	6	9	15	20	34
B. OPERATED	2,547	12.8	165	2	4	9	17	28	39	74
TOTAL										
0–19 Years	1,010	7.7	101	1	2	4	10	18	28	49
20–34	1,656	6.5	57	1	2	4	8	14	21	39
35–49	3,969	7.6	72	2	3	5	9	16	23	46
50–64	10,557	8.2	66	2	3	6	10	17	23	43
65+	22,290	7.8	48	2	4	6	9	15	20	34
GRAND TOTAL	39,482	7.8	57	2	3	6	10	16	21	39

518.0: PULMONARY COLLAPSE

Type of Patients	Observed Patients	Avg. Stay	Vari-ance	Percentiles						
				10th	25th	50th	75th	90th	95th	99th
1. SINGLE DX										
A. Not Operated										
0–19 Years	1	2.0	0	2	2	2	2	2	2	2
20–34	0									
35–49	0									
50–64	0									
65+	0									
B. Operated										
0–19 Years	0									
20–34	0									
35–49	0									
50–64	0									
65+	0									
2. MULTIPLE DX										
A. Not Operated										
0–19 Years	40	4.9	48	1	2	4	5	8	23	41
20–34	16	3.7	8	1	1	2	6	7	10	10
35–49	51	3.8	13	1	2	3	4	7	11	19
50–64	86	4.6	43	1	2	3	5	9	15	52
65+	222	4.3	15	1	2	3	5	8	11	22
B. Operated										
0–19 Years	0									
20–34	2	16.9	285	5	5	5	29	29	29	29
35–49	4	5.5	27	1	1	3	5	13	13	13
50–64	12	3.7	4	1	2	3	4	6	7	7
65+	19	6.9	31	1	2	6	11	18	20	20
SUBTOTALS:										
1. SINGLE DX										
A. Not Operated	1	2.0	0	2	2	2	2	2	2	2
B. Operated	0									
2. MULTIPLE DX										
A. Not Operated	415	4.3	23	1	2	3	5	8	12	22
B. Operated	37	6.2	36	1	3	5	7	13	20	29
1. SINGLE DX	1	2.0	0	2	2	2	2	2	2	2
2. MULTIPLE DX	452	4.5	24	1	2	3	5	8	12	23
A. NOT OPERATED	416	4.3	23	1	2	3	5	8	12	22
B. OPERATED	37	6.2	36	1	3	5	7	13	20	29
TOTAL										
0–19 Years	41	4.8	47	1	2	4	5	8	9	41
20–34	18	5.1	42	1	1	3	6	10	29	29
35–49	55	3.9	13	1	2	3	4	9	13	19
50–64	98	4.5	38	1	2	3	5	8	15	52
65+	241	4.5	17	1	2	3	5	8	12	22
GRAND TOTAL	453	4.5	24	1	2	3	5	8	12	23

518.1: INTERSTITIAL EMPHYSEMA

Type of Patients	Observed Patients	Avg. Stay	Vari-ance	Percentiles						
				10th	25th	50th	75th	90th	95th	99th
1. SINGLE DX										
A. Not Operated										
0–19 Years	14	1.7	1	1	1	1	2	3	5	5
20–34	6	1.2	<1	1	1	1	1	2	2	2
35–49	0									
50–64	0									
65+	0									
B. Operated										
0–19 Years	0									
20–34	0									
35–49	0									
50–64	0									
65+	0									
2. MULTIPLE DX										
A. Not Operated										
0–19 Years	71	2.2	3	1	1	2	3	5	6	9
20–34	109	2.7	5	1	1	2	3	5	7	11
35–49	14	4.3	6	2	2	3	6	8	10	10
50–64	12	3.0	5	1	2	2	3	5	9	9
65+	22	5.1	17	1	3	4	6	11	12	18
B. Operated										
0–19 Years	2	5.0	8	3	3	3	7	7	7	7
20–34	1	2.0	0	2	2	2	2	2	2	2
35–49	1	22.0	0	22	22	22	22	22	22	22
50–64	3	14.5	438	2	2	3	39	39	39	39
65+	1	20.0	0	20	20	20	20	20	20	20
SUBTOTALS:										
1. SINGLE DX										
A. Not Operated	20	1.6	1	1	1	1	2	3	5	5
B. Operated	0									
2. MULTIPLE DX										
A. Not Operated	228	2.9	6	1	1	2	3	6	8	12
B. Operated	8	12.2	181	2	3	3	20	39	39	39
1. SINGLE DX	20	1.6	1	1	1	1	2	3	5	5
2. MULTIPLE DX	236	3.2	14	1	1	2	3	6	9	20
A. NOT OPERATED	248	2.8	6	1	1	2	3	6	8	12
B. OPERATED	8	12.2	181	2	3	3	20	39	39	39
TOTAL										
0–19 Years	87	2.2	3	1	1	2	3	5	6	9
20–34	116	2.6	5	1	1	2	3	5	7	11
35–49	15	5.5	27	2	2	4	6	10	22	22
50–64	15	5.3	90	1	2	2	5	12	39	39
65+	23	5.7	26	1	3	4	7	12	18	20
GRAND TOTAL	256	3.1	13	1	1	2	3	6	9	20

Length of Stay by Diagnosis and Operation, Western Region, 2008

Western Region, October 2006–September 2007 Data, by Diagnosis

518.3: PULMONARY EOSINOPHILIA

Type of Patients	Observed Patients	Avg. Stay	Variance	10th	25th	50th	75th	90th	95th	99th
1. SINGLE DX										
A. Not Operated										
0–19 Years	0									
20–34	2	4.5	4	3	3	5	6	6	6	6
35–49	1	1.0	0	1	1	1	1	1	1	1
50–64	1	1.0	0	1	1	1	1	1	1	1
65+	1	2.0	0	2	2	2	2	2	2	2
B. Operated										
0–19 Years	0									
20–34	1	3.0	0	3	3	3	3	3	3	3
35–49	0									
50–64	2	2.5	<1	2	2	3	3	3	3	3
65+	1	3.0	0	3	3	3	3	3	3	3
2. MULTIPLE DX										
A. Not Operated										
0–19 Years	7	3.4	6	1	2	3	5	8	8	8
20–34	20	4.5	11	2	2	3	7	11	12	12
35–49	56	5.0	17	2	3	4	6	10	11	27
50–64	76	5.7	16	2	3	5	8	11	14	19
65+	208	5.7	24	2	3	4	7	11	16	22
B. Operated										
0–19 Years	3	8.0	0	8	8	8	8	8	8	8
20–34	11	4.5	4	2	3	4	6	7	8	8
35–49	30	7.4	19	3	4	7	10	14	15	17
50–64	32	6.5	15	3	4	6	8	12	16	16
65+	66	6.4	23	3	3	5	9	13	16	20
SUBTOTALS:										
1. SINGLE DX										
A. Not Operated	5	2.6	4	1	1	2	3	6	6	6
B. Operated	4	2.8	<1	2	3	3	3	3	3	3
2. MULTIPLE DX										
A. Not Operated	367	5.5	20	2	3	4	7	11	14	22
B. Operated	142	6.5	19	2	3	6	8	13	15	20
1. SINGLE DX	9	2.7	2	1	2	3	3	6	6	6
2. MULTIPLE DX	509	5.8	20	2	3	5	7	11	15	20
A. NOT OPERATED	372	5.5	20	2	3	4	7	11	14	22
B. OPERATED	146	6.4	19	2	3	5	8	13	15	20
TOTAL										
0–19 Years	10	4.8	9	1	2	3	8	8	8	8
20–34	34	4.4	8	2	2	3	6	8	11	12
35–49	87	5.8	18	2	3	5	8	11	14	27
50–64	111	5.8	15	2	3	5	8	11	15	17
65+	276	5.9	24	2	3	4	7	12	16	22
GRAND TOTAL	518	5.7	20	2	3	5	7	11	15	20

518.4: ACUTE LUNG EDEMA NOS

Type of Patients	Observed Patients	Avg. Stay	Variance	10th	25th	50th	75th	90th	95th	99th
1. SINGLE DX										
A. Not Operated										
0–19 Years	0									
20–34	0									
35–49	2	1.5	<1	1		2	2	2	2	2
50–64	0									
65+	0									
B. Operated										
0–19 Years	0									
20–34	0									
35–49	0									
50–64	0									
65+	0									
2. MULTIPLE DX										
A. Not Operated										
0–19 Years	11	3.2	5	1	1	2	5	6	8	8
20–34	42	2.8	8	1	1	2	3	6	8	14
35–49	75	2.7	4	1	1	2	3	5	8	10
50–64	147	3.6	14	1	2	3	4	7	9	23
65+	259	3.5	8	1	1	3	4	7	9	15
B. Operated										
0–19 Years	6	2.2	1	1	1	2	3	4	4	4
20–34	7	6.3	161	1	1	1	3	35	35	35
35–49	11	5.9	72	2	2	3	5	7	31	31
50–64	15	4.3	9	1	3	3	6	7	13	13
65+	16	4.9	24	1	2	4	4	16	17	17
SUBTOTALS:										
1. SINGLE DX										
A. Not Operated	2	1.5	<1	1		2	2	2	2	2
B. Operated	0									
2. MULTIPLE DX										
A. Not Operated	534	3.3	9	1	1	2	4	7	9	15
B. Operated	55	4.8	42	1	2	3	5	8	17	35
1. SINGLE DX	2	1.5	<1	1		2	2	2	2	2
2. MULTIPLE DX	589	3.5	12	1	1	3	4	7	9	19
A. NOT OPERATED	536	3.3	9	1	1	2	4	7	9	15
B. OPERATED	55	4.8	42	1	2	3	5	8	17	35
TOTAL										
0–19 Years	17	2.8	4	1	1	2	4	6	8	8
20–34	49	3.3	28	1	1	2	3	6	10	35
35–49	88	3.1	13	1	1	2	4	5	8	31
50–64	162	3.7	13	1	2	3	4	7	9	23
65+	275	3.6	9	1	2	3	4	7	10	16
GRAND TOTAL	591	3.5	12	1	1	3	4	7	9	19

518.5: POSTTR PULMON INSUFF

Type of Patients	Observed Patients	Avg. Stay	Variance	10th	25th	50th	75th	90th	95th	99th
1. SINGLE DX										
A. Not Operated										
0–19 Years	2	1.0	0	1	1	1	1	1	1	1
20–34	0									
35–49	0									
50–64	0									
65+	0									
B. Operated										
0–19 Years	0									
20–34	0									
35–49	0									
50–64	0									
65+	0									
2. MULTIPLE DX										
A. Not Operated										
0–19 Years	33	4.8	58	1	1	2	4	15	20	37
20–34	37	4.7	18	1	1	3	6	11	14	19
35–49	58	6.1	56	1	2	3	8	14	16	49
50–64	72	7.6	50	1	2	5	10	21	24	26
65+	120	9.7	139	1	2	6	14	21	33	59
B. Operated										
0–19 Years	17	10.8	173	1	2	5	17	31	49	49
20–34	17	15.8	379	2	3	6	22	56	63	63
35–49	23	11.8	275	1	2	7	13	27	35	75
50–64	56	9.5	329	1	1	4	7	23	69	96
65+	81	6.9	64	1	2	4	9	15	21	48
SUBTOTALS:										
1. SINGLE DX										
A. Not Operated	2	1.0	0	1	1	1	1	1	1	1
B. Operated	0									
2. MULTIPLE DX										
A. Not Operated	320	7.5	85	1	2	4	10	18	24	37
B. Operated	194	9.3	205	1	2	4	10	22	38	75
1. SINGLE DX	2	1.0	0	1	1	1	1	1	1	1
2. MULTIPLE DX	514	8.2	131	1	2	4	10	20	27	63
A. NOT OPERATED	322	7.4	84	1	2	4	10	18	23	37
B. OPERATED	194	9.3	205	1	2	4	10	22	38	75
TOTAL										
0–19 Years	52	6.6	100	1	2	2	7	19	31	49
20–34	54	8.2	154	1	2	3	9	19	38	63
35–49	81	7.7	122	1	2	3	9	15	26	75
50–64	128	8.4	172	1	2	4	9	21	25	71
65+	201	8.5	110	1	2	5	12	21	28	48
GRAND TOTAL	516	8.1	130	1	2	4	10	20	27	63

Length of Stay by Diagnosis and Operation, Western Region, 2008

Western Region, October 2006–September 2007 Data, by Diagnosis

518.81: AC RESPIRATORY FAILURE

Type of Patients	Observed Patients	Avg. Stay	Variance	Percentiles						
				10th	25th	50th	75th	90th	95th	99th
1. SINGLE DX										
A. Not Operated										
0–19 Years	0									
20–34	0									
35–49	1	5.0	0	5	5	5	5	5	5	5
50–64	1	3.0	0	3	3	3	3	3	3	3
65+	2	4.5	13	2	2	5	7	7	7	7
B. Operated										
0–19 Years	0									
20–34	0									
35–49	0									
50–64	0									
65+	0									
2. MULTIPLE DX										
A. Not Operated										
0–19 Years	493	9.4	96	2	3	7	12	20	28	49
20–34	1,082	6.5	49	1	2	4	8	14	21	38
35–49	2,780	7.4	61	2	3	5	9	15	20	41
50–64	7,160	8.1	57	2	4	6	10	16	21	39
65+	15,764	7.7	40	2	4	6	10	15	19	30
B. Operated										
0–19 Years	28	25.2	328	5	13	21	31	54	71	75
20–34	48	17.0	153	4	10	13	22	37	39	58
35–49	144	18.4	233	4	8	15	25	37	57	>99
50–64	366	16.3	152	5	8	13	21	34	44	68
65+	665	16.5	154	5	8	13	21	31	42	74
SUBTOTALS:										
1. SINGLE DX										
A. Not Operated	4	4.3	5	2	3	4	5	7	7	7
B. Operated	0									
2. MULTIPLE DX										
A. Not Operated	27,279	7.7	48	2	4	6	10	15	20	34
B. Operated	1,251	16.9	167	5	8	13	22	34	45	75
1. SINGLE DX	4	4.3	5	2	3	4	5	7	7	7
2. MULTIPLE DX	28,530	8.1	57	2	4	6	10	16	22	38
A. NOT OPERATED	27,283	7.7	48	2	4	6	10	15	20	34
B. OPERATED	1,251	16.9	167	5	8	13	22	34	45	75
TOTAL										
0–19 Years	521	10.3	121	2	3	7	13	23	31	57
20–34	1,130	6.9	58	1	3	5	8	15	22	39
35–49	2,925	8.0	75	2	3	5	9	17	23	48
50–64	7,527	8.5	65	2	4	6	10	17	23	43
65+	16,431	8.0	47	2	4	6	10	16	20	33
GRAND TOTAL	28,534	8.1	57	2	4	6	10	16	22	38

518.82: OTHER PULMONARY INSUFF

Type of Patients	Observed Patients	Avg. Stay	Variance	Percentiles						
				10th	25th	50th	75th	90th	95th	99th
1. SINGLE DX										
A. Not Operated										
0–19 Years	6	2.2	2	1	1	2	4	4	4	4
20–34	0									
35–49	0									
50–64	0									
65+	0									
B. Operated										
0–19 Years	0									
20–34	0									
35–49	0									
50–64	0									
65+	0									
2. MULTIPLE DX										
A. Not Operated										
0–19 Years	143	3.9	43	1	1	2	4	7	11	32
20–34	23	4.4	15	1	1	4	5	12	13	13
35–49	52	6.2	39	1	2	4	9	15	18	31
50–64	97	8.2	84	1	3	6	10	17	23	59
65+	165	5.9	23	2	3	5	8	12	16	22
B. Operated										
0–19 Years	4	6.5	14	4	4	5	6	12	12	12
20–34	1	45.0	0	45	45	45	45	45	45	45
35–49	2	8.0	2	7	7	7	9	9	9	9
50–64	10	8.4	58	1	1	7	13	18	23	23
65+	12	10.5	146	3	3	7	11	19	46	46
SUBTOTALS:										
1. SINGLE DX										
A. Not Operated	6	2.2	2	1	1	2	4	4	4	4
B. Operated	0									
2. MULTIPLE DX										
A. Not Operated	480	5.7	45	1	2	4	7	13	17	32
B. Operated	29	10.2	124	1	4	7	11	23	45	46
1. SINGLE DX	6	2.2	2	1	1	2	4	4	4	4
2. MULTIPLE DX	509	6.0	50	1	2	4	7	13	17	32
A. NOT OPERATED	486	5.7	44	1	2	4	7	13	17	32
B. OPERATED	29	10.2	124	1	4	7	11	23	45	46
TOTAL										
0–19 Years	153	3.9	41	1	1	2	4	7	12	32
20–34	24	6.1	83	1	1	4	7	13	13	45
35–49	54	6.3	38	1	2	4	9	15	18	31
50–64	107	8.2	81	1	3	6	10	18	23	54
65+	177	6.2	32	2	3	5	8	12	16	31
GRAND TOTAL	515	5.9	50	1	2	4	7	13	17	32

518.83: CHR RESPIRATORY FAILURE

Type of Patients	Observed Patients	Avg. Stay	Variance	Percentiles						
				10th	25th	50th	75th	90th	95th	99th
1. SINGLE DX										
A. Not Operated										
0–19 Years	0									
20–34	0									
35–49	0									
50–64	0									
65+	0									
B. Operated										
0–19 Years	0									
20–34	0									
35–49	0									
50–64	0									
65+	0									
2. MULTIPLE DX										
A. Not Operated										
0–19 Years	20	8.5	188	1	1	2	9	22	42	49
20–34	17	5.3	31	1	3	4	6	9	25	25
35–49	28	10.0	345	1	3	5	9	22	33	98
50–64	118	9.0	163	2	3	5	10	22	27	91
65+	209	7.8	105	2	3	5	9	19	31	>99
B. Operated										
0–19 Years	2	33.9	945	12	12	12	56	56	56	56
20–34	0									
35–49	4	10.3	82	2	2	16	20	20	20	20
50–64	10	11.4	95	1	2	9	18	31	31	31
65+	6	15.4	94	2	10	15	25	28	28	28
SUBTOTALS:										
1. SINGLE DX										
A. Not Operated	0									
B. Operated	0									
2. MULTIPLE DX										
A. Not Operated	392	8.3	140	2	3	5	9	20	31	>99
B. Operated	22	14.3	165	2	3	13	19	28	31	56
1. SINGLE DX	0									
2. MULTIPLE DX	414	8.6	143	2	3	5	9	21	31	>99
A. NOT OPERATED	392	8.3	140	2	3	5	9	20	31	>99
B. OPERATED	22	14.3	165	2	3	13	19	28	31	56
TOTAL										
0–19 Years	22	10.8	272	1	1	4	11	42	49	56
20–34	17	5.3	31	1	3	4	6	9	25	25
35–49	32	10.0	308	2	3	5	10	22	33	98
50–64	128	9.2	158	2	3	5	11	22	27	91
65+	215	8.0	106	2	3	5	9	20	31	>99
GRAND TOTAL	414	8.6	143	2	3	5	9	21	31	>99

Length of Stay by Diagnosis and Operation, Western Region, 2008

Western Region, October 2006–September 2007 Data, by Diagnosis

518.84: AC & CHR RESP FAILURE

Type of Patients	Observed Patients	Avg. Stay	Vari-ance	10th	25th	50th	75th	90th	95th	99th
1. SINGLE DX										
A. *Not Operated*										
0–19 Years	0									
20–34	0									
35–49	0									
50–64	0									
65+	1	8.0	0	8	8	8	8	8	8	8
B. *Operated*										
0–19 Years	0									
20–34	0									
35–49	0									
50–64	0									
65+	0									
2. MULTIPLE DX										
A. *Not Operated*										
0–19 Years	33	12.0	113	2	3	9	15	28	35	41
20–34	105	8.1	49	2	4	6	11	17	22	37
35–49	381	8.2	63	2	3	6	10	19	25	39
50–64	1,763	8.1	51	3	4	6	10	15	20	38
65+	3,751	7.7	44	2	4	6	9	14	19	35
B. *Operated*										
0–19 Years	1	72.0	0	72	72	72	72	72	72	72
20–34	10	19.3	214	7	12	14	22	57	72	72
35–49	19	23.2	183	8	11	20	34	46	48	57
50–64	84	22.6	332	5	11	18	29	48	65	>99
65+	106	19.6	199	7	11	16	23	41	43	92
SUBTOTALS:										
1. SINGLE DX										
A. *Not Operated*	1	8.0	0	8	8	8	8	8	8	8
B. *Operated*	0									
2. MULTIPLE DX										
A. *Not Operated*	6,033	7.9	48	2	4	6	10	15	20	37
B. *Operated*	220	21.2	259	7	11	17	27	43	56	93
1. SINGLE DX	1	8.0	0	8	8	8	8	8	8	8
2. MULTIPLE DX	6,253	8.4	61	2	4	6	10	16	22	42
A. NOT OPERATED	6,034	7.9	48	2	4	6	10	15	20	37
B. OPERATED	220	21.2	259	7	11	17	27	43	56	93
TOTAL										
0–19 Years	34	13.7	215	2	3	10	18	30	41	72
20–34	115	9.1	72	2	4	6	12	20	23	39
35–49	400	9.0	79	2	3	6	11	21	29	45
50–64	1,847	8.8	72	3	4	6	11	17	23	46
65+	3,858	8.0	52	2	4	6	10	15	21	40
GRAND TOTAL	6,254	8.4	61	2	4	6	10	16	22	42

518.89: OTHER LUNG DISEASE NEC

Type of Patients	Observed Patients	Avg. Stay	Vari-ance	10th	25th	50th	75th	90th	95th	99th
1. SINGLE DX										
A. *Not Operated*										
0–19 Years	2	1.0	0	1	1	1	1	1	1	1
20–34	2	1.5	<1	1	1	2	2	2	2	2
35–49	4	2.5	2	1	2	3	4	4	4	4
50–64	1	1.0	0	1	1	1	1	1	1	1
65+	1	1.0	0	1	1	1	1	1	1	1
B. *Operated*										
0–19 Years	2	2.0	2	1	1	1	3	3	3	3
20–34	5	4.0	5	1	3	4	5	7	7	7
35–49	4	2.0	<1	1	1	2	3	3	3	3
50–64	11	3.4	5	1	2	3	4	6	8	8
65+	2	2.5	<1	2	2	3	3	3	3	3
2. MULTIPLE DX										
A. *Not Operated*										
0–19 Years	51	4.6	25	1	1	3	6	10	19	23
20–34	52	3.2	5	1	2	3	5	5	8	11
35–49	110	4.3	16	1	2	3	5	9	10	17
50–64	209	4.0	13	1	2	3	5	8	11	21
65+	336	4.2	13	1	2	3	5	9	10	18
B. *Operated*										
0–19 Years	13	5.8	14	2	2	5	9	11	12	12
20–34	34	6.6	45	2	3	5	8	13	17	37
35–49	95	4.0	12	1	2	3	6	7	10	23
50–64	195	4.7	23	1	2	3	6	9	13	45
65+	214	4.8	14	1	2	4	6	9	14	18
SUBTOTALS:										
1. SINGLE DX										
A. *Not Operated*	10	1.7	1	1	1	1	2	4	4	4
B. *Operated*	24	3.1	4	1	2	3	4	6	7	8
2. MULTIPLE DX										
A. *Not Operated*	758	4.1	14	1	2	3	5	8	11	20
B. *Operated*	551	4.7	19	1	2	4	6	9	13	24
1. SINGLE DX	34	2.7	3	1	1	2	4	5	7	8
2. MULTIPLE DX	1,309	4.4	16	1	2	3	5	9	11	21
A. NOT OPERATED	768	4.1	14	1	2	3	5	8	10	20
B. OPERATED	575	4.7	18	1	2	4	6	9	13	24
TOTAL										
0–19 Years	68	4.6	22	1	2	3	6	11	12	23
20–34	93	4.5	22	1	2	3	5	9	11	37
35–49	213	4.1	14	1	2	3	5	8	10	17
50–64	416	4.3	18	1	2	3	5	8	11	24
65+	553	4.4	13	1	2	3	5	9	11	18
GRAND TOTAL	1,343	4.3	16	1	2	3	5	9	11	21

519: OTH RESP SYSTEM DISEASES

Type of Patients	Observed Patients	Avg. Stay	Vari-ance	10th	25th	50th	75th	90th	95th	99th
1. SINGLE DX										
A. *Not Operated*										
0–19 Years	32	1.6	<1	1	1	1	2	3	3	3
20–34	2	2.0	0	2	2	2	2	2	2	2
35–49	3	1.3	<1	1	1	1	2	2	2	2
50–64	0									
65+	0									
B. *Operated*										
0–19 Years	2	3.0	8	1	1	1	5	5	5	5
20–34	5	1.8	2	1	1	1	2	4	4	4
35–49	5	2.2	5	1	1	1	2	6	6	6
50–64	7	1.9	2	1	1	2	3	5	5	5
65+	2	1.5	<1	1	1	2	2	2	2	2
2. MULTIPLE DX										
A. *Not Operated*										
0–19 Years	255	3.0	16	1	1	2	3	6	8	15
20–34	76	4.0	11	1	2	3	6	8	11	18
35–49	164	4.3	37	1	2	5	5	9	16	38
50–64	284	4.4	25	1	3	3	6	10	14	35
65+	471	4.6	17	1	3	3	6	10	14	20
B. *Operated*										
0–19 Years	56	6.0	78	2	4	7	9	19	26	45
20–34	66	7.1	112	2	4	9	11	15	20	77
35–49	88	7.9	151	1	4	8	13	19	36	62
50–64	153	6.0	46	2	4	7	9	13	19	30
65+	148	7.2	65	2	5	7	10	15	21	51
SUBTOTALS:										
1. SINGLE DX										
A. *Not Operated*	37	1.6	<1	1	1	1	2	3	3	3
B. *Operated*	21	2.0	3	1	1	2	2	5	5	6
2. MULTIPLE DX										
A. *Not Operated*	1,250	4.2	21	1	1	3	5	9	13	21
B. *Operated*	511	6.8	82	1	2	4	8	15	23	55
1. SINGLE DX	58	1.7	1	1	1	1	2	3	5	6
2. MULTIPLE DX	1,761	4.9	40	1	1	3	6	11	15	32
A. NOT OPERATED	1,287	4.1	21	1	1	3	5	9	13	21
B. OPERATED	532	6.6	79	1	2	4	8	14	22	55
TOTAL										
0–19 Years	345	3.4	26	1	1	2	3	7	11	26
20–34	149	5.3	58	1	2	3	7	11	15	26
35–49	260	5.5	78	1	1	3	6	12	18	58
50–64	444	4.9	33	1	2	3	6	11	15	30
65+	621	5.2	30	1	2	3	6	12	15	26
GRAND TOTAL	1,819	4.8	39	1	1	3	6	11	15	32

Length of Stay by Diagnosis and Operation, Western Region, 2008

519.02: TRACHEOSTOMY MECH COMP

Type of Patients	Observed Patients	Avg. Stay	Variance	Percentiles 10th	25th	50th	75th	90th	95th	99th
1. SINGLE DX										
A. Not Operated										
0–19 Years	0									
20–34	0									
35–49	1	1.0	0		1	1	1	1	1	1
50–64	0									
65+	0									
B. Operated										
0–19 Years	1	5.0	0	5	5	5	5	5	5	5
20–34	0									
35–49	2	4.0	8	2	2	4	6	6	6	6
50–64	1	5.0	0	5	5	5	5	5	5	5
65+	1	1.0	0	1	1	1	1	1	1	1
2. MULTIPLE DX										
A. Not Operated										
0–19 Years	6	6.1	92	1	1	1	8	25	25	25
20–34	9	3.1	12	1	1	2	3	12	12	12
35–49	22	6.7	96	1	1	2	7	21	25	38
50–64	35	5.9	33	1	2	4	8	16	25	>99
65+	42	5.8	29	1	1	3	8	14	15	21
B. Operated										
0–19 Years	13	5.3	28	1	1	3	7	11	19	19
20–34	19	6.9	32	1	2	7	9	20	20	20
35–49	26	10.3	190	1	1	5	12	26	42	58
50–64	40	4.9	23	1	2	3	7	9	9	23
65+	42	5.9	25	1	2	4	10	12	13	24
SUBTOTALS:										
1. SINGLE DX										
A. Not Operated	1	1.0	0	1	1	1	1	1	1	1
B. Operated	5	3.8	5	1	2	5	5	6	6	6
2. MULTIPLE DX										
A. Not Operated	114	5.8	44	1	1	3	8	15	21	38
B. Operated	140	6.5	59	1	2	4	9	13	22	42
1. SINGLE DX	6	3.3	5	1	1	2	5	6	6	6
2. MULTIPLE DX	254	6.2	52	1	1	3	8	15	21	42
A. NOT OPERATED	115	5.8	44	1	1	3	8	15	21	38
B. OPERATED	145	6.4	57	2	2	4	9	12	20	42
TOTAL										
0–19 Years	20	5.5	42	1	1	3	7	11	19	25
20–34	28	5.7	28	1	1	3	7	12	20	20
35–49	51	8.3	141	1	1	3	11	23	38	58
50–64	76	5.4	27	1	2	4	7	14	22	>99
65+	85	5.8	27	1	2	3	10	13	15	24
GRAND TOTAL	260	6.1	51	1	1	3	8	14	21	42

519.09: TRACHEOSTOMY COMP NEC

Type of Patients	Observed Patients	Avg. Stay	Variance	Percentiles 10th	25th	50th	75th	90th	95th	99th
1. SINGLE DX										
A. Not Operated										
0–19 Years	0									
20–34	0									
35–49	0									
50–64	0									
65+	0									
B. Operated										
0–19 Years	1	1.0	0	1	1	1	1	1	1	1
20–34	0									
35–49	0									
50–64	1	1.0	0	1	1	1	1	1	1	1
65+	0									
2. MULTIPLE DX										
A. Not Operated										
0–19 Years	24	6.0	88	1	1	3	4	13	14	46
20–34	11	4.2	14	1	1	2	7	10	11	11
35–49	37	5.2	66	1	1	3	5	13	20	46
50–64	82	5.3	47	1	2	3	6	12	15	45
65+	99	5.6	33	1	2	4	7	13	18	32
B. Operated										
0–19 Years	23	3.2	28	1	1	3	2	8	19	19
20–34	8	4.9	21	1	1	4	6	14	14	14
35–49	8	5.0	20	1	2	3	11	13	13	13
50–64	34	6.5	115	1	2	3	6	13	24	59
65+	39	8.2	113	1	2	5	10	23	32	55
SUBTOTALS:										
1. SINGLE DX										
A. Not Operated	0									
B. Operated	2	1.0	0	1	1	1	1	1	1	1
2. MULTIPLE DX										
A. Not Operated	253	5.4	46	1	1	3	6	13	17	45
B. Operated	112	6.2	84	1	1	3	7	14	23	55
1. SINGLE DX	2	1.0	0	1	1	1	1	1	1	1
2. MULTIPLE DX	365	5.6	58	1	1	3	6	13	18	46
A. NOT OPERATED	253	5.4	46	1	1	3	6	13	17	45
B. OPERATED	114	6.1	83	1	1	3	7	14	23	55
TOTAL										
0–19 Years	48	4.6	59	1	1	3	4	13	19	46
20–34	19	4.5	16	1	1	3	7	11	14	14
35–49	45	5.2	57	1	1	3	5	13	15	46
50–64	117	5.6	66	1	2	3	6	13	18	45
65+	138	6.3	56	1	2	4	8	15	22	32
GRAND TOTAL	367	5.6	58	1	1	3	6	13	18	46

519.11: ACUTE BRONCHOSPASM

Type of Patients	Observed Patients	Avg. Stay	Variance	Percentiles 10th	25th	50th	75th	90th	95th	99th
1. SINGLE DX										
A. Not Operated										
0–19 Years	11	1.4	<1	1	1	1	2	2	3	3
20–34	0									
35–49	0									
50–64	0									
65+	0									
B. Operated										
0–19 Years	0									
20–34	0									
35–49	1	1.0	0	1	1	1	1	1	1	1
50–64	1	1.0	0	1	1	1	1	1	1	1
65+	0									
2. MULTIPLE DX										
A. Not Operated										
0–19 Years	30	1.8	1	1	1	1	2	4	4	4
20–34	14	2.9	5	1	1	2	3	7	7	7
35–49	24	1.9	1	1	1	2	3	3	5	5
50–64	46	2.2	3	1	1	2	2	4	6	8
65+	93	3.3	7	1	2	3	4	6	7	16
B. Operated										
0–19 Years	0									
20–34	3	2.3	5	1	1	1	5	5	5	5
35–49	1	1.0	0	1	1	1	1	1	1	1
50–64	1	4.0	0	4	4	4	4	4	4	4
65+	0									
SUBTOTALS:										
1. SINGLE DX										
A. Not Operated	11	1.4	<1	1	1	1	2	2	3	3
B. Operated	2	1.0	0	1	1	1	1	1	1	1
2. MULTIPLE DX										
A. Not Operated	207	2.6	5	1	1	2	3	5	7	11
B. Operated	5	2.4	4	1	1	1	4	5	5	5
1. SINGLE DX	13	1.3	<1	1	1	1	1	2	3	3
2. MULTIPLE DX	212	2.6	5	1	1	2	3	5	7	11
A. NOT OPERATED	218	2.6	4	1	1	2	3	5	7	11
B. OPERATED	7	2.0	3	1	1	1	4	5	5	5
TOTAL										
0–19 Years	41	1.7	<1	1	1	1	2	3	4	4
20–34	17	2.8	5	1	1	2	3	7	7	7
35–49	26	1.9	1	1	1	2	3	3	5	5
50–64	48	2.2	3	1	1	2	3	4	6	8
65+	93	3.3	7	1	2	3	4	6	7	16
GRAND TOTAL	225	2.6	4	1	1	2	3	5	6	11

Length of Stay by Diagnosis and Operation, Western Region, 2008

Western Region, October 2006–September 2007 Data, by Diagnosis

519.19: TRACHEA/BRONCHUS DIS NEC

Type of Patients	Observed Patients	Avg. Stay	Vari- ance	10th	25th	50th	75th	90th	95th	99th
1. SINGLE DX										
A. Not Operated										
0–19 Years	4	1.8	<1	1	1	2	3	3	3	3
20–34	2	2.0	0	2	2	2	2	2	2	2
35–49	0									
50–64	0									
65+	0									
B. Operated										
0–19 Years	0									
20–34	5	1.8	2	1	1	1	2	4	4	4
35–49	2	1.0	0	1	1	1	1	1	1	1
50–64	4	1.5	1	1	1	1	3	3	3	3
65+	1	2.0	0	2	2	2	2	2	2	2
2. MULTIPLE DX										
A. Not Operated										
0–19 Years	31	2.5	4	1	1	2	3	6	7	7
20–34	14	4.9	21	2	2	3	6	10	18	18
35–49	23	4.9	29	1	1	2	8	15	16	18
50–64	37	3.9	15	1	1	2	4	10	13	16
65+	51	4.7	16	2	2	4	6	10	15	20
B. Operated										
0–19 Years	13	7.3	62	1	1	5	8	20	26	26
20–34	26	6.3	42	1	1	3	10	15	17	26
35–49	31	6.9	126	1	1	4	8	11	28	60
50–64	40	4.9	12	1	3	4	7	9	13	13
65+	36	7.1	96	1	2	4	8	17	28	51
SUBTOTALS:										
1. SINGLE DX										
A. Not Operated	6	1.8	<1	1	1	2	2	3	3	3
B. Operated	12	1.6	1	1	1	1	2	3	4	4
2. MULTIPLE DX										
A. Not Operated	156	4.1	16	1	1	3	5	10	15	18
B. Operated	146	6.3	66	1	2	4	8	13	20	51
1. SINGLE DX	18	1.7	<1	1	1	1	2	3	4	4
2. MULTIPLE DX	302	5.2	41	1	1	3	7	12	15	28
A. NOT OPERATED	162	4.0	16	1	1	3	5	9	13	18
B. OPERATED	158	6.0	62	2	2	3	7	13	20	51
TOTAL										
0–19 Years	48	3.7	23	1	1	2	5	7	13	26
20–34	47	5.2	31	1	2	3	8	15	17	26
35–49	56	5.9	82	1	1	3	8	12	18	60
50–64	81	4.3	13	1	1	3	7	9	12	16
65+	88	5.6	49	1	2	4	6	12	17	51
GRAND TOTAL	320	5.0	39	1	1	3	6	11	15	28

519.8: RESP SYSTEM DISEASE NEC

Type of Patients	Observed Patients	Avg. Stay	Vari- ance	10th	25th	50th	75th	90th	95th	99th
1. SINGLE DX										
A. Not Operated										
0–19 Years	7	2.0	<1	1	1	2	3	3	3	3
20–34	0									
35–49	2	1.5	<1	1	1	1	2	2	2	2
50–64	0									
65+	0									
B. Operated										
0–19 Years	0									
20–34	0									
35–49	0									
50–64	0									
65+	0									
2. MULTIPLE DX										
A. Not Operated										
0–19 Years	116	2.7	7	1	1	2	3	6	8	15
20–34	11	3.4	6	1	1	3	5	6	9	9
35–49	36	3.2	5	1	2	3	5	6	8	8
50–64	46	3.8	9	1	2	3	5	9	10	14
65+	132	4.1	9	2	2	3	5	7	10	16
B. Operated										
0–19 Years	3	5.0	21	1	1	4	4	10	10	10
20–34	1	25.0	0	25	25	25	25	25	25	25
35–49	3	21.1	>999	1	1	1	62	62	62	62
50–64	10	8.0	42	2	3	6	13	21	21	21
65+	1	13.0	0	13	13	13	13	13	13	13
SUBTOTALS:										
1. SINGLE DX										
A. Not Operated	9	1.9	<1	1	1	2	2	3	3	3
B. Operated	0									
2. MULTIPLE DX										
A. Not Operated	341	3.5	8	1	2	3	4	7	9	15
B. Operated	18	10.9	210	1	2	6	13	25	62	62
1. SINGLE DX	9	1.9	<1	1	1	2	2	3	3	3
2. MULTIPLE DX	359	3.8	20	1	2	3	5	7	10	19
A. NOT OPERATED	350	3.4	8	1	2	3	4	7	9	15
B. OPERATED	18	10.9	210	1	2	6	13	25	62	62
TOTAL										
0–19 Years	126	2.8	7	1	1	2	3	6	8	15
20–34	12	5.2	45	1	1	3	6	9	25	25
35–49	41	4.5	88	1	2	3	5	6	8	62
50–64	56	4.6	17	1	2	3	6	10	14	21
65+	133	4.1	9	2	2	3	5	7	11	16
GRAND TOTAL	368	3.8	20	1	2	3	4	7	10	19

520: TOOTH DEVELOP/ERUPT PBX

Type of Patients	Observed Patients	Avg. Stay	Vari- ance	10th	25th	50th	75th	90th	95th	99th
1. SINGLE DX										
A. Not Operated										
0–19 Years	1	1.0	0	1	1	1	1	1	1	1
20–34	2	1.0	0	1	1	1	1	1	1	1
35–49	0									
50–64	0									
65+										
B. Operated										
0–19 Years	1	1.0	0	1	1	1	1	1	1	1
20–34	0									
35–49	0									
50–64	0									
65+	0									
2. MULTIPLE DX										
A. Not Operated										
0–19 Years	12	1.2	<1	1	1	1	1	2	2	2
20–34	13	1.7	<1	1	1	2	2	3	3	3
35–49	2	2.0	2	1	2	1	3	3	3	3
50–64	0									
65+	0									
B. Operated										
0–19 Years	3	1.7	1	1	1	2	3	3	3	3
20–34	2	2.0	2	1	1	2	3	3	3	3
35–49	0									
50–64	0									
65+	0									
SUBTOTALS:										
1. SINGLE DX										
A. Not Operated	3	1.0	0	1	1	1	1	1	1	1
B. Operated	1	1.0	0	1	1	1	1	1	1	1
2. MULTIPLE DX										
A. Not Operated	27	1.5	<1	1	1	1	2	2	3	3
B. Operated	5	1.8	1	1	1	1	3	3	3	3
1. SINGLE DX	4	1.0	0	1	1	1	1	1	1	1
2. MULTIPLE DX	32	1.5	<1	1	1	1	2	3	3	3
A. NOT OPERATED	30	1.4	<1	1	1	1	2	2	2	3
B. OPERATED	6	1.7	1	1	1	1	3	3	3	3
TOTAL										
0–19 Years	17	1.2	<1	1	1	1	1	2	2	3
20–34	17	1.7	<1	1	1	2	2	3	3	3
35–49	2	2.0	2	1	1	1	3	3	3	3
50–64	0									
65+	0									
GRAND TOTAL	36	1.5	<1	1	1	1	2	2	3	3

Length of Stay by Diagnosis and Operation, Western Region, 2008

Western Region, October 2006–September 2007 Data, by Diagnosis

521: HARD TISSUE DIS OF TEETH

Type of Patients	Observed Patients	Avg. Stay	Variance	10th	25th	50th	75th	90th	95th	99th
1. SINGLE DX										
A. *Not Operated*										
0–19 Years	0									
20–34	4	1.5	<1	1	1	1	2	2	2	2
35–49	1	1.0	0	1	1	1	1	1	1	1
50–64	0									
65+	0									
B. *Operated*										
0–19 Years	0									
20–34	0									
35–49	0									
50–64	0									
65+	0									
2. MULTIPLE DX										
A. *Not Operated*										
0–19 Years	25	1.4	1	1	1	1	1	2	2	6
20–34	24	1.8	<1	1	1	2	2	3	4	4
35–49	18	3.1	12	1	1	2	4	12	12	12
50–64	14	1.6	1	1	1	1	2	2	5	5
65+	13	2.3	2	1	2	2	3	5	5	5
B. *Operated*										
0–19 Years	4	1.5	1	1	1	1	3	3	3	3
20–34	9	2.2	2	1	1	2	2	5	5	5
35–49	15	2.6	5	1	1	2	4	7	8	8
50–64	10	2.2	3	1	1	1	3	4	6	6
65+	9	1.4	<1	1	1	1	2	3	3	3
SUBTOTALS:										
1. SINGLE DX										
A. *Not Operated*	5	1.4	<1	1	1	1	2	2	2	2
B. *Operated*	0									
2. MULTIPLE DX										
A. *Not Operated*	94	2.0	3	1	1	1	2	4	5	12
B. *Operated*	47	2.1	3	1	1	2	2	4	6	8
1. SINGLE DX	5	1.4	<1	1	1	1	2	2	2	2
2. MULTIPLE DX	141	2.0	3	1	1	1	2	4	5	12
A. NOT OPERATED	99	1.9	3	1	1	1	2	4	5	12
B. OPERATED	47	2.1	3	1	1	2	2	4	6	8
TOTAL										
0–19 Years	29	1.4	1	1	1	1	1	2	3	6
20–34	37	1.9	1	1	1	2	2	4	4	5
35–49	34	2.8	8	1	1	2	4	7	12	12
50–64	24	1.9	2	1	1	1	2	4	5	6
65+	22	2.0	2	1	1	2	2	4	5	5
GRAND TOTAL	146	2.0	3	1	1	1	2	4	5	12

522: PULP & PERIAPICAL DIS

Type of Patients	Observed Patients	Avg. Stay	Variance	10th	25th	50th	75th	90th	95th	99th
1. SINGLE DX										
A. *Not Operated*										
0–19 Years	39	2.0	<1	1	1	2	2	3	3	4
20–34	16	1.8	1	1	1	2	2	4	4	4
35–49	9	2.2	<1	2	2	2	3	3	3	3
50–64	4	1.8	<1	1	1	2	2	3	3	3
65+	3	2.0	3	1	1	1	4	4	4	4
B. *Operated*										
0–19 Years	4	1.8	<1	1	1	2	3	3	3	3
20–34	9	3.3	3	1	2	3	5	6	6	6
35–49	2	1.5	<1	1	1	1	2	2	2	2
50–64	2	3.0	2	2	2	3	4	4	4	4
65+	0									
2. MULTIPLE DX										
A. *Not Operated*										
0–19 Years	131	2.2	2	1	1	2	3	4	4	7
20–34	186	2.5	2	1	1	2	3	4	5	8
35–49	225	2.8	3	1	1	2	4	5	6	9
50–64	141	2.8	6	1	2	2	3	5	6	14
65+	116	3.4	7	2	2	3	4	6	8	13
B. *Operated*										
0–19 Years	28	2.4	1	1	2	2	3	4	5	5
20–34	62	3.2	6	1	2	2	4	5	7	15
35–49	65	3.3	6	1	2	2	4	7	7	14
50–64	27	4.9	14	2	2	3	7	12	12	15
65+	18	5.7	12	2	3	5	8	11	13	13
SUBTOTALS:										
1. SINGLE DX										
A. *Not Operated*	71	1.9	<1	1	1	1	2	3	4	4
B. *Operated*	17	2.7	2	1	2	2	4	5	6	6
2. MULTIPLE DX										
A. *Not Operated*	799	2.7	4	1	1	2	3	5	6	12
B. *Operated*	200	3.5	8	1	2	2	4	7	9	15
1. SINGLE DX	88	2.1	1	1	1	2	3	4	4	6
2. MULTIPLE DX	999	2.9	5	1	2	2	3	5	7	12
A. NOT OPERATED	870	2.7	4	1	1	2	3	4	6	12
B. OPERATED	217	3.5	7	1	2	2	4	7	9	14
TOTAL										
0–19 Years	202	2.2	1	1	1	2	3	3	4	7
20–34	273	2.6	3	1	1	2	3	5	5	10
35–49	301	2.8	4	1	1	2	4	5	7	10
50–64	174	3.1	7	2	2	2	4	6	9	15
65+	137	3.7	8	1	2	3	4	7	10	13
GRAND TOTAL	1,087	2.8	4	1	2	2	3	5	7	12

522.5: PERIAPICAL ABSCESS

Type of Patients	Observed Patients	Avg. Stay	Variance	10th	25th	50th	75th	90th	95th	99th
1. SINGLE DX										
A. *Not Operated*										
0–19 Years	37	1.9	<1	1	1	2	2	3	3	3
20–34	14	1.9	1	1	1	2	2	4	4	4
35–49	8	2.3	<1	1	1	3	3	3	3	3
50–64	3	2.0	<1	1	1	2	2	3	3	3
65+	3	2.0	3	1	1	1	4	4	4	4
B. *Operated*										
0–19 Years	2	2.0	2	1	1	3	3	3	3	3
20–34	9	3.3	3	1	2	3	5	6	6	6
35–49	2	1.5	<1	1	1	1	2	2	2	2
50–64	1	2.0	0	2	2	2	2	2	2	2
65+	0									
2. MULTIPLE DX										
A. *Not Operated*										
0–19 Years	116	2.3	2	1	2	2	3	4	5	7
20–34	161	2.5	2	1	1	2	3	4	5	8
35–49	182	2.7	3	1	1	2	3	5	6	10
50–64	123	2.8	6	1	2	2	3	5	6	14
65+	88	3.3	6	2	2	3	4	6	8	13
B. *Operated*										
0–19 Years	23	2.4	1	1	2	2	3	4	5	5
20–34	55	3.2	6	1	2	2	4	5	7	15
35–49	57	3.2	6	1	2	2	4	7	7	14
50–64	23	5.0	16	2	2	3	8	12	12	15
65+	13	5.9	11	2	3	5	8	10	13	13
SUBTOTALS:										
1. SINGLE DX										
A. *Not Operated*	65	2.0	<1	1	1	2	3	3	3	4
B. *Operated*	14	2.8	3	2	2	2	4	5	6	6
2. MULTIPLE DX										
A. *Not Operated*	670	2.7	4	1	1	2	3	5	6	12
B. *Operated*	171	3.6	8	1	2	3	4	7	10	15
1. SINGLE DX	79	2.1	1	1	1	2	3	3	4	6
2. MULTIPLE DX	841	2.9	5	1	2	2	3	5	7	13
A. NOT OPERATED	735	2.6	4	1	1	2	3	4	6	12
B. OPERATED	185	3.5	8	1	2	3	4	7	9	15
TOTAL										
0–19 Years	178	2.2	1	1	1	2	3	3	4	7
20–34	239	2.7	3	1	1	2	3	5	5	10
35–49	249	2.8	4	1	1	2	3	5	7	10
50–64	150	3.1	8	1	2	2	4	6	9	15
65+	104	3.6	7	1	2	3	4	7	10	13
GRAND TOTAL	920	2.8	4	1	2	2	3	5	7	12

Length of Stay by Diagnosis and Operation, Western Region, 2008

Western Region, October 2006–September 2007 Data, by Diagnosis

523: GINGIVAL/PERIODONTAL DIS

Type of Patients	Observed Patients	Avg. Stay	Variance	10th	25th	50th	75th	90th	95th	99th
1. SINGLE DX										
A. Not Operated										
0–19 Years	3	2.3	<1	2	2	2	3	3	3	3
20–34	6	1.3	<1	1	1	1	2	2	2	2
35–49	4	2.2	2	1	1	1	3	4	4	4
50–64	0									
65+	0									
B. Operated										
0–19 Years	0									
20–34	0									
35–49	0									
50–64	0									
65+	0									
2. MULTIPLE DX										
A. Not Operated										
0–19 Years	42	2.7	2	1	2	2	4	5	6	6
20–34	28	2.0	2	1	1	2	3	3	5	6
35–49	38	2.6	4	1	1	2	3	4	8	11
50–64	42	3.1	5	1	1	3	4	5	7	11
65+	53	4.1	12	1	2	3	6	8	10	18
B. Operated										
0–19 Years	2	3.5	4	2	2	4	5	5	5	5
20–34	7	2.9	5	1	1	3	4	7	7	7
35–49	5	2.0	1	1	1	2	2	4	4	4
50–64	6	2.0	<1	1	1	2	3	3	3	3
65+	1	1.0	0	1	1	1	1	1	1	1
SUBTOTALS:										
1. SINGLE DX										
A. Not Operated	13	1.8	<1	1	1	2	2	3	4	4
B. Operated	0									
2. MULTIPLE DX										
A. Not Operated	203	3.0	6	1	1	2	4	6	8	11
B. Operated	21	2.4	3	1	2	2	3	4	5	7
1. SINGLE DX	13	1.8	<1	1	1	2	2	3	4	4
2. MULTIPLE DX	224	3.0	6	1	1	2	4	6	7	11
A. NOT OPERATED	216	3.0	6	1	1	2	4	6	8	11
B. OPERATED	21	2.4	3	1	1	2	3	4	5	7
TOTAL										
0–19 Years	47	2.7	2	1	2	2	4	5	6	6
20–34	41	2.1	2	1	1	2	3	3	5	7
35–49	47	2.5	4	1	1	2	3	4	6	11
50–64	48	2.9	4	1	2	3	4	5	7	11
65+	54	4.0	12	1	2	3	6	8	10	18
GRAND TOTAL	237	2.9	5	1	1	2	4	6	7	11

524: DENTOFACIAL ANOMALIES

Type of Patients	Observed Patients	Avg. Stay	Variance	10th	25th	50th	75th	90th	95th	99th
1. SINGLE DX										
A. Not Operated										
0–19 Years	0									
20–34	1	1.0	0	1	1	1	1	1	1	1
35–49	1	1.0	0	1	1	1	1	1	1	1
50–64	0									
65+	0									
B. Operated										
0–19 Years	81	1.3	<1	1	1	1	1	2	2	6
20–34	121	1.3	<1	1	1	1	1	2	2	3
35–49	52	1.3	<1	1	1	1	2	2	2	3
50–64	27	1.1	<1	1	1	1	1	2	2	2
65+	0									
2. MULTIPLE DX										
A. Not Operated										
0–19 Years	1	1.0	0	1	1	1	1	1	1	1
20–34	7	1.4	<1	1	1	1	2	2	2	2
35–49	16	1.9	<1	1	1	2	2	3	3	3
50–64	6	3.3	18	1	1	2	4	12	12	12
65+	21	2.4	2	1	2	2	3	3	6	7
B. Operated										
0–19 Years	341	1.6	1	1	1	1	2	2	3	6
20–34	530	1.5	<1	1	1	1	2	2	3	4
35–49	228	1.8	4	1	1	2	2	2	3	10
50–64	149	1.6	1	1	1	1	2	3	3	8
65+	15	2.1	2	1	1	2	3	4	6	6
SUBTOTALS:										
1. SINGLE DX										
A. Not Operated	2	1.0	0	1	1	1	1	1	1	1
B. Operated	281	1.3	<1	1	1	1	1	2	2	5
2. MULTIPLE DX										
A. Not Operated	51	2.2	3	1	1	2	2	3	6	12
B. Operated	1,263	1.6	1	1	1	1	2	2	3	6
1. SINGLE DX	283	1.3	<1	1	1	1	1	2	2	5
2. MULTIPLE DX	1,314	1.6	1	1	1	1	2	2	3	6
A. NOT OPERATED	53	2.2	3	1	1	2	2	3	6	12
B. OPERATED	1,544	1.5	1	1	1	1	2	2	3	6
TOTAL										
0–19 Years	423	1.5	1	1	1	1	2	2	3	6
20–34	659	1.4	<1	1	1	1	2	2	3	4
35–49	297	1.7	3	1	1	2	2	2	3	7
50–64	182	1.6	2	1	1	1	2	2	3	9
65+	36	2.3	2	1	1	2	3	4	6	7
GRAND TOTAL	1,597	1.5	1	1	1	1	2	2	3	6

524.03: MAXILLARY HYPOPLASIA

Type of Patients	Observed Patients	Avg. Stay	Variance	10th	25th	50th	75th	90th	95th	99th
1. SINGLE DX										
A. Not Operated										
0–19 Years	0									
20–34	0									
35–49	0									
50–64	0									
65+	0									
B. Operated										
0–19 Years	14	1.1	<1	1	1	1	1	2	2	2
20–34	23	1.2	<1	1	1	1	1	2	2	2
35–49	5	1.0	0	1	1	1	1	1	1	1
50–64	3	1.0	0	1	1	1	1	1	1	1
65+	0									
2. MULTIPLE DX										
A. Not Operated										
0–19 Years	0									
20–34	0									
35–49	0									
50–64	0									
65+	0									
B. Operated										
0–19 Years	113	1.5	<1	1	1	1	2	2	2	3
20–34	184	1.5	<1	1	1	1	2	2	3	4
35–49	54	1.6	<1	1	1	2	2	2	3	4
50–64	27	1.3	<1	1	1	1	2	2	2	2
65+	0									
SUBTOTALS:										
1. SINGLE DX										
A. Not Operated	0									
B. Operated	45	1.1	<1	1	1	1	1	2	2	2
2. MULTIPLE DX										
A. Not Operated	0									
B. Operated	378	1.5	<1	1	1	1	2	2	3	4
1. SINGLE DX	45	1.1	<1	1	1	1	1	2	2	2
2. MULTIPLE DX	378	1.5	<1	1	1	2	2	2	3	4
A. NOT OPERATED	0									
B. OPERATED	423	1.5	<1	1	1	1	2	2	2	3
TOTAL										
0–19 Years	127	1.5	<1	1	1	1	2	2	2	3
20–34	207	1.5	<1	1	1	1	2	2	3	3
35–49	59	1.6	<1	1	1	1	2	2	3	4
50–64	30	1.3	<1	1	1	1	2	2	2	2
65+	0									
GRAND TOTAL	423	1.5	<1	1	1	1	2	2	2	3

Length of Stay by Diagnosis and Operation, Western Region, 2008

525: OTHER DENTAL DISORDER

Type of Patients	Observed Patients	Avg. Stay	Variance	10th	25th	50th	75th	90th	95th	99th
1. SINGLE DX										
A. *Not Operated*										
0–19 Years	0									
20–34	0									
35–49	0									
50–64	0									
65+	0									
B. *Operated*										
0–19 Years	6	1.0	0	1	1	1	1	1	1	1
20–34	1	2.0	0	2	2	2	2	2	2	2
35–49	1	1.0	0	1	1	1	1	1	1	1
50–64	3	1.3	<1	1	1	1	2	2	2	2
65+	0									
2. MULTIPLE DX										
A. *Not Operated*										
0–19 Years	0									
20–34	3	1.0	0	1	1	1	1	1	1	1
35–49	3	1.7	<1	1	1	2	2	2	2	2
50–64	3	3.0	7	1	1	2	6	6	6	6
65+	2	2.5	4	1	1	3	4	4	4	4
B. *Operated*										
0–19 Years	25	1.2	<1	1	1	1	1	2	2	2
20–34	4	1.0	0	1	1	1	1	1	1	1
35–49	2	1.5	<1	1	1	2	2	2	2	2
50–64	10	1.5	<1	1	1	1	2	2	3	3
65+	6	2.2	4	1	1	1	3	6	6	6
SUBTOTALS:										
1. SINGLE DX										
A. *Not Operated*	0									
B. *Operated*	11	1.2	<1	1	1	1	1	2	2	2
2. MULTIPLE DX										
A. *Not Operated*	11	2.0	3	1	1	1	2	4	6	6
B. *Operated*	47	1.4	<1	1	1	1	1	2	3	6
1. SINGLE DX	11	1.2	<1	1	1	1	1	2	2	2
2. MULTIPLE DX	58	1.5	1	1	1	1	2	2	4	6
A. NOT OPERATED	11	2.0	3	1	1	1	2	4	6	6
B. OPERATED	58	1.3	<1	1	1	1	1	2	3	6
TOTAL										
0–19 Years	31	1.1	<1	1	1	1	1	2	2	2
20–34	8	1.1	<1	1	1	1	1	2	2	2
35–49	6	1.5	<1	1	1	2	2	2	2	2
50–64	16	1.8	2	1	1	1	2	3	6	6
65+	8	2.3	4	1	1	1	4	6	6	6
GRAND TOTAL	69	1.4	<1	1	1	1	2	2	3	6

526: JAW DISEASES

Type of Patients	Observed Patients	Avg. Stay	Variance	10th	25th	50th	75th	90th	95th	99th
1. SINGLE DX										
A. *Not Operated*										
0–19 Years	1	3.0	0	3	3	3	3	3	3	3
20–34	6	2.5	1	1	2	2	3	4	4	4
35–49	1	2.0	0	2	2	2	2	2	2	2
50–64	0									
65+	1	2.0	0	2	2	2	2	2	2	2
B. *Operated*										
0–19 Years	5	2.6	4	1	1	2	3	6	6	6
20–34	12	1.9	1	1	1	2	3	3	4	4
35–49	6	2.0	2	1	1	1	3	4	4	4
50–64	6	3.5	32	1	1	1	2	15	15	15
65+	1	1.0	0	1	1	1	1	1	1	1
2. MULTIPLE DX										
A. *Not Operated*										
0–19 Years	11	6.0	153	1	1	2	4	5	43	43
20–34	25	2.7	3	1	1	2	4	5	6	6
35–49	46	4.4	51	1	2	3	4	6	14	42
50–64	68	2.4	5	1	1	2	3	5	8	14
65+	69	3.2	5	1	1	2	5	6	8	10
B. *Operated*										
0–19 Years	24	3.5	10	2	2	2	5	7	9	15
20–34	44	5.2	60	1	3	3	6	10	18	48
35–49	48	5.2	27	1	1	3	7	13	19	22
50–64	70	5.5	33	1	1	4	7	12	15	29
65+	55	6.1	43	1	1	5	8	15	17	36
SUBTOTALS:										
1. SINGLE DX										
A. *Not Operated*	9	2.4	<1	1	2	2	3	4	4	4
B. *Operated*	30	2.3	7	1	1	1	3	4	6	15
2. MULTIPLE DX										
A. *Not Operated*	219	3.3	22	1	1	2	4	6	8	28
B. *Operated*	241	5.3	37	1	3	3	7	12	16	29
1. SINGLE DX	39	2.4	6	1	1	2	3	4	6	15
2. MULTIPLE DX	460	4.4	31	1	1	2	5	9	14	29
A. NOT OPERATED	228	3.2	21	1	1	2	4	6	8	28
B. OPERATED	271	5.0	34	1	1	3	7	12	16	29
TOTAL										
0–19 Years	41	4.1	46	1	1	2	4	6	9	43
20–34	87	3.8	33	1	1	2	4	7	10	48
35–49	101	4.6	36	1	1	3	5	9	14	42
50–64	144	4.0	22	1	1	2	5	8	13	26
65+	126	4.5	23	1	1	3	6	9	15	19
GRAND TOTAL	499	4.2	29	1	1	2	5	8	14	29

526.4: JAW INFLAMMATION

Type of Patients	Observed Patients	Avg. Stay	Variance	10th	25th	50th	75th	90th	95th	99th
1. SINGLE DX										
A. *Not Operated*										
0–19 Years	1	3.0	0	3	3	3	3	3	3	3
20–34	6	2.5	1	1	2	2	3	4	4	4
35–49	1	2.0	0	2	2	2	2	2	2	2
50–64	0									
65+	1	2.0	0	2	2	2	2	2	2	2
B. *Operated*										
0–19 Years	2	4.5	4	3	3	3	6	6	6	6
20–34	1	2.0	0	2	2	2	2	2	2	2
35–49	3	2.7	2	1	1	3	4	4	4	4
50–64	3	5.7	65	1	1	1	15	15	15	15
65+	0									
2. MULTIPLE DX										
A. *Not Operated*										
0–19 Years	5	11.6	310	2	4	4	5	43	43	43
20–34	20	2.7	3	1	1	2	4	5	6	6
35–49	29	5.6	76	1	2	3	5	14	28	42
50–64	34	3.3	8	1	1	3	4	8	8	14
65+	29	4.1	5	2	2	4	6	8	8	10
B. *Operated*										
0–19 Years	10	4.9	18	1	2	3	6	15	15	15
20–34	20	7.6	107	1	2	5	7	12	18	48
35–49	22	7.9	38	2	4	6	12	19	19	22
50–64	27	4.9	12	1	2	4	7	10	12	13
65+	21	8.6	69	1	3	6	11	17	19	36
SUBTOTALS:										
1. SINGLE DX										
A. *Not Operated*	9	2.4	<1	1	2	2	3	4	4	4
B. *Operated*	9	4.0	20	1	3	3	4	15	15	15
2. MULTIPLE DX										
A. *Not Operated*	117	4.3	36	1	2	3	5	6	10	42
B. *Operated*	100	6.9	50	1	2	5	8	15	19	36
1. SINGLE DX	18	3.2	10	1	2	2	3	6	15	15
2. MULTIPLE DX	217	5.5	44	1	2	4	6	12	17	42
A. NOT OPERATED	126	4.2	34	1	2	3	5	6	8	42
B. OPERATED	109	6.6	48	1	2	5	8	15	19	36
TOTAL										
0–19 Years	18	6.6	93	2	3	3	6	15	43	43
20–34	47	4.7	52	1	2	3	5	7	12	48
35–49	55	6.3	57	1	2	4	6	14	22	42
50–64	64	4.1	12	1	2	3	6	8	12	15
65+	51	5.9	36	2	2	5	6	11	17	36
GRAND TOTAL	235	5.3	42	1	2	3	6	11	16	42

Length of Stay by Diagnosis and Operation, Western Region, 2008

Western Region, October 2006–September 2007 Data, by Diagnosis

527: SALIVARY GLAND DISEASES

Type of Patients	Observed Patients	Avg. Stay	Variance	10th	25th	50th	75th	90th	95th	99th
1. SINGLE DX										
A. Not Operated										
0–19 Years	46	2.3	2	1	1	2	3	4	5	7
20–34	13	2.4	2	1	1	2	3	5	5	5
35–49	8	2.1	<1	1	1	2	3	3	3	3
50–64	9	2.4	<1	2	2	2	3	4	4	4
65+	4	1.8	<1	1	1	2	3	3	3	3
B. Operated										
0–19 Years	13	1.5	<1	1	1	1	1	3	3	3
20–34	13	1.9	1	1	1	1	2	3	5	5
35–49	25	1.6	<1	1	1	1	2	3	3	4
50–64	13	1.6	2	1	1	1	1	4	5	5
65+	3	1.0	0	1	1	1	1	1	1	1
2. MULTIPLE DX										
A. Not Operated										
0–19 Years	69	2.6	3	1	2	2	3	6	6	7
20–34	85	2.8	4	1	2	2	3	5	8	10
35–49	139	3.4	7	1	2	2	4	7	9	11
50–64	193	3.8	7	1	2	3	5	7	9	12
65+	436	5.3	16	2	3	4	7	9	12	25
B. Operated										
0–19 Years	21	3.1	21	1	1	2	2	5	12	20
20–34	32	2.4	3	1	1	2	4	5	5	7
35–49	60	2.9	6	1	1	2	5	8	8	9
50–64	97	2.1	5	1	1	1	2	5	8	12
65+	75	4.4	40	1	2	2	5	11	19	36
SUBTOTALS:										
1. SINGLE DX										
A. Not Operated	80	2.3	1	1	1	2	3	4	5	7
B. Operated	67	1.6	1	1	1	1	2	3	4	5
2. MULTIPLE DX										
A. Not Operated	922	4.3	12	1	2	3	5	8	10	16
B. Operated	285	3.0	16	1	1	1	3	7	9	21
1. SINGLE DX	147	2.0	1	1	1	2	3	4	4	5
2. MULTIPLE DX	1,207	3.9	13	1	2	3	5	8	10	19
A. NOT OPERATED	1,002	4.1	11	1	2	3	5	8	10	16
B. OPERATED	352	2.7	13	1	1	1	3	6	8	20
TOTAL										
0–19 Years	149	2.5	5	1	1	2	3	5	6	12
20–34	143	2.6	3	1	1	2	3	5	5	10
35–49	232	3.0	6	1	1	2	4	7	8	11
50–64	312	3.1	7	1	2	2	4	7	8	12
65+	518	5.1	20	1	2	4	6	10	12	25
GRAND TOTAL	1,354	3.7	12	1	1	3	5	8	10	19

527.2: SIALOADENITIS

Type of Patients	Observed Patients	Avg. Stay	Variance	10th	25th	50th	75th	90th	95th	99th
1. SINGLE DX										
A. Not Operated										
0–19 Years	39	2.2	<1	1	1	2	3	4	4	5
20–34	10	1.7	<1	1	1	2	2	3	3	3
35–49	5	1.8	<1	1	2	2	3	3	3	3
50–64	6	2.2	<1	1	2	2	3	4	4	4
65+	2	1.0	0	1	1	1	1	1	1	1
B. Operated										
0–19 Years	2	2.0	2	1	2	2	3	3	3	3
20–34	2	2.5	<1	2	2	2	3	3	3	3
35–49	12	1.3	<1	1	1	1	2	3	3	3
50–64	5	2.4	4	1	1	1	4	5	5	5
65+	2	1.0	0	1	1	1	1	1	1	1
2. MULTIPLE DX										
A. Not Operated										
0–19 Years	60	2.5	2	1	2	2	3	5	6	7
20–34	63	2.7	3	1	2	2	3	4	5	10
35–49	101	3.2	8	1	2	2	4	7	8	11
50–64	154	3.7	6	1	2	3	5	7	9	12
65+	387	5.2	14	2	3	4	6	9	12	20
B. Operated										
0–19 Years	5	1.8	<1	1	1	1	2	3	3	3
20–34	11	2.5	5	1	1	1	5	5	7	7
35–49	22	2.9	7	1	1	1	5	7	8	8
50–64	43	1.9	4	1	1	1	2	5	6	10
65+	39	5.4	62	1	1	2	7	17	27	36
SUBTOTALS:										
1. SINGLE DX										
A. Not Operated	62	2.0	<1	1	1	2	2	3	4	7
B. Operated	23	1.7	1	1	1	1	2	3	4	5
2. MULTIPLE DX										
A. Not Operated	765	4.2	11	1	2	3	5	8	11	16
B. Operated	120	3.3	25	1	1	1	3	7	12	27
1. SINGLE DX	85	1.9	<1	1	1	2	2	3	4	5
2. MULTIPLE DX	885	4.1	13	1	2	3	5	8	11	19
A. NOT OPERATED	827	4.1	10	1	2	3	5	8	10	16
B. OPERATED	143	3.0	22	1	1	1	3	7	10	20
TOTAL										
0–19 Years	106	2.3	2	1	1	2	3	4	6	7
20–34	86	2.6	3	1	2	2	3	5	5	10
35–49	140	3.0	7	1	1	2	4	7	8	11
50–64	208	3.3	6	1	2	2	4	7	9	12
65+	430	5.2	18	1	3	4	6	9	13	25
GRAND TOTAL	970	3.9	12	1	2	3	5	8	10	19

528: ORAL SOFT TISSUE DISEASE

Type of Patients	Observed Patients	Avg. Stay	Variance	10th	25th	50th	75th	90th	95th	99th
1. SINGLE DX										
A. Not Operated										
0–19 Years	26	2.1	2	1	1	2	2	4	4	8
20–34	8	1.5	<1	1	1	2	2	2	2	2
35–49	12	2.4	2	1	1	2	3	4	6	6
50–64	7	3.9	6	2	2	3	4	9	9	9
65+	1	4.0	0	4	4	4	4	4	4	4
B. Operated										
0–19 Years	15	1.3	<1	1	1	1	1	3	3	3
20–34	17	2.1	1	1	1	2	3	3	4	4
35–49	8	3.1	9	1	1	3	6	9	9	9
50–64	4	1.8	<1	1	1	2	2	2	2	2
65+	0									
2. MULTIPLE DX										
A. Not Operated										
0–19 Years	128	3.3	7	1	2	3	4	6	10	12
20–34	125	3.5	11	1	2	3	4	6	10	17
35–49	200	4.5	18	1	2	3	6	9	12	25
50–64	242	5.7	27	2	3	4	7	11	18	31
65+	272	5.9	45	2	3	4	7	11	16	38
B. Operated										
0–19 Years	63	2.4	2	1	1	2	3	4	5	9
20–34	129	3.7	8	1	2	3	5	6	9	13
35–49	126	3.8	14	1	2	3	4	6	10	15
50–64	96	4.0	13	1	2	3	5	8	10	28
65+	35	4.8	21	1	3	4	6	8	8	28
SUBTOTALS:										
1. SINGLE DX										
A. Not Operated	54	2.3	3	1	1	2	3	4	6	9
B. Operated	44	2.0	2	1	1	1	3	3	4	9
2. MULTIPLE DX										
A. Not Operated	967	4.9	27	1	2	3	6	10	13	28
B. Operated	449	3.7	11	1	2	3	5	6	8	15
1. SINGLE DX	98	2.2	3	1	1	2	3	4	6	9
2. MULTIPLE DX	1,416	4.5	22	1	2	3	5	9	12	25
A. NOT OPERATED	1,021	4.8	26	1	2	3	6	10	13	25
B. OPERATED	493	3.5	11	1	2	3	4	6	8	15
TOTAL										
0–19 Years	232	2.8	5	1	1	2	3	5	8	11
20–34	279	3.4	9	1	2	3	4	6	9	17
35–49	346	4.2	16	1	2	3	5	8	11	23
50–64	349	5.1	23	1	2	4	6	10	14	29
65+	308	5.8	42	2	3	4	7	11	16	33
GRAND TOTAL	1,514	4.4	21	1	2	3	5	8	12	25

528.3: CELLULITIS/ABSCESS MOUTH

Type of Patients	Observed Patients	Avg. Stay	Variance	Percentiles						
				10th	25th	50th	75th	90th	95th	99th
1. SINGLE DX										
A. Not Operated										
0-19 Years	9	1.9	<1	1	1	2	2	4	4	4
20-34	5	1.6	<1	1	1	2	2	2	2	2
35-49	8	2.0	3	1	1	2	2	6	6	6
50-64	3	4.3	16	2	2	2	9	9	9	9
65+	1	4.0	0	4	4	4	4	4	4	4
B. Operated										
0-19 Years	5	1.6	<1	1	1	1	2	3	3	3
20-34	12	2.1	<1	1	1	2	3	3	4	4
35-49	5	4.0	12	1	1	3	6	9	9	9
50-64	3	2.0	0	2	2	2	2	2	2	2
65+	0									
2. MULTIPLE DX										
A. Not Operated										
0-19 Years	39	2.3	1	1	2	2	3	4	5	6
20-34	59	3.1	13	1	2	2	3	5	7	28
35-49	71	3.8	18	1	2	3	5	6	9	30
50-64	54	3.9	6	2	2	3	5	7	9	13
65+	53	3.6	7	1	2	3	4	6	9	16
B. Operated										
0-19 Years	25	2.9	4	1	2	2	3	6	7	9
20-34	85	3.7	9	1	2	3	5	6	10	19
35-49	71	4.4	22	1	2	3	5	9	14	34
50-64	54	4.2	10	1	2	3	6	8	10	15
65+	16	4.5	4	2	3	5	6	7	8	8
SUBTOTALS:										
1. SINGLE DX										
A. Not Operated	26	2.2	3	1	1	2	2	4	6	9
B. Operated	25	2.4	3	1	1	2	3	4	6	9
2. MULTIPLE DX										
A. Not Operated	276	3.4	10	1	2	3	4	6	8	20
B. Operated	251	4.0	12	1	2	3	5	7	10	15
1. SINGLE DX	51	2.3	3	1	1	2	2	4	6	9
2. MULTIPLE DX	527	3.7	11	1	2	3	5	6	9	16
A. NOT OPERATED	302	3.3	10	1	2	2	4	6	7	16
B. OPERATED	276	3.8	12	1	2	3	5	7	10	15
TOTAL										
0-19 Years	78	2.4	2	1	1	2	3	4	6	9
20-34	161	3.3	10	1	2	2	4	6	7	19
35-49	155	4.0	19	1	2	3	5	8	10	30
50-64	114	4.0	8	1	2	3	5	8	10	14
65+	70	3.8	7	2	2	3	5	7	8	16
GRAND TOTAL	578	3.6	11	1	2	3	4	6	9	16

528.5: LIP DISEASES

Type of Patients	Observed Patients	Avg. Stay	Variance	Percentiles						
				10th	25th	50th	75th	90th	95th	99th
1. SINGLE DX										
A. Not Operated										
0-19 Years	6	1.7	<1	1	1	2	2	2	2	2
20-34	3	1.3	<1	1	1	1	2	2	2	2
35-49	3	3.0	1	2	2	3	4	4	4	4
50-64	4	3.5	<1	3	3	3	4	4	4	4
65+	0									
B. Operated										
0-19 Years	0									
20-34	3	2.0	3	1	1	1	4	4	4	4
35-49	2	2.0	2	1	1	3	3	3	3	3
50-64	0									
65+	0									
2. MULTIPLE DX										
A. Not Operated										
0-19 Years	14	3.2	6	1	2	2	3	4	5	6
20-34	32	3.1	1	2	2	3	4	5	5	28
35-49	42	3.2	4	1	2	3	4	6	7	11
50-64	22	3.3	3	1	2	3	4	5	6	7
65+	6	4.5	9	2	2	3	6	6	10	10
B. Operated										
0-19 Years	7	2.7	<1	2	2	3	3	3	3	3
20-34	34	3.7	4	1	2	3	4	6	8	9
35-49	38	3.3	2	1	2	3	4	5	6	7
50-64	29	3.2	3	1	2	3	4	6	6	7
65+	8	4.5	5	1	3	4	6	8	8	8
SUBTOTALS:										
1. SINGLE DX										
A. Not Operated	16	2.3	1	1	1	2	3	4	4	4
B. Operated	5	2.0	2	1	1	2	3	4	4	4
2. MULTIPLE DX										
A. Not Operated	116	3.3	3	1	2	3	4	5	7	10
B. Operated	116	3.4	3	1	2	3	4	6	7	8
1. SINGLE DX	21	2.2	1	1	1	2	3	4	6	9
2. MULTIPLE DX	232	3.3	3	1	2	3	4	6	7	10
A. NOT OPERATED	132	3.1	3	1	2	3	4	5	6	10
B. OPERATED	121	3.4	3	1	2	3	4	6	6	8
TOTAL										
0-19 Years	27	2.7	3	1	2	3	3	4	6	9
20-34	72	3.2	3	1	2	3	4	6	7	19
35-49	85	3.2	3	1	2	3	4	5	6	11
50-64	55	3.3	2	2	2	3	5	5	6	7
65+	14	4.5	6	2	3	4	6	8	10	10
GRAND TOTAL	253	3.3	3	1	2	3	4	6	6	10

529: TONGUE DISORDERS

Type of Patients	Observed Patients	Avg. Stay	Variance	Percentiles						
				10th	25th	50th	75th	90th	95th	99th
1. SINGLE DX										
A. Not Operated										
0-19 Years	3	2.0	0	2	2	2	2	2	2	2
20-34	2	3.0	0	3	3	3	3	3	3	3
35-49	2	1.5	<1	1	1	2	2	2	2	2
50-64	1	4.0	0	4	4	4	4	4	4	4
65+	0									
B. Operated										
0-19 Years	0									
20-34	2	1.0	0	1	1	1	1	1	1	1
35-49	1	1.0	0	1	1	1	1	1	1	1
50-64	0									
65+	0									
2. MULTIPLE DX										
A. Not Operated										
0-19 Years	4	2.8	2	2	2	2	2	5	5	5
20-34	8	3.3	9	1	1	2	7	9	9	9
35-49	10	2.5	1	1	1	3	3	4	4	4
50-64	22	4.9	29	1	2	3	6	8	15	24
65+	29	3.4	13	1	1	2	4	7	13	17
B. Operated										
0-19 Years	3	1.0	0	1	1	1	1	1	1	1
20-34	4	4.5	6	1	1	5	5	7	7	7
35-49	14	2.7	3	1	1	2	4	5	6	6
50-64	23	3.6	50	1	1	2	2	6	8	35
65+	11	4.1	14	2	2	3	6	7	14	14
SUBTOTALS:										
1. SINGLE DX										
A. Not Operated	8	2.4	<1	1	2	2	3	4	4	4
B. Operated	3	1.0	0	1	1	1	1	1	1	1
2. MULTIPLE DX										
A. Not Operated	73	3.7	15	1	1	2	4	7	13	24
B. Operated	55	3.4	25	1	2	2	4	6	8	35
1. SINGLE DX	11	2.0	1	1	1	2	3	3	4	4
2. MULTIPLE DX	128	3.5	19	1	1	2	4	7	9	24
A. NOT OPERATED	81	3.5	14	1	2	2	4	7	9	24
B. OPERATED	58	3.3	24	1	1	2	4	6	8	35
TOTAL										
0-19 Years	10	2.0	1	1	1	2	2	2	5	5
20-34	16	3.3	7	1	1	2	5	7	9	9
35-49	27	2.5	2	1	1	3	4	5	5	6
50-64	46	4.2	38	1	1	2	5	8	15	35
65+	40	3.6	13	1	1	2	4	7	14	17
GRAND TOTAL	139	3.4	18	1	1	2	4	7	9	24

Length of Stay by Diagnosis and Operation, Western Region, 2008

Western Region, October 2006–September 2007 Data, by Diagnosis

530: DISEASES OF ESOPHAGUS

Type of Patients	Observed Patients	Avg. Stay	Vari-ance	10th	25th	50th	75th	90th	95th	99th
1. SINGLE DX										
A. Not Operated										
0–19 Years	291	2.0	3	1	1	2	2	3	4	12
20–34	16	2.7	12	1	1	2	2	5	15	15
35–49	50	1.5	1	1	1	1	2	2	4	8
50–64	48	1.4	<1	1	1	1	1	3	3	4
65+	19	2.0	3	1	1	1	2	6	6	6
B. Operated										
0–19 Years	41	2.2	1	1	1	2	3	3	4	5
20–34	53	1.9	1	1	1	2	2	3	4	5
35–49	69	2.0	7	1	1	1	2	2	4	22
50–64	57	2.1	2	1	1	1	2	3	4	11
65+	16	1.3	<1	1	1	1	2	2	2	2
2. MULTIPLE DX										
A. Not Operated										
0–19 Years	1,143	3.1	15	1	1	2	3	6	9	16
20–34	1,269	2.5	5	1	1	2	3	5	6	11
35–49	3,682	2.7	7	1	1	2	3	5	7	12
50–64	5,778	2.9	8	1	1	2	3	6	7	14
65+	8,648	3.3	10	1	1	2	4	6	9	15
B. Operated										
0–19 Years	349	7.2	85	1	2	4	8	16	24	52
20–34	267	3.3	35	1	1	2	3	6	11	29
35–49	802	3.5	37	1	1	2	3	7	10	34
50–64	1,222	4.3	49	1	1	2	4	10	16	39
65+	918	5.5	54	1	2	3	7	12	20	34
SUBTOTALS:										
1. SINGLE DX										
A. Not Operated	424	1.9	3	1	1	1	2	3	4	11
B. Operated	236	2.0	3	1	1	2	2	3	4	7
2. MULTIPLE DX										
A. Not Operated	20,520	3.0	9	1	1	2	4	6	8	14
B. Operated	3,558	4.6	51	1	1	2	5	10	17	37
1. SINGLE DX	660	1.9	3	1	1	1	2	3	4	11
2. MULTIPLE DX	24,078	3.2	15	1	1	2	4	6	9	19
A. NOT OPERATED	20,944	3.0	9	1	1	2	4	6	8	14
B. OPERATED	3,794	4.5	49	1	1	2	4	10	16	36
TOTAL										
0–19 Years	1,824	3.7	29	1	1	2	4	8	12	25
20–34	1,605	2.6	10	1	1	2	3	5	6	14
35–49	4,603	2.8	12	1	1	2	3	5	7	15
50–64	7,105	3.1	16	1	1	2	4	6	9	19
65+	9,601	3.5	14	1	1	2	4	7	10	19
GRAND TOTAL	24,738	3.2	15	1	1	2	4	6	9	19

530.0: ACHALASIA & CARDIOSPASM

Type of Patients	Observed Patients	Avg. Stay	Vari-ance	10th	25th	50th	75th	90th	95th	99th
1. SINGLE DX										
A. Not Operated										
0–19 Years	0									
20–34	1	5.0	0	5	5	5	5	5	5	5
35–49	1	8.0	0	8	8	8	8	8	8	8
50–64	0									
65+	0									
B. Operated										
0–19 Years	6	2.5	3	1	1	1	4	5	5	5
20–34	18	2.5	2	1	2	2	3	4	5	5
35–49	21	2.1	3	1	1	1	2	4	5	7
50–64	17	2.1	<1	1	1	2	2	3	4	4
65+	4	1.3	<1	1	1	1	1	2	2	2
2. MULTIPLE DX										
A. Not Operated										
0–19 Years	2	2.5	4	1	1	2	3	4	4	4
20–34	18	3.8	12	1	2	3	4	8	15	15
35–49	30	3.3	3	2	2	3	4	6	7	9
50–64	48	4.0	7	1	2	3	6	7	10	11
65+	135	5.0	18	1	2	4	6	10	12	20
B. Operated										
0–19 Years	10	4.2	25	1	1	2	4	12	15	15
20–34	46	3.5	10	1	2	2	5	8	11	13
35–49	92	3.0	9	1	1	2	3	7	8	23
50–64	157	4.2	35	1	2	2	4	10	21	39
65+	101	4.5	25	1	1	3	7	12	14	21
SUBTOTALS:										
1. SINGLE DX										
A. Not Operated	2	6.5	4	5	5	5	8	8	8	8
B. Operated	66	2.2	2	1	1	2	3	4	5	7
2. MULTIPLE DX										
A. Not Operated	233	4.5	13	1	2	3	6	9	11	19
B. Operated	406	3.9	23	1	1	2	4	9	13	26
1. SINGLE DX	68	2.3	2	1	1	2	3	5	5	8
2. MULTIPLE DX	639	4.1	20	1	2	3	5	9	12	25
A. NOT OPERATED	235	4.5	13	1	2	3	6	9	11	19
B. OPERATED	472	3.7	21	1	1	2	4	8	12	26
TOTAL										
0–19 Years	18	3.4	15	1	1	2	4	8	15	25
20–34	83	3.4	8	1	1	2	4	8	11	14
35–49	144	3.0	7	1	1	2	3	6	8	11
50–64	222	4.0	26	1	2	2	4	8	11	32
65+	240	4.7	21	1	2	3	6	10	14	21
GRAND TOTAL	707	4.0	18	1	2	2	5	8	11	24

530.10: ESOPHAGITIS NOS

Type of Patients	Observed Patients	Avg. Stay	Vari-ance	10th	25th	50th	75th	90th	95th	99th
1. SINGLE DX										
A. Not Operated										
0–19 Years	1	1.0	0	1	1	1	1	1	1	1
20–34	0									
35–49	1	1.0	0	1	1	1	1	1	1	1
50–64	1	1.0	0	1	1	1	1	1	1	1
65+	1	1.0	0	1	1	1	1	1	1	1
B. Operated										
0–19 Years	0									
20–34	0									
35–49	0									
50–64	0									
65+	0									
2. MULTIPLE DX										
A. Not Operated										
0–19 Years	26	3.4	7	1	1	3	5	5	11	11
20–34	75	2.2	2	1	1	2	3	3	5	6
35–49	167	2.7	5	1	1	2	3	5	6	11
50–64	218	2.9	5	1	1	2	4	6	7	10
65+	291	3.5	10	1	2	3	4	6	9	21
B. Operated										
0–19 Years	2	9.5	40	5	5	5	14	14	14	14
20–34	8	3.0	0	3	3	3	3	3	3	3
35–49	8	3.6	4	1	2	4	6	6	7	7
50–64	6	3.3	33	1	1	1	1	15	15	15
65+	3	4.3	6	2	2	4	7	7	7	7
SUBTOTALS:										
1. SINGLE DX										
A. Not Operated	4	1.0	0	1	1	1	1	1	1	1
B. Operated	0									
2. MULTIPLE DX										
A. Not Operated	777	3.0	7	1	1	2	4	6	7	11
B. Operated	20	4.2	16	1	1	3	6	7	15	15
1. SINGLE DX	4	1.0	0	1	1	1	1	1	1	1
2. MULTIPLE DX	797	3.1	7	1	1	2	4	6	7	14
A. NOT OPERATED	781	3.0	7	1	1	2	4	6	7	11
B. OPERATED	20	4.2	16	1	1	3	6	7	15	15
TOTAL										
0–19 Years	29	3.7	11	1	1	3	5	11	11	14
20–34	76	2.2	2	1	1	2	3	4	5	6
35–49	176	2.7	5	1	1	2	3	5	7	11
50–64	225	3.0	6	1	1	2	4	6	7	13
65+	295	3.5	10	1	2	3	4	6	9	21
GRAND TOTAL	801	3.1	7	1	1	2	4	6	7	14

530.11: REFLUX ESOPHAGITIS

Type of Patients	Observed Patients	Avg. Stay	Vari-ance	Percentiles 10th	25th	50th	75th	90th	95th	99th
1. SINGLE DX										
A. Not Operated										
0–19 Years	1	4.0	0	4	4	4	4	4	4	4
20–34	1	2.0	0	2	2	2	2	2	2	2
35–49	2	1.0	0	1	1	1	1	1	1	1
50–64	0									
65+	0									
B. Operated										
0–19 Years	2	2.5	<1	2	2	2	3	3	3	3
20–34	2	1.5	<1	1	1	1	2	2	2	2
35–49	2	2.5	4	1	1	4	4	4	4	4
50–64	5	2.2	<1	1	2	2	3	3	4	4
65+	0									
2. MULTIPLE DX										
A. Not Operated										
0–19 Years	33	3.6	13	1	2	3	4	6	14	18
20–34	69	2.6	6	1	1	2	3	5	7	15
35–49	203	3.5	15	1	2	3	4	6	8	15
50–64	259	3.2	5	1	2	3	4	6	7	12
65+	344	3.3	10	1	2	2	4	6	8	14
B. Operated										
0–19 Years	14	4.9	22	1	2	3	8	12	16	16
20–34	21	4.2	62	1	1	2	2	7	9	37
35–49	64	2.3	3	1	1	2	3	5	6	7
50–64	93	3.2	13	1	1	2	4	7	10	22
65+	49	3.4	9	1	2	2	5	9	11	12
SUBTOTALS:										
1. SINGLE DX										
A. Not Operated	4	2.0	2	1	1	1	2	4	4	4
B. Operated	11	2.2	<1	1	1	2	3	3	4	4
2. MULTIPLE DX										
A. Not Operated	908	3.3	10	1	2	2	4	6	8	14
B. Operated	241	3.2	15	1	1	2	4	7	10	19
1. SINGLE DX	15	2.1	1	1	1	2	3	4	4	4
2. MULTIPLE DX	1,149	3.2	11	1	1	2	4	6	8	15
A. NOT OPERATED	912	3.2	10	1	2	2	4	6	8	14
B. OPERATED	252	3.2	14	1	1	2	4	7	10	19
TOTAL										
0–19 Years	50	4.0	15	1	2	3	4	10	14	18
20–34	93	3.0	19	1	1	2	3	6	8	37
35–49	271	3.2	12	1	1	2	4	6	8	15
50–64	357	3.2	7	1	1	2	4	6	8	14
65+	393	3.3	10	1	2	2	4	6	8	14
GRAND TOTAL	1,164	3.2	11	1	1	2	4	6	8	15

530.12: ACUTE ESOPHAGITIS

Type of Patients	Observed Patients	Avg. Stay	Vari-ance	Percentiles 10th	25th	50th	75th	90th	95th	99th
1. SINGLE DX										
A. Not Operated										
0–19 Years	0									
20–34	0									
35–49	0									
50–64	0									
65+	0									
B. Operated										
0–19 Years	0									
20–34	0									
35–49	0									
50–64	0									
65+	0									
2. MULTIPLE DX										
A. Not Operated										
0–19 Years	7	2.6	3	1	1	3	3	6	6	6
20–34	23	2.7	1	1	2	3	4	4	4	5
35–49	59	2.8	4	1	1	2	4	6	8	8
50–64	74	2.8	5	1	1	2	3	5	6	16
65+	104	3.4	5	1	2	3	4	6	8	10
B. Operated										
0–19 Years	0									
20–34	1	5.0	0	5	5	5	5	5	5	5
35–49	0									
50–64	0									
65+	5	16.6	74	4	12	19	23	25	25	25
SUBTOTALS:										
1. SINGLE DX										
A. Not Operated	0									
B. Operated	0									
2. MULTIPLE DX										
A. Not Operated	267	3.0	4	1	1	3	4	6	7	10
B. Operated	6	14.6	82	4	5	12	23	25	25	25
1. SINGLE DX	0									
2. MULTIPLE DX	273	3.3	9	1	2	3	4	6	8	19
A. NOT OPERATED	267	3.0	4	1	1	3	4	6	7	10
B. OPERATED	6	14.6	82	4	5	12	23	25	25	25
TOTAL										
0–19 Years	7	2.6	3	1	1	3	3	6	6	6
20–34	24	2.8	2	1	2	3	4	4	5	5
35–49	59	2.8	4	1	1	2	4	6	8	8
50–64	74	2.8	5	1	1	2	3	5	6	16
65+	109	4.0	15	1	2	3	5	8	10	23
GRAND TOTAL	273	3.3	9	1	2	3	4	6	8	19

530.19: ESOPHAGITIS NEC

Type of Patients	Observed Patients	Avg. Stay	Vari-ance	Percentiles 10th	25th	50th	75th	90th	95th	99th
1. SINGLE DX										
A. Not Operated										
0–19 Years	4	2.0	<1	1	2	2	3	3	3	3
20–34	1	2.0	0	2	2	2	2	2	2	2
35–49	0									
50–64	1	4.0	0	4	4	4	4	4	4	4
65+	2	6.0	0	6	6	6	6	6	6	6
B. Operated										
0–19 Years	0									
20–34	0									
35–49	0									
50–64	0									
65+	0									
2. MULTIPLE DX										
A. Not Operated										
0–19 Years	60	3.3	14	1	1	2	3	6	11	22
20–34	183	3.4	14	1	2	3	4	6	8	16
35–49	417	3.4	7	1	2	3	4	7	8	14
50–64	579	3.8	9	1	2	3	5	7	10	16
65+	875	4.1	17	1	2	3	5	8	10	18
B. Operated										
0–19 Years	2	2.0	0	2	2	2	2	2	2	2
20–34	3	27.1	>999	3	3	5	73	73	73	73
35–49	11	16.5	543	1	1	6	24	61	62	62
50–64	18	8.9	44	4	4	7	13	20	23	23
65+	27	12.7	156	3	4	9	17	27	36	59
SUBTOTALS:										
1. SINGLE DX										
A. Not Operated	8	3.2	4	1	2	2	4	6	6	6
B. Operated	0									
2. MULTIPLE DX										
A. Not Operated	2,114	3.8	12	1	2	3	5	7	9	17
B. Operated	61	12.6	245	1	3	7	16	24	59	73
1. SINGLE DX	8	3.2	4	1	2	2	4	6	6	6
2. MULTIPLE DX	2,175	4.0	21	1	2	3	5	8	10	20
A. NOT OPERATED	2,122	3.8	12	1	2	3	5	7	9	17
B. OPERATED	61	12.6	245	1	3	7	16	24	59	73
TOTAL										
0–19 Years	66	3.2	13	1	1	2	3	6	8	22
20–34	187	3.8	39	1	2	3	4	6	9	42
35–49	428	3.7	24	1	2	3	4	7	9	18
50–64	598	3.9	11	1	2	3	5	7	10	19
65+	904	4.4	23	1	2	3	5	8	11	21
GRAND TOTAL	2,183	4.0	21	1	2	3	5	8	10	20

Length of Stay by Diagnosis and Operation, Western Region, 2008

Western Region, October 2006–September 2007 Data, by Diagnosis

530.20: ESOPH ULCER W/O BLEEDING

Type of Patients	Observed Patients	Avg. Stay	Vari-ance	Percentiles						
				10th	25th	50th	75th	90th	95th	99th
1. SINGLE DX										
A. *Not Operated*										
0–19 Years	0									
20–34	1	3.0	0	3	3	3	3	3	3	3
35–49	0									
50–64	0									
65+	0									
B. *Operated*										
0–19 Years	0									
20–34	0									
35–49	0									
50–64	0									
65+	0									
2. MULTIPLE DX										
A. *Not Operated*										
0–19 Years	14	2.9	4	1	1	3	3	4	9	9
20–34	69	2.9	4	1	2	3	3	6	7	11
35–49	105	3.1	3	1	2	3	4	6	7	8
50–64	155	4.5	47	1	2	3	5	8	11	42
65+	298	4.4	13	2	2	3	5	9	11	20
B. *Operated*										
0–19 Years	0									
20–34	0									
35–49	3	6.0	36	2	2	3	13	13	13	13
50–64	3	7.7	17	3	3	9	11	11	11	11
65+	2	9.0	8	7	7	7	11	11	11	11
SUBTOTALS:										
1. SINGLE DX										
A. *Not Operated*	1	3.0	0	3	3	3	3	3	3	3
B. *Operated*	0									
2. MULTIPLE DX										
A. *Not Operated*	641	4.0	19	1	2	3	5	7	9	19
B. *Operated*	8	7.4	18	2	3	7	11	13	13	13
1. SINGLE DX	1	3.0	0	3	3	3	3	3	3	3
2. MULTIPLE DX	649	4.1	19	1	2	3	5	8	10	19
A. NOT OPERATED	642	4.0	19	1	2	3	5	7	9	19
B. OPERATED	8	7.4	18	2	3	7	11	13	13	13
TOTAL										
0–19 Years	14	2.9	4	1	1	3	3	4	9	9
20–34	70	2.9	4	1	2	3	3	5	7	11
35–49	108	3.2	4	1	2	3	4	6	8	10
50–64	158	4.6	46	1	2	3	6	8	11	42
65+	300	4.4	14	2	2	3	5	9	11	19
GRAND TOTAL	650	4.1	19	1	2	3	5	8	10	19

530.21: ESOPH ULCER W BLEEDING

Type of Patients	Observed Patients	Avg. Stay	Vari-ance	Percentiles						
				10th	25th	50th	75th	90th	95th	99th
1. SINGLE DX										
A. *Not Operated*										
0–19 Years	0									
20–34	0									
35–49	0									
50–64	0									
65+	1	1.0	0	1	1	1	1	1	1	1
B. *Operated*										
0–19 Years	0									
20–34	0									
35–49	0									
50–64	0									
65+	0									
2. MULTIPLE DX										
A. *Not Operated*										
0–19 Years	3	3.7	4	2	2	3	6	6	6	6
20–34	72	2.8	6	1	1	2	3	4	5	16
35–49	276	3.2	7	1	2	3	4	6	8	12
50–64	500	3.8	11	1	2	3	5	7	9	15
65+	1,081	4.2	9	2	2	3	5	8	10	16
B. *Operated*										
0–19 Years	1	24.0	0	24	24	24	24	24	24	24
20–34	0									
35–49	5	7.6	13	4	5	7	9	13	13	13
50–64	10	12.3	113	3	6	9	12	38	38	38
65+	33	10.7	52	4	6	8	13	23	27	29
SUBTOTALS:										
1. SINGLE DX										
A. *Not Operated*	1	1.0	0	1	1	1	1	1	1	1
B. *Operated*	0									
2. MULTIPLE DX										
A. *Not Operated*	1,932	3.9	9	1	2	3	5	7	10	15
B. *Operated*	49	11.0	62	4	6	9	13	24	27	38
1. SINGLE DX	1	1.0	0	1	1	1	1	1	1	1
2. MULTIPLE DX	1,981	4.1	12	1	2	3	5	8	10	17
A. NOT OPERATED	1,933	3.9	9	1	2	3	5	7	10	15
B. OPERATED	49	11.0	62	4	6	9	13	24	27	38
TOTAL										
0–19 Years	4	8.7	105	2	3	6	6	24	24	24
20–34	72	2.8	6	1	1	2	3	4	5	16
35–49	281	3.3	8	1	2	3	4	7	8	13
50–64	510	3.9	14	1	2	3	5	7	10	20
65+	1,115	4.4	12	2	2	3	5	8	11	17
GRAND TOTAL	1,982	4.1	12	1	2	3	5	8	10	17

530.3: ESOPHAGEAL STRICTURE

Type of Patients	Observed Patients	Avg. Stay	Vari-ance	Percentiles						
				10th	25th	50th	75th	90th	95th	99th
1. SINGLE DX										
A. *Not Operated*										
0–19 Years	4	5.0	64	1	1	1	1	17	17	17
20–34	1	1.0	0	1	1	1	1	1	1	1
35–49	3	2.7	2	1	1	3	4	4	4	4
50–64	3	1.7	0	1	1	1	3	3	3	3
65+	2	1.0	0	1	1	1	1	1	1	1
B. *Operated*										
0–19 Years	1	1.0	0	1	1	1	1	1	1	1
20–34	0									
35–49	0									
50–64	0									
65+	0									
2. MULTIPLE DX										
A. *Not Operated*										
0–19 Years	14	4.1	13	1	1	3	7	9	13	13
20–34	34	3.4	5	1	2	3	5	5	8	8
35–49	101	3.5	7	1	2	3	5	7	9	12
50–64	217	3.9	20	1	3	3	4	8	11	23
65+	603	3.8	12	1	2	3	5	7	10	20
B. *Operated*										
0–19 Years	5	15.9	247	3	4	14	16	42	42	42
20–34	5	9.0	34	5	5	7	9	19	19	19
35–49	11	17.1	223	6	7	11	27	42	46	46
50–64	30	17.4	433	2	2	10	22	41	56	96
65+	29	9.0	49	2	4	8	10	17	22	34
SUBTOTALS:										
1. SINGLE DX										
A. *Not Operated*	13	2.8	19	1	1	1	3	4	17	17
B. *Operated*	1	1.0	0	1	1	1	1	1	1	1
2. MULTIPLE DX										
A. *Not Operated*	969	3.8	13	1	2	3	5	8	10	20
B. *Operated*	80	13.7	235	2	4	9	16	34	42	96
1. SINGLE DX	14	2.6	18	1	1	1	3	4	17	17
2. MULTIPLE DX	1,049	4.5	37	1	2	3	5	9	13	29
A. NOT OPERATED	982	3.8	13	1	2	3	5	8	10	20
B. OPERATED	81	13.5	234	2	4	9	16	34	42	96
TOTAL										
0–19 Years	24	6.6	83	1	1	3	7	16	17	42
20–34	40	4.1	11	1	2	3	6	8	8	19
35–49	115	4.7	42	1	2	3	6	9	12	42
50–64	250	5.5	87	1	3	3	5	11	18	51
65+	634	4.0	15	1	2	3	5	8	12	20
GRAND TOTAL	1,063	4.5	37	1	2	3	5	9	13	29

530.5: ESOPHAGEAL DYSKINESIA

Type of Patients	Observed Patients	Avg. Stay	Vari-ance	Percentiles						
				10th	25th	50th	75th	90th	95th	99th
1. SINGLE DX										
A. Not Operated										
0–19 Years	0									
20–34	0									
35–49	5	1.0	0	1	1	1	1	1	1	1
50–64	3	1.0	0	1	1	1	1	1	1	1
65+	0									
B. Operated										
0–19 Years	0									
20–34	0									
35–49	0									
50–64	0									
65+	0									
2. MULTIPLE DX										
A. Not Operated										
0–19 Years	9	5.0	19	1	1	4	8	12	12	12
20–34	23	1.7	1	1	1	1	2	3	4	4
35–49	117	2.0	4	1	1	1	2	4	4	12
50–64	227	2.4	9	1	1	1	3	5	7	13
65+	426	2.9	12	1	1	2	3	5	7	13
B. Operated										
0–19 Years	1	8.0	0	8	8	8	8	8	8	8
20–34	1	1.0	0	1	1	1	1	1	1	1
35–49	6	3.2	8	1	1	2	5	8	8	8
50–64	7	6.1	22	2	3	4	7	16	16	16
65+	10	8.1	89	1	2	6	10	33	33	33
SUBTOTALS:										
1. SINGLE DX										
A. Not Operated	8	1.0	0	1	1	1	1	1	1	1
B. Operated	0									
2. MULTIPLE DX										
A. Not Operated	802	2.6	10	1	1	2	3	5	7	13
B. Operated	25	6.1	46	1	2	4	7	12	16	33
1. SINGLE DX	**8**	**1.0**	**0**	**1**	**1**	**1**	**1**	**1**	**1**	**1**
2. MULTIPLE DX	**827**	**2.7**	**11**	**1**	**1**	**2**	**3**	**5**	**8**	**13**
A. NOT OPERATED	**810**	**2.6**	**10**	**1**	**1**	**2**	**3**	**5**	**7**	**13**
B. OPERATED	**25**	**6.1**	**46**	**1**	**2**	**4**	**7**	**12**	**16**	**33**
TOTAL										
0–19 Years	10	5.3	18	1	1	4	8	12	12	12
20–34	24	1.7	1	1	1	1	2	3	4	4
35–49	128	2.0	4	1	1	1	2	4	4	12
50–64	237	2.5	9	1	1	2	3	5	7	16
65+	436	3.0	14	1	1	2	3	5	8	16
GRAND TOTAL	**835**	**2.7**	**11**	**1**	**1**	**2**	**3**	**5**	**8**	**13**

530.6: ACQ ESOPH DIVERTICULUM

Type of Patients	Observed Patients	Avg. Stay	Vari-ance	Percentiles						
				10th	25th	50th	75th	90th	95th	99th
1. SINGLE DX										
A. Not Operated										
0–19 Years	0									
20–34	0									
35–49	1	1.0	0	1	1	1	1	1	1	1
50–64	2	1.0	0	1	1	1	1	1	1	1
65+	3	3.0	7	1	1	2	6	6	6	6
B. Operated										
0–19 Years	1	4.0	0	4	4	4	4	4	4	4
20–34	0									
35–49	3	1.0	0	1	1	1	1	1	1	1
50–64	3	2.7	4	1	1	2	5	5	5	5
65+	8	1.3	<1	1	1	1	1	2	2	2
2. MULTIPLE DX										
A. Not Operated										
0–19 Years	0									
20–34	0									
35–49	4	2.0	1	1	1	1	3	3	3	3
50–64	18	2.6	7	1	1	1	3	8	10	10
65+	90	3.8	17	1	1	3	5	9	12	27
B. Operated										
0–19 Years	0									
20–34	0									
35–49	7	4.0	24	2	2	2	3	15	15	15
50–64	73	4.0	20	1	1	3	5	10	16	>99
65+	192	4.0	17	1	1	2	5	10	15	20
SUBTOTALS:										
1. SINGLE DX										
A. Not Operated	6	2.0	4	1	1	1	2	6	6	6
B. Operated	15	1.7	2	1	1	1	2	4	5	5
2. MULTIPLE DX										
A. Not Operated	112	3.5	15	1	1	2	5	8	12	15
B. Operated	272	4.0	18	1	1	2	5	10	15	21
1. SINGLE DX	**21**	**1.8**	**2**	**1**	**1**	**1**	**2**	**4**	**5**	**6**
2. MULTIPLE DX	**384**	**3.9**	**17**	**1**	**1**	**2**	**5**	**10**	**13**	**21**
A. NOT OPERATED	**118**	**3.5**	**15**	**1**	**1**	**2**	**5**	**8**	**12**	**15**
B. OPERATED	**287**	**3.9**	**17**	**1**	**1**	**2**	**5**	**10**	**15**	**21**
TOTAL										
0–19 Years	1	4.0	0	4	4	4	4	4	4	4
20–34	0									
35–49	15	2.7	12	1	1	2	3	3	15	15
50–64	96	3.6	17	1	1	2	4	8	15	>99
65+	293	3.9	17	1	1	2	5	9	12	20
GRAND TOTAL	**405**	**3.8**	**17**	**1**	**1**	**2**	**5**	**9**	**12**	**21**

530.7: MALLORY-WEISS SYNDROME

Type of Patients	Observed Patients	Avg. Stay	Vari-ance	Percentiles						
				10th	25th	50th	75th	90th	95th	99th
1. SINGLE DX										
A. Not Operated										
0–19 Years	6	1.0	0	1	1	1	1	1	1	1
20–34	1	2.0	0	2	2	2	2	2	2	2
35–49	2	1.5	<1	1	1	2	2	2	2	2
50–64	4	2.0	1	1	1	3	3	3	3	3
65+	0									
B. Operated										
0–19 Years	0									
20–34	0									
35–49	0									
50–64	0									
65+	0									
2. MULTIPLE DX										
A. Not Operated										
0–19 Years	59	1.8	2	1	1	1	2	3	5	9
20–34	402	2.2	2	1	1	2	3	4	5	7
35–49	757	3.0	10	1	2	2	3	5	7	13
50–64	872	3.5	9	1	2	3	4	7	9	16
65+	1,050	3.6	8	1	2	3	4	6	8	14
B. Operated										
0–19 Years	0									
20–34	4	7.0	31	2	2	6	9	14	14	14
35–49	11	7.9	13	4	5	7	11	11	15	15
50–64	12	10.0	67	4	5	8	11	21	31	31
65+	27	10.2	73	3	6	7	12	21	33	36
SUBTOTALS:										
1. SINGLE DX										
A. Not Operated	13	1.5	<1	1	1	1	2	3	3	3
B. Operated	0									
2. MULTIPLE DX										
A. Not Operated	3,140	3.2	8	1	2	2	4	6	8	14
B. Operated	54	9.5	55	3	5	7	11	20	31	36
1. SINGLE DX	**13**	**1.5**	**<1**	**1**	**1**	**1**	**2**	**3**	**3**	**3**
2. MULTIPLE DX	**3,194**	**3.3**	**9**	**1**	**2**	**3**	**4**	**6**	**8**	**15**
A. NOT OPERATED	**3,153**	**3.2**	**8**	**1**	**2**	**2**	**4**	**6**	**8**	**14**
B. OPERATED	**54**	**9.5**	**55**	**3**	**5**	**7**	**11**	**20**	**31**	**36**
TOTAL										
0–19 Years	65	1.8	2	1	1	1	2	3	4	9
20–34	407	2.2	2	1	1	2	3	3	5	8
35–49	770	3.1	10	1	2	2	4	5	8	13
50–64	888	3.5	10	1	2	3	4	7	9	18
65+	1,077	3.7	10	1	2	3	4	7	9	19
GRAND TOTAL	**3,207**	**3.3**	**9**	**1**	**2**	**3**	**4**	**6**	**8**	**15**

Length of Stay by Diagnosis and Operation, Western Region, 2008

Western Region, October 2006–September 2007 Data, by Diagnosis

530.81: ESOPHAGEAL REFLUX

Type of Patients	Observed Patients	Avg. Stay	Variance	10th	25th	50th	75th	90th	95th	99th
1. SINGLE DX										
A. Not Operated										
0–19 Years	274	1.9	3	1	1	2	2	3	4	11
20–34	7	1.1	<1	1	1	1	1	2	2	2
35–49	34	1.3	<1	1	1	1	1	2	3	3
50–64	32	1.3	<1	1	1	1	1	2	2	4
65+	10	1.2	<1	1	1	1	1	2	2	2
B. Operated										
0–19 Years	29	2.0	<1	1	1	2	3	3	3	4
20–34	33	1.6	<1	1	1	1	2	3	4	4
35–49	41	1.6	<1	1	1	1	2	3	3	4
50–64	31	1.7	<1	1	1	2	2	3	3	4
65+	4	1.5	<1	1	1	2	2	2	3	2
2. MULTIPLE DX										
A. Not Operated										
0–19 Years	901	3.1	17	1	2	2	3	6	9	16
20–34	214	2.1	4	1	1	1	2	4	5	11
35–49	1,180	1.8	2	1	1	1	2	3	4	8
50–64	2,186	1.7	2	1	1	1	2	3	4	6
65+	2,590	2.0	2	1	1	1	2	4	5	8
B. Operated										
0–19 Years	305	7.3	88	2	2	4	8	17	25	52
20–34	173	2.1	4	1	1	2	2	4	5	17
35–49	543	2.4	7	1	1	2	3	4	6	10
50–64	743	2.7	8	1	2	2	3	5	8	15
65+	365	3.2	12	1	2	2	4	6	9	24
SUBTOTALS:										
1. SINGLE DX										
A. Not Operated	357	1.8	2	1	1	1	2	3	4	6
B. Operated	138	1.7	<1	1	1	1	2	3	3	4
2. MULTIPLE DX										
A. Not Operated	7,071	2.0	4	1	1	1	2	4	5	10
B. Operated	2,129	3.3	22	1	1	2	3	6	10	25
1. SINGLE DX	495	1.8	2	1	1	1	2	3	4	5
2. MULTIPLE DX	9,200	2.3	9	1	1	2	3	4	6	13
A. NOT OPERATED	7,428	2.0	4	1	1	1	2	4	5	10
B. OPERATED	2,267	3.2	21	1	1	2	3	6	9	25
TOTAL										
0–19 Years	1,509	3.7	32	1	2	2	4	8	12	26
20–34	427	2.0	4	1	1	1	2	4	5	11
35–49	1,798	2.0	4	1	1	1	2	4	5	9
50–64	2,992	2.0	3	1	1	1	2	4	5	9
65+	2,969	2.1	4	1	1	1	2	4	5	10
GRAND TOTAL	9,695	2.3	8	1	1	2	2	4	6	13

530.82: ESOPHAGEAL HEMORRHAGE

Type of Patients	Observed Patients	Avg. Stay	Variance	10th	25th	50th	75th	90th	95th	99th
1. SINGLE DX										
A. Not Operated										
0–19 Years	0									
20–34	0									
35–49	0									
50–64	0									
65+	0									
B. Operated										
0–19 Years	0									
20–34	0									
35–49	0									
50–64	0									
65+	0									
2. MULTIPLE DX										
A. Not Operated										
0–19 Years	5	3.2	1	2	2	4	4	4	4	4
20–34	38	2.4	2	1	1	2	3	5	5	7
35–49	113	3.7	10	1	2	3	4	5	8	20
50–64	201	3.9	10	1	2	3	5	5	10	17
65+	382	4.3	12	2	2	3	5	8	11	19
B. Operated										
0–19 Years	1	12.0	0	12	12	12	12	12	12	12
20–34	0									
35–49	5	10.0	56	2	6	10	10	22	22	22
50–64	4	11.2	33	6	6	12	12	19	19	19
65+	9	12.6	109	3	7	9	14	34	34	34
SUBTOTALS:										
1. SINGLE DX										
A. Not Operated	0									
B. Operated	0									
2. MULTIPLE DX										
A. Not Operated	739	4.0	11	1	2	3	5	7	10	18
B. Operated	19	11.6	67	3	6	10	14	25	34	34
1. SINGLE DX	0									
2. MULTIPLE DX	758	4.2	14	1	2	3	5	8	11	20
A. NOT OPERATED	739	4.0	11	1	2	3	5	7	10	18
B. OPERATED	19	11.6	67	3	6	10	14	25	34	34
TOTAL										
0–19 Years	6	4.7	14	2	2	4	4	8	12	26
20–34	38	2.4	2	1	1	2	3	4	5	7
35–49	118	3.9	13	1	2	3	4	6	10	21
50–64	205	4.0	12	1	2	3	5	7	11	18
65+	391	4.5	16	2	2	3	5	8	13	25
GRAND TOTAL	758	4.2	14	1	2	3	5	8	11	20

530.85: BARRETT'S ESOPHAGUS

Type of Patients	Observed Patients	Avg. Stay	Variance	10th	25th	50th	75th	90th	95th	99th
1. SINGLE DX										
A. Not Operated										
0–19 Years	0									
20–34	0									
35–49	0									
50–64	0									
65+	0									
B. Operated										
0–19 Years	0									
20–34	0									
35–49	0									
50–64	0									
65+	0									
2. MULTIPLE DX										
A. Not Operated										
0–19 Years	2	10.0	97	3	3	10	17	17	17	17
20–34	26	2.9	2	1	2	3	4	5	5	5
35–49	97	3.4	4	1	2	3	4	6	7	12
50–64	157	3.5	7	1	2	3	5	7	8	15
65+	251	3.4	7	1	2	3	4	6	8	14
B. Operated										
0–19 Years	2	3.5	12	1	1	1	6	6	6	6
20–34	3	1.3	<1	1	1	1	2	2	2	2
35–49	12	7.8	149	1	1	3	8	16	44	44
50–64	31	6.1	107	1	1	2	9	13	25	53
65+	28	9.7	120	2	2	7	10	19	37	51
SUBTOTALS:										
1. SINGLE DX										
A. Not Operated	0									
B. Operated	0									
2. MULTIPLE DX										
A. Not Operated	533	3.4	7	1	2	3	4	6	8	14
B. Operated	76	7.4	113	1	2	3	8	16	37	53
1. SINGLE DX	0									
2. MULTIPLE DX	609	3.9	21	1	2	3	4	7	10	19
A. NOT OPERATED	533	3.4	7	1	2	3	4	6	8	14
B. OPERATED	76	7.4	113	1	2	3	8	16	37	53
TOTAL										
0–19 Years	4	6.7	51	1	3	3	17	17	17	17
20–34	29	2.7	2	1	2	3	3	5	5	5
35–49	109	3.9	21	1	2	3	4	7	8	16
50–64	188	3.9	24	1	2	3	5	7	11	25
65+	279	4.1	22	2	2	3	5	7	10	23
GRAND TOTAL	609	3.9	21	1	2	3	4	7	10	19

531: GASTRIC ULCER

Type of Patients	Observed Patients	Avg. Stay	Variance	Percentiles 10th	25th	50th	75th	90th	95th	99th
1. SINGLE DX										
A. Not Operated										
0–19 Years	6	2.7	3	1	1	2	4	5	5	5
20–34	4	3.3	7	1	1	3	7	7	7	7
35–49	11	1.9	<1	1	1	2	3	3	3	3
50–64	12	2.9	3	2	2	3	3	4	8	8
65+	7	3.7	14	1	1	2	6	11	11	11
B. Operated										
0–19 Years	2	3.5	<1	3	3	4	4	4	4	4
20–34	7	4.6	1	3	4	4	6	6	6	6
35–49	6	5.5	<1	5	5	5	6	6	6	6
50–64	8	6.0	3	4	5	6	7	8	8	8
65+	0									
2. MULTIPLE DX										
A. Not Operated										
0–19 Years	60	3.5	8	1	2	3	4	6	8	16
20–34	439	2.9	4	1	2	2	3	5	7	12
35–49	1,435	3.2	7	1	2	3	4	6	7	13
50–64	3,134	3.3	7	1	2	3	4	6	8	14
65+	6,990	3.8	8	2	2	3	5	7	9	15
B. Operated										
0–19 Years	7	7.4	29	4	4	5	9	19	19	19
20–34	81	7.7	50	4	4	6	8	10	22	43
35–49	201	9.5	57	4	5	7	11	19	24	40
50–64	382	12.0	119	4	6	8	14	23	35	56
65+	526	12.3	84	5	7	10	15	22	28	47
SUBTOTALS:										
1. SINGLE DX										
A. Not Operated	40	2.8	4	1	1	2	3	5	7	11
B. Operated	23	5.2	2	4	4	5	6	7	8	8
2. MULTIPLE DX										
A. Not Operated	12,058	3.6	8	1	2	3	4	6	8	15
B. Operated	1,197	11.4	90	4	6	8	14	21	29	50
1. SINGLE DX	63	3.7	5	1	2	3	5	6	8	11
2. MULTIPLE DX	13,255	4.3	20	1	2	3	5	8	11	23
A. NOT OPERATED	12,098	3.6	8	1	2	3	4	6	8	15
B. OPERATED	1,220	11.3	89	4	6	8	14	21	28	49
TOTAL										
0–19 Years	75	3.8	10	1	2	3	4	7	9	19
20–34	531	3.7	14	1	2	3	4	7	8	20
35–49	1,653	3.9	18	1	2	3	4	7	10	21
50–64	3,536	4.3	26	1	2	3	5	8	12	26
65+	7,523	4.4	18	2	2	3	5	8	11	22
GRAND TOTAL	13,318	4.3	20	1	2	3	5	8	11	22

531.00: AGU W HEMORRHAGE S OBSTR

Type of Patients	Observed Patients	Avg. Stay	Variance	Percentiles 10th	25th	50th	75th	90th	95th	99th
1. SINGLE DX										
A. Not Operated										
0–19 Years	0									
20–34	0									
35–49	0									
50–64	2	5.0	18	2	2	8	8	8	8	8
65+	2	1.5	<1	1	1	2	2	2	2	2
B. Operated										
0–19 Years	0									
20–34	0									
35–49	0									
50–64	0									
65+	0									
2. MULTIPLE DX										
A. Not Operated										
0–19 Years	5	3.6	<1	3	3	3	4	5	5	5
20–34	50	2.5	1	1	2	2	3	4	5	6
35–49	166	2.9	3	1	2	3	4	5	6	10
50–64	422	3.4	6	1	2	3	4	6	8	13
65+	902	4.0	7	2	2	3	5	7	9	16
B. Operated										
0–19 Years	0									
20–34	2	22.1	282	10	10	34	34	34	34	34
35–49	4	11.0	9	7	11	12	14	14	14	14
50–64	18	16.1	173	5	8	11	19	31	56	56
65+	30	12.3	266	6	7	9	12	13	17	97
SUBTOTALS:										
1. SINGLE DX										
A. Not Operated	4	3.3	10	1	2	2	8	8	8	8
B. Operated	0									
2. MULTIPLE DX										
A. Not Operated	1,545	3.7	7	2	2	3	4	7	9	15
B. Operated	54	13.8	213	6	7	10	13	29	34	97
1. SINGLE DX	4	3.3	10	1	2	2	8	8	8	8
2. MULTIPLE DX	1,599	4.0	17	2	2	3	5	7	10	16
A. NOT OPERATED	1,549	3.7	7	2	2	3	4	7	9	15
B. OPERATED	54	13.8	213	6	7	10	13	29	34	97
TOTAL										
0–19 Years	5	3.6	<1	3	3	3	4	5	5	5
20–34	52	3.2	21	1	2	2	3	5	6	34
35–49	170	3.1	5	1	2	3	4	6	7	12
50–64	442	3.9	19	1	2	3	4	8	9	20
65+	934	4.3	18	2	2	3	5	8	10	16
GRAND TOTAL	1,603	4.0	17	2	2	3	5	7	10	16

531.30: ACUTE GASTRIC ULCER NOS

Type of Patients	Observed Patients	Avg. Stay	Variance	Percentiles 10th	25th	50th	75th	90th	95th	99th
1. SINGLE DX										
A. Not Operated										
0–19 Years	1	1.0	0	1	1	1	1	1	1	1
20–34	0									
35–49	0									
50–64	0									
65+										
B. Operated										
0–19 Years	0									
20–34	0									
35–49	0									
50–64	0									
65+	0									
2. MULTIPLE DX										
A. Not Operated										
0–19 Years	1	4.0	0	4	4	4	4	4	4	4
20–34	14	3.8	9	1	2	3	5	6	12	12
35–49	37	3.3	5	1	2	3	4	7	9	9
50–64	35	3.0	3	1	2	2	4	5	6	9
65+	74	3.5	3	2	2	3	4	6	7	10
B. Operated										
0–19 Years	0									
20–34	2	3.0	0	3	3	3	3	3	3	3
35–49	1	21.0	0	21	21	21	21	21	21	21
50–64	4	7.3	62	2	4	4	19	19	19	19
65+	0									
SUBTOTALS:										
1. SINGLE DX										
A. Not Operated	1	1.0	0	1	1	1	1	1	1	1
B. Operated	0									
2. MULTIPLE DX										
A. Not Operated	161	3.4	4	1	2	3	4	6	7	10
B. Operated	7	8.0	68	2	3	4	19	21	21	21
1. SINGLE DX	1	1.0	0	1	1	1	1	1	1	1
2. MULTIPLE DX	168	3.6	7	1	2	3	4	6	8	19
A. NOT OPERATED	162	3.4	4	1	2	3	4	6	7	10
B. OPERATED	7	8.0	68	2	3	4	19	21	21	21
TOTAL										
0–19 Years	2	2.5	4	1	1	3	4	4	4	4
20–34	16	3.7	8	1	2	3	5	5	12	12
35–49	38	3.8	13	1	2	3	4	8	9	21
50–64	39	3.4	10	2	2	3	4	5	9	19
65+	74	3.5	3	2	2	3	4	6	7	10
GRAND TOTAL	169	3.6	7	2	2	3	4	6	8	19

Length of Stay by Diagnosis and Operation, Western Region, 2008

Western Region, October 2006–September 2007 Data, by Diagnosis

531.40: CGU W HEMOR W/O OBSTRUCT

Type of Patients	Observed Patients	Avg. Stay	Vari-ance	10th	25th	50th	75th	90th	95th	99th
1. SINGLE DX										
A. *Not Operated*										
0–19 Years	1	3.0	0	3	3	3	3	3	3	3
20–34	1	2.0	0	2	2	2	2	2	2	2
35–49	5	1.6	<1	1	1	2	2	2	2	2
50–64	7	2.4	<1	1	2	3	3	3	4	4
65+	5	4.6	17	1	1	4	6	11	11	11
B. *Operated*										
0–19 Years	0									
20–34	0									
35–49	0									
50–64	1	4.0	0	4	4	4	4	4	4	4
65+	0									
2. MULTIPLE DX										
A. *Not Operated*										
0–19 Years	25	3.0	9	1	2	2	3	5	5	16
20–34	226	2.7	4	1	2	2	3	4	7	8
35–49	853	3.1	9	1	2	2	3	6	7	13
50–64	2,127	3.2	6	1	2	3	4	6	8	14
65+	5,158	3.8	9	1	2	3	4	7	9	15
B. *Operated*										
0–19 Years	0									
20–34	7	8.9	15	5	6	8	10	17	17	17
35–49	19	13.6	123	4	7	9	19	29	49	49
50–64	78	14.5	169	4	6	11	19	34	46	70
65+	162	12.3	60	5	7	11	16	22	27	46
SUBTOTALS:										
1. SINGLE DX										
A. *Not Operated*	19	2.8	6	1	1	2	3	3	3	11
B. *Operated*	1	4.0	0	4	4	4	4	4	4	4
2. MULTIPLE DX										
A. *Not Operated*	8,389	3.5	8	1	2	3	4	6	8	14
B. *Operated*	266	13.0	96	4	6	11	17	23	29	49
1. SINGLE DX	20	2.8	5	1	1	2	3	4	6	11
2. MULTIPLE DX	8,655	3.8	13	1	2	3	4	7	9	19
A. NOT OPERATED	8,408	3.5	8	1	2	3	4	6	8	14
B. OPERATED	267	12.9	96	4	6	10	17	23	29	49
TOTAL										
0–19 Years	26	3.0	8	1	2	2	3	5	5	16
20–34	234	2.9	5	1	2	2	3	5	7	12
35–49	877	3.3	14	1	2	2	4	6	8	19
50–64	2,213	3.6	16	1	2	3	4	6	9	19
65+	5,325	4.0	12	1	2	3	5	7	10	19
GRAND TOTAL	8,675	3.8	13	1	2	3	4	7	9	19

531.50: CGU W PERF W/O OBSTRUCT

Type of Patients	Observed Patients	Avg. Stay	Vari-ance	10th	25th	50th	75th	90th	95th	99th
1. SINGLE DX										
A. *Not Operated*										
0–19 Years	1	5.0	0	5	5	5	5	5	5	5
20–34	0									
35–49	0									
50–64	0									
65+	0									
B. *Operated*										
0–19 Years	2	3.5	<1	3	3	4	4	4	4	4
20–34	5	4.0	<1	3	4	4	4	5	5	5
35–49	5	5.4	<1	5	5	5	6	6	6	6
50–64	4	7.0	1	6	6	6	8	8	8	8
65+	0									
2. MULTIPLE DX										
A. *Not Operated*										
0–19 Years	0									
20–34	1	9.0	0	9	9	9	9	9	9	9
35–49	6	3.2	2	1	3	3	4	5	6	7
50–64	13	4.5	2	3	4	5	5	6	7	7
65+	18	5.5	17	2	3	5	7	19	>99	>99
B. *Operated*										
0–19 Years	4	5.0	2	4	4	5	5	7	7	7
20–34	48	6.7	29	4	4	5	7	7	18	35
35–49	96	8.1	46	4	5	6	8	15	20	51
50–64	170	9.8	52	4	6	7	11	18	23	43
65+	183	11.8	67	5	7	9	14	21	29	50
SUBTOTALS:										
1. SINGLE DX										
A. *Not Operated*	1	5.0	0	5	5	5	5	5	5	5
B. *Operated*	16	5.1	2	3	4	5	6	8	8	8
2. MULTIPLE DX										
A. *Not Operated*	38	4.9	10	2	3	5	6	9	19	>99
B. *Operated*	501	9.9	56	4	6	9	11	18	25	41
1. SINGLE DX	17	5.1	2	3	4	5	6	8	8	8
2. MULTIPLE DX	539	9.5	55	4	5	7	11	18	24	43
A. NOT OPERATED	39	4.9	10	2	3	5	6	9	19	>99
B. OPERATED	517	9.7	55	4	5	7	11	18	25	41
TOTAL										
0–19 Years	7	4.6	2	3	4	4	5	7	7	7
20–34	54	6.5	27	4	4	5	7	9	18	35
35–49	107	7.7	43	3	5	6	8	15	19	34
50–64	187	9.4	49	4	5	7	10	18	23	43
65+	201	11.2	65	5	6	9	14	21	29	50
GRAND TOTAL	556	9.4	54	4	5	7	11	18	24	43

531.90: GASTRIC ULCER NOS

Type of Patients	Observed Patients	Avg. Stay	Vari-ance	10th	25th	50th	75th	90th	95th	99th
1. SINGLE DX										
A. *Not Operated*										
0–19 Years	3	2.3	2	1	1	2	4	4	4	4
20–34	1	1.0	0	1	1	1	1	1	1	1
35–49	5	2.0	1	1	1	2	3	3	3	3
50–64	3	2.7	<1	2	2	3	3	3	3	3
65+	0									
B. *Operated*										
0–19 Years	0									
20–34	1	6.0	0	6	6	6	6	6	6	6
35–49	0									
50–64	0									
65+	0									
2. MULTIPLE DX										
A. *Not Operated*										
0–19 Years	26	3.5	4	1	2	3	4	7	7	9
20–34	127	3.1	4	1	2	2	4	6	7	11
35–49	318	3.2	4	1	2	3	4	6	7	10
50–64	430	3.3	6	1	2	3	4	6	7	12
65+	639	3.7	7	1	2	3	4	7	8	13
B. *Operated*										
0–19 Years	0									
20–34	5	3.5	<1	3	3	3	4	4	4	4
35–49	9	7.6	21	3	5	6	9	18	18	18
50–64	18	8.9	54	1	4	7	12	22	27	27
65+	19	8.3	17	3	5	8	12	14	18	18
SUBTOTALS:										
1. SINGLE DX										
A. *Not Operated*	12	2.2	1	1	1	2	3	3	4	4
B. *Operated*	1	6.0	0	6	6	6	6	6	6	6
2. MULTIPLE DX										
A. *Not Operated*	1,540	3.4	6	1	2	3	4	6	7	12
B. *Operated*	48	8.2	31	3	4	7	11	18	19	27
1. SINGLE DX	13	2.5	2	1	1	2	3	4	6	6
2. MULTIPLE DX	1,588	3.6	7	1	2	3	4	6	8	14
A. NOT OPERATED	1,552	3.4	6	1	2	3	4	6	7	12
B. OPERATED	49	8.1	30	3	4	7	10	18	19	27
TOTAL										
0–19 Years	29	3.3	4	1	2	3	4	7	7	9
20–34	131	3.2	4	1	2	2	4	6	7	11
35–49	332	3.3	5	1	2	3	4	6	7	11
50–64	451	3.5	9	1	2	3	4	6	8	18
65+	658	3.8	7	1	2	3	5	7	9	15
GRAND TOTAL	1,601	3.6	7	1	2	3	4	6	8	14

Length of Stay by Diagnosis and Operation, Western Region, 2008

532: DUODENAL ULCER

Type of Patients	Observed Patients	Avg. Stay	Variance	10th	25th	50th	75th	90th	95th	99th
1. SINGLE DX										
A. Not Operated										
0–19 Years	2	4.0	8	2	2	4	6	6	6	6
20–34	17	2.0	2	1	1	2	2	4	5	5
35–49	16	2.6	1	1	2	3	3	4	5	5
50–64	13	2.0	1	1	1	2	2	4	4	4
65+	8	2.4	3	1	1	2	3	6	6	6
B. Operated										
0–19 Years	2	6.0	2	5	5	6	7	7	7	7
20–34	7	5.4	2	4	4	5	7	7	7	7
35–49	7	4.9	<1	4	4	5	6	6	6	6
50–64	14	5.3	5	3	4	5	7	8	11	11
65+	2	5.5	5	4	4	6	7	7	7	7
2. MULTIPLE DX										
A. Not Operated										
0–19 Years	62	3.0	3	1	2	2	4	6	6	8
20–34	479	2.7	3	1	2	2	3	5	6	10
35–49	1,144	3.2	5	1	2	3	4	6	7	12
50–64	2,237	3.6	10	1	2	3	4	6	9	14
65+	4,343	4.3	10	2	2	3	5	8	10	17
B. Operated										
0–19 Years	18	7.0	10	4	5	6	10	12	14	14
20–34	88	7.5	64	4	5	6	8	9	15	61
35–49	263	8.5	50	4	5	6	10	15	22	58
50–64	416	13.4	169	5	6	9	15	26	42	82
65+	661	12.3	70	5	7	10	15	23	28	44
SUBTOTALS:										
1. SINGLE DX										
A. Not Operated	56	2.3	2	1	1	2	3	4	5	6
B. Operated	32	5.3	3	4	4	5	6	7	8	11
2. MULTIPLE DX										
A. Not Operated	8,265	3.8	9	1	2	3	5	7	9	16
B. Operated	1,446	11.6	98	5	6	9	14	21	29	61
1. SINGLE DX	88	3.4	4	1	2	3	5	6	7	11
2. MULTIPLE DX	9,711	5.0	30	2	2	3	6	10	14	27
A. NOT OPERATED	8,321	3.8	9	1	2	3	5	7	9	16
B. OPERATED	1,478	11.4	96	4	6	9	13	21	28	61
TOTAL										
0–19 Years	84	4.0	7	1	2	3	5	7	10	14
20–34	591	3.4	15	1	2	3	4	6	8	14
35–49	1,430	4.2	18	1	2	3	5	8	11	21
50–64	2,680	5.1	47	2	3	4	6	10	14	36
65+	5,014	5.3	25	2	3	4	6	11	15	25
GRAND TOTAL	9,799	5.0	30	2	2	3	6	10	14	27

532.00: AC DU W HEMOR W/O OBSTR

Type of Patients	Observed Patients	Avg. Stay	Variance	10th	25th	50th	75th	90th	95th	99th
1. SINGLE DX										
A. Not Operated										
0–19 Years	0									
20–34	3	1.0	0	1	1	1	1	1	1	1
35–49	4	2.8	3	1	1	3	3	5	5	5
50–64	2	1.5	<1	1	1	1	2	2	2	2
65+	3	1.3	<1	1	1	1	2	2	2	2
B. Operated										
0–19 Years	0									
20–34	0									
35–49	0									
50–64	0									
65+	0									
2. MULTIPLE DX										
A. Not Operated										
0–19 Years	8	2.8	1	2	2	2	3	5	5	5
20–34	68	2.5	2	1	2	2	3	5	5	7
35–49	152	3.1	5	1	2	3	4	6	6	13
50–64	300	3.5	9	1	2	3	4	6	9	14
65+	635	4.6	12	2	3	4	6	8	11	17
B. Operated										
0–19 Years	0									
20–34	3	6.3	9	3	3	7	9	9	9	9
35–49	7	11.1	18	6	6	10	16	16	16	16
50–64	33	12.3	52	6	9	11	13	21	25	42
65+	56	11.8	43	5	7	10	15	20	25	35
SUBTOTALS:										
1. SINGLE DX										
A. Not Operated	12	1.8	1	1	1	1	2	3	5	5
B. Operated	0									
2. MULTIPLE DX										
A. Not Operated	1,163	4.0	10	2	2	3	5	7	9	16
B. Operated	99	11.8	43	5	7	10	14	20	25	42
1. SINGLE DX	12	1.8	1	1	1	1	2	3	5	5
2. MULTIPLE DX	1,262	4.6	17	2	2	3	5	9	13	23
A. NOT OPERATED	1,175	4.0	10	2	2	3	5	7	9	16
B. OPERATED	99	11.8	43	5	7	10	14	20	25	42
TOTAL										
0–19 Years	8	2.8	1	2	2	2	3	5	5	5
20–34	74	2.6	3	1	2	2	3	4	6	9
35–49	163	3.5	8	1	2	3	4	6	10	16
50–64	335	4.4	20	1	2	3	5	9	13	24
65+	694	5.2	18	2	3	4	6	10	14	23
GRAND TOTAL	1,274	4.6	17	2	2	3	5	9	13	23

532.40: CHR DU W HEMOR W/O OBSTR

Type of Patients	Observed Patients	Avg. Stay	Variance	10th	25th	50th	75th	90th	95th	99th
1. SINGLE DX										
A. Not Operated										
0–19 Years	2	4.0	8	2	2	4	6	6	6	6
20–34	7	1.9	1	1	1	2	2	4	4	4
35–49	9	2.7	1	1	2	2	3	4	4	4
50–64	7	2.1	2	1	1	3	4	4	4	4
65+	4	3.5	3	2	3	3	5	6	6	6
B. Operated										
0–19 Years	0									
20–34	0									
35–49	0									
50–64	0									
65+	0									
2. MULTIPLE DX										
A. Not Operated										
0–19 Years	36	3.1	3	2	2	3	4	4	6	6
20–34	336	2.6	2	1	2	2	3	4	6	8
35–49	750	3.0	4	1	2	2	4	5	7	10
50–64	1,547	3.5	11	1	2	3	4	6	8	14
65+	3,079	4.2	9	2	2	3	5	8	10	17
B. Operated										
0–19 Years	7	10.0	0	10	10	10	10	10	10	10
20–34	7	9.1	27	5	5	7	9	18	18	18
35–49	27	11.7	129	3	5	9	13	20	30	58
50–64	83	15.4	175	6	9	11	18	27	43	94
65+	192	12.4	62	4	7	11	16	21	25	44
SUBTOTALS:										
1. SINGLE DX										
A. Not Operated	29	2.6	2	1	1	2	3	4	6	6
B. Operated	0									
2. MULTIPLE DX										
A. Not Operated	5,748	3.8	9	2	2	3	5	7	9	15
B. Operated	310	13.1	99	4	7	11	16	22	30	48
1. SINGLE DX	29	2.6	2	1	1	2	3	4	6	6
2. MULTIPLE DX	6,058	4.2	18	1	2	3	5	8	11	20
A. NOT OPERATED	5,777	3.8	9	1	2	3	4	7	9	15
B. OPERATED	310	13.1	99	4	7	11	16	22	30	48
TOTAL										
0–19 Years	39	3.3	4	1	2	3	3	5	6	10
20–34	350	2.7	3	1	2	2	3	3	6	9
35–49	786	3.3	10	1	2	3	4	6	8	13
50–64	1,637	4.1	26	2	2	3	4	8	11	24
65+	3,275	4.7	16	2	2	4	5	9	12	21
GRAND TOTAL	6,087	4.2	18	1	2	3	5	8	11	20

Length of Stay by Diagnosis and Operation, Western Region, 2008

Western Region, October 2006–September 2007 Data, by Diagnosis

532.50: CHR DU W PERF W/O OBSTR

Type of Patients	Observed Patients	Avg. Stay	Vari-ance	10th	25th	50th	75th	90th	95th	99th
1. SINGLE DX										
A. Not Operated										
0–19 Years	0									
20–34	2	1.5	<1	1	1	2	2	2	2	2
35–49	2	2.0	2	1	1	2	3	3	3	3
50–64	1	3.0	0	3	3	3	3	3	3	3
65+	0									
B. Operated										
0–19 Years	2	6.0	2	5	5	6	7	7	7	7
20–34	6	5.7	1	4	4	6	7	7	7	7
35–49	6	5.0	<1	4	4	5	6	6	6	6
50–64	11	5.3	6	3	3	5	7	8	11	11
65+	0									
2. MULTIPLE DX										
A. Not Operated										
0–19 Years	0									
20–34	6	5.5	8	3	4	5	5	11	11	11
35–49	19	5.4	8	1	4	6	7	10	10	10
50–64	23	7.1	15	3	4	6	10	13	14	15
65+	50	6.8	20	3	4	6	8	11	14	30
B. Operated										
0–19 Years	14	7.3	10	4	5	6	10	12	14	14
20–34	51	5.9	2	4	5	6	7	8	9	9
35–49	141	7.3	39	4	5	6	8	11	15	34
50–64	181	10.8	95	5	6	8	11	19	29	54
65+	244	11.5	55	5	7	9	14	23	28	44
SUBTOTALS:										
1. SINGLE DX A. Not Operated	5	2.0	<1	1	1	2	3	3	3	3
1. SINGLE DX B. Operated	25	5.4	3	3	4	5	6	7	8	11
2. MULTIPLE DX A. Not Operated	98	6.5	16	3	4	6	8	11	14	30
2. MULTIPLE DX B. Operated	631	9.8	62	4	6	7	11	18	26	44
1. SINGLE DX	30	4.8	4	3	3	5	6	7	8	11
2. MULTIPLE DX	729	9.4	57	4	5	7	11	16	24	41
A. NOT OPERATED	103	6.3	16	2	4	6	8	11	14	16
B. OPERATED	656	9.7	60	4	6	7	11	17	26	44
TOTAL										
0–19 Years	16	7.1	9	4	5	6	7	12	14	14
20–34	65	5.7	3	4	5	6	7	8	9	11
35–49	168	7.0	34	4	4	6	8	11	14	34
50–64	216	10.1	84	4	5	7	11	18	29	52
65+	294	10.7	52	5	6	9	13	21	27	44
GRAND TOTAL	759	9.2	56	4	5	7	10	16	23	41

532.90: DU NOS W/O COMP

Type of Patients	Observed Patients	Avg. Stay	Vari-ance	10th	25th	50th	75th	90th	95th	99th
1. SINGLE DX										
A. Not Operated										
0–19 Years	0									
20–34	1	2.0	0	2	2	2	2	2	2	2
35–49	1	3.0	0	3	3	3	3	3	3	3
50–64	3	1.7	<1	1	1	2	2	2	2	2
65+	0									
B. Operated										
0–19 Years	0									
20–34	0									
35–49	0									
50–64	0									
65+	0									
2. MULTIPLE DX										
A. Not Operated										
0–19 Years	11	2.8	3	1	2	2	4	5	6	6
20–34	49	2.8	5	1	1	2	3	5	5	14
35–49	159	3.3	8	1	1	3	4	5	8	20
50–64	242	3.2	4	1	2	3	4	6	7	10
65+	334	3.4	5	2	2	3	4	6	7	12
B. Operated										
0–19 Years	0									
20–34	1	8.0	0	8	8	8	8	8	8	8
35–49	0									
50–64	3	27.7	982	9	9	10	64	64	64	64
65+	7	5.3	13	1	3	5	7	12	12	12
SUBTOTALS:										
1. SINGLE DX A. Not Operated	5	2.0	<1	1	2	2	2	3	3	3
1. SINGLE DX B. Operated	0									
2. MULTIPLE DX A. Not Operated	795	3.3	5	1	2	3	4	6	7	12
2. MULTIPLE DX B. Operated	11	11.6	312	3	3	7	10	12	64	64
1. SINGLE DX	5	2.0	<1	1	2	2	2	3	3	3
2. MULTIPLE DX	806	3.4	10	1	2	3	4	6	8	12
A. NOT OPERATED	800	3.3	5	1	2	3	4	6	7	12
B. OPERATED	11	11.6	312	3	3	7	10	12	64	64
TOTAL										
0–19 Years	11	2.8	3	1	1	2	4	5	6	6
20–34	51	2.9	6	1	1	2	3	5	8	14
35–49	160	3.3	8	1	2	3	4	5	8	20
50–64	248	3.5	19	2	2	3	4	6	8	10
65+	341	3.5	5	2	2	3	4	6	7	12
GRAND TOTAL	811	3.4	10	1	2	3	4	6	8	12

533: PEPTIC ULCER SITE NOS

Type of Patients	Observed Patients	Avg. Stay	Vari-ance	10th	25th	50th	75th	90th	95th	99th
1. SINGLE DX										
A. Not Operated										
0–19 Years	4	2.3	4	1	1	2	5	5	5	5
20–34	8	1.8	<1	1	1	2	2	2	3	3
35–49	3	1.0	0	1	1	2	1	1	1	1
50–64	4	2.0	1	1	1	2	3	3	3	3
65+	4	2.8	5	1	2	3	6	6	6	6
B. Operated										
0–19 Years	0									
20–34	0									
35–49	0									
50–64	0									
65+	0									
2. MULTIPLE DX										
A. Not Operated										
0–19 Years	11	2.4	3	1	1	2	4	5	6	6
20–34	71	2.3	5	1	1	2	3	5	6	12
35–49	214	2.7	7	1	1	2	3	5	6	18
50–64	327	3.2	9	1	1	3	4	6	8	15
65+	510	3.5	10	1	2	3	4	6	9	17
B. Operated										
0–19 Years	0									
20–34	6	7.7	77	2	2	5	8	25	25	25
35–49	8	7.1	10	3	6	6	11	11	11	11
50–64	21	11.5	111	4	5	10	13	17	21	52
65+	38	11.5	97	4	6	9	13	25	42	47
SUBTOTALS:										
1. SINGLE DX A. Not Operated	23	2.0	2	1	1	2	2	3	5	6
1. SINGLE DX B. Operated	0									
2. MULTIPLE DX A. Not Operated	1,133	3.2	9	1	1	2	4	6	8	17
2. MULTIPLE DX B. Operated	73	10.7	90	4	5	9	12	19	30	52
1. SINGLE DX	23	2.0	2	1	1	2	2	3	5	6
2. MULTIPLE DX	1,206	3.6	17	1	1	2	4	7	10	21
A. NOT OPERATED	1,156	3.1	9	1	1	2	4	6	8	17
B. OPERATED	73	10.7	90	4	5	9	12	19	30	52
TOTAL										
0–19 Years	15	2.3	3	1	1	2	2	5	6	6
20–34	85	2.7	11	1	1	2	3	5	6	25
35–49	225	2.9	7	1	1	2	4	6	7	18
50–64	352	3.6	19	1	2	3	4	7	10	21
65+	552	4.0	20	1	2	3	4	8	11	24
GRAND TOTAL	1,229	3.6	17	1	1	2	4	7	10	21

Length of Stay by Diagnosis and Operation, Western Region, 2008

Western Region, October 2006–September 2007 Data, by Diagnosis

533.40: CHR PEPTIC ULCER W HEMOR

Type of Patients	Observed Patients	Avg. Stay	Vari-ance	Percentiles						
				10th	25th	50th	75th	90th	95th	99th
1. SINGLE DX										
A. Not Operated										
0–19 Years	0									
20–34	1	2.0	0	2	2	2	2	2	2	2
35–49	0									
50–64	1	3.0	0	3	3	3	3	3	3	3
65+	1	6.0	0	6	6	6	6	6	6	6
B. Operated										
0–19 Years	0									
20–34	0									
35–49	0									
50–64	0									
65+	0									
2. MULTIPLE DX										
A. Not Operated										
0–19 Years	2	3.5	12	1	1	1	6	6	6	6
20–34	17	2.9	13	1	1	1	3	12	12	12
35–49	62	3.0	7	1	1	2	4	6	7	18
50–64	147	3.6	13	1	2	2	4	7	9	22
65+	285	3.7	11	1	2	3	4	7	9	22
B. Operated										
0–19 Years	0									
20–34	0									
35–49	1	3.0	0	3	3	3	3	3	3	3
50–64	2	11.5	59	6	6	17	17	17	17	17
65+	11	14.0	147	4	6	13	16	19	47	47
SUBTOTALS:										
1. SINGLE DX										
A. Not Operated	3	3.7	4	2	2	3	3	6	6	6
B. Operated	0									
2. MULTIPLE DX										
A. Not Operated	513	3.5	11	1	2	3	4	7	9	19
B. Operated	14	12.9	126	3	6	13	16	19	47	47
1. SINGLE DX	3	3.7	4	2	2	3	3	6	6	6
2. MULTIPLE DX	527	3.8	17	1	2	3	4	7	10	22
A. NOT OPERATED	516	3.5	11	1	2	3	4	7	9	19
B. OPERATED	14	12.9	126	3	6	13	16	19	47	47
TOTAL										
0–19 Years	2	3.5	12	1	1	1	6	6	6	6
20–34	18	2.9	12	1	1	1	3	12	12	12
35–49	63	3.0	7	1	1	2	4	6	7	18
50–64	150	3.7	14	1	2	2	4	7	9	22
65+	297	4.1	20	1	2	3	4	8	12	22
GRAND TOTAL	530	3.8	16	1	2	3	4	7	10	22

533.90: PEPTIC ULCER NOS S COMP

Type of Patients	Observed Patients	Avg. Stay	Vari-ance	Percentiles						
				10th	25th	50th	75th	90th	95th	99th
1. SINGLE DX										
A. Not Operated										
0–19 Years	3	2.7	4	1	1	2	5	5	5	5
20–34	5	1.4	<1	1	1	1	2	2	2	2
35–49	3	1.0	0	1	1	1	1	1	1	1
50–64	3	1.7	1	1	1	1	3	3	3	3
65+	1	2.0	0	2	2	2	2	2	2	2
B. Operated										
0–19 Years	0									
20–34	0									
35–49	0									
50–64	0									
65+	0									
2. MULTIPLE DX										
A. Not Operated										
0–19 Years	8	2.3	2	1	1	2	4	5	5	5
20–34	48	2.2	2	1	1	2	3	4	6	6
35–49	129	2.4	4	1	1	2	3	4	6	7
50–64	142	2.4	3	1	1	2	3	5	6	8
65+	169	2.8	4	1	1	2	3	5	6	9
B. Operated										
0–19 Years	0									
20–34	1	8.0	0	8	8	8	8	8	8	8
35–49	2	8.5	13	6	6	9	11	11	11	11
50–64	1	15.0	0	15	15	15	15	15	15	15
65+	5	7.0	6	5	5	7	7	11	11	11
SUBTOTALS:										
1. SINGLE DX										
A. Not Operated	15	1.7	1	1	1	1	2	3	5	5
B. Operated	0									
2. MULTIPLE DX										
A. Not Operated	496	2.5	4	1	1	2	3	5	6	9
B. Operated	9	8.3	11	5	6	7	11	15	15	15
1. SINGLE DX	15	1.7	1	1	1	1	2	3	5	5
2. MULTIPLE DX	505	2.6	4	1	1	2	3	5	6	9
A. NOT OPERATED	511	2.5	4	1	1	2	3	5	6	8
B. OPERATED	9	8.3	11	5	6	7	11	15	15	15
TOTAL										
0–19 Years	11	2.4	2	1	1	2	4	5	5	5
20–34	54	2.2	3	1	1	2	3	4	6	8
35–49	134	2.5	5	1	1	2	3	4	6	11
50–64	146	2.4	4	1	1	2	3	5	6	8
65+	175	2.9	5	1	1	2	4	5	7	11
GRAND TOTAL	520	2.6	4	1	1	2	3	5	6	9

534: GASTROJEJUNAL ULCER

Type of Patients	Observed Patients	Avg. Stay	Vari-ance	Percentiles						
				10th	25th	50th	75th	90th	95th	99th
1. SINGLE DX										
A. Not Operated										
0–19 Years	0									
20–34	2	5.5	24	2	2	9	9	9	9	9
35–49	0									
50–64	0									
65+	2	1.5	<1	1	1	2	2	2	2	2
B. Operated										
0–19 Years	0									
20–34	1	6.0	0	6	6	6	6	6	6	6
35–49	1	2.0	0	2	2	2	2	2	2	2
50–64	0									
65+	0									
2. MULTIPLE DX										
A. Not Operated										
0–19 Years	5	2.2	1	1	2	2	2	4	4	4
20–34	93	3.4	8	1	2	3	4	7	9	17
35–49	206	3.6	11	1	2	3	4	6	10	13
50–64	298	3.8	12	1	2	3	4	6	9	22
65+	218	4.3	14	2	2	3	5	7	10	21
B. Operated										
0–19 Years	1	13.0	0	13	13	13	13	13	13	13
20–34	27	7.2	26	3	3	6	9	14	20	21
35–49	60	8.6	60	2	4	7	9	16	27	41
50–64	61	8.4	46	3	4	7	11	15	17	46
65+	34	13.7	196	6	6	11	15	31	40	75
SUBTOTALS:										
1. SINGLE DX										
A. Not Operated	4	3.5	14	1	1	2	6	9	9	9
B. Operated	2	4.0	8	2	2	6	6	6	6	6
2. MULTIPLE DX										
A. Not Operated	820	3.8	12	1	2	3	4	7	9	18
B. Operated	183	9.3	79	3	4	7	12	16	21	46
1. SINGLE DX	6	3.7	10	1	2	2	6	9	9	9
2. MULTIPLE DX	1,003	4.8	29	2	2	3	5	10	14	29
A. NOT OPERATED	824	3.8	12	1	2	3	4	7	9	18
B. OPERATED	185	9.3	78	3	4	7	11	16	21	46
TOTAL										
0–19 Years	6	4.0	20	1	2	2	4	13	13	13
20–34	123	4.3	14	1	2	3	5	5	13	20
35–49	267	4.7	26	1	2	3	6	9	12	34
50–64	359	4.6	21	2	2	3	5	10	14	22
65+	254	5.5	48	2	2	4	6	11	16	38
GRAND TOTAL	1,009	4.8	28	2	2	3	5	10	14	27

Length of Stay by Diagnosis and Operation, Western Region, 2008

Western Region, October 2006–September 2007 Data, by Diagnosis

534.40: CHR GJU W HEMOR S OBSTR

Type of Patients	Observed Patients	Avg. Stay	Variance	10th	25th	50th	75th	90th	95th	99th
1. SINGLE DX										
A. Not Operated										
0–19 Years	0									
20–34	1	9.0	0	9	9	9	9	9	9	9
35–49	0									
50–64	0									
65+	2	1.5	<1	1	1	2	2	2	2	2
B. Operated										
0–19 Years	0									
20–34	0									
35–49	0									
50–64	0									
65+	0									
2. MULTIPLE DX										
A. Not Operated										
0–19 Years	1	1.0	0	1	1	1	1	1	1	1
20–34	37	3.1	4	1	2	3	3	5	7	12
35–49	113	3.6	15	1	2	3	4	6	10	17
50–64	175	3.6	10	1	2	3	4	6	8	22
65+	156	4.3	16	2	2	3	5	7	9	23
B. Operated										
0–19 Years	0									
20–34	3	11.0	75	5	5	7	21	21	21	21
35–49	7	6.1	44	1	1	2	9	19	19	19
50–64	12	9.6	27	4	4	8	13	16	19	19
65+	13	16.6	395	4	6	11	14	40	75	75
SUBTOTALS:										
1. SINGLE DX										
A. Not Operated	3	4.0	19	1	1	2	9	9	9	9
B. Operated	0									
2. MULTIPLE DX										
A. Not Operated	482	3.8	13	1	2	3	4	6	8	22
B. Operated	35	11.6	178	2	4	9	14	19	40	75
1. SINGLE DX	3	4.0	19	1	1	2	9	9	9	9
2. MULTIPLE DX	517	4.3	28	1	2	3	5	7	12	23
A. NOT OPERATED	485	3.8	13	1	2	3	4	6	8	22
B. OPERATED	35	11.6	178	2	4	9	14	19	40	75
TOTAL										
0–19 Years	1	1.0	0	1	1	1	1	1	1	1
20–34	41	3.8	13	1	2	3	4	7	9	21
35–49	120	3.8	17	1	2	3	4	7	11	19
50–64	187	4.0	13	1	2	3	5	7	12	22
65+	171	5.2	54	2	2	3	5	8	15	40
GRAND TOTAL	520	4.3	28	1	2	3	5	7	12	23

534.90: GJU NOS W/O COMP

Type of Patients	Observed Patients	Avg. Stay	Variance	10th	25th	50th	75th	90th	95th	99th
1. SINGLE DX										
A. Not Operated										
0–19 Years	0									
20–34	0									
35–49	0									
50–64	0									
65+	0									
B. Operated										
0–19 Years	0									
20–34	0									
35–49	0									
50–64	0									
65+	0									
2. MULTIPLE DX										
A. Not Operated										
0–19 Years	2	2.0	0	2	2	2	2	2	2	2
20–34	32	3.1	5	2	2	3	3	6	9	10
35–49	52	3.7	6	1	2	3	4	7	9	12
50–64	50	3.8	6	1	2	3	6	8	9	10
65+	21	4.1	7	2	3	3	5	7	10	11
B. Operated										
0–19 Years	0									
20–34	3	6.0	37	2	2	3	13	13	13	13
35–49	8	7.1	36	1	5	6	7	21	21	21
50–64	5	4.8	13	2	3	3	5	11	11	11
65+	3	8.7	40	5	5	5	16	16	16	16
SUBTOTALS:										
1. SINGLE DX										
A. Not Operated	0									
B. Operated	0									
2. MULTIPLE DX										
A. Not Operated	157	3.6	6	1	2	3	4	7	9	11
B. Operated	19	6.6	27	2	3	5	7	16	21	21
1. SINGLE DX	0									
2. MULTIPLE DX	176	4.0	9	1	2	3	5	8	10	16
A. NOT OPERATED	157	3.6	6	1	2	3	4	7	9	11
B. OPERATED	19	6.6	27	2	3	5	7	16	21	21
TOTAL										
0–19 Years	2	2.0	0	2	2	2	2	2	2	2
20–34	35	3.4	8	2	2	3	4	8	10	13
35–49	60	4.1	11	1	2	3	5	7	9	21
50–64	55	3.9	6	1	3	3	6	8	9	11
65+	24	4.7	12	2	3	4	5	10	11	16
GRAND TOTAL	176	4.0	9	1	2	3	5	8	10	16

535: GASTRITIS & DUODENITIS

Type of Patients	Observed Patients	Avg. Stay	Variance	10th	25th	50th	75th	90th	95th	99th
1. SINGLE DX										
A. Not Operated										
0–19 Years	58	1.8	<1	1	1	2	2	3	4	4
20–34	53	1.9	1	1	1	2	2	3	4	7
35–49	43	1.8	1	1	1	1	3	3	4	6
50–64	15	2.3	3	1	1	2	2	5	7	7
65+	8	2.3	1	1	1	2	3	4	4	4
B. Operated										
0–19 Years	0									
20–34	0									
35–49	0									
50–64	0									
65+	0									
2. MULTIPLE DX										
A. Not Operated										
0–19 Years	442	2.6	8	1	1	2	3	5	6	10
20–34	1,509	2.7	5	1	1	2	3	5	6	10
35–49	3,034	3.0	8	1	2	2	4	5	7	12
50–64	3,929	3.3	8	1	2	3	4	6	8	13
65+	6,298	3.7	9	1	2	3	5	7	9	15
B. Operated										
0–19 Years	6	8.9	106	1	1	3	19	25	25	25
20–34	21	7.2	32	2	2	6	9	17	19	>99
35–49	47	9.1	93	2	4	7	12	17	20	63
50–64	59	9.3	39	3	5	8	11	18	23	29
65+	124	8.6	42	3	4	7	10	16	22	32
SUBTOTALS:										
1. SINGLE DX										
A. Not Operated	177	1.9	1	1	1	2	2	3	4	7
B. Operated	0									
2. MULTIPLE DX										
A. Not Operated	15,212	3.4	8	1	2	3	4	6	8	14
B. Operated	257	8.7	51	2	4	7	11	17	23	42
1. SINGLE DX	177	1.9	1	1	1	2	2	3	4	7
2. MULTIPLE DX	15,469	3.4	9	1	2	3	4	6	8	15
A. NOT OPERATED	15,389	3.3	8	1	2	3	4	6	8	14
B. OPERATED	257	8.7	51	2	4	7	11	17	23	42
TOTAL										
0–19 Years	506	2.5	8	1	1	2	3	5	6	11
20–34	1,583	2.8	6	1	1	2	3	5	7	12
35–49	3,124	3.1	9	1	2	2	4	6	7	14
50–64	4,003	3.4	8	1	2	3	4	6	9	15
65+	6,430	3.8	10	1	2	3	5	7	9	16
GRAND TOTAL	15,646	3.4	9	1	2	3	4	6	8	15

535.00: ACUTE GASTRITIS S HEMOR

Type of Patients	Observed Patients	Avg. Stay	Variance	10th	25th	50th	75th	90th	95th	99th
1. SINGLE DX										
A. Not Operated										
0–19 Years	14	1.2	<1	1	1	1	1	2	2	2
20–34	9	1.8	<1	1	1	2	2	3	3	3
35–49	5	1.6	<1	1	1	1	2	3	3	3
50–64	1	7.0	0	7	7	7	7	7	7	7
65+	2	2.5	<1	2	2	3	3	3	3	3
B. Operated										
0–19 Years	0									
20–34	0									
35–49	0									
50–64	0									
65+	0									
2. MULTIPLE DX										
A. Not Operated										
0–19 Years	97	2.6	19	1	1	2	3	4	7	41
20–34	165	2.5	3	1	1	2	3	5	6	10
35–49	289	2.7	3	1	1	2	4	5	6	8
50–64	296	3.0	8	1	1	2	4	6	8	15
65+	397	3.3	8	1	2	3	4	6	7	11
B. Operated										
0–19 Years	0									
20–34	1	4.0	0	4	4	4	4	4	4	4
35–49	6	5.3	9	1	4	4	7	10	10	10
50–64	4	6.8	34	2	2	6	14	14	14	14
65+	4	6.5	3	4	7	7	8	8	8	8
SUBTOTALS:										
1. SINGLE DX										
A. Not Operated	31	1.7	1	1	1	1	2	3	3	7
B. Operated	0									
2. MULTIPLE DX										
A. Not Operated	1,244	2.9	7	1	1	2	4	6	7	11
B. Operated	15	5.9	12	2	4	6	8	10	14	14
1. SINGLE DX	31	1.7	1	1	1	1	2	3	3	7
2. MULTIPLE DX	1,259	3.0	7	1	1	2	4	6	7	11
A. NOT OPERATED	1,275	2.9	7	1	1	2	4	5	7	11
B. OPERATED	15	5.9	12	2	4	6	8	14	14	14
TOTAL										
0–19 Years	111	2.4	17	1	1	1	3	4	7	11
20–34	175	2.5	3	1	1	2	3	5	6	10
35–49	300	2.7	3	1	1	2	4	5	6	8
50–64	301	3.1	8	1	1	2	4	6	8	14
65+	403	3.3	8	1	2	3	4	6	7	10
GRAND TOTAL	1,290	2.9	7	1	1	2	4	6	7	11

535.01: ACUTE GASTRITIS W HEMOR

Type of Patients	Observed Patients	Avg. Stay	Variance	10th	25th	50th	75th	90th	95th	99th
1. SINGLE DX										
A. Not Operated										
0–19 Years	1	2.0	0	2	2	2	2	2	2	2
20–34	3	3.7	8	2	2	2	7	7	7	7
35–49	2	1.0	0	1	1	1	1	1	1	1
50–64	0									
65+	0									
B. Operated										
0–19 Years	0									
20–34	0									
35–49	0									
50–64	0									
65+	0									
2. MULTIPLE DX										
A. Not Operated										
0–19 Years	7	3.3	4	2	2	2	6	6	6	6
20–34	53	2.7	9	1	1	2	3	5	7	21
35–49	91	2.9	3	1	2	3	4	5	7	9
50–64	171	3.6	7	1	2	3	4	6	9	13
65+	361	4.4	14	2	2	3	5	8	10	23
B. Operated										
0–19 Years	1	19.0	0	19	19	19	19	19	19	19
20–34	3	9.0	49	19	2	9	16	16	16	16
35–49	3	14.3	36	8	8	15	20	20	20	20
50–64	2	11.0	49	6	6	16	16	16	16	16
65+	7	13.6	104	5	5	9	24	31	31	31
SUBTOTALS:										
1. SINGLE DX										
A. Not Operated	6	2.5	5	1	1	2	2	7	7	7
B. Operated	0									
2. MULTIPLE DX										
A. Not Operated	683	3.9	11	1	2	3	5	7	9	17
B. Operated	16	12.9	63	5	7	14	16	24	31	31
1. SINGLE DX	6	2.5	5	1	1	2	2	2	7	7
2. MULTIPLE DX	699	4.1	13	1	2	3	5	8	10	20
A. NOT OPERATED	689	3.9	11	1	2	3	5	7	9	17
B. OPERATED	16	12.9	63	5	7	14	16	24	31	31
TOTAL										
0–19 Years	9	4.9	31	2	2	2	6	19	19	19
20–34	59	3.1	12	1	1	2	3	7	10	21
35–49	96	3.3	8	1	2	3	4	6	8	20
50–64	173	3.7	8	1	2	3	4	7	10	16
65+	368	4.6	17	2	2	3	6	9	11	24
GRAND TOTAL	705	4.1	13	1	2	3	5	8	10	20

535.10: ATROPH GASTRITIS S HEMOR

Type of Patients	Observed Patients	Avg. Stay	Variance	10th	25th	50th	75th	90th	95th	99th
1. SINGLE DX										
A. Not Operated										
0–19 Years	1	1.0	0	1	1	1	1	1	1	1
20–34	3	2.0	1	1	1	2	3	3	3	3
35–49	5	1.4	<1	1	1	1	1	3	3	3
50–64	2	2.0	0	2	2	2	2	2	2	2
65+	1	2.0	0	2	2	2	2	2	2	*
B. Operated										
0–19 Years	0									
20–34	0									
35–49	0									
50–64	0									
65+	0									
2. MULTIPLE DX										
A. Not Operated										
0–19 Years	20	2.4	2	1	1	2	3	5	5	6
20–34	79	3.7	6	1	2	3	4	6	10	14
35–49	152	3.7	9	1	2	3	4	7	10	15
50–64	176	3.9	8	2	2	3	5	7	10	13
65+	296	3.9	6	1	2	3	5	7	8	14
B. Operated										
0–19 Years	1	1.0	0	1	1	1	1	1	1	1
20–34	1	5.0	0	5	5	5	5	5	5	5
35–49	1	63.0	0	63	63	63	63	63	63	63
50–64	4	12.5	66	5	6	18	18	21	21	21
65+	2	8.5	<1	8	8	8	9	9	9	9
SUBTOTALS:										
1. SINGLE DX										
A. Not Operated	12	1.7	<1	1	1	1	2	3	3	3
B. Operated	0									
2. MULTIPLE DX										
A. Not Operated	723	3.8	7	1	2	3	5	7	9	14
B. Operated	9	15.1	363	1	5	8	18	63	63	63
1. SINGLE DX	12	1.7	<1	1	1	1	2	3	3	3
2. MULTIPLE DX	732	3.9	13	1	2	3	5	7	9	15
A. NOT OPERATED	735	3.8	7	1	2	3	5	7	9	14
B. OPERATED	9	15.1	363	1	5	8	18	63	63	63
TOTAL										
0–19 Years	22	2.2	2	1	2	2	3	5	5	6
20–34	83	3.6	6	2	2	3	4	6	8	14
35–49	158	4.0	31	1	2	3	4	6	10	21
50–64	182	4.1	10	2	2	3	5	7	10	18
65+	299	3.9	7	2	2	3	5	7	8	14
GRAND TOTAL	744	3.9	12	1	2	3	5	7	9	15

Length of Stay by Diagnosis and Operation, Western Region, 2008

Western Region, October 2006–September 2007 Data, by Diagnosis

Type of Patients	535.11: ATROPH GASTRITIS W HEMOR										535.30: ALC GASTRITIS W/O HEMOR										535.31: ALC GASTRITIS W HEMOR									
	Observed Patients	Avg. Stay	Variance	Percentiles							Observed Patients	Avg. Stay	Variance	Percentiles							Observed Patients	Avg. Stay	Variance	Percentiles						
				10th	25th	50th	75th	90th	95th	99th				10th	25th	50th	75th	90th	95th	99th				10th	25th	50th	75th	90th	95th	99th
1. SINGLE DX																														
A. Not Operated																														
0–19 Years	1	3.0	0	3	3	3	3	3	3	3	0										0									
20–34	0										2	1.0	0	1	1	1	1	1	1	1	0									
35–49	0										1	1.0	0	1	1	1	1	1	1	1	0									
50–64	0										0										0									
65+	0										0										0									
B. Operated																														
0–19 Years	0										0										0									
20–34	0										0										0									
35–49	0										0										0									
50–64	0										0										0									
65+	0										0										0									
2. MULTIPLE DX																														
A. Not Operated																														
0–19 Years	7	3.0	4	1	1	3	4	7	7	7	6	3.0	16	1	1	2	2	7	11	11	1	1.0	0	1	1	1	1	1	1	1
20–34	20	2.6	7	1	1	2	2	6	11	11	103	2.4	3	1	1	2	3	5	6	9	83	2.2	2	1	1	2	3	3	5	11
35–49	66	3.8	13	1	2	3	5	6	7	21	255	2.3	2	1	1	2	3	4	5	8	272	3.6	35	1	2	3	4	6	8	17
50–64	105	4.2	13	1	2	3	5	8	10	22	209	2.8	5	1	1	2	3	5	6	12	225	4.0	14	1	2	3	5	8	10	25
65+	274	4.0	9	1	2	3	5	8	9	13	64	4.0	38	1	2	3	4	6	8	49	61	4.7	13	2	2	4	6	8	12	23
B. Operated																														
0–19 Years	0										0										0									
20–34	1	11.0	0	11	11	11	11	11	11	11	0										1	16.0	0	16	16	16	16	16	16	16
35–49	1	10.0	0	10	10	10	10	10	10	10	1	3.0	0	3	3	3	3	3	3	3	4	7.2	13	3	4	5	8	12	12	12
50–64	0										0										1	3.0	0	3	3	3	3	3	3	3
65+	7	7.4	8	4	4	7	9	12	12	13	1	7.0	0	7	7	7	7	7	7	7	2	14.5	217	4	4	15	25	25	25	25
SUBTOTALS:																														
1. SINGLE DX																														
A. Not Operated	1	3.0	0	3	3	3	3	3	3	3	3	1.0	0	1	1	1	1	1	1	1	0									
B. Operated	0										0										0									
2. MULTIPLE DX																														
A. Not Operated	472	3.9	10	1	2	3	5	7	9	19	637	2.7	7	1	1	2	3	5	6	11	642	3.6	21	1	2	3	4	7	8	17
B. Operated	9	8.1	8	4	7	9	11	>99	>99	>99	2	5.0	8	3	7	7	7	7	7	7	8	9.6	59	3	4	5	16	25	25	25
1. SINGLE DX	1	3.0	0	3	3	3	3	3	3	3	3	1.0	0	1	1	1	1	1	1	1	0									
2. MULTIPLE DX	481	4.0	11	1	2	3	5	8	10	21	639	2.7	7	1	1	2	3	5	6	11	650	3.7	22	1	2	3	4	7	9	23
A. NOT OPERATED	473	3.9	10	1	2	3	5	7	9	19	640	2.7	7	1	1	2	3	5	6	11	642	3.6	21	1	2	3	4	7	8	17
B. OPERATED	9	8.1	8	4	7	9	11	>99	>99	>99	2	5.0	8	3	7	7	7	7	7	7	8	9.6	59	3	4	5	16	25	25	25
TOTAL																														
0–19 Years	8	3.0	4	1	2	3	3	7	7	7	6	3.0	16	1	1	2	3	7	11	11	1	1.0	0	1	1	1	1	1	1	1
20–34	20	2.6	7	1	1	2	3	8	11	>99	105	2.4	3	1	1	2	3	5	6	9	84	2.3	5	1	1	2	3	4	5	16
35–49	67	3.9	14	1	2	3	5	7	11	21	257	2.3	2	1	1	2	3	4	5	8	276	3.7	35	1	2	2	4	6	8	17
50–64	106	4.2	13	1	2	3	5	9	10	22	209	2.8	5	1	1	2	3	5	6	12	226	4.0	14	2	2	3	5	8	10	25
65+	281	4.1	9	1	2	3	5	8	9	13	65	4.0	37	1	2	3	4	7	8	49	63	5.0	19	2	2	4	6	8	12	25
GRAND TOTAL	482	4.0	11	1	2	3	5	8	10	21	642	2.7	7	1	1	2	3	5	6	11	650	3.7	22	1	2	3	4	7	9	23

Length of Stay by Diagnosis and Operation, Western Region, 2008

Western Region, October 2006–September 2007 Data, by Diagnosis

535.40: GASTRITIS NEC W/O HEMOR

Type of Patients	Observed Patients	Avg. Stay	Vari-ance	10th	25th	50th	75th	90th	95th	99th
1. SINGLE DX										
A. Not Operated										
0–19 Years	7	2.1	<1	1	1	2	3	3	3	3
20–34	13	2.2	1	1	1	2	3	4	4	4
35–49	2	3.5	<1	3	3	4	4	4	4	4
50–64	3	2.0	0	2	2	2	2	2	2	2
65+	1	2.0	0	2	2	2	2	2	2	2
B. Operated										
0–19 Years	0									
20–34	0									
35–49	0									
50–64	0									
65+	0									
2. MULTIPLE DX										
A. Not Operated										
0–19 Years	92	2.3	2	1	1	2	3	4	6	9
20–34	294	3.2	5	1	2	2	4	6	8	11
35–49	552	3.0	4	1	2	3	4	6	7	9
50–64	635	3.4	5	1	2	3	4	6	8	13
65+	815	3.5	7	1	2	3	4	6	8	14
B. Operated										
0–19 Years	1	1.0	0	1	1	1	1	1	1	1
20–34	7	6.6	37	2	2	6	8	19	19	19
35–49	8	4.1	4	2	2	3	6	7	7	7
50–64	12	9.3	27	5	6	8	11	14	23	23
65+	11	6.7	5	4	4	6	8	9	11	11
SUBTOTALS:										
1. SINGLE DX										
A. Not Operated	26	2.3	<1	1	2	2	3	4	4	4
B. Operated	0									
2. MULTIPLE DX										
A. Not Operated	2,388	3.3	5	1	2	3	4	6	8	12
B. Operated	39	6.8	20	2	4	6	8	11	19	23
1. SINGLE DX	26	2.3	<1	1	2	2	3	4	4	4
2. MULTIPLE DX	2,427	3.3	6	1	2	3	4	6	8	12
A. NOT OPERATED	2,414	3.3	5	1	2	3	4	6	7	11
B. OPERATED	39	6.8	20	2	4	6	8	11	19	23
TOTAL										
0–19 Years	100	2.3	2	1	1	2	3	4	6	7
20–34	314	3.2	6	1	2	2	4	6	8	11
35–49	562	3.0	4	1	2	3	4	6	7	9
50–64	650	3.5	6	2	2	3	4	6	8	14
65+	827	3.6	7	1	2	3	4	7	8	14
GRAND TOTAL	2,453	3.3	6	1	2	3	4	6	8	12

535.41: GASTRITIS NEC W HEMOR

Type of Patients	Observed Patients	Avg. Stay	Vari-ance	10th	25th	50th	75th	90th	95th	99th
1. SINGLE DX										
A. Not Operated										
0–19 Years	1	3.0	0	3	3	3	3	3	3	3
20–34	3	1.7	<1	1	1	2	2	2	2	2
35–49	0									
50–64	3	1.7	<1	1	1	2	2	2	2	2
65+	0									
B. Operated										
0–19 Years	0									
20–34	0									
35–49	0									
50–64	0									
65+	0									
2. MULTIPLE DX										
A. Not Operated										
0–19 Years	22	2.6	4	1	1	2	3	4	5	10
20–34	126	2.6	4	1	1	2	3	5	6	10
35–49	309	3.1	5	1	2	3	4	6	7	11
50–64	643	3.4	9	1	2	3	4	6	8	16
65+	1,549	3.9	10	1	2	3	5	7	10	16
B. Operated										
0–19 Years	1	25.0	0	25	25	25	25	25	25	25
20–34	3	6.4	14	2	2	8	8	9	9	9
35–49	8	10.5	52	1	7	8	17	23	23	23
50–64	14	11.6	71	4	6	9	16	28	29	29
65+	42	7.4	24	2	4	8	9	12	17	24
SUBTOTALS:										
1. SINGLE DX										
A. Not Operated	7	1.9	<1	1	1	2	2	3	3	3
B. Operated	0									
2. MULTIPLE DX										
A. Not Operated	2,649	3.6	9	1	2	3	4	7	9	15
B. Operated	68	8.8	42	2	4	8	10	18	24	29
1. SINGLE DX	7	1.9	<1	1	1	2	2	3	3	3
2. MULTIPLE DX	2,717	3.7	11	1	2	3	4	7	10	16
A. NOT OPERATED	2,656	3.6	9	1	2	3	4	7	9	15
B. OPERATED	68	8.8	42	2	4	8	10	18	24	29
TOTAL										
0–19 Years	24	3.5	24	1	1	2	3	5	10	25
20–34	132	2.6	4	1	1	2	3	5	7	10
35–49	317	3.3	7	1	2	3	4	6	8	15
50–64	660	3.6	12	1	2	3	4	6	10	18
65+	1,591	4.0	11	1	2	3	5	8	10	16
GRAND TOTAL	2,724	3.7	11	1	2	3	4	7	10	16

535.50: GASTRODUODENITIS NOS

Type of Patients	Observed Patients	Avg. Stay	Vari-ance	10th	25th	50th	75th	90th	95th	99th
1. SINGLE DX										
A. Not Operated										
0–19 Years	30	1.9	<1	1	1	2	2	3	4	4
20–34	13	1.3	<1	1	1	1	2	2	2	2
35–49	19	1.6	1	1	1	1	2	4	4	4
50–64	4	2.2	4	1	1	1	2	5	5	5
65+	3	2.0	3	1	1	1	4	4	4	4
B. Operated										
0–19 Years	0									
20–34	0									
35–49	0									
50–64	0									
65+	0									
2. MULTIPLE DX										
A. Not Operated										
0–19 Years	154	2.4	3	1	1	2	3	5	6	10
20–34	409	2.5	4	1	1	2	3	5	5	8
35–49	615	2.8	6	1	1	2	3	5	7	12
50–64	815	2.7	4	1	1	2	3	5	6	11
65+	1,001	3.2	7	2	2	3	4	6	8	13
B. Operated										
0–19 Years	0									
20–34	4	4.2	15	1	3	7	15	16	16	16
35–49	7	7.7	32	2	3	7	10	18	18	18
50–64	9	7.9	30	1	3	7	10	18	18	18
65+	11	8.5	35	2	3	6	14	15	20	20
SUBTOTALS:										
1. SINGLE DX										
A. Not Operated	69	1.7	1	1	1	1	2	4	4	5
B. Operated	0									
2. MULTIPLE DX										
A. Not Operated	2,994	2.9	5	1	1	2	4	5	7	11
B. Operated	31	7.6	30	2	3	7	11	15	18	20
1. SINGLE DX	69	1.7	1	1	1	1	2	4	4	5
2. MULTIPLE DX	3,025	2.9	6	1	1	2	4	5	7	13
A. NOT OPERATED	3,063	2.8	5	1	1	2	4	5	7	11
B. OPERATED	31	7.6	30	2	3	7	11	15	18	20
TOTAL										
0–19 Years	184	2.3	3	1	1	2	3	4	5	10
20–34	426	2.5	4	1	1	2	3	5	5	9
35–49	641	2.8	6	1	1	2	3	5	7	12
50–64	828	2.8	5	1	1	2	3	5	7	12
65+	1,015	3.3	7	2	2	3	4	6	8	14
GRAND TOTAL	3,094	2.9	6	1	1	2	4	5	7	12

Length of Stay by Diagnosis and Operation, Western Region, 2008

Western Region, October 2006–September 2007 Data, by Diagnosis

535.51: GASTRITIS NOS W HEMOR

Type of Patients	Observed Patients	Avg. Stay	Vari- ance	10th	25th	50th	75th	90th	95th	99th
1. SINGLE DX										
A. Not Operated										
0–19 Years	2	1.0	0	1	1		1	1	1	1
20–34	5	1.8	<1	1	2	2	2	2	2	2
35–49	4	1.3	<1	1	1	1	1	1	1	2
50–64	1	1.0	0	1	1	1	1	1	1	1
65+	0									
B. Operated										
0–19 Years	0									
20–34	0									
35–49	0									
50–64	0									
65+	0									
2. MULTIPLE DX										
A. Not Operated										
0–19 Years	20	4.2	23	1	1	3	5	9	9	22
20–34	110	2.6	14	1	1	2	3	4	6	8
35–49	287	3.1	6	1	2	2	4	5	6	14
50–64	441	3.7	11	1	2	3	4	7	9	16
65+	1,122	4.0	10	1	2	3	5	7	10	16
B. Operated										
0–19 Years	1	3.0	0	3	3	3	3	3	3	3
20–34	1	17.0	0	17	17	17	17	17	17	17
35–49	3	9.4	10	7	7	8	13	13	13	13
50–64	10	8.0	21	2	3	9	11	16	16	16
65+	26	10.5	91	3	4	7	16	22	32	42
SUBTOTALS:										
1. SINGLE DX										
A. Not Operated	12	1.4	<1	1	1	1	2	2	2	2
B. Operated	0									
2. MULTIPLE DX										
A. Not Operated	1,980	3.7	10	1	2	3	4	7	9	16
B. Operated	41	9.8	66	3	4	8	12	17	22	42
1. SINGLE DX	12	1.4	<1	1	1	1	2	2	2	2
2. MULTIPLE DX	2,021	3.8	12	1	2	3	4	7	9	17
A. NOT OPERATED	1,992	3.7	10	1	2	3	4	7	9	16
B. OPERATED	41	9.8	66	3	4	8	12	17	22	42
TOTAL										
0–19 Years	23	3.9	21	1	1	3	5	7	9	22
20–34	116	2.7	15	1	1	2	3	4	6	17
35–49	294	3.1	7	1	2	2	4	5	7	14
50–64	452	3.8	11	1	2	3	4	6	10	16
65+	1,148	4.1	12	1	2	3	5	8	10	18
GRAND TOTAL	2,033	3.8	12	1	2	3	4	7	9	17

535.60: DUODENITIS W/O HEMOR

Type of Patients	Observed Patients	Avg. Stay	Vari- ance	10th	25th	50th	75th	90th	95th	99th
1. SINGLE DX										
A. Not Operated										
0–19 Years	0									
20–34	2	2.0	0	2	2	2	2	2	2	2
35–49	5	3.0	4	1	2	3	3	6	6	6
50–64	1	3.0	0	3	3	3	3	3	3	3
65+	1	3.0	0	3	3	3	3	3	3	3
B. Operated										
0–19 Years	0									
20–34	0									
35–49	0									
50–64	0									
65+	0									
2. MULTIPLE DX										
A. Not Operated										
0–19 Years	13	3.2	6	1	2	3	4	5	10	10
20–34	48	3.1	3	1	2	3	4	6	7	7
35–49	90	2.9	3	1	2	3	4	5	6	9
50–64	98	3.5	6	1	2	3	5	6	9	12
65+	98	3.0	5	1	1	2	4	6	7	15
B. Operated										
0–19 Years	1	5.0	0	5	5	5	5	5	5	5
20–34	0									
35–49	3	5.0	3	4	4	4	7	7	7	7
50–64	1	7.0	0	7	7	7	7	7	7	7
65+	2	9.0	71	3	3	7	15	15	15	15
SUBTOTALS:										
1. SINGLE DX										
A. Not Operated	9	2.8	2	1	2	3	3	6	6	6
B. Operated	0									
2. MULTIPLE DX										
A. Not Operated	347	3.2	4	1	2	3	4	6	7	10
B. Operated	7	6.4	16	3	4	5	7	15	15	15
1. SINGLE DX	9	2.8	2	1	2	3	3	6	6	6
2. MULTIPLE DX	354	3.2	5	1	2	3	4	6	7	11
A. NOT OPERATED	356	3.1	4	1	2	3	4	6	7	10
B. OPERATED	7	6.4	16	3	4	5	7	15	15	15
TOTAL										
0–19 Years	14	3.4	6	1	2	3	3	5	10	10
20–34	50	3.1	3	1	2	2	4	6	7	7
35–49	98	3.0	3	1	2	3	4	5	6	9
50–64	100	3.5	6	1	2	3	5	6	9	12
65+	101	3.2	6	1	2	3	4	6	7	15
GRAND TOTAL	363	3.2	5	1	2	3	4	6	7	11

535.61: DUODENITIS W HEMORRHAGE

Type of Patients	Observed Patients	Avg. Stay	Vari- ance	10th	25th	50th	75th	90th	95th	99th
1. SINGLE DX										
A. Not Operated										
0–19 Years	0									
20–34	0									
35–49	0									
50–64	0									
65+	0									
B. Operated										
0–19 Years	0									
20–34	0									
35–49	0									
50–64	0									
65+	0									
2. MULTIPLE DX										
A. Not Operated										
0–19 Years	2	3.0	2	2	2	3	4	4	4	4
20–34	18	2.8	2	1	2	3	3	4	7	7
35–49	48	2.8	4	1	2	2	3	5	6	11
50–64	112	3.4	5	1	2	3	4	7	8	11
65+	255	3.9	12	2	2	3	5	7	9	15
B. Operated										
0–19 Years	0									
20–34	0									
35–49	2	15.5	24	12	12	12	19	19	19	19
50–64	1	3.0	0	3	3	3	3	3	3	3
65+	8	7.0	7	2	6	8	9	11	11	11
SUBTOTALS:										
1. SINGLE DX										
A. Not Operated	0									
B. Operated	0									
2. MULTIPLE DX										
A. Not Operated	435	3.6	9	1	2	3	4	7	8	14
B. Operated	11	8.2	22	3	6	8	11	12	19	19
1. SINGLE DX	0									
2. MULTIPLE DX	446	3.7	10	1	2	3	4	7	9	15
A. NOT OPERATED	435	3.6	9	1	2	3	4	7	8	14
B. OPERATED	11	8.2	22	3	6	8	11	12	19	19
TOTAL										
0–19 Years	2	3.0	2	2	2	3	4	4	4	4
20–34	18	2.8	2	1	2	3	3	4	7	7
35–49	50	3.3	10	1	2	2	3	6	11	19
50–64	113	3.4	5	1	2	3	4	7	8	11
65+	263	4.0	12	2	2	3	5	7	9	15
GRAND TOTAL	446	3.7	10	1	2	3	4	7	9	15

536: STOMACH FUNCTION DISORD

Type of Patients	Observed Patients	Avg. Stay	Vari-ance	Percentiles 10th	25th	50th	75th	90th	95th	99th
1. SINGLE DX										
A. Not Operated										
0–19 Years	35	2.5	7	1	1	1	3	7	8	12
20–34	12	2.3	2	1	1	2	4	4	5	5
35–49	12	2.3	1	1	2	2	3	4	5	5
50–64	5	2.0	1	1	1	2	2	4	4	4
65+	0									
B. Operated										
0–19 Years	1	1.0	0	1	1	1	1	1	1	1
20–34	1	3.0	0	3	3	3	3	3	3	3
35–49	1	2.0	0	2	2	2	2	2	2	2
50–64	0									
65+	0									
2. MULTIPLE DX										
A. Not Operated										
0–19 Years	504	3.7	20	1	1	2	5	7	10	20
20–34	940	3.8	16	1	2	3	5	8	10	18
35–49	1,241	3.8	13	1	2	3	5	8	11	21
50–64	1,500	4.4	22	1	2	3	6	9	12	22
65+	2,183	4.9	22	2	2	4	6	10	14	23
B. Operated										
0–19 Years	52	10.3	232	2	3	5	9	25	60	>99
20–34	43	9.1	226	1	2	5	10	21	24	95
35–49	87	9.7	144	2	3	7	12	21	29	82
50–64	111	9.1	100	1	3	7	12	20	38	>99
65+	170	11.5	82	3	5	9	15	23	29	56
SUBTOTALS:										
1. SINGLE DX										
A. Not Operated	64	2.4	5	1	1	2	3	5	7	12
B. Operated	3	2.0	<1	1	1	2	3	3	3	3
2. MULTIPLE DX										
A. Not Operated	6,368	4.3	19	1	2	3	5	9	12	22
B. Operated	463	10.2	128	2	4	7	13	23	29	88
1. SINGLE DX	67	2.3	4	1	1	2	3	5	7	12
2. MULTIPLE DX	6,831	4.7	29	1	2	3	6	10	14	26
A. NOT OPERATED	6,432	4.3	19	1	2	3	5	9	12	22
B. OPERATED	466	10.2	128	2	4	7	13	23	29	88
TOTAL										
0–19 Years	592	4.2	41	1	1	2	5	8	12	35
20–34	996	4.0	26	1	2	3	5	8	11	23
35–49	1,341	4.2	24	1	2	3	5	8	13	22
50–64	1,616	4.7	29	1	2	3	6	10	14	29
65+	2,353	5.4	29	2	2	4	7	11	16	26
GRAND TOTAL	6,898	4.7	29	1	2	3	6	10	14	25

536.2: PERSISTENT VOMITING

Type of Patients	Observed Patients	Avg. Stay	Vari-ance	Percentiles 10th	25th	50th	75th	90th	95th	99th
1. SINGLE DX										
A. Not Operated										
0–19 Years	27	2.2	5	1	1	1	2	7	7	8
20–34	7	1.6	<1	1	1	2	2	2	2	2
35–49	8	2.3	<1	1	2	2	3	4	4	4
50–64	3	2.7	1	2	2	2	4	4	4	4
65+	0									
B. Operated										
0–19 Years	0									
20–34	0									
35–49	0									
50–64	0									
65+	0									
2. MULTIPLE DX										
A. Not Operated										
0–19 Years	254	3.1	20	1	1	2	4	6	7	15
20–34	446	3.1	10	1	1	2	4	6	8	17
35–49	505	3.2	8	1	1	2	4	6	8	16
50–64	407	3.8	11	1	2	3	5	7	10	19
65+	326	3.7	9	2	2	3	5	7	10	14
B. Operated										
0–19 Years	3	9.7	63	2	2	9	18	18	18	18
20–34	5	5.8	40	2	2	2	8	16	16	16
35–49	6	7.8	90	1	1	1	12	25	25	25
50–64	9	8.9	26	4	5	12	14	>99	>99	>99
65+	5	8.6	14	3	8	8	12	12	12	12
SUBTOTALS:										
1. SINGLE DX										
A. Not Operated	45	2.1	3	1	1	2	2	4	7	8
B. Operated	0									
2. MULTIPLE DX										
A. Not Operated	1,938	3.4	11	1	1	2	4	6	9	17
B. Operated	28	8.2	39	1	2	8	12	18	25	>99
1. SINGLE DX	45	2.1	3	1	1	2	2	4	7	8
2. MULTIPLE DX	1,966	3.5	11	1	2	2	4	7	9	18
A. NOT OPERATED	1,983	3.4	11	1	1	2	4	6	9	17
B. OPERATED	28	8.2	39	1	2	8	12	18	25	>99
TOTAL										
0–19 Years	284	3.1	19	1	1	2	4	6	7	18
20–34	458	3.1	10	1	1	2	4	6	8	17
35–49	519	3.2	9	1	1	2	4	6	8	17
50–64	419	3.9	12	1	2	3	5	7	12	19
65+	331	3.8	9	2	2	3	5	7	10	14
GRAND TOTAL	2,011	3.4	11	1	1	2	4	7	9	18

536.3: GASTROPARESIS

Type of Patients	Observed Patients	Avg. Stay	Vari-ance	Percentiles 10th	25th	50th	75th	90th	95th	99th
1. SINGLE DX										
A. Not Operated										
0–19 Years	3	4.0	7	2	2	3	3	7	7	7
20–34	4	3.8	2	2	4	4	5	5	5	5
35–49	2	3.5	4	2	2	4	4	5	5	5
50–64	0									
65+	0									
B. Operated										
0–19 Years	0									
20–34	1	3.0	0	3	3	3	3	3	3	3
35–49	1	2.0	0	2	2	2	2	2	2	2
50–64	0									
65+	0									
2. MULTIPLE DX										
A. Not Operated										
0–19 Years	28	4.9	15	1	2	4	7	10	12	18
20–34	280	4.5	12	1	2	3	6	9	12	16
35–49	393	4.8	19	1	2	3	6	9	14	22
50–64	377	4.6	14	2	3	4	6	8	10	17
65+	295	5.7	23	2	3	4	7	12	15	23
B. Operated										
0–19 Years	5	8.2	36	2	5	5	13	16	16	16
20–34	19	6.2	61	1	1	2	2	23	25	25
35–49	32	7.6	76	2	2	4	8	17	32	33
50–64	21	7.7	53	1	3	6	8	14	26	26
65+	21	11.6	91	3	5	7	16	28	30	31
SUBTOTALS:										
1. SINGLE DX										
A. Not Operated	9	3.8	3	2	2	4	5	7	7	7
B. Operated	2	2.5	<1	2	2	3	3	3	3	3
2. MULTIPLE DX										
A. Not Operated	1,373	4.9	17	1	2	4	6	9	13	21
B. Operated	98	8.3	70	1	2	5	11	25	29	33
1. SINGLE DX	11	3.6	3	2	2	3	5	5	7	7
2. MULTIPLE DX	1,471	5.1	21	1	2	4	6	10	14	25
A. NOT OPERATED	1,382	4.9	17	1	2	4	6	9	13	21
B. OPERATED	100	8.1	70	1	2	5	11	25	28	32
TOTAL										
0–19 Years	36	5.3	18	1	2	4	7	12	16	18
20–34	304	4.6	15	1	2	3	6	9	12	20
35–49	428	5.0	23	1	2	3	6	10	15	26
50–64	398	4.8	17	2	2	4	6	9	12	26
65+	316	6.1	29	2	3	4	8	14	16	28
GRAND TOTAL	1,482	5.1	21	1	2	4	6	10	14	25

Length of Stay by Diagnosis and Operation, Western Region, 2008

Western Region, October 2006–September 2007 Data, by Diagnosis

536.41: GASTROSTOMY INFECTION

Type of Patients	Observed Patients	Avg. Stay	Variance	10th	25th	50th	75th	90th	95th	99th
1. SINGLE DX										
A. Not Operated										
0–19 Years	0									
20–34	0									
35–49	0									
50–64	1	1.0	0	1	1	1	1	1	1	1
65+	0									
B. Operated										
0–19 Years	0									
20–34	0									
35–49	0									
50–64	0									
65+	0									
2. MULTIPLE DX										
A. Not Operated										
0–19 Years	66	5.4	20	2	3	4	6	12	17	25
20–34	38	6.4	31	1	3	5	7	16	19	27
35–49	54	7.0	30	2	3	5	10	15	19	26
50–64	186	6.5	26	2	3	5	9	14	16	25
65+	513	7.2	38	2	3	5	9	15	18	28
B. Operated										
0–19 Years	2	5.0	2	4	4	5	6	6	6	6
20–34	1	24.0	0	24	24	24	24	24	24	24
35–49	12	11.0	64	3	7	9	17	24	27	27
50–64	21	12.0	175	5	5	7	13	18	37	59
65+	53	12.0	58	5	7	9	15	25	29	33
SUBTOTALS:										
1. SINGLE DX										
A. Not Operated	1	1.0	0	1	1	1	1	1	1	1
B. Operated	0									
2. MULTIPLE DX										
A. Not Operated	857	6.8	33	2	3	5	9	14	18	27
B. Operated	89	11.8	85	4	6	9	14	25	29	59
1. SINGLE DX	1	1.0	0	1	1	1	1	1	1	1
2. MULTIPLE DX	946	7.3	40	2	3	5	9	15	19	29
A. NOT OPERATED	858	6.8	33	2	3	5	9	14	18	27
B. OPERATED	89	11.8	85	4	6	9	14	25	29	59
TOTAL										
0–19 Years	68	5.4	19	2	3	4	6	12	17	25
20–34	39	6.8	38	1	3	5	8	18	24	27
35–49	66	7.7	37	2	3	6	10	17	21	26
50–64	208	7.0	43	2	3	5	9	14	19	30
65+	566	7.6	41	2	4	6	9	15	20	29
GRAND TOTAL	947	7.3	40	2	3	5	9	15	19	29

536.42: GASTROSTOMY MECH COMP

Type of Patients	Observed Patients	Avg. Stay	Variance	10th	25th	50th	75th	90th	95th	99th
1. SINGLE DX										
A. Not Operated										
0–19 Years	1	1.0	0	1	1	1	1	1	1	1
20–34	0									
35–49	0									
50–64	1	1.0	0	1	1	1	1	1	1	1
65+	0									
B. Operated										
0–19 Years	1	1.0	0	1	1	1	1	1	1	1
20–34	0									
35–49	0									
50–64	0									
65+	0									
2. MULTIPLE DX										
A. Not Operated										
0–19 Years	66	3.6	10	1	1	2	5	8	11	14
20–34	45	4.2	23	1	2	3	4	8	16	23
35–49	70	3.5	10	1	1	3	6	6	11	19
50–64	164	4.9	38	1	2	3	6	11	14	52
65+	457	4.2	12	1	2	3	5	8	11	19
B. Operated										
0–19 Years	10	7.9	53	3	4	5	8	25	25	25
20–34	10	16.6	789	4	4	8	10	95	95	95
35–49	21	10.8	291	3	3	7	10	14	21	82
50–64	23	7.4	101	2	3	5	10	11	12	51
65+	53	10.7	90	2	4	8	14	19	28	56
SUBTOTALS:										
1. SINGLE DX										
A. Not Operated	2	1.0	0	1	1	1	1	1	1	1
B. Operated	1	1.0	0	1	1	1	1	1	1	1
2. MULTIPLE DX										
A. Not Operated	802	4.2	17	1	2	3	5	8	11	21
B. Operated	117	10.3	181	2	4	7	11	19	28	82
1. SINGLE DX	3	1.0	0	1	1	1	1	1	1	1
2. MULTIPLE DX	919	5.0	42	1	2	3	6	10	14	26
A. NOT OPERATED	804	4.2	17	1	2	3	5	8	11	21
B. OPERATED	118	10.2	180	2	4	7	11	19	28	82
TOTAL										
0–19 Years	78	4.1	17	1	2	3	5	9	13	25
20–34	55	6.4	173	1	2	3	7	10	21	95
35–49	91	5.2	82	1	2	3	6	9	14	82
50–64	188	5.2	45	1	2	4	6	11	14	52
65+	510	4.9	24	1	2	4	6	9	14	23
GRAND TOTAL	922	5.0	42	1	2	3	6	10	14	26

536.49: GASTROSTOMY COMP NEC

Type of Patients	Observed Patients	Avg. Stay	Variance	10th	25th	50th	75th	90th	95th	99th
1. SINGLE DX										
A. Not Operated										
0–19 Years	2	1.0	0	1	1	1	1	1	1	1
20–34	0									
35–49	0									
50–64	0									
65+	0									
B. Operated										
0–19 Years	0									
20–34	0									
35–49	0									
50–64	0									
2. MULTIPLE DX										
A. Not Operated										
0–19 Years	34	3.4	37	1	1	1	3	6	20	32
20–34	23	4.0	15	1	1	2	5	10	11	15
35–49	39	3.9	11	1	2	3	5	9	12	16
50–64	84	6.3	90	1	2	4	6	12	17	60
65+	228	5.1	24	1	2	4	6	10	13	23
B. Operated										
0–19 Years	21	9.4	351	3	3	4	8	25	88	>99
20–34	7	7.3	13	3	4	6	11	12	12	12
35–49	10	16.7	234	2	9	14	17	57	57	57
50–64	23	10.1	85	2	3	8	19	29	38	>99
65+	31	12.1	131	2	5	9	19	23	28	58
SUBTOTALS:										
1. SINGLE DX										
A. Not Operated	2	1.0	0	1	1	1	1	1	1	1
B. Operated	0									
2. MULTIPLE DX										
A. Not Operated	408	5.0	37	1	2	3	6	10	14	26
B. Operated	92	11.1	171	2	4	8	14	23	57	>99
1. SINGLE DX	2	1.0	0	1	1	1	1	1	1	1
2. MULTIPLE DX	500	6.1	67	1	2	4	7	13	20	58
A. NOT OPERATED	410	5.0	37	1	2	3	6	10	14	26
B. OPERATED	92	11.1	171	2	4	8	14	23	57	>99
TOTAL										
0–19 Years	57	5.5	156	1	2	2	5	11	32	>99
20–34	30	4.7	16	1	2	3	7	11	12	15
35–49	49	6.5	80	1	2	4	7	16	17	57
50–64	107	7.1	91	1	2	4	9	15	26	60
65+	259	5.9	42	2	2	4	7	12	20	28
GRAND TOTAL	502	6.1	67	1	2	4	7	13	20	58

536.8: STOMACH FUNCT DISORD NEC

Type of Patients	Observed Patients	Avg. Stay	Variance	Percentiles 10th	25th	50th	75th	90th	95th	99th
1. SINGLE DX										
A. Not Operated										
0–19 Years	2	6.6	60	1	1	12	12	12	12	12
20–34	1	1.0	0	1	1	1	1	1	1	1
35–49	1	1.0	0	1	1	1	1	1	1	1
50–64	0									
65+	0									
B. Operated										
0–19 Years	0									
20–34	0									
35–49	0									
50–64	0									
65+	0									
2. MULTIPLE DX										
A. Not Operated										
0–19 Years	52	4.2	25	1	2	3	5	8	11	35
20–34	92	3.4	9	1	1	1	5	7	8	14
35–49	162	2.8	6	1	1	2	3	5	7	13
50–64	246	2.9	10	1	1	2	3	6	8	17
65+	309	2.7	7	1	1	2	3	5	7	12
B. Operated										
0–19 Years	11	16.1	354	3	4	6	27	39	60	60
20–34		5.0	0	5	5	5	5	5	5	5
35–49	4	7.8	33	3	5	6	16	16	16	16
50–64	9	11.0	190	1	2	8	11	46	46	46
65+	5	12.3	42	3	11	13	14	21	21	21
SUBTOTALS:										
1. SINGLE DX										
A. Not Operated	4	3.8	31	1	1	1	12	12	12	12
B. Operated	0									
2. MULTIPLE DX										
A. Not Operated	861	2.9	9	1	1	2	4	6	8	14
B. Operated	30	12.5	195	2	4	7	14	27	46	60
1. SINGLE DX	4	3.8	31	1	1	1	12	12	12	12
2. MULTIPLE DX	891	3.3	18	1	1	2	4	7	8	22
A. NOT OPERATED	865	2.9	9	1	1	2	4	6	8	14
B. OPERATED	30	12.5	195	2	4	7	14	27	46	60
TOTAL										
0–19 Years	65	6.3	96	1	2	3	6	11	27	60
20–34	94	3.4	9	1	1	2	5	7	7	14
35–49	167	2.9	7	1	1	2	3	5	5	16
50–64	255	3.2	18	1	1	2	3	7	9	22
65+	314	2.8	9	1	1	2	3	6	8	14
GRAND TOTAL	895	3.3	18	1	1	2	4	7	8	22

537: OTH GASTRODUODENAL DIS

Type of Patients	Observed Patients	Avg. Stay	Variance	Percentiles 10th	25th	50th	75th	90th	95th	99th
1. SINGLE DX										
A. Not Operated										
0–19 Years	2	1.5	<1	1	1	2	2	2	2	2
20–34	1	2.0		2	2	2	2	2	2	2
35–49	2	5.0	8	3	3	5	7	7	7	7
50–64	6	2.8	3	1	1	2	5	5	5	5
65+	1	5.0	0	5	5	5	5	5	5	5
B. Operated										
0–19 Years	56	2.3	1	1	2	2	3	3	4	7
20–34	3	4.3	4	2	2	5	6	6	6	6
35–49	4	7.7	13	3	3	7	11	11	11	11
50–64	2	5.0	2	4	4	5	6	6	6	6
65+	0									
2. MULTIPLE DX										
A. Not Operated										
0–19 Years	26	3.9	28	1	1	3	4	9	9	27
20–34	78	5.4	38	1	2	4	6	10	22	38
35–49	233	4.7	20	1	2	5	6	10	14	23
50–64	670	4.2	18	2	2	3	5	8	10	18
65+	2,482	4.4	12	2	2	3	5	8	11	18
B. Operated										
0–19 Years	79	4.0	21	1	2	2	4	9	15	28
20–34	30	8.4	36	1	5	5	13	15	22	23
35–49	81	8.1	44	2	3	6	11	18	22	32
50–64	216	10.2	114	3	4	7	13	20	28	62
65+	261	12.3	106	3	6	10	16	22	31	67
SUBTOTALS:										
1. SINGLE DX										
A. Not Operated	12	3.1	4	1	1	2	5	5	7	7
B. Operated	65	2.8	4	1	2	2	3	5	7	11
2. MULTIPLE DX										
A. Not Operated	3,489	4.4	14	2	2	3	5	8	11	20
B. Operated	667	10.0	94	2	4	7	13	20	26	62
1. SINGLE DX	77	2.8	4	1	2	2	3	5	7	11
2. MULTIPLE DX	4,156	5.3	31	2	2	4	6	11	15	27
A. NOT OPERATED	3,501	4.4	14	2	2	3	5	8	11	20
B. OPERATED	732	9.3	91	2	3	7	12	19	26	59
TOTAL										
0–19 Years	163	3.4	15	1	2	2	3	5	9	27
20–34	112	6.2	38	1	2	4	7	14	22	26
35–49	320	5.6	28	1	2	3	7	13	18	25
50–64	894	5.7	47	2	3	4	6	12	16	33
65+	2,744	5.2	26	2	2	4	6	10	14	26
GRAND TOTAL	4,233	5.3	31	2	2	4	6	10	15	26

537.0: ACQ PYLORIC STENOSIS

Type of Patients	Observed Patients	Avg. Stay	Variance	Percentiles 10th	25th	50th	75th	90th	95th	99th
1. SINGLE DX										
A. Not Operated										
0–19 Years	1	1.0	0	1	1	1	1	1	1	1
20–34	1	2.0	0	2	2	2	2	2	2	2
35–49	1	7.0	0	7	7	7	7	7	7	7
50–64	2	3.0	8	1	1	1	5	5	5	5
65+	1	5.0	0	5	5	5	5	5	5	5
B. Operated										
0–19 Years	52	2.3	1	1	2	2	2	3	4	7
20–34	1	6.0	0	6	6	6	6	6	6	6
35–49	1	10.0	0	10	10	10	10	10	10	10
50–64	2	5.0	2	4	4	5	5	6	6	6
65+	0									
2. MULTIPLE DX										
A. Not Operated										
0–19 Years	7	3.0	8	1	1	2	4	5	6	9
20–34	29	7.4	68	1	3	5	8	22	26	38
35–49	71	5.1	29	1	2	3	7	10	17	25
50–64	156	5.0	18	2	2	4	6	9	13	25
65+	238	6.1	25	2	3	5	7	13	18	24
B. Operated										
0–19 Years	52	3.0	5	2	2	2	3	5	6	12
20–34	10	9.2	17	4	6	7	13	14	15	15
35–49	36	9.7	46	3	3	8	13	22	24	27
50–64	118	10.5	122	4	5	7	12	21	26	68
65+	102	15.6	181	6	7	11	18	34	46	79
SUBTOTALS:										
1. SINGLE DX										
A. Not Operated	6	3.5	6	1	1	2	5	7	7	7
B. Operated	56	2.6	2	1	2	2	3	4	6	10
2. MULTIPLE DX										
A. Not Operated	501	5.7	26	1	2	4	7	12	15	26
B. Operated	318	10.8	127	2	4	7	13	21	33	68
1. SINGLE DX	62	2.7	3	1	2	2	3	5	6	10
2. MULTIPLE DX	819	7.6	71	2	3	5	9	16	22	46
A. NOT OPERATED	507	5.6	26	1	2	4	7	12	15	25
B. OPERATED	374	9.6	117	2	3	7	12	19	27	68
TOTAL										
0–19 Years	112	2.6	3	2	2	2	3	4	5	12
20–34	41	7.6	53	1	3	6	8	15	22	38
35–49	109	6.7	38	1	2	5	8	14	22	25
50–64	278	7.3	70	2	3	5	8	14	21	62
65+	341	8.9	90	2	4	6	11	18	24	66
GRAND TOTAL	881	7.3	68	2	3	5	8	15	21	46

Length of Stay by Diagnosis and Operation, Western Region, 2008

405

Western Region, October 2006–September 2007 Data, by Diagnosis

537.83: UP GI ANGIODYSPLAS W HEM

Type of Patients	Observed Patients	Avg. Stay	Variance	Percentiles						
				10th	25th	50th	75th	90th	95th	99th
1. SINGLE DX										
A. Not Operated										
0–19 Years	1	2.0	0	2	2	2	2	2	2	2
20–34	0									
35–49	0									
50–64	1	1.0	0	1	1	1	1	1	1	1
65+	0									
B. Operated										
0–19 Years	0									
20–34	0									
35–49	0									
50–64	0									
65+	0									
2. MULTIPLE DX										
A. Not Operated										
0–19 Years	1	3.0	0	3	3	3	3	3	3	3
20–34	12	6.2	47	1	3	4	7	10	26	26
35–49	38	3.4	7	1	2	3	4	7	12	12
50–64	246	3.7	7	1	2	3	4	7	9	12
65+	1,672	4.0	8	2	2	3	5	7	9	16
B. Operated										
0–19 Years	0									
20–34	1	7.0	0	7	7	7	7	7	7	7
35–49	1	4.0	0	4	4	4	4	4	4	4
50–64	11	10.0	41	6	6	8	13	17	24	24
65+	47	9.8	39	4	6	10	11	18	26	30
SUBTOTALS:										
1. SINGLE DX										
A. Not Operated	2	1.5	<1	1	1	2	2	2	2	2
B. Operated	0									
2. MULTIPLE DX										
A. Not Operated	1,969	4.0	8	2	2	3	5	7	9	16
B. Operated	60	9.7	38	4	6	9	11	18	26	30
1. SINGLE DX	2	1.5	<1	1	2	2	2	2	2	2
2. MULTIPLE DX	2,029	4.1	10	2	2	3	5	8	10	17
A. NOT OPERATED	1,971	4.0	8	2	2	3	5	7	9	16
B. OPERATED	60	9.7	38	4	6	9	11	18	26	30
TOTAL										
0–19 Years	2	2.5	<1	2	2	3	3	3	3	3
20–34	13	6.2	43	1	3	4	7	10	26	26
35–49	39	3.4	7	1	2	3	4	7	12	12
50–64	258	4.0	10	1	2	3	5	8	10	17
65+	1,719	4.2	10	2	2	3	5	8	10	17
GRAND TOTAL	2,031	4.1	10	2	2	3	5	8	10	17

537.84: UP GI DIEULAFOY LESION

Type of Patients	Observed Patients	Avg. Stay	Variance	Percentiles						
				10th	25th	50th	75th	90th	95th	99th
1. SINGLE DX										
A. Not Operated										
0–19 Years	0									
20–34	0									
35–49	0									
50–64	1	2.0	0	2	2	2	2	2	2	2
65+	0									
B. Operated										
0–19 Years	0									
20–34	0									
35–49	0									
50–64	0									
65+	0									
2. MULTIPLE DX										
A. Not Operated										
0–19 Years	2	3.0	0	3	3	3	3	3	3	3
20–34	15	2.8	1	1	2	3	4	4	5	5
35–49	33	4.8	14	2	2	3	6	12	13	14
50–64	103	4.1	7	2	2	3	5	7	9	13
65+	355	4.8	13	2	3	4	6	9	11	20
B. Operated										
0–19 Years	1	17.0	0	17	17	17	17	17	17	17
20–34	1	9.0	0	9	9	9	9	9	9	9
35–49	4	18.5	131	4	9	19	32	32	32	32
50–64	9	12.0	119	1	4	9	19	34	34	34
65+	23	13.2	52	5	9	11	19	21	26	31
SUBTOTALS:										
1. SINGLE DX										
A. Not Operated	1	2.0	0	2	2	2	2	2	2	2
B. Operated	0									
2. MULTIPLE DX										
A. Not Operated	508	4.6	12	2	3	4	5	8	11	17
B. Operated	38	13.5	72	4	8	12	19	26	32	34
1. SINGLE DX	1	2.0	0	2	2	2	2	2	2	2
2. MULTIPLE DX	546	5.2	21	2	3	4	6	10	15	26
A. NOT OPERATED	509	4.6	12	2	3	4	5	8	11	17
B. OPERATED	38	13.5	72	4	8	12	19	26	32	34
TOTAL										
0–19 Years	3	7.7	65	3	3	3	17	17	17	17
20–34	16	3.2	4	1	2	3	4	5	9	9
35–49	37	6.3	42	2	2	4	7	14	20	32
50–64	113	4.7	20	2	2	4	5	9	13	19
65+	378	5.3	20	2	3	4	6	10	15	26
GRAND TOTAL	547	5.2	21	2	3	4	6	10	15	26

537.89: GASTRODUODENAL DIS NEC

Type of Patients	Observed Patients	Avg. Stay	Variance	Percentiles						
				10th	25th	50th	75th	90th	95th	99th
1. SINGLE DX										
A. Not Operated										
0–19 Years	0									
20–34	0									
35–49	0									
50–64	0									
65+	0									
B. Operated										
0–19 Years	1	5.0	0	5	5	5	5	5	5	5
20–34	0									
35–49	2	5.0	8	3	3	7	7	7	7	7
50–64	0									
65+	0									
2. MULTIPLE DX										
A. Not Operated										
0–19 Years	8	2.5	3	1	1	2	4	5	5	5
20–34	7	3.0	<1	2	3	3	3	4	4	4
35–49	50	4.7	19	2	3	3	5	11	15	19
50–64	94	4.5	62	2	3	3	5	8	9	75
65+	83	4.0	13	1	2	3	5	8	12	21
B. Operated										
0–19 Years	6	4.7	9	1	3	5	7	9	9	9
20–34	6	8.4	75	1	2	4	15	23	23	23
35–49	14	5.1	10	1	3	5	6	11	12	12
50–64	26	9.3	138	2	3	5	13	17	28	58
65+	34	7.8	30	3	3	6	12	14	16	26
SUBTOTALS:										
1. SINGLE DX										
A. Not Operated	0									
B. Operated	3	5.0	4	3	3	5	7	7	7	7
2. MULTIPLE DX										
A. Not Operated	242	4.3	32	1	2	3	5	8	11	19
B. Operated	86	7.6	61	2	3	6	9	15	17	58
1. SINGLE DX	3	5.0	4	3	3	5	7	7	7	7
2. MULTIPLE DX	328	5.1	42	1	2	3	6	11	15	26
A. NOT OPERATED	242	4.3	32	1	2	3	5	8	11	19
B. OPERATED	89	7.6	59	2	3	6	9	15	17	58
TOTAL										
0–19 Years	15	3.5	6	1	1	3	5	7	9	9
20–34	13	5.5	39	2	3	3	4	15	23	23
35–49	66	4.8	16	1	2	3	6	10	14	19
50–64	120	5.5	81	2	2	3	5	9	16	58
65+	117	5.1	21	1	2	3	6	12	14	21
GRAND TOTAL	331	5.1	42	1	2	3	6	11	15	26

Length of Stay by Diagnosis and Operation, Western Region, 2008

538: GI MUCOSITIS

Type of Patients	Observed Patients	Avg. Stay	Vari-ance	10th	25th	50th	75th	90th	95th	99th
1. SINGLE DX										
A. Not Operated										
0–19 Years	0									
20–34	0									
35–49	0									
50–64	0									
65+	0									
B. Operated										
0–19 Years	0									
20–34	0									
35–49	0									
50–64	0									
65+	0									
2. MULTIPLE DX										
A. Not Operated										
0–19 Years	0									
20–34	1	3.0	0	3	3	3	3	3	3	3
35–49	1	2.0	0	2	2	2	2	2	2	2
50–64	1	9.0	0	9	9	9	9	9	9	9
65+	6	7.9	122	1	3	5	5	30	30	30
B. Operated										
0–19 Years	0									
20–34	0									
35–49	0									
50–64	0									
65+	0									
SUBTOTALS:										
1. SINGLE DX										
A. Not Operated	0									
B. Operated	0									
2. MULTIPLE DX										
A. Not Operated	9	6.8	82	1	3	3	5	30	30	30
B. Operated	0									
1. SINGLE DX	0									
2. MULTIPLE DX	9	6.8	82	1	3	3	5	30	30	30
A. NOT OPERATED	9	6.8	82	1	3	3	5	30	30	30
B. OPERATED	0									
TOTAL										
0–19 Years	0									
20–34	1	3.0	0	3	3	3	3	3	3	3
35–49	1	2.0	0	2	2	2	2	2	2	2
50–64	1	9.0	0	9	9	9	9	9	9	9
65+	6	7.9	122	1	3	5	5	30	30	30
GRAND TOTAL	9	6.8	82	1	3	3	5	30	30	30

540: ACUTE APPENDICITIS

Type of Patients	Observed Patients	Avg. Stay	Vari-ance	10th	25th	50th	75th	90th	95th	99th
1. SINGLE DX										
A. Not Operated										
0–19 Years	168	4.7	10	1	2	4	6	8	11	17
20–34	123	3.6	5	1	2	3	5	6	7	10
35–49	69	3.1	4	1	2	3	4	5	8	9
50–64	42	3.1	3	1	2	3	4	5	6	9
65+	10	4.2	3	3	3	4	6	7	7	7
B. Operated										
0–19 Years	9,636	2.1	3	1	1	1	2	4	5	8
20–34	8,660	1.7	1	1	1	1	2	3	4	6
35–49	4,084	1.8	2	1	1	1	2	3	4	6
50–64	1,499	2.0	2	1	1	2	2	4	5	7
65+	208	2.1	2	1	1	2	3	4	5	7
2. MULTIPLE DX										
A. Not Operated										
0–19 Years	162	5.7	14	2	3	5	8	10	13	20
20–34	130	4.2	11	1	2	3	6	9	10	13
35–49	164	4.2	7	1	2	4	6	7	9	12
50–64	165	4.4	11	1	2	4	6	8	10	18
65+	146	5.3	13	2	3	5	6	10	12	18
B. Operated										
0–19 Years	6,544	3.6	12	1	1	2	5	7	10	16
20–34	8,162	2.5	7	1	1	2	3	5	7	13
35–49	7,812	2.8	8	1	1	2	3	6	8	14
50–64	6,884	3.4	13	1	2	2	4	7	9	17
65+	3,913	4.8	21	1	2	3	6	10	14	24
SUBTOTALS:										
1. SINGLE DX										
A. Not Operated	412	3.9	7	1	2	3	5	7	9	13
B. Operated	24,087	1.9	2	1	1	1	2	4	5	7
2. MULTIPLE DX										
A. Not Operated	767	4.8	12	1	3	4	6	9	11	18
B. Operated	33,315	3.3	12	1	1	2	4	7	9	17
1. SINGLE DX	24,499	1.9	2	1	1	1	2	4	5	7
2. MULTIPLE DX	34,082	3.3	12	1	1	2	4	7	9	17
A. NOT OPERATED	1,179	4.5	10	1	2	4	6	8	10	17
B. OPERATED	57,402	2.7	8	1	1	2	3	6	8	14
TOTAL										
0–19 Years	16,510	2.7	7	1	1	2	3	6	8	13
20–34	17,075	2.1	4	1	1	2	3	4	6	11
35–49	12,129	2.5	6	1	1	2	3	5	7	12
50–64	8,590	3.2	12	1	1	2	4	6	9	16
65+	4,277	4.7	21	1	2	3	6	10	13	24
GRAND TOTAL	58,581	2.7	8	1	1	2	3	6	8	14

540.0: AC APPEND W PERITONITIS

Type of Patients	Observed Patients	Avg. Stay	Vari-ance	10th	25th	50th	75th	90th	95th	99th
1. SINGLE DX										
A. Not Operated										
0–19 Years	47	4.5	5	2	3	4	6	7	8	11
20–34	30	3.4	3	1	2	3	5	6	6	6
35–49	17	3.9	4	2	3	4	5	8	9	9
50–64	6	4.9	5	2	4	5	5	9	9	9
65+	2	2.0	2	1	1	3	3	3	3	3
B. Operated										
0–19 Years	1,414	3.7	4	1	2	3	5	6	7	9
20–34	735	3.0	3	1	2	3	4	5	6	9
35–49	484	2.9	3	1	2	3	4	5	6	9
50–64	255	3.1	3	1	2	3	4	5	6	10
65+	52	3.3	3	1	2	3	4	6	7	7
2. MULTIPLE DX										
A. Not Operated										
0–19 Years	40	6.1	13	3	4	5	8	11	13	21
20–34	21	4.1	8	1	2	3	6	7	10	11
35–49	27	3.9	4	1	3	4	5	7	8	8
50–64	26	4.3	3	3	3	4	5	6	7	9
65+	26	4.7	9	2	3	4	6	12	12	12
B. Operated										
0–19 Years	1,541	5.5	13	2	3	5	7	9	12	17
20–34	1,135	4.3	10	1	2	4	5	8	10	19
35–49	1,405	4.4	10	1	2	4	5	8	10	16
50–64	1,728	4.7	15	2	3	4	6	8	11	16
65+	1,243	6.0	21	2	3	5	7	11	14	25
SUBTOTALS:										
1. SINGLE DX										
A. Not Operated	102	4.0	4	2	2	4	5	6	8	11
B. Operated	2,940	3.3	3	1	2	3	4	6	7	9
2. MULTIPLE DX										
A. Not Operated	140	4.8	9	2	3	4	6	8	11	13
B. Operated	7,052	5.0	14	2	3	4	6	9	11	19
1. SINGLE DX	3,042	3.4	4	1	2	3	4	6	7	9
2. MULTIPLE DX	7,192	5.0	14	2	3	4	6	9	11	19
A. NOT OPERATED	242	4.5	7	2	3	4	6	8	9	12
B. OPERATED	9,992	4.5	12	1	2	4	6	8	10	17
TOTAL										
0–19 Years	3,042	4.7	10	2	3	4	6	8	10	15
20–34	1,921	3.8	8	1	2	3	5	6	9	15
35–49	1,933	4.0	8	1	2	4	5	7	9	15
50–64	2,015	4.5	13	2	3	4	6	8	10	15
65+	1,323	5.8	20	2	3	5	7	11	14	24
GRAND TOTAL	10,234	4.5	12	1	2	4	6	8	10	17

Length of Stay by Diagnosis and Operation, Western Region, 2008

407

Western Region, October 2006–September 2007 Data, by Diagnosis

540.1: APPENDICEAL ABSCESS

Type of Patients	Observed Patients	Avg. Stay	Variance	10th	25th	50th	75th	90th	95th	99th
1. SINGLE DX										
A. Not Operated										
0–19 Years	90	5.8	11	2	4	5	7	10	13	17
20–34	63	4.5	5	2	3	4	6	7	9	12
35–49	38	3.3	3	1	2	3	4	5	9	9
50–64	29	3.1	2	1	2	3	4	5	6	7
65+	8	4.8	2	3	4	4	6	7	7	7
B. Operated										
0–19 Years	567	4.5	8	1	3	4	6	8	10	16
20–34	350	3.6	5	1	3	3	4	6	8	12
35–49	244	3.6	4	1	2	3	4	6	7	10
50–64	111	3.8	4	1	2	3	5	6	8	10
65+	16	2.6	2	1	1	3	3	5	6	6
2. MULTIPLE DX										
A. Not Operated										
0–19 Years	100	6.4	14	3	4	5	8	12	15	18
20–34	65	5.7	13	2	3	5	8	9	11	23
35–49	95	4.9	7	2	3	4	7	8	10	17
50–64	108	5.1	15	2	2	4	6	10	14	18
65+	95	5.9	15	2	3	5	7	11	13	24
B. Operated										
0–19 Years	1,015	7.0	23	3	4	6	9	13	16	25
20–34	790	6.1	22	2	3	5	8	11	14	25
35–49	973	5.7	17	2	3	5	7	10	13	23
50–64	1,163	6.3	29	2	3	5	8	12	15	30
65+	799	7.8	34	2	4	6	10	15	21	29
SUBTOTALS:										
1. SINGLE DX										
A. Not Operated	228	4.6	7	2	3	4	6	8	9	14
B. Operated	1,288	4.0	6	1	2	4	5	7	9	13
2. MULTIPLE DX										
A. Not Operated	463	5.6	13	2	3	5	7	10	13	18
B. Operated	4,740	6.6	25	2	3	5	8	12	16	27
1. SINGLE DX	1,516	4.1	7	1	2	4	5	7	9	13
2. MULTIPLE DX	5,203	6.5	24	2	3	5	8	12	15	25
A. NOT OPERATED	691	5.3	11	2	3	4	7	9	12	18
B. OPERATED	6,028	6.0	22	2	3	5	7	11	15	25
TOTAL										
0–19 Years	1,772	6.1	18	2	3	5	7	11	14	21
20–34	1,268	5.3	17	2	3	4	7	10	13	20
35–49	1,350	5.2	14	2	3	4	6	10	12	20
50–64	1,411	6.0	26	2	3	5	7	11	14	28
65+	918	7.4	32	2	4	6	9	15	19	28
GRAND TOTAL	6,719	5.9	21	2	3	5	7	11	14	24

540.9: ACUTE APPENDICITIS NOS

Type of Patients	Observed Patients	Avg. Stay	Variance	10th	25th	50th	75th	90th	95th	99th
1. SINGLE DX										
A. Not Operated										
0–19 Years	31	1.7	2	1	1	1	2	3	4	7
20–34	30	1.8	1	1	1	1	2	3	4	5
35–49	14	1.6	1	1	1	1	2	3	4	4
50–64	7	1.6	1	1	1	1	2	4	4	4
65+	0									
B. Operated										
0–19 Years	7,655	1.6	<1	1	1	1	2	3	3	5
20–34	7,575	1.4	<1	1	1	1	2	2	3	4
35–49	3,356	1.5	<1	1	1	1	2	2	3	4
50–64	1,133	1.6	<1	1	1	1	2	2	3	5
65+	140	1.6	<1	1	1	1	2	3	3	5
2. MULTIPLE DX										
A. Not Operated										
0–19 Years	22	2.2	5	1	1	1	3	5	8	8
20–34	44	2.0	2	1	1	1	3	4	5	7
35–49	42	2.8	3	1	1	2	4	5	7	8
50–64	31	2.3	1	1	1	2	3	4	4	5
65+	25	3.7	7	1	1	3	5	8	8	10
B. Operated										
0–19 Years	3,988	2.0	2	1	1	2	2	4	5	8
20–34	6,237	1.8	2	1	1	1	2	3	4	7
35–49	5,434	1.9	3	1	1	1	3	4	4	8
50–64	3,993	2.0	3	1	1	2	3	4	5	8
65+	1,871	2.8	8	1	2	2	3	5	7	14
SUBTOTALS:										
1. SINGLE DX										
A. Not Operated	82	1.7	1	1	1	1	2	3	4	7
B. Operated	19,859	1.5	<1	1	1	1	2	2	3	4
2. MULTIPLE DX										
A. Not Operated	164	2.5	4	1	1	2	3	5	7	8
B. Operated	21,523	2.0	3	1	1	1	2	4	5	9
1. SINGLE DX	19,941	1.5	<1	1	1	1	2	2	3	4
2. MULTIPLE DX	21,687	2.0	3	1	1	1	2	4	5	9
A. NOT OPERATED	246	2.3	3	1	1	2	3	5	6	8
B. OPERATED	41,382	1.8	2	1	1	1	2	3	4	7
TOTAL										
0–19 Years	11,696	1.7	1	1	1	1	2	3	4	6
20–34	13,886	1.6	1	1	1	1	2	3	3	5
35–49	8,846	1.8	2	1	1	1	2	3	3	7
50–64	5,164	1.9	3	1	1	2	3	5	5	7
65+	2,036	2.7	8	1	2	2	3	5	7	14
GRAND TOTAL	41,628	1.8	2	1	1	1	2	3	4	7

541: APPENDICITIS NOS

Type of Patients	Observed Patients	Avg. Stay	Variance	10th	25th	50th	75th	90th	95th	99th
1. SINGLE DX										
A. Not Operated										
0–19 Years	13	1.5	<1	1	1	1	2	2	3	3
20–34	8	1.8	1	1	1	2	2	2	4	4
35–49	5	2.0	1	1	1	2	3	3	3	3
50–64	7	2.3	2	1	1	2	3	5	5	5
65+	0									
B. Operated										
0–19 Years	215	1.5	<1	1	1	1	2	3	3	4
20–34	167	1.5	<1	1	1	1	2	2	3	4
35–49	75	1.6	<1	1	1	1	2	2	3	6
50–64	30	1.5	<1	1	1	1	2	2	3	4
65+	3	2.3	2	1	1	2	4	4	4	4
2. MULTIPLE DX										
A. Not Operated										
0–19 Years	19	4.2	35	1	1	1	7	11	24	24
20–34	24	2.3	4	1	1	2	3	5	5	10
35–49	36	2.4	2	1	1	2	3	5	5	6
50–64	21	3.0	4	1	2	2	4	5	6	8
65+	42	5.1	8	2	3	5	7	8	10	14
B. Operated										
0–19 Years	159	2.0	2	1	1	2	2	3	4	7
20–34	206	2.1	3	1	1	1	2	4	5	10
35–49	175	2.2	3	1	1	1	3	3	6	8
50–64	116	2.2	4	1	1	2	3	4	5	11
65+	50	2.6	4	2	3	2	3	5	6	10
SUBTOTALS:										
1. SINGLE DX										
A. Not Operated	33	1.8	1	1	1	1	2	3	4	5
B. Operated	490	1.5	<1	1	1	1	2	3	3	4
2. MULTIPLE DX										
A. Not Operated	142	3.5	10	1	1	3	5	8	9	14
B. Operated	706	2.1	3	1	1	2	3	4	5	10
1. SINGLE DX	523	1.5	<1	1	1	1	2	3	3	4
2. MULTIPLE DX	848	2.4	4	1	1	2	3	5	6	11
A. NOT OPERATED	175	3.2	9	1	1	2	4	7	9	14
B. OPERATED	1,196	1.9	2	1	1	1	2	3	4	8
TOTAL										
0–19 Years	406	1.8	3	1	1	1	2	3	4	9
20–34	405	1.8	2	1	1	1	2	3	4	10
35–49	291	2.0	2	1	1	2	2	4	5	7
50–64	174	2.2	3	1	2	2	3	4	5	11
65+	95	3.7	7	1	2	3	5	8	10	14
GRAND TOTAL	1,371	2.1	3	1	1	1	2	4	5	10

542: OTHER APPENDICITIS

Type of Patients	Observed Patients	Avg. Stay	Vari-ance	10th	25th	50th	75th	90th	95th	99th
1. SINGLE DX										
A. Not Operated										
0–19 Years	5	3.8	1	3	3	3	5	5	5	5
20–34	3	2.0	0	2	2	2	2	2	2	2
35–49	4	1.5	<1	1	1	1	1	3	3	3
50–64	4	2.7	<1	2	2	2	3	4	4	4
65+	1	2.0	0	2	2	2	2	2	2	2
B. Operated										
0–19 Years	52	1.4	<1	1	1	1	2	2	3	4
20–34	27	1.3	<1	1	1	1	1	2	2	3
35–49	18	1.3	<1	1	1	1	2	2	2	2
50–64	7	1.6	1	1	1	1	2	4	4	4
65+	1	1.0	0	1	1	1	1	1	1	1
2. MULTIPLE DX										
A. Not Operated										
0–19 Years	2	5.5	24	2	2	6	9	9	9	9
20–34	9	2.5	2	1	1	3	3	5	5	5
35–49	8	3.1	4	1	2	3	4	7	7	7
50–64	7	3.3	5	1	1	3	5	7	7	7
65+	6	4.2	5	3	3	5	6	7	7	7
B. Operated										
0–19 Years	51	2.2	4	1	1	1	2	4	7	12
20–34	55	3.0	5	1	1	2	4	7	8	10
35–49	59	2.6	6	1	1	2	3	5	9	14
50–64	40	2.4	4	1	1	2	3	5	6	10
65+	27	3.0	8	1	1	2	4	6	8	13
SUBTOTALS:										
1. SINGLE DX										
A. Not Operated	17	2.6	2	1	2	2	3	5	5	5
B. Operated	105	1.4	<1	1	1	1	2	2	3	4
2. MULTIPLE DX										
A. Not Operated	32	3.3	5	1	2	3	5	7	7	9
B. Operated	232	2.6	5	1	1	2	3	6	7	12
1. SINGLE DX	122	1.5	<1	1	1	1	2	3	3	5
2. MULTIPLE DX	264	2.7	5	1	1	2	3	6	7	12
A. NOT OPERATED	49	3.1	4	1	2	3	4	6	7	9
B. OPERATED	337	2.2	4	1	1	1	2	4	7	11
TOTAL										
0–19 Years	110	2.0	3	1	1	1	2	4	5	9
20–34	94	2.4	4	1	1	2	3	5	7	10
35–49	89	2.3	5	1	1	2	3	4	5	14
50–64	58	2.4	4	1	1	2	3	5	7	10
65+	35	3.1	7	1	1	2	5	6	8	13
GRAND TOTAL	386	2.3	4	1	1	2	3	5	7	11

543: OTH DISEASES OF APPENDIX

Type of Patients	Observed Patients	Avg. Stay	Vari-ance	10th	25th	50th	75th	90th	95th	99th
1. SINGLE DX										
A. Not Operated										
0–19 Years	2	1.0	0	1	1	1	1	1	1	1
20–34	4	1.3	<1	1	1	1	1	2	2	2
35–49	2	1.0	0	1	1	1	1	1	1	1
50–64	0									
65+	0									
B. Operated										
0–19 Years	47	1.6	1	1	1	1	2	3	3	7
20–34	20	1.7	<1	1	1	2	2	4	4	4
35–49	7	2.0	2	1	1	2	2	5	5	5
50–64	12	2.7	3	1	1	3	4	5	6	6
65+	3	2.3	2	1	1	2	4	4	4	4
2. MULTIPLE DX										
A. Not Operated										
0–19 Years	13	1.7	3	1	1	1	2	2	7	7
20–34	4	1.5	<1	1	1	2	2	2	2	2
35–49	3	1.3	<1	1	1	1	1	2	2	2
50–64	5	1.6	<1	1	1	1	2	3	3	3
65+	5	1.8	<1	1	1	2	2	3	3	3
B. Operated										
0–19 Years	58	2.2	3	1	1	1	2	4	6	12
20–34	56	2.2	6	1	1	2	3	5	7	8
35–49	51	2.3	3	1	1	2	3	4	6	9
50–64	68	2.4	3	1	1	2	3	5	6	7
65+	35	5.1	26	1	1	3	6	11	20	21
SUBTOTALS:										
1. SINGLE DX										
A. Not Operated	8	1.1	<1	1	1	1	1	2	2	2
B. Operated	89	1.8	2	1	1	2	2	4	4	7
2. MULTIPLE DX										
A. Not Operated	30	1.6	1	1	1	1	2	2	3	7
B. Operated	268	2.6	7	1	1	2	3	5	7	15
1. SINGLE DX	97	1.8	1	1	1	1	2	3	4	7
2. MULTIPLE DX	298	2.5	6	1	1	2	3	5	7	15
A. NOT OPERATED	38	1.5	1	1	1	1	2	2	3	7
B. OPERATED	357	2.4	6	1	1	2	3	5	6	12
TOTAL										
0–19 Years	120	1.9	2	1	1	1	2	3	4	7
20–34	84	2.0	3	1	1	2	3	5	5	8
35–49	63	2.2	3	1	1	2	3	4	5	9
50–64	85	2.4	3	1	1	2	3	5	6	7
65+	43	4.6	23	1	1	3	5	11	15	21
GRAND TOTAL	395	2.4	5	1	1	2	3	5	6	12

543.9: APPENDIX DISEASE NEC

Type of Patients	Observed Patients	Avg. Stay	Vari-ance	10th	25th	50th	75th	90th	95th	99th
1. SINGLE DX										
A. Not Operated										
0–19 Years	2	1.0	0	1	1	1	1	1	1	1
20–34	4	1.3	<1	1	1	1	1	2	2	2
35–49	2	1.0	0	1	1	1	1	1	1	1
50–64	0									
65+	0									
B. Operated										
0–19 Years	25	1.5	2	1	1	1	1	3	3	7
20–34	15	1.8	1	1	1	2	2	4	4	4
35–49	6	2.2	2	1	1	2	2	5	5	5
50–64	12	2.7	3	1	1	3	4	5	6	6
65+	3	2.3	2	1	1	2	4	4	4	4
2. MULTIPLE DX										
A. Not Operated										
0–19 Years	13	1.7	3	1	1	1	2	2	7	7
20–34	4	1.5	<1	1	1	2	2	2	2	2
35–49	3	1.3	<1	1	1	1	1	2	2	2
50–64	5	1.6	<1	1	1	1	2	3	3	3
65+	5	1.8	<1	1	1	2	2	3	3	3
B. Operated										
0–19 Years	40	2.4	4	1	1	2	3	4	6	12
20–34	47	2.2	3	1	1	2	3	5	7	8
35–49	49	2.3	3	1	1	2	3	5	6	9
50–64	66	2.4	3	1	1	2	3	5	6	7
65+	34	5.1	27	1	1	3	6	11	20	21
SUBTOTALS:										
1. SINGLE DX										
A. Not Operated	8	1.1	<1	1	1	1	1	2	2	2
B. Operated	61	1.9	2	1	1	2	2	4	5	7
2. MULTIPLE DX										
A. Not Operated	30	1.6	1	1	1	1	2	2	3	7
B. Operated	236	2.7	7	1	1	2	3	6	7	15
1. SINGLE DX	69	1.8	2	1	1	1	2	4	5	7
2. MULTIPLE DX	266	2.6	7	1	1	2	3	5	7	15
A. NOT OPERATED	38	1.5	1	1	1	1	2	2	3	7
B. OPERATED	297	2.6	6	1	1	2	3	5	7	15
TOTAL										
0–19 Years	80	2.0	3	1	1	1	2	4	6	12
20–34	70	2.0	2	1	1	2	3	5	6	8
35–49	60	2.2	2	1	1	2	3	4	5	9
50–64	83	2.4	3	1	1	2	3	5	6	7
65+	42	4.5	23	1	1	3	5	11	15	21
GRAND TOTAL	335	2.5	6	1	1	2	3	5	7	12

Length of Stay by Diagnosis and Operation, Western Region, 2008

Western Region, October 2006–September 2007 Data, by Diagnosis

550: INGUINAL HERNIA

Type of Patients	Observed Patients	Avg. Stay	Variance	10th	25th	50th	75th	90th	95th	99th
1. SINGLE DX										
A. Not Operated										
0–19 Years	12	1.1	<1	1	1	1	1	1	2	2
20–34	4	1.0	0	1	1	1	1	1	1	1
35–49	4	2.0	4	1	1	1	1	5	5	5
50–64	6	1.0	0	1	1	1	1	1	1	1
65+	0									
B. Operated										
0–19 Years	165	1.2	<1	1	1	1	1	2	2	2
20–34	139	1.5	<1	1	1	1	2	2	4	4
35–49	159	1.7	1	1	1	1	2	3	4	5
50–64	146	1.7	2	1	1	1	2	3	4	6
65+	75	1.6	1	1	1	1	2	3	4	5
2. MULTIPLE DX										
A. Not Operated										
0–19 Years	18	1.6	<1	1	1	1	2	4	4	4
20–34	15	2.5	15	1	1	1	2	4	16	16
35–49	38	1.9	2	1	1	1	2	5	6	6
50–64	85	2.3	5	1	1	1	3	5	6	14
65+	235	3.0	8	1	1	2	4	6	8	14
B. Operated										
0–19 Years	218	2.2	30	1	1	1	2	3	5	26
20–34	196	2.0	4	1	1	2	3	5	5	14
35–49	543	2.5	6	1	1	2	3	5	7	10
50–64	900	2.8	9	1	1	2	3	6	9	15
65+	2,277	3.9	19	1	1	2	5	8	12	22
SUBTOTALS:										
1. SINGLE DX										
A. Not Operated	26	1.2	<1	1	1	1	1	1	2	2
B. Operated	684	1.5	1	1	1	1	2	3	3	6
2. MULTIPLE DX										
A. Not Operated	391	2.6	7	1	1	2	3	6	7	14
B. Operated	4,134	3.3	15	1	1	2	4	7	10	19
1. SINGLE DX	710	1.5	1	1	1	1	2	3	3	6
2. MULTIPLE DX	4,525	3.2	15	1	1	2	4	7	10	18
A. NOT OPERATED	417	2.5	6	1	1	1	3	5	7	14
B. OPERATED	4,818	3.0	14	1	1	2	3	7	9	18
TOTAL										
0–19 Years	413	1.8	16	1	1	1	2	2	4	14
20–34	354	1.8	3	1	1	1	2	3	4	9
35–49	744	2.3	5	1	1	2	2	5	6	10
50–64	1,137	2.6	8	1	1	2	2	6	8	14
65+	2,587	3.7	18	1	1	2	5	8	11	21
GRAND TOTAL	5,235	3.0	13	1	1	2	3	6	9	17

550.10: UNILAT IH W OBSTRUCTION

Type of Patients	Observed Patients	Avg. Stay	Variance	10th	25th	50th	75th	90th	95th	99th
1. SINGLE DX										
A. Not Operated										
0–19 Years	5	1.2	<1	1	1	1	1	2	2	2
20–34	2	1.0	0	1	1	1	1	1	1	1
35–49	0									
50–64	2	1.0	0	1	1	1	1	1	1	1
65+	0									
B. Operated										
0–19 Years	47	1.2	<1	1	1	1	1	2	2	2
20–34	92	1.5	<1	1	1	1	2	2	3	4
35–49	93	1.7	1	1	1	1	2	3	4	6
50–64	75	1.8	3	1	1	1	2	3	5	9
65+	31	1.9	1	1	1	1	3	4	4	5
2. MULTIPLE DX										
A. Not Operated										
0–19 Years	3	1.7	<1	1	1	2	2	2	2	4
20–34	8	3.5	27	1	1	1	4	16	16	16
35–49	12	1.3	<1	1	1	1	1	3	3	3
50–64	33	2.1	3	1	1	1	3	5	7	8
65+	123	3.2	9	1	1	2	4	6	9	14
B. Operated										
0–19 Years	49	2.1	9	1	1	1	2	4	4	20
20–34	114	2.0	2	1	1	2	3	4	5	9
35–49	250	2.8	8	1	1	2	3	6	8	14
50–64	431	3.0	10	1	1	2	4	6	9	14
65+	1,011	4.5	21	1	2	3	6	9	13	21
SUBTOTALS:										
1. SINGLE DX										
A. Not Operated	9	1.1	<1	1	1	1	1	2	2	2
B. Operated	338	1.6	1	1	1	1	2	3	4	6
2. MULTIPLE DX										
A. Not Operated	179	2.9	8	1	1	2	4	6	8	16
B. Operated	1,855	3.7	16	1	1	2	4	8	11	19
1. SINGLE DX	347	1.6	1	1	1	1	2	3	4	6
2. MULTIPLE DX	2,034	3.6	15	1	1	2	4	8	11	19
A. NOT OPERATED	188	2.8	8	1	1	2	3	6	8	16
B. OPERATED	2,193	3.4	14	1	1	2	4	7	10	18
TOTAL										
0–19 Years	104	1.6	4	1	1	1	2	2	3	8
20–34	216	1.8	3	1	1	1	2	3	4	9
35–49	355	2.5	6	1	1	2	3	5	7	12
50–64	541	2.8	9	1	1	2	3	6	8	14
65+	1,165	4.3	19	1	1	3	5	9	12	21
GRAND TOTAL	2,381	3.3	14	1	1	2	4	7	10	18

550.11: RECUR UNILAT IH W OBSTR

Type of Patients	Observed Patients	Avg. Stay	Variance	10th	25th	50th	75th	90th	95th	99th
1. SINGLE DX										
A. Not Operated										
0–19 Years	0									
20–34	0									
35–49	0	1.0	0	1	1	1	1	1	1	1
50–64	0									
65+	0									
B. Operated										
0–19 Years	5	1.6	2	1	1	1	2	4	4	4
20–34	7	1.9	2	1	1	1	2	5	5	5
35–49	16	1.9	5	1	1	1	2	3	10	10
50–64	14	2.1	3	1	1	1	3	5	6	6
65+	11	1.6	1	1	1	1	3	3	4	4
2. MULTIPLE DX										
A. Not Operated										
0–19 Years	1	1.0	0	1	1	1	1	1	1	1
20–34	0									
35–49	3	3.3	6	1	1	3	3	6	6	6
50–64	3	3.0	1	2	2	3	4	4	4	4
65+	13	4.1	29	1	1	3	4	6	21	21
B. Operated										
0–19 Years	5	4.2	10	2	2	4	5	9	9	9
20–34	9	2.0	<1	1	1	2	2	3	3	3
35–49	61	2.8	6	1	1	2	3	5	6	18
50–64	72	3.2	12	1	1	2	4	6	11	21
65+	274	4.4	20	2	2	3	5	8	13	22
SUBTOTALS:										
1. SINGLE DX										
A. Not Operated	1	1.0	0	1	1	1	1	1	1	1
B. Operated	53	1.9	3	1	1	1	2	4	5	10
2. MULTIPLE DX										
A. Not Operated	20	3.7	19	1	1	3	4	6	21	21
B. Operated	421	3.9	16	1	2	3	5	7	11	22
1. SINGLE DX	54	1.9	3	1	1	1	2	4	5	10
2. MULTIPLE DX	441	3.9	16	1	1	3	4	7	11	22
A. NOT OPERATED	21	3.5	19	1	1	3	4	6	6	21
B. OPERATED	474	3.7	15	1	1	2	4	7	11	22
TOTAL										
0–19 Years	11	2.7	7	1	1	1	2	5	9	9
20–34	16	1.9	1	1	1	2	2	3	5	5
35–49	81	2.6	6	1	1	2	3	5	6	18
50–64	89	3.0	10	1	2	2	3	6	8	21
65+	298	4.2	19	2	2	3	5	8	13	22
GRAND TOTAL	495	3.6	15	1	1	2	4	7	11	22

Length of Stay by Diagnosis and Operation, Western Region, 2008

550.90: UNILAT INGUINAL HERNIA

Type of Patients	Observed Patients	Avg. Stay	Variance	10th	25th	50th	75th	90th	95th	99th
1. SINGLE DX										
A. Not Operated										
0–19 Years	6	1.0	0	1	1	1	1	1	1	1
20–34	2	1.0	0	1	1	1	1	1	1	1
35–49	3	2.3	5	1	1	1	5	5	5	5
50–64	2	1.0	0	1	1	1	1	1	1	1
65+	0									
B. Operated										
0–19 Years	41	1.1	<1	1	1	1	1	1	2	2
20–34	25	1.3	<1	1	1	1	1	2	2	5
35–49	34	1.6	1	1	1	1	2	3	4	6
50–64	29	1.5	<1	1	1	1	2	3	3	4
65+	21	1.3	<1	1	1	1	1	3	3	3
2. MULTIPLE DX										
A. Not Operated										
0–19 Years	10	1.4	<1	1	1	1	1	2	4	4
20–34	5	1.2	<1	1	1	1	1	2	2	2
35–49	16	1.8	2	1	1	1	2	5	6	6
50–64	36	2.3	6	1	1	1	3	5	6	14
65+	60	2.3	3	1	1	2	3	4	7	8
B. Operated										
0–19 Years	53	1.3	<1	1	1	1	1	2	3	5
20–34	51	1.8	2	1	1	1	2	3	4	8
35–49	157	2.1	3	1	1	1	3	4	6	9
50–64	229	2.4	7	1	1	1	3	6	7	13
65+	522	2.5	8	1	1	1	3	5	7	13
SUBTOTALS:										
1. SINGLE DX										
A. Not Operated	13	1.3	<1	1	1	1	1	1	5	5
B. Operated	150	1.4	<1	1	1	1	1	2	3	5
2. MULTIPLE DX										
A. Not Operated	127	2.1	4	1	1	1	3	4	6	8
B. Operated	1,012	2.3	6	1	1	1	3	5	7	13
1. SINGLE DX	163	1.4	<1	1	1	1	1	2	3	5
2. MULTIPLE DX	1,139	2.3	6	1	1	1	3	5	7	13
A. NOT OPERATED	140	2.1	3	1	1	1	2	4	6	8
B. OPERATED	1,162	2.2	6	1	1	1	3	5	6	13
TOTAL										
0–19 Years	110	1.2	<1	1	1	1	1	2	2	4
20–34	83	1.6	3	1	1	1	2	3	4	8
35–49	210	2.0	3	1	1	1	3	4	5	9
50–64	296	2.3	6	1	1	1	3	5	7	14
65+	603	2.4	7	1	1	1	3	5	7	13
GRAND TOTAL	1,302	2.2	5	1	1	1	2	5	6	13

550.91: RECUR UNILAT IH

Type of Patients	Observed Patients	Avg. Stay	Variance	10th	25th	50th	75th	90th	95th	99th
1. SINGLE DX										
A. Not Operated										
0–19 Years	0									
20–34	0									
35–49	0									
50–64	1	1.0	0	1	1	1	1	1	1	1
65+	0									
B. Operated										
0–19 Years	2	1.5	<1	1	1	1	2	2	2	2
20–34	4	1.3	<1	1	1	1	1	2	2	2
35–49	6	1.3	<1	1	1	1	2	2	2	2
50–64	4	1.3	<1	1	1	1	2	2	2	2
65+	1	1.0	0	1	1	1	1	1	1	1
2. MULTIPLE DX										
A. Not Operated										
0–19 Years	0									
20–34	1	2.0	0	2	2	2	2	2	2	2
35–49	4	2.5	6	1	1	2	6	6	6	6
50–64	3	2.0	<1	1	1	2	3	3	3	3
65+	12	2.8	7	1	1	2	3	7	7	7
B. Operated										
0–19 Years	4	1.5	<1	1	1	1	1	3	3	3
20–34	6	2.2	2	1	2	1	2	5	5	5
35–49	17	2.1	5	1	1	1	2	5	9	9
50–64	35	1.9	2	1	1	1	2	4	5	7
65+	133	2.3	4	1	1	1	3	5	6	10
SUBTOTALS:										
1. SINGLE DX										
A. Not Operated	1	1.0	0	1	1	1	1	1	1	1
B. Operated	17	1.3	<1	1	1	1	2	2	2	2
2. MULTIPLE DX										
A. Not Operated	20	2.6	5	1	1	1	3	7	7	7
B. Operated	195	2.2	3	1	1	1	3	5	5	10
1. SINGLE DX	18	1.3	<1	1	1	1	2	2	2	2
2. MULTIPLE DX	215	2.2	3	1	1	1	3	5	7	10
A. NOT OPERATED	21	2.5	5	1	1	1	3	7	7	7
B. OPERATED	212	2.1	3	1	1	1	3	5	7	10
TOTAL										
0–19 Years	6	1.5	<1	1	1	1	1	3	3	3
20–34	11	1.8	1	1	1	1	2	3	5	5
35–49	27	2.0	4	1	1	1	2	5	6	9
50–64	43	1.8	2	1	1	1	2	3	5	7
65+	146	2.4	4	1	1	1	3	5	7	10
GRAND TOTAL	233	2.2	3	1	1	1	3	5	6	10

550.92: BILAT INGUINAL HERNIA

Type of Patients	Observed Patients	Avg. Stay	Variance	10th	25th	50th	75th	90th	95th	99th
1. SINGLE DX										
A. Not Operated										
0–19 Years	1	1.0	0			1	1	1	1	1
20–34	0									
35–49	0									
50–64	1	1.0	0			1	1	1	1	1
65+	0									
B. Operated										
0–19 Years	50	1.1	<1	1	1	1	1	1	2	3
20–34	9	2.1	4	1	1	1	2	7	7	7
35–49	8	1.0	0	1	1	1	1	1	1	1
50–64	14	1.3	<1	1	1	1	1	2	2	2
65+	4	1.0	0	1	1	1	1	1	1	1
2. MULTIPLE DX										
A. Not Operated										
0–19 Years	3	2.3	2	1	1	2	4	4	4	4
20–34	0									
35–49	1	3.0	0	3	3	3	3	3	3	3
50–64	5	3.4	11	1	1	3	3	9	9	9
65+	9	2.2	2	1	1	2	3	3	5	5
B. Operated										
0–19 Years	86	2.8	69	1	1	1	1	2	5	53
20–34	11	2.8	17	1	1	2	2	7	15	15
35–49	39	2.3	7	1	1	2	3	5	5	6
50–64	70	2.5	7	1	1	2	2	5	10	13
65+	159	2.2	4	1	1	1	2	4	8	11
SUBTOTALS:										
1. SINGLE DX										
A. Not Operated	2	1.0	0	1	1	1	1	1	1	1
B. Operated	85	1.2	<1	1	1	1	1	2	2	7
2. MULTIPLE DX										
A. Not Operated	18	2.6	4	1	1	2	3	5	9	9
B. Operated	365	2.4	20	1	1	1	2	4	7	15
1. SINGLE DX	87	1.2	<1	1	1	1	1	2	2	7
2. MULTIPLE DX	383	2.4	19	1	1	1	2	4	7	15
A. NOT OPERATED	20	2.5	4	1	1	1	3	5	5	9
B. OPERATED	450	2.2	17	1	1	1	2	4	6	14
TOTAL										
0–19 Years	140	2.2	43	1	1	1	2	2	3	52
20–34	20	2.5	11	1	1	1	2	5	15	15
35–49	48	2.1	7	1	1	2	2	5	5	6
50–64	90	2.4	7	1	1	1	2	5	9	13
65+	172	2.1	4	1	1	1	2	4	7	11
GRAND TOTAL	470	2.2	16	1	1	1	2	4	6	14

Length of Stay by Diagnosis and Operation, Western Region, 2008

Western Region, October 2006–September 2007 Data, by Diagnosis

551: OTH ABD HERNIA W GANGR

Type of Patients	Observed Patients	Avg. Stay	Vari-ance	10th	25th	50th	75th	90th	95th	99th
1. SINGLE DX										
A. Not Operated										
0–19 Years	0									
20–34	0									
35–49	0									
50–64	0									
65+	1	1.0	0					1	1	1
B. Operated										
0–19 Years	0									
20–34	2	2.5	<1	2	2	3	3	3	3	3
35–49	4	3.8	10	1	1	6	7	7	7	7
50–64	2	3.0	8	1	1	5	5	5	5	5
65+	0									
2. MULTIPLE DX										
A. Not Operated										
0–19 Years	0									
20–34	1	2.0	0	2	2	2	2	2	2	2
35–49	0									
50–64	0									
65+	0									
B. Operated										
0–19 Years	0									
20–34	4	7.5	48	1	1	8	17	17	17	17
35–49	34	8.2	54	2	3	5	13	18	27	31
50–64	57	6.6	15	2	4	6	9	13	15	>99
65+	113	9.7	55	3	5	8	13	17	25	35
SUBTOTALS:										
1. SINGLE DX										
A. Not Operated	1	1.0	0	1	1	1	1	1	1	1
B. Operated	8	3.3	6	1	1	3	5	7	7	7
2. MULTIPLE DX										
A. Not Operated	1	2.0	0	2	2	2	2	2	2	2
B. Operated	208	8.5	45	2	3	4	6	11	21	35
1. SINGLE DX	9	3.0	6	1	1	2	5	7	7	7
2. MULTIPLE DX	209	8.5	45	3	4	6	11	17	21	35
A. NOT OPERATED	2	1.5	<1	1	1	1	2	2	2	2
B. OPERATED	216	8.3	44	3	4	6	11	17	21	35
TOTAL										
0–19 Years	0									
20–34	7	5.3	32	1	2	3	8	17	17	17
35–49	38	7.7	51	2	3	5	9	18	27	31
50–64	59	6.5	15	2	4	6	9	12	15	>99
65+	114	9.6	55	3	5	8	13	17	25	35
GRAND TOTAL	218	8.3	44	2	4	6	11	17	21	35

552: OTH ABD HERNIA W OBSTR

Type of Patients	Observed Patients	Avg. Stay	Vari-ance	10th	25th	50th	75th	90th	95th	99th
1. SINGLE DX										
A. Not Operated										
0–19 Years	1	1.0	0	1	1	1	1	1	1	1
20–34	4	1.0	0	1	1	1	1	1	1	1
35–49	14	2.0	3	1	1	1	2	3	8	8
50–64	6	2.3	3	1	1	1	4	5	5	5
65+	5	2.6	4	1	1	2	3	6	6	6
B. Operated										
0–19 Years	9	1.2	<1	1	1	1	1	2	2	2
20–34	101	1.6	1	1	1	1	2	3	4	6
35–49	223	2.0	3	1	1	1	2	3	4	6
50–64	149	2.2	2	1	1	2	3	4	5	7
65+	63	2.7	4	1	1	2	4	5	6	10
2. MULTIPLE DX										
A. Not Operated										
0–19 Years	3	2.0	1	1	1	2	3	3	3	3
20–34	20	1.7	<1	1	1	2	2	3	3	3
35–49	127	2.9	10	1	1	2	4	5	7	12
50–64	279	3.2	12	1	2	2	4	6	8	12
65+	464	4.0	12	1	2	3	5	8	10	17
B. Operated										
0–19 Years	33	3.9	11	1	2	3	6	7	8	18
20–34	441	3.3	16	2	2	3	5	6	9	16
35–49	1,817	4.1	25	2	2	3	5	8	10	24
50–64	2,797	4.9	27	2	3	4	6	10	13	26
65+	3,466	6.2	36	2	3	5	8	13	17	29
SUBTOTALS:										
1. SINGLE DX										
A. Not Operated	30	2.0	3	1	1	1	2	4	6	8
B. Operated	545	2.0	2	1	1	2	2	4	5	7
2. MULTIPLE DX										
A. Not Operated	893	3.5	12	1	2	3	4	7	9	17
B. Operated	8,554	5.2	31	2	2	4	6	10	14	27
1. SINGLE DX	575	2.0	2	1	1	2	2	4	5	7
2. MULTIPLE DX	9,447	5.0	29	2	2	4	6	10	14	27
A. NOT OPERATED	923	3.5	11	1	1	3	4	7	9	16
B. OPERATED	9,099	5.0	29	2	2	4	6	10	14	27
TOTAL										
0–19 Years	46	3.2	9	1	1	2	4	6	8	18
20–34	566	2.9	13	1	1	2	3	6	7	15
35–49	2,181	3.8	22	1	1	3	5	7	10	22
50–64	3,231	4.7	25	2	3	3	6	9	12	25
65+	3,998	5.9	33	2	2	4	7	12	17	29
GRAND TOTAL	10,022	4.9	28	2	2	3	6	10	14	26

552.00: UNILAT FH W OBSTRUCTION

Type of Patients	Observed Patients	Avg. Stay	Vari-ance	10th	25th	50th	75th	90th	95th	99th
1. SINGLE DX										
A. Not Operated										
0–19 Years	0									
20–34	0									
35–49	0									
50–64	0									
65+	1	6.0	0	6	6	6	6	6	6	6
B. Operated										
0–19 Years	1	1.0	0	1	1	1	1	1	1	1
20–34	5	1.0	0	1	1	1	1	1	1	1
35–49	13	1.9	1	1	1	2	2	2	5	5
50–64	14	1.4	<1	1	1	1	2	2	4	4
65+	16	1.9	1	1	1	1	3	4	4	4
2. MULTIPLE DX										
A. Not Operated										
0–19 Years	0									
20–34	0									
35–49	2	3.0	2	2	2	4	4	4	4	4
50–64	1	1.0	0	1	1	1	1	1	1	1
65+	11	6.4	33	1	2	5	10	11	20	20
B. Operated										
0–19 Years	4	1.5	<1	1	1	2	2	2	2	2
20–34	4	1.0	0	1	1	1	1	1	1	1
35–49	34	2.5	6	1	1	2	3	5	10	11
50–64	84	3.9	11	1	2	3	5	7	10	17
65+	440	5.3	21	1	2	4	7	11	15	23
SUBTOTALS:										
1. SINGLE DX										
A. Not Operated	1	6.0	0	6	6	6	6	6	6	6
B. Operated	49	1.7	1	1	1	1	2	4	4	5
2. MULTIPLE DX										
A. Not Operated	14	5.5	29	1	2	3	8	11	20	20
B. Operated	564	4.9	20	1	2	4	6	10	14	22
1. SINGLE DX	50	1.7	1	1	1	1	2	4	4	6
2. MULTIPLE DX	578	4.9	20	1	2	4	6	10	14	22
A. NOT OPERATED	15	5.5	27	1	2	4	8	11	20	20
B. OPERATED	613	4.7	19	1	2	3	6	10	14	21
TOTAL										
0–19 Years	3	1.3	<1	1	1	1	2	2	2	2
20–34	9	1.0	0	1	1	1	1	1	1	1
35–49	49	2.3	5	1	1	2	2	5	8	11
50–64	99	3.5	10	1	2	2	5	7	10	17
65+	468	5.3	21	1	2	4	7	11	14	23
GRAND TOTAL	628	4.7	19	1	2	3	6	10	14	21

Western Region, October 2006–September 2007 Data, by Diagnosis

552.1: UMBILICAL HERNIA W OBSTR

Type of Patients	Observed Patients	Avg. Stay	Variance	10th	25th	50th	75th	90th	95th	99th
1. SINGLE DX										
A. Not Operated										
0–19 Years	1	1.0	0	1	1	1	1	1	1	1
20–34	1	1.0	0	1	1	1	1	1	1	1
35–49	6	1.3	<1	1	1	1	2	2	2	2
50–64	1	1.0	0	1	1	1	1	1	1	1
65+	1	3.0	0	3	3	3	3	3	3	3
B. Operated										
0–19 Years	6	1.2	<1	1	1	1	1	2	2	2
20–34	53	1.4	<1	1	1	1	2	2	3	4
35–49	84	1.6	2	1	1	1	2	3	4	10
50–64	33	1.8	1	1	1	1	2	4	4	5
65+	2	1.0	0	1	1	1	1	1	1	1
2. MULTIPLE DX										
A. Not Operated										
0–19 Years	2	2.5	<1	2	2	3	3	3	3	3
20–34	4	1.3	<1	1	1	1	1	2	2	2
35–49	27	2.6	6	1	1	2	3	5	7	12
50–64	54	2.4	5	1	1	2	3	5	7	12
65+	69	3.6	16	1	2	2	5	7	8	29
B. Operated										
0–19 Years	14	2.1	1	1	1	2	3	4	4	4
20–34	122	2.1	2	1	1	2	3	4	5	6
35–49	428	3.0	17	1	1	2	4	6	9	24
50–64	563	3.8	15	1	1	2	5	8	11	19
65+	426	4.9	24	2	2	4	6	10	14	25
SUBTOTALS:										
1. SINGLE DX										
A. Not Operated	10	1.4	<1	1	1	1	2	2	3	3
B. Operated	178	1.6	1	1	1	1	2	3	4	5
2. MULTIPLE DX										
A. Not Operated	156	2.9	10	1	1	2	4	6	8	14
B. Operated	1,553	3.8	17	1	1	2	5	8	11	23
1. SINGLE DX	188	1.6	1	1	1	1	2	3	4	5
2. MULTIPLE DX	1,709	3.7	17	1	1	2	5	8	11	19
A. NOT OPERATED	166	2.8	10	1	1	2	3	6	7	14
B. OPERATED	1,731	3.5	16	1	1	2	4	8	10	19
TOTAL										
0–19 Years	23	1.8	<1	1	1	2	2	3	4	4
20–34	180	1.9	2	1	1	1	2	4	5	6
35–49	545	2.8	14	1	1	2	3	5	8	15
50–64	651	3.6	14	1	1	2	5	8	11	19
65+	498	4.7	23	1	2	4	6	9	14	25
GRAND TOTAL	1,897	3.5	16	1	1	2	4	7	10	19

552.20: OBSTR VENTRAL HERNIA NOS

Type of Patients	Observed Patients	Avg. Stay	Variance	10th	25th	50th	75th	90th	95th	99th
1. SINGLE DX										
A. Not Operated										
0–19 Years	0									
20–34	1	1.0	0	1	1	1	1	1	1	1
35–49	3	3.3	16	1	1	1	8	8	8	8
50–64	1	1.0	0	1	1	1	1	1	1	1
65+	2	1.5	<1	1	1	1	2	2	2	2
B. Operated										
0–19 Years	0									
20–34	8	1.8	1	1	1	2	2	4	4	4
35–49	27	1.6	<1	1	1	1	2	3	4	4
50–64	17	1.9	2	1	1	2	2	5	5	5
65+	8	2.1	2	1	1	2	4	4	4	4
2. MULTIPLE DX										
A. Not Operated										
0–19 Years	0									
20–34	4	1.5	<1	1	1	1	2	2	2	2
35–49	26	3.7	32	1	1	2	4	7	10	29
50–64	69	3.2	5	1	2	2	4	6	8	11
65+	97	4.1	12	2	2	3	5	8	12	17
B. Operated										
0–19 Years	2	3.0	0	3	3	3	3	3	3	3
20–34	47	2.6	2	1	1	2	3	5	6	6
35–49	198	3.8	24	1	1	3	5	7	8	22
50–64	318	4.8	29	1	2	3	6	9	13	29
65+	342	5.9	23	3	3	5	8	13	15	23
SUBTOTALS:										
1. SINGLE DX										
A. Not Operated	7	2.1	7	1	1	1	2	8	8	8
B. Operated	60	1.8	1	1	1	1	2	4	4	5
2. MULTIPLE DX										
A. Not Operated	196	3.7	12	2	2	3	4	7	10	17
B. Operated	907	4.9	25	2	2	4	6	10	14	23
1. SINGLE DX	67	1.8	2	1	1	1	2	4	4	8
2. MULTIPLE DX	1,103	4.7	23	2	2	3	6	9	13	23
A. NOT OPERATED	203	3.6	12	2	2	3	4	7	10	16
B. OPERATED	967	4.7	24	2	2	3	6	9	13	23
TOTAL										
0–19 Years	2	3.0	0	3	3	3	3	3	3	3
20–34	60	2.4	2	1	1	2	3	4	6	6
35–49	254	3.5	23	1	1	3	4	7	8	22
50–64	405	4.4	25	2	2	3	5	8	11	26
65+	449	5.5	21	2	2	4	7	12	15	22
GRAND TOTAL	1,170	4.5	22	2	2	3	6	9	13	23

552.21: OBSTR INCISIONAL HERNIA

Type of Patients	Observed Patients	Avg. Stay	Variance	10th	25th	50th	75th	90th	95th	99th
1. SINGLE DX										
A. Not Operated										
0–19 Years	0									
20–34	1	1.0	0	1	1	1	1	1	1	1
35–49	4	2.0	<1	1	2	2	3	3	3	3
50–64	4	3.0	3	1	1	2	4	5	5	5
65+	0									
B. Operated										
0–19 Years	1	1.0	0	1	1	1	1	1	1	1
20–34	18	2.0	2	1	1	1	2	5	6	6
35–49	62	2.3	1	1	1	2	3	4	5	6
50–64	60	2.5	2	1	1	2	3	5	5	7
65+	18	3.7	6	1	1	3	5	7	10	10
2. MULTIPLE DX										
A. Not Operated										
0–19 Years	0									
20–34	8	1.9	<1	1	1	2	3	3	3	3
35–49	55	2.8	5	1	1	2	4	6	8	11
50–64	100	2.8	4	1	1	3	4	5	7	10
65+	156	3.7	8	1	2	3	5	7	10	14
B. Operated										
0–19 Years	6	6.3	35	3	3	3	6	18	18	18
20–34	165	3.7	17	1	1	3	4	7	11	18
35–49	810	4.3	19	2	2	3	5	8	10	20
50–64	1,337	5.0	23	1	2	4	6	9	13	25
65+	1,402	5.9	27	1	2	4	7	12	16	29
SUBTOTALS:										
1. SINGLE DX										
A. Not Operated	9	2.3	2	1	1	2	3	5	5	5
B. Operated	159	2.5	3	1	1	2	3	5	5	7
2. MULTIPLE DX										
A. Not Operated	319	3.3	6	1	1	3	4	6	8	12
B. Operated	3,720	5.1	24	1	2	4	6	10	14	27
1. SINGLE DX	168	2.5	2	1	1	2	3	5	5	7
2. MULTIPLE DX	4,039	5.0	23	1	2	4	6	10	13	26
A. NOT OPERATED	328	3.2	6	1	1	3	4	6	8	12
B. OPERATED	3,879	5.0	23	1	2	4	6	10	14	27
TOTAL										
0–19 Years	7	5.6	34	1	2	3	6	18	18	18
20–34	192	3.4	15	1	1	2	4	6	11	18
35–49	931	4.1	17	1	2	3	5	7	10	18
50–64	1,501	4.8	21	1	2	4	6	9	12	23
65+	1,576	5.6	26	1	2	4	7	11	16	28
GRAND TOTAL	4,207	4.9	22	1	2	4	6	10	13	25

Length of Stay by Diagnosis and Operation, Western Region, 2008

Western Region, October 2006–September 2007 Data, by Diagnosis

552.29: OBSTR VENTRAL HERNIA NEC

Type of Patients	Observed Patients	Avg. Stay	Vari-ance	Percentiles 10th	25th	50th	75th	90th	95th	99th
1. SINGLE DX										
A. Not Operated										
0–19 Years	0									
20–34	0									
35–49	0									
50–64	0									
65+	1	1.0	0			1	1	1	1	1
B. Operated										
0–19 Years	1	2.0	0	2	2	2	2	2	2	2
20–34	12	1.3	<1	1	1	1	1	2	3	3
35–49	26	1.8	1	1	1	1	2	3	4	5
50–64	18	2.1	2	1	1	1	2	3	7	7
65+	12	2.5	3	1	1	2	4	5	6	6
2. MULTIPLE DX										
A. Not Operated										
0–19 Years	0									
20–34	1	1.0	0	1	1	1	1	1	1	1
35–49	12	2.1	1	1	1	2	3	4	4	4
50–64	31	4.0	15	1	1	3	5	9	9	20
65+	55	3.8	8	2	2	3	5	9	9	12
B. Operated										
0–19 Years	0									
20–34	41	2.7	4	1	1	2	4	6	6	10
35–49	186	3.7	28	1	1	3	5	7	9	44
50–64	263	5.5	54	1	2	3	6	11	16	34
65+	318	5.4	26	1	2	4	7	10	15	28
SUBTOTALS:										
1. SINGLE DX										
A. Not Operated	1	1.0	0	1	1	1	1	1	1	1
B. Operated	69	1.9	2	1	1	2	3	3	5	7
2. MULTIPLE DX										
A. Not Operated	99	3.6	10	1	2	3	4	9	9	20
B. Operated	808	4.9	35	1	2	3	6	9	13	32
1. SINGLE DX	70	1.9	2	1	1	1	2	3	5	7
2. MULTIPLE DX	907	4.8	33	1	2	3	6	9	13	29
A. NOT OPERATED	100	3.6	10	1	2	3	4	8	9	20
B. OPERATED	877	4.7	33	1	2	3	6	9	13	32
TOTAL										
0–19 Years	1	2.0	0	2	2	2	2	2	2	2
20–34	54	2.3	4	1	1	1	3	5	6	10
35–49	224	3.4	24	1	1	2	4	6	8	21
50–64	312	5.1	48	2	2	3	6	10	14	33
65+	386	5.1	23	1	2	4	6	10	14	28
GRAND TOTAL	977	4.6	31	1	2	3	5	9	12	29

552.3: DIAPHRAGM HERNIA W OBSTR

Type of Patients	Observed Patients	Avg. Stay	Vari-ance	Percentiles 10th	25th	50th	75th	90th	95th	99th
1. SINGLE DX										
A. Not Operated										
0–19 Years	0									
20–34	0									
35–49	0									
50–64	0									
65+	0									
B. Operated										
0–19 Years	0									
20–34	3	5.7	1	5	5	5	7	7	7	7
35–49	3	3.7	2	2	1	4	5	5	5	5
50–64	1	1.0	0	1	1	1	1	1	1	1
65+	1	4.0	0	4	4	4	4	4	4	4
2. MULTIPLE DX										
A. Not Operated										
0–19 Years	0									
20–34	0									
35–49	2	3.5	12	1	1	6	6	6	6	6
50–64	4	14.2	457	3	3	4	46	46	46	46
65+	46	4.9	21	2	3	4	6	9	10	28
B. Operated										
0–19 Years	6	5.3	5	2	3	6	7	8	8	8
20–34	17	8.6	86	3	4	6	8	15	41	41
35–49	50	6.2	16	3	3	5	9	12	15	19
50–64	124	7.5	28	2	4	6	10	15	20	25
65+	312	9.4	109	2	4	6	11	18	26	55
SUBTOTALS:										
1. SINGLE DX										
A. Not Operated	0									
B. Operated	8	4.1	4	1	4	5	5	7	7	7
2. MULTIPLE DX										
A. Not Operated	52	5.5	52	2	3	4	6	9	17	46
B. Operated	509	8.5	79	2	4	6	10	16	21	45
1. SINGLE DX	8	4.1	4	1	4	5	5	7	7	7
2. MULTIPLE DX	561	8.2	77	2	3	6	10	16	21	46
A. NOT OPERATED	52	5.5	52	2	3	4	6	9	17	46
B. OPERATED	517	8.4	78	2	4	6	10	16	21	45
TOTAL										
0–19 Years	6	5.3	5	2	3	6	7	8	8	8
20–34	20	8.2	74	3	4	6	8	15	41	41
35–49	55	6.0	16	2	3	5	9	10	15	19
50–64	129	7.6	39	2	4	6	9	15	20	27
65+	359	8.8	99	2	3	6	11	17	25	55
GRAND TOTAL	569	8.2	76	2	3	6	10	16	21	46

552.8: HERNIA SITE NEC W OBSTR

Type of Patients	Observed Patients	Avg. Stay	Vari-ance	Percentiles 10th	25th	50th	75th	90th	95th	99th
1. SINGLE DX										
A. Not Operated										
0–19 Years	0									
20–34	1	1.0	0	1	1	1	1	1	1	1
35–49	1	2.0	0	2	2	2	2	2	2	2
50–64	0									
65+	0									
B. Operated										
0–19 Years	0									
20–34	3	2.5	4	1	1	1	1	4	4	4
35–49	6	5.1	40	1	2	3	4	18	18	18
50–64	5	3.2	<1	2	3	3	4	4	4	4
65+	3	4.3	<1	4	4	4	5	5	5	5
2. MULTIPLE DX										
A. Not Operated										
0–19 Years	0									
20–34	3	2.3	<1	2	2	2	3	3	3	3
35–49	2	2.5	4	1	1	1	1	4	4	4
50–64	14	3.2	3	2	2	2	4	6	6	6
65+	26	3.8	5	1	2	3	5	8	8	8
B. Operated										
0–19 Years	6	6.0	0	6	6	6	6	6	6	6
20–34	41	4.1	12	1	1	3	5	8	11	16
35–49	94	7.7	103	2	3	5	7	13	28	54
50–64	94	6.9	69	2	3	5	8	11	13	65
65+	172	10.2	52	3	6	8	13	19	25	39
SUBTOTALS:										
1. SINGLE DX										
A. Not Operated	2	1.5	<1	1	1	2	2	2	2	2
B. Operated	16	4.1	15	1	2	3	4	5	18	18
2. MULTIPLE DX										
A. Not Operated	45	3.4	4	1	2	3	5	6	8	8
B. Operated	403	8.2	67	2	3	6	10	15	22	46
1. SINGLE DX	18	3.8	14	1	2	3	4	5	18	18
2. MULTIPLE DX	448	7.7	62	2	3	6	9	15	22	46
A. NOT OPERATED	47	3.4	4	1	2	3	5	6	8	8
B. OPERATED	419	8.0	65	2	3	6	10	15	22	46
TOTAL										
0–19 Years	2	6.0	0	6	6	6	6	6	6	6
20–34	47	3.9	11	1	2	3	5	8	11	16
35–49	103	7.4	97	1	3	4	7	13	21	53
50–64	113	6.3	59	2	3	5	7	11	13	46
65+	201	9.2	50	2	5	8	11	18	23	36
GRAND TOTAL	466	7.6	61	2	3	6	9	15	22	46

553: OTHER ABDOMINAL HERNIA

Type of Patients	Observed Patients	Avg. Stay	Variance	10th	25th	50th	75th	90th	95th	99th
1. SINGLE DX										
A. Not Operated										
0–19 Years	2	2.5	4	1	1	1	4	4	4	4
20–34	9	1.1	<1	1	1	1	1	1	2	2
35–49	11	1.2	<1	1	1	1	1	1	2	2
50–64	6	1.5	<1	1	1	2	2	2	2	2
65+	3	1.7	1	1	1	1	3	3	3	3
B. Operated										
0–19 Years	18	1.7	2	1	1	1	2	5	5	5
20–34	65	2.2	2	1	1	2	3	4	5	6
35–49	192	2.1	2	1	1	2	2	4	5	9
50–64	194	1.9	1	1	1	2	2	3	4	6
65+	100	2.2	2	1	1	2	3	4	6	7
2. MULTIPLE DX										
A. Not Operated										
0–19 Years	12	2.0	<1	1	1	2	3	3	3	3
20–34	58	2.4	3	1	1	2	3	5	6	10
35–49	178	2.6	5	1	1	2	3	5	7	14
50–64	312	2.7	5	1	1	2	4	5	7	10
65+	550	2.9	6	1	1	2	4	5	7	12
B. Operated										
0–19 Years	90	3.8	15	1	2	3	5	7	9	31
20–34	534	3.1	11	1	1	2	4	6	8	14
35–49	2,088	3.3	13	1	1	2	4	6	8	18
50–64	3,789	3.5	15	1	2	3	4	7	8	19
65+	3,846	4.0	18	1	2	3	5	8	11	20
SUBTOTALS:										
1. SINGLE DX										
A. Not Operated	31	1.4	<1	1	1	1	2	2	3	4
B. Operated	569	2.1	2	1	1	2	3	4	5	6
2. MULTIPLE DX										
A. Not Operated	1,110	2.8	5	1	1	2	4	5	7	10
B. Operated	10,347	3.6	16	1	2	3	4	7	9	19
1. SINGLE DX	600	2.0	2	1	2	2	3	4	5	6
2. MULTIPLE DX	11,457	3.6	15	1	2	3	4	7	9	18
A. NOT OPERATED	1,141	2.7	5	1	1	2	3	5	7	10
B. OPERATED	10,916	3.6	15	1	2	3	4	7	9	19
TOTAL										
0–19 Years	122	3.3	12	1	1	2	4	6	8	17
20–34	666	2.9	9	1	1	2	3	6	7	14
35–49	2,469	3.2	12	1	1	2	4	6	8	16
50–64	4,301	3.4	14	1	1	2	4	6	8	18
65+	4,499	3.9	16	1	2	3	5	7	10	20
GRAND TOTAL	12,057	3.5	14	1	1	3	4	7	9	18

553.1: UMBILICAL HERNIA

Type of Patients	Observed Patients	Avg. Stay	Variance	10th	25th	50th	75th	90th	95th	99th
1. SINGLE DX										
A. Not Operated										
0–19 Years	1	4.0	0	4	4	4	4	4	4	4
20–34	3	1.0	0	1	1	1	1	1	1	1
35–49	3	1.3	<1	1	1	1	1	2	2	2
50–64	0									
65+	0									
B. Operated										
0–19 Years	10	1.0	0	1	1	1	1	1	1	1
20–34	10	1.5	<1	1	1	1	2	3	3	3
35–49	13	1.9	1	1	1	2	2	3	5	5
50–64	13	1.3	<1	1	1	1	1	2	3	3
65+	3	2.0	<1	1	1	2	3	3	3	3
2. MULTIPLE DX										
A. Not Operated										
0–19 Years	4	2.0	1	1	1	2	3	3	3	3
20–34	4	1.3	<1	1	1	1	1	2	2	2
35–49	21	2.1	2	1	1	2	3	4	4	5
50–64	23	2.0	2	1	1	2	3	4	5	5
65+	22	1.9	1	1	1	2	2	4	4	4
B. Operated										
0–19 Years	10	1.9	<1	1	1	2	3	3	3	3
20–34	49	2.1	2	1	1	2	2	4	4	7
35–49	141	2.4	3	1	1	2	3	4	6	10
50–64	162	2.8	7	1	1	2	3	5	7	16
65+	136	3.0	16	1	1	3	5	6	8	18
SUBTOTALS:										
1. SINGLE DX										
A. Not Operated	7	1.6	1	1	1	1	2	4	4	4
B. Operated	49	1.5	<1	1	1	2	2	3	3	5
2. MULTIPLE DX										
A. Not Operated	74	2.0	1	1	1	2	3	4	4	5
B. Operated	498	2.6	8	1	1	2	3	5	7	14
1. SINGLE DX	56	1.5	<1	1	1	2	2	3	3	5
2. MULTIPLE DX	572	2.6	7	1	1	2	3	5	6	13
A. NOT OPERATED	81	1.9	1	1	1	2	3	4	4	5
B. OPERATED	547	2.5	7	1	1	2	3	5	7	13
TOTAL										
0–19 Years	25	1.6	<1	1	1	2	3	3	3	4
20–34	66	1.9	2	1	1	2	3	4	4	7
35–49	178	2.3	3	1	1	2	3	4	6	10
50–64	198	2.6	6	1	1	2	3	5	7	16
65+	161	2.8	14	1	1	3	3	6	8	18
GRAND TOTAL	628	2.5	7	1	1	2	3	5	6	12

553.20: VENTRAL HERNIA NOS

Type of Patients	Observed Patients	Avg. Stay	Variance	10th	25th	50th	75th	90th	95th	99th
1. SINGLE DX										
A. Not Operated										
0–19 Years	0									
20–34	0									
35–49	2	1.0	0	1	1	1	1	1	1	1
50–64	0									
65+	1	1.0	0	1	1	1	1	1	1	1
B. Operated										
0–19 Years	3	2.0	<1	1	1	2	3	3	3	3
20–34	5	2.4	3	1	1	3	3	5	5	5
35–49	22	1.6	2	1	1	1	2	2	2	7
50–64	19	1.9	<1	1	1	2	3	3	3	3
65+	6	1.7	<1	1	1	2	2	3	3	3
2. MULTIPLE DX										
A. Not Operated										
0–19 Years	0									
20–34	3	2.0	<1	1	1	2	3	3	3	3
35–49	32	2.3	4	1	1	2	3	4	7	9
50–64	53	2.9	9	1	1	2	3	6	10	18
65+	54	2.9	4	1	1	2	4	6	6	9
B. Operated										
0–19 Years	5	3.4	5	2	2	3	4	7	7	7
20–34	57	2.7	3	1	1	2	4	6	8	8
35–49	198	3.4	9	1	1	2	4	6	9	18
50–64	316	3.1	8	1	1	2	4	6	7	18
65+	292	3.7	13	2	2	3	5	7	10	15
SUBTOTALS:										
1. SINGLE DX										
A. Not Operated	3	1.0	0	1	1	1	1	1	1	1
B. Operated	55	1.8	1	1	1	2	2	3	3	7
2. MULTIPLE DX										
A. Not Operated	142	2.8	6	1	1	2	3	6	7	10
B. Operated	868	3.3	10	1	1	2	4	6	8	16
1. SINGLE DX	58	1.8	1	1	1	1	2	3	3	7
2. MULTIPLE DX	1,010	3.3	9	1	1	2	4	6	8	15
A. NOT OPERATED	145	2.7	6	1	1	2	3	6	7	10
B. OPERATED	923	3.3	10	1	1	2	4	6	8	15
TOTAL										
0–19 Years	8	2.9	4	1	2	3	4	7	7	7
20–34	65	2.7	4	1	1	2	4	5	7	8
35–49	254	3.1	8	1	1	2	4	6	9	15
50–64	388	3.0	8	1	1	2	4	6	7	14
65+	353	3.5	12	1	1	3	4	7	9	14
GRAND TOTAL	1,068	3.2	9	1	1	2	4	6	8	15

Length of Stay by Diagnosis and Operation, Western Region, 2008

Western Region, October 2006–September 2007 Data, by Diagnosis

553.21: INCISIONAL HERNIA

Type of Patients	Observed Patients	Avg. Stay	Vari- ance	10th	25th	50th	75th	90th	95th	99th
1. SINGLE DX										
A. Not Operated										
0–19 Years	0									
20–34	2	1.0	0	1	1	1	1	1	1	1
35–49	5	1.2	<1	1	1	1	1	1	2	2
50–64	4	1.5	<1	1	1	2	2	2	2	2
65+	0									
B. Operated										
0–19 Years	2	1.5	<1	1	1	2	2	2	2	2
20–34	35	2.2	1	1	1	2	3	3	5	6
35–49	126	2.0	1	1	1	2	3	4	4	5
50–64	125	1.9	<1	1	1	2	2	3	4	5
65+	71	2.2	2	1	1	2	3	4	5	6
2. MULTIPLE DX										
A. Not Operated										
0–19 Years	0									
20–34	14	2.6	7	1	1	1	3	6	10	10
35–49	39	2.8	8	1	1	2	4	6	9	15
50–64	91	2.7	5	1	1	3	4	5	7	11
65+	63	3.4	7	1	1	3	4	7	9	13
B. Operated										
0–19 Years	35	3.4	10	1	1	2	5	6	8	17
20–34	285	3.1	7	1	1	2	4	7	8	14
35–49	1,275	3.5	13	2	2	3	4	6	8	20
50–64	2,428	3.6	16	2	2	3	4	6	8	20
65+	2,332	3.7	14	2	2	3	5	7	9	18
SUBTOTALS:										
1. SINGLE DX										
A. Not Operated	11	1.3	<1	1	1	1	1	2	2	2
B. Operated	359	2.0	1	1	1	2	3	3	4	5
2. MULTIPLE DX										
A. Not Operated	207	2.9	6	1	1	2	4	6	9	11
B. Operated	6,355	3.6	14	1	2	3	4	7	8	19
1. SINGLE DX	370	2.0	1	1	2	2	3	3	4	5
2. MULTIPLE DX	6,562	3.6	14	2	2	3	4	7	8	18
A. NOT OPERATED	218	2.9	6	1	1	2	4	6	9	11
B. OPERATED	6,714	3.5	14	1	2	3	4	6	8	18
TOTAL										
0–19 Years	37	3.3	9	1	1	2	4	6	8	17
20–34	336	2.9	6	1	1	2	4	6	8	14
35–49	1,445	3.3	12	2	2	3	4	6	8	16
50–64	2,648	3.5	15	2	2	3	4	6	8	19
65+	2,466	3.7	13	2	2	3	4	7	9	18
GRAND TOTAL	6,932	3.5	13	2	2	3	4	6	8	18

553.29: VENTRAL HERNIA NEC

Type of Patients	Observed Patients	Avg. Stay	Vari- ance	10th	25th	50th	75th	90th	95th	99th
1. SINGLE DX										
A. Not Operated										
0–19 Years	0									
20–34	1	1.0	0	1	1	1	1	1	1	1
35–49	0									
50–64	2	1.5	<1	1	1	1	2	2	2	2
65+	1	1.0	0	1	1	1	1	1	1	1
B. Operated										
0–19 Years	1	2.0	0	2	2	2	2	2	2	2
20–34	5	2.4	1	1	2	2	3	4	4	4
35–49	12	2.1	1	1	1	2	3	3	5	5
50–64	22	1.9	2	1	1	2	3	3	3	6
65+	5	1.6	<1	1	1	1	2	3	3	3
2. MULTIPLE DX										
A. Not Operated										
0–19 Years	0									
20–34	4	1.0	0	1	1	1	2	2	2	2
35–49	17	2.1	2	1	1	2	2	3	3	7
50–64	21	2.0	2	1	1	2	2	3	5	6
65+	22	2.7	4	1	1	2	4	6	7	7
B. Operated										
0–19 Years	8	3.5	7	1	1	3	6	8	8	8
20–34	39	4.0	53	1	1	2	5	6	8	47
35–49	134	3.2	14	1	1	2	4	6	7	16
50–64	182	3.5	12	1	2	2	4	7	9	20
65+	179	3.8	16	1	2	2	5	8	10	20
SUBTOTALS:										
1. SINGLE DX										
A. Not Operated	4	1.3	<1	1	1	1	1	2	2	2
B. Operated	45	2.0	1	1	1	2	3	3	4	6
2. MULTIPLE DX										
A. Not Operated	64	2.2	3	1	1	2	3	4	6	7
B. Operated	542	3.6	16	1	2	2	4	7	9	20
1. SINGLE DX	49	1.9	1	1	1	2	2	3	4	6
2. MULTIPLE DX	606	3.4	15	1	2	2	4	7	9	17
A. NOT OPERATED	68	2.2	2	1	1	2	3	4	6	7
B. OPERATED	587	3.4	15	1	2	2	4	7	9	20
TOTAL										
0–19 Years	9	3.3	6	1	1	2	5	6	8	8
20–34	49	3.6	43	1	1	2	4	5	6	47
35–49	163	3.0	12	1	1	2	4	6	7	16
50–64	227	3.2	10	1	2	2	4	7	8	16
65+	207	3.6	14	1	2	2	4	8	10	17
GRAND TOTAL	655	3.3	14	1	1	2	4	7	9	17

553.3: DIAPHRAGMATIC HERNIA

Type of Patients	Observed Patients	Avg. Stay	Vari- ance	10th	25th	50th	75th	90th	95th	99th
1. SINGLE DX										
A. Not Operated										
0–19 Years	0									
20–34	2	1.0	0	1	1	1	1	1	1	1
35–49	1	1.0	0	1	1	1	1	1	1	1
50–64	0									
65+	1	3.0	0	3	3	3	3	3	3	3
B. Operated										
0–19 Years	6	5.0	0	5	5	5	5	5	5	5
20–34	6	4.0	2	2	3	5	5	6	6	6
35–49	15	3.0	4	1	3	3	4	5	9	9
50–64	13	3.1	2	1	2	3	4	4	6	6
65+	14	3.1	5	1	1	3	4	7	7	7
2. MULTIPLE DX										
A. Not Operated										
0–19 Years	7	2.0	1	1	1	2	3	3	3	3
20–34	29	2.6	3	1	2	2	3	5	5	9
35–49	63	2.8	5	1	1	2	3	5	7	14
50–64	116	2.9	4	1	1	2	4	5	7	10
65+	378	3.0	6	1	2	2	4	5	7	14
B. Operated										
0–19 Years	28	5.5	30	2	3	4	6	9	9	31
20–34	78	3.5	18	1	1	2	4	7	11	32
35–49	273	3.3	24	1	1	2	4	6	8	18
50–64	634	3.6	15	1	2	4	4	7	9	18
65+	869	5.2	29	2	4	4	6	11	15	25
SUBTOTALS:										
1. SINGLE DX										
A. Not Operated	4	1.5	1	1	1	1	3	3	3	3
B. Operated	50	3.2	3	1	2	3	4	6	7	9
2. MULTIPLE DX										
A. Not Operated	593	2.9	5	1	1	2	4	5	7	12
B. Operated	1,882	4.3	24	1	2	3	5	8	12	24
1. SINGLE DX	54	3.1	3	1	2	3	4	6	7	9
2. MULTIPLE DX	2,475	4.0	20	1	2	3	5	8	11	20
A. NOT OPERATED	597	2.9	5	1	1	2	4	5	7	12
B. OPERATED	1,932	4.3	23	1	2	3	5	8	12	23
TOTAL										
0–19 Years	37	4.8	25	2	2	4	5	9	9	31
20–34	115	3.3	13	1	1	2	4	6	9	15
35–49	352	3.2	19	1	1	2	4	6	8	17
50–64	763	3.5	13	1	2	3	4	7	9	16
65+	1,262	4.5	23	1	2	3	5	9	13	24
GRAND TOTAL	2,529	4.0	19	1	2	3	5	8	11	20

553.8: HERNIA NEC

Type of Patients	Observed Patients	Avg. Stay	Variance	10th	25th	50th	75th	90th	95th	99th
1. SINGLE DX										
A. Not Operated										
0–19 Years	1	1.0	0		1	1	1	1	1	1
20–34	1	2.0	0	2	2	2	2	2	2	2
35–49	0									
50–64	0									
65+	0									
B. Operated										
0–19 Years	0									
20–34	0									
35–49	1	1.0	0	1	1	1	1	1	1	1
50–64	1	3.0	0	3	3	3	3	3	3	3
65+	0									
2. MULTIPLE DX										
A. Not Operated										
0–19 Years	1	2.0	0	2	2	2	2	2	2	2
20–34	3	2.7	2	1	1	3	4	4	4	4
35–49	5	2.6	1	1	2	3	3	4	4	4
50–64	5	2.8	1	1	3	3	3	4	4	4
65+	8	1.8	1	1	1	1	3	4	4	4
B. Operated										
0–19 Years	3	2.0	<1	1	1	2	3	3	3	3
20–34	20	3.1	4	1	2	3	4	6	9	9
35–49	60	2.8	6	1	1	2	3	6	6	18
50–64	52	3.6	16	1	1	2	4	6	14	21
65+	25	4.9	20	2	2	2	6	14	15	16
SUBTOTALS:										
1. SINGLE DX										
A. Not Operated	2	1.5	<1	1	1	1	2	2	2	2
B. Operated	2	2.0	2	1	1	2	3	3	3	3
2. MULTIPLE DX										
A. Not Operated	22	2.3	1	1	1	3	3	4	4	4
B. Operated	160	3.4	12	1	2	2	4	6	9	18
1. SINGLE DX	4	1.8	<1	1	1	1	2	3	3	3
2. MULTIPLE DX	182	3.3	10	1	1	2	4	6	9	18
A. NOT OPERATED	24	2.3	1	1	1	2	3	4	4	4
B. OPERATED	162	3.4	11	1	2	2	4	6	9	18
TOTAL										
0–19 Years	5	1.8	<1	1	1	2	2	3	3	3
20–34	24	3.0	3	1	2	2	4	5	6	9
35–49	66	2.8	6	1	1	2	3	6	6	18
50–64	58	3.6	14	2	2	3	4	6	14	21
65+	33	4.1	17	1	2	3	5	10	15	16
GRAND TOTAL	186	3.3	10	1	1	2	4	6	9	18

555: REGIONAL ENTERITIS

Type of Patients	Observed Patients	Avg. Stay	Variance	10th	25th	50th	75th	90th	95th	99th
1. SINGLE DX										
A. Not Operated										
0–19 Years	65	2.6	5	1	1	1	4	6	6	11
20–34	77	2.7	4	1	1	2	3	5	6	13
35–49	28	2.8	2	2	2	3	4	5	6	6
50–64	17	2.8	3	1	2	2	5	6	7	7
65+	3	2.7	4	1	1	2	5	5	5	5
B. Operated										
0–19 Years	7	3.9	3	2	2	3	5	7	7	7
20–34	16	6.3	9	4	5	5	7	11	14	14
35–49	4	5.2	3	3	3	5	7	7	7	7
50–64	3	3.3	6	1	1	3	6	6	6	6
65+	0									
2. MULTIPLE DX										
A. Not Operated										
0–19 Years	306	5.2	19	1	2	4	7	12	14	21
20–34	1,539	4.2	13	1	2	3	5	8	10	17
35–49	1,360	4.6	17	1	2	4	6	8	11	20
50–64	1,001	4.6	15	2	2	3	5	9	11	23
65+	655	5.2	19	2	3	4	6	10	13	23
B. Operated										
0–19 Years	52	9.1	59	3	5	7	9	19	28	37
20–34	349	8.7	48	3	4	7	10	18	22	38
35–49	320	9.2	46	4	5	7	10	17	25	39
50–64	254	10.0	77	4	5	7	11	19	26	55
65+	148	9.2	39	4	5	7	11	16	22	34
SUBTOTALS:										
1. SINGLE DX										
A. Not Operated	190	2.7	4	1	1	2	4	6	6	11
B. Operated	30	5.3	8	2	3	5	6	8	11	14
2. MULTIPLE DX										
A. Not Operated	4,861	4.6	16	1	2	4	6	9	11	21
B. Operated	1,123	9.2	53	4	5	7	11	18	24	39
1. SINGLE DX	220	3.0	5	1	1	2	4	6	7	11
2. MULTIPLE DX	5,984	5.5	26	2	2	4	7	10	14	27
A. NOT OPERATED	5,051	4.5	16	1	2	3	5	9	11	21
B. OPERATED	1,153	9.1	52	3	5	7	10	18	24	39
TOTAL										
0–19 Years	430	5.2	25	1	2	4	7	11	14	24
20–34	1,981	5.0	22	1	2	4	6	9	13	27
35–49	1,712	5.4	26	2	2	4	7	10	14	27
50–64	1,275	5.6	32	2	2	4	7	11	15	28
65+	806	5.9	25	2	3	4	8	11	15	25
GRAND TOTAL	6,204	5.4	26	1	2	4	6	10	14	27

555.0: REG ENTERITIS SM INTEST

Type of Patients	Observed Patients	Avg. Stay	Variance	10th	25th	50th	75th	90th	95th	99th
1. SINGLE DX										
A. Not Operated										
0–19 Years	9	3.1	3	1	2	3	4	6	6	6
20–34	29	2.9	6	1	2	2	3	6	7	13
35–49	11	3.2	2	1	2	3	4	5	6	6
50–64	2	3.0	2	2	2	4	4	4	4	4
65+	0									
B. Operated										
0–19 Years	3	3.7	8	2	2	2	7	7	7	7
20–34	4	4.5	6	1	5	6	6	6	6	6
35–49	2	5.0	8	3	3	3	7	7	7	7
50–64	2	2.0	2	1	1	1	3	3	3	3
65+	0									
2. MULTIPLE DX										
A. Not Operated										
0–19 Years	71	5.0	23	1	2	4	7	9	16	24
20–34	408	4.0	8	2	2	3	5	7	9	16
35–49	352	4.3	9	2	2	4	5	8	10	15
50–64	270	4.2	11	1	2	3	5	8	11	16
65+	165	5.1	18	2	3	4	6	9	12	23
B. Operated										
0–19 Years	25	8.8	37	4	5	7	9	15	25	28
20–34	146	8.2	35	3	4	6	10	16	22	31
35–49	131	9.2	34	4	5	8	12	16	21	27
50–64	108	9.4	59	4	5	7	11	19	22	33
65+	75	9.0	36	4	5	8	11	15	19	44
SUBTOTALS:										
1. SINGLE DX										
A. Not Operated	51	3.0	4	1	2	3	4	5	6	13
B. Operated	11	3.9	5	1	2	3	6	7	7	7
2. MULTIPLE DX										
A. Not Operated	1,266	4.3	11	2	2	3	5	8	10	18
B. Operated	485	8.9	40	4	5	7	11	17	22	33
1. SINGLE DX	62	3.2	5	1	2	3	4	6	7	13
2. MULTIPLE DX	1,751	5.6	23	2	3	4	7	11	15	24
A. NOT OPERATED	1,317	4.3	11	1	2	3	5	8	10	18
B. OPERATED	496	8.8	40	3	5	7	10	17	22	33
TOTAL										
0–19 Years	108	5.7	27	1	2	4	7	12	16	25
20–34	587	5.0	18	1	2	4	6	10	13	22
35–49	496	5.6	20	2	3	4	7	11	14	23
50–64	382	5.6	30	2	3	4	7	11	16	25
65+	240	6.3	27	2	3	5	8	12	16	24
GRAND TOTAL	1,813	5.5	23	2	3	4	7	11	14	23

Length of Stay by Diagnosis and Operation, Western Region, 2008

Western Region, October 2006–September 2007 Data, by Diagnosis

555.1: REG ENTERITIS LG INTEST

Type of Patients	Observed Patients	Avg. Stay	Vari-ance	Percentiles 10th	25th	50th	75th	90th	95th	99th
1. SINGLE DX										
A. Not Operated										
0–19 Years	12	4.3	11	1	2	4	6	9	11	11
20–34	13	2.2	2	1	1	2	3	4	5	5
35–49	4	1.7	<1	1	1	1	2	3	3	3
50–64	4	2.0	<1	1	2	2	3	3	3	3
65+	0									
B. Operated										
0–19 Years	0									
20–34	3	6.3	6	4	4	6	9	9	9	9
35–49	0									
50–64	0									
65+	0									
2. MULTIPLE DX										
A. Not Operated										
0–19 Years	67	6.5	25	1	3	5	9	16	17	19
20–34	317	4.7	14	2	2	4	6	9	11	16
35–49	290	5.2	17	2	3	4	7	11	13	20
50–64	227	5.5	25	2	3	4	6	11	14	27
65+	213	5.9	23	2	3	4	8	12	14	25
B. Operated										
0–19 Years	8	10.8	138	1	6	6	18	37	37	37
20–34	60	10.2	73	4	5	7	12	19	33	46
35–49	84	8.9	53	4	5	7	10	16	26	45
50–64	57	10.5	114	3	7	7	11	22	39	55
65+	32	9.9	50	4	5	7	14	22	27	29
SUBTOTALS:										
1. SINGLE DX										
A. Not Operated	33	2.9	6	1	1	2	4	6	6	11
B. Operated	3	6.3	6	4	4	6	9	9	9	9
2. MULTIPLE DX										
A. Not Operated	1,114	5.4	19	2	3	4	7	10	14	23
B. Operated	241	9.8	74	3	5	7	11	20	27	46
1. SINGLE DX	36	3.1	7	1	1	2	4	6	9	11
2. MULTIPLE DX	1,355	6.1	32	2	3	5	7	12	17	30
A. NOT OPERATED	1,147	5.3	19	2	2	4	7	10	13	23
B. OPERATED	244	9.8	73	3	5	7	11	20	27	46
TOTAL										
0–19 Years	87	6.6	34	1	2	5	8	16	18	37
20–34	393	5.5	26	2	3	4	7	10	15	30
35–49	378	6.0	27	2	3	5	7	11	16	28
50–64	288	6.5	46	2	3	5	7	12	20	39
65+	245	6.4	28	2	3	5	8	12	17	27
GRAND TOTAL	1,391	6.1	31	2	3	4	7	12	16	30

555.2: REG ENTERIT SM/LG INTEST

Type of Patients	Observed Patients	Avg. Stay	Vari-ance	Percentiles 10th	25th	50th	75th	90th	95th	99th
1. SINGLE DX										
A. Not Operated										
0–19 Years	10	2.9	5	1	1	2	4	6	7	7
20–34	8	3.4	3	2	2	3	4	6	6	6
35–49	2	3.5	4	2	2	4	5	5	5	5
50–64	2	3.0	2	2	2	3	4	4	4	4
65+	0									
B. Operated										
0–19 Years	4	4.0	1	3	3	5	5	5	5	5
20–34	6	7.3	12	5	5	5	8	14	14	14
35–49	1	5.0	0	5	5	5	5	5	5	5
50–64	1	6.0	0	6	6	6	6	6	6	6
65+	0									
2. MULTIPLE DX										
A. Not Operated										
0–19 Years	54	5.6	16	2	3	5	6	12	14	21
20–34	172	5.4	26	2	2	4	6	11	13	31
35–49	124	6.1	44	3	3	4	7	12	16	34
50–64	78	5.4	26	2	3	3	6	10	20	25
65+	39	5.3	24	1	2	4	7	10	19	26
B. Operated										
0–19 Years	13	10.6	80	5	5	6	12	23	33	33
20–34	95	8.9	48	4	5	7	10	17	24	40
35–49	55	8.8	37	4	5	7	12	18	28	>99
50–64	53	10.7	83	5	6	8	12	16	35	56
65+	23	9.2	53	4	5	7	10	20	23	34
SUBTOTALS:										
1. SINGLE DX										
A. Not Operated	22	3.1	3	1	2	3	4	6	6	7
B. Operated	12	5.9	8	3	5	5	7	8	14	14
2. MULTIPLE DX										
A. Not Operated	467	5.6	29	2	3	4	6	11	14	29
B. Operated	239	9.4	55	4	5	7	10	18	25	40
1. SINGLE DX	34	4.1	7	1	2	4	5	7	8	14
2. MULTIPLE DX	706	6.9	41	2	3	5	8	13	19	35
A. NOT OPERATED	489	5.5	28	2	3	4	6	11	14	29
B. OPERATED	251	9.2	53	4	5	7	10	17	25	40
TOTAL										
0–19 Years	81	6.0	28	2	3	5	8	12	14	33
20–34	281	6.5	35	2	3	5	7	13	17	38
35–49	182	6.9	42	3	3	5	8	13	22	50
50–64	134	7.4	54	2	3	6	9	14	20	39
65+	62	6.8	38	2	3	5	8	11	20	34
GRAND TOTAL	740	6.8	40	2	3	5	8	13	19	35

555.9: REGIONAL ENTERITIS NOS

Type of Patients	Observed Patients	Avg. Stay	Vari-ance	Percentiles 10th	25th	50th	75th	90th	95th	99th
1. SINGLE DX										
A. Not Operated										
0–19 Years	34	1.7	2	1	1	1	2	4	6	6
20–34	27	2.4	3	1	1	2	3	4	6	7
35–49	11	2.6	2	2	1	2	3	4	6	6
50–64	9	3.0	5	1	1	2	4	7	7	7
65+	3	2.7	4	1	1	2	5	5	5	5
B. Operated										
0–19 Years	0									
20–34	3	6.7	14	4	4	5	11	11	11	11
35–49	1	6.0	0	6	6	6	6	6	6	6
50–64	0									
65+	0									
2. MULTIPLE DX										
A. Not Operated										
0–19 Years	114	4.2	14	1	2	3	6	10	12	14
20–34	642	3.8	12	1	2	3	5	7	9	17
35–49	594	4.2	16	1	2	3	5	8	10	19
50–64	426	4.2	10	1	2	3	5	8	10	16
65+	238	4.6	16	1	2	4	5	9	12	15
B. Operated										
0–19 Years	6	5.2	7	3	3	6	7	9	9	9
20–34	48	8.3	52	3	5	6	10	20	24	29
35–49	50	10.1	74	3	5	7	12	21	35	39
50–64	36	9.8	68	4	5	7	13	17	32	44
65+	18	9.0	21	4	6	9	14	16	16	16
SUBTOTALS:										
1. SINGLE DX										
A. Not Operated	84	2.2	3	1	1	2	3	5	6	7
B. Operated	4	6.5	10	4	4	5	6	11	11	11
2. MULTIPLE DX										
A. Not Operated	2,014	4.1	13	1	2	3	5	8	10	16
B. Operated	158	9.2	58	3	4	7	11	18	26	39
1. SINGLE DX	88	2.4	4	1	1	2	3	6	6	11
2. MULTIPLE DX	2,172	4.5	18	1	2	3	5	8	11	23
A. NOT OPERATED	2,098	4.0	13	1	2	3	5	8	10	16
B. OPERATED	162	9.1	57	3	4	6	11	18	24	39
TOTAL										
0–19 Years	154	3.7	12	1	1	3	5	9	11	14
20–34	720	4.1	15	1	2	3	5	7	11	24
35–49	656	4.6	23	1	2	3	5	9	11	26
50–64	471	4.6	17	1	2	4	5	8	12	23
65+	259	4.9	17	1	2	4	6	9	13	16
GRAND TOTAL	2,260	4.4	18	1	2	3	5	8	11	22

Length of Stay by Diagnosis and Operation, Western Region, 2008

Western Region, October 2006–September 2007 Data, by Diagnosis

556: ULCERATIVE COLITIS

Type of Patients	Observed Patients	Avg. Stay	Variance	10th	25th	50th	75th	90th	95th	99th
1. SINGLE DX										
A. Not Operated										
0–19 Years	38	4.0	6	1	2	3	5	7	9	11
20–34	68	3.6	4	1	2	3	4	6	7	10
35–49	46	3.4	4	1	2	3	4	7	7	9
50–64	17	3.7	11	1	1	3	5	7	14	14
65+	1	1.0	0	1	1	1	1	1	1	1
B. Operated										
0–19 Years	8	5.3	<1	4	5	5	6	6	6	6
20–34	29	5.3	3	4	4	5	6	7	9	12
35–49	19	6.5	5	4	5	6	8	11	11	11
50–64	7	6.1	4	3	4	7	9	9	9	9
65+	1	5.0	0	5	5	5	5	5	5	5
2. MULTIPLE DX										
A. Not Operated										
0–19 Years	283	5.9	31	1	3	4	7	12	15	29
20–34	1,063	4.7	14	2	2	4	6	9	12	20
35–49	964	5.1	20	2	3	4	6	10	12	20
50–64	819	5.2	17	2	3	4	7	10	13	22
65+	958	5.5	17	2	3	4	7	10	14	22
B. Operated										
0–19 Years	31	13.0	70	5	6	9	20	25	26	33
20–34	139	10.9	91	4	5	8	13	22	28	41
35–49	189	11.2	74	4	6	8	14	23	25	49
50–64	224	12.8	146	4	6	8	15	26	36	57
65+	149	12.3	104	4	6	8	16	25	33	56
SUBTOTALS:										
1. SINGLE DX										
A. Not Operated	170	3.6	5	1	2	3	5	7	8	11
B. Operated	64	5.7	4	4	4	5	6	9	9	12
2. MULTIPLE DX										
A. Not Operated	4,087	5.2	18	2	3	4	6	10	13	22
B. Operated	732	11.9	105	4	6	8	14	24	31	56
1. SINGLE DX	234	4.2	6	1	2	4	6	7	9	11
2. MULTIPLE DX	4,819	6.2	37	2	3	4	7	12	17	30
A. NOT OPERATED	4,257	5.1	17	2	3	4	6	10	13	21
B. OPERATED	796	11.4	100	4	5	8	14	23	29	56
TOTAL										
0–19 Years	360	6.3	35	2	3	4	8	13	19	29
20–34	1,299	5.3	25	2	3	4	6	10	14	26
35–49	1,218	6.0	33	2	3	5	7	12	15	25
50–64	1,067	6.8	54	2	3	5	8	13	19	39
65+	1,109	6.4	34	2	3	5	6	12	17	31
GRAND TOTAL	5,053	6.1	36	2	3	4	7	12	16	29

556.2: ULCERATIVE PROCTITIS

Type of Patients	Observed Patients	Avg. Stay	Variance	10th	25th	50th	75th	90th	95th	99th
1. SINGLE DX										
A. Not Operated										
0–19 Years	1	3.0	0	3	3	3	3	3	3	3
20–34	1	3.0	0	3	3	3	3	3	3	3
35–49	4	1.8	<1	1	1	2	3	3	3	3
50–64	0									
65+	0									
B. Operated										
0–19 Years	1	5.0	0	5	5	5	5	5	5	5
20–34	0									
35–49	1	6.0	0	6	6	6	6	6	6	6
50–64	0									
65+	0									
2. MULTIPLE DX										
A. Not Operated										
0–19 Years	9	3.1	7	1	2	3	3	10	10	10
20–34	24	4.6	14	1	2	4	7	9	12	15
35–49	36	4.4	12	1	2	4	6	8	12	18
50–64	20	5.0	15	1	3	4	9	12	13	13
65+	82	4.8	12	2	3	4	6	7	9	26
B. Operated										
0–19 Years	0									
20–34	12	7.7	22	4	6	7	7	15	19	19
35–49	9	8.3	35	4	5	6	8	19	19	19
50–64	10	7.0	16	3	4	5	11	11	15	15
65+	10	12.5	77	4	6	11	18	33	33	33
SUBTOTALS:										
1. SINGLE DX										
A. Not Operated	6	2.2	<1	1	1	2	3	3	3	3
B. Operated	2	5.5	<1	5	5	6	6	6	6	6
2. MULTIPLE DX										
A. Not Operated	171	4.6	12	1	2	4	6	9	12	18
B. Operated	41	8.8	39	4	5	6	11	18	19	33
1. SINGLE DX	8	3.0	3	1	2	3	3	6	6	6
2. MULTIPLE DX	212	5.4	20	2	3	4	7	11	15	19
A. NOT OPERATED	177	4.5	12	1	2	4	6	9	12	18
B. OPERATED	43	8.7	37	4	5	6	11	18	19	33
TOTAL										
0–19 Years	11	3.3	6	1	2	3	3	5	10	10
20–34	37	5.6	18	2	2	5	6	12	15	19
35–49	50	4.9	17	1	2	4	7	10	18	19
50–64	30	5.7	16	2	3	4	8	12	13	15
65+	92	5.6	24	2	3	4	6	10	14	33
GRAND TOTAL	220	5.3	19	2	3	4	6	11	15	19

556.3: ULCERATIVE PROCTOSIGMOID

Type of Patients	Observed Patients	Avg. Stay	Variance	10th	25th	50th	75th	90th	95th	99th
1. SINGLE DX										
A. Not Operated										
0–19 Years	3	2.0	1	1	1	2	3	3	3	3
20–34	1	3.0	0	3	3	3	3	3	3	3
35–49	1	5.0	0	5	5	5	5	5	5	5
50–64	0									
65+	0									
B. Operated										
0–19 Years	0									
20–34	1	6.0	0	6	6	6	6	6	6	6
35–49	2	7.0	8	5	5	9	9	9	9	9
50–64	0									
65+	0									
2. MULTIPLE DX										
A. Not Operated										
0–19 Years	2	2.5	<1	2	2	2	3	3	3	3
20–34	31	4.9	14	2	2	4	6	10	11	19
35–49	38	6.6	20	2	4	6	8	12	17	24
50–64	30	4.1	9	2	2	3	5	8	10	14
65+	54	5.8	24	2	3	4	7	13	16	27
B. Operated										
0–19 Years	1	9.0	0	9	9	9	9	9	9	9
20–34	4	11.0	34	6	6	15	17	17	17	17
35–49	4	10.7	18	6	6	9	12	16	16	16
50–64	8	10.3	71	4	5	9	12	30	30	30
65+	14	15.1	220	4	7	8	16	45	51	51
SUBTOTALS:										
1. SINGLE DX										
A. Not Operated	5	2.8	2	1	2	3	3	5	5	5
B. Operated	3	6.7	4	5	5	6	9	9	9	9
2. MULTIPLE DX										
A. Not Operated	155	5.4	19	3	3	4	7	10	14	24
B. Operated	31	12.6	123	5	6	9	15	23	45	51
1. SINGLE DX	8	4.3	7	1	3	5	6	9	9	9
2. MULTIPLE DX	186	6.6	42	2	3	5	8	13	17	45
A. NOT OPERATED	160	5.4	18	2	2	4	7	10	14	24
B. OPERATED	34	12.0	115	5	6	9	12	23	45	51
TOTAL										
0–19 Years	6	3.4	8	1	2	3	3	9	9	9
20–34	37	5.5	19	2	2	5	6	11	17	19
35–49	45	6.9	20	2	4	6	9	12	16	24
50–64	38	5.4	27	2	3	4	8	10	14	30
65+	68	7.7	76	2	3	5	8	16	23	51
GRAND TOTAL	194	6.5	41	2	3	5	8	12	17	45

Length of Stay by Diagnosis and Operation, Western Region, 2008

Western Region, October 2006–September 2007 Data, by Diagnosis

556.5: LEFT-SIDED UC

Type of Patients	Observed Patients	Avg. Stay	Variance	10th	25th	50th	75th	90th	95th	99th
1. SINGLE DX										
A. Not Operated										
0–19 Years	1	3.0	0	3	3	3	3	3	3	3
20–34	4	4.3	2	3	3	5	6	6	6	6
35–49	3	2.7	<1	2	2	3	3	3	3	3
50–64	5	3.4	6	1	2	2	5	7	7	7
65+	0									
B. Operated										
0–19 Years	0									
20–34	0									
35–49	0									
50–64	1	6.0	0	6	6	6	6	6	6	6
65+	1	6.0	0	6	6	6	6	6	6	6
2. MULTIPLE DX										
A. Not Operated										
0–19 Years	14	6.5	20	2	3	4	9	13	16	16
20–34	78	5.3	27	2	3	4	6	10	14	31
35–49	54	5.4	12	2	3	4	8	10	12	14
50–64	56	5.3	10	2	3	5	7	11	13	15
65+	52	5.0	11	2	3	5	6	8	9	22
B. Operated										
0–19 Years	0									
20–34	6	10.2	42	4	4	9	16	19	19	19
35–49	9	13.6	100	3	6	14	16	36	36	36
50–64	7	8.9	65	3	3	6	11	26	26	26
65+	6	18.1	188	3	11	12	31	39	39	39
SUBTOTALS:										
1. SINGLE DX										
A. Not Operated	13	3.5	3	2	2	3	5	6	7	7
B. Operated	2	6.0	0	6	6	6	6	6	6	6
2. MULTIPLE DX										
A. Not Operated	254	5.3	16	2	3	4	7	10	13	23
B. Operated	28	12.7	99	3	5	11	16	31	36	39
1. SINGLE DX	15	3.8	3	2	2	3	6	6	7	7
2. MULTIPLE DX	282	6.1	29	2	3	5	7	12	15	31
A. NOT OPERATED	267	5.3	16	2	3	4	7	10	12	23
B. OPERATED	30	12.2	95	3	5	11	16	36	36	39
TOTAL										
0–19 Years	15	6.3	20	2	3	4	9	13	16	16
20–34	88	5.6	28	2	3	4	6	11	16	31
35–49	67	6.4	30	2	3	5	9	13	15	36
50–64	69	5.6	16	2	3	5	7	11	13	26
65+	58	6.4	43	2	3	5	7	11	22	39
GRAND TOTAL	297	6.0	28	2	3	4	7	11	15	31

556.6: UNIVERSAL UC

Type of Patients	Observed Patients	Avg. Stay	Variance	10th	25th	50th	75th	90th	95th	99th
1. SINGLE DX										
A. Not Operated										
0–19 Years	7	6.0	12	2	2	7	9	11	11	11
20–34	23	3.0	3	1	2	3	4	5	5	8
35–49	3	2.0	3	1	1	1	4	4	4	4
50–64	0									
65+	0									
B. Operated										
0–19 Years	3	5.7	<1	5	5	6	6	6	6	6
20–34	5	7.0	8	5	5	6	7	12	12	12
35–49	1	11.0	0	11	11	11	11	11	11	11
50–64	0									
65+	0									
2. MULTIPLE DX										
A. Not Operated										
0–19 Years	85	7.0	52	2	3	5	9	14	23	45
20–34	213	5.6	20	2	3	4	7	12	15	21
35–49	217	5.4	22	2	3	4	7	10	14	23
50–64	164	5.9	21	2	3	5	8	12	14	28
65+	201	6.1	19	3	3	5	8	10	14	32
B. Operated										
0–19 Years	10	14.0	41	6	9	14	19	26	26	26
20–34	36	12.5	76	4	5	9	19	26	32	36
35–49	52	12.7	121	6	6	9	17	24	29	68
50–64	55	14.2	137	5	6	11	18	29	39	57
65+	35	16.1	159	5	8	12	21	28	56	56
SUBTOTALS:										
1. SINGLE DX										
A. Not Operated	33	3.6	6	1	2	3	4	7	9	11
B. Operated	9	7.0	7	5	5	6	7	12	12	12
2. MULTIPLE DX										
A. Not Operated	880	5.9	24	2	3	4	7	11	14	28
B. Operated	188	13.8	119	5	6	11	18	27	32	57
1. SINGLE DX	42	4.3	8	1	2	4	6	8	11	12
2. MULTIPLE DX	1,068	7.3	49	2	3	5	8	14	21	34
A. NOT OPERATED	913	5.8	23	2	3	4	7	11	14	27
B. OPERATED	197	13.5	116	5	6	10	18	26	32	57
TOTAL										
0–19 Years	105	7.6	51	2	3	5	9	16	23	29
20–34	277	6.3	32	2	3	5	7	13	19	28
35–49	273	6.8	48	2	3	5	9	13	20	38
50–64	219	8.0	62	2	3	5	7	15	25	39
65+	236	7.6	52	3	4	5	8	14	21	34
GRAND TOTAL	1,110	7.1	48	2	3	5	8	14	21	32

556.8: OTHER ULCERATIVE COLITIS

Type of Patients	Observed Patients	Avg. Stay	Variance	10th	25th	50th	75th	90th	95th	99th
1. SINGLE DX										
A. Not Operated										
0–19 Years	5	4.2	2	2	4	4	5	6	6	6
20–34	8	4.3	5	1	2	4	4	6	7	7
35–49	8	3.4	2	2	2	3	3	6	6	6
50–64	3	4.4	8	1	1	6	6	6	6	6
65+	0									
B. Operated										
0–19 Years	1	5.0	0	5	5	5	5	5	5	5
20–34	7	5.4	3	4	4	5	6	9	9	9
35–49	3	5.7	2	4	4	6	7	7	7	7
50–64	2	7.0	0	7	7	7	7	7	7	7
65+	0									
2. MULTIPLE DX										
A. Not Operated										
0–19 Years	35	5.4	14	1	3	4	7	12	13	15
20–34	166	5.1	15	2	3	4	6	10	13	20
35–49	147	5.2	13	2	3	4	7	10	13	18
50–64	152	5.4	22	2	3	4	7	10	15	26
65+	147	5.3	14	2	3	4	7	9	15	18
B. Operated										
0–19 Years	6	9.4	60	5	6	7	7	25	25	25
20–34	22	17.0	323	4	5	8	22	41	41	77
35–49	40	10.1	52	4	5	8	8	24	29	30
50–64	44	15.8	203	5	6	12	20	33	44	79
65+	29	10.3	52	4	5	7	14	24	27	29
SUBTOTALS:										
1. SINGLE DX										
A. Not Operated	24	4.0	3	2	2	4	6	6	7	7
B. Operated	13	5.7	2	4	4	6	7	7	9	9
2. MULTIPLE DX										
A. Not Operated	647	5.2	16	2	3	4	7	10	13	20
B. Operated	141	12.9	147	5	6	8	16	28	33	77
1. SINGLE DX	37	4.6	4	2	3	4	6	7	7	9
2. MULTIPLE DX	788	6.6	48	2	3	5	8	13	18	35
A. NOT OPERATED	671	5.2	16	2	3	4	6	10	13	20
B. OPERATED	154	12.3	139	4	6	8	15	27	33	77
TOTAL										
0–19 Years	47	5.8	19	2	3	5	7	12	13	25
20–34	203	6.4	60	2	3	4	7	11	19	41
35–49	198	6.1	24	2	3	5	8	11	16	29
50–64	201	7.7	79	2	3	5	8	15	22	44
65+	176	6.1	23	2	3	5	7	13	17	27
GRAND TOTAL	825	6.5	46	2	3	5	7	13	18	33

Length of Stay by Diagnosis and Operation, Western Region, 2008

556.9: ULCERATIVE COLITIS NOS

Type of Patients	Observed Patients	Avg. Stay	Vari-ance	Percentiles 10th	25th	50th	75th	90th	95th	99th
1. SINGLE DX										
A. Not Operated										
0–19 Years	20	3.6	5	1	2	3	5	7	8	8
20–34	27	3.7	5	1	2	3	5	7	8	10
35–49	24	3.9	6	1	2	3	5	7	9	9
50–64	8	3.9	18	1	1	3	4	14	14	14
65+	1	1.0	0	1	1	1	1	1	1	1
B. Operated										
0–19 Years	3	5.0	<1	4	5	5	6	6	6	6
20–34	14	4.7	<1	4	4	5	5	6	6	6
35–49	10	6.6	6	2	5	6	8	9	11	11
50–64	3	5.3	10	3	3	4	9	9	9	9
65+	1	5.0	0	5	5	5	5	5	5	5
2. MULTIPLE DX										
A. Not Operated										
0–19 Years	127	5.0	18	1	2	4	7	9	12	23
20–34	513	4.2	9	1	2	3	5	8	10	16
35–49	447	4.8	23	1	2	4	6	9	12	15
50–64	360	4.9	15	2	2	3	6	9	11	21
65+	390	5.3	17	2	3	4	7	10	13	21
B. Operated										
0–19 Years	11	13.1	122	4	4	7	24	26	33	33
20–34	51	8.2	21	4	5	7	10	13	18	23
35–49	64	10.1	38	5	6	7	13	21	23	25
50–64	82	12.2	167	4	6	8	12	24	39	77
65+	48	9.7	53	4	5	8	11	22	25	36
SUBTOTALS:										
1. SINGLE DX										
A. Not Operated	80	3.7	6	1	2	3	5	7	9	14
B. Operated	31	5.4	4	4	4	5	6	8	9	11
2. MULTIPLE DX										
A. Not Operated	1,837	4.8	16	2	2	4	6	9	11	18
B. Operated	256	10.4	84	4	5	7	12	22	25	56
1. SINGLE DX	111	4.2	6	1	2	4	5	7	9	11
2. MULTIPLE DX	2,093	5.5	28	2	3	4	7	10	14	24
A. NOT OPERATED	1,917	4.7	16	2	2	4	6	9	11	18
B. OPERATED	287	9.9	77	4	5	7	11	21	24	56
TOTAL										
0–19 Years	161	5.4	27	1	2	4	7	9	14	29
20–34	605	4.5	11	1	2	4	6	8	11	17
35–49	545	5.5	27	2	3	4	7	10	13	23
50–64	453	6.2	50	2	3	4	8	11	16	39
65+	440	5.8	22	2	3	4	7	11	15	25
GRAND TOTAL	2,204	5.4	27	2	3	4	7	10	14	24

557: VASC INSUFF INTESTINE

Type of Patients	Observed Patients	Avg. Stay	Vari-ance	Percentiles 10th	25th	50th	75th	90th	95th	99th
1. SINGLE DX										
A. Not Operated										
0–19 Years	8	3.6	13	1	1	3	3	11	11	11
20–34	13	1.7	<1	1	1	2	2	3	3	3
35–49	8	2.4	2	1	1	2	3	3	4	4
50–64	13	2.3	<1	1	2	2	3	3	4	4
65+	6	3.0	6	1	2	2	3	8	8	8
B. Operated										
0–19 Years	4	1.3	<1	1	1	1	1	2	2	2
20–34	11	2.4	1	1	2	2	3	4	4	4
35–49	8	1.3	<1	1	1	1	1	3	3	3
50–64	3	5.3	2	4	4	5	7	7	7	7
65+	4	1.0	0	1	1	1	1	1	1	1
2. MULTIPLE DX										
A. Not Operated										
0–19 Years	27	9.5	74	1	3	7	13	25	29	30
20–34	126	4.0	9	1	2	3	5	7	9	15
35–49	472	4.1	9	2	2	3	5	8	10	18
50–64	1,635	4.1	10	2	2	3	5	7	9	17
65+	4,332	4.9	14	2	3	4	6	9	12	20
B. Operated										
0–19 Years	23	10.0	166	1	2	6	14	42	51	>99
20–34	56	12.8	238	2	4	7	14	36	42	76
35–49	153	11.3	139	2	4	8	14	22	32	56
50–64	391	13.7	189	4	6	9	16	27	43	74
65+	1,102	12.8	100	5	7	10	16	23	31	55
SUBTOTALS:										
1. SINGLE DX										
A. Not Operated	48	2.5	4	1	1	2	3	4	7	11
B. Operated	30	2.0	2	1	1	1	3	4	5	7
2. MULTIPLE DX										
A. Not Operated	6,592	4.6	13	2	2	4	6	8	11	19
B. Operated	1,725	12.8	129	4	6	10	16	24	35	69
1. SINGLE DX	78	2.3	3	1	1	2	3	4	7	11
2. MULTIPLE DX	8,317	6.3	48	2	3	4	7	13	18	36
A. NOT OPERATED	6,640	4.6	13	2	2	4	6	8	11	19
B. OPERATED	1,755	12.6	129	3	6	10	16	24	34	69
TOTAL										
0–19 Years	62	8.4	101	1	2	5	11	23	30	>99
20–34	206	6.2	87	2	2	4	6	12	21	42
35–49	641	5.8	50	2	3	4	7	12	17	32
50–64	2,042	5.9	58	2	3	4	8	12	17	42
65+	5,444	6.5	42	2	3	5	8	13	18	33
GRAND TOTAL	8,395	6.3	48	2	3	4	7	13	18	36

557.0: AC VASC INSUFF INTESTINE

Type of Patients	Observed Patients	Avg. Stay	Vari-ance	Percentiles 10th	25th	50th	75th	90th	95th	99th
1. SINGLE DX										
A. Not Operated										
0–19 Years	5	3.8	17	1	1	3	3	11	11	11
20–34	11	1.6	<1	1	1	2	3	3	3	3
35–49	5	2.2	2	1	1	2	3	4	4	4
50–64	5	2.0	1	1	1	2	3	3	3	3
65+	2	2.0	0	2	2	2	2	2	2	2
B. Operated										
0–19 Years	3	1.3	<1	1	1	1	2	2	2	2
20–34	10	2.4	1	1	2	2	3	4	4	4
35–49	8	1.3	<1	1	1	1	1	3	3	3
50–64	2	4.5	<1	4	4	5	5	5	5	5
65+	0									
2. MULTIPLE DX										
A. Not Operated										
0–19 Years	14	13.2	112	1	2	10	23	29	30	30
20–34	47	4.3	12	2	2	3	5	7	8	21
35–49	168	4.4	13	2	2	3	5	8	11	21
50–64	509	4.4	13	2	2	4	5	8	10	20
65+	1,210	5.2	18	2	3	4	6	10	12	21
B. Operated										
0–19 Years	15	7.2	113	1	2	4	14	42	>99	>99
20–34	39	10.8	212	1	3	6	11	36	42	76
35–49	109	11.3	139	2	4	8	15	23	29	56
50–64	269	14.9	230	4	6	10	18	31	46	85
65+	650	13.6	108	5	7	11	17	24	33	55
SUBTOTALS:										
1. SINGLE DX										
A. Not Operated	28	2.2	4	1	1	2	3	3	4	11
B. Operated	23	2.0	2	1	1	2	3	3	4	5
2. MULTIPLE DX										
A. Not Operated	1,948	5.0	17	2	3	4	6	9	12	21
B. Operated	1,082	13.5	147	4	6	10	16	26	37	72
1. SINGLE DX	51	2.1	3	1	1	2	3	4	4	11
2. MULTIPLE DX	3,030	8.0	80	2	3	5	9	16	23	47
A. NOT OPERATED	1,976	4.9	17	2	3	4	6	9	12	21
B. OPERATED	1,105	13.2	146	4	6	10	16	25	37	71
TOTAL										
0–19 Years	37	8.5	103	1	1	4	4	29	42	>99
20–34	107	6.2	94	1	2	4	8	12	21	42
35–49	290	6.9	72	1	2	4	8	15	21	51
50–64	785	8.0	112	2	3	5	9	16	27	56
65+	1,862	8.1	65	2	3	6	10	17	22	43
GRAND TOTAL	3,081	7.9	79	3	3	5	9	16	23	47

Length of Stay by Diagnosis and Operation, Western Region, 2008

Western Region, October 2006–September 2007 Data, by Diagnosis

557.1: CHR VASC INSUFF INTEST

Type of Patients	Observed Patients	Avg. Stay	Variance	10th	25th	50th	75th	90th	95th	99th
1. SINGLE DX										
A. Not Operated										
0–19 Years	2	4.0	18	1	1	4	7	7	7	7
20–34	1	2.0	0	2	2	2	2	2	2	2
35–49	0									
50–64	1	2.0	0	2	2	2	2	2	2	2
65+	0									
B. Operated										
0–19 Years	0									
20–34	0									
35–49	0									
50–64	0									
65+	4	1.0	0	1	1	1	1	1	1	1
2. MULTIPLE DX										
A. Not Operated										
0–19 Years	13	5.4	6	2	4	5	7	9	9	9
20–34	31	4.9	13	2	2	4	6	12	13	14
35–49	24	5.0	15	2	2	4	7	13	13	17
50–64	92	5.6	23	1	3	4	6	13	17	24
65+	321	5.1	18	2	3	4	6	10	13	22
B. Operated										
0–19 Years	7	16.6	273	5	5	11	20	51	51	51
20–34	7	30.7	354	12	22	23	36	70	70	70
35–49	24	11.0	104	3	5	8	16	19	21	50
50–64	48	10.0	71	1	3	8	14	20	20	44
65+	193	11.3	131	2	4	9	14	22	35	93
SUBTOTALS:										
1. SINGLE DX — A. Not Operated	4	3.0	7	1	2	2	2	7	7	7
1. SINGLE DX — B. Operated	4	1.0	0	1	1	1	1	1	1	1
2. MULTIPLE DX — A. Not Operated	481	5.2	18	2	3	4	6	10	13	22
2. MULTIPLE DX — B. Operated	279	11.6	135	2	4	9	16	23	36	70
1. SINGLE DX	8	2.0	4	1	1	1	2	7	7	7
2. MULTIPLE DX	760	7.6	70	2	3	5	9	16	21	44
A. NOT OPERATED	485	5.2	18	2	3	4	6	10	13	22
B. OPERATED	283	11.5	135	1	4	9	15	22	35	70
TOTAL										
0–19 Years	22	8.9	111	2	4	5	9	19	20	51
20–34	39	9.5	168	2	3	4	12	23	36	70
35–49	48	8.0	68	2	3	5	12	17	19	50
50–64	141	7.1	43	1	3	5	10	16	19	32
65+	518	7.4	69	2	3	5	9	16	21	43
GRAND TOTAL	768	7.5	70	2	3	5	9	16	21	44

557.9: VASC INSUFF INTEST NOS

Type of Patients	Observed Patients	Avg. Stay	Variance	10th	25th	50th	75th	90th	95th	99th
1. SINGLE DX										
A. Not Operated										
0–19 Years	1	2.0	0	2	2	2	2	2	2	2
20–34	1	2.0	0	2	2	2	2	2	2	2
35–49	3	2.7	2	1	1	3	4	4	4	4
50–64	7	2.6	<1	1	2	3	3	4	4	4
65+	4	3.5	10	1	1	2	3	8	8	8
B. Operated										
0–19 Years	1	1.0	0	1	1	1	1	1	1	1
20–34	1	2.0	0	2	2	2	2	2	2	2
35–49	0									
50–64	1	7.0	0	7	7	7	7	7	7	7
65+	0									
2. MULTIPLE DX										
A. Not Operated										
0–19 Years	0									
20–34	48	3.1	4	1	2	3	5	6	6	9
35–49	280	3.9	6	2	2	3	5	7	8	16
50–64	1,034	3.8	7	2	2	3	5	7	8	14
65+	2,801	4.7	12	2	3	4	6	9	11	19
B. Operated										
0–19 Years	1	8.0	0	8	8	8	8	8	8	8
20–34	10	7.8	31	4	5	6	7	19	19	19
35–49	20	11.7	193	3	4	6	10	25	41	56
50–64	74	11.4	99	5	6	9	14	22	23	69
65+	259	12.1	55	5	7	10	16	22	29	50
SUBTOTALS:										
1. SINGLE DX — A. Not Operated	16	2.8	3	1	2	2	3	4	8	8
1. SINGLE DX — B. Operated	3	3.3	10	1	1	2	7	7	7	7
2. MULTIPLE DX — A. Not Operated	4,163	4.4	10	2	2	3	5	8	10	17
2. MULTIPLE DX — B. Operated	364	11.8	70	5	6	9	15	22	28	56
1. SINGLE DX	19	2.8	4	1	2	2	3	7	8	8
2. MULTIPLE DX	4,527	5.0	19	2	2	4	6	9	13	23
A. NOT OPERATED	4,179	4.4	10	2	2	3	5	8	10	17
B. OPERATED	367	11.7	70	5	6	9	14	22	28	56
TOTAL										
0–19 Years	3	3.7	14	1	1	2	3	5	5	9
20–34	60	3.9	11	1	2	3	5	6	8	19
35–49	303	4.4	22	2	2	3	5	8	10	20
50–64	1,116	4.3	16	2	3	3	5	8	10	19
65+	3,064	5.3	20	2	3	4	6	10	14	25
GRAND TOTAL	4,546	5.0	19	2	2	4	6	9	13	23

558: OTH NONINF GASTROENT

Type of Patients	Observed Patients	Avg. Stay	Variance	10th	25th	50th	75th	90th	95th	99th
1. SINGLE DX										
A. Not Operated										
0–19 Years	667	1.6	<1	1	1	1	2	3	3	4
20–34	239	1.8	1	1	1	1	2	3	4	5
35–49	134	1.8	2	1	1	1	2	3	4	7
50–64	75	2.0	3	1	1	1	2	4	5	14
65+	24	1.8	1	1	1	2	2	3	5	5
B. Operated										
0–19 Years	9	1.8	<1	1	1	1	3	3	3	3
20–34	7	3.0	8	1	1	2	3	9	9	9
35–49	7	1.6	<1	1	1	1	2	3	3	3
50–64	1	1.0	0	1	1	1	1	1	1	1
65+	1	3.0	0	3	3	3	3	3	3	3
2. MULTIPLE DX										
A. Not Operated										
0–19 Years	3,260	2.1	3	1	1	2	2	4	5	9
20–34	1,845	2.4	3	1	1	2	3	4	6	9
35–49	2,903	2.8	6	1	1	2	3	5	7	12
50–64	3,654	3.0	6	1	1	2	4	6	7	12
65+	6,225	3.3	7	1	2	3	4	6	8	13
B. Operated										
0–19 Years	29	2.9	9	1	1	2	3	5	11	15
20–34	45	4.6	24	1	2	3	5	8	14	26
35–49	59	6.6	31	1	3	5	9	14	21	25
50–64	94	9.9	59	3	5	8	14	21	29	>99
65+	112	10.7	77	2	5	8	14	23	31	49
SUBTOTALS:										
1. SINGLE DX — A. Not Operated	1,139	1.7	1	1	1	1	2	3	4	5
1. SINGLE DX — B. Operated	25	2.1	3	1	1	2	3	3	3	9
2. MULTIPLE DX — A. Not Operated	17,887	2.9	6	1	1	2	3	5	7	12
2. MULTIPLE DX — B. Operated	339	8.3	58	2	3	6	11	20	25	41
1. SINGLE DX	1,164	1.7	1	1	1	1	2	3	4	5
2. MULTIPLE DX	18,226	3.0	7	1	1	2	4	6	7	14
A. NOT OPERATED	19,026	2.8	6	1	1	2	3	5	7	12
B. OPERATED	364	7.9	57	2	3	5	11	19	24	41
TOTAL										
0–19 Years	3,965	2.0	3	1	1	2	2	3	4	8
20–34	2,136	2.4	4	1	1	2	3	4	6	9
35–49	3,103	2.8	7	1	1	2	3	5	7	13
50–64	3,824	3.2	9	1	1	3	4	6	8	15
65+	6,362	3.5	9	1	2	3	4	6	8	15
GRAND TOTAL	19,390	2.9	7	1	1	2	3	5	7	13

Length of Stay by Diagnosis and Operation, Western Region, 2008

Western Region, October 2006–September 2007 Data, by Diagnosis

558.1: RADIATION GASTROENT

Type of Patients	Observed Patients	Avg. Stay	Variance	Percentiles						
				10th	25th	50th	75th	90th	95th	99th
1. SINGLE DX										
A. Not Operated										
0–19 Years	0									
20–34	0									
35–49	0									
50–64	1	14.0	0	14	14	14	14	14	14	14
65+	0									
B. Operated										
0–19 Years	0									
20–34	0									
35–49	0									
50–64	0									
65+	0									
2. MULTIPLE DX										
A. Not Operated										
0–19 Years	0									
20–34	8	4.8	9	1	1	4	8	9	9	9
35–49	35	5.4	13	2	3	5	7	9	15	16
50–64	115	5.3	18	2	3	4	6	10	14	22
65+	232	5.3	24	1	2	4	6	11	16	20
B. Operated										
0–19 Years	0									
20–34	1	9.0	0	9	9	9	9	9	9	9
35–49	4	14.7	48	10	11	13	13	25	25	25
50–64	22	14.5	79	5	8	13	21	31	31	>99
65+	29	14.2	92	5	7	12	19	35	41	>99
SUBTOTALS:										
1. SINGLE DX										
A. Not Operated	1	14.0	0	14	14	14	14	14	14	14
B. Operated	0									
2. MULTIPLE DX										
A. Not Operated	390	5.3	21	2	2	4	6	11	16	22
B. Operated	56	14.3	80	5	8	12	19	31	41	>99
1. SINGLE DX	1	14.0	0	14	14	14	14	14	14	14
2. MULTIPLE DX	446	6.4	37	2	3	5	8	15	19	35
A. NOT OPERATED	391	5.3	21	2	2	4	6	11	16	22
B. OPERATED	56	14.3	80	5	8	12	19	31	41	>99
TOTAL										
0–19 Years	0									
20–34	9	5.2	9	1	4	5	8	9	9	9
35–49	39	6.4	23	2	3	5	7	13	16	25
50–64	138	6.8	39	2	3	5	8	15	22	31
65+	261	6.3	39	2	2	4	8	15	18	40
GRAND TOTAL	447	6.4	37	2	3	5	8	15	19	35

558.9: NONINF GASTROENT NEC&NOS

Type of Patients	Observed Patients	Avg. Stay	Variance	Percentiles						
				10th	25th	50th	75th	90th	95th	99th
1. SINGLE DX										
A. Not Operated										
0–19 Years	654	1.6	<1	1	1	1	2	3	3	4
20–34	239	1.8	1	1	1	1	2	3	4	5
35–49	134	1.8	2	1	1	1	2	3	4	7
50–64	74	1.9	1	1	1	1	2	3	5	5
65+	24	1.8	1	1	1	2	2	3	5	5
B. Operated										
0–19 Years	9	1.8	<1	1	1	1	3	3	3	3
20–34	7	3.0	8	1	1	2	3	9	9	9
35–49	7	1.6	<1	1	1	1	2	3	3	3
50–64	1	1.0	0	1	1	1	1	1	1	1
65+	1	3.0	0	3	3	3	3	3	3	3
2. MULTIPLE DX										
A. Not Operated										
0–19 Years	3,173	2.1	3	1	1	2	2	4	5	8
20–34	1,829	2.4	3	1	1	2	3	4	6	9
35–49	2,847	2.7	5	1	1	2	3	5	6	11
50–64	3,496	2.9	5	1	1	2	4	5	7	12
65+	5,932	3.2	6	1	2	3	4	6	8	12
B. Operated										
0–19 Years	28	2.6	7	1	1	2	3	4	5	15
20–34	44	4.5	24	1	2	3	5	8	14	26
35–49	53	5.7	23	1	2	4	8	12	17	22
50–64	70	7.9	29	2	4	7	11	16	20	22
65+	82	9.5	68	2	4	7	12	22	24	49
SUBTOTALS:										
1. SINGLE DX										
A. Not Operated	1,125	1.7	1	1	1	1	2	3	4	5
B. Operated	25	2.1	3	1	1	2	3	3	3	9
2. MULTIPLE DX										
A. Not Operated	17,277	2.8	5	1	1	2	3	5	7	11
B. Operated	277	6.9	41	1	2	5	9	15	21	30
1. SINGLE DX	1,150	1.7	1	1	1	1	2	3	4	5
2. MULTIPLE DX	17,554	2.8	6	1	1	2	3	5	7	12
A. NOT OPERATED	18,402	2.7	5	1	1	2	3	5	7	11
B. OPERATED	302	6.5	40	1	2	4	8	14	21	26
TOTAL										
0–19 Years	3,864	2.0	3	1	1	2	2	3	4	8
20–34	2,119	2.4	4	1	1	2	3	4	6	9
35–49	3,041	2.8	5	1	1	2	3	5	7	12
50–64	3,641	3.0	6	1	1	2	4	6	7	13
65+	6,039	3.3	7	1	2	3	4	6	8	13
GRAND TOTAL	18,704	2.8	6	1	1	2	3	5	7	12

560: INTESTINAL OBSTRUCTION

Type of Patients	Observed Patients	Avg. Stay	Variance	Percentiles						
				10th	25th	50th	75th	90th	95th	99th
1. SINGLE DX										
A. Not Operated										
0–19 Years	241	1.9	3	1	1	1	2	3	4	9
20–34	211	2.4	2	1	1	2	3	4	4	6
35–49	308	2.4	2	1	1	2	3	4	5	9
50–64	271	2.5	3	1	1	2	3	4	6	9
65+	131	2.4	2	1	1	2	3	4	4	6
B. Operated										
0–19 Years	85	3.5	7	2	2	3	4	7	8	16
20–34	67	5.3	14	1	3	5	7	10	13	18
35–49	75	4.6	8	2	3	4	5	7	8	21
50–64	84	5.1	8	2	3	5	5	8	10	16
65+	26	5.3	11	2	4	5	7	7	9	18
2. MULTIPLE DX										
A. Not Operated										
0–19 Years	887	2.9	11	1	1	2	3	5	8	16
20–34	1,575	3.7	15	1	2	3	4	7	9	18
35–49	4,298	3.7	10	1	2	3	4	7	9	17
50–64	8,114	3.8	11	1	2	3	5	7	10	16
65+	17,772	4.3	13	1	2	3	5	8	11	18
B. Operated										
0–19 Years	369	8.2	64	2	4	6	10	16	23	51
20–34	669	8.5	58	3	5	7	10	14	20	40
35–49	1,703	9.6	69	3	5	7	11	18	23	45
50–64	3,067	10.4	65	4	6	8	13	20	24	46
65+	5,667	11.9	58	5	7	10	15	21	26	40
SUBTOTALS:										
1. SINGLE DX										
A. Not Operated	1,162	2.3	2	1	1	2	3	4	5	9
B. Operated	337	4.6	10	2	2	4	6	8	10	18
2. MULTIPLE DX										
A. Not Operated	32,646	4.0	12	1	2	3	5	8	10	18
B. Operated	11,475	10.8	63	4	6	9	13	20	25	42
1. SINGLE DX	1,499	2.8	5	1	2	2	4	5	7	11
2. MULTIPLE DX	44,121	5.8	34	1	2	4	7	12	16	28
A. NOT OPERATED	33,808	4.0	12	1	2	3	5	7	10	17
B. OPERATED	11,812	10.7	63	4	6	9	13	20	25	41
TOTAL										
0–19 Years	1,582	4.0	27	1	1	2	5	8	12	25
20–34	2,522	4.9	30	1	2	3	6	10	13	23
35–49	6,384	5.2	33	1	2	3	6	11	15	27
50–64	11,536	5.6	34	1	2	4	7	12	16	28
65+	23,596	6.1	34	2	2	4	8	13	17	28
GRAND TOTAL	45,620	5.7	34	1	2	4	7	12	16	28

Length of Stay by Diagnosis and Operation, Western Region, 2008

560.0: INTUSSUSCEPTION

Type of Patients	Observed Patients	Avg. Stay	Vari- ance	Percentiles 10th	25th	50th	75th	90th	95th	99th
1. SINGLE DX										
A. Not Operated										
0–19 Years	108	1.4	<1	1	1	1	2	2	3	4
20–34	2	1.5	<1	1	1	2	2	2	2	2
35–49	4	2.0	<1	1	1	2	2	3	3	3
50–64	2	1.0	0	1	1	1	1	1	1	1
65+	0									
B. Operated										
0–19 Years	49	2.3	2	1	1	2	3	4	4	7
20–34	9	4.0	2	2	3	4	5	7	7	7
35–49	2	4.5	4	3	3	6	6	6	6	6
50–64	0									
65+	0									
2. MULTIPLE DX										
A. Not Operated										
0–19 Years	78	1.9	2	1	1	2	2	3	4	9
20–34	27	2.2	3	1	1	2	2	5	5	8
35–49	35	3.4	9	1	2	2	4	7	11	14
50–64	25	3.4	12	1	2	2	4	8	11	16
65+	24	3.4	5	1	2	3	5	6	7	10
B. Operated										
0–19 Years	116	4.2	9	2	2	3	5	7	8	17
20–34	57	5.3	6	3	4	5	8	8	8	16
35–49	75	7.0	21	3	4	6	8	13	15	26
50–64	60	6.4	17	3	4	5	8	12	17	21
65+	53	11.0	124	4	6	8	12	16	28	71
SUBTOTALS:										
1. SINGLE DX										
A. Not Operated	116	1.5	<1	1	1	1	2	2	3	4
B. Operated	60	2.7	2	1	2	2	3	4	7	7
2. MULTIPLE DX										
A. Not Operated	189	2.6	5	1	1	2	3	5	8	14
B. Operated	361	6.3	34	2	3	5	7	12	15	26
1. SINGLE DX	176	1.9	2	1	1	1	2	3	4	7
2. MULTIPLE DX	550	5.0	27	2	2	4	6	10	13	22
A. NOT OPERATED	305	2.2	4	1	1	2	2	4	5	11
B. OPERATED	421	5.8	31	2	3	5	7	11	14	25
TOTAL										
0–19 Years	351	2.6	5	1	1	2	3	5	7	11
20–34	95	4.2	6	1	2	4	6	7	8	16
35–49	116	5.7	20	2	3	5	7	11	14	25
50–64	87	5.4	18	2	2	5	7	11	15	21
65+	77	8.6	98	4	4	6	10	15	22	71
GRAND TOTAL	726	4.3	23	2	2	3	5	8	12	21

560.1: PARALYTIC ILEUS

Type of Patients	Observed Patients	Avg. Stay	Vari- ance	Percentiles 10th	25th	50th	75th	90th	95th	99th
1. SINGLE DX										
A. Not Operated										
0–19 Years	21	1.8	<1	1	1	2	2	3	3	4
20–34	15	2.2	1	1	1	2	3	4	5	5
35–49	25	2.9	8	1	1	2	3	6	9	12
50–64	12	2.2	2	1	2	2	4	4	4	4
65+	7	2.0	2	1	1	2	3	5	5	5
B. Operated										
0–19 Years	0									
20–34	2	4.5	<1	4	4	5	5	5	5	5
35–49	1	7.0	0	7	7	7	7	7	7	7
50–64	0									
65+	0									
2. MULTIPLE DX										
A. Not Operated										
0–19 Years	240	2.5	5	1	1	2	3	5	6	11
20–34	367	3.7	10	1	2	3	5	7	9	18
35–49	944	3.9	17	1	2	3	5	7	10	21
50–64	1,502	4.3	17	1	2	3	5	8	12	19
65+	3,501	4.8	16	1	2	4	6	10	12	20
B. Operated										
0–19 Years	4	14.5	110	1	7	20	25	25	25	25
20–34	7	10.6	35	4	7	8	13	22	22	22
35–49	38	10.6	137	3	5	8	12	19	39	66
50–64	65	13.8	227	3	6	10	16	27	46	87
65+	109	11.9	44	4	6	12	16	21	24	27
SUBTOTALS:										
1. SINGLE DX										
A. Not Operated	80	2.3	3	1	1	2	3	4	6	12
B. Operated	3	5.3	2	4	4	5	7	7	7	7
2. MULTIPLE DX										
A. Not Operated	6,554	4.4	16	1	2	3	5	9	12	20
B. Operated	223	12.3	114	3	5	10	16	21	26	63
1. SINGLE DX	83	2.4	4	1	1	2	3	4	6	12
2. MULTIPLE DX	6,777	4.7	21	1	2	3	6	9	13	21
A. NOT OPERATED	6,634	4.4	16	1	2	3	5	9	12	20
B. OPERATED	226	12.2	113	3	5	10	16	21	26	63
TOTAL										
0–19 Years	265	2.7	8	1	1	2	3	5	7	20
20–34	391	3.8	11	1	2	3	5	7	10	19
35–49	1,008	4.2	23	1	2	3	5	8	11	22
50–64	1,579	4.6	29	1	2	4	5	9	13	24
65+	3,617	5.0	19	1	2	4	6	10	13	21
GRAND TOTAL	6,860	4.6	21	1	2	3	6	9	13	21

560.2: INTESTINAL VOLVULUS

Type of Patients	Observed Patients	Avg. Stay	Vari- ance	Percentiles 10th	25th	50th	75th	90th	95th	99th
1. SINGLE DX										
A. Not Operated										
0–19 Years	1	8.0	0	8	8	8	8	8	8	8
20–34	4	1.5	<1	1	1	2	2	2	2	2
35–49	7	1.6	2	1	1	1	1	5	5	5
50–64	0									
65+	2	1.5	<1	1	1	2	2	2	2	2
B. Operated										
0–19 Years	6	3.5	5	1	2	3	5	6	6	6
20–34	12	4.2	9	1	2	4	5	6	12	12
35–49	10	3.3	6	2	2	3	4	6	6	6
50–64	13	4.5	5	3	3	4	6	7	10	10
65+	4	9.3	35	5	7	7	18	18	18	18
2. MULTIPLE DX										
A. Not Operated										
0–19 Years	8	2.0	2	1	1	2	3	5	5	5
20–34	18	2.8	4	1	1	2	5	6	7	7
35–49	22	3.0	4	1	1	2	4	6	7	8
50–64	54	3.2	10	1	2	3	4	5	7	21
65+	207	4.5	12	1	2	4	6	9	10	17
B. Operated										
0–19 Years	28	9.9	140	3	5	7	9	16	30	63
20–34	78	7.1	20	3	5	7	9	13	15	26
35–49	162	8.2	84	3	4	6	9	13	20	64
50–64	282	9.1	57	3	5	7	10	17	21	44
65+	661	11.5	85	5	7	9	14	19	24	54
SUBTOTALS:										
1. SINGLE DX										
A. Not Operated	14	2.0	4	1	1	2	2	5	8	8
B. Operated	45	4.5	10	1	3	4	6	7	10	18
2. MULTIPLE DX										
A. Not Operated	309	4.0	11	1	2	3	5	8	10	17
B. Operated	1,211	10.2	77	4	6	8	12	18	23	49
1. SINGLE DX	59	3.9	10	1	1	3	5	7	10	18
2. MULTIPLE DX	1,520	8.9	70	2	4	7	11	17	21	44
A. NOT OPERATED	323	3.9	11	1	2	3	5	8	10	17
B. OPERATED	1,256	10.0	76	4	5	8	12	18	22	49
TOTAL										
0–19 Years	43	7.5	102	1	3	6	8	13	16	63
20–34	112	5.9	19	1	3	5	7	11	13	25
35–49	201	7.1	73	2	3	5	8	12	16	41
50–64	349	8.0	53	2	4	6	10	16	19	34
65+	874	9.8	76	3	5	8	12	18	22	48
GRAND TOTAL	1,579	8.7	69	2	4	7	10	16	21	44

560.39: INTESTINE IMPACTION NEC

Type of Patients	Observed Patients	Avg. Stay	Vari-ance	Percentiles 10th	25th	50th	75th	90th	95th	99th
1. SINGLE DX										
A. Not Operated										
0–19 Years	51	1.9	1	1	1	1	2	3	4	7
20–34	4	2.0	2	1	1	2	2	4	4	4
35–49	7	1.3	<1	1	1	1	2	2	2	2
50–64	1	4.0	0	4	4	4	4	4	4	4
65+	8	1.7	1	1	1	1	2	4	4	4
B. Operated										
0–19 Years	0									
20–34	0									
35–49	0									
50–64	0									
65+	0									
2. MULTIPLE DX										
A. Not Operated										
0–19 Years	322	2.4	3	1	1	2	3	4	6	9
20–34	114	3.8	12	1	2	3	5	7	10	18
35–49	182	3.4	9	1	2	3	4	6	9	19
50–64	362	3.9	9	1	2	3	5	8	9	15
65+	1,836	4.1	12	1	2	3	5	8	11	16
B. Operated										
0–19 Years	7	4.5	7	1	2	4	8	8	8	8
20–34	4	8.7	17	5	5	6	10	14	14	14
35–49	4	8.3	5	6	7	9	11	11	11	11
50–64	18	12.5	124	3	8	10	13	20	53	53
65+	60	10.3	57	2	6	9	13	21	25	38
SUBTOTALS:										
1. SINGLE DX										
A. Not Operated	71	1.8	1	1	1	1	2	3	4	7
B. Operated	0									
2. MULTIPLE DX										
A. Not Operated	2,816	3.8	11	1	2	3	5	7	10	15
B. Operated	93	10.1	64	3	6	8	12	20	25	53
1. SINGLE DX	71	1.8	1	1	1	1	2	3	4	7
2. MULTIPLE DX	2,909	4.0	14	1	2	3	5	8	11	19
A. NOT OPERATED	2,887	3.8	11	1	2	3	5	7	10	15
B. OPERATED	93	10.1	64	3	6	8	12	20	25	53
TOTAL										
0–19 Years	380	2.4	3	1	1	2	3	4	6	9
20–34	122	3.9	12	1	1	2	3	5	10	18
35–49	193	3.4	9	1	2	3	4	7	9	19
50–64	381	4.3	18	1	2	3	5	8	11	20
65+	1,904	4.3	15	1	2	3	5	8	11	19
GRAND TOTAL	2,980	4.0	14	1	2	3	5	8	10	19

560.81: INTESTINAL ADHES W OBSTR

Type of Patients	Observed Patients	Avg. Stay	Vari-ance	Percentiles 10th	25th	50th	75th	90th	95th	99th
1. SINGLE DX										
A. Not Operated										
0–19 Years	6	4.9	43	1	2	3	3	3	18	18
20–34	36	2.4	1	1	2	3	3	4	4	5
35–49	43	2.4	2	1	1	2	3	4	5	6
50–64	43	2.5	2	1	1	2	3	5	5	7
65+	19	2.7	6	1	1	2	3	4	12	12
B. Operated										
0–19 Years	28	5.6	11	2	3	6	8	9	10	16
20–34	41	6.3	17	2	4	5	7	11	16	18
35–49	60	4.8	9	2	3	4	5	8	8	21
50–64	64	5.3	9	2	3	5	7	9	11	16
65+	19	4.5	3	2	3	4	6	7	7	7
2. MULTIPLE DX										
A. Not Operated										
0–19 Years	25	3.0	3	1	2	3	4	4	5	10
20–34	153	3.6	6	1	2	3	4	7	9	11
35–49	557	3.8	9	1	2	3	4	7	10	17
50–64	1,144	3.8	9	1	2	3	5	7	9	16
65+	2,411	4.3	11	2	2	4	5	7	10	17
B. Operated										
0–19 Years	172	9.6	48	4	5	8	12	17	25	30
20–34	432	8.9	65	3	5	7	12	16	21	41
35–49	1,148	9.7	62	3	5	8	12	18	23	39
50–64	2,063	10.3	55	4	6	8	13	19	24	40
65+	3,847	12.0	52	5	7	10	15	21	26	39
SUBTOTALS:										
1. SINGLE DX										
A. Not Operated	147	2.6	4	1	1	2	3	4	5	12
B. Operated	212	5.3	10	2	3	5	7	8	11	18
2. MULTIPLE DX										
A. Not Operated	4,290	4.1	10	1	2	3	5	7	10	17
B. Operated	7,662	11.0	56	4	6	9	13	20	25	39
1. SINGLE DX	359	4.2	9	1	2	3	5	8	10	18
2. MULTIPLE DX	11,952	8.5	50	2	4	7	11	17	22	34
A. NOT OPERATED	4,437	4.0	10	1	2	3	5	7	10	17
B. OPERATED	7,874	10.8	56	4	6	9	13	20	25	39
TOTAL										
0–19 Years	231	8.3	43	2	4	6	10	16	21	30
20–34	662	7.2	51	2	3	6	9	13	18	36
35–49	1,808	7.5	50	2	3	6	10	15	20	33
50–64	3,314	7.9	48	2	3	6	10	16	21	34
65+	6,296	9.0	50	2	4	7	12	18	22	34
GRAND TOTAL	12,311	8.4	50	2	4	7	11	17	22	34

560.89: INTESTINAL OBSTR NEC

Type of Patients	Observed Patients	Avg. Stay	Vari-ance	Percentiles 10th	25th	50th	75th	90th	95th	99th
1. SINGLE DX										
A. Not Operated										
0–19 Years	7	2.4	<1	1	2	2	3	4	4	4
20–34	19	2.5	1	1	2	2	4	4	5	5
35–49	41	2.5	4	1	1	2	3	5	5	9
50–64	32	2.8	5	1	1	3	3	5	8	12
65+	13	2.6	<1	2	2	2	3	4	4	4
B. Operated										
0–19 Years	2	1.5	<1	1	1	2	2	2	2	2
20–34	1	3.0	0	3	3	3	3	3	3	3
35–49	0									
50–64	1	5.0	0	5	5	5	5	5	5	5
65+	0									
2. MULTIPLE DX										
A. Not Operated										
0–19 Years	50	4.3	11	1	2	3	6	8	10	18
20–34	168	4.8	65	1	2	3	5	7	14	56
35–49	484	3.9	10	1	2	3	5	8	10	18
50–64	985	4.4	13	1	2	3	5	9	12	18
65+	1,850	4.9	22	1	2	4	6	10	13	21
B. Operated										
0–19 Years	19	11.5	85	3	7	9	13	30	38	38
20–34	40	8.6	28	3	6	8	14	14	27	27
35–49	139	11.3	128	3	5	8	14	20	28	73
50–64	270	11.7	99	4	6	9	14	23	31	66
65+	448	12.4	60	5	7	10	16	22	27	40
SUBTOTALS:										
1. SINGLE DX										
A. Not Operated	112	2.6	3	1	1	2	3	4	5	9
B. Operated	4	2.8	3	1	2	3	5	5	5	5
2. MULTIPLE DX										
A. Not Operated	3,537	4.6	20	1	2	3	6	9	12	20
B. Operated	916	11.8	81	4	6	9	15	22	28	50
1. SINGLE DX	116	2.6	3	1	1	2	3	5	5	9
2. MULTIPLE DX	4,453	6.1	41	1	2	4	8	13	18	30
A. NOT OPERATED	3,649	4.6	19	1	2	3	5	9	12	20
B. OPERATED	920	11.8	81	4	6	9	15	22	28	50
TOTAL										
0–19 Years	78	5.8	38	1	2	4	7	10	18	38
20–34	228	5.2	56	1	2	3	6	11	14	27
35–49	664	5.4	44	1	2	3	7	11	15	28
50–64	1,288	5.9	40	1	3	4	7	13	17	32
65+	2,311	6.4	38	2	3	4	8	13	18	30
GRAND TOTAL	4,569	6.0	40	1	2	4	7	13	18	30

Length of Stay by Diagnosis and Operation, Western Region, 2008

425

Western Region, October 2006–September 2007 Data, by Diagnosis

560.9: INTESTINAL OBSTR NOS

Type of Patients	Observed Patients	Avg. Stay	Vari-ance	10th	25th	50th	75th	90th	95th	99th
1. SINGLE DX										
A. Not Operated										
0–19 Years	46	2.5	5	1	1	2	3	5	7	11
20–34	130	2.4	2	1	1	2	3	4	5	6
35–49	181	2.4	2	1	1	2	3	4	5	6
50–64	180	2.5	3	1	1	2	3	4	6	9
65+	82	2.4	1	1	2	2	3	4	4	6
B. Operated										
0–19 Years	0									
20–34	2	1.0	0	1	1	1	1	1	1	1
35–49	2	2.5	<1	2	2	3	3	3	3	3
50–64	6	3.7	5	1	2	5	5	7	7	7
65+	3	5.0	16	1	1	5	9	9	9	9
2. MULTIPLE DX										
A. Not Operated										
0–19 Years	159	4.4	39	1	2	3	5	9	13	38
20–34	726	3.5	10	1	2	3	4	7	8	18
35–49	2,070	3.4	8	1	2	3	4	6	8	14
50–64	4,033	3.5	9	1	2	3	4	6	9	15
65+	7,909	4.0	9	1	2	3	5	7	10	16
B. Operated										
0–19 Years	22	13.3	251	3	5	10	12	22	55	64
20–34	51	9.9	132	3	5	7	12	15	26	81
35–49	136	9.7	55	4	5	7	13	18	23	38
50–64	294	11.1	78	4	6	8	13	21	28	61
65+	439	11.6	73	4	6	9	14	22	29	42
SUBTOTALS:										
1. SINGLE DX										
A. Not Operated	619	2.5	2	1	1	2	3	4	5	8
B. Operated	13	3.4	7	1	1	2	5	7	8	9
2. MULTIPLE DX										
A. Not Operated	14,897	3.8	9	1	2	3	5	7	9	16
B. Operated	942	11.1	79	4	6	9	13	21	28	55
1. SINGLE DX	632	2.5	2	1	1	2	3	4	5	8
2. MULTIPLE DX	15,839	4.2	16	1	2	3	5	8	11	21
A. NOT OPERATED	15,516	3.7	9	1	2	3	4	7	9	16
B. OPERATED	955	11.0	79	4	6	9	13	21	28	55
TOTAL										
0–19 Years	227	4.9	60	1	2	3	5	10	16	55
20–34	909	3.7	18	1	2	3	4	7	10	20
35–49	2,389	3.7	12	1	2	3	4	7	9	18
50–64	4,513	4.0	17	1	2	3	5	8	11	21
65+	8,433	4.3	15	1	2	3	5	8	11	20
GRAND TOTAL	16,471	4.1	16	1	2	3	5	8	11	20

562: DIVERTICULA OF INTESTINE

Type of Patients	Observed Patients	Avg. Stay	Vari-ance	10th	25th	50th	75th	90th	95th	99th
1. SINGLE DX										
A. Not Operated										
0–19 Years	7	2.4	3	1	1	2	4	5	5	5
20–34	208	2.9	2	1	2	2	4	5	6	9
35–49	508	2.7	2	1	2	2	3	4	5	8
50–64	297	2.8	2	1	2	2	3	5	5	8
65+	73	2.3	2	1	1	2	3	4	5	7
B. Operated										
0–19 Years	5	3.2	2	2	2	3	4	5	5	5
20–34	48	4.3	5	2	3	4	5	7	8	14
35–49	195	4.3	3	2	3	4	5	6	8	10
50–64	154	4.6	4	3	3	4	5	7	8	14
65+	29	4.8	2	3	4	4	6	7	8	8
2. MULTIPLE DX										
A. Not Operated										
0–19 Years	25	3.7	15	1	2	3	4	9	13	20
20–34	990	3.4	6	1	2	3	4	6	7	12
35–49	4,169	3.4	5	1	2	3	4	6	8	12
50–64	7,192	3.4	6	1	2	3	4	6	8	12
65+	16,637	3.8	8	1	2	3	5	7	9	14
B. Operated										
0–19 Years	15	8.1	107	2	3	4	7	19	40	40
20–34	390	7.6	27	3	5	6	9	13	18	28
35–49	2,105	7.3	23	3	4	6	9	13	16	24
50–64	3,606	8.0	38	3	4	6	9	15	19	33
65+	3,554	10.4	58	4	6	8	13	19	24	42
SUBTOTALS:										
1. SINGLE DX										
A. Not Operated	1,093	2.7	2	1	2	2	3	4	5	8
B. Operated	431	4.4	4	2	3	4	5	7	8	11
2. MULTIPLE DX										
A. Not Operated	29,013	3.6	7	1	2	3	4	6	8	13
B. Operated	9,670	8.7	43	4	5	7	10	16	21	35
1. SINGLE DX	1,524	3.2	3	1	2	3	4	5	6	8
2. MULTIPLE DX	38,683	4.9	21	2	2	4	6	9	13	23
A. NOT OPERATED	30,106	3.6	7	1	2	3	4	6	8	13
B. OPERATED	10,101	8.5	43	3	5	7	10	16	21	34
TOTAL										
0–19 Years	52	4.7	42	1	2	3	4	7	19	40
20–34	1,636	4.3	14	1	2	3	5	8	10	20
35–49	6,977	4.5	13	2	2	4	6	9	12	18
50–64	11,249	4.9	20	2	2	4	6	9	13	22
65+	20,293	5.0	23	2	3	4	6	10	14	24
GRAND TOTAL	40,207	4.8	20	2	2	4	6	9	13	23

562.10: COLON DIVERTICULOSIS

Type of Patients	Observed Patients	Avg. Stay	Vari-ance	10th	25th	50th	75th	90th	95th	99th
1. SINGLE DX										
A. Not Operated										
0–19 Years	0									
20–34	9	2.7	2	1	2	2	3	6	6	6
35–49	9	2.2	<1	1	2	3	3	3	3	3
50–64	10	3.0	5	1	1	3	3	8	8	8
65+	6	2.3	1	1	2	2	3	4	4	4
B. Operated										
0–19 Years	1	4.0	0	4	4	4	4	4	4	4
20–34	2	4.5	4	3	3	3	6	6	6	6
35–49	16	3.9	1	2	4	4	4	5	6	6
50–64	17	4.8	2	3	4	5	5	8	8	8
65+	4	4.3	4	3	3	4	7	7	7	7
2. MULTIPLE DX										
A. Not Operated										
0–19 Years	0									
20–34	39	2.5	2	1	2	3	3	4	5	9
35–49	147	3.2	4	1	2	3	4	5	7	11
50–64	346	3.4	6	1	2	3	4	6	7	12
65+	800	3.6	9	1	2	3	4	7	8	11
B. Operated										
0–19 Years	0									
20–34	28	5.9	13	3	3	5	7	9	10	20
35–49	183	6.4	20	3	4	5	7	12	15	21
50–64	328	6.7	26	3	4	5	7	12	16	26
65+	316	8.6	31	4	5	7	10	16	20	27
SUBTOTALS:										
1. SINGLE DX										
A. Not Operated	34	2.6	2	1	2	2	3	4	6	8
B. Operated	40	4.4	2	3	3	4	5	6	7	8
2. MULTIPLE DX										
A. Not Operated	1,332	3.5	7	1	2	3	4	6	8	12
B. Operated	855	7.3	27	3	4	6	8	14	18	27
1. SINGLE DX	74	3.6	3	2	2	3	5	6	7	8
2. MULTIPLE DX	2,187	5.0	19	2	2	4	6	9	13	21
A. NOT OPERATED	1,366	3.5	7	1	2	3	4	6	8	12
B. OPERATED	895	7.2	27	3	4	6	8	14	18	27
TOTAL										
0–19 Years	1	4.0	0	4	4	4	4	4	4	4
20–34	78	3.8	8	1	2	3	5	7	9	20
35–49	355	4.9	15	2	3	4	6	9	13	19
50–64	701	4.9	18	2	3	4	6	9	12	21
65+	1,126	5.0	20	1	2	4	6	9	13	22
GRAND TOTAL	2,261	4.9	18	2	2	4	6	9	13	21

Length of Stay by Diagnosis and Operation, Western Region, 2008

Western Region, October 2006–September 2007 Data, by Diagnosis

562.11: COLON DIVERTICULITIS

Type of Patients	Observed Patients	Avg. Stay	Vari-ance	Percentiles						
				10th	25th	50th	75th	90th	95th	99th
1. SINGLE DX										
A. Not Operated										
0–19 Years	6	2.5	3	1	1	3	4	5	5	5
20–34	195	2.8	2	1	2	3	3	5	6	9
35–49	487	2.7	2	1	2	2	3	5	5	8
50–64	278	2.8	2	1	2	3	4	4	5	7
65+	57	2.5	2	1	1	2	3	5	5	7
B. Operated										
0–19 Years	4	3.0	2	2	2	3	5	5	5	5
20–34	45	4.3	5	2	3	4	5	7	8	14
35–49	176	4.3	3	2	3	4	5	7	8	10
50–64	136	4.5	4	2	3	4	5	7	8	12
65+	24	4.7	2	3	4	5	6	7	7	8
2. MULTIPLE DX										
A. Not Operated										
0–19 Years	23	3.8	16	2	2	3	4	4	10	20
20–34	911	3.4	6	1	2	3	4	6	8	12
35–49	3,694	3.4	5	1	2	3	4	6	7	12
50–64	5,296	3.5	6	1	2	3	4	6	8	13
65+	7,338	4.0	9	1	2	3	5	7	9	15
B. Operated										
0–19 Years	12	9.1	130	2	3	4	18	19	40	40
20–34	354	7.6	27	4	5	6	9	13	16	28
35–49	1,869	7.4	21	3	4	6	9	13	16	24
50–64	3,089	8.0	36	3	4	6	9	14	19	33
65+	2,527	10.1	55	4	5	8	13	18	23	39
SUBTOTALS:										
1. SINGLE DX										
A. Not Operated	1,023	2.7	2	1	2	2	4	5	5	8
B. Operated	385	4.4	3	2	3	4	5	7	8	11
2. MULTIPLE DX										
A. Not Operated	17,262	3.7	7	1	2	3	4	7	8	14
B. Operated	7,851	8.5	40	4	5	7	10	16	20	34
1. SINGLE DX	1,408	3.2	3	1	2	3	4	5	6	9
2. MULTIPLE DX	25,113	5.2	22	2	2	4	6	10	14	24
A. NOT OPERATED	18,285	3.6	7	1	2	3	4	6	8	13
B. OPERATED	8,236	8.3	39	3	5	6	10	15	20	33
TOTAL										
0–19 Years	45	5.0	47	1	2	3	4	10	19	40
20–34	1,505	4.4	14	1	2	3	5	8	10	20
35–49	6,226	4.6	13	2	2	3	6	9	12	18
50–64	8,799	5.1	21	2	2	4	6	10	13	23
65+	9,946	5.5	28	2	2	4	7	11	15	26
GRAND TOTAL	26,521	5.1	21	2	2	4	6	10	13	23

562.12: COLON DIVERTICULOS W HEM

Type of Patients	Observed Patients	Avg. Stay	Vari-ance	Percentiles						
				10th	25th	50th	75th	90th	95th	99th
1. SINGLE DX										
A. Not Operated										
0–19 Years	0									
20–34	0									
35–49	5	1.8	<1	2	2	2	2	2	2	2
50–64	7	1.3	<1	1	1	1	2	2	2	2
65+	9	1.7	<1	1	1	2	2	2	2	2
B. Operated										
0–19 Years	0									
20–34	1	3.0	0	3	3	3	3	3	3	3
35–49	0									
50–64	1	15.0	0	15	15	15	15	15	15	15
65+	0									
2. MULTIPLE DX										
A. Not Operated										
0–19 Years	1	1.0	0	1	1	1	1	1	1	1
20–34	14	2.9	3	1	2	2	4	5	7	7
35–49	224	2.6	3	1	2	2	3	4	5	8
50–64	1,232	2.9	5	1	2	2	4	5	6	11
65+	7,269	3.5	6	1	2	3	4	6	8	13
B. Operated										
0–19 Years	0									
20–34	2	14.9	125	7	7	7	23	23	23	23
35–49	19	12.9	238	4	7	8	14	19	74	74
50–64	99	11.6	104	4	6	9	13	20	24	92
65+	453	12.9	81	5	7	10	15	24	32	47
SUBTOTALS:										
1. SINGLE DX										
A. Not Operated	21	1.6	<1	1	1	2	2	2	2	2
B. Operated	2	9.0	71	3	3	9	15	15	15	15
2. MULTIPLE DX										
A. Not Operated	8,740	3.4	6	1	2	3	4	6	8	13
B. Operated	573	12.6	90	5	7	10	15	23	29	49
1. SINGLE DX	23	2.2	8	1	1	2	2	2	3	15
2. MULTIPLE DX	9,313	4.0	16	1	2	3	5	7	10	20
A. NOT OPERATED	8,761	3.4	6	1	2	3	4	6	8	13
B. OPERATED	575	12.6	89	5	7	10	15	23	29	49
TOTAL										
0–19 Years	1	1.0	0	1	1	1	1	1	1	1
20–34	17	4.4	26	1	2	3	4	7	23	23
35–49	248	3.4	27	1	2	2	4	6	8	16
50–64	1,339	3.6	17	1	2	2	4	7	10	20
65+	7,731	4.1	15	1	2	3	5	7	10	20
GRAND TOTAL	9,336	4.0	16	1	2	3	5	7	10	20

562.13: COLON DIVERTICULIT W HEM

Type of Patients	Observed Patients	Avg. Stay	Vari-ance	Percentiles						
				10th	25th	50th	75th	90th	95th	99th
1. SINGLE DX										
A. Not Operated										
0–19 Years	1	2.0	0	2	2	2	2	2	2	2
20–34	2	4.0	8	2	2	2	6	6	6	6
35–49	6	2.5	5	1	1	2	2	7	7	7
50–64	2	6.0	32	2	2	6	10	10	10	10
65+	0									
B. Operated										
0–19 Years	0									
20–34	0									
35–49	3	4.0	<1	3	3	4	5	5	5	5
50–64	0									
65+	0									
2. MULTIPLE DX										
A. Not Operated										
0–19 Years	1	3.0	0	3	3	3	3	3	3	3
20–34	19	3.3	2	2	2	3	4	6	7	7
35–49	87	4.0	7	1	2	3	5	7	9	14
50–64	279	3.6	7	1	2	3	5	7	9	11
65+	1,073	4.2	9	2	2	3	5	8	9	14
B. Operated										
0–19 Years	2	2.0	0	2	2	2	2	2	2	2
20–34	2	17.0	49	12	12	17	22	22	22	22
35–49	21	8.9	23	4	6	8	11	16	16	22
50–64	54	10.8	28	6	7	10	13	21	24	>99
65+	146	12.9	86	5	7	10	16	24	30	62
SUBTOTALS:										
1. SINGLE DX										
A. Not Operated	11	3.4	9	1	2	2	6	7	10	10
B. Operated	3	4.0	<1	3	3	4	5	5	5	5
2. MULTIPLE DX										
A. Not Operated	1,459	4.0	8	1	2	3	5	7	9	14
B. Operated	224	12.0	67	5	7	10	16	22	27	62
1. SINGLE DX	14	3.5	7	1	2	2	5	7	10	10
2. MULTIPLE DX	1,683	5.1	23	2	2	4	6	10	13	24
A. NOT OPERATED	1,470	4.0	8	2	2	3	5	7	9	14
B. OPERATED	227	11.9	67	5	7	10	15	22	27	62
TOTAL										
0–19 Years	3	2.3	<1	2	2	2	3	3	3	3
20–34	23	4.5	20	2	2	3	5	7	12	22
35–49	117	4.8	13	1	2	4	6	10	11	16
50–64	335	4.8	17	1	2	3	6	10	12	23
65+	1,219	5.2	26	2	2	3	6	10	14	27
GRAND TOTAL	1,697	5.1	23	2	2	4	6	10	13	24

Length of Stay by Diagnosis and Operation, Western Region, 2008

Western Region, October 2006–September 2007 Data, by Diagnosis

564: FUNCT DIGESTIVE DIS NEC

Type of Patients	Observed Patients	Avg. Stay	Variance	10th	25th	50th	75th	90th	95th	99th
1. SINGLE DX										
A. Not Operated										
0–19 Years	199	1.5	<1	1	1	1	2	3	4	5
20–34	36	2.1	2	1	1	2	2	4	7	7
35–49	29	2.2	2	1	1	2	3	4	6	7
50–64	20	2.0	2	1	1	2	3	4	5	6
65+	13	2.1	1	1	1	2	3	3	5	5
B. Operated										
0–19 Years	4	1.8	<1	1	1	2	3	3	3	3
20–34	2	5.0	8	3	3	7	7	7	7	7
35–49	1	6.0	0	6	6	6	6	6	6	6
50–64	0									
65+	1	2.0	0	2	2	2	2	2	2	2
2. MULTIPLE DX										
A. Not Operated										
0–19 Years	733	2.4	5	1	1	2	3	4	6	11
20–34	874	3.3	8	1	2	3	4	7	8	13
35–49	1,343	3.3	7	1	2	3	4	6	8	14
50–64	1,611	3.3	8	1	1	3	4	6	8	14
65+	3,300	3.3	8	1	2	3	4	6	8	14
B. Operated										
0–19 Years	28	4.9	11	1	2	4	6	11	11	12
20–34	55	8.9	50	1	5	6	12	17	26	34
35–49	106	8.5	42	3	5	6	10	17	22	28
50–64	121	8.7	50	3	4	7	10	18	25	32
65+	108	10.7	83	2	5	8	12	22	32	44
SUBTOTALS:										
1. SINGLE DX										
A. Not Operated	297	1.7	1	1	1	1	2	3	4	7
B. Operated	8	3.1	5	1	2	3	6	7	7	7
2. MULTIPLE DX										
A. Not Operated	7,861	3.2	7	1	1	2	4	6	8	14
B. Operated	418	8.9	56	2	4	7	11	19	25	39
1. SINGLE DX	305	1.8	2	1	1	1	2	3	4	7
2. MULTIPLE DX	8,279	3.5	11	1	2	3	4	7	9	18
A. NOT OPERATED	8,158	3.2	7	1	1	2	4	6	8	14
B. OPERATED	426	8.8	55	2	4	7	11	19	25	39
TOTAL										
0–19 Years	964	2.3	5	1	1	2	3	4	6	11
20–34	967	3.6	12	1	2	3	4	7	9	17
35–49	1,479	3.7	12	1	2	3	5	7	9	19
50–64	1,752	3.7	12	1	2	3	4	7	9	18
65+	3,422	3.5	12	1	2	3	4	7	9	17
GRAND TOTAL	8,584	3.4	11	1	1	3	4	7	9	17

564.00: CONSTIPATION NOS

Type of Patients	Observed Patients	Avg. Stay	Variance	10th	25th	50th	75th	90th	95th	99th
1. SINGLE DX										
A. Not Operated										
0–19 Years	138	1.6	1	1	1	1	2	3	4	7
20–34	13	2.2	3	1	1	2	2	4	7	7
35–49	9	1.8	<1	1	1	2	2	3	3	3
50–64	7	1.1	<1	1	1	1	1	2	2	2
65+	7	2.2	2	1	1	2	3	3	5	5
B. Operated										
0–19 Years	2	2.0	2	1	1	3	3	3	3	3
20–34	0									
35–49	0									
50–64	0									
65+	0									
2. MULTIPLE DX										
A. Not Operated										
0–19 Years	429	2.1	3	1	1	2	2	4	5	8
20–34	192	2.9	12	1	1	3	3	6	8	10
35–49	354	2.7	5	1	1	3	3	5	6	12
50–64	560	2.7	5	1	1	2	4	5	7	10
65+	1,566	2.9	5	1	1	2	4	5	7	11
B. Operated										
0–19 Years	9	4.6	12	1	2	4	6	12	12	12
20–34	3	5.0	12	1	2	7	7	7	7	7
35–49	6	6.1	14	2	2	5	9	11	11	11
50–64	10	7.6	22	2	3	7	11	14	14	14
65+	18	6.2	28	2	4	5	7	11	24	24
SUBTOTALS:										
1. SINGLE DX										
A. Not Operated	174	1.7	1	1	1	1	2	3	4	7
B. Operated	2	2.0	2	1	1	3	3	3	3	3
2. MULTIPLE DX										
A. Not Operated	3,101	2.7	5	1	1	2	3	5	7	10
B. Operated	46	6.1	20	2	2	5	7	11	14	24
1. SINGLE DX	176	1.7	1	1	1	1	2	3	4	7
2. MULTIPLE DX	3,147	2.8	5	1	1	2	3	5	7	11
A. NOT OPERATED	3,275	2.7	5	1	1	2	3	5	7	10
B. OPERATED	48	5.9	20	2	2	5	7	11	14	24
TOTAL										
0–19 Years	578	2.0	3	1	1	2	2	4	6	11
20–34	208	2.9	11	1	1	2	3	6	7	17
35–49	369	2.7	5	1	1	3	3	5	6	9
50–64	577	2.8	5	1	1	2	4	5	7	11
65+	1,591	2.9	5	1	1	2	4	5	7	11
GRAND TOTAL	3,323	2.7	5	1	1	2	3	5	7	11

564.09: CONSTIPATION NEC

Type of Patients	Observed Patients	Avg. Stay	Variance	10th	25th	50th	75th	90th	95th	99th
1. SINGLE DX										
A. Not Operated										
0–19 Years	48	1.4	<1	1	1	1	2	2	2	3
20–34	3	1.3	<1	1	1	1	2	2	2	2
35–49	3	1.3	<1	1	1	1	2	2	2	2
50–64	4	1.0	0	1	1	1	1	1	1	1
65+	3	2.0	<1	1	1	2	3	3	3	3
B. Operated										
0–19 Years	2	1.5	<1	1	1	2	2	2	2	2
20–34	0									
35–49	0									
50–64	0									
65+	0									
2. MULTIPLE DX										
A. Not Operated										
0–19 Years	213	2.5	4	1	1	2	3	4	5	10
20–34	137	2.8	5	1	1	2	3	5	7	12
35–49	253	2.8	6	1	1	2	3	5	6	15
50–64	390	2.9	5	1	1	2	4	6	7	12
65+	1,009	3.1	6	1	2	2	4	6	7	12
B. Operated										
0–19 Years	13	5.4	11	2	3	4	4	8	11	11
20–34	6	6.0	34	1	2	3	13	14	14	14
35–49	11	8.0	38	2	4	5	9	17	22	22
50–64	10	5.0	7	1	3	5	6	9	9	9
65+	19	7.1	22	1	4	6	10	16	19	19
SUBTOTALS:										
1. SINGLE DX										
A. Not Operated	61	1.4	<1	1	1	1	2	2	2	3
B. Operated	2	1.5	<1	1	1	2	2	2	2	2
2. MULTIPLE DX										
A. Not Operated	2,002	2.9	5	1	1	2	4	5	7	12
B. Operated	59	6.4	21	2	3	5	9	13	17	22
1. SINGLE DX	63	1.4	<1	1	1	1	2	2	2	3
2. MULTIPLE DX	2,061	3.0	6	1	1	2	4	6	8	14
A. NOT OPERATED	2,063	2.9	5	1	1	2	4	5	7	12
B. OPERATED	61	6.3	21	2	3	5	8	11	16	22
TOTAL										
0–19 Years	276	2.4	4	1	1	2	3	4	6	11
20–34	146	2.9	6	1	1	2	3	5	7	14
35–49	267	3.0	9	1	1	2	3	5	7	18
50–64	404	3.0	6	1	1	2	4	6	7	12
65+	1,031	3.2	6	1	2	2	4	6	8	13
GRAND TOTAL	2,124	3.0	6	1	1	2	4	6	7	14

Length of Stay by Diagnosis and Operation, Western Region, 2008

564.1: IRRITABLE BOWEL SYNDROME

Type of Patients	Observed Patients	Avg. Stay	Vari-ance	10th	25th	50th	75th	90th	95th	99th
1. SINGLE DX										
A. Not Operated										
0–19 Years	6	1.7	1	1	1	1	2	4	4	4
20–34	16	1.9	1	1	1	2	2	4	4	4
35–49	11	2.6	4	1	1	3	4	4	7	7
50–64	3	2.3	2	1	1	2	4	4	4	4
65+	2	1.5	<1	1	1	1	2	2	2	2
B. Operated										
0–19 Years	0									
20–34	0									
35–49	0									
50–64	0									
65+	0									
2. MULTIPLE DX										
A. Not Operated										
0–19 Years	50	3.3	6	1	2	3	4	6	10	11
20–34	436	3.4	6	1	2	3	4	7	8	12
35–49	562	3.6	7	1	2	3	4	7	8	13
50–64	427	3.7	7	1	2	3	5	7	9	14
65+	416	3.8	7	1	2	3	5	7	9	14
B. Operated										
0–19 Years	1	7.0	0	7	7	7	7	7	7	7
20–34	11	6.5	7	3	6	6	9	9	10	10
35–49	7	7.9	58	1	4	5	10	24	24	24
50–64	11	8.6	56	3	4	7	9	19	26	26
65+	6	6.3	6	5	5	7	7	8	8	8
SUBTOTALS:										
1. SINGLE DX										
A. Not Operated	38	2.1	2	1	1	2	3	4	4	7
B. Operated	0									
2. MULTIPLE DX										
A. Not Operated	1,891	3.6	7	1	2	3	4	7	8	13
B. Operated	36	7.4	30	2	5	7	8	10	24	26
1. SINGLE DX	38	2.1	2	1	1	2	3	4	4	7
2. MULTIPLE DX	1,927	3.7	8	1	2	3	5	7	9	14
A. NOT OPERATED	1,929	3.6	7	1	2	3	4	7	8	13
B. OPERATED	36	7.4	30	2	5	7	8	10	24	26
TOTAL										
0–19 Years	57	3.2	6	1	1	3	4	6	10	11
20–34	463	3.4	6	1	2	3	4	7	8	12
35–49	580	3.6	8	1	2	3	4	7	8	14
50–64	441	3.9	9	1	2	3	5	7	9	16
65+	424	3.8	7	1	2	3	5	7	9	14
GRAND TOTAL	1,965	3.6	7	1	2	3	5	7	8	14

564.89: OTH FUNCT DIS INTESTINE

Type of Patients	Observed Patients	Avg. Stay	Vari-ance	10th	25th	50th	75th	90th	95th	99th
1. SINGLE DX										
A. Not Operated										
0–19 Years	2	1.0	0	1	1	1	1	1	1	1
20–34	2	2.5	<1	2	2	3	3	3	3	3
35–49	1	6.0	0	6	6	6	6	6	6	6
50–64	1	6.0	0	6	6	6	6	6	6	6
65+	1	3.0	0	3	3	3	3	3	3	3
B. Operated										
0–19 Years	0									
20–34	1	3.0	0	3	3	3	3	3	3	3
35–49	0									
50–64	0									
65+	1	2.0	0	2	2	2	2	2	2	2
2. MULTIPLE DX										
A. Not Operated										
0–19 Years	21	5.2	48	1	1	4	6	8	10	33
20–34	45	4.2	14	1	2	3	5	7	13	19
35–49	56	5.4	20	1	2	4	8	11	18	19
50–64	114	4.9	19	1	2	4	6	9	12	17
65+	159	5.7	31	1	3	4	6	12	16	30
B. Operated										
0–19 Years	1	3.0	0	3	3	3	3	3	3	3
20–34	18	12.1	76	4	6	9	16	27	34	34
35–49	33	9.9	40	5	5	7	11	19	24	28
50–64	44	9.5	64	3	5	7	12	18	28	41
65+	30	12.2	55	8	8	10	15	20	22	41
SUBTOTALS:										
1. SINGLE DX										
A. Not Operated	7	3.2	4	1	2	3	6	6	6	6
B. Operated	2	2.5	<1	2	2	3	3	3	3	3
2. MULTIPLE DX										
A. Not Operated	395	5.2	25	1	2	4	6	11	15	30
B. Operated	126	10.6	57	4	5	8	13	21	27	41
1. SINGLE DX	9	3.0	4	1	2	3	3	6	6	6
2. MULTIPLE DX	521	6.5	38	2	3	5	8	14	19	33
A. NOT OPERATED	402	5.2	24	1	2	4	6	10	14	27
B. OPERATED	128	10.5	57	5	5	8	13	21	27	41
TOTAL										
0–19 Years	24	4.8	43	1	1	3	6	8	10	33
20–34	66	6.3	42	1	2	4	7	16	19	34
35–49	90	7.1	31	2	3	5	9	17	19	28
50–64	159	6.2	35	2	3	5	7	12	17	34
65+	191	6.7	40	2	3	4	8	14	20	37
GRAND TOTAL	530	6.5	37	2	3	5	8	14	19	33

565: ANAL FISSURE & FISTULA

Type of Patients	Observed Patients	Avg. Stay	Vari-ance	10th	25th	50th	75th	90th	95th	99th
1. SINGLE DX										
A. Not Operated										
0–19 Years	3	1.0	0	1	1	1	1	1	1	1
20–34	1	2.0	0	2	2	2	2	2	2	2
35–49	2	6.0	32	2	2	10	10	10	10	10
50–64	0									
65+	0									
B. Operated										
0–19 Years	4	1.0	0	1	1	1	1	1	1	1
20–34	12	1.4	<1	1	1	1	2	2	4	4
35–49	21	1.4	<1	1	1	1	2	2	2	3
50–64	9	1.8	2	1	1	1	2	5	5	5
65+	2	1.5	<1	1	1	1	2	2	2	2
2. MULTIPLE DX										
A. Not Operated										
0–19 Years	16	1.8	<1	1	1	2	2	3	3	3
20–34	32	3.4	8	1	1	3	5	6	10	12
35–49	57	2.7	8	1	1	2	3	4	7	20
50–64	51	2.3	3	1	2	2	3	5	6	7
65+	70	3.6	12	1	2	2	5	7	9	24
B. Operated										
0–19 Years	19	2.8	5	1	1	2	3	6	10	10
20–34	69	2.9	11	1	1	2	3	7	8	22
35–49	162	2.9	11	1	1	2	3	6	8	21
50–64	129	3.3	21	1	1	2	3	8	11	25
65+	63	3.8	16	1	2	2	4	10	14	18
SUBTOTALS:										
1. SINGLE DX										
A. Not Operated	6	2.8	13	1	1	2	2	2	10	10
B. Operated	48	1.4	<1	1	1	1	1	2	3	5
2. MULTIPLE DX										
A. Not Operated	226	2.9	8	1	1	2	4	6	7	14
B. Operated	442	3.1	14	1	2	3	3	7	10	22
1. SINGLE DX	54	1.6	2	1	1	1	2	2	4	10
2. MULTIPLE DX	668	3.1	12	1	1	2	3	6	9	21
A. NOT OPERATED	232	2.9	8	1	1	2	4	6	7	14
B. OPERATED	490	3.0	13	1	1	2	3	7	10	22
TOTAL										
0–19 Years	42	2.1	3	1	1	2	3	3	5	10
20–34	114	2.9	9	1	1	2	4	6	8	12
35–49	242	2.8	10	1	1	2	3	5	8	20
50–64	189	3.0	15	1	2	2	3	7	9	25
65+	135	3.7	14	1	2	2	4	8	11	18
GRAND TOTAL	722	3.0	12	1	1	2	3	6	9	20

Length of Stay by Diagnosis and Operation, Western Region, 2008

Western Region, October 2006–September 2007 Data, by Diagnosis

565.0: ANAL FISSURE

Type of Patients	Observed Patients	Avg. Stay	Variance	Percentiles 10th	25th	50th	75th	90th	95th	99th
1. SINGLE DX										
A. Not Operated										
0–19 Years	3	1.0	0	1	1	1	1	1	1	1
20–34	0									
35–49	0									
50–64	0									
65+	0									
B. Operated										
0–19 Years	0									
20–34	2	1.0	0	1	1	1	1	1	1	1
35–49	1	1.0	0	1	1	1	1	1	1	1
50–64	2	2.0	2	1	1	3	3	3	3	3
65+	0									
2. MULTIPLE DX										
A. Not Operated										
0–19 Years	15	1.7	<1	1	1	2	2	3	3	3
20–34	17	3.1	8	1	1	2	5	7	10	10
35–49	45	2.5	8	1	1	2	3	4	4	20
50–64	30	2.0	1	1	1	2	2	4	5	6
65+	55	3.5	14	1	1	2	4	7	8	24
B. Operated										
0–19 Years	2	1.5	<1	1	1	1	2	2	2	2
20–34	14	1.8	<1	1	1	2	2	3	4	4
35–49	38	2.5	7	1	1	2	3	7	9	13
50–64	38	2.0	2	1	1	2	2	3	5	7
65+	23	4.0	23	1	1	2	3	11	15	18
SUBTOTALS:										
1. SINGLE DX A. Not Operated	3	1.0	0	1	1	1	1	1	1	1
B. Operated	5	1.4	<1	1	1	1	1	3	3	3
2. MULTIPLE DX A. Not Operated	162	2.7	8	1	1	2	3	5	7	20
B. Operated	115	2.5	8	1	1	2	3	5	9	15
1. SINGLE DX	8	1.3	<1	1	1	1	1	3	3	3
2. MULTIPLE DX	277	2.7	8	1	1	2	3	5	7	18
A. NOT OPERATED	165	2.7	8	1	1	2	3	5	7	20
B. OPERATED	120	2.5	8	1	1	2	3	5	9	15
TOTAL										
0–19 Years	20	1.6	<1	1	1	2	2	3	3	3
20–34	33	2.4	5	1	1	1	3	6	7	10
35–49	84	2.5	8	1	1	2	3	4	7	20
50–64	70	2.0	2	1	1	2	2	3	5	7
65+	78	3.6	16	1	1	2	4	8	14	24
GRAND TOTAL	285	2.6	8	1	1	2	3	5	7	18

565.1: ANAL FISTULA

Type of Patients	Observed Patients	Avg. Stay	Variance	Percentiles 10th	25th	50th	75th	90th	95th	99th
1. SINGLE DX										
A. Not Operated										
0–19 Years	0									
20–34	1	2.0	0	2	2	2	2	2	2	2
35–49	2	6.0	32	2	2	10	10	10	10	10
50–64	0									
65+	0									
B. Operated										
0–19 Years	4	1.0	0	1	1	1	1	1	1	1
20–34	10	1.5	<1	1	1	1	2	4	4	4
35–49	20	1.4	<1	1	1	1	2	2	3	3
50–64	7	1.7	2	1	1	1	2	5	5	5
65+	2	1.5	<1	1	1	1	2	2	2	2
2. MULTIPLE DX										
A. Not Operated										
0–19 Years	1	3.0	0	3	3	3	3	3	3	3
20–34	15	3.7	8	1	1	4	5	6	8	12
35–49	12	3.3	6	1	2	3	5	7	9	9
50–64	21	2.7	4	1	1	2	2	6	7	7
65+	15	4.2	8	1	2	3	6	9	10	10
B. Operated										
0–19 Years	17	2.9	5	1	1	2	3	6	10	10
20–34	55	3.2	14	1	1	2	4	7	12	22
35–49	124	3.1	13	1	1	2	3	6	8	21
50–64	91	3.8	28	1	1	2	4	9	12	32
65+	40	3.7	13	1	1	3	4	10	14	15
SUBTOTALS:										
1. SINGLE DX A. Not Operated	3	4.7	21	2	2	2	10	10	10	10
B. Operated	43	1.4	<1	1	1	1	2	2	3	5
2. MULTIPLE DX A. Not Operated	64	3.4	6	1	1	3	5	7	9	12
B. Operated	327	3.4	17	1	1	2	4	8	11	22
1. SINGLE DX	46	1.7	2	1	1	1	2	2	4	10
2. MULTIPLE DX	391	3.4	15	1	1	2	4	7	10	22
A. NOT OPERATED	67	3.5	7	1	1	3	5	7	9	12
B. OPERATED	370	3.1	15	1	1	2	3	7	10	22
TOTAL										
0–19 Years	22	2.6	5	1	1	2	3	5	6	10
20–34	81	3.0	11	1	1	2	4	6	8	22
35–49	158	2.9	11	1	1	2	3	6	8	21
50–64	119	3.5	22	1	1	2	4	8	11	25
65+	57	3.7	11	1	2	3	4	10	11	15
GRAND TOTAL	437	3.2	14	1	1	2	4	7	10	22

566: ANAL & RECTAL ABSCESS

Type of Patients	Observed Patients	Avg. Stay	Variance	Percentiles 10th	25th	50th	75th	90th	95th	99th
1. SINGLE DX										
A. Not Operated										
0–19 Years	11	3.5	4	2	2	3	4	7	7	7
20–34	14	2.6	4	1	1	2	3	5	8	8
35–49	17	2.1	1	1	1	2	3	3	4	4
50–64	9	1.2	<1	1	1	1	1	2	2	2
65+	0									
B. Operated										
0–19 Years	61	2.3	3	1	1	2	3	4	6	10
20–34	219	1.8	2	1	1	1	2	4	4	6
35–49	197	1.9	2	1	1	2	2	3	4	8
50–64	72	2.1	2	1	1	2	2	4	6	9
65+	8	1.9	2	1	1	1	3	4	4	4
2. MULTIPLE DX										
A. Not Operated										
0–19 Years	28	2.5	4	1	1	2	3	6	7	8
20–34	57	3.6	5	1	2	3	5	7	8	10
35–49	126	3.6	17	1	1	2	4	7	10	25
50–64	120	4.5	27	1	2	3	5	7	11	24
65+	123	5.0	17	1	2	4	6	10	12	24
B. Operated										
0–19 Years	114	3.4	6	1	1	3	4	5	8	12
20–34	528	2.6	4	1	1	2	3	5	6	11
35–49	1,064	3.2	9	1	1	2	4	6	8	16
50–64	851	4.0	34	1	1	3	4	8	11	26
65+	427	5.3	26	1	2	4	6	11	15	27
SUBTOTALS:										
1. SINGLE DX A. Not Operated	51	2.4	3	1	1	2	3	4	7	8
B. Operated	557	1.9	2	1	1	2	2	4	4	8
2. MULTIPLE DX A. Not Operated	454	4.2	18	1	1	3	5	8	11	24
B. Operated	2,984	3.6	18	1	1	2	4	7	10	21
1. SINGLE DX	608	2.0	2	1	1	2	2	4	4	8
2. MULTIPLE DX	3,438	3.7	18	1	1	3	4	7	10	21
A. NOT OPERATED	505	4.0	16	1	2	3	5	7	10	24
B. OPERATED	3,541	3.3	16	1	1	2	4	7	9	20
TOTAL										
0–19 Years	214	2.9	5	1	1	2	4	5	7	11
20–34	818	2.5	4	1	1	2	3	5	6	11
35–49	1,404	3.0	9	1	1	2	4	6	8	16
50–64	1,052	3.9	31	1	2	2	4	7	10	26
65+	558	5.2	24	1	2	4	6	11	14	27
GRAND TOTAL	4,046	3.4	16	1	1	2	4	7	10	20

Length of Stay by Diagnosis and Operation, Western Region, 2008

567: PERITON/RETROPERIT INF

Type of Patients	Observed Patients	Avg. Stay	Vari-ance	10th	25th	50th	75th	90th	95th	99th
1. SINGLE DX										
A. *Not Operated*										
0–19 Years	26	3.9	3	2	2	3	5	6	7	7
20–34	41	3.6	6	1	2	3	5	6	8	13
35–49	17	3.4	8	1	2	3	4	6	13	13
50–64	18	3.9	4	2	2	3	5	7	9	9
65+	3	5.0	7	3	3	4	8	8	8	8
B. *Operated*										
0–19 Years	7	3.9	7	1	1	4	6	8	8	8
20–34	8	5.6	29	1	1	6	7	17	17	17
35–49	4	5.2	8	3	3	3	6	9	9	9
50–64	5	4.8	13	1	5	6	8	8	8	8
65+	1	5.0	0	5	5	5	5	5	5	5
2. MULTIPLE DX										
A. *Not Operated*										
0–19 Years	102	6.0	26	2	3	5	8	11	12	16
20–34	278	5.4	18	1	3	4	7	10	12	22
35–49	754	6.2	38	2	3	5	7	11	14	34
50–64	1,182	6.2	30	2	3	5	8	12	15	27
65+	747	7.3	33	2	4	6	9	14	18	27
B. *Operated*										
0–19 Years	45	8.5	34	2	3	8	12	17	21	23
20–34	109	10.2	89	2	4	8	13	23	28	47
35–49	178	10.8	80	3	5	9	13	20	24	53
50–64	230	12.4	98	4	6	10	16	25	33	42
65+	228	12.3	93	3	6	10	16	27	32	49
SUBTOTALS:										
1. SINGLE DX										
A. *Not Operated*	105	3.8	5	1	2	3	5	6	8	13
B. *Operated*	25	4.9	14	1	1	5	7	8	9	17
2. MULTIPLE DX										
A. *Not Operated*	3,063	6.4	31	2	3	5	8	13	16	27
B. *Operated*	790	11.5	88	3	5	9	15	23	30	50
1. SINGLE DX	130	4.0	7	1	2	3	5	7	8	13
2. MULTIPLE DX	3,853	7.4	47	2	3	6	9	15	19	36
A. NOT OPERATED	3,168	6.3	31	2	3	5	8	12	15	27
B. OPERATED	815	11.3	87	3	5	8	15	23	30	49
TOTAL										
0–19 Years	180	6.2	26	2	3	5	8	12	15	23
20–34	436	6.5	40	1	3	5	8	13	18	30
35–49	953	7.0	48	2	3	5	8	13	19	41
50–64	1,435	7.2	45	2	3	5	9	14	19	34
65+	979	8.5	51	2	4	7	10	16	22	38
GRAND TOTAL	3,983	7.3	46	2	3	5	9	15	19	35

567.22: PERITONEAL ABSCESS

Type of Patients	Observed Patients	Avg. Stay	Vari-ance	10th	25th	50th	75th	90th	95th	99th
1. SINGLE DX										
A. *Not Operated*										
0–19 Years	22	3.8	3	2	2	3	5	6	7	7
20–34	27	3.4	3	1	2	3	5	6	6	8
35–49	12	3.3	11	1	2	2	4	6	13	13
50–64	12	3.9	3	2	3	4	5	7	7	7
65+	3	5.0	7	3	3	4	8	8	8	8
B. *Operated*										
0–19 Years	4	5.8	3	4	5	6	6	8	8	8
20–34	6	7.2	29	1	4	7	7	17	17	17
35–49	4	5.2	8	3	3	3	6	9	9	9
50–64	0									
65+	0									
2. MULTIPLE DX										
A. *Not Operated*										
0–19 Years	56	5.8	11	2	3	5	8	9	12	16
20–34	104	5.6	16	2	3	5	7	11	14	22
35–49	215	6.6	54	2	3	5	7	12	16	34
50–64	316	6.3	22	2	3	5	8	12	15	27
65+	295	8.2	34	2	4	7	10	14	18	29
B. *Operated*										
0–19 Years	22	8.0	21	3	5	8	12	17	21	23
20–34	45	10.3	67	3	5	8	13	24	28	47
35–49	78	11.1	78	3	6	9	13	20	23	53
50–64	98	11.6	45	4	6	10	15	25	26	42
65+	95	12.9	99	3	6	11	16	27	38	>99
SUBTOTALS:										
1. SINGLE DX										
A. *Not Operated*	76	3.7	4	2	2	3	5	6	8	13
B. *Operated*	14	6.2	15	3	4	6	7	9	17	17
2. MULTIPLE DX										
A. *Not Operated*	986	6.8	32	2	3	6	8	13	16	28
B. *Operated*	338	11.4	70	3	6	9	15	21	26	50
1. SINGLE DX	90	4.0	7	2	2	3	5	7	8	17
2. MULTIPLE DX	1,324	8.0	46	2	4	6	10	16	20	33
A. NOT OPERATED	1,062	6.6	31	2	3	5	8	12	16	27
B. OPERATED	352	11.2	69	3	6	9	15	20	26	50
TOTAL										
0–19 Years	104	5.9	13	2	3	5	8	11	14	23
20–34	182	6.5	32	2	3	5	8	12	18	30
35–49	309	7.6	62	2	3	6	9	13	20	50
50–64	426	7.5	32	2	3	6	10	15	18	28
65+	393	9.3	53	2	4	7	12	18	24	41
GRAND TOTAL	1,414	7.8	44	2	4	6	10	15	19	31

567.23: SPONT BACT PERITONITIS

Type of Patients	Observed Patients	Avg. Stay	Vari-ance	10th	25th	50th	75th	90th	95th	99th
1. SINGLE DX										
A. *Not Operated*										
0–19 Years	0									
20–34	0									
35–49	0									
50–64	0									
65+	0									
B. *Operated*										
0–19 Years	0									
20–34	0									
35–49	0									
50–64	0									
65+	0									
2. MULTIPLE DX										
A. *Not Operated*										
0–19 Years	8	5.0	4	2	4	5	7	8	8	8
20–34	43	5.3	24	2	3	4	6	10	15	24
35–49	275	6.1	33	2	3	4	7	11	16	40
50–64	488	5.9	23	2	3	5	7	12	14	27
65+	174	6.2	18	2	3	5	8	12	15	20
B. *Operated*										
0–19 Years	0									
20–34	2	9.5	40	5	5	5	14	14	14	14
35–49	9	10.2	38	3	7	8	13	22	22	22
50–64	18	15.5	73	6	9	15	19	26	40	40
65+	1	12.0	0	12	12	12	12	12	12	12
SUBTOTALS:										
1. SINGLE DX										
A. *Not Operated*	0									
B. *Operated*	0									
2. MULTIPLE DX										
A. *Not Operated*	988	6.0	25	2	3	5	7	11	15	25
B. *Operated*	30	13.4	61	4	8	12	17	22	26	40
1. SINGLE DX	0									
2. MULTIPLE DX	1,018	6.2	27	2	3	5	7	12	16	26
A. NOT OPERATED	988	6.0	25	2	3	5	7	11	15	25
B. OPERATED	30	13.4	61	4	8	12	17	22	26	40
TOTAL										
0–19 Years	8	5.0	4	2	4	5	7	8	8	8
20–34	45	5.5	24	2	3	4	6	10	15	24
35–49	284	6.2	33	2	3	5	7	11	16	40
50–64	506	6.3	27	2	3	5	8	13	16	27
65+	175	6.2	18	2	3	5	8	12	15	20
GRAND TOTAL	1,018	6.2	27	2	3	5	7	12	16	26

Length of Stay by Diagnosis and Operation, Western Region, 2008

Western Region, October 2006–September 2007 Data, by Diagnosis

567.29: OTH SUPPURAT PERITONITIS

Type of Patients	Observed Patients	Avg. Stay	Variance	10th	25th	50th	75th	90th	95th	99th
1. SINGLE DX										
A. Not Operated										
0–19 Years	0									
20–34	0									
35–49	0									
50–64	1	9.0	0	9	9	9	9	9	9	9
65+	0									
B. Operated										
0–19 Years	0									
20–34	0									
35–49	0									
50–64	0									
65+	0									
2. MULTIPLE DX										
A. Not Operated										
0–19 Years	7	5.7	23	3	3	3	6	16	16	16
20–34	25	4.0	4	2	3	4	5	7	8	8
35–49	72	5.3	16	2	3	4	6	11	15	22
50–64	115	6.4	26	2	3	5	7	18	18	24
65+	51	8.1	114	2	3	5	9	11	21	65
B. Operated										
0–19 Years	4	13.3	103	4	5	21	23	23	23	23
20–34	8	17.7	424	1	4	12	47	52	52	52
35–49	13	11.7	62	4	8	10	12	16	34	34
50–64	18	14.7	151	4	6	8	23	35	37	37
65+	12	12.7	95	5	8	8	18	18	40	40
SUBTOTALS:										
1. SINGLE DX										
A. Not Operated	1	9.0	0	9	9	9	9	9	9	9
B. Operated	0									
2. MULTIPLE DX										
A. Not Operated	270	6.2	39	2	3	5	7	10	16	35
B. Operated	55	13.9	146	4	6	10	18	35	40	52
1. SINGLE DX	1	9.0	0	9	9	9	9	9	9	9
2. MULTIPLE DX	325	7.5	65	2	3	5	8	15	21	47
A. NOT OPERATED	271	6.2	39	2	3	5	7	10	16	35
B. OPERATED	55	13.9	146	4	6	10	18	35	40	52
TOTAL										
0–19 Years	11	8.5	59	3	3	5	16	21	23	23
20–34	33	7.3	131	1	3	4	5	12	47	52
35–49	85	6.2	28	2	3	4	8	12	16	34
50–64	134	7.5	50	2	4	6	9	16	23	35
65+	63	8.9	112	3	4	6	9	16	21	65
GRAND TOTAL	326	7.5	65	2	3	5	8	15	21	47

567.31: PSOAS MUSCLE ABSCESS

Type of Patients	Observed Patients	Avg. Stay	Variance	10th	25th	50th	75th	90th	95th	99th
1. SINGLE DX										
A. Not Operated										
0–19 Years	1	2.0	0	2	2	2	2	2	2	2
20–34	2	3.5	12	1	1	6	6	6	6	6
35–49	0									
50–64	0									
65+	0									
B. Operated										
0–19 Years	0									
20–34	0									
35–49	0									
50–64	0									
65+	0									
2. MULTIPLE DX										
A. Not Operated										
0–19 Years	12	9.4	137	3	3	7	8	10	46	46
20–34	34	7.5	21	3	4	7	9	15	17	21
35–49	57	7.8	42	3	4	6	6	17	21	34
50–64	68	10.0	146	3	4	7	12	18	23	87
65+	65	8.4	16	4	5	8	11	14	14	21
B. Operated										
0–19 Years	3	8.7	42	2	2	9	15	15	15	15
20–34	15	10.9	40	2	5	10	16	23	24	24
35–49	20	12.3	125	6	7	13	13	16	24	56
50–64	24	9.2	51	3	4	8	11	21	23	31
65+	19	15.0	125	3	6	13	21	35	38	38
SUBTOTALS:										
1. SINGLE DX										
A. Not Operated	3	3.0	7	1	1	2	2	6	6	6
B. Operated	0									
2. MULTIPLE DX										
A. Not Operated	236	8.6	66	3	4	7	10	16	19	46
B. Operated	81	11.6	85	4	6	9	15	23	31	56
1. SINGLE DX	3	3.0	7	1	1	2	2	6	6	6
2. MULTIPLE DX	317	9.4	73	3	5	7	11	17	23	46
A. NOT OPERATED	239	8.6	66	3	4	7	10	16	19	46
B. OPERATED	81	11.6	85	4	6	9	15	23	31	56
TOTAL										
0–19 Years	16	8.8	110	2	3	7	9	15	46	46
20–34	51	8.4	28	3	5	7	10	16	21	24
35–49	77	9.0	66	3	5	6	11	17	24	56
50–64	92	9.8	120	3	4	7	12	18	23	87
65+	84	9.9	47	3	5	8	12	16	21	38
GRAND TOTAL	320	9.3	72	3	4	7	11	17	23	46

568: OTH PERITONEAL DISORDERS

Type of Patients	Observed Patients	Avg. Stay	Variance	10th	25th	50th	75th	90th	95th	99th
1. SINGLE DX										
A. Not Operated										
0–19 Years	2	2.5	<1	2	2	3	3	3	3	3
20–34	2	3.5	4	2	2	5	5	5	5	5
35–49	0									
50–64	0									
65+	2	1.0	0	1	1	1	1	1	1	1
B. Operated										
0–19 Years	5	4.2	9	2	2	3	5	9	9	9
20–34	17	2.0	1	1	1	2	2	4	5	5
35–49	20	2.2	2	1	1	2	3	4	5	5
50–64	13	2.1	2	1	1	2	3	3	6	6
65+	2	3.5	<1	3	3	4	4	4	4	4
2. MULTIPLE DX										
A. Not Operated										
0–19 Years	10	2.3	1	1	1	2	3	4	4	4
20–34	74	3.8	19	1	2	3	4	7	9	29
35–49	112	4.5	11	1	2	4	6	8	10	14
50–64	155	4.8	12	2	2	4	6	9	12	17
65+	215	4.7	12	1	2	4	6	9	11	18
B. Operated										
0–19 Years	31	2.8	3	1	1	2	4	5	7	7
20–34	202	4.0	17	1	2	3	5	7	9	21
35–49	431	4.1	14	1	2	3	5	7	12	17
50–64	340	5.0	36	1	2	3	6	10	14	30
65+	223	7.3	56	1	3	5	9	14	21	35
SUBTOTALS:										
1. SINGLE DX										
A. Not Operated	6	2.3	2	1	1	2	3	5	5	5
B. Operated	57	2.3	2	1	1	2	3	5	5	9
2. MULTIPLE DX										
A. Not Operated	566	4.6	13	1	2	4	6	9	11	18
B. Operated	1,227	4.9	29	1	2	3	6	10	14	27
1. SINGLE DX	63	2.3	2	1	1	2	3	5	5	9
2. MULTIPLE DX	1,793	4.8	24	1	2	3	6	9	13	25
A. NOT OPERATED	572	4.5	12	1	2	3	6	9	11	18
B. OPERATED	1,284	4.8	28	1	2	3	6	10	14	27
TOTAL										
0–19 Years	48	2.8	3	1	2	2	4	5	7	9
20–34	295	3.8	16	1	2	3	4	7	9	25
35–49	563	4.1	13	1	2	3	5	8	11	17
50–64	508	4.9	28	1	2	4	6	10	13	21
65+	442	6.0	36	1	2	4	8	12	16	30
GRAND TOTAL	1,856	4.7	23	1	2	3	6	9	13	24

Length of Stay by Diagnosis and Operation, Western Region, 2008

568.0: PERITONEAL ADHESIONS

Type of Patients	Observed Patients	Avg. Stay	Vari-ance	Percentiles						
				10th	25th	50th	75th	90th	95th	99th
1. SINGLE DX										
A. Not Operated										
0–19 Years	0									
20–34	0									
35–49	0									
50–64	0									
65+	0									
B. Operated										
0–19 Years	2	4.0	2	3	3	4	5	5	5	5
20–34	6	2.2	<1	1	2	2	2	4	4	4
35–49	17	2.3	2	1	1	2	3	5	5	5
50–64	10	1.9	3	1	1	1	2	6	6	6
65+	0									
2. MULTIPLE DX										
A. Not Operated										
0–19 Years	0									
20–34	33	4.0	18	1	2	3	4	8	10	24
35–49	59	5.1	15	1	3	4	7	10	13	24
50–64	78	4.8	13	1	2	4	6	10	12	19
65+	42	4.2	14	1	2	3	5	8	12	18
B. Operated										
0–19 Years	13	2.5	3	1	1	2	4	4	6	6
20–34	117	4.1	21	1	2	3	5	7	9	25
35–49	307	4.0	15	1	2	3	5	8	11	17
50–64	214	4.8	36	1	1	3	6	10	14	30
65+	132	6.2	29	2	2	5	9	12	16	27
SUBTOTALS:										
1. SINGLE DX *A. Not Operated*	0									
B. Operated	35	2.3	2	1	1	2	3	5	5	6
2. MULTIPLE DX *A. Not Operated*	212	4.6	15	1	2	4	6	9	12	19
B. Operated	783	4.6	24	1	2	3	6	10	13	24
1. SINGLE DX	35	2.3	2	1	1	2	3	5	5	6
2. MULTIPLE DX	995	4.6	22	1	2	3	6	9	13	24
A. NOT OPERATED	212	4.6	15	1	2	4	6	9	12	19
B. OPERATED	818	4.5	24	1	2	3	5	9	13	25
TOTAL										
0–19 Years	15	2.7	3	1	1	2	4	5	6	6
20–34	156	4.0	19	1	2	3	4	7	9	25
35–49	383	4.1	14	1	2	3	5	8	11	17
50–64	302	4.7	30	1	2	3	6	10	13	30
65+	174	5.7	26	1	2	4	8	12	15	27
GRAND TOTAL	1,030	4.5	22	1	2	3	6	9	13	24

568.81: HEMOPERITONEUM

Type of Patients	Observed Patients	Avg. Stay	Vari-ance	Percentiles						
				10th	25th	50th	75th	90th	95th	99th
1. SINGLE DX										
A. Not Operated										
0–19 Years	0									
20–34	1	2.0	0	2	2	2	2	2	2	2
35–49	0									
50–64	0									
65+	0									
B. Operated										
0–19 Years	0									
20–34	6	2.3	2	1	1	2	3	5	5	5
35–49	0									
50–64	0									
65+	0									
2. MULTIPLE DX										
A. Not Operated										
0–19 Years	5	2.6	2	2	2	2	4	4	4	4
20–34	27	4.1	29	1	1	3	5	6	9	29
35–49	33	4.1	6	1	2	4	5	8	9	12
50–64	53	4.7	10	2	3	4	5	9	12	17
65+	105	5.6	12	2	3	5	7	10	11	18
B. Operated										
0–19 Years	13	2.9	4	1	2	2	4	5	6	7
20–34	45	3.6	14	1	2	3	4	8	11	19
35–49	33	5.4	19	2	2	4	7	11	17	19
50–64	27	8.3	95	3	3	5	9	18	21	51
65+	44	10.7	105	3	5	8	12	24	28	57
SUBTOTALS:										
1. SINGLE DX *A. Not Operated*	1	2.0	0	2	2	2	2	2	2	2
B. Operated	6	2.3	2	1	1	2	3	5	5	5
2. MULTIPLE DX *A. Not Operated*	223	4.9	13	2	3	4	6	9	11	18
B. Operated	162	6.6	60	1	2	4	8	14	19	51
1. SINGLE DX	7	2.3	2	1	1	2	3	5	5	5
2. MULTIPLE DX	385	5.6	34	1	2	4	7	11	15	29
A. NOT OPERATED	224	4.9	13	2	3	4	6	9	11	18
B. OPERATED	168	6.5	59	1	2	4	8	14	19	51
TOTAL										
0–19 Years	18	2.8	3	1	2	2	4	5	7	7
20–34	79	3.7	18	1	2	3	4	7	9	29
35–49	66	4.8	13	1	2	4	6	9	12	19
50–64	80	5.9	41	2	3	4	7	10	17	51
65+	149	7.1	45	2	3	6	8	12	18	35
GRAND TOTAL	392	5.6	33	1	2	4	7	10	15	29

568.89: PERITONEAL DISORDER NEC

Type of Patients	Observed Patients	Avg. Stay	Vari-ance	Percentiles						
				10th	25th	50th	75th	90th	95th	99th
1. SINGLE DX										
A. Not Operated										
0–19 Years	2	2.5	<1	2	2	3	3	3	3	3
20–34	1	5.0	0	5	5	5	5	5	5	5
35–49	0									
50–64	0									
65+	2	1.0	0	1	1	1	1	1	1	1
B. Operated										
0–19 Years	3	4.3	16	2	2	2	2	9	9	9
20–34	5	1.4	<1	1	1	1	1	3	3	3
35–49	3	1.7	<1	1	1	2	2	2	2	2
50–64	3	2.7	<1	2	2	3	3	3	3	3
65+	2	3.5	<1	3	3	4	4	4	4	4
2. MULTIPLE DX										
A. Not Operated										
0–19 Years	5	2.0	<1	1	1	2	3	3	3	3
20–34	13	2.5	3	1	1	2	3	5	7	7
35–49	19	3.5	5	1	2	3	5	7	8	8
50–64	23	5.0	10	2	3	4	8	9	12	12
65+	62	3.8	8	1	2	3	5	7	8	14
B. Operated										
0–19 Years	5	3.2	5	1	2	3	3	7	7	7
20–34	37	3.7	7	1	2	3	5	7	9	12
35–49	91	4.0	10	1	2	3	5	7	8	16
50–64	98	4.4	15	1	2	3	5	10	13	25
65+	46	7.4	76	2	3	5	8	19	24	49
SUBTOTALS:										
1. SINGLE DX *A. Not Operated*	5	2.4	3	1	1	2	3	5	5	5
B. Operated	16	2.5	4	1	1	2	3	4	9	9
2. MULTIPLE DX *A. Not Operated*	122	3.8	8	1	2	3	5	8	9	14
B. Operated	277	4.7	24	1	2	3	5	9	13	25
1. SINGLE DX	21	2.5	3	1	1	2	3	4	5	9
2. MULTIPLE DX	399	4.4	19	1	2	3	5	8	12	24
A. NOT OPERATED	127	3.7	7	1	2	3	5	8	9	14
B. OPERATED	293	4.5	23	1	2	3	5	9	13	25
TOTAL										
0–19 Years	15	2.9	5	1	2	2	3	7	9	9
20–34	56	3.2	6	1	1	3	5	7	7	12
35–49	113	3.9	9	1	2	3	5	7	9	15
50–64	124	4.5	14	1	2	3	5	9	12	18
65+	112	5.2	39	1	2	4	6	9	14	30
GRAND TOTAL	420	4.3	18	1	2	3	5	8	12	20

Length of Stay by Diagnosis and Operation, Western Region, 2008

Western Region, October 2006–September 2007 Data, by Diagnosis

569: OTH INTESTINAL DISORDERS

Type of Patients	Observed Patients	Avg. Stay	Variance	10th	25th	50th	75th	90th	95th	99th
1. SINGLE DX										
A. Not Operated										
0–19 Years	21	1.5	<1	1	1	1	2	2	2	2
20–34	15	2.9	4	1	2	2	4	7	7	7
35–49	19	1.9	1	1	1	2	3	4	4	4
50–64	17	2.1	2	1	1	2	3	4	5	5
65+	8	2.1	4	1	1	2	2	7	7	7
B. Operated										
0–19 Years	15	3.3	3	2	2	3	4	6	6	6
20–34	19	3.2	4	1	3	3	4	6	7	7
35–49	37	4.6	8	2	3	4	5	9	11	14
50–64	30	4.1	7	1	2	4	5	8	9	11
65+	36	3.1	5	1	2	2	4	7	8	10
2. MULTIPLE DX										
A. Not Operated										
0–19 Years	132	4.7	51	1	1	3	5	10	15	38
20–34	404	3.7	18	1	1	3	4	7	11	21
35–49	1,010	4.1	19	1	2	3	5	8	10	25
50–64	1,783	4.5	27	1	2	3	5	9	12	24
65+	5,292	4.1	12	1	2	3	5	8	10	18
B. Operated										
0–19 Years	103	9.6	130	1	3	6	11	20	27	57
20–34	288	8.3	92	2	4	6	9	15	25	63
35–49	783	8.8	72	3	4	7	11	18	25	43
50–64	1,592	9.0	93	2	4	6	10	19	28	55
65+	2,654	8.9	73	2	4	6	11	18	24	46
SUBTOTALS:										
1. SINGLE DX										
A. Not Operated	80	2.1	2	1	1	2	2	4	4	7
B. Operated	137	3.8	6	1	2	3	5	7	9	11
2. MULTIPLE DX										
A. Not Operated	8,621	4.2	17	1	2	3	5	8	11	20
B. Operated	5,420	8.9	81	2	4	6	11	19	25	49
1. SINGLE DX	217	3.1	5	1	1	3	4	6	8	11
2. MULTIPLE DX	14,041	6.0	47	1	2	4	7	12	18	35
A. NOT OPERATED	8,701	4.1	17	1	2	3	5	8	11	20
B. OPERATED	5,557	8.8	80	2	4	6	11	18	25	49
TOTAL										
0–19 Years	271	6.3	82	1	2	3	7	14	21	57
20–34	726	5.5	52	1	2	4	6	11	15	38
35–49	1,849	6.1	47	1	2	4	7	12	19	32
50–64	3,422	6.6	62	1	2	4	8	13	20	44
65+	7,990	5.7	37	1	2	4	7	12	17	30
GRAND TOTAL	14,258	5.9	46	1	2	4	7	12	18	35

569.1: RECTAL PROLAPSE

Type of Patients	Observed Patients	Avg. Stay	Variance	10th	25th	50th	75th	90th	95th	99th
1. SINGLE DX										
A. Not Operated										
0–19 Years	3	1.3	<1	1	1	1	2	2	2	2
20–34	1	4.0	0	4	4	4	4	4	4	4
35–49	1	1.0	0	1	1	1	1	1	1	1
50–64	1	1.0	0	1	1	1	1	1	1	1
65+	1	1.0	0	1	1	1	1	1	1	1
B. Operated										
0–19 Years	1	6.0	0	6	6	6	6	6	6	6
20–34	8	2.3	1	1	1	3	3	4	4	4
35–49	10	4.4	7	3	3	4	5	5	11	11
50–64	11	4.6	5	3	3	4	5	8	9	9
65+	20	2.2	1	1	2	2	3	4	4	4
2. MULTIPLE DX										
A. Not Operated										
0–19 Years	5	1.2	<1	1	1	1	1	2	2	2
20–34	5	1.6	<1	1	1	1	2	3	3	3
35–49	15	4.9	10	1	2	4	8	9	11	11
50–64	25	3.4	8	1	2	3	5	7	10	12
65+	111	3.2	5	1	2	2	4	6	7	12
B. Operated										
0–19 Years	10	3.1	3	1	2	3	6	7	7	7
20–34	58	6.0	36	3	3	5	6	9	13	40
35–49	156	5.6	21	2	3	4	7	10	15	28
50–64	344	4.8	12	2	3	4	6	9	11	20
65+	791	5.1	18	1	2	4	6	10	14	22
SUBTOTALS:										
1. SINGLE DX										
A. Not Operated	7	1.6	1	1	1	1	2	4	4	4
B. Operated	50	3.2	4	1	2	3	5	7	8	11
2. MULTIPLE DX										
A. Not Operated	161	3.3	6	1	1	2	4	7	8	12
B. Operated	1,359	5.1	18	2	3	4	6	10	12	23
1. SINGLE DX	57	3.0	4	1	1	3	4	5	8	11
2. MULTIPLE DX	1,520	4.9	17	1	2	4	6	9	12	22
A. NOT OPERATED	168	3.2	6	1	1	2	4	7	8	12
B. OPERATED	1,409	5.1	17	2	3	4	6	9	12	22
TOTAL										
0–19 Years	19	2.5	3	1	1	2	3	6	7	7
20–34	72	5.2	32	1	3	4	6	8	12	40
35–49	182	5.5	20	2	3	4	6	10	12	32
50–64	381	4.7	11	2	3	4	6	8	11	20
65+	923	4.8	17	1	2	4	6	12	13	22
GRAND TOTAL	1,577	4.9	17	1	2	4	6	9	12	22

569.3: RECTAL & ANAL HEMORRHAGE

Type of Patients	Observed Patients	Avg. Stay	Variance	10th	25th	50th	75th	90th	95th	99th
1. SINGLE DX										
A. Not Operated										
0–19 Years	8	1.5	<1	1	1	1	2	2	2	2
20–34	2	1.0	0	1	1	1	1	1	1	1
35–49	4	1.0	0	1	1	1	1	1	1	1
50–64	3	1.0	0	1	1	1	1	1	1	1
65+	1	1.0	0	1	1	1	1	1	1	1
B. Operated										
0–19 Years	0									
20–34	0									
35–49	0									
50–64	0									
2. MULTIPLE DX										
A. Not Operated										
0–19 Years	33	2.2	2	1	1	2	3	4	5	5
20–34	122	2.4	4	1	1	2	4	5	5	11
35–49	279	3.1	9	1	1	2	4	6	8	18
50–64	481	3.1	6	1	1	2	4	6	8	12
65+	1,462	3.3	8	1	2	3	4	6	9	14
B. Operated										
0–19 Years	2	5.5	40	2	2	5	10	10	10	10
20–34	3	6.3	26	2	2	5	12	12	12	12
35–49	10	7.9	27	2	3	8	13	14	16	16
50–64	19	7.1	52	1	2	4	10	15	30	30
65+	44	7.7	31	2	4	7	10	15	19	29
SUBTOTALS:										
1. SINGLE DX										
A. Not Operated	18	1.2	<1	1	1	2	1	2	2	2
B. Operated	0									
2. MULTIPLE DX										
A. Not Operated	2,377	3.2	8	1	2	2	4	6	8	14
B. Operated	78	7.5	34	2	3	7	10	15	19	30
1. SINGLE DX	18	1.2	<1	1	1	1	1	2	2	2
2. MULTIPLE DX	2,455	3.3	9	1	2	2	4	6	9	15
A. NOT OPERATED	2,395	3.2	8	1	2	2	4	6	8	14
B. OPERATED	78	7.5	34	2	3	7	10	15	19	30
TOTAL										
0–19 Years	43	2.2	3	1	1	2	3	4	5	10
20–34	127	2.5	4	1	1	2	3	5	6	12
35–49	293	3.2	10	1	2	2	4	7	9	18
50–64	503	3.3	9	1	2	2	4	7	9	15
65+	1,507	3.5	9	1	2	3	4	7	9	15
GRAND TOTAL	2,473	3.3	9	1	2	2	4	6	9	15

434

Length of Stay by Diagnosis and Operation, Western Region 2008

Western Region, October 2006–September 2007 Data, by Diagnosis

569.41: RECTAL & ANAL ULCER

Type of Patients	Observed Patients	Avg. Stay	Variance	10th	25th	50th	75th	90th	95th	99th
1. SINGLE DX										
A. Not Operated										
0–19 Years	0									
20–34	0									
35–49	1	1.0	0	1	1	1	1	1	1	1
50–64	0									
65+	0									
B. Operated										
0–19 Years	1	2.0	0	2	2	2	2	2	2	2
20–34	0									
35–49	1	2.0	0	2	2	2	2	2	2	2
50–64	0									
65+	0									
2. MULTIPLE DX										
A. Not Operated										
0–19 Years	5	3.4	1	2	3	3	4	5	5	5
20–34	22	4.1	24	1	2	3	4	6	7	25
35–49	53	3.9	7	1	2	3	5	8	9	10
50–64	71	5.0	35	2	2	3	5	8	11	39
65+	374	4.5	11	2	2	4	6	9	10	16
B. Operated										
0–19 Years	1	5.0	0	5	5	5	5	5	5	5
20–34	1	3.0	0	3	3	3	3	3	3	3
35–49	14	5.2	13	1	3	4	7	12	13	13
50–64	17	8.0	46	1	3	6	10	18	25	25
65+	38	9.2	103	2	4	5	12	20	35	52
SUBTOTALS:										
1. SINGLE DX										
A. Not Operated	1	1.0	0	1	1	1	1	1	1	1
B. Operated	2	2.0	0	2	2	2	2	2	2	2
2. MULTIPLE DX										
A. Not Operated	525	4.5	14	2	2	3	5	9	10	16
B. Operated	71	8.0	70	2	3	5	10	18	20	52
1. SINGLE DX	3	1.7	<1	1	1	2	2	2	2	2
2. MULTIPLE DX	596	4.9	22	2	2	4	6	9	12	25
A. NOT OPERATED	526	4.5	14	2	2	3	5	9	10	16
B. OPERATED	73	7.8	69	2	3	5	9	18	20	52
TOTAL										
0–19 Years	7	3.4	2	2	2	3	5	5	5	5
20–34	23	4.1	23	2	2	3	4	6	7	25
35–49	69	4.1	8	1	2	3	5	9	10	13
50–64	88	5.6	38	2	3	4	6	10	15	39
65+	412	5.0	21	2	3	4	6	9	12	20
GRAND TOTAL	599	4.9	22	2	2	4	6	9	12	25

569.49: RECTAL & ANAL DISORD NEC

Type of Patients	Observed Patients	Avg. Stay	Variance	10th	25th	50th	75th	90th	95th	99th
1. SINGLE DX										
A. Not Operated										
0–19 Years	0									
20–34	3	4.3	5	3	3	3	7	7	7	7
35–49	1	2.0	0	2	2	2	2	2	2	2
50–64	1	4.0	0	4	4	4	4	4	4	4
65+	1	2.0	0	2	2	2	2	2	2	2
B. Operated										
0–19 Years	1	1.0	0	1	1	1	1	1	1	1
20–34	3	3.7	9	1	1	3	7	7	7	7
35–49	3	3.3	1	2	2	4	4	4	4	4
50–64	0									
65+	0									
2. MULTIPLE DX										
A. Not Operated										
0–19 Years	4	3.5	14	1	1	1	3	5	9	9
20–34	31	3.2	2	1	2	3	4	6	6	6
35–49	69	3.2	6	1	2	3	4	6	8	16
50–64	77	3.9	9	1	2	3	6	7	9	20
65+	321	3.8	11	2	2	3	4	8	10	17
B. Operated										
0–19 Years	1	1.0	0	1	1	1	1	1	1	1
20–34	14	2.6	2	1	2	2	4	5	5	5
35–49	24	6.7	103	1	2	3	4	13	31	43
50–64	43	7.5	103	1	2	4	8	19	22	52
65+	65	8.2	87	1	2	6	11	17	20	56
SUBTOTALS:										
1. SINGLE DX										
A. Not Operated	6	3.5	3	2	2	3	4	7	7	7
B. Operated	7	3.1	4	1	1	3	4	7	7	7
2. MULTIPLE DX										
A. Not Operated	502	3.7	9	1	2	3	4	7	9	16
B. Operated	147	7.2	87	1	2	4	8	16	22	52
1. SINGLE DX	13	3.3	4	1	2	3	4	7	7	7
2. MULTIPLE DX	649	4.5	29	1	2	3	5	9	13	27
A. NOT OPERATED	508	3.7	9	1	2	3	4	7	9	16
B. OPERATED	154	7.0	84	1	2	4	8	16	22	52
TOTAL										
0–19 Years	6	2.7	10	1	1	1	3	9	9	9
20–34	51	3.1	3	1	2	3	4	6	6	7
35–49	97	4.0	31	1	2	3	4	8	13	43
50–64	121	5.2	45	2	2	3	6	9	15	40
65+	387	4.5	26	2	3	3	5	9	13	27
GRAND TOTAL	662	4.4	29	2	2	3	5	9	12	27

569.5: INTESTINAL ABSCESS

Type of Patients	Observed Patients	Avg. Stay	Variance	10th	25th	50th	75th	90th	95th	99th
1. SINGLE DX										
A. Not Operated										
0–19 Years	1	2.0	0	2	2	2	2	2	2	2
20–34	1	2.0	0	2	2	2	2	2	2	2
35–49	0									
50–64	1	2.0	0	2	2	2	2	2	2	2
65+	0									
B. Operated										
0–19 Years	0									
20–34	1	7.0	0	7	7	7	7	7	7	7
35–49	3	5.3	6	3	3	5	5	8	8	8
50–64	0									
65+	0									
2. MULTIPLE DX										
A. Not Operated										
0–19 Years	6	4.3	3	3	3	4	6	7	7	7
20–34	17	4.4	16	1	2	3	4	10	17	17
35–49	76	5.0	10	2	3	4	7	9	11	16
50–64	109	5.5	13	2	3	5	7	10	11	18
65+	126	6.1	19	2	3	5	7	12	14	24
B. Operated										
0–19 Years	3	6.3	6	4	4	6	9	9	9	9
20–34	10	8.7	19	2	6	6	12	13	15	15
35–49	32	10.4	36	4	6	10	13	19	21	29
50–64	38	11.7	93	5	6	8	12	29	39	41
65+	42	12.2	59	6	7	11	15	22	23	47
SUBTOTALS:										
1. SINGLE DX										
A. Not Operated	3	2.0	0	2	2	2	2	2	2	2
B. Operated	4	5.8	5	3	3	6	8	8	8	8
2. MULTIPLE DX										
A. Not Operated	334	5.6	15	2	3	5	7	10	13	20
B. Operated	125	11.2	59	5	6	10	12	21	27	41
1. SINGLE DX	7	4.1	6	2	2	3	7	8	8	8
2. MULTIPLE DX	459	7.1	33	2	4	6	9	13	17	29
A. NOT OPERATED	337	5.5	15	2	3	4	7	10	13	20
B. OPERATED	129	11.0	58	5	6	9	12	21	27	41
TOTAL										
0–19 Years	10	4.7	5	3	3	4	6	7	9	9
20–34	29	5.9	20	2	3	4	8	13	15	17
35–49	111	6.6	23	2	3	5	8	12	16	21
50–64	148	7.1	40	2	4	5	8	12	19	39
65+	168	7.6	36	2	4	6	10	15	18	27
GRAND TOTAL	466	7.0	33	2	4	6	9	13	17	29

Length of Stay by Diagnosis and Operation, Western Region, 2008

Western Region, October 2006–September 2007 Data, by Diagnosis

569.61: COLO/ENTERSTMY INFECTION

Type of Patients	Observed Patients	Avg. Stay	Vari-ance	10th	25th	50th	75th	90th	95th	99th
1. SINGLE DX										
A. Not Operated										
0–19 Years	0									
20–34	0									
35–49	0									
50–64	0									
65+	0									
B. Operated										
0–19 Years	0									
20–34	0									
35–49	0									
50–64	0									
65+	0									
2. MULTIPLE DX										
A. Not Operated										
0–19 Years	6	13.1	216	1	2	2	21	38	38	38
20–34	20	4.5	9	1	2	4	6	9	12	12
35–49	43	5.4	20	1	3	4	8	11	14	22
50–64	87	6.7	64	2	3	4	8	10	24	56
65+	84	6.0	16	2	3	4	8	12	14	18
B. Operated										
0–19 Years	3	26.3	210	12	12	26	41	41	41	41
20–34	4	5.8	14	2	5	5	11	11	11	11
35–49	12	13.5	153	4	5	7	14	34	36	36
50–64	27	12.0	74	4	7	10	15	21	22	43
65+	23	12.7	325	3	6	7	11	16	49	83
SUBTOTALS:										
1. SINGLE DX										
A. Not Operated	0									
B. Operated	0									
2. MULTIPLE DX										
A. Not Operated	240	6.2	39	2	3	4	8	11	15	36
B. Operated	69	12.7	176	3	5	8	14	30	41	83
1. SINGLE DX	0									
2. MULTIPLE DX	309	7.6	77	2	3	5	9	14	22	43
A. NOT OPERATED	240	6.2	39	2	3	4	8	11	15	36
B. OPERATED	69	12.7	176	3	5	8	14	30	41	83
TOTAL										
0–19 Years	9	17.5	231	1	2	15	26	41	41	41
20–34	24	4.7	10	1	2	4	6	9	11	12
35–49	55	7.2	58	1	3	5	8	14	30	36
50–64	114	7.9	70	2	3	5	9	15	24	43
65+	107	7.4	88	2	3	6	9	13	16	49
GRAND TOTAL	309	7.6	77	2	3	5	9	14	22	43

569.62: COLO/ENTERSTMY MECH COMP

Type of Patients	Observed Patients	Avg. Stay	Vari-ance	10th	25th	50th	75th	90th	95th	99th
1. SINGLE DX										
A. Not Operated										
0–19 Years	0									
20–34	0									
35–49	0									
50–64	0									
65+	1	1.0	0	1	1	1	1	1	1	1
B. Operated										
0–19 Years	0									
20–34	1	1.0	0	1	1	1	1	1	1	1
35–49	0									
50–64	0									
65+	1	4.0	0	4	4	4	4	4	4	4
2. MULTIPLE DX										
A. Not Operated										
0–19 Years	20	5.6	34	1	2	3	8	12	16	22
20–34	21	4.6	9	2	2	4	6	7	10	14
35–49	48	4.6	33	1	2	3	5	8	10	38
50–64	63	4.9	18	1	3	4	5	9	12	23
65+	97	4.5	21	1	2	3	5	9	15	27
B. Operated										
0–19 Years	9	18.5	541	2	6	11	20	77	77	77
20–34	10	7.5	29	3	3	6	8	11	21	21
35–49	43	10.0	127	2	3	7	12	22	25	61
50–64	83	8.3	39	2	4	6	11	16	21	29
65+	90	8.9	77	1	3	6	11	22	24	48
SUBTOTALS:										
1. SINGLE DX										
A. Not Operated	1	1.0	0	1	1	1	1	1	1	1
B. Operated	2	2.5	4	1	1	1	4	4	4	4
2. MULTIPLE DX										
A. Not Operated	249	4.7	22	1	2	3	5	9	14	23
B. Operated	235	9.2	90	2	3	6	11	21	25	48
1. SINGLE DX	3	2.0	3	1	1	1	4	4	4	4
2. MULTIPLE DX	484	6.9	60	1	2	5	8	15	22	38
A. NOT OPERATED	250	4.7	22	1	2	3	5	9	14	23
B. OPERATED	237	9.2	89	2	3	6	11	21	25	48
TOTAL										
0–19 Years	29	9.6	215	1	2	5	11	22	27	77
20–34	32	5.4	17	2	2	5	6	9	14	21
35–49	91	7.1	84	1	2	4	8	15	23	61
50–64	146	6.8	33	2	3	5	8	15	19	28
65+	189	6.6	53	1	2	4	8	18	23	35
GRAND TOTAL	487	6.9	60	2	2	5	8	15	22	38

569.69: COLO/ENTERSTMY COMP NEC

Type of Patients	Observed Patients	Avg. Stay	Vari-ance	10th	25th	50th	75th	90th	95th	99th
1. SINGLE DX										
A. Not Operated										
0–19 Years	1	1.0	0	1	1	1	1	1	1	1
20–34	0									
35–49	3	2.7	2	1	1	3	4	4	4	4
50–64	2	1.5	<1	1	1	1	2	2	2	2
65+	0									
B. Operated										
0–19 Years	2	4.0	8	2	2	2	6	6	6	6
20–34	2	3.5	4	2	2	2	5	5	5	5
35–49	8	3.6	2	2	3	3	4	6	6	6
50–64	7	3.7	12	1	1	3	5	11	11	11
65+	8	2.2	2	1	2	2	2	5	5	5
2. MULTIPLE DX										
A. Not Operated										
0–19 Years	11	3.1	9	1	1	2	2	6	10	10
20–34	39	6.1	75	1	2	3	6	20	24	46
35–49	86	4.2	35	1	2	3	5	7	10	54
50–64	175	4.9	34	1	3	3	6	11	16	30
65+	247	4.2	17	1	2	3	5	8	11	26
B. Operated										
0–19 Years	33	8.3	53	2	3	6	11	18	26	32
20–34	56	8.6	85	3	4	6	9	15	35	51
35–49	165	7.0	25	3	4	6	9	12	16	27
50–64	400	7.7	57	2	4	6	9	15	21	46
65+	617	8.4	78	2	4	6	10	17	25	46
SUBTOTALS:										
1. SINGLE DX										
A. Not Operated	6	2.0	2	1	1	1	3	3	4	4
B. Operated	27	3.3	5	1	2	3	5	6	6	11
2. MULTIPLE DX										
A. Not Operated	558	4.5	29	1	2	3	5	9	13	30
B. Operated	1,271	8.0	64	2	4	6	9	16	22	46
1. SINGLE DX	33	3.0	4	1	2	3	4	5	6	11
2. MULTIPLE DX	1,829	6.9	56	1	3	5	8	14	20	42
A. NOT OPERATED	564	4.5	29	1	2	3	5	9	13	30
B. OPERATED	1,298	7.9	63	2	3	6	9	15	22	46
TOTAL										
0–19 Years	47	6.8	45	1	2	5	5	17	19	32
20–34	97	7.5	80	1	2	5	8	15	25	51
35–49	262	5.9	29	1	3	4	7	11	14	27
50–64	584	6.8	51	1	3	5	8	14	20	46
65+	872	7.2	64	1	3	5	8	14	21	42
GRAND TOTAL	1,862	6.9	55	1	3	5	8	14	20	42

Length of Stay by Diagnosis and Operation, Western Region, 2008

Western Region, October 2006–September 2007 Data, by Diagnosis

569.81: INTESTINAL FISTULA

Type of Patients	Observed Patients	Avg. Stay	Vari-ance	Percentiles						
				10th	25th	50th	75th	90th	95th	99th
1. SINGLE DX										
A. Not Operated										
0–19 Years	0									
20–34	2	5.5	4	4	4	4	7	7	7	7
35–49	2	2.5	4	1	1	1	4	4	4	4
50–64	1	1.0	0	1	1	1	1	1	1	1
65+	2	4.5	12	2	2	2	7	7	7	7
B. Operated										
0–19 Years	2	3.5	<1	3	3	3	4	4	4	4
20–34	0									
35–49	1	9.0	0	9	9	9	9	9	9	9
50–64	1	1.0	0	1	1	1	1	1	1	1
65+	1	7.0	0	7	7	7	7	7	7	7
2. MULTIPLE DX										
A. Not Operated										
0–19 Years	3	22.4	>999	1	1	6	60	60	60	60
20–34	27	6.3	44	2	2	4	7	19	20	27
35–49	72	8.6	67	2	3	6	10	23	26	35
50–64	109	8.6	70	2	4	7	11	17	22	34
65+	104	7.7	39	2	4	6	9	15	21	32
B. Operated										
0–19 Years	5	20.7	496	1	7	12	26	57	57	57
20–34	31	17.5	396	3	4	10	19	35	73	78
35–49	85	13.8	148	5	6	10	19	26	30	83
50–64	126	14.4	157	5	6	10	19	35	43	>99
65+	128	15.2	184	5	7	12	18	28	60	>99
SUBTOTALS:										
1. SINGLE DX										
A. Not Operated	7	3.7	7	1	1	4	7	7	7	7
B. Operated	5	4.8	10	1	3	4	7	9	9	9
2. MULTIPLE DX										
A. Not Operated	315	8.2	65	2	3	6	10	18	25	35
B. Operated	375	14.9	187	5	6	10	19	29	55	>99
1. SINGLE DX	12	4.2	8	1	2	4	7	7	9	9
2. MULTIPLE DX	690	11.8	142	3	5	8	15	26	35	78
A. NOT OPERATED	322	8.1	64	2	3	6	10	17	25	35
B. OPERATED	380	14.7	186	4	6	10	19	29	55	>99
TOTAL										
0–19 Years	10	17.7	515	1	3	7	26	57	60	60
20–34	60	12.1	253	2	3	6	14	27	63	78
35–49	160	11.3	116	3	5	8	14	25	28	50
50–64	237	11.6	125	3	5	8	15	27	37	>99
65+	235	11.7	131	3	5	8	14	24	34	76
GRAND TOTAL	702	11.7	140	3	5	8	15	26	35	76

569.82: INTESTINAL ULCERATION

Type of Patients	Observed Patients	Avg. Stay	Vari-ance	Percentiles						
				10th	25th	50th	75th	90th	95th	99th
1. SINGLE DX										
A. Not Operated										
0–19 Years	0									
20–34	0									
35–49	1	2.0	0	2	2	2	2	2	2	2
50–64	0									
65+	0									
B. Operated										
0–19 Years	0									
20–34	0									
35–49	0									
50–64	0									
65+	0									
2. MULTIPLE DX										
A. Not Operated										
0–19 Years	3	3.3	<1	3	3	3	4	4	4	4
20–34	20	2.8	2	1	2	3	4	5	5	5
35–49	61	3.0	4	1	2	3	4	5	5	13
50–64	155	3.4	5	1	2	3	4	6	7	10
65+	378	4.4	13	2	2	3	5	8	10	22
B. Operated										
0–19 Years	0									
20–34	1	7.0	0	7	7	7	7	7	7	7
35–49	7	10.9	39	3	7	10	15	22	22	22
50–64	30	9.2	29	4	6	8	10	21	22	23
65+	45	10.3	71	4	4	8	14	18	21	48
SUBTOTALS:										
1. SINGLE DX										
A. Not Operated	1	2.0	0	2	2	2	2	2	2	2
B. Operated	0									
2. MULTIPLE DX										
A. Not Operated	617	4.0	10	1	2	3	5	7	9	20
B. Operated	83	9.9	52	4	5	8	13	18	22	48
1. SINGLE DX	1	2.0	0	2	2	2	2	2	2	2
2. MULTIPLE DX	700	4.7	19	2	2	3	5	9	12	22
A. NOT OPERATED	618	4.0	10	1	2	3	5	7	9	20
B. OPERATED	83	9.9	52	4	5	8	13	18	22	48
TOTAL										
0–19 Years	3	3.3	<1	3	3	3	4	4	4	4
20–34	21	3.0	3	1	2	3	4	5	5	7
35–49	69	3.8	13	1	2	3	4	7	12	22
50–64	185	4.4	13	1	2	3	6	9	10	22
65+	423	5.0	22	2	2	4	6	9	14	23
GRAND TOTAL	701	4.7	19	2	2	3	5	9	12	22

569.83: INTESTINAL PERFORATION

Type of Patients	Observed Patients	Avg. Stay	Vari-ance	Percentiles						
				10th	25th	50th	75th	90th	95th	99th
1. SINGLE DX										
A. Not Operated										
0–19 Years	1	4.0	0	4	4	4	4	4	4	4
20–34	1	2.0	0	2	2	2	2	2	2	2
35–49	3	2.0	1	1	1	2	3	3	3	3
50–64	4	3.7	2	2	2	4	4	5	5	5
65+	0									
B. Operated										
0–19 Years	1	2.0	0	2	2	2	2	2	2	2
20–34	3	4.3	<1	4	4	4	5	5	5	5
35–49	4	9.3	13	6	6	9	10	14	14	14
50–64	3	6.7	6	4	4	7	7	9	9	9
65+	3	8.3	2	7	7	8	10	10	10	10
2. MULTIPLE DX										
A. Not Operated										
0–19 Years	3	9.4	36	3	3	10	15	15	15	15
20–34	8	5.3	12	1	2	6	8	10	10	10
35–49	16	9.4	90	2	3	7	13	31	31	31
50–64	35	4.5	9	1	2	3	6	8	12	13
65+	85	6.0	20	1	3	5	8	12	16	22
B. Operated										
0–19 Years	17	12.2	77	6	6	9	18	21	38	38
20–34	71	9.4	42	4	5	8	11	16	19	38
35–49	168	12.0	99	5	7	9	14	22	26	50
50–64	282	14.3	173	5	7	10	17	30	44	93
65+	489	13.4	80	6	8	11	16	25	34	46
SUBTOTALS:										
1. SINGLE DX										
A. Not Operated	9	3.0	2	2	2	3	4	5	5	5
B. Operated	14	6.9	10	4	4	7	9	10	14	14
2. MULTIPLE DX										
A. Not Operated	147	6.0	26	2	3	5	8	12	16	31
B. Operated	1,027	13.1	107	5	7	10	16	25	35	51
1. SINGLE DX	23	5.4	10	2	3	4	7	10	10	14
2. MULTIPLE DX	1,174	12.3	102	4	6	9	15	24	32	50
A. NOT OPERATED	156	5.9	25	2	3	4	7	12	16	31
B. OPERATED	1,041	13.1	106	5	7	10	16	25	35	51
TOTAL										
0–19 Years	22	11.0	70	3	6	9	15	19	21	38
20–34	83	8.7	40	4	5	7	13	15	18	38
35–49	191	11.6	96	5	6	9	13	22	27	50
50–64	324	13.0	162	4	6	9	15	28	37	68
65+	577	12.3	78	5	7	10	15	22	30	44
GRAND TOTAL	1,197	12.1	101	4	6	9	15	23	31	50

Length of Stay by Diagnosis and Operation, Western Region, 2008

Western Region, October 2006–September 2007 Data, by Diagnosis

569.85: INTEST ANGIODYSPL W HEM

Type of Patients	Observed Patients	Avg. Stay	Variance	10th	25th	50th	75th	90th	95th	99th
1. SINGLE DX										
A. Not Operated										
0–19 Years	0									
20–34	1	3.0	0	3	3	3	3	3	3	3
35–49	0									
50–64	0									
65+	0									
B. Operated										
0–19 Years	0									
20–34	0									
35–49	0									
50–64	0									
65+	0									
2. MULTIPLE DX										
A. Not Operated										
0–19 Years	0									
20–34	9	3.8	19	1	2	3	3	15	15	15
35–49	52	4.0	9	1	2	3	5	8	10	13
50–64	215	4.2	11	2	2	3	5	8	11	20
65+	1,481	4.1	9	2	2	3	5	8	10	15
B. Operated										
0–19 Years	0									
20–34	0	9.0	0	9	9	9	9	9	9	9
35–49	6	13.8	35	7	8	13	16	23	23	23
50–64	33	10.3	92	2	5	8	12	19	26	54
65+	119	10.5	55	3	5	9	13	23	26	29
SUBTOTALS:										
1. SINGLE DX										
A. Not Operated	1	3.0	0	3	3	3	3	3	3	3
B. Operated	0									
2. MULTIPLE DX										
A. Not Operated	1,757	4.1	9	2	2	3	5	8	10	16
B. Operated	159	10.6	61	3	5	9	13	22	26	30
1. SINGLE DX	1	3.0	0	3	3	3	3	3	3	3
2. MULTIPLE DX	1,916	4.6	17	2	2	3	5	9	12	22
A. NOT OPERATED	1,758	4.1	9	2	2	3	5	8	10	16
B. OPERATED	159	10.6	61	3	5	9	13	22	26	30
TOTAL										
0–19 Years	0									
20–34	11	4.2	18	1	2	3	4	9	15	15
35–49	58	5.0	20	1	2	3	7	12	16	23
50–64	248	5.0	26	2	2	3	6	10	14	22
65+	1,600	4.6	15	2	2	3	5	9	12	22
GRAND TOTAL	1,917	4.6	17	2	2	3	5	9	12	22

569.89: INTESTINAL DISORDER NEC

Type of Patients	Observed Patients	Avg. Stay	Variance	10th	25th	50th	75th	90th	95th	99th
1. SINGLE DX										
A. Not Operated										
0–19 Years	2	1.0	0	1	1	1	1	1	1	1
20–34	3	2.0	0	2	2	2	2	2	2	2
35–49	0									
50–64	1	1.0	0	1	1	1	1	1	1	1
65+	0									
B. Operated										
0–19 Years	5	3.4	2	2	2	3	5	5	5	5
20–34	1	3.0	0	3	3	3	3	3	3	3
35–49	5	4.0	6	2	2	4	4	8	8	8
50–64	3	4.3	<1	4	4	4	5	5	5	5
65+	2	4.5	<1	4	4	5	5	5	5	5
2. MULTIPLE DX										
A. Not Operated										
0–19 Years	19	5.9	34	1	2	3	9	14	24	24
20–34	33	3.8	17	1	1	3	3	12	13	17
35–49	63	3.6	5	1	2	4	5	7	9	10
50–64	79	6.8	155	1	2	4	6	12	17	83
65+	157	4.4	13	1	2	3	5	9	12	19
B. Operated										
0–19 Years	13	5.4	12	1	3	5	6	9	14	14
20–34	17	3.8	5	1	2	4	7	7	7	7
35–49	34	5.1	22	1	3	4	6	8	11	28
50–64	77	7.3	136	2	3	5	8	13	19	97
65+	76	8.5	30	3	5	7	10	16	19	30
SUBTOTALS:										
1. SINGLE DX										
A. Not Operated	6	1.5	<1	1	1	2	2	2	2	2
B. Operated	16	3.9	3	2	3	4	5	5	8	8
2. MULTIPLE DX										
A. Not Operated	351	4.8	46	1	2	3	5	9	13	24
B. Operated	217	7.0	65	2	3	5	8	13	18	30
1. SINGLE DX	22	3.2	3	1	2	3	4	5	5	8
2. MULTIPLE DX	568	5.7	54	1	2	4	7	11	14	30
A. NOT OPERATED	357	4.8	45	1	2	3	5	9	13	24
B. OPERATED	233	6.8	61	2	3	5	8	13	17	30
TOTAL										
0–19 Years	39	5.2	22	1	2	5	6	10	14	24
20–34	54	3.6	12	1	1	3	4	7	13	17
35–49	102	4.1	11	1	2	3	5	7	9	11
50–64	160	6.9	142	2	2	4	7	12	17	83
65+	235	5.8	22	2	3	4	8	12	16	24
GRAND TOTAL	590	5.6	53	1	2	4	6	10	14	30

570: ACUTE LIVER NECROSIS

Type of Patients	Observed Patients	Avg. Stay	Variance	10th	25th	50th	75th	90th	95th	99th
1. SINGLE DX										
A. Not Operated										
0–19 Years	2	3.5	4	2	2	4	5	5	5	5
20–34	9	2.2	1	1	1	2	3	4	4	4
35–49	4	4.0	3	2	3	4	4	6	6	6
50–64	2	3.0	0	3	3	3	3	3	3	3
65+	0									
B. Operated										
0–19 Years	0									
20–34	0									
35–49	0									
50–64	0									
65+	0									
2. MULTIPLE DX										
A. Not Operated										
0–19 Years	32	5.4	34	2	3	4	7	9	13	34
20–34	113	4.6	14	2	2	4	5	10	14	17
35–49	201	5.7	32	2	2	4	7	13	18	28
50–64	216	6.4	37	2	3	4	8	13	17	26
65+	151	5.1	11	2	3	4	7	9	12	17
B. Operated										
0–19 Years	1	14.0	0	14	14	85	>99	>99	>99	>99
20–34	2	12.5	41	8	8	13	13	17	17	17
35–49	7	13.4	27	10	10	12	13	25	25	25
50–64	8	14.7	53	5	12	17	22	25	25	25
65+	2	8.0	18	5	5	5	11	11	11	11
SUBTOTALS:										
1. SINGLE DX										
A. Not Operated	17	2.9	2	1	2	3	4	5	6	6
B. Operated	0									
2. MULTIPLE DX										
A. Not Operated	713	5.6	26	2	2	4	7	11	16	26
B. Operated	20	13.3	35	5	10	12	17	25	25	>99
1. SINGLE DX	17	2.9	2	1	2	3	4	5	6	6
2. MULTIPLE DX	733	5.8	28	2	2	4	7	12	17	26
A. NOT OPERATED	730	5.5	26	2	2	4	7	11	15	26
B. OPERATED	20	13.3	35	5	10	12	17	25	25	>99
TOTAL										
0–19 Years	35	5.6	34	2	3	4	7	13	34	>99
20–34	124	4.6	15	2	2	3	5	10	14	17
35–49	212	5.9	33	2	2	4	7	13	18	28
50–64	226	6.6	39	2	3	5	8	14	18	26
65+	153	5.1	11	2	3	4	7	9	12	17
GRAND TOTAL	750	5.7	28	2	2	4	7	12	17	26

Western Region, October 2006–September 2007 Data, by Diagnosis

571: CHR LIVER DIS/CIRRHOSIS

Type of Patients	Observed Patients	Avg. Stay	Vari-ance	10th	25th	50th	75th	90th	95th	99th
1. SINGLE DX										
A. Not Operated										
0–19 Years	6	2.0	6	1	1	1	1	7	7	7
20–34	4	4.8	8	1	4	4	7	7	7	7
35–49	5	2.4	4	1	1	2	2	6	6	6
50–64	11	2.6	4	1	1	2	2	4	8	8
65+	1	2.0	0	2	2	2	2	2	2	2
B. Operated										
0–19 Years	1	1.0	0	1	1	1	1	1	1	1
20–34	0									
35–49	0									
50–64	0									
65+	0									
2. MULTIPLE DX										
A. Not Operated										
0–19 Years	54	3.6	7	1	1	3	5	8	9	11
20–34	700	5.1	24	1	2	4	6	10	14	27
35–49	5,266	5.4	31	1	2	4	6	11	15	26
50–64	7,472	5.2	25	1	2	4	6	10	14	25
65+	3,169	5.3	21	2	3	4	7	10	13	22
B. Operated										
0–19 Years	6	14.7	182	2	2	26	27	28	28	28
20–34	27	16.1	157	4	8	11	22	42	44	49
35–49	236	11.4	107	2	5	9	14	27	34	58
50–64	582	10.7	103	2	5	8	13	23	32	60
65+	200	10.2	93	1	4	8	13	21	30	54
SUBTOTALS:										
1. SINGLE DX										
A. Not Operated	27	2.7	5	1	1	2	4	7	7	8
B. Operated	1	1.0	0	1	1	1	1	1	1	1
2. MULTIPLE DX										
A. Not Operated	16,661	5.2	26	1	2	4	6	10	14	25
B. Operated	1,051	10.9	104	2	4	8	14	24	32	58
1. SINGLE DX	28	2.7	5	1	1	2	4	7	7	8
2. MULTIPLE DX	17,712	5.6	32	1	2	4	7	11	15	29
A. NOT OPERATED	16,688	5.2	26	1	2	4	6	10	14	25
B. OPERATED	1,052	10.9	104	2	4	8	14	24	32	58
TOTAL										
0–19 Years	67	4.4	31	1	1	3	5	9	11	28
20–34	731	5.5	32	1	2	4	7	11	16	34
35–49	5,507	5.6	36	1	2	4	7	12	16	30
50–64	8,065	5.6	33	1	2	4	7	11	15	29
65+	3,370	5.6	26	2	3	4	7	10	14	26
GRAND TOTAL	17,740	5.6	32	1	2	4	7	11	15	29

571.1: AC ALCOHOLIC HEPATITIS

Type of Patients	Observed Patients	Avg. Stay	Vari-ance	10th	25th	50th	75th	90th	95th	99th
1. SINGLE DX										
A. Not Operated										
0–19 Years	0									
20–34	1	4.0	0	4	4	4	4	4	4	4
35–49	1	2.0	0	2	2	2	2	2	2	2
50–64	2	2.0	0	2	2	2	2	2	2	2
65+	0									
B. Operated										
0–19 Years	0									
20–34	0									
35–49	0									
50–64	0									
65+	0									
2. MULTIPLE DX										
A. Not Operated										
0–19 Years	2	5.5	40	1	1	4	10	10	10	10
20–34	242	5.0	27	1	2	4	6	9	13	35
35–49	909	6.2	35	2	3	4	7	13	18	30
50–64	683	6.2	38	2	3	4	8	13	16	29
65+	114	6.1	31	2	3	4	7	13	15	29
B. Operated										
0–19 Years	0									
20–34	1	11.0	0	11	11	11	11	11	11	11
35–49	9	18.9	411	3	4	9	37	58	58	58
50–64	8	12.6	11	9	9	11	17	17	17	17
65+	0									
SUBTOTALS:										
1. SINGLE DX										
A. Not Operated	4	2.5	1	2	2	2	4	4	4	4
B. Operated	0									
2. MULTIPLE DX										
A. Not Operated	1,950	6.0	35	2	3	4	7	13	17	29
B. Operated	18	15.7	210	4	9	11	17	39	58	58
1. SINGLE DX	4	2.5	1	2	2	2	4	4	4	4
2. MULTIPLE DX	1,968	6.1	37	2	3	4	7	13	17	30
A. NOT OPERATED	1,954	6.0	35	2	3	4	7	13	17	29
B. OPERATED	18	15.7	210	4	9	11	17	39	58	58
TOTAL										
0–19 Years	2	5.5	40	1	1	4	10	10	10	10
20–34	244	5.0	27	1	2	4	6	9	13	35
35–49	919	6.3	39	2	3	4	8	14	18	31
50–64	693	6.2	38	2	3	4	8	13	17	29
65+	114	6.1	31	2	3	4	7	13	15	29
GRAND TOTAL	1,972	6.1	37	2	3	4	7	13	17	30

571.2: ALCOHOL LIVER CIRRHOSIS

Type of Patients	Observed Patients	Avg. Stay	Vari-ance	10th	25th	50th	75th	90th	95th	99th
1. SINGLE DX										
A. Not Operated										
0–19 Years	0									
20–34	0									
35–49	1	1.0	0	1	1	1	1	1	1	1
50–64	5	2.0	2	1	1	1	3	4	4	4
65+	0									
B. Operated										
0–19 Years	0									
20–34	0									
35–49	0									
50–64	0									
65+	0									
2. MULTIPLE DX										
A. Not Operated										
0–19 Years	0									
20–34	280	5.7	24	2	3	4	7	11	14	27
35–49	3,076	5.5	34	1	2	4	6	11	15	28
50–64	4,106	5.2	25	1	2	4	6	10	14	26
65+	1,077	5.4	22	2	3	4	7	10	14	25
B. Operated										
0–19 Years	0									
20–34	9	19.8	183	4	12	16	23	49	49	49
35–49	139	11.6	96	2	5	9	14	29	34	42
50–64	254	10.7	104	2	4	8	13	22	34	54
65+	70	10.0	92	1	3	8	13	22	30	46
SUBTOTALS:										
1. SINGLE DX										
A. Not Operated	6	1.8	2	1	1	1	3	4	4	4
B. Operated	0									
2. MULTIPLE DX										
A. Not Operated	8,539	5.4	28	2	2	4	6	10	15	27
B. Operated	472	11.0	102	2	4	8	14	26	34	49
1. SINGLE DX	6	1.8	2	1	1	1	3	4	4	4
2. MULTIPLE DX	9,011	5.7	33	2	2	4	7	11	16	30
A. NOT OPERATED	8,545	5.4	28	2	2	4	6	10	15	27
B. OPERATED	472	11.0	102	2	4	8	14	26	34	49
TOTAL										
0–19 Years	0									
20–34	289	6.1	35	2	3	4	8	13	16	30
35–49	3,216	5.8	38	1	2	4	7	12	17	31
50–64	4,365	5.5	31	1	2	4	7	11	15	30
65+	1,147	5.7	27	2	3	4	7	10	15	27
GRAND TOTAL	9,017	5.7	33	2	2	4	7	11	16	30

Length of Stay by Diagnosis and Operation, Western Region, 2008

571.3: ALCOHOL LIVER DAMAGE NOS

Type of Patients	Observed Patients	Avg. Stay	Vari-ance	Percentiles						
				10th	25th	50th	75th	90th	95th	99th
1. SINGLE DX										
A. Not Operated										
0–19 Years	0									
20–34	0									
35–49	0									
50–64	0									
65+	0									
B. Operated										
0–19 Years	0									
20–34	0									
35–49	0									
50–64	0									
65+	0									
2. MULTIPLE DX										
A. Not Operated										
0–19 Years	0									
20–34	21	5.8	58	1	2	3	5	13	17	34
35–49	141	3.7	10	1	2	3	4	7	8	14
50–64	177	4.4	18	1	2	3	5	9	11	28
65+	49	5.0	16	1	3	4	5	12	15	18
B. Operated										
0–19 Years	0									
20–34	0									
35–49	1	14.0	0	14	14	14	14	14	14	14
50–64	5	3.6	28	1	1	1	2	2	13	13
65+	1	4.0	0	4	4	4	4	4	4	4
SUBTOTALS:										
1. SINGLE DX										
A. Not Operated	0									
B. Operated	0									
2. MULTIPLE DX										
A. Not Operated	388	4.3	17	1	2	3	5	8	12	26
B. Operated	7	5.2	34	1	1	2	13	14	14	14
1. SINGLE DX	0									
2. MULTIPLE DX	395	4.3	17	1	2	3	5	8	12	26
A. NOT OPERATED	388	4.3	17	1	2	3	5	8	12	26
B. OPERATED	7	5.2	34	1	1	2	13	14	14	14
TOTAL										
0–19 Years	0									
20–34	21	5.8	58	1	2	3	5	13	17	34
35–49	142	3.8	11	1	2	3	5	8	8	14
50–64	182	4.4	18	1	2	3	5	9	11	28
65+	50	5.0	15	2	3	4	5	12	15	18
GRAND TOTAL	395	4.3	17	1	2	3	5	8	12	26

571.49: CHRONIC HEPATITIS NEC

Type of Patients	Observed Patients	Avg. Stay	Vari-ance	Percentiles						
				10th	25th	50th	75th	90th	95th	99th
1. SINGLE DX										
A. Not Operated										
0–19 Years	2	4.0	18	1	1	1	7	7	7	7
20–34	2	7.0	0	7	7	7	7	7	7	7
35–49	2	4.0	8	2	2	6	6	6	6	6
50–64	1	8.0	0	8	8	8	8	8	8	8
65+	0									
B. Operated										
0–19 Years	0									
20–34	0									
35–49	0									
50–64	0									
65+	0									
2. MULTIPLE DX										
A. Not Operated										
0–19 Years	20	2.8	4	1	1	3	5	6	6	6
20–34	36	5.1	12	2	3	4	7	9	11	19
35–49	50	5.5	42	2	2	5	7	8	11	47
50–64	88	6.6	75	2	3	4	7	13	18	68
65+	52	6.0	16	2	3	5	7	13	15	18
B. Operated										
0–19 Years	1	2.0	0	2	2	2	2	2	2	2
20–34	4	8.5	11	4	4	8	11	11	11	11
35–49	3	5.7	16	2	2	5	10	10	10	10
50–64	8	14.0	396	1	3	9	23	60	60	60
65+	0									
SUBTOTALS:										
1. SINGLE DX										
A. Not Operated	7	5.4	8	1	2	7	7	8	8	8
B. Operated	0									
2. MULTIPLE DX										
A. Not Operated	246	5.7	41	2	3	4	7	10	15	39
B. Operated	16	10.3	207	1	3	8	11	23	60	60
1. SINGLE DX	7	5.4	8	2	2	7	7	8	8	8
2. MULTIPLE DX	262	6.0	52	2	3	4	7	11	15	47
A. NOT OPERATED	253	5.7	41	2	3	4	7	10	15	39
B. OPERATED	16	10.3	207	1	3	8	11	23	60	60
TOTAL										
0–19 Years	23	2.9	4	1	1	2	5	6	6	7
20–34	42	5.5	12	2	3	4	7	10	11	19
35–49	55	5.4	39	2	2	5	7	8	11	47
50–64	97	7.2	101	2	3	4	8	15	20	68
65+	52	6.0	16	2	3	5	7	13	15	18
GRAND TOTAL	269	6.0	51	2	3	4	7	11	15	47

571.5: LIVER CIRRHOSIS W/O ALC

Type of Patients	Observed Patients	Avg. Stay	Vari-ance	Percentiles						
				10th	25th	50th	75th	90th	95th	99th
1. SINGLE DX										
A. Not Operated										
0–19 Years	0									
20–34	0									
35–49	0									
50–64	2	1.5	<1	1	1	1	2	2	2	2
65+	1	2.0	0	2	2	2	2	2	2	2
B. Operated										
0–19 Years	0									
20–34	0									
35–49	0									
50–64	0									
65+	0									
2. MULTIPLE DX										
A. Not Operated										
0–19 Years	21	4.8	8	2	3	4	6	9	9	11
20–34	87	4.5	15	1	2	3	6	10	12	20
35–49	953	4.4	17	1	2	3	5	8	11	21
50–64	2,192	4.8	20	1	2	4	6	9	12	22
65+	1,706	5.2	20	2	3	4	7	10	12	21
B. Operated										
0–19 Years	3	11.0	214	2	2	3	28	28	28	28
20–34	10	18.9	207	3	8	12	27	44	44	44
35–49	71	10.5	102	2	4	8	13	19	25	71
50–64	273	10.4	92	2	5	8	13	23	30	59
65+	115	10.4	105	1	3	8	14	22	30	54
SUBTOTALS:										
1. SINGLE DX										
A. Not Operated	3	1.7	<1	1	1	2	2	2	2	2
B. Operated	0									
2. MULTIPLE DX										
A. Not Operated	4,959	4.8	19	1	2	4	6	9	12	21
B. Operated	472	10.6	100	2	4	8	13	22	30	59
1. SINGLE DX	3	1.7	<1	1	1	2	2	2	2	2
2. MULTIPLE DX	5,431	5.3	29	1	2	4	6	10	14	27
A. NOT OPERATED	4,962	4.8	19	1	2	4	6	9	12	21
B. OPERATED	472	10.6	100	2	4	8	13	22	30	59
TOTAL										
0–19 Years	24	5.6	30	2	3	4	8	9	11	28
20–34	97	6.0	52	1	2	4	7	12	19	44
35–49	1,024	4.8	25	1	2	3	6	9	14	24
50–64	2,467	5.4	31	1	2	4	6	11	15	28
65+	1,822	5.6	27	2	3	4	7	10	14	24
GRAND TOTAL	5,434	5.3	29	1	2	4	6	10	14	27

Length of Stay by Diagnosis and Operation, Western Region, 2008

571.8: CHRONIC LIVER DIS NEC

Type of Patients	Observed Patients	Avg. Stay	Vari-ance	Percentiles						
				10th	25th	50th	75th	90th	95th	99th
1. SINGLE DX										
A. *Not Operated*										
0–19 Years	4	1.0	0	1	1	1	1	1	1	1
20–34	1	1.0	0	1	1	1	1	1	1	1
35–49	1	1.0	0	1	1	1	1	1	1	1
50–64	0									
65+	0									
B. *Operated*										
0–19 Years	1	1.0	0	1	1	1	1	1	1	1
20–34	0									
35–49	0									
50–64	0									
65+	0									
2. MULTIPLE DX										
A. *Not Operated*										
0–19 Years	7	2.1	1	1	1	2	3	4	4	4
20–34	24	2.9	3	1	1	3	4	5	5	6
35–49	65	5.0	43	1	2	3	5	9	13	45
50–64	101	4.1	7	1	2	3	6	8	9	11
65+	68	4.8	19	1	3	4	6	9	10	32
B. *Operated*										
0–19 Years	1	26.0	0	26	26	26	26	26	26	26
20–34	2	6.5	<1	6	6	6	7	7	7	7
35–49	9	8.6	48	1	5	6	12	23	23	23
50–64	15	12.7	272	1	3	8	11	34	64	64
65+	6	7.5	13	2	6	7	11	12	12	12
SUBTOTALS:										
1. SINGLE DX										
A. *Not Operated*	6	1.0	0	1	1	1	1	1	1	1
B. *Operated*	1	1.0	0	1	1	1	1	1	1	1
2. MULTIPLE DX										
A. *Not Operated*	265	4.3	19	1	2	3	5	8	10	26
B. *Operated*	33	10.7	147	1	5	7	11	23	34	64
1. SINGLE DX	7	1.0	0	1	1	1	1	1	1	1
2. MULTIPLE DX	298	5.0	36	1	2	3	6	9	12	34
A. NOT OPERATED	271	4.3	18	1	2	3	5	8	10	26
B. OPERATED	34	10.4	145	1	5	7	11	23	34	64
TOTAL										
0–19 Years	13	3.6	47	1	1	1	3	4	26	26
20–34	27	3.1	3	1	1	3	4	6	6	7
35–49	75	5.3	44	1	2	3	6	12	18	45
50–64	116	5.2	48	1	2	3	6	9	11	34
65+	74	5.1	18	2	3	4	7	9	12	32
GRAND TOTAL	305	4.9	36	1	2	3	6	9	12	32

572: SEQUELA OF CHR LIVER DIS

Type of Patients	Observed Patients	Avg. Stay	Vari-ance	Percentiles						
				10th	25th	50th	75th	90th	95th	99th
1. SINGLE DX										
A. *Not Operated*										
0–19 Years	1	7.0	0	7	7	7	7	7	7	7
20–34	8	5.0	8	1	2	5	5	10	10	10
35–49	4	3.0	3	1	2	4	5	5	5	5
50–64	6	2.2	1	1	1	2	3	4	4	4
65+	1	12.0	0	12	12	12	12	12	12	12
B. *Operated*										
0–19 Years	0									
20–34	0									
35–49	2	9.5	12	7	7	12	12	12	12	12
50–64	0									
65+	0									
2. MULTIPLE DX										
A. *Not Operated*										
0–19 Years	33	5.8	38	1	2	4	7	11	17	33
20–34	200	6.8	58	2	3	5	8	13	17	31
35–49	2,150	5.2	29	1	2	4	6	11	14	27
50–64	4,922	5.1	31	1	2	3	6	10	14	28
65+	2,854	5.1	19	2	2	4	6	10	13	23
B. *Operated*										
0–19 Years	5	12.6	68	2	9	10	20	22	22	22
20–34	16	8.4	30	2	5	8	10	19	20	20
35–49	57	12.9	121	3	5	10	18	26	43	52
50–64	127	15.0	221	3	6	11	21	36	56	>99
65+	66	12.4	76	3	6	10	18	27	31	33
SUBTOTALS:										
1. SINGLE DX										
A. *Not Operated*	20	4.2	9	1	2	4	5	7	10	12
B. *Operated*	2	9.5	12	7	7	12	12	12	12	12
2. MULTIPLE DX										
A. *Not Operated*	10,159	5.1	28	1	2	3	6	10	14	26
B. *Operated*	271	13.5	152	3	6	10	18	27	38	>99
1. SINGLE DX	22	4.7	11	1	2	4	7	10	12	12
2. MULTIPLE DX	10,430	5.3	33	1	2	4	6	11	15	29
A. NOT OPERATED	10,179	5.1	28	1	2	4	6	10	14	26
B. OPERATED	273	13.5	151	3	6	10	18	27	38	>99
TOTAL										
0–19 Years	39	6.7	44	1	2	5	9	17	22	33
20–34	224	6.9	55	2	3	5	9	14	18	30
35–49	2,213	5.4	33	1	2	4	7	11	16	29
50–64	5,055	5.3	38	1	2	3	6	11	15	31
65+	2,921	5.2	22	2	2	4	6	10	14	24
GRAND TOTAL	10,452	5.3	33	1	2	4	6	11	15	29

572.0: LIVER ABSCESS

Type of Patients	Observed Patients	Avg. Stay	Vari-ance	Percentiles						
				10th	25th	50th	75th	90th	95th	99th
1. SINGLE DX										
A. *Not Operated*										
0–19 Years	1	7.0	0	7	7	7	7	7	7	7
20–34	8	5.0	8	1	2	5	5	10	10	10
35–49	3	3.7	2	2	2	4	5	5	5	5
50–64	5	2.4	1	1	2	2	3	4	4	4
65+	1	12.0	0	12	12	12	12	12	12	12
B. *Operated*										
0–19 Years	0									
20–34	0									
35–49	2	9.5	12	7	7	12	12	12	12	12
50–64	0									
65+	0									
2. MULTIPLE DX										
A. *Not Operated*										
0–19 Years	18	6.4	17	1	3	6	8	12	17	17
20–34	63	9.0	124	2	4	7	11	15	22	84
35–49	136	8.3	34	3	4	7	11	17	20	30
50–64	224	8.8	38	3	5	7	11	16	19	31
65+	276	9.1	40	3	5	8	12	19	22	33
B. *Operated*										
0–19 Years	1	10.0	0	10	10	10	10	10	10	10
20–34	8	10.8	43	2	7	12	14	20	20	20
35–49	11	12.4	165	1	4	9	17	19	47	47
50–64	34	17.4	220	5	8	13	23	27	56	71
65+	23	17.2	100	3	8	18	26	31	32	33
SUBTOTALS:										
1. SINGLE DX										
A. *Not Operated*	18	4.5	9	1	2	4	5	10	12	12
B. *Operated*	2	9.5	12	7	7	12	12	12	12	12
2. MULTIPLE DX										
A. *Not Operated*	717	8.8	45	3	4	7	11	17	21	31
B. *Operated*	77	15.8	157	3	8	13	22	28	45	71
1. SINGLE DX	20	5.1	11	1	2	5	7	12	12	12
2. MULTIPLE DX	794	9.5	60	3	5	8	12	18	24	36
A. NOT OPERATED	735	8.7	45	3	4	7	11	17	21	31
B. OPERATED	79	15.7	154	3	8	13	22	28	45	71
TOTAL										
0–19 Years	20	6.6	15	1	3	6	9	12	17	17
20–34	79	8.8	105	2	4	7	11	16	22	84
35–49	152	8.6	43	2	4	7	11	17	20	34
50–64	263	9.8	70	3	5	8	12	18	24	45
65+	300	9.7	49	3	5	8	12	20	25	33
GRAND TOTAL	814	9.4	59	3	5	7	12	18	24	34

Length of Stay by Diagnosis and Operation, Western Region, 2008

Western Region, October 2006–September 2007 Data, by Diagnosis

572.2: HEPATIC COMA

Type of Patients	Observed Patients	Avg. Stay	Vari-ance	Percentiles						
				10th	25th	50th	75th	90th	95th	99th
1. SINGLE DX										
A. Not Operated										
0–19 Years	0									
20–34	0									
35–49	1	1.0	0	1	1	1	1	1	1	1
50–64	1	1.0	0	1	1	1	1	1	1	1
65+	0									
B. Operated										
0–19 Years	0									
20–34	0									
35–49	0									
50–64	0									
65+	0									
2. MULTIPLE DX										
A. Not Operated										
0–19 Years	3	4.0	7	2	2	3	7	7	7	7
20–34	99	5.7	24	1	2	4	8	13	18	20
35–49	1,772	5.0	29	1	2	3	6	10	14	26
50–64	4,285	4.9	31	1	2	3	6	10	14	29
65+	2,394	4.6	15	1	2	4	6	9	11	20
B. Operated										
0–19 Years	0									
20–34	1	9.0	0	9	9	9	9	9	9	9
35–49	29	14.8	120	9	7	12	21	29	31	52
50–64	45	18.2	356	3	12	12	25	59	>99	>99
65+	27	10.3	49	3	6	9	13	17	28	33
SUBTOTALS:										
1. SINGLE DX										
A. Not Operated	2	1.0	0	1	1	1	1	1	1	1
B. Operated	0									
2. MULTIPLE DX										
A. Not Operated	8,553	4.8	26	1	2	3	6	9	13	26
B. Operated	102	15.1	212	3	6	11	21	36	56	>99
1. SINGLE DX	2	1.0	0	1	1	1	1	1	1	1
2. MULTIPLE DX	8,655	5.0	29	1	2	3	6	10	14	28
A. NOT OPERATED	8,555	4.8	26	1	2	3	6	9	13	26
B. OPERATED	102	15.1	212	3	6	11	21	36	56	>99
TOTAL										
0–19 Years	3	4.0	7	2	2	3	7	7	7	7
20–34	100	5.7	24	1	2	4	8	12	17	20
35–49	1,802	5.1	32	1	2	3	6	10	15	28
50–64	4,331	5.0	36	1	2	3	6	10	14	31
65+	2,421	4.7	16	1	2	4	6	9	12	20
GRAND TOTAL	8,657	5.0	29	1	2	3	6	10	14	28

572.3: PORTAL HYPERTENSION

Type of Patients	Observed Patients	Avg. Stay	Vari-ance	Percentiles						
				10th	25th	50th	75th	90th	95th	99th
1. SINGLE DX										
A. Not Operated										
0–19 Years	0									
20–34	0									
35–49	0									
50–64	0									
65+	0									
B. Operated										
0–19 Years	0									
20–34	0									
35–49	0									
50–64	0									
65+	0									
2. MULTIPLE DX										
A. Not Operated										
0–19 Years	9	1.9	<1	1	1	2	2	3	3	3
20–34	24	4.7	9	2	3	4	6	10	10	13
35–49	124	3.7	6	2	2	3	5	6	8	14
50–64	214	3.9	10	1	2	3	5	7	9	14
65+	93	3.9	6	2	2	4	5	6	8	18
B. Operated										
0–19 Years	3	11.1	103	2	2	9	22	22	22	22
20–34	3	5.0	7	3	3	4	4	8	8	8
35–49	8	6.3	16	3	3	5	10	13	13	13
50–64	15	4.1	7	2	2	3	7	8	8	8
65+	9	8.9	32	6	6	7	13	18	18	18
SUBTOTALS:										
1. SINGLE DX										
A. Not Operated	0									
B. Operated	0									
2. MULTIPLE DX										
A. Not Operated	464	3.8	8	1	2	3	5	7	9	14
B. Operated	38	6.3	24	2	2	6	8	13	18	22
1. SINGLE DX	0									
2. MULTIPLE DX	502	4.0	10	1	2	3	5	7	10	18
A. NOT OPERATED	464	3.8	8	1	2	3	5	7	9	14
B. OPERATED	38	6.3	24	2	2	6	8	13	18	22
TOTAL										
0–19 Years	12	4.2	37	1	2	2	3	7	7	7
20–34	27	4.7	8	2	3	4	6	10	10	13
35–49	132	3.8	7	2	2	3	5	7	9	14
50–64	229	3.9	10	1	2	3	5	7	8	14
65+	102	4.4	10	2	2	4	5	7	10	18
GRAND TOTAL	502	4.0	10	1	2	3	5	7	10	18

572.8: OTH SEQUELA CHR LIV DIS

Type of Patients	Observed Patients	Avg. Stay	Vari-ance	Percentiles						
				10th	25th	50th	75th	90th	95th	99th
1. SINGLE DX										
A. Not Operated										
0–19 Years	0									
20–34	0									
35–49	0									
50–64	0									
65+	0									
B. Operated										
0–19 Years	0									
20–34	0									
35–49	0									
50–64	0									
65+	0									
2. MULTIPLE DX										
A. Not Operated										
0–19 Years	1	5.0	0	5	5	5	5	5	5	5
20–34	12	7.8	74	2	2	5	10	16	31	31
35–49	90	6.0	37	1	2	5	8	11	15	39
50–64	142	5.3	23	1	2	4	6	12	14	22
65+	51	4.0	7	1	2	4	4	7	10	14
B. Operated										
0–19 Years	1	20.0	0	20	20	20	20	20	20	20
20–34	4	6.3	12	2	5	8	10	10	10	10
35–49	9	13.6	152	2	7	13	16	43	43	43
50–64	29	11.1	42	5	6	9	14	23	24	27
65+	5	4.8	8	1	3	6	6	8	8	8
SUBTOTALS:										
1. SINGLE DX										
A. Not Operated	0									
B. Operated	0									
2. MULTIPLE DX										
A. Not Operated	296	5.4	27	1	2	4	6	11	14	31
B. Operated	48	10.7	61	3	6	8	14	20	24	43
1. SINGLE DX	0									
2. MULTIPLE DX	344	6.1	35	1	2	4	8	13	18	31
A. NOT OPERATED	296	5.4	27	1	2	4	6	11	14	31
B. OPERATED	48	10.7	61	3	6	8	14	20	24	43
TOTAL										
0–19 Years	2	12.5	113	5	5	13	20	20	20	20
20–34	16	7.4	57	2	2	5	5	10	16	31
35–49	99	6.7	50	1	2	5	9	14	17	43
50–64	171	6.3	31	1	2	5	8	14	19	27
65+	56	4.0	7	1	2	4	5	7	10	14
GRAND TOTAL	344	6.1	35	1	2	4	8	13	18	31

Length of Stay by Diagnosis and Operation, Western Region, 2008

Western Region, October 2006–September 2007 Data, by Diagnosis

573: OTH LIVER DISORDERS

Type of Patients	Observed Patients	Avg. Stay	Vari-ance	Percentiles 10th	25th	50th	75th	90th	95th	99th
1. SINGLE DX										
A. Not Operated										
0–19 Years	5	2.8	2	1	2	3	3	5	5	5
20–34	9	2.9	10	1	1	2	2	10	10	10
35–49	6	1.0	0	1	1	1	1	1	1	1
50–64	10	3.2	11	1	1	2	5	11	11	11
65+	5	3.4	3	2	2	3	4	6	6	6
B. Operated										
0–19 Years	1	2.0	0	2	2	2	2	2	2	2
20–34	1	4.0	0	4	4	4	4	4	4	4
35–49	5	3.0	3	1	2	3	3	6	6	6
50–64	8	2.4	5	1	1	2	2	7	7	7
65+	2	1.5	<1	1	1	1	2	2	2	2
2. MULTIPLE DX										
A. Not Operated										
0–19 Years	59	6.2	137	1	2	3	4	9	29	78
20–34	163	4.0	9	1	2	3	6	7	10	18
35–49	284	4.3	11	1	2	3	6	8	10	16
50–64	379	4.1	12	1	2	3	5	8	10	19
65+	461	4.7	13	1	2	4	6	9	12	17
B. Operated										
0–19 Years	4	6.5	22	2	2	5	13	13	13	13
20–34	18	6.7	23	3	4	5	9	13	21	21
35–49	40	4.6	21	1	2	4	5	7	13	26
50–64	77	6.5	60	2	2	4	7	13	23	45
65+	66	5.0	28	1	2	4	6	10	17	28
SUBTOTALS:										
1. SINGLE DX										
A. Not Operated	35	2.7	6	1	1	2	3	6	10	11
B. Operated	17	2.5	3	1	1	2	3	6	7	7
2. MULTIPLE DX										
A. Not Operated	1,346	4.5	17	1	2	3	6	9	11	19
B. Operated	205	5.7	38	1	2	4	6	12	17	31
1. SINGLE DX	52	2.7	5	1	1	2	3	6	7	11
2. MULTIPLE DX	1,551	4.6	20	1	2	3	6	9	11	22
A. NOT OPERATED	1,381	4.4	17	1	2	3	6	9	11	19
B. OPERATED	222	5.4	36	1	2	4	6	11	16	31
TOTAL										
0–19 Years	69	5.9	119	1	2	3	5	9	26	78
20–34	191	4.2	11	1	2	3	6	8	10	20
35–49	335	4.3	12	1	2	3	6	8	11	16
50–64	474	4.5	20	1	2	3	5	8	11	25
65+	534	4.7	15	1	2	4	6	9	12	19
GRAND TOTAL	1,603	4.5	20	1	2	3	6	9	11	21

573.3: HEPATITIS NOS

Type of Patients	Observed Patients	Avg. Stay	Vari-ance	Percentiles 10th	25th	50th	75th	90th	95th	99th
1. SINGLE DX										
A. Not Operated										
0–19 Years	3	2.3	1	1	1	3	3	3	3	3
20–34	7	3.3	12	1	1	2	6	10	10	10
35–49	3	1.0	0	1	1	1	1	1	1	1
50–64	5	5.0	15	1	2	5	6	11	11	11
65+	0									
B. Operated										
0–19 Years	0									
20–34	0									
35–49	0									
50–64	0									
65+	0									
2. MULTIPLE DX										
A. Not Operated										
0–19 Years	42	3.7	20	1	2	3	4	7	8	29
20–34	122	3.9	8	1	2	3	5	7	9	12
35–49	176	4.1	8	2	2	3	5	8	10	14
50–64	183	3.9	8	1	2	3	5	8	9	15
65+	209	4.6	10	1	2	4	6	9	11	14
B. Operated										
0–19 Years	1	2.0	0	2	2	2	2	2	2	2
20–34	3	6.0	19	3	3	5	11	11	11	11
35–49	2	8.5	40	4	4	4	13	13	13	13
50–64	2	5.0	0	5	5	5	5	5	5	5
65+	4	13.2	39	7	7	9	17	20	20	20
SUBTOTALS:										
1. SINGLE DX										
A. Not Operated	18	3.2	10	1	1	2	5	10	11	11
B. Operated	0									
2. MULTIPLE DX										
A. Not Operated	732	4.1	9	1	2	3	5	8	10	14
B. Operated	12	8.4	34	3	4	7	11	17	20	20
1. SINGLE DX	18	3.2	10	1	1	2	5	10	11	11
2. MULTIPLE DX	744	4.2	10	1	2	3	5	8	10	15
A. NOT OPERATED	750	4.1	9	1	2	3	5	8	10	14
B. OPERATED	12	8.4	34	3	4	7	11	17	20	20
TOTAL										
0–19 Years	46	3.6	18	1	2	3	4	7	8	29
20–34	132	3.9	8	1	2	3	5	7	10	12
35–49	181	4.1	9	2	2	3	5	8	10	14
50–64	190	3.9	8	1	2	3	5	8	10	15
65+	213	4.8	12	2	2	4	6	9	11	17
GRAND TOTAL	762	4.2	10	1	2	3	5	8	10	15

573.8: LIVER DISORDERS NEC

Type of Patients	Observed Patients	Avg. Stay	Vari-ance	Percentiles 10th	25th	50th	75th	90th	95th	99th
1. SINGLE DX										
A. Not Operated										
0–19 Years	1	5.0	0	5	5	5	5	5	5	5
20–34	2	1.5	<1	1	1	2	2	2	2	2
35–49	0									
50–64	2	1.5	<1	1	1	1	2	2	2	2
65+	3	2.3	<1	2	2	2	3	3	3	3
B. Operated										
0–19 Years	0									
20–34	1	4.0	0	4	4	4	4	4	4	4
35–49	5	3.0	3	1	2	3	3	6	6	6
50–64	8	2.4	5	1	1	2	2	7	7	7
65+	2	1.5	<1	1	1	1	2	2	2	2
2. MULTIPLE DX										
A. Not Operated										
0–19 Years	14	14.6	446	2	3	6	17	40	78	78
20–34	30	3.5	6	1	2	3	4	4	9	10
35–49	55	5.2	20	1	2	4	7	10	12	25
50–64	115	4.3	13	1	2	3	5	8	11	16
65+	147	5.2	19	1	2	4	6	11	13	26
B. Operated										
0–19 Years	2	5.5	<1	5	5	5	6	6	6	6
20–34	10	6.5	33	2	3	4	9	21	21	21
35–49	37	4.4	21	1	2	4	4	7	15	26
50–64	72	6.2	62	2	2	4	6	11	23	45
65+	55	4.3	20	1	2	3	5	8	13	28
SUBTOTALS:										
1. SINGLE DX										
A. Not Operated	8	2.3	2	1	2	3	3	5	5	5
B. Operated	16	2.6	3	1	1	2	3	6	7	7
2. MULTIPLE DX										
A. Not Operated	361	5.1	36	1	2	4	6	10	13	26
B. Operated	176	5.2	38	1	2	4	5	10	15	40
1. SINGLE DX	24	2.5	3	1	1	2	3	5	6	7
2. MULTIPLE DX	537	5.2	36	1	2	4	6	10	13	28
A. NOT OPERATED	369	5.1	35	1	2	4	6	10	13	26
B. OPERATED	192	5.0	36	1	2	4	5	9	15	40
TOTAL										
0–19 Years	17	13.0	376	2	3	6	9	40	78	78
20–34	43	4.1	13	1	2	3	5	9	10	21
35–49	97	4.7	19	1	2	4	6	8	12	26
50–64	197	4.9	32	1	2	3	6	9	13	40
65+	207	4.9	19	1	2	4	6	10	13	26
GRAND TOTAL	561	5.0	35	1	2	4	6	9	13	28

Length of Stay by Diagnosis and Operation, Western Region, 2008

Western Region, October 2006–September 2007 Data, by Diagnosis

574: CHOLELITHIASIS

Type of Patients	Observed Patients	Avg. Stay	Variance	10th	25th	50th	75th	90th	95th	99th
1. SINGLE DX										
A. Not Operated										
0–19 Years	73	1.8	1	1	1	1	2	3	3	9
20–34	474	2.2	3	1	1	2	3	4	5	7
35–49	265	2.1	2	1	1	2	3	3	5	6
50–64	142	2.4	3	1	1	2	3	5	6	8
65+	45	2.1	2	1	1	2	2	4	4	8
B. Operated										
0–19 Years	548	2.2	2	1	1	2	3	4	5	7
20–34	3,045	2.1	2	1	1	2	2	4	5	7
35–49	1,763	2.0	2	1	1	2	2	4	5	7
50–64	855	2.0	2	1	1	1	3	4	5	7
65+	230	2.0	2	1	1	1	3	3	5	7
2. MULTIPLE DX										
A. Not Operated										
0–19 Years	191	2.5	3	1	1	2	3	5	6	9
20–34	1,346	2.8	5	1	1	2	3	5	7	11
35–49	1,634	3.0	6	1	1	2	4	6	7	13
50–64	2,334	3.5	9	1	2	3	4	7	9	16
65+	4,690	4.2	11	1	2	3	5	8	10	16
B. Operated										
0–19 Years	1,028	3.2	9	1	2	2	4	6	7	14
20–34	8,914	2.9	6	1	1	2	4	6	7	11
35–49	10,026	3.1	8	1	1	2	4	6	8	14
50–64	11,069	3.7	11	1	2	3	5	7	9	17
65+	13,172	5.1	22	1	2	4	7	10	13	23
SUBTOTALS:										
1. SINGLE DX										
A. Not Operated	999	2.2	2	1	1	2	3	4	5	7
B. Operated	6,441	2.1	2	1	1	2	3	4	5	7
2. MULTIPLE DX										
A. Not Operated	10,195	3.6	9	1	2	3	5	7	9	15
B. Operated	44,209	3.8	13	1	2	3	5	8	10	18
1. SINGLE DX	7,440	2.1	2	1	1	2	3	4	5	7
2. MULTIPLE DX	54,404	3.8	13	1	2	3	5	7	9	18
A. NOT OPERATED	11,194	3.5	9	1	2	3	4	7	9	15
B. OPERATED	50,650	3.6	12	1	1	3	4	7	10	18
TOTAL										
0–19 Years	1,840	2.8	7	1	1	2	3	5	7	12
20–34	13,779	2.7	5	1	1	2	3	5	6	10
35–49	13,688	3.0	7	1	1	2	4	6	7	13
50–64	14,400	3.5	10	1	1	3	4	7	9	16
65+	18,137	4.8	19	1	2	4	6	10	13	21
GRAND TOTAL	61,844	3.6	12	1	2	3	4	7	9	17

574.00: GB CAL W ACUTE CHOL

Type of Patients	Observed Patients	Avg. Stay	Variance	10th	25th	50th	75th	90th	95th	99th
1. SINGLE DX										
A. Not Operated										
0–19 Years	10	2.5	6	1	1	2	3	3	9	9
20–34	106	2.2	2	1	1	2	3	3	6	6
35–49	76	2.1	1	1	1	2	3	4	5	6
50–64	38	2.6	3	1	1	2	3	5	5	8
65+	9	3.3	7	1	1	2	4	8	8	8
B. Operated										
0–19 Years	161	1.9	1	1	1	2	2	3	4	6
20–34	1,052	2.0	1	1	1	2	2	3	4	6
35–49	679	2.0	1	1	1	2	2	3	4	7
50–64	301	2.2	2	1	1	2	3	4	5	7
65+	61	2.3	1	2	2	2	3	3	5	7
2. MULTIPLE DX										
A. Not Operated										
0–19 Years	24	2.4	4	1	1	2	3	6	8	8
20–34	188	2.8	4	1	1	2	4	5	6	11
35–49	260	2.8	5	1	1	3	4	5	7	11
50–64	364	3.7	9	1	2	3	5	7	10	15
65+	707	4.8	12	1	2	4	6	9	11	18
B. Operated										
0–19 Years	415	2.7	5	1	1	2	3	5	6	12
20–34	4,199	2.6	4	1	1	2	3	5	6	9
35–49	4,867	2.9	7	1	2	2	4	5	7	12
50–64	5,130	3.6	10	1	2	3	4	7	9	15
65+	5,547	5.3	19	2	3	4	7	10	13	21
SUBTOTALS:										
1. SINGLE DX										
A. Not Operated	239	2.3	2	1	1	2	3	4	6	8
B. Operated	2,254	2.0	1	1	1	2	3	3	4	6
2. MULTIPLE DX										
A. Not Operated	1,543	3.9	10	1	2	3	5	7	8	16
B. Operated	20,158	3.7	11	1	2	3	5	7	9	17
1. SINGLE DX	2,493	2.1	2	1	1	2	3	3	4	7
2. MULTIPLE DX	21,701	3.7	11	1	2	3	5	7	9	17
A. NOT OPERATED	1,782	3.7	9	1	2	3	5	7	9	15
B. OPERATED	22,412	3.5	10	1	2	3	4	7	9	17
TOTAL										
0–19 Years	610	2.5	4	1	1	2	3	4	5	11
20–34	5,545	2.5	3	1	1	2	3	5	6	9
35–49	5,882	2.8	6	1	1	2	3	5	7	12
50–64	5,833	3.5	9	1	2	3	4	7	9	15
65+	6,324	5.2	18	2	2	4	7	10	13	21
GRAND TOTAL	24,194	3.5	10	1	2	3	4	7	9	17

574.01: GB CAL W AC CHOL-OBSTR

Type of Patients	Observed Patients	Avg. Stay	Variance	10th	25th	50th	75th	90th	95th	99th
1. SINGLE DX										
A. Not Operated										
0–19 Years	0									
20–34	6	2.5	<1	2	2	2	3	4	4	4
35–49	3	2.7	2	1	1	3	4	4	4	4
50–64	0									
65+	1	1.0	0	1	1	1	1	1	1	1
B. Operated										
0–19 Years	8	1.8	1	1	1	2	3	4	4	4
20–34	51	2.2	3	1	1	2	3	5	5	8
35–49	34	2.2	1	1	1	2	3	4	4	5
50–64	19	1.9	2	1	1	2	3	6	6	6
65+	1	1.0	0	1	1	1	1	1	1	1
2. MULTIPLE DX										
A. Not Operated										
0–19 Years	0									
20–34	8	3.6	6	1	1	3	6	7	7	7
35–49	14	5.0	15	2	3	4	5	9	16	16
50–64	32	5.7	26	2	3	4	5	11	16	26
65+	44	6.3	37	1	3	5	7	13	14	37
B. Operated										
0–19 Years	37	3.1	6	1	1	3	3	5	12	12
20–34	273	3.2	5	1	2	2	3	7	8	10
35–49	342	3.6	8	1	1	3	4	7	9	16
50–64	399	4.4	15	1	2	3	5	8	12	19
65+	471	6.0	22	2	3	5	8	12	16	23
SUBTOTALS:										
1. SINGLE DX										
A. Not Operated	10	2.4	1	1	2	3	3	4	4	4
B. Operated	113	2.1	2	1	1	2	3	4	5	7
2. MULTIPLE DX										
A. Not Operated	98	5.7	28	1	3	4	6	12	16	37
B. Operated	1,522	4.5	15	1	2	3	6	9	12	21
1. SINGLE DX	123	2.1	2	1	1	2	3	4	5	7
2. MULTIPLE DX	1,620	4.5	16	1	2	3	6	9	12	21
A. NOT OPERATED	108	5.4	26	1	3	4	6	11	14	26
B. OPERATED	1,635	4.3	15	1	2	3	5	9	12	21
TOTAL										
0–19 Years	45	2.9	6	1	1	3	3	4	7	12
20–34	338	3.0	5	1	2	2	4	6	8	10
35–49	393	3.5	8	1	2	3	4	7	9	16
50–64	450	4.4	15	2	3	5	7	8	12	19
65+	517	6.0	24	2	3	5	7	12	16	23
GRAND TOTAL	1,743	4.4	15	1	2	3	5	9	12	21

Length of Stay by Diagnosis and Operation, Western Region, 2008

TOOLS TO GROW YOUR BUSINESS

FROM BENCHMARKING TOOLS FOR INDUSTRY-WIDE INFORMATION TO CUSTOMIZED HOSPITAL-SPECIFIC REPORTS, CHOOSE FROM A VARIETY OF PUBLICATIONS TO MEET YOUR NEEDS. AVAILABLE IN SOFTBOUND, PDF, AND DATA FILE FORMATS.

Hospital Benchmarking Tools and Guides

The Sourcebook—Hospital data by comparison group
The gold standard for measuring hospital operations and financial performance—with five years of proprietary comparative and historical data on nearly 60 key performance measures for 150+ hospital comparison groups. This guide gives true apples-to-apples comparisons.

Profiles of U.S. Hospitals—Individual data on 6,000+ hospitals
Current and in-depth data available on the financial, operational, and clinical performance of nearly every hospital in the United States. The perfect resource for hospital CEOs and CFOs, industry consultants and suppliers, investment bankers, and more.

The DRG Handbook—Six pages of data for each DRG
Detailed clinical, financial, and statistical data on 100 of the most significant diagnosis-related groups (DRGs) for both all-payer and Medicare patient groups.

Length of Stay Series—Data-based LOS norms trusted for more than 40 years
On-target length of stay (LOS) and benchmark information for every ICD-9-CM code. Compiled from an all-payer database representing approximately 20 million discharges.

Thomson Reuters 100 Top Hospitals® Benchmarks Reports

100 Top Hospitals Study Benchmarks Reports
An attractive printed document that lists award winners; describes the program, including database details, criteria, and methodologies; and outlines exciting findings on how the 100 Top Hospitals are setting performance benchmarks.

100 Top Hospitals: National Benchmarks Reports
These new reports are an affordable way to view a snapshot of a hospital's performance—individually, in relation to its peers, and in comparison to the 100 Top Hospitals winners. Reports help to assess current performance and five-year direction and speed of change against the latest benchmarks and peers, and to identify strengths and weaknesses to set performance targets.

100 Top Hospitals: Cardiovascular Benchmarks Reports
Performance measure scores and graphical analysis help you assess your performance against the latest 100 Top Hospitals cardiovascular benchmarks. Performance is evaluated in four key cardiovascular treatment areas for Medicare patients: heart failure, heart attack, angioplasty, and bypass surgery.

100 Top Hospitals Unlimited Access
Includes unlimited access to the most recent 100 Top Hospitals National and Cardiovascular Results Reports, 10 Performance Improvement Leaders Reports, all other 100 Top Hospitals study results released within 12 months, and free PDFs of study publications.

FOR MORE INFORMATION Visit http://provider.thomsonhealthcare.com/Hospitals/Publications/

To place an order with our Sales Department, please complete the information on the back and submit via:

- Fax +1 866 314 9717
- Ph +1 616 248 4645
- E-mail healthcare.pubs@thomsonreuters.com
- Invoice will be mailed separately from shipment.

HEALTHCARE

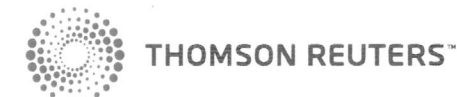

THOMSON REUTERS™

<table>
<tr><td colspan="2">**SHIP-TO INFORMATION**</td><td colspan="2">**BILL-TO INFORMATION (IF DIFFERENT FROM SHIP-TO)**</td></tr>
<tr><td colspan="2">Name:</td><td colspan="2">Name:</td></tr>
<tr><td colspan="2">Title:</td><td colspan="2">Title:</td></tr>
<tr><td colspan="2">Organization:</td><td colspan="2">Organization:</td></tr>
<tr><td colspan="2">Address:</td><td colspan="2">Address:</td></tr>
<tr><td colspan="2">City:</td><td colspan="2">City:</td></tr>
<tr><td colspan="2">State:</td><td colspan="2">State:</td></tr>
<tr><td colspan="2">ZIP Code:</td><td colspan="2">ZIP Code:</td></tr>
<tr><td colspan="2">Phone:</td><td colspan="2">Phone:</td></tr>
<tr><td colspan="2">Fax:</td><td colspan="2">Fax:</td></tr>
<tr><td colspan="2">E-Mail:</td><td colspan="2">E-Mail:</td></tr>
</table>

SHIPPING (PLEASE CHECK ONE)

If you have a FedEx or UPS account that you prefer to use, please indicate here:

☐ Ground: $8.95 (covers up to 5 books to one location)

☐ Priority: $18.25 (covers one book or one CD, $4.00 for each additional book)

☐ Standard: $17.25 (covers one book or one CD, $4.00 for each additional book)

☐ 2-Day: $9.25 (covers one book or one CD, $4.00 for each additional book)

SOURCEBOOK

Format	Price	Quantity
Softbound Book	$799	
PDF CD-ROM (1-2 users)	$849	
PDF CD-ROM (3-5 users)	$1,200	
PDF CD-ROM (6 or more users)	$3,000	
ASCII Data File CD (1 user)	$1,399	
Each additional user ASCII	$300	
	Subtotal*	

LENGTH OF STAY

Format	Version	Regular Price	Quantity
Softbound	United States	$599	
	Western Region	$599	
	Southern Region	$599	
	North Central Region	$599	
	Northeastern Region	$599	
	Pediatric	$599	
	Complete Set (includes all versions above)	$1,549	
CD-ROM (PDF file)	1-2 users	$535	
	3-5 users	$1,035	
	6 or more users	$3,000	
		Subtotal*	

PAYMENT METHOD (PLEASE CHECK ONE)

☐ If you have a purchase order #, please indicate here: _____

☐ Invoice me now (payment due in 30 days)

	SUBTOTAL
Sourcebook	
Length of Stay	
DRG Handbook	
Profiles of U.S. Hospitals	
100 Top Hospitals	
Shipping Subtotal	
TOTAL	

DRG HANDBOOK

100 Top DRGs	Price	Quantity
Softbound Book	$649	
PDF CD-ROM (1-2 users)	$657	
PDF CD-ROM (3-5 users)	$1,255	
PDF CD-ROM (6 or more users)	$3,000	

Prices for All DRGs (543)	Price	Quantity
ASCII Data File All DRGs (1 user)	$1,464	
Each additional user	$315	
	Subtotal*	

PROFILES OF U.S. HOSPITALS

Format	Price	Quantity
Softbound Book	$559	
PDF (1-2 users)	$549	
PDF (3-5 users)	$950	
PDF (6 or more users)	$3,000	
ASCII Data File (1 user)	$1,399	
Each additional user	$300	
	Subtotal*	

To place an order with our Sales Department, please complete this form and submit via:

- Fax +1 866 314 9717
- Ph +1 616 248 4645
- E-mail healthcare.pubs@ thomsonreuters.com

THOMSON REUTERS 100 TOP HOSPITALS® REPORTS

Please Indicate Hospital Name, City/State, and Type (National or Cardiovascular)

	Type	Price	Quantity
1) Hospital Name, City/State, Type:	National	$1,700	
2) Hospital Name, City/State, Type:	Cardiovascular	$1,195	
3) Hospital Name, City/State, Type:			
4) Unlimited Access			
		Subtotal*	

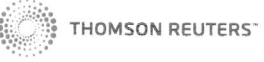 THOMSON REUTERS™

574.10: GB CALCULUS W CHOL NEC

Type of Patients	Observed Patients	Avg. Stay	Vari-ance	10th	25th	50th	75th	90th	95th	99th
1. SINGLE DX										
A. Not Operated										
0–19 Years	5	1.4	<1	1	1	1	2	2	2	2
20–34	52	1.6	<1	1	1	1	2	3	4	4
35–49	30	1.8	2	1	1	1	2	4	5	5
50–64	9	1.8	2	1	1	1	2	5	5	5
65+	1	1.0	0	1	1	1	1	1	1	1
B. Operated										
0–19 Years	190	1.7	<1	1	1	1	2	3	4	5
20–34	1,107	1.7	<1	1	1	1	2	3	4	5
35–49	675	1.5	1	1	1	1	2	3	3	6
50–64	361	1.5	<1	1	1	1	2	3	3	6
65+	105	1.6	2	1	1	1	2	3	4	5
2. MULTIPLE DX										
A. Not Operated										
0–19 Years	19	1.6	<1	1	1	1	2	3	4	4
20–34	116	2.4	3	1	1	2	3	5	7	9
35–49	156	2.7	5	1	1	2	3	6	8	10
50–64	219	3.4	12	1	1	2	4	7	9	12
65+	385	3.6	8	1	2	3	4	7	10	14
B. Operated										
0–19 Years	226	2.7	11	1	1	2	3	5	6	11
20–34	2,259	2.5	4	1	1	2	3	5	6	10
35–49	2,797	2.8	7	1	1	2	3	5	7	13
50–64	3,194	3.0	8	1	1	2	4	6	8	15
65+	3,700	3.6	15	1	1	2	5	7	10	18
SUBTOTALS:										
1. SINGLE DX										
A. Not Operated	97	1.7	1	1	1	1	2	3	4	5
B. Operated	2,438	1.6	1	1	1	1	2	3	4	5
2. MULTIPLE DX										
A. Not Operated	895	3.2	8	1	1	2	4	7	9	13
B. Operated	12,176	3.0	9	1	1	2	4	6	8	15
1. SINGLE DX	2,535	1.6	1	1	1	1	2	3	4	5
2. MULTIPLE DX	13,071	3.0	9	1	1	2	4	6	8	15
A. NOT OPERATED	992	3.0	7	1	1	2	4	6	8	12
B. OPERATED	14,614	2.8	8	1	1	2	3	6	8	14
TOTAL										
0–19 Years	440	2.2	7	1	1	2	3	4	5	8
20–34	3,534	2.2	3	1	1	2	3	4	5	9
35–49	3,658	2.5	6	1	1	2	3	5	7	12
50–64	3,783	2.8	8	1	1	2	4	6	8	14
65+	4,191	3.5	14	1	2	2	5	7	10	17
GRAND TOTAL	15,606	2.8	8	1	1	2	3	6	8	14

574.11: GB CAL W CHOL NEC-OBSTR

Type of Patients	Observed Patients	Avg. Stay	Vari-ance	10th	25th	50th	75th	90th	95th	99th
1. SINGLE DX										
A. Not Operated										
0–19 Years	0									
20–34	3	1.3	<1	1	1	1	2	2	2	2
35–49	2	1.5	<1	1	1	2	2	2	2	2
50–64	0									
65+	0									
B. Operated										
0–19 Years	5	3.0	2	2	2	4	4	4	4	4
20–34	20	1.7	1	1	1	1	2	3	4	5
35–49	12	1.9	1	1	1	2	3	3	4	4
50–64	3	2.0	<1	1	1	2	2	3	3	3
65+	4	1.5	<1	1	1	2	2	2	2	2
2. MULTIPLE DX										
A. Not Operated										
0–19 Years	1	3.0	0	3	3	3	3	3	3	3
20–34	1	3.0	0	3	3	3	3	3	3	3
35–49	8	5.1	17	2	3	4	4	15	15	15
50–64	8	8.0	24	2	4	8	13	16	16	16
65+	22	5.8	15	1	4	5	7	12	13	16
B. Operated										
0–19 Years	4	3.0	7	1	2	2	7	7	7	7
20–34	86	3.4	8	1	2	3	4	6	7	22
35–49	91	3.2	8	1	1	3	4	6	8	22
50–64	100	4.1	13	1	2	3	6	8	10	23
65+	111	6.0	24	1	2	5	8	13	17	22
SUBTOTALS:										
1. SINGLE DX										
A. Not Operated	5	1.4	<1	1	1	1	2	2	2	2
B. Operated	44	1.9	1	1	1	1	3	4	4	5
2. MULTIPLE DX										
A. Not Operated	40	6.0	17	2	3	4	8	13	16	16
B. Operated	392	4.3	15	1	2	3	5	8	12	22
1. SINGLE DX	49	1.8	1	1	1	1	2	4	4	5
2. MULTIPLE DX	432	4.4	15	1	2	3	6	9	13	22
A. NOT OPERATED	45	5.5	17	1	3	4	7	13	15	16
B. OPERATED	436	4.0	14	1	2	3	5	8	11	22
TOTAL										
0–19 Years	10	3.0	3	1	2	3	4	4	7	7
20–34	110	3.0	7	1	1	3	4	5	5	14
35–49	113	3.2	8	1	1	3	4	6	8	15
50–64	111	4.3	14	1	2	3	6	9	10	18
65+	137	5.8	22	1	2	5	8	13	16	22
GRAND TOTAL	481	4.1	15	1	2	3	5	8	12	22

574.20: GB CALCULUS W/O CHOL

Type of Patients	Observed Patients	Avg. Stay	Vari-ance	10th	25th	50th	75th	90th	95th	99th
1. SINGLE DX										
A. Not Operated										
0–19 Years	21	1.1	<1	1	1	1	1	1	2	2
20–34	101	1.3	<1	1	1	1	1	2	2	3
35–49	61	1.5	<1	1	1	1	2	3	3	4
50–64	31	1.6	2	1	1	1	2	2	5	8
65+	13	1.5	<1	1	1	1	2	3	3	3
B. Operated										
0–19 Years	44	1.7	2	1	1	1	2	4	5	6
20–34	179	1.8	2	1	1	1	2	4	5	6
35–49	134	1.8	2	1	1	1	2	4	5	8
50–64	57	1.5	<1	1	1	1	2	3	4	5
65+	23	1.1	<1	1	1	1	1	2	2	2
2. MULTIPLE DX										
A. Not Operated										
0–19 Years	56	1.7	1	1	1	1	2	3	3	7
20–34	333	2.0	2	1	1	2	3	4	4	7
35–49	450	2.5	5	1	1	2	3	5	6	10
50–64	628	2.7	6	1	1	2	3	5	6	13
65+	1,021	3.1	7	1	1	2	4	6	8	14
B. Operated										
0–19 Years	70	2.7	4	1	1	2	3	5	6	12
20–34	356	2.6	3	1	1	2	3	5	6	9
35–49	460	2.5	4	1	1	2	3	5	7	9
50–64	516	2.7	7	1	1	2	4	5	7	13
65+	498	3.3	12	1	2	2	4	7	9	16
SUBTOTALS:										
1. SINGLE DX										
A. Not Operated	227	1.4	<1	1	1	1	2	2	3	4
B. Operated	437	1.7	2	1	1	1	2	3	5	6
2. MULTIPLE DX										
A. Not Operated	2,488	2.7	6	1	1	2	3	5	7	13
B. Operated	1,900	2.8	7	1	1	2	4	6	7	13
1. SINGLE DX	664	1.6	1	1	1	1	2	3	4	6
2. MULTIPLE DX	4,388	2.8	6	1	1	2	3	5	7	13
A. NOT OPERATED	2,715	2.6	5	1	1	2	3	5	7	12
B. OPERATED	2,337	2.6	6	1	1	2	3	5	7	11
TOTAL										
0–19 Years	191	2.0	2	1	1	1	3	4	5	7
20–34	969	2.1	2	1	1	2	3	4	5	8
35–49	1,105	2.3	4	1	1	2	3	5	6	9
50–64	1,232	2.7	6	1	1	2	3	5	7	13
65+	1,555	3.1	8	1	2	2	4	6	8	15
GRAND TOTAL	5,052	2.6	6	1	1	2	3	5	7	12

Length of Stay by Diagnosis and Operation, Western Region, 2008

Western Region, October 2006–September 2007 Data, by Diagnosis

574.30: BD CAL W ACUTE CHOL

Type of Patients	Observed Patients	Avg. Stay	Vari-ance	Percentiles						
				10th	25th	50th	75th	90th	95th	99th
1. SINGLE DX										
A. Not Operated										
0–19 Years	2	3.0	2	2	2	3	4	4	4	4
20–34	2	3.0	8	1	1	1	5	5	5	5
35–49	5	4.6	9	1	2	6	6	8	8	8
50–64	6	3.5	2	2	2	4	4	6	6	6
65+	2	2.0	2	1	1	1	3	3	3	3
B. Operated										
0–19 Years	5	3.6	2	2	3	3	5	5	5	5
20–34	35	3.2	3	1	2	3	4	6	6	9
35–49	17	4.2	10	2	2	4	4	9	14	14
50–64	3	5.0	4	3	3	5	7	7	7	7
65+	1	4.0	0	4	4	4	4	4	4	4
2. MULTIPLE DX										
A. Not Operated										
0–19 Years	3	3.7	4	2	2	3	6	6	6	6
20–34	15	4.0	4	2	3	3	5	7	9	9
35–49	17	3.4	4	1	2	3	4	6	9	9
50–64	15	3.8	7	1	2	3	5	7	11	11
65+	60	5.1	14	2	3	4	6	9	11	22
B. Operated										
0–19 Years	14	5.4	13	2	2	5	10	11	11	11
20–34	111	4.5	10	2	3	4	5	7	10	18
35–49	74	4.6	6	2	3	4	6	8	10	12
50–64	117	4.8	11	2	3	4	6	8	12	14
65+	159	6.6	20	2	4	6	8	13	17	23
SUBTOTALS:										
1. SINGLE DX										
A. Not Operated	17	3.5	4	1	2	3	5	6	8	8
B. Operated	61	3.6	5	1	2	3	4	6	7	14
2. MULTIPLE DX										
A. Not Operated	110	4.5	10	2	3	4	5	9	9	16
B. Operated	475	5.3	14	2	3	4	6	10	13	20
1. SINGLE DX	78	3.6	5	1	2	3	5	6	8	14
2. MULTIPLE DX	585	5.2	13	2	3	4	6	10	12	20
A. NOT OPERATED	127	4.3	9	2	2	4	5	9	9	16
B. OPERATED	536	5.1	13	2	3	4	6	10	12	19
TOTAL										
0–19 Years	24	4.6	9	2	2	3	6	10	11	11
20–34	163	4.1	8	1	2	3	5	6	9	18
35–49	113	4.4	6	2	3	4	6	8	9	12
50–64	141	4.7	10	2	2	4	6	9	11	14
65+	222	6.2	19	2	3	5	8	12	14	22
GRAND TOTAL	663	5.0	13	2	3	4	6	9	12	19

574.31: BD CAL W AC CHOL-OBSTR

Type of Patients	Observed Patients	Avg. Stay	Vari-ance	Percentiles						
				10th	25th	50th	75th	90th	95th	99th
1. SINGLE DX										
A. Not Operated										
0–19 Years	0									
20–34	1	2.0	0	2	2	2	2	2	2	2
35–49	0									
50–64	0									
65+	0									
B. Operated										
0–19 Years	1	6.0	0	6	6	6	6	6	6	6
20–34	14	3.0	4	2	2	2	3	4	4	9
35–49	4	2.5	4	1	1	2	4	5	5	5
50–64	3	2.7	2	1	1	3	4	4	4	4
65+	1	1.0	0	1	1	1	1	1	1	1
2. MULTIPLE DX										
A. Not Operated										
0–19 Years	2	6.5	<1	6	6	6	7	7	7	7
20–34	10	4.7	8	1	3	4	6	7	11	11
35–49	14	3.3	2	2	2	3	5	6	6	6
50–64	19	5.1	16	2	3	4	6	10	19	19
65+	41	6.2	44	2	2	4	7	11	16	40
B. Operated										
0–19 Years	2	5.0	2	4	4	5	6	6	6	6
20–34	51	4.4	6	2	3	4	5	7	10	13
35–49	47	5.0	10	2	3	5	7	11	11	16
50–64	76	6.0	14	3	4	5	7	10	11	19
65+	141	7.4	29	3	4	6	9	15	16	28
SUBTOTALS:										
1. SINGLE DX										
A. Not Operated	1	2.0	0	2	2	2	2	2	2	2
B. Operated	23	2.9	3	1	2	2	4	5	6	9
2. MULTIPLE DX										
A. Not Operated	86	5.3	26	2	3	4	6	10	11	40
B. Operated	317	6.2	20	3	3	5	7	11	16	24
1. SINGLE DX	24	2.9	3	1	2	2	3	5	6	9
2. MULTIPLE DX	403	6.0	21	2	3	5	7	11	15	24
A. NOT OPERATED	87	5.3	26	2	2	4	6	10	11	40
B. OPERATED	340	6.0	20	2	3	5	7	11	15	24
TOTAL										
0–19 Years	5	5.8	1	4	6	6	6	7	7	7
20–34	76	4.1	6	2	2	3	5	7	10	13
35–49	65	4.5	9	2	3	4	5	8	11	16
50–64	98	5.7	14	2	3	5	7	10	16	19
65+	183	7.1	32	2	4	6	8	15	16	33
GRAND TOTAL	427	5.9	21	2	3	5	7	11	15	24

574.40: BD CALCULUS W CHOL NEC

Type of Patients	Observed Patients	Avg. Stay	Vari-ance	Percentiles						
				10th	25th	50th	75th	90th	95th	99th
1. SINGLE DX										
A. Not Operated										
0–19 Years	1	3.0	0	3	3	3	3	3	3	3
20–34	3	4.3	1	3	3	5	5	5	5	5
35–49	2	3.5	12	1	1	4	4	6	6	6
50–64	2	4.0	2	3	3	3	5	5	5	5
65+	0									
B. Operated										
0–19 Years	5	3.0	2	1	2	4	4	4	4	4
20–34	22	3.4	5	2	2	3	3	6	8	9
35–49	8	3.1	2	1	1	3	3	6	6	6
50–64	4	1.5	<1	1	1	1	2	2	2	2
65+	3	2.0	<1	1	1	2	3	3	3	3
2. MULTIPLE DX										
A. Not Operated										
0–19 Years	5	2.4	1	1	1	2	3	3	4	4
20–34	9	2.1	2	1	1	2	3	5	5	5
35–49	10	5.1	22	1	2	4	8	16	16	16
50–64	16	3.0	3	1	2	3	3	6	7	7
65+	50	4.6	4	2	3	5	6	7	8	10
B. Operated										
0–19 Years	8	4.4	10	1	3	4	5	11	11	11
20–34	62	4.5	10	1	2	4	5	8	9	17
35–49	52	4.2	6	1	2	4	5	6	9	10
50–64	55	4.8	11	1	2	4	6	10	13	14
65+	96	5.9	22	2	3	4	7	11	16	25
SUBTOTALS:										
1. SINGLE DX										
A. Not Operated	8	3.9	3	1	3	3	5	6	6	6
B. Operated	42	3.0	3	1	2	2	4	5	6	9
2. MULTIPLE DX										
A. Not Operated	90	4.0	6	1	2	3	6	7	8	16
B. Operated	273	5.0	14	2	2	4	6	9	11	20
1. SINGLE DX	50	3.1	3	1	2	3	4	6	6	9
2. MULTIPLE DX	363	4.7	12	2	2	4	6	9	11	17
A. NOT OPERATED	98	4.0	6	1	2	3	5	7	8	16
B. OPERATED	315	4.7	13	2	2	4	6	9	11	17
TOTAL										
0–19 Years	19	3.4	5	1	2	3	4	6	6	11
20–34	96	4.0	8	2	2	3	5	8	9	17
35–49	72	4.2	8	1	2	4	5	8	9	16
50–64	77	4.2	9	1	2	3	5	10	11	14
65+	149	5.4	16	2	3	4	7	9	11	24
GRAND TOTAL	413	4.5	11	1	2	4	6	8	11	17

Length of Stay by Diagnosis and Operation, Western Region, 2008

Western Region, October 2006–September 2007 Data, by Diagnosis

574.41: BD CAL W CHOL NEC-OBSTR

Type of Patients	Observed Patients	Avg. Stay	Vari-ance	10th	25th	50th	75th	90th	95th	99th
1. SINGLE DX										
A. Not Operated										
0–19 Years	1	2.0	0	2	2	2	2	2	2	2
20–34	0									
35–49	1	5.0	0	5	5	5	5	5	5	5
50–64	2	3.0	2	2	2	3	4	5	5	4
65+	0									
B. Operated										
0–19 Years	2	4.0	2	3	3	3	5	5	5	5
20–34	5	3.4	3	2	2	3	4	6	6	6
35–49	6	4.7	12	1	2	4	8	9	9	9
50–64	0									
65+	0									
2. MULTIPLE DX										
A. Not Operated										
0–19 Years	0									
20–34	7	3.9	7	1	2	3	5	6	9	9
35–49	3	4.0	0	4	4	4	4	4	4	4
50–64	12	6.7	39	2	2	4	8	16	21	21
65+	44	4.8	9	2	3	4	6	8	10	16
B. Operated										
0–19 Years	2	13.9	198	4	4	4	24	24	24	24
20–34	36	4.7	14	2	3	4	5	8	10	23
35–49	32	5.1	12	2	3	4	6	10	13	16
50–64	39	8.1	47	2	3	6	11	20	24	31
65+	64	7.3	20	3	4	6	9	13	15	23
SUBTOTALS:										
1. SINGLE DX										
A. Not Operated	4	3.3	2	2	2	2	5	5	5	5
B. Operated	13	4.1	6	2	2	3	6	8	9	9
2. MULTIPLE DX										
A. Not Operated	66	5.0	14	2	3	4	6	9	13	21
B. Operated	173	6.6	27	2	3	5	8	13	18	24
1. SINGLE DX	17	3.9	5	2	2	3	5	8	9	9
2. MULTIPLE DX	239	6.2	24	2	3	5	8	13	16	24
A. NOT OPERATED	70	4.9	13	2	3	4	6	8	13	21
B. OPERATED	186	6.4	26	2	3	5	8	13	16	24
TOTAL										
0–19 Years	5	7.5	84	2	3	4	5	24	24	24
20–34	48	4.4	12	2	3	4	5	8	9	23
35–49	42	4.9	11	2	3	4	6	9	12	16
50–64	53	7.6	44	2	3	6	10	18	21	31
65+	108	6.3	17	2	3	5	8	13	14	21
GRAND TOTAL	256	6.0	23	2	3	4	7	12	16	24

574.50: BD CAL W/O CHOLECYSTITIS

Type of Patients	Observed Patients	Avg. Stay	Vari-ance	10th	25th	50th	75th	90th	95th	99th
1. SINGLE DX										
A. Not Operated										
0–19 Years	17	1.9	1	1	1	2	2	3	5	5
20–34	103	2.7	6	1	2	2	3	4	5	7
35–49	45	2.5	2	1	2	2	3	5	5	8
50–64	28	2.7	3	1	2	2	4	6	6	7
65+	14	1.8	<1	1	2	2	2	3	4	4
B. Operated										
0–19 Years	5	4.0	8	1	1	5	6	7	7	7
20–34	20	5.0	12	1	2	4	7	9	14	14
35–49	8	5.0	15	1	2	3	10	11	14	11
50–64	7	3.4	8	1	1	3	6	8	8	8
65+	3	5.0	4	3	3	5	7	7	7	7
2. MULTIPLE DX										
A. Not Operated										
0–19 Years	37	3.0	3	1	2	2	3	6	7	9
20–34	312	3.1	5	1	2	3	4	5	7	12
35–49	318	3.1	3	1	2	3	4	6	7	8
50–64	457	3.5	7	1	2	3	4	7	8	13
65+	848	4.0	8	1	2	3	5	7	9	13
B. Operated										
0–19 Years	3	2.7	<1	2	2	3	3	3	3	3
20–34	37	4.1	6	2	3	3	5	7	8	13
35–49	44	5.0	15	1	2	4	6	10	14	19
50–64	38	5.6	15	2	3	5	7	10	13	21
65+	70	5.9	13	2	4	5	8	9	12	18
SUBTOTALS:										
1. SINGLE DX										
A. Not Operated	207	2.6	4	1	2	2	3	4	5	7
B. Operated	43	4.6	10	1	2	4	7	9	10	14
2. MULTIPLE DX										
A. Not Operated	1,972	3.6	6	1	2	3	5	7	8	13
B. Operated	192	5.2	12	2	3	4	8	9	12	19
1. SINGLE DX	250	2.9	6	1	2	2	3	5	7	11
2. MULTIPLE DX	2,164	3.7	7	1	2	3	5	7	8	13
A. NOT OPERATED	2,179	3.5	6	1	2	3	4	6	8	12
B. OPERATED	235	5.1	12	2	3	4	7	9	11	18
TOTAL										
0–19 Years	62	2.8	3	1	2	2	3	5	6	9
20–34	472	3.2	6	1	2	3	4	6	7	13
35–49	415	3.3	5	1	2	3	4	6	7	11
50–64	530	3.6	7	1	2	3	5	7	9	13
65+	935	4.1	8	1	2	3	5	7	9	14
GRAND TOTAL	2,414	3.7	7	1	2	3	5	7	8	13

574.51: BD CAL W/O CHOL-OBSTR

Type of Patients	Observed Patients	Avg. Stay	Vari-ance	10th	25th	50th	75th	90th	95th	99th
1. SINGLE DX										
A. Not Operated										
0–19 Years	3	2.0	0	2	2	2	2	2	2	2
20–34	26	2.5	1	1	2	2	3	4	4	5
35–49	16	2.6	2	1	2	2	3	4	6	6
50–64	11	2.5	3	1	1	2	4	4	6	6
65+	2	2.0	0	2	2	2	2	2	2	2
B. Operated										
0–19 Years	1	3.0	0	3	3	3	3	3	3	3
20–34	6	4.2	4	2	2	4	6	7	7	7
35–49	3	4.0	<1	3	3	4	5	5	5	5
50–64	2	5.5	5	4	4	6	6	7	7	7
65+	1	2.0	0	2	2	2	2	2	2	2
2. MULTIPLE DX										
A. Not Operated										
0–19 Years	16	2.8	2	2	2	3	3	5	6	6
20–34	170	3.4	5	2	2	3	4	7	8	11
35–49	183	3.8	12	2	3	3	4	6	8	22
50–64	296	4.0	9	2	3	3	5	8	9	17
65+	794	4.7	11	3	3	4	6	9	11	17
B. Operated										
0–19 Years	4	3.0	2	2	2	3	3	5	5	5
20–34	28	7.8	231	2	3	4	8	9	15	84
35–49	21	6.0	17	2	3	5	7	13	14	14
50–64	33	8.0	38	3	5	7	9	11	23	33
65+	74	9.9	57	3	5	8	13	20	26	44
SUBTOTALS:										
1. SINGLE DX										
A. Not Operated	58	2.5	1	1	2	2	3	4	5	6
B. Operated	13	4.1	3	2	3	4	5	7	7	7
2. MULTIPLE DX										
A. Not Operated	1,459	4.3	10	2	3	3	5	8	10	17
B. Operated	160	8.4	78	3	4	6	9	17	23	44
1. SINGLE DX	71	2.8	2	1	2	2	4	4	6	7
2. MULTIPLE DX	1,619	4.7	18	2	3	4	6	9	11	21
A. NOT OPERATED	1,517	4.2	10	2	3	3	5	8	10	16
B. OPERATED	173	8.1	73	2	4	6	9	16	23	44
TOTAL										
0–19 Years	24	2.7	2	2	2	2	3	5	5	6
20–34	230	3.9	34	2	2	3	4	7	8	15
35–49	223	3.9	12	1	2	3	5	7	12	20
50–64	342	4.3	13	1	3	4	6	8	10	19
65+	871	5.1	17	2	3	4	6	9	13	21
GRAND TOTAL	1,690	4.6	18	2	2	3	6	9	11	21

Length of Stay by Diagnosis and Operation, Western Region, 2008

Western Region, October 2006–September 2007 Data, by Diagnosis

574.60: GB & BD CAL W AC CHOL

Type of Patients	Observed Patients	Avg. Stay	Vari-ance	10th	25th	50th	75th	90th	95th	99th
1. SINGLE DX										
A. Not Operated										
0–19 Years	2	1.5	<1	1	1	1	2	2	2	2
20–34	10	2.6	2	1	2	2	3	6	6	6
35–49	6	2.7	2	1	2	2	3	5	5	5
50–64	3	3.7	6	1	1	4	6	6	6	6
65+	0									
B. Operated										
0–19 Years	14	3.2	2	2	2	3	4	5	7	7
20–34	108	3.4	3	2	2	3	4	4	6	7
35–49	42	3.2	3	2	2	3	4	5	6	8
50–64	20	4.0	5	2	3	4	5	7	11	11
65+	6	2.3	1	1	1	2	3	4	4	4
2. MULTIPLE DX										
A. Not Operated										
0–19 Years	3	4.0	3	3	3	3	5	6	6	6
20–34	14	2.9	3	1	1	3	5	6	6	6
35–49	18	4.7	20	1	2	4	6	9	20	20
50–64	31	4.9	11	2	3	4	6	8	11	18
65+	70	4.6	11	2	3	4	6	8	9	22
B. Operated										
0–19 Years	32	3.8	4	2	2	3	5	7	8	10
20–34	235	4.0	6	1	2	4	5	7	9	13
35–49	229	4.4	11	2	3	4	5	8	10	18
50–64	254	5.1	14	2	3	4	6	9	12	20
65+	341	6.9	34	3	4	5	8	12	15	32
SUBTOTALS:										
1. SINGLE DX										
A. Not Operated	21	2.7	2	1	2	2	3	5	6	6
B. Operated	190	3.4	3	2	2	3	4	6	7	9
2. MULTIPLE DX										
A. Not Operated	136	4.5	11	2	3	4	5	8	9	20
B. Operated	1,091	5.2	19	2	3	4	6	10	12	24
1. SINGLE DX	211	3.3	3	1	2	3	4	5	6	8
2. MULTIPLE DX	1,227	5.2	18	2	3	4	6	9	12	24
A. NOT OPERATED	157	4.3	10	1	2	4	5	8	9	20
B. OPERATED	1,281	5.0	17	2	3	4	6	9	11	24
TOTAL										
0–19 Years	51	3.5	4	2	2	3	4	6	7	10
20–34	367	3.7	5	1	2	3	5	6	7	11
35–49	295	4.2	11	2	2	4	5	7	9	20
50–64	308	5.0	13	2	3	4	6	9	11	18
65+	417	6.4	30	2	3	5	8	12	15	32
GRAND TOTAL	1,438	4.9	16	2	3	4	6	9	11	20

574.61: GB&BD CAL/AC CHOL-OBSTR

Type of Patients	Observed Patients	Avg. Stay	Vari-ance	10th	25th	50th	75th	90th	95th	99th
1. SINGLE DX										
A. Not Operated										
0–19 Years	0									
20–34	5	4.6	3	2	4	5	5	7	7	7
35–49	1	1.0	0	1	1	1	1	1	1	1
50–64	2	1.5	<1	1	1	2	2	2	2	2
65+	0									
B. Operated										
0–19 Years	15	2.9	2	2	2	3	3	5	6	6
20–34	40	2.9	2	2	2	3	4	5	6	7
35–49	14	3.1	2	1	2	3	5	5	6	6
50–64	7	4.0	6	1	3	3	5	9	9	9
65+	0									
2. MULTIPLE DX										
A. Not Operated										
0–19 Years	1	2.0	0	2	2	2	2	2	2	2
20–34	14	4.2	7	2	3	3	5	8	11	11
35–49	12	2.9	4	1	1	2	4	6	7	7
50–64	18	6.0	20	1	3	5	8	14	16	16
65+	45	5.4	14	2	3	4	6	11	12	19
B. Operated										
0–19 Years	29	4.2	5	2	3	3	5	9	9	9
20–34	125	4.1	5	2	3	4	6	7	7	13
35–49	125	5.1	19	2	3	4	6	8	14	22
50–64	155	5.5	30	2	3	4	6	9	14	32
65+	247	7.5	40	3	4	6	9	13	19	37
SUBTOTALS:										
1. SINGLE DX										
A. Not Operated	8	3.4	5	1	2	4	5	7	7	7
B. Operated	76	3.1	2	1	2	3	4	5	6	9
2. MULTIPLE DX										
A. Not Operated	90	5.0	13	2	2	4	6	11	12	19
B. Operated	681	5.9	28	2	3	4	7	10	14	32
1. SINGLE DX	84	3.1	3	1	2	3	4	5	6	9
2. MULTIPLE DX	771	5.7	26	2	3	4	7	11	14	29
A. NOT OPERATED	98	4.8	13	2	2	4	6	11	12	19
B. OPERATED	757	5.6	26	2	3	4	6	10	13	29
TOTAL										
0–19 Years	45	3.7	4	2	2	3	4	7	9	9
20–34	184	3.9	5	2	2	3	5	7	7	13
35–49	152	4.8	17	2	2	4	6	8	13	22
50–64	182	5.4	28	2	3	4	6	9	14	32
65+	292	7.2	36	3	4	6	9	13	19	37
GRAND TOTAL	855	5.5	24	2	3	4	6	10	13	29

574.70: GB&BD CAL W CHOL NEC

Type of Patients	Observed Patients	Avg. Stay	Vari-ance	10th	25th	50th	75th	90th	95th	99th
1. SINGLE DX										
A. Not Operated										
0–19 Years	1	2.0	0	2	2	2	2	2	2	2
20–34	10	2.8	3	1	2	2	4	5	6	6
35–49	2	1.5	<1	1	1	1	2	2	2	2
50–64	0									
65+	0									
B. Operated										
0–19 Years	30	2.9	2	1	2	3	3	5	6	7
20–34	151	3.1	3	1	2	3	3	5	6	8
35–49	48	3.0	4	1	2	3	4	5	6	10
50–64	17	2.8	3	1	2	3	3	5	7	7
65+	4	1.5	1	1	1	1	3	3	3	3
2. MULTIPLE DX										
A. Not Operated										
0–19 Years	4	5.5	14	2	3	5	10	10	10	10
20–34	14	2.4	1	1	2	2	3	4	4	4
35–49	21	3.6	5	2	2	3	4	5	8	10
50–64	28	3.5	4	1	2	3	5	6	7	9
65+	76	4.7	12	2	2	4	6	9	12	18
B. Operated										
0–19 Years	69	5.0	32	2	3	3	6	8	11	45
20–34	381	3.8	4	2	2	3	5	5	8	10
35–49	238	4.0	6	2	2	3	5	6	10	13
50–64	313	4.6	12	1	2	4	6	8	12	17
65+	493	5.8	21	2	3	5	7	10	13	26
SUBTOTALS:										
1. SINGLE DX										
A. Not Operated	13	2.5	2	1	2	2	3	3	6	6
B. Operated	250	3.0	3	1	2	3	4	5	6	9
2. MULTIPLE DX										
A. Not Operated	143	4.1	9	1	2	3	5	8	10	18
B. Operated	1,494	4.7	14	2	3	4	6	9	11	21
1. SINGLE DX	263	3.0	3	1	2	3	4	5	6	9
2. MULTIPLE DX	1,637	4.6	13	2	2	4	6	8	11	19
A. NOT OPERATED	156	4.0	9	1	2	3	5	8	10	18
B. OPERATED	1,744	4.5	12	2	2	4	5	8	10	19
TOTAL										
0–19 Years	104	4.4	23	2	2	3	5	7	10	18
20–34	556	3.6	4	2	2	3	4	6	7	10
35–49	309	3.8	6	1	2	3	5	6	9	13
50–64	358	4.4	11	2	3	3	5	8	11	17
65+	573	5.6	20	2	3	4	7	10	13	26
GRAND TOTAL	1,900	4.4	12	2	2	3	5	8	10	19

Western Region, October 2006–September 2007 Data, by Diagnosis

574.71: GB&BD CAL&CHOL NEC-OBSTR

Type of Patients	Observed Patients	Avg. Stay	Vari-ance	10th	25th	50th	75th	90th	95th	99th
1. SINGLE DX										
A. Not Operated										
0–19 Years	1	1.0	0	1	1	1	1	1	1	1
20–34	5	3.2	3	1	2	4	4	5	5	5
35–49	2	3.0	2	2	2	2	4	4	4	4
50–64	0									
65+	0									
B. Operated										
0–19 Years	24	3.1	2	2	2	3	4	5	5	6
20–34	65	3.1	2	1	2	3	4	5	6	7
35–49	24	2.8	2	1	2	2	4	4	5	5
50–64	15	2.8	1	1	2	3	5	5	6	5
65+	3	2.3	<1	2	2	2	3	3	3	3
2. MULTIPLE DX										
A. Not Operated										
0–19 Years	2	5.5	<1	5	5	5	6	6	6	6
20–34	10	4.1	4	1	3	5	5	8	8	8
35–49	14	4.1	5	2	2	4	6	8	8	8
50–64	18	3.6	3	2	2	3	5	6	6	6
65+	60	5.3	12	3	3	4	7	10	13	18
B. Operated										
0–19 Years	37	4.4	10	2	2	3	5	7	15	15
20–34	186	4.6	8	2	2	4	6	8	11	16
35–49	157	4.6	9	2	2	4	6	9	12	15
50–64	159	5.3	13	2	3	4	6	10	11	23
65+	299	7.9	52	3	3	6	10	17	21	37
SUBTOTALS:										
1. SINGLE DX										
A. Not Operated	8	2.9	2	1	1	2	4	5	5	5
B. Operated	131	3.0	2	1	2	3	4	5	6	6
2. MULTIPLE DX										
A. Not Operated	104	4.8	9	2	3	4	6	8	10	16
B. Operated	838	5.9	27	2	3	5	7	11	15	29
1. SINGLE DX	139	3.0	2	2	2	3	4	5	6	6
2. MULTIPLE DX	942	5.8	25	3	3	4	7	11	15	25
A. NOT OPERATED	112	4.6	9	2	3	4	6	8	10	16
B. OPERATED	969	5.5	25	3	3	4	6	10	14	25
TOTAL										
0–19 Years	64	3.9	7	2	2	4	5	6	7	15
20–34	266	4.2	7	2	2	4	5	7	9	15
35–49	197	4.3	8	2	2	4	6	8	10	15
50–64	192	4.9	12	2	3	4	6	9	11	23
65+	362	7.5	46	2	3	6	9	14	21	37
GRAND TOTAL	1,081	5.4	23	3	3	4	6	10	14	24

574.80: GB & BD CAL W ACCHR CHOL

Type of Patients	Observed Patients	Avg. Stay	Vari-ance	10th	25th	50th	75th	90th	95th	99th
1. SINGLE DX										
A. Not Operated										
0–19 Years	1	1.0	0	1	1	1	1	1	1	1
20–34	2	1.5	<1	1	1	2	2	2	2	2
35–49	0									
50–64	0									
65+	0									
B. Operated										
0–19 Years	18	3.3	3	2	2	3	4	6	6	8
20–34	79	2.8	2	1	2	3	3	5	6	8
35–49	25	3.2	1	2	2	3	4	5	5	6
50–64	13	2.5	2	1	2	3	3	4	5	5
65+	5	3.2	2	1	3	3	4	5	5	5
2. MULTIPLE DX										
A. Not Operated										
0–19 Years	1	7.0	0	7	7	7	7	7	7	7
20–34	2	2.0	0	2	2	2	2	2	2	2
35–49	2	4.0	18	1	1	7	7	7	7	7
50–64	3	7.3	20	3	3	7	12	12	12	12
65+	11	4.8	5	2	3	5	6	7	12	9
B. Operated										
0–19 Years	30	4.0	5	2	2	4	5	9	9	9
20–34	223	4.0	9	2	2	4	5	7	8	13
35–49	234	4.6	22	2	3	4	5	8	9	15
50–64	216	5.4	18	2	3	5	7	10	13	22
65+	428	6.8	27	2	3	5	8	13	16	26
SUBTOTALS:										
1. SINGLE DX										
A. Not Operated	3	1.3	<1	1	1	1	2	2	2	2
B. Operated	140	2.9	2	1	2	3	4	5	6	8
2. MULTIPLE DX										
A. Not Operated	19	5.0	8	1	2	5	7	9	12	12
B. Operated	1,131	5.5	21	2	3	4	7	10	14	22
1. SINGLE DX	143	2.9	2	1	2	3	3	5	6	8
2. MULTIPLE DX	1,150	5.5	21	2	3	4	7	10	13	22
A. NOT OPERATED	22	4.5	9	1	2	5	7	7	9	12
B. OPERATED	1,271	5.2	20	2	3	4	6	10	13	22
TOTAL										
0–19 Years	50	3.7	4	2	2	3	5	7	9	9
20–34	306	3.7	7	2	2	3	4	7	8	13
35–49	261	4.5	20	2	3	4	5	8	9	15
50–64	232	5.3	17	2	3	4	7	10	13	22
65+	444	6.7	26	2	3	5	8	13	16	26
GRAND TOTAL	1,293	5.2	19	2	3	4	6	10	13	22

574.81: GBBD CAL/ACCHR CHOL-OBST

Type of Patients	Observed Patients	Avg. Stay	Vari-ance	10th	25th	50th	75th	90th	95th	99th
1. SINGLE DX										
A. Not Operated										
0–19 Years	0									
20–34	0									
35–49	0									
50–64	0									
65+	0									
B. Operated										
0–19 Years	8	4.7	11	1	3	4	5	12	12	12
20–34	39	3.7	4	2	2	3	4	7	8	10
35–49	14	3.4	3	1	2	4	4	6	6	6
50–64	12	4.4	19	3	2	3	4	10	16	16
65+	4	5.2	3	3	3	5	6	7	7	7
2. MULTIPLE DX										
A. Not Operated										
0–19 Years	0									
20–34	1	7.0	0	7	7	7	7	7	7	7
35–49	2	3.5	13	1	1	4	6	6	6	6
50–64	1	4.0	0	4	4	4	4	4	4	4
65+	10	10.1	147	1	4	8	12	12	43	43
B. Operated										
0–19 Years	30	4.6	8	2	3	4	7	9	11	12
20–34	142	5.0	10	2	3	4	6	10	12	15
35–49	129	5.9	21	2	3	4	7	10	14	23
50–64	180	5.9	20	2	3	5	7	10	13	29
65+	270	8.0	34	3	4	7	10	14	20	31
SUBTOTALS:										
1. SINGLE DX										
A. Not Operated	0									
B. Operated	77	3.9	6	2	2	3	4	7	10	16
2. MULTIPLE DX										
A. Not Operated	14	8.5	111	1	4	6	8	12	43	43
B. Operated	751	6.4	24	2	3	5	8	11	14	28
1. SINGLE DX	77	3.9	6	2	2	3	4	7	10	16
2. MULTIPLE DX	765	6.4	26	2	3	5	8	11	14	28
A. NOT OPERATED	14	8.5	111	1	4	6	8	12	43	43
B. OPERATED	828	6.2	23	2	3	5	8	11	14	27
TOTAL										
0–19 Years	38	4.6	8	1	3	4	6	9	9	12
20–34	182	4.7	9	2	3	4	6	9	11	15
35–49	145	5.6	19	2	3	4	7	10	13	23
50–64	193	5.8	19	2	3	5	7	10	13	29
65+	284	8.0	38	3	4	7	10	13	20	37
GRAND TOTAL	842	6.2	24	2	3	5	8	11	14	28

Length of Stay by Diagnosis and Operation, Western Region, 2008

Western Region, October 2006–September 2007 Data, by Diagnosis

574.90: GB&BD CAL W/O CHOL

Type of Patients	Observed Patients	Avg. Stay	Vari-ance	Percentiles						
				10th	25th	50th	75th	90th	95th	99th
1. SINGLE DX										
A. Not Operated										
0–19 Years	6	2.3	<1	1	2	3	3	3	3	3
20–34	29	2.4	2	1	1	2	3	4	5	5
35–49	7	2.0	1	1	1	2	3	4	4	4
50–64	6	2.3	2	1	1	2	4	4	4	4
65+	2	3.0	2	2	2	4	4	4	4	4
B. Operated										
0–19 Years	9	3.0	6	1	2	2	3	9	9	9
20–34	38	3.5	6	1	2	3	4	8	9	11
35–49	12	3.8	8	2	2	3	5	8	10	10
50–64	10	3.0	2	1	2	3	4	5	5	5
65+	4	3.7	5	2	2	3	4	7	7	7
2. MULTIPLE DX										
A. Not Operated										
0–19 Years	9	1.9	1	1	1	1	3	4	4	4
20–34	68	3.9	15	1	2	3	4	8	10	25
35–49	80	3.1	5	1	2	2	4	6	9	12
50–64	89	3.5	8	1	2	2	4	8	9	17
65+	169	4.0	19	1	2	3	5	8	9	14
B. Operated										
0–19 Years	10	3.7	3	2	2	4	4	7	7	7
20–34	76	3.6	5	2	2	3	4	7	8	12
35–49	50	4.1	11	2	2	3	6	8	10	17
50–64	51	4.8	23	1	2	4	6	8	16	28
65+	106	5.6	17	2	3	4	7	11	15	20
SUBTOTALS:										
1. SINGLE DX										
A. Not Operated	50	2.3	1	1	1	2	3	4	4	4
B. Operated	73	3.4	5	2	2	3	4	7	9	9
2. MULTIPLE DX										
A. Not Operated	415	3.7	13	1	2	3	4	8	9	14
B. Operated	293	4.6	14	1	2	4	6	9	12	20
1. SINGLE DX	**123**	**3.0**	**4**	**2**	**2**	**2**	**4**	**5**	**8**	**10**
2. MULTIPLE DX	**708**	**4.1**	**14**	**1**	**2**	**3**	**5**	**8**	**10**	**17**
A. NOT OPERATED	**465**	**3.5**	**12**	**1**	**2**	**3**	**4**	**7**	**9**	**14**
B. OPERATED	**366**	**4.4**	**13**	**1**	**2**	**3**	**6**	**8**	**11**	**19**
TOTAL										
0–19 Years	34	2.8	3	1	2	3	3	4	7	9
20–34	211	3.5	8	1	2	3	4	7	9	12
35–49	149	3.4	7	1	2	2	4	7	9	13
50–64	156	3.9	13	1	2	3	5	7	9	19
65+	281	4.6	18	2	2	4	6	9	11	20
GRAND TOTAL	**831**	**3.9**	**12**	**1**	**2**	**3**	**5**	**8**	**9**	**17**

574.91: GB&BD CAL W/O CHOL-OBSTR

Type of Patients	Observed Patients	Avg. Stay	Vari-ance	Percentiles						
				10th	25th	50th	75th	90th	95th	99th
1. SINGLE DX										
A. Not Operated										
0–19 Years	2	2.0	0	2	2	2	2	2	2	2
20–34	5	2.0	<1	1	2	2	2	3	3	3
35–49	4	3.3	5	1	2	2	4	6	6	6
50–64	3	1.7	<1	1	1	2	2	2	2	2
65+	1	3.0	0	3	3	3	3	3	3	3
B. Operated										
0–19 Years	2	3.5	4	2	2	5	5	5	5	5
20–34	11	4.1	2	3	3	4	5	6	7	7
35–49	2	2.5	<1	2	2	2	3	3	3	3
50–64	1	3.0	0	3	3	3	3	3	3	3
65+	1	3.0	0	3	3	3	3	3	3	3
2. MULTIPLE DX										
A. Not Operated										
0–19 Years	5	2.6	4	1	2	2	2	6	6	6
20–34	38	3.2	7	1	2	2	5	6	9	16
35–49	38	3.4	3	1	3	3	4	6	7	7
50–64	48	3.9	12	1	2	3	6	8	11	19
65+	184	4.9	11	2	3	4	6	9	11	21
B. Operated										
0–19 Years	5	3.6	5	1	3	3	4	7	7	7
20–34	35	4.4	5	2	2	4	6	7	9	11
35–49	24	5.0	29	2	3	4	5	7	7	29
50–64	23	5.7	26	2	3	4	7	8	8	27
65+	44	9.4	94	3	4	7	11	15	19	64
SUBTOTALS:										
1. SINGLE DX										
A. Not Operated	15	2.3	2	1	2	2	3	4	6	6
B. Operated	17	3.7	2	2	3	3	4	6	7	7
2. MULTIPLE DX										
A. Not Operated	313	4.3	10	2	2	3	5	8	10	19
B. Operated	131	6.4	47	2	3	4	7	11	15	29
1. SINGLE DX	**32**	**3.1**	**2**	**2**	**2**	**3**	**4**	**5**	**6**	**7**
2. MULTIPLE DX	**444**	**4.9**	**22**	**2**	**3**	**4**	**6**	**9**	**12**	**21**
A. NOT OPERATED	**328**	**4.2**	**10**	**2**	**2**	**3**	**5**	**8**	**9**	**19**
B. OPERATED	**148**	**6.1**	**43**	**2**	**3**	**4**	**7**	**11**	**15**	**29**
TOTAL										
0–19 Years	14	3.0	3	1	2	2	4	6	7	7
20–34	89	3.7	6	2	2	3	5	7	8	16
35–49	68	3.9	13	1	2	3	5	6	7	29
50–64	75	4.3	16	1	2	3	5	8	11	27
65+	230	5.7	30	2	3	4	7	10	15	21
GRAND TOTAL	**476**	**4.8**	**21**	**2**	**2**	**4**	**6**	**9**	**11**	**21**

575: OTH GALLBLADDER DISORDER

Type of Patients	Observed Patients	Avg. Stay	Vari-ance	Percentiles						
				10th	25th	50th	75th	90th	95th	99th
1. SINGLE DX										
A. Not Operated										
0–19 Years	9	2.0	<1	1	2	2	2	3	3	3
20–34	65	2.2	2	1	1	2	3	4	5	8
35–49	45	2.2	2	1	1	2	3	5	5	7
50–64	27	2.8	1	1	2	2	3	5	5	5
65+	7	2.0	1	1	1	2	3	4	4	4
B. Operated										
0–19 Years	69	2.1	2	1	1	2	3	4	5	10
20–34	367	2.1	2	1	1	2	3	4	5	7
35–49	261	2.0	1	1	1	2	2	4	4	6
50–64	142	2.2	2	1	1	2	3	4	5	8
65+	32	1.9	1	1	1	2	2	4	4	5
2. MULTIPLE DX										
A. Not Operated										
0–19 Years	42	3.0	3	1	2	2	4	6	7	8
20–34	195	2.9	4	1	1	2	4	6	7	11
35–49	345	3.1	6	1	2	3	4	7	8	13
50–64	425	4.0	11	1	2	3	5	8	10	18
65+	733	4.5	11	1	3	4	6	8	10	17
B. Operated										
0–19 Years	171	3.5	7	1	2	3	5	7	9	18
20–34	1,229	3.3	8	1	2	3	5	6	8	15
35–49	1,799	3.6	12	1	2	3	4	7	9	16
50–64	1,816	4.0	16	1	2	3	5	8	10	17
65+	2,123	5.6	25	3	3	4	7	11	14	24
SUBTOTALS:										
1. SINGLE DX										
A. Not Operated	153	2.3	2	1	1	2	3	4	5	7
B. Operated	871	2.1	2	1	1	2	3	4	5	7
2. MULTIPLE DX										
A. Not Operated	1,740	3.9	9	1	2	3	5	7	9	15
B. Operated	7,138	4.2	17	2	3	4	7	8	11	20
1. SINGLE DX	**1,024**	**2.1**	**2**	**1**	**1**	**2**	**3**	**4**	**5**	**7**
2. MULTIPLE DX	**8,878**	**4.2**	**15**	**1**	**2**	**3**	**5**	**8**	**11**	**19**
A. NOT OPERATED	**1,893**	**3.8**	**9**	**1**	**2**	**3**	**5**	**7**	**9**	**15**
B. OPERATED	**8,009**	**4.0**	**16**	**1**	**2**	**3**	**5**	**8**	**11**	**19**
TOTAL										
0–19 Years	291	3.0	6	1	1	2	4	6	7	15
20–34	1,856	3.0	6	1	1	2	4	6	7	14
35–49	2,450	3.4	10	1	1	3	4	7	9	15
50–64	2,410	3.9	15	1	2	3	5	7	10	17
65+	2,895	5.3	21	1	2	4	7	10	13	24
GRAND TOTAL	**9,902**	**4.0**	**14**	**1**	**2**	**3**	**5**	**8**	**10**	**18**

Length of Stay by Diagnosis and Operation, Western Region, 2008

Western Region, October 2006–September 2007 Data, by Diagnosis

575.0: ACUTE CHOLECYSTITIS

Type of Patients	Observed Patients	Avg. Stay	Variance	10th	25th	50th	75th	90th	95th	99th
1. SINGLE DX										
A. Not Operated										
0–19 Years	4	2.0	<1	1	1	2	3	3	3	3
20–34	43	2.4	2	1	1	2	3	4	5	8
35–49	35	2.3	2	1	1	2	3	5	5	7
50–64	21	3.0	1	2	2	3	3	5	5	5
65+	4	2.5	2	1	2	3	4	4	4	4
B. Operated										
0–19 Years	22	1.8	<1	1	1	2	2	3	4	4
20–34	201	2.2	2	1	1	2	3	4	5	7
35–49	142	2.1	2	1	1	2	3	4	4	6
50–64	76	2.5	3	1	1	2	3	4	5	9
65+	15	2.4	2	2	2	4	4	4	4	5
2. MULTIPLE DX										
A. Not Operated										
0–19 Years	9	3.1	3	1	2	3	3	7	7	7
20–34	79	2.7	4	1	1	2	3	5	7	13
35–49	156	3.2	6	1	1	2	4	7	8	13
50–64	225	4.3	12	1	2	4	5	8	11	20
65+	429	4.7	10	2	3	4	6	9	11	15
B. Operated										
0–19 Years	37	3.9	11	1	2	3	5	9	18	>99
20–34	403	3.0	6	1	2	2	4	5	7	14
35–49	626	3.8	14	1	2	3	4	7	9	19
50–64	763	4.5	22	1	2	4	6	8	11	20
65+	1,140	6.1	26	2	3	5	7	11	15	24
SUBTOTALS:										
1. SINGLE DX										
A. Not Operated	107	2.5	2	1	1	2	3	4	5	7
B. Operated	456	2.2	2	1	1	2	3	4	5	8
2. MULTIPLE DX										
A. Not Operated	898	4.2	10	1	2	3	5	8	10	14
B. Operated	2,969	4.7	21	1	2	4	6	9	12	21
1. SINGLE DX	563	2.3	2	1	1	2	3	4	5	8
2. MULTIPLE DX	3,867	4.6	18	1	2	4	6	9	12	21
A. NOT OPERATED	1,005	4.0	9	1	2	3	5	8	10	14
B. OPERATED	3,425	4.4	19	1	2	3	5	9	12	21
TOTAL										
0–19 Years	72	3.1	7	1	1	2	4	6	9	>99
20–34	726	2.7	4	1	1	2	3	5	6	12
35–49	959	3.4	11	1	1	3	4	7	8	16
50–64	1,085	4.3	18	1	2	3	5	8	11	20
65+	1,588	5.7	22	2	3	5	7	10	13	24
GRAND TOTAL	4,430	4.3	17	1	2	3	5	8	11	20

575.10: CHOLECYSTITIS NOS

Type of Patients	Observed Patients	Avg. Stay	Variance	10th	25th	50th	75th	90th	95th	99th
1. SINGLE DX										
A. Not Operated										
0–19 Years	2	1.5	<1	1	1	2	2	2	2	2
20–34	8	1.4	<1	1	1	1	2	3	3	3
35–49	5	1.8	<1	1	1	2	2	3	3	3
50–64	5	1.6	<1	1	1	2	2	3	3	3
65+	3	1.3	<1	1	1	1	2	2	2	2
B. Operated										
0–19 Years	4	3.3	2	2	3	3	3	5	5	5
20–34	15	1.9	2	1	1	2	2	3	6	6
35–49	11	1.6	<1	1	1	2	2	2	3	3
50–64	4	1.5	<1	1	1	1	1	3	3	3
65+	2	1.5	<1	1	1	2	2	2	2	2
2. MULTIPLE DX										
A. Not Operated										
0–19 Years	9	2.9	4	1	2	3	3	7	8	8
20–34	42	2.3	3	1	1	2	3	5	6	6
35–49	68	2.8	4	1	2	2	4	6	6	10
50–64	65	3.4	5	1	2	4	5	7	8	12
65+	100	4.1	17	1	2	3	6	9	13	27
B. Operated										
0–19 Years	5	3.4	3	1	3	3	4	6	6	6
20–34	64	3.2	4	1	2	2	4	6	7	9
35–49	69	3.5	8	1	2	3	4	7	9	15
50–64	70	4.0	8	1	2	3	6	8	9	14
65+	45	4.3	10	1	2	5	7	9	10	14
SUBTOTALS:										
1. SINGLE DX										
A. Not Operated	23	1.5	<1	1	1	2	2	3	3	3
B. Operated	36	1.9	1	1	1	2	2	3	5	6
2. MULTIPLE DX										
A. Not Operated	284	3.3	9	1	2	3	4	6	8	17
B. Operated	253	3.7	7	1	2	3	5	7	9	14
1. SINGLE DX	59	1.8	1	1	1	2	3	3	3	6
2. MULTIPLE DX	537	3.5	8	1	2	3	5	6	8	14
A. NOT OPERATED	307	3.2	9	1	1	3	4	6	8	13
B. OPERATED	289	3.5	7	1	2	3	5	7	8	14
TOTAL										
0–19 Years	20	3.0	3	1	2	3	3	5	6	6
20–34	129	2.6	3	1	1	2	3	5	6	12
35–49	153	3.0	6	1	2	2	4	6	7	14
50–64	144	3.6	6	1	2	3	5	7	8	12
65+	150	4.1	14	1	2	3	7	10	10	25
GRAND TOTAL	596	3.3	8	1	1	3	4	6	8	14

575.11: CHRONIC CHOLECYSTITIS

Type of Patients	Observed Patients	Avg. Stay	Variance	10th	25th	50th	75th	90th	95th	99th
1. SINGLE DX										
A. Not Operated										
0–19 Years	0									
20–34	3	3.7	9	1	1	3	7	7	7	7
35–49	4	1.3	<1	1	1	1	1	1	2	2
50–64	1	4.0	0	4	4	4	4	4	4	4
65+	0									
B. Operated										
0–19 Years	18	1.6	1	1	1	1	2	3	3	5
20–34	87	2.0	2	1	1	2	2	4	5	8
35–49	60	1.8	1	1	1	2	2	3	5	6
50–64	29	1.6	1	1	1	1	2	3	4	5
65+	9	1.4	<1	1	1	1	2	3	3	3
2. MULTIPLE DX										
A. Not Operated										
0–19 Years	3	3.7	8	2	2	2	3	7	7	7
20–34	22	3.6	4	2	2	3	3	7	7	8
35–49	44	3.0	4	1	2	3	4	6	7	9
50–64	38	3.5	9	1	1	3	5	6	7	18
65+	74	4.1	8	2	2	3	5	8	9	17
B. Operated										
0–19 Years	71	3.3	6	1	2	3	4	6	9	14
20–34	431	3.5	9	1	2	3	4	7	8	17
35–49	635	3.4	7	1	1	3	4	7	9	13
50–64	512	3.2	13	1	1	2	4	6	9	13
65+	419	4.1	14	1	2	3	5	9	11	20
SUBTOTALS:										
1. SINGLE DX										
A. Not Operated	8	2.5	5	1	1	1	4	7	7	7
B. Operated	203	1.8	1	1	1	2	2	3	4	6
2. MULTIPLE DX										
A. Not Operated	181	3.6	7	1	2	3	5	7	8	17
B. Operated	2,068	3.5	11	1	1	3	4	7	9	15
1. SINGLE DX	211	1.9	2	1	1	1	2	3	5	6
2. MULTIPLE DX	2,249	3.5	10	1	1	3	5	7	9	15
A. NOT OPERATED	189	3.6	7	1	1	3	5	7	8	17
B. OPERATED	2,271	3.4	10	1	1	2	4	7	9	15
TOTAL										
0–19 Years	92	3.0	6	1	1	2	3	4	6	8
20–34	543	3.3	8	1	2	2	4	6	8	17
35–49	743	3.2	7	1	1	2	4	6	7	12
50–64	580	3.2	13	1	1	2	4	6	9	14
65+	502	4.0	13	1	2	3	5	8	11	18
GRAND TOTAL	2,460	3.4	10	1	2	2	4	7	9	15

Length of Stay by Diagnosis and Operation, Western Region, 2008

Western Region, October 2006–September 2007 Data, by Diagnosis

575.12: AC & CHR CHOLECYSTITIS

Type of Patients	Observed Patients	Avg. Stay	Vari- ance	Percentiles						
				10th	25th	50th	75th	90th	95th	99th
1. SINGLE DX										
A. Not Operated										
0–19 Years	0									
20–34	4	1.8	<1	1	1	2	2	2	2	2
35–49	1	3.0	0	3	3	3	3	3	3	3
50–64	0									
65+	0									
B. Operated										
0–19 Years	5	3.8	14	1	1	3	4	10	10	10
20–34	41	1.9	1	1	1	2	2	3	4	5
35–49	28	2.2	1	1	1	2	3	4	5	5
50–64	19	2.5	1	1	2	3	3	3	5	5
65+	3	2.0	<1	1	1	2	3	3	3	3
2. MULTIPLE DX										
A. Not Operated										
0–19 Years	1	5.0	0	5	5	5	5	5	5	5
20–34	5	5.0	11	3	3	4	4	11	11	11
35–49	6	2.8	3	1	2	3	3	6	6	6
50–64	17	5.5	12	2	2	4	7	11	14	14
65+	28	5.0	18	1	2	4	7	9	12	21
B. Operated										
0–19 Years	19	2.8	3	1	2	3	3	7	7	7
20–34	136	3.3	9	1	2	2	4	6	7	16
35–49	217	4.0	13	1	2	3	5	8	10	20
50–64	276	4.3	9	1	2	3	6	8	10	15
65+	351	6.2	31	2	3	5	7	12	17	32
SUBTOTALS:										
1. SINGLE DX										
A. Not Operated	5	2.0	<1	1	2	2	2	3	3	3
B. Operated	96	2.2	2	1	1	2	3	4	5	10
2. MULTIPLE DX										
A. Not Operated	57	4.9	14	1	3	4	6	9	12	21
B. Operated	999	4.7	19	1	2	4	6	9	12	21
1. SINGLE DX	101	2.2	2	1	1	2	3	4	4	5
2. MULTIPLE DX	1,056	4.7	18	1	2	4	6	9	12	21
A. NOT OPERATED	62	4.7	13	1	2	3	6	9	11	21
B. OPERATED	1,095	4.5	18	1	2	3	6	9	12	21
TOTAL										
0–19 Years	25	3.1	5	1	2	3	3	7	7	10
20–34	186	3.0	8	1	1	2	4	5	7	16
35–49	252	3.8	12	1	2	3	4	7	9	20
50–64	312	4.2	9	1	2	3	5	8	10	15
65+	382	6.1	30	2	3	5	7	12	17	32
GRAND TOTAL	1,157	4.5	17	1	2	3	6	9	12	21

575.8: GB DISORDER NEC

Type of Patients	Observed Patients	Avg. Stay	Vari- ance	Percentiles						
				10th	25th	50th	75th	90th	95th	99th
1. SINGLE DX										
A. Not Operated										
0–19 Years	3	2.3	<1	2	2	2	2	3	3	3
20–34	5	1.6	<1	1	1	1	2	3	3	3
35–49	0									
50–64	0									
65+										
B. Operated										
0–19 Years	19	2.3	2	1	1	2	3	4	4	6
20–34	20	1.7	1	1	1	1	2	3	3	5
35–49	17	1.5	<1	1	1	1	2	2	3	3
50–64	12	2.0	2	1	1	1	3	4	5	5
65+	1	1.0	0	1	1	1	1	1	1	1
2. MULTIPLE DX										
A. Not Operated										
0–19 Years	13	2.5	1	2	2	2	3	4	4	5
20–34	41	3.1	3	2	2	3	4	5	7	8
35–49	66	3.3	11	2	2	3	4	6	8	22
50–64	53	3.1	4	1	2	2	4	6	8	9
65+	73	4.2	6	2	3	4	6	7	8	16
B. Operated										
0–19 Years	36	3.5	8	1	1	3	5	6	8	15
20–34	177	3.7	11	1	2	3	5	7	8	21
35–49	220	3.4	7	1	2	3	4	7	9	12
50–64	151	3.0	8	1	2	3	4	7	9	13
65+	103	4.8	23	2	3	4	7	9	12	24
SUBTOTALS:										
1. SINGLE DX										
A. Not Operated	8	1.9	<1	1	1	2	2	3	3	3
B. Operated	69	1.8	1	1	1	1	3	4	4	6
2. MULTIPLE DX										
A. Not Operated	246	3.5	6	2	2	3	4	6	8	15
B. Operated	687	3.6	11	1	1	3	5	7	9	18
1. SINGLE DX	77	1.8	1	1	1	1	2	3	4	6
2. MULTIPLE DX	933	3.6	10	1	2	3	4	6	7	16
A. NOT OPERATED	254	3.4	6	1	2	3	4	6	8	15
B. OPERATED	756	3.5	10	1	1	3	4	6	7	17
TOTAL										
0–19 Years	71	3.0	5	1	1	3	4	5	6	15
20–34	243	3.4	9	1	1	3	4	6	8	15
35–49	303	3.3	8	1	1	3	4	6	8	13
50–64	216	3.0	7	1	2	3	4	5	7	12
65+	177	4.6	16	2	3	4	6	8	10	24
GRAND TOTAL	1,010	3.5	9	1	1	3	4	7	9	15

576: OTH DISORD BILIARY TRACT

Type of Patients	Observed Patients	Avg. Stay	Vari- ance	Percentiles						
				10th	25th	50th	75th	90th	95th	99th
1. SINGLE DX										
A. Not Operated										
0–19 Years	9	4.9	33	1	2	3	4	19	19	19
20–34	24	2.6	1	1	2	3	3	4	5	5
35–49	28	3.0	9	1	1	2	3	7	9	15
50–64	23	2.1	2	1	1	2	3	4	4	6
65+	8	1.6	<1	1	1	2	2	3	3	3
B. Operated										
0–19 Years	5	6.0	31	1	2	5	7	15	15	15
20–34	7	5.5	12	1	2	5	10	10	10	10
35–49	2	5.5	4	4	4	4	7	7	7	7
50–64	0									
65+	0									
2. MULTIPLE DX										
A. Not Operated										
0–19 Years	103	4.5	13	1	2	3	6	10	13	15
20–34	296	4.2	12	1	2	3	5	8	11	19
35–49	646	4.3	13	1	2	3	5	8	11	17
50–64	1,031	4.5	18	1	2	3	5	8	11	21
65+	1,918	4.8	15	2	2	4	6	9	12	20
B. Operated										
0–19 Years	12	5.3	24	1	2	5	7	8	19	19
20–34	56	7.8	70	2	3	6	8	15	25	54
35–49	92	7.2	24	3	4	6	10	13	16	>99
50–64	146	9.2	52	3	4	7	11	20	24	37
65+	189	9.4	53	3	5	8	11	18	23	32
SUBTOTALS:										
1. SINGLE DX										
A. Not Operated	92	2.8	7	1	1	2	3	4	7	19
B. Operated	14	5.7	16	1	2	5	7	10	15	15
2. MULTIPLE DX										
A. Not Operated	3,994	4.6	15	1	2	4	6	8	11	20
B. Operated	495	8.6	49	3	4	7	10	17	22	37
1. SINGLE DX	106	3.1	9	1	1	2	4	6	9	15
2. MULTIPLE DX	4,489	5.0	20	1	2	4	6	10	13	23
A. NOT OPERATED	4,086	4.5	15	1	2	3	6	8	11	20
B. OPERATED	509	8.6	48	3	4	7	10	17	22	34
TOTAL										
0–19 Years	129	4.7	16	1	2	4	6	10	14	19
20–34	383	4.6	21	1	2	3	6	8	11	25
35–49	768	4.6	15	1	2	3	6	9	12	21
50–64	1,200	5.0	24	2	2	4	6	10	13	24
65+	2,115	5.2	20	2	2	4	6	10	13	23
GRAND TOTAL	4,595	5.0	20	1	2	4	6	10	13	22

452

Length of Stay by Diagnosis and Operation, Western Region, 2008

Western Region, October 2006–September 2007 Data, by Diagnosis

576.1: CHOLANGITIS

Type of Patients	Observed Patients	Avg. Stay	Vari-ance	10th	25th	50th	75th	90th	95th	99th
1. SINGLE DX										
A. Not Operated										
0–19 Years	3	10.3	59	4	4	8	19	19	19	19
20–34	4	3.5	2	2	3	4	5	5	5	5
35–49	8	3.0	4	1	1	3	3	7	7	7
50–64	4	3.0	6	1	1	4	4	6	6	6
65+	2	2.5	<1	2	2	3	3	3	3	3
B. Operated										
0–19 Years	0									
20–34	0									
35–49	1	4.0	0	4	4	4	4	4	4	4
50–64	0									
65+	0									
2. MULTIPLE DX										
A. Not Operated										
0–19 Years	47	5.1	16	1	2	4	8	12	14	16
20–34	67	3.9	8	2	2	3	5	8	11	15
35–49	189	4.3	12	1	2	3	5	8	10	16
50–64	344	4.5	15	2	2	3	5	8	11	21
65+	737	4.8	15	2	3	4	6	8	11	21
B. Operated										
0–19 Years	3	4.7	6	2	2	5	7	7	7	7
20–34	17	7.7	46	2	3	6	9	15	30	30
35–49	24	8.2	43	3	4	6	11	13	16	34
50–64	53	9.6	70	2	4	6	12	21	26	41
65+	93	8.3	24	4	5	7	10	15	18	27
SUBTOTALS:										
1. SINGLE DX										
A. Not Operated	21	4.1	15	1	2	3	4	7	8	19
B. Operated	1	4.0	0	4	4	4	4	4	4	4
2. MULTIPLE DX										
A. Not Operated	1,384	4.6	14	1	2	4	6	8	11	21
B. Operated	190	8.5	41	3	5	7	10	16	21	34
1. SINGLE DX	22	4.1	15	1	2	3	4	7	8	19
2. MULTIPLE DX	1,574	5.1	19	2	3	4	6	10	13	24
A. NOT OPERATED	1,405	4.6	14	2	2	4	6	8	11	21
B. OPERATED	191	8.5	41	3	4	7	10	16	21	34
TOTAL										
0–19 Years	53	5.4	18	1	2	4	4	8	12	14
20–34	88	4.6	17	2	2	3	5	9	11	30
35–49	222	4.7	17	1	2	3	6	8	12	16
50–64	401	5.1	25	2	2	4	6	10	16	26
65+	832	5.2	17	2	3	4	6	10	12	21
GRAND TOTAL	1,596	5.1	19	2	2	4	6	10	13	24

576.2: BILE DUCT OBSTRUCTION

Type of Patients	Observed Patients	Avg. Stay	Vari-ance	10th	25th	50th	75th	90th	95th	99th
1. SINGLE DX										
A. Not Operated										
0–19 Years	3	2.7	2	1	1	3	4	4	4	4
20–34	4	3.3	2	2	3	3	5	5	5	5
35–49	9	3.0	21	1	1	1	2	15	15	15
50–64	12	1.8	1	1	1	1	2	3	4	4
65+	4	1.3	<1	1	1	1	2	2	2	2
B. Operated										
0–19 Years	0									
20–34	1	10.0	0	10	10	10	10	10	10	10
35–49	0									
50–64	0									
65+	0									
2. MULTIPLE DX										
A. Not Operated										
0–19 Years	18	4.5	20	1	2	3	4	14	15	15
20–34	86	4.6	17	1	2	3	6	8	12	29
35–49	219	4.5	10	1	2	4	6	8	11	18
50–64	434	4.7	22	1	2	4	6	9	11	20
65+	743	4.7	14	2	2	4	6	9	11	19
B. Operated										
0–19 Years	4	6.5	71	1	1	5	19	19	19	19
20–34	24	10.1	116	3	5	7	11	19	25	54
35–49	40	7.9	21	4	5	6	10	13	21	>99
50–64	69	8.7	47	3	4	7	10	18	24	37
65+	70	11.7	96	4	6	9	14	24	28	67
SUBTOTALS:										
1. SINGLE DX										
A. Not Operated	32	2.3	7	1	1	2	3	4	5	15
B. Operated	1	10.0	0	10	10	10	10	10	10	10
2. MULTIPLE DX										
A. Not Operated	1,500	4.7	16	1	2	4	6	9	11	19
B. Operated	207	9.7	68	3	5	7	11	20	25	54
1. SINGLE DX	33	2.5	8	1	1	2	3	4	10	15
2. MULTIPLE DX	1,707	5.3	25	1	2	4	7	10	13	24
A. NOT OPERATED	1,532	4.6	16	1	2	4	6	8	11	19
B. OPERATED	208	9.7	68	3	5	8	11	20	25	54
TOTAL										
0–19 Years	25	4.6	25	1	2	3	4	8	15	19
20–34	115	5.7	42	2	2	4	7	11	16	29
35–49	268	5.0	14	1	2	4	6	10	12	23
50–64	515	5.1	27	1	2	4	6	10	13	24
65+	817	5.3	25	1	2	4	7	10	14	24
GRAND TOTAL	1,740	5.2	25	1	2	4	6	10	13	24

576.8: BILIARY TRACT DISORD NEC

Type of Patients	Observed Patients	Avg. Stay	Vari-ance	10th	25th	50th	75th	90th	95th	99th
1. SINGLE DX										
A. Not Operated										
0–19 Years	3	1.7	<1	1	1	2	2	2	2	2
20–34	13	2.4	1	1	2	2	3	4	4	4
35–49	9	3.3	5	1	2	3	3	9	9	9
50–64	6	2.2	<1	1	2	2	3	3	3	3
65+	1	1.0	0	1	1	1	1	1	1	1
B. Operated										
0–19 Years	5	6.0	31	1	2	5	7	15	15	15
20–34	5	5.4	8	2	5	5	5	10	10	10
35–49	1	7.0	0	7	7	7	7	7	7	7
50–64	0									
65+	0									
2. MULTIPLE DX										
A. Not Operated										
0–19 Years	34	3.7	6	1	2	3	5	7	8	11
20–34	116	4.0	10	2	2	3	5	8	9	18
35–49	210	4.0	17	1	2	3	5	8	10	17
50–64	220	4.1	13	1	2	3	5	8	10	16
65+	414	4.8	16	1	2	4	6	9	13	21
B. Operated										
0–19 Years	5	4.6	6	1	4	5	5	8	8	8
20–34	15	4.3	7	1	1	5	7	8	8	8
35–49	26	5.1	8	2	3	5	6	8	8	15
50–64	20	8.3	22	3	6	7	8	17	18	18
65+	22	6.5	17	2	3	6	9	11	15	15
SUBTOTALS:										
1. SINGLE DX										
A. Not Operated	32	2.5	2	1	2	2	3	4	4	9
B. Operated	11	5.8	16	2	2	5	7	10	15	15
2. MULTIPLE DX										
A. Not Operated	994	4.3	15	1	2	3	5	8	11	20
B. Operated	88	6.0	15	1	3	6	7	11	15	18
1. SINGLE DX	43	3.4	8	1	2	3	4	7	9	15
2. MULTIPLE DX	1,082	4.5	15	1	2	3	6	9	11	20
A. NOT OPERATED	1,026	4.3	14	1	2	3	5	8	11	20
B. OPERATED	99	6.0	15	1	3	6	7	11	15	18
TOTAL										
0–19 Years	47	3.9	9	1	2	3	5	8	8	15
20–34	149	4.0	9	1	2	3	5	8	9	18
35–49	246	4.1	15	1	2	3	5	8	10	17
50–64	246	4.4	15	1	2	3	6	8	11	18
65+	437	4.9	16	1	2	4	6	10	13	21
GRAND TOTAL	1,125	4.4	15	1	2	3	6	9	11	18

Length of Stay by Diagnosis and Operation, Western Region, 2008

Western Region, October 2006–September 2007 Data, by Diagnosis

577: DISEASES OF PANCREAS

Type of Patients	Observed Patients	Avg. Stay	Variance	10th	25th	50th	75th	90th	95th	99th
1. SINGLE DX										
A. Not Operated										
0–19 Years	148	3.5	5	1	2	3	4	6	7	13
20–34	230	2.6	3	1	1	2	3	5	5	8
35–49	159	2.9	4	1	1	2	4	5	6	11
50–64	103	2.6	4	1	1	2	3	5	5	10
65+	32	3.3	4	1	2	3	4	5	8	11
B. Operated										
0–19 Years	3	11.7	94	1	1	14	20	20	20	20
20–34	9	4.5	24	1	2	2	3	14	14	14
35–49	9	5.2	2	3	5	5	6	6	8	8
50–64	5	4.4	1	3	8	4	5	6	6	6
65+	1	8.0	0	8	8	8	8	8	8	8
2. MULTIPLE DX										
A. Not Operated										
0–19 Years	733	4.9	17	1	2	4	6	10	13	21
20–34	5,539	4.5	19	1	2	3	5	9	12	22
35–49	10,995	4.6	20	1	2	3	5	9	12	23
50–64	9,878	4.8	23	1	2	3	6	9	13	24
65+	8,093	4.8	19	2	2	4	6	9	12	22
B. Operated										
0–19 Years	289	5.7	30	2	3	4	7	9	14	37
20–34	1,739	5.8	42	2	3	4	6	10	15	32
35–49	1,731	6.8	53	2	3	5	7	13	20	39
50–64	2,085	7.3	52	2	4	5	8	14	20	46
65+	2,379	8.0	52	3	4	6	9	15	21	40
SUBTOTALS:										
1. SINGLE DX										
A. Not Operated	672	2.9	4	1	2	2	4	5	6	12
B. Operated	27	5.6	21	2	2	5	6	14	14	20
2. MULTIPLE DX										
A. Not Operated	35,238	4.7	20	1	2	3	5	9	12	23
B. Operated	8,223	7.0	50	2	3	5	8	13	19	39
1. SINGLE DX	699	3.0	5	1	2	2	4	5	7	14
2. MULTIPLE DX	43,461	5.1	27	2	2	4	6	10	14	26
A. NOT OPERATED	35,910	4.7	20	1	2	3	5	9	12	23
B. OPERATED	8,250	7.0	50	2	3	5	8	13	19	39
TOTAL										
0–19 Years	1,173	4.9	19	2	2	4	6	9	13	23
20–34	7,517	4.8	24	2	2	3	5	9	13	23
35–49	12,894	4.9	25	2	2	4	6	9	13	25
50–64	12,071	5.2	29	2	2	4	6	10	14	27
65+	10,505	5.5	29	2	3	4	6	10	14	27
GRAND TOTAL	44,160	5.1	27	2	2	4	6	10	14	26

577.0: ACUTE PANCREATITIS

Type of Patients	Observed Patients	Avg. Stay	Variance	10th	25th	50th	75th	90th	95th	99th
1. SINGLE DX										
A. Not Operated										
0–19 Years	126	3.4	5	1	2	3	4	5	7	10
20–34	203	2.5	2	1	1	2	3	4	5	7
35–49	139	2.9	3	1	2	3	4	5	6	10
50–64	80	2.6	3	1	2	2	3	5	5	10
65+	28	3.4	5	1	2	3	4	5	8	11
B. Operated										
0–19 Years	0									
20–34	3	6.0	47	2	2	2	14	14	14	14
35–49	0									
50–64	0									
65+	0									
2. MULTIPLE DX										
A. Not Operated										
0–19 Years	646	4.9	17	2	2	4	6	10	13	21
20–34	5,035	4.5	18	1	2	3	5	9	12	22
35–49	9,806	4.7	20	2	2	3	5	9	12	23
50–64	8,786	4.8	23	2	2	4	6	9	13	24
65+	7,404	4.8	19	2	2	4	6	9	12	22
B. Operated										
0–19 Years	266	5.2	17	2	3	4	6	9	12	21
20–34	1,613	5.5	39	2	3	4	6	10	13	27
35–49	1,485	6.4	52	2	3	5	7	11	18	40
50–64	1,799	6.9	48	2	3	5	7	13	19	46
65+	2,195	7.8	50	3	4	6	9	14	20	38
SUBTOTALS:										
1. SINGLE DX										
A. Not Operated	576	2.8	3	1	2	2	4	5	6	10
B. Operated	3	6.0	47	2	2	2	14	14	14	14
2. MULTIPLE DX										
A. Not Operated	31,657	4.7	21	2	2	3	5	9	12	23
B. Operated	7,358	6.7	47	2	3	5	7	12	18	38
1. SINGLE DX	579	2.9	4	1	2	2	4	5	6	10
2. MULTIPLE DX	39,015	5.1	26	2	2	4	6	10	13	26
A. NOT OPERATED	32,233	4.7	20	2	2	3	5	9	12	23
B. OPERATED	7,361	6.7	47	2	3	5	7	12	18	38
TOTAL										
0–19 Years	1,038	4.8	16	2	2	4	6	9	12	21
20–34	6,854	4.7	23	2	2	3	5	9	12	23
35–49	11,430	4.9	25	2	2	4	6	9	13	25
50–64	10,645	5.2	28	2	2	4	6	10	14	27
65+	9,627	5.5	28	2	3	4	6	10	14	27
GRAND TOTAL	39,594	5.1	26	2	2	4	6	10	13	26

577.1: CHRONIC PANCREATITIS

Type of Patients	Observed Patients	Avg. Stay	Variance	10th	25th	50th	75th	90th	95th	99th
1. SINGLE DX										
A. Not Operated										
0–19 Years	17	3.5	4	1	2	4	5	6	7	7
20–34	23	2.3	2	1	1	2	3	4	4	6
35–49	15	2.1	1	1	1	2	3	4	5	5
50–64	14	1.6	<1	1	1	1	2	3	4	4
65+	0									
B. Operated										
0–19 Years	1	14.0	0	14	14	14	14	14	14	14
20–34	2	2.5	<1	2	2	2	3	3	3	3
35–49	0									
50–64	1	4.0	0	4	4	4	4	4	4	4
65+	1	8.0	0	8	8	8	8	8	8	8
2. MULTIPLE DX										
A. Not Operated										
0–19 Years	71	5.0	15	2	3	4	6	10	12	23
20–34	403	4.3	19	1	2	3	5	8	10	19
35–49	996	4.2	16	1	2	3	5	8	10	19
50–64	830	4.6	16	1	2	3	6	9	12	21
65+	332	4.4	15	1	2	4	5	8	11	26
B. Operated										
0–19 Years	11	6.2	13	3	4	5	8	9	15	15
20–34	50	7.4	28	2	4	7	8	14	15	34
35–49	89	8.9	64	2	4	7	10	19	26	44
50–64	108	10.0	74	3	5	8	13	19	25	29
65+	66	8.1	32	3	4	7	11	17	20	28
SUBTOTALS:										
1. SINGLE DX										
A. Not Operated	69	2.4	2	1	1	2	3	5	5	7
B. Operated	5	6.2	24	2	3	4	8	14	14	14
2. MULTIPLE DX										
A. Not Operated	2,632	4.4	16	1	2	3	5	8	11	21
B. Operated	324	8.8	54	3	4	7	11	16	23	35
1. SINGLE DX	74	2.7	4	1	1	2	3	5	6	14
2. MULTIPLE DX	2,956	4.9	22	1	2	4	6	9	13	25
A. NOT OPERATED	2,701	4.3	16	1	2	3	5	8	11	20
B. OPERATED	329	8.8	54	3	4	7	10	16	23	35
TOTAL										
0–19 Years	100	5.0	14	2	3	4	6	10	14	23
20–34	478	4.5	20	1	2	3	6	9	11	19
35–49	1,100	4.5	21	1	2	3	5	9	12	27
50–64	953	5.2	25	1	2	4	6	10	14	23
65+	399	5.1	20	1	3	4	6	10	14	27
GRAND TOTAL	3,030	4.8	22	1	2	4	6	9	13	25

Length of Stay by Diagnosis and Operation, Western Region, 2008

Western Region, October 2006–September 2007 Data, by Diagnosis

577.2: PANCREAS CYST/PSEUDOCYST

Type of Patients	Observed Patients	Avg. Stay	Variance	10th	25th	50th	75th	90th	95th	99th
1. SINGLE DX										
A. Not Operated										
0–19 Years	5	6.4	32	1	2	4	12	13	13	13
20–34	4	7.7	32	4	4	4	7	16	16	16
35–49	3	7.0	43	1	1	6	14	14	14	14
50–64	4	6.5	33	3	3	3	5	15	15	15
65+	1	1.0	0	1	1	1	1	1	1	1
B. Operated										
0–19 Years	1	1.0	0	1	1	1	1	1	1	1
20–34	4	4.3	27	1	2	2	12	12	12	12
35–49	7	4.7	<1	3	4	5	5	6	6	6
50–64	4	4.5	2	3	3	4	5	6	6	6
65+	0									
2. MULTIPLE DX										
A. Not Operated										
0–19 Years	13	5.1	25	1	1	4	6	10	19	19
20–34	69	6.6	78	1	2	4	8	13	16	68
35–49	113	4.7	12	1	2	4	6	8	13	16
50–64	129	6.5	50	1	2	4	8	15	22	29
65+	113	6.7	37	1	3	5	8	16	22	25
B. Operated										
0–19 Years	12	15.1	252	4	5	9	14	37	51	51
20–34	72	11.7	82	4	5	10	15	20	33	50
35–49	142	9.8	48	3	5	8	13	20	22	39
50–64	149	10.2	76	4	5	7	12	21	26	44
65+	88	10.6	98	3	5	7	12	20	33	55
SUBTOTALS:										
1. SINGLE DX										
A. Not Operated	17	6.5	28	1	3	4	12	15	16	16
B. Operated	16	4.3	7	1	3	5	5	6	12	12
2. MULTIPLE DX										
A. Not Operated	437	6.1	41	1	2	4	7	13	19	27
B. Operated	463	10.5	77	4	5	8	13	21	27	50
1. SINGLE DX	33	5.5	18	1	3	4	6	13	15	16
2. MULTIPLE DX	900	8.4	64	2	4	6	10	18	23	44
A. NOT OPERATED	454	6.1	40	1	2	4	7	13	19	27
B. OPERATED	479	10.3	76	4	5	8	13	20	26	50
TOTAL										
0–19 Years	31	9.1	132	1	2	5	10	19	37	51
20–34	149	9.1	83	2	4	7	12	17	24	50
35–49	265	7.5	38	2	3	6	10	17	21	35
50–64	286	8.4	66	2	4	6	10	18	24	44
65+	202	8.3	67	3	4	6	10	18	23	45
GRAND TOTAL	933	8.3	63	2	4	6	10	18	23	44

577.8: PANCREATIC DISEASE NEC

Type of Patients	Observed Patients	Avg. Stay	Variance	10th	25th	50th	75th	90th	95th	99th
1. SINGLE DX										
A. Not Operated										
0–19 Years	0									
20–34	0									
35–49	1	8.0	0	8	8	8	8	8	8	8
50–64	4	2.3	2	1	1	1	4	4	4	4
65+	0									
B. Operated										
0–19 Years	1	20.0	0	20	20	20	20	20	20	20
20–34	0									
35–49	0									
50–64	0									
65+	0									
2. MULTIPLE DX										
A. Not Operated										
0–19 Years	3	3.3	2	2	2	3	5	5	5	5
20–34	23	3.9	6	2	2	3	5	8	9	10
35–49	52	3.9	15	1	2	3	4	6	9	26
50–64	77	4.8	46	1	2	3	5	9	19	47
65+	106	4.5	13	1	2	4	6	8	10	12
B. Operated										
0–19 Years	0									
20–34	2	9.0	18	6	6	6	12	12	12	12
35–49	9	7.2	5	5	5	6	10	10	10	10
50–64	23	7.6	22	2	5	6	11	15	17	18
65+	17	11.2	95	4	5	9	13	41	>99	>99
SUBTOTALS:										
1. SINGLE DX										
A. Not Operated	5	3.4	8	1	1	3	4	8	8	8
B. Operated	1	20.0	0	20	20	20	20	20	20	20
2. MULTIPLE DX										
A. Not Operated	261	4.4	22	1	2	3	5	8	10	28
B. Operated	51	8.8	44	4	5	6	10	16	28	>99
1. SINGLE DX	6	6.2	53	1	1	4	8	20	20	20
2. MULTIPLE DX	312	5.1	28	1	2	4	6	10	13	29
A. NOT OPERATED	266	4.4	22	1	2	3	5	8	10	28
B. OPERATED	52	9.0	46	4	5	7	11	17	28	>99
TOTAL										
0–19 Years	4	7.5	71	2	2	5	20	20	20	20
20–34	25	4.3	9	2	2	3	6	9	10	12
35–49	62	4.5	14	1	2	3	6	9	10	26
50–64	104	5.3	40	1	2	4	6	12	17	29
65+	123	5.4	29	1	2	4	7	10	13	41
GRAND TOTAL	318	5.1	29	1	2	4	6	10	13	29

577.9: PANCREATIC DISEASE NOS

Type of Patients	Observed Patients	Avg. Stay	Variance	10th	25th	50th	75th	90th	95th	99th
1. SINGLE DX										
A. Not Operated										
0–19 Years	0									
20–34	0									
35–49	1	1.0	0	1	1	1	1	1	1	1
50–64	1	2.0	0	2	2	2	2	2	2	2
65+	3	2.7	1	2	2	2	4	4	4	4
B. Operated										
0–19 Years	0									
20–34	0									
35–49	2	7.0	2	6	6	8	8	8	8	8
50–64	0									
65+	0									
2. MULTIPLE DX										
A. Not Operated										
0–19 Years	0									
20–34	9	3.1	3	1	2	3	4	7	7	7
35–49	28	3.8	10	1	1	3	5	8	8	16
50–64	76	3.8	11	1	2	3	5	8	9	19
65+	138	4.0	9	1	2	3	5	8	10	14
B. Operated										
0–19 Years	0									
20–34	2	8.5	4	7	7	7	10	10	10	10
35–49	6	6.0	20	2	3	4	10	13	13	13
50–64	6	10.2	63	5	6	7	10	26	26	26
65+	13	11.6	58	4	7	10	15	21	29	29
SUBTOTALS:										
1. SINGLE DX										
A. Not Operated	5	2.2	1	1	2	2	2	4	4	4
B. Operated	2	7.0	2	6	6	8	8	8	8	8
2. MULTIPLE DX										
A. Not Operated	251	3.9	9	1	2	3	5	8	9	16
B. Operated	27	9.8	48	3	4	8	12	21	26	29
1. SINGLE DX	7	3.6	7	1	2	2	6	8	8	8
2. MULTIPLE DX	278	4.5	16	1	2	3	6	9	11	21
A. NOT OPERATED	256	3.9	9	1	2	3	5	8	9	16
B. OPERATED	29	9.6	45	3	5	8	11	21	26	29
TOTAL										
0–19 Years	0									
20–34	11	4.1	8	1	2	3	7	7	10	10
35–49	37	4.2	12	1	2	3	6	8	13	16
50–64	83	4.2	16	1	2	3	6	9	10	26
65+	154	4.7	17	1	2	3	6	9	11	21
GRAND TOTAL	285	4.5	16	1	2	3	6	9	10	21

Length of Stay by Diagnosis and Operation, Western Region, 2008

Western Region, October 2006–September 2007 Data, by Diagnosis

578: GASTROINTESTINAL HEMOR

Type of Patients	Observed Patients	Avg. Stay	Variance	10th	25th	50th	75th	90th	95th	99th
1. SINGLE DX										
A. Not Operated										
0–19 Years	21	1.5	<1	1	1	1	2	2	3	3
20–34	16	1.8	2	1	1	1	3	4	5	5
35–49	10	1.7	<1	1	1	2	2	2	4	4
50–64	17	2.2	7	1	1	1	2	4	12	12
65+	6	2.7	5	1	2	2	2	7	7	7
B. Operated										
0–19 Years	0									
20–34	0									
35–49	0									
50–64	0									
65+	1	11.0	0	11	11	11	11	11	11	11
2. MULTIPLE DX										
A. Not Operated										
0–19 Years	296	2.7	6	1	1	2	3	5	8	14
20–34	891	2.8	5	1	1	2	3	5	7	11
35–49	2,658	3.3	9	1	2	2	4	6	8	14
50–64	4,937	3.5	11	1	2	3	4	7	8	15
65+	14,148	3.9	9	1	2	3	5	7	9	15
B. Operated										
0–19 Years	6	6.0	56	2	2	3	6	21	21	21
20–34	21	9.4	46	2	5	8	12	19	24	24
35–49	73	10.2	72	3	5	8	13	20	30	45
50–64	120	10.1	115	3	4	7	12	18	30	60
65+	398	9.1	55	3	4	7	12	18	24	38
SUBTOTALS:										
1. SINGLE DX										
A. Not Operated	70	1.9	3	1	1	1	2	3	4	12
B. Operated	1	11.0	0	11	11	11	11	11	11	11
2. MULTIPLE DX										
A. Not Operated	22,930	3.7	9	1	2	3	4	7	9	15
B. Operated	618	9.4	68	3	4	7	12	18	25	38
1. SINGLE DX	71	2.0	4	1	1	1	2	3	5	12
2. MULTIPLE DX	23,548	3.8	12	1	2	3	5	7	9	17
A. NOT OPERATED	23,000	3.7	9	1	2	3	4	7	9	15
B. OPERATED	619	9.4	68	3	4	7	12	18	25	38
TOTAL										
0–19 Years	323	2.6	6	1	1	2	3	5	7	14
20–34	928	2.9	6	1	1	2	3	5	8	13
35–49	2,741	3.4	12	1	2	3	4	6	9	17
50–64	5,074	3.6	14	1	2	3	4	7	9	17
65+	14,553	4.0	11	1	2	3	5	7	10	17
GRAND TOTAL	23,619	3.8	12	2	3	3	5	7	9	17

578.0: HEMATEMESIS

Type of Patients	Observed Patients	Avg. Stay	Variance	10th	25th	50th	75th	90th	95th	99th
1. SINGLE DX										
A. Not Operated										
0–19 Years	9	1.1	<1	1	1	1	1	2	2	2
20–34	4	1.8	2	1	1	1	4	4	4	4
35–49	0									
50–64	0									
65+	0									
B. Operated										
0–19 Years	0									
20–34	0									
35–49	0									
50–64	0									
65+	0									
2. MULTIPLE DX										
A. Not Operated										
0–19 Years	104	2.5	6	1	1	2	3	5	7	10
20–34	263	2.7	5	1	1	2	4	5	8	12
35–49	621	3.1	6	2	2	2	4	6	8	13
50–64	668	3.5	9	1	2	3	4	7	9	14
65+	1,238	3.7	8	1	2	3	5	7	9	16
B. Operated										
0–19 Years	3	8.3	119	2	2	2	21	21	21	21
20–34	2	11.0	49	6	6	6	16	16	16	16
35–49	12	8.3	38	3	3	5	12	13	23	23
50–64	13	10.7	28	5	6	10	16	17	18	18
65+	26	8.9	81	2	3	6	11	20	29	38
SUBTOTALS:										
1. SINGLE DX										
A. Not Operated	13	1.3	<1	1	1	1	1	2	4	4
B. Operated	0									
2. MULTIPLE DX										
A. Not Operated	2,894	3.4	8	1	2	3	4	6	9	14
B. Operated	56	9.2	57	2	4	6	13	18	23	38
1. SINGLE DX	13	1.3	<1	1	1	1	1	2	4	4
2. MULTIPLE DX	2,950	3.5	9	1	2	3	4	7	9	16
A. NOT OPERATED	2,907	3.4	8	1	2	3	4	6	9	14
B. OPERATED	56	9.2	57	2	4	6	13	18	23	38
TOTAL										
0–19 Years	116	2.5	8	1	1	2	3	5	8	17
20–34	269	2.8	6	1	1	2	3	5	9	12
35–49	633	3.2	7	2	2	3	4	6	9	14
50–64	681	3.6	10	1	2	3	4	7	9	17
65+	1,264	3.8	10	1	2	3	5	7	9	17
GRAND TOTAL	2,963	3.5	9	1	2	3	4	7	9	16

578.1: BLOOD IN STOOL

Type of Patients	Observed Patients	Avg. Stay	Variance	10th	25th	50th	75th	90th	95th	99th
1. SINGLE DX										
A. Not Operated										
0–19 Years	8	2.0	<1	1	1	2	3	3	3	3
20–34	5	1.6	<1	1	1	1	2	3	3	3
35–49	2	1.5	<1	1	2	2	2	2	2	2
50–64	6	1.7	1	1	1	1	2	4	4	4
65+	0									
B. Operated										
0–19 Years	0									
20–34	0									
35–49	0									
50–64	0									
2. MULTIPLE DX										
A. Not Operated										
0–19 Years	136	2.5	3	1	1	2	3	5	6	9
20–34	176	2.7	5	1	2	2	3	5	6	13
35–49	499	2.9	5	1	2	2	3	5	7	11
50–64	1,061	3.1	5	1	2	2	4	6	7	13
65+	3,381	3.6	8	1	2	3	4	7	8	14
B. Operated										
0–19 Years	0									
20–34	5	4.2	10	1	2	3	7	8	8	8
35–49	17	11.2	104	2	5	7	17	30	37	37
50–64	20	6.4	20	2	3	6	8	11	22	22
65+	96	8.4	48	2	4	7	11	15	18	57
SUBTOTALS:										
1. SINGLE DX										
A. Not Operated	21	1.8	<1	1	1	2	2	3	3	4
B. Operated	0									
2. MULTIPLE DX										
A. Not Operated	5,253	3.4	7	1	2	3	4	6	8	14
B. Operated	138	8.3	51	2	4	7	11	16	20	37
1. SINGLE DX	21	1.8	<1	1	1	2	2	3	3	4
2. MULTIPLE DX	5,391	3.5	9	1	2	3	4	7	8	15
A. NOT OPERATED	5,274	3.4	7	1	2	3	4	6	8	14
B. OPERATED	138	8.3	51	2	4	7	11	16	20	37
TOTAL										
0–19 Years	144	2.4	3	1	1	2	3	4	6	9
20–34	186	2.7	5	1	1	2	3	5	7	13
35–49	518	3.2	11	2	2	2	4	6	8	17
50–64	1,087	3.1	6	2	2	2	4	6	7	13
65+	3,477	3.7	10	2	3	3	4	7	9	15
GRAND TOTAL	5,412	3.5	9	1	2	3	4	7	8	15

Length of Stay by Diagnosis and Operation, Western Region, 2008

Western Region, October 2006–September 2007 Data, by Diagnosis

578.9: GI HEMORRHAGE NOS

Type of Patients	Observed Patients	Avg. Stay	Variance	10th	25th	50th	75th	90th	95th	99th
1. SINGLE DX										
A. Not Operated										
0–19 Years	4	1.3	<1	1	1	1	1	2	2	2
20–34	7	2.0	2	1	1	1	3	5	5	5
35–49	8	1.8	1	1	1	1	2	4	4	4
50–64	11	2.4	10	1	1	1	2	3	12	12
65+	6	2.7	5	1	2	2	2	7	7	7
B. Operated										
0–19 Years	0									
20–34	0									
35–49	0									
50–64	0									
65+	1	11.0	0	11	11	11	11	11	11	11
2. MULTIPLE DX										
A. Not Operated										
0–19 Years	56	3.5	10	1	1	3	4	8	11	17
20–34	452	2.8	4	1	1	2	3	5	7	11
35–49	1,538	3.4	11	1	2	3	4	6	9	16
50–64	3,208	3.6	13	1	2	3	4	7	9	16
65+	9,529	4.0	9	1	2	3	5	7	10	15
B. Operated										
0–19 Years	3	3.7	4	2	2	3	6	6	6	6
20–34	14	11.1	50	3	5	11	13	24	24	24
35–49	44	10.3	72	3	5	8	13	18	26	45
50–64	87	10.9	146	3	4	8	13	18	33	85
65+	276	9.4	54	3	4	7	12	19	25	38
SUBTOTALS:										
1. SINGLE DX										
A. Not Operated	36	2.1	4	1	1	1	2	4	7	12
B. Operated	1	11.0	0	11	11	11	11	11	11	11
2. MULTIPLE DX										
A. Not Operated	14,783	3.8	10	1	2	3	5	7	9	16
B. Operated	424	9.8	75	3	5	7	12	19	25	42
1. SINGLE DX	37	2.4	7	1	1	2	2	5	11	12
2. MULTIPLE DX	15,207	4.0	13	1	2	3	5	7	10	18
A. NOT OPERATED	14,819	3.8	10	1	2	3	5	7	9	16
B. OPERATED	425	9.8	74	3	5	7	12	19	25	42
TOTAL										
0–19 Years	63	3.3	10	1	1	2	4	6	8	17
20–34	473	3.0	7	1	1	2	3	5	8	13
35–49	1,590	3.6	14	1	2	3	4	7	9	18
50–64	3,306	3.8	18	1	2	3	4	7	9	18
65+	9,812	4.1	11	1	2	3	5	8	10	18
GRAND TOTAL	15,244	4.0	13	1	2	3	5	7	10	18

579: INTESTINAL MALABSORPTION

Type of Patients	Observed Patients	Avg. Stay	Variance	10th	25th	50th	75th	90th	95th	99th
1. SINGLE DX										
A. Not Operated										
0–19 Years	1	1.0	0	1	1	1	1	1	1	1
20–34	0									
35–49	0									
50–64	0									
65+	0									
B. Operated										
0–19 Years	0									
20–34	0									
35–49	1	4.0	0	4	4	4	4	4	4	4
50–64	1	8.0	0	8	8	8	8	8	8	8
65+	0									
2. MULTIPLE DX										
A. Not Operated										
0–19 Years	113	7.8	191	1	2	3	7	18	26	85
20–34	42	5.5	33	2	3	4	6	9	11	38
35–49	105	6.3	39	2	2	5	8	14	19	29
50–64	139	7.0	54	2	3	5	8	14	21	30
65+	143	6.9	54	2	3	5	8	12	19	35
B. Operated										
0–19 Years	6	13.7	73	3	6	16	27	>99	>99	>99
20–34	12	11.0	90	4	5	6	11	23	33	33
35–49	19	7.2	41	1	4	5	8	18	27	27
50–64	43	9.7	98	2	4	6	10	29	30	39
65+	14	16.9	367	6	6	8	20	32	78	78
SUBTOTALS:										
1. SINGLE DX										
A. Not Operated	1	1.0	0	1	1	1	1	1	1	1
B. Operated	2	6.0	8	4	4	8	8	8	8	8
2. MULTIPLE DX										
A. Not Operated	542	6.9	78	2	2	4	8	14	20	45
B. Operated	94	10.7	128	3	4	7	13	29	32	>99
1. SINGLE DX	3	4.4	12	1	1	4	4	8	8	8
2. MULTIPLE DX	636	7.5	87	2	3	5	8	16	25	57
A. NOT OPERATED	543	6.9	78	2	2	4	8	14	20	45
B. OPERATED	96	10.6	126	3	4	7	13	29	32	>99
TOTAL										
0–19 Years	120	8.1	185	1	2	3	8	18	27	88
20–34	54	6.7	50	2	3	5	8	11	23	38
35–49	125	6.4	39	2	2	5	8	14	19	29
50–64	183	7.6	65	2	3	5	8	15	27	39
65+	157	7.8	88	2	3	5	9	17	22	61
GRAND TOTAL	639	7.4	87	2	3	5	8	16	25	57

579.3: INTEST POSTOP NONABSORP

Type of Patients	Observed Patients	Avg. Stay	Variance	10th	25th	50th	75th	90th	95th	99th
1. SINGLE DX										
A. Not Operated										
0–19 Years	0									
20–34	0									
35–49	0									
50–64	0									
65+	0									
B. Operated										
0–19 Years	0									
20–34	0									
35–49	1	4.0	0	4	4	4	4	4	4	4
50–64	1	8.0	0	8	8	8	8	8	8	8
65+	0									
2. MULTIPLE DX										
A. Not Operated										
0–19 Years	40	12.9	399	2	2	5	16	39	85	88
20–34	7	11.4	150	4	4	6	13	38	38	38
35–49	55	7.1	57	2	2	4	8	19	25	37
50–64	86	7.4	68	2	3	6	8	14	21	64
65+	46	7.0	36	2	4	5	9	12	19	29
B. Operated										
0–19 Years	5	15.8	57	6	13	16	27	>99	>99	>99
20–34	9	11.1	95	3	5	7	11	33	33	33
35–49	18	7.4	43	1	4	5	9	18	27	27
50–64	34	10.8	116	2	4	6	12	30	31	39
65+	12	18.0	423	6	6	8	22	32	78	78
SUBTOTALS:										
1. SINGLE DX										
A. Not Operated	0									
B. Operated	2	6.0	8	4	4	8	8	8	8	8
2. MULTIPLE DX										
A. Not Operated	234	8.3	120	2	3	5	9	19	27	64
B. Operated	78	11.5	145	3	4	7	17	30	33	>99
1. SINGLE DX	2	6.0	8	4	4	8	8	8	8	8
2. MULTIPLE DX	312	9.1	128	2	3	6	10	21	29	78
A. NOT OPERATED	234	8.3	120	2	3	5	9	19	27	64
B. OPERATED	80	11.3	142	3	4	7	16	29	32	>99
TOTAL										
0–19 Years	45	13.2	360	2	2	5	17	39	85	>99
20–34	16	11.2	111	4	5	6	11	33	38	38
35–49	74	7.1	53	2	2	4	8	18	25	37
50–64	121	8.4	82	2	4	6	9	20	29	39
65+	58	9.3	130	2	4	6	10	20	29	78
GRAND TOTAL	314	9.1	127	2	3	6	10	21	29	78

Length of Stay by Diagnosis and Operation, Western Region, 2008

Western Region, October 2006–September 2007 Data, by Diagnosis

580: ACUTE NEPHRITIS

Type of Patients	Observed Patients	Avg. Stay	Vari-ance	10th	25th	50th	75th	90th	95th	99th
1. SINGLE DX										
A. Not Operated										
0–19 Years	5	2.6	1		2	3	3	4	4	4
20–34	0									
35–49	0									
50–64	1	1.0	0	1	1	1	1	1	1	1
65+	0									
B. Operated										
0–19 Years	0									
20–34	0									
35–49	0									
50–64	0									
65+	0									
2. MULTIPLE DX										
A. Not Operated										
0–19 Years	56	4.1	7	1	2	3	5	8	10	12
20–34	21	5.5	12	3	3	4	6	9	10	17
35–49	17	5.5	8	2	3	4	8	10	10	10
50–64	38	8.3	64	2	3	6	11	16	23	44
65+	55	7.1	24	3	4	6	9	14	17	23
B. Operated										
0–19 Years	2	4.0	8	2	2	4	6	6	6	6
20–34	1	7.0	0	7	7	7	7	7	7	7
35–49	2	10.5	40	6	6	11	15	15	15	15
50–64										
65+	5	13.2	143	2	5	10	17	32	32	32
SUBTOTALS:										
1. SINGLE DX										
A. Not Operated	6	2.3	1	1	1	3	3	4	4	4
B. Operated	0									
2. MULTIPLE DX										
A. Not Operated	187	6.1	26	2	3	5	8	12	16	23
B. Operated	10	10.2	84	2	5	6	15	32	32	32
1. SINGLE DX	6	2.3	1	1	1	3	3	4	4	4
2. MULTIPLE DX	197	6.3	30	2	3	5	8	12	17	32
A. NOT OPERATED	193	6.0	26	2	3	5	8	12	16	23
B. OPERATED	10	10.2	84	2	5	6	15	32	32	32
TOTAL										
0–19 Years	63	3.9	7	1	2	3	5	7	10	12
20–34	21	5.5	12	3	3	4	6	9	10	17
35–49	18	5.6	8	2	3	4	8	10	10	10
50–64	41	8.2	61	2	3	6	11	15	21	44
65+	60	7.6	34	2	4	6	10	17	21	32
GRAND TOTAL	203	6.2	29	2	3	5	8	12	16	23

581: NEPHROTIC SYNDROME

Type of Patients	Observed Patients	Avg. Stay	Vari-ance	10th	25th	50th	75th	90th	95th	99th
1. SINGLE DX										
A. Not Operated										
0–19 Years	61	2.1	2	1	1	2	3	4	4	7
20–34	2	2.0	2	1	1	2	3	3	3	3
35–49	1	1.0	0	1	1	1	1	1	1	1
50–64	2	5.6	24	2	2	9	9	9	9	9
65+	0									
B. Operated										
0–19 Years	0									
20–34	0									
35–49	0									
50–64	0									
65+	0									
2. MULTIPLE DX										
A. Not Operated										
0–19 Years	174	3.3	9	1	2	2	4	7	9	17
20–34	87	3.8	9	1	2	3	5	8	11	>99
35–49	110	4.9	27	1	2	4	6	9	13	27
50–64	134	5.3	25	1	2	4	7	11	14	31
65+	105	5.8	20	1	2	5	7	13	15	20
B. Operated										
0–19 Years	0									
20–34	7	6.7	28	2	3	4	13	15	15	15
35–49	3	4.3	1	3	3	5	5	5	5	5
50–64	7	10.2	47	5	5	8	14	24	24	24
65+	4	11.8	4	10	10	13	14	14	14	14
SUBTOTALS:										
1. SINGLE DX										
A. Not Operated	66	2.2	2	1	1	2	3	4	5	9
B. Operated	0									
2. MULTIPLE DX										
A. Not Operated	610	4.5	18	1	2	3	6	9	13	21
B. Operated	21	8.5	30	3	5	7	13	14	15	24
1. SINGLE DX	66	2.2	2	1	1	2	3	4	5	9
2. MULTIPLE DX	631	4.7	19	1	2	3	6	10	13	22
A. NOT OPERATED	676	4.3	17	1	2	3	5	9	13	21
B. OPERATED	21	8.5	30	3	5	7	13	14	15	24
TOTAL										
0–19 Years	235	3.0	7	1	2	2	3	6	8	15
20–34	96	4.0	10	1	2	3	5	8	12	>99
35–49	114	4.8	26	1	2	4	6	9	13	27
50–64	143	5.5	27	1	2	4	7	11	14	31
65+	109	6.0	20	1	2	5	8	13	15	20
GRAND TOTAL	697	4.4	18	1	2	3	6	9	13	21

581.9: NEPHROTIC SYNDROME NOS

Type of Patients	Observed Patients	Avg. Stay	Vari-ance	10th	25th	50th	75th	90th	95th	99th
1. SINGLE DX										
A. Not Operated										
0–19 Years	53	2.1	2	1	1	2	3	4	5	7
20–34	2	2.0	2	1	1	2	3	3	3	3
35–49	1	1.0	0	1	1	1	1	1	1	1
50–64	1	2.0	0	2	2	2	2	2	2	2
65+	0									
B. Operated										
0–19 Years	0									
20–34	0									
35–49	0									
50–64	0									
65+	0									
2. MULTIPLE DX										
A. Not Operated										
0–19 Years	132	3.1	5	1	2	2	4	6	8	11
20–34	52	3.6	8	1	2	3	5	7	11	12
35–49	83	3.8	10	1	2	3	5	8	10	17
50–64	96	4.6	20	1	2	3	6	9	14	31
65+	81	5.4	16	1	2	4	7	11	14	17
B. Operated										
0–19 Years	0									
20–34	3	7.0	48	3	3	3	15	15	15	15
35–49	3	4.3	1	3	3	5	5	5	5	5
50–64	3	6.7	2	5	5	7	8	8	8	8
65+	2	11.5	5	10	10	12	13	13	13	13
SUBTOTALS:										
1. SINGLE DX										
A. Not Operated	57	2.1	2	1	1	2	3	4	5	7
B. Operated	0									
2. MULTIPLE DX										
A. Not Operated	444	4.0	12	1	2	3	5	8	11	15
B. Operated	11	7.0	17	3	3	5	10	13	15	15
1. SINGLE DX	57	2.1	2	1	1	2	3	4	5	7
2. MULTIPLE DX	455	4.1	12	1	2	3	5	8	11	15
A. NOT OPERATED	501	3.8	11	1	2	3	5	8	11	15
B. OPERATED	11	7.0	17	3	3	5	10	13	15	15
TOTAL										
0–19 Years	185	2.8	4	1	1	2	3	5	7	11
20–34	57	3.7	10	1	2	3	5	8	12	15
35–49	87	3.8	9	1	2	3	5	8	10	17
50–64	100	4.6	20	1	2	3	6	9	14	31
65+	83	5.6	16	1	2	4	7	12	14	17
GRAND TOTAL	512	3.9	12	1	2	3	5	8	11	15

Western Region, October 2006–September 2007 Data, by Diagnosis

582: CHRONIC NEPHRITIS

Type of Patients	Observed Patients	Avg. Stay	Vari-ance	10th	25th	50th	75th	90th	95th	99th
1. SINGLE DX										
A. Not Operated										
0–19 Years	0									
20–34	0									
35–49	1	1.0	0	1	1	1	1	1	1	1
50–64	0									
65+	0									
B. Operated										
0–19 Years	0									
20–34	0									
35–49	0									
50–64	0									
65+	0									
2. MULTIPLE DX										
A. Not Operated										
0–19 Years	18	1.9	2	1	1	1	2	5	6	6
20–34	10	3.4	11	1	1	3	4	12	12	12
35–49	7	2.6	2	1	1	3	3	5	5	5
50–64	9	4.7	15	1	2	3	6	13	13	13
65+	5	4.8	10	2	3	4	5	10	10	10
B. Operated										
0–19 Years	2	10.9	97	4	4	18	18	18	18	18
20–34	7	4.4	4	2	3	4	5	8	8	8
35–49	11	6.0	36	1	2	4	6	16	19	19
50–64	10	4.4	14	2	2	3	5	14	14	14
65+	2	6.0	0	6	6	6	6	6	6	6
SUBTOTALS:										
1. SINGLE DX										
A. Not Operated	1	1.0	0	1	1	1	1	1	1	1
B. Operated	0									
2. MULTIPLE DX										
A. Not Operated	49	3.1	8	1	1	2	2	6	10	13
B. Operated	32	5.5	22	2	3	3	4	14	18	19
1. SINGLE DX	1	1.0	0	1	1	1	1	1	1	1
2. MULTIPLE DX	81	4.1	15	1	2	3	5	7	13	19
A. NOT OPERATED	50	3.1	8	1	1	2	2	6	10	13
B. OPERATED	32	5.5	22	2	3	4	6	14	18	19
TOTAL										
0–19 Years	20	2.8	15	1	1	1	2	5	6	18
20–34	17	3.8	8	1	2	3	5	8	12	12
35–49	19	4.5	24	1	1	3	5	16	19	19
50–64	19	4.5	13	1	2	3	6	13	14	14
65+	7	5.1	7	2	3	5	6	10	10	10
GRAND TOTAL	82	4.0	14	1	2	3	5	7	13	19

583: NEPHRITIS NOS

Type of Patients	Observed Patients	Avg. Stay	Vari-ance	10th	25th	50th	75th	90th	95th	99th
1. SINGLE DX										
A. Not Operated										
0–19 Years	4	1.8	<1	1	1	1	2	3	3	3
20–34	1	1.0	0	1	1	1	1	1	1	1
35–49	2	1.0	0	1	1	1	1	1	1	1
50–64	0									
65+	0									
B. Operated										
0–19 Years	0									
20–34	0									
35–49	0									
50–64	0									
65+	0									
2. MULTIPLE DX										
A. Not Operated										
0–19 Years	42	3.5	12	1	1	2	4	8	12	15
20–34	59	4.0	20	1	1	3	4	9	18	24
35–49	47	6.1	46	1	2	4	9	12	16	38
50–64	46	7.3	54	1	2	5	10	19	23	31
65+	45	7.4	39	1	3	5	10	18	19	26
B. Operated										
0–19 Years	3	5.6	17	1	1	7	9	9	9	9
20–34	8	5.8	2	4	5	5	7	8	8	8
35–49	6	9.8	63	2	5	6	16	23	23	23
50–64	12	4.6	4	3	3	4	7	7	8	8
65+	4	5.0	<1	4	5	5	6	6	6	6
SUBTOTALS:										
1. SINGLE DX										
A. Not Operated	7	1.4	<1	1	1	1	2	3	3	3
B. Operated	0									
2. MULTIPLE DX										
A. Not Operated	239	5.6	36	1	2	3	7	13	19	26
B. Operated	33	6.0	16	3	4	5	7	8	16	23
1. SINGLE DX	7	1.4	<1	1	1	1	2	3	3	3
2. MULTIPLE DX	272	5.7	34	1	2	4	7	12	18	26
A. NOT OPERATED	246	5.5	35	1	1	3	7	13	18	26
B. OPERATED	33	6.0	16	3	4	5	7	8	16	23
TOTAL										
0–19 Years	49	3.5	12	1	1	2	4	5	6	15
20–34	68	4.2	18	1	2	3	5	8	13	24
35–49	55	6.4	48	1	2	5	9	16	19	38
50–64	58	6.8	45	1	3	5	8	13	23	31
65+	49	7.2	36	1	3	5	10	18	19	26
GRAND TOTAL	279	5.6	33	1	2	4	7	12	18	26

584: ACUTE RENAL FAILURE

Type of Patients	Observed Patients	Avg. Stay	Vari-ance	10th	25th	50th	75th	90th	95th	99th
1. SINGLE DX										
A. Not Operated										
0–19 Years	4	5.5	25	3	3	3	13	13	13	13
20–34	3	3.3	10	1	1	2	6	7	7	7
35–49	3	1.3	<1	1	1	1	1	2	2	2
50–64	3	2.0	3	1	1	1	1	4	4	4
65+	5	8.6	29	4	7	7	7	18	18	18
B. Operated										
0–19 Years	0									
20–34	0									
35–49	0									
50–64	0									
65+	0									
2. MULTIPLE DX										
A. Not Operated										
0–19 Years	234	5.0	17	1	2	4	6	11	14	20
20–34	1,450	4.9	21	1	2	3	6	11	14	22
35–49	3,849	5.4	31	1	2	4	6	11	15	27
50–64	9,995	5.5	28	2	2	4	7	11	15	27
65+	29,691	5.5	20	2	3	4	7	10	13	22
B. Operated										
0–19 Years	18	17.6	330	6	8	12	15	57	74	74
20–34	85	11.9	169	3	6	8	13	24	35	95
35–49	229	11.5	80	4	6	10	14	22	29	69
50–64	672	11.3	85	4	6	9	14	22	28	54
65+	1,548	11.2	70	4	6	9	14	21	26	43
SUBTOTALS:										
1. SINGLE DX										
A. Not Operated	18	4.7	21	1	1	3	7	13	18	18
B. Operated	0									
2. MULTIPLE DX										
A. Not Operated	45,219	5.4	23	2	3	4	7	10	14	23
B. Operated	2,552	11.3	80	4	6	9	14	21	27	46
1. SINGLE DX	18	4.7	21	1	1	3	7	13	18	18
2. MULTIPLE DX	47,771	5.8	28	2	3	4	7	11	15	26
A. NOT OPERATED	45,237	5.4	23	2	3	4	7	10	14	23
B. OPERATED	2,552	11.3	80	4	6	9	14	21	27	46
TOTAL										
0–19 Years	256	5.9	48	1	2	4	7	12	16	23
20–34	1,538	5.3	31	2	2	4	7	11	15	27
35–49	4,081	5.7	36	2	2	4	7	12	16	32
50–64	10,670	5.9	34	2	3	4	7	12	16	29
65+	31,244	5.7	24	2	3	4	7	11	14	25
GRAND TOTAL	47,789	5.8	28	2	3	4	7	11	15	26

Length of Stay by Diagnosis and Operation, Western Region, 2008

Western Region, October 2006–September 2007 Data, by Diagnosis

584.5: AC RF W TUBULAR NEPHR

Type of Patients	Observed Patients	Avg. Stay	Vari-ance	Percentiles						
				10th	25th	50th	75th	90th	95th	99th
1. SINGLE DX										
A. Not Operated										
0–19 Years	1	3.0	0	3	3	3	3	3	3	3
20–34	2	4.0	18	1	1	1	1	7	7	7
35–49	1	1.0	0	1	1	1	1	1	1	1
50–64	0									
65+	0									
B. Operated										
0–19 Years	0									
20–34	0									
35–49	0									
50–64	0									
65+	0									
2. MULTIPLE DX										
A. Not Operated										
0–19 Years	30	5.2	9	3	3	4	7	10	10	16
20–34	155	7.0	34	2	3	5	9	15	22	27
35–49	348	7.2	29	2	3	5	10	14	19	27
50–64	868	7.9	43	2	4	6	10	16	21	35
65+	1,792	8.0	40	3	4	6	10	16	20	32
B. Operated										
0–19 Years	2	31.5	>999	6	6	32	57	57	57	57
20–34	7	16.5	300	2	2	10	24	52	52	52
35–49	20	20.7	272	7	9	15	23	41	52	69
50–64	52	18.3	186	6	9	14	27	34	54	63
65+	117	14.9	84	6	9	12	20	29	34	45
SUBTOTALS:										
1. SINGLE DX										
A. Not Operated	4	3.0	8	1	1	1	3	7	7	7
B. Operated	0									
2. MULTIPLE DX										
A. Not Operated	3,193	7.8	39	2	4	6	10	15	20	32
B. Operated	198	16.6	146	6	9	12	22	30	43	63
1. SINGLE DX	4	3.0	8	1	1	1	3	7	7	7
2. MULTIPLE DX	3,391	8.4	50	3	4	6	10	16	22	35
A. NOT OPERATED	3,197	7.8	39	2	4	6	10	15	20	31
B. OPERATED	198	16.6	146	6	9	12	22	30	43	63
TOTAL										
0–19 Years	33	6.8	90	3	3	4	7	10	16	16
20–34	164	7.4	47	2	3	5	10	16	22	27
35–49	369	7.9	51	2	3	6	10	16	20	31
50–64	920	8.5	57	2	4	6	11	17	23	36
65+	1,909	8.5	45	3	4	7	11	16	21	33
GRAND TOTAL	3,395	8.3	50	3	4	6	10	16	22	34

584.8: ACUTE RENAL FAILURE NEC

Type of Patients	Observed Patients	Avg. Stay	Vari-ance	Percentiles						
				10th	25th	50th	75th	90th	95th	99th
1. SINGLE DX										
A. Not Operated										
0–19 Years	0									
20–34	0									
35–49	0									
50–64	0									
65+	0									
B. Operated										
0–19 Years	0									
20–34	0									
35–49	0									
50–64	0									
65+	0									
2. MULTIPLE DX										
A. Not Operated										
0–19 Years	6	6.2	25	2	3	5	9	15	15	15
20–34	22	5.5	8	2	4	4	8	9	10	11
35–49	42	7.7	90	2	3	4	8	18	25	43
50–64	129	5.9	20	2	2	5	8	11	13	23
65+	189	6.8	38	2	3	5	8	13	17	34
B. Operated										
0–19 Years	1	74.0	0	74	74	74	74	74	74	74
20–34	4	6.5	4	5	5	7	9	9	9	9
35–49	4	8.3	29	3	3	8	12	15	15	15
50–64	10	10.1	27	4	8	9	12	14	22	22
65+	16	12.5	100	2	4	9	17	30	34	34
SUBTOTALS:										
1. SINGLE DX										
A. Not Operated	0									
B. Operated	0									
2. MULTIPLE DX										
A. Not Operated	388	6.5	36	2	3	5	8	12	16	34
B. Operated	35	12.4	174	4	5	9	15	24	34	74
1. SINGLE DX	0									
2. MULTIPLE DX	423	7.0	49	2	3	5	9	13	18	34
A. NOT OPERATED	388	6.5	36	2	3	5	8	12	16	34
B. OPERATED	35	12.4	174	4	5	9	15	24	34	74
TOTAL										
0–19 Years	7	15.9	677	2	3	5	15	74	74	74
20–34	26	5.6	7	2	4	5	8	9	10	11
35–49	46	7.8	84	2	3	5	9	18	25	43
50–64	139	6.2	22	2	3	5	8	12	14	23
65+	205	7.2	45	2	3	5	9	15	18	34
GRAND TOTAL	423	7.0	49	2	3	5	9	13	18	34

584.9: ACUTE RENAL FAILURE NOS

Type of Patients	Observed Patients	Avg. Stay	Vari-ance	Percentiles						
				10th	25th	50th	75th	90th	95th	99th
1. SINGLE DX										
A. Not Operated										
0–19 Years	3	6.4	33	3	3	3	3	13	13	13
20–34	1	2.0	0	1	2	2	2	2	2	2
35–49	2	1.5	<1	1	1	1	1	2	2	2
50–64	3	2.0	3	1	1	1	4	4	4	4
65+	5	8.6	29	4	7	7	7	18	18	18
B. Operated										
0–19 Years	0									
20–34	0									
35–49	0									
50–64	0									
65+	0									
2. MULTIPLE DX										
A. Not Operated										
0–19 Years	198	4.9	18	1	2	4	6	11	14	23
20–34	1,273	4.6	18	2	2	3	6	10	13	21
35–49	3,459	5.1	30	1	2	4	6	10	15	27
50–64	8,995	5.3	27	2	2	4	6	10	14	25
65+	27,701	5.3	18	2	3	4	7	10	13	21
B. Operated										
0–19 Years	15	12.0	19	7	8	12	14	17	23	23
20–34	74	11.8	166	3	6	8	13	23	35	95
35–49	205	10.7	54	4	6	9	13	21	26	45
50–64	608	10.7	73	4	6	9	13	20	26	39
65+	1,413	10.8	67	4	6	9	13	20	25	42
SUBTOTALS:										
1. SINGLE DX										
A. Not Operated	14	5.2	25	1	2	3	7	13	18	18
B. Operated	0									
2. MULTIPLE DX										
A. Not Operated	41,626	5.2	21	2	3	4	8	10	13	22
B. Operated	2,315	10.8	70	4	6	9	13	20	25	43
1. SINGLE DX	14	5.2	25	1	2	3	7	13	18	18
2. MULTIPLE DX	43,941	5.5	25	2	3	4	7	11	14	25
A. NOT OPERATED	41,640	5.2	21	2	3	4	6	10	13	22
B. OPERATED	2,315	10.8	70	4	6	9	13	20	25	43
TOTAL										
0–19 Years	216	5.4	21	1	2	4	7	12	15	23
20–34	1,348	5.0	29	1	2	3	6	11	14	26
35–49	3,666	5.5	33	1	2	4	7	11	16	32
50–64	9,606	5.6	31	2	2	4	7	11	15	28
65+	29,119	5.5	22	2	3	4	7	11	14	23
GRAND TOTAL	43,955	5.5	25	2	3	4	7	11	14	25

Length of Stay by Diagnosis and Operation, Western Region, 2008

Western Region, October 2006–September 2007 Data, by Diagnosis

585: CHRONIC KIDNEY DISEASE

Type of Patients	Observed Patients	Avg. Stay	Vari-ance	10th	25th	50th	75th	90th	95th	99th
1. SINGLE DX										
A. *Not Operated*										
0–19 Years	2	1.0	0	1	1	1	1	1	1	1
20–34	1	1.0	0	1	1	1	1	1	1	1
35–49	8	1.1	<1	1	1	1	1	2	2	2
50–64	4	1.0	0	1	1	1	1	1	1	1
65+	4	3.3	11	1	1	3	8	8	8	8
B. *Operated*										
0–19 Years	1	1.0	0	1	1	1	1	1	1	1
20–34	0									
35–49	0									
50–64	4	1.5	<1	1	1	2	2	2	2	2
65+	3	1.0	0	1	1	1	1	1	1	1
2. MULTIPLE DX										
A. *Not Operated*										
0–19 Years	42	4.5	22	1	2	4	5	9	14	23
20–34	142	4.1	16	1	1	3	5	10	12	18
35–49	294	3.8	19	1	1	2	5	8	10	23
50–64	463	4.4	24	1	2	3	5	9	12	23
65+	726	4.9	19	1	2	4	6	10	13	22
B. *Operated*										
0–19 Years	44	7.1	39	2	4	6	8	12	14	38
20–34	120	5.4	12	2	3	5	7	10	12	16
35–49	166	5.1	14	1	3	5	6	10	11	23
50–64	237	6.2	44	1	3	5	7	11	14	29
65+	226	5.5	36	1	1	4	7	11	15	28
SUBTOTALS:										
1. SINGLE DX										
A. *Not Operated*	19	1.5	3	1	1	1	1	3	8	8
B. *Operated*	8	1.3	<1	1	1	1	2	2	2	2
2. MULTIPLE DX										
A. *Not Operated*	1,667	4.5	20	1	2	3	6	9	13	22
B. *Operated*	793	5.7	30	1	3	5	7	10	14	25
1. SINGLE DX	27	1.5	2	1	1	1	1	2	3	8
2. MULTIPLE DX	2,460	4.9	24	1	2	4	6	10	13	23
A. NOT OPERATED	1,686	4.5	20	1	2	3	6	9	13	22
B. OPERATED	801	5.7	30	1	3	5	7	10	14	24
TOTAL										
0–19 Years	89	5.7	31	1	2	4	7	12	14	38
20–34	263	4.7	14	1	2	3	6	10	12	18
35–49	468	4.2	17	1	1	3	6	9	10	23
50–64	708	5.0	31	1	2	4	6	9	13	23
65+	959	5.0	23	1	2	4	6	10	14	24
GRAND TOTAL	2,487	4.8	24	1	2	4	6	10	13	23

585.6: ESRD

Type of Patients	Observed Patients	Avg. Stay	Vari-ance	10th	25th	50th	75th	90th	95th	99th
1. SINGLE DX										
A. *Not Operated*										
0–19 Years	2	1.0	0	1	1	1	1	1	1	1
20–34	1	1.0	0	1	1	1	1	1	1	1
35–49	5	1.2	<1	1	1	1	1	2	2	2
50–64	4	1.0	0	1	1	1	1	1	1	1
65+	2	1.0	0	1	1	1	1	1	1	1
B. *Operated*										
0–19 Years	1	1.0	0	1	1	1	1	1	1	1
20–34	0									
35–49	0									
50–64	4	1.5	<1	1	1	2	2	2	2	2
65+	2	1.0	0	1	1	1	1	1	1	1
2. MULTIPLE DX										
A. *Not Operated*										
0–19 Years	29	4.8	27	1	2	4	5	14	18	23
20–34	116	4.2	16	1	1	3	5	10	13	18
35–49	249	3.8	21	1	1	2	5	8	11	23
50–64	353	4.3	20	1	1	3	5	9	12	22
65+	462	5.1	23	1	2	4	6	11	14	24
B. *Operated*										
0–19 Years	35	7.6	46	2	4	6	9	13	22	38
20–34	114	5.4	12	2	3	5	6	10	13	16
35–49	152	5.3	14	1	3	5	6	9	11	23
50–64	222	6.2	46	1	3	5	7	11	14	29
65+	197	5.5	39	1	1	4	7	11	15	32
SUBTOTALS:										
1. SINGLE DX										
A. *Not Operated*	14	1.1	<1	1	1	1	1	1	2	2
B. *Operated*	7	1.3	<1	1	1	1	2	2	2	2
2. MULTIPLE DX										
A. *Not Operated*	1,209	4.5	22	1	1	3	6	9	13	23
B. *Operated*	720	5.7	32	1	3	5	7	10	14	25
1. SINGLE DX	21	1.1	<1	1	1	1	1	2	2	2
2. MULTIPLE DX	1,929	5.0	26	1	2	4	6	10	14	24
A. NOT OPERATED	1,223	4.5	21	1	1	3	6	9	13	23
B. OPERATED	727	5.7	32	1	3	5	7	10	14	25
TOTAL										
0–19 Years	67	6.1	38	1	2	4	7	13	18	38
20–34	231	4.8	14	1	2	3	6	10	13	18
35–49	406	4.3	19	1	1	3	6	9	11	23
50–64	583	5.0	31	1	2	4	6	9	13	23
65+	663	5.2	28	1	2	4	6	11	15	25
GRAND TOTAL	1,950	4.9	26	1	2	4	6	10	14	24

585.9: CHRONIC KIDNEY DIS NOS

Type of Patients	Observed Patients	Avg. Stay	Vari-ance	10th	25th	50th	75th	90th	95th	99th
1. SINGLE DX										
A. *Not Operated*										
0–19 Years	0									
20–34	0									
35–49	2	1.0	0	1	1	1	1	1	1	1
50–64	0									
65+	1	3.0	0	3	3	3	3	3	3	3
B. *Operated*										
0–19 Years	0									
20–34	0									
35–49	0									
50–64	0									
65+	1	1.0	0	1	1	1	1	1	1	1
2. MULTIPLE DX										
A. *Not Operated*										
0–19 Years	6	4.7	4	2	4	4	5	8	8	8
20–34	11	3.1	9	1	1	2	4	5	11	11
35–49	19	3.3	4	1	1	3	5	7	8	8
50–64	40	4.5	15	1	2	3	6	12	15	16
65+	133	4.2	7	1	2	3	6	8	9	13
B. *Operated*										
0–19 Years	0									
20–34	0									
35–49	2	2.5	4	1	1	1	4	4	4	4
50–64	3	10.0	12	6	6	12	12	12	12	12
65+	7	3.9	12	1	2	2	9	9	9	9
SUBTOTALS:										
1. SINGLE DX										
A. *Not Operated*	3	1.7	1	1	1	1	3	3	3	3
B. *Operated*	1	1.0	0	1	1	1	1	1	1	1
2. MULTIPLE DX										
A. *Not Operated*	209	4.1	9	1	2	3	5	8	10	14
B. *Operated*	12	5.2	18	1	2	4	9	12	12	12
1. SINGLE DX	4	1.5	1	1	1	1	3	3	3	3
2. MULTIPLE DX	221	4.2	9	1	2	3	5	8	10	14
A. NOT OPERATED	212	4.1	8	1	2	3	5	8	10	14
B. OPERATED	13	4.9	18	1	2	2	9	12	12	12
TOTAL										
0–19 Years	6	4.7	4	2	4	4	5	8	8	8
20–34	11	3.1	9	1	1	2	4	5	11	11
35–49	23	3.1	4	1	1	3	4	5	7	8
50–64	43	4.9	17	1	2	4	6	12	12	16
65+	142	4.2	7	1	2	3	6	8	9	13
GRAND TOTAL	225	4.1	9	1	2	3	5	8	10	14

Length of Stay by Diagnosis and Operation, Western Region, 2008

Western Region, October 2006–September 2007 Data, by Diagnosis

586: RENAL FAILURE NOS

Type of Patients	Observed Patients	Avg. Stay	Variance	10th	25th	50th	75th	90th	95th	99th
1. SINGLE DX										
A. Not Operated										
0–19 Years	0									
20–34	0									
35–49	0									
50–64	1	1.0	0	1	1	1	1	1	1	1
65+	0									
B. Operated										
0–19 Years	0									
20–34	1	1.0	0	1	1	1	1	1	1	1
35–49	0									
50–64	0									
65+	0									
2. MULTIPLE DX										
A. Not Operated										
0–19 Years	0									
20–34	6	2.0	2	1	1	2	3	4	4	4
35–49	13	3.1	7	1	2	2	3	8	9	9
50–64	33	4.1	15	1	2	3	4	12	14	15
65+	121	3.8	6	1	2	3	5	7	8	11
B. Operated										
0–19 Years	0									
20–34	0									
35–49	1	4.0	0	4	4	4	4	4	4	4
50–64	2	3.0	8	1	1	5	5	5	5	5
65+	3	9.3	25	4	4	10	14	14	14	14
SUBTOTALS:										
1. SINGLE DX										
A. Not Operated	1	1.0	0	1	1	1	1	1	1	1
B. Operated	1	1.0	0	1	1	1	1	1	1	1
2. MULTIPLE DX										
A. Not Operated	173	3.8	8	1	2	3	5	8	9	14
B. Operated	6	6.4	23	1	4	5	10	14	14	14
1. SINGLE DX	2	1.0	0	1	1	1	1	1	1	1
2. MULTIPLE DX	179	3.9	8	1	2	3	5	8	10	14
A. NOT OPERATED	174	3.8	8	1	2	3	5	8	9	14
B. OPERATED	7	5.6	23	1	1	4	10	14	14	14
TOTAL										
0–19 Years	0									
20–34	7	1.9	1	1	1	1	3	4	4	4
35–49	14	3.2	7	1	1	3	4	8	9	9
50–64	36	4.0	15	1	2	3	4	12	14	15
65+	124	4.0	7	1	2	3	5	8	9	12
GRAND TOTAL	181	3.8	8	1	2	3	5	8	9	14

587: RENAL SCLEROSIS NOS

Type of Patients	Observed Patients	Avg. Stay	Variance	10th	25th	50th	75th	90th	95th	99th
1. SINGLE DX										
A. Not Operated										
0–19 Years	0									
20–34	0									
35–49	0									
50–64	0									
65+	0									
B. Operated										
0–19 Years	0									
20–34	1	4.0	0	4	4	4	4	4	4	4
35–49	2	2.5	<1	2	2	2	3	3	3	3
50–64	0									
65+	0									
2. MULTIPLE DX										
A. Not Operated										
0–19 Years	1	1.0	0	1	1	1	1	1	1	1
20–34	0									
35–49	1	1.0	0	1	1	1	1	1	1	1
50–64	0									
65+	0									
B. Operated										
0–19 Years	2	2.5	<1	2	2	2	3	3	3	3
20–34	8	3.0	1	2	2	3	4	5	5	5
35–49	6	3.3	4	2	3	3	5	6	6	6
50–64	11	3.6	2	2	3	3	4	5	7	7
65+	7	3.7	10	1	1	3	6	9	9	9
SUBTOTALS:										
1. SINGLE DX										
A. Not Operated	0									
B. Operated	3	3.0	1	2	2	3	4	4	4	4
2. MULTIPLE DX										
A. Not Operated	2	1.0	0	1	1	1	1	1	1	1
B. Operated	34	3.4	4	1	2	3	4	6	7	9
1. SINGLE DX	3	3.0	1	2	2	3	4	4	4	4
2. MULTIPLE DX	36	3.2	4	1	2	3	4	6	7	9
A. NOT OPERATED	2	1.0	0	1	1	1	1	1	1	1
B. OPERATED	37	3.3	3	1	2	3	4	6	7	9
TOTAL										
0–19 Years	3	2.0	<1	1	1	2	3	3	3	3
20–34	9	3.1	1	2	2	3	4	5	5	5
35–49	9	2.9	3	1	2	2	4	6	6	6
50–64	11	3.6	2	2	3	3	4	5	7	7
65+	7	3.7	10	1	1	3	6	9	9	9
GRAND TOTAL	39	3.2	3	1	2	3	4	6	7	9

588: IMPAIRED RENAL FUNCTION

Type of Patients	Observed Patients	Avg. Stay	Variance	10th	25th	50th	75th	90th	95th	99th
1. SINGLE DX										
A. Not Operated										
0–19 Years	1	1.0	0	1	1	1	1	1	1	1
20–34	2	2.0	0	2	2	2	2	2	2	2
35–49	0									
50–64	0									
B. Operated										
0–19 Years	0									
20–34	0									
35–49	0									
50–64	0									
2. MULTIPLE DX										
A. Not Operated										
0–19 Years	15	2.2	2	1	1	2	3	4	5	5
20–34	14	3.6	10	1	1	2	5	9	11	11
35–49	34	7.2	107	1	2	4	8	11	34	55
50–64	54	8.3	101	1	3	5	9	20	26	58
65+	53	7.3	63	1	3	5	8	15	26	39
B. Operated										
0–19 Years	2	7.5	4	6	6	9	9	9	9	9
20–34	57	5.2	15	2	3	4	7	10	15	19
35–49	109	4.8	14	1	2	4	6	9	12	23
50–64	104	3.8	8	1	2	3	5	7	10	15
65+	35	5.5	23	2	2	4	6	12	20	20
SUBTOTALS:										
1. SINGLE DX										
A. Not Operated	3	1.7	<1	1	1	2	2	2	2	2
B. Operated	0									
2. MULTIPLE DX										
A. Not Operated	170	6.9	76	1	2	4	8	14	26	55
B. Operated	307	4.6	13	1	2	4	6	9	12	20
1. SINGLE DX	3	1.7	<1	1	1	2	2	2	2	2
2. MULTIPLE DX	477	5.4	37	2	2	4	6	10	15	34
A. NOT OPERATED	173	6.8	76	1	2	4	8	13	26	55
B. OPERATED	307	4.6	13	1	2	4	6	9	12	20
TOTAL										
0–19 Years	18	2.7	5	1	1	2	4	6	9	9
20–34	73	4.8	14	1	2	4	6	9	13	19
35–49	143	5.4	36	2	2	4	7	9	13	34
50–64	158	5.4	44	1	2	3	6	10	16	35
65+	88	6.6	47	2	2	4	8	12	20	39
GRAND TOTAL	480	5.4	37	1	2	4	6	10	15	34

462

Length of Stay by Diagnosis and Operation, Western Region, 2008

Western Region, October 2006–September 2007 Data, by Diagnosis

588.81: 2ND RENAL HYPERPARA

Type of Patients	Observed Patients	Avg. Stay	Variance	10th	25th	50th	75th	90th	95th	99th
1. SINGLE DX										
A. Not Operated										
0–19 Years	0									
20–34	0									
35–49	0									
50–64	0									
65+	0									
B. Operated										
0–19 Years	0									
20–34	0									
35–49	0									
50–64	0									
65+	0									
2. MULTIPLE DX										
A. Not Operated										
0–19 Years	0									
20–34	2	5.0	31	1	1	1	9	9	9	9
35–49	7	5.4	15	1	1	6	8	11	11	11
50–64	10	5.5	14	1	2	5	9	12	12	12
65+	7	6.2	16	1	1	8	8	12	12	12
B. Operated										
0–19 Years	2	7.5	4	6	6	9	9	9	9	9
20–34	56	5.2	15	2	3	4	7	10	15	19
35–49	108	4.8	14	2	2	4	6	9	12	23
50–64	102	3.7	7	1	2	3	5	6	9	15
65+	35	5.5	23	2	2	4	6	12	20	20
SUBTOTALS:										
1. SINGLE DX										
A. Not Operated	0									
B. Operated	0									
2. MULTIPLE DX										
A. Not Operated	26	5.6	14	1	2	5	8	11	12	12
B. Operated	303	4.6	13	1	2	4	6	9	12	20
1. SINGLE DX	0									
2. MULTIPLE DX	329	4.7	13	1	2	4	6	9	12	20
A. NOT OPERATED	26	5.6	14	1	2	5	8	11	12	12
B. OPERATED	303	4.6	13	1	2	4	6	9	12	20
TOTAL										
0–19 Years	2	7.5	4	6	6	9	9	9	9	9
20–34	58	5.2	15	2	3	4	7	10	15	19
35–49	115	4.8	14	2	2	4	6	9	12	23
50–64	112	3.9	8	1	2	3	5	7	10	15
65+	42	5.6	21	2	2	4	8	12	12	20
GRAND TOTAL	329	4.7	13	1	2	4	6	9	12	20

589: SMALL KIDNEY

Type of Patients	Observed Patients	Avg. Stay	Variance	10th	25th	50th	75th	90th	95th	99th
1. SINGLE DX										
A. Not Operated										
0–19 Years	0									
20–34	0									
35–49	0									
50–64	0									
65+	0									
B. Operated										
0–19 Years	0									
20–34	0									
35–49	0									
50–64	0									
65+	0									
2. MULTIPLE DX										
A. Not Operated										
0–19 Years	0									
20–34	0									
35–49	0									
50–64	0									
65+	0									
B. Operated										
0–19 Years	0									
20–34	0									
35–49	0									
50–64	0									
65+	0									
SUBTOTALS:										
1. SINGLE DX										
A. Not Operated	0									
B. Operated	0									
2. MULTIPLE DX										
A. Not Operated	0									
B. Operated	0									
1. SINGLE DX	0									
2. MULTIPLE DX	0									
A. NOT OPERATED	0									
B. OPERATED	0									
TOTAL										
0–19 Years	0									
20–34	0									
35–49	0									
50–64	0									
65+	0									
GRAND TOTAL	0									

590: KIDNEY INFECTION

Type of Patients	Observed Patients	Avg. Stay	Variance	10th	25th	50th	75th	90th	95th	99th
1. SINGLE DX										
A. Not Operated										
0–19 Years	417	2.5	2	1	2	2	3	4	5	7
20–34	220	2.1	1	1	1	2	3	3	4	5
35–49	94	2.0	1	1	1	2	2	4	4	6
50–64	33	2.3	2	1	1	2	3	4	4	7
65+	7	2.4	<1	1	2	2	3	4	4	4
B. Operated										
0–19 Years	1	3.0	0	3	3	3	3	3	3	3
20–34	3	1.0	0	1	1	1	1	1	1	1
35–49	1	2.0	0	2	2	2	2	2	2	2
50–64	3	3.3	6	1	1	3	6	6	6	6
65+	0									
2. MULTIPLE DX										
A. Not Operated										
0–19 Years	3,485	3.3	6	1	2	3	4	6	7	13
20–34	3,855	3.0	4	1	2	3	4	5	6	11
35–49	3,818	3.3	6	1	2	3	4	6	7	13
50–64	3,745	3.6	8	1	2	3	4	6	8	14
65+	5,115	3.9	8	1	2	3	5	7	9	15
B. Operated										
0–19 Years	25	6.7	28	2	4	5	8	11	15	26
20–34	129	6.5	34	2	3	5	8	13	15	26
35–49	168	8.1	60	2	4	6	10	18	26	43
50–64	220	8.4	62	3	4	6	10	19	22	47
65+	241	9.1	76	3	4	7	11	17	22	40
SUBTOTALS:										
1. SINGLE DX										
A. Not Operated	771	2.3	2	1	1	2	3	4	5	6
B. Operated	8	2.3	3	1	1	3	3	6	6	6
2. MULTIPLE DX										
A. Not Operated	20,018	3.5	7	1	2	3	4	6	8	13
B. Operated	783	8.2	61	2	4	6	10	17	22	43
1. SINGLE DX	779	2.3	2	1	1	2	3	4	5	6
2. MULTIPLE DX	20,801	3.7	9	1	2	3	4	6	8	16
A. NOT OPERATED	20,789	3.4	6	1	2	3	4	6	8	13
B. OPERATED	791	8.1	60	2	4	6	10	17	22	43
TOTAL										
0–19 Years	3,928	3.2	6	1	2	3	4	6	7	13
20–34	4,207	3.0	5	1	2	3	4	6	6	12
35–49	4,081	3.5	9	1	2	3	4	6	8	15
50–64	4,001	3.9	12	1	2	3	5	7	9	18
65+	5,363	4.2	12	2	2	3	5	8	10	18
GRAND TOTAL	21,580	3.6	9	1	2	3	4	6	8	15

Length of Stay by Diagnosis and Operation, Western Region, 2008

Western Region, October 2006–September 2007 Data, by Diagnosis

590.10: AC PYELONEPHRITIS NOS

Type of Patients	Observed Patients	Avg. Stay	Variance	10th	25th	50th	75th	90th	95th	99th
1. SINGLE DX										
A. Not Operated										
0–19 Years	177	2.6	2	1	2	2	3	4	5	7
20–34	113	2.2	1	1	1	2	3	3	4	6
35–49	44	2.1	1	1	1	2	2	4	4	5
50–64	14	1.9	<1	1	1	2	2	3	4	4
65+	2	2.0	2	1	1	3	3	3	4	3
B. Operated										
0–19 Years	1	3.0	0	3	3	3	3	3	3	3
20–34	0									
35–49	0									
50–64	0									
65+	0									
2. MULTIPLE DX										
A. Not Operated										
0–19 Years	1,522	3.3	5	1	2	3	4	6	7	12
20–34	1,815	3.0	4	1	2	3	4	5	6	10
35–49	1,740	3.2	4	1	2	3	4	5	7	12
50–64	1,598	3.6	6	1	2	3	4	6	8	14
65+	2,299	4.0	8	2	2	3	5	7	9	15
B. Operated										
0–19 Years	6	4.7	5	2	2	4	7	7	7	7
20–34	42	6.0	16	3	4	5	7	10	11	22
35–49	61	8.6	57	3	6	6	11	18	24	43
50–64	91	8.3	39	3	4	6	11	18	20	30
65+	75	8.1	25	3	4	7	10	16	19	25
SUBTOTALS:										
1. SINGLE DX										
A. Not Operated	350	2.4	2	1	2	2	3	4	5	6
B. Operated	1	3.0	0	3	3	3	3	3	3	3
2. MULTIPLE DX										
A. Not Operated	8,974	3.5	6	1	2	3	4	6	8	13
B. Operated	275	7.9	36	3	4	6	10	16	19	30
1. SINGLE DX	351	2.4	2	1	1	2	3	4	5	6
2. MULTIPLE DX	9,249	3.6	7	1	2	3	4	6	8	14
A. NOT OPERATED	9,324	3.4	6	1	2	3	4	6	7	13
B. OPERATED	276	7.9	36	3	4	6	10	16	19	30
TOTAL										
0–19 Years	1,706	3.3	5	1	2	3	4	6	7	12
20–34	1,970	3.0	4	1	2	3	4	5	6	10
35–49	1,845	3.4	7	1	2	3	4	6	7	13
50–64	1,703	3.8	9	1	2	3	5	7	9	17
65+	2,376	4.2	9	2	2	3	5	7	9	16
GRAND TOTAL	9,600	3.6	7	1	2	3	4	6	8	14

590.2: RENAL/PERIRENAL ABSCESS

Type of Patients	Observed Patients	Avg. Stay	Variance	10th	25th	50th	75th	90th	95th	99th
1. SINGLE DX										
A. Not Operated										
0–19 Years	0									
20–34	3	2.7	4	1	1	2	5	5	5	5
35–49	1	5.0	0	5	5	5	5	5	5	5
50–64	3	2.7	2	1	2	3	4	4	4	4
65+	1	2.0	0	2	2	2	2	2	2	2
B. Operated										
0–19 Years	0									
20–34	1	1.0	0	1	1	1	1	1	1	1
35–49	0									
50–64	1	1.0	0	1	1	1	1	1	1	1
65+	0									
2. MULTIPLE DX										
A. Not Operated										
0–19 Years	16	7.2	32	2	3	4	10	17	20	20
20–34	42	5.7	17	2	3	4	7	10	15	19
35–49	50	8.0	39	2	4	6	10	19	22	29
50–64	59	8.1	36	3	4	6	9	15	23	35
65+	32	7.1	23	2	3	6	11	13	18	19
B. Operated										
0–19 Years	4	8.8	10	4	10	10	10	11	11	11
20–34	7	9.7	26	5	6	8	14	19	19	19
35–49	22	12.6	122	3	6	9	18	28	35	41
50–64	33	13.1	154	5	5	8	19	28	47	54
65+	29	11.2	55	4	6	8	15	25	26	30
SUBTOTALS:										
1. SINGLE DX										
A. Not Operated	8	2.9	3	1	2	2	5	5	5	5
B. Operated	2	1.0	0	1	1	1	1	1	1	1
2. MULTIPLE DX										
A. Not Operated	199	7.3	31	2	3	6	10	15	19	25
B. Operated	95	12.0	100	4	5	8	17	26	35	54
1. SINGLE DX	10	2.5	3	1	1	2	4	5	5	5
2. MULTIPLE DX	294	8.8	57	2	4	6	10	19	24	41
A. NOT OPERATED	207	7.2	30	2	3	6	10	15	19	25
B. OPERATED	97	11.8	100	3	5	8	15	26	35	54
TOTAL										
0–19 Years	20	7.5	27	3	3	5	10	14	17	20
20–34	53	5.9	20	2	3	5	8	12	16	19
35–49	73	9.4	67	2	4	7	11	21	28	41
50–64	96	9.6	82	3	5	6	10	19	28	54
65+	62	9.0	42	2	4	7	12	19	20	30
GRAND TOTAL	304	8.6	57	2	4	6	10	19	23	35

590.80: PYELONEPHRITIS NOS

Type of Patients	Observed Patients	Avg. Stay	Variance	10th	25th	50th	75th	90th	95th	99th
1. SINGLE DX										
A. Not Operated										
0–19 Years	239	2.4	2	1	1	2	3	4	5	8
20–34	102	2.0	<1	1	1	2	3	3	4	5
35–49	47	1.9	1	1	1	2	2	3	4	6
50–64	16	2.6	2	2	2	3	3	4	7	7
65+	4	2.8	<1	2	2	3	4	4	4	4
B. Operated										
0–19 Years	0									
20–34	2	1.0	0	1	1	1	1	1	1	1
35–49	0									
50–64	1	3.0	0	3	3	3	3	3	3	3
65+	0									
2. MULTIPLE DX										
A. Not Operated										
0–19 Years	1,929	3.2	6	1	2	3	4	6	7	12
20–34	1,953	2.9	4	1	2	3	3	5	6	11
35–49	1,978	3.3	6	1	2	3	4	6	7	13
50–64	2,059	3.5	7	1	2	3	4	6	8	13
65+	2,754	3.8	8	1	2	3	5	7	9	15
B. Operated										
0–19 Years	14	7.2	42	2	4	5	8	15	26	26
20–34	58	7.5	53	3	3	6	8	15	17	49
35–49	55	7.1	50	2	3	5	8	14	18	45
50–64	66	6.3	19	2	3	5	8	13	15	21
65+	111	8.9	56	3	4	7	11	16	24	40
SUBTOTALS:										
1. SINGLE DX										
A. Not Operated	408	2.2	2	1	1	2	3	4	5	6
B. Operated	3	1.7	1	1	1	1	1	1	3	3
2. MULTIPLE DX										
A. Not Operated	10,673	3.4	6	1	2	3	4	6	8	13
B. Operated	304	7.7	46	2	4	6	9	15	18	40
1. SINGLE DX	411	2.2	2	1	1	2	3	4	5	6
2. MULTIPLE DX	10,977	3.5	8	1	2	3	4	6	8	14
A. NOT OPERATED	11,081	3.3	6	1	2	3	4	6	7	13
B. OPERATED	307	7.6	46	2	4	6	9	15	18	40
TOTAL										
0–19 Years	2,182	3.2	6	1	2	3	4	5	7	12
20–34	2,115	3.0	6	1	2	3	4	5	6	12
35–49	2,080	3.4	7	1	2	3	4	6	8	13
50–64	2,142	3.6	7	2	2	3	5	6	8	15
65+	2,869	4.0	10	1	2	3	5	7	9	17
GRAND TOTAL	11,388	3.5	8	1	2	3	4	6	8	14

Length of Stay by Diagnosis and Operation, Western Region, 2008

Western Region, October 2006–September 2007 Data, by Diagnosis

591: HYDRONEPHROSIS

Type of Patients	Observed Patients	Avg. Stay	Vari- ance	10th	25th	50th	75th	90th	95th	99th
1. SINGLE DX										
A. Not Operated										
0–19 Years	5	1.4	<1	1	1	1	2	2	2	2
20–34	2	2.0	2	1	1	1	3	3	3	3
35–49	2	3.5	12	1	1	4	6	6	6	6
50–64	2	1.5	<1	1	1	2	2	2	2	2
65+	3	1.0	0	1	1	1	1	1	1	1
B. Operated										
0–19 Years	1	4.0	0	4	4	4	4	4	4	4
20–34	4	2.7	0	1	1	2	2	4	4	4
35–49	2	2.0	0	2	2	2	2	2	2	2
50–64	0									
65+	0									
2. MULTIPLE DX										
A. Not Operated										
0–19 Years	24	3.0	6	1	2	2	3	7	7	12
20–34	57	2.2	3	1	1	2	3	5	6	8
35–49	81	3.2	10	1	1	2	4	7	10	20
50–64	119	2.9	4	1	1	2	4	6	7	9
65+	186	3.5	8	1	2	3	4	7	9	14
B. Operated										
0–19 Years	11	2.5	1	1	2	2	3	4	5	5
20–34	30	4.2	30	1	3	3	4	11	16	28
35–49	66	3.9	9	1	2	3	5	7	9	17
50–64	87	4.6	16	1	2	3	6	9	13	23
65+	138	5.3	18	1	2	4	7	11	14	20
SUBTOTALS:										
1. SINGLE DX										
A. Not Operated	14	1.7	2	1	1	1	2	3	3	6
B. Operated	7	2.7	2	1	2	2	4	4	4	4
2. MULTIPLE DX										
A. Not Operated	467	3.1	7	1	1	2	4	7	8	13
B. Operated	332	4.7	16	1	2	3	6	9	13	22
1. SINGLE DX	21	2.1	2	1	1	2	2	4	4	6
2. MULTIPLE DX	799	3.7	12	1	2	3	5	8	10	18
A. NOT OPERATED	481	3.1	7	1	1	2	4	6	8	13
B. OPERATED	339	4.6	16	1	2	3	6	9	13	22
TOTAL										
0–19 Years	41	2.7	4	1	2	2	3	4	7	12
20–34	93	2.9	12	1	1	3	3	5	7	28
35–49	151	3.5	9	1	1	3	4	5	10	17
50–64	208	3.6	10	1	1	3	5	7	9	15
65+	327	4.2	13	1	2	3	6	9	12	18
GRAND TOTAL	820	3.7	11	1	2	3	5	8	10	17

592: RENAL/URETERAL CALCULUS

Type of Patients	Observed Patients	Avg. Stay	Vari- ance	10th	25th	50th	75th	90th	95th	99th
1. SINGLE DX										
A. Not Operated										
0–19 Years	38	1.5	<1	1	1	1	2	3	4	4
20–34	177	1.5	<1	1	1	1	2	3	3	4
35–49	183	1.4	<1	1	1	1	2	2	3	4
50–64	143	1.3	<1	1	1	1	1	2	2	4
65+	34	1.4	1	1	1	1	1	2	4	6
B. Operated										
0–19 Years	26	1.7	<1	1	1	2	2	2	2	5
20–34	173	2.0	2	1	1	2	3	4	4	7
35–49	205	2.1	2	1	1	2	3	4	5	9
50–64	146	1.9	1	1	1	2	3	3	4	6
65+	36	1.6	<1	1	1	2	2	3	4	5
2. MULTIPLE DX										
A. Not Operated										
0–19 Years	293	2.1	4	1	1	2	3	4	5	8
20–34	1,807	2.0	2	1	1	2	3	4	5	7
35–49	2,905	2.1	3	1	1	2	3	4	5	9
50–64	3,083	2.1	4	1	1	2	3	4	5	9
65+	2,160	2.7	8	1	1	2	3	5	7	13
B. Operated										
0–19 Years	117	3.3	6	1	1	3	4	6	9	11
20–34	1,055	2.7	12	1	1	2	4	5	6	13
35–49	1,988	2.8	6	1	1	2	3	5	7	13
50–64	2,353	2.8	7	1	1	2	3	5	7	14
65+	1,604	3.4	10	1	1	2	4	7	10	15
SUBTOTALS:										
1. SINGLE DX										
A. Not Operated	575	1.4	<1	1	1	1	2	2	3	4
B. Operated	586	2.0	2	1	1	2	2	4	4	7
2. MULTIPLE DX										
A. Not Operated	10,248	2.2	4	1	1	2	3	4	5	10
B. Operated	7,117	2.9	8	1	1	2	4	6	8	14
1. SINGLE DX	1,161	1.7	1	1	1	1	2	3	4	6
2. MULTIPLE DX	17,365	2.5	6	1	1	2	3	5	6	12
A. NOT OPERATED	10,823	2.2	4	1	1	2	3	4	5	10
B. OPERATED	7,703	2.8	8	1	1	2	3	5	8	14
TOTAL										
0–19 Years	474	2.3	4	1	1	2	3	4	6	11
20–34	3,212	2.2	5	1	1	2	3	4	5	9
35–49	5,281	2.3	4	1	1	2	3	4	6	11
50–64	5,725	2.4	5	1	1	2	3	5	6	12
65+	3,834	3.0	9	1	1	2	4	6	8	15
GRAND TOTAL	18,526	2.5	6	1	1	2	3	5	6	12

592.0: KIDNEY CALCULUS

Type of Patients	Observed Patients	Avg. Stay	Vari- ance	10th	25th	50th	75th	90th	95th	99th
1. SINGLE DX										
A. Not Operated										
0–19 Years	14	1.6	<1	1	1	1	2	3	4	4
20–34	63	1.7	1	1	1	1	2	3	3	7
35–49	60	1.5	<1	1	1	1	2	2	3	7
50–64	37	1.3	<1	1	1	1	1	2	3	3
65+	5	1.0	0	1	1	1	1	1	1	1
B. Operated										
0–19 Years	8	2.5	2	2	2	2	2	5	5	5
20–34	71	2.5	2	1	1	2	3	4	5	8
35–49	85	2.8	4	1	2	2	3	5	6	10
50–64	71	2.3	1	1	1	2	3	4	5	6
65+	18	2.1	1	1	1	2	3	4	5	5
2. MULTIPLE DX										
A. Not Operated										
0–19 Years	129	2.3	6	1	1	2	3	4	5	8
20–34	661	2.2	3	1	1	2	3	4	5	8
35–49	1,029	2.4	4	1	1	2	3	5	6	12
50–64	947	2.3	4	1	1	2	3	4	6	12
65+	719	2.8	13	1	1	2	3	5	7	15
B. Operated										
0–19 Years	33	4.6	7	2	3	4	6	8	11	11
20–34	337	3.4	10	1	2	3	4	5	8	15
35–49	679	3.5	11	1	2	3	4	7	9	17
50–64	984	3.4	9	1	2	3	4	6	9	18
65+	611	3.6	11	1	2	3	4	7	11	16
SUBTOTALS:										
1. SINGLE DX										
A. Not Operated	179	1.5	<1	1	1	1	2	2	3	7
B. Operated	253	2.5	2	1	1	2	3	4	5	9
2. MULTIPLE DX										
A. Not Operated	3,485	2.4	6	1	1	2	3	5	6	12
B. Operated	2,644	3.5	10	1	2	3	4	7	9	16
1. SINGLE DX	432	2.1	2	1	1	2	3	4	5	7
2. MULTIPLE DX	6,129	2.9	8	1	1	2	3	5	7	14
A. NOT OPERATED	3,664	2.4	6	1	1	2	3	4	6	12
B. OPERATED	2,897	3.4	10	1	2	2	4	6	9	16
TOTAL										
0–19 Years	184	2.7	6	1	1	2	3	5	7	11
20–34	1,132	2.6	5	1	1	2	3	5	6	11
35–49	1,853	2.8	7	1	1	2	3	5	7	14
50–64	2,039	2.8	7	1	1	2	3	5	7	14
65+	1,353	3.1	12	1	1	2	4	6	9	16
GRAND TOTAL	6,561	2.8	8	1	1	2	3	5	7	14

Length of Stay by Diagnosis and Operation, Western Region, 2008

Western Region, October 2006–September 2007 Data, by Diagnosis

592.1: URETERAL CALCULUS

Type of Patients	Observed Patients	Avg. Stay	Vari- ance	10th	25th	50th	75th	90th	95th	99th
1. SINGLE DX										
A. Not Operated										
0–19 Years	23	1.4	<1	1	1	1	2	3	3	4
20–34	114	1.3	<1	1	1	1	2	2	3	3
35–49	122	1.3	<1	1	1	1	1	2	2	3
50–64	105	1.4	<1	1	1	1	2	3	3	4
65+	29	1.5	1	1	1	1	2	2	4	6
B. Operated										
0–19 Years	18	1.4	<1	1	1	1	2	2	2	2
20–34	102	1.6	<1	1	1	1	2	3	4	5
35–49	120	1.6	<1	1	1	1	2	3	4	4
50–64	75	1.5	<1	1	1	1	2	3	3	6
65+	18	1.2	<1	1	1	1	1	2	3	3
2. MULTIPLE DX										
A. Not Operated										
0–19 Years	163	2.0	2	1	1	2	3	4	4	6
20–34	1,140	1.9	2	1	1	2	3	3	4	7
35–49	1,862	2.0	2	1	1	2	2	4	5	7
50–64	2,132	2.0	3	1	1	2	3	4	5	8
65+	1,431	2.6	5	1	1	2	3	5	7	12
B. Operated										
0–19 Years	84	2.7	4	1	2	2	3	5	6	11
20–34	716	2.4	12	1	1	2	3	4	5	10
35–49	1,307	2.4	3	1	1	2	3	4	5	10
50–64	1,368	2.4	5	1	1	2	3	4	6	12
65+	993	3.3	9	1	1	2	4	7	9	15
SUBTOTALS:										
1. SINGLE DX										
A. Not Operated	393	1.4	<1	1	1	1	2	2	3	4
B. Operated	333	1.5	<1	1	1	1	2	3	3	5
2. MULTIPLE DX										
A. Not Operated	6,728	2.1	3	1	1	2	3	4	5	9
B. Operated	4,468	2.6	7	1	1	2	3	5	7	12
1. SINGLE DX	726	1.4	<1	1	1	1	2	2	3	4
2. MULTIPLE DX	11,196	2.3	5	1	1	2	3	4	6	10
A. NOT OPERATED	7,121	2.1	3	1	1	2	3	4	5	8
B. OPERATED	4,801	2.5	6	1	1	2	3	5	6	12
TOTAL										
0–19 Years	288	2.1	3	1	1	2	3	4	5	9
20–34	2,072	2.0	5	1	1	2	2	4	5	8
35–49	3,411	2.1	3	1	1	2	3	4	5	8
50–64	3,680	2.1	4	1	1	2	3	4	5	10
65+	2,471	2.9	7	1	1	2	3	6	8	13
GRAND TOTAL	11,922	2.3	4	1	1	2	3	4	5	10

593: DISORD KIDNEY/URETER NEC

Type of Patients	Observed Patients	Avg. Stay	Vari- ance	10th	25th	50th	75th	90th	95th	99th
1. SINGLE DX										
A. Not Operated										
0–19 Years	9	1.8	<1	1	1	1	2	4	4	4
20–34	3	2.0	<1	1	1	2	2	3	3	3
35–49	13	1.2	<1	1	1	1	1	2	2	2
50–64	5	2.0	2	1	1	1	3	4	4	4
65+	3	2.4	5	1	2	1	5	5	5	5
B. Operated										
0–19 Years	121	2.3	1	1	1	2	3	3	3	6
20–34	39	2.4	2	1	2	2	3	5	6	6
35–49	45	2.5	1	1	2	2	3	4	4	5
50–64	23	2.4	<1	1	1	2	3	4	4	5
65+	8	1.6	<1	1	1	1	2	3	3	3
2. MULTIPLE DX										
A. Not Operated										
0–19 Years	90	3.0	12	1	1	2	3	6	9	27
20–34	149	3.2	7	1	1	2	4	6	8	15
35–49	390	3.3	10	1	1	2	4	6	8	14
50–64	578	3.4	9	1	1	2	4	7	9	16
65+	1,255	3.7	9	1	2	3	5	7	9	16
B. Operated										
0–19 Years	370	2.6	2	1	2	2	3	4	5	8
20–34	205	3.9	9	1	2	2	4	7	10	15
35–49	382	4.0	22	1	2	3	4	7	8	16
50–64	576	4.0	18	1	2	3	5	7	11	27
65+	547	4.5	15	1	2	3	6	9	12	19
SUBTOTALS:										
1. SINGLE DX										
A. Not Operated	33	1.7	1	1	1	1	2	3	4	5
B. Operated	236	2.3	1	1	1	2	3	4	4	6
2. MULTIPLE DX										
A. Not Operated	2,462	3.5	9	1	2	3	4	7	9	16
B. Operated	2,080	3.9	15	1	2	3	4	7	9	18
1. SINGLE DX	269	2.2	1	1	1	2	3	4	4	6
2. MULTIPLE DX	4,542	3.7	12	1	2	3	4	7	9	16
A. NOT OPERATED	2,495	3.5	9	1	2	3	4	7	9	15
B. OPERATED	2,316	3.7	13	1	2	3	4	7	9	17
TOTAL										
0–19 Years	590	2.6	3	1	2	2	3	4	5	9
20–34	396	3.5	8	1	2	3	4	6	9	15
35–49	830	3.5	15	1	2	3	4	7	8	14
50–64	1,182	3.7	13	1	2	3	4	7	9	18
65+	1,813	4.0	11	1	2	3	5	8	10	18
GRAND TOTAL	4,811	3.6	11	1	2	3	4	7	9	16

593.2: ACQUIRED KIDNEY CYST

Type of Patients	Observed Patients	Avg. Stay	Vari- ance	10th	25th	50th	75th	90th	95th	99th
1. SINGLE DX										
A. Not Operated										
0–19 Years	0									
20–34	1	2.0	0	2	2	2	2	2	2	2
35–49	0									
50–64	1	3.0	0	3	3	3	3	3	3	3
65+	0									
B. Operated										
0–19 Years	4	3.2	3	1	1	3	4	5	5	5
20–34	0									
35–49	6	3.0	1	2	2	3	3	5	5	5
50–64	3	2.7	1	2	2	2	4	4	4	4
65+	1	1.0	0	1	1	1	1	1	1	1
2. MULTIPLE DX										
A. Not Operated										
0–19 Years	2	2.0	0	2	2	2	2	2	2	2
20–34	6	3.5	12	1	1	1	1	6	6	6
35–49	12	4.1	13	1	2	3	3	4	8	14
50–64	27	2.6	3	1	1	2	3	5	7	7
65+	36	4.3	17	1	2	3	5	11	14	19
B. Operated										
0–19 Years	1	3.0	0	3	3	3	3	3	3	3
20–34	8	3.1	1	1	3	3	3	5	5	5
35–49	20	3.0	3	1	2	3	4	6	7	7
50–64	75	3.0	4	1	2	3	4	5	6	11
65+	68	3.5	8	2	2	3	4	7	8	15
SUBTOTALS:										
1. SINGLE DX										
A. Not Operated	2	2.5	<1	2	2	2	3	3	3	3
B. Operated	14	2.9	2	1	1	3	4	5	5	5
2. MULTIPLE DX										
A. Not Operated	79	3.6	11	1	1	3	4	8	11	19
B. Operated	172	3.2	5	1	2	3	4	6	8	13
1. SINGLE DX	16	2.8	1	1	2	3	3	5	5	5
2. MULTIPLE DX	251	3.4	7	1	2	3	4	6	8	14
A. NOT OPERATED	81	3.6	11	1	1	3	4	7	11	19
B. OPERATED	186	3.2	5	1	2	3	4	6	7	13
TOTAL										
0–19 Years	7	2.9	2	1	2	3	3	4	5	5
20–34	11	3.1	2	1	2	3	3	5	6	6
35–49	38	3.3	6	1	2	3	3	6	8	14
50–64	106	2.9	3	1	2	3	3	5	6	9
65+	105	3.8	11	1	2	3	5	8	11	15
GRAND TOTAL	267	3.3	7	1	2	3	4	6	8	14

Western Region, October 2006–September 2007 Data, by Diagnosis

593.3: URETERAL STRICTURE/KINK

Type of Patients	Observed Patients	Avg. Stay	Variance	Percentiles 10th	25th	50th	75th	90th	95th	99th
1. SINGLE DX										
A. Not Operated										
0–19 Years	0									
20–34	0									
35–49	3	1.3	<1	1	1	1	2	2	2	2
50–64	1	1.0	0	1	1	1	1	1	1	1
65+	0									
B. Operated										
0–19 Years	2	5.5	12	3	3	8	8	8	8	8
20–34	1	1.0	0	1	1	1	1	1	1	1
35–49	8	2.6	<1	1	2	3	3	4	4	4
50–64	1	1.0	0	1	1	1	1	1	1	1
65+	0									
2. MULTIPLE DX										
A. Not Operated										
0–19 Years	2	1.5	<1	1	1	2	2	2	2	2
20–34	19	2.4	2	1	1	2	3	5	6	6
35–49	57	2.2	3	1	1	1	3	5	6	6
50–64	62	3.1	8	1	1	2	4	6	8	18
65+	55	3.2	6	1	1	3	4	5	10	13
B. Operated										
0–19 Years	20	2.8	2	2	2	3	3	4	7	7
20–34	32	3.6	5	1	2	3	4	7	8	10
35–49	68	3.5	4	1	2	3	4	6	7	10
50–64	72	3.7	7	1	2	3	5	7	9	16
65+	57	4.7	13	1	2	3	6	10	11	17
SUBTOTALS:										
1. SINGLE DX										
A. Not Operated	4	1.3	<1	1	1	1	2	2	2	2
B. Operated	12	2.8	4	1	1	3	3	4	8	8
2. MULTIPLE DX										
A. Not Operated	195	2.8	5	1	1	2	4	6	7	13
B. Operated	249	3.8	7	1	2	3	5	7	9	16
1. SINGLE DX	16	2.4	3	1	1	2	3	4	8	8
2. MULTIPLE DX	444	3.3	7	1	2	3	4	6	8	13
A. NOT OPERATED	199	2.7	5	1	1	2	4	6	7	11
B. OPERATED	261	3.7	7	1	2	3	4	7	9	16
TOTAL										
0–19 Years	24	2.9	3	2	2	2	3	4	7	8
20–34	52	3.1	4	1	2	3	4	5	8	10
35–49	136	2.9	3	1	1	3	4	5	6	9
50–64	136	3.4	8	1	1	3	4	7	9	16
65+	112	3.9	10	1	2	3	5	7	11	17
GRAND TOTAL	460	3.3	7	1	2	3	4	6	8	13

593.4: URETERIC OBSTRUCTION NEC

Type of Patients	Observed Patients	Avg. Stay	Variance	Percentiles 10th	25th	50th	75th	90th	95th	99th
1. SINGLE DX										
A. Not Operated										
0–19 Years	1	2.0	0	2	2	2	2	2	2	2
20–34	1	1.0	0	1	1	1	1	1	1	1
35–49	1	1.0	0	1	1	1	1	1	1	1
50–64	0									
65+	0									
B. Operated										
0–19 Years	14	2.6	2	2	2	2	3	4	6	6
20–34	36	2.4	2	1	1	2	3	5	6	6
35–49	20	2.2	1	1	1	2	3	4	4	4
50–64	5	2.4	1	1	2	2	3	4	4	4
65+	3	1.3	<1	1	1	1	2	2	2	2
2. MULTIPLE DX										
A. Not Operated										
0–19 Years	19	2.2	3	1	1	2	3	6	7	7
20–34	41	2.8	3	1	1	2	4	5	6	8
35–49	63	2.9	15	1	1	2	3	5	6	30
50–64	77	3.2	5	1	1	2	4	6	8	11
65+	132	3.3	7	1	2	3	4	6	9	11
B. Operated										
0–19 Years	75	2.7	2	1	2	2	3	4	6	8
20–34	119	3.7	8	1	2	3	4	6	12	15
35–49	164	4.1	8	1	2	3	5	8	9	13
50–64	191	4.7	28	1	2	3	5	8	15	36
65+	180	5.0	16	1	2	4	7	10	13	21
SUBTOTALS:										
1. SINGLE DX										
A. Not Operated	3	1.3	<1	1	1	1	2	2	2	2
B. Operated	78	2.3	2	1	1	2	3	4	5	6
2. MULTIPLE DX										
A. Not Operated	332	3.1	7	1	1	2	4	6	8	11
B. Operated	729	4.3	15	1	2	3	5	8	12	21
1. SINGLE DX	81	2.3	2	1	1	2	3	4	5	6
2. MULTIPLE DX	1,061	3.9	13	1	2	3	5	8	10	19
A. NOT OPERATED	335	3.1	7	1	1	2	4	6	8	11
B. OPERATED	807	4.1	14	1	2	3	5	8	11	19
TOTAL										
0–19 Years	109	2.6	2	1	1	2	3	4	6	8
20–34	197	3.3	6	1	2	3	4	5	8	13
35–49	248	3.6	10	1	2	3	4	7	9	13
50–64	273	4.2	22	1	2	3	5	8	13	28
65+	315	4.3	13	1	2	3	6	9	11	19
GRAND TOTAL	1,142	3.8	12	1	2	3	4	7	10	17

593.70: VUR NOS

Type of Patients	Observed Patients	Avg. Stay	Variance	Percentiles 10th	25th	50th	75th	90th	95th	99th
1. SINGLE DX										
A. Not Operated										
0–19 Years	4	1.5	<1	1	1	2	2	2	2	2
20–34	0									
35–49	0									
50–64	0									
65+	0									
B. Operated										
0–19 Years	77	2.1	<1	1	1	2	2	3	4	5
20–34	0									
35–49	1	2.0	0	2	2	2	2	2	2	2
50–64	0									
65+	0									
2. MULTIPLE DX										
A. Not Operated										
0–19 Years	28	3.6	9	1	1	3	4	9	10	12
20–34	1	5.0	0	5	5	5	5	5	5	5
35–49	1	2.0	0	2	2	2	2	2	2	2
50–64	0									
65+	6	4.8	8	1	3	6	6	9	9	9
B. Operated										
0–19 Years	193	2.5	1	1	2	2	3	4	4	6
20–34	6	4.2	4	3	3	4	4	8	8	8
35–49	6	3.2	4	2	2	2	4	7	7	7
50–64	4	5.0	17	2	2	4	11	11	11	11
65+	3	5.3	9	2	2	6	8	8	8	8
SUBTOTALS:										
1. SINGLE DX										
A. Not Operated	4	1.5	<1	1	1	2	2	2	2	2
B. Operated	78	2.1	<1	1	1	2	3	3	4	5
2. MULTIPLE DX										
A. Not Operated	36	3.8	8	1	2	3	5	9	10	12
B. Operated	212	2.6	2	1	2	2	3	4	5	8
1. SINGLE DX	82	2.0	<1	1	1	2	3	3	5	5
2. MULTIPLE DX	248	2.8	3	1	2	2	3	4	6	10
A. NOT OPERATED	40	3.6	8	1	1	3	5	8	9	12
B. OPERATED	290	2.5	2	1	2	2	3	4	4	8
TOTAL										
0–19 Years	302	2.4	2	1	2	2	3	4	4	8
20–34	7	4.3	3	3	3	4	5	8	8	8
35–49	8	2.9	3	2	2	2	4	7	7	7
50–64	4	5.0	17	2	2	4	11	11	11	11
65+	9	5.0	7	1	3	6	6	9	9	9
GRAND TOTAL	330	2.6	3	1	2	2	3	4	6	9

Length of Stay by Diagnosis and Operation, Western Region, 2008

Western Region, October 2006–September 2007 Data, by Diagnosis

593.81: RENAL VASCULAR DISORDER

Type of Patients	Observed Patients	Avg. Stay	Vari-ance	Percentiles 10th	25th	50th	75th	90th	95th	99th
1. SINGLE DX										
A. Not Operated										
0–19 Years	1	1.0	0	1	1	1	1	1	1	1
20–34	0									
35–49	2	2.0	0	2	2	2	2	2	2	2
50–64	0									
65+	0									
B. Operated										
0–19 Years	0									
20–34	0									
35–49	0									
50–64	0									
65+	0									
2. MULTIPLE DX										
A. Not Operated										
0–19 Years	6	1.8	<1	1	2	2	2	2	2	2
20–34	25	5.0	13	1	2	5	6	8	10	18
35–49	101	4.6	13	2	2	4	6	8	11	16
50–64	85	4.9	12	1	3	4	6	9	11	21
65+	148	5.0	11	2	3	4	7	9	10	19
B. Operated										
0–19 Years	0									
20–34	4	8.5	94	2	2	4	5	23	23	23
35–49	9	7.4	36	2	3	5	7	19	19	19
50–64	12	9.4	63	5	5	6	11	13	33	33
65+	28	7.6	35	2	3	6	11	18	18	23
SUBTOTALS:										
1. SINGLE DX										
A. Not Operated	3	1.7	<1	1	1	2	2	2	2	2
B. Operated	0									
2. MULTIPLE DX										
A. Not Operated	365	4.8	12	2	2	4	6	9	11	19
B. Operated	53	8.0	43	2	4	6	11	18	23	33
1. SINGLE DX	3	1.7	<1	1	1	2	2	2	2	2
2. MULTIPLE DX	418	5.2	17	2	3	4	6	9	13	23
A. NOT OPERATED	368	4.8	12	2	2	4	6	9	11	19
B. OPERATED	53	8.0	43	2	4	6	11	18	23	33
TOTAL										
0–19 Years	7	1.7	<1	1	1	2	2	2	2	2
20–34	29	5.5	23	1	2	5	6	10	18	23
35–49	112	4.7	15	2	2	4	6	8	13	19
50–64	97	5.5	20	1	3	5	7	11	13	33
65+	176	5.4	15	2	3	6	7	9	14	23
GRAND TOTAL	421	5.2	17	2	3	4	6	9	13	23

593.89: RENAL/URETER DISORD NEC

Type of Patients	Observed Patients	Avg. Stay	Vari-ance	Percentiles 10th	25th	50th	75th	90th	95th	99th
1. SINGLE DX										
A. Not Operated										
0–19 Years	0									
20–34	0									
35–49	0									
50–64	0									
65+	0									
B. Operated										
0–19 Years	3	2.3	<1	2	2	2	3	3	3	3
20–34	0									
35–49	0									
50–64	0									
65+	0									
2. MULTIPLE DX										
A. Not Operated										
0–19 Years	6	1.8	1	1	1	2	2	2	4	4
20–34	14	3.2	9	1	1	2	3	10	10	10
35–49	31	3.0	11	1	1	2	3	6	13	14
50–64	33	3.2	10	1	2	2	4	7	9	16
65+	32	3.1	3	1	2	3	4	6	7	7
B. Operated										
0–19 Years	9	3.2	2	1	3	3	4	5	5	5
20–34	13	3.9	6	2	3	3	4	8	10	10
35–49	23	3.5	3	2	2	3	5	5	7	7
50–64	33	3.7	8	1	2	3	5	8	11	12
65+	24	5.6	30	1	3	4	8	10	11	27
SUBTOTALS:										
1. SINGLE DX										
A. Not Operated	0									
B. Operated	3	2.3	<1	2	2	2	3	3	3	3
2. MULTIPLE DX										
A. Not Operated	116	3.0	7	1	1	2	4	6	9	14
B. Operated	102	4.1	12	1	2	3	5	8	10	12
1. SINGLE DX	3	2.3	<1	2	2	2	3	3	3	3
2. MULTIPLE DX	218	3.5	10	1	2	3	4	7	10	14
A. NOT OPERATED	116	3.0	7	1	1	2	4	6	9	14
B. OPERATED	105	4.0	11	1	2	3	5	8	10	12
TOTAL										
0–19 Years	18	2.6	2	1	2	2	3	5	5	5
20–34	27	3.6	7	1	2	3	4	10	10	10
35–49	54	3.2	7	1	2	2	4	6	9	14
50–64	66	3.4	9	1	2	3	4	7	9	16
65+	56	4.2	16	1	3	3	5	8	10	27
GRAND TOTAL	221	3.5	10	1	2	3	4	7	9	14

593.9: RENAL/URETER DISORD NOS

Type of Patients	Observed Patients	Avg. Stay	Vari-ance	Percentiles 10th	25th	50th	75th	90th	95th	99th
1. SINGLE DX										
A. Not Operated										
0–19 Years	2	1.5	<1	1	1	2	2	2	2	2
20–34	0									
35–49	6	1.0	0	1	1	1	1	1	1	1
50–64	3	2.0	3	1	1	1	4	4	4	4
65+	3	2.4	5	1	1	1	5	5	5	5
B. Operated										
0–19 Years	3	1.7	1	1	1	1	1	3	3	3
20–34	2	3.0	8	1	1	1	5	5	5	5
35–49	9	2.4	2	1	1	3	4	4	4	5
50–64	14	2.4	<1	2	2	2	3	3	4	4
65+	4	2.0	1	1	1	1	1	3	3	3
2. MULTIPLE DX										
A. Not Operated										
0–19 Years	19	4.0	37	1	1	2	3	11	27	27
20–34	44	2.8	7	1	1	2	3	5	7	15
35–49	120	2.9	5	1	1	2	4	6	8	12
50–64	291	3.2	9	1	1	2	4	6	8	16
65+	841	3.6	9	2	2	3	4	6	9	16
B. Operated										
0–19 Years	13	2.6	3	1	1	3	3	3	7	7
20–34	18	3.7	11	1	1	2	5	10	13	13
35–49	83	3.4	5	1	2	3	3	6	7	14
50–64	178	3.2	4	1	2	3	4	6	7	11
65+	176	3.4	9	1	2	3	4	6	8	14
SUBTOTALS:										
1. SINGLE DX										
A. Not Operated	14	1.6	2	1	1	1	1	1	4	5
B. Operated	32	2.3	1	1	1	2	3	4	4	5
2. MULTIPLE DX										
A. Not Operated	1,315	3.4	9	1	2	3	4	6	9	16
B. Operated	468	3.3	6	1	2	3	4	6	7	13
1. SINGLE DX	46	2.1	2	1	1	2	3	4	4	5
2. MULTIPLE DX	1,783	3.4	8	1	2	3	4	6	8	15
A. NOT OPERATED	1,329	3.4	9	1	2	3	4	6	9	16
B. OPERATED	500	3.3	6	1	2	3	4	6	7	13
TOTAL										
0–19 Years	37	3.2	20	1	1	2	3	7	11	27
20–34	64	3.1	8	1	1	2	4	6	10	15
35–49	218	3.0	5	1	1	3	4	6	7	12
50–64	486	3.2	7	1	2	3	4	6	7	13
65+	1,024	3.6	9	1	2	3	4	6	9	16
GRAND TOTAL	1,829	3.4	8	1	2	3	4	6	8	14

Length of Stay by Diagnosis and Operation, Western Region, 2008

Western Region, October 2006–September 2007 Data, by Diagnosis

594: LOWER URINARY CALCULUS

Type of Patients	Observed Patients	Avg. Stay	Vari-ance	10th	25th	50th	75th	90th	95th	99th
1. SINGLE DX										
A. Not Operated										
0–19 Years	3	1.3	<1	1	1	1	2	2	2	2
20–34	2	1.0	0	1	1	1	1	1	1	1
35–49	2	1.5	<1	1	1	1	2	2	2	2
50–64	2	1.0	0	1	1	1	1	1	1	1
65+	3	1.0	0	1	1	1	1	1	1	1
B. Operated										
0–19 Years	0									
20–34	1	1.0	0	1	1	1	1	1	1	1
35–49	0									
50–64	1	1.0	0	1	1	1	1	1	1	1
65+	2	2.5	4	1	1	4	4	4	4	4
2. MULTIPLE DX										
A. Not Operated										
0–19 Years	10	4.8	23	1	2	2	8	11	15	15
20–34	27	2.2	2	1	1	2	3	5	5	7
35–49	45	2.5	2	1	1	2	3	4	4	9
50–64	101	2.2	4	1	1	2	3	4	5	15
65+	148	2.3	4	1	1	1	3	5	7	11
B. Operated										
0–19 Years	5	3.6	9	1	1	3	5	8	8	8
20–34	26	3.1	6	1	1	2	5	7	8	8
35–49	36	3.4	13	1	1	2	4	6	11	20
50–64	94	2.4	4	1	1	2	3	5	7	12
65+	324	2.8	8	1	1	2	3	6	8	14
SUBTOTALS:										
1. SINGLE DX										
A. Not Operated	12	1.2	<1	1	1	1	1	2	2	2
B. Operated	4	1.8	2	1	1	1	1	4	4	4
2. MULTIPLE DX										
A. Not Operated	331	2.4	4	1	1	2	3	5	7	11
B. Operated	485	2.8	7	1	1	2	3	6	8	14
1. SINGLE DX	16	1.3	<1	1	1	1	1	2	4	4
2. MULTIPLE DX	816	2.6	6	1	1	2	3	6	7	14
A. NOT OPERATED	343	2.3	4	1	1	2	3	5	6	11
B. OPERATED	489	2.8	7	1	1	2	3	6	8	14
TOTAL										
0–19 Years	18	3.9	16	1	1	2	5	11	15	15
20–34	56	2.6	4	1	1	2	3	5	7	8
35–49	83	2.9	7	1	1	2	3	4	6	20
50–64	198	2.2	4	1	1	2	3	4	6	12
65+	477	2.6	7	1	1	2	3	6	8	14
GRAND TOTAL	832	2.6	6	1	1	2	3	5	7	14

594.1: BLADDER CALCULUS NEC

Type of Patients	Observed Patients	Avg. Stay	Vari-ance	10th	25th	50th	75th	90th	95th	99th
1. SINGLE DX										
A. Not Operated										
0–19 Years	1	2.0	0	2	2	2	2	2	2	2
20–34	0									
35–49	0									
50–64	1	1.0	0	1	1	1	1	1	1	1
65+	3	1.0	0	1	1	1	1	1	1	1
B. Operated										
0–19 Years	0									
20–34	1	1.0	0	1	1	1	1	1	1	1
35–49	0									
50–64	1	1.0	0	1	1	1	1	1	1	1
65+	2	2.5	4	1	1	4	4	4	4	4
2. MULTIPLE DX										
A. Not Operated										
0–19 Years	7	4.7	25	1	2	2	8	15	15	15
20–34	16	1.9	2	1	1	1	2	3	7	7
35–49	30	2.8	3	1	2	3	3	4	6	9
50–64	76	2.3	5	1	1	2	3	4	6	15
65+	134	2.3	5	1	1	1	3	5	7	11
B. Operated										
0–19 Years	5	3.6	9	1	1	3	5	8	8	8
20–34	23	3.4	6	1	1	3	6	7	8	8
35–49	25	3.9	17	1	2	3	4	8	11	20
50–64	83	2.1	3	1	1	2	3	5	6	7
65+	302	2.7	6	1	1	2	3	6	8	14
SUBTOTALS:										
1. SINGLE DX										
A. Not Operated	5	1.2	<1	1	1	1	1	2	2	2
B. Operated	4	1.8	2	1	1	1	4	4	4	4
2. MULTIPLE DX										
A. Not Operated	263	2.4	5	1	1	2	3	5	7	12
B. Operated	438	2.7	6	1	1	2	3	6	8	12
1. SINGLE DX	9	1.5	1	1	1	1	1	4	4	4
2. MULTIPLE DX	701	2.6	6	1	1	2	3	6	7	12
A. NOT OPERATED	268	2.4	5	1	1	2	3	5	7	12
B. OPERATED	442	2.7	6	1	1	2	3	6	7	12
TOTAL										
0–19 Years	13	4.1	16	1	2	2	5	8	15	15
20–34	40	2.7	5	1	1	2	3	7	7	8
35–49	55	3.3	9	1	2	3	4	6	9	20
50–64	161	2.2	4	1	1	2	3	4	6	8
65+	441	2.5	5	1	1	2	3	6	7	12
GRAND TOTAL	710	2.6	6	1	1	2	3	6	7	12

595: CYSTITIS

Type of Patients	Observed Patients	Avg. Stay	Vari-ance	10th	25th	50th	75th	90th	95th	99th
1. SINGLE DX										
A. Not Operated										
0–19 Years	8	2.3	<1	2	2	2	2	4	4	4
20–34	5	1.6	<1	1	1	2	2	2	2	2
35–49	3	2.3	2	1	1	2	4	4	4	4
50–64	2	1.0	0	1	1	1	1	1	1	1
65+	0									
B. Operated										
0–19 Years	0									
20–34	1	2.0	0	2	2	2	2	2	2	2
35–49	1	4.0	0	4	4	4	4	4	4	4
50–64	0									
65+	1	1.0	0	1	1	1	1	1	1	1
2. MULTIPLE DX										
A. Not Operated										
0–19 Years	42	3.0	3	1	2	2	4	5	7	9
20–34	110	3.6	8	1	2	3	4	7	9	12
35–49	172	3.5	5	1	2	3	4	7	9	11
50–64	266	4.3	34	1	2	3	5	8	11	25
65+	1,157	4.2	9	1	2	3	5	8	10	15
B. Operated										
0–19 Years	3	5.7	<1	5	5	6	6	6	6	6
20–34	19	3.4	13	1	2	3	5	7	16	16
35–49	41	6.2	105	1	2	4	6	10	15	66
50–64	117	6.5	59	1	2	4	8	12	22	35
65+	430	6.4	41	1	2	5	8	13	18	39
SUBTOTALS:										
1. SINGLE DX										
A. Not Operated	18	1.9	<1	1	1	2	2	4	4	4
B. Operated	3	2.3	2	1	1	4	4	4	4	4
2. MULTIPLE DX										
A. Not Operated	1,747	4.0	12	1	2	3	5	8	10	15
B. Operated	610	6.3	48	1	2	4	8	12	18	39
1. SINGLE DX	21	2.0	<1	1	1	2	2	4	4	4
2. MULTIPLE DX	2,357	4.6	22	1	2	3	6	9	11	23
A. NOT OPERATED	1,765	4.0	12	1	2	3	5	8	10	15
B. OPERATED	613	6.3	48	1	2	4	8	12	18	39
TOTAL										
0–19 Years	53	3.0	3	1	2	2	4	6	7	9
20–34	135	3.5	8	1	2	3	4	7	9	16
35–49	217	4.0	25	1	2	3	5	8	9	15
50–64	385	5.0	42	1	2	3	6	10	13	35
65+	1,588	4.8	19	1	2	4	6	9	12	21
GRAND TOTAL	2,378	4.6	22	1	2	3	6	9	11	23

Length of Stay by Diagnosis and Operation, Western Region, 2008

Western Region, October 2006–September 2007 Data, by Diagnosis

595.0: ACUTE CYSTITIS

Type of Patients	Observed Patients	Avg. Stay	Variance	10th	25th	50th	75th	90th	95th	99th
1. SINGLE DX										
A. Not Operated										
0–19 Years	4	2.5	<1	2	2	2	2	4	4	4
20–34	2	1.5	<1	1	1	1	2	2	2	2
35–49	1	1.0	0	1	1	1	1	1	1	1
50–64	0									
65+	0									
B. Operated										
0–19 Years	0									
20–34	0									
35–49	0									
50–64	0									
65+	0									
2. MULTIPLE DX										
A. Not Operated										
0–19 Years	14	3.1	4	1	2	3	4	6	8	8
20–34	35	4.0	14	1	2	3	5	8	10	20
35–49	49	3.8	7	1	2	3	5	9	9	11
50–64	87	4.2	38	1	2	3	5	7	11	55
65+	391	3.9	7	1	2	3	5	7	9	14
B. Operated										
0–19 Years	0									
20–34	1	7.0	0	7	7	7	7	7	7	7
35–49	9	6.3	12	2	4	6	7	14	14	14
50–64	20	7.7	141	1	2	4	6	18	54	54
65+	64	7.0	36	2	3	6	8	13	18	39
SUBTOTALS:										
1. SINGLE DX										
A. Not Operated	7	2.0	<1	1	1	2	2	4	4	4
B. Operated	0									
2. MULTIPLE DX										
A. Not Operated	576	4.0	12	1	2	3	5	8	9	14
B. Operated	94	7.0	54	2	3	6	8	14	18	54
1. SINGLE DX	7	2.0	<1	1	1	2	2	4	4	4
2. MULTIPLE DX	670	4.4	19	1	2	3	5	8	10	18
A. NOT OPERATED	583	3.9	12	1	2	3	5	7	9	14
B. OPERATED	94	7.0	54	2	3	6	8	14	18	54
TOTAL										
0–19 Years	18	3.0	3	1	2	2	4	6	8	8
20–34	38	3.9	13	1	2	3	5	8	10	20
35–49	59	4.1	8	1	2	3	6	9	10	14
50–64	107	4.9	58	1	2	3	5	9	13	54
65+	455	4.4	12	1	2	3	5	8	10	18
GRAND TOTAL	677	4.4	19	1	2	3	5	8	10	18

595.82: IRRADIATION CYSTITIS

Type of Patients	Observed Patients	Avg. Stay	Variance	10th	25th	50th	75th	90th	95th	99th
1. SINGLE DX										
A. Not Operated										
0–19 Years	0									
20–34	0									
35–49	0									
50–64	0									
65+	0									
B. Operated										
0–19 Years	0									
20–34	0									
35–49	0									
50–64	0									
65+	0									
2. MULTIPLE DX										
A. Not Operated										
0–19 Years	1	1.0	0	1	1	1	1	1	1	1
20–34	0									
35–49	7	4.7	7	1	3	5	7	9	9	9
50–64	32	6.3	116	1	3	3	6	10	15	62
65+	175	4.3	14	1	2	3	5	8	11	22
B. Operated										
0–19 Years	0									
20–34	0									
35–49	6	6.8	22	3	4	5	10	15	15	15
50–64	28	6.9	64	2	3	4	9	11	31	35
65+	199	6.2	42	1	2	5	7	12	17	44
SUBTOTALS:										
1. SINGLE DX										
A. Not Operated	0									
B. Operated	0									
2. MULTIPLE DX										
A. Not Operated	215	4.6	29	1	2	3	5	8	11	22
B. Operated	233	6.3	44	1	3	4	8	11	17	40
1. SINGLE DX	0									
2. MULTIPLE DX	448	5.5	37	1	2	4	6	11	15	35
A. NOT OPERATED	215	4.6	29	1	2	3	5	8	11	22
B. OPERATED	233	6.3	44	1	3	4	8	11	17	40
TOTAL										
0–19 Years	1	1.0	0	1	1	1	1	1	1	1
20–34	0									
35–49	13	5.7	14	3	3	5	7	10	15	15
50–64	60	6.6	90	2	3	4	7	11	31	62
65+	374	5.3	30	1	2	4	6	11	15	26
GRAND TOTAL	448	5.5	37	1	2	4	6	11	15	35

595.9: CYSTITIS NOS

Type of Patients	Observed Patients	Avg. Stay	Variance	10th	25th	50th	75th	90th	95th	99th
1. SINGLE DX										
A. Not Operated										
0–19 Years	4	2.0	0	2	2	2	2	2	2	2
20–34	1	1.0	0	1	1	1	1	1	1	1
35–49	1	2.0	0	2	2	2	2	2	2	2
50–64	0									
65+	0									
B. Operated										
0–19 Years	0									
20–34	0									
35–49	0									
50–64	0									
65+	0									
2. MULTIPLE DX										
A. Not Operated										
0–19 Years	24	2.8	3	2	2	2	3	5	5	9
20–34	44	3.0	3	2	2	3	4	5	6	9
35–49	78	3.1	4	2	2	3	4	6	8	11
50–64	102	3.6	10	2	2	3	4	6	8	16
65+	454	4.2	10	2	2	3	5	8	10	17
B. Operated										
0–19 Years	1	6.0	0	6	6	6	6	6	6	6
20–34	2	2.5	<1	2	2	3	3	3	3	3
35–49	5	18.2	739	2	3	5	15	66	66	66
50–64	17	7.7	33	2	4	6	6	20	23	23
65+	68	7.6	43	2	3	5	9	17	20	31
SUBTOTALS:										
1. SINGLE DX										
A. Not Operated	6	1.8	<1	1	2	2	2	2	2	2
B. Operated	0									
2. MULTIPLE DX										
A. Not Operated	702	3.8	9	1	2	3	5	7	9	14
B. Operated	93	8.0	76	2	3	5	9	17	23	66
1. SINGLE DX	6	1.8	<1	1	2	2	2	2	2	2
2. MULTIPLE DX	795	4.3	19	1	2	3	5	8	11	23
A. NOT OPERATED	708	3.8	9	1	2	3	5	7	9	14
B. OPERATED	93	8.0	76	2	3	5	9	17	23	66
TOTAL										
0–19 Years	29	2.8	3	2	2	2	3	5	5	9
20–34	47	2.9	3	2	2	3	4	5	6	9
35–49	84	4.0	53	1	2	3	4	6	8	66
50–64	119	4.2	15	2	2	3	5	8	12	23
65+	522	4.6	16	2	3	3	6	9	12	20
GRAND TOTAL	801	4.3	19	1	2	3	5	8	11	20

Western Region, October 2006–September 2007 Data, by Diagnosis

596: OTHER BLADDER DISORDERS

Type of Patients	Observed Patients	Avg. Stay	Variance	Percentiles						
				10th	25th	50th	75th	90th	95th	99th
1. SINGLE DX										
A. Not Operated										
0–19 Years	1	4.0	0	4	4	4	4	4	4	4
20–34	1	3.0	0	3	3	3	3	3	3	3
35–49	1	1.0	0	1	1	1	1	1	1	1
50–64	0									
65+	1	1.0	0	1	1	1	1	1	1	1
B. Operated										
0–19 Years	3	4.0	19	1	1	2	9	9	9	9
20–34	1	1.0	0	1	1	1	1	1	1	1
35–49	9	2.9	3	1	1	3	4	6	6	6
50–64	4	2.0	4	1	1	1	5	5	5	5
65+	9	1.5	<1	1	1	1	2	3	3	3
2. MULTIPLE DX										
A. Not Operated										
0–19 Years	19	2.3	2	1	1	2	3	4	7	7
20–34	39	4.4	13	1	2	3	6	11	13	16
35–49	81	4.5	10	1	2	4	6	9	10	15
50–64	146	3.6	8	1	2	3	5	7	8	12
65+	457	4.2	16	2	2	3	5	8	12	22
B. Operated										
0–19 Years	51	7.9	61	2	5	7	9	13	14	55
20–34	86	7.9	39	2	4	6	10	17	23	31
35–49	183	7.1	64	1	2	6	8	14	20	57
50–64	416	5.6	33	1	2	4	7	12	15	27
65+	987	4.8	31	1	1	3	6	11	15	29
SUBTOTALS:										
1. SINGLE DX										
A. Not Operated	4	2.3	2	1	1	1	4	4	4	4
B. Operated	26	2.3	4	1	1	3	3	5	6	9
2. MULTIPLE DX										
A. Not Operated	742	4.1	14	1	2	3	5	8	11	20
B. Operated	1,723	5.5	37	1	2	4	7	12	17	30
1. SINGLE DX	30	2.3	4	1	1	1	3	5	6	9
2. MULTIPLE DX	2,465	5.1	31	1	2	3	7	11	15	27
A. NOT OPERATED	746	4.1	13	1	2	3	5	8	11	20
B. OPERATED	1,749	5.5	37	1	2	3	7	12	16	30
TOTAL										
0–19 Years	74	6.3	49	1	2	5	7	11	14	55
20–34	127	6.7	33	2	3	6	7	13	18	26
35–49	274	6.1	47	1	2	5	7	12	19	38
50–64	566	5.1	27	1	2	4	7	11	14	27
65+	1,454	4.6	27	1	1	3	6	11	15	27
GRAND TOTAL	2,495	5.0	30	1	1	3	7	11	15	27

596.0: BLADDER NECK OBSTRUCTION

Type of Patients	Observed Patients	Avg. Stay	Variance	Percentiles						
				10th	25th	50th	75th	90th	95th	99th
1. SINGLE DX										
A. Not Operated										
0–19 Years	0									
20–34	1	3.0	0	3	3	3	3	3	3	3
35–49	1	1.0	0	1	1	1	1	1	1	1
50–64	0									
65+	0									
B. Operated										
0–19 Years	0									
20–34	1	1.0	0	1	1	1	1	1	1	1
35–49	3	1.3	<1	1	1	1	1	2	2	2
50–64	2	1.0	0	1	1	1	1	1	1	1
65+	8	1.3	<1	1	1	1	2	2	2	2
2. MULTIPLE DX										
A. Not Operated										
0–19 Years	2	5.0	8	3	3	7	7	7	7	7
20–34	4	3.8	<1	3	3	4	4	4	4	4
35–49	18	3.0	3	1	1	3	4	6	6	6
50–64	39	3.2	6	1	2	2	5	7	8	12
65+	160	3.5	8	1	2	3	4	5	7	15
B. Operated										
0–19 Years	0									
20–34	2	1.5	<1	1	1	1	2	2	2	2
35–49	22	2.2	4	1	1	1	2	6	7	8
50–64	105	2.0	4	1	1	1	2	3	3	11
65+	408	2.1	5	1	1	1	2	4	4	12
SUBTOTALS:										
1. SINGLE DX										
A. Not Operated	2	2.0	2	1	1	1	3	3	3	3
B. Operated	14	1.2	<1	1	1	1	1	2	2	2
2. MULTIPLE DX										
A. Not Operated	223	3.4	7	1	2	3	4	6	8	14
B. Operated	537	2.1	5	1	1	1	2	4	6	12
1. SINGLE DX	16	1.3	<1	1	1	1	2	2	3	3
2. MULTIPLE DX	760	2.5	6	1	1	2	3	5	7	13
A. NOT OPERATED	225	3.4	7	1	2	3	4	6	8	14
B. OPERATED	551	2.1	5	1	1	1	2	4	6	12
TOTAL										
0–19 Years	2	5.0	8	3	3	7	7	7	7	7
20–34	8	2.8	2	1	1	3	3	4	4	4
35–49	44	2.4	4	1	1	1	4	6	6	8
50–64	146	2.3	5	1	1	1	2	5	7	12
65+	576	2.5	7	1	1	2	3	5	7	14
GRAND TOTAL	776	2.4	6	1	1	2	3	5	7	13

596.1: INTESTINOVESICAL FISTULA

Type of Patients	Observed Patients	Avg. Stay	Variance	Percentiles						
				10th	25th	50th	75th	90th	95th	99th
1. SINGLE DX										
A. Not Operated										
0–19 Years	0									
20–34	0									
35–49	0									
50–64	0									
65+	0									
B. Operated										
0–19 Years	0									
20–34	0									
35–49	2	5.0	2	4	4	5	6	6	6	6
50–64	1	5.0	0	5	5	5	5	5	5	5
65+	1	3.0	0	3	3	3	3	3	3	3
2. MULTIPLE DX										
A. Not Operated										
0–19 Years	0									
20–34	12	7.6	25	2	2	7	13	13	16	16
35–49	15	4.9	12	2	2	4	7	11	12	12
50–64	24	4.5	7	1	2	5	6	8	8	10
65+	65	6.4	35	1	3	4	8	14	20	25
B. Operated										
0–19 Years	3	10.0	7	7	7	11	12	12	12	12
20–34	24	8.8	57	3	5	7	10	24	26	31
35–49	82	8.2	49	4	5	7	9	13	20	57
50–64	153	8.6	43	4	5	7	9	15	19	36
65+	251	10.4	48	4	6	9	12	19	25	36
SUBTOTALS:										
1. SINGLE DX										
A. Not Operated	0									
B. Operated	4	4.5	2	3	4	5	5	6	6	6
2. MULTIPLE DX										
A. Not Operated	116	6.0	25	1	2	4	8	13	19	23
B. Operated	513	9.4	47	4	6	7	11	17	23	36
1. SINGLE DX	4	4.5	2	3	4	5	5	6	6	6
2. MULTIPLE DX	629	8.8	45	3	5	7	11	16	22	35
A. NOT OPERATED	116	6.0	25	1	2	4	8	13	19	23
B. OPERATED	517	9.4	47	4	6	7	11	17	23	36
TOTAL										
0–19 Years	3	10.0	7	7	7	11	12	12	12	12
20–34	36	8.4	45	3	4	7	11	16	26	31
35–49	99	7.6	44	3	4	6	9	12	20	57
50–64	178	8.0	40	3	5	7	9	14	19	36
65+	317	9.5	47	3	5	8	12	19	23	35
GRAND TOTAL	633	8.8	45	3	5	7	11	16	22	35

Length of Stay by Diagnosis and Operation, Western Region, 2008

Western Region, October 2006–September 2007 Data, by Diagnosis

596.54: NEUROGENIC BLADDER NOS

Type of Patients	Observed Patients	Avg. Stay	Variance	Percentiles						
				10th	25th	50th	75th	90th	95th	99th
1. SINGLE DX										
A. Not Operated										
0–19 Years	0									
20–34	0									
35–49	0									
50–64	0									
65+	0									
B. Operated										
0–19 Years	1	9.0	0	9	9	9	9	9	9	9
20–34	0									
35–49	0									
50–64	0									
65+	0									
2. MULTIPLE DX										
A. Not Operated										
0–19 Years	9	2.0	<1	1	1	2	2	4	4	4
20–34	7	2.0	<1	1	1	2	3	3	3	3
35–49	20	5.1	12	1	3	5	7	9	15	15
50–64	26	4.7	12	1	2	4	6	12	12	17
65+	52	4.3	8	1	2	4	6	7	10	15
B. Operated										
0–19 Years	39	7.4	16	3	5	7	9	13	14	22
20–34	36	8.2	23	2	5	8	12	15	17	23
35–49	35	9.2	146	1	2	6	12	20	38	63
50–64	46	6.2	19	1	3	4	10	13	13	18
65+	37	4.3	13	1	2	4	6	8	11	18
SUBTOTALS:										
1. SINGLE DX										
A. Not Operated	0									
B. Operated	1	9.0	0	9	9	9	9	9	9	9
2. MULTIPLE DX										
A. Not Operated	114	4.2	10	1	2	3	6	8	10	15
B. Operated	193	7.0	43	1	3	6	9	13	16	38
1. SINGLE DX	1	9.0	0	9	9	9	9	9	9	9
2. MULTIPLE DX	307	5.9	32	1	2	5	8	12	15	22
A. NOT OPERATED	114	4.2	10	1	2	3	6	8	10	15
B. OPERATED	194	7.0	43	1	3	6	9	13	16	38
TOTAL										
0–19 Years	49	6.4	17	1	3	6	8	13	14	22
20–34	43	7.2	25	2	3	7	11	13	16	23
35–49	55	7.7	100	1	2	5	9	15	21	63
50–64	72	5.7	17	1	3	4	8	11	13	18
65+	89	4.3	10	1	2	4	6	8	10	18
GRAND TOTAL	308	6.0	32	1	2	5	8	12	15	22

596.7: BLADDER WALL HEMORRHAGE

Type of Patients	Observed Patients	Avg. Stay	Variance	Percentiles						
				10th	25th	50th	75th	90th	95th	99th
1. SINGLE DX										
A. Not Operated										
0–19 Years	0									
20–34	0									
35–49	0									
50–64	0									
65+	1	1.0	0	1	1	1	1	1	1	1
B. Operated										
0–19 Years	0									
20–34	0									
35–49	0									
50–64	0									
65+	0									
2. MULTIPLE DX										
A. Not Operated										
0–19 Years	1	1.0	0	1	1	1	1	1	1	1
20–34	1	4.0	0	4	4	4	4	4	4	4
35–49	3	3.3	4	1	1	1	5	5	5	5
50–64	15	2.5	6	1	1	1	3	6	10	10
65+	67	3.3	10	1	1	2	5	7	10	22
B. Operated										
0–19 Years	0									
20–34	1	2.0	0	2	2	2	2	2	2	2
35–49	3	11.3	25	6	6	12	16	16	16	16
50–64	11	4.1	9	1	1	3	3	9	9	9
65+	60	4.2	16	1	2	3	5	8	9	24
SUBTOTALS:										
1. SINGLE DX										
A. Not Operated	1	1.0	0	1	1	1	1	1	1	1
B. Operated	0									
2. MULTIPLE DX										
A. Not Operated	87	3.1	9	1	1	2	4	7	9	22
B. Operated	75	4.5	17	1	2	3	6	9	12	24
1. SINGLE DX	1	1.0	0	1	1	1	1	1	1	1
2. MULTIPLE DX	162	3.8	13	1	1	3	5	8	9	22
A. NOT OPERATED	88	3.1	9	1	1	2	4	7	9	22
B. OPERATED	75	4.5	17	1	2	3	6	9	12	24
TOTAL										
0–19 Years	1	1.0	0	1	1	1	1	1	1	1
20–34	2	3.0	2	2	2	3	4	4	4	4
35–49	6	7.3	31	1	4	5	12	16	16	16
50–64	26	3.2	8	1	1	2	5	9	10	10
65+	128	3.7	13	1	2	3	5	8	9	22
GRAND TOTAL	163	3.7	13	1	1	3	5	8	9	22

596.8: BLADDER DISORDER NEC

Type of Patients	Observed Patients	Avg. Stay	Variance	Percentiles						
				10th	25th	50th	75th	90th	95th	99th
1. SINGLE DX										
A. Not Operated										
0–19 Years	1	4.0	0	4	4	4	4	4	4	4
20–34	0									
35–49	0									
50–64	0									
65+	0									
B. Operated										
0–19 Years	0									
20–34	0									
35–49	0									
50–64	1	1.0	0	1	1	1	1	1	1	1
65+	0									
2. MULTIPLE DX										
A. Not Operated										
0–19 Years	5	1.6	<1	1	1	1	2	3	3	3
20–34	11	3.6	2	2	2	3	3	4	6	6
35–49	10	4.1	8	1	1	5	5	6	10	10
50–64	25	2.8	5	1	1	2	3	6	7	9
65+	67	4.5	22	1	2	3	5	10	16	29
B. Operated										
0–19 Years	1	2.0	0	2	2	2	2	2	2	2
20–34	4	8.5	103	1	1	2	23	23	23	23
35–49	6	7.7	92	1	1	3	19	21	21	21
50–64	29	3.4	12	1	1	2	2	4	11	15
65+	87	3.2	10	1	1	2	3	8	11	16
SUBTOTALS:										
1. SINGLE DX										
A. Not Operated	1	4.0	0	4	4	4	4	4	4	4
B. Operated	1	1.0	0	1	1	1	1	1	1	1
2. MULTIPLE DX										
A. Not Operated	118	3.9	15	1	2	3	3	7	10	18
B. Operated	127	3.6	18	1	1	2	4	10	11	21
1. SINGLE DX	2	2.5	4	1	1	1	4	4	4	4
2. MULTIPLE DX	245	3.8	16	1	1	2	4	8	11	21
A. NOT OPERATED	119	3.9	15	1	2	3	5	7	10	18
B. OPERATED	128	3.6	17	1	1	2	4	10	11	21
TOTAL										
0–19 Years	7	2.0	1	1	1	2	3	4	4	4
20–34	15	4.9	29	2	2	3	6	8	23	23
35–49	16	5.5	39	1	1	3	6	19	21	21
50–64	55	3.1	9	1	1	2	3	7	10	15
65+	154	3.8	16	1	1	2	4	9	11	18
GRAND TOTAL	247	3.7	16	1	1	2	4	8	11	21

Length of Stay by Diagnosis and Operation, Western Region, 2008

597: URETHRITIS/URETHRAL SYND

Type of Patients	Observed Patients	Avg. Stay	Vari-ance	Percentiles						
				10th	25th	50th	75th	90th	95th	99th
1. SINGLE DX										
A. *Not Operated*										
0–19 Years	1	1.0	0	1	1	1	1	1	1	1
20–34	0									
35–49	1	1.0	0	1	1	1	1	1	1	1
50–64	0									
65+	0									
B. *Operated*										
0–19 Years	1	1.0	0	1	1	1	1	1	1	1
20–34	1	4.0	0	4	4	4	4	4	4	4
35–49	0									
50–64	0									
65+	0									
2. MULTIPLE DX										
A. *Not Operated*										
0–19 Years	0									
20–34	4	2.0	<1	1	1	2	2	3	3	3
35–49	8	2.9	6	1	1	2	3	8	8	8
50–64	13	4.0	6	2	2	3	5	8	9	9
65+	24	3.8	6	2	2	3	6	8	8	9
B. *Operated*										
0–19 Years	0									
20–34	3	4.7	30	1	1	2	11	11	11	11
35–49	3	8.7	85	1	1	6	19	19	19	19
50–64	2	2.5	<1	2	2	2	3	3	3	3
65+	7	4.1	21	1	1	2	5	14	14	14
SUBTOTALS:										
1. SINGLE DX										
A. *Not Operated*	2	1.0	0	1	1	1	1	1	1	1
B. *Operated*	2	2.5	4	1	1	1	4	4	4	4
2. MULTIPLE DX										
A. *Not Operated*	49	3.6	6	1	2	3	5	8	8	9
B. *Operated*	15	4.9	30	1	1	2	6	14	19	19
1. SINGLE DX	4	1.8	2	1	1	1	1	4	4	4
2. MULTIPLE DX	64	3.9	11	1	2	3	5	8	9	19
A. NOT OPERATED	51	3.5	6	1	2	3	5	8	8	9
B. OPERATED	17	4.7	27	1	1	2	5	14	19	19
TOTAL										
0–19 Years	2	1.0	0	1	1	1	1	1	1	1
20–34	8	3.2	11	1	1	2	3	11	11	11
35–49	12	4.2	27	1	1	2	6	11	19	19
50–64	15	3.8	5	2	2	3	5	8	9	9
65+	31	3.9	9	1	2	3	6	8	9	14
GRAND TOTAL	68	3.8	11	1	2	3	5	8	9	19

598: URETHRAL STRICTURE

Type of Patients	Observed Patients	Avg. Stay	Vari-ance	Percentiles						
				10th	25th	50th	75th	90th	95th	99th
1. SINGLE DX										
A. *Not Operated*										
0–19 Years	0									
20–34	1	1.0	0	1	1	1	1	1	1	1
35–49	3	2.0	3	1	1	1	4	4	4	4
50–64	1	1.0	0	1	1	1	1	1	1	1
65+	0									
B. *Operated*										
0–19 Years	4	1.5	<1	1	1	1	2	2	2	2
20–34	19	2.1	2	1	1	1	2	2	6	6
35–49	19	1.6	<1	1	1	1	2	3	5	5
50–64	15	1.4	<1	1	1	1	2	2	3	3
65+	13	1.6	1	1	1	1	2	3	4	4
2. MULTIPLE DX										
A. *Not Operated*										
0–19 Years	2	1.5	<1	1	1	1	2	2	2	2
20–34	27	2.0	1	1	1	2	3	4	4	4
35–49	28	2.7	4	1	1	2	4	6	7	8
50–64	35	2.6	4	1	1	2	4	5	7	10
65+	76	2.5	5	1	1	2	3	5	7	12
B. *Operated*										
0–19 Years	17	3.1	2	2	2	3	3	5	6	6
20–34	74	2.5	5	1	1	2	3	5	6	15
35–49	78	2.7	5	1	1	2	4	5	7	13
50–64	109	3.1	14	1	1	2	4	7	11	15
65+	185	2.9	9	1	1	2	4	6	7	18
SUBTOTALS:										
1. SINGLE DX										
A. *Not Operated*	5	1.6	2	1	1	1	1	4	4	4
B. *Operated*	70	1.7	1	1	1	1	2	3	4	6
2. MULTIPLE DX										
A. *Not Operated*	168	2.4	4	1	1	2	3	5	7	10
B. *Operated*	463	2.8	8	1	1	2	4	6	7	15
1. SINGLE DX	75	1.7	1	1	1	1	2	3	4	6
2. MULTIPLE DX	631	2.7	7	1	1	2	4	6	7	13
A. NOT OPERATED	173	2.4	4	1	1	2	3	5	7	10
B. OPERATED	533	2.7	7	1	1	2	3	5	7	15
TOTAL										
0–19 Years	23	2.7	2	1	1	2	4	5	5	6
20–34	121	2.3	4	1	1	2	3	5	6	7
35–49	128	2.5	4	1	1	2	3	6	6	8
50–64	160	2.8	10	1	1	2	3	6	9	15
65+	274	2.7	7	1	1	2	3	5	7	17
GRAND TOTAL	706	2.6	7	1	1	2	3	5	7	12

598.8: URETHRAL STRICTURE NEC

Type of Patients	Observed Patients	Avg. Stay	Vari-ance	Percentiles						
				10th	25th	50th	75th	90th	95th	99th
1. SINGLE DX										
A. *Not Operated*										
0–19 Years	0									
20–34	1	1.0	0	1	1	1	1	1	1	1
35–49	3	2.0	3	1	1	1	4	4	4	4
50–64	1	1.0	0	1	1	1	1	1	1	1
65+	0									
B. *Operated*										
0–19 Years	3	1.7	<1	1	1	1	2	2	2	2
20–34	14	1.9	2	1	1	1	2	2	6	6
35–49	12	1.6	<1	1	1	1	2	3	5	5
50–64	9	1.5	<1	1	1	1	2	3	3	3
65+	12	1.7	1	1	1	1	2	3	4	4
2. MULTIPLE DX										
A. *Not Operated*										
0–19 Years	1	1.0	0	1	1	1	1	1	1	1
20–34	21	1.9	1	1	1	2	2	4	4	4
35–49	19	2.8	5	1	1	2	4	7	8	8
50–64	27	2.6	5	1	1	2	4	5	7	10
65+	53	2.6	5	1	1	2	3	5	8	12
B. *Operated*										
0–19 Years	14	3.2	2	2	2	3	3	5	6	6
20–34	54	2.4	5	1	1	2	3	5	6	15
35–49	56	2.7	5	1	1	2	4	5	7	13
50–64	86	3.2	14	1	1	2	4	7	10	28
65+	157	3.0	10	1	1	2	4	6	8	18
SUBTOTALS:										
1. SINGLE DX										
A. *Not Operated*	5	1.6	2	1	1	1	1	4	4	4
B. *Operated*	50	1.7	1	1	1	1	2	3	4	6
2. MULTIPLE DX										
A. *Not Operated*	121	2.5	4	1	1	2	3	5	7	10
B. *Operated*	367	2.9	9	1	1	2	4	6	7	17
1. SINGLE DX	55	1.7	1	1	1	1	2	3	4	6
2. MULTIPLE DX	488	2.8	8	1	1	2	4	6	7	15
A. NOT OPERATED	126	2.4	4	1	1	2	3	5	7	10
B. OPERATED	417	2.8	8	1	1	2	3	5	7	15
TOTAL										
0–19 Years	18	2.8	2	1	2	2	4	5	6	6
20–34	90	2.2	4	1	1	2	3	4	5	15
35–49	90	2.5	4	1	1	2	3	5	7	13
50–64	123	3.0	11	1	1	2	4	6	9	12
65+	222	2.8	8	1	1	2	4	6	8	17
GRAND TOTAL	543	2.7	7	1	1	2	3	5	7	13

Length of Stay by Diagnosis and Operation, Western Region, 2008

Western Region, October 2006–September 2007 Data, by Diagnosis

599: OTH URINARY TRACT DISORD

Type of Patients	Observed Patients	Avg. Stay	Variance	10th	25th	50th	75th	90th	95th	99th
1. SINGLE DX										
A. Not Operated										
0–19 Years	303	2.4	2	1	1	2	3	4	5	7
20–34	44	1.9	2	1	1	1	2	4	4	7
35–49	20	2.1	2	1	1	2	2	4	6	6
50–64	23	1.8	<1	1	1	1	2	3	3	3
65+	21	2.4	8	1	1	1	3	3	9	12
B. Operated										
0–19 Years	0									
20–34	1	1.0	0	1	1	1	1	1	1	1
35–49	2	1.0	0	1	1	1	1	1	1	
50–64	0									
65+	6	1.8	<1	1	1	2	3	3	3	3
2. MULTIPLE DX										
A. Not Operated										
0–19 Years	2,610	3.4	7	1	2	3	4	6	7	12
20–34	1,489	3.3	10	1	2	3	4	6	8	17
35–49	2,821	3.8	15	1	2	3	5	7	9	18
50–64	6,346	4.0	14	1	2	3	5	7	10	18
65+	36,435	4.0	10	1	2	3	5	7	9	16
B. Operated										
0–19 Years	22	6.0	28	2	2	5	7	13	18	21
20–34	63	7.7	75	1	2	4	10	19	26	45
35–49	216	5.5	70	1	2	4	6	15	20	32
50–64	416	4.7	38	1	1	2	6	11	15	25
65+	1,106	6.9	48	2	2	5	9	15	21	32
SUBTOTALS:										
1. SINGLE DX										
A. Not Operated	411	2.3	2	1	1	2	3	4	5	7
B. Operated	9	1.6	<1	1	1	1	2	3	3	3
2. MULTIPLE DX										
A. Not Operated	49,701	4.0	11	1	2	3	5	7	9	16
B. Operated	1,823	6.3	50	1	2	4	8	14	19	32
1. SINGLE DX	420	2.3	2	1	2	2	3	4	5	7
2. MULTIPLE DX	51,524	4.0	12	1	2	3	5	7	10	17
A. NOT OPERATED	50,112	4.0	11	1	2	3	5	7	9	16
B. OPERATED	1,832	6.2	50	1	2	4	8	14	19	32
TOTAL										
0–19 Years	2,935	3.3	6	1	2	3	4	6	7	12
20–34	1,597	3.4	13	1	2	3	4	6	9	19
35–49	3,059	3.9	19	1	2	3	5	7	10	20
50–64	6,785	4.0	15	1	2	3	5	8	10	19
65+	37,568	4.1	11	1	2	3	5	7	10	17
GRAND TOTAL	51,944	4.0	12	1	2	3	5	7	10	17

599.0: URINARY TRACT INF NOS

Type of Patients	Observed Patients	Avg. Stay	Variance	10th	25th	50th	75th	90th	95th	99th
1. SINGLE DX										
A. Not Operated										
0–19 Years	291	2.4	2	1	1	2	3	4	5	7
20–34	40	1.7	<1	1	1	1	2	4	4	4
35–49	15	1.9	<1	1	1	2	2	3	4	4
50–64	14	1.8	<1	1	1	2	2	3	3	3
65+	13	3.2	12	1	2	2	3	9	12	12
B. Operated										
0–19 Years	0									
20–34	0									
35–49	0									
50–64	0									
65+	1	3.0	0	3	3	3	3	3	3	3
2. MULTIPLE DX										
A. Not Operated										
0–19 Years	2,562	3.4	7	1	2	3	4	6	8	12
20–34	1,425	3.3	10	1	2	3	4	6	8	17
35–49	2,681	3.9	16	1	2	3	5	7	9	18
50–64	5,973	4.1	14	1	2	3	5	7	10	18
65+	34,824	4.1	10	1	2	3	5	7	9	16
B. Operated										
0–19 Years	16	7.2	33	2	2	6	9	18	21	21
20–34	33	11.2	98	3	4	9	14	26	32	45
35–49	73	10.9	133	3	5	7	13	22	31	67
50–64	127	9.5	71	3	5	8	12	17	20	49
65+	518	10.1	58	3	5	8	13	20	27	35
SUBTOTALS:										
1. SINGLE DX										
A. Not Operated	373	2.3	2	1	1	2	3	4	5	7
B. Operated	1	3.0	0	3	3	3	3	3	3	3
2. MULTIPLE DX										
A. Not Operated	47,465	4.0	11	1	2	3	5	7	9	16
B. Operated	767	10.1	69	3	5	8	12	20	27	46
1. SINGLE DX	374	2.3	2	1	1	2	3	4	5	7
2. MULTIPLE DX	48,232	4.1	12	1	2	3	5	7	10	17
A. NOT OPERATED	47,838	4.0	11	1	2	3	5	7	9	16
B. OPERATED	768	10.1	69	3	5	8	12	20	27	46
TOTAL										
0–19 Years	2,869	3.3	6	1	2	3	4	6	7	12
20–34	1,498	3.4	13	1	2	3	4	6	9	19
35–49	2,769	4.1	20	1	2	3	5	7	10	21
50–64	6,114	4.2	16	1	2	3	5	8	11	19
65+	35,356	4.2	11	1	2	3	5	7	10	17
GRAND TOTAL	48,606	4.1	12	1	2	3	5	7	10	17

599.7: HEMATURIA

Type of Patients	Observed Patients	Avg. Stay	Variance	10th	25th	50th	75th	90th	95th	99th
1. SINGLE DX										
A. Not Operated										
0–19 Years	10	1.7	<1	1	1	2	2	2	3	3
20–34	2	6.5	<1	6	6	6	6	7	7	7
35–49	4	3.0	4	2	2	2	6	6	6	6
50–64	8	1.8	<1	1	1	1	2	2	3	3
65+	7	1.3	<1	1	1	1	1	2	2	2
B. Operated										
0–19 Years	0									
20–34	0									
35–49	1	1.0	0	1	1	1	1	1	1	1
50–64	0									
65+	2	1.5	<1	1	1	2	2	2	2	2
2. MULTIPLE DX										
A. Not Operated										
0–19 Years	40	2.0	1	1	1	2	2	3	4	5
20–34	48	2.9	7	1	1	2	3	7	9	15
35–49	111	3.2	8	1	1	2	4	6	8	14
50–64	293	3.0	18	1	2	2	3	5	7	13
65+	1,364	3.1	7	1	2	2	4	6	8	13
B. Operated										
0–19 Years	2	2.5	<1	2	2	2	3	3	3	3
20–34	4	3.3	2	3	3	4	4	7	4	4
35–49	8	5.6	21	1	3	4	10	15	15	15
50–64	59	5.2	20	1	2	4	7	8	11	24
65+	310	5.2	22	1	2	4	7	10	13	20
SUBTOTALS:										
1. SINGLE DX										
A. Not Operated	31	2.1	2	1	1	2	2	3	6	7
B. Operated	3	1.3	<1	1	1	2	2	2	2	2
2. MULTIPLE DX										
A. Not Operated	1,856	3.1	9	1	2	2	4	6	8	13
B. Operated	383	5.2	21	1	2	4	7	10	14	24
1. SINGLE DX	34	2.0	2	1	1	2	2	3	6	7
2. MULTIPLE DX	2,239	3.4	11	1	2	3	4	7	9	15
A. NOT OPERATED	1,887	3.1	8	1	1	2	4	6	8	13
B. OPERATED	386	5.1	21	1	2	4	7	10	14	24
TOTAL										
0–19 Years	52	1.9	<1	1	1	2	2	3	4	5
20–34	54	3.1	7	1	1	2	4	7	9	15
35–49	124	3.3	9	1	1	2	4	6	9	15
50–64	360	3.3	19	1	1	2	4	6	10	15
65+	1,683	3.5	10	1	2	3	4	7	9	16
GRAND TOTAL	2,273	3.4	11	1	2	3	4	7	9	15

Length of Stay by Diagnosis and Operation, Western Region, 2008

Western Region, October 2006–September 2007 Data, by Diagnosis

600: HYPERPLASIA OF PROSTATE

Type of Patients	Observed Patients	Avg. Stay	Variance	10th	25th	50th	75th	90th	95th	99th
1. SINGLE DX										
A. Not Operated										
0–19 Years	0									
20–34	0									
35–49	0									
50–64	0									
65+	5	1.8	2	1	1	1	2	4	4	4
B. Operated										
0–19 Years	0									
20–34	0									
35–49	10	1.1	<1	1	1	1	1	1	2	2
50–64	124	1.3	<1	1	1	1	2	2	2	3
65+	242	1.6	<1	1	1	1	2	3	3	5
2. MULTIPLE DX										
A. Not Operated										
0–19 Years	0									
20–34	1	1.0	0	1	1	1	1	1	1	1
35–49	23	3.1	4	1	1	3	4	7	7	7
50–64	187	2.8	5	1	1	2	4	5	7	12
65+	923	3.3	10	1	1	2	4	6	8	15
B. Operated										
0–19 Years	0									
20–34	2	1.5	<1	1	1	2	2	2	2	2
35–49	97	1.6	1	1	1	1	2	3	4	7
50–64	2,241	1.9	3	1	1	1	2	3	5	9
65+	8,497	2.3	6	1	1	2	2	4	6	12
SUBTOTALS:										
1. SINGLE DX — A. Not Operated	5	1.8	2	1	1	1	2	4	4	4
1. SINGLE DX — B. Operated	376	1.5	<1	1	1	1	2	3	3	5
2. MULTIPLE DX — A. Not Operated	1,134	3.2	9	1	1	2	4	6	8	15
2. MULTIPLE DX — B. Operated	10,837	2.2	5	1	1	2	2	4	6	11
1. SINGLE DX	381	1.5	<1	1	1	1	2	3	3	5
2. MULTIPLE DX	11,971	2.3	6	1	1	2	2	4	6	12
A. NOT OPERATED	1,139	3.2	9	1	1	2	4	6	8	15
B. OPERATED	11,213	2.1	5	1	1	2	2	4	6	11
TOTAL										
0–19 Years	0									
20–34	3	1.3	<1	1	1	1	2	2	2	2
35–49	130	1.9	2	1	1	1	2	4	5	7
50–64	2,552	1.9	3	1	1	1	2	3	5	9
65+	9,667	2.3	6	1	1	2	3	4	6	12
GRAND TOTAL	12,352	2.2	5	1	1	2	2	4	6	11

600.00: PROS HYPERTR S OBST/LUTS

Type of Patients	Observed Patients	Avg. Stay	Variance	10th	25th	50th	75th	90th	95th	99th
1. SINGLE DX										
A. Not Operated										
0–19 Years	0									
20–34	0									
35–49	0									
50–64	0									
65+	2	2.5	4	1	1	1	4	4	4	4
B. Operated										
0–19 Years	0									
20–34	0									
35–49	0									
50–64	28	1.3	<1	1	1	1	2	2	3	3
65+	44	1.6	<1	1	1	1	2	3	3	5
2. MULTIPLE DX										
A. Not Operated										
0–19 Years	0									
20–34	0									
35–49	4	2.3	4	1	1	2	2	5	5	5
50–64	14	2.0	<1	1	1	2	3	3	4	4
65+	103	3.1	15	1	1	2	4	6	7	11
B. Operated										
0–19 Years	0									
20–34	0									
35–49	9	1.6	<1	1	1	1	2	3	3	3
50–64	251	1.7	1	1	1	1	2	3	3	8
65+	868	2.2	5	1	1	2	2	4	6	10
SUBTOTALS:										
1. SINGLE DX — A. Not Operated	2	2.5	4	1	1	1	4	4	4	4
1. SINGLE DX — B. Operated	72	1.5	<1	1	1	1	2	3	3	5
2. MULTIPLE DX — A. Not Operated	121	3.0	13	1	1	2	4	6	7	11
2. MULTIPLE DX — B. Operated	1,128	2.1	4	1	1	2	2	4	5	9
1. SINGLE DX	74	1.5	<1	1	1	1	2	3	3	5
2. MULTIPLE DX	1,249	2.2	5	1	1	2	2	4	5	9
A. NOT OPERATED	123	3.0	13	1	1	2	4	6	7	11
B. OPERATED	1,200	2.0	4	1	1	2	2	4	5	9
TOTAL										
0–19 Years	0									
20–34	0									
35–49	13	1.8	1	1	1	1	2	3	5	5
50–64	293	1.7	1	1	1	1	2	3	3	8
65+	1,017	2.3	6	1	1	2	3	4	6	10
GRAND TOTAL	1,323	2.1	5	1	1	1	2	4	5	9

600.01: PROS HYPERTR W OBST/LUTS

Type of Patients	Observed Patients	Avg. Stay	Variance	10th	25th	50th	75th	90th	95th	99th
1. SINGLE DX										
A. Not Operated										
0–19 Years	0									
20–34	0									
35–49	0									
50–64	0									
65+	2	1.5	<1	1	1	1	2	2	2	2
B. Operated										
0–19 Years	0									
20–34	0									
35–49	6	1.0	0	1	1	1	1	1	1	1
50–64	85	1.3	<1	1	1	1	2	2	2	4
65+	170	1.6	<1	1	1	1	2	3	3	6
2. MULTIPLE DX										
A. Not Operated										
0–19 Years	0									
20–34	1	1.0	0	1	1	1	1	1	1	1
35–49	16	3.5	5	1	2	3	6	7	7	7
50–64	154	2.9	5	1	1	2	4	6	8	12
65+	755	3.3	10	1	1	2	4	6	8	16
B. Operated										
0–19 Years	0									
20–34	2	1.5	<1	1	1	2	2	2	2	2
35–49	75	1.6	1	1	1	1	2	3	4	6
50–64	1,774	1.9	3	1	1	1	2	3	5	9
65+	6,770	2.3	6	1	1	2	2	4	6	12
SUBTOTALS:										
1. SINGLE DX — A. Not Operated	2	1.5	<1	1	1	1	2	2	2	2
1. SINGLE DX — B. Operated	261	1.5	<1	1	1	1	2	2	3	5
2. MULTIPLE DX — A. Not Operated	926	3.2	9	1	1	2	4	6	8	15
2. MULTIPLE DX — B. Operated	8,621	2.2	5	1	1	2	2	4	6	12
1. SINGLE DX	263	1.5	<1	1	1	1	2	2	3	5
2. MULTIPLE DX	9,547	2.3	6	1	1	2	2	4	6	12
A. NOT OPERATED	928	3.2	9	1	1	2	4	6	8	15
B. OPERATED	8,882	2.2	5	1	1	2	2	4	6	12
TOTAL										
0–19 Years	0									
20–34	2	1.3	<1	1	1	1	2	2	2	2
35–49	97	1.9	2	1	1	1	2	4	6	7
50–64	2,013	2.0	3	1	1	2	3	4	5	9
65+	7,697	2.4	6	1	1	2	3	5	6	13
GRAND TOTAL	9,810	2.3	6	1	1	2	2	4	6	12

Length of Stay by Diagnosis and Operation, Western Region, 2008

Western Region, October 2006–September 2007 Data, by Diagnosis

600.21: BEN PROS HYPERPL W LUTS

Type of Patients	Observed Patients	Avg. Stay	Variance	10th	25th	50th	75th	90th	95th	99th
1. SINGLE DX										
A. Not Operated										
0–19 Years	0									
20–34	0									
35–49	0									
50–64	0									
65+	0									
B. Operated										
0–19 Years	0									
20–34	0									
35–49	0									
50–64	2	1.0	0	1	1	1	1	1	1	1
65+	5	2.0	2	1	1	2	2	4	4	4
2. MULTIPLE DX										
A. Not Operated										
0–19 Years	0									
20–34	0									
35–49	1	2.0	0	2	2	2	2	2	2	2
50–64	0									
65+	7	3.0	3	1	1	3	5	5	5	5
B. Operated										
0–19 Years	0									
20–34	0									
35–49	5	2.8	6	1	1	2	3	7	7	7
50–64	49	1.9	2	1	1	2	2	3	3	3
65+	241	2.4	4	1	1	2	3	5	6	11
SUBTOTALS:										
1. SINGLE DX — A. Not Operated	0									
1. SINGLE DX — B. Operated	7	1.7	1	1	1	1	2	4	4	4
2. MULTIPLE DX — A. Not Operated	8	2.9	3	1	2	3	5	5	5	5
2. MULTIPLE DX — B. Operated	295	2.3	4	1	1	2	3	5	6	11
1. SINGLE DX	7	1.7	1	1	1	1	2	4	4	4
2. MULTIPLE DX	303	2.3	3	1	1	2	3	5	6	11
A. NOT OPERATED	8	2.9	3	1	2	3	5	5	5	5
B. OPERATED	302	2.3	3	1	1	2	3	5	6	11
TOTAL										
0–19 Years	0									
20–34	0									
35–49	6	2.7	5	1	1	2	3	7	7	7
50–64	51	1.9	2	1	1	2	2	3	6	7
65+	253	2.4	4	1	1	2	3	5	6	11
GRAND TOTAL	310	2.3	3	1	1	2	3	5	6	11

600.91: PROS HYPERPL W OBST/LUTS

Type of Patients	Observed Patients	Avg. Stay	Variance	10th	25th	50th	75th	90th	95th	99th
1. SINGLE DX										
A. Not Operated										
0–19 Years	0									
20–34	0									
35–49	0									
50–64	0									
65+	0									
B. Operated										
0–19 Years	0									
20–34	0									
35–49	2	1.0	0	1	1	1	1	1	1	1
50–64	4	1.3	<1	1	1	1	2	2	2	2
65+	7	1.7	1	1	1	1	2	4	4	4
2. MULTIPLE DX										
A. Not Operated										
0–19 Years	0									
20–34	0									
35–49	2	3.0	2	2	2	3	4	4	4	4
50–64	15	2.7	13	1	1	2	3	4	15	15
65+	49	3.4	7	1	1	3	4	7	8	14
B. Operated										
0–19 Years	0									
20–34	0									
35–49	3	1.7	<1	1	1	1	2	2	2	2
50–64	101	1.8	3	1	1	1	2	3	4	10
65+	360	2.0	3	1	1	2	2	3	5	10
SUBTOTALS:										
1. SINGLE DX — A. Not Operated	0									
1. SINGLE DX — B. Operated	13	1.5	<1	1	1	1	2	2	4	4
2. MULTIPLE DX — A. Not Operated	66	3.2	8	1	1	3	4	6	8	15
2. MULTIPLE DX — B. Operated	464	2.0	3	1	1	2	2	3	5	10
1. SINGLE DX	13	1.5	<1	1	1	1	2	2	4	4
2. MULTIPLE DX	530	2.1	4	1	1	2	2	4	6	11
A. NOT OPERATED	66	3.2	8	1	1	3	4	6	8	15
B. OPERATED	477	2.0	3	1	1	2	2	3	5	10
TOTAL										
0–19 Years	0									
20–34	0									
35–49	7	1.9	1	1	1	2	2	3	4	4
50–64	120	1.9	4	1	1	1	2	3	4	15
65+	416	2.2	3	1	1	2	2	4	6	10
GRAND TOTAL	543	2.1	4	1	1	2	2	4	6	11

601: PROSTATIC INFLAMMATION

Type of Patients	Observed Patients	Avg. Stay	Variance	10th	25th	50th	75th	90th	95th	99th
1. SINGLE DX										
A. Not Operated										
0–19 Years	0									
20–34	0									
35–49	3	2.4	2	1	1	2	4	4	4	4
50–64	4	1.5	<1	1	1	1	3	3	3	3
65+	3	1.3	<1	1	1	1	2	2	2	2
B. Operated										
0–19 Years	0									
20–34	0									
35–49	0									
50–64	0									
65+	0									
2. MULTIPLE DX										
A. Not Operated										
0–19 Years	5	2.8	4	1	2	2	3	6	6	6
20–34	24	2.6	2	1	1	2	3	5	5	6
35–49	90	2.9	5	1	2	3	3	5	6	14
50–64	222	3.1	5	1	2	3	4	6	7	12
65+	271	3.5	7	1	2	3	4	6	8	17
B. Operated										
0–19 Years	0									
20–34	6	6.3	35	2	3	4	6	18	18	18
35–49	11	7.2	66	2	2	3	13	14	28	28
50–64	44	5.6	49	1	1	3	7	18	20	34
65+	49	2.7	4	1	1	2	4	5	8	10
SUBTOTALS:										
1. SINGLE DX — A. Not Operated	10	1.7	1	1	1	1	2	4	4	4
1. SINGLE DX — B. Operated	0									
2. MULTIPLE DX — A. Not Operated	612	3.2	6	1	2	3	4	6	7	13
2. MULTIPLE DX — B. Operated	110	4.5	32	1	2	3	5	10	18	28
1. SINGLE DX	10	1.7	1	1	1	1	2	4	4	4
2. MULTIPLE DX	722	3.4	10	1	2	3	4	6	9	18
A. NOT OPERATED	622	3.2	6	1	2	3	4	6	7	13
B. OPERATED	110	4.5	32	1	2	3	5	10	18	28
TOTAL										
0–19 Years	5	2.8	4	1	2	2	3	6	6	6
20–34	30	3.4	10	1	2	3	4	6	6	18
35–49	104	3.4	12	1	2	3	4	6	7	14
50–64	270	3.5	13	1	2	3	4	6	9	20
65+	323	3.3	7	1	2	3	4	6	8	12
GRAND TOTAL	732	3.4	10	1	2	3	4	6	9	18

Length of Stay by Diagnosis and Operation, Western Region, 2008

Western Region, October 2006–September 2007 Data, by Diagnosis

601.0: ACUTE PROSTATITIS

Type of Patients	Observed Patients	Avg. Stay	Vari-ance	10th	25th	50th	75th	90th	95th	99th
1. SINGLE DX										
A. Not Operated										
0–19 Years	0									
20–34	0									
35–49	1	2.0	0	2	2	2	2	2	2	2
50–64	2	2.0	2	1	1	2	3	3	3	3
65+	2	1.5	<1	1	1	2	2	2	2	2
B. Operated										
0–19 Years	0									
20–34	0									
35–49	0									
50–64	0									
65+	0									
2. MULTIPLE DX										
A. Not Operated										
0–19 Years	2	2.5	<1	2	2	3	3	3	3	3
20–34	10	3.0	3	1	2	2	5	6	6	6
35–49	50	2.9	4	1	2	3	3	5	6	14
50–64	136	3.3	5	1	2	3	4	6	8	12
65+	150	3.7	10	1	2	3	4	6	9	18
B. Operated										
0–19 Years	0									
20–34	1	18.0	0	18	18	18	18	18	18	18
35–49	2	4.5	4	3	3	6	6	6	6	6
50–64	10	1.9	4	1	1	1	1	7	7	7
65+	19	2.8	4	1	1	2	4	5	8	8
SUBTOTALS:										
1. SINGLE DX										
A. Not Operated	5	1.8	<1	1	1	2	2	3	3	3
B. Operated	0									
2. MULTIPLE DX										
A. Not Operated	348	3.4	7	1	2	3	4	6	8	14
B. Operated	32	3.1	11	1	1	2	4	6	8	18
1. SINGLE DX	5	1.8	<1	1	2	2	2	3	3	3
2. MULTIPLE DX	380	3.4	7	1	2	3	4	6	8	17
A. NOT OPERATED	353	3.4	7	1	2	3	4	6	8	14
B. OPERATED	32	3.1	11	1	1	2	4	6	8	18
TOTAL										
0–19 Years	2	2.5	<1	2	2	3	3	3	3	3
20–34	11	4.4	23	1	2	3	5	6	18	18
35–49	53	3.0	4	1	2	3	3	5	6	14
50–64	148	3.2	5	1	2	3	4	6	8	12
65+	171	3.6	9	1	2	3	4	6	9	18
GRAND TOTAL	385	3.4	7	1	2	3	4	6	8	17

601.9: PROSTATITIS NOS

Type of Patients	Observed Patients	Avg. Stay	Vari-ance	10th	25th	50th	75th	90th	95th	99th
1. SINGLE DX										
A. Not Operated										
0–19 Years	0									
20–34	0									
35–49	0									
50–64	2	1.0	0	1	1	1	1	1	1	1
65+	0									
B. Operated										
0–19 Years	0									
20–34	0									
35–49	0									
50–64	0									
65+	0									
2. MULTIPLE DX										
A. Not Operated										
0–19 Years	2	1.5	<1	1	1	1	2	2	2	2
20–34	9	2.0	<1	1	1	2	3	3	3	3
35–49	28	2.5	2	1	1	2	3	4	6	6
50–64	62	2.5	3	1	1	2	3	4	6	9
65+	87	3.0	3	1	2	3	4	5	6	9
B. Operated										
0–19 Years	0									
20–34	1	6.0	0	6	6	6	6	6	6	6
35–49	1	13.0	0	13	13	13	13	13	13	13
50–64	4	2.5	4	1	1	2	4	5	5	5
65+	4	2.2	2	1	1	3	3	4	4	4
SUBTOTALS:										
1. SINGLE DX										
A. Not Operated	2	1.0	0	1	1	1	1	1	1	1
B. Operated	0									
2. MULTIPLE DX										
A. Not Operated	188	2.7	3	1	1	2	3	5	6	9
B. Operated	10	3.8	14	1	1	3	5	13	13	13
1. SINGLE DX	2	1.0	0	1	1	1	1	1	1	1
2. MULTIPLE DX	198	2.7	3	1	1	2	3	5	6	9
A. NOT OPERATED	190	2.7	3	1	1	2	3	5	6	9
B. OPERATED	10	3.8	14	1	1	3	5	13	13	13
TOTAL										
0–19 Years	2	1.5	<1	1	1	1	2	2	2	2
20–34	10	2.4	2	1	1	2	3	6	6	6
35–49	29	2.8	6	1	1	2	3	5	6	13
50–64	68	2.4	3	1	1	2	3	5	6	9
65+	91	3.0	3	1	2	3	4	5	6	9
GRAND TOTAL	200	2.7	3	1	1	2	3	5	6	9

602: OTH PROSTATIC DISORDERS

Type of Patients	Observed Patients	Avg. Stay	Vari-ance	10th	25th	50th	75th	90th	95th	99th
1. SINGLE DX										
A. Not Operated										
0–19 Years	0									
20–34	0									
35–49	0									
50–64	0									
65+	0									
B. Operated										
0–19 Years	0									
20–34	0									
35–49	0									
50–64	0									
65+	0									
2. MULTIPLE DX										
A. Not Operated										
0–19 Years	0									
20–34	0									
35–49	2	1.5	<1	1	1	2	2	2	2	2
50–64	9	2.3	1	1	1	3	3	4	4	4
65+	34	3.7	8	1	2	3	5	9	10	10
B. Operated										
0–19 Years	0									
20–34	0									
35–49	1	11.0	0	11	11	11	11	11	11	11
50–64	16	3.4	14	1	2	2	3	5	17	17
65+	122	3.8	19	1	1	2	4	8	14	21
SUBTOTALS:										
1. SINGLE DX										
A. Not Operated	0									
B. Operated	0									
2. MULTIPLE DX										
A. Not Operated	45	3.4	7	1	1	3	4	8	9	10
B. Operated	139	3.8	18	1	1	2	4	8	16	21
1. SINGLE DX	0									
2. MULTIPLE DX	184	3.7	16	1	1	2	4	8	11	21
A. NOT OPERATED	45	3.4	7	1	1	3	4	8	9	10
B. OPERATED	139	3.8	18	1	1	2	4	8	16	21
TOTAL										
0–19 Years	0									
20–34	0									
35–49	3	4.7	30	1	1	2	11	11	11	11
50–64	25	3.0	10	1	2	2	3	4	5	17
65+	156	3.8	16	1	1	2	4	8	11	21
GRAND TOTAL	184	3.7	16	1	1	2	4	8	11	21

Length of Stay by Diagnosis and Operation, Western Region, 2008

Western Region, October 2006–September 2007 Data, by Diagnosis

603: HYDROCELE

Type of Patients	Observed Patients	Avg. Stay	Variance	Percentiles 10th	25th	50th	75th	90th	95th	99th
1. SINGLE DX										
A. Not Operated										
0–19 Years	3	1.0	0	1	1	1	1	1	1	1
20–34	0									
35–49	0									
50–64	2	1.5	<1	1	1	1	2	2	2	2
65+	0									
B. Operated										
0–19 Years	3	1.0	0	1	1	1	1	1	1	1
20–34	3	1.0	0	1	1	1	1	1	1	1
35–49	5	1.6	<1	1	1	1	2	3	3	3
50–64	3	2.0	<1	1	1	2	3	3	3	3
65+	0									
2. MULTIPLE DX										
A. Not Operated										
0–19 Years	4	2.7	4	1	1	1	4	5	5	5
20–34	9	2.1	3	1	1	1	2	6	6	6
35–49	9	3.4	3	1	2	4	4	6	6	6
50–64	19	1.8	2	1	1	1	2	3	7	7
65+	17	3.3	6	1	2	3	4	7	10	10
B. Operated										
0–19 Years	9	1.4	1	1	1	1	1	4	4	4
20–34	8	1.6	1	1	1	1	2	4	4	4
35–49	15	2.7	5	1	1	2	3	5	9	9
50–64	32	2.7	10	1	1	1	3	6	10	15
65+	38	2.2	4	1	1	1	3	5	6	9
SUBTOTALS:										
1. SINGLE DX										
A. Not Operated	5	1.2	<1	1	1	1	1	2	2	2
B. Operated	14	1.4	<1	1	1	1	2	3	3	3
2. MULTIPLE DX										
A. Not Operated	58	2.6	4	1	1	2	4	6	7	10
B. Operated	102	2.3	5	1	1	1	3	5	6	10
1. SINGLE DX	19	1.4	<1	1	1	1	2	3	3	3
2. MULTIPLE DX	160	2.4	5	1	1	1	3	5	7	10
A. NOT OPERATED	63	2.5	4	1	1	2	3	5	6	10
B. OPERATED	116	2.2	5	1	1	1	3	5	6	10
TOTAL										
0–19 Years	19	1.6	2	1	1	1	1	4	5	5
20–34	20	1.8	2	1	1	1	2	4	6	6
35–49	29	2.7	4	1	1	2	4	5	6	9
50–64	56	2.3	6	1	1	1	2	5	7	15
65+	55	2.5	4	1	1	2	3	5	7	10
GRAND TOTAL	179	2.3	4	1	1	1	3	5	6	10

604: ORCHITIS & EPIDIDYMITIS

Type of Patients	Observed Patients	Avg. Stay	Variance	Percentiles 10th	25th	50th	75th	90th	95th	99th
1. SINGLE DX										
A. Not Operated										
0–19 Years	20	2.3	3	1	2	2	3	3	7	7
20–34	25	2.4	2	1	2	2	3	4	4	7
35–49	26	2.4	3	1	1	2	3	5	5	9
50–64	11	2.0	1	1	1	2	3	3	4	4
65+	2	2.0	0	2	2	2	2	2	2	2
B. Operated										
0–19 Years	2	2.5	4	1	1	1	4	4	4	4
20–34	9	2.7	3	1	1	3	4	6	6	6
35–49	6	3.3	13	1	1	2	5	10	10	10
50–64	1	2.0	0	2	2	2	2	2	2	2
65+	0									
2. MULTIPLE DX										
A. Not Operated										
0–19 Years	34	2.9	11	1	1	2	3	5	7	20
20–34	132	3.0	5	1	2	3	4	6	6	15
35–49	283	3.4	6	1	2	3	4	7	8	12
50–64	267	3.6	14	1	2	3	4	6	8	15
65+	269	4.1	6	2	2	4	5	7	9	14
B. Operated										
0–19 Years	5	2.6	4	1	1	2	2	4	6	6
20–34	13	4.3	16	1	2	3	5	12	13	13
35–49	35	5.0	10	2	2	4	7	11	11	12
50–64	27	6.2	17	1	3	5	10	13	14	15
65+	39	6.6	60	1	2	4	6	16	31	37
SUBTOTALS:										
1. SINGLE DX										
A. Not Operated	84	2.3	2	1	1	2	3	4	5	9
B. Operated	18	2.8	6	1	1	2	4	6	10	10
2. MULTIPLE DX										
A. Not Operated	985	3.6	8	1	2	3	4	6	8	14
B. Operated	119	5.6	29	1	2	4	6	12	14	31
1. SINGLE DX	102	2.4	3	1	1	2	3	4	5	9
2. MULTIPLE DX	1,104	3.8	11	1	2	3	5	7	9	15
A. NOT OPERATED	1,069	3.5	8	1	2	3	4	6	8	14
B. OPERATED	137	5.3	27	1	2	4	6	11	13	31
TOTAL										
0–19 Years	61	2.7	7	1	1	2	3	4	6	20
20–34	179	3.0	6	1	2	3	3	6	6	15
35–49	350	3.5	6	1	2	3	4	7	9	12
50–64	306	3.8	14	1	2	3	4	7	10	15
65+	310	4.4	14	2	2	4	5	7	10	18
GRAND TOTAL	1,206	3.7	10	1	2	3	4	7	9	15

604.0: ORCHITIS W ABSCESS

Type of Patients	Observed Patients	Avg. Stay	Variance	Percentiles 10th	25th	50th	75th	90th	95th	99th
1. SINGLE DX										
A. Not Operated										
0–19 Years	1	3.0	0	3	3	3	3	3	3	3
20–34	3	2.0	1	1	1	2	3	3	3	3
35–49	1	9.0	0	9	9	9	9	9	9	9
50–64	1	3.0	0	3	3	3	3	3	3	3
65+	0									
B. Operated										
0–19 Years	0									
20–34	7	3.2	3	1	1	3	5	6	6	6
35–49	5	3.8	15	1	1	2	5	10	10	10
50–64	1	2.0	0	2	2	2	2	2	2	2
65+	0									
2. MULTIPLE DX										
A. Not Operated										
0–19 Years	4	3.3	4	2	2	2	3	6	6	6
20–34	17	3.5	5	2	2	3	4	6	8	10
35–49	41	4.7	11	2	3	4	6	8	9	18
50–64	33	5.1	14	1	2	4	7	10	15	16
65+	32	5.2	7	2	3	5	6	8	11	12
B. Operated										
0–19 Years	1	2.0	0	2	2	2	2	2	2	2
20–34	4	6.5	15	2	5	5	6	12	12	12
35–49	24	5.0	10	2	2	4	7	7	11	12
50–64	17	6.4	23	1	3	5	10	14	15	15
65+	22	7.1	63	2	3	5	8	11	20	37
SUBTOTALS:										
1. SINGLE DX										
A. Not Operated	6	3.5	8	1	2	3	3	9	9	9
B. Operated	13	3.3	7	1	1	3	5	6	10	10
2. MULTIPLE DX										
A. Not Operated	127	4.7	10	2	2	4	6	8	11	16
B. Operated	68	6.1	30	2	3	5	7	12	14	37
1. SINGLE DX	19	3.4	7	1	1	3	5	9	10	10
2. MULTIPLE DX	195	5.2	17	2	3	5	6	10	12	20
A. NOT OPERATED	133	4.7	10	2	2	4	6	8	11	16
B. OPERATED	81	5.6	27	1	2	5	6	11	13	37
TOTAL										
0–19 Years	6	3.0	2	2	2	3	3	6	6	6
20–34	31	3.7	6	1	2	3	5	6	10	12
35–49	71	4.8	10	2	2	4	4	9	11	18
50–64	52	5.4	17	1	2	4	4	13	15	16
65+	54	6.0	30	2	3	5	5	11	12	37
GRAND TOTAL	214	5.0	16	1	2	4	4	10	12	18

Length of Stay by Diagnosis and Operation, Western Region, 2008

478

Western Region, October 2006–September 2007 Data, by Diagnosis

604.90: ORCHITIS/EPIDIDYMIT NOS

Type of Patients	Observed Patients	Avg. Stay	Variance	10th	25th	50th	75th	90th	95th	99th
1. SINGLE DX										
A. Not Operated										
0–19 Years	15	2.2	3	1	1	1	3	5	7	7
20–34	18	2.6	2	1	1	2	3	4	7	7
35–49	18	2.2	1	1	1	2	3	5	5	5
50–64	4	2.2	2	1	1	2	2	4	4	4
65+	1	2.0	0	2	2	2	2	2	2	2
B. Operated										
0–19 Years	1	1.0	0	1	1	1	1	1	1	1
20–34	1	1.0	0	1	1	1	1	1	1	1
35–49	1	1.0	0	1	1	1	1	1	1	1
50–64	0									
65+	0									
2. MULTIPLE DX										
A. Not Operated										
0–19 Years	17	2.4	3	1	1	2	3	4	7	7
20–34	73	2.8	4	1	2	2	3	5	6	15
35–49	163	3.1	4	1	2	3	4	5	7	10
50–64	158	3.3	17	1	2	3	4	6	7	9
65+	146	4.0	6	2	2	4	5	6	9	17
B. Operated										
0–19 Years	3	3.4	6	1	1	3	6	6	6	6
20–34	8	3.6	16	1	1	2	5	13	13	13
35–49	6	5.7	16	2	2	6	10	11	11	11
50–64	7	5.6	12	1	3	5	10	10	10	10
65+	13	6.0	73	1	1	3	6	16	31	31
SUBTOTALS:										
1. SINGLE DX										
A. Not Operated	56	2.3	2	1	1	2	3	4	5	7
B. Operated	3	1.0	0	1	1	1	1	1	1	1
2. MULTIPLE DX										
A. Not Operated	557	3.3	9	1	2	3	4	6	7	11
B. Operated	37	5.1	33	1	2	3	6	11	16	31
1. SINGLE DX	59	2.3	2	1	1	2	3	4	5	7
2. MULTIPLE DX	594	3.4	10	1	2	3	4	6	7	15
A. NOT OPERATED	613	3.2	8	1	2	3	4	5	7	11
B. OPERATED	40	4.8	32	1	1	3	6	11	13	31
TOTAL										
0–19 Years	36	2.4	3	1	1	2	3	5	7	7
20–34	100	2.8	5	1	2	2	3	5	6	15
35–49	188	3.1	4	1	2	3	4	5	7	11
50–64	169	3.4	17	1	2	3	4	6	7	10
65+	160	4.1	12	2	2	3	5	6	9	18
GRAND TOTAL	653	3.3	10	1	2	3	4	6	7	13

604.99: OTH ORCHITIS/EPIDIDYMIT

Type of Patients	Observed Patients	Avg. Stay	Variance	10th	25th	50th	75th	90th	95th	99th
1. SINGLE DX										
A. Not Operated										
0–19 Years	4	2.5	2	1	1	3	4	4	4	4
20–34	4	2.0	0	2	2	2	2	2	2	2
35–49	7	2.0	1	1	1	2	3	4	4	4
50–64	6	1.7	<1	1	1	2	2	3	3	3
65+	1	2.0	0	2	2	2	2	2	2	2
B. Operated										
0–19 Years	1	4.0	0	4	4	4	4	4	4	4
20–34	1	1.0	0	1	1	1	1	1	1	1
35–49	0									
50–64	0									
65+	0									
2. MULTIPLE DX										
A. Not Operated										
0–19 Years	13	3.5	25	1	2	2	3	3	20	20
20–34	42	3.2	8	1	1	3	4	6	6	17
35–49	79	3.5	5	1	2	3	4	7	8	11
50–64	76	3.6	5	1	2	3	4	6	8	14
65+	91	4.1	6	2	2	4	5	7	9	14
B. Operated										
0–19 Years	1	1.0	0	1	1	1	1	1	1	1
20–34	1	1.0	0	1	1	1	1	1	1	1
35–49	5	4.2	9	1	3	3	5	9	9	9
50–64	3	7.0	7	5	5	6	10	10	10	10
65+	4	5.5	27	1	1	4	4	13	13	13
SUBTOTALS:										
1. SINGLE DX										
A. Not Operated	22	2.0	<1	1	1	2	2	3	4	4
B. Operated	2	2.5	5	1	1	3	4	4	4	4
2. MULTIPLE DX										
A. Not Operated	301	3.6	7	1	2	3	4	7	8	14
B. Operated	14	4.7	14	1	2	4	6	10	13	13
1. SINGLE DX	24	2.0	1	1	1	2	2	4	4	4
2. MULTIPLE DX	315	3.7	7	1	2	3	4	7	9	14
A. NOT OPERATED	323	3.5	6	1	2	3	4	7	8	14
B. OPERATED	16	4.5	13	1	1	4	6	10	13	13
TOTAL										
0–19 Years	19	3.2	18	1	1	2	3	4	20	20
20–34	48	3.0	7	1	1	3	3	6	6	17
35–49	91	3.4	5	1	2	3	4	7	8	11
50–64	85	3.5	6	1	2	3	4	6	8	14
65+	96	4.1	6	2	2	4	5	7	9	14
GRAND TOTAL	339	3.6	7	1	2	3	4	7	8	14

605: REDUN PREPUCE & PHIMOSIS

Type of Patients	Observed Patients	Avg. Stay	Variance	10th	25th	50th	75th	90th	95th	99th
1. SINGLE DX										
A. Not Operated										
0–19 Years	4	1.8	2		1	1	1	4	4	4
20–34	1	1.0	0	1	1	1	1	1	1	1
35–49	0									
50–64	1	1.0	0	1	1	1	1	1	1	1
65+	0									
B. Operated										
0–19 Years	9	1.1	<1	1	1	1	1	2	2	2
20–34	1	1.0	0	1	1	1	1	1	1	1
35–49	0									
50–64	0									
65+	0									
2. MULTIPLE DX										
A. Not Operated										
0–19 Years	11	2.0	4	1	1	1	2	2	8	8
20–34	2	2.0	0	1	1	1	1	1	1	1
35–49	5	1.2	<1	1	1	1	1	2	2	2
50–64	7	1.6	<1	1	1	1	2	3	3	3
65+	9	3.6	7	1	2	3	6	8	8	8
B. Operated										
0–19 Years	13	1.3	<1	1	1	1	1	2	3	3
20–34	4	1.8	<1	1	1	1	4	4	4	4
35–49	6	3.2	3	1	2	4	4	6	6	6
50–64	6	5.5	63	1	1	1	7	21	21	21
65+	18	2.0	1	1	1	2	2	4	5	5
SUBTOTALS:										
1. SINGLE DX										
A. Not Operated	6	1.5	1	1	1	1	1	4	4	4
B. Operated	10	1.1	<1	1	1	1	1	1	2	2
2. MULTIPLE DX										
A. Not Operated	34	2.2	4	1	1	1	2	6	8	8
B. Operated	47	2.4	10	1	1	1	2	4	6	21
1. SINGLE DX	16	1.3	<1	1	1	1	1	2	4	4
2. MULTIPLE DX	81	2.3	7	1	1	1	2	4	6	21
A. NOT OPERATED	40	2.1	4	1	1	1	2	6	8	8
B. OPERATED	57	2.1	8	1	1	1	2	4	6	21
TOTAL										
0–19 Years	37	1.5	2	1	1	1	1	2	4	8
20–34	8	1.4	1	1	1	1	1	4	4	4
35–49	11	2.3	3	1	1	2	4	4	6	6
50–64	14	3.2	29	1	1	2	2	7	21	21
65+	27	2.5	6	2	2	3	3	6	6	8
GRAND TOTAL	97	2.1	6	1	1	1	2	4	6	21

Length of Stay by Diagnosis and Operation, Western Region, 2008

Western Region, October 2006–September 2007 Data, by Diagnosis

606: MALE INFERTILITY

Type of Patients	Observed Patients	Avg. Stay	Variance	Percentiles						
				10th	25th	50th	75th	90th	95th	99th
1. SINGLE DX										
A. Not Operated										
0–19 Years	0									
20–34	0									
35–49	0									
50–64	0									
65+	0									
B. Operated										
0–19 Years	0									
20–34	1	1.0	0	1	1	1	1	1	1	1
35–49	0									
50–64	1	1.0	0	1	1	1	1	1	1	1
65+	0									
2. MULTIPLE DX										
A. Not Operated										
0–19 Years	0									
20–34	0									
35–49	0									
50–64	0									
65+	0									
B. Operated										
0–19 Years	0									
20–34	1	1.0	0	1	1	1	1	1	1	1
35–49	0									
50–64	0									
65+	0									
SUBTOTALS:										
1. SINGLE DX										
A. Not Operated	0									
B. Operated	2	1.0	0	1	1	1	1	1	1	1
2. MULTIPLE DX										
A. Not Operated	0									
B. Operated	1	1.0	0	1	1	1	1	1	1	1
1. SINGLE DX	2	1.0	0	1	1	1	1	1	1	1
2. MULTIPLE DX	1	1.0	0	1	1	1	1	1	1	1
A. NOT OPERATED	0									
B. OPERATED	3	1.0	0	1	1	1	1	1	1	1
TOTAL										
0–19 Years	0									
20–34	1	1.0	0	1	1	1	1	1	1	1
35–49	1	1.0	0	1	1	1	1	1	1	1
50–64	1	1.0	0	1	1	1	1	1	1	1
65+	0									
GRAND TOTAL	3	1.0	0	1	1	1	1	1	1	1

607: DISORDERS OF PENIS

Type of Patients	Observed Patients	Avg. Stay	Variance	Percentiles						
				10th	25th	50th	75th	90th	95th	99th
1. SINGLE DX										
A. Not Operated										
0–19 Years	19	1.7	<1	1	1	2	2	3	3	3
20–34	2	1.5	<1	1	1	2	2	2	2	2
35–49	4	2.0	2	1	1	1	4	4	4	4
50–64	1	2.0	0	2	2	2	2	2	2	2
65+	0									
B. Operated										
0–19 Years	2	1.5	<1	1	1	2	2	2	2	2
20–34	10	2.5	2	1	1	1	4	4	4	4
35–49	19	1.6	<1	1	1	1	2	3	3	3
50–64	25	1.2	<1	1	1	1	1	2	2	2
65+	22	1.1	<1	1	1	1	1	1	2	2
2. MULTIPLE DX										
A. Not Operated										
0–19 Years	74	1.8	<1	1	1	2	2	3	3	6
20–34	47	3.5	12	1	2	3	4	6	8	22
35–49	49	2.7	4	1	1	2	4	6	7	8
50–64	42	4.3	21	1	1	4	5	8	11	28
65+	36	4.3	12	1	2	3	6	8	14	16
B. Operated										
0–19 Years	16	2.6	2	1	1	3	3	5	5	5
20–34	49	4.2	23	1	1	3	6	8	9	30
35–49	113	2.9	10	1	1	2	4	6	8	15
50–64	268	1.8	4	1	1	1	2	3	5	12
65+	268	2.0	10	1	1	1	1	3	9	22
SUBTOTALS:										
1. SINGLE DX										
A. Not Operated	26	1.7	<1	1	1	2	2	3	3	4
B. Operated	78	1.4	<1	1	1	1	2	2	3	4
2. MULTIPLE DX										
A. Not Operated	248	3.1	9	1	1	2	4	6	8	16
B. Operated	714	2.2	9	1	1	1	2	5	7	15
1. SINGLE DX	104	1.5	<1	1	1	1	2	3	3	4
2. MULTIPLE DX	962	2.5	9	1	1	1	3	5	8	16
A. NOT OPERATED	274	3.0	9	1	1	2	4	6	8	16
B. OPERATED	792	2.2	8	1	1	1	2	4	7	15
TOTAL										
0–19 Years	111	1.9	1	1	1	2	3	3	4	5
20–34	108	3.7	16	1	1	3	4	7	9	22
35–49	185	2.7	7	1	1	2	3	5	7	15
50–64	336	2.0	6	1	1	1	2	4	6	12
65+	326	2.2	10	1	1	1	2	4	9	16
GRAND TOTAL	1,066	2.4	8	1	1	1	3	5	7	15

607.84: IMPOTENCE ORGANIC ORIGIN

Type of Patients	Observed Patients	Avg. Stay	Variance	Percentiles						
				10th	25th	50th	75th	90th	95th	99th
1. SINGLE DX										
A. Not Operated										
0–19 Years	0									
20–34	0									
35–49	0									
50–64	0									
65+	0									
B. Operated										
0–19 Years	0									
20–34	0									
35–49	3	1.0	0	1	1	1	1	1	1	1
50–64	8	1.3	<1	1	1	1	2	2	2	2
65+	20	1.1	<1	1	1	1	1	2	2	2
2. MULTIPLE DX										
A. Not Operated										
0–19 Years	0									
20–34	0									
35–49	0									
50–64	4	1.0	0	1	1	1	1	1	1	1
65+	2	1.0	0	1	1	1	1	1	1	1
B. Operated										
0–19 Years	0									
20–34	2	1.5	<1	1	1	1	1	2	2	2
35–49	23	1.5	<1	1	1	1	1	2	3	4
50–64	170	1.3	<1	1	1	1	1	2	3	5
65+	231	1.6	5	1	1	1	1	2	3	11
SUBTOTALS:										
1. SINGLE DX										
A. Not Operated	0									
B. Operated	31	1.1	<1	1	1	1	1	2	2	2
2. MULTIPLE DX										
A. Not Operated	6	1.0	0	1	1	1	1	1	1	1
B. Operated	426	1.5	3	1	1	1	1	2	3	9
1. SINGLE DX	31	1.1	<1	1	1	1	1	2	2	2
2. MULTIPLE DX	432	1.5	3	1	1	1	1	2	3	9
A. NOT OPERATED	6	1.0	0	1	1	1	1	1	1	1
B. OPERATED	457	1.4	3	1	1	1	1	2	3	9
TOTAL										
0–19 Years	0									
20–34	2	1.5	<1	1	1	1	1	2	2	2
35–49	26	1.4	<1	1	1	1	1	2	3	4
50–64	182	1.3	<1	1	1	1	1	2	3	5
65+	253	1.5	5	1	1	1	1	2	3	11
GRAND TOTAL	463	1.4	3	1	1	1	1	2	3	9

Length of Stay by Diagnosis and Operation, Western Region, 2008

Western Region, October 2006–September 2007 Data, by Diagnosis

608: OTH DISORD MALE GENITAL

Type of Patients	Observed Patients	Avg. Stay	Vari-ance	10th	25th	50th	75th	90th	95th	99th
1. SINGLE DX										
A. Not Operated										
0–19 Years	19	1.3	<1	1	1	1	2	2	2	2
20–34	20	2.2	1	1	1	2	3	4	4	4
35–49	21	2.2	2	1	1	2	3	4	4	6
50–64	5	2.2	3	1	1	1	3	5	5	5
65+	3	2.3	<1	2	2	2	3	3	3	3
B. Operated										
0–19 Years	107	1.1	<1	1	1	1	1	1	2	2
20–34	41	1.0	<1	1	1	1	1	1	1	2
35–49	12	1.3	<1	1	1	1	2	2	4	4
50–64	3	1.3	<1	1	1	1	2	2	2	2
65+	1	1.0	0	2						1
2. MULTIPLE DX										
A. Not Operated										
0–19 Years	43	3.1	23	1	1	2	3	3	7	31
20–34	232	4.1	13	1	2	3	5	8	12	20
35–49	472	4.5	13	1	2	3	6	8	11	19
50–64	424	5.2	26	1	2	4	7	10	13	25
65+	222	4.5	11	2	2	4	5	8	10	15
B. Operated										
0–19 Years	89	1.5	1	1	1	1	1	2	3	10
20–34	85	4.0	62	1	1	1	4	9	19	60
35–49	88	6.8	59	1	1	4	9	16	20	48
50–64	107	10.2	125	1	2	6	16	25	30	45
65+	66	7.9	87	2	2	4	10	19	25	58
SUBTOTALS:										
1. SINGLE DX										
A. Not Operated	68	2.0	1	1	1	1	2	2	4	6
B. Operated	164	1.1	<1	1	1	1	1	1	2	3
2. MULTIPLE DX										
A. Not Operated	1,393	4.6	17	1	2	3	6	9	12	21
B. Operated	435	6.2	78	1	1	2	8	17	23	45
1. SINGLE DX	232	1.3	<1	1	1	1	1	2	3	4
2. MULTIPLE DX	1,828	5.0	32	1	2	3	6	10	15	28
A. NOT OPERATED	1,461	4.5	17	1	2	3	5	9	11	20
B. OPERATED	599	4.8	62	1	1	1	5	14	21	36
TOTAL										
0–19 Years	258	1.6	5	1	1	1	2	3	3	10
20–34	378	3.6	23	1	1	2	4	6	11	21
35–49	593	4.7	20	1	2	3	6	9	14	23
50–64	539	6.1	49	1	2	4	7	13	19	36
65+	292	5.2	30	2	2	4	6	10	14	31
GRAND TOTAL	2,060	4.6	30	1	1	3	5	9	14	27

608.20: TESTICULAR TORSION NOS

Type of Patients	Observed Patients	Avg. Stay	Vari-ance	10th	25th	50th	75th	90th	95th	99th
1. SINGLE DX										
A. Not Operated										
0–19 Years	3	1.3	<1	1	1	1	2	2	2	2
20–34	0									
35–49	1	1.0	0	1	1	1	1	1	1	1
50–64	1	1.0	0	1	1	1	1	1	1	1
65+	0									
B. Operated										
0–19 Years	82	1.1	<1	1	1	1	1	1	2	3
20–34	29	1.0	0	1	1	1	1	1	1	1
35–49	5	1.0	0	1	1	1	1	1	1	1
50–64	1	1.0	0	1	1	1	1	1	1	1
65+	0									
2. MULTIPLE DX										
A. Not Operated										
0–19 Years	2	1.0	0	1	1	1	1	1	1	1
20–34	3	1.0	0	1	1	1	1	1	1	1
35–49	1	3.0	0	3	3	3	3	3	3	3
50–64	0									
65+	2	2.5	4	1	1	1	4	4	4	4
B. Operated										
0–19 Years	57	1.4	<1	1	1	1	2	3	3	4
20–34	40	1.4	<1	1	1	1	2	2	2	4
35–49	9	2.7	8	1	1	3	3	9	9	9
50–64	11	1.8	3	1	1	1	2	3	7	7
65+	2	1.5	<1	1	1	2	2	2	2	2
SUBTOTALS:										
1. SINGLE DX										
A. Not Operated	5	1.2	<1	1	1	1	1	2	2	2
B. Operated	117	1.0	<1	1	1	1	1	1	1	2
2. MULTIPLE DX										
A. Not Operated	8	1.6	1	1	1	1	2	4	4	4
B. Operated	119	1.5	1	1	1	1	2	3	4	7
1. SINGLE DX	122	1.1	<1	1	1	1	1	1	1	2
2. MULTIPLE DX	127	1.5	1	1	1	1	2	3	4	7
A. NOT OPERATED	13	1.5	<1	1	1	1	1	3	4	4
B. OPERATED	236	1.3	<1	1	1	1	1	2	3	6
TOTAL										
0–19 Years	144	1.2	<1	1	1	1	1	2	2	4
20–34	72	1.2	<1	1	1	1	1	2	2	4
35–49	16	2.1	5	1	1	1	1	6	9	9
50–64	13	1.7	3	1	1	1	2	4	7	7
65+	4	2.0	2	1	1	1	2	4	4	4
GRAND TOTAL	249	1.3	<1	1	1	1	1	2	3	6

608.4: MALE GEN INFLAM DIS NEC

Type of Patients	Observed Patients	Avg. Stay	Vari-ance	10th	25th	50th	75th	90th	95th	99th
1. SINGLE DX										
A. Not Operated										
0–19 Years	9	1.3	<1	1	1	1	2	2	2	2
20–34	15	2.3	2	1	1	2	3	4	4	4
35–49	18	2.3	2	1	1	2	4	4	6	6
50–64	3	3.0	4	1	1	3	5	5	5	5
65+	2	2.5	<1	2	2	3	3	3	3	3
B. Operated										
0–19 Years	0									
20–34	0									
35–49	0									
50–64	0									
65+	0									
2. MULTIPLE DX										
A. Not Operated										
0–19 Years	31	3.7	30	1	2	3	3	3	12	31
20–34	193	4.1	10	1	2	3	5	8	10	20
35–49	412	4.3	12	1	2	3	5	8	11	19
50–64	344	5.0	18	2	2	4	6	9	12	21
65+	172	4.6	11	2	3	4	5	8	10	20
B. Operated										
0–19 Years	2	2.5	4	1	1	3	4	4	4	4
20–34	12	6.3	20	2	4	6	10	10	18	18
35–49	37	7.7	32	2	3	7	10	16	19	23
50–64	33	7.2	21	3	4	6	9	13	15	23
65+	27	7.3	32	3	3	6	10	16	17	25
SUBTOTALS:										
1. SINGLE DX										
A. Not Operated	47	2.2	2	1	1	2	3	4	4	6
B. Operated	0									
2. MULTIPLE DX										
A. Not Operated	1,152	4.5	14	2	2	3	5	8	11	19
B. Operated	111	7.2	27	2	3	6	9	15	18	23
1. SINGLE DX	47	2.2	2	1	1	2	3	4	4	6
2. MULTIPLE DX	1,263	4.7	16	1	2	4	6	9	12	20
A. NOT OPERATED	1,199	4.4	14	1	2	3	5	8	11	19
B. OPERATED	111	7.2	27	2	3	6	9	15	18	23
TOTAL										
0–19 Years	42	3.1	23	1	1	2	3	3	7	31
20–34	220	4.1	11	1	2	3	5	8	10	18
35–49	467	4.5	14	1	2	3	6	8	12	19
50–64	380	5.1	18	2	3	4	7	9	13	23
65+	201	4.9	15	2	3	4	6	9	10	20
GRAND TOTAL	1,310	4.6	15	1	2	4	6	9	12	20

Length of Stay by Diagnosis and Operation, Western Region, 2008

Western Region, October 2006–September 2007 Data, by Diagnosis

610: BENIGN MAMMARY DYSPLASIA

Type of Patients	Observed Patients	Avg. Stay	Vari-ance	10th	25th	50th	75th	90th	95th	99th
1. SINGLE DX										
A. Not Operated										
0–19 Years	0									
20–34	1	1.0	0	1	1	1	1	1	1	1
35–49	1	1.0	0	1	1	1	1	1	1	1
50–64	0									
65+	0									
B. Operated										
0–19 Years	0									
20–34	2	1.0	0	1	1	1	1	1	1	1
35–49	7	1.3	<1	1	1	1	2	2	2	2
50–64	4	1.5	<1	1	1	2	2	2	2	2
65+	1	2.0	0	2	2	2	2	2	2	2
2. MULTIPLE DX										
A. Not Operated										
0–19 Years	0									
20–34	1	3.0	0	3	3	3	3	3	3	3
35–49	2	2.5	4	1	1	1	4	4	4	4
50–64	5	3.6	7	1	2	3	4	8	8	8
65+	0									
B. Operated										
0–19 Years	7	1.0	0	1	1	1	1	1	1	1
20–34	7	3.3	27	1	1	1	3	15	15	15
35–49	39	2.0	1	1	1	2	2	3	4	6
50–64	55	2.2	2	1	1	2	3	4	6	8
65+	25	1.7	2	1	1	1	2	3	4	8
SUBTOTALS:										
1. SINGLE DX										
A. Not Operated	2	1.0	0	1	1	1	1	1	1	1
B. Operated	14	1.4	<1	1	1	1	2	2	2	2
2. MULTIPLE DX										
A. Not Operated	8	3.2	5	1	2	3	4	8	8	8
B. Operated	127	2.1	3	1	1	1	2	4	5	8
1. SINGLE DX	16	1.3	<1	1	1	1	2	2	2	2
2. MULTIPLE DX	135	2.1	3	1	1	2	3	4	6	8
A. NOT OPERATED	10	2.8	5	1	1	2	4	4	8	8
B. OPERATED	141	2.0	3	1	1	1	2	4	5	8
TOTAL										
0–19 Years	1	1.0	0	1	1	1	1	1	1	1
20–34	11	2.6	17	1	1	1	3	3	15	15
35–49	49	1.9	1	1	1	2	3	3	4	6
50–64	64	2.2	3	1	1	2	3	4	6	8
65+	26	1.7	2	1	2	1	2	3	4	8
GRAND TOTAL	151	2.1	3	1	1	1	2	4	5	8

611: OTHER BREAST DISORDERS

Type of Patients	Observed Patients	Avg. Stay	Vari-ance	10th	25th	50th	75th	90th	95th	99th
1. SINGLE DX										
A. Not Operated										
0–19 Years	33	2.3	3	1	1	2	3	4	7	7
20–34	135	2.3	2	1	1	2	3	4	5	6
35–49	56	2.1	1	1	1	2	3	4	5	5
50–64	17	2.5	2	1	1	2	4	4	5	5
65+	4	4.3	14	1	1	7	8	8	8	8
B. Operated										
0–19 Years	24	1.0	0	1	1	1	1	1	1	1
20–34	118	1.8	5	1	1	1	2	4	5	11
35–49	90	1.3	<1	1	1	1	2	2	3	5
50–64	59	1.4	<1	1	1	1	1	2	4	6
65+	4	1.5	1	1	1	1	3	3	3	3
2. MULTIPLE DX										
A. Not Operated										
0–19 Years	84	3.6	8	1	2	3	4	6	8	18
20–34	249	3.2	6	1	1	3	4	6	7	13
35–49	324	3.4	5	1	2	3	5	6	8	10
50–64	282	3.8	13	1	2	3	5	7	8	16
65+	139	4.0	6	1	2	4	5	7	8	14
B. Operated										
0–19 Years	33	1.5	2	1	1	1	1	2	6	7
20–34	220	1.8	2	1	1	1	2	4	5	7
35–49	512	2.2	7	1	1	2	2	4	7	16
50–64	687	1.9	4	1	1	2	2	4	5	11
65+	212	2.3	8	1	1	1	2	6	7	17
SUBTOTALS:										
1. SINGLE DX										
A. Not Operated	245	2.3	2	1	1	2	3	4	5	7
B. Operated	295	1.5	2	1	1	1	1	2	4	7
2. MULTIPLE DX										
A. Not Operated	1,078	3.5	8	2	2	3	5	6	8	14
B. Operated	1,664	2.1	5	1	1	1	2	4	6	12
1. SINGLE DX	540	1.9	2	1	1	1	2	4	5	7
2. MULTIPLE DX	2,742	2.6	7	1	1	2	3	5	7	13
A. NOT OPERATED	1,323	3.3	7	2	2	3	4	6	8	12
B. OPERATED	1,959	2.0	5	1	1	1	2	4	5	12
TOTAL										
0–19 Years	174	2.6	6	1	1	2	3	3	7	15
20–34	722	2.4	4	1	1	2	3	5	6	11
35–49	982	2.6	6	1	1	2	3	5	7	12
50–64	1,045	2.4	7	1	1	1	4	4	6	12
65+	359	3.0	8	1	2	2	4	4	8	15
GRAND TOTAL	3,282	2.5	6	1	2	2	3	5	7	12

611.0: INFLAM BREAST DISEASE

Type of Patients	Observed Patients	Avg. Stay	Vari-ance	10th	25th	50th	75th	90th	95th	99th
1. SINGLE DX										
A. Not Operated										
0–19 Years	31	2.4	3	1	1	2	3	4	7	7
20–34	132	2.3	2	1	1	2	3	4	5	6
35–49	53	2.2	1	1	1	2	3	4	5	5
50–64	16	2.6	2	1	1	2	4	4	5	5
65+	4	4.3	14	1	1	7	8	8	8	8
B. Operated										
0–19 Years	1	1.0	0	1	1	1	1	1	1	1
20–34	33	3.4	13	1	1	2	4	5	11	20
35–49	13	2.5	<1	2	2	3	3	3	5	5
50–64	3	3.3	4	1	1	4	5	5	5	5
65+	2	2.0	2	1	1	3	3	3	3	3
2. MULTIPLE DX										
A. Not Operated										
0–19 Years	82	3.6	8	1	2	3	4	6	8	18
20–34	243	3.2	6	1	1	3	4	6	7	13
35–49	303	3.5	5	1	2	3	5	6	8	10
50–64	249	4.0	14	1	2	3	5	7	9	16
65+	119	4.0	6	2	2	4	5	7	8	14
B. Operated										
0–19 Years	5	3.4	8	1	1	2	6	7	7	7
20–34	45	3.2	3	1	2	3	4	6	7	8
35–49	95	4.9	19	1	2	3	6	11	17	19
50–64	76	4.5	17	1	2	3	5	10	12	24
65+	52	4.9	18	1	2	4	6	8	15	23
SUBTOTALS:										
1. SINGLE DX										
A. Not Operated	236	2.3	2	1	1	2	3	4	5	7
B. Operated	52	3.1	9	1	2	2	3	5	7	20
2. MULTIPLE DX										
A. Not Operated	996	3.6	8	1	2	3	5	6	8	14
B. Operated	273	4.5	16	1	2	3	6	9	13	20
1. SINGLE DX	288	2.5	3	1	1	2	3	4	5	8
2. MULTIPLE DX	1,269	3.8	10	1	2	3	5	7	9	16
A. NOT OPERATED	1,232	3.4	7	1	2	3	4	6	8	12
B. OPERATED	325	4.3	15	1	2	3	5	8	12	20
TOTAL										
0–19 Years	119	3.3	7	1	2	3	4	6	8	15
20–34	453	2.9	5	1	1	2	4	6	7	12
35–49	464	3.6	8	2	2	3	5	7	9	17
50–64	344	4.1	14	1	2	3	5	7	10	20
65+	177	4.3	9	1	2	4	6	8	8	17
GRAND TOTAL	1,557	3.6	9	1	2	3	4	7	8	16

Length of Stay by Diagnosis and Operation, Western Region, 2008

Western Region, October 2006–September 2007 Data, by Diagnosis

611.1: BREAST HYPERTROPHY

Type of Patients	Observed Patients	Avg. Stay	Variance	10th	25th	50th	75th	90th	95th	99th
1. SINGLE DX										
A. Not Operated										
0–19 Years	2	1.5	<1	1	1	2	2	2	2	2
20–34	0									
35–49	0									
50–64	0									
65+	0									
B. Operated										
0–19 Years	21	1.0	0	1	1	1	1	1	1	1
20–34	83	1.2	<1	1	1	1	1	2	2	4
35–49	73	1.2	<1	1	1	1	1	2	2	4
50–64	54	1.2	<1	1	1	1	1	2	2	2
65+	2	1.0	0	1	1	1	1	1	1	1
2. MULTIPLE DX										
A. Not Operated										
0–19 Years	1	1.0	0	1	1	1	1	1	1	1
20–34	1	1.0	0	1	1	1	1	1	1	1
35–49	4	1.0	0	1	1	1	1	1	1	1
50–64	8	1.3	<1	1	1	1	2	2	2	2
65+	1	2.0	0	2	2	2	2	2	2	2
B. Operated										
0–19 Years	25	1.1	<1	1	1	1	1	2	2	2
20–34	145	1.3	<1	1	1	1	1	2	2	4
35–49	295	1.4	1	1	1	1	2	2	3	9
50–64	420	1.4	<1	1	1	1	2	2	3	5
65+	105	1.3	<1	1	1	1	1	2	3	5
SUBTOTALS:										
1. SINGLE DX										
A. Not Operated	2	1.5	<1	1	1	2	2	2	2	2
B. Operated	233	1.1	<1	1	1	1	1	2	2	2
2. MULTIPLE DX										
A. Not Operated	15	1.2	<1	1	1	1	1	2	2	2
B. Operated	990	1.4	<1	1	1	1	2	2	3	5
1. SINGLE DX	235	1.1	<1	1	1	1	1	2	2	2
2. MULTIPLE DX	1,005	1.4	<1	1	1	1	2	2	3	5
A. NOT OPERATED	17	1.2	<1	1	1	1	1	2	2	2
B. OPERATED	1,223	1.3	<1	1	1	1	2	2	3	5
TOTAL										
0–19 Years	49	1.1	<1	1	1	1	1	1	2	2
20–34	229	1.2	<1	1	1	1	1	2	2	4
35–49	372	1.4	1	1	1	1	2	2	3	6
50–64	482	1.3	<1	1	1	1	2	2	3	5
65+	108	1.3	<1	1	1	1	1	2	3	5
GRAND TOTAL	1,240	1.3	<1	1	1	1	2	2	3	5

611.8: BREAST DISORDERS NEC

Type of Patients	Observed Patients	Avg. Stay	Variance	10th	25th	50th	75th	90th	95th	99th
1. SINGLE DX										
A. Not Operated										
0–19 Years	0									
20–34	0									
35–49	1	1.0	0	1	1		1	1	1	1
50–64	0									
65+	0									
B. Operated										
0–19 Years	1	1.0	0	1	1	1	1	1	1	1
20–34	1	6.0	0	6	6	6	6	6	6	6
35–49	2	1.0	0	1	1	1	1	1	1	1
50–64	2	4.0	8	2	2	4	6	6	6	6
65+	0									
2. MULTIPLE DX										
A. Not Operated										
0–19 Years	0									
20–34	0									
35–49	0									
50–64	3	2.0	<1	1	1	2	3	3	3	3
65+	7	5.0	7	1	3	5	7	9	9	9
B. Operated										
0–19 Years	3	1.0	0	1	1	1	1	1	1	1
20–34	22	2.3	3	1	1	1	4	5	5	6
35–49	97	2.2	2	1	1	2	3	4	5	8
50–64	159	2.2	3	1	1	1	3	4	5	8
65+	31	2.2	8	1	1	1	2	3	4	17
SUBTOTALS:										
1. SINGLE DX										
A. Not Operated	1	1.0	0	1	1	1	1	1	1	1
B. Operated	6	2.8	6	1	1	2	6	6	6	6
2. MULTIPLE DX										
A. Not Operated	10	4.1	7	1	2	3	6	9	9	9
B. Operated	312	2.2	3	1	1	1	3	4	5	8
1. SINGLE DX	7	2.6	6	1	1	1	6	6	6	6
2. MULTIPLE DX	322	2.2	3	1	1	2	3	4	5	8
A. NOT OPERATED	11	3.8	7	1	1	3	6	7	9	9
B. OPERATED	318	2.2	3	1	1	1	3	4	5	8
TOTAL										
0–19 Years	4	1.0	0	1	1	1	1	1	1	1
20–34	23	2.4	4	1	1	2	5	5	6	6
35–49	100	2.1	2	1	1	2	3	4	5	8
50–64	164	2.2	3	1	1	1	3	4	5	8
65+	38	2.7	9	1	1	2	3	6	9	17
GRAND TOTAL	329	2.2	4	1	1	2	3	4	5	8

614: FEMALE PELVIC INFLAM DIS

Type of Patients	Observed Patients	Avg. Stay	Variance	10th	25th	50th	75th	90th	95th	99th
1. SINGLE DX										
A. Not Operated										
0–19 Years	72	2.3	2	1	1	2	3	4	5	6
20–34	209	2.4	2	1	2	2	3	4	5	7
35–49	107	2.8	2	1	2	2	3	5	6	6
50–64	15	2.2	<1	1	2	2	2	4	4	4
65+	0									
B. Operated										
0–19 Years	12	2.5	4	1	1	2	3	3	8	8
20–34	41	2.2	2	1	1	2	3	4	5	6
35–49	43	2.8	2	1	2	2	3	5	6	8
50–64	8	2.9	3	1	2	2	4	7	7	7
65+	2	4.0	8	2	2	6	6	6	6	6
2. MULTIPLE DX										
A. Not Operated										
0–19 Years	243	2.9	4	1	2	2	4	5	6	12
20–34	810	2.9	3	1	2	3	4	5	6	9
35–49	589	3.7	6	1	2	3	5	7	8	13
50–64	200	4.9	14	2	3	4	6	9	13	21
65+	48	7.4	38	2	4	5	10	20	22	27
B. Operated										
0–19 Years	66	5.4	108	1	2	3	5	9	10	86
20–34	648	3.6	8	1	2	3	4	5	7	15
35–49	1,224	4.1	15	1	2	3	5	8	11	19
50–64	421	4.0	13	1	2	3	5	8	10	21
65+	93	5.6	48	2	2	3	7	12	14	55
SUBTOTALS:										
1. SINGLE DX										
A. Not Operated	403	2.5	2	1	2	2	3	4	5	7
B. Operated	106	2.6	2	1	2	2	3	5	6	8
2. MULTIPLE DX										
A. Not Operated	1,890	3.5	7	1	2	3	4	6	8	14
B. Operated	2,452	4.0	16	1	2	3	5	8	11	19
1. SINGLE DX	509	2.5	2	1	2	2	3	4	5	7
2. MULTIPLE DX	4,342	3.8	12	1	2	3	4	7	10	17
A. NOT OPERATED	2,293	3.3	6	1	2	3	4	6	7	13
B. OPERATED	2,558	4.0	16	1	2	3	5	8	10	19
TOTAL										
0–19 Years	393	3.2	22	1	2	2	4	5	7	12
20–34	1,708	3.1	5	1	2	3	4	5	7	12
35–49	1,963	3.9	11	1	2	3	5	8	10	17
50–64	644	4.2	13	1	2	3	5	8	11	21
65+	143	6.2	44	1	2	4	8	13	21	27
GRAND TOTAL	4,851	3.7	11	1	2	3	4	7	9	17

Length of Stay by Diagnosis and Operation, Western Region, 2008

Western Region, October 2006–September 2007 Data, by Diagnosis

614.0: AC SALPINGO-OOPHORITIS

Type of Patients	Observed Patients	Avg. Stay	Variance	10th	25th	Percentiles 50th	75th	90th	95th	99th
1. SINGLE DX										
A. Not Operated										
0–19 Years	7	2.4	<1	2	2	2	3	3	3	3
20–34	13	3.3	3	2	2	3	4	4	8	8
35–49	10	3.8	3	2	2	5	5	6	6	6
50–64	3	2.7	1	2	2	2	4	4	4	4
65+	0									
B. Operated										
0–19 Years	2	2.0	0	2	2	2	2	2	2	2
20–34	1	2.0	0	2	2	2	2	2	2	2
35–49	2	3.5	13	1	1	4	6	6	6	6
50–64	1	7.0	0	7	7	7	7	7	7	7
65+	0									
2. MULTIPLE DX										
A. Not Operated										
0–19 Years	7	4.0	7	1	2	3	6	9	9	9
20–34	25	3.7	5	2	3	3	4	6	9	11
35–49	34	4.3	5	2	3	4	5	8	9	9
50–64	15	4.7	6	2	3	4	6	9	11	11
65+	0									
B. Operated										
0–19 Years	10	6.0	11	2	3	4	8	10	12	12
20–34	43	5.4	18	2	3	5	7	7	10	26
35–49	90	6.6	19	3	4	5	8	11	13	30
50–64	29	7.3	28	2	4	6	8	18	21	21
65+	2	10.5	24	7	7	14	14	14	14	14
SUBTOTALS:										
1. SINGLE DX										
A. Not Operated	33	3.2	2	2	2	3	4	5	6	8
B. Operated	6	3.3	6	1	2	2	6	7	7	7
2. MULTIPLE DX										
A. Not Operated	81	4.2	5	2	3	4	5	8	9	11
B. Operated	174	6.4	20	3	4	5	8	12	14	26
1. SINGLE DX	39	3.2	3	2	2	3	4	6	7	8
2. MULTIPLE DX	255	5.7	16	2	3	5	7	10	12	21
A. NOT OPERATED	114	3.9	5	2	2	3	5	7	9	11
B. OPERATED	180	6.3	20	2	3	5	8	11	14	26
TOTAL										
0–19 Years	26	4.2	8	2	2	3	6	9	10	12
20–34	82	4.5	12	2	3	3	5	9	9	26
35–49	136	5.8	15	2	3	5	7	10	12	20
50–64	48	6.2	21	2	3	5	7	12	18	21
65+	2	10.5	24	7	7	14	14	14	14	14
GRAND TOTAL	294	5.4	15	2	3	4	7	9	12	21

614.1: CHR SALPINGO-OOPHORITIS

Type of Patients	Observed Patients	Avg. Stay	Variance	10th	25th	Percentiles 50th	75th	90th	95th	99th
1. SINGLE DX										
A. Not Operated										
0–19 Years	0									
20–34	3	2.7	1	2	2	2	4	4	4	4
35–49	4	2.5	2	1	1	2	4	4	6	6
50–64	1	2.0	0	2	2	2	2	2	2	2
65+	0									
B. Operated										
0–19 Years	1	8.0	0	8	8	8	8	8	8	8
20–34	1	1.0	0	1	1	1	1	1	1	1
35–49	7	2.1	<1	1	2	2	3	3	3	3
50–64	2	2.0	0	2	2	2	2	2	2	2
65+	1	2.0	0	2	2	2	2	2	2	2
2. MULTIPLE DX										
A. Not Operated										
0–19 Years	3	3.0	<1	2	2	3	4	4	4	4
20–34	13	2.6	2	1	2	2	3	5	6	6
35–49	28	2.9	4	1	1	2	3	7	7	7
50–64	6	5.3	42	1	1	4	6	18	18	18
65+	1	2.0	0	2	2	2	2	2	2	2
B. Operated										
0–19 Years	7	3.3	2	1	2	3	5	5	5	5
20–34	90	2.7	2	1	2	2	3	4	6	9
35–49	254	2.9	6	1	2	2	3	5	8	15
50–64	137	2.4	2	1	2	2	3	4	5	7
65+	28	3.2	5	2	2	3	4	5	8	12
SUBTOTALS:										
1. SINGLE DX										
A. Not Operated	8	2.5	1	1	2	2	3	4	4	4
B. Operated	12	2.5	3	1	2	2	2	3	8	8
2. MULTIPLE DX										
A. Not Operated	51	3.1	8	1	2	2	4	6	7	18
B. Operated	516	2.8	4	1	2	2	3	5	6	11
1. SINGLE DX	20	2.5	2	1	2	2	3	4	4	8
2. MULTIPLE DX	567	2.8	5	1	2	2	3	5	7	12
A. NOT OPERATED	59	3.0	7	1	2	2	4	6	7	18
B. OPERATED	528	2.8	4	1	2	2	3	5	6	11
TOTAL										
0–19 Years	11	3.6	4	2	2	3	5	6	8	8
20–34	107	2.7	2	1	2	2	3	5	6	7
35–49	293	2.9	6	1	1	2	3	5	7	15
50–64	146	2.5	4	1	1	2	3	4	5	10
65+	30	3.1	5	2	2	3	4	5	8	12
GRAND TOTAL	587	2.8	4	1	2	2	3	5	7	12

614.2: SALPINGO-OOPHORITIS NOS

Type of Patients	Observed Patients	Avg. Stay	Variance	10th	25th	Percentiles 50th	75th	90th	95th	99th
1. SINGLE DX										
A. Not Operated										
0–19 Years	10	2.5	3	1	1	2	3	6	6	6
20–34	60	2.8	2	1	2	2	3	5	7	8
35–49	38	2.9	1	2	2	3	3	5	6	6
50–64	9	2.2	<1	1	2	2	2	4	4	4
65+	0									
B. Operated										
0–19 Years	1	3.0	0	3	3	3	3	3	3	3
20–34	9	3.4	3	1	2	4	5	6	6	6
35–49	9	4.1	3	2	4	4	5	8	8	8
50–64	1	4.0	0	4	4	4	4	4	4	4
65+	0									
2. MULTIPLE DX										
A. Not Operated										
0–19 Years	34	2.9	5	1	2	2	3	4	6	13
20–34	147	3.3	3	2	2	3	4	6	7	9
35–49	182	4.0	4	2	2	4	5	7	8	11
50–64	37	4.3	6	1	3	4	5	8	10	11
65+	0									
B. Operated										
0–19 Years	108	6.1	7	3	4	5	9	10	10	10
20–34	212	5.1	13	2	3	4	7	10	13	17
35–49	212	6.5	18	2	3	5	8	12	14	21
50–64	71	6.3	18	2	3	5	8	12	15	23
65+	13	6.8	13	3	4	6	8	13	14	14
SUBTOTALS:										
1. SINGLE DX										
A. Not Operated	117	2.7	2	1	2	2	3	5	6	7
B. Operated	20	3.7	3	1	3	4	5	5	6	8
2. MULTIPLE DX										
A. Not Operated	400	3.7	4	2	2	3	5	7	7	11
B. Operated	411	6.1	16	2	3	5	8	12	14	19
1. SINGLE DX	137	2.9	2	1	2	3	4	5	6	8
2. MULTIPLE DX	811	4.9	12	2	3	4	6	9	12	17
A. NOT OPERATED	517	3.5	4	1	2	3	4	6	7	11
B. OPERATED	431	6.0	16	2	3	5	8	12	14	19
TOTAL										
0–19 Years	52	3.2	6	2	2	3	4	6	9	13
20–34	324	3.8	7	1	2	3	5	7	9	15
35–49	441	5.1	12	2	3	4	7	10	12	16
50–64	118	5.3	14	2	3	4	8	10	12	19
65+	13	6.8	13	3	4	6	8	13	14	14
GRAND TOTAL	948	4.6	11	2	2	4	6	9	11	16

Length of Stay by Diagnosis and Operation, Western Region, 2008

614.3: ACUTE PARAMETRITIS

Type of Patients	Observed Patients	Avg. Stay	Variance	10th	25th	50th	75th	90th	95th	99th
1. SINGLE DX										
A. *Not Operated*										
0–19 Years	10	2.2	<1	1	2	2	3	3	3	3
20–34	24	2.2	<1	1	2	2	3	3	4	4
35–49	13	2.8	2	1	2	2	3	5	6	6
50–64	0									
65+	0									
B. *Operated*										
0–19 Years	0									
20–34	3	1.0	0	1	1	1	1	1	1	1
35–49	0									
50–64	0									
65+	0									
2. MULTIPLE DX										
A. *Not Operated*										
0–19 Years	43	3.1	2	1	2	3	4	5	6	7
20–34	125	3.0	4	1	2	3	3	5	7	10
35–49	67	4.3	11	1	2	3	5	9	12	17
50–64	24	5.3	22	2	2	4	7	14	14	19
65+	13	8.1	48	2	4	6	11	13	27	27
B. *Operated*										
0–19 Years	5	5.4	8	3	4	4	6	10	10	10
20–34	26	5.4	8	2	3	5	7	10	10	13
35–49	22	6.6	13	2	4	6	9	11	14	14
50–64	12	7.8	50	3	4	5	7	21	24	24
65+	7	19.7	311	2	7	21	23	55	55	55
SUBTOTALS:										
1. SINGLE DX										
A. *Not Operated*	47	2.3	1	1	2	2	3	4	4	6
B. *Operated*	3	1.0	0	1	1	1	1	1	1	1
2. MULTIPLE DX										
A. *Not Operated*	272	3.8	10	1	2	3	4	7	10	17
B. *Operated*	72	7.6	58	2	4	6	8	14	22	55
1. SINGLE DX	50	2.3	1	1	1	2	3	4	4	6
2. MULTIPLE DX	344	4.6	22	1	2	3	5	9	13	23
A. NOT OPERATED	319	3.6	9	1	2	3	4	6	10	16
B. OPERATED	75	7.3	58	2	3	5	8	14	22	55
TOTAL										
0–19 Years	58	3.1	3	1	2	3	4	5	7	10
20–34	178	3.2	5	1	2	3	4	6	8	12
35–49	102	4.6	12	2	2	4	5	9	12	16
50–64	36	6.1	31	2	2	4	7	14	21	24
65+	20	12.2	162	2	4	8	21	27	27	55
GRAND TOTAL	394	4.3	20	1	2	3	5	8	12	23

614.4: CHRONIC PARAMETRITIS

Type of Patients	Observed Patients	Avg. Stay	Variance	10th	25th	50th	75th	90th	95th	99th
1. SINGLE DX										
A. *Not Operated*										
0–19 Years	4	3.8	4	1	1	4	6	6	6	6
20–34	3	3.7	<1	3	3	4	4	4	4	4
35–49	6	3.5	4	2	2	2	5	7	7	7
50–64	1	2.0	0	2	2	2	2	2	2	2
65+	0									
B. *Operated*										
0–19 Years	0									
20–34	1	3.0	0	3	3	3	3	3	3	3
35–49	2	3.5	<1	3	3	3	4	4	4	4
50–64	0									
65+	1	6.0	0	6	6	6	6	6	6	6
2. MULTIPLE DX										
A. *Not Operated*										
0–19 Years	8	6.9	14	2	4	8	11	12	12	12
20–34	35	4.4	12	1	2	3	5	8	13	18
35–49	66	5.1	11	2	3	4	6	10	13	17
50–64	70	5.6	19	2	3	5	6	9	14	24
65+	30	7.9	37	3	4	5	10	21	22	23
B. *Operated*										
0–19 Years	7	16.1	951	1	2	5	10	86	86	86
20–34	25	5.3	16	2	3	4	7	12	15	17
35–49	53	5.9	38	2	3	4	8	10	14	42
50–64	24	4.4	6	2	2	4	6	7	10	11
65+	13	6.8	17	2	4	7	9	13	14	14
SUBTOTALS:										
1. SINGLE DX										
A. *Not Operated*	14	3.5	3	2	2	4	4	6	7	7
B. *Operated*	4	4.0	2	3	3	3	4	6	6	6
2. MULTIPLE DX										
A. *Not Operated*	209	5.6	19	2	3	4	7	11	14	22
B. *Operated*	122	6.2	76	2	3	4	7	11	14	42
1. SINGLE DX	18	3.6	3	2	2	3	4	6	7	7
2. MULTIPLE DX	331	5.8	40	2	3	4	7	11	14	23
A. NOT OPERATED	223	5.5	18	2	3	4	6	11	13	22
B. OPERATED	126	6.1	74	2	3	4	7	11	14	42
TOTAL										
0–19 Years	19	9.6	350	1	3	5	9	12	86	86
20–34	64	4.7	13	2	3	4	6	8	13	18
35–49	127	5.3	22	2	3	4	7	10	13	17
50–64	95	5.2	16	2	3	4	6	9	13	24
65+	44	7.5	30	2	4	6	10	14	21	23
GRAND TOTAL	349	5.7	38	2	3	4	7	11	14	23

614.6: FE PELVIC PERITON ADHES

Type of Patients	Observed Patients	Avg. Stay	Variance	10th	25th	50th	75th	90th	95th	99th
1. SINGLE DX										
A. *Not Operated*										
0–19 Years	0									
20–34	2	1.5	<1	1	1	2	2	2	2	2
35–49	0									
50–64	0									
65+	0									
B. *Operated*										
0–19 Years	3	1.3	<1	1	1	1	2	2	2	2
20–34	19	2.0	<1	1	1	2	3	3	3	3
35–49	20	2.3	<1	1	2	2	3	3	4	4
50–64	3	2.0	0	2	2	2	2	2	2	2
65+	0									
2. MULTIPLE DX										
A. *Not Operated*										
0–19 Years	0									
20–34	9	2.4	2	1	1	3	3	4	4	4
35–49	7	2.4	<1	2	2	2	3	3	3	3
50–64	6	3.3	19	1	1	1	3	12	12	12
65+	1	4.0	0	4	4	4	4	4	4	4
B. *Operated*										
0–19 Years	6	2.7	2	1	1	3	3	5	5	5
20–34	277	2.5	2	1	2	2	3	4	5	9
35–49	532	2.8	9	1	2	2	3	4	6	16
50–64	132	3.1	7	1	2	2	3	5	8	18
65+	29	3.0	6	2	2	2	3	9	9	11
SUBTOTALS:										
1. SINGLE DX										
A. *Not Operated*	2	1.5	<1	1	1	2	2	2	2	2
B. *Operated*	45	2.1	<1	1	1	2	3	3	3	4
2. MULTIPLE DX										
A. *Not Operated*	23	2.7	5	1	1	2	3	4	4	12
B. *Operated*	976	2.8	6	1	2	2	3	4	6	14
1. SINGLE DX	47	2.0	<1	1	1	2	3	3	3	4
2. MULTIPLE DX	999	2.8	6	1	2	2	3	4	6	12
A. NOT OPERATED	25	2.6	5	1	1	2	3	4	4	12
B. OPERATED	1,021	2.7	6	1	2	2	3	4	6	12
TOTAL										
0–19 Years	9	2.2	2	1	1	2	3	5	5	5
20–34	307	2.5	2	1	2	2	3	4	5	9
35–49	559	2.8	8	1	2	2	3	4	6	16
50–64	141	3.1	8	1	2	2	3	5	8	18
65+	30	3.1	6	2	2	2	3	5	9	11
GRAND TOTAL	1,046	2.7	6	1	2	2	3	4	6	12

Length of Stay by Diagnosis and Operation, Western Region, 2008

Western Region, October 2006–September 2007 Data, by Diagnosis

614.9: FE PELV INFLAM DIS NOS

Type of Patients	Observed Patients	Avg. Stay	Vari-ance	Percentiles 10th	25th	50th	75th	90th	95th	99th
1. SINGLE DX										
A. Not Operated										
0–19 Years	40	2.1	1	1	1	2	3	4	5	5
20–34	100	2.2	1	1	1	2	3	4	4	6
35–49	36	2.4	1	1	2	2	3	4	5	6
50–64	1	1.0	0	1	1	1	1	1	1	1
65+	0									
B. Operated										
0–19 Years	4	2.0	<1	1	2	2	2	3	3	3
20–34	7	2.2	<1	1	1	2	3	3	3	3
35–49	3	3.3	10	1	1	2	7	7	7	7
50–64	1	2.0	0	2	2	2	2	2	2	2
65+	0									
2. MULTIPLE DX										
A. Not Operated										
0–19 Years	144	2.6	2	1	2	2	3	5	5	7
20–34	444	2.7	2	1	2	2	3	5	5	8
35–49	199	2.9	3	1	2	3	4	5	6	9
50–64	38	4.0	6	2	2	3	5	7	8	14
65+	2	1.5	<1	1	1	2	2	2	2	2
B. Operated										
0–19 Years	20	3.0	3	1	2	3	4	5	6	7
20–34	72	3.6	5	1	2	3	5	6	9	12
35–49	53	4.3	12	1	2	3	5	9	12	18
50–64	15	5.3	10	2	2	5	9	9	11	11
65+	1	8.0	0	8	8	8	8	8	8	8
SUBTOTALS:										
1. SINGLE DX										
A. Not Operated	177	2.2	1	1	1	2	3	4	5	6
B. Operated	15	2.3	2	1	1	2	3	3	5	7
2. MULTIPLE DX										
A. Not Operated	827	2.8	3	1	2	2	3	5	6	8
B. Operated	161	3.9	8	1	2	3	5	8	9	13
1. SINGLE DX	192	2.2	1	1	1	2	3	4	5	6
2. MULTIPLE DX	988	3.0	4	1	2	3	4	5	7	11
A. NOT OPERATED	1,004	2.7	3	1	2	2	3	5	6	8
B. OPERATED	176	3.8	8	1	2	3	5	8	9	13
TOTAL										
0–19 Years	208	2.5	2	1	2	2	3	5	5	7
20–34	623	2.7	3	1	2	2	3	5	6	9
35–49	291	3.1	5	1	2	3	4	5	7	13
50–64	55	4.3	8	2	2	4	6	8	9	14
65+	3	3.6	14	1	1	2	2	8	8	8
GRAND TOTAL	1,180	2.8	3	1	2	2	3	5	6	10

615: UTERINE INFLAMMATORY DIS

Type of Patients	Observed Patients	Avg. Stay	Vari-ance	Percentiles 10th	25th	50th	75th	90th	95th	99th
1. SINGLE DX										
A. Not Operated										
0–19 Years	3	2.3	<1	2	2	2	3	3	3	3
20–34	16	2.1	2	2	1	2	3	5	5	5
35–49	4	2.8	2	2	2	2	5	5	5	5
50–64	2	2.0	2	1	1	1	3	3	3	3
65+	0									
B. Operated										
0–19 Years	1	2.0	0	2	2	2	2	2	2	2
20–34	1	1.0	0	1	1	1	1	1	1	1
35–49	2	3.0	2	2	2	2	4	4	4	4
50–64	0									
65+	0									
2. MULTIPLE DX										
A. Not Operated										
0–19 Years	11	2.1	<1	1	1	2	3	3	4	4
20–34	69	2.4	2	1	2	2	3	4	5	7
35–49	58	3.0	4	1	2	2	4	6	8	11
50–64	12	2.6	1	2	2	2	3	4	5	5
65+	10	3.5	12	1	3	2	4	11	11	11
B. Operated										
0–19 Years	1	1.0	0	1	1	1	1	1	1	1
20–34	27	3.7	10	1	2	3	4	8	9	15
35–49	29	3.1	5	1	2	3	4	5	7	10
50–64	13	5.2	18	2	2	3	6	11	16	16
65+	19	4.7	20	1	2	4	5	12	19	19
SUBTOTALS:										
1. SINGLE DX										
A. Not Operated	25	2.2	2	1	1	2	3	5	5	5
B. Operated	4	2.2	2	1	1	2	2	4	4	4
2. MULTIPLE DX										
A. Not Operated	160	2.7	3	1	2	2	3	5	6	11
B. Operated	89	3.9	12	1	2	3	5	8	11	19
1. SINGLE DX	29	2.2	1	1	1	2	3	5	5	5
2. MULTIPLE DX	249	3.1	7	1	2	2	4	6	8	15
A. NOT OPERATED	185	2.6	3	1	2	2	3	5	6	11
B. OPERATED	93	3.8	11	1	2	3	5	8	11	19
TOTAL										
0–19 Years	16	2.1	<1	1	1	2	2	3	4	4
20–34	113	2.7	4	1	2	2	3	5	7	9
35–49	93	3.0	4	1	2	2	4	6	8	11
50–64	27	3.8	11	1	2	3	5	7	11	16
65+	29	4.3	17	1	2	3	5	11	12	19
GRAND TOTAL	278	3.0	6	1	2	2	3	5	8	15

616: OTH FEMALE GENIT INFLAM

Type of Patients	Observed Patients	Avg. Stay	Vari-ance	Percentiles 10th	25th	50th	75th	90th	95th	99th
1. SINGLE DX										
A. Not Operated										
0–19 Years	8	2.8	1	1	2	3	3	3	5	5
20–34	10	2.7	1	2	2	2	3	5	5	5
35–49	10	1.9	1	1	1	2	2	3	4	4
50–64	2	4.0	8	2	2	4	6	6	6	6
65+	1	1.0	0	1	1	1	1	1	1	1
B. Operated										
0–19 Years	28	2.2	2	1	1	2	2	4	6	6
20–34	38	2.0	2	1	1	2	2	4	6	6
35–49	19	1.7	1	1	2	2	2	4	4	4
50–64	4	2.3	<1	2	2	2	3	3	3	3
65+	2	2.0	2	1	1	3	3	3	3	3
2. MULTIPLE DX										
A. Not Operated										
0–19 Years	71	3.0	3	1	2	3	4	5	7	11
20–34	98	3.0	5	1	2	3	4	6	6	14
35–49	124	3.0	4	1	2	3	4	6	7	9
50–64	89	4.2	6	2	2	4	5	8	9	12
65+	83	4.7	8	1	3	4	6	8	10	16
B. Operated										
0–19 Years	89	3.8	4	2	3	3	4	6	8	12
20–34	139	2.7	5	1	1	2	3	6	8	9
35–49	322	3.2	7	1	2	2	4	6	8	11
50–64	182	4.4	25	2	2	3	5	8	12	33
65+	89	4.5	13	1	2	4	5	9	11	20
SUBTOTALS:										
1. SINGLE DX										
A. Not Operated	31	2.5	2	1	2	2	3	4	5	6
B. Operated	91	2.0	2	1	1	2	2	4	4	6
2. MULTIPLE DX										
A. Not Operated	465	3.5	5	1	2	3	4	7	8	11
B. Operated	821	3.6	11	1	2	3	4	7	9	15
1. SINGLE DX	122	2.1	2	1	1	2	3	4	5	6
2. MULTIPLE DX	1,286	3.6	9	1	2	3	4	7	9	14
A. NOT OPERATED	496	3.5	5	1	2	3	4	7	8	11
B. OPERATED	912	3.4	10	1	2	3	4	7	9	14
TOTAL										
0–19 Years	196	3.3	4	1	2	3	4	6	7	11
20–34	285	2.7	4	1	1	2	3	5	7	11
35–49	475	3.1	6	1	2	3	4	6	7	11
50–64	277	4.3	19	1	2	3	5	8	11	25
65+	175	4.5	11	1	2	4	6	8	10	19
GRAND TOTAL	1,408	3.4	9	1	2	3	4	7	8	14

Length of Stay by Diagnosis and Operation, Western Region, 2008

Western Region, October 2006–September 2007 Data, by Diagnosis

616.0: CERVICITIS

Type of Patients	Observed Patients	Avg. Stay	Variance	10th	25th	50th	75th	90th	95th	99th
1. SINGLE DX										
A. Not Operated										
0–19 Years	0									
20–34	1	2.0	0	2	2	2	2	2	2	2
35–49	0									
50–64	0									
65+	0									
B. Operated										
0–19 Years	0									
20–34	1	6.0	0	6	6	6	6	6	6	6
35–49	1	1.0	0	1	1	1	1	1	1	1
50–64	0									
65+	0									
2. MULTIPLE DX										
A. Not Operated										
0–19 Years	2	2.0	2	1	1	2	3	3	3	3
20–34	13	2.0	1	1	1	2	2	4	4	4
35–49	10	1.9	2	1	1	1	3	5	5	5
50–64	5	2.2	2	1	2	2	3	4	4	4
65+	1	1.0	0	1	1	1	1	1	1	1
B. Operated										
0–19 Years	0									
20–34	55	2.1	2	1	1	2	2	3	7	8
35–49	172	2.5	2	1	2	2	3	4	5	9
50–64	48	2.4	1	1	2	2	3	4	4	8
65+	5	4.2	6	1	3	4	6	7	7	7
SUBTOTALS:										
1. SINGLE DX										
A. Not Operated	1	2.0	0	2	2	2	2	2	2	2
B. Operated	2	3.5	12	1	1	6	6	6	6	6
2. MULTIPLE DX										
A. Not Operated	31	2.0	1	1	1	2	3	4	4	5
B. Operated	280	2.4	2	1	2	2	3	4	5	9
1. SINGLE DX	3	3.0	7	1	1	2	6	6	6	6
2. MULTIPLE DX	311	2.4	2	1	1	2	3	4	5	8
A. NOT OPERATED	32	2.0	1	1	1	2	2	4	4	5
B. OPERATED	282	2.4	2	1	2	2	3	4	5	9
TOTAL										
0–19 Years	2	2.0	2	1	1	2	3	3	3	3
20–34	70	2.1	2	1	1	2	2	4	6	8
35–49	183	2.5	2	1	2	2	3	4	5	9
50–64	53	2.3	1	1	2	2	3	4	4	8
65+	6	3.7	6	1	1	4	6	7	7	7
GRAND TOTAL	314	2.4	2	1	2	2	3	4	5	8

616.10: VAGINITIS NOS

Type of Patients	Observed Patients	Avg. Stay	Variance	10th	25th	50th	75th	90th	95th	99th
1. SINGLE DX										
A. Not Operated										
0–19 Years	5	3.0	1	2	2	3	3	5	5	5
20–34	4	2.8	<1	2	2	3	4	4	4	4
35–49	4	1.3	<1	1	1	1	1	2	2	2
50–64	2	4.0	8	2	2	4	6	6	6	6
65+	0									
B. Operated										
0–19 Years	1	3.0	0	3	3	3	3	3	3	3
20–34	4	2.5	6	1	1	2	6	6	6	6
35–49	4	2.5	<1	2	2	2	2	4	4	4
50–64	0									
65+	0									
2. MULTIPLE DX										
A. Not Operated										
0–19 Years	33	2.9	3	1	2	2	3	5	7	8
20–34	46	2.8	2	1	1	3	4	5	5	7
35–49	61	3.2	5	1	2	3	4	7	8	11
50–64	51	4.2	8	2	2	3	6	8	10	12
65+	46	4.4	7	3	2	4	6	8	10	11
B. Operated										
0–19 Years	14	3.7	7	2	3	3	4	4	12	12
20–34	9	2.9	3	1	1	3	4	6	6	6
35–49	22	3.4	4	1	2	3	4	7	7	8
50–64	21	7.5	89	2	3	4	7	12	25	42
65+	16	5.3	18	4	4	4	6	8	20	20
SUBTOTALS:										
1. SINGLE DX										
A. Not Operated	15	2.6	2	1	2	2	3	5	6	6
B. Operated	9	2.6	3	1	2	3	3	6	6	6
2. MULTIPLE DX										
A. Not Operated	237	3.5	5	1	2	3	4	7	8	11
B. Operated	82	4.8	31	1	3	4	5	8	12	42
1. SINGLE DX	24	2.6	2	1	2	2	3	5	6	6
2. MULTIPLE DX	319	3.9	12	1	2	3	5	7	9	12
A. NOT OPERATED	252	3.5	5	1	2	3	4	7	8	11
B. OPERATED	91	4.6	28	1	2	3	5	7	12	42
TOTAL										
0–19 Years	53	3.1	4	1	2	3	4	5	7	12
20–34	63	2.8	2	1	1	3	4	5	6	7
35–49	91	3.1	4	1	2	3	4	7	8	11
50–64	74	5.1	32	2	2	4	6	9	12	42
65+	62	4.6	10	2	3	4	6	8	10	20
GRAND TOTAL	343	3.8	12	1	2	3	4	7	8	12

616.4: VULVAR ABSCESS NEC

Type of Patients	Observed Patients	Avg. Stay	Variance	10th	25th	50th	75th	90th	95th	99th
1. SINGLE DX										
A. Not Operated										
0–19 Years	1	3.0	0	3	3	3	3	3	3	3
20–34	4	3.0	2	2	2	2	3	5	5	5
35–49	5	2.6	1	1	2	3	3	4	4	4
50–64	0									
65+	1	1.0	0	1	1	1	1	1	1	1
B. Operated										
0–19 Years	20	2.1	2	1	1	2	2	4	6	6
20–34	14	2.4	1	1	1	2	3	4	4	4
35–49	5	1.8	2	1	1	1	2	4	4	4
50–64	1	2.0	0	2	2	2	2	2	2	2
65+	1	3.0	0	3	3	3	3	3	3	3
2. MULTIPLE DX										
A. Not Operated										
0–19 Years	33	3.2	4	2	2	3	4	4	7	11
20–34	31	4.0	9	1	2	3	5	5	11	14
35–49	43	3.1	8	1	2	3	4	5	6	8
50–64	25	4.7	5	2	3	5	5	8	9	11
65+	35	5.3	8	3	4	4	6	9	11	16
B. Operated										
0–19 Years	71	3.8	3	2	2	3	5	6	7	11
20–34	43	4.0	8	1	2	3	6	8	9	14
35–49	96	4.6	14	1	2	4	6	9	11	29
50–64	92	5.2	23	1	2	4	6	11	14	33
65+	55	4.6	10	1	2	4	6	10	11	15
SUBTOTALS:										
1. SINGLE DX										
A. Not Operated	11	2.6	1	1	2	3	3	4	5	5
B. Operated	41	2.2	1	1	1	2	3	4	4	6
2. MULTIPLE DX										
A. Not Operated	167	4.0	6	2	2	3	5	7	9	14
B. Operated	357	4.5	13	1	2	4	6	8	11	16
1. SINGLE DX	52	2.3	1	1	1	2	3	4	4	6
2. MULTIPLE DX	524	4.4	11	1	2	4	5	8	11	15
A. NOT OPERATED	178	3.9	6	2	2	3	5	7	9	14
B. OPERATED	398	4.3	12	1	2	3	5	8	11	16
TOTAL										
0–19 Years	125	3.3	4	1	2	3	4	6	7	11
20–34	92	3.7	7	1	2	3	4	7	9	14
35–49	149	4.0	10	1	2	3	5	7	9	12
50–64	118	5.1	19	1	3	4	6	10	13	22
65+	92	4.8	10	2	3	4	6	9	11	16
GRAND TOTAL	576	4.2	10	1	2	3	5	7	10	15

Length of Stay by Diagnosis and Operation, Western Region, 2008

Western Region, October 2006–September 2007 Data, by Diagnosis

617: ENDOMETRIOSIS

Type of Patients	Observed Patients	Avg. Stay	Variance	10th	25th	50th	75th	90th	95th	99th
1. SINGLE DX										
A. Not Operated										
0–19 Years	2	1.5	<1	1	1	1	1	2	2	2
20–34	12	2.8	5	1	1	2	2	5	6	8
35–49	4	2.5	2	1	2	3	4	4	4	4
50–64	2	2.5	<1	2	2	2	3	3	3	3
65+	0									
B. Operated										
0–19 Years	1	4.0	0	4	4	4	4	4	4	4
20–34	94	1.9	<1	1	1	2	2	3	3	4
35–49	132	2.0	<1	1	1	2	3	3	3	4
50–64	25	2.2	1	1	1	2	3	4	4	4
65+	0									
2. MULTIPLE DX										
A. Not Operated										
0–19 Years	9	2.3	3	1	1	1	3	6	6	6
20–34	93	2.4	2	1	1	2	3	5	5	8
35–49	67	2.6	3	1	1	2	3	5	6	8
50–64	10	2.4	5	1	1	1	3	4	8	8
65+	1	2.0	0	2	2	2	2	2	2	2
B. Operated										
0–19 Years	29	2.7	3	1	1	2	3	6	7	7
20–34	2,120	2.4	2	1	2	2	3	4	5	8
35–49	6,205	2.4	2	1	2	2	3	4	4	7
50–64	1,260	2.6	4	1	2	2	3	4	5	10
65+	75	3.1	7	1	2	3	4	5	7	16
SUBTOTALS:										
1. SINGLE DX										
A. Not Operated	20	2.6	4	1	1	2	3	6	8	8
B. Operated	252	2.0	<1	1	1	2	2	3	3	4
2. MULTIPLE DX										
A. Not Operated	180	2.4	3	1	1	2	3	4	6	8
B. Operated	9,689	2.4	2	1	2	2	3	4	5	8
1. SINGLE DX	272	2.0	<1	1	1	2	3	3	4	5
2. MULTIPLE DX	9,869	2.4	2	1	2	2	3	4	5	8
A. NOT OPERATED	200	2.5	3	1	1	2	3	4	6	8
B. OPERATED	9,941	2.4	2	1	2	2	3	4	5	8
TOTAL										
0–19 Years	41	2.6	3	1	1	2	3	5	6	7
20–34	2,319	2.3	2	1	1	2	3	4	5	8
35–49	6,408	2.4	2	2	2	2	3	4	4	7
50–64	1,297	2.6	4	1	2	3	3	4	5	9
65+	76	3.1	7	1	2	3	4	5	7	16
GRAND TOTAL	10,141	2.4	2	1	2	2	3	4	5	8

617.0: UTERINE ENDOMETRIOSIS

Type of Patients	Observed Patients	Avg. Stay	Variance	10th	25th	50th	75th	90th	95th	99th
1. SINGLE DX										
A. Not Operated										
0–19 Years	0									
20–34	0									
35–49	2	2.5	4	1	1	2	4	4	4	4
50–64	1	2.0	0	2	2	2	2	2	2	2
65+	0									
B. Operated										
0–19 Years	0									
20–34	28	1.9	<1	1	1	2	2	3	3	3
35–49	59	2.0	<1	1	1	2	3	3	3	3
50–64	12	2.1	<1	1	1	2	3	4	4	4
65+	0									
2. MULTIPLE DX										
A. Not Operated										
0–19 Years	2	2.5	4	1	1	2	4	4	4	4
20–34	22	2.5	2	1	1	2	3	4	4	7
35–49	23	3.1	4	2	2	2	4	6	7	8
50–64	5	1.6	<1	1	1	1	2	3	3	3
65+	0									
B. Operated										
0–19 Years	10	2.9	5	1	1	2	3	6	7	7
20–34	927	2.3	1	1	1	2	3	3	4	7
35–49	3,793	2.3	1	1	1	2	3	3	4	6
50–64	857	2.4	3	1	2	2	3	4	5	7
65+	48	2.7	5	1	1	3	3	5	5	16
SUBTOTALS:										
1. SINGLE DX										
A. Not Operated	3	2.3	2	1	1	2	4	4	4	4
B. Operated	99	2.0	<1	1	1	2	2	3	3	4
2. MULTIPLE DX										
A. Not Operated	52	2.7	3	1	1	2	4	5	7	8
B. Operated	5,635	2.3	2	1	2	2	3	3	4	6
1. SINGLE DX	102	2.0	<1	1	1	2	3	3	3	4
2. MULTIPLE DX	5,687	2.3	2	1	2	2	3	4	5	6
A. NOT OPERATED	55	2.6	3	1	1	2	4	5	7	8
B. OPERATED	5,734	2.3	2	1	2	2	3	4	5	6
TOTAL										
0–19 Years	12	2.8	5	1	1	2	3	5	6	7
20–34	977	2.2	1	1	1	2	3	3	4	7
35–49	3,877	2.3	1	1	1	2	3	3	4	6
50–64	875	2.4	3	1	2	2	3	4	5	7
65+	48	2.7	5	1	1	3	3	5	5	16
GRAND TOTAL	5,789	2.3	2	1	2	2	3	3	4	6

617.1: OVARIAN ENDOMETRIOSIS

Type of Patients	Observed Patients	Avg. Stay	Variance	10th	25th	50th	75th	90th	95th	99th
1. SINGLE DX										
A. Not Operated										
0–19 Years	0									
20–34	4	2.0	<1	1	2	2	3	3	3	3
35–49	0									
50–64	0									
65+	0									
B. Operated										
0–19 Years	1	4.0	0	4	4	4	4	4	4	4
20–34	46	2.0	<1	1	1	2	2	3	3	4
35–49	46	2.0	<1	1	1	2	2	3	3	4
50–64	8	2.1	<1	1	1	2	3	3	3	3
65+	0									
2. MULTIPLE DX										
A. Not Operated										
0–19 Years	0									
20–34	6	1.5	<1	1	1	1	2	3	3	3
35–49	9	1.8	<1	1	1	2	2	3	3	3
50–64	1	1.0	0	1	1	1	1	1	1	1
65+	0									
B. Operated										
0–19 Years	11	2.4	1	1	1	2	3	4	4	4
20–34	555	2.4	2	1	2	2	3	3	4	8
35–49	1,205	2.6	4	1	2	2	3	4	5	8
50–64	247	3.0	6	1	2	3	3	5	7	13
65+	17	3.1	3	1	2	3	4	5	7	7
SUBTOTALS:										
1. SINGLE DX										
A. Not Operated	4	2.0	<1	1	2	2	3	3	3	3
B. Operated	101	2.0	<1	1	1	2	2	3	3	4
2. MULTIPLE DX										
A. Not Operated	16	1.6	<1	1	1	1	2	3	3	3
B. Operated	2,035	2.6	4	1	2	2	3	4	5	9
1. SINGLE DX	105	2.0	<1	1	1	2	2	3	3	4
2. MULTIPLE DX	2,051	2.6	4	1	2	2	3	4	5	9
A. NOT OPERATED	20	1.7	<1	1	1	1	2	3	3	3
B. OPERATED	2,136	2.6	4	1	2	2	3	4	5	9
TOTAL										
0–19 Years	12	2.5	1	1	1	2	2	4	4	4
20–34	611	2.4	2	1	2	2	3	4	4	7
35–49	1,260	2.6	4	1	2	2	3	4	5	8
50–64	256	3.0	6	1	2	3	3	5	7	13
65+	17	3.1	3	1	2	3	4	5	7	7
GRAND TOTAL	2,156	2.6	3	1	2	2	3	4	5	9

Length of Stay by Diagnosis and Operation, Western Region, 2008

617.3: PELV PERIT ENDOMETRIOSIS

Type of Patients	Observed Patients	Avg. Stay	Vari- ance	Percentiles						
				10th	25th	50th	75th	90th	95th	99th
1. SINGLE DX										
A. Not Operated										
0–19 Years	0									
20–34	3	1.0	0	1	1	1	1	1	1	1
35–49	1	3.0	0	3	3	3	3	3	3	3
50–64	0									
65+	0									
B. Operated										
0–19 Years	0									
20–34	14	1.5	<1	1	1	1	2	2	3	3
35–49	13	1.9	<1	1	1	2	2	3	4	4
50–64	2	2.5	4	1	1	1	4	4	4	4
65+	0									
2. MULTIPLE DX										
A. Not Operated										
0–19 Years	2	1.0	0	1	1	1	1	1	1	1
20–34	23	2.8	2	1	2	3	4	5	5	5
35–49	18	2.5	2	1	1	2	4	4	6	6
50–64	0									
65+	1	2.0	0	2	2	2	2	2	2	2
B. Operated										
0–19 Years	7	3.3	4	2	2	3	5	7	7	7
20–34	468	2.3	2	1	1	2	3	4	5	9
35–49	873	2.3	2	1	1	2	3	4	5	7
50–64	103	2.7	2	1	2	2	3	5	5	7
65+	8	5.9	22	2	4	4	9	16	16	16
SUBTOTALS:										
1. SINGLE DX *A. Not Operated*	4	1.5	<1	1	1	1	1	3	3	3
B. Operated	29	1.7	<1	1	1	1	2	3	4	4
2. MULTIPLE DX *A. Not Operated*	44	2.6	2	1	1	2	3	4	5	6
B. Operated	1,459	2.4	2	1	1	2	3	4	5	8
1. SINGLE DX	33	1.7	<1	1	1	1	2	3	4	4
2. MULTIPLE DX	1,503	2.4	2	1	1	2	3	4	5	8
A. NOT OPERATED	48	2.5	2	1	1	2	3	4	5	6
B. OPERATED	1,488	2.4	2	1	1	2	3	4	5	8
TOTAL										
0–19 Years	9	2.8	4	1	1	2	3	7	7	7
20–34	508	2.3	2	1	1	2	3	4	5	9
35–49	905	2.3	2	1	1	2	3	4	5	7
50–64	105	2.7	2	1	2	2	3	5	5	7
65+	9	5.5	21	2	2	4	6	16	16	16
GRAND TOTAL	1,536	2.4	2	1	1	2	3	4	5	8

617.9: ENDOMETRIOSIS NOS

Type of Patients	Observed Patients	Avg. Stay	Vari- ance	Percentiles						
				10th	25th	50th	75th	90th	95th	99th
1. SINGLE DX										
A. Not Operated										
0–19 Years	2	1.5	<1	1	1	1	2	2	2	2
20–34	4	5.3	6	2	5	6	6	8	8	8
35–49	0									
50–64	0									
65+	0									
B. Operated										
0–19 Years	0									
20–34	4	2.8	<1	2	2	2	3	4	4	4
35–49	8	2.1	<1	1	2	2	2	3	3	3
50–64	0									
65+	0									
2. MULTIPLE DX										
A. Not Operated										
0–19 Years	5	2.8	4	1	1	3	3	6	6	6
20–34	38	2.3	2	1	1	2	3	4	5	8
35–49	10	2.0	2	1	1	2	2	6	6	6
50–64	3	4.7	9	2	2	4	8	8	8	8
65+	0									
B. Operated										
0–19 Years	0									
20–34	71	2.3	2	1	1	2	3	4	5	6
35–49	103	2.1	1	1	1	2	3	3	4	7
50–64	13	1.9	<1	1	2	2	2	3	3	3
65+	1	2.0	0	2	2	2	2	2	2	2
SUBTOTALS:										
1. SINGLE DX *A. Not Operated*	6	4.0	8	1	2	5	6	8	8	8
B. Operated	12	2.3	<1	2	2	2	3	3	4	4
2. MULTIPLE DX *A. Not Operated*	56	2.4	3	1	1	2	3	4	6	8
B. Operated	188	2.2	1	1	1	2	3	3	4	7
1. SINGLE DX	18	2.9	3	1	2	2	3	6	8	8
2. MULTIPLE DX	244	2.2	2	1	1	2	3	4	5	8
A. NOT OPERATED	62	2.6	3	1	1	2	3	5	6	8
B. OPERATED	200	2.2	1	1	1	2	3	3	4	7
TOTAL										
0–19 Years	7	2.4	3	1	1	2	3	6	6	6
20–34	117	2.4	2	1	1	2	3	4	5	8
35–49	121	2.1	1	1	1	2	3	3	4	7
50–64	16	2.4	3	1	2	2	3	4	8	8
65+	1	2.0	0	2	2	2	2	2	2	2
GRAND TOTAL	262	2.3	2	1	1	2	3	4	5	8

618: GENITAL PROLAPSE

Type of Patients	Observed Patients	Avg. Stay	Vari- ance	Percentiles						
				10th	25th	50th	75th	90th	95th	99th
1. SINGLE DX										
A. Not Operated										
0–19 Years	0									
20–34	0									
35–49	2	1.0	0	1	1	1	1	1	1	1
50–64	2	2.0	0	2	2	2	2	2	2	2
65+	1	1.0	0	1	1	1	1	1	1	1
B. Operated										
0–19 Years	0									
20–34	42	1.6	<1	1	1	2	2	2	2	3
35–49	201	1.7	<1	1	1	2	2	3	3	4
50–64	478	1.7	<1	1	1	2	2	3	3	4
65+	291	1.7	<1	1	1	2	2	3	3	4
2. MULTIPLE DX										
A. Not Operated										
0–19 Years	0									
20–34	1	2.0	0	2	2	2	2	2	2	2
35–49	24	2.2	11	1	1	1	2	3	4	17
50–64	50	1.6	2	1	1	1	2	3	4	8
65+	76	2.1	8	1	1	1	2	4	5	23
B. Operated										
0–19 Years	0									
20–34	675	1.9	<1	1	1	2	2	3	3	4
35–49	4,604	1.9	<1	1	1	2	2	3	3	5
50–64	8,485	1.9	1	1	1	2	2	3	3	5
65+	8,402	2.0	2	1	1	2	2	3	4	7
SUBTOTALS:										
1. SINGLE DX *A. Not Operated*	5	1.4	<1	1	1	1	2	2	2	2
B. Operated	1,012	1.7	<1	1	1	2	2	3	3	4
2. MULTIPLE DX *A. Not Operated*	151	2.0	6	1	1	2	2	3	5	17
B. Operated	22,166	2.0	1	1	1	2	2	3	4	6
1. SINGLE DX	1,017	1.7	<1	1	1	2	2	3	3	4
2. MULTIPLE DX	22,317	2.0	1	1	1	2	2	3	4	6
A. NOT OPERATED	156	2.0	6	1	1	1	2	3	5	17
B. OPERATED	23,178	1.9	1	1	1	2	2	3	4	6
TOTAL										
0–19 Years	0									
20–34	718	1.8	<1	1	1	2	2	3	3	4
35–49	4,831	1.9	<1	1	1	2	2	3	3	5
50–64	9,015	1.9	<1	1	1	2	2	3	3	5
65+	8,770	2.0	2	1	1	2	2	3	4	7
GRAND TOTAL	23,334	1.9	1	1	1	2	2	3	4	6

Length of Stay by Diagnosis and Operation, Western Region, 2008

Western Region, October 2006–September 2007 Data, by Diagnosis

618.01: MIDLINE CYSTOCELE

Type of Patients	Observed Patients	Avg. Stay	Vari-ance	Percentiles						
				10th	25th	50th	75th	90th	95th	99th
1. SINGLE DX										
A. Not Operated										
0–19 Years	0									
20–34	0									
35–49	0									
50–64	0									
65+	0									
B. Operated										
0–19 Years	0									
20–34	1	1.0	0	1	1	1	1	1	1	1
35–49	10	1.5	<1	1	1	1	2	2	3	3
50–64	43	1.3	<1	1	1	1	1	2	2	3
65+	30	1.4	<1	1	1	1	2	2	2	4
2. MULTIPLE DX										
A. Not Operated										
0–19 Years	0									
20–34	0									
35–49	4	1.3	<1	1	1	1	1	2	2	2
50–64	7	1.7	<1	1	1	2	2	3	3	3
65+	7	2.3	3	1	1	1	4	5	5	5
B. Operated										
0–19 Years	0									
20–34	93	1.6	<1	1	1	2	2	2	3	4
35–49	603	1.6	<1	1	1	1	2	3	3	4
50–64	1,158	1.6	<1	1	1	1	2	3	3	4
65+	1,232	1.7	1	1	1	1	2	3	3	6
SUBTOTALS:										
1. SINGLE DX										
A. Not Operated	0									
B. Operated	84	1.4	<1	1	1	1	2	2	2	4
2. MULTIPLE DX										
A. Not Operated	18	1.8	1	1	1	1	2	4	5	5
B. Operated	3,086	1.7	<1	1	1	1	2	3	3	5
1. SINGLE DX	84	1.4	<1	1	1	1	2	2	2	4
2. MULTIPLE DX	3,104	1.7	<1	1	1	1	2	3	3	5
A. NOT OPERATED	18	1.8	1	1	1	1	2	4	5	5
B. OPERATED	3,170	1.7	<1	1	1	1	2	3	3	5
TOTAL										
0–19 Years	0									
20–34	94	1.6	<1	1	1	2	2	2	3	4
35–49	617	1.6	<1	1	1	1	2	3	3	4
50–64	1,208	1.6	<1	1	1	1	2	3	3	4
65+	1,269	1.7	1	1	1	1	2	3	3	6
GRAND TOTAL	3,188	1.7	<1	1	1	1	2	3	3	5

618.04: RECTOCELE

Type of Patients	Observed Patients	Avg. Stay	Vari-ance	Percentiles						
				10th	25th	50th	75th	90th	95th	99th
1. SINGLE DX										
A. Not Operated										
0–19 Years	0									
20–34	0									
35–49	1	1.0	0	1	1	1	1	1	1	1
50–64	0									
65+	0									
B. Operated										
0–19 Years	0									
20–34	8	1.4	<1	1	1	1	2	2	2	2
35–49	14	1.2	<1	1	1	1	1	2	2	2
50–64	39	1.3	<1	1	1	1	2	2	2	3
65+	15	1.3	<1	1	1	1	1	2	3	3
2. MULTIPLE DX										
A. Not Operated										
0–19 Years	0									
20–34	0									
35–49	0									
50–64	4	3.3	10	1	1	2	8	8	8	8
65+	2	1.0	0	1	1	1	1	1	1	1
B. Operated										
0–19 Years	0									
20–34	45	1.7	<1	1	1	1	2	2	3	4
35–49	297	1.7	<1	1	1	1	2	3	3	5
50–64	511	1.5	<1	1	1	1	2	2	3	5
65+	475	1.7	1	1	1	1	2	3	4	5
SUBTOTALS:										
1. SINGLE DX										
A. Not Operated	1	1.0	0	1	1	1	1	1	1	1
B. Operated	76	1.3	<1	1	1	1	2	2	2	3
2. MULTIPLE DX										
A. Not Operated	6	2.5	8	1	1	2	2	8	8	8
B. Operated	1,328	1.6	<1	1	1	1	2	3	3	5
1. SINGLE DX	77	1.3	<1	1	1	1	2	2	2	3
2. MULTIPLE DX	1,334	1.6	1	1	1	1	2	3	3	5
A. NOT OPERATED	7	2.3	7	1	1	1	2	8	8	8
B. OPERATED	1,404	1.6	<1	1	1	1	2	3	3	5
TOTAL										
0–19 Years	0									
20–34	53	1.6	<1	1	1	1	2	2	3	4
35–49	312	1.7	1	1	1	1	2	3	3	5
50–64	554	1.5	<1	1	1	1	2	2	3	5
65+	492	1.6	<1	1	1	1	2	3	3	5
GRAND TOTAL	1,411	1.6	<1	1	1	1	2	3	3	5

618.1: UTERINE PROLAPSE

Type of Patients	Observed Patients	Avg. Stay	Vari-ance	Percentiles						
				10th	25th	50th	75th	90th	95th	99th
1. SINGLE DX										
A. Not Operated										
0–19 Years	0									
20–34	0									
35–49	0									
50–64	0									
65+	0									
B. Operated										
0–19 Years	0									
20–34	10	1.8	<1	1	1	2	2	3	3	3
35–49	38	1.7	<1	1	1	2	2	3	3	4
50–64	39	1.6	<1	1	1	1	2	2	3	3
65+	11	1.5	<1	1	1	1	2	2	2	2
2. MULTIPLE DX										
A. Not Operated										
0–19 Years	0									
20–34	1	2.0	0	2	2	2	2	2	2	2
35–49	9	2.0	1	1	1	1	3	4	4	4
50–64	7	1.4	<1	1	1	1	2	3	3	3
65+	16	2.2	2	1	1	2	3	4	6	6
B. Operated										
0–19 Years	0									
20–34	140	1.8	<1	1	1	2	2	3	3	5
35–49	498	1.9	<1	1	1	2	2	3	3	5
50–64	392	2.0	<1	1	1	1	2	3	4	5
65+	215	2.2	2	1	1	2	3	4	4	8
SUBTOTALS:										
1. SINGLE DX										
A. Not Operated	0									
B. Operated	98	1.6	<1	1	1	2	2	2	3	4
2. MULTIPLE DX										
A. Not Operated	33	2.0	1	1	1	2	3	4	4	6
B. Operated	1,245	1.9	1	1	1	2	2	3	3	5
1. SINGLE DX	98	1.6	<1	1	1	2	2	2	3	4
2. MULTIPLE DX	1,278	1.9	1	1	1	2	2	3	4	5
A. NOT OPERATED	33	2.0	1	1	1	2	3	4	4	6
B. OPERATED	1,343	1.9	<1	1	1	2	2	3	4	5
TOTAL										
0–19 Years	0									
20–34	151	1.8	<1	1	1	2	2	3	3	5
35–49	545	1.9	<1	1	1	2	2	3	3	5
50–64	438	1.9	<1	1	1	2	2	3	4	5
65+	242	2.1	2	1	1	2	3	4	4	8
GRAND TOTAL	1,376	1.9	<1	1	1	2	2	3	4	5

Length of Stay by Diagnosis and Operation, Western Region, 2008

Western Region, October 2006–September 2007 Data, by Diagnosis

618.2: UTEROVAG PROLAP-INCOMPL

Type of Patients	Observed Patients	Avg. Stay	Vari- ance	10th	25th	50th	75th	90th	95th	99th
1. SINGLE DX										
A. Not Operated										
0–19 Years	0									
20–34	0									
35–49	0									
50–64	0									
65+	0									
B. Operated										
0–19 Years	0									
20–34	7	1.7	<1	1	1	2	2	2	2	2
35–49	37	1.8	<1	1	1	2	2	2	3	5
50–64	80	1.8	<1	1	1	2	2	3	3	4
65+	44	1.8	<1	1	1	2	2	3	3	3
2. MULTIPLE DX										
A. Not Operated										
0–19 Years	0									
20–34	0									
35–49	3	1.3	<1	1	1	1	2	2	2	2
50–64	2	1.0	0	1	1	1	2	1	1	1
65+	2	1.0	0	1	1	1	2	1	1	1
B. Operated										
0–19 Years	0									
20–34	161	2.0	<1	1	1	2	3	3	3	6
35–49	1,043	2.0	<1	1	1	2	2	3	3	5
50–64	1,439	2.0	<1	1	1	2	2	3	4	5
65+	886	2.2	2	1	1	2	3	3	4	6
SUBTOTALS:										
1. SINGLE DX										
A. Not Operated	0									
B. Operated	168	1.8	<1	1	1	2	2	3	3	4
2. MULTIPLE DX										
A. Not Operated	7	1.1	<1	1	1	1	1	2	2	2
B. Operated	3,529	2.1	1	1	1	2	2	3	4	5
1. SINGLE DX	168	1.8	<1	1	1	2	2	3	3	4
2. MULTIPLE DX	3,536	2.1	1	1	1	2	2	3	4	5
A. NOT OPERATED	7	1.1	<1	1	1	1	1	2	2	2
B. OPERATED	3,697	2.0	1	1	1	2	2	3	4	5
TOTAL										
0–19 Years	0									
20–34	168	2.0	<1	1	1	2	3	3	3	6
35–49	1,083	2.0	<1	1	1	2	2	3	3	5
50–64	1,521	2.0	<1	1	1	2	2	3	3	5
65+	932	2.1	2	1	1	2	3	3	4	6
GRAND TOTAL	3,704	2.0	1	1	1	2	2	3	4	5

618.3: UTEROVAG PROLAPSE-COMPL

Type of Patients	Observed Patients	Avg. Stay	Vari- ance	10th	25th	50th	75th	90th	95th	99th
1. SINGLE DX										
A. Not Operated										
0–19 Years	0									
20–34	0									
35–49	0									
50–64	0									
65+	1	1.0	0	1	1	1	1	1	1	1
B. Operated										
0–19 Years	0									
20–34	2	2.0	0	2	2	2	2	2	2	2
35–49	31	1.9	<1	1	1	2	2	3	3	4
50–64	66	1.9	<1	1	1	2	2	3	3	4
65+	49	1.8	<1	1	1	2	2	2	3	3
2. MULTIPLE DX										
A. Not Operated										
0–19 Years	0									
20–34	0									
35–49	2	8.9	127	1	1	1	17	17	17	17
50–64	4	2.0	2	1	1	2	2	4	4	4
65+	11	4.4	41	1	1	2	5	6	23	23
B. Operated										
0–19 Years	0									
20–34	36	2.1	1	1	1	2	3	3	3	6
35–49	340	2.1	<1	1	2	2	3	3	4	5
50–64	845	2.1	1	1	1	2	3	3	4	6
65+	1,069	2.4	2	1	2	2	3	4	4	9
SUBTOTALS:										
1. SINGLE DX										
A. Not Operated	1	1.0	0	1	1	1	1	1	1	1
B. Operated	148	1.8	<1	1	1	2	2	3	3	4
2. MULTIPLE DX										
A. Not Operated	17	4.4	38	1	1	2	4	17	23	23
B. Operated	2,290	2.3	2	1	2	2	3	3	4	7
1. SINGLE DX	149	1.8	<1	1	1	2	2	3	3	4
2. MULTIPLE DX	2,307	2.3	2	1	2	2	3	4	4	7
A. NOT OPERATED	18	4.2	36	1	1	2	4	17	23	23
B. OPERATED	2,438	2.2	2	1	2	2	3	3	4	7
TOTAL										
0–19 Years	0									
20–34	38	2.1	1	1	1	2	2	3	3	6
35–49	373	2.2	1	1	1	2	2	3	4	5
50–64	915	2.1	1	1	1	2	3	3	4	6
65+	1,130	2.4	3	1	2	2	3	4	4	9
GRAND TOTAL	2,456	2.2	2	1	2	2	3	4	4	7

618.4: UTEROVAG PROLAPSE NOS

Type of Patients	Observed Patients	Avg. Stay	Vari- ance	10th	25th	50th	75th	90th	95th	99th
1. SINGLE DX										
A. Not Operated										
0–19 Years	0									
20–34	0									
35–49	1	1.0	0	1	1	1	1	1	1	1
50–64	1	2.0	0	2	2	2	2	2	2	2
65+	0									
B. Operated										
0–19 Years	0									
20–34	6	1.7	<1	1	1	2	2	2	2	2
35–49	42	1.7	<1	1	1	2	2	3	3	4
50–64	78	1.9	<1	1	1	2	3	3	3	4
65+	47	1.9	<1	1	1	2	3	3	3	4
2. MULTIPLE DX										
A. Not Operated										
0–19 Years	0									
20–34	0									
35–49	1	1.0	0	1	1	1	1	1	1	1
50–64	7	1.0	0	1	1	1	1	1	1	1
65+	14	1.7	2	1	1	1	2	4	5	5
B. Operated										
0–19 Years	0									
20–34	76	1.9	<1	1	1	2	2	3	3	4
35–49	698	2.1	<1	1	2	2	3	3	4	5
50–64	1,126	2.1	1	1	1	2	3	3	4	5
65+	789	2.2	2	1	1	2	3	3	4	7
SUBTOTALS:										
1. SINGLE DX										
A. Not Operated	2	1.5	<1	1	1	2	2	2	2	2
B. Operated	173	1.8	<1	1	1	2	2	3	3	4
2. MULTIPLE DX										
A. Not Operated	22	1.5	1	1	1	1	2	3	4	5
B. Operated	2,689	2.1	1	1	1	2	3	3	4	5
1. SINGLE DX	175	1.8	<1	1	1	2	2	3	3	4
2. MULTIPLE DX	2,711	2.1	1	1	2	2	3	3	4	5
A. NOT OPERATED	24	1.5	1	1	1	1	1	3	3	5
B. OPERATED	2,862	2.1	1	1	1	2	3	3	4	5
TOTAL										
0–19 Years	0									
20–34	82	1.9	<1	1	1	2	2	3	3	4
35–49	742	2.1	<1	1	2	2	3	3	4	5
50–64	1,212	2.1	1	1	1	2	3	3	4	5
65+	850	2.1	1	1	1	2	3	3	4	5
GRAND TOTAL	2,886	2.1	1	1	1	2	3	3	4	5

Length of Stay by Diagnosis and Operation, Western Region, 2008

Western Region, October 2006–September 2007 Data, by Diagnosis

618.5: POSTOP VAGINAL PROLAPSE

Type of Patients	Observed Patients	Avg. Stay	Variance	10th	25th	50th	75th	90th	95th	99th
1. SINGLE DX										
A. Not Operated										
0–19 Years	0									
20–34	0									
35–49	0									
50–64	1	2.0	0	2	2	2	2	2	2	2
65+	0									
B. Operated										
0–19 Years	0									
20–34	3	1.3	<1	1	1	1	2	2	2	2
35–49	17	1.6	<1	1	1	2	2	2	3	3
50–64	98	1.6	<1	1	1	1	2	3	3	4
65+	75	1.5	<1	1	1	1	2	2	3	3
2. MULTIPLE DX										
A. Not Operated										
0–19 Years	0									
20–34	0									
35–49	0									
50–64	10	1.4	<1	1	1	1	2	2	3	3
65+	14	1.4	<1	1	1	1	2	2	4	4
B. Operated										
0–19 Years	0									
20–34	26	1.8	<1	1	1	2	2	3	3	5
35–49	446	1.8	<1	1	1	2	2	3	3	5
50–64	1,839	1.9	1	1	1	2	2	3	4	6
65+	2,699	1.9	2	1	1	2	2	3	4	7
SUBTOTALS:										
1. SINGLE DX										
A. Not Operated	1	2.0	0	2	2	2	2	2	2	2
B. Operated	193	1.6	<1	1	1	1	2	2	3	4
2. MULTIPLE DX										
A. Not Operated	24	1.4	<1	1	1	1	2	2	3	4
B. Operated	5,010	1.9	1	1	1	2	2	3	4	6
1. SINGLE DX	194	1.6	<1	1	1	1	2	2	3	4
2. MULTIPLE DX	5,034	1.9	1	1	1	2	2	3	4	6
A. NOT OPERATED	25	1.4	<1	1	1	1	2	2	3	4
B. OPERATED	5,203	1.9	1	1	1	2	2	3	4	6
TOTAL										
0–19 Years	0									
20–34	29	1.7	1	1	1	2	2	3	3	5
35–49	463	1.8	<1	1	1	2	2	3	3	5
50–64	1,948	1.9	1	1	1	2	2	3	3	6
65+	2,788	1.9	2	1	1	2	2	3	4	7
GRAND TOTAL	5,228	1.9	1	1	1	2	2	3	4	6

618.6: VAGINAL ENTEROCELE

Type of Patients	Observed Patients	Avg. Stay	Variance	10th	25th	50th	75th	90th	95th	99th
1. SINGLE DX										
A. Not Operated										
0–19 Years	0									
20–34	0									
35–49	0									
50–64	0									
65+	0									
B. Operated										
0–19 Years	0									
20–34	1	1.0	0	1	1	1	1	1	1	1
35–49	1	1.0	0	1	1	1	1	1	1	1
50–64	5	1.2	<1	1	1	1	1	2	2	2
65+	1	2.0	0	2	2	2	2	2	2	2
2. MULTIPLE DX										
A. Not Operated										
0–19 Years	0									
20–34	0									
35–49	0									
50–64	0									
65+	1	1.0	0	1	1	1	1	1	1	1
B. Operated										
0–19 Years	0									
20–34	11	1.5	<1	1	1	1	2	2	3	3
35–49	80	2.0	1	1	1	2	2	3	4	7
50–64	235	1.9	1	1	1	2	2	3	4	6
65+	316	1.9	2	1	2	2	2	3	4	7
SUBTOTALS:										
1. SINGLE DX										
A. Not Operated	0									
B. Operated	8	1.3	<1	1	1	1	2	2	2	2
2. MULTIPLE DX										
A. Not Operated	1	1.0	0	1	1	1	1	1	1	1
B. Operated	642	1.9	1	1	1	2	2	3	4	6
1. SINGLE DX	8	1.3	<1	1	1	1	2	2	2	2
2. MULTIPLE DX	643	1.9	1	1	1	2	2	3	4	6
A. NOT OPERATED	1	1.0	0	1	1	1	1	1	1	1
B. OPERATED	650	1.9	1	1	1	2	2	3	4	6
TOTAL										
0–19 Years	0									
20–34	12	1.5	<1	1	1	1	2	2	3	3
35–49	81	2.0	1	1	1	2	3	3	4	7
50–64	240	1.9	<1	1	1	2	2	3	3	6
65+	318	1.9	2	1	1	2	2	3	4	7
GRAND TOTAL	651	1.9	1	1	1	2	2	3	4	6

618.89: OTHER GENITAL PROLAPSE

Type of Patients	Observed Patients	Avg. Stay	Variance	10th	25th	50th	75th	90th	95th	99th
1. SINGLE DX										
A. Not Operated										
0–19 Years	0									
20–34	0									
35–49	0									
50–64	0									
65+	0									
B. Operated										
0–19 Years	0									
20–34	3	1.3	<1	1	1	1	2	2	2	2
35–49	8	1.9	<1	1	2	2	2	3	3	3
50–64	23	2.1	<1	1	1	2	3	3	4	4
65+	6	1.7	<1	1	1	1	2	3	3	3
2. MULTIPLE DX										
A. Not Operated										
0–19 Years	0									
20–34	0									
35–49	1	1.0	0	1	1	1	1	1	1	1
50–64	6	1.8	2	1	1	1	3	4	4	4
65+	3	2.0	<1	1	1	2	3	3	3	3
B. Operated										
0–19 Years	0									
20–34	71	2.0	<1	1	1	2	2	3	4	4
35–49	435	2.1	1	1	1	2	3	3	4	5
50–64	645	2.0	<1	1	1	2	2	3	4	5
65+	443	2.3	6	1	1	2	3	3	4	8
SUBTOTALS:										
1. SINGLE DX										
A. Not Operated	0									
B. Operated	40	1.9	<1	1	1	2	2	3	4	4
2. MULTIPLE DX										
A. Not Operated	10	1.8	1	1	1	1	3	3	4	6
B. Operated	1,594	2.1	2	1	1	2	3	3	4	6
1. SINGLE DX	40	1.9	<1	1	1	2	2	3	4	4
2. MULTIPLE DX	1,604	2.1	2	1	1	2	3	3	4	6
A. NOT OPERATED	10	1.8	1	1	1	1	3	3	4	4
B. OPERATED	1,634	2.1	2	1	1	2	3	3	4	6
TOTAL										
0–19 Years	0									
20–34	74	1.9	<1	1	1	2	2	3	4	4
35–49	444	2.1	1	1	1	2	3	3	4	5
50–64	674	2.0	<1	1	1	2	2	3	4	5
65+	452	2.3	6	1	1	2	3	3	4	8
GRAND TOTAL	1,644	2.1	2	1	1	2	3	3	4	6

Length of Stay by Diagnosis and Operation, Western Region, 2008

619: FEMALE GENITAL FISTULA

Type of Patients	Observed Patients	Avg. Stay	Variance	Percentiles						
				10th	25th	50th	75th	90th	95th	99th
1. SINGLE DX										
A. *Not Operated*										
0–19 Years	1	1.0	0	1	1	1	1	1	1	1
20–34	1	2.0	0	2	2	2	2	2	2	2
35–49	1	2.0	0	2	2	2	2	2	2	2
50–64	0									
65+	1	1.0	0	1	1	1	1	1	1	1
B. *Operated*										
0–19 Years	0									
20–34	9	2.3	2	1	1	2	4	5	5	5
35–49	20	2.3	2	1	1	2	3	4	4	7
50–64	8	2.0	1	1	1	2	3	4	4	4
65+	1	1.0	0	1	1	1	1	1	1	1
2. MULTIPLE DX										
A. *Not Operated*										
0–19 Years	0									
20–34	6	2.5	4	1	1	2	3	6	6	6
35–49	16	3.2	7	1	1	3	5	7	10	10
50–64	24	4.7	17	1	2	3	6	12	13	17
65+	60	5.8	22	1	3	5	7	12	19	21
B. *Operated*										
0–19 Years	6	6.2	48	1	1	2	7	19	19	19
20–34	75	4.0	27	1	2	3	5	6	10	42
35–49	169	5.0	65	1	2	3	5	9	14	28
50–64	207	6.8	43	2	3	5	8	14	19	37
65+	203	9.7	55	4	5	7	11	20	25	36
SUBTOTALS:										
1. SINGLE DX										
A. *Not Operated*	4	1.5	<1	1	1	2	2	2	2	2
B. *Operated*	38	2.2	2	1	1	2	3	4	5	7
2. MULTIPLE DX										
A. *Not Operated*	106	5.0	19	1	2	4	6	11	15	20
B. *Operated*	660	6.9	55	1	3	5	8	14	20	37
1. SINGLE DX	42	2.1	2	1	1	2	3	4	4	7
2. MULTIPLE DX	766	6.6	50	1	3	5	8	14	19	36
A. NOT OPERATED	110	4.9	19	1	2	4	6	11	15	20
B. OPERATED	698	6.6	53	1	3	5	8	14	20	37
TOTAL										
0–19 Years	7	5.4	44	1	1	2	7	19	19	19
20–34	91	3.7	23	1	1	3	4	6	10	42
35–49	206	4.6	55	1	2	3	5	8	13	27
50–64	239	6.4	40	1	3	5	8	13	18	37
65+	265	8.7	50	3	4	7	10	19	24	36
GRAND TOTAL	808	6.4	49	1	2	5	8	14	19	35

619.1: FE DIGEST-GENIT FISTULA

Type of Patients	Observed Patients	Avg. Stay	Variance	Percentiles						
				10th	25th	50th	75th	90th	95th	99th
1. SINGLE DX										
A. *Not Operated*										
0–19 Years	1	1.0	0	1	1	1	1	1	1	1
20–34	0									
35–49	1	2.0	0	2	2	2	2	2	2	2
50–64	0									
65+	1	1.0	0	1	1	1	1	1	1	1
B. *Operated*										
0–19 Years	0									
20–34	9	2.3	2	1	1	2	4	5	5	5
35–49	10	2.5	4	1	1	2	4	4	7	7
50–64	1	1.0	0	1	1	1	1	1	1	1
65+	1	1.0	0	1	1	1	1	1	1	1
2. MULTIPLE DX										
A. *Not Operated*										
0–19 Years	0									
20–34	5	2.6	4	1	1	2	3	6	6	6
35–49	11	4.1	8	1	2	4	6	7	10	10
50–64	17	5.3	21	1	2	4	6	13	17	17
65+	57	5.7	22	2	2	4	7	12	19	21
B. *Operated*										
0–19 Years	3	7.4	101	1	1	2	19	19	19	19
20–34	60	4.2	33	1	2	3	5	8	10	42
35–49	101	5.8	103	1	2	3	7	11	17	28
50–64	173	7.3	45	2	4	6	9	14	19	52
65+	195	9.8	55	4	5	7	12	20	26	40
SUBTOTALS:										
1. SINGLE DX										
A. *Not Operated*	3	1.3	<1	1	1	1	2	2	2	2
B. *Operated*	21	2.3	3	1	1	2	4	4	5	7
2. MULTIPLE DX										
A. *Not Operated*	90	5.2	19	1	2	4	6	12	15	21
B. *Operated*	532	7.6	62	2	3	6	9	16	22	40
1. SINGLE DX	24	2.2	3	1	1	2	2	4	5	7
2. MULTIPLE DX	622	7.3	56	2	3	5	9	15	21	37
A. NOT OPERATED	93	5.1	19	1	2	4	6	11	15	21
B. OPERATED	553	7.4	61	1	3	5	9	15	22	40
TOTAL										
0–19 Years	4	5.8	78	1	1	2	2	19	19	19
20–34	74	3.9	27	1	1	3	4	6	10	42
35–49	123	5.4	87	1	2	3	5	9	14	28
50–64	191	7.1	43	2	3	5	9	14	19	52
65+	254	8.8	50	3	4	7	10	19	24	36
GRAND TOTAL	646	7.1	55	1	3	5	8	15	20	37

620: NONINFL DISORD OV/FALL

Type of Patients	Observed Patients	Avg. Stay	Variance	Percentiles						
				10th	25th	50th	75th	90th	95th	99th
1. SINGLE DX										
A. *Not Operated*										
0–19 Years	133	1.5	<1	1	1	1	2	2	3	5
20–34	197	1.4	<1	1	1	1	2	2	3	4
35–49	57	1.4	<1	1	1	1	2	2	3	6
50–64	8	1.9	3	1	1	1	2	6	6	6
65+	0									
B. *Operated*										
0–19 Years	149	1.8	<1	1	1	2	2	3	3	4
20–34	333	1.8	1	1	1	2	2	3	4	5
35–49	180	2.0	1	1	1	2	3	3	4	6
50–64	64	2.1	1	1	1	2	3	3	3	8
65+	10	2.0	2	1	1	2	2	3	6	6
2. MULTIPLE DX										
A. *Not Operated*										
0–19 Years	196	1.8	2	1	1	1	2	3	5	6
20–34	619	1.9	2	1	1	1	2	4	5	8
35–49	462	2.1	2	1	1	2	3	4	5	8
50–64	88	2.5	5	1	1	2	3	5	5	14
65+	43	3.4	6	1	2	3	4	7	8	13
B. *Operated*										
0–19 Years	479	2.3	3	1	1	2	3	4	4	7
20–34	1,984	2.3	3	1	2	2	3	4	5	8
35–49	2,880	2.6	4	1	2	2	3	4	5	10
50–64	1,204	2.6	4	1	2	2	3	4	5	10
65+	500	3.2	7	1	2	3	4	5	8	14
SUBTOTALS:										
1. SINGLE DX										
A. *Not Operated*	395	1.4	<1	1	1	1	2	2	3	5
B. *Operated*	736	1.9	1	1	1	2	2	3	4	5
2. MULTIPLE DX										
A. *Not Operated*	1,408	2.0	2	1	1	2	3	4	5	8
B. *Operated*	7,047	2.6	4	1	2	2	3	4	5	10
1. SINGLE DX	1,131	1.7	<1	1	1	1	2	3	3	5
2. MULTIPLE DX	8,455	2.5	4	1	2	2	3	4	5	9
A. NOT OPERATED	1,803	1.9	2	1	1	1	2	4	5	8
B. OPERATED	7,783	2.5	3	1	1	2	3	4	5	9
TOTAL										
0–19 Years	957	2.0	2	1	1	2	2	3	4	6
20–34	3,133	2.1	2	1	1	2	3	4	5	7
35–49	3,579	2.5	4	1	1	2	3	4	5	10
50–64	1,364	2.6	4	1	2	2	3	4	5	10
65+	553	3.2	7	1	2	3	4	6	8	13
GRAND TOTAL	9,586	2.4	3	1	1	2	3	4	5	9

Length of Stay by Diagnosis and Operation, Western Region, 2008

Western Region, October 2006–September 2007 Data, by Diagnosis

620.0: OVARIAN FOLLICULAR CYST

Type of Patients	Observed Patients	Avg. Stay	Variance	10th	25th	50th	75th	90th	95th	99th
1. SINGLE DX										
A. Not Operated										
0–19 Years	4	2.0	<1	1	2	2	3	3	3	3
20–34	3	1.3	<1	1	1	1	2	2	2	2
35–49	2	1.0	0	1	1	1	1	1	1	1
50–64	0									
65+	0									
B. Operated										
0–19 Years	6	2.5	1	1	2	2	4	4	4	4
20–34	9	2.5	5	1	1	1	3	7	7	7
35–49	10	2.0	<1	1	2	2	2	3	3	3
50–64	0									
65+	0									
2. MULTIPLE DX										
A. Not Operated										
0–19 Years	10	3.0	4	1	1	2	5	6	6	6
20–34	15	2.8	4	1	2	2	3	6	9	9
35–49	7	2.9	6	1	1	2	4	8	8	8
50–64	0									
65+	0									
B. Operated										
0–19 Years	10	1.7	<1	1	1	1	2	3	3	3
20–34	110	2.4	2	1	2	2	3	4	6	6
35–49	211	3.0	12	1	2	2	3	4	7	17
50–64	43	2.8	13	1	2	2	3	3	3	24
65+	5	2.0	<1	1	1	2	3	3	3	3
SUBTOTALS:										
1. SINGLE DX										
A. Not Operated	9	1.6	<1	1	1	1	2	3	3	3
B. Operated	25	2.3	2	1	1	2	3	4	5	7
2. MULTIPLE DX										
A. Not Operated	32	2.9	5	1	1	2	4	6	8	9
B. Operated	379	2.7	8	1	2	2	3	4	6	17
1. SINGLE DX	34	2.1	2	1	1	2	2	4	5	7
2. MULTIPLE DX	411	2.7	8	1	2	2	3	4	6	14
A. NOT OPERATED	41	2.6	4	1	1	2	3	6	6	9
B. OPERATED	404	2.7	8	1	2	2	3	4	6	14
TOTAL										
0–19 Years	30	2.3	2	1	1	2	2	3	6	6
20–34	137	2.4	2	1	1	2	3	4	6	7
35–49	230	2.9	11	1	2	2	3	4	7	17
50–64	43	2.8	13	1	2	2	3	3	3	24
65+	5	2.0	<1	1	1	2	3	3	3	3
GRAND TOTAL	445	2.7	8	1	2	2	3	4	6	14

620.1: CORPUS LUTEUM CYST

Type of Patients	Observed Patients	Avg. Stay	Variance	10th	25th	50th	75th	90th	95th	99th
1. SINGLE DX										
A. Not Operated										
0–19 Years	6	1.3	<1	1	1	1	1	3	3	3
20–34	24	1.3	<1	1	1	1	2	2	2	3
35–49	5	2.0	1	1	1	2	2	4	4	4
50–64	1	2.0	0	2	2	2	2	2	2	2
65+	0									
B. Operated										
0–19 Years	16	1.8	<1	1	1	2	2	3	4	4
20–34	58	1.7	<1	1	1	1	2	3	4	4
35–49	17	2.3	2	1	1	2	3	3	6	6
50–64	6	1.7	<1	1	2	2	2	3	3	3
65+	0									
2. MULTIPLE DX										
A. Not Operated										
0–19 Years	21	1.7	<1	1	1	1	2	3	3	3
20–34	62	1.8	1	1	1	1	2	3	4	5
35–49	33	1.9	3	1	1	2	2	3	5	9
50–64	0									
65+	0									
B. Operated										
0–19 Years	65	2.7	12	1	1	2	3	5	6	27
20–34	400	2.3	3	1	1	2	3	4	4	7
35–49	537	2.6	3	1	2	2	3	4	6	10
50–64	84	2.8	6	1	2	2	3	5	6	20
65+	1	3.0	0	3	3	3	3	3	3	3
SUBTOTALS:										
1. SINGLE DX										
A. Not Operated	36	1.4	<1	1	1	1	2	3	3	4
B. Operated	97	1.8	<1	1	1	2	2	3	4	6
2. MULTIPLE DX										
A. Not Operated	116	1.8	1	1	1	2	2	3	4	5
B. Operated	1,087	2.5	4	1	1	2	3	4	5	10
1. SINGLE DX	133	1.7	<1	1	1	2	2	3	3	4
2. MULTIPLE DX	1,203	2.5	4	1	1	2	3	4	5	9
A. NOT OPERATED	152	1.7	1	1	1	1	2	3	4	5
B. OPERATED	1,184	2.5	4	1	1	2	3	4	5	10
TOTAL										
0–19 Years	108	2.3	8	1	1	2	3	4	5	10
20–34	544	2.2	2	1	1	2	3	4	4	6
35–49	592	2.6	3	1	2	2	3	4	6	10
50–64	91	2.7	5	1	2	2	3	4	6	20
65+	1	3.0	0	3	3	3	3	3	3	3
GRAND TOTAL	1,336	2.4	3	1	1	2	3	4	5	9

620.2: OVARIAN CYST NEC & NOS

Type of Patients	Observed Patients	Avg. Stay	Variance	10th	25th	50th	75th	90th	95th	99th
1. SINGLE DX										
A. Not Operated										
0–19 Years	120	1.5	<1	1	1	1	2	2	3	5
20–34	160	1.4	<1	1	1	1	2	2	3	4
35–49	48	1.4	<1	1	1	1	2	2	2	6
50–64	7	1.9	3	1	1	1	2	6	6	6
65+	0									
B. Operated										
0–19 Years	81	1.7	<1	1	1	2	2	3	3	3
20–34	202	1.8	<1	1	1	2	2	3	4	5
35–49	109	1.9	<1	1	1	2	2	3	3	4
50–64	47	2.2	<1	1	1	2	3	3	3	8
65+	8	1.6	<1	1	1	2	2	3	3	3
2. MULTIPLE DX										
A. Not Operated										
0–19 Years	160	1.7	1	1	1	2	2	3	4	5
20–34	513	1.9	2	1	1	2	2	4	5	8
35–49	384	2.1	2	1	1	2	3	4	5	7
50–64	69	2.5	5	1	1	2	3	5	6	14
65+	30	3.4	6	1	2	3	4	6	7	13
B. Operated										
0–19 Years	202	2.2	2	1	1	2	3	4	4	7
20–34	1,089	2.3	2	1	1	2	3	4	5	8
35–49	1,641	2.6	4	1	2	2	3	4	5	10
50–64	850	2.6	4	1	2	2	3	4	5	8
65+	395	3.0	6	1	2	3	4	5	7	13
SUBTOTALS:										
1. SINGLE DX										
A. Not Operated	335	1.4	<1	1	1	1	2	2	3	5
B. Operated	447	1.8	<1	1	1	2	2	3	3	5
2. MULTIPLE DX										
A. Not Operated	1,156	2.0	2	1	1	2	3	4	5	8
B. Operated	4,177	2.5	3	1	1	2	3	4	5	10
1. SINGLE DX	782	1.7	<1	1	1	1	2	3	3	5
2. MULTIPLE DX	5,333	2.4	3	1	1	2	3	4	5	9
A. NOT OPERATED	1,491	1.9	2	1	1	1	2	3	5	7
B. OPERATED	4,624	2.5	3	1	1	2	3	4	5	9
TOTAL										
0–19 Years	563	1.8	1	1	1	2	2	3	4	6
20–34	1,964	2.1	2	1	1	2	3	4	5	8
35–49	2,182	2.5	3	1	1	2	3	4	5	10
50–64	973	2.5	4	1	2	2	3	4	5	9
65+	433	3.0	6	1	2	3	4	5	7	13
GRAND TOTAL	6,115	2.3	3	1	1	2	3	4	5	9

Length of Stay by Diagnosis and Operation, Western Region, 2008

Western Region, October 2006–September 2007 Data, by Diagnosis

620.5: OVARY OR TUBE TORSION

Type of Patients	Observed Patients	Avg. Stay	Variance	10th	25th	50th	75th	90th	95th	99th
1. SINGLE DX										
A. Not Operated										
0–19 Years	0									
20–34	3	1.0	0		1	1	1	1	1	1
35–49	0									
50–64	0									
65+	0									
B. Operated										
0–19 Years	26	2.0	<1	1	1	2	3	3	3	3
20–34	33	1.8	<1	1	1	2	2	3	3	3
35–49	24	1.9	<1	1	1	2	3	3	3	4
50–64	5	2.6	1	1	2	3	3	4	4	4
65+	1	6.0	0	6	6	6	6	6	6	6
2. MULTIPLE DX										
A. Not Operated										
0–19 Years	2	3.5	12	1	1	1	1	6	6	6
20–34	4	1.5	<1	1	1	1	1	3	3	3
35–49	6	1.5	<1	1	1	1	2	3	3	3
50–64	0									
65+	0									
B. Operated										
0–19 Years	157	2.3	1	1	1	2	3	4	4	7
20–34	242	2.4	2	1	1	2	3	4	5	8
35–49	237	2.5	3	1	1	2	3	4	5	8
50–64	90	3.2	5	1	2	3	4	6	7	15
65+	41	5.3	12	2	3	4	6	10	11	17
SUBTOTALS:										
1. SINGLE DX *A. Not Operated*	3	1.0	0	1	1	1	1	1	1	1
1. SINGLE DX *B. Operated*	89	2.0	<1	1	1	2	3	3	3	6
2. MULTIPLE DX *A. Not Operated*	12	1.8	2	1	1	1	2	3	6	6
2. MULTIPLE DX *B. Operated*	767	2.7	3	1	1	2	3	4	6	9
1. SINGLE DX	92	1.9	<1	1	1	2	3	3	3	6
2. MULTIPLE DX	779	2.6	3	1	1	2	3	4	6	9
A. NOT OPERATED	15	1.7	2	1	1	1	2	3	6	6
B. OPERATED	856	2.6	3	1	1	2	3	4	6	9
TOTAL										
0–19 Years	185	2.2	1	1	1	2	2	3	4	7
20–34	282	2.3	2	1	1	2	3	4	5	8
35–49	267	2.4	2	1	1	2	3	4	5	8
50–64	95	3.2	4	1	2	3	4	6	7	15
65+	42	5.3	11	2	3	4	6	10	11	17
GRAND TOTAL	871	2.6	3	1	1	2	3	4	6	9

620.8: NONINFL DIS OV/FALL NEC

Type of Patients	Observed Patients	Avg. Stay	Variance	10th	25th	50th	75th	90th	95th	99th
1. SINGLE DX										
A. Not Operated										
0–19 Years	3	1.0	0	1	1	1	1	1	1	1
20–34	6	1.2	<1	1	1	1	1	2	2	2
35–49	1	2.0	0	2	2	2	2	2	2	2
50–64	0									
65+	0									
B. Operated										
0–19 Years	19	1.6	<1	1	1	2	2	3	3	3
20–34	30	2.3	2	1	1	2	3	4	6	6
35–49	17	2.4	3	1	2	2	3	4	8	8
50–64	6	1.8	<1	1	1	2	3	3	3	3
65+	1	1.0	0	1	1	1	1	1	1	1
2. MULTIPLE DX										
A. Not Operated										
0–19 Years	2	2.0	2	1	1	1	3	3	3	3
20–34	17	1.9	1	1	1	1	2	4	5	5
35–49	12	1.5	<1	1	2	2	2	2	3	3
50–64	5	2.0	2	1	1	2	3	4	4	4
65+	7	3.0	7	1	1	2	5	8	8	8
B. Operated										
0–19 Years	45	2.2	1	1	1	2	3	4	4	6
20–34	128	2.5	1	1	2	2	3	4	6	8
35–49	233	2.5	4	1	2	2	3	4	5	8
50–64	124	2.5	3	1	2	2	3	4	5	9
65+	51	2.5	4	1	1	2	3	4	8	9
SUBTOTALS:										
1. SINGLE DX *A. Not Operated*	10	1.2	<1	1	1	1	1	2	2	2
1. SINGLE DX *B. Operated*	73	2.1	2	1	1	2	3	3	4	8
2. MULTIPLE DX *A. Not Operated*	43	2.0	2	1	1	1	2	4	5	8
2. MULTIPLE DX *B. Operated*	581	2.5	3	1	2	2	3	4	5	9
1. SINGLE DX	83	2.0	2	1	1	2	2	3	4	8
2. MULTIPLE DX	624	2.5	3	1	1	2	3	4	5	9
A. NOT OPERATED	53	1.8	2	1	1	1	2	3	5	8
B. OPERATED	654	2.4	3	1	1	2	3	4	5	9
TOTAL										
0–19 Years	69	2.0	1	1	1	2	2	4	4	6
20–34	181	2.4	2	1	1	2	3	4	5	8
35–49	263	2.5	4	1	2	2	3	4	5	8
50–64	135	2.4	3	1	1	2	3	4	4	9
65+	59	2.6	4	1	1	2	3	5	8	9
GRAND TOTAL	707	2.4	3	1	1	2	3	4	5	8

621: DISORDERS OF UTERUS NEC

Type of Patients	Observed Patients	Avg. Stay	Variance	10th	25th	50th	75th	90th	95th	99th
1. SINGLE DX										
A. Not Operated										
0–19 Years	1	1.0	0	1	1	1	1	1	1	1
20–34	2	2.5	4	1	1	1	4	4	4	4
35–49	0									
50–64	1	3.0	0	3	3	3	3	3	3	3
65+	1	1.0	0	1	1	1	1	1	1	1
B. Operated										
0–19 Years	0									
20–34	8	1.9	<1	1	1	2	2	3	3	3
35–49	30	1.6	<1	1	1	2	2	3	3	3
50–64	26	1.9	<1	1	1	2	2	3	4	4
65+	3	2.0	<1	1	2	2	3	3	3	3
2. MULTIPLE DX										
A. Not Operated										
0–19 Years	4	1.3	<1	1	1	1	1	2	2	2
20–34	8	2.8	4	1	2	3	3	7	7	7
35–49	23	2.0	2	1	1	2	2	4	4	6
50–64	14	1.4	<1	1	1	1	1	2	4	4
65+	9	2.0	1	1	1	2	2	3	3	3
B. Operated										
0–19 Years	2	1.5	<1	1	1	1	2	2	2	2
20–34	145	2.1	4	1	1	2	2	4	5	6
35–49	856	2.2	2	1	1	2	3	3	4	6
50–64	830	2.4	5	1	1	2	3	4	4	11
65+	318	2.6	3	1	1	2	3	5	5	9
SUBTOTALS:										
1. SINGLE DX *A. Not Operated*	5	2.0	2	1	1	1	3	4	4	4
1. SINGLE DX *B. Operated*	67	1.8	<1	1	1	2	2	3	3	4
2. MULTIPLE DX *A. Not Operated*	58	1.9	2	1	1	2	2	3	3	7
2. MULTIPLE DX *B. Operated*	2,151	2.3	3	1	1	2	3	4	4	8
1. SINGLE DX	72	1.8	<1	1	1	2	2	3	3	4
2. MULTIPLE DX	2,209	2.3	3	1	1	2	3	4	4	8
A. NOT OPERATED	63	1.9	2	1	1	1	2	3	4	7
B. OPERATED	2,218	2.3	3	1	1	2	3	4	4	8
TOTAL										
0–19 Years	7	1.3	<1	1	1	1	1	2	2	2
20–34	163	2.1	2	1	1	2	3	3	5	6
35–49	909	2.1	2	1	1	2	3	3	4	6
50–64	871	2.4	5	1	1	2	3	4	4	11
65+	331	2.6	3	1	1	2	3	5	5	9
GRAND TOTAL	2,281	2.3	3	1	1	2	3	4	4	8

Length of Stay by Diagnosis and Operation, Western Region, 2008

Western Region, October 2006–September 2007 Data, by Diagnosis

621.0: CORPUS UTERI POLYP

Type of Patients	Observed Patients	Avg. Stay	Vari-ance	10th	25th	50th	75th	90th	95th	99th
1. SINGLE DX										
A. Not Operated										
0–19 Years	0									
20–34	0									
35–49	0									
50–64	0									
65+	0									
B. Operated										
0–19 Years	0									
20–34	1	1.0	0		1	1	1	1	1	1
35–49	6	1.3	<1		1	1	2	2	2	2
50–64	1	2.0	0		2	2	2	2	2	2
65+	0									
2. MULTIPLE DX										
A. Not Operated										
0–19 Years	0									
20–34	1	1.0	0	1	1	1	1	1	1	1
35–49	3	1.0	0	1	1	1	1	1	1	1
50–64	2	1.0	0	1	1	1	1	1	1	1
65+	3	2.0	<1	1	1	2	3	3	3	3
B. Operated										
0–19 Years	1	2.0	0	2	2	2	2	2	2	2
20–34	31	1.5	<1	1	1	1	2	2	3	3
35–49	187	2.0	1	1	1	2	2	3	4	6
50–64	145	2.5	4	1	1	2	3	4	6	11
65+	101	2.8	3	1	1	3	4	5	5	7
SUBTOTALS:										
1. SINGLE DX A. Not Operated	0									
1. SINGLE DX B. Operated	8	1.4	<1	1	1	1	2	2	2	2
2. MULTIPLE DX A. Not Operated	9	1.3	<1	1	1	1	2	3	3	3
2. MULTIPLE DX B. Operated	465	2.3	3	1	1	2	3	4	5	10
1. SINGLE DX	8	1.4	<1	1	1	1	2	2	2	2
2. MULTIPLE DX	474	2.2	3	1	1	2	3	4	5	10
A. NOT OPERATED	9	1.3	<1	1	1	1	2	3	3	3
B. OPERATED	473	2.3	3	1	1	2	3	4	5	10
TOTAL										
0–19 Years	1	2.0	0	2	2	2	2	2	2	2
20–34	33	1.5	<1	1	1	1	2	2	3	3
35–49	196	1.9	1	1	1	2	2	3	4	7
50–64	148	2.4	4	1	1	2	3	4	6	11
65+	104	2.7	3	1	2	3	4	5	5	7
GRAND TOTAL	482	2.2	3	1	1	2	3	4	5	10

621.2: UTERINE HYPERTROPHY

Type of Patients	Observed Patients	Avg. Stay	Vari-ance	10th	25th	50th	75th	90th	95th	99th
1. SINGLE DX										
A. Not Operated										
0–19 Years	0									
20–34	0									
35–49	0									
50–64	0									
65+	0									
B. Operated										
0–19 Years	0									
20–34	0									
35–49	0									
50–64	0									
65+	0									
2. MULTIPLE DX										
A. Not Operated										
0–19 Years	0									
20–34	0									
35–49	7	2.3	4	1	1	1	4	6	6	6
50–64	1	2.0	0	2	2	2	2	2	2	2
65+	1	1.0	0	1	1	1	1	1	1	1
B. Operated										
0–19 Years	0									
20–34	25	2.4	1	1	2	2	3	3	3	6
35–49	174	2.2	1	1	1	2	3	3	4	6
50–64	49	2.2	1	1	2	2	3	3	4	6
65+	3	2.3	1	1	3	3	3	3	3	3
SUBTOTALS:										
1. SINGLE DX A. Not Operated	0									
1. SINGLE DX B. Operated	0									
2. MULTIPLE DX A. Not Operated	9	2.1	3	1	1	1	2	6	6	6
2. MULTIPLE DX B. Operated	251	2.2	1	1	2	2	3	3	4	6
1. SINGLE DX	0									
2. MULTIPLE DX	260	2.2	1	1	1	2	3	3	4	6
A. NOT OPERATED	9	2.1	3	1	1	1	2	6	6	6
B. OPERATED	251	2.2	1	1	2	2	3	3	4	6
TOTAL										
0–19 Years	0									
20–34	25	2.4	1	1	2	2	3	3	3	6
35–49	181	2.2	1	1	1	2	3	3	4	6
50–64	50	2.2	1	1	2	2	3	3	4	6
65+	4	2.0	1	1	1	2	3	3	3	3
GRAND TOTAL	260	2.2	1	1	1	2	3	3	4	6

621.30: ENDOMET HYPERPLASIA NOS

Type of Patients	Observed Patients	Avg. Stay	Vari-ance	10th	25th	50th	75th	90th	95th	99th
1. SINGLE DX										
A. Not Operated										
0–19 Years	0									
20–34	0									
35–49	0									
50–64	0									
65+	0									
B. Operated										
0–19 Years	0									
20–34	2	2.5	<1	2	2	2	3	3	3	3
35–49	5	1.8	<1	1	1	2	2	3	3	3
50–64	3	2.0	<1	1	1	2	3	3	3	3
65+	0									
2. MULTIPLE DX										
A. Not Operated										
0–19 Years	0									
20–34	0									
35–49	2	1.0	0	1	1	1	1	1	1	1
50–64	5	1.8	2	1	1	1	2	4	4	4
65+	0									
B. Operated										
0–19 Years	0									
20–34	10	2.1	<1	1	1	1	2	3	3	3
35–49	76	2.1	1	1	1	2	3	3	4	6
50–64	102	2.2	2	1	1	2	3	3	4	6
65+	33	2.5	2	1	1	2	4	5	5	6
SUBTOTALS:										
1. SINGLE DX A. Not Operated	0									
1. SINGLE DX B. Operated	10	2.0	<1	1	1	2	2	3	3	3
2. MULTIPLE DX A. Not Operated	7	1.6	1	1	1	1	2	4	4	4
2. MULTIPLE DX B. Operated	221	2.2	2	1	1	2	3	4	4	6
1. SINGLE DX	10	2.0	<1	1	1	2	2	3	3	3
2. MULTIPLE DX	228	2.2	2	1	1	2	3	4	5	6
A. NOT OPERATED	7	1.6	1	1	1	1	2	4	4	4
B. OPERATED	231	2.2	2	1	1	2	3	4	5	6
TOTAL										
0–19 Years	0									
20–34	12	2.2	<1	1	1	2	3	3	3	3
35–49	83	2.1	1	1	1	2	3	3	4	6
50–64	110	2.2	2	1	1	2	3	3	4	6
65+	33	2.5	2	1	1	2	4	5	6	6
GRAND TOTAL	238	2.2	2	1	1	2	3	4	5	6

Length of Stay by Diagnosis and Operation, Western Region, 2008

Western Region, October 2006–September 2007 Data, by Diagnosis

621.31: SIMPLE EH W/O ATYPIA

Type of Patients	Observed Patients	Avg. Stay	Vari-ance	Percentiles						
				10th	25th	50th	75th	90th	95th	99th
1. SINGLE DX										
A. Not Operated										
0–19 Years	0									
20–34	0									
35–49	0									
50–64	0									
65+	0									
B. Operated										
0–19 Years	0									
20–34	1	1.0	0	1	1	1	1	1	1	1
35–49	2	1.5	<1	1	1	2	2	2	2	2
50–64	2	1.5	<1	1	1	1	2	2	2	2
65+	1	2.0	0	2	2	2	2	2	2	2
2. MULTIPLE DX										
A. Not Operated										
0–19 Years	0									
20–34	0									
35–49	0									
50–64	1	2.0	0	2	2	2	2	2	2	2
65+	0									
B. Operated										
0–19 Years	0									
20–34	11	1.7	<1	1	1	2	2	2	3	3
35–49	73	2.0	<1	1	1	2	3	3	3	4
50–64	53	2.2	2	1	1	2	3	3	4	8
65+	22	2.5	1	2	2	2	3	4	4	5
SUBTOTALS:										
1. SINGLE DX										
A. Not Operated	0									
B. Operated	6	1.5	<1	1	1	2	2	2	2	2
2. MULTIPLE DX										
A. Not Operated	1	2.0	0	2	2	2	2	2	2	2
B. Operated	159	2.1	1	1	1	2	3	3	4	5
1. SINGLE DX	6	1.5	<1	1	1	2	2	2	2	2
2. MULTIPLE DX	160	2.1	1	1	1	2	3	3	4	5
A. NOT OPERATED	1	2.0	0	2	2	2	2	2	2	2
B. OPERATED	165	2.1	1	1	1	2	3	3	4	5
TOTAL										
0–19 Years	0									
20–34	12	1.7	<1	1	1	2	2	2	3	3
35–49	75	2.0	<1	1	1	2	3	3	3	4
50–64	56	2.2	2	1	1	2	3	3	4	8
65+	23	2.4	1	2	2	2	3	4	4	5
GRAND TOTAL	166	2.1	1	1	1	2	3	3	4	5

621.32: COMPLEX EH W/O ATYPIA

Type of Patients	Observed Patients	Avg. Stay	Vari-ance	Percentiles						
				10th	25th	50th	75th	90th	95th	99th
1. SINGLE DX										
A. Not Operated										
0–19 Years	0									
20–34	0									
35–49	0									
50–64	0									
65+	0									
B. Operated										
0–19 Years	0									
20–34	1	1.0	0	1	1	1	1	1	1	1
35–49	4	1.3	<1	1	1	1	2	2	2	2
50–64	4	1.8	<1	1	2	2	2	2	2	2
65+	1	1.0	0	1	1	1	1	1	1	1
2. MULTIPLE DX										
A. Not Operated										
0–19 Years	0									
20–34	0									
35–49	0									
50–64	0									
65+	0									
B. Operated										
0–19 Years	0									
20–34	11	1.6	<1	1	1	2	2	2	3	3
35–49	75	2.3	2	1	2	2	3	3	5	8
50–64	91	2.7	15	1	1	2	3	3	5	27
65+	25	2.3	1	1	1	2	3	4	4	5
SUBTOTALS:										
1. SINGLE DX										
A. Not Operated	0									
B. Operated	10	1.4	<1	1	1	1	2	2	2	2
2. MULTIPLE DX										
A. Not Operated	0									
B. Operated	202	2.5	8	1	1	2	3	3	5	17
1. SINGLE DX	10	1.4	<1	1	1	1	2	2	2	2
2. MULTIPLE DX	202	2.5	8	1	1	2	3	3	5	17
A. NOT OPERATED	0									
B. OPERATED	212	2.4	7	1	1	2	3	3	5	17
TOTAL										
0–19 Years	0									
20–34	12	1.6	<1	1	1	2	2	2	3	3
35–49	79	2.3	2	1	1	2	3	3	5	8
50–64	95	2.7	15	1	1	2	3	3	5	27
65+	26	2.2	1	1	1	2	3	4	4	5
GRAND TOTAL	212	2.4	7	1	1	2	3	3	5	17

621.33: AEH

Type of Patients	Observed Patients	Avg. Stay	Vari-ance	Percentiles						
				10th	25th	50th	75th	90th	95th	99th
1. SINGLE DX										
A. Not Operated										
0–19 Years	0									
20–34	0									
35–49	0									
50–64	1	3.0	0	3	3	3	3	3	3	3
65+	0									
B. Operated										
0–19 Years	0									
20–34	2	2.5	<1	2	2	2	3	3	3	3
35–49	10	1.9	<1	1	1	2	2	3	3	3
50–64	16	2.0	<1	1	1	2	2	4	4	4
65+	1	3.0	0	3	3	3	3	3	3	3
2. MULTIPLE DX										
A. Not Operated										
0–19 Years	0									
20–34	0									
35–49	2	1.5	<1	1	1	1	1	2	2	2
50–64	5	1.0	0	1	1	1	1	1	1	1
65+	2	1.0	0	1	1	1	1	1	1	1
B. Operated										
0–19 Years	0									
20–34	21	2.7	2	1	2	3	3	4	5	6
35–49	184	2.3	2	1	1	2	3	3	4	11
50–64	341	2.4	5	1	2	2	3	4	4	10
65+	118	2.4	3	1	1	2	3	4	5	9
SUBTOTALS:										
1. SINGLE DX										
A. Not Operated	1	3.0	0	3	3	3	3	3	3	3
B. Operated	29	2.0	<1	1	1	2	2	3	4	4
2. MULTIPLE DX										
A. Not Operated	9	1.1	<1	1	1	1	1	2	2	2
B. Operated	664	2.4	4	1	1	2	3	3	4	10
1. SINGLE DX	30	2.1	<1	1	1	2	2	3	4	4
2. MULTIPLE DX	673	2.4	4	1	1	2	3	3	4	10
A. NOT OPERATED	10	1.3	<1	1	1	1	1	3	3	3
B. OPERATED	693	2.4	4	1	1	2	3	3	4	10
TOTAL										
0–19 Years	0									
20–34	23	2.7	2	1	2	3	3	4	5	6
35–49	196	2.3	2	1	1	2	3	3	4	11
50–64	363	2.4	5	1	1	2	3	4	4	10
65+	121	2.4	3	1	1	2	3	4	5	9
GRAND TOTAL	703	2.4	4	1	1	2	3	3	4	9

Length of Stay by Diagnosis and Operation, Western Region, 2008

Western Region, October 2006–September 2007 Data, by Diagnosis

622: NONINFL DISORDER CERVIX

Type of Patients	Observed Patients	Avg. Stay	Vari-ance	10th	25th	50th	75th	90th	95th	99th
1. SINGLE DX										
A. Not Operated										
0–19 Years	0									
20–34	0									
35–49	0									
50–64	0									
65+	0									
B. Operated										
0–19 Years	0									
20–34	26	1.4	<1	1	1	1	2	2	2	3
35–49	37	1.5	<1	1	1	1	2	2	3	3
50–64	14	1.9	<1	1	1	2	2	3	3	3
65+	4	2.0	<1	1	2	2	2	3	3	3
2. MULTIPLE DX										
A. Not Operated										
0–19 Years	0									
20–34	5	3.2	7	1	1	2	5	7	7	7
35–49	4	2.3	2	1	1	1	3	4	4	4
50–64	7	2.9	4	1	2	2	3	7	7	7
65+	1	3.0	0	3	3	3	3	3	3	3
B. Operated										
0–19 Years	2	4.0	8	2	2	2	6	6	6	6
20–34	145	1.8	<1	1	1	2	2	3	3	4
35–49	345	1.9	<1	1	1	2	2	3	3	4
50–64	256	2.1	1	1	1	2	3	3	3	8
65+	59	2.3	4	1	1	2	3	3	5	16
SUBTOTALS:										
1. SINGLE DX										
A. Not Operated	0									
B. Operated	81	1.5	<1	1	1	1	2	2	3	3
2. MULTIPLE DX										
A. Not Operated	17	2.8	4	1	1	2	3	7	7	7
B. Operated	807	2.0	1	1	1	2	2	3	3	5
1. SINGLE DX	**81**	**1.5**	**<1**	**1**	**1**	**1**	**2**	**2**	**3**	**3**
2. MULTIPLE DX	**824**	**2.0**	**1**	**1**	**1**	**2**	**2**	**3**	**4**	**6**
A. NOT OPERATED	**17**	**2.8**	**4**	**1**	**1**	**2**	**3**	**7**	**7**	**7**
B. OPERATED	**888**	**1.9**	**1**	**1**	**1**	**2**	**2**	**3**	**3**	**5**
TOTAL										
0–19 Years	2	4.0	8	2	2	2	6	6	6	6
20–34	176	1.8	1	1	1	2	2	3	3	7
35–49	386	1.9	<1	1	1	2	2	3	3	4
50–64	277	2.1	1	1	1	2	3	3	3	8
65+	64	2.3	4	1	1	2	3	3	4	16
GRAND TOTAL	**905**	**2.0**	**1**	**1**	**1**	**2**	**2**	**3**	**3**	**6**

622.10: CERVICAL DYSPLASIA NOS

Type of Patients	Observed Patients	Avg. Stay	Vari-ance	10th	25th	50th	75th	90th	95th	99th
1. SINGLE DX										
A. Not Operated										
0–19 Years	0									
20–34	0									
35–49	0									
50–64	0									
65+	0									
B. Operated										
0–19 Years	0									
20–34	7	1.6	<1	1	1	2	2	2	2	2
35–49	13	1.5	<1	1	1	1	2	2	3	3
50–64	7	2.0	<1	1	1	2	3	3	3	3
65+	1	1.0	0	1	1	1	1	1	1	1
2. MULTIPLE DX										
A. Not Operated										
0–19 Years	0									
20–34	0									
35–49	1	3.0	0	3	3	3	3	3	3	3
50–64	1	2.0	0	2	2	2	2	2	2	2
65+	0									
B. Operated										
0–19 Years	0									
20–34	45	1.8	<1	1	1	2	2	3	3	4
35–49	117	1.9	<1	1	1	2	2	3	3	4
50–64	84	1.9	<1	1	1	2	2	3	3	8
65+	21	2.3	2	1	2	2	2	3	5	6
SUBTOTALS:										
1. SINGLE DX										
A. Not Operated	0									
B. Operated	28	1.6	<1	1	1	2	2	3	3	3
2. MULTIPLE DX										
A. Not Operated	2	2.5	<1	2	3	3	3	3	3	3
B. Operated	267	1.9	<1	1	1	2	2	3	3	5
1. SINGLE DX	**28**	**1.6**	**<1**	**1**	**1**	**2**	**2**	**3**	**3**	**3**
2. MULTIPLE DX	**269**	**2.0**	**<1**	**1**	**1**	**2**	**2**	**3**	**3**	**5**
A. NOT OPERATED	**2**	**2.5**	**<1**	**2**	**3**	**3**	**3**	**3**	**3**	**3**
B. OPERATED	**295**	**1.9**	**<1**	**1**	**1**	**2**	**2**	**3**	**3**	**5**
TOTAL										
0–19 Years	0									
20–34	52	1.8	<1	1	1	2	2	3	3	4
35–49	131	1.9	<1	1	1	2	2	3	3	4
50–64	92	1.9	<1	1	1	2	2	3	3	8
65+	22	2.2	2	1	2	2	2	3	5	6
GRAND TOTAL	**297**	**1.9**	**<1**	**1**	**1**	**2**	**2**	**3**	**3**	**5**

622.11: MILD CERVICAL DYSPLASIA

Type of Patients	Observed Patients	Avg. Stay	Vari-ance	10th	25th	50th	75th	90th	95th	99th
1. SINGLE DX										
A. Not Operated										
0–19 Years	0									
20–34	0									
35–49	0									
50–64	0									
65+	0									
B. Operated										
0–19 Years	0									
20–34	3	2.0	<1	1	1	2	3	3	3	3
35–49	6	2.0	<1	1	2	2	2	3	3	3
50–64	2	2.0	0	2	2	2	2	2	2	2
65+	2	2.5	<1	2	2	2	3	3	3	3
2. MULTIPLE DX										
A. Not Operated										
0–19 Years	0									
20–34	2	1.5	<1	1	1	2	2	2	2	2
35–49	0									
50–64	1	3.0	0	3	3	3	3	3	3	3
65+	0									
B. Operated										
0–19 Years	0									
20–34	34	1.9	<1	1	1	2	3	3	4	4
35–49	78	1.9	<1	1	1	2	3	3	3	4
50–64	58	2.1	<1	1	2	2	3	3	3	4
65+	12	1.7	<1	1	2	2	2	3	3	3
SUBTOTALS:										
1. SINGLE DX										
A. Not Operated	0									
B. Operated	13	2.1	<1	1	2	2	2	3	3	3
2. MULTIPLE DX										
A. Not Operated	3	2.0	<1	1	1	2	3	3	3	3
B. Operated	182	1.9	<1	1	1	2	2	3	3	4
1. SINGLE DX	**13**	**2.1**	**<1**	**1**	**2**	**2**	**2**	**3**	**3**	**3**
2. MULTIPLE DX	**185**	**1.9**	**<1**	**1**	**1**	**2**	**2**	**3**	**3**	**4**
A. NOT OPERATED	**3**	**2.0**	**<1**	**1**	**1**	**2**	**3**	**3**	**3**	**3**
B. OPERATED	**195**	**1.9**	**<1**	**1**	**1**	**2**	**2**	**3**	**3**	**4**
TOTAL										
0–19 Years	0									
20–34	39	1.9	<1	1	1	2	3	3	4	4
35–49	84	1.9	<1	1	1	2	2	3	3	4
50–64	61	2.1	<1	1	2	2	3	3	3	4
65+	14	1.8	<1	1	1	2	2	3	3	3
GRAND TOTAL	**198**	**1.9**	**<1**	**1**	**1**	**2**	**2**	**3**	**3**	**4**

Length of Stay by Diagnosis and Operation, Western Region, 2008

Western Region, October 2006–September 2007 Data, by Diagnosis

622.12: MOD CERVICAL DYSPLASIA

Type of Patients	Observed Patients	Avg. Stay	Variance	10th	25th	50th	75th	90th	95th	99th
1. SINGLE DX										
A. Not Operated										
0–19 Years	0									
20–34	0									
35–49	0									
50–64	0									
65+	0									
B. Operated										
0–19 Years	0									
20–34	15	1.1	<1	1	1	1	1	2	2	2
35–49	16	1.4	<1	1	1	1	2	2	3	3
50–64	4	1.3	<1	1	1	1	2	2	2	2
65+	1	2.0	0	2	2	2	2	2	2	2
2. MULTIPLE DX										
A. Not Operated										
0–19 Years	0									
20–34	1	1.0	0	1	1	1	1	1	1	1
35–49	0									
50–64	0									
65+	0									
B. Operated										
0–19 Years	0									
20–34	52	2.0	1	1	1	2	3	3	4	8
35–49	106	1.9	<1	1	1	2	2	3	3	4
50–64	78	2.2	2	1	1	2	3	3	4	12
65+	18	2.8	12	2	2	2	3	4	16	16
SUBTOTALS:										
1. SINGLE DX										
A. Not Operated	0									
B. Operated	36	1.3	<1	1	1	1	2	2	2	3
2. MULTIPLE DX										
A. Not Operated	1	1.0		1	1	1	1	1	1	1
B. Operated	254	2.1	2	1	1	2	2	3	4	9
1. SINGLE DX	36	1.3	<1	1	1	1	2	2	2	3
2. MULTIPLE DX	255	2.1	2	1	1	2	2	3	4	9
A. NOT OPERATED	1	1.0	0	1	1	1	1	1	1	1
B. OPERATED	290	2.0	2	1	1	2	2	3	3	9
TOTAL										
0–19 Years	0									
20–34	68	1.8	1	1	1	1	2	3	3	8
35–49	122	1.8	<1	1	1	2	2	3	3	4
50–64	82	2.2	2	1	1	2	3	3	3	12
65+	19	2.8	11	2	2	2	3	4	16	16
GRAND TOTAL	291	2.0	2	1	1	2	2	3	3	9

623: NONINFLAM DISORD VAGINA

Type of Patients	Observed Patients	Avg. Stay	Variance	10th	25th	50th	75th	90th	95th	99th
1. SINGLE DX										
A. Not Operated										
0–19 Years	0									
20–34	2	1.0	0	1	1	1	1	1	1	1
35–49	3	1.3	<1	1	1	1	2	2	2	2
50–64	1	1.0	0	1	1	1	1	1	1	1
65+	0									
B. Operated										
0–19 Years	0									
20–34	7	1.0	0	1	1	1	1	1	1	1
35–49	9	1.1	<1	1	1	1	1	2	2	2
50–64	0									
65+	1	1.0	0	1	1	1	1	1	1	1
2. MULTIPLE DX										
A. Not Operated										
0–19 Years	15	1.7	<1	1	1	1	3	3	3	3
20–34	30	1.9	2	1	1	1	2	5	5	6
35–49	79	2.0	2	1	1	1	2	4	5	8
50–64	50	2.4	3	1	1	2	3	5	5	9
65+	67	2.9	3	1	1	3	4	5	7	10
B. Operated										
0–19 Years	4	1.5	<1	1	1	2	2	3	3	3
20–34	25	2.3	3	1	1	2	3	4	6	7
35–49	47	2.6	3	1	1	2	3	6	6	7
50–64	47	2.6	10	1	1	2	3	4	10	18
65+	19	3.0	6	1	2	2	4	7	8	8
SUBTOTALS:										
1. SINGLE DX										
A. Not Operated	6	1.2	<1	1	1	1	1	2	2	2
B. Operated	17	1.1	<1	1	1	1	1	1	2	2
2. MULTIPLE DX										
A. Not Operated	241	2.3	3	1	1	2	3	4	5	8
B. Operated	142	2.6	6	1	1	2	3	6	7	13
1. SINGLE DX	23	1.1	<1	1	1	1	1	2	2	2
2. MULTIPLE DX	383	2.4	4	1	1	2	3	5	6	10
A. NOT OPERATED	247	2.3	3	1	1	2	3	4	5	8
B. OPERATED	159	2.4	5	1	1	2	3	6	7	13
TOTAL										
0–19 Years	19	1.7	<1	1	1	1	3	3	3	3
20–34	64	1.9	2	1	1	1	3	4	5	7
35–49	138	2.1	2	1	1	1	3	4	6	7
50–64	98	2.5	6	1	1	2	3	5	8	18
65+	87	2.9	4	1	1	3	4	6	7	10
GRAND TOTAL	406	2.3	4	1	1	2	3	5	6	9

623.8: NONINFL DISORDER VAG NEC

Type of Patients	Observed Patients	Avg. Stay	Variance	10th	25th	50th	75th	90th	95th	99th
1. SINGLE DX										
A. Not Operated										
0–19 Years	0									
20–34	2	1.0	0	1	1	1	1	1	1	1
35–49	3	1.3	<1	1	1	1	2	2	2	2
50–64	1	1.0	0	1	1	1	1	1	1	1
65+	0									
B. Operated										
0–19 Years	0									
20–34	4	1.0	0	1	1	1	1	1	1	1
35–49	7	1.1	<1	1	1	1	1	2	2	2
50–64	0									
65+	1	1.0	0	1	1	1	1	1	1	1
2. MULTIPLE DX										
A. Not Operated										
0–19 Years	14	1.7	<1	1	1	1	2	3	3	3
20–34	29	1.9	2	1	1	1	2	5	5	6
35–49	76	1.9	2	1	1	1	2	4	5	8
50–64	48	2.5	3	1	1	2	3	5	5	9
65+	64	2.9	4	1	1	3	4	5	7	10
B. Operated										
0–19 Years	4	1.5	<1	1	1	1	2	3	3	3
20–34	20	2.3	3	1	1	2	3	3	7	7
35–49	40	2.4	3	1	1	2	3	5	6	7
50–64	31	3.1	15	1	1	2	3	6	13	18
65+	12	4.0	7	2	2	3	4	7	8	8
SUBTOTALS:										
1. SINGLE DX										
A. Not Operated	6	1.2	<1	1	1	1	1	2	2	2
B. Operated	12	1.1	<1	1	1	1	1	1	2	2
2. MULTIPLE DX										
A. Not Operated	231	2.3	3	1	1	2	3	5	5	8
B. Operated	107	2.7	7	1	1	2	3	6	7	13
1. SINGLE DX	18	1.1	<1	1	1	1	1	2	2	2
2. MULTIPLE DX	338	2.4	4	1	1	2	3	5	6	10
A. NOT OPERATED	237	2.3	3	1	1	2	3	5	5	8
B. OPERATED	119	2.6	6	1	1	2	3	6	7	13
TOTAL										
0–19 Years	18	1.6	<1	1	1	1	2	3	3	3
20–34	55	1.9	2	1	1	1	3	4	6	7
35–49	126	2.0	2	1	1	1	3	4	5	7
50–64	80	2.7	8	1	1	2	3	5	8	18
65+	77	3.1	4	1	2	3	4	7	7	10
GRAND TOTAL	356	2.4	4	1	1	2	3	5	6	10

Length of Stay by Diagnosis and Operation, Western Region, 2008

Western Region, October 2006–September 2007 Data, by Diagnosis

Length of Stay by Diagnosis and Operation, Western Region, 2008

Type of Patients	624: NONINFL DISORDER VULVA										625: FEMALE GENITAL SYMPTOMS										625.0: DYSPAREUNIA									
	Observed Patients	Avg. Stay	Vari-ance	10th	25th	50th	75th	90th	95th	99th	Observed Patients	Avg. Stay	Vari-ance	10th	25th	50th	75th	90th	95th	99th	Observed Patients	Avg. Stay	Vari-ance	10th	25th	50th	75th	90th	95th	99th
1. SINGLE DX																														
A. Not Operated																														
0–19 Years	0										28	1.4	<1	1	1	1	2	2	2	3	0									
20–34	2	1.5	<1	1	1	2	2	2	2	2	30	1.6	<1	1	1	1	2	3	3	3	0									
35–49	0										14	1.3	<1	1	1	1	1	2	2	2	0									
50–64	0										4	1.3	<1	1	1	1	1	2	2	2	0									
65+	0										1	3.0	0	3	3	3	3	3	3	3	0									
B. Operated																														
0–19 Years	2	1.5	<1	1	1	2	2	2	2	2	3	2.0	1	1	1	1	3	3	3	3	0									
20–34	2	1.5	<1	1	1	1	2	2	2	2	56	1.4	<1	1	1	1	2	3	3	3	1	3.0	0	3	3	3	3	3	3	3
35–49	0										207	1.4	<1	1	1	1	2	2	3	3	1	1.0	0	1	1	1	1	1	1	1
50–64	0										122	1.4	<1	1	1	1	2	2	3	3	0									
65+	3	1.0	0	1	1	1	1	1	1	1	29	1.2	<1	1	1	1	1	2	2	2	0									
2. MULTIPLE DX																														
A. Not Operated																														
0–19 Years	0										48	1.9	1	1	1	2	2	3	4	5	0									
20–34	4	1.0	0	1	1	1	1	1	1	1	215	2.3	3	1	1	2	3	4	6	8	1	2.0	0	2	2	2	2	2	2	2
35–49	1	1.5	1	1	1	1	3	3	3	3	171	1.9	2	1	1	1	2	4	4	9	0									
50–64	2	4.0	18	1	1	1	7	7	7	7	70	2.9	9	1	1	2	4	6	8	19	0									
65+	3	4.3	1	3	3	5	5	5	5	5	38	2.6	5	1	1	2	4	7	8	9	0									
B. Operated																														
0–19 Years	1	4.0	0	4	4	4	4	4	4	4	24	2.1	2	1	1	1	2	4	5	7	0									
20–34	5	2.2	<1	1	2	2	3	3	3	3	1,410	2.0	1	1	1	1	2	3	4	6	79	2.0	<1	1	1	2	2	3	3	4
35–49	17	2.2	4	1	1	2	2	4	9	9	3,554	1.9	1	1	1	1	2	3	4	5	89	1.9	1	1	1	2	2	3	3	7
50–64	13	1.4	2	1	1	1	1	1	6	6	1,588	1.7	1	1	1	1	2	3	3	5	26	1.5	<1	1	1	2	2	2	2	3
65+	19	1.6	1	1	1	1	2	3	6	6	768	1.6	2	1	1	1	2	3	3	6	3	1.0	0	1	1	1	1	1	1	1
SUBTOTALS:																														
1. SINGLE DX																														
A. Not Operated	2	1.5	<1	1	1	2	2	2	2	2	77	1.4	<1	1	1	1	2	2	3	3	0									
B. Operated	7	1.3	<1	1	1	1	2	2	2	2	417	1.4	<1	1	1	1	2	2	3	3	2	2.0	2	1	1	2	2	3	3	3
2. MULTIPLE DX																														
A. Not Operated	10	2.8	5	1	1	3	5	5	7	7	542	2.2	3	1	1	2	3	4	6	9	0									
B. Operated	55	1.8	2	1	1	1	2	3	6	9	7,344	1.9	1	1	1	1	2	3	4	6	197	1.9	<1	1	1	2	2	3	3	4
1. SINGLE DX	9	1.3	<1	1	1	1	2	2	2	2	494	1.4	<1	1	1	1	2	2	3	3	2	2.0	2	1	1	2	2	3	3	3
2. MULTIPLE DX	65	2.0	3	1	1	1	2	4	6	9	7,886	1.9	1	1	1	2	2	3	4	6	198	1.9	<1	1	1	2	2	3	3	4
A. NOT OPERATED	12	2.6	4	1	1	2	3	5	7	7	619	2.1	3	1	1	2	3	4	5	9	1	2.0	0	2	2	2	2	2	2	2
B. OPERATED	62	1.8	2	1	1	1	2	3	4	9	7,761	1.8	1	1	1	2	2	3	4	6	199	1.9	<1	1	1	2	2	3	3	4
TOTAL																														
0–19 Years	3	2.3	2	1	1	2	2	4	4	4	103	1.8	<1	1	1	2	2	3	4	5	0									
20–34	10	1.8	<1	1	1	2	2	3	3	3	1,711	2.0	1	1	1	2	2	3	4	6	81	2.0	<1	1	1	2	2	3	3	4
35–49	21	2.1	3	1	1	2	2	3	4	9	3,946	1.9	1	1	1	1	2	3	4	5	90	1.9	1	1	1	2	2	3	3	7
50–64	15	1.7	4	1	1	1	1	6	7	7	1,784	1.7	1	1	1	1	2	3	4	6	26	1.5	<1	1	1	2	2	2	2	3
65+	25	1.9	2	1	1	1	2	5	5	6	836	1.6	2	1	1	1	2	3	4	7	3	1.0	0	1	1	1	1	1	1	1
GRAND TOTAL	74	1.9	2	1	1	1	2	4	6	9	8,380	1.9	1	1	1	2	2	3	4	6	200	1.9	<1	1	1	2	2	3	3	4

Western Region, October 2006–September 2007 Data, by Diagnosis

625.3: DYSMENORRHEA

Type of Patients	Observed Patients	Avg. Stay	Vari-ance	10th	25th	50th	75th	90th	95th	99th
1. SINGLE DX										
A. Not Operated										
0–19 Years	8	1.1	<1	1	1	1	1	2	2	2
20–34	0									
35–49	4	1.3	<1	1	1	1	2	2	2	2
50–64	0									
65+	0									
B. Operated										
0–19 Years	0									
20–34	10	1.2	<1	1	1	1	1	2	2	2
35–49	34	1.7	<1	1	1	1	2	3	3	4
50–64	1	1.0	0	1	1	1	1	1	1	1
65+	0									
2. MULTIPLE DX										
A. Not Operated										
0–19 Years	13	1.6	<1	1	1	1	1	3	4	4
20–34	23	2.3	7	1	1	1	1	5	8	12
35–49	16	1.4	<1	1	1	1	1	2	4	4
50–64	2	2.0	0	2	2	2	2	2	2	2
65+	0									
B. Operated										
0–19 Years	0									
20–34	565	1.9	<1	1	1	2	2	3	3	5
35–49	1,469	1.9	1	1	1	2	2	3	3	5
50–64	141	2.1	2	1	1	2	3	3	4	7
65+	1	1.0	0	1	1	1	1	1	1	1
SUBTOTALS:										
1. SINGLE DX										
A. Not Operated	12	1.2	<1	1	1	1	1	2	2	2
B. Operated	45	1.5	<1	1	1	1	2	3	3	4
2. MULTIPLE DX										
A. Not Operated	54	1.9	4	1	1	1	2	3	5	12
B. Operated	2,176	1.9	1	1	1	2	2	3	3	5
1. SINGLE DX	57	1.5	<1	1	1	1	2	2	3	4
2. MULTIPLE DX	2,230	1.9	1	1	1	2	2	3	3	5
A. NOT OPERATED	66	1.7	3	1	1	1	2	3	4	12
B. OPERATED	2,221	1.9	1	1	1	2	2	3	3	5
TOTAL										
0–19 Years	21	1.4	<1	1	1	1	1	2	3	4
20–34	598	1.9	1	1	1	2	2	3	3	5
35–49	1,523	1.9	1	1	1	2	2	3	3	5
50–64	144	2.1	2	1	1	2	3	3	4	7
65+	1	1.0	0	1	1	1	1	1	1	1
GRAND TOTAL	2,287	1.9	1	1	1	2	2	3	3	5

625.6: FE STRESS INCONTINENCE

Type of Patients	Observed Patients	Avg. Stay	Vari-ance	10th	25th	50th	75th	90th	95th	99th
1. SINGLE DX										
A. Not Operated										
0–19 Years	0									
20–34	0									
35–49	0									
50–64	0									
65+	1	3.0	0	3	3	3	3	3	3	3
B. Operated										
0–19 Years	0									
20–34	18	1.3	<1	1	1	1	2	2	2	3
35–49	140	1.2	<1	1	1	1	1	2	2	3
50–64	111	1.3	<1	1	1	1	2	2	2	2
65+	29	1.2	<1	1	1	1	1	2	2	2
2. MULTIPLE DX										
A. Not Operated										
0–19 Years	0									
20–34	0									
35–49	11	1.0	0	1	1	1	1	1	1	1
50–64	5	1.0	0	1	1	1	1	1	1	1
65+	7	1.0	0	1	1	1	1	1	1	1
B. Operated										
0–19 Years	0									
20–34	125	1.7	1	1	1	1	2	3	4	5
35–49	985	1.6	<1	1	1	1	2	3	3	5
50–64	1,156	1.5	<1	1	1	1	2	3	3	5
65+	724	1.5	<1	1	1	1	2	3	3	6
SUBTOTALS:										
1. SINGLE DX										
A. Not Operated	1	3.0	0	3	3	3	3	3	3	3
B. Operated	298	1.3	<1	1	1	1	1	2	2	3
2. MULTIPLE DX										
A. Not Operated	23	1.0	0	1	1	1	1	1	1	1
B. Operated	2,990	1.6	<1	1	1	1	2	3	3	5
1. SINGLE DX	299	1.3	<1	1	1	1	2	2	2	3
2. MULTIPLE DX	3,013	1.6	<1	1	1	1	2	3	3	5
A. NOT OPERATED	24	1.1	<1	1	1	1	1	1	3	3
B. OPERATED	3,288	1.5	<1	1	1	1	2	3	3	5
TOTAL										
0–19 Years	0									
20–34	143	1.7	1	1	1	1	2	3	3	5
35–49	1,136	1.6	<1	1	1	1	2	3	3	5
50–64	1,272	1.5	<1	1	1	1	2	3	3	5
65+	761	1.5	<1	1	1	1	2	3	3	6
GRAND TOTAL	3,312	1.5	<1	1	1	1	2	3	3	5

625.8: FE GENITAL SYMPTOMS NEC

Type of Patients	Observed Patients	Avg. Stay	Vari-ance	10th	25th	50th	75th	90th	95th	99th
1. SINGLE DX										
A. Not Operated										
0–19 Years	1	3.0	0	3	3	3	3	3	3	3
20–34	7	1.3	<1	1	1	1	2	2	2	2
35–49	4	1.5	<1	1	1	2	2	2	2	2
50–64	1	1.0	0	1	1	1	1	1	1	1
65+	0									
B. Operated										
0–19 Years	0									
20–34	2	1.0	0	1	1	1	1	1	1	1
35–49	5	2.0	<1	1	1	2	3	3	3	3
50–64	5	2.4	1	2	2	2	3	4	4	4
65+	0									
2. MULTIPLE DX										
A. Not Operated										
0–19 Years	1	1.0	0	1	1	1	1	1	1	1
20–34	15	2.9	8	1	1	2	4	5	12	12
35–49	38	2.1	3	1	1	2	3	5	6	9
50–64	30	3.1	12	1	1	2	4	6	8	19
65+	14	3.1	7	1	1	1	5	7	8	8
B. Operated										
0–19 Years	4	1.5	<1	1	1	2	2	2	2	2
20–34	41	2.4	3	1	1	2	3	5	6	8
35–49	96	2.5	3	1	2	2	3	4	5	15
50–64	70	2.6	2	1	2	2	3	4	5	6
65+	26	3.3	5	2	2	3	4	6	6	12
SUBTOTALS:										
1. SINGLE DX										
A. Not Operated	13	1.5	<1	1	1	1	2	2	2	3
B. Operated	12	2.0	1	1	1	2	3	3	3	4
2. MULTIPLE DX										
A. Not Operated	98	2.7	7	1	2	2	3	6	8	19
B. Operated	237	2.6	3	1	2	2	3	4	5	9
1. SINGLE DX	25	1.7	<1	1	1	1	2	3	3	4
2. MULTIPLE DX	335	2.6	4	1	1	2	3	5	6	12
A. NOT OPERATED	111	2.5	7	1	1	2	3	5	7	12
B. OPERATED	249	2.6	3	1	2	3	3	4	5	9
TOTAL										
0–19 Years	6	1.7	<1	1	1	1	2	3	3	3
20–34	65	2.3	4	1	1	2	3	5	6	12
35–49	143	2.4	3	1	1	2	3	5	5	9
50–64	106	2.7	5	1	1	2	3	5	5	8
65+	40	3.2	6	1	1	3	4	6	8	12
GRAND TOTAL	360	2.6	4	1	1	2	3	5	6	12

Length of Stay by Diagnosis and Operation, Western Region, 2008

Western Region, October 2006–September 2007 Data, by Diagnosis

625.9: FE GENITAL SYMPTOMS NOS

Type of Patients	Observed Patients	Avg. Stay	Vari-ance	10th	25th	50th	75th	90th	95th	99th
1. SINGLE DX										
A. Not Operated										
0–19 Years	6	1.7	<1	1	1	2	2	2	2	2
20–34	22	1.6	<1	1	1	1	2	2	3	3
35–49	4	1.0	0	1	1	1	1	1	1	1
50–64	1	1.0	0	1	1	1	1	1	1	1
65+	0									
B. Operated										
0–19 Years	3	2.0	1	1	1	2	3	3	3	3
20–34	21	1.6	<1	1	1	2	2	2	3	3
35–49	26	1.9	<1	1	1	2	3	3	3	3
50–64	5	2.0	<1	1	2	2	2	3	3	3
65+	0									
2. MULTIPLE DX										
A. Not Operated										
0–19 Years	24	2.2	1	1	1	2	3	4	4	5
20–34	157	2.2	2	1	1	2	3	4	5	7
35–49	98	2.0	2	1	1	2	3	4	4	10
50–64	30	3.1	7	1	1	2	5	8	8	9
65+	17	2.7	5	1	1	2	4	5	9	9
B. Operated										
0–19 Years	16	2.3	3	1	1	2	2	4	7	7
20–34	539	2.1	1	1	1	2	3	3	4	6
35–49	863	2.2	2	1	1	2	3	3	4	6
50–64	182	2.2	1	1	2	2	3	3	4	7
65+	14	2.7	4	1	1	2	4	6	7	7
SUBTOTALS:										
1. SINGLE DX										
A. Not Operated	33	1.5	<1	1	1	1	2	3	3	3
B. Operated	55	1.8	<1	1	1	2	2	3	3	3
2. MULTIPLE DX										
A. Not Operated	326	2.2	3	1	1	2	3	4	5	8
B. Operated	1,614	2.2	2	1	1	2	3	3	4	6
1. SINGLE DX	88	1.7	<1	1	1	2	2	3	3	3
2. MULTIPLE DX	1,940	2.2	2	1	1	2	3	3	4	7
A. NOT OPERATED	359	2.2	2	1	1	2	3	4	5	8
B. OPERATED	1,669	2.2	2	1	1	2	3	3	4	6
TOTAL										
0–19 Years	49	2.1	2	1	1	2	2	3	4	7
20–34	739	2.1	1	1	1	2	3	3	4	6
35–49	991	2.2	2	1	1	2	3	3	4	6
50–64	218	2.3	2	1	1	2	2	4	5	8
65+	31	2.7	4	1	1	2	4	5	7	9
GRAND TOTAL	2,028	2.2	2	1	1	2	3	3	4	7

626: DISORDER OF MENSTRUATION

Type of Patients	Observed Patients	Avg. Stay	Vari-ance	10th	25th	50th	75th	90th	95th	99th
1. SINGLE DX										
A. Not Operated										
0–19 Years	1	2.0	0	2	2	2	2	2	2	2
20–34	20	1.3	<1	1	1	1	1	2	3	3
35–49	32	1.5	1	1	1	1	2	3	3	6
50–64	3	1.3	<1	1	1	1	2	2	2	2
65+	0									
B. Operated										
0–19 Years	0	1.0	0	1	1	1	1	1	1	1
20–34	80	1.6	<1	1	1	1	2	3	3	3
35–49	231	1.7	<1	1	1	1	2	3	3	4
50–64	48	1.7	<1	1	1	1	2	3	3	4
65+	0									
2. MULTIPLE DX										
A. Not Operated										
0–19 Years	120	1.7	1	1	1	1	2	3	3	5
20–34	298	1.6	<1	1	1	1	2	3	4	4
35–49	626	1.7	1	1	1	1	2	3	4	7
50–64	129	1.8	2	1	1	1	2	3	4	8
65+	13	2.5	2	1	1	2	4	5	5	5
B. Operated										
0–19 Years	22	2.5	1	2	2	2	3	4	5	7
20–34	1,893	2.1	2	1	1	2	3	3	4	6
35–49	10,095	2.1	1	1	1	2	3	3	4	6
50–64	1,988	2.2	2	1	1	2	3	3	4	7
65+	9	2.6	3	1	2	2	4	6	6	6
SUBTOTALS:										
1. SINGLE DX										
A. Not Operated	56	1.5	<1	1	1	1	2	3	3	6
B. Operated	360	1.6	<1	1	1	1	2	3	3	4
2. MULTIPLE DX										
A. Not Operated	1,186	1.7	1	1	1	1	2	3	4	7
B. Operated	14,007	2.1	1	1	1	2	3	3	4	6
1. SINGLE DX	416	1.6	<1	1	1	1	2	3	3	4
2. MULTIPLE DX	15,193	2.1	1	1	1	2	3	3	4	6
A. NOT OPERATED	1,242	1.7	1	1	1	1	2	3	4	7
B. OPERATED	14,367	2.1	1	1	1	2	3	3	4	6
TOTAL										
0–19 Years	144	1.9	1	1	1	2	2	3	4	7
20–34	2,291	2.0	2	1	1	1	3	3	4	6
35–49	10,984	2.0	1	1	1	2	3	3	4	6
50–64	2,168	2.2	2	1	1	2	3	3	5	7
65+	22	2.6	3	1	1	2	4	5	5	6
GRAND TOTAL	15,609	2.0	1	1	1	2	3	3	4	6

626.2: EXCESSIVE MENSTRUATION

Type of Patients	Observed Patients	Avg. Stay	Vari-ance	10th	25th	50th	75th	90th	95th	99th
1. SINGLE DX										
A. Not Operated										
0–19 Years	0									
20–34	10	1.1	<1	1	1	1	1	1	2	2
35–49	20	1.8	2	1	1	2	2	3	6	6
50–64	0	1.5	<1	1	1	2	2	2	2	2
65+	0									
B. Operated										
0–19 Years	0									
20–34	51	1.7	<1	1	1	2	2	3	3	3
35–49	163	1.6	<1	1	1	1	2	3	3	4
50–64	36	1.7	<1	1	1	2	2	3	3	3
65+	0									
2. MULTIPLE DX										
A. Not Operated										
0–19 Years	70	1.6	<1	1	1	1	2	3	3	5
20–34	175	1.6	<1	1	1	1	2	3	4	4
35–49	426	1.7	1	1	1	1	2	3	4	6
50–64	85	1.5	<1	1	1	1	2	3	3	6
65+	1	4.0	0	4	4	4	4	4	4	4
B. Operated										
0–19 Years	16	2.4	1	1	2	2	3	4	5	5
20–34	1,443	2.1	2	1	1	2	3	3	4	6
35–49	8,232	2.1	1	1	1	2	3	3	4	5
50–64	1,534	2.2	2	1	1	2	3	3	4	7
65+	3	1.3	<1	1	1	1	2	2	2	2
SUBTOTALS:										
1. SINGLE DX										
A. Not Operated	32	1.5	1	1	1	1	2	3	3	6
B. Operated	250	1.6	<1	1	1	1	2	3	3	4
2. MULTIPLE DX										
A. Not Operated	757	1.7	<1	1	1	1	2	3	4	6
B. Operated	11,228	2.1	1	1	1	2	3	3	4	6
1. SINGLE DX	282	1.6	<1	1	1	1	2	3	3	4
2. MULTIPLE DX	11,985	2.1	1	1	1	2	3	3	4	6
A. NOT OPERATED	789	1.7	1	1	1	1	2	3	4	6
B. OPERATED	11,478	2.1	1	1	1	2	3	3	4	6
TOTAL										
0–19 Years	86	1.8	<1	1	1	1	2	3	3	5
20–34	1,679	2.0	2	1	1	2	3	3	4	6
35–49	8,841	2.0	1	1	1	2	3	3	4	5
50–64	1,657	2.2	2	1	1	2	3	3	4	6
65+	4	2.0	2	1	1	2	3	4	4	4
GRAND TOTAL	12,267	2.0	1	1	1	2	3	3	4	6

Western Region, October 2006–September 2007 Data, by Diagnosis

626.8: MENSTRUAL DISORDER NEC

Type of Patients	Observed Patients	Avg. Stay	Variance	10th	25th	50th	75th	90th	95th	99th
1. SINGLE DX										
A. Not Operated										
0–19 Years	1	2.0	0	2	2	2	2	2	2	2
20–34	9	1.6	<1	1	1	1	2	2	3	3
35–49	8	1.1	<1	1	1	1	1	2	2	2
50–64	1	1.0	0	1	1	1	1	1	1	1
65+	0									
B. Operated										
0–19 Years	0									
20–34	21	1.4	<1	1	1	1	2	2	3	3
35–49	55	1.8	<1	1	1	2	2	3	3	4
50–64	10	1.8	1	1	1	1	2	3	4	4
65+	0									
2. MULTIPLE DX										
A. Not Operated										
0–19 Years	45	1.9	2	1	1	1	2	3	4	8
20–34	116	1.6	<1	1	1	1	2	3	4	4
35–49	173	1.7	1	1	1	1	2	3	3	8
50–64	38	2.3	4	1	1	2	2	5	8	10
65+	11	2.6	2	1	2	2	4	5	5	5
B. Operated										
0–19 Years	5	3.0	2	2	2	2	4	5	5	5
20–34	352	2.1	2	1	1	2	2	3	4	7
35–49	1,561	2.1	1	1	1	2	3	3	4	7
50–64	388	2.2	2	1	1	2	3	3	4	8
65+	6	3.2	4	1	2	4	4	6	6	6
SUBTOTALS:										
1. SINGLE DX										
A. Not Operated	19	1.4	<1	1	1	1	2	2	3	3
B. Operated	86	1.7	<1	1	1	1	2	3	3	4
2. MULTIPLE DX										
A. Not Operated	383	1.8	2	1	1	1	2	3	4	8
B. Operated	2,312	2.1	2	1	1	2	3	3	4	7
1. SINGLE DX	105	1.6	<1	1	1	1	2	3	3	4
2. MULTIPLE DX	2,695	2.1	2	1	1	2	3	3	4	7
A. NOT OPERATED	402	1.7	2	1	1	1	2	3	4	8
B. OPERATED	2,398	2.1	2	1	1	2	3	3	4	7
TOTAL										
0–19 Years	51	2.0	2	1	1	2	2	4	5	8
20–34	498	2.0	2	1	1	1	2	3	4	6
35–49	1,797	2.1	1	1	1	2	3	3	4	7
50–64	437	2.2	2	1	1	2	3	3	4	8
65+	17	2.8	3	1	1	2	4	5	6	6
GRAND TOTAL	2,800	2.1	2	1	1	2	3	3	4	7

627: MENOPAUSAL DISORDERS

Type of Patients	Observed Patients	Avg. Stay	Variance	10th	25th	50th	75th	90th	95th	99th
1. SINGLE DX										
A. Not Operated										
0–19 Years	0									
20–34	0									
35–49	0									
50–64	0									
65+	0									
B. Operated										
0–19 Years	0									
20–34	1	2.0	0	2	2	2	2	2	2	2
35–49	5	1.0	0	1	1	1	1	1	1	1
50–64	17	1.7	<1	1	1	1	2	3	3	3
65+	5	1.2	<1	1	1	1	1	2	2	2
2. MULTIPLE DX										
A. Not Operated										
0–19 Years	3	2.0	3	1	1	1	2	3	4	4
20–34	11	1.6	<1	1	1	2	2	2	2	2
35–49	33	1.6	<1	1	1	1	2	3	3	4
50–64	48	1.7	1	1	1	1	2	3	4	5
65+	69	3.6	8	1	2	3	4	8	10	13
B. Operated										
0–19 Years	0									
20–34	57	2.5	5	1	1	2	3	4	7	15
35–49	335	2.2	2	1	1	2	3	3	4	8
50–64	874	2.3	3	1	1	2	3	4	4	8
65+	297	2.9	7	1	1	2	3	6	8	15
SUBTOTALS:										
1. SINGLE DX										
A. Not Operated	0									
B. Operated	28	1.5	<1	1	1	1	2	3	3	3
2. MULTIPLE DX										
A. Not Operated	164	2.5	5	1	1	2	3	5	7	11
B. Operated	1,563	2.4	4	1	1	2	3	4	5	11
1. SINGLE DX	28	1.5	<1	1	1	1	2	3	3	3
2. MULTIPLE DX	1,727	2.4	4	1	1	2	3	4	5	11
A. NOT OPERATED	164	2.5	5	1	1	2	3	5	7	11
B. OPERATED	1,591	2.4	4	1	1	2	3	4	5	11
TOTAL										
0–19 Years	3	2.0	3	1	1	1	2	4	4	4
20–34	69	2.3	5	1	1	2	3	4	5	15
35–49	373	2.1	2	1	1	2	3	3	4	8
50–64	939	2.2	3	1	1	2	3	3	4	7
65+	371	3.0	7	1	1	2	4	6	8	15
GRAND TOTAL	1,755	2.4	4	1	1	2	3	4	5	11

627.0: PREMENOPAUSE MENORRHAGIA

Type of Patients	Observed Patients	Avg. Stay	Variance	10th	25th	50th	75th	90th	95th	99th
1. SINGLE DX										
A. Not Operated										
0–19 Years	0									
20–34	0									
35–49	0									
50–64	0									
65+	0									
B. Operated										
0–19 Years	0									
20–34	1	2.0	0	2	2	2	2	2	2	2
35–49	4	1.0	0	1	1	1	1	1	1	1
50–64	2	2.0	2	1	1	1	3	3	3	3
65+	0									
2. MULTIPLE DX										
A. Not Operated										
0–19 Years	2	2.5	4	1	1	4	4	4	4	4
20–34	11	1.6	<1	1	1	1	2	2	2	2
35–49	24	1.6	<1	1	1	1	2	3	3	4
50–64	10	1.0	0	1	1	1	1	1	1	1
65+	0									
B. Operated										
0–19 Years	0									
20–34	56	2.5	5	1	1	2	3	4	7	15
35–49	242	2.3	3	1	1	2	3	3	5	8
50–64	79	2.2	2	1	1	2	3	4	4	9
65+	3	3.0	7	1	1	2	3	6	6	6
SUBTOTALS:										
1. SINGLE DX										
A. Not Operated	0									
B. Operated	7	1.4	<1	1	1	1	2	3	3	3
2. MULTIPLE DX										
A. Not Operated	47	1.5	<1	1	1	1	2	2	3	4
B. Operated	380	2.3	3	1	1	2	3	4	5	9
1. SINGLE DX	7	1.4	<1	1	1	1	2	3	3	3
2. MULTIPLE DX	427	2.2	3	1	1	2	3	4	4	9
A. NOT OPERATED	47	1.5	<1	1	1	1	2	2	3	4
B. OPERATED	387	2.3	3	1	1	2	3	4	5	9
TOTAL										
0–19 Years	2	2.5	4	1	1	4	4	4	4	4
20–34	68	2.3	5	1	1	2	3	4	5	15
35–49	270	2.2	2	1	1	2	3	3	5	8
50–64	91	2.1	2	1	1	2	3	3	4	9
65+	3	3.0	7	1	1	2	3	6	6	6
GRAND TOTAL	434	2.2	3	1	1	2	3	4	4	9

Length of Stay by Diagnosis and Operation, Western Region, 2008

Western Region, October 2006–September 2007 Data, by Diagnosis

627.1: POSTMENOPAUSAL BLEEDING

Type of Patients	Observed Patients	Avg. Stay	Vari-ance	10th	25th	50th	75th	90th	95th	99th
1. SINGLE DX										
A. Not Operated										
0–19 Years	0									
20–34	0									
35–49	0									
50–64	0									
65+	0									
B. Operated										
0–19 Years	0									
20–34	0									
35–49	1	1.0	0	1	1	1	1	1	1	1
50–64	15	1.6	<1	1	1	1	2	3	3	3
65+	5	1.2	<1	1	1	1	1	2	2	2
2. MULTIPLE DX										
A. Not Operated										
0–19 Years	0									
20–34	0									
35–49	6	1.7	1	1	1	1	3	3	3	3
50–64	36	1.9	1	1	1	2	3	4	5	5
65+	59	3.5	8	1	2	3	4	8	11	13
B. Operated										
0–19 Years	0									
20–34	1	3.0	0	3	3	3	3	3	3	3
35–49	89	2.0	<1	1	1	2	3	3	4	5
50–64	786	2.3	3	1	1	2	3	4	4	8
65+	292	2.9	7	1	1	2	3	6	8	15
SUBTOTALS:										
1. SINGLE DX										
A. Not Operated	0									
B. Operated	21	1.5	<1	1	1	1	2	2	3	3
2. MULTIPLE DX										
A. Not Operated	101	2.8	6	1	1	2	4	5	8	11
B. Operated	1,168	2.4	4	1	1	2	3	4	5	11
1. SINGLE DX	21	1.5	<1	1	1	1	2	2	3	3
2. MULTIPLE DX	1,269	2.5	4	1	1	2	3	4	5	11
A. NOT OPERATED	101	2.8	6	1	1	2	4	5	8	11
B. OPERATED	1,189	2.4	4	1	1	2	3	4	5	11
TOTAL										
0–19 Years	0									
20–34	1	3.0	0	3	3	3	3	3	3	3
35–49	96	2.0	<1	1	1	2	3	3	4	5
50–64	837	2.3	3	1	1	2	3	4	4	7
65+	356	3.0	7	1	1	2	3	6	8	15
GRAND TOTAL	1,290	2.5	4	1	1	2	3	4	5	11

628: FEMALE INFERTILITY

Type of Patients	Observed Patients	Avg. Stay	Vari-ance	10th	25th	50th	75th	90th	95th	99th
1. SINGLE DX										
A. Not Operated										
0–19 Years	1	2.0	0	2	2	2	2	2	2	2
20–34	1	1.0	0	1	1	1	1	1	1	1
35–49	0									
50–64	0									
65+	0									
B. Operated										
0–19 Years	0									
20–34	2	2.0	0	2	2	2	2	2	2	2
35–49	4	1.5	<1	1	1	1	2	2	2	2
50–64	0									
65+	0									
2. MULTIPLE DX										
A. Not Operated										
0–19 Years	2	1.0	0	1	1	1	1	1	1	1
20–34	6	1.5	<1	1	1	1	2	3	3	3
35–49	1	1.0	0	1	1	1	1	1	1	1
50–64	0									
65+	0									
B. Operated										
0–19 Years	0									
20–34	13	1.4	<1	1	1	1	1	3	3	3
35–49	13	2.2	3	1	1	2	2	3	7	7
50–64	1	15.0	0	15	15	15	15	15	15	15
65+	0									
SUBTOTALS:										
1. SINGLE DX										
A. Not Operated	2	1.5	<1	1	1	1	2	2	2	2
B. Operated	6	1.7	<1	1	1	1	2	2	2	2
2. MULTIPLE DX										
A. Not Operated	9	1.3	<1	1	1	1	1	3	3	3
B. Operated	27	2.3	8	1	1	1	2	3	7	15
1. SINGLE DX	8	1.6	<1	1	1	1	2	2	3	3
2. MULTIPLE DX	36	2.0	6	1	1	1	3	3	7	15
A. NOT OPERATED	11	1.4	<1	1	1	1	2	2	3	3
B. OPERATED	33	2.2	7	1	1	1	2	3	7	15
TOTAL										
0–19 Years	3	1.3	<1	1	1	1	2	2	2	2
20–34	22	1.5	<1	1	1	1	2	3	3	3
35–49	18	1.9	2	1	1	2	3	3	7	7
50–64	1	15.0	0	15	15	15	15	15	15	15
65+	0									
GRAND TOTAL	44	2.0	5	1	1	1	2	3	3	15

629: OTH FEMALE GENITAL DIS

Type of Patients	Observed Patients	Avg. Stay	Vari-ance	10th	25th	50th	75th	90th	95th	99th
1. SINGLE DX										
A. Not Operated										
0–19 Years	0									
20–34	0									
35–49	1	1.0	0	1	1	1	1	1	1	1
50–64	0									
65+	0									
B. Operated										
0–19 Years	0									
20–34	0									
35–49	1	2.0	0	2	2	2	2	2	2	2
50–64	0									
65+	0									
2. MULTIPLE DX										
A. Not Operated										
0–19 Years	1	1.0	0	1	1	1	1	1	1	1
20–34	1	1.0	0	1	1	1	1	1	1	1
35–49	5	2.4	2	1	1	2	4	4	4	4
50–64	2	4.5	<1	4	4	5	5	5	5	5
65+	1	7.0	0	7	7	7	7	7	7	7
B. Operated										
0–19 Years	1	2.0	0	2	2	2	2	2	2	2
20–34	5	2.6	2	1	1	3	4	4	4	4
35–49	8	2.5	2	1	1	3	3	4	4	4
50–64	10	2.0	1	1	1	2	3	4	4	4
65+	0									
SUBTOTALS:										
1. SINGLE DX										
A. Not Operated	1	1.0	0	1	1	1	1	1	1	1
B. Operated	1	2.0	0	2	2	2	2	2	2	2
2. MULTIPLE DX										
A. Not Operated	10	3.0	4	1	1	4	4	5	7	7
B. Operated	24	2.3	1	1	1	2	3	4	4	4
1. SINGLE DX	2	1.5	<1	1	1	2	2	2	2	2
2. MULTIPLE DX	34	2.5	2	1	1	2	4	4	5	7
A. NOT OPERATED	11	2.8	4	1	1	2	4	5	7	7
B. OPERATED	25	2.3	1	1	1	2	3	4	4	4
TOTAL										
0–19 Years	2	1.5	<1	1	1	1	2	2	2	2
20–34	6	2.3	2	1	1	1	4	4	4	4
35–49	15	2.3	1	1	1	2	3	4	5	7
50–64	12	2.4	2	1	2	2	4	4	5	15
65+	1	7.0	0	7	7	7	7	7	7	7
GRAND TOTAL	36	2.4	2	1	1	2	4	4	5	7

Length of Stay by Diagnosis and Operation, Western Region, 2008

630: HYDATIDIFORM MOLE

Type of Patients	Observed Patients	Avg. Stay	Vari-ance	10th	25th	50th	75th	90th	95th	99th
1. SINGLE DX										
A. Not Operated										
0–19 Years	9	1.3	<1	1	1	1	1	3	3	3
20–34	16	1.7	2	1	1	1	2	3	6	6
35–49	6	1.3	<1	1	1	1	2	2	2	2
50–64	1	2.0	0	2	2	2	2	2	2	2
65+	0									
B. Operated										
0–19 Years	5	1.4	<1	1	1	1	2	2	2	2
20–34	15	1.4	1	1	1	1	1	2	5	5
35–49	8	1.8	<1	1	1	1	3	3	3	3
50–64	3	2.0	1	2	2	2	3	3	3	3
65+	0									
2. MULTIPLE DX										
A. Not Operated										
0–19 Years	6	2.2	2	1	1	2	2	5	5	5
20–34	16	1.5	<1	1	1	1	2	3	4	4
35–49	4	1.0	0	1	1	1	1	1	1	1
50–64	2	3.0	8	1	1	1	5	5	5	5
65+	0									
B. Operated										
0–19 Years	4	1.8	<1	1	1	1	3	3	3	3
20–34	11	1.6	1	1	1	1	2	2	5	5
35–49	10	3.1	2	2	2	3	4	5	6	6
50–64	1	2.0	0	2	2	2	2	2	2	2
65+	0									
SUBTOTALS:										
1. SINGLE DX										
A. Not Operated	32	1.5	<1	1	1	1	2	2	3	3
B. Operated	31	1.6	<1	1	1	1	2	3	3	5
2. MULTIPLE DX										
A. Not Operated	28	1.7	1	1	1	2	2	4	5	5
B. Operated	26	2.2	2	1	1	2	3	5	5	6
1. SINGLE DX	63	1.5	<1	1	1	1	2	3	3	6
2. MULTIPLE DX	54	1.9	2	1	1	1	2	4	5	6
A. NOT OPERATED	60	1.6	1	1	1	1	2	3	4	6
B. OPERATED	57	1.9	1	1	1	1	2	3	5	6
TOTAL										
0–19 Years	24	1.6	<1	1	1	1	2	3	3	5
20–34	58	1.6	1	1	1	1	2	3	5	6
35–49	28	2.0	2	1	1	2	3	4	5	6
50–64	7	2.3	2	1	1	2	3	5	5	5
65+	0									
GRAND TOTAL	117	1.7	1	1	1	1	2	3	5	6

631: ABNORMAL POC NEC

Type of Patients	Observed Patients	Avg. Stay	Vari-ance	10th	25th	50th	75th	90th	95th	99th
1. SINGLE DX										
A. Not Operated										
0–19 Years	16	1.1	<1	1	1	1	1	2	2	2
20–34	52	1.2	<1	1	1	1	1	2	2	3
35–49	13	1.2	<1	1	1	1	2	2	2	3
50–64	1	1.0	0	1	1	1	1	1	1	1
65+	0									
B. Operated										
0–19 Years	6	1.0	0	1	1	1	1	1	1	1
20–34	18	1.4	<1	1	1	1	2	3	3	3
35–49	5	1.2	<1	1	1	1	2	2	2	2
50–64	1	4.0	0	4	4	4	4	4	4	4
65+	0									
2. MULTIPLE DX										
A. Not Operated										
0–19 Years	15	1.5	<1	1	1	1	2	2	4	4
20–34	44	1.4	<1	1	1	1	2	2	3	4
35–49	22	1.8	1	1	1	1	2	4	4	4
50–64	4	1.7	2	1	1	1	1	4	4	4
65+	0									
B. Operated										
0–19 Years	8	1.5	<1	1	1	1	2	3	3	3
20–34	30	2.2	5	1	1	1	3	3	4	13
35–49	12	1.9	2	1	1	1	2	3	6	6
50–64	5	3.0	4	1	1	4	4	6	6	6
65+	0									
SUBTOTALS:										
1. SINGLE DX										
A. Not Operated	82	1.2	<1	1	1	1	1	2	2	3
B. Operated	30	1.4	<1	1	1	1	1	3	3	4
2. MULTIPLE DX										
A. Not Operated	85	1.5	<1	1	1	1	2	3	4	4
B. Operated	55	2.1	4	1	1	2	3	4	6	13
1. SINGLE DX	112	1.2	<1	1	1	1	2	2	2	3
2. MULTIPLE DX	140	1.8	2	1	1	1	2	3	4	6
A. NOT OPERATED	167	1.4	<1	1	1	1	2	2	3	4
B. OPERATED	85	1.8	3	1	1	1	2	3	4	13
TOTAL										
0–19 Years	45	1.3	<1	1	1	1	1	2	2	4
20–34	144	1.5	1	1	1	1	2	3	3	4
35–49	52	1.6	1	1	1	1	2	3	4	6
50–64	11	2.5	3	1	1	1	4	4	6	6
65+	0									
GRAND TOTAL	252	1.5	1	1	1	1	2	3	4	6

632: MISSED ABORTION

Type of Patients	Observed Patients	Avg. Stay	Vari-ance	10th	25th	50th	75th	90th	95th	99th
1. SINGLE DX										
A. Not Operated										
0–19 Years	80	1.4	<1	1	1	1	2	2	2	5
20–34	659	1.3	<1	1	1	1	1	2	2	3
35–49	157	1.2	<1	1	1	1	1	2	3	3
50–64	2	1.0	0	1	1	1	1	1	1	1
65+	0									
B. Operated										
0–19 Years	58	1.2	<1	1	1	1	1	2	2	4
20–34	441	1.3	<1	1	1	1	1	2	2	3
35–49	151	1.2	<1	1	1	1	1	2	3	3
50–64	14	1.7	1	1	1	1	2	2	5	5
65+	0									
2. MULTIPLE DX										
A. Not Operated										
0–19 Years	108	1.7	2	1	1	1	2	3	3	10
20–34	594	1.7	1	1	1	1	2	3	3	6
35–49	236	1.6	<1	1	1	1	2	2	4	7
50–64	14	1.3	<1	1	1	1	2	2	2	2
65+	0									
B. Operated										
0–19 Years	48	1.5	<1	1	1	1	2	3	4	4
20–34	578	1.8	3	1	1	1	2	3	4	9
35–49	276	1.7	2	1	1	1	2	3	4	8
50–64	15	2.2	2	1	2	2	3	5	5	5
65+	0									
SUBTOTALS:										
1. SINGLE DX										
A. Not Operated	898	1.3	<1	1	1	1	1	2	2	3
B. Operated	664	1.3	<1	1	1	1	1	2	2	4
2. MULTIPLE DX										
A. Not Operated	952	1.6	1	1	1	1	2	3	3	6
B. Operated	917	1.8	3	1	1	1	2	3	4	8
1. SINGLE DX	1,562	1.3	<1	1	1	1	1	2	2	3
2. MULTIPLE DX	1,869	1.7	2	1	1	1	2	3	4	8
A. NOT OPERATED	1,850	1.5	<1	1	1	1	2	2	3	5
B. OPERATED	1,581	1.6	2	1	1	1	2	3	3	8
TOTAL										
0–19 Years	294	1.5	1	1	1	1	2	2	3	6
20–34	2,272	1.5	1	1	1	1	2	2	3	6
35–49	820	1.5	1	1	1	1	2	2	3	6
50–64	45	1.7	1	1	1	1	2	3	5	5
65+	0									
GRAND TOTAL	3,431	1.5	1	1	1	1	2	3	3	6

505

Length of Stay by Diagnosis and Operation, Western Region, 2008

Western Region, October 2006–September 2007 Data, by Diagnosis

633: ECTOPIC PREGNANCY

Type of Patients	Observed Patients	Avg. Stay	Variance	10th	25th	50th	75th	90th	95th	99th
1. SINGLE DX										
A. Not Operated										
0–19 Years	11	2.0	4	1	1	1	2	2	8	8
20–34	175	1.4	<1	1	1	1	2	2	3	4
35–49	31	1.2	<1	1	1	1	1	2	2	3
50–64	0									
65+	0									
B. Operated										
0–19 Years	74	1.7	<1	1	1	1	2	2	3	5
20–34	1,044	1.7	<1	1	1	1	2	2	3	4
35–49	258	1.7	<1	1	1	1	2	2	3	4
50–64	15	2.1	1	1	1	2	2	4	5	5
65+	0									
2. MULTIPLE DX										
A. Not Operated										
0–19 Years	20	1.6	<1	1	1	1	3	3	3	3
20–34	155	1.5	1	1	1	1	2	2	3	7
35–49	46	1.9	1	1	1	2	2	2	3	8
50–64	4	2.7	8	1	1	1	2	7	7	7
65+	0									
B. Operated										
0–19 Years	207	1.8	<1	1	1	2	2	2	3	5
20–34	2,634	2.1	4	1	1	2	3	3	4	6
35–49	835	2.1	2	1	1	2	3	3	4	7
50–64	45	2.0	1	1	1	2	3	4	4	6
65+	0									
SUBTOTALS:										
1. SINGLE DX										
A. Not Operated	217	1.4	<1	1	1	1	1	2	3	4
B. Operated	1,391	1.7	<1	1	1	1	2	2	3	4
2. MULTIPLE DX										
A. Not Operated	225	1.6	1	1	1	1	2	2	3	7
B. Operated	3,721	2.1	4	1	1	2	3	3	4	6
1. SINGLE DX	1,608	1.7	<1	1	1	1	2	2	3	4
2. MULTIPLE DX	3,946	2.0	3	1	1	2	3	3	4	6
A. NOT OPERATED	442	1.5	1	1	1	1	2	2	3	7
B. OPERATED	5,112	2.0	3	1	1	2	3	3	4	6
TOTAL										
0–19 Years	312	1.8	1	1	1	2	2	2	3	5
20–34	4,008	1.9	3	1	1	2	2	3	4	6
35–49	1,170	2.0	2	1	1	2	3	3	4	6
50–64	64	2.1	2	1	1	2	3	4	5	7
65+	0									
GRAND TOTAL	5,554	1.9	3	1	1	2	2	3	4	6

633.10: TUBAL PREG W/O IU PREG

Type of Patients	Observed Patients	Avg. Stay	Variance	10th	25th	50th	75th	90th	95th	99th
1. SINGLE DX										
A. Not Operated										
0–19 Years	3	1.7	<1	1	1	1	2	2	2	2
20–34	71	1.4	<1	1	1	1	1	2	2	3
35–49	10	1.2	<1	1	1	1	1	2	2	2
50–64	0									
65+	0									
B. Operated										
0–19 Years	69	1.7	<1	1	1	1	2	3	3	5
20–34	947	1.7	<1	1	1	1	2	3	3	4
35–49	226	1.7	<1	1	1	1	2	3	3	4
50–64	12	2.1	2	1	1	2	2	4	5	5
2. MULTIPLE DX										
A. Not Operated										
0–19 Years	7	1.9	1	1	1	1	3	3	3	3
20–34	56	1.4	<1	1	1	1	2	2	3	3
35–49	16	2.2	3	1	2	2	2	3	8	8
50–64	1	2.0	0	2	2	1	2	2	2	2
65+	0									
B. Operated										
0–19 Years	187	1.9	<1	1	1	2	2	3	4	5
20–34	2,307	2.0	5	1	1	2	3	3	4	6
35–49	737	2.0	2	1	1	2	3	3	4	5
50–64	39	2.1	2	1	1	2	3	4	5	6
65+	0									
SUBTOTALS:										
1. SINGLE DX										
A. Not Operated	84	1.4	<1	1	1	1	2	2	2	4
B. Operated	1,254	1.7	<1	1	1	1	2	3	3	5
2. MULTIPLE DX										
A. Not Operated	80	1.6	1	1	1	1	2	3	3	7
B. Operated	3,270	2.0	4	1	1	2	3	3	4	6
1. SINGLE DX	1,338	1.7	<1	1	1	1	2	3	3	4
2. MULTIPLE DX	3,350	2.0	4	1	1	2	3	3	4	6
A. NOT OPERATED	164	1.5	<1	1	1	1	2	2	3	4
B. OPERATED	4,524	1.9	3	1	1	2	3	3	4	6
TOTAL										
0–19 Years	266	1.8	<1	1	1	1	2	2	3	5
20–34	3,381	1.9	4	1	1	2	2	3	4	6
35–49	989	2.0	1	1	1	2	2	3	4	5
50–64	52	2.1	1	1	2	2	3	4	5	6
65+	0									
GRAND TOTAL	4,688	1.9	3	1	1	2	2	3	4	6

633.80: ECTOPIC NEC W/O IU PREG

Type of Patients	Observed Patients	Avg. Stay	Variance	10th	25th	50th	75th	90th	95th	99th
1. SINGLE DX										
A. Not Operated										
0–19 Years	2	5.0	18	2	2	2	8	8	8	8
20–34	19	1.7	2	1	1	1	2	4	7	7
35–49	4	1.0	0	1	1	1	1	1	1	1
50–64	0									
65+	0									
B. Operated										
0–19 Years	3	1.7	1	1	1	1	3	3	3	3
20–34	32	2.1	<1	1	2	2	3	3	4	4
35–49	16	2.4	<1	1	2	2	3	4	4	4
50–64	2	2.5	<1	2	2	2	3	3	3	3
65+	0									
2. MULTIPLE DX										
A. Not Operated										
0–19 Years	3	1.7	1	1	1	1	3	3	3	3
20–34	22	1.7	2	1	1	2	2	2	3	3
35–49	7	2.3	<1	2	2	2	3	4	4	4
50–64	1	7.0	0	7	7	7	7	7	7	7
65+	0									
B. Operated										
0–19 Years	6	1.5	<1	1	1	1	2	2	2	2
20–34	128	2.7	2	1	2	3	4	4	5	7
35–49	47	3.2	3	1	2	3	4	6	7	9
50–64	2	2.5	<1	2	2	2	3	3	3	3
65+	0									
SUBTOTALS:										
1. SINGLE DX										
A. Not Operated	25	1.8	3	1	1	1	2	4	7	8
B. Operated	53	2.2	<1	1	1	2	3	3	4	4
2. MULTIPLE DX										
A. Not Operated	33	2.0	2	1	1	1	2	3	7	7
B. Operated	183	2.8	2	1	2	3	4	5	5	8
1. SINGLE DX	78	2.1	2	1	1	2	3	4	4	8
2. MULTIPLE DX	216	2.7	2	1	2	3	3	5	5	7
A. NOT OPERATED	58	1.9	3	1	1	1	2	4	7	8
B. OPERATED	236	2.7	2	1	2	3	3	4	5	7
TOTAL										
0–19 Years	14	2.1	3	1	1	1	2	3	8	8
20–34	201	2.4	2	1	2	2	3	4	5	7
35–49	74	2.8	3	1	2	2	3	5	6	9
50–64	5	3.4	4	2	3	3	3	7	7	7
65+	0									
GRAND TOTAL	294	2.5	2	1	1	2	3	4	5	8

Length of Stay by Diagnosis and Operation, Western Region, 2008

Western Region, October 2006–September 2007 Data, by Diagnosis

633.90: ECTOPIC NOS W/O IU PREG

Type of Patients	Observed Patients	Avg. Stay	Variance	10th	25th	50th	75th	90th	95th	99th
1. SINGLE DX										
A. Not Operated										
0–19 Years	4	1.3	<1	1	1	1	2	2	2	2
20–34	73	1.2	<1	1	1	1	1	2	3	3
35–49	14	1.2	<1	1	1	1	1	2	3	3
50–64	0									
65+	0									
B. Operated										
0–19 Years	1	2.0	0	2	2	2	2	2	2	2
20–34	29	1.6	<1	1	1	1	2	2	3	3
35–49	6	1.7	<1	1	1	2	2	3	3	3
50–64	0									
65+	0									
2. MULTIPLE DX										
A. Not Operated										
0–19 Years	9	1.3	<1	1	1	1	1	3	3	3
20–34	60	1.4	<1	1	1	1	1	2	4	5
35–49	16	1.6	<1	1	1	1	2	3	3	3
50–64	2	1.0	0	1	1	1	1	1	1	1
65+	0									
B. Operated										
0–19 Years	6	1.5	<1	1	1	1	2	2	2	2
20–34	55	2.0	2	1	1	1	3	4	5	7
35–49	14	2.4	1	1	2	2	3	4	5	5
50–64	0									
65+	0									
SUBTOTALS:										
1. SINGLE DX										
A. Not Operated	91	1.2	<1	1	1	1	1	2	3	3
B. Operated	36	1.6	<1	1	1	1	2	3	3	3
2. MULTIPLE DX										
A. Not Operated	87	1.4	<1	1	1	1	2	2	3	5
B. Operated	75	2.1	2	1	1	2	3	4	5	7
1. SINGLE DX	127	1.3	<1	1	1	1	2	2	3	3
2. MULTIPLE DX	162	1.7	1	1	1	1	2	3	4	5
A. NOT OPERATED	178	1.3	<1	1	1	1	1	2	3	4
B. OPERATED	111	1.9	1	1	1	2	3	3	4	5
TOTAL										
0–19 Years	20	1.4	<1	1	1	1	2	2	3	3
20–34	217	1.5	<1	1	1	1	2	3	4	5
35–49	50	1.7	<1	1	1	1	2	3	3	5
50–64	2	1.0	0	1	1	1	1	1	1	1
65+	0									
GRAND TOTAL	289	1.6	<1	1	1	1	2	3	3	5

634: SPONTANEOUS ABORTION

Type of Patients	Observed Patients	Avg. Stay	Variance	10th	25th	50th	75th	90th	95th	99th
1. SINGLE DX										
A. Not Operated										
0–19 Years	77	1.3	<1	1	1	1	1	2	2	3
20–34	383	1.3	<1	1	1	1	1	2	3	4
35–49	91	1.2	<1	1	1	1	1	2	2	3
50–64	3	1.7	1	1	1	1	3	3	3	3
65+	0									
B. Operated										
0–19 Years	122	1.1	<1	1	1	1	1	2	2	2
20–34	820	1.2	<1	1	1	1	1	2	2	3
35–49	251	1.2	<1	1	1	1	2	2	2	3
50–64	21	1.1	<1	1	1	1	1	1	2	2
65+	0									
2. MULTIPLE DX										
A. Not Operated										
0–19 Years	81	2.1	7	1	1	1	2	3	5	19
20–34	436	1.7	2	1	1	1	2	3	4	7
35–49	157	1.8	3	1	1	1	2	3	5	12
50–64	7	1.7	<1	1	1	2	2	3	3	3
65+	0									
B. Operated										
0–19 Years	96	1.7	4	1	1	1	2	3	4	17
20–34	798	1.8	4	1	1	1	2	3	4	9
35–49	365	1.8	3	1	1	1	2	3	4	10
50–64	25	2.0	7	1	1	1	2	2	8	13
65+	0									
SUBTOTALS:										
1. SINGLE DX										
A. Not Operated	554	1.3	<1	1	1	1	1	2	2	4
B. Operated	1,214	1.2	<1	1	1	1	2	2	2	3
2. MULTIPLE DX										
A. Not Operated	681	1.8	3	1	1	1	2	3	4	9
B. Operated	1,284	1.8	4	1	1	1	3	3	4	11
1. SINGLE DX	1,768	1.2	<1	1	1	1	1	2	2	3
2. MULTIPLE DX	1,965	1.8	3	1	1	1	2	3	4	11
A. NOT OPERATED	1,235	1.5	2	1	1	1	2	3	3	7
B. OPERATED	2,498	1.5	2	1	1	2	3	3	4	8
TOTAL										
0–19 Years	376	1.5	3	1	1	1	2	2	3	12
20–34	2,437	1.5	2	1	1	1	2	3	3	6
35–49	864	1.6	2	1	1	1	2	3	4	10
50–64	56	1.6	4	1	1	1	2	3	3	13
65+	0									
GRAND TOTAL	3,733	1.5	2	1	1	1	2	2	3	7

634.11: SAB W HEMORRHAGE-INCOMPL

Type of Patients	Observed Patients	Avg. Stay	Variance	10th	25th	50th	75th	90th	95th	99th
1. SINGLE DX										
A. Not Operated										
0–19 Years	8	1.4	<1	1	1	1	2	2	2	2
20–34	11	1.3	<1	1	1	1	2	2	2	2
35–49	5	1.6	<1	1	1	1	2	3	3	3
50–64	0									
65+	0									
B. Operated										
0–19 Years	13	1.2	<1	1	1	1	1	2	2	2
20–34	162	1.1	<1	1	1	1	1	2	2	3
35–49	47	1.1	<1	1	1	1	1	1	2	3
50–64	2	1.0	0	1	1	1	1	1	1	1
65+	0									
2. MULTIPLE DX										
A. Not Operated										
0–19 Years	7	1.4	<1	1	1	1	2	2	2	2
20–34	39	1.4	<1	1	1	1	2	3	3	4
35–49	25	1.5	<1	1	1	1	2	3	3	3
50–64	0									
65+	0									
B. Operated										
0–19 Years	22	1.2	<1	1	1	1	1	2	2	3
20–34	273	1.6	3	1	1	1	2	3	4	9
35–49	132	1.7	2	1	1	1	2	3	4	9
50–64	13	1.2	<1	1	1	1	1	2	2	2
65+	0									
SUBTOTALS:										
1. SINGLE DX										
A. Not Operated	24	1.4	<1	1	1	1	2	2	2	3
B. Operated	224	1.1	<1	1	1	1	1	2	2	3
2. MULTIPLE DX										
A. Not Operated	71	1.5	<1	1	1	1	2	3	3	4
B. Operated	440	1.6	2	1	1	1	2	3	4	9
1. SINGLE DX	248	1.2	<1	1	1	1	1	2	2	3
2. MULTIPLE DX	511	1.6	2	1	1	1	2	3	4	11
A. NOT OPERATED	95	1.4	<1	1	1	1	2	2	3	7
B. OPERATED	664	1.4	2	1	1	1	2	3	3	8
TOTAL										
0–19 Years	50	1.2	<1	1	1	1	1	2	2	3
20–34	485	1.4	2	1	1	1	2	2	3	7
35–49	209	1.5	2	1	1	1	2	3	4	8
50–64	15	1.1	<1	1	1	1	1	2	2	2
65+	0									
GRAND TOTAL	759	1.4	2	1	1	1	1	2	3	7

Length of Stay by Diagnosis and Operation, Western Region, 2008

Western Region, October 2006–September 2007 Data, by Diagnosis

634.91: INCOMPLETE SAB W/O COMP

Type of Patients	Observed Patients	Avg. Stay	Variance	10th	25th	50th	75th	90th	95th	99th
1. SINGLE DX										
A. Not Operated										
0–19 Years	25	1.3	<1	1	1	1	1	2	3	3
20–34	145	1.4	2	1	1	1	1	2	3	4
35–49	30	1.2	<1	1	1	1	1	2	2	3
50–64	0									
65+										
B. Operated										
0–19 Years	96	1.1	<1	1	1	1	1	1	2	2
20–34	554	1.1	<1	1	1	1	1	1	2	3
35–49	179	1.1	<1	1	1	1	1	1	2	3
50–64	18	1.1	<1	1	1	1	1	1	2	2
65+	0									
2. MULTIPLE DX										
A. Not Operated										
0–19 Years	17	1.6	1	1	1	1	2	3	5	5
20–34	102	1.6	2	1	1	1	2	2	3	11
35–49	28	1.4	1	1	1	1	1	2	5	6
50–64	0									
65+										
B. Operated										
0–19 Years	40	1.2	<1	1	1	1	1	2	2	2
20–34	331	1.6	3	1	1	1	2	3	4	6
35–49	151	1.4	2	1	1	1	1	3	3	10
50–64	6	2.3	8	1	1	1	2	8	8	8
65+	0									
SUBTOTALS:										
1. SINGLE DX										
A. Not Operated	200	1.3	1	1	1	1	1	2	3	4
B. Operated	847	1.1	<1	1	1	1	1	1	2	2
2. MULTIPLE DX										
A. Not Operated	147	1.6	2	1	1	1	2	2	3	11
B. Operated	528	1.5	2	1	1	1	1	2	3	6
1. SINGLE DX	1,047	1.1	<1	1	1	1	1	2	2	3
2. MULTIPLE DX	675	1.5	2	1	1	1	2	2	3	8
A. NOT OPERATED	347	1.4	2	1	1	1	1	2	3	7
B. OPERATED	1,375	1.3	1	1	1	1	1	2	2	5
TOTAL										
0–19 Years	178	1.2	<1	1	1	1	1	2	2	3
20–34	1,132	1.3	1	1	1	1	1	2	3	5
35–49	388	1.3	<1	1	1	1	1	2	2	6
50–64	24	1.4	2	1	1	1	2	2	2	8
65+	0									
GRAND TOTAL	1,722	1.3	1	1	1	1	1	2	2	5

634.92: COMPLETE SAB W/O COMP

Type of Patients	Observed Patients	Avg. Stay	Variance	10th	25th	50th	75th	90th	95th	99th
1. SINGLE DX										
A. Not Operated										
0–19 Years	28	1.2	<1	1	1	1	1	2	2	2
20–34	132	1.2	<1	1	1	1	1	2	2	4
35–49	30	1.0	<1	1	1	1	1	1	1	2
50–64	3	1.7	1	1	1	1	3	3	3	3
65+	0									
B. Operated										
0–19 Years	3	1.3	<1	1	1	1	1	2	2	2
20–34	10	1.1	<1	1	1	1	1	1	1	2
35–49	5	1.2	<1	1	1	1	1	2	2	2
50–64	0									
65+	0									
2. MULTIPLE DX										
A. Not Operated										
0–19 Years	17	1.2	<1	1	1	1	1	2	2	2
20–34	96	1.6	<1	1	1	1	2	3	4	6
35–49	26	1.4	<1	1	1	1	2	3	3	4
50–64	2	2.0	0	2	2	2	2	2	2	2
65+	0									
B. Operated										
0–19 Years	3	4.7	40	1	1	1	12	12	12	12
20–34	14	1.6	<1	1	1	1	2	3	4	4
35–49	5	1.2	<1	1	1	1	1	2	2	2
50–64	1	1.0	0	1	1	1	1	1	1	1
65+	0									
SUBTOTALS:										
1. SINGLE DX										
A. Not Operated	193	1.2	<1	1	1	1	1	2	2	4
B. Operated	18	1.2	<1	1	1	1	1	2	2	2
2. MULTIPLE DX										
A. Not Operated	141	1.5	<1	1	1	1	2	2	3	5
B. Operated	23	1.9	5	1	1	1	2	3	4	12
1. SINGLE DX	211	1.2	<1	1	1	1	1	2	2	4
2. MULTIPLE DX	164	1.6	1	1	1	1	2	2	4	6
A. NOT OPERATED	334	1.3	<1	1	1	1	1	2	3	5
B. OPERATED	41	1.6	3	1	1	1	2	2	3	12
TOTAL										
0–19 Years	51	1.4	2	1	1	1	1	2	2	12
20–34	252	1.4	<1	1	1	1	1	2	3	5
35–49	66	1.2	<1	1	1	1	1	2	2	4
50–64	6	1.7	<1	1	1	2	2	3	3	3
65+	0									
GRAND TOTAL	375	1.3	<1	1	1	1	1	2	3	5

635: LEGALLY INDUCED ABORTION

Type of Patients	Observed Patients	Avg. Stay	Variance	10th	25th	50th	75th	90th	95th	99th
1. SINGLE DX										
A. Not Operated										
0–19 Years	10	1.3	<1	1	1	1	2	2	2	2
20–34	56	1.4	<1	1	1	1	2	2	2	4
35–49	13	1.5	<1	1	1	1	2	2	2	2
50–64	2	1.5	<1	1	1	2	2	2	2	2
65+	0									
B. Operated										
0–19 Years	13	1.4	<1	1	1	1	2	2	3	3
20–34	67	1.2	<1	1	1	1	1	2	3	4
35–49	22	1.4	<1	1	1	1	2	2	3	4
50–64	5	1.2	<1	1	1	1	1	2	2	2
65+	0									
2. MULTIPLE DX										
A. Not Operated										
0–19 Years	29	1.8	2	1	1	1	2	4	5	8
20–34	255	1.7	2	1	1	1	2	3	4	7
35–49	81	1.6	3	1	1	1	2	2	3	15
50–64	10	1.2	<1	1	1	1	1	2	2	2
65+	0									
B. Operated										
0–19 Years	26	2.1	1	1	1	2	3	4	4	5
20–34	212	2.2	3	1	1	2	3	3	5	9
35–49	73	2.4	5	1	1	2	3	4	7	16
50–64	3	2.3	<1	2	2	2	3	3	3	3
65+	0									
SUBTOTALS:										
1. SINGLE DX										
A. Not Operated	81	1.4	<1	1	1	1	2	2	2	4
B. Operated	107	1.3	<1	1	1	1	1	2	3	4
2. MULTIPLE DX										
A. Not Operated	375	1.7	2	1	1	1	2	3	4	7
B. Operated	314	2.3	3	1	2	2	3	4	5	9
1. SINGLE DX	188	1.3	<1	1	1	1	2	2	2	4
2. MULTIPLE DX	689	2.0	3	1	1	1	2	3	5	8
A. NOT OPERATED	456	1.6	2	1	1	1	2	3	4	7
B. OPERATED	421	2.0	3	1	1	1	3	4	5	7
TOTAL										
0–19 Years	78	1.8	2	1	1	1	2	3	4	8
20–34	590	1.8	2	1	1	1	2	3	4	7
35–49	189	1.8	3	1	1	1	2	3	4	15
50–64	20	1.4	<1	1	1	1	2	2	2	3
65+	0									
GRAND TOTAL	877	1.8	2	1	1	1	2	3	4	7

Length of Stay by Diagnosis and Operation, Western Region, 2008

Western Region, October 2006–September 2007 Data, by Diagnosis

635.92: COMPL LEGAL AB W/O COMP

Type of Patients	Observed Patients	Avg. Stay	Variance	10th	25th	50th	75th	90th	95th	99th
1. SINGLE DX										
A. Not Operated										
0–19 Years	7	1.1	<1	1	1	1	1	2	2	2
20–34	27	1.3	<1	1	1	1	2	2	2	2
35–49	9	1.6	<1	1	1	2	2	2	2	2
50–64	2	1.5	<1	1	1	2	2	2	2	2
65+	0									
B. Operated										
0–19 Years	1	1.0	0	1	1	1	1	1	1	1
20–34	4	1.0	0	1	1	1	1	1	1	1
35–49	2	3.0	2	2	2	4	4	4	4	4
50–64	1	1.0	0	1	1	1	1	1	1	1
65+	0									
2. MULTIPLE DX										
A. Not Operated										
0–19 Years	9	1.1	<1	1	1	1	1	2	2	2
20–34	149	1.7	2	1	1	1	2	3	4	7
35–49	55	1.6	4	1	1	1	2	2	3	15
50–64	8	1.3	<1	1	1	1	1	2	2	2
65+	0									
B. Operated										
0–19 Years	7	2.0	1	1	1	2	3	4	4	4
20–34	52	2.5	6	1	1	2	3	3	7	16
35–49	17	2.3	1	1	1	2	3	4	5	6
50–64	1	3.0	0	3	3	3	3	3	3	3
65+	0									
SUBTOTALS:										
1. SINGLE DX										
A. Not Operated	45	1.3	<1	1	1	1	2	2	2	2
B. Operated	8	1.5	1	1	1	1	1	2	2	2
2. MULTIPLE DX										
A. Not Operated	221	1.7	2	1	1	1	2	2	4	7
B. Operated	77	2.4	4	1	1	2	3	3	6	16
1. SINGLE DX	53	1.3	<1	1	1	1	2	2	2	4
2. MULTIPLE DX	298	1.9	3	1	1	1	2	3	4	12
A. NOT OPERATED	266	1.6	2	1	1	1	2	2	3	7
B. OPERATED	85	2.3	4	1	1	2	3	3	5	16
TOTAL										
0–19 Years	24	1.4	<1	1	1	1	1	2	3	4
20–34	232	1.8	3	1	1	1	2	3	4	7
35–49	83	1.8	3	1	1	1	2	3	3	15
50–64	12	1.4	<1	1	1	1	2	2	3	3
65+	0									
GRAND TOTAL	351	1.8	3	1	1	1	2	3	4	7

636: ILLEGAL INDUCED ABORTION

Type of Patients	Observed Patients	Avg. Stay	Variance	10th	25th	50th	75th	90th	95th	99th
1. SINGLE DX										
A. Not Operated										
0–19 Years	0									
20–34	0									
35–49	0									
50–64	0									
65+	0									
B. Operated										
0–19 Years	0									
20–34	0									
35–49	0									
50–64	0									
65+	0									
2. MULTIPLE DX										
A. Not Operated										
0–19 Years	0									
20–34	1	1.0	0		1	1	1	1	1	1
35–49	0									
50–64	0									
65+	0									
B. Operated										
0–19 Years	1	2.0	0	2	2	2	2	2	2	2
20–34	2	4.0	8	2	2	6	6	6	6	6
35–49	0									
50–64	0									
65+	0									
SUBTOTALS:										
1. SINGLE DX										
A. Not Operated	0									
B. Operated	0									
2. MULTIPLE DX										
A. Not Operated	1	1.0	0	1	1	1	1	1	1	1
B. Operated	3	3.3	5	1	2	2	6	6	6	6
1. SINGLE DX	0									
2. MULTIPLE DX	4	2.8	5	1	2	2	6	6	6	6
A. NOT OPERATED	1	1.0	0	1	1	1	1	1	1	1
B. OPERATED	3	3.3	5	2	2	2	6	6	6	6
TOTAL										
0–19 Years	1	2.0	0	2	2	2	2	2	2	2
20–34	3	3.0	7	1	1	2	6	6	6	6
35–49	0									
50–64	0									
65+	0									
GRAND TOTAL	4	2.8	5	1	2	2	6	6	6	6

637: UNSPECIFIED ABORTION

Type of Patients	Observed Patients	Avg. Stay	Variance	10th	25th	50th	75th	90th	95th	99th
1. SINGLE DX										
A. Not Operated										
0–19 Years	2	1.5	<1	1	1	2	2	2	2	2
20–34	21	1.1	<1	1	1	1	1	2	2	2
35–49	4	1.5	1	1	1	1	3	3	3	3
50–64	1	1.0	0	1	1	1	1	1	1	1
65+	0									
B. Operated										
0–19 Years	15	1.0	0	1	1	1	1	1	1	1
20–34	110	1.2	<1	1	1	1	1	2	2	4
35–49	33	1.2	<1	1	1	1	1	2	2	3
50–64	3	1.0	0	1	1	1	1	1	1	1
65+	0									
2. MULTIPLE DX										
A. Not Operated										
0–19 Years	4	2.7	2	1	1	3	3	4	4	4
20–34	16	1.8	2	1	1	1	2	4	6	6
35–49	6	1.3	<1	1	1	1	1	3	3	3
50–64	0									
65+	0									
B. Operated										
0–19 Years	12	2.2	4	1	1	1	2	6	6	6
20–34	73	1.7	2	1	1	1	2	3	4	8
35–49	28	1.4	<1	1	1	1	2	3	3	3
50–64	3	1.3	<1	1	1	1	2	2	2	2
65+	0									
SUBTOTALS:										
1. SINGLE DX										
A. Not Operated	28	1.2	<1	1	1	1	1	2	2	3
B. Operated	161	1.2	<1	1	1	1	1	2	2	4
2. MULTIPLE DX										
A. Not Operated	26	1.9	2	1	1	1	3	4	4	6
B. Operated	116	1.7	2	1	1	1	2	3	4	6
1. SINGLE DX	189	1.2	<1	1	1	1	1	2	2	4
2. MULTIPLE DX	142	1.7	2	1	1	1	2	3	4	6
A. NOT OPERATED	54	1.5	1	1	1	1	2	3	4	6
B. OPERATED	277	1.4	<1	1	1	1	1	2	3	6
TOTAL										
0–19 Years	33	1.7	2	1	1	1	2	3	6	6
20–34	220	1.4	<1	1	1	1	1	2	3	6
35–49	71	1.3	<1	1	1	1	1	2	3	3
50–64	7	1.1	<1	1	1	1	1	2	2	2
65+	0									
GRAND TOTAL	331	1.4	<1	1	1	1	1	2	3	6

Length of Stay by Diagnosis and Operation, Western Region, 2008

Western Region, October 2006–September 2007 Data, by Diagnosis

638: FAILED ATTEMPTED AB

Type of Patients	Observed Patients	Avg. Stay	Variance	Percentiles						
				10th	25th	50th	75th	90th	95th	99th
1. SINGLE DX										
A. Not Operated										
0–19 Years	0									
20–34	1	2.0	0	2	2	2	2	2	2	2
35–49	0									
50–64	0									
65+	0									
B. Operated										
0–19 Years	1	1.0	0	1	1	1	1	1	1	1
20–34	6	1.0	0	1	1	1	1	1	1	1
35–49	0									
50–64	0									
65+	0									
2. MULTIPLE DX										
A. Not Operated										
0–19 Years	0									
20–34	0									
35–49	1	1.0	0	1	1	1	1	1	1	1
50–64	0									
65+	0									
B. Operated										
0–19 Years	1	1.0	0	1	1	1	1	1	1	1
20–34	6	3.3	23	1	1	2	2	13	13	13
35–49	1	1.0	0	1	1	1	1	1	1	1
50–64	0									
65+	0									
SUBTOTALS:										
1. SINGLE DX										
A. Not Operated	1	2.0	0	2	2	2	2	2	2	2
B. Operated	7	1.0	0	1	1	1	1	1	1	1
2. MULTIPLE DX										
A. Not Operated	1	1.0	0	1	1	1	1	1	1	1
B. Operated	8	2.8	17	1	1	1	2	13	13	13
1. SINGLE DX	8	1.1	<1	1	1	1	1	2	2	2
2. MULTIPLE DX	9	2.6	15	1	1	1	2	13	13	13
A. NOT OPERATED	2	1.5	<1	1	1	1	2	2	2	2
B. OPERATED	15	1.9	10	1	1	1	1	2	13	13
TOTAL										
0–19 Years	2	1.0	0	1	1	1	1	1	1	1
20–34	13	2.2	11	1	1	1	2	2	13	13
35–49	2	1.0	0	1	1	1	1	1	1	1
50–64	0									
65+	0									
GRAND TOTAL	17	1.9	8	1	1	1	1	2	13	13

639: COMP FOLLOWING ABORTION

Type of Patients	Observed Patients	Avg. Stay	Variance	Percentiles						
				10th	25th	50th	75th	90th	95th	99th
1. SINGLE DX										
A. Not Operated										
0–19 Years	7	1.6	<1	1	1	1	3	3	3	3
20–34	35	1.8	<1	1	1	1	2	3	4	4
35–49	4	2.0	<1	2	2	2	3	3	3	3
50–64	1	1.0	0	1	1	1	1	1	1	1
65+	0									
B. Operated										
0–19 Years	1	2.0	0	2	2	2	2	2	2	2
20–34	15	1.4	1	1	1	1	1	2	2	5
35–49	1	1.0	0	1	1	1	1	1	1	1
50–64	1	2.0	0	2	2	2	2	2	2	2
65+	0									
2. MULTIPLE DX										
A. Not Operated										
0–19 Years	35	2.3	2	1	1	2	3	4	5	6
20–34	236	2.5	3	1	1	2	3	4	5	10
35–49	49	2.3	2	1	1	2	3	3	6	7
50–64	4	2.5	3	1	2	2	5	5	5	5
65+	0									
B. Operated										
0–19 Years	8	3.9	15	1	1	2	3	10	10	10
20–34	65	2.8	6	1	2	2	3	5	7	14
35–49	20	3.1	5	1	2	3	3	4	10	10
50–64	1	4.0	0	4	4	4	4	4	4	4
65+	0									
SUBTOTALS:										
1. SINGLE DX										
A. Not Operated	47	1.8	<1	1	1	1	2	3	4	4
B. Operated	18	1.4	<1	1	1	1	2	2	5	5
2. MULTIPLE DX										
A. Not Operated	324	2.4	3	1	1	2	3	4	5	9
B. Operated	94	2.9	6	1	1	2	3	6	10	14
1. SINGLE DX	65	1.7	<1	1	1	1	2	3	4	5
2. MULTIPLE DX	418	2.5	4	1	1	2	3	5	6	10
A. NOT OPERATED	371	2.3	3	1	1	2	3	4	5	9
B. OPERATED	112	2.7	6	1	1	2	3	5	8	10
TOTAL										
0–19 Years	51	2.4	4	1	1	2	3	4	6	10
20–34	351	2.4	4	1	1	2	3	4	5	10
35–49	74	2.5	3	1	1	2	3	4	6	10
50–64	7	2.4	2	1	2	2	4	5	5	5
65+	0									
GRAND TOTAL	483	2.4	3	1	1	2	3	4	6	10

639.0: POSTABORTION GU INFECT

Type of Patients	Observed Patients	Avg. Stay	Variance	Percentiles						
				10th	25th	50th	75th	90th	95th	99th
1. SINGLE DX										
A. Not Operated										
0–19 Years	3	1.7	1	1	1	1	3	3	3	3
20–34	17	2.0	1	1	1	2	2	4	4	4
35–49	3	2.3	<1	2	2	2	3	3	3	3
50–64	0									
65+	0									
B. Operated										
0–19 Years	0									
20–34	5	2.0	3	1	1	1	2	5	5	5
35–49	1	1.0	0	1	1	1	1	1	1	1
50–64	1	2.0	0	2	2	2	2	2	2	2
65+	0									
2. MULTIPLE DX										
A. Not Operated										
0–19 Years	28	2.3	2	1	1	2	3	4	5	6
20–34	154	2.5	3	1	2	2	3	4	5	9
35–49	27	2.1	<1	1	1	2	3	3	3	5
50–64	4	2.5	3	1	2	2	5	5	5	5
65+	0									
B. Operated										
0–19 Years	4	6.2	19	2	2	3	10	10	10	10
20–34	17	3.4	6	1	2	3	5	7	7	14
35–49	5	5.0	14	2	2	3	8	10	10	10
50–64	0									
65+	0									
SUBTOTALS:										
1. SINGLE DX										
A. Not Operated	23	2.0	<1	1	1	2	3	3	4	4
B. Operated	7	1.9	2	1	1	1	2	5	5	5
2. MULTIPLE DX										
A. Not Operated	213	2.4	3	1	2	2	3	4	5	8
B. Operated	26	4.1	10	1	2	3	6	10	10	10
1. SINGLE DX	30	2.0	1	1	1	2	2	3	4	5
2. MULTIPLE DX	239	2.6	4	1	2	2	3	5	7	10
A. NOT OPERATED	236	2.4	2	1	1	2	3	4	5	8
B. OPERATED	33	3.7	9	1	2	2	5	10	10	10
TOTAL										
0–19 Years	35	2.7	5	1	1	2	3	5	10	10
20–34	193	2.6	3	1	2	2	3	4	5	10
35–49	36	2.5	3	1	2	2	2	3	8	10
50–64	5	2.4	2	1	2	2	2	5	5	5
65+	0									
GRAND TOTAL	269	2.6	3	1	1	2	3	5	6	10

Length of Stay by Diagnosis and Operation, Western Region, 2008

©2009 Thomson Reuters. All rights reserved.

640: HEMORRHAGE IN EARLY PREG

Type of Patients	Observed Patients	Avg. Stay	Variance	10th	25th	50th	75th	90th	95th	99th
1. SINGLE DX										
A. Not Operated										
0–19 Years	22	2.0	4	1	1	1	2	3	4	10
20–34	178	1.6	2	1	1	1	2	3	4	9
35–49	24	1.6	1	1	1	1	2	3	5	5
50–64	1	1.0	0	1	1	1	1	1	1	1
65+	0									
B. Operated										
0–19 Years	0									
20–34	3	1.3	<1	1	1	1	2	2	2	2
35–49	0									
50–64	0									
65+	0									
2. MULTIPLE DX										
A. Not Operated										
0–19 Years	44	2.0	3	1	1	1	3	5	5	8
20–34	301	2.5	19	1	1	2	3	5	6	10
35–49	85	3.0	20	1	1	2	3	7	9	37
50–64	4	3.7	10	1	1	1	7	7	7	7
65+	0									
B. Operated										
0–19 Years	1	2.0	0	2	2	2	2	2	2	2
20–34	27	3.6	8	1	1	3	5	9	9	9
35–49	11	7.2	192	1	2	3	6	6	49	49
50–64	0									
65+	0									
SUBTOTALS:										
1. SINGLE DX										
A. Not Operated	225	1.7	2	1	1	1	2	3	4	9
B. Operated	3	1.3	<1	1	1	1	2	2	2	2
2. MULTIPLE DX										
A. Not Operated	434	2.6	18	1	1	2	3	5	7	11
B. Operated	39	4.6	58	1	1	3	5	9	9	49
1. SINGLE DX	228	1.7	2	1	1	1	2	3	4	9
2. MULTIPLE DX	473	2.7	21	1	1	2	3	5	7	12
A. NOT OPERATED	659	2.3	12	1	1	1	2	5	6	10
B. OPERATED	42	4.3	55	1	1	2	5	7	9	49
TOTAL										
0–19 Years	67	2.0	3	1	1	1	2	4	5	10
20–34	509	2.3	13	1	1	1	3	4	6	10
35–49	120	3.1	32	1	1	2	3	6	9	37
50–64	5	3.2	9	1	1	1	6	7	7	7
65+	0									
GRAND TOTAL	701	2.4	15	1	1	1	3	5	7	10

640.03: THREATENED AB-AP

Type of Patients	Observed Patients	Avg. Stay	Variance	10th	25th	50th	75th	90th	95th	99th
1. SINGLE DX										
A. Not Operated										
0–19 Years	15	2.4	5	1	1	2	3	4	10	10
20–34	116	1.6	2	1	1	1	2	3	4	9
35–49	14	1.6	1	1	1	1	2	3	5	5
50–64	1	1.0	0	1	1	1	1	1	1	1
65+	0									
B. Operated										
0–19 Years	0									
20–34	2	1.5	<1	1	1	2	2	2	2	2
35–49	0									
50–64	0									
65+	0									
2. MULTIPLE DX										
A. Not Operated										
0–19 Years	28	1.9	2	1	1	1	3	5	5	6
20–34	177	2.6	30	1	1	2	3	5	6	12
35–49	49	3.2	29	1	1	2	3	8	9	37
50–64	2	6.5	<1	6	6	7	7	7	7	7
65+	0									
B. Operated										
0–19 Years	0									
20–34	13	2.8	5	1	2	3	3	7	7	7
35–49	6	10.7	348	1	2	3	6	49	49	49
50–64	0									
65+	0									
SUBTOTALS:										
1. SINGLE DX										
A. Not Operated	146	1.7	3	1	1	1	2	3	4	10
B. Operated	2	1.5	<1	1	1	2	2	2	2	2
2. MULTIPLE DX										
A. Not Operated	256	2.7	27	1	1	2	3	5	6	12
B. Operated	19	5.3	114	1	1	2	5	7	49	49
1. SINGLE DX	148	1.7	3	1	1	1	2	3	4	10
2. MULTIPLE DX	275	2.9	33	1	1	2	3	5	7	37
A. NOT OPERATED	402	2.3	18	1	1	1	2	4	6	10
B. OPERATED	21	4.9	104	1	1	2	4	7	7	49
TOTAL										
0–19 Years	43	2.1	3	1	1	1	3	4	5	10
20–34	308	2.3	18	1	1	1	3	4	6	9
35–49	69	3.6	52	1	1	2	3	6	9	49
50–64	3	4.7	10	1	1	6	6	7	7	7
65+	0									
GRAND TOTAL	423	2.5	22	1	1	1	3	5	6	11

641: AP HEMOR & PLAC PREV

Type of Patients	Observed Patients	Avg. Stay	Variance	10th	25th	50th	75th	90th	95th	99th
1. SINGLE DX										
A. Not Operated										
0–19 Years	84	1.6	<1	1	1	1	2	3	4	4
20–34	818	2.2	5	1	1	2	3	4	6	11
35–49	86	2.8	14	1	1	2	3	5	7	27
50–64	4	1.3	<1	1	1	1	1	2	2	2
65+	0									
B. Operated										
0–19 Years	31	2.9	<1	2	3	3	3	4	4	4
20–34	416	3.3	9	2	3	3	3	4	4	13
35–49	38	2.9	<1	2	2	3	3	4	4	5
50–64	1	3.0	0	3	3	3	3	3	3	3
65+	0									
2. MULTIPLE DX										
A. Not Operated										
0–19 Years	249	2.9	10	1	1	2	3	5	8	16
20–34	2,336	3.3	18	1	1	2	3	6	10	23
35–49	820	3.7	23	1	1	2	4	7	12	25
50–64	27	5.4	82	2	2	2	7	21	24	41
65+	0									
B. Operated										
0–19 Years	239	4.5	31	2	3	3	4	6	11	36
20–34	3,167	5.1	51	2	3	3	4	8	17	38
35–49	1,408	5.8	66	2	3	4	4	10	21	42
50–64	73	5.9	50	2	3	4	5	18	25	>99
65+	0									
SUBTOTALS:										
1. SINGLE DX										
A. Not Operated	992	2.2	5	1	1	2	2	4	6	12
B. Operated	486	3.2	8	2	3	3	3	4	4	13
2. MULTIPLE DX										
A. Not Operated	3,432	3.4	19	1	1	2	3	7	10	24
B. Operated	4,887	5.3	55	2	3	3	5	8	18	40
1. SINGLE DX	1,478	2.5	6	1	1	2	3	4	5	12
2. MULTIPLE DX	8,319	4.5	41	1	2	3	4	7	14	34
A. NOT OPERATED	4,424	3.1	17	1	1	2	3	6	9	23
B. OPERATED	5,373	5.1	51	2	3	3	4	8	17	39
TOTAL										
0–19 Years	603	3.3	17	1	2	3	4	5	8	22
20–34	6,737	4.0	33	1	2	3	4	6	11	31
35–49	2,352	4.9	49	1	2	3	4	9	17	36
50–64	105	5.6	56	2	2	3	4	18	24	42
65+	0									
GRAND TOTAL	9,797	4.2	36	1	2	3	4	7	13	32

Length of Stay by Diagnosis and Operation, Western Region, 2008

Western Region, October 2006–September 2007 Data, by Diagnosis

641.01: PLACENTA PREVIA-DEL

Type of Patients	Observed Patients	Avg. Stay	Vari-ance	10th	25th	50th	75th	90th	95th	99th
1. SINGLE DX										
A. Not Operated										
0–19 Years	3	1.0	0	1	1	1	1	1	1	1
20–34	28	1.8	<1	1	1	2	2	3	3	3
35–49	0									
50–64	0									
65+	0									
B. Operated										
0–19 Years	5	3.2	<1	2	3	3	4	4	4	4
20–34	192	3.0	<1	2	2	3	3	4	4	5
35–49	18	2.8	<1	2	2	3	3	4	4	4
50–64	1	3.0	0	3	3	3	3	3	3	3
65+	0									
2. MULTIPLE DX										
A. Not Operated										
0–19 Years	8	2.1	2	1	1	2	2	5	5	5
20–34	120	2.1	<1	1	1	2	3	3	3	4
35–49	17	2.0	<1	1	2	2	2	3	3	3
50–64	0									
65+	0									
B. Operated										
0–19 Years	16	2.8	<1	2	2	3	3	4	4	4
20–34	588	3.5	8	2	2	3	4	4	5	20
35–49	401	3.5	6	2	3	3	4	4	5	15
50–64	26	3.8	16	2	2	3	4	4	4	23
65+	0									
SUBTOTALS:										
1. SINGLE DX										
A. Not Operated	31	1.7	<1	1	1	2	2	3	3	3
B. Operated	216	3.0	<1	1	2	3	3	4	4	5
2. MULTIPLE DX										
A. Not Operated	145	2.1	<1	1	1	2	3	3	3	5
B. Operated	1,031	3.5	7	2	3	3	4	4	5	18
1. SINGLE DX	247	2.8	1	2	2	3	3	4	4	5
2. MULTIPLE DX	1,176	3.3	7	2	2	3	4	4	5	18
A. NOT OPERATED	176	2.0	<1	1	1	2	2	3	3	5
B. OPERATED	1,247	3.4	6	2	3	3	4	4	5	17
TOTAL										
0–19 Years	32	2.5	1	1	2	2	3	4	4	5
20–34	928	3.2	6	2	2	3	3	4	5	13
35–49	436	3.4	5	2	2	3	4	4	5	15
50–64	27	3.8	15	2	2	3	4	4	4	23
65+	0									
GRAND TOTAL	1,423	3.2	6	2	2	3	4	4	5	14

641.11: PLACENTA PREV HEMOR-DEL

Type of Patients	Observed Patients	Avg. Stay	Vari-ance	10th	25th	50th	75th	90th	95th	99th
1. SINGLE DX										
A. Not Operated										
0–19 Years	0									
20–34	7	2.4	4	1	1	2	2	7	7	7
35–49	0									
50–64	0									
65+	0									
B. Operated										
0–19 Years	5	2.8	<1	2	3	3	3	3	3	3
20–34	114	4.0	30	2	3	3	4	4	6	39
35–49	12	3.1	<1	2	2	3	4	4	5	5
50–64	0									
65+	0									
2. MULTIPLE DX										
A. Not Operated										
0–19 Years	6	1.8	<1	1	1	2	2	3	3	3
20–34	46	3.6	22	1	2	3	3	9	12	29
35–49	19	4.2	27	1	2	3	4	9	24	24
50–64	1	2.0	0	2	2	2	2	2	2	2
65+	0									
B. Operated										
0–19 Years	39	6.6	82	2	3	3	5	19	22	52
20–34	928	7.4	120	2	3	4	5	19	28	62
35–49	491	8.7	148	2	3	4	8	22	33	67
50–64	21	8.5	113	2	3	4	9	27	42	>99
65+	0									
SUBTOTALS:										
1. SINGLE DX										
A. Not Operated	7	2.4	4	1	1	2	2	7	7	7
B. Operated	131	3.8	26	2	3	3	4	4	6	39
2. MULTIPLE DX										
A. Not Operated	72	3.6	21	1	2	3	3	8	12	29
B. Operated	1,479	7.8	128	2	3	4	6	20	30	63
1. SINGLE DX	138	3.8	25	2	2	3	4	4	6	39
2. MULTIPLE DX	1,551	7.6	124	2	3	4	6	20	30	62
A. NOT OPERATED	79	3.5	20	1	2	2	3	8	12	29
B. OPERATED	1,610	7.5	121	2	3	4	5	20	30	62
TOTAL										
0–19 Years	50	5.6	67	2	2	3	4	12	21	52
20–34	1,095	6.9	107	2	3	3	5	18	27	62
35–49	522	8.4	142	2	3	4	7	22	32	62
50–64	22	8.2	110	2	3	4	9	27	42	>99
65+	0									
GRAND TOTAL	1,689	7.3	117	2	3	4	5	19	28	62

641.13: PLACENTA PREV HEMOR-AP

Type of Patients	Observed Patients	Avg. Stay	Vari-ance	10th	25th	50th	75th	90th	95th	99th
1. SINGLE DX										
A. Not Operated										
0–19 Years	8	1.6	1	1	1	1	2	4	4	4
20–34	254	2.7	7	1	2	2	3	6	8	14
35–49	48	3.5	23	1	2	2	4	7	9	27
50–64	3	1.3	<1	1	1	1	2	2	2	2
65+	0									
B. Operated										
0–19 Years	0									
20–34	0									
35–49	0									
50–64	0									
65+	0									
2. MULTIPLE DX										
A. Not Operated										
0–19 Years	16	3.1	4	1	1	2	4	7	7	7
20–34	429	4.4	25	1	2	3	5	8	13	29
35–49	266	4.5	29	1	3	3	5	9	16	30
50–64	11	6.6	133	2	2	3	6	6	41	41
65+	0									
B. Operated										
0–19 Years	0									
20–34	1	6.0	0	6	6	6	6	6	6	6
35–49	0									
50–64	1	9.0	0	9	9	9	9	9	9	9
65+	0									
SUBTOTALS:										
1. SINGLE DX										
A. Not Operated	313	2.8	10	1	1	2	3	6	8	17
B. Operated	0									
2. MULTIPLE DX										
A. Not Operated	722	4.5	27	1	2	3	5	8	14	30
B. Operated	2	7.5	4	6	6	9	9	9	9	9
1. SINGLE DX	313	2.8	10	1	1	2	3	6	8	17
2. MULTIPLE DX	724	4.5	27	1	2	3	5	8	14	30
A. NOT OPERATED	1,035	4.0	23	1	1	2	5	8	12	28
B. OPERATED	2	7.5	4	6	6	9	9	9	9	9
TOTAL										
0–19 Years	24	2.6	4	1	1	2	4	6	7	7
20–34	684	3.8	19	1	1	2	4	8	11	23
35–49	314	4.3	28	1	1	3	5	8	16	30
50–64	15	5.7	100	1	2	2	6	9	41	41
65+	0									
GRAND TOTAL	1,037	4.0	23	1	1	2	5	8	12	28

641.21: PREMATURE SEP PLAC-DEL

Type of Patients	Observed Patients	Avg. Stay	Variance	10th	25th	50th	75th	90th	95th	99th
1. SINGLE DX										
A. Not Operated										
0–19 Years	17	1.8	<1	1	1	2	2	3	3	3
20–34	179	1.9	6	1	1	2	2	3	3	4
35–49	8	2.0	<1	1	2	2	2	3	3	3
50–64	0									
65+	0									
B. Operated										
0–19 Years	18	2.9	<1	2	3	3	3	4	4	4
20–34	106	3.2	2	2	2	3	3	4	5	8
35–49	6	2.7	<1	2	2	3	3	3	3	3
50–64	0									
65+	0									
2. MULTIPLE DX										
A. Not Operated										
0–19 Years	119	2.7	11	1	2	2	2	3	5	16
20–34	915	2.5	7	1	1	2	2	3	6	13
35–49	195	2.8	8	1	2	2	3	5	10	15
50–64	9	6.7	82	1	2	3	3	24	24	24
65+	0									
B. Operated										
0–19 Years	177	4.1	22	2	3	3	4	5	8	36
20–34	1,562	4.4	24	2	3	3	4	6	10	27
35–49	475	4.7	23	2	3	4	4	7	11	29
50–64	25	5.9	29	3	3	4	6	9	22	23
65+	0									
SUBTOTALS:										
1. SINGLE DX — A. Not Operated	204	1.9	5	1	1	2	2	3	3	4
1. SINGLE DX — B. Operated	130	3.1	2	2	2	3	3	4	4	8
2. MULTIPLE DX — A. Not Operated	1,238	2.6	9	1	1	2	3	4	6	15
2. MULTIPLE DX — B. Operated	2,239	4.5	24	2	3	3	4	6	10	28
1. SINGLE DX	334	2.4	4	1	2	2	3	3	4	7
2. MULTIPLE DX	3,477	3.8	19	2	3	3	4	6	9	25
A. NOT OPERATED	1,442	2.5	8	1	1	2	3	3	6	15
B. OPERATED	2,369	4.4	23	2	3	3	4	6	10	28
TOTAL										
0–19 Years	331	3.4	16	2	2	3	4	5	6	28
20–34	2,762	3.6	18	1	2	3	4	5	8	23
35–49	684	4.1	19	2	2	3	4	7	10	28
50–64	34	6.1	41	2	3	4	6	21	23	24
65+	0									
GRAND TOTAL	3,811	3.7	18	1	2	3	4	5	9	24

641.23: PREMATURE SEP PLAC-AP

Type of Patients	Observed Patients	Avg. Stay	Variance	10th	25th	50th	75th	90th	95th	99th
1. SINGLE DX										
A. Not Operated										
0–19 Years	14	2.1	2	1	1	1	2	3	4	4
20–34	104	2.7	6	1	1	2	3	5	7	13
35–49	7	1.9	1	1	1	1	3	4	4	4
50–64	0									
65+	0									
B. Operated										
0–19 Years	0									
20–34	0									
35–49	0									
50–64	0									
65+	0									
2. MULTIPLE DX										
A. Not Operated										
0–19 Years	39	4.1	17	1	1	3	5	8	10	24
20–34	291	5.8	51	1	2	4	7	13	19	41
35–49	129	5.3	49	1	2	3	6	12	16	36
50–64	1	2.0	0	2	2	2	2	2	2	2
65+	0									
B. Operated										
0–19 Years	0									
20–34	2	2.0	2	1	1	2	3	3	3	3
35–49	0									
50–64	0									
65+	0									
SUBTOTALS:										
1. SINGLE DX — A. Not Operated	125	2.6	5	1	1	2	3	5	7	13
1. SINGLE DX — B. Operated	0									
2. MULTIPLE DX — A. Not Operated	460	5.5	48	1	2	3	6	12	17	38
2. MULTIPLE DX — B. Operated	2	2.0	2	1	1	2	3	3	3	3
1. SINGLE DX	125	2.6	5	1	1	2	3	5	7	13
2. MULTIPLE DX	462	5.5	48	1	2	3	6	12	17	38
A. NOT OPERATED	585	4.9	40	1	2	3	6	11	15	36
B. OPERATED	2	2.0	2	1	2	3	3	3	3	3
TOTAL										
0–19 Years	53	3.6	13	1	1	3	4	7	9	24
20–34	397	5.0	41	1	2	3	6	11	16	38
35–49	136	5.2	47	1	2	3	5	12	16	36
50–64	1	2.0	0	2	2	2	2	2	2	2
65+	0									
GRAND TOTAL	587	4.9	40	1	2	3	6	11	15	36

641.83: AP HEMORRHAGE NEC-AP

Type of Patients	Observed Patients	Avg. Stay	Variance	10th	25th	50th	75th	90th	95th	99th
1. SINGLE DX										
A. Not Operated										
0–19 Years	10	1.3	<1	1	1	1	2	2	2	2
20–34	38	1.5	<1	1	1	1	2	3	3	4
35–49	3	1.3	<1	1	1	1	2	2	2	2
50–64	1	1.0	0	1	1	1	1	1	1	1
65+	0									
B. Operated										
0–19 Years	0									
20–34	0									
35–49	0									
50–64	0									
65+	0									
2. MULTIPLE DX										
A. Not Operated										
0–19 Years	16	1.7	<1	1	1	2	2	3	4	4
20–34	112	3.1	16	1	1	2	3	6	11	22
35–49	40	3.0	9	1	1	2	4	5	10	16
50–64	0									
65+	0									
B. Operated										
0–19 Years	0									
20–34	2	1.5	<1	1	1	2	2	2	2	2
35–49	1	2.0	0	2	2	2	2	2	2	2
50–64	0									
65+	0									
SUBTOTALS:										
1. SINGLE DX — A. Not Operated	52	1.5	<1	1	1	1	2	2	3	4
1. SINGLE DX — B. Operated	0									
2. MULTIPLE DX — A. Not Operated	168	2.9	13	1	1	2	3	6	7	22
2. MULTIPLE DX — B. Operated	3	1.7	<1	1	1	2	2	2	2	2
1. SINGLE DX	52	1.5	<1	1	1	1	2	2	3	4
2. MULTIPLE DX	171	2.9	13	1	1	2	3	5	7	22
A. NOT OPERATED	220	2.6	10	1	1	2	3	5	7	18
B. OPERATED	3	1.7	<1	1	1	2	2	2	2	2
TOTAL										
0–19 Years	26	1.5	<1	1	1	1	2	2	3	4
20–34	152	2.7	12	1	1	2	3	5	6	22
35–49	44	2.8	8	1	1	2	4	5	7	16
50–64	1	1.0	0	1	1	1	1	1	1	1
65+	0									
GRAND TOTAL	223	2.6	10	1	1	2	3	5	6	18

Length of Stay by Diagnosis and Operation, Western Region, 2008

Western Region, October 2006–September 2007 Data, by Diagnosis

641.91: ANTEPARTUM HEMOR NOS-DEL

Type of Patients	Observed Patients	Avg. Stay	Variance	10th	25th	50th	75th	90th	95th	99th
1. SINGLE DX										
A. Not Operated										
0–19 Years	3	2.3	2	1	1	2	4	4	4	4
20–34	30	1.9	<1	1	1	2	2	3	3	4
35–49	2	1.5	<1	1	1	1	2	2	2	2
50–64	0									
65+	0									
B. Operated										
0–19 Years	3	2.7	<1	2	2	3	3	3	3	3
20–34	1	3.0	0	3	3	3	3	3	3	3
35–49	0									
50–64	0									
65+	0									
2. MULTIPLE DX										
A. Not Operated										
0–19 Years	8	2.5	3	1	2	2	2	7	7	7
20–34	111	2.3	5	1	1	2	3	3	3	4
35–49	19	2.1	1	1	1	2	3	3	6	6
50–64	1	2.0	0	2	2	2	2	2	2	2
65+	0									
B. Operated										
0–19 Years	5	2.6	1	1	2	3	3	4	4	4
20–34	45	3.3	3	2	3	3	4	5	5	10
35–49	20	4.3	15	2	3	3	4	6	20	20
50–64	0									
65+	0									
SUBTOTALS:										
1. SINGLE DX										
A. Not Operated	35	1.9	<1	1	1	2	2	3	4	4
B. Operated	4	2.8	<1	2	2	3	3	3	3	3
2. MULTIPLE DX										
A. Not Operated	139	2.3	5	1	2	2	3	3	4	7
B. Operated	70	3.5	6	2	2	3	4	5	6	20
1. SINGLE DX	39	2.0	<1	1	1	2	2	3	4	4
2. MULTIPLE DX	209	2.7	5	1	2	2	3	4	5	10
A. NOT OPERATED	174	2.2	4	1	1	2	3	3	4	7
B. OPERATED	74	3.5	6	2	2	3	4	5	6	20
TOTAL										
0–19 Years	19	2.5	2	1	2	2	3	4	4	7
20–34	187	2.5	4	1	2	2	3	4	4	10
35–49	41	3.1	9	1	2	3	4	4	6	20
50–64	1	2.0	0	2	2	2	2	2	2	2
65+	0									
GRAND TOTAL	248	2.6	5	1	2	2	3	4	4	10

641.93: ANTEPARTUM HEMOR NOS-AP

Type of Patients	Observed Patients	Avg. Stay	Variance	10th	25th	50th	75th	90th	95th	99th
1. SINGLE DX										
A. Not Operated										
0–19 Years	24	1.2	<1	1	1	1	1	2	2	3
20–34	136	1.6	2	1	1	1	2	3	3	9
35–49	17	1.8	<1	1	1	2	2	3	4	4
50–64	0									
65+	0									
B. Operated										
0–19 Years	0									
20–34	0									
35–49	0									
50–64	0									
65+	0									
2. MULTIPLE DX										
A. Not Operated										
0–19 Years	26	2.3	8	1	1	1	2	4	9	13
20–34	202	3.0	14	1	1	2	3	6	8	17
35–49	95	2.6	10	1	1	2	3	6	7	18
50–64	4	1.3	<1	1	1	2	2	2	2	2
65+	0									
B. Operated										
0–19 Years	0									
20–34	0									
35–49	0									
50–64	0									
65+	0									
SUBTOTALS:										
1. SINGLE DX										
A. Not Operated	177	1.6	2	1	1	1	2	3	3	9
B. Operated	0									
2. MULTIPLE DX										
A. Not Operated	327	2.8	12	1	1	2	3	6	8	17
B. Operated	0									
1. SINGLE DX	177	1.6	2	1	1	1	2	3	3	9
2. MULTIPLE DX	327	2.8	12	1	1	2	3	6	8	17
A. NOT OPERATED	504	2.4	9	1	1	1	3	4	7	17
B. OPERATED	0									
TOTAL										
0–19 Years	50	1.8	4	1	1	1	2	3	4	7
20–34	338	2.4	9	1	1	2	3	5	7	17
35–49	112	2.5	8	1	1	2	3	5	7	17
50–64	4	1.3	<1	1	1	2	2	2	2	2
65+	0									
GRAND TOTAL	504	2.4	9	1	1	1	3	4	7	17

642: HYPERTENSION COMP PREG

Type of Patients	Observed Patients	Avg. Stay	Variance	10th	25th	50th	75th	90th	95th	99th
1. SINGLE DX										
A. Not Operated										
0–19 Years	415	2.3	1	1	2	2	3	3	4	7
20–34	2,397	2.1	2	1	1	2	3	3	4	6
35–49	221	2.0	2	1	1	2	3	3	3	8
50–64	5	2.0	<1	1	1	2	3	3	3	3
65+	0									
B. Operated										
0–19 Years	79	3.4	1	2	3	3	4	5	6	7
20–34	245	3.8	2	3	3	4	4	5	6	10
35–49	14	3.9	2	2	3	4	4	5	7	7
50–64	1	4.0	0	4	4	4	4	4	4	4
65+	0									
2. MULTIPLE DX										
A. Not Operated										
0–19 Years	2,354	3.0	3	1	2	3	3	4	5	10
20–34	14,211	2.8	4	1	2	3	3	4	5	11
35–49	3,088	2.8	7	1	2	2	3	4	6	13
50–64	112	3.4	39	1	2	2	3	4	5	21
65+	0									
B. Operated										
0–19 Years	1,079	4.7	7	3	3	4	5	7	9	15
20–34	8,255	4.7	12	3	3	4	5	7	9	20
35–49	2,510	5.1	18	3	3	4	5	8	11	23
50–64	138	5.6	22	3	3	4	6	9	13	29
65+	0									
SUBTOTALS:										
1. SINGLE DX										
A. Not Operated	3,038	2.2	2	1	2	2	3	3	4	7
B. Operated	339	3.7	2	2	3	4	4	5	6	9
2. MULTIPLE DX										
A. Not Operated	19,765	2.8	5	1	2	2	3	4	5	11
B. Operated	11,982	4.8	13	3	3	4	5	7	10	21
1. SINGLE DX	3,377	2.3	2	1	2	2	3	4	4	7
2. MULTIPLE DX	31,747	3.6	9	2	2	3	4	6	7	16
A. NOT OPERATED	22,803	2.7	5	1	2	2	3	4	5	11
B. OPERATED	12,321	4.8	13	3	3	4	5	7	10	21
TOTAL										
0–19 Years	3,927	3.4	5	2	2	3	4	5	7	12
20–34	25,108	3.4	8	1	2	3	4	5	7	15
35–49	5,833	3.8	13	1	2	3	4	6	9	19
50–64	256	4.6	30	2	2	4	5	7	10	29
65+	0									
GRAND TOTAL	35,124	3.5	8	1	2	3	4	6	7	15

Length of Stay by Diagnosis and Operation, Western Region, 2008

642.01: BEH COMP PREGNANCY-DEL

Type of Patients	Observed Patients	Avg. Stay	Variance	Percentiles						
				10th	25th	50th	75th	90th	95th	99th
1. SINGLE DX										
A. Not Operated										
0–19 Years	2	2.0	0	2	2	2	2	2	2	2
20–34	21	2.0	<1	1	1	2	2	3	3	4
35–49	9	1.4	<1	1	1	1	2	2	2	2
50–64	0									
65+	0									
B. Operated										
0–19 Years	1	3.0	0	3	3	3	3	3	3	3
20–34	1	3.0	0	3	3	3	3	3	3	3
35–49	0									
50–64	0									
65+	0									
2. MULTIPLE DX										
A. Not Operated										
0–19 Years	22	2.4	<1	1	2	2	3	3	4	4
20–34	1,001	2.2	<1	1	2	2	3	3	4	5
35–49	343	2.3	2	1	2	2	3	3	4	6
50–64	13	2.5	<1	2	2	2	3	4	4	4
65+	0									
B. Operated										
0–19 Years	10	3.3	<1	3	3	3	4	4	5	5
20–34	390	3.8	6	2	3	3	4	6	7	12
35–49	222	3.7	3	2	3	3	4	6	7	10
50–64	9	3.9	<1	3	4	4	4	5	5	5
65+	0									
SUBTOTALS:										
1. SINGLE DX										
A. Not Operated	32	1.8	<1	1	1	2	2	3	3	4
B. Operated	2	3.0	0	3	3	3	3	3	3	3
2. MULTIPLE DX										
A. Not Operated	1,379	2.2	1	1	2	2	3	3	4	5
B. Operated	631	3.8	5	2	3	3	4	6	7	12
1. SINGLE DX	34	1.9	<1	1	1	2	2	3	3	4
2. MULTIPLE DX	2,010	2.7	3	1	2	2	3	4	5	9
A. NOT OPERATED	1,411	2.2	1	1	2	2	3	3	4	5
B. OPERATED	633	3.7	5	2	3	3	4	6	7	12
TOTAL										
0–19 Years	35	2.6	<1	2	2	3	3	4	4	5
20–34	1,413	2.7	3	1	2	2	3	4	5	8
35–49	574	2.8	3	1	2	2	3	4	6	10
50–64	22	3.1	1	2	2	3	4	4	4	5
65+	0									
GRAND TOTAL	2,044	2.7	3	1	2	2	3	4	5	9

642.03: BEH COMP PREGNANCY-AP

Type of Patients	Observed Patients	Avg. Stay	Variance	Percentiles						
				10th	25th	50th	75th	90th	95th	99th
1. SINGLE DX										
A. Not Operated										
0–19 Years	0									
20–34	26	1.4	<1	1	1	1	2	2	3	3
35–49	8	1.1	<1	1	1	1	1	2	2	2
50–64	0									
65+	0									
B. Operated										
0–19 Years	0									
20–34	0									
35–49	0									
50–64	0									
65+	0									
2. MULTIPLE DX										
A. Not Operated										
0–19 Years	6	2.0	1	1	1	2	2	4	4	4
20–34	295	2.3	5	1	1	2	2	4	6	14
35–49	151	2.3	4	1	1	2	3	4	6	9
50–64	4	2.5	2	1	1	2	3	4	4	4
65+	0									
B. Operated										
0–19 Years	0									
20–34	0									
35–49	0									
50–64	0									
65+	0									
SUBTOTALS:										
1. SINGLE DX										
A. Not Operated	34	1.3	<1	1	1	1	2	2	3	3
B. Operated	0									
2. MULTIPLE DX										
A. Not Operated	456	2.3	5	1	1	2	3	4	6	14
B. Operated	0									
1. SINGLE DX	34	1.3	<1	1	1	1	2	2	3	3
2. MULTIPLE DX	456	2.3	5	1	1	2	3	4	6	14
A. NOT OPERATED	490	2.2	4	1	1	2	3	4	6	14
B. OPERATED	0									
TOTAL										
0–19 Years	6	2.0	1	1	1	2	2	4	4	4
20–34	321	2.2	5	1	1	2	2	4	6	14
35–49	159	2.2	4	1	1	2	3	4	6	9
50–64	4	2.5	2	1	1	2	3	4	4	5
65+	0									
GRAND TOTAL	490	2.2	4	1	1	2	3	4	6	14

642.31: TRANSIENT HTN PREG-DEL

Type of Patients	Observed Patients	Avg. Stay	Variance	Percentiles						
				10th	25th	50th	75th	90th	95th	99th
1. SINGLE DX										
A. Not Operated										
0–19 Years	125	2.3	<1	1	2	2	3	3	3	4
20–34	773	2.2	<1	1	2	2	3	3	4	5
35–49	26	2.1	<1	1	1	2	3	3	3	3
50–64	0									
65+	0									
B. Operated										
0–19 Years	16	3.5	2	2	3	3	4	5	7	7
20–34	63	3.7	2	2	3	3	4	5	5	11
35–49	4	3.8	<1	3	4	4	4	4	4	4
50–64	0									
65+	0									
2. MULTIPLE DX										
A. Not Operated										
0–19 Years	734	2.6	1	2	2	2	3	4	4	7
20–34	4,708	2.4	1	1	2	2	3	3	4	5
35–49	778	2.5	2	1	2	2	3	3	4	8
50–64	28	2.4	<1	2	2	2	3	4	4	4
65+	0									
B. Operated										
0–19 Years	224	4.0	3	3	3	4	5	5	6	11
20–34	1,849	3.7	3	2	3	3	4	5	6	10
35–49	488	3.9	<1	2	3	4	5	5	7	12
50–64	26	4.5	4	3	3	4	5	6	7	13
65+	0									
SUBTOTALS:										
1. SINGLE DX										
A. Not Operated	924	2.2	<1	1	2	2	3	3	3	5
B. Operated	83	3.6	2	2	3	3	4	5	5	11
2. MULTIPLE DX										
A. Not Operated	6,248	2.4	1	1	2	2	3	3	4	5
B. Operated	2,587	3.8	3	2	3	4	4	5	6	11
1. SINGLE DX	1,007	2.4	1	1	2	2	3	3	4	5
2. MULTIPLE DX	8,835	2.8	2	2	2	3	3	4	5	8
A. NOT OPERATED	7,172	2.4	1	1	2	2	3	3	4	5
B. OPERATED	2,670	3.8	3	2	3	4	4	5	6	11
TOTAL										
0–19 Years	1,099	2.9	2	2	2	3	3	4	5	8
20–34	7,393	2.7	2	1	2	3	3	4	5	7
35–49	1,296	3.0	3	2	2	3	4	4	5	10
50–64	54	3.4	4	3	3	3	4	5	6	13
65+	0									
GRAND TOTAL	9,842	2.8	2	2	2	3	3	4	5	7

Length of Stay by Diagnosis and Operation, Western Region, 2008

Western Region, October 2006–September 2007 Data, by Diagnosis

642.33: TRANSIENT HTN PREG-AP

Type of Patients	Observed Patients	Avg. Stay	Vari-ance	10th	25th	50th	75th	90th	95th	99th
1. SINGLE DX										
A. Not Operated										
0–19 Years	51	1.6	<1	1	1	1	2	3	3	4
20–34	349	1.5	1	1	1	1	2	3	3	6
35–49	40	1.5	1	1	1	1	2	3	4	6
50–64	1	1.0	0	1	1	1	1	1	1	1
65+	0									
B. Operated										
0–19 Years	0									
20–34	0									
35–49	0									
50–64	0									
65+	0									
2. MULTIPLE DX										
A. Not Operated										
0–19 Years	62	2.0	3	1	1	1	2	3	4	9
20–34	547	1.9	3	1	1	1	2	3	5	9
35–49	201	1.9	3	1	1	1	2	3	4	9
50–64	4	1.7	2	1	1	1	1	4	4	4
65+	0									
B. Operated										
0–19 Years	0									
20–34	2	9.0	49	4	4	14	14	14	14	14
35–49	0									
50–64	0									
65+	0									
SUBTOTALS:										
1. SINGLE DX										
A. Not Operated	441	1.5	1	1	1	1	2	2	3	6
B. Operated	0									
2. MULTIPLE DX										
A. Not Operated	814	1.9	3	1	1	1	2	3	5	9
B. Operated	2	9.0	49	4	4	14	14	14	14	14
1. SINGLE DX	441	1.5	1	1	1	1	2	2	3	6
2. MULTIPLE DX	816	1.9	3	1	1	1	2	3	5	9
A. NOT OPERATED	1,255	1.8	2	1	1	1	2	3	4	9
B. OPERATED	2	9.0	49	4	4	14	14	14	14	14
TOTAL										
0–19 Years	113	1.8	2	1	1	1	2	3	3	9
20–34	898	1.8	3	1	1	1	2	3	4	9
35–49	241	1.8	2	1	1	1	2	3	4	9
50–64	5	1.6	2	1	1	1	1	4	4	4
65+	0									
GRAND TOTAL	1,257	1.8	2	1	1	1	2	3	4	9

642.41: MILD/NOS PRE-ECLAM-DEL

Type of Patients	Observed Patients	Avg. Stay	Vari-ance	10th	25th	50th	75th	90th	95th	99th
1. SINGLE DX										
A. Not Operated										
0–19 Years	128	2.5	<1	2	2	2	3	3	4	6
20–34	500	2.4	<1	1	2	2	3	3	4	5
35–49	13	2.2	<1	1	2	2	3	3	3	3
50–64	0									
65+	0									
B. Operated										
0–19 Years	20	3.4	1	2	3	3	4	4	4	7
20–34	41	3.5	1	2	3	3	5	5	6	6
35–49	2	4.5	<1	4	4	5	5	5	5	5
50–64	0									
65+	0									
2. MULTIPLE DX										
A. Not Operated										
0–19 Years	987	3.1	4	2	2	3	3	5	5	14
20–34	4,067	2.9	4	2	2	3	3	4	5	10
35–49	576	3.3	15	2	2	3	3	4	6	21
50–64	24	2.8	2	1	2	3	3	4	5	8
65+	0									
B. Operated										
0–19 Years	359	4.2	5	2	3	4	5	6	7	14
20–34	2,356	4.5	11	2	3	4	5	6	9	19
35–49	623	4.6	12	2	3	4	5	7	10	21
50–64	26	4.2	2	3	3	4	5	6	6	10
65+	0									
SUBTOTALS:										
1. SINGLE DX										
A. Not Operated	641	2.4	<1	1	2	2	3	3	4	5
B. Operated	63	3.5	1	2	3	3	4	5	5	7
2. MULTIPLE DX										
A. Not Operated	5,654	3.0	5	2	2	3	3	4	5	12
B. Operated	3,364	4.5	10	2	3	4	5	6	9	19
1. SINGLE DX	704	2.5	1	1	2	2	3	4	4	6
2. MULTIPLE DX	9,018	3.6	8	2	2	3	4	5	7	16
A. NOT OPERATED	6,295	2.9	5	2	2	3	3	4	5	11
B. OPERATED	3,427	4.5	10	2	3	4	5	6	9	19
TOTAL										
0–19 Years	1,494	3.3	5	2	2	3	4	5	6	12
20–34	6,964	3.4	7	2	2	3	4	5	6	15
35–49	1,214	4.0	14	2	2	3	4	6	9	21
50–64	50	3.5	3	2	3	3	4	5	6	10
65+	0									
GRAND TOTAL	9,722	3.5	7	2	2	3	4	5	6	15

642.43: MILD/NOS PRE-ECLAM-AP

Type of Patients	Observed Patients	Avg. Stay	Vari-ance	10th	25th	50th	75th	90th	95th	99th
1. SINGLE DX										
A. Not Operated										
0–19 Years	35	2.4	3	1	1	2	3	4	7	8
20–34	265	2.1	5	1	1	2	3	3	5	11
35–49	18	1.4	<1	1	1	1	2	2	3	3
50–64	0									
65+	0									
B. Operated										
0–19 Years	0									
20–34	0									
35–49	0									
50–64	0									
65+	0									
2. MULTIPLE DX										
A. Not Operated										
0–19 Years	51	2.4	3	1	1	2	3	4	5	9
20–34	456	2.9	10	1	1	2	3	6	9	16
35–49	159	3.1	17	1	1	2	3	7	10	28
50–64	2	17.0	31	13	13	13	21	21	21	21
65+	0									
B. Operated										
0–19 Years	0									
20–34	0									
35–49	0									
50–64	0									
65+	0									
SUBTOTALS:										
1. SINGLE DX										
A. Not Operated	318	2.1	5	1	1	2	2	4	5	11
B. Operated	0									
2. MULTIPLE DX										
A. Not Operated	668	2.9	12	1	1	2	3	6	9	18
B. Operated	0									
1. SINGLE DX	318	2.1	5	1	1	2	2	4	5	11
2. MULTIPLE DX	668	2.9	12	1	1	2	3	6	9	18
A. NOT OPERATED	986	2.7	10	1	1	2	3	5	7	16
B. OPERATED	0									
TOTAL										
0–19 Years	86	2.4	3	1	1	2	3	4	6	9
20–34	721	2.6	8	1	1	2	3	5	7	14
35–49	177	2.9	16	1	1	2	3	7	9	28
50–64	2	17.0	31	13	13	13	21	21	21	21
65+	0									
GRAND TOTAL	986	2.7	10	1	1	2	3	5	7	16

Length of Stay by Diagnosis and Operation, Western Region, 2008

Western Region, October 2006–September 2007 Data, by Diagnosis

642.44: MILD/NOS PRE-ECLAM-PP

Type of Patients	Observed Patients	Avg. Stay	Variance	10th	25th	50th	75th	90th	95th	99th
1. SINGLE DX										
A. Not Operated										
0–19 Years	10	2.1	<1	1	1	3	3	3	3	3
20–34	86	1.9	<1	1	1	2	2	3	3	4
35–49	33	1.9	<1	1	1	2	2	3	3	3
50–64	0									
65+	0									
B. Operated										
0–19 Years	0									
20–34	0									
35–49	0									
50–64	0									
65+	0									
2. MULTIPLE DX										
A. Not Operated										
0–19 Years	7	2.6	<1	2	2	2	3	4	4	4
20–34	119	2.4	3	1	2	2	3	4	5	8
35–49	44	2.8	4	2	2	2	3	4	5	13
50–64	0									
65+	0									
B. Operated										
0–19 Years	0									
20–34	0									
35–49	0									
50–64	0									
65+	0									
SUBTOTALS:										
1. SINGLE DX A. Not Operated	129	1.9	<1	1	1	2	2	3	3	4
1. SINGLE DX B. Operated	0									
2. MULTIPLE DX A. Not Operated	170	2.5	3	1	2	2	3	4	5	13
2. MULTIPLE DX B. Operated	0									
1. SINGLE DX	129	1.9	<1	1	1	2	2	3	3	4
2. MULTIPLE DX	170	2.5	3	1	2	2	3	4	5	13
A. NOT OPERATED	299	2.3	2	1	2	2	3	3	4	7
B. OPERATED	0									
TOTAL										
0–19 Years	17	2.3	<1	1	2	2	3	3	4	4
20–34	205	2.2	2	1	1	2	3	4	4	7
35–49	77	2.4	2	1	2	2	3	3	5	13
50–64	0									
65+	0									
GRAND TOTAL	299	2.3	2	1	2	2	3	3	4	7

642.51: SEVERE PRE-ECLAM-DEL

Type of Patients	Observed Patients	Avg. Stay	Variance	10th	25th	50th	75th	90th	95th	99th
1. SINGLE DX										
A. Not Operated										
0–19 Years	19	2.8	1	1	2	3	4	5	5	5
20–34	85	3.3	2	2	2	3	4	5	6	9
35–49	3	6.6	22	3	3	5	12	12	12	12
50–64	1	2.0	0	2	2	2	2	2	2	2
65+	0									
B. Operated										
0–19 Years	32	3.2	<1	2	3	3	4	4	5	5
20–34	119	4.0	2	3	3	4	4	5	7	10
35–49	7	3.9	3	2	2	4	4	7	7	7
50–64	1	4.0	0	4	4	4	4	4	4	4
65+	0									
2. MULTIPLE DX										
A. Not Operated										
0–19 Years	317	3.8	4	2	3	3	4	6	7	10
20–34	1,352	4.1	10	2	3	3	4	6	8	17
35–49	271	3.8	4	2	3	3	4	6	8	13
50–64	11	3.1	1	2	2	3	4	4	5	5
65+	0									
B. Operated										
0–19 Years	376	5.3	8	3	4	5	6	8	11	17
20–34	2,703	5.4	14	3	4	5	6	8	10	22
35–49	751	6.1	29	3	4	5	6	10	14	26
50–64	46	6.2	20	3	4	5	8	10	13	29
65+	0									
SUBTOTALS:										
1. SINGLE DX A. Not Operated	108	3.3	3	2	2	3	4	5	6	9
1. SINGLE DX B. Operated	159	3.9	2	2	3	4	4	5	7	10
2. MULTIPLE DX A. Not Operated	1,951	4.0	8	2	3	3	4	6	8	16
2. MULTIPLE DX B. Operated	3,876	5.6	17	3	4	5	6	8	11	23
1. SINGLE DX	267	3.6	2	2	3	3	4	5	6	10
2. MULTIPLE DX	5,827	5.0	14	3	3	4	6	8	10	21
A. NOT OPERATED	2,059	3.9	8	2	3	3	4	6	8	15
B. OPERATED	4,035	5.5	16	3	4	4	6	8	11	22
TOTAL										
0–19 Years	744	4.5	7	2	3	4	5	7	9	14
20–34	4,259	4.9	13	3	3	4	6	8	9	20
35–49	1,032	5.5	24	3	3	4	6	9	12	25
50–64	59	5.5	17	2	3	4	6	9	13	29
65+	0									
GRAND TOTAL	6,094	5.0	14	3	3	4	6	8	10	21

642.61: ECLAMPSIA-DEL

Type of Patients	Observed Patients	Avg. Stay	Variance	10th	25th	50th	75th	90th	95th	99th
1. SINGLE DX										
A. Not Operated										
0–19 Years	0									
20–34	9	2.2	<1	2	2	2	2	3	3	3
35–49	0									
50–64	0									
65+	0									
B. Operated										
0–19 Years	8	3.5	2	2	3	3	5	6	6	6
20–34	11	4.1	3	3	3	4	4	5	9	9
35–49	0									
50–64	0									
65+	0									
2. MULTIPLE DX										
A. Not Operated										
0–19 Years	19	3.3	<1	2	3	3	4	4	5	5
20–34	55	3.4	5	2	2	3	4	5	7	16
35–49	8	3.1	<1	2	2	3	4	4	4	4
50–64	0									
65+	0									
B. Operated										
0–19 Years	75	4.8	4	3	4	5	6	7	10	>99
20–34	135	4.8	7	3	4	5	5	7	8	18
35–49	20	4.2	2	3	3	4	5	6	8	8
50–64	0									
65+	0									
SUBTOTALS:										
1. SINGLE DX A. Not Operated	9	2.2	<1	2	2	2	2	3	3	3
1. SINGLE DX B. Operated	19	3.8	3	2	3	3	4	6	9	9
2. MULTIPLE DX A. Not Operated	82	3.4	3	2	3	3	4	5	5	16
2. MULTIPLE DX B. Operated	230	4.8	5	3	4	4	5	7	8	18
1. SINGLE DX	28	3.3	2	2	2	3	4	5	6	9
2. MULTIPLE DX	312	4.4	5	2	3	4	5	7	8	16
A. NOT OPERATED	91	3.3	3	2	3	3	4	4	5	16
B. OPERATED	249	4.7	5	3	3	4	5	7	8	18
TOTAL										
0–19 Years	102	4.4	3	2	3	4	5	7	8	13
20–34	210	4.3	6	2	3	4	5	7	8	16
35–49	28	3.9	2	2	3	4	5	6	6	8
50–64	0									
65+	0									
GRAND TOTAL	340	4.3	5	2	3	4	5	7	8	16

Length of Stay by Diagnosis and Operation, Western Region, 2008

Western Region, October 2006–September 2007 Data, by Diagnosis

642.71: TOX W PRE-EXIST HTN-DEL

Type of Patients	Observed Patients	Avg. Stay	Variance	10th	25th	50th	75th	90th	95th	99th
1. SINGLE DX										
A. Not Operated										
0–19 Years	0									
20–34	7	3.4	3	2	2	3	4	7	7	7
35–49	2	4.0	0	4	4	4	4	4	4	4
50–64	0									
65+	0									
B. Operated										
0–19 Years	1	7.0	0	7	7	7	7	7	7	7
20–34	4	3.5	<1	3	3	4	4	4	4	4
35–49	0									
50–64	0									
65+	0									
2. MULTIPLE DX										
A. Not Operated										
0–19 Years	22	3.6	4	2	3	3	4	5	7	10
20–34	404	4.5	20	2	2	3	5	7	12	24
35–49	150	3.7	5	2	2	3	4	7	8	12
50–64	5	3.2	<1	2	3	3	3	4	4	4
65+	0									
B. Operated										
0–19 Years	25	8.1	63	3	4	6	8	13	25	39
20–34	599	6.5	30	3	4	5	7	11	19	28
35–49	334	6.4	28	3	4	5	7	11	16	27
50–64	30	7.4	58	3	4	6	7	13	20	43
65+	0									
SUBTOTALS:										
1. SINGLE DX — A. Not Operated	9	3.6	2	2	3	3	4	7	7	7
B. Operated	5	4.2	3	3	3	4	4	7	7	7
2. MULTIPLE DX — A. Not Operated	581	4.2	15	2	3	3	4	7	10	23
B. Operated	988	6.6	31	3	4	5	7	11	19	30
1. SINGLE DX	14	3.8	2	2	3	4	4	7	7	7
2. MULTIPLE DX	1,569	5.7	26	2	3	4	6	10	15	28
A. NOT OPERATED	590	4.2	15	2	3	3	4	7	10	23
B. OPERATED	993	6.6	30	3	4	5	7	11	19	30
TOTAL										
0–19 Years	48	6.0	39	2	3	4	7	10	13	39
20–34	1,014	5.7	27	2	3	4	6	10	17	28
35–49	486	5.6	22	2	3	4	6	9	13	26
50–64	35	6.8	52	3	3	5	7	12	20	43
65+	0									
GRAND TOTAL	1,583	5.7	26	2	3	4	6	10	15	28

642.73: TOX W PRE-EXIST HTN-AP

Type of Patients	Observed Patients	Avg. Stay	Variance	10th	25th	50th	75th	90th	95th	99th
1. SINGLE DX										
A. Not Operated										
0–19 Years	0									
20–34	12	2.9	20	1	1	2	2	3	17	17
35–49	2	6.0	8	4	4	4	8	8	8	8
50–64	0									
65+	0									
B. Operated										
0–19 Years	0									
20–34	0									
35–49	0									
50–64	0									
65+	0									
2. MULTIPLE DX										
A. Not Operated										
0–19 Years	3	2.3	<1	2	2	2	3	3	3	3
20–34	170	3.9	19	1	2	3	4	7	14	27
35–49	80	3.5	11	1	1	3	4	6	12	19
50–64	4	2.0	2	1	1	2	2	4	4	4
65+	0									
B. Operated										
0–19 Years	0									
20–34	0									
35–49	0									
50–64	0									
65+	0									
SUBTOTALS:										
1. SINGLE DX — A. Not Operated	14	3.4	19	1	1	2	3	8	17	17
B. Operated	0									
2. MULTIPLE DX — A. Not Operated	257	3.7	16	1	1	2	4	7	13	20
B. Operated	0									
1. SINGLE DX	14	3.4	19	1	1	2	3	8	17	17
2. MULTIPLE DX	257	3.7	16	1	1	2	4	7	13	20
A. NOT OPERATED	271	3.7	16	1	1	2	4	7	13	20
B. OPERATED	0									
TOTAL										
0–19 Years	3	2.3	<1	2	2	2	3	3	3	3
20–34	182	3.8	19	1	1	2	4	7	14	27
35–49	82	3.5	11	1	1	3	4	6	11	19
50–64	4	2.0	2	1	1	2	2	4	4	4
65+	0									
GRAND TOTAL	271	3.7	16	1	1	2	4	7	13	20

642.91: HYPERTENSION NOS-DEL

Type of Patients	Observed Patients	Avg. Stay	Variance	10th	25th	50th	75th	90th	95th	99th
1. SINGLE DX										
A. Not Operated										
0–19 Years	15	2.0	<1	1	2	2	2	3	3	3
20–34	85	2.0	<1	1	2	2	2	3	3	4
35–49	5	2.0	<1	1	2	2	2	3	3	3
50–64	0									
65+	0									
B. Operated										
0–19 Years	5	4.0	2	3	3	4	4	6	6	6
20–34	1	3.0	0	3	3	3	3	3	3	3
35–49	0									
50–64	0									
65+	0									
2. MULTIPLE DX										
A. Not Operated										
0–19 Years	63	2.3	<1	1	2	2	3	3	3	5
20–34	479	2.3	<1	1	2	2	3	3	4	5
35–49	109	2.8	21	1	2	2	3	3	4	19
50–64	8	2.3	<1	1	2	2	2	4	4	4
65+	0									
B. Operated										
0–19 Years	8	3.9	<1	3	3	4	4	6	6	6
20–34	148	3.7	5	2	3	3	4	5	6	16
35–49	48	3.8	2	2	3	3	5	6	7	8
50–64	1	3.0	0	3	3	3	3	3	3	3
65+	0									
SUBTOTALS:										
1. SINGLE DX — A. Not Operated	105	2.0	<1	1	2	2	2	3	3	3
B. Operated	6	3.8	1	3	3	4	4	6	6	6
2. MULTIPLE DX — A. Not Operated	659	2.3	4	1	2	2	3	3	4	5
B. Operated	205	3.7	4	2	3	3	4	5	6	14
1. SINGLE DX	111	2.1	<1	1	2	2	2	3	3	4
2. MULTIPLE DX	864	2.7	4	1	2	2	3	4	5	8
A. NOT OPERATED	764	2.3	4	1	2	2	3	3	4	5
B. OPERATED	211	3.7	4	2	3	3	4	5	6	14
TOTAL										
0–19 Years	86	2.4	<1	1	2	2	3	3	3	6
20–34	717	2.5	2	1	2	2	3	4	5	6
35–49	163	3.1	15	1	2	2	3	5	5	19
50–64	9	2.3	<1	1	2	2	3	4	4	4
65+	0									
GRAND TOTAL	975	2.6	4	1	2	2	3	4	5	7

Length of Stay by Diagnosis and Operation, Western Region, 2008

Western Region, October 2006–September 2007 Data, by Diagnosis

642.93: HYPERTENSION NOS-AP

Type of Patients	Observed Patients	Avg. Stay	Variance	10th	25th	50th	75th	90th	95th	99th
1. SINGLE DX										
A. Not Operated										
0–19 Years	6	1.2	<1	1	1	1	1	2	2	2
20–34	53	1.6	<1	1	1	1	2	2	3	5
35–49	11	2.0	4	1	1	1	2	3	8	8
50–64	0									
65+	0									
B. Operated										
0–19 Years	0									
20–34	0									
35–49	0									
50–64	0									
65+	0									
2. MULTIPLE DX										
A. Not Operated										
0–19 Years	10	1.5	<1	1	1	2	2	2	2	2
20–34	81	1.8	3	1	1	1	2	3	3	16
35–49	52	1.9	2	1	1	1	2	4	6	8
50–64	0									
65+	0									
B. Operated										
0–19 Years	0									
20–34	1	6.0	0	6	6	6	6	6	6	6
35–49	0									
50–64	0									
65+	0									
SUBTOTALS:										
1. SINGLE DX										
A. Not Operated	70	1.7	1	1	1	1	2	2	3	8
B. Operated	0									
2. MULTIPLE DX										
A. Not Operated	143	1.8	3	1	1	1	2	3	4	8
B. Operated	1	6.0	0	6	6	6	6	6	6	6
1. SINGLE DX	70	1.7	1	1	1	1	2	2	3	8
2. MULTIPLE DX	144	1.8	3	1	1	1	2	3	4	8
A. NOT OPERATED	213	1.8	2	1	1	1	2	3	4	8
B. OPERATED	1	6.0	0	6	6	6	6	6	6	6
TOTAL										
0–19 Years	16	1.4	<1	1	1	1	2	2	2	2
20–34	135	1.8	2	1	1	1	2	3	4	6
35–49	63	1.9	3	1	1	1	2	4	6	8
50–64	0									
65+	0									
GRAND TOTAL	214	1.8	2	1	1	1	2	3	4	8

643: EXCESS VOMITING IN PREG

Type of Patients	Observed Patients	Avg. Stay	Variance	10th	25th	50th	75th	90th	95th	99th
1. SINGLE DX										
A. Not Operated										
0–19 Years	118	2.3	3	1	1	2	3	4	7	8
20–34	868	2.4	4	1	1	2	3	4	5	10
35–49	48	2.6	3	1	2	2	3	4	5	9
50–64	2	1.0	0	1	1	1	1	1	1	1
65+	0									
B. Operated										
0–19 Years	1	2.0	0	2	2	2	2	2	2	2
20–34	1	3.0	0	3	3	3	3	3	3	3
35–49	1	4.0	0	4	4	4	4	4	4	4
50–64	0									
65+	0									
2. MULTIPLE DX										
A. Not Operated										
0–19 Years	405	3.0	7	1	2	2	3	5	9	14
20–34	2,726	3.2	13	1	1	2	4	6	8	18
35–49	343	2.8	7	1	1	2	3	5	7	13
50–64	16	3.6	9	1	1	3	5	7	12	12
65+	0									
B. Operated										
0–19 Years	5	10.2	192	3	3	4	6	35	35	35
20–34	47	9.2	173	2	3	4	8	30	33	68
35–49	4	5.5	14	3	3	4	11	11	11	11
50–64	0									
65+	0									
SUBTOTALS:										
1. SINGLE DX										
A. Not Operated	1,036	2.4	4	1	1	2	3	4	5	10
B. Operated	3	3.0	1	2	2	3	4	4	4	4
2. MULTIPLE DX										
A. Not Operated	3,490	3.2	12	1	2	2	4	6	8	17
B. Operated	56	9.0	161	2	3	4	8	30	35	68
1. SINGLE DX	1,039	2.4	4	1	1	2	3	4	5	10
2. MULTIPLE DX	3,546	3.2	15	1	1	2	4	6	8	18
A. NOT OPERATED	4,526	3.0	10	1	1	2	3	5	7	15
B. OPERATED	59	8.7	154	2	3	4	7	30	35	68
TOTAL										
0–19 Years	529	2.9	8	1	1	2	3	5	8	14
20–34	3,642	3.1	14	1	1	2	4	6	8	18
35–49	396	2.8	6	1	1	2	3	5	7	13
50–64	18	3.3	9	1	1	3	5	7	12	12
65+	0									
GRAND TOTAL	4,585	3.1	12	1	1	2	3	6	8	17

643.03: MILD HG-ANTEPARTUM

Type of Patients	Observed Patients	Avg. Stay	Variance	10th	25th	50th	75th	90th	95th	99th
1. SINGLE DX										
A. Not Operated										
0–19 Years	82	2.2	2	1	1	2	2	4	5	8
20–34	588	2.4	4	1	1	2	3	4	5	9
35–49	40	2.5	3	1	2	2	3	4	8	9
50–64	2	1.0	0	1	1	1	1	1	1	1
65+	0									
B. Operated										
0–19 Years	1	2.0	0	2	2	2	2	2	2	2
20–34	0									
35–49	0									
50–64	0									
65+	0									
2. MULTIPLE DX										
A. Not Operated										
0–19 Years	101	3.2	6	1	2	2	4	5	8	13
20–34	764	3.4	15	1	2	2	4	6	9	20
35–49	95	2.9	5	1	1	2	3	6	8	12
50–64	9	5.2	10	1	3	5	6	12	12	12
65+	0									
B. Operated										
0–19 Years	1	3.0	0	3	3	3	3	3	3	3
20–34	4	3.0	11	1	1	1	2	8	8	8
35–49	0									
50–64	0									
65+	0									
SUBTOTALS:										
1. SINGLE DX										
A. Not Operated	712	2.4	3	1	1	2	3	4	5	8
B. Operated	1	2.0	0	2	2	2	2	2	2	2
2. MULTIPLE DX										
A. Not Operated	969	3.4	13	1	2	2	4	6	9	18
B. Operated	5	3.0	8	1	2	2	3	8	8	8
1. SINGLE DX	713	2.4	3	1	1	2	3	4	5	8
2. MULTIPLE DX	974	3.4	13	1	2	2	4	6	9	18
A. NOT OPERATED	1,681	2.9	9	1	1	2	3	5	7	13
B. OPERATED	6	2.8	7	1	2	2	3	8	8	8
TOTAL										
0–19 Years	185	2.7	4	1	2	2	3	5	7	13
20–34	1,356	3.0	10	1	1	2	3	5	7	14
35–49	135	2.8	4	1	1	2	3	5	8	10
50–64	11	4.5	11	1	1	4	6	7	12	12
65+	0									
GRAND TOTAL	1,687	2.9	9	1	1	2	3	5	7	13

Length of Stay by Diagnosis and Operation, Western Region, 2008

Western Region, October 2006–September 2007 Data, by Diagnosis

643.13: HG W METABOL DISTURB-AP

Type of Patients	Observed Patients	Avg. Stay	Variance	10th	25th	50th	75th	90th	95th	99th
1. SINGLE DX										
A. Not Operated										
0–19 Years	22	3.0	6	1	2	3	3	5	8	11
20–34	178	3.0	7	1	1	2	4	5	8	15
35–49	7	2.7	2	1	2	3	3	5	5	5
50–64	0									
65+	0									
B. Operated										
0–19 Years	0									
20–34	0									
35–49	0									
50–64	0									
65+	0									
2. MULTIPLE DX										
A. Not Operated										
0–19 Years	233	3.0	7	1	2	2	3	5	9	15
20–34	1,457	3.2	9	1	2	2	4	6	8	16
35–49	177	3.0	8	1	1	2	4	5	7	21
50–64	7	1.6	1	1	1	1	2	4	4	4
65+	0									
B. Operated										
0–19 Years	0									
20–34	9	7.5	51	3	5	5	6	26	26	26
35–49	2	4.0	0	4	4	4	4	4	4	4
50–64	0									
65+	0									
SUBTOTALS:										
1. SINGLE DX										
A. Not Operated	207	3.0	7	1	1	2	4	5	8	14
B. Operated	0									
2. MULTIPLE DX										
A. Not Operated	1,874	3.1	9	1	2	2	4	6	8	16
B. Operated	11	6.9	43	3	4	5	6	8	26	26
1. SINGLE DX	207	3.0	7	1	1	2	4	5	8	14
2. MULTIPLE DX	1,885	3.2	9	1	2	2	4	6	8	16
A. NOT OPERATED	2,081	3.1	9	1	2	2	4	6	8	15
B. OPERATED	11	6.9	43	3	4	5	6	8	26	26
TOTAL										
0–19 Years	255	3.0	7	1	2	2	3	5	9	15
20–34	1,644	3.2	9	1	2	2	4	6	8	16
35–49	186	3.0	8	1	1	2	4	5	7	21
50–64	7	1.6	1	1	1	1	2	4	4	4
65+	0									
GRAND TOTAL	2,092	3.1	9	1	2	2	4	6	8	16

643.23: LATE VOMITING PREG-AP

Type of Patients	Observed Patients	Avg. Stay	Variance	10th	25th	50th	75th	90th	95th	99th
1. SINGLE DX										
A. Not Operated										
0–19 Years	8	1.9	4	1	1	1	1	7	7	7
20–34	59	1.7	1	1	1	1	2	3	4	6
35–49	0									
50–64	0									
65+	0									
B. Operated										
0–19 Years	0									
20–34	0									
35–49	0									
50–64	0									
65+	0									
2. MULTIPLE DX										
A. Not Operated										
0–19 Years	50	2.8	6	1	1	2	4	6	8	11
20–34	287	3.0	16	1	1	2	3	6	9	17
35–49	40	2.3	7	1	1	2	2	4	6	16
50–64	0									
65+	0									
B. Operated										
0–19 Years	0									
20–34	0									
35–49	0									
50–64	0									
65+	0									
SUBTOTALS:										
1. SINGLE DX										
A. Not Operated	67	1.7	1	1	1	1	2	3	4	7
B. Operated	0									
2. MULTIPLE DX										
A. Not Operated	377	2.9	14	1	1	2	3	6	8	17
B. Operated	0									
1. SINGLE DX	67	1.7	1	1	1	1	2	3	4	7
2. MULTIPLE DX	377	2.9	14	1	1	2	3	6	8	17
A. NOT OPERATED	444	2.7	12	1	1	2	3	5	7	16
B. OPERATED	0									
TOTAL										
0–19 Years	58	2.6	6	1	1	2	4	6	8	11
20–34	346	2.8	14	1	1	2	3	5	7	17
35–49	40	2.3	7	1	1	2	2	4	6	16
50–64	0									
65+	0									
GRAND TOTAL	444	2.7	12	1	1	2	3	5	7	16

644: EARLY/THREATENED LABOR

Type of Patients	Observed Patients	Avg. Stay	Variance	10th	25th	50th	75th	90th	95th	99th
1. SINGLE DX										
A. Not Operated										
0–19 Years	1,361	2.2	5	1	1	2	2	3	5	12
20–34	6,401	2.0	4	1	1	2	2	3	4	10
35–49	357	1.7	3	1	1	1	2	3	4	11
50–64	12	1.7	<1	1	1	2	2	2	4	4
65+	0									
B. Operated										
0–19 Years	2	3.0	0	3	3	3	3	3	3	3
20–34	52	3.8	17	2	3	3	3	5	7	30
35–49	4	3.3	<1	3	3	3	4	4	4	4
50–64	0									
65+	0									
2. MULTIPLE DX										
A. Not Operated										
0–19 Years	3,218	2.9	13	1	1	2	3	5	8	19
20–34	16,087	3.1	21	1	1	2	3	5	8	24
35–49	3,068	3.6	34	1	1	2	3	6	12	32
50–64	118	4.4	124	1	1	2	3	5	12	74
65+	0									
B. Operated										
0–19 Years	445	4.7	26	2	3	3	5	8	12	32
20–34	4,590	5.2	49	2	3	3	5	8	15	43
35–49	1,259	6.0	64	2	3	4	5	10	22	45
50–64	57	7.3	136	2	3	4	6	14	35	67
65+	0									
SUBTOTALS:										
1. SINGLE DX										
A. Not Operated	8,131	2.0	4	1	1	2	2	3	4	11
B. Operated	58	3.7	15	2	2	3	4	5	7	30
2. MULTIPLE DX										
A. Not Operated	22,491	3.1	22	1	1	2	3	5	9	25
B. Operated	6,351	5.3	51	2	3	4	5	8	16	43
1. SINGLE DX	8,189	2.0	4	1	1	2	2	3	4	11
2. MULTIPLE DX	28,842	3.6	29	1	2	2	3	6	10	29
A. NOT OPERATED	30,622	2.8	18	1	1	2	3	5	7	22
B. OPERATED	6,409	5.3	51	2	3	4	5	8	16	43
TOTAL										
0–19 Years	5,026	2.9	12	1	1	2	3	5	7	18
20–34	27,130	3.2	23	1	1	2	3	5	8	25
35–49	4,688	4.1	41	1	2	2	4	7	13	35
50–64	187	5.1	121	1	2	2	4	6	15	74
65+	0									
GRAND TOTAL	37,031	3.3	24	1	1	2	3	5	9	26

Western Region, October 2006–September 2007 Data, by Diagnosis

644.03: THREAT PREMAT LABOR-AP

Type of Patients	Observed Patients	Avg. Stay	Variance	10th	25th	50th	75th	90th	95th	99th
1. SINGLE DX										
A. Not Operated										
0–19 Years	748	2.4	7	1	1	2	3	4	6	14
20–34	3,295	2.2	6	1	1	1	2	4	5	14
35–49	218	1.9	4	1	1	1	2	3	4	11
50–64	5	2.0	1	1	1	2	2	4	4	4
65+	0									
B. Operated										
0–19 Years	0									
20–34	0									
35–49	0									
50–64	0									
65+	0									
2. MULTIPLE DX										
A. Not Operated										
0–19 Years	1,072	3.6	24	1	1	2	4	7	12	25
20–34	5,709	3.9	37	1	1	2	4	7	13	32
35–49	1,347	4.3	53	1	1	2	4	8	17	38
50–64	37	6.0	229	1	1	1	3	11	44	83
65+	0									
B. Operated										
0–19 Years	1	6.0	0	6	6	6	6	6	6	6
20–34	17	4.0	10	1	2	3	4	9	13	13
35–49	5	8.4	15	5	5	7	12	13	13	13
50–64	0									
65+	0									
SUBTOTALS:										
1. SINGLE DX										
A. Not Operated	4,266	2.2	6	1	1	1	2	4	6	14
B. Operated	0									
2. MULTIPLE DX										
A. Not Operated	8,165	3.9	39	1	1	2	4	7	13	33
B. Operated	23	5.1	14	2	2	4	7	12	13	13
1. SINGLE DX	4,266	2.2	6	1	1	1	2	4	6	14
2. MULTIPLE DX	8,188	3.9	39	1	1	2	4	8	13	33
A. NOT OPERATED	12,431	3.3	28	1	1	2	3	6	11	27
B. OPERATED	23	5.1	14	2	2	4	7	12	13	13
TOTAL										
0–19 Years	1,821	3.1	18	1	1	2	3	6	9	23
20–34	9,021	3.2	27	1	1	2	3	6	10	26
35–49	1,570	4.0	47	1	1	2	4	8	14	35
50–64	42	5.5	203	1	1	3	8	21	83	83
65+	0									
GRAND TOTAL	12,454	3.3	28	1	1	2	3	6	11	27

644.13: THREAT LABOR NEC-AP

Type of Patients	Observed Patients	Avg. Stay	Variance	10th	25th	50th	75th	90th	95th	99th
1. SINGLE DX										
A. Not Operated										
0–19 Years	155	1.1	<1	1	1	1	1	1	2	3
20–34	811	1.1	<1	1	1	1	1	1	2	3
35–49	79	1.1	<1	1	1	1	1	1	2	4
50–64	3	1.0	0	1	1	1	1	1	1	1
65+	0									
B. Operated										
0–19 Years	0									
20–34	0									
35–49	0									
50–64	0									
65+	0									
2. MULTIPLE DX										
A. Not Operated										
0–19 Years	87	1.5	4	1	1	1	1	2	3	19
20–34	582	1.3	1	1	1	1	1	2	3	8
35–49	154	1.6	7	1	1	1	2	2	5	12
50–64	2	1.0	0	1	1	1	1	1	1	1
65+	0									
B. Operated										
0–19 Years	0									
20–34	4	2.5	<1	2	2	2	2	4	4	4
35–49	0									
50–64	0									
65+	0									
SUBTOTALS:										
1. SINGLE DX										
A. Not Operated	1,048	1.1	<1	1	1	1	1	1	2	3
B. Operated	0									
2. MULTIPLE DX										
A. Not Operated	825	1.4	3	1	1	1	1	2	3	8
B. Operated	4	2.5	<1	2	2	2	2	4	4	4
1. SINGLE DX	1,048	1.1	<1	1	1	1	1	1	2	3
2. MULTIPLE DX	829	1.4	3	1	1	1	1	2	3	8
A. NOT OPERATED	1,873	1.2	2	1	1	1	1	2	3	6
B. OPERATED	4	2.5	<1	2	2	2	2	4	4	4
TOTAL										
0–19 Years	242	1.2	2	1	1	1	1	2	2	4
20–34	1,397	1.2	1	1	1	1	1	2	3	5
35–49	233	1.5	4	1	1	1	1	2	3	8
50–64	5	1.0	0	1	1	1	1	1	1	1
65+	0									
GRAND TOTAL	1,877	1.2	2	1	1	1	1	2	2	6

644.21: EARLY ONSET DELIVERY-DEL

Type of Patients	Observed Patients	Avg. Stay	Variance	10th	25th	50th	75th	90th	95th	99th
1. SINGLE DX										
A. Not Operated										
0–19 Years	456	2.1	2	1	1	2	2	3	4	8
20–34	2,293	2.0	3	1	1	2	2	3	3	5
35–49	60	2.0	<1	1	1	2	2	3	3	5
50–64	4	1.8	<1	1	2	2	2	2	2	2
65+	0									
B. Operated										
0–19 Years	2	3.0	0	3	3	3	3	3	3	3
20–34	52	3.8	17	2	2	3	4	5	7	30
35–49	4	3.3	<1	3	3	3	4	4	4	4
50–64	0									
65+	0									
2. MULTIPLE DX										
A. Not Operated										
0–19 Years	2,059	2.6	7	1	2	2	3	4	6	14
20–34	9,795	2.7	12	1	2	2	3	4	6	19
35–49	1,567	3.1	19	1	2	2	3	5	8	26
50–64	79	3.8	78	1	2	2	3	5	6	74
65+	0									
B. Operated										
0–19 Years	444	4.7	26	2	3	3	5	8	12	32
20–34	4,569	5.2	49	2	3	3	5	8	15	43
35–49	1,254	6.0	65	2	3	4	5	10	22	45
50–64	57	7.3	136	2	3	4	6	14	35	67
65+	0									
SUBTOTALS:										
1. SINGLE DX										
A. Not Operated	2,813	2.0	3	1	1	2	2	3	3	5
B. Operated	58	3.7	15	2	2	3	4	5	7	30
2. MULTIPLE DX										
A. Not Operated	13,500	2.8	12	1	2	2	3	4	6	19
B. Operated	6,324	5.3	51	2	3	4	5	8	16	43
1. SINGLE DX	2,871	2.1	3	1	1	2	2	3	3	6
2. MULTIPLE DX	19,824	3.6	26	1	2	2	3	5	9	28
A. NOT OPERATED	16,313	2.6	11	1	2	2	3	4	6	17
B. OPERATED	6,382	5.3	51	2	3	4	5	8	16	43
TOTAL										
0–19 Years	2,961	2.9	9	1	2	2	3	5	7	16
20–34	16,709	3.3	22	1	2	2	3	5	8	25
35–49	2,885	4.3	41	1	2	3	4	7	13	37
50–64	140	5.2	102	1	2	3	4	6	14	67
65+	0									
GRAND TOTAL	22,695	3.4	23	1	2	2	3	5	8	26

Length of Stay by Diagnosis and Operation, Western Region, 2008

Western Region, October 2006–September 2007 Data, by Diagnosis

645: LATE PREGNANCY

Type of Patients	Observed Patients	Avg. Stay	Variance	10th	25th	50th	75th	90th	95th	99th
1. SINGLE DX										
A. Not Operated										
0–19 Years	1,022	2.0	<1	1	2	2	2	3	3	4
20–34	7,328	1.8	<1	1	1	2	2	3	3	4
35–49	169	1.8	<1	1	1	2	2	3	3	3
50–64	7	1.9	<1	1	1	2	2	3	3	3
65+	0									
B. Operated										
0–19 Years	12	3.1	<1	2	3	3	4	4	4	4
20–34	85	3.2	<1	2	3	3	4	4	4	7
35–49	3	3.0	<1	2	2	3	4	4	4	4
50–64	0									
65+	0									
2. MULTIPLE DX										
A. Not Operated										
0–19 Years	4,482	2.2	<1	1	2	2	3	3	3	5
20–34	28,861	2.0	<1	1	1	2	2	3	3	4
35–49	4,034	2.0	<1	1	1	2	2	3	3	4
50–64	182	2.1	<1	2	2	2	3	3	3	4
65+	0									
B. Operated										
0–19 Years	924	3.5	1	2	3	3	4	5	5	7
20–34	6,563	3.3	2	2	2	3	4	5	5	6
35–49	1,016	3.3	1	2	2	3	4	5	5	6
50–64	52	3.3	1	2	2	3	4	5	5	6
65+	0									
SUBTOTALS:										
1. SINGLE DX										
A. Not Operated	8,526	1.9	<1	1	1	2	2	3	3	4
B. Operated	100	3.2	<1	2	3	3	4	4	4	7
2. MULTIPLE DX										
A. Not Operated	37,559	2.0	<1	1	2	2	3	3	3	4
B. Operated	8,555	3.3	2	2	3	3	4	5	5	6
1. SINGLE DX	8,626	1.9	<1	1	1	2	2	3	3	4
2. MULTIPLE DX	46,114	2.3	1	2	2	3	3	4	4	5
A. NOT OPERATED	46,085	2.0	<1	1	1	2	2	3	3	4
B. OPERATED	8,655	3.3	2	2	3	3	4	5	5	6
TOTAL										
0–19 Years	6,440	2.4	<1	1	2	2	3	3	4	5
20–34	42,837	2.2	1	1	2	2	3	3	4	5
35–49	5,222	2.3	1	1	2	2	3	4	4	5
50–64	241	2.3	1	1	2	2	3	4	4	5
65+	0									
GRAND TOTAL	54,740	2.2	1	1	2	2	3	3	4	5

645.11: POST TERM PREG-DEL

Type of Patients	Observed Patients	Avg. Stay	Variance	10th	25th	50th	75th	90th	95th	99th
1. SINGLE DX										
A. Not Operated										
0–19 Years	994	2.0	<1	1		2	2	3	3	4
20–34	7,134	1.8	<1	1		2	2	3	3	4
35–49	165	1.8	<1	1		2	2	3	3	3
50–64	7	1.9	<1	1		2	2	3	3	3
65+	0									
B. Operated										
0–19 Years	10	3.1	<1	2	3	3	3	4	4	4
20–34	80	3.2	<1	2	3	3	4	4	5	7
35–49	3	3.0	<1	2	2	3	4	4	4	4
50–64	0									
65+	0									
2. MULTIPLE DX										
A. Not Operated										
0–19 Years	4,377	2.2	<1	1	2	2	3	3	3	5
20–34	28,180	2.0	<1	1	1	2	2	3	3	4
35–49	3,920	2.0	<1	1	1	2	2	3	3	4
50–64	180	2.1	<1	1	2	2	3	3	3	4
65+	0									
B. Operated										
0–19 Years	902	3.5	1	2	3	3	4	5	5	7
20–34	6,433	3.3	1	2	2	3	4	5	5	6
35–49	983	3.3	1	2	2	3	4	5	5	6
50–64	50	3.3	1	2	2	3	4	5	5	6
65+	0									
SUBTOTALS:										
1. SINGLE DX										
A. Not Operated	8,300	1.9	<1	1	1	2	2	3	3	4
B. Operated	93	3.2	<1	2	3	3	4	4	4	7
2. MULTIPLE DX										
A. Not Operated	36,657	2.0	<1	1	2	2	3	3	3	4
B. Operated	8,368	3.3	1	2	2	3	4	5	5	6
1. SINGLE DX	8,393	1.9	<1	1	1	2	2	3	3	4
2. MULTIPLE DX	45,025	2.3	<1	1	2	2	3	3	4	5
A. NOT OPERATED	44,957	2.0	<1	1	2	2	3	3	3	4
B. OPERATED	8,461	3.3	1	2	3	3	4	5	5	6
TOTAL										
0–19 Years	6,283	2.4	<1	1	2	2	3	3	4	5
20–34	41,827	2.2	<1	1	2	2	3	4	4	5
35–49	5,071	2.3	1	1	2	2	3	4	4	5
50–64	237	2.3	1	1	2	2	3	4	4	5
65+	0									
GRAND TOTAL	53,418	2.2	<1	1	2	2	3	4	4	5

645.13: POST TERM PREG-AP

Type of Patients	Observed Patients	Avg. Stay	Variance	10th	25th	50th	75th	90th	95th	99th
1. SINGLE DX										
A. Not Operated										
0–19 Years	18	1.1	<1	1	1	1	1	1	2	2
20–34	112	1.1	<1	1	1	1	1	1	2	2
35–49	1	1.0	0	1	1	1	1	1	1	1
50–64	0									
65+	0									
B. Operated										
0–19 Years	0									
20–34	0									
35–49	0									
50–64	0									
65+	0									
2. MULTIPLE DX										
A. Not Operated										
0–19 Years	50	1.1	<1	1	1	1	1	2	2	2
20–34	283	1.2	<1	1	1	1	1	2	2	3
35–49	54	1.3	<1	1	1	1	1	2	3	3
50–64	0									
65+	0									
B. Operated										
0–19 Years	1	3.0	0	3	3	3	3	3	3	3
20–34	1	5.0	0	5	5	5	5	5	5	5
35–49	1	3.0	0	3	3	3	3	3	3	3
50–64	0									
65+	0									
SUBTOTALS:										
1. SINGLE DX										
A. Not Operated	131	1.1	<1	1	1	1	1	1	2	2
B. Operated	0									
2. MULTIPLE DX										
A. Not Operated	387	1.2	<1	1	1	1	2	2	2	3
B. Operated	3	3.7	1	3	3	3	5	5	5	6
1. SINGLE DX	131	1.1	<1	1	1	1	1	1	2	2
2. MULTIPLE DX	390	1.2	<1	1	1	1	2	2	2	3
A. NOT OPERATED	518	1.2	<1	1	1	1	1	2	2	3
B. OPERATED	3	3.7	1	3	3	3	5	5	5	6
TOTAL										
0–19 Years	69	1.2	<1	1	1	1	1	2	2	3
20–34	396	1.2	<1	1	1	1	1	2	2	3
35–49	56	1.3	<1	1	1	1	1	2	3	3
50–64	0									
65+	0									
GRAND TOTAL	521	1.2	<1	1	1	1	1	2	2	3

Western Region, October 2006–September 2007 Data, by Diagnosis

645.21: PROLONGED PREGNANCY-DEL

Type of Patients	Observed Patients	Avg. Stay	Vari-ance	Percentiles						
				10th	25th	50th	75th	90th	95th	99th
1. SINGLE DX										
A. *Not Operated*										
0–19 Years	10	2.1	<1	1	2	2	2	4	4	4
20–34	79	1.8	<1	1	1	2	2	3	3	4
35–49	3	2.0	0	2	2	2	2	2	2	2
50–64	0									
65+	0									
B. *Operated*										
0–19 Years	2	3.0	2	2	2	4	4	4	4	4
20–34	5	3.2	<1	2	3	3	4	4	4	4
35–49	0									
50–64	0									
65+	0									
2. MULTIPLE DX										
A. *Not Operated*										
0–19 Years	53	2.3	<1	1	2	2	3	3	3	4
20–34	389	2.1	<1	1	2	2	3	3	3	4
35–49	56	2.4	2	1	2	2	3	4	5	8
50–64	2	2.5	<1	2	2	2	3	3	3	3
65+	0									
B. *Operated*										
0–19 Years	21	3.9	6	2	3	3	4	6	6	13
20–34	129	3.9	40	2	3	3	4	5	6	8
35–49	32	3.5	<1	2	3	3	4	5	5	5
50–64	2	3.0	0	3	3	3	3	3	3	3
65+	0									
SUBTOTALS:										
1. SINGLE DX										
A. *Not Operated*	92	1.8	<1	1	1	2	2	3	3	3
B. *Operated*	7	3.2	<1	2	2	3	4	4	4	4
2. MULTIPLE DX										
A. *Not Operated*	500	2.1	<1	1	2	2	3	3	3	4
B. *Operated*	184	3.8	29	2	3	3	4	5	6	13
1. SINGLE DX	99	1.9	<1	1	1	2	2	3	4	4
2. MULTIPLE DX	684	2.6	9	1	2	2	3	4	4	6
A. NOT OPERATED	592	2.1	<1	1	2	2	3	3	3	4
B. OPERATED	191	3.8	28	2	3	3	4	5	6	13
TOTAL										
0–19 Years	86	2.7	2	1	2	2	3	4	4	13
20–34	602	2.5	10	1	2	2	3	4	5	6
35–49	91	2.7	2	1	2	2	3	4	5	8
50–64	4	2.8	<1	2	3	3	3	3	3	3
65+	0									
GRAND TOTAL	783	2.5	8	1	2	2	3	4	4	6

646: OTHER COMP OF PREGNANCY

Type of Patients	Observed Patients	Avg. Stay	Vari-ance	Percentiles						
				10th	25th	50th	75th	90th	95th	99th
1. SINGLE DX										
A. *Not Operated*										
0–19 Years	95	1.9	<1	1	1	2	3	3	4	4
20–34	483	1.8	<1	1	1	2	2	3	3	4
35–49	13	1.9	<1	1	1	2	2	3	3	3
50–64	0									
65+	0									
B. *Operated*										
0–19 Years	2	3.5	<1	3	3	4	4	4	4	4
20–34	25	3.0	<1	2	2	3	4	4	4	4
35–49	0									
50–64	0									
65+	0									
2. MULTIPLE DX										
A. *Not Operated*										
0–19 Years	2,740	2.7	3	1	2	2	3	4	5	8
20–34	10,322	2.4	3	1	2	2	3	4	5	8
35–49	1,054	2.5	3	1	2	2	3	4	5	9
50–64	43	1.9	1	1	2	2	2	3	5	5
65+	0									
B. *Operated*										
0–19 Years	191	3.8	8	1	2	3	5	7	8	18
20–34	1,306	3.5	8	2	2	3	4	6	8	15
35–49	207	3.6	6	2	2	3	4	5	8	14
50–64	9	4.7	24	1	2	3	5	17	17	17
65+	0									
SUBTOTALS:										
1. SINGLE DX										
A. *Not Operated*	591	1.8	<1	1	1	2	2	3	3	4
B. *Operated*	27	3.1	<1	2	2	3	4	4	4	4
2. MULTIPLE DX										
A. *Not Operated*	14,159	2.5	3	1	2	2	3	4	5	8
B. *Operated*	1,713	3.6	8	1	2	3	4	6	8	16
1. SINGLE DX	618	1.8	<1	1	1	2	2	3	3	4
2. MULTIPLE DX	15,872	2.6	4	1	2	2	3	4	5	9
A. NOT OPERATED	14,750	2.5	3	1	2	2	3	4	5	8
B. OPERATED	1,740	3.6	8	1	2	3	4	6	8	16
TOTAL										
0–19 Years	3,028	2.7	3	1	2	2	3	5	5	9
20–34	12,136	2.5	3	1	2	2	3	4	5	9
35–49	1,274	2.6	4	1	2	2	3	4	6	11
50–64	52	2.4	6	1	2	2	3	5	5	17
65+	0									
GRAND TOTAL	16,490	2.6	3	1	2	2	3	4	5	9

646.21: RENAL DIS PREG NOS-DEL

Type of Patients	Observed Patients	Avg. Stay	Vari-ance	Percentiles						
				10th	25th	50th	75th	90th	95th	99th
1. SINGLE DX										
A. *Not Operated*										
0–19 Years	6	2.2	<1	1	2	2	3	3	3	3
20–34	17	2.1	<1	1	2	2	2	3	3	3
35–49	1	1.0	0	1	1	1	1	1	1	1
50–64	0									
65+	0									
B. *Operated*										
0–19 Years	0									
20–34	0									
35–49	0									
50–64	0									
65+	0									
2. MULTIPLE DX										
A. *Not Operated*										
0–19 Years	31	2.8	4	2	2	2	3	3	5	12
20–34	175	2.3	1	1	2	2	3	4	4	7
35–49	19	3.0	5	1	2	2	3	4	11	11
50–64	1	2.0	0	2	2	2	2	2	2	2
65+	0									
B. *Operated*										
0–19 Years	9	6.4	25	2	4	5	6	19	19	19
20–34	40	4.1	11	2	3	4	4	6	6	22
35–49	11	3.4	7	2	2	3	4	4	7	7
50–64	2	9.4	111	2	2	2	17	17	17	17
65+	0									
SUBTOTALS:										
1. SINGLE DX										
A. *Not Operated*	24	2.0	<1	1	2	2	2	3	3	3
B. *Operated*	0									
2. MULTIPLE DX										
A. *Not Operated*	226	2.4	2	1	2	2	3	4	4	11
B. *Operated*	62	4.5	14	2	3	4	5	6	9	22
1. SINGLE DX	24	2.0	<1	1	2	2	2	3	3	3
2. MULTIPLE DX	288	2.9	5	1	2	2	3	4	6	17
A. NOT OPERATED	250	2.4	2	1	2	2	3	4	4	11
B. OPERATED	62	4.5	14	2	3	4	5	6	9	22
TOTAL										
0–19 Years	46	3.4	9	2	2	3	3	5	7	19
20–34	232	2.6	3	1	2	2	3	4	5	9
35–49	31	3.0	4	2	2	3	4	4	7	11
50–64	3	6.9	74	2	2	2	17	17	17	17
65+	0									
GRAND TOTAL	312	2.8	5	1	2	2	3	4	6	12

523

Length of Stay by Diagnosis and Operation, Western Region, 2008

Western Region, October 2006–September 2007 Data, by Diagnosis

646.23: RENAL DIS PREG NOS-AP

Type of Patients	Observed Patients	Avg. Stay	Variance	10th	25th	50th	75th	90th	95th	99th
1. SINGLE DX										
A. Not Operated										
0–19 Years	2	2.5	<1	2	2	2	3	3	3	3
20–34	15	1.4	<1	1	1	1	2	2	2	2
35–49	0									
50–64	0									
65+	0									
B. Operated										
0–19 Years	0									
20–34	0									
35–49	0									
50–64	0									
65+	0									
2. MULTIPLE DX										
A. Not Operated										
0–19 Years	63	3.7	24	1	1	2	4	5	13	33
20–34	491	2.6	4	1	1	2	3	5	6	12
35–49	45	1.9	3	1	1	1	2	4	5	9
50–64	1	5.0	0	5	5	5	5	5	5	5
65+	0									
B. Operated										
0–19 Years	3	10.0	31	4	4	11	15	15	15	15
20–34	35	2.8	4	1	2	2	3	5	9	9
35–49	9	3.6	6	1	2	3	4	9	9	9
50–64	0									
65+	0									
SUBTOTALS:										
1. SINGLE DX A. Not Operated	17	1.5	<1	1	1	1	2	2	3	3
B. Operated	0									
2. MULTIPLE DX A. Not Operated	600	2.7	6	1	1	2	3	5	6	14
B. Operated	47	3.4	8	1	2	3	4	9	9	15
1. SINGLE DX	17	1.5	<1	1	1	1	2	2	3	3
2. MULTIPLE DX	647	2.7	6	1	1	2	3	5	6	14
A. NOT OPERATED	617	2.7	6	1	1	2	3	5	6	13
B. OPERATED	47	3.4	8	2	2	3	4	9	9	15
TOTAL										
0–19 Years	68	3.9	24	1	1	3	4	10	14	33
20–34	541	2.6	4	1	1	2	3	5	6	11
35–49	54	2.2	3	1	1	2	3	4	6	9
50–64	1	5.0	0	5	5	5	5	5	5	5
65+	0									
GRAND TOTAL	664	2.7	6	1	1	2	3	5	6	14

646.61: GU INFECT IN PREG-DEL

Type of Patients	Observed Patients	Avg. Stay	Variance	10th	25th	50th	75th	90th	95th	99th
1. SINGLE DX										
A. Not Operated										
0–19 Years	0									
20–34	10	1.7	<1	1	1	2	2	2	2	2
35–49	0									
50–64	0									
65+	0									
B. Operated										
0–19 Years	0									
20–34	0									
35–49	0									
50–64	0									
65+	0									
2. MULTIPLE DX										
A. Not Operated										
0–19 Years	166	2.7	2	1	2	2	3	4	6	9
20–34	669	2.4	4	1	2	2	3	3	5	8
35–49	32	2.3	1	1	2	2	3	3	4	6
50–64	5	2.6	2	1	2	2	3	5	5	5
65+	0									
B. Operated										
0–19 Years	25	4.3	5	2	3	4	6	8	8	8
20–34	130	4.2	20	2	2	3	5	8	9	12
35–49	16	4.7	18	2	2	3	4	10	18	18
50–64	0									
65+	0									
SUBTOTALS:										
1. SINGLE DX A. Not Operated	10	1.7	<1	1	1	2	2	2	2	2
B. Operated	0									
2. MULTIPLE DX A. Not Operated	872	2.4	3	1	2	2	3	4	5	9
B. Operated	171	4.2	18	2	2	3	5	8	9	18
1. SINGLE DX	10	1.7	<1	1	1	2	2	2	2	2
2. MULTIPLE DX	1,043	2.7	6	1	2	2	3	4	6	10
A. NOT OPERATED	882	2.4	3	1	2	2	3	4	5	9
B. OPERATED	171	4.2	18	2	2	3	5	8	9	18
TOTAL										
0–19 Years	191	2.9	3	1	2	2	3	5	6	9
20–34	809	2.7	7	1	2	2	3	4	6	10
35–49	48	3.1	8	1	2	2	3	5	9	18
50–64	5	2.6	2	1	2	2	3	5	5	5
65+	0									
GRAND TOTAL	1,053	2.7	6	1	2	2	3	4	6	10

646.63: GU INFECT IN PREG-AP

Type of Patients	Observed Patients	Avg. Stay	Variance	10th	25th	50th	75th	90th	95th	99th
1. SINGLE DX										
A. Not Operated										
0–19 Years	28	2.1	1	1	1	2	3	4	4	4
20–34	49	1.9	<1	1	1	2	3	3	3	5
35–49	2	1.5	<1	1	1	2	2	2	2	2
50–64	0									
65+	0									
B. Operated										
0–19 Years	0									
20–34	0									
35–49	0									
50–64	0									
65+	0									
2. MULTIPLE DX										
A. Not Operated										
0–19 Years	1,879	2.7	2	1	2	2	3	4	5	7
20–34	5,086	2.6	2	1	2	2	3	4	5	7
35–49	413	2.6	2	1	2	2	3	4	5	7
50–64	17	1.7	<1	1	1	2	2	3	3	3
65+	0									
B. Operated										
0–19 Years	13	2.6	3	1	2	2	3	5	7	7
20–34	63	5.0	25	1	3	4	5	9	17	30
35–49	9	3.9	3	2	3	4	5	7	7	7
50–64	1	1.0	0	1	1	1	1	1	1	1
65+	0									
SUBTOTALS:										
1. SINGLE DX A. Not Operated	79	1.9	<1	1	1	2	2	3	3	5
B. Operated	0									
2. MULTIPLE DX A. Not Operated	7,395	2.6	2	1	2	2	3	4	5	7
B. Operated	86	4.5	20	1	2	4	5	7	10	30
1. SINGLE DX	79	1.9	<1	1	1	2	2	3	3	5
2. MULTIPLE DX	7,481	2.6	2	1	2	2	3	4	5	7
A. NOT OPERATED	7,474	2.6	2	1	2	2	3	4	5	7
B. OPERATED	86	4.5	20	1	2	4	5	7	10	30
TOTAL										
0–19 Years	1,920	2.7	2	1	2	2	3	4	5	7
20–34	5,198	2.6	2	1	2	2	3	4	5	8
35–49	424	2.6	2	1	2	2	3	4	5	7
50–64	18	1.6	<1	1	1	2	2	3	3	3
65+	0									
GRAND TOTAL	7,560	2.6	2	1	2	2	3	4	5	7

Length of Stay by Diagnosis and Operation, Western Region, 2008

Western Region, October 2006–September 2007 Data, by Diagnosis

646.64: GU INFECT IN PREG-PP

Type of Patients	Observed Patients	Avg. Stay	Vari-ance	10th	25th	50th	75th	90th	95th	99th
1. SINGLE DX										
A. Not Operated										
0–19 Years	4	3.0	<1	2	2	3	3	4	4	4
20–34	14	2.1	1	1	1	2	3	3	5	5
35–49	0									
50–64	0									
65+	0									
B. Operated										
0–19 Years	0									
20–34	0									
35–49	0									
50–64	0									
65+	0									
2. MULTIPLE DX										
A. Not Operated										
0–19 Years	81	3.1	4	1	2	3	4	5	7	14
20–34	355	2.8	3	1	2	2	3	5	6	9
35–49	42	2.2	<1	1	1	2	3	4	4	4
50–64	1	5.0	0	5	5	5	5	5	5	5
65+	0									
B. Operated										
0–19 Years	3	3.3	10	1	1	2	7	7	7	7
20–34	13	4.2	7	2	2	4	4	9	10	10
35–49	1	5.0	0	5	5	5	5	5	5	5
50–64	0									
65+	0									
SUBTOTALS:										
1. SINGLE DX										
A. Not Operated	18	2.3	1	1	1	2	3	4	5	5
B. Operated	0									
2. MULTIPLE DX										
A. Not Operated	479	2.8	3	1	2	2	3	5	6	9
B. Operated	17	4.1	7	2	2	4	5	9	10	10
1. SINGLE DX	18	2.3	1	1	1	2	3	4	5	5
2. MULTIPLE DX	496	2.8	3	1	2	2	3	5	6	10
A. NOT OPERATED	497	2.8	3	1	2	2	3	4	6	9
B. OPERATED	17	4.1	7	2	2	4	5	9	10	10
TOTAL										
0–19 Years	88	3.1	4	1	2	3	4	5	7	14
20–34	382	2.8	3	1	2	2	3	5	6	10
35–49	43	2.3	1	1	1	2	3	4	4	5
50–64	1	5.0	0	5	5	5	5	5	5	5
65+	0									
GRAND TOTAL	514	2.8	3	1	2	2	3	5	6	9

646.81: PREG COMP NEC-DEL

Type of Patients	Observed Patients	Avg. Stay	Vari-ance	10th	25th	50th	75th	90th	95th	99th
1. SINGLE DX										
A. Not Operated										
0–19 Years	23	1.9	<1	1	1	2	3	3	3	3
20–34	191	1.8	<1	1	1	2	2	3	3	3
35–49	6	2.5	<1	2	2	3	3	3	3	3
50–64	0									
65+	0									
B. Operated										
0–19 Years	2	3.5	<1	3	3	4	4	4	4	4
20–34	20	3.1	<1	2	3	3	4	4	4	4
35–49	0									
50–64	0									
65+	0									
2. MULTIPLE DX										
A. Not Operated										
0–19 Years	171	2.2	<1	1	2	2	3	3	4	5
20–34	1,363	2.2	2	1	2	2	3	3	4	6
35–49	133	2.2	1	1	2	2	3	3	4	7
50–64	6	2.3	1	1	2	2	3	4	4	4
65+	0									
B. Operated										
0–19 Years	28	4.3	10	2	3	3	5	8	8	18
20–34	379	3.5	5	2	2	3	4	5	6	13
35–49	84	3.7	6	2	3	3	4	5	7	18
50–64	3	4.3	1	3	3	5	5	5	5	5
65+	0									
SUBTOTALS:										
1. SINGLE DX										
A. Not Operated	220	1.9	<1	1	1	2	2	3	3	3
B. Operated	22	3.1	<1	3	3	3	4	4	4	4
2. MULTIPLE DX										
A. Not Operated	1,673	2.2	2	1	2	2	3	3	4	6
B. Operated	494	3.6	6	2	2	3	5	9	10	16
1. SINGLE DX	242	2.0	<1	1	1	2	2	3	3	4
2. MULTIPLE DX	2,167	2.5	3	1	2	2	3	4	4	9
A. NOT OPERATED	1,893	2.1	2	1	2	2	3	3	4	5
B. OPERATED	516	3.5	5	2	2	3	4	5	7	14
TOTAL										
0–19 Years	224	2.4	3	1	2	2	3	4	4	8
20–34	1,953	2.4	3	1	2	2	3	4	4	7
35–49	223	2.8	4	1	2	3	3	4	5	11
50–64	9	3.0	2	2	2	3	4	5	5	5
65+	0									
GRAND TOTAL	2,409	2.4	3	1	2	2	3	4	4	8

646.83: PREG COMP NEC-AP

Type of Patients	Observed Patients	Avg. Stay	Vari-ance	10th	25th	50th	75th	90th	95th	99th
1. SINGLE DX										
A. Not Operated										
0–19 Years	12	1.3	<1	1	1	1	1	2	3	3
20–34	47	1.2	<1	1	1	1	1	1	2	6
35–49	0									
50–64	0									
65+	0									
B. Operated										
0–19 Years	0									
20–34	1	2.0	0	2	2	2	2	2	2	2
35–49	0									
50–64	0									
65+	0									
2. MULTIPLE DX										
A. Not Operated										
0–19 Years	284	2.3	5	1	1	2	3	4	6	9
20–34	1,605	2.2	4	1	1	2	3	4	5	9
35–49	284	2.6	6	1	1	2	3	5	6	13
50–64	10	1.1	<1	1	1	1	1	1	2	2
65+	0									
B. Operated										
0–19 Years	66	3.6	5	1	2	3	5	7	7	12
20–34	407	3.7	8	1	2	3	5	9	9	15
35–49	48	3.4	6	1	2	3	4	7	8	14
50–64	2	4.0	8	2	2	2	6	6	6	6
65+	0									
SUBTOTALS:										
1. SINGLE DX										
A. Not Operated	59	1.2	<1	1	1	1	1	1	2	6
B. Operated	1	2.0	0	2	2	2	2	2	2	2
2. MULTIPLE DX										
A. Not Operated	2,183	2.3	4	1	1	2	3	4	6	9
B. Operated	523	3.6	7	1	2	3	5	7	8	14
1. SINGLE DX	60	1.2	<1	1	1	1	1	1	2	6
2. MULTIPLE DX	2,706	2.5	5	1	1	2	3	5	7	11
A. NOT OPERATED	2,242	2.2	4	1	1	2	3	4	6	9
B. OPERATED	524	3.6	7	1	2	3	5	7	8	14
TOTAL										
0–19 Years	362	2.5	5	1	1	2	3	5	6	10
20–34	2,060	2.5	5	1	1	2	3	5	7	11
35–49	332	2.7	6	1	1	2	3	5	6	13
50–64	12	1.6	2	1	1	1	1	2	2	6
65+	0									
GRAND TOTAL	2,766	2.5	5	1	1	2	3	5	6	11

Length of Stay by Diagnosis and Operation, Western Region, 2008

Western Region, October 2006–September 2007 Data, by Diagnosis

646.84: PREG COMP NEC-PP

Type of Patients	Observed Patients	Avg. Stay	Variance	10th	25th	50th	75th	90th	95th	99th
1. SINGLE DX										
A. Not Operated										
0–19 Years	0									
20–34	1	1.0	0	1	1	1	1	1	1	1
35–49	0									
50–64	0									
65+	0									
B. Operated										
0–19 Years	0									
20–34	0									
35–49	0									
50–64	0									
65+	0									
2. MULTIPLE DX										
A. Not Operated										
0–19 Years	12	2.9	4	1	2	2	3	5	8	8
20–34	74	2.4	4	1	1	2	3	4	7	10
35–49	18	2.2	2	1	1	2	3	4	7	7
50–64	0									
65+										
B. Operated										
0–19 Years	39	2.9	3	1	2	3	3	5	7	10
20–34	161	2.4	2	1	1	2	3	4	5	6
35–49	7	2.1	<1	2	2	2	2	3	3	3
50–64	1	1.0	0	1	1	1	1	1	1	1
65+	0									
SUBTOTALS:										
1. SINGLE DX										
A. Not Operated	1	1.0	0	1	1	1	1	1	1	1
B. Operated	0									
2. MULTIPLE DX										
A. Not Operated	104	2.4	3	1	1	2	3	4	7	10
B. Operated	208	2.5	2	1	1	2	3	4	5	6
1. SINGLE DX	1	1.0	0	1	1	1	1	1	1	1
2. MULTIPLE DX	312	2.4	2	1	1	2	3	4	6	8
A. NOT OPERATED	105	2.4	3	1	1	2	3	4	7	10
B. OPERATED	208	2.5	2	1	1	2	3	4	5	6
TOTAL										
0–19 Years	51	2.9	3	1	2	3	3	5	7	10
20–34	236	2.4	2	1	1	2	3	4	6	7
35–49	25	2.2	2	1	2	2	3	4	7	7
50–64	1	1.0	0	1	1	1	1	1	1	1
65+	0									
GRAND TOTAL	313	2.4	2	1	1	2	3	4	6	8

647: INFECTIVE DIS IN PREG

Type of Patients	Observed Patients	Avg. Stay	Variance	10th	25th	50th	75th	90th	95th	99th
1. SINGLE DX										
A. Not Operated										
0–19 Years	9	2.0	<1	1	2	2	2	3	3	3
20–34	75	2.3	5	1	2	2	2	3	3	20
35–49	4	2.5	3	1	2	2	2	5	5	5
50–64	0									
65+	0									
B. Operated										
0–19 Years	4	3.0	0	3	3	3	3	3	3	3
20–34	11	2.8	<1	2	2	3	3	3	4	4
35–49	0									
50–64	0									
65+	0									
2. MULTIPLE DX										
A. Not Operated										
0–19 Years	361	2.5	3	1	2	2	3	5	6	10
20–34	2,228	2.4	4	1	1	2	3	4	6	11
35–49	279	2.8	6	1	1	2	3	5	7	15
50–64	8	2.8	2	2	2	2	3	6	6	6
65+	0									
B. Operated										
0–19 Years	205	3.0	<1	2	2	3	3	4	4	6
20–34	1,213	3.2	13	2	2	3	3	4	5	11
35–49	250	3.3	3	2	3	3	4	4	5	13
50–64	15	4.9	61	2	2	3	4	4	33	33
65+	0									
SUBTOTALS:										
1. SINGLE DX										
A. Not Operated	88	2.2	4	1	2	2	2	3	3	20
B. Operated	15	2.9	<1	2	3	3	3	3	4	4
2. MULTIPLE DX										
A. Not Operated	2,876	2.5	4	1	1	2	3	4	6	11
B. Operated	1,683	3.2	11	2	2	3	3	4	4	11
1. SINGLE DX	103	2.3	4	1	2	2	3	3	3	5
2. MULTIPLE DX	4,559	2.7	7	1	2	2	3	4	5	11
A. NOT OPERATED	2,964	2.5	4	1	1	2	3	4	6	11
B. OPERATED	1,698	3.2	11	2	2	3	3	4	5	11
TOTAL										
0–19 Years	579	2.7	3	1	2	2	3	5	7	10
20–34	3,527	2.7	7	1	2	2	3	4	5	11
35–49	533	3.0	5	1	2	2	3	4	6	13
50–64	23	4.1	41	2	2	3	4	4	6	33
65+	0									
GRAND TOTAL	4,662	2.7	7	1	2	2	3	4	5	11

647.61: OTH VIRUS IN PREG-DEL

Type of Patients	Observed Patients	Avg. Stay	Variance	10th	25th	50th	75th	90th	95th	99th
1. SINGLE DX										
A. Not Operated										
0–19 Years	1	2.0	0	2	2	2	2	2	2	2
20–34	9	1.8	<1	1	1	2	2	3	3	3
35–49	0									
50–64	0									
65+	0									
B. Operated										
0–19 Years	4	3.0	0	3	3	3	3	3	3	3
20–34	10	2.9	<1	2	3	3	3	4	4	4
35–49	0									
50–64	0									
65+	0									
2. MULTIPLE DX										
A. Not Operated										
0–19 Years	120	1.9	<1	1	1	2	2	3	3	4
20–34	961	1.8	<1	1	1	2	2	3	3	3
35–49	83	1.9	<1	1	1	2	2	3	4	4
50–64	6	2.2	<1	2	2	2	3	3	3	3
65+	0									
B. Operated										
0–19 Years	184	2.9	<1	2	2	3	3	4	4	4
20–34	1,102	2.9	<1	2	3	3	3	4	4	5
35–49	228	3.2	2	2	3	3	4	4	4	6
50–64	13	2.8	<1	2	2	3	3	4	4	4
65+	0									
SUBTOTALS:										
1. SINGLE DX										
A. Not Operated	10	1.8	<1	1	1	2	2	3	3	3
B. Operated	14	2.9	<1	2	3	3	3	3	4	4
2. MULTIPLE DX										
A. Not Operated	1,170	1.8	<1	1	1	2	2	3	3	4
B. Operated	1,527	2.9	<1	2	3	3	3	4	4	5
1. SINGLE DX	24	2.5	<1	1	2	3	3	3	3	4
2. MULTIPLE DX	2,697	2.5	1	1	2	3	3	4	4	5
A. NOT OPERATED	1,180	1.8	<1	1	1	2	2	3	3	4
B. OPERATED	1,541	2.9	<1	2	2	3	3	4	4	5
TOTAL										
0–19 Years	309	2.5	<1	1	2	3	3	4	4	4
20–34	2,082	2.4	<1	1	2	2	3	4	4	5
35–49	311	2.9	2	2	2	3	3	4	4	5
50–64	19	2.6	<1	2	2	3	3	4	4	4
65+	0									
GRAND TOTAL	2,721	2.5	1	1	2	3	3	4	4	5

Length of Stay by Diagnosis and Operation, Western Region, 2008

647.63: OTH VIRUS IN PREG-AP

Type of Patients	Observed Patients	Avg. Stay	Variance	Percentiles 10th	25th	50th	75th	90th	95th	99th
1. SINGLE DX										
A. Not Operated										
0–19 Years	0									
20–34	2	2.0	2	1	1	3	3	3	3	3
35–49	0									
50–64	0									
65+	0									
B. Operated										
0–19 Years	0									
20–34	0									
35–49	0									
50–64	0									
65+	0									
2. MULTIPLE DX										
A. Not Operated										
0–19 Years	23	2.6	5	1	1	2	4	5	6	10
20–34	157	2.6	6	1	1	2	3	5	6	9
35–49	28	2.2	2	1	1	2	3	4	5	6
50–64	0									
65+	0									
B. Operated										
0–19 Years	2	1.5	<1	1	1	2	2	2	2	2
20–34	5	5.0	46	1	1	2	4	17	17	17
35–49	1	8.0	0	8	8	8	8	8	8	8
50–64	0									
65+	0									
SUBTOTALS:										
1. SINGLE DX										
A. Not Operated	2	2.0	2	1	1	3	3	3	3	3
B. Operated	0									
2. MULTIPLE DX										
A. Not Operated	208	2.5	6	1	1	2	3	5	6	9
B. Operated	8	4.5	31	1	1	2	4	17	17	17
1. SINGLE DX	2	2.0	2	1	1	3	3	3	3	3
2. MULTIPLE DX	216	2.6	7	1	1	2	3	5	6	10
A. NOT OPERATED	210	2.5	6	1	1	2	3	5	6	9
B. OPERATED	8	4.5	31	1	1	2	4	17	17	17
TOTAL										
0–19 Years	25	2.5	5	1	1	2	3	5	6	10
20–34	164	2.6	7	1	1	2	3	5	6	9
35–49	29	2.4	3	1	1	2	3	5	6	8
50–64	0									
65+	0									
GRAND TOTAL	218	2.6	7	1	1	2	3	5	6	10

647.81: OTH INFECT DIS PREG-DEL

Type of Patients	Observed Patients	Avg. Stay	Variance	Percentiles 10th	25th	50th	75th	90th	95th	99th
1. SINGLE DX										
A. Not Operated										
0–19 Years	8	2.0	<1	1	1	2	2	3	3	3
20–34	56	2.1	<1	1	2	2	3	3	3	4
35–49	3	1.7	<1	1	1	2	2	2	2	2
50–64	0									
65+	0									
B. Operated										
0–19 Years	0									
20–34	1	2.0	0	2	2	2	2	2	2	2
35–49	0									
50–64	0									
65+	0									
2. MULTIPLE DX										
A. Not Operated										
0–19 Years	64	2.2	<1	2	2	2	2	3	3	4
20–34	374	2.2	2	1	2	2	2	3	4	7
35–49	35	2.4	3	1	2	2	2	3	4	12
50–64	0									
65+	0									
B. Operated										
0–19 Years	5	4.0	1	3	3	4	4	6	6	6
20–34	67	7.0	198	2	2	3	6	11	23	93
35–49	9	2.4	<1	2	2	3	3	4	4	4
50–64	1	4.0	0	4	4	4	4	4	4	4
65+	0									
SUBTOTALS:										
1. SINGLE DX										
A. Not Operated	67	2.1	<1	1	2	2	3	3	3	4
B. Operated	1	2.0	0	2	2	2	2	2	2	2
2. MULTIPLE DX										
A. Not Operated	473	2.2	2	1	2	2	3	3	4	7
B. Operated	82	6.3	164	2	3	3	4	9	13	93
1. SINGLE DX	68	2.1	<1	1	2	2	3	3	3	4
2. MULTIPLE DX	555	2.8	27	1	2	2	3	4	6	13
A. NOT OPERATED	540	2.2	1	1	2	2	3	3	4	7
B. OPERATED	83	6.3	162	2	2	3	5	9	13	93
TOTAL										
0–19 Years	77	2.3	<1	1	2	2	3	3	4	6
20–34	498	2.8	30	1	2	2	3	3	6	15
35–49	47	2.4	3	1	2	2	3	4	4	12
50–64	1	4.0	0	4	4	4	4	4	4	4
65+	0									
GRAND TOTAL	623	2.7	25	1	2	2	3	5	5	12

647.83: OTH INFECT DIS PREG-AP

Type of Patients	Observed Patients	Avg. Stay	Variance	Percentiles 10th	25th	50th	75th	90th	95th	99th
1. SINGLE DX										
A. Not Operated										
0–19 Years	0									
20–34	1	1.0	0	1	1	1	1	1	1	1
35–49	0									
50–64	0									
65+	0									
B. Operated										
0–19 Years	0									
20–34	0									
35–49	0									
50–64	0									
65+	0									
2. MULTIPLE DX										
A. Not Operated										
0–19 Years	92	3.7	5	1	2	4	5	6	8	14
20–34	456	3.8	9	1	2	3	5	7	10	16
35–49	101	3.7	9	1	2	3	5	7	8	19
50–64	2	4.5	4	3	3	6	6	6	6	6
65+	0									
B. Operated										
0–19 Years	1	3.0	0	3	3	3	3	3	3	3
20–34	10	6.2	28	1	1	5	11	14	14	14
35–49	6	7.5	43	2	3	7	8	20	20	20
50–64	0									
65+	0									
SUBTOTALS:										
1. SINGLE DX										
A. Not Operated	1	1.0	0	1	1	1	1	1	1	1
B. Operated	0									
2. MULTIPLE DX										
A. Not Operated	651	3.7	8	1	2	3	5	7	9	15
B. Operated	17	6.5	30	1	2	5	8	14	20	20
1. SINGLE DX	1	1.0	0	1	1	1	1	1	1	1
2. MULTIPLE DX	668	3.8	9	1	2	3	5	7	10	16
A. NOT OPERATED	652	3.7	8	1	2	3	5	7	9	15
B. OPERATED	17	6.5	30	1	2	5	8	14	20	20
TOTAL										
0–19 Years	93	3.7	5	1	2	4	5	6	8	14
20–34	467	3.8	9	1	2	3	5	7	10	16
35–49	107	3.9	11	1	3	3	5	7	10	19
50–64	2	4.5	4	3	3	6	6	6	6	6
65+	0									
GRAND TOTAL	669	3.8	9	1	2	3	5	7	10	16

Length of Stay by Diagnosis and Operation, Western Region, 2008

Western Region, October 2006–September 2007 Data, by Diagnosis

648: OTH CURRENT COND IN PREG

Type of Patients	Observed Patients	Avg. Stay	Vari-ance	10th	25th	50th	75th	90th	95th	99th
1. SINGLE DX										
A. Not Operated										
0–19 Years	153	1.8	<1	1	1	2	2	3	3	4
20–34	2,524	1.8	<1	1	1	2	2	3	3	4
35–49	174	1.8	<1	1	1	2	2	3	3	5
50–64	8	1.6	<1	1	1	2	2	3	3	3
65+	0									
B. Operated										
0–19 Years	3	3.0	0	3	3	3	3	3	3	3
20–34	101	2.8	<1	2	2	3	3	4	4	5
35–49	14	2.9	<1	2	2	3	3	4	4	4
50–64	0									
65+	0									
2. MULTIPLE DX										
A. Not Operated										
0–19 Years	5,661	2.2	4	1	1	2	2	3	4	8
20–34	48,174	2.1	4	1	1	2	2	3	4	7
35–49	6,753	2.2	4	1	1	2	2	3	4	9
50–64	291	2.2	2	1	2	2	3	3	4	8
65+	0									
B. Operated										
0–19 Years	551	3.4	12	1	2	3	4	5	7	15
20–34	8,110	3.2	9	2	2	3	4	5	6	13
35–49	2,097	3.3	7	2	2	3	4	5	6	18
50–64	109	3.2	2	2	2	3	4	4	5	8
65+	0									
SUBTOTALS:										
1. SINGLE DX										
A. Not Operated	2,859	1.8	<1	1	1	2	2	3	3	4
B. Operated	118	2.8	<1	2	2	3	3	4	4	5
2. MULTIPLE DX										
A. Not Operated	60,879	2.1	4	1	1	2	2	3	4	8
B. Operated	10,867	3.2	9	2	2	3	4	5	6	14
1. SINGLE DX	2,977	1.9	<1	1	1	2	2	3	3	4
2. MULTIPLE DX	71,746	2.3	5	1	1	2	3	3	4	9
A. NOT OPERATED	63,738	2.1	4	1	1	2	2	3	4	7
B. OPERATED	10,985	3.2	9	2	2	3	4	5	6	14
TOTAL										
0–19 Years	6,368	2.3	5	1	2	2	3	3	4	8
20–34	58,909	2.2	5	1	1	2	2	3	4	8
35–49	9,038	2.5	5	1	2	2	3	4	5	11
50–64	408	2.5	2	1	2	2	3	4	5	8
65+	0									
GRAND TOTAL	74,723	2.3	5	1	1	2	3	3	4	8

648.01: DM IN PREG-DELIVERED

Type of Patients	Observed Patients	Avg. Stay	Vari-ance	10th	25th	50th	75th	90th	95th	99th
1. SINGLE DX										
A. Not Operated										
0–19 Years	1	2.0	0	2	2	2	2	2	2	2
20–34	8	2.4	1	2	2	3	3	4	4	4
35–49	4	2.2	<1	1	1	2	3	3	3	3
50–64	0									
65+	0									
B. Operated										
0–19 Years	0									
20–34	0									
35–49	0									
50–64	0									
65+	0									
2. MULTIPLE DX										
A. Not Operated										
0–19 Years	50	3.3	6	2	2	2	3	3	4	8
20–34	740	2.4	3	1	2	2	3	3	4	7
35–49	193	2.2	1	1	2	2	3	3	4	9
50–64	14	2.3	<1	1	2	2	3	3	4	8
65+	0									
B. Operated										
0–19 Years	20	6.5	66	3	3	4	4	13	34	34
20–34	530	4.6	27	2	3	3	4	6	11	36
35–49	192	4.0	7	2	3	3	4	6	7	21
50–64	0	3.3	<1	2	3	3	4	5	5	5
65+	0									
SUBTOTALS:										
1. SINGLE DX										
A. Not Operated	13	2.3	<1	1	2	2	3	3	4	4
B. Operated	0									
2. MULTIPLE DX										
A. Not Operated	997	2.4	2	1	2	2	3	3	4	8
B. Operated	751	4.5	22	1	3	3	4	6	10	36
1. SINGLE DX	13	2.3	<1	1	2	2	3	3	4	4
2. MULTIPLE DX	1,748	3.3	12	1	2	3	4	5	6	19
A. NOT OPERATED	1,010	2.4	2	1	2	2	3	3	4	8
B. OPERATED	751	4.5	22	2	3	3	4	6	10	36
TOTAL										
0–19 Years	71	4.2	25	2	2	2	3	5	13	34
20–34	1,278	3.3	14	1	2	3	4	5	6	22
35–49	389	3.1	5	2	2	2	4	5	6	11
50–64	23	2.7	1	2	2	2	3	4	5	5
65+	0									
GRAND TOTAL	1,761	3.3	12	1	2	3	4	5	6	19

648.03: DM IN PREG-AP

Type of Patients	Observed Patients	Avg. Stay	Vari-ance	10th	25th	50th	75th	90th	95th	99th
1. SINGLE DX										
A. Not Operated										
0–19 Years	5	3.0	3	1	2	3	4	5	5	5
20–34	13	2.9	1	2	2	3	3	4	5	5
35–49	4	2.0	0	2	2	2	2	2	2	2
50–64	0									
65+	0									
B. Operated										
0–19 Years	0									
20–34	0									
35–49	0									
50–64	0									
65+	0									
2. MULTIPLE DX										
A. Not Operated										
0–19 Years	104	4.0	12	1	2	3	5	8	9	12
20–34	951	3.6	10	1	2	3	4	6	8	15
35–49	260	3.5	7	1	2	3	4	7	8	12
50–64	10	3.3	2	2	2	3	4	5	5	5
65+	0									
B. Operated										
0–19 Years	0									
20–34	7	6.3	33	1	2	3	13	15	15	15
35–49	1	2.0	0	2	2	2	2	2	2	2
50–64	0									
65+	0									
SUBTOTALS:										
1. SINGLE DX										
A. Not Operated	19	2.8	1	1	2	3	4	5	5	5
B. Operated	0									
2. MULTIPLE DX										
A. Not Operated	1,325	3.6	10	1	2	3	5	6	8	15
B. Operated	8	5.8	31	1	2	3	13	15	15	15
1. SINGLE DX	19	2.8	1	1	2	3	4	5	5	5
2. MULTIPLE DX	1,333	3.6	10	1	2	3	4	6	8	15
A. NOT OPERATED	1,344	3.6	10	1	2	3	4	6	8	15
B. OPERATED	8	5.8	31	1	2	3	13	15	15	15
TOTAL										
0–19 Years	109	4.0	12	1	2	3	5	8	9	12
20–34	971	3.6	10	1	2	3	4	6	8	15
35–49	262	3.5	7	1	2	3	4	7	8	12
50–64	10	3.3	2	2	2	3	4	5	5	5
65+	0									
GRAND TOTAL	1,352	3.6	10	1	2	3	5	6	8	15

Length of Stay by Diagnosis and Operation, Western Region, 2008

Western Region, October 2006–September 2007 Data, by Diagnosis

648.11: THYROID DYSF IN PREG-DEL

Type of Patients	Observed Patients	Avg. Stay	Variance	10th	25th	50th	75th	90th	95th	99th
1. SINGLE DX										
A. Not Operated										
0–19 Years	0									
20–34	12	2.1	<1	1	1	2	2	3	3	3
35–49	3	2.0	<1	1	1	2	3	3	3	3
50–64	0									
65+	0									
B. Operated										
0–19 Years	0									
20–34	0									
35–49	1	2.0	0	2	2	2	2	2	2	2
50–64	0									
65+	0									
2. MULTIPLE DX										
A. Not Operated										
0–19 Years	36	1.9	<1	1	1	2	2	3	3	3
20–34	1,111	1.8	<1	1	1	2	2	3	3	3
35–49	164	1.9	<1	1	1	2	2	3	3	3
50–64	8	1.8	<1	1	1	2	2	2	2	2
65+	0									
B. Operated										
0–19 Years	2	3.0	2	2	2	4	4	4	4	4
20–34	146	2.9	3	2	2	3	3	4	5	8
35–49	42	3.0	1	2	2	3	4	4	5	5
50–64	1	3.0	0	3	3	3	3	3	3	3
65+	0									
SUBTOTALS:										
1. SINGLE DX										
A. Not Operated	15	2.1	<1	1	2	2	3	3	3	3
B. Operated	1	2.0	0	2	2	2	2	2	2	2
2. MULTIPLE DX										
A. Not Operated	1,319	1.8	<1	1	1	2	2	3	3	3
B. Operated	191	2.9	3	2	2	3	3	4	5	8
1. SINGLE DX	16	2.1	<1	1	2	2	3	3	3	3
2. MULTIPLE DX	1,510	1.9	<1	1	1	2	2	3	3	4
A. NOT OPERATED	1,334	1.8	<1	1	1	2	2	3	3	3
B. OPERATED	192	2.9	3	2	2	3	3	4	5	8
TOTAL										
0–19 Years	38	2.0	<1	1	1	2	2	3	3	3
20–34	1,269	1.9	<1	1	1	2	2	3	3	3
35–49	210	2.1	<1	1	2	2	2	3	4	5
50–64	9	1.9	<1	1	2	2	2	3	3	3
65+	0									
GRAND TOTAL	1,526	1.9	<1	1	1	2	2	3	3	4

648.21: ANEMIA IN PREG-DELIVERED

Type of Patients	Observed Patients	Avg. Stay	Variance	10th	25th	50th	75th	90th	95th	99th
1. SINGLE DX										
A. Not Operated										
0–19 Years	25	1.9	<1	1	1	2	2	3	3	3
20–34	115	1.7	<1	1	1	2	2	2	3	3
35–49	4	1.8	<1	1	1	2	3	3	3	3
50–64	0									
65+	0									
B. Operated										
0–19 Years	0									
20–34	2	2.5	<1	2	2	2	3	3	3	3
35–49	1	3.0	0	3	3	3	3	3	3	3
50–64	0									
65+	0									
2. MULTIPLE DX										
A. Not Operated										
0–19 Years	841	2.0	5	1	1	2	2	3	3	4
20–34	3,855	1.8	1	1	1	2	2	3	3	4
35–49	231	2.0	<1	1	1	2	2	3	3	5
50–64	8	2.4	3	1	2	2	3	6	6	6
65+	0									
B. Operated										
0–19 Years	29	2.9	1	2	2	3	4	4	5	6
20–34	458	2.8	2	2	2	3	3	4	5	8
35–49	48	3.0	6	1	2	3	4	4	5	18
50–64	6	3.7	<1	3	3	4	4	4	4	4
65+	0									
SUBTOTALS:										
1. SINGLE DX										
A. Not Operated	144	1.7	<1	1	1	2	2	3	3	3
B. Operated	3	2.7	<1	2	2	3	3	3	3	3
2. MULTIPLE DX										
A. Not Operated	4,935	1.9	2	1	1	2	2	3	3	4
B. Operated	541	2.9	2	2	2	3	3	4	5	8
1. SINGLE DX	147	1.7	<1	1	1	2	2	3	3	3
2. MULTIPLE DX	5,476	2.0	2	1	1	2	2	3	3	5
A. NOT OPERATED	5,079	1.9	2	1	1	2	2	3	3	4
B. OPERATED	544	2.9	2	2	2	3	3	4	5	8
TOTAL										
0–19 Years	895	2.1	4	1	1	2	2	3	3	4
20–34	4,430	1.9	1	1	1	2	2	3	3	4
35–49	284	2.1	2	1	2	2	2	3	4	5
50–64	14	2.9	2	2	2	3	3	4	6	6
65+	0									
GRAND TOTAL	5,623	2.0	2	1	1	2	2	3	3	5

648.22: ANEMIA IN PREG-DEL PP

Type of Patients	Observed Patients	Avg. Stay	Variance	10th	25th	50th	75th	90th	95th	99th
1. SINGLE DX										
A. Not Operated										
0–19 Years	9	1.9	<1	1	2	2	2	2	2	2
20–34	34	2.0	<1	1	2	2	2	3	3	3
35–49	1	2.0	0	2	2	2	2	2	2	2
50–64	0									
65+	0									
B. Operated										
0–19 Years	0									
20–34	0									
35–49	0									
50–64	0									
65+	0									
2. MULTIPLE DX										
A. Not Operated										
0–19 Years	160	2.0	<1	1	2	2	3	3	4	4
20–34	650	1.9	<1	1	1	2	2	3	3	4
35–49	28	1.8	<1	1	1	2	2	3	3	3
50–64	1	1.0	0	1	1	1	1	1	1	1
65+	0									
B. Operated										
0–19 Years	4	2.8	<1	2	2	2	4	4	4	4
20–34	65	2.8	3	1	2	2	3	4	5	14
35–49	11	2.8	<1	2	2	3	4	4	4	4
50–64	2	3.5	<1	3	3	3	4	4	4	4
65+	0									
SUBTOTALS:										
1. SINGLE DX										
A. Not Operated	44	2.0	<1	1	2	2	2	3	3	3
B. Operated	0									
2. MULTIPLE DX										
A. Not Operated	839	1.9	<1	1	1	2	2	3	3	4
B. Operated	82	2.8	3	2	2	3	3	4	5	14
1. SINGLE DX	44	2.0	<1	1	2	2	2	3	3	3
2. MULTIPLE DX	921	2.0	<1	1	2	2	2	3	3	4
A. NOT OPERATED	883	1.9	<1	1	2	2	2	3	3	4
B. OPERATED	82	2.8	3	2	2	3	3	4	5	14
TOTAL										
0–19 Years	173	2.0	<1	1	2	2	2	3	3	4
20–34	749	2.0	<1	1	1	2	2	3	3	5
35–49	40	2.1	<1	1	1	2	3	3	4	4
50–64	3	2.7	2	2	3	3	4	4	4	4
65+	0									
GRAND TOTAL	965	2.0	<1	1	2	2	2	3	3	4

Length of Stay by Diagnosis and Operation, Western Region, 2008

Western Region, October 2006–September 2007 Data, by Diagnosis

648.23: ANEMIA IN PREG-AP

Type of Patients	Observed Patients	Avg. Stay	Variance	10th	25th	50th	75th	90th	95th	99th
1. SINGLE DX										
A. Not Operated										
0–19 Years	0									
20–34	2	1.0	0	1	1	1	1	1	1	1
35–49	0									
50–64	0									
65+	0									
B. Operated										
0–19 Years	0									
20–34	0									
35–49	0									
50–64	0									
65+	0									
2. MULTIPLE DX										
A. Not Operated										
0–19 Years	30	2.3	4	1	1	1	3	4	6	11
20–34	231	3.8	28	1	1	2	4	9	11	26
35–49	33	1.9	1	1	1	1	2	4	5	5
50–64	3	1.0	0	1	1	1	1	1	1	1
65+	0									
B. Operated										
0–19 Years	0									
20–34	2	21.1	573	4	4	38	38	38	38	38
35–49	0									
50–64	0									
65+	0									
SUBTOTALS:										
1. SINGLE DX										
A. Not Operated	2	1.0	0	1	1	1	1	1	1	1
B. Operated	0									
2. MULTIPLE DX										
A. Not Operated	297	3.4	23	1	1	2	4	7	11	26
B. Operated	2	21.1	573	4	4	38	38	38	38	38
1. SINGLE DX	2	1.0	0	1	1	1	1	1	1	1
2. MULTIPLE DX	299	3.5	27	1	1	2	4	8	11	27
A. NOT OPERATED	299	3.4	23	1	1	2	4	7	11	26
B. OPERATED	2	21.1	573	4	4	38	38	38	38	38
TOTAL										
0–19 Years	30	2.3	4	1	1	1	3	4	6	11
20–34	235	3.9	33	1	1	2	4	9	12	27
35–49	33	1.9	1	1	1	1	2	4	5	5
50–64	3	1.0	0	1	1	1	1	1	1	1
65+	0									
GRAND TOTAL	301	3.5	27	1	1	2	4	7	11	26

648.31: DRUG DEPEND IN PREG-DEL

Type of Patients	Observed Patients	Avg. Stay	Variance	10th	25th	50th	75th	90th	95th	99th
1. SINGLE DX										
A. Not Operated										
0–19 Years	0									
20–34	2	2.0	0	2	2	2	2	2	2	2
35–49	0									
50–64	0									
65+	0									
B. Operated										
0–19 Years	0									
20–34	0									
35–49	0									
50–64	0									
65+	0									
2. MULTIPLE DX										
A. Not Operated										
0–19 Years	15	2.0	<1	1	1	2	3	3	3	3
20–34	181	2.1	<1	1	2	2	2	3	3	4
35–49	20	2.2	<1	1	2	2	2	3	3	5
50–64	0									
65+	0									
B. Operated										
0–19 Years	2	2.0	0	2	2	2	2	2	2	2
20–34	30	4.6	75	2	2	3	4	5	5	50
35–49	7	3.6	<1	2	3	4	4	5	5	5
50–64	0									
65+	0									
SUBTOTALS:										
1. SINGLE DX										
A. Not Operated	2	2.0	0	2	2	2	2	2	2	2
B. Operated	0									
2. MULTIPLE DX										
A. Not Operated	216	2.1	<1	1	2	2	2	3	3	4
B. Operated	39	4.3	58	2	2	3	4	5	5	50
1. SINGLE DX	2	2.0	0	2	2	2	2	2	2	2
2. MULTIPLE DX	255	2.4	10	1	2	2	3	3	4	5
A. NOT OPERATED	218	2.1	<1	1	2	2	2	3	3	4
B. OPERATED	39	4.3	58	2	2	3	4	5	5	50
TOTAL										
0–19 Years	17	2.0	<1	1	2	2	2	3	3	3
20–34	213	2.4	12	1	2	2	3	3	4	5
35–49	27	2.6	1	2	2	2	3	4	5	5
50–64	0									
65+	0									
GRAND TOTAL	257	2.4	10	1	2	2	3	4	4	5

648.33: DRUG DEPEND IN PREG-AP

Type of Patients	Observed Patients	Avg. Stay	Variance	10th	25th	50th	75th	90th	95th	99th
1. SINGLE DX										
A. Not Operated										
0–19 Years	0									
20–34	0									
35–49	0									
50–64	0									
65+	0									
B. Operated										
0–19 Years	0									
20–34	0									
35–49	0									
50–64	0									
65+	0									
2. MULTIPLE DX										
A. Not Operated										
0–19 Years	11	10.8	128	1	2	5	22	24	32	32
20–34	172	12.6	220	1	2	4	25	32	40	63
35–49	13	16.6	388	1	4	10	25	30	73	73
50–64	0									
65+	0									
B. Operated										
0–19 Years	0									
20–34	1	55.0	0	55	55	55	55	55	55	55
35–49	0									
50–64	0									
65+	0									
SUBTOTALS:										
1. SINGLE DX										
A. Not Operated	0									
B. Operated	0									
2. MULTIPLE DX										
A. Not Operated	196	12.8	225	1	2	4	24	32	40	65
B. Operated	1	55.0	0	55	55	55	55	55	55	55
1. SINGLE DX	0									
2. MULTIPLE DX	197	13.0	233	1	2	4	25	32	41	65
A. NOT OPERATED	196	12.8	225	1	2	4	24	32	40	65
B. OPERATED	1	55.0	0	55	55	55	55	55	55	55
TOTAL										
0–19 Years	11	10.8	128	1	2	5	22	24	32	32
20–34	173	12.8	229	1	2	4	25	33	41	63
35–49	13	16.6	388	1	4	10	25	30	73	73
50–64	0									
65+	0									
GRAND TOTAL	197	13.0	233	1	2	4	25	32	41	65

Length of Stay by Diagnosis and Operation, Western Region, 2008

Western Region, October 2006–September 2007 Data, by Diagnosis

648.41: MENTAL DISORD PREG-DEL

Type of Patients	Observed Patients	Avg. Stay	Variance	10th	25th	50th	75th	90th	95th	99th
1. SINGLE DX										
A. Not Operated										
0–19 Years	0									
20–34	10	1.9	<1	1	2	2	2	3	3	3
35–49	0									
50–64	0									
65+	0									
B. Operated										
0–19 Years	0									
20–34	0									
35–49	0									
50–64	0									
65+	0									
2. MULTIPLE DX										
A. Not Operated										
0–19 Years	253	2.0	<1	1	2	2	2	3	3	4
20–34	1,811	1.9	3	1	1	2	2	3	3	4
35–49	106	2.4	19	1	2	2	2	3	3	4
50–64	2	1.5	<1	1	1	2	2	2	2	2
65+	0									
B. Operated										
0–19 Years	16	3.1	<1	2	3	3	3	4	6	6
20–34	210	2.8	4	2	2	3	3	4	4	9
35–49	40	2.8	<1	2	2	3	3	4	5	5
50–64	0									
65+	0									
SUBTOTALS:										
1. SINGLE DX										
A. Not Operated	10	1.9	<1	1	2	2	2	3	3	3
B. Operated	0									
2. MULTIPLE DX										
A. Not Operated	2,172	1.9	3	1	1	2	2	3	3	4
B. Operated	266	2.9	3	2	2	3	3	4	4	9
1. SINGLE DX	10	1.9	<1	1	2	2	2	3	3	3
2. MULTIPLE DX	2,438	2.0	3	1	2	2	2	3	3	4
A. NOT OPERATED	2,182	1.9	3	1	1	2	2	3	3	4
B. OPERATED	266	2.9	3	2	2	3	3	4	4	9
TOTAL										
0–19 Years	269	2.1	<1	1	2	2	3	3	3	5
20–34	2,031	2.0	3	1	1	2	2	3	3	4
35–49	146	2.5	14	1	2	2	3	3	4	5
50–64	2	1.5	<1	1	1	2	2	2	2	2
65+	0									
GRAND TOTAL	2,448	2.0	3	1	1	2	2	3	3	4

648.43: MENTAL DISORD PREG-AP

Type of Patients	Observed Patients	Avg. Stay	Variance	10th	25th	50th	75th	90th	95th	99th
1. SINGLE DX										
A. Not Operated										
0–19 Years	0									
20–34	0									
35–49	0									
50–64	0									
65+	0									
B. Operated										
0–19 Years	0									
20–34	0									
35–49	0									
50–64	0									
65+	0									
2. MULTIPLE DX										
A. Not Operated										
0–19 Years	54	5.0	46	1	1	3	6	10	16	45
20–34	424	4.4	36	1	1	3	4	10	15	35
35–49	79	5.2	27	1	2	3	6	15	19	22
50–64	6	5.2	13	2	3	5	6	12	12	12
65+	0									
B. Operated										
0–19 Years	0									
20–34	2	14.0	31	10	10	18	18	18	18	18
35–49	1	4.0	0	4	4	4	4	4	4	4
50–64	0									
65+	0									
SUBTOTALS:										
1. SINGLE DX										
A. Not Operated	0									
B. Operated	0									
2. MULTIPLE DX										
A. Not Operated	563	4.6	35	1	1	3	5	10	16	35
B. Operated	3	10.7	49	4	4	10	18	18	18	18
1. SINGLE DX	0									
2. MULTIPLE DX	566	4.6	36	1	1	3	5	10	16	35
A. NOT OPERATED	563	4.6	35	1	1	3	5	10	16	35
B. OPERATED	3	10.7	49	4	4	10	18	18	18	18
TOTAL										
0–19 Years	54	5.0	46	1	1	3	6	10	16	45
20–34	426	4.5	36	1	1	3	4	10	15	35
35–49	80	5.2	27	1	2	3	6	12	19	22
50–64	6	5.2	13	2	3	5	6	12	12	12
65+	0									
GRAND TOTAL	566	4.6	36	1	1	3	5	10	16	35

648.44: MENTAL DISORD PREG-PP

Type of Patients	Observed Patients	Avg. Stay	Variance	10th	25th	50th	75th	90th	95th	99th
1. SINGLE DX										
A. Not Operated										
0–19 Years	1	1.0	0	1	1	1	1	1	1	1
20–34	1	1.0	0	1	1	1	1	1	1	1
35–49	0									
50–64	0									
65+	0									
B. Operated										
0–19 Years	0									
20–34	0									
35–49	0									
50–64	0									
65+	0									
2. MULTIPLE DX										
A. Not Operated										
0–19 Years	21	4.7	16	1	2	3	8	9	13	14
20–34	222	4.0	20	1	2	2	4	8	14	24
35–49	53	4.5	42	1	2	2	4	7	25	35
50–64	2	4.5	25	1	1	5	8	8	8	8
65+	0									
B. Operated										
0–19 Years	1	7.0	0	7	7	7	7	7	7	7
20–34	4	2.3	<1	2	2	2	3	3	3	3
35–49	0									
50–64	0									
65+	0									
SUBTOTALS:										
1. SINGLE DX										
A. Not Operated	2	1.0	0	1	1	1	1	1	1	1
B. Operated	0									
2. MULTIPLE DX										
A. Not Operated	298	4.1	24	1	2	2	4	8	14	27
B. Operated	5	3.2	5	2	2	2	3	7	7	7
1. SINGLE DX	2	1.0	0	1	1	1	1	1	1	1
2. MULTIPLE DX	303	4.1	23	1	2	2	4	8	14	26
A. NOT OPERATED	300	4.1	24	1	2	2	4	8	14	26
B. OPERATED	5	3.2	5	2	2	2	3	7	7	7
TOTAL										
0–19 Years	23	4.6	15	1	2	3	8	9	13	14
20–34	227	3.9	20	1	2	2	4	8	14	24
35–49	53	4.5	42	1	2	2	4	7	25	35
50–64	2	4.5	25	1	1	5	8	8	8	8
65+	0									
GRAND TOTAL	305	4.1	23	1	2	2	4	8	14	26

Length of Stay by Diagnosis and Operation, Western Region, 2008

Western Region, October 2006–September 2007 Data, by Diagnosis

648.61: CV DIS NEC IN PREG-DEL

Type of Patients	Observed Patients	Avg. Stay	Variance	10th	25th	50th	75th	90th	95th	99th
1. SINGLE DX										
A. Not Operated										
0–19 Years	0									
20–34	4	1.8	<1	1	1	2	2	2	2	2
35–49	0									
50–64	0									
65+	0									
B. Operated										
0–19 Years	0									
20–34	1	2.0	0	2	2	2	2	2	2	2
35–49	0									
50–64	0									
65+	0									
2. MULTIPLE DX										
A. Not Operated										
0–19 Years	32	1.9	<1	1	1	2	2	3	3	4
20–34	400	2.1	2	1	1	2	2	3	4	7
35–49	59	2.1	2	1	1	2	2	3	5	9
50–64	3	2.0	0	2	2	2	2	2	2	2
65+	0									
B. Operated										
0–19 Years	5	3.4	1	2	3	3	4	5	5	5
20–34	113	4.1	14	2	3	3	4	6	11	26
35–49	32	5.1	24	2	3	4	5	10	18	25
50–64	1	3.0	0	3	3	3	3	3	3	3
65+	0									
SUBTOTALS:										
1. SINGLE DX										
A. Not Operated	4	1.8	<1	1	1	2	2	2	2	2
B. Operated	1	2.0	0	2	2	2	2	2	2	2
2. MULTIPLE DX										
A. Not Operated	494	2.1	2	1	1	2	2	3	4	7
B. Operated	151	4.3	16	2	2	3	5	7	11	26
1. SINGLE DX	5	1.8	<1	1	2	2	2	2	2	2
2. MULTIPLE DX	645	2.6	6	1	2	2	3	4	6	14
A. NOT OPERATED	498	2.1	2	1	1	2	2	3	4	7
B. OPERATED	152	4.3	16	2	2	3	5	7	11	26
TOTAL										
0–19 Years	37	2.1	<1	1	1	2	2	3	4	5
20–34	518	2.5	5	1	2	2	3	4	6	13
35–49	91	3.2	11	1	2	2	3	5	9	25
50–64	4	2.3	<1	2	2	2	2	3	3	3
65+	0									
GRAND TOTAL	650	2.6	6	1	2	2	3	4	6	14

648.63: CV DIS NEC IN PREG-AP

Type of Patients	Observed Patients	Avg. Stay	Variance	10th	25th	50th	75th	90th	95th	99th
1. SINGLE DX										
A. Not Operated										
0–19 Years	0									
20–34	0									
35–49	0									
50–64	0									
65+	0									
B. Operated										
0–19 Years	0									
20–34	0									
35–49	0									
50–64	0									
65+	0									
2. MULTIPLE DX										
A. Not Operated										
0–19 Years	12	1.8	<1	1	1	1	2	3	4	4
20–34	149	2.5	13	1	1	2	2	4	6	14
35–49	37	1.8	1	1	1	1	2	3	4	5
50–64	1	2.0	0	2	2	2	2	2	2	2
65+	0									
B. Operated										
0–19 Years	1	2.0	0	2	2	2	2	2	2	2
20–34	5	7.6	13	3	5	8	11	11	11	11
35–49	0									
50–64	0									
65+	0									
SUBTOTALS:										
1. SINGLE DX										
A. Not Operated	0									
B. Operated	0									
2. MULTIPLE DX										
A. Not Operated	199	2.3	10	1	1	2	2	4	6	14
B. Operated	6	6.7	15	2	3	8	11	11	11	11
1. SINGLE DX	0									
2. MULTIPLE DX	205	2.4	11	1	1	2	3	4	6	12
A. NOT OPERATED	199	2.3	10	1	1	2	2	4	6	14
B. OPERATED	6	6.7	15	2	3	8	11	11	11	11
TOTAL										
0–19 Years	13	1.8	<1	1	1	1	2	3	4	4
20–34	154	2.7	14	1	1	2	3	5	8	14
35–49	37	1.8	1	1	1	1	2	3	4	5
50–64	1	2.0	0	2	2	2	2	2	2	2
65+	0									
GRAND TOTAL	205	2.4	11	1	1	2	3	4	6	12

648.71: BONE DISORD IN PREG-DEL

Type of Patients	Observed Patients	Avg. Stay	Variance	10th	25th	50th	75th	90th	95th	99th
1. SINGLE DX										
A. Not Operated										
0–19 Years	0									
20–34	6	2.0	2	1	2	2	3	4	4	4
35–49	0									
50–64	0									
65+	0									
B. Operated										
0–19 Years	0									
20–34	8	2.9	<1	2	3	3	3	4	4	4
35–49	0									
50–64	0									
65+	0									
2. MULTIPLE DX										
A. Not Operated										
0–19 Years	3	1.7	<1	1	1	2	2	2	2	2
20–34	136	2.0	<1	1	1	2	2	3	3	3
35–49	13	2.1	<1	1	2	2	3	3	3	3
50–64	1	3.0	0	3	3	3	3	3	3	3
65+	0									
B. Operated										
0–19 Years	5	3.4	<1	3	3	3	3	4	4	4
20–34	101	2.9	<1	2	2	3	3	4	4	5
35–49	19	3.1	<1	2	2	3	4	4	4	4
50–64	1	4.0	0	4	4	4	4	4	4	4
65+	0									
SUBTOTALS:										
1. SINGLE DX										
A. Not Operated	6	2.0	2	1	2	2	3	4	4	4
B. Operated	8	2.9	<1	2	3	3	3	4	4	4
2. MULTIPLE DX										
A. Not Operated	153	2.0	<1	1	1	2	2	3	3	3
B. Operated	126	2.9	<1	2	2	3	3	4	4	5
1. SINGLE DX	14	2.5	1	1	2	2	3	4	4	4
2. MULTIPLE DX	279	2.4	<1	1	2	2	3	4	4	5
A. NOT OPERATED	159	2.0	<1	1	1	2	2	3	3	4
B. OPERATED	134	2.9	<1	2	2	3	3	4	4	5
TOTAL										
0–19 Years	8	2.8	1	1	2	3	3	4	4	4
20–34	251	2.4	<1	1	2	3	3	4	5	5
35–49	32	2.7	<1	2	3	3	4	4	4	4
50–64	2	3.5	<1	3	3	3	4	4	4	4
65+	0									
GRAND TOTAL	293	2.4	<1	1	2	3	3	4	4	5

Length of Stay by Diagnosis and Operation, Western Region, 2008

Western Region, October 2006–September 2007 Data, by Diagnosis

648.81: ABN GTT IN PREG-DEL

Type of Patients	Observed Patients	Avg. Stay	Vari-ance	Percentiles 10th	25th	50th	75th	90th	95th	99th
1. SINGLE DX										
A. Not Operated										
0–19 Years	51	2.1	<1	1	2	2	3	3	3	3
20–34	1,757	1.8	<1	1	1	2	2	3	3	4
35–49	121	1.8	<1	1	1	2	2	3	3	5
50–64	6	1.7	<1	1	1	2	2	3	3	3
65+	0									
B. Operated										
0–19 Years	0									
20–34	50	2.9	<1	2	2	3	3	4	4	5
35–49	6	3.0	<1	2	2	3	4	4	4	4
50–64	0									
65+	0									
2. MULTIPLE DX										
A. Not Operated										
0–19 Years	283	2.4	2	1	2	2	3	3	4	6
20–34	7,214	2.0	<1	1	2	2	3	3	3	4
35–49	2,327	2.0	<1	1	1	2	3	3	3	4
50–64	101	2.2	<1	1	2	2	3	3	3	5
65+	0									
B. Operated										
0–19 Years	76	3.7	2	2	3	3	4	5	7	10
20–34	2,488	3.1	4	2	2	3	4	4	5	8
35–49	1,056	3.1	2	2	2	3	4	4	5	8
50–64	49	3.1	1	2	2	3	4	4	5	6
65+	0									
SUBTOTALS:										
1. SINGLE DX										
A. Not Operated	1,935	1.8	<1	1	1	2	2	3	3	4
B. Operated	56	2.9	<1	2	2	3	3	4	4	5
2. MULTIPLE DX										
A. Not Operated	9,925	2.0	<1	1	2	2	3	3	3	4
B. Operated	3,669	3.1	3	2	2	3	4	4	5	8
1. SINGLE DX	1,991	1.8	<1	1	1	2	2	3	3	4
2. MULTIPLE DX	13,594	2.3	2	1	2	2	3	3	4	6
A. NOT OPERATED	11,860	2.0	<1	1	1	2	2	3	3	4
B. OPERATED	3,725	3.1	3	2	2	3	4	4	5	8
TOTAL										
0–19 Years	410	2.6	2	1	2	2	3	4	5	7
20–34	11,509	2.2	2	1	2	2	3	3	4	5
35–49	3,510	2.3	1	1	2	2	3	4	4	6
50–64	156	2.5	1	2	2	2	3	4	4	6
65+	0									
GRAND TOTAL	15,585	2.3	2	1	2	2	3	3	4	6

648.83: ABN GTT IN PREG-AP

Type of Patients	Observed Patients	Avg. Stay	Vari-ance	Percentiles 10th	25th	50th	75th	90th	95th	99th
1. SINGLE DX										
A. Not Operated										
0–19 Years	9	1.6	<1	1	1	1	2	3	3	3
20–34	192	2.3	2	1	2	2	3	4	5	7
35–49	18	2.3	1	1	2	2	3	4	4	4
50–64	2	1.5	<1	1	1	1	2	2	2	2
65+	0									
B. Operated										
0–19 Years	0									
20–34	0									
35–49	0									
50–64	0									
65+	0									
2. MULTIPLE DX										
A. Not Operated										
0–19 Years	27	2.7	4	1	1	2	4	6	6	9
20–34	504	2.6	4	1	2	2	3	5	6	8
35–49	214	2.6	3	1	2	2	3	5	6	8
50–64	3	5.0	13	1	3	6	8	8	8	8
65+	0									
B. Operated										
0–19 Years	0									
20–34	1	2.0	0	2	2	2	2	2	2	2
35–49	1	4.0	0	4	4	4	4	4	4	4
50–64	0									
65+	0									
SUBTOTALS:										
1. SINGLE DX										
A. Not Operated	221	2.3	2	1	1	2	3	4	5	7
B. Operated	0									
2. MULTIPLE DX										
A. Not Operated	748	2.6	4	1	1	2	3	5	6	8
B. Operated	2	3.0	2	2	2	3	4	4	4	4
1. SINGLE DX	221	2.3	2	1	1	2	3	4	5	7
2. MULTIPLE DX	750	2.6	4	1	1	2	3	5	6	8
A. NOT OPERATED	969	2.5	3	1	1	2	3	5	6	8
B. OPERATED	2	3.0	2	2	2	3	4	4	5	4
TOTAL										
0–19 Years	36	2.5	3	1	1	2	3	4	5	9
20–34	697	2.5	3	1	1	2	3	5	6	8
35–49	233	2.5	3	1	1	2	3	5	6	8
50–64	5	3.6	10	1	1	2	6	8	8	8
65+	0									
GRAND TOTAL	971	2.5	3	1	1	2	3	5	6	8

648.91: OTH CCE COMP PREG-DEL

Type of Patients	Observed Patients	Avg. Stay	Vari-ance	Percentiles 10th	25th	50th	75th	90th	95th	99th
1. SINGLE DX										
A. Not Operated										
0–19 Years	33	1.8	<1	1	2	2	2	2	2	3
20–34	237	1.8	<1	1	1	2	2	3	3	3
35–49	7	1.7	<1	1	1	1	3	3	3	3
50–64	0									
65+	0									
B. Operated										
0–19 Years	2									
20–34	34	3.0	0	3	3	3	3	3	3	3
35–49	6	2.7	<1	2	2	3	3	4	4	4
50–64	0	2.8	<1	2	2	3	3	4	4	4
65+	0									
2. MULTIPLE DX										
A. Not Operated										
0–19 Years	2,798	2.1	1	1	2	2	2	3	3	4
20–34	23,220	1.9	<1	1	2	2	2	3	3	4
35–49	1,893	2.0	<1	1	2	2	2	3	3	4
50–64	93	2.0	<1	1	2	2	2	3	3	4
65+	0									
B. Operated										
0–19 Years	187	3.2	4	2	2	3	3	4	5	12
20–34	2,791	3.0	9	2	2	3	3	4	5	11
35–49	448	3.6	16	2	3	3	4	4	8	27
50–64	25	2.6	<1	2	2	2	3	4	4	5
65+	0									
SUBTOTALS:										
1. SINGLE DX										
A. Not Operated	277	1.8	<1	1	1	2	2	3	3	3
B. Operated	42	2.8	<1	2	2	3	3	4	4	4
2. MULTIPLE DX										
A. Not Operated	28,004	2.0	<1	1	2	2	3	3	4	8
B. Operated	3,451	3.1	10	2	2	3	4	5	6	16
1. SINGLE DX	319	1.9	<1	1	1	2	2	3	3	4
2. MULTIPLE DX	31,455	2.1	2	1	2	2	3	3	5	8
A. NOT OPERATED	28,281	2.0	<1	1	2	2	3	3	4	8
B. OPERATED	3,493	3.1	10	2	3	3	4	5	6	16
TOTAL										
0–19 Years	3,020	2.1	1	1	2	2	3	3	5	9
20–34	26,282	2.0	2	1	2	2	3	3	4	8
35–49	2,354	2.3	4	1	2	2	3	4	9	8
50–64	118	2.2	<1	1	2	2	3	3	4	8
65+	0									
GRAND TOTAL	31,774	2.1	2	1	2	2	3	3	5	8

Length of Stay by Diagnosis and Operation, Western Region, 2008

Western Region, October 2006–September 2007 Data, by Diagnosis

648.93: OTH CCE COMP PREG-AP

Type of Patients	Observed Patients	Avg. Stay	Variance	10th	25th	50th	75th	90th	95th	99th
1. SINGLE DX										
A. Not Operated										
0–19 Years	18	1.1	<1	1	1	1	1	1	2	2
20–34	113	1.2	<1	1	1	1	1	2	2	3
35–49	12	1.1	<1	1	1	1	1	1	2	2
50–64	0									
65+	0									
B. Operated										
0–19 Years	0									
20–34	2	3.0	8		1	1	5	5	5	5
35–49	0									
50–64	0									
65+	0									
2. MULTIPLE DX										
A. Not Operated										
0–19 Years	852	2.2	11	1	1	1	2	4	5	8
20–34	5,460	2.3	7	1	1	2	3	5	6	12
35–49	860	2.5	8	1	1	2	3	5	6	15
50–64	28	1.8	3	1	1	1	2	3	4	10
65+	0									
B. Operated										
0–19 Years	177	3.2	19	1	1	2	4	6	7	15
20–34	984	3.2	10	1	1	2	4	6	9	16
35–49	154	3.3	11	1	1	2	4	6	9	21
50–64	8	4.6	11	1	2	4	5	11	11	11
65+	0									
SUBTOTALS:										
1. SINGLE DX										
A. Not Operated	143	1.2	<1	1	1	1	1	2	2	3
B. Operated	2	3.0	8	1	1	1	5	5	5	5
2. MULTIPLE DX										
A. Not Operated	7,200	2.3	7	1	1	2	3	4	6	12
B. Operated	1,323	3.2	12	1	1	2	4	6	8	15
1. SINGLE DX	145	1.2	<1	1	1	1	1	2	2	5
2. MULTIPLE DX	8,523	2.4	8	1	1	2	3	5	6	13
A. NOT OPERATED	7,343	2.3	7	1	1	1	3	4	6	12
B. OPERATED	1,325	3.2	12	1	1	2	4	6	8	15
TOTAL										
0–19 Years	1,047	2.3	12	1	1	2	3	4	6	9
20–34	6,559	2.4	7	1	1	2	3	5	6	12
35–49	1,026	2.6	8	1	1	2	3	5	7	15
50–64	36	2.4	6	1	1	1	2	5	10	11
65+	0									
GRAND TOTAL	8,668	2.4	8	1	1	2	3	5	6	13

648.94: OTH CCE COMP PREG-PP

Type of Patients	Observed Patients	Avg. Stay	Variance	10th	25th	50th	75th	90th	95th	99th
1. SINGLE DX										
A. Not Operated										
0–19 Years	0									
20–34	1	3.0	0	3	3	3	3	3	3	3
35–49	1	2.0	0	2	2	2	2	2	2	2
50–64	0									
65+	0									
B. Operated										
0–19 Years	0									
20–34	0									
35–49	0									
50–64	0									
65+	0									
2. MULTIPLE DX										
A. Not Operated										
0–19 Years	27	3.3	6	1	1	2	5	6	9	10
20–34	201	3.0	16	1	1	2	3	5	8	20
35–49	54	2.4	3	1	1	2	3	4	5	9
50–64	1	2.0	0	2	2	2	2	2	2	2
65+	0									
B. Operated										
0–19 Years	19	3.2	10	1	1	2	4	8	13	13
20–34	127	2.9	6	1	1	2	3	5	8	14
35–49	27	3.0	9	1	1	2	3	9	10	12
50–64	1	3.0	0	3	3	3	3	3	3	3
65+	0									
SUBTOTALS:										
1. SINGLE DX										
A. Not Operated	2	2.5	<1	2	2	2	3	3	3	3
B. Operated	0									
2. MULTIPLE DX										
A. Not Operated	283	2.9	12	1	1	2	3	5	6	14
B. Operated	174	2.9	7	1	1	2	3	6	9	14
1. SINGLE DX	2	2.5	<1	2	2	2	3	3	3	3
2. MULTIPLE DX	457	2.9	10	1	1	2	3	5	8	14
A. NOT OPERATED	285	2.9	12	1	1	2	3	5	6	14
B. OPERATED	174	2.9	7	1	1	2	3	6	9	14
TOTAL										
0–19 Years	46	3.3	8	1	1	2	3	4	7	13
20–34	329	2.9	12	1	1	2	3	5	8	14
35–49	82	2.6	5	1	1	2	3	5	8	12
50–64	2	2.5	<1	2	2	3	3	3	3	3
65+	0									
GRAND TOTAL	459	2.9	10	1	1	2	3	5	8	14

649: OTH COND/STATUS IN PREG

Type of Patients	Observed Patients	Avg. Stay	Variance	10th	25th	50th	75th	90th	95th	99th
1. SINGLE DX										
A. Not Operated										
0–19 Years	80	1.5	<1	1	1	1	2	2	3	3
20–34	625	1.6	<1	1	1	1	2	2	3	3
35–49	17	1.8	4	1	1	1	2	2	9	9
50–64	0									
65+	0									
B. Operated										
0–19 Years	0									
20–34	5	2.8	<1	2	2	3	3	4	4	4
35–49	0									
50–64	0									
65+	0									
2. MULTIPLE DX										
A. Not Operated										
0–19 Years	294	2.2	3	1	1	2	2	3	4	10
20–34	2,376	2.0	2	1	1	2	2	3	3	7
35–49	203	2.1	2	1	1	2	2	3	4	6
50–64	4	1.8	<1	1	1	2	2	2	2	2
65+	0									
B. Operated										
0–19 Years	31	3.7	6	2	2	3	4	6	7	14
20–34	476	2.9	3	1	2	3	3	4	5	8
35–49	74	3.3	3	2	2	3	3	4	5	12
50–64	5	3.8	<1	3	3	4	4	5	5	5
65+	0									
SUBTOTALS:										
1. SINGLE DX										
A. Not Operated	722	1.6	<1	1	1	1	2	2	3	3
B. Operated	5	2.8	<1	2	2	3	3	4	4	4
2. MULTIPLE DX										
A. Not Operated	2,877	2.0	2	1	1	2	2	3	4	7
B. Operated	586	3.0	3	2	2	3	3	4	5	8
1. SINGLE DX	727	1.6	<1	1	1	1	2	2	3	3
2. MULTIPLE DX	3,463	2.2	3	1	1	2	3	3	4	8
A. NOT OPERATED	3,599	1.9	2	1	1	2	2	3	3	6
B. OPERATED	591	3.0	3	2	2	3	3	4	5	8
TOTAL										
0–19 Years	405	2.2	3	1	1	2	2	3	4	9
20–34	3,482	2.0	2	1	1	2	2	3	4	7
35–49	294	2.4	3	1	1	2	2	4	5	9
50–64	9	2.9	2	2	2	3	3	5	5	5
65+	0									
GRAND TOTAL	4,190	2.1	2	1	1	2	2	3	4	7

Length of Stay by Diagnosis and Operation, Western Region, 2008

534

Western Region, October 2006–September 2007 Data, by Diagnosis

649.01: TOBAC USE COMP PREG-DEL

Type of Patients	Observed Patients	Avg. Stay	Vari- ance	10th	25th	50th	75th	90th	95th	99th
1. SINGLE DX										
A. Not Operated										
0–19 Years	71	1.5	<1	1	1	1	2	2	3	3
20–34	507	1.6	<1	1	1	2	2	2	2	3
35–49	6	1.5	<1	1	1	2	2	2	2	2
50–64	0									
65+	0									
B. Operated										
0–19 Years	0									
20–34	2	2.5	<1	2	2	3	3	3	3	3
35–49	0									
50–64	0									
65+	0									
2. MULTIPLE DX										
A. Not Operated										
0–19 Years	112	1.8	<1	1	1	2	2	2	3	4
20–34	669	1.7	<1	1	1	2	2	2	3	3
35–49	24	1.8	<1	1	1	2	2	3	3	3
50–64	0									
65+	0									
B. Operated										
0–19 Years	4	3.5	6	2	2	3	7	7	7	7
20–34	105	2.1	<1	1	1	2	2	3	4	4
35–49	9	1.9	1	1	1	2	2	4	4	4
50–64	0									
65+	0									
SUBTOTALS:										
1. SINGLE DX										
A. Not Operated	584	1.6	<1	1	1	1	2	2	3	3
B. Operated	2	2.5	<1	2	2	3	3	3	3	3
2. MULTIPLE DX										
A. Not Operated	805	1.7	<1	1	1	2	2	2	3	3
B. Operated	118	2.1	<1	1	2	2	2	3	4	6
1. SINGLE DX	586	1.6	<1	1	1	1	2	2	3	3
2. MULTIPLE DX	923	1.8	<1	1	1	2	2	3	3	4
A. NOT OPERATED	1,389	1.6	<1	1	1	2	2	3	3	3
B. OPERATED	120	2.1	<1	1	2	2	2	3	3	6
TOTAL										
0–19 Years	187	1.7	<1	1	1	2	2	2	3	5
20–34	1,283	1.7	<1	1	1	2	2	2	2	3
35–49	39	1.8	<1	1	1	2	2	3	3	4
50–64	0									
65+	0									
GRAND TOTAL	1,509	1.7	<1	1	1	2	2	2	3	3

649.11: OBESITY COMP PREG-DEL

Type of Patients	Observed Patients	Avg. Stay	Vari- ance	10th	25th	50th	75th	90th	95th	99th
1. SINGLE DX										
A. Not Operated										
0–19 Years	3	1.7	1	1	1	1	3	3	3	3
20–34	29	1.6	<1	1	1	2	2	2	3	3
35–49	0									
50–64	0									
65+	0									
B. Operated										
0–19 Years	0									
20–34	1	2.0	0	2	2	2	2	2	2	2
35–49	0									
50–64	0									
65+	0									
2. MULTIPLE DX										
A. Not Operated										
0–19 Years	48	2.0	<1	1	2	2	3	3	3	4
20–34	634	1.9	<1	1	1	2	2	3	3	4
35–49	30	1.6	<1	1	1	2	2	2	3	3
50–64	1	2.0	0	2	2	2	2	2	2	2
65+	0									
B. Operated										
0–19 Years	7	3.3	<1	2	3	3	3	4	4	4
20–34	142	2.6	<1	2	2	3	3	4	5	5
35–49	14	3.4	<1	2	3	3	4	5	5	5
50–64	1	4.0	0	4	4	4	4	4	4	4
65+	0									
SUBTOTALS:										
1. SINGLE DX										
A. Not Operated	32	1.6	<1	1	1	1	2	3	3	3
B. Operated	1	2.0	0	2	2	2	2	2	2	2
2. MULTIPLE DX										
A. Not Operated	713	1.9	<1	1	1	2	2	3	3	4
B. Operated	164	2.7	<1	2	2	3	3	4	4	5
1. SINGLE DX	33	1.6	<1	1	1	2	2	3	3	3
2. MULTIPLE DX	877	2.0	<1	1	1	2	2	3	4	4
A. NOT OPERATED	745	1.9	<1	1	1	2	2	3	3	4
B. OPERATED	165	2.7	<1	2	2	3	3	4	4	5
TOTAL										
0–19 Years	58	2.2	<1	1	2	2	3	3	3	4
20–34	806	2.0	<1	1	1	2	2	3	3	3
35–49	44	2.2	1	1	2	2	3	3	4	5
50–64	4	3.0	2	2	2	3	4	4	4	4
65+	0									
GRAND TOTAL	910	2.0	<1	1	1	2	2	3	4	4

649.31: COAG DEFECT IN PREG-DEL

Type of Patients	Observed Patients	Avg. Stay	Vari- ance	10th	25th	50th	75th	90th	95th	99th
1. SINGLE DX										
A. Not Operated										
0–19 Years	0									
20–34	1	1.0	0	1	1	1	1	1	1	1
35–49	0									
50–64	0									
65+	0									
B. Operated										
0–19 Years	0									
20–34	1	4.0	0	4	4	4	4	4	4	4
35–49	0									
50–64	0									
65+	0									
2. MULTIPLE DX										
A. Not Operated										
0–19 Years	40	2.7	2	2	2	2	3	4	6	10
20–34	468	2.2	3	1	2	2	3	3	4	6
35–49	63	2.4	3	1	2	2	3	3	4	13
50–64	1	2.0	0	2	2	2	2	2	2	2
65+	0									
B. Operated										
0–19 Years	11	4.2	13	2	2	3	4	7	14	14
20–34	112	3.5	5	2	3	3	4	5	5	11
35–49	31	3.5	2	2	2	3	5	5	5	8
50–64	3	3.3	<1	3	3	3	4	4	4	4
65+	0									
SUBTOTALS:										
1. SINGLE DX										
A. Not Operated	1	1.0	0	1	1	1	1	1	1	1
B. Operated	1	4.0	0	4	4	4	4	4	4	4
2. MULTIPLE DX										
A. Not Operated	572	2.3	3	1	2	2	3	3	4	6
B. Operated	157	3.6	3	2	3	3	4	5	5	11
1. SINGLE DX	2	2.5	4	1	1	3	4	4	4	4
2. MULTIPLE DX	729	2.5	3	1	2	2	3	4	5	10
A. NOT OPERATED	573	2.3	3	1	2	2	3	3	4	6
B. OPERATED	158	3.6	3	2	3	3	4	5	5	11
TOTAL										
0–19 Years	51	3.0	5	2	2	2	3	4	7	14
20–34	582	2.5	3	1	2	2	3	4	4	7
35–49	94	2.7	3	1	2	2	3	4	5	13
50–64	4	3.0	<1	2	2	3	4	4	4	4
65+	0									
GRAND TOTAL	731	2.5	3	1	2	2	3	4	5	10

Length of Stay by Diagnosis and Operation, Western Region, 2008

Western Region, October 2006–September 2007 Data, by Diagnosis

649.41: EPILEPSY IN PREG-DEL

Type of Patients	Observed Patients	Avg. Stay	Variance	10th	25th	50th	75th	90th	95th	99th
1. SINGLE DX										
A. Not Operated										
0–19 Years	0									
20–34	2	2.0	0	2	2	2	2	2	2	2
35–49	0									
50–64	0									
65+	0									
B. Operated										
0–19 Years	0									
20–34	0									
35–49	0									
50–64	0									
65+	0									
2. MULTIPLE DX										
A. Not Operated										
0–19 Years	28	2.9	19	1	2	2	2	4	4	25
20–34	198	2.1	5	1	1	2	2	3	3	8
35–49	20	2.0	<1	1	2	2	3	3	3	3
50–64	1	2.0	0	2	2	2	2	2	2	2
65+	0									
B. Operated										
0–19 Years	9	3.3	2	2	2	3	4	6	6	6
20–34	69	3.5	10	2	2	3	4	5	7	27
35–49	10	2.8	2	2	2	3	3	5	5	5
50–64	0									
65+	0									
SUBTOTALS:										
1. SINGLE DX										
A. Not Operated	2	2.0	0	2	2	2	2	2	2	2
B. Operated	0									
2. MULTIPLE DX										
A. Not Operated	247	2.2	6	1	1	2	2	3	3	8
B. Operated	88	3.4	8	2	2	3	4	5	6	27
1. SINGLE DX	2	2.0	0	2	2	2	2	2	2	2
2. MULTIPLE DX	335	2.5	7	1	2	2	3	4	5	8
A. NOT OPERATED	249	2.2	6	1	1	2	2	3	3	8
B. OPERATED	88	3.4	8	2	2	3	4	5	6	27
TOTAL										
0–19 Years	37	3.0	15	1	2	2	3	4	6	25
20–34	269	2.5	7	1	2	2	3	4	5	8
35–49	30	2.3	1	1	2	2	3	3	5	5
50–64	1	2.0	0	2	2	2	2	2	2	2
65+	0									
GRAND TOTAL	337	2.5	7	1	2	2	3	4	5	8

650: NORMAL DELIVERY

Type of Patients	Observed Patients	Avg. Stay	Variance	10th	25th	50th	75th	90th	95th	99th
1. SINGLE DX										
A. Not Operated										
0–19 Years	6,831	1.8	<1	1	1	2	2	3	3	3
20–34	47,627	1.7	<1	1	1	2	2	2	3	3
35–49	465	1.7	<1	1	1	2	2	2	3	3
50–64	21	1.8	<1	1	2	2	2	2	2	3
65+	0									
B. Operated										
0–19 Years	1	1.0	0	1	1	1	1	1	1	1
20–34	31	2.0	<1	1	2	2	2	3	3	3
35–49	2	2.5	<1	2	2	2	3	3	3	3
50–64	0									
65+	0									
2. MULTIPLE DX										
A. Not Operated										
0–19 Years	601	1.8	<1	1	1	2	2	3	3	3
20–34	3,584	1.6	<1	1	1	2	2	2	3	3
35–49	56	1.8	<1	1	1	2	2	2	3	3
50–64	3	1.7	<1	1	1	2	2	2	2	2
65+	0									
B. Operated										
0–19 Years	0									
20–34	1,974	2.0	<1	1	2	2	2	3	3	4
35–49	63	2.0	<1	1	2	2	2	3	3	3
50–64	4	1.8	<1	2	2	2	2	2	2	2
65+	0									
SUBTOTALS:										
1. SINGLE DX										
A. Not Operated	54,944	1.7	<1	1	1	2	2	2	3	3
B. Operated	34	2.0	<1	1	2	2	2	3	3	3
2. MULTIPLE DX										
A. Not Operated	4,244	1.7	<1	1	1	2	2	2	3	3
B. Operated	2,041	2.0	<1	1	2	2	2	3	3	3
1. SINGLE DX	54,978	1.7	<1	1	1	2	2	2	3	3
2. MULTIPLE DX	6,285	1.8	<1	1	1	2	2	2	3	3
A. NOT OPERATED	59,188	1.7	<1	1	1	2	2	2	3	3
B. OPERATED	2,075	2.0	<1	2	2	2	2	3	3	3
TOTAL										
0–19 Years	7,433	1.8	<1	1	1	2	2	3	3	3
20–34	53,216	1.7	<1	1	1	2	2	2	3	3
35–49	586	1.8	<1	1	1	2	2	2	3	3
50–64	28	1.8	<1	1	1	2	2	2	2	3
65+	0									
GRAND TOTAL	61,263	1.7	<1	1	1	2	2	2	3	3

651: MULTIPLE GESTATION

Type of Patients	Observed Patients	Avg. Stay	Variance	10th	25th	50th	75th	90th	95th	99th
1. SINGLE DX										
A. Not Operated										
0–19 Years	7	2.4	3	1	1	2	3	6	6	6
20–34	107	2.0	1	1	2	2	2	3	3	4
35–49	9	1.8	<1	1	1	2	2	3	3	3
50–64	0									
65+	0									
B. Operated										
0–19 Years	10	3.2	<1	2	3	3	4	4	4	4
20–34	130	3.2	<1	2	3	3	4	4	4	4
35–49	2	2.5	<1	2	2	3	3	3	3	3
50–64	0									
65+	0									
2. MULTIPLE DX										
A. Not Operated										
0–19 Years	63	2.9	5	1	2	2	3	5	6	16
20–34	927	3.1	22	1	2	2	3	4	7	22
35–49	278	3.2	19	1	2	2	3	4	7	27
50–64	12	3.1	3	2	2	2	4	4	8	8
65+	0									
B. Operated										
0–19 Years	120	5.7	55	2	3	3	4	10	25	39
20–34	1,648	4.5	28	2	3	3	4	6	9	36
35–49	681	5.0	41	3	3	4	4	6	12	41
50–64	40	6.7	187	3	4	4	4	8	10	88
65+	0									
SUBTOTALS:										
1. SINGLE DX										
A. Not Operated	123	2.0	1	1	1	2	2	2	3	6
B. Operated	142	3.2	<1	2	3	3	4	4	4	4
2. MULTIPLE DX										
A. Not Operated	1,280	3.1	21	1	2	2	3	4	7	24
B. Operated	2,489	4.7	35	2	3	4	4	6	10	38
1. SINGLE DX	265	2.6	1	1	2	3	3	4	4	5
2. MULTIPLE DX	3,769	4.2	31	2	2	3	3	5	9	34
A. NOT OPERATED	1,403	3.0	19	1	2	2	3	4	6	20
B. OPERATED	2,631	4.7	34	2	3	4	4	6	10	36
TOTAL										
0–19 Years	200	4.6	37	2	2	3	4	6	14	39
20–34	2,812	3.9	24	2	2	3	4	5	8	32
35–49	970	4.5	35	2	3	3	4	5	11	31
50–64	52	5.9	146	2	3	4	4	7	10	88
65+	0									
GRAND TOTAL	4,034	4.1	29	2	2	3	4	5	9	33

Length of Stay by Diagnosis and Operation, Western Region, 2008

651.01: TWIN PREGNANCY-DELIVERED

Type of Patients	Observed Patients	Avg. Stay	Vari-ance	Percentiles 10th	25th	50th	75th	90th	95th	99th
1. SINGLE DX										
A. Not Operated										
0–19 Years	6	2.7	3	1	2	2	3	6	6	6
20–34	90	2.0	<1	1	2	2	2	3	3	4
35–49	6	2.0	<1	1	2	2	2	3	3	3
50–64	0									
65+	0									
B. Operated										
0–19 Years	10	3.2	<1	2	3	3	4	4	4	4
20–34	129	3.2	<1	2	3	3	4	4	4	4
35–49	2	2.5	<1	2	2	3	3	3	3	3
50–64	0									
65+	0									
2. MULTIPLE DX										
A. Not Operated										
0–19 Years	43	3.0	3	2	2	2	2	5	6	9
20–34	691	2.9	18	2	2	2	2	3	4	17
35–49	203	3.1	19	2	2	2	3	4	5	24
50–64	8	3.4	4	2	2	3	3	8	8	8
65+	0									
B. Operated										
0–19 Years	115	5.7	54	2	3	3	4	10	23	39
20–34	1,514	4.2	20	2	3	3	4	5	7	30
35–49	611	4.5	24	2	3	3	4	5	9	26
50–64	31	4.8	15	3	4	4	4	5	8	25
65+	0									
SUBTOTALS:										
1. SINGLE DX										
A. Not Operated	102	2.1	<1	1	2	2	2	3	3	4
B. Operated	141	3.2	<1	2	3	3	4	4	4	4
2. MULTIPLE DX										
A. Not Operated	945	2.9	17	2	2	2	3	4	5	17
B. Operated	2,271	4.4	23	2	3	3	4	5	8	31
1. SINGLE DX	243	2.7	<1	2	2	3	3	4	4	4
2. MULTIPLE DX	3,216	3.9	22	2	2	3	4	5	7	28
A. NOT OPERATED	1,047	2.8	16	2	2	2	3	3	4	13
B. OPERATED	2,412	4.3	22	2	3	4	4	5	8	30
TOTAL										
0–19 Years	174	4.7	38	2	3	3	4	6	12	39
20–34	2,424	3.7	18	2	2	3	4	4	6	26
35–49	822	4.1	23	2	3	3	4	5	7	26
50–64	39	4.5	13	2	3	4	4	7	8	25
65+	0									
GRAND TOTAL	3,459	3.9	21	2	2	3	4	5	7	27

652: MALPOSITION OF FETUS

Type of Patients	Observed Patients	Avg. Stay	Vari-ance	Percentiles 10th	25th	50th	75th	90th	95th	99th
1. SINGLE DX										
A. Not Operated										
0–19 Years	73	1.7	<1	1	1	2	2	2	3	4
20–34	646	1.7	<1	1	1	2	2	2	3	4
35–49	28	1.5	<1	1	1	2	2	2	2	3
50–64	3	1.7	<1	1	1	2	2	2	2	2
65+	0									
B. Operated										
0–19 Years	397	2.8	<1	2	2	3	3	4	4	5
20–34	3,824	3.0	<1	2	2	3	3	4	4	5
35–49	207	3.0	<1	2	2	3	4	4	4	5
50–64	9	3.3	<1	2	3	4	4	4	4	4
65+	0									
2. MULTIPLE DX										
A. Not Operated										
0–19 Years	310	2.1	<1	1	2	2	2	3	3	4
20–34	2,434	2.0	2	1	1	2	2	3	3	4
35–49	455	2.0	2	1	1	2	2	3	3	4
50–64	19	2.2	<1	1	2	2	2	3	5	5
65+	0									
B. Operated										
0–19 Years	1,261	3.6	11	2	3	3	3	4	5	14
20–34	13,343	3.5	7	2	3	3	4	4	5	12
35–49	4,702	3.6	8	2	3	3	4	4	5	14
50–64	275	4.0	29	2	3	3	4	4	5	30
65+	0									
SUBTOTALS:										
1. SINGLE DX										
A. Not Operated	750	1.7	<1	1	1	2	2	2	3	4
B. Operated	4,437	3.0	<1	2	2	3	3	4	4	5
2. MULTIPLE DX										
A. Not Operated	3,218	2.0	2	1	1	2	2	3	3	4
B. Operated	19,581	3.5	8	2	3	3	4	4	5	13
1. SINGLE DX	5,187	2.8	<1	2	2	3	3	4	4	5
2. MULTIPLE DX	22,799	3.3	7	2	2	3	4	4	5	11
A. NOT OPERATED	3,968	1.9	1	1	1	2	2	3	3	4
B. OPERATED	24,018	3.4	6	2	3	3	4	4	5	10
TOTAL										
0–19 Years	2,041	3.1	7	2	2	3	3	4	5	8
20–34	20,247	3.1	5	2	2	3	4	4	5	9
35–49	5,392	3.4	8	2	3	3	4	5	5	12
50–64	306	3.8	26	2	3	3	4	4	5	28
65+	0									
GRAND TOTAL	27,986	3.2	6	2	2	3	4	4	5	9

652.01: UNSTABLE LIE-DELIVERED

Type of Patients	Observed Patients	Avg. Stay	Vari-ance	Percentiles 10th	25th	50th	75th	90th	95th	99th
1. SINGLE DX										
A. Not Operated										
0–19 Years	0									
20–34	14	2.0	<1	1	2	2	2	3	3	3
35–49	2	1.0	0	1	1	1	1	1	1	1
50–64	0									
65+	0									
B. Operated										
0–19 Years	2	3.0	0	3	3	3	3	3	3	3
20–34	16	3.1	<1	2	3	3	3	4	4	4
35–49	0									
50–64	0									
65+	0									
2. MULTIPLE DX										
A. Not Operated										
0–19 Years	3	2.7	<1	2	2	3	3	3	3	3
20–34	107	2.1	<1	1	2	2	2	3	3	4
35–49	35	2.3	<1	1	2	2	3	4	4	4
50–64	0									
65+	0									
B. Operated										
0–19 Years	8	2.6	<1	2	2	3	3	4	4	4
20–34	115	3.5	23	2	2	3	4	4	5	7
35–49	57	3.2	2	2	2	3	4	4	5	9
50–64	3	3.7	<1	3	3	4	4	4	4	4
65+	0									
SUBTOTALS:										
1. SINGLE DX										
A. Not Operated	16	1.9	<1	1	1	2	2	3	3	3
B. Operated	18	3.1	<1	2	3	3	3	4	4	4
2. MULTIPLE DX										
A. Not Operated	145	2.1	<1	1	2	2	2	3	3	4
B. Operated	183	3.4	15	2	2	3	4	4	5	9
1. SINGLE DX	34	2.5	<1	1	2	3	3	3	4	4
2. MULTIPLE DX	328	2.8	9	2	2	2	3	4	4	6
A. NOT OPERATED	161	2.1	<1	1	2	2	2	3	3	4
B. OPERATED	201	3.3	14	2	2	3	4	4	5	7
TOTAL										
0–19 Years	13	2.7	<1	2	2	3	3	3	4	4
20–34	252	2.8	11	2	2	2	3	4	4	6
35–49	94	2.8	1	2	3	3	3	4	5	9
50–64	3	3.7	<1	3	3	4	4	4	4	4
65+	0									
GRAND TOTAL	362	2.8	8	2	2	2	3	4	4	6

Length of Stay by Diagnosis and Operation, Western Region, 2008

Western Region, October 2006–September 2007 Data, by Diagnosis

652.11: CEPHALIC VERSION-DEL

Type of Patients	Observed Patients	Avg. Stay	Variance	10th	25th	50th	75th	90th	95th	99th
1. SINGLE DX										
A. Not Operated										
0–19 Years	3	2.3	<1	2	2	2	3	3	3	3
20–34	35	1.7	<1	1	1	2	2	2	3	4
35–49	4	2.0	0	2	2	2	2	2	2	2
50–64	0									
65+	0									
B. Operated										
0–19 Years	0									
20–34	8	2.8	1	1	2	3	4	4	4	4
35–49	0									
50–64	0									
65+	0									
2. MULTIPLE DX										
A. Not Operated										
0–19 Years	18	2.1	<1	1	1	2	3	3	4	4
20–34	186	2.0	<1	1	1	2	2	3	4	4
35–49	60	2.1	<1	1	2	2	3	3	4	4
50–64	2	1.5	<1	1	1	2	2	2	2	2
65+	0									
B. Operated										
0–19 Years	5	10.2	208	3	4	4	4	36	36	36
20–34	53	3.2	1	2	2	3	4	4	5	8
35–49	24	3.1	1	2	2	3	4	4	5	6
50–64	4	2.8	<1	2	2	3	3	3	3	3
65+	0									
SUBTOTALS:										
1. SINGLE DX										
A. Not Operated	42	1.8	<1	1	1	2	2	2	2	2
B. Operated	8	2.8	1	1	2	3	3	4	4	4
2. MULTIPLE DX										
A. Not Operated	266	2.0	<1	1	1	2	2	2	3	4
B. Operated	86	3.5	14	2	2	3	4	4	5	36
1. SINGLE DX	50	1.9	<1	1	1	2	2	3	4	4
2. MULTIPLE DX	352	2.4	4	1	2	2	3	4	4	6
A. NOT OPERATED	308	2.0	<1	1	1	2	2	3	4	4
B. OPERATED	94	3.5	13	2	2	3	3	4	5	36
TOTAL										
0–19 Years	26	3.7	44	1	2	2	3	4	4	36
20–34	282	2.2	1	1	2	2	3	4	4	6
35–49	88	2.4	1	1	2	2	3	4	4	6
50–64	6	2.3	<1	1	2	2	3	3	3	3
65+	0									
GRAND TOTAL	402	2.3	4	1	2	2	3	4	4	6

652.21: BREECH PRESENTATION-DEL

Type of Patients	Observed Patients	Avg. Stay	Variance	10th	25th	50th	75th	90th	95th	99th
1. SINGLE DX										
A. Not Operated										
0–19 Years	7	1.6	<1	1	1	2	2	2	2	2
20–34	37	1.9	<1	1	1	2	2	3	4	4
35–49	0									
50–64	0									
65+	0									
B. Operated										
0–19 Years	291	2.8	<1	2	2	3	3	4	4	5
20–34	2,841	2.9	<1	2	2	3	3	4	4	4
35–49	134	2.9	<1	2	2	3	3	4	4	4
50–64	5	3.4	<1	2	3	4	4	4	4	4
65+	0									
2. MULTIPLE DX										
A. Not Operated										
0–19 Years	11	1.5	<1	1	1	2	2	3	4	4
20–34	162	2.0	2	1	1	2	2	3	4	6
35–49	38	2.1	<1	1	2	2	3	3	4	4
50–64	0	1.0	0	1	1	1	1	1	1	1
65+	0									
B. Operated										
0–19 Years	650	3.5	15	2	2	3	3	4	5	13
20–34	7,135	3.2	4	2	3	3	4	4	5	9
35–49	2,596	3.4	6	2	3	3	4	4	5	11
50–64	162	3.7	11	2	3	3	4	4	4	28
65+	0									
SUBTOTALS:										
1. SINGLE DX										
A. Not Operated	44	1.9	<1	1	1	2	2	2	3	4
B. Operated	3,271	2.9	<1	2	2	3	3	4	4	4
2. MULTIPLE DX										
A. Not Operated	212	2.0	2	1	1	2	2	3	4	5
B. Operated	10,543	3.3	6	2	3	3	4	4	5	9
1. SINGLE DX	3,315	2.9	<1	2	2	3	3	4	4	4
2. MULTIPLE DX	10,755	3.3	6	2	3	3	4	4	5	9
A. NOT OPERATED	256	2.0	1	1	1	2	2	3	4	5
B. OPERATED	13,814	3.2	4	2	3	3	4	4	4	8
TOTAL										
0–19 Years	959	3.2	11	2	2	3	3	4	4	9
20–34	10,175	3.1	3	2	2	3	3	4	4	7
35–49	2,768	3.4	6	2	3	3	4	4	4	10
50–64	168	3.6	11	2	3	3	4	4	4	28
65+	0									
GRAND TOTAL	14,070	3.2	4	2	2	3	3	4	4	8

652.31: TRANS/OBLIQUE LIE-DEL

Type of Patients	Observed Patients	Avg. Stay	Variance	10th	25th	50th	75th	90th	95th	99th
1. SINGLE DX										
A. Not Operated										
0–19 Years	4	1.3	<1	1	1	1	2	2	2	2
20–34	40	1.8	<1	1	1	2	2	3	3	3
35–49	1	1.0	0	1	1	1	1	1	1	1
50–64	0									
65+	0									
B. Operated										
0–19 Years	7	2.9	<1	2	2	3	3	4	4	4
20–34	121	3.0	<1	2	3	3	3	4	4	5
35–49	15	2.8	<1	2	3	3	4	4	4	4
50–64	0	3.5		3	3	4	4	4	4	4
65+	0									
2. MULTIPLE DX										
A. Not Operated										
0–19 Years	17	1.9	<1	1	1	2	2	3	3	3
20–34	117	2.0	<1	1	2	2	2	3	3	4
35–49	23	1.8	<1	1	1	2	2	3	3	4
50–64	0	3.0	0	3	3	3	3	3	3	3
65+	0									
B. Operated										
0–19 Years	55	3.2	<1	2	3	3	3	4	4	5
20–34	726	3.4	5	2	3	3	4	4	5	10
35–49	372	3.3	2	2	3	3	4	4	4	9
50–64	20	3.5	2	2	3	3	4	5	5	7
65+	0									
SUBTOTALS:										
1. SINGLE DX										
A. Not Operated	45	1.7	<1	1	1	2	2	3	3	3
B. Operated	145	2.9	<1	2	2	3	3	4	4	5
2. MULTIPLE DX										
A. Not Operated	158	2.0	<1	1	1	2	2	3	3	4
B. Operated	1,173	3.4	4	2	3	3	4	4	5	9
1. SINGLE DX	190	2.7	<1	1	2	3	3	4	4	5
2. MULTIPLE DX	1,331	3.2	3	2	3	3	4	4	5	9
A. NOT OPERATED	203	1.9	<1	1	1	2	2	3	3	4
B. OPERATED	1,318	3.3	3	2	3	3	4	4	5	9
TOTAL										
0–19 Years	83	2.8	<1	2	2	3	3	4	4	5
20–34	1,004	3.1	4	2	2	3	4	4	5	9
35–49	411	3.2	2	2	3	3	4	4	5	8
50–64	23	3.4	1	2	3	3	4	5	5	7
65+	0									
GRAND TOTAL	1,521	3.1	3	2	2	3	4	4	5	9

Length of Stay by Diagnosis and Operation, Western Region, 2008

Western Region, October 2006–September 2007 Data, by Diagnosis

652.41: FACE/BROW PRESENT-DEL

Type of Patients	Observed Patients	Avg. Stay	Vari-ance	Percentiles						
				10th	25th	50th	75th	90th	95th	99th
1. SINGLE DX										
A. Not Operated										
0–19 Years	1	2.0	0	2	2	2	2	2	2	2
20–34	22	1.6	<1	1	1	2	2	2	2	3
35–49	0									
50–64	0									
65+	0									
B. Operated										
0–19 Years	9	2.7	<1	2	2	3	3	4	4	4
20–34	18	3.2	<1	2	3	3	4	5	5	5
35–49	4	3.3	<1	2	2	3	4	4	4	4
50–64	0									
65+	0									
2. MULTIPLE DX										
A. Not Operated										
0–19 Years	7	1.9	<1	1	2	2	2	2	2	2
20–34	61	1.8	<1	1	1	2	2	3	3	3
35–49	8	1.6	<1	1	1	1	2	3	3	3
50–64	2	2.0	0	2	2	2	2	2	2	2
65+	0									
B. Operated										
0–19 Years	17	3.4	2	2	3	3	4	4	8	8
20–34	132	3.1	<1	2	3	3	4	4	4	5
35–49	35	3.0	<1	2	2	3	4	4	4	5
50–64	2	3.0	2	2	2	2	4	4	4	4
65+	0									
SUBTOTALS:										
1. SINGLE DX										
A. Not Operated	23	1.7	<1	1	2	2	2	2	2	2
B. Operated	31	3.1	<1	2	2	3	3	4	5	5
2. MULTIPLE DX										
A. Not Operated	78	1.8	<1	1	1	2	2	3	3	3
B. Operated	186	3.1	1	2	2	3	4	4	4	8
1. SINGLE DX	54	2.5	1	1	2	2	3	4	4	5
2. MULTIPLE DX	264	2.7	1	1	2	3	3	4	4	5
A. NOT OPERATED	101	1.8	<1	1	1	2	2	3	3	3
B. OPERATED	217	3.1	<1	2	2	3	4	4	4	5
TOTAL										
0–19 Years	34	2.9	2	2	2	3	3	4	4	8
20–34	233	2.6	1	1	2	3	3	4	4	5
35–49	47	2.8	1	1	2	3	4	4	4	5
50–64	4	2.5	<1	2	2	3	2	4	4	4
65+	0									
GRAND TOTAL	318	2.7	1	1	2	3	3	4	4	5

652.51: HIGH HEAD AT TERM-DEL

Type of Patients	Observed Patients	Avg. Stay	Vari-ance	Percentiles						
				10th	25th	50th	75th	90th	95th	99th
1. SINGLE DX										
A. Not Operated										
0–19 Years	3	2.7	1	2	2	2	4	4	4	4
20–34	30	2.2	<1	1	2	2	3	3	4	4
35–49	1	2.0	0	2	2	2	2	2	2	2
50–64	0									
65+	0									
B. Operated										
0–19 Years	28	3.3	<1	3	3	3	4	4	4	5
20–34	211	3.5	<1	3	3	3	4	4	5	5
35–49	17	3.5	<1	2	3	3	4	5	5	5
50–64	1	4.0	0	4	4	4	4	4	4	4
65+	0									
2. MULTIPLE DX										
A. Not Operated										
0–19 Years	29	2.3	<1	1	2	2	3	4	4	4
20–34	223	2.2	<1	1	2	2	3	3	3	4
35–49	41	2.3	<1	1	2	2	3	3	3	5
50–64	0									
65+	0									
B. Operated										
0–19 Years	277	3.7	<1	3	3	4	4	5	5	7
20–34	2,133	3.7	1	3	3	4	4	5	5	6
35–49	496	3.8	1	3	3	4	4	5	5	7
50–64	22	3.8	<1	3	3	4	4	5	5	5
65+	0									
SUBTOTALS:										
1. SINGLE DX										
A. Not Operated	34	2.2	<1	1	2	2	3	3	4	4
B. Operated	257	3.5	<1	3	3	3	4	4	5	5
2. MULTIPLE DX										
A. Not Operated	293	2.3	<1	1	2	2	3	3	3	5
B. Operated	2,928	3.7	1	3	3	4	4	5	5	6
1. SINGLE DX	291	3.3	<1	2	3	3	4	4	5	5
2. MULTIPLE DX	3,221	3.6	1	2	3	4	4	5	5	6
A. NOT OPERATED	327	2.2	<1	1	2	2	3	3	4	4
B. OPERATED	3,185	3.7	<1	3	3	4	4	5	5	6
TOTAL										
0–19 Years	337	3.5	<1	2	3	3	4	5	5	7
20–34	2,597	3.5	1	2	3	3	4	5	6	6
35–49	555	3.7	1	2	3	4	4	5	5	6
50–64	23	3.8	<1	3	3	4	4	5	5	5
65+	0									
GRAND TOTAL	3,512	3.5	1	2	3	3	4	5	5	6

652.61: MULT GEST MALPRESENT-DEL

Type of Patients	Observed Patients	Avg. Stay	Vari-ance	Percentiles						
				10th	25th	50th	75th	90th	95th	99th
1. SINGLE DX										
A. Not Operated										
0–19 Years	1	2.0	0	2	2	2	2	2	2	2
20–34	17	2.0	<1	2	2	2	2	2	3	3
35–49	1	2.0	0	2	2	2	2	2	2	2
50–64	0									
65+	0									
B. Operated										
0–19 Years	19	2.8	<1	2	3	3	3	4	5	5
20–34	187	3.3	<1	2	3	3	4	4	4	5
35–49	12	3.4	<1	2	3	4	4	4	5	5
50–64	0									
65+	0									
2. MULTIPLE DX										
A. Not Operated										
0–19 Years	12	3.1	2	2	2	3	3	5	5	5
20–34	158	2.6	4	1	2	2	3	4	4	10
35–49	40	2.9	12	1	2	3	3	4	4	24
50–64	0									
65+	0									
B. Operated										
0–19 Years	94	4.0	9	2	3	3	4	5	7	24
20–34	1,550	4.5	27	2	3	4	4	5	9	30
35–49	620	4.8	29	3	3	4	4	5	9	30
50–64	39	6.2	152	3	3	4	4	5	30	77
65+	0									
SUBTOTALS:										
1. SINGLE DX										
A. Not Operated	19	2.0	<1	2	2	2	2	2	3	3
B. Operated	218	3.2	<1	2	3	3	4	4	4	5
2. MULTIPLE DX										
A. Not Operated	214	2.7	6	1	2	3	3	4	4	10
B. Operated	2,303	4.6	29	2	3	4	4	5	9	30
1. SINGLE DX	237	3.1	<1	2	3	3	4	4	4	5
2. MULTIPLE DX	2,517	4.4	27	2	3	4	4	5	9	30
A. NOT OPERATED	233	2.6	5	1	2	3	3	4	4	10
B. OPERATED	2,521	4.5	27	2	3	4	4	5	8	30
TOTAL										
0–19 Years	126	3.7	7	2	3	3	4	5	7	18
20–34	1,912	4.2	23	2	3	3	4	5	8	28
35–49	673	4.7	28	2	3	4	4	5	8	30
50–64	43	5.9	138	3	3	4	4	5	5	77
65+	0									
GRAND TOTAL	2,754	4.3	25	2	3	3	4	5	8	29

Length of Stay by Diagnosis and Operation, Western Region, 2008

Western Region, October 2006–September 2007 Data, by Diagnosis

652.81: MALPOSITION NEC-DEL

Type of Patients	Observed Patients	Avg. Stay	Variance	10th	25th	50th	75th	90th	95th	99th
1. SINGLE DX										
A. Not Operated										
0–19 Years	42	1.8	<1	1	1	2	2	2	2	3
20–34	366	1.7	<1	1	1	2	2	2	2	3
35–49	14	1.6	<1	1	1	1	2	2	2	3
50–64	3	1.7	<1	1	1	2	2	2	2	2
65+	0									
B. Operated										
0–19 Years	41	2.8	<1	2	2	3	3	3	3	5
20–34	414	2.9	<1	2	2	3	3	4	4	5
35–49	23	3.0	<1	2	2	3	3	3	4	4
50–64	1	2.0	0	2	2	2	2	2	2	2
65+	0									
2. MULTIPLE DX										
A. Not Operated										
0–19 Years	196	2.1	<1	1	2	2	2	2	3	4
20–34	1,278	1.9	<1	1	1	2	2	3	3	4
35–49	167	1.8	<1	1	1	2	2	2	3	4
50–64	8	2.0	0	2	2	2	2	2	2	2
65+	0									
B. Operated										
0–19 Years	154	3.5	9	2	2	3	3	5	7	23
20–34	1,460	3.3	5	2	2	3	4	4	5	14
35–49	494	3.3	3	2	2	3	4	4	4	10
50–64	23	3.4	2	3	3	3	4	4	5	8
65+	0									
SUBTOTALS:										
1. SINGLE DX										
A. Not Operated	425	1.7	<1	1	1	2	2	2	3	3
B. Operated	479	2.9	<1	2	2	3	3	3	4	5
2. MULTIPLE DX										
A. Not Operated	1,649	1.9	<1	1	1	2	2	3	3	4
B. Operated	2,131	3.3	5	2	2	3	4	4	5	13
1. SINGLE DX	904	2.3	<1	1	2	2	3	3	4	4
2. MULTIPLE DX	3,780	2.7	3	2	2	2	3	4	4	9
A. NOT OPERATED	2,074	1.8	<1	1	2	2	2	3	3	4
B. OPERATED	2,610	3.2	4	2	2	3	4	4	5	11
TOTAL										
0–19 Years	433	2.6	4	1	2	2	3	4	4	9
20–34	3,518	2.6	3	2	2	2	3	4	4	7
35–49	698	2.9	2	2	2	3	3	4	4	9
50–64	35	2.9	2	2	2	3	3	4	5	8
65+	0									
GRAND TOTAL	4,684	2.6	3	2	2	2	3	4	4	7

653: DISPROPORTION

Type of Patients	Observed Patients	Avg. Stay	Variance	10th	25th	50th	75th	90th	95th	99th
1. SINGLE DX										
A. Not Operated										
0–19 Years	6	1.8	<1	1	1	2	2	3	3	3
20–34	28	1.8	<1	1	1	2	2	3	3	3
35–49	2	4.5	4	3	3	3	6	6	6	6
50–64	0									
65+	0									
B. Operated										
0–19 Years	82	3.1	<1	3	3	3	3	4	4	6
20–34	534	3.2	<1	2	3	3	4	4	4	5
35–49	27	3.6	1	2	3	3	4	5	5	5
50–64	0									
65+	0									
2. MULTIPLE DX										
A. Not Operated										
0–19 Years	14	2.5	<1	2	2	2	3	4	4	4
20–34	148	2.2	2	1	1	2	3	3	4	5
35–49	25	2.9	7	2	2	3	3	4	6	15
50–64	0	3.0	0	3	3	3	3	3	3	3
65+	0									
B. Operated										
0–19 Years	538	3.5	1	2	3	3	4	5	5	8
20–34	3,504	3.5	2	2	3	3	4	5	5	6
35–49	720	3.6	<1	3	3	3	4	5	5	6
50–64	37	3.7	1	3	3	4	4	5	6	7
65+	0									
SUBTOTALS:										
1. SINGLE DX										
A. Not Operated	36	2.0	1	1	1	2	2	3	3	3
B. Operated	643	3.2	<1	3	3	3	4	4	4	5
2. MULTIPLE DX										
A. Not Operated	188	2.3	3	1	2	2	3	3	4	4
B. Operated	4,799	3.5	2	2	3	3	4	5	5	6
1. SINGLE DX	679	3.1	<1	2	3	3	4	4	4	5
2. MULTIPLE DX	4,987	3.5	2	2	3	3	4	5	5	6
A. NOT OPERATED	224	2.2	2	1	1	2	3	3	4	6
B. OPERATED	5,442	3.5	2	2	3	3	4	5	5	6
TOTAL										
0–19 Years	640	3.4	1	2	3	3	4	5	5	7
20–34	4,214	3.4	2	2	3	3	4	5	5	6
35–49	774	3.5	1	2	3	3	4	4	5	6
50–64	38	3.7	<1	3	3	4	4	5	6	7
65+	0									
GRAND TOTAL	5,666	3.4	2	2	3	3	4	5	5	6

653.41: FPD-DELIVERED

Type of Patients	Observed Patients	Avg. Stay	Variance	10th	25th	50th	75th	90th	95th	99th
1. SINGLE DX										
A. Not Operated										
0–19 Years	2	1.5	<1	1	1	2	2	2	2	2
20–34	10	1.9	<1	1	1	2	2	3	3	3
35–49	0									
50–64	0									
65+	0									
B. Operated										
0–19 Years	66	3.1	<1	3	3	3	4	4	4	6
20–34	413	3.2	<1	3	3	3	4	4	4	5
35–49	23	3.7	1	3	3	3	5	5	5	5
50–64	0									
65+	0									
2. MULTIPLE DX										
A. Not Operated										
0–19 Years	6	2.8	1	1	1	3	4	4	4	4
20–34	40	2.3	<1	1	2	2	3	3	3	5
35–49	11	2.4	<1	2	2	2	3	3	4	4
50–64	0	3.0	0	3	3	3	3	3	3	3
65+										
B. Operated										
0–19 Years	492	3.5	1	2	3	3	4	5	5	8
20–34	3,009	3.5	1	2	3	3	4	5	5	6
35–49	574	3.6	<1	3	3	4	4	5	5	6
50–64	31	3.8	1	3	3	4	4	5	6	7
65+	0									
SUBTOTALS:										
1. SINGLE DX										
A. Not Operated	12	1.8	<1	1	1	2	2	2	3	3
B. Operated	502	3.2	<1	3	3	3	4	4	5	5
2. MULTIPLE DX										
A. Not Operated	58	2.4	<1	1	2	2	3	3	4	5
B. Operated	4,106	3.5	1	2	3	3	4	5	5	6
1. SINGLE DX	514	3.2	<1	2	3	3	4	4	5	5
2. MULTIPLE DX	4,164	3.5	1	2	3	3	4	5	5	6
A. NOT OPERATED	70	2.3	<1	1	2	2	3	3	4	5
B. OPERATED	4,608	3.5	<1	2	3	3	4	5	5	6
TOTAL										
0–19 Years	566	3.5	1	2	3	3	4	5	5	8
20–34	3,472	3.5	<1	2	3	3	4	5	5	6
35–49	608	3.6	<1	2	3	3	4	5	5	6
50–64	32	3.8	1	3	3	3	4	5	6	7
65+	0									
GRAND TOTAL	4,678	3.5	1	2	3	3	4	5	5	6

Western Region, October 2006–September 2007 Data, by Diagnosis

653.51: FPD LARGE FETUS-DEL

Type of Patients	Observed Patients	Avg. Stay	Vari-ance	10th	25th	50th	75th	90th	95th	99th
1. SINGLE DX										
A. Not Operated										
0–19 Years	0									
20–34	10	1.7	<1	1	1	2	2	2	2	2
35–49	0									
50–64	0									
65+	0									
B. Operated										
0–19 Years	9	2.8	<1	2	3	3	3	3	3	3
20–34	79	2.9	<1	2	2	3	3	4	4	5
35–49	2	3.5	<1	3	3	3	4	4	4	4
50–64	0									
65+	0									
2. MULTIPLE DX										
A. Not Operated										
0–19 Years	4	2.0	0	2	2	2	2	2	2	2
20–34	56	2.0	<1	1	1	2	2	3	4	5
35–49	7	1.9	<1	1	1	2	3	3	3	3
50–64	0									
65+	0									
B. Operated										
0–19 Years	23	3.1	<1	2	3	3	4	4	4	5
20–34	321	3.1	<1	2	2	3	3	4	4	5
35–49	92	3.2	<1	2	3	3	4	4	5	5
50–64	5	3.2	<1	3	3	3	4	4	4	4
65+	0									
SUBTOTALS:										
1. SINGLE DX										
A. Not Operated	10	1.7	<1	1	1	2	2	2	2	2
B. Operated	90	2.9	<1	2	2	3	3	4	4	5
2. MULTIPLE DX										
A. Not Operated	67	2.0	<1	1	1	2	2	3	3	5
B. Operated	441	3.1	<1	2	3	3	4	4	4	5
1. SINGLE DX	100	2.8	<1	2	2	3	3	4	4	4
2. MULTIPLE DX	508	3.0	<1	2	3	3	4	4	4	5
A. NOT OPERATED	77	1.9	<1	1	1	2	2	3	3	5
B. OPERATED	531	3.1	<1	2	3	3	4	4	4	5
TOTAL										
0–19 Years	36	2.9	<1	2	2	3	3	4	4	5
20–34	466	2.9	<1	2	2	3	3	4	4	5
35–49	101	3.1	<1	2	3	3	4	4	5	5
50–64	5	3.2	<1	2	3	3	4	4	4	4
65+	0									
GRAND TOTAL	608	2.9	<1	2	2	3	3	4	4	5

654: ABN PELVIC ORGAN IN PREG

Type of Patients	Observed Patients	Avg. Stay	Vari-ance	10th	25th	50th	75th	90th	95th	99th
1. SINGLE DX										
A. Not Operated										
0–19 Years	43	3.4	17	1	1	2	3	8	10	20
20–34	1,047	2.0	10	1	1	2	2	3	3	10
35–49	84	1.8	1	1	1	2	2	3	3	8
50–64	1	2.0	0	2	2	2	2	2	2	2
65+	0									
B. Operated										
0–19 Years	856	2.7	<1	2	2	3	3	4	4	4
20–34	20,876	2.7	<1	2	2	3	3	4	4	4
35–49	1,177	2.8	<1	2	2	3	3	4	4	5
50–64	55	2.9	<1	2	2	3	3	4	4	6
65+	0									
2. MULTIPLE DX										
A. Not Operated										
0–19 Years	234	3.4	56	1	1	2	3	4	9	37
20–34	4,636	2.6	30	1	1	2	2	3	4	29
35–49	1,245	3.0	46	1	1	2	2	3	5	44
50–64	64	4.3	144	1	1	2	2	4	11	92
65+	0									
B. Operated										
0–19 Years	1,412	3.0	11	2	2	3	3	4	4	7
20–34	54,032	2.9	3	2	2	3	3	4	4	6
35–49	20,807	3.0	3	2	2	3	3	4	4	6
50–64	1,211	3.3	8	2	3	3	4	4	4	6
65+	0									
SUBTOTALS:										
1. SINGLE DX										
A. Not Operated	1,175	2.0	10	1	1	2	2	3	3	11
B. Operated	22,964	2.7	<1	2	2	3	3	4	4	4
2. MULTIPLE DX										
A. Not Operated	6,179	2.8	35	1	1	2	3	3	4	35
B. Operated	77,462	2.9	3	2	2	3	3	4	4	6
1. SINGLE DX	24,139	2.7	1	2	2	3	3	4	4	4
2. MULTIPLE DX	83,641	2.9	5	2	2	3	3	4	4	6
A. NOT OPERATED	7,354	2.6	31	1	1	2	2	3	4	30
B. OPERATED	100,426	2.9	2	2	2	3	3	4	4	5
TOTAL										
0–19 Years	2,545	2.9	12	2	2	3	3	4	4	9
20–34	80,591	2.8	4	2	2	3	3	4	4	6
35–49	23,313	3.0	5	2	2	3	3	4	4	6
50–64	1,331	3.3	14	2	2	3	4	4	4	7
65+	0									
GRAND TOTAL	107,780	2.9	4	2	2	3	3	4	4	6

654.11: UTERINE TUMOR-DELIVERED

Type of Patients	Observed Patients	Avg. Stay	Vari-ance	10th	25th	50th	75th	90th	95th	99th
1. SINGLE DX										
A. Not Operated										
0–19 Years	2	2.5	<1	2	2	2	2	3	3	3
20–34	12	1.7	<1	1	1	2	2	2	3	3
35–49	0									
50–64	0									
65+	0									
B. Operated										
0–19 Years	0									
20–34	3	3.0	<1	2	2	3		4	4	4
35–49	0									
50–64	0									
65+	0									
2. MULTIPLE DX										
A. Not Operated										
0–19 Years	5	2.0	<1	1	2	2	2	3	3	3
20–34	130	1.9	<1	1	1	2	2	3	3	4
35–49	45	2.0	<1	1	1	2	2	3	3	5
50–64	1	2.0	0	2	2	2	2	2	2	2
65+	0									
B. Operated										
0–19 Years	0									
20–34	161	3.2	6	2	2	3	3	4	4	10
35–49	173	3.3	1	2	3	3	3	4	5	7
50–64	13	3.4	<1	3	3	3	4	4	4	4
65+	0									
SUBTOTALS:										
1. SINGLE DX										
A. Not Operated	14	1.8	<1	1	1	2	2	3	3	3
B. Operated	3	3.0		2	2	3	4	4	4	4
2. MULTIPLE DX										
A. Not Operated	181	1.9	3	1	1	2	2	3	3	5
B. Operated	347	3.3	3	2	3	3	3	4	5	9
1. SINGLE DX	17	2.0	<1	1	1	2	2	3	4	4
2. MULTIPLE DX	528	2.8	3	1	2	3	3	4	4	7
A. NOT OPERATED	195	1.9	<1	1	1	2	2	3	3	5
B. OPERATED	350	3.3	3	2	3	3	3	4	5	9
TOTAL										
0–19 Years	7	2.1	<1	1	2	2	2	3	3	3
20–34	306	2.6	4	1	2	2	3	4	4	7
35–49	218	3.0	1	2	2	3	3	4	5	7
50–64	14	3.3	<1	2	3	3	3	4	4	4
65+	0									
GRAND TOTAL	545	2.8	3	1	2	3	3	4	4	7

Length of Stay by Diagnosis and Operation, Western Region, 2008

Western Region, October 2006–September 2007 Data, by Diagnosis

654.21: PREVIOUS CD NOS-DEL

Type of Patients	Observed Patients	Avg. Stay	Vari-ance	10th	25th	50th	75th	90th	95th	99th
1. SINGLE DX										
A. Not Operated										
0–19 Years	17	1.9	<1	1	1	2	2	3	3	3
20–34	811	1.7	1	1	1	2	2	2	3	3
35–49	65	1.7	1	1	1	2	2	2	3	3
50–64	1	2.0	0	2	2	2	2	2	2	2
65+	0									
B. Operated										
0–19 Years	834	2.7	<1	2	2	3	3	4	4	4
20–34	20,406	2.7	<1	2	2	3	3	4	4	4
35–49	1,130	2.8	<1	2	2	3	3	4	4	4
50–64	51	2.9	<1	2	2	3	3	4	4	4
65+	0									
2. MULTIPLE DX										
A. Not Operated										
0–19 Years	97	2.0	<1	1	2	2	2	3	3	6
20–34	3,223	1.9	<1	1	1	2	2	3	3	4
35–49	867	1.8	<1	1	1	2	2	3	3	4
50–64	47	1.9	<1	1	1	2	2	3	3	4
65+	0									
B. Operated										
0–19 Years	1,303	2.9	8	2	2	3	3	4	4	6
20–34	52,302	2.9	1	2	2	3	3	4	4	5
35–49	19,930	3.0	1	2	2	3	3	4	4	5
50–64	1,146	3.2	3	2	3	3	4	4	4	5
65+	0									
SUBTOTALS:										
1. SINGLE DX										
A. Not Operated	894	1.7	<1	1	1	2	2	2	3	3
B. Operated	22,421	2.7	<1	2	2	3	3	4	4	4
2. MULTIPLE DX										
A. Not Operated	4,234	1.9	<1	1	1	2	2	3	3	4
B. Operated	74,681	2.9	1	2	2	3	3	4	4	5
1. SINGLE DX	23,315	2.7	<1	2	2	3	3	4	4	4
2. MULTIPLE DX	78,915	2.8	2	2	2	3	3	4	4	5
A. NOT OPERATED	5,128	1.8	<1	1	1	2	2	3	3	4
B. OPERATED	97,102	2.9	1	2	2	3	3	4	4	5
TOTAL										
0–19 Years	2,251	2.8	5	2	2	3	3	4	4	5
20–34	76,742	2.8	1	2	2	3	3	4	4	5
35–49	21,992	2.9	1	2	2	3	3	4	4	5
50–64	1,245	3.1	3	2	3	3	4	4	4	5
65+	0									
GRAND TOTAL	102,230	2.8	1	2	2	3	3	4	4	5

654.41: ABN GRAVID UTER NEC-DEL

Type of Patients	Observed Patients	Avg. Stay	Vari-ance	10th	25th	50th	75th	90th	95th	99th
1. SINGLE DX										
A. Not Operated										
0–19 Years	0									
20–34	12	1.8	<1	1	1	2	2	3	3	3
35–49	0									
50–64	0									
65+	0									
B. Operated										
0–19 Years	28	3.1	<1	2	3	3	4	4	4	4
20–34	3	3.0	1	2	2	3	4	4	4	4
35–49	0									
50–64	0									
65+	0									
2. MULTIPLE DX										
A. Not Operated										
0–19 Years	6	1.8	<1	1	1	2	2	2	2	2
20–34	84	1.7	<1	1	1	2	2	3	3	3
35–49	10	1.7	<1	1	1	2	2	3	3	3
50–64	0									
65+	0									
B. Operated										
0–19 Years	7	2.4	<1	2	2	2	3	3	3	3
20–34	186	3.1	1	2	2	3	4	4	5	7
35–49	70	3.6	7	2	3	3	4	4	4	23
50–64	7	3.0	<1	2	3	3	3	4	4	4
65+	0									
SUBTOTALS:										
1. SINGLE DX										
A. Not Operated	12	1.8	<1	1	1	2	2	3	3	3
B. Operated	31	3.1	<1	2	3	3	4	4	4	4
2. MULTIPLE DX										
A. Not Operated	100	1.7	<1	1	1	2	2	3	3	3
B. Operated	270	3.2	3	2	2	3	4	4	5	9
1. SINGLE DX	43	2.7	<1	1	2	3	3	4	4	4
2. MULTIPLE DX	370	2.8	3	1	2	3	3	4	4	7
A. NOT OPERATED	112	1.7	<1	1	1	2	2	3	3	3
B. OPERATED	301	3.2	2	2	2	3	4	4	4	7
TOTAL										
0–19 Years	13	2.2	<1	2	2	2	3	3	3	3
20–34	310	2.7	1	1	2	3	3	4	4	6
35–49	83	3.3	6	2	2	3	4	4	4	23
50–64	7	3.0	<1	2	3	3	3	4	4	4
65+	0									
GRAND TOTAL	413	2.8	2	1	2	3	3	4	4	6

654.43: ABN GRAVID UTERUS NEC-AP

Type of Patients	Observed Patients	Avg. Stay	Vari-ance	10th	25th	50th	75th	90th	95th	99th
1. SINGLE DX										
A. Not Operated										
0–19 Years	0									
20–34	2	1.0	0	1	1	1	1	1	1	1
35–49	0									
50–64	0									
65+	0									
B. Operated										
0–19 Years	3	2.3	1	1	1	3	3	3	3	3
20–34	0									
35–49	0									
50–64	0									
65+	0									
2. MULTIPLE DX										
A. Not Operated										
0–19 Years	14	1.2	<1	1	1	1	2	3	3	3
20–34	124	1.7	1	1	1	1	2	3	3	5
35–49	14	1.2	<1	1	1	1	1	2	2	2
50–64	0	2.0	0	1	1	1	1	1	1	1
65+	0									
B. Operated										
0–19 Years	41	2.3	<1	1	2	2	3	4	4	5
20–34	282	2.6	2	2	2	2	3	4	5	9
35–49	42	2.7	3	1	2	2	3	4	5	10
50–64	1	4.0	0	4	4	4	4	4	4	4
65+	0									
SUBTOTALS:										
1. SINGLE DX										
A. Not Operated	2	1.0	0	1	1	1	1	1	1	1
B. Operated	3	2.3	1	1	1	3	3	3	3	3
2. MULTIPLE DX										
A. Not Operated	154	1.6	<1	1	1	1	2	3	3	5
B. Operated	366	2.6	2	1	2	2	3	4	5	9
1. SINGLE DX	5	1.8	1	1	1	1	3	3	3	3
2. MULTIPLE DX	520	2.3	2	1	1	2	3	4	5	8
A. NOT OPERATED	156	1.6	<1	1	1	1	2	3	3	5
B. OPERATED	369	2.6	2	1	2	2	3	4	5	9
TOTAL										
0–19 Years	55	2.0	1	1	1	2	3	3	4	5
20–34	411	2.3	2	1	1	2	3	4	5	8
35–49	56	2.3	3	1	1	2	3	3	5	10
50–64	3	2.0	3	1	1	1	4	4	4	4
65+	0									
GRAND TOTAL	525	2.3	2	1	1	2	3	4	5	8

Length of Stay by Diagnosis and Operation, Western Region, 2008

Western Region, October 2006–September 2007 Data, by Diagnosis

654.51: CERV INCOMPETENCE-DEL

Type of Patients	Observed Patients	Avg. Stay	Variance	10th	25th	50th	75th	90th	95th	99th
1. SINGLE DX										
A. Not Operated										
0–19 Years	1	2.0	0	2	2	2	2	2	2	2
20–34	48	1.7	<1	1	1	2	2	3	3	4
35–49	1	2.0	0	2	2	2	2	2	2	2
50–64	0									
65+	0									
B. Operated										
0–19 Years	0									
20–34	11	3.8	3	3	3	3	4	4	9	9
35–49	1	2.0	0	2	2	2	2	2	2	2
50–64	0									
65+	0									
2. MULTIPLE DX										
A. Not Operated										
0–19 Years	37	3.6	26	1	1	2	3	8	14	28
20–34	293	3.7	40	1	1	2	3	7	14	35
35–49	58	5.3	173	1	2	2	3	5	29	81
50–64	5	14.0	118	2	7	11	21	29	29	29
65+	0									
B. Operated										
0–19 Years	12	11.5	326	3	3	4	17	19	66	66
20–34	198	8.9	185	2	3	3	8	24	36	75
35–49	65	9.1	281	2	3	4	6	54	94	>99
50–64	11	12.4	490	2	3	3	7	29	75	75
65+	0									
SUBTOTALS:										
1. SINGLE DX										
A. Not Operated	50	1.7	<1	1	1	2	2	2	2	2
B. Operated	12	3.7	3	2	3	3	4	4	9	9
2. MULTIPLE DX										
A. Not Operated	393	4.1	60	1	1	2	3	7	16	39
B. Operated	286	9.2	221	2	3	4	7	27	48	>99
1. SINGLE DX	62	2.1	2	1	1	2	2	2	3	9
2. MULTIPLE DX	679	6.2	134	1	2	3	4	15	29	75
A. NOT OPERATED	443	3.8	54	1	1	2	3	6	14	35
B. OPERATED	298	9.0	214	2	3	4	7	25	44	98
TOTAL										
0–19 Years	50	5.5	104	1	2	2	4	14	19	66
20–34	550	5.4	95	1	2	2	4	12	25	50
35–49	125	7.2	229	1	2	3	4	16	59	>99
50–64	16	12.9	359	2	3	5	21	29	75	75
65+	0									
GRAND TOTAL	741	5.9	125	1	2	2	4	13	28	75

654.53: CERV INCOMPETENCE-AP

Type of Patients	Observed Patients	Avg. Stay	Variance	10th	25th	50th	75th	90th	95th	99th
1. SINGLE DX										
A. Not Operated										
0–19 Years										
20–34	12	7.1	41	2	3	5	10	18	20	20
35–49	48	5.6	157	1	1	2	3	11	22	64
50–64	6	3.5	9	1	1	4	6	8	8	8
65+	0									
B. Operated										
0–19 Years	0									
20–34	9	1.6	2	1	1	1	1	5	5	5
35–49	248	2.0	2	1	1	1	2	4	4	9
50–64	29	2.0	4	1	1	2	2	6	7	8
65+	3	3.0	7	1	1	2	6	6	6	6
2. MULTIPLE DX										
A. Not Operated										
0–19 Years	19	15.4	483	2	2	7	21	39	90	90
20–34	223	11.5	333	1	1	3	11	39	57	83
35–49	101	11.0	278	1	1	2	12	37	46	71
50–64	4	24.3	>999	1	2	2	92	92	92	92
65+	0									
B. Operated										
0–19 Years	16	4.8	19	2	2	4	5	8	19	19
20–34	382	3.8	26	1	1	2	4	7	9	35
35–49	196	4.2	85	1	1	2	4	7	9	60
50–64	11	2.1	2	1	1	2	4	5	>99	>99
65+	0									
SUBTOTALS:										
1. SINGLE DX										
A. Not Operated	66	5.7	122	1	1	2	5	11	20	64
B. Operated	289	2.0	3	1	1	1	2	4	6	9
2. MULTIPLE DX										
A. Not Operated	347	11.7	340	1	1	3	12	39	57	84
B. Operated	605	3.9	45	1	1	2	4	7	9	>99
1. SINGLE DX	355	2.7	27	1	1	1	3	4	8	20
2. MULTIPLE DX	952	6.8	166	1	1	2	5	16	37	71
A. NOT OPERATED	413	10.7	310	1	1	3	10	37	56	83
B. OPERATED	894	3.3	32	1	1	2	4	6	8	40
TOTAL										
0–19 Years	56	8.4	200	1	2	4	8	20	37	90
20–34	901	5.3	116	1	1	2	4	9	23	61
35–49	332	6.1	146	1	1	2	4	12	37	60
50–64	18	7.2	450	1	1	2	4	92	>99	>99
65+	0									
GRAND TOTAL	1,307	5.6	131	1	1	2	4	10	28	61

654.61: ABN CERVIX NEC PREG-DEL

Type of Patients	Observed Patients	Avg. Stay	Variance	10th	25th	50th	75th	90th	95th	99th
1. SINGLE DX										
A. Not Operated										
0–19 Years										
20–34	2	2.0	0	2	2	2	2	2	2	2
35–49	23	1.8	<1	1	2	2	2	2	2	3
50–64	0									
65+	0									
B. Operated										
0–19 Years	0									
20–34	1	3.0	0	3	3	3	3	3	3	3
35–49	8	2.5	<1	1	2	3	3	4	4	4
50–64	0									
65+	0									
2. MULTIPLE DX										
A. Not Operated										
0–19 Years	27	2.0	<1	1	2	2	3	3	3	3
20–34	171	2.4	15	1	1	2	2	3	3	22
35–49	9	1.6	<1	1	1	2	2	2	2	2
50–64	2	2.0	0	2	2	2	2	2	2	2
65+	0									
B. Operated										
0–19 Years	8	5.3	41	2	3	3	4	21	21	21
20–34	79	4.4	83	2	2	3	4	4	8	78
35–49	27	9.3	212	3	3	4	4	40	47	52
50–64	1	2.0	0	2	2	2	2	2	2	2
65+	0									
SUBTOTALS:										
1. SINGLE DX										
A. Not Operated	25	1.8	<1	1	2	2	2	2	2	3
B. Operated	9	2.6	<1	1	2	3	3	4	4	4
2. MULTIPLE DX										
A. Not Operated	209	2.3	13	1	1	2	2	3	3	20
B. Operated	115	5.6	112	2	2	3	4	5	33	52
1. SINGLE DX	34	2.0	<1	1	2	2	2	3	3	4
2. MULTIPLE DX	324	3.5	50	1	2	2	3	4	5	40
A. NOT OPERATED	234	2.3	11	1	1	2	2	3	3	20
B. OPERATED	124	5.4	105	2	2	3	4	5	21	52
TOTAL										
0–19 Years	38	2.7	10	1	2	2	3	3	4	21
20–34	281	2.9	33	1	2	2	3	3	4	33
35–49	36	7.4	169	1	2	3	4	33	47	52
50–64	2	2.0	0	2	2	2	2	2	2	2
65+	0									
GRAND TOTAL	358	3.4	46	1	2	2	3	4	5	40

Length of Stay by Diagnosis and Operation, Western Region, 2008

Western Region, October 2006–September 2007 Data, by Diagnosis

654.63: ABN CERVIX NEC PREG-AP

Type of Patients	Observed Patients	Avg. Stay	Vari-ance	10th	25th	50th	75th	90th	95th	99th
1. SINGLE DX										
A. Not Operated										
0–19 Years	5	2.0	1	1	1	2	2	4	4	4
20–34	30	4.3	52	1	1	2	3	7	20	36
35–49	3	2.0	0	2	2	2	2	2	2	2
50–64	0									
65+	0									
B. Operated										
0–19 Years	2	3.0	2	2	2	3	4	4	4	4
20–34	5	2.4	2	2	1	2	2	5	5	5
35–49	0									
50–64	0									
65+	0									
2. MULTIPLE DX										
A. Not Operated										
0–19 Years	12	4.8	26	1	2	3	7	9	19	19
20–34	143	7.9	158	1	2	3	7	24	42	58
35–49	56	8.4	160	1	2	3	7	27	42	57
50–64	1	11.0	0	11	11	11	11	11	11	11
65+	0									
B. Operated										
0–19 Years	2	2.0	2	1	1	1	3	3	3	3
20–34	22	3.5	27	1	1	2	3	4	6	26
35–49	15	3.1	9	1	1	2	3	8	12	12
50–64	0									
65+	0									
SUBTOTALS:										
1. SINGLE DX										
A. Not Operated	38	3.8	42	1	1	2	3	7	20	36
B. Operated	7	2.6	2	1	2	2	4	5	5	5
2. MULTIPLE DX										
A. Not Operated	212	7.9	150	1	2	3	7	24	42	57
B. Operated	39	3.3	19	1	1	2	3	6	12	26
1. SINGLE DX	45	3.6	36	1	1	2	3	6	13	36
2. MULTIPLE DX	251	7.1	132	1	2	3	6	19	36	57
A. NOT OPERATED	250	7.2	135	1	2	3	6	22	36	57
B. OPERATED	46	3.2	16	1	1	2	3	5	8	26
TOTAL										
0–19 Years	21	3.7	16	1	2	3	4	7	9	19
20–34	200	6.7	127	1	2	2	5	17	32	58
35–49	74	7.1	128	1	2	3	6	22	40	57
50–64	1	11.0	0	11	11	11	11	11	11	11
65+	0									
GRAND TOTAL	296	6.6	119	1	2	2	5	17	32	57

654.81: ABN VULVA IN PREG-DEL

Type of Patients	Observed Patients	Avg. Stay	Vari-ance	10th	25th	50th	75th	90th	95th	99th
1. SINGLE DX										
A. Not Operated										
0–19 Years	0									
20–34	6	1.7	<1	1	1	2	2	2	2	2
35–49	0									
50–64	0									
65+	0									
B. Operated										
0–19 Years	2	2.5	<1	2	2	3	3	3	3	3
20–34	57	2.6	<1	2	2	3	3	4	4	4
35–49	5	3.2	<1	3	3	3	3	4	4	4
50–64	1	2.0	0	2	2	2	2	2	2	2
65+	0									
2. MULTIPLE DX										
A. Not Operated										
0–19 Years	2	2.0	0	2	2	2	2	2	2	2
20–34	22	1.7	<1	1	1	1	2	3	3	4
35–49	2	2.0	0	2	2	2	2	2	2	2
50–64	0									
65+	0									
B. Operated										
0–19 Years	4	2.3	<1	2	2	2	3	3	3	3
20–34	112	2.6	<1	2	2	3	3	4	4	4
35–49	45	3.2	1	3	3	3	4	4	8	8
50–64	1	3.0	0	3	3	3	3	3	3	3
65+	0									
SUBTOTALS:										
1. SINGLE DX										
A. Not Operated	6	1.7	<1	1	1	2	2	2	2	2
B. Operated	65	2.7	<1	2	2	3	3	4	4	4
2. MULTIPLE DX										
A. Not Operated	26	1.8	<1	1	1	2	2	3	3	4
B. Operated	162	2.7	<1	2	2	3	3	4	4	5
1. SINGLE DX	71	2.6	<1	2	2	3	3	4	4	4
2. MULTIPLE DX	188	2.6	<1	1	2	3	3	4	4	5
A. NOT OPERATED	32	1.8	<1	1	1	2	2	3	3	4
B. OPERATED	227	2.7	<1	2	2	3	3	4	4	4
TOTAL										
0–19 Years	8	2.3	<1	2	2	2	3	3	3	3
20–34	197	2.5	<1	1	2	2	3	4	4	4
35–49	52	3.2	1	2	3	3	4	4	8	8
50–64	2	2.5	<1	2	2	3	3	3	3	3
65+	0									
GRAND TOTAL	259	2.6	<1	2	2	3	3	4	4	4

654.91: ABN PELVIC TISS NEC-DEL

Type of Patients	Observed Patients	Avg. Stay	Vari-ance	10th	25th	50th	75th	90th	95th	99th
1. SINGLE DX										
A. Not Operated										
0–19 Years	0									
20–34	1	1.0	0	1	1	1	1	1	1	1
35–49	0									
50–64	0									
65+	0									
B. Operated										
0–19 Years	5	2.2	<1	2	2	2	2	3	3	3
20–34	66	3.0	<1	2	3	3	3	4	4	5
35–49	9	3.0	<1	2	2	3	4	4	4	4
50–64	0									
65+	0									
2. MULTIPLE DX										
A. Not Operated										
0–19 Years	0									
20–34	6	1.8	<1	1	1	2	2	3	3	3
35–49	2	2.5	4	1	1	4	4	4	4	4
50–64	0									
65+	0									
B. Operated										
0–19 Years	3	3.0	0	3	3	3	3	3	3	3
20–34	132	3.2	4	2	3	3	3	4	4	10
35–49	188	3.4	2	2	3	3	4	4	4	5
50–64	17	3.8	3	3	3	3	4	5	9	9
65+	0									
SUBTOTALS:										
1. SINGLE DX										
A. Not Operated	1	1.0	0	1	1	1	1	1	1	1
B. Operated	80	3.0	<1	2	2	3	3	4	4	5
2. MULTIPLE DX										
A. Not Operated	8	2.0	1	1	1	2	3	4	4	4
B. Operated	340	3.3	3	2	3	3	4	4	4	9
1. SINGLE DX	81	3.0	<1	2	2	3	3	4	4	5
2. MULTIPLE DX	348	3.3	3	2	3	3	3	4	4	9
A. NOT OPERATED	9	1.9	1	1	1	2	2	4	4	4
B. OPERATED	420	3.3	3	2	3	3	3	4	4	5
TOTAL										
0–19 Years	8	2.5	<1	2	2	3	3	3	3	3
20–34	205	3.1	3	2	2	3	3	4	4	5
35–49	199	3.4	2	2	3	3	3	4	4	5
50–64	17	3.8	2	3	3	3	4	5	9	9
65+	0									
GRAND TOTAL	429	3.2	3	2	3	3	3	4	4	5

Length of Stay by Diagnosis and Operation, Western Region, 2008

655: FETAL ABN AFFECT MOTHER

Type of Patients	Observed Patients	Avg. Stay	Vari-ance	Percentiles 10th	25th	50th	75th	90th	95th	99th
1. SINGLE DX										
A. Not Operated										
0–19 Years	36	2.3	5	1	1	2	3	3	3	14
20–34	405	1.8	<1	1	1	2	2	3	3	4
35–49	15	1.9	<1	1	1	2	3	3	3	3
50–64	0									
65+	0									
B. Operated										
0–19 Years	21	3.1	<1	2	3	3	4	4	4	4
20–34	85	3.2	<1	2	3	3	4	4	4	6
35–49	3	3.3	<1	3	3	3	4	4	4	4
50–64	0									
65+	0									
2. MULTIPLE DX										
A. Not Operated										
0–19 Years	229	2.2	2	1	1	2	3	3	4	8
20–34	1,356	2.2	6	1	2	2	3	3	3	9
35–49	270	2.1	6	1	1	2	3	3	4	4
50–64	11	2.2	<1	1	2	2	3	3	4	4
65+	0									
B. Operated										
0–19 Years	106	4.1	32	2	3	3	4	5	7	9
20–34	748	3.6	9	2	3	3	4	5	5	18
35–49	179	3.8	4	2	3	3	4	6	7	12
50–64	12	3.1	2	1	2	3	4	5	6	6
65+	0									
SUBTOTALS:										
1. SINGLE DX										
A. Not Operated	456	1.8	<1	1	1	2	2	3	3	4
B. Operated	109	3.2	<1	2	3	3	4	4	4	5
2. MULTIPLE DX										
A. Not Operated	1,866	2.2	5	1	1	2	3	3	4	8
B. Operated	1,045	3.7	10	2	3	3	4	5	6	14
1. SINGLE DX	565	2.1	1	1	2	2	3	3	4	4
2. MULTIPLE DX	2,911	2.8	8	1	2	2	3	4	5	11
A. NOT OPERATED	2,322	2.2	4	1	1	2	3	3	3	6
B. OPERATED	1,154	3.6	10	2	3	3	4	5	6	13
TOTAL										
0–19 Years	392	2.8	11	1	2	2	3	4	5	10
20–34	2,594	2.6	6	1	2	2	3	4	4	10
35–49	467	2.8	5	1	2	2	3	4	5	11
50–64	23	2.7	2	1	2	2	4	4	5	6
65+	0									
GRAND TOTAL	3,476	2.6	7	1	2	2	3	4	5	10

655.71: DECR FETAL MOVEMENT-DEL

Type of Patients	Observed Patients	Avg. Stay	Vari-ance	Percentiles 10th	25th	50th	75th	90th	95th	99th
1. SINGLE DX										
A. Not Operated										
0–19 Years	10	2.5	<1	2	2	2	3	3	3	3
20–34	151	2.0	<1	1	2	2	2	3	3	4
35–49	2	2.5	<1	2	2	3	3	3	3	3
50–64	0									
65+	0									
B. Operated										
0–19 Years	2	3.0	0	3	3	3	4	5	5	5
20–34	15	3.3	<1	3	3	3	4	5	5	5
35–49	1	4.0	0	4	4	4	4	4	4	4
50–64	0									
65+	0									
2. MULTIPLE DX										
A. Not Operated										
0–19 Years	90	2.4	<1	1	2	2	3	3	4	5
20–34	634	2.2	1	1	2	2	3	3	3	4
35–49	110	2.2	<1	1	2	2	3	3	4	4
50–64	3	2.3	<1	2	2	2	3	3	3	3
65+	0									
B. Operated										
0–19 Years	38	3.5	1	2	3	3	4	5	5	7
20–34	361	3.3	4	1	3	3	4	4	5	7
35–49	76	3.8	3	2	3	3	4	6	6	12
50–64	2	3.0	2	2	2	3	4	4	4	4
65+	0									
SUBTOTALS:										
1. SINGLE DX										
A. Not Operated	163	2.1	<1	1	2	2	2	3	3	4
B. Operated	18	3.3	<1	3	3	3	4	4	5	5
2. MULTIPLE DX										
A. Not Operated	837	2.2	1	1	2	2	3	3	3	4
B. Operated	477	3.4	3	2	3	3	4	5	5	10
1. SINGLE DX	181	2.2	<1	1	2	2	3	3	3	5
2. MULTIPLE DX	1,314	2.7	2	1	2	2	3	4	4	6
A. NOT OPERATED	1,000	2.2	1	1	2	2	3	3	3	4
B. OPERATED	495	3.4	3	2	3	3	4	5	5	10
TOTAL										
0–19 Years	140	2.7	1	2	2	2	3	4	5	5
20–34	1,161	2.5	2	1	2	2	3	4	4	6
35–49	189	2.8	2	1	2	3	3	4	5	11
50–64	5	2.6	<1	2	2	2	4	4	4	4
65+	0									
GRAND TOTAL	1,495	2.6	2	1	2	2	3	4	4	6

655.81: FET ABNORMALITY NEC-DEL

Type of Patients	Observed Patients	Avg. Stay	Vari-ance	Percentiles 10th	25th	50th	75th	90th	95th	99th
1. SINGLE DX										
A. Not Operated										
0–19 Years	11	2.1	<1	1	2	2	3	3	3	3
20–34	130	2.0	<1	1	1	2	2	3	3	4
35–49	4	2.8	<1	2	3	3	3	3	3	3
50–64	0									
65+	0									
B. Operated										
0–19 Years	14	3.3	<1	2	3	3	4	4	4	4
20–34	41	3.3	<1	2	3	3	4	4	4	5
35–49	2	3.0	0	3	3	3	3	3	3	3
50–64	0									
65+	0									
2. MULTIPLE DX										
A. Not Operated										
0–19 Years	70	2.3	2	1	1	2	3	3	5	10
20–34	409	2.2	2	1	2	2	3	3	3	6
35–49	70	2.1	<1	1	2	2	3	3	3	4
50–64	2	3.0	2	2	2	2	4	4	4	4
65+	0									
B. Operated										
0–19 Years	43	4.9	77	2	3	3	4	6	8	60
20–34	248	4.2	19	2	3	3	4	5	9	25
35–49	71	3.9	5	2	3	3	4	5	10	14
50–64	5	4.4	1	3	4	4	5	6	6	6
65+	0									
SUBTOTALS:										
1. SINGLE DX										
A. Not Operated	145	2.0	<1	1	1	2	2	3	3	4
B. Operated	57	3.3	<1	2	3	3	4	4	4	4
2. MULTIPLE DX										
A. Not Operated	551	2.2	2	1	2	2	3	3	3	6
B. Operated	367	4.3	23	2	3	3	4	5	9	25
1. SINGLE DX	202	2.3	<1	1	2	2	3	3	4	4
2. MULTIPLE DX	918	3.0	11	1	2	3	3	4	5	15
A. NOT OPERATED	696	2.2	1	1	2	2	3	3	3	6
B. OPERATED	424	4.1	20	2	3	3	4	5	8	24
TOTAL										
0–19 Years	138	3.2	26	1	2	3	3	5	6	10
20–34	828	2.8	8	1	2	2	3	4	5	15
35–49	147	3.0	4	1	2	3	3	4	5	11
50–64	7	4.0	2	2	3	4	5	6	6	6
65+	0									
GRAND TOTAL	1,120	2.9	9	1	2	2	3	4	5	12

Length of Stay by Diagnosis and Operation, Western Region, 2008

Western Region, October 2006–September 2007 Data, by Diagnosis

656: OTH FETAL PBX AFF MOTHER

Type of Patients	Observed Patients	Avg. Stay	Vari-ance	10th	25th	50th	75th	90th	95th	99th
1. SINGLE DX										
A. Not Operated										
0–19 Years	394	1.9	<1	1	1	2	2	3	3	4
20–34	2,706	1.7	<1	1	1	2	2	3	3	4
35–49	106	1.7	<1	1	1	2	2	3	3	4
50–64	3	1.3	<1	1	1	1	2	2	2	2
65+	0									
B. Operated										
0–19 Years	98	2.9	<1	2	2	3	3	4	4	4
20–34	840	3.0	<1	2	3	3	3	4	4	5
35–49	37	3.1	<1	2	3	3	3	5	5	5
50–64	0									
65+	0									
2. MULTIPLE DX										
A. Not Operated										
0–19 Years	1,234	2.3	4	1	2	2	2	3	4	5
20–34	8,223	2.0	2	1	1	2	2	3	3	5
35–49	1,380	2.2	6	1	2	2	2	3	4	6
50–64	61	2.2	1	1	2	2	2	3	4	7
65+	0									
B. Operated										
0–19 Years	514	3.5	5	2	3	3	4	4	5	15
20–34	5,326	3.3	5	2	3	3	4	4	6	10
35–49	1,489	3.7	11	2	3	3	4	5	6	16
50–64	77	3.8	4	2	3	3	4	6	9	12
65+	0									
SUBTOTALS:										
1. SINGLE DX										
A. Not Operated	3,209	1.8	<1	1	1	2	2	3	3	4
B. Operated	975	3.0	<1	2	2	3	3	4	4	5
2. MULTIPLE DX										
A. Not Operated	10,898	2.1	2	1	1	2	2	3	3	5
B. Operated	7,406	3.4	6	2	3	3	4	4	5	11
1. SINGLE DX	4,184	2.1	1	1	1	2	3	3	4	4
2. MULTIPLE DX	18,304	2.6	4	1	2	2	3	4	4	8
A. NOT OPERATED	14,107	2.0	2	1	1	2	2	3	3	5
B. OPERATED	8,381	3.4	6	2	3	3	4	4	5	11
TOTAL										
0–19 Years	2,240	2.5	3	1	2	2	3	4	4	7
20–34	17,095	2.4	3	1	2	2	3	4	4	7
35–49	3,012	2.9	9	1	2	3	3	4	5	11
50–64	141	3.1	3	1	2	3	4	4	6	11
65+	0									
GRAND TOTAL	22,488	2.5	4	1	2	2	3	4	4	7

656.11: RH ISOIMMUNIZATION-DEL

Type of Patients	Observed Patients	Avg. Stay	Vari-ance	10th	25th	50th	75th	90th	95th	99th
1. SINGLE DX										
A. Not Operated										
0–19 Years	79	1.8	<1	1	1	2	2	2	3	3
20–34	591	1.7	<1	1	1	2	2	3	3	3
35–49	14	2.0	<1	1	2	2	2	3	3	3
50–64	2	1.5	<1	1	1	2	2	2	2	2
65+	0									
B. Operated										
0–19 Years	0									
20–34	6	2.5	<1	2	2	2	3	3	3	3
35–49	0									
50–64	0									
65+	0									
2. MULTIPLE DX										
A. Not Operated										
0–19 Years	165	1.9	<1	1	1	2	2	3	3	3
20–34	1,005	1.8	<1	1	1	2	2	3	3	3
35–49	94	1.9	<1	1	1	2	2	3	3	4
50–64	6	1.8	<1	2	2	2	2	2	2	2
65+	0									
B. Operated										
0–19 Years	10	2.7	<1	2	2	3	3	3	4	4
20–34	141	2.6	2	1	2	3	3	4	4	4
35–49	20	2.9	1	2	2	3	3	4	6	6
50–64	3	6.3	24	3	3	4	12	12	12	12
65+	0									
SUBTOTALS:										
1. SINGLE DX										
A. Not Operated	686	1.7	<1	1	1	2	2	2	3	3
B. Operated	6	2.5	<1	2	2	2	3	3	3	3
2. MULTIPLE DX										
A. Not Operated	1,270	1.8	<1	1	1	2	2	3	3	4
B. Operated	174	2.7	2	2	2	3	3	4	5	9
1. SINGLE DX	692	1.7	<1	1	1	2	2	2	3	3
2. MULTIPLE DX	1,444	1.9	<1	1	1	2	2	3	3	4
A. NOT OPERATED	1,956	1.8	<1	1	1	2	2	3	3	3
B. OPERATED	180	2.7	2	2	2	3	3	4	5	9
TOTAL										
0–19 Years	254	1.9	<1	1	1	2	2	3	3	3
20–34	1,743	1.8	<1	1	1	2	2	3	3	4
35–49	128	2.1	<1	1	2	2	2	3	4	4
50–64	11	3.0	10	2	2	2	3	4	12	12
65+	0									
GRAND TOTAL	2,136	1.8	<1	1	1	2	2	3	3	4

656.31: FETAL DISTRESS-DELIVERED

Type of Patients	Observed Patients	Avg. Stay	Vari-ance	10th	25th	50th	75th	90th	95th	99th
1. SINGLE DX										
A. Not Operated										
0–19 Years	14	1.9	<1	1	1	2	2	3	3	3
20–34	48	1.8	<1	1	1	2	2	3	3	3
35–49	4	2.3	<1	1	2	3	3	3	3	3
50–64	0									
65+	0									
B. Operated										
0–19 Years	7	3.0	<1	2	3	3	3	4	4	4
20–34	55	3.4	<1	2	3	3	4	4	5	5
35–49	3	3.3	<1	3	3	3	4	4	4	4
50–64	0									
65+	0									
2. MULTIPLE DX										
A. Not Operated										
0–19 Years	31	2.2	<1	1	2	2	2	3	4	5
20–34	203	2.0	<1	1	2	2	2	3	3	3
35–49	39	2.3	<1	1	2	2	3	3	4	4
50–64	0	2.5	<1	2	2	3	3	3	3	2
65+	0									
B. Operated										
0–19 Years	72	3.4	1	2	3	3	3	5	5	8
20–34	449	3.4	2	2	3	3	4	5	5	10
35–49	89	3.7	2	3	3	3	4	5	5	15
50–64	8	3.9	2	2	3	3	6	6	6	6
65+	0									
SUBTOTALS:										
1. SINGLE DX										
A. Not Operated	66	1.9	<1	1	1	2	2	3	3	3
B. Operated	65	3.4	<1	2	3	3	4	4	5	5
2. MULTIPLE DX										
A. Not Operated	275	2.1	<1	1	2	2	2	3	3	4
B. Operated	618	3.4	2	2	3	3	4	5	5	8
1. SINGLE DX	131	2.6	1	1	2	3	3	4	4	5
2. MULTIPLE DX	893	3.0	2	2	2	3	4	4	5	8
A. NOT OPERATED	341	2.0	<1	1	2	2	2	3	3	4
B. OPERATED	683	3.4	2	2	3	3	4	5	5	8
TOTAL										
0–19 Years	124	2.9	1	2	2	3	3	4	5	6
20–34	755	2.9	2	2	2	3	4	4	5	7
35–49	135	3.2	2	2	3	3	4	4	5	6
50–64	10	3.6	2	2	2	3	5	6	6	6
65+	0									
GRAND TOTAL	1,024	3.0	2	2	2	3	4	4	5	7

Western Region, October 2006–September 2007 Data, by Diagnosis

656.41: INTRAUTERINE DEATH-DEL

Type of Patients	Observed Patients	Avg. Stay	Variance	Percentiles						
				10th	25th	50th	75th	90th	95th	99th
1. SINGLE DX										
A. Not Operated										
0–19 Years	69	1.6	<1	1	1	1	2	3		4
20–34	298	1.5	<1	1	1	1	2	2	3	4
35–49	33	1.7	<1	1	1	1	2	2	4	5
50–64	1	1.0	0	1	1	1	1	1	1	1
65+	0									
B. Operated										
0–19 Years	1	1.0	0	1	1	1	1	1	1	1
20–34	14	2.8	1	2	2	3	3	4	5	5
35–49	0									
50–64	0									
65+	0									
2. MULTIPLE DX										
A. Not Operated										
0–19 Years	185	1.8	<1	1	1	2	2	3	3	7
20–34	1,183	1.8	2	1	1	2	2	3	4	7
35–49	323	2.1	14	1	1	2	2	3	5	8
50–64	15	1.6	<1	1	1	1	2	3	3	3
65+	0									
B. Operated										
0–19 Years	29	2.9	3	1	2	3	4	4	5	9
20–34	293	3.0	4	1	2	3	3	5	6	13
35–49	127	3.3	6	2	2	3	4	5	6	10
50–64	7	4.4	15	1	2	3	9	11	11	11
65+	0									
SUBTOTALS:										
1. SINGLE DX										
A. Not Operated	401	1.5	<1	1	1	1	2	2	3	4
B. Operated	15	2.7	1	1	2	3	3	4	5	6
2. MULTIPLE DX										
A. Not Operated	1,706	1.9	4	1	1	2	2	3	4	7
B. Operated	456	3.1	5	1	2	3	4	5	7	12
1. SINGLE DX	**416**	**1.6**	**<1**	**1**	**1**	**1**	**2**	**2**	**3**	**4**
2. MULTIPLE DX	**2,162**	**2.1**	**4**	**1**	**1**	**2**	**3**	**4**	**5**	**8**
A. NOT OPERATED	**2,107**	**1.8**	**3**	**1**	**1**	**2**	**2**	**3**	**4**	**7**
B. OPERATED	**471**	**3.1**	**5**	**1**	**2**	**3**	**4**	**5**	**6**	**12**
TOTAL										
0–19 Years	284	1.9	1	1	1	1	2	3	4	7
20–34	1,788	2.0	2	1	1	2	2	3	4	8
35–49	483	2.4	12	1	1	2	3	4	5	10
50–64	23	2.4	6	1	1	2	3	3	9	11
65+	0									
GRAND TOTAL	**2,578**	**2.1**	**4**	**1**	**1**	**2**	**2**	**3**	**4**	**8**

656.51: POOR FETAL GROWTH-DEL

Type of Patients	Observed Patients	Avg. Stay	Variance	Percentiles						
				10th	25th	50th	75th	90th	95th	99th
1. SINGLE DX										
A. Not Operated										
0–19 Years	95	2.3	<1	2	2	2	3	3	3	4
20–34	413	2.0	<1	1	2	2	2	3	3	4
35–49	6	2.0	<1	1	2	2	2	3	4	3
50–64	0									
65+	0									
B. Operated										
0–19 Years	6	2.5	<1	2	2	3	3	3	3	3
20–34	20	3.6	<1	2	3	3	4	5	5	6
35–49	4	2.8	<1	2	2	2	4	4	4	4
50–64	0									
65+	0									
2. MULTIPLE DX										
A. Not Operated										
0–19 Years	444	2.7	8	2	2	2	3	4	4	6
20–34	2,012	2.3	1	1	2	2	3	3	4	5
35–49	274	2.3	<1	1	2	2	3	3	4	5
50–64	7	2.9	2	2	2	2	3	6	6	6
65+	0									
B. Operated										
0–19 Years	93	4.6	18	2	3	4	4	7	15	29
20–34	899	4.4	19	2	3	4	4	6	10	29
35–49	273	5.4	45	2	3	4	5	8	12	41
50–64	12	4.0	<1	3	3	4	5	5	6	6
65+	0									
SUBTOTALS:										
1. SINGLE DX										
A. Not Operated	514	2.1	<1	1	2	2	3	3	3	4
B. Operated	30	3.3	1	2	3	3	4	4	5	6
2. MULTIPLE DX										
A. Not Operated	2,737	2.4	2	1	2	2	3	3	4	5
B. Operated	1,277	4.7	24	2	3	4	4	7	11	30
1. SINGLE DX	**544**	**2.1**	**<1**	**1**	**2**	**2**	**3**	**3**	**3**	**4**
2. MULTIPLE DX	**4,014**	**3.1**	**10**	**1**	**2**	**3**	**3**	**4**	**5**	**17**
A. NOT OPERATED	**3,251**	**2.3**	**2**	**1**	**2**	**2**	**3**	**3**	**4**	**5**
B. OPERATED	**1,307**	**4.6**	**24**	**2**	**3**	**4**	**4**	**7**	**11**	**29**
TOTAL										
0–19 Years	638	2.9	9	2	2	3	3	4	4	15
20–34	3,344	2.9	7	1	2	2	3	5	5	14
35–49	557	3.8	25	2	3	3	4	5	8	29
50–64	19	3.6	2	2	3	3	4	6	6	6
65+	0									
GRAND TOTAL	**4,558**	**3.0**	**9**	**2**	**2**	**2**	**3**	**4**	**5**	**16**

656.61: EXCESS FETAL GROWTH-DEL

Type of Patients	Observed Patients	Avg. Stay	Variance	Percentiles						
				10th	25th	50th	75th	90th	95th	99th
1. SINGLE DX										
A. Not Operated										
0–19 Years	26	2.0	<1	1	2	2	2	3	3	4
20–34	516	1.8	2	1	1	2	2	3	3	4
35–49	15	1.7	<1	1	1	2	2	2	3	3
50–64	0									
65+	0									
B. Operated										
0–19 Years	51	3.0	<1	2	2	3	4	4	4	4
20–34	622	2.9	<1	2	2	3	3	4	4	4
35–49	23	2.9	<1	2	2	3	3	4	4	5
50–64	0									
65+	0									
2. MULTIPLE DX										
A. Not Operated										
0–19 Years	115	2.3	<1	1	2	2	3	3	4	4
20–34	1,878	2.0	<1	1	2	2	2	3	3	4
35–49	347	2.2	<1	1	2	2	3	3	3	4
50–64	19	2.4	<1	1	2	2	3	4	4	4
65+	0									
B. Operated										
0–19 Years	198	3.2	2	2	3	3	4	4	4	9
20–34	2,676	3.1	<1	2	2	3	4	4	4	5
35–49	780	3.2	<1	2	3	3	4	4	4	5
50–64	30	3.5	2	3	3	4	4	5	5	11
65+	0									
SUBTOTALS:										
1. SINGLE DX										
A. Not Operated	557	1.8	2	1	2	2	2	3	3	4
B. Operated	696	2.9	<1	2	2	3	3	4	4	6
2. MULTIPLE DX										
A. Not Operated	2,359	2.1	<1	1	2	2	3	3	3	5
B. Operated	3,684	3.1	1	2	3	3	4	4	5	30
1. SINGLE DX	**1,253**	**2.5**	**1**	**1**	**2**	**2**	**3**	**3**	**4**	**4**
2. MULTIPLE DX	**6,043**	**2.7**	**<1**	**2**	**2**	**3**	**3**	**4**	**4**	**5**
A. NOT OPERATED	**2,916**	**2.0**	**<1**	**1**	**2**	**2**	**3**	**3**	**3**	**4**
B. OPERATED	**4,380**	**3.1**	**<1**	**2**	**3**	**3**	**4**	**4**	**4**	**5**
TOTAL										
0–19 Years	390	2.8	1	2	2	3	3	4	4	5
20–34	5,692	2.6	1	1	2	2	3	4	4	4
35–49	1,165	2.9	<1	2	2	3	3	4	4	5
50–64	49	3.1	2	2	2	3	4	4	4	11
65+	0									
GRAND TOTAL	**7,296**	**2.7**	**1**	**1**	**2**	**3**	**3**	**4**	**4**	**5**

Length of Stay by Diagnosis and Operation, Western Region, 2008

Western Region, October 2006–September 2007 Data, by Diagnosis

656.71: OTHER PLACENTAL COND-DEL

Type of Patients	Observed Patients	Avg. Stay	Variance	10th	25th	50th	75th	90th	95th	99th
1. SINGLE DX										
A. Not Operated										
0–19 Years	5	2.0	1	1	1	2	3	3	3	3
20–34	61	1.7	<1	1	1	2	2	2	3	4
35–49	3	1.3	<1	1	1	1	2	2	2	2
50–64	0									
65+	0									
B. Operated										
0–19 Years	0									
20–34	1	2.0	0	2	2	2	2	2	2	2
35–49	0									
50–64	0									
65+	0									
2. MULTIPLE DX										
A. Not Operated										
0–19 Years	25	2.0	<1	1	2	2	2	3	3	3
20–34	147	1.8	<1	1	1	2	2	3	3	4
35–49	23	1.9	<1	1	1	2	2	3	3	3
50–64	3	1.7	<1	1	1	2	2	2	2	2
65+	0									
B. Operated										
0–19 Years	3	1.7	<1	1	1	2	2	2	2	2
20–34	44	3.0	2	2	2	3	3	4	6	10
35–49	14	3.2	2	2	2	3	4	5	6	6
50–64	0									
65+	0									
SUBTOTALS:										
1. SINGLE DX										
A. Not Operated	69	1.7	<1	1	1	2	2	2	3	3
B. Operated	1	2.0	0	2	2	2	2	2	2	2
2. MULTIPLE DX										
A. Not Operated	198	1.8	<1	1	1	2	2	2	3	3
B. Operated	61	3.0	2	2	2	3	3	4	6	10
1. SINGLE DX	70	1.7	<1	1	1	2	2	2	3	3
2. MULTIPLE DX	259	2.1	1	1	1	2	3	3	4	6
A. NOT OPERATED	267	1.8	<1	1	1	2	2	3	3	4
B. OPERATED	62	3.0	2	2	2	3	3	4	6	10
TOTAL										
0–19 Years	33	2.0	<1	2	2	2	2	3	3	3
20–34	253	2.0	1	1	1	2	2	3	3	6
35–49	40	2.3	1	1	2	2	3	4	5	6
50–64	3	1.7	<1	1	1	2	2	2	2	2
65+	0									
GRAND TOTAL	329	2.0	<1	1	1	2	2	3	3	6

656.81: FET/PLAC PROBLEM NEC-DEL

Type of Patients	Observed Patients	Avg. Stay	Variance	10th	25th	50th	75th	90th	95th	99th
1. SINGLE DX										
A. Not Operated										
0–19 Years	94	1.9	<1	1	2	2	2	3	3	3
20–34	707	1.7	<1	1	1	2	2	3	3	3
35–49	21	1.7	<1	1	1	2	2	2	3	3
50–64	0									
65+	0									
B. Operated										
0–19 Years	32	2.8	<1	2	2	3	3	4	4	4
20–34	118	3.2	<1	3	3	3	3	4	5	5
35–49	7	4.0	1	3	3	4	5	5	5	5
50–64	0									
65+	0									
2. MULTIPLE DX										
A. Not Operated										
0–19 Years	230	2.0	<1	1	1	2	2	3	3	4
20–34	1,511	1.8	<1	1	1	2	2	3	3	4
35–49	182	1.8	<1	1	1	2	2	3	3	4
50–64	7	1.7	<1	1	1	2	2	2	2	2
65+	0									
B. Operated										
0–19 Years	109	3.3	1	2	3	3	4	5	5	6
20–34	801	3.3	6	2	3	3	4	4	5	6
35–49	182	3.8	5	2	3	3	4	5	6	16
50–64	17	3.4	1	2	3	3	4	4	6	6
65+	0									
SUBTOTALS:										
1. SINGLE DX										
A. Not Operated	822	1.7	<1	1	1	2	2	3	3	3
B. Operated	157	3.2	<1	2	3	3	4	4	5	5
2. MULTIPLE DX										
A. Not Operated	1,930	1.9	<1	1	1	2	2	3	3	4
B. Operated	1,109	3.4	5	2	3	3	4	4	5	7
1. SINGLE DX	979	2.0	<1	1	1	2	2	3	4	5
2. MULTIPLE DX	3,039	2.4	3	1	2	2	3	4	4	6
A. NOT OPERATED	2,752	1.8	<1	1	1	2	2	3	3	4
B. OPERATED	1,266	3.4	5	2	3	3	4	4	5	7
TOTAL										
0–19 Years	465	2.3	<1	1	2	2	3	4	4	5
20–34	3,137	2.2	2	1	1	2	3	4	4	5
35–49	392	2.8	3	1	2	2	3	4	5	10
50–64	24	2.9	1	2	2	3	4	4	4	6
65+	0									
GRAND TOTAL	4,018	2.3	2	1	2	2	3	4	4	5

657: POLYHYDRAMNIOS

Type of Patients	Observed Patients	Avg. Stay	Variance	10th	25th	50th	75th	90th	95th	99th
1. SINGLE DX										
A. Not Operated										
0–19 Years	6	1.5	<1	1	1	1	2	3	3	3
20–34	101	1.8	<1	1	1	2	2	3	3	3
35–49	6	1.7	<1	1	1	2	2	2	2	2
50–64	0									
65+	0									
B. Operated										
0–19 Years	0									
20–34	5	3.2	<1	2	3	3	4	4	4	4
35–49	2	3.5	<1	3	3	3	4	4	4	4
50–64	0									
65+	0									
2. MULTIPLE DX										
A. Not Operated										
0–19 Years	43	2.4	2	1	2	2	3	4	4	7
20–34	540	2.3	5	1	2	2	3	3	4	10
35–49	124	2.2	2	1	1	2	2	3	4	10
50–64	4	1.8	<1	1	1	2	2	2	2	2
65+	0									
B. Operated										
0–19 Years	19	4.4	12	2	2	4	5	7	17	17
20–34	305	3.5	5	2	2	3	4	5	5	13
35–49	103	3.9	32	2	2	3	4	5	6	9
50–64	0	3.8	<1	3	4	4	4	4	4	4
65+	0									
SUBTOTALS:										
1. SINGLE DX										
A. Not Operated	113	1.8	<1	1	1	2	2	3	3	3
B. Operated	7	3.3	<1	2	3	3	4	4	4	4
2. MULTIPLE DX										
A. Not Operated	711	2.3	4	1	2	2	3	3	4	10
B. Operated	431	3.6	12	2	2	3	4	5	6	14
1. SINGLE DX	120	1.9	<1	1	1	2	2	3	3	4
2. MULTIPLE DX	1,142	2.8	7	1	2	2	3	4	5	11
A. NOT OPERATED	824	2.2	4	1	2	2	3	4	4	10
B. OPERATED	438	3.6	12	2	3	3	4	5	6	14
TOTAL										
0–19 Years	68	2.9	5	1	2	2	3	6	7	17
20–34	951	2.6	5	1	2	2	3	4	5	11
35–49	235	2.9	16	1	2	2	3	4	5	10
50–64	8	2.7	1	2	2	2	4	4	4	4
65+	0									
GRAND TOTAL	1,262	2.7	7	1	2	2	3	4	5	11

Length of Stay by Diagnosis and Operation, Western Region, 2008

Western Region, October 2006–September 2007 Data, by Diagnosis

657.01: POLYHYDRAMNIOS-DELIVERED

Type of Patients	Observed Patients	Avg. Stay	Vari- ance	10th	25th	50th	75th	90th	95th	99th
1. SINGLE DX										
A. Not Operated										
0–19 Years	5	1.6	<1	1	1	1	2	3	3	3
20–34	90	1.8	<1	1	1	2	2	3	3	4
35–49	5	1.8	<1	1	2	2	2	2	2	2
50–64	0									
65+	0									
B. Operated										
0–19 Years	0									
20–34	5	3.2	<1	2	3	3	4	4	4	4
35–49	2	3.5	<1	3	3	3	4	4	4	4
50–64	0									
65+	0									
2. MULTIPLE DX										
A. Not Operated										
0–19 Years	37	2.5	2	1	2	2	3	4	6	7
20–34	486	2.2	3	1	2	2	2	3	3	5
35–49	108	2.1	1	1	2	2	3	3	3	4
50–64	4	1.8	<1	1	1	2	2	2	2	2
65+	0									
B. Operated										
0–19 Years	19	4.4	12	2	2	4	5	7	17	17
20–34	303	3.5	5	2	2	3	4	5	5	13
35–49	102	3.9	32	2	2	3	4	5	6	9
50–64	4	3.8	<1	3	4	4	4	4	4	4
65+	0									
SUBTOTALS:										
1. SINGLE DX										
A. Not Operated	100	1.8	<1	1	1	2	2	3	3	4
B. Operated	7	3.3	<1	2	3	3	4	4	4	4
2. MULTIPLE DX										
A. Not Operated	635	2.2	3	1	2	2	3	3	3	6
B. Operated	428	3.6	12	2	2	3	4	5	6	14
1. SINGLE DX	107	1.9	<1	1	1	2	2	3	3	4
2. MULTIPLE DX	1,063	2.8	7	1	2	2	3	4	5	11
A. NOT OPERATED	735	2.2	2	1	2	2	2	3	3	5
B. OPERATED	435	3.6	12	2	2	3	4	5	6	14
TOTAL										
0–19 Years	61	3.0	6	1	2	2	3	5	7	17
20–34	884	2.6	4	1	2	2	3	4	5	9
35–49	217	3.0	16	1	2	2	3	4	5	9
50–64	8	2.7	1	1	2	2	4	4	4	4
65+	0									
GRAND TOTAL	1,170	2.7	6	1	2	2	3	4	5	9

658: OTH AMNIOTIC CAVITY PROB

Type of Patients	Observed Patients	Avg. Stay	Vari- ance	10th	25th	50th	75th	90th	95th	99th
1. SINGLE DX										
A. Not Operated										
0–19 Years	380	2.3	2	1	2	2	3	3	4	10
20–34	2,324	2.2	2	1	2	2	2	3	3	8
35–49	96	2.4	10	1	1	2	3	3	6	26
50–64	2	1.5	<1	1	1	2	2	2	2	2
65+	0									
B. Operated										
0–19 Years	8	3.4	<1	3	3	3	4	4	4	4
20–34	66	3.3	<1	2	3	3	4	4	5	6
35–49	2	3.5	<1	3	3	4	4	4	4	4
50–64	0									
65+	0									
2. MULTIPLE DX										
A. Not Operated										
0–19 Years	2,464	2.8	7	1	2	2	3	4	5	15
20–34	14,870	2.8	9	1	2	2	3	4	5	16
35–49	2,610	2.9	11	1	2	2	3	4	6	18
50–64	119	3.2	24	1	2	2	3	4	8	24
65+	0									
B. Operated										
0–19 Years	619	4.4	24	2	3	3	4	5	7	27
20–34	5,478	4.5	22	2	3	3	4	6	11	27
35–49	1,493	4.8	27	2	3	4	5	7	11	29
50–64	89	6.5	75	2	3	4	5	16	22	47
65+	0									
SUBTOTALS:										
1. SINGLE DX										
A. Not Operated	2,802	2.2	3	1	2	2	2	3	3	9
B. Operated	76	3.3	<1	3	3	3	4	5	6	
2. MULTIPLE DX										
A. Not Operated	20,063	2.8	9	1	2	2	3	4	5	16
B. Operated	7,679	4.6	24	2	3	3	4	6	11	28
1. SINGLE DX	2,878	2.2	3	1	2	2	3	3	4	9
2. MULTIPLE DX	27,742	3.3	14	1	2	3	3	5	7	21
A. NOT OPERATED	22,865	2.7	9	1	2	2	3	4	5	15
B. OPERATED	7,755	4.5	23	2	3	3	4	6	11	28
TOTAL										
0–19 Years	3,471	3.1	10	2	2	2	3	4	6	16
20–34	22,738	3.1	12	2	2	3	3	4	6	19
35–49	4,201	3.5	18	1	2	3	4	5	8	24
50–64	210	4.6	48	1	2	3	4	7	16	44
65+	0									
GRAND TOTAL	30,620	3.2	13	1	2	3	3	5	6	20

658.01: OLIGOHYDRAMNIOS-DEL

Type of Patients	Observed Patients	Avg. Stay	Vari- ance	10th	25th	50th	75th	90th	95th	99th
1. SINGLE DX										
A. Not Operated										
0–19 Years	88	2.3	<1	1	2	2	3	3	3	4
20–34	653	2.1	<1	1	2	2	3	3	3	4
35–49	19	2.3	<1	1	2	2	3	3	4	4
50–64	0									
65+	0									
B. Operated										
0–19 Years	3	3.3	<1	3	3	3	4	4	4	4
20–34	37	3.3	<1	2	3	3	4	4	5	5
35–49	1	3.0	0	3	3	3	3	3	3	3
50–64	0									
65+	0									
2. MULTIPLE DX										
A. Not Operated										
0–19 Years	728	2.6	1	2	2	2	3	3	4	6
20–34	4,367	2.5	2	1	2	2	3	3	4	6
35–49	777	2.5	2	1	2	2	3	3	4	6
50–64	36	2.6	<1	2	2	3	3	3	3	4
65+	0									
B. Operated										
0–19 Years	207	3.9	14	2	3	3	4	5	5	8
20–34	1,963	3.8	8	2	3	3	4	5	6	17
35–49	532	4.2	15	1	3	4	4	5	6	21
50–64	29	3.6	<1	2	3	3	4	5	5	6
65+	0									
SUBTOTALS:										
1. SINGLE DX										
A. Not Operated	760	2.1	<1	1	2	2	3	3	3	4
B. Operated	41	3.3	<1	3	3	3	4	4	4	5
2. MULTIPLE DX										
A. Not Operated	5,908	2.5	2	1	2	2	3	3	4	6
B. Operated	2,731	3.9	10	2	3	3	4	5	6	18
1. SINGLE DX	801	2.2	<1	1	2	2	3	3	3	4
2. MULTIPLE DX	8,639	2.9	5	2	2	3	3	4	5	9
A. NOT OPERATED	6,668	2.5	2	1	2	2	3	3	4	6
B. OPERATED	2,772	3.9	9	2	3	3	4	5	6	18
TOTAL										
0–19 Years	1,026	2.8	4	2	2	3	3	4	5	6
20–34	7,020	2.8	4	2	2	3	3	4	5	8
35–49	1,329	3.2	8	2	2	3	3	4	5	13
50–64	65	3.1	<1	2	3	3	3	5	6	
65+	0									
GRAND TOTAL	9,440	2.9	5	2	2	3	3	4	5	9

Length of Stay by Diagnosis and Operation, Western Region, 2008

Western Region, October 2006–September 2007 Data, by Diagnosis

658.03: OLIGOHYDRAMNIOS-AP

Type of Patients	Observed Patients	Avg. Stay	Variance	10th	25th	50th	75th	90th	95th	99th
1. SINGLE DX										
A. Not Operated										
0–19 Years	24	3.0	7	1	1	2	3	6	10	11
20–34	122	2.3	6	1	1	1	2	5	7	12
35–49	11	1.9	3	1	1	1	3	4	6	6
50–64	0									
65+	0									
B. Operated										
0–19 Years	0									
20–34	0									
35–49	0									
50–64	0									
65+	0									
2. MULTIPLE DX										
A. Not Operated										
0–19 Years	52	2.9	13	1	1	2	3	5	11	20
20–34	373	3.1	14	1	1	2	4	7	9	21
35–49	130	3.5	15	1	1	2	4	8	11	21
50–64	2	1.0	0	1	1	1	1	1	1	1
65+	0									
B. Operated										
0–19 Years	0									
20–34	1	5.0	0	5	5	5	5	5	5	5
35–49	0									
50–64	0									
65+	0									
SUBTOTALS:										
1. SINGLE DX — A. Not Operated	157	2.4	6	1	1	1	2	6	8	12
1. SINGLE DX — B. Operated	0									
2. MULTIPLE DX — A. Not Operated	557	3.2	14	1	1	2	4	7	10	21
2. MULTIPLE DX — B. Operated	1	5.0	0	5	5	5	5	5	5	5
1. SINGLE DX	157	2.4	6	1	1	1	2	6	8	12
2. MULTIPLE DX	558	3.2	14	1	1	2	4	7	10	21
A. NOT OPERATED	714	3.0	12	1	1	2	3	7	10	20
B. OPERATED	1	5.0	0	5	5	5	5	5	5	5
TOTAL										
0–19 Years	76	2.9	11	1	1	2	3	6	11	20
20–34	496	2.9	12	1	1	2	3	7	9	20
35–49	141	3.4	14	1	1	2	4	7	9	21
50–64	2	1.0	0	1	1	1	1	1	1	1
65+	0									
GRAND TOTAL	715	3.0	12	1	1	2	3	7	10	20

658.11: PREMATURE RUPT MEMB-DEL

Type of Patients	Observed Patients	Avg. Stay	Variance	10th	25th	50th	75th	90th	95th	99th
1. SINGLE DX										
A. Not Operated										
0–19 Years	159	2.0	<1	1	2	2	2	3	3	3
20–34	957	1.9	<1	1	1	2	2	3	3	4
35–49	39	1.8	<1	1	1	2	2	3	3	3
50–64	2	1.5	<1	1	1	2	2	2	2	2
65+	0									
B. Operated										
0–19 Years	5	3.4	<1	3	3	3	4	4	4	4
20–34	14	3.1	<1	2	3	3	4	4	4	4
35–49	1	4.0	0	4	4	4	4	4	4	4
50–64	0									
65+	0									
2. MULTIPLE DX										
A. Not Operated										
0–19 Years	941	2.4	3	1	2	2	3	3	3	9
20–34	6,402	2.3	4	1	2	2	3	3	4	10
35–49	1,131	2.5	6	1	2	2	3	3	4	14
50–64	48	2.2	3	1	1	2	2	3	3	13
65+	0									
B. Operated										
0–19 Years	201	4.1	30	2	3	3	4	5	7	25
20–34	2,016	3.7	9	2	3	3	4	5	7	20
35–49	641	4.2	17	2	3	4	4	6	8	22
50–64	41	5.3	36	2	3	4	4	8	20	33
65+	0									
SUBTOTALS:										
1. SINGLE DX — A. Not Operated	1,157	1.9	<1	1	1	2	2	3	3	4
1. SINGLE DX — B. Operated	20	3.3	<1	3	3	3	4	4	4	4
2. MULTIPLE DX — A. Not Operated	8,522	2.3	4	1	2	2	3	3	4	10
2. MULTIPLE DX — B. Operated	2,899	3.9	13	2	3	3	4	5	8	21
1. SINGLE DX	1,177	2.0	<1	1	1	2	2	3	3	4
2. MULTIPLE DX	11,421	2.7	7	1	2	2	3	4	5	13
A. NOT OPERATED	9,679	2.3	4	1	2	2	3	3	3	10
B. OPERATED	2,919	3.9	13	2	3	3	4	5	8	21
TOTAL										
0–19 Years	1,306	2.6	7	1	2	2	3	3	4	11
20–34	9,389	2.6	5	1	2	2	3	4	5	11
35–49	1,812	3.1	11	1	2	2	3	4	6	18
50–64	91	3.5	20	2	3	3	4	5	8	33
65+	0									
GRAND TOTAL	12,598	2.7	6	1	2	2	3	4	5	12

658.13: PREMATURE RUPT MEMB-AP

Type of Patients	Observed Patients	Avg. Stay	Variance	10th	25th	50th	75th	90th	95th	99th
1. SINGLE DX										
A. Not Operated										
0–19 Years	18	3.2	9	1	1	3	3	8	13	13
20–34	125	2.7	12	1	1	2	3	5	8	16
35–49	11	4.6	61	1	1	1	3	12	26	26
50–64	0									
65+	0									
B. Operated										
0–19 Years	0									
20–34	0									
35–49	0									
50–64	0									
65+	0									
2. MULTIPLE DX										
A. Not Operated										
0–19 Years	44	3.5	15	1	1	2	5	8	13	16
20–34	189	4.7	42	1	1	2	5	13	19	32
35–49	61	2.9	18	1	1	2	3	5	8	28
50–64	1	2.0	0	2	2	2	2	2	2	2
65+	0									
B. Operated										
0–19 Years	0									
20–34	4	1.5	<1	1	1	1	2	2	2	2
35–49	1	2.0	0	2	2	2	2	2	2	2
50–64	0									
65+	0									
SUBTOTALS:										
1. SINGLE DX — A. Not Operated	154	2.9	15	1	1	2	3	5	11	26
1. SINGLE DX — B. Operated	0									
2. MULTIPLE DX — A. Not Operated	295	4.1	34	1	1	2	4	9	17	31
2. MULTIPLE DX — B. Operated	5	1.6	<1	1	1	2	2	2	2	2
1. SINGLE DX	154	2.9	15	1	1	2	3	5	11	26
2. MULTIPLE DX	300	4.1	33	1	1	2	4	9	16	31
A. NOT OPERATED	449	3.7	27	1	1	2	4	8	15	28
B. OPERATED	5	1.6	<1	1	1	2	2	2	2	2
TOTAL										
0–19 Years	62	3.4	13	1	1	2	4	8	13	16
20–34	318	3.9	31	1	1	2	4	8	16	30
35–49	73	3.2	24	1	2	2	3	5	13	28
50–64	1	2.0	0	2	2	2	2	2	2	2
65+	0									
GRAND TOTAL	454	3.7	27	1	1	2	4	8	15	28

Length of Stay by Diagnosis and Operation. Western Region, 2008

Western Region, October 2006–September 2007 Data, by Diagnosis

658.21: PROLONG RUPT MEMB-DEL

Type of Patients	Observed Patients	Avg. Stay	Variance	Percentiles 10th	25th	50th	75th	90th	95th	99th
1. SINGLE DX										
A. Not Operated										
0–19 Years	40	2.8	6	2	2	2	3	3	7	16
20–34	237	2.6	6	1	2	2	3	3	5	11
35–49	6	4.8	23	2	2	2	6	14	14	14
50–64	0									
65+	0									
B. Operated										
0–19 Years	0									
20–34	6	3.3	2	2	3	3	3	6	6	6
35–49	0									
50–64	0									
65+	0									
2. MULTIPLE DX										
A. Not Operated										
0–19 Years	347	4.5	33	2	2	3	4	8	15	33
20–34	2,112	4.4	35	2	2	3	4	8	14	30
35–49	352	4.8	39	2	2	3	4	11	14	31
50–64	22	6.9	109	1	2	3	7	13	24	47
65+	0									
B. Operated										
0–19 Years	104	5.9	41	3	3	4	5	13	19	36
20–34	904	7.8	76	3	3	4	8	17	25	46
35–49	215	8.2	82	3	4	5	9	18	27	40
50–64	17	14.9	227	4	4	8	18	44	47	47
65+	0									
SUBTOTALS:										
1. SINGLE DX										
A. Not Operated	283	2.7	7	1	2	2	3	3	5	15
B. Operated	6	3.3	2	2	3	3	3	6	6	6
2. MULTIPLE DX										
A. Not Operated	2,833	4.5	36	2	2	3	4	8	14	31
B. Operated	1,240	7.8	77	3	3	4	8	17	26	46
1. SINGLE DX	289	2.7	7	1	2	2	3	3	6	15
2. MULTIPLE DX	4,073	5.5	51	2	2	3	5	12	19	39
A. NOT OPERATED	3,116	4.3	33	2	2	3	4	8	14	31
B. OPERATED	1,246	7.8	77	3	3	4	8	17	26	46
TOTAL										
0–19 Years	491	4.6	33	2	2	3	4	8	16	35
20–34	3,259	5.2	47	2	2	3	5	11	18	37
35–49	573	6.1	58	2	2	3	6	13	23	40
50–64	39	10.4	172	2	2	5	13	42	47	47
65+	0									
GRAND TOTAL	4,362	5.3	48	2	2	3	5	11	18	39

658.41: AMNIOTIC INFECTION-DEL

Type of Patients	Observed Patients	Avg. Stay	Variance	Percentiles 10th	25th	50th	75th	90th	95th	99th
1. SINGLE DX										
A. Not Operated										
0–19 Years	36	2.3	<1	2	2	2	3	3	4	4
20–34	167	2.2	<1	1	2	2	3	3	3	4
35–49	3	2.0	<1	1	1	2	3	3	3	3
50–64	0									
65+	0									
B. Operated										
0–19 Years	0									
20–34	9	3.7	<1	3	3	3	4	5	5	5
35–49	0									
50–64	0									
65+	0									
2. MULTIPLE DX										
A. Not Operated										
0–19 Years	329	2.7	<1	2	2	3	4	4	4	6
20–34	1,301	2.6	3	2	2	3	3	4	4	6
35–49	132	2.9	16	2	2	3	3	4	4	6
50–64	10	2.5	<1	2	2	3	3	4	4	4
65+	0									
B. Operated										
0–19 Years	105	4.4	11	3	3	4	5	6	7	24
20–34	569	4.2	6	3	3	4	4	5	7	18
35–49	98	4.3	5	3	3	4	5	7	8	19
50–64	2	3.5	<1	3	3	4	4	4	4	4
65+	0									
SUBTOTALS:										
1. SINGLE DX										
A. Not Operated	206	2.2	<1	2	2	2	3	3	3	4
B. Operated	9	3.7	<1	3	3	3	4	5	5	5
2. MULTIPLE DX										
A. Not Operated	1,772	2.6	4	2	2	3	3	4	4	6
B. Operated	774	4.2	7	3	3	4	5	6	7	19
1. SINGLE DX	215	2.3	<1	1	2	2	3	3	4	4
2. MULTIPLE DX	2,546	3.1	5	2	2	3	3	4	5	9
A. NOT OPERATED	1,978	2.6	3	2	2	3	3	4	4	6
B. OPERATED	783	4.2	7	3	3	4	5	6	7	19
TOTAL										
0–19 Years	470	3.0	3	2	2	3	3	4	5	7
20–34	2,046	3.0	4	2	2	3	3	5	5	8
35–49	233	3.5	12	2	2	3	3	5	6	11
50–64	12	2.7	<1	2	2	3	3	4	4	4
65+	0									
GRAND TOTAL	2,761	3.1	5	2	2	3	3	4	5	8

659: OTH INDICATION CARE-DEL

Type of Patients	Observed Patients	Avg. Stay	Variance	Percentiles 10th	25th	50th	75th	90th	95th	99th
1. SINGLE DX										
A. Not Operated										
0–19 Years	1,314	1.9	<1	1	1	2	2	2	3	3
20–34	5,460	1.8	<1	1	1	2	2	3	3	3
35–49	5,205	1.7	<1	1	1	2	2	2	3	3
50–64	311	1.9	<1	1	1	2	2	3	3	3
65+	0									
B. Operated										
0–19 Years	301	3.1	<1	2	3	3	4	4	4	5
20–34	1,781	3.2	<1	2	3	3	4	4	4	5
35–49	219	3.1	<1	2	3	3	4	4	4	5
50–64	17	3.0	1	2	2	3	4	4	5	5
65+	0									
2. MULTIPLE DX										
A. Not Operated										
0–19 Years	4,749	2.2	<1	1	2	2	3	3	3	5
20–34	22,842	2.0	<1	1	1	2	2	3	3	4
35–49	15,977	1.9	<1	1	1	2	2	3	3	4
50–64	838	2.0	<1	1	1	2	2	3	3	4
65+	0									
B. Operated										
0–19 Years	2,670	3.5	3	2	3	3	4	5	5	11
20–34	18,598	3.5	4	2	3	3	4	5	5	8
35–49	9,328	3.3	5	2	3	3	4	5	5	9
50–64	568	3.5	6	3	3	3	4	5	5	13
65+	0									
SUBTOTALS:										
1. SINGLE DX										
A. Not Operated	12,290	1.8	<1	1	1	2	2	3	3	3
B. Operated	2,318	3.1	<1	2	3	3	4	4	4	5
2. MULTIPLE DX										
A. Not Operated	44,406	2.0	<1	1	1	2	2	3	3	4
B. Operated	31,164	3.5	4	2	3	3	4	5	5	9
1. SINGLE DX	14,608	2.0	<1	1	2	2	3	3	4	4
2. MULTIPLE DX	75,570	2.6	3	2	2	3	3	4	5	7
A. NOT OPERATED	56,696	1.9	<1	1	1	2	3	3	3	4
B. OPERATED	33,482	3.5	4	2	3	3	4	5	5	9
TOTAL										
0–19 Years	9,034	2.6	2	1	2	2	3	4	4	6
20–34	48,681	2.6	3	1	2	3	3	4	5	6
35–49	30,729	2.3	2	1	2	3	3	4	4	6
50–64	1,734	2.5	3	1	2	2	3	4	4	6
65+	0									
GRAND TOTAL	90,178	2.5	2	1	2	2	3	3	4	6

Length of Stay by Diagnosis and Operation, Western Region, 2008

Western Region, October 2006–September 2007 Data, by Diagnosis

659.11: FAIL INDUCTION NOS-DEL

Type of Patients	Observed Patients	Avg. Stay	Variance	10th	25th	50th	75th	90th	95th	99th
1. SINGLE DX										
A. Not Operated										
0–19 Years	0									
20–34	3	2.3	<1	2	2	2	3	3	3	3
35–49	0									
50–64	0									
65+	0									
B. Operated										
0–19 Years	13	3.1	<1	2	2	3	4	4	5	5
20–34	52	3.7	<1	3	3	4	4	5	5	5
35–49	0									
50–64	0									
65+	0									
2. MULTIPLE DX										
A. Not Operated										
0–19 Years	5	2.4	1	1	2	2	3	4	4	4
20–34	11	2.3	<1	1	1	3	3	3	3	3
35–49	1	3.0	0	3	3	3	3	3	3	3
50–64	0									
65+	0									
B. Operated										
0–19 Years	144	3.9	1	3	3	4	5	5	6	7
20–34	1,085	4.1	3	3	3	4	5	5	6	8
35–49	218	4.4	2	3	3	4	5	6	7	8
50–64	15	4.2	1	3	3	4	5	5	7	7
65+	0									
SUBTOTALS:										
1. SINGLE DX										
A. Not Operated	3	2.3	<1	2	2	2	3	3	3	3
B. Operated	65	3.5	<1	2	3	4	4	5	5	5
2. MULTIPLE DX										
A. Not Operated	17	2.4	<1	1	2	3	3	3	4	4
B. Operated	1,462	4.1	3	3	3	4	5	6	6	8
1. SINGLE DX	68	3.5	<1	2	3	4	4	5	5	5
2. MULTIPLE DX	1,479	4.1	3	3	3	4	5	6	6	8
A. NOT OPERATED	20	2.4	<1	1	2	3	3	3	4	4
B. OPERATED	1,527	4.1	2	3	3	4	5	6	6	8
TOTAL										
0–19 Years	162	3.8	1	2	3	4	4	5	6	7
20–34	1,151	4.1	3	3	3	4	5	6	6	8
35–49	219	4.4	2	3	3	4	5	6	6	8
50–64	15	4.2	1	3	3	4	5	5	7	7
65+	0									
GRAND TOTAL	1,547	4.1	2	3	3	4	5	5	6	8

659.13: FAIL INDUCTION NOS-AP

Type of Patients	Observed Patients	Avg. Stay	Variance	10th	25th	50th	75th	90th	95th	99th
1. SINGLE DX										
A. Not Operated										
0–19 Years	65	1.1	<1	1	1	1	1	1	2	3
20–34	380	1.1	<1	1	1	1	1	2	2	2
35–49	46	1.0	<1	1	1	1	1	1	1	2
50–64	0									
65+	0									
B. Operated										
0–19 Years	0									
20–34	0									
35–49	0									
50–64	0									
65+	0									
2. MULTIPLE DX										
A. Not Operated										
0–19 Years	48	1.2	<1	1	1	1	1	2	2	2
20–34	407	1.2	<1	1	1	1	1	2	2	3
35–49	98	1.2	0	1	1	1	1	2	2	3
50–64	0	1.0		1	1	1	1	1	1	1
65+	0									
B. Operated										
0–19 Years	0									
20–34	1	5.0	0	5	5	5	5	5	5	5
35–49	0									
50–64	0									
65+	0									
SUBTOTALS:										
1. SINGLE DX										
A. Not Operated	491	1.1	<1	1	1	1	1	1	2	2
B. Operated	0									
2. MULTIPLE DX										
A. Not Operated	554	1.2	<1	1	1	1	1	2	2	3
B. Operated	1	5.0	0	5	5	5	5	5	5	5
1. SINGLE DX	491	1.1	<1	1	1	1	1	1	2	2
2. MULTIPLE DX	555	1.2	<1	1	1	1	2	2	2	3
A. NOT OPERATED	1,045	1.1	<1	1	1	1	1	2	2	3
B. OPERATED	1	5.0	0	5	5	5	5	5	5	5
TOTAL										
0–19 Years	113	1.2	<1	1	1	1	2	2	2	2
20–34	788	1.1	<1	1	1	1	1	2	2	3
35–49	144	1.2	<1	1	1	1	1	2	2	2
50–64	1	1.0	0	1	1	1	1	1	1	1
65+	0									
GRAND TOTAL	1,046	1.1	<1	1	1	1	1	2	2	3

659.21: PYREXIA IN LABOR-DEL

Type of Patients	Observed Patients	Avg. Stay	Variance	10th	25th	50th	75th	90th	95th	99th
1. SINGLE DX										
A. Not Operated										
0–19 Years	55	2.3	<1	1	2	2	3	3	3	5
20–34	217	2.2	<1	1	2	2	3	3	3	4
35–49	3	2.0	<1	1	1	2	3	3	3	3
50–64	0									
65+	0									
B. Operated										
0–19 Years	0									
20–34	2	3.5	<1	3	3	4	4	4	4	4
35–49	0									
50–64	0									
65+	0									
2. MULTIPLE DX										
A. Not Operated										
0–19 Years	184	2.3	<1	2	2	2	3	3	3	4
20–34	795	2.2	<1	1	2	2	3	3	3	4
35–49	64	2.4	<1	2	2	2	3	3	4	4
50–64	0	2.3		2	2	2	3	3	3	3
65+	0									
B. Operated										
0–19 Years	10	3.1	<1	2	3	3	4	4	4	4
20–34	106	3.4	4	2	3	3	4	5	5	13
35–49	13	3.7	2	3	3	4	4	5	7	7
50–64	0									
65+	0									
SUBTOTALS:										
1. SINGLE DX										
A. Not Operated	275	2.2	<1	1	2	2	3	3	3	5
B. Operated	2	3.5	<1	3	4	4	4	4	4	4
2. MULTIPLE DX										
A. Not Operated	1,046	2.3	<1	2	2	2	3	3	3	4
B. Operated	129	3.4	3	2	3	3	4	5	5	13
1. SINGLE DX	277	2.2	<1	1	2	2	3	3	3	5
2. MULTIPLE DX	1,175	2.4	<1	2	2	2	3	3	4	5
A. NOT OPERATED	1,321	2.3	<1	1	2	2	3	3	3	4
B. OPERATED	131	3.4	3	2	3	3	4	5	5	13
TOTAL										
0–19 Years	249	2.4	<1	2	2	2	3	3	3	4
20–34	1,120	2.3	<1	1	2	2	3	3	4	5
35–49	80	2.6	1	2	2	2	3	4	4	7
50–64	3	2.3	<1	2	2	2	3	3	3	3
65+	0									
GRAND TOTAL	1,452	2.4	<1	1	2	2	3	3	4	5

Length of Stay by Diagnosis and Operation, Western Region, 2008

Western Region, October 2006–September 2007 Data, by Diagnosis

659.41: GRAND MULTIPARITY-DEL

Type of Patients	Observed Patients	Avg. Stay	Variance	10th	25th	50th	75th	90th	95th	99th
1. SINGLE DX										
A. Not Operated										
0–19 Years	0									
20–34	297	1.6	<1	1	1	2	2	2	3	3
35–49	31	1.5	<1	1	1	2	2	2	3	2
50–64	2	2.5	<1	2	2	3	3	3	3	3
65+	0									
B. Operated										
0–19 Years	0									
20–34	7	2.3	<1	1	2	2	3	4	4	4
35–49	0									
50–64	0									
65+	0									
2. MULTIPLE DX										
A. Not Operated										
0–19 Years	0									
20–34	491	1.8	<1	1	1	2	2	3	3	3
35–49	206	1.7	<1	1	1	2	2	3	3	3
50–64	10	1.5	<1	1	1	2	2	2	2	2
65+	0									
B. Operated										
0–19 Years	0									
20–34	358	2.4	3	1	2	2	3	3	4	5
35–49	85	2.5	<1	2	2	3	3	4	4	4
50–64	5	2.8	1	2	2	4	4	4	4	4
65+	0									
SUBTOTALS:										
1. SINGLE DX										
A. Not Operated	330	1.6	<1	1	1	2	2	2	3	3
B. Operated	7	2.3	<1	2	2	3	3	4	4	4
2. MULTIPLE DX										
A. Not Operated	707	1.7	<1	1	1	2	2	3	3	3
B. Operated	448	2.5	3	2	2	2	3	4	4	5
1. SINGLE DX	337	1.6	<1	1	1	2	2	2	3	3
2. MULTIPLE DX	1,155	2.0	1	1	1	2	2	3	3	4
A. NOT OPERATED	1,037	1.7	<1	1	1	2	2	3	3	3
B. OPERATED	455	2.5	3	2	2	2	3	4	4	5
TOTAL										
0–19 Years	0									
20–34	1,153	1.9	1	1	1	2	2	3	3	4
35–49	322	1.9	<1	1	1	2	2	3	3	4
50–64	17	2.0	<1	1	1	2	2	3	3	4
65+	0									
GRAND TOTAL	1,492	1.9	1	1	1	2	2	3	3	4

659.51: ELDERLY PRIMIGRAVIDA-DEL

Type of Patients	Observed Patients	Avg. Stay	Variance	10th	25th	50th	75th	90th	95th	99th
1. SINGLE DX										
A. Not Operated										
0–19 Years	1	3.0	0	3	3	3	3	3	3	3
20–34	6	1.5	<1	1	1	1	2	3	3	3
35–49	399	2.0	<1	1	2	2	2	3	3	3
50–64	31	2.0	<1	1	1	2	2	3	3	4
65+	0									
B. Operated										
0–19 Years	0									
20–34	0									
35–49	61	3.3	<1	2	3	3	4	4	4	5
50–64	6	3.0	<1	2	2	3	4	4	4	4
65+	0									
2. MULTIPLE DX										
A. Not Operated										
0–19 Years	4	2.0	<1	1	2	2	3	3	3	3
20–34	15	2.3	<1	2	2	3	3	3	4	4
35–49	1,462	2.2	<1	1	2	3	3	3	4	4
50–64	102	2.3	<1	2	2	3	3	3	3	4
65+	0									
B. Operated										
0–19 Years	0									
20–34	8	3.4	2	2	3	3	4	6	6	6
35–49	773	3.6	3	2	3	3	4	5	5	8
50–64	64	4.0	13	2	3	4	4	5	5	31
65+	0									
SUBTOTALS:										
1. SINGLE DX										
A. Not Operated	437	2.0	<1	1	2	2	2	3	3	3
B. Operated	67	3.3	<1	2	3	3	4	4	4	5
2. MULTIPLE DX										
A. Not Operated	1,583	2.2	<1	1	2	2	3	3	3	4
B. Operated	845	3.6	4	2	3	3	4	5	5	8
1. SINGLE DX	504	2.2	<1	1	2	2	3	3	4	4
2. MULTIPLE DX	2,428	2.7	2	2	2	2	3	4	5	6
A. NOT OPERATED	2,020	2.2	<1	1	2	2	3	3	4	4
B. OPERATED	912	3.6	4	2	3	3	4	5	5	8
TOTAL										
0–19 Years	5	2.2	<1	1	2	2	3	3	3	3
20–34	29	2.4	1	1	2	2	3	4	4	6
35–49	2,695	2.6	2	1	2	2	3	4	4	6
50–64	203	2.8	5	2	2	2	3	4	5	5
65+	0									
GRAND TOTAL	2,932	2.6	2	1	2	2	3	4	4	6

659.61: ELDERLY MULTIGRAVIDA-DEL

Type of Patients	Observed Patients	Avg. Stay	Variance	10th	25th	50th	75th	90th	95th	99th
1. SINGLE DX										
A. Not Operated										
0–19 Years	1	2.0	0	2	2	2	2	2	2	2
20–34	37	1.6	<1	1	1	2	2	2	2	3
35–49	4,549	1.7	<1	1	1	2	2	2	3	3
50–64	274	1.8	<1	1	1	2	2	3	3	3
65+	0									
B. Operated										
0–19 Years	0									
20–34	0									
35–49	73	2.9	<1	2	2	3	3	4	4	4
50–64	6	2.0	<1	1	2	2	3	3	3	3
65+	0									
2. MULTIPLE DX										
A. Not Operated										
0–19 Years	0									
20–34	61	1.8	<1	1	1	2	2	3	3	4
35–49	10,479	1.8	<1	1	1	2	3	3	3	4
50–64	563	1.9	<1	1	1	2	2	3	3	3
65+	0									
B. Operated										
0–19 Years	0									
20–34	24	2.8	2	2	2	2	3	4	5	8
35–49	4,019	2.8	3	2	2	3	3	4	4	6
50–64	277	3.1	3	2	2	3	4	4	5	11
65+	0									
SUBTOTALS:										
1. SINGLE DX										
A. Not Operated	4,861	1.7	<1	1	1	2	2	2	3	3
B. Operated	79	2.9	<1	2	2	3	3	4	4	4
2. MULTIPLE DX										
A. Not Operated	11,103	1.8	<1	1	1	2	3	3	3	4
B. Operated	4,320	2.8	3	2	2	3	3	4	5	6
1. SINGLE DX	4,940	1.7	<1	1	1	2	2	2	3	3
2. MULTIPLE DX	15,423	2.1	1	1	2	2	3	3	4	5
A. NOT OPERATED	15,964	1.8	<1	1	1	2	2	3	3	3
B. OPERATED	4,399	2.8	3	2	2	3	3	4	4	6
TOTAL										
0–19 Years	1	2.0	0	2	2	2	2	2	2	2
20–34	122	1.9	<1	1	1	2	2	3	3	5
35–49	19,120	2.0	1	1	2	2	3	3	4	5
50–64	1,120	2.2	1	2	2	3	3	4	4	6
65+	0									
GRAND TOTAL	20,363	2.0	1	1	1	2	3	4	4	5

553

Length of Stay by Diagnosis and Operation, Western Region, 2008

Western Region, October 2006–September 2007 Data, by Diagnosis

Type of Patients	659.71: ABN FHR/RHYTHM-DEL Observed Patients	Avg. Stay	Vari-ance	10th	25th	50th	75th	90th	95th	99th	659.73: ABN FHR/RHYTHM-AP Observed Patients	Avg. Stay	Vari-ance	10th	25th	50th	75th	90th	95th	99th	659.81: COMP LABOR NEC-DEL Observed Patients	Avg. Stay	Vari-ance	10th	25th	50th	75th	90th	95th	99th
1. SINGLE DX																														
A. Not Operated																														
0–19 Years	628	1.9	<1	1	1	2	2	3	3	3	13	1.1	<1	1	1	1	1	1	2	2	523	2.0	<1	1	2	2	2	3	3	3
20–34	3,563	1.8	<1	1	1	2	2	3	3	3	87	1.6	1	1	1	1	2	3	4	6	702	1.8	<1	1	1	2	2	3	3	3
35–49	117	2.0	<1	1	1	2	2	3	3	3	6	1.5	2	1	1	1	1	4	4	4	19	1.8	<1	1	1	2	2	3	3	3
50–64	4	2.0	<1	1	1	2	2	3	3	3	0										0									
65+	0										0										0									
B. Operated																														
0–19 Years	278	3.1	<1	2	3	3	4	4	4	5	0										8	2.4	<1	2	2	2	3	4	4	4
20–34	1,613	3.2	<1	2	3	3	4	4	4	5	3	2.0	1	1	1	2	3	3	3	3	102	2.8	<1	2	2	3	3	3	4	5
35–49	74	3.1	<1	2	3	3	4	4	4	5	0										10	2.8	<1	2	2	3	3	4	4	4
50–64	4	4.0	<1	3	4	4	5	5	5	5	0										1	4.0	0	4	4	4	4	4	4	4
65+	0										0										0									
2. MULTIPLE DX																														
A. Not Operated																														
0–19 Years	3,270	2.2	<1	1	2	2	2	3	3	5	41	2.2	5	1	1	1	2	3	3	11	1,142	2.1	<1	1	2	2	2	3	3	4
20–34	18,737	2.0	<1	1	2	2	2	3	3	4	246	2.4	9	1	1	1	2	5	8	15	1,811	1.9	<1	1	1	2	2	3	3	4
35–49	3,056	2.1	<1	1	2	2	2	3	4	4	81	2.3	7	1	1	1	2	6	8	14	374	2.0	<1	1	2	2	2	3	3	3
50–64	143	2.1	<1	1	2	2	3	3	3	5	0										14	2.1	<1	1	2	2	2	3	3	3
65+	0										0										0									
B. Operated																														
0–19 Years	2,369	3.5	3	2	3	3	4	5	5	11	0										137	3.4	7	2	2	3	4	4	5	7
20–34	16,376	3.5	4	2	3	3	4	5	5	9	3	3.3	2	2	2	3	5	5	5	5	551	2.8	<1	2	2	3	3	4	4	5
35–49	4,027	3.8	7	2	3	3	4	5	6	15	0										176	3.1	1	2	2	3	4	4	5	6
50–64	193	4.0	10	2	3	4	4	5	5	28	0										12	3.2	<1	3	3	3	3	4	5	5
65+	0										0										0									
SUBTOTALS:																														
1. SINGLE DX																														
A. Not Operated	4,312	1.9	<1	1	1	2	2	3	3	3	106	1.5	1	1	1	1	2	3	4	6	1,244	1.9	<1	1	1	2	2	3	3	3
B. Operated	1,969	3.2	<1	2	3	3	4	4	4	5	3	2.0	1	1	1	2	3	3	3	3	121	2.8	<1	2	2	3	3	4	4	5
2. MULTIPLE DX																														
A. Not Operated	25,206	2.0	<1	1	2	2	2	3	3	4	368	2.4	8	1	1	1	2	5	8	14	3,341	2.0	<1	1	2	2	2	3	3	4
B. Operated	22,965	3.6	4	2	3	3	4	5	5	10	3	3.3	2	2	2	3	5	5	5	5	876	2.9	2	2	2	3	3	4	5	6
1. SINGLE DX	6,281	2.3	<1	2	2	2	3	4	4	5	109	1.5	1	1	1	1	2	3	4	6	1,365	2.0	<1	1	2	2	2	3	3	4
2. MULTIPLE DX	48,171	2.8	3	2	2	3	3	4	5	7	371	2.4	8	1	1	1	2	5	8	14	4,217	2.2	<1	1	2	2	3	3	4	5
A. NOT OPERATED	29,518	2.0	<1	1	2	2	2	3	3	4	474	2.2	6	1	1	1	2	4	7	14	4,585	2.0	<1	1	2	2	2	3	3	4
B. OPERATED	24,934	3.6	4	2	3	3	4	5	5	9	6	2.7	2	2	2	3	4	5	5	5	997	2.9	2	2	3	3	3	4	5	6
TOTAL																														
0–19 Years	6,545	2.7	2	1	2	2	3	4	4	7	54	1.9	4	1	1	1	2	3	4	7	1,810	2.2	1	1	2	2	3	3	3	4
20–34	40,289	2.7	3	1	2	2	3	4	5	6	339	2.2	7	1	1	1	2	5	7	14	3,166	2.1	<1	1	2	2	3	3	3	4
35–49	7,274	3.0	5	2	2	3	4	4	5	9	87	2.3	7	1	1	1	2	6	8	14	579	2.3	<1	1	2	2	3	4	4	5
50–64	344	3.2	7	2	2	3	4	5	5	11	0										27	2.6	<1	2	2	3	3	4	4	5
65+	0										0										0									
GRAND TOTAL	54,452	2.7	3	1	2	2	3	4	5	7	480	2.2	6	1	1	1	2	5	7	14	5,582	2.1	<1	1	2	2	3	3	4	5

Length of Stay by Diagnosis and Operation, Western Region, 2008

Western Region, October 2006–September 2007 Data, by Diagnosis

660: OBSTRUCTED LABOR

Type of Patients	Observed Patients	Avg. Stay	Variance	Percentiles						
				10th	25th	50th	75th	90th	95th	99th
1. SINGLE DX										
A. *Not Operated*										
0–19 Years	62	1.7	<1	1	1	2	2	2	3	3
20–34	843	1.7	<1	1	1	2	2	2	3	3
35–49	35	1.6	<1	1	1	1	2	2	3	3
50–64	0									
65+	0									
B. *Operated*										
0–19 Years	17	3.1	<1	2	3	3	3	4	5	5
20–34	132	3.2	<1	2	3	3	4	4	5	5
35–49	4	3.8	<1	3	3	4	4	5	5	5
50–64	1	4.0	0	4	4	4	4	4	4	4
65+	0									
2. MULTIPLE DX										
A. *Not Operated*										
0–19 Years	430	2.1	<1	1	2	2	2	3	3	4
20–34	3,573	1.9	<1	1	1	2	3	3	3	4
35–49	581	1.9	<1	1	1	2	3	3	3	4
50–64	24	2.0	2	1	1	2	2	3	3	8
65+	0									
B. *Operated*										
0–19 Years	1,516	3.5	3	2	3	3	4	5	5	8
20–34	11,304	3.5	3	2	3	3	4	5	5	7
35–49	2,419	3.8	6	2	3	4	4	5	5	10
50–64	143	3.8	1	3	3	4	4	5	6	7
65+	0									
SUBTOTALS:										
1. SINGLE DX										
A. *Not Operated*	940	1.7	<1	1	1	2	2	2	3	3
B. *Operated*	154	3.2	<1	2	3	3	4	4	5	5
2. MULTIPLE DX										
A. *Not Operated*	4,608	2.0	<1	1	1	2	2	3	3	4
B. *Operated*	15,382	3.5	3	2	3	3	4	5	5	7
1. SINGLE DX	1,094	1.9	<1	1	2	2	2	3	4	4
2. MULTIPLE DX	19,990	3.2	3	2	3	3	4	5	5	7
A. NOT OPERATED	5,548	1.9	<1	1	1	2	2	3	3	4
B. OPERATED	15,536	3.5	3	2	3	3	4	5	5	7
TOTAL										
0–19 Years	2,025	3.2	2	2	2	3	4	4	5	7
20–34	15,852	3.0	3	2	2	3	4	4	5	6
35–49	3,039	3.4	6	2	2	4	4	5	5	9
50–64	168	3.6	2	2	3	4	4	5	6	8
65+	0									
GRAND TOTAL	21,084	3.1	3	2	3	3	4	4	5	7

660.01: OBSTR/FETAL MALPOS-DEL

Type of Patients	Observed Patients	Avg. Stay	Variance	Percentiles						
				10th	25th	50th	75th	90th	95th	99th
1. SINGLE DX										
A. *Not Operated*										
0–19 Years	1	3.0	0	3	3	3	3	3	3	3
20–34	0									
35–49	0									
50–64	0									
65+	0									
B. *Operated*										
0–19 Years	1	4.0	0	4	4	4	4	4	4	4
20–34	18	3.4	<1	2	3	3	4	4	5	5
35–49	1	5.0	0	5	5	5	5	5	5	5
50–64	1	4.0	0	4	4	4	4	4	4	4
65+	0									
2. MULTIPLE DX										
A. *Not Operated*										
0–19 Years	20	2.1	<1	2	2	2	2	3	3	3
20–34	220	2.1	<1	1	2	2	3	3	3	4
35–49	33	2.3	<1	1	2	2	3	3	4	4
50–64	1	8.0	0	8	8	8	8	8	8	8
65+	0									
B. *Operated*										
0–19 Years	556	3.5	4	2	3	3	4	5	5	8
20–34	4,602	3.4	4	2	3	3	4	5	5	8
35–49	1,008	3.8	10	2	3	4	4	5	5	14
50–64	59	3.9	2	3	3	4	4	5	7	10
65+	0									
SUBTOTALS:										
1. SINGLE DX										
A. *Not Operated*	1	3.0	0	3	3	3	3	3	3	3
B. *Operated*	21	3.5	<1	3	3	4	4	4	5	5
2. MULTIPLE DX										
A. *Not Operated*	274	2.1	<1	1	2	2	3	3	3	4
B. *Operated*	6,225	3.5	5	2	3	3	4	5	5	9
1. SINGLE DX	22	3.5	<1	3	3	3	4	4	5	5
2. MULTIPLE DX	6,499	3.4	5	2	3	3	4	5	5	9
A. NOT OPERATED	275	2.2	<1	1	2	2	3	3	3	4
B. OPERATED	6,246	3.5	5	2	3	3	4	5	5	9
TOTAL										
0–19 Years	578	3.4	4	2	3	3	4	5	5	8
20–34	4,840	3.4	4	2	3	3	4	5	5	8
35–49	1,042	3.7	10	2	3	3	4	5	5	14
50–64	61	4.0	2	3	3	4	4	5	7	10
65+	0									
GRAND TOTAL	6,521	3.4	5	2	3	3	4	5	5	9

660.11: BONY PELVIS OBSTR-DEL

Type of Patients	Observed Patients	Avg. Stay	Variance	Percentiles						
				10th	25th	50th	75th	90th	95th	99th
1. SINGLE DX										
A. *Not Operated*										
0–19 Years	0									
20–34	0									
35–49	0									
50–64	0									
65+	0									
B. *Operated*										
0–19 Years	4	3.0	<1	2	2	3	4	4	4	4
20–34	15	3.5	<1	2	3	4	4	4	5	5
35–49	0									
50–64	0									
65+	0									
2. MULTIPLE DX										
A. *Not Operated*										
0–19 Years	13	2.1	<1	1	2	2	2	3	3	3
20–34	78	2.4	<1	2	2	2	3	3	4	4
35–49	16	2.7	<1	2	2	3	3	4	4	4
50–64	0									
65+	0									
B. *Operated*										
0–19 Years	721	3.5	2	2	3	3	4	5	5	8
20–34	4,392	3.5	1	2	3	3	4	5	5	6
35–49	816	3.8	2	2	3	3	4	5	5	6
50–64	43	3.9	1	3	3	4	4	5	5	7
65+	0									
SUBTOTALS:										
1. SINGLE DX										
A. *Not Operated*	0									
B. *Operated*	19	3.4	<1	2	3	3	4	4	5	5
2. MULTIPLE DX										
A. *Not Operated*	107	2.4	<1	2	2	2	3	3	4	4
B. *Operated*	5,972	3.6	2	2	3	3	4	5	5	6
1. SINGLE DX	19	3.4	<1	2	3	3	4	4	5	5
2. MULTIPLE DX	6,079	3.6	2	2	3	4	4	5	5	6
A. NOT OPERATED	107	2.4	<1	2	2	2	3	3	4	4
B. OPERATED	5,991	3.6	2	2	3	3	4	5	5	6
TOTAL										
0–19 Years	738	3.5	2	2	3	3	4	5	5	8
20–34	4,485	3.5	1	2	3	3	4	5	5	6
35–49	832	3.8	2	2	3	4	4	5	5	6
50–64	43	3.9	1	3	3	4	4	5	5	7
65+	0									
GRAND TOTAL	6,098	3.6	2	2	3	3	4	5	5	6

Length of Stay by Diagnosis and Operation, Western Region, 2008

Western Region, October 2006–September 2007 Data, by Diagnosis

660.21: ABN PELV TISS OBSTR-DEL

Type of Patients	Observed Patients	Avg. Stay	Vari-ance	10th	25th	50th	75th	90th	95th	99th
1. SINGLE DX										
A. Not Operated										
0–19 Years	0									
20–34	2	1.5	<1	1	1	2	2	2	2	2
35–49	0									
50–64	0									
65+	0									
B. Operated										
0–19 Years	0									
20–34	0									
35–49	1	3.0	0	3	3	3	3	3	3	3
50–64	0									
65+	0									
2. MULTIPLE DX										
A. Not Operated										
0–19 Years	3	1.3	<1	1	1	1	2	2	2	2
20–34	26	1.8	<1	1	1	2	2	3	3	4
35–49	2	2.5	<1	2	2	3	3	3	3	3
50–64	0									
65+	0									
B. Operated										
0–19 Years	9	3.2	<1	2	3	3	4	5	5	5
20–34	255	3.4	11	2	3	3	4	4	5	9
35–49	96	3.6	6	2	3	3	4	4	9	17
50–64	11	2.9	<1	2	2	3	3	3	5	5
65+	0									
SUBTOTALS:										
1. SINGLE DX										
A. Not Operated	2	1.5	<1	1	1	2	2	2	2	2
B. Operated	1	3.0	0	3	3	3	3	3	3	3
2. MULTIPLE DX										
A. Not Operated	31	1.8	<1	1	1	2	2	2	3	4
B. Operated	371	3.5	9	2	3	3	4	4	5	15
1. SINGLE DX	3	2.0	<1	1	1	2	3	3	3	3
2. MULTIPLE DX	402	3.3	9	2	2	3	4	4	5	11
A. NOT OPERATED	33	1.8	<1	1	1	2	2	3	3	4
B. OPERATED	372	3.5	9	2	3	3	4	4	5	15
TOTAL										
0–19 Years	12	2.8	1	1	2	3	3	3	5	5
20–34	283	3.3	10	2	2	3	4	4	4	9
35–49	99	3.6	6	2	3	3	4	4	9	17
50–64	11	2.9	<1	2	2	3	3	3	5	5
65+	0									
GRAND TOTAL	405	3.3	9	2	2	3	4	4	5	11

660.31: DTA & POP-DELIVERED

Type of Patients	Observed Patients	Avg. Stay	Vari-ance	10th	25th	50th	75th	90th	95th	99th
1. SINGLE DX										
A. Not Operated										
0–19 Years	16	1.9	<1	1	2	2	2	3	3	3
20–34	152	1.8	<1	1	1	2	2	2	3	3
35–49	5	1.2	<1	1	1	1	1	2	2	2
50–64	0									
65+	0									
B. Operated										
0–19 Years	10	2.7	<1	2	2	3	3	3	3	3
20–34	70	3.2	<1	2	3	3	4	4	5	5
35–49	2	3.5	<1	3	3	4	4	4	4	4
50–64	0									
65+	0									
2. MULTIPLE DX										
A. Not Operated										
0–19 Years	107	2.3	<1	1	1	2	3	3	3	5
20–34	771	2.0	<1	1	1	2	2	3	3	4
35–49	112	1.9	<1	1	1	2	2	2	3	3
50–64	4	1.8	<1	1	2	2	2	2	2	2
65+	0									
B. Operated										
0–19 Years	177	3.6	1	2	3	4	4	5	5	7
20–34	1,379	3.6	1	2	3	4	4	5	5	6
35–49	341	3.8	1	3	3	4	4	5	5	7
50–64	27	3.7	<1	3	3	4	4	5	5	6
65+	0									
SUBTOTALS:										
1. SINGLE DX										
A. Not Operated	173	1.8	<1	1	1	2	2	2	3	3
B. Operated	82	3.1	<1	2	3	3	4	4	5	5
2. MULTIPLE DX										
A. Not Operated	994	2.0	<1	1	1	2	2	3	3	4
B. Operated	1,924	3.7	1	2	3	4	4	5	5	7
1. SINGLE DX	255	2.2	<1	1	2	2	3	3	4	5
2. MULTIPLE DX	2,918	3.1	2	2	2	3	4	5	5	6
A. NOT OPERATED	1,167	2.0	<1	1	1	2	2	3	3	4
B. OPERATED	2,006	3.6	1	2	3	4	4	5	5	6
TOTAL										
0–19 Years	310	3.0	1	2	2	3	3	4	5	7
20–34	2,372	3.0	2	1	2	3	4	4	5	6
35–49	460	3.3	2	2	2	3	4	5	5	6
50–64	31	3.4	1	2	3	3	4	5	5	6
65+	0									
GRAND TOTAL	3,173	3.0	2	2	2	3	4	5	5	6

660.41: SHOULDER DYSTOCIA-DEL

Type of Patients	Observed Patients	Avg. Stay	Vari-ance	10th	25th	50th	75th	90th	95th	99th
1. SINGLE DX										
A. Not Operated										
0–19 Years	44	1.7	<1	1	1	2	2	2	3	3
20–34	663	1.7	<1	1	1	2	2	2	3	3
35–49	30	1.6	<1	1	1	2	2	2	3	3
50–64	0									
65+	0									
B. Operated										
0–19 Years	0									
20–34	10	2.4	<1	2	2	2	3	3	3	3
35–49	0									
50–64	0									
65+	0									
2. MULTIPLE DX										
A. Not Operated										
0–19 Years	268	2.1	<1	1	2	2	3	3	3	4
20–34	2,390	1.9	<1	1	1	2	2	3	3	4
35–49	398	1.8	<1	1	1	2	2	3	3	4
50–64	19	1.8	<1	1	1	2	2	3	3	3
65+	0									
B. Operated										
0–19 Years	6	3.3	8	2	2	2	3	9	9	9
20–34	192	2.3	<1	1	2	2	3	3	4	6
35–49	53	2.7	2	2	2	2	3	4	4	12
50–64	1	4.0	0	4	4	4	4	4	4	4
65+	0									
SUBTOTALS:										
1. SINGLE DX										
A. Not Operated	737	1.7	<1	1	1	2	2	2	3	3
B. Operated	10	2.4	<1	2	2	2	3	3	3	3
2. MULTIPLE DX										
A. Not Operated	3,075	1.9	<1	1	1	2	2	3	3	4
B. Operated	252	2.4	1	1	2	2	3	3	4	8
1. SINGLE DX	747	1.7	<1	1	1	2	2	2	3	3
2. MULTIPLE DX	3,327	2.0	<1	1	1	2	2	3	3	4
A. NOT OPERATED	3,812	1.9	<1	1	1	2	2	3	3	4
B. OPERATED	262	2.4	1	2	2	2	3	3	4	8
TOTAL										
0–19 Years	318	2.1	<1	1	2	2	2	3	3	4
20–34	3,255	1.9	<1	1	1	2	2	3	3	4
35–49	481	1.9	<1	1	1	2	2	3	3	4
50–64	20	1.9	<1	1	1	2	2	3	4	4
65+	0									
GRAND TOTAL	4,074	1.9	<1	1	1	2	2	3	3	4

Length of Stay by Diagnosis and Operation, Western Region, 2008

Western Region, October 2006–September 2007 Data, by Diagnosis

660.61: FAIL TRIAL LABOR NOS-DEL

Type of Patients	Observed Patients	Avg. Stay	Variance	10th	25th	50th	75th	90th	95th	99th
1. SINGLE DX										
A. Not Operated										
0–19 Years	0									
20–34	1	2.0	0	2	2	2	2	2	2	2
35–49	0									
50–64	0									
65+	0									
B. Operated										
0–19 Years	1	5.0	0	5	5	5	5	5	5	5
20–34	7	3.1	<1	2	3	3	3	5	5	5
35–49	0									
50–64	0									
65+	0									
2. MULTIPLE DX										
A. Not Operated										
0–19 Years	0									
20–34	4	1.5	<1	1	1	2	2	2	2	2
35–49	2	4.0	0	4	4	4	4	4	4	4
50–64	0									
65+	0									
B. Operated										
0–19 Years	15	3.7	1	2	3	4	4	5	6	6
20–34	219	3.6	<1	3	3	3	4	5	5	6
35–49	43	3.6	<1	2	3	4	4	5	5	6
50–64	1	4.0	0	4	4	4	4	4	4	4
65+	0									
SUBTOTALS:										
1. SINGLE DX										
A. Not Operated	1	2.0	0	2	2	2	2	2	2	2
B. Operated	8	3.4	1	2	3	3	4	5	5	5
2. MULTIPLE DX										
A. Not Operated	6	2.3	2	1	1	2	4	4	4	4
B. Operated	278	3.6	<1	3	3	4	4	5	5	6
1. SINGLE DX	9	3.2	1	2	3	3	4	5	5	5
2. MULTIPLE DX	284	3.6	<1	3	3	4	4	5	5	6
A. NOT OPERATED	7	2.3	2	1	1	2	4	4	4	4
B. OPERATED	286	3.6	<1	3	3	4	4	5	5	6
TOTAL										
0–19 Years	16	3.8	1	2	3	4	4	5	6	6
20–34	231	3.6	<1	2	3	3	4	5	5	6
35–49	45	3.6	<1	2	3	3	4	5	5	6
50–64	0	4.0	0	4	4	4	4	4	4	4
65+	0									
GRAND TOTAL	293	3.6	<1	2	3	3	4	5	5	6

660.71: FAIL FORCEPS/VED NOS-DEL

Type of Patients	Observed Patients	Avg. Stay	Variance	10th	25th	50th	75th	90th	95th	99th
1. SINGLE DX										
A. Not Operated										
0–19 Years	0									
20–34	4	1.8	<1	1	1	2	2	2	2	3
35–49	0									
50–64	0									
65+	0									
B. Operated										
0–19 Years	1	4.0	0	4	4	4	4	4	4	4
20–34	4	3.3	<1	2	3	3	4	4	4	4
35–49	0									
50–64	0									
65+	0									
2. MULTIPLE DX										
A. Not Operated										
0–19 Years	5	2.2	1	1	1	3	3	3	3	3
20–34	17	2.2	<1	1	2	2	3	3	3	3
35–49	1	3.0	0	3	3	3	3	3	3	3
50–64	0									
65+	0									
B. Operated										
0–19 Years	20	4.5	7	3	4	4	4	5	15	15
20–34	181	3.7	1	2	3	4	4	5	5	7
35–49	43	4.3	4	3	3	5	5	5	5	16
50–64	1	6.0	0	6	6	6	6	6	6	6
65+	0									
SUBTOTALS:										
1. SINGLE DX										
A. Not Operated	4	1.8	<1	1	1	2	2	2	2	3
B. Operated	5	3.4	<1	2	3	4	4	5	5	4
2. MULTIPLE DX										
A. Not Operated	23	2.2	<1	1	2	2	2	3	3	3
B. Operated	245	3.8	2	2	3	4	4	5	5	7
1. SINGLE DX	9	2.7	1	1	2	3	3	4	4	4
2. MULTIPLE DX	268	3.7	2	2	3	4	4	5	5	7
A. NOT OPERATED	27	2.2	<1	1	2	2	2	3	3	3
B. OPERATED	250	3.8	2	2	3	4	4	5	5	7
TOTAL										
0–19 Years	26	4.0	6	3	3	4	4	5	5	15
20–34	206	3.5	1	2	3	3	4	5	5	6
35–49	44	4.2	4	3	3	4	5	5	5	16
50–64	0	6.0	0	6	6	6	6	6	6	6
65+	0									
GRAND TOTAL	277	3.7	2	2	3	4	4	5	5	7

661: ABNORMAL FORCES OF LABOR

Type of Patients	Observed Patients	Avg. Stay	Variance	10th	25th	50th	75th	90th	95th	99th
1. SINGLE DX										
A. Not Operated										
0–19 Years	296	1.7	<1	1	1	2	2	2	3	3
20–34	3,302	1.5	<1	1	1	1	1	2	3	3
35–49	123	1.6	<1	1	1	2	2	2	2	3
50–64	7	1.6	<1	1	1	2	2	2	2	2
65+	0									
B. Operated										
0–19 Years	358	3.4	<1	2	3	3	4	4	5	5
20–34	1,830	3.4	<1	2	3	3	4	4	5	5
35–49	72	3.8	<1	3	3	4	4	5	5	7
50–64	4	3.8	<1	3	4	4	4	4	4	4
65+	0									
2. MULTIPLE DX										
A. Not Operated										
0–19 Years	1,073	2.0	<1	1	1	2	2	3	3	5
20–34	10,189	1.8	<1	1	1	2	3	3	3	4
35–49	1,956	1.9	<1	1	1	2	3	3	3	4
50–64	83	1.9	<1	1	1	2	2	3	3	3
65+	0									
B. Operated										
0–19 Years	2,673	3.7	1	3	3	4	4	5	5	8
20–34	17,028	3.7	1	3	3	4	4	5	5	7
35–49	3,527	3.9	3	3	3	4	4	5	6	7
50–64	197	3.8	<1	3	3	4	4	5	5	6
65+	0									
SUBTOTALS:										
1. SINGLE DX										
A. Not Operated	3,728	1.6	<1	1	1	1	2	2	3	3
B. Operated	2,264	3.4	<1	2	3	3	4	4	5	5
2. MULTIPLE DX										
A. Not Operated	13,301	1.8	<1	1	1	2	2	3	3	4
B. Operated	23,425	3.7	2	2	3	4	4	5	5	7
1. SINGLE DX	5,992	2.3	1	1	1	2	3	4	4	5
2. MULTIPLE DX	36,726	3.0	2	1	2	3	4	5	5	6
A. NOT OPERATED	17,029	1.7	<1	1	1	2	2	3	3	4
B. OPERATED	25,689	3.7	2	2	3	4	4	5	5	7
TOTAL										
0–19 Years	4,400	3.1	2	2	2	3	4	5	5	7
20–34	32,349	2.9	2	1	2	3	4	5	5	6
35–49	5,678	3.1	3	1	2	3	4	5	5	7
50–64	291	3.2	2	1	2	3	4	5	5	6
65+	0									
GRAND TOTAL	42,718	2.9	2	1	2	3	4	5	5	6

Length of Stay by Diagnosis and Operation, Western Region, 2008

Western Region, October 2006–September 2007 Data, by Diagnosis

661.01: PRIM UTERINE INERTIA-DEL

Type of Patients	Observed Patients	Avg. Stay	Variance	10th	25th	50th	75th	90th	95th	99th
1. SINGLE DX										
A. Not Operated										
0–19 Years	27	1.9	<1	1	1	2	3	3	3	3
20–34	189	1.8	<1	1	1	2	2	3	3	3
35–49	6	1.5	<1	1	1	1	2	2	2	2
50–64	0									
65+	0									
B. Operated										
0–19 Years	130	3.5	<1	2	3	3	4	5	5	5
20–34	636	3.5	<1	2	3	3	4	5	5	5
35–49	21	3.8	<1	3	3	4	4	5	6	5
50–64	1	4.0	0	4	4	4	4	4	4	4
65+	0									
2. MULTIPLE DX										
A. Not Operated										
0–19 Years	168	2.2	<1	1	2	2	3	3	4	5
20–34	989	2.0	<1	1	1	2	2	3	3	4
35–49	122	2.1	<1	1	2	2	3	3	3	4
50–64	7	2.1	<1	1	2	2	3	3	3	3
65+	0									
B. Operated										
0–19 Years	1,076	3.7	1	2	3	4	4	5	5	7
20–34	6,404	3.7	1	3	3	4	4	5	5	7
35–49	1,292	4.0	4	3	3	4	5	5	6	7
50–64	56	3.8	<1	3	3	4	4	5	5	5
65+	0									
SUBTOTALS:										
1. SINGLE DX A. Not Operated	222	1.8	<1	1	1	2	2	3	3	3
1. SINGLE DX B. Operated	788	3.5	<1	2	3	3	4	5	5	5
2. MULTIPLE DX A. Not Operated	1,286	2.1	<1	1	2	2	3	3	3	4
2. MULTIPLE DX B. Operated	8,828	3.8	2	3	3	4	4	5	5	7
1. SINGLE DX	1,010	3.1	1	2	2	3	4	4	5	5
2. MULTIPLE DX	10,114	3.5	2	2	3	4	4	5	5	7
A. NOT OPERATED	1,508	2.0	<1	1	2	2	2	3	3	4
B. OPERATED	9,616	3.7	2	3	3	4	4	5	5	7
TOTAL										
0–19 Years	1,401	3.4	1	2	3	3	4	5	5	7
20–34	8,218	3.5	2	2	3	3	4	5	5	7
35–49	1,441	3.8	4	2	3	4	4	5	6	7
50–64	64	3.6	<1	2	3	4	4	5	5	5
65+	0									
GRAND TOTAL	11,124	3.5	2	2	3	3	4	5	5	7

661.11: 2ND UTERINE INERTIA-DEL

Type of Patients	Observed Patients	Avg. Stay	Variance	10th	25th	50th	75th	90th	95th	99th
1. SINGLE DX										
A. Not Operated										
0–19 Years	19	2.2	<1	2	2	2	2	3	3	3
20–34	138	2.0	<1	1	2	2	2	3	3	4
35–49	3	2.0	<1	1	1	2	3	3	3	3
50–64	0									
65+	0									
B. Operated										
0–19 Years	129	3.2	<1	2	3	3	4	4	5	5
20–34	712	3.4	<1	2	3	3	4	4	5	5
35–49	29	4.0	1	3	3	4	5	6	6	7
50–64	1	4.0	0	4	4	4	4	4	4	4
65+	0									
2. MULTIPLE DX										
A. Not Operated										
0–19 Years	128	2.2	<1	1	2	2	3	3	4	5
20–34	679	2.2	<1	1	2	2	3	3	4	5
35–49	100	2.1	<1	1	2	2	3	3	3	4
50–64	3	2.0	<1	1	1	2	3	3	3	3
65+	0									
B. Operated										
0–19 Years	955	3.8	2	3	3	4	4	5	5	9
20–34	6,518	3.8	1	3	3	4	4	5	5	7
35–49	1,456	3.9	2	3	3	4	5	5	6	7
50–64	96	4.0	<1	3	3	4	4	5	5	6
65+	0									
SUBTOTALS:										
1. SINGLE DX A. Not Operated	160	2.0	<1	1	2	2	2	3	3	4
1. SINGLE DX B. Operated	871	3.4	<1	2	3	3	4	4	5	6
2. MULTIPLE DX A. Not Operated	910	2.2	<1	1	2	2	3	3	3	5
2. MULTIPLE DX B. Operated	9,025	3.8	1	3	3	4	4	5	5	7
1. SINGLE DX	1,031	3.2	<1	2	3	3	4	4	5	5
2. MULTIPLE DX	9,935	3.7	2	2	3	4	4	5	5	7
A. NOT OPERATED	1,070	2.2	<1	1	2	2	3	3	3	5
B. OPERATED	9,896	3.8	1	3	3	4	4	5	5	7
TOTAL										
0–19 Years	1,231	3.5	2	2	3	3	4	5	5	8
20–34	8,047	3.6	1	2	3	4	4	5	5	7
35–49	1,588	3.8	2	2	3	4	4	5	6	7
50–64	100	4.0	1	3	3	4	5	5	5	6
65+	0									
GRAND TOTAL	10,966	3.6	2	3	3	4	4	5	5	7

661.21: UTERINE INERTIA NEC-DEL

Type of Patients	Observed Patients	Avg. Stay	Variance	10th	25th	50th	75th	90th	95th	99th
1. SINGLE DX										
A. Not Operated										
0–19 Years	53	2.0	<1	1	2	2	2	3	3	3
20–34	449	1.8	<1	1	1	2	2	3	3	3
35–49	17	2.0	<1	2	2	2	2	3	3	3
50–64	0									
65+	0									
B. Operated										
0–19 Years	99	3.4	<1	2	3	3	4	4	5	5
20–34	474	3.4	<1	3	3	3	4	4	5	5
35–49	22	3.4	<1	2	3	3	4	4	5	5
50–64	0	3.5	<1	3	3	4	4	4	4	4
65+	0									
2. MULTIPLE DX										
A. Not Operated										
0–19 Years	247	2.2	<1	1	2	2	3	3	3	5
20–34	1,970	2.1	<1	1	2	2	3	3	3	4
35–49	490	2.3	<1	1	2	2	3	3	3	5
50–64	21	2.3	<1	2	2	2	3	3	3	3
65+	0									
B. Operated										
0–19 Years	620	3.6	1	2	3	4	4	5	5	8
20–34	3,615	3.7	2	2	3	4	4	5	5	7
35–49	665	3.8	1	3	3	4	4	5	5	7
50–64	41	3.7	1	2	3	4	4	5	5	6
65+	0									
SUBTOTALS:										
1. SINGLE DX A. Not Operated	519	1.9	<1	1	1	2	2	3	3	3
1. SINGLE DX B. Operated	597	3.4	<1	2	3	3	4	4	5	5
2. MULTIPLE DX A. Not Operated	2,728	2.1	<1	1	2	2	3	3	3	4
2. MULTIPLE DX B. Operated	4,941	3.7	2	2	3	4	4	5	5	7
1. SINGLE DX	1,116	2.7	1	1	2	3	3	4	4	5
2. MULTIPLE DX	7,669	3.1	2	2	2	3	4	5	5	6
A. NOT OPERATED	3,247	2.1	<1	1	2	2	2	3	3	4
B. OPERATED	5,538	3.6	2	2	3	3	4	5	5	7
TOTAL										
0–19 Years	1,019	3.2	2	2	2	3	4	5	5	7
20–34	6,508	3.0	2	2	2	3	4	4	5	6
35–49	1,194	3.1	1	2	2	3	4	5	5	6
50–64	64	3.2	1	2	2	3	4	5	5	6
65+	0									
GRAND TOTAL	8,785	3.1	2	2	2	3	4	5	5	6

Length of Stay by Diagnosis and Operation, Western Region, 2008

Western Region, October 2006–September 2007 Data, by Diagnosis

661.31: PRECIPITATE LABOR-DEL

Type of Patients	Observed Patients	Avg. Stay	Variance	10th	25th	50th	75th	90th	95th	99th
1. SINGLE DX										
A. Not Operated										
0–19 Years	176	1.6	<1	1	1	2	2	2	3	3
20–34	2,394	1.4	<1	1	1	1	2	2	3	3
35–49	86	1.5	<1	1	1	1	2	2	3	3
50–64	7	1.6	<1	1	1	2	2	2	2	2
65+	0									
B. Operated										
0–19 Years	0									
20–34	3	1.7	<1	1		2	2	2	2	2
35–49	0									
50–64	0									
65+	0									
2. MULTIPLE DX										
A. Not Operated										
0–19 Years	492	1.7	<1	1	1	2	2	2	3	4
20–34	6,317	1.6	<1	1	1	2	2	2	3	3
35–49	1,209	1.6	<1	1	1	2	2	2	3	3
50–64	52	1.7	<1	1	1	2	2	3	3	3
65+	0									
B. Operated										
0–19 Years	17	1.8	<1	1	2	2	2	2	3	3
20–34	443	1.9	<1	1	1	2	2	3	3	4
35–49	108	2.0	<1	1	2	2	3	3	4	4
50–64	4	1.8	<1	1	1	1	2	3	3	3
65+	0									
SUBTOTALS:										
1. SINGLE DX — A. Not Operated	2,663	1.5	<1	1	1	1	2	2	2	3
1. SINGLE DX — B. Operated	3	1.7	<1	1	1	2	2	2	2	2
2. MULTIPLE DX — A. Not Operated	8,070	1.6	<1	1	1	2	2	2	3	3
2. MULTIPLE DX — B. Operated	572	1.9	<1	1	1	2	2	3	3	4
1. SINGLE DX	2,666	1.5	<1	1	1	1	2	2	2	3
2. MULTIPLE DX	8,642	1.6	<1	1	1	2	2	2	3	3
A. NOT OPERATED	10,733	1.6	<1	1	1	2	2	2	3	3
B. OPERATED	575	1.9	<1	1	1	2	2	3	4	4
TOTAL										
0–19 Years	685	1.7	<1	1	1	2	2	2	3	3
20–34	9,157	1.6	<1	1	1	2	2	2	3	3
35–49	1,403	1.6	<1	1	1	2	2	2	3	4
50–64	63	1.7	<1	1	1	2	2	3	3	3
65+	0									
GRAND TOTAL	11,308	1.6	<1	1	1	2	2	2	2	3

662: LONG LABOR

Type of Patients	Observed Patients	Avg. Stay	Variance	10th	25th	50th	75th	90th	95th	99th
1. SINGLE DX										
A. Not Operated										
0–19 Years	42	2.3	<1	2	2	2	3	3	3	3
20–34	223	2.1	<1	1	2	2	2	3	3	3
35–49	5	1.8	<1	1	1	2	2	3	3	3
50–64	1	1.0	0	1	1	1	1	1	1	1
65+	0									
B. Operated										
0–19 Years	1	4.0	0	4	4	4	4	4	4	4
20–34	12	3.3	<1	3	3	3	4	4	4	4
35–49	1	4.0	0	4	4	4	4	4	4	4
50–64	0									
65+	0									
2. MULTIPLE DX										
A. Not Operated										
0–19 Years	243	2.4	1	1	2	2	3	3	3	5
20–34	1,609	2.3	<1	1	2	2	3	3	3	4
35–49	278	2.5	2	1	2	2	3	3	4	5
50–64	11	2.6	<1	2	2	3	3	4	4	4
65+	0									
B. Operated										
0–19 Years	44	3.6	1	2	3	3	4	5	6	7
20–34	361	3.6	1	3	3	4	4	5	5	8
35–49	67	3.7	1	2	3	4	4	5	5	8
50–64	5	4.2	<1	3	4	4	5	5	5	5
65+	0									
SUBTOTALS:										
1. SINGLE DX — A. Not Operated	271	2.1	<1	1	2	2	3	3	3	3
1. SINGLE DX — B. Operated	14	3.4	<1	3	3	4	4	4	4	4
2. MULTIPLE DX — A. Not Operated	2,141	2.3	<1	1	2	2	3	3	3	4
2. MULTIPLE DX — B. Operated	477	3.6	1	2	3	4	4	5	5	8
1. SINGLE DX	285	2.2	<1	1	2	2	3	3	3	4
2. MULTIPLE DX	2,618	2.6	1	1	2	2	3	4	4	5
A. NOT OPERATED	2,412	2.3	<1	1	2	2	3	3	4	4
B. OPERATED	491	3.6	1	2	3	4	4	5	5	8
TOTAL										
0–19 Years	330	2.6	1	2	2	2	3	3	4	6
20–34	2,205	2.5	1	1	2	2	3	4	4	5
35–49	351	2.7	2	1	2	3	4	4	5	5
50–64	17	3.0	1	1	2	3	4	5	5	5
65+	0									
GRAND TOTAL	2,903	2.5	1	1	2	2	3	4	4	5

662.01: PROLONGED 1ST STAGE-DEL

Type of Patients	Observed Patients	Avg. Stay	Variance	10th	25th	50th	75th	90th	95th	99th
1. SINGLE DX										
A. Not Operated										
0–19 Years	15	2.3	<1	1	2	2	3	3	3	3
20–34	61	2.3	<1	2	2	2	3	3	3	3
35–49	0									
50–64	0									
65+	0									
B. Operated										
0–19 Years	0									
20–34	1	4.0	0	4	4	4	4	4	4	4
35–49	0									
50–64	0									
65+	0									
2. MULTIPLE DX										
A. Not Operated										
0–19 Years	47	2.4	<1	2	2	2	3	3	3	4
20–34	235	2.2	<1	1	2	2	3	3	3	4
35–49	26	2.1	<1	1	2	2	3	4	4	5
50–64	2	2.5	<1	2	2	3	3	4	4	4
65+	0									
B. Operated										
0–19 Years	4	3.8	3	2	2	4	4	5	6	6
20–34	64	3.6	1	2	3	4	4	5	5	6
35–49	11	3.7	<1	3	3	4	4	5	5	5
50–64	0									
65+	0									
SUBTOTALS:										
1. SINGLE DX — A. Not Operated	76	2.3	<1	2	2	2	3	3	3	3
1. SINGLE DX — B. Operated	1	4.0	0	4	4	4	4	4	4	4
2. MULTIPLE DX — A. Not Operated	310	2.2	<1	1	2	2	3	3	3	4
2. MULTIPLE DX — B. Operated	79	3.6	1	2	3	4	4	5	6	6
1. SINGLE DX	77	2.4	<1	2	2	2	3	3	3	4
2. MULTIPLE DX	389	2.5	1	1	2	2	3	4	4	6
A. NOT OPERATED	386	2.3	<1	1	2	2	3	3	3	4
B. OPERATED	80	3.6	1	2	3	4	4	5	5	6
TOTAL										
0–19 Years	66	2.5	<1	1	2	2	3	3	3	6
20–34	361	2.5	1	1	2	2	3	4	4	6
35–49	37	2.6	1	1	2	3	4	4	5	5
50–64	2	2.5	<1	2	2	3	3	4	5	5
65+	0									
GRAND TOTAL	466	2.5	<1	1	2	2	3	4	4	6

Length of Stay by Diagnosis and Operation, Western Region, 2008

Western Region, October 2006–September 2007 Data, by Diagnosis

662.11: PROLONGED LABOR NOS-DEL

Type of Patients	Observed Patients	Avg. Stay	Vari-ance	10th	25th	50th	75th	90th	95th	99th
1. SINGLE DX										
A. Not Operated										
0–19 Years	14	2.5	<1	2	2	3	3	3	3	3
20–34	41	2.0	<1	1	2	2	2	3	3	3
35–49	1	2.0	0	2		2	2	2	2	2
50–64	0									
65+	0									
B. Operated										
0–19 Years	0									
20–34	5	3.0	<1	2	3	3	3	4	4	4
35–49	0									
50–64	0									
65+	0									
2. MULTIPLE DX										
A. Not Operated										
0–19 Years	25	2.3	<1	2	2	2	3	3	3	3
20–34	182	2.2	<1	1	2	2	3	3	3	4
35–49	18	2.5	<1	1	2	3	3	3	4	4
50–64	1	1.0	0	1	1	1	1	1	1	1
65+	0									
B. Operated										
0–19 Years	8	3.3	1	1	3	3	4	5	5	5
20–34	39	3.2	2	2	2	3	4	5	5	6
35–49	3	3.7	2	2	2	4	5	5	5	5
50–64	4	4.2	<1	3	3	4	5	5	5	5
65+	0									
SUBTOTALS:										
1. SINGLE DX										
A. Not Operated	56	2.1	<1	1	2	2	3	3	3	3
B. Operated	5	3.0	<1	2	3	3	3	4	4	4
2. MULTIPLE DX										
A. Not Operated	226	2.2	<1	1	2	2	3	3	3	4
B. Operated	54	3.3	2	2	2	3	4	5	5	6
1. SINGLE DX	61	2.2	<1	1	2	2	3	3	3	4
2. MULTIPLE DX	280	2.5	<1	2	2	2	3	4	4	5
A. NOT OPERATED	282	2.2	<1	1	2	2	3	3	3	4
B. OPERATED	59	3.3	1	2	2	3	4	5	5	6
TOTAL										
0–19 Years	47	2.5	<1	2	2	2	3	3	4	5
20–34	267	2.4	<1	1	2	2	3	3	4	5
35–49	22	2.6	<1	2	2	3	4	4	4	5
50–64	5	3.6	3	1	3	4	5	5	5	5
65+	0									
GRAND TOTAL	341	2.4	<1	1	2	2	3	3	4	5

662.21: PROLONGED 2ND STAGE-DEL

Type of Patients	Observed Patients	Avg. Stay	Vari-ance	10th	25th	50th	75th	90th	95th	99th
1. SINGLE DX										
A. Not Operated										
0–19 Years	13	2.2	<1	2	2	2	2	3	3	3
20–34	117	2.0	<1	1	2	2	2	3	3	3
35–49	4	1.8	<1	1	1	2	3	3	3	3
50–64	0	1.0	0	1	1	1	1	1	1	1
65+	0									
B. Operated										
0–19 Years	1	4.0	0	4	4	4	4	4	4	4
20–34	6	3.5	<1	3	3	4	4	4	4	4
35–49	1	4.0	0	4	4	4	4	4	4	4
50–64	0									
65+	0									
2. MULTIPLE DX										
A. Not Operated										
0–19 Years	169	2.4	<1	1	2	2	3	3	3	3
20–34	1,187	2.3	<1	1	2	2	3	3	3	4
35–49	233	2.5	3	1	2	3	4	4	5	5
50–64	8	2.9	<1	2	2	3	3	4	4	4
65+	0									
B. Operated										
0–19 Years	32	3.7	1	2	3	4	5	6	6	7
20–34	253	3.6	1	2	3	4	4	5	5	8
35–49	53	3.7	1	2	3	4	4	5	5	8
50–64	1	4.0	0	4	4	4	4	4	4	4
65+	0									
SUBTOTALS:										
1. SINGLE DX										
A. Not Operated	135	2.0	<1	1	2	2	2	3	3	3
B. Operated	8	3.6	<1	3	3	3	4	4	4	4
2. MULTIPLE DX										
A. Not Operated	1,597	2.3	<1	1	2	2	3	3	3	4
B. Operated	339	3.6	1	2	3	4	4	5	5	8
1. SINGLE DX	143	2.1	<1	1	2	2	2	3	3	4
2. MULTIPLE DX	1,936	2.6	1	1	2	2	3	4	4	5
A. NOT OPERATED	1,732	2.3	<1	1	2	2	3	3	3	4
B. OPERATED	347	3.6	1	2	3	4	4	5	5	8
TOTAL										
0–19 Years	215	2.6	<1	2	2	2	3	3	4	5
20–34	1,563	2.5	1	1	2	2	3	3	4	5
35–49	291	2.7	3	1	2	3	3	4	5	8
50–64	10	2.8	1	2	2	3	4	4	4	4
65+	0									
GRAND TOTAL	2,079	2.5	1	2	2	2	3	4	4	5

663: UMBILICAL CORD COMP

Type of Patients	Observed Patients	Avg. Stay	Vari-ance	10th	25th	50th	75th	90th	95th	99th
1. SINGLE DX										
A. Not Operated										
0–19 Years	1,757	1.9	<1	1	1	2	2	3	3	3
20–34	14,185	1.7	<1	1	1	2	2	3	3	3
35–49	471	1.7	<1	1	1	2	3	3	3	3
50–64	25	1.8	<1	1	1	2	3	3	3	3
65+	0									
B. Operated										
0–19 Years	13	3.3	<1	2	3	3	4	4	5	5
20–34	135	2.8	<1	2	3	3	4	4	4	4
35–49	12	2.7	<1	2	3	3	3	3	3	3
50–64	1	4.0	0	4	4	4	4	4	4	4
65+	0									
2. MULTIPLE DX										
A. Not Operated										
0–19 Years	2,498	2.0	<1	1	2	2	3	3	3	4
20–34	19,016	1.8	<1	1	1	2	3	3	3	4
35–49	2,707	1.8	<1	1	1	2	3	3	3	3
50–64	135	2.0	<1	2	2	2	3	3	3	3
65+	0									
B. Operated										
0–19 Years	166	3.0	1	2	2	3	5	5	5	6
20–34	2,651	2.8	11	1	2	3	4	4	4	8
35–49	556	3.4	21	2	2	3	4	4	5	20
50–64	24	2.8	3	2	2	4	5	5	5	10
65+	0									
SUBTOTALS:										
1. SINGLE DX										
A. Not Operated	16,438	1.7	<1	1	1	2	2	3	3	3
B. Operated	161	2.9	<1	2	3	3	4	4	5	5
2. MULTIPLE DX										
A. Not Operated	24,356	1.9	<1	1	1	2	3	3	3	4
B. Operated	3,397	2.9	12	1	2	3	4	4	4	12
1. SINGLE DX	16,599	1.7	<1	1	1	2	2	3	3	3
2. MULTIPLE DX	27,753	2.0	2	1	2	2	3	4	4	4
A. NOT OPERATED	40,794	1.8	<1	1	1	2	3	3	3	3
B. OPERATED	3,558	2.9	12	1	2	3	4	4	4	11
TOTAL										
0–19 Years	4,434	2.0	<1	1	1	2	3	3	3	4
20–34	35,987	1.9	1	1	1	2	3	3	3	4
35–49	3,746	2.1	4	1	1	3	3	4	3	5
50–64	185	2.1	<1	2	2	2	3	3	5	5
65+	0									
GRAND TOTAL	44,352	1.9	1	1	2	2	3	3	3	4

Length of Stay by Diagnosis and Operation, Western Region, 2008

Western Region, October 2006–September 2007 Data, by Diagnosis

663.01: CORD PROLAPSE-DELIVERED

Type of Patients	Observed Patients	Avg. Stay	Variance	Percentiles						
				10th	25th	50th	75th	90th	95th	99th
1. SINGLE DX										
A. Not Operated										
0–19 Years	3	2.3	<1	2	2	2	3	3	3	3
20–34	32	1.8	<1	1	1	2	2	2	3	3
35–49	1	2.0	0	2	2	2	2	2	2	2
50–64	0									
65+	0									
B. Operated										
0–19 Years	5	3.6	<1	3	3	3	4	5	5	5
20–34	37	3.0	<1	2	2	3	3	4	4	4
35–49	4	3.0	0	3	3	3	3	3	3	3
50–64	0									
65+	0									
2. MULTIPLE DX										
A. Not Operated										
0–19 Years	10	2.3	<1	1	1	2	2	3	3	3
20–34	89	1.9	<1	1	1	2	2	3	3	6
35–49	22	1.7	<1	1	1	2	2	2	3	3
50–64	2	2.0	2	1	1	3	3	3	3	3
65+	0									
B. Operated										
0–19 Years	34	3.5	<1	3	3	3	4	5	5	6
20–34	370	3.5	6	2	2	3	4	4	5	17
35–49	109	3.8	6	2	3	3	4	5	8	16
50–64	4	4.3	15	2	10	10	10	10	10	10
65+	0									
SUBTOTALS:										
1. SINGLE DX										
A. Not Operated	36	1.9	<1	1	2	2	2	3	3	3
B. Operated	46	3.0	<1	2	3	3	3	4	4	5
2. MULTIPLE DX										
A. Not Operated	123	1.9	<1	1	1	2	2	3	3	3
B. Operated	517	3.6	5	2	3	3	4	5	5	17
1. SINGLE DX	82	2.5	<1	1	2	2	3	4	4	5
2. MULTIPLE DX	640	3.3	5	2	2	3	4	4	5	16
A. NOT OPERATED	159	1.9	<1	1	1	2	2	3	3	3
B. OPERATED	563	3.5	5	2	3	3	4	5	5	17
TOTAL										
0–19 Years	52	3.2	<1	2	3	3	4	4	5	6
20–34	528	3.1	5	2	2	3	4	4	5	15
35–49	136	3.4	5	2	2	3	4	5	7	16
50–64	6	3.5	11	1	2	3	3	10	10	10
65+	0									
GRAND TOTAL	722	3.2	5	2	2	3	4	4	5	15

663.11: CORD AROUND NECK-DEL

Type of Patients	Observed Patients	Avg. Stay	Variance	Percentiles						
				10th	25th	50th	75th	90th	95th	99th
1. SINGLE DX										
A. Not Operated										
0–19 Years	339	1.9	<1	1	1	2	2	3	3	3
20–34	2,907	1.7	<1	1	1	2	2	3	3	3
35–49	96	1.7	<1	1	1	2	2	3	3	4
50–64	8	2.1	<1	1	2	2	2	3	3	3
65+	0									
B. Operated										
0–19 Years	4	3.0	<1	2	2	3	4	4	4	4
20–34	22	2.8	<1	2	2	3	3	4	4	4
35–49	1	2.0	0	2	2	2	2	2	2	2
50–64	0									
65+	0									
2. MULTIPLE DX										
A. Not Operated										
0–19 Years	626	2.0	<1	1	2	2	2	3	3	4
20–34	4,372	1.8	<1	1	1	2	2	3	3	4
35–49	677	1.9	<1	1	1	2	2	3	3	4
50–64	30	2.0	<1	1	2	3	3	3	3	3
65+	0									
B. Operated										
0–19 Years	33	2.6	<1	2	2	3	3	4	4	4
20–34	543	2.6	2	1	2	2	3	4	4	8
35–49	92	2.6	1	1	2	2	3	4	4	7
50–64	5	2.4	1	1	2	2	3	4	4	4
65+	0									
SUBTOTALS:										
1. SINGLE DX										
A. Not Operated	3,350	1.7	<1	1	1	2	2	3	3	3
B. Operated	27	2.8	<1	2	3	3	3	4	4	4
2. MULTIPLE DX										
A. Not Operated	5,705	1.9	<1	1	1	2	2	3	3	4
B. Operated	673	2.6	2	1	2	3	3	4	4	7
1. SINGLE DX	3,377	1.7	<1	1	1	2	2	3	3	3
2. MULTIPLE DX	6,378	1.9	<1	1	1	2	2	3	3	4
A. NOT OPERATED	9,055	1.8	<1	1	1	2	2	3	3	3
B. OPERATED	700	2.6	2	1	2	3	3	4	4	7
TOTAL										
0–19 Years	1,002	2.0	<1	1	1	2	2	3	3	4
20–34	7,844	1.9	<1	1	1	2	2	3	3	4
35–49	866	1.9	<1	1	1	2	2	3	3	4
50–64	43	2.1	<1	1	2	2	3	3	3	4
65+	0									
GRAND TOTAL	9,755	1.9	<1	1	1	2	2	3	3	4

663.21: CORD COMPRESS NEC-DEL

Type of Patients	Observed Patients	Avg. Stay	Variance	Percentiles						
				10th	25th	50th	75th	90th	95th	99th
1. SINGLE DX										
A. Not Operated										
0–19 Years	53	1.9	<1	1	1	2	2	3	3	3
20–34	557	1.6	<1	1	1	2	2	3	3	3
35–49	27	1.7	<1	1	1	2	2	3	3	3
50–64	0									
65+	0									
B. Operated										
0–19 Years	1	4.0	0	4	4	4	4	4	4	4
20–34	2	3.5	<1	3	3	3	4	4	4	4
35–49	1	1.0	0	1	1	1	1	1	1	1
50–64	0									
65+	0									
2. MULTIPLE DX										
A. Not Operated										
0–19 Years	108	2.1	<1	1	2	2	2	3	3	4
20–34	965	1.9	<1	1	1	2	2	3	3	3
35–49	167	1.9	<1	1	1	2	2	3	3	3
50–64	7	2.0	<1	1	2	2	2	3	3	3
65+	0									
B. Operated										
0–19 Years	10	3.6	4	2	2	3	3	6	8	8
20–34	113	3.1	30	1	2	2	3	4	5	30
35–49	35	2.5	<1	1	2	2	3	4	4	4
50–64	0									
65+	0									
SUBTOTALS:										
1. SINGLE DX										
A. Not Operated	637	1.6	<1	1	1	2	2	3	3	3
B. Operated	4	3.0	2	1	3	4	4	4	4	4
2. MULTIPLE DX										
A. Not Operated	1,247	1.9	<1	1	1	2	2	3	3	3
B. Operated	158	3.0	22	1	2	2	3	4	5	30
1. SINGLE DX	641	1.7	<1	1	1	2	2	3	3	3
2. MULTIPLE DX	1,405	2.0	3	1	1	2	2	3	4	4
A. NOT OPERATED	1,884	1.8	<1	1	1	2	2	3	3	3
B. OPERATED	162	3.0	22	1	2	2	3	4	5	30
TOTAL										
0–19 Years	172	2.2	<1	1	2	2	3	3	3	6
20–34	1,637	1.9	<1	1	1	2	2	3	3	4
35–49	230	1.9	<1	1	1	2	2	3	3	4
50–64	7	2.0	<1	1	2	2	2	3	3	3
65+	0									
GRAND TOTAL	2,046	1.9	2	1	1	2	2	3	3	4

561

Length of Stay by Diagnosis and Operation, Western Region, 2008

Western Region, October 2006–September 2007 Data, by Diagnosis

663.31: CORD ENTANGLE NEC-DEL

Type of Patients	Observed Patients	Avg. Stay	Vari-ance	10th	25th	50th	75th	90th	95th	99th
1. SINGLE DX										
A. Not Operated										
0–19 Years	1,299	1.9	<1	1	1	2	2	3	3	3
20–34	10,193	1.7	<1	1	1	2	2	2	3	3
35–49	333	1.7	<1	1	1	2	2	2	3	3
50–64	17	1.7		1	1	2	2	2	3	3
65+	0									
B. Operated										
0–19 Years	3	3.0	<1	2	2	3	4	4	4	4
20–34	62	2.7	<1	2	2	3	3	4	4	4
35–49	4	2.8	<1	2	2	3	3	3	3	3
50–64	1	4.0	0	4	4	4	4	4	4	4
65+	0									
2. MULTIPLE DX										
A. Not Operated										
0–19 Years	1,656	2.0	<1	1	2	2	2	3	3	4
20–34	12,824	1.8	<1	1	1	2	2	3	3	3
35–49	1,742	1.8	<1	1	1	2	2	3	3	3
50–64	93	2.0	<1	1	2	2	2	3	3	3
65+	0									
B. Operated										
0–19 Years	80	2.9	<1	1	2	3	4	4	5	6
20–34	1,474	2.4	1	1	2	2	3	4	4	5
35–49	252	2.7	1	2	2	2	3	4	4	5
50–64	11	2.4	<1	2	2	2	2	3	5	5
65+	0									
SUBTOTALS:										
1. SINGLE DX										
A. Not Operated	11,842	1.7	<1	1	1	2	2	3	3	3
B. Operated	70	2.7	<1	2	2	3	3	4	4	4
2. MULTIPLE DX										
A. Not Operated	16,315	1.9	<1	1	1	2	2	3	3	4
B. Operated	1,817	2.4	1	1	2	2	3	4	4	5
1. SINGLE DX	11,912	1.7	<1	1	1	2	2	3	3	3
2. MULTIPLE DX	18,132	1.9	<1	1	1	2	2	3	3	4
A. NOT OPERATED	28,157	1.8	<1	1	1	2	2	3	3	3
B. OPERATED	1,887	2.4	1	1	2	2	3	4	4	5
TOTAL										
0–19 Years	3,038	2.0	<1	1	1	2	2	3	3	4
20–34	24,553	1.8	<1	1	1	2	2	3	3	3
35–49	2,331	1.9	<1	1	1	2	2	3	3	3
50–64	122	2.0	<1	1	2	2	2	3	3	3
65+	0									
GRAND TOTAL	30,044	1.8	<1	1	1	2	2	3	3	4

663.41: SHORT CORD-DELIVERED

Type of Patients	Observed Patients	Avg. Stay	Vari-ance	10th	25th	50th	75th	90th	95th	99th
1. SINGLE DX										
A. Not Operated										
0–19 Years	33	2.0	<1	1	2	2	3	3	3	3
20–34	260	1.8	<1	1	1	2	3	3	3	4
35–49	2	2.5	<1	2	2	3	3	3	3	3
50–64	0									
65+	0									
B. Operated										
0–19 Years	0									
20–34	1	2.0	0	2	2	2	2	2	2	2
35–49	0									
50–64	0									
65+	0									
2. MULTIPLE DX										
A. Not Operated										
0–19 Years	50	2.0	<1	1	2	2	2	3	3	4
20–34	313	1.9	<1	1	1	2	2	3	3	3
35–49	35	2.0	<1	1	2	2	2	3	3	3
50–64	0	1.5	<1	1	2	1	2	2	2	2
65+	0									
B. Operated										
0–19 Years	4	2.8	<1	2	2	3	4	4	5	6
20–34	32	2.2	<1	1	1	2	2	3	4	5
35–49	3	2.0	<1	1	1	2	3	3	4	5
50–64	1	2.0	0	2	2	2	2	2	2	2
65+	0									
SUBTOTALS:										
1. SINGLE DX										
A. Not Operated	295	1.8	<1	1	1	2	2	3	3	4
B. Operated	1	2.0	0	2	2	3	3	2	2	2
2. MULTIPLE DX										
A. Not Operated	400	1.9	<1	1	1	2	2	3	3	3
B. Operated	40	2.2	<1	1	2	2	3	3	4	5
1. SINGLE DX	296	1.8	<1	1	1	2	2	3	3	4
2. MULTIPLE DX	440	1.9	<1	1	1	2	2	3	3	4
A. NOT OPERATED	695	1.9	<1	1	1	2	2	3	3	3
B. OPERATED	41	2.2	3	1	2	2	3	4	4	5
TOTAL										
0–19 Years	87	2.1	<1	1	2	2	2	3	3	4
20–34	606	1.8	<1	1	1	2	2	3	3	3
35–49	40	2.0	<1	1	2	2	3	3	3	3
50–64	3	1.7	<1	1	1	2	2	2	2	2
65+	0									
GRAND TOTAL	736	1.9	<1	1	1	2	2	3	3	4

663.81: CORD COMP NEC-DELIVERED

Type of Patients	Observed Patients	Avg. Stay	Vari-ance	10th	25th	50th	75th	90th	95th	99th
1. SINGLE DX										
A. Not Operated										
0–19 Years	24	2.0	<1	1	1	2	2	3	3	3
20–34	210	1.7	<1	1	1	2	2	3	3	3
35–49	12	1.9	<1	1	1	2	2	3	3	3
50–64	0									
65+	0									
B. Operated										
0–19 Years	0									
20–34	3	3.0	1	2	2	3	4	4	4	4
35–49	2	3.0	0	3	3	3	3	3	3	3
50–64	0									
65+	0									
2. MULTIPLE DX										
A. Not Operated										
0–19 Years	48	1.9	<1	1	1	2	2	3	3	4
20–34	406	1.8	<1	1	1	2	2	3	3	3
35–49	56	2.0	<1	1	2	2	2	4	4	6
50–64	0	4.0	0	4	4	4	4	4	4	4
65+	0									
B. Operated										
0–19 Years	4	2.3	<1	1	2	3	3	4	4	6
20–34	67	2.5	<1	1	2	3	3	4	4	6
35–49	22	4.0	10	2	2	3	4	5	9	16
50–64	0									
65+	0									
SUBTOTALS:										
1. SINGLE DX										
A. Not Operated	246	1.7	<1	1	1	2	2	3	3	3
B. Operated	5	3.0		2	3	3	3	4	4	4
2. MULTIPLE DX										
A. Not Operated	511	1.9	<1	1	1	2	2	3	3	4
B. Operated	93	2.8	3	1	2	3	3	4	4	16
1. SINGLE DX	251	1.7	<1	1	1	2	2	3	3	3
2. MULTIPLE DX	604	2.0	1	1	1	2	2	3	3	5
A. NOT OPERATED	757	1.8	<1	1	1	2	2	3	3	4
B. OPERATED	98	2.8	3	1	2	3	3	4	4	16
TOTAL										
0–19 Years	76	2.0	<1	1	1	2	2	3	3	4
20–34	686	1.9	<1	1	1	2	2	3	3	4
35–49	92	2.5	3	1	2	2	3	4	4	16
50–64	1	4.0	0	4	4	4	4	4	4	4
65+	0									
GRAND TOTAL	855	1.9	<1	1	1	2	2	3	3	4

Western Region, October 2006–September 2007 Data, by Diagnosis

664: PERINEAL TRAUMA W DEL

Type of Patients	Observed Patients	Avg. Stay	Variance	10th	25th	50th	75th	90th	95th	99th
1. SINGLE DX										
A. Not Operated										
0–19 Years	6,543	1.9	<1	1	1	2	2	3	3	3
20–34	46,518	1.8	<1	1	1	2	2	3	3	3
35–49	2,077	1.7	<1	1	1	2	2	2	3	3
50–64	99	1.9	<1	1	2	2	2	3	3	4
65+	0									
B. Operated										
0–19 Years	5	2.0	<1	1	2	2	2	3	3	3
20–34	40	1.9	<1	1	1	2	2	3	3	3
35–49	3	1.7	<1	1	1	2	2	2	2	2
50–64	0									
65+	0									
2. MULTIPLE DX										
A. Not Operated										
0–19 Years	12,319	2.1	<1	1	2	2	3	3	3	4
20–34	84,635	2.0	<1	1	1	2	2	3	3	4
35–49	16,856	2.0	<1	1	1	2	2	3	3	4
50–64	781	2.0	<1	1	1	2	2	3	3	4
65+	0									
B. Operated										
0–19 Years	210	2.4	1	2	2	2	3	3	4	5
20–34	4,110	2.1	<1	1	2	2	2	3	3	5
35–49	1,172	2.1	<1	1	2	2	2	3	3	4
50–64	69	2.3	<1	2	2	2	2	3	4	6
65+	0									
SUBTOTALS:										
1. SINGLE DX										
A. Not Operated	55,237	1.8	<1	1	1	2	2	3	3	3
B. Operated	48	1.9	<1	1	1	2	2	3	3	3
2. MULTIPLE DX										
A. Not Operated	114,591	2.0	<1	1	1	2	2	3	3	4
B. Operated	5,561	2.1	<1	1	2	2	2	3	3	5
1. SINGLE DX	55,285	1.8	<1	1	1	2	2	2	3	3
2. MULTIPLE DX	120,152	2.0	<1	1	2	2	2	3	3	4
A. NOT OPERATED	169,828	1.9	<1	1	1	2	2	3	3	4
B. OPERATED	5,609	2.1	<1	1	2	2	2	3	3	5
TOTAL										
0–19 Years	19,077	2.0	<1	1	1	2	2	3	3	4
20–34	135,303	1.9	<1	1	1	2	2	3	3	4
35–49	20,108	1.9	<1	1	1	2	2	3	3	4
50–64	949	2.0	<1	2	2	2	2	3	3	4
65+	0									
GRAND TOTAL	175,437	1.9	<1	1	1	2	2	3	3	4

664.01: DEL W 1 DEGREE LAC-DEL

Type of Patients	Observed Patients	Avg. Stay	Variance	10th	25th	50th	75th	90th	95th	99th
1. SINGLE DX										
A. Not Operated										
0–19 Years	3,389	1.8	<1	1	1	2	2	3	3	3
20–34	22,356	1.7	<1	1	1	2	2	2	3	3
35–49	972	1.7	<1	1	1	2	2	2	3	3
50–64	52	1.9	<1	1	2	2	2	3	3	4
65+	0									
B. Operated										
0–19 Years	3	2.0	<1	1	1	2	2	3	3	3
20–34	18	1.7	<1	1	1	2	2	3	3	3
35–49	1	1.0	0	1	1	1	1	1	1	1
50–64	0									
65+	0									
2. MULTIPLE DX										
A. Not Operated										
0–19 Years	5,834	2.1	1	1	2	2	3	3	3	4
20–34	35,680	1.9	<1	1	1	2	2	3	3	4
35–49	6,877	1.9	1	1	1	2	2	3	3	4
50–64	337	1.9	<1	1	1	2	2	3	3	4
65+	0									
B. Operated										
0–19 Years	98	2.4	2	2	2	2	3	3	4	13
20–34	2,152	2.1	<1	1	1	2	2	3	3	4
35–49	602	2.1	<1	1	1	2	2	3	3	4
50–64	38	2.3	<1	2	2	2	3	3	4	6
65+	0									
SUBTOTALS:										
1. SINGLE DX										
A. Not Operated	26,769	1.7	<1	1	1	2	2	2	3	3
B. Operated	22	1.7	<1	1	1	2	2	3	3	3
2. MULTIPLE DX										
A. Not Operated	48,728	1.9	<1	1	1	2	2	3	3	4
B. Operated	2,890	2.1	<1	1	2	2	2	3	3	5
1. SINGLE DX	26,791	1.7	<1	1	1	2	2	2	3	3
2. MULTIPLE DX	51,618	1.9	<1	1	1	2	2	3	3	4
A. NOT OPERATED	75,497	1.9	<1	1	1	2	2	3	3	4
B. OPERATED	2,912	2.1	<1	1	2	2	2	3	3	4
TOTAL										
0–19 Years	9,324	2.0	<1	1	1	2	2	3	3	4
20–34	60,206	1.8	<1	1	1	2	2	3	3	4
35–49	8,452	1.9	<1	1	1	2	2	3	3	4
50–64	427	2.0	<1	1	2	2	2	3	3	4
65+	0									
GRAND TOTAL	78,409	1.9	<1	1	1	2	2	3	3	4

664.11: DEL W 2 DEGREE LAC-DEL

Type of Patients	Observed Patients	Avg. Stay	Variance	10th	25th	50th	75th	90th	95th	99th
1. SINGLE DX										
A. Not Operated										
0–19 Years	2,682	1.9	<1	1	1	2	2	2	3	3
20–34	21,536	1.8	<1	1	1	2	2	3	3	3
35–49	988	1.8	<1	1	1	2	2	2	3	3
50–64	44	1.9	<1	1	2	2	2	3	3	3
65+	0									
B. Operated										
0–19 Years	0									
20–34	15	1.9	<1	1	2	2	2	3	3	3
35–49	2	2.0	0	2	2	2	2	2	2	2
50–64	0									
65+	0									
2. MULTIPLE DX										
A. Not Operated										
0–19 Years	5,467	2.1	<1	1	2	2	3	3	3	4
20–34	42,462	2.0	<1	1	2	2	2	3	3	4
35–49	8,979	2.0	<1	1	1	2	2	3	3	4
50–64	408	2.0	<1	1	1	2	2	3	3	4
65+	0									
B. Operated										
0–19 Years	92	2.3	<1	2	2	2	3	3	4	5
20–34	1,767	2.1	<1	1	2	2	2	3	3	5
35–49	524	2.2	<1	1	2	2	2	3	3	5
50–64	31	2.2	<1	2	2	2	2	3	4	4
65+	0									
SUBTOTALS:										
1. SINGLE DX										
A. Not Operated	25,250	1.8	<1	1	1	2	2	3	3	3
B. Operated	17	1.9	<1	1	2	2	2	3	3	3
2. MULTIPLE DX										
A. Not Operated	57,316	2.0	<1	1	1	2	2	3	3	4
B. Operated	2,414	2.1	<1	1	2	2	2	3	3	5
1. SINGLE DX	25,267	1.8	<1	1	1	2	2	3	3	3
2. MULTIPLE DX	59,730	2.0	<1	1	1	2	2	3	3	4
A. NOT OPERATED	82,566	1.9	<1	1	1	2	2	3	3	4
B. OPERATED	2,431	2.1	<1	1	2	2	2	3	3	5
TOTAL										
0–19 Years	8,241	2.1	<1	1	2	2	2	3	3	4
20–34	65,780	1.9	<1	1	1	2	2	3	3	4
35–49	10,493	2.0	<1	1	1	2	2	3	3	4
50–64	483	2.0	<1	1	2	2	2	3	3	4
65+	0									
GRAND TOTAL	84,997	2.0	<1	1	1	2	2	3	3	4

Length of Stay by Diagnosis and Operation, Western Region, 2008

Western Region, October 2006–September 2007 Data, by Diagnosis

664.14: DEL W 2 DEGREE LAC-PP

Type of Patients	Observed Patients	Avg. Stay	Vari-ance	10th	25th	50th	75th	90th	95th	99th
1. SINGLE DX										
A. Not Operated										
0–19 Years	12	1.8	<1	1	1	2	2	2	3	3
20–34	102	1.4	<1	1	1	1	2	2	2	2
35–49	27	1.4	<1	1	1	2	2	2	2	2
50–64	2	1.5	<1	1	1	2	2	2	2	2
65+	0									
B. Operated										
0–19 Years	0									
20–34	1	2.0	0	2	2	2	2	2	2	2
35–49	0									
50–64	0									
65+	0									
2. MULTIPLE DX										
A. Not Operated										
0–19 Years	21	1.8	<1	1	2	2	2	2	2	3
20–34	87	1.7	<1	1	1	2	2	2	3	4
35–49	33	1.5	<1	1	1	1	2	2	2	3
50–64	2	1.5	<1	1	1	2	2	2	2	2
65+	0									
B. Operated										
0–19 Years	0									
20–34	3	2.0	0	2	2	2	2	2	2	2
35–49	4	2.3	<1	2	2	2	3	3	3	3
50–64	0									
65+	0									
SUBTOTALS:										
1. SINGLE DX										
A. Not Operated	143	1.5	<1	1	1	1	2	2	2	3
B. Operated	1	2.0	0	2	2	2	2	2	2	2
2. MULTIPLE DX										
A. Not Operated	143	1.7	<1	1	1	2	2	2	3	3
B. Operated	7	2.2	<1	2	2	2	2	3	3	3
1. SINGLE DX	144	1.5	<1	1	1	1	2	2	2	3
2. MULTIPLE DX	150	1.7	<1	1	1	2	2	2	3	3
A. NOT OPERATED	286	1.6	<1	1	1	2	2	2	2	3
B. OPERATED	8	2.1	<1	2	2	2	2	3	3	3
TOTAL										
0–19 Years	33	1.8	<1	1	1	2	2	2	3	3
20–34	193	1.6	<1	1	1	2	2	2	2	3
35–49	64	1.5	<1	1	1	1	2	2	2	3
50–64	4	1.5	<1	1	1	2	2	2	2	2
65+	0									
GRAND TOTAL	294	1.6	<1	1	1	2	2	2	2	3

664.21: DEL W 3 DEGREE LAC-DEL

Type of Patients	Observed Patients	Avg. Stay	Vari-ance	10th	25th	50th	75th	90th	95th	99th
1. SINGLE DX										
A. Not Operated										
0–19 Years	279	1.9	<1	1	2	2	2	3	3	3
20–34	1,638	1.9	<1	1	2	2	2	3	3	3
35–49	50	1.9	<1	1	2	2	2	3	3	3
50–64	1	2.0	0	2	2	2	2	2	2	2
65+	0									
B. Operated										
0–19 Years	0									
20–34	1	3.0	0	3	3	3	3	3	3	3
35–49	0									
50–64	0									
65+	0									
2. MULTIPLE DX										
A. Not Operated										
0–19 Years	646	2.2	<1	1	2	2	3	3	3	4
20–34	4,579	2.2	<1	1	2	2	3	3	3	4
35–49	732	2.3	2	1	2	2	3	4	4	5
50–64	23	2.0	<1	1	2	2	2	3	3	3
65+	0									
B. Operated										
0–19 Years	10	2.6	<1	1	2	2	3	3	5	5
20–34	106	2.4	<1	1	2	2	3	3	4	5
35–49	25	2.5	<1	1	2	2	3	4	4	4
50–64	0									
65+	0									
SUBTOTALS:										
1. SINGLE DX										
A. Not Operated	1,968	1.9	<1	1	2	2	2	3	3	3
B. Operated	1	3.0	0	3	3	3	3	3	3	3
2. MULTIPLE DX										
A. Not Operated	5,980	2.2	<1	1	2	2	3	3	3	4
B. Operated	141	2.4	<1	1	2	2	3	3	4	5
1. SINGLE DX	1,969	1.9	<1	1	2	2	2	3	3	3
2. MULTIPLE DX	6,121	2.2	<1	1	2	2	3	3	3	4
A. NOT OPERATED	7,948	2.2	<1	1	2	2	3	3	3	4
B. OPERATED	142	2.4	<1	1	2	2	3	3	4	5
TOTAL										
0–19 Years	935	2.2	<1	1	2	2	3	3	3	4
20–34	6,324	2.1	<1	1	2	2	3	3	3	4
35–49	807	2.3	2	1	2	2	3	3	4	5
50–64	24	2.0	<1	1	2	2	2	3	3	3
65+	0									
GRAND TOTAL	8,090	2.2	<1	1	2	2	3	3	3	4

664.31: DEL W 4 DEGREE LAC-DEL

Type of Patients	Observed Patients	Avg. Stay	Vari-ance	10th	25th	50th	75th	90th	95th	99th
1. SINGLE DX										
A. Not Operated										
0–19 Years	105	2.1	<1	1	2	2	2	3	3	3
20–34	415	2.0	<1	1	2	2	2	3	3	3
35–49	9	2.0	<1	1	2	2	2	3	3	3
50–64	0									
65+	0									
B. Operated										
0–19 Years	1	2.0	0	2	2	2	2	2	2	2
20–34	2	2.5	<1	2	2	3	3	3	3	3
35–49	0									
50–64	0									
65+	0									
2. MULTIPLE DX										
A. Not Operated										
0–19 Years	238	2.3	<1	1	2	2	3	3	4	5
20–34	1,168	2.3	<1	1	2	2	3	3	3	4
35–49	140	2.5	<1	2	2	3	3	3	4	6
50–64	4	3.3	4	2	2	3	6	6	6	6
65+	0									
B. Operated										
0–19 Years	5	2.4	<1	2	2	2	3	3	3	3
20–34	39	2.4	1	1	2	2	3	3	5	7
35–49	10	2.4	<1	2	2	2	3	3	4	4
50–64	0									
65+	0									
SUBTOTALS:										
1. SINGLE DX										
A. Not Operated	529	2.0	<1	1	2	2	2	3	3	3
B. Operated	3	2.3	<1	2	3	3	3	3	3	3
2. MULTIPLE DX										
A. Not Operated	1,550	2.3	<1	1	2	2	3	3	4	5
B. Operated	54	2.4	1	1	2	2	3	3	4	7
1. SINGLE DX	532	2.0	<1	1	2	2	2	3	3	3
2. MULTIPLE DX	1,604	2.3	<1	1	2	2	3	3	4	5
A. NOT OPERATED	2,079	2.3	<1	1	2	2	3	3	3	4
B. OPERATED	57	2.4	1	1	2	2	3	3	4	7
TOTAL										
0–19 Years	349	2.2	<1	1	2	2	3	3	3	4
20–34	1,624	2.2	<1	1	2	2	3	3	3	4
35–49	159	2.4	<1	2	2	2	3	3	4	6
50–64	4	3.3	4	2	2	2	6	6	6	6
65+	0									
GRAND TOTAL	2,136	2.3	<1	1	2	2	3	3	3	4

Length of Stay by Diagnosis and Operation, Western Region, 2008

Western Region, October 2006–September 2007 Data, by Diagnosis

664.41: OB PERINEAL LAC NOS-DEL

Type of Patients	Observed Patients	Avg. Stay	Vari-ance	10th	25th	50th	75th	90th	95th	99th
1. SINGLE DX										
A. *Not Operated*										
0–19 Years	20	1.6	<1	1	1	2	2	2	2	2
20–34	108	1.7	<1	1	1	2	2	2	3	3
35–49	7	1.4	<1	1	1	1	2	2	2	2
50–64	0									
65+	0									
B. *Operated*										
0–19 Years	0									
20–34	0									
35–49	0									
50–64	0									
65+	0									
2. MULTIPLE DX										
A. *Not Operated*										
0–19 Years	28	1.9	<1	1	1	2	2	2	3	3
20–34	124	1.9	<1	1	1	2	2	3	3	3
35–49	22	2.0	<1	1	2	2	2	3	3	4
50–64	1	2.0	0	2	2	2	2	2	2	2
65+	0									
B. *Operated*										
0–19 Years	0									
20–34	9	2.2	<1	2	2	2	2	3	3	3
35–49	2	2.0	0	2	2	2	2	2	2	2
50–64	0									
65+	0									
SUBTOTALS:										
1. SINGLE DX										
A. *Not Operated*	135	1.7	<1	1	1	2	2	2	3	3
B. *Operated*	0									
2. MULTIPLE DX										
A. *Not Operated*	175	1.9	<1	1	1	2	2	3	3	3
B. *Operated*	11	2.2	<1	2	2	2	2	3	3	3
1. SINGLE DX	135	1.7	<1	1	1	2	2	2	3	3
2. MULTIPLE DX	186	1.9	<1	1	1	2	2	3	3	3
A. NOT OPERATED	310	1.8	<1	1	1	2	2	3	3	3
B. OPERATED	11	2.2	<1	2	2	2	2	3	3	3
TOTAL										
0–19 Years	48	1.8	<1	1	1	2	2	3	3	3
20–34	241	1.8	<1	1	1	2	2	3	3	3
35–49	31	1.9	<1	1	1	2	2	3	3	4
50–64	1	2.0	0	2	2	2	2	2	2	2
65+	0									
GRAND TOTAL	321	1.8	<1	1	1	2	2	3	3	3

664.81: OB PERI TRAUMA NEC-DEL

Type of Patients	Observed Patients	Avg. Stay	Vari-ance	10th	25th	50th	75th	90th	95th	99th
1. SINGLE DX										
A. *Not Operated*										
0–19 Years	22	2.0	<1	2	2	2	2	3	3	4
20–34	171	1.7	2	1	1	2	2	2	3	3
35–49	5	1.6	<1	1	1	1	2	3	3	3
50–64	0									
65+	0									
B. *Operated*										
0–19 Years	0									
20–34	1	2.0	0	2	2	2	2	2	2	2
35–49	0									
50–64	0									
65+	0									
2. MULTIPLE DX										
A. *Not Operated*										
0–19 Years	50	2.0	<1	1	1	2	2	3	3	4
20–34	334	1.8	<1	1	1	2	2	3	3	4
35–49	38	1.8	<1	1	1	2	2	3	3	3
50–64	3	2.0	0	2	2	2	2	2	2	2
65+	0									
B. *Operated*										
0–19 Years	0									
20–34	14	1.9	<1	1	1	2	2	3	3	3
35–49	2	1.5	<1	1	1	2	2	2	2	2
50–64	0									
65+	0									
SUBTOTALS:										
1. SINGLE DX										
A. *Not Operated*	198	1.7	2	1	1	2	2	2	3	4
B. *Operated*	1	2.0	0	2	2	2	2	2	2	2
2. MULTIPLE DX										
A. *Not Operated*	425	1.9	<1	1	1	2	2	3	3	4
B. *Operated*	16	1.9	<1	1	1	2	2	3	3	3
1. SINGLE DX	199	1.7	2	1	1	2	2	2	3	4
2. MULTIPLE DX	441	1.9	<1	1	1	2	2	3	3	4
A. NOT OPERATED	623	1.8	<1	1	1	2	2	3	3	4
B. OPERATED	17	1.9	<1	2	2	2	2	3	3	3
TOTAL										
0–19 Years	72	2.0	<1	1	2	2	2	3	3	4
20–34	520	1.8	<1	1	1	2	2	3	3	4
35–49	45	1.8	<1	1	1	2	2	3	3	4
50–64	3	2.0	0	2	2	2	2	2	2	2
65+	0									
GRAND TOTAL	640	1.8	<1	1	1	2	2	3	3	4

665: OTHER OBSTETRICAL TRAUMA

Type of Patients	Observed Patients	Avg. Stay	Vari-ance	10th	25th	50th	75th	90th	95th	99th
1. SINGLE DX										
A. *Not Operated*										
0–19 Years	647	1.8	<1	1	1	2	2	3	3	3
20–34	2,665	1.7	<1	1	1	2	2	3	3	3
35–49	62	1.6	<1	1	1	1	2	3	3	3
50–64	4	1.8	<1	1	2	2	2	2	2	2
65+	0									
B. *Operated*										
0–19 Years	121	1.8	<1	1	1	2	2	3	3	3
20–34	523	1.7	<1	1	1	2	2	2	3	3
35–49	11	1.9	<1	1	2	2	2	2	3	3
50–64	2	2.0	0	2	2	2	2	2	2	2
65+	0									
2. MULTIPLE DX										
A. *Not Operated*										
0–19 Years	1,277	2.1	<1	1	2	2	2	3	3	4
20–34	5,190	2.0	1	1	1	2	2	3	3	4
35–49	576	2.1	2	1	2	2	2	3	3	5
50–64	30	2.2	1	1	2	2	3	3	3	7
65+	0									
B. *Operated*										
0–19 Years	364	2.3	<1	1	2	2	3	3	4	6
20–34	1,978	2.2	1	1	2	2	3	3	4	6
35–49	258	2.6	3	1	2	2	3	4	5	10
50–64	17	3.1	6	2	2	2	3	5	12	12
65+	0									
SUBTOTALS:										
1. SINGLE DX										
A. *Not Operated*	3,378	1.7	<1	1	1	2	2	3	3	3
B. *Operated*	657	1.7	<1	1	1	2	2	3	3	3
2. MULTIPLE DX										
A. *Not Operated*	7,073	2.0	1	1	2	2	2	3	3	4
B. *Operated*	2,617	2.2	1	1	2	2	3	3	4	6
1. SINGLE DX	4,035	1.7	<1	1	1	2	2	3	3	3
2. MULTIPLE DX	9,690	2.1	1	1	2	2	3	3	4	5
A. NOT OPERATED	10,451	1.9	<1	1	1	2	2	3	3	4
B. OPERATED	3,274	2.1	1	1	2	2	2	3	4	6
TOTAL										
0–19 Years	2,409	2.0	<1	1	2	2	2	3	3	4
20–34	10,356	2.0	1	1	1	2	2	3	3	4
35–49	907	2.2	2	1	1	2	3	3	4	7
50–64	53	2.5	3	1	2	2	3	3	5	12
65+	0									
GRAND TOTAL	13,725	2.0	1	1	1	2	2	3	3	4

Length of Stay by Diagnosis and Operation, Western Region, 2008

Western Region, October 2006–September 2007 Data, by Diagnosis

665.31: LACERATION OF CERVIX-DEL

Type of Patients	Observed Patients	Avg. Stay	Variance	10th	25th	50th	75th	90th	95th	99th
1. SINGLE DX										
A. Not Operated										
0–19 Years	0									
20–34	19	1.7	<1	1	1	2	2	3	3	3
35–49	0									
50–64	0									
65+	0									
B. Operated										
0–19 Years	8	1.8	<1	1	1	2	2	3	3	3
20–34	32	2.0	<1	1	2	2	2	2	3	5
35–49	0									
50–64	0									
65+	0									
2. MULTIPLE DX										
A. Not Operated										
0–19 Years	7	2.7	1	2	2	2	3	5	5	5
20–34	35	2.1	<1	1	2	2	3	3	3	4
35–49	6	2.3	<1	1	2	3	3	3	3	3
50–64	0									
65+	0									
B. Operated										
0–19 Years	33	2.8	1	2	2	3	3	4	4	7
20–34	238	2.4	1	1	2	2	3	4	4	6
35–49	33	2.8	4	2	2	2	3	4	10	11
50–64	0									
65+	0									
SUBTOTALS:										
1. SINGLE DX A. Not Operated	19	1.7	<1	1	1	2	2	3	3	3
B. Operated	40	1.9	<1	1	2	2	2	3	3	5
2. MULTIPLE DX A. Not Operated	48	2.2	<1	1	2	2	3	3	3	5
B. Operated	304	2.5	2	1	2	2	3	4	4	7
1. SINGLE DX	59	1.9	<1	1	1	2	2	3	3	5
2. MULTIPLE DX	352	2.4	2	1	2	2	3	4	4	7
A. NOT OPERATED	67	2.1	<1	1	2	2	3	3	3	5
B. OPERATED	344	2.4	2	1	2	2	3	4	4	7
TOTAL										
0–19 Years	48	2.6	1	1	2	2	3	4	4	7
20–34	324	2.3	1	1	2	2	3	3	4	6
35–49	39	2.8	4	2	2	2	3	4	10	11
50–64	0									
65+	0									
GRAND TOTAL	411	2.4	2	1	2	2	3	3	4	6

665.41: HIGH VAGINAL LAC-DEL

Type of Patients	Observed Patients	Avg. Stay	Variance	10th	25th	50th	75th	90th	95th	99th
1. SINGLE DX										
A. Not Operated										
0–19 Years	346	1.9	<1	1	1	2	2	3	3	4
20–34	1,341	1.8	<1	1	1	2	2	3	3	3
35–49	33	1.7	<1	1	1	2	2	3	3	3
50–64	4	1.8	<1	1	2	2	2	2	2	2
65+	0									
B. Operated										
0–19 Years	0									
20–34	0									
35–49	0									
50–64	0									
65+	0									
2. MULTIPLE DX										
A. Not Operated										
0–19 Years	690	2.1	<1	1	2	2	2	3	3	4
20–34	2,471	2.1	2	1	2	2	3	3	3	4
35–49	292	2.0	<1	1	2	2	3	3	3	4
50–64	23	2.1	<1	2	2	3	3	3	3	3
65+	0									
B. Operated										
0–19 Years	18	2.4	<1	1	2	3	3	4	5	5
20–34	91	2.2	2	1	2	2	3	3	4	14
35–49	24	2.1	<1	1	2	2	2	3	3	3
50–64	2	2.5	<1	2	2	2	3	3	3	3
65+	0									
SUBTOTALS:										
1. SINGLE DX A. Not Operated	1,724	1.8	<1	1	1	2	2	3	3	3
B. Operated	0									
2. MULTIPLE DX A. Not Operated	3,476	2.1	2	1	2	2	2	3	3	4
B. Operated	135	2.2	2	1	2	2	3	3	3	5
1. SINGLE DX	1,724	1.8	<1	1	1	2	2	3	3	3
2. MULTIPLE DX	3,611	2.1	2	1	2	2	2	3	3	4
A. NOT OPERATED	5,200	2.0	1	1	1	2	2	3	3	4
B. OPERATED	135	2.2	2	1	2	2	3	3	3	5
TOTAL										
0–19 Years	1,054	2.1	<1	1	2	2	2	3	3	4
20–34	3,903	2.0	1	1	1	2	2	3	3	4
35–49	349	2.0	<1	1	1	2	2	3	3	4
50–64	29	2.1	<1	2	2	2	2	3	3	3
65+	0									
GRAND TOTAL	5,335	2.0	1	1	1	2	2	3	3	4

665.51: OB INJ PELV ORG NEC-DEL

Type of Patients	Observed Patients	Avg. Stay	Variance	10th	25th	50th	75th	90th	95th	99th
1. SINGLE DX										
A. Not Operated										
0–19 Years	287	1.8	<1	1	1	2	2	2	3	3
20–34	1,198	1.6	<1	1	1	2	2	2	3	3
35–49	26	1.5	<1	1	1	1	2	2	3	3
50–64	0									
65+	0									
B. Operated										
0–19 Years	111	1.8	<1	1	1	2	2	3	3	3
20–34	480	1.7	<1	1	1	2	2	2	3	3
35–49	9	1.8	<1	1	2	2	2	2	2	2
50–64	2	2.0	0	2	2	2	2	2	2	2
65+	0									
2. MULTIPLE DX										
A. Not Operated										
0–19 Years	540	2.0	<1	1	2	2	2	3	3	4
20–34	2,464	1.9	<1	1	1	2	2	3	3	4
35–49	258	2.0	<1	1	2	2	2	3	3	4
50–64	0									
65+	0									
B. Operated										
0–19 Years	304	2.2	<1	1	2	2	2	3	3	5
20–34	1,510	2.0	<1	1	2	2	2	3	3	4
35–49	161	2.1	<1	1	2	2	2	3	4	5
50–64	11	2.2	<1	2	2	2	3	3	3	3
65+	0									
SUBTOTALS:										
1. SINGLE DX A. Not Operated	1,511	1.7	<1	1	1	2	2	2	3	3
B. Operated	602	1.7	<1	1	1	2	2	2	3	3
2. MULTIPLE DX A. Not Operated	3,266	2.0	<1	1	1	2	2	3	3	4
B. Operated	1,986	2.0	<1	1	2	2	2	3	3	5
1. SINGLE DX	2,113	1.7	<1	1	1	2	2	2	3	3
2. MULTIPLE DX	5,252	2.0	<1	1	2	2	2	3	3	4
A. NOT OPERATED	4,777	1.9	<1	1	1	2	2	3	3	4
B. OPERATED	2,588	2.0	<1	1	1	2	2	3	3	4
TOTAL										
0–19 Years	1,242	2.0	<1	1	2	2	2	3	3	4
20–34	5,652	1.9	<1	1	1	2	2	3	3	4
35–49	454	2.0	<1	1	2	2	2	3	3	5
50–64	17	2.0	<1	1	2	2	2	3	3	3
65+	0									
GRAND TOTAL	7,365	1.9	<1	1	1	2	2	3	3	4

Length of Stay by Diagnosis and Operation, Western Region, 2008

Western Region, October 2006–September 2007 Data, by Diagnosis

666: POSTPARTUM HEMORRHAGE

Type of Patients	Observed Patients	Avg. Stay	Vari-ance	Percentiles						
				10th	25th	50th	75th	90th	95th	99th
1. SINGLE DX										
A. Not Operated										
0–19 Years	90	1.9	<1	1	1	2	2	3	3	5
20–34	645	1.7	<1	1	1	2	2	3	3	4
35–49	31	1.7	<1	1	1	2	2	2	3	5
50–64	0									
65+	0									
B. Operated										
0–19 Years	19	2.0	<1	1	1	2	2	4	5	5
20–34	167	1.7	<1	1	1	2	2	3	3	4
35–49	31	1.6	1	1	1	1	2	3	4	5
50–64	0									
65+	0									
2. MULTIPLE DX										
A. Not Operated										
0–19 Years	306	2.2	<1	1	2	2	3	3	4	4
20–34	1,715	2.1	2	1	2	2	2	3	3	5
35–49	205	2.0	<1	1	1	2	2	4	4	5
50–64	16	2.0	<1	1	2	2	2	3	3	3
65+	0									
B. Operated										
0–19 Years	101	2.6	4	1	2	2	3	4	5	17
20–34	831	2.5	3	1	2	2	3	4	5	8
35–49	200	3.5	22	1	2	3	4	5	7	28
50–64	9	3.1	<1	2	3	3	4	4	4	4
65+	0									
SUBTOTALS:										
1. SINGLE DX										
A. Not Operated	766	1.7	<1	1	1	2	2	3	3	4
B. Operated	217	1.7	<1	1	1	2	2	3	3	4
2. MULTIPLE DX										
A. Not Operated	2,242	2.1	2	1	2	2	2	3	3	5
B. Operated	1,141	2.7	7	1	2	2	3	4	6	12
1. SINGLE DX	983	1.7	<1	1	1	2	2	3	3	4
2. MULTIPLE DX	3,383	2.3	3	1	2	2	3	3	4	7
A. NOT OPERATED	3,008	2.0	1	1	1	2	2	3	3	5
B. OPERATED	1,358	2.6	6	1	1	2	3	4	5	11
TOTAL										
0–19 Years	516	2.2	1	1	2	2	3	3	4	6
20–34	3,358	2.1	2	1	1	2	2	3	3	6
35–49	467	2.6	10	1	1	2	3	4	5	16
50–64	25	2.4	<1	2	2	2	3	4	4	4
65+	0									
GRAND TOTAL	4,366	2.2	3	1	1	2	2	3	4	6

666.02: 3RD STAGE PP HEMOR-DEL

Type of Patients	Observed Patients	Avg. Stay	Vari-ance	Percentiles						
				10th	25th	50th	75th	90th	95th	99th
1. SINGLE DX										
A. Not Operated										
0–19 Years	7	1.7	<1	1	1	2	2	2	2	2
20–34	42	1.8	<1	1	1	2	2	3	3	3
35–49	3	2.0	0	2	2	2	2	2	2	2
50–64	0									
65+	0									
B. Operated										
0–19 Years	2	2.0	0	2	2	2	2	2	2	2
20–34	10	2.2	<1	2	2	2	2	3	3	3
35–49	0									
50–64	0									
65+	0									
2. MULTIPLE DX										
A. Not Operated										
0–19 Years	18	2.1	<1	1	1	2	3	3	4	4
20–34	136	2.1	2	1	2	2	2	3	4	5
35–49	27	2.3	<1	1	2	2	3	4	4	4
50–64	3	2.0	0	2	2	2	2	2	2	2
65+	0									
B. Operated										
0–19 Years	11	2.5	1	1	2	3	3	4	4	4
20–34	140	3.2	4	2	2	3	4	5	6	13
35–49	39	6.6	87	2	2	4	5	16	28	51
50–64	2	3.5	<1	3	3	4	4	4	4	4
65+	0									
SUBTOTALS:										
1. SINGLE DX										
A. Not Operated	52	1.8	<1	1	1	2	2	3	3	3
B. Operated	12	2.2	<1	2	2	2	2	3	3	3
2. MULTIPLE DX										
A. Not Operated	184	2.2	2	1	2	2	2	3	3	5
B. Operated	192	3.8	22	2	2	3	4	5	11	28
1. SINGLE DX	64	1.9	<1	1	2	2	2	3	3	3
2. MULTIPLE DX	376	3.0	13	1	2	2	3	4	5	18
A. NOT OPERATED	236	2.1	2	1	2	2	2	3	3	4
B. OPERATED	204	3.7	21	2	2	3	4	5	7	22
TOTAL										
0–19 Years	38	2.1	<1	1	2	2	3	3	4	4
20–34	328	2.5	3	1	2	2	3	4	5	12
35–49	69	4.7	54	2	2	3	4	11	16	51
50–64	5	2.6	<1	2	2	3	3	4	4	4
65+	0									
GRAND TOTAL	440	2.8	11	1	2	2	3	4	5	17

666.12: IMMED PP HEMOR NEC-DEL

Type of Patients	Observed Patients	Avg. Stay	Vari-ance	Percentiles						
				10th	25th	50th	75th	90th	95th	99th
1. SINGLE DX										
A. Not Operated										
0–19 Years	65	1.9	<1	1	1	2	2	2	3	5
20–34	494	1.7	<1	1	1	2	2	3	3	3
35–49	11	1.8	<1	1	1	2	2	2	3	3
50–64	0									
65+	0									
B. Operated										
0–19 Years	5	1.8	<1	1	2	2	2	2	2	2
20–34	32	1.9	<1	1	2	2	2	3	3	4
35–49	0									
50–64	0									
65+	0									
2. MULTIPLE DX										
A. Not Operated										
0–19 Years	239	2.2	<1	1	2	2	3	3	4	4
20–34	1,237	2.1	<1	1	2	2	2	3	3	4
35–49	107	2.0	<1	1	2	2	3	3	3	5
50–64	9	2.0	<1	2	2	2	3	3	3	3
65+	0									
B. Operated										
0–19 Years	36	2.7	1	2	2	2	3	4	5	6
20–34	263	2.8	4	2	2	2	3	4	5	7
35–49	37	3.6	3	2	2	3	5	6	7	7
50–64	5	3.2	<1	3	3	3	4	4	4	4
65+	0									
SUBTOTALS:										
1. SINGLE DX										
A. Not Operated	570	1.8	<1	1	1	2	2	3	3	3
B. Operated	37	1.9	<1	2	2	2	2	3	3	4
2. MULTIPLE DX										
A. Not Operated	1,592	2.1	<1	1	2	2	2	3	3	4
B. Operated	341	2.9	4	2	2	3	4	4	6	7
1. SINGLE DX	607	1.8	<1	1	1	2	2	3	3	3
2. MULTIPLE DX	1,933	2.2	1	1	2	2	3	3	4	6
A. NOT OPERATED	2,162	2.0	<1	1	2	2	2	3	3	4
B. OPERATED	378	2.8	4	2	2	2	3	4	5	7
TOTAL										
0–19 Years	345	2.2	<1	1	2	2	3	3	4	5
20–34	2,026	2.1	1	1	2	2	3	3	3	5
35–49	155	2.4	2	1	2	2	3	4	5	7
50–64	14	2.4	<1	1	2	2	3	4	4	4
65+	0									
GRAND TOTAL	2,540	2.1	1	1	2	2	2	3	4	5

Length of Stay by Diagnosis and Operation, Western Region, 2008

Western Region, October 2006–September 2007 Data, by Diagnosis

Type of Patients	666.22: DELAYED PP HEMOR-DEL PP										666.24: DELAYED PP HEMOR-PP										667: RET PLAC/MEMB W/O HEMOR									
	Observed Patients	Avg. Stay	Vari-ance	10th	25th	50th	75th	90th	95th	99th	Observed Patients	Avg. Stay	Vari-ance	10th	25th	50th	75th	90th	95th	99th	Observed Patients	Avg. Stay	Vari-ance	10th	25th	50th	75th	90th	95th	99th
1. SINGLE DX																														
A. Not Operated																														
0–19 Years	8	2.3	<1	1	2	2	3	3	3	3	5	1.2	<1	1	1	1	1	2	2	2	19	1.7	<1	1	1	2	2	2	3	3
20–34	34	1.8	<1	1	1	2	2	2	3	3	46	1.3	<1	1	1	1	1	2	3	5	193	1.7	<1	1	1	2	2	2	3	4
35–49	2	2.0	0	2	2	2	2	2	2	2	9	1.2	<1	1	1	1	1	2	2	2	12	1.7	<1	1	1	2	2	2	2	2
50–64	0										0										0									
65+	0										0										0									
B. Operated																														
0–19 Years	5	2.4	<1	2	2	2	2	4	4	4	5	2.0	3	1	1	2	2	5	5	5	11	1.5	<1	1	1	1	2	2	3	3
20–34	35	2.0	<1	1	1	2	3	3	4	4	84	1.4	<1	1	1	1	2	2	3	4	44	1.8	<1	1	1	2	2	3	3	4
35–49	1	3.0	0	3	3	3	3	3	3	3	30	1.5	1	1	1	2	2	3	4	5	9	1.8	<1	1	1	2	2	3	3	3
50–64	0										0										0									
65+	0										0										0									
2. MULTIPLE DX																														
A. Not Operated																														
0–19 Years	25	2.2	<1	1	2	2	3	4	4	4	13	1.7	<1	1	1	2	2	3	4	4	43	1.9	<1	1	1	2	2	3	3	4
20–34	127	2.2	<1	1	1	2	3	3	3	4	126	1.8	1	1	1	2	2	3	3	6	318	1.8	<1	1	1	2	2	3	3	4
35–49	16	1.7	<1	1	1	2	2	2	3	3	30	1.9	2	1	1	2	2	3	4	7	75	1.9	<1	1	1	2	2	3	3	4
50–64	2	2.5	<1	2	2	2	3	3	3	3	0										4	2.3	<1	2	2	2	3	3	3	3
65+	0										0										0									
B. Operated																														
0–19 Years	21	2.7	<1	2	2	3	3	4	4	4	27	1.8	1	1	1	2	2	4	4	5	21	2.1	1	1	2	2	3	3	3	5
20–34	114	2.7	2	2	2	2	3	4	5	8	276	2.0	2	1	1	2	3	3	4	8	149	2.4	4	1	2	2	3	3	5	8
35–49	27	2.7	2	2	2	2	3	4	4	8	82	2.4	4	1	1	2	3	4	5	17	47	4.8	74	2	2	2	4	6	30	41
50–64	1	2.0	0	2	2	2	2	2	2	2	1	3.0	0	3	3	3	3	3	3	3	2	2.0	0	2	2	2	2	2	2	2
65+	0										0										0									
SUBTOTALS:																														
1. SINGLE DX																														
A. Not Operated	44	1.9	<1	1	1	2	2	3	3	3	60	1.3	<1	1	1	1	1	2	3	5	224	1.7	<1	1	1	2	2	2	3	4
B. Operated	41	2.1	<1	1	1	2	3	3	4	4	119	1.4	<1	1	1	1	2	3	3	5	64	1.8	<1	1	1	2	2	3	3	4
2. MULTIPLE DX																														
A. Not Operated	170	2.1	<1	1	2	2	3	3	3	4	169	1.8	1	1	1	2	2	3	4	7	440	1.8	<1	1	1	2	2	3	3	4
B. Operated	163	2.7	2	2	2	2	3	4	4	8	386	2.1	2	1	1	2	3	4	4	8	219	2.9	19	1	2	2	3	4	6	30
1. SINGLE DX	85	2.0	<1	1	1	2	2	3	3	4	179	1.4	<1	1	1	1	1	2	3	5	288	1.7	<1	1	1	2	2	2	3	4
2. MULTIPLE DX	333	2.4	1	1	2	2	3	3	4	6	555	2.0	2	1	1	2	3	3	4	8	659	2.2	7	1	1	2	2	3	4	8
A. NOT OPERATED	214	2.1	<1	1	2	2	3	3	3	4	229	1.7	1	1	1	1	2	3	4	6	664	1.8	<1	1	1	2	2	3	3	4
B. OPERATED	204	2.5	2	1	2	2	3	4	4	8	505	1.9	2	1	1	2	3	4	4	7	283	2.6	15	1	1	2	3	3	5	30
TOTAL																														
0–19 Years	59	2.4	<1	1	2	2	3	4	4	4	50	1.7	1	1	1	2	2	3	4	5	94	1.8	<1	1	1	2	2	3	3	5
20–34	310	2.3	1	1	2	2	3	3	4	6	532	1.8	1	1	1	2	2	3	4	7	704	1.9	1	1	1	2	2	3	3	5
35–49	46	2.3	1	1	2	2	3	4	4	8	151	2.1	3	1	1	2	3	4	4	8	143	2.9	26	1	1	2	2	3	4	36
50–64	3	2.3	<1	2	2	2	3	3	3	3	1	3.0	0	3	3	3	3	3	3	3	6	2.2	<1	2	2	2	3	3	3	3
65+	0										0										0									
GRAND TOTAL	418	2.3	1	1	2	2	3	3	4	6	734	1.8	2	1	1	2	2	3	4	7	947	2.0	5	1	1	2	2	3	3	6

Length of Stay by Diagnosis and Operation, Western Region, 2008

Western Region, October 2006–September 2007 Data, by Diagnosis

667.02: RET PLAC S HEMOR-DEL PP

Type of Patients	Observed Patients	Avg. Stay	Vari- ance	10th	25th	50th	75th	90th	95th	99th
1. SINGLE DX										
A. Not Operated										
0–19 Years	10	1.8	<1	1	1	2	2	2	3	3
20–34	106	1.8	<1	1	1	2	2	3	3	4
35–49	3	1.7	<1	1	1	2	2	2	2	2
50–64	0									
65+	0									
B. Operated										
0–19 Years	3	2.3	<1	2	2	3	3	3	3	3
20–34	10	1.9	<1	1	1	2	2	3	3	3
35–49	1	3.0	0	3	3	3	3	3	3	3
50–64	0									
65+	0									
2. MULTIPLE DX										
A. Not Operated										
0–19 Years	18	1.7	<1	1	1	2	2	3	3	3
20–34	166	1.9	1	1	1	2	2	3	3	5
35–49	43	1.9	<1	1	1	2	2	3	3	4
50–64	2	2.5	<1	2	2	3	3	3	3	3
65+	0									
B. Operated										
0–19 Years	3	2.0	<1	1	1	2	2	3	3	3
20–34	64	2.5	1	1	2	2	3	4	5	6
35–49	26	6.9	125	1	2	3	4	30	36	41
50–64	1	2.0	0	2	2	2	2	2	2	2
65+	0									
SUBTOTALS:										
1. SINGLE DX										
A. Not Operated	119	1.8	<1	1	1	2	2	3	3	4
B. Operated	14	2.1	<1	1	2	2	3	3	3	3
2. MULTIPLE DX										
A. Not Operated	229	1.9	<1	1	1	2	2	3	3	4
B. Operated	94	3.7	38	1	2	2	3	5	6	41
1. SINGLE DX	133	1.8	<1	1	1	2	2	3	3	4
2. MULTIPLE DX	323	2.4	12	1	1	2	2	3	4	17
A. NOT OPERATED	348	1.9	<1	1	1	2	2	3	3	4
B. OPERATED	108	3.5	34	1	2	2	3	4	6	36
TOTAL										
0–19 Years	34	1.8	<1	1	1	2	2	3	3	3
20–34	346	2.0	4	1	1	2	2	3	3	6
35–49	73	3.7	50	1	2	2	3	4	17	41
50–64	3	2.3	<1	2	2	2	3	3	3	3
65+	0									
GRAND TOTAL	456	2.3	9	1	1	2	2	3	4	12

668: COMP ANES IN DELIVERY

Type of Patients	Observed Patients	Avg. Stay	Vari- ance	10th	25th	50th	75th	90th	95th	99th
1. SINGLE DX										
A. Not Operated										
0–19 Years	2	2.0	2	1	1	3	3	3	3	3
20–34	12	1.7	<1	1	1	1	2	3	3	3
35–49	1	1.0	0	1	1	1	1	1	1	1
50–64	0									
65+	0									
B. Operated										
0–19 Years	0									
20–34	0									
35–49	0									
50–64	0									
65+	0									
2. MULTIPLE DX										
A. Not Operated										
0–19 Years	20	2.3	2	1	1	2	3	4	6	6
20–34	199	2.3	2	1	2	2	3	5	7	7
35–49	9	2.6	5	1	1	2	3	8	8	8
50–64	0									
65+	0									
B. Operated										
0–19 Years	1	3.0	0	3	3	3	3	3	3	3
20–34	17	3.7	4	2	3	4	4	5	10	10
35–49	1	4.0	0	4	4	4	4	4	4	4
50–64	0									
65+	0									
SUBTOTALS:										
1. SINGLE DX										
A. Not Operated	15	1.7	<1	1	1	1	2	3	3	3
B. Operated	0									
2. MULTIPLE DX										
A. Not Operated	228	2.3	2	1	2	2	3	4	5	7
B. Operated	19	3.7	3	2	3	3	4	5	10	10
1. SINGLE DX	15	1.7	<1	1	1	1	2	3	3	3
2. MULTIPLE DX	247	2.4	2	1	2	2	3	4	5	8
A. NOT OPERATED	243	2.3	2	1	1	2	3	4	5	7
B. OPERATED	19	3.7	3	2	3	3	4	5	10	10
TOTAL										
0–19 Years	23	2.3	2	1	1	2	3	4	6	6
20–34	228	2.4	2	1	2	2	3	4	5	7
35–49	11	2.6	4	1	1	2	3	4	8	8
50–64	0									
65+	0									
GRAND TOTAL	262	2.4	2	1	1	2	3	4	5	8

669: OTH COMP LABOR/DELIVERY

Type of Patients	Observed Patients	Avg. Stay	Vari- ance	10th	25th	50th	75th	90th	95th	99th
1. SINGLE DX										
A. Not Operated										
0–19 Years	485	2.0	<1	1	2	2	2	3	3	4
20–34	2,200	1.9	<1	1	1	2	2	3	3	4
35–49	63	2.0	<1	1	2	2	2	3	3	4
50–64	6	2.3	<1	2	2	2	3	3	3	3
65+	0									
B. Operated										
0–19 Years	29	2.8	<1	2	2	3	3	4	4	4
20–34	423	2.9	<1	2	2	3	3	4	4	4
35–49	20	3.1	<1	2	3	3	4	4	4	4
50–64	1	4.0	0	4	4	4	4	4	4	4
65+	0									
2. MULTIPLE DX										
A. Not Operated										
0–19 Years	1,034	2.1	<1	1	2	2	3	3	3	4
20–34	5,829	2.2	<1	1	2	2	3	3	3	4
35–49	896	2.1	<1	1	2	2	3	3	3	4
50–64	57	2.3	<1	1	2	2	3	3	3	4
65+	0									
B. Operated										
0–19 Years	69	3.1	4	3	3	3	4	4	6	16
20–34	873	3.0	2	2	2	3	3	4	4	7
35–49	387	3.3	4	2	3	3	4	4	4	7
50–64	16	3.3	<1	2	3	4	4	4	4	4
65+	0									
SUBTOTALS:										
1. SINGLE DX										
A. Not Operated	2,754	1.9	<1	1	1	2	2	3	3	4
B. Operated	473	2.9	<1	2	2	3	3	4	4	4
2. MULTIPLE DX										
A. Not Operated	7,816	2.2	<1	1	2	2	3	3	4	4
B. Operated	1,345	3.1	3	2	2	3	4	4	4	7
1. SINGLE DX	3,227	2.1	<1	1	2	2	3	3	3	4
2. MULTIPLE DX	9,161	2.3	1	1	2	2	3	4	4	5
A. NOT OPERATED	10,570	2.1	<1	1	2	2	3	3	3	4
B. OPERATED	1,818	3.0	2	2	2	3	4	4	4	6
TOTAL										
0–19 Years	1,617	2.2	<1	1	2	2	3	3	3	4
20–34	9,325	2.2	<1	1	2	2	3	4	4	5
35–49	1,366	2.5	2	1	2	2	3	3	4	5
50–64	80	2.5	<1	2	2	2	3	4	4	4
65+	0									
GRAND TOTAL	12,388	2.2	1	1	2	2	3	3	4	5

Length of Stay by Diagnosis and Operation, Western Region, 2008

Western Region, October 2006–September 2007 Data, by Diagnosis

669.51: FORCEPS/VED NOS-DEL

Type of Patients	Observed Patients	Avg. Stay	Variance	10th	25th	50th	75th	90th	95th	99th
1. SINGLE DX										
A. Not Operated										
0–19 Years	337	2.0	<1	1	2	2	2	3	3	4
20–34	1,356	1.9	<1	1	2	2	2	3	3	4
35–49	43	2.0	<1	1	2	2	2	3	3	4
50–64	5	2.2	<1	2	2	2	2	3	3	3
65+	0									
B. Operated										
0–19 Years	0									
20–34	1	2.0	0	2	2	2	2	2	2	2
35–49	0									
50–64	0									
65+	0									
2. MULTIPLE DX										
A. Not Operated										
0–19 Years	528	2.1	<1	1	2	2	2	3	3	4
20–34	2,532	2.0	<1	1	2	2	2	3	3	4
35–49	375	2.0	<1	1	2	2	2	3	3	3
50–64	25	2.0	<1	1	2	2	2	3	3	3
65+	0									
B. Operated										
0–19 Years	9	2.3	<1	2	2	2	2	4	4	4
20–34	106	2.4	<1	2	2	2	3	4	4	4
35–49	21	2.4	<1	1	2	2	3	3	4	4
50–64	0									
65+	0									
SUBTOTALS:										
1. SINGLE DX										
A. Not Operated	1,741	2.0	<1	1	1	2	2	3	3	4
B. Operated	1	2.0	0	2	2	2	2	2	2	2
2. MULTIPLE DX										
A. Not Operated	3,460	2.1	<1	1	2	2	2	3	3	4
B. Operated	136	2.4	<1	2	2	2	3	4	4	4
1. SINGLE DX	1,742	2.0	<1	1	1	2	2	3	3	4
2. MULTIPLE DX	3,596	2.1	<1	2	2	2	3	3	3	4
A. NOT OPERATED	5,201	2.0	<1	1	2	2	2	3	3	4
B. OPERATED	137	2.4	<1	2	2	2	3	4	4	4
TOTAL										
0–19 Years	874	2.1	<1	1	2	2	2	3	3	4
20–34	3,995	2.0	<1	1	2	2	2	3	3	4
35–49	439	2.0	<1	1	2	2	2	3	3	3
50–64	30	2.1	<1	1	2	2	2	3	3	3
65+	0									
GRAND TOTAL	5,338	2.0	<1	1	2	2	2	3	3	4

669.71: CESAREAN DEL NOS-DEL

Type of Patients	Observed Patients	Avg. Stay	Variance	10th	25th	50th	75th	90th	95th	99th
1. SINGLE DX										
A. Not Operated										
0–19 Years	0									
20–34	0									
35–49	0									
50–64	0									
65+	0									
B. Operated										
0–19 Years	22	2.7	<1	2	2	3	3	4	4	4
20–34	386	2.9	<1	2	2	3	3	4	4	5
35–49	18	3.0	<1	2	2	3	3	4	4	4
50–64	1	4.0	0	4	4	4	4	4	4	4
65+	0									
2. MULTIPLE DX										
A. Not Operated										
0–19 Years	0									
20–34	2	2.0	2	1	1	1	3	3	3	3
35–49	0									
50–64	0									
65+	0									
B. Operated										
0–19 Years	28	2.9	1	2	2	2	3	4	6	6
20–34	471	3.0	<1	2	2	3	3	4	4	5
35–49	295	3.2	<1	2	3	3	4	4	4	5
50–64	11	3.6	<1	3	3	4	4	4	4	4
65+	0									
SUBTOTALS:										
1. SINGLE DX										
A. Not Operated	0									
B. Operated	427	2.9	<1	2	2	3	3	4	4	4
2. MULTIPLE DX										
A. Not Operated	2	2.0	2	1	1	1	3	3	3	3
B. Operated	805	3.1	<1	2	2	3	4	4	4	5
1. SINGLE DX	427	2.9	<1	2	2	3	3	4	4	4
2. MULTIPLE DX	807	3.1	<1	2	2	3	4	4	4	5
A. NOT OPERATED	2	2.0	2	1	1	1	3	3	3	3
B. OPERATED	1,232	3.0	<1	2	2	3	4	4	4	5
TOTAL										
0–19 Years	50	2.8	<1	2	2	2	3	4	4	6
20–34	859	3.0	<1	2	2	3	3	4	4	5
35–49	313	3.2	<1	2	2	3	4	4	4	5
50–64	12	3.7	<1	3	3	4	4	4	4	4
65+	0									
GRAND TOTAL	1,234	3.0	<1	2	2	3	4	4	4	5

669.81: COMP LABOR/DEL NEC-DEL

Type of Patients	Observed Patients	Avg. Stay	Variance	10th	25th	50th	75th	90th	95th	99th
1. SINGLE DX										
A. Not Operated										
0–19 Years	123	2.1	<1	1	2	2	2	3	3	3
20–34	614	1.9	<1	1	2	2	2	3	3	3
35–49	13	1.9	<1	1	2	2	2	3	3	3
50–64	1	3.0	0	3	3	3	3	3	3	3
65+	0									
B. Operated										
0–19 Years	3	2.7	<1	2	2	2	3	3	3	3
20–34	28	3.0	<1	2	3	3	3	4	4	4
35–49	1	3.0	0	3	3	3	3	3	3	3
50–64	0									
65+	0									
2. MULTIPLE DX										
A. Not Operated										
0–19 Years	459	2.2	<1	1	2	2	3	3	3	4
20–34	2,932	2.2	<1	1	2	2	3	3	3	4
35–49	468	2.2	<1	1	2	2	3	3	3	4
50–64	29	2.5	<1	2	2	3	3	4	4	4
65+	0									
B. Operated										
0–19 Years	25	3.0	1	1	2	3	4	4	4	4
20–34	207	2.9	1	2	2	3	3	4	5	7
35–49	44	3.0	2	2	2	3	4	4	5	7
50–64	4	2.5	1	2	2	2	4	4	4	4
65+	0									
SUBTOTALS:										
1. SINGLE DX										
A. Not Operated	751	2.0	<1	1	2	2	2	3	3	3
B. Operated	32	2.9	<1	2	3	3	3	4	4	4
2. MULTIPLE DX										
A. Not Operated	3,888	2.2	<1	1	2	2	3	3	3	4
B. Operated	280	2.9	1	2	2	3	4	4	5	7
1. SINGLE DX	783	2.0	<1	1	2	2	3	3	3	4
2. MULTIPLE DX	4,168	2.3	<1	1	2	3	3	4	4	5
A. NOT OPERATED	4,639	2.2	<1	1	2	2	3	3	3	4
B. OPERATED	312	2.9	1	2	2	3	4	4	4	7
TOTAL										
0–19 Years	610	2.2	<1	1	2	2	3	3	3	4
20–34	3,781	2.2	<1	1	2	2	3	3	3	4
35–49	526	2.3	<1	1	2	2	3	3	4	5
50–64	34	2.5	<1	2	2	2	3	4	4	4
65+	0									
GRAND TOTAL	4,951	2.2	<1	1	2	2	3	3	3	4

Length of Stay by Diagnosis and Operation, Western Region, 2008

Western Region, October 2006–September 2007 Data, by Diagnosis

669.82: COMP LABOR/DEL NEC-DELPP

Type of Patients	Observed Patients	Avg. Stay	Variance	10th	25th	50th	75th	90th	95th	99th
1. SINGLE DX										
A. Not Operated										
0–19 Years	14	1.8	<1	1	1	2	2	3	3	3
20–34	165	1.7	<1	1	1	2	2	2	3	3
35–49	3	2.3	<1	2	2	2	3	3	3	3
50–64	0									
65+	0									
B. Operated										
0–19 Years	0									
20–34	0									
35–49	0									
50–64	0									
65+	0									
2. MULTIPLE DX										
A. Not Operated										
0–19 Years	26	2.1	<1	1	2	2	3	3	3	4
20–34	187	2.0	<1	1	1	2	2	3	3	5
35–49	20	2.1	<1	1	2	2	2	3	3	4
50–64	2	2.0	0	2	2	2	2	2	2	2
65+	0									
B. Operated										
0–19 Years	1	4.0	0	4	4	4	4	4	4	4
20–34	20	2.3	<1	1	2	2	3	3	3	4
35–49	2	2.5	<1	2	2	2	3	3	3	3
50–64	0									
65+	0									
SUBTOTALS:										
1. SINGLE DX										
A. Not Operated	182	1.7	<1	1	1	2	2	2	3	3
B. Operated	0									
2. MULTIPLE DX										
A. Not Operated	235	2.0	<1	1	2	2	2	3	3	5
B. Operated	23	2.4	<1	2	2	2	3	3	4	4
1. SINGLE DX	182	1.7	<1	1	1	2	2	2	3	3
2. MULTIPLE DX	258	2.0	<1	1	2	2	2	3	3	5
A. NOT OPERATED	417	1.9	<1	1	1	2	2	3	3	4
B. OPERATED	23	2.4	<1	2	2	3	3	3	4	4
TOTAL										
0–19 Years	41	2.1	<1	1	1	2	3	3	3	4
20–34	372	1.9	<1	1	1	2	2	3	3	4
35–49	25	2.1	<1	1	2	2	3	3	3	4
50–64	2	2.0	0	2	2	2	2	2	2	2
65+	0									
GRAND TOTAL	440	1.9	<1	1	2	2	2	3	3	4

670: MAJ PUERPERAL INFECTION

Type of Patients	Observed Patients	Avg. Stay	Variance	10th	25th	50th	75th	90th	95th	99th
1. SINGLE DX										
A. Not Operated										
0–19 Years	25	2.1	<1	1	2	2	3	3	3	3
20–34	87	2.3	<1	1	2	2	3	4	4	4
35–49	16	1.9	<1	1	1	2	2	3	4	4
50–64	0									
65+	0									
B. Operated										
0–19 Years	0									
20–34	1	3.0	0	3	3	3	3	3	3	3
35–49	0									
50–64	0									
65+	0									
2. MULTIPLE DX										
A. Not Operated										
0–19 Years	213	3.1	3	1	2	3	4	5	6	8
20–34	1,021	3.0	4	1	2	3	3	5	6	10
35–49	145	3.4	6	1	2	3	4	7	9	13
50–64	3	4.0	3	3	3	3	6	6	6	6
65+	0									
B. Operated										
0–19 Years	22	6.1	21	3	3	4	8	13	17	18
20–34	153	6.2	79	2	2	4	7	12	15	34
35–49	22	8.1	74	2	3	6	9	17	23	39
50–64	1	4.0	0	4	4	4	4	4	4	4
65+	0									
SUBTOTALS:										
1. SINGLE DX										
A. Not Operated	128	2.2	<1	1	2	2	3	3	4	4
B. Operated	1	3.0	0	3	3	3	3	3	3	3
2. MULTIPLE DX										
A. Not Operated	1,382	3.0	4	1	2	3	3	5	7	10
B. Operated	198	6.4	72	2	3	4	7	13	17	39
1. SINGLE DX	129	2.2	<1	1	2	2	3	3	4	4
2. MULTIPLE DX	1,580	3.5	14	1	2	3	4	6	8	15
A. NOT OPERATED	1,510	3.0	4	1	2	3	3	5	7	10
B. OPERATED	199	6.4	71	2	3	4	7	13	17	39
TOTAL										
0–19 Years	260	3.3	5	1	2	3	4	6	8	13
20–34	1,262	3.3	14	1	2	3	4	6	8	14
35–49	183	3.9	16	1	2	3	4	7	10	23
50–64	4	4.0	2	3	3	3	6	6	6	6
65+	0									
GRAND TOTAL	1,709	3.4	13	1	2	3	4	6	8	14

670.04: MAJOR PP INFECT-PP

Type of Patients	Observed Patients	Avg. Stay	Variance	10th	25th	50th	75th	90th	95th	99th
1. SINGLE DX										
A. Not Operated										
0–19 Years	25	2.1	<1	1	2	2	3	3	3	3
20–34	86	2.3	<1	1	2	2	3	4	4	4
35–49	16	1.9	<1	1	1	2	2	3	4	4
50–64	0									
65+	0									
B. Operated										
0–19 Years	0									
20–34	1	3.0	0	3	3	3	3	3	3	3
35–49	0									
50–64	0									
65+	0									
2. MULTIPLE DX										
A. Not Operated										
0–19 Years	195	3.0	3	1	2	3	4	5	6	8
20–34	970	2.9	4	1	2	3	3	5	6	10
35–49	141	3.5	6	1	2	3	4	7	9	13
50–64	3	4.0	3	3	3	3	6	6	6	6
65+	0									
B. Operated										
0–19 Years	21	6.1	22	3	3	4	8	13	17	18
20–34	134	5.6	25	2	2	4	7	12	15	27
35–49	19	7.6	73	2	2	7	9	17	39	39
50–64	1	4.0	0	4	4	4	4	4	4	4
65+	0									
SUBTOTALS:										
1. SINGLE DX										
A. Not Operated	127	2.2	<1	1	2	2	3	3	4	4
B. Operated	1	3.0	0	3	3	3	3	3	3	3
2. MULTIPLE DX										
A. Not Operated	1,309	3.0	4	1	2	3	3	5	7	10
B. Operated	175	5.8	29	2	2	4	7	13	17	29
1. SINGLE DX	128	2.2	<1	1	2	2	3	3	4	4
2. MULTIPLE DX	1,484	3.3	8	1	2	3	4	6	8	14
A. NOT OPERATED	1,436	2.9	4	1	2	3	3	5	7	10
B. OPERATED	176	5.8	29	2	2	4	7	13	17	29
TOTAL										
0–19 Years	241	3.2	5	1	2	3	4	5	8	13
20–34	1,191	3.2	7	1	2	3	4	5	8	13
35–49	176	3.8	15	1	2	3	4	6	10	17
50–64	4	4.0	2	3	3	3	6	6	6	6
65+	0									
GRAND TOTAL	1,612	3.2	7	1	2	3	4	6	8	13

Length of Stay by Diagnosis and Operation, Western Region, 2008

Western Region, October 2006–September 2007 Data, by Diagnosis

671: VENOUS COMP IN PREG & PP

Type of Patients	Observed Patients	Avg. Stay	Vari-ance	10th	25th	50th	75th	90th	95th	99th
1. SINGLE DX										
A. Not Operated										
0–19 Years	9	2.3	2	1	2	2	3	5	5	5
20–34	133	2.4	3	1	1	2	3	5	7	9
35–49	15	3.5	5	1	2	3	5	7	8	8
50–64	2	2.0	2	1	1	1	3	3	3	3
65+	0									
B. Operated										
0–19 Years	0									
20–34	8	2.4	<1	2	2	2	2	4	4	4
35–49	0									
50–64	0									
65+	0									
2. MULTIPLE DX										
A. Not Operated										
0–19 Years	39	3.4	6	1	2	3	5	8	8	10
20–34	521	3.1	10	1	2	3	3	6	8	15
35–49	127	2.8	5	1	1	2	3	6	7	11
50–64	0									
65+	0									
B. Operated										
0–19 Years	9	6.9	14	1	6	7	9	14	14	14
20–34	132	4.1	12	2	2	3	4	9	11	20
35–49	39	3.7	14	1	1	3	4	7	12	21
50–64	0									
65+	0									
SUBTOTALS:										
1. SINGLE DX										
A. Not Operated	159	2.5	3	1	1	2	3	5	7	9
B. Operated	8	2.4	<1	2	2	2	2	4	4	4
2. MULTIPLE DX										
A. Not Operated	687	3.1	9	1	2	2	3	6	8	14
B. Operated	180	4.2	13	1	2	3	5	9	11	21
1. SINGLE DX	167	2.5	3	1	1	2	3	5	7	9
2. MULTIPLE DX	867	3.3	10	1	2	2	4	6	9	15
A. NOT OPERATED	846	3.0	8	1	2	2	3	6	7	13
B. OPERATED	188	4.1	13	1	2	3	4	9	11	21
TOTAL										
0–19 Years	57	3.8	8	1	2	3	6	8	9	14
20–34	794	3.2	9	1	2	2	4	6	9	15
35–49	181	3.0	7	1	1	2	4	6	7	13
50–64	2	2.0	2	1	1	1	3	3	3	3
65+	0									
GRAND TOTAL	1,034	3.2	9	1	2	2	4	6	8	14

672: PUERPERAL PYREXIA NOS

Type of Patients	Observed Patients	Avg. Stay	Vari-ance	10th	25th	50th	75th	90th	95th	99th
1. SINGLE DX										
A. Not Operated										
0–19 Years	19	2.2	<1	1	2	2	3	3	4	4
20–34	70	2.2	<1	1	2	2	3	3	4	4
35–49	3	1.7	1	1	1	1	3	3	3	3
50–64	0									
65+	0									
B. Operated										
0–19 Years	0									
20–34	0									
35–49	0									
50–64	0									
65+	0									
2. MULTIPLE DX										
A. Not Operated										
0–19 Years	35	2.8	4	1	2	2	3	5	8	11
20–34	121	2.7	3	1	2	2	3	5	6	8
35–49	18	2.4	3	1	1	2	3	5	6	6
50–64	0									
65+	0									
B. Operated										
0–19 Years	0									
20–34	10	3.9	5	1	3	3	5	9	9	9
35–49	1	3.0	0	3	3	3	3	3	3	3
50–64	0									
65+	0									
SUBTOTALS:										
1. SINGLE DX										
A. Not Operated	92	2.2	<1	1	2	2	3	3	4	4
B. Operated	0									
2. MULTIPLE DX										
A. Not Operated	174	2.7	3	1	2	2	3	5	6	9
B. Operated	11	3.8	4	2	3	3	5	5	9	9
1. SINGLE DX	92	2.2	<1	1	2	2	3	3	4	4
2. MULTIPLE DX	185	2.7	3	1	2	2	3	5	6	9
A. NOT OPERATED	266	2.5	2	1	2	2	3	4	5	8
B. OPERATED	11	3.8	4	2	3	3	5	5	9	9
TOTAL										
0–19 Years	54	2.6	3	1	2	2	3	4	6	11
20–34	201	2.6	2	1	2	2	3	4	5	9
35–49	22	2.3	2	1	1	2	3	5	5	6
50–64	0									
65+	0									
GRAND TOTAL	277	2.6	2	1	2	2	3	4	5	9

673: OB PULMONARY EMBOLISM

Type of Patients	Observed Patients	Avg. Stay	Vari-ance	10th	25th	50th	75th	90th	95th	99th
1. SINGLE DX										
A. Not Operated										
0–19 Years	0									
20–34	24	3.1	5	1	2	2	3	5	8	9
35–49	6	4.2	3	2	2	5	6	6	6	6
50–64	0									
65+	0									
B. Operated										
0–19 Years	0									
20–34	0									
35–49	0									
50–64	0									
65+	0									
2. MULTIPLE DX										
A. Not Operated										
0–19 Years	7	3.6	2	2	2	3	5	5	5	5
20–34	153	4.0	9	1	2	3	5	7	8	15
35–49	44	3.9	7	1	2	3	5	7	9	13
50–64	0									
65+	0									
B. Operated										
0–19 Years	2	12.5	4	11	11	11	14	14	14	14
20–34	24	7.8	23	4	5	6	8	14	17	22
35–49	7	9.0	24	2	5	10	13	16	16	16
50–64	0									
65+	0									
SUBTOTALS:										
1. SINGLE DX										
A. Not Operated	30	3.3	5	1	2	2	4	7	8	9
B. Operated	0									
2. MULTIPLE DX										
A. Not Operated	204	4.0	8	1	2	3	5	7	8	15
B. Operated	33	8.3	23	4	5	7	11	14	17	22
1. SINGLE DX	30	3.3	5	1	2	2	4	7	8	9
2. MULTIPLE DX	237	4.6	12	1	2	4	5	8	13	17
A. NOT OPERATED	234	3.9	8	1	2	3	5	7	8	15
B. OPERATED	33	8.3	23	4	5	7	11	14	17	22
TOTAL										
0–19 Years	9	5.6	18	2	3	5	5	14	14	14
20–34	201	4.4	11	1	2	4	5	8	10	22
35–49	57	4.6	11	1	2	4	6	10	13	16
50–64	0									
65+	0									
GRAND TOTAL	267	4.4	12	1	2	4	5	8	12	17

Length of Stay by Diagnosis and Operation, Western Region. 2008

Western Region, October 2006–September 2007 Data, by Diagnosis

674: PUERPERAL COMP NEC & NOS

Type of Patients	Observed Patients	Avg. Stay	Variance	10th	25th	50th	75th	90th	95th	99th
1. SINGLE DX										
A. Not Operated										
0–19 Years	26	2.5	1	1	2	2	3	5	5	5
20–34	160	2.5	2	1	1	2	3	4	6	8
35–49	37	2.1	2	1	1	2	2	4	6	6
50–64	0									
65+	0									
B. Operated										
0–19 Years	1	1.0	0	1	1	1	1	1	1	1
20–34	22	3.2	11	1	1	2	4	5	7	16
35–49	11	2.7	3	1	1	2	4	4	7	7
50–64	0									
65+	0									
2. MULTIPLE DX										
A. Not Operated										
0–19 Years	155	3.1	7	1	2	2	4	5	7	18
20–34	1,166	3.1	5	1	2	3	4	6	8	12
35–49	291	3.4	7	1	2	3	4	6	8	11
50–64	9	4.5	14	2	2	3	5	14	14	14
65+	0									
B. Operated										
0–19 Years	161	3.4	7	1	2	3	4	6	9	12
20–34	786	3.9	20	1	2	3	4	7	10	19
35–49	124	5.0	34	1	2	3	6	9	13	37
50–64	3	2.7	1	2	2	2	4	4	4	4
65+	0									
SUBTOTALS:										
1. SINGLE DX										
A. Not Operated	223	2.4	2	1	1	2	3	4	5	7
B. Operated	34	3.0	8	1	1	2	4	5	7	16
2. MULTIPLE DX										
A. Not Operated	1,621	3.2	6	1	2	3	4	6	8	12
B. Operated	1,074	4.0	20	1	2	3	4	7	10	20
1. SINGLE DX	257	2.5	3	1	1	2	3	5	6	8
2. MULTIPLE DX	2,695	3.5	11	1	2	3	4	6	9	17
A. NOT OPERATED	1,844	3.1	5	1	2	2	4	6	7	11
B. OPERATED	1,108	3.9	19	1	2	3	4	7	10	19
TOTAL										
0–19 Years	343	3.2	7	1	2	3	4	6	7	12
20–34	2,134	3.4	11	1	2	3	4	6	9	15
35–49	463	3.7	15	1	2	3	4	7	9	22
50–64	12	4.0	11	2	2	3	5	5	14	14
65+	0									
GRAND TOTAL	2,952	3.4	11	1	2	3	4	6	9	16

674.34: OB SURG COMP NEC-PP

Type of Patients	Observed Patients	Avg. Stay	Variance	10th	25th	50th	75th	90th	95th	99th
1. SINGLE DX										
A. Not Operated										
0–19 Years	19	2.5	2	1	2	2	3	5	5	5
20–34	118	2.5	2	1	1	2	3	4	6	8
35–49	35	2.0	1	1	1	2	2	3	4	6
50–64	0									
65+	0									
B. Operated										
0–19 Years	0									
20–34	11	3.1	4	1	1	3	5	5	7	7
35–49	6	3.7	4	1	3	4	4	7	7	7
50–64	0									
65+	0									
2. MULTIPLE DX										
A. Not Operated										
0–19 Years	72	3.0	3	2	2	3	4	5	6	8
20–34	534	3.4	4	2	2	3	4	6	8	10
35–49	130	3.4	6	2	2	3	4	6	7	9
50–64	6	4.7	22	2	2	3	4	14	14	14
65+	0									
B. Operated										
0–19 Years	14	7.0	24	3	4	5	9	12	21	21
20–34	113	5.7	16	2	3	5	7	11	13	17
35–49	35	6.7	45	2	3	5	8	13	18	37
50–64	1	4.0	0	4	4	4	4	4	4	4
65+	0									
SUBTOTALS:										
1. SINGLE DX										
A. Not Operated	172	2.4	2	1	1	2	3	4	5	8
B. Operated	17	3.3	4	1	2	3	4	7	7	7
2. MULTIPLE DX										
A. Not Operated	742	3.4	5	1	2	3	4	6	8	10
B. Operated	163	6.0	23	2	3	5	8	11	13	26
1. SINGLE DX	189	2.5	2	1	1	2	3	5	5	8
2. MULTIPLE DX	905	3.9	9	1	2	3	5	7	9	14
A. NOT OPERATED	914	3.2	4	1	2	3	4	6	7	10
B. OPERATED	180	5.8	21	2	3	5	7	11	13	26
TOTAL										
0–19 Years	105	3.4	7	1	2	3	4	6	8	12
20–34	776	3.6	7	1	2	3	5	7	9	13
35–49	206	3.8	14	1	2	3	5	7	8	18
50–64	7	4.6	18	2	4	5	5	14	14	14
65+	0									
GRAND TOTAL	1,094	3.6	8	1	2	3	5	7	9	13

674.84: PP COMP NEC-PP

Type of Patients	Observed Patients	Avg. Stay	Variance	10th	25th	50th	75th	90th	95th	99th
1. SINGLE DX										
A. Not Operated										
0–19 Years	0									
20–34	3	1.3	<1	1	1	1	2	2	2	2
35–49	0									
50–64	0									
65+	0									
B. Operated										
0–19 Years	0									
20–34	0									
35–49	1	2.0	0	2	2	2	2	2	2	2
50–64	0									
65+	0									
2. MULTIPLE DX										
A. Not Operated										
0–19 Years	47	3.5	16	1	1	2	3	3	7	20
20–34	287	2.6	4	1	1	2	3	5	6	10
35–49	74	2.7	4	1	1	2	3	5	6	11
50–64	0									
65+										
B. Operated										
0–19 Years	139	2.9	4	1	2	3	3	5	7	11
20–34	578	3.2	6	1	2	2	4	6	8	14
35–49	53	3.0	4	1	2	2	4	6	7	11
50–64	0									
65+										
SUBTOTALS:										
1. SINGLE DX										
A. Not Operated	3	1.3	<1	1	1	1	2	2	2	2
B. Operated	1	2.0	0	2	2	2	2	2	2	2
2. MULTIPLE DX										
A. Not Operated	408	2.7	6	1	2	2	3	5	7	11
B. Operated	770	3.1	6	1	2	2	4	6	7	13
1. SINGLE DX	4	1.5	<1	1	1	1	2	2	2	2
2. MULTIPLE DX	1,178	3.0	6	1	2	2	4	5	7	13
A. NOT OPERATED	411	2.7	5	1	1	2	3	5	7	11
B. OPERATED	771	3.1	6	1	2	2	4	6	7	13
TOTAL										
0–19 Years	186	3.1	7	1	2	2	3	5	7	18
20–34	868	3.0	6	1	1	2	4	5	7	13
35–49	128	2.8	4	1	1	2	4	5	7	11
50–64	0									
65+										
GRAND TOTAL	1,182	3.0	6	1	2	2	4	5	7	13

Length of Stay by Diagnosis and Operation, Western Region, 2008

Western Region, October 2006–September 2007 Data, by Diagnosis

675: INFECT BREAST IN PREG

Type of Patients	Observed Patients	Avg. Stay	Vari-ance	10th	25th	50th	75th	90th	95th	99th
1. SINGLE DX										
A. Not Operated										
0–19 Years	40	2.5	2	1	1	2	3	5	6	6
20–34	124	2.0	1	1	1	2	3	3	4	5
35–49	20	1.9	1	1	1	2	2	4	4	4
50–64	0									
65+	0									
B. Operated										
0–19 Years	3	1.3	<1	1	1	1	2	2	2	2
20–34	12	1.8	<1	1	1	2	2	2	3	3
35–49	0									
50–64	0									
65+	0									
2. MULTIPLE DX										
A. Not Operated										
0–19 Years	42	3.4	5	1	2	3	4	6	8	10
20–34	233	3.0	4	1	1	3	4	5	7	10
35–49	47	2.7	2	1	1	3	3	5	6	7
50–64	2	2.0	2	1	1	3	3	3	3	3
65+	0									
B. Operated										
0–19 Years	4	8.5	41	3	3	3	15	15	15	15
20–34	23	5.1	11	2	2	5	6	9	12	15
35–49	2	3.0	2	2	2	4	4	4	4	4
50–64	0									
65+	0									
SUBTOTALS:										
1. SINGLE DX										
A. Not Operated	184	2.1	1	1	1	2	3	4	5	6
B. Operated	15	1.7	<1	1	1	2	2	2	3	3
2. MULTIPLE DX										
A. Not Operated	324	3.0	4	1	2	2	4	6	7	10
B. Operated	29	5.4	15	2	3	4	6	13	15	15
1. SINGLE DX	199	2.1	1	1	1	2	3	3	5	6
2. MULTIPLE DX	353	3.2	5	1	2	3	4	6	8	12
A. NOT OPERATED	508	2.7	3	1	1	2	3	5	6	9
B. OPERATED	44	4.1	13	1	2	3	5	9	13	15
TOTAL										
0–19 Years	89	3.1	6	1	1	3	4	6	8	15
20–34	392	2.8	4	1	2	2	3	5	6	11
35–49	69	2.5	2	1	1	2	3	4	6	7
50–64	2	2.0	2	1	1	3	3	3	3	3
65+	0									
GRAND TOTAL	552	2.8	4	1	1	2	3	5	6	11

675.24: MASTITIS IN PREG-PP

Type of Patients	Observed Patients	Avg. Stay	Vari-ance	10th	25th	50th	75th	90th	95th	99th
1. SINGLE DX										
A. Not Operated										
0–19 Years	24	2.6	2	1	1	2	3	5	5	6
20–34	74	2.0	1	1	1	2	3	3	4	7
35–49	15	1.8	1	1	1	1	3	3	4	4
50–64	0									
65+	0									
B. Operated										
0–19 Years	0									
20–34	0									
35–49	0									
50–64	0									
65+	0									
2. MULTIPLE DX										
A. Not Operated										
0–19 Years	19	3.0	5	1	1	2	4	6	10	10
20–34	133	2.5	2	1	2	2	3	4	5	7
35–49	25	2.7	2	1	1	3	3	4	5	6
50–64	2	2.0	2	1	1	3	3	3	3	3
65+	0									
B. Operated										
0–19 Years	1	3.0	0	3	3	3	3	3	3	3
20–34	5	4.8	19	2	2	2	6	12	12	12
35–49	0									
50–64	0									
65+	0									
SUBTOTALS:										
1. SINGLE DX										
A. Not Operated	113	2.1	1	1	1	2	3	3	5	6
B. Operated	0									
2. MULTIPLE DX										
A. Not Operated	179	2.6	2	1	2	2	3	4	5	7
B. Operated	6	4.5	16	2	2	3	6	12	12	12
1. SINGLE DX	113	2.1	1	1	1	2	3	3	5	6
2. MULTIPLE DX	185	2.7	2	1	2	2	3	5	6	10
A. NOT OPERATED	292	2.4	2	1	1	2	3	4	5	7
B. OPERATED	6	4.5	16	2	3	3	6	12	12	12
TOTAL										
0–19 Years	44	2.8	3	1	1	2	3	5	6	10
20–34	212	2.4	2	1	1	2	3	4	5	7
35–49	40	2.4	2	1	1	2	3	4	5	6
50–64	2	2.0	2	1	1	3	3	3	3	3
65+	0									
GRAND TOTAL	298	2.4	2	1	1	2	3	4	5	7

676: OTH BREAST/LACT DIS PREG

Type of Patients	Observed Patients	Avg. Stay	Vari-ance	10th	25th	50th	75th	90th	95th	99th
1. SINGLE DX										
A. Not Operated										
0–19 Years	4	2.0	<1	1	2	2	2	3	3	3
20–34	23	1.9	<1	1	1	2	2	3	3	3
35–49	2	2.5	<1	2	2	2	3	3	3	3
50–64	0									
65+	0									
B. Operated										
0–19 Years	0									
20–34	0									
35–49	0									
50–64	0									
65+	0									
2. MULTIPLE DX										
A. Not Operated										
0–19 Years	3	2.3	2	1	1	2	4	4	4	4
20–34	12	2.2	1	1	1	2	2	4	4	4
35–49	0									
50–64	0									
65+	0									
B. Operated										
0–19 Years	0									
20–34	3	2.0	<1	1	1	2	3	3	3	3
35–49	1	1.0	0	1	1	1	1	1	1	1
50–64	0									
65+	0									
SUBTOTALS:										
1. SINGLE DX										
A. Not Operated	29	1.9	<1	1	1	2	2	3	3	3
B. Operated	0									
2. MULTIPLE DX										
A. Not Operated	15	2.2	1	1	1	2	3	4	4	4
B. Operated	4	1.7	<1	1	1	1	2	3	3	3
1. SINGLE DX	29	1.9	<1	1	1	2	2	3	3	3
2. MULTIPLE DX	19	2.1	1	1	1	2	3	4	4	4
A. NOT OPERATED	44	2.0	<1	1	1	2	3	3	4	4
B. OPERATED	4	1.7	<1	1	1	1	2	3	3	3
TOTAL										
0–19 Years	7	2.2	1	1	1	2	3	4	4	4
20–34	38	2.0	<1	1	1	2	2	3	4	4
35–49	3	2.0	<1	1	1	2	3	3	3	3
50–64	0									
65+	0									
GRAND TOTAL	48	2.0	<1	1	1	2	3	3	4	4

Length of Stay by Diagnosis and Operation, Western Region, 2008

Western Region, October 2006–September 2007 Data, by Diagnosis

677: LATE EFFECT OB COMP

Type of Patients	Observed Patients	Avg. Stay	Variance	10th	25th	50th	75th	90th	95th	99th
1. SINGLE DX										
A. Not Operated										
0–19 Years	0									
20–34	0									
35–49	0									
50–64	0									
65+	0									
B. Operated										
0–19 Years	0									
20–34	0									
35–49	0									
50–64	0									
65+	0									
2. MULTIPLE DX										
A. Not Operated										
0–19 Years	0									
20–34	0									
35–49	0									
50–64	0									
65+	0									
B. Operated										
0–19 Years	0									
20–34	0									
35–49	0									
50–64	0									
65+	0									
SUBTOTALS:										
1. SINGLE DX — A. Not Operated	0									
B. Operated	0									
2. MULTIPLE DX — A. Not Operated	0									
B. Operated	0									
1. SINGLE DX	0									
2. MULTIPLE DX	0									
A. NOT OPERATED	0									
B. OPERATED	0									
TOTAL										
0–19 Years	0									
20–34	0									
35–49	0									
50–64	0									
65+	0									
GRAND TOTAL	0									

680: CARBUNCLE & FURUNCLE

Type of Patients	Observed Patients	Avg. Stay	Variance	10th	25th	50th	75th	90th	95th	99th
1. SINGLE DX										
A. Not Operated										
0–19 Years	0									
20–34	4	2.5	2	1	1	2	3	4	4	4
35–49	2	1.5	<1	1	1	2	2	2	2	2
50–64	1	4.0	0	4	4	4	4	4	4	4
65+	0									
B. Operated										
0–19 Years	0									
20–34	0									
35–49	0									
50–64	0									
65+	0									
2. MULTIPLE DX										
A. Not Operated										
0–19 Years	18	2.7	2	1	2	3	3	5	5	5
20–34	37	2.8	5	1	1	2	3	5	6	14
35–49	62	4.0	7	2	2	3	5	6	9	16
50–64	64	4.5	15	1	2	3	5	9	12	21
65+	33	4.4	8	1	2	4	6	8	10	12
B. Operated										
0–19 Years	1	13.0	0	13	13	13	13	13	13	13
20–34	3	3.3	2	2	2	3	5	5	5	5
35–49	8	5.0	12	2	2	4	5	13	13	13
50–64	11	7.9	25	3	4	7	9	13	20	20
65+	8	11.5	210	3	4	4	19	45	45	45
SUBTOTALS:										
1. SINGLE DX — A. Not Operated	7	2.4	2	1	1	2	4	4	4	4
B. Operated	0									
2. MULTIPLE DX — A. Not Operated	214	3.9	9	1	2	3	5	7	10	16
B. Operated	31	7.8	69	3	3	5	9	13	20	45
1. SINGLE DX	7	2.4	2	1	1	2	4	4	4	4
2. MULTIPLE DX	245	4.4	18	1	2	3	5	8	12	20
A. NOT OPERATED	221	3.8	9	1	2	3	5	7	10	16
B. OPERATED	31	7.8	69	3	3	5	9	13	20	45
TOTAL										
0–19 Years	19	3.2	7	1	2	3	4	5	13	13
20–34	44	2.8	5	1	1	2	3	5	5	14
35–49	72	4.0	8	2	2	3	5	6	10	16
50–64	76	5.0	18	1	2	4	6	9	14	21
65+	41	5.8	51	1	3	4	7	9	12	45
GRAND TOTAL	252	4.3	18	1	2	3	5	8	12	20

681: FINGER & TOE CELLULITIS

Type of Patients	Observed Patients	Avg. Stay	Variance	10th	25th	50th	75th	90th	95th	99th
1. SINGLE DX										
A. Not Operated										
0–19 Years	56	2.0	1	1	1	2	2	4	4	6
20–34	55	2.0	1	1	1	2	3	3	4	6
35–49	58	2.3	2	1	1	2	3	4	6	7
50–64	27	2.6	2	1	2	2	3	5	5	7
65+	5	3.8	4	2	3	3	4	7	7	7
B. Operated										
0–19 Years	6	2.7	3	1	1	3	4	5	5	5
20–34	12	2.7	5	1	1	3	4	7	7	7
35–49	6	2.8	2	1	2	3	3	5	5	5
50–64	6	3.7	3	2	2	4	5	6	6	6
65+	1	3.0	0	3	3	3	3	3	3	3
2. MULTIPLE DX										
A. Not Operated										
0–19 Years	273	2.7	3	1	2	3	3	4	6	9
20–34	430	3.1	3	1	2	3	4	6	7	10
35–49	774	3.5	8	1	2	3	4	6	8	13
50–64	823	3.5	7	1	2	3	4	6	8	14
65+	624	3.9	7	1	2	3	5	7	9	13
B. Operated										
0–19 Years	59	3.8	4	2	3	4	5	6	8	10
20–34	221	4.4	12	2	3	4	5	7	10	23
35–49	350	4.7	14	2	3	4	6	9	11	21
50–64	257	5.9	19	2	3	5	7	11	15	24
65+	195	5.8	23	3	3	5	7	10	13	29
SUBTOTALS:										
1. SINGLE DX — A. Not Operated	201	2.2	2	1	1	2	3	4	5	7
B. Operated	31	2.9	3	1	1	3	4	5	7	7
2. MULTIPLE DX — A. Not Operated	2,924	3.4	6	1	2	3	4	6	8	13
B. Operated	1,082	5.1	16	2	3	4	6	9	12	23
1. SINGLE DX	232	2.3	2	1	1	2	3	4	5	7
2. MULTIPLE DX	4,006	3.9	10	1	2	3	5	7	9	16
A. NOT OPERATED	3,125	3.4	6	1	2	3	4	6	8	13
B. OPERATED	1,113	5.0	16	2	3	4	6	9	12	23
TOTAL										
0–19 Years	394	2.8	3	1	2	3	4	5	6	9
20–34	718	3.4	7	1	2	3	4	6	8	12
35–49	1,188	3.8	10	1	2	3	5	7	9	16
50–64	1,113	4.0	11	1	2	3	5	7	10	17
65+	825	4.3	11	2	2	3	5	8	10	16
GRAND TOTAL	4,238	3.8	9	1	2	3	5	7	9	15

Length of Stay by Diagnosis and Operation, Western Region, 2008

Western Region, October 2006–September 2007 Data, by Diagnosis

681.00: FINGER CELLULITIS NOS

Type of Patients	Observed Patients	Avg. Stay	Variance	10th	25th	50th	75th	90th	95th	99th
1. SINGLE DX										
A. Not Operated										
0–19 Years	30	2.0	1	1	1	2	2	4	4	4
20–34	40	2.1	1	1	1	2	3	4	4	6
35–49	44	2.4	2	1	1	2	3	4	6	7
50–64	24	2.4	2	1	2	2	3	4	5	7
65+	4	3.8	5	2	2	3	7	7	7	7
B. Operated										
0–19 Years	5	2.2	2	1	1	2	3	4	4	4
20–34	12	2.7	5	1	1	2	4	7	7	7
35–49	6	2.8	2	1	2	3	3	5	5	5
50–64	6	3.7	3	2	2	4	5	6	6	6
65+	0									
2. MULTIPLE DX										
A. Not Operated										
0–19 Years	134	2.5	2	1	1	2	3	4	5	6
20–34	302	3.0	3	1	2	3	4	6	7	9
35–49	527	3.3	5	1	2	3	4	6	7	12
50–64	464	3.4	7	1	2	3	4	6	7	14
65+	252	3.6	6	1	2	3	4	7	9	12
B. Operated										
0–19 Years	41	3.6	4	2	2	3	5	5	8	10
20–34	173	4.3	11	2	3	3	5	7	10	24
35–49	277	4.5	12	2	3	4	5	8	11	21
50–64	147	5.4	16	2	3	4	6	10	15	23
65+	93	4.7	7	2	3	4	6	8	10	14
SUBTOTALS:										
1. SINGLE DX										
A. Not Operated	142	2.3	2	1	1	2	3	4	5	7
B. Operated	29	2.8	3	1	1	2	4	6	7	7
2. MULTIPLE DX										
A. Not Operated	1,679	3.3	5	1	2	3	4	6	7	12
B. Operated	731	4.6	12	2	3	4	5	8	11	17
1. SINGLE DX	171	2.4	2	1	1	2	3	4	6	7
2. MULTIPLE DX	2,410	3.7	8	1	2	3	4	7	8	14
A. NOT OPERATED	1,821	3.2	5	1	2	3	4	6	7	12
B. OPERATED	760	4.5	12	2	3	4	5	8	11	17
TOTAL										
0–19 Years	210	2.7	3	1	2	2	3	5	5	9
20–34	527	3.4	6	1	2	3	4	6	7	11
35–49	854	3.7	8	1	2	3	4	7	9	14
50–64	641	3.8	9	1	2	3	5	7	10	16
65+	349	3.9	7	1	2	3	5	7	9	13
GRAND TOTAL	2,581	3.6	7	1	2	3	4	6	8	14

681.10: TOE CELLULITIS NOS

Type of Patients	Observed Patients	Avg. Stay	Variance	10th	25th	50th	75th	90th	95th	99th
1. SINGLE DX										
A. Not Operated										
0–19 Years	21	2.1	2	1	1	2	2	3	4	6
20–34	5	2.0	<1	1	1	2	3	3	3	3
35–49	6	1.7	<1	1	1	2	3	3	3	3
50–64	2	3.5	5	2	2	4	5	5	5	5
65+	0									
B. Operated										
0–19 Years	1	5.0	0	5	5	5	5	5	5	5
20–34	0									
35–49	0									
50–64	0									
65+	0									
2. MULTIPLE DX										
A. Not Operated										
0–19 Years	102	2.9	3	1	2	2	4	5	6	8
20–34	77	3.1	4	1	2	3	4	6	7	12
35–49	194	3.9	16	1	2	3	5	7	9	16
50–64	305	3.6	7	1	2	3	4	6	8	14
65+	336	4.2	7	2	2	3	5	8	9	15
B. Operated										
0–19 Years	11	4.9	4	2	4	5	6	6	8	8
20–34	31	4.6	8	2	3	4	5	7	13	13
35–49	52	6.0	23	2	3	5	7	10	17	28
50–64	87	7.0	23	3	4	6	8	11	17	26
65+	95	6.9	32	2	3	6	8	12	16	43
SUBTOTALS:										
1. SINGLE DX										
A. Not Operated	34	2.1	1	1	1	2	3	4	5	6
B. Operated	1	5.0	0	5	5	5	5	5	5	5
2. MULTIPLE DX										
A. Not Operated	1,014	3.7	8	1	2	3	5	7	8	15
B. Operated	276	6.4	24	2	3	5	8	11	15	28
1. SINGLE DX	35	2.1	2	1	1	2	3	4	5	6
2. MULTIPLE DX	1,290	4.3	13	1	2	3	5	8	10	18
A. NOT OPERATED	1,048	3.7	8	1	2	3	4	7	8	15
B. OPERATED	277	6.4	24	2	3	5	8	11	15	28
TOTAL										
0–19 Years	135	2.9	3	1	2	2	4	5	5	8
20–34	113	3.4	6	1	2	3	4	6	7	13
35–49	252	4.3	18	1	2	3	5	7	10	18
50–64	394	4.3	12	1	2	3	5	8	10	23
65+	431	4.8	14	2	3	4	6	8	10	18
GRAND TOTAL	1,325	4.3	13	1	2	3	5	8	10	18

682: CELLULITIS & ABSCESS NEC

Type of Patients	Observed Patients	Avg. Stay	Variance	10th	25th	50th	75th	90th	95th	99th
1. SINGLE DX										
A. Not Operated										
0–19 Years	1,150	2.5	2	1	2	2	3	4	5	7
20–34	577	2.3	2	1	2	2	3	4	5	6
35–49	596	2.4	3	1	2	2	3	5	5	8
50–64	273	2.5	3	1	2	2	3	4	6	9
65+	66	2.8	3	1	2	2	4	5	6	7
B. Operated										
0–19 Years	61	3.1	3	1	2	3	4	5	5	10
20–34	66	3.0	4	1	2	2	4	6	7	8
35–49	66	3.0	7	1	2	2	4	5	7	18
50–64	33	3.3	3	2	2	3	4	6	7	18
65+	4	1.8	<1	1	1	1	2	3	3	3
2. MULTIPLE DX										
A. Not Operated										
0–19 Years	4,938	3.2	4	1	2	3	4	6	7	10
20–34	7,419	3.6	7	1	2	3	4	6	8	14
35–49	15,385	4.1	11	1	2	3	5	7	10	16
50–64	16,823	4.5	14	2	2	4	5	8	11	18
65+	17,794	4.7	12	2	3	4	6	8	11	17
B. Operated										
0–19 Years	463	4.6	16	2	3	4	6	8	10	16
20–34	1,257	5.5	23	2	3	4	6	10	14	24
35–49	2,593	6.8	40	2	3	5	8	13	18	31
50–64	2,279	7.9	60	3	4	6	9	15	21	40
65+	1,635	7.9	37	3	4	6	10	15	18	30
SUBTOTALS:										
1. SINGLE DX										
A. Not Operated	2,662	2.5	2	1	2	2	3	4	5	7
B. Operated	230	3.0	4	1	2	3	4	5	7	10
2. MULTIPLE DX										
A. Not Operated	62,359	4.2	11	1	2	3	5	8	10	16
B. Operated	8,227	7.0	42	2	3	5	8	13	18	33
1. SINGLE DX	2,892	2.5	2	1	1	2	3	4	5	8
2. MULTIPLE DX	70,586	4.6	16	1	2	3	5	8	11	19
A. NOT OPERATED	65,021	4.2	11	1	2	3	5	8	10	16
B. OPERATED	8,457	6.9	41	2	3	5	8	13	18	33
TOTAL										
0–19 Years	6,612	3.2	5	1	2	3	4	5	7	10
20–34	9,319	3.8	10	1	2	3	5	7	9	16
35–49	18,640	4.4	15	1	2	3	5	8	11	20
50–64	19,408	4.9	21	2	2	4	6	9	12	22
65+	19,499	4.9	15	2	3	4	6	9	12	19
GRAND TOTAL	73,478	4.5	15	1	2	3	5	8	11	19

Length of Stay by Diagnosis and Operation, Western Region, 2008

Western Region, October 2006–September 2007 Data, by Diagnosis

682.0: FACE CELLULITIS

Type of Patients	Observed Patients	Avg. Stay	Variance	10th	25th	50th	75th	90th	95th	99th
1. SINGLE DX										
A. Not Operated										
0–19 Years	246	2.4	2	1	2	2	3	4	5	7
20–34	77	2.2	2	1	1	2	3	4	4	5
35–49	79	2.2	1	1	2	2	3	4	5	6
50–64	39	2.6	2	1	2	2	3	5	5	6
65+	8	2.9	2	1	2	3	3	6	6	6
B. Operated										
0–19 Years	16	3.2	5	1	1	3	4	4	10	10
20–34	17	2.6	3	1	1	2	3	5	7	7
35–49	13	3.8	19	2	2	2	3	5	18	18
50–64	7	4.0	5	2	2	3	5	8	8	8
65+	0									
2. MULTIPLE DX										
A. Not Operated										
0–19 Years	972	2.8	3	1	2	2	3	5	6	8
20–34	1,103	3.2	4	1	2	3	4	5	7	9
35–49	1,532	3.4	5	1	2	3	4	6	7	12
50–64	1,160	3.6	6	1	2	3	4	6	8	13
65+	854	4.2	12	2	2	3	5	7	10	18
B. Operated										
0–19 Years	79	4.1	11	2	2	4	5	7	10	27
20–34	174	4.1	8	1	2	3	5	7	9	15
35–49	195	5.7	35	2	3	4	6	10	15	29
50–64	122	5.7	36	2	3	4	6	9	13	24
65+	57	6.5	14	2	4	5	9	12	13	17
SUBTOTALS:										
1. SINGLE DX										
A. Not Operated	449	2.4	1	1	2	2	3	4	5	6
B. Operated	53	3.2	8	1	2	3	4	5	8	18
2. MULTIPLE DX										
A. Not Operated	5,621	3.5	6	1	2	3	4	6	7	13
B. Operated	627	5.1	23	2	3	4	6	9	12	22
1. SINGLE DX	502	2.5	2	1	2	2	3	4	5	7
2. MULTIPLE DX	6,248	3.6	8	1	2	3	4	6	8	14
A. NOT OPERATED	6,070	3.4	6	1	2	3	4	6	7	12
B. OPERATED	680	5.0	22	2	3	4	6	9	11	22
TOTAL										
0–19 Years	1,313	2.8	3	1	2	2	3	5	6	9
20–34	1,371	3.3	4	1	2	3	4	6	7	10
35–49	1,819	3.6	9	1	2	3	4	6	8	14
50–64	1,328	3.8	9	1	2	3	5	7	8	14
65+	919	4.4	12	2	2	3	5	8	10	17
GRAND TOTAL	6,750	3.5	8	1	2	3	4	6	8	13

682.1: NECK CELLULITIS

Type of Patients	Observed Patients	Avg. Stay	Variance	10th	25th	50th	75th	90th	95th	99th
1. SINGLE DX										
A. Not Operated										
0–19 Years	79	3.4	2	2	2	3	4	5	6	10
20–34	33	2.6	3	2	1	2	4	5	6	7
35–49	22	3.0	3	1	2	3	4	5	6	7
50–64	10	2.3	<1	1	2	2	3	4	4	4
65+	3	5.3	2	4	4	5	7	7	7	7
B. Operated										
0–19 Years	5	3.8	1	3	3	3	5	5	5	5
20–34	5	3.4	4	1	2	4	4	6	6	6
35–49	1	4.0	0	4	4	4	4	4	4	4
50–64	0									
65+	0									
2. MULTIPLE DX										
A. Not Operated										
0–19 Years	246	4.2	8	2	2	3	5	7	10	13
20–34	213	3.9	8	1	2	3	5	5	8	16
35–49	360	4.2	8	1	2	3	5	8	10	15
50–64	304	4.7	15	1	2	3	6	9	11	20
65+	176	5.1	13	2	3	4	6	10	11	20
B. Operated										
0–19 Years	49	4.6	7	2	3	4	6	9	11	13
20–34	37	5.3	17	2	3	4	7	7	17	21
35–49	75	6.7	42	3	4	5	7	11	15	53
50–64	63	6.6	47	2	3	5	7	12	16	41
65+	35	7.5	42	2	4	6	11	14	17	36
SUBTOTALS:										
1. SINGLE DX										
A. Not Operated	147	3.1	3	1	2	3	4	5	6	8
B. Operated	11	3.6	2	2	3	4	5	5	6	6
2. MULTIPLE DX										
A. Not Operated	1,299	4.4	10	1	2	4	6	8	10	16
B. Operated	259	6.2	34	2	3	5	7	11	15	36
1. SINGLE DX	158	3.2	3	1	2	3	4	5	6	8
2. MULTIPLE DX	1,558	4.7	15	2	2	4	6	9	11	20
A. NOT OPERATED	1,446	4.3	10	1	2	4	5	8	10	15
B. OPERATED	270	6.1	33	2	3	5	7	11	15	36
TOTAL										
0–19 Years	379	4.1	7	2	3	3	5	7	9	13
20–34	288	4.0	9	1	2	3	4	7	8	20
35–49	458	4.6	14	1	2	4	5	8	11	16
50–64	377	5.0	20	1	2	4	6	8	12	27
65+	214	5.5	18	2	3	5	7	10	13	20
GRAND TOTAL	1,716	4.6	14	1	2	4	6	8	11	18

682.2: TRUNK CELLULITIS

Type of Patients	Observed Patients	Avg. Stay	Variance	10th	25th	50th	75th	90th	95th	99th
1. SINGLE DX										
A. Not Operated										
0–19 Years	114	2.6	3	1	1	2	3	5	6	7
20–34	64	2.5	3	1	1	2	3	5	6	7
35–49	55	2.8	7	1	1	2	3	4	9	15
50–64	24	3.0	5	1	1	2	4	6	7	9
65+	5	2.6	<1	2	2	3	3	3	3	3
B. Operated										
0–19 Years	18	2.7	3	1	1	3	3	6	6	6
20–34	14	2.2	2	1	1	2	2	4	6	6
35–49	17	1.9	1	1	1	2	2	4	5	5
50–64	6	2.5	<1	2	2	2	3	4	4	4
65+	3	1.7	1	1	1	1	3	3	3	3
2. MULTIPLE DX										
A. Not Operated										
0–19 Years	608	3.7	6	2	2	3	4	6	8	13
20–34	744	3.7	7	1	2	3	5	6	8	14
35–49	1,701	4.5	14	1	2	3	5	8	11	19
50–64	1,646	4.8	16	1	2	4	6	9	11	21
65+	984	4.9	11	2	3	4	6	9	11	17
B. Operated										
0–19 Years	80	3.9	7	1	2	4	6	9	14	16
20–34	201	5.5	24	1	3	4	7	11	14	26
35–49	410	6.4	36	2	4	5	8	13	17	29
50–64	435	7.6	74	2	3	6	8	15	23	49
65+	250	7.1	35	4	4	6	9	13	16	33
SUBTOTALS:										
1. SINGLE DX										
A. Not Operated	262	2.6	4	1	1	2	3	5	6	10
B. Operated	58	2.3	2	1	1	2	3	4	6	6
2. MULTIPLE DX										
A. Not Operated	5,683	4.5	12	1	2	4	5	8	11	18
B. Operated	1,376	6.6	45	2	3	5	8	13	18	33
1. SINGLE DX	320	2.6	3	1	1	2	3	5	6	9
2. MULTIPLE DX	7,059	4.9	20	2	2	4	6	9	12	23
A. NOT OPERATED	5,945	4.4	12	1	2	3	5	8	10	17
B. OPERATED	1,434	6.4	44	2	3	5	8	13	17	33
TOTAL										
0–19 Years	820	3.5	6	1	2	3	4	6	7	13
20–34	1,023	4.0	10	1	2	3	5	7	9	16
35–49	2,183	4.8	18	1	2	4	6	8	13	22
50–64	2,111	5.3	29	2	2	4	6	10	14	25
65+	1,242	5.3	17	2	3	4	7	10	12	18
GRAND TOTAL	7,379	4.8	19	1	2	4	6	9	12	23

Length of Stay by Diagnosis and Operation, Western Region, 2008

Western Region, October 2006–September 2007 Data, by Diagnosis

682.3: ARM CELLULITIS

Type of Patients	Observed Patients	Avg. Stay	Vari-ance	10th	25th	50th	75th	90th	95th	99th
1. SINGLE DX										
A. Not Operated										
0–19 Years	88	2.4	3	1	1	2	3	4	5	11
20–34	72	2.2	1	1	1	2	3	4	4	6
35–49	75	2.3	2	1	1	2	3	4	5	6
50–64	35	2.9	6	1	1	2	3	6	7	14
65+	11	3.4	3	2	2	3	5	5	6	6
B. Operated										
0–19 Years	3	2.7	4	1	1	2	5	4	5	5
20–34	5	3.2	<1	2	3	4	4	5	5	5
35–49	4	4.0	<1	3	4	4	5	5	5	5
50–64	4	3.5	<1	3	3	3	5	5	5	5
65+	0									
2. MULTIPLE DX										
A. Not Operated										
0–19 Years	441	3.0	4	1	2	3	4	6	6	10
20–34	1,077	3.5	7	1	2	3	4	6	8	14
35–49	2,082	3.9	9	1	2	3	5	7	9	15
50–64	1,782	4.0	8	1	2	3	5	7	9	16
65+	1,633	4.2	9	2	2	3	5	8	10	16
B. Operated										
0–19 Years	29	6.3	58	2	3	4	6	9	15	43
20–34	205	5.3	17	2	3	4	6	10	14	22
35–49	418	6.2	29	2	3	5	8	13	16	28
50–64	253	7.4	48	2	3	5	8	15	21	36
65+	131	7.4	23	3	4	6	10	14	17	23
SUBTOTALS:										
1. SINGLE DX A. Not Operated	281	2.4	3	1	1	2	3	4	5	8
B. Operated	16	3.4	1	2	3	3	4	5	5	5
2. MULTIPLE DX A. Not Operated	7,015	3.9	8	1	2	3	4	6	8	15
B. Operated	1,036	6.5	32	2	3	5	7	10	13	32
1. SINGLE DX	297	2.5	3	1	2	2	3	4	5	8
2. MULTIPLE DX	8,051	4.2	12	2	2	3	5	8	10	18
A. NOT OPERATED	7,296	3.8	8	1	2	3	5	7	9	15
B. OPERATED	1,052	6.4	32	2	3	5	8	13	17	32
TOTAL										
0–19 Years	561	3.1	7	1	2	3	4	5	7	11
20–34	1,359	3.7	9	1	2	3	5	7	9	16
35–49	2,579	4.3	13	1	2	3	5	8	10	18
50–64	2,074	4.4	14	1	2	4	5	8	11	20
65+	1,775	4.4	11	2	3	4	5	8	11	17
GRAND TOTAL	8,348	4.2	12	2	3	3	5	8	10	17

682.4: HAND CELLULITIS

Type of Patients	Observed Patients	Avg. Stay	Vari-ance	10th	25th	50th	75th	90th	95th	99th
1. SINGLE DX										
A. Not Operated										
0–19 Years	77	2.2	2	1	1	2	3	4	5	7
20–34	72	2.5	2	1	1	2	3	4	5	6
35–49	76	2.4	3	1	1	2	3	5	6	8
50–64	41	2.7	3	1	1	2	3	4	6	8
65+	11	2.0	1	1	1	2	3	3	4	4
B. Operated										
0–19 Years	3	3.3	1	2	2	4	4	4	4	4
20–34	6	5.0	3	3	3	6	6	7	7	7
35–49	7	2.3	2	1	1	2	4	4	6	7
50–64	6	3.7	4	2	2	3	5	7	7	7
65+	0									
2. MULTIPLE DX										
A. Not Operated										
0–19 Years	251	2.4	2	1	2	3	3	4	5	7
20–34	590	3.3	5	1	2	3	4	6	7	10
35–49	1,013	3.5	8	1	2	3	4	6	8	14
50–64	887	3.7	10	1	2	3	4	7	9	16
65+	961	3.9	8	1	2	3	5	7	9	15
B. Operated										
0–19 Years	36	4.2	6	1	3	4	6	8	10	10
20–34	158	5.2	20	2	3	4	6	9	12	27
35–49	313	5.5	14	2	3	4	7	10	12	19
50–64	181	6.5	56	2	3	5	7	10	17	49
65+	95	5.8	14	2	3	5	8	11	15	17
SUBTOTALS:										
1. SINGLE DX A. Not Operated	277	2.4	2	1	1	2	3	4	6	7
B. Operated	22	3.5	3	2	2	3	5	6	7	7
2. MULTIPLE DX A. Not Operated	3,702	3.5	8	1	2	3	4	6	8	14
B. Operated	783	5.7	25	2	3	4	7	10	13	22
1. SINGLE DX	299	2.5	2	1	1	2	3	5	6	7
2. MULTIPLE DX	4,485	3.9	11	1	2	3	5	7	9	16
A. NOT OPERATED	3,979	3.5	7	1	2	3	4	6	8	14
B. OPERATED	805	5.6	24	2	3	4	7	10	13	21
TOTAL										
0–19 Years	367	2.6	3	1	2	3	4	6	6	9
20–34	826	3.6	8	1	2	3	4	6	8	14
35–49	1,409	3.9	10	1	2	3	5	7	9	16
50–64	1,115	4.1	18	1	2	3	5	7	10	19
65+	1,067	4.1	8	1	2	3	5	8	9	16
GRAND TOTAL	4,784	3.8	11	1	2	3	5	7	9	16

682.5: BUTTOCK CELLULITIS

Type of Patients	Observed Patients	Avg. Stay	Vari-ance	10th	25th	50th	75th	90th	95th	99th
1. SINGLE DX										
A. Not Operated										
0–19 Years	199	2.4	2	1	1	2	3	4	4	7
20–34	32	2.3	2	1	1	2	2	5	5	6
35–49	37	2.3	1	1	1	2	3	4	4	5
50–64	8	1.5	<1	1	1	1	2	3	3	3
65+	3	1.7		1	1	3	3	3	3	3
B. Operated										
0–19 Years	2	2.7	2	1	1	3	4	4	4	4
20–34	2	3.5	12	1	2	4	6	6	6	6
35–49	6	4.2	16	1	2	3	4	12	12	12
50–64	1	3.0	0	3	3	3	3	3	3	3
65+	1	2.0	0	2	2	2	2	2	2	2
2. MULTIPLE DX										
A. Not Operated										
0–19 Years	826	3.3	3	1	2	3	4	6	7	9
20–34	344	3.7	7	1	2	3	5	6	8	16
35–49	728	4.4	12	1	2	4	6	8	10	19
50–64	618	4.5	13	2	3	4	6	8	11	16
65+	354	5.0	11	2	3	4	6	10	11	17
B. Operated										
0–19 Years	49	3.6	4	1	2	3	4	6	7	10
20–34	70	5.4	63	1	3	4	6	9	12	63
35–49	184	6.8	48	2	3	5	8	12	21	43
50–64	182	7.8	37	2	4	6	11	15	20	31
65+	122	6.8	24	2	4	6	8	12	15	28
SUBTOTALS:										
1. SINGLE DX A. Not Operated	279	2.3	2	1	1	2	3	4	5	6
B. Operated	13	3.5	9	1	2	3	4	6	12	12
2. MULTIPLE DX A. Not Operated	2,870	4.1	9	1	2	3	5	7	10	16
B. Operated	607	6.7	39	2	3	5	8	13	19	30
1. SINGLE DX	292	2.3	2	1	1	3	3	4	5	7
2. MULTIPLE DX	3,477	4.5	16	1	2	4	6	8	11	20
A. NOT OPERATED	3,149	3.9	9	1	2	3	5	7	9	16
B. OPERATED	620	6.6	39	2	3	5	8	13	19	30
TOTAL										
0–19 Years	1,077	3.2	3	1	2	3	4	6	7	9
20–34	448	3.9	16	1	2	3	5	7	9	16
35–49	955	4.8	20	2	2	4	6	9	12	22
50–64	809	5.2	21	2	3	4	6	10	14	24
65+	480	5.4	15	2	3	4	7	10	13	20
GRAND TOTAL	3,769	4.4	15	1	2	3	5	8	11	19

Length of Stay by Diagnosis and Operation, Western Region, 2008

Western Region, October 2006–September 2007 Data, by Diagnosis

682.6: LEG CELLULITIS

Type of Patients	Observed Patients	Avg. Stay	Variance	10th	25th	50th	75th	90th	95th	99th
1. SINGLE DX										
A. Not Operated										
0–19 Years	268	2.6	2	1	2	2	3	4	5	7
20–34	184	2.2	1	1	1	2	3	4	4	8
35–49	216	2.5	2	1	2	2	3	5	6	7
50–64	90	2.4	3	1	1	2	3	4	6	10
65+	18	2.3	2	1	1	2	3	5	6	6
B. Operated										
0–19 Years	12	3.3	1	2	2	3	4	4	5	5
20–34	11	3.7	7	1	2	3	6	8	8	8
35–49	16	3.2	5	1	2	3	4	7	9	9
50–64	7	1.9	<1	1	1	2	3	3	3	3
65+	0									
2. MULTIPLE DX										
A. Not Operated										
0–19 Years	1,231	3.3	4	1	2	3	4	6	7	12
20–34	2,814	3.8	9	1	2	3	5	7	9	14
35–49	6,751	4.3	12	1	2	3	5	8	10	17
50–64	8,903	4.7	16	2	2	4	6	9	11	19
65+	11,151	4.8	12	2	3	4	6	9	11	18
B. Operated										
0–19 Years	113	5.2	10	2	3	4	7	9	10	14
20–34	314	6.4	27	2	3	5	8	12	17	27
35–49	741	7.9	57	2	4	6	9	16	22	37
50–64	749	8.8	64	3	4	7	11	17	22	40
65+	674	8.8	47	3	5	7	11	16	21	36
SUBTOTALS:										
1. SINGLE DX										
A. Not Operated	776	2.5	2	1	2	2	3	4	5	8
B. Operated	46	3.1	4	1	2	3	4	6	8	9
2. MULTIPLE DX										
A. Not Operated	30,850	4.5	13	2	2	4	6	8	11	18
B. Operated	2,591	8.1	52	2	4	6	10	16	20	36
1. SINGLE DX	822	2.5	2	1	2	2	3	4	5	8
2. MULTIPLE DX	33,441	4.8	17	2	2	4	6	9	12	20
A. NOT OPERATED	31,626	4.5	13	2	2	4	5	8	11	18
B. OPERATED	2,637	8.0	51	2	4	6	10	15	20	36
TOTAL										
0–19 Years	1,624	3.3	4	1	2	3	4	6	7	12
20–34	3,323	4.0	11	1	2	3	5	7	10	17
35–49	7,724	4.6	17	1	2	4	6	8	11	21
50–64	9,749	5.0	21	2	3	4	6	9	12	22
65+	11,843	5.0	15	2	3	4	6	9	12	19
GRAND TOTAL	34,263	4.7	17	2	2	4	6	9	12	20

682.7: FOOT CELLULITIS

Type of Patients	Observed Patients	Avg. Stay	Variance	10th	25th	50th	75th	90th	95th	99th
1. SINGLE DX										
A. Not Operated										
0–19 Years	72	2.2	2	1	1	2	3	3	4	9
20–34	41	2.5	3	1	1	2	3	5	6	8
35–49	35	2.2	3	1	1	2	3	5	6	6
50–64	23	2.0	2	1	1	2	3	3	5	7
65+	6	3.8	4	3	3	4	4	7	7	7
B. Operated										
0–19 Years	1	3.0	0	3	3	3	3	3	3	3
20–34	5	2.0	0	1	1	3	3	3	3	3
35–49	2	2.5	<1	2	2	3	4	3	3	3
50–64	2	6.5	<1	6	6	7	7	7	7	7
65+	0									
2. MULTIPLE DX										
A. Not Operated										
0–19 Years	308	3.1	4	1	2	3	4	5	6	10
20–34	481	3.9	10	1	2	3	5	7	10	16
35–49	1,105	4.1	12	1	2	3	5	8	10	14
50–64	1,403	4.4	14	1	2	4	5	8	10	18
65+	1,581	4.6	11	2	2	4	6	8	10	18
B. Operated										
0–19 Years	25	6.8	80	2	3	5	7	9	9	48
20–34	91	6.2	16	2	3	5	8	12	15	17
35–49	233	7.8	38	3	4	6	10	16	19	28
50–64	278	8.7	56	3	5	7	10	15	21	45
65+	255	7.9	25	3	4	7	10	15	18	27
SUBTOTALS:										
1. SINGLE DX										
A. Not Operated	177	2.3	2	1	1	2	3	4	6	8
B. Operated	10	3.1	4	1	2	3	4	6	7	9
2. MULTIPLE DX										
A. Not Operated	4,878	4.3	12	1	2	3	5	8	10	16
B. Operated	882	7.9	39	3	4	6	10	15	18	33
1. SINGLE DX	187	2.3	2	1	1	2	3	4	6	8
2. MULTIPLE DX	5,760	4.8	18	2	2	4	6	9	12	21
A. NOT OPERATED	5,055	4.2	12	1	2	3	5	8	10	16
B. OPERATED	892	7.9	39	3	4	6	10	15	18	33
TOTAL										
0–19 Years	406	3.2	9	1	2	3	4	6	7	10
20–34	618	4.1	11	1	2	3	5	7	8	17
35–49	1,375	4.7	18	1	2	4	6	9	12	20
50–64	1,706	5.1	23	2	3	4	6	9	13	25
65+	1,842	5.0	14	2	3	4	6	9	12	20
GRAND TOTAL	5,947	4.7	17	2	2	4	6	9	12	20

682.8: CELLULITIS NEC

Type of Patients	Observed Patients	Avg. Stay	Variance	10th	25th	50th	75th	90th	95th	99th
1. SINGLE DX										
A. Not Operated										
0–19 Years	7	3.3	<1	2	3	3	4	4	4	4
20–34	2	4.0	8	2	2	3	6	6	6	6
35–49	1	1.0	0	1	1	1	1	1	1	1
50–64	3	2.0	<1	1	1	2	3	3	3	3
65+	1	2.0	0	2	2	2	2	2	2	2
B. Operated										
0–19 Years	0									
20–34	1	1.0	0	1	1	1	1	1	1	1
35–49	0									
50–64	0									
65+	0									
2. MULTIPLE DX										
A. Not Operated										
0–19 Years	51	3.4	2	2	2	3	4	5	6	7
20–34	46	4.4	9	2	2	3	6	10	10	14
35–49	101	4.3	8	2	2	3	5	8	11	13
50–64	109	4.6	8	2	3	4	6	8	9	15
65+	87	5.1	19	2	3	4	6	10	11	35
B. Operated										
0–19 Years	3	3.3	1	2	2	4	4	4	4	4
20–34	7	5.4	22	1	2	4	7	15	15	15
35–49	22	6.8	35	1	3	5	8	10	13	29
50–64	16	8.4	148	3	4	5	7	9	53	53
65+	16	9.5	133	2	4	6	14	20	48	48
SUBTOTALS:										
1. SINGLE DX										
A. Not Operated	14	2.9	2	1	2	3	4	4	6	6
B. Operated	1	1.0	0	1	1	1	1	1	1	1
2. MULTIPLE DX										
A. Not Operated	394	4.4	10	2	2	4	5	8	10	15
B. Operated	64	7.6	83	2	4	5	7	14	20	53
1. SINGLE DX	15	2.7	2	1	2	3	4	4	6	6
2. MULTIPLE DX	458	4.9	21	2	3	4	6	9	11	20
A. NOT OPERATED	408	4.4	10	2	2	4	5	8	10	14
B. OPERATED	65	7.5	83	2	4	5	7	14	20	53
TOTAL										
0–19 Years	61	3.4	2	2	2	3	4	5	5	7
20–34	56	4.4	10	2	2	3	6	10	10	15
35–49	124	4.7	14	2	3	4	6	8	11	14
50–64	128	5.0	26	2	3	4	6	8	9	15
65+	104	5.7	38	2	3	4	6	11	14	35
GRAND TOTAL	473	4.8	21	2	2	4	6	8	11	20

Percentiles

579

Length of Stay by Diagnosis and Operation, Western Region, 2008

Western Region, October 2006–September 2007 Data, by Diagnosis

683: ACUTE LYMPHADENITIS

Type of Patients	Observed Patients	Avg. Stay	Variance	10th	25th	50th	75th	90th	95th	99th
1. SINGLE DX										
A. Not Operated										
0–19 Years	57	3.3	6	1	2	3	4	6	9	14
20–34	3	3.0	7	1	1	2	6	6	6	6
35–49	1	2.0	0	2	2	2	2	2	2	2
50–64	0									
65+	0									
B. Operated										
0–19 Years	13	2.9	4	1	1	2	4	6	7	7
20–34	5	1.6	<1	1	1	2	2	2	2	2
35–49	1	1.0	0	1	1	1	1	1	1	1
50–64	0									
65+	0									
2. MULTIPLE DX										
A. Not Operated										
0–19 Years	166	3.7	5	1	2	3	5	6	10	11
20–34	24	3.4	6	1	1	3	5	7	8	10
35–49	24	4.7	18	1	2	3	8	10	11	18
50–64	21	3.1	2	1	2	3	4	5	6	6
65+	19	5.9	17	2	3	5	8	10	19	19
B. Operated										
0–19 Years	45	5.2	10	2	3	4	7	9	11	15
20–34	14	4.9	6	2	3	5	7	9	10	10
35–49	20	5.8	12	3	3	4	9	12	12	12
50–64	19	5.5	17	2	3	4	6	12	17	17
65+	12	3.8	8	1	1	4	5	7	10	10
SUBTOTALS:										
1. SINGLE DX										
A. Not Operated	61	3.3	6	1	2	3	4	6	8	14
B. Operated	19	2.4	3	1	1	2	3	6	7	7
2. MULTIPLE DX										
A. Not Operated	254	3.9	8	1	2	3	5	7	10	13
B. Operated	110	5.2	11	2	3	4	7	10	12	15
1. SINGLE DX	80	3.1	5	1	2	3	4	6	7	14
2. MULTIPLE DX	364	4.3	9	1	2	4	5	8	10	15
A. NOT OPERATED	315	3.8	7	1	2	3	5	7	10	13
B. OPERATED	129	4.8	11	1	3	4	7	9	12	15
TOTAL										
0–19 Years	281	3.8	7	1	2	3	5	7	10	14
20–34	46	3.6	6	1	2	3	5	7	8	10
35–49	46	5.0	15	1	2	4	8	11	12	18
50–64	40	4.2	10	2	3	5	8	12	12	17
65+	31	5.1	14	3	3	4	7	10	10	19
GRAND TOTAL	444	4.1	8	1	2	3	5	8	10	15

684: IMPETIGO

Type of Patients	Observed Patients	Avg. Stay	Variance	10th	25th	50th	75th	90th	95th	99th
1. SINGLE DX										
A. Not Operated										
0–19 Years	27	2.2	1	1	1	2	3	4	4	4
20–34	0									
35–49	1	1.0	0	1	1	1	1	1	1	1
50–64	1	2.0	0	2	2	2	2	2	2	2
65+	0									
B. Operated										
0–19 Years	0									
20–34	0									
35–49	0									
50–64	0									
65+	0									
2. MULTIPLE DX										
A. Not Operated										
0–19 Years	80	2.9	3	1	2	3	4	5	6	10
20–34	13	3.9	5	2	3	3	5	7	9	9
35–49	21	3.7	5	1	2	3	6	7	7	8
50–64	14	3.7	4	2	2	3	4	5	6	8
65+	19	5.0	12	1	2	5	7	11	12	12
B. Operated										
0–19 Years	0									
20–34	0									
35–49	0									
50–64	1	11.0	0	11	11	11	11	11	11	11
65+	0									
SUBTOTALS:										
1. SINGLE DX										
A. Not Operated	29	2.2	1	1	1	2	3	4	4	4
B. Operated	0									
2. MULTIPLE DX										
A. Not Operated	147	3.5	5	1	2	3	5	7	8	13
B. Operated	1	11.0	0	11	11	11	11	11	11	11
1. SINGLE DX	29	2.2	1	1	1	2	3	4	4	4
2. MULTIPLE DX	148	3.5	5	1	2	3	5	7	8	15
A. NOT OPERATED	176	3.3	4	1	2	3	5	7	8	13
B. OPERATED	1	11.0	0	11	11	11	11	11	11	11
TOTAL										
0–19 Years	107	2.8	2	1	2	3	4	5	5	7
20–34	13	3.9	5	2	3	3	5	7	9	9
35–49	22	3.6	5	1	2	3	6	7	7	8
50–64	16	4.1	7	2	2	3	5	8	11	11
65+	19	5.0	12	1	2	5	7	11	12	12
GRAND TOTAL	177	3.3	5	1	2	3	4	6	8	11

685: PILONIDAL CYST

Type of Patients	Observed Patients	Avg. Stay	Variance	10th	25th	50th	75th	90th	95th	99th
1. SINGLE DX										
A. Not Operated										
0–19 Years	28	1.8	<1	1	1	2	2	3	3	4
20–34	25	2.1	2	1	1	2	2	5	6	6
35–49	5	1.6	2	1	1	1	1	4	4	4
50–64	2	2.5	<1	2	2	3	3	3	3	3
65+	0									
B. Operated										
0–19 Years	37	2.3	5	1	1	1	3	5	7	12
20–34	38	2.0	2	1	1	1	2	4	6	7
35–49	8	1.5	<1	1	1	1	2	3	3	3
50–64	1	6.0	0	6	6	6	6	6	6	6
65+	0									
2. MULTIPLE DX										
A. Not Operated										
0–19 Years	38	2.2	1	1	1	2	3	4	5	5
20–34	43	2.7	7	1	1	2	3	5	7	15
35–49	22	3.3	8	1	1	2	4	8	8	10
50–64	10	5.9	38	3	3	3	6	22	22	22
65+	5	3.0	1	2	2	3	3	4	4	4
B. Operated										
0–19 Years	27	3.2	8	1	1	3	3	5	8	13
20–34	54	2.7	3	1	1	2	3	5	6	9
35–49	27	2.9	7	1	1	2	3	6	10	11
50–64	12	4.3	15	1	1	3	7	9	13	13
65+	8	6.6	47	1	1	4	8	19	19	19
SUBTOTALS:										
1. SINGLE DX										
A. Not Operated	60	1.9	1	1	1	2	2	3	5	6
B. Operated	84	2.1	3	1	1	1	3	4	6	12
2. MULTIPLE DX										
A. Not Operated	118	3.0	8	1	1	2	3	6	8	15
B. Operated	128	3.2	9	1	1	2	4	7	9	15
1. SINGLE DX	144	2.0	3	1	1	2	2	4	6	7
2. MULTIPLE DX	246	3.1	9	1	1	2	4	6	9	15
A. NOT OPERATED	178	2.6	6	1	1	2	3	5	7	15
B. OPERATED	212	2.8	7	1	1	2	3	6	8	13
TOTAL										
0–19 Years	130	2.4	4	1	1	2	3	5	6	12
20–34	160	2.4	4	1	1	2	3	5	6	9
35–49	62	2.8	6	1	1	2	3	6	8	11
50–64	25	4.9	23	2	2	3	6	22	13	22
65+	13	5.2	31	1	2	3	4	15	19	19
GRAND TOTAL	390	2.7	7	1	1	2	3	6	8	15

Length of Stay by Diagnosis and Operation, Western Region, 2008

685.0: PILONIDAL CYST W ABSCESS

Type of Patients	Observed Patients	Avg. Stay	Variance	Percentiles						
				10th	25th	50th	75th	90th	95th	99th
1. SINGLE DX										
A. Not Operated										
0–19 Years	25	1.8	<1	1	1	2	2	3	3	4
20–34	23	2.2	2	1	1	2	3	5	6	6
35–49	5	1.6	2	1	1	1	1	4	4	6
50–64	2	2.5	<1	2	2	3	3	3	3	3
65+	0									
B. Operated										
0–19 Years	19	2.1	2	1	1	2	3	4	7	7
20–34	22	2.0	2	1	1	1	3	3	4	7
35–49	6	1.7	<1	1	1	1	2	3	3	3
50–64	1	6.0	0	6	6	6	6	6	6	6
65+	0									
2. MULTIPLE DX										
A. Not Operated										
0–19 Years	29	2.4	1	1	1	2	3	4	4	5
20–34	37	2.8	8	1	1	2	3	6	9	15
35–49	22	3.3	8	1	1	2	4	8	8	10
50–64	8	4.3	8	1	1	3	6	9	9	9
65+	5	3.0	1	2	2	3	4	4	4	4
B. Operated										
0–19 Years	15	3.3	10	1	1	2	5	6	13	13
20–34	34	2.6	4	1	1	2	4	5	6	9
35–49	19	3.0	7	1	1	2	4	6	11	11
50–64	8	4.4	19	1	2	3	9	13	13	13
65+	5	9.4	55	2	3	8	15	19	19	19
SUBTOTALS:										
1. SINGLE DX										
A. Not Operated	55	2.0	1	1	1	2	2	3	5	6
B. Operated	48	2.1	2	1	1	2	3	4	6	7
2. MULTIPLE DX										
A. Not Operated	101	2.9	6	1	1	2	3	6	8	10
B. Operated	81	3.4	12	1	1	2	4	6	11	19
1. SINGLE DX	103	2.0	2	1	1	2	2	3	5	7
2. MULTIPLE DX	182	3.1	8	1	1	2	4	6	9	15
A. NOT OPERATED	156	2.6	4	1	1	2	3	5	7	10
B. OPERATED	129	2.9	9	1	1	2	3	6	9	15
TOTAL										
0–19 Years	88	2.3	3	1	1	2	3	4	5	13
20–34	116	2.5	4	1	1	2	3	5	6	9
35–49	52	2.8	6	1	1	2	3	6	8	11
50–64	19	4.2	11	2	2	3	6	9	13	13
65+	10	6.2	36	2	2	4	8	15	19	19
GRAND TOTAL	285	2.7	6	1	1	2	3	5	8	15

686: OTH LOCAL SKIN INFECTION

Type of Patients	Observed Patients	Avg. Stay	Variance	Percentiles						
				10th	25th	50th	75th	90th	95th	99th
1. SINGLE DX										
A. Not Operated										
0–19 Years	7	1.6	<1	1	1	1	2	3	3	3
20–34	8	2.3	2	1	1	2	3	5	5	5
35–49	9	2.3	2	1	1	2	3	6	6	6
50–64	2	3.0	2	2	2	3	4	4	4	4
65+	1	3.0	0	3	3	3	3	3	3	3
B. Operated										
0–19 Years	4	1.3	<1	1	1	1	3	4	4	7
20–34	2	3.5	12	1	1	2	3	3	6	6
35–49	2	2.0	2	1	1	2	3	3	3	3
50–64	3	2.0	<1	1	1	2	2	3	3	3
65+	0									
2. MULTIPLE DX										
A. Not Operated										
0–19 Years	49	3.3	5	1	2	3	4	8	8	9
20–34	56	3.9	10	1	2	3	5	9	9	18
35–49	80	4.1	13	1	2	3	5	9	12	21
50–64	110	4.7	30	1	2	3	5	10	15	28
65+	71	4.9	22	1	2	4	6	10	13	30
B. Operated										
0–19 Years	4	3.3	7	1	1	5	6	6	6	6
20–34	16	3.8	12	1	1	4	5	5	15	15
35–49	14	7.9	55	2	3	6	9	17	29	29
50–64	36	5.1	17	1	2	4	7	11	16	17
65+	20	5.0	15	1	3	4	7	9	17	17
SUBTOTALS:										
1. SINGLE DX										
A. Not Operated	27	2.2	2	1	1	2	3	4	5	6
B. Operated	11	2.0	2	1	1	1	3	3	6	6
2. MULTIPLE DX										
A. Not Operated	366	4.3	18	1	2	3	5	9	11	26
B. Operated	90	5.2	22	1	2	4	6	11	16	29
1. SINGLE DX	38	2.1	2	1	1	2	3	4	5	6
2. MULTIPLE DX	456	4.5	19	1	2	3	5	9	12	26
A. NOT OPERATED	393	4.2	18	1	2	3	5	8	11	26
B. OPERATED	101	4.9	21	1	2	4	6	9	15	17
TOTAL										
0–19 Years	64	3.0	5	1	1	2	3	4	5	9
20–34	82	3.7	9	1	2	3	5	7	9	18
35–49	105	4.5	19	1	2	3	5	6	12	21
50–64	151	4.7	26	1	2	3	5	9	15	28
65+	92	4.9	20	1	2	4	6	9	13	30
GRAND TOTAL	494	4.3	18	1	2	3	5	9	11	26

690: ERYTHEMATOSQUAMOUS DERM

Type of Patients	Observed Patients	Avg. Stay	Variance	Percentiles						
				10th	25th	50th	75th	90th	95th	99th
1. SINGLE DX										
A. Not Operated										
0–19 Years	6	1.3	<1	1	1	1	2	2	2	2
20–34	0									
35–49	0									
50–64	0									
65+	0									
B. Operated										
0–19 Years	0									
20–34	0									
35–49	0									
50–64	0									
65+	0									
2. MULTIPLE DX										
A. Not Operated										
0–19 Years	6	1.7	<1	1	1	2	2	3	3	3
20–34	2	7.0	8	5	5	9	9	9	9	9
35–49	4	4.7	10	2	2	3	5	9	9	9
50–64	4	4.5	12	1	2	7	8	8	8	8
65+	4	4.5	10	2	2	4	9	9	9	9
B. Operated										
0–19 Years	0									
20–34	0									
35–49	0									
50–64	0									
65+	0									
SUBTOTALS:										
1. SINGLE DX										
A. Not Operated	6	1.3	<1	1	1	1	2	2	2	2
B. Operated	0									
2. MULTIPLE DX										
A. Not Operated	20	4.0	8	1	2	3	3	9	9	9
B. Operated	0									
1. SINGLE DX	6	1.3	<1	1	1	1	2	2	2	2
2. MULTIPLE DX	20	4.0	8	1	2	3	7	9	9	9
A. NOT OPERATED	26	3.4	8	1	1	2	5	9	9	9
B. OPERATED	0									
TOTAL										
0–19 Years	12	1.5	<1	1	1	1	2	2	3	3
20–34	2	7.0	8	5	5	9	9	9	9	9
35–49	4	4.7	10	2	2	3	5	9	9	9
50–64	4	4.5	12	1	2	7	8	8	8	8
65+	4	4.5	10	2	2	4	9	9	9	9
GRAND TOTAL	26	3.4	8	1	1	2	5	9	9	9

Length of Stay by Diagnosis and Operation, Western Region, 2008

Western Region, October 2006–September 2007 Data, by Diagnosis

691: ATOPIC DERMATITIS

Type of Patients	Observed Patients	Avg. Stay	Variance	10th	25th	50th	75th	90th	95th	99th
1. SINGLE DX										
A. Not Operated										
0–19 Years	7	3.0	5	1	1	2	5	7	7	7
20–34	1	2.0	0	2	2	2	2	2	2	2
35–49	0									
50–64	0									
65+	0									
B. Operated										
0–19 Years	0									
20–34	0									
35–49	0									
50–64	0									
65+	0									
2. MULTIPLE DX										
A. Not Operated										
0–19 Years	44	2.7	4	1	1	2	4	4	6	12
20–34	5	2.2	<1	1	2	2	3	3	3	3
35–49	14	2.2	2	1	1	2	3	4	5	5
50–64	6	3.0	2	1	3	3	3	5	5	5
65+	6	4.2	3	2	3	4	6	6	6	6
B. Operated										
0–19 Years	0									
20–34	1	6.0	0	6	6	6	6	6	6	6
35–49	0									
50–64	0									
65+	0									
SUBTOTALS:										
1. SINGLE DX										
A. Not Operated	8	2.9	4	1	2	2	5	7	7	7
B. Operated	0									
2. MULTIPLE DX										
A. Not Operated	75	2.7	3	1	1	3	3	5	6	12
B. Operated	1	6.0	0	6	6	6	6	6	6	6
1. SINGLE DX	8	2.9	4	1	2	2	5	7	7	7
2. MULTIPLE DX	76	2.8	3	1	1	3	4	5	6	12
A. NOT OPERATED	83	2.8	3	1	1	2	3	5	6	12
B. OPERATED	1	6.0	0	6	6	6	6	6	6	6
TOTAL										
0–19 Years	51	2.8	4	1	1	2	4	5	6	12
20–34	6	2.2	<1	1	2	2	3	3	3	3
35–49	15	2.5	2	1	1	2	3	5	6	6
50–64	6	3.0	2	1	3	3	3	5	5	5
65+	6	4.2	3	2	3	4	6	6	6	6
GRAND TOTAL	84	2.8	3	1	1	3	4	5	6	12

692: CONTACT DERMATITIS

Type of Patients	Observed Patients	Avg. Stay	Variance	10th	25th	50th	75th	90th	95th	99th
1. SINGLE DX										
A. Not Operated										
0–19 Years	21	1.8	2	1	1	2	2	2	3	7
20–34	5	2.6	5	1	1	1	4	6	6	6
35–49	4	1.8	2	1	1	1	2	4	4	4
50–64	6	2.3	5	1	1	2	2	7	7	7
65+	0									
B. Operated										
0–19 Years	0									
20–34	0									
35–49	0									
50–64	0									
65+	0									
2. MULTIPLE DX										
A. Not Operated										
0–19 Years	60	2.5	5	1	1	2	3	4	5	17
20–34	52	2.6	4	1	1	2	3	5	6	10
35–49	82	2.8	4	1	1	2	3	5	7	12
50–64	82	2.7	3	1	2	2	3	5	5	12
65+	95	3.6	19	1	2	2	4	7	8	38
B. Operated										
0–19 Years	0									
20–34	1	7.0	0	7	7	7	7	7	7	7
35–49	3	5.3	9	2	2	6	8	8	8	8
50–64	3	2.7	2	1	1	3	4	4	4	4
65+	3	5.3	9	2	2	6	8	8	8	8
SUBTOTALS:										
1. SINGLE DX										
A. Not Operated	36	2.0	3	1	1	1	2	4	7	7
B. Operated	0									
2. MULTIPLE DX										
A. Not Operated	371	2.9	8	1	1	2	4	5	7	13
B. Operated	10	4.7	7	2	2	4	7	8	8	8
1. SINGLE DX	36	2.0	3	1	1	1	2	4	7	7
2. MULTIPLE DX	381	3.0	8	1	1	2	4	5	7	13
A. NOT OPERATED	407	2.8	7	1	1	2	3	5	7	12
B. OPERATED	10	4.7	7	2	2	4	7	8	8	8
TOTAL										
0–19 Years	81	2.3	4	1	1	2	3	4	5	17
20–34	58	2.7	4	1	1	2	4	5	6	10
35–49	89	2.9	5	1	1	2	3	6	8	12
50–64	91	2.7	3	1	1	2	3	5	6	12
65+	98	3.7	18	1	2	2	5	7	8	38
GRAND TOTAL	417	2.9	7	1	1	2	3	5	7	12

692.9: DERMATITIS NOS

Type of Patients	Observed Patients	Avg. Stay	Variance	10th	25th	50th	75th	90th	95th	99th
1. SINGLE DX										
A. Not Operated										
0–19 Years	13	1.6	<1	1	1	2	2	2	3	3
20–34	3	2.7	8	1	1	1	1	6	6	6
35–49	3	2.0	3	1	1	1	1	4	4	4
50–64	4	2.7	8	1	1	2	2	7	7	7
65+	0									
B. Operated										
0–19 Years	0									
20–34	0									
35–49	0									
50–64	0									
65+	0									
2. MULTIPLE DX										
A. Not Operated										
0–19 Years	44	2.8	6	1	2	2	3	5	5	17
20–34	32	2.9	5	1	1	2	3	5	6	10
35–49	43	2.4	2	1	1	2	3	4	4	7
50–64	53	2.6	3	1	1	2	3	4	5	12
65+	57	3.4	7	1	2	2	4	7	8	13
B. Operated										
0–19 Years	0									
20–34	1	7.0	0	7	7	7	7	7	7	7
35–49	1	8.0	0	8	8	8	8	8	8	8
50–64	1	4.0	0	4	4	4	4	4	4	4
65+	1	6.0	0	6	6	6	6	6	6	6
SUBTOTALS:										
1. SINGLE DX										
A. Not Operated	23	2.0	3	1	1	1	2	4	6	7
B. Operated	0									
2. MULTIPLE DX										
A. Not Operated	229	2.9	5	1	1	2	4	5	7	13
B. Operated	4	6.2	3	4	4	6	7	8	8	8
1. SINGLE DX	23	2.0	3	1	1	1	2	4	6	7
2. MULTIPLE DX	233	2.9	5	1	1	2	4	5	7	13
A. NOT OPERATED	252	2.8	5	1	1	2	3	5	7	12
B. OPERATED	4	6.2	3	4	4	6	7	8	8	8
TOTAL										
0–19 Years	57	2.6	5	1	1	2	3	4	5	17
20–34	36	3.0	5	1	1	2	5	6	7	10
35–49	47	2.5	2	1	1	2	3	4	6	8
50–64	58	2.7	4	1	2	2	5	5	7	12
65+	58	3.5	7	1	2	2	5	7	8	13
GRAND TOTAL	256	2.9	5	1	1	2	4	5	7	13

Western Region, October 2006–September 2007 Data, by Diagnosis

693: DERM D/T INTERNAL AGENT

Type of Patients	Observed Patients	Avg. Stay	Vari-ance	10th	25th	50th	75th	90th	95th	99th
1. SINGLE DX										
A. Not Operated										
0–19 Years	15	1.3	<1	1	1	1	1	3	3	3
20–34	6	1.5	<1	1	1	2	2	2	2	2
35–49	3	2.7	2	1	1	3	4	4	4	4
50–64	3	1.3	<1	1	1	1	2	2	2	2
65+	0									
B. Operated										
0–19 Years	0									
20–34	0									
35–49	0									
50–64	0									
65+	0									
2. MULTIPLE DX										
A. Not Operated										
0–19 Years	72	2.8	6	1	1	3	3	5	8	15
20–34	132	2.7	5	1	1	2	3	4	6	9
35–49	195	2.9	4	1	1	2	4	6	7	11
50–64	206	3.4	9	1	1	3	4	7	8	14
65+	323	3.8	11	1	2	3	5	6	10	18
B. Operated										
0–19 Years	0									
20–34	2	5.5	40	1	1	6	10	10	10	10
35–49	3	10.7	42	6	6	8	18	18	18	18
50–64	3	11.0	7	9	9	10	14	14	14	14
65+	1	3.0	0	3	3	3	3	3	3	3
SUBTOTALS:										
1. SINGLE DX										
A. Not Operated	27	1.5	<1	1	1	1	2	2	3	3
B. Operated	0									
2. MULTIPLE DX										
A. Not Operated	928	3.3	8	1	2	3	4	6	8	15
B. Operated	9	8.8	27	1	6	9	10	18	18	18
1. SINGLE DX	**27**	**1.5**	**<1**	**1**	**1**	**1**	**2**	**3**	**3**	**4**
2. MULTIPLE DX	**937**	**3.4**	**9**	**1**	**2**	**3**	**4**	**6**	**8**	**17**
A. NOT OPERATED	**955**	**3.3**	**8**	**1**	**1**	**3**	**4**	**6**	**8**	**15**
B. OPERATED	**9**	**8.8**	**27**	**1**	**6**	**9**	**10**	**18**	**18**	**18**
TOTAL										
0–19 Years	87	2.6	5	1	1	2	3	5	7	15
20–34	140	2.7	5	1	1	2	3	4	6	10
35–49	201	3.1	6	1	1	2	4	6	8	11
50–64	212	3.5	10	1	1	3	4	7	9	14
65+	324	3.8	11	1	2	3	5	6	10	18
GRAND TOTAL	**964**	**3.3**	**9**	**1**	**2**	**3**	**4**	**6**	**8**	**17**

693.0: DRUG DERMATITIS NOS

Type of Patients	Observed Patients	Avg. Stay	Vari-ance	10th	25th	50th	75th	90th	95th	99th
1. SINGLE DX										
A. Not Operated										
0–19 Years	3	2.0	<1	1	1	2	3	3	3	3
20–34	5	1.6	<1	1	1	2	2	2	2	2
35–49	3	2.7	2	1	1	3	3	4	4	4
50–64	2	1.5	<1	1	1	1	2	2	2	2
65+	0									
B. Operated										
0–19 Years	0									
20–34	0									
35–49	0									
50–64	0									
65+	0									
2. MULTIPLE DX										
A. Not Operated										
0–19 Years	65	3.0	6	1	1	3	3	6	8	15
20–34	127	2.7	5	1	1	2	3	5	6	9
35–49	187	3.0	4	1	1	2	4	6	7	11
50–64	199	3.5	9	1	2	3	4	7	8	18
65+	308	3.8	12	1	2	3	5	6	10	18
B. Operated										
0–19 Years	0									
20–34	2	5.5	40	1	6	6	10	10	10	10
35–49	3	10.7	42	6	6	8	18	18	18	18
50–64	3	11.0	7	9	9	10	14	14	14	14
65+	1	3.0	0	3	3	3	3	3	3	3
SUBTOTALS:										
1. SINGLE DX										
A. Not Operated	13	1.9	<1	1	1	2	2	3	4	4
B. Operated	0									
2. MULTIPLE DX										
A. Not Operated	886	3.4	8	1	2	3	4	6	8	17
B. Operated	9	8.8	27	1	6	9	10	18	18	18
1. SINGLE DX	**13**	**1.9**	**<1**	**1**	**1**	**2**	**2**	**3**	**4**	**4**
2. MULTIPLE DX	**895**	**3.4**	**9**	**1**	**2**	**3**	**4**	**6**	**8**	**18**
A. NOT OPERATED	**899**	**3.3**	**8**	**1**	**2**	**3**	**4**	**6**	**8**	**17**
B. OPERATED	**9**	**8.8**	**27**	**1**	**6**	**9**	**10**	**18**	**18**	**18**
TOTAL										
0–19 Years	68	3.0	6	1	1	3	3	6	8	15
20–34	134	2.7	5	1	1	2	3	5	7	10
35–49	193	3.1	6	1	1	2	4	6	8	11
50–64	204	3.6	10	1	2	3	5	7	9	14
65+	309	3.8	12	1	2	3	5	6	10	18
GRAND TOTAL	**908**	**3.4**	**9**	**1**	**2**	**3**	**4**	**6**	**8**	**17**

694: BULLOUS DERMATOSES

Type of Patients	Observed Patients	Avg. Stay	Vari-ance	10th	25th	50th	75th	90th	95th	99th
1. SINGLE DX										
A. Not Operated										
0–19 Years	1	2.0	0	2	2	2	2	2	2	2
20–34	1	1.0	0	1	1	1	1	1	1	1
35–49	2	2.0	2	1	1	3	3	3	3	3
50–64	0									
65+	0									
B. Operated										
0–19 Years	0									
20–34	0									
35–49	0									
50–64	0									
65+	0									
2. MULTIPLE DX										
A. Not Operated										
0–19 Years	4	9.0	27	2	8	11	13	13	13	13
20–34	13	5.7	20	2	2	2	8	13	15	15
35–49	30	8.5	73	2	3	6	8	26	30	30
50–64	38	7.0	33	2	3	5	8	17	21	25
65+	116	6.8	34	2	3	5	8	15	21	26
B. Operated										
0–19 Years	0									
20–34	0									
35–49	0									
50–64	2	12.5	25	9	9	13	16	16	16	16
65+	4	11.0	55	4	4	12	21	21	21	21
SUBTOTALS:										
1. SINGLE DX										
A. Not Operated	4	1.8	<1	1	1	2	3	3	3	3
B. Operated	0									
2. MULTIPLE DX										
A. Not Operated	201	7.1	39	2	3	5	8	16	21	30
B. Operated	6	11.5	39	4	7	12	16	21	21	21
1. SINGLE DX	**4**	**1.8**	**<1**	**1**	**1**	**2**	**3**	**3**	**3**	**3**
2. MULTIPLE DX	**207**	**7.2**	**39**	**2**	**3**	**5**	**9**	**16**	**21**	**30**
A. NOT OPERATED	**205**	**7.0**	**38**	**2**	**3**	**5**	**8**	**16**	**21**	**30**
B. OPERATED	**6**	**11.5**	**39**	**4**	**7**	**12**	**16**	**21**	**21**	**21**
TOTAL										
0–19 Years	5	7.6	30	2	2	8	13	13	13	13
20–34	14	5.4	20	1	3	3	8	13	15	15
35–49	32	8.1	71	2	3	5	8	26	30	30
50–64	40	7.3	33	2	3	5	9	15	21	25
65+	120	6.9	35	2	3	5	8	15	21	26
GRAND TOTAL	**211**	**7.1**	**39**	**2**	**3**	**5**	**8**	**16**	**21**	**30**

Length of Stay by Diagnosis and Operation, Western Region, 2008

Western Region, October 2006–September 2007 Data, by Diagnosis

695: ERYTHEMATOUS CONDITIONS

Type of Patients	Observed Patients	Avg. Stay	Variance	10th	25th	50th	75th	90th	95th	99th
1. SINGLE DX										
A. Not Operated										
0–19 Years	40	1.9	1	1	1	2	2	4	4	5
20–34	11	4.2	13	1	2	3	4	11	11	11
35–49	7	2.0	0	1	1	2	3	4	4	4
50–64	3	1.0	0	1	1	1	1	1	1	1
65+	0									
B. Operated										
0–19 Years	0									
20–34	0									
35–49	0									
50–64	0									
65+	0									
2. MULTIPLE DX										
A. Not Operated										
0–19 Years	147	3.7	19	1	1	2	4	9	12	23
20–34	111	4.5	12	2	2	3	6	9	11	15
35–49	154	5.4	26	1	2	4	6	11	16	25
50–64	150	5.1	28	1	2	4	6	11	14	29
65+	181	5.3	16	1	3	4	7	11	14	17
B. Operated										
0–19 Years	0									
20–34	10	11.5	45	3	5	14	16	20	21	21
35–49	5	5.6	40	1	1	3	7	16	16	16
50–64	10	12.2	423	1	1	6	13	14	69	69
65+	7	11.1	107	3	3	9	17	32	32	32
SUBTOTALS:										
1. SINGLE DX										
A. Not Operated	61	2.3	4	1	1	2	2	4	4	5
B. Operated	0									
2. MULTIPLE DX										
A. Not Operated	743	4.8	21	1	2	3	6	11	13	23
B. Operated	32	10.7	168	1	3	8	14	19	32	69
1. SINGLE DX	61	2.3	4	1	1	2	2	4	4	11
2. MULTIPLE DX	775	5.1	28	1	2	3	6	11	14	25
A. NOT OPERATED	804	4.6	20	1	2	3	6	10	13	23
B. OPERATED	32	10.7	168	1	3	8	14	19	32	69
TOTAL										
0–19 Years	187	3.3	16	1	1	2	4	7	11	23
20–34	132	5.0	17	2	2	3	7	11	14	21
35–49	166	5.2	26	1	2	4	6	11	16	25
50–64	163	5.4	53	1	2	3	6	11	14	37
65+	188	5.5	20	1	3	4	7	12	14	24
GRAND TOTAL	836	4.9	27	1	2	3	6	11	14	24

695.1: ERYTHEMA MULTIFORME

Type of Patients	Observed Patients	Avg. Stay	Variance	10th	25th	50th	75th	90th	95th	99th
1. SINGLE DX										
A. Not Operated										
0–19 Years	37	1.9	1	1	1	2	2	2	4	5
20–34	9	4.6	14	1	2	3	3	4	11	11
35–49	2	1.5	<1	1	1	2	2	2	2	2
50–64	0									
65+	0									
B. Operated										
0–19 Years	0									
20–34	0									
35–49	0									
50–64	0									
65+	0									
2. MULTIPLE DX										
A. Not Operated										
0–19 Years	129	3.8	19	1	1	2	4	9	12	23
20–34	78	4.9	14	2	2	4	7	9	12	23
35–49	104	5.5	28	2	2	4	6	12	16	22
50–64	96	5.8	33	2	2	4	7	12	17	37
65+	124	5.6	17	2	3	5	7	13	14	17
B. Operated										
0–19 Years	0									
20–34	4	17.7	8	15	15	16	19	21	21	21
35–49	0									
50–64	3	30.9	>999	10	10	14	69	69	69	69
65+	3	9.6	49	3	3	9	17	17	17	17
SUBTOTALS:										
1. SINGLE DX										
A. Not Operated	48	2.4	4	1	1	2	2	4	5	11
B. Operated	0									
2. MULTIPLE DX										
A. Not Operated	531	5.1	23	1	2	4	6	11	14	23
B. Operated	10	19.3	332	3	10	15	19	21	69	69
1. SINGLE DX	48	2.4	4	1	1	2	2	4	5	11
2. MULTIPLE DX	541	5.3	31	1	2	4	6	12	15	24
A. NOT OPERATED	579	4.9	22	1	2	3	6	11	13	23
B. OPERATED	10	19.3	332	3	10	15	19	21	69	69
TOTAL										
0–19 Years	166	3.4	16	1	1	2	4	7	11	23
20–34	91	5.4	20	2	2	4	7	11	15	23
35–49	106	5.4	28	2	2	4	6	12	16	22
50–64	99	6.5	73	1	2	4	8	13	19	69
65+	127	5.7	18	2	3	5	7	13	14	17
GRAND TOTAL	589	5.1	30	1	2	3	6	11	15	24

696: PSORIASIS/LIKE DISORDERS

Type of Patients	Observed Patients	Avg. Stay	Variance	10th	25th	50th	75th	90th	95th	99th
1. SINGLE DX										
A. Not Operated										
0–19 Years	1	1.0	0	1	1	1	1	1	1	1
20–34	4	4.0	2	2	2	4	5	5	5	5
35–49	4	2.3	4	1	1	2	2	5	5	5
50–64	1	2.0	0	2	2	2	2	2	2	2
65+	1	4.0	0	4	4	4	4	4	4	4
B. Operated										
0–19 Years	0									
20–34	0									
35–49	0									
50–64	2	2.5	<1	2	2	2	3	3	3	3
65+	0									
2. MULTIPLE DX										
A. Not Operated										
0–19 Years	6	4.2	5	1	3	4	4	7	7	7
20–34	26	4.5	11	1	3	4	5	8	12	15
35–49	66	5.3	41	1	3	4	6	9	13	38
50–64	80	4.5	17	1	2	4	5	9	11	26
65+	60	5.0	12	2	3	5	6	9	11	17
B. Operated										
0–19 Years	0									
20–34	4	3.0	3	1	1	3	5	5	5	5
35–49	13	3.5	2	3	3	3	3	6	7	7
50–64	35	3.7	6	2	2	3	4	6	10	13
65+	7	5.1	33	2	2	4	4	18	18	18
SUBTOTALS:										
1. SINGLE DX										
A. Not Operated	11	2.9	3	1	1	2	2	5	5	5
B. Operated	2	2.5	<1	2	2	2	2	3	3	3
2. MULTIPLE DX										
A. Not Operated	238	4.8	21	1	2	4	6	9	12	26
B. Operated	59	3.8	8	2	3	3	4	6	10	18
1. SINGLE DX	13	2.8	2	1	2	2	4	5	5	5
2. MULTIPLE DX	297	4.6	19	1	2	3	5	9	12	26
A. NOT OPERATED	249	4.7	20	1	2	4	5	9	12	26
B. OPERATED	61	3.7	8	2	3	3	4	6	8	18
TOTAL										
0–19 Years	7	3.7	5	1	1	4	6	7	7	7
20–34	34	4.2	9	1	3	4	5	7	12	15
35–49	83	4.8	34	1	2	3	5	8	12	38
50–64	118	4.2	13	2	2	3	5	9	10	20
65+	68	5.0	14	2	3	4	6	10	15	18
GRAND TOTAL	310	4.5	18	1	2	3	5	8	11	23

697: LICHEN

Type of Patients	Observed Patients	Avg. Stay	Variance	10th	25th	50th	75th	90th	95th	99th
1. SINGLE DX										
A. Not Operated										
0–19 Years	0									
20–34	0									
35–49	0									
50–64	0									
65+	0									
B. Operated										
0–19 Years	0									
20–34	0									
35–49	0									
50–64	0									
65+	0									
2. MULTIPLE DX										
A. Not Operated										
0–19 Years	0									
20–34	0									
35–49	2	2.0	2	1	1	2	3	3	3	3
50–64	1	2.0	0	2	2	2	2	2	2	2
65+	2	2.0	0	2	2	2	2	2	2	2
B. Operated										
0–19 Years	0									
20–34	0									
35–49	0									
50–64	0									
65+	0									
SUBTOTALS:										
1. SINGLE DX										
A. Not Operated	0									
B. Operated	0									
2. MULTIPLE DX										
A. Not Operated	5	2.0	<1	1	2	2	2	3	3	3
B. Operated	0									
1. SINGLE DX	0									
2. MULTIPLE DX	5	2.0	<1	1	2	2	2	3	3	3
A. NOT OPERATED	5	2.0	<1	1	2	2	2	3	3	3
B. OPERATED	0									
TOTAL										
0–19 Years	0									
20–34	0									
35–49	2	2.0	2	1	1	2	3	3	3	3
50–64	1	2.0	0	2	2	2	2	2	2	2
65+	2	2.0	0	2	2	2	2	2	2	2
GRAND TOTAL	5	2.0	<1	1	2	2	2	3	3	3

698: PRURITUS & LIKE COND

Type of Patients	Observed Patients	Avg. Stay	Variance	10th	25th	50th	75th	90th	95th	99th
1. SINGLE DX										
A. Not Operated										
0–19 Years	0									
20–34	0									
35–49	0									
50–64	1	1.0	0	1	1	1	1	1	1	1
65+	1	1.0	0	1	1	1	1	1	1	1
B. Operated										
0–19 Years	0									
20–34	0									
35–49	0									
50–64	0									
65+	0									
2. MULTIPLE DX										
A. Not Operated										
0–19 Years	6	1.7	<1	1	1	2	2	3	3	3
20–34	5	3.2	5	1	1	3	5	6	6	6
35–49	18	3.0	7	1	1	2	4	6	11	11
50–64	23	4.0	16	1	1	3	5	6	10	19
65+	25	4.1	11	1	2	3	6	7	10	15
B. Operated										
0–19 Years	0									
20–34	1	1.0	0	1	1	1	1	1	1	1
35–49	0									
50–64	1	8.0	0	8	8	8	8	8	8	8
65+	1	12.0	0	12	12	12	12	12	12	12
SUBTOTALS:										
1. SINGLE DX										
A. Not Operated	2	1.0	0	1	1	1	1	1	1	1
B. Operated	0									
2. MULTIPLE DX										
A. Not Operated	77	3.5	10	1	1	3	5	6	10	19
B. Operated	3	7.0	31	1	1	8	12	12	12	12
1. SINGLE DX	2	1.0	0	1	1	1	1	1	1	1
2. MULTIPLE DX	80	3.7	11	1	1	3	5	7	11	19
A. NOT OPERATED	79	3.5	10	1	1	3	5	6	10	19
B. OPERATED	3	7.0	31	1	1	8	12	12	12	12
TOTAL										
0–19 Years	6	1.7	<1	1	1	2	2	3	3	3
20–34	6	2.8	5	1	1	3	4	6	6	6
35–49	18	3.0	7	1	1	2	4	6	11	11
50–64	25	4.1	16	1	1	3	5	8	10	19
65+	27	4.2	13	1	2	3	6	8	12	15
GRAND TOTAL	82	3.6	11	1	1	3	5	7	10	19

700: CORNS & CALLOSITIES

Type of Patients	Observed Patients	Avg. Stay	Variance	10th	25th	50th	75th	90th	95th	99th
1. SINGLE DX										
A. Not Operated										
0–19 Years	0									
20–34	0									
35–49	0									
50–64	0									
65+	0									
B. Operated										
0–19 Years	0									
20–34	0									
35–49	0									
50–64	0									
65+	0									
2. MULTIPLE DX										
A. Not Operated										
0–19 Years	0									
20–34	0									
35–49	0									
50–64	1	6.0	0	6	6	6	6	6	6	6
65+	0									
B. Operated										
0–19 Years	0									
20–34	0									
35–49	0									
50–64	0									
65+	0									
SUBTOTALS:										
1. SINGLE DX										
A. Not Operated	0									
B. Operated	0									
2. MULTIPLE DX										
A. Not Operated	1	6.0	0	6	6	6	6	6	6	6
B. Operated	0									
1. SINGLE DX	0									
2. MULTIPLE DX	1	6.0	0	6	6	6	6	6	6	6
A. NOT OPERATED	1	6.0	0	6	6	6	6	6	6	6
B. OPERATED	0									
TOTAL										
0–19 Years	0									
20–34	0									
35–49	0									
50–64	1	6.0	0	6	6	6	6	6	6	6
65+	0									
GRAND TOTAL	1	6.0	0	6	6	6	6	6	6	6

Length of Stay by Diagnosis and Operation, Western Region, 2008

Western Region, October 2006–September 2007 Data, by Diagnosis

701: OTH SKIN HYPERTR/ATROPHY

Type of Patients	Observed Patients	Avg. Stay	Variance	10th	25th	50th	75th	90th	95th	99th
1. SINGLE DX										
A. Not Operated										
0–19 Years	4	2.0	<1	1	1	2	2	3	3	3
20–34	1	1.0	0	1	1	1	1	1	1	1
35–49	1	1.0	0	1	1	1	1	1	1	1
50–64	0									
65+	0									
B. Operated										
0–19 Years	0									
20–34	6	1.3	<1	1	1	1	2	2	2	2
35–49	15	2.0	4	1	1	2	2	6	8	8
50–64	37	1.1	<1	1	1	1	1	2	2	2
65+	7	1.0	0	1	1	1	1	1	1	1
2. MULTIPLE DX										
A. Not Operated										
0–19 Years	10	1.3	<1	1	1	1	1	2	2	2
20–34	7	9.0	360	1	1	2	3	52	52	52
35–49	8	3.5	5	1	2	3	4	8	8	8
50–64	15	2.4	4	1	1	2	3	6	7	7
65+	7	2.3	<1	1	1	3	3	3	3	3
B. Operated										
0–19 Years	6	3.8	15	1	1	4	5	11	11	11
20–34	27	2.3	4	1	1	2	3	5	7	9
35–49	103	2.0	3	1	1	1	2	4	6	7
50–64	167	1.7	5	1	1	1	2	3	4	11
65+	53	1.7	3	1	1	1	2	3	5	10
SUBTOTALS:										
1. SINGLE DX *A. Not Operated*	6	1.7	<1	1	1	1	1	2	3	3
B. Operated	65	1.3	1	1	1	1	1	2	2	8
2. MULTIPLE DX *A. Not Operated*	47	3.3	55	1	1	2	2	5	7	52
B. Operated	356	1.9	4	1	1	1	2	4	5	11
1. SINGLE DX	71	1.4	1	1	1	1	1	2	2	8
2. MULTIPLE DX	403	2.1	10	1	1	1	2	4	5	11
A. NOT OPERATED	53	3.1	49	1	1	1	2	4	7	52
B. OPERATED	421	1.8	4	1	1	1	2	3	5	10
TOTAL										
0–19 Years	20	2.2	6	1	1	1	2	5	11	11
20–34	41	3.3	64	1	1	1	2	4	7	52
35–49	127	2.1	3	1	1	1	2	5	6	8
50–64	219	1.7	4	1	1	1	2	3	4	9
65+	67	1.7	2	1	1	1	2	3	4	10
GRAND TOTAL	474	2.0	9	1	1	1	2	3	5	11

701.8: SKIN HYPERTR/ATROPHY NEC

Type of Patients	Observed Patients	Avg. Stay	Variance	10th	25th	50th	75th	90th	95th	99th
1. SINGLE DX										
A. Not Operated										
0–19 Years	0									
20–34	0									
35–49	0									
50–64	0									
65+	0									
B. Operated										
0–19 Years	0									
20–34	2	1.0	0	1	1	1	1	1	1	1
35–49	11	1.2	<1	1	1	1	2	2	2	2
50–64	37	1.1	<1	1	1	1	1	1	2	2
65+	7	1.0	0	1	1	1	1	1	1	1
2. MULTIPLE DX										
A. Not Operated										
0–19 Years	0									
20–34	1	1.0	0	1	1	1	1	1	1	1
35–49	0									
50–64	6	1.3	<1	1	1	1	2	2	2	2
65+	1	1.0	0	1	1	1	1	1	1	1
B. Operated										
0–19 Years	0									
20–34	7	1.3	<1	1	1	1	2	2	2	2
35–49	69	1.6	<1	1	1	1	2	3	3	5
50–64	117	1.3	<1	1	1	1	1	2	2	4
65+	42	1.5	2	1	1	1	1	3	3	10
SUBTOTALS:										
1. SINGLE DX *A. Not Operated*	0									
B. Operated	57	1.1	<1	1	1	1	1	2	2	2
2. MULTIPLE DX *A. Not Operated*	8	1.3	<1	1	1	1	1	2	2	2
B. Operated	235	1.4	<1	1	1	1	2	2	3	5
1. SINGLE DX	57	1.1	<1	1	1	1	1	2	2	2
2. MULTIPLE DX	243	1.4	<1	1	1	1	2	2	3	5
A. NOT OPERATED	8	1.3	<1	1	1	1	1	2	2	2
B. OPERATED	292	1.4	<1	1	1	1	2	2	3	5
TOTAL										
0–19 Years	0									
20–34	10	1.2	<1	1	1	1	1	2	2	2
35–49	80	1.5	<1	1	1	1	2	2	3	5
50–64	160	1.3	<1	1	1	1	1	2	3	4
65+	50	1.5	2	1	1	1	1	3	3	10
GRAND TOTAL	300	1.4	<1	1	1	1	2	2	3	5

702: OTHER DERMATOSES

Type of Patients	Observed Patients	Avg. Stay	Variance	10th	25th	50th	75th	90th	95th	99th
1. SINGLE DX										
A. Not Operated										
0–19 Years	0									
20–34	0									
35–49	0									
50–64	0									
65+	0									
B. Operated										
0–19 Years	0									
20–34	0									
35–49	0									
50–64	0									
65+	0									
2. MULTIPLE DX										
A. Not Operated										
0–19 Years	0									
20–34	0									
35–49	2	10.0	0	10	10	10	10	10	10	10
50–64	3	4.3	6	2	2	4	7	7	7	7
65+	2	2.0	0	2	2	2	2	2	2	2
B. Operated										
0–19 Years	0									
20–34	0									
35–49	0									
50–64	1	2.0	0	2	2	2	2	2	2	2
65+	1	2.0	0	2	2	2	2	2	2	2
SUBTOTALS:										
1. SINGLE DX *A. Not Operated*	0									
B. Operated	0									
2. MULTIPLE DX *A. Not Operated*	7	5.3	13	2	2	4	10	10	10	10
B. Operated	2	2.0	0	2	2	2	2	2	2	2
1. SINGLE DX	0									
2. MULTIPLE DX	9	4.6	12	2	2	4	7	10	10	10
A. NOT OPERATED	7	5.3	13	2	2	4	10	10	10	10
B. OPERATED	2	2.0	0	2	2	2	2	2	2	2
TOTAL										
0–19 Years	0									
20–34	0									
35–49	2	10.0	0	10	10	10	10	10	10	10
50–64	4	3.8	6	2	2	4	7	7	7	7
65+	3	2.0	0	2	2	2	2	2	2	2
GRAND TOTAL	9	4.6	12	2	2	4	7	10	10	10

Length of Stay by Diagnosis and Operation, Western Region, 2008

Western Region, October 2006–September 2007 Data, by Diagnosis

703: DISEASES OF NAIL

Type of Patients	Observed Patients	Avg. Stay	Vari-ance	10th	25th	50th	75th	90th	95th	99th
1. SINGLE DX										
A. Not Operated										
0–19 Years	4	1.8	2	1	1	1		4	4	4
20–34	0									
35–49	0									
50–64	0									
65+	0									
B. Operated										
0–19 Years	0									
20–34	0									
35–49	0									
50–64	0									
65+	0									
2. MULTIPLE DX										
A. Not Operated										
0–19 Years	8	1.8	<1	1	1	2	2	3	3	3
20–34	2	1.5	<1	1	1	2	2	2	2	2
35–49	2	1.5	<1	1	1	2	2	2	2	2
50–64	2	1.5	<1	1	1	2	2	2	2	2
65+	0									
B. Operated										
0–19 Years	0									
20–34	0									
35–49	0									
50–64	0									
65+	0									
SUBTOTALS:										
1. SINGLE DX										
A. Not Operated	4	1.8	2	1	1	1		4	4	4
B. Operated	0									
2. MULTIPLE DX										
A. Not Operated	14	1.7	<1	1	1	2	2	2	3	3
B. Operated	0									
1. SINGLE DX	4	1.8	2	1	1	1		4	4	4
2. MULTIPLE DX	14	1.7	2	1	1	2	2	2	3	3
A. NOT OPERATED	18	1.7	<1	1	1	2	2	3	4	4
B. OPERATED	0									
TOTAL										
0–19 Years	12	1.8	<1	1	1	2	2	3	4	4
20–34	2	1.5	<1	1	1	2	2	2	2	2
35–49	2	1.5	<1	1	1	2	2	2	2	2
50–64	2	1.5	<1	1	1	2	2	2	2	2
65+	0									
GRAND TOTAL	18	1.7	<1	1	1	2	2	3	4	4

704: HAIR & FOLLICLE DISEASE

Type of Patients	Observed Patients	Avg. Stay	Vari-ance	10th	25th	50th	75th	90th	95th	99th
1. SINGLE DX										
A. Not Operated										
0–19 Years	0									
20–34	1	1.0	0	1	1	1	1	1	1	1
35–49	2	2.5	<1	2	2	3	3	3	3	3
50–64	1	1.0	0	1	1	1	1	1	1	1
65+	0									
B. Operated										
0–19 Years	0									
20–34	0									
35–49	0									
50–64	0									
65+	0									
2. MULTIPLE DX										
A. Not Operated										
0–19 Years	7	1.9	<1	1	1	2	2	3	3	3
20–34	16	3.0	3	2	2	3	3	4	9	9
35–49	27	2.8	2	1	2	3	4	5	6	6
50–64	10	3.4	3	2	2	2	4	7	7	7
65+	6	3.3	4	2	2	3	4	7	7	7
B. Operated										
0–19 Years	0									
20–34	7	2.3	5	1	1	1	3	7	7	7
35–49	1	5.0	0	5	5	5	5	5	5	5
50–64	0									
65+	1	5.0	0	5	5	5	5	5	5	5
SUBTOTALS:										
1. SINGLE DX										
A. Not Operated	4	1.8	<1	1	1	2	2	3	3	3
B. Operated	0									
2. MULTIPLE DX										
A. Not Operated	66	2.9	3	1	2	2	3	5	6	9
B. Operated	9	2.9	5	1	1	2	5	7	7	7
1. SINGLE DX	4	1.8	<1	1	1	2	2	3	3	3
2. MULTIPLE DX	75	2.9	3	1	2	2	3	5	7	9
A. NOT OPERATED	70	2.8	3	1	2	2	3	5	6	9
B. OPERATED	9	2.9	5	1	2	2	5	7	7	7
TOTAL										
0–19 Years	7	1.9	<1	1	1	2	2	3	3	3
20–34	24	2.7	4	1	2	2	3	4	7	9
35–49	30	2.9	2	1	2	3	4	5	6	6
50–64	11	3.2	4	2	2	2	4	6	7	7
65+	7	3.6	4	2	2	3	5	7	7	7
GRAND TOTAL	79	2.8	3	1	2	2	3	5	7	9

705: DISORDERS OF SWEAT GLAND

Type of Patients	Observed Patients	Avg. Stay	Vari-ance	10th	25th	50th	75th	90th	95th	99th
1. SINGLE DX										
A. Not Operated										
0–19 Years	3	2.3	2	1	1	2	4	4	4	4
20–34	3	2.0	<1	1	1	2	3	3	3	3
35–49	4	1.7	2	1	1	1	1	4	4	4
50–64	2	2.0	2	1	1	3	3	3	3	3
65+	1	4.0	0	4	4	4	4	4	4	4
B. Operated										
0–19 Years	9	1.1	<1	1	1	1	1	2	2	2
20–34	35	2.2	10	1	1	1	2	5	12	16
35–49	14	2.1	2	1	1	1	3	4	5	5
50–64	4	1.3	<1	1	1	1	1	2	2	2
65+	0									
2. MULTIPLE DX										
A. Not Operated										
0–19 Years	5	2.0	2	1	1	1	3	4	4	4
20–34	42	3.9	20	1	1	2	4	8	13	24
35–49	52	4.2	11	1	2	3	5	8	11	17
50–64	59	4.2	17	1	1	3	5	9	16	20
65+	7	10.1	454	1	1	2	4	59	59	59
B. Operated										
0–19 Years	10	3.7	42	1	1	2	2	4	22	22
20–34	49	3.7	27	1	1	2	4	10	12	29
35–49	54	4.3	23	1	2	2	5	9	17	22
50–64	39	6.0	46	1	2	4	7	16	25	33
65+	7	14.5	292	1	1	12	23	49	49	49
SUBTOTALS:										
1. SINGLE DX										
A. Not Operated	13	2.2	2	1	1	2	3	4	4	4
B. Operated	62	2.0	6	1	1	1	2	4	5	16
2. MULTIPLE DX										
A. Not Operated	165	4.3	33	1	2	3	5	9	14	24
B. Operated	159	4.9	45	1	2	2	5	12	20	33
1. SINGLE DX	75	2.0	5	1	1	1	2	4	5	16
2. MULTIPLE DX	324	4.6	39	1	1	2	5	11	16	29
A. NOT OPERATED	178	4.2	31	1	1	3	4	9	14	24
B. OPERATED	221	4.1	36	1	1	2	4	10	16	29
TOTAL										
0–19 Years	27	2.4	16	1	1	2	2	4	4	22
20–34	129	3.3	20	1	1	2	3	7	12	24
35–49	124	3.9	15	1	1	3	5	8	11	21
50–64	104	4.7	28	1	1	3	5	11	16	25
65+	15	11.8	329	1	3	3	13	49	59	59
GRAND TOTAL	399	4.1	34	1	1	2	4	9	14	25

Length of Stay by Diagnosis and Operation, Western Region, 2008

Western Region, October 2006–September 2007 Data, by Diagnosis

705.83: HIDRADENITIS

Type of Patients	Observed Patients	Avg. Stay	Variance	10th	25th	50th	75th	90th	95th	99th
1. SINGLE DX										
A. Not Operated										
0–19 Years	2	3.0	2	2	2	4	4	4	4	4
20–34	3	2.0	<1		1	2	3	3	3	3
35–49	4	1.7	2	1	1	1	1	4	4	4
50–64	2	2.0	2	1	1	3	3	3	3	3
65+	1	4.0	0	4	4	4	4	4	4	4
B. Operated										
0–19 Years	1	1.0	0	1	1	1	1	1	1	1
20–34	6	7.5	27	3	4	5	12	16	16	16
35–49	8	3.0	1	1	3	3	4	5	5	5
50–64	0									
65+	0									
2. MULTIPLE DX										
A. Not Operated										
0–19 Years	3	2.0	3	1	1	1	4	4	4	4
20–34	37	4.2	22	1	1	3	5	12	14	24
35–49	48	4.5	11	1	2	3	5	10	11	17
50–64	54	4.4	18	1	2	3	5	9	16	20
65+	5	13.6	630	1	2	3	4	59	59	59
B. Operated										
0–19 Years	3	9.3	120	2	2	4	22	22	22	22
20–34	20	6.1	50	1	2	7	7	11	20	29
35–49	45	4.9	25	1	2	3	6	11	17	22
50–64	32	7.1	50	2	3	5	8	16	25	33
65+	5	19.5	328	1	12	13	23	49	49	49
SUBTOTALS:										
1. SINGLE DX										
A. Not Operated	12	2.3	2	1	1	2	2	4	4	4
B. Operated	15	4.7	16	1	3	3	5	12	16	16
2. MULTIPLE DX										
A. Not Operated	147	4.6	36	1	2	3	5	10	14	24
B. Operated	105	6.6	59	1	2	4	7	17	22	33
1. SINGLE DX	27	3.6	11	1	1	3	4	5	12	16
2. MULTIPLE DX	252	5.5	47	1	2	3	6	12	17	33
A. NOT OPERATED	159	4.5	34	1	2	3	5	9	14	24
B. OPERATED	120	6.3	54	1	2	4	7	16	22	33
TOTAL										
0–19 Years	9	4.5	44	1	1	2	4	22	22	22
20–34	66	5.0	31	1	2	3	6	12	16	29
35–49	105	4.4	16	1	2	3	5	9	14	21
50–64	88	5.3	31	1	2	4	7	14	16	33
65+	11	15.4	406	1	2	4	23	49	59	59
GRAND TOTAL	279	5.3	43	2	2	3	6	12	17	33

706: SEBACEOUS GLAND DISEASE

Type of Patients	Observed Patients	Avg. Stay	Variance	10th	25th	50th	75th	90th	95th	99th
1. SINGLE DX										
A. Not Operated										
0–19 Years	13	1.6	<1	1	1	1	1	2	3	3
20–34	7	1.7	4	1	1	1	1	6	6	6
35–49	6	1.3	<1	1	1	1	1	3	3	3
50–64	0									
65+	0									
B. Operated										
0–19 Years	0									
20–34	2	1.0	0	1	1	1	1	1	1	1
35–49	3	1.0	0	1	1	1	1	1	1	1
50–64	1	1.0	0	1	1	1	1	1	1	1
65+	0									
2. MULTIPLE DX										
A. Not Operated										
0–19 Years	9	2.3	<1	1	2	2	3	4	4	4
20–34	12	2.3	2	1	1	2	3	4	5	5
35–49	22	1.8	1	1	1	1	3	3	4	4
50–64	34	3.0	8	1	1	2	4	7	7	15
65+	30	2.7	5	1	1	2	4	7	8	8
B. Operated										
0–19 Years	1	3.0	0	3	3	3	3	3	3	3
20–34	3	1.9	0	1	1	1	1	1	1	1
35–49	11	1.9	<1	1	1	2	3	3	3	3
50–64	10	5.3	58	1	2	2	6	26	26	26
65+	9	3.0	4	2	2	2	4	7	7	7
SUBTOTALS:										
1. SINGLE DX										
A. Not Operated	26	1.6	1	1	1	1	2	3	3	6
B. Operated	6	1.0	0	1	1	1	1	1	1	1
2. MULTIPLE DX										
A. Not Operated	107	2.6	5	1	1	2	3	5	7	8
B. Operated	34	3.2	19	1	1	2	3	6	8	26
1. SINGLE DX	32	1.5	1	1	1	1	1	3	3	6
2. MULTIPLE DX	141	2.7	8	1	1	2	3	5	7	15
A. NOT OPERATED	133	2.4	4	1	1	2	3	5	7	8
B. OPERATED	40	2.8	17	1	1	2	3	6	8	26
TOTAL										
0–19 Years	23	2.0	<1	1	1	2	3	3	3	4
20–34	24	1.9	2	1	1	1	2	4	5	6
35–49	42	1.7	<1	1	1	1	3	3	3	4
50–64	45	3.5	19	1	1	2	4	7	8	26
65+	39	2.8	5	1	2	2	4	7	8	8
GRAND TOTAL	173	2.5	7	1	1	2	3	5	7	15

707: CHRONIC ULCER OF SKIN

Type of Patients	Observed Patients	Avg. Stay	Variance	10th	25th	50th	75th	90th	95th	99th
1. SINGLE DX										
A. Not Operated										
0–19 Years	0									
20–34	1	2.0	0			2	2	2	2	2
35–49	0									
50–64	4	4.0	22		2	2	11	11	11	11
65+	1	4.0	0	4	4	4	4	4	4	4
B. Operated										
0–19 Years	2	8.5	59	3	3	3	14	14	14	14
20–34	2	3.0	8	1	1	5	5	5	5	5
35–49	6	4.7	10	2	1	2	8	9	9	9
50–64	4	4.5	17	1	1	4	9	9	9	9
65+	2	5.0	2	4	4	6	6	6	6	6
2. MULTIPLE DX										
A. Not Operated										
0–19 Years	47	7.4	84	2	3	4	7	13	18	51
20–34	286	7.1	107	1	3	4	7	13	25	59
35–49	772	6.8	50	2	3	5	8	14	20	41
50–64	1,275	6.7	49	2	3	5	8	13	18	43
65+	2,408	6.1	24	2	3	5	7	11	15	27
B. Operated										
0–19 Years	41	10.4	167	1	3	5	13	28	41	56
20–34	231	10.9	141	1	4	7	14	22	34	61
35–49	595	10.9	135	3	4	7	14	22	32	77
50–64	955	10.6	138	2	4	7	12	23	34	87
65+	1,689	8.5	57	3	4	7	10	17	22	39
SUBTOTALS:										
1. SINGLE DX										
A. Not Operated	6	3.7	14	1	2	2	4	11	11	11
B. Operated	16	5.0	14	1	2	5	8	9	14	14
2. MULTIPLE DX										
A. Not Operated	4,788	6.4	40	2	3	5	7	12	17	37
B. Operated	3,511	9.7	100	2	4	7	11	20	28	52
1. SINGLE DX	22	4.6	14	1	2	4	7	9	11	14
2. MULTIPLE DX	8,299	7.8	68	2	3	6	9	16	22	46
A. NOT OPERATED	4,794	6.4	40	2	3	5	7	12	17	37
B. OPERATED	3,527	9.6	100	2	4	7	11	20	28	52
TOTAL										
0–19 Years	90	8.8	121	1	3	4	9	21	41	56
20–34	520	8.7	125	2	3	5	10	18	27	59
35–49	1,373	8.5	91	2	3	6	10	18	25	50
50–64	2,238	8.3	91	2	3	6	8	17	26	57
65+	4,100	7.1	39	2	3	5	8	14	19	33
GRAND TOTAL	8,321	7.8	68	2	3	6	9	16	22	46

Length of Stay by Diagnosis and Operation, Western Region, 2008

Western Region, October 2006–September 2007 Data, by Diagnosis

707.03: DECUBITUS ULCER-LOW BACK

Type of Patients	Observed Patients	Avg. Stay	Variance	10th	25th	50th	75th	90th	95th	99th
1. SINGLE DX										
A. Not Operated										
0–19 Years	0									
20–34	0									
35–49	0									
50–64	1	1.0	0	1	1	1	1	1	1	1
65+	0									
B. Operated										
0–19 Years	0									
20–34	0									
35–49	0									
50–64	0									
65+	0									
2. MULTIPLE DX										
A. Not Operated										
0–19 Years	8	16.1	369	1	2	6	13	51	51	51
20–34	63	8.6	172	2	3	4	10	15	23	88
35–49	143	8.9	64	2	4	7	11	19	24	>99
50–64	237	8.9	107	2	4	6	10	18	28	65
65+	574	6.5	27	2	3	5	8	12	17	29
B. Operated										
0–19 Years	9	11.9	208	1	3	7	13	46	46	46
20–34	85	11.9	135	2	5	8	15	24	39	61
35–49	154	13.6	231	3	5	9	17	27	49	86
50–64	259	12.8	185	3	5	8	16	29	42	>99
65+	558	10.2	81	3	5	8	13	20	25	47
SUBTOTALS:										
1. SINGLE DX										
A. Not Operated	1	1.0	0	1	1	1	1	1	1	1
B. Operated	0									
2. MULTIPLE DX										
A. Not Operated	1,025	7.6	63	2	3	6	9	15	21	55
B. Operated	1,065	11.5	135	3	5	8	14	23	34	81
1. SINGLE DX	1	1.0	0	1	1	1	1	1	1	1
2. MULTIPLE DX	2,090	9.6	103	2	4	7	11	20	27	69
A. NOT OPERATED	1,026	7.6	63	2	3	6	9	15	21	55
B. OPERATED	1,065	11.5	135	3	5	8	14	23	34	81
TOTAL										
0–19 Years	17	13.9	271	1	3	7	13	46	51	51
20–34	148	10.5	152	2	3	6	13	22	39	61
35–49	297	11.3	156	2	5	8	15	23	33	86
50–64	497	10.9	151	2	4	7	13	24	39	88
65+	1,132	8.4	57	3	4	6	10	17	22	39
GRAND TOTAL	2,091	9.6	103	2	4	7	11	20	27	69

707.04: DECUBITUS ULCER-HIP

Type of Patients	Observed Patients	Avg. Stay	Variance	10th	25th	50th	75th	90th	95th	99th
1. SINGLE DX										
A. Not Operated										
0–19 Years	0									
20–34	0									
35–49	0									
50–64	0									
65+	1	14.0	0	14	14	14	14	14	14	14
B. Operated										
0–19 Years	0									
20–34	0									
35–49	1	5.0	0	5	5	5	5	5	5	5
50–64	1	7.0	0	7	7	7	7	7	7	7
65+	0									
2. MULTIPLE DX										
A. Not Operated										
0–19 Years	3	6.7	6	4	4	7	9	9	9	9
20–34	13	11.7	328	3	4	5	12	16	70	70
35–49	35	9.9	77	2	4	7	13	19	34	41
50–64	37	8.5	55	2	4	6	10	24	28	30
65+	123	6.3	21	2	3	5	7	10	15	25
B. Operated										
0–19 Years	7	8.2	53	1	2	7	14	21	21	21
20–34	36	14.1	359	2	5	9	16	25	77	94
35–49	109	11.4	109	3	4	8	15	23	42	48
50–64	118	13.9	218	3	5	8	21	34	44	>99
65+	150	8.1	46	2	4	6	9	17	22	38
SUBTOTALS:										
1. SINGLE DX										
A. Not Operated	0									
B. Operated	3	8.7	22	5	5	7	14	14	14	14
2. MULTIPLE DX										
A. Not Operated	211	7.6	56	2	4	6	8	14	24	34
B. Operated	420	11.1	142	2	4	7	14	25	36	77
1. SINGLE DX	3	8.7	22	5	5	7	14	14	14	14
2. MULTIPLE DX	631	9.9	116	2	4	7	11	22	30	70
A. NOT OPERATED	211	7.6	56	2	4	6	8	14	24	34
B. OPERATED	423	11.1	142	2	4	7	14	25	36	77
TOTAL										
0–19 Years	11	8.3	37	2	3	7	14	14	21	21
20–34	49	13.5	345	2	4	9	14	25	70	94
35–49	145	11.0	101	3	4	8	14	22	34	48
50–64	156	12.5	183	3	5	7	17	31	42	>99
65+	273	7.3	35	2	4	6	8	14	20	30
GRAND TOTAL	634	9.9	116	2	4	7	11	22	30	70

707.05: DECUBITUS ULCER-BUTTOCK

Type of Patients	Observed Patients	Avg. Stay	Variance	10th	25th	50th	75th	90th	95th	99th
1. SINGLE DX										
A. Not Operated										
0–19 Years	0									
20–34	0									
35–49	0									
50–64	0									
65+	0									
B. Operated										
0–19 Years	0									
20–34	0									
35–49	1	2.0	0	2	2	2	2	2	2	2
50–64	0									
65+	0									
2. MULTIPLE DX										
A. Not Operated										
0–19 Years	9	6.2	18	1	3	6	7	13	13	13
20–34	46	7.7	108	1	2	5	7	17	25	59
35–49	98	7.6	51	2	3	6	9	15	22	39
50–64	127	7.3	65	2	3	5	8	14	20	43
65+	205	6.4	26	2	3	5	7	12	17	30
B. Operated										
0–19 Years	9	17.7	387	1	1	10	28	56	56	56
20–34	37	11.0	109	3	5	7	15	23	45	49
35–49	93	11.1	125	3	5	7	14	21	29	88
50–64	108	10.7	139	3	5	7	12	21	27	53
65+	148	8.8	50	3	4	7	11	19	27	33
SUBTOTALS:										
1. SINGLE DX										
A. Not Operated	0									
B. Operated	1	2.0	0	2	2	2	2	2	2	2
2. MULTIPLE DX										
A. Not Operated	485	7.0	48	2	3	5	8	14	19	39
B. Operated	395	10.3	106	3	5	7	12	21	29	53
1. SINGLE DX	1	2.0	0	2	2	2	2	2	2	2
2. MULTIPLE DX	880	8.5	77	2	4	6	10	17	25	45
A. NOT OPERATED	485	7.0	48	2	3	5	8	14	19	39
B. OPERATED	396	10.3	106	3	5	7	12	21	29	53
TOTAL										
0–19 Years	18	12.0	226	1	3	7	13	41	56	56
20–34	83	9.2	110	2	4	6	9	17	26	59
35–49	192	9.2	89	2	4	7	11	20	26	39
50–64	235	8.9	101	2	4	6	10	17	23	53
65+	353	7.4	37	2	4	6	9	14	21	31
GRAND TOTAL	881	8.5	77	2	4	6	10	17	25	45

Length of Stay by Diagnosis and Operation, Western Region, 2008

Western Region, October 2006–September 2007 Data, by Diagnosis

Type of Patients	707.07: DECUBITUS ULCER-HEEL Observed Patients	Avg. Stay	Vari-ance	10th	25th	50th	75th	90th	95th	99th	707.09: DECUBITUS ULCER-SITE NEC Observed Patients	Avg. Stay	Vari-ance	10th	25th	50th	75th	90th	95th	99th	707.10: LOWER LIMB ULCER NOS Observed Patients	Avg. Stay	Vari-ance	10th	25th	50th	75th	90th	95th	99th
1. SINGLE DX																													
A. Not Operated																													
0–19 Years	0										0										0									
20–34	0										0										0									
35–49	0										0										0									
50–64	0										0										0									
65+	0										0										0									
B. Operated																													
0–19 Years	0										0										0									
20–34	0										0										0									
35–49	0										2	5.5	24	2	2	9	9	9	9	9	0									
50–64	0										0										0									
65+	0										0										0									
2. MULTIPLE DX																													
A. Not Operated																													
0–19 Years	0										6	4.2	11	2	3	2	6	10	10	10	1	11.0	0	11	11	11	11	11	11	11
20–34	14	6.7	120	2	2	4	7	8	44	44	14	9.9	156	2	3	7	12	26	47	47	6	4.3	7	1	2	4	6	7	8	8
35–49	14	6.9	45	1	3	5	8	11	28	28	31	5.6	27	1	3	4	6	12	20	22	16	4.4	6	2	4	5	6	6	10	10
50–64	45	6.6	40	2	3	4	8	13	23	31	55	6.1	38	1	3	5	7	12	18	41	36	6.6	27	2	4	5	8	12	15	30
65+	230	6.1	33	2	3	4	7	10	17	28	111	6.2	37	2	3	5	7	12	18	46	62	5.6	12	2	3	5	7	12	14	>99
B. Operated																													
0–19 Years	2	4.0	2	3	3	4	5	5	5	5	5	7.8	61	3	3	3	9	21	21	21	0									
20–34	7	8.6	35	2	3	8	14	18	18	18	19	7.9	54	1	4	5	10	23	24	24	0									
35–49	6	11.8	43	6	6	7	16	22	22	22	50	10.5	162	2	4	6	13	29	36	71	5	11.2	120	1	3	7	18	27	27	27
50–64	41	8.2	49	2	3	6	10	15	21	31	80	10.9	166	2	3	7	12	22	29	80	6	5.7	24	1	1	7	7	14	14	14
65+	154	8.2	43	3	4	6	10	15	20	35	71	9.4	94	3	4	6	10	24	32	53	16	6.1	11	3	4	5	5	10	14	14
SUBTOTALS:																													
1. SINGLE DX																													
A. Not Operated	0										0										0									
B. Operated	0										2	5.5	24	2	2	9	9	9	9	9	0									
2. MULTIPLE DX																													
A. Not Operated	303	6.2	38	2	3	4	7	11	18	31	217	6.3	43	2	3	5	7	12	19	46	121	5.7	16	2	3	5	7	11	13	30
B. Operated	210	8.3	43	3	4	6	10	16	21	31	225	10.0	129	2	4	6	11	23	29	54	27	7.0	34	1	3	6	8	14	18	27
1. SINGLE DX	0										2	5.5	24	2	2	9	9	9	9	9	0									
2. MULTIPLE DX	513	7.1	41	2	3	5	8	14	20	31	442	8.2	90	2	3	5	9	19	28	53	148	5.9	19	2	3	5	7	12	14	30
A. NOT OPERATED	303	6.2	38	2	3	4	7	11	18	31	217	6.3	43	2	3	5	7	12	19	46	121	5.7	16	2	3	5	7	11	13	30
B. OPERATED	210	8.3	43	3	4	6	10	16	21	31	227	10.0	129	2	4	6	11	23	29	54	27	7.0	34	1	3	6	8	14	18	27
TOTAL																													
0–19 Years	2	4.0	2	3	3	4	5	5	5	5	11	5.8	33	2	3	3	9	10	21	21	1	11.0	0	11	11	11	11	11	11	11
20–34	21	7.3	89	2	3	4	8	14	18	44	33	8.8	95	2	3	5	10	23	26	47	6	4.3	7	1	2	4	7	8	8	8
35–49	20	8.4	48	3	4	6	9	16	22	28	83	8.6	113	2	3	5	9	20	29	71	21	6.1	38	1	2	5	6	10	18	27
50–64	86	7.3	44	2	3	6	8	16	23	31	135	8.9	119	2	3	6	9	21	29	54	42	6.5	26	2	4	5	7	12	14	30
65+	384	6.9	38	2	3	5	8	13	18	33	182	7.5	61	2	4	5	8	16	26	53	78	5.7	12	2	3	5	7	12	14	>99
GRAND TOTAL	513	7.1	41	2	3	5	8	14	20	31	444	8.2	90	2	3	5	9	19	28	53	148	5.9	19	2	3	5	7	12	14	30

Length of Stay by Diagnosis and Operation, Western Region, 2008

Western Region, October 2006–September 2007 Data, by Diagnosis

707.12: CALF ULCER

Type of Patients	Observed Patients	Avg. Stay	Variance	10th	25th	50th	75th	90th	95th	99th
1. SINGLE DX										
A. Not Operated										
0–19 Years	0									
20–34	0									
35–49	0									
50–64	0									
65+	0									
B. Operated										
0–19 Years	0									
20–34	0									
35–49	0									
50–64	0									
65+	1	1.0	0	1	1	1	1	1	1	1
2. MULTIPLE DX										
A. Not Operated										
0–19 Years	0									
20–34	14	6.4	63	1	1	3	8	9	32	32
35–49	54	8.4	107	2	4	6	9	14	20	69
50–64	99	6.4	31	2	3	5	8	13	19	27
65+	164	5.8	19	2	3	5	7	10	15	25
B. Operated										
0–19 Years	1	28.0	0	28	28	28	28	28	28	28
20–34	2	4.5	<1	4	4	5	5	5	5	5
35–49	11	8.8	48	4	4	8	9	15	27	27
50–64	30	9.3	67	2	4	7	10	18	29	36
65+	63	7.7	24	3	4	7	10	15	19	24
SUBTOTALS:										
1. SINGLE DX										
A. Not Operated	0									
B. Operated	1	1.0	0	1	1	1	1	1	1	1
2. MULTIPLE DX										
A. Not Operated	331	6.4	39	2	3	5	8	13	17	30
B. Operated	107	8.4	41	3	4	7	10	18	20	29
1. SINGLE DX	1	1.0	0	1	1	1	1	1	1	1
2. MULTIPLE DX	438	6.9	40	2	3	5	8	14	19	30
A. NOT OPERATED	331	6.4	39	2	3	5	8	13	17	30
B. OPERATED	108	8.3	41	3	4	6	10	18	20	29
TOTAL										
0–19 Years	1	28.0	0	28	28	28	28	28	28	28
20–34	16	6.2	55	1	4	4	8	9	32	32
35–49	65	8.4	96	3	4	6	9	15	20	69
50–64	130	7.0	41	2	3	5	8	16	20	30
65+	227	6.4	21	2	3	5	8	13	16	24
GRAND TOTAL	439	6.9	40	2	3	5	8	14	19	30

707.13: ANKLE ULCER

Type of Patients	Observed Patients	Avg. Stay	Variance	10th	25th	50th	75th	90th	95th	99th
1. SINGLE DX										
A. Not Operated										
0–19 Years	0									
20–34	1	2.0	0	2	2	2	2	2	2	2
35–49	0									
50–64	0									
65+	0									
B. Operated										
0–19 Years	0									
20–34	1	1.0	0	1	1	1	1	1	1	1
35–49	0									
50–64	0									
65+	1	4.0	0	4	4	4	4	4	4	4
2. MULTIPLE DX										
A. Not Operated										
0–19 Years	5	6.0	19	2	4	4	7	13	13	13
20–34	9	3.3	3	2	2	3	3	7	7	7
35–49	38	5.6	60	1	2	4	6	8	22	46
50–64	72	5.3	13	2	2	5	7	10	13	19
65+	140	6.0	18	2	3	5	7	10	12	20
B. Operated										
0–19 Years	0									
20–34	7	9.0	32	2	4	8	14	18	18	18
35–49	13	8.6	48	4	5	7	9	11	30	30
50–64	39	7.5	35	2	4	6	9	13	26	30
65+	71	7.2	31	2	3	6	9	15	20	28
SUBTOTALS:										
1. SINGLE DX										
A. Not Operated	1	2.0	0	2	2	2	2	2	2	2
B. Operated	2	2.5	4	1	1	4	4	4	4	4
2. MULTIPLE DX										
A. Not Operated	264	5.6	22	2	3	5	7	10	12	22
B. Operated	130	7.5	34	2	4	6	9	14	20	30
1. SINGLE DX	3	2.3	2	1	1	2	4	4	4	4
2. MULTIPLE DX	394	6.3	27	2	3	5	8	11	15	30
A. NOT OPERATED	265	5.6	22	2	3	5	7	10	12	22
B. OPERATED	132	7.5	34	2	4	6	9	14	20	30
TOTAL										
0–19 Years	5	6.0	19	2	4	4	7	13	13	13
20–34	18	5.3	22	2	2	3	4	14	18	18
35–49	51	6.4	58	2	2	5	7	10	22	46
50–64	111	6.0	22	2	3	5	8	10	13	26
65+	212	6.4	23	2	3	5	8	11	16	23
GRAND TOTAL	397	6.2	26	2	3	5	8	11	15	30

707.14: HEEL & MIDFOOT ULCER

Type of Patients	Observed Patients	Avg. Stay	Variance	10th	25th	50th	75th	90th	95th	99th
1. SINGLE DX										
A. Not Operated										
0–19 Years	0									
20–34	0									
35–49	0									
50–64	0									
65+	0									
B. Operated										
0–19 Years	0									
20–34	1	5.0	0	5	5	5	5	5	5	5
35–49	0									
50–64	0									
65+	0									
2. MULTIPLE DX										
A. Not Operated										
0–19 Years	1	4.0	0	4	4	4	4	4	4	4
20–34	12	4.7	19	1	2	3	6	12	15	15
35–49	28	5.1	41	1	2	3	6	11	11	35
50–64	72	5.8	56	2	3	4	7	9	12	63
65+	95	5.6	18	2	3	4	7	11	15	25
B. Operated										
0–19 Years	2	2.5	5	1	1	3	4	4	4	4
20–34	8	5.7	13	2	2	5	7	13	13	13
35–49	15	8.4	51	3	4	6	8	19	29	29
50–64	46	7.4	25	4	4	7	9	14	20	23
65+	75	6.6	36	3	3	6	8	11	16	45
SUBTOTALS:										
1. SINGLE DX										
A. Not Operated	0									
B. Operated	1	5.0	0	5	5	5	5	5	5	5
2. MULTIPLE DX										
A. Not Operated	208	5.5	34	2	3	4	7	10	13	25
B. Operated	146	6.9	32	2	3	6	8	13	17	29
1. SINGLE DX	1	5.0	0	5	5	5	5	5	5	5
2. MULTIPLE DX	354	6.1	34	2	3	5	7	11	15	29
A. NOT OPERATED	208	5.5	34	2	3	4	7	10	13	25
B. OPERATED	147	6.9	32	2	3	6	8	13	17	29
TOTAL										
0–19 Years	3	3.0	3	1	1	4	4	4	4	4
20–34	21	5.1	16	2	3	4	7	12	13	15
35–49	43	6.2	46	2	3	4	6	11	19	35
50–64	118	6.4	44	2	3	5	7	11	15	23
65+	170	6.0	26	2	3	5	7	11	15	25
GRAND TOTAL	355	6.1	34	2	3	5	7	11	15	29

Length of Stay by Diagnosis and Operation, Western Region, 2008

Western Region, October 2006–September 2007 Data, by Diagnosis

707.15: OTHER FOOT ULCER

Type of Patients	Observed Patients	Avg. Stay	Vari-ance	10th	25th	50th	75th	90th	95th	99th
1. SINGLE DX										
A. Not Operated										
0–19 Years	0									
20–34	0									
35–49	0									
50–64	0									
65+	1	4.0	0	4	4	4	4	4	4	4
B. Operated										
0–19 Years	1	3.0	0	3	3	3	3	3	3	3
20–34	0									
35–49	1	8.0	0	8	8	8	8	8	8	8
50–64	1	1.0	0	1	1	1	1	1	1	1
65+	1	6.0	0	6	6	6	6	6	6	6
2. MULTIPLE DX										
A. Not Operated										
0–19 Years	6	5.3	2	4	4	6	7	7	7	7
20–34	34	5.0	27	1	3	4	6	9	9	31
35–49	112	5.1	23	2	2	4	6	9	15	21
50–64	199	5.0	16	1	2	4	6	9	11	26
65+	268	5.5	18	2	3	5	7	9	13	23
B. Operated										
0–19 Years	13	4.5	2	3	4	5	6	6	6	6
20–34	13	6.7	42	1	4	5	8	11	26	26
35–49	47	6.0	15	2	4	5	8	9	12	24
50–64	124	7.8	56	2	3	5	10	16	23	30
65+	176	6.4	26	2	3	5	8	11	15	35
SUBTOTALS:										
1. SINGLE DX										
A. Not Operated	1	4.0	0	4	4	4	4	4	4	4
B. Operated	4	4.5	10	1	1	3	6	8	8	8
2. MULTIPLE DX										
A. Not Operated	619	5.2	18	2	3	4	6	9	12	23
B. Operated	364	6.8	36	2	3	5	8	13	18	30
1. SINGLE DX	5	4.4	7	1	3	4	6	8	8	8
2. MULTIPLE DX	983	5.8	25	2	3	4	7	11	14	28
A. NOT OPERATED	620	5.2	18	2	3	4	6	9	12	23
B. OPERATED	368	6.8	35	2	3	5	8	13	18	30
TOTAL										
0–19 Years	11	4.8	2	3	4	4	6	7	7	7
20–34	47	5.4	31	1	3	4	6	9	11	31
35–49	160	5.4	21	2	3	4	6	10	12	24
50–64	324	6.0	33	2	3	4	7	11	16	28
65+	446	5.9	21	2	3	5	7	10	13	27
GRAND TOTAL	988	5.8	25	2	3	4	7	11	14	28

707.19: LOWER LIMB ULCER NEC

Type of Patients	Observed Patients	Avg. Stay	Vari-ance	10th	25th	50th	75th	90th	95th	99th
1. SINGLE DX										
A. Not Operated										
0–19 Years	0									
20–34	0									
35–49	0									
50–64	1	2.0	0	2	2	2	2	2	2	2
65+	0									
B. Operated										
0–19 Years	0									
20–34	0									
35–49	1	2.0	0	2	2	2	2	2	2	2
50–64	1	9.0	0	9	9	9	9	9	9	9
65+	0									
2. MULTIPLE DX										
A. Not Operated										
0–19 Years	3	8.0	75	2	2	4	18	18	18	18
20–34	21	6.8	82	1	2	4	7	12	23	39
35–49	112	6.3	46	2	3	5	8	11	21	26
50–64	186	6.1	21	2	3	5	8	12	14	26
65+	299	5.9	20	2	3	5	7	10	14	24
B. Operated										
0–19 Years	5	1.0	0	1	1	1	1	1	1	1
20–34	5	18.4	175	7	12	14	18	41	41	41
35–49	40	9.8	93	2	4	7	14	20	20	50
50–64	45	9.1	202	2	4	7	9	15	19	98
65+	114	7.3	25	3	4	6	9	15	18	22
SUBTOTALS:										
1. SINGLE DX										
A. Not Operated	1	2.0	0	2	2	2	2	2	2	2
B. Operated	2	5.5	24	2	2	6	9	9	9	9
2. MULTIPLE DX										
A. Not Operated	621	6.1	27	2	3	5	7	11	15	26
B. Operated	205	8.4	82	2	4	6	10	17	20	41
1. SINGLE DX	3	4.3	16	2	2	2	2	9	9	9
2. MULTIPLE DX	826	6.7	42	2	3	5	8	13	17	27
A. NOT OPERATED	622	6.1	27	2	3	5	7	11	14	26
B. OPERATED	207	8.4	82	2	4	6	10	17	20	41
TOTAL										
0–19 Years	4	6.2	62	1	1	2	4	18	18	18
20–34	26	9.1	115	1	2	5	12	23	39	41
35–49	153	7.2	60	2	3	5	8	15	21	50
50–64	233	6.7	57	2	3	5	8	12	15	26
65+	413	6.3	21	2	3	5	8	13	15	22
GRAND TOTAL	829	6.7	42	2	3	5	8	13	17	27

707.8: CHRONIC SKIN ULCER NEC

Type of Patients	Observed Patients	Avg. Stay	Vari-ance	10th	25th	50th	75th	90th	95th	99th
1. SINGLE DX										
A. Not Operated										
0–19 Years	0									
20–34	0									
35–49	0									
50–64	2	6.6	40	2	2	11	11	11	11	11
65+	0									
B. Operated										
0–19 Years	0									
20–34	0									
35–49	0									
50–64	0									
65+	0									
2. MULTIPLE DX										
A. Not Operated										
0–19 Years	3	4.3	5	3	3	3	7	7	7	7
20–34	25	4.9	18	1	2	3	6	13	14	16
35–49	62	4.7	18	1	2	3	6	10	13	24
50–64	68	5.3	14	2	2	5	7	13	14	>99
65+	67	5.4	13	2	2	5	7	10	13	17
B. Operated										
0–19 Years	8	4.0	0	4	4	4	4	4	4	4
20–34	8	4.5	14	1	1	2	6	6	10	10
35–49	33	8.1	62	2	3	6	9	18	29	34
50–64	37	5.6	20	1	3	4	6	10	15	23
65+	48	5.0	18	1	2	4	7	10	13	22
SUBTOTALS:										
1. SINGLE DX										
A. Not Operated	2	6.6	40	2	2	11	11	11	11	11
B. Operated	0									
2. MULTIPLE DX										
A. Not Operated	225	5.1	15	1	2	4	7	10	14	17
B. Operated	127	5.9	31	1	2	4	7	11	16	29
1. SINGLE DX	2	6.6	40	2	2	11	11	11	11	11
2. MULTIPLE DX	352	5.4	21	1	2	4	7	11	14	24
A. NOT OPERATED	227	5.1	15	1	2	4	7	11	14	17
B. OPERATED	127	5.9	31	1	2	4	7	11	16	29
TOTAL										
0–19 Years	4	4.3	4	3	3	3	4	7	7	7
20–34	33	4.8	17	1	2	3	6	10	14	16
35–49	95	5.9	35	1	2	4	7	11	18	34
50–64	107	5.4	16	2	2	5	7	12	14	23
65+	115	5.2	15	1	2	4	7	10	13	17
GRAND TOTAL	354	5.4	21	1	2	4	7	11	14	24

708: URTICARIA

Type of Patients	Observed Patients	Avg. Stay	Variance	Percentiles 10th	25th	50th	75th	90th	95th	99th
1. SINGLE DX										
A. Not Operated										
0–19 Years	22	1.5	<1	1	1	1	2	2	3	3
20–34	8	1.9	2	1	1	1	2	5	5	5
35–49	3	1.3	<1	1	1	1	2	2	2	2
50–64	2	1.5	<1	1	1	2	2	2	2	2
65+	1	2.0	0	2	2	2	2	2	2	2
B. Operated										
0–19 Years	0									
20–34	0									
35–49	0									
50–64	0									
65+	0									
2. MULTIPLE DX										
A. Not Operated										
0–19 Years	67	1.9	2	1	1	1	2	3	6	6
20–34	56	2.3	2	1	1	2	3	5	5	7
35–49	73	2.1	2	1	1	2	2	5	5	8
50–64	71	2.4	2	1	1	2	3	4	6	8
65+	88	3.1	4	2	2	3	4	6	7	11
B. Operated										
0–19 Years	1	1.0	0	1	1	1	1	1	1	1
20–34	0									
35–49	1	4.0	0	4	4	4	4	4	4	4
50–64	0									
65+	2	2.0	0	2	2	2	2	2	2	2
SUBTOTALS:										
1. SINGLE DX										
A. Not Operated	36	1.6	<1	1	1	1	2	2	3	5
B. Operated	0									
2. MULTIPLE DX										
A. Not Operated	355	2.4	3	1	1	2	3	5	6	8
B. Operated	4	2.3	2	1	1	2	4	4	4	4
1. SINGLE DX	36	1.6	<1	1	1	1	2	2	3	5
2. MULTIPLE DX	359	2.4	3	1	1	2	3	5	6	8
A. NOT OPERATED	391	2.3	3	1	1	2	3	5	6	8
B. OPERATED	4	2.3	2	1	1	2	4	4	4	4
TOTAL										
0–19 Years	90	1.8	2	1	1	1	2	3	5	6
20–34	64	2.2	2	1	1	2	2	5	5	7
35–49	77	2.1	2	1	1	2	2	4	5	8
50–64	73	2.4	2	1	1	2	3	4	6	8
65+	91	3.1	4	1	2	2	4	6	7	11
GRAND TOTAL	395	2.3	3	1	1	2	3	5	6	8

708.0: ALLERGIC URTICARIA

Type of Patients	Observed Patients	Avg. Stay	Variance	Percentiles 10th	25th	50th	75th	90th	95th	99th
1. SINGLE DX										
A. Not Operated										
0–19 Years	10	1.4	<1	1	1	1	2	3	3	3
20–34	4	2.5	3	1	1	2	5	5	5	5
35–49	2	1.5	<1	1	1	2	2	2	2	2
50–64	1	1.0	0	1	1	2	2	2	1	1
65+	1	2.0	0	2	2	2	2	2	2	2
B. Operated										
0–19 Years	0									
20–34	0									
35–49	0									
50–64	0									
65+	0									
2. MULTIPLE DX										
A. Not Operated										
0–19 Years	39	2.1	3	1	1	1	2	3	6	6
20–34	38	2.3	2	1	1	2	3	5	5	7
35–49	53	2.2	2	1	1	2	3	5	5	8
50–64	59	2.4	2	1	1	2	3	4	6	8
65+	58	3.2	4	2	2	3	4	6	8	11
B. Operated										
0–19 Years	1	1.0	0	1	1	1	1	1	1	1
20–34	0									
35–49	1	4.0	0	4	4	4	4	4	4	4
50–64	0									
65+	2	2.0	0	2	2	2	2	2	2	2
SUBTOTALS:										
1. SINGLE DX										
A. Not Operated	18	1.7	1	1	1	1	2	3	5	5
B. Operated	0									
2. MULTIPLE DX										
A. Not Operated	247	2.5	3	1	1	2	3	5	6	8
B. Operated	4	2.3	2	1	1	2	4	4	4	4
1. SINGLE DX	18	1.7	1	1	1	1	2	3	5	5
2. MULTIPLE DX	251	2.5	3	1	1	2	3	5	6	8
A. NOT OPERATED	265	2.4	3	1	1	2	3	5	6	8
B. OPERATED	4	2.3	2	1	1	2	4	4	4	4
TOTAL										
0–19 Years	50	1.9	2	1	1	1	2	3	5	6
20–34	42	2.3	2	1	1	2	3	5	5	7
35–49	56	2.2	2	1	1	2	3	5	5	8
50–64	60	2.4	2	1	1	2	3	4	6	8
65+	61	3.1	4	1	2	3	4	6	7	11
GRAND TOTAL	269	2.4	3	1	1	2	3	5	6	8

709: OTHER SKIN DISORDERS

Type of Patients	Observed Patients	Avg. Stay	Variance	Percentiles 10th	25th	50th	75th	90th	95th	99th
1. SINGLE DX										
A. Not Operated										
0–19 Years	3	2.0	<1	1	1	2	3	3	3	3
20–34	1	2.0	0	2	2	2	2	2	2	2
35–49	0									
50–64	3	4.0	27	1	1	1	10	10	10	10
65+	0									
B. Operated										
0–19 Years	4	1.3	<1	1	1	1	2	2	2	2
20–34	5	3.0	5	1	1	2	5	6	6	6
35–49	3	3.0	3	2	2	2	5	5	5	5
50–64	1	1.0	0	1	1	1	1	1	1	1
65+	1	1.0	0	1	1	1	1	1	1	1
2. MULTIPLE DX										
A. Not Operated										
0–19 Years	14	2.4	4	1	1	2	3	5	8	8
20–34	14	3.0	4	1	2	3	4	5	9	9
35–49	30	3.9	27	1	1	2	5	9	19	23
50–64	40	3.4	11	1	2	2	4	9	10	17
65+	26	3.7	10	1	2	2	6	9	11	12
B. Operated										
0–19 Years	43	5.0	51	1	1	1	6	12	25	28
20–34	48	4.8	16	1	2	4	7	10	11	22
35–49	85	5.9	75	1	1	3	6	17	26	46
50–64	86	4.0	21	1	1	2	6	10	14	26
65+	47	3.4	13	1	1	2	4	7	8	23
SUBTOTALS:										
1. SINGLE DX										
A. Not Operated	7	2.9	11	1	1	2	3	10	10	10
B. Operated	14	2.2	3	1	1	2	2	5	6	6
2. MULTIPLE DX										
A. Not Operated	124	3.4	13	1	1	2	4	8	10	19
B. Operated	309	4.7	39	1	1	2	6	10	18	30
1. SINGLE DX	21	2.4	5	1	1	2	2	5	6	10
2. MULTIPLE DX	433	4.3	32	1	1	2	5	9	14	28
A. NOT OPERATED	131	3.4	13	1	1	2	4	8	10	19
B. OPERATED	323	4.6	37	1	1	2	6	9	17	30
TOTAL										
0–19 Years	64	4.1	37	1	1	2	4	9	22	28
20–34	68	4.3	13	1	2	3	6	9	11	22
35–49	118	5.3	62	1	1	2	5	11	25	41
50–64	130	3.8	17	1	1	2	5	10	11	19
65+	74	3.5	12	1	1	2	5	7	9	23
GRAND TOTAL	454	4.3	30	1	1	2	5	9	14	28

Length of Stay by Diagnosis and Operation, Western Region, 2008

Western Region, October 2006–September 2007 Data, by Diagnosis

710: DIF CONNECTIVE TISS DIS

Type of Patients	Observed Patients	Avg. Stay	Variance	10th	25th	50th	75th	90th	95th	99th
1. SINGLE DX										
A. Not Operated										
0–19 Years	43	1.8	1	1	1	2	2	3	4	5
20–34	17	2.1	2	1	1	2	2	4	5	5
35–49	11	2.1	3	1	1	3	3	4	6	6
50–64	4	3.0	11	1	1	2	2	8	8	8
65+	1	1.0	0	1	1	1	1	1	1	1
B. Operated										
0–19 Years	0									
20–34	0									
35–49	1	6.0	0	6	6	6	6	6	6	6
50–64	1	5.0	0	5	5	5	5	5	5	5
65+	0									
2. MULTIPLE DX										
A. Not Operated										
0–19 Years	286	4.4	23	1	1	3	5	10	15	23
20–34	913	6.0	43	1	2	4	7	13	20	34
35–49	709	5.8	47	1	2	4	7	12	18	33
50–64	560	6.0	50	1	2	4	7	13	17	42
65+	255	6.9	50	2	3	5	8	15	19	35
B. Operated										
0–19 Years	19	10.0	70	2	4	9	12	26	35	35
20–34	70	12.0	124	3	5	9	15	26	33	73
35–49	76	10.4	83	2	5	9	15	21	31	46
50–64	84	9.8	94	2	4	7	11	27	27	70
65+	36	8.2	33	3	4	7	10	15	17	33
SUBTOTALS:										
1. SINGLE DX										
A. Not Operated	76	2.0	2	1	1	1	2	4	5	8
B. Operated	2	5.5	<1	5	5	6	6	6	6	6
2. MULTIPLE DX										
A. Not Operated	2,723	5.9	44	1	2	4	7	13	18	34
B. Operated	285	10.3	89	3	4	7	13	21	28	46
1. SINGLE DX	78	2.0	2	1	1	1	3	4	5	8
2. MULTIPLE DX	3,008	6.3	50	1	2	4	7	14	19	35
A. NOT OPERATED	2,799	5.8	43	1	2	4	7	12	18	34
B. OPERATED	287	10.3	89	3	4	7	13	21	28	46
TOTAL										
0–19 Years	348	4.3	25	1	1	2	5	10	15	26
20–34	1,000	6.4	50	1	2	4	7	14	21	34
35–49	797	6.2	52	1	2	4	7	14	19	35
50–64	649	6.5	56	1	3	4	8	14	19	42
65+	292	7.1	48	2	3	5	9	15	19	35
GRAND TOTAL	**3,086**	**6.2**	**49**	**1**	**2**	**4**	**7**	**14**	**19**	**35**

710.0: SYST LUPUS ERYTHEMATOSUS

Type of Patients	Observed Patients	Avg. Stay	Variance	10th	25th	50th	75th	90th	95th	99th
1. SINGLE DX										
A. Not Operated										
0–19 Years	22	2.1	1	1	1	2	3	3	4	5
20–34	13	2.1	2	1	1	2	3	4	5	5
35–49	9	2.3	3	1	1	2	3	4	6	6
50–64	2	4.5	24	1	1	8	8	8	8	8
65+	0									
B. Operated										
0–19 Years	0									
20–34	0									
35–49	0									
50–64	0									
65+	0									
2. MULTIPLE DX										
A. Not Operated										
0–19 Years	232	4.7	25	1	1	3	5	10	16	23
20–34	827	6.2	45	1	2	4	7	14	20	34
35–49	544	5.7	38	1	2	4	7	12	18	30
50–64	334	5.9	42	1	2	4	7	12	18	34
65+	100	6.6	49	2	3	4	8	13	18	58
B. Operated										
0–19 Years	14	10.1	67	4	5	9	12	14	35	35
20–34	52	11.7	136	3	5	9	15	25	33	73
35–49	48	9.7	76	2	4	7	15	19	21	46
50–64	40	9.8	128	2	4	9	13	18	23	70
65+	7	6.7	14	3	3	6	11	12	12	12
SUBTOTALS:										
1. SINGLE DX										
A. Not Operated	46	2.2	2	1	1	2	3	4	5	8
B. Operated	0									
2. MULTIPLE DX										
A. Not Operated	2,037	5.8	41	1	2	4	7	12	18	33
B. Operated	161	10.3	104	3	4	7	13	19	26	70
1. SINGLE DX	46	2.2	2	1	1	2	3	4	5	8
2. MULTIPLE DX	2,198	6.2	47	1	2	4	7	14	19	34
A. NOT OPERATED	2,083	5.8	40	1	2	4	7	12	18	33
B. OPERATED	161	10.3	104	3	4	7	13	19	26	70
TOTAL										
0–19 Years	268	4.7	27	1	1	3	5	10	16	26
20–34	892	6.4	52	1	2	4	7	14	21	35
35–49	601	5.9	42	1	2	4	7	13	18	31
50–64	376	6.3	52	2	2	4	8	14	18	35
65+	107	6.6	47	3	3	4	8	12	18	21
GRAND TOTAL	**2,244**	**6.1**	**46**	**1**	**2**	**4**	**7**	**14**	**19**	**34**

710.1: SYSTEMIC SCLEROSIS

Type of Patients	Observed Patients	Avg. Stay	Variance	10th	25th	50th	75th	90th	95th	99th
1. SINGLE DX										
A. Not Operated										
0–19 Years	3	1.0	0	1	1	1	1	1	1	1
20–34	0									
35–49	0									
50–64	0									
65+	0									
B. Operated										
0–19 Years	0									
20–34	0									
35–49	0									
50–64	0									
65+	0									
2. MULTIPLE DX										
A. Not Operated										
0–19 Years	5	2.4	10	1	1	1	1	8	8	8
20–34	15	6.6	34	2	3	5	7	17	21	21
35–49	52	6.5	52	2	4	5	7	13	19	48
50–64	82	7.4	67	2	3	5	8	15	20	48
65+	72	6.8	32	2	3	5	8	14	17	35
B. Operated										
0–19 Years	0									
20–34	8	12.0	96	5	5	5	19	19	19	19
35–49	8	8.9	77	2	2	5	8	27	27	27
50–64	8	12.3	76	1	6	7	19	27	27	27
65+	2	6.5	40	2	2	11	11	11	11	11
SUBTOTALS:										
1. SINGLE DX										
A. Not Operated	3	1.0	0	1	1	1	1	1	1	1
B. Operated	0									
2. MULTIPLE DX										
A. Not Operated	226	6.8	49	2	3	5	8	14	19	42
B. Operated	20	10.3	68	2	5	7	19	27	27	27
1. SINGLE DX	3	1.0	0	1	1	1	1	1	1	1
2. MULTIPLE DX	246	7.1	51	2	3	5	8	16	19	42
A. NOT OPERATED	229	6.8	49	1	3	5	7	14	19	42
B. OPERATED	20	10.3	68	2	5	7	19	27	27	27
TOTAL										
0–19 Years	8	1.9	6	1	1	1	1	8	8	8
20–34	17	7.2	39	2	3	5	7	19	21	21
35–49	60	6.8	55	2	3	5	7	16	21	48
50–64	90	7.8	69	2	3	5	10	18	21	48
65+	74	6.8	31	2	3	5	8	14	17	35
GRAND TOTAL	**249**	**7.0**	**51**	**1**	**3**	**5**	**8**	**16**	**19**	**42**

Length of Stay by Diagnosis and Operation, Western Region, 2008

710.4: POLYMYOSITIS

Type of Patients	Observed Patients	Avg. Stay	Vari-ance	Percentiles						
				10th	25th	50th	75th	90th	95th	99th
1. SINGLE DX										
A. Not Operated										
0–19 Years	0									
20–34	0									
35–49	1	1.0	0	1	1	1	1	1	1	1
50–64	0									
65+	1	1.0	0	1	1	1	1	1	1	1
B. Operated										
0–19 Years	0									
20–34	0									
35–49	1	6.0	0	6	6	6	6	6	6	6
50–64	1	5.0	0	5	5	5	5	5	5	5
65+	0									
2. MULTIPLE DX										
A. Not Operated										
0–19 Years	4	5.7	6	4	4	5	6	9	9	9
20–34	14	4.7	18	1	1	4	5	8	17	17
35–49	31	6.4	114	1	2	5	7	8	12	62
50–64	49	5.2	23	2	2	4	6	13	16	25
65+	38	6.3	19	1	3	5	8	12	18	19
B. Operated										
0–19 Years	1	2.0	0	2	2	2	2	2	2	2
20–34	10	15.0	116	7	9	9	19	39	39	39
35–49	8	11.6	97	1	5	8	14	31	31	31
50–64	19	8.7	52	3	4	7	8	25	31	31
65+	12	7.2	8	3	6	8	10	10	10	10
SUBTOTALS:										
1. SINGLE DX										
A. Not Operated	2	1.0	0	1	1	1	1	1	1	1
B. Operated	2	5.5	<1	5	5	6	6	6	6	6
2. MULTIPLE DX										
A. Not Operated	136	5.8	41	1	2	4	7	10	16	25
B. Operated	50	9.9	66	3	5	8	10	20	31	39
1. SINGLE DX	4	3.2	7	1	1	1	5	6	6	6
2. MULTIPLE DX	186	6.9	51	2	3	5	8	13	19	39
A. NOT OPERATED	138	5.7	41	1	2	4	7	10	16	25
B. OPERATED	52	9.8	64	3	5	8	10	20	31	39
TOTAL										
0–19 Years	5	5.0	7	2	4	4	6	9	9	9
20–34	24	9.0	82	1	2	4	9	19	28	39
35–49	41	7.3	108	1	2	5	7	12	20	62
50–64	69	6.2	32	2	3	4	7	13	19	31
65+	51	6.4	16	2	3	6	8	10	14	19
GRAND TOTAL	190	6.8	50	2	3	5	8	12	19	39

711: ARTHROPATHY W INFECTION

Type of Patients	Observed Patients	Avg. Stay	Vari-ance	Percentiles						
				10th	25th	50th	75th	90th	95th	99th
1. SINGLE DX										
A. Not Operated										
0–19 Years	23	3.6	9	1	1	2	4	9	10	11
20–34	4	2.8	<1	2	2	3	4	4	4	4
35–49	6	2.5	2	1	2	2	3	5	5	5
50–64	8	2.4	3	1	1	2	3	5	5	5
65+	2	1.5	<1	1	1	1	2	2	2	2
B. Operated										
0–19 Years	55	4.5	6	2	3	4	6	8	10	12
20–34	25	3.4	2	1	3	3	4	5	6	8
35–49	23	4.2	8	1	2	4	5	9	9	11
50–64	11	3.3	1	2	2	3	5	5	5	5
65+	6	7.9	19	4	4	7	11	15	15	15
2. MULTIPLE DX										
A. Not Operated										
0–19 Years	56	5.8	19	1	3	4	7	12	15	20
20–34	88	4.3	11	2	3	4	6	7	9	27
35–49	171	6.0	39	2	3	4	7	12	19	40
50–64	236	6.5	45	2	3	4	8	13	20	29
65+	375	6.1	27	2	3	5	7	12	14	25
B. Operated										
0–19 Years	174	6.9	42	2	3	5	8	13	19	37
20–34	322	6.2	41	2	3	4	7	14	20	29
35–49	603	6.9	39	2	3	5	8	14	19	29
50–64	777	7.8	59	2	4	6	9	15	22	39
65+	773	7.6	32	3	4	6	9	15	19	29
SUBTOTALS:										
1. SINGLE DX										
A. Not Operated	43	3.0	6	1	1	2	4	6	9	11
B. Operated	120	4.3	7	2	3	4	5	8	9	12
2. MULTIPLE DX										
A. Not Operated	926	6.0	32	2	3	4	7	12	15	27
B. Operated	2,649	7.3	43	2	3	5	9	15	20	32
1. SINGLE DX	163	4.0	7	1	2	3	5	8	9	12
2. MULTIPLE DX	3,575	6.9	41	2	3	5	8	14	19	30
A. NOT OPERATED	969	5.9	31	2	3	4	7	12	14	27
B. OPERATED	2,769	7.1	42	2	3	5	9	14	20	31
TOTAL										
0–19 Years	308	6.0	30	2	3	5	7	11	15	29
20–34	439	5.7	34	2	3	4	6	12	17	27
35–49	803	6.6	38	2	3	5	7	14	19	29
50–64	1,032	7.4	55	2	3	5	9	15	21	38
65+	1,156	7.1	31	2	4	5	9	13	18	28
GRAND TOTAL	3,738	6.8	40	2	3	5	8	13	19	29

711.01: PYOGEN ARTHRITIS-SHOULD

Type of Patients	Observed Patients	Avg. Stay	Vari-ance	Percentiles						
				10th	25th	50th	75th	90th	95th	99th
1. SINGLE DX										
A. Not Operated										
0–19 Years	0									
20–34	0									
35–49	0									
50–64	0									
65+	0									
B. Operated										
0–19 Years	1	10.0	0	10	10	10	10	10	10	10
20–34	0									
35–49	1	1.0	0	1	1	1	1	1	1	1
50–64	0									
65+	1	7.0	0	7	7	7	7	7	7	7
2. MULTIPLE DX										
A. Not Operated										
0–19 Years	2	3.0	8	1	1	3	5	5	5	5
20–34	4	3.2	4	2	2	2	3	6	6	6
35–49	11	12.3	172	2	4	5	25	26	42	42
50–64	24	6.6	28	2	3	5	7	13	16	24
65+	34	6.6	26	3	4	5	6	13	22	22
B. Operated										
0–19 Years	2	7.5	4	6	6	9	9	9	9	9
20–34	12	10.7	63	3	6	7	15	22	24	24
35–49	49	9.7	58	2	5	7	13	18	21	43
50–64	72	8.2	41	3	5	6	10	14	20	46
65+	130	7.6	30	3	4	6	9	13	21	26
SUBTOTALS:										
1. SINGLE DX										
A. Not Operated	0									
B. Operated	3	6.0	21	1	1	7	10	10	10	10
2. MULTIPLE DX										
A. Not Operated	75	7.2	49	2	3	5	7	16	24	42
B. Operated	265	8.3	40	3	4	6	11	17	21	29
1. SINGLE DX	3	6.0	21	1	1	7	10	10	10	10
2. MULTIPLE DX	340	8.0	42	3	4	6	10	17	22	29
A. NOT OPERATED	75	7.2	49	2	3	5	7	16	24	42
B. OPERATED	268	8.3	40	3	4	6	11	17	21	29
TOTAL										
0–19 Years	5	6.2	13	1	5	6	9	10	10	10
20–34	16	8.9	58	2	3	6	13	22	24	24
35–49	61	10.0	77	2	4	7	13	19	26	43
50–64	96	7.8	38	3	4	6	9	13	20	46
65+	165	7.4	29	3	4	6	9	13	21	26
GRAND TOTAL	343	8.0	42	3	4	6	10	17	22	29

Length of Stay by Diagnosis and Operation, Western Region, 2008

Western Region, October 2006–September 2007 Data, by Diagnosis

711.04: PYOGEN ARTHRITIS-HAND

Type of Patients	Observed Patients	Avg. Stay	Variance	Percentiles						
				10th	25th	50th	75th	90th	95th	99th
1. SINGLE DX										
A. Not Operated										
0–19 Years	1	11.0	0	11	11	11	11	11	11	11
20–34	0									
35–49	0									
50–64	0									
65+	1	2.0	0	2	2	2	2	2	2	2
B. Operated										
0–19 Years	2	2.5	<1	2	2	3	3	3	3	3
20–34	6	3.3	2	1	3	3	3	5	5	5
35–49	9	3.0	2	1	2	3	4	5	5	5
50–64	0									
65+	1	4.0	0	4	4	4	4	4	4	4
2. MULTIPLE DX										
A. Not Operated										
0–19 Years	3	5.3	10	3	3	4	4	9	9	9
20–34	10	3.2	2	1	2	3	4	5	6	6
35–49	7	3.6	<1	2	3	3	4	5	5	5
50–64	8	4.0	4	2	3	3	6	6	6	6
65+	10	5.1	14	1	2	5	7	14	14	14
B. Operated										
0–19 Years	17	3.5	5	1	2	3	4	7	10	10
20–34	102	4.0	8	1	2	3	5	7	9	15
35–49	80	4.4	14	2	2	3	5	8	13	27
50–64	60	4.0	5	2	2	3	5	7	8	15
65+	44	4.2	10	2	2	3	5	7	7	18
SUBTOTALS:										
1. SINGLE DX										
A. Not Operated	2	6.5	41	2	2	7	11	11	11	11
B. Operated	18	3.1	2	1	2	3	4	5	5	5
2. MULTIPLE DX										
A. Not Operated	38	4.1	6	2	2	4	5	7	9	14
B. Operated	303	4.1	9	2	2	3	5	7	9	17
1. SINGLE DX	20	3.4	5	1	2	3	4	5	5	5
2. MULTIPLE DX	341	4.1	9	2	2	3	5	7	9	17
A. NOT OPERATED	40	4.2	7	2	2	4	5	7	9	14
B. OPERATED	321	4.0	9	2	2	3	5	7	9	17
TOTAL										
0–19 Years	23	4.0	8	2	2	3	4	9	10	11
20–34	118	3.9	7	1	2	3	5	7	9	15
35–49	96	4.2	12	2	2	3	5	7	9	27
50–64	68	4.0	5	2	2	3	5	6	8	15
65+	56	4.3	10	2	2	3	5	7	14	18
GRAND TOTAL	361	4.1	9	2	2	3	5	7	9	17

711.05: PYOGEN ARTHRITIS-PELVIS

Type of Patients	Observed Patients	Avg. Stay	Variance	Percentiles						
				10th	25th	50th	75th	90th	95th	99th
1. SINGLE DX										
A. Not Operated										
0–19 Years	5	1.8	2	1	1	1	2	4	4	4
20–34	1	2.0	0	2	2	2	2	2	2	2
35–49	0									
50–64	0									
65+	0									
B. Operated										
0–19 Years	19	5.6	8	2	3	5	8	10	12	12
20–34	3	4.7	1	4	4	4	6	6	6	6
35–49	2	5.5	12	3	3	3	8	8	8	8
50–64	1	3.0	0	3	3	3	3	3	3	3
65+	0									
2. MULTIPLE DX										
A. Not Operated										
0–19 Years	13	6.2	16	2	3	5	9	12	14	14
20–34	5	7.0	1	6	6	7	8	8	8	8
35–49	19	9.7	89	2	3	6	13	24	40	40
50–64	29	7.6	50	2	3	5	10	20	28	29
65+	26	6.9	24	2	3	5	10	14	18	19
B. Operated										
0–19 Years	55	8.6	61	3	4	7	10	14	19	49
20–34	19	8.3	43	4	5	6	10	20	26	26
35–49	42	8.9	48	4	5	6	10	19	27	32
50–64	56	11.5	124	4	5	8	14	21	38	67
65+	62	8.7	19	4	6	8	11	14	17	20
SUBTOTALS:										
1. SINGLE DX										
A. Not Operated	6	1.8	1	1	1	2	2	4	4	4
B. Operated	25	5.4	7	3	3	5	7	9	10	12
2. MULTIPLE DX										
A. Not Operated	92	7.6	43	2	3	6	9	14	20	40
B. Operated	234	9.3	62	3	5	7	11	17	21	39
1. SINGLE DX	31	4.7	8	2	3	4	6	8	10	12
2. MULTIPLE DX	326	8.9	57	3	4	7	11	17	21	39
A. NOT OPERATED	98	7.3	43	2	3	5	9	14	20	40
B. OPERATED	259	9.0	58	3	5	7	10	17	20	39
TOTAL										
0–19 Years	92	7.3	43	2	3	6	9	12	14	49
20–34	28	7.5	31	2	4	6	9	16	20	26
35–49	63	9.0	58	3	4	6	10	19	27	40
50–64	86	10.1	101	3	4	7	12	21	29	67
65+	88	8.2	21	3	5	7	11	14	18	20
GRAND TOTAL	357	8.5	54	3	4	7	10	16	20	39

711.06: PYOGEN ARTHRITIS-LOW LEG

Type of Patients	Observed Patients	Avg. Stay	Variance	Percentiles						
				10th	25th	50th	75th	90th	95th	99th
1. SINGLE DX										
A. Not Operated										
0–19 Years	10	2.2	<1	1	2	2	3	4	4	4
20–34	3	3.0	<1	2	2	3	4	4	4	4
35–49	5	2.6	2	1	2	2	3	5	5	5
50–64	6	2.2	3	1	1	2	3	5	5	5
65+	0									
B. Operated										
0–19 Years	20	3.9	4	1	2	3	6	7	7	7
20–34	10	3.9	3	2	3	4	7	7	8	8
35–49	7	6.9	8	4	4	7	9	11	11	11
50–64	6	3.3	2	2	2	3	5	5	5	5
65+	2	10.5	40	6	6	15	15	15	15	15
2. MULTIPLE DX										
A. Not Operated										
0–19 Years	23	5.3	19	1	3	4	6	10	15	19
20–34	44	4.6	17	2	2	4	5	7	9	27
35–49	90	4.9	16	1	2	4	6	9	13	27
50–64	115	7.3	64	2	3	4	9	14	23	39
65+	179	6.4	33	2	3	5	8	11	13	42
B. Operated										
0–19 Years	66	6.1	27	2	3	5	7	13	19	24
20–34	132	7.4	59	2	3	5	9	15	24	31
35–49	302	7.2	36	2	3	5	9	15	22	28
50–64	432	8.2	66	3	4	6	9	16	23	49
65+	367	8.3	41	3	4	6	11	17	22	32
SUBTOTALS:										
1. SINGLE DX										
A. Not Operated	24	2.4	1	1	2	2	3	4	5	5
B. Operated	45	4.6	7	2	3	4	6	8	9	15
2. MULTIPLE DX										
A. Not Operated	451	6.1	36	2	3	5	7	12	14	27
B. Operated	1,299	7.8	50	3	4	5	9	16	23	32
1. SINGLE DX	69	3.8	6	1	2	3	5	7	9	15
2. MULTIPLE DX	1,750	7.4	47	2	3	5	9	15	21	32
A. NOT OPERATED	475	5.9	35	2	3	4	7	12	14	27
B. OPERATED	1,344	7.7	49	3	4	5	9	16	22	32
TOTAL										
0–19 Years	119	5.2	21	2	2	4	6	11	16	23
20–34	189	6.5	47	2	3	5	7	13	23	31
35–49	404	6.6	32	2	3	5	8	14	19	28
50–64	559	7.9	65	3	4	5	9	16	23	49
65+	548	7.7	39	3	4	6	10	15	20	32
GRAND TOTAL	1,819	7.2	46	2	3	5	9	15	21	32

Length of Stay by Diagnosis and Operation, Western Region, 2008

Western Region, October 2006–September 2007 Data, by Diagnosis

711.07: PYOGEN ARTHRITIS-ANKLE

Type of Patients	Observed Patients	Avg. Stay	Variance	10th	25th	50th	75th	90th	95th	99th
1. SINGLE DX										
A. *Not Operated*										
0–19 Years	1	6.0	0	6	6	6	6	6	6	6
20–34	0									
35–49	0									
50–64	0									
65+	0									
B. *Operated*										
0–19 Years	9	4.1	4	2	3	4	5	8	8	8
20–34	3	2.3	2	1	1	2	4	4	4	4
35–49	1	4.0	0	4	4	4	4	4	4	4
50–64	0									
65+	1	4.0	0	4	4	4	4	4	4	4
2. MULTIPLE DX										
A. *Not Operated*										
0–19 Years	6	8.0	44	2	2	7	10	20	20	20
20–34	8	4.3	12	1	2	4	6	12	12	12
35–49	12	5.6	22	2	3	4	6	9	19	19
50–64	10	3.5	3	2	3	3	4	8	8	8
65+	27	7.2	37	3	4	5	9	17	20	28
B. *Operated*										
0–19 Years	18	6.7	29	3	4	5	7	13	26	26
20–34	17	6.7	73	1	3	3	6	14	36	36
35–49	53	6.7	27	2	3	5	9	14	17	28
50–64	61	6.7	31	2	3	5	8	11	18	29
65+	54	6.6	22	3	4	5	8	11	14	26
SUBTOTALS:										
1. SINGLE DX										
A. *Not Operated*	1	6.0	0	6	6	6	6	6	6	6
B. *Operated*	14	3.7	3	2	2	4	5	5	8	8
2. MULTIPLE DX										
A. *Not Operated*	63	6.0	27	2	3	4	7	12	19	28
B. *Operated*	203	6.7	30	2	3	5	8	13	17	28
1. SINGLE DX	15	3.9	3	2	2	4	5	6	8	8
2. MULTIPLE DX	266	6.5	29	2	3	5	8	13	18	28
A. NOT OPERATED	64	6.0	27	2	3	4	7	12	19	28
B. OPERATED	217	6.5	29	2	3	5	8	13	17	28
TOTAL										
0–19 Years	34	6.2	24	2	4	5	7	10	20	26
20–34	28	5.5	49	1	2	3	4	13	14	36
35–49	66	6.5	26	2	3	4	8	14	17	28
50–64	71	6.3	28	2	3	5	8	10	18	29
65+	82	6.8	26	3	4	5	8	12	17	28
GRAND TOTAL	281	6.4	28	2	3	5	7	12	17	28

712: CRYSTAL ARTHROPATHIES

Type of Patients	Observed Patients	Avg. Stay	Variance	10th	25th	50th	75th	90th	95th	99th
1. SINGLE DX										
A. *Not Operated*										
0–19 Years	0									
20–34	0									
35–49	0									
50–64	0									
65+	0									
B. *Operated*										
0–19 Years	0									
20–34	0									
35–49	0									
50–64	0									
65+	0									
2. MULTIPLE DX										
A. *Not Operated*										
0–19 Years	0									
20–34	0									
35–49	0									
50–64	0									
65+	1	4.0	0	4	4	4	4	4	4	4
B. *Operated*										
0–19 Years	0									
20–34	0									
35–49	0									
50–64	0									
65+	0									
SUBTOTALS:										
1. SINGLE DX										
A. *Not Operated*	0									
B. *Operated*	0									
2. MULTIPLE DX										
A. *Not Operated*	1	4.0	0	4	4	4	4	4	4	4
B. *Operated*	0									
1. SINGLE DX	0									
2. MULTIPLE DX	1	4.0	0	4	4	4	4	4	4	4
A. NOT OPERATED	1	4.0	0	4	4	4	4	4	4	4
B. OPERATED	0									
TOTAL										
0–19 Years	0									
20–34	0									
35–49	0									
50–64	0									
65+	1	4.0	0	4	4	4	4	4	4	4
GRAND TOTAL	1	4.0	0	4	4	4	4	4	4	4

713: ARTHROPATHY IN CCE

Type of Patients	Observed Patients	Avg. Stay	Variance	10th	25th	50th	75th	90th	95th	99th
1. SINGLE DX										
A. *Not Operated*										
0–19 Years	0									
20–34	0									
35–49	0									
50–64	0									
65+	0									
B. *Operated*										
0–19 Years	0									
20–34	0									
35–49	0									
50–64	0									
65+	0									
2. MULTIPLE DX										
A. *Not Operated*										
0–19 Years	0									
20–34	0									
35–49	0									
50–64	0									
65+	0									
B. *Operated*										
0–19 Years	0									
20–34	0									
35–49	0									
50–64	0									
65+	0									
SUBTOTALS:										
1. SINGLE DX										
A. *Not Operated*	0									
B. *Operated*	0									
2. MULTIPLE DX										
A. *Not Operated*	0									
B. *Operated*	0									
1. SINGLE DX	0									
2. MULTIPLE DX	0									
A. NOT OPERATED	0									
B. OPERATED	0									
TOTAL										
0–19 Years	0									
20–34	0									
35–49	0									
50–64	0									
65+	0									
GRAND TOTAL	0									

Length of Stay by Diagnosis and Operation, Western Region, 2008

Western Region, October 2006–September 2007 Data, by Diagnosis

714: RA & INFLAM POLYARTHROP

Type of Patients	Observed Patients	Avg. Stay	Vari-ance	10th	25th	50th	75th	90th	95th	99th
1. SINGLE DX										
A. Not Operated										
0–19 Years	12	2.4	5	1	1	1	3	5	5	8
20–34	5	3.4	3	2	2	3	4	6	6	6
35–49	7	2.4	5	1	2	1	3	7	7	7
50–64	9	5.5	93	1	1	2	4	31	31	31
65+	2	3.5	4	2	2	4	5	5	5	5
B. Operated										
0–19 Years	3	2.3	<1	2	2	2	3	3	3	3
20–34	11	2.4	2	2	1	2	3	4	6	6
35–49	11	2.9	<1	2	2	3	3	4	4	4
50–64	24	3.0	2	2	2	3	3	5	5	7
65+	22	3.1	1	2	2	3	4	4	4	5
2. MULTIPLE DX										
A. Not Operated										
0–19 Years	53	3.5	9	1	1	3	4	8	8	14
20–34	86	4.9	30	1	2	3	6	9	11	43
35–49	159	4.0	36	1	2	3	5	7	10	27
50–64	315	4.3	27	1	2	3	5	8	11	24
65+	501	4.7	16	2	2	4	6	9	11	19
B. Operated										
0–19 Years	10	5.5	12	2	3	4	7	13	13	13
20–34	70	3.5	3	2	3	3	4	5	7	9
35–49	219	3.4	3	2	3	3	4	5	7	9
50–64	604	3.4	4	2	3	3	4	5	6	12
65+	526	3.6	8	2	3	3	4	5	7	14
SUBTOTALS:										
1. SINGLE DX										
A. Not Operated	35	3.4	27	1	1	2	4	7	8	31
B. Operated	71	2.9	1	2	2	3	4	4	5	7
2. MULTIPLE DX										
A. Not Operated	1,114	4.4	23	1	2	3	5	9	11	20
B. Operated	1,429	3.5	5	2	3	3	4	5	6	13
1. SINGLE DX	106	3.1	10	1	2	3	4	5	5	8
2. MULTIPLE DX	2,543	3.9	13	1	2	3	4	7	9	17
A. NOT OPERATED	1,149	4.4	23	1	2	3	5	8	11	21
B. OPERATED	1,500	3.5	5	2	2	3	4	5	7	13
TOTAL										
0–19 Years	78	3.6	9	1	1	3	4	8	11	14
20–34	172	4.1	17	2	2	3	5	8	9	21
35–49	396	3.6	17	1	2	3	4	6	8	15
50–64	952	3.7	12	2	2	3	4	6	9	17
65+	1,051	4.1	12	2	3	3	5	7	9	18
GRAND TOTAL	2,649	3.9	13	1	2	3	4	7	9	17

714.0: RHEUMATOID ARTHRITIS

Type of Patients	Observed Patients	Avg. Stay	Vari-ance	10th	25th	50th	75th	90th	95th	99th
1. SINGLE DX										
A. Not Operated										
0–19 Years	3	3.0	4	1	1	3	3	5	5	5
20–34	1	2.0	0	2	2	2	2	2	2	2
35–49	4	1.0	0	1	1	1	1	1	1	1
50–64	5	1.8	2	1	1	1	2	4	4	4
65+	2	3.5	4	2	2	4	5	5	5	5
B. Operated										
0–19 Years	0									
20–34	7	2.1	1	1	1	2	3	4	4	4
35–49	10	2.8	<1	2	3	3	3	3	4	4
50–64	21	3.0	2	2	2	3	3	4	5	7
65+	22	3.1	1	2	2	3	4	4	4	5
2. MULTIPLE DX										
A. Not Operated										
0–19 Years	3	3.7	14	1	2	2	2	8	8	8
20–34	42	5.0	50	1	2	3	4	9	11	43
35–49	108	3.2	7	1	1	2	4	7	9	10
50–64	236	3.9	25	1	2	3	5	7	10	19
65+	375	4.3	9	1	2	3	5	9	10	16
B. Operated										
0–19 Years	0									
20–34	41	3.4	2	2	3	3	4	5	7	8
35–49	193	3.4	3	2	2	3	4	5	7	10
50–64	546	3.2	2	2	2	3	4	5	5	10
65+	497	3.5	6	2	3	3	4	5	6	13
SUBTOTALS:										
1. SINGLE DX										
A. Not Operated	15	2.1	2	1	1	2	3	5	5	5
B. Operated	60	2.9	1	2	2	3	3	4	5	7
2. MULTIPLE DX										
A. Not Operated	764	4.1	16	1	2	3	5	8	10	19
B. Operated	1,277	3.4	4	2	2	3	4	5	6	10
1. SINGLE DX	75	2.7	2	1	2	3	3	4	5	7
2. MULTIPLE DX	2,041	3.6	9	1	2	3	4	6	8	13
A. NOT OPERATED	779	4.0	16	1	2	3	5	8	10	19
B. OPERATED	1,337	3.3	4	2	2	3	4	5	6	10
TOTAL										
0–19 Years	6	3.3	7	1	1	2	2	8	8	8
20–34	91	4.0	25	1	2	3	4	7	9	43
35–49	315	3.3	4	1	2	3	4	6	8	10
50–64	808	3.4	9	1	2	3	4	5	7	12
65+	896	3.8	8	2	2	3	4	6	9	14
GRAND TOTAL	2,116	3.6	9	1	2	3	4	6	8	13

715: OSTEOARTHROSIS ET AL

Type of Patients	Observed Patients	Avg. Stay	Vari-ance	10th	25th	50th	75th	90th	95th	99th
1. SINGLE DX										
A. Not Operated										
0–19 Years	0									
20–34	0									
35–49	2	2.0	2	1	1	2	3	3	3	3
50–64	34	2.0	1	1	1	1	3	3	3	5
65+	17	2.5	6	1	1	2	3	4	11	11
B. Operated										
0–19 Years	3	2.7	2	1	1	3	3	4	4	4
20–34	43	2.5	2	1	2	2	3	3	4	11
35–49	756	2.9	1	2	2	3	3	4	5	7
50–64	2,977	2.9	1	2	3	3	3	4	5	6
65+	2,241	3.1	1	2	3	3	4	4	5	6
2. MULTIPLE DX										
A. Not Operated										
0–19 Years	0									
20–34	10	3.6	10	1	1	3	7	7	9	9
35–49	77	3.4	7	1	1	3	4	8	10	10
50–64	412	2.7	8	1	1	3	3	6	8	13
65+	1,537	3.4	10	1	1	3	4	7	9	15
B. Operated										
0–19 Years	10	2.4	<1	1	2	3	3	3	3	3
20–34	312	3.2	5	2	2	3	4	5	6	9
35–49	5,531	3.2	2	2	2	3	4	5	5	8
50–64	39,523	3.3	2	2	3	3	4	5	5	8
65+	70,167	3.6	3	2	3	3	4	5	6	9
SUBTOTALS:										
1. SINGLE DX										
A. Not Operated	53	2.2	3	1	1	1	3	3	4	11
B. Operated	6,020	3.0	1	2	2	3	3	4	5	6
2. MULTIPLE DX										
A. Not Operated	2,036	3.3	10	1	1	3	4	7	9	15
B. Operated	115,543	3.5	3	2	3	3	4	5	6	9
1. SINGLE DX	6,073	3.0	1	2	2	3	3	4	5	6
2. MULTIPLE DX	117,579	3.5	3	2	3	3	4	5	6	9
A. NOT OPERATED	2,089	3.3	9	1	1	3	4	7	9	15
B. OPERATED	121,563	3.5	3	2	3	3	4	5	6	9
TOTAL										
0–19 Years	13	2.5	<1	1	2	3	3	3	4	4
20–34	365	3.1	5	1	2	3	4	5	6	10
35–49	6,366	3.2	2	2	2	3	4	5	5	8
50–64	42,946	3.3	2	2	3	3	4	5	5	8
65+	73,962	3.6	3	2	3	3	4	5	6	9
GRAND TOTAL	123,652	3.5	3	2	3	3	4	5	6	9

Length of Stay by Diagnosis and Operation, Western Region, 2008

Western Region, October 2006–September 2007 Data, by Diagnosis

715.11: LOC PRIMARY OA-SHOULDER

Type of Patients	Observed Patients	Avg. Stay	Vari-ance	10th	25th	50th	75th	90th	95th	99th
1. SINGLE DX										
A. Not Operated										
0–19 Years	0									
20–34	0									
35–49	0									
50–64	0									
65+	0									
B. Operated										
0–19 Years	0									
20–34	0									
35–49	0									
50–64	12	2.0	<1	1	1	2	2	3	4	4
65+	13	1.9	<1	1	1	2	2	3	4	4
2. MULTIPLE DX										
A. Not Operated										
0–19 Years	0									
20–34	0									
35–49	1	2.0	0	2	2	2	2	2	2	2
50–64	0									
65+	5	2.6	3	1	1	2	4	5	5	5
B. Operated										
0–19 Years	1	1.0	0	1	1	1	1	1	1	1
20–34	0									
35–49	16	2.1	<1	1	2	2	3	3	3	3
50–64	78	2.2	1	1	2	2	3	4	4	6
65+	228	2.5	5	1	2	2	3	4	5	7
SUBTOTALS:										
1. SINGLE DX										
A. Not Operated	0									
B. Operated	25	2.0	<1	1	1	2	2	3	4	4
2. MULTIPLE DX										
A. Not Operated	6	2.5	3	1	1	2	4	5	5	5
B. Operated	323	2.4	4	1	2	2	3	3	4	7
1. SINGLE DX	25	2.0	<1	1	1	2	2	3	4	4
2. MULTIPLE DX	329	2.4	4	1	2	2	3	4	4	7
A. NOT OPERATED	6	2.5	3	1	1	2	4	5	5	5
B. OPERATED	348	2.4	4	1	2	2	3	3	4	7
TOTAL										
0–19 Years	1	1.0	0	1	1	1	1	1	1	1
20–34	0									
35–49	17	2.1	<1	1	2	2	3	3	3	3
50–64	90	2.2	1	1	2	2	3	4	4	6
65+	246	2.5	5	1	2	2	3	4	5	7
GRAND TOTAL	354	2.4	4	1	2	2	3	4	4	7

715.15: LOC PRIMARY OA-PELVIS

Type of Patients	Observed Patients	Avg. Stay	Vari-ance	10th	25th	50th	75th	90th	95th	99th
1. SINGLE DX										
A. Not Operated										
0–19 Years	0									
20–34	0									
35–49	0									
50–64	1	2.0	0	2	2	2	2	2	2	2
65+	1	4.0	0	4	4	4	4	4	4	4
B. Operated										
0–19 Years	0									
20–34	2	7.0	32	3	3	7	11	11	11	11
35–49	37	2.9	<1	2	2	3	3	4	4	5
50–64	77	3.3	2	2	3	3	4	5	6	10
65+	34	3.2	<1	2	3	3	4	4	5	5
2. MULTIPLE DX										
A. Not Operated										
0–19 Years	0									
20–34	0									
35–49	3	3.7	14	1	1	2	8	8	8	8
50–64	4	3.5	19	1	1	1	10	10	10	10
65+	20	2.8	4	1	1	3	3	4	5	10
B. Operated										
0–19 Years	0									
20–34	13	3.2	2	2	2	3	4	5	6	6
35–49	139	3.3	1	2	3	3	4	5	6	7
50–64	743	3.4	2	2	3	3	4	5	6	8
65+	1,232	3.7	3	2	3	3	4	5	6	9
SUBTOTALS:										
1. SINGLE DX										
A. Not Operated	2	3.0	2	2	2	3	4	4	4	4
B. Operated	150	3.2	2	2	3	3	4	4	5	10
2. MULTIPLE DX										
A. Not Operated	27	3.0	7	1	1	2	3	8	10	10
B. Operated	2,127	3.5	2	2	3	3	4	5	6	9
1. SINGLE DX	152	3.2	2	2	3	3	4	4	5	10
2. MULTIPLE DX	2,154	3.5	2	2	3	3	4	5	6	9
A. NOT OPERATED	29	3.0	6	1	1	2	3	8	10	10
B. OPERATED	2,277	3.5	2	2	3	3	4	5	6	9
TOTAL										
0–19 Years	0									
20–34	15	3.7	6	2	2	3	4	6	11	11
35–49	179	3.2	1	2	3	3	4	5	5	8
50–64	825	3.4	2	2	3	3	4	5	6	10
65+	1,287	3.6	3	2	3	3	4	5	6	10
GRAND TOTAL	2,306	3.5	2	2	3	3	4	5	6	9

715.16: LOC PRIMARY OA-LOWER LEG

Type of Patients	Observed Patients	Avg. Stay	Vari-ance	10th	25th	50th	75th	90th	95th	99th
1. SINGLE DX										
A. Not Operated										
0–19 Years	0									
20–34	0									
35–49	0									
50–64	0									
65+	0									
B. Operated										
0–19 Years	1	4.0	0	4	4	4	4	4	4	4
20–34	0									
35–49	26	2.9	2	1	2	3	3	4	6	7
50–64	152	3.2	1	2	3	3	4	5	5	6
65+	115	3.0	1	2	3	3	4	4	5	6
2. MULTIPLE DX										
A. Not Operated										
0–19 Years	0									
20–34	0									
35–49	5	4.2	5	1	4	4	5	7	7	7
50–64	15	1.8	2	1	1	1	2	4	6	6
65+	43	3.8	22	1	1	2	4	7	10	28
B. Operated										
0–19 Years	0									
20–34	1	4.0	0	4	4	4	4	4	4	4
35–49	187	3.0	1	2	2	3	4	4	5	7
50–64	1,763	3.3	2	2	3	3	4	5	6	8
65+	3,144	3.5	2	2	3	3	4	5	6	9
SUBTOTALS:										
1. SINGLE DX										
A. Not Operated	0									
B. Operated	294	3.1	1	2	3	3	4	5	5	7
2. MULTIPLE DX										
A. Not Operated	63	3.3	17	1	1	2	4	7	7	28
B. Operated	5,095	3.4	2	2	3	3	4	5	6	8
1. SINGLE DX	294	3.1	1	2	3	3	4	5	5	7
2. MULTIPLE DX	5,158	3.4	2	2	3	3	4	5	6	8
A. NOT OPERATED	63	3.3	17	1	1	2	4	7	7	28
B. OPERATED	5,389	3.4	2	2	3	3	4	5	6	8
TOTAL										
0–19 Years	1	4.0	0	4	4	4	4	4	4	4
20–34	1	4.0	0	4	4	4	4	4	4	4
35–49	218	3.1	1	2	3	3	4	5	5	7
50–64	1,930	3.3	2	2	3	3	4	5	6	8
65+	3,302	3.5	3	2	3	3	4	5	6	9
GRAND TOTAL	5,452	3.4	2	2	3	3	4	5	6	8

Length of Stay by Diagnosis and Operation, Western Region, 2008

599

Western Region, October 2006–September 2007 Data, by Diagnosis

715.25: LOC SECONDARY OA-PELVIS

Type of Patients	Observed Patients	Avg. Stay	Variance	10th	25th	50th	75th	90th	95th	99th
1. SINGLE DX										
A. Not Operated										
0–19 Years	0									
20–34	0									
35–49	0									
50–64	0									
65+	0									
B. Operated										
0–19 Years	0									
20–34	0									
35–49	4	3.3	<1	3	3	3	3	4	4	4
50–64	2	3.5	<1	3	3	3	4	4	4	4
65+	3	3.0	<1	2	2	3	4	4	4	4
2. MULTIPLE DX										
A. Not Operated										
0–19 Years	0									
20–34	0									
35–49	0									
50–64	1	1.0	0	1	1	1	1	1	1	1
65+	1	4.0	0	4	4	4	4	4	4	4
B. Operated										
0–19 Years	2	3.0	0	3	3	3	3	3	3	3
20–34	20	5.0	47	2	2	3	4	10	33	33
35–49	92	3.2	1	2	2	3	4	5	5	7
50–64	144	3.5	2	2	3	3	4	5	6	7
65+	89	3.8	2	3	3	3	4	5	6	12
SUBTOTALS:										
1. SINGLE DX										
A. Not Operated	0									
B. Operated	9	3.2	<1	2	3	3	4	4	4	4
2. MULTIPLE DX										
A. Not Operated	2	2.5	4	1	1	3	4	4	4	4
B. Operated	347	3.6	4	2	3	3	4	4	6	8
1. SINGLE DX	9	3.2	<1	2	3	3	4	4	4	4
2. MULTIPLE DX	349	3.6	4	2	3	3	4	5	6	8
A. NOT OPERATED	2	2.5	4	1	1	3	4	4	4	4
B. OPERATED	356	3.6	4	2	3	3	4	5	6	8
TOTAL										
0–19 Years	2	3.0	0	3	3	3	3	3	3	3
20–34	20	5.0	47	2	3	3	4	10	33	33
35–49	96	3.2	1	2	3	3	4	4	5	7
50–64	147	3.4	2	2	3	3	4	4	6	7
65+	93	3.8	2	3	3	3	4	5	6	12
GRAND TOTAL	358	3.6	4	2	3	3	4	5	6	8

715.26: LOC SECONDARY OA-LOW LEG

Type of Patients	Observed Patients	Avg. Stay	Variance	10th	25th	50th	75th	90th	95th	99th
1. SINGLE DX										
A. Not Operated										
0–19 Years	0									
20–34	0									
35–49	0									
50–64	0									
65+	0									
B. Operated										
0–19 Years	0									
20–34	0									
35–49	4	3.3	<1	3	3	3	4	4	4	4
50–64	14	3.2	<1	3	3	3	4	4	4	4
65+	3	2.7	<1	2	2	3	3	3	3	3
2. MULTIPLE DX										
A. Not Operated										
0–19 Years	0									
20–34	0									
35–49	0									
50–64	1	3.0	0	3	3	3	3	3	3	3
65+	1	2.0	0	2	2	2	2	2	2	2
B. Operated										
0–19 Years	0									
20–34	4	3.3	2	3	3	3	5	5	5	5
35–49	103	3.3	2	2	3	3	4	5	5	7
50–64	256	3.3	1	2	3	3	4	4	5	7
65+	116	3.7	2	2	3	3	4	5	6	8
SUBTOTALS:										
1. SINGLE DX										
A. Not Operated	0									
B. Operated	21	3.1	<1	3	3	3	4	4	4	4
2. MULTIPLE DX										
A. Not Operated	2	2.5	<1	2	2	3	3	3	3	3
B. Operated	479	3.4	1	2	3	3	4	5	5	8
1. SINGLE DX	21	3.1	<1	3	3	3	4	4	4	4
2. MULTIPLE DX	481	3.4	1	2	3	3	4	5	5	8
A. NOT OPERATED	2	2.5	<1	2	2	3	3	3	3	3
B. OPERATED	500	3.4	1	2	3	3	4	5	5	8
TOTAL										
0–19 Years	0									
20–34	4	3.3	2	2	3	3	5	5	5	5
35–49	107	3.3	2	2	3	3	4	4	5	7
50–64	271	3.3	<1	2	3	3	4	4	5	7
65+	120	3.7	2	2	3	3	4	5	6	8
GRAND TOTAL	502	3.4	1	2	3	3	4	5	5	8

715.31: LOC OA NOS-SHOULDER

Type of Patients	Observed Patients	Avg. Stay	Variance	10th	25th	50th	75th	90th	95th	99th
1. SINGLE DX										
A. Not Operated										
0–19 Years	0									
20–34	0									
35–49	0									
50–64	0									
65+	0									
B. Operated										
0–19 Years	0									
20–34	2	2.0	0	2	2	2	2	2	2	2
35–49	17	1.4	<1	1	1	1	2	2	2	2
50–64	89	1.8	<1	1	1	2	2	3	3	8
65+	75	1.8	<1	1	1	2	2	3	3	5
2. MULTIPLE DX										
A. Not Operated										
0–19 Years	0									
20–34	0									
35–49	0									
50–64	21	2.0	2	1	1	2	2	3	4	7
65+	52	2.2	3	1	1	1	3	6	6	8
B. Operated										
0–19 Years	0									
20–34	11	2.5	1	1	2	2	3	4	4	4
35–49	101	2.0	3	1	1	2	2	3	3	15
50–64	811	2.1	3	1	1	2	2	3	4	6
65+	2,037	2.3	2	1	2	2	3	3	4	6
SUBTOTALS:										
1. SINGLE DX										
A. Not Operated	0									
B. Operated	183	1.8	<1	1	1	2	2	3	3	5
2. MULTIPLE DX										
A. Not Operated	73	2.1	3	1	1	1	3	4	6	8
B. Operated	2,960	2.2	3	1	1	2	2	4	6	8
1. SINGLE DX	183	1.8	<1	1	1	2	2	3	3	5
2. MULTIPLE DX	3,033	2.2	2	1	1	2	3	3	4	7
A. NOT OPERATED	73	2.1	3	1	1	1	3	4	6	8
B. OPERATED	3,143	2.2	2	1	1	2	3	3	4	6
TOTAL										
0–19 Years	0									
20–34	13	2.4	<1	1	2	2	3	4	4	4
35–49	118	2.0	3	1	1	2	2	3	3	8
50–64	921	2.0	2	1	1	2	2	3	4	6
65+	2,164	2.3	2	1	1	2	3	3	4	7
GRAND TOTAL	3,216	2.2	2	1	1	2	3	3	4	7

Length of Stay by Diagnosis and Operation, Western Region, 2008

Western Region, October 2006–September 2007 Data, by Diagnosis

715.35: LOC OA NOS-PELVIS

Type of Patients	Observed Patients	Avg. Stay	Variance	Percentiles						
				10th	25th	50th	75th	90th	95th	99th
1. SINGLE DX										
A. Not Operated										
0–19 Years	0									
20–34	0									
35–49	0									
50–64	0									
65+	2	6.1	49		1	11	11	11	11	11
B. Operated										
0–19 Years	1	3.0	0	3	3	3	3	3	3	3
20–34	15	2.9	<1	2	2	3	3	4	4	4
35–49	267	2.9	<1	2	2	3	3	4	4	7
50–64	800	2.9	1	2	2	3	3	4	5	6
65+	430	3.2	<1	2	3	3	4	4	5	6
2. MULTIPLE DX										
A. Not Operated										
0–19 Years	0									
20–34	2	4.0	18	1	1	7	7	7	7	7
35–49	13	3.4	6	1	2	3	4	7	9	9
50–64	73	3.0	7	1	1	2	4	7	10	12
65+	302	3.6	10	1	1	3	5	7	10	14
B. Operated										
0–19 Years	3	2.7	<1	2	2	3	3	3	3	3
20–34	117	3.2	2	2	2	3	4	4	6	8
35–49	1,594	3.3	2	2	3	3	4	4	5	8
50–64	8,315	3.3	2	2	3	3	4	5	5	8
65+	13,662	3.7	3	2	3	3	4	5	6	10
SUBTOTALS:										
1. SINGLE DX										
A. Not Operated	2	6.1	49		1	11	11	11	11	11
B. Operated	1,513	3.0	<1	2	2	3	3	4	5	6
2. MULTIPLE DX										
A. Not Operated	390	3.5	9	1	1	3	5	7	10	14
B. Operated	23,691	3.5	3	2	3	3	4	5	6	9
1. SINGLE DX	1,515	3.0	1	2	2	3	3	4	5	6
2. MULTIPLE DX	24,081	3.5	3	2	3	3	4	5	6	9
A. NOT OPERATED	392	3.5	9	1	2	3	5	7	10	14
B. OPERATED	25,204	3.5	3	2	3	3	4	5	6	9
TOTAL										
0–19 Years	4	2.8	<1	2	3	3	3	3	3	3
20–34	134	3.2	2	2	2	3	4	4	6	8
35–49	1,874	3.2	2	2	3	3	4	4	5	8
50–64	9,188	3.3	2	2	3	3	4	5	5	8
65+	14,396	3.7	3	2	3	3	4	5	6	10
GRAND TOTAL	25,596	3.5	3	2	3	3	4	5	6	9

715.36: LOC OA NOS-LOWER LEG

Type of Patients	Observed Patients	Avg. Stay	Variance	Percentiles						
				10th	25th	50th	75th	90th	95th	99th
1. SINGLE DX										
A. Not Operated										
0–19 Years	0									
20–34	0									
35–49	0									
50–64	1	5.0	0	5	5	5	5	5	5	5
65+	6	2.2	<1	1	1	3	3	3	3	3
B. Operated										
0–19 Years	1	1.0	0	1	1	1	1	1	1	1
20–34	7	1.9	<1	1	1	2	2	3	3	3
35–49	205	2.9	1	2	2	3	3	4	5	6
50–64	1,077	3.1	<1	2	3	3	4	4	5	6
65+	1,011	3.2	<1	2	3	3	4	4	5	6
2. MULTIPLE DX										
A. Not Operated										
0–19 Years	0									
20–34	1	1.0	0	1	1	1	1	1	1	1
35–49	25	3.1	8	1	1	2	4	7	9	10
50–64	134	2.8	6	1	1	2	4	6	8	10
65+	512	3.5	12	1	1	3	4	7	9	17
B. Operated										
0–19 Years	0									
20–34	40	2.9	2	1	2	3	4	4	5	8
35–49	1,869	3.3	2	2	3	3	4	5	5	8
50–64	17,286	3.4	2	2	3	3	4	5	5	8
65+	31,812	3.7	3	2	3	3	4	5	6	9
SUBTOTALS:										
1. SINGLE DX										
A. Not Operated	7	2.6	2	1	1	3	3	5	5	5
B. Operated	2,301	3.1	<1	2	3	3	4	4	5	6
2. MULTIPLE DX										
A. Not Operated	672	3.3	11	1	1	3	4	7	9	16
B. Operated	51,007	3.6	3	2	3	3	4	5	6	9
1. SINGLE DX	2,308	3.1	<1	2	3	3	4	4	5	6
2. MULTIPLE DX	51,679	3.6	3	2	3	3	4	5	6	9
A. NOT OPERATED	679	3.3	11	1	1	3	4	7	9	16
B. OPERATED	53,308	3.5	2	2	3	3	4	5	6	9
TOTAL										
0–19 Years	1	1.0	0	1	1	1	1	1	1	1
20–34	48	2.7	2	1	2	3	4	4	5	8
35–49	2,099	3.3	2	2	2	3	4	5	5	8
50–64	18,498	3.4	2	2	3	3	4	5	5	8
65+	33,341	3.6	3	2	3	3	4	5	6	10
GRAND TOTAL	53,987	3.5	3	2	3	3	4	5	6	9

715.37: LOC OA NOS-ANKLE

Type of Patients	Observed Patients	Avg. Stay	Variance	Percentiles						
				10th	25th	50th	75th	90th	95th	99th
1. SINGLE DX										
A. Not Operated										
0–19 Years	0									
20–34	0									
35–49	0									
50–64	0									
65+	0									
B. Operated										
0–19 Years	0									
20–34	3	1.7	<1	1	1	2	2	2	2	2
35–49	14	1.9	1	1	1	2	2	3	5	5
50–64	26	1.7	<1	1	1	2	2	3	3	4
65+	15	1.7	<1	1	1	1	2	3	3	3
2. MULTIPLE DX										
A. Not Operated										
0–19 Years	0									
20–34	1	1.0	0	1	1	1	1	1	1	1
35–49	1	2.0	0	2	2	2	2	2	2	2
50–64	2	5.0	18	2	2	8	8	8	8	8
65+	9	4.3	22	1	2	3	4	16	16	16
B. Operated										
0–19 Years	0									
20–34	12	2.1	1	1	1	2	3	3	5	5
35–49	91	2.4	2	1	2	2	3	4	5	7
50–64	234	2.3	1	1	2	2	3	3	4	6
65+	281	2.6	2	1	2	2	3	4	5	8
SUBTOTALS:										
1. SINGLE DX										
A. Not Operated	0									
B. Operated	58	1.7	<1	1	1	2	2	3	3	5
2. MULTIPLE DX										
A. Not Operated	13	4.0	17	1	1	2	4	8	16	16
B. Operated	618	2.4	2	1	2	2	3	4	5	7
1. SINGLE DX	58	1.7	<1	1	1	2	2	3	3	5
2. MULTIPLE DX	631	2.5	2	1	2	2	3	4	5	8
A. NOT OPERATED	13	4.0	17	1	1	2	4	8	16	16
B. OPERATED	676	2.4	2	1	2	2	3	4	5	7
TOTAL										
0–19 Years	0									
20–34	16	1.9	1	1	1	2	2	3	3	5
35–49	106	2.4	2	1	2	2	3	4	5	8
50–64	262	2.2	1	1	1	2	3	3	4	8
65+	305	2.6	3	1	2	2	3	4	5	8
GRAND TOTAL	689	2.4	2	1	2	2	3	4	5	8

Length of Stay by Diagnosis and Operation, Western Region, 2008

Western Region, October 2006–September 2007 Data, by Diagnosis

715.89: OA MULT SITES NOT GEN

Type of Patients	Observed Patients	Avg. Stay	Variance	10th	25th	50th	75th	90th	95th	99th
1. SINGLE DX										
A. Not Operated										
0–19 Years	0									
20–34	0									
35–49	0									
50–64	0									
65+	0									
B. Operated										
0–19 Years	0									
20–34	0									
35–49	0									
50–64	2	2.5	<1	2	2	3	3	3	3	3
65+	2	2.5	4	1	1	4	4	4	4	4
2. MULTIPLE DX										
A. Not Operated										
0–19 Years	0									
20–34	1	1.0	0	1	1	1	1	1	1	1
35–49	0									
50–64	7	9.5	84	1	3	6	13	28	28	28
65+	68	4.4	12	1	2	4	6	10	12	>99
B. Operated										
0–19 Years	0									
20–34	1	3.0	0	3	3	3	3	3	3	3
35–49	15	2.8	<1	2	2	3	3	4	4	4
50–64	123	3.3	2	2	2	3	4	5	6	7
65+	314	4.0	7	2	3	3	4	6	7	19
SUBTOTALS:										
1. SINGLE DX										
A. Not Operated	0									
B. Operated	4	2.5	2	1	1	3	4	4	4	4
2. MULTIPLE DX										
A. Not Operated	76	4.8	20	1	2	4	6	10	14	>99
B. Operated	453	3.7	6	2	3	3	4	5	6	18
1. SINGLE DX	4	2.5	2	1	1	3	4	4	4	4
2. MULTIPLE DX	529	3.9	8	2	3	3	4	6	7	20
A. NOT OPERATED	76	4.8	20	1	2	4	6	10	14	>99
B. OPERATED	457	3.7	6	2	3	3	4	5	6	18
TOTAL										
0–19 Years	0									
20–34	2	2.0	2	1	1	2	3	3	3	3
35–49	15	2.8	<1	2	2	3	3	4	4	4
50–64	132	3.6	7	2	2	3	4	5	6	13
65+	384	4.0	8	2	3	3	4	6	8	21
GRAND TOTAL	533	3.9	8	2	3	3	4	6	7	20

715.91: OSTEOARTHOSIS NOS-SHOULD

Type of Patients	Observed Patients	Avg. Stay	Variance	10th	25th	50th	75th	90th	95th	99th
1. SINGLE DX										
A. Not Operated										
0–19 Years	0									
20–34	0									
35–49	0									
50–64	0									
65+	0									
B. Operated										
0–19 Years	0									
20–34	0									
35–49	8	1.8	<1	1	2	2	2	2	2	2
50–64	27	1.5	<1	1	1	2	2	2	2	2
65+	19	1.9	<1	1	1	2	2	4	4	4
2. MULTIPLE DX										
A. Not Operated										
0–19 Years	0									
20–34	0									
35–49	2	3.5	<1	3	3	4	4	4	4	4
50–64	8	2.4	8	1	1	1	3	9	9	9
65+	38	2.4	3	1	1	2	3	6	7	7
B. Operated										
0–19 Years	0									
20–34	7	1.7	<1	1	1	2	2	2	2	2
35–49	43	1.8	<1	1	1	2	2	3	3	3
50–64	285	2.0	2	1	1	2	3	3	4	6
65+	691	2.3	1	1	1	2	3	4	5	6
SUBTOTALS:										
1. SINGLE DX										
A. Not Operated	0									
B. Operated	54	1.7	<1	1	1	2	2	2	2	4
2. MULTIPLE DX										
A. Not Operated	48	2.4	4	1	1	2	3	6	7	9
B. Operated	1,026	2.2	1	1	1	2	3	3	4	6
1. SINGLE DX	54	1.7	<1	1	1	2	2	2	3	4
2. MULTIPLE DX	1,074	2.2	2	1	1	2	3	3	4	6
A. NOT OPERATED	48	2.4	4	1	1	2	3	6	7	9
B. OPERATED	1,080	2.2	1	1	1	2	3	3	4	6
TOTAL										
0–19 Years	0									
20–34	7	1.7	<1	1	1	2	2	2	3	4
35–49	53	1.9	<1	1	1	2	2	3	3	4
50–64	320	1.9	2	1	1	2	3	3	4	6
65+	748	2.3	1	1	1	2	3	4	5	6
GRAND TOTAL	1,128	2.2	2	1	1	2	3	3	4	6

715.95: OSTEOARTHOSIS NOS-PELVIS

Type of Patients	Observed Patients	Avg. Stay	Variance	10th	25th	50th	75th	90th	95th	99th
1. SINGLE DX										
A. Not Operated										
0–19 Years	0									
20–34	0									
35–49	0									
50–64	0									
65+	0									
B. Operated										
0–19 Years	0									
20–34	5	2.6	<1	2	2	3	3	3	3	3
35–49	81	3.1	1	2	2	3	4	5	5	7
50–64	235	2.8	<1	2	2	3	3	4	4	6
65+	149	3.0	<1	2	3	3	3	4	4	5
2. MULTIPLE DX										
A. Not Operated										
0–19 Years	0									
20–34	2	5.0	32	1	1	1	9	9	9	9
35–49	9	3.7	10	1	1	3	5	10	10	10
50–64	42	2.5	8	1	1	1	3	5	8	16
65+	178	3.4	10	1	2	3	4	6	9	22
B. Operated										
0–19 Years	0									
20–34	42	3.4	1	2	3	3	4	5	5	6
35–49	519	3.2	2	2	3	3	4	5	5	8
50–64	2,930	3.4	2	2	3	3	4	5	5	8
65+	4,881	3.6	2	2	3	3	4	5	6	9
SUBTOTALS:										
1. SINGLE DX										
A. Not Operated	0									
B. Operated	470	2.9	1	2	2	3	3	4	5	6
2. MULTIPLE DX										
A. Not Operated	231	3.3	10	1	1	2	4	6	9	16
B. Operated	8,372	3.5	2	2	3	3	4	5	6	9
1. SINGLE DX	470	2.9	1	2	2	3	3	4	5	6
2. MULTIPLE DX	8,603	3.5	2	2	3	3	4	5	6	9
A. NOT OPERATED	231	3.3	10	1	1	2	4	6	9	16
B. OPERATED	8,842	3.5	2	2	3	3	4	5	6	9
TOTAL										
0–19 Years	0									
20–34	49	3.4	2	2	3	3	4	5	5	9
35–49	609	3.2	2	2	3	3	4	5	5	8
50–64	3,207	3.3	2	2	3	3	4	5	5	8
65+	5,208	3.6	3	2	3	3	4	5	6	9
GRAND TOTAL	9,073	3.5	2	2	3	3	4	5	6	9

Western Region, October 2006–September 2007 Data, by Diagnosis

715.96: OSTEOARTHROSIS NOS-LOW LE

Type of Patients	Observed Patients	Avg. Stay	Vari-ance	10th	25th	50th	75th	90th	95th	99th
1. SINGLE DX										
A. Not Operated										
0–19 Years	0									
20–34	0									
35–49	2	2.0	2	1	1		3	3	3	3
50–64	31	1.9	1	1	1		3	3	3	3
65+	7	1.9	1	1	1		3	3	3	3
B. Operated										
0–19 Years	0									
20–34	2	2.5	<1	2	2	3	3	3	3	3
35–49	75	3.1	<1	2	2	3	3	4	5	6
50–64	437	3.1	<1	2	3	3	4	4	5	6
65+	362	3.1	<1	2	3	3	4	4	4	6
2. MULTIPLE DX										
A. Not Operated										
0–19 Years	0									
20–34	0									
35–49	13	3.2	6	1	1	3	4	7	8	8
50–64	83	2.3	6	1	1	1	3	4	6	18
65+	205	3.1	8	1	1	2	4	6	8	14
B. Operated										
0–19 Years	1	1.0	0	1	1	1	1	1	1	1
20–34	20	3.3	3	2	2	3	3	6	6	9
35–49	647	3.4	2	2	3	3	4	5	6	10
50–64	6,259	3.4	3	2	3	3	4	5	5	8
65+	11,336	3.7	3	2	3	3	4	5	6	9
SUBTOTALS:										
1. SINGLE DX A. Not Operated	40	1.9	1	1	1	1	3	3	3	3
1. SINGLE DX B. Operated	876	3.1	<1	2	3	3	4	4	5	6
2. MULTIPLE DX A. Not Operated	301	2.9	7	1	1	2	4	6	8	14
2. MULTIPLE DX B. Operated	18,263	3.6	3	2	3	3	4	5	6	9
1. SINGLE DX	916	3.1	<1	2	3	3	4	5	6	6
2. MULTIPLE DX	18,564	3.6	3	2	3	3	4	5	6	9
A. NOT OPERATED	341	2.8	7	1	1	2	3	5	8	14
B. OPERATED	19,139	3.5	3	2	3	3	4	5	6	9
TOTAL										
0–19 Years	1	1.0	0	1	1	1	1	1	1	1
20–34	22	3.2	2	2	2	3	3	4	6	9
35–49	737	3.3	2	2	3	3	4	5	6	8
50–64	6,810	3.4	3	2	3	3	4	5	6	8
65+	11,910	3.6	3	2	3	3	4	5	6	9
GRAND TOTAL	19,480	3.5	3	2	3	3	4	5	6	9

715.97: OSTEOARTHROSIS NOS-ANKLE

Type of Patients	Observed Patients	Avg. Stay	Vari-ance	10th	25th	50th	75th	90th	95th	99th
1. SINGLE DX										
A. Not Operated										
0–19 Years	0									
20–34	0									
35–49	0									
50–64	0									
65+	0									
B. Operated										
0–19 Years	0									
20–34	4	1.8	<1	1	1	1	3	3	3	3
35–49	7	2.1	3	1	1	1	4	5	5	5
50–64	13	1.8	1	1	1	1	2	3	4	4
65+	4	1.3	<1	1	1	1	2	2	2	2
2. MULTIPLE DX										
A. Not Operated										
0–19 Years	0									
20–34	0									
35–49	1	9.0	0	9	9	9	9	9	9	9
50–64	2	2.5	<1	2	2	2	3	3	3	3
65+	3	2.7	8	1	1	1	6	6	6	6
B. Operated										
0–19 Years	1	3.0	0	3	3	3	3	3	3	3
20–34	8	2.6	5	1	1	2	5	7	7	7
35–49	42	2.2	2	1	1	2	3	4	5	6
50–64	87	2.2	1	1	1	2	3	4	4	7
65+	96	2.2	1	1	1	2	3	3	4	7
SUBTOTALS:										
1. SINGLE DX A. Not Operated	0									
1. SINGLE DX B. Operated	28	1.8	1	1	1	1	2	4	4	5
2. MULTIPLE DX A. Not Operated	6	3.6	10	1	1	2	6	9	9	9
2. MULTIPLE DX B. Operated	234	2.2	2	1	1	2	3	4	5	7
1. SINGLE DX	28	1.8	1	1	1	1	2	4	4	5
2. MULTIPLE DX	240	2.3	2	1	1	2	3	4	5	7
A. NOT OPERATED	6	3.6	10	1	1	2	6	9	9	9
B. OPERATED	262	2.2	2	1	1	2	3	4	4	7
TOTAL										
0–19 Years	1	3.0	0	3	3	3	3	3	3	3
20–34	12	2.3	4	1	1	2	3	5	7	7
35–49	50	2.4	3	1	1	2	3	5	5	9
50–64	102	2.1	1	1	1	2	3	4	4	6
65+	103	2.2	1	1	1	2	3	3	4	6
GRAND TOTAL	268	2.2	2	1	1	2	3	4	5	7

716: ARTHROPATHIES NEC & NOS

Type of Patients	Observed Patients	Avg. Stay	Vari-ance	10th	25th	50th	75th	90th	95th	99th
1. SINGLE DX										
A. Not Operated										
0–19 Years	8	2.0	2	1	1	2	2	5	5	5
20–34	3	4.3	10	2	2	3	8	8	8	8
35–49	7	3.2	3	1	2	3	4	6	6	6
50–64	2	2.5	4	1	1	3	4	4	4	4
65+	0									
B. Operated										
0–19 Years	3	2.7	<1	2	2	3	3	3	3	3
20–34	22	1.6	<1	1	1	1	2	3	3	3
35–49	77	2.5	1	1	2	2	3	4	4	5
50–64	93	2.7	1	1	2	3	3	4	4	5
65+	35	2.8	1	2	2	3	3	4	5	5
2. MULTIPLE DX										
A. Not Operated										
0–19 Years	28	2.6	3	1	1	2	3	5	5	7
20–34	34	2.7	3	1	1	2	4	5	7	8
35–49	76	3.8	11	1	2	3	5	7	10	20
50–64	123	2.9	5	1	1	3	4	5	6	12
65+	174	3.4	12	2	1	3	4	7	9	25
B. Operated										
0–19 Years	12	5.7	41	2	2	3	6	11	24	24
20–34	109	2.8	5	1	2	2	3	5	5	8
35–49	438	3.0	4	1	2	3	4	4	6	8
50–64	1,146	3.1	3	1	2	3	4	5	6	8
65+	1,129	3.3	5	2	2	3	4	5	6	9
SUBTOTALS:										
1. SINGLE DX A. Not Operated	20	2.8	4	1	2	2	3	5	6	8
1. SINGLE DX B. Operated	230	2.5	1	1	2	3	3	4	4	5
2. MULTIPLE DX A. Not Operated	435	3.2	8	1	2	3	4	6	8	15
2. MULTIPLE DX B. Operated	2,834	3.2	4	1	2	3	4	5	6	9
1. SINGLE DX	250	2.6	1	1	2	3	3	4	5	5
2. MULTIPLE DX	3,269	3.2	5	1	2	3	4	5	6	10
A. NOT OPERATED	455	3.2	8	1	1	3	4	6	8	15
B. OPERATED	3,064	3.1	4	1	2	3	4	5	6	9
TOTAL										
0–19 Years	51	3.2	13	1	1	2	4	5	7	24
20–34	168	2.7	3	1	2	3	3	5	6	8
35–49	598	3.0	5	1	2	3	4	5	6	10
50–64	1,364	3.1	3	1	2	3	4	5	6	8
65+	1,338	3.3	6	2	2	3	4	5	6	10
GRAND TOTAL	3,519	3.1	4	1	2	3	4	5	6	10

Length of Stay by Diagnosis and Operation, Western Region, 2008

Western Region, October 2006–September 2007 Data, by Diagnosis

716.15: TRAUM ARTHROPATHY-PELVIS · 716.16: TRAUM ARTHROPATHY-LOW LE · 716.17: TRAUM ARTHROPATHY-ANKLE

Type of Patients	716.15 Obs. Pts	Avg. Stay	Vari-ance	10th	25th	50th	75th	90th	95th	99th	716.16 Obs. Pts	Avg. Stay	Vari-ance	10th	25th	50th	75th	90th	95th	99th	716.17 Obs. Pts	Avg. Stay	Vari-ance	10th	25th	50th	75th	90th	95th	99th
1. SINGLE DX																															
A. Not Operated																															
0–19 Years	0										0										0									
20–34	0										0										0									
35–49	0										0										0									
50–64	0										0										0									
65+	0										0										0									
B. Operated																															
0–19 Years	1	3.0	0	3	3	3	3	3	3	3	0										1	2.0	0	2	2	2	2	2	2	2
20–34	4	2.3	<1	1	2	3	3	3	3	3	2	2.0	0	2	2	2	2	2	2	2	9	1.5	<1	1	1	1	2	2	3	3
35–49	9	3.7	<1	3	3	3	4	5	5	5	19	2.8	<1	1	2	3	3	4	4	4	15	1.6	<1	1	1	1	2	3	4	4
50–64	6	3.3	<1	3	3	3	4	4	4	4	22	3.2	<1	2	3	3	4	4	4	4	10	1.9	2	1	1	2	2	5	5	5
65+	1	2.0	0	2	2	2	2	2	2	2	2	3.5	<1	3	3	3	4	4	4	4	1	2.0	0	2	2	2	2	2	2	2
2. MULTIPLE DX																															
A. Not Operated																															
0–19 Years	0										0										0									
20–34	1	3.0	0	3	3	3	3	3	3	3	1	3.0	0	3	3	3	3	3	3	3	0									
35–49	2	5.0	2	4	4	4	6	6	6	6	2	2.0	2	1	1	1	3	3	3	3	0									
50–64	2	5.0	31	1	1	9	9	9	9	9	4	2.2	<1	1	1	2	3	3	3	3	3	2.0	1	1	1	2	3	3	3	3
65+											5	2.8	2	1	2	3	4	4	4	4	0									
B. Operated																															
0–19 Years	2	4.5	4	3	3	5	6	6	6	6	1	3.0	0	3	3	3	3	3	3	3	3	2.3	<1	2	2	2	3	3	3	3
20–34	22	3.5	2	2	3	3	4	5	6	8	16	4.2	7	2	3	3	4	8	12	12	30	2.0	<1	1	1	2	3	3	4	4
35–49	66	3.4	1	2	3	3	4	5	6	7	149	3.2	2	2	3	3	4	5	6	8	84	2.0	<1	1	1	2	3	3	4	4
50–64	119	3.8	4	2	3	3	4	6	7	14	337	3.4	3	2	3	3	4	5	6	8	174	2.3	2	1	1	2	3	4	4	7
65+	84	3.8	2	3	3	3	4	5	6	9	152	3.7	2	2	3	3	4	5	7	10	92	2.5	1	2	2	2	3	4	5	6
SUBTOTALS:																															
1. SINGLE DX																															
A. Not Operated	0										0										0									
B. Operated	21	3.2	<1	2	3	3	4	4	5	5	45	3.0	<1	2	2	3	4	4	4	4	36	1.7	<1	1	1	1	2	3	4	5
2. MULTIPLE DX																															
A. Not Operated	5	4.6	9	1	1	3	6	9	9	9	12	2.5	1	1	1	3	3	4	4	4	3	2.0	1	1	1	2	3	3	3	3
B. Operated	293	3.7	2	2	3	3	4	5	6	9	655	3.5	3	2	3	3	4	5	6	9	383	2.2	1	1	1	2	3	3	4	6
1. SINGLE DX	21	3.2	<1	2	3	3	4	4	5	5	45	3.0	<1	2	2	3	4	4	4	4	36	1.7	<1	1	1	1	2	3	4	5
2. MULTIPLE DX	298	3.7	3	2	3	3	4	5	6	9	667	3.4	3	2	3	3	4	5	6	9	386	2.2	2	1	1	2	3	4	4	6
A. NOT OPERATED	5	4.6	9	1	3	4	6	9	9	9	12	2.5	1	1	1	3	3	4	4	4	3	2.0	1	1	1	2	3	3	3	3
B. OPERATED	314	3.6	2	2	3	3	4	5	6	8	700	3.4	3	2	3	3	4	5	6	9	419	2.2	2	1	1	2	3	4	4	6
TOTAL																															
0–19 Years	3	4.0	3	3	3	3	6	6	6	6	1	3.0	0	3	3	3	3	3	3	3	4	2.3	<1	2	2	2	2	3	3	3
20–34	26	3.3	2	2	2	3	4	5	6	8	19	3.9	6	2	3	3	4	8	12	12	39	1.9	<1	1	1	2	2	3	3	4
35–49	76	3.4	1	2	3	3	4	5	6	7	170	3.2	2	2	2	3	4	4	5	8	99	1.9	<1	1	1	2	3	3	4	4
50–64	127	3.8	3	2	3	3	4	6	7	14	363	3.4	3	2	3	3	4	5	6	8	187	2.2	2	1	1	2	3	4	4	7
65+	87	3.8	2	3	3	3	4	5	6	9	159	3.7	2	2	3	3	4	5	7	10	93	2.5	1	2	2	3	4	4	5	6
GRAND TOTAL	319	3.7	2	2	3	3	4	5	6	9	712	3.4	3	2	3	3	4	5	6	9	422	2.2	2	1	1	2	3	4	4	6

Length of Stay by Diagnosis and Operation, Western Region, 2008

Western Region, October 2006–September 2007 Data, by Diagnosis

716.91: ARTHROPATHY NOS-SHOULDER

Type of Patients	Observed Patients	Avg. Stay	Variance	Percentiles 10th	25th	50th	75th	90th	95th	99th
1. SINGLE DX										
A. Not Operated										
0–19 Years	1	1.0	0	1	1	1	1	1	1	1
20–34	0									
35–49	0									
50–64	0									
65+	0									
B. Operated										
0–19 Years	0									
20–34	0									
35–49	0									
50–64	5	1.8	<1	1	2	2	2	2	2	2
65+	4	1.5	<1	1	1	1	2	2	2	2
2. MULTIPLE DX										
A. Not Operated										
0–19 Years	0									
20–34	1	2.0	0	2	2	2	2	2	2	2
35–49	4	2.0	2	1	1	1	1	4	4	4
50–64	2	3.5	4	2	2	2	5	5	5	5
65+	16	2.3	6	1	1	2	2	3	11	11
B. Operated										
0–19 Years	0									
20–34	3	2.0	3	1	1	1	4	4	4	4
35–49	5	1.2	<1	1	1	1	1	2	2	2
50–64	46	1.8	<1	1	1	2	2	3	4	6
65+	173	2.7	15	2	2	2	3	4	5	20
SUBTOTALS:										
1. SINGLE DX										
A. Not Operated	1	1.0	0	1	1	1	1	1	1	1
B. Operated	9	1.7	<1	1	1	2	2	2	2	2
2. MULTIPLE DX										
A. Not Operated	23	2.3	5	1	1	2	2	4	5	11
B. Operated	227	2.5	12	1	1	2	3	4	4	9
1. SINGLE DX	10	1.6	<1	1	1	2	2	2	2	2
2. MULTIPLE DX	250	2.5	11	1	1	2	3	4	5	11
A. NOT OPERATED	24	2.2	5	1	1	2	2	4	5	11
B. OPERATED	236	2.5	11	1	1	2	3	4	5	11
TOTAL										
0–19 Years	1	1.0	0	1	1	1	1	1	1	1
20–34	4	2.0	2	1	1	1	2	4	4	4
35–49	9	1.6	1	1	1	1	2	4	4	4
50–64	53	1.9	1	1	1	2	2	3	4	6
65+	193	2.7	14	1	2	2	3	4	5	20
GRAND TOTAL	260	2.4	10	1	1	2	3	4	4	11

716.95: ARTHROPATHY NOS-PELVIS

Type of Patients	Observed Patients	Avg. Stay	Variance	Percentiles 10th	25th	50th	75th	90th	95th	99th
1. SINGLE DX										
A. Not Operated										
0–19 Years	1	1.0	0	1	1	1	1	1	1	1
20–34	0									
35–49	1	2.0	0	2	2	2	2	2	2	2
50–64	1	1.0	0	1	1	1	1	1	1	1
65+	0									
B. Operated										
0–19 Years	0									
20–34	0									
35–49	8	3.4	<1	3	3	3	3	5	5	5
50–64	11	2.8	1	2	2	3	3	4	5	5
65+	9	3.2	<1	3	3	3	4	5	5	5
2. MULTIPLE DX										
A. Not Operated										
0–19 Years	5	2.4	1	1	2	2	3	4	4	4
20–34	0									
35–49	3	5.3	16	1	1	6	9	9	9	9
50–64	9	2.0	1	1	1	2	2	4	4	4
65+	12	2.5	2	1	1	3	4	4	4	4
B. Operated										
0–19 Years	1	4.0	0	4	4	4	4	4	4	4
20–34	5	3.6	2	2	3	3	4	6	6	6
35–49	18	3.4	<1	2	3	3	4	5	5	5
50–64	78	3.5	1	2	3	3	4	5	6	8
65+	120	3.8	4	2	3	3	4	5	7	12
SUBTOTALS:										
1. SINGLE DX										
A. Not Operated	3	1.3	<1	1	1	1	1	2	2	2
B. Operated	28	3.1	<1	3	3	3	3	5	5	5
2. MULTIPLE DX										
A. Not Operated	29	2.6	3	1	1	2	3	4	6	9
B. Operated	222	3.6	3	2	3	3	4	5	6	9
1. SINGLE DX	31	2.9	1	2	2	3	3	4	5	5
2. MULTIPLE DX	251	3.5	3	3	3	3	4	5	6	9
A. NOT OPERATED	32	2.5	3	1	1	2	3	4	6	9
B. OPERATED	250	3.6	2	2	3	3	4	5	6	9
TOTAL										
0–19 Years	7	2.4	2	1	1	2	2	3	4	4
20–34	5	3.6	2	3	3	3	4	6	6	6
35–49	30	3.5	2	3	3	3	4	5	6	9
50–64	99	3.2	3	2	3	3	4	5	6	8
65+	141	3.6	3	2	3	3	4	5	7	12
GRAND TOTAL	282	3.5	3	3	3	3	4	5	6	9

716.96: ARTHROPATHY NOS-LOW LEG

Type of Patients	Observed Patients	Avg. Stay	Variance	Percentiles 10th	25th	50th	75th	90th	95th	99th
1. SINGLE DX										
A. Not Operated										
0–19 Years	1	5.0	0	5	5	5	5	5	5	5
20–34	1	2.0		2	2	2	2	2	2	2
35–49	0									
50–64	0									
65+	0									
B. Operated										
0–19 Years	0									
20–34	1	2.0	0	2	2	2	2	2	2	2
35–49	12	2.4	1	1	2	2	3	4	4	4
50–64	26	2.9	<1	2	2	3	3	4	5	5
65+	12	3.1	<1	3	3	3	3	4	5	5
2. MULTIPLE DX										
A. Not Operated										
0–19 Years	1	4.0	0	4	4	4	4	4	4	4
20–34	5	1.8	2	1	1	1	2	4	4	4
35–49	6	3.5	3	1	2	5	5	5	5	5
50–64	12	1.8	2	1	1	1	1	3	6	6
65+	31	3.2	8	1	1	2	3	7	7	15
B. Operated										
0–19 Years	1	6.0	0	6	6	6	6	6	6	6
20–34	3	1.7	1	1	1	1	1	3	3	3
35–49	36	3.9	20	2	2	3	4	6	6	29
50–64	211	3.5	2	2	3	3	3	5	6	8
65+	314	3.7	2	2	3	3	4	6	7	9
SUBTOTALS:										
1. SINGLE DX										
A. Not Operated	2	3.5	4	2	2	5	5	5	5	5
B. Operated	51	2.8	<1	2	2	3	3	4	4	5
2. MULTIPLE DX										
A. Not Operated	55	2.8	6	1	1	2	3	6	7	15
B. Operated	565	3.6	3	2	3	3	4	5	7	8
1. SINGLE DX	53	2.8	1	2	2	3	3	4	5	5
2. MULTIPLE DX	620	3.5	3	3	3	3	4	5	7	8
A. NOT OPERATED	57	2.9	6	1	1	2	3	6	7	15
B. OPERATED	616	3.5	3	2	3	3	4	5	7	8
TOTAL										
0–19 Years	3	5.0	<1	4	4	5	6	6	6	6
20–34	10	1.8	1	1	1	2	2	4	4	4
35–49	54	3.5	14	2	3	3	4	5	6	29
50–64	249	3.3	3	2	3	3	3	5	6	8
65+	357	3.6	3	2	3	3	4	6	7	9
GRAND TOTAL	673	3.5	3	3	3	3	4	5	7	8

Length of Stay by Diagnosis and Operation, Western Region, 2008

Western Region, October 2006–September 2007 Data, by Diagnosis

717: INTERNAL DERANG KNEE

Type of Patients	Observed Patients	Avg. Stay	Variance	10th	25th	50th	75th	90th	95th	99th
1. SINGLE DX										
A. Not Operated										
0–19 Years	0									
20–34	0									
35–49	1	1.0	0	1	1	1	1	1	1	1
50–64	0									
65+	0									
B. Operated										
0–19 Years	18	1.2	<1	1	1	1	1	2	2	2
20–34	29	1.5	<1	1	1	1	1	3	4	4
35–49	22	1.7	2	1	1	1	2	3	4	6
50–64	10	1.5	<1	1	1	1	2	3	3	3
65+	2	1.0	0	1	1	1	1	1	1	1
2. MULTIPLE DX										
A. Not Operated										
0–19 Years	3	1.7	1	1	1	1	3	3	3	3
20–34	0									
35–49	8	3.6	1	2	3	4	4	6	6	6
50–64	8	5.2	28	1	2	5	5	17	17	17
65+	24	3.5	5	2	2	3	4	8	8	9
B. Operated										
0–19 Years	59	1.3	<1	1	1	1	1	2	3	5
20–34	174	1.8	3	1	1	1	2	3	4	9
35–49	242	1.6	1	1	1	1	2	3	4	6
50–64	202	1.9	3	1	1	1	2	3	5	9
65+	116	2.6	4	1	1	2	3	5	7	11
SUBTOTALS:										
1. SINGLE DX										
A. Not Operated	1	1.0	0	1	1	1	1	1	1	1
B. Operated	81	1.5	<1	1	1	1	2	2	3	6
2. MULTIPLE DX										
A. Not Operated	43	3.7	8	1	2	3	5	7	8	17
B. Operated	793	1.9	3	1	1	1	2	3	4	9
1. SINGLE DX	82	1.5	<1	1	1	1	2	2	3	6
2. MULTIPLE DX	836	2.0	3	1	1	1	2	3	5	9
A. NOT OPERATED	44	3.7	8	1	2	3	5	7	8	17
B. OPERATED	874	1.8	2	1	1	1	2	3	4	9
TOTAL										
0–19 Years	80	1.3	<1	1	1	1	1	2	3	5
20–34	203	1.7	3	1	1	1	2	3	4	7
35–49	273	1.7	2	1	1	1	2	3	4	6
50–64	220	2.0	4	1	1	1	2	4	5	10
65+	142	2.7	4	1	1	2	3	5	7	11
GRAND TOTAL	918	1.9	3	1	1	1	2	3	5	9

717.83: OLD DISRUPTION ACL

Type of Patients	Observed Patients	Avg. Stay	Variance	10th	25th	50th	75th	90th	95th	99th
1. SINGLE DX										
A. Not Operated										
0–19 Years	0									
20–34	0									
35–49	0									
50–64	0									
65+	0									
B. Operated										
0–19 Years	13	1.2	<1	1	1	1	1	2	2	2
20–34	16	1.1	<1	1	1	1	1	2	2	2
35–49	11	1.2	<1	1	1	1	2	2	2	2
50–64	4	1.3	<1	1	1	1	2	2	2	2
65+	1	1.0	0	1	1	1	1	1	1	1
2. MULTIPLE DX										
A. Not Operated										
0–19 Years	2	1.0	0	1	1	1	1	1	1	1
20–34	0									
35–49	0									
50–64	1	1.0	0	1	1	1	1	1	1	1
65+	2	7.0	8	5	5	5	9	9	9	9
B. Operated										
0–19 Years	43	1.2	<1	1	1	1	1	2	3	3
20–34	107	1.5	<1	1	1	1	2	3	3	4
35–49	113	1.5	<1	1	1	1	2	3	3	4
50–64	39	1.9	3	1	1	1	2	3	4	9
65+	1	1.0	0	1	1	1	1	1	1	1
SUBTOTALS:										
1. SINGLE DX										
A. Not Operated	0									
B. Operated	45	1.2	<1	1	1	1	1	2	2	2
2. MULTIPLE DX										
A. Not Operated	5	3.4	13	1	1	1	5	9	9	9
B. Operated	303	1.5	1	1	1	1	2	3	3	6
1. SINGLE DX	45	1.2	<1	1	1	1	1	2	2	2
2. MULTIPLE DX	308	1.5	1	1	1	1	2	3	4	6
A. NOT OPERATED	5	3.4	13	1	1	1	5	9	9	9
B. OPERATED	348	1.5	<1	1	1	1	2	3	3	6
TOTAL										
0–19 Years	58	1.2	<1	1	1	1	1	2	2	3
20–34	123	1.5	<1	1	1	1	2	3	3	4
35–49	124	1.5	<1	1	1	1	2	3	3	4
50–64	44	1.8	3	1	1	1	2	4	5	6
65+	4	4.0	15	1	1	5	5	9	9	9
GRAND TOTAL	353	1.5	1	1	1	1	2	3	3	6

718: OTHER JOINT DERANGEMENT

Type of Patients	Observed Patients	Avg. Stay	Variance	10th	25th	50th	75th	90th	95th	99th
1. SINGLE DX										
A. Not Operated										
0–19 Years	4	1.5	1	1	1	1	3	3	3	3
20–34	19	1.7	3	1	1	1	2	3	3	8
35–49	7	2.4	5	1	1	1	3	3	7	7
50–64	5	3.6	18	1	1	2	3	11	11	11
65+	0									
B. Operated										
0–19 Years	75	1.6	1	1	1	1	2	3	3	8
20–34	87	1.8	2	1	1	1	2	3	5	8
35–49	52	1.9	1	1	1	2	2	3	4	5
50–64	30	1.7	<1	1	1	1	2	3	3	4
65+	6	1.5	<1	1	1	2	2	2	2	2
2. MULTIPLE DX										
A. Not Operated										
0–19 Years	16	3.0	22	1	1	1	3	4	20	20
20–34	30	2.1	6	1	1	1	2	5	5	14
35–49	51	3.0	9	1	1	2	4	6	7	17
50–64	104	2.3	5	1	1	2	3	5	6	11
65+	137	3.2	7	1	1	3	4	6	8	16
B. Operated										
0–19 Years	185	2.4	5	1	1	2	3	4	5	16
20–34	333	2.2	3	1	1	2	3	3	5	11
35–49	343	2.4	5	1	1	2	3	4	6	13
50–64	443	2.7	5	1	1	2	3	5	6	11
65+	245	3.3	8	1	1	3	4	6	8	14
SUBTOTALS:										
1. SINGLE DX										
A. Not Operated	35	2.1	5	1	1	1	2	3	3	11
B. Operated	250	1.7	1	1	1	1	2	3	4	7
2. MULTIPLE DX										
A. Not Operated	338	2.8	7	1	1	2	3	5	8	16
B. Operated	1,549	2.6	5	1	1	2	3	5	7	13
1. SINGLE DX	285	1.8	2	1	1	1	2	3	4	8
2. MULTIPLE DX	1,887	2.6	6	1	1	2	3	5	7	13
A. NOT OPERATED	373	2.7	7	1	1	2	3	5	8	16
B. OPERATED	1,799	2.5	5	1	1	2	3	4	6	12
TOTAL										
0–19 Years	280	2.2	5	1	1	2	3	3	5	16
20–34	469	2.1	3	1	1	1	3	4	5	11
35–49	453	2.4	5	1	1	2	3	4	6	14
50–64	582	2.6	5	1	1	3	3	5	6	11
65+	388	3.2	7	1	1	3	4	6	8	14
GRAND TOTAL	2,172	2.5	5	1	1	2	3	5	7	13

Length of Stay by Diagnosis and Operation, Western Region, 2008

Western Region, October 2006–September 2007 Data, by Diagnosis

718.31: RECUR DISLOCAT-SHOULDER

Type of Patients	Observed Patients	Avg. Stay	Vari-ance	10th	25th	50th	75th	90th	95th	99th
1. SINGLE DX										
A. Not Operated										
0–19 Years	1	1.0	0	1	1	1	1	1	1	1
20–34	12	1.8	4	1	1	1	2	2	8	8
35–49	2	1.0	0	1	1	1	1	1	1	1
50–64	1	1.0	0	1	1	1	1	1	1	1
65+	0									
B. Operated										
0–19 Years	14	1.1	<1	1	1	1	1	2	2	2
20–34	29	1.6	2	1	1	1	2	3	3	8
35–49	13	1.3	<1	1	1	1	1	2	3	3
50–64	6	1.0	0	1	1	1	1	1	1	1
65+	1	1.0	0	1	1	1	1	1	1	1
2. MULTIPLE DX										
A. Not Operated										
0–19 Years	3	1.3	<1	1	1	1	2	2	2	2
20–34	9	2.5	18	1	1	1	1	2	14	14
35–49	9	4.2	18	1	1	4	5	14	14	14
50–64	4	2.8	4	1	1	4	5	5	5	5
65+	35	3.4	8	1	2	3	4	6	9	16
B. Operated										
0–19 Years	13	2.6	19	1	1	2	2	4	17	17
20–34	57	2.0	5	1	1	1	2	3	4	14
35–49	33	2.1	3	1	1	1	3	4	7	8
50–64	46	3.4	15	1	1	2	4	6	8	24
65+	45	2.9	5	1	2	2	4	6	7	10
SUBTOTALS:										
1. SINGLE DX										
A. Not Operated	16	1.6	3	1	1	1	1	2	8	8
B. Operated	63	1.4	<1	1	1	1	1	2	3	8
2. MULTIPLE DX										
A. Not Operated	60	3.3	10	1	1	3	4	6	9	16
B. Operated	194	2.6	8	1	1	2	3	5	7	17
1. SINGLE DX	79	1.4	1	1	1	1	2	2	3	8
2. MULTIPLE DX	254	2.7	9	1	1	2	3	5	8	16
A. NOT OPERATED	76	2.9	9	1	1	2	4	6	9	16
B. OPERATED	257	2.3	7	1	1	1	3	5	7	14
TOTAL										
0–19 Years	31	1.8	8	1	1	1	1	2	4	17
20–34	107	1.9	5	1	1	1	2	3	4	14
35–49	57	2.2	5	1	1	1	3	5	7	14
50–64	57	3.0	13	1	1	2	4	5	8	24
65+	81	3.1	6	1	1	3	4	6	7	16
GRAND TOTAL	333	2.4	7	1	1	1	3	5	7	14

718.56: ANKYLOSIS-LOWER LEG

Type of Patients	Observed Patients	Avg. Stay	Vari-ance	10th	25th	50th	75th	90th	95th	99th
1. SINGLE DX										
A. Not Operated										
0–19 Years	0									
20–34	4	1.8	<1	1	1	2	2	3	3	3
35–49	2	2.0	2	1	1	1	3	3	3	3
50–64	3	2.0	<1	1	1	2	3	3	3	3
65+	0									
B. Operated										
0–19 Years	1	2.0	0	2	2	2	2	2	2	2
20–34	4	2.3	2	2	1	2	2	4	4	4
35–49	9	2.2	2	2	1	2	2	5	5	5
50–64	3	2.3	1	1	1	3	3	3	5	3
65+	0									
2. MULTIPLE DX										
A. Not Operated										
0–19 Years	6	2.2	1	1	1	2	3	4	4	4
20–34	5	2.2	3	1	1	1	2	5	5	5
35–49	11	2.6	2	2	2	2	3	4	6	6
50–64	53	2.0	1	2	1	2	3	3	5	6
65+	34	2.0	2	1	1	1	3	4	5	7
B. Operated										
0–19 Years	7	4.7	15	1	1	3	7	12	17	12
20–34	7	2.4	<1	2	2	2	3	3	3	3
35–49	29	2.6	10	1	1	2	3	4	4	18
50–64	43	2.7	1	1	2	2	3	4	5	6
65+	33	2.9	2	2	2	3	3	5	6	6
SUBTOTALS:										
1. SINGLE DX										
A. Not Operated	9	1.9	<1	1	1	1	2	3	3	3
B. Operated	17	2.2	1	1	1	2	3	4	5	5
2. MULTIPLE DX										
A. Not Operated	109	2.1	2	1	1	2	3	4	5	6
B. Operated	119	2.8	4	1	2	3	3	4	6	12
1. SINGLE DX	26	2.1	1	1	1	2	3	3	4	5
2. MULTIPLE DX	228	2.5	3	1	1	2	3	4	5	7
A. NOT OPERATED	118	2.1	2	1	1	2	3	4	5	6
B. OPERATED	136	2.7	4	2	2	2	3	4	6	12
TOTAL										
0–19 Years	14	3.4	9	1	1	1	4	7	12	12
20–34	20	2.2	1	1	1	2	3	3	4	5
35–49	51	2.5	6	1	1	2	3	5	7	18
50–64	102	2.3	1	1	1	2	3	4	5	6
65+	67	2.4	2	2	1	2	3	5	5	7
GRAND TOTAL	254	2.4	3	1	1	2	3	4	5	7

719: JOINT DISORDER NEC & NOS

Type of Patients	Observed Patients	Avg. Stay	Vari-ance	10th	25th	50th	75th	90th	95th	99th
1. SINGLE DX										
A. Not Operated										
0–19 Years	41	1.4	<1	1	1	1	2	2	3	4
20–34	14	2.1	4	1	1	2	2	4	8	8
35–49	13	1.6	<1	1	1	1	2	3	4	4
50–64	14	1.6	1	1	1	1	2	3	4	4
65+	4	1.7	<1	1	1	1	2	3	3	3
B. Operated										
0–19 Years	8	2.1	6	1	1	1	2	8	8	8
20–34	19	1.8	<1	1	1	2	3	3	3	3
35–49	13	2.3	1	2	2	2	3	4	4	4
50–64	10	2.8	3	2	2	2	3	6	6	6
65+	2	3.0	8	1	1	1	5	5	5	5
2. MULTIPLE DX										
A. Not Operated										
0–19 Years	128	2.3	3	1	1	2	3	4	6	9
20–34	155	3.0	6	1	1	2	4	6	8	13
35–49	318	2.7	5	1	1	2	3	6	8	11
50–64	560	3.0	12	1	1	2	4	6	7	21
65+	1,883	3.2	6	1	2	3	4	6	7	13
B. Operated										
0–19 Years	28	2.3	4	1	1	2	3	5	6	10
20–34	57	2.6	<1	1	2	2	3	5	7	11
35–49	102	3.2	24	1	1	2	4	6	6	9
50–64	136	2.9	5	1	2	3	4	5	6	13
65+	156	4.5	21	2	2	3	5	8	15	25
SUBTOTALS:										
1. SINGLE DX										
A. Not Operated	86	1.6	1	1	1	1	2	3	4	8
B. Operated	52	2.2	2	1	1	2	3	4	6	8
2. MULTIPLE DX										
A. Not Operated	3,044	3.0	7	1	1	2	4	6	7	13
B. Operated	479	3.4	15	1	1	3	4	6	8	18
1. SINGLE DX	138	1.8	2	1	1	1	2	3	4	8
2. MULTIPLE DX	3,523	3.1	8	1	1	2	4	6	7	13
A. NOT OPERATED	3,130	3.0	7	1	1	2	4	6	7	13
B. OPERATED	531	3.3	13	1	1	3	4	6	8	18
TOTAL										
0–19 Years	205	2.1	3	1	1	2	3	4	6	9
20–34	245	2.8	5	1	1	2	3	6	7	11
35–49	446	2.8	9	1	1	2	3	6	7	11
50–64	720	2.9	10	1	1	2	3	6	7	16
65+	2,045	3.3	7	2	2	3	4	6	8	15
GRAND TOTAL	3,661	3.0	8	1	1	2	4	6	7	13

Length of Stay by Diagnosis and Operation, Western Region, 2008

Western Region, October 2006–September 2007 Data, by Diagnosis

719.06: JOINT EFFUSION-LOWER LEG

Type of Patients	Observed Patients	Avg. Stay	Variance	10th	25th	50th	75th	90th	95th	99th
1. SINGLE DX										
A. Not Operated										
0–19 Years	6	1.7	<1	1	1	2	2	2	3	3
20–34	4	3.0	11	1	1	1	2	2	8	8
35–49	3	2.3	2	1	1	2	4	4	4	4
50–64	1	1.0	0	1	1	1	1	1	1	1
65+	0									
B. Operated										
0–19 Years	1	8.0	0	8	8	8	8	8	8	8
20–34	0									
35–49	2	2.5	<1	2	2	3	3	3	3	3
50–64	0									
65+	0									
2. MULTIPLE DX										
A. Not Operated										
0–19 Years	13	3.4	6	1	2	2	4	6	9	9
20–34	16	3.9	4	2	2	4	6	6	7	7
35–49	43	2.8	6	1	1	2	3	5	9	13
50–64	77	3.2	5	1	2	3	4	7	8	11
65+	215	3.5	5	1	2	3	4	6	8	12
B. Operated										
0–19 Years	4	4.5	14	2	3	3	10	10	10	10
20–34	3	5.3	24	2	2	3	11	11	11	11
35–49	2	4.0	8	2	2	4	6	6	6	6
50–64	6	3.5	2	2	3	3	4	6	6	6
65+	12	5.0	6	2	3	4	6	8	9	9
SUBTOTALS:										
1. SINGLE DX										
A. Not Operated	14	2.1	4	1	1	1	2	2	8	8
B. Operated	3	4.4	10	2	2	3	6	8	8	8
2. MULTIPLE DX										
A. Not Operated	364	3.4	5	1	2	3	4	6	8	12
B. Operated	27	4.6	7	2	3	3	6	9	10	11
1. SINGLE DX	17	2.5	5	1	1	2	3	8	8	8
2. MULTIPLE DX	391	3.5	5	1	2	3	4	6	8	12
A. NOT OPERATED	378	3.3	5	1	2	3	4	6	8	12
B. OPERATED	30	4.5	7	2	3	3	6	9	10	11
TOTAL										
0–19 Years	24	3.3	7	1	2	2	4	8	9	10
20–34	23	4.0	7	1	2	4	6	7	8	11
35–49	50	2.8	6	1	1	2	3	5	9	13
50–64	84	3.2	5	1	2	3	4	7	7	11
65+	227	3.6	5	1	2	3	4	6	8	12
GRAND TOTAL	408	3.4	5	1	2	3	4	7	8	11

719.16: HEMARTHROSIS-LOWER LEG

Type of Patients	Observed Patients	Avg. Stay	Variance	10th	25th	50th	75th	90th	95th	99th
1. SINGLE DX										
A. Not Operated										
0–19 Years	0									
20–34	0									
35–49	1	2.0	0	2	2	2	2	2	2	2
50–64	0									
65+	0									
B. Operated										
0–19 Years	0									
20–34	0									
35–49	0									
50–64	0									
65+	0									
2. MULTIPLE DX										
A. Not Operated										
0–19 Years	6	3.5	4	1	3	3	4	7	7	7
20–34	20	3.9	8	1	2	3	5	8	11	11
35–49	15	3.8	8	1	1	3	6	8	11	11
50–64	33	3.4	4	1	2	3	5	6	7	7
65+	133	4.0	6	1	2	3	5	7	9	11
B. Operated										
0–19 Years	1	2.0	0	2	2	2	2	2	2	2
20–34	1	3.0	0	3	3	3	3	3	3	3
35–49	3	4.7	12	1	1	5	8	8	8	8
50–64	6	5.2	17	2	3	3	6	13	13	13
65+	20	7.4	49	3	3	4	10	18	30	30
SUBTOTALS:										
1. SINGLE DX										
A. Not Operated	1	2.0	0	2	2	2	2	2	2	2
B. Operated	0									
2. MULTIPLE DX										
A. Not Operated	207	3.9	6	1	2	3	5	7	8	11
B. Operated	31	6.4	37	2	3	4	8	13	18	30
1. SINGLE DX	1	2.0	0	2	2	2	2	2	2	2
2. MULTIPLE DX	238	4.2	11	1	2	3	5	7	11	16
A. NOT OPERATED	208	3.8	6	1	2	3	5	7	8	11
B. OPERATED	31	6.4	37	2	3	4	8	13	18	30
TOTAL										
0–19 Years	7	3.3	4	1	2	3	4	7	7	7
20–34	21	3.9	8	1	2	3	5	8	8	11
35–49	19	3.8	8	1	1	3	6	8	11	11
50–64	39	3.7	6	2	2	3	5	7	7	13
65+	153	4.4	13	2	2	3	5	8	11	18
GRAND TOTAL	239	4.2	10	1	2	3	5	7	11	16

719.41: JOINT PAIN-SHOULDER

Type of Patients	Observed Patients	Avg. Stay	Variance	10th	25th	50th	75th	90th	95th	99th
1. SINGLE DX										
A. Not Operated										
0–19 Years	3	1.3	<1	1	1	1	1	2	2	2
20–34	1	2.0	0	2	2	2	2	2	2	2
35–49	2	1.0	0	1	1	1	1	1	1	1
50–64	1	1.0	0	1	1	1	1	1	1	1
65+	0									
B. Operated										
0–19 Years	0	1.0	0	1	1	1	1	1	1	1
20–34	0									
35–49	0									
50–64	0									
65+	0									
2. MULTIPLE DX										
A. Not Operated										
0–19 Years	13	1.8	<1	1	1	2	2	3	4	4
20–34	16	1.7	3	1	1	1	2	4	7	7
35–49	69	2.0	4	1	1	1	2	4	5	13
50–64	114	1.9	5	1	1	1	2	3	5	9
65+	232	2.1	3	1	2	2	3	4	5	6
B. Operated										
0–19 Years	0									
20–34	0									
35–49	5	1.6	<1	1	1	1	2	3	3	3
50–64	8	1.6	<1	1	1	2	2	3	3	3
65+	12	3.5	46	1	1	2	2	2	25	25
SUBTOTALS:										
1. SINGLE DX										
A. Not Operated	7	1.3	<1	1	1	1	2	2	2	2
B. Operated	1	1.0	0	1	1	1	1	1	1	1
2. MULTIPLE DX										
A. Not Operated	444	2.0	4	1	1	1	2	4	5	8
B. Operated	25	2.5	22	1	1	2	2	3	3	25
1. SINGLE DX	8	1.3	<1	1	1	1	2	2	2	2
2. MULTIPLE DX	469	2.0	5	1	1	1	2	4	5	9
A. NOT OPERATED	451	2.0	4	1	1	1	2	4	5	8
B. OPERATED	26	2.5	22	1	1	2	2	3	3	25
TOTAL										
0–19 Years	17	1.7	<1	1	1	1	2	3	4	4
20–34	17	1.8	2	1	1	1	2	4	7	7
35–49	76	1.9	4	1	1	1	2	3	5	13
50–64	123	1.9	5	1	1	1	2	3	5	9
65+	244	2.1	5	1	1	1	2	4	5	6
GRAND TOTAL	477	2.0	5	1	1	1	2	4	5	9

Length of Stay by Diagnosis and Operation, Western Region, 2008

719.45: JOINT PAIN-PELVIS

Type of Patients	Observed Patients	Avg. Stay	Variance	10th	25th	50th	75th	90th	95th	99th
1. SINGLE DX										
A. Not Operated										
0–19 Years	12	1.7	<1	1	1	1	2	3	4	4
20–34	2	1.0	0	1	1	1	1	1	1	1
35–49	2	1.5	<1	1	1	1	2	2	2	2
50–64	1	1.0	0	1	1	2	2	2	2	2
65+	1	3.0	0	3	3	3	3	3	3	3
B. Operated										
0–19 Years	0									
20–34	1	1.0	0	1	1	1	1	1	1	1
35–49	0									
50–64	2	4.5	4	3	3	6	6	6	6	6
65+	0									
2. MULTIPLE DX										
A. Not Operated										
0–19 Years	34	2.1	3	1	1	2	2	4	4	9
20–34	25	2.2	2	1	1	2	2	4	4	7
35–49	56	3.2	7	1	1	2	4	7	10	11
50–64	150	3.7	22	1	1	3	4	7	8	22
65+	875	3.2	5	1	2	3	4	6	7	13
B. Operated										
0–19 Years	2	3.5	12	1	1	1	6	6	6	6
20–34	2	2.5	<1	2	2	2	3	3	3	3
35–49	4	15.3	509	1	1	5	49	49	49	49
50–64	16	4.1	15	1	3	4	4	5	18	18
65+	25	4.7	16	2	3	3	5	9	15	17
SUBTOTALS:										
1. SINGLE DX										
A. Not Operated	18	1.6	<1	1	1	1	2	3	4	4
B. Operated	3	3.4	6	1	1	3	6	6	6	6
2. MULTIPLE DX										
A. Not Operated	1,140	3.2	8	1	2	3	4	6	8	13
B. Operated	49	5.2	54	1	2	3	5	9	17	49
1. SINGLE DX	21	1.9	2	1	1	1	2	3	4	6
2. MULTIPLE DX	1,189	3.3	10	1	2	3	4	6	8	17
A. NOT OPERATED	1,158	3.2	7	1	2	3	4	6	7	13
B. OPERATED	52	5.1	51	2	2	3	5	7	17	49
TOTAL										
0–19 Years	48	2.0	2	1	1	2	2	4	4	9
20–34	30	2.1	2	1	1	2	2	4	6	7
35–49	62	3.9	40	1	1	2	5	7	10	49
50–64	169	3.7	21	1	2	3	4	6	8	22
65+	901	3.2	6	1	2	3	4	6	7	13
GRAND TOTAL	1,210	3.3	9	1	2	3	4	6	8	16

719.46: JOINT PAIN-LOWER LEG

Type of Patients	Observed Patients	Avg. Stay	Variance	10th	25th	50th	75th	90th	95th	99th
1. SINGLE DX										
A. Not Operated										
0–19 Years	4	1.0	0	1	1	1	1	1	1	1
20–34	2	2.0	0	2	2	2	2	2	2	2
35–49	1	1.0	0	1	1	1	1	1	1	1
50–64	3	1.7	1	1	1	1	3	3	3	3
65+	0									
B. Operated										
0–19 Years	2	1.0	0	1	1	1	1	1	1	1
20–34	0									
35–49	0									
50–64	0									
65+	0									
2. MULTIPLE DX										
A. Not Operated										
0–19 Years	16	2.8	4	1	1	2	2	4	6	8
20–34	12	1.8	<1	1	1	2	2	3	4	4
35–49	44	2.3	4	1	1	2	2	4	7	11
50–64	55	3.5	16	1	2	3	4	6	9	29
65+	144	3.7	12	2	2	3	4	7	9	19
B. Operated										
0–19 Years	0									
20–34	6	2.7	7	1	1	2	2	8	8	8
35–49	12	3.4	2	2	2	3	4	5	7	7
50–64	17	2.7	3	1	1	3	3	6	7	7
65+	17	4.2	18	1	1	3	4	11	17	17
SUBTOTALS:										
1. SINGLE DX										
A. Not Operated	10	1.4	<1	1	1	1	2	3	3	3
B. Operated	2	1.0	0	1	1	1	1	1	1	1
2. MULTIPLE DX										
A. Not Operated	271	3.3	11	1	1	3	4	6	8	19
B. Operated	52	3.4	8	1	1	3	4	7	8	17
1. SINGLE DX	12	1.3	<1	1	1	1	2	2	3	3
2. MULTIPLE DX	323	3.3	10	1	1	3	4	7	8	18
A. NOT OPERATED	281	3.2	10	1	1	3	4	6	8	19
B. OPERATED	54	3.3	8	1	1	3	4	7	8	17
TOTAL										
0–19 Years	22	2.3	4	1	1	2	3	5	6	8
20–34	20	2.1	3	1	1	2	2	3	4	8
35–49	57	2.5	4	1	1	2	3	5	7	11
50–64	75	3.2	13	1	1	3	4	6	8	29
65+	161	3.7	12	2	2	3	4	7	11	19
GRAND TOTAL	335	3.2	10	1	1	2	4	6	8	18

719.7: DIFFICULTY WALKING

Type of Patients	Observed Patients	Avg. Stay	Variance	10th	25th	50th	75th	90th	95th	99th
1. SINGLE DX										
A. Not Operated										
0–19 Years	1	1.0	0	1	1	1	1	1	1	1
20–34	0									
35–49	0									
50–64	1	1.0	0	1	1	1	1	1	1	1
65+	0									
B. Operated										
0–19 Years	0									
20–34	0									
35–49	0									
50–64	0									
65+	0									
2. MULTIPLE DX										
A. Not Operated										
0–19 Years	3	1.3	<1	1	1	1	2	2	2	2
20–34	4	4.0	9	1	1	2	6	7	7	7
35–49	4	3.8	4	2	2	5	6	6	6	6
50–64	7	4.3	6	1	3	4	7	8	8	8
65+	58	2.8	2	1	2	3	4	4	5	9
B. Operated										
0–19 Years	0									
20–34	0									
35–49	0									
50–64	1	1.0	0	1	1	1	1	1	1	1
65+	0									
SUBTOTALS:										
1. SINGLE DX										
A. Not Operated	2	1.0	0	1	1	1	1	1	1	1
B. Operated	0									
2. MULTIPLE DX										
A. Not Operated	76	3.0	3	1	2	3	4	5	7	9
B. Operated	1	1.0	0	1	1	1	1	1	1	1
1. SINGLE DX	2	1.0	0	1	1	1	1	1	1	1
2. MULTIPLE DX	77	3.0	3	1	1	3	4	5	7	9
A. NOT OPERATED	78	2.9	3	1	2	3	4	5	7	9
B. OPERATED	1	1.0	0	1	1	1	1	1	1	1
TOTAL										
0–19 Years	4	1.3	<1	1	1	1	2	2	2	2
20–34	4	4.0	9	1	1	2	6	7	7	7
35–49	4	3.8	4	2	2	5	6	6	6	6
50–64	9	3.6	7	2	2	3	4	8	8	8
65+	58	2.8	2	1	2	3	4	4	5	9
GRAND TOTAL	79	2.9	3	1	1	3	4	5	7	9

609

Length of Stay by Diagnosis and Operation, Western Region, 2008

Western Region, October 2006–September 2007 Data, by Diagnosis

720: INFLAM SPONDYLOPATHIES

Type of Patients	Observed Patients	Avg. Stay	Variance	10th	25th	50th	75th	90th	95th	99th
1. SINGLE DX										
A. Not Operated										
0–19 Years	3	2.7	8	1	1	1	6	6	6	6
20–34	4	1.0	0	1	1	1	1	1	1	1
35–49	0									
50–64	2	1.0	0	1	1	1	1	1	1	1
65+	0									
B. Operated										
0–19 Years	0									
20–34	1	3.0	0	3	3	3	3	3	3	3
35–49	0									
50–64	0									
65+	0									
2. MULTIPLE DX										
A. Not Operated										
0–19 Years	10	8.7	41	1	4	8	16	16	19	19
20–34	24	6.5	90	2	3	4	5	11	11	49
35–49	17	3.4	3	1	2	3	5	7	7	7
50–64	30	5.8	72	1	2	3	6	11	14	47
65+	70	4.8	18	1	2	3	6	9	12	24
B. Operated										
0–19 Years	0									
20–34	7	4.2	20	1	2	3	4	14	14	14
35–49	11	7.6	15	3	4	8	10	12	15	15
50–64	35	4.9	39	1	2	3	5	8	24	31
65+	21	4.3	15	1	2	3	6	10	10	15
SUBTOTALS:										
1. SINGLE DX *A. Not Operated*	9	1.6	3	1	1	1	1	6	6	6
B. Operated	1	3.0	0	3	3	3	3	3	3	3
2. MULTIPLE DX *A. Not Operated*	151	5.4	40	1	2	4	6	10	14	47
B. Operated	74	5.1	27	1	2	3	6	10	15	31
1. SINGLE DX	10	1.7	3	1	1	1	1	6	6	6
2. MULTIPLE DX	225	5.3	36	1	2	3	6	10	14	31
A. NOT OPERATED	160	5.2	39	1	2	3	6	10	13	47
B. OPERATED	75	5.1	27	1	2	3	6	10	15	31
TOTAL										
0–19 Years	13	7.3	39	1	1	6	10	16	19	19
20–34	36	5.3	66	1	2	3	5	11	14	49
35–49	28	5.0	12	1	3	4	7	10	12	15
50–64	67	5.2	53	1	2	3	5	11	14	47
65+	91	4.7	17	1	2	3	6	10	12	24
GRAND TOTAL	235	5.1	35	1	2	3	6	10	14	31

721: SPONDYLOSIS ET AL

Type of Patients	Observed Patients	Avg. Stay	Variance	10th	25th	50th	75th	90th	95th	99th
1. SINGLE DX										
A. Not Operated										
0–19 Years	0									
20–34	1	1.0	0	1	1	1	1	1	1	1
35–49	10	2.0	2	1	1	2	3	4	5	6
50–64	13	2.9	2	1	2	3	4	5	6	7
65+	8	2.1	1	1	1	2	3	4	4	6
B. Operated										
0–19 Years	2	2.5	<1	2	2	3	3	3	3	3
20–34	39	2.3	2	1	1	2	3	4	5	7
35–49	355	1.8	2	1	1	1	2	3	3	5
50–64	436	1.9	2	1	1	2	2	4	4	5
65+	138	2.1	2	1	1	2	2	4	5	5
2. MULTIPLE DX										
A. Not Operated										
0–19 Years	3	2.7	<1	2	2	3	3	3	3	3
20–34	53	3.6	12	2	2	3	3	4	10	20
35–49	263	3.8	17	1	2	3	5	7	10	28
50–64	561	3.9	12	1	2	3	5	8	10	17
65+	1,715	4.1	12	1	2	3	5	7	10	16
B. Operated										
0–19 Years	12	3.4	4	2	2	3	5	5	7	7
20–34	209	2.7	11	1	1	2	3	5	6	12
35–49	2,261	2.5	5	1	1	2	3	5	6	12
50–64	5,219	2.9	10	1	1	2	4	6	8	15
65+	4,735	3.8	17	1	1	3	5	7	10	20
SUBTOTALS:										
1. SINGLE DX *A. Not Operated*	32	2.4	2	1	1	2	3	4	5	6
B. Operated	970	1.9	2	1	1	1	2	4	5	7
2. MULTIPLE DX *A. Not Operated*	2,595	4.0	12	2	2	3	5	7	10	16
B. Operated	12,436	3.2	12	1	1	2	4	6	8	16
1. SINGLE DX	1,002	1.9	2	1	1	1	2	4	5	7
2. MULTIPLE DX	15,031	3.3	12	1	1	2	4	6	8	16
A. NOT OPERATED	2,627	4.0	12	2	2	3	5	7	10	16
B. OPERATED	13,406	3.1	11	1	1	2	4	6	8	16
TOTAL										
0–19 Years	17	3.2	3	1	2	3	5	5	7	7
20–34	302	2.8	10	1	1	2	3	5	6	14
35–49	2,889	2.5	6	1	1	2	3	5	6	12
50–64	6,229	3.0	10	1	2	3	5	6	8	15
65+	6,596	3.9	15	1	2	3	5	7	10	19
GRAND TOTAL	16,033	3.2	12	1	1	2	4	6	8	16

721.0: CERVICAL SPONDYLOSIS

Type of Patients	Observed Patients	Avg. Stay	Variance	10th	25th	50th	75th	90th	95th	99th
1. SINGLE DX										
A. Not Operated										
0–19 Years	0									
20–34	0									
35–49	2	1.0	0	1	1	1	1	1	1	1
50–64	2	1.5	<1	1	1	2	2	2	2	2
65+	1	2.0	0	2	2	2	2	2	2	2
B. Operated										
0–19 Years	0									
20–34	7	1.3	<1	1	1	1	1	2	2	2
35–49	167	1.3	<1	1	1	1	1	2	2	4
50–64	189	1.5	<1	1	1	2	2	2	3	4
65+	26	1.7	<1	1	1	2	2	3	3	4
2. MULTIPLE DX										
A. Not Operated										
0–19 Years	0									
20–34	10	2.1	1	1	1	2	3	4	4	4
35–49	66	3.1	4	1	1	3	5	6	7	10
50–64	166	3.4	16	1	1	3	4	6	8	29
65+	324	3.3	6	1	2	3	4	6	8	13
B. Operated										
0–19 Years	0									
20–34	51	1.4	<1	1	1	1	2	2	3	4
35–49	940	1.7	3	1	1	1	2	3	4	6
50–64	1,682	1.9	3	1	1	2	3	3	4	8
65+	694	2.6	13	1	1	2	3	5	7	15
SUBTOTALS:										
1. SINGLE DX *A. Not Operated*	5	1.4	<1	1	1	1	2	2	2	2
B. Operated	389	1.4	<1	1	1	1	2	2	3	4
2. MULTIPLE DX *A. Not Operated*	566	3.3	9	1	1	2	4	6	7	16
B. Operated	3,367	2.0	5	1	1	1	2	3	5	9
1. SINGLE DX	394	1.4	<1	1	1	1	2	2	3	4
2. MULTIPLE DX	3,933	2.1	5	1	1	2	4	4	6	10
A. NOT OPERATED	571	3.2	9	1	1	2	4	6	7	16
B. OPERATED	3,756	1.9	4	1	1	1	2	3	4	8
TOTAL										
0–19 Years	0									
20–34	68	1.5	<1	1	1	1	2	3	3	4
35–49	1,175	1.7	1	1	1	1	2	3	4	6
50–64	2,039	2.0	4	1	1	1	3	3	5	9
65+	1,045	2.8	11	1	1	2	3	5	7	15
GRAND TOTAL	4,327	2.1	5	1	1	1	2	4	5	9

721.1: CERV SPONDYL W MYELOP

Type of Patients	Observed Patients	Avg. Stay	Vari-ance	Percentiles						
				10th	25th	50th	75th	90th	95th	99th
1. SINGLE DX										
A. Not Operated										
0–19 Years	0									
20–34	0									
35–49	3	1.7	<1	1	1	2	2	2	2	2
50–64	3	2.7	<1	2	2	3	3	3	3	3
65+	3	2.0	1	1	2	2	3	3	3	3
B. Operated										
0–19 Years	0									
20–34	5	1.6	<1	1	1	1	2	3	3	3
35–49	106	1.8	2	1	1	1	2	3	5	7
50–64	149	2.1	3	1	1	1	2	4	5	9
65+	61	2.0	2	1	1	2	2	4	5	8
2. MULTIPLE DX										
A. Not Operated										
0–19 Years	0									
20–34	1	2.0	0	2	2	2	2	2	2	2
35–49	26	3.8	30	1	1	2	4	7	10	28
50–64	67	4.1	14	1	2	3	5	7	14	20
65+	152	4.9	30	1	2	3	5	10	15	32
B. Operated										
0–19 Years	3	3.0	4	1	1	3	5	5	5	7
20–34	38	2.7	10	1	1	1	3	6	12	15
35–49	602	2.6	9	1	1	2	3	5	7	15
50–64	1,699	3.3	17	1	1	2	4	7	10	21
65+	1,576	4.3	25	2	2	3	5	8	13	27
SUBTOTALS:										
1. SINGLE DX										
A. Not Operated	9	2.1	<1	2	2	2	3	3	3	3
B. Operated	321	2.0	2	1	1	1	2	4	5	8
2. MULTIPLE DX										
A. Not Operated	246	4.5	26	2	2	3	5	9	14	28
B. Operated	3,918	3.6	19	1	1	2	4	7	11	23
1. SINGLE DX	330	2.0	2	1	1	1	2	4	5	8
2. MULTIPLE DX	4,164	3.6	20	1	1	2	4	7	11	23
A. NOT OPERATED	255	4.4	25	1	2	3	5	9	14	28
B. OPERATED	4,239	3.5	18	1	1	2	4	7	10	21
TOTAL										
0–19 Years	3	3.0	4	1	1	3	5	5	5	5
20–34	44	2.6	9	1	1	1	3	6	9	15
35–49	737	2.5	9	1	1	2	3	5	7	15
50–64	1,918	3.2	16	1	1	2	4	6	10	20
65+	1,792	4.3	25	2	2	3	5	8	13	27
GRAND TOTAL	4,494	3.5	19	1	1	2	4	7	11	22

721.3: LUMBOSACRAL SPONDYLOSIS

Type of Patients	Observed Patients	Avg. Stay	Vari-ance	Percentiles						
				10th	25th	50th	75th	90th	95th	99th
1. SINGLE DX										
A. Not Operated										
0–19 Years	0									
20–34	1	1.0	0	1	1	1	1	1	1	1
35–49	2	2.0	2	1	1	3	3	3	3	3
50–64	6	3.3	3	2	2	3	5	6	6	6
65+	3	2.7	2	1	1	3	4	4	4	4
B. Operated										
0–19 Years	2	2.5	<1	2	2	3	3	3	3	3
20–34	23	2.7	2	1	1	3	3	4	5	7
35–49	73	2.8	3	1	2	3	4	5	6	9
50–64	83	2.4	2	1	1	2	3	4	5	8
65+	44	2.4	4	1	1	2	3	5	6	10
2. MULTIPLE DX										
A. Not Operated										
0–19 Years	3	2.7	<1	2	2	3	3	3	3	3
20–34	36	3.4	7	1	2	3	4	5	9	14
35–49	133	3.7	9	1	2	3	5	7	11	16
50–64	272	3.8	8	1	2	3	5	8	9	16
65+	1,042	4.2	8	1	2	3	5	8	10	15
B. Operated										
0–19 Years	9	3.6	4	1	2	3	5	7	7	7
20–34	96	3.1	3	1	2	3	4	5	6	12
35–49	598	3.4	5	1	2	3	4	6	7	12
50–64	1,567	3.6	7	1	2	3	4	6	8	14
65+	2,126	3.8	9	1	2	3	4	7	8	15
SUBTOTALS:										
1. SINGLE DX										
A. Not Operated	12	2.8	3	2	2	3	4	5	6	6
B. Operated	225	2.6	3	1	1	2	3	4	5	8
2. MULTIPLE DX										
A. Not Operated	1,486	4.1	8	1	2	3	5	8	10	15
B. Operated	4,396	3.7	8	1	2	3	5	7	8	14
1. SINGLE DX	237	2.6	3	1	1	2	3	5	6	8
2. MULTIPLE DX	5,882	3.8	8	1	2	3	5	7	8	14
A. NOT OPERATED	1,498	4.1	8	1	2	3	5	8	10	15
B. OPERATED	4,621	3.6	7	1	2	3	5	6	8	14
TOTAL										
0–19 Years	14	3.2	3	2	2	3	5	5	7	7
20–34	156	3.1	4	1	2	3	4	5	7	12
35–49	806	3.4	5	1	2	3	4	6	7	12
50–64	1,928	3.6	7	1	2	3	4	6	8	14
65+	3,215	3.9	9	1	2	3	5	7	9	15
GRAND TOTAL	6,119	3.7	8	1	2	3	5	7	8	14

721.42: L SPONDYL W MYELOPATHY

Type of Patients	Observed Patients	Avg. Stay	Vari-ance	Percentiles						
				10th	25th	50th	75th	90th	95th	99th
1. SINGLE DX										
A. Not Operated										
0–19 Years	0									
20–34	0									
35–49	1	4.0	0	4	4	4	4	4	4	4
50–64	1	5.0	0	5	5	5	5	5	5	5
65+	1	1.0	0	1	1	1	1	1	1	1
B. Operated										
0–19 Years	0									
20–34	2	2.0	2	1	1	1	3	3	3	3
35–49	4	1.3	<1	1	1	1	1	2	2	2
50–64	11	2.0	1	1	1	2	3	4	4	4
65+	4	2.3	2	1	2	2	4	4	4	4
2. MULTIPLE DX										
A. Not Operated										
0–19 Years	0									
20–34	0									
35–49	14	6.0	39	2	2	4	5	12	25	25
50–64	8	4.8	15	2	2	4	7	12	12	12
65+	57	4.3	6	2	3	4	6	7	10	14
B. Operated										
0–19 Years	0									
20–34	7	2.3	4	1	1	1	4	4	6	6
35–49	37	3.5	6	1	2	3	4	7	9	12
50–64	119	3.4	10	1	1	3	5	6	9	18
65+	222	4.1	18	1	1	3	5	8	12	21
SUBTOTALS:										
1. SINGLE DX										
A. Not Operated	3	3.3	4	1	1	4	5	5	5	5
B. Operated	21	1.9	1	1	1	2	2	4	4	4
2. MULTIPLE DX										
A. Not Operated	79	4.7	13	2	2	4	6	8	12	25
B. Operated	385	3.8	14	1	1	3	5	7	11	21
1. SINGLE DX	24	2.1	2	1	1	2	3	4	4	5
2. MULTIPLE DX	464	3.9	14	1	1	3	5	7	11	21
A. NOT OPERATED	82	4.6	13	2	2	4	6	8	10	25
B. OPERATED	406	3.7	14	1	1	3	5	7	10	20
TOTAL										
0–19 Years	0									
20–34	9	2.2	3	1	1	3	3	6	6	6
35–49	56	4.0	15	2	2	3	5	8	12	25
50–64	139	3.4	10	1	1	3	4	6	9	18
65+	284	4.1	15	1	1	3	5	8	11	21
GRAND TOTAL	488	3.8	14	1	1	3	5	7	10	21

Length of Stay by Diagnosis and Operation, Western Region, 2008

Western Region, October 2006–September 2007 Data, by Diagnosis

722: INTERVERTEBRAL DISC DIS

Type of Patients	Observed Patients	Avg. Stay	Vari-ance	Percentiles						
				10th	25th	50th	75th	90th	95th	99th
1. SINGLE DX										
A. Not Operated										
0–19 Years	8	3.5	7	1	1	3	7	8	8	8
20–34	69	2.8	9	1	1	2	3	5	6	23
35–49	157	2.4	2	1	1	2	3	4	6	8
50–64	70	1.9	2	1	1	2	2	3	5	9
65+	16	2.6	1	1	2	2	4	4	4	4
B. Operated										
0–19 Years	70	1.4	<1	1	1	1	1	3	4	4
20–34	1,366	1.6	1	1	1	1	2	3	4	5
35–49	2,884	1.7	1	1	1	1	2	3	4	6
50–64	1,831	1.7	2	1	1	1	2	3	4	6
65+	350	1.7	2	1	1	1	2	3	4	6
2. MULTIPLE DX										
A. Not Operated										
0–19 Years	24	3.8	10	1	2	3	4	7	7	15
20–34	482	3.3	7	1	2	3	4	6	8	14
35–49	1,354	3.5	9	1	2	3	4	7	8	15
50–64	1,732	3.7	10	1	2	3	5	7	9	16
65+	2,530	4.2	9	1	2	3	5	8	10	15
B. Operated										
0–19 Years	104	2.4	6	1	1	2	3	3	6	9
20–34	3,324	2.5	4	1	1	2	3	5	6	11
35–49	12,153	2.5	7	1	1	2	3	5	6	12
50–64	15,911	2.9	8	1	1	2	4	6	7	14
65+	9,291	3.5	13	1	1	3	4	7	9	17
SUBTOTALS:										
1. SINGLE DX										
A. Not Operated	320	2.4	4	1	1	2	3	4	6	9
B. Operated	6,501	1.7	1	1	1	1	2	3	4	6
2. MULTIPLE DX										
A. Not Operated	6,122	3.8	9	1	2	3	5	7	9	15
B. Operated	40,783	2.9	9	1	1	2	4	6	7	14
1. SINGLE DX	6,821	1.7	2	1	1	1	2	3	4	6
2. MULTIPLE DX	46,905	3.0	9	1	1	2	4	6	8	14
A. NOT OPERATED	6,442	3.8	9	1	2	3	5	7	9	15
B. OPERATED	47,284	2.7	8	1	1	2	4	5	7	13
TOTAL										
0–19 Years	206	2.2	5	1	1	1	3	4	6	9
20–34	5,241	2.3	4	1	1	2	3	5	6	10
35–49	16,548	2.5	6	1	1	2	3	5	6	11
50–64	19,544	2.8	8	1	1	2	4	6	7	13
65+	12,187	3.6	12	1	1	3	5	7	9	17
GRAND TOTAL	53,726	2.8	8	1	1	2	4	6	7	14

722.0: CERV DISC DISPLACEMENT

Type of Patients	Observed Patients	Avg. Stay	Vari-ance	Percentiles						
				10th	25th	50th	75th	90th	95th	99th
1. SINGLE DX										
A. Not Operated										
0–19 Years	1	7.0	0	7	7	7	7	7	7	7
20–34	1	5.0	0	5	5	5	5	5	5	5
35–49	8	2.0	<1	1	1	2	3	3	3	3
50–64	2	1.0	0	1	1	1	1	1	1	1
65+	0									
B. Operated										
0–19 Years	0									
20–34	120	1.5	1	1	1	1	2	3	4	5
35–49	560	1.4	<1	1	1	1	1	2	3	6
50–64	325	1.4	<1	1	1	1	2	2	3	4
65+	25	1.4	<1	1	1	1	2	3	3	3
2. MULTIPLE DX										
A. Not Operated										
0–19 Years	0									
20–34	17	3.4	9	1	1	2	4	8	12	12
35–49	101	3.1	11	1	1	2	4	6	7	28
50–64	99	2.9	5	1	1	2	4	6	7	8
65+	38	3.2	5	1	1	3	4	7	8	10
B. Operated										
0–19 Years	1	3.0	0	3	3	3	3	3	3	3
20–34	289	1.6	1	1	1	1	2	3	3	6
35–49	2,383	1.7	2	1	1	1	2	3	4	7
50–64	2,244	1.8	3	1	1	1	2	3	4	8
65+	468	2.3	8	1	1	1	3	4	6	16
SUBTOTALS:										
1. SINGLE DX										
A. Not Operated	12	2.5	4	1	1	2	3	7	7	7
B. Operated	1,030	1.4	<1	1	1	1	2	2	3	5
2. MULTIPLE DX										
A. Not Operated	255	3.0	7	1	1	2	4	6	8	15
B. Operated	5,385	1.8	3	1	1	1	2	3	4	8
1. SINGLE DX	1,042	1.4	<1	1	1	1	2	2	3	5
2. MULTIPLE DX	5,640	1.8	3	1	1	1	2	3	4	9
A. NOT OPERATED	267	3.0	7	1	1	2	4	6	8	11
B. OPERATED	6,415	1.7	3	1	1	1	2	3	4	8
TOTAL										
0–19 Years	2	5.0	8	3	3	7	7	7	7	9
20–34	427	1.7	2	1	1	1	2	3	4	7
35–49	3,052	1.7	2	1	1	1	2	3	4	7
50–64	2,670	1.8	3	1	1	1	2	3	4	8
65+	531	2.4	8	1	1	3	5	5	7	15
GRAND TOTAL	6,682	1.8	3	1	1	1	2	3	4	8

722.10: LUMBAR DISC DISPLACEMENT

Type of Patients	Observed Patients	Avg. Stay	Vari-ance	Percentiles						
				10th	25th	50th	75th	90th	95th	99th
1. SINGLE DX										
A. Not Operated										
0–19 Years	4	1.5	<1	1	1	1	1	3	3	3
20–34	51	2.7	4	1	1	2	4	5	6	12
35–49	100	2.5	3	1	1	2	3	6	6	8
50–64	42	2.0	2	1	1	2	2	3	5	7
65+	5	2.8	2	1	2	3	4	4	4	4
B. Operated										
0–19 Years	61	1.3	<1	1	1	1	1	2	4	4
20–34	1,041	1.4	<1	1	1	1	2	3	3	5
35–49	1,656	1.5	1	1	1	1	2	3	4	6
50–64	940	1.5	<1	1	1	1	2	3	3	5
65+	214	1.6	2	1	1	2	2	3	4	6
2. MULTIPLE DX										
A. Not Operated										
0–19 Years	11	3.4	6	1	1	3	4	7	7	7
20–34	281	3.1	5	1	2	2	4	6	7	12
35–49	630	3.4	6	1	2	3	4	6	8	13
50–64	621	3.5	8	1	2	3	4	7	9	14
65+	644	4.0	8	1	2	3	5	7	9	14
B. Operated										
0–19 Years	81	1.9	2	1	1	1	2	4	5	9
20–34	2,117	2.2	4	1	1	1	3	5	6	10
35–49	5,170	2.4	4	1	1	2	3	5	6	10
50–64	6,222	2.5	5	1	1	2	3	5	6	11
65+	3,975	2.8	8	1	1	2	4	6	8	13
SUBTOTALS:										
1. SINGLE DX										
A. Not Operated	202	2.4	3	1	1	2	3	4	6	8
B. Operated	3,912	1.5	1	1	1	1	2	3	4	5
2. MULTIPLE DX										
A. Not Operated	2,187	3.6	7	1	2	3	4	7	8	14
B. Operated	17,565	2.5	5	1	1	1	3	5	7	11
1. SINGLE DX	4,114	1.5	1	1	1	1	2	3	4	6
2. MULTIPLE DX	19,752	2.6	6	1	1	2	3	5	7	12
A. NOT OPERATED	2,389	3.5	7	1	2	3	4	6	8	13
B. OPERATED	21,477	2.3	5	1	1	1	3	5	6	11
TOTAL										
0–19 Years	157	1.8	2	1	1	1	2	4	5	8
20–34	3,490	2.1	3	1	1	1	3	4	5	9
35–49	7,556	2.3	4	1	1	1	3	4	6	10
50–64	7,825	2.4	5	1	2	2	3	5	6	11
65+	4,838	2.9	8	1	2	3	4	6	8	13
GRAND TOTAL	23,866	2.4	5	1	1	2	3	5	6	11

Length of Stay by Diagnosis and Operation, Western Region, 2008

722.11: THOR DISC DISPLACEMENT

Type of Patients	Observed Patients	Avg. Stay	Vari-ance	10th	25th	50th	75th	90th	95th	99th
1. SINGLE DX										
A. *Not Operated*										
0–19 Years	0									
20–34	2	1.0	0	1	1	1	1	1	1	1
35–49	2	2.5	4	1	1	1	4	4	4	4
50–64	0									
65+	0									
B. *Operated*										
0–19 Years	0									
20–34	6	1.8	1	1	1	1	2	4	4	4
35–49	8	2.6	3	1	1	1	4	5	5	5
50–64	8	2.0	1	1	1	2	3	4	4	4
65+	3	2.0	3	1	1	1	4	4	4	4
2. MULTIPLE DX										
A. *Not Operated*										
0–19 Years	1	4.0	0	4	4	4	4	4	4	4
20–34	8	2.5	<1	1	2	2	3	4	4	4
35–49	18	4.1	18	1	2	3	4	12	18	18
50–64	17	4.4	37	1	2	3	7	27	27	27
65+	16	4.6	5	2	3	5	6	11	11	11
B. *Operated*										
0–19 Years	1	4.0	0	4	4	4	4	4	4	4
20–34	18	6.5	54	2	2	4	8	12	33	33
35–49	41	4.5	8	2	3	4	6	7	7	16
50–64	60	4.8	17	1	2	4	6	11	12	20
65+	54	3.7	11	1	3	3	5	9	10	15
SUBTOTALS:										
1. SINGLE DX										
A. *Not Operated*	4	1.8	2	1	1	1	1	4	4	4
B. *Operated*	25	2.2	2	1	1	1	4	4	4	5
2. MULTIPLE DX										
A. *Not Operated*	60	4.1	17	1	2	3	5	6	12	27
B. *Operated*	174	4.6	17	1	2	3	6	9	12	20
1. SINGLE DX	29	2.1	2	1	1	1	4	4	4	5
2. MULTIPLE DX	234	4.4	17	1	2	3	6	9	12	20
A. NOT OPERATED	64	3.9	17	1	2	3	4	6	11	27
B. OPERATED	199	4.3	15	1	2	3	6	9	11	16
TOTAL										
0–19 Years	2	4.0	0	4	4	4	4	4	4	4
20–34	34	4.4	33	1	2	3	5	8	12	33
35–49	69	4.1	10	1	2	3	6	7	9	18
50–64	85	4.5	19	1	1	3	6	10	12	27
65+	73	3.8	9	1	1	3	5	8	10	15
GRAND TOTAL	263	4.2	16	1	2	3	5	8	11	20

722.4: CERVICAL DISC DEGEN

Type of Patients	Observed Patients	Avg. Stay	Vari-ance	10th	25th	50th	75th	90th	95th	99th
1. SINGLE DX										
A. *Not Operated*										
0–19 Years	0									
20–34	1	2.0	0	2	2	2	2	2	2	2
35–49	3	1.7	1	1	1	1	3	3	3	3
50–64	1	1.0	0	1	1	1	1	1	1	1
65+	1	2.0	0	2	2	2	2	2	2	2
B. *Operated*										
0–19 Years	0									
20–34	11	1.5	<1	1	1	1	2	2	3	3
35–49	88	1.5	<1	1	1	1	2	3	3	4
50–64	106	1.4	<1	1	1	1	2	2	3	4
65+	19	1.5	<1	1	1	2	2	3	3	3
2. MULTIPLE DX										
A. *Not Operated*										
0–19 Years	0									
20–34	5	5.6	43	1	2	3	5	17	17	17
35–49	59	2.9	5	1	1	2	4	6	8	10
50–64	110	2.7	4	1	1	2	4	5	7	10
65+	171	3.4	6	2	2	3	5	6	8	14
B. *Operated*										
0–19 Years	2	1.0	0	1	1	1	1	1	1	1
20–34	42	1.7	<1	1	1	1	2	3	3	4
35–49	672	1.8	2	1	1	1	2	3	4	7
50–64	1,148	2.0	3	1	2	2	3	3	4	9
65+	371	2.5	6	1	2	2	3	5	6	17
SUBTOTALS:										
1. SINGLE DX										
A. *Not Operated*	6	1.7	<1	1	1	1	2	3	3	3
B. *Operated*	224	1.4	<1	1	1	1	2	2	3	4
2. MULTIPLE DX										
A. *Not Operated*	345	3.2	6	1	1	2	4	6	8	12
B. *Operated*	2,235	2.0	3	1	1	2	2	3	5	9
1. SINGLE DX	230	1.4	<1	1	1	1	2	2	3	4
2. MULTIPLE DX	2,580	2.2	4	1	1	2	3	4	5	10
A. NOT OPERATED	351	3.1	6	1	1	2	4	6	8	12
B. OPERATED	2,459	2.0	3	1	1	2	2	3	4	9
TOTAL										
0–19 Years	2	1.0	0	1	1	1	1	1	1	1
20–34	59	2.0	5	1	1	1	2	3	4	17
35–49	822	1.8	2	1	1	1	2	3	4	8
50–64	1,365	2.0	3	1	1	2	3	3	5	9
65+	562	2.8	6	1	2	2	3	5	7	14
GRAND TOTAL	2,810	2.1	4	1	1	2	2	4	5	9

722.52: LUMBAR/LS DISC DEGEN

Type of Patients	Observed Patients	Avg. Stay	Vari-ance	10th	25th	50th	75th	90th	95th	99th
1. SINGLE DX										
A. *Not Operated*										
0–19 Years	0									
20–34	7	4.9	66	1	1	2	3	23	23	23
35–49	19	2.9	2	2	2	2	4	5	6	6
50–64	7	1.9	1	1	1	2	2	4	4	4
65+	3	1.3	<1	1	1	1	2	2	2	2
B. *Operated*										
0–19 Years	3	2.0	<1	1	1	2	3	3	3	3
20–34	81	2.9	2	1	2	3	4	4	5	6
35–49	253	3.1	2	1	2	3	4	5	5	7
50–64	192	2.9	2	1	2	3	4	5	6	8
65+	45	2.2	1	1	1	2	3	4	4	5
2. MULTIPLE DX										
A. *Not Operated*										
0–19 Years	3	3.0	<1	2	2	3	4	4	4	4
20–34	95	3.4	6	2	2	3	4	6	8	16
35–49	266	3.6	10	1	2	3	4	6	8	17
50–64	475	3.8	9	1	2	3	5	7	9	15
65+	1,124	4.3	7	2	2	4	5	8	10	15
B. *Operated*										
0–19 Years	10	3.6	2	2	3	3	4	6	6	6
20–34	520	3.5	3	2	2	3	4	5	6	9
35–49	2,108	3.8	7	2	2	3	4	6	7	12
50–64	3,564	4.0	7	2	2	4	5	7	8	13
65+	2,653	4.1	9	2	2	4	5	7	9	15
SUBTOTALS:										
1. SINGLE DX										
A. *Not Operated*	36	3.0	14	1	1	2	3	5	6	23
B. *Operated*	574	2.9	2	1	2	3	4	5	5	6
2. MULTIPLE DX										
A. *Not Operated*	1,963	4.0	8	1	2	3	5	7	9	15
B. *Operated*	8,855	3.9	7	1	2	3	5	7	8	13
1. SINGLE DX	610	2.9	3	1	2	3	4	5	5	6
2. MULTIPLE DX	10,818	4.0	7	1	2	3	5	7	8	14
A. NOT OPERATED	1,999	4.0	8	1	2	3	5	7	9	15
B. OPERATED	9,429	3.9	7	1	2	3	5	6	8	13
TOTAL										
0–19 Years	16	3.2	2	2	2	3	4	5	6	6
20–34	703	3.4	4	2	2	3	4	5	6	10
35–49	2,646	3.7	7	2	2	3	4	6	7	12
50–64	4,238	3.9	7	2	2	3	5	7	8	13
65+	3,825	4.2	9	1	2	4	5	7	9	15
GRAND TOTAL	11,428	3.9	7	1	2	3	5	7	8	13

Length of Stay by Diagnosis and Operation, Western Region, 2008

Western Region, October 2006–September 2007 Data, by Diagnosis

722.71: CERV DISC DIS W MYELOP

Type of Patients	Observed Patients	Avg. Stay	Variance	Percentiles 10th	25th	50th	75th	90th	95th	99th
1. SINGLE DX										
A. Not Operated										
0–19 Years	0									
20–34	0									
35–49	3	1.7	<1	1	1		2	2	2	2
50–64	1	9.0	0	9	9		9	9	9	9
65+	0									
B. Operated										
0–19 Years	0									
20–34	27	2.1	5	1	1	1	2	4	6	11
35–49	175	1.6	1	1	1	1	2	3	3	5
50–64	148	1.6	1	1	1	1	2	3	4	6
65+	21	1.8	2	1	1	1	2	3	3	7
2. MULTIPLE DX										
A. Not Operated										
0–19 Years	0									
20–34	3	2.0	0	2	2	2	2	2	2	2
35–49	31	4.2	17	1	1	3	5	7	16	20
50–64	56	3.6	8	1	2	3	4	8	10	14
65+	58	4.4	12	1	2	3	6	10	12	16
B. Operated										
0–19 Years	3	2.7	4	1	1	2	5	5	5	5
20–34	96	2.1	5	1	1	1	3	4	5	15
35–49	876	2.3	8	1	1	1	2	4	7	17
50–64	1,379	3.0	16	1	1	2	3	6	9	24
65+	787	4.4	34	1	1	3	5	10	14	25
SUBTOTALS:										
1. SINGLE DX — A. Not Operated	4	3.5	14	1	2	2	2	9	9	9
1. SINGLE DX — B. Operated	371	1.7	1	1	1	1	2	2	2	6
2. MULTIPLE DX — A. Not Operated	148	4.0	11	1	2	3	5	9	11	16
2. MULTIPLE DX — B. Operated	3,141	3.1	19	1	1	2	3	6	10	22
1. SINGLE DX	375	1.7	2	1	1	1	2	3	4	7
2. MULTIPLE DX	3,289	3.1	18	1	1	2	3	6	10	22
A. NOT OPERATED	152	4.0	11	1	2	3	5	9	11	16
B. OPERATED	3,512	3.0	17	1	1	2	3	6	9	21
TOTAL										
0–19 Years	3	2.7	4	1	1	2	2	5	5	5
20–34	126	2.1	5	1	1	1	2	4	5	13
35–49	1,085	2.2	8	1	1	1	2	4	6	17
50–64	1,584	2.9	15	1	1	2	3	6	9	23
65+	866	4.3	31	1	1	3	5	10	14	24
GRAND TOTAL	3,664	3.0	17	1	1	2	3	6	9	20

722.73: LUMBAR DISC DIS W MYELOP

Type of Patients	Observed Patients	Avg. Stay	Variance	Percentiles 10th	25th	50th	75th	90th	95th	99th
1. SINGLE DX										
A. Not Operated										
0–19 Years	0									
20–34	2	2.0	0	2	2	2	2	2	2	2
35–49	6	2.8	<1	1	3	3	3	4	4	4
50–64	4	1.3	<1	1	1	1	2	2	2	2
65+	1	4.0	0	4	4	4	4	4	4	4
B. Operated										
0–19 Years	4	1.5	<1	1	1	1	2	2	2	2
20–34	64	1.6	1	1	1	1	2	2	3	5
35–49	79	1.7	1	1	1	1	2	3	4	6
50–64	56	2.3	14	1	1	1	2	4	4	28
65+	8	2.5	3	1	1	2	3	6	6	6
2. MULTIPLE DX										
A. Not Operated										
0–19 Years	0									
20–34	23	3.2	3	1	2	3	4	6	6	7
35–49	29	4.1	6	1	2	4	5	8	9	11
50–64	46	4.2	10	2	2	3	6	9	11	15
65+	90	4.3	7	2	3	4	6	8	10	14
B. Operated										
0–19 Years	3	1.7	<1	1	1	2	2	2	2	2
20–34	141	2.7	5	1	1	2	3	5	6	12
35–49	394	3.3	24	1	1	2	4	5	7	19
50–64	455	3.2	14	1	1	2	4	6	7	22
65+	318	3.8	11	1	1	3	5	9	10	16
SUBTOTALS:										
1. SINGLE DX — A. Not Operated	13	2.3	1	1	1	2	3	4	4	4
1. SINGLE DX — B. Operated	211	1.8	5	1	1	1	2	3	4	6
2. MULTIPLE DX — A. Not Operated	188	4.1	7	2	2	3	5	7	10	14
2. MULTIPLE DX — B. Operated	1,311	3.3	15	1	1	2	4	6	8	16
1. SINGLE DX	224	1.9	4	1	1	1	2	4	4	6
2. MULTIPLE DX	1,499	3.4	14	1	1	3	4	6	9	15
A. NOT OPERATED	201	4.0	7	1	2	3	5	7	9	14
B. OPERATED	1,522	3.1	14	1	1	2	4	6	8	15
TOTAL										
0–19 Years	7	1.6	<1	1	1	1	2	2	2	2
20–34	230	2.4	4	1	1	2	3	4	6	11
35–49	508	3.1	20	1	1	2	4	5	7	13
50–64	561	3.2	14	1	1	2	4	6	7	22
65+	417	3.9	10	1	2	3	5	8	10	14
GRAND TOTAL	1,723	3.2	13	1	1	2	4	6	8	14

722.83: POSTLAMINEC SYND-LUMBAR

Type of Patients	Observed Patients	Avg. Stay	Variance	Percentiles 10th	25th	50th	75th	90th	95th	99th
1. SINGLE DX										
A. Not Operated										
0–19 Years	0									
20–34	1	1.0	0	1	1	1	1	1	1	1
35–49	7	1.6	<1	1	1	2	2	2	2	2
50–64	5	1.6	<1	1	1	1	2	3	3	3
65+	4	2.7	<1	2	2	2	3	4	4	4
B. Operated										
0–19 Years	0									
20–34	3	3.0	3	2	2	2	5	5	5	5
35–49	19	2.0	2	1	1	2	2	3	7	7
50–64	16	2.3	1	1	1	2	3	4	5	5
65+	11	2.1	2	1	1	2	3	3	5	5
2. MULTIPLE DX										
A. Not Operated										
0–19 Years	0									
20–34	9	4.0	6	1	3	3	6	8	8	8
35–49	68	3.4	7	1	2	3	4	7	10	14
50–64	85	3.6	11	1	1	2	4	9	11	17
65+	77	3.0	6	1	1	2	4	7	8	13
B. Operated										
0–19 Years	0									
20–34	32	3.6	6	1	2	3	4	6	10	11
35–49	183	3.5	8	1	2	3	5	6	9	16
50–64	320	4.0	11	1	2	3	5	7	9	20
65+	301	4.3	17	1	2	3	5	7	11	21
SUBTOTALS:										
1. SINGLE DX — A. Not Operated	17	1.8	<1	1	1	2	2	3	4	4
1. SINGLE DX — B. Operated	49	2.2	2	1	1	2	3	4	5	7
2. MULTIPLE DX — A. Not Operated	239	3.4	8	1	1	3	4	7	10	13
2. MULTIPLE DX — B. Operated	836	4.0	12	1	2	3	5	7	9	19
1. SINGLE DX	66	2.1	1	1	1	2	3	3	5	7
2. MULTIPLE DX	1,075	3.9	11	1	2	3	5	7	10	18
A. NOT OPERATED	256	3.3	8	1	1	2	4	7	10	13
B. OPERATED	885	3.9	12	1	2	3	5	7	9	19
TOTAL										
0–19 Years	0									
20–34	45	3.6	5	1	1	3	4	7	8	11
35–49	277	3.4	7	1	1	3	4	6	9	14
50–64	426	3.8	11	1	2	3	5	7	10	18
65+	393	4.0	14	1	2	3	5	7	9	21
GRAND TOTAL	1,141	3.8	11	1	2	3	5	7	9	17

Length of Stay by Diagnosis and Operation, Western Region, 2008

Western Region, October 2006—September 2007 Data, by Diagnosis

722.91: DISC DISORD NEC&NOS-CERV

Type of Patients	Observed Patients	Avg. Stay	Variance	10th	25th	50th	75th	90th	95th	99th
1. SINGLE DX										
A. Not Operated										
0–19 Years	0									
20–34	0									
35–49	1	1.0	0	1	1	1	1	1	1	1
50–64	0									
65+	0									
B. Operated										
0–19 Years	0									
20–34	2	1.0	0	1	1	1	1	1	1	1
35–49	13	1.2	<1	1	1	1	1	2	3	3
50–64	15	2.7	11	1	1	2	3	4	14	14
65+	1	1.0	0	1	1	1	1	1	1	1
2. MULTIPLE DX										
A. Not Operated										
0–19 Years	0									
20–34	0									
35–49	18	3.2	7	1	1	2	5	8	10	10
50–64	27	4.3	26	1	2	3	5	11	13	25
65+	28	5.1	17	1	3	4	5	12	15	17
B. Operated										
0–19 Years	0									
20–34	6	2.5	4	1	1	1	4	6	6	6
35–49	76	2.0	3	1	1	1	2	4	6	11
50–64	117	3.7	34	1	1	2	3	8	12	34
65+	48	3.7	61	1	1	2	3	6	11	54
SUBTOTALS:										
1. SINGLE DX										
A. Not Operated	1	1.0	0	1	1	1	1	1	1	1
B. Operated	31	1.9	6	1	1	1	2	3	4	14
2. MULTIPLE DX										
A. Not Operated	73	4.3	18	1	2	3	5	10	13	25
B. Operated	247	3.1	29	1	1	2	3	6	11	34
1. SINGLE DX	32	1.9	5	1	1	1	2	3	4	14
2. MULTIPLE DX	320	3.4	27	1	2	3	6	11	11	27
A. NOT OPERATED	74	4.3	18	1	2	3	5	10	13	25
B. OPERATED	278	3.0	27	1	1	2	3	6	11	34
TOTAL										
0–19 Years	0									
20–34	8	2.1	4	1	1	1	2	6	6	6
35–49	108	2.1	4	1	1	1	2	5	6	10
50–64	159	3.7	30	1	1	2	3	8	13	34
65+	77	4.2	44	1	1	3	4	11	12	54
GRAND TOTAL	352	3.3	25	1	1	2	3	6	11	27

722.93: DISC DISORD NEC&NOS-LUMB

Type of Patients	Observed Patients	Avg. Stay	Variance	10th	25th	50th	75th	90th	95th	99th
1. SINGLE DX										
A. Not Operated										
0–19 Years	1	8.0	0	8	8	8	8	8	8	8
20–34	4	2.2	2	1	1	1	3	4	4	4
35–49	6	2.8	2	1	1	3	4	4	4	4
50–64	4	1.5	<1	1	1	2	2	2	2	2
65+	1	4.0	0	4	4	4	4	4	4	4
B. Operated										
0–19 Years	1	1.0	0	1	1	1	1	1	1	1
20–34	9	3.1	<1	2	2	3	4	4	4	4
35–49	21	2.9	2	2	2	3	4	4	5	6
50–64	17	3.0	8	1	1	2	4	7	12	12
65+	0									
2. MULTIPLE DX										
A. Not Operated										
0–19 Years	7	5.1	25	1	1	3	7	15	15	15
20–34	32	4.7	23	2	2	4	5	9	14	26
35–49	95	4.7	12	1	2	4	6	9	14	17
50–64	129	5.0	13	1	2	4	7	10	12	16
65+	181	5.4	20	1	2	4	7	10	13	24
B. Operated										
0–19 Years	2	12.5	177	3	3	3	22	22	22	22
20–34	42	3.7	9	1	3	3	5	7	9	13
35–49	155	4.9	19	3	3	4	5	9	12	21
50–64	227	5.9	47	1	2	4	7	12	21	39
65+	184	7.2	57	2	2	5	9	16	20	40
SUBTOTALS:										
1. SINGLE DX										
A. Not Operated	16	2.7	4	1	1	2	4	4	8	8
B. Operated	48	2.9	4	1	2	3	4	5	6	12
2. MULTIPLE DX										
A. Not Operated	444	5.1	17	1	2	4	7	10	13	20
B. Operated	610	5.9	41	1	2	4	7	12	19	39
1. SINGLE DX	64	2.9	4	1	2	3	4	4	6	12
2. MULTIPLE DX	1,054	5.6	31	1	2	4	7	11	15	29
A. NOT OPERATED	460	5.0	16	1	2	4	6	10	13	20
B. OPERATED	658	5.7	39	1	2	4	7	12	18	39
TOTAL										
0–19 Years	11	6.4	45	1	1	3	8	15	22	22
20–34	87	3.9	13	2	2	3	4	7	10	26
35–49	277	4.6	15	1	2	4	5	9	12	20
50–64	377	5.4	34	2	2	4	7	13	15	29
65+	366	6.3	39	2	2	4	8	13	19	31
GRAND TOTAL	1,118	5.4	30	1	2	4	7	11	15	28

723: OTHER CERV SPINE DISORD

Type of Patients	Observed Patients	Avg. Stay	Variance	10th	25th	50th	75th	90th	95th	99th
1. SINGLE DX										
A. Not Operated										
0–19 Years	15	1.3	<1	1	1	1	1	3	3	3
20–34	7	1.7	<1	1	1	1	3	3	3	3
35–49	12	1.5	<1	1	1	1	2	2	2	3
50–64	6	2.5	2	2	1	3	3	5	5	5
65+	3	2.3	<1	2	2	2	3	3	3	3
B. Operated										
0–19 Years	2	1.0	0	1	1	1	1	1	1	1
20–34	6	1.5	<1	1	1	1	2	3	3	3
35–49	90	1.7	5	1	1	1	2	3	3	22
50–64	128	1.7	1	1	1	1	2	3	4	6
65+	33	1.8	1	1	1	1	2	3	3	6
2. MULTIPLE DX										
A. Not Operated										
0–19 Years	39	1.8	3	1	1	2	2	4	4	10
20–34	116	2.4	7	1	1	2	3	4	6	15
35–49	330	2.6	12	1	2	2	3	5	7	10
50–64	411	2.8	6	1	2	3	3	6	7	13
65+	504	2.8	5	1	2	3	3	6	7	11
B. Operated										
0–19 Years	9	3.8	4	1	3	4	4	8	8	8
20–34	42	1.9	1	1	1	2	2	3	3	5
35–49	628	2.2	5	1	1	2	2	4	6	11
50–64	1,283	2.7	9	1	1	2	3	5	7	17
65+	720	3.7	20	2	2	2	4	8	11	23
SUBTOTALS:										
1. SINGLE DX										
A. Not Operated	43	1.7	<1	1	1	1	2	3	3	5
B. Operated	259	1.7	3	1	1	1	2	3	3	6
2. MULTIPLE DX										
A. Not Operated	1,400	2.7	5	1	2	3	3	5	7	12
B. Operated	2,682	2.9	11	1	2	4	4	6	8	17
1. SINGLE DX	302	1.7	2	1	1	2	2	3	3	6
2. MULTIPLE DX	4,082	2.8	9	1	2	3	4	5	8	15
A. NOT OPERATED	1,443	2.6	5	1	1	2	3	5	7	12
B. OPERATED	2,941	2.8	10	1	2	3	4	5	8	17
TOTAL										
0–19 Years	65	1.9	3	1	1	1	2	4	4	10
20–34	171	2.2	5	1	1	2	3	4	5	15
35–49	1,060	2.3	5	1	1	2	3	5	6	11
50–64	1,828	2.7	7	1	1	2	3	5	7	14
65+	1,260	3.3	14	1	2	3	4	7	9	18
GRAND TOTAL	4,384	2.7	9	1	1	2	3	5	7	15

Length of Stay by Diagnosis and Operation, Western Region, 2008

Western Region, October 2006–September 2007 Data, by Diagnosis

723.0: CERVICAL SPINAL STENOSIS

Type of Patients	Observed Patients	Avg. Stay	Variance	10th	25th	50th	75th	90th	95th	99th
1. SINGLE DX										
A. Not Operated										
0–19 Years	0									
20–34	1	1.0	0	1	1	1	1	1	1	1
35–49	1	2.0	0	2	2	2	2	2	2	2
50–64	4	2.3	4	2	2	2	5	5	5	5
65+	2	2.5	<1	2	2	3	3	3	3	3
B. Operated										
0–19 Years	0									
20–34	2	1.5	<1	1	1	2	2	2	2	2
35–49	68	1.8	7	1	1	1	2	2	3	22
50–64	98	1.7	2	1	1	2	2	3	4	9
65+	30	1.9	1	1	1	2	2	3	3	6
2. MULTIPLE DX										
A. Not Operated										
0–19 Years	1	1.0	0	1	1	1	1	1	1	1
20–34	4	3.3	2	2	2	4	5	5	5	5
35–49	59	3.3	7	1	2	3	4	6	7	15
50–64	92	3.4	6	1	2	3	4	6	8	13
65+	129	3.5	6	1	2	3	5	7	9	11
B. Operated										
0–19 Years	3	3.0	<1	2	2	3	4	4	4	4
20–34	27	1.8	<1	1	1	2	2	2	3	5
35–49	498	2.2	5	1	1	2	3	4	5	12
50–64	1,082	2.8	9	1	1	2	3	5	6	18
65+	656	3.8	20	1	1	3	4	8	11	25
SUBTOTALS:										
1. SINGLE DX										
A. Not Operated	8	2.1	2	1	1	2	2	3	5	5
B. Operated	198	1.8	3	1	1	1	2	3	4	9
2. MULTIPLE DX										
A. Not Operated	285	3.4	6	1	2	3	4	7	8	11
B. Operated	2,266	2.9	12	1	1	2	3	6	8	18
1. SINGLE DX	206	1.8	3	1	1	1	2	3	4	6
2. MULTIPLE DX	2,551	3.0	11	1	1	2	4	6	8	17
A. NOT OPERATED	293	3.4	6	2	2	3	4	6	8	11
B. OPERATED	2,464	2.8	11	1	1	2	3	5	8	18
TOTAL										
0–19 Years	4	2.5	2	1	1	2	3	4	4	4
20–34	34	1.9	1	1	1	2	2	3	5	5
35–49	626	2.2	5	1	1	2	3	4	6	12
50–64	1,276	2.7	8	1	1	2	3	5	7	17
65+	817	3.7	18	1	1	3	4	7	10	19
GRAND TOTAL	2,757	2.9	10	1	1	2	3	6	8	17

723.1: CERVICALGIA

Type of Patients	Observed Patients	Avg. Stay	Variance	10th	25th	50th	75th	90th	95th	99th
1. SINGLE DX										
A. Not Operated										
0–19 Years	10	1.1	<1	1	1	1	1	1	2	2
20–34	4	1.3	<1	1	1	1	1	2	2	2
35–49	4	1.5	<1	1	1	1	2	3	3	3
50–64	1	3.0	0	3	3	3	3	3	3	3
65+	0									
B. Operated										
0–19 Years	0									
20–34	0									
35–49	1	1.0	0	1	1	1	1	1	1	1
50–64	0									
65+	0									
2. MULTIPLE DX										
A. Not Operated										
0–19 Years	30	1.7	3	1	1	1	2	3	4	10
20–34	89	2.1	4	1	1	2	3	4	6	15
35–49	152	2.3	4	1	1	2	3	4	6	10
50–64	173	2.5	5	1	1	2	3	4	6	13
65+	214	2.5	6	1	1	2	3	5	7	15
B. Operated										
0–19 Years	0									
20–34	4	1.8	<1	1	1	2	2	3	3	3
35–49	12	2.2	8	1	1	2	4	11	11	11
50–64	21	2.7	2	1	1	3	4	4	5	5
65+	7	3.2	6	1	1	3	5	7	7	7
SUBTOTALS:										
1. SINGLE DX										
A. Not Operated	19	1.3	<1	1	1	1	1	3	3	3
B. Operated	1	1.0	0	1	1	1	1	1	1	1
2. MULTIPLE DX										
A. Not Operated	658	2.3	5	1	1	2	3	4	6	13
B. Operated	44	2.5	4	1	1	2	3	5	5	11
1. SINGLE DX	20	1.3	<1	1	1	1	1	2	3	3
2. MULTIPLE DX	702	2.4	5	1	1	2	3	4	6	13
A. NOT OPERATED	677	2.3	5	1	1	2	3	4	6	13
B. OPERATED	45	2.5	4	1	1	2	3	5	5	11
TOTAL										
0–19 Years	40	1.6	2	1	1	1	2	2	4	4
20–34	97	2.0	3	1	1	2	2	4	6	15
35–49	169	2.2	4	1	1	2	3	4	6	11
50–64	195	2.5	4	1	1	2	3	4	6	13
65+	221	2.5	6	1	1	2	3	5	7	15
GRAND TOTAL	722	2.3	5	1	1	2	3	4	6	13

723.4: BRACHIAL NEURITIS NOS

Type of Patients	Observed Patients	Avg. Stay	Variance	10th	25th	50th	75th	90th	95th	99th
1. SINGLE DX										
A. Not Operated										
0–19 Years	0									
20–34	0									
35–49	2	1.5	<1	1	1	2	2	2	2	2
50–64	1	3.0	0	3	3	3	3	3	3	3
65+	0									
B. Operated										
0–19 Years	0									
20–34	3	3.0	0	1	1	1	1	1	1	1
35–49	16	1.3	<1	1	1	1	1	2	3	3
50–64	28	1.5	<1	1	1	1	2	3	3	4
65+	3	1.0	0	1	1	1	1	1	1	1
2. MULTIPLE DX										
A. Not Operated										
0–19 Years	1	4.0	0	4	4	4	4	4	4	4
20–34	13	4.1	37	1	2	3	3	5	24	24
35–49	70	2.7	4	1	1	2	3	5	7	11
50–64	110	2.5	3	1	1	2	3	5	6	16
65+	98	2.5	3	1	1	2	3	5	6	9
B. Operated										
0–19 Years	0									
20–34	7	1.9	2	1	1	1	2	5	5	5
35–49	93	1.9	3	1	1	1	2	3	5	11
50–64	128	1.9	3	1	1	1	2	3	5	13
65+	39	2.1	4	1	1	1	2	4	7	11
SUBTOTALS:										
1. SINGLE DX										
A. Not Operated	3	2.0	<1	1	1	2	2	3	3	3
B. Operated	50	1.4	<1	1	1	1	2	2	3	4
2. MULTIPLE DX										
A. Not Operated	292	2.6	6	1	1	2	3	5	6	16
B. Operated	267	1.9	3	1	1	1	2	3	5	11
1. SINGLE DX	53	1.4	<1	1	1	1	2	2	3	4
2. MULTIPLE DX	559	2.3	5	1	1	2	3	5	6	11
A. NOT OPERATED	295	2.6	6	1	1	2	3	5	6	16
B. OPERATED	317	1.8	3	1	1	1	2	3	5	11
TOTAL										
0–19 Years	1	4.0	0	4	4	4	4	4	4	4
20–34	23	3.0	22	1	1	2	3	4	5	24
35–49	181	2.1	3	1	1	2	2	4	6	11
50–64	267	2.1	4	1	1	1	2	4	5	13
65+	140	2.4	3	1	1	2	3	5	6	9
GRAND TOTAL	612	2.2	4	1	1	2	3	4	6	11

Length of Stay by Diagnosis and Operation, Western Region, 2008

Western Region, October 2006–September 2007 Data, by Diagnosis

724: OTHER/UNSPEC BACK DISORD

Type of Patients	Observed Patients	Avg. Stay	Vari-ance	Percentiles 10th	25th	50th	75th	90th	95th	99th
1. SINGLE DX										
A. Not Operated										
0–19 Years	8	1.5	<1	1	1	1	2	3	3	3
20–34	32	1.5	<1	1	1	1	2	2	4	4
35–49	48	2.2	2	1	1	2	3	4	5	7
50–64	33	2.4	3	1	1	2	3	4	5	10
65+	22	2.2	2	1	1	2	3	4	4	7
B. Operated										
0–19 Years	1	1.0	0	1	1	1	1	1	1	1
20–34	35	2.1	2	1	1	2	3	4	5	6
35–49	138	2.1	3	1	1	1	3	4	5	9
50–64	300	1.8	2	1	1	1	2	3	4	7
65+	263	1.9	1	1	1	2	2	4	4	6
2. MULTIPLE DX										
A. Not Operated										
0–19 Years	89	2.8	6	1	1	2	3	6	9	12
20–34	476	2.8	5	1	1	2	3	6	7	12
35–49	1,070	3.1	8	1	1	2	4	6	7	14
50–64	1,543	3.3	8	1	1	3	4	7	9	13
65+	3,727	3.7	9	1	2	3	5	7	9	15
B. Operated										
0–19 Years	8	3.7	19	1	1	2	4	14	14	14
20–34	151	2.8	5	1	1	2	4	5	5	13
35–49	1,045	2.9	8	1	1	2	4	5	7	14
50–64	4,438	2.9	8	1	1	2	4	5	7	13
65+	9,006	3.1	8	1	1	3	4	6	7	13
SUBTOTALS:										
1. SINGLE DX *A. Not Operated*	143	2.0	2	1	1	2	2	4	4	7
B. Operated	737	1.9	2	1	1	1	3	4	5	7
2. MULTIPLE DX *A. Not Operated*	6,905	3.4	8	1	2	3	4	7	8	14
B. Operated	14,648	3.0	8	1	1	2	4	6	7	13
1. SINGLE DX	880	1.9	2	1	1	1	2	4	5	7
2. MULTIPLE DX	21,553	3.2	8	1	1	3	4	6	8	13
A. NOT OPERATED	7,048	3.4	8	1	2	3	4	7	8	14
B. OPERATED	15,385	3.0	8	1	1	2	4	5	7	13
TOTAL										
0–19 Years	106	2.8	6	1	1	2	3	6	9	12
20–34	694	2.7	5	1	1	2	3	5	7	12
35–49	2,301	2.9	7	1	1	2	4	5	7	14
50–64	6,314	2.9	8	1	1	2	4	6	7	13
65+	13,018	3.2	9	1	1	3	4	6	8	14
GRAND TOTAL	22,433	3.1	8	1	1	2	4	6	7	13

724.02: SPINAL STENOSIS-LUMBAR

Type of Patients	Observed Patients	Avg. Stay	Vari-ance	Percentiles 10th	25th	50th	75th	90th	95th	99th
1. SINGLE DX										
A. Not Operated										
0–19 Years	0									
20–34	1	4.0	0	4	4	4	4	4	4	4
35–49	2	3.0	2	2	2	2	4	4	4	4
50–64	5	2.6	1	1	2	3	3	4	4	4
65+	6	2.7	<1	2	2	2	3	4	4	4
B. Operated										
0–19 Years	1	1.0	0	1	1	1	1	1	1	1
20–34	19	2.0	2	1	1	2	2	4	4	6
35–49	111	2.3	4	1	1	2	3	4	6	9
50–64	273	1.8	2	1	1	1	2	3	4	7
65+	257	1.9	1	1	1	1	2	4	4	6
2. MULTIPLE DX										
A. Not Operated										
0–19 Years	0									
20–34	17	3.1	3	2	2	3	4	6	7	7
35–49	66	3.6	12	1	1	2	4	8	13	17
50–64	197	3.8	10	1	1	3	5	9	11	14
65+	971	4.3	11	2	2	4	5	8	11	16
B. Operated										
0–19 Years	5	2.6	2	1	1	2	3	4	4	4
20–34	95	2.6	4	1	1	2	3	5	6	13
35–49	836	2.9	7	1	1	2	4	5	7	13
50–64	4,084	2.9	6	1	1	2	4	5	7	12
65+	8,716	3.1	8	1	1	3	4	6	7	13
SUBTOTALS:										
1. SINGLE DX *A. Not Operated*	14	2.8	<1	2	2	3	4	4	4	4
B. Operated	661	1.9	2	1	1	1	2	4	5	7
2. MULTIPLE DX *A. Not Operated*	1,251	4.2	11	1	2	3	5	8	11	16
B. Operated	13,736	3.0	7	1	1	2	4	5	7	13
1. SINGLE DX	675	1.9	2	1	1	2	2	4	5	7
2. MULTIPLE DX	14,987	3.1	8	1	1	2	4	6	7	13
A. NOT OPERATED	1,265	4.1	11	1	2	3	5	8	11	16
B. OPERATED	14,397	3.0	7	1	1	2	4	5	7	13
TOTAL										
0–19 Years	6	2.3	2	1	1	2	3	4	4	4
20–34	132	2.6	3	1	1	2	3	5	6	8
35–49	1,015	2.9	7	1	1	2	3	5	7	13
50–64	4,559	2.8	6	1	1	2	4	5	7	12
65+	9,950	3.2	8	1	1	3	4	6	7	13
GRAND TOTAL	15,662	3.0	8	1	2	2	4	6	7	13

724.2: LUMBAGO

Type of Patients	Observed Patients	Avg. Stay	Vari-ance	Percentiles 10th	25th	50th	75th	90th	95th	99th
1. SINGLE DX										
A. Not Operated										
0–19 Years	2	1.0	0	1	1	1	1	1	1	1
20–34	20	1.5	<1	1	1	1	2	2	4	4
35–49	29	2.0	3	1	1	2	2	4	7	7
50–64	17	2.5	5	1	1	2	2	5	10	10
65+	4	1.8	<1	1	1	2	2	3	3	3
B. Operated										
0–19 Years	0									
20–34	3	1.7	1	1	1	1	3	3	3	3
35–49	4	1.8	<1	1	1	1	3	3	3	3
50–64	3	1.0	0	1	1	1	1	1	1	1
65+	0									
2. MULTIPLE DX										
A. Not Operated										
0–19 Years	33	3.0	5	1	1	2	4	6	8	11
20–34	279	2.9	5	1	1	2	3	6	7	13
35–49	578	3.2	9	1	1	3	4	6	8	18
50–64	659	3.4	7	1	2	3	4	7	8	13
65+	1,342	3.6	10	1	2	3	4	7	8	14
B. Operated										
0–19 Years	16	5.6	52	1	1	2	14	14	14	14
20–34	16	3.4	3	1	2	2	3	5	7	7
35–49	60	3.0	5	1	2	2	4	6	8	11
50–64	81	3.1	6	1	1	2	4	6	7	13
65+	51	4.9	40	1	1	3	6	11	16	36
SUBTOTALS:										
1. SINGLE DX *A. Not Operated*	72	1.9	2	1	1	1	2	3	5	10
B. Operated	10	1.5	<1	1	1	1	2	3	3	3
2. MULTIPLE DX *A. Not Operated*	2,891	3.4	9	1	2	3	4	6	8	14
B. Operated	211	3.6	15	1	1	3	4	7	11	16
1. SINGLE DX	82	1.9	2	1	1	1	2	3	4	10
2. MULTIPLE DX	3,102	3.4	9	1	2	3	4	6	8	14
A. NOT OPERATED	2,963	3.4	9	1	2	3	4	6	8	14
B. OPERATED	221	3.5	14	1	1	3	4	7	10	16
TOTAL										
0–19 Years	38	3.1	8	1	1	2	4	6	11	14
20–34	318	2.8	5	1	1	2	3	6	7	12
35–49	671	3.1	8	1	1	2	4	6	8	18
50–64	760	3.3	7	1	2	3	4	6	8	13
65+	1,397	3.7	11	1	2	3	4	7	8	15
GRAND TOTAL	3,184	3.4	9	1	2	3	4	6	8	14

Length of Stay by Diagnosis and Operation, Western Region, 2008

Western Region, October 2006–September 2007 Data, by Diagnosis

724.3: SCIATICA

Type of Patients	Observed Patients	Avg. Stay	Variance	10th	25th	50th	75th	90th	95th	99th
1. SINGLE DX										
A. Not Operated										
0–19 Years	0									
20–34	3	1.0	0	1	1	1	1	1	1	1
35–49	6	1.0	0	1	1	1	1	1	1	1
50–64	1	2.0	0	2	2	2	2	2	2	2
65+	3	3.0	12	1	1	1	7	7	7	7
B. Operated										
0–19 Years	0									
20–34	0									
35–49	0									
50–64	2	3.0	8	1	1	5	5	5	5	5
65+	0									
2. MULTIPLE DX										
A. Not Operated										
0–19 Years	2	6.5	59	1	1	12	12	12	12	12
20–34	16	2.1	2	1	1	1	3	4	6	6
35–49	62	3.1	5	1	1	2	5	6	7	9
50–64	106	3.2	10	1	1	2	4	6	13	16
65+	223	3.7	6	1	2	3	5	7	8	12
B. Operated										
0–19 Years	0									
20–34	1	2.0	0	2	2	2	2	2	2	2
35–49	4	4.0	6	2	2	5	7	7	7	7
50–64	13	3.2	15	1	1	2	2	9	14	14
65+	6	5.8	44	1	1	2	9	18	18	18
SUBTOTALS:										
1. SINGLE DX										
A. Not Operated	8	1.9	4	1	1	1	1	7	7	7
B. Operated	2	3.0	8	1	1	5	5	5	5	5
2. MULTIPLE DX										
A. Not Operated	409	3.4	7	1	2	3	4	6	8	13
B. Operated	24	3.9	19	1	1	2	4	9	14	18
1. SINGLE DX	10	2.1	4	1	1	1	2	5	7	7
2. MULTIPLE DX	433	3.5	7	1	2	3	4	6	8	15
A. NOT OPERATED	417	3.4	7	1	2	3	4	6	8	13
B. OPERATED	26	3.9	18	1	1	2	5	9	14	18
TOTAL										
0–19 Years	2	6.5	59	1	1	12	12	12	12	12
20–34	20	1.9	2	1	1	1	2	3	4	6
35–49	67	3.1	5	1	1	2	5	6	7	9
50–64	122	3.2	10	1	1	2	4	6	13	16
65+	232	3.8	6	1	2	3	5	7	8	13
GRAND TOTAL	443	3.4	7	1	2	3	4	6	8	15

724.4: LUMBOSACRAL NEURITIS NOS

Type of Patients	Observed Patients	Avg. Stay	Variance	10th	25th	50th	75th	90th	95th	99th
1. SINGLE DX										
A. Not Operated										
0–19 Years	0									
20–34	1	1.0	0	1	1	1	1	1	1	1
35–49	6	2.5	2	1	1	3	4	4	4	4
50–64	4	2.8	3	1	2	3	5	5	5	5
65+	3	1.0	0	1	1	1	1	1	1	1
B. Operated										
0–19 Years	0									
20–34	7	2.6	2	1	1	3	3	5	5	5
35–49	12	1.8	1	1	1	1	3	3	3	3
50–64	16	1.6	<1	1	1	1	2	3	4	4
65+	4	1.8	<1	1	2	2	2	2	2	2
2. MULTIPLE DX										
A. Not Operated										
0–19 Years	1	2.0	0	2	2	2	2	2	2	2
20–34	38	3.6	8	1	2	2	4	10	10	11
35–49	106	3.2	6	1	2	2	4	6	7	11
50–64	159	3.8	10	1	2	3	5	7	8	12
65+	224	4.3	12	1	2	3	6	8	10	20
B. Operated										
0–19 Years	0									
20–34	21	2.6	5	1	1	2	2	4	7	7
35–49	68	2.5	4	1	1	2	3	5	6	11
50–64	138	2.4	7	1	1	1	3	5	7	10
65+	120	2.5	5	2	2	2	3	5	7	12
SUBTOTALS:										
1. SINGLE DX										
A. Not Operated	14	2.2	2	1	1	2	3	4	5	5
B. Operated	39	1.9	1	1	1	1	3	3	4	5
2. MULTIPLE DX										
A. Not Operated	528	3.8	10	1	2	3	5	7	10	15
B. Operated	347	2.5	5	1	1	2	3	5	7	11
1. SINGLE DX	53	1.9	1	1	1	1	3	3	4	5
2. MULTIPLE DX	875	3.3	9	1	1	2	4	6	8	14
A. NOT OPERATED	542	3.8	10	1	2	3	5	7	10	15
B. OPERATED	386	2.4	5	1	1	2	3	5	6	11
TOTAL										
0–19 Years	1	2.0	0	2	2	2	2	2	2	2
20–34	67	3.1	7	1	2	2	3	8	10	11
35–49	192	2.8	5	1	1	2	4	6	6	11
50–64	317	3.1	8	1	1	3	4	6	8	12
65+	351	3.6	10	1	1	3	5	7	10	15
GRAND TOTAL	928	3.2	8	1	1	2	4	6	8	14

724.5: BACKACHE NOS

Type of Patients	Observed Patients	Avg. Stay	Variance	10th	25th	50th	75th	90th	95th	99th
1. SINGLE DX										
A. Not Operated										
0–19 Years	5	1.4	<1	1	1	1	2	2	2	2
20–34	4	1.5	<1	1	1	2	2	2	2	2
35–49	8	2.3	2	1	2	2	4	5	5	5
50–64	5	2.0	<1	2	2	2	2	3	3	3
65+	5	2.0	2	1	1	1	3	4	4	4
B. Operated										
0–19 Years	0									
20–34	0									
35–49	1	4.0	0	4	4	4	4	4	4	4
50–64	0									
65+	0									
2. MULTIPLE DX										
A. Not Operated										
0–19 Years	36	2.9	6	1	1	2	3	6	9	11
20–34	94	2.4	4	1	1	2	3	5	6	15
35–49	183	2.7	6	1	1	2	3	5	6	11
50–64	313	2.8	5	1	1	2	3	5	8	11
65+	704	3.0	4	1	2	2	4	6	7	10
B. Operated										
0–19 Years	0									
20–34	1	1.0	0	1	1	1	1	1	1	1
35–49	17	3.4	36	1	1	1	3	6	26	26
50–64	21	3.5	13	1	1	2	4	8	10	14
65+	21	4.8	18	1	1	4	8	9	11	17
SUBTOTALS:										
1. SINGLE DX										
A. Not Operated	27	1.9	1	1	1	2	2	2	4	5
B. Operated	1	4.0	0	4	4	4	4	4	4	4
2. MULTIPLE DX										
A. Not Operated	1,330	2.8	5	1	1	2	4	5	7	11
B. Operated	60	3.9	21	1	1	2	5	9	14	26
1. SINGLE DX	28	2.0	1	1	1	2	3	4	4	5
2. MULTIPLE DX	1,390	2.9	6	1	1	2	4	5	7	11
A. NOT OPERATED	1,357	2.8	5	1	1	2	4	5	7	11
B. OPERATED	61	3.9	20	1	1	2	4	9	11	26
TOTAL										
0–19 Years	41	2.7	6	1	1	2	3	6	9	11
20–34	99	2.4	4	1	1	2	3	5	6	15
35–49	209	2.7	8	1	1	2	3	5	6	11
50–64	339	2.8	6	1	1	2	4	5	8	11
65+	730	3.0	5	1	2	2	4	6	7	11
GRAND TOTAL	1,418	2.9	5	1	2	2	4	5	7	11

Length of Stay by Diagnosis and Operation, Western Region, 2008

724.8: OTHER BACK SYMPTOMS

Type of Patients	Observed Patients	Avg. Stay	Variance	Percentiles 10th	25th	50th	75th	90th	95th	99th
1. SINGLE DX										
A. Not Operated										
0–19 Years	1	3.0	0	3	3	3	3	3	3	3
20–34	3	1.3	<1	1	1	1	2	2	2	2
35–49	1	2.0	0	2	2	2	2	2	2	2
50–64	1	1.0	0	1	1	1	1	1	1	1
65+	0									
B. Operated										
0–19 Years	0									
20–34	0									
35–49	1	1.0	0	1	1	1	1	1	1	1
50–64	0									
65+	0									
2. MULTIPLE DX										
A. Not Operated										
0–19 Years	11	2.1	1	1	1	2	2	4	4	4
20–34	18	2.6	4	1	1	2	3	5	9	9
35–49	44	2.6	2	1	1	2	4	4	4	7
50–64	54	2.9	7	1	1	2	3	7	8	15
65+	73	3.3	3	1	2	3	4	6	7	10
B. Operated										
0–19 Years	0									
20–34	0									
35–49	5	2.0	1	1	1	2	3	3	3	3
50–64	16	1.7	1	1	1	1	2	4	4	4
65+	9	2.9	6	1	1	2	4	8	8	8
SUBTOTALS:										
1. SINGLE DX										
A. Not Operated	6	1.7	<1	1	1	2	2	3	3	3
B. Operated	1	1.0	0	1	1	1	1	1	1	1
2. MULTIPLE DX										
A. Not Operated	200	2.9	4	1	2	2	4	5	7	9
B. Operated	30	2.1	3	1	1	1	3	4	5	8
1. SINGLE DX	7	1.6	<1	1	1	1	2	3	3	3
2. MULTIPLE DX	230	2.8	4	1	1	2	4	5	7	9
A. NOT OPERATED	206	2.9	4	1	1	2	4	5	7	9
B. OPERATED	31	2.1	3	1	1	1	3	4	5	8
TOTAL										
0–19 Years	12	2.2	1	1	1	2	3	4	4	4
20–34	21	2.4	4	1	1	2	3	4	5	9
35–49	51	2.5	2	1	1	2	4	4	4	7
50–64	71	2.6	6	1	1	2	3	5	8	15
65+	82	3.3	4	1	2	3	4	6	7	10
GRAND TOTAL	237	2.8	4	1	1	2	4	5	7	9

725: POLYMYALGIA RHEUMATICA

Type of Patients	Observed Patients	Avg. Stay	Variance	Percentiles 10th	25th	50th	75th	90th	95th	99th
1. SINGLE DX										
A. Not Operated										
0–19 Years	0									
20–34	0									
35–49	0									
50–64	0									
65+	0									
B. Operated										
0–19 Years	0									
20–34	0									
35–49	0									
50–64	0									
65+	0									
2. MULTIPLE DX										
A. Not Operated										
0–19 Years	0									
20–34	3	7.3	4	5	5	8	9	9	9	9
35–49	5	4.0	13	1	1	4	4	10	10	10
50–64	37	4.0	9	1	2	3	5	9	11	13
65+	307	4.5	11	2	2	4	6	8	10	17
B. Operated										
0–19 Years	0									
20–34	0									
35–49	0									
50–64	6	4.3	8	1	2	4	6	9	9	9
65+	21	6.5	16	3	4	5	10	12	13	16
SUBTOTALS:										
1. SINGLE DX										
A. Not Operated	0									
B. Operated	0									
2. MULTIPLE DX										
A. Not Operated	352	4.5	10	2	2	4	6	8	10	17
B. Operated	27	6.0	15	2	3	5	9	12	13	16
1. SINGLE DX	0									
2. MULTIPLE DX	379	4.6	11	2	2	4	6	8	11	17
A. NOT OPERATED	352	4.5	10	2	2	4	6	8	10	17
B. OPERATED	27	6.0	15	3	3	5	9	12	13	16
TOTAL										
0–19 Years	0									
20–34	3	7.3	4	5	5	8	9	9	9	9
35–49	5	4.0	13	1	1	4	4	10	10	10
50–64	43	4.1	9	1	2	3	5	9	10	13
65+	328	4.7	11	2	3	4	6	8	11	17
GRAND TOTAL	379	4.6	11	2	2	4	6	8	11	17

726: PERIPH ENTHESOPATHIES

Type of Patients	Observed Patients	Avg. Stay	Variance	Percentiles 10th	25th	50th	75th	90th	95th	99th
1. SINGLE DX										
A. Not Operated										
0–19 Years	5	2.2	1	1	1	3	3	3	3	3
20–34	10	2.1	<1	1	2	2	2	3	3	4
35–49	15	2.0	1	1	1	2	2	3	4	5
50–64	15	2.3	3	1	1	2	2	5	7	7
65+	3	1.7	<1	1	1	2	2	2	2	2
B. Operated										
0–19 Years	7	2.3	<1	1	2	2	3	3	3	3
20–34	28	2.0	2	1	1	2	3	4	5	5
35–49	55	1.7	<1	1	1	1	2	3	4	5
50–64	74	1.5	<1	1	1	1	2	3	3	4
65+	40	1.3	<1	1	1	1	1	2	3	4
2. MULTIPLE DX										
A. Not Operated										
0–19 Years	37	3.5	5	1	2	3	4	6	9	11
20–34	116	3.3	5	1	2	3	4	5	6	13
35–49	303	3.2	4	1	2	3	4	6	7	9
50–64	396	3.4	7	1	2	3	4	6	9	14
65+	593	3.5	7	1	2	3	4	7	8	14
B. Operated										
0–19 Years	50	3.4	4	1	2	3	4	7	7	9
20–34	206	4.0	11	1	2	3	5	8	9	17
35–49	616	3.2	8	1	1	2	4	6	9	14
50–64	1,269	2.5	7	1	1	2	3	5	7	13
65+	1,479	2.5	7	1	2	2	3	5	7	13
SUBTOTALS:										
1. SINGLE DX										
A. Not Operated	48	2.1	1	1	1	2	2	3	5	7
B. Operated	204	1.6	<1	1	1	1	2	3	3	5
2. MULTIPLE DX										
A. Not Operated	1,445	3.4	6	1	2	3	4	6	8	13
B. Operated	3,620	2.7	7	1	2	2	3	6	8	14
1. SINGLE DX	252	1.7	1	1	1	1	2	3	4	5
2. MULTIPLE DX	5,065	2.9	7	1	2	2	4	6	8	13
A. NOT OPERATED	1,493	3.4	6	1	2	3	4	6	8	13
B. OPERATED	3,824	2.6	7	1	1	2	3	5	7	13
TOTAL										
0–19 Years	99	3.3	4	1	2	3	4	6	7	11
20–34	360	3.5	8	1	2	3	5	6	8	16
35–49	989	3.1	6	1	1	2	4	5	8	13
50–64	1,754	2.6	7	1	1	2	3	5	7	13
65+	2,115	2.8	7	1	1	2	3	6	8	13
GRAND TOTAL	5,317	2.8	7	1	1	2	4	6	8	13

Length of Stay by Diagnosis and Operation, Western Region, 2008

Western Region, October 2006–September 2007 Data, by Diagnosis

726.10: ROTATOR CUFF SYND NOS

Type of Patients	Observed Patients	Avg. Stay	Vari-ance	10th	25th	50th	75th	90th	95th	99th
1. SINGLE DX										
A. Not Operated										
0–19 Years	0									
20–34	0									
35–49	2	1.5	<1	1	1	2	2	2	2	2
50–64	0									
65+	1	2.0	0	2	2	2	2	2	2	2
B. Operated										
0–19 Years	0									
20–34	3	1.0	0	1	1	1	1	1	1	1
35–49	21	1.2	<1	1	1	1	1	2	2	3
50–64	36	1.3	<1	1	1	1	1	3	3	3
65+	33	1.3	<1	1	1	1	1	2	3	4
2. MULTIPLE DX										
A. Not Operated										
0–19 Years	0									
20–34	9	2.8	2	1	2	3	4	5	5	5
35–49	28	2.6	7	1	1	2	4	6	8	13
50–64	49	2.7	8	1	1	2	3	6	8	16
65+	117	3.1	7	1	1	2	2	6	8	15
B. Operated										
0–19 Years	0									
20–34	12	1.3	<1	1	1	1	1	2	2	2
35–49	140	1.7	4	1	1	1	2	3	3	3
50–64	591	1.6	2	1	1	1	2	3	3	3
65+	920	1.8	2	1	1	1	2	3	4	7
SUBTOTALS:										
1. SINGLE DX A. Not Operated	3	1.7	<1	1	1	2	2	2	2	2
1. SINGLE DX B. Operated	93	1.3	<1	1	1	1	1	2	3	4
2. MULTIPLE DX A. Not Operated	203	3.0	7	1	1	2	4	6	8	16
2. MULTIPLE DX B. Operated	1,663	1.8	2	1	1	1	2	3	3	7
1. SINGLE DX	96	1.3	<1	1	1	1	1	2	3	4
2. MULTIPLE DX	1,866	1.9	3	1	1	1	2	3	4	9
A. NOT OPERATED	206	2.9	7	1	1	2	4	6	8	15
B. OPERATED	1,756	1.7	2	1	1	1	2	3	4	7
TOTAL										
0–19 Years	0									
20–34	24	1.8	1	1	1	1	2	4	4	5
35–49	191	1.8	4	1	1	1	2	3	4	13
50–64	676	1.7	2	1	1	1	2	3	5	8
65+	1,071	2.0	3	1	1	1	2	4	5	8
GRAND TOTAL	1,962	1.9	3	1	1	1	2	3	4	8

726.2: SHOULD REGION DISORD NEC

Type of Patients	Observed Patients	Avg. Stay	Vari-ance	10th	25th	50th	75th	90th	95th	99th
1. SINGLE DX										
A. Not Operated										
0–19 Years	0									
20–34	0									
35–49	0									
50–64	0									
65+	0									
B. Operated										
0–19 Years	0									
20–34	2	1.0	0	1	1	1	1	1	1	1
35–49	7	1.1	<1	1	1	1	1	2	2	2
50–64	4	1.0	0	1	1	1	1	1	1	1
65+	1	2.0	0	2	2	2	2	2	2	2
2. MULTIPLE DX										
A. Not Operated										
0–19 Years	1	2.0	0	2	2	2	2	2	2	2
20–34	1	13.0	0	13	13	13	13	13	13	13
35–49	11	2.8	4	1	1	2	3	5	7	7
50–64	10	2.3	3	1	1	2	3	5	6	6
65+	24	2.3	7	2	2	2	3	4	5	13
B. Operated										
0–19 Years	2	1.0	0	1	1	1	1	1	1	1
20–34	8	1.1	<1	1	1	1	1	2	2	2
35–49	84	1.5	<1	1	1	1	2	2	3	4
50–64	199	1.5	2	1	1	1	2	3	3	6
65+	141	1.6	1	1	1	2	2	3	3	8
SUBTOTALS:										
1. SINGLE DX A. Not Operated	0									
1. SINGLE DX B. Operated	14	1.1	<1	1	1	1	1	2	2	2
2. MULTIPLE DX A. Not Operated	47	2.7	7	1	1	2	3	5	7	13
2. MULTIPLE DX B. Operated	434	1.5	2	1	1	1	2	3	3	6
1. SINGLE DX	14	1.1	<1	1	1	1	1	2	2	2
2. MULTIPLE DX	481	1.7	2	1	1	1	2	3	4	8
A. NOT OPERATED	47	2.7	7	1	1	2	3	5	7	13
B. OPERATED	448	1.5	2	1	1	1	2	3	3	6
TOTAL										
0–19 Years	3	1.3	<1	1	1	1	2	2	2	2
20–34	11	2.2	13	1	1	1	1	2	13	13
35–49	102	1.6	1	1	1	1	2	3	4	5
50–64	213	1.5	2	1	1	1	2	3	4	6
65+	166	1.7	2	1	1	2	2	3	4	9
GRAND TOTAL	495	1.6	2	1	1	1	2	3	4	8

726.33: OLECRANON BURSITIS

Type of Patients	Observed Patients	Avg. Stay	Vari-ance	10th	25th	50th	75th	90th	95th	99th
1. SINGLE DX										
A. Not Operated										
0–19 Years	2	1.0	0	1	1	1	1	1	1	1
20–34	3	2.0	<1	1	1	3	3	3	3	3
35–49	3	1.7	<1	1	1	2	2	2	2	2
50–64	3	1.0	0	1	1	1	1	1	1	1
65+	1	2.0	0	2	2	2	2	2	2	2
B. Operated										
0–19 Years	2	2.0	0	2	2	2	2	2	2	2
20–34	3	3.0	4	1	1	3	5	5	5	5
35–49	9	2.4	2	1	1	2	3	5	5	5
50–64	5	3.2	<1	2	3	3	4	4	4	4
65+	2	1.0	0	1	1	1	1	1	1	1
2. MULTIPLE DX										
A. Not Operated										
0–19 Years	8	2.8	2	1	2	3	4	5	5	5
20–34	40	3.1	3	1	2	3	4	5	5	10
35–49	107	3.4	4	1	2	3	4	6	7	10
50–64	137	3.6	6	1	2	3	5	7	9	12
65+	130	3.6	5	1	2	3	4	6	7	14
B. Operated										
0–19 Years	13	2.7	2	1	2	3	3	4	5	5
20–34	43	5.1	22	2	3	4	6	8	17	23
35–49	109	4.3	6	1	2	4	5	8	9	12
50–64	145	4.0	5	2	2	4	5	7	8	11
65+	164	5.1	18	2	2	4	6	9	11	25
SUBTOTALS:										
1. SINGLE DX A. Not Operated	12	1.5	<1	1	1	1	2	2	3	3
1. SINGLE DX B. Operated	21	2.5	2	1	1	2	3	4	5	5
2. MULTIPLE DX A. Not Operated	422	3.5	5	1	2	3	4	6	8	11
2. MULTIPLE DX B. Operated	474	4.5	12	2	2	4	5	8	10	21
1. SINGLE DX	33	2.2	2	1	1	2	3	4	5	5
2. MULTIPLE DX	896	4.0	9	1	2	3	5	7	9	16
A. NOT OPERATED	434	3.4	5	1	2	3	4	6	8	11
B. OPERATED	495	4.4	11	2	2	4	5	8	10	21
TOTAL										
0–19 Years	25	2.5	2	1	2	2	3	4	5	5
20–34	89	4.1	13	1	2	3	5	6	8	23
35–49	228	3.8	5	1	2	3	5	7	9	11
50–64	290	3.7	6	2	2	3	5	7	8	11
65+	297	4.4	13	1	2	4	5	8	10	24
GRAND TOTAL	929	4.0	9	1	2	3	5	7	9	16

Length of Stay by Diagnosis and Operation, Western Region, 2008

Western Region, October 2006–September 2007 Data, by Diagnosis

726.5: HIP ENTHESOPATHY

Type of Patients	Observed Patients	Avg. Stay	Vari-ance	10th	25th	50th	75th	90th	95th	99th
1. SINGLE DX										
A. Not Operated										
0–19 Years	0									
20–34	0									
35–49	0									
50–64	1	2.0	0	2	2	2	2	2	2	2
65+	1	1.0	0	1	1	1	1	1	1	1
B. Operated										
0–19 Years	0									
20–34	9	1.3	<1	1	1	1	1	2	2	2
35–49	3	1.3	<1	1	1	1	1	2	2	2
50–64	7	1.4	<1	1	1	1	1	2	2	2
65+	0									
2. MULTIPLE DX										
A. Not Operated										
0–19 Years	1	5.0	0	5	5	5	5	5	5	5
20–34	7	4.3	28	1	1	2	5	16	16	16
35–49	19	3.7	5	1	1	4	5	7	8	8
50–64	39	4.5	10	1	2	3	6	10	12	14
65+	205	3.8	9	1	2	3	4	7	8	12
B. Operated										
0–19 Years	3	3.3	2	2	2	3	3	5	5	5
20–34	7	1.3	<1	1	1	1	1	2	2	2
35–49	34	1.7	1	1	1	1	2	4	4	4
50–64	28	2.4	3	1	1	2	3	4	6	6
65+	59	3.4	10	1	1	4	4	8	12	14
SUBTOTALS:										
1. SINGLE DX										
A. Not Operated	2	1.5	<1	1	1	2	2	2	2	2
B. Operated	19	1.4	<1	1	1	1	1	2	2	3
2. MULTIPLE DX										
A. Not Operated	271	3.9	9	1	2	3	5	7	9	16
B. Operated	131	2.6	6	1	1	2	3	5	8	13
1. SINGLE DX	21	1.4	<1	1	1	1	2	2	2	3
2. MULTIPLE DX	402	3.5	9	1	2	3	4	7	9	14
A. NOT OPERATED	273	3.9	9	1	2	3	5	7	9	16
B. OPERATED	150	2.5	5	1	1	2	3	5	8	13
TOTAL										
0–19 Years	4	3.7	2	2	2	3	3	5	5	5
20–34	23	2.2	10	1	1	1	2	5	5	16
35–49	56	2.4	8	1	1	1	4	5	7	8
50–64	75	3.4	8	1	1	3	4	8	10	14
65+	265	3.7	9	1	2	3	4	7	9	14
GRAND TOTAL	423	3.4	8	1	1	3	4	7	8	14

726.65: PREPATELLAR BURSITIS

Type of Patients	Observed Patients	Avg. Stay	Vari-ance	10th	25th	50th	75th	90th	95th	99th
1. SINGLE DX										
A. Not Operated										
0–19 Years	3	3.0	0	3	3	3	3	3	3	3
20–34	4	2.3	2	1	1	2	4	4	4	4
35–49	7	2.4	2	1	2	2	3	5	5	5
50–64	5	3.6	5	2	2	2	5	7	7	7
65+	0									
B. Operated										
0–19 Years	4	2.5	<1	3	3	3	3	3	3	3
20–34	7	3.0	<1	2	2	3	3	5	5	5
35–49	3	2.7	<1	2	2	3	3	3	3	3
50–64	1	3.0	0	3	3	3	3	3	3	3
65+	1	1.0	0	1	1	1	1	1	1	1
2. MULTIPLE DX										
A. Not Operated										
0–19 Years	19	3.9	8	2	2	3	4	9	11	11
20–34	43	3.0	2	2	2	3	4	5	5	7
35–49	87	3.2	3	1	2	3	4	6	6	9
50–64	76	3.5	5	1	2	3	5	7	8	12
65+	40	4.0	5	2	2	3	5	8	9	10
B. Operated										
0–19 Years	26	4.3	4	2	3	4	6	7	7	9
20–34	93	4.5	8	2	3	4	5	8	11	16
35–49	151	5.2	12	2	3	4	6	10	13	18
50–64	138	5.8	24	2	3	4	7	11	14	34
65+	79	5.4	15	2	2	5	7	10	12	22
SUBTOTALS:										
1. SINGLE DX										
A. Not Operated	19	2.8	2	2	2	2	3	5	7	7
B. Operated	16	2.7	<1	1	2	3	3	3	5	5
2. MULTIPLE DX										
A. Not Operated	265	3.4	4	1	2	3	4	6	8	11
B. Operated	487	5.2	15	2	3	4	6	10	13	20
1. SINGLE DX	35	2.7	2	1	2	3	3	5	5	7
2. MULTIPLE DX	752	4.6	12	2	2	4	6	8	11	18
A. NOT OPERATED	284	3.4	4	1	2	3	4	6	7	11
B. OPERATED	503	5.1	15	2	3	4	6	10	12	20
TOTAL										
0–19 Years	52	3.9	5	2	3	3	4	7	9	11
20–34	147	3.9	7	1	2	3	5	7	9	14
35–49	248	4.4	9	1	2	4	5	8	12	16
50–64	220	5.0	18	2	3	4	6	9	12	20
65+	120	4.9	12	2	2	4	7	8	11	21
GRAND TOTAL	787	4.5	12	2	2	4	5	8	11	18

727: OTH DIS SYNOV/TEND/BURSA

Type of Patients	Observed Patients	Avg. Stay	Vari-ance	10th	25th	50th	75th	90th	95th	99th
1. SINGLE DX										
A. Not Operated										
0–19 Years	62	1.8	2	1	1	1	2	3	4	8
20–34	6	1.8	<1	1	1	2	3	3	3	3
35–49	6	2.2	3	1	1	1	3	5	5	5
50–64	5	1.8	<1	1	1	2	2	3	3	3
65+	1	2.0	0	2	2	2	2	2	2	2
B. Operated										
0–19 Years	14	2.4	5	1	1	1	4	5	8	8
20–34	37	2.1	1	1	1	2	3	3	4	5
35–49	52	2.2	2	1	1	2	3	4	5	6
50–64	59	1.6	<1	1	1	1	2	3	3	4
65+	29	1.5	<1	2	1	2	2	3	3	4
2. MULTIPLE DX										
A. Not Operated										
0–19 Years	101	1.9	1	1	1	2	2	3	4	5
20–34	70	3.1	8	1	2	3	3	6	7	21
35–49	96	3.8	13	1	2	3	4	7	10	27
50–64	126	3.2	6	1	2	2	4	6	8	11
65+	177	3.3	5	1	2	3	4	6	9	11
B. Operated										
0–19 Years	78	3.1	11	1	2	4	4	5	8	25
20–34	219	4.0	15	2	2	3	4	7	13	18
35–49	441	3.6	10	1	2	3	4	8	10	15
50–64	833	2.5	5	1	2	2	3	5	6	10
65+	861	2.4	5	1	2	2	3	4	6	10
SUBTOTALS:										
1. SINGLE DX										
A. Not Operated	80	1.8	2	1	1	1	2	3	4	8
B. Operated	191	1.9	1	1	1	2	2	3	4	6
2. MULTIPLE DX										
A. Not Operated	570	3.1	6	1	1	2	4	6	8	12
B. Operated	2,432	2.8	7	1	2	2	3	6	7	14
1. SINGLE DX	271	1.9	1	1	1	1	2	3	4	6
2. MULTIPLE DX	3,002	2.9	7	1	1	2	4	6	8	14
A. NOT OPERATED	650	2.9	6	1	1	2	4	6	7	11
B. OPERATED	2,623	2.7	7	1	1	2	3	5	7	14
TOTAL										
0–19 Years	255	2.3	5	1	1	2	3	4	5	8
20–34	332	3.6	12	2	2	3	4	7	9	18
35–49	595	3.5	10	1	1	3	4	7	9	16
50–64	1,068	2.5	5	1	1	2	3	5	6	10
65+	1,063	2.5	5	1	2	2	3	5	7	11
GRAND TOTAL	3,273	2.8	7	1	1	2	3	5	7	14

Length of Stay by Diagnosis and Operation, Western Region, 2008

Western Region, October 2006–September 2007 Data, by Diagnosis

727.00: SYNOVITIS NOS

Type of Patients	Observed Patients	Avg. Stay	Variance	10th	25th	50th	75th	90th	95th	99th
1. SINGLE DX										
A. Not Operated										
0–19 Years	51	1.9	2	1	1	1	3	4	5	8
20–34	0									
35–49	1	1.0	0	1	1	1	1	1	1	1
50–64	0									
65+	0									
B. Operated										
0–19 Years	1	8.0	0	8	8	8	8	8	8	8
20–34	2	2.5	<1	2	2	3	3	3	3	3
35–49	3	2.3	2	1	1	2	4	4	4	4
50–64	0									
65+	0									
2. MULTIPLE DX										
A. Not Operated										
0–19 Years	67	1.8	<1	1	1	2	2	3	4	5
20–34	8	3.8	6	1	2	3	6	6	8	8
35–49	11	5.5	54	2	2	3	6	7	27	27
50–64	9	3.7	10	1	2	4	4	11	11	11
65+	27	4.3	9	1	2	4	7	9	9	11
B. Operated										
0–19 Years	6	3.7	7	1	1	4	5	8	8	8
20–34	10	3.8	9	1	1	4	7	9	9	9
35–49	27	4.3	24	1	1	2	6	12	15	20
50–64	34	3.1	10	1	1	2	4	6	10	17
65+	26	3.5	8	2	2	3	5	7	9	13
SUBTOTALS:										
1. SINGLE DX										
A. Not Operated	52	1.9	2	1	1	1	2	4	5	8
B. Operated	6	3.3	6	1	2	3	4	8	8	8
2. MULTIPLE DX										
A. Not Operated	122	2.9	10	1	1	2	3	6	8	11
B. Operated	103	3.6	12	1	2	2	4	8	10	17
1. SINGLE DX	58	2.1	3	1	1	1	3	4	5	8
2. MULTIPLE DX	225	3.2	11	1	2	2	4	7	9	17
A. NOT OPERATED	174	2.6	8	1	1	2	3	5	8	11
B. OPERATED	109	3.6	12	1	1	2	4	8	10	17
TOTAL										
0–19 Years	125	2.0	2	1	1	1	2	4	5	8
20–34	20	3.7	6	1	2	3	6	7	8	9
35–49	42	4.4	29	1	1	2	4	9	15	27
50–64	43	3.2	9	1	1	2	4	6	10	17
65+	53	3.9	8	1	2	3	5	8	9	13
GRAND TOTAL	283	3.0	10	1	1	2	3	6	8	17

727.05: TENOSYNOV HAND/WRIST NEC

Type of Patients	Observed Patients	Avg. Stay	Variance	10th	25th	50th	75th	90th	95th	99th
1. SINGLE DX										
A. Not Operated										
0–19 Years	1	3.0	0	3	3	3	3	3	3	3
20–34	5	2.0	1	1	1	2	3	3	3	3
35–49	2	3.0	8	1	1	3	5	5	5	5
50–64	3	2.0	1	1	1	2	3	3	3	3
65+	0									
B. Operated										
0–19 Years	4	3.5	2	2	3	4	5	5	5	5
20–34	16	2.6	1	2	2	2	3	4	5	5
35–49	18	3.0	2	1	2	3	4	5	5	5
50–64	8	2.4	<1	1	2	3	3	3	3	3
65+	2	2.5	<1	2	2	3	3	3	3	3
2. MULTIPLE DX										
A. Not Operated										
0–19 Years	9	2.9	2	1	2	2	4	6	6	6
20–34	46	2.9	3	1	2	3	5	6	6	8
35–49	46	3.7	10	1	1	3	5	7	10	16
50–64	61	3.4	6	1	1	3	4	6	8	15
65+	37	2.8	4	1	1	2	3	5	5	10
B. Operated										
0–19 Years	20	4.0	8	2	2	4	4	5	5	15
20–34	141	4.6	17	2	2	3	5	8	14	18
35–49	189	4.4	8	2	3	4	5	8	10	13
50–64	142	4.4	11	2	3	4	5	7	9	19
65+	92	3.9	8	2	3	3	5	6	8	21
SUBTOTALS:										
1. SINGLE DX										
A. Not Operated	11	2.3	2	1	1	2	3	3	5	5
B. Operated	48	2.8	1	2	2	3	4	5	5	5
2. MULTIPLE DX										
A. Not Operated	199	3.2	6	1	2	3	4	6	8	15
B. Operated	584	4.4	11	2	3	4	5	7	10	17
1. SINGLE DX	59	2.7	1	1	2	3	3	5	5	5
2. MULTIPLE DX	783	4.1	10	2	2	3	5	7	10	17
A. NOT OPERATED	210	3.2	6	1	2	3	4	6	8	14
B. OPERATED	632	4.3	10	2	3	4	5	7	10	17
TOTAL										
0–19 Years	34	3.6	5	2	2	3	4	5	6	15
20–34	208	4.0	13	2	2	3	4	7	13	17
35–49	255	4.2	8	2	2	4	5	8	10	14
50–64	214	4.0	9	2	2	3	5	7	8	16
65+	131	3.6	7	1	2	3	4	6	8	11
GRAND TOTAL	842	4.0	9	2	2	3	5	7	9	16

727.40: SYNOVIAL CYST NOS

Type of Patients	Observed Patients	Avg. Stay	Variance	10th	25th	50th	75th	90th	95th	99th
1. SINGLE DX										
A. Not Operated										
0–19 Years	0									
20–34	0									
35–49	0									
50–64	0									
65+	0									
B. Operated										
0–19 Years	0									
20–34	0									
35–49	9	1.1	<1	1	1	1	1	2	2	2
50–64	24	1.5	<1	1	1	1	2	3	3	4
65+	9	1.2	<1	1	1	1	1	2	2	2
2. MULTIPLE DX										
A. Not Operated										
0–19 Years	0									
20–34	0									
35–49	3	6.6	17	2	2	8	10	10	10	10
50–64	8	2.9	4	1	2	2	5	7	7	7
65+	11	3.1	4	1	1	3	5	5	7	7
B. Operated										
0–19 Years	0									
20–34	5	1.0	0	1	1	1	1	1	1	1
35–49	45	2.7	10	1	1	1	3	7	8	19
50–64	276	1.9	2	1	1	1	2	4	5	8
65+	270	2.0	5	1	1	1	2	4	6	9
SUBTOTALS:										
1. SINGLE DX										
A. Not Operated	0									
B. Operated	42	1.4	<1	1	1	1	2	2	3	4
2. MULTIPLE DX										
A. Not Operated	22	3.5	7	1	2	3	5	7	8	10
B. Operated	596	2.0	4	1	1	1	2	4	6	9
1. SINGLE DX	42	1.4	<1	1	1	1	2	2	3	4
2. MULTIPLE DX	618	2.0	4	1	1	1	2	4	6	9
A. NOT OPERATED	22	3.5	7	1	2	3	5	7	8	10
B. OPERATED	638	1.9	4	1	1	1	2	4	6	8
TOTAL										
0–19 Years	0									
20–34	5	1.0	0	1	1	1	1	1	1	1
35–49	57	2.6	10	1	1	1	3	7	8	19
50–64	308	1.9	2	1	1	1	2	4	5	7
65+	290	2.0	5	1	1	1	2	4	6	9
GRAND TOTAL	660	2.0	4	1	1	1	2	4	6	9

Length of Stay by Diagnosis and Operation, Western Region, 2008

Western Region, October 2006–September 2007 Data, by Diagnosis

727.61: ROTATOR CUFF RUPTURE

Type of Patients	Observed Patients	Avg. Stay	Variance	Percentiles						
				10th	25th	50th	75th	90th	95th	99th
1. SINGLE DX										
A. Not Operated										
0–19 Years	0									
20–34	0									
35–49	0									
50–64	0									
65+	0									
B. Operated										
0–19 Years	0									
20–34	0									
35–49	6	1.5	<1		1	2	2	2	2	2
50–64	10	1.4	<1	1	1	1	1	2	4	4
65+	11	1.1	<1	1	1	1	1	1	2	2
2. MULTIPLE DX										
A. Not Operated										
0–19 Years	0									
20–34	0									
35–49	2	3.5	<1	3	3	4	4	4	4	4
50–64	4	4.8	<1	4	4	5	5	6	6	6
65+	11	2.5	4	1	1	1	5	5	6	6
B. Operated										
0–19 Years	0									
20–34	1	1.0	0	1	1	1	1	1	1	1
35–49	32	1.6	2	1	1	1	2	2	4	8
50–64	139	1.5	<1	1	1	1	2	3	3	5
65+	225	1.7	1	1	1	1	2	3	3	5
SUBTOTALS:										
1. SINGLE DX										
A. Not Operated	0									
B. Operated	27	1.3	<1	1	1	1	1	2	2	4
2. MULTIPLE DX										
A. Not Operated	17	3.1	4	1	1	3	5	6	6	6
B. Operated	397	1.6	<1	1	1	1	2	3	3	5
1. SINGLE DX	27	1.3	<1	1	1	1	1	2	2	4
2. MULTIPLE DX	414	1.7	1	1	1	1	2	3	4	6
A. NOT OPERATED	17	3.1	4	1	1	3	5	6	6	6
B. OPERATED	424	1.6	<1	1	1	1	2	3	3	5
TOTAL										
0–19 Years	0									
20–34	1	1.0	0	1	1	1	1	1	1	1
35–49	40	1.7	2	1	1	1	2	3	4	8
50–64	153	1.6	1	1	1	1	2	3	4	6
65+	247	1.7	1	1	1	1	2	3	4	5
GRAND TOTAL	441	1.7	1	1	1	1	2	3	4	6

728: MUSCLE/LIG/FASCIA DISORD

Type of Patients	Observed Patients	Avg. Stay	Variance	Percentiles						
				10th	25th	50th	75th	90th	95th	99th
1. SINGLE DX										
A. Not Operated										
0–19 Years	31	2.7	3	1	1	2	4	5	6	6
20–34	51	2.8	3	1	1	2	4	5	5	7
35–49	14	2.4	2	1	1	2	3	4	5	5
50–64	4	2.8	12	1	1	1	1	8	8	8
65+	1	3.0	0	3	3	3	3	3	3	3
B. Operated										
0–19 Years	9	2.8	2	2	2	3	3	6	6	6
20–34	8	5.2	36	1	2	3	3	19	19	19
35–49	15	2.0	2	1	1	2	2	3	3	7
50–64	8	2.6	5	1	1	2	2	8	8	8
65+	1	1.0	0	1	1	1	1	1	1	1
2. MULTIPLE DX										
A. Not Operated										
0–19 Years	154	3.4	6	1	2	3	5	7	9	11
20–34	578	3.8	11	1	2	3	5	7	10	15
35–49	772	3.6	12	1	2	3	4	7	9	16
50–64	845	4.5	29	1	2	3	5	9	12	23
65+	2,090	4.5	12	2	2	4	5	8	10	17
B. Operated										
0–19 Years	39	7.8	92	1	2	4	10	23	28	48
20–34	188	9.9	132	3	3	6	13	23	34	65
35–49	404	12.8	189	2	4	9	17	28	42	80
50–64	413	14.5	226	2	4	10	21	38	46	>99
65+	255	11.4	135	2	4	8	14	25	39	53
SUBTOTALS:										
1. SINGLE DX										
A. Not Operated	101	2.7	3	1	1	2	4	5	5	7
B. Operated	41	2.9	10	1	1	2	3	6	8	19
2. MULTIPLE DX										
A. Not Operated	4,439	4.2	15	1	2	3	5	8	10	18
B. Operated	1,299	12.5	182	2	4	8	17	29	42	77
1. SINGLE DX	142	2.8	5	1	2	2	4	5	6	9
2. MULTIPLE DX	5,738	6.1	65	1	2	4	7	12	20	45
A. NOT OPERATED	4,540	4.2	15	1	2	3	5	8	10	17
B. OPERATED	1,340	12.2	179	1	3	8	16	28	42	77
TOTAL										
0–19 Years	233	4.0	22	1	2	3	5	7	10	23
20–34	825	5.2	45	1	2	3	7	10	16	37
35–49	1,205	6.7	90	1	2	3	7	16	23	50
50–64	1,270	7.7	115	2	3	4	8	19	29	66
65+	2,347	5.2	30	2	3	4	6	9	13	27
GRAND TOTAL	5,880	6.0	64	2	2	4	6	12	20	45

728.85: MUSCLE SPASM

Type of Patients	Observed Patients	Avg. Stay	Variance	Percentiles						
				10th	25th	50th	75th	90th	95th	99th
1. SINGLE DX										
A. Not Operated										
0–19 Years	2	1.5	<1	1	1	2	2	2	2	2
20–34	2	1.0	0	1	1	1	1	1	1	1
35–49	3	2.0	3	1	1	1	1	4	4	4
50–64	0									
65+	0									
B. Operated										
0–19 Years	0									
20–34	0									
35–49	0									
50–64	0									
65+	1	1.0	0	1	1	1	1	1	1	1
2. MULTIPLE DX										
A. Not Operated										
0–19 Years	11	2.5	8	1	1	1	3	7	9	9
20–34	28	2.9	9	1	1	2	2	9	10	11
35–49	39	2.8	7	1	1	2	3	7	8	15
50–64	52	2.6	5	1	1	2	3	5	8	10
65+	52	2.5	3	1	1	2	3	4	5	10
B. Operated										
0–19 Years	2	3.5	<1	3	3	4	4	4	4	4
20–34	13	3.6	4	2	3	3	4	7	8	8
35–49	11	3.8	31	1	1	2	3	6	20	20
50–64	6	4.0	25	1	1	2	4	14	14	14
65+	2	5.0	8	3	3	7	7	7	7	7
SUBTOTALS:										
1. SINGLE DX										
A. Not Operated	7	1.6	1	1	1	1	2	4	4	4
B. Operated	1	1.0	0	1	1	1	1	1	1	1
2. MULTIPLE DX										
A. Not Operated	182	2.7	6	1	1	2	3	5	8	11
B. Operated	34	3.8	15	2	2	3	4	7	14	20
1. SINGLE DX	8	1.5	1	1	1	1	2	4	4	4
2. MULTIPLE DX	216	2.8	7	1	1	2	3	6	9	14
A. NOT OPERATED	189	2.6	5	1	1	2	3	5	8	11
B. OPERATED	35	3.8	15	1	1	3	4	7	14	20
TOTAL										
0–19 Years	15	2.5	6	1	1	2	3	7	9	9
20–34	43	3.0	7	1	1	2	3	8	9	11
35–49	53	3.0	12	1	1	2	3	6	8	20
50–64	58	2.7	7	1	1	2	3	5	10	14
65+	55	2.6	4	1	1	2	3	5	7	10
GRAND TOTAL	224	2.8	7	1	1	2	3	5	8	14

Length of Stay by Diagnosis and Operation, Western Region, 2008

Western Region, October 2006–September 2007 Data, by Diagnosis

728.86: NECROTIZING FASCIITIS

Type of Patients	Observed Patients	Avg. Stay	Variance	10th	25th	50th	75th	90th	95th	99th
1. SINGLE DX										
A. Not Operated										
0–19 Years	0									
20–34	0									
35–49	0									
50–64	1	8.0		8	8	8	8	8		8
65+	0									
B. Operated										
0–19 Years	2	3.0	0	3	3	3		3	3	3
20–34	3	8.0	90	2	2	3	19	19	19	19
35–49	2	1.5	<1	1	1	1	2	2	2	2
50–64	2	5.5	13	3	3	6	8	8	8	8
65+	0									
2. MULTIPLE DX										
A. Not Operated										
0–19 Years	1	6.0	0	6	6	6	6	6	6	6
20–34	6	15.2	170	5	7	12	21	39	39	39
35–49	8	11.1	41	2	6	8	14	20	20	20
50–64	18	7.0	21	1	4	6	10	15	17	17
65+	8	7.4	36	1	3	5	9	19	19	19
B. Operated										
0–19 Years	7	19.9	201	8	8	15	28	48	48	48
20–34	87	16.5	189	4	6	13	22	34	43	71
35–49	249	17.0	211	5	8	13	22	33	49	88
50–64	238	19.7	257	5	8	15	28	45	60	>99
65+	96	16.9	222	4	6	13	24	41	51	70
SUBTOTALS:										
1. SINGLE DX										
A. Not Operated	1	8.0	0	8	8	8	8	8	8	8
B. Operated	9	4.9	32	1	2	3	3	19	19	19
2. MULTIPLE DX										
A. Not Operated	41	9.0	53	2	5	7	12	19	20	39
B. Operated	677	17.9	226	4	8	14	24	40	50	98
1. SINGLE DX	10	5.2	29	1	2	3	8	8	19	19
2. MULTIPLE DX	718	17.4	220	4	7	13	23	40	49	88
A. NOT OPERATED	42	9.0	52	2	5	7	12	19	20	39
B. OPERATED	686	17.7	226	4	7	13	24	40	50	98
TOTAL										
0–19 Years	10	15.1	193	3	6	8	19	28	48	48
20–34	96	16.2	184	3	6	13	21	34	43	71
35–49	259	16.7	207	4	8	13	21	32	47	88
50–64	259	18.7	250	5	8	14	26	43	55	>99
65+	104	16.1	213	4	6	11	21	40	49	65
GRAND TOTAL	728	17.2	220	4	7	13	22	39	49	88

728.87: MUSCLE WEAKNESS

Type of Patients	Observed Patients	Avg. Stay	Variance	10th	25th	50th	75th	90th	95th	99th
1. SINGLE DX										
A. Not Operated										
0–19 Years	2	3.0	8	1	1	1	5	5	5	5
20–34	2	2.0	0	2	2	2	2	2	2	2
35–49	0									
50–64	1	1.0	0	1	1	1	1	1	1	1
65+	0									
B. Operated										
0–19 Years	1	2.0	0	2	2	2	2	2	2	2
20–34	0									
35–49	0									
50–64	1	2.0	0	2	2	2	2	2	2	2
65+	0									
2. MULTIPLE DX										
A. Not Operated										
0–19 Years	1	3.0	0	3	3	3	3	3	3	3
20–34	29	2.6	3	1	1	2	4	5	6	8
35–49	48	2.5	3	1	1	2	4	5	6	7
50–64	70	3.1	7	1	1	2	4	8	10	12
65+	146	3.2	4	1	2	3	4	6	7	11
B. Operated										
0–19 Years	3	5.7	52	1	1	2	14	14	14	14
20–34	1	1.0	0	1	1	1	1	1	1	1
35–49	1	7.0	0	7	7	7	7	7	7	7
50–64	1	3.0	0	3	3	3	3	3	3	3
65+	6	9.1	54	1	3	7	14	19	19	19
SUBTOTALS:										
1. SINGLE DX										
A. Not Operated	5	2.2	3	1	1	2	2	5	5	5
B. Operated	2	2.0	0	2	2	2	2	2	2	2
2. MULTIPLE DX										
A. Not Operated	294	3.0	5	1	1	2	4	6	7	12
B. Operated	12	6.9	42	1	1	7	14	14	19	19
1. SINGLE DX	7	2.1	2	1	1	2	2	5	5	5
2. MULTIPLE DX	306	3.2	7	1	1	2	4	6	8	13
A. NOT OPERATED	299	3.0	5	1	1	2	4	6	7	12
B. OPERATED	14	6.2	39	1	1	3	13	14	19	19
TOTAL										
0–19 Years	7	4.0	21	1	1	1	5	14	14	14
20–34	32	2.5	3	1	1	2	3	4	6	8
35–49	49	2.6	3	1	1	2	4	6	7	7
50–64	73	3.1	7	1	1	2	3	7	10	12
65+	152	3.5	7	1	2	3	4	7	7	14
GRAND TOTAL	313	3.2	7	1	1	2	4	6	8	13

728.88: RHABDOMYOLYSIS

Type of Patients	Observed Patients	Avg. Stay	Variance	10th	25th	50th	75th	90th	95th	99th
1. SINGLE DX										
A. Not Operated										
0–19 Years	17	3.1	3	1	1	3	4	6	6	6
20–34	44	3.0	3	1	2	3	4	5	5	7
35–49	9	2.7	2	1	2	3	3	5	5	5
50–64	2	1.0	0	1	1	1	1	1	1	1
65+	1	3.0	0	3	3	3	3	3	3	3
B. Operated										
0–19 Years	0									
20–34	0									
35–49	0									
50–64	0									
65+	0									
2. MULTIPLE DX										
A. Not Operated										
0–19 Years	98	3.0	4	1	2	2	4	6	7	9
20–34	477	3.7	7	1	2	3	5	7	9	14
35–49	584	3.4	8	1	2	3	4	7	9	15
50–64	594	4.6	33	1	2	3	5	8	12	27
65+	1,606	4.5	12	2	3	4	5	8	10	16
B. Operated										
0–19 Years	1	13.0	0	13	13	13	13	13	13	13
20–34	12	7.0	19	3	4	7	9	13	17	17
35–49	13	16.0	443	5	6	10	15	20	84	84
50–64	17	18.0	107	5	9	19	24	31	42	42
65+	45	12.8	87	5	8	10	14	22	31	53
SUBTOTALS:										
1. SINGLE DX										
A. Not Operated	73	3.0	3	1	2	3	4	5	6	7
B. Operated	0									
2. MULTIPLE DX										
A. Not Operated	3,359	4.2	14	1	2	3	5	8	10	17
B. Operated	88	13.5	138	4	7	10	17	25	31	84
1. SINGLE DX	73	3.0	3	1	2	3	4	5	6	7
2. MULTIPLE DX	3,447	4.4	19	1	2	3	5	8	11	21
A. NOT OPERATED	3,432	4.1	14	1	2	3	5	8	10	16
B. OPERATED	88	13.5	138	4	7	10	17	25	31	84
TOTAL										
0–19 Years	116	3.1	4	1	2	2	4	6	7	9
20–34	533	3.7	7	1	2	3	5	7	9	14
35–49	606	3.7	20	1	2	3	4	7	9	17
50–64	613	4.9	40	2	3	3	5	9	14	29
65+	1,652	4.7	15	2	3	4	6	8	11	20
GRAND TOTAL	3,520	4.4	19	1	2	3	5	8	10	21

Western Region, October 2006–September 2007 Data, by Diagnosis

728.89: MUSCLE/LIGAMENT DIS NEC

Type of Patients	Observed Patients	Avg. Stay	Vari-ance	Percentiles						
				10th	25th	50th	75th	90th	95th	99th
1. SINGLE DX										
A. Not Operated										
0–19 Years	1	2.0	0	2	2	2	2	2	2	2
20–34	2	1.5	<1	1	1	2	2	2	2	2
35–49	0									
50–64	0									
65+	0									
B. Operated										
0–19 Years	3	3.0	7	1	1	2	6	6	6	6
20–34	1	2.0	0	2	2	2	2	2	2	2
35–49	3	1.3	<1	1	1	1	2	2	2	2
50–64	0									
65+	0									
2. MULTIPLE DX										
A. Not Operated										
0–19 Years	6	4.8	14	2	2	4	9	10	10	10
20–34	16	5.2	12	2	3	4	6	12	13	13
35–49	51	4.4	9	2	2	4	6	8	11	15
50–64	72	4.8	15	2	2	3	6	9	14	20
65+	227	5.4	19	1	2	5	7	9	13	27
B. Operated										
0–19 Years	8	4.5	12	1	1	5	8	10	10	10
20–34	34	4.7	15	1	2	3	6	11	14	14
35–49	66	4.9	20	1	2	4	6	11	15	25
50–64	71	7.9	142	1	2	4	8	16	25	89
65+	69	7.1	28	2	4	7	9	13	20	26
SUBTOTALS:										
1. SINGLE DX										
A. Not Operated	3	1.7	<1	1	1	2	2	2	2	2
B. Operated	7	2.1	3	1	1	2	2	6	6	6
2. MULTIPLE DX										
A. Not Operated	372	5.1	16	2	2	4	6	9	13	21
B. Operated	248	6.3	57	1	2	4	8	13	18	27
1. SINGLE DX	10	2.0	2	1	1	2	2	2	2	6
2. MULTIPLE DX	620	5.6	33	1	2	4	7	11	14	26
A. NOT OPERATED	375	5.1	16	2	2	4	6	9	13	21
B. OPERATED	255	6.2	56	2	2	4	8	13	18	27
TOTAL										
0–19 Years	18	4.2	10	1	2	2	6	10	10	10
20–34	53	4.7	14	1	2	3	6	11	13	14
35–49	120	4.6	15	2	2	4	6	9	12	19
50–64	143	6.3	80	2	2	4	7	14	18	35
65+	296	5.8	21	1	3	5	7	10	14	27
GRAND TOTAL	630	5.5	33	1	2	4	7	11	14	26

729: DISORD SOFT TISS NEC

Type of Patients	Observed Patients	Avg. Stay	Vari-ance	Percentiles						
				10th	25th	50th	75th	90th	95th	99th
1. SINGLE DX										
A. Not Operated										
0–19 Years	43	1.7	2	1	1	1	2	3	4	7
20–34	11	1.8	<1	1	1	2	3	3	3	3
35–49	20	2.0	4	1	1	1	2	3	4	10
50–64	16	1.3	<1	1	1	1	1	2	3	3
65+	7	1.4	<1	1	1	1	2	3	3	3
B. Operated										
0–19 Years	9	2.2	2	1	1	2	3	5	5	5
20–34	12	2.1	2	1	1	1	3	5	5	5
35–49	7	1.1	<1	1	1	1	1	2	2	2
50–64	3	1.7	1	1	1	1	3	3	3	3
65+	0									
2. MULTIPLE DX										
A. Not Operated										
0–19 Years	129	2.6	7	1	1	2	3	6	8	10
20–34	321	3.0	13	1	1	2	3	6	8	23
35–49	686	2.9	7	1	1	2	4	6	7	13
50–64	938	3.0	10	1	1	2	3	6	8	17
65+	1,318	2.9	6	1	1	2	4	5	7	12
B. Operated										
0–19 Years	25	3.7	10	1	1	3	4	8	11	13
20–34	66	6.0	66	1	2	3	7	15	21	44
35–49	128	5.5	41	1	1	3	7	12	19	27
50–64	151	5.5	34	1	2	3	7	11	18	29
65+	107	6.4	47	2	2	5	9	12	16	40
SUBTOTALS:										
1. SINGLE DX										
A. Not Operated	97	1.7	2	1	1	1	2	3	4	10
B. Operated	31	1.9	2	1	2	2	2	4	5	5
2. MULTIPLE DX										
A. Not Operated	3,392	2.9	8	1	1	2	4	6	8	15
B. Operated	477	5.7	42	1	2	3	7	12	18	39
1. SINGLE DX	128	1.8	2	1	1	1	2	3	4	7
2. MULTIPLE DX	3,869	3.3	13	1	1	2	4	7	9	19
A. NOT OPERATED	3,489	2.9	8	1	1	2	3	6	8	14
B. OPERATED	508	5.5	41	2	2	3	7	12	17	38
TOTAL										
0–19 Years	206	2.5	6	1	1	2	3	6	8	11
20–34	410	3.5	22	1	1	2	4	7	9	27
35–49	841	3.3	13	1	1	2	4	6	9	19
50–64	1,108	3.3	14	1	1	2	4	7	10	22
65+	1,432	3.2	10	1	2	2	4	6	8	13
GRAND TOTAL	3,997	3.2	13	1	1	2	4	7	9	18

729.1: MYALGIA & MYOSITIS NOS

Type of Patients	Observed Patients	Avg. Stay	Vari-ance	Percentiles						
				10th	25th	50th	75th	90th	95th	99th
1. SINGLE DX										
A. Not Operated										
0–19 Years	15	2.1	3	1	1	1	3	5	7	7
20–34		2.0	2	1	1	3	3	3	3	3
35–49	4	2.5	2	2	2	2	3	4	4	4
50–64	4	1.0	0	1	1	1	1	1	1	1
65+	0									
B. Operated										
0–19 Years	0									
20–34	0									
35–49	0									
50–64	0									
65+	0									
2. MULTIPLE DX										
A. Not Operated										
0–19 Years	49	3.4	12	1	1	2	4	8	10	19
20–34	88	4.5	34	1	2	3	5	8	14	38
35–49	161	3.2	8	1	1	2	4	6	8	11
50–64	224	2.9	7	1	1	2	3	7	8	13
65+	205	2.9	6	1	1	2	4	6	7	11
B. Operated										
0–19 Years	8	6.0	2	5	5	5	7	7	7	7
20–34	8	8.8	26	2	6	7	11	17	17	17
35–49	18	5.7	14	2	4	5	6	10	10	17
50–64	15	8.3	40	3	6	7	9	12	29	29
65+	21	8.2	25	3	5	7	11	13	16	22
SUBTOTALS:										
1. SINGLE DX										
A. Not Operated	25	2.0	3	1	1	1	3	4	5	7
B. Operated	0									
2. MULTIPLE DX										
A. Not Operated	727	3.2	10	1	1	2	4	6	8	15
B. Operated	64	7.5	25	3	5	7	9	13	17	29
1. SINGLE DX	25	2.0	3	1	1	1	3	4	5	7
2. MULTIPLE DX	791	3.5	13	1	1	2	4	7	9	19
A. NOT OPERATED	752	3.1	10	1	1	2	4	6	8	15
B. OPERATED	64	7.5	25	3	5	7	9	13	17	29
TOTAL										
0–19 Years	66	3.2	10	1	1	2	4	7	9	19
20–34	98	4.8	34	1	2	3	6	9	17	38
35–49	183	3.4	9	1	1	3	4	6	8	17
50–64	243	3.2	11	1	1	3	4	7	9	14
65+	226	3.4	10	1	1	3	4	7	9	16
GRAND TOTAL	816	3.5	13	1	2	2	4	7	9	18

Length of Stay by Diagnosis and Operation, Western Region, 2008

Western Region, October 2006–September 2007 Data, by Diagnosis

729.39: PANNICULITIS SITE NEC

Type of Patients	Observed Patients	Avg. Stay	Vari-ance	10th	25th	50th	75th	90th	95th	99th
1. SINGLE DX										
A. Not Operated										
0–19 Years	0									
20–34	0									
35–49	0									
50–64	0									
65+	0									
B. Operated										
0–19 Years	0									
20–34	2	1.0	0	1	1	1	1	1	1	1
35–49	1	1.0	0	1	1	1	1	1	1	1
50–64	1	1.0	0	1	1	1	1	1	1	1
65+	0									
2. MULTIPLE DX										
A. Not Operated										
0–19 Years	1	9.0	0	9	9	9	9	9	9	9
20–34	9	4.7	4	2	4	4	5	8	8	8
35–49	52	5.1	13	2	3	4	6	9	11	21
50–64	45	5.7	17	3	3	5	7	11	14	23
65+	20	5.8	44	2	2	3	7	10	12	30
B. Operated										
0–19 Years	0									
20–34	18	3.0	5	1	1	2	5	7	7	7
35–49	28	3.9	76	1	1	2	3	5	10	47
50–64	43	3.7	14	1	2	2	4	7	9	22
65+	9	5.0	13	1	2	4	6	12	12	12
SUBTOTALS:										
1. SINGLE DX										
A. Not Operated	0									
B. Operated	4	1.0	0	1	1	1	1	1	1	1
2. MULTIPLE DX										
A. Not Operated	127	5.4	18	2	3	4	6	10	12	23
B. Operated	98	3.7	29	1	1	2	4	7	10	47
1. SINGLE DX	4	1.0	0	1	1	1	1	1	1	1
2. MULTIPLE DX	225	4.7	24	1	2	3	6	9	11	23
A. NOT OPERATED	127	5.4	18	2	3	4	6	10	12	23
B. OPERATED	102	3.6	29	1	1	2	4	7	9	22
TOTAL										
0–19 Years	1	9.0	0	9	9	9	9	9	9	9
20–34	29	3.4	5	1	1	3	5	7	8	8
35–49	81	4.6	34	1	2	3	5	9	11	47
50–64	89	4.7	17	1	2	3	6	11	11	23
65+	29	5.5	34	1	2	3	7	12	12	30
GRAND TOTAL	229	4.6	24	1	2	3	6	9	11	23

729.5: PAIN IN LIMB

Type of Patients	Observed Patients	Avg. Stay	Vari-ance	10th	25th	50th	75th	90th	95th	99th
1. SINGLE DX										
A. Not Operated										
0–19 Years	9	1.7	<1	1	1	1	2	3	3	3
20–34	3	2.3	<1	2	2	2	3	3	3	3
35–49	4	1.3	<1	1	1	1	2	2	2	2
50–64	7	1.3	<1	1	1	1	2	2	2	2
65+	1	1.0	0	1	1	1	1	1	1	1
B. Operated										
0–19 Years	2	1.5	<1	1	1	2	2	2	2	2
20–34	2	2.0	0	2	2	2	2	2	2	2
35–49	0									
50–64	0									
65+	0									
2. MULTIPLE DX										
A. Not Operated										
0–19 Years	36	1.6	<1	1	1	1	2	3	3	4
20–34	71	2.2	2	1	1	2	3	4	5	7
35–49	165	2.3	3	1	1	2	3	4	7	8
50–64	271	2.6	10	1	1	3	3	5	8	22
65+	418	2.7	5	1	1	2	3	5	7	12
B. Operated										
0–19 Years	5	1.8	<1	1	1	2	2	3	3	3
20–34	7	4.3	9	2	3	3	6	10	10	10
35–49	12	2.4	3	1	1	1	3	5	5	5
50–64	15	4.1	10	1	1	3	6	8	13	13
65+	10	5.9	25	1	2	3	8	16	16	16
SUBTOTALS:										
1. SINGLE DX										
A. Not Operated	24	1.5	<1	1	1	1	2	3	3	3
B. Operated	4	1.8	<1	1	2	2	2	2	2	2
2. MULTIPLE DX										
A. Not Operated	961	2.5	6	1	1	2	3	5	7	14
B. Operated	49	3.8	11	1	1	3	5	8	12	16
1. SINGLE DX	28	1.6	<1	1	1	1	2	3	3	3
2. MULTIPLE DX	1,010	2.6	6	1	1	2	3	5	7	14
A. NOT OPERATED	985	2.5	6	1	1	2	3	5	7	14
B. OPERATED	53	3.7	11	1	1	3	5	8	12	16
TOTAL										
0–19 Years	52	1.6	<1	1	1	1	2	3	3	4
20–34	83	2.4	3	1	1	2	3	5	6	10
35–49	181	2.3	3	1	1	2	3	4	6	8
50–64	293	2.6	10	1	1	2	3	5	8	22
65+	429	2.8	6	1	1	2	3	5	7	13
GRAND TOTAL	1,038	2.6	6	1	1	2	3	5	7	14

729.81: LIMB SWELLING

Type of Patients	Observed Patients	Avg. Stay	Vari-ance	10th	25th	50th	75th	90th	95th	99th
1. SINGLE DX										
A. Not Operated										
0–19 Years	2	2.0	2	1	1	3	3	3	3	3
20–34	1	1.0	0	1	1	1	1	1	1	1
35–49	2	1.5	<1	1	1	1	2	2	2	2
50–64	2	2.0	<1	1	1	1	3	3	3	3
65+	2	1.5	<1	1	1	2	2	2	2	2
B. Operated										
0–19 Years	0									
20–34	0									
35–49	0									
50–64	0									
65+	0									
2. MULTIPLE DX										
A. Not Operated										
0–19 Years	9	2.3	3	1	1	2	2	7	7	7
20–34	26	1.9	3	1	1	1	2	3	4	9
35–49	58	2.2	3	1	1	2	3	4	6	9
50–64	75	2.5	3	1	1	2	3	5	6	12
65+	111	2.3	2	1	1	2	3	4	5	7
B. Operated										
0–19 Years	1	2.0	0	2	2	2	2	2	2	2
20–34	0									
35–49	0									
50–64	1	2.0	0	2	2	2	2	2	2	2
65+	0									
SUBTOTALS:										
1. SINGLE DX										
A. Not Operated	9	1.7	<1	1	1	1	2	3	3	3
B. Operated	0									
2. MULTIPLE DX										
A. Not Operated	279	2.3	3	1	1	2	3	4	6	9
B. Operated	2	2.0	0	2	2	2	2	2	2	2
1. SINGLE DX	9	1.7	<1	1	1	1	2	3	3	3
2. MULTIPLE DX	281	2.3	3	1	1	2	3	4	6	9
A. NOT OPERATED	288	2.3	3	1	1	2	3	4	6	9
B. OPERATED	2	2.0	0	2	2	2	2	2	2	2
TOTAL										
0–19 Years	12	2.3	3	1	1	2	3	3	3	7
20–34	27	1.9	3	1	1	1	2	3	3	9
35–49	60	2.2	3	1	1	2	3	4	5	9
50–64	78	2.5	3	1	1	2	3	5	6	12
65+	113	2.3	2	1	1	2	3	4	5	7
GRAND TOTAL	290	2.3	3	1	1	2	3	4	6	9

729.89: MS SYMPTOMS LIMB NEC

Type of Patients	Observed Patients	Avg. Stay	Vari- ance	Percentiles						
				10th	25th	50th	75th	90th	95th	99th
1. SINGLE DX										
A. *Not Operated*										
0–19 Years	11	1.2	<1	1	1	1	1	2	2	2
20–34	4	1.8	<1	1	1	2	2	3	3	3
35–49	7	2.4	11	1	1	1	2	10	10	10
50–64	2	1.5	<1	1	1	2	2	2	2	2
65+	2	2.0	2	1	1	1	3	3	3	3
B. *Operated*										
0–19 Years	1	3.0	0	3	3	3	3	3	3	3
20–34	0									
35–49	0									
50–64	0									
65+	0									
2. MULTIPLE DX										
A. *Not Operated*										
0–19 Years	25	2.5	4	1	1	2	3	6	7	8
20–34	101	2.6	5	1	1	2	3	5	7	10
35–49	203	2.8	5	1	1	2	3	5	7	12
50–64	265	3.0	8	1	1	2	3	6	8	16
65+	506	3.0	4	1	2	3	4	5	7	12
B. *Operated*										
0–19 Years	1	13.0	0	13	13	13	13	13	13	13
20–34	2	1.5	<1	1	1	2	2	2	2	2
35–49	2	4.6	24	1	1	8	8	8	8	8
50–64	5	5.4	13	2	2	5	8	10	10	10
65+	9	5.0	12	1	2	6	8	9	9	9
SUBTOTALS:										
1. SINGLE DX										
A. *Not Operated*	26	1.7	3	1	1	1	2	3	3	3
B. *Operated*	1	3.0	0	3	3	3	3	3	3	3
2. MULTIPLE DX										
A. *Not Operated*	1,100	2.9	5	1	1	2	4	5	7	13
B. *Operated*	19	5.1	15	1	2	5	8	10	13	13
1. SINGLE DX	27	1.7	3	1	1	1	2	3	3	3
2. MULTIPLE DX	1,119	3.0	6	1	1	2	4	6	7	13
A. NOT OPERATED	1,126	2.9	5	1	1	2	3	5	7	13
B. OPERATED	20	5.0	14	1	2	5	8	10	13	13
TOTAL										
0–19 Years	38	2.4	6	1	1	1	3	6	8	13
20–34	107	2.6	5	1	1	2	3	5	7	10
35–49	212	2.8	6	1	1	2	3	5	7	12
50–64	272	3.0	8	1	1	2	3	6	8	16
65+	517	3.1	4	1	2	3	4	6	7	12
GRAND TOTAL	1,146	2.9	6	1	1	2	4	6	7	13

730: OSTEOMYELITIS

Type of Patients	Observed Patients	Avg. Stay	Vari- ance	Percentiles						
				10th	25th	50th	75th	90th	95th	99th
1. SINGLE DX										
A. *Not Operated*										
0–19 Years	31	5.6	20	1	2	5	7	10	15	21
20–34	4	3.8	4	1	4	4	4	6	6	6
35–49	7	2.4	7	1	1	1	3	8	8	8
50–64	8	3.5	5	1	3	3	5	8	8	8
65+	2	3.5	12	1	1	1	6	6	6	6
B. *Operated*										
0–19 Years	16	4.2	17	1	1	3	5	10	14	14
20–34	11	4.6	32	1	2	3	5	6	21	21
35–49	19	3.3	5	1	1	3	5	7	8	8
50–64	14	4.9	27	1	2	3	5	12	20	20
65+	4	4.3	10	1	1	2	7	7	7	7
2. MULTIPLE DX										
A. *Not Operated*										
0–19 Years	187	6.0	19	2	3	5	8	12	15	21
20–34	245	8.6	84	2	4	6	9	18	27	55
35–49	682	8.1	66	2	3	6	9	16	24	45
50–64	891	8.3	76	2	3	6	10	17	24	46
65+	911	6.9	27	2	3	6	8	12	16	26
B. *Operated*										
0–19 Years	182	9.6	86	2	4	7	11	21	29	48
20–34	377	9.1	86	2	4	7	11	20	26	55
35–49	964	9.6	86	2	4	7	12	19	30	50
50–64	1,417	9.9	104	2	4	7	12	21	29	54
65+	1,365	8.5	61	2	4	7	10	17	23	47
SUBTOTALS:										
1. SINGLE DX										
A. *Not Operated*	52	4.6	16	1	2	4	6	8	14	21
B. *Operated*	64	4.1	17	1	1	3	5	8	12	21
2. MULTIPLE DX										
A. *Not Operated*	2,916	7.7	56	2	3	6	9	15	21	41
B. *Operated*	4,305	9.3	84	2	4	7	11	19	27	50
1. SINGLE DX	116	4.4	16	1	1	3	6	8	14	21
2. MULTIPLE DX	7,221	8.7	73	2	4	6	10	17	25	47
A. NOT OPERATED	2,968	7.6	55	2	3	6	9	15	21	41
B. OPERATED	4,369	9.2	84	2	4	7	11	19	27	50
TOTAL										
0–19 Years	416	7.5	52	2	3	6	9	15	21	43
20–34	637	8.8	85	2	4	6	10	20	26	55
35–49	1,672	8.9	77	2	3	6	10	18	27	48
50–64	2,330	9.2	93	2	4	6	11	19	28	51
65+	2,282	7.9	48	2	4	6	10	15	20	36
GRAND TOTAL	7,337	8.6	73	2	4	6	10	17	25	47

730.07: AC OSTEOMYELITIS-ANKLE

Type of Patients	Observed Patients	Avg. Stay	Vari- ance	Percentiles						
				10th	25th	50th	75th	90th	95th	99th
1. SINGLE DX										
A. *Not Operated*										
0–19 Years	2	4.5	24	1	1	8	8	8	8	8
20–34	1	4.0	0	4	4	4	4	4	4	4
35–49	0									
50–64	0									
65+	0									
B. *Operated*										
0–19 Years	0									
20–34	0									
35–49	0									
50–64	0									
65+	0									
2. MULTIPLE DX										
A. *Not Operated*										
0–19 Years	7	5.6	12	2	3	5	8	12	12	12
20–34	10	6.6	20	2	2	6	12	12	13	13
35–49	42	8.3	42	3	4	7	12	16	17	37
50–64	68	7.2	27	3	4	6	9	16	21	>99
65+	74	6.6	32	2	3	5	7	13	20	37
B. *Operated*										
0–19 Years	12	8.3	90	3	4	5	8	13	37	37
20–34	28	11.4	103	2	4	8	16	27	28	43
35–49	95	9.5	85	3	4	7	11	16	34	50
50–64	182	9.5	74	3	4	7	11	19	28	47
65+	206	7.6	37	2	4	6	10	14	22	25
SUBTOTALS:										
1. SINGLE DX										
A. *Not Operated*	3	4.3	12	1	1	4	8	8	8	8
B. *Operated*	0									
2. MULTIPLE DX										
A. *Not Operated*	201	7.1	31	2	4	6	9	14	17	37
B. *Operated*	523	8.8	64	3	4	7	10	17	25	45
1. SINGLE DX	3	4.3	12	1	1	4	8	8	8	8
2. MULTIPLE DX	724	8.3	55	2	4	6	10	16	23	43
A. NOT OPERATED	204	7.1	31	2	4	6	9	14	17	37
B. OPERATED	523	8.8	64	3	4	7	10	17	25	45
TOTAL										
0–19 Years	21	7.0	56	2	3	5	8	12	13	37
20–34	39	10.0	84	2	4	7	13	26	28	43
35–49	137	9.2	72	3	4	7	11	16	29	47
50–64	250	8.9	62	3	4	7	10	16	27	47
65+	280	7.3	36	2	3	6	9	14	20	28
GRAND TOTAL	727	8.3	55	2	4	6	10	16	23	43

627

Length of Stay by Diagnosis and Operation, Western Region, 2008

Western Region, October 2006–September 2007 Data, by Diagnosis

730.08: AC OSTEOMYELITIS NEC

Type of Patients	Observed Patients	Avg. Stay	Variance	10th	25th	50th	75th	90th	95th	99th
1. SINGLE DX										
A. Not Operated										
0–19 Years	0									
20–34	0									
35–49	0									
50–64	1	1.0	0	1	1	1	1	1	1	1
65+	0									
B. Operated										
0–19 Years	0									
20–34	0									
35–49	1	5.0	0	5	5	5	5	5	5	5
50–64	0									
65+	0									
2. MULTIPLE DX										
A. Not Operated										
0–19 Years	11	7.3	29	1	4	6	12	13	18	18
20–34	6	12.5	226	1	5	8	14	42	42	42
35–49	28	9.3	93	3	4	8	11	15	16	54
50–64	45	8.6	56	2	4	6	9	16	23	36
65+	45	7.8	19	3	5	7	11	15	16	18
B. Operated										
0–19 Years	2	8.5	4	7	7	7	10	10	10	10
20–34	4	7.7	9	5	5	7	7	12	12	12
35–49	37	14.8	130	5	6	11	17	34	42	44
50–64	71	16.2	157	4	8	13	19	33	40	73
65+	55	12.6	86	3	6	9	17	29	31	41
SUBTOTALS:										
1. SINGLE DX										
A. Not Operated	1	1.0	0	1	1	1	1	1	1	1
B. Operated	1	5.0	0	5	5	5	5	5	5	5
2. MULTIPLE DX										
A. Not Operated	135	8.6	55	3	4	7	11	16	19	42
B. Operated	169	14.4	125	4	7	11	18	30	39	49
1. SINGLE DX	2	3.0	8	1	1	1	5	5	5	5
2. MULTIPLE DX	304	11.8	102	3	5	9	15	26	33	44
A. NOT OPERATED	136	8.5	55	2	4	6	11	16	19	42
B. OPERATED	170	14.4	125	4	7	11	18	30	39	49
TOTAL										
0–19 Years	13	7.4	24	1	4	6	10	13	18	18
20–34	10	10.6	134	5	5	7	12	14	42	42
35–49	66	12.3	119	3	5	10	14	30	39	54
50–64	117	13.2	131	3	6	10	17	28	37	49
65+	100	10.4	61	3	5	8	14	22	29	32
GRAND TOTAL	306	11.8	102	3	5	9	15	26	33	44

730.16: CHR OSTEOMYELITIS-LOW LE

Type of Patients	Observed Patients	Avg. Stay	Variance	10th	25th	50th	75th	90th	95th	99th
1. SINGLE DX										
A. Not Operated										
0–19 Years	0									
20–34	0									
35–49	1	3.0	0	3	3	3	3	3	3	3
50–64	0									
65+	0									
B. Operated										
0–19 Years	1	2.0	0	2	2	2	2	2	2	2
20–34	1	1.0	0	1	1	1	1	1	1	1
35–49	4	2.0	2	1	1	2	4	4	4	4
50–64	3	2.0	<1	1	2	2	3	3	3	3
65+	1	1.0	0	1	1	1	1	1	1	1
2. MULTIPLE DX										
A. Not Operated										
0–19 Years	7	9.3	65	3	4	7	7	25	25	25
20–34	14	7.4	104	1	2	5	6	13	13	41
35–49	28	5.5	24	1	1	3	6	14	15	22
50–64	24	9.0	47	3	3	8	12	19	23	29
65+	14	7.2	25	2	3	5	11	15	16	16
B. Operated										
0–19 Years	10	19.8	333	1	7	10	44	48	48	48
20–34	28	9.2	131	2	4	6	7	24	30	57
35–49	59	8.1	79	2	4	6	10	17	19	61
50–64	65	8.8	84	2	4	6	10	17	22	52
65+	37	6.3	16	1	3	5	8	13	14	15
SUBTOTALS:										
1. SINGLE DX										
A. Not Operated	1	3.0	0	3	3	3	3	3	3	3
B. Operated	10	1.8	1	1	1	1	2	3	3	4
2. MULTIPLE DX										
A. Not Operated	87	7.4	46	3	5	5	10	15	22	41
B. Operated	199	8.7	94	2	3	6	10	17	25	57
1. SINGLE DX	11	1.9	1	1	1	2	3	3	4	4
2. MULTIPLE DX	286	8.3	79	2	3	6	10	16	23	52
A. NOT OPERATED	88	7.3	46	1	3	5	9	15	22	41
B. OPERATED	209	8.4	91	2	3	6	9	17	24	52
TOTAL										
0–19 Years	18	14.7	236	2	4	10	16	44	48	48
20–34	43	8.5	118	2	4	5	7	20	30	57
35–49	92	7.0	61	2	3	5	8	14	19	61
50–64	92	8.6	72	1	3	6	10	17	23	52
65+	52	6.4	18	2	3	5	9	13	15	16
GRAND TOTAL	297	8.1	78	3	3	6	9	16	23	52

730.17: CHR OSTEOMYELITIS-ANKLE

Type of Patients	Observed Patients	Avg. Stay	Variance	10th	25th	50th	75th	90th	95th	99th
1. SINGLE DX										
A. Not Operated										
0–19 Years	0									
20–34	0									
35–49	1	1.0	0	1	1	1	1	1	1	1
50–64	0									
65+	0									
B. Operated										
0–19 Years	1	10.0	0	10	10	10	10	10	10	10
20–34	0									
35–49	1	1.0	0	1	1	1	1	1	1	1
50–64	2	16.0	32	12	12	16	20	20	20	20
65+	0									
2. MULTIPLE DX										
A. Not Operated										
0–19 Years	3	4.3	2	2	3	4	6	6	6	6
20–34	13	7.7	16	3	5	8	11	13	15	15
35–49	49	7.5	55	2	2	3	9	18	21	40
50–64	56	7.4	96	1	2	5	8	16	24	63
65+	58	5.7	16	2	3	5	7	11	14	23
B. Operated										
0–19 Years	5	4.6	22	2	2	3	3	13	13	13
20–34	25	7.3	35	1	1	6	10	11	16	29
35–49	90	7.2	46	2	3	6	8	15	19	50
50–64	147	7.2	36	2	3	6	9	13	20	41
65+	149	7.2	44	1	3	5	8	16	19	54
SUBTOTALS:										
1. SINGLE DX										
A. Not Operated	1	1.0	0	1	1	1	1	1	1	1
B. Operated	4	10.8	60	10	10	12	20	20	20	20
2. MULTIPLE DX										
A. Not Operated	179	6.8	52	2	3	5	8	14	20	40
B. Operated	416	7.2	40	2	3	6	9	15	19	41
1. SINGLE DX	5	8.8	64	1	1	10	12	20	20	20
2. MULTIPLE DX	595	7.1	44	2	3	5	9	14	19	40
A. NOT OPERATED	180	6.8	52	2	3	5	8	14	18	40
B. OPERATED	420	7.2	41	2	3	6	9	15	19	41
TOTAL										
0–19 Years	9	5.1	15	2	3	3	6	13	13	13
20–34	38	7.4	28	2	4	6	11	13	16	29
35–49	141	7.2	49	2	3	5	8	15	19	40
50–64	205	7.3	53	2	3	6	9	15	20	41
65+	207	6.8	36	2	3	5	8	14	18	28
GRAND TOTAL	600	7.1	44	2	3	5	9	14	19	40

730.24: OSTEOMYELITIS NOS-HAND

Type of Patients	Observed Patients	Avg. Stay	Vari-ance	10th	25th	50th	75th	90th	95th	99th
1. SINGLE DX										
A. Not Operated										
0–19 Years	0									
20–34	1	4.0	0	4	4	4	4	4	4	4
35–49	0									
50–64	0									
65+	0									
B. Operated										
0–19 Years	0									
20–34	1	3.0	0	3	3	3	3	3	3	3
35–49	2	4.5	4	3	3	6	6	6	6	6
50–64	1	5.0	0	5	5	5	5	5	5	5
65+	0									
2. MULTIPLE DX										
A. Not Operated										
0–19 Years	8	4.4	8	1	4	4	5	10	10	10
20–34	13	9.9	72	3	4	7	10	27	28	28
35–49	51	7.2	57	2	3	5	9	13	25	45
50–64	30	4.5	17	1	2	3	6	8	11	21
65+	27	5.7	16	1	4	5	7	11	14	19
B. Operated										
0–19 Years	4	5.3	43	2	2	2	15	15	15	15
20–34	36	5.4	15	2	3	4	7	11	12	20
35–49	60	5.7	36	2	3	4	6	9	14	44
50–64	47	7.4	49	2	3	6	10	14	15	43
65+	35	5.5	11	2	3	5	7	11	13	16
SUBTOTALS:										
1. SINGLE DX										
A. Not Operated	1	4.0	0	4	4	4	4	4	4	4
B. Operated	4	4.3	2	3	3	5	6	6	6	6
2. MULTIPLE DX										
A. Not Operated	129	6.4	39	1	3	4	8	11	19	28
B. Operated	182	6.0	31	2	3	5	7	11	14	43
1. SINGLE DX	**5**	**4.2**	**2**	**3**	**3**	**4**	**5**	**6**	**6**	**6**
2. MULTIPLE DX	**311**	**6.2**	**34**	**2**	**3**	**5**	**7**	**11**	**15**	**28**
A. NOT OPERATED	**130**	**6.4**	**39**	**1**	**3**	**4**	**8**	**11**	**19**	**28**
B. OPERATED	**186**	**6.0**	**30**	**2**	**3**	**5**	**7**	**11**	**14**	**43**
TOTAL										
0–19 Years	12	4.7	17	1	2	4	6	10	15	15
20–34	51	6.5	32	2	3	4	9	11	20	28
35–49	113	6.4	45	2	3	5	7	13	18	44
50–64	78	6.3	38	2	3	5	8	13	15	43
65+	62	5.6	13	2	3	5	7	10	13	19
GRAND TOTAL	**316**	**6.1**	**34**	**2**	**3**	**5**	**7**	**11**	**15**	**28**

730.25: OSTEOMYELITIS NOS-PELVIS

Type of Patients	Observed Patients	Avg. Stay	Vari-ance	10th	25th	50th	75th	90th	95th	99th
1. SINGLE DX										
A. Not Operated										
0–19 Years	9	6.6	20	1	4	7	9	15	15	15
20–34	1	1.0	0	1	1	1	1	1	1	1
35–49	2	1.0	0	1	1	1	1	1	1	1
50–64	0									
65+	0									
B. Operated										
0–19 Years	2	6.5	24	3	3	10	10	10	10	10
20–34	1	1.0	0	1	1	1	1	1	1	1
35–49	1	2.0	0	2	2	2	2	2	2	2
50–64	0									
65+	1	7.0	0	7	7	7	7	7	7	7
2. MULTIPLE DX										
A. Not Operated										
0–19 Years	22	7.3	20	4	4	6	9	13	14	21
20–34	26	13.8	207	4	5	8	15	28	55	60
35–49	46	8.3	53	2	4	7	9	16	21	42
50–64	39	12.0	170	2	3	7	15	31	45	56
65+	22	7.3	21	3	5	6	8	11	17	22
B. Operated										
0–19 Years	8	19.1	195	3	11	21	32	43	43	43
20–34	37	11.7	127	3	4	9	17	22	24	64
35–49	61	12.3	135	2	4	7	16	28	35	47
50–64	51	15.0	194	3	6	9	18	31	50	65
65+	48	12.6	192	3	5	8	16	29	37	85
SUBTOTALS:										
1. SINGLE DX										
A. Not Operated	12	5.2	21	1	1	5	7	10	15	15
B. Operated	5	4.6	14	1	2	3	7	10	10	10
2. MULTIPLE DX										
A. Not Operated	155	9.9	103	2	4	7	12	21	30	56
B. Operated	205	13.2	164	3	5	9	18	28	42	64
1. SINGLE DX	**17**	**5.0**	**18**	**1**	**1**	**4**	**7**	**10**	**15**	**15**
2. MULTIPLE DX	**360**	**11.8**	**140**	**3**	**5**	**8**	**15**	**25**	**37**	**60**
A. NOT OPERATED	**167**	**9.5**	**98**	**2**	**4**	**7**	**11**	**20**	**30**	**56**
B. OPERATED	**210**	**13.0**	**162**	**3**	**5**	**9**	**17**	**28**	**42**	**64**
TOTAL										
0–19 Years	41	9.4	72	3	4	7	11	21	25	43
20–34	65	12.2	158	3	5	8	16	23	28	64
35–49	110	10.3	103	2	4	7	15	24	31	47
50–64	90	13.7	184	2	4	9	18	31	45	65
65+	71	10.9	141	3	5	7	11	20	32	85
GRAND TOTAL	**377**	**11.5**	**136**	**2**	**4**	**7**	**15**	**25**	**37**	**60**

730.26: OSTEOMYELITIS NOS-LOW LE

Type of Patients	Observed Patients	Avg. Stay	Vari-ance	10th	25th	50th	75th	90th	95th	99th
1. SINGLE DX										
A. Not Operated										
0–19 Years	2	4.0	2	3	3	4	5	5	5	5
20–34	0									
35–49	0									
50–64	1	4.0	0	4	4	4	4	4	4	4
65+	0									
B. Operated										
0–19 Years	1	8.0	0	8	8	8	8	8	8	8
20–34	2	4.0	8	2	2	2	6	6	6	6
35–49	2	3.5	12	1	1	6	6	6	6	6
50–64	2	1.5	<1	1	1	1	2	2	2	2
65+	1	7.0	0	7	7	7	7	7	7	7
2. MULTIPLE DX										
A. Not Operated										
0–19 Years	34	4.6	5	2	3	5	6	7	8	10
20–34	19	5.3	10	1	2	5	8	11	11	11
35–49	41	8.5	47	3	4	6	10	19	24	28
50–64	53	7.9	37	2	4	6	9	18	21	32
65+	55	7.7	22	3	5	7	8	15	22	22
B. Operated										
0–19 Years	30	10.8	124	2	4	7	15	22	40	48
20–34	31	7.1	28	3	3	5	10	14	17	25
35–49	51	7.3	52	2	3	4	9	16	26	28
50–64	68	6.9	29	3	3	5	9	15	17	28
65+	53	7.3	33	3	3	6	10	13	24	28
SUBTOTALS:										
1. SINGLE DX										
A. Not Operated	3	4.0	1	3	3	4	5	5	5	5
B. Operated	8	4.1	8	1	2	6	7	8	8	8
2. MULTIPLE DX										
A. Not Operated	202	7.2	28	2	4	6	8	13	21	28
B. Operated	233	7.6	48	2	3	5	9	16	24	29
1. SINGLE DX	**11**	**4.1**	**6**	**1**	**2**	**4**	**6**	**7**	**8**	**8**
2. MULTIPLE DX	**435**	**7.4**	**39**	**2**	**4**	**6**	**9**	**15**	**22**	**28**
A. NOT OPERATED	**205**	**7.1**	**28**	**2**	**4**	**6**	**8**	**13**	**21**	**28**
B. OPERATED	**241**	**7.5**	**47**	**2**	**3**	**5**	**9**	**15**	**22**	**29**
TOTAL										
0–19 Years	67	7.4	67	2	3	6	8	15	22	48
20–34	52	6.3	21	3	3	5	9	12	14	25
35–49	94	7.7	49	2	3	5	9	19	26	28
50–64	124	7.2	32	2	4	6	9	15	20	28
65+	109	7.5	27	3	4	7	9	14	22	24
GRAND TOTAL	**446**	**7.3**	**38**	**2**	**3**	**6**	**8**	**15**	**22**	**28**

Length of Stay by Diagnosis and Operation, Western Region, 2008

Western Region, October 2006–September 2007 Data, by Diagnosis

730.27: OSTEOMYELITIS NOS-ANKLE

Type of Patients	Observed Patients	Avg. Stay	Variance	Percentiles						
				10th	25th	50th	75th	90th	95th	99th
1. SINGLE DX										
A. Not Operated										
0–19 Years	5	3.8	4	1	3	4	5	6	6	6
20–34	1	6.0	0		6	6	6	6	6	6
35–49	0									
50–64	2	3.0	0	3	3	3	3	3	3	3
65+	0									
B. Operated										
0–19 Years	1	3.0	0	3	3	3	3	3	3	3
20–34	1	4.0	0	3	3	4	4	4	4	4
35–49	2	6.5	4	5	5	8	8	8	8	8
50–64	1	4.0	0	4	4	4	4	4	4	4
65+	1	2.0	0	2	2	2	2	2	2	2
2. MULTIPLE DX										
A. Not Operated										
0–19 Years	29	4.7	11	2	2	4	7	9	9	15
20–34	59	5.2	9	2	3	5	7	9	12	14
35–49	162	6.5	36	2	3	5	8	12	16	34
50–64	300	7.8	81	2	3	5	9	15	22	41
65+	369	6.0	16	2	3	5	8	11	13	20
B. Operated										
0–19 Years	21	8.3	32	3	4	7	10	16	17	23
20–34	56	8.2	76	3	4	7	9	15	21	61
35–49	197	7.8	35	2	4	7	10	15	18	34
50–64	413	8.4	71	2	4	6	10	16	22	49
65+	471	7.6	30	2	4	6	10	15	19	29
SUBTOTALS:										
1. SINGLE DX										
A. Not Operated	8	3.9	3	1	3	3	6	6	6	6
B. Operated	6	4.3	4	2	3	4	5	8	8	8
2. MULTIPLE DX										
A. Not Operated	919	6.6	41	2	3	5	8	12	16	34
B. Operated	1,158	7.9	48	2	4	6	10	15	19	44
1. SINGLE DX	14	4.1	3	2	3	4	5	6	8	8
2. MULTIPLE DX	2,077	7.3	45	2	3	6	9	14	18	34
A. NOT OPERATED	927	6.6	41	2	3	5	8	12	15	34
B. OPERATED	1,164	7.9	47	2	4	6	10	15	19	44
TOTAL										
0–19 Years	56	5.9	21	2	2	4	8	11	16	23
20–34	117	6.6	43	2	4	5	8	11	15	29
35–49	361	7.2	35	2	3	6	9	14	17	34
50–64	716	8.1	75	2	4	6	9	16	22	47
65+	841	6.9	24	2	4	6	9	13	16	27
GRAND TOTAL	2,091	7.3	45	2	3	6	9	14	18	34

730.28: OSTEOMYELITIS NOS-NEC

Type of Patients	Observed Patients	Avg. Stay	Variance	Percentiles						
				10th	25th	50th	75th	90th	95th	99th
1. SINGLE DX										
A. Not Operated										
0–19 Years	1	6.0	0	6	6	6	6	6	6	6
20–34	0									
35–49	2	4.5	24	1	1	8	8	8	8	8
50–64	2	6.5	4	5	5	7	8	8	8	8
65+	0									
B. Operated										
0–19 Years	1	1.0	0	1	1	1	1	1	1	1
20–34	0									
35–49	1	7.0	0	7	7	7	7	7	7	7
50–64	0									
65+	0									
2. MULTIPLE DX										
A. Not Operated										
0–19 Years	20	7.5	29	2	3	7	10	19	20	20
20–34	26	9.8	79	2	4	7	10	25	32	34
35–49	87	9.1	73	2	4	7	11	15	27	49
50–64	156	9.9	75	2	4	7	12	19	26	46
65+	170	9.3	52	3	4	8	11	18	23	38
B. Operated										
0–19 Years	9	9.1	54	3	4	6	16	21	21	23
20–34	14	13.0	264	3	4	7	12	48	53	53
35–49	105	13.9	135	3	6	10	17	32	43	48
50–64	124	13.7	177	3	6	9	16	30	41	80
65+	142	11.7	71	4	6	9	15	22	26	47
SUBTOTALS:										
1. SINGLE DX										
A. Not Operated	5	5.6	8	1	5	6	6	8	8	8
B. Operated	2	4.0	18	1	1	7	7	7	7	7
2. MULTIPLE DX										
A. Not Operated	459	9.4	64	3	4	7	12	18	26	45
B. Operated	394	12.9	128	4	6	9	16	26	39	68
1. SINGLE DX	7	5.2	9	1	1	6	8	8	8	8
2. MULTIPLE DX	853	11.0	96	3	5	8	14	22	31	49
A. NOT OPERATED	464	9.3	64	3	4	7	12	18	26	45
B. OPERATED	396	12.9	127	4	6	9	16	26	39	68
TOTAL										
0–19 Years	31	7.7	35	2	3	6	11	19	20	21
20–34	40	10.9	141	3	4	7	12	25	34	53
35–49	195	11.6	111	3	5	8	14	26	41	49
50–64	282	11.5	123	3	5	8	14	24	32	77
65+	312	10.4	62	3	5	8	13	21	26	41
GRAND TOTAL	860	11.0	96	3	5	8	14	22	31	49

731: OSTEITIS DEFORMANS

Type of Patients	Observed Patients	Avg. Stay	Variance	Percentiles						
				10th	25th	50th	75th	90th	95th	99th
1. SINGLE DX										
A. Not Operated										
0–19 Years	0									
20–34	1	3.0	0	3	3	3	3	3	3	3
35–49	0									
50–64	0									
65+	0									
B. Operated										
0–19 Years	0									
20–34	1	3.0	0	3	3	3	3	3	3	3
35–49	0									
50–64	0									
65+	0									
2. MULTIPLE DX										
A. Not Operated										
0–19 Years	1	1.0	0	1	1	1	1	1	1	1
20–34	0									
35–49	1	11.0	0	11	11	11	11	11	11	11
50–64	3	2.3	<1	2	2	2	3	3	3	3
65+	17	3.8	6	2	2	4	4	8	11	11
B. Operated										
0–19 Years	1	4.0	0	4	4	4	4	4	4	4
20–34	2	3.5	<1	3	3	4	4	4	4	4
35–49	2	11.5	175	1	2	12	21	21	21	21
50–64	4	4.3	8	1	3	6	6	6	7	7
65+	5	7.2	23	1	6	6	9	14	14	14
SUBTOTALS:										
1. SINGLE DX										
A. Not Operated	1	3.0	0	3	3	3	3	3	3	3
B. Operated	1	3.0	0	3	3	3	3	3	3	3
2. MULTIPLE DX										
A. Not Operated	22	3.8	8	2	2	3	3	4	8	11
B. Operated	14	6.2	30	1	3	6	7	14	21	21
1. SINGLE DX	2	3.0	0	3	3	3	3	3	3	3
2. MULTIPLE DX	36	4.8	17	1	2	4	6	11	14	21
A. NOT OPERATED	23	3.8	8	2	2	3	4	8	11	11
B. OPERATED	15	6.0	29	1	3	4	7	14	21	21
TOTAL										
0–19 Years	2	2.5	4	1	1	4	4	4	4	4
20–34	4	3.3	<1	3	3	3	4	4	4	4
35–49	3	11.3	89	2	2	11	21	21	21	21
50–64	7	3.4	5	1	2	3	6	7	7	7
65+	22	4.6	11	2	2	4	6	9	11	14
GRAND TOTAL	38	4.7	17	1	2	4	6	11	14	21

Length of Stay by Diagnosis and Operation, Western Region, 2008

Western Region, October 2006–September 2007 Data, by Diagnosis

732: OSTEOCHONDROPATHIES

Type of Patients	Observed Patients	Avg. Stay	Variance	10th	25th	50th	75th	90th	95th	99th
1. SINGLE DX										
A. Not Operated										
0–19 Years	0									
20–34	0									
35–49	0									
50–64	0									
65+	0									
B. Operated										
0–19 Years	143	1.9	2		1	1	2	3	4	6
20–34	20	2.7	4	1	1	2	4	5	9	9
35–49	4	1.5	1	1	1	1	3	3	3	3
50–64	2	2.0	0	2	2	2	2	2	2	2
65+	0									
2. MULTIPLE DX										
A. Not Operated										
0–19 Years	9	2.2	1	1	1	2	3	4	4	4
20–34	0									
35–49	1	2.0	0	2	2	2	2	2	2	2
50–64	4	2.5	3	1	2	2	5	5	5	5
65+	3	3.0	4	1	3	3	5	5	5	5
B. Operated										
0–19 Years	155	2.3	3	1	1	2	3	5	6	8
20–34	34	3.9	10	1	1	3	5	7	11	15
35–49	56	3.0	3	1	2	3	3	5	7	10
50–64	41	2.6	2	1	2	3	3	4	6	7
65+	11	3.5	3	2	2	3	4	6	7	7
SUBTOTALS:										
1. SINGLE DX										
A. Not Operated	0									
B. Operated	169	2.0	2	1	1	1	2	4	4	9
2. MULTIPLE DX										
A. Not Operated	17	2.4	2	1	1	2	3	5	5	5
B. Operated	297	2.7	4	1	1	2	3	5	7	10
1. SINGLE DX	169	2.0	2	1	1	1	2	4	4	9
2. MULTIPLE DX	314	2.7	4	1	1	2	3	5	7	10
A. NOT OPERATED	17	2.4	2	1	1	2	3	5	5	5
B. OPERATED	466	2.4	3	1	1	2	3	5	6	9
TOTAL										
0–19 Years	307	2.1	2	1	1	2	3	4	5	8
20–34	54	3.5	8	1	1	2	5	7	10	15
35–49	61	2.9	3	1	2	3	3	5	6	10
50–64	47	2.6	2	1	2	2	3	4	6	7
65+	14	3.4	3	2	2	3	4	6	7	7
GRAND TOTAL	483	2.4	3	1	1	2	3	5	6	9

733: OTH BONE/CART DISORDER

Type of Patients	Observed Patients	Avg. Stay	Variance	10th	25th	50th	75th	90th	95th	99th
1. SINGLE DX										
A. Not Operated										
0–19 Years	12	1.4	1	1	1	1	1	2	5	5
20–34	8	1.9	3	1	1	1	4	5	5	5
35–49	27	1.2	<1	1	1	1	1	2	2	2
50–64	18	1.6	<1	1	1	1	2	3	4	4
65+	12	1.5	<1	1	1	1	3	3	3	3
B. Operated										
0–19 Years	87	1.9	2	1	1	1	2	4	5	8
20–34	167	2.1	2	1	1	2	3	3	4	8
35–49	186	2.2	2	1	1	2	3	4	4	7
50–64	153	2.3	2	1	1	2	3	4	5	6
65+	85	1.7	1	1	1	1	2	3	4	6
2. MULTIPLE DX										
A. Not Operated										
0–19 Years	68	2.6	6	1	1	2	3	5	7	15
20–34	216	2.5	9	1	1	2	3	5	8	13
35–49	795	2.5	9	1	1	2	3	5	7	14
50–64	1,375	3.2	13	1	2	2	4	7	9	18
65+	4,559	4.4	13	2	2	3	5	8	11	18
B. Operated										
0–19 Years	306	2.6	6	1	1	2	3	5	7	14
20–34	929	3.1	17	1	1	2	4	6	7	19
35–49	2,098	3.8	20	1	2	3	4	7	11	20
50–64	3,838	4.1	18	1	2	3	4	8	12	22
65+	7,762	4.5	19	1	2	3	6	9	12	21
SUBTOTALS:										
1. SINGLE DX										
A. Not Operated	77	1.4	<1	1	1	1	2	3	4	5
B. Operated	678	2.1	2	1	1	2	3	4	4	7
2. MULTIPLE DX										
A. Not Operated	7,013	3.8	13	1	2	3	5	8	10	18
B. Operated	14,933	4.2	19	1	2	3	5	8	11	21
1. SINGLE DX	755	2.0	2	1	1	2	3	4	4	7
2. MULTIPLE DX	21,946	4.1	17	1	2	3	5	8	11	20
A. NOT OPERATED	7,090	3.8	13	1	2	3	5	8	10	18
B. OPERATED	15,611	4.1	18	1	2	3	5	8	11	21
TOTAL										
0–19 Years	473	2.5	5	1	1	2	3	4	7	14
20–34	1,320	2.9	14	1	1	2	3	5	7	17
35–49	3,106	3.3	16	1	1	2	4	6	9	19
50–64	5,384	3.8	17	1	1	3	4	7	11	21
65+	12,418	4.4	17	1	2	3	6	9	11	20
GRAND TOTAL	22,701	4.0	17	1	2	3	5	8	11	20

733.11: PATH FX HUMERUS

Type of Patients	Observed Patients	Avg. Stay	Variance	10th	25th	50th	75th	90th	95th	99th
1. SINGLE DX										
A. Not Operated										
0–19 Years	0									
20–34	0									
35–49	1	1.0	0	1	1	1	1	1	1	1
50–64	0									
65+	0									
B. Operated										
0–19 Years	0									
20–34	0									
35–49	0									
50–64	1	2.0	0	2	2	2	2	2	2	2
65+	1	2.0	0	2	2	2	2	2	2	2
2. MULTIPLE DX										
A. Not Operated										
0–19 Years	3	4.7	12	1	1	5	8	8	8	8
20–34	2	1.5	<1	1	1	1	2	2	2	2
35–49	5	5.6	7	1	6	7	7	7	7	7
50–64	16	8.0	67	1	2	5	12	20	30	30
65+	59	4.3	10	1	2	3	5	9	13	16
B. Operated										
0–19 Years	5	1.6	<1	1	1	1	2	3	3	3
20–34	4	3.3	4	1	2	5	5	5	5	5
35–49	15	4.3	11	1	2	3	6	9	13	13
50–64	68	3.5	11	1	1	3	4	9	12	16
65+	152	5.4	21	1	2	4	7	11	13	22
SUBTOTALS:										
1. SINGLE DX										
A. Not Operated	1	1.0	0	1	1	1	1	1	1	1
B. Operated	2	2.0	0	2	2	2	2	2	2	2
2. MULTIPLE DX										
A. Not Operated	85	5.0	22	1	2	4	6	9	13	30
B. Operated	244	4.7	18	1	2	3	7	10	13	18
1. SINGLE DX	3	1.7	<1	1	1	2	2	2	2	2
2. MULTIPLE DX	329	4.8	19	1	2	3	6	10	13	20
A. NOT OPERATED	86	5.0	22	1	2	4	6	9	13	30
B. OPERATED	246	4.7	18	1	2	3	6	10	13	18
TOTAL										
0–19 Years	8	2.8	6	1	1	2	5	8	8	8
20–34	6	2.7	3	1	1	3	5	5	5	5
35–49	21	4.4	10	1	2	3	7	9	9	13
50–64	85	4.3	24	1	1	3	4	11	13	30
65+	212	5.1	18	1	2	4	7	10	13	18
GRAND TOTAL	332	4.8	19	1	2	3	6	10	13	20

Length of Stay by Diagnosis and Operation, Western Region, 2008

Western Region, October 2006–September 2007 Data, by Diagnosis

733.13: PATH FX VERTEBRAE

Type of Patients	Observed Patients	Avg. Stay	Vari-ance	10th	25th	50th	75th	90th	95th	99th
1. SINGLE DX										
A. Not Operated										
0–19 Years	0									
20–34	0									
35–49	0									
50–64	0									
65+	4	2.0	1	1	1	3	3	3	3	3
B. Operated										
0–19 Years	1	1.0	0	1	1	1	1	1	1	1
20–34	0									
35–49	1	1.0	0	1	1	1	1	1	1	1
50–64	8	1.0	0	1	1	1	1	1	1	1
65+	48	1.3	<1	1	1	1	1	2	2	6
2. MULTIPLE DX										
A. Not Operated										
0–19 Years	5	2.8	6	1	1	2	3	7	7	7
20–34	7	4.7	18	1	2	3	7	13	13	13
35–49	68	5.9	21	2	3	5	7	12	14	25
50–64	256	5.6	27	2	3	4	7	9	16	25
65+	2,871	4.9	15	2	3	4	6	9	11	20
B. Operated										
0–19 Years	3	2.7	<1	2	2	3	3	3	3	3
20–34	6	9.7	148	1	1	6	12	33	33	33
35–49	111	7.1	55	1	1	5	11	16	19	33
50–64	545	5.5	45	1	1	3	8	13	18	29
65+	3,979	4.2	23	1	1	3	6	10	12	22
SUBTOTALS:										
1. SINGLE DX										
A. Not Operated	4	2.0	1	1	1	3	3	3	3	3
B. Operated	58	1.2	<1	1	1	1	1	2	2	6
2. MULTIPLE DX										
A. Not Operated	3,207	5.0	16	2	3	4	6	9	12	21
B. Operated	4,644	4.5	27	1	1	3	6	10	13	24
1. SINGLE DX	62	1.3	<1	1	1	1	1	2	3	6
2. MULTIPLE DX	7,851	4.7	22	1	1	3	6	10	13	22
A. NOT OPERATED	3,211	5.0	16	2	3	4	6	9	12	21
B. OPERATED	4,702	4.4	26	1	1	3	6	10	13	24
TOTAL										
0–19 Years	9	2.6	4	1	1	2	3	7	7	7
20–34	13	7.0	77	1	2	4	7	13	33	33
35–49	180	6.6	42	1	2	5	9	14	18	33
50–64	809	5.5	39	1	1	4	7	13	17	29
65+	6,902	4.5	19	1	1	3	6	9	12	21
GRAND TOTAL	7,913	4.7	22	1	1	3	6	10	13	22

733.14: PATH FX FEMUR NECK

Type of Patients	Observed Patients	Avg. Stay	Vari-ance	10th	25th	50th	75th	90th	95th	99th
1. SINGLE DX										
A. Not Operated										
0–19 Years	0									
20–34	0									
35–49	0									
50–64	1	4.0	0	4	4	4	4	4	4	4
65+	0									
B. Operated										
0–19 Years	1	1.0	0	1	1	1	1	1	1	1
20–34	1	6.0	0	6	6	6	6	6	6	6
35–49	0									
50–64	0									
65+	0									
2. MULTIPLE DX										
A. Not Operated										
0–19 Years	3	6.0	61	1	1	2	15	15	15	15
20–34	2	7.5	4	6	6	6	9	9	9	9
35–49	8	5.0	6	1	4	5	7	8	8	8
50–64	20	7.0	43	1	3	5	10	18	19	23
65+	98	5.0	16	2	3	4	7	9	13	23
B. Operated										
0–19 Years	10	4.7	9	1	2	4	5	9	9	9
20–34	14	5.6	12	3	4	5	5	7	9	17
35–49	67	8.7	76	3	4	6	9	17	22	48
50–64	241	7.2	46	3	4	5	8	14	18	31
65+	734	6.4	17	3	4	5	8	11	15	22
SUBTOTALS:										
1. SINGLE DX										
A. Not Operated	1	4.0	0	4	4	4	4	4	4	4
B. Operated	2	3.5	12	1	1	4	6	6	6	6
2. MULTIPLE DX										
A. Not Operated	131	5.4	20	1	3	4	7	10	15	23
B. Operated	1,066	6.7	27	3	4	5	8	12	16	25
1. SINGLE DX	3	3.7	6	1	1	4	6	6	6	6
2. MULTIPLE DX	1,197	6.6	27	3	4	5	8	12	16	25
A. NOT OPERATED	132	5.4	20	1	3	4	7	10	15	23
B. OPERATED	1,068	6.7	27	3	4	5	8	12	16	25
TOTAL										
0–19 Years	14	4.7	17	1	1	4	8	9	15	15
20–34	17	5.8	10	3	4	5	6	9	17	17
35–49	75	8.3	69	3	4	6	8	17	22	48
50–64	262	7.2	45	2	4	5	7	15	19	31
65+	832	6.3	17	3	4	5	7	11	14	22
GRAND TOTAL	1,200	6.6	27	3	4	5	8	12	16	25

733.15: PATH FX FEMUR NEC

Type of Patients	Observed Patients	Avg. Stay	Vari-ance	10th	25th	50th	75th	90th	95th	99th
1. SINGLE DX										
A. Not Operated										
0–19 Years	0									
20–34	0									
35–49	0									
50–64	0									
65+	0									
B. Operated										
0–19 Years	2	5.0	8	3	3	5	7	7	7	7
20–34	0									
35–49	1	1.0	0	1	1	1	1	1	1	1
50–64	0									
65+	1	5.0	0	5	5	5	5	5	5	5
2. MULTIPLE DX										
A. Not Operated										
0–19 Years	12	3.3	10	1	1	2	5	5	12	12
20–34	3	4.7	6	2	2	5	7	7	7	7
35–49	2	4.0	6	2	2	3	6	6	6	6
50–64	17	4.2	16	1	2	3	4	7	18	18
65+	56	4.7	15	1	3	4	6	8	11	22
B. Operated										
0–19 Years	22	3.6	8	1	2	3	3	4	7	14
20–34	8	10.2	86	1	4	6	6	28	28	28
35–49	31	7.5	70	3	4	5	9	11	21	47
50–64	136	7.4	40	2	4	5	8	14	23	32
65+	238	6.9	34	3	4	5	7	12	19	34
SUBTOTALS:										
1. SINGLE DX										
A. Not Operated	0									
B. Operated	4	4.0	7	1	3	5	5	7	7	7
2. MULTIPLE DX										
A. Not Operated	90	4.4	14	1	2	4	5	8	11	22
B. Operated	435	7.0	39	3	4	5	8	13	21	34
1. SINGLE DX	4	4.0	7	1	3	5	5	7	7	7
2. MULTIPLE DX	525	6.5	35	2	3	5	7	12	19	32
A. NOT OPERATED	90	4.4	14	1	2	4	5	8	11	22
B. OPERATED	439	7.0	38	3	4	5	8	13	21	34
TOTAL										
0–19 Years	36	3.6	8	1	2	3	5	7	12	14
20–34	11	8.7	68	2	4	5	14	19	28	28
35–49	34	7.1	65	2	3	5	8	11	21	47
50–64	153	7.0	38	2	3	5	8	13	22	32
65+	295	6.5	31	3	4	5	7	10	18	34
GRAND TOTAL	529	6.5	35	2	3	5	7	12	19	32

Length of Stay by Diagnosis and Operation, Western Region, 2008

733.19: PATHOLOGIC FRACTURE NEC

Type of Patients	Observed Patients	Avg. Stay	Variance	Percentiles						
				10th	25th	50th	75th	90th	95th	99th
1. SINGLE DX										
A. Not Operated										
0–19 Years	0									
20–34	0									
35–49	0									
50–64	0									
65+	0									
B. Operated										
0–19 Years	0									
20–34	1	3.0	0	3	3	3	3	3	3	3
35–49	0									
50–64	0									
65+	0									
2. MULTIPLE DX										
A. Not Operated										
0–19 Years	2	3.0	0	3	3	3	3	3	3	3
20–34	3	5.7	20	1	1	6	10	10	10	10
35–49	12	3.8	9	1	1	3	7	8	10	10
50–64	64	5.2	21	2	2	4	8	10	15	22
65+	258	4.8	11	2	3	4	6	8	11	21
B. Operated										
0–19 Years	3	1.3	<1	1	1	1	2	2	2	2
20–34	4	5.7	58	1	1	1	4	17	17	17
35–49	7	5.7	12	1	3	5	8	11	11	11
50–64	30	5.6	19	1	2	4	8	14	14	16
65+	42	5.2	15	1	2	4	7	10	13	16
SUBTOTALS:										
1. SINGLE DX										
A. Not Operated	0									
B. Operated	1	3.0	0	3	3	3	3	3	3	3
2. MULTIPLE DX										
A. Not Operated	339	4.9	13	2	3	4	6	9	11	22
B. Operated	86	5.3	17	1	2	4	7	11	14	17
1. SINGLE DX	1	3.0	0	3	3	3	3	3	3	3
2. MULTIPLE DX	425	4.9	14	2	3	4	6	9	12	21
A. NOT OPERATED	339	4.9	13	2	3	4	6	9	11	22
B. OPERATED	87	5.2	17	1	2	4	7	11	14	17
TOTAL										
0–19 Years	5	2.0	1	1	1	2	3	3	3	3
20–34	8	5.4	32	1	1	4	10	17	17	17
35–49	19	4.5	11	1	1	3	8	10	11	11
50–64	94	5.4	20	2	2	4	8	11	15	22
65+	300	4.9	11	2	3	4	6	9	11	21
GRAND TOTAL	426	4.9	14	2	3	4	6	9	12	21

733.41: ASEPTIC NECROSIS HUMERUS

Type of Patients	Observed Patients	Avg. Stay	Variance	Percentiles						
				10th	25th	50th	75th	90th	95th	99th
1. SINGLE DX										
A. Not Operated										
0–19 Years	0									
20–34	0									
35–49	0									
50–64	0									
65+	0									
B. Operated										
0–19 Years	0									
20–34	1	1.0	0	1	1	1	1	1	1	1
35–49	3	2.0	<1	1	1	2	3	3	3	3
50–64	5	1.8	<1	1	1	2	2	3	3	3
65+	0									
2. MULTIPLE DX										
A. Not Operated										
0–19 Years	0									
20–34	1	1.0	0	1	1	1	1	1	1	1
35–49	1	1.0	0	1	1	1	1	1	1	1
50–64	3	4.3	5	3	3	3	7	7	7	7
65+	3	5.3	26	1	1	4	11	11	11	11
B. Operated										
0–19 Years	1	2.0	0	2	2	2	2	2	2	2
20–34	11	2.6	2	1	1	2	4	4	5	5
35–49	48	2.5	1	1	1	2	3	4	5	6
50–64	100	2.4	3	1	1	2	3	4	5	9
65+	103	2.7	3	1	1	2	3	5	5	10
SUBTOTALS:										
1. SINGLE DX										
A. Not Operated	0									
B. Operated	9	1.8	<1	1	1	2	2	3	3	3
2. MULTIPLE DX										
A. Not Operated	8	3.9	12	1	1	3	4	11	11	11
B. Operated	263	2.6	3	1	1	2	3	4	5	9
1. SINGLE DX	9	1.8	<1	1	1	2	2	3	3	3
2. MULTIPLE DX	271	2.6	3	1	1	2	3	4	5	10
A. NOT OPERATED	8	3.9	12	1	1	3	4	11	11	11
B. OPERATED	272	2.5	3	1	1	2	3	4	5	9
TOTAL										
0–19 Years	1	2.0	0	2	2	2	2	2	2	2
20–34	13	2.3	2	1	1	2	3	4	5	5
35–49	52	2.4	1	1	1	2	3	4	5	6
50–64	108	2.5	3	1	1	2	3	4	5	9
65+	106	2.8	4	1	1	2	3	5	6	11
GRAND TOTAL	280	2.6	3	1	1	2	3	4	5	10

733.42: ASEPTIC NECROSIS FEMUR

Type of Patients	Observed Patients	Avg. Stay	Variance	Percentiles						
				10th	25th	50th	75th	90th	95th	99th
1. SINGLE DX										
A. Not Operated										
0–19 Years	1	1.0	0	1	1	1	1	1	1	1
20–34	1	4.0	0	4	4	4	4	4	4	4
35–49	0									
50–64	0									
65+	1	1.0	0	1	1	1	1	1	1	1
B. Operated										
0–19 Years	2	4.5	<1	4	4	4	5	5	5	5
20–34	19	2.6	<1	1	2	3	3	4	4	4
35–49	49	2.8	1	2	2	3	3	4	4	5
50–64	47	3.0	1	1	3	3	3	5	5	5
65+	5	2.8	1	1	3	3	3	4	4	4
2. MULTIPLE DX										
A. Not Operated										
0–19 Years	5	1.8	<1	1	1	2	2	3	3	3
20–34	9	3.7	15	1	1	3	4	13	13	13
35–49	27	5.4	28	1	2	3	6	14	14	24
50–64	40	4.4	12	2	2	4	6	10	11	16
65+	68	4.3	8	2	2	4	5	8	10	16
B. Operated										
0–19 Years	19	3.5	4	1	2	4	5	6	8	8
20–34	202	3.6	9	2	2	3	4	5	6	12
35–49	663	3.6	4	2	3	3	4	5	6	14
50–64	1,079	3.7	5	2	3	3	4	6	7	12
65+	783	4.4	11	3	3	4	5	7	9	15
SUBTOTALS:										
1. SINGLE DX										
A. Not Operated	3	2.0	3	1	1	1	4	4	4	4
B. Operated	122	2.9	1	1	2	3	3	4	5	5
2. MULTIPLE DX										
A. Not Operated	149	4.4	13	1	2	3	5	10	11	16
B. Operated	2,746	3.9	7	2	3	3	4	6	7	13
1. SINGLE DX	125	2.8	1	1	2	3	3	4	5	5
2. MULTIPLE DX	2,895	3.9	7	2	3	3	4	6	8	14
A. NOT OPERATED	152	4.3	13	1	2	3	5	9	11	16
B. OPERATED	2,868	3.8	7	2	3	3	4	6	7	13
TOTAL										
0–19 Years	27	3.2	4	1	1	3	3	6	6	8
20–34	231	3.5	8	1	2	3	4	5	6	13
35–49	739	3.6	5	2	3	3	4	5	7	14
50–64	1,166	3.7	6	2	3	3	4	6	7	12
65+	857	4.4	10	2	3	4	5	7	9	15
GRAND TOTAL	3,020	3.8	7	2	3	3	4	6	8	14

Length of Stay by Diagnosis and Operation, Western Region, 2008

Western Region, October 2006–September 2007 Data, by Diagnosis

733.49: ASEPT NECROSIS BONE NEC

Type of Patients	Observed Patients	Avg. Stay	Variance	10th	25th	50th	75th	90th	95th	99th
1. SINGLE DX										
A. Not Operated										
0–19 Years	0									
20–34	0									
35–49	0									
50–64	0									
65+	0									
B. Operated										
0–19 Years	0									
20–34	2	1.5	<1	1	1	2	2	2	2	2
35–49	1	3.0	0	3	3	3	3	3	3	3
50–64	0									
65+	0									
2. MULTIPLE DX										
A. Not Operated										
0–19 Years	1	4.0	0	4	4	4	4	4	4	4
20–34	7	3.7	8	1	1	4	5	5	9	9
35–49	9	2.0	11	1	1	2	3	4	4	4
50–64	7	4.6	11	1	2	4	6	11	11	11
65+	14	4.1	7	1	2	4	5	7	10	10
B. Operated										
0–19 Years	2	1.5	<1	1	1	2	2	2	2	2
20–34	13	4.3	6	2	3	4	5	6	11	11
35–49	44	4.6	41	1	3	3	4	5	12	42
50–64	68	3.4	6	1	2	3	4	5	6	19
65+	69	4.3	11	2	3	3	4	6	12	21
SUBTOTALS:										
1. SINGLE DX										
A. Not Operated	0									
B. Operated	3	2.0	<1	1	1	2	3	3	3	3
2. MULTIPLE DX										
A. Not Operated	38	3.6	7	1	1	3	5	7	10	11
B. Operated	196	4.0	16	2	2	3	4	6	10	21
1. SINGLE DX	3	2.0	<1	1	1	2	3	3	3	3
2. MULTIPLE DX	234	3.9	14	2	3	3	4	6	10	19
A. NOT OPERATED	38	3.6	7	1	1	3	5	7	10	11
B. OPERATED	199	4.0	16	2	2	3	4	6	10	21
TOTAL										
0–19 Years	3	2.3	2	1	1	2	4	4	4	4
20–34	22	3.8	6	2	2	4	5	6	9	11
35–49	54	4.1	35	2	3	3	4	7	12	42
50–64	75	3.5	7	2	3	3	4	6	7	19
65+	83	4.3	11	3	3	3	5	7	10	21
GRAND TOTAL	237	3.9	14	2	3	3	4	6	10	19

733.6: TIETZE'S DISEASE

Type of Patients	Observed Patients	Avg. Stay	Variance	10th	25th	50th	75th	90th	95th	99th
1. SINGLE DX										
A. Not Operated										
0–19 Years	6	1.0	0	1	1	1	1	1	1	1
20–34	5	1.0	0	1	1	1	1	1	1	1
35–49	24	1.1	<1	1	1	1	1	1	2	2
50–64	13	1.4	<1	1	1	1	2	2	2	2
65+	5	1.0	0	1	1	1	1	1	1	1
B. Operated										
0–19 Years	0									
20–34	0									
35–49	0									
50–64	0									
65+	0									
2. MULTIPLE DX										
A. Not Operated										
0–19 Years	20	1.8	1	1	1	1	2	3	4	4
20–34	150	2.0	7	1	1	1	2	4	5	10
35–49	605	1.8	1	1	1	1	2	3	4	6
50–64	853	1.9	2	1	1	1	2	4	4	7
65+	855	2.2	5	1	1	2	3	4	5	10
B. Operated										
0–19 Years	0									
20–34	0									
35–49	2	3.5	<1	3	3	4	4	4	4	4
50–64	4	10.0	58	2	5	16	17	17	17	17
65+	6	12.0	130	1	3	9	21	30	30	30
SUBTOTALS:										
1. SINGLE DX										
A. Not Operated	53	1.1	<1	1	1	1	1	2	2	2
B. Operated	0									
2. MULTIPLE DX										
A. Not Operated	2,483	2.0	3	1	1	1	2	4	5	8
B. Operated	12	9.9	85	2	3	5	16	21	30	30
1. SINGLE DX	53	1.1	<1	1	1	1	1	2	2	2
2. MULTIPLE DX	2,495	2.0	4	1	1	1	2	4	5	9
A. NOT OPERATED	2,536	2.0	3	1	1	1	2	4	5	8
B. OPERATED	12	9.9	85	2	3	5	16	21	30	30
TOTAL										
0–19 Years	26	1.6	<1	1	1	1	2	3	4	4
20–34	155	2.0	6	1	1	1	2	4	5	10
35–49	631	1.8	1	1	1	1	2	3	4	6
50–64	870	1.9	2	1	1	1	2	4	5	7
65+	866	2.3	7	1	1	2	3	4	5	11
GRAND TOTAL	2,548	2.0	4	1	1	1	2	4	5	8

733.81: FRACTURE MALUNION

Type of Patients	Observed Patients	Avg. Stay	Variance	10th	25th	50th	75th	90th	95th	99th
1. SINGLE DX										
A. Not Operated										
0–19 Years	0									
20–34	0									
35–49	0									
50–64	2	1.5	<1	1	1	2	2	2	2	2
65+	1	1.0	0	1	1	1	1	1	1	1
B. Operated										
0–19 Years	18	1.8	2	1	1	2	2	4	7	7
20–34	23	1.9	2	1	1	2	2	3	3	8
35–49	21	1.9	2	1	1	2	2	3	3	7
50–64	14	2.0	2	1	1	3	3	4	4	4
65+	3	2.7	<1	2	2	3	3	3	3	3
2. MULTIPLE DX										
A. Not Operated										
0–19 Years	1	1.0	0	1	1	1	1	1	1	1
20–34	3	3.3	16	1	1	1	8	8	8	8
35–49	3	1.7	<1	1	1	2	2	2	2	2
50–64	10	2.9	16	1	1	2	2	14	14	14
65+	12	3.6	16	1	1	2	3	7	15	15
B. Operated										
0–19 Years	69	1.6	<1	1	1	1	1	3	4	5
20–34	120	3.4	53	1	1	2	3	7	11	15
35–49	226	3.1	15	1	1	2	3	5	8	19
50–64	279	2.9	6	1	1	2	4	5	8	15
65+	247	3.6	8	2	2	3	4	7	9	15
SUBTOTALS:										
1. SINGLE DX										
A. Not Operated	3	1.3	<1	1	1	1	2	2	2	2
B. Operated	79	1.9	2	1	1	2	2	3	4	8
2. MULTIPLE DX										
A. Not Operated	29	3.0	13	1	1	1	3	8	14	15
B. Operated	941	3.1	14	1	1	2	4	6	8	16
1. SINGLE DX	82	1.9	2	1	1	1	2	3	4	8
2. MULTIPLE DX	970	3.1	14	1	1	2	4	6	8	16
A. NOT OPERATED	32	2.9	12	1	1	1	3	7	14	15
B. OPERATED	1,020	3.0	14	1	1	2	3	5	8	15
TOTAL										
0–19 Years	88	1.7	1	1	1	1	2	3	4	7
20–34	146	3.2	44	1	1	2	3	6	8	15
35–49	250	2.9	14	1	1	2	3	5	7	19
50–64	305	2.9	6	1	1	3	3	5	7	15
65+	263	3.5	8	2	2	3	4	7	9	15
GRAND TOTAL	1,052	3.0	14	1	1	2	3	5	8	15

Western Region, October 2006–September 2007 Data, by Diagnosis

733.82: FRACTURE NONUNION

Type of Patients	Observed Patients	Avg. Stay	Vari-ance	10th	25th	50th	75th	90th	95th	99th
1. SINGLE DX										
A. Not Operated										
0–19 Years	0									
20–34	1	5.0	0	5	5	5	5	5	5	5
35–49	1	2.0	0	2	2	2	2	2	2	2
50–64	0									
65+	1	3.0	0	3	3	3	3	3	3	3
B. Operated										
0–19 Years	18	1.9	1	1	1	1	3	3	4	4
20–34	83	1.7	<1	1	1	1	2	3	3	4
35–49	95	2.0	2	1	1	2	2	4	5	4
50–64	62	2.3	2	1	1	2	3	4	6	8
65+	16	2.3	2	1	2	2	3	5	6	6
2. MULTIPLE DX										
A. Not Operated										
0–19 Years	3	1.7	1	1	1	1	3	3	3	3
20–34	6	2.3	1	1	1	2	3	4	4	4
35–49	12	2.8	3	1	2	3	3	6	6	6
50–64	32	4.5	17	1	1	3	6	11	15	17
65+	50	3.8	6	1	2	3	5	7	8	12
B. Operated										
0–19 Years	111	2.7	9	1	1	2	3	5	8	16
20–34	439	2.5	9	1	1	2	3	5	7	16
35–49	720	3.3	22	1	1	2	3	6	8	19
50–64	1,010	3.1	9	1	2	2	4	5	7	15
65+	1,081	4.0	11	1	2	3	5	7	10	16
SUBTOTALS:										
1. SINGLE DX										
A. Not Operated	3	3.3	2	2	2	3	3	5	5	5
B. Operated	274	2.0	2	1	1	2	2	4	4	6
2. MULTIPLE DX										
A. Not Operated	103	3.7	9	1	2	3	5	7	8	15
B. Operated	3,361	3.4	12	1	2	3	4	6	10	16
1. SINGLE DX	277	2.0	2	1	1	2	3	4	4	6
2. MULTIPLE DX	3,464	3.4	12	1	2	3	4	6	8	16
A. NOT OPERATED	106	3.7	9	1	2	3	5	7	8	15
B. OPERATED	3,635	3.3	12	1	1	3	4	6	8	16
TOTAL										
0–19 Years	132	2.6	8	1	1	2	3	4	5	16
20–34	529	2.4	8	1	1	2	3	4	6	13
35–49	828	3.1	19	1	1	2	3	6	7	17
50–64	1,104	3.1	9	1	1	2	4	5	7	15
65+	1,148	4.0	11	1	2	3	5	7	9	16
GRAND TOTAL	3,741	3.3	12	1	1	3	4	6	8	16

733.90: DISORDER BONE & CART NOS

Type of Patients	Observed Patients	Avg. Stay	Vari-ance	10th	25th	50th	75th	90th	95th	99th
1. SINGLE DX										
A. Not Operated										
0–19 Years	3	2.7	4	1	1	2	5	5	5	5
20–34	0									
35–49	1	2.0	0	2	2	2	2	2	2	2
50–64	0									
65+	0									
B. Operated										
0–19 Years	6	2.0	2	1	1	1	3	4	4	4
20–34	5	2.0	2	1	1	2	3	4	4	4
35–49	2	2.0	0	2	2	2	2	2	2	2
50–64	8	1.3	<1	1	1	1	2	2	1	1
65+	1	1.0	0	1	1	1	1	1	1	1
2. MULTIPLE DX										
A. Not Operated										
0–19 Years	6	1.7	<1	1	1	2	2	2	2	2
20–34	10	2.1	1	1	1	2	3	4	4	4
35–49	14	2.8	3	1	1	2	5	5	6	6
50–64	19	3.4	10	1	2	2	4	8	14	14
65+	43	3.6	12	1	2	3	4	6	11	19
B. Operated										
0–19 Years	4	2.7	2	1	1	3	3	4	4	4
20–34	14	1.9	1	1	1	2	2	2	5	5
35–49	24	2.2	6	1	1	1	2	3	7	12
50–64	38	3.4	19	1	1	2	4	7	20	20
65+	32	4.0	19	1	1	3	5	9	15	20
SUBTOTALS:										
1. SINGLE DX										
A. Not Operated	4	2.5	3	1	1	2	2	5	5	5
B. Operated	22	1.6	1	1	1	2	2	3	4	4
2. MULTIPLE DX										
A. Not Operated	92	3.2	9	1	1	2	4	6	8	19
B. Operated	112	3.1	14	1	1	2	3	7	10	20
1. SINGLE DX	26	1.7	1	1	1	2	2	4	4	5
2. MULTIPLE DX	204	3.1	11	1	1	2	4	6	9	20
A. NOT OPERATED	96	3.1	8	1	1	2	4	6	8	19
B. OPERATED	134	2.9	12	1	1	2	3	6	9	20
TOTAL										
0–19 Years	19	2.2	1	1	1	2	3	4	5	5
20–34	29	2.0	1	1	1	2	3	3	4	5
35–49	41	2.4	5	1	1	2	3	6	6	12
50–64	65	3.2	14	1	1	2	4	5	8	20
65+	76	3.7	15	1	1	3	4	7	13	20
GRAND TOTAL	230	3.0	10	1	1	2	3	6	8	20

733.95: STRESS FX-BONE NEC

Type of Patients	Observed Patients	Avg. Stay	Vari-ance	10th	25th	50th	75th	90th	95th	99th
1. SINGLE DX										
A. Not Operated										
0–19 Years	0									
20–34	0									
35–49	0									
50–64	0									
65+	0									
B. Operated										
0–19 Years	1	2.0	0	2	2	2	2	2	2	2
20–34	5	1.4	<1	1	1	1	1	2	2	2
35–49	3	2.0	<1	1	1	2	3	3	3	3
50–64	0									
65+	3	2.3	<1	2	2	2	3	3	3	3
2. MULTIPLE DX										
A. Not Operated										
0–19 Years	0									
20–34	1	13.0	0	13	13	13	13	13	13	13
35–49	6	8.8	264	1	3	3	3	42	42	42
50–64	6	6.0	18	2	3	5	6	14	14	14
65+	80	4.4	6	2	3	4	6	8	9	12
B. Operated										
0–19 Years	2	3.5	4	2	2	2	4	5	5	5
20–34	8	3.5	14	1	1	1	4	12	12	12
35–49	14	4.7	16	1	2	4	6	11	15	15
50–64	46	3.6	12	1	3	3	4	6	8	20
65+	88	5.4	25	2	3	4	6	8	10	42
SUBTOTALS:										
1. SINGLE DX										
A. Not Operated	0									
B. Operated	12	1.8	<1	1	1	2	2	3	3	3
2. MULTIPLE DX										
A. Not Operated	93	4.9	22	2	3	4	6	8	12	42
B. Operated	158	4.7	20	1	2	4	4	6	12	20
1. SINGLE DX	12	1.8	<1	1	1	2	2	2	3	3
2. MULTIPLE DX	251	4.7	21	2	3	4	6	8	12	20
A. NOT OPERATED	93	4.9	22	2	3	4	6	8	12	42
B. OPERATED	170	4.5	19	1	2	3	4	6	11	20
TOTAL										
0–19 Years	3	3.0	3	2	2	2	5	5	5	5
20–34	14	3.5	16	1	1	3	4	12	13	13
35–49	23	5.4	75	1	2	3	6	11	15	42
50–64	52	3.9	13	2	3	4	5	8	14	20
65+	171	4.9	16	2	3	4	6	8	9	20
GRAND TOTAL	263	4.6	20	1	2	3	6	8	11	20

Length of Stay by Diagnosis and Operation, Western Region, 2008

Western Region, October 2006–September 2007 Data, by Diagnosis

734: FLAT FOOT

Type of Patients	Observed Patients	Avg. Stay	Vari-ance	10th	25th	50th	75th	90th	95th	99th
1. SINGLE DX										
A. Not Operated										
0–19 Years	0									
20–34	0									
35–49	0									
50–64	0									
65+	0									
B. Operated										
0–19 Years	7	1.6	<1	1	1	1	2			3
20–34	0									
35–49	3	2.7	<1	2	2	3	3	3	3	3
50–64	1	2.0	0	2	2	2	2	2	2	2
65+	1	3.0	0	3	3	3	3	3	3	3
2. MULTIPLE DX										
A. Not Operated										
0–19 Years	0									
20–34	0									
35–49	0									
50–64	0									
65+	4	1.8	<1	1	1	1	3	3	3	3
B. Operated										
0–19 Years	16	2.8	6	1	1	2	2	4	11	11
20–34	24	2.0	<1	1	1	2	3	3	4	4
35–49	32	1.9	2	1	1	1	2	3	5	6
50–64	119	2.4	2	1	1	2	3	4	5	8
65+	92	2.7	2	1	2	3	3	4	5	7
SUBTOTALS:										
1. SINGLE DX										
A. Not Operated	0									
B. Operated	12	2.0	<1	1	1	2	3	3	3	3
2. MULTIPLE DX										
A. Not Operated	4	1.8	<1	1	1	1	3	3	3	3
B. Operated	283	2.4	2	1	1	2	3	3	5	8
1. SINGLE DX	12	2.0	<1	1	1	2	3	3	3	3
2. MULTIPLE DX	287	2.4	2	1	1	2	3	4	5	8
A. NOT OPERATED	4	1.8	<1	1	1	1	3	3	3	3
B. OPERATED	295	2.4	2	1	1	2	3	4	5	8
TOTAL										
0–19 Years	23	2.4	5	1	1	2	3	4	4	11
20–34	24	2.0	<1	1	1	2	3	3	4	4
35–49	35	2.0	2	1	1	2	3	3	5	6
50–64	120	2.4	2	1	1	2	3	4	5	8
65+	97	2.6	2	2	2	3	3	4	5	7
GRAND TOTAL	299	2.4	2	1	1	2	3	4	5	7

735: ACQ DEFORMITIES OF TOE

Type of Patients	Observed Patients	Avg. Stay	Vari-ance	10th	25th	50th	75th	90th	95th	99th
1. SINGLE DX										
A. Not Operated										
0–19 Years	0									
20–34	0									
35–49	0									
50–64	0									
65+	0									
B. Operated										
0–19 Years	0									
20–34	1	1.0	0	1	1	1	1	1	1	1
35–49	3	1.0	0	1	1	1	1	1	1	1
50–64	2	1.0	0	1	1	1	1	1	1	1
65+	2	3.0	2	2	2	2	4	4	4	4
2. MULTIPLE DX										
A. Not Operated										
0–19 Years	0									
20–34	2	1.0	0	1	1	1	1	1	1	1
35–49	1	1.0	0	1	1	1	1	1	1	1
50–64	0									
65+	0									
B. Operated										
0–19 Years	6	2.0	0	2	2	2	2	2	2	2
20–34	9	2.1	<1	1	1	2	2	3	4	4
35–49	39	1.9	1	1	1	2	2	3	3	6
50–64	107	1.9	1	1	1	2	3	3	4	5
65+	112	2.4	3	2	2	2	3	4	5	9
SUBTOTALS:										
1. SINGLE DX										
A. Not Operated	0									
B. Operated	8	1.5	1	1	1	2	1	4	4	4
2. MULTIPLE DX										
A. Not Operated	3	1.0	0	1	1	1	1	1	1	1
B. Operated	273	2.1	2	1	1	2	3	4	4	9
1. SINGLE DX	8	1.5	1	1	1	2	1	4	4	4
2. MULTIPLE DX	276	2.1	2	1	1	2	3	4	4	9
A. NOT OPERATED	3	1.0	0	1	1	1	1	1	1	1
B. OPERATED	281	2.1	2	1	1	2	3	4	4	9
TOTAL										
0–19 Years	6	2.0	0	2	2	2	2	2	2	2
20–34	12	1.8	<1	1	1	2	2	3	4	4
35–49	43	1.8	1	1	1	2	2	3	4	6
50–64	109	1.9	1	1	1	2	3	3	4	5
65+	114	2.4	3	2	1	2	3	4	5	9
GRAND TOTAL	284	2.1	2	1	1	2	3	4	4	9

736: OTH ACQ LIMB DEFORMITIES

Type of Patients	Observed Patients	Avg. Stay	Vari-ance	10th	25th	50th	75th	90th	95th	99th
1. SINGLE DX										
A. Not Operated										
0–19 Years	0									
20–34	1	2.0	0	2	2	2	2	2	2	2
35–49	2	1.0	0	1	1	1	1	1	1	1
50–64	2	3.0	2	2	2	3	4	4	4	4
65+	0									
B. Operated										
0–19 Years	34	1.7	<1	1	1	2	2	3	3	4
20–34	9	2.3	2	1	2	2	2	6	6	6
35–49	5	2.2	3	1	1	2	2	5	5	5
50–64	12	3.0	1	1	2	3	4	4	5	5
65+	1	1.0	0	1	1	1	1	1	1	1
2. MULTIPLE DX										
A. Not Operated										
0–19 Years	4	1.8	2	1	1	3	4	4	4	4
20–34	6	2.8	3	1	1	3	4	5	5	5
35–49	21	3.4	7	1	1	3	4	8	9	9
50–64	27	3.0	7	1	1	2	4	7	7	12
65+	37	3.3	8	1	1	3	4	7	8	15
B. Operated										
0–19 Years	187	2.3	11	2	2	2	3	4	5	10
20–34	126	3.2	8	1	2	3	4	6	7	12
35–49	185	3.4	8	1	2	3	4	6	8	16
50–64	379	3.7	8	1	2	3	4	6	9	14
65+	415	4.2	8	2	3	3	5	7	9	15
SUBTOTALS:										
1. SINGLE DX										
A. Not Operated	5	2.0	1	1	1	2	2	4	4	4
B. Operated	61	2.1	1	1	1	2	3	4	4	6
2. MULTIPLE DX										
A. Not Operated	95	3.1	7	1	1	2	4	7	8	15
B. Operated	1,292	3.5	9	2	2	3	4	6	8	15
1. SINGLE DX	66	2.1	1	1	1	2	3	4	4	6
2. MULTIPLE DX	1,387	3.5	9	1	2	3	4	6	8	15
A. NOT OPERATED	100	3.1	7	1	1	2	4	7	8	12
B. OPERATED	1,353	3.5	9	1	2	3	4	6	8	15
TOTAL										
0–19 Years	225	2.2	9	1	1	2	2	4	5	7
20–34	142	3.1	7	1	2	3	4	6	7	12
35–49	213	3.3	7	1	2	3	4	6	9	14
50–64	420	3.6	8	1	2	3	4	6	8	13
65+	453	4.1	8	2	3	3	5	7	9	15
GRAND TOTAL	1,453	3.5	9	1	2	3	4	6	8	15

Western Region, October 2006–September 2007 Data, by Diagnosis

736.6: ACQ KNEE DEFORMITY NEC

Type of Patients	Observed Patients	Avg. Stay	Variance	10th	25th	50th	75th	90th	95th	99th
1. SINGLE DX										
A. Not Operated										
0–19 Years	0									
20–34	0									
35–49	0									
50–64	0									
65+	0									
B. Operated										
0–19 Years	1	2.0	0		2	2	2	2		2
20–34	0									
35–49	0									
50–64	5	3.2	<1	2	3	3	4	4	4	4
65+	0									
2. MULTIPLE DX										
A. Not Operated										
0–19 Years	0									
20–34	0									
35–49	0									
50–64	1	1.0	0	1	1	1	1	1	1	1
65+	5	1.0	0	1	1	1	1	1	1	1
B. Operated										
0–19 Years	0									
20–34	3	4.0	1	3	3	4	5	5	5	5
35–49	24	4.3	9	2	2	3	5	8	9	14
50–64	117	4.5	6	3	3	4	5	8	10	13
65+	163	4.8	8	3	3	4	6	7	11	15
SUBTOTALS:										
1. SINGLE DX										
A. Not Operated	0									
B. Operated	6	3.0	<1	2	2	3	4	4	4	4
2. MULTIPLE DX										
A. Not Operated	6	1.0	0	1	1	1	1	1	1	1
B. Operated	307	4.6	7	3	3	4	5	8	11	15
1. SINGLE DX	6	3.0	<1	2	2	3	4	4	4	4
2. MULTIPLE DX	313	4.5	7	2	3	4	5	8	11	15
A. NOT OPERATED	6	1.0	0	1	1	1	1	1	1	1
B. OPERATED	313	4.6	7	3	3	4	5	8	11	15
TOTAL										
0–19 Years	1	2.0	0	2	2	2	2	2	2	2
20–34	3	4.0	1	3	3	4	5	5	5	5
35–49	24	4.3	9	2	2	3	5	8	9	14
50–64	123	4.4	6	3	3	4	5	8	10	13
65+	168	4.7	8	3	3	4	6	7	11	15
GRAND TOTAL	319	4.5	7	2	3	4	5	8	10	15

736.79: ACQ ANKLE-FOOT DEF NEC

Type of Patients	Observed Patients	Avg. Stay	Variance	10th	25th	50th	75th	90th	95th	99th
1. SINGLE DX										
A. Not Operated										
0–19 Years	0									
20–34	0									
35–49	2	1.0	0	1	1	1	1	1	1	1
50–64	2	3.0	2	2	2	3	4	4	4	4
65+	0									
B. Operated										
0–19 Years	5	2.2	2	1	1	2	3	4	4	4
20–34	2	1.5	<1	1	1	1	2	2	2	2
35–49	1	2.0	0	2	2	2	2	2	2	2
50–64	1	1.0	0	1	1	1	1	1	1	1
65+	0									
2. MULTIPLE DX										
A. Not Operated										
0–19 Years	2	2.5	4	1	1	1	4	4	4	4
20–34	2	4.0	2	3	3	5	5	5	5	5
35–49	13	3.1	7	1	1	2	3	8	9	9
50–64	18	3.3	8	1	1	2	5	7	12	12
65+	21	3.8	4	2	2	3	4	7	7	8
B. Operated										
0–19 Years	32	1.8	2	1	1	1	2	3	4	7
20–34	25	2.5	3	1	2	2	3	5	7	8
35–49	39	2.9	8	1	1	2	3	6	9	16
50–64	62	2.8	6	1	2	2	3	4	7	18
65+	69	2.5	2	2	2	2	3	4	5	6
SUBTOTALS:										
1. SINGLE DX										
A. Not Operated	4	2.0	2	1	1	1	2	4	4	4
B. Operated	9	1.9	1	1	1	2	2	4	4	4
2. MULTIPLE DX										
A. Not Operated	56	3.4	6	1	2	3	4	7	8	12
B. Operated	227	2.6	4	1	1	2	3	4	6	9
1. SINGLE DX	13	1.9	1	1	1	2	2	4	4	4
2. MULTIPLE DX	283	2.7	5	1	1	2	3	5	7	12
A. NOT OPERATED	60	3.3	6	1	1	3	4	7	8	12
B. OPERATED	236	2.5	4	1	1	2	3	4	6	9
TOTAL										
0–19 Years	39	1.9	2	1	1	1	2	4	4	7
20–34	29	2.6	3	1	2	2	3	5	7	8
35–49	55	2.9	7	1	1	2	3	6	9	16
50–64	83	2.9	6	1	1	2	3	5	7	18
65+	90	2.8	2	2	2	3	3	5	6	8
GRAND TOTAL	296	2.7	4	1	1	2	3	5	7	12

737: CURVATURE OF SPINE

Type of Patients	Observed Patients	Avg. Stay	Variance	10th	25th	50th	75th	90th	95th	99th
1. SINGLE DX										
A. Not Operated										
0–19 Years	2	1.0	0	1	1	1	1	1	1	1
20–34	0									
35–49	0									
50–64	0									
65+	0									
B. Operated										
0–19 Years	139	4.7	2	3	4	5	5	6	7	9
20–34	27	5.1	3	4	4	5	6	6	6	12
35–49	3	8.3	30	3	3	8	14	14	14	14
50–64	4	3.8	5	1	3	5	5	6	6	6
65+	1	3.0	0	3	3	3	3	3	3	3
2. MULTIPLE DX										
A. Not Operated										
0–19 Years	10	1.6	2	1	1	1	1	2	6	6
20–34	5	2.2	2	1	1	2	3	4	4	4
35–49	5	2.0	3	1	1	1	2	5	5	5
50–64	11	3.6	9	1	1	3	7	7	10	10
65+	52	3.9	6	1	2	3	6	7	8	12
B. Operated										
0–19 Years	330	6.0	11	4	4	5	7	8	10	23
20–34	94	6.3	14	3	4	5	7	10	13	25
35–49	119	7.4	76	3	4	6	8	12	14	54
50–64	471	7.1	20	3	4	6	9	13	16	22
65+	585	6.8	27	3	4	6	8	11	15	28
SUBTOTALS:										
1. SINGLE DX										
A. Not Operated	2	1.0	0	1	1	1	1	1	1	1
B. Operated	174	4.8	3	3	4	5	5	6	7	12
2. MULTIPLE DX										
A. Not Operated	83	3.4	6	1	1	3	5	7	7	12
B. Operated	1,599	6.7	25	3	4	6	8	11	15	25
1. SINGLE DX	176	4.8	3	3	4	5	5	6	7	12
2. MULTIPLE DX	1,682	6.6	24	3	4	6	8	11	14	25
A. NOT OPERATED	85	3.3	6	1	1	3	5	7	7	12
B. OPERATED	1,773	6.5	23	3	4	5	8	11	14	25
TOTAL										
0–19 Years	481	5.5	9	3	4	5	6	8	9	23
20–34	126	5.9	12	3	4	5	6	9	12	20
35–49	127	7.2	73	2	4	5	8	12	14	54
50–64	486	7.0	20	3	4	6	9	13	16	22
65+	638	6.6	26	3	4	6	8	11	14	26
GRAND TOTAL	1,858	6.4	22	3	4	5	7	11	14	24

Length of Stay by Diagnosis and Operation, Western Region, 2008

737.30: IDIOPATHIC SCOLIOSIS

Type of Patients	Observed Patients	Avg. Stay	Variance	10th	25th	50th	75th	90th	95th	99th
1. SINGLE DX										
A. Not Operated										
0–19 Years	0									
20–34	0									
35–49	0									
50–64	0									
65+	0									
B. Operated										
0–19 Years	114	4.8	2	3	4	4	5	6	7	9
20–34	21	5.4	3	4	3	5	6	6	7	12
35–49	3	8.3	30	3	3	8	14	14	14	14
50–64	1	3.0	0	3	3	3	3	3	3	3
65+	1	3.0	0	3	3	3	3	3	3	3
2. MULTIPLE DX										
A. Not Operated										
0–19 Years	6	1.8	4	1	1	1	1	6	6	6
20–34	3	1.3	<1	1	1	1	2	2	2	2
35–49	3	1.3	<1	1	1	1	2	2	2	2
50–64	6	2.2	<1	1	1	2	3	3	3	3
65+	30	3.9	5	1	2	3	6	7	8	9
B. Operated										
0–19 Years	213	5.8	6	4	4	5	6	8	9	15
20–34	59	6.1	7	4	5	6	7	8	10	20
35–49	55	7.6	49	4	4	6	8	11	14	54
50–64	232	7.4	21	3	4	7	9	14	16	25
65+	312	6.5	22	3	4	5	8	11	14	25
SUBTOTALS:										
1. SINGLE DX										
A. Not Operated	0									
B. Operated	140	4.9	3	3	4	5	5	6	7	12
2. MULTIPLE DX										
A. Not Operated	48	3.1	5	1	1	2	4	6	7	9
B. Operated	871	6.6	19	4	4	6	8	11	14	25
1. SINGLE DX	140	4.9	3	3	4	5	5	6	7	12
2. MULTIPLE DX	919	6.4	19	3	4	5	8	10	14	24
A. NOT OPERATED	48	3.1	5	1	1	2	4	6	7	9
B. OPERATED	1,011	6.4	17	3	4	5	7	10	13	24
TOTAL										
0–19 Years	333	5.3	5	4	4	5	6	7	8	14
20–34	83	5.8	7	4	4	5	6	9	9	20
35–49	61	7.3	47	3	4	6	8	11	14	54
50–64	239	7.3	21	3	4	7	9	14	16	25
65+	343	6.3	21	2	3	5	8	11	14	25
GRAND TOTAL	1,059	6.2	17	3	4	5	7	10	13	24

737.39: SCOLIOSIS NEC

Type of Patients	Observed Patients	Avg. Stay	Variance	10th	25th	50th	75th	90th	95th	99th
1. SINGLE DX										
A. Not Operated										
0–19 Years	0									
20–34	0									
35–49	0									
50–64	0									
65+	0									
B. Operated										
0–19 Years	7	4.0	2	3	3	3	5	6	7	7
20–34	1	1.0	0	1	1	1	1	1	1	1
35–49	0									
50–64	0									
65+	0									
2. MULTIPLE DX										
A. Not Operated										
0–19 Years	1	1.0	0	1	1	1	1	1	1	1
20–34	1	3.0	0	3	3	3	3	3	3	3
35–49	1	5.0	0	5	5	5	5	5	5	5
50–64	3	6.0	21	1	1	7	10	10	10	10
65+	10	4.9	10	3	3	4	7	12	12	12
B. Operated										
0–19 Years	56	7.4	30	4	5	6	8	13	22	35
20–34	9	5.4	10	4	4	4	7	13	13	13
35–49	14	4.6	5	3	3	5	5	7	9	9
50–64	124	6.5	16	2	4	6	8	13	14	18
65+	187	6.6	33	3	4	5	8	11	14	46
SUBTOTALS:										
1. SINGLE DX										
A. Not Operated	0									
B. Operated	8	3.6	3	3	3	3	4	7	7	7
2. MULTIPLE DX										
A. Not Operated	16	4.8	11	1	2	4	7	10	12	25
B. Operated	390	6.6	26	3	4	5	8	11	14	25
1. SINGLE DX	8	3.6	3	3	3	3	4	7	7	7
2. MULTIPLE DX	406	6.5	25	3	4	5	8	11	14	23
A. NOT OPERATED	16	4.8	11	1	2	4	7	10	12	25
B. OPERATED	398	6.5	25	3	4	5	8	11	14	25
TOTAL										
0–19 Years	64	6.9	28	3	4	5	7	11	16	35
20–34	11	4.8	10	3	3	4	7	7	13	13
35–49	15	4.6	5	1	3	5	5	7	9	9
50–64	127	6.5	16	2	4	6	8	13	14	18
65+	197	6.5	32	3	4	5	8	11	14	46
GRAND TOTAL	414	6.5	25	3	4	5	8	11	14	23

738: OTHER ACQUIRED DEFORMITY

Type of Patients	Observed Patients	Avg. Stay	Variance	10th	25th	50th	75th	90th	95th	99th
1. SINGLE DX										
A. Not Operated										
0–19 Years	0									
20–34	0									
35–49	1	1.0	0	1	1	1	1	1	1	1
50–64	2	2.0	2	1	1	2	3	3	3	3
65+	1	1.0	0	1	1	1	1	1	1	1
B. Operated										
0–19 Years	32	2.1	2	1	1	2	3	4	5	5
20–34	50	2.4	2	1	1	2	3	5	6	6
35–49	72	3.3	8	1	2	3	4	5	6	23
50–64	61	3.1	3	1	2	3	4	5	6	8
65+	16	3.1	3	1	2	3	4	6	6	6
2. MULTIPLE DX										
A. Not Operated										
0–19 Years	6	4.2	7	1	2	4	6	8	8	8
20–34	12	3.2	8	1	1	2	5	6	10	10
35–49	19	3.9	26	1	1	2	4	13	22	22
50–64	47	2.4	4	1	1	2	3	5	7	9
65+	95	4.3	11	1	2	4	5	8	12	17
B. Operated										
0–19 Years	119	3.3	6	1	1	3	4	6	8	12
20–34	389	3.3	6	1	2	3	4	6	8	13
35–49	857	4.0	13	1	2	3	5	6	8	16
50–64	2,179	4.0	8	2	2	3	5	6	8	14
65+	2,263	4.2	9	1	3	4	5	7	8	16
SUBTOTALS:										
1. SINGLE DX										
A. Not Operated	4	1.5	<1	1	1	1	1	3	3	3
B. Operated	231	2.9	4	1	2	3	4	5	6	8
2. MULTIPLE DX										
A. Not Operated	179	3.7	11	1	1	3	5	7	10	17
B. Operated	5,807	4.0	9	2	2	4	5	7	8	15
1. SINGLE DX	235	2.8	4	1	1	2	4	5	6	8
2. MULTIPLE DX	5,986	4.0	9	1	2	4	5	7	8	15
A. NOT OPERATED	183	3.6	11	1	1	3	5	7	10	17
B. OPERATED	6,038	4.0	9	1	2	3	5	7	8	15
TOTAL										
0–19 Years	157	3.1	5	1	1	2	4	6	8	12
20–34	451	3.2	6	1	1	3	4	6	8	12
35–49	949	3.9	13	2	2	3	5	6	8	16
50–64	2,289	3.9	8	2	3	3	5	6	8	14
65+	2,375	4.2	9	1	3	4	5	7	8	16
GRAND TOTAL	6,221	4.0	9	1	2	3	5	7	8	15

Length of Stay by Diagnosis and Operation, Western Region, 2008

Western Region, October 2006–September 2007 Data, by Diagnosis

738.19: OTH ACQ HEAD DEFORMITY

Type of Patients	Observed Patients	Avg. Stay	Vari-ance	Percentiles						
				10th	25th	50th	75th	90th	95th	99th
1. SINGLE DX										
A. Not Operated										
0–19 Years	0									
20–34	0									
35–49	0									
50–64	1	1.0	0		1	1			1	1
65+	0									
B. Operated										
0–19 Years	16	1.9	1	1	1	2	2	4	5	5
20–34	25	1.7	1	1	1	1	2	3	3	6
35–49	13	3.1	36	1	1	1	2	3	23	23
50–64	12	2.5	4	1	1	2	5	6	6	6
65+	1	1.0	0	1	1	1	1	1	1	1
2. MULTIPLE DX										
A. Not Operated										
0–19 Years	3	3.0	4	1	1	3	5	5	5	5
20–34	1	2.0	0	2	2	2	2	2	2	2
35–49	3	8.7	134	1	1	3	22	22	22	22
50–64	2	2.0	2	1	1	2	3	3	3	3
65+	3	1.7	1	1	1	1	3	3	3	3
B. Operated										
0–19 Years	87	3.3	6	1	1	3	4	7	8	12
20–34	173	3.1	9	1	1	2	3	7	10	14
35–49	166	4.2	45	1	1	2	4	8	15	31
50–64	192	3.6	16	1	2	2	4	7	10	27
65+	72	3.4	18	1	1	2	4	7	8	32
SUBTOTALS:										
1. SINGLE DX										
A. Not Operated	1	1.0	0	1	1	1	1	1	1	1
B. Operated	67	2.2	8	1	1	1	2	4	6	23
2. MULTIPLE DX										
A. Not Operated	12	3.8	34	1	1	2	3	5	22	22
B. Operated	690	3.5	20	1	1	2	4	8	10	19
1. SINGLE DX	68	2.1	8	1	1	1	2	4	6	23
2. MULTIPLE DX	702	3.5	20	1	1	2	4	8	10	19
A. NOT OPERATED	13	3.6	32	1	1	2	3	5	22	22
B. OPERATED	757	3.4	19	1	1	2	4	7	10	19
TOTAL										
0–19 Years	106	3.0	6	1	1	2	4	6	8	12
20–34	199	2.9	8	1	1	2	3	7	10	14
35–49	182	4.2	45	1	1	2	4	8	15	31
50–64	207	3.5	15	1	1	2	4	7	9	19
65+	76	3.3	17	1	1	2	4	7	8	32
GRAND TOTAL	770	3.4	19	1	1	2	4	7	10	21

738.4: ACQ SPONDYLOLISTHESIS

Type of Patients	Observed Patients	Avg. Stay	Vari-ance	Percentiles						
				10th	25th	50th	75th	90th	95th	99th
1. SINGLE DX										
A. Not Operated										
0–19 Years	0									
20–34	0									
35–49	1	1.0	0	1	1	1	1	1	1	1
50–64	1	3.0	0	3	3	3	3	3	3	3
65+	1	1.0	0	1	1	1	1	1	1	1
B. Operated										
0–19 Years	2	3.0	2	2	2	2	4	4	4	4
20–34	17	3.5	3	3	3	3	4	6	6	6
35–49	51	3.5	3	2	2	3	4	5	6	9
50–64	48	3.3	2	2	2	3	4	5	6	8
65+	15	3.2	3	2	2	3	4	6	6	6
2. MULTIPLE DX										
A. Not Operated										
0–19 Years	2	7.0	2	6	6	6	8	8	8	8
20–34	8	3.6	10	1	2	2	6	10	10	10
35–49	14	3.1	9	1	2	2	3	4	13	13
50–64	41	2.6	4	1	1	2	3	5	7	9
65+	89	4.4	11	1	2	4	5	8	12	17
B. Operated										
0–19 Years	17	3.7	2	3	3	4	4	5	6	6
20–34	174	3.8	3	2	2	3	5	6	7	9
35–49	642	4.0	6	2	3	4	5	6	7	12
50–64	1,926	4.0	8	2	3	4	5	6	8	13
65+	2,150	4.2	9	1	3	4	5	7	8	16
SUBTOTALS:										
1. SINGLE DX										
A. Not Operated	3	1.7	1	1	1	1	3	3	3	3
B. Operated	133	3.4	2	2	2	3	4	5	6	8
2. MULTIPLE DX										
A. Not Operated	154	3.8	9	1	2	3	5	7	10	15
B. Operated	4,909	4.1	8	2	3	4	5	7	8	14
1. SINGLE DX	136	3.3	2	1	2	3	4	5	6	8
2. MULTIPLE DX	5,063	4.1	8	2	3	4	5	7	8	14
A. NOT OPERATED	157	3.7	9	1	2	3	5	7	10	15
B. OPERATED	5,042	4.1	8	2	3	4	5	7	8	14
TOTAL										
0–19 Years	21	4.0	3	2	3	4	4	6	6	8
20–34	199	3.8	3	2	3	4	5	6	7	10
35–49	708	3.9	5	2	3	4	5	6	7	12
50–64	2,016	4.0	7	2	3	4	5	6	8	13
65+	2,255	4.2	9	1	3	4	5	7	8	16
GRAND TOTAL	5,199	4.1	8	2	3	4	5	7	8	14

739: NONALLOPATHIC LESIONS

Type of Patients	Observed Patients	Avg. Stay	Vari-ance	Percentiles						
				10th	25th	50th	75th	90th	95th	99th
1. SINGLE DX										
A. Not Operated										
0–19 Years	0									
20–34	0									
35–49	0									
50–64	0									
65+	0									
B. Operated										
0–19 Years	1	1.0	0		1	1	1	1	1	1
20–34	0									
35–49	1	1.0	0	1	1	1	1	1	1	1
50–64	0									
65+	0									
2. MULTIPLE DX										
A. Not Operated										
0–19 Years	0									
20–34	1	3.0	0	3	3	3	3	3	3	3
35–49	2	2.0	0	2	2	2	2	2	2	2
50–64	1	1.0	0	1	1	1	1	1	1	1
65+	0									
B. Operated										
0–19 Years	0									
20–34	0									
35–49	1	3.0	0	3	3	3	3	3	3	3
50–64	0									
65+	1	2.0	0	2	2	2	2	2	2	2
SUBTOTALS:										
1. SINGLE DX										
A. Not Operated	0									
B. Operated	2	1.0	0	1	1	1	1	1	1	1
2. MULTIPLE DX										
A. Not Operated	4	2.0	<1	1	1	2	3	3	3	3
B. Operated	2	2.5	<1	2	2	3	3	3	3	3
1. SINGLE DX	2	1.0	0	1	1	1	1	1	1	1
2. MULTIPLE DX	6	2.2	<1	1	2	2	3	3	3	3
A. NOT OPERATED	4	2.0	<1	1	1	2	3	3	3	3
B. OPERATED	4	1.8	<1	1	1	2	3	3	3	3
TOTAL										
0–19 Years	1	1.0	0	1	1	1	1	1	1	1
20–34	1	3.0	0	3	3	3	3	3	3	3
35–49	4	2.0	<1	1	1	2	3	3	3	3
50–64	1	1.0	0	1	1	1	1	1	1	1
65+	1	2.0	0	2	2	2	2	2	2	2
GRAND TOTAL	8	1.9	<1	1	1	2	3	3	3	3

Length of Stay by Diagnosis and Operation, Western Region, 2008

Western Region, October 2006–September 2007 Data, by Diagnosis

740: ANENCEPHALUS ET AL

Type of Patients	Observed Patients	Avg. Stay	Variance	10th	25th	50th	75th	90th	95th	99th
1. SINGLE DX										
A. Not Operated										
0–19 Years	0									
20–34	0									
35–49	0									
50–64	0									
65+	0									
B. Operated										
0–19 Years	0									
20–34	0									
35–49	0									
50–64	0									
65+	0									
2. MULTIPLE DX										
A. Not Operated										
0–19 Years	0									
20–34	0									
35–49	0									
50–64	0									
65+	0									
B. Operated										
0–19 Years	0									
20–34	0									
35–49	0									
50–64	0									
65+	0									
SUBTOTALS:										
1. SINGLE DX										
A. Not Operated	0									
B. Operated	0									
2. MULTIPLE DX										
A. Not Operated	0									
B. Operated	0									
1. SINGLE DX	0									
2. MULTIPLE DX	0									
A. NOT OPERATED	0									
B. OPERATED	0									
TOTAL										
0–19 Years	0									
20–34	0									
35–49	0									
50–64	0									
65+	0									
GRAND TOTAL	0									

741: SPINA BIFIDA

Type of Patients	Observed Patients	Avg. Stay	Variance	10th	25th	50th	75th	90th	95th	99th
1. SINGLE DX										
A. Not Operated										
0–19 Years	0									
20–34	0									
35–49	0									
50–64	0									
65+	0									
B. Operated										
0–19 Years	9	2.5	4	1	1	2	2	7	7	7
20–34	3	3.0	3	1	1	3	3	4	4	4
35–49	3	2.3	1	1	1	3	3	3	3	3
50–64	1	4.0	0	4	4	4	4	4	4	4
65+	0									
2. MULTIPLE DX										
A. Not Operated										
0–19 Years	13	2.9	5	1	1	2	5	5	5	8
20–34	8	3.3	5	1	1	3	5	6	6	6
35–49	5	5.8	64	1	1	3	4	20	20	20
50–64	3	3.7	8	2	2	2	7	7	7	7
65+	0									
B. Operated										
0–19 Years	60	6.2	39	2	3	4	7	11	21	31
20–34	28	9.1	222	3	3	5	8	18	22	82
35–49	21	4.5	14	2	2	4	5	9	9	17
50–64	8	5.0	4	3	4	4	7	8	8	8
65+	1	16.0	0	16	16	16	16	16	16	16
SUBTOTALS:										
1. SINGLE DX										
A. Not Operated	0									
B. Operated	16	2.6	3	1	1	2	4	4	7	7
2. MULTIPLE DX										
A. Not Operated	29	3.6	14	1	1	3	5	7	8	20
B. Operated	118	6.6	77	2	3	4	7	11	21	31
1. SINGLE DX	16	2.6	3	1	1	2	4	4	7	7
2. MULTIPLE DX	147	6.0	66	2	2	4	7	10	18	31
A. NOT OPERATED	29	3.6	14	1	1	3	5	7	8	20
B. OPERATED	134	6.1	69	2	3	4	7	10	18	31
TOTAL										
0–19 Years	82	5.3	32	1	2	3	6	10	16	31
20–34	39	7.4	166	1	3	4	7	10	22	82
35–49	29	4.5	20	1	2	3	5	9	17	20
50–64	12	4.6	4	2	3	4	7	7	8	8
65+	1	16.0	0	16	16	16	16	16	16	16
GRAND TOTAL	163	5.7	60	1	2	4	6	10	17	31

742: OTH NERV SYST ANOMALIES

Type of Patients	Observed Patients	Avg. Stay	Variance	10th	25th	50th	75th	90th	95th	99th
1. SINGLE DX										
A. Not Operated										
0–19 Years	4	1.0	0	1	1	1	1	1	1	1
20–34	0									
35–49	1	1.0	0	1	1	1	1	1	1	1
50–64	0									
65+	0									
B. Operated										
0–19 Years	109	1.8	2	1	1	2	2	3	4	5
20–34	11	2.5	1	1	2	3	3	4	4	4
35–49	2	3.5	<1	3	3	4	4	4	4	4
50–64	8	3.0	3	1	2	2	4	7	7	7
65+	2	1.5	<1	1	1	2	2	2	2	2
2. MULTIPLE DX										
A. Not Operated										
0–19 Years	52	3.9	23	1	1	2	5	8	12	30
20–34	11	2.8	5	1	1	2	4	5	8	8
35–49	8	5.8	15	3	3	5	9	12	12	12
50–64	7	1.9	1	1	1	1	3	4	4	4
65+	8	4.5	5	2	3	3	6	8	8	8
B. Operated										
0–19 Years	276	2.9	11	1	1	2	3	6	9	18
20–34	49	5.4	16	2	3	4	7	10	10	22
35–49	67	5.6	35	1	2	4	6	12	18	39
50–64	80	5.5	37	1	3	4	6	14	14	48
65+	24	5.8	18	3	3	4	10	12	13	15
SUBTOTALS:										
1. SINGLE DX										
A. Not Operated	5	1.0	0	1	1	1	1	1	1	1
B. Operated	132	2.0	2	1	1	2	2	3	4	7
2. MULTIPLE DX										
A. Not Operated	86	3.8	17	1	1	2	5	8	9	30
B. Operated	496	4.1	21	1	1	3	5	9	13	22
1. SINGLE DX	137	2.0	2	1	1	2	2	3	4	7
2. MULTIPLE DX	582	4.1	20	1	1	3	5	9	12	22
A. NOT OPERATED	91	3.6	16	1	1	2	5	8	9	30
B. OPERATED	628	3.7	18	1	1	2	4	8	11	19
TOTAL										
0–19 Years	441	2.8	11	1	1	2	3	5	8	16
20–34	71	4.6	14	1	2	4	6	8	10	22
35–49	78	5.5	32	1	2	4	6	12	18	39
50–64	95	5.0	33	1	2	4	6	9	14	48
65+	34	5.2	15	3	3	4	7	12	13	15
GRAND TOTAL	719	3.7	17	1	1	2	4	8	11	19

Western Region, October 2006–September 2007 Data, by Diagnosis

742.59: OTH SPINAL CORD ANOMALY

Type of Patients	Observed Patients	Avg. Stay	Vari-ance	10th	25th	50th	75th	90th	95th	99th
1. SINGLE DX										
A. Not Operated										
0–19 Years	1	1.0	0	1	1	1	1	1	1	1
20–34	0									
35–49	0									
50–64	0									
65+	0									
B. Operated										
0–19 Years	83	1.8	3	1	1	1	2	3	4	14
20–34	4	2.5	2	1	1	2	3	4	4	4
35–49	1	4.0	0	4	4	4	4	4	4	4
50–64	4	2.5	2	1	2	2	3	4	4	4
65+	1	1.0	0	1	1	1	1	1	1	1
2. MULTIPLE DX										
A. Not Operated										
0–19 Years	7	1.0	0	1	1	1	1	1	1	1
20–34	0									
35–49	1	5.0	0	5	5	5	5	5	5	5
50–64	0									
65+	2	4.5	4	3	3	5	6	6	6	6
B. Operated										
0–19 Years	215	2.4	5	1	1	2	3	5	7	14
20–34	23	4.7	14	2	3	4	6	7	10	19
35–49	26	4.5	19	2	2	3	5	8	18	18
50–64	28	4.6	8	1	3	4	6	7	9	15
65+	3	5.3	<1	5	5	5	6	6	6	6
SUBTOTALS:										
1. SINGLE DX										
A. Not Operated	1	1.0	0	1	1	1	1	1	1	1
B. Operated	93	1.9	3	1	1	1	2	4	4	14
2. MULTIPLE DX										
A. Not Operated	10	2.1	4	1	1	1	3	6	6	6
B. Operated	295	3.0	8	1	1	2	4	6	7	18
1. SINGLE DX	94	1.9	3	1	1	1	2	4	4	14
2. MULTIPLE DX	305	3.0	8	1	1	2	4	6	7	18
A. NOT OPERATED	11	2.0	3	1	1	1	3	5	6	6
B. OPERATED	388	2.7	7	1	1	2	3	5	7	18
TOTAL										
0–19 Years	306	2.2	5	1	1	2	3	4	6	14
20–34	27	4.4	13	1	2	4	5	7	10	19
35–49	28	4.5	18	2	2	4	5	8	18	18
50–64	32	4.3	7	1	3	4	5	7	9	15
65+	6	4.3	4	1	3	5	6	6	6	6
GRAND TOTAL	399	2.7	7	1	1	2	3	5	7	15

743: CONGENITAL EYE ANOMALY

Type of Patients	Observed Patients	Avg. Stay	Vari-ance	10th	25th	50th	75th	90th	95th	99th
1. SINGLE DX										
A. Not Operated										
0–19 Years	2	2.0	0	2	2	2	2	2	2	2
20–34	0									
35–49	0									
50–64	0									
65+	0									
B. Operated										
0–19 Years	8	1.0	0	1	1	1	1	1	1	1
20–34	0									
35–49	1	2.0	0	2	2	2	2	2	2	2
50–64	0									
65+	0									
2. MULTIPLE DX										
A. Not Operated										
0–19 Years	4	4.0	11	2	2	2	3	9	9	9
20–34	0									
35–49	1	1.0	0	1	1	1	1	1	1	1
50–64	0									
65+	0									
B. Operated										
0–19 Years	20	3.3	40	1	1	1	2	3	15	27
20–34	0									
35–49	0									
50–64	0									
65+	0									
SUBTOTALS:										
1. SINGLE DX										
A. Not Operated	2	2.0	0	2	2	2	2	2	2	2
B. Operated	9	1.1	<1	1	1	1	1	2	2	2
2. MULTIPLE DX										
A. Not Operated	5	3.4	10	1	2	2	3	9	9	9
B. Operated	20	3.3	40	1	1	1	2	3	15	27
1. SINGLE DX	11	1.3	<1	1	1	1	2	2	2	2
2. MULTIPLE DX	25	3.4	34	1	1	1	2	9	15	27
A. NOT OPERATED	7	3.0	7	1	2	2	3	9	9	9
B. OPERATED	29	2.7	29	1	1	1	2	3	15	27
TOTAL										
0–19 Years	34	2.8	26	1	1	1	2	3	15	27
20–34	0									
35–49	2	1.5	<1	1	1	2	2	2	2	2
50–64	0									
65+	0									
GRAND TOTAL	36	2.7	24	1	1	1	2	3	15	27

744: CONG ANOMAL EAR/FACE/NK

Type of Patients	Observed Patients	Avg. Stay	Vari-ance	10th	25th	50th	75th	90th	95th	99th
1. SINGLE DX										
A. Not Operated										
0–19 Years	5	1.6	<1	1	1	1	2	3	3	3
20–34	3	3.3	1	2	2	4	4	4	4	4
35–49	3	1.0	0	1	1	1	1	1	1	1
50–64	1	3.0	0	3	3	3	3	3	3	3
65+	0									
B. Operated										
0–19 Years	62	1.6	2	1	1	1	2	3	5	6
20–34	20	1.9	3	1	1	1	2	3	8	8
35–49	18	1.1	<1	1	1	1	1	2	2	2
50–64	7	1.1	<1	1	1	1	1	2	2	2
65+	0									
2. MULTIPLE DX										
A. Not Operated										
0–19 Years	10	2.6	4	1	1	2	3	7	7	7
20–34	8	2.9	4	1	2	2	3	7	7	7
35–49	1	2.0	0	2	2	2	2	2	2	2
50–64	3	1.7	<1	1	1	2	2	2	2	2
65+	0									
B. Operated										
0–19 Years	67	2.1	4	1	1	2	3	4	4	14
20–34	29	2.1	3	1	1	2	2	5	6	8
35–49	19	1.5	<1	1	1	1	2	3	4	4
50–64	12	1.8	1	1	1	2	3	3	4	4
65+	5	1.2	<1	1	1	1	1	2	2	2
SUBTOTALS:										
1. SINGLE DX										
A. Not Operated	12	2.0	1	1	1	2	3	4	4	4
B. Operated	107	1.6	2	1	1	1	2	3	5	6
2. MULTIPLE DX										
A. Not Operated	22	2.5	3	1	2	2	3	5	7	7
B. Operated	132	2.0	3	1	1	1	2	3	4	10
1. SINGLE DX	119	1.6	2	1	1	1	2	3	5	6
2. MULTIPLE DX	154	2.0	3	1	1	1	2	4	5	10
A. NOT OPERATED	34	2.4	2	1	1	2	3	4	7	7
B. OPERATED	239	1.8	2	1	1	1	2	3	5	8
TOTAL										
0–19 Years	144	1.9	3	1	1	1	2	3	5	10
20–34	60	2.2	3	1	1	2	2	5	7	8
35–49	41	1.3	<1	1	1	1	1	2	3	4
50–64	23	1.7	<1	1	1	1	2	3	3	4
65+	5	1.2	<1	1	1	1	1	2	2	2
GRAND TOTAL	273	1.9	2	1	1	1	2	3	5	8

Length of Stay by Diagnosis and Operation, Western Region, 2008

Western Region, October 2006–September 2007 Data, by Diagnosis

745: CARD SEPTAL CLOSE ANOMAL

Type of Patients	Observed Patients	Avg. Stay	Vari-ance	10th	25th	50th	75th	90th	95th	99th
1. SINGLE DX										
A. Not Operated										
0–19 Years	16	1.3	<1	1	1	1	1	2	3	3
20–34	2	2.5	4	1	1	1	4	4	4	4
35–49	0									
50–64	3	1.0	0	1	1	1	1	1	1	1
65+	0									
B. Operated										
0–19 Years	89	2.1	2	1	1	1	3	4	5	8
20–34	17	1.5	1	1	1	1	2	2	4	4
35–49	16	1.4	1	1	1	1	1	4	5	5
50–64	15	1.4	1	1	1	1	1	4	4	4
65+	8	1.0	0	1	1	1	1	1	1	1
2. MULTIPLE DX										
A. Not Operated										
0–19 Years	145	3.9	33	1	1	2	4	8	19	25
20–34	30	4.0	13	1	2	3	5	12	13	13
35–49	35	3.8	11	1	1	2	6	9	11	15
50–64	33	5.0	64	1	1	2	6	9	16	45
65+	21	3.7	7	1	2	2	6	8	9	9
B. Operated										
0–19 Years	737	7.3	65	2	3	5	8	15	22	45
20–34	113	4.2	34	1	1	3	5	9	13	16
35–49	195	2.9	9	1	1	1	4	6	7	19
50–64	229	2.5	11	1	1	1	2	7	9	17
65+	146	2.9	21	1	1	1	2	8	10	28
SUBTOTALS:										
1. SINGLE DX										
A. Not Operated	21	1.3	<1	1	1	1	1	2	3	4
B. Operated	145	1.8	2	1	1	1	2	4	4	4
2. MULTIPLE DX										
A. Not Operated	264	4.0	29	1	1	2	5	9	13	25
B. Operated	1,420	5.2	46	1	1	3	6	11	16	36
1. SINGLE DX	166	1.8	2	1	1	1	2	4	4	7
2. MULTIPLE DX	1,684	5.0	44	1	1	3	6	11	16	35
A. NOT OPERATED	285	3.8	28	1	1	2	4	9	13	25
B. OPERATED	1,565	4.9	43	1	1	3	6	11	16	35
TOTAL										
0–19 Years	987	6.2	57	1	2	4	7	14	20	44
20–34	162	3.8	26	1	1	3	5	9	13	16
35–49	246	2.9	9	1	1	1	4	6	8	16
50–64	280	2.7	17	1	1	1	3	7	9	21
65+	175	2.9	19	1	1	1	2	8	10	28
GRAND TOTAL	1,850	4.7	41	1	1	3	6	10	16	31

745.4: VENTRICULAR SEPT DEFECT

Type of Patients	Observed Patients	Avg. Stay	Vari-ance	10th	25th	50th	75th	90th	95th	99th
1. SINGLE DX										
A. Not Operated										
0–19 Years	5	1.2	<1	1	1	1	1	2	2	2
20–34	1	1.0	0	1	1	1	1	1	1	1
35–49	0									
50–64	0									
65+	0									
B. Operated										
0–19 Years	12	3.1	2	2	2	3	3	6	6	6
20–34	1	2.0	0	2	2	2	2	2	2	2
35–49	0									
50–64	0									
65+	0									
2. MULTIPLE DX										
A. Not Operated										
0–19 Years	48	5.2	46	1	1	3	5	13	23	31
20–34	4	5.0	29	2	2	3	13	13	13	13
35–49	8	5.9	22	2	2	3	13	15	15	15
50–64	2	9.0	97	2	2	9	16	16	16	16
65+	2	5.5	24	2	2	2	9	9	9	9
B. Operated										
0–19 Years	228	6.0	43	2	3	4	6	9	14	28
20–34	16	8.4	159	3	3	4	6	16	53	53
35–49	14	6.9	24	3	3	5	9	14	19	19
50–64	7	6.5	63	1	1	3	10	23	23	23
65+	0									
SUBTOTALS:										
1. SINGLE DX										
A. Not Operated	6	1.2	<1	1	1	1	1	2	2	2
B. Operated	13	3.0	2	2	2	3	3	6	6	6
2. MULTIPLE DX										
A. Not Operated	64	5.4	41	1	2	3	7	13	17	31
B. Operated	265	6.2	49	2	3	4	6	11	16	37
1. SINGLE DX	19	2.4	2	1	1	2	3	6	6	6
2. MULTIPLE DX	329	6.0	47	2	3	4	6	12	16	31
A. NOT OPERATED	70	5.0	39	1	1	2	5	13	17	31
B. OPERATED	278	6.0	47	2	3	4	6	11	16	37
TOTAL										
0–19 Years	293	5.6	42	2	3	4	6	10	14	31
20–34	22	7.1	123	2	3	3	6	13	16	53
35–49	22	6.5	22	2	3	5	9	14	15	19
50–64	9	7.0	61	1	2	3	10	23	23	23
65+	2	5.5	24	2	2	2	9	9	9	9
GRAND TOTAL	348	5.8	46	2	3	4	6	12	16	31

745.5: OSTIUM SECUNDUM TYPE ASD

Type of Patients	Observed Patients	Avg. Stay	Vari-ance	10th	25th	50th	75th	90th	95th	99th
1. SINGLE DX										
A. Not Operated										
0–19 Years	2	1.0	0	1	1	1	1	1	1	1
20–34	4	4.0	0	4	4	4	4	4	4	4
35–49	0									
50–64	3	1.0	0	1	1	1	1	1	1	1
65+	0									
B. Operated										
0–19 Years	67	1.6	<1	1	1	2	2	3	3	4
20–34	16	1.5	1	1	1	1	1	4	4	4
35–49	16	1.4	1	1	1	1	1	4	5	5
50–64	15	1.4	1	1	1	1	1	4	4	4
65+	7	1.0	0	1	1	1	1	1	1	1
2. MULTIPLE DX										
A. Not Operated										
0–19 Years	23	3.7	40	1	1	2	3	4	22	25
20–34	13	3.3	9	1	1	2	3	6	12	12
35–49	20	3.1	8	1	1	2	4	6	9	11
50–64	26	2.8	5	1	1	2	5	6	7	9
65+	18	3.6	7	1	1	3	6	8	9	9
B. Operated										
0–19 Years	129	4.5	42	1	1	3	4	8	13	45
20–34	78	3.1	10	1	1	1	4	8	11	15
35–49	166	2.2	4	1	1	1	4	5	6	7
50–64	217	2.2	9	1	1	1	1	6	8	15
65+	143	2.6	15	1	1	2	2	7	10	23
SUBTOTALS:										
1. SINGLE DX										
A. Not Operated	6	1.5	1	1	1	1	1	4	4	4
B. Operated	121	1.5	<1	1	1	1	1	3	4	4
2. MULTIPLE DX										
A. Not Operated	100	3.3	14	1	1	2	4	6	9	22
B. Operated	733	2.8	16	1	1	1	3	6	9	19
1. SINGLE DX	127	1.5	<1	1	1	1	1	3	4	4
2. MULTIPLE DX	833	2.8	15	1	1	2	4	6	9	21
A. NOT OPERATED	106	3.2	14	1	1	2	4	6	9	22
B. OPERATED	854	2.6	14	1	1	1	3	6	8	19
TOTAL										
0–19 Years	221	3.5	31	1	1	2	4	6	11	26
20–34	108	2.9	9	1	1	1	4	6	9	13
35–49	202	2.3	4	1	1	1	3	5	6	9
50–64	261	2.2	8	1	1	1	2	6	8	15
65+	168	2.6	14	1	1	2	2	7	9	23
GRAND TOTAL	960	2.7	14	1	1	1	3	6	8	19

Length of Stay by Diagnosis and Operation, Western Region, 2008

Western Region, October 2006–September 2007 Data, by Diagnosis

746: OTHER CONG ANOMALY HEART

Type of Patients	Observed Patients	Avg. Stay	Variance	10th	25th	50th	75th	90th	95th	99th
1. SINGLE DX										
A. Not Operated										
0–19 Years	12	1.5	<1	1	1	1	2	3	3	3
20–34	1	1.0	0	1	1	1	1	1	1	1
35–49	1	2.0	0	2	2	2	2	2	2	2
50–64	2	2.0	2	1	1	1	3	3	3	3
65+	1	1.0	0	1	1	1	1	1	1	1
B. Operated										
0–19 Years	25	3.1	9	1	1	2	4	5	9	14
20–34	6	3.5	6	1	2	4	4	8	8	8
35–49	2	2.0	2	1	1	1	3	3	3	3
50–64	3	5.3	<1	5	5	5	6	6	6	6
65+	0									
2. MULTIPLE DX										
A. Not Operated										
0–19 Years	93	2.8	27	1	1	1	2	6	10	34
20–34	25	4.4	26	1	1	3	5	10	17	22
35–49	31	3.3	6	1	2	2	4	7	9	10
50–64	32	2.4	5	1	1	2	3	4	9	11
65+	18	2.6	3	1	1	3	3	4	7	7
B. Operated										
0–19 Years	286	7.8	101	1	3	5	9	16	28	73
20–34	72	7.3	51	3	4	5	7	15	21	46
35–49	128	5.7	18	2	4	5	7	9	11	18
50–64	176	6.6	35	3	4	5	7	10	14	31
65+	88	7.8	33	4	5	6	9	14	17	38
SUBTOTALS:										
1. SINGLE DX										
A. Not Operated	17	1.5	<1	1	1	1	2	3	3	3
B. Operated	36	3.3	8	1	1	3	5	6	9	14
2. MULTIPLE DX										
A. Not Operated	199	3.0	18	1	1	2	3	7	10	22
B. Operated	750	7.1	59	2	4	5	8	12	18	49
1. SINGLE DX	53	2.7	6	1	1	2	4	5	8	14
2. MULTIPLE DX	949	6.2	53	1	3	5	7	11	17	42
A. NOT OPERATED	216	2.9	17	1	1	2	3	6	10	22
B. OPERATED	786	6.9	57	1	4	5	8	12	18	49
TOTAL										
0–19 Years	416	6.2	81	1	1	4	7	13	22	64
20–34	104	6.3	44	1	3	4	7	13	20	28
35–49	162	5.2	16	1	3	4	6	9	10	18
50–64	213	5.9	32	1	4	5	7	10	11	28
65+	107	6.8	31	2	4	6	8	13	16	35
GRAND TOTAL	1,002	6.0	51	1	2	5	7	11	16	42

746.4: CONGENITAL AVI

Type of Patients	Observed Patients	Avg. Stay	Variance	10th	25th	50th	75th	90th	95th	99th
1. SINGLE DX										
A. Not Operated										
0–19 Years	1	2.0	0	2	2	2	2	2	2	2
20–34	0									
35–49	0									
50–64	1	1.0	0	1	1	1	1	1	1	1
65+	0									
B. Operated										
0–19 Years	0									
20–34	1	4.0	0	4	4	4	4	4	4	4
35–49	0									
50–64	3	5.3	<1	5	5	5	6	6	6	6
65+	0									
2. MULTIPLE DX										
A. Not Operated										
0–19 Years	0									
20–34	2	13.6	141	5	5	22	22	22	22	22
35–49	4	4.0	11	2	2	3	9	9	9	9
50–64	8	2.8	11	1	1	2	2	4	11	11
65+	1	1.0	0	1	1	1	1	1	1	1
B. Operated										
0–19 Years	15	4.9	7	1	3	5	7	11	>99	>99
20–34	33	6.2	21	4	4	5	6	10	13	28
35–49	62	5.9	6	3	4	5	7	9	10	18
50–64	107	6.7	15	4	5	5	8	10	16	21
65+	73	7.4	23	4	5	6	8	12	16	38
SUBTOTALS:										
1. SINGLE DX										
A. Not Operated	2	1.5	<1	1	1	1	2	2	2	2
B. Operated	4	5.0	<1	4	5	5	6	6	6	6
2. MULTIPLE DX										
A. Not Operated	15	4.4	33	1	1	2	5	7	22	22
B. Operated	290	6.6	16	4	4	6	7	10	13	31
1. SINGLE DX	6	3.8	4	1	2	5	5	6	6	6
2. MULTIPLE DX	305	6.5	17	4	4	5	7	10	13	28
A. NOT OPERATED	17	4.1	30	1	1	2	3	6	10	22
B. OPERATED	294	6.5	16	4	4	5	7	10	13	31
TOTAL										
0–19 Years	16	4.8	7	1	3	4	5	7	13	22
20–34	36	6.6	26	3	4	5	6	9	10	28
35–49	66	5.8	7	3	4	5	7	9	10	18
50–64	119	6.3	16	4	5	5	7	10	16	21
65+	74	7.3	24	4	5	6	8	12	16	38
GRAND TOTAL	311	6.4	17	3	4	5	7	10	13	28

747: OTH CONG CIRC SYST ANOM

Type of Patients	Observed Patients	Avg. Stay	Variance	10th	25th	50th	75th	90th	95th	99th
1. SINGLE DX										
A. Not Operated										
0–19 Years	43	1.5	2	1	1	1	1	2	5	8
20–34	15	1.5	<1	1	1	1	2	2	4	4
35–49	7	1.6	1	1	1	1	2	2	4	4
50–64	2	2.5	4	1	1	4	4	4	4	4
65+	2	2.0	2	1	1	1	1	3	3	3
B. Operated										
0–19 Years	71	1.9	3	1	1	1	2	4	7	9
20–34	27	2.1	2	1	1	2	3	5	5	6
35–49	18	2.2	2	1	1	2	3	5	6	6
50–64	20	2.6	4	1	1	1	4	6	6	6
65+	2	1.0	0	1	1	1	1	1	1	1
2. MULTIPLE DX										
A. Not Operated										
0–19 Years	127	4.8	99	1	1	1	3	14	18	50
20–34	42	2.3	5	1	1	2	3	4	5	8
35–49	67	2.7	5	1	1	2	3	5	7	12
50–64	62	2.7	4	1	1	2	3	6	6	10
65+	92	4.2	14	1	2	3	5	7	10	23
B. Operated										
0–19 Years	339	7.1	126	1	3	4	7	13	25	82
20–34	142	5.0	34	4	4	5	6	8	17	50
35–49	169	4.3	14	3	4	5	6	8	12	20
50–64	178	5.3	25	4	5	5	7	13	14	30
65+	74	6.1	32	4	5	6	8	12	17	34
SUBTOTALS:										
1. SINGLE DX										
A. Not Operated	69	1.5	2	1	1	1	1	3	4	8
B. Operated	138	2.1	3	1	1	1	3	5	6	8
2. MULTIPLE DX										
A. Not Operated	390	3.7	38	1	1	2	4	6	12	30
B. Operated	902	5.8	64	1	4	4	7	12	17	48
1. SINGLE DX	207	1.9	3	1	1	1	2	4	6	8
2. MULTIPLE DX	1,292	5.2	57	1	3	4	6	10	16	48
A. NOT OPERATED	459	3.4	33	1	1	2	3	6	11	23
B. OPERATED	1,040	5.3	57	1	3	4	6	10	15	46
TOTAL										
0–19 Years	580	5.5	100	1	1	2	6	12	19	66
20–34	226	3.9	24	1	3	3	5	8	10	27
35–49	261	3.7	11	1	3	3	5	7	9	18
50–64	262	4.5	20	1	4	4	6	10	13	24
65+	170	4.9	23	2	5	6	6	10	14	24
GRAND TOTAL	1,499	4.7	51	1	3	4	6	9	14	41

Length of Stay by Diagnosis and Operation, Western Region, 2008

Western Region, October 2006–September 2007 Data, by Diagnosis

747.81: CEREBROVASCULAR ANOMALY

Type of Patients	Observed Patients	Avg. Stay	Variance	Percentiles						
				10th	25th	50th	75th	90th	95th	99th
1. SINGLE DX										
A. Not Operated										
0–19 Years	5	1.0	0	1	1	1	1	1	1	1
20–34	6	1.3	<1	1	1	1	2	2	2	2
35–49	4	2.0	2	1	1	1	2	4	4	4
50–64	0									
65+	2	2.0	2	1	1	1	3	3	3	3
B. Operated										
0–19 Years	22	2.6	4	1	1	2	3	5	7	9
20–34	17	2.6	2	1	1	2	3	5	6	6
35–49	13	2.2	2	1	1	2	3	4	5	5
50–64	18	2.8	4	1	1	2	4	6	6	6
65+	2	1.0	0	1	1	1	1	1	1	1
2. MULTIPLE DX										
A. Not Operated										
0–19 Years	17	3.6	24	1	1	2	2	13	16	16
20–34	19	2.1	2	1	1	2	3	4	5	5
35–49	41	2.4	3	1	1	2	3	4	5	10
50–64	29	3.1	5	1	1	2	4	6	6	10
65+	17	2.9	3	1	2	3	4	5	7	7
B. Operated										
0–19 Years	46	5.8	45	1	2	3	7	11	24	34
20–34	91	4.7	20	1	2	3	6	8	17	>99
35–49	108	4.2	13	1	2	3	6	8	12	18
50–64	120	4.7	21	1	2	3	6	11	13	24
65+	41	5.4	32	1	2	4	7	10	12	34
SUBTOTALS:										
1. SINGLE DX										
A. Not Operated	17	1.5	<1	1	1	1	2	3	4	4
B. Operated	72	2.6	3	1	1	2	4	5	6	9
2. MULTIPLE DX										
A. Not Operated	123	2.8	6	1	1	2	3	5	6	13
B. Operated	406	4.7	23	1	2	3	6	9	13	27
1. SINGLE DX	89	2.4	3	1	1	2	3	5	6	9
2. MULTIPLE DX	529	4.3	19	1	2	3	5	9	13	25
A. NOT OPERATED	140	2.6	6	1	1	2	3	5	6	13
B. OPERATED	478	4.4	20	1	2	3	6	9	13	27
TOTAL										
0–19 Years	90	4.4	31	1	1	2	5	10	14	34
20–34	133	3.9	16	1	2	3	5	8	13	27
35–49	166	3.5	10	1	1	2	4	7	9	18
50–64	167	4.2	17	1	1	3	5	9	12	24
65+	62	4.5	23	1	2	3	6	11	11	34
GRAND TOTAL	618	4.0	18	1	1	3	5	8	12	24

748: RESPIRATORY SYST ANOMALY

Type of Patients	Observed Patients	Avg. Stay	Variance	Percentiles						
				10th	25th	50th	75th	90th	95th	99th
1. SINGLE DX										
A. Not Operated										
0–19 Years	31	1.5	<1	1	1	1	2	2	3	3
20–34	0									
35–49	0									
50–64	0									
65+	1	7.0	0	7	7	7	7	7	7	7
B. Operated										
0–19 Years	27	2.2	2	1	1	2	3	4	6	6
20–34	1	3.0	0	3	3	3	3	3	3	3
35–49	0									
50–64	0									
65+	0									
2. MULTIPLE DX										
A. Not Operated										
0–19 Years	114	4.2	23	1	1	2	5	10	12	21
20–34	2	2.5	4	1	1	4	4	4	4	4
35–49	3	2.0	1	1	1	2	3	3	3	3
50–64	2	6.0	2	5	5	6	7	7	7	7
65+	3	5.0	28	1	1	3	11	11	11	11
B. Operated										
0–19 Years	62	5.7	66	1	1	3	5	14	18	44
20–34	16	4.6	5	1	4	4	7	7	8	8
35–49	6	3.3	4	1	1	3	5	6	6	6
50–64	30	4.8	38	1	1	4	5	8	10	35
65+	6	3.8	5	1	3	3	4	8	8	8
SUBTOTALS:										
1. SINGLE DX										
A. Not Operated	32	1.7	1	1	1	1	2	3	3	7
B. Operated	28	2.2	2	1	1	2	3	4	6	6
2. MULTIPLE DX										
A. Not Operated	124	4.2	22	1	1	2	5	10	12	21
B. Operated	120	5.1	44	1	1	3	5	9	16	35
1. SINGLE DX	60	1.9	2	1	1	1	2	3	6	7
2. MULTIPLE DX	244	4.6	33	1	1	3	5	10	14	35
A. NOT OPERATED	156	3.6	19	1	1	2	4	9	11	21
B. OPERATED	148	4.6	38	1	1	3	5	8	14	35
TOTAL										
0–19 Years	234	4.0	31	1	1	2	4	9	14	33
20–34	19	4.3	5	1	3	4	7	7	8	8
35–49	9	2.9	3	1	1	3	4	6	6	6
50–64	32	4.9	36	1	4	4	5	8	10	35
65+	10	4.5	10	1	3	3	7	8	11	11
GRAND TOTAL	304	4.1	28	1	1	3	5	8	12	33

749: CLEFT PALATE & CLEFT LIP

Type of Patients	Observed Patients	Avg. Stay	Variance	Percentiles						
				10th	25th	50th	75th	90th	95th	99th
1. SINGLE DX										
A. Not Operated										
0–19 Years	4	2.0	<1	1	1	2	2	3	3	3
20–34	0									
35–49	0									
50–64	0									
65+	0									
B. Operated										
0–19 Years	287	1.2	<1	1	1	1	1	2	2	3
20–34	6	1.7	1	1	1	1	2	4	4	4
35–49	1	1.0	0	1	1	1	1	1	1	1
50–64	1	2.0	0	2	2	2	2	2	2	2
65+	0									
2. MULTIPLE DX										
A. Not Operated										
0–19 Years	13	4.6	54	1	1	2	5	7	28	28
20–34	0	8.0	0	8	8	8	8	8	8	8
35–49	0									
50–64	0									
65+	0									
B. Operated										
0–19 Years	595	1.5	2	1	1	2	2	2	3	7
20–34	27	1.4	<1	1	1	1	2	2	2	4
35–49	4	1.3	<1	1	1	1	1	1	2	2
50–64	2	1.0	0	1	1	1	1	1	1	1
65+	1	2.0	0	2	2	2	2	2	2	2
SUBTOTALS:										
1. SINGLE DX										
A. Not Operated	4	2.0	<1	1	1	2	2	3	3	3
B. Operated	295	1.2	<1	1	1	1	1	2	2	4
2. MULTIPLE DX										
A. Not Operated	14	4.9	50	1	1	2	6	8	28	28
B. Operated	629	1.5	2	1	1	1	2	2	3	7
1. SINGLE DX	299	1.2	<1	1	1	1	1	2	2	4
2. MULTIPLE DX	643	1.6	3	1	1	1	2	2	3	7
A. NOT OPERATED	18	4.2	40	1	1	1	5	8	28	28
B. OPERATED	924	1.4	2	1	1	1	2	2	3	6
TOTAL										
0–19 Years	899	1.4	2	1	1	1	2	2	3	6
20–34	34	1.7	2	1	1	1	2	2	4	8
35–49	5	1.2	<1	1	1	1	2	2	2	2
50–64	3	1.3	<1	2	2	2	2	2	2	2
65+	1	2.0	0	2	2	2	2	2	2	2
GRAND TOTAL	942	1.5	2	1	1	1	1	2	3	7

Length of Stay by Diagnosis and Operation, Western Region, 2008

Western Region, October 2006–September 2007 Data, by Diagnosis

750: OTHER UPPER GI ANOMALY

Type of Patients	Observed Patients	Avg. Stay	Variance	10th	25th	50th	75th	90th	95th	99th
1. SINGLE DX										
A. Not Operated										
0–19 Years	18	1.2	<1	1	1	1	1	2	2	3
20–34	0									
35–49	0									
50–64	0									
65+	0									
B. Operated										
0–19 Years	451	2.3	<1	1	2	2	3	3	4	5
20–34	1	1.0	0	1	1	1	1	1	1	1
35–49	0									
50–64	0									
65+	0									
2. MULTIPLE DX										
A. Not Operated										
0–19 Years	41	2.7	5	1	1	2	3	7	7	10
20–34	4	7.0	33	1	3	7	12	14	14	14
35–49	2	5.6	40	1	1	10	10	10	10	10
50–64	12	3.3	3	1	2	4	4	5	7	7
65+	24	5.2	25	2	2	3	6	12	12	23
B. Operated										
0–19 Years	470	3.8	37	1	2	3	4	6	8	45
20–34	4	1.5	<1	1	1	1	1	3	3	3
35–49	3	1.7	<1	1	1	2	2	2	2	2
50–64	2	4.0	2	3	3	4	5	5	5	5
65+	3	6.0	31	1	1	5	12	12	12	12
SUBTOTALS:										
1. SINGLE DX										
A. Not Operated	18	1.2	<1	1	1	1	1	2	2	3
B. Operated	452	2.3	<1	1	2	2	3	3	4	5
2. MULTIPLE DX										
A. Not Operated	83	3.8	14	1	1	3	4	8	11	23
B. Operated	482	3.8	36	1	2	3	4	6	8	45
1. SINGLE DX	470	2.2	<1	1	2	2	3	3	4	5
2. MULTIPLE DX	565	3.8	33	1	2	3	4	6	9	35
A. NOT OPERATED	101	3.3	12	1	1	2	4	7	10	14
B. OPERATED	934	3.1	20	1	2	2	3	4	6	25
TOTAL										
0–19 Years	980	3.0	19	1	1	2	3	4	6	25
20–34	9	3.9	21	1	1	1	4	14	14	14
35–49	5	3.2	15	1	1	2	2	10	10	10
50–64	14	3.4	3	1	2	4	4	5	7	7
65+	27	5.3	25	2	2	3	7	12	12	23
GRAND TOTAL	1,035	3.1	19	1	2	2	3	5	7	23

750.5: CONG PYLORIC STENOSIS

Type of Patients	Observed Patients	Avg. Stay	Variance	10th	25th	50th	75th	90th	95th	99th
1. SINGLE DX										
A. Not Operated										
0–19 Years	12	1.3	<1	1	1	1	1	2	2	3
20–34	0									
35–49	0									
50–64	0									
65+	0									
B. Operated										
0–19 Years	437	2.3	<1	2	2	2	3	3	4	5
20–34	0									
35–49	0									
50–64	0									
65+	0									
2. MULTIPLE DX										
A. Not Operated										
0–19 Years	20	2.0	2	1	1	2	2	3	4	7
20–34	0									
35–49	0									
50–64	0									
65+	0									
B. Operated										
0–19 Years	389	3.0	3	2	2	3	4	5	6	8
20–34	0									
35–49	0									
50–64	0									
65+	0									
SUBTOTALS:										
1. SINGLE DX										
A. Not Operated	12	1.3	<1	1	1	1	1	2	3	3
B. Operated	437	2.3	<1	2	2	2	3	3	4	5
2. MULTIPLE DX										
A. Not Operated	20	2.0	2	1	1	2	2	3	4	7
B. Operated	389	3.0	3	2	2	3	4	5	6	8
1. SINGLE DX	449	2.3	<1	2	2	2	3	3	4	5
2. MULTIPLE DX	409	3.0	3	1	2	3	4	5	6	8
A. NOT OPERATED	32	1.8	2	1	1	1	2	3	4	7
B. OPERATED	826	2.6	2	1	2	2	3	4	5	7
TOTAL										
0–19 Years	858	2.6	2	1	2	2	3	4	5	7
20–34	0									
35–49	0									
50–64	0									
65+	0									
GRAND TOTAL	858	2.6	2	1	2	2	3	4	5	7

751: OTH ANOM DIGESTIVE SYST

Type of Patients	Observed Patients	Avg. Stay	Variance	10th	25th	50th	75th	90th	95th	99th
1. SINGLE DX										
A. Not Operated										
0–19 Years	17	2.9	7	1	1	2	3	6	12	12
20–34	1	1.0	0	1	1	1	1	1	1	1
35–49	1	1.0	0	1	1	1	1	1	1	1
50–64	0									
65+	1	1.0	0	1	1	1	1	1	1	1
B. Operated										
0–19 Years	92	4.0	8	2	3	4	4	6	9	21
20–34	13	3.8	3	2	3	3	4	6	8	8
35–49	5	3.0	3	1	2	3	4	5	5	5
50–64	8	3.9	5	1	1	4	6	7	7	7
65+	0									
2. MULTIPLE DX										
A. Not Operated										
0–19 Years	76	3.7	13	1	1	2	5	8	9	24
20–34	18	3.1	7	1	1	2	4	6	11	11
35–49	25	5.0	35	1	2	3	5	13	23	23
50–64	23	3.7	16	1	1	2	4	11	14	14
65+	31	3.0	4	1	1	3	4	6	7	7
B. Operated										
0–19 Years	355	8.0	114	2	3	5	9	16	25	66
20–34	80	5.4	9	2	3	5	7	9	11	13
35–49	120	6.3	21	2	3	5	8	13	16	23
50–64	94	7.8	68	2	3	5	9	14	27	56
65+	47	7.4	22	3	4	7	9	14	15	24
SUBTOTALS:										
1. SINGLE DX										
A. Not Operated	20	2.7	7	1	1	2	3	4	6	12
B. Operated	118	3.9	7	1	3	4	4	6	8	14
2. MULTIPLE DX										
A. Not Operated	173	3.7	14	1	1	3	4	7	11	23
B. Operated	696	7.3	74	2	3	5	8	13	20	56
1. SINGLE DX	138	3.7	7	2	2	3	4	6	8	14
2. MULTIPLE DX	869	6.6	64	1	3	5	7	13	19	45
A. NOT OPERATED	193	3.6	14	1	1	2	4	7	11	23
B. OPERATED	814	6.8	66	2	3	5	8	13	19	45
TOTAL										
0–19 Years	540	6.5	82	1	2	4	7	12	21	59
20–34	112	4.8	9	1	2	4	4	9	11	12
35–49	151	5.9	23	2	3	5	7	13	18	23
50–64	125	6.8	57	1	3	5	7	13	19	40
65+	79	5.6	19	1	3	5	7	11	15	24
GRAND TOTAL	1,007	6.2	57	1	3	4	7	12	18	40

Length of Stay by Diagnosis and Operation, Western Region, 2008

Western Region, October 2006–September 2007 Data, by Diagnosis

751.0: MECKEL'S DIVERTICULUM

Type of Patients	Observed Patients	Avg. Stay	Variance	10th	25th	50th	75th	90th	95th	99th
1. SINGLE DX										
A. Not Operated										
0–19 Years	0									
20–34	1	1.0	0	1	1	1		1	1	1
35–49	0									
50–64	0									
65+	0									
B. Operated										
0–19 Years	18	3.2	4	1	2	3	3	6	9	9
20–34	11	4.0	4	2	2	4	6	6	8	8
35–49	1	2.0	0	2	2	2	2	2	2	2
50–64	2	3.5	<1	3	3	4	4	4	4	4
65+	0									
2. MULTIPLE DX										
A. Not Operated										
0–19 Years	3	2.3	1	1	1	3	3	3	3	3
20–34	3	4.4	33	1	1	1	11	11	11	11
35–49	2	2.0	0	2	2	2	2	2	2	2
50–64	2	3.5	12	1	1	1	6	6	6	6
65+	0									
B. Operated										
0–19 Years	65	5.4	14	2	3	5	6	9	11	25
20–34	46	5.3	8	2	3	4	7	10	10	12
35–49	67	6.7	23	2	3	6	8	13	18	26
50–64	45	7.3	80	2	3	5	7	11	19	56
65+	29	8.3	28	3	6	7	10	15	20	24
SUBTOTALS:										
1. SINGLE DX										
A. Not Operated	1	1.0	0	1	1	1	1	1	1	1
B. Operated	32	3.5	4	2	2	3	3	6	8	9
2. MULTIPLE DX										
A. Not Operated	10	3.1	10	1	1	2	3	6	11	11
B. Operated	252	6.4	30	2	3	5	8	11	15	26
1. SINGLE DX	33	3.4	4	1	2	3	4	6	8	9
2. MULTIPLE DX	262	6.2	29	2	3	5	7	11	15	26
A. NOT OPERATED	11	2.9	9	1	1	2	3	6	11	11
B. OPERATED	284	6.0	27	2	3	5	7	10	14	26
TOTAL										
0–19 Years	86	4.8	13	2	3	4	6	9	11	25
20–34	61	4.9	8	2	3	4	7	9	10	12
35–49	70	6.5	23	2	3	6	8	13	18	26
50–64	49	7.0	74	2	3	5	7	11	19	56
65+	29	8.3	28	3	6	7	10	15	20	24
GRAND TOTAL	295	5.9	27	2	3	5	7	10	14	26

752: GENITAL ORGAN ANOMALIES

Type of Patients	Observed Patients	Avg. Stay	Variance	10th	25th	50th	75th	90th	95th	99th
1. SINGLE DX										
A. Not Operated										
0–19 Years	2	4.0	18	1	1	7	7	7	7	7
20–34	1	1.0	0	1	1	1	1	1	1	1
35–49	0									
50–64	0									
65+	0									
B. Operated										
0–19 Years	39	1.9	2	1	1	2	2	3	4	8
20–34	5	1.6	<1	1	1	1	2	3	3	3
35–49	3	1.3	<1	1	1	1	2	2	2	2
50–64	2	2.0	0	2	2	2	2	2	2	2
65+	0									
2. MULTIPLE DX										
A. Not Operated										
0–19 Years	14	4.6	40	1	1	2	3	15	19	19
20–34	2	1.5	<1	1	1	1	3	2	2	2
35–49	1	3.0	0	3	3	3	3	3	3	3
50–64	0									
65+	1	2.0	0	2	2	2	2	2	2	2
B. Operated										
0–19 Years	132	2.4	9	1	1	2	3	5	7	11
20–34	51	2.4	4	1	1	2	3	4	8	10
35–49	39	2.3	2	1	1	2	2	5	6	7
50–64	23	2.0	<1	1	1	2	3	3	4	4
65+	6	3.7	8	2	2	3	4	9	9	9
SUBTOTALS:										
1. SINGLE DX										
A. Not Operated	3	3.0	12	1	1	1	7	7	7	7
B. Operated	49	1.8	1	1	1	2	2	3	3	8
2. MULTIPLE DX										
A. Not Operated	18	4.0	32	1	1	2	2	15	19	19
B. Operated	251	2.4	6	1	1	2	3	4	7	10
1. SINGLE DX	52	1.9	2	1	1	2	2	3	4	8
2. MULTIPLE DX	269	2.5	8	1	1	2	3	5	7	15
A. NOT OPERATED	21	3.9	28	1	1	2	3	14	15	19
B. OPERATED	300	2.3	5	1	1	2	2	4	6	10
TOTAL										
0–19 Years	187	2.5	10	1	1	2	2	5	7	19
20–34	59	2.3	4	1	1	2	2	4	8	10
35–49	43	2.2	2	1	1	2	2	4	6	7
50–64	25	2.0	<1	1	1	2	3	3	4	4
65+	7	3.4	7	2	2	3	4	9	9	9
GRAND TOTAL	321	2.4	7	1	1	2	2	4	7	14

753: URINARY SYSTEM ANOMALIES

Type of Patients	Observed Patients	Avg. Stay	Variance	10th	25th	50th	75th	90th	95th	99th
1. SINGLE DX										
A. Not Operated										
0–19 Years	11	1.9	<1	1	1	2	2	3	4	4
20–34	4	2.3	2	1	2	2	2	4	4	4
35–49	2	1.5	<1	1	2	2	2	2	2	2
50–64	1	2.0	0	2	2	2	2	2	2	2
65+	0									
B. Operated										
0–19 Years	81	2.0	1	1	1	2	3	3	4	8
20–34	21	2.1	<1	1	2	2	3	3	3	3
35–49	13	2.4	2	1	2	3	3	4	5	5
50–64	7	2.4	2	1	1	2	4	4	4	4
65+	1	2.0	0	2	2	2	2	2	2	2
2. MULTIPLE DX										
A. Not Operated										
0–19 Years	43	4.3	27	1	2	4	4	14	16	23
20–34	38	3.4	4	2	2	3	3	6	7	8
35–49	93	4.0	16	1	2	3	5	8	15	20
50–64	88	3.4	7	1	1	3	5	7	9	11
65+	53	4.2	7	2	2	4	5	8	10	13
B. Operated										
0–19 Years	236	2.9	7	1	1	2	3	5	8	13
20–34	97	3.5	7	2	3	3	4	5	7	18
35–49	121	4.9	11	2	3	4	6	9	11	18
50–64	140	6.0	77	1	3	4	6	11	13	38
65+	59	5.0	16	1	2	4	7	9	12	24
SUBTOTALS:										
1. SINGLE DX										
A. Not Operated	18	1.9	<1	1	1	2	2	4	4	4
B. Operated	123	2.1	1	1	2	2	3	3	4	5
2. MULTIPLE DX										
A. Not Operated	315	3.9	12	1	2	3	5	8	11	18
B. Operated	653	4.2	25	1	2	3	5	8	10	18
1. SINGLE DX	141	2.1	1	1	1	2	3	3	4	5
2. MULTIPLE DX	968	4.1	21	1	2	3	5	8	10	18
A. NOT OPERATED	333	3.8	12	1	2	3	5	8	10	18
B. OPERATED	776	3.9	22	1	2	3	5	7	10	18
TOTAL										
0–19 Years	371	2.9	8	1	1	2	3	5	8	16
20–34	160	3.3	5	1	2	3	4	6	6	17
35–49	229	4.4	13	1	2	3	6	9	11	18
50–64	236	4.9	50	1	2	4	6	9	11	32
65+	113	4.6	12	1	2	4	6	9	11	16
GRAND TOTAL	1,109	3.9	19	1	2	3	5	7	10	18

Length of Stay by Diagnosis and Operation, Western Region. 2008

Western Region, October 2006–September 2007 Data, by Diagnosis

753.21: CONG OBSTRUCTION UPJ

Type of Patients	Observed Patients	Avg. Stay	Vari-ance	Percentiles 10th	25th	50th	75th	90th	95th	99th
1. SINGLE DX										
A. Not Operated										
0–19 Years	1	1.0	0	1	1	1	1	1	1	1
20–34	0									
35–49	0									
50–64	1	2.0	0	2	2	2	2	2	2	2
65+	0									
B. Operated										
0–19 Years	34	2.0	<1	1	1	2	3	3	3	4
20–34	7	2.3	<1	2	2	2	3	3	3	3
35–49	8	2.3	1	2	2	2	4	4	4	4
50–64	1	1.0	0	1	1	1	1	1	1	1
65+	1	2.0	0	2	2	2	2	2	2	2
2. MULTIPLE DX										
A. Not Operated										
0–19 Years	5	2.0	<1	1	2	2	2	3	3	3
20–34	2	2.0	0	2	2	2	2	2	2	2
35–49	4	1.3	<1	1	1	1	2	2	2	2
50–64	3	4.0	19	1	1	9	9	9	9	9
65+	3	3.7	2	2	2	5	5	5	5	5
B. Operated										
0–19 Years	76	2.4	2	1	1	2	3	4	5	6
20–34	39	3.0	7	1	2	4	4	5	6	17
35–49	22	3.4	6	1	2	3	3	7	8	11
50–64	17	3.2	3	1	2	3	4	6	6	6
65+	14	3.6	5	1	2	3	5	7	8	8
SUBTOTALS:										
1. SINGLE DX										
A. Not Operated	2	1.5	<1	1	1	2	2	2	2	2
B. Operated	51	2.0	<1	1	1	2	3	3	3	4
2. MULTIPLE DX										
A. Not Operated	17	2.5	4	1	1	2	2	5	9	9
B. Operated	168	2.9	4	1	2	3	3	5	6	11
1. SINGLE DX	53	2.0	<1	1	1	2	3	3	4	4
2. MULTIPLE DX	185	2.8	4	1	2	3	3	5	6	11
A. NOT OPERATED	19	2.4	4	1	1	2	3	5	9	9
B. OPERATED	219	2.7	3	1	2	3	3	4	6	8
TOTAL										
0–19 Years	116	2.3	1	1	1	2	3	4	5	6
20–34	48	2.8	6	1	2	3	3	4	5	17
35–49	34	2.9	4	1	2	3	3	4	8	11
50–64	22	3.1	4	1	2	3	4	6	6	9
65+	18	3.5	4	2	2	5	5	7	8	8
GRAND TOTAL	238	2.6	3	1	2	3	3	4	6	9

754: CONG MS DEFORMITIES

Type of Patients	Observed Patients	Avg. Stay	Vari-ance	Percentiles 10th	25th	50th	75th	90th	95th	99th
1. SINGLE DX										
A. Not Operated										
0–19 Years	17	1.2	<1	1	1	1	1	2	3	3
20–34	0									
35–49	0									
50–64	0									
65+	0									
B. Operated										
0–19 Years	225	2.2	2	1	1	1	3	5	5	7
20–34	21	2.8	2	1	1	3	4	4	5	5
35–49	9	4.2	4	1	3	5	5	7	7	7
50–64	2	2.0	2	1	1	2	3	3	3	3
65+	0									
2. MULTIPLE DX										
A. Not Operated										
0–19 Years	18	2.3	8	1	1	1	2	7	7	12
20–34	3	1.7	1	1	1	1	3	3	3	3
35–49	2	3.0	2	2	2	2	4	4	4	4
50–64	0									
65+	0									
B. Operated										
0–19 Years	359	3.2	8	1	1	3	4	6	7	17
20–34	56	4.4	9	1	2	3	5	8	11	16
35–49	41	3.7	3	1	2	4	5	6	7	7
50–64	45	3.3	4	1	2	3	4	6	6	11
65+	17	3.5	4	3	3	3	4	7	9	9
SUBTOTALS:										
1. SINGLE DX										
A. Not Operated	17	1.2	<1	1	1	1	1	2	3	3
B. Operated	257	2.3	3	1	1	3	3	5	5	7
2. MULTIPLE DX										
A. Not Operated	23	2.3	7	1	1	1	3	4	7	12
B. Operated	518	3.4	7	1	1	3	5	6	7	14
1. SINGLE DX	274	2.3	2	1	1	2	3	5	5	7
2. MULTIPLE DX	541	3.4	7	1	1	3	4	6	7	14
A. NOT OPERATED	40	1.8	4	1	1	1	2	4	7	12
B. OPERATED	775	3.0	6	1	1	3	4	6	7	13
TOTAL										
0–19 Years	619	2.8	6	1	1	2	4	5	6	13
20–34	80	3.8	7	1	2	3	5	6	10	16
35–49	52	3.8	3	1	2	4	5	6	7	7
50–64	47	3.2	4	1	2	3	4	6	6	11
65+	17	3.5	4	3	3	3	4	7	9	9
GRAND TOTAL	815	3.0	6	1	2	3	4	6	7	12

755: OTH CONG LIMB ANOMALY

Type of Patients	Observed Patients	Avg. Stay	Vari-ance	Percentiles 10th	25th	50th	75th	90th	95th	99th
1. SINGLE DX										
A. Not Operated										
0–19 Years	2	1.0	0	1	1	1	1	1	1	1
20–34	0									
35–49	0									
50–64	0									
65+	0									
B. Operated										
0–19 Years	100	1.8	1	1	1	1	2	3	5	6
20–34	12	3.5	4	1	1	3	5	6	6	6
35–49	3	2.3	1	1	1	3	3	3	3	3
50–64	3	2.3	5	1	1	1	5	5	5	5
65+	0									
2. MULTIPLE DX										
A. Not Operated										
0–19 Years	5	2.0	<1	1	1	2	2	3	3	3
20–34	1	2.0	0	2	2	2	2	2	2	2
35–49	1	2.0	0	2	2	2	2	2	2	2
50–64	2	3.0	8	1	1	1	5	5	5	5
65+	1	3.0	0	3	3	3	3	3	3	3
B. Operated										
0–19 Years	155	2.7	12	1	1	2	3	4	6	22
20–34	82	3.3	3	2	2	3	4	6	6	10
35–49	109	3.4	3	2	3	3	4	5	6	11
50–64	88	3.5	3	2	3	3	4	6	6	12
65+	21	3.0	1	3	2	3	3	4	5	6
SUBTOTALS:										
1. SINGLE DX										
A. Not Operated	2	1.0	0	1	1	1	1	1	1	1
B. Operated	118	2.0	2	1	1	1	2	5	5	6
2. MULTIPLE DX										
A. Not Operated	10	2.3	2	1	1	1	3	5	5	5
B. Operated	455	3.2	6	1	2	3	4	5	6	11
1. SINGLE DX	120	1.9	2	1	1	1	2	4	5	6
2. MULTIPLE DX	465	3.1	6	1	2	3	4	5	6	11
A. NOT OPERATED	12	2.1	2	1	1	2	3	3	5	5
B. OPERATED	573	2.9	6	1	2	3	4	5	6	11
TOTAL										
0–19 Years	262	2.3	8	1	1	2	3	4	5	8
20–34	95	3.3	3	2	2	3	4	5	6	10
35–49	113	3.4	3	2	3	3	4	5	6	11
50–64	93	3.5	3	2	3	3	4	5	6	12
65+	22	3.0	1	2	2	3	3	4	5	6
GRAND TOTAL	585	2.9	5	1	2	3	4	5	6	11

647

Length of Stay by Diagnosis and Operation, Western Region, 2008

Western Region, October 2006–September 2007 Data, by Diagnosis

755.63: CONG HIP DEFORMITY NEC

Type of Patients	Observed Patients	Avg. Stay	Variance	10th	25th	50th	75th	90th	95th	99th
1. SINGLE DX										
A. *Not Operated*										
0–19 Years	0									
20–34	0									
35–49	0									
50–64	0									
65+	0									
B. *Operated*										
0–19 Years	33	2.5	2	1	2	2	3	5	5	6
20–34	8	4.6	1	3	4	5	6	6	6	6
35–49	1	3.0	0	3	3	3	3	3	3	3
50–64	2	3.0	8	1	1	3	5	5	5	5
65+	0									
2. MULTIPLE DX										
A. *Not Operated*										
0–19 Years	0									
20–34	0									
35–49	1	2.0	0	2	2	2	2	2	2	2
50–64	1	5.0	0	5	5	5	5	5	5	5
65+	1	3.0	0	3	3	3	3	3	3	3
B. *Operated*										
0–19 Years	54	3.6	24	1	2	3	4	5	7	37
20–34	59	3.8	3	2	3	3	4	6	7	10
35–49	96	3.6	3	2	3	3	4	5	6	14
50–64	83	3.6	3	2	3	3	4	6	6	12
65+	20	3.1	1	2	3	3	3	4	6	6
SUBTOTALS:										
1. SINGLE DX										
A. *Not Operated*	0									
B. *Operated*	44	3.0	3	1	2	3	4	5	5	6
2. MULTIPLE DX										
A. *Not Operated*	3	3.3	2	2	2	3	3	5	5	5
B. *Operated*	312	3.6	6	2	3	3	4	5	6	11
1. SINGLE DX	**44**	**3.0**	**3**	**1**	**2**	**3**	**4**	**5**	**5**	**6**
2. MULTIPLE DX	**315**	**3.6**	**6**	**2**	**3**	**3**	**5**	**5**	**6**	**11**
A. NOT OPERATED	**3**	**3.3**	**2**	**2**	**2**	**3**	**5**	**5**	**5**	**5**
B. OPERATED	**356**	**3.5**	**6**	**2**	**3**	**3**	**4**	**5**	**6**	**11**
TOTAL										
0–19 Years	87	3.2	16	1	2	2	4	5	6	37
20–34	67	3.9	3	2	3	4	5	6	6	10
35–49	98	3.6	3	2	3	3	4	5	6	14
50–64	86	3.6	3	2	3	3	4	6	6	15
65+	21	3.1	1	2	3	3	3	4	5	6
GRAND TOTAL	**359**	**3.5**	**6**	**2**	**3**	**3**	**4**	**5**	**6**	**11**

756: OTHER MS ANOMALIES

Type of Patients	Observed Patients	Avg. Stay	Variance	10th	25th	50th	75th	90th	95th	99th
1. SINGLE DX										
A. *Not Operated*										
0–19 Years	14	2.5	4	1	2	2	3	3	3	9
20–34	1	3.0	0	3	3	3	3	3	3	3
35–49	2	1.5	<1	1	1	1	2	2	2	2
50–64	0									
65+	0									
B. *Operated*										
0–19 Years	143	2.9	2	1	2	2	4	4	5	6
20–34	17	2.9	3	1	2	3	4	4	8	8
35–49	20	3.3	<1	2	3	3	4	4	5	5
50–64	21	3.5	3	2	2	3	4	6	6	8
65+	10	3.0	3	1	2	3	4	7	7	7
2. MULTIPLE DX										
A. *Not Operated*										
0–19 Years	52	6.6	82	1	2	3	8	16	23	49
20–34	9	3.7	8	1	2	2	5	8	8	8
35–49	18	2.5	6	1	1	2	3	4	11	11
50–64	26	3.2	10	1	1	2	3	6	11	14
65+	51	3.1	6	1	2	2	4	6	8	12
B. *Operated*										
0–19 Years	295	5.2	54	1	2	4	5	10	14	63
20–34	93	3.8	5	1	2	3	5	6	8	13
35–49	238	3.9	9	2	2	3	4	6	9	16
50–64	489	4.2	13	2	3	4	5	7	9	17
65+	449	4.3	9	2	3	4	5	7	9	15
SUBTOTALS:										
1. SINGLE DX										
A. *Not Operated*	17	2.4	3	1	2	2	3	3	3	9
B. *Operated*	211	3.0	2	1	2	3	4	4	5	7
2. MULTIPLE DX										
A. *Not Operated*	156	4.3	34	1	1	2	5	9	12	34
B. *Operated*	1,564	4.4	19	1	3	4	5	7	10	21
1. SINGLE DX	**228**	**2.9**	**2**	**1**	**2**	**3**	**4**	**4**	**5**	**8**
2. MULTIPLE DX	**1,720**	**4.4**	**20**	**1**	**2**	**4**	**5**	**7**	**10**	**23**
A. NOT OPERATED	**173**	**4.1**	**32**	**1**	**1**	**3**	**4**	**9**	**12**	**34**
B. OPERATED	**1,775**	**4.2**	**17**	**1**	**2**	**4**	**5**	**7**	**9**	**19**
TOTAL										
0–19 Years	504	4.6	42	1	2	3	4	8	13	42
20–34	120	3.6	5	1	2	3	4	7	8	12
35–49	278	3.8	9	1	2	3	4	6	9	16
50–64	536	4.2	13	1	3	4	5	6	9	15
65+	510	4.1	9	1	2	4	5	7	9	12
GRAND TOTAL	**1,948**	**4.2**	**18**	**1**	**2**	**3**	**5**	**7**	**9**	**21**

756.0: ANOMALY SKULL/FACE BONES

Type of Patients	Observed Patients	Avg. Stay	Variance	10th	25th	50th	75th	90th	95th	99th
1. SINGLE DX										
A. *Not Operated*										
0–19 Years	1	1.0	0	1	1	1	1	1	1	1
20–34	0									
35–49	0									
50–64	0									
65+	0									
B. *Operated*										
0–19 Years	104	3.0	1	1	2	3	4	5	5	5
20–34	1	2.0	0	2	2	2	2	2	2	2
35–49	1	3.0	0	3	3	3	3	3	3	3
50–64	0									
65+	0									
2. MULTIPLE DX										
A. *Not Operated*										
0–19 Years	14	8.7	154	1	1	6	11	12	49	49
20–34	0									
35–49	0									
50–64	1	1.0	0	1	1	1	1	1	1	1
65+	1	3.0	0	3	3	3	3	3	3	3
B. *Operated*										
0–19 Years	149	4.0	25	1	2	3	4	6	8	54
20–34	6	2.3	3	1	1	1	4	5	5	5
35–49	2	1.5	<1	1	1	2	2	2	2	2
50–64	2	12.0	18	9	9	12	15	15	15	15
65+	0									
SUBTOTALS:										
1. SINGLE DX										
A. *Not Operated*	1	1.0	0	1	1	1	1	1	1	1
B. *Operated*	106	3.0	1	1	2	3	4	5	5	5
2. MULTIPLE DX										
A. *Not Operated*	16	7.8	139	1	1	3	3	12	49	49
B. *Operated*	159	4.0	24	1	2	3	4	5	8	54
1. SINGLE DX	**107**	**3.0**	**1**	**1**	**2**	**3**	**4**	**5**	**5**	**5**
2. MULTIPLE DX	**175**	**4.4**	**35**	**1**	**2**	**3**	**4**	**7**	**11**	**54**
A. NOT OPERATED	**17**	**7.4**	**133**	**1**	**1**	**3**	**8**	**12**	**49**	**49**
B. OPERATED	**265**	**3.6**	**15**	**1**	**2**	**3**	**4**	**5**	**6**	**28**
TOTAL										
0–19 Years	268	3.8	23	1	2	3	4	6	8	49
20–34	7	2.3	3	1	1	2	3	5	5	5
35–49	3	2.0	<1	1	1	2	3	3	3	3
50–64	3	8.3	49	1	1	9	15	15	15	15
65+	1	3.0	0	3	3	3	3	3	3	3
GRAND TOTAL	**282**	**3.8**	**23**	**1**	**2**	**3**	**4**	**6**	**8**	**49**

Length of Stay by Diagnosis and Operation, Western Region, 2008

756.12: SPONDYLOLISTHESIS

Type of Patients	Observed Patients	Avg. Stay	Vari-ance	10th	25th	50th	75th	90th	95th	99th
1. SINGLE DX										
A. *Not Operated*										
0–19 Years	0									
20–34	0									
35–49	1	2.0	0	2	2	2	2	2	2	2
50–64	0									
65+	0									
B. *Operated*										
0–19 Years	4	3.0	0	3	3	3	3	3	3	3
20–34	9	3.3	4	2	2	3	4	8	8	8
35–49	19	3.3	1	2	3	4	4	4	5	5
50–64	21	3.5	3	2	2	3	4	6	6	8
65+	10	3.0	3	1	2	3	4	7	7	7
2. MULTIPLE DX										
A. *Not Operated*										
0–19 Years	1	2.0	0	2	2	2	2	2	2	2
20–34	3	4.4	12	1	1	4	8	8	8	8
35–49	10	1.7	1	1	1	1	2	4	4	4
50–64	18	3.5	13	1	1	2	4	11	14	14
65+	37	3.2	5	1	1	3	5	8	8	9
B. *Operated*										
0–19 Years	22	4.1	7	2	3	4	4	5	11	13
20–34	49	3.8	2	2	3	4	5	5	6	9
35–49	193	3.9	8	2	3	3	4	6	7	16
50–64	438	4.2	10	2	3	4	5	6	8	13
65+	428	4.3	9	2	3	4	5	7	9	15
SUBTOTALS:										
1. SINGLE DX										
A. *Not Operated*	1	2.0	0	2	2	2	2	2	2	2
B. *Operated*	63	3.3	2	2	2	3	4	5	6	8
2. MULTIPLE DX										
A. *Not Operated*	69	3.1	7	1	1	2	4	6	8	14
B. *Operated*	1,130	4.2	9	2	3	4	5	6	8	13
1. SINGLE DX	64	3.3	2	2	2	3	4	5	6	8
2. MULTIPLE DX	1,199	4.1	9	2	3	4	5	6	8	14
A. NOT OPERATED	70	3.1	7	1	1	2	4	6	8	14
B. OPERATED	1,193	4.1	9	2	3	4	5	6	8	13
TOTAL										
0–19 Years	27	3.9	6	2	3	3	4	5	11	13
20–34	61	3.7	3	2	3	3	4	5	7	9
35–49	223	3.8	7	2	3	3	4	6	7	13
50–64	477	4.1	10	2	3	4	5	6	8	14
65+	475	4.2	9	1	3	4	5	7	9	15
GRAND TOTAL	1,263	4.1	8	2	3	4	5	6	8	13

757: CONG SKIN ANOMALIES

Type of Patients	Observed Patients	Avg. Stay	Vari-ance	10th	25th	50th	75th	90th	95th	99th
1. SINGLE DX										
A. *Not Operated*										
0–19 Years	5	1.4	<1	1	1	1	1	1	3	3
20–34	2	9.0	128	1	1	9	17	17	17	17
35–49	0									
50–64	1	3.0		3	3	3	3	3	3	3
65+	0									
B. *Operated*										
0–19 Years	3	1.0	0	1	1	1	1	1	1	1
20–34	2	1.0	0	1	1	1	1	1	1	1
35–49	0									
50–64	1	1.0	0	1	1	1	1	1	1	1
65+	0									
2. MULTIPLE DX										
A. *Not Operated*										
0–19 Years	12	3.8	11	1	2	3	3	10	11	11
20–34	10	5.0	9	2	3	4	8	8	11	11
35–49	1	6.0	0	6	6	6	6	6	6	6
50–64	4	3.0	2	1	3	4	4	4	4	4
65+	2	2.0	2	1	1	3	5	8	8	9
B. *Operated*										
0–19 Years	2	2.5	4	1	1	4	4	5	5	4
20–34	4	4.3	12	1	1	3	5	5	9	9
35–49	6	3.2	4	1	1	3	5	6	6	6
50–64	4	1.0	0	1	1	1	1	1	1	1
65+	0									
SUBTOTALS:										
1. SINGLE DX										
A. *Not Operated*	8	3.5	30	1	1	1	2	2	17	17
B. *Operated*	6	1.0	0	1	1	1	1	1	1	1
2. MULTIPLE DX										
A. *Not Operated*	29	4.1	8	1	2	3	4	6	10	11
B. *Operated*	16	2.8	5	1	1	1	4	6	9	9
1. SINGLE DX	14	2.4	18	1	1	1	1	5	6	8
2. MULTIPLE DX	45	3.6	8	1	1	3	5	6	10	11
A. NOT OPERATED	37	4.0	12	1	1	3	4	6	11	17
B. OPERATED	22	2.3	5	1	1	1	3	5	6	9
TOTAL										
0–19 Years	22	2.8	7	1	1	2	4	5	10	11
20–34	18	4.8	18	1	2	4	4	5	17	17
35–49	7	3.6	5	1	3	3	6	6	6	6
50–64	10	2.0	2	1	1	1	3	4	4	4
65+	2	2.0	2	1	1	3	3	3	3	3
GRAND TOTAL	59	3.3	10	1	1	3	4	6	11	17

758: CHROMOSOMAL ANOMALIES

Type of Patients	Observed Patients	Avg. Stay	Vari-ance	10th	25th	50th	75th	90th	95th	99th
1. SINGLE DX										
A. *Not Operated*										
0–19 Years	1	1.0	0	1	1	1	1	1	1	1
20–34	0									
35–49	0									
50–64	0									
65+										
B. *Operated*										
0–19 Years	1	1.0	0	1	1	1	1	1	1	1
20–34	0									
35–49	0									
50–64	0									
65+	0									
2. MULTIPLE DX										
A. *Not Operated*										
0–19 Years	20	6.3	60	1	1	3	8	12	12	36
20–34	1	12.0	0	12	12	12	12	12	12	12
35–49	3	3.3	10	1	1	2	7	7	7	7
50–64	4	6.0	25	1	1	5	13	13	13	13
65+	0									
B. *Operated*										
0–19 Years	12	11.7	297	1	1	2	28	37	50	50
20–34	0									
35–49	0									
50–64	1	3.0	0	3	3	3	3	3	3	3
65+	1	3.0	0	3	3	3	3	3	3	3
SUBTOTALS:										
1. SINGLE DX										
A. *Not Operated*	1	1.0	0	1	1	1	1	1	1	1
B. *Operated*	1	1.0	0	1	1	1	1	1	1	1
2. MULTIPLE DX										
A. *Not Operated*	28	6.1	48	1	1	5	8	12	13	36
B. *Operated*	14	10.5	261	1	1	2	15	37	50	50
1. SINGLE DX	2	1.0	0	1	1	1	1	1	1	1
2. MULTIPLE DX	42	7.6	119	1	1	3	8	15	36	50
A. NOT OPERATED	29	6.0	47	1	1	5	8	12	13	36
B. OPERATED	15	9.8	249	1	1	2	15	37	50	50
TOTAL										
0–19 Years	34	7.9	144	1	1	3	8	28	37	50
20–34	2	12.0	0	12	12	12	12	12	12	12
35–49	3	3.3	10	1	1	2	7	7	7	7
50–64	5	5.4	21	1	3	5	5	13	13	13
65+	1	3.0	0	3	3	3	3	3	3	3
GRAND TOTAL	44	7.3	115	1	1	3	8	15	36	50

Length of Stay by Diagnosis and Operation, Western Region, 2008

Western Region, October 2006–September 2007 Data, by Diagnosis

759: CONG ANOMALIES NEC & NOS

Type of Patients	Observed Patients	Avg. Stay	Vari-ance	10th	25th	50th	75th	90th	95th	99th
1. SINGLE DX										
A. Not Operated										
0–19 Years	7	1.7	<1	1	1	2	2	3	3	3
20–34	0									
35–49	0									
50–64	1	5.0	0	5	5	5	5	5	5	5
65+	0									
B. Operated										
0–19 Years	72	1.3	<1	1	1	1	1	2	2	7
20–34	13	1.4	<1	1	1	1	1	3	4	4
35–49	20	1.6	<1	1	1	1	2	2	4	4
50–64	13	1.3	<1	1	1	1	2	2	2	2
65+	4	1.3	<1	1	1	1	1	2	2	2
2. MULTIPLE DX										
A. Not Operated										
0–19 Years	69	3.4	13	1	2	3	4	7	10	23
20–34	23	4.7	26	1	1	3	6	16	17	17
35–49	16	3.3	5	1	1	3	5	6	9	9
50–64	18	6.0	73	1	2	3	6	16	37	37
65+	3	2.3	1	1	1	3	3	3	3	3
B. Operated										
0–19 Years	58	6.4	96	1	1	4	7	16	27	63
20–34	37	5.5	96	1	1	3	6	13	16	58
35–49	48	4.3	48	1	1	2	5	8	13	46
50–64	63	3.7	11	1	1	2	5	8	10	18
65+	31	3.3	32	1	1	2	3	4	5	33
SUBTOTALS:										
1. SINGLE DX										
A. Not Operated	8	2.1	2	1	1	2	2	3	5	5
B. Operated	122	1.4	<1	1	1	1	1	2	2	5
2. MULTIPLE DX										
A. Not Operated	129	4.0	23	1	1	3	4	7	15	23
B. Operated	237	4.7	56	1	1	3	5	10	16	46
1. SINGLE DX	130	1.4	<1	1	1	1	2	2	3	5
2. MULTIPLE DX	366	4.5	44	1	1	3	5	9	15	37
A. NOT OPERATED	137	3.9	22	1	1	3	4	7	15	23
B. OPERATED	359	3.6	40	1	1	2	4	7	12	33
TOTAL										
0–19 Years	206	3.5	36	1	1	2	3	7	13	27
20–34	73	4.5	59	1	1	2	5	11	16	58
35–49	84	3.5	29	1	1	2	4	7	9	46
50–64	95	3.8	22	1	1	2	5	7	10	37
65+	38	3.0	26	1	1	2	3	4	5	33
GRAND TOTAL	496	3.7	35	1	1	2	4	7	13	33

760: MTL COND AFF FETUS/NB

Type of Patients	Observed Patients	Avg. Stay	Vari-ance	10th	25th	50th	75th	90th	95th	99th
1. SINGLE DX										
A. Not Operated										
0–19 Years	2	2.0	2	1	1	3	3	3	3	3
20–34	0									
35–49	0									
50–64	0									
65+	0									
B. Operated										
0–19 Years	0									
20–34	0									
35–49	0									
50–64	0									
2. MULTIPLE DX										
A. Not Operated										
0–19 Years	7	6.1	27	2	2	4	8	17	17	17
20–34	1	12.0	0	12	12	12	12	12	12	12
35–49	1	5.0	0	5	5	5	5	5	5	5
50–64	0									
65+	0									
B. Operated										
0–19 Years	0									
20–34	0									
35–49	0									
50–64	0									
65+	0									
SUBTOTALS:										
1. SINGLE DX										
A. Not Operated	2	2.0	2	1	1	3	3	3	3	3
B. Operated	0									
2. MULTIPLE DX										
A. Not Operated	9	6.7	25	2	4	5	8	17	17	17
B. Operated	0									
1. SINGLE DX	2	2.0	2	1	1	3	3	3	3	3
2. MULTIPLE DX	9	6.7	25	2	4	5	8	17	17	17
A. NOT OPERATED	11	5.8	23	2	2	4	8	12	17	17
B. OPERATED	0									
TOTAL										
0–19 Years	9	5.2	24	1	2	4	6	17	17	17
20–34	1	12.0	0	12	12	12	12	12	12	12
35–49	1	5.0	0	5	5	5	5	5	5	5
50–64	0									
65+	0									
GRAND TOTAL	11	5.8	23	2	2	4	8	12	17	17

761: MATERNAL COMP AFF NB

Type of Patients	Observed Patients	Avg. Stay	Vari-ance	10th	25th	50th	75th	90th	95th	99th
1. SINGLE DX										
A. Not Operated										
0–19 Years	0									
20–34	0									
35–49	0									
50–64	0									
65+	0									
B. Operated										
0–19 Years	0									
20–34	0									
35–49	0									
50–64	0									
2. MULTIPLE DX										
A. Not Operated										
0–19 Years	0									
20–34	0									
35–49	0									
50–64	0									
65+	0									
B. Operated										
0–19 Years	0									
20–34	0									
35–49	0									
50–64	0									
65+	0									
SUBTOTALS:										
1. SINGLE DX										
A. Not Operated	0									
B. Operated	0									
2. MULTIPLE DX										
A. Not Operated	0									
B. Operated	0									
1. SINGLE DX	0									
2. MULTIPLE DX	0									
A. NOT OPERATED	0									
B. OPERATED	0									
TOTAL										
0–19 Years	0									
20–34	0									
35–49	0									
50–64	0									
65+	0									
GRAND TOTAL	0									

Length of Stay by Diagnosis and Operation, Western Region, 2008

Western Region, October 2006–September 2007 Data, by Diagnosis

762: COMP PLAC/CORD AFF NB

Type of Patients	Observed Patients	Avg. Stay	Variance	Percentiles						
				10th	25th	50th	75th	90th	95th	99th
1. SINGLE DX										
A. Not Operated										
0–19 Years	0									
20–34	0									
35–49	0									
50–64	0									
B. Operated										
0–19 Years	0									
20–34	0									
35–49	0									
50–64	0									
2. MULTIPLE DX										
A. Not Operated										
0–19 Years	0									
20–34	0									
35–49	0									
50–64	0									
B. Operated										
0–19 Years	0									
20–34	0									
35–49	0									
50–64	0									
SUBTOTALS:										
1. SINGLE DX A. Not Operated	0									
B. Operated	0									
2. MULTIPLE DX A. Not Operated	0									
B. Operated	0									
1. SINGLE DX	0									
2. MULTIPLE DX	0									
A. NOT OPERATED	0									
B. OPERATED	0									
TOTAL										
0–19 Years	0									
20–34	0									
35–49	0									
50–64	0									
65+	0									
GRAND TOTAL	0									

763: OTH COMP DEL AFF NB

Type of Patients	Observed Patients	Avg. Stay	Variance	Percentiles						
				10th	25th	50th	75th	90th	95th	99th
1. SINGLE DX										
A. Not Operated										
0–19 Years	1	1.0	0	1	1	1	1	1	1	1
20–34	0									
35–49	0									
50–64	0									
B. Operated										
0–19 Years	0									
20–34	0									
35–49	0									
50–64	0									
2. MULTIPLE DX										
A. Not Operated										
0–19 Years	0									
20–34	0									
35–49	0									
50–64	0									
B. Operated										
0–19 Years	0									
20–34	0									
35–49	0									
50–64	0									
SUBTOTALS:										
1. SINGLE DX A. Not Operated	1	1.0	0	1	1	1	1	1	1	1
B. Operated	0									
2. MULTIPLE DX A. Not Operated	0									
B. Operated	0									
1. SINGLE DX	1	1.0	0	1	1	1	1	1	1	1
2. MULTIPLE DX	0									
A. NOT OPERATED	1	1.0	0	1	1	1	1	1	1	1
B. OPERATED	0									
TOTAL										
0–19 Years	1	1.0	0	1	1	1	1	1	1	1
20–34	0									
35–49	0									
50–64	0									
65+	0									
GRAND TOTAL	1	1.0	0	1	1	1	1	1	1	1

764: SLOW FETAL GROWTH/MALNUT

Type of Patients	Observed Patients	Avg. Stay	Variance	Percentiles						
				10th	25th	50th	75th	90th	95th	99th
1. SINGLE DX										
A. Not Operated										
0–19 Years	2	2.0	0	2	2	2	2	2	2	2
20–34	0									
35–49	0									
50–64	0									
B. Operated										
0–19 Years	0									
20–34	0									
35–49	0									
50–64	0									
2. MULTIPLE DX										
A. Not Operated										
0–19 Years	31	8.2	34	2	3	8	11	16	21	24
20–34	0									
35–49	0									
50–64	0									
B. Operated										
0–19 Years	3	23.0	587	7	7	11	51	51	51	51
20–34	0									
35–49	0									
50–64	0									
SUBTOTALS:										
1. SINGLE DX A. Not Operated	2	2.0	0	2	2	2	2	2	2	2
B. Operated	0									
2. MULTIPLE DX A. Not Operated	31	8.2	34	2	3	8	11	16	21	24
B. Operated	3	23.0	587	7	7	11	51	51	51	51
1. SINGLE DX	2	2.0	0	2	2	2	2	2	2	2
2. MULTIPLE DX	34	9.5	85	2	3	8	11	17	24	51
A. NOT OPERATED	33	7.8	34	2	3	7	10	16	21	24
B. OPERATED	3	23.0	587	7	7	11	51	51	51	51
TOTAL										
0–19 Years	36	9.1	83	2	3	8	11	17	24	51
20–34	0									
35–49	0									
50–64	0									
65+	0									
GRAND TOTAL	36	9.1	83	2	3	8	11	17	24	51

Length of Stay by Diagnosis and Operation, Western Region, 2008

Western Region, October 2006–September 2007 Data, by Diagnosis

765: SHORT GESTATION/LOW BWT

Type of Patients	Observed Patients	Avg. Stay	Variance	10th	25th	50th	75th	90th	95th	99th
1. SINGLE DX										
A. Not Operated										
0–19 Years	1	4.0	0	4	4	4	4	4	4	4
20–34	0									
35–49	0									
50–64	0									
65+	0									
B. Operated										
0–19 Years	1	5.0	0	5	5	5	5	5	5	5
20–34	0									
35–49	0									
50–64	0									
65+	0									
2. MULTIPLE DX										
A. Not Operated										
0–19 Years	719	17.9	272	3	7	13	24	40	55	87
20–34	0									
35–49	0									
50–64	0									
65+	0									
B. Operated										
0–19 Years	88	30.9	860	4	7	25	56	92	>99	>99
20–34	0									
35–49	0									
50–64	0									
65+	0									
SUBTOTALS:										
1. SINGLE DX										
A. Not Operated	1	4.0	0	4	4	4	4	4	4	4
B. Operated	1	5.0	0	5	5	5	5	5	5	5
2. MULTIPLE DX										
A. Not Operated	719	17.9	272	3	7	13	24	40	55	87
B. Operated	88	30.9	860	4	7	25	56	92	>99	>99
1. SINGLE DX	2	4.5	<1	4	4	5	5	5	5	5
2. MULTIPLE DX	807	19.3	352	3	7	13	26	45	68	>99
A. NOT OPERATED	720	17.9	272	3	7	13	24	40	55	87
B. OPERATED	89	30.6	858	4	7	24	56	92	>99	>99
TOTAL										
0–19 Years	809	19.3	351	3	7	13	25	45	68	>99
20–34	0									
35–49	0									
50–64	0									
65+	0									
GRAND TOTAL	809	19.3	351	3	7	13	25	45	68	>99

765.18: PRETERM NB NEC 2-2.5 KG

Type of Patients	Observed Patients	Avg. Stay	Variance	10th	25th	50th	75th	90th	95th	99th
1. SINGLE DX										
A. Not Operated										
0–19 Years	0									
20–34	0									
35–49	0									
50–64	0									
65+	0									
B. Operated										
0–19 Years	0									
20–34	0									
35–49	0									
50–64	0									
65+	0									
2. MULTIPLE DX										
A. Not Operated										
0–19 Years	188	10.8	75	2	5	9	15	22	26	42
20–34	0									
35–49	0									
50–64	0									
65+	0									
B. Operated										
0–19 Years	18	16.8	424	3	4	7	18	56	79	79
20–34	0									
35–49	0									
50–64	0									
65+	0									
SUBTOTALS:										
1. SINGLE DX										
A. Not Operated	0									
B. Operated	0									
2. MULTIPLE DX										
A. Not Operated	188	10.8	75	2	5	9	15	22	26	42
B. Operated	18	16.8	424	3	4	7	18	56	79	79
1. SINGLE DX	0									
2. MULTIPLE DX	206	11.3	107	3	5	8	15	23	28	56
A. NOT OPERATED	188	10.8	75	2	5	9	15	22	26	42
B. OPERATED	18	16.8	424	3	4	7	18	56	79	79
TOTAL										
0–19 Years	206	11.3	107	3	5	8	15	23	28	56
20–34	0									
35–49	0									
50–64	0									
65+	0									
GRAND TOTAL	206	11.3	107	3	5	8	15	23	28	56

766: LONG GESTATION/HIGH BWT

Type of Patients	Observed Patients	Avg. Stay	Variance	10th	25th	50th	75th	90th	95th	99th
1. SINGLE DX										
A. Not Operated										
0–19 Years	10	1.7	2	1	1	1	2	2	6	6
20–34	0									
35–49	0									
50–64	0									
65+	0									
B. Operated										
0–19 Years	0									
20–34	0									
35–49	0									
50–64	0									
65+	0									
2. MULTIPLE DX										
A. Not Operated										
0–19 Years	18	3.4	9	1	2	2	4	9	11	11
20–34	0									
35–49	0									
50–64	0									
65+	0									
B. Operated										
0–19 Years	1	2.0	0	2	2	2	2	2	2	2
20–34	0									
35–49	0									
50–64	0									
65+	0									
SUBTOTALS:										
1. SINGLE DX										
A. Not Operated	10	1.7	2	1	1	1	2	2	6	6
B. Operated	0									
2. MULTIPLE DX										
A. Not Operated	18	3.4	9	1	2	2	4	9	11	11
B. Operated	1	2.0	0	2	2	2	2	2	2	2
1. SINGLE DX	10	1.7	2	1	1	1	2	2	6	6
2. MULTIPLE DX	19	3.3	8	1	2	2	4	9	11	11
A. NOT OPERATED	28	2.8	7	1	1	2	3	7	9	11
B. OPERATED	1	2.0	0	2	2	2	2	2	2	2
TOTAL										
0–19 Years	29	2.8	7	1	1	2	3	7	9	11
20–34	0									
35–49	0									
50–64	0									
65+	0									
GRAND TOTAL	29	2.8	7	1	1	2	3	7	9	11

Length of Stay by Diagnosis and Operation, Western Region, 2008

Western Region, October 2006–September 2007 Data, by Diagnosis

767: BIRTH TRAUMA

Type of Patients	Observed Patients	Avg. Stay	Vari-ance	Percentiles						
				10th	25th	50th	75th	90th	95th	99th
1. SINGLE DX										
A. *Not Operated*										
0–19 Years	10	1.2	<1	1	1	1	1	2	2	2
20–34	0									
35–49	0									
50–64	0									
65+	0									
B. *Operated*										
0–19 Years	2	1.0	0	1	1	1	1	1	1	1
20–34	0									
35–49	0									
50–64	0									
65+	0									
2. MULTIPLE DX										
A. *Not Operated*										
0–19 Years	35	5.7	87	1	2	3	6	13	20	53
20–34	0									
35–49	0									
50–64	0									
65+	0									
B. *Operated*										
0–19 Years	3	6.7	32	2	2	5	13	13	13	13
20–34	0									
35–49	0									
50–64	0									
65+	0									
SUBTOTALS:										
1. SINGLE DX										
A. *Not Operated*	10	1.2	<1	1	1	1	1	2	2	2
B. *Operated*	2	1.0	0	1	1	1	1	1	1	1
2. MULTIPLE DX										
A. *Not Operated*	35	5.7	87	1	2	3	6	13	20	53
B. *Operated*	3	6.7	32	2	2	5	13	13	13	13
1. SINGLE DX	12	1.2	<1	1	1	1	2	2	2	2
2. MULTIPLE DX	38	5.8	81	1	2	3	6	13	20	53
A. NOT OPERATED	45	4.7	71	1	1	2	3	10	13	53
B. OPERATED	5	4.4	26	1	1	2	5	13	13	13
TOTAL										
0–19 Years	50	4.7	66	1	1	2	4	13	13	53
20–34	0									
35–49	0									
50–64	0									
65+	0									
GRAND TOTAL	50	4.7	66	1	1	2	4	13	13	53

768: INTRAUTERINE ASPHYXIA

Type of Patients	Observed Patients	Avg. Stay	Vari-ance	Percentiles						
				10th	25th	50th	75th	90th	95th	99th
1. SINGLE DX										
A. *Not Operated*										
0–19 Years	0									
20–34	0									
35–49	0									
50–64	0									
65+	0									
B. *Operated*										
0–19 Years	0									
20–34	0									
35–49	0									
50–64	0									
65+	0									
2. MULTIPLE DX										
A. *Not Operated*										
0–19 Years	11	12.2	57	3	5	10	18	22	25	25
20–34	0									
35–49	0									
50–64	0									
65+	0									
B. *Operated*										
0–19 Years	2	24.5	24	21	21	25	28	28	28	28
20–34	0									
35–49	0									
50–64	0									
65+	0									
SUBTOTALS:										
1. SINGLE DX										
A. *Not Operated*	0									
B. *Operated*	0									
2. MULTIPLE DX										
A. *Not Operated*	11	12.2	57	3	5	10	18	22	25	25
B. *Operated*	2	24.5	24	21	21	25	28	28	28	28
1. SINGLE DX	0									
2. MULTIPLE DX	13	14.1	71	3	8	14	21	25	28	28
A. NOT OPERATED	11	12.2	57	3	5	10	18	22	25	25
B. OPERATED	2	24.5	24	21	21	25	28	28	28	28
TOTAL										
0–19 Years	13	14.1	71	3	8	14	21	25	28	28
20–34	0									
35–49	0									
50–64	0									
65+	0									
GRAND TOTAL	13	14.1	71	3	8	14	21	25	28	28

769: RESP DISTRESS SYNDROME

Type of Patients	Observed Patients	Avg. Stay	Vari-ance	Percentiles						
				10th	25th	50th	75th	90th	95th	99th
1. SINGLE DX										
A. *Not Operated*										
0–19 Years	2	9.0	8	7	7	9	11	11	11	11
20–34	0									
35–49	0									
50–64	0									
65+	0									
B. *Operated*										
0–19 Years	0									
20–34	0									
35–49	0									
50–64	0									
65+	0									
2. MULTIPLE DX										
A. *Not Operated*										
0–19 Years	213	17.3	308	4	7	12	20	45	67	97
20–34	0									
35–49	0									
50–64	0									
65+	0									
B. *Operated*										
0–19 Years	25	30.9	845	6	9	19	39	97	97	>99
20–34	0									
35–49	0									
50–64	0									
65+	0									
SUBTOTALS:										
1. SINGLE DX										
A. *Not Operated*	2	9.0	8	7	7	9	11	11	11	11
B. *Operated*	0									
2. MULTIPLE DX										
A. *Not Operated*	213	17.3	308	4	7	12	20	45	67	97
B. *Operated*	25	30.9	845	6	9	19	39	97	97	>99
1. SINGLE DX	2	9.0	8	7	7	9	11	11	11	11
2. MULTIPLE DX	238	18.7	379	5	7	12	21	46	70	>99
A. NOT OPERATED	215	17.2	306	4	7	12	20	45	67	97
B. OPERATED	25	30.9	845	6	9	19	39	97	97	>99
TOTAL										
0–19 Years	240	18.6	376	5	7	12	21	46	70	>99
20–34	0									
35–49	0									
50–64	0									
65+	0									
GRAND TOTAL	240	18.6	376	5	7	12	21	46	70	>99

Length of Stay by Diagnosis and Operation, Western Region, 2008

Western Region, October 2006–September 2007 Data, by Diagnosis

770: OTH NB RESPIRATORY COND

Type of Patients	Observed Patients	Avg. Stay	Vari-ance	Percentiles						
				10th	25th	50th	75th	90th	95th	99th
1. SINGLE DX										
A. Not Operated										
0–19 Years	279	2.1	3	1	1	2	2	4	6	9
20–34	0									
35–49	0									
50–64	0									
65+	0									
B. Operated										
0–19 Years	2	3.0	8	1	1	1	5	5	5	5
20–34	0									
35–49	0									
50–64	0									
65+	0									
2. MULTIPLE DX										
A. Not Operated										
0–19 Years	1,337	5.6	52	1	2	3	7	11	17	35
20–34	1	4.0	0	4	4	4	4	4	4	4
35–49	0									
50–64	0									
65+	0									
B. Operated										
0–19 Years	40	15.4	402	3	4	7	25	74	>99	>99
20–34	0									
35–49	0									
50–64	0									
65+	0									
SUBTOTALS:										
1. SINGLE DX										
A. Not Operated	279	2.1	3	1	1	2	2	4	6	9
B. Operated	2	3.0	8	1	1	1	5	5	5	5
2. MULTIPLE DX										
A. Not Operated	1,338	5.6	52	1	2	3	7	11	17	35
B. Operated	40	15.4	402	3	4	7	25	74	>99	>99
1. SINGLE DX	281	2.1	3	1	1	2	2	4	6	9
2. MULTIPLE DX	1,378	5.9	65	1	2	4	7	12	19	51
A. NOT OPERATED	1,617	5.0	45	1	2	3	6	10	15	34
B. OPERATED	42	14.8	389	2	4	6	20	74	>99	>99
TOTAL										
0–19 Years	1,658	5.2	56	1	2	3	6	11	16	45
20–34	1	4.0	0	4	4	4	4	4	4	4
35–49	0									
50–64	0									
65+	0									
GRAND TOTAL	1,659	5.2	56	1	2	3	6	11	16	45

770.81: NB PRIMARY APNEA

Type of Patients	Observed Patients	Avg. Stay	Vari-ance	Percentiles						
				10th	25th	50th	75th	90th	95th	99th
1. SINGLE DX										
A. Not Operated										
0–19 Years	95	2.2	3	1	1	2	3	4	6	10
20–34	0									
35–49	0									
50–64	0									
65+	0									
B. Operated										
0–19 Years	0									
20–34	0									
35–49	0									
50–64	0									
65+	0									
2. MULTIPLE DX										
A. Not Operated										
0–19 Years	265	4.5	32	2	2	3	5	10	13	31
20–34	0									
35–49	0									
50–64	0									
65+	0									
B. Operated										
0–19 Years	2	12.4	111	5	5	5	20	20	20	20
20–34	0									
35–49	0									
50–64	0									
65+	0									
SUBTOTALS:										
1. SINGLE DX										
A. Not Operated	95	2.2	3	1	1	2	3	4	6	10
B. Operated	0									
2. MULTIPLE DX										
A. Not Operated	265	4.5	32	2	2	3	5	10	13	31
B. Operated	2	12.4	111	5	5	5	20	20	20	20
1. SINGLE DX	95	2.2	3	1	1	2	3	4	6	10
2. MULTIPLE DX	267	4.6	33	1	2	3	5	11	14	31
A. NOT OPERATED	360	3.9	26	1	1	2	4	9	12	26
B. OPERATED	2	12.4	111	5	5	5	20	20	20	20
TOTAL										
0–19 Years	362	4.0	26	1	2	2	4	9	12	26
20–34	0									
35–49	0									
50–64	0									
65+	0									
GRAND TOTAL	362	4.0	26	1	2	2	4	9	12	26

770.89: NB RESPIRATORY PBX NEC

Type of Patients	Observed Patients	Avg. Stay	Vari-ance	Percentiles						
				10th	25th	50th	75th	90th	95th	99th
1. SINGLE DX										
A. Not Operated										
0–19 Years	87	1.9	3	1	1	1	2	3	6	10
20–34	0									
35–49	0									
50–64	0									
65+	0									
B. Operated										
0–19 Years	0									
20–34	0									
35–49	0									
50–64	0									
65+	0									
2. MULTIPLE DX										
A. Not Operated										
0–19 Years	412	5.5	49	1	2	3	6	11	15	34
20–34	0									
35–49	0									
50–64	0									
65+	0									
B. Operated										
0–19 Years	15	21.8	609	2	5	19	45	>99	>99	>99
20–34	0									
35–49	0									
50–64	0									
65+	0									
SUBTOTALS:										
1. SINGLE DX										
A. Not Operated	87	1.9	3	1	1	1	2	3	6	10
B. Operated	0									
2. MULTIPLE DX										
A. Not Operated	412	5.5	49	1	2	3	6	11	15	34
B. Operated	15	21.8	609	2	5	19	45	>99	>99	>99
1. SINGLE DX	87	1.9	3	1	1	1	2	3	6	10
2. MULTIPLE DX	427	6.1	76	1	2	4	7	12	21	74
A. NOT OPERATED	499	4.9	43	1	2	3	6	10	14	28
B. OPERATED	15	21.8	609	2	5	19	45	>99	>99	>99
TOTAL										
0–19 Years	514	5.4	66	1	2	3	6	10	18	60
20–34	0									
35–49	0									
50–64	0									
65+	0									
GRAND TOTAL	514	5.4	66	1	2	3	6	10	18	60

Length of Stay by Diagnosis and Operation, Western Region, 2008

Western Region, October 2006–September 2007 Data, by Diagnosis

771: PERINATAL INFECTION

Type of Patients	Observed Patients	Avg. Stay	Vari-ance	Percentiles						
				10th	25th	50th	75th	90th	95th	99th
1. SINGLE DX										
A. Not Operated										
0–19 Years	254	3.4	5	2	2	3	4	7	8	13
20–34	0									
35–49	0									
50–64	0									
65+	0									
B. Operated										
0–19 Years	0									
20–34	0									
35–49	0									
50–64	0									
65+	0									
2. MULTIPLE DX										
A. Not Operated										
0–19 Years	1,694	5.7	24	2	2	4	7	11	14	22
20–34	0									
35–49	0									
50–64	0									
65+	0									
B. Operated										
0–19 Years	53	8.4	44	2	4	8	10	17	30	>99
20–34	0									
35–49	0									
50–64	0									
65+	0									
SUBTOTALS:										
1. SINGLE DX										
A. Not Operated	254	3.4	5	2	2	3	4	7	8	13
B. Operated	0									
2. MULTIPLE DX										
A. Not Operated	1,694	5.7	24	2	2	4	7	11	14	22
B. Operated	53	8.4	44	2	4	8	10	17	30	>99
1. SINGLE DX	254	3.4	5	2	2	3	4	7	8	13
2. MULTIPLE DX	1,747	5.7	25	2	3	4	7	11	14	24
A. NOT OPERATED	1,948	5.4	22	2	2	4	7	10	14	21
B. OPERATED	53	8.4	44	2	4	8	10	17	30	>99
TOTAL										
0–19 Years	2,001	5.5	23	2	2	4	7	10	14	22
20–34	0									
35–49	0									
50–64	0									
65+	0									
GRAND TOTAL	2,001	5.5	23	2	2	4	7	10	14	22

771.81: NB SEPTICEMIA

Type of Patients	Observed Patients	Avg. Stay	Vari-ance	Percentiles						
				10th	25th	50th	75th	90th	95th	99th
1. SINGLE DX										
A. Not Operated										
0–19 Years	103	3.2	4	2	2	3	4	7	7	10
20–34	0									
35–49	0									
50–64	0									
65+	0									
B. Operated										
0–19 Years	0									
20–34	0									
35–49	0									
50–64	0									
65+	0									
2. MULTIPLE DX										
A. Not Operated										
0–19 Years	531	6.5	39	2	3	5	8	13	16	29
20–34	0									
35–49	0									
50–64	0									
65+	0									
B. Operated										
0–19 Years	19	11.2	84	3	5	9	17	30	30	>99
20–34	0									
35–49	0									
50–64	0									
65+	0									
SUBTOTALS:										
1. SINGLE DX										
A. Not Operated	103	3.2	4	2	2	3	4	7	7	10
B. Operated	0									
2. MULTIPLE DX										
A. Not Operated	531	6.5	39	2	3	5	8	13	16	29
B. Operated	19	11.2	84	3	5	9	17	30	30	>99
1. SINGLE DX	103	3.2	4	2	2	3	4	7	7	10
2. MULTIPLE DX	550	6.7	41	2	3	5	9	14	18	38
A. NOT OPERATED	634	6.0	35	2	2	4	7	11	15	27
B. OPERATED	19	11.2	84	3	5	9	17	30	30	>99
TOTAL										
0–19 Years	653	6.1	37	2	2	4	8	13	16	30
20–34	0									
35–49	0									
50–64	0									
65+	0									
GRAND TOTAL	653	6.1	37	2	2	4	8	13	16	30

771.82: NB URINARY TRACT INFECT

Type of Patients	Observed Patients	Avg. Stay	Vari-ance	Percentiles						
				10th	25th	50th	75th	90th	95th	99th
1. SINGLE DX										
A. Not Operated										
0–19 Years	51	3.9	3	2	3	4	5	6	7	7
20–34	0									
35–49	0									
50–64	0									
65+	0									
B. Operated										
0–19 Years	0									
20–34	0									
35–49	0									
50–64	0									
65+	0									
2. MULTIPLE DX										
A. Not Operated										
0–19 Years	526	5.9	13	2	3	5	8	10	13	15
20–34	0									
35–49	0									
50–64	0									
65+	0									
B. Operated										
0–19 Years	14	8.1	4	7	7	8	10	10	10	10
20–34	0									
35–49	0									
50–64	0									
65+	0									
SUBTOTALS:										
1. SINGLE DX										
A. Not Operated	51	3.9	3	2	3	4	5	6	7	7
B. Operated	0									
2. MULTIPLE DX										
A. Not Operated	526	5.9	13	2	3	5	8	10	13	15
B. Operated	14	8.1	4	7	7	8	10	10	10	10
1. SINGLE DX	51	3.9	3	2	3	4	5	6	7	7
2. MULTIPLE DX	540	6.0	12	2	3	5	8	10	13	15
A. NOT OPERATED	577	5.7	12	2	3	5	7	10	13	15
B. OPERATED	14	8.1	4	7	7	8	10	10	10	10
TOTAL										
0–19 Years	591	5.8	12	2	3	5	8	10	13	15
20–34	0									
35–49	0									
50–64	0									
65+	0									
GRAND TOTAL	591	5.8	12	2	3	5	8	10	13	15

Length of Stay by Diagnosis and Operation, Western Region, 2008

Western Region, October 2006–September 2007 Data, by Diagnosis

771.89: PERINATAL INFECTION NEC

Type of Patients	Observed Patients	Avg. Stay	Vari-ance	10th	25th	50th	75th	90th	95th	99th
1. SINGLE DX										
A. Not Operated										
0–19 Years	16	3.2	10	1	2	2	3	5	14	14
20–34	0									
35–49	0									
50–64	0									
65+	0									
B. Operated										
0–19 Years	0									
20–34	0									
35–49	0									
50–64	0									
65+	0									
2. MULTIPLE DX										
A. Not Operated										
0–19 Years	376	4.2	16	1	2	3	5	8	11	22
20–34	0									
35–49	0									
50–64	0									
65+	0									
B. Operated										
0–19 Years	6	3.3	8	1	2	3	9	>99	>99	>99
20–34	0									
35–49	0									
50–64	0									
65+	0									
SUBTOTALS:										
1. SINGLE DX A. Not Operated	16	3.2	10	1	2	2	3	5	14	14
B. Operated	0									
2. MULTIPLE DX A. Not Operated	376	4.2	16	1	2	3	5	8	11	22
B. Operated	6	3.3	8	1	2	3	9	>99	>99	>99
1. SINGLE DX	16	3.2	10	1	2	2	3	5	14	14
2. MULTIPLE DX	382	4.2	16	1	2	3	5	8	11	26
A. NOT OPERATED	392	4.2	16	1	2	3	5	8	11	22
B. OPERATED	6	3.3	8	1	2	3	9	>99	>99	>99
TOTAL										
0–19 Years	398	4.2	16	1	2	3	5	8	11	26
20–34	0									
35–49	0									
50–64	0									
65+	0									
GRAND TOTAL	398	4.2	16	1	2	3	5	8	11	26

772: FETAL/NEONATAL HEMOR

Type of Patients	Observed Patients	Avg. Stay	Vari-ance	10th	25th	50th	75th	90th	95th	99th
1. SINGLE DX										
A. Not Operated										
0–19 Years	10	1.6	<1	1	1	1	2	3	3	3
20–34	0									
35–49	0									
50–64	0									
65+	0									
B. Operated										
0–19 Years	0									
20–34	0									
35–49	0									
50–64	0									
65+	0									
2. MULTIPLE DX										
A. Not Operated										
0–19 Years	49	5.1	53	1	1	2	5	14	20	42
20–34	0									
35–49	0									
50–64	0									
65+	0									
B. Operated										
0–19 Years	5	37.0	550	12	28	30	40	75	75	75
20–34	0									
35–49	0									
50–64	0									
65+	0									
SUBTOTALS:										
1. SINGLE DX A. Not Operated	10	1.6	<1	1	1	1	2	3	3	3
B. Operated	0									
2. MULTIPLE DX A. Not Operated	49	5.1	53	1	1	2	5	14	20	42
B. Operated	5	37.0	550	12	28	30	40	75	75	75
1. SINGLE DX	10	1.6	<1	1	1	1	2	3	3	3
2. MULTIPLE DX	54	8.1	177	1	1	3	7	22	40	75
A. NOT OPERATED	59	4.5	46	1	1	2	5	9	20	42
B. OPERATED	5	37.0	550	12	28	30	40	75	75	75
TOTAL										
0–19 Years	64	7.0	155	1	1	2	5	20	30	75
20–34	0									
35–49	0									
50–64	0									
65+	0									
GRAND TOTAL	64	7.0	155	1	1	2	5	20	30	75

773: NB HEMOLY DIS-ISOIMMUN

Type of Patients	Observed Patients	Avg. Stay	Vari-ance	10th	25th	50th	75th	90th	95th	99th
1. SINGLE DX										
A. Not Operated										
0–19 Years	377	1.8	<1	1	1	2	2	3	3	5
20–34	0									
35–49	0									
50–64	0									
65+	0									
B. Operated										
0–19 Years	1	3.0	0	3	3	3	3	3	3	3
20–34	0									
35–49	0									
50–64	0									
65+	0									
2. MULTIPLE DX										
A. Not Operated										
0–19 Years	251	2.5	4	1	1	2	3	4	6	13
20–34	0									
35–49	0									
50–64	0									
65+	0									
B. Operated										
0–19 Years	2	6.0	8	4	4	8	8	8	8	8
20–34	0									
35–49	0									
50–64	0									
65+	0									
SUBTOTALS:										
1. SINGLE DX A. Not Operated	377	1.8	<1	1	1	2	2	3	3	5
B. Operated	1	3.0	0	3	3	3	3	3	3	3
2. MULTIPLE DX A. Not Operated	251	2.5	4	1	1	2	3	4	6	13
B. Operated	2	6.0	8	4	4	8	8	8	8	8
1. SINGLE DX	378	1.8	<1	1	1	2	2	3	3	5
2. MULTIPLE DX	253	2.5	4	1	1	2	3	4	7	13
A. NOT OPERATED	628	2.1	2	1	1	2	2	3	4	8
B. OPERATED	3	5.0	7	3	3	4	8	8	8	8
TOTAL										
0–19 Years	631	2.1	2	1	1	2	2	3	4	8
20–34	0									
35–49	0									
50–64	0									
65+	0									
GRAND TOTAL	631	2.1	2	1	1	2	2	3	4	8

Western Region, October 2006–September 2007 Data, by Diagnosis

773.1: NB HEMOLY DIS-ABO ISOIMM

Type of Patients	Observed Patients	Avg. Stay	Vari-ance	Percentiles						
				10th	25th	50th	75th	90th	95th	99th
1. SINGLE DX										
A. Not Operated										
0–19 Years	311	1.8	<1	1	1	2	2	3	3	4
20–34	0									
35–49	0									
50–64	0									
65+	0									
B. Operated										
0–19 Years	1	3.0	0	3	3	3	3	3	3	3
20–34	0									
35–49	0									
50–64	0									
65+	0									
2. MULTIPLE DX										
A. Not Operated										
0–19 Years	189	2.3	2	1	1	2	3	4	4	9
20–34	0									
35–49	0									
50–64	0									
65+	0									
B. Operated										
0–19 Years	0									
20–34	0									
35–49	0									
50–64	0									
65+	0									
SUBTOTALS:										
1. SINGLE DX										
A. Not Operated	311	1.8	<1	1	1	2	2	3	3	4
B. Operated	1	3.0	0	3	3	3	3	3	3	3
2. MULTIPLE DX										
A. Not Operated	189	2.3	2	1	1	2	3	4	4	9
B. Operated	0									
1. SINGLE DX	312	1.8	<1	1	1	2	2	3	3	4
2. MULTIPLE DX	189	2.3	2	1	1	2	3	4	4	9
A. NOT OPERATED	500	2.0	1	1	1	2	2	3	4	7
B. OPERATED	1	3.0	0	3	3	3	3	3	3	3
TOTAL										
0–19 Years	501	2.0	1	1	1	2	2	3	4	7
20–34	0									
35–49	0									
50–64	0									
65+	0									
GRAND TOTAL	501	2.0	1	1	1	2	2	3	4	7

774: OTHER PERINATAL JAUNDICE

Type of Patients	Observed Patients	Avg. Stay	Vari-ance	Percentiles						
				10th	25th	50th	75th	90th	95th	99th
1. SINGLE DX										
A. Not Operated										
0–19 Years	6,248	1.6	<1	1	1	1	2	2	2	3
20–34	0									
35–49	0									
50–64	0									
65+	0									
B. Operated										
0–19 Years	11	1.9	<1	1	2	2	2	2	3	3
20–34	0									
35–49	0									
50–64	0									
65+	0									
2. MULTIPLE DX										
A. Not Operated										
0–19 Years	3,035	2.1	3	1	1	2	2	3	4	9
20–34	0									
35–49	0									
50–64	0									
65+	0									
B. Operated										
0–19 Years	26	4.1	21	1	1	2	5	12	13	20
20–34	0									
35–49	0									
50–64	0									
65+	0									
SUBTOTALS:										
1. SINGLE DX										
A. Not Operated	6,248	1.6	<1	1	1	1	2	2	3	3
B. Operated	11	1.9	<1	2	2	2	2	3	3	3
2. MULTIPLE DX										
A. Not Operated	3,035	2.1	3	1	1	2	2	3	4	9
B. Operated	26	4.1	21	1	1	2	5	12	13	20
1. SINGLE DX	6,259	1.6	<1	1	1	1	2	2	3	3
2. MULTIPLE DX	3,061	2.1	3	1	1	2	2	3	4	9
A. NOT OPERATED	9,283	1.7	1	1	1	2	2	3	3	6
B. OPERATED	37	3.5	16	1	2	2	3	9	13	20
TOTAL										
0–19 Years	9,320	1.7	1	1	1	2	2	3	3	6
20–34	0									
35–49	0									
50–64	0									
65+	0									
GRAND TOTAL	9,320	1.7	1	1	1	2	2	3	3	6

774.2: NB JAUNDICE-PRETERM DEL

Type of Patients	Observed Patients	Avg. Stay	Vari-ance	Percentiles						
				10th	25th	50th	75th	90th	95th	99th
1. SINGLE DX										
A. Not Operated										
0–19 Years	376	1.6	<1	1	1	1	2	2	3	4
20–34	0									
35–49	0									
50–64	0									
65+	0									
B. Operated										
0–19 Years	2	2.0	2	1	1	1	3	3	3	3
20–34	0									
35–49	0									
50–64	0									
65+	0									
2. MULTIPLE DX										
A. Not Operated										
0–19 Years	357	2.3	4	1	1	2	2	4	6	13
20–34	0									
35–49	0									
50–64	0									
65+	0									
B. Operated										
0–19 Years	7	7.3	44	1	3	6	12	20	20	20
20–34	0									
35–49	0									
50–64	0									
65+	0									
SUBTOTALS:										
1. SINGLE DX										
A. Not Operated	376	1.6	<1	1	1	1	2	2	3	4
B. Operated	2	2.0	2	1	1	1	3	3	3	3
2. MULTIPLE DX										
A. Not Operated	357	2.3	4	1	1	2	2	4	6	13
B. Operated	7	7.3	44	1	3	6	12	20	20	20
1. SINGLE DX	378	1.6	<1	1	1	1	2	2	3	4
2. MULTIPLE DX	364	2.4	5	1	1	2	2	4	6	13
A. NOT OPERATED	733	1.9	3	1	1	2	2	3	4	8
B. OPERATED	9	6.1	38	1	3	3	6	20	20	20
TOTAL										
0–19 Years	742	2.0	3	1	1	2	2	3	4	10
20–34	0									
35–49	0									
50–64	0									
65+	0									
GRAND TOTAL	742	2.0	3	1	1	2	2	3	4	10

Length of Stay by Diagnosis and Operation, Western Region, 2008

Western Region, October 2006–September 2007 Data, by Diagnosis

774.39: DELAY CONJ JAUNDICE NEC

Type of Patients	Observed Patients	Avg. Stay	Vari-ance	10th	25th	50th	75th	90th	95th	99th
1. SINGLE DX										
A. Not Operated										
0–19 Years	272	1.7	<1	1	1	2	2	2	3	4
20–34	0									
35–49	0									
50–64	0									
65+	0									
B. Operated										
0–19 Years	0									
20–34	0									
35–49	0									
50–64	0									
65+	0									
2. MULTIPLE DX										
A. Not Operated										
0–19 Years	176	2.3	5	1	1	2	2	4	6	11
20–34	0									
35–49	0									
50–64	0									
65+	0									
B. Operated										
0–19 Years	0									
20–34	0									
35–49	0									
50–64	0									
65+	0									
SUBTOTALS:										
1. SINGLE DX										
A. Not Operated	272	1.7	<1	1	1	2	2	2	3	4
B. Operated	0									
2. MULTIPLE DX										
A. Not Operated	176	2.3	5	1	1	2	2	4	6	11
B. Operated	0									
1. SINGLE DX	272	1.7	<1	1	1	2	2	2	3	4
2. MULTIPLE DX	176	2.3	5	1	1	2	2	4	6	11
A. NOT OPERATED	448	1.9	3	1	1	2	2	3	4	8
B. OPERATED	0									
TOTAL										
0–19 Years	448	1.9	3	1	1	2	2	3	4	8
20–34	0									
35–49	0									
50–64	0									
65+	0									
GRAND TOTAL	448	1.9	3	1	1	2	2	3	4	8

774.6: FETAL/NN JAUNDICE NOS

Type of Patients	Observed Patients	Avg. Stay	Vari-ance	10th	25th	50th	75th	90th	95th	99th
1. SINGLE DX										
A. Not Operated										
0–19 Years	5,562	1.6	<1	1	1	1	2	2	3	3
20–34	0									
35–49	0									
50–64	0									
65+	0									
B. Operated										
0–19 Years	9	1.9	<1	1	2	2	2	2	2	2
20–34	0									
35–49	0									
50–64	0									
65+	0									
2. MULTIPLE DX										
A. Not Operated										
0–19 Years	2,452	2.0	2	1	1	2	2	3	4	8
20–34	0									
35–49	0									
50–64	0									
65+	0									
B. Operated										
0–19 Years	18	2.4	4	1	1	2	3	5	9	9
20–34	0									
35–49	0									
50–64	0									
65+	0									
SUBTOTALS:										
1. SINGLE DX										
A. Not Operated	5,562	1.6	<1	1	1	1	2	2	3	3
B. Operated	9	1.9	<1	1	2	2	2	2	2	2
2. MULTIPLE DX										
A. Not Operated	2,452	2.0	2	1	1	2	2	3	4	8
B. Operated	18	2.4	4	1	1	2	3	5	9	9
1. SINGLE DX	5,571	1.6	<1	1	1	1	2	2	3	3
2. MULTIPLE DX	2,470	2.0	2	1	1	2	2	3	4	8
A. NOT OPERATED	8,014	1.7	1	1	1	2	2	3	3	5
B. OPERATED	27	2.2	3	1	1	2	2	3	5	9
TOTAL										
0–19 Years	8,041	1.7	1	1	1	2	2	3	3	5
20–34	0									
35–49	0									
50–64	0									
65+	0									
GRAND TOTAL	8,041	1.7	1	1	1	2	2	3	3	5

775: NB ENDOCR/METABOL DIS

Type of Patients	Observed Patients	Avg. Stay	Vari-ance	10th	25th	50th	75th	90th	95th	99th
1. SINGLE DX										
A. Not Operated										
0–19 Years	14	2.5	5	1	1	2	3	6	8	8
20–34	0									
35–49	0									
50–64	0									
65+	0									
B. Operated										
0–19 Years	0									
20–34	0									
35–49	0									
50–64	0									
65+	0									
2. MULTIPLE DX										
A. Not Operated										
0–19 Years	440	3.2	11	1	1	2	4	7	9	18
20–34	0									
35–49	0									
50–64	0									
65+	0									
B. Operated										
0–19 Years	9	11.7	114	1	3	9	21	29	29	29
20–34	0									
35–49	0									
50–64	0									
65+	0									
SUBTOTALS:										
1. SINGLE DX										
A. Not Operated	14	2.5	5	1	1	2	3	6	8	8
B. Operated	0									
2. MULTIPLE DX										
A. Not Operated	440	3.2	11	1	1	2	4	7	9	18
B. Operated	9	11.7	114	1	3	9	21	29	29	29
1. SINGLE DX	14	2.5	5	1	1	2	3	6	8	8
2. MULTIPLE DX	449	3.4	14	1	1	2	4	7	10	24
A. NOT OPERATED	454	3.2	11	1	1	2	4	7	9	18
B. OPERATED	9	11.7	114	1	3	9	21	29	29	29
TOTAL										
0–19 Years	463	3.4	14	1	1	2	4	7	9	24
20–34	0									
35–49	0									
50–64	0									
65+	0									
GRAND TOTAL	463	3.4	14	1	1	2	4	7	9	24

Length of Stay by Diagnosis and Operation, Western Region, 2008

658

Western Region, October 2006–September 2007 Data, by Diagnosis

775.5: NEONATAL DEHYDRATION

Type of Patients	Observed Patients	Avg. Stay	Variance	Percentiles 10th	25th	50th	75th	90th	95th	99th
1. SINGLE DX										
A. Not Operated										
0–19 Years	7	1.9	1	1	1	2	2	4	4	4
20–34	0									
35–49	0									
50–64	0									
65+	0									
B. Operated										
0–19 Years	0									
20–34	0									
35–49	0									
50–64	0									
65+	0									
2. MULTIPLE DX										
A. Not Operated										
0–19 Years	342	2.5	5	1	1	2	3	4	5	10
20–34	0									
35–49	0									
50–64	0									
65+	0									
B. Operated										
0–19 Years	4	7.5	81	2	3	4	21	21	21	21
20–34	0									
35–49	0									
50–64	0									
65+	0									
SUBTOTALS:										
1. SINGLE DX										
A. Not Operated	7	1.9	1	1	1	2	2	4	4	4
B. Operated	0									
2. MULTIPLE DX										
A. Not Operated	342	2.5	5	1	1	2	3	4	5	10
B. Operated	4	7.5	81	2	3	4	21	21	21	21
1. SINGLE DX	7	1.9	1	1	1	2	2	4	4	4
2. MULTIPLE DX	346	2.5	6	1	1	2	3	4	6	10
A. NOT OPERATED	349	2.5	5	1	1	2	3	4	5	10
B. OPERATED	4	7.5	81	2	3	4	21	21	21	21
TOTAL										
0–19 Years	353	2.5	6	1	1	2	3	4	6	10
20–34	0									
35–49	0									
50–64	0									
65+	0									
GRAND TOTAL	353	2.5	6	1	1	2	3	4	6	10

776: HEMATOLOGICAL DIS OF NB

Type of Patients	Observed Patients	Avg. Stay	Variance	Percentiles 10th	25th	50th	75th	90th	95th	99th
1. SINGLE DX										
A. Not Operated										
0–19 Years	7	2.0	1	1	1	2	3	4	4	4
20–34	0									
35–49	0									
50–64	0									
65+	0									
B. Operated										
0–19 Years	0									
20–34	0									
35–49	0									
50–64	0									
65+	0									
2. MULTIPLE DX										
A. Not Operated										
0–19 Years	47	6.8	66	1	2	5	8	16	22	44
20–34	0									
35–49	0									
50–64	0									
65+	0									
B. Operated										
0–19 Years	2	11.0	18	8	8	11	14	14	14	14
20–34	0									
35–49	0									
50–64	0									
65+	0									
SUBTOTALS:										
1. SINGLE DX										
A. Not Operated	7	2.0	1	1	1	2	3	4	4	4
B. Operated	0									
2. MULTIPLE DX										
A. Not Operated	47	6.8	66	1	2	5	8	16	22	44
B. Operated	2	11.0	18	8	8	11	14	14	14	14
1. SINGLE DX	7	2.0	1	1	1	2	3	4	4	4
2. MULTIPLE DX	49	7.0	64	1	2	5	8	16	22	44
A. NOT OPERATED	54	6.2	60	1	2	4	6	14	22	44
B. OPERATED	2	11.0	18	8	8	11	14	14	14	14
TOTAL										
0–19 Years	56	6.4	59	1	2	4	8	14	22	44
20–34	0									
35–49	0									
50–64	0									
65+	0									
GRAND TOTAL	56	6.4	59	1	2	4	8	14	22	44

777: PERINATAL GI SYSTEM DIS

Type of Patients	Observed Patients	Avg. Stay	Variance	Percentiles 10th	25th	50th	75th	90th	95th	99th
1. SINGLE DX										
A. Not Operated										
0–19 Years	18	1.8	2	1	1	1	2	5	5	5
20–34	0									
35–49	0									
50–64	0									
65+	0									
B. Operated										
0–19 Years	0									
20–34	0									
35–49	0									
50–64	0									
65+	0									
2. MULTIPLE DX										
A. Not Operated										
0–19 Years	143	4.8	55	1	1	2	4	14	19	44
20–34	0									
35–49	0									
50–64	0									
65+	0									
B. Operated										
0–19 Years	20	37.9	978	5	13	48	84	>99	>99	>99
20–34	0									
35–49	0									
50–64	0									
65+	0									
SUBTOTALS:										
1. SINGLE DX										
A. Not Operated	18	1.8	2	1	1	1	2	5	5	5
B. Operated	0									
2. MULTIPLE DX										
A. Not Operated	143	4.8	55	1	1	2	4	14	19	44
B. Operated	20	37.9	978	5	13	48	84	>99	>99	>99
1. SINGLE DX	18	1.8	2	1	1	1	2	5	5	5
2. MULTIPLE DX	163	8.9	282	1	2	2	7	42	77	>99
A. NOT OPERATED	161	4.5	49	1	1	2	4	11	18	44
B. OPERATED	20	37.9	978	5	13	48	84	>99	>99	>99
TOTAL										
0–19 Years	181	8.2	258	1	1	2	6	30	70	>99
20–34	0									
35–49	0									
50–64	0									
65+	0									
GRAND TOTAL	181	8.2	258	1	1	2	6	30	70	>99

Length of Stay by Diagnosis and Operation, Western Region, 2008

Western Region, October 2006–September 2007 Data, by Diagnosis

778: INTEGUMENT/TEMP COND NB

Type of Patients	Observed Patients	Avg. Stay	Variance	10th	25th	50th	75th	90th	95th	99th
1. SINGLE DX										
A. Not Operated										
0–19 Years	272	2.5	1	2	2	2	3	3	5	7
20–34	0									
35–49	0									
50–64	0									
65+	0									
B. Operated										
0–19 Years	2	2.0	0	2	2	2	2	2	2	2
20–34	0									
35–49	0									
50–64	0									
65+	0									
2. MULTIPLE DX										
A. Not Operated										
0–19 Years	549	3.0	6	2	2	2	3	5	7	14
20–34	0									
35–49	0									
50–64	0									
65+	0									
B. Operated										
0–19 Years	4	1.3	<1	1	1	1	1	2	2	2
20–34	0									
35–49	0									
50–64	0									
65+	0									
SUBTOTALS:										
1. SINGLE DX										
A. Not Operated	272	2.5	1	2	2	2	3	3	5	7
B. Operated	2	2.0	0	2	2	2	2	2	2	2
2. MULTIPLE DX										
A. Not Operated	549	3.0	6	2	2	2	3	5	7	14
B. Operated	4	1.3	<1	1	1	1	1	2	2	2
1. SINGLE DX	274	2.5	1	2	2	2	3	3	5	7
2. MULTIPLE DX	553	3.0	6	2	2	2	3	5	7	14
A. NOT OPERATED	821	2.9	4	2	2	2	3	4	6	10
B. OPERATED	6	1.5	<1	1	1	1	2	2	2	2
TOTAL										
0–19 Years	827	2.8	4	2	2	2	3	4	6	10
20–34	0									
35–49	0									
50–64	0									
65+	0									
GRAND TOTAL	827	2.8	4	2	2	2	3	4	6	10

778.4: NB TEMP REGUL DISTURBNEC

Type of Patients	Observed Patients	Avg. Stay	Variance	10th	25th	50th	75th	90th	95th	99th
1. SINGLE DX										
A. Not Operated										
0–19 Years	251	2.5	<1	2	2	2	3	3	4	6
20–34	0									
35–49	0									
50–64	0									
65+	0									
B. Operated										
0–19 Years	2	2.0	0	2	2	2	2	2	2	2
20–34	0									
35–49	0									
50–64	0									
65+	0									
2. MULTIPLE DX										
A. Not Operated										
0–19 Years	414	2.8	2	2	2	2	3	4	6	8
20–34	0									
35–49	0									
50–64	0									
65+	0									
B. Operated										
0–19 Years	0									
20–34	0									
35–49	0									
50–64	0									
65+	0									
SUBTOTALS:										
1. SINGLE DX										
A. Not Operated	251	2.5	<1	2	2	2	3	3	4	6
B. Operated	2	2.0	0	2	2	2	2	2	2	2
2. MULTIPLE DX										
A. Not Operated	414	2.8	2	2	2	2	3	4	6	8
B. Operated	0									
1. SINGLE DX	253	2.5	<1	2	2	2	3	3	4	6
2. MULTIPLE DX	414	2.8	2	2	2	2	3	4	6	8
A. NOT OPERATED	665	2.7	2	2	2	2	3	4	5	8
B. OPERATED	2	2.0	0	2	2	2	2	2	2	2
TOTAL										
0–19 Years	667	2.7	2	2	2	2	3	4	5	8
20–34	0									
35–49	0									
50–64	0									
65+	0									
GRAND TOTAL	667	2.7	2	2	2	2	3	4	5	8

779: OTH PERINATAL CONDITION

Type of Patients	Observed Patients	Avg. Stay	Variance	10th	25th	50th	75th	90th	95th	99th
1. SINGLE DX										
A. Not Operated										
0–19 Years	143	2.6	5	1	1	2	3	5	7	12
20–34	0									
35–49	0									
50–64	0									
65+	0									
B. Operated										
0–19 Years	2	1.5	<1	1	1	2	2	2	2	2
20–34	0									
35–49	0									
50–64	0									
65+	0									
2. MULTIPLE DX										
A. Not Operated										
0–19 Years	2,063	3.7	14	1	2	3	4	7	10	20
20–34	0									
35–49	0									
50–64	0									
65+	1	5.0	0	5	5	5	5	5	5	5
B. Operated										
0–19 Years	68	8.2	144	2	2	4	8	27	44	>99
20–34	0									
35–49	0									
50–64	0									
65+	0									
SUBTOTALS:										
1. SINGLE DX										
A. Not Operated	143	2.6	5	1	1	2	3	5	7	12
B. Operated	2	1.5	<1	1	1	2	2	2	2	2
2. MULTIPLE DX										
A. Not Operated	2,064	3.7	14	1	2	3	4	7	10	20
B. Operated	68	8.2	144	2	2	4	8	27	44	>99
1. SINGLE DX	145	2.6	5	1	1	2	3	5	7	12
2. MULTIPLE DX	2,132	3.9	18	1	2	3	4	8	11	23
A. NOT OPERATED	2,207	3.7	13	1	2	3	4	7	10	20
B. OPERATED	70	8.0	141	2	2	4	8	21	44	>99
TOTAL										
0–19 Years	2,276	3.8	18	1	2	3	4	7	10	22
20–34	0									
35–49	0									
50–64	0									
65+	1	5.0	0	5	5	5	5	5	5	5
GRAND TOTAL	2,277	3.8	18	1	2	3	4	7	10	22

Length of Stay by Diagnosis and Operation, Western Region, 2008

Western Region, October 2006–September 2007 Data, by Diagnosis

779.3: NB FEEDING PROBLEMS

Type of Patients	Observed Patients	Avg. Stay	Variance	Percentiles 10th	25th	50th	75th	90th	95th	99th
1. SINGLE DX										
A. Not Operated										
0–19 Years	79	2.1	3	1	1	2	3	4	5	11
20–34	0									
35–49	0									
50–64	0									
65+	0									
B. Operated										
0–19 Years	1	2.0	0	2	2	2	2	2	2	2
20–34	0									
35–49	0									
50–64	0									
65+	0									
2. MULTIPLE DX										
A. Not Operated										
0–19 Years	391	4.0	23	1	1	2	4	8	14	26
20–34	0									
35–49	0									
50–64	0									
65+	0									
B. Operated										
0–19 Years	11	21.3	443	2	2	15	34	51	65	65
20–34	0									
35–49	0									
50–64	0									
65+	0									
SUBTOTALS:										
1. SINGLE DX										
A. Not Operated	79	2.1	3	1	1	2	3	4	5	11
B. Operated	1	2.0	0	2	2	2	2	2	2	2
2. MULTIPLE DX										
A. Not Operated	391	4.0	23	1	1	2	4	8	14	26
B. Operated	11	21.3	443	2	2	15	34	51	65	65
1. SINGLE DX	80	2.1	3	1	1	2	2	4	5	11
2. MULTIPLE DX	402	4.4	41	1	1	2	5	10	15	28
A. NOT OPERATED	470	3.6	20	1	1	2	4	8	12	26
B. OPERATED	12	19.7	434	2	2	12	28	51	65	65
TOTAL										
0–19 Years	482	4.0	36	1	1	2	4	8	14	28
20–34	0									
35–49	0									
50–64	0									
65+	0									
GRAND TOTAL	482	4.0	36	1	1	2	4	8	14	28

779.89: PERINATAL CONDITION NEC

Type of Patients	Observed Patients	Avg. Stay	Variance	Percentiles 10th	25th	50th	75th	90th	95th	99th
1. SINGLE DX										
A. Not Operated										
0–19 Years	5	2.4	2	1	2	2	2	5	5	5
20–34	0									
35–49	0									
50–64	0									
65+	0									
B. Operated										
0–19 Years	0									
20–34	0									
35–49	0									
50–64	0									
65+	0									
2. MULTIPLE DX										
A. Not Operated										
0–19 Years	1,508	3.4	7	1	2	3	4	7	9	15
20–34	0									
35–49	0									
50–64	0									
65+	0									
B. Operated										
0–19 Years	55	5.3	47	1	2	3	5	11	21	>99
20–34	0									
35–49	0									
50–64	0									
65+	0									
SUBTOTALS:										
1. SINGLE DX										
A. Not Operated	5	2.4	2	1	2	2	2	5	5	5
B. Operated	0									
2. MULTIPLE DX										
A. Not Operated	1,508	3.4	7	1	2	3	4	7	9	15
B. Operated	55	5.3	47	1	2	3	5	11	21	>99
1. SINGLE DX	5	2.4	2	1	2	2	2	5	5	5
2. MULTIPLE DX	1,563	3.4	9	1	2	3	4	7	9	16
A. NOT OPERATED	1,513	3.4	7	1	2	3	4	7	9	15
B. OPERATED	55	5.3	47	1	2	3	5	11	21	>99
TOTAL										
0–19 Years	1,568	3.4	9	1	2	3	4	7	9	16
20–34	0									
35–49	0									
50–64	0									
65+	0									
GRAND TOTAL	1,568	3.4	9	1	2	3	4	7	9	16

780: GENERAL SYMPTOMS

Type of Patients	Observed Patients	Avg. Stay	Variance	Percentiles 10th	25th	50th	75th	90th	95th	99th
1. SINGLE DX										
A. Not Operated										
0–19 Years	1,648	2.0	1	1	1	2	2	3	4	7
20–34	234	2.3	4	1	1	2	3	4	6	11
35–49	201	2.4	4	1	1	2	3	5	6	7
50–64	160	2.0	2	1	1	1	2	4	6	8
65+	102	1.5	<1	1	1	1	2	2	3	5
B. Operated										
0–19 Years	6	1.7	1	1	1	1	1	3	3	3
20–34	2	2.0	0	2	2	2	2	2	2	2
35–49	7	3.0	8	1	1	2	3	9	9	9
50–64	2	1.0	0	1	1	1	1	1	1	1
65+	2	1.0	0	1	1	1	1	1	1	1
2. MULTIPLE DX										
A. Not Operated										
0–19 Years	5,413	2.3	4	1	1	2	3	4	5	9
20–34	3,870	2.7	7	1	1	2	3	5	7	12
35–49	8,082	2.8	8	1	1	2	3	5	7	13
50–64	14,989	2.9	8	1	1	2	3	5	7	14
65+	36,998	2.9	6	1	1	2	4	5	7	12
B. Operated										
0–19 Years	41	6.2	80	1	2	3	8	12	17	52
20–34	73	6.0	88	1	1	3	6	12	20	68
35–49	132	6.2	60	1	1	3	8	15	20	65
50–64	249	6.8	51	1	2	5	5	15	21	35
65+	609	6.5	30	1	3	5	5	13	16	32
SUBTOTALS:										
1. SINGLE DX										
A. Not Operated	2,345	2.0	2	1	1	2	2	4	5	7
B. Operated	19	2.1	4	1	1	1	3	3	9	9
2. MULTIPLE DX										
A. Not Operated	69,352	2.8	7	1	1	2	3	5	7	13
B. Operated	1,104	6.5	44	1	2	5	8	13	17	33
1. SINGLE DX	2,364	2.0	2	1	1	2	2	4	5	7
2. MULTIPLE DX	70,456	2.9	7	1	1	2	3	5	7	13
A. NOT OPERATED	71,697	2.8	7	1	1	2	3	5	7	13
B. OPERATED	1,123	6.4	44	1	2	5	8	13	17	33
TOTAL										
0–19 Years	7,108	2.3	4	1	1	2	3	4	5	9
20–34	4,179	2.8	9	1	1	2	3	5	7	13
35–49	8,422	2.9	9	1	1	2	3	6	7	14
50–64	15,400	2.9	9	1	1	2	3	6	8	15
65+	37,711	3.0	7	1	1	2	4	6	7	13
GRAND TOTAL	72,820	2.9	7	1	1	2	3	5	7	13

Length of Stay by Diagnosis and Operation, Western Region, 2008

Western Region, October 2006–September 2007 Data, by Diagnosis

780.02: TRANS ALTER AWARENESS

Type of Patients	Observed Patients	Avg. Stay	Variance	10th	25th	50th	75th	90th	95th	99th
1. SINGLE DX										
A. Not Operated										
0–19 Years	4	2.3	<1	2	2	2	2	3	3	3
20–34	4	2.8	5	1	1	2	6	6	6	6
35–49	3	2.7	<1	2	2	3	3	3	3	3
50–64	3	1.7	<1	1	1	2	2	2	2	2
65+	0									
B. Operated										
0–19 Years	0									
20–34	0									
35–49	0									
50–64	0									
65+	0									
2. MULTIPLE DX										
A. Not Operated										
0–19 Years	34	2.0	<1	1	1	2	3	3	4	4
20–34	22	3.1	1	2	2	3	4	4	5	6
35–49	31	3.1	3	1	2	3	4	4	7	8
50–64	55	3.1	9	1	2	2	3	5	8	21
65+	174	3.2	20	1	2	2	4	5	6	24
B. Operated										
0–19 Years	0									
20–34	0									
35–49	0									
50–64	0									
65+	1	2.0	0	2	2	2	2	2	2	2
SUBTOTALS:										
1. SINGLE DX										
A. Not Operated	14	2.4	1	1	2	2	2	3	3	6
B. Operated	0									
2. MULTIPLE DX										
A. Not Operated	316	3.0	13	1	2	2	4	5	6	17
B. Operated	1	2.0	0	2	2	2	2	2	2	2
1. SINGLE DX	14	2.4	1	1	2	2	2	3	3	6
2. MULTIPLE DX	317	3.0	13	1	2	2	4	5	6	17
A. NOT OPERATED	330	3.0	13	1	2	2	3	5	6	17
B. OPERATED	1	2.0	0	2	2	2	2	2	2	2
TOTAL										
0–19 Years	38	2.0	<1	1	1	2	3	3	4	4
20–34	26	3.0	2	2	2	3	4	5	6	6
35–49	34	3.1	3	1	2	3	4	6	7	8
50–64	58	3.0	9	1	2	2	3	5	6	21
65+	175	3.2	20	1	2	2	4	5	6	24
GRAND TOTAL	331	3.0	13	1	2	2	3	5	6	17

780.09: ALTER CONSCIOUSNESS NEC

Type of Patients	Observed Patients	Avg. Stay	Variance	10th	25th	50th	75th	90th	95th	99th
1. SINGLE DX										
A. Not Operated										
0–19 Years	25	1.7	<1	1	1	1	2	2	3	4
20–34	6	1.3	<1	1	1	1	1	3	3	3
35–49	4	1.0	0	1	1	1	1	1	1	1
50–64	4	1.8	<1	1	1	2	2	3	3	3
65+	8	1.6	<1	1	1	2	2	3	3	3
B. Operated										
0–19 Years	0									
20–34	0									
35–49	1	1.0	0	1	1	1	1	1	1	1
50–64	0									
65+	0									
2. MULTIPLE DX										
A. Not Operated										
0–19 Years	121	2.1	4	1	1	1	2	4	6	10
20–34	220	2.5	15	1	1	2	3	4	5	21
35–49	542	3.0	7	1	2	2	4	6	8	15
50–64	1,112	3.4	13	1	2	3	4	6	9	20
65+	2,927	3.6	10	1	2	3	4	7	9	16
B. Operated										
0–19 Years	1	1.0	0	1	1	1	1	1	1	1
20–34	1	10.0	0	10	10	10	10	10	10	10
35–49	8	5.4	24	1	2	2	7	12	12	12
50–64	15	8.0	39	1	2	7	13	16	22	22
65+	43	10.9	68	3	5	8	16	21	30	33
SUBTOTALS:										
1. SINGLE DX										
A. Not Operated	47	1.6	<1	1	1	1	2	3	3	4
B. Operated	1	1.0	0	1	1	1	1	1	1	1
2. MULTIPLE DX										
A. Not Operated	4,922	3.4	10	1	2	3	4	6	8	16
B. Operated	68	9.4	58	1	4	8	13	21	23	33
1. SINGLE DX	48	1.6	<1	1	1	2	2	3	3	4
2. MULTIPLE DX	4,990	3.5	12	1	2	3	4	7	9	17
A. NOT OPERATED	4,969	3.4	10	1	2	3	4	6	8	16
B. OPERATED	69	9.3	58	1	4	8	13	21	23	33
TOTAL										
0–19 Years	147	2.0	3	1	1	1	2	3	5	10
20–34	227	2.5	15	1	1	1	3	4	6	21
35–49	555	3.0	8	1	1	2	4	6	8	15
50–64	1,131	3.5	14	1	2	2	4	7	9	21
65+	2,978	3.7	11	2	2	3	4	7	9	17
GRAND TOTAL	5,038	3.5	11	1	2	3	4	7	9	17

780.2: SYNCOPE & COLLAPSE

Type of Patients	Observed Patients	Avg. Stay	Variance	10th	25th	50th	75th	90th	95th	99th
1. SINGLE DX										
A. Not Operated										
0–19 Years	69	1.5	1	1	1	1	2	2	3	7
20–34	43	1.5	1	1	1	1	2	3	4	6
35–49	49	1.5	1	1	1	1	2	2	4	5
50–64	63	1.5	<1	1	1	1	2	2	3	6
65+	51	1.2	<1	1	1	1	1	2	2	3
B. Operated										
0–19 Years	1	1.0	0	1	1	1	1	1	1	1
20–34	0									
35–49	1	1.0	0	1	1	1	1	1	1	1
50–64	2	1.0	0	1	1	1	1	1	1	1
2. MULTIPLE DX										
A. Not Operated										
0–19 Years	294	1.7	1	1	1	1	2	3	4	7
20–34	799	2.0	2	1	1	2	2	4	5	7
35–49	2,273	2.1	3	1	1	2	3	4	5	8
50–64	5,734	2.2	3	1	1	2	3	4	5	8
65+	19,124	2.5	4	1	1	2	3	5	6	9
B. Operated										
0–19 Years	2	11.0	70	5	5	5	17	17	17	17
20–34	11	3.2	4	1	2	3	4	6	7	7
35–49	33	4.8	16	1	2	4	6	10	14	17
50–64	98	5.6	28	1	2	4	6	12	16	35
65+	374	5.3	17	1	3	4	6	10	13	19
SUBTOTALS:										
1. SINGLE DX										
A. Not Operated	275	1.5	<1	1	1	1	2	2	3	6
B. Operated	4	1.0	0	1	1	1	1	1	1	1
2. MULTIPLE DX										
A. Not Operated	28,224	2.4	4	1	1	2	3	4	6	9
B. Operated	518	5.3	19	1	3	4	6	10	14	21
1. SINGLE DX	279	1.5	<1	1	1	1	2	2	3	6
2. MULTIPLE DX	28,742	2.4	4	1	1	2	3	5	6	10
A. NOT OPERATED	28,499	2.4	4	1	1	2	3	4	6	9
B. OPERATED	522	5.3	19	1	3	4	6	10	13	21
TOTAL										
0–19 Years	366	1.7	2	1	1	1	2	3	4	7
20–34	853	2.0	2	1	1	2	2	4	5	7
35–49	2,355	2.2	3	1	1	2	3	4	5	9
50–64	5,896	2.2	4	1	2	3	3	4	5	9
65+	19,551	2.5	4	1	1	3	3	5	6	10
GRAND TOTAL	29,021	2.4	4	1	2	3	3	5	6	10

Length of Stay by Diagnosis and Operation, Western Region, 2008

Western Region, October 2006–September 2007 Data, by Diagnosis

780.31: FEBRILE CONVULSIONS NOS

Type of Patients	Observed Patients	Avg. Stay	Vari-ance	10th	25th	50th	75th	90th	95th	99th
1. SINGLE DX										
A. Not Operated										
0–19 Years	158	1.7	<1	1	1	1	2	3	4	5
20–34	0									
35–49	0									
50–64	0									
65+	0									
B. Operated										
0–19 Years	0									
20–34	0									
35–49	0									
50–64	0									
65+	0									
2. MULTIPLE DX										
A. Not Operated										
0–19 Years	681	2.0	4	1	1	2	2	3	4	7
20–34	1	3.0	0	3	3	3	3	3	3	3
35–49	3	4.0	3	3	3	3	6	6	6	6
50–64	11	3.0	3	1	2	2	4	5	7	7
65+	5	3.6	3	1	3	4	4	6	6	6
B. Operated										
0–19 Years	1	3.0	0	3	3	3	3	3	3	3
20–34	0									
35–49	0									
50–64	0									
65+	0									
SUBTOTALS:										
1. SINGLE DX										
A. Not Operated	158	1.7	<1	1	1	1	2	3	4	5
B. Operated	0									
2. MULTIPLE DX										
A. Not Operated	701	2.1	4	1	1	2	2	3	5	7
B. Operated	1	3.0	0	3	3	3	3	3	3	3
1. SINGLE DX	158	1.7	<1	1	1	1	2	3	4	5
2. MULTIPLE DX	702	2.1	4	1	1	2	2	3	4	7
A. NOT OPERATED	859	2.0	3	1	1	2	2	3	4	7
B. OPERATED	1	3.0	0	3	3	3	3	3	3	3
TOTAL										
0–19 Years	840	2.0	3	1	1	2	2	3	4	7
20–34	1	3.0	0	3	3	3	3	3	3	3
35–49	3	4.0	3	3	3	3	6	6	6	6
50–64	11	3.0	3	1	2	2	4	5	7	7
65+	5	3.6	3	1	3	4	4	6	6	6
GRAND TOTAL	860	2.0	3	1	1	2	2	3	4	7

780.32: COMPLEX FEBRILE CONVULS

Type of Patients	Observed Patients	Avg. Stay	Vari-ance	10th	25th	50th	75th	90th	95th	99th
1. SINGLE DX										
A. Not Operated										
0–19 Years	82	1.6	<1	1	1	1	2	3	4	4
20–34	1	1.0	0	1	1	1	1	1	1	1
35–49	0									
50–64	1	1.0	0	1	1	1	1	1	1	1
65+	0									
B. Operated										
0–19 Years	1	3.0	0	3	3	3	3	3	3	3
20–34	0									
35–49	0									
50–64	0									
65+	0									
2. MULTIPLE DX										
A. Not Operated										
0–19 Years	226	2.2	2	1	1	2	3	4	5	7
20–34	1	1.5	<1	1	1	1	2	2	2	2
35–49	1	2.0	0	2	2	2	2	2	2	2
50–64	1	1.0	0	1	1	1	1	1	1	1
65+	2	2.0	2	1	1	1	3	3	3	3
B. Operated										
0–19 Years	0									
20–34	0									
35–49	0									
50–64	0									
65+	0									
SUBTOTALS:										
1. SINGLE DX										
A. Not Operated	84	1.6	<1	1	1	1	2	3	4	4
B. Operated	1	3.0	0	3	3	3	3	3	3	3
2. MULTIPLE DX										
A. Not Operated	232	2.2	2	1	1	2	3	4	5	7
B. Operated	0									
1. SINGLE DX	85	1.6	<1	1	1	1	2	3	4	4
2. MULTIPLE DX	232	2.2	2	1	1	2	3	4	5	7
A. NOT OPERATED	316	2.0	2	1	1	2	3	4	4	7
B. OPERATED	1	3.0	0	3	3	3	3	3	3	3
TOTAL										
0–19 Years	309	2.0	2	1	1	2	3	4	4	7
20–34	3	1.3	<1	1	1	1	2	2	2	2
35–49	1	2.0	0	2	2	2	2	2	2	2
50–64	2	1.0	0	1	1	1	1	1	1	1
65+	2	2.0	2	1	1	1	3	3	3	3
GRAND TOTAL	317	2.0	2	1	1	2	3	4	4	7

780.39: OTHER CONVULSIONS

Type of Patients	Observed Patients	Avg. Stay	Vari-ance	10th	25th	50th	75th	90th	95th	99th
1. SINGLE DX										
A. Not Operated										
0–19 Years	564	1.8	1	1	1	1	2	3	4	7
20–34	155	2.6	5	1	1	2	3	6	7	12
35–49	124	2.9	4	1	1	2	4	5	7	12
50–64	62	2.6	4	1	1	2	4	5	7	8
65+	17	1.5	<1	1	1	1	2	3	3	3
B. Operated										
0–19 Years	1	1.0	0	1	1	1	1	1	1	1
20–34	1	2.0	0	2	2	2	2	2	2	2
35–49	3	2.3	<1	2	2	2	3	3	3	3
50–64	1	1.0	0	1	1	1	1	1	1	1
65+	0									
2. MULTIPLE DX										
A. Not Operated										
0–19 Years	1,733	2.3	4	1	1	2	3	4	6	10
20–34	1,919	2.9	7	1	1	2	4	6	7	14
35–49	3,108	3.2	12	1	2	2	4	6	8	14
50–64	3,677	3.5	12	1	2	3	4	7	9	17
65+	4,268	3.7	10	1	2	3	5	7	9	16
B. Operated										
0–19 Years	14	8.4	203	1	1	3	6	27	52	52
20–34	30	5.9	54	1	1	3	6	13	30	30
35–49	35	10.0	141	2	3	7	13	26	65	>99
50–64	39	11.8	113	3	5	8	15	31	32	52
65+	62	9.3	59	3	4	8	12	15	23	45
SUBTOTALS:										
1. SINGLE DX										
A. Not Operated	922	2.1	3	1	1	2	2	4	5	8
B. Operated	6	1.8	<1	1	1	2	2	3	3	3
2. MULTIPLE DX										
A. Not Operated	14,705	3.3	10	1	2	2	4	6	8	15
B. Operated	180	9.3	98	1	3	7	12	22	30	65
1. SINGLE DX	928	2.1	3	1	1	2	2	4	5	8
2. MULTIPLE DX	14,885	3.4	12	1	2	2	4	6	9	16
A. NOT OPERATED	15,627	3.2	10	1	1	2	4	6	8	15
B. OPERATED	186	9.1	96	1	3	6	12	22	30	65
TOTAL										
0–19 Years	2,312	2.2	5	1	1	2	3	4	5	10
20–34	2,105	2.9	7	1	1	2	4	6	7	14
35–49	3,270	3.3	13	1	1	2	4	6	8	15
50–64	3,779	3.6	14	1	2	3	4	7	9	19
65+	4,347	3.8	12	1	2	3	5	7	10	17
GRAND TOTAL	15,813	3.3	11	1	1	2	4	6	9	16

Length of Stay by Diagnosis and Operation, Western Region, 2008

Western Region, October 2006–September 2007 Data, by Diagnosis

780.4: DIZZINESS & GIDDINESS

Type of Patients	Observed Patients	Avg. Stay	Variance	10th	25th	50th	75th	90th	95th	99th
1. SINGLE DX										
A. Not Operated										
0–19 Years	3	2.0	1	1	1	2	3	3	3	3
20–34	7	2.3	2	1	1	2	4	4	4	4
35–49	9	1.2	<1	1	1	1	1	2	2	2
50–64	12	1.3	<1	1	1	1	1	2	3	3
65+	9	1.1	<1	1	1	1	1	2	2	2
B. Operated										
0–19 Years	0									
20–34	0									
35–49	0									
50–64	0									
65+	0									
2. MULTIPLE DX										
A. Not Operated										
0–19 Years	19	2.9	6	1	1	2	4	7	9	9
20–34	106	2.0	2	1	1	2	2	3	5	8
35–49	433	2.1	3	1	1	2	3	4	5	10
50–64	1,065	2.0	2	1	1	2	2	4	5	8
65+	2,946	2.3	3	1	1	2	3	4	5	8
B. Operated										
0–19 Years	1	2.0	0	2	2	2	2	2	2	2
20–34	1	4.0	0	4	4	4	4	4	4	4
35–49	3	6.7	80	1	1	4	17	17	17	17
50–64	10	3.4	11	1	1	2	5	12	12	12
65+	17	6.1	55	3	3	4	7	10	33	33
SUBTOTALS:										
1. SINGLE DX										
A. Not Operated	40	1.5	<1	1	1	1	2	3	3	4
B. Operated	0									
2. MULTIPLE DX										
A. Not Operated	4,569	2.2	2	1	1	2	3	4	5	8
B. Operated	32	5.1	39	1	2	3	5	10	17	33
1. SINGLE DX	40	1.5	<1	1	1	1	2	3	3	4
2. MULTIPLE DX	4,601	2.2	3	1	1	2	3	4	5	8
A. NOT OPERATED	4,609	2.2	2	1	1	2	3	4	5	8
B. OPERATED	32	5.1	39	1	2	3	5	10	17	33
TOTAL										
0–19 Years	23	2.8	5	1	1	2	3	4	6	9
20–34	114	2.1	2	1	1	2	3	4	5	8
35–49	445	2.1	4	1	1	2	3	4	5	10
50–64	1,087	2.0	2	1	1	2	2	4	5	8
65+	2,972	2.3	3	1	1	2	3	4	5	8
GRAND TOTAL	4,641	2.2	3	1	1	2	3	4	5	8

780.6: FEVER

Type of Patients	Observed Patients	Avg. Stay	Variance	10th	25th	50th	75th	90th	95th	99th
1. SINGLE DX										
A. Not Operated										
0–19 Years	685	2.4	1	1	2	2	3	3	4	7
20–34	8	2.9	5	1	2	2	3	8	8	8
35–49	6	3.5	4	2	2	3	6	6	6	6
50–64	4	5.2	7	3	3	4	5	9	9	9
65+	4	2.0	<1	1	1	2	2	3	3	3
B. Operated										
0–19 Years	2	2.0	2	1	1	3	3	3	3	3
20–34	0									
35–49	1	9.0	0	9	9	9	9	9	9	9
50–64	0									
65+	0									
2. MULTIPLE DX										
A. Not Operated										
0–19 Years	2,119	2.5	3	1	2	2	3	4	5	9
20–34	529	3.6	8	1	2	3	4	7	9	17
35–49	947	3.5	9	1	2	3	4	6	8	16
50–64	1,502	3.6	8	1	2	3	4	7	9	15
65+	2,389	3.7	8	1	2	3	5	7	9	15
B. Operated										
0–19 Years	18	5.7	14	2	3	4	9	12	13	13
20–34	15	11.0	278	2	3	5	12	20	68	68
35–49	22	8.3	35	3	4	8	15	23	23	23
50–64	46	8.0	42	1	4	7	9	16	20	32
65+	53	7.6	19	3	5	7	9	13	16	24
SUBTOTALS:										
1. SINGLE DX										
A. Not Operated	707	2.4	1	1	2	2	3	4	5	7
B. Operated	3	4.3	17	1	1	3	9	9	9	9
2. MULTIPLE DX										
A. Not Operated	7,486	3.3	7	1	2	3	4	6	8	14
B. Operated	154	7.9	52	2	4	7	9	15	20	32
1. SINGLE DX	710	2.4	1	1	2	2	3	4	5	7
2. MULTIPLE DX	7,640	3.4	9	1	2	3	4	6	8	15
A. NOT OPERATED	8,193	3.2	7	1	2	3	4	6	8	13
B. OPERATED	157	7.9	52	2	4	7	9	15	20	32
TOTAL										
0–19 Years	2,824	2.5	3	2	2	2	3	4	5	9
20–34	552	3.7	17	1	2	3	4	7	9	17
35–49	976	3.6	10	1	2	3	4	7	9	16
50–64	1,552	3.8	10	1	2	3	5	7	9	16
65+	2,446	3.8	9	1	2	3	5	7	9	16
GRAND TOTAL	8,350	3.3	8	2	3	3	4	6	8	15

780.79: MALAISE & FATIGUE NEC

Type of Patients	Observed Patients	Avg. Stay	Variance	10th	25th	50th	75th	90th	95th	99th
1. SINGLE DX										
A. Not Operated										
0–19 Years	4	1.0	0	1	1	1	1	1	1	1
20–34	4	1.3	<1	1	1	1	1	2	2	2
35–49	1	1.0	0	1	1	1	1	1	1	1
50–64	0									
65+	5	3.2	7	1	1	2	5	7	7	7
B. Operated										
0–19 Years	0									
20–34	0									
35–49	0									
50–64	0									
65+	0									
2. MULTIPLE DX										
A. Not Operated										
0–19 Years	34	2.1	5	1	1	2	2	3	5	13
20–34	61	2.5	4	1	1	2	3	5	5	13
35–49	173	2.9	9	1	1	2	4	5	9	19
50–64	485	3.0	6	1	1	2	4	5	7	14
65+	2,322	3.0	6	1	2	3	4	5	7	11
B. Operated										
0–19 Years	0									
20–34	0									
35–49	2	3.0	2	2	2	3	4	4	4	4
50–64	8	7.5	166	1	1	2	5	39	39	39
65+	26	7.4	46	1	1	6	10	20	21	25
SUBTOTALS:										
1. SINGLE DX										
A. Not Operated	14	1.9	3	1	1	1	2	5	7	7
B. Operated	0									
2. MULTIPLE DX										
A. Not Operated	3,075	3.0	6	1	1	2	4	5	7	12
B. Operated	36	7.2	67	1	1	5	8	20	25	39
1. SINGLE DX	14	1.9	3	1	1	1	2	5	7	7
2. MULTIPLE DX	3,111	3.0	7	1	1	2	4	5	7	12
A. NOT OPERATED	3,089	3.0	6	1	1	2	4	5	7	12
B. OPERATED	36	7.2	67	1	1	5	8	20	25	39
TOTAL										
0–19 Years	38	2.0	4	1	1	1	2	3	5	13
20–34	65	2.4	4	1	1	2	3	5	5	13
35–49	176	2.9	9	1	2	2	4	5	9	19
50–64	493	3.1	8	1	2	3	4	5	7	15
65+	2,353	3.0	7	1	2	3	4	5	7	12
GRAND TOTAL	3,125	3.0	7	1	2	2	4	5	7	12

Length of Stay by Diagnosis and Operation, Western Region, 2008

Western Region, October 2006–September 2007 Data, by Diagnosis

780.97: ALTERED MENTAL STATUS

Type of Patients	Observed Patients	Avg. Stay	Variance	Percentiles						
				10th	25th	50th	75th	90th	95th	99th
1. SINGLE DX										
A. Not Operated										
0–19 Years	17	1.5	1	1	1	1	2	2	5	5
20–34	4	1.5	<1	1	1	2	2	2	2	2
35–49	3	1.0	0	1	1	1	1	1	1	1
50–64	11	1.2	<1	1	1	1	1	1	3	3
65+	5	1.6	<1	1	1	2	2	2	2	2
B. Operated										
0–19 Years	0									
20–34	0									
35–49	0									
50–64	0									
65+	0									
2. MULTIPLE DX										
A. Not Operated										
0–19 Years	76	2.3	9	1	1	1	2	4	6	24
20–34	174	2.6	27	1	1	2	3	5	6	11
35–49	466	3.1	12	1	1	2	4	6	9	18
50–64	1,146	3.3	12	1	1	2	4	6	9	18
65+	2,572	3.6	9	1	2	3	4	7	9	16
B. Operated										
0–19 Years	0									
20–34	2	8.5	59	3	3	14	14	14	14	14
35–49	2	9.0	126	1	1	9	17	17	17	17
50–64	10	5.4	6	2	4	5	7	10	10	10
65+	27	7.3	20	2	4	6	10	15	17	17
SUBTOTALS:										
1. SINGLE DX										
A. Not Operated	40	1.4	<1	1	1	1	2	2	3	5
B. Operated	0									
2. MULTIPLE DX										
A. Not Operated	4,434	3.4	11	1	2	3	4	6	9	16
B. Operated	41	7.0	20	2	4	6	9	14	17	17
1. SINGLE DX	40	1.4	<1	1	1	1	2	2	3	5
2. MULTIPLE DX	4,475	3.5	11	1	2	3	4	7	9	16
A. NOT OPERATED	4,474	3.4	11	1	2	3	4	6	9	16
B. OPERATED	41	7.0	20	2	4	6	9	14	17	17
TOTAL										
0–19 Years	93	2.1	8	1	1	1	2	4	5	24
20–34	180	2.6	27	1	1	2	3	5	6	14
35–49	471	3.1	12	1	1	2	4	6	9	18
50–64	1,167	3.3	12	1	1	2	4	6	9	18
65+	2,604	3.7	9	1	2	3	5	7	9	16
GRAND TOTAL	4,515	3.4	11	1	2	3	4	7	9	16

780.99: GENERAL SYMPTOMS NEC

Type of Patients	Observed Patients	Avg. Stay	Variance	Percentiles						
				10th	25th	50th	75th	90th	95th	99th
1. SINGLE DX										
A. Not Operated										
0–19 Years	7	1.4	<1	1	1	1	2	2	2	2
20–34	0									
35–49	0									
50–64	0									
65+	1	2.0	0	2	2	2	2	2	2	2
B. Operated										
0–19 Years	0									
20–34	0									
35–49	0									
50–64	0									
65+	0									
2. MULTIPLE DX										
A. Not Operated										
0–19 Years	13	2.8	9	1	1	2	3	4	9	12
20–34	7	1.9	<1	1	1	2	2	3	3	3
35–49	24	1.9	1	1	1	2	2	3	3	6
50–64	51	3.7	28	1	1	2	4	6	8	36
65+	78	3.4	9	1	2	3	4	6	13	16
B. Operated										
0–19 Years	0									
20–34	0									
35–49	0									
50–64	0									
65+	1	4.0	0	4	4	4	4	4	4	4
SUBTOTALS:										
1. SINGLE DX										
A. Not Operated	8	1.5	<1	1	1	2	2	2	2	2
B. Operated	0									
2. MULTIPLE DX										
A. Not Operated	173	3.1	13	1	1	2	3	5	9	16
B. Operated	1	4.0	0	4	4	4	4	4	4	4
1. SINGLE DX	8	1.5	<1	1	1	2	2	2	2	2
2. MULTIPLE DX	174	3.2	13	1	1	2	4	5	9	16
A. NOT OPERATED	181	3.1	13	1	1	2	3	5	8	16
B. OPERATED	1	4.0	0	4	4	4	4	4	4	4
TOTAL										
0–19 Years	20	2.3	6	1	1	2	3	4	4	12
20–34	7	1.9	<1	1	1	2	2	3	3	3
35–49	24	1.9	1	1	1	2	2	3	3	6
50–64	51	3.7	28	1	1	2	4	6	8	36
65+	80	3.3	9	1	2	3	4	6	9	16
GRAND TOTAL	182	3.1	13	1	1	2	3	5	8	16

781: NERVOUS/MS SYST SYMPTOMS

Type of Patients	Observed Patients	Avg. Stay	Variance	Percentiles						
				10th	25th	50th	75th	90th	95th	99th
1. SINGLE DX										
A. Not Operated										
0–19 Years	31	1.5	<1	1	1	1	2	2	4	5
20–34	4	2.3	2	1	2	2	3	4	4	4
35–49	4	1.8	<1	1	1	2	2	3	3	3
50–64	5	3.4	6	1	1	4	4	7	7	7
65+	1	1.0	0	1	1	1	1	1	1	1
B. Operated										
0–19 Years	0									
20–34	0									
35–49	0									
50–64	1	2.0	0	2	2	2	2	2	2	2
65+	0									
2. MULTIPLE DX										
A. Not Operated										
0–19 Years	148	2.5	5	1	1	2	3	5	8	11
20–34	131	3.0	19	1	1	2	3	5	7	15
35–49	317	2.9	5	1	1	2	3	6	7	11
50–64	584	3.2	10	1	1	2	4	6	8	17
65+	1,492	3.2	7	2	2	3	4	5	7	12
B. Operated										
0–19 Years	0									
20–34	6	2.6	5	1	1	2	3	7	7	7
35–49	2	2.0	0	2	2	2	2	4	4	4
50–64	11	3.8	19	2	2	2	6	8	15	15
65+	17	5.2	28	2	2	3	5	14	21	21
SUBTOTALS:										
1. SINGLE DX										
A. Not Operated	45	1.8	2	1	1	1	2	4	4	7
B. Operated	1	2.0	0	2	2	2	2	2	2	2
2. MULTIPLE DX										
A. Not Operated	2,672	3.1	8	1	1	2	4	6	7	13
B. Operated	43	3.8	18	1	1	2	4	8	14	21
1. SINGLE DX	46	1.8	2	1	1	1	2	4	4	7
2. MULTIPLE DX	2,715	3.1	8	1	1	2	4	6	7	14
A. NOT OPERATED	2,717	3.1	8	1	1	2	4	5	7	13
B. OPERATED	44	3.8	17	1	2	2	4	8	14	21
TOTAL										
0–19 Years	186	2.3	4	1	1	1	3	4	6	11
20–34	141	2.9	18	1	1	2	3	5	6	15
35–49	323	2.8	5	1	1	2	3	6	7	11
50–64	601	3.2	10	1	1	2	4	6	8	15
65+	1,510	3.2	7	2	2	3	4	5	7	13
GRAND TOTAL	2,761	3.1	8	1	1	2	4	6	7	14

Length of Stay by Diagnosis and Operation, Western Region, 2008

Western Region, October 2006–September 2007 Data, by Diagnosis

781.0: ABN INVOL MOVEMENT NEC

Type of Patients	Observed Patients	Avg. Stay	Vari-ance	Percentiles						
				10th	25th	50th	75th	90th	95th	99th
1. SINGLE DX										
A. Not Operated										
0–19 Years	18	1.5	<1	1	1	1	2	2		4
20–34	4	2.3	2	1	2	2	3	4		4
35–49	1	2.0	0	2	2	2	2	2		2
50–64	1	1.0	0	1	1	1	1	1		1
65+	0									
B. Operated										
0–19 Years	0									
20–34	0									
35–49	0									
50–64	1	2.0	0	2	2	2	2	2		2
65+	0									
2. MULTIPLE DX										
A. Not Operated										
0–19 Years	66	1.9	2	1	1	1	2	3	4	8
20–34	40	3.2	9	1	1	2	4	6	8	15
35–49	54	2.8	4	1	1	2	4	6	7	9
50–64	80	2.5	4	1	1	2	3	6	6	9
65+	179	3.0	6	1	1	2	4	5	8	15
B. Operated										
0–19 Years	6	2.8	5	1	1	2	3	7	7	7
20–34	4	1.5	<1	1	1	2	2	2	2	2
35–49	1	2.0	0	2	2	2	2	2	2	2
50–64	6	1.5	<1	1	1	1	2	3	3	3
65+	4	4.0	17	1	2	3	7	10	10	10
SUBTOTALS:										
1. SINGLE DX										
A. Not Operated	24	1.6	<1	1	1	1	2	2	4	4
B. Operated	1	2.0	0	2	2	2	2	2	2	2
2. MULTIPLE DX										
A. Not Operated	419	2.7	5	1	1	2	3	5	7	12
B. Operated	21	2.4	5	1	1	2	3	3	7	10
1. SINGLE DX	25	1.6	<1	1	1	1	2	2	4	4
2. MULTIPLE DX	440	2.7	5	1	1	2	3	5	6	12
A. NOT OPERATED	443	2.7	5	1	1	2	3	5	6	12
B. OPERATED	22	2.4	5	1	1	2	3	3	7	10
TOTAL										
0–19 Years	90	1.9	2	1	1	1	2	3	4	8
20–34	48	3.0	8	1	1	2	3	6	8	15
35–49	56	2.8	4	1	1	2	3	6	7	9
50–64	88	2.4	3	1	1	2	3	5	6	9
65+	183	3.0	7	1	1	2	4	5	8	15
GRAND TOTAL	465	2.6	5	1	1	2	3	5	7	12

781.2: ABNORMALITY OF GAIT

Type of Patients	Observed Patients	Avg. Stay	Vari-ance	Percentiles						
				10th	25th	50th	75th	90th	95th	99th
1. SINGLE DX										
A. Not Operated										
0–19 Years	2	1.0	0	1	1	1	1	1	1	1
20–34	0									
35–49	0									
50–64	1	7.0	0	7	7	7	7	7	7	7
65+	1	1.0	0	1	1	1	1	1	1	1
B. Operated										
0–19 Years	0									
20–34	0									
35–49	0									
50–64	0									
65+	0									
2. MULTIPLE DX										
A. Not Operated										
0–19 Years	13	3.6	8	1	1	3	6	8	9	9
20–34	12	3.6	8	1	1	3	4	6	11	11
35–49	54	2.8	5	1	1	2	3	6	7	10
50–64	139	3.4	14	1	2	2	4	7	9	14
65+	674	3.2	7	1	2	3	4	5	7	12
B. Operated										
0–19 Years	1	1.0	0	1	1	1	1	1	1	1
20–34	0									
35–49	0									
50–64	3	9.7	22	6	6	8	15	15	15	15
65+	10	5.3	33	2	3	3	5	7	21	21
SUBTOTALS:										
1. SINGLE DX										
A. Not Operated	4	2.5	9	1	1	1	7	7	7	7
B. Operated	0									
2. MULTIPLE DX										
A. Not Operated	892	3.2	8	1	2	3	4	5	7	12
B. Operated	14	5.9	31	2	3	4	7	15	21	21
1. SINGLE DX	4	2.5	9	1	1	1	7	7	7	7
2. MULTIPLE DX	906	3.3	9	1	2	3	4	6	7	14
A. NOT OPERATED	896	3.2	8	1	2	3	4	5	7	12
B. OPERATED	14	5.9	31	2	3	4	7	15	21	21
TOTAL										
0–19 Years	16	3.1	8	1	1	3	6	8	9	9
20–34	12	3.6	8	1	1	3	4	6	11	11
35–49	54	2.8	5	1	1	2	3	6	7	10
50–64	143	3.6	15	1	2	3	4	7	9	15
65+	685	3.2	7	1	2	3	4	5	7	12
GRAND TOTAL	910	3.3	9	1	2	3	4	6	7	12

781.3: LACK OF COORDINATION

Type of Patients	Observed Patients	Avg. Stay	Vari-ance	Percentiles						
				10th	25th	50th	75th	90th	95th	99th
1. SINGLE DX										
A. Not Operated										
0–19 Years	10	1.6	2	1	1	1	2	5	5	5
20–34	0									
35–49	1	1.0	0	1	1	1	1	1	1	1
50–64	1	4.0	0	4	4	4	4	4	4	4
65+	0									
B. Operated										
0–19 Years	0									
20–34	0									
35–49	0									
50–64	0									
65+	0									
2. MULTIPLE DX										
A. Not Operated										
0–19 Years	49	2.7	7	1	1	2	3	6	10	13
20–34	40	3.4	49	1	2	2	3	5	5	46
35–49	119	2.9	5	1	2	2	3	6	7	10
50–64	258	3.2	8	1	2	3	4	6	7	17
65+	533	3.2	5	1	2	3	4	6	7	12
B. Operated										
0–19 Years	0									
20–34	0									
35–49	0									
50–64	1	4.0	0	4	4	4	4	4	4	4
65+	2	8.5	60	3	3	14	14	14	14	14
SUBTOTALS:										
1. SINGLE DX										
A. Not Operated	12	1.8	2	1	1	1	2	4	5	5
B. Operated	0									
2. MULTIPLE DX										
A. Not Operated	999	3.1	8	1	2	3	4	6	7	13
B. Operated	4	5.8	31	2	2	4	7	14	14	14
1. SINGLE DX	12	1.8	2	1	1	1	2	4	5	5
2. MULTIPLE DX	1,003	3.2	8	1	2	3	4	6	7	13
A. NOT OPERATED	1,011	3.1	8	1	2	3	4	6	7	13
B. OPERATED	4	5.8	31	2	2	4	7	14	14	14
TOTAL										
0–19 Years	59	2.5	6	1	1	1	3	5	10	13
20–34	41	3.4	48	1	1	2	3	4	5	46
35–49	120	2.9	5	1	2	2	3	5	7	10
50–64	260	3.2	7	1	2	3	4	6	7	17
65+	535	3.2	6	1	2	3	4	6	7	13
GRAND TOTAL	1,015	3.1	8	1	2	3	4	6	7	13

Length of Stay by Diagnosis and Operation, Western Region, 2008

Western Region, October 2006–September 2007 Data, by Diagnosis

782: SKIN & INTEGUMENT NEC SX

Type of Patients	Observed Patients	Avg. Stay	Variance	Percentiles 10th	25th	50th	75th	90th	95th	99th
1. SINGLE DX										
A. Not Operated										
0–19 Years	45	1.7	1	1	1	1	2	2	4	6
20–34	12	1.8	1	1	1	1	2	4	4	4
35–49	13	1.5	<1	1	1	1	1	3	3	3
50–64	9	1.1	<1	1	1	1	1	2	2	2
65+	2	1.5	<1	1	1	1	2	2	2	2
B. Operated										
0–19 Years	0									
20–34	2	1.0	0	1	1	1	1	1	1	1
35–49	0									
50–64	1	4.0	0	4	4	4	4	4	4	4
65+	0									
2. MULTIPLE DX										
A. Not Operated										
0–19 Years	178	2.2	6	1	1	2	2	4	6	18
20–34	265	2.2	2	1	1	2	3	4	5	8
35–49	693	2.4	5	1	1	2	3	4	7	13
50–64	898	2.5	5	1	1	2	3	5	6	11
65+	1,048	2.9	7	1	1	2	4	6	7	13
B. Operated										
0–19 Years	4	9.6	61	6	6	7	21	21	21	21
20–34	2	2.0	0	2	2	2	2	2	2	2
35–49	7	6.2	5	3	4	6	8	9	9	9
50–64	13	3.9	12	1	1	3	5	9	12	12
65+	13	6.5	49	1	1	5	9	15	25	25
SUBTOTALS:										
1. SINGLE DX										
A. Not Operated	81	1.6	1	1	1	1	2	3	4	6
B. Operated	3	2.0	3	1	1	1	4	4	4	4
2. MULTIPLE DX										
A. Not Operated	3,082	2.6	5	1	1	2	3	5	7	12
B. Operated	38	5.8	29	1	2	4	8	12	21	25
1. SINGLE DX	84	1.6	1	1	1	1	2	3	4	6
2. MULTIPLE DX	3,120	2.6	6	1	1	2	3	5	7	12
A. NOT OPERATED	3,163	2.6	5	1	1	2	3	5	7	12
B. OPERATED	41	5.5	28	1	1	4	7	11	15	25
TOTAL										
0–19 Years	227	2.3	6	1	1	2	2	4	6	18
20–34	280	2.2	2	1	1	2	3	4	5	8
35–49	713	2.5	5	1	1	2	3	5	8	12
50–64	921	2.5	5	1	1	2	3	5	7	11
65+	1,063	3.0	7	1	1	2	4	6	8	15
GRAND TOTAL	3,204	2.6	6	1	1	2	3	5	7	12

782.0: SKIN SENSATION DISTURB

Type of Patients	Observed Patients	Avg. Stay	Variance	Percentiles 10th	25th	50th	75th	90th	95th	99th
1. SINGLE DX										
A. Not Operated										
0–19 Years	7	1.3	<1	1	1	1	2	2	2	2
20–34	9	1.4	1	1	1	1	1	4	4	4
35–49	8	1.3	<1	1	1	1	1	3	3	3
50–64	7	1.1	<1	1	1	1	1	2	2	2
65+	0									
B. Operated										
0–19 Years	0									
20–34	0									
35–49	0									
50–64	0									
65+	0									
2. MULTIPLE DX										
A. Not Operated										
0–19 Years	24	1.5	<1	1	1	1	2	2	3	4
20–34	166	1.9	1	1	1	1	2	3	4	7
35–49	468	2.0	2	1	1	1	2	3	5	9
50–64	508	1.8	1	1	1	2	2	3	4	6
65+	412	2.1	2	1	1	2	3	4	5	7
B. Operated										
0–19 Years	0									
20–34	0									
35–49	1	8.0	0	8	8	8	8	8	8	8
50–64	2	1.0	0	1	1	1	1	1	1	1
65+	0									
SUBTOTALS:										
1. SINGLE DX										
A. Not Operated	31	1.3	<1	1	1	1	1	2	3	4
B. Operated	0									
2. MULTIPLE DX										
A. Not Operated	1,578	1.9	2	1	1	2	2	3	4	7
B. Operated	3	3.3	16	1	1	1	8	8	8	8
1. SINGLE DX	31	1.3	<1	1	1	1	1	2	3	4
2. MULTIPLE DX	1,581	1.9	2	1	1	2	2	3	4	8
A. NOT OPERATED	1,609	1.9	2	1	1	1	2	3	4	7
B. OPERATED	3	3.3	16	1	1	1	8	8	8	8
TOTAL										
0–19 Years	31	1.4	<1	1	1	1	2	2	3	4
20–34	175	1.9	1	1	1	1	2	3	4	7
35–49	477	2.0	2	1	1	1	2	3	5	9
50–64	517	1.8	1	1	1	2	2	3	4	6
65+	412	2.1	2	1	1	2	3	4	5	7
GRAND TOTAL	1,612	1.9	2	1	1	1	2	3	4	7

782.1: NONSP SKIN ERUPTION NEC

Type of Patients	Observed Patients	Avg. Stay	Variance	Percentiles 10th	25th	50th	75th	90th	95th	99th
1. SINGLE DX										
A. Not Operated										
0–19 Years	4	1.0	0	1	1	1	1	1	1	1
20–34	1	2.0	0	2	2	2	2	2	2	2
35–49	0									
50–64	0									
65+	0									
B. Operated										
0–19 Years	0									
20–34	0									
35–49	0									
50–64	0									
65+	0									
2. MULTIPLE DX										
A. Not Operated										
0–19 Years	29	1.8	2	1	1	1	2	3	4	7
20–34	30	2.5	2	1	1	2	3	4	5	7
35–49	26	3.3	17	1	1	2	3	7	15	18
50–64	45	3.2	6	2	2	3	4	5	6	12
65+	51	3.7	6	2	2	3	5	6	9	13
B. Operated										
0–19 Years	0									
20–34	0									
35–49	0									
50–64	3	4.0	1	3	3	4	5	5	5	5
65+	0									
SUBTOTALS:										
1. SINGLE DX										
A. Not Operated	5	1.2	<1	1	1	1	1	2	2	2
B. Operated	0									
2. MULTIPLE DX										
A. Not Operated	181	3.0	6	1	3	4	4	5	7	15
B. Operated	3	4.0	1	3	3	4	5	5	5	5
1. SINGLE DX	5	1.2	<1	1	1	1	1	2	2	2
2. MULTIPLE DX	184	3.0	6	1	1	3	4	5	7	15
A. NOT OPERATED	186	2.9	6	1	1	2	4	5	7	15
B. OPERATED	3	4.0	1	3	3	4	5	5	5	5
TOTAL										
0–19 Years	33	1.7	1	1	1	1	2	3	4	7
20–34	31	2.5	2	1	1	2	3	4	5	7
35–49	26	3.3	17	1	1	2	3	7	15	18
50–64	48	3.3	3	2	2	3	4	5	6	12
65+	51	3.7	6	2	2	3	5	6	9	13
GRAND TOTAL	189	3.0	6	1	1	2	4	5	7	15

Length of Stay by Diagnosis and Operation, Western Region, 2008

Western Region, October 2006–September 2007 Data, by Diagnosis

782.3: EDEMA

Type of Patients	Observed Patients	Avg. Stay	Vari-ance	10th	25th	50th	75th	90th	95th	99th
1. SINGLE DX										
A. Not Operated										
0–19 Years	0									
20–34	1	4.0	0	4	4	4	4	4	4	4
35–49	0									
50–64	1	1.0	0	1	1	1	1	1	1	1
65+	0									
B. Operated										
0–19 Years	0									
20–34	0									
35–49	0									
50–64	0									
65+	0									
2. MULTIPLE DX										
A. Not Operated										
0–19 Years	18	2.7	3	1	1	2	4	5	7	7
20–34	31	2.8	3	1	1	2	4	5	7	8
35–49	127	3.2	6	1	2	3	4	6	8	14
50–64	255	3.2	6	1	2	3	4	6	8	13
65+	350	3.5	9	1	2	3	4	6	8	17
B. Operated										
0–19 Years	0									
20–34	0									
35–49	1	4.0	0	4	4	4	4	4	4	4
50–64	2	6.5	59	1	1	7	12	12	12	12
65+	3	3.7	5	1	1	5	5	5	5	5
SUBTOTALS:										
1. SINGLE DX — A. Not Operated	2	2.5	4	1	1	3	4	4	4	4
1. SINGLE DX — B. Operated	0									
2. MULTIPLE DX — A. Not Operated	781	3.3	7	1	2	3	4	6	8	14
2. MULTIPLE DX — B. Operated	6	4.7	16	1	1	5	5	12	12	12
1. SINGLE DX	2	2.5	4	1	1	3	4	4	4	4
2. MULTIPLE DX	787	3.3	7	1	2	3	4	6	8	14
A. NOT OPERATED	783	3.3	7	1	2	3	4	6	8	14
B. OPERATED	6	4.7	16	1	1	5	5	12	12	12
TOTAL										
0–19 Years	18	2.7	3	1	1	2	4	5	7	7
20–34	32	2.9	3	1	1	3	4	5	7	8
35–49	128	3.2	6	1	2	3	4	6	8	14
50–64	258	3.2	6	1	2	3	4	6	8	13
65+	353	3.5	9	1	2	3	4	6	8	17
GRAND TOTAL	789	3.3	7	1	2	3	4	6	8	14

782.4: JAUNDICE NOS

Type of Patients	Observed Patients	Avg. Stay	Vari-ance	10th	25th	50th	75th	90th	95th	99th
1. SINGLE DX										
A. Not Operated										
0–19 Years	17	1.8	<1	1	1	2	2	2	4	4
20–34	0									
35–49	2	2.0	2	1	1	3	3	3	3	3
50–64	1	1.0	0	1	1	1	1	1	1	1
65+	0									
B. Operated										
0–19 Years	0									
20–34	0									
35–49	0									
50–64	0									
65+	0									
2. MULTIPLE DX										
A. Not Operated										
0–19 Years	31	3.6	21	1	1	2	3	5	8	19
20–34	26	2.8	5	2	2	3	6	6	8	10
35–49	45	4.3	13	1	2	3	6	11	12	14
50–64	44	4.4	18	1	2	3	6	8	10	25
65+	89	4.0	9	1	2	3	5	9	11	15
B. Operated										
0–19 Years	2	12.6	143	4	4	21	21	21	21	21
20–34	0									
35–49	2	5.5	12	3	3	3	8	8	8	8
50–64	1	7.0	0	7	7	7	7	7	7	7
65+	0									
SUBTOTALS:										
1. SINGLE DX — A. Not Operated	20	1.8	<1	1	1	2	2	3	3	4
1. SINGLE DX — B. Operated	0									
2. MULTIPLE DX — A. Not Operated	235	4.0	13	1	2	3	5	9	11	18
2. MULTIPLE DX — B. Operated	5	8.6	52	3	4	7	8	21	21	21
1. SINGLE DX	20	1.8	<1	1	1	2	2	3	3	4
2. MULTIPLE DX	240	4.1	14	2	2	3	5	9	12	19
A. NOT OPERATED	255	3.8	12	1	2	3	4	9	11	18
B. OPERATED	5	8.6	52	3	4	7	8	21	21	21
TOTAL										
0–19 Years	50	3.4	21	1	1	2	3	5	8	21
20–34	26	2.8	5	2	2	2	3	6	8	10
35–49	49	4.3	13	1	2	3	6	11	12	14
50–64	46	4.4	18	1	2	3	6	8	10	25
65+	89	4.0	9	1	2	3	5	9	11	15
GRAND TOTAL	260	3.9	13	2	2	3	4	9	11	19

782.7: SPONTANEOUS ECCHYMOSES

Type of Patients	Observed Patients	Avg. Stay	Vari-ance	10th	25th	50th	75th	90th	95th	99th
1. SINGLE DX										
A. Not Operated										
0–19 Years	2	1.5	<1	1	1	1	2	2	2	2
20–34	0									
35–49	0									
50–64	0									
65+	1	2.0	0	2	2	2	2	2	2	2
B. Operated										
0–19 Years	0									
20–34	0									
35–49	0									
50–64	0									
65+	0									
2. MULTIPLE DX										
A. Not Operated										
0–19 Years	14	1.8	<1	1	1	2	2	3	4	4
20–34	5	2.2	<1	1	2	2	3	3	3	3
35–49	20	3.1	3	1	2	3	4	6	6	7
50–64	37	3.6	9	1	2	2	5	8	11	12
65+	128	3.5	9	1	2	3	4	6	9	16
B. Operated										
0–19 Years	0									
20–34	0									
35–49	2	7.0	8	5	5	9	9	9	9	9
50–64	0									
65+	5	12.6	67	3	9	11	15	25	25	25
SUBTOTALS:										
1. SINGLE DX — A. Not Operated	3	1.7	<1	1	1	2	2	2	2	2
1. SINGLE DX — B. Operated	0									
2. MULTIPLE DX — A. Not Operated	204	3.3	8	1	2	3	4	6	8	12
2. MULTIPLE DX — B. Operated	7	11.0	53	3	5	9	15	25	25	25
1. SINGLE DX	3	1.7	<1	1	1	2	2	2	2	2
2. MULTIPLE DX	211	3.6	11	1	2	3	4	7	9	16
A. NOT OPERATED	207	3.3	8	1	2	3	4	6	8	12
B. OPERATED	7	11.0	53	3	5	9	15	25	25	25
TOTAL										
0–19 Years	16	1.8	<1	1	1	2	2	3	4	4
20–34	5	2.2	<1	1	2	2	3	3	3	3
35–49	22	3.4	5	1	2	3	5	6	7	9
50–64	37	3.6	9	1	2	2	5	8	11	12
65+	134	3.8	13	1	2	3	4	7	10	25
GRAND TOTAL	214	3.6	11	1	2	3	4	7	9	16

Length of Stay by Diagnosis and Operation, Western Region, 2008

Western Region, October 2006–September 2007 Data, by Diagnosis

783: NUTRIT/METABOL/DEVEL SX

Type of Patients	Observed Patients	Avg. Stay	Vari-ance	10th	25th	50th	75th	90th	95th	99th
1. SINGLE DX										
A. Not Operated										
0–19 Years	113	3.0	6	1	2	2	4	6	7	12
20–34	0									
35–49	1	5.0	0	5	5	5	5	5	5	5
50–64	0									
65+	1	1.0	0	1	1	1	1	1	1	1
B. Operated										
0–19 Years	0									
20–34	0									
35–49	0									
50–64	0									
65+	0									
2. MULTIPLE DX										
A. Not Operated										
0–19 Years	816	5.1	28	1	2	3	6	10	15	27
20–34	42	6.4	74	1	2	4	7	12	32	>99
35–49	68	4.4	22	1	2	3	6	8	11	27
50–64	277	5.1	18	1	2	4	6	9	15	23
65+	1,872	4.5	18	2	2	3	5	8	10	21
B. Operated										
0–19 Years	39	11.6	146	2	4	9	15	23	47	57
20–34	0									
35–49	4	4.8	13	2	2	3	10	10	10	10
50–64	10	10.0	53	3	4	9	17	23	23	23
65+	25	7.9	25	3	5	7	10	12	14	27
SUBTOTALS:										
1. SINGLE DX										
A. Not Operated	115	3.0	6	1	2	2	4	6	7	12
B. Operated	0									
2. MULTIPLE DX										
A. Not Operated	3,075	4.7	21	1	2	3	6	9	12	26
B. Operated	78	9.9	91	2	4	8	11	19	27	57
1. SINGLE DX	115	3.0	6	1	2	2	4	6	7	12
2. MULTIPLE DX	3,153	4.8	24	1	2	4	6	9	12	26
A. NOT OPERATED	3,190	4.7	21	1	2	3	6	8	12	25
B. OPERATED	78	9.9	91	2	4	8	11	19	27	57
TOTAL										
0–19 Years	968	5.1	32	1	2	3	6	10	15	28
20–34	42	6.4	74	1	2	4	7	12	32	>99
35–49	73	4.4	21	1	2	3	5	8	11	27
50–64	287	5.3	20	1	2	4	6	9	16	23
65+	1,898	4.5	18	2	2	4	5	8	10	21
GRAND TOTAL	3,268	4.8	23	1	2	3	6	9	12	26

783.0: ANOREXIA

Type of Patients	Observed Patients	Avg. Stay	Vari-ance	10th	25th	50th	75th	90th	95th	99th
1. SINGLE DX										
A. Not Operated										
0–19 Years	1	2.0	0	2	2	2	2	2	2	2
20–34	0									
35–49	0									
50–64	0									
65+	0									
B. Operated										
0–19 Years	0									
20–34	0									
35–49	0									
50–64	0									
65+	0									
2. MULTIPLE DX										
A. Not Operated										
0–19 Years	17	3.5	4	1	2	3	5	7	8	8
20–34	11	6.2	34	1	2	6	7	7	22	22
35–49	11	3.1	5	1	2	2	4	4	9	9
50–64	21	4.3	7	2	2	3	5	9	9	11
65+	112	4.1	8	1	2	3	5	7	8	15
B. Operated										
0–19 Years	0									
20–34	0									
35–49	1	2.0	0	2	2	2	2	2	2	2
50–64	1	7.0	0	7	7	7	7	7	7	7
65+	1	8.0	0	8	8	8	8	8	8	8
SUBTOTALS:										
1. SINGLE DX										
A. Not Operated	1	2.0	0	2	2	2	2	2	2	2
B. Operated	0									
2. MULTIPLE DX										
A. Not Operated	172	4.1	9	1	2	3	5	7	9	17
B. Operated	3	5.7	10	2	2	7	8	8	8	8
1. SINGLE DX	1	2.0	0	2	2	2	2	2	2	2
2. MULTIPLE DX	175	4.1	9	1	2	3	6	7	9	17
A. NOT OPERATED	173	4.1	9	1	2	3	5	7	9	17
B. OPERATED	3	5.7	10	2	2	7	8	8	8	8
TOTAL										
0–19 Years	18	3.5	4	1	2	3	5	7	8	8
20–34	11	6.2	34	1	2	6	7	7	22	22
35–49	12	3.0	5	1	2	2	3	4	9	9
50–64	22	4.4	7	2	2	4	6	9	9	11
65+	113	4.1	8	1	2	3	5	7	8	15
GRAND TOTAL	176	4.1	9	1	2	3	6	7	9	17

783.41: FAILURE TO THRIVE

Type of Patients	Observed Patients	Avg. Stay	Vari-ance	10th	25th	50th	75th	90th	95th	99th
1. SINGLE DX										
A. Not Operated										
0–19 Years	90	3.2	6	1	2	3	4	6	7	17
20–34	0									
35–49	0									
50–64	0									
65+	0									
B. Operated										
0–19 Years	0									
20–34	0									
35–49	0									
50–64	0									
65+	0									
2. MULTIPLE DX										
A. Not Operated										
0–19 Years	611	5.5	29	2	2	4	7	11	15	27
20–34	0									
35–49	0									
50–64	0									
65+	0									
B. Operated										
0–19 Years	27	13.2	186	3	4	9	15	37	47	57
20–34	0									
35–49	0									
50–64	0									
65+	0									
SUBTOTALS:										
1. SINGLE DX										
A. Not Operated	90	3.2	6	1	2	3	4	6	7	17
B. Operated	0									
2. MULTIPLE DX										
A. Not Operated	611	5.5	29	2	2	4	7	11	15	27
B. Operated	27	13.2	186	3	4	9	15	37	47	57
1. SINGLE DX	90	3.2	6	1	2	3	4	6	7	17
2. MULTIPLE DX	638	5.8	38	2	2	4	7	12	17	34
A. NOT OPERATED	701	5.2	27	1	2	4	6	10	15	27
B. OPERATED	27	13.2	186	3	4	9	15	37	47	57
TOTAL										
0–19 Years	728	5.5	35	1	2	4	7	11	15	33
20–34	0									
35–49	0									
50–64	0									
65+	0									
GRAND TOTAL	728	5.5	35	1	2	4	7	11	15	33

Length of Stay by Diagnosis and Operation, Western Region, 2008

Western Region, October 2006–September 2007 Data, by Diagnosis

783.7: ADULT FAILURE TO THRIVE

Type of Patients	Observed Patients	Avg. Stay	Variance	10th	25th	50th	75th	90th	95th	99th
1. SINGLE DX										
A. Not Operated										
0–19 Years	0									
20–34	0									
35–49	1	5.0	0	5	5	5	5	5	5	5
50–64	0									
65+	1	1.0	0	1	1	1	1	1	1	1
B. Operated										
0–19 Years	0									
20–34	0									
35–49	0									
50–64	0									
65+	0									
2. MULTIPLE DX										
A. Not Operated										
0–19 Years	4	4.8	8	3	3	3	9	9	9	9
20–34	14	10.8	165	2	3	7	12	46	>99	>99
35–49	38	5.5	33	1	2	3	7	11	26	27
50–64	218	5.3	20	2	3	4	6	11	16	23
65+	1,633	4.5	19	2	3	4	5	8	10	21
B. Operated										
0–19 Years	0									
20–34	0									
35–49	1	4.0	0	4	4	4	4	4	4	4
50–64	5	11.6	71	2	6	10	17	23	23	23
65+	19	8.3	32	2	4	7	10	14	27	27
SUBTOTALS:										
1. SINGLE DX										
A. Not Operated	2	3.0	8	1	1	1	5	5	5	5
B. Operated	0									
2. MULTIPLE DX										
A. Not Operated	1,907	4.7	20	2	3	4	6	8	11	25
B. Operated	25	8.8	39	2	4	7	10	17	23	27
1. SINGLE DX	2	3.0	8	1	1	1	5	5	5	5
2. MULTIPLE DX	1,932	4.7	21	2	3	4	6	8	11	26
A. NOT OPERATED	1,909	4.7	20	2	3	4	6	8	11	25
B. OPERATED	25	8.8	39	2	4	7	10	17	23	27
TOTAL										
0–19 Years	4	4.8	8	3	3	3	9	9	9	9
20–34	14	10.8	165	2	3	7	12	46	>99	>99
35–49	40	5.5	31	1	2	3	7	8	12	27
50–64	223	5.5	22	2	3	4	6	12	17	23
65+	1,653	4.6	19	2	3	4	5	8	10	21
GRAND TOTAL	1,934	4.7	21	2	3	4	6	8	11	26

784: SX INVOLVING HEAD/NECK

Type of Patients	Observed Patients	Avg. Stay	Vari-ance	10th	25th	50th	75th	90th	95th	99th
1. SINGLE DX										
A. Not Operated										
0–19 Years	61	1.6	1	1	1	1	2	3	4	6
20–34	37	2.1	2	1	1	1	2	5	6	6
35–49	39	1.5	<1	1	1	1	2	3	4	4
50–64	29	2.0	5	1	1	1	2	4	6	11
65+	15	1.9	2	1	1	1	3	3	5	5
B. Operated										
0–19 Years	5	1.6	<1	1	1	1	2	3	3	3
20–34	13	2.1	3	1	1	1	3	5	5	5
35–49	8	1.1	<1	1	1	1	1	2	2	2
50–64	13	1.7	<1	1	1	1	2	2	5	5
65+	5	1.8	<1	1	1	2	2	3	3	3
2. MULTIPLE DX										
A. Not Operated										
0–19 Years	358	2.2	5	1	1	2	3	4	5	13
20–34	789	2.6	6	1	1	2	3	5	7	11
35–49	1,174	2.7	5	1	1	2	3	5	7	12
50–64	1,567	2.6	4	1	1	2	3	5	6	10
65+	2,338	2.7	5	1	1	2	3	5	7	12
B. Operated										
0–19 Years	18	3.6	12	1	1	3	4	6	16	16
20–34	44	4.5	17	1	1	3	5	11	12	15
35–49	73	4.0	17	1	1	3	7	7	13	27
50–64	146	3.7	19	1	1	3	5	7	9	28
65+	213	4.4	17	2	2	3	5	9	12	24
SUBTOTALS:										
1. SINGLE DX										
A. Not Operated	181	1.8	2	1	1	1	2	4	4	6
B. Operated	44	1.7	1	1	1	2	2	3	5	5
2. MULTIPLE DX										
A. Not Operated	6,226	2.6	5	1	1	2	3	5	6	11
B. Operated	494	4.1	17	1	1	3	5	8	11	25
1. SINGLE DX	225	1.8	2	1	1	1	2	4	4	6
2. MULTIPLE DX	6,720	2.8	6	1	1	2	3	5	7	12
A. NOT OPERATED	6,407	2.6	5	1	1	2	3	5	6	11
B. OPERATED	538	3.9	16	1	1	3	5	8	10	24
TOTAL										
0–19 Years	442	2.2	5	1	1	2	3	4	5	13
20–34	883	2.7	6	1	1	2	3	5	7	12
35–49	1,294	2.7	6	1	1	2	3	5	7	13
50–64	1,755	2.7	6	1	1	2	3	5	6	11
65+	2,571	2.9	6	1	1	2	4	5	7	13
GRAND TOTAL	6,945	2.7	6	1	1	2	3	5	7	12

784.0: HEADACHE

Type of Patients	Observed Patients	Avg. Stay	Vari-ance	10th	25th	50th	75th	90th	95th	99th
1. SINGLE DX										
A. Not Operated										
0–19 Years	25	1.8	2	1	1	1	2	3	4	6
20–34	24	2.0	3	1	1	1	2	5	6	6
35–49	32	1.6	<1	1	1	1	2	3	4	4
50–64	16	2.0	2	1	1	1	3	4	6	6
65+	1	1.0	0	1	1	1	1	1	1	1
B. Operated										
0–19 Years	1	1.0	0	1	1	1	1	1	1	1
20–34	2	3.0	8	1	1	5	5	5	5	5
35–49	0									
50–64	0									
65+	0									
2. MULTIPLE DX										
A. Not Operated										
0–19 Years	245	2.4	6	1	1	2	3	4	6	13
20–34	641	2.7	6	1	1	2	3	5	7	11
35–49	827	2.7	5	1	1	2	3	5	6	12
50–64	831	2.5	3	1	1	2	3	5	6	9
65+	715	2.5	5	1	1	2	3	5	6	11
B. Operated										
0–19 Years	3	6.3	69	1	1	2	16	16	16	16
20–34	12	3.9	11	1	2	5	6	9	10	10
35–49	21	6.4	34	2	3	5	7	13	13	27
50–64	36	6.2	58	2	3	4	6	10	28	40
65+	57	5.0	24	1	2	4	6	8	16	28
SUBTOTALS:										
1. SINGLE DX										
A. Not Operated	98	1.8	2	1	1	1	2	4	5	6
B. Operated	3	2.4	5	1	1	2	5	5	5	5
2. MULTIPLE DX										
A. Not Operated	3,259	2.6	5	1	1	2	3	5	6	11
B. Operated	129	5.5	34	1	2	4	6	10	16	28
1. SINGLE DX	101	1.8	2	1	1	1	2	4	5	6
2. MULTIPLE DX	3,388	2.7	6	1	1	2	3	5	7	12
A. NOT OPERATED	3,357	2.6	5	1	1	2	3	5	6	11
B. OPERATED	132	5.4	34	2	2	4	6	9	16	28
TOTAL										
0–19 Years	274	2.3	6	1	1	2	3	4	6	16
20–34	679	2.7	6	1	1	2	3	5	7	11
35–49	880	2.7	6	1	1	2	3	5	6	13
50–64	883	2.6	6	1	1	2	3	5	6	10
65+	773	2.7	6	1	1	2	3	5	7	13
GRAND TOTAL	3,489	2.7	6	1	1	2	3	5	7	12

Length of Stay by Diagnosis and Operation, Western Region, 2008

Western Region, October 2006–September 2007 Data, by Diagnosis

784.2: SWELLING IN HEAD & NECK

Type of Patients	Observed Patients	Avg. Stay	Variance	10th	25th	50th	75th	90th	95th	99th
1. SINGLE DX										
A. Not Operated										
0–19 Years	9	1.1	<1	1	1	1	1		2	2
20–34	3	1.7	<1	1	1	2	2		2	2
35–49	0									
50–64	4	3.8	24	1	1	2	11	11	11	11
65+	3	1.7	1	1	1	1	3	3	3	3
B. Operated										
0–19 Years	4	1.7	<1	1	1	1	2	3	3	3
20–34	6	2.0	3	1	1	1	3	5	5	5
35–49	6	1.0	0	1	1	1	1	1	1	1
50–64	11	1.6	1	1	1	1	2	2	5	5
65+	2	2.5		2	2	3	3	3	3	3
2. MULTIPLE DX										
A. Not Operated										
0–19 Years	31	1.9	1	1	1	2	2	3	4	5
20–34	31	2.3	6	1	1	1	3	5	5	13
35–49	55	2.3	6	1	1	1	3	4	8	15
50–64	68	2.1	2	1	1	1	3	5	6	6
65+	68	2.6	6	1	1	2	3	5	6	15
B. Operated										
0–19 Years	11	3.4	3	1	2	3	5	6	6	6
20–34	15	4.6	25	1	1	2	9	14	15	15
35–49	17	2.5	6	1	1	1	3	5	10	10
50–64	39	2.2	4	1	1	1	3	5	7	9
65+	26	3.3	11	1	2	2	5	6	10	15
SUBTOTALS:										
1. SINGLE DX										
A. Not Operated	19	1.9	5	1	1	1	2	3	11	11
B. Operated	29	1.7	1	1	1	2	2	3	5	5
2. MULTIPLE DX										
A. Not Operated	253	2.3	5	1	1	2	3	5	6	13
B. Operated	108	3.0	9	1	1	2	4	6	10	15
1. SINGLE DX	48	1.7	3	1	1	1	2	3	5	11
2. MULTIPLE DX	361	2.5	6	1	1	2	3	5	6	15
A. NOT OPERATED	272	2.3	5	1	1	1	3	5	6	13
B. OPERATED	137	2.7	8	1	1	1	3	6	9	15
TOTAL										
0–19 Years	55	2.1	2	1	1	2	3	4	5	6
20–34	55	2.8	11	1	1	1	3	5	13	15
35–49	78	2.3	5	1	1	1	3	4	8	15
50–64	122	2.1	3	1	1	1	3	5	6	9
65+	99	2.7	7	1	1	2	3	6	7	15
GRAND TOTAL	409	2.4	6	1	1	1	3	5	6	14

784.5: SPEECH DISTURBANCE NEC

Type of Patients	Observed Patients	Avg. Stay	Variance	10th	25th	50th	75th	90th	95th	99th
1. SINGLE DX										
A. Not Operated										
0–19 Years	0									
20–34	0									
35–49	0									
50–64	1	1.0	0	1	1	1	1	1	1	1
65+	0									
B. Operated										
0–19 Years	0									
20–34	0									
35–49	0									
50–64	0									
65+	0									
2. MULTIPLE DX										
A. Not Operated										
0–19 Years	3	1.3	<1	1	1	1	2	2	2	2
20–34	26	2.5	6	1	1	2	3	4	8	11
35–49	65	2.1	2	1	1	2	2	4	4	9
50–64	130	2.7	6	1	1	2	3	5	7	14
65+	203	2.6	3	1	1	2	3	5	5	10
B. Operated										
0–19 Years	0									
20–34	0									
35–49	0									
50–64	1	1.0	0	1	1	1	1	1	1	1
65+	1	10.0	0	10	10	10	10	10	10	10
SUBTOTALS:										
1. SINGLE DX										
A. Not Operated	1	1.0	0	1	1	1	1	1	1	1
B. Operated	0									
2. MULTIPLE DX										
A. Not Operated	427	2.6	4	1	1	2	3	5	6	11
B. Operated	2	5.5	40	1	1	10	10	10	10	10
1. SINGLE DX	1	1.0	0	1	1	1	1	1	1	1
2. MULTIPLE DX	429	2.6	4	1	1	2	3	5	6	11
A. NOT OPERATED	428	2.6	4	1	1	2	3	5	6	11
B. OPERATED	2	5.5	40	1	1	10	10	10	10	10
TOTAL										
0–19 Years	3	1.3	<1	1	1	1	2	2	2	2
20–34	26	2.5	6	1	1	2	3	4	8	11
35–49	65	2.1	2	1	1	2	2	4	4	9
50–64	132	2.7	6	1	1	2	3	5	7	14
65+	204	2.7	4	1	1	2	3	5	5	10
GRAND TOTAL	430	2.6	4	1	1	2	3	5	6	11

784.7: EPISTAXIS

Type of Patients	Observed Patients	Avg. Stay	Variance	10th	25th	50th	75th	90th	95th	99th
1. SINGLE DX										
A. Not Operated										
0–19 Years	5	1.6	2	1	1	1	1	4	4	4
20–34	8	2.6	2	1	2	2	4	5	5	5
35–49	7	1.3	<1	1	1	1	2	2	2	2
50–64	8	1.4	1	1	1	1	1	4	4	4
65+	11	2.0	2	1	1	1	3	3	5	5
B. Operated										
0–19 Years	0									
20–34	5	1.8	2	1	2	2	4	4	4	4
35–49	2	1.5	<1	2	2	2	2	2	2	2
50–64	2	2.0	0	2	2	2	2	2	2	2
65+	3	1.3	<1	1	1	1	1	2	2	2
2. MULTIPLE DX										
A. Not Operated										
0–19 Years	43	2.1	2	1	1	1	3	4	4	7
20–34	64	2.3	2	1	1	2	3	4	4	8
35–49	185	2.9	5	1	1	2	4	6	7	10
50–64	468	2.8	5	1	1	2	4	5	7	12
65+	1,204	2.9	5	1	1	2	4	5	7	12
B. Operated										
0–19 Years	3	2.0	3	1	2	3	5	4	4	4
20–34	14	4.3	11	2	3	5	11	11	12	12
35–49	35	3.2	7	1	3	3	4	6	7	15
50–64	67	3.4	4	2	3	5	5	6	7	10
65+	127	4.3	14	2	3	5	9	12	12	17
SUBTOTALS:										
1. SINGLE DX										
A. Not Operated	39	1.8	2	1	1	1	2	4	5	5
B. Operated	12	1.7	<1	1	1	2	2	2	4	4
2. MULTIPLE DX										
A. Not Operated	1,964	2.8	5	1	1	2	4	5	7	11
B. Operated	246	3.9	10	1	2	3	5	7	10	16
1. SINGLE DX	51	1.8	1	1	1	1	2	4	4	5
2. MULTIPLE DX	2,210	2.9	6	1	2	2	4	6	7	12
A. NOT OPERATED	2,003	2.8	5	1	1	2	4	5	7	11
B. OPERATED	258	3.8	10	2	2	3	5	7	10	16
TOTAL										
0–19 Years	51	2.0	2	1	1	2	3	4	5	7
20–34	91	2.6	4	1	1	2	4	6	5	12
35–49	229	2.9	5	1	1	2	4	6	7	10
50–64	545	2.9	6	1	2	2	4	5	7	11
65+	1,345	3.0	6	1	2	2	4	6	7	13
GRAND TOTAL	2,261	2.9	6	1	1	2	4	5	7	12

Length of Stay by Diagnosis and Operation, Western Region, 2008

Western Region, October 2006–September 2007 Data, by Diagnosis

785: CARDIOVASCULAR SYST SX

Type of Patients	Observed Patients	Avg. Stay	Variance	Percentiles						
				10th	25th	50th	75th	90th	95th	99th
1. SINGLE DX										
A. Not Operated										
0–19 Years	14	2.1	2	1	1	2	3	4	6	6
20–34	6	1.2	<1	1	1	1	1	2	2	2
35–49	14	1.3	<1	1	1	1	1	2	3	3
50–64	7	1.6	<1	1	1	1	2	4	4	4
65+	4	1.0	0	1	1	1	1	1	1	1
B. Operated										
0–19 Years	15	2.5	11	1	1	2	2	5	14	14
20–34	14	1.9	1	1	1	1	3	3	5	5
35–49	9	1.1	<1	1	1	1	1	2	2	2
50–64	10	2.9	10	1	1	1	4	9	9	9
65+	1	1.0	0	1	1	1	1	1	1	1
2. MULTIPLE DX										
A. Not Operated										
0–19 Years	84	2.7	8	1	1	2	3	5	7	17
20–34	178	2.5	10	1	1	1	3	5	7	23
35–49	370	2.4	9	1	1	1	2	4	8	18
50–64	612	2.3	7	1	1	1	2	4	6	12
65+	844	2.5	7	1	2	2	3	5	7	14
B. Operated										
0–19 Years	26	3.0	4	1	1	3	4	7	7	7
20–34	79	5.1	23	1	2	4	7	11	16	25
35–49	136	4.8	24	1	1	3	6	11	16	26
50–64	234	5.0	24	1	1	4	7	12	15	22
65+	287	6.3	28	1	2	5	9	13	16	27
SUBTOTALS:										
1. SINGLE DX										
A. Not Operated	45	1.6	1	1	1	1	2	3	4	6
B. Operated	49	2.1	6	1	1	1	2	5	8	14
2. MULTIPLE DX										
A. Not Operated	2,088	2.4	7	1	1	1	3	5	7	15
B. Operated	762	5.4	25	1	1	4	7	12	15	24
1. SINGLE DX	94	1.9	4	1	1	1	2	3	5	14
2. MULTIPLE DX	2,850	3.2	14	1	1	2	4	7	11	19
A. NOT OPERATED	2,133	2.4	7	1	1	1	3	5	7	15
B. OPERATED	811	5.2	25	1	1	4	7	12	15	24
TOTAL										
0–19 Years	139	2.7	7	1	1	2	3	5	7	14
20–34	277	3.2	14	1	1	2	4	7	10	23
35–49	529	3.0	14	1	1	2	3	7	10	18
50–64	863	3.0	13	1	1	2	4	7	10	20
65+	1,136	3.4	15	1	1	2	4	8	11	18
GRAND TOTAL	2,944	3.2	14	1	1	2	4	7	10	19

785.0: TACHYCARDIA NOS

Type of Patients	Observed Patients	Avg. Stay	Variance	Percentiles						
				10th	25th	50th	75th	90th	95th	99th
1. SINGLE DX										
A. Not Operated										
0–19 Years	2	4.0	8	2	2	2	6	6	6	6
20–34	1	1.0	0	1	1	1	1	1	1	1
35–49	2	1.0	0	1	1	1	1	1	1	1
50–64	0									
65+	1	1.0	0	1	1	1	1	1	1	1
B. Operated										
0–19 Years	0									
20–34	2	1.0	0	1	1	1	1	1	1	1
35–49	0									
50–64	0									
65+	0									
2. MULTIPLE DX										
A. Not Operated										
0–19 Years	27	2.7	9	1	1	1	3	7	12	12
20–34	66	2.4	13	1	1	2	2	4	8	23
35–49	85	2.0	2	1	1	2	2	4	5	9
50–64	110	2.2	4	1	1	2	2	3	5	12
65+	166	2.3	5	1	1	2	3	4	6	9
B. Operated										
0–19 Years	1	1.0	0	1	1	1	1	1	1	1
20–34	2	16.5	142	8	8	17	25	25	25	25
35–49	4	2.3	2	1	1	2	4	4	4	4
50–64	3	5.0	37	1	1	2	12	12	12	12
65+	5	4.6	16	2	2	2	9	9	9	9
SUBTOTALS:										
1. SINGLE DX										
A. Not Operated	6	2.0	4	1	1	1	2	6	6	6
B. Operated	2	1.0	0	1	1	1	1	1	1	1
2. MULTIPLE DX										
A. Not Operated	454	2.3	6	1	1	2	3	4	6	12
B. Operated	15	5.4	43	1	1	2	9	12	25	25
1. SINGLE DX	8	1.8	3	1	1	1	2	6	6	6
2. MULTIPLE DX	469	2.4	7	1	1	2	3	4	7	13
A. NOT OPERATED	460	2.3	6	1	1	2	3	4	6	12
B. OPERATED	17	4.9	40	1	1	2	8	12	25	25
TOTAL										
0–19 Years	30	2.7	9	1	1	2	3	5	7	14
20–34	71	2.7	20	1	1	2	4	7	10	23
35–49	91	2.0	2	1	1	2	3	4	5	9
50–64	113	2.3	5	1	1	2	3	3	7	12
65+	172	2.4	6	1	1	2	3	4	6	9
GRAND TOTAL	477	2.4	7	1	1	2	3	4	7	13

785.1: PALPITATIONS

Type of Patients	Observed Patients	Avg. Stay	Variance	Percentiles						
				10th	25th	50th	75th	90th	95th	99th
1. SINGLE DX										
A. Not Operated										
0–19 Years	2	1.0	0	1	1	1	1	1	1	1
20–34	3	1.0	0	1	1	1	1	1	1	1
35–49	9	1.1	<1	1	1	1	1	2	2	2
50–64	5	1.2	<1	1	1	1	1	2	2	2
65+	2	1.0	0	1	1	1	1	1	1	1
B. Operated										
0–19 Years	0									
20–34	1	1.0	0	1	1	1	1	1	1	1
35–49	0									
50–64	0									
65+	0									
2. MULTIPLE DX										
A. Not Operated										
0–19 Years	11	1.2	<1	1	1	1	1	1	3	3
20–34	61	1.5	<1	1	1	1	2	2	3	6
35–49	202	1.5	1	1	1	1	2	2	3	5
50–64	376	1.6	1	1	1	1	2	3	3	6
65+	482	1.6	<1	1	1	1	2	3	3	5
B. Operated										
0–19 Years	2	2.5	5	1	1	3	4	4	4	4
20–34	1	4.0	0	4	4	4	4	4	4	4
35–49	3	4.0	13	1	1	3	8	8	8	8
50–64	1	1.0	0	1	1	1	1	1	1	1
65+	2	1.5	<1	1	1	2	2	2	2	2
SUBTOTALS:										
1. SINGLE DX										
A. Not Operated	21	1.1	<1	1	1	1	1	1	2	2
B. Operated	1	1.0	0	1	1	1	1	1	1	1
2. MULTIPLE DX										
A. Not Operated	1,132	1.5	<1	1	1	1	2	3	3	5
B. Operated	9	2.8	5	1	2	2	4	8	8	8
1. SINGLE DX	22	1.1	<1	1	1	1	1	1	2	2
2. MULTIPLE DX	1,141	1.6	<1	1	1	1	2	3	3	5
A. NOT OPERATED	1,153	1.5	<1	1	1	1	2	3	3	5
B. OPERATED	10	2.6	5	1	1	1	4	8	8	8
TOTAL										
0–19 Years	15	1.3	<1	1	1	1	1	3	4	4
20–34	66	1.5	<1	1	1	1	2	2	3	6
35–49	214	1.5	1	1	1	1	2	2	3	6
50–64	382	1.6	<1	1	1	1	2	3	3	6
65+	486	1.6	<1	1	1	1	2	3	3	5
GRAND TOTAL	1,163	1.5	<1	1	1	1	2	3	3	5

Length of Stay by Diagnosis and Operation, Western Region, 2008

Western Region, October 2006–September 2007 Data, by Diagnosis

785.4: GANGRENE

Type of Patients	Observed Patients	Avg. Stay	Variance	10th	25th	50th	75th	90th	95th	99th
1. SINGLE DX										
A. Not Operated										
0–19 Years	0									
20–34	0									
35–49	2	1.5	<1	1	1	2	2	2	2	2
50–64	0									
65+	0									
B. Operated										
0–19 Years	2	8.0	71	2	2	14	14	14	14	14
20–34	1	2.0	0	2	2	2	2	2	2	2
35–49	0									
50–64	1	8.0	0	8	8	8	8	8	8	8
65+	0									
2. MULTIPLE DX										
A. Not Operated										
0–19 Years	0									
20–34	2	3.5	12	1	1	1	6	6	6	6
35–49	24	6.9	35	1	2	4	9	16	18	19
50–64	23	4.5	12	1	1	5	6	10	11	13
65+	55	5.4	21	1	2	4	6	11	15	22
B. Operated										
0–19 Years	2	5.0	8	3	3	3	7	7	7	7
20–34	11	9.1	60	1	2	10	16	17	24	24
35–49	53	6.7	37	1	2	5	10	16	17	27
50–64	92	7.7	31	2	4	6	10	15	20	30
65+	164	8.3	32	3	4	7	11	15	18	29
SUBTOTALS:										
1. SINGLE DX										
A. Not Operated	2	1.5	<1	1	1	2	2	2	2	2
B. Operated	4	6.5	33	2	2	8	14	14	14	14
2. MULTIPLE DX										
A. Not Operated	104	5.5	22	1	2	4	6	13	15	21
B. Operated	322	7.9	34	2	4	7	10	16	19	27
1. SINGLE DX	6	4.9	27	1	2	2	8	14	14	14
2. MULTIPLE DX	426	7.3	32	1	3	6	10	15	18	27
A. NOT OPERATED	106	5.4	22	1	2	4	6	13	15	21
B. OPERATED	326	7.8	33	2	4	7	10	16	19	27
TOTAL										
0–19 Years	4	6.5	30	2	3	3	14	14	14	14
20–34	14	7.8	54	1	2	6	12	17	24	24
35–49	79	6.6	36	1	2	4	10	16	18	27
50–64	116	7.1	28	1	4	6	9	13	20	24
65+	219	7.5	31	2	4	6	10	15	18	27
GRAND TOTAL	432	7.2	32	1	3	6	10	15	18	27

785.6: ENLARGEMENT LYMPH NODES

Type of Patients	Observed Patients	Avg. Stay	Variance	10th	25th	50th	75th	90th	95th	99th
1. SINGLE DX										
A. Not Operated										
0–19 Years	9	1.9	1	1	1	2	2	4	4	4
20–34	2	1.5	<1	1	1	2	2	2	2	2
35–49	1	3.0	0	3	3	3	3	3	3	3
50–64	2	2.5	4	1	1	1	4	4	4	4
65+	1	1.0	0	1	1	1	1	1	1	1
B. Operated										
0–19 Years	13	1.7	1	1	1	1	2	2	5	5
20–34	10	2.2	2	1	1	2	3	3	5	5
35–49	8	1.0	0	1	1	1	1	1	1	1
50–64	9	2.3	7	1	1	1	2	9	9	9
65+	1	1.0	0	1	1	1	1	1	1	1
2. MULTIPLE DX										
A. Not Operated										
0–19 Years	37	2.5	2	1	1	2	4	4	5	5
20–34	41	3.4	6	1	2	3	4	7	8	11
35–49	38	3.9	16	1	2	3	4	9	14	21
50–64	57	3.4	11	1	1	2	4	7	10	21
65+	44	3.4	7	1	1	2	4	8	8	12
B. Operated										
0–19 Years	21	3.0	3	2	2	3	3	5	7	7
20–34	65	4.1	8	1	2	4	6	8	10	11
35–49	75	3.4	11	1	1	2	5	7	12	16
50–64	133	3.2	10	1	1	2	4	6	8	18
65+	110	3.4	9	1	2	2	5	8	10	12
SUBTOTALS:										
1. SINGLE DX										
A. Not Operated	15	1.9	1	1	1	2	3	4	4	4
B. Operated	41	1.8	2	1	1	1	2	3	5	9
2. MULTIPLE DX										
A. Not Operated	217	3.3	9	1	1	2	4	7	9	14
B. Operated	404	3.4	9	1	1	2	5	7	10	14
1. SINGLE DX	56	1.8	2	1	1	1	2	4	5	9
2. MULTIPLE DX	621	3.4	9	1	1	2	4	7	9	14
A. NOT OPERATED	232	3.3	8	1	1	2	4	7	9	14
B. OPERATED	445	3.3	9	1	1	2	5	7	9	14
TOTAL										
0–19 Years	80	2.4	2	1	1	2	3	4	5	7
20–34	118	3.6	7	1	2	3	5	8	9	11
35–49	122	3.4	12	1	1	2	4	7	10	16
50–64	201	3.2	10	1	1	2	4	6	9	18
65+	156	3.3	8	1	2	2	5	8	10	12
GRAND TOTAL	677	3.3	9	1	1	2	4	7	9	14

786: RESP SYST/OTH CHEST SX

Type of Patients	Observed Patients	Avg. Stay	Variance	10th	25th	50th	75th	90th	95th	99th
1. SINGLE DX										
A. Not Operated										
0–19 Years	231	1.5	<1	1	1	1	2	3	3	4
20–34	140	1.2	<1	1	1	1	1	2	3	3
35–49	631	1.2	<1	1	1	1	1	2	2	4
50–64	602	1.2	<1	1	1	1	1	2	2	3
65+	182	1.3	<1	1	1	1	1	2	3	4
B. Operated										
0–19 Years	1	2.0	0	2	2	2	2	2	2	2
20–34	5	3.4	3	1	3	3	5	5	5	5
35–49	1	3.0	0	3	3	3	3	3	3	3
50–64	2	1.5	<1	1	1	2	3	3	3	3
65+	4	2.5	<1	2	2	3	3	3	3	3
2. MULTIPLE DX										
A. Not Operated										
0–19 Years	957	2.5	9	1	1	2	3	5	7	13
20–34	3,369	1.8	5	1	1	1	2	3	4	8
35–49	24,651	1.8	2	1	1	1	2	3	4	7
50–64	42,290	1.8	2	1	1	1	2	3	4	7
65+	41,877	2.0	2	1	1	1	2	4	5	8
B. Operated										
0–19 Years	17	4.1	19	1	1	2	7	13	14	14
20–34	53	6.1	45	2	3	4	8	14	18	41
35–49	154	4.6	23	1	2	3	6	9	13	32
50–64	372	5.2	24	1	2	4	7	12	15	25
65+	449	5.1	25	1	2	4	6	10	14	25
SUBTOTALS:										
1. SINGLE DX										
A. Not Operated	1,786	1.2	<1	1	1	1	2	2	3	4
B. Operated	13	2.7	2	1	2	3	5	5	5	5
2. MULTIPLE DX										
A. Not Operated	113,144	1.9	2	1	1	1	2	3	4	7
B. Operated	1,045	5.1	26	1	2	4	6	11	14	26
1. SINGLE DX	1,799	1.3	<1	1	1	1	1	2	3	4
2. MULTIPLE DX	114,189	1.9	3	1	1	1	2	3	4	8
A. NOT OPERATED	114,930	1.9	2	1	1	1	2	3	4	7
B. OPERATED	1,058	5.1	25	1	2	4	6	11	14	26
TOTAL										
0–19 Years	1,206	2.3	8	1	1	2	3	4	6	12
20–34	3,567	1.9	6	1	1	1	2	3	4	9
35–49	25,437	1.8	2	1	1	1	2	3	4	7
50–64	43,266	1.8	2	1	1	1	2	3	4	7
65+	42,512	2.0	3	1	1	1	2	4	5	8
GRAND TOTAL	115,988	1.9	3	1	1	1	2	3	4	8

Length of Stay by Diagnosis and Operation, Western Region, 2008

Western Region, October 2006–September 2007 Data, by Diagnosis

786.03: APNEA

Type of Patients	Observed Patients	Avg. Stay	Variance	10th	25th	50th	75th	90th	95th	99th
1. SINGLE DX										
A. Not Operated										
0–19 Years	98	1.7	<1	1	1	1	2	3	4	6
20–34	0									
35–49	0									
50–64	0									
65+	0									
B. Operated										
0–19 Years	0									
20–34	0									
35–49	0									
50–64	0									
65+	0									
2. MULTIPLE DX										
A. Not Operated										
0–19 Years	238	3.5	22	1	1	2	4	7	11	26
20–34	3	1.7	<1	1	1	2	2	2	2	2
35–49	4	3.3	2	2	3	3	5	5	5	5
50–64	6	1.8	<1	1	1	1	2	3	5	3
65+	7	2.0	2	1	1	1	3	5	5	5
B. Operated										
0–19 Years	4	3.7	8	1	1	2	5	7	7	7
20–34	0									
35–49	1	2.0	0	2	2	2	2	2	2	2
50–64	1	8.0	0	8	8	8	8	8	8	8
65+	1	3.0	0	3	3	3	3	3	3	3
SUBTOTALS:										
1. SINGLE DX A. Not Operated	98	1.7	<1	1	1	1	2	3	4	6
B. Operated	0									
2. MULTIPLE DX A. Not Operated	258	3.4	20	1	1	2	4	7	11	26
B. Operated	7	4.0	7	1	2	3	7	8	8	8
1. SINGLE DX	98	1.7	<1	1	1	1	2	3	4	6
2. MULTIPLE DX	265	3.4	20	1	1	2	4	7	10	26
A. NOT OPERATED	356	2.9	16	1	1	2	3	5	9	24
B. OPERATED	7	4.0	7	1	2	3	7	8	8	8
TOTAL										
0–19 Years	340	3.0	16	1	1	2	3	6	9	24
20–34	3	1.7	<1	1	1	2	2	2	2	2
35–49	5	3.0	2	2	2	3	3	5	5	5
50–64	7	2.7	6	1	1	2	3	5	8	8
65+	8	2.1	2	1	1	2	3	5	5	5
GRAND TOTAL	363	3.0	15	1	1	2	3	6	8	24

786.05: SHORTNESS OF BREATH

Type of Patients	Observed Patients	Avg. Stay	Variance	10th	25th	50th	75th	90th	95th	99th
1. SINGLE DX										
A. Not Operated										
0–19 Years	1	1.0	0	1	1	1	1	1	1	1
20–34	2	2.5	<1	2	2	3	3	3	3	3
35–49	1	2.0	0	2	2	2	2	2	2	2
50–64	2	1.0	0	1	1	1	1	1	1	1
65+	1	3.0	0	3	3	3	3	3	3	3
B. Operated										
0–19 Years	0									
20–34	0									
35–49	0									
50–64	0									
65+	0									
2. MULTIPLE DX										
A. Not Operated										
0–19 Years	13	1.7	2	1	1	1	2	2	6	6
20–34	41	1.7	<1	1	1	2	2	3	3	4
35–49	141	2.1	3	1	1	2	2	4	5	9
50–64	360	2.2	6	1	1	1	3	4	5	13
65+	736	2.3	4	1	1	2	3	4	5	8
B. Operated										
0–19 Years	0									
20–34	1	2.0	0	2	2	2	2	2	2	2
35–49	1	2.0	0	2	2	2	2	2	2	2
50–64	5	3.8	11	1	1	3	5	9	9	9
65+	7	7.8	75	1	1	5	15	24	24	24
SUBTOTALS:										
1. SINGLE DX A. Not Operated	7	1.9	<1	1	1	2	2	3	3	3
B. Operated	0									
2. MULTIPLE DX A. Not Operated	1,291	2.2	4	1	1	2	3	4	5	9
B. Operated	14	5.5	44	1	1	3	5	15	24	24
1. SINGLE DX	7	1.9	<1	1	1	2	2	3	3	3
2. MULTIPLE DX	1,305	2.3	5	1	1	2	3	4	5	9
A. NOT OPERATED	1,298	2.2	4	1	1	2	3	4	5	9
B. OPERATED	14	5.5	44	1	1	3	5	15	24	24
TOTAL										
0–19 Years	14	1.6	2	1	1	1	2	2	2	6
20–34	44	1.8	<1	1	1	2	2	3	3	4
35–49	143	2.1	3	1	1	2	2	4	5	9
50–64	367	2.2	6	1	1	1	3	4	5	13
65+	744	2.4	5	1	1	2	3	4	6	9
GRAND TOTAL	1,312	2.3	5	1	1	2	3	4	5	9

786.09: RESP ABNORMALITY NEC

Type of Patients	Observed Patients	Avg. Stay	Variance	10th	25th	50th	75th	90th	95th	99th
1. SINGLE DX										
A. Not Operated										
0–19 Years	57	1.3	<1	1	1	1	1	2	3	4
20–34	1	1.0	0	1	1	1	1	1	1	1
35–49	1	1.0	0	1	1	1	1	1	1	1
50–64	0									
65+	2	2.0	2	1	1	3	3	3	3	3
B. Operated										
0–19 Years	0									
20–34	0									
35–49	0									
50–64	0									
65+	0									
2. MULTIPLE DX										
A. Not Operated										
0–19 Years	275	2.4	6	1	1	2	3	4	6	12
20–34	38	2.2	1	1	1	2	3	4	4	4
35–49	141	2.3	4	1	1	2	3	4	6	11
50–64	350	2.1	4	1	1	2	3	4	5	8
65+	752	2.4	4	1	1	2	3	5	6	10
B. Operated										
0–19 Years	7	5.0	26	1	1	2	9	14	14	14
20–34	0									
35–49	5	2.6	6	1	1	2	2	7	7	7
50–64	5	9.3	196	1	2	4	5	34	34	34
65+	10	4.7	12	1	1	3	8	9	10	10
SUBTOTALS:										
1. SINGLE DX A. Not Operated	61	1.3	<1	1	1	1	1	2	3	4
B. Operated	0									
2. MULTIPLE DX A. Not Operated	1,556	2.3	4	1	1	2	3	4	6	10
B. Operated	27	5.2	46	1	1	2	7	10	14	34
1. SINGLE DX	61	1.3	<1	1	1	1	1	2	3	4
2. MULTIPLE DX	1,583	2.4	5	1	1	2	3	5	6	10
A. NOT OPERATED	1,617	2.3	4	1	1	2	3	4	6	10
B. OPERATED	27	5.2	46	1	1	2	7	10	14	34
TOTAL										
0–19 Years	339	2.3	6	1	1	1	3	4	6	12
20–34	39	2.2	1	1	1	2	3	4	4	4
35–49	147	2.3	4	1	1	2	3	5	6	11
50–64	355	2.2	5	1	1	2	3	4	5	8
65+	764	2.5	4	1	1	2	3	5	6	10
GRAND TOTAL	1,644	2.3	4	1	1	2	3	4	6	10

Length of Stay by Diagnosis and Operation, Western Region, 2008

Western Region, October 2006–September 2007 Data, by Diagnosis

786.2: COUGH

Type of Patients	Observed Patients	Avg. Stay	Variance	10th	25th	50th	75th	90th	95th	99th
1. SINGLE DX										
A. Not Operated										
0–19 Years	8	1.8	<1	1	1	1	2	3	3	3
20–34	0									
35–49	1	1.0	0	1	1	1	1	1	1	1
50–64	0									
65+	0									
B. Operated										
0–19 Years	0									
20–34	0									
35–49	0									
50–64	0									
65+	0									
2. MULTIPLE DX										
A. Not Operated										
0–19 Years	40	2.1	2	1	1	2	3	4	6	6
20–34	12	2.1	1	1	1	2	3	4	4	4
35–49	31	3.5	7	1	2	3	5	6	8	13
50–64	41	3.7	28	1	1	2	3	7	13	31
65+	80	2.6	4	1	1	2	3	5	6	11
B. Operated										
0–19 Years	1	1.0	0	1	1	1	1	1	1	1
20–34	1	9.0	0	9	9	9	9	9	9	9
35–49	3	4.7	2	3	3	5	6	6	6	6
50–64	1	2.0	0	2	2	2	2	2	2	2
65+	1	3.0	0	3	3	3	3	3	3	3
SUBTOTALS:										
1. SINGLE DX										
A. Not Operated	9	1.7	<1	1	1	1	2	3	3	3
B. Operated	0									
2. MULTIPLE DX										
A. Not Operated	204	2.8	9	1	1	2	3	6	7	13
B. Operated	7	4.1	7	1	2	3	6	9	9	9
1. SINGLE DX	9	1.7	<1	1	1	1	2	3	3	3
2. MULTIPLE DX	211	2.9	9	1	1	2	3	6	7	13
A. NOT OPERATED	213	2.8	9	1	1	2	3	5	7	13
B. OPERATED	7	4.1	7	1	2	3	6	9	9	9
TOTAL										
0–19 Years	49	2.0	2	1	1	2	3	4	4	6
20–34	13	2.6	5	1	1	2	3	4	9	9
35–49	35	3.5	7	1	2	3	5	6	8	13
50–64	42	3.7	27	1	1	2	3	7	13	31
65+	81	2.6	4	1	1	2	3	5	6	11
GRAND TOTAL	220	2.8	9	1	1	2	3	6	7	13

786.3: HEMOPTYSIS

Type of Patients	Observed Patients	Avg. Stay	Variance	10th	25th	50th	75th	90th	95th	99th
1. SINGLE DX										
A. Not Operated										
0–19 Years	0									
20–34	4	1.8	<1	1	1	2	3	3	3	3
35–49	1	4.0	0	4	4	4	4	4	4	4
50–64	2	3.5	4	2	2	2	5	5	5	5
65+	0									
B. Operated										
0–19 Years	0									
20–34	0									
35–49	0									
50–64	0									
65+	0									
2. MULTIPLE DX										
A. Not Operated										
0–19 Years	23	4.1	17	1	1	2	7	11	13	13
20–34	60	6.3	165	1	2	3	6	9	16	94
35–49	91	4.6	32	1	2	3	6	7	9	39
50–64	211	3.4	8	1	2	3	4	6	8	18
65+	392	3.5	7	2	2	3	5	7	8	12
B. Operated										
0–19 Years	0									
20–34	9	10.0	38	3	4	10	15	18	18	18
35–49	11	3.7	11	2	2	2	4	6	13	13
50–64	23	8.7	50	2	3	5	14	18	19	28
65+	40	6.5	37	1	2	4	8	14	19	26
SUBTOTALS:										
1. SINGLE DX										
A. Not Operated	7	2.6	2	1	1	2	4	5	5	5
B. Operated	0									
2. MULTIPLE DX										
A. Not Operated	777	3.8	23	1	2	3	5	7	9	21
B. Operated	83	7.1	39	2	2	4	11	17	19	28
1. SINGLE DX	7	2.6	2	1	1	2	4	5	5	5
2. MULTIPLE DX	860	4.1	25	1	2	3	5	8	11	23
A. NOT OPERATED	784	3.8	23	1	2	3	5	7	9	21
B. OPERATED	83	7.1	39	2	2	4	11	17	19	28
TOTAL										
0–19 Years	23	4.1	17	1	1	2	7	11	13	13
20–34	73	6.5	142	1	1	3	6	14	18	94
35–49	103	4.5	29	1	2	3	6	7	9	29
50–64	236	3.9	15	1	2	3	5	7	12	21
65+	432	3.8	10	1	2	3	5	7	9	17
GRAND TOTAL	867	4.1	25	1	2	3	5	8	11	23

786.50: CHEST PAIN NOS

Type of Patients	Observed Patients	Avg. Stay	Variance	10th	25th	50th	75th	90th	95th	99th
1. SINGLE DX										
A. Not Operated										
0–19 Years	5	1.0	0	1	1	1	1	1	1	1
20–34	31	1.1	<1	1	1	1	1	1	2	3
35–49	177	1.2	<1	1	1	1	1	2	2	4
50–64	160	1.3	<1	1	1	1	1	2	3	7
65+	68	1.2	<1	1	1	1	1	2	2	3
B. Operated										
0–19 Years	0									
20–34	0									
35–49	0									
50–64	0									
65+	0									
2. MULTIPLE DX										
A. Not Operated										
0–19 Years	52	1.7	<1	1	1	1	2	3	3	5
20–34	687	1.7	2	1	1	1	2	3	4	7
35–49	5,520	1.7	1	1	1	1	2	3	4	6
50–64	10,178	1.7	2	1	1	1	2	3	4	7
65+	10,442	2.0	2	1	1	1	2	4	5	7
B. Operated										
0–19 Years	0									
20–34	5	7.0	34	2	4	5	7	17	17	17
35–49	20	4.7	15	1	2	3	6	12	13	13
50–64	59	5.3	24	1	1	3	9	13	16	20
65+	101	4.9	38	1	1	3	5	10	14	28
SUBTOTALS:										
1. SINGLE DX										
A. Not Operated	441	1.2	<1	1	1	1	1	2	2	4
B. Operated	0									
2. MULTIPLE DX										
A. Not Operated	26,879	1.8	2	1	1	1	2	3	4	7
B. Operated	185	5.1	31	1	1	3	7	11	14	28
1. SINGLE DX	441	1.2	<1	1	1	1	1	2	2	4
2. MULTIPLE DX	27,064	1.8	2	1	1	1	2	3	4	7
A. NOT OPERATED	27,320	1.8	2	1	1	1	2	3	4	7
B. OPERATED	185	5.1	31	1	1	3	7	11	14	28
TOTAL										
0–19 Years	57	1.6	<1	1	1	1	2	3	3	5
20–34	723	1.7	2	1	1	1	2	3	4	7
35–49	5,717	1.7	1	1	1	1	2	3	4	6
50–64	10,397	1.8	2	1	1	1	2	3	4	7
65+	10,611	2.0	3	1	1	1	2	4	5	8
GRAND TOTAL	27,505	1.8	2	1	1	1	2	3	4	7

Length of Stay by Diagnosis and Operation, Western Region, 2008

Western Region, October 2006–September 2007 Data, by Diagnosis

786.51: PRECORDIAL PAIN

Type of Patients	Observed Patients	Avg. Stay	Vari-ance	10th	25th	50th	75th	90th	95th	99th
1. SINGLE DX										
A. Not Operated										
0–19 Years	0									
20–34	4	1.0	0	1	1	1	1	1	1	1
35–49	4	2.0	4	1	1	1	3	5	5	5
50–64	10	1.1	<1	1	1	1	1	1	2	2
65+	8	1.9	2	1	1	2	2	5	5	5
B. Operated										
0–19 Years	0									
20–34	0									
35–49	0									
50–64	0									
65+	0									
2. MULTIPLE DX										
A. Not Operated										
0–19 Years	5	2.0	3	1	1	1	2	5	5	5
20–34	70	1.7	1	1	1	1	2	4	5	5
35–49	603	1.8	3	1	1	1	2	3	4	7
50–64	1,072	1.7	1	1	1	1	2	3	4	6
65+	1,041	2.0	2	1	1	1	2	4	5	8
B. Operated										
0–19 Years	0									
20–34	2	2.0	2	1	1	3	3	3	3	3
35–49	3	6.0	7	4	4	5	9	9	9	9
50–64	12	3.7	9	1	1	2	5	8	9	9
65+	14	4.3	7	1	2	4	6	8	9	9
SUBTOTALS:										
1. SINGLE DX										
A. Not Operated	26	1.5	1	1	1	1	1	2	5	5
B. Operated	0									
2. MULTIPLE DX										
A. Not Operated	2,791	1.8	2	1	1	1	2	3	4	7
B. Operated	31	4.1	8	1	1	4	6	8	9	9
1. SINGLE DX	26	1.5	1	1	1	1	1	2	5	5
2. MULTIPLE DX	2,822	1.8	2	1	1	1	2	3	4	7
A. NOT OPERATED	2,817	1.8	2	1	1	1	2	3	4	7
B. OPERATED	31	4.1	8	1	1	4	6	8	9	9
TOTAL										
0–19 Years	5	2.0	3	1	1	1	2	5	5	5
20–34	76	1.7	1	1	1	1	2	3	5	5
35–49	610	1.8	3	1	1	1	2	3	4	7
50–64	1,094	1.7	1	1	1	1	2	3	4	6
65+	1,063	2.0	2	1	1	1	2	4	5	8
GRAND TOTAL	2,848	1.8	2	1	1	1	2	3	4	7

786.52: PAINFUL RESPIRATION

Type of Patients	Observed Patients	Avg. Stay	Vari-ance	10th	25th	50th	75th	90th	95th	99th
1. SINGLE DX										
A. Not Operated										
0–19 Years	2	1.0	0	1	1	1	1	1	1	1
20–34	7	1.1	<1	1	1	1	1	2	2	2
35–49	9	1.2	<1	1	1	1	1	2	2	2
50–64	7	1.0	0	1	1	1	1	1	1	1
65+	2	1.0	0	1	1	1	1	1	1	1
B. Operated										
0–19 Years	0									
20–34	0									
35–49	0									
50–64	0									
65+	0									
2. MULTIPLE DX										
A. Not Operated										
0–19 Years	14	2.8	5	1	1	2	4	6	8	8
20–34	155	2.2	4	1	1	1	3	4	8	10
35–49	542	2.0	3	1	1	1	2	4	5	10
50–64	821	2.0	2	1	1	1	2	4	5	7
65+	1,039	2.2	3	1	1	2	3	4	5	8
B. Operated										
0–19 Years	0									
20–34	4	7.3	33	2	2	10	14	14	14	14
35–49	4	3.3	10	1	2	2	2	8	8	8
50–64	8	8.5	35	3	3	8	16	18	18	18
65+	8	7.2	34	2	2	7	10	19	19	19
SUBTOTALS:										
1. SINGLE DX										
A. Not Operated	27	1.1	<1	1	1	1	1	2	2	2
B. Operated	0									
2. MULTIPLE DX										
A. Not Operated	2,571	2.1	3	1	1	1	2	4	5	9
B. Operated	24	7.0	30	2	2	5	10	16	18	19
1. SINGLE DX	27	1.1	<1	1	1	1	1	2	2	2
2. MULTIPLE DX	2,595	2.1	3	1	1	2	3	4	5	10
A. NOT OPERATED	2,598	2.1	3	1	1	1	2	4	5	9
B. OPERATED	24	7.0	30	2	2	5	10	16	18	19
TOTAL										
0–19 Years	16	2.6	5	1	1	2	4	6	8	8
20–34	166	2.3	5	1	1	1	3	5	8	11
35–49	555	2.0	3	1	1	1	2	4	5	10
50–64	836	2.0	3	1	1	1	2	4	5	9
65+	1,049	2.2	3	1	2	2	3	4	5	9
GRAND TOTAL	2,622	2.1	3	1	1	1	3	4	5	10

786.59: CHEST PAIN NEC

Type of Patients	Observed Patients	Avg. Stay	Vari-ance	10th	25th	50th	75th	90th	95th	99th
1. SINGLE DX										
A. Not Operated										
0–19 Years	14	1.4	<1	1	1	1	2	2	3	3
20–34	87	1.2	<1	1	1	1	1	2	3	3
35–49	434	1.2	<1	1	1	1	1	2	2	3
50–64	417	1.2	<1	1	1	1	1	2	2	3
65+	95	1.3	<1	1	1	1	1	2	3	4
B. Operated										
0–19 Years	0									
20–34	0									
35–49	0									
50–64	0									
65+	0									
2. MULTIPLE DX										
A. Not Operated										
0–19 Years	125	1.8	1	1	1	1	2	3	4	5
20–34	2,269	1.7	2	1	1	1	2	3	4	6
35–49	17,494	1.7	2	1	1	1	2	3	4	7
50–64	29,069	1.8	2	1	1	1	2	3	4	7
65+	27,090	1.9	2	1	1	1	2	3	4	7
B. Operated										
0–19 Years	0									
20–34	11	7.0	134	2	2	3	7	9	41	41
35–49	62	5.4	43	1	1	4	6	9	14	33
50–64	168	5.1	21	1	2	4	7	10	14	25
65+	168	4.8	19	2	2	4	6	9	12	25
SUBTOTALS:										
1. SINGLE DX										
A. Not Operated	1,047	1.2	<1	1	1	1	1	2	2	3
B. Operated	0									
2. MULTIPLE DX										
A. Not Operated	76,047	1.8	2	1	1	1	2	3	4	7
B. Operated	409	5.0	26	2	2	4	6	10	14	30
1. SINGLE DX	1,047	1.2	<1	1	1	1	1	2	2	3
2. MULTIPLE DX	76,456	1.8	2	1	1	1	2	3	4	7
A. NOT OPERATED	77,094	1.8	2	1	1	1	2	3	4	7
B. OPERATED	409	5.0	26	2	2	4	6	10	14	30
TOTAL										
0–19 Years	139	1.8	1	1	1	1	2	3	4	5
20–34	2,367	1.7	2	1	1	1	2	3	4	6
35–49	17,990	1.7	2	1	1	1	2	3	4	7
50–64	29,654	1.8	2	1	1	1	2	3	4	7
65+	27,353	1.9	2	1	1	1	2	4	5	7
GRAND TOTAL	77,503	1.8	2	1	1	1	2	3	4	7

Western Region, October 2006–September 2007 Data, by Diagnosis

786.6: CHEST SWELLING/MASS/LUMP

Type of Patients	Observed Patients	Avg. Stay	Variance	10th	25th	50th	75th	90th	95th	99th
1. SINGLE DX										
A. Not Operated										
0–19 Years	0									
20–34	4	1.8	<1	1	1	2	3	3	3	3
35–49	3	2.0	3	1	1	1	4	4	4	4
50–64	4	2.0	<1	1	2	2	3	3	4	4
65+	6	2.2	2	1	1	1	4	4	4	4
B. Operated										
0–19 Years	1	2.0	0	2	2	2	2	2	2	2
20–34	5	3.4	3	1	3	3	5	5	5	5
35–49	1	3.0	0	3	3	3	3	3	3	3
50–64	2	1.5	<1	1	1	2	2	2	2	2
65+	3	2.3	<1	2	2	2	3	3	3	3
2. MULTIPLE DX										
A. Not Operated										
0–19 Years	4	3.5	2	2	2	4	4	5	5	5
20–34	16	3.1	3	1	2	3	4	5	8	8
35–49	51	2.9	4	1	1	3	4	6	7	8
50–64	130	3.1	8	1	1	2	4	6	7	15
65+	207	2.9	4	1	1	2	4	6	7	9
B. Operated										
0–19 Years	3	1.7	1	1	1	1	3	3	3	3
20–34	20	3.9	6	1	3	3	4	8	11	11
35–49	42	4.2	8	2	2	3	6	8	10	13
50–64	88	4.4	15	1	2	3	5	8	14	20
65+	98	5.1	18	1	2	4	7	10	14	21
SUBTOTALS:										
1. SINGLE DX										
A. Not Operated	17	2.0	1	1	1	2	3	4	4	4
B. Operated	12	2.7	2	1	2	3	3	5	5	5
2. MULTIPLE DX										
A. Not Operated	408	3.0	5	1	1	2	4	6	7	10
B. Operated	251	4.6	14	1	2	3	6	9	13	20
1. SINGLE DX	29	2.3	2	1	1	2	3	4	5	5
2. MULTIPLE DX	659	3.6	9	1	1	3	5	7	9	19
A. NOT OPERATED	425	2.9	5	1	1	2	4	6	7	10
B. OPERATED	263	4.5	14	1	2	3	5	9	13	20
TOTAL										
0–19 Years	8	2.6	2	1	1	2	4	5	5	5
20–34	45	3.4	4	1	2	3	4	5	8	11
35–49	97	3.4	6	1	1	3	5	7	8	13
50–64	224	3.5	11	1	1	3	5	7	8	20
65+	314	3.6	9	1	1	3	5	7	9	15
GRAND TOTAL	688	3.5	9	1	1	3	5	7	8	19

787: GI SYSTEM SYMPTOMS

Type of Patients	Observed Patients	Avg. Stay	Variance	10th	25th	50th	75th	90th	95th	99th
1. SINGLE DX										
A. Not Operated										
0–19 Years	86	1.4	<1	1	1	1	2	3	3	4
20–34	13	1.5	<1	1	1	1	2	3	3	3
35–49	21	2.1	3	1	1	1	2	4	5	7
50–64	8	1.3	<1	1	1	1	1	2	2	2
65+	7	2.3	2	1	1	2	4	4	4	4
B. Operated										
0–19 Years	1	4.0	0	4	4	4	4	4	4	4
20–34	7	1.6	<1	1	1	1	2	3	3	3
35–49	11	2.3	1	1	1	2	3	4	4	4
50–64	5	3.0	4	1	2	2	4	6	6	6
65+	2	4.0	2	3	3	5	5	5	5	5
2. MULTIPLE DX										
A. Not Operated										
0–19 Years	763	2.3	6	1	1	2	3	4	6	16
20–34	952	3.0	6	1	2	2	4	6	7	13
35–49	1,592	3.3	13	1	2	3	4	6	8	14
50–64	2,276	3.3	8	1	2	3	4	6	8	14
65+	4,435	3.6	11	1	2	3	4	7	9	16
B. Operated										
0–19 Years	26	7.7	265	2	2	3	6	10	28	83
20–34	43	2.9	5	1	2	2	4	7	7	7
35–49	96	4.6	29	1	2	3	5	12	15	30
50–64	149	4.2	20	1	1	3	5	9	12	22
65+	146	7.1	69	2	2	4	8	16	22	32
SUBTOTALS:										
1. SINGLE DX										
A. Not Operated	135	1.6	1	1	1	1	2	3	4	5
B. Operated	26	2.4	2	1	1	2	3	4	5	6
2. MULTIPLE DX										
A. Not Operated	10,018	3.3	10	1	2	3	4	6	8	15
B. Operated	460	5.3	51	1	2	3	6	11	16	31
1. SINGLE DX	161	1.7	1	1	1	1	2	3	4	6
2. MULTIPLE DX	10,478	3.4	12	1	1	3	4	6	9	16
A. NOT OPERATED	10,153	3.3	10	1	1	2	4	6	8	15
B. OPERATED	486	5.1	49	1	2	3	6	11	15	31
TOTAL										
0–19 Years	876	2.4	14	1	1	2	3	4	6	16
20–34	1,015	2.9	6	1	1	2	4	6	7	12
35–49	1,720	3.3	13	1	2	3	4	7	8	15
50–64	2,438	3.3	9	1	2	3	4	6	9	15
65+	4,590	3.7	13	1	2	3	5	7	9	17
GRAND TOTAL	10,639	3.4	12	1	1	2	4	6	9	16

787.01: NAUSEA W VOMITING

Type of Patients	Observed Patients	Avg. Stay	Variance	10th	25th	50th	75th	90th	95th	99th
1. SINGLE DX										
A. Not Operated										
0–19 Years	8	1.9	2	1	1	1	3	4	4	4
20–34	5	1.8	1	1	1	1	3	3	3	3
35–49	11	1.7	1	1	1	1	2	3	4	4
50–64	5	1.2	<1	1	1	1	1	2	2	2
65+	2	2.0	2	1	2	2	3	3	3	3
B. Operated										
0–19 Years	0									
20–34	0									
35–49	0									
50–64	0									
65+	0									
2. MULTIPLE DX										
A. Not Operated										
0–19 Years	172	2.6	8	1	1	2	3	5	8	17
20–34	698	3.0	7	1	1	2	4	6	7	13
35–49	1,066	3.2	15	1	1	2	4	6	8	14
50–64	1,291	3.1	7	1	1	2	4	6	8	13
65+	1,857	3.2	8	1	1	3	4	6	8	13
B. Operated										
0–19 Years	16	5.0	31	1	1	1	9	9	9	9
20–34	16	2.2	3	1	1	1	3	5	7	7
35–49	32	4.4	17	1	1	3	6	10	15	15
50–64	20	5.7	40	1	1	3	9	14	22	22
65+	36	7.6	66	1	2	4	9	20	28	32
SUBTOTALS:										
1. SINGLE DX										
A. Not Operated	31	1.7	1	1	1	1	3	3	4	4
B. Operated	0									
2. MULTIPLE DX										
A. Not Operated	5,084	3.1	9	1	1	2	4	6	8	13
B. Operated	106	5.4	38	1	1	3	7	14	19	28
1. SINGLE DX	31	1.7	1	1	1	1	3	3	4	4
2. MULTIPLE DX	5,190	3.1	10	1	1	3	4	6	8	14
A. NOT OPERATED	5,115	3.1	9	1	1	2	4	6	8	13
B. OPERATED	106	5.4	38	1	1	3	7	14	19	28
TOTAL										
0–19 Years	182	2.6	8	1	1	2	3	5	8	17
20–34	719	3.0	7	1	1	2	4	6	7	13
35–49	1,109	3.2	15	1	1	2	4	6	8	14
50–64	1,316	3.1	7	1	1	2	4	6	8	13
65+	1,895	3.3	10	1	1	3	4	6	8	14
GRAND TOTAL	5,221	3.1	10	1	1	2	4	6	8	14

Length of Stay by Diagnosis and Operation, Western Region, 2008

Western Region, October 2006–September 2007 Data, by Diagnosis

787.02: NAUSEA ALONE

Type of Patients	Observed Patients	Avg. Stay	Variance	Percentiles 10th	25th	50th	75th	90th	95th	99th
1. SINGLE DX										
A. Not Operated										
0–19 Years	0									
20–34	0									
35–49	1	1.0	0	1	1	1	1	1	1	1
50–64	0									
65+	0									
B. Operated										
0–19 Years	0									
20–34	0									
35–49	0									
50–64	0									
65+	0									
2. MULTIPLE DX										
A. Not Operated										
0–19 Years	5	1.4	<1	1	1	1	1	3	3	3
20–34	15	2.6	2	1	1	2	4	5	5	5
35–49	34	3.1	7	1	1	2	6	7	8	8
50–64	69	2.7	5	1	1	2	3	6	8	13
65+	185	3.0	9	1	1	2	3	6	8	18
B. Operated										
0–19 Years	1	4.0	0	4	4	4	4	4	4	4
20–34	10	1.8	3	1	1	1	2	2	7	7
35–49	11	1.3	<1	1	1	1	2	2	2	2
50–64	17	1.8	5	1	1	1	1	3	10	10
65+	13	3.9	34	1	1	2	3	9	22	22
SUBTOTALS:										
1. SINGLE DX										
A. Not Operated	1	1.0	0	1	1	1	1	1	1	1
B. Operated	0									
2. MULTIPLE DX										
A. Not Operated	308	2.9	7	1	1	2	3	6	8	12
B. Operated	52	2.2	11	1	1	1	2	4	9	22
1. SINGLE DX	**1**	**1.0**	**0**	**1**	**1**	**1**	**1**	**1**	**1**	**1**
2. MULTIPLE DX	**360**	**2.8**	**8**	**1**	**1**	**2**	**3**	**6**	**8**	**13**
A. NOT OPERATED	**309**	**2.9**	**7**	**1**	**1**	**2**	**3**	**6**	**8**	**12**
B. OPERATED	**52**	**2.2**	**11**	**1**	**1**	**1**	**2**	**4**	**9**	**22**
TOTAL										
0–19 Years	6	1.8	2	1	1	1	1	3	4	4
20–34	25	2.3	3	1	1	2	3	5	5	7
35–49	46	2.6	6	1	1	2	2	7	7	8
50–64	86	2.5	5	1	1	2	3	5	8	13
65+	198	3.1	10	1	1	2	3	7	9	22
GRAND TOTAL	**361**	**2.8**	**8**	**1**	**1**	**2**	**3**	**6**	**8**	**13**

787.03: VOMITING ALONE

Type of Patients	Observed Patients	Avg. Stay	Variance	Percentiles 10th	25th	50th	75th	90th	95th	99th
1. SINGLE DX										
A. Not Operated										
0–19 Years	51	1.3	<1	1	1	1	1	1	3	4
20–34	1	1.0	0	1	1	1	1	1	1	1
35–49	0									
50–64	1	1.0	0	1	1	1	1	1	1	1
65+	1	4.0	0	4	4	4	4	4	4	4
B. Operated										
0–19 Years	1	4.0	0	4	4	4	4	4	4	4
20–34	0									
35–49	0									
50–64	0									
65+	0									
2. MULTIPLE DX										
A. Not Operated										
0–19 Years	335	1.8	2	1	1	1	2	3	3	9
20–34	43	2.9	5	1	1	2	4	6	7	9
35–49	48	2.9	7	1	1	2	4	6	9	12
50–64	61	2.5	2	1	1	2	3	5	5	7
65+	101	2.7	4	1	1	2	3	5	6	13
B. Operated										
0–19 Years	3	11.3	210	1	1	5	28	28	28	28
20–34	0									
35–49	0									
50–64	1	5.0	0	5	5	5	5	5	5	5
65+	1	1.0	0	1	1	1	1	1	1	1
SUBTOTALS:										
1. SINGLE DX										
A. Not Operated	54	1.4	<1	1	1	1	1	3	3	4
B. Operated	1	4.0	0	4	4	4	4	4	4	4
2. MULTIPLE DX										
A. Not Operated	588	2.2	3	1	1	2	3	4	6	10
B. Operated	5	8.0	128	1	1	5	5	28	28	28
1. SINGLE DX	**55**	**1.4**	**<1**	**1**	**1**	**1**	**1**	**3**	**4**	**4**
2. MULTIPLE DX	**593**	**2.3**	**4**	**1**	**1**	**2**	**3**	**4**	**6**	**10**
A. NOT OPERATED	**642**	**2.1**	**3**	**1**	**1**	**2**	**3**	**4**	**5**	**9**
B. OPERATED	**6**	**7.3**	**105**	**4**	**1**	**4**	**5**	**28**	**28**	**28**
TOTAL										
0–19 Years	390	1.8	4	1	1	1	2	3	4	4
20–34	44	2.9	5	1	1	2	4	6	7	9
35–49	48	2.9	7	1	1	2	4	6	9	12
50–64	63	2.5	2	1	1	2	3	5	5	7
65+	103	2.7	4	1	1	2	3	5	6	7
GRAND TOTAL	**648**	**2.2**	**4**	**1**	**1**	**2**	**3**	**4**	**6**	**10**

787.2: DYSPHAGIA

Type of Patients	Observed Patients	Avg. Stay	Variance	Percentiles 10th	25th	50th	75th	90th	95th	99th
1. SINGLE DX										
A. Not Operated										
0–19 Years	6	1.0	0	1	1	1	1	1	1	1
20–34	2	1.0	0	1	1	1	1	1	1	1
35–49	2	1.5	<1	1	2	2	2	2	2	2
50–64	1	2.0	0	2	2	2	2	2	2	2
65+	2	1.0	0	1	1	1	1	1	1	1
B. Operated										
0–19 Years	0	1.0	0	1	1	1	1	1	1	1
20–34	0									
35–49	0									
50–64	0									
65+	1	3.0	0	3	3	3	3	3	3	3
2. MULTIPLE DX										
A. Not Operated										
0–19 Years	47	3.3	11	1	1	2	4	7	11	16
20–34	48	2.6	3	1	1	2	3	6	7	7
35–49	109	3.4	8	1	1	2	4	6	8	12
50–64	204	3.5	8	2	2	3	5	7	10	12
65+	588	4.2	11	1	2	3	5	8	11	17
B. Operated										
0–19 Years	7	3.0	8	1	1	2	3	9	9	9
20–34	0	2.0	0	2	2	2	2	2	2	2
35–49	6	10.9	120	2	2	14	14	30	30	30
50–64	9	4.1	9	1	2	3	4	4	10	10
65+	24	9.6	201	2	2	4	10	20	30	68
SUBTOTALS:										
1. SINGLE DX										
A. Not Operated	13	1.2	<1	1	1	1	1	1	2	2
B. Operated	2	2.0	2	1	2	2	3	3	3	3
2. MULTIPLE DX										
A. Not Operated	996	3.8	10	1	2	3	5	8	10	16
B. Operated	49	7.4	122	2	2	3	8	15	30	68
1. SINGLE DX	**15**	**1.3**	**<1**	**1**	**1**	**1**	**1**	**2**	**3**	**3**
2. MULTIPLE DX	**1,045**	**4.0**	**16**	**2**	**2**	**3**	**5**	**8**	**11**	**17**
A. NOT OPERATED	**1,009**	**3.8**	**10**	**1**	**2**	**3**	**5**	**8**	**10**	**16**
B. OPERATED	**51**	**7.2**	**118**	**2**	**2**	**3**	**8**	**14**	**30**	**68**
TOTAL										
0–19 Years	60	3.1	10	1	1	2	4	7	11	16
20–34	54	2.5	3	1	1	2	3	5	7	7
35–49	117	3.7	15	1	1	2	5	8	12	14
50–64	214	3.5	8	2	3	3	4	7	10	12
65+	615	4.4	19	2	2	3	5	8	11	19
GRAND TOTAL	**1,060**	**3.9**	**15**	**2**	**2**	**3**	**5**	**8**	**11**	**17**

Length of Stay by Diagnosis and Operation, Western Region, 2008

787.6: INCONTINENCE OF FECES

Type of Patients	Observed Patients	Avg. Stay	Vari-ance	Percentiles						
				10th	25th	50th	75th	90th	95th	99th
1. SINGLE DX										
A. Not Operated										
0–19 Years	2	2.0	2	1	1	3	3	3	3	3
20–34	0									
35–49	0									
50–64	0									
65+	0									
B. Operated										
0–19 Years	0									
20–34	5	1.8	<1	1	1	2	2	3	3	3
35–49	10	2.4	1	1	1	3	3	4	4	4
50–64	5	3.0	4	1	2	2	4	6	6	6
65+	1	5.0	0	5	5	5	5	5	5	5
2. MULTIPLE DX										
A. Not Operated										
0–19 Years	32	2.4	1	1	2	2	3	4	5	5
20–34	2	3.5	<1	3	3	4	4	4	4	4
35–49	2	5.0	32	1	1	5	9	9	9	9
50–64	9	4.5	50	1	2	2	2	23	23	23
65+	8	5.9	34	1	1	4	14	16	16	16
B. Operated										
0–19 Years	12	4.0	6	2	2	3	6	7	7	10
20–34	11	4.4	4	1	3	4	7	7	7	7
35–49	40	3.1	3	2	2	3	4	5	5	8
50–64	82	3.6	8	1	2	3	5	7	9	15
65+	51	5.9	31	2	3	5	6	11	16	31
SUBTOTALS:										
1. SINGLE DX										
A. Not Operated	2	2.0	2	1	1	3	3	3	3	3
B. Operated	21	2.5	2	1	1	2	3	4	5	6
2. MULTIPLE DX										
A. Not Operated	53	3.4	15	1	2	2	4	5	14	23
B. Operated	196	4.2	13	1	2	3	5	7	10	24
1. SINGLE DX	23	2.5	2	1	1	2	3	4	5	6
2. MULTIPLE DX	249	4.0	14	1	2	3	5	7	10	23
A. NOT OPERATED	55	3.4	15	1	2	2	4	5	14	23
B. OPERATED	217	4.0	12	1	2	3	5	7	10	16
TOTAL										
0–19 Years	46	2.8	3	1	2	3	3	5	6	10
20–34	18	3.6	4	1	2	3	5	7	7	7
35–49	52	3.1	11	1	2	3	4	5	7	9
50–64	96	3.7	11	1	3	3	5	7	10	23
65+	60	5.9	30	2	3	5	6	14	16	31
GRAND TOTAL	272	3.9	13	1	2	3	5	7	10	23

787.91: DIARRHEA

Type of Patients	Observed Patients	Avg. Stay	Vari-ance	Percentiles						
				10th	25th	50th	75th	90th	95th	99th
1. SINGLE DX										
A. Not Operated										
0–19 Years	14	1.8	<1	1	1	2	2	3	3	3
20–34	4	1.5	<1	1	1	2	2	2	2	2
35–49	5	2.6	3	1	1	2	4	5	5	5
50–64	1	1.0	0	1	1	1	1	1	1	1
65+	2	3.0	2	2	2	2	4	4	4	4
B. Operated										
0–19 Years	0									
20–34	0									
35–49	1	1.0	0	1	1	1	1	1	1	1
50–64	0									
65+	0									
2. MULTIPLE DX										
A. Not Operated										
0–19 Years	151	2.7	11	1	1	2	3	4	6	20
20–34	136	2.9	5	1	2	2	3	5	7	13
35–49	308	3.5	8	1	2	3	4	7	8	15
50–64	601	3.9	10	1	2	3	5	7	9	19
65+	1,610	4.1	14	1	2	3	5	8	10	17
B. Operated										
0–19 Years	1	83.0	0	83	83	83	83	83	83	83
20–34	2	7.0	0	7	7	7	7	7	7	7
35–49	6	15.7	63	6	7	19	21	26	26	26
50–64	15	8.5	64	2	4	6	12	13	34	34
65+	18	8.1	30	2	4	8	9	17	21	21
SUBTOTALS:										
1. SINGLE DX										
A. Not Operated	26	2.0	1	1	1	2	2	4	4	5
B. Operated	1	1.0	0	1	1	1	1	1	1	1
2. MULTIPLE DX										
A. Not Operated	2,806	3.8	12	1	2	3	5	7	9	17
B. Operated	42	11.1	178	3	4	7	13	21	26	83
1. SINGLE DX	27	1.9	1	1	1	2	2	4	4	5
2. MULTIPLE DX	2,848	3.9	15	1	2	3	5	7	10	19
A. NOT OPERATED	2,832	3.8	12	1	2	3	5	7	9	17
B. OPERATED	43	10.8	176	2	4	7	13	21	26	83
TOTAL										
0–19 Years	166	3.1	49	1	1	2	3	4	6	29
20–34	142	2.9	5	1	2	2	4	6	7	13
35–49	320	3.7	11	1	2	3	4	7	9	19
50–64	617	4.0	12	1	2	3	5	7	10	19
65+	1,630	4.1	14	1	2	3	5	8	10	17
GRAND TOTAL	2,875	3.9	15	1	2	3	5	7	10	19

788: URINARY SYSTEM SYMPTOMS

Type of Patients	Observed Patients	Avg. Stay	Vari-ance	Percentiles						
				10th	25th	50th	75th	90th	95th	99th
1. SINGLE DX										
A. Not Operated										
0–19 Years	4	1.3	<1	1	1	1	1	1	2	2
20–34	6	1.3	<1	1	1	1	2	2	2	2
35–49	10	1.3	<1	1	1	1	2	2	2	2
50–64	7	1.4	<1	1	1	1	2	3	3	3
65+	2	2.0	2	1	1	1	3	3	3	3
B. Operated										
0–19 Years	0									
20–34	3	1.0	0	1	1	1	1	1	1	1
35–49	5	1.0	0	1	1	1	1	1	1	1
50–64	19	1.1	<1	1	1	1	1	1	2	2
65+	13	1.4	<1	1	1	1	1	2	4	4
2. MULTIPLE DX										
A. Not Operated										
0–19 Years	31	2.3	2	1	1	2	3	4	5	7
20–34	67	2.9	5	1	1	2	4	6	7	10
35–49	124	2.6	4	1	2	2	3	5	6	12
50–64	154	2.6	6	1	2	3	3	5	6	14
65+	401	2.8	4	1	2	2	3	5	7	11
B. Operated										
0–19 Years	3	2.0	<1	1	2	2	3	3	3	3
20–34	28	3.1	8	1	2	3	3	9	11	11
35–49	139	2.2	14	1	1	1	2	3	5	17
50–64	274	1.6	1	1	1	1	2	3	4	7
65+	477	1.9	5	1	1	1	1	3	6	13
SUBTOTALS:										
1. SINGLE DX										
A. Not Operated	29	1.4	<1	1	1	1	2	2	3	3
B. Operated	40	1.2	<1	1	1	1	1	2	2	4
2. MULTIPLE DX										
A. Not Operated	777	2.7	4	1	2	2	3	5	7	12
B. Operated	921	1.9	5	1	1	1	2	3	5	11
1. SINGLE DX	69	1.3	<1	1	1	1	1	2	2	4
2. MULTIPLE DX	1,698	2.3	5	1	1	2	3	4	6	12
A. NOT OPERATED	806	2.6	4	1	1	2	3	5	7	11
B. OPERATED	961	1.9	5	1	1	1	2	3	4	11
TOTAL										
0–19 Years	38	2.1	2	1	1	2	3	4	5	7
20–34	104	2.8	5	1	1	2	3	6	8	11
35–49	278	2.3	9	1	2	2	2	4	6	14
50–64	454	1.9	3	1	1	1	2	4	5	9
65+	893	2.3	5	1	2	2	3	4	6	12
GRAND TOTAL	1,767	2.2	5	1	1	2	3	4	6	11

Length of Stay by Diagnosis and Operation, Western Region, 2008

Western Region, October 2006–September 2007 Data, by Diagnosis

788.0: RENAL COLIC

Type of Patients	Observed Patients	Avg. Stay	Vari-ance	10th	25th	50th	75th	90th	95th	99th
1. SINGLE DX										
A. Not Operated										
0–19 Years	2	1.0	0	1	1	1	1	1	1	1
20–34	4	1.3	<1	1	1	1	2	2	2	2
35–49	6	1.5	<1	1	1	2	2	2	2	2
50–64	5	1.4	<1	1	1	1	1	1	3	3
65+	1	3.0	0	3	3	3	3	3	3	3
B. Operated										
0–19 Years	0									
20–34	0									
35–49	0									
50–64	0									
65+	0									
2. MULTIPLE DX										
A. Not Operated										
0–19 Years	4	1.3	<1	1	1	1	2	2	2	2
20–34	35	3.0	5	1	1	2	4	7	7	10
35–49	58	2.0	1	1	1	2	2	4	5	6
50–64	44	2.1	2	1	1	2	3	4	4	7
65+	14	1.9	<1	1	1	2	2	3	4	4
B. Operated										
0–19 Years	0									
20–34	1	6.0	0	6	6	6	6	6	6	6
35–49	3	1.0	0	1	1	1	1	1	1	1
50–64	2	3.5	4	2	2	4	5	5	5	5
65+	1	5.0	0	5	5	5	5	5	5	5
SUBTOTALS:										
1. SINGLE DX										
A. Not Operated	18	1.5	<1	1	1	1	2	2	2	3
B. Operated	0									
2. MULTIPLE DX										
A. Not Operated	155	2.2	2	1	1	2	3	4	5	7
B. Operated	7	3.0	5	1	1	2	5	6	6	6
1. SINGLE DX	18	1.5	<1	1	1	1	2	2	2	3
2. MULTIPLE DX	162	2.3	2	1	1	2	3	4	5	7
A. NOT OPERATED	173	2.1	2	1	1	2	3	4	5	7
B. OPERATED	7	3.0	5	1	1	2	5	6	6	6
TOTAL										
0–19 Years	6	1.2	<1	1	1	1	1	2	2	2
20–34	40	2.9	5	1	1	2	4	6	7	10
35–49	67	1.9	1	1	1	2	2	4	4	6
50–64	51	2.1	2	1	1	2	3	4	5	7
65+	16	2.1	1	1	1	2	3	4	5	5
GRAND TOTAL	180	2.2	2	1	1	2	3	4	5	7

788.20: RETENTION OF URINE NOS

Type of Patients	Observed Patients	Avg. Stay	Vari-ance	10th	25th	50th	75th	90th	95th	99th
1. SINGLE DX										
A. Not Operated										
0–19 Years	2	1.5	<1	1	1	2	2	2	2	2
20–34	1	1.0	0	1	1	1	1	1	1	1
35–49	2	1.0	0	1	1	1	1	1	1	1
50–64	1	1.0	0	1	1	1	1	1	1	1
65+	1	1.0	0	1	1	1	1	1	1	1
B. Operated										
0–19 Years	0									
20–34	0									
35–49	0									
50–64	2	1.5	<1	1	1	2	2	2	2	2
65+	1	4.0	0	4	4	4	4	4	4	4
2. MULTIPLE DX										
A. Not Operated										
0–19 Years	9	2.9	3	1	2	2	3	7	7	7
20–34	22	3.1	6	1	2	2	4	6	8	10
35–49	41	3.0	7	1	1	2	4	6	7	12
50–64	61	2.5	5	1	1	2	3	5	5	14
65+	228	2.8	4	1	1	2	3	5	6	12
B. Operated										
0–19 Years	1	3.0	0	3	3	3	3	3	3	3
20–34	5	2.0	<1	1	2	2	2	3	3	3
35–49	8	3.8	19	1	2	2	5	14	14	14
50–64	18	1.9	2	1	1	1	3	4	5	5
65+	66	2.2	5	1	1	2	2	4	6	14
SUBTOTALS:										
1. SINGLE DX										
A. Not Operated	7	1.1	<1	1	1	1	1	2	2	2
B. Operated	3	2.3	2	1	1	2	4	4	4	4
2. MULTIPLE DX										
A. Not Operated	361	2.8	5	1	1	2	3	5	7	12
B. Operated	98	2.3	5	1	1	2	2	4	6	14
1. SINGLE DX	10	1.5	<1	1	1	1	2	2	4	4
2. MULTIPLE DX	459	2.7	5	1	1	2	3	5	6	14
A. NOT OPERATED	368	2.8	5	1	1	2	3	5	6	12
B. OPERATED	101	2.3	5	1	1	1	2	4	6	14
TOTAL										
0–19 Years	12	2.7	3	1	2	2	3	4	7	7
20–34	28	2.9	5	1	2	2	4	6	8	10
35–49	51	3.1	8	1	1	2	4	6	12	14
50–64	82	2.3	4	1	1	2	3	5	5	14
65+	296	2.6	5	1	1	2	3	5	6	14
GRAND TOTAL	469	2.6	5	1	1	2	3	5	6	14

788.33: URGE & STRESS INCONT

Type of Patients	Observed Patients	Avg. Stay	Vari-ance	10th	25th	50th	75th	90th	95th	99th
1. SINGLE DX										
A. Not Operated										
0–19 Years	0									
20–34	0									
35–49	0									
50–64	0									
65+	0									
B. Operated										
0–19 Years	0									
20–34	2	1.0	0	1	1	1	1	1	1	1
35–49	4	1.0	0	1	1	1	1	1	1	1
50–64	17	1.1	<1	1	1	1	1	1	2	2
65+	3	1.3	<1	1	1	1	2	2	2	2
2. MULTIPLE DX										
A. Not Operated										
0–19 Years	0									
20–34	0									
35–49	0									
50–64	0									
65+	1	1.0	0	1	1	1	1	1	1	1
B. Operated										
0–19 Years	0									
20–34	12	1.9	<1	1	1	2	2	3	3	3
35–49	105	1.7	1	1	1	1	2	3	3	7
50–64	173	1.5	<1	1	1	1	1	2	2	4
65+	179	1.7	2	1	1	1	2	3	4	9
SUBTOTALS:										
1. SINGLE DX										
A. Not Operated	0									
B. Operated	26	1.1	<1	1	1	1	1	1	2	2
2. MULTIPLE DX										
A. Not Operated	1	1.0	0	1	1	1	1	1	1	1
B. Operated	469	1.7	1	1	1	1	2	3	3	8
1. SINGLE DX	26	1.1	<1	1	1	1	1	1	2	2
2. MULTIPLE DX	470	1.7	1	1	1	1	2	3	3	8
A. NOT OPERATED	1	1.0	0	1	1	1	1	1	1	1
B. OPERATED	495	1.6	1	1	1	1	2	3	3	8
TOTAL										
0–19 Years	0									
20–34	14	1.8	<1	1	1	2	2	3	3	3
35–49	109	1.7	1	1	1	1	2	3	3	7
50–64	190	1.5	<1	1	1	1	1	2	3	4
65+	183	1.7	2	1	1	1	2	3	4	9
GRAND TOTAL	496	1.6	1	1	1	1	2	3	3	8

Length of Stay by Diagnosis and Operation, Western Region, 2008

789: OTH ABDOMEN/PELVIS SX

Type of Patients	Observed Patients	Avg. Stay	Variance	Percentiles						
				10th	25th	50th	75th	90th	95th	99th
1. SINGLE DX										
A. Not Operated										
0–19 Years	629	1.3	<1	1	1	1	2	2	3	4
20–34	376	1.5	<1	1	1	1	2	3	3	5
35–49	224	1.5	<1	1	1	1	2	3	3	6
50–64	123	1.7	1	1	1	1	2	3	4	5
65+	39	2.2	5	1	1	2	3	3	5	14
B. Operated										
0–19 Years	81	1.5	<1	1	1	1	2	2	3	4
20–34	70	1.9	2	1	1	2	2	3	4	11
35–49	28	1.8	1	1	1	1	2	3	5	5
50–64	19	2.2	4	1	1	2	2	5	9	9
65+	3	1.7	1	1	1	1	3	3	3	3
2. MULTIPLE DX										
A. Not Operated										
0–19 Years	1,777	2.0	3	1	1	1	2	3	5	9
20–34	3,974	2.7	5	1	1	1	3	5	7	12
35–49	5,605	2.9	6	1	1	2	4	6	7	12
50–64	5,310	3.0	7	1	1	2	4	6	7	12
65+	6,205	3.1	6	1	1	2	4	6	8	13
B. Operated										
0–19 Years	185	2.6	4	1	1	2	4	5	7	11
20–34	456	3.2	12	1	1	2	4	7	9	20
35–49	404	3.9	16	1	2	3	5	7	10	20
50–64	307	4.8	21	1	2	4	6	10	14	21
65+	220	6.1	29	1	2	4	8	14	16	23
SUBTOTALS:										
1. SINGLE DX										
A. Not Operated	1,391	1.5	<1	1	1	1	2	2	3	5
B. Operated	201	1.8	1	1	1	1	2	3	3	5
2. MULTIPLE DX										
A. Not Operated	22,871	2.9	6	1	1	2	4	6	7	12
B. Operated	1,572	4.0	17	1	1	3	5	8	11	21
1. SINGLE DX	1,592	1.5	<1	1	1	1	2	3	3	5
2. MULTIPLE DX	24,443	2.9	7	1	1	2	4	6	8	13
A. NOT OPERATED	24,262	2.8	6	1	1	2	4	5	7	12
B. OPERATED	1,773	3.8	16	1	1	2	5	8	11	20
TOTAL										
0–19 Years	2,672	1.8	3	1	1	1	2	3	4	8
20–34	4,876	2.6	5	1	1	2	3	5	7	12
35–49	6,261	2.9	7	1	1	2	4	6	8	13
50–64	5,759	3.0	8	1	1	2	4	6	8	13
65+	6,467	3.2	7	1	1	2	4	6	8	14
GRAND TOTAL	26,035	2.9	7	1	1	2	4	6	7	13

789.00: ABDOMINAL PAIN-SITE NOS

Type of Patients	Observed Patients	Avg. Stay	Variance	Percentiles						
				10th	25th	50th	75th	90th	95th	99th
1. SINGLE DX										
A. Not Operated										
0–19 Years	150	1.4	<1	1	1	1	2	2	3	4
20–34	63	1.4	<1	1	1	1	2	2	3	5
35–49	51	1.5	<1	1	1	1	2	2	3	5
50–64	25	1.6	<1	1	1	1	2	2	3	5
65+	10	2.0	2	1	1	1	3	3	5	5
B. Operated										
0–19 Years	9	1.6	<1	1	1	1	2	3	3	3
20–34	1	1.0	0	1	1	1	1	1	1	1
35–49	1	1.0	0	1	1	1	1	1	1	1
50–64	1	1.0	0	1	1	1	1	1	1	1
65+	0									
2. MULTIPLE DX										
A. Not Operated										
0–19 Years	452	1.9	2	1	1	1	2	3	4	7
20–34	787	2.7	4	1	1	2	3	5	7	11
35–49	1,116	2.9	6	1	1	2	3	6	8	13
50–64	1,130	3.0	7	1	1	2	4	6	8	11
65+	1,392	3.2	6	1	2	3	4	6	7	13
B. Operated										
0–19 Years	14	2.8	5	1	1	2	4	5	7	8
20–34	34	3.9	20	1	1	3	4	7	12	24
35–49	50	5.0	50	1	2	3	5	7	15	48
50–64	31	4.3	9	1	2	4	6	10	10	11
65+	36	5.6	22	1	2	5	8	12	16	20
SUBTOTALS:										
1. SINGLE DX										
A. Not Operated	299	1.4	<1	1	1	1	2	2	3	5
B. Operated	12	1.4	<1	1	1	1	2	3	3	3
2. MULTIPLE DX										
A. Not Operated	4,877	2.9	6	1	1	2	4	6	7	12
B. Operated	165	4.6	26	1	2	3	6	10	12	24
1. SINGLE DX	311	1.4	<1	1	1	1	2	3	3	5
2. MULTIPLE DX	5,042	2.9	7	1	1	2	4	6	7	12
A. NOT OPERATED	5,176	2.8	6	1	1	2	3	5	7	11
B. OPERATED	177	4.4	25	1	1	3	6	9	12	24
TOTAL										
0–19 Years	625	1.8	2	1	1	1	2	3	4	7
20–34	885	2.7	5	1	1	2	3	5	7	12
35–49	1,218	2.9	8	1	1	2	4	6	8	13
50–64	1,187	3.0	7	1	1	2	4	6	8	11
65+	1,438	3.2	7	1	2	3	4	6	8	13
GRAND TOTAL	5,353	2.8	6	1	1	2	4	6	7	12

789.01: RUQ ABDOMINAL PAIN

Type of Patients	Observed Patients	Avg. Stay	Variance	Percentiles						
				10th	25th	50th	75th	90th	95th	99th
1. SINGLE DX										
A. Not Operated										
0–19 Years	18	1.6	<1	1	1	1	2	3	3	3
20–34	36	1.6	<1	1	1	1	2	3	3	5
35–49	21	1.7	<1	1	1	1	2	3	3	4
50–64	7	2.6	6	1	1	2	3	8	8	8
65+	3	1.3	<1	1	1	1	2	2	2	2
B. Operated										
0–19 Years	2	1.0	0	1	1	1	1	1	1	1
20–34	3	5.3	24	2	2	3	11	11	11	11
35–49	0									
50–64	0									
65+	0									
2. MULTIPLE DX										
A. Not Operated										
0–19 Years	113	2.2	4	1	1	2	2	4	6	11
20–34	477	2.8	4	1	1	2	3	5	7	11
35–49	715	3.1	6	1	1	2	4	6	6	12
50–64	590	3.0	6	1	1	2	4	6	8	12
65+	527	3.1	7	1	1	2	4	6	7	11
B. Operated										
0–19 Years	6	4.5	13	1	1	3	4	8	8	10
20–34	28	4.6	11	1	2	4	6	9	12	14
35–49	28	4.8	11	1	2	4	7	9	12	13
50–64	12	4.4	8	2	3	4	6	8	10	10
65+	17	5.6	22	1	3	5	8	15	17	17
SUBTOTALS:										
1. SINGLE DX										
A. Not Operated	85	1.7	1	1	1	1	2	3	4	8
B. Operated	5	3.6	18	1	2	2	3	11	11	11
2. MULTIPLE DX										
A. Not Operated	2,422	3.0	6	1	1	2	4	6	7	11
B. Operated	91	4.8	12	1	2	4	7	10	12	17
1. SINGLE DX	90	1.8	2	1	1	1	2	3	4	11
2. MULTIPLE DX	2,513	3.0	6	1	1	2	4	6	8	12
A. NOT OPERATED	2,507	2.9	6	1	1	2	4	6	7	11
B. OPERATED	96	4.8	13	1	2	4	6	10	12	17
TOTAL										
0–19 Years	139	2.2	4	1	1	2	2	4	6	11
20–34	544	2.8	5	1	1	2	3	5	7	12
35–49	764	3.1	7	1	1	2	4	6	8	12
50–64	609	3.0	6	1	1	2	4	6	8	11
65+	547	3.2	8	1	2	3	4	6	8	12
GRAND TOTAL	2,603	3.0	6	1	1	2	4	6	8	12

Length of Stay by Diagnosis and Operation, Western Region, 2008

Western Region, October 2006–September 2007 Data, by Diagnosis

789.02: LUQ ABDOMINAL PAIN

Type of Patients	Observed Patients	Avg. Stay	Variance	10th	25th	50th	75th	90th	95th	99th
1. SINGLE DX										
A. Not Operated										
0–19 Years	4	2.0	<1	1	2	2	3	3	3	3
20–34	3	1.3	<1	1	1	1	2	2	2	2
35–49	3	1.3	<1	1	1	1	2	2	2	2
50–64	2	1.0	0	1	1	1	1	1	1	1
65+	0									
B. Operated										
0–19 Years	0									
20–34	0									
35–49	0									
50–64	0									
65+	0									
2. MULTIPLE DX										
A. Not Operated										
0–19 Years	29	1.8	1	1	1	1	2	3	4	5
20–34	80	3.0	5	1	1	2	4	6	8	12
35–49	173	3.2	9	1	1	2	4	5	8	17
50–64	178	2.8	5	1	1	2	3	5	7	15
65+	162	3.1	5	1	2	3	4	6	7	11
B. Operated										
0–19 Years	0									
20–34	6	2.3	2	1	2	2	3	5	5	5
35–49	7	3.4	3	1	2	3	5	6	6	6
50–64	6	5.8	12	1	2	7	9	9	9	9
65+	0									
SUBTOTALS:										
1. SINGLE DX										
A. Not Operated	12	1.5	<1	1	1	1	2	2	3	3
B. Operated	0									
2. MULTIPLE DX										
A. Not Operated	622	3.0	6	1	1	2	4	5	7	13
B. Operated	19	3.8	7	1	2	3	6	9	9	9
1. SINGLE DX	12	1.5	<1	1	1	1	2	2	3	3
2. MULTIPLE DX	641	3.0	6	1	1	2	4	5	7	13
A. NOT OPERATED	634	2.9	6	1	1	2	4	5	7	13
B. OPERATED	19	3.8	7	2	2	3	6	9	9	9
TOTAL										
0–19 Years	33	1.9	1	1	1	2	2	3	4	5
20–34	89	2.9	5	1	1	2	4	6	8	12
35–49	183	3.1	8	1	1	2	4	5	8	17
50–64	186	2.9	5	1	1	2	4	6	7	15
65+	162	3.1	5	1	2	3	4	6	7	11
GRAND TOTAL	653	3.0	6	1	1	2	4	5	7	13

789.03: RLQ ABDOMINAL PAIN

Type of Patients	Observed Patients	Avg. Stay	Variance	10th	25th	50th	75th	90th	95th	99th
1. SINGLE DX										
A. Not Operated										
0–19 Years	253	1.2	<1	1	1	1	1	2	2	3
20–34	142	1.4	<1	1	1	1	2	2	3	5
35–49	69	1.3	<1	1	1	1	2	2	3	3
50–64	30	1.8	1	1	1	2	2	4	4	4
65+	5	2.0	<1	1	2	2	2	3	3	3
B. Operated										
0–19 Years	61	1.5	<1	1	1	1	2	2	2	4
20–34	50	1.7	<1	1	1	1	2	3	3	3
35–49	19	1.4	<1	1	1	1	2	2	3	3
50–64	7	1.6	<1	1	1	2	2	2	2	2
65+	1	1.0	0	1	1	1	1	1	1	1
2. MULTIPLE DX										
A. Not Operated										
0–19 Years	450	1.7	2	1	1	1	2	3	4	7
20–34	732	2.3	4	1	1	2	3	5	6	10
35–49	579	2.6	5	1	1	2	3	5	7	12
50–64	444	2.9	20	1	1	2	3	5	7	15
65+	456	3.0	5	1	1	2	4	6	8	11
B. Operated										
0–19 Years	132	2.2	3	1	1	2	3	4	5	11
20–34	259	2.4	4	1	1	2	3	5	7	11
35–49	137	2.6	5	1	1	2	3	5	7	10
50–64	62	2.7	5	1	1	2	4	5	8	10
65+	30	5.2	26	1	1	3	7	13	14	18
SUBTOTALS:										
1. SINGLE DX										
A. Not Operated	499	1.3	<1	1	1	1	1	2	3	4
B. Operated	138	1.5	<1	1	1	1	2	2	3	3
2. MULTIPLE DX										
A. Not Operated	2,661	2.5	7	1	1	2	3	5	7	11
B. Operated	620	2.6	6	1	1	2	3	5	7	13
1. SINGLE DX	637	1.4	<1	1	1	1	2	2	3	4
2. MULTIPLE DX	3,281	2.5	7	1	1	2	3	5	7	11
A. NOT OPERATED	3,160	2.3	6	1	1	2	3	4	6	10
B. OPERATED	758	2.4	5	1	1	2	3	5	7	12
TOTAL										
0–19 Years	896	1.6	1	1	1	1	2	3	4	7
20–34	1,183	2.2	4	1	1	2	3	4	6	10
35–49	804	2.5	5	1	1	2	3	5	6	11
50–64	543	2.8	17	1	1	2	4	5	7	13
65+	492	3.1	6	1	1	2	4	7	8	13
GRAND TOTAL	3,918	2.3	6	1	1	2	3	4	6	11

789.04: LLQ ABDOMINAL PAIN

Type of Patients	Observed Patients	Avg. Stay	Variance	10th	25th	50th	75th	90th	95th	99th
1. SINGLE DX										
A. Not Operated										
0–19 Years	22	1.5	2	1	1	1	1	1	4	6
20–34	22	1.9	2	1	1	1	3	3	4	6
35–49	15	1.5	<1	1	1	1	2	3	3	3
50–64	6	1.7	1	1	1	1	2	4	4	4
65+	4	2.3	<1	1	1	2	3	3	3	3
B. Operated										
0–19 Years	0									
20–34	3	2.0	0	2	2	2	2	2	2	2
35–49	0									
50–64	0									
65+	1	1.0	0	1	1	1	1	1	1	1
2. MULTIPLE DX										
A. Not Operated										
0–19 Years	64	2.4	9	1	1	2	3	4	5	23
20–34	203	2.6	4	1	1	2	3	4	6	10
35–49	352	3.1	7	1	1	3	4	6	8	13
50–64	319	3.2	6	1	2	3	4	6	7	14
65+	392	3.3	7	1	1	3	4	6	8	14
B. Operated										
0–19 Years	4	4.2	11	1	2	2	3	8	8	8
20–34	15	2.3	4	1	1	2	2	5	7	7
35–49	14	3.4	7	1	2	3	5	6	6	6
50–64	17	4.7	16	1	2	4	7	10	15	15
65+	7	9.3	36	3	4	7	13	20	20	20
SUBTOTALS:										
1. SINGLE DX										
A. Not Operated	69	1.7	1	1	1	1	2	3	4	6
B. Operated	5	1.6	<1	1	2	2	2	2	2	2
2. MULTIPLE DX										
A. Not Operated	1,330	3.1	6	1	1	2	4	6	8	13
B. Operated	57	4.3	15	1	2	3	6	9	13	20
1. SINGLE DX	74	1.7	1	1	1	1	2	3	4	6
2. MULTIPLE DX	1,387	3.1	7	1	1	2	4	6	8	14
A. NOT OPERATED	1,399	3.0	6	1	1	2	4	6	8	13
B. OPERATED	62	4.1	14	1	1	2	6	9	12	20
TOTAL										
0–19 Years	90	2.3	8	1	1	1	3	4	6	23
20–34	243	2.5	4	1	1	2	3	4	6	10
35–49	382	3.0	7	1	1	2	4	6	8	13
50–64	342	3.2	7	1	1	3	4	7	8	15
65+	404	3.4	8	1	2	3	4	7	9	14
GRAND TOTAL	1,461	3.0	7	1	1	2	4	6	8	14

Length of Stay by Diagnosis and Operation, Western Region, 2008

Western Region, October 2006–September 2007 Data, by Diagnosis

789.05: PERIUMBILIC ABD PAIN

Type of Patients	Observed Patients	Avg. Stay	Variance	10th	25th	50th	75th	90th	95th	99th
1. SINGLE DX										
A. *Not Operated*										
0–19 Years	41	1.3	<1	1	1	1	1	2	2	3
20–34	15	1.3	<1	1	1	1	1	3	3	3
35–49	3	4.6	10	1	1	6	7	7	7	7
50–64	3	1.0	0	1	1	1	1	1	1	1
65+	2	1.0	0	1	1	1	1	1	1	1
B. *Operated*										
0–19 Years	0									
20–34	0									
35–49	1	2.0	0	2	2	2	2	2	2	2
50–64	0									
65+	0									
2. MULTIPLE DX										
A. *Not Operated*										
0–19 Years	71	1.6	1	1	1	1	2	2	2	7
20–34	79	2.2	2	1	1	2	3	4	5	8
35–49	79	2.8	4	1	1	2	4	6	7	10
50–64	60	2.5	3	1	1	2	3	5	6	9
65+	106	2.8	5	1	1	2	4	5	6	9
B. *Operated*										
0–19 Years	2	3.0	2	2	2	2	4	4	4	4
20–34	6	3.0	12	2	1	2	3	10	10	10
35–49	5	4.6	6	1	4	4	7	7	7	7
50–64	4	2.3	<1	1	1	2	3	3	3	3
65+	1	14.0	0	14	14	14	14	14	14	14
SUBTOTALS:										
1. SINGLE DX										
A. *Not Operated*	64	1.4	1	1	1	1	1	2	2	3
B. *Operated*	1	2.0	0	2	2	2	2	2	2	2
2. MULTIPLE DX										
A. *Not Operated*	395	2.4	3	1	1	2	3	5	6	9
B. *Operated*	18	3.9	13	1	1	3	4	10	14	14
1. SINGLE DX	65	1.4	1	1	1	1	1	2	3	3
2. MULTIPLE DX	413	2.5	4	1	1	2	3	5	6	9
A. NOT OPERATED	459	2.3	3	1	1	2	3	5	6	9
B. OPERATED	19	3.8	12	1	1	3	4	10	14	14
TOTAL										
0–19 Years	114	1.5	<1	1	1	1	2	2	4	6
20–34	100	2.1	3	1	1	1	3	4	5	10
35–49	88	2.9	4	1	1	2	4	7	7	10
50–64	67	2.4	3	1	1	2	3	4	6	9
65+	109	2.9	6	1	1	2	4	5	6	14
GRAND TOTAL	478	2.3	4	1	1	2	3	5	6	9

789.06: EPIGASTRIC ABD PAIN

Type of Patients	Observed Patients	Avg. Stay	Variance	10th	25th	50th	75th	90th	95th	99th
1. SINGLE DX										
A. *Not Operated*										
0–19 Years	24	1.6	1	1	1	1	2	3	3	6
20–34	24	1.6	<1	1	1	1	2	3	3	4
35–49	12	1.8	1	1	1	1	2	3	5	5
50–64	11	2.0	<1	1	1	2	3	3	4	4
65+	5	2.2	3	1	1	1	3	5	5	5
B. *Operated*										
0–19 Years	1	2.0	0	2	2	2	2	2	2	2
20–34	1	5.0	0	5	5	5	5	5	5	5
35–49	0									
50–64	0									
65+	0									
2. MULTIPLE DX										
A. *Not Operated*										
0–19 Years	143	2.2	2	1	1	2	3	4	5	8
20–34	623	2.8	5	1	1	2	4	5	7	11
35–49	994	2.9	6	1	1	2	4	6	7	13
50–64	1,011	2.6	5	1	1	2	3	5	6	11
65+	1,250	2.7	5	1	1	2	3	5	7	12
B. *Operated*										
0–19 Years	3	2.7	4	1	1	2	5	5	5	5
20–34	26	5.1	30	1	2	5	7	8	8	29
35–49	28	4.2	8	2	2	3	6	7	9	14
50–64	25	7.4	40	1	3	5	9	20	21	21
65+	12	5.3	13	3	3	4	7	9	14	14
SUBTOTALS:										
1. SINGLE DX										
A. *Not Operated*	76	1.7	1	1	1	1	2	3	4	6
B. *Operated*	2	3.5	4	2	2	2	5	5	5	5
2. MULTIPLE DX										
A. *Not Operated*	4,021	2.7	5	1	1	2	3	5	7	12
B. *Operated*	94	5.4	24	1	2	4	7	9	16	29
1. SINGLE DX	78	1.8	1	1	1	1	2	3	5	6
2. MULTIPLE DX	4,115	2.8	6	1	1	2	3	5	7	13
A. NOT OPERATED	4,097	2.7	5	1	1	2	3	5	7	12
B. OPERATED	96	5.3	24	1	2	4	7	9	16	29
TOTAL										
0–19 Years	171	2.1	2	1	1	2	3	4	5	8
20–34	674	2.9	6	1	1	2	4	5	7	11
35–49	1,034	2.9	6	1	1	2	4	6	7	13
50–64	1,047	2.7	6	1	1	2	3	5	7	13
65+	1,267	2.7	5	1	1	2	3	5	7	13
GRAND TOTAL	4,193	2.8	6	1	1	2	3	5	7	13

789.07: GENERALIZED ABD PAIN

Type of Patients	Observed Patients	Avg. Stay	Variance	10th	25th	50th	75th	90th	95th	99th
1. SINGLE DX										
A. *Not Operated*										
0–19 Years	19	1.2	<1	1	1	1	1	2	2	2
20–34	11	2.3	5	1	1	1	3	4	8	8
35–49	3	1.7	<1	1	1	2	2	2	2	2
50–64	6	1.7	<1	1	1	2	2	3	3	3
65+	1	3.0	0	3	3	3	3	3	3	3
B. *Operated*										
0–19 Years	0									
20–34	0									
35–49	0									
50–64	0									
65+	0									
2. MULTIPLE DX										
A. *Not Operated*										
0–19 Years	91	2.1	5	1	1	1	2	4	6	15
20–34	165	3.5	11	1	2	3	5	7	10	18
35–49	241	3.3	7	1	1	3	4	7	8	12
50–64	204	3.4	8	1	2	3	4	6	8	10
65+	282	3.5	8	1	2	3	4	7	8	15
B. *Operated*										
0–19 Years	3	2.7	<1	2	2	3	3	3	3	3
20–34	13	3.6	7	1	2	3	5	7	7	10
35–49	11	7.9	23	5	5	6	10	11	20	20
50–64	7	8.8	178	1	3	5	6	39	39	39
65+	13	12.3	72	1	8	11	15	23	32	32
SUBTOTALS:										
1. SINGLE DX										
A. *Not Operated*	40	1.7	2	1	1	1	2	3	3	8
B. *Operated*	0									
2. MULTIPLE DX										
A. *Not Operated*	983	3.3	8	1	1	3	4	7	8	14
B. *Operated*	47	7.8	62	1	3	5	10	16	23	39
1. SINGLE DX	40	1.7	2	1	1	1	2	3	3	8
2. MULTIPLE DX	1,030	3.5	11	1	1	3	4	7	9	16
A. NOT OPERATED	1,023	3.2	8	1	1	2	4	7	8	14
B. OPERATED	47	7.8	62	1	3	5	10	16	23	39
TOTAL										
0–19 Years	113	2.0	4	1	1	1	2	3	6	11
20–34	189	3.5	10	1	1	3	4	7	10	18
35–49	255	3.5	8	1	1	3	4	7	10	14
50–64	217	3.5	14	1	2	3	4	6	8	17
65+	296	3.9	13	1	2	3	4	8	10	20
GRAND TOTAL	1,070	3.4	11	1	1	3	4	7	9	16

Length of Stay by Diagnosis and Operation, Western Region, 2008

Western Region, October 2006–September 2007 Data, by Diagnosis

789.09: ABDOMINAL PAIN-SITE NEC

Type of Patients	Observed Patients	Avg. Stay	Variance	10th	25th	50th	75th	90th	95th	99th
1. SINGLE DX										
A. Not Operated										
0–19 Years	91	1.3	<1	1	1	1	1	2	3	4
20–34	51	1.7	<1	1	1	1	2	3	4	5
35–49	36	1.4	<1	1	1	1	2	2	3	3
50–64	22	1.4	<1	1	1	1	1	3	3	3
65+	7	1.7	<1	1	1	2	2	3	3	3
B. Operated										
0–19 Years	5	1.6	<1	1	1	2	2	2	2	2
20–34	4	1.3	<1	1	1	1	1	2	2	2
35–49	1	2.0	0	2	2	2	2	2	2	2
50–64	0									
65+	0									
2. MULTIPLE DX										
A. Not Operated										
0–19 Years	338	2.1	3	1	1	1	2	4	5	9
20–34	745	2.8	5	1	1	2	3	5	7	13
35–49	1,061	3.0	5	1	1	2	4	6	7	12
50–64	944	3.1	6	1	1	2	4	6	8	13
65+	1,217	3.1	6	1	1	2	4	6	8	13
B. Operated										
0–19 Years	15	3.7	6	1	2	4	6	7	8	8
20–34	37	4.9	42	1	2	3	5	10	22	32
35–49	48	4.3	15	1	2	4	5	10	11	22
50–64	35	6.0	26	2	2	5	7	14	18	19
65+	33	7.6	35	3	3	7	9	16	21	23
SUBTOTALS:										
1. SINGLE DX										
A. Not Operated	207	1.4	<1	1	1	1	2	2	3	4
B. Operated	10	1.5	<1	1	1	1	2	2	2	2
2. MULTIPLE DX										
A. Not Operated	4,305	2.9	6	1	1	2	4	6	8	12
B. Operated	168	5.4	28	1	2	4	7	12	18	23
1. SINGLE DX	217	1.4	<1	1	1	1	2	2	3	4
2. MULTIPLE DX	4,473	3.0	7	1	1	2	4	6	8	14
A. NOT OPERATED	4,512	2.9	6	1	1	2	4	6	7	12
B. OPERATED	178	5.2	27	1	2	4	6	11	18	23
TOTAL										
0–19 Years	449	2.0	3	1	1	1	2	4	5	9
20–34	837	2.8	7	1	1	2	3	5	7	13
35–49	1,146	3.0	6	1	1	2	4	6	8	12
50–64	1,001	3.1	7	1	1	2	4	6	8	14
65+	1,257	3.2	8	1	1	3	4	6	8	14
GRAND TOTAL	4,690	2.9	7	1	1	2	4	6	8	13

789.39: ABD/PELV SWELL-SITE NEC

Type of Patients	Observed Patients	Avg. Stay	Variance	10th	25th	50th	75th	90th	95th	99th
1. SINGLE DX										
A. Not Operated										
0–19 Years	1	1.0	0	1	1	1	1	1	1	1
20–34	2	3.0	2	2	2	2	4	4	4	4
35–49	2	1.5	<1	1	1	1	2	2	2	2
50–64	1	3.0	0	3	3	3	3	3	3	3
65+	0									
B. Operated										
0–19 Years	0									
20–34	3	2.7	2	1	1	3	4	4	4	4
35–49	1	5.0	0	5	5	5	5	5	5	5
50–64	3	3.0	3	2	2	2	5	5	5	5
65+	0									
2. MULTIPLE DX										
A. Not Operated										
0–19 Years	4	1.3	<1	1	1	1	2	2	2	2
20–34	8	2.5	4	1	1	2	2	6	6	6
35–49	26	2.8	5	1	1	2	5	6	7	7
50–64	28	3.6	7	1	2	3	4	9	9	12
65+	57	3.6	6	1	2	3	5	7	9	12
B. Operated										
0–19 Years	0									
20–34	4	4.5	3	3	4	4	4	7	7	7
35–49	27	3.9	6	1	2	3	6	7	9	10
50–64	28	4.9	16	2	2	3	7	10	11	19
65+	19	4.6	37	1	2	3	4	8	29	29
SUBTOTALS:										
1. SINGLE DX										
A. Not Operated	6	2.2	1	1	1	2	3	4	4	4
B. Operated	7	3.1	2	1	2	3	5	5	5	5
2. MULTIPLE DX										
A. Not Operated	123	3.3	6	1	1	3	5	6	7	12
B. Operated	78	4.5	17	1	2	3	6	9	10	29
1. SINGLE DX	13	2.7	2	1	2	2	4	5	5	5
2. MULTIPLE DX	201	3.7	10	1	2	3	5	7	9	12
A. NOT OPERATED	129	3.2	6	1	1	3	4	6	7	12
B. OPERATED	85	4.4	16	1	2	3	5	8	10	29
TOTAL										
0–19 Years	5	1.2	<1	1	1	1	1	2	2	2
20–34	17	3.1	3	1	2	3	4	6	7	7
35–49	56	3.3	5	1	1	3	5	6	7	10
50–64	60	4.2	11	1	2	3	5	10	10	19
65+	76	3.8	14	1	2	3	5	7	9	29
GRAND TOTAL	214	3.7	10	1	2	3	5	7	9	12

789.5: ASCITES

Type of Patients	Observed Patients	Avg. Stay	Variance	10th	25th	50th	75th	90th	95th	99th
1. SINGLE DX										
A. Not Operated										
0–19 Years	1	5.0	0	5	5	5	5	5	5	5
20–34	1	2.0	0	2	2	2	2	2	2	2
35–49	4	3.5	7	1	2	4	4	7	7	7
50–64	2	1.5	<1	1	1	2	2	2	2	2
65+	1	2.0	0	2	2	2	2	2	2	2
B. Operated										
0–19 Years	0									
20–34	1	1.5	<1	1	1	2	2	2	2	2
35–49	0									
50–64	1	1.0	0	1	1	1	1	1	1	1
65+	0									
2. MULTIPLE DX										
A. Not Operated										
0–19 Years	15	4.3	36	1	1	2	5	10	24	24
20–34	39	3.4	12	1	1	2	4	8	13	18
35–49	181	3.1	8	1	1	2	4	6	7	18
50–64	311	3.3	9	1	1	3	4	6	8	11
65+	267	3.6	10	1	2	3	4	7	11	18
B. Operated										
0–19 Years	0									
20–34	11	3.0	2	2	2	2	4	4	4	4
35–49	11	7.1	73	1	2	4	7	20	27	27
50–64	21	6.2	33	1	2	5	7	13	17	24
65+	11	6.3	26	1	1	6	10	13	16	16
SUBTOTALS:										
1. SINGLE DX										
A. Not Operated	9	2.9	4	1	2	2	4	7	7	7
B. Operated	3	1.3	<1	1	1	1	2	2	2	2
2. MULTIPLE DX										
A. Not Operated	813	3.4	10	1	1	2	4	7	9	18
B. Operated	45	6.3	38	1	2	4	7	16	20	27
1. SINGLE DX	12	2.5	4	1	1	2	4	5	7	7
2. MULTIPLE DX	858	3.5	12	1	1	3	4	7	10	18
A. NOT OPERATED	822	3.4	10	1	1	2	4	7	9	18
B. OPERATED	48	6.0	37	1	2	4	7	16	20	27
TOTAL										
0–19 Years	16	4.4	34	1	1	2	5	10	24	24
20–34	44	3.2	11	1	1	2	4	5	10	18
35–49	196	3.3	12	1	1	2	4	6	8	20
50–64	335	3.4	11	1	2	3	4	7	9	17
65+	279	3.7	11	1	2	3	5	8	11	18
GRAND TOTAL	870	3.5	12	1	1	2	4	7	10	18

Length of Stay by Diagnosis and Operation, Western Region, 2008

790: ABNORMAL BLOOD FINDINGS

Type of Patients	Observed Patients	Avg. Stay	Vari-ance	Percentiles						
				10th	25th	50th	75th	90th	95th	99th
1. SINGLE DX										
A. *Not Operated*										
0–19 Years	20	1.8	<1	1	1	2	3	3	4	4
20–34	5	2.4	3	1	1	2	3	5	5	5
35–49	0									
50–64	0									
65+	2	2.0	2	1	1	2	3	3	3	3
B. *Operated*										
0–19 Years	0									
20–34	0									
35–49	0									
50–64	0									
65+	0									
2. MULTIPLE DX										
A. *Not Operated*										
0–19 Years	391	4.3	10	1	2	3	6	9	11	17
20–34	226	5.5	33	1	2	4	6	12	19	29
35–49	573	6.1	40	2	2	4	7	12	18	34
50–64	1,049	5.4	22	1	2	4	7	10	14	25
65+	2,274	5.0	17	1	2	4	7	9	12	18
B. *Operated*										
0–19 Years	6	8.3	7	6	6	7	11	12	12	12
20–34	5	13.6	70	6	10	12	12	28	28	28
35–49	25	11.9	54	4	8	9	16	22	27	29
50–64	53	13.6	214	3	6	9	16	26	32	95
65+	97	11.1	93	4	6	9	14	20	27	72
SUBTOTALS:										
1. SINGLE DX										
A. *Not Operated*	27	1.9	1	1	1	2	3	3	4	5
B. *Operated*	0									
2. MULTIPLE DX										
A. *Not Operated*	4,513	5.2	21	1	2	4	7	10	13	24
B. *Operated*	186	11.9	119	4	6	9	14	23	29	72
1. SINGLE DX	27	1.9	1	1	1	2	3	3	4	5
2. MULTIPLE DX	4,699	5.5	27	1	2	4	7	11	14	27
A. NOT OPERATED	4,540	5.2	21	1	2	4	7	10	13	24
B. OPERATED	186	11.9	119	4	6	9	14	23	29	72
TOTAL										
0–19 Years	417	4.3	10	1	2	3	6	9	11	15
20–34	236	5.6	35	1	2	4	7	12	19	29
35–49	598	6.3	41	2	2	4	8	13	20	34
50–64	1,102	5.8	34	1	2	4	7	11	16	28
65+	2,373	5.3	22	1	2	4	7	10	12	22
GRAND TOTAL	4,726	5.5	27	1	2	4	7	11	14	27

790.7: BACTEREMIA

Type of Patients	Observed Patients	Avg. Stay	Vari-ance	Percentiles						
				10th	25th	50th	75th	90th	95th	99th
1. SINGLE DX										
A. *Not Operated*										
0–19 Years	8	2.3	1	1	1	3	3	3	4	4
20–34	0									
35–49	0									
50–64	0									
65+	1	3.0	0	3	3	3	3	3	3	3
B. *Operated*										
0–19 Years	0									
20–34	0									
35–49	0									
50–64	0									
65+	0									
2. MULTIPLE DX										
A. *Not Operated*										
0–19 Years	333	4.7	11	2	2	4	6	9	11	17
20–34	170	6.5	39	2	3	4	8	15	20	30
35–49	446	6.9	44	2	3	5	8	13	21	35
50–64	798	6.1	24	2	3	5	7	12	15	27
65+	1,620	5.9	19	2	3	5	7	10	13	20
B. *Operated*										
0–19 Years	6	8.3	7	6	6	7	11	12	12	12
20–34	5	13.6	70	6	10	12	12	28	28	28
35–49	22	12.8	53	4	8	12	16	22	27	29
50–64	49	14.6	220	5	7	10	16	29	32	95
65+	78	11.6	56	5	6	9	14	22	27	41
SUBTOTALS:										
1. SINGLE DX										
A. *Not Operated*	9	2.3	1	1	1	3	3	4	4	4
B. *Operated*	0									
2. MULTIPLE DX										
A. *Not Operated*	3,367	6.0	24	2	3	5	7	11	14	27
B. *Operated*	160	12.6	105	5	6	10	15	25	29	49
1. SINGLE DX	9	2.3	1	1	1	3	3	4	4	4
2. MULTIPLE DX	3,527	6.3	29	2	3	5	8	12	15	28
A. NOT OPERATED	3,376	6.0	24	2	3	5	7	11	14	27
B. OPERATED	160	12.6	105	5	6	10	15	25	29	49
TOTAL										
0–19 Years	347	4.7	11	2	2	4	6	9	11	17
20–34	175	6.7	41	2	3	4	8	15	21	30
35–49	468	7.2	46	2	3	5	8	13	21	35
50–64	847	6.6	39	2	3	5	8	13	16	30
65+	1,699	6.2	22	2	3	5	8	11	14	24
GRAND TOTAL	3,536	6.3	29	2	3	5	8	12	15	28

790.92: ABN COAGULATION PROFILE

Type of Patients	Observed Patients	Avg. Stay	Vari-ance	Percentiles						
				10th	25th	50th	75th	90th	95th	99th
1. SINGLE DX										
A. *Not Operated*										
0–19 Years	0									
20–34	0									
35–49	0									
50–64	0									
65+	1	1.0	0	1	1	1	1	1	1	1
B. *Operated*										
0–19 Years	0									
20–34	0									
35–49	0									
50–64	0									
65+	0									
2. MULTIPLE DX										
A. *Not Operated*										
0–19 Years	7	3.0	4	1	1	3	5	6	6	6
20–34	19	2.4	3	1	1	2	3	6	7	7
35–49	71	3.4	14	1	1	2	4	7	10	24
50–64	166	2.9	7	1	1	2	4	6	7	13
65+	523	2.9	7	1	1	2	4	6	8	14
B. *Operated*										
0–19 Years	0									
20–34	0									
35–49	3	5.0	13	2	2	4	9	9	9	9
50–64	3	2.0	0	2	2	2	2	2	2	2
65+	11	8.0	21	4	5	7	10	12	19	19
SUBTOTALS:										
1. SINGLE DX										
A. *Not Operated*	1	1.0	0	1	1	1	1	1	1	1
B. *Operated*	0									
2. MULTIPLE DX										
A. *Not Operated*	786	3.0	7	1	1	2	4	6	8	14
B. *Operated*	17	6.4	21	2	2	6	9	12	19	19
1. SINGLE DX	1	1.0	0	1	1	1	1	1	1	1
2. MULTIPLE DX	803	3.0	8	1	1	2	4	6	8	14
A. NOT OPERATED	787	3.0	7	1	1	2	4	6	8	14
B. OPERATED	17	6.4	21	2	2	6	9	12	19	19
TOTAL										
0–19 Years	7	3.0	4	1	1	3	5	6	6	6
20–34	19	2.4	3	1	1	2	3	6	7	7
35–49	74	3.4	14	1	2	2	4	7	10	24
50–64	169	2.9	6	1	1	2	4	6	7	13
65+	535	3.0	8	1	1	2	4	6	8	14
GRAND TOTAL	804	3.0	8	1	1	2	4	6	8	14

Length of Stay by Diagnosis and Operation, Western Region, 2008

Western Region, October 2006–September 2007 Data, by Diagnosis

791: ABNORMAL URINE FINDINGS

Type of Patients	Observed Patients	Avg. Stay	Vari-ance	10th	25th	50th	75th	90th	95th	99th
1. SINGLE DX										
A. Not Operated										
0–19 Years	6	1.5	<1	1	1	1	2	3	3	3
20–34	1	1.0	0	1	1	1	1	1	1	1
35–49	1	1.0	0	1	1	1	1	1	1	1
50–64	1	1.0	0	1	1	1	1	1	1	1
65+	0									
B. Operated										
0–19 Years	0									
20–34	0									
35–49	0									
50–64	0									
65+	0									
2. MULTIPLE DX										
A. Not Operated										
0–19 Years	16	1.4	<1	1	1	1	2	2	3	3
20–34	10	1.6	<1	1	1	1	2	2	3	3
35–49	10	2.5	6	1	1	2	3	3	9	9
50–64	17	1.4	<1	1	1	1	2	3	3	3
65+	19	3.6	5	1	1	3	6	7	8	8
B. Operated										
0–19 Years	0									
20–34	0									
35–49	0									
50–64	0									
65+	1	1.0	0	1	1	1	1	1	1	1
SUBTOTALS:										
1. SINGLE DX										
A. Not Operated	9	1.3	<1	1	1	1	1	1	3	3
B. Operated	0									
2. MULTIPLE DX										
A. Not Operated	72	2.2	3	1	1	1	2	5	6	9
B. Operated	1	1.0	0	1	1	1	1	1	1	1
1. SINGLE DX	9	1.3	<1	1	1	1	1	3	3	3
2. MULTIPLE DX	73	2.2	3	1	1	1	2	5	6	9
A. NOT OPERATED	81	2.1	3	1	1	1	2	4	6	9
B. OPERATED	1	1.0	0	1	1	1	1	1	1	1
TOTAL										
0–19 Years	22	1.5	<1	1	1	1	2	2	3	3
20–34	11	1.5	<1	1	1	1	2	2	3	3
35–49	11	2.4	5	1	1	2	3	3	9	9
50–64	18	1.4	<1	1	1	1	2	3	3	3
65+	20	3.5	5	1	1	3	5	6	7	8
GRAND TOTAL	82	2.1	3	1	1	1	2	4	6	9

792: ABN FIND-OTH BODY SUBST

Type of Patients	Observed Patients	Avg. Stay	Vari-ance	10th	25th	50th	75th	90th	95th	99th
1. SINGLE DX										
A. Not Operated										
0–19 Years	2	1.5	<1	1	1	1	1	2	2	2
20–34	3	2.0	0	2	2	2	2	2	2	2
35–49	0									
50–64	0									
65+	0									
B. Operated										
0–19 Years	0									
20–34	0									
35–49	0									
50–64	0									
65+	0									
2. MULTIPLE DX										
A. Not Operated										
0–19 Years	4	2.0	2	1	1	1	2	4	4	4
20–34	14	1.9	1	1	1	2	2	3	5	5
35–49	8	3.9	25	1	2	2	3	16	16	16
50–64	17	2.7	7	1	1	1	3	8	8	8
65+	45	2.5	5	1	1	2	3	4	6	12
B. Operated										
0–19 Years	0									
20–34	0									
35–49	1	4.0	0	4	4	4	4	4	4	4
50–64	0									
65+	2	7.5	24	4	4	4	11	11	11	11
SUBTOTALS:										
1. SINGLE DX										
A. Not Operated	5	1.8	<1	1	2	2	2	2	2	2
B. Operated	0									
2. MULTIPLE DX										
A. Not Operated	88	2.5	6	1	1	2	3	4	8	16
B. Operated	3	6.3	16	4	4	4	11	11	11	11
1. SINGLE DX	5	1.8	<1	1	2	2	2	2	2	2
2. MULTIPLE DX	91	2.7	7	1	1	2	3	4	8	16
A. NOT OPERATED	93	2.5	6	1	1	2	3	4	8	16
B. OPERATED	3	6.3	16	4	4	4	11	11	11	11
TOTAL										
0–19 Years	6	1.8	1	1	1	1	2	4	4	4
20–34	17	1.9	1	1	1	2	2	3	5	5
35–49	9	3.9	22	1	2	2	3	16	16	16
50–64	17	2.7	7	1	1	1	3	8	8	8
65+	47	2.7	6	1	1	2	3	4	11	12
GRAND TOTAL	96	2.6	7	1	1	2	3	4	8	16

793: ABN FIND-BODY STRUCT NOS

Type of Patients	Observed Patients	Avg. Stay	Vari-ance	10th	25th	50th	75th	90th	95th	99th
1. SINGLE DX										
A. Not Operated										
0–19 Years	2	2.0	2	1	1	1	3	3	3	3
20–34		4.0	0	4	4	4	4	4	4	4
35–49	0									
50–64	0									
65+	0									
B. Operated										
0–19 Years	0									
20–34	0									
35–49	0									
50–64	1	3.0	0	3	3	3	3	3	3	3
65+	2	1.0	0	1	1	1	1	1	1	1
2. MULTIPLE DX										
A. Not Operated										
0–19 Years	4	1.8	<1	1	1	2	2	2	2	2
20–34	5	2.8	6	1	1	3	3	5	7	7
35–49	11	2.8	7	1	1	2	5	5	5	9
50–64	11	3.1	5	1	1	3	5	6	7	7
65+	29	2.4	4	1	1	1	3	6	6	9
B. Operated										
0–19 Years	1	4.0	0	4	4	4	4	4	4	4
20–34	4	4.2	15	2	2	2	3	10	10	10
35–49	5	4.8	14	1	1	5	8	8	9	9
50–64	9	2.7	4	1	1	3	3	6	6	6
65+	10	2.1	4	1	1	1	3	7	7	7
SUBTOTALS:										
1. SINGLE DX										
A. Not Operated	3	2.7	2	1	1	3	3	4	4	4
B. Operated	3	1.7	1	1	1	1	1	3	3	3
2. MULTIPLE DX										
A. Not Operated	60	2.6	4	1	1	2	3	6	7	9
B. Operated	29	3.1	7	1	1	2	4	8	9	10
1. SINGLE DX	6	2.2	2	1	1	1	2	4	4	4
2. MULTIPLE DX	89	2.8	5	1	1	2	3	6	8	10
A. NOT OPERATED	63	2.6	4	1	1	2	3	6	7	9
B. OPERATED	32	3.0	7	1	1	2	3	7	9	10
TOTAL										
0–19 Years	7	2.1	1	1	1	2	2	4	4	4
20–34	10	3.5	8	1	2	2	4	7	10	10
35–49	16	3.4	9	1	1	2	5	9	9	9
50–64	21	2.9	4	1	1	3	3	6	6	7
65+	41	2.3	4	1	1	1	3	6	6	9
GRAND TOTAL	95	2.7	5	1	1	2	3	6	8	10

Western Region, October 2006–September 2007 Data, by Diagnosis

794: ABNORMAL FUNCTION STUDY

Type of Patients	Observed Patients	Avg. Stay	Variance	10th	25th	50th	75th	90th	95th	99th
1. SINGLE DX										
A. Not Operated										
0–19 Years	2	2.5	4	1	1	4	4	4	4	4
20–34	1	2.0	0	2	2	2	2	2	2	2
35–49	0									
50–64	1	1.0	0	1	1	1	1	1	1	1
65+	0									
B. Operated										
0–19 Years	0									
20–34	0									
35–49	0									
50–64	0									
65+	0									
2. MULTIPLE DX										
A. Not Operated										
0–19 Years	4	1.3	<1	1	1	1	2	2	2	2
20–34	22	2.6	7	1	1	2	3	5	6	13
35–49	62	2.1	4	1	1	2	2	3	5	14
50–64	138	2.5	46	1	1	1	2	4	6	8
65+	171	2.4	3	1	1	2	3	5	6	8
B. Operated										
0–19 Years	0									
20–34	2	3.5	4	2	2	5	5	5	5	5
35–49	2	1.0	0	1	1	1	1	1	1	1
50–64	7	2.3	6	1	1	1	4	7	7	7
65+	10	3.7	21	1	1	1	4	8	15	15
SUBTOTALS:										
1. SINGLE DX										
A. Not Operated	4	2.0	2	1	1	2	4	4	4	4
B. Operated	0									
2. MULTIPLE DX										
A. Not Operated	397	2.4	18	1	1	2	3	5	6	8
B. Operated	21	3.0	12	1	1	1	4	7	8	15
1. SINGLE DX	4	2.0	2	1	1	2	4	4	4	4
2. MULTIPLE DX	418	2.4	18	1	1	2	3	5	6	8
A. NOT OPERATED	401	2.4	18	1	1	2	3	5	6	8
B. OPERATED	21	3.0	12	1	1	1	4	7	8	15
TOTAL										
0–19 Years	6	1.7	1	1	1	1	2	4	4	4
20–34	25	2.6	7	1	1	2	3	5	6	13
35–49	64	2.0	3	1	1	2	2	3	5	14
50–64	146	2.5	43	1	1	1	2	4	6	8
65+	181	2.5	4	1	1	2	3	5	7	8
GRAND TOTAL	422	2.4	18	1	1	2	3	5	6	8

794.31: NONSPECIFIC ABN EKG/ECG

Type of Patients	Observed Patients	Avg. Stay	Variance	10th	25th	50th	75th	90th	95th	99th
1. SINGLE DX										
A. Not Operated										
0–19 Years	0									
20–34	0									
35–49	0									
50–64	0									
65+	0									
B. Operated										
0–19 Years	0									
20–34	0									
35–49	0									
50–64	0									
65+	0									
2. MULTIPLE DX										
A. Not Operated										
0–19 Years	0									
20–34	9	3.9	15	1	1	2	5	13	13	13
35–49	34	1.7	<1	1	1	2	2	3	3	4
50–64	65	2.8	94	1	1	1	2	4	5	80
65+	93	2.2	3	1	1	2	3	5	6	8
B. Operated										
0–19 Years	0									
20–34	0									
35–49	2	1.0	0	1	1	1	1	1	1	1
50–64	5	2.8	7	1	1	1	4	7	7	7
65+	3	1.3	<1	1	1	1	2	2	2	2
SUBTOTALS:										
1. SINGLE DX										
A. Not Operated	0									
B. Operated	0									
2. MULTIPLE DX										
A. Not Operated	201	2.4	32	1	1	1	2	4	5	8
B. Operated	10	2.0	4	1	1	1	2	7	7	7
1. SINGLE DX	0									
2. MULTIPLE DX	211	2.4	31	1	1	1	2	4	5	8
A. NOT OPERATED	201	2.4	32	1	1	1	2	4	5	8
B. OPERATED	10	2.0	4	1	1	1	2	7	7	7
TOTAL										
0–19 Years	0									
20–34	9	3.9	15	1	1	2	5	13	13	13
35–49	36	1.6	<1	1	1	1	2	3	3	4
50–64	70	2.8	88	1	1	1	2	4	5	80
65+	96	2.2	3	1	1	2	3	5	6	8
GRAND TOTAL	211	2.4	31	1	1	1	2	4	5	8

795: ABN CYTOLOG/HIST/DNA

Type of Patients	Observed Patients	Avg. Stay	Variance	10th	25th	50th	75th	90th	95th	99th
1. SINGLE DX										
A. Not Operated										
0–19 Years	6	2.5	2	1	2	2	3	5	5	5
20–34	2	1.0	0	1	1	1	1	1	1	1
35–49	1	1.0	0	1	1	1	1	1	1	1
50–64	1	1.0	0	1	1	1	1	1	1	1
65+	1	1.0	0	1	1	1	1	1	1	1
B. Operated										
0–19 Years	0									
20–34	1	3.0	0	3	3	3	3	3	3	3
35–49	9	1.6	<1	1	1	1	2	3	3	3
50–64	2	2.0	2	1	1	3	3	3	3	3
65+	0									
2. MULTIPLE DX										
A. Not Operated										
0–19 Years	10	1.9	<1	1	1	2	2	3	3	3
20–34	10	6.2	50	1	1	5	9	10	24	24
35–49	25	5.6	21	1	2	4	7	13	13	17
50–64	24	4.3	28	1	1	3	5	7	8	27
65+	32	5.8	24	1	3	4	8	11	18	19
B. Operated										
0–19 Years	0									
20–34	15	1.6	<1	1	1	1	2	2	3	3
35–49	44	2.2	1	1	1	2	3	4	5	5
50–64	38	2.1	1	1	1	2	3	4	4	4
65+	17	2.8	3	1	2	2	3	5	8	8
SUBTOTALS:										
1. SINGLE DX										
A. Not Operated	11	1.8	2	1	1	1	2	3	5	5
B. Operated	12	1.8	<1	1	1	2	2	3	3	3
2. MULTIPLE DX										
A. Not Operated	101	5.0	25	1	2	3	6	11	17	24
B. Operated	114	2.2	1	1	1	2	3	4	4	5
1. SINGLE DX	23	1.8	1	1	1	1	2	3	3	5
2. MULTIPLE DX	215	3.5	15	1	1	2	4	7	11	19
A. NOT OPERATED	112	4.7	24	1	1	3	6	11	17	24
B. OPERATED	126	2.1	1	1	1	2	3	4	4	5
TOTAL										
0–19 Years	16	2.1	1	1	1	2	3	3	5	5
20–34	28	3.3	22	1	1	2	3	9	10	24
35–49	79	3.2	10	1	1	2	3	6	12	17
50–64	65	2.9	12	1	1	2	3	5	6	27
65+	50	4.7	19	2	2	3	7	11	17	19
GRAND TOTAL	238	3.3	14	1	1	2	4	7	11	19

Length of Stay by Diagnosis and Operation, Western Region, 2008

Western Region, October 2006–September 2007 Data, by Diagnosis

796: OTHER ABNORMAL FINDINGS

Type of Patients	Observed Patients	Avg. Stay	Variance	10th	25th	50th	75th	90th	95th	99th
1. SINGLE DX										
A. Not Operated										
0–19 Years	3	1.3	<1	1	1	1	2	2	2	2
20–34	0									
35–49	0									
50–64	0									
65+	0									
B. Operated										
0–19 Years	0									
20–34	0									
35–49	0									
50–64	0									
65+	0									
2. MULTIPLE DX										
A. Not Operated										
0–19 Years	10	3.6	15	1	2	2	4	14	14	14
20–34	13	3.2	10	1	2	2	3	5	13	13
35–49	16	2.4	3	1	1	2	3	4	7	7
50–64	41	2.9	4	1	1	2	3	6	7	8
65+	107	3.1	7	1	1	2	4	6	9	12
B. Operated										
0–19 Years	0									
20–34	0									
35–49	3	1.3	<1	1	1	1	2	2	2	2
50–64	1	2.0	0	2	2	2	2	2	2	2
65+	2	1.0	0	1	1	1	1	1	1	1
SUBTOTALS:										
1. SINGLE DX										
A. Not Operated	3	1.3	<1	1	1	1	2	2	2	2
B. Operated	0									
2. MULTIPLE DX										
A. Not Operated	187	3.0	7	1	1	2	4	6	8	14
B. Operated	6	1.3	<1	1	1	1	2	2	2	2
1. SINGLE DX	3	1.3	<1	1	1	1	2	2	2	2
2. MULTIPLE DX	193	3.0	7	1	1	2	4	6	8	14
A. NOT OPERATED	190	3.0	7	1	1	2	4	6	8	14
B. OPERATED	6	1.3	<1	1	1	1	2	2	2	2
TOTAL										
0–19 Years	13	3.1	12	1	1	2	3	5	14	14
20–34	13	3.2	10	1	2	2	3	5	13	13
35–49	19	2.2	3	1	1	2	3	4	7	7
50–64	42	2.9	4	1	1	2	3	6	7	8
65+	109	3.1	7	1	1	2	4	6	9	12
GRAND TOTAL	196	2.9	7	1	1	2	4	6	8	14

796.0: ABN TOXICOLOGIC FINDING

Type of Patients	Observed Patients	Avg. Stay	Variance	10th	25th	50th	75th	90th	95th	99th
1. SINGLE DX										
A. Not Operated										
0–19 Years	0									
20–34	0									
35–49	0									
50–64	0									
65+	0									
B. Operated										
0–19 Years	0									
20–34	0									
35–49	0									
50–64	0									
65+	0									
2. MULTIPLE DX										
A. Not Operated										
0–19 Years	1	2.0	0	2	2	2	2	2	2	2
20–34	11	3.4	12	1	2	2	4	5	13	13
35–49	11	2.7	3	1	1	2	4	4	7	7
50–64	25	3.6	5	1	2	3	5	5	8	8
65+	55	3.8	10	1	2	3	5	8	9	17
B. Operated										
0–19 Years	0									
20–34	0									
35–49	0									
50–64	0									
65+	0									
SUBTOTALS:										
1. SINGLE DX										
A. Not Operated	0									
B. Operated	0									
2. MULTIPLE DX										
A. Not Operated	103	3.6	8	1	2	3	5	7	9	13
B. Operated	0									
1. SINGLE DX	0									
2. MULTIPLE DX	103	3.6	8	1	2	3	5	7	9	13
A. NOT OPERATED	103	3.6	8	1	2	3	5	7	9	13
B. OPERATED	0									
TOTAL										
0–19 Years	1	2.0	0	2	2	2	2	2	2	2
20–34	11	3.4	12	1	2	2	4	5	13	13
35–49	11	2.7	3	1	1	2	4	4	7	7
50–64	25	3.6	5	1	2	3	5	5	8	8
65+	55	3.8	10	1	1	3	5	8	9	17
GRAND TOTAL	103	3.6	8	1	2	3	5	7	9	13

797: SENILITY W/O PSYCHOSIS

Type of Patients	Observed Patients	Avg. Stay	Variance	10th	25th	50th	75th	90th	95th	99th
1. SINGLE DX										
A. Not Operated										
0–19 Years	0									
20–34	0									
35–49	0									
50–64	0									
65+	0									
B. Operated										
0–19 Years	0									
20–34	0									
35–49	0									
50–64	0									
65+	0									
2. MULTIPLE DX										
A. Not Operated										
0–19 Years	0									
20–34	0									
35–49	0									
50–64	0									
65+	29	4.4	10	1	3	3	5	10	13	14
B. Operated										
0–19 Years	0									
20–34	0									
35–49	0									
50–64	0									
65+	0									
SUBTOTALS:										
1. SINGLE DX										
A. Not Operated	0									
B. Operated	0									
2. MULTIPLE DX										
A. Not Operated	29	4.4	10	1	3	3	5	10	13	14
B. Operated	0									
1. SINGLE DX	0									
2. MULTIPLE DX	29	4.4	10	1	3	3	5	10	13	14
A. NOT OPERATED	29	4.4	10	1	3	3	5	10	13	14
B. OPERATED	0									
TOTAL										
0–19 Years	0									
20–34	0									
35–49	0									
50–64	0									
65+	29	4.4	10	1	3	3	5	10	13	14
GRAND TOTAL	29	4.4	10	1	3	3	5	10	13	14

Length of Stay by Diagnosis and Operation, Western Region, 2008

Western Region, October 2006–September 2007 Data, by Diagnosis

689

798: SUDDEN DEATH CAUSE UNKN

Type of Patients	Observed Patients	Avg. Stay	Vari-ance	10th	25th	50th	75th	90th	95th	99th
1. SINGLE DX										
A. Not Operated										
0–19 Years	0									
20–34	0									
35–49	0									
50–64	0									
65+	0									
B. Operated										
0–19 Years	0									
20–34	0									
35–49	0									
50–64	0									
65+	0									
2. MULTIPLE DX										
A. Not Operated										
0–19 Years	0									
20–34	0									
35–49	0									
50–64	0									
65+	0									
B. Operated										
0–19 Years	0									
20–34	0									
35–49	0									
50–64	0									
65+	0									
SUBTOTALS:										
1. SINGLE DX A. Not Operated	0									
B. Operated	0									
2. MULTIPLE DX A. Not Operated	0									
B. Operated	0									
1. SINGLE DX	0									
2. MULTIPLE DX	0									
A. NOT OPERATED	0									
B. OPERATED	0									
TOTAL 0–19 Years	0									
20–34	0									
35–49	0									
50–64	0									
65+	0									
GRAND TOTAL	0									

799: OTH ILL-DEF MORB/MORT

Type of Patients	Observed Patients	Avg. Stay	Vari-ance	10th	25th	50th	75th	90th	95th	99th
1. SINGLE DX A. Not Operated 0–19 Years	13	1.6	<1	1	1	1	2	3	3	3
20–34	5	30.0	>999	1	1	1	72	76	76	76
35–49	4	1.3	<1	1	1	1	1	2	2	2
50–64	7	1.1	<1	1	1	1	2	>99	>99	>99
65+	7	2.7	11	1	1	1	3	>99	>99	>99
B. Operated 0–19 Years	0									
20–34	0									
35–49	0									
50–64	0									
65+	0									
2. MULTIPLE DX A. Not Operated 0–19 Years	102	2.5	9	1	1	2	3	4	5	8
20–34	39	2.2	4	1	1	1	2	6	6	9
35–49	125	3.1	10	1	1	2	3	7	9	17
50–64	243	3.1	9	1	1	2	4	6	8	17
65+	683	3.5	9	1	2	3	4	7	9	16
B. Operated 0–19 Years	4	14.8	114	14	17	27	27	27	27
20–34	2	3.5	12	1	1	4	6	6	6
35–49	13	4.7	25	1	1	2	7	12	15	15
50–64	20	4.3	54	1	1	2	3	16	32	32
65+	40	3.2	8	1	1	2	4	6	9	14
SUBTOTALS:										
1. SINGLE DX A. Not Operated	36	5.6	284	1	1	1	2	76	>99	>99
B. Operated	0									
2. MULTIPLE DX A. Not Operated	1,192	3.3	9	1	1	2	4	6	8	16
B. Operated	79	4.3	32	1	1	2	5	12	16	32
1. SINGLE DX	36	5.6	284	1	1	1	2	76	>99	>99
2. MULTIPLE DX	1,271	3.3	10	1	1	2	4	6	9	17
A. NOT OPERATED	1,228	3.3	17	1	1	2	4	6	9	19
B. OPERATED	79	4.3	32	1	1	2	5	12	16	32
TOTAL 0–19 Years	119	2.8	16	1	1	2	3	4	7	27
20–34	46	5.3	221	1	1	1	3	6	9	76
35–49	142	3.2	11	1	1	2	3	7	11	17
50–64	270	3.2	12	1	1	2	4	6	8	32
65+	730	3.5	9	1	2	3	4	7	9	16
GRAND TOTAL	1,307	3.4	18	1	1	2	4	6	9	20

799.02: HYPOXEMIA

Type of Patients	Observed Patients	Avg. Stay	Vari-ance	10th	25th	50th	75th	90th	95th	99th
1. SINGLE DX A. Not Operated 0–19 Years	9	1.8	<1	1	1	2	2	3	3	3
20–34	0									
35–49	1	1.0	0	1	1	1	1	1	1
50–64	1	1.0	0	1	1	1	1	1	1
65+	0									
B. Operated 0–19 Years	0									
20–34	0									
35–49	0									
50–64	0									
65+	0									
2. MULTIPLE DX A. Not Operated 0–19 Years	89	2.6	10	1	1	2	3	4	5	29
20–34	32	1.9	2	1	1	1	2	4	6	6
35–49	108	3.1	10	1	1	2	3	7	9	17
50–64	211	2.9	7	1	1	2	4	5	6	14
65+	482	2.9	4	1	2	3	4	5	7	9
B. Operated 0–19 Years	3	15.1	170	1	1	17	27	27	27	27
20–34	1	1.0	0	1	1	1	1	1	1
35–49	10	2.3	4	1	1	1	2	7	7	7
50–64	18	4.5	60	1	1	2	3	16	32	32
65+	35	3.1	9	1	1	2	4	7	9	14
SUBTOTALS:										
1. SINGLE DX A. Not Operated	11	1.6	<1	1	1	1	2	3	3	3
B. Operated	0									
2. MULTIPLE DX A. Not Operated	922	2.9	6	1	1	2	4	5	7	11
B. Operated	67	3.9	32	1	1	2	4	9	16	32
1. SINGLE DX	11	1.6	<1	1	1	1	2	3	3	3
2. MULTIPLE DX	989	2.9	8	1	1	2	4	6	7	14
A. NOT OPERATED	933	2.9	6	1	1	2	4	5	7	11
B. OPERATED	67	3.9	32	1	1	2	4	9	16	32
TOTAL 0–19 Years	101	2.9	17	1	1	2	3	4	6	27
20–34	33	1.9	2	1	1	1	2	4	6	6
35–49	119	3.0	9	1	1	2	3	7	9	17
50–64	230	3.0	11	1	1	2	4	6	7	17
65+	517	2.9	4	1	1	2	4	6	7	9
GRAND TOTAL	1,000	2.9	8	1	1	2	4	6	7	14

Length of Stay by Diagnosis and Operation, Western Region, 2008

Western Region, October 2006–September 2007 Data, by Diagnosis

799.3: DEBILITY NOS

Type of Patients	Observed Patients	Avg. Stay	Variance	10th	25th	50th	75th	90th	95th	99th
1. SINGLE DX										
A. Not Operated										
0–19 Years	0									
20–34	0									
35–49	0									
50–64	0									
65+	0									
B. Operated										
0–19 Years	0									
20–34	0									
35–49	0									
50–64	0									
65+	0									
2. MULTIPLE DX										
A. Not Operated										
0–19 Years	0									
20–34	1	9.0		9	9	9	9	9	9	9
35–49	4	3.0	3	1	3	3	5	5	5	5
50–64	10	4.1	8	1	2	4	7	8	8	8
65+	152	4.9	20	1	2	3	6	11	15	25
B. Operated										
0–19 Years	0									
20–34	0									
35–49	0									
50–64	0									
65+	1	6.0	0	6	6	6	6	6	6	6
SUBTOTALS:										
1. SINGLE DX										
A. Not Operated	0									
B. Operated	0									
2. MULTIPLE DX										
A. Not Operated	167	4.8	18	1	2	3	6	10	14	25
B. Operated	1	6.0	0	6	6	6	6	6	6	6
1. SINGLE DX	0									
2. MULTIPLE DX	168	4.8	18	1	2	3	6	10	14	25
A. NOT OPERATED	167	4.8	18	1	2	3	6	10	14	25
B. OPERATED	1	6.0	0	6	6	6	6	6	6	6
TOTAL										
0–19 Years	0									
20–34	1	9.0		9	9	9	9	9	9	9
35–49	4	3.0	3	1	3	3	5	5	5	5
50–64	10	4.1	8	1	2	4	7	8	8	8
65+	153	4.9	19	1	2	3	6	11	15	25
GRAND TOTAL	168	4.8	18	1	2	3	6	10	14	25

800: SKULL VAULT FRACTURE

Type of Patients	Observed Patients	Avg. Stay	Variance	10th	25th	50th	75th	90th	95th	99th
1. SINGLE DX										
A. Not Operated										
0–19 Years	224	1.4	<1	1	1	1	2	2	3	4
20–34	12	2.0	1	1	1	2	3	3	4	4
35–49	11	1.7	<1	1	1	2	2	3	3	3
50–64	0									
65+	3	2.0	1	1	2	2	3	3	3	3
B. Operated										
0–19 Years	24	3.1	2	2	2	3	4	6	6	6
20–34	12	3.1	13	1	1	2	3	5	14	14
35–49	2	2.5	<1	2	2	3	3	3	3	3
50–64	0									
65+	1	3.0	0	3	3	3	3	3	3	3
2. MULTIPLE DX										
A. Not Operated										
0–19 Years	398	2.6	8	1	1	2	3	5	6	19
20–34	181	3.3	11	1	1	2	4	6	10	18
35–49	129	4.5	35	1	2	3	5	14	14	39
50–64	108	6.0	57	1	2	3	7	12	17	36
65+	81	5.5	30	1	2	4	6	11	15	32
B. Operated										
0–19 Years	172	11.4	162	2	3	6	15	27	37	78
20–34	181	13.6	242	2	4	8	17	33	47	76
35–49	116	17.5	294	3	5	11	23	49	60	>99
50–64	66	18.7	362	2	5	13	24	58	63	>99
65+	28	18.4	161	4	8	16	22	37	49	56
SUBTOTALS:										
1. SINGLE DX										
A. Not Operated	250	1.5	<1	1	1	1	2	2	3	4
B. Operated	39	3.1	5	1	2	3	3	6	6	14
2. MULTIPLE DX										
A. Not Operated	897	3.7	22	1	1	2	4	7	11	26
B. Operated	563	14.6	244	2	4	9	19	37	53	80
1. SINGLE DX	289	1.7	2	1	1	2	2	3	4	6
2. MULTIPLE DX	1,460	7.9	135	1	2	4	9	20	31	64
A. NOT OPERATED	1,147	3.2	18	1	1	2	3	6	10	21
B. OPERATED	602	13.8	237	2	4	8	18	35	52	78
TOTAL										
0–19 Years	818	4.2	52	1	1	2	4	9	17	37
20–34	386	8.1	145	1	2	4	9	18	31	71
35–49	258	10.2	193	1	2	5	12	28	46	80
50–64	174	10.8	209	2	2	5	13	30	52	69
65+	113	8.6	92	2	3	5	11	20	26	49
GRAND TOTAL	1,749	6.9	119	1	2	3	6	17	28	60

800.01: CL VAULT FX S INJ S LOC

Type of Patients	Observed Patients	Avg. Stay	Variance	10th	25th	50th	75th	90th	95th	99th
1. SINGLE DX										
A. Not Operated										
0–19 Years	99	1.3	<1	1	1	1	1	2	2	7
20–34	1	1.0	0	1	1	1	1	1	1	1
35–49	0									
50–64	0									
65+	0									
B. Operated										
0–19 Years	2	2.5	4	1	1	1	4	4	4	4
20–34	0									
35–49	0									
50–64	0									
65+	0									
2. MULTIPLE DX										
A. Not Operated										
0–19 Years	100	1.6	2	1	1	1	2	3	3	7
20–34	16	1.6	<1	1	1	1	2	3	4	4
35–49	16	2.0	<1	1	1	2	3	3	4	4
50–64	13	3.1	7	1	1	2	4	8	9	9
65+	4	4.8	9	1	1	4	8	8	8	8
B. Operated										
0–19 Years	7	4.3	19	1	1	4	6	13	13	13
20–34	6	5.5	19	2	2	4	10	12	12	12
35–49	2	4.0	8	2	2	6	6	6	6	6
50–64	1	2.0	0	2	2	2	2	2	2	2
65+	0									
SUBTOTALS:										
1. SINGLE DX										
A. Not Operated	100	1.3	<1	1	1	1	1	2	2	7
B. Operated	2	2.5	4	1	1	1	4	4	4	4
2. MULTIPLE DX										
A. Not Operated	149	1.9	3	1	1	1	2	3	4	9
B. Operated	16	4.6	15	1	2	4	6	12	13	13
1. SINGLE DX	102	1.3	<1	1	1	1	1	2	2	4
2. MULTIPLE DX	165	2.1	4	1	1	1	2	4	6	12
A. NOT OPERATED	249	1.6	2	1	1	1	2	3	4	8
B. OPERATED	18	4.3	14	1	2	3	6	12	13	13
TOTAL										
0–19 Years	208	1.6	2	1	1	1	2	2	2	7
20–34	23	2.6	8	1	1	2	3	4	10	12
35–49	18	2.2	2	1	1	2	3	4	6	6
50–64	14	3.0	6	1	1	2	4	8	9	9
65+	14	4.8	9	2	3	4	8	8	8	8
GRAND TOTAL	267	1.8	3	1	1	1	2	3	4	11

690

Length of Stay by Diagnosis and Operation, Western Region, 2008

Western Region, October 2006–September 2007 Data, by Diagnosis

801: SKULL BASE FRACTURE

Type of Patients	Observed Patients	Avg. Stay	Variance	10th	25th	50th	75th	90th	95th	99th
1. SINGLE DX										
A. *Not Operated*										
0–19 Years	222	1.6	1	1	1	1	2	3	4	5
20–34	53	2.3	3	1	1	2	3	5	6	7
35–49	24	2.0	3	1	1	1	2	3	7	7
50–64	11	3.4	12	1	1	2	4	5	13	13
65+	4	2.3	4	1	1	2	2	5	5	5
B. *Operated*										
0–19 Years	22	3.6	8	1	2	3	4	5	9	14
20–34	16	3.1	6	1	1	2	3	8	8	8
35–49	8	4.6	11	1	2	5	9	10	10	10
50–64	1	5.0	0	5	5	5	5	5	5	5
65+	0									
2. MULTIPLE DX										
A. *Not Operated*										
0–19 Years	769	3.1	10	1	1	2	4	6	8	17
20–34	966	3.6	17	1	1	2	4	7	10	23
35–49	702	4.7	27	1	2	3	6	11	15	24
50–64	517	5.8	73	1	2	3	6	12	17	36
65+	596	5.4	33	1	2	4	7	11	15	29
B. *Operated*										
0–19 Years	291	12.9	195	3	4	8	17	29	42	78
20–34	513	14.3	214	3	4	9	19	33	48	77
35–49	383	16.3	249	3	5	11	23	36	48	>99
50–64	219	18.2	261	3	7	14	24	44	62	>99
65+	138	15.6	155	4	7	12	22	33	41	62
SUBTOTALS:										
1. SINGLE DX										
A. *Not Operated*	314	1.8	2	1	1	1	2	3	5	7
B. *Operated*	47	3.6	8	1	2	3	4	8	9	14
2. MULTIPLE DX										
A. *Not Operated*	3,550	4.3	29	1	2	3	5	9	13	27
B. *Operated*	1,544	15.2	223	3	5	11	21	35	49	85
1. SINGLE DX	**361**	**2.1**	**3**	**1**	**1**	**1**	**2**	**4**	**5**	**9**
2. MULTIPLE DX	**5,094**	**7.6**	**113**	**1**	**2**	**4**	**9**	**19**	**29**	**62**
A. NOT OPERATED	**3,864**	**4.1**	**28**	**1**	**1**	**3**	**5**	**9**	**13**	**25**
B. OPERATED	**1,591**	**14.9**	**220**	**3**	**5**	**10**	**21**	**34**	**48**	**85**
TOTAL										
0–19 Years	1,304	5.0	68	1	2	2	5	12	19	45
20–34	1,548	7.1	107	1	2	3	7	18	27	54
35–49	1,117	8.6	133	1	2	4	11	22	33	69
50–64	748	9.4	159	1	2	5	12	23	33	77
65+	738	7.3	72	1	3	4	9	16	23	43
GRAND TOTAL	**5,455**	**7.3**	**108**	**1**	**2**	**3**	**8**	**18**	**28**	**60**

801.01: CL BASE FX S IC INJ SLOC

Type of Patients	Observed Patients	Avg. Stay	Variance	10th	25th	50th	75th	90th	95th	99th
1. SINGLE DX										
A. *Not Operated*										
0–19 Years	71	1.2	<1	1	1	1	1	2	2	3
20–34	10	1.8	<1	1	1	2	2	4	5	5
35–49	2	1.0	0	1	1	1	1	1	1	1
50–64	0									
65+	0									
B. *Operated*										
0–19 Years	1	5.0	0	5	5	5	5	5	5	5
20–34	2	2.0	2	1	1	2	3	3	3	3
35–49	2	4.0	2	3	5	5	5	5	5	5
50–64	0									
65+	0									
2. MULTIPLE DX										
A. *Not Operated*										
0–19 Years	136	1.7	1	1	1	2	2	3	4	4
20–34	106	1.9	1	1	1	2	2	4	4	5
35–49	84	2.5	4	1	2	2	3	4	7	12
50–64	61	3.2	12	1	2	3	4	6	8	19
65+	116	3.3	8	1	2	3	4	6	9	16
B. *Operated*										
0–19 Years	18	4.7	26	1	1	3	5	17	18	18
20–34	31	3.8	8	1	2	3	5	8	11	12
35–49	24	4.2	10	1	2	3	5	8	12	12
50–64	11	11.1	242	1	6	14	14	16	55	55
65+	12	9.6	44	2	8	8	15	18	21	21
SUBTOTALS:										
1. SINGLE DX										
A. *Not Operated*	83	1.2	<1	1	1	1	1	2	2	3
B. *Operated*	5	3.4	3	1	3	3	5	5	5	5
2. MULTIPLE DX										
A. *Not Operated*	503	2.4	5	1	1	2	3	5	6	13
B. *Operated*	96	5.6	48	1	2	3	6	12	17	55
1. SINGLE DX	**88**	**1.4**	**<1**	**1**	**1**	**1**	**1**	**2**	**3**	**5**
2. MULTIPLE DX	**599**	**3.0**	**13**	**1**	**1**	**2**	**3**	**6**	**8**	**17**
A. NOT OPERATED	**586**	**2.3**	**4**	**1**	**1**	**2**	**3**	**5**	**6**	**13**
B. OPERATED	**101**	**5.5**	**46**	**1**	**2**	**3**	**6**	**12**	**16**	**21**
TOTAL										
0–19 Years	226	1.8	4	1	1	1	2	3	4	9
20–34	149	2.3	3	1	1	2	3	5	6	11
35–49	112	2.9	5	1	1	2	3	5	8	12
50–64	72	4.4	53	1	2	3	4	11	16	55
65+	128	3.9	14	1	2	3	4	8	13	18
GRAND TOTAL	**687**	**2.8**	**12**	**1**	**1**	**2**	**3**	**5**	**8**	**17**

801.02: CL BASE FX S IC INJ-BRF

Type of Patients	Observed Patients	Avg. Stay	Variance	10th	25th	50th	75th	90th	95th	99th
1. SINGLE DX										
A. *Not Operated*										
0–19 Years	20	1.3	<1	1	1	1	1	3	3	3
20–34	3	1.7	<1	1	1	2	2	2	2	2
35–49	0									
50–64	0									
65+	0									
B. *Operated*										
0–19 Years	0									
20–34	1	8.0	0	8	8	8	8	8	8	8
35–49	1	2.0	0	2	2	2	2	2	2	2
50–64	0									
65+	0									
2. MULTIPLE DX										
A. *Not Operated*										
0–19 Years	68	2.2	6	1	1	2	2	4	5	19
20–34	64	2.1	6	1	1	2	2	4	8	13
35–49	62	2.5	10	1	1	2	3	4	6	24
50–64	33	3.1	13	1	1	2	4	4	10	20
65+	22	3.0	3	1	1	3	4	5	6	6
B. *Operated*										
0–19 Years	9	4.2	5	2	3	5	5	8	8	8
20–34	22	5.4	30	2	2	5	7	10	11	26
35–49	11	7.5	22	3	3	7	11	11	18	18
50–64	9	8.8	94	2	2	5	8	27	27	27
65+	6	4.3	5	2	3	3	5	8	8	8
SUBTOTALS:										
1. SINGLE DX										
A. *Not Operated*	23	1.3	<1	1	1	1	1	2	3	3
B. *Operated*	2	5.0	18	2	2	5	8	8	8	8
2. MULTIPLE DX										
A. *Not Operated*	249	2.4	7	1	1	2	3	4	6	19
B. *Operated*	57	6.1	32	2	3	4	8	11	24	27
1. SINGLE DX	**25**	**1.6**	**2**	**1**	**1**	**1**	**1**	**3**	**3**	**8**
2. MULTIPLE DX	**306**	**3.1**	**14**	**1**	**1**	**2**	**4**	**6**	**9**	**24**
A. NOT OPERATED	**272**	**2.4**	**7**	**1**	**1**	**2**	**3**	**4**	**6**	**19**
B. OPERATED	**59**	**6.0**	**32**	**2**	**2**	**4**	**8**	**11**	**24**	**27**
TOTAL										
0–19 Years	97	2.2	5	1	1	2	3	4	6	19
20–34	90	3.0	13	1	1	2	3	8	10	26
35–49	74	3.2	14	1	2	2	4	7	11	24
50–64	42	4.3	34	2	2	4	4	8	20	27
65+	28	3.3	3	1	2	3	5	6	6	8
GRAND TOTAL	**331**	**3.0**	**13**	**1**	**1**	**2**	**3**	**6**	**9**	**24**

Length of Stay by Diagnosis and Operation, Western Region, 2008

Western Region, October 2006–September 2007 Data, by Diagnosis

801.06: CL BASE FX S IC INJ-NEC

Type of Patients	Observed Patients	Avg. Stay	Variance	10th	25th	50th	75th	90th	95th	99th
1. SINGLE DX										
A. Not Operated										
0–19 Years	4	1.7	<1	1	1	1	2	3	3	3
20–34	1	1.0	0	1	1	1	1	1	1	1
35–49	1	1.0	0	1	1	1	1	1	1	1
50–64	0									
65+	0									
B. Operated										
0–19 Years	0									
20–34	0									
35–49	0									
50–64	0									
65+	0									
2. MULTIPLE DX										
A. Not Operated										
0–19 Years	63	2.3	3	1	1	2	3	4	5	10
20–34	96	2.5	4	1	1	2	3	5	7	14
35–49	69	2.9	6	1	1	2	5	6	8	13
50–64	27	3.2	3	1	2	3	5	6	6	7
65+	31	3.7	8	1	1	3	5	7	11	11
B. Operated										
0–19 Years	11	6.1	13	3	3	5	8	12	13	13
20–34	31	10.1	151	2	3	7	10	22	24	67
35–49	16	20.8	270	4	11	18	28	49	63	63
50–64	7	15.4	141	3	6	10	31	31	31	31
65+	4	11.5	14	7	10	14	15	15	15	15
SUBTOTALS:										
1. SINGLE DX										
A. Not Operated	6	1.5	<1	1	1	1	2	3	3	3
B. Operated	0									
2. MULTIPLE DX										
A. Not Operated	286	2.7	5	1	1	2	3	5	7	11
B. Operated	69	12.6	167	3	5	8	15	28	33	67
1. SINGLE DX	6	1.5	<1	1	1	1	2	3	3	3
2. MULTIPLE DX	355	4.6	51	1	1	2	5	10	15	33
A. NOT OPERATED	292	2.7	5	1	1	2	3	5	7	11
B. OPERATED	69	12.6	167	3	5	8	15	28	33	67
TOTAL										
0–19 Years	78	2.8	6	1	1	2	3	6	8	13
20–34	128	4.3	50	1	1	2	5	8	13	24
35–49	86	6.2	102	1	2	2	5	16	25	63
50–64	34	5.7	54	1	2	3	6	10	31	31
65+	35	4.6	14	1	2	3	6	11	14	15
GRAND TOTAL	361	4.6	51	1	1	2	5	9	14	33

801.20: CL BASE FX SAH/SDH-NOS

Type of Patients	Observed Patients	Avg. Stay	Variance	10th	25th	50th	75th	90th	95th	99th
1. SINGLE DX										
A. Not Operated										
0–19 Years	8	2.2	2	1	1	2	3	5	5	5
20–34	2	3.0	8	1	1	5	5	5	5	5
35–49	1	2.0	0	2	2	2	2	2	2	2
50–64	1	4.0	0	4	4	4	4	4	4	4
65+	0									
B. Operated										
0–19 Years	0									
20–34	2	7.0	2	6	6	8	8	8	8	8
35–49	1	10.0	0	10	10	10	10	10	10	10
50–64	0									
65+	0									
2. MULTIPLE DX										
A. Not Operated										
0–19 Years	21	2.6	2	1	1	3	4	4	5	6
20–34	53	4.4	22	1	2	3	6	9	11	31
35–49	57	5.3	31	1	2	3	6	14	20	22
50–64	40	6.4	39	2	2	5	9	14	17	35
65+	40	7.2	25	2	4	7	10	14	16	22
B. Operated										
0–19 Years	17	16.7	417	4	5	11	20	38	85	85
20–34	26	13.6	133	3	6	11	19	31	33	48
35–49	29	14.3	114	8	6	11	18	33	35	37
50–64	18	23.8	397	8	12	15	28	77	>99	>99
65+	13	13.9	115	4	8	9	14	32	36	36
SUBTOTALS:										
1. SINGLE DX										
A. Not Operated	12	2.5	2	1	1	2	3	5	5	5
B. Operated	3	8.0	4	6	6	8	10	10	10	10
2. MULTIPLE DX										
A. Not Operated	211	5.4	28	1	2	3	7	11	16	22
B. Operated	103	16.1	223	4	6	11	22	33	48	85
1. SINGLE DX	15	3.6	7	1	1	3	5	8	10	10
2. MULTIPLE DX	314	8.9	116	1	3	5	11	20	32	59
A. NOT OPERATED	223	5.2	27	1	2	3	7	11	16	22
B. OPERATED	106	15.9	218	4	6	11	20	33	48	85
TOTAL										
0–19 Years	46	7.7	197	1	2	4	5	20	30	85
20–34	83	7.3	73	1	2	5	9	18	30	48
35–49	88	8.3	75	1	2	5	11	20	32	37
50–64	59	11.6	209	2	3	7	14	26	57	>99
65+	53	8.8	53	3	4	7	11	16	27	36
GRAND TOTAL	329	8.7	113	1	2	5	11	20	31	59

801.21: CL BASE FX SAH/SDH S LOC

Type of Patients	Observed Patients	Avg. Stay	Variance	10th	25th	50th	75th	90th	95th	99th
1. SINGLE DX										
A. Not Operated										
0–19 Years	36	1.8	2	1	1	1	2	3	5	9
20–34	4	2.5	3	1	1	2	2	5	5	5
35–49	3	2.0	1	1	1	2	3	3	3	3
50–64	0									
65+	1	1.0	0	1	1	1	1	1	1	1
B. Operated										
0–19 Years	7	2.9	1	1	2	3	4	4	4	4
20–34	0									
35–49	0									
50–64	0									
2. MULTIPLE DX										
A. Not Operated										
0–19 Years	82	2.7	3	1	2	2	3	4	7	11
20–34	65	4.0	14	1	2	3	5	8	9	23
35–49	56	6.6	40	1	2	4	10	14	21	29
50–64	58	4.9	26	1	2	3	5	10	17	29
65+	89	5.0	19	1	2	4	7	10	12	23
B. Operated										
0–19 Years	21	10.6	221	2	3	5	9	24	40	62
20–34	25	11.6	89	3	5	9	14	27	32	35
35–49	21	12.4	130	4	5	8	13	29	30	48
50–64	19	12.5	107	3	5	12	17	28	44	44
65+	15	16.3	248	4	7	10	21	37	62	62
SUBTOTALS:										
1. SINGLE DX										
A. Not Operated	44	1.8	2	1	1	1	2	3	5	9
B. Operated	7	2.9	1	1	2	3	4	4	4	4
2. MULTIPLE DX										
A. Not Operated	350	4.5	20	1	2	3	5	10	13	23
B. Operated	101	12.4	149	3	4	8	15	29	37	62
1. SINGLE DX	51	2.0	2	1	1	2	2	4	5	9
2. MULTIPLE DX	451	6.3	60	1	2	4	7	14	21	40
A. NOT OPERATED	394	4.2	19	1	2	3	5	9	13	23
B. OPERATED	108	11.8	145	2	4	7	15	29	37	62
TOTAL										
0–19 Years	146	3.6	41	1	1	2	4	6	9	40
20–34	94	6.0	44	1	2	3	7	14	23	35
35–49	80	8.0	69	1	3	5	10	20	24	48
50–64	77	6.8	56	2	2	4	8	17	20	44
65+	105	6.6	65	1	2	4	8	12	21	37
GRAND TOTAL	502	5.8	56	1	2	3	7	13	20	37

Western Region, October 2006–September 2007 Data, by Diagnosis

801.22: CL BASE FX SAH/SDH-BRIEF

Type of Patients	Observed Patients	Avg. Stay	Variance	Percentiles 10th	25th	50th	75th	90th	95th	99th
1. SINGLE DX										
A. Not Operated										
0–19 Years	12	1.9	<1	1	1	2	2	3	4	4
20–34	9	3.1	3	1	2	2	5	6	6	6
35–49	4	2.7	8	1	1	1	2	7	7	7
50–64	1	4.0	0	4	4	4	4	4	4	4
65+	1	2.0	0	2	2	2	2	2	2	2
B. Operated										
0–19 Years	4	2.5	<1	2	2	2	3	3	3	3
20–34	1	3.0	0	3	3	3	3	3	3	3
35–49	1	2.0	0	2	2	2	2	2	2	2
50–64	1	5.0	0	5	5	5	5	5	5	5
65+	0									
2. MULTIPLE DX										
A. Not Operated										
0–19 Years	71	3.6	8	1	2	3	4	7	8	18
20–34	112	3.6	14	1	2	2	5	6	10	21
35–49	71	5.2	25	1	2	3	7	11	14	31
50–64	66	5.9	25	2	2	4	8	12	14	29
65+	63	6.2	35	2	3	4	7	11	14	31
B. Operated										
0–19 Years	27	10.6	75	3	4	6	19	24	26	30
20–34	42	9.6	139	2	4	6	13	18	22	74
35–49	32	16.1	171	4	6	15	23	29	30	69
50–64	23	13.6	32	5	8	14	19	20	21	23
65+	14	13.8	76	4	7	12	22	28	29	29
SUBTOTALS:										
1. SINGLE DX										
A. Not Operated	27	2.5	3	1	1	2	3	5	6	7
B. Operated	7	2.9	1	2	2	3	3	5	5	5
2. MULTIPLE DX										
A. Not Operated	383	4.7	21	1	2	3	6	10	13	29
B. Operated	138	12.4	114	3	5	10	18	24	29	69
1. SINGLE DX	34	2.6	2	1	2	2	3	5	6	7
2. MULTIPLE DX	521	6.7	57	1	2	4	8	16	22	30
A. NOT OPERATED	410	4.6	20	1	2	3	6	10	12	28
B. OPERATED	145	11.9	112	3	4	9	18	24	28	69
TOTAL										
0–19 Years	114	5.0	33	1	2	3	5	12	20	26
20–34	164	5.1	52	1	2	3	6	11	15	28
35–49	108	8.3	92	1	3	4	10	21	27	31
50–64	91	7.8	37	2	3	6	12	17	20	29
65+	78	7.5	50	2	3	5	11	16	28	31
GRAND TOTAL	555	6.5	55	1	2	4	8	15	21	30

801.26: CL BASE FX SAH/SDH-NEC

Type of Patients	Observed Patients	Avg. Stay	Variance	Percentiles 10th	25th	50th	75th	90th	95th	99th
1. SINGLE DX										
A. Not Operated										
0–19 Years	11	2.6	3	1	1	2	2	5	5	5
20–34	4	1.5	<1	1	1	1	1	3	3	3
35–49	0									
50–64	6	4.2	21	1	1	3	5	13	13	13
65+	0									
B. Operated										
0–19 Years	2	2.5	4	1	1	1	1	4	4	4
20–34	2	2.5	4	1	1	1	1	4	4	4
35–49	1	9.0	0	9	9	9	9	9	9	9
50–64	0									
65+	0									
2. MULTIPLE DX										
A. Not Operated										
0–19 Years	73	5.4	31	2	2	4	6	11	16	35
20–34	141	4.8	26	1	2	3	5	11	16	25
35–49	86	6.4	28	2	3	5	9	14	18	28
50–64	70	9.4	188	1	3	4	10	29	36	73
65+	59	7.6	74	2	3	5	8	20	29	48
B. Operated										
0–19 Years	54	15.2	224	4	5	12	18	28	46	77
20–34	83	17.2	237	3	5	13	24	35	48	91
35–49	68	22.6	303	5	10	19	33	46	64	>99
50–64	38	19.5	264	6	7	14	25	51	63	>99
65+	22	14.9	70	6	9	12	23	25	28	33
SUBTOTALS:										
1. SINGLE DX										
A. Not Operated	21	2.9	8	1	1	2	4	5	5	13
B. Operated	5	3.8	11	1	1	4	4	9	9	9
2. MULTIPLE DX										
A. Not Operated	429	6.3	62	2	2	4	7	13	21	36
B. Operated	265	18.3	246	4	6	14	25	39	51	92
1. SINGLE DX	26	3.1	8	1	1	2	4	5	9	13
2. MULTIPLE DX	694	10.9	166	2	3	6	14	28	36	70
A. NOT OPERATED	450	6.2	60	1	2	4	7	13	20	36
B. OPERATED	270	18.1	246	4	6	13	25	38	51	92
TOTAL										
0–19 Years	140	8.9	127	2	3	5	11	21	28	67
20–34	230	9.2	138	1	4	8	12	24	31	49
35–49	155	13.5	212	2	4	8	18	34	45	92
50–64	114	12.5	228	2	3	7	15	23	51	73
65+	81	9.6	83	2	3	7	12	23	28	48
GRAND TOTAL	720	10.6	163	2	3	6	13	27	36	68

802: FRACTURE OF FACE BONES

Type of Patients	Observed Patients	Avg. Stay	Variance	Percentiles 10th	25th	50th	75th	90th	95th	99th
1. SINGLE DX										
A. Not Operated										
0–19 Years	46	1.6	<1	1	1	1	2	3	3	4
20–34	57	2.0	2	1	1	1	2	5	6	7
35–49	23	2.3	7	1	1	1	2	3	9	12
50–64	6	2.7	4	1	3	3	4	6	6	6
65+	2	5.0	8	3	3	5	7	7	7	7
B. Operated										
0–19 Years	58	2.2	5	1	1	1	3	4	6	16
20–34	164	2.1	5	1	1	1	2	3	4	17
35–49	67	2.1	2	1	1	2	3	4	5	7
50–64	22	2.5	6	1	2	2	3	5	8	10
65+	3	1.0	0	1	1	1	1	1	1	1
2. MULTIPLE DX										
A. Not Operated										
0–19 Years	339	1.8	2	1	1	1	2	3	5	7
20–34	711	2.1	4	1	1	1	2	4	6	11
35–49	523	2.6	13	1	1	2	3	5	7	11
50–64	330	2.7	9	1	1	2	3	5	7	19
65+	542	3.3	10	2	2	3	4	6	7	14
B. Operated										
0–19 Years	434	3.5	18	1	1	2	4	7	11	25
20–34	1,415	3.5	18	1	1	2	4	7	11	22
35–49	839	4.2	27	1	1	3	5	8	11	24
50–64	440	4.6	34	1	2	3	5	10	16	29
65+	216	5.4	28	1	2	4	8	12	17	26
SUBTOTALS:										
1. SINGLE DX										
A. Not Operated	134	2.0	3	1	1	1	2	4	6	9
B. Operated	314	2.1	4	1	1	2	2	4	5	13
2. MULTIPLE DX										
A. Not Operated	2,445	2.5	8	1	1	2	3	5	6	12
B. Operated	3,344	4.0	23	1	1	2	5	8	12	25
1. SINGLE DX	448	2.1	4	1	1	1	2	4	6	12
2. MULTIPLE DX	5,789	3.3	17	1	1	2	4	7	10	21
A. NOT OPERATED	2,579	2.5	8	1	1	2	3	5	6	12
B. OPERATED	3,658	3.8	22	1	1	2	4	8	12	24
TOTAL										
0–19 Years	877	2.7	10	1	1	2	3	5	7	20
20–34	2,347	3.0	13	1	1	2	3	6	9	18
35–49	1,452	3.5	21	1	1	2	4	7	10	23
50–64	798	3.8	24	1	2	2	4	8	11	26
65+	763	3.9	16	2	2	3	5	8	11	20
GRAND TOTAL	6,237	3.3	16	1	1	2	4	7	9	20

Length of Stay by Diagnosis and Operation, Western Region, 2008

Western Region, October 2006–September 2007 Data, by Diagnosis

802.0: CLOSED NASAL BONE FX

Type of Patients	Observed Patients	Avg. Stay	Variance	Percentiles						
				10th	25th	50th	75th	90th	95th	99th
1. SINGLE DX										
A. Not Operated										
0–19 Years	4	1.0	0	1	1	1	1		1	1
20–34	5	1.2	<1	1	1	1	1	2	2	2
35–49	1	1.0	0	1	1	1	1		1	1
50–64	0									
65+	2	5.0	8	3	3	5	7	7	7	7
B. Operated										
0–19 Years	1	1.0	0	1	1	1	1		1	1
20–34	3	3.0	0	3	3	3	3	3	3	3
35–49	3	2.3	<1	2	2	2	3	3	3	3
50–64	0									
65+	0									
2. MULTIPLE DX										
A. Not Operated										
0–19 Years	80	1.7	2	1	1	1	2	3	4	8
20–34	143	1.9	4	1	1	1	2	3	6	10
35–49	97	2.1	7	1	1	2	2	4	5	25
50–64	56	2.6	3	1	1	2	4	5	6	11
65+	164	3.1	5	1	2	3	4	5	7	14
B. Operated										
0–19 Years	9	4.0	42	1	1	1	3	21	21	21
20–34	24	2.3	3	1	1	2	4	5	6	6
35–49	24	3.0	5	1	1	2	4	6	7	10
50–64	16	3.6	15	2	2	2	4	8	16	16
65+	7	5.5	22	1	1	4	9	13	13	13
SUBTOTALS:										
1. SINGLE DX										
A. Not Operated	12	1.8	3	1	1	1	1	3	7	7
B. Operated	5	2.2	<1	1	2	2	3	3	3	3
2. MULTIPLE DX										
A. Not Operated	540	2.3	5	1	1	2	3	4	6	11
B. Operated	80	3.2	12	1	1	2	4	7	10	21
1. SINGLE DX	17	1.9	2	1	1	1	2	3	7	7
2. MULTIPLE DX	620	2.5	6	1	1	2	3	5	6	13
A. NOT OPERATED	552	2.3	5	1	1	2	3	4	6	11
B. OPERATED	85	3.2	11	1	1	2	4	7	9	21
TOTAL										
0–19 Years	94	1.9	5	1	1	1	2	3	5	21
20–34	173	1.9	4	1	1	1	2	4	6	10
35–49	125	2.3	6	1	1	2	3	4	5	10
50–64	72	2.8	6	1	1	2	4	5	7	16
65+	173	3.2	6	1	2	3	4	6	7	14
GRAND TOTAL	637	2.4	6	1	1	2	3	5	6	13

802.22: CLSD SUBCONDYLAR FX MAND

Type of Patients	Observed Patients	Avg. Stay	Variance	Percentiles						
				10th	25th	50th	75th	90th	95th	99th
1. SINGLE DX										
A. Not Operated										
0–19 Years	3	1.3	<1	1	1	1	1	2	2	2
20–34	4	2.5	6	1	1	2	6	6	6	6
35–49	0									
50–64	0									
65+	0									
B. Operated										
0–19 Years	1	1.0	0	1	1	1	1		1	1
20–34	12	1.4	<1	1	1	1	2	2	3	3
35–49	2	1.5	<1	1	1	2	2	2	2	2
50–64	3	1.7	<1	1	1	2	2	2	2	2
65+	0									
2. MULTIPLE DX										
A. Not Operated										
0–19 Years	19	1.5	<1	1	1	1	2	2	2	2
20–34	38	2.7	4	1	2	2	3	5	9	9
35–49	29	2.6	4	1	1	2	3	7	8	8
50–64	15	3.3	8	1	1	2	5	8	10	10
65+	7	5.4	22	1	1	4	12	12	12	12
B. Operated										
0–19 Years	25	3.6	13	1	2	3	4	5	6	20
20–34	66	3.1	11	1	1	2	4	7	11	16
35–49	30	3.5	10	1	2	2	4	6	9	9
50–64	16	2.2	2	1	1	2	2	4	6	6
65+	5	11.0	26	4	9	12	12	18	18	18
SUBTOTALS:										
1. SINGLE DX										
A. Not Operated	7	2.0	3	1	1	1	2	6	6	6
B. Operated	18	1.4	<1	1	1	2	2	2	3	3
2. MULTIPLE DX										
A. Not Operated	108	2.7	6	1	1	2	3	5	9	11
B. Operated	142	3.4	13	1	1	2	3	7	12	18
1. SINGLE DX	25	1.6	1	1	1	1	2	2	3	6
2. MULTIPLE DX	250	3.1	10	1	1	2	3	7	10	16
A. NOT OPERATED	115	2.7	6	1	1	2	3	5	9	11
B. OPERATED	160	3.2	12	1	1	2	3	7	11	18
TOTAL										
0–19 Years	48	2.6	8	1	1	2	3	4	5	20
20–34	120	2.8	8	1	1	2	3	5	8	15
35–49	61	3.0	7	1	1	2	3	7	8	16
50–64	34	2.6	5	1	1	2	3	5	8	10
65+	12	7.7	30	1	4	12	12	18	18	18
GRAND TOTAL	275	3.0	9	1	1	2	3	6	9	16

802.25: CLOSED FX ANGLE OF JAW

Type of Patients	Observed Patients	Avg. Stay	Variance	Percentiles						
				10th	25th	50th	75th	90th	95th	99th
1. SINGLE DX										
A. Not Operated										
0–19 Years	8	1.5	1	1	1	2	2	4	4	4
20–34	15	1.9	2	1	1	2	2	3	6	6
35–49	6	1.5	<1	1	1	1	2	2	3	3
50–64	1	4.0	0	4	4	4	4	4	4	4
65+	0									
B. Operated										
0–19 Years	15	2.3	2	1	1	2	3	3	4	6
20–34	30	2.3	9	1	1	2	3	4	4	18
35–49	14	2.4	3	1	1	2	3	6	7	7
50–64	2	1.5	<1	1	1	2	2	2	2	2
65+	0									
2. MULTIPLE DX										
A. Not Operated										
0–19 Years	12	1.8	<1	1	1	1	2	3	4	4
20–34	57	1.9	2	1	1	2	3	3	4	9
35–49	21	3.4	42	1	1	2	5	5	6	31
50–64	11	4.0	35	1	2	5	6	6	21	21
65+	2	5.5	<1	5	5	5	6	6	6	6
B. Operated										
0–19 Years	64	2.4	5	1	1	2	3	4	6	15
20–34	196	2.8	6	1	1	3	3	6	9	12
35–49	81	3.4	10	1	2	3	5	7	9	15
50–64	28	4.4	27	2	3	3	4	8	20	23
65+	4	6.2	56	1	9	12	6	17	17	17
SUBTOTALS:										
1. SINGLE DX										
A. Not Operated	30	1.8	1	1	1	2	2	4	4	6
B. Operated	61	2.3	6	1	2	2	3	4	6	18
2. MULTIPLE DX										
A. Not Operated	103	2.5	14	1	1	2	3	4	5	21
B. Operated	373	3.1	9	1	1	2	4	6	9	15
1. SINGLE DX	91	2.1	4	1	1	2	2	4	6	18
2. MULTIPLE DX	476	2.9	10	1	1	2	3	6	8	17
A. NOT OPERATED	133	2.3	11	1	1	2	3	4	5	21
B. OPERATED	434	2.9	8	1	1	2	3	6	8	15
TOTAL										
0–19 Years	99	2.2	4	1	1	2	3	4	6	15
20–34	298	2.6	5	1	1	2	3	5	7	12
35–49	122	3.2	14	1	1	2	4	7	8	15
50–64	42	4.1	26	1	3	5	6	17	20	23
65+	6	6.0	34	1	5	6	17	17	17	17
GRAND TOTAL	567	2.8	9	1	1	2	3	6	8	17

Length of Stay by Diagnosis and Operation, Western Region, 2008

802.26: CLSD FX SYMPH MAND BODY

Type of Patients	Observed Patients	Avg. Stay	Variance	10th	25th	50th	75th	90th	95th	99th
1. SINGLE DX										
A. *Not Operated*										
0–19 Years	2	1.5	<1	1	1	2	2	2	2	2
20–34	5	1.8	<1	1	1	2	2	2	3	3
35–49	1	1.0	0	1	1	1	1	1	1	1
50–64	0									
65+	0									
B. *Operated*										
0–19 Years	7	2.0	2	1	1	2	2	5	5	5
20–34	7	1.7	1	1	1	1	2	4	4	4
35–49	5	2.6	2	2	2	2	2	5	5	5
50–64	0									
65+	0									
2. MULTIPLE DX										
A. *Not Operated*										
0–19 Years	14	1.9	1	1	1	2	2	3	5	5
20–34	18	2.3	2	1	1	2	4	4	5	5
35–49	5	1.8	<1	1	1	2	2	3	3	3
50–64	0									
65+	1	1.0	0	1	1	1	1	1	1	1
B. *Operated*										
0–19 Years	51	3.7	30	1	1	2	4	6	16	30
20–34	133	3.0	8	1	1	2	4	6	8	12
35–49	55	4.7	16	1	2	3	6	11	14	18
50–64	15	3.6	11	1	1	5	5	8	13	13
65+	8	5.4	9	3	3	5	6	12	12	12
SUBTOTALS:										
1. SINGLE DX										
A. *Not Operated*	8	1.6	<1	1	1	2	2	2	2	3
B. *Operated*	19	2.1	2	1	1	2	2	5	5	5
2. MULTIPLE DX										
A. *Not Operated*	38	2.1	2	1	1	2	3	4	5	5
B. *Operated*	262	3.6	14	1	1	2	4	8	10	22
1. SINGLE DX	27	1.9	1	1	1	2	2	4	5	5
2. MULTIPLE DX	300	3.4	13	1	1	2	4	7	9	18
A. NOT OPERATED	46	2.0	1	1	1	2	3	4	4	5
B. OPERATED	281	3.5	14	1	1	2	4	7	10	22
TOTAL										
0–19 Years	74	3.1	22	1	1	2	3	5	8	30
20–34	163	2.8	7	1	1	2	3	5	6	12
35–49	66	4.2	15	2	2	3	5	10	14	18
50–64	15	3.6	11	1	1	2	5	8	13	13
65+	9	4.9	10	1	3	4	6	12	12	12
GRAND TOTAL	327	3.3	12	1	1	2	4	6	9	18

802.28: CLSD FX MANDIBLE BDY NEC

Type of Patients	Observed Patients	Avg. Stay	Variance	10th	25th	50th	75th	90th	95th	99th
1. SINGLE DX										
A. *Not Operated*										
0–19 Years	6	1.7	<1	1	1	2	2	2	2	2
20–34	1	6.0	0	6	6	6	6	6	6	6
35–49	3	5.3	34	1	1	3	12	12	12	12
50–64	1	1.0	0	1	1	1	1	1	1	1
65+	0									
B. *Operated*										
0–19 Years	4	1.5	<1	1	1	2	2	2	2	2
20–34	11	2.5	5	1	1	1	3	7	7	7
35–49	5	3.4	4	1	2	3	5	6	6	6
50–64	4	4.0	9	1	3	3	4	8	8	8
65+	1	1.0	0	1	1	1	1	1	1	1
2. MULTIPLE DX										
A. *Not Operated*										
0–19 Years	6	2.3	3	1	1	1	3	5	5	5
20–34	20	1.7	<1	1	1	1	2	3	3	4
35–49	14	2.2	2	1	1	2	2	4	6	6
50–64	4	13.0	66	5	7	7	19	21	21	21
65+	4	2.3	<1	1	1	2	3	3	3	3
B. *Operated*										
0–19 Years	20	2.9	5	1	2	2	3	6	6	11
20–34	64	2.2	3	1	1	2	3	5	5	8
35–49	54	4.9	70	1	1	3	5	8	11	62
50–64	21	3.3	4	1	2	3	5	5	5	8
65+	16	7.2	59	1	2	5	10	16	30	30
SUBTOTALS:										
1. SINGLE DX										
A. *Not Operated*	11	3.0	11	1	1	2	3	6	12	12
B. *Operated*	25	2.7	5	1	1	2	3	7	7	8
2. MULTIPLE DX										
A. *Not Operated*	48	2.9	15	1	1	2	3	5	7	21
B. *Operated*	175	3.7	31	1	1	2	5	7	10	30
1. SINGLE DX	36	2.8	6	1	1	2	3	4	8	12
2. MULTIPLE DX	223	3.5	28	1	1	2	4	7	10	21
A. NOT OPERATED	59	2.9	14	1	1	2	3	6	12	21
B. OPERATED	200	3.6	28	1	1	2	4	7	10	16
TOTAL										
0–19 Years	36	2.5	4	1	1	2	3	5	6	11
20–34	96	2.1	3	1	1	2	3	5	6	8
35–49	76	4.3	52	1	1	3	5	10	11	62
50–64	30	4.6	22	1	2	4	5	8	19	21
65+	21	5.9	50	1	2	4	7	14	16	30
GRAND TOTAL	259	3.4	25	1	1	2	4	7	10	21

802.4: CLSD FX MALAR/MAXILLARY

Type of Patients	Observed Patients	Avg. Stay	Variance	10th	25th	50th	75th	90th	95th	99th
1. SINGLE DX										
A. *Not Operated*										
0–19 Years	2	1.0	0	1	1	1	1	1	1	1
20–34	4	1.3	<1	1	1	1	1	2	2	2
35–49	3	2.0	0	2	2	2	2	2	2	2
50–64	0									
65+	0									
B. *Operated*										
0–19 Years	5	4.4	43	1	1	1	3	16	16	16
20–34	25	2.1	2	1	1	2	2	4	5	7
35–49	12	1.8	1	1	1	1	3	4	4	4
50–64	4	3.5	19	1	2	2	10	10	10	10
65+	2	1.0	0	1	1	1	1	1	1	1
2. MULTIPLE DX										
A. *Not Operated*										
0–19 Years	28	1.9	3	1	1	1	2	3	7	8
20–34	115	2.0	3	1	1	2	2	4	6	11
35–49	88	2.4	6	1	1	2	3	5	7	19
50–64	78	2.3	3	1	1	2	3	4	6	12
65+	116	3.5	12	1	2	3	5	6	8	16
B. *Operated*										
0–19 Years	37	3.4	13	1	1	3	5	6	10	20
20–34	245	3.5	17	1	1	2	4	7	11	20
35–49	197	4.2	24	1	1	2	5	9	11	29
50–64	122	4.6	41	1	2	3	5	10	12	23
65+	53	5.9	32	1	2	4	8	12	20	29
SUBTOTALS:										
1. SINGLE DX										
A. *Not Operated*	9	1.4	<1	1	1	1	2	2	2	2
B. *Operated*	48	2.4	7	1	1	1	2	4	7	16
2. MULTIPLE DX										
A. *Not Operated*	425	2.5	7	1	1	2	3	5	7	11
B. *Operated*	654	4.1	25	1	1	3	5	9	12	25
1. SINGLE DX	57	2.2	6	1	1	1	2	4	7	16
2. MULTIPLE DX	1,079	3.5	18	1	1	2	4	7	10	23
A. NOT OPERATED	434	2.5	6	1	1	2	3	5	7	11
B. OPERATED	702	4.0	24	1	1	2	5	8	11	24
TOTAL										
0–19 Years	72	2.8	11	1	1	1	3	5	9	20
20–34	389	2.9	12	1	1	2	3	6	8	17
35–49	300	3.6	18	1	1	2	5	8	10	25
50–64	204	3.7	27	1	1	2	4	8	11	21
65+	171	4.2	19	1	2	3	5	8	11	29
GRAND TOTAL	1,136	3.4	18	1	1	2	4	7	10	21

695

Length of Stay by Diagnosis and Operation, Western Region, 2008

Western Region, October 2006–September 2007 Data, by Diagnosis

802.6: CLOSED FX ORBITAL FLOOR

Type of Patients	Observed Patients	Avg. Stay	Variance	10th	25th	50th	75th	90th	95th	99th
1. SINGLE DX										
A. Not Operated										
0–19 Years	3	1.0	0	1	1	1	1	1	1	1
20–34	2	2.5	4	1	1	4	4	4	4	4
35–49	0									
50–64	1	6.0	0	6	6	6	6	6	6	6
65+	0									
B. Operated										
0–19 Years	11	1.5	1	1	1	1	3	3	4	4
20–34	20	3.3	19	1	1	2	3	13	17	17
35–49	6	1.3	<1	1	1	1	1	1	3	3
50–64	6	1.7	3	1	1	1	1	5	5	5
65+	0									
2. MULTIPLE DX										
A. Not Operated										
0–19 Years	44	1.4	<1	1	1	1	2	2	3	4
20–34	84	2.1	6	1	1	1	2	3	4	21
35–49	72	3.1	44	1	1	2	3	4	6	57
50–64	59	2.6	4	1	1	2	3	5	8	10
65+	111	2.8	3	1	2	2	4	5	6	8
B. Operated										
0–19 Years	42	3.2	9	1	1	2	3	7	8	16
20–34	169	3.3	11	1	1	3	4	9	9	16
35–49	117	4.6	18	2	2	3	5	10	14	19
50–64	66	3.8	21	1	1	2	4	10	15	26
65+	59	3.9	17	1	1	2	5	10	12	22
SUBTOTALS:										
1. SINGLE DX										
A. Not Operated	6	2.3	5	1	1	1	4	6	6	6
B. Operated	43	2.3	10	1	1	1	2	4	8	17
2. MULTIPLE DX										
A. Not Operated	370	2.5	12	1	1	2	3	5	6	10
B. Operated	453	3.8	15	1	1	2	4	8	12	19
1. SINGLE DX	49	2.3	9	1	1	1	2	5	8	17
2. MULTIPLE DX	823	3.2	14	1	1	2	4	6	9	18
A. NOT OPERATED	376	2.5	12	1	1	2	3	5	6	10
B. OPERATED	496	3.6	15	1	1	2	4	8	12	19
TOTAL										
0–19 Years	100	2.2	5	1	1	1	2	4	6	11
20–34	275	2.9	10	1	1	2	3	6	8	17
35–49	195	3.9	28	1	1	3	4	8	12	24
50–64	132	3.2	13	1	1	2	4	6	10	17
65+	170	3.2	8	1	1	3	4	6	9	12
GRAND TOTAL	872	3.1	14	1	1	2	4	6	9	18

802.8: CLSD FX FACIAL BONE NEC

Type of Patients	Observed Patients	Avg. Stay	Variance	10th	25th	50th	75th	90th	95th	99th
1. SINGLE DX										
A. Not Operated										
0–19 Years	1	1.0	0	1	1	1	1	1	1	1
20–34	1	2.0	0	2	2	2	2	2	2	2
35–49	0									
50–64	1	3.0	0	3	3	3	3	3	3	3
65+	0									
B. Operated										
0–19 Years	0									
20–34	3	1.3	<1	1	1	1	2	2	2	2
35–49	1	1.0	0	1	1	1	1	1	1	1
50–64	0									
65+	0									
2. MULTIPLE DX										
A. Not Operated										
0–19 Years	69	1.8	1	1	1	1	2	3	4	7
20–34	89	2.0	3	1	1	1	3	4	5	12
35–49	91	2.3	3	1	1	2	3	4	6	10
50–64	56	2.7	4	1	1	2	3	5	8	10
65+	86	3.9	28	1	2	3	4	7	9	46
B. Operated										
0–19 Years	33	2.9	12	1	1	1	3	5	14	15
20–34	79	3.7	10	1	2	3	3	7	12	18
35–49	56	3.9	14	1	2	3	5	8	12	22
50–64	35	5.6	37	1	2	4	7	12	23	29
65+	10	6.0	23	2	2	6	9	10	17	17
SUBTOTALS:										
1. SINGLE DX										
A. Not Operated	3	2.0	<1	1	1	1	3	3	3	3
B. Operated	4	1.3	<1	1	1	1	2	2	2	2
2. MULTIPLE DX										
A. Not Operated	391	2.5	9	1	1	2	3	5	6	10
B. Operated	213	4.1	17	1	1	3	5	8	12	22
1. SINGLE DX	7	1.6	<1	1	1	1	2	3	3	3
2. MULTIPLE DX	604	3.1	12	1	1	2	4	6	9	17
A. NOT OPERATED	394	2.5	9	1	1	2	3	5	6	10
B. OPERATED	217	4.0	17	1	1	3	5	8	12	22
TOTAL										
0–19 Years	103	2.1	5	1	1	1	2	4	5	14
20–34	172	2.8	7	1	1	2	3	5	7	16
35–49	148	2.9	8	1	1	2	3	6	8	12
50–64	92	3.8	19	1	1	3	4	7	11	29
65+	96	4.1	27	1	2	3	5	8	10	46
GRAND TOTAL	611	3.1	12	1	1	2	4	6	9	17

803: OTHER SKULL FRACTURE

Type of Patients	Observed Patients	Avg. Stay	Variance	10th	25th	50th	75th	90th	95th	99th
1. SINGLE DX										
A. Not Operated										
0–19 Years	47	1.6	3	1	1	1	2	2	3	11
20–34	11	2.0	3	1	1	1	3	3	7	7
35–49	5	2.0	2	1	1	1	3	4	4	4
50–64	1	2.0	0	2	2	2	2	2	2	2
65+	0									
B. Operated										
0–19 Years	5	3.2	2	1	3	3	4	5	5	5
20–34	5	2.6	2	1	2	2	3	5	5	5
35–49	1	9.0	0	9	9	9	9	9	9	9
50–64	1	3.0	0	3	3	3	3	3	3	3
65+	1	11.0	0	11	11	11	11	11	11	11
2. MULTIPLE DX										
A. Not Operated										
0–19 Years	86	3.3	10	1	1	2	4	7	9	21
20–34	80	3.6	15	1	1	3	4	10	10	24
35–49	64	6.0	46	1	2	3	7	12	24	35
50–64	63	5.7	23	1	2	4	7	12	15	24
65+	55	5.0	14	1	3	4	6	8	11	25
B. Operated										
0–19 Years	38	10.7	103	2	3	6	15	26	32	44
20–34	65	15.5	222	3	4	9	24	33	44	67
35–49	37	19.8	262	4	8	16	28	54	61	>99
50–64	32	19.3	288	5	7	12	22	48	61	65
65+	19	17.8	78	8	10	17	26	34	34	34
SUBTOTALS:										
1. SINGLE DX										
A. Not Operated	64	1.7	3	1	1	1	2	3	4	11
B. Operated	13	4.0	9	1	2	3	5	9	11	11
2. MULTIPLE DX										
A. Not Operated	348	4.6	22	1	2	3	6	9	13	24
B. Operated	191	16.2	210	3	5	12	23	34	53	67
1. SINGLE DX	77	2.1	4	1	1	1	2	4	7	11
2. MULTIPLE DX	539	8.7	119	1	2	5	10	23	31	61
A. NOT OPERATED	412	4.1	20	1	1	3	5	8	12	24
B. OPERATED	204	15.4	206	3	5	11	22	33	48	65
TOTAL										
0–19 Years	176	4.5	39	1	1	2	5	11	17	32
20–34	161	8.3	132	1	2	4	8	24	31	61
35–49	107	10.6	162	1	3	5	13	28	47	61
50–64	97	10.1	150	1	3	6	12	22	33	65
65+	75	8.3	61	2	4	6	10	21	27	34
GRAND TOTAL	616	7.9	109	1	2	4	9	21	30	59

Length of Stay by Diagnosis and Operation, Western Region, 2008

804: MULT FX SKULL W OTH BONE

Type of Patients	Observed Patients	Avg. Stay	Variance	Percentiles						
				10th	25th	50th	75th	90th	95th	99th
1. SINGLE DX										
A. Not Operated										
0–19 Years	2	2.0	0	2	2	2	2	2	2	2
20–34	2	3.0	8	1	1	5	5	5	5	5
35–49	1	2.0	0	2	2	2	2	2	2	2
50–64	0									
65+	0									
B. Operated										
0–19 Years	2	2.0	2	1	1	3	3	3	3	3
20–34	0									
35–49	0									
50–64	0									
65+	0									
2. MULTIPLE DX										
A. Not Operated										
0–19 Years	6	5.7	45	1	2	3	6	19	19	19
20–34	8	3.8	7	1	2	2	7	8	8	8
35–49	9	3.9	7	1	1	4	5	9	9	9
50–64	11	9.3	73	1	4	7	11	19	30	30
65+	13	6.9	33	2	3	6	10	12	22	22
B. Operated										
0–19 Years	9	12.3	51	3	7	11	16	25	25	25
20–34	20	20.3	557	3	6	10	21	66	73	79
35–49	14	18.2	260	3	6	12	21	45	50	50
50–64	10	17.1	102	3	7	19	24	26	36	36
65+	6	19.8	63	8	15	17	27	29	29	29
SUBTOTALS:										
1. SINGLE DX										
A. Not Operated	5	2.4	2	1	2	2	2	5	5	5
B. Operated	2	2.0	2	1	1	3	3	3	3	3
2. MULTIPLE DX										
A. Not Operated	47	6.2	36	1	2	5	8	12	19	30
B. Operated	59	18.0	277	3	7	13	21	43	66	79
1. SINGLE DX	7	2.3	2	1	1	2	3	5	5	5
2. MULTIPLE DX	106	12.8	204	2	3	8	17	26	43	73
A. NOT OPERATED	52	5.8	34	1	2	4	7	11	19	30
B. OPERATED	61	17.5	276	3	7	13	21	36	50	79
TOTAL										
0–19 Years	19	8.0	54	1	2	5	14	20	25	25
20–34	30	14.8	432	2	3	8	15	66	73	79
35–49	24	12.2	203	1	3	6	17	43	45	50
50–64	21	13.0	98	3	5	10	19	26	30	36
65+	19	10.9	78	2	3	8	17	27	29	29
GRAND TOTAL	113	12.1	198	2	3	7	16	26	43	73

805: VERT FX W/O CORD INJ

Type of Patients	Observed Patients	Avg. Stay	Variance	Percentiles						
				10th	25th	50th	75th	90th	95th	99th
1. SINGLE DX										
A. Not Operated										
0–19 Years	78	2.0	2	1	1	2	2	4	5	7
20–34	177	2.4	3	1	1	2	3	4	5	11
35–49	115	2.6	4	1	1	2	3	6	6	9
50–64	67	2.4	2	1	1	2	3	4	6	7
65+	29	2.6	2	1	1	3	3	5	6	7
B. Operated										
0–19 Years	25	4.8	8	1	3	4	6	9	10	11
20–34	53	4.1	6	1	2	3	5	8	9	13
35–49	42	3.9	9	1	2	3	5	8	11	11
50–64	40	2.8	7	1	1	1	4	6	8	14
65+	41	1.5	2	1	1	1	1	2	5	7
2. MULTIPLE DX										
A. Not Operated										
0–19 Years	428	2.6	5	1	1	2	3	5	6	10
20–34	1,049	3.1	7	1	2	2	4	6	8	14
35–49	1,018	3.5	12	2	2	3	4	7	9	18
50–64	1,255	4.1	21	2	2	3	5	8	10	19
65+	4,675	4.5	11	3	3	4	5	8	10	18
B. Operated										
0–19 Years	183	7.5	26	3	4	6	9	14	18	29
20–34	537	7.9	66	2	4	6	9	15	21	39
35–49	591	8.3	69	2	4	6	10	17	23	40
50–64	785	8.2	78	1	3	6	10	18	24	47
65+	2,878	6.2	36	2	3	5	8	13	18	31
SUBTOTALS:										
1. SINGLE DX										
A. Not Operated	466	2.4	3	1	1	2	3	4	6	7
B. Operated	201	3.3	8	1	1	2	5	7	9	13
2. MULTIPLE DX										
A. Not Operated	8,425	4.1	12	2	2	3	5	7	10	18
B. Operated	4,974	7.0	51	2	3	5	9	14	20	34
1. SINGLE DX	667	2.7	4	1	1	2	4	5	7	11
2. MULTIPLE DX	13,399	5.1	28	1	2	4	6	10	14	27
A. NOT OPERATED	8,891	4.0	12	1	2	3	5	7	10	17
B. OPERATED	5,175	6.9	49	1	3	5	8	14	20	34
TOTAL										
0–19 Years	714	3.9	15	1	1	3	5	8	11	20
20–34	1,816	4.5	29	1	2	3	5	9	12	29
35–49	1,766	5.1	36	1	2	3	6	10	15	30
50–64	2,147	5.5	45	1	2	4	7	12	16	32
65+	7,623	5.1	21	2	3	4	6	10	13	24
GRAND TOTAL	14,066	5.0	28	1	2	4	6	10	14	26

805.01: FX C1 VERTEBRA-CLOSED

Type of Patients	Observed Patients	Avg. Stay	Variance	Percentiles						
				10th	25th	50th	75th	90th	95th	99th
1. SINGLE DX										
A. Not Operated										
0–19 Years	3	1.3	<1	1	1	1	2	2	2	2
20–34	2	2.0	0	2	2	2	2	2	2	2
35–49	4	2.5	2	1	1	3	4	4	4	4
50–64	1	2.0	0	2	2	2	2	2	2	2
65+	2	4.5	4	3	3	3	6	6	6	6
B. Operated										
0–19 Years	1	3.0	0	3	3	3	3	3	3	3
20–34	2	4.5	12	2	2	7	7	7	7	7
35–49	1	2.0	0	2	2	2	2	2	2	2
50–64	0									
65+	0									
2. MULTIPLE DX										
A. Not Operated										
0–19 Years	15	2.2	1	1	1	2	3	3	5	5
20–34	37	3.1	6	1	1	2	4	7	10	10
35–49	36	3.8	26	1	1	2	3	9	16	27
50–64	39	4.0	11	1	2	3	5	8	14	15
65+	162	4.8	17	1	2	4	6	9	14	19
B. Operated										
0–19 Years	10	5.5	6	1	4	5	8	9	9	9
20–34	23	10.2	168	2	3	5	10	21	39	54
35–49	30	7.1	49	2	2	5	7	18	25	31
50–64	35	8.5	59	2	4	6	9	18	27	38
65+	65	10.6	48	3	5	9	16	20	23	32
SUBTOTALS:										
1. SINGLE DX										
A. Not Operated	12	2.4	2	1	2	2	3	4	6	6
B. Operated	4	3.5	6	2	2	3	7	7	7	7
2. MULTIPLE DX										
A. Not Operated	289	4.2	15	1	2	3	5	9	13	19
B. Operated	163	9.1	66	2	4	6	12	20	24	39
1. SINGLE DX	16	2.7	3	1	2	2	3	6	7	7
2. MULTIPLE DX	452	6.0	39	1	2	4	7	14	19	31
A. NOT OPERATED	301	4.1	15	1	2	3	5	8	12	19
B. OPERATED	167	9.0	65	2	4	6	11	20	24	39
TOTAL										
0–19 Years	29	3.3	6	1	1	3	4	8	8	9
20–34	64	5.6	74	1	2	3	5	10	20	54
35–49	71	5.1	36	1	2	3	6	13	18	31
50–64	75	6.1	38	2	2	4	8	13	18	38
65+	229	6.4	32	1	3	5	8	15	19	27
GRAND TOTAL	468	5.9	38	1	2	4	7	14	18	31

Length of Stay by Diagnosis and Operation, Western Region, 2008

Western Region, October 2006–September 2007 Data, by Diagnosis

805.02: FX C2 VERTEBRA-CLOSED

Type of Patients	Observed Patients	Avg. Stay	Vari-ance	10th	25th	50th	75th	90th	95th	99th
1. SINGLE DX										
A. Not Operated										
0–19 Years	4	1.0	0	1	1	1	1	1	1	1
20–34	5	2.0	2	1	1	1	3	4	4	4
35–49	4	2.0	<1	1	1	2	3	3	3	3
50–64	1	1.0	0	1	1	1	1	1	1	1
65+	8	2.9	4	1	2	3	3	7	7	7
B. Operated										
0–19 Years	4	6.8	5	5	5	6	10	10	10	10
20–34	10	3.9	7	1	2	3	5	7	9	9
35–49	6	3.2	2	1	1	2	4	5	5	5
50–64	7	3.3	6	1	1	3	6	6	6	6
65+	3	3.7	6	1	5	4	6	6	6	6
2. MULTIPLE DX										
A. Not Operated										
0–19 Years	29	2.4	2	1	1	2	3	4	5	7
20–34	41	3.2	6	1	1	2	4	6	7	11
35–49	67	3.8	19	1	2	3	4	8	10	30
50–64	82	4.2	27	1	2	3	4	8	14	33
65+	407	4.7	13	1	2	4	6	9	11	16
B. Operated										
0–19 Years	25	7.6	37	2	4	6	8	15	18	29
20–34	55	5.8	32	2	3	5	6	11	20	35
35–49	60	7.2	80	2	4	5	8	14	17	67
50–64	95	8.6	87	2	3	5	11	18	25	62
65+	321	9.7	71	3	5	7	11	20	25	42
SUBTOTALS:										
1. SINGLE DX										
A. Not Operated	22	2.1	2	1	1	2	3	3	4	7
B. Operated	30	4.0	6	1	2	4	6	6	9	10
2. MULTIPLE DX										
A. Not Operated	626	4.3	15	1	2	3	5	8	11	19
B. Operated	556	8.7	70	2	4	6	10	18	24	47
1. SINGLE DX	52	3.2	5	1	1	3	4	6	7	10
2. MULTIPLE DX	1,182	6.4	46	1	3	4	8	13	18	33
A. NOT OPERATED	648	4.2	14	1	2	3	5	8	11	19
B. OPERATED	586	8.5	68	2	4	6	10	18	24	47
TOTAL										
0–19 Years	62	4.7	23	2	2	3	6	10	12	29
20–34	111	4.5	20	1	2	4	6	8	11	21
35–49	137	5.2	47	1	2	3	6	10	15	30
50–64	185	6.4	62	1	3	4	7	15	19	47
65+	739	6.8	44	2	3	5	8	14	19	32
GRAND TOTAL	1,234	6.3	44	1	3	4	7	13	18	32

805.05: FX C5 VERTEBRA-CLOSED

Type of Patients	Observed Patients	Avg. Stay	Vari-ance	10th	25th	50th	75th	90th	95th	99th
1. SINGLE DX										
A. Not Operated										
0–19 Years	2	1.5	<1	1	1	1	2	2	2	2
20–34	9	1.3	<1	1	1	1	1	2	2	2
35–49	2	1.0	0	1	1	1	1	1	1	1
50–64	2	1.0	0	1	1	1	1	1	1	1
65+	0									
B. Operated										
0–19 Years	4	3.3	<1	2	3	3	4	4	4	4
20–34	5	3.2	2	2	3	3	4	5	5	5
35–49	2	3.0	2	2	2	4	4	4	4	4
50–64	0									
65+	0									
2. MULTIPLE DX										
A. Not Operated										
0–19 Years	11	2.6	5	1	1	2	4	6	7	7
20–34	35	3.0	3	1	2	3	4	6	6	9
35–49	27	2.6	5	1	2	2	4	7	7	8
50–64	22	4.0	23	1	2	3	4	8	10	23
65+	35	3.0	5	1	1	3	4	5	5	13
B. Operated										
0–19 Years	8	6.5	30	1	4	5	7	19	19	19
20–34	35	5.2	14	1	3	4	7	10	14	16
35–49	31	5.5	13	2	3	4	8	11	12	13
50–64	18	6.9	29	1	3	5	11	16	21	21
65+	19	10.7	126	1	3	7	12	33	41	41
SUBTOTALS:										
1. SINGLE DX										
A. Not Operated	15	1.3	<1	1	1	1	2	2	2	2
B. Operated	11	3.2	1	2	2	3	4	4	5	5
2. MULTIPLE DX										
A. Not Operated	130	3.1	8	1	1	2	4	6	7	13
B. Operated	111	6.6	39	1	3	5	8	12	18	33
1. SINGLE DX	26	2.1	2	1	1	2	3	4	4	5
2. MULTIPLE DX	241	4.7	25	1	2	3	6	10	12	26
A. NOT OPERATED	145	2.9	7	1	1	2	4	6	7	13
B. OPERATED	122	6.3	36	1	3	4	8	12	16	33
TOTAL										
0–19 Years	25	3.9	14	1	1	3	5	7	8	19
20–34	84	3.8	9	1	2	3	4	8	10	16
35–49	62	4.0	11	1	1	3	6	9	11	13
50–64	42	5.1	27	1	2	3	7	12	16	23
65+	54	5.7	60	1	2	3	5	12	26	41
GRAND TOTAL	267	4.4	23	1	2	3	5	10	12	26

805.06: FX C6 VERTEBRA-CLOSED

Type of Patients	Observed Patients	Avg. Stay	Vari-ance	10th	25th	50th	75th	90th	95th	99th
1. SINGLE DX										
A. Not Operated										
0–19 Years	0									
20–34	9	1.5	<1	1	1	1	2	2	2	2
35–49	3	1.0	0	1	1	1	1	1	1	1
50–64	0									
65+	1	1.0	0	1	1	1	1	1	1	1
B. Operated										
0–19 Years	2	4.5	24	1	1	2	3	8	8	8
20–34	5	2.6	<1	2	2	3	3	3	3	3
35–49	4	1.5	<1	1	1	2	2	2	2	2
50–64	1	1.0	0	1	1	1	1	1	1	1
65+	0									
2. MULTIPLE DX										
A. Not Operated										
0–19 Years	21	1.9	1	1	1	2	3	3	4	4
20–34	61	2.3	2	1	1	2	3	5	5	9
35–49	59	3.0	32	1	1	3	5	10	18	43
50–64	21	3.9	12	2	2	3	6	7	11	15
65+	45	4.6	9	1	2	4	6	9	9	15
B. Operated										
0–19 Years	11	6.0	13	3	3	5	8	9	15	15
20–34	36	5.2	13	2	3	4	6	10	15	16
35–49	62	7.2	173	2	3	4	7	13	18	99
50–64	44	7.4	98	1	3	4	8	13	29	46
65+	28	9.7	109	3	4	6	11	20	34	49
SUBTOTALS:										
1. SINGLE DX										
A. Not Operated	8	1.3	<1	1	1	1	1	2	2	2
B. Operated	12	2.4	4	1	1	2	3	3	8	8
2. MULTIPLE DX										
A. Not Operated	207	3.1	14	1	1	2	4	6	9	15
B. Operated	181	7.2	103	2	3	4	7	14	20	49
1. SINGLE DX	20	2.0	3	1	1	1	2	3	3	8
2. MULTIPLE DX	388	5.0	60	1	2	3	5	9	15	45
A. NOT OPERATED	215	3.0	14	1	1	2	4	6	9	15
B. OPERATED	193	6.9	99	2	3	4	7	13	20	49
TOTAL										
0–19 Years	34	3.4	9	1	1	3	4	8	9	15
20–34	106	3.3	8	1	1	3	4	6	8	15
35–49	128	4.9	103	1	1	2	4	8	14	43
50–64	66	6.2	72	1	2	4	6	13	16	46
65+	74	6.5	53	1	3	5	7	11	20	49
GRAND TOTAL	408	4.8	57	1	2	3	5	9	14	43

Length of Stay by Diagnosis and Operation, Western Region, 2008

Western Region, October 2006–September 2007 Data, by Diagnosis

805.07: FX C7 VERTEBRA-CLOSED

Type of Patients	Observed Patients	Avg. Stay	Vari-ance	10th	25th	50th	75th	90th	95th	99th
1. SINGLE DX										
A. Not Operated										
0–19 Years	5	1.4	<1	1	1	1	2	2	2	2
20–34	4	1.0	0	1	1	1	1	1	1	1
35–49	7	2.1	3	1	1	2	2	6	6	6
50–64	1	1.0	0	1	1	1	1	1	1	1
65+	0									
B. Operated										
0–19 Years	1	1.0	0	1	1	1	1	1	1	1
20–34	3	6.3	34	1	2	4	13	13	13	13
35–49	2	4.6	24	2	1	8	8	8	8	8
50–64	0									
65+	0									
2. MULTIPLE DX										
A. Not Operated										
0–19 Years	29	2.5	3	1	1	2	3	6	6	7
20–34	78	2.5	6	1	1	2	3	5	6	18
35–49	67	3.4	17	1	1	2	4	6	9	27
50–64	47	3.3	6	1	1	3	5	8	9	11
65+	41	3.2	5	2	2	3	4	5	7	13
B. Operated										
0–19 Years	3	3.7	4	2	2	3	6	6	6	6
20–34	28	5.7	26	2	2	5	6	16	17	23
35–49	34	6.8	22	2	3	6	9	14	19	21
50–64	26	6.6	37	2	2	5	8	14	17	28
65+	22	9.9	93	1	4	6	11	24	31	33
SUBTOTALS:										
1. SINGLE DX										
A. Not Operated	17	1.6	2	1	1	1	2	2	5	6
B. Operated	6	4.8	23	1	1	4	8	13	13	13
2. MULTIPLE DX										
A. Not Operated	262	3.0	8	1	1	2	3	5	8	18
B. Operated	113	7.0	41	2	3	5	8	16	22	31
1. SINGLE DX	23	2.4	8	1	1	1	2	6	8	13
2. MULTIPLE DX	375	4.2	21	1	2	3	5	8	14	27
A. NOT OPERATED	279	2.9	8	1	1	2	3	5	8	18
B. OPERATED	119	6.9	40	2	3	5	8	16	22	31
TOTAL										
0–19 Years	38	2.4	3	1	1	2	3	6	7	7
20–34	113	3.4	13	1	1	2	4	6	8	18
35–49	110	4.4	20	1	1	3	6	9	14	21
50–64	74	4.4	19	1	2	3	5	9	14	28
65+	63	5.5	45	1	2	3	6	11	22	33
GRAND TOTAL	398	4.1	21	1	1	3	5	8	13	27

805.2: FX DORSAL VERTEBRA-CLOSE

Type of Patients	Observed Patients	Avg. Stay	Vari-ance	10th	25th	50th	75th	90th	95th	99th
1. SINGLE DX										
A. Not Operated										
0–19 Years	20	2.5	3	1	1	2	4	5	5	7
20–34	59	2.5	3	1	1	2	3	4	6	11
35–49	39	2.7	3	1	1	2	4	5	6	9
50–64	20	2.2	2	1	1	2	3	4	5	5
65+	2	2.0	2	1	1	2	3	3	3	3
B. Operated										
0–19 Years	4	6.5	15	2	5	5	8	11	11	11
20–34	9	4.5	7	1	3	4	5	6	9	9
35–49	10	3.1	5	1	1	2	6	6	6	6
50–64	7	1.6	1	1	1	1	2	4	4	4
65+	11	1.4	1	1	1	2	1	1	5	5
2. MULTIPLE DX										
A. Not Operated										
0–19 Years	115	2.5	3	1	1	3	3	4	6	7
20–34	295	3.1	7	1	1	3	4	6	7	15
35–49	222	3.5	7	1	2	3	5	7	9	12
50–64	296	3.9	12	1	2	3	5	7	9	17
65+	1,191	4.4	9	2	3	4	6	8	10	17
B. Operated										
0–19 Years	39	8.8	36	3	5	7	11	18	25	29
20–34	118	8.4	72	3	4	6	10	15	27	48
35–49	108	8.7	54	1	4	7	9	16	24	36
50–64	189	8.1	73	1	3	6	11	18	24	48
65+	935	5.2	29	1	1	4	7	10	14	27
SUBTOTALS:										
1. SINGLE DX										
A. Not Operated	140	2.5	3	1	1	2	3	4	5	9
B. Operated	41	3.0	7	1	1	2	5	6	8	11
2. MULTIPLE DX										
A. Not Operated	2,119	4.0	9	1	2	3	5	7	9	15
B. Operated	1,389	6.2	43	1	2	5	8	13	17	34
1. SINGLE DX	181	2.6	4	1	1	2	4	5	6	11
2. MULTIPLE DX	3,508	4.9	24	1	2	4	6	9	13	26
A. NOT OPERATED	2,259	3.9	9	1	2	3	5	7	9	15
B. OPERATED	1,430	6.2	42	1	2	5	8	13	17	34
TOTAL										
0–19 Years	178	4.0	17	1	1	3	3	6	12	25
20–34	481	4.4	28	1	2	3	5	8	11	29
35–49	379	4.9	26	1	2	3	6	10	14	27
50–64	512	5.4	38	1	2	4	6	11	16	33
65+	2,139	4.7	18	1	2	4	6	9	12	21
GRAND TOTAL	3,689	4.8	23	1	2	4	6	9	13	26

805.4: FX LUMBAR VERTEBRA-CLSD

Type of Patients	Observed Patients	Avg. Stay	Vari-ance	10th	25th	50th	75th	90th	95th	99th
1. SINGLE DX										
A. Not Operated										
0–19 Years	38	2.0	1	1	1	2	2	4	5	5
20–34	85	2.5	2	1	1	2	4	5	5	7
35–49	48	2.9	5	1	1	2	4	6	6	12
50–64	40	2.6	2	2	2	2	3	6	6	7
65+	16	2.4	2	1	1	2	3	5	5	5
B. Operated										
0–19 Years	7	4.9	9	1	2	5	8	9	9	9
20–34	17	4.4	5	1	3	4	5	8	9	9
35–49	15	5.8	12	1	3	5	9	11	11	11
50–64	23	3.1	10	1	1	2	4	7	8	14
65+	26	1.3	1	1	1	1	1	1	2	7
2. MULTIPLE DX										
A. Not Operated										
0–19 Years	131	2.8	5	1	1	2	3	5	6	10
20–34	357	3.0	6	1	1	2	4	5	7	11
35–49	428	3.5	7	1	2	3	4	6	8	14
50–64	573	4.1	17	1	2	3	5	8	10	17
65+	2,089	4.5	10	2	3	4	5	8	10	16
B. Operated										
0–19 Years	54	7.3	21	3	4	6	10	13	17	22
20–34	148	8.3	39	3	5	7	11	14	19	35
35–49	195	9.0	58	2	4	7	11	20	25	40
50–64	303	7.5	80	1	2	5	10	15	20	45
65+	1,381	5.5	22	1	2	4	7	11	14	23
SUBTOTALS:										
1. SINGLE DX										
A. Not Operated	227	2.5	3	1	1	2	3	5	6	7
B. Operated	88	3.4	9	1	1	2	5	8	9	14
2. MULTIPLE DX										
A. Not Operated	3,578	4.1	10	1	2	3	5	7	10	16
B. Operated	2,081	6.4	36	1	3	5	8	13	17	29
1. SINGLE DX	315	2.8	5	1	1	2	4	6	7	11
2. MULTIPLE DX	5,659	4.9	21	1	2	4	6	10	13	22
A. NOT OPERATED	3,805	4.0	10	1	2	3	5	7	9	15
B. OPERATED	2,169	6.2	35	1	2	5	8	13	17	27
TOTAL										
0–19 Years	230	3.8	12	1	1	3	5	8	10	17
20–34	607	4.3	19	1	2	3	5	9	11	27
35–49	686	5.1	28	1	2	3	6	10	15	27
50–64	939	5.1	39	1	2	3	6	10	14	26
65+	3,512	4.8	15	1	2	4	6	9	12	21
GRAND TOTAL	5,974	4.8	20	1	2	4	6	9	13	22

Length of Stay by Diagnosis and Operation, Western Region, 2008

Western Region, October 2006–September 2007 Data, by Diagnosis

805.6: FX SACRUM/COCCYX-CLOSED

Type of Patients	Observed Patients	Avg. Stay	Variance	10th	25th	50th	75th	90th	95th	99th
1. SINGLE DX										
A. Not Operated										
0–19 Years	1	2.0	0	2	2	2	2	2	2	2
20–34	2	2.5	4	1	1	2	4	4	4	4
35–49	4	2.5	2	1	1	2	3	4	4	4
50–64	1	1.0	0	1	1	1	1	1	1	1
65+	0									
B. Operated										
0–19 Years	0									
20–34	0									
35–49	0									
50–64	0									
65+	1	1.0	0	1	1	1	1	1	1	1
2. MULTIPLE DX										
A. Not Operated										
0–19 Years	61	2.7	6	1	1	2	4	5	7	14
20–34	80	3.7	5	1	2	4	5	7	9	12
35–49	72	4.6	20	2	2	3	6	11	13	28
50–64	117	5.5	76	1	2	3	6	11	16	22
65+	558	4.7	16	2	3	4	5	8	11	22
B. Operated										
0–19 Years	16	8.3	22	4	5	8	10	15	21	21
20–34	43	13.5	238	3	5	8	16	30	35	80
35–49	24	10.1	45	4	6	8	14	20	23	28
50–64	33	11.4	41	5	7	9	16	16	22	26
65+	51	9.5	41	3	5	8	12	18	26	29
SUBTOTALS:										
1. SINGLE DX										
A. Not Operated	8	2.3	2	1	1	2	2	4	4	4
B. Operated	1	1.0	0	1	1	1	1	1	1	1
2. MULTIPLE DX										
A. Not Operated	888	4.5	23	1	3	3	5	8	11	22
B. Operated	167	10.9	92	4	5	8	14	20	26	64
1. SINGLE DX	9	2.1	2	1	1	2	3	4	4	4
2. MULTIPLE DX	1,055	5.5	39	2	3	4	6	11	16	28
A. NOT OPERATED	896	4.5	22	1	3	3	5	8	11	22
B. OPERATED	168	10.8	92	3	5	8	14	20	26	64
TOTAL										
0–19 Years	78	3.9	14	1	1	3	4	8	12	21
20–34	125	7.0	106	1	3	4	7	12	22	64
35–49	100	5.9	31	2	2	4	7	13	20	28
50–64	151	6.7	74	1	2	4	8	16	19	26
65+	610	5.1	19	2	3	4	6	9	13	26
GRAND TOTAL	1,064	5.5	39	2	3	4	6	11	15	28

806: VERTEBRAL FX W CORD INJ

Type of Patients	Observed Patients	Avg. Stay	Variance	10th	25th	50th	75th	90th	95th	99th
1. SINGLE DX										
A. Not Operated										
0–19 Years	1	2.0	0	2	2	2	2	2	2	2
20–34	4	3.5	9	2	2	2	2	8	8	8
35–49	4	3.3	5	2	2	4	6	6	6	6
50–64	2	1.0	0	1	1	1	1	1	1	1
65+	0									
B. Operated										
0–19 Years	5	6.0	0	6	6	6	6	6	6	6
20–34	5	6.8	24	3	3	5	11	13	13	13
35–49	5	5.0	3	2	5	5	6	7	7	7
50–64	2	6.5	12	4	4	4	9	9	9	9
65+	0									
2. MULTIPLE DX										
A. Not Operated										
0–19 Years	22	7.1	33	1	2	6	11	14	17	21
20–34	40	7.7	54	2	3	5	10	17	25	>99
35–49	32	7.0	39	2	3	5	11	17	21	23
50–64	41	6.7	45	1	2	4	7	17	22	26
65+	80	5.6	24	2	3	4	7	10	14	29
B. Operated										
0–19 Years	86	15.9	149	5	8	12	19	36	40	58
20–34	259	16.7	211	8	8	12	21	37	58	>99
35–49	202	17.3	178	5	8	13	24	39	45	>99
50–64	167	16.9	254	4	7	12	21	38	54	>99
65+	140	14.8	186	5	7	11	20	29	38	99
SUBTOTALS:										
1. SINGLE DX										
A. Not Operated	11	2.8	5	1	1	2	4	6	8	8
B. Operated	13	6.0	11	2	4	5	7	11	13	13
2. MULTIPLE DX										
A. Not Operated	215	6.6	36	2	3	5	8	15	21	29
B. Operated	854	16.5	201	5	7	12	21	36	49	>99
1. SINGLE DX	24	4.5	11	1	2	4	6	9	11	13
2. MULTIPLE DX	1,069	14.5	184	3	6	10	19	33	44	>99
A. NOT OPERATED	226	6.4	36	1	2	5	8	14	20	29
B. OPERATED	867	16.4	200	5	7	12	21	36	49	>99
TOTAL										
0–19 Years	110	13.9	137	3	6	11	17	29	40	52
20–34	308	15.2	197	4	6	11	19	36	55	>99
35–49	243	15.5	170	3	7	11	22	36	44	>99
50–64	212	14.7	227	3	5	10	18	35	50	>99
65+	220	11.5	146	3	5	8	15	25	32	96
GRAND TOTAL	1,093	14.3	182	3	6	10	18	32	44	>99

807: FX RIB/STERN/LAR/TRACH

Type of Patients	Observed Patients	Avg. Stay	Variance	10th	25th	50th	75th	90th	95th	99th
1. SINGLE DX										
A. Not Operated										
0–19 Years	9	1.2	<1	1	1	1	1	2	2	2
20–34	18	1.2	<1	1	1	1	1	2	2	2
35–49	38	2.0	3	1	1	1	2	4	5	10
50–64	35	2.1	4	1	1	1	3	4	7	10
65+	15	1.5	<1	1	1	1	2	2	4	4
B. Operated										
0–19 Years	0									
20–34	1	5.0	0	5	5	5	5	5	5	5
35–49	4	2.7	2	1	1	2	4	4	4	4
50–64	0									
65+	1	5.0	0	5	5	5	5	5	5	5
2. MULTIPLE DX										
A. Not Operated										
0–19 Years	136	2.7	7	1	1	2	3	5	9	14
20–34	496	3.2	11	1	1	2	4	6	9	14
35–49	1,055	3.4	14	1	2	3	4	7	9	23
50–64	1,474	4.0	14	1	2	3	5	8	11	20
65+	2,755	4.4	16	1	2	3	5	8	11	21
B. Operated										
0–19 Years	4	24.8	25	20	21	28	30	30	30	30
20–34	47	11.7	86	3	5	9	16	26	32	38
35–49	72	10.9	84	4	6	9	14	21	29	56
50–64	81	15.4	223	4	6	11	18	29	43	79
65+	70	12.7	123	4	6	9	18	26	32	60
SUBTOTALS:										
1. SINGLE DX										
A. Not Operated	115	1.8	2	1	1	1	2	3	4	10
B. Operated	6	3.5	3	1	2	4	5	5	5	5
2. MULTIPLE DX										
A. Not Operated	5,916	4.0	15	1	2	3	5	8	10	19
B. Operated	274	13.1	138	3	6	9	17	26	36	60
1. SINGLE DX	121	1.8	2	1	1	1	2	4	4	10
2. MULTIPLE DX	6,190	4.4	24	1	2	3	5	9	12	25
A. NOT OPERATED	6,031	3.9	15	1	2	3	5	8	10	19
B. OPERATED	280	12.9	137	3	5	9	17	26	36	60
TOTAL										
0–19 Years	149	3.2	20	1	1	2	3	6	12	28
20–34	562	3.8	22	1	1	2	4	8	11	26
35–49	1,169	3.8	21	1	1	3	4	8	11	27
50–64	1,590	4.5	31	1	2	3	5	9	13	26
65+	2,841	4.6	20	1	2	3	5	9	12	23
GRAND TOTAL	6,311	4.3	24	1	2	3	5	9	12	25

Length of Stay by Diagnosis and Operation, Western Region, 2008

Western Region, October 2006–September 2007 Data, by Diagnosis

807.00: FRACTURE RIB NOS-CLOSED

Type of Patients	Observed Patients	Avg. Stay	Variance	10th	25th	50th	75th	90th	95th	99th
1. SINGLE DX										
A. *Not Operated*										
0–19 Years	3	1.0	0	1	1	1	1	1	1	1
20–34	4	1.3	<1	1	1	1	1	2	2	2
35–49	2	1.0	0	1	1	1	1	1	1	1
50–64	4	3.3	20	1	1	1	10	10	10	10
65+	2	1.5	<1	1	1	2	2	2	2	2
B. *Operated*										
0–19 Years	0									
20–34	0									
35–49	0									
50–64	0									
65+	0									
2. MULTIPLE DX										
A. *Not Operated*										
0–19 Years	7	1.4	<1	1	1	1	2	2	2	2
20–34	25	2.2	2	1	1	2	3	4	5	6
35–49	53	3.2	13	1	1	2	4	5	7	23
50–64	63	2.9	6	1	1	2	4	5	7	15
65+	134	3.3	4	1	2	3	4	6	7	10
B. *Operated*										
0–19 Years	0									
20–34	0									
35–49	0									
50–64	0									
65+	1	3.0	0	3	3	3	3	3	3	3
SUBTOTALS:										
1. SINGLE DX										
A. *Not Operated*	15	1.7	5	1	1	1	1	2	10	10
B. *Operated*	0									
2. MULTIPLE DX										
A. *Not Operated*	282	3.0	6	1	1	2	4	6	7	15
B. *Operated*	1	3.0	0	3	3	3	3	3	3	3
1. SINGLE DX	15	1.7	5	1	1	1	1	2	10	10
2. MULTIPLE DX	283	3.0	6	1	1	2	4	6	7	15
A. NOT OPERATED	297	3.0	6	1	1	2	4	6	7	15
B. OPERATED	1	3.0	0	3	3	3	3	3	3	3
TOTAL										
0–19 Years	10	1.3	<1	1	1	1	2	2	2	2
20–34	29	2.1	2	1	1	1	3	4	5	6
35–49	55	3.1	13	1	1	2	4	5	7	23
50–64	67	3.0	6	1	1	2	4	6	7	15
65+	137	3.2	4	1	2	3	4	6	7	10
GRAND TOTAL	298	3.0	6	1	1	2	4	6	7	15

807.01: FRACTURE ONE RIB-CLOSED

Type of Patients	Observed Patients	Avg. Stay	Variance	10th	25th	50th	75th	90th	95th	99th
1. SINGLE DX										
A. *Not Operated*										
0–19 Years	2	1.5	<1	1	1	1	2	2	2	2
20–34	2	1.0	0	1	1	1	1	1	1	1
35–49	3	3.3	1	2	2	4	4	4	4	4
50–64	5	1.4	<1	1	1	1	2	2	2	2
65+	4	1.0	0	1	1	1	1	1	1	1
B. *Operated*										
0–19 Years	0									
20–34	0									
35–49	0									
50–64	0									
65+	0									
2. MULTIPLE DX										
A. *Not Operated*										
0–19 Years	27	1.8	<1	1	1	2	2	3	3	4
20–34	99	2.3	3	1	1	2	3	4	6	10
35–49	165	2.4	3	1	1	2	3	5	6	9
50–64	165	2.8	5	1	1	2	4	6	7	11
65+	474	3.7	8	1	2	3	4	6	9	15
B. *Operated*										
0–19 Years	0									
20–34	4	3.8	2	3	3	3	5	6	6	6
35–49	5	6.4	7	5	5	7	7	10	10	10
50–64	0									
65+	4	5.3	17	1	4	5	5	11	11	11
SUBTOTALS:										
1. SINGLE DX										
A. *Not Operated*	16	1.6	1	1	1	1	2	4	4	4
B. *Operated*	0									
2. MULTIPLE DX										
A. *Not Operated*	930	3.1	6	1	1	2	4	6	8	12
B. *Operated*	13	5.2	9	3	3	5	7	10	11	11
1. SINGLE DX	16	1.6	1	1	1	1	2	4	4	4
2. MULTIPLE DX	943	3.1	7	1	1	3	4	6	8	12
A. NOT OPERATED	946	3.1	6	1	1	2	4	6	8	12
B. OPERATED	13	5.2	9	3	3	5	7	10	11	11
TOTAL										
0–19 Years	29	1.8	<1	1	1	2	2	3	3	4
20–34	105	2.3	3	1	1	2	3	4	6	10
35–49	173	2.5	4	1	1	2	3	5	7	10
50–64	170	2.7	5	1	1	2	3	6	7	11
65+	482	3.7	8	1	2	3	4	6	9	15
GRAND TOTAL	959	3.1	7	1	1	2	4	6	8	12

807.02: FRACTURE TWO RIBS-CLOSED

Type of Patients	Observed Patients	Avg. Stay	Variance	10th	25th	50th	75th	90th	95th	99th
1. SINGLE DX										
A. *Not Operated*										
0–19 Years	2	1.0	0	1	1	1	1	1	1	1
20–34	2	1.0	0	1	1	1	1	1	1	1
35–49	4	1.0	0	1	1	1	1	1	1	1
50–64	2	2.5	4	1	1	4	4	4	4	4
65+	2	1.5	<1	1	1	1	2	2	2	2
B. *Operated*										
0–19 Years	0									
20–34	0									
35–49	0									
50–64	0									
65+	0									
2. MULTIPLE DX										
A. *Not Operated*										
0–19 Years	32	1.7	1	1	1	2	2	3	4	6
20–34	51	3.1	9	1	1	2	3	7	9	14
35–49	131	2.8	5	1	1	2	4	5	7	12
50–64	178	3.7	20	1	1	3	4	7	9	26
65+	482	4.0	11	1	2	3	5	7	9	17
B. *Operated*										
0–19 Years	0									
20–34	0									
35–49	1	10.0	0	10	10	10	10	10	10	10
50–64	2	8.0	49	3	3	8	13	13	13	13
65+	3	7.0	7	4	4	8	9	9	9	9
SUBTOTALS:										
1. SINGLE DX										
A. *Not Operated*	12	1.3	<1	1	1	1	1	2	4	4
B. *Operated*	0									
2. MULTIPLE DX										
A. *Not Operated*	874	3.6	11	1	2	3	4	7	9	16
B. *Operated*	6	7.8	14	3	4	9	10	13	13	13
1. SINGLE DX	12	1.3	<1	1	1	1	1	2	4	4
2. MULTIPLE DX	880	3.6	12	1	2	3	4	7	9	16
A. NOT OPERATED	886	3.6	11	1	2	3	4	6	9	16
B. OPERATED	6	7.8	14	3	4	9	10	13	13	13
TOTAL										
0–19 Years	34	1.7	1	1	1	2	2	3	4	6
20–34	53	3.1	8	1	1	2	3	7	9	14
35–49	136	2.8	5	1	1	2	4	5	7	12
50–64	182	3.7	20	1	1	3	4	7	9	26
65+	487	4.0	11	2	2	3	5	7	9	17
GRAND TOTAL	892	3.6	11	2	2	3	4	7	9	16

Length of Stay by Diagnosis and Operation, Western Region, 2008

Western Region, October 2006–September 2007 Data, by Diagnosis

807.03: FRACTURE THREE RIBS-CLSD

Type of Patients	Observed Patients	Avg. Stay	Variance	10th	25th	50th	75th	90th	95th	99th
1. SINGLE DX										
A. Not Operated										
0–19 Years	0									
20–34	1	1.0	0					1	1	1
35–49	4	2.5	3	1	1	2	2	5	5	5
50–64	4	2.3	2	1	2	2	4	4	4	4
65+	3	1.3	<1	1	1	1	2	2	2	2
B. Operated										
0–19 Years	0									
20–34	0									
35–49	0									
50–64	0									
65+	0									
2. MULTIPLE DX										
A. Not Operated										
0–19 Years	18	2.5	2	1	1	2	4	5	5	5
20–34	74	2.9	5	1	1	2	4	6	8	14
35–49	157	2.7	3	1	1	2	3	5	7	9
50–64	246	3.6	9	1	2	3	4	7	9	16
65+	457	4.1	10	1	2	3	5	8	10	15
B. Operated										
0–19 Years	0									
20–34	4	6.0	7	3	5	5	7	9	9	9
35–49	7	8.0	13	3	5	8	12	13	13	13
50–64	5	6.2	12	1	5	7	8	10	10	10
65+	6	9.5	17	5	6	8	14	15	15	15
SUBTOTALS:										
1. SINGLE DX *A. Not Operated*	12	2.0	2	1	1	2	2	4	5	5
B. Operated	0									
2. MULTIPLE DX *A. Not Operated*	952	3.6	9	1	2	3	4	7	9	15
B. Operated	22	7.6	13	3	5	7	9	13	14	15
1. SINGLE DX	12	2.0	2	1	1	2	2	4	5	5
2. MULTIPLE DX	974	3.7	9	1	2	3	5	7	9	15
A. NOT OPERATED	964	3.6	9	1	2	3	4	7	9	15
B. OPERATED	22	7.6	13	3	5	7	9	13	14	15
TOTAL										
0–19 Years	18	2.5	2	1	1	2	4	5	5	5
20–34	79	3.0	5	1	1	3	4	6	8	14
35–49	168	2.9	5	1	1	2	4	6	8	12
50–64	255	3.6	9	1	2	3	5	7	9	16
65+	466	4.2	11	1	2	3	5	8	11	15
GRAND TOTAL	986	3.7	9	1	2	3	5	7	9	15

807.04: FRACTURE FOUR RIBS-CLSD

Type of Patients	Observed Patients	Avg. Stay	Variance	10th	25th	50th	75th	90th	95th	99th
1. SINGLE DX										
A. Not Operated										
0–19 Years	0									
20–34	0									
35–49	3	2.0	3	1	1	1	4	4	4	4
50–64	4	1.0	0	1	1	1	1	1	1	1
65+	1	1.0	0	1	1	1	1	1	1	1
B. Operated										
0–19 Years	0									
20–34	0									
35–49	0									
50–64	0									
65+	0									
2. MULTIPLE DX										
A. Not Operated										
0–19 Years	11	3.5	7	1	2	3	5	6	10	10
20–34	45	3.2	5	1	2	3	4	6	7	11
35–49	105	3.6	13	1	2	3	4	7	9	14
50–64	164	3.8	10	1	2	3	5	7	9	22
65+	286	4.8	20	1	2	4	6	9	12	25
B. Operated										
0–19 Years	0									
20–34	3	5.3	6	3	3	5	8	8	8	8
35–49	7	8.4	30	1	3	8	13	16	16	16
50–64	6	8.3	40	4	5	6	8	21	21	21
65+	6	6.7	47	1	3	6	7	20	20	20
SUBTOTALS:										
1. SINGLE DX *A. Not Operated*	8	1.4	1	1	1	1	1	4	4	4
B. Operated	0									
2. MULTIPLE DX *A. Not Operated*	611	4.2	15	1	2	3	5	8	11	22
B. Operated	22	7.5	31	3	3	6	8	16	20	21
1. SINGLE DX	8	1.4	1	1	1	1	1	4	4	4
2. MULTIPLE DX	633	4.3	16	1	2	3	5	8	11	22
A. NOT OPERATED	619	4.2	15	1	2	3	5	8	11	22
B. OPERATED	22	7.5	31	3	3	6	8	16	20	21
TOTAL										
0–19 Years	11	3.5	7	1	2	3	5	6	10	10
20–34	48	3.3	6	1	2	3	4	7	8	11
35–49	115	3.8	15	1	1	3	5	8	11	16
50–64	174	3.9	12	1	2	3	5	7	9	22
65+	293	4.8	21	1	2	4	6	9	12	25
GRAND TOTAL	641	4.3	16	1	2	3	5	8	11	22

807.05: FRACTURE FIVE RIBS-CLSD

Type of Patients	Observed Patients	Avg. Stay	Variance	10th	25th	50th	75th	90th	95th	99th
1. SINGLE DX										
A. Not Operated										
0–19 Years	0									
20–34	1	1.0	0	1	1	1	1	1	1	1
35–49	2	2.5	4	1	1	4	4	4	4	4
50–64	5	2.0	1	1	1	2	3	3	3	3
65+	0									
B. Operated										
0–19 Years	0									
20–34	0									
35–49	0									
50–64	0									
65+	0									
2. MULTIPLE DX										
A. Not Operated										
0–19 Years	4	2.8	5	1	1	2	6	6	6	6
20–34	21	3.1	4	1	2	3	4	5	6	9
35–49	68	3.6	6	1	2	3	4	7	9	12
50–64	109	4.4	10	1	2	4	5	9	10	15
65+	152	4.3	7	2	3	4	6	8	9	15
B. Operated										
0–19 Years	1	28.0	0	28	28	28	28	28	28	28
20–34	4	5.5	4	4	5	6	6	7	7	7
35–49	4	8.0	28	2	5	12	13	13	13	13
50–64	11	15.7	142	5	6	14	22	24	43	43
65+	8	15.1	358	4	4	8	19	60	60	60
SUBTOTALS:										
1. SINGLE DX *A. Not Operated*	8	2.0	1	1	1	2	3	4	4	4
B. Operated	0									
2. MULTIPLE DX *A. Not Operated*	354	4.1	8	1	2	3	5	8	9	15
B. Operated	26	14.0	182	4	5	8	19	28	43	60
1. SINGLE DX	8	2.0	1	1	1	2	3	4	4	4
2. MULTIPLE DX	380	4.8	25	1	2	4	6	9	12	24
A. NOT OPERATED	362	4.1	8	1	2	3	5	8	9	15
B. OPERATED	26	14.0	182	4	5	8	19	28	43	60
TOTAL										
0–19 Years	5	7.8	131	1	2	2	6	28	28	28
20–34	24	3.3	4	1	2	3	4	6	7	9
35–49	74	3.8	8	1	2	3	5	7	10	13
50–64	125	5.3	31	2	2	4	6	10	15	24
65+	160	4.9	28	2	3	4	6	8	11	19
GRAND TOTAL	388	4.7	25	1	2	4	6	9	12	24

Length of Stay by Diagnosis and Operation, Western Region, 2008

Western Region, October 2006—September 2007 Data, by Diagnosis

807.06: FRACTURE SIX RIBS-CLOSED

Type of Patients	Observed Patients	Avg. Stay	Variance	10th	25th	50th	75th	90th	95th	99th
1. SINGLE DX										
A. Not Operated										
0–19 Years	0									
20–34	0									
35–49	0									
50–64	2	5.0	8	3	3	3	7	7	7	7
65+	0									
B. Operated										
0–19 Years	0									
20–34	0									
35–49	0									
50–64	0									
65+	0									
2. MULTIPLE DX										
A. Not Operated										
0–19 Years	3	3.3	<1	3	3	3	4	4	4	4
20–34	12	7.9	119	2	3	5	6	11	42	42
35–49	62	4.5	18	1	2	3	5	9	10	23
50–64	68	4.9	16	1	2	3	7	11	14	16
65+	87	5.4	20	1	2	4	7	10	13	24
B. Operated										
0–19 Years	0									
20–34	3	14.6	99	7	7	11	26	26	26	26
35–49	5	4.8	10	1	3	7	7	9	9	9
50–64	2	12.0	49	7	7	12	17	17	17	17
65+	2	12.5	40	8	8	8	17	17	17	17
SUBTOTALS:										
1. SINGLE DX										
A. Not Operated	2	5.0	8	3	3	3	7	7	7	7
B. Operated	0									
2. MULTIPLE DX										
A. Not Operated	232	5.1	23	2	2	4	6	10	14	23
B. Operated	12	9.8	50	3	7	8	11	17	26	26
1. SINGLE DX	2	5.0	8	3	3	3	7	7	7	7
2. MULTIPLE DX	244	5.3	25	1	2	4	7	10	16	24
A. NOT OPERATED	234	5.1	23	1	2	4	7	10	14	23
B. OPERATED	12	9.8	50	3	7	8	11	16	26	26
TOTAL										
0–19 Years	3	3.3	<1	3	3	3	4	4	4	4
20–34	15	9.3	115	2	3	6	11	26	42	42
35–49	67	4.5	17	1	2	3	5	9	10	23
50–64	72	5.1	17	2	3	3	7	11	16	17
65+	89	5.5	21	1	2	4	7	11	15	24
GRAND TOTAL	246	5.3	25	1	2	4	7	10	16	24

807.09: FX MULT RIBS NOS-CLOSED

Type of Patients	Observed Patients	Avg. Stay	Variance	10th	25th	50th	75th	90th	95th	99th
1. SINGLE DX										
A. Not Operated										
0–19 Years	0									
20–34	2	1.0	0	1	1	1	1	1	1	1
35–49	5	1.4	<1	1	1	1	2	2	2	2
50–64	2	1.0	0	1	1	1	1	1	1	1
65+	2	3.0	2	2	2	3	4	4	4	4
B. Operated										
0–19 Years	0									
20–34	0									
35–49	0									
50–64	0									
65+	0									
2. MULTIPLE DX										
A. Not Operated										
0–19 Years	8	4.8	27	1	2	3	6	17	17	17
20–34	52	3.2	5	1	1	3	4	6	7	12
35–49	110	3.6	11	1	2	3	4	7	10	17
50–64	208	4.6	16	1	2	3	6	9	11	21
65+	272	5.2	18	2	3	4	6	10	13	25
B. Operated										
0–19 Years	0									
20–34	6	13.0	63	5	5	13	19	25	25	25
35–49	5	15.2	116	6	7	9	27	27	27	27
50–64	10	11.3	17	6	7	11	15	17	17	17
65+	12	16.1	54	7	8	16	22	26	26	26
SUBTOTALS:										
1. SINGLE DX										
A. Not Operated	11	1.5	<1	1	1	1	2	2	4	4
B. Operated	0									
2. MULTIPLE DX										
A. Not Operated	650	4.6	16	1	2	3	6	9	12	22
B. Operated	33	13.9	52	6	7	12	19	26	27	27
1. SINGLE DX	11	1.5	<1	1	1	1	2	2	4	4
2. MULTIPLE DX	683	5.0	21	1	2	4	6	10	14	26
A. NOT OPERATED	661	4.5	15	1	2	3	6	9	12	22
B. OPERATED	33	13.9	52	6	7	12	19	26	27	27
TOTAL										
0–19 Years	8	4.8	27	1	2	3	6	17	17	17
20–34	60	4.1	19	1	1	3	5	7	12	25
35–49	120	4.0	19	1	2	3	5	7	11	27
50–64	220	4.9	18	1	2	4	6	10	14	21
65+	286	5.7	24	2	3	4	7	10	16	26
GRAND TOTAL	694	5.0	21	1	2	4	6	10	14	26

807.2: FRACTURE OF STERNUM-CLSD

Type of Patients	Observed Patients	Avg. Stay	Variance	10th	25th	50th	75th	90th	95th	99th
1. SINGLE DX										
A. Not Operated										
0–19 Years	1	1.0	0	1	1	1	1	1	1	1
20–34	5	1.4	<1	1	1	1	2	2	2	2
35–49	11	1.3	<1	1	1	1	1	2	3	3
50–64	7	2.0	<1	1	1	2	3	3	3	3
65+	1	1.0	0	1	1	1	1	1	1	1
B. Operated										
0–19 Years	0									
20–34	0									
35–49	2	3.0	2	2	2	2	4	4	4	4
50–64	0									
65+	0									
2. MULTIPLE DX										
A. Not Operated										
0–19 Years	14	3.3	12	1	1	2	3	9	13	13
20–34	62	2.5	4	1	1	2	3	4	6	12
35–49	103	2.5	4	1	1	2	3	5	6	10
50–64	127	3.0	7	1	2	2	4	6	8	15
65+	258	4.0	12	1	2	3	5	8	11	18
B. Operated										
0–19 Years	2	25.5	39	21	21	26	30	30	30	30
20–34	2	12.4	179	3	4	22	22	22	22	22
35–49	5	6.0	7	3	4	6	7	10	10	10
50–64	7	15.9	701	1	1	8	13	75	75	75
65+	6	6.2	15	2	2	6	8	12	12	12
SUBTOTALS:										
1. SINGLE DX										
A. Not Operated	25	1.5	<1	1	1	1	2	3	3	3
B. Operated	2	3.0	2	2	2	4	4	4	4	4
2. MULTIPLE DX										
A. Not Operated	564	3.3	9	1	1	2	4	7	9	16
B. Operated	22	11.6	258	2	3	7	12	22	30	75
1. SINGLE DX	27	1.6	<1	1	1	1	2	3	3	4
2. MULTIPLE DX	586	3.6	21	1	1	2	4	7	10	21
A. NOT OPERATED	589	3.3	9	1	1	2	4	7	9	16
B. OPERATED	24	10.9	241	2	3	6	12	22	30	75
TOTAL										
0–19 Years	17	5.8	69	1	1	2	5	21	30	30
20–34	69	2.7	9	1	1	2	3	5	8	22
35–49	121	2.6	4	1	1	2	3	5	7	10
50–64	141	3.6	45	1	2	2	4	5	9	15
65+	265	4.1	12	1	2	3	5	8	11	18
GRAND TOTAL	613	3.6	20	1	1	2	4	7	10	18

Length of Stay by Diagnosis and Operation, Western Region, 2008

Western Region, October 2006–September 2007 Data, by Diagnosis

808: PELVIC FRACTURE

Type of Patients	Observed Patients	Avg. Stay	Variance	10th	25th	50th	75th	90th	95th	99th
1. SINGLE DX										
A. Not Operated										
0–19 Years	39	2.0	2	1	1	1	3	4	4	5
20–34	36	2.4	4	1	1	2	3	4	7	11
35–49	26	2.9	3	1	1	3	4	5	6	6
50–64	31	2.1	1	1	1	2	3	3	5	5
65+	19	2.2	2	1	1	2	3	5	5	5
B. Operated										
0–19 Years	8	3.4	4	1	1	3	5	5	6	6
20–34	22	6.2	10	3	4	6	7	11	12	14
35–49	18	4.9	7	2	3	4	7	9	10	10
50–64	5	5.4	7	3	3	5	7	9	9	9
65+	0									
2. MULTIPLE DX										
A. Not Operated										
0–19 Years	239	3.2	7	1	2	3	5	7	8	11
20–34	385	3.6	9	1	2	3	5	7	9	16
35–49	328	4.6	37	1	2	3	5	8	11	21
50–64	638	5.0	23	1	2	4	6	9	15	24
65+	5,512	4.0	8	2	3	3	5	7	9	15
B. Operated										
0–19 Years	128	9.7	78	3	5	8	11	17	31	47
20–34	381	10.7	92	3	6	9	13	19	27	66
35–49	330	11.3	63	5	6	9	13	22	27	38
50–64	309	13.3	116	4	6	10	16	26	35	54
65+	277	10.7	84	4	6	8	13	19	27	49
SUBTOTALS:										
1. SINGLE DX										
A. Not Operated	151	2.3	2	1	1	2	3	4	5	7
B. Operated	53	5.3	8	2	3	5	7	9	11	14
2. MULTIPLE DX										
A. Not Operated	7,102	4.1	11	2	3	3	5	7	9	16
B. Operated	1,425	11.3	89	4	6	9	13	22	30	51
1. SINGLE DX	204	3.1	6	1	1	2	4	6	8	11
2. MULTIPLE DX	8,527	5.3	31	2	3	4	6	10	14	29
A. NOT OPERATED	7,253	4.1	11	1	2	3	5	7	9	16
B. OPERATED	1,478	11.1	87	4	6	9	13	21	29	51
TOTAL										
0–19 Years	414	5.1	38	1	2	3	6	10	14	38
20–34	824	6.9	60	1	2	5	9	14	19	42
35–49	702	7.7	59	2	3	5	10	15	22	36
50–64	983	7.5	67	2	3	5	9	16	23	46
65+	5,808	4.4	14	2	3	3	5	7	10	18
GRAND TOTAL	8,731	5.3	31	2	3	4	6	10	14	29

808.0: FRACTURE ACETABULUM-CLSD

Type of Patients	Observed Patients	Avg. Stay	Variance	10th	25th	50th	75th	90th	95th	99th
1. SINGLE DX										
A. Not Operated										
0–19 Years	6	1.5	1	1	1	1	1	4	4	4
20–34	14	2.2	2	1	1	2	3	4	6	6
35–49	12	2.6	2	1	1	2	2	4	6	6
50–64	13	1.8	<1	1	1	2	2	3	3	3
65+	5	2.4	3	1	1	2	3	5	5	5
B. Operated										
0–19 Years	4	3.7	5	1	1	3	5	6	6	6
20–34	21	6.3	10	4	4	6	7	11	12	14
35–49	14	5.5	8	3	3	5	8	9	10	10
50–64	3	5.0	4	3	3	5	7	7	7	7
65+	0									
2. MULTIPLE DX										
A. Not Operated										
0–19 Years	41	3.0	5	1	1	2	2	4	6	11
20–34	99	3.5	10	1	1	2	5	8	10	19
35–49	84	5.5	104	1	2	4	5	9	10	72
50–64	141	5.1	27	1	2	3	6	12	16	24
65+	730	4.5	15	2	3	3	5	8	11	20
B. Operated										
0–19 Years	42	7.5	15	3	5	7	9	12	15	21
20–34	212	9.3	28	4	6	8	12	17	19	23
35–49	182	11.0	62	5	6	9	13	20	25	36
50–64	178	12.4	92	5	6	10	14	22	35	54
65+	145	11.6	100	4	6	9	14	20	31	49
SUBTOTALS:										
1. SINGLE DX										
A. Not Operated	50	2.1	2	1	1	2	3	4	5	6
B. Operated	42	5.7	8	2	3	5	7	9	11	14
2. MULTIPLE DX										
A. Not Operated	1,095	4.5	23	1	2	3	5	8	12	22
B. Operated	759	10.8	66	4	6	9	13	19	25	46
1. SINGLE DX	92	3.8	8	1	2	3	5	7	9	14
2. MULTIPLE DX	1,854	7.1	50	2	3	5	9	14	19	35
A. NOT OPERATED	1,145	4.4	22	1	2	3	5	8	11	22
B. OPERATED	801	10.5	64	4	6	9	13	19	24	46
TOTAL										
0–19 Years	93	5.0	14	1	2	3	5	9	12	21
20–34	346	7.2	28	1	3	6	10	14	18	22
35–49	292	8.8	77	2	4	7	10	16	24	63
50–64	335	8.8	75	2	3	6	12	19	23	46
65+	880	5.7	36	2	3	4	6	11	15	33
GRAND TOTAL	1,946	6.9	48	2	3	5	9	14	19	35

808.2: FRACTURE OF PUBIS-CLOSED

Type of Patients	Observed Patients	Avg. Stay	Variance	10th	25th	50th	75th	90th	95th	99th
1. SINGLE DX										
A. Not Operated										
0–19 Years	13	2.0	1	1	1	2	3	3	4	4
20–34	16	2.4	6	1	1	2	3	4	11	11
35–49	12	3.1	3	1	1	4	5	5	6	6
50–64	13	2.3	2	1	1	2	3	5	5	5
65+	10	2.0	<1	1	1	2	3	3	3	3
B. Operated										
0–19 Years	0									
20–34	1	4.0	0	4	4	4	4	4	4	4
35–49	0									
50–64	0									
65+	0									
2. MULTIPLE DX										
A. Not Operated										
0–19 Years	119	3.7	10	2	2	3	4	8	9	18
20–34	207	3.9	10	1	2	3	5	8	9	16
35–49	197	4.1	12	1	2	3	5	8	9	18
50–64	408	5.0	23	2	2	4	6	9	14	24
65+	4,180	4.0	7	2	3	3	5	7	8	14
B. Operated										
0–19 Years	40	9.6	62	3	5	8	12	17	24	47
20–34	66	10.1	61	4	5	7	12	18	27	36
35–49	62	10.2	41	5	5	8	13	19	21	37
50–64	60	11.8	67	4	6	9	15	23	29	39
65+	95	9.8	63	3	5	8	13	18	21	62
SUBTOTALS:										
1. SINGLE DX										
A. Not Operated	64	2.4	3	1	1	2	3	4	5	11
B. Operated	1	4.0	0	4	4	4	4	4	4	4
2. MULTIPLE DX										
A. Not Operated	5,111	4.0	9	2	3	3	5	7	9	16
B. Operated	323	10.3	59	4	5	8	13	18	25	38
1. SINGLE DX	65	2.4	3	1	1	2	3	4	5	11
2. MULTIPLE DX	5,434	4.4	14	2	3	3	5	8	10	19
A. NOT OPERATED	5,175	4.0	9	2	3	3	5	7	9	16
B. OPERATED	324	10.3	59	4	5	8	13	18	25	38
TOTAL										
0–19 Years	172	5.0	28	1	2	3	7	10	14	24
20–34	289	5.2	28	1	2	4	6	10	16	35
35–49	272	5.4	25	1	2	4	6	11	16	25
50–64	481	5.8	34	2	3	4	7	12	16	29
65+	4,285	4.1	9	2	3	3	5	7	9	16
GRAND TOTAL	5,499	4.4	14	2	3	3	5	8	10	19

Length of Stay by Diagnosis and Operation, Western Region, 2008

Western Region, October 2006–September 2007 Data, by Diagnosis

808.41: FRACTURE OF ILIUM-CLOSED

Type of Patients	Observed Patients	Avg. Stay	Variance	Percentiles 10th	25th	50th	75th	90th	95th	99th
1. SINGLE DX										
A. Not Operated										
0–19 Years	10	1.6	1	1	1	1	2	4		4
20–34	3	4.4	6	2	2	4	7	7		7
35–49	0									
50–64	2	2.0	2	1	1	1	3	3		3
65+	0									
B. Operated										
0–19 Years	1	1.0	0	1	1	1	1	1		1
20–34	1	5.0	0	5	5	5	5	5		5
35–49	2	3.0	0	3	3	3	3	3		3
50–64	0									
65+	0									
2. MULTIPLE DX										
A. Not Operated										
0–19 Years	47	2.6	4	1	1	2	3	5	8	9
20–34	31	2.4	2	1	1	2	3	4	5	5
35–49	23	4.4	13	2	2	3	5	10	13	15
50–64	32	4.2	7	1	2	4	6	8	10	10
65+	135	3.9	7	1	3	3	5	6	9	11
B. Operated										
0–19 Years	12	5.7	9	3	3	6	6	11	12	12
20–34	13	5.9	10	2	3	7	9	10	10	10
35–49	16	11.5	67	5	6	10	14	29	29	29
50–64	16	10.0	83	2	4	8	14	32	>99	>99
65+	6	7.7	14	2	5	8	11	12	12	12
SUBTOTALS:										
1. SINGLE DX										
A. Not Operated	15	2.2	3	1	1	1	3	4	7	7
B. Operated	4	3.0	3	1	1	3	5	5	5	5
2. MULTIPLE DX										
A. Not Operated	268	3.6	7	1	2	3	5	6	9	13
B. Operated	63	8.5	47	2	4	7	11	17	29	>99
1. SINGLE DX	19	2.4	3	1	1	2	3	5	7	7
2. MULTIPLE DX	331	4.5	18	1	2	3	5	9	11	29
A. NOT OPERATED	283	3.5	7	1	2	3	5	6	8	13
B. OPERATED	67	8.2	46	2	3	6	11	17	29	>99
TOTAL										
0–19 Years	70	3.0	6	1	1	2	3	6	8	12
20–34	48	3.5	6	1	1	3	5	9	9	10
35–49	41	7.1	45	2	3	5	10	14	21	29
50–64	50	6.0	38	1	2	4	8	12	29	>99
65+	141	4.1	8	1	3	3	5	7	9	12
GRAND TOTAL	350	4.4	18	1	2	3	5	9	11	29

808.8: PELVIC FRACTURE NOS-CLSD

Type of Patients	Observed Patients	Avg. Stay	Variance	Percentiles 10th	25th	50th	75th	90th	95th	99th
1. SINGLE DX										
A. Not Operated										
0–19 Years	0									
20–34	0									
35–49	0									
50–64	1	3.0	0	3	3	3	3	3	3	3
65+	2	3.0	8	1	1	1	5	5	5	5
B. Operated										
0–19 Years	0									
20–34	0									
35–49	0									
50–64	0									
65+	0									
2. MULTIPLE DX										
A. Not Operated										
0–19 Years	4	1.7	<1	1	1	2	2	3	3	3
20–34	10	2.2	<1	1	2	2	3	4	4	4
35–49	3	2.7	1	2	2	2	4	4	4	4
50–64	21	5.3	24	2	3	4	5	9	15	22
65+	221	3.9	5	2	3	3	5	6	8	12
B. Operated										
0–19 Years	2	10.5	<1	10	10	10	11	11	11	11
20–34	8	15.3	79	5	5	12	20	31	31	31
35–49	4	9.7	7	7	7	10	12	12	12	12
50–64	5	20.3	355	3	9	18	20	52	52	52
65+	9	7.0	7	5	5	6	8	13	13	13
SUBTOTALS:										
1. SINGLE DX										
A. Not Operated	3	3.0	4	1	1	3	5	5	5	5
B. Operated	0									
2. MULTIPLE DX										
A. Not Operated	259	3.9	6	2	3	3	5	6	8	14
B. Operated	28	12.4	101	5	6	10	13	22	31	52
1. SINGLE DX	3	3.0	4	1	1	3	5	5	5	5
2. MULTIPLE DX	287	4.7	21	2	3	5	5	8	12	22
A. NOT OPERATED	262	3.9	6	2	3	3	5	6	8	14
B. OPERATED	28	12.4	101	5	6	10	13	22	31	52
TOTAL										
0–19 Years	6	4.7	21	1	1	2	3	6	8	11
20–34	18	8.0	78	1	2	3	5	9	22	31
35–49	7	6.7	17	2	2	7	10	14	12	12
50–64	27	8.0	109	2	3	4	8	12	29	52
65+	232	4.0	5	2	3	3	5	7	9	13
GRAND TOTAL	290	4.7	21	2	3	5	5	8	12	22

809: FRACTURE OF TRUNK BONES

Type of Patients	Observed Patients	Avg. Stay	Variance	Percentiles 10th	25th	50th	75th	90th	95th	99th
1. SINGLE DX										
A. Not Operated										
0–19 Years	1	3.0	0	3	3	3	3	3	3	3
20–34	0									
35–49	0									
50–64	0									
65+	0									
B. Operated										
0–19 Years	0									
20–34	0									
35–49	0									
50–64	0									
65+	0									
2. MULTIPLE DX										
A. Not Operated										
0–19 Years	1	1.0	0	1	1	1	1	1	1	1
20–34	0									
35–49	0									
50–64	1	4.0	0	4	4	4	4	4	4	4
65+	1	1.0	0	1	1	1	1	1	1	1
B. Operated										
0–19 Years	0									
20–34	0									
35–49	0									
50–64	0									
65+	0									
SUBTOTALS:										
1. SINGLE DX										
A. Not Operated	1	3.0	0	3	3	3	3	3	3	3
B. Operated	0									
2. MULTIPLE DX										
A. Not Operated	3	2.0	3	1	1	1	1	4	4	4
B. Operated	0									
1. SINGLE DX	1	3.0	0	3	3	3	3	3	3	3
2. MULTIPLE DX	3	2.0	3	1	1	1	1	4	4	4
A. NOT OPERATED	4	2.3	2	1	1	3	4	4	4	4
B. OPERATED	0									
TOTAL										
0–19 Years	2	2.0	2	1	1	3	3	3	3	3
20–34	0									
35–49	0									
50–64	1	4.0	0	4	4	4	4	4	4	4
65+	1	1.0	0	1	1	1	1	1	1	1
GRAND TOTAL	4	2.3	2	1	1	3	4	4	4	4

Length of Stay by Diagnosis and Operation, Western Region, 2008

Western Region, October 2006–September 2007 Data, by Diagnosis

810: CLAVICLE FRACTURE

Type of Patients	Observed Patients	Avg. Stay	Variance	10th	25th	50th	75th	90th	95th	99th
1. SINGLE DX										
A. Not Operated										
0–19 Years	12	1.3	<1	1	1	1	1	2	3	3
20–34	9	1.3	<1	1	1	1	1	3	3	3
35–49	4	1.3	<1	1	1	1	1	1	2	2
50–64	2	1.5	<1	1	1	2	2	2	2	2
65+	0									
B. Operated										
0–19 Years	37	1.2	<1	1	1	1	1	2	2	3
20–34	52	1.7	5	1	1	1	1	3	6	14
35–49	37	1.3	<1	1	1	1	1	2	3	4
50–64	24	1.1	<1	1	1	1	1	1	2	2
65+	2	1.0	0	1	1	1	1	1	1	1
2. MULTIPLE DX										
A. Not Operated										
0–19 Years	83	1.8	2	1	1	1	2	3	4	7
20–34	122	2.1	3	1	1	1	2	4	5	8
35–49	143	2.6	5	1	1	2	3	5	7	9
50–64	152	3.1	7	1	1	2	4	6	8	14
65+	242	3.7	6	1	2	3	4	7	8	11
B. Operated										
0–19 Years	36	3.1	7	1	1	2	4	6	9	13
20–34	74	3.1	15	1	1	2	4	7	11	28
35–49	109	3.3	13	1	1	2	4	7	10	14
50–64	114	3.5	26	1	1	2	5	7	10	22
65+	27	6.0	71	1	1	2	5	24	25	30
SUBTOTALS:										
1. SINGLE DX										
A. Not Operated	27	1.3	<1	1	1	1	1	2	3	3
B. Operated	152	1.4	2	1	1	1	1	2	3	10
2. MULTIPLE DX										
A. Not Operated	742	2.9	5	1	1	2	4	6	7	12
B. Operated	360	3.5	22	1	1	2	4	7	11	26
1. SINGLE DX	179	1.4	2	1	1	1	1	2	3	10
2. MULTIPLE DX	1,102	3.1	11	1	1	2	4	6	8	15
A. NOT OPERATED	769	2.8	5	1	1	2	4	6	7	12
B. OPERATED	512	2.9	17	1	1	2	3	6	9	24
TOTAL										
0–19 Years	168	1.9	3	1	1	1	2	4	5	9
20–34	257	2.3	7	1	1	1	2	4	7	14
35–49	293	2.7	7	1	1	2	3	6	7	14
50–64	292	3.1	14	1	2	3	4	6	8	16
65+	271	3.9	13	1	2	3	4	7	9	24
GRAND TOTAL	1,281	2.9	10	1	1	2	3	6	8	14

810.00: CLSD FX CLAVICLE NOS

Type of Patients	Observed Patients	Avg. Stay	Variance	10th	25th	50th	75th	90th	95th	99th
1. SINGLE DX										
A. Not Operated										
0–19 Years	6	1.3	<1	1	1	1	1	2	3	3
20–34	5	1.6	<1	1	1	1	2	3	3	3
35–49	2	1.0	0	1	1	1	1	1	1	1
50–64	0									
65+	0									
B. Operated										
0–19 Years	9	1.2	<1	1	1	1	1	2	2	2
20–34	20	2.3	12	1	1	1	1	3	10	14
35–49	9	1.6	1	1	1	1	1	3	4	4
50–64	9	1.1	<1	1	1	1	1	1	2	2
65+	0									
2. MULTIPLE DX										
A. Not Operated										
0–19 Years	33	2.0	2	1	1	1	2	3	4	7
20–34	61	2.0	2	1	1	1	2	4	5	8
35–49	51	2.5	4	1	1	2	3	5	7	9
50–64	65	3.3	7	1	1	2	5	6	8	14
65+	93	3.7	8	1	2	3	4	7	8	11
B. Operated										
0–19 Years	4	2.7	3	1	2	2	3	5	5	5
20–34	22	4.2	38	1	1	2	4	11	12	28
35–49	20	3.4	9	1	1	3	5	10	11	11
50–64	31	5.3	75	1	1	2	6	8	22	46
65+	7	2.0	3	1	1	2	2	5	5	5
SUBTOTALS:										
1. SINGLE DX										
A. Not Operated	13	1.4	<1	1	1	1	1	2	3	3
B. Operated	47	1.7	5	1	1	1	1	3	4	14
2. MULTIPLE DX										
A. Not Operated	303	2.9	6	1	1	2	4	6	7	12
B. Operated	84	4.1	40	1	1	2	5	8	11	46
1. SINGLE DX	60	1.6	4	1	1	1	1	2	3	14
2. MULTIPLE DX	387	3.2	14	1	1	2	4	6	8	22
A. NOT OPERATED	316	2.8	6	1	1	2	4	6	7	12
B. OPERATED	131	3.3	29	1	1	1	3	6	11	28
TOTAL										
0–19 Years	52	1.8	2	1	1	1	2	4	5	7
20–34	108	2.5	12	1	1	1	2	4	8	14
35–49	82	2.6	5	1	1	2	3	5	7	11
50–64	105	3.7	28	1	2	2	4	6	10	22
65+	100	3.6	8	1	2	3	4	6	9	12
GRAND TOTAL	447	3.0	13	1	1	2	3	6	8	14

810.02: CLSD FX CLAVICLE SHAFT

Type of Patients	Observed Patients	Avg. Stay	Variance	10th	25th	50th	75th	90th	95th	99th
1. SINGLE DX										
A. Not Operated										
0–19 Years	5	1.2	<1	1	1	1	1	2	2	2
20–34	1	1.0	0	1	1	1	1	1	1	1
35–49	2	1.5	<1	1	1	2	2	2	2	2
50–64	2	1.5	<1	1	1	2	2	2	2	2
65+	0									
B. Operated										
0–19 Years	25	1.2	<1	1	1	1	1	2	2	3
20–34	24	1.2	<1	1	1	1	1	2	2	3
35–49	18	1.1	<1	1	1	1	1	2	2	2
50–64	11	1.1	<1	1	1	1	1	1	2	2
65+	0									
2. MULTIPLE DX										
A. Not Operated										
0–19 Years	41	1.6	1	1	1	1	2	3	3	6
20–34	43	2.3	6	1	1	2	2	4	7	14
35–49	65	2.7	6	1	1	2	3	5	7	16
50–64	65	3.0	7	1	2	2	3	6	7	16
65+	68	3.8	5	1	2	3	5	7	7	11
B. Operated										
0–19 Years	17	2.7	6	1	1	2	3	5	9	9
20–34	32	2.7	5	1	1	2	3	5	8	9
35–49	52	2.8	8	1	1	2	3	6	9	14
50–64	45	2.7	5	1	1	2	3	6	7	11
65+	10	7.5	74	1	2	3	14	25	25	25
SUBTOTALS:										
1. SINGLE DX										
A. Not Operated	10	1.3	<1	1	1	1	1	2	2	2
B. Operated	78	1.2	<1	1	1	1	1	2	2	3
2. MULTIPLE DX										
A. Not Operated	282	2.8	6	1	1	2	3	6	7	14
B. Operated	156	3.1	11	1	1	2	4	7	9	19
1. SINGLE DX	88	1.2	<1	1	1	1	1	2	2	3
2. MULTIPLE DX	438	2.9	8	1	1	2	4	6	7	14
A. NOT OPERATED	292	2.8	6	1	1	2	3	6	7	14
B. OPERATED	234	2.4	8	1	1	1	3	5	7	14
TOTAL										
0–19 Years	88	1.7	2	1	1	1	2	3	3	9
20–34	100	2.2	4	1	1	1	2	4	7	9
35–49	137	2.5	6	1	1	1	3	6	7	14
50–64	123	2.7	6	1	2	2	5	6	7	14
65+	78	4.3	14	1	2	3	5	7	11	25
GRAND TOTAL	526	2.6	7	1	1	2	3	6	7	14

706

Western Region, October 2006–September 2007 Data, by Diagnosis

811: SCAPULA FRACTURE

Type of Patients	Observed Patients	Avg. Stay	Variance	10th	25th	50th	75th	90th	95th	99th
1. SINGLE DX										
A. Not Operated										
0–19 Years	2	1.0	0	1	1	1	1	1	1	1
20–34	3	2.7	8	1	1	1	6	6	6	6
35–49	1	1.0	0	1	1	1	1	1	1	1
50–64	1	1.0	0	1	1	1	1	1	1	1
65+	0									
B. Operated										
0–19 Years	0									
20–34	7	2.7	3	1	2	2	3	6	6	6
35–49	6	2.0	<1	1	1	2	3	3	3	3
50–64	4	1.7	<1	1	1	1	2	3	3	3
65+	0									
2. MULTIPLE DX										
A. Not Operated										
0–19 Years	32	2.2	2	1	1	2	3	4	5	5
20–34	78	2.2	4	1	1	2	3	4	5	12
35–49	66	2.9	7	1	1	2	4	6	8	15
50–64	80	3.1	8	1	1	3	4	6	8	20
65+	85	3.6	6	1	2	3	5	7	9	13
B. Operated										
0–19 Years	6	6.0	43	1	3	4	6	19	19	19
20–34	30	4.8	34	1	2	3	5	11	16	30
35–49	27	4.3	11	1	1	3	7	9	10	12
50–64	35	6.3	117	1	2	3	6	10	35	56
65+	26	3.4	13	1	2	3	3	9	11	16
SUBTOTALS:										
1. SINGLE DX										
A. Not Operated	7	1.7	4	1	1	1	1	6	6	6
B. Operated	17	2.2	2	1	1	2	3	3	6	6
2. MULTIPLE DX										
A. Not Operated	341	2.9	6	1	1	2	4	6	7	12
B. Operated	124	4.9	48	1	2	3	6	10	16	35
1. SINGLE DX	24	2.1	2	1	1	2	3	3	6	6
2. MULTIPLE DX	465	3.4	18	1	1	2	4	7	10	20
A. NOT OPERATED	348	2.9	6	1	1	2	4	6	7	12
B. OPERATED	141	4.6	43	1	2	3	5	9	12	35
TOTAL										
0–19 Years	40	2.7	9	1	1	2	3	5	5	19
20–34	118	2.9	12	1	1	2	3	5	10	16
35–49	100	3.2	8	1	1	2	4	7	9	15
50–64	120	4.0	41	1	1	3	4	7	10	35
65+	111	3.6	8	1	2	3	5	7	10	13
GRAND TOTAL	489	3.4	17	1	2	2	4	6	9	20

812: HUMERUS FRACTURE

Type of Patients	Observed Patients	Avg. Stay	Variance	10th	25th	50th	75th	90th	95th	99th
1. SINGLE DX										
A. Not Operated										
0–19 Years	166	1.3	<1	1	1	1	1	2	2	6
20–34	33	1.3	<1	1	1	1	2	2	2	6
35–49	17	2.1	4	1	1	1	2	5	8	8
50–64	25	1.8	1	1	1	1	2	3	5	5
65+	14	1.5	<1	1	1	1	2	3	3	3
B. Operated										
0–19 Years	1,609	1.3	<1	1	1	1	1	2	2	3
20–34	185	2.0	2	1	1	2	2	3	4	7
35–49	143	1.8	<1	1	1	2	2	3	4	4
50–64	142	2.1	3	1	1	2	2	3	5	7
65+	74	2.7	5	1	1	2	3	4	7	15
2. MULTIPLE DX										
A. Not Operated										
0–19 Years	106	2.2	7	1	1	2	2	4	8	13
20–34	158	2.2	5	1	1	2	3	4	6	16
35–49	149	2.7	5	1	1	2	4	5	6	15
50–64	466	4.3	31	1	1	3	5	8	14	26
65+	2,296	3.6	6	1	2	3	4	6	8	13
B. Operated										
0–19 Years	676	2.1	6	1	1	2	2	4	6	15
20–34	564	4.4	26	1	2	3	5	9	15	25
35–49	595	4.2	24	1	2	3	5	9	13	30
50–64	1,460	4.0	17	1	2	3	5	8	12	21
65+	2,885	4.3	13	1	2	3	5	8	10	18
SUBTOTALS:										
1. SINGLE DX										
A. Not Operated	255	1.4	<1	1	1	1	1	2	3	6
B. Operated	2,153	1.5	<1	1	1	2	2	3	3	5
2. MULTIPLE DX										
A. Not Operated	3,175	3.6	10	1	2	3	4	6	8	16
B. Operated	6,180	4.0	16	1	2	3	5	8	11	21
1. SINGLE DX	2,408	1.5	<1	1	1	2	2	3	3	5
2. MULTIPLE DX	9,355	3.8	14	1	2	3	5	7	10	19
A. NOT OPERATED	3,430	3.4	10	1	2	3	4	6	8	15
B. OPERATED	8,333	3.3	13	1	2	3	4	7	9	18
TOTAL										
0–19 Years	2,557	1.5	2	1	1	2	2	3	3	8
20–34	940	3.5	18	1	1	2	4	7	11	22
35–49	904	3.6	18	1	1	2	4	7	10	23
50–64	2,093	3.9	19	1	2	3	5	8	11	23
65+	5,269	4.0	10	1	2	3	5	7	9	16
GRAND TOTAL	11,763	3.4	12	1	2	3	4	7	9	18

812.00: CL FX UP END HUMERUS NOS

Type of Patients	Observed Patients	Avg. Stay	Variance	10th	25th	50th	75th	90th	95th	99th
1. SINGLE DX										
A. Not Operated										
0–19 Years	7	1.4	<1	1	1	1	2	3	3	3
20–34	2	2.0	0	2	2	2	2	2	2	2
35–49	2	1.0	0	1	1	1	1	1	1	1
50–64	3	1.7	<1	1	1	2	2	2	2	2
65+	3	1.7	1	1	1	1	3	3	3	3
B. Operated										
0–19 Years	14	1.4	<1	1	1	1	2	2	2	3
20–34	11	1.9	1	1	1	2	2	3	4	7
35–49	16	1.7	<1	1	1	2	2	3	3	4
50–64	29	1.8	<1	1	1	2	2	3	3	3
65+	19	2.4	3	1	1	2	3	5	7	7
2. MULTIPLE DX										
A. Not Operated										
0–19 Years	6	1.2	<1	1	1	1	2	2	2	2
20–34	2	1.5	<1	1	1	2	2	2	2	2
35–49	15	2.9	4	1	1	2	4	5	9	9
50–64	55	5.8	52	1	1	3	7	14	25	36
65+	335	3.4	4	1	2	3	4	6	8	10
B. Operated										
0–19 Years	6	2.0	2	1	1	2	2	4	4	4
20–34	21	3.3	9	1	2	3	4	9	9	10
35–49	39	2.6	3	1	1	2	4	5	7	7
50–64	246	3.7	14	1	2	3	4	7	12	20
65+	476	3.8	10	1	2	3	4	7	9	18
SUBTOTALS:										
1. SINGLE DX										
A. Not Operated	17	1.5	<1	1	1	1	2	3	3	3
B. Operated	89	1.9	1	1	1	2	2	3	4	7
2. MULTIPLE DX										
A. Not Operated	413	3.7	11	1	2	3	4	6	9	18
B. Operated	788	3.7	11	1	2	3	4	7	9	18
1. SINGLE DX	106	1.8	1	1	1	2	2	3	4	5
2. MULTIPLE DX	1,201	3.7	11	1	2	3	4	7	9	18
A. NOT OPERATED	430	3.6	11	1	2	3	4	6	9	18
B. OPERATED	877	3.5	10	1	2	3	4	7	9	18
TOTAL										
0–19 Years	33	1.5	<1	1	1	1	2	2	3	4
20–34	36	2.7	6	1	1	2	3	7	9	10
35–49	72	2.4	3	1	1	2	3	4	6	9
50–64	333	3.9	20	1	2	3	4	8	12	23
65+	833	3.6	15	1	2	3	4	6	8	15
GRAND TOTAL	1,307	3.5	11	1	2	3	4	7	9	18

Length of Stay by Diagnosis and Operation, Western Region, 2008

Western Region, October 2006–September 2007 Data, by Diagnosis

812.01: CL FX SURG NECK HUMERUS

Type of Patients	Observed Patients	Avg. Stay	Variance	10th	25th	50th	75th	90th	95th	99th
1. SINGLE DX										
A. Not Operated										
0–19 Years	3	1.0	0	1	1	1	1	1	1	1
20–34	2	1.0	0	1	1	1	1	1	1	1
35–49		1.0	0	1	1	1	1	1	1	1
50–64	7	2.0	2	1	1	1	3	5	5	5
65+	4	1.0	0	1	1	1	1	1	1	1
B. Operated										
0–19 Years	14	1.4	<1	1	1	1	2	2	2	2
20–34	11	2.7	8	1	1	2	3	4	11	11
35–49	18	1.4	<1	1	1	1	2	2	2	2
50–64	24	1.9	<1	1	1	2	2	3	3	6
65+	14	2.4	<1	1	2	2	3	3	4	4
2. MULTIPLE DX										
A. Not Operated										
0–19 Years	7	1.7	1	1	1	1	2	4	4	4
20–34	3	1.3	<1	1	1	1	2	2	2	2
35–49	16	3.3	6	1	1	3	5	7	8	8
50–64	121	4.3	20	1	2	3	5	8	14	25
65+	809	3.7	6	1	2	3	5	6	8	13
B. Operated										
0–19 Years	12	2.8	5	1	1	2	4	5	8	8
20–34	44	3.3	3	1	2	3	4	6	7	8
35–49	64	4.2	14	1	2	3	6	8	10	22
50–64	235	4.3	24	1	2	3	5	9	12	25
65+	611	4.6	14	1	2	4	6	8	11	17
SUBTOTALS:										
1. SINGLE DX A. Not Operated	17	1.4	1	1	1	1	2	3	5	5
B. Operated	81	1.9	2	1	1	2	2	3	3	11
2. MULTIPLE DX A. Not Operated	956	3.7	8	1	2	3	5	6	8	15
B. Operated	966	4.4	16	1	2	3	6	8	11	21
1. SINGLE DX	98	1.8	2	1	1	1	2	3	4	11
2. MULTIPLE DX	1,922	4.1	12	1	2	3	5	7	10	18
A. NOT OPERATED	973	3.7	8	1	2	3	4	6	8	15
B. OPERATED	1,047	4.2	15	1	2	3	5	8	10	19
TOTAL										
0–19 Years	36	1.9	2	1	1	1	2	4	5	8
20–34	60	3.0	4	1	2	2	4	6	8	11
35–49	99	3.5	11	1	1	2	5	7	9	22
50–64	387	4.1	21	1	2	3	5	8	12	25
65+	1,438	4.0	9	1	2	3	5	7	9	15
GRAND TOTAL	2,020	4.0	12	1	2	3	5	7	10	18

812.03: CL FX GR TUBEROS HUMERUS

Type of Patients	Observed Patients	Avg. Stay	Variance	10th	25th	50th	75th	90th	95th	99th
1. SINGLE DX										
A. Not Operated										
0–19 Years	3	1.0	0	1	1	1	2	1	1	1
20–34	3	1.3	<1	1	1	1	2	2	2	2
35–49	2	3.0	8	1	1	1	5	5	5	5
50–64	4	1.3	<1	1	1	1	1	1	2	2
65+	2	1.0	0	1	1	1	1	1	1	1
B. Operated										
0–19 Years	0									
20–34	2	1.5	<1	1	1	1	2	2	2	2
35–49	13	1.2	<1	1	1	1	1	2	2	2
50–64	7	1.4	<1	1	1	1	2	2	2	2
65+	5	2.0	<1	1	2	2	2	3	3	3
2. MULTIPLE DX										
A. Not Operated										
0–19 Years	1	2.0	0	2	2	2	2	2	2	2
20–34	20	2.2	1	1	1	2	3	4	4	4
35–49	19	2.2	2	1	1	2	3	5	5	5
50–64	56	3.7	24	1	2	3	4	7	9	36
65+	149	3.6	5	1	2	3	4	7	8	11
B. Operated										
0–19 Years	2	2.5	4	1	1	2	4	4	4	4
20–34	37	2.5	7	1	1	2	3	6	9	14
35–49	56	2.8	6	1	1	2	3	7	7	14
50–64	147	2.9	7	1	1	2	4	6	9	15
65+	190	3.6	10	2	2	3	4	8	11	16
SUBTOTALS:										
1. SINGLE DX A. Not Operated	14	1.4	1	1	1	1	1	2	5	5
B. Operated	27	1.4	<1	1	1	1	2	2	3	3
2. MULTIPLE DX A. Not Operated	245	3.4	9	2	2	3	4	7	8	11
B. Operated	432	3.2	8	1	1	2	4	7	9	15
1. SINGLE DX	41	1.4	<1	1	1	1	2	2	3	5
2. MULTIPLE DX	677	3.3	9	1	1	2	4	7	9	14
A. NOT OPERATED	259	3.3	9	1	1	3	4	7	8	11
B. OPERATED	459	3.1	8	1	1	2	4	7	9	15
TOTAL										
0–19 Years	6	1.7	1	1	1	2	2	4	4	4
20–34	62	2.3	5	1	1	2	3	4	6	14
35–49	90	2.5	4	1	1	2	3	5	7	14
50–64	214	3.0	11	1	1	2	4	6	9	15
65+	346	3.6	8	2	2	3	4	7	10	14
GRAND TOTAL	718	3.1	8	1	1	2	4	7	9	14

812.09: CL FX UPPER HUMERUS NEC

Type of Patients	Observed Patients	Avg. Stay	Variance	10th	25th	50th	75th	90th	95th	99th
1. SINGLE DX										
A. Not Operated										
0–19 Years	8	1.3	<1	1	1	1	1	3	3	3
20–34	0									
35–49	4	3.5	10	1	2	3	8	8	8	8
50–64	4	1.8	<1	1	1	2	3	3	3	3
65+	3	1.7	1	1	1	1	3	3	3	3
B. Operated										
0–19 Years	13	1.2	<1	1	1	2	2	2	2	2
20–34	4	1.5	<1	1	1	2	2	2	2	2
35–49	23	1.9	<1	1	1	2	3	3	4	4
50–64	27	1.8	<1	1	1	2	3	3	3	3
65+	19	4.1	12	1	2	3	5	8	15	15
2. MULTIPLE DX										
A. Not Operated										
0–19 Years	9	4.2	16	1	1	2	8	12	12	12
20–34	9	2.5	9	1	1	1	3	10	10	10
35–49	37	2.4	3	1	1	2	3	5	6	7
50–64	102	4.5	54	1	2	3	5	8	11	26
65+	508	3.8	9	1	2	3	5	7	9	13
B. Operated										
0–19 Years	22	3.9	15	1	2	3	5	11	12	13
20–34	33	5.2	26	2	2	3	5	16	16	20
35–49	89	3.3	7	1	2	3	4	7	10	15
50–64	310	3.8	16	1	2	3	4	8	10	21
65+	680	4.2	10	1	2	4	5	7	9	15
SUBTOTALS:										
1. SINGLE DX A. Not Operated	19	1.9	3	1	1	2	3	3	8	8
B. Operated	86	2.2	4	1	1	2	3	4	5	15
2. MULTIPLE DX A. Not Operated	665	3.8	16	1	2	3	5	7	9	17
B. Operated	1,134	4.1	12	1	2	3	5	8	10	17
1. SINGLE DX	105	2.2	4	1	1	2	3	4	5	8
2. MULTIPLE DX	1,799	4.0	14	1	2	3	5	8	10	17
A. NOT OPERATED	684	3.8	16	1	2	3	4	7	9	17
B. OPERATED	1,220	3.9	12	1	2	3	5	8	10	16
TOTAL										
0–19 Years	52	2.9	11	1	1	2	2	8	12	13
20–34	46	4.4	22	1	1	3	5	13	16	20
35–49	153	2.9	5	1	1	2	3	6	8	11
50–64	443	3.9	24	1	2	3	4	8	10	26
65+	1,210	4.0	10	1	2	3	5	7	9	15
GRAND TOTAL	1,904	3.9	13	1	2	3	5	7	10	16

Length of Stay by Diagnosis and Operation, Western Region, 2008

Western Region, October 2006–September 2007 Data, by Diagnosis

812.20: CLOSED FX HUMERUS NOS

Type of Patients	Observed Patients	Avg. Stay	Variance	10th	25th	50th	75th	90th	95th	99th
1. SINGLE DX										
A. Not Operated										
0–19 Years	5	1.2	<1	1	1	1	1	2	2	2
20–34	0									
35–49	1	1.0	0	1	1	1	1	1	1	1
50–64	1	2.0	0	2	2	2	2	2	2	2
65+	0									
B. Operated										
0–19 Years	1	1.0	0	1	1	1	1	1	1	1
20–34	3	1.0	0	1	1	1	1	1	1	1
35–49	2	1.0	0	1	1	1	1	1	1	1
50–64	2	1.0	0	1	1	1	1	1	1	1
65+	0									
2. MULTIPLE DX										
A. Not Operated										
0–19 Years	5	1.2	<1	1	1	1	1	2	2	2
20–34	8	2.3	3	1	1	2	4	6	6	6
35–49	6	5.3	59	1	2	2	3	21	21	21
50–64	12	4.4	33	1	1	2	4	13	19	19
65+	81	3.5	7	1	2	3	4	6	7	16
B. Operated										
0–19 Years	3	1.3	<1	1	1	1	2	2	2	2
20–34	6	2.6	8	1	1	1	4	8	8	8
35–49	2	1.5	<1	1	1	1	2	2	2	2
50–64	10	3.6	10	1	1	3	5	11	11	11
65+	26	5.9	47	1	2	4	6	16	23	30
SUBTOTALS:										
1. SINGLE DX										
A. Not Operated	7	1.3	<1	1	1	1	2	2	2	2
B. Operated	8	1.0	0	1	1	1	1	1	1	1
2. MULTIPLE DX										
A. Not Operated	112	3.5	12	1	1	3	4	6	8	19
B. Operated	47	4.5	31	1	1	3	5	8	16	30
1. SINGLE DX	15	1.1	<1	1	1	1	1	2	2	2
2. MULTIPLE DX	159	3.8	17	1	1	3	4	7	13	23
A. NOT OPERATED	119	3.4	11	1	1	3	4	6	8	19
B. OPERATED	55	4.0	28	1	1	2	5	7	16	30
TOTAL										
0–19 Years	14	1.2	<1	1	1	1	1	2	2	2
20–34	17	2.2	4	1	1	1	2	6	8	8
35–49	11	3.4	34	1	1	2	3	3	21	21
50–64	25	3.7	20	1	1	2	4	11	13	19
65+	107	4.1	17	1	2	3	4	7	8	23
GRAND TOTAL	174	3.6	17	1	1	3	4	7	11	23

812.21: CLOSED FX HUMERUS SHAFT

Type of Patients	Observed Patients	Avg. Stay	Variance	10th	25th	50th	75th	90th	95th	99th
1. SINGLE DX										
A. Not Operated										
0–19 Years	18	1.8	3	1	1	1	2	6	6	6
20–34	10	1.1	<1	1	1	1	1	2	2	2
35–49	1	3.0	0	3	3	3	3	3	3	3
50–64	3	2.7	4	1	1	2	5	5	5	5
65+	0									
B. Operated										
0–19 Years	19	1.4	<1	1	1	1	1	2	5	5
20–34	60	1.6	<1	1	1	1	2	3	4	5
35–49	25	1.8	<1	1	1	2	2	3	3	4
50–64	19	1.9	1	1	1	2	3	3	5	5
65+	8	1.3	<1	1	1	1	2	2	2	2
2. MULTIPLE DX										
A. Not Operated										
0–19 Years	32	2.5	11	1	1	2	2	4	11	18
20–34	51	2.5	11	1	1	1	3	4	9	18
35–49	27	2.3	3	1	1	2	3	5	5	7
50–64	84	3.4	11	1	1	2	4	7	9	19
65+	215	3.5	5	2	2	3	4	6	8	11
B. Operated										
0–19 Years	43	3.8	12	1	2	2	5	7	8	16
20–34	140	4.5	23	1	2	3	5	10	17	25
35–49	121	3.8	15	1	2	2	4	8	11	23
50–64	207	4.5	21	1	2	3	5	9	12	25
65+	350	4.4	11	2	2	4	5	8	11	20
SUBTOTALS:										
1. SINGLE DX										
A. Not Operated	32	1.7	2	1	1	1	2	3	6	6
B. Operated	131	1.6	<1	1	1	1	2	3	3	5
2. MULTIPLE DX										
A. Not Operated	409	3.2	8	1	1	2	4	6	8	15
B. Operated	861	4.3	16	1	2	3	5	9	12	21
1. SINGLE DX	163	1.6	1	1	1	1	2	3	4	6
2. MULTIPLE DX	1,270	4.0	13	1	2	3	5	8	11	20
A. NOT OPERATED	441	3.1	7	1	1	2	4	6	8	15
B. OPERATED	992	4.0	15	2	2	3	5	8	11	21
TOTAL										
0–19 Years	112	2.7	9	1	1	2	3	6	7	16
20–34	261	3.3	16	1	1	2	3	7	11	19
35–49	174	3.2	12	1	1	2	4	6	10	23
50–64	313	4.0	17	1	2	3	5	8	12	24
65+	573	4.0	9	2	2	3	5	8	10	15
GRAND TOTAL	1,433	3.7	13	1	1	3	5	7	10	19

812.40: CLSD FX LOW HUMERUS NOS

Type of Patients	Observed Patients	Avg. Stay	Variance	10th	25th	50th	75th	90th	95th	99th
1. SINGLE DX										
A. Not Operated										
0–19 Years	9	1.2	<1	1	1	1	1	1	3	3
20–34	7	1.3	<1	1	1	1	2	2	2	2
35–49	2	1.5	<1	1	1	1	2	2	2	2
50–64	0									
65+	0									
B. Operated										
0–19 Years	12	1.1	<1	1	1	1	1	1	2	2
20–34	29	1.9	1	1	1	2	2	4	4	6
35–49	6	1.7	<1	1	2	2	2	2	2	2
50–64	4	1.7	2	1	1	1	1	4	4	4
65+	1	1.0	0	1	1	1	1	1	1	1
2. MULTIPLE DX										
A. Not Operated										
0–19 Years	4	3.0	3	3	3	3	3	5	5	5
20–34	16	2.1	3	1	2	2	2	5	6	6
35–49	5	3.2	3	2	2	2	4	6	6	6
50–64	11	2.6	4	1	1	2	4	4	8	8
65+	45	3.9	10	1	2	3	4	8	12	14
B. Operated										
0–19 Years	18	2.6	3	1	1	2	3	6	7	7
20–34	30	3.1	6	1	2	3	4	6	8	12
35–49	21	3.2	5	2	2	3	5	5	6	10
50–64	39	3.9	15	1	2	3	4	8	12	23
65+	81	5.3	39	2	2	4	5	11	15	48
SUBTOTALS:										
1. SINGLE DX										
A. Not Operated	18	1.3	<1	1	1	1	1	2	3	3
B. Operated	52	1.6	1	1	1	1	2	3	4	6
2. MULTIPLE DX										
A. Not Operated	81	3.3	7	1	1	3	4	6	8	14
B. Operated	189	4.2	23	1	2	3	5	8	11	25
1. SINGLE DX	70	1.5	<1	1	1	1	2	3	4	6
2. MULTIPLE DX	270	3.9	18	1	2	3	5	7	11	23
A. NOT OPERATED	99	2.9	6	1	1	2	4	6	8	14
B. OPERATED	241	3.6	19	1	1	2	4	7	10	23
TOTAL										
0–19 Years	43	1.9	2	1	1	2	2	3	6	7
20–34	82	2.3	3	1	2	2	3	4	6	12
35–49	34	2.9	4	1	2	2	4	5	6	10
50–64	54	3.5	12	1	2	3	4	6	8	23
65+	127	4.8	29	1	2	3	5	9	14	25
GRAND TOTAL	340	3.4	16	1	1	2	4	6	9	16

Length of Stay by Diagnosis and Operation, Western Region, 2008

Western Region, October 2006–September 2007 Data, by Diagnosis

812.41: CLSD SUPRACONDYL FX HUM

Type of Patients	Observed Patients	Avg. Stay	Vari- ance	10th	25th	50th	75th	90th	95th	99th
1. SINGLE DX										
A. Not Operated										
0–19 Years	84	1.1	<1	1	1	1	1	1	2	2
20–34	1	1.0	0			1			1	1
35–49	2	2.0	0	2	2	2	2	2	2	2
50–64	0									
65+	1	2.0	0	2	2	2	2	2	2	2
B. Operated										
0–19 Years	1,266	1.2	<1	1	1	1	1	2	2	3
20–34	24	2.2	2	1	1	2	3	3	5	7
35–49	11	2.2	2	1	1	2	3	4	4	4
50–64	9	2.3	1	1	2	3	3	4	4	4
65+	3	2.7	<1	2	2	3	3	3	3	3
2. MULTIPLE DX										
A. Not Operated										
0–19 Years	20	1.7	7	1	1	1	1	2	2	13
20–34	9	1.7	2	1	1	1	1	5	5	5
35–49	4	3.0	1	2	2	4	4	4	4	4
50–64	2	5.0	2	4	4	4	6	6	6	6
65+	67	3.7	6	1	2	3	5	6	9	13
B. Operated										
0–19 Years	388	1.5	1	1	1	1	2	2	3	5
20–34	71	2.6	3	1	2	2	3	4	7	11
35–49	43	2.9	3	1	2	3	4	5	5	5
50–64	75	4.2	13	1	2	3	6	9	12	20
65+	222	4.3	16	1	2	3	5	8	10	20
SUBTOTALS:										
1. SINGLE DX — A. Not Operated	88	1.1	<1	1	1	1	1	1	2	2
1. SINGLE DX — B. Operated	1,313	1.3	<1	1	1	1	2	2	2	3
2. MULTIPLE DX — A. Not Operated	102	3.1	7	1	1	3	4	6	9	13
2. MULTIPLE DX — B. Operated	799	2.7	8	1	1	2	3	5	8	15
1. SINGLE DX	1,401	1.2	<1	1	1	1	1	2	2	3
2. MULTIPLE DX	901	2.8	8	1	1	2	3	5	8	14
A. NOT OPERATED	190	2.2	5	1	1	1	3	5	6	13
B. OPERATED	2,112	1.8	4	1	1	1	2	3	5	10
TOTAL										
0–19 Years	1,758	1.3	<1	1	1	1	1	2	2	3
20–34	105	2.4	3	1	1	2	3	4	6	8
35–49	60	2.7	1	2	2	3	4	4	5	5
50–64	86	4.1	12	1	2	3	6	9	10	20
65+	293	4.1	13	1	2	3	5	8	10	20
GRAND TOTAL	2,302	1.8	4	1	1	1	2	3	5	10

812.42: CLSD FX HUM LAT CONDYL

Type of Patients	Observed Patients	Avg. Stay	Vari- ance	10th	25th	50th	75th	90th	95th	99th
1. SINGLE DX										
A. Not Operated										
0–19 Years	8	1.3	<1	1	1	1	1	2	2	2
20–34	0									
35–49	0									
50–64	1	2.0	0	2	2	2	2	2	2	2
65+	0									
B. Operated										
0–19 Years	151	1.4	<1	1	1	1	2	2	2	3
20–34	5	1.8	<1	1	1	2	2	3	3	3
35–49	4	1.5	<1	1	1	1	3	3	3	3
50–64	0									
65+	1	2.0	0	2	2	2	2	2	2	2
2. MULTIPLE DX										
A. Not Operated										
0–19 Years	8	1.5	1	1	1	1	1	4	4	4
20–34	2	3.0	2	2	2	2	4	4	4	4
35–49	0									
50–64	5	3.6	22	1	1	2	2	12	12	12
65+	12	3.2	6	1	3	3	4	8	8	8
B. Operated										
0–19 Years	61	1.5	<1	1	1	1	2	2	2	5
20–34	9	3.6	10	1	1	2	3	9	9	9
35–49	8	4.2	13	1	2	2	6	11	11	11
50–64	10	2.2	1	1	2	2	3	4	4	4
65+	34	3.0	2	2	2	3	4	5	6	7
SUBTOTALS:										
1. SINGLE DX — A. Not Operated	9	1.3	<1	1	1	1	2	2	2	2
1. SINGLE DX — B. Operated	161	1.4	<1	1	1	1	2	2	2	3
2. MULTIPLE DX — A. Not Operated	27	2.8	7	1	1	2	4	8	8	12
2. MULTIPLE DX — B. Operated	122	2.3	3	1	1	2	3	4	6	9
1. SINGLE DX	170	1.4	<1	1	1	1	2	2	2	3
2. MULTIPLE DX	149	2.4	4	1	1	2	3	4	7	11
A. NOT OPERATED	36	2.4	6	1	1	2	3	4	8	12
B. OPERATED	283	1.8	2	1	1	2	2	3	4	9
TOTAL										
0–19 Years	228	1.4	<1	1	1	1	2	2	2	3
20–34	16	2.9	7	1	1	2	3	9	9	9
35–49	12	3.3	11	1	1	2	3	8	11	11
50–64	16	2.6	7	1	2	2	3	4	12	12
65+	47	3.0	3	2	2	3	4	5	7	8
GRAND TOTAL	319	1.9	2	1	1	2	2	3	4	9

813: RADIUS & ULNA FRACTURE

Type of Patients	Observed Patients	Avg. Stay	Vari- ance	10th	25th	50th	75th	90th	95th	99th
1. SINGLE DX										
A. Not Operated										
0–19 Years	377	1.1	<1	1	1	1	1	1	2	3
20–34	55	1.6	1	1	1	1	2	4	4	6
35–49	48	1.6	<1	1	1	1	2	3	4	5
50–64	32	1.8	5	1	1	1	1	3	9	10
65+	8	1.1	<1	1	1	1	1	2	2	2
B. Operated										
0–19 Years	812	1.5	<1	1	1	2	2	2	3	4
20–34	439	2.1	4	1	1	2	2	4	5	10
35–49	330	2.0	3	1	1	1	2	4	5	9
50–64	264	2.1	3	1	1	1	2	4	6	8
65+	79	1.7	<1	1	1	1	2	3	4	5
2. MULTIPLE DX										
A. Not Operated										
0–19 Years	220	1.5	2	1	1	1	2	2	3	7
20–34	159	2.2	4	1	1	1	3	4	6	12
35–49	185	2.3	5	1	1	1	3	4	7	11
50–64	228	2.7	9	1	1	2	3	5	7	20
65+	664	3.5	10	1	2	3	4	6	8	18
B. Operated										
0–19 Years	587	2.4	5	1	1	2	3	5	6	12
20–34	1,214	3.5	20	1	1	2	4	7	10	19
35–49	1,232	3.4	18	1	2	2	6	7	10	20
50–64	1,633	3.1	12	1	1	2	4	7	9	17
65+	2,275	3.3	10	1	1	2	4	6	8	14
SUBTOTALS:										
1. SINGLE DX — A. Not Operated	520	1.3	<1	1	1	1	1	2	3	5
1. SINGLE DX — B. Operated	1,924	1.8	2	1	1	1	2	3	4	8
2. MULTIPLE DX — A. Not Operated	1,456	2.8	8	1	1	2	3	5	7	14
2. MULTIPLE DX — B. Operated	6,941	3.2	13	1	1	2	4	6	9	17
1. SINGLE DX	2,444	1.7	2	1	1	1	2	3	4	8
2. MULTIPLE DX	8,397	3.2	12	1	1	2	4	6	8	17
A. NOT OPERATED	1,976	2.4	7	1	1	1	3	5	6	13
B. OPERATED	8,865	2.9	11	1	1	2	3	6	8	16
TOTAL										
0–19 Years	1,996	1.7	2	1	1	1	2	3	4	8
20–34	1,867	3.0	15	1	1	2	3	6	9	18
35–49	1,795	3.0	14	1	1	2	3	6	9	18
50–64	2,157	2.9	10	1	1	2	3	6	8	17
65+	3,026	3.3	10	1	1	3	5	6	8	14
GRAND TOTAL	10,841	2.8	10	1	1	2	3	6	8	15

Length of Stay by Diagnosis and Operation, Western Region, 2008

Western Region, October 2006–September 2007 Data, by Diagnosis

813.01: CL FX OLECRAN PROC ULNA

Type of Patients	Observed Patients	Avg. Stay	Variance	Percentiles 10th	25th	50th	75th	90th	95th	99th
1. SINGLE DX										
A. Not Operated										
0–19 Years	2	1.5	<1	1	1	2	2	2	2	2
20–34	3	2.0	3	1	1	1	4	4	4	4
35–49	2	2.0	2	1	1	3	3	3	3	3
50–64	1	1.0	0	1	1	1	1	1	1	1
65+	0									
B. Operated										
0–19 Years	24	1.3	<1	1	1	1	2	2	2	2
20–34	29	2.2	7	1	1	1	2	5	5	15
35–49	26	2.5	6	1	1	2	2	8	9	9
50–64	30	2.2	5	1	1	2	2	4	7	12
65+	12	1.7	1	1	2	2	2	4	4	4
2. MULTIPLE DX										
A. Not Operated										
0–19 Years	4	1.8	2	1	1	1	4	4	4	4
20–34	13	2.8	6	1	1	2	3	7	8	8
35–49	13	3.2	21	1	1	2	3	4	18	18
50–64	9	3.0	5	1	1	2	4	8	8	8
65+	44	4.0	27	1	2	3	4	5	13	31
B. Operated										
0–19 Years	24	2.0	2	1	1	1	2	4	5	6
20–34	59	3.7	38	1	2	2	3	6	18	37
35–49	90	3.3	14	1	1	2	4	7	12	26
50–64	168	2.9	8	1	1	2	4	6	7	16
65+	445	3.7	13	1	2	3	4	7	9	16
SUBTOTALS:										
1. SINGLE DX										
A. Not Operated	8	1.8	1	1	1	1	2	4	4	4
B. Operated	121	2.1	5	1	1	1	2	4	6	12
2. MULTIPLE DX										
A. Not Operated	83	3.5	19	1	1	2	4	5	13	31
B. Operated	786	3.4	13	1	1	2	4	7	9	18
1. SINGLE DX	129	2.0	4	1	1	1	2	4	6	12
2. MULTIPLE DX	869	3.4	14	1	1	2	4	7	9	18
A. NOT OPERATED	91	3.3	18	1	1	2	4	5	13	31
B. OPERATED	907	3.2	12	1	1	2	4	6	9	16
TOTAL										
0–19 Years	54	1.7	1	1	1	1	2	3	4	6
20–34	104	3.1	24	1	1	1	3	5	8	29
35–49	131	3.2	13	1	1	2	4	7	9	18
50–64	208	2.8	7	1	1	1	3	6	7	15
65+	501	3.7	14	1	1	3	4	7	9	16
GRAND TOTAL	998	3.3	13	1	1	2	4	6	9	18

813.05: CL FX RADIUS HEAD

Type of Patients	Observed Patients	Avg. Stay	Variance	Percentiles 10th	25th	50th	75th	90th	95th	99th
1. SINGLE DX										
A. Not Operated										
0–19 Years	6	1.3	<1	1	1	1	2	2	2	2
20–34	10	2.6	3	1	1	1	4	6	6	6
35–49	7	2.0	2	1	1	2	2	5	5	5
50–64	2	7.0	18	4	4	10	10	10	10	10
65+	0									
B. Operated										
0–19 Years	13	1.2	<1	1	1	1	1	2	2	2
20–34	23	2.2	5	1	1	1	2	4	5	9
35–49	19	2.1	4	1	1	1	2	6	8	9
50–64	9	2.0	3	1	1	1	2	4	6	12
65+	0									
2. MULTIPLE DX										
A. Not Operated										
0–19 Years	5	2.0	3	1	1	1	2	5	5	5
20–34	17	2.4	2	1	1	2	3	5	6	6
35–49	19	1.6	2	1	1	2	3	5	5	5
50–64	19	3.1	20	1	1	2	3	5	21	21
65+	36	2.8	2	2	2	3	3	4	6	8
B. Operated										
0–19 Years	14	1.9	2	1	1	1	2	5	5	5
20–34	60	4.1	110	1	1	2	3	6	9	76
35–49	80	3.3	25	1	1	2	3	7	9	40
50–64	79	2.7	5	1	1	2	3	6	8	16
65+	47	3.6	16	2	2	3	5	7	7	27
SUBTOTALS:										
1. SINGLE DX										
A. Not Operated	25	2.5	5	1	1	2	4	5	6	10
B. Operated	64	1.9	4	1	1	1	2	3	3	9
2. MULTIPLE DX										
A. Not Operated	96	2.5	6	1	1	2	3	4	5	21
B. Operated	280	3.3	35	1	1	2	3	6	8	34
1. SINGLE DX	89	2.1	4	1	1	1	2	4	6	10
2. MULTIPLE DX	376	3.1	27	1	1	2	3	6	7	27
A. NOT OPERATED	121	2.5	5	1	1	2	3	4	5	10
B. OPERATED	344	3.0	29	1	1	2	3	6	8	27
TOTAL										
0–19 Years	38	1.6	1	1	1	1	2	3	4	6
20–34	110	3.3	62	1	1	2	3	5	6	34
35–49	125	2.8	17	1	1	2	3	7	9	18
50–64	109	2.8	8	1	1	2	3	6	7	15
65+	83	3.2	10	1	2	3	4	7	9	27
GRAND TOTAL	465	2.9	23	1	1	2	3	5	7	21

813.11: OPN FX OLECRAN PROC ULNA

Type of Patients	Observed Patients	Avg. Stay	Variance	Percentiles 10th	25th	50th	75th	90th	95th	99th
1. SINGLE DX										
A. Not Operated										
0–19 Years	0									
20–34	1	3.0	0	3	3	3	3	3	3	3
35–49	1	1.0	0	1	1	1	1	1	1	1
50–64	0									
65+	0									
B. Operated										
0–19 Years	5	1.8	2	1	1	1	2	4	4	4
20–34	12	2.4	<1	1	2	2	3	3	4	4
35–49	13	1.9	1	1	1	2	2	4	4	4
50–64	10	2.0	1	1	1	2	3	3	4	4
65+	0									
2. MULTIPLE DX										
A. Not Operated										
0–19 Years	2	1.0	0	1	1	1	1	1	1	1
20–34	1	6.0	0	6	6	6	6	6	6	6
35–49	1	2.0	0	2	2	2	2	2	2	2
50–64	2	13.5	307	1	1	14	26	26	26	26
65+	1	6.0	0	6	6	6	6	6	6	6
B. Operated										
0–19 Years	17	2.8	3	1	2	3	3	6	7	7
20–34	63	6.0	83	1	2	3	7	14	23	58
35–49	60	4.7	24	1	2	3	6	10	18	26
50–64	55	4.6	52	1	2	3	5	9	12	52
65+	67	3.9	9	1	2	3	5	8	9	18
SUBTOTALS:										
1. SINGLE DX										
A. Not Operated	2	2.0	2	1	1	3	3	3	3	3
B. Operated	40	2.1	1	1	1	2	3	4	4	4
2. MULTIPLE DX										
A. Not Operated	7	6.1	82	1	1	2	6	26	26	26
B. Operated	262	4.7	39	1	2	3	5	9	14	30
1. SINGLE DX	42	2.1	1	1	1	2	3	4	4	4
2. MULTIPLE DX	269	4.7	40	1	2	3	5	9	14	30
A. NOT OPERATED	9	5.2	65	1	1	2	6	26	26	26
B. OPERATED	302	4.3	35	1	2	3	5	9	13	26
TOTAL										
0–19 Years	24	2.5	3	1	1	2	3	5	6	7
20–34	77	5.4	69	1	2	3	5	13	23	58
35–49	75	4.2	21	1	1	2	4	10	14	26
50–64	67	4.5	51	1	1	2	4	8	12	52
65+	68	3.9	9	1	2	3	5	8	9	18
GRAND TOTAL	311	4.3	36	1	2	3	5	9	13	26

Length of Stay by Diagnosis and Operation, Western Region, 2008

Western Region, October 2006–September 2007 Data, by Diagnosis

813.21: CL FX RADIUS SHAFT

Type of Patients	Observed Patients	Avg. Stay	Variance	10th	25th	50th	75th	90th	95th	99th
1. SINGLE DX										
A. Not Operated										
0–19 Years	7	1.9	3	1	1	1	2	6	6	6
20–34	3	2.0	<1	1	1	2	3	3	3	3
35–49	1	1.0	0	1	1	1	1	1	1	1
50–64	0									
65+	0									
B. Operated										
0–19 Years	18	1.2	<1	1	1	1	1	2	2	2
20–34	34	2.4	5	1	1	2	3	5	9	10
35–49	11	1.3	<1	1	1	1	2	2	2	2
50–64	3	1.7	<1	1	1	2	2	2	2	2
65+	4	1.3	<1	1	1	1	2	2	2	2
2. MULTIPLE DX										
A. Not Operated										
0–19 Years	3	1.3	<1	1	1	1	2	2	2	2
20–34	2	3.0	8	1	1	5	5	5	5	5
35–49	3	1.7	1	1	1	1	3	3	3	3
50–64	1	2.0	0	2	2	2	2	2	2	2
65+	7	2.7	<1	2	2	2	4	4	4	4
B. Operated										
0–19 Years	31	2.7	7	1	1	2	3	6	9	10
20–34	79	3.0	6	1	1	2	4	6	9	13
35–49	46	2.9	9	1	1	2	3	5	6	15
50–64	45	3.7	11	1	1	3	5	8	12	14
65+	24	2.6	5	1	1	2	3	4	7	11
SUBTOTALS:										
1. SINGLE DX										
A. Not Operated	11	1.8	2	1	1	1	1	3	6	6
B. Operated	70	1.8	3	1	1	1	2	3	5	10
2. MULTIPLE DX										
A. Not Operated	16	2.3	2	1	1	2	3	4	5	5
B. Operated	225	3.0	8	1	1	2	4	6	9	14
1. SINGLE DX	81	1.8	3	1	1	1	2	3	5	10
2. MULTIPLE DX	241	3.0	7	1	1	2	4	6	9	14
A. NOT OPERATED	27	2.1	2	1	1	2	3	4	5	6
B. OPERATED	295	2.7	7	1	1	2	3	6	9	14
TOTAL										
0–19 Years	59	2.1	4	1	1	1	2	5	9	10
20–34	118	2.8	5	1	1	2	3	6	9	10
35–49	61	2.5	7	1	1	2	3	4	6	15
50–64	49	3.5	10	1	1	2	5	8	12	14
65+	35	2.5	4	1	1	2	3	4	7	11
GRAND TOTAL	322	2.7	6	1	1	2	3	6	8	13

813.23: CL FX SHAFT RAD W ULNA

Type of Patients	Observed Patients	Avg. Stay	Variance	10th	25th	50th	75th	90th	95th	99th
1. SINGLE DX										
A. Not Operated										
0–19 Years	84	1.1	<1	1	1	1	1	1	2	6
20–34	1	1.0	0	1	1	1	1	1	1	1
35–49	0									
50–64	1	1.0	0	1	1	1	1	1	1	1
65+	0									
B. Operated										
0–19 Years	164	1.4	<1	1	1	2	2	2	3	4
20–34	55	2.1	2	1	1	2	2	3	6	9
35–49	17	1.7	<1	1	1	2	2	3	3	3
50–64	6	1.7	<1	1	1	2	2	3	3	3
65+	0									
2. MULTIPLE DX										
A. Not Operated										
0–19 Years	31	1.2	<1	1	1	1	2	2	2	4
20–34	1	2.0	0	2	2	2	2	2	2	2
35–49	0									
50–64	3	2.3	2	1	2	2	4	4	4	4
65+	4	3.5	6	1	5	5	6	6	6	6
B. Operated										
0–19 Years	83	2.0	2	1	1	2	2	3	5	8
20–34	110	3.0	12	1	1	2	4	6	7	15
35–49	58	3.7	13	1	2	2	4	8	11	20
50–64	54	3.6	21	1	2	2	3	6	13	30
65+	37	4.6	13	2	2	3	7	9	14	17
SUBTOTALS:										
1. SINGLE DX										
A. Not Operated	86	1.1	<1	1	1	1	1	1	2	6
B. Operated	242	1.6	<1	1	1	2	2	3	5	9
2. MULTIPLE DX										
A. Not Operated	39	1.5	<1	1	1	1	3	4	5	6
B. Operated	342	3.1	12	1	2	2	3	6	9	17
1. SINGLE DX	328	1.5	<1	1	1	1	2	3	5	9
2. MULTIPLE DX	381	3.0	11	1	1	2	3	6	8	17
A. NOT OPERATED	125	1.3	<1	1	1	1	2	4	5	6
B. OPERATED	584	2.5	8	1	1	2	3	5	7	15
TOTAL										
0–19 Years	362	1.4	<1	1	1	1	2	2	2	6
20–34	167	2.7	9	1	1	2	3	5	7	15
35–49	75	3.2	11	1	2	2	3	7	10	20
50–64	64	3.4	19	1	2	2	3	6	9	30
65+	41	4.5	12	2	2	3	6	7	11	17
GRAND TOTAL	709	2.3	7	1	1	1	2	4	7	14

813.33: OPN FX SHAFT RAD W ULNA

Type of Patients	Observed Patients	Avg. Stay	Variance	10th	25th	50th	75th	90th	95th	99th
1. SINGLE DX										
A. Not Operated										
0–19 Years	9	1.2	<1	1	1	1	1	3	3	3
20–34	0									
35–49	0									
50–64	0									
65+	0									
B. Operated										
0–19 Years	127	1.7	<1	1	1	2	2	3	3	4
20–34	29	2.1	3	1	1	2	2	4	5	10
35–49	11	2.0	1	1	1	2	3	3	4	4
50–64	3	2.0	0	2	2	2	2	2	2	2
65+	1	4.0	0	4	4	4	4	4	4	4
2. MULTIPLE DX										
A. Not Operated										
0–19 Years	3	1.3	<1	1	1	2	2	2	2	2
20–34	1	3.0	0	3	3	3	3	3	3	3
35–49	1	1.0	0	1	1	1	1	1	1	1
50–64	0									
65+	0									
B. Operated										
0–19 Years	69	2.6	5	1	1	2	3	5	7	16
20–34	98	4.5	21	1	2	3	5	12	16	22
35–49	41	5.9	72	1	2	3	5	15	20	45
50–64	41	4.6	25	1	1	3	6	10	13	24
65+	40	4.7	19	1	2	3	5	11	14	23
SUBTOTALS:										
1. SINGLE DX										
A. Not Operated	9	1.2	<1	1	1	1	1	3	3	3
B. Operated	171	1.8	1	1	1	2	2	3	3	5
2. MULTIPLE DX										
A. Not Operated	5	1.6	<1	1	1	1	1	3	3	3
B. Operated	289	4.3	25	1	2	3	4	10	14	24
1. SINGLE DX	180	1.8	1	1	1	1	2	3	3	5
2. MULTIPLE DX	294	4.3	25	1	1	3	4	10	14	24
A. NOT OPERATED	14	1.4	<1	1	1	1	1	3	3	3
B. OPERATED	460	3.4	18	1	1	2	3	7	11	22
TOTAL										
0–19 Years	208	2.0	2	1	1	2	2	3	4	7
20–34	128	4.0	18	1	1	2	4	10	14	20
35–49	53	5.0	58	1	2	2	4	11	20	45
50–64	44	4.4	23	1	1	2	5	10	13	24
65+	41	4.7	19	1	2	4	5	11	11	23
GRAND TOTAL	474	3.3	17	1	1	2	3	7	11	22

Length of Stay by Diagnosis and Operation, Western Region, 2008

Western Region, October 2006–September 2007 Data, by Diagnosis

813.41: CL COLLES' FRACTURE

Type of Patients	Observed Patients	Avg. Stay	Variance	10th	25th	50th	75th	90th	95th	99th
1. SINGLE DX										
A. Not Operated										
0–19 Years	15	1.1	<1	1	1	1	1	1	2	2
20–34	5	1.0	0	1	1	1	1	1	1	1
35–49	4	1.0	0	1	1	1	1	1	1	1
50–64	4	1.3	<1	1	1	1	2	2	2	2
65+	2	1.0	0	1	1	1	1	1	1	1
B. Operated										
0–19 Years	21	1.2	<1	1	1	1	1	2	2	2
20–34	26	1.6	<1	1	1	1	2	3	3	5
35–49	29	1.9	2	1	1	2	2	5	5	6
50–64	33	2.2	3	1	1	2	3	5	6	7
65+	6	1.3	<1	1	1	1	2	2	2	2
2. MULTIPLE DX										
A. Not Operated										
0–19 Years	14	1.3	<1	1	1	1	2	2	2	2
20–34	17	2.2	2	1	1	1	3	4	6	6
35–49	25	2.3	5	1	1	1	2	6	7	10
50–64	38	2.5	3	1	1	2	3	4	7	9
65+	120	3.4	7	1	2	3	4	5	8	18
B. Operated										
0–19 Years	12	1.5	<1	1	1	1	2	2	2	2
20–34	42	3.4	11	1	1	2	5	7	11	15
35–49	69	2.7	5	1	1	2	3	6	9	10
50–64	142	2.9	9	1	1	2	3	6	8	19
65+	217	3.0	7	1	2	2	4	7	8	12
SUBTOTALS:										
1. SINGLE DX										
A. Not Operated	30	1.1	<1	1	1	1	1	1	2	2
B. Operated	115	1.8	2	1	1	1	2	4	5	6
2. MULTIPLE DX										
A. Not Operated	214	2.9	6	1	1	2	4	5	7	10
B. Operated	482	3.0	8	1	1	2	4	6	8	15
1. SINGLE DX	145	1.6	1	1	1	1	2	2	5	6
2. MULTIPLE DX	696	2.9	7	1	1	2	4	6	8	15
A. NOT OPERATED	244	2.7	5	1	1	2	3	5	7	10
B. OPERATED	597	2.7	7	1	1	2	3	6	8	15
TOTAL										
0–19 Years	62	1.2	<1	1	1	1	1	2	2	2
20–34	90	2.5	6	1	1	1	3	5	7	15
35–49	127	2.4	4	1	1	2	3	5	7	10
50–64	217	2.7	7	1	1	2	3	5	7	16
65+	345	3.1	7	1	2	3	4	6	8	15
GRAND TOTAL	841	2.7	6	1	1	2	3	5	7	12

813.42: CL FX DISTAL RADIUS NEC

Type of Patients	Observed Patients	Avg. Stay	Variance	10th	25th	50th	75th	90th	95th	99th
1. SINGLE DX										
A. Not Operated										
0–19 Years	59	1.0	<1	1	1	1	1	1	1	2
20–34	15	1.1	<1	1	1	1	1	1	2	2
35–49	21	1.4	<1	1	1	1	2	2	2	4
50–64	12	1.2	<1	1	1	1	1	1	3	3
65+	4	1.0	0	1	1	1	1	1	1	1
B. Operated										
0–19 Years	60	1.5	<1	1	1	1	1	2	3	6
20–34	90	1.6	1	1	1	1	2	3	4	6
35–49	93	1.7	2	1	1	1	2	3	5	8
50–64	80	1.8	2	1	1	1	3	3	5	7
65+	27	1.2	<1	1	1	1	1	2	2	3
2. MULTIPLE DX										
A. Not Operated										
0–19 Years	45	1.6	4	1	1	1	2	2	3	14
20–34	43	2.0	4	1	1	1	2	3	4	12
35–49	54	2.4	5	1	1	2	3	7	8	9
50–64	82	2.4	3	1	1	2	3	5	6	9
65+	223	3.6	9	1	2	3	4	6	8	19
B. Operated										
0–19 Years	71	2.2	4	1	1	1	3	5	6	10
20–34	192	2.9	6	1	1	2	4	6	8	13
35–49	256	2.8	18	1	1	2	3	6	8	14
50–64	407	2.5	7	1	1	2	3	5	7	16
65+	548	2.7	5	1	2	2	3	6	8	10
SUBTOTALS:										
1. SINGLE DX										
A. Not Operated	111	1.1	<1	1	1	1	1	1	2	3
B. Operated	350	1.6	1	1	1	1	2	3	4	6
2. MULTIPLE DX										
A. Not Operated	447	2.9	7	1	1	2	3	6	7	14
B. Operated	1,474	2.7	8	1	1	2	3	5	8	12
1. SINGLE DX	461	1.5	1	1	1	1	2	2	4	6
2. MULTIPLE DX	1,921	2.7	8	1	1	2	3	5	7	12
A. NOT OPERATED	558	2.5	6	1	1	2	3	5	6	12
B. OPERATED	1,824	2.5	7	1	1	2	3	5	7	11
TOTAL										
0–19 Years	235	1.6	2	1	1	1	2	3	4	9
20–34	340	2.4	5	1	1	2	3	5	7	11
35–49	424	2.5	12	1	1	2	3	5	8	12
50–64	581	2.4	5	1	1	2	3	5	7	14
65+	802	2.9	6	1	2	2	4	6	7	11
GRAND TOTAL	2,382	2.5	7	1	1	2	3	5	7	12

813.44: CL FX LOW RADIUS W ULNA

Type of Patients	Observed Patients	Avg. Stay	Variance	10th	25th	50th	75th	90th	95th	99th
1. SINGLE DX										
A. Not Operated										
0–19 Years	142	1.1	<1	1	1	1	1	1	2	2
20–34	6	1.0	0	1	1	1	1	1	1	1
35–49	5	2.2	1	1	1	3	3	3	3	3
50–64	5	1.2	<1	1	1	1	1	2	2	2
65+	2	1.5	<1	1	1	2	2	2	2	2
B. Operated										
0–19 Years	162	1.3	<1	1	1	1	1	2	2	4
20–34	34	1.7	1	1	1	1	2	3	5	5
35–49	45	1.7	2	1	1	1	2	4	4	7
50–64	31	1.6	<1	1	1	1	2	2	3	6
65+	9	2.3	2	1	2	2	2	5	5	5
2. MULTIPLE DX										
A. Not Operated										
0–19 Years	62	1.6	1	1	1	1	2	2	4	7
20–34	24	1.6	<1	1	1	1	2	3	3	4
35–49	31	2.2	1	1	1	2	3	4	4	5
50–64	41	3.0	17	1	1	2	3	6	7	20
65+	138	3.7	15	1	2	3	4	7	8	13
B. Operated										
0–19 Years	105	2.3	7	1	1	2	3	4	6	16
20–34	151	3.2	6	1	1	2	4	6	8	10
35–49	149	3.1	13	1	1	2	4	7	9	20
50–64	216	2.9	6	1	1	2	4	7	8	11
65+	345	3.1	5	1	1	3	4	6	7	13
SUBTOTALS:										
1. SINGLE DX										
A. Not Operated	160	1.1	<1	1	1	1	1	2	2	3
B. Operated	281	1.5	<1	1	1	1	2	2	3	5
2. MULTIPLE DX										
A. Not Operated	296	2.8	11	1	1	2	3	5	7	19
B. Operated	966	3.0	7	1	1	2	4	5	8	13
1. SINGLE DX	441	1.3	<1	1	1	1	1	2	3	5
2. MULTIPLE DX	1,262	3.0	8	1	1	2	4	6	8	13
A. NOT OPERATED	456	2.2	8	1	1	1	3	4	6	13
B. OPERATED	1,247	2.6	6	1	1	2	3	6	7	11
TOTAL										
0–19 Years	471	1.5	2	1	1	1	2	2	3	7
20–34	215	2.7	5	1	1	2	3	5	7	10
35–49	230	2.7	9	1	1	2	3	5	8	14
50–64	293	2.8	8	1	1	2	4	6	8	11
65+	494	3.3	8	1	2	3	4	6	8	13
GRAND TOTAL	1,703	2.5	6	1	1	2	3	5	7	11

Length of Stay by Diagnosis and Operation, Western Region, 2008

Western Region, October 2006–September 2007 Data, by Diagnosis

813.52: OPN FX DISTAL RADIUS NEC

Type of Patients	Observed Patients	Avg. Stay	Vari- ance	10th	25th	50th	75th	90th	95th	99th
1. SINGLE DX										
A. Not Operated										
0–19 Years	2	1.5	<1	1	1	1	2	2	2	2
20–34	1	1.0	0	1	1	1	1	1	1	1
35–49	1	1.0	0	1	1	1	1	1	1	1
50–64	1	1.0	0	1	1	1	1	1	1	1
65+	0									
B. Operated										
0–19 Years	3	1.3	<1	1	1	1	2	2	2	2
20–34	12	2.1	2	1	1	1	2	4	6	6
35–49	14	1.9	2	1	1	1	2	4	6	6
50–64	5	1.6	<1	1	1	2	2	2	2	2
65+	6	2.0	<1	1	2	2	2	3	3	3
2. MULTIPLE DX										
A. Not Operated										
0–19 Years	4	1.5	<1	1	1	1	1	3	3	3
20–34	1	4.0	0	4	4	4	4	4	4	4
35–49	2	1.5	<1	1	1	1	1	2	2	2
50–64	1	5.0	0	5	5	5	5	5	5	5
65+	2	4.0	8	2	2	4	6	6	6	6
B. Operated										
0–19 Years	7	2.4	2	1	2	2	3	4	5	5
20–34	40	3.6	6	1	1	3	5	7	8	12
35–49	48	4.4	21	1	1	3	5	8	14	22
50–64	43	3.6	21	1	1	3	4	6	15	22
65+	69	3.2	16	1	2	2	4	5	6	33
SUBTOTALS:										
1. SINGLE DX										
A. Not Operated	5	1.2	<1	1	1	1	1	2	2	2
B. Operated	40	1.9	2	1	1	1	2	3	6	6
2. MULTIPLE DX										
A. Not Operated	10	2.6	3	1	1	2	4	6	6	6
B. Operated	207	3.6	16	1	2	2	4	6	8	22
1. SINGLE DX	45	1.8	1	1	1	1	2	3	4	6
2. MULTIPLE DX	217	3.5	15	1	1	2	4	6	8	22
A. NOT OPERATED	15	2.1	3	1	1	1	3	5	6	6
B. OPERATED	247	3.3	14	1	1	2	4	6	8	22
TOTAL										
0–19 Years	16	1.9	1	1	1	2	2	3	5	5
20–34	54	3.2	6	1	1	3	5	6	8	12
35–49	65	3.7	17	1	1	2	5	7	13	22
50–64	50	3.3	19	1	1	2	3	6	15	22
65+	77	3.1	15	1	2	2	3	5	6	33
GRAND TOTAL	262	3.2	13	1	1	2	4	6	7	22

813.54: OPN FX LOW RADIUS W ULNA

Type of Patients	Observed Patients	Avg. Stay	Vari- ance	10th	25th	50th	75th	90th	95th	99th
1. SINGLE DX										
A. Not Operated										
0–19 Years	6	1.3	<1	1	1	1	1	3	3	3
20–34	1	3.0	0	3	3	3	3	3	3	3
35–49	0									
50–64	0									
65+	0									
B. Operated										
0–19 Years	91	1.7	2	1	1	2	2	3	4	11
20–34	28	3.2	16	1	2	2	3	4	10	22
35–49	12	3.3	15	1	2	2	3	4	15	15
50–64	14	2.5	5	1	1	2	3	5	8	8
65+	5	1.6	<1	1	1	2	2	2	2	2
2. MULTIPLE DX										
A. Not Operated										
0–19 Years	8	1.5	<1	2	2	2	2	2	2	2
20–34	1	2.0	0	2	2	2	2	2	2	2
35–49	2	1.0	0	1	1	1	1	1	1	1
50–64	4	2.5	<1	2	2	2	3	3	3	3
65+	7	2.3	3	1	1	2	4	5	5	5
B. Operated										
0–19 Years	52	2.5	10	1	2	2	3	4	5	23
20–34	53	3.9	11	1	2	3	4	8	11	18
35–49	82	4.1	11	1	2	3	5	9	11	17
50–64	107	3.5	14	1	2	3	4	7	12	17
65+	213	3.6	25	1	2	3	4	6	8	21
SUBTOTALS:										
1. SINGLE DX										
A. Not Operated	7	1.6	<1	1	1	1	1	3	3	3
B. Operated	150	2.2	6	1	1	2	2	3	4	15
2. MULTIPLE DX										
A. Not Operated	22	1.9	1	1	1	2	2	3	4	5
B. Operated	507	3.6	17	1	2	3	4	7	10	18
1. SINGLE DX	157	2.2	6	1	1	2	2	3	4	15
2. MULTIPLE DX	529	3.5	17	1	2	3	4	7	10	18
A. NOT OPERATED	29	1.8	1	1	1	2	2	3	4	5
B. OPERATED	657	3.3	15	1	2	3	4	6	9	18
TOTAL										
0–19 Years	157	2.0	5	1	1	2	2	3	4	11
20–34	83	3.6	12	1	2	3	4	7	11	22
35–49	96	3.9	11	1	2	3	5	9	11	17
50–64	125	3.4	13	1	1	3	4	6	10	17
65+	225	3.5	24	1	2	3	4	6	7	21
GRAND TOTAL	686	3.2	15	1	2	3	4	6	9	18

814: CARPAL FRACTURE

Type of Patients	Observed Patients	Avg. Stay	Vari- ance	10th	25th	50th	75th	90th	95th	99th
1. SINGLE DX										
A. Not Operated										
0–19 Years	0									
20–34	5	1.0	0	1	1	1	1	1	1	1
35–49	0									
50–64	1	2.0	0	2	2	2	2	2	2	2
65+	0									
B. Operated										
0–19 Years	5	1.0	0	1	1	1	1	1	1	1
20–34	6	1.5	<1	1	1	1	2	3	3	3
35–49	4	1.0	0	1	1	1	1	1	1	1
50–64	1	3.0	0	3	3	3	3	3	3	3
65+	0									
2. MULTIPLE DX										
A. Not Operated										
0–19 Years	5	1.6	2	1	1	1	1	4	4	4
20–34	15	2.2	2	1	1	2	3	4	6	6
35–49	15	2.3	3	1	1	2	3	5	6	6
50–64	12	2.7	6	1	1	3	3	3	10	10
65+	31	4.2	23	1	2	3	5	7	11	27
B. Operated										
0–19 Years	30	2.8	7	1	1	2	2	3	9	13
20–34	74	2.6	6	1	1	2	3	6	9	11
35–49	38	3.1	5	1	1	3	4	7	8	9
50–64	21	2.8	5	1	2	2	5	5	7	8
65+	11	2.5	1	1	2	2	3	4	5	5
SUBTOTALS:										
1. SINGLE DX										
A. Not Operated	6	1.2	<1	1	1	1	1	2	2	2
B. Operated	16	1.3	<1	1	1	1	1	3	3	3
2. MULTIPLE DX										
A. Not Operated	78	3.0	12	1	1	2	4	6	7	27
B. Operated	174	2.8	5	1	1	2	3	6	8	11
1. SINGLE DX	22	1.3	<1	1	1	1	1	2	3	3
2. MULTIPLE DX	252	2.8	7	1	1	2	3	6	8	11
A. NOT OPERATED	84	2.9	11	1	1	2	3	5	7	27
B. OPERATED	190	2.6	5	1	1	2	3	6	8	11
TOTAL										
0–19 Years	40	2.5	6	1	1	2	2	5	9	13
20–34	100	2.4	5	1	1	2	3	6	9	11
35–49	57	2.7	4	1	1	2	4	6	7	9
50–64	35	2.7	5	1	2	3	5	6	8	10
65+	42	3.7	18	1	2	3	4	6	7	27
GRAND TOTAL	274	2.7	7	1	1	2	3	6	8	11

Length of Stay by Diagnosis and Operation, Western Region, 2008

Western Region, October 2006–September 2007 Data, by Diagnosis

815: METACARPAL FRACTURE

Type of Patients	Observed Patients	Avg. Stay	Vari-ance	Percentiles						
				10th	25th	50th	75th	90th	95th	99th
1. SINGLE DX										
A. Not Operated										
0–19 Years	4	1.0	0	1	1	1	1	1	1	1
20–34	10	1.3	<1	1	1	1	2	2	2	2
35–49	4	1.5	<1	1	1	1	2	2	2	2
50–64	3	2.7	2	1	1	3	4	4	4	4
65+	1	1.0	0	1	1	1	1	1	1	1
B. Operated										
0–19 Years	18	1.6	<1	1	1	1	2	3	3	3
20–34	45	1.5	<1	1	1	1	2	2	3	5
35–49	26	2.1	4	1	1	1	2	4	7	10
50–64	11	2.3	3	1	1	2	3	4	6	6
65+	2	1.0	0	1	1	1	1	1	1	1
2. MULTIPLE DX										
A. Not Operated										
0–19 Years	20	1.3	<1	1	1	1	1	2	4	4
20–34	36	1.7	1	1	1	1	2	4	5	5
35–49	18	2.7	2	1	2	2	3	5	5	5
50–64	22	2.1	3	1	1	2	2	4	5	8
65+	25	3.6	12	1	1	3	4	7	13	14
B. Operated										
0–19 Years	52	3.0	17	1	1	2	3	5	9	25
20–34	171	2.9	9	1	1	2	3	6	9	18
35–49	120	2.7	8	1	1	2	3	5	7	15
50–64	87	3.0	6	1	1	2	4	6	7	18
65+	30	3.4	8	1	2	2	5	7	10	13
SUBTOTALS:										
1. SINGLE DX										
A. Not Operated	22	1.5	<1	1	1	1	2	2	3	4
B. Operated	102	1.7	2	1	1	1	2	3	4	7
2. MULTIPLE DX										
A. Not Operated	121	2.3	4	1	1	2	3	4	5	13
B. Operated	460	2.9	9	1	1	2	3	6	7	18
1. SINGLE DX	124	1.7	2	1	1	1	2	3	4	7
2. MULTIPLE DX	581	2.8	8	1	1	2	3	5	7	17
A. NOT OPERATED	143	2.1	4	1	1	1	2	4	5	13
B. OPERATED	562	2.7	8	1	1	2	3	5	7	17
TOTAL										
0–19 Years	94	2.3	10	1	1	1	2	4	7	25
20–34	262	2.5	6	1	1	2	3	4	6	15
35–49	168	2.6	6	1	1	2	3	5	7	15
50–64	123	2.8	5	1	1	2	4	5	7	8
65+	58	3.4	10	1	1	2	4	7	13	14
GRAND TOTAL	705	2.6	7	1	1	2	3	5	7	15

816: FRACTURE PHALANGES HAND

Type of Patients	Observed Patients	Avg. Stay	Vari-ance	Percentiles						
				10th	25th	50th	75th	90th	95th	99th
1. SINGLE DX										
A. Not Operated										
0–19 Years	5	1.2	<1	1	1	1	1	2	2	2
20–34	5	1.2	<1	1	1	1	1	2	2	2
35–49	7	1.4	<1	1	1	1	2	3	3	3
50–64	1	2.0	0	2	2	2	2	2	2	2
65+	0									
B. Operated										
0–19 Years	41	1.6	1	1	1	1	2	2	3	7
20–34	58	1.8	1	1	1	1	2	3	4	6
35–49	46	1.7	2	1	1	1	2	4	5	7
50–64	14	1.4	<1	1	1	1	2	2	3	3
65+	4	1.5	<1	1	2	2	2	2	2	2
2. MULTIPLE DX										
A. Not Operated										
0–19 Years	9	2.2	3	1	1	1	3	6	6	6
20–34	32	1.7	1	1	1	1	2	3	4	5
35–49	26	2.1	2	1	2	2	3	4	6	7
50–64	24	2.3	2	1	2	2	3	5	6	6
65+	26	2.7	3	1	2	2	4	5	6	8
B. Operated										
0–19 Years	97	2.3	5	1	1	2	2	4	7	17
20–34	284	2.2	6	1	1	2	2	5	5	15
35–49	228	2.4	6	1	1	2	3	5	6	15
50–64	192	2.1	4	1	1	1	2	4	7	11
65+	106	2.3	4	1	1	2	3	5	6	8
SUBTOTALS:										
1. SINGLE DX										
A. Not Operated	18	1.3	<1	1	1	1	2	2	3	3
B. Operated	163	1.7	1	1	1	1	2	3	4	7
2. MULTIPLE DX										
A. Not Operated	117	2.2	2	1	1	2	3	4	6	7
B. Operated	907	2.2	5	1	1	2	3	5	6	15
1. SINGLE DX	181	1.6	1	1	1	1	2	3	4	7
2. MULTIPLE DX	1,024	2.2	5	1	1	2	3	5	6	14
A. NOT OPERATED	135	2.0	2	1	1	1	3	4	6	7
B. OPERATED	1,070	2.2	5	1	1	2	3	5	6	14
TOTAL										
0–19 Years	152	2.0	4	1	1	1	2	4	5	10
20–34	379	2.1	5	1	1	1	2	4	5	15
35–49	307	2.2	5	1	1	1	2	5	6	15
50–64	231	2.1	4	1	1	2	3	5	6	10
65+	136	2.4	4	1	2	2	3	5	6	8
GRAND TOTAL	1,205	2.1	5	1	1	1	2	4	5	13

816.11: OP FX MID/PROX PHAL HAND

Type of Patients	Observed Patients	Avg. Stay	Vari-ance	Percentiles						
				10th	25th	50th	75th	90th	95th	99th
1. SINGLE DX										
A. Not Operated										
0–19 Years	1	1.0	0	1	1	1	1	1	1	1
20–34	2	1.5	<1	1	1	2	2	2	2	2
35–49	2	2.5	<1	2	2	2	3	3	3	3
50–64	0									
65+	0									
B. Operated										
0–19 Years	14	1.2	<1	1	1	1	2	2	2	2
20–34	33	1.7	<1	1	1	1	2	3	4	4
35–49	19	1.7	2	1	1	1	2	4	6	6
50–64	6	1.7	<1	1	1	2	2	3	3	3
65+	3	1.7	<1	1	1	2	2	2	2	2
2. MULTIPLE DX										
A. Not Operated										
0–19 Years	2	1.0	0	1	1	1	1	1	1	1
20–34	9	1.3	<1	1	1	1	1	3	3	3
35–49	5	3.4	5	1	2	3	4	7	7	7
50–64	4	2.0	<1	1	2	2	3	3	3	3
65+	2	1.5	<1	1	1	2	2	2	2	2
B. Operated										
0–19 Years	47	2.3	4	1	1	2	2	4	5	10
20–34	148	2.2	6	1	1	1	2	4	5	15
35–49	114	2.4	6	1	1	2	3	5	6	15
50–64	90	2.1	3	1	1	1	3	4	6	8
65+	53	2.6	5	1	1	2	3	5	7	14
SUBTOTALS:										
1. SINGLE DX										
A. Not Operated	5	1.8	<1	1	1	2	2	2	3	3
B. Operated	75	1.6	<1	1	1	1	2	3	4	6
2. MULTIPLE DX										
A. Not Operated	22	1.9	2	1	1	1	2	3	4	7
B. Operated	452	2.3	5	1	1	1	3	4	6	14
1. SINGLE DX	80	1.6	<1	1	1	1	2	3	3	6
2. MULTIPLE DX	474	2.2	5	1	1	1	3	4	6	14
A. NOT OPERATED	27	1.9	2	1	1	1	2	3	4	7
B. OPERATED	527	2.2	4	1	1	1	2	4	5	13
TOTAL										
0–19 Years	64	2.0	3	1	1	1	2	4	5	10
20–34	192	2.0	5	1	1	1	2	4	5	15
35–49	140	2.3	5	1	1	1	3	4	6	15
50–64	100	2.1	4	1	1	1	2	4	6	8
65+	58	2.5	5	1	2	2	3	5	7	14
GRAND TOTAL	554	2.2	4	1	1	1	2	4	5	13

Length of Stay by Diagnosis and Operation, Western Region, 2008

Western Region, October 2006–September 2007 Data, by Diagnosis

816.12: OP FX DISTAL PHAL HAND

Type of Patients	Observed Patients	Avg. Stay	Vari-ance	10th	25th	50th	75th	90th	95th	99th
1. SINGLE DX										
A. Not Operated										
0–19 Years	0									
20–34	0									
35–49	1	1.0	0	1	1	1	1	1	1	1
50–64	1	2.0	0	2	2	2	2	2	2	2
65+	0									
B. Operated										
0–19 Years	9	1.4	<1	1	1	1	2	2	2	2
20–34	6	1.2	<1	1	1	1	1	1	2	2
35–49	10	1.8	2	1	1	1	2	4	5	5
50–64	4	1.3	<1	1	1	1	1	2	2	2
65+	0									
2. MULTIPLE DX										
A. Not Operated										
0–19 Years	2	2.5	4	1	1	1	1	4	4	4
20–34	5	2.4	3	1	1	2	2	3	5	5
35–49	6	1.5	<1	1	1	1	1	2	3	3
50–64	5	1.4	<1	1	1	1	1	2	2	2
65+	2	1.5	<1	1	1	2	2	2	2	2
B. Operated										
0–19 Years	32	2.0	8	1	1	1	1	2	3	17
20–34	66	2.3	8	1	1	1	2	3	4	19
35–49	64	1.8	2	1	1	1	2	2	4	7
50–64	68	1.6	1	1	1	1	2	3	4	5
65+	25	1.8	2	1	1	1	2	4	5	5
SUBTOTALS:										
1. SINGLE DX — A. Not Operated	2	1.5	<1	1	1	2	2	2	2	2
1. SINGLE DX — B. Operated	29	1.5	<1	1	2	1	1	2	4	5
2. MULTIPLE DX — A. Not Operated	20	1.8	1	1	1	1	2	2	3	4
2. MULTIPLE DX — B. Operated	255	1.9	4	1	1	1	2	4	5	13
1. SINGLE DX	31	1.5	<1	1	1	1	2	2	4	5
2. MULTIPLE DX	275	1.9	4	1	1	1	2	4	5	13
A. NOT OPERATED	22	1.8	1	1	1	1	2	3	4	5
B. OPERATED	284	1.9	4	1	1	1	2	4	5	13
TOTAL										
0–19 Years	43	1.9	6	1	1	1	2	3	4	17
20–34	77	2.2	7	1	1	1	2	4	5	19
35–49	81	1.8	2	1	1	1	2	4	5	7
50–64	78	1.6	<1	1	1	1	2	3	4	5
65+	27	1.8	1	1	1	1	2	4	5	5
GRAND TOTAL	306	1.9	4	1	1	1	2	4	5	8

817: MULTIPLE HAND FRACTURES

Type of Patients	Observed Patients	Avg. Stay	Vari-ance	10th	25th	50th	75th	90th	95th	99th
1. SINGLE DX										
A. Not Operated										
0–19 Years	2	2.0	2		1		2	3	3	3
20–34	0									
35–49	1	2.0	0		2		2	2	2	2
50–64	0									
65+	0									
B. Operated										
0–19 Years	4	2.5	3	1	2	2	5	5	5	5
20–34	5	1.4	<1	1	1	1	2	2	2	2
35–49	3	2.3	<1	2	2	2	3	3	3	3
50–64	0									
65+	1	1.0	0	1	1	1	1	1	1	1
2. MULTIPLE DX										
A. Not Operated										
0–19 Years	1	1.0	0	1	1	1	1	1	1	1
20–34	1	1.0	0	1	1	1	1	1	1	1
35–49	0									
50–64	1	1.0	0	1	1	1	1	1	1	1
65+	3	2.0	<1	1	1	2	3	3	3	3
B. Operated										
0–19 Years	12	5.1	22	2	2	3	5	13	14	14
20–34	25	6.7	79	1	2	4	6	18	30	35
35–49	16	3.5	24	1	1	2	2	6	21	21
50–64	10	2.2	2	1	1	2	3	5	5	5
65+	6	7.2	105	2	2	3	5	28	28	28
SUBTOTALS:										
1. SINGLE DX — A. Not Operated	3	2.0	<1	1	1	2	3	3	3	3
1. SINGLE DX — B. Operated	13	1.9	1	1	1	2	2	3	5	5
2. MULTIPLE DX — A. Not Operated	6	1.5	<1	1	1	1	1	2	3	3
2. MULTIPLE DX — B. Operated	69	5.1	48	1	2	3	5	14	21	35
1. SINGLE DX	16	1.9	1	1	1	2	2	3	5	5
2. MULTIPLE DX	75	4.8	45	1	1	2	5	13	21	35
A. NOT OPERATED	9	1.7	<1	1	1	1	2	3	3	3
B. OPERATED	82	4.6	42	1	1	2	4	11	18	35
TOTAL										
0–19 Years	19	4.0	16	1	2	3	5	13	14	14
20–34	31	5.7	68	1	1	2	5	16	30	35
35–49	20	3.3	19	1	1	2	3	5	6	21
50–64	11	2.1	2	1	1	2	3	4	5	5
65+	10	5.0	66	1	2	2	3	5	28	28
GRAND TOTAL	91	4.3	38	1	1	2	4	10	18	35

818: FRACTURE ARM MULT/NOS

Type of Patients	Observed Patients	Avg. Stay	Vari-ance	10th	25th	50th	75th	90th	95th	99th
1. SINGLE DX										
A. Not Operated										
0–19 Years	0									
20–34	0									
35–49	0									
50–64	0									
65+										
B. Operated										
0–19 Years	0									
20–34	0									
35–49	0									
50–64										
65+	0									
2. MULTIPLE DX										
A. Not Operated										
0–19 Years	0									
20–34	0									
35–49	0									
50–64										
65+	0									
B. Operated										
0–19 Years	0									
20–34	0									
35–49	0									
50–64	0									
65+	0									
SUBTOTALS:										
1. SINGLE DX — A. Not Operated	0									
1. SINGLE DX — B. Operated	0									
2. MULTIPLE DX — A. Not Operated	0									
2. MULTIPLE DX — B. Operated	0									
1. SINGLE DX	0									
2. MULTIPLE DX	0									
A. NOT OPERATED	0									
B. OPERATED	0									
TOTAL										
0–19 Years	0									
20–34	0									
35–49	0									
50–64	0									
65+	0									
GRAND TOTAL	0									

Length of Stay by Diagnosis and Operation, Western Region, 2008

819: FX ARMS W RIB/STERNUM

Type of Patients	Observed Patients	Avg. Stay	Vari- ance	Percentiles						
				10th	25th	50th	75th	90th	95th	99th
1. SINGLE DX										
A. *Not Operated*										
0–19 Years	0									
20–34	0									
35–49	0									
50–64	0									
65+	0									
B. *Operated*										
0–19 Years	0									
20–34	0									
35–49	0									
50–64	0									
65+	0									
2. MULTIPLE DX										
A. *Not Operated*										
0–19 Years	0									
20–34	0									
35–49	0									
50–64	0									
65+	0									
B. *Operated*										
0–19 Years	0									
20–34	0									
35–49	0									
50–64	0									
65+	0									
SUBTOTALS:										
1. SINGLE DX										
A. *Not Operated*	0									
B. *Operated*	0									
2. MULTIPLE DX										
A. *Not Operated*	0									
B. *Operated*	0									
1. SINGLE DX	0									
2. MULTIPLE DX	0									
A. NOT OPERATED	0									
B. OPERATED	0									
TOTAL										
0–19 Years	0									
20–34	0									
35–49	0									
50–64	0									
65+	0									
GRAND TOTAL	0									

820: FRACTURE NECK OF FEMUR

Type of Patients	Observed Patients	Avg. Stay	Vari- ance	Percentiles						
				10th	25th	50th	75th	90th	95th	99th
1. SINGLE DX										
A. *Not Operated*										
0–19 Years	20	2.4	8	1	1	2	3	3	4	14
20–34	4	1.5	<1	1	1	2	2	2	2	2
35–49	7	2.4	3	1	1	2	3	6	6	6
50–64	4	1.3	<1	1	1	1	1	2	2	2
65+	12	3.2	5	1	1	3	5	5	8	8
B. *Operated*										
0–19 Years	95	2.5	2	1	1	2	3	4	5	9
20–34	83	2.8	2	1	2	3	3	5	5	9
35–49	111	3.0	3	1	2	3	4	5	6	10
50–64	187	3.4	4	1	2	3	4	5	7	11
65+	195	3.9	2	3	3	4	4	5	6	9
2. MULTIPLE DX										
A. *Not Operated*										
0–19 Years	28	4.2	38	1	2	2	4	9	17	31
20–34	24	2.6	1	1	2	3	3	4	4	6
35–49	73	4.4	14	1	2	3	6	10	12	21
50–64	193	5.5	32	1	2	3	7	12	17	28
65+	2,067	4.7	25	1	2	3	5	9	14	24
B. *Operated*										
0–19 Years	151	4.4	10	1	2	4	6	8	10	16
20–34	398	6.4	32	2	3	5	8	12	18	29
35–49	906	6.1	34	2	3	4	7	12	16	27
50–64	4,061	6.1	24	3	4	5	7	11	14	25
65+	37,215	5.7	13	3	4	5	7	9	11	20
SUBTOTALS:										
1. SINGLE DX										
A. *Not Operated*	47	2.5	5	1	1	2	3	5	6	14
B. *Operated*	671	3.3	3	1	2	3	4	5	6	9
2. MULTIPLE DX										
A. *Not Operated*	2,385	4.8	25	1	2	3	5	9	14	24
B. *Operated*	42,731	5.8	14	3	4	5	7	9	12	20
1. SINGLE DX	718	3.2	3	1	2	3	4	5	6	9
2. MULTIPLE DX	45,116	5.7	15	3	4	5	7	9	12	21
A. NOT OPERATED	2,432	4.7	25	1	2	3	5	9	14	24
B. OPERATED	43,402	5.7	14	3	4	5	7	9	12	20
TOTAL										
0–19 Years	294	3.6	11	1	2	3	4	7	9	17
20–34	509	5.6	28	2	3	4	6	11	14	23
35–49	1,097	5.6	30	2	3	4	6	11	15	26
50–64	4,445	5.9	24	2	3	5	7	11	14	25
65+	39,489	5.7	13	3	4	5	6	9	12	20
GRAND TOTAL	45,834	5.7	15	3	4	5	6	9	12	21

820.00: CLSD FX FEM INTRACAP NOS

Type of Patients	Observed Patients	Avg. Stay	Vari- ance	Percentiles						
				10th	25th	50th	75th	90th	95th	99th
1. SINGLE DX										
A. *Not Operated*										
0–19 Years	0									
20–34	0									
35–49	0									
50–64	0									
65+	0									
B. *Operated*										
0–19 Years	0									
20–34	1	3.0	0	3	3	3	3	3	3	3
35–49	1	2.0	0	2	2	2	2	2	2	2
50–64	6	3.8	3	3	3	3	4	7	7	7
65+	3	3.0	0	3	3	3	3	3	3	3
2. MULTIPLE DX										
A. *Not Operated*										
0–19 Years	0									
20–34	0									
35–49	0									
50–64	0									
65+	3	4.7	9	2	2	4	8	8	8	8
B. *Operated*										
0–19 Years	0									
20–34	3	3.0	4	1	1	3	5	5	5	5
35–49	2	2.5	<1	2	2	2	3	3	3	3
50–64	32	5.7	15	2	3	5	6	10	17	17
65+	346	5.4	8	3	4	5	6	8	11	16
SUBTOTALS:										
1. SINGLE DX										
A. *Not Operated*	0									
B. *Operated*	11	3.4	2	3	3	3	3	4	7	7
2. MULTIPLE DX										
A. *Not Operated*	3	4.7	9	2	2	4	8	8	8	8
B. *Operated*	383	5.4	9	3	4	5	6	8	11	17
1. SINGLE DX	11	3.4	2	3	3	3	3	4	7	7
2. MULTIPLE DX	386	5.4	9	3	4	5	6	8	11	17
A. NOT OPERATED	3	4.7	9	2	2	4	8	8	8	8
B. OPERATED	394	5.4	8	3	4	5	6	8	11	17
TOTAL										
0–19 Years	0									
20–34	4	3.0	3	1	1	2	3	5	5	5
35–49	3	2.3	<1	2	2	2	3	3	3	3
50–64	38	5.4	14	2	3	5	6	10	17	17
65+	352	5.4	8	3	4	5	5	8	11	16
GRAND TOTAL	397	5.4	8	3	4	5	6	8	11	17

Length of Stay by Diagnosis and Operation, Western Region, 2008

Western Region, October 2006–September 2007 Data, by Diagnosis

820.02: CL FX MIDCERVICAL FEMUR

Type of Patients	Observed Patients	Avg. Stay	Variance	10th	25th	50th	75th	90th	95th	99th
1. SINGLE DX										
A. Not Operated										
0–19 Years	0									
20–34	0									
35–49	0									
50–64	0									
65+	0									
B. Operated										
0–19 Years	3	1.3	<1	1	1	1	2	2	2	2
20–34	2	1.5	<1	1	1	1	2	2	2	2
35–49	3	3.7	1	3	3	3	5	5	5	5
50–64	4	4.0	3	2	4	4	6	6	6	6
65+	5	5.6	7	3	4	5	6	10	10	10
2. MULTIPLE DX										
A. Not Operated										
0–19 Years	0									
20–34	0									
35–49	2	7.5	83	1	1	1	14	14	14	14
50–64	0									
65+	17	6.1	85	1	2	4	5	12	14	40
B. Operated										
0–19 Years	2	3.5	<1	3	3	3	4	4	4	4
20–34	7	4.4	7	2	3	4	5	10	10	10
35–49	27	5.4	25	2	3	4	6	11	16	25
50–64	96	5.5	16	2	3	4	6	12	15	21
65+	725	6.0	19	3	4	5	7	10	12	21
SUBTOTALS:										
1. SINGLE DX										
A. Not Operated	0									
B. Operated	17	3.7	5	1	2	3	5	5	6	10
2. MULTIPLE DX										
A. Not Operated	19	6.3	80	1	1	3	7	14	14	40
B. Operated	857	5.9	19	3	4	5	7	10	12	21
1. SINGLE DX	17	3.7	5	1	2	3	5	6	6	10
2. MULTIPLE DX	876	5.9	20	3	4	5	7	10	12	22
A. NOT OPERATED	19	6.3	80	1	1	3	7	14	40	40
B. OPERATED	874	5.8	19	3	4	5	6	10	12	21
TOTAL										
0–19 Years	5	2.2	2	1	1	2	3	4	4	4
20–34	9	3.8	7	1	2	3	4	10	10	10
35–49	32	5.4	24	2	2	4	5	11	16	25
50–64	100	5.5	15	2	3	4	6	11	15	21
65+	747	6.0	21	3	4	5	7	10	12	22
GRAND TOTAL	893	5.8	20	3	4	5	6	10	12	22

820.03: CLSD FX BASE FEMORAL NK

Type of Patients	Observed Patients	Avg. Stay	Variance	10th	25th	50th	75th	90th	95th	99th
1. SINGLE DX										
A. Not Operated										
0–19 Years	0									
20–34	0									
35–49	0									
50–64	0									
65+	2	5.0	18	2	2	8	8	8	8	8
B. Operated										
0–19 Years	4	2.3	<1	1	1	2	3	3	3	3
20–34	8	3.6	1	2	3	3	4	5	5	5
35–49	10	4.0	17	1	1	3	4	6	15	15
50–64	10	4.8	24	1	2	3	5	7	18	18
65+	9	4.1	4	3	3	3	4	9	9	9
2. MULTIPLE DX										
A. Not Operated										
0–19 Years	1	1.0	0	1	1	1	1	1	1	1
20–34	0									
35–49	2	11.6	179	2	2	21	21	21	21	21
50–64	9	8.2	66	1	3	4	14	24	24	24
65+	43	4.3	21	1	2	3	5	6	12	24
B. Operated										
0–19 Years	7	4.6	6	1	3	4	7	8	8	8
20–34	8	15.8	167	2	3	18	29	38	38	38
35–49	42	5.4	24	2	3	4	5	11	14	27
50–64	146	5.7	14	3	4	5	7	9	11	22
65+	972	5.8	15	3	4	5	7	9	12	22
SUBTOTALS:										
1. SINGLE DX										
A. Not Operated	2	5.0	18	2	2	8	8	8	8	8
B. Operated	41	4.0	11	2	2	3	4	6	9	18
2. MULTIPLE DX										
A. Not Operated	55	5.1	33	1	2	3	5	14	21	24
B. Operated	1,175	5.9	16	3	4	5	7	9	13	24
1. SINGLE DX	43	4.0	11	2	2	3	4	7	9	18
2. MULTIPLE DX	1,230	5.8	17	3	4	5	7	9	13	24
A. NOT OPERATED	57	5.1	32	1	2	3	5	14	21	24
B. OPERATED	1,216	5.8	16	3	4	5	7	9	13	24
TOTAL										
0–19 Years	12	3.5	5	1	1	3	3	7	8	8
20–34	16	9.7	118	2	3	4	18	29	38	38
35–49	54	5.3	27	2	3	3	5	12	20	27
50–64	165	5.8	17	3	3	5	7	9	15	24
65+	1,026	5.8	15	3	4	5	7	9	12	22
GRAND TOTAL	1,273	5.8	17	3	4	5	7	9	13	24

820.09: CL FX FEM TRANSCERV NEC

Type of Patients	Observed Patients	Avg. Stay	Variance	10th	25th	50th	75th	90th	95th	99th
1. SINGLE DX										
A. Not Operated										
0–19 Years	4	1.3	<1	1	1	1	2	2	2	2
20–34	0									
35–49	2	2.0	2	1	1	2	3	3	3	3
50–64	1	1.0	0	1	1	1	1	1	1	1
65+	1	1.0	0	1	1	1	1	1	1	1
B. Operated										
0–19 Years	14	2.7	5	1	1	2	4	5	9	9
20–34	9	2.3	3	1	2	2	3	6	6	6
35–49	18	2.1	<1	1	2	2	3	3	4	4
50–64	46	2.9	2	2	2	3	3	5	5	7
65+	53	4.0	2	3	4	4	5	6	6	9
2. MULTIPLE DX										
A. Not Operated										
0–19 Years	6	1.5	<1	1	1	1	2	3	3	3
20–34	6	2.8	1	1	3	3	4	4	4	4
35–49	19	3.4	7	1	3	3	5	7	10	10
50–64	32	5.5	26	1	2	4	6	12	17	22
65+	369	4.5	15	1	2	3	5	9	12	22
B. Operated										
0–19 Years	12	4.5	12	2	2	3	5	8	14	14
20–34	49	6.0	12	2	3	5	9	11	13	14
35–49	147	5.8	29	2	3	4	7	12	18	30
50–64	860	5.9	38	2	3	4	7	10	14	29
65+	8,449	5.6	11	3	4	5	7	9	11	19
SUBTOTALS:										
1. SINGLE DX										
A. Not Operated	8	1.4	<1	1	1	1	2	3	3	3
B. Operated	140	3.2	2	1	2	3	4	5	6	9
2. MULTIPLE DX										
A. Not Operated	432	4.4	15	1	2	3	5	9	12	22
B. Operated	9,517	5.7	14	3	4	5	7	9	12	20
1. SINGLE DX	148	3.1	3	1	2	3	4	5	6	9
2. MULTIPLE DX	9,949	5.6	14	3	4	5	6	9	12	20
A. NOT OPERATED	440	4.4	15	1	2	3	5	9	12	22
B. OPERATED	9,657	5.6	14	3	4	5	6	9	12	20
TOTAL										
0–19 Years	36	2.9	7	1	2	2	4	5	9	14
20–34	64	5.2	12	2	3	4	8	10	12	14
35–49	186	5.2	25	1	2	4	6	10	14	30
50–64	939	5.7	36	2	3	4	6	10	14	26
65+	8,872	5.6	11	3	4	5	6	9	11	19
GRAND TOTAL	10,097	5.6	14	3	4	5	6	9	12	20

Length of Stay by Diagnosis and Operation, Western Region, 2008

Western Region, October 2006–September 2007 Data, by Diagnosis

820.20: CLSD TROCHANTERIC FX NOS

Type of Patients	Observed Patients	Avg. Stay	Variance	10th	25th	50th	75th	90th	95th	99th
1. SINGLE DX										
A. Not Operated										
0–19 Years	0									
20–34	0									
35–49	2	4.0	8	2	2	6	6	6	6	6
50–64	2	1.5	<1	1	1	1	2	2	2	2
65+	4	2.8	2	1	3	3	4	4	4	4
B. Operated										
0–19 Years	3	3.3	4	1	1	4	5	5	5	5
20–34	3	2.7	2	1	1	3	4	4	4	4
35–49	2	2.5	<1	2	2	2	3	3	3	3
50–64	3	3.0	3	2	2	2	5	5	5	5
65+	1	4.0	0	4	4	4	4	4	4	4
2. MULTIPLE DX										
A. Not Operated										
0–19 Years	0									
20–34	3	1.7	<1	1	1	2	2	2	2	2
35–49	15	4.1	16	1	1	2	7	12	13	13
50–64	71	4.0	9	1	2	3	5	8	12	15
65+	633	3.9	8	2	2	3	4	6	9	16
B. Operated										
0–19 Years	2	4.5	4	3	3	3	6	6	6	6
20–34	16	8.3	59	3	3	6	12	19	31	31
35–49	23	12.1	178	2	5	7	16	21	44	56
50–64	89	6.6	34	2	4	5	7	13	15	44
65+	621	6.0	13	3	4	5	7	10	14	21
SUBTOTALS:										
1. SINGLE DX										
A. Not Operated	8	2.8	3	1	2	3	4	6	6	6
B. Operated	12	3.0	2	1	2	3	4	5	5	5
2. MULTIPLE DX										
A. Not Operated	722	3.9	8	2	2	3	5	6	9	15
B. Operated	751	6.3	23	3	4	5	7	11	14	25
1. SINGLE DX	20	2.9	2	1	2	3	4	5	6	6
2. MULTIPLE DX	1,473	5.1	17	2	3	4	6	9	13	21
A. NOT OPERATED	730	3.9	8	1	2	3	5	6	9	15
B. OPERATED	763	6.3	23	3	4	5	7	11	14	25
TOTAL										
0–19 Years	5	3.8	4	1	3	4	5	6	6	6
20–34	22	6.6	50	2	2	4	9	12	19	31
35–49	42	8.4	118	2	2	6	8	18	21	56
50–64	165	5.4	24	1	2	4	6	8	14	28
65+	1,259	4.9	12	2	3	4	6	8	11	20
GRAND TOTAL	1,493	5.1	17	3	3	4	6	9	13	21

820.21: CL INTERTROCHANTERIC FX

Type of Patients	Observed Patients	Avg. Stay	Variance	10th	25th	50th	75th	90th	95th	99th
1. SINGLE DX										
A. Not Operated										
0–19 Years	4	2.5	2	1	1	3	4	4	4	4
20–34	1	1.0	0	1	1	1	1	1	1	1
35–49	2	1.5	<1	1	1	2	2	2	2	2
50–64	0									
65+	3	3.7	5	1	1	5	5	5	5	5
B. Operated										
0–19 Years	7	3.0	2	1	2	3	4	5	5	5
20–34	24	2.9	3	1	1	3	4	5	6	7
35–49	35	3.1	3	2	2	3	4	5	6	6
50–64	43	3.8	4	2	2	4	5	5	7	11
65+	48	4.0	1	3	3	4	5	5	6	7
2. MULTIPLE DX										
A. Not Operated										
0–19 Years	5	3.8	9	2	2	2	4	9	9	9
20–34	2	2.5	<1	2	2	3	3	3	3	3
35–49	18	4.6	11	2	2	4	6	11	12	12
50–64	44	7.3	75	1	2	3	9	19	26	42
65+	491	5.4	33	1	2	3	6	11	17	29
B. Operated										
0–19 Years	19	6.0	18	2	3	5	7	16	18	18
20–34	115	5.1	13	2	3	4	7	9	11	18
35–49	343	6.0	20	3	3	5	7	11	15	26
50–64	1,559	6.5	24	3	4	5	7	12	16	28
65+	15,756	5.8	12	3	4	5	7	9	11	20
SUBTOTALS:										
1. SINGLE DX										
A. Not Operated	10	2.5	3	1	1	2	4	5	5	5
B. Operated	157	3.6	2	2	2	3	4	5	6	9
2. MULTIPLE DX										
A. Not Operated	560	5.5	36	1	2	3	6	12	17	29
B. Operated	17,792	5.8	13	3	4	5	7	9	12	20
1. SINGLE DX	167	3.5	3	2	2	3	4	5	6	9
2. MULTIPLE DX	18,352	5.8	14	3	4	5	7	9	12	21
A. NOT OPERATED	570	5.4	35	1	2	3	6	11	17	29
B. OPERATED	17,949	5.8	13	3	4	5	7	9	12	20
TOTAL										
0–19 Years	35	4.7	14	2	2	4	6	8	16	18
20–34	142	4.6	12	2	3	4	7	8	10	18
35–49	398	5.7	19	3	3	5	7	11	15	25
50–64	1,646	6.5	25	3	4	5	7	12	16	28
65+	16,298	5.8	13	3	4	5	7	9	12	20
GRAND TOTAL	18,519	5.8	14	3	4	5	7	9	12	21

820.22: CLSD SUBTROCHANTERIC FX

Type of Patients	Observed Patients	Avg. Stay	Variance	10th	25th	50th	75th	90th	95th	99th
1. SINGLE DX										
A. Not Operated										
0–19 Years	5	2.0	1	1	1	2	3	3	3	3
20–34	0									
35–49	0									
50–64	0									
65+	1	4.0	0	4	4	4	4	4	4	4
B. Operated										
0–19 Years	24	3.0	2	1	2	3	4	4	6	6
20–34	11	2.7	3	1	1	2	5	5	5	5
35–49	12	4.2	6	2	2	4	4	7	10	10
50–64	11	3.7	3	2	2	3	6	6	7	7
65+	8	3.3	1	2	3	3	4	5	5	5
2. MULTIPLE DX										
A. Not Operated										
0–19 Years	8	8.7	104	2	2	5	17	31	31	31
20–34	0									
35–49	3	7.7	6	5	5	8	10	10	10	10
50–64	7	3.4	6	1	1	3	6	7	7	7
65+	66	4.8	20	1	2	4	6	8	16	24
B. Operated										
0–19 Years	43	4.7	7	1	3	4	6	8	9	13
20–34	107	6.7	18	3	4	6	9	12	18	20
35–49	134	6.8	30	3	4	5	8	11	15	22
50–64	345	6.0	13	3	4	5	7	10	12	21
65+	1,627	6.2	15	3	4	5	7	10	13	22
SUBTOTALS:										
1. SINGLE DX										
A. Not Operated	6	2.3	1	1	1	3	3	4	4	4
B. Operated	66	3.3	3	1	2	3	4	6	6	10
2. MULTIPLE DX										
A. Not Operated	84	5.1	27	1	2	4	6	9	17	31
B. Operated	2,256	6.2	15	3	4	5	7	10	13	22
1. SINGLE DX	72	3.2	3	1	2	3	4	5	6	10
2. MULTIPLE DX	2,340	6.2	16	3	4	5	7	10	13	22
A. NOT OPERATED	90	4.9	26	1	2	4	6	9	17	31
B. OPERATED	2,322	6.1	15	3	4	5	7	10	13	22
TOTAL										
0–19 Years	80	4.4	16	1	2	4	5	7	9	31
20–34	118	6.3	18	3	3	5	8	12	18	20
35–49	149	6.6	28	3	4	5	8	12	15	22
50–64	363	5.9	13	3	4	5	7	10	12	21
65+	1,702	6.2	15	3	4	5	7	10	13	22
GRAND TOTAL	2,412	6.1	16	4	4	5	7	10	13	22

Length of Stay by Diagnosis and Operation, Western Region, 2008

Western Region, October 2006–September 2007 Data, by Diagnosis

820.8: CL FX NECK OF FEMUR NOS

Type of Patients	Observed Patients	Avg. Stay	Variance	10th	25th	50th	75th	90th	95th	99th
1. SINGLE DX										
A. Not Operated										
0–19 Years	3	6.0	49	1		3	14	14	14	14
20–34	1	2.0	0	2	2	2	2	2	2	2
35–49	0									
50–64	1	1.0	0	1	1	1	1	1	1	1
65+	1	1.0	0	1	1	1	1	1	1	1
B. Operated										
0–19 Years	11	1.8	2	1	1	3	3	4	4	4
20–34	18	2.6	1	1	2	3	3	4	4	4
35–49	28	2.5	<1	1	2	3	3	4	4	4
50–64	62	3.1	3	1	2	3	4	5	6	9
65+	68	3.6	2	2	3	3	4	5	5	9
2. MULTIPLE DX										
A. Not Operated										
0–19 Years	4	2.3	2	1	2	3	4	4	4	4
20–34	3	3.0	<1	2	3	3	4	4	4	4
35–49	11	4.0	3	2	3	5	5	6	7	7
50–64	28	6.0	21	1	3	6	8	11	14	21
65+	431	5.6	47	1	2	4	6	13	16	30
B. Operated										
0–19 Years	22	4.4	16	1	1	3	7	10	10	16
20–34	51	4.7	15	1	2	4	6	6	13	17
35–49	170	4.4	10	2	2	4	5	7	10	17
50–64	905	5.5	17	2	3	4	6	10	13	20
65+	8,618	5.6	14	3	4	5	6	9	11	19
SUBTOTALS:										
1. SINGLE DX										
A. Not Operated	6	3.6	26	1	1	1	3	14	14	14
B. Operated	187	3.0	2	2	2	3	4	5	5	9
2. MULTIPLE DX										
A. Not Operated	477	5.6	44	1	2	4	6	12	16	30
B. Operated	9,766	5.6	14	3	4	5	6	9	11	19
1. SINGLE DX	193	3.1	3	1	2	3	4	5	5	9
2. MULTIPLE DX	10,243	5.6	15	3	4	5	6	9	12	20
A. NOT OPERATED	483	5.6	44	1	2	4	6	12	16	30
B. OPERATED	9,953	5.5	14	3	4	5	6	9	11	19
TOTAL										
0–19 Years	40	3.6	14	1	1	2	4	9	10	16
20–34	73	4.1	11	1	2	3	5	9	13	17
35–49	209	4.1	9	2	2	3	5	7	10	17
50–64	996	5.3	16	2	3	4	6	9	13	20
65+	9,118	5.6	15	3	4	5	6	9	11	20
GRAND TOTAL	10,436	5.5	15	3	4	5	6	9	11	20

821: OTHER FEMORAL FRACTURE

Type of Patients	Observed Patients	Avg. Stay	Variance	10th	25th	50th	75th	90th	95th	99th
1. SINGLE DX										
A. Not Operated										
0–19 Years	340	1.8	4	1	1	1	2	3	4	11
20–34	8	1.9	1	1	1	1	2	4	4	4
35–49	1	2.0	0	2	2	2	2	2	2	2
50–64	0									
65+	1	4.0	0	4	4	4	4	4	4	4
B. Operated										
0–19 Years	404	2.6	2	1	2	2	3	4	5	8
20–34	173	3.0	2	2	2	3	4	5	6	9
35–49	59	2.8	3	1	2	3	3	5	6	11
50–64	28	3.4	3	2	2	3	4	6	7	8
65+	14	4.9	5	3	3	5	5	8	10	10
2. MULTIPLE DX										
A. Not Operated										
0–19 Years	191	2.9	9	1	1	2	3	5	8	20
20–34	44	3.2	6	1	1	3	4	5	7	14
35–49	44	4.8	17	1	2	3	7	10	12	22
50–64	142	5.8	34	2	3	5	7	10	14	35
65+	573	4.5	10	2	3	4	5	8	11	18
B. Operated										
0–19 Years	763	5.1	27	2	2	4	6	9	13	24
20–34	1,055	6.7	45	2	3	5	8	13	20	35
35–49	608	7.9	81	2	3	5	8	16	23	53
50–64	966	7.9	69	3	4	6	9	15	22	50
65+	2,457	6.5	22	3	4	5	7	9	14	24
SUBTOTALS:										
1. SINGLE DX										
A. Not Operated	350	1.8	4	1	1	1	2	3	4	11
B. Operated	678	2.8	3	1	2	3	3	5	5	9
2. MULTIPLE DX										
A. Not Operated	994	4.3	14	1	2	3	5	8	11	20
B. Operated	5,849	6.7	41	2	4	5	8	12	17	35
1. SINGLE DX	1,028	2.5	3	1	1	2	3	4	5	9
2. MULTIPLE DX	6,843	6.4	38	2	3	5	7	11	16	34
A. NOT OPERATED	1,344	3.7	13	1	2	3	4	7	10	19
B. OPERATED	6,527	6.3	39	2	3	5	7	11	16	34
TOTAL										
0–19 Years	1,698	3.6	17	1	2	2	4	7	10	19
20–34	1,280	6.1	40	2	3	4	7	12	18	35
35–49	712	7.2	73	2	3	5	8	15	22	47
50–64	1,136	7.5	64	3	4	6	8	14	21	47
65+	3,045	6.1	20	3	4	5	7	10	13	23
GRAND TOTAL	7,871	5.9	35	2	3	4	7	11	15	31

821.00: CLSD FX FEMUR NOS

Type of Patients	Observed Patients	Avg. Stay	Variance	10th	25th	50th	75th	90th	95th	99th
1. SINGLE DX										
A. Not Operated										
0–19 Years	32	1.7	3	1	1	1	2	3	4	11
20–34	0									
35–49	0									
50–64	0									
65+	0									
B. Operated										
0–19 Years	15	2.7	3	1	2	2	3	4	8	8
20–34	5	2.0	0	2	2	2	2	2	2	2
35–49	0									
50–64	2	2.5	<1	2	2	3	3	3	3	3
65+	0									
2. MULTIPLE DX										
A. Not Operated										
0–19 Years	15	1.9	2	1	1	1	2	4	5	5
20–34	3	6.0	12	4	4	4	10	10	10	10
35–49	3	3.0	7	1	2	2	6	6	6	6
50–64	9	6.8	32	1	2	5	13	15	15	15
65+	21	4.1	12	1	2	4	4	7	8	16
B. Operated										
0–19 Years	18	4.3	9	2	3	4	5	6	15	15
20–34	21	4.9	12	2	3	4	8	10	10	16
35–49	18	6.0	16	2	3	4	8	14	15	15
50–64	14	6.4	65	3	3	5	6	7	34	34
65+	93	5.6	6	3	4	5	7	9	10	15
SUBTOTALS:										
1. SINGLE DX										
A. Not Operated	32	1.7	3	1	1	1	2	3	4	11
B. Operated	18	2.7	2	1	2	2	3	4	8	8
2. MULTIPLE DX										
A. Not Operated	51	4.0	14	1	1	2	5	8	14	16
B. Operated	164	5.5	13	3	3	5	6	9	12	16
1. SINGLE DX	50	2.1	3	1	1	2	2	3	4	11
2. MULTIPLE DX	215	5.1	14	2	3	4	6	9	12	16
A. NOT OPERATED	83	3.1	11	1	1	2	4	7	11	16
B. OPERATED	182	5.2	13	2	3	4	6	9	10	16
TOTAL										
0–19 Years	80	2.5	5	1	2	2	3	5	6	15
20–34	25	4.9	12	2	3	4	6	10	10	16
35–49	21	5.6	16	2	3	4	6	12	14	15
50–64	25	6.2	47	2	3	4	7	14	15	34
65+	114	5.3	7	2	3	5	7	9	10	15
GRAND TOTAL	265	4.5	13	2	3	4	6	9	10	16

Length of Stay by Diagnosis and Operation, Western Region, 2008

Western Region, October 2006–September 2007 Data, by Diagnosis

821.01: CLSD FX FEMUR SHAFT

Type of Patients	Observed Patients	Avg. Stay	Variance	10th	25th	50th	75th	90th	95th	99th
1. SINGLE DX										
A. Not Operated										
0–19 Years	269	1.8	3	1	1	1	2	3	4	8
20–34	0									
35–49	0									
50–64	0									
65+	1	4.0	0	4	4	4	4	4	4	4
B. Operated										
0–19 Years	284	2.7	2	1	2	2	3	5	5	8
20–34	120	2.9	2	1	2	3	4	5	5	8
35–49	35	2.8	3	1	2	3	3	4	5	11
50–64	15	2.8	1	2	2	3	4	4	5	5
65+	5	5.6	11	3	3	5	8	10	10	10
2. MULTIPLE DX										
A. Not Operated										
0–19 Years	130	2.9	10	1	1	2	3	5	8	16
20–34	14	3.1	2	1	2	3	4	4	7	7
35–49	7	6.7	24	1	2	7	10	15	15	15
50–64	12	4.2	7	2	3	3	5	8	9	9
65+	98	4.8	11	2	3	4	6	8	13	19
B. Operated										
0–19 Years	549	4.7	13	2	2	4	6	9	12	20
20–34	675	5.9	30	2	3	4	7	11	15	25
35–49	287	6.8	30	2	3	5	8	14	19	29
50–64	352	7.2	76	3	3	5	8	12	17	53
65+	925	6.4	23	3	4	5	7	10	13	23
SUBTOTALS:										
1. SINGLE DX										
A. Not Operated	270	1.8	3	1	1	1	2	3	4	8
B. Operated	459	2.8	2	1	2	3	4	5	5	9
2. MULTIPLE DX										
A. Not Operated	261	3.8	11	1	2	3	4	7	11	18
B. Operated	2,788	6.1	31	2	3	5	7	11	14	25
1. SINGLE DX	729	2.4	3	1	1	2	3	4	5	8
2. MULTIPLE DX	3,049	5.9	29	2	3	5	7	10	14	25
A. NOT OPERATED	531	2.8	8	1	2	2	3	6	8	16
B. OPERATED	3,247	5.6	28	2	3	4	7	10	13	24
TOTAL										
0–19 Years	1,232	3.4	9	1	2	2	4	7	9	16
20–34	809	5.4	26	2	3	4	6	10	13	23
35–49	329	6.3	28	2	3	5	8	13	18	25
50–64	379	7.0	72	2	3	5	8	12	16	53
65+	1,029	6.2	22	3	4	5	7	10	13	22
GRAND TOTAL	3,778	5.2	26	2	3	4	6	10	13	23

821.11: OPEN FX FEMUR SHAFT

Type of Patients	Observed Patients	Avg. Stay	Variance	10th	25th	50th	75th	90th	95th	99th
1. SINGLE DX										
A. Not Operated										
0–19 Years	1	2.0	0	2	2	2	2	2	2	2
20–34	0									
35–49	0									
50–64	0									
65+	0									
B. Operated										
0–19 Years	14	3.4	3	2	2	3	4	6	7	7
20–34	16	4.0	3	2	3	3	5	7	8	8
35–49	1	3.0	0	3	3	3	3	3	3	3
50–64	0									
65+	0									
2. MULTIPLE DX										
A. Not Operated										
0–19 Years	1	2.0	0	2	2	2	2	2	2	2
20–34	2	3.0	8	1	1	1	5	5	5	5
35–49	1	4.0	0	4	4	4	4	4	4	4
50–64	0									
65+	0									
B. Operated										
0–19 Years	75	8.4	98	2	3	5	10	17	20	65
20–34	159	9.9	78	3	4	6	13	21	30	40
35–49	64	11.0	163	3	4	7	13	25	32	73
50–64	39	15.0	221	3	5	11	19	43	69	>99
65+	19	9.9	59	4	5	9	13	16	37	37
SUBTOTALS:										
1. SINGLE DX										
A. Not Operated	1	2.0	0	2	2	2	2	2	2	2
B. Operated	31	3.7	3	2	3	3	4	6	7	8
2. MULTIPLE DX										
A. Not Operated	4	3.0	3	1	1	3	4	5	5	5
B. Operated	356	10.3	114	3	4	7	13	22	32	65
1. SINGLE DX	32	3.6	3	2	3	3	4	6	7	8
2. MULTIPLE DX	360	10.3	114	3	4	6	12	22	32	65
A. NOT OPERATED	5	2.8	3	1	2	2	4	5	5	5
B. OPERATED	387	9.8	109	3	4	6	12	21	30	65
TOTAL										
0–19 Years	91	7.5	85	2	3	5	9	15	17	65
20–34	177	9.3	74	3	4	6	11	21	28	40
35–49	66	10.8	160	3	4	7	13	25	32	73
50–64	39	15.0	221	3	5	11	19	43	69	>99
65+	19	9.9	59	4	5	9	13	16	37	37
GRAND TOTAL	392	9.7	108	2	4	6	11	20	30	65

821.20: CLSD FX LOW END FEM NOS

Type of Patients	Observed Patients	Avg. Stay	Variance	10th	25th	50th	75th	90th	95th	99th
1. SINGLE DX										
A. Not Operated										
0–19 Years	15	1.4	<1	1	1	1	2	2	3	3
20–34	0									
35–49	0									
50–64	0									
65+	0									
B. Operated										
0–19 Years	23	2.2	2	1	1	2	3	5	5	6
20–34	6	3.8	7	2	2	3	4	9	9	9
35–49	6	3.3	2	2	2	3	5	5	5	5
50–64	1	3.0	0	3	3	3	3	3	3	3
65+	2	3.5	<1	3	3	3	4	4	4	4
2. MULTIPLE DX										
A. Not Operated										
0–19 Years	9	2.8	5	1	1	2	5	7	7	7
20–34	2	4.5	4	3	3	6	6	6	6	6
35–49	6	6.0	20	1	2	4	10	12	12	12
50–64	24	5.4	13	2	3	5	6	11	14	15
65+	116	4.5	13	1	2	4	5	9	13	20
B. Operated										
0–19 Years	23	3.7	5	1	2	3	5	7	7	7
20–34	18	5.6	15	3	3	5	8	13	13	13
35–49	21	5.7	20	3	4	4	6	7	16	21
50–64	78	6.9	46	3	4	5	7	11	18	43
65+	222	6.7	25	4	4	5	8	11	13	23
SUBTOTALS:										
1. SINGLE DX										
A. Not Operated	15	1.4	<1	1	1	1	2	2	3	3
B. Operated	38	2.7	3	1	1	3	3	5	6	9
2. MULTIPLE DX										
A. Not Operated	157	4.6	13	1	2	4	6	9	13	20
B. Operated	362	6.4	28	3	4	5	7	11	13	35
1. SINGLE DX	53	2.4	3	1	1	2	3	5	5	9
2. MULTIPLE DX	519	5.9	24	2	3	5	7	10	13	22
A. NOT OPERATED	172	4.3	13	1	2	3	5	9	12	20
B. OPERATED	400	6.1	26	2	3	5	7	10	13	23
TOTAL										
0–19 Years	70	2.6	4	1	2	2	3	6	7	7
20–34	26	5.1	13	2	3	3	8	11	13	13
35–49	33	5.3	17	2	3	4	6	10	16	21
50–64	103	6.5	38	2	3	5	7	11	15	42
65+	340	5.9	22	2	3	5	7	10	13	22
GRAND TOTAL	572	5.5	23	2	3	5	7	10	13	22

Length of Stay by Diagnosis and Operation, Western Region, 2008

Western Region, October 2006–September 2007 Data, by Diagnosis

821.21: CLSD FX FEMORAL CONDYLE

Type of Patients	Observed Patients	Avg. Stay	Variance	10th	25th	50th	75th	90th	95th	99th
1. SINGLE DX										
A. Not Operated										
0–19 Years	2	1.5	<1	1	1	2	2	2	2	2
20–34	4	2.3	2	1	2	2	2	4	4	4
35–49	1	2.0	0	2	2	2	2	2	2	2
50–64	0									
65+	0									
B. Operated										
0–19 Years	10	1.5	<1	1	1	1	2	2	3	3
20–34	7	3.0	3	2	2	2	5	6	6	6
35–49	6	1.8	<1	1	1	2	2	3	3	3
50–64	0									
65+	0									
2. MULTIPLE DX										
A. Not Operated										
0–19 Years	2	3.5	4	2	2	5	5	5	5	5
20–34	7	1.4	1	1	1	1	1	4	4	4
35–49	5	2.8	6	1	1	5	5	6	6	6
50–64	37	3.9	6	1	2	3	5	7	8	14
65+	109	4.5	9	2	3	4	5	8	10	16
B. Operated										
0–19 Years	17	5.1	101	1	1	2	3	9	43	43
20–34	28	5.7	18	2	3	4	7	15	16	17
35–49	53	5.1	13	2	3	4	7	12	14	>99
50–64	76	6.8	38	2	3	5	8	14	16	39
65+	196	6.5	24	3	4	5	8	10	18	29
SUBTOTALS:										
1. SINGLE DX										
A. Not Operated	7	2.0	<1	1	1	2	2	2	4	4
B. Operated	23	2.0	2	1	1	2	2	3	5	6
2. MULTIPLE DX										
A. Not Operated	160	4.2	8	1	2	3	5	8	10	16
B. Operated	370	6.2	28	2	3	5	7	11	17	31
1. SINGLE DX	30	2.0	1	1	1	2	2	3	5	6
2. MULTIPLE DX	530	5.6	23	2	3	4	7	10	14	29
A. NOT OPERATED	167	4.1	8	1	2	3	5	7	9	16
B. OPERATED	393	6.0	28	2	3	4	7	11	16	31
TOTAL										
0–19 Years	31	3.6	57	1	1	2	2	5	9	43
20–34	46	4.3	15	1	2	3	6	9	15	17
35–49	65	4.5	12	1	2	3	6	9	13	>99
50–64	113	5.8	29	2	3	4	6	11	14	31
65+	305	5.8	19	3	3	4	7	10	13	24
GRAND TOTAL	560	5.4	23	3	3	4	6	10	14	29

821.23: CLSD SUPRACONDYL FX FEM

Type of Patients	Observed Patients	Avg. Stay	Variance	10th	25th	50th	75th	90th	95th	99th
1. SINGLE DX										
A. Not Operated										
0–19 Years	3	1.0	0	1	1	1	1	1	1	1
20–34	0									
35–49	0									
50–64	0									
65+	0									
B. Operated										
0–19 Years	18	1.8	1	1	1	1	2	4	4	4
20–34	5	3.0	1	2	2	3	3	5	5	5
35–49	2	4.0	8	2	2	6	6	6	6	6
50–64	5	3.6	3	2	2	3	5	6	6	6
65+	4	5.3	2	4	5	5	5	7	7	7
2. MULTIPLE DX										
A. Not Operated										
0–19 Years	11	2.1	1	1	2	2	2	4	4	4
20–34	6	4.5	22	2	2	3	5	14	14	14
35–49	14	3.9	4	2	2	3	5	7	8	8
50–64	42	7.9	82	2	3	5	8	20	28	44
65+	157	4.3	9	2	3	3	5	8	10	16
B. Operated										
0–19 Years	21	4.0	10	1	2	3	5	8	8	14
20–34	35	6.3	27	2	3	5	8	11	14	30
35–49	86	8.1	161	2	3	5	8	14	16	88
50–64	247	7.5	33	3	4	6	9	15	19	47
65+	724	6.6	19	3	4	5	8	11	14	23
SUBTOTALS:										
1. SINGLE DX										
A. Not Operated	3	1.0	0	1	1	1	1	1	1	1
B. Operated	34	2.8	3	1	1	2	4	5	6	7
2. MULTIPLE DX										
A. Not Operated	230	4.8	24	2	2	4	5	8	12	28
B. Operated	1,113	6.8	34	3	4	5	8	12	15	29
1. SINGLE DX	37	2.6	3	1	1	2	4	5	6	7
2. MULTIPLE DX	1,343	6.5	32	3	4	5	7	11	15	29
A. NOT OPERATED	233	4.8	24	2	2	3	5	8	12	28
B. OPERATED	1,147	6.7	33	3	4	5	8	11	15	31
TOTAL										
0–19 Years	53	2.7	6	1	1	2	3	5	8	14
20–34	46	5.7	25	2	3	4	8	11	14	30
35–49	102	7.4	139	2	3	4	8	12	15	77
50–64	294	7.5	39	3	4	6	9	15	21	47
65+	885	6.2	18	3	4	5	7	10	13	23
GRAND TOTAL	1,380	6.4	32	3	4	5	7	11	15	29

821.29: CLSD FX LOW END FEM NEC

Type of Patients	Observed Patients	Avg. Stay	Variance	10th	25th	50th	75th	90th	95th	99th
1. SINGLE DX										
A. Not Operated										
0–19 Years	12	3.6	45	1	1	1	2	3	25	25
20–34	1	3.0	0	3	3	3	3	3	3	3
35–49	0									
50–64	0									
65+	0									
B. Operated										
0–19 Years	14	2.5	6	1	1	2	2	5	10	10
20–34	4	2.5	<1	2	2	3	3	3	3	3
35–49	3	2.3	6	1	1	2	4	4	4	4
50–64	2	5.0	8	3	3	5	7	7	7	7
65+	1	4.0	0	4	4	4	4	4	4	4
2. MULTIPLE DX										
A. Not Operated										
0–19 Years	11	4.8	31	1	1	3	7	8	20	20
20–34	1	4.0	0	4	4	4	5	7	4	4
35–49	5	4.0	6	2	2	4	5	5	7	7
50–64	10	4.7	5	3	3	4	6	7	9	9
65+	51	5.0	9	3	3	4	7	8	11	13
B. Operated										
0–19 Years	15	2.3	1	1	1	2	2	4	4	4
20–34	15	6.1	31	3	3	4	6	14	22	22
35–49	11	8.3	161	4	4	5	6	14	53	53
50–64	61	8.0	52	4	4	6	9	15	22	48
65+	155	6.1	12	3	4	5	7	9	11	22
SUBTOTALS:										
1. SINGLE DX										
A. Not Operated	13	3.5	42	1	1	2	3	3	25	25
B. Operated	24	2.7	4	1	2	3	3	5	7	10
2. MULTIPLE DX										
A. Not Operated	78	4.8	11	1	3	4	7	8	11	20
B. Operated	257	6.5	32	3	4	5	7	11	15	34
1. SINGLE DX	37	3.0	17	1	1	2	3	5	10	25
2. MULTIPLE DX	335	6.1	27	3	4	5	7	10	13	26
A. NOT OPERATED	91	4.6	15	1	2	4	7	8	11	25
B. OPERATED	281	6.2	30	3	4	5	7	10	14	34
TOTAL										
0–19 Years	48	3.2	20	1	1	2	3	7	10	25
20–34	21	5.2	24	2	3	4	5	11	14	22
35–49	23	6.6	109	2	2	5	5	7	14	53
50–64	73	7.5	45	3	4	6	8	15	22	48
65+	207	5.8	12	3	4	5	7	9	11	15
GRAND TOTAL	372	5.8	27	2	3	5	7	10	13	26

Length of Stay by Diagnosis and Operation, Western Region, 2008

Western Region, October 2006–September 2007 Data, by Diagnosis

822: PATELLA FRACTURE

Type of Patients	Observed Patients	Avg. Stay	Vari-ance	10th	25th	50th	75th	90th	95th	99th
1. SINGLE DX										
A. Not Operated										
0–19 Years	0									
20–34	3	1.0	0	1	1	1	1	1	1	1
35–49	5	1.4	<1	1	1	1	2	2	2	2
50–64	10	1.5	<1	1	1	1	2	3	3	3
65+	2	2.0	0	2	2	2	2	2	2	2
B. Operated										
0–19 Years	23	1.8	1	1	1	2	2	3	5	5
20–34	73	2.4	6	1	1	2	2	4	8	14
35–49	59	1.7	<1	1	1	2	2	3	3	4
50–64	63	2.3	2	1	1	2	3	4	5	9
65+	21	1.7	<1	1	2	2	2	3	3	3
2. MULTIPLE DX										
A. Not Operated										
0–19 Years	5	2.4	7	1	1	2	2	7	7	7
20–34	23	1.8	1	1	1	2	2	4	4	4
35–49	23	3.1	10	1	1	2	4	5	9	15
50–64	45	3.9	14	1	2	3	5	6	7	23
65+	280	3.8	19	1	2	3	4	6	9	15
B. Operated										
0–19 Years	48	4.1	27	1	1	2	5	7	14	26
20–34	177	3.8	11	1	2	3	5	8	9	19
35–49	220	3.7	13	1	2	3	4	7	10	21
50–64	487	3.8	15	1	2	3	4	7	11	23
65+	728	3.6	6	1	2	3	4	6	8	11
SUBTOTALS:										
1. SINGLE DX										
A. Not Operated	20	1.5	<1	1	1	1	2	3	3	3
B. Operated	239	2.1	3	1	1	2	2	3	5	9
2. MULTIPLE DX										
A. Not Operated	376	3.6	17	1	2	3	4	6	9	15
B. Operated	1,660	3.7	11	1	2	3	4	7	9	19
1. SINGLE DX	259	2.0	3	1	1	2	2	3	5	9
2. MULTIPLE DX	2,036	3.7	12	1	2	3	4	7	9	18
A. NOT OPERATED	396	3.5	16	1	2	3	4	6	9	15
B. OPERATED	1,899	3.5	10	1	2	3	4	6	8	18
TOTAL										
0–19 Years	76	3.3	19	1	1	2	3	6	11	26
20–34	276	3.2	9	1	1	2	3	4	9	17
35–49	307	3.2	11	1	1	3	3	6	9	20
50–64	605	3.6	13	1	2	3	4	6	9	20
65+	1,031	3.6	10	1	2	3	4	6	8	13
GRAND TOTAL	2,295	3.5	11	1	2	3	4	6	8	18

822.0: CLOSED FRACTURE PATELLA

Type of Patients	Observed Patients	Avg. Stay	Vari-ance	10th	25th	50th	75th	90th	95th	99th
1. SINGLE DX										
A. Not Operated										
0–19 Years	0									
20–34	3	1.0	0	1	1	1	1	1	1	1
35–49	4	1.3	<1	1	1	1	2	2	2	2
50–64	10	1.5	<1	1	1	1	2	3	3	3
65+	2	2.0	0	2	2	2	2	2	2	2
B. Operated										
0–19 Years	16	1.3	<1	1	1	1	1	3	3	3
20–34	60	2.5	7	1	1	2	2	5	8	14
35–49	51	1.6	<1	1	1	2	2	3	3	4
50–64	60	2.3	2	1	1	2	3	4	5	9
65+	21	1.7	<1	1	1	2	2	3	3	3
2. MULTIPLE DX										
A. Not Operated										
0–19 Years	2	1.5	<1	1	1	2	2	2	2	2
20–34	22	1.8	1	1	1	1	2	4	4	4
35–49	22	3.2	11	1	1	2	4	5	9	15
50–64	42	3.9	15	1	1	3	6	6	7	23
65+	279	3.8	19	1	2	3	4	6	9	15
B. Operated										
0–19 Years	27	2.6	3	1	1	2	3	5	6	7
20–34	93	3.1	7	1	2	3	4	8	8	17
35–49	162	3.0	5	1	1	2	4	6	7	11
50–64	443	3.5	12	1	2	3	4	6	8	18
65+	703	3.6	6	1	2	3	4	6	8	11
SUBTOTALS:										
1. SINGLE DX										
A. Not Operated	19	1.4	<1	1	1	1	2	3	3	3
B. Operated	208	2.0	3	1	1	2	2	3	5	9
2. MULTIPLE DX										
A. Not Operated	367	3.6	17	1	2	3	4	6	9	15
B. Operated	1,428	3.5	8	1	2	3	4	6	8	14
1. SINGLE DX	227	2.0	3	1	1	2	2	3	4	9
2. MULTIPLE DX	1,795	3.5	10	1	2	3	4	6	8	15
A. NOT OPERATED	386	3.5	16	1	2	3	4	6	9	15
B. OPERATED	1,636	3.3	8	1	2	3	4	6	8	13
TOTAL										
0–19 Years	45	2.1	2	1	1	2	3	4	5	7
20–34	178	2.7	6	1	1	2	3	5	8	14
35–49	239	2.7	5	1	1	2	3	5	7	11
50–64	555	3.4	11	1	2	3	4	6	8	18
65+	1,005	3.6	10	1	2	3	4	6	8	13
GRAND TOTAL	2,022	3.3	9	1	2	3	4	6	8	14

822.1: OPEN FRACTURE PATELLA

Type of Patients	Observed Patients	Avg. Stay	Vari-ance	10th	25th	50th	75th	90th	95th	99th
1. SINGLE DX										
A. Not Operated										
0–19 Years	0									
20–34	0									
35–49	1	2.0	0	2	2	2	2	2	2	2
50–64	0									
65+	0									
B. Operated										
0–19 Years	7	2.9	2	1	2	2	5	5	5	5
20–34	13	1.8	<1	1	1	1	2	3	4	4
35–49	8	2.0	<1	1	1	1	2	3	3	3
50–64	3	2.3	1	1	1	3	3	3	3	3
65+	0									
2. MULTIPLE DX										
A. Not Operated										
0–19 Years	3	3.0	12	1	1	1	1	7	7	7
20–34	1	2.0	0	2	2	2	2	2	2	2
35–49	1	2.0	0	2	2	2	2	2	2	2
50–64	3	3.0	3	2	2	2	5	5	5	5
65+	1	1.0	0	1	1	1	1	1	1	1
B. Operated										
0–19 Years	21	6.0	54	1	2	3	6	14	25	26
20–34	84	4.5	14	1	2	3	6	8	12	21
35–49	58	5.7	30	2	2	3	6	17	21	24
50–64	44	6.4	35	2	3	4	8	12	20	26
65+	25	3.7	6	1	2	3	4	8	10	10
SUBTOTALS:										
1. SINGLE DX										
A. Not Operated	1	2.0	0	2	2	2	2	2	2	2
B. Operated	31	2.2	1	1	1	2	3	3	5	5
2. MULTIPLE DX										
A. Not Operated	9	2.6	4	1	1	2	2	7	7	7
B. Operated	232	5.2	25	2	2	3	6	11	18	25
1. SINGLE DX	32	2.2	1	1	1	2	2	3	5	5
2. MULTIPLE DX	241	5.1	25	1	2	3	6	11	17	25
A. NOT OPERATED	10	2.5	4	1	1	2	2	5	7	7
B. OPERATED	263	4.8	23	1	2	3	5	10	17	25
TOTAL										
0–19 Years	31	5.0	39	1	2	3	6	11	25	26
20–34	98	4.1	13	1	2	3	5	8	12	21
35–49	68	5.1	28	2	2	3	5	11	18	24
50–64	50	5.9	32	2	2	4	7	12	20	26
65+	26	3.6	6	1	2	3	4	8	10	10
GRAND TOTAL	273	4.8	23	1	2	3	5	10	17	25

Length of Stay by Diagnosis and Operation, Western Region, 2008

Western Region, October 2006–September 2007 Data, by Diagnosis

823: TIBIA & FIBULA FRACTURE

Type of Patients	Observed Patients	Avg. Stay	Vari- ance	10th	25th	50th	75th	90th	95th	99th
1. SINGLE DX										
A. Not Operated										
0–19 Years	190	1.6	<1	1	1	1	2	3	3	4
20–34	81	1.8	1	1	1	1	2	3	4	8
35–49	52	2.1	3	1	1	2	2	4	7	10
50–64	23	2.4	3	1	1	2	3	4	8	8
65+	10	2.7	3	1	1	3	3	5	6	6
B. Operated										
0–19 Years	448	2.3	2	1	1	2	3	4	5	7
20–34	667	2.6	4	1	1	2	3	4	5	11
35–49	548	3.0	7	1	2	2	3	5	7	17
50–64	288	3.0	6	1	2	2	4	5	7	13
65+	32	3.3	5	2	2	3	4	4	8	12
2. MULTIPLE DX										
A. Not Operated										
0–19 Years	144	2.0	2	1	1	2	2	4	5	7
20–34	198	2.7	5	1	1	2	3	5	7	13
35–49	262	3.7	23	1	1	3	4	7	10	31
50–64	460	4.4	27	1	2	3	5	9	13	27
65+	881	4.0	8	1	2	3	5	7	9	16
B. Operated										
0–19 Years	566	4.7	30	1	2	3	5	10	14	28
20–34	1,730	5.3	38	1	2	3	6	11	16	29
35–49	2,198	5.6	44	1	2	4	6	12	18	38
50–64	2,202	6.2	58	2	2	4	7	12	19	40
65+	1,137	5.8	26	2	3	4	7	10	14	32
SUBTOTALS:										
1. SINGLE DX										
A. Not Operated	356	1.8	2	1	1	1	2	3	4	8
B. Operated	1,983	2.7	5	1	2	2	3	5	6	13
2. MULTIPLE DX										
A. Not Operated	1,945	3.8	14	1	2	3	4	7	9	21
B. Operated	7,833	5.7	43	1	2	4	6	11	17	35
1. SINGLE DX	2,339	2.6	5	1	1	2	3	4	6	12
2. MULTIPLE DX	9,778	5.3	38	1	2	4	6	10	16	32
A. NOT OPERATED	2,301	3.5	13	1	1	3	4	6	9	19
B. OPERATED	9,816	5.1	37	1	2	3	6	10	15	32
TOTAL										
0–19 Years	1,348	3.2	15	1	1	2	3	6	9	21
20–34	2,676	4.4	27	1	2	3	5	9	14	26
35–49	3,060	4.9	37	1	2	3	5	10	16	33
50–64	2,973	5.6	49	1	3	4	6	11	17	37
65+	2,060	5.0	19	2	3	4	6	8	11	26
GRAND TOTAL	12,117	4.8	33	1	2	3	5	9	14	29

823.00: CLSD FX UPPER END TIBIA

Type of Patients	Observed Patients	Avg. Stay	Vari- ance	10th	25th	50th	75th	90th	95th	99th
1. SINGLE DX										
A. Not Operated										
0–19 Years	27	1.9	2	1	1	1	3	3	3	7
20–34	20	2.1	1	1	1	2	3	4	5	5
35–49	22	2.5	5	1	1	2	3	5	7	10
50–64	15	2.5	3	1	1	2	3	4	8	8
65+	7	2.4	2	1	1	3	3	5	5	5
B. Operated										
0–19 Years	77	2.1	2	1	1	2	3	4	5	7
20–34	162	2.6	3	1	1	2	3	4	6	11
35–49	192	3.2	10	1	2	2	3	5	7	21
50–64	133	3.3	8	1	2	3	4	6	8	13
65+	18	2.9	2	1	2	3	3	4	8	8
2. MULTIPLE DX										
A. Not Operated										
0–19 Years	23	1.7	1	1	1	1	2	3	4	5
20–34	69	3.0	6	1	1	2	4	6	8	13
35–49	109	3.4	8	1	1	3	4	7	8	13
50–64	218	4.6	36	1	2	3	5	10	15	28
65+	464	4.0	7	2	3	3	5	7	8	14
B. Operated										
0–19 Years	89	3.3	9	1	2	3	4	7	9	17
20–34	417	4.7	29	1	2	3	6	9	13	23
35–49	747	5.1	29	1	2	4	6	10	15	31
50–64	901	5.2	24	2	2	4	6	10	14	24
65+	466	5.4	14	2	3	5	7	9	11	20
SUBTOTALS:										
1. SINGLE DX										
A. Not Operated	91	2.2	3	1	1	2	3	3	5	10
B. Operated	582	2.9	7	1	2	2	3	5	7	16
2. MULTIPLE DX										
A. Not Operated	883	3.9	14	1	2	3	5	7	10	20
B. Operated	2,620	5.0	24	1	2	4	6	9	13	24
1. SINGLE DX	673	2.8	6	1	2	2	3	5	7	14
2. MULTIPLE DX	3,503	4.8	22	1	2	4	6	9	12	23
A. NOT OPERATED	974	3.8	13	1	2	3	4	7	9	19
B. OPERATED	3,202	4.7	21	1	2	3	6	9	12	23
TOTAL										
0–19 Years	216	2.5	5	1	1	2	3	5	7	11
20–34	668	4.0	21	2	2	3	4	8	10	22
35–49	1,070	4.5	24	1	2	3	5	9	13	23
50–64	1,267	4.8	24	2	3	4	6	10	13	25
65+	955	4.6	11	2	3	4	6	8	10	18
GRAND TOTAL	4,176	4.4	20	1	2	3	5	8	12	22

823.01: CLSD FX UPPER END FIBULA

Type of Patients	Observed Patients	Avg. Stay	Vari- ance	10th	25th	50th	75th	90th	95th	99th
1. SINGLE DX										
A. Not Operated										
0–19 Years	0									
20–34	3	1.0	0	1	1	1	1	1	1	1
35–49	0									
50–64	0									
65+	0									
B. Operated										
0–19 Years	1	1.0	0	1	1	1	1	1	1	1
20–34	3	3.0	3	1	1	4	4	4	4	4
35–49	0									
50–64	1	4.0	0	4	4	4	4	4	4	4
65+	0									
2. MULTIPLE DX										
A. Not Operated										
0–19 Years	3	2.3	<1	2	2	2	3	3	3	3
20–34	19	2.4	4	1	1	2	3	5	8	8
35–49	26	3.0	6	1	2	2	4	8	9	9
50–64	39	4.3	22	1	2	3	5	9	22	22
65+	46	3.9	7	2	2	3	5	7	9	14
B. Operated										
0–19 Years	17	1.0	0	1	1	1	1	1	1	1
20–34	20	3.4	9	1	1	2	4	10	11	11
35–49	20	2.6	5	1	1	2	3	5	10	10
50–64	19	10.2	292	1	2	5	11	25	76	76
65+	9	3.4	6	1	2	3	5	7	8	8
SUBTOTALS:										
1. SINGLE DX										
A. Not Operated	3	1.0	0	1	1	1	1	1	1	1
B. Operated	5	2.8	3	1	1	4	4	4	4	4
2. MULTIPLE DX										
A. Not Operated	133	3.6	11	1	2	3	4	7	9	22
B. Operated	66	5.1	96	1	1	2	5	10	15	76
1. SINGLE DX	8	2.1	2	1	1	1	4	4	4	4
2. MULTIPLE DX	199	4.1	39	1	1	3	5	8	11	22
A. NOT OPERATED	136	3.5	11	1	1	3	4	7	9	22
B. OPERATED	71	4.9	89	1	1	3	5	10	15	76
TOTAL										
0–19 Years	5	1.8	<1	1	1	2	2	3	3	3
20–34	42	2.7	6	1	1	2	4	5	8	11
35–49	46	2.8	6	1	1	2	4	6	9	10
50–64	59	6.2	113	1	2	3	6	15	22	76
65+	55	3.8	6	1	2	3	5	7	9	14
GRAND TOTAL	207	4.0	38	1	1	3	4	8	10	22

823.02: CLSD FX UP TIB W FIBULA

Type of Patients	Observed Patients	Avg. Stay	Variance	10th	25th	50th	75th	90th	95th	99th
1. SINGLE DX										
A. Not Operated										
0–19 Years	7	1.3	<1	1	1	1	1	3	3	3
20–34	4	1.7	2	1	1	1	1	4	4	4
35–49	8	2.4	5	1	1	1	3	7	7	7
50–64	2	1.0	0	1	1	1	1	1	1	1
65+	0									
B. Operated										
0–19 Years	8	1.9	1	1	1	1	2	4	4	4
20–34	18	3.1	7	2	2	2	3	5	13	13
35–49	21	4.2	17	1	2	3	4	9	12	17
50–64	7	3.7	5	1	2	4	4	8	8	8
65+	4	4.5	26	1	1	3	12	12	12	12
2. MULTIPLE DX										
A. Not Operated										
0–19 Years	8	2.1	<1	1	1	2	3	4	4	4
20–34	16	2.4	2	1	1	2	3	4	5	5
35–49	31	4.9	30	2	3	3	4	9	10	31
50–64	81	5.0	35	1	2	3	5	10	12	38
65+	175	4.2	12	1	2	3	5	8	9	18
B. Operated										
0–19 Years	21	3.6	8	1	2	3	5	7	8	12
20–34	68	6.2	32	1	2	4	9	15	19	23
35–49	147	7.2	57	2	3	5	9	15	22	45
50–64	205	7.4	60	2	3	5	8	14	19	40
65+	136	6.2	17	3	3	5	8	11	14	25
SUBTOTALS:										
1. SINGLE DX										
A. Not Operated	21	1.8	3	1	1	1	1	4	4	7
B. Operated	58	3.5	11	1	2	2	4	8	12	17
2. MULTIPLE DX										
A. Not Operated	311	4.4	19	1	2	3	5	8	10	27
B. Operated	577	6.8	44	2	3	5	8	13	19	38
1. SINGLE DX	79	3.0	9	1	1	2	3	7	12	17
2. MULTIPLE DX	888	5.9	37	2	3	4	7	11	16	31
A. NOT OPERATED	332	4.2	19	1	2	3	5	8	10	27
B. OPERATED	635	6.5	42	2	3	5	8	12	18	30
TOTAL										
0–19 Years	44	2.7	5	1	1	2	3	5	6	12
20–34	106	4.9	25	1	1	3	5	13	15	23
35–49	207	6.4	48	1	2	4	8	12	21	38
50–64	295	6.6	53	2	3	5	8	12	19	40
65+	315	5.1	15	2	3	4	6	9	12	21
GRAND TOTAL	967	5.7	35	1	3	4	7	11	15	30

823.20: CLSD FX SHAFT TIBIA

Type of Patients	Observed Patients	Avg. Stay	Variance	10th	25th	50th	75th	90th	95th	99th
1. SINGLE DX										
A. Not Operated										
0–19 Years	48	1.4	<1	1	1	1	2	2	3	3
20–34	12	1.7	<1	1	1	2	2	3	3	3
35–49	4	1.3	<1	1	1	1	1	2	2	2
50–64	2	1.5	<1	1	1	2	2	2	2	2
65+	0									
B. Operated										
0–19 Years	52	1.8	<1	1	1	2	2	3	3	4
20–34	64	2.0	1	1	1	2	3	3	4	5
35–49	38	2.2	3	1	1	2	3	4	5	10
50–64	14	1.9	1	1	1	2	3	4	4	4
65+	2	2.5	<1	2	2	3	3	3	3	3
2. MULTIPLE DX										
A. Not Operated										
0–19 Years	34	2.3	3	1	1	2	3	5	6	7
20–34	15	2.5	3	1	1	2	4	5	6	6
35–49	9	1.9	<1	1	1	2	2	3	3	3
50–64	13	4.0	23	1	1	3	4	9	18	31
65+	20	5.2	33	1	2	3	5	10	14	26
B. Operated										
0–19 Years	48	4.2	26	1	2	3	4	7	10	33
20–34	118	3.7	10	1	2	3	4	6	11	15
35–49	175	4.2	39	1	2	3	4	8	9	42
50–64	175	4.5	26	1	2	3	5	8	12	32
65+	80	4.7	6	2	3	4	6	8	10	>99
SUBTOTALS:										
1. SINGLE DX										
A. Not Operated	66	1.5	<1	1	1	1	2	2	3	3
B. Operated	170	2.0	1	1	1	2	3	3	4	5
2. MULTIPLE DX										
A. Not Operated	91	3.2	13	1	1	2	4	6	9	26
B. Operated	596	4.3	24	1	2	3	5	8	10	32
1. SINGLE DX	236	1.8	1	1	1	2	2	3	4	5
2. MULTIPLE DX	687	4.1	23	1	2	3	5	7	10	27
A. NOT OPERATED	157	2.5	8	1	1	2	3	5	6	18
B. OPERATED	766	3.8	20	1	2	3	4	6	9	27
TOTAL										
0–19 Years	182	2.4	9	1	1	2	3	4	6	18
20–34	209	3.0	7	1	1	2	4	5	6	15
35–49	226	3.7	32	1	2	3	4	6	9	27
50–64	204	4.3	24	1	2	3	5	7	11	27
65+	102	4.7	11	2	3	4	6	8	10	26
GRAND TOTAL	923	3.5	18	1	2	3	4	6	9	26

823.22: CLSD FX SHAFT FIB W TIB

Type of Patients	Observed Patients	Avg. Stay	Variance	10th	25th	50th	75th	90th	95th	99th
1. SINGLE DX										
A. Not Operated										
0–19 Years	65	1.6	<1	1	1	1	2	3	3	4
20–34	17	1.8	1	1	1	2	2	3	5	5
35–49	9	1.8	<1	1	1	2	2	3	3	3
50–64	3	3.6	14	1	1	2	8	8	8	8
65+	0									
B. Operated										
0–19 Years	138	2.3	1	1	2	2	3	4	4	6
20–34	181	2.5	2	1	2	2	3	4	5	7
35–49	138	2.5	3	1	1	2	3	4	6	8
50–64	56	2.6	3	1	1	2	3	5	7	8
65+	2	3.5	<1	3	3	4	4	4	4	4
2. MULTIPLE DX										
A. Not Operated										
0–19 Years	34	2.0	1	1	1	2	3	4	4	6
20–34	29	2.7	3	1	1	2	4	5	6	7
35–49	36	6.2	101	1	2	3	5	12	35	51
50–64	43	3.6	11	1	2	3	5	6	7	21
65+	64	3.7	7	1	2	3	5	7	8	16
B. Operated										
0–19 Years	161	4.0	9	1	2	3	5	7	11	15
20–34	376	4.0	13	1	2	3	5	6	10	22
35–49	415	3.9	12	1	2	3	5	7	10	20
50–64	315	4.9	49	2	2	3	5	9	13	34
65+	195	5.0	11	2	3	4	6	8	11	22
SUBTOTALS:										
1. SINGLE DX										
A. Not Operated	94	1.7	1	1	1	1	2	3	4	8
B. Operated	515	2.5	2	1	1	2	3	4	5	7
2. MULTIPLE DX										
A. Not Operated	206	3.7	24	1	2	3	4	6	8	21
B. Operated	1,462	4.3	20	1	2	3	5	8	10	22
1. SINGLE DX	609	2.4	2	1	1	2	3	4	5	7
2. MULTIPLE DX	1,668	4.2	21	1	2	3	5	8	10	22
A. NOT OPERATED	300	3.1	18	1	1	2	3	5	7	21
B. OPERATED	1,977	3.8	16	1	2	3	4	7	10	20
TOTAL										
0–19 Years	398	2.8	5	1	2	3	3	5	7	14
20–34	603	3.4	10	1	2	3	4	6	8	16
35–49	598	3.7	16	1	2	3	4	7	10	20
50–64	417	4.5	39	2	2	3	5	8	11	26
65+	261	4.7	10	2	3	4	6	8	10	16
GRAND TOTAL	2,277	3.7	16	1	2	3	4	7	9	20

Length of Stay by Diagnosis and Operation, Western Region, 2008

Western Region, October 2006–September 2007 Data, by Diagnosis

823.30: OPN FX TIBIA SHAFT

Type of Patients	Observed Patients	Avg. Stay	Variance	10th	25th	50th	75th	90th	95th	99th
1. SINGLE DX										
A. Not Operated										
0–19 Years	2	1.0	0	1	1	1	1	1	1	1
20–34	6	1.8	<1	1	1	2	2	3	3	3
35–49	1	1.0	0	1	1	1	1	1	1	1
50–64	0									
65+	0									
B. Operated										
0–19 Years	29	2.4	2	1	2	2	3	4	4	8
20–34	25	2.5	<1	1	2	3	3	4	4	4
35–49	17	3.5	2	2	3	3	4	6	6	6
50–64	4	2.0	<1	1	2	2	2	3	3	3
65+	0									
2. MULTIPLE DX										
A. Not Operated										
0–19 Years	2	1.0	0	1	1	1	1	1	1	1
20–34	6	4.4	19	2	2	3	4	13	13	13
35–49	3	1.7	<1	1	1	2	2	2	2	2
50–64	0									
65+	0									
B. Operated										
0–19 Years	46	4.1	8	1	3	4	4	7	8	17
20–34	82	6.9	50	2	2	4	9	16	18	46
35–49	63	8.5	142	2	3	5	9	16	21	72
50–64	47	10.0	147	3	3	5	10	25	37	56
65+	13	4.5	7	2	4	4	5	6	12	12
SUBTOTALS:										
1. SINGLE DX										
A. Not Operated	9	1.6	<1	1	1	1	2	3	3	3
B. Operated	75	2.7	2	1	2	2	3	4	6	8
2. MULTIPLE DX										
A. Not Operated	11	3.0	12	1	1	2	3	4	13	13
B. Operated	251	7.2	84	2	3	4	8	16	22	56
1. SINGLE DX	84	2.5	2	1	2	2	3	4	5	8
2. MULTIPLE DX	262	7.0	82	2	3	4	8	16	22	56
A. NOT OPERATED	20	2.4	7	1	1	2	2	4	13	13
B. OPERATED	326	6.2	69	2	2	4	6	13	19	51
TOTAL										
0–19 Years	79	3.3	6	1	2	3	4	6	8	17
20–34	119	5.6	39	1	2	3	6	13	18	25
35–49	84	7.1	112	1	2	4	9	15	19	72
50–64	51	9.4	140	2	3	5	9	22	37	56
65+	13	4.5	7	2	4	4	5	6	12	12
GRAND TOTAL	346	5.9	66	1	2	4	6	13	19	51

823.32: OPN FX SHAFT TIBIA W FIB

Type of Patients	Observed Patients	Avg. Stay	Variance	10th	25th	50th	75th	90th	95th	99th
1. SINGLE DX										
A. Not Operated										
0–19 Years	4	2.3	2	1	1	3	3	4	4	4
20–34	2	1.5	<1	1	1	2	2	2	2	2
35–49	0									
50–64	0									
65+	0									
B. Operated										
0–19 Years	66	3.1	6	2	2	3	3	4	6	16
20–34	73	2.8	3	1	2	3	3	4	5	13
35–49	40	3.8	6	2	2	3	4	7	8	13
50–64	12	2.5	1	1	2	3	3	3	4	4
65+	1	3.0	0	3	3	3	3	3	3	3
2. MULTIPLE DX										
A. Not Operated										
0–19 Years	5	2.0	<1	1	2	2	2	3	3	3
20–34	5	1.5	<1	1	1	2	2	3	3	3
35–49	1	3.0	0	3	3	3	3	3	3	3
50–64	3	4.7	<1	4	4	5	5	5	5	5
65+	2	2.5	<1	2	2	3	3	3	3	3
B. Operated										
0–19 Years	100	6.8	54	2	2	4	8	18	26	29
20–34	284	7.3	71	2	3	4	8	16	21	47
35–49	192	8.8	104	2	3	5	10	22	27	59
50–64	167	10.2	128	2	3	6	13	25	39	>99
65+	66	9.6	106	3	3	5	10	30	36	39
SUBTOTALS:										
1. SINGLE DX										
A. Not Operated	6	2.0	2	1	1	2	3	4	4	4
B. Operated	192	3.1	5	2	2	3	4	5	6	15
2. MULTIPLE DX										
A. Not Operated	13	2.7	2	1	2	2	3	5	5	5
B. Operated	809	8.4	92	2	3	5	10	19	29	47
1. SINGLE DX	198	3.1	4	1	2	3	4	5	6	15
2. MULTIPLE DX	822	8.3	91	2	3	5	10	19	28	47
A. NOT OPERATED	19	2.5	2	1	1	2	3	5	5	5
B. OPERATED	1,001	7.4	80	2	3	4	8	17	26	45
TOTAL										
0–19 Years	175	5.2	37	2	2	3	5	12	18	29
20–34	361	6.3	60	2	2	4	7	14	19	45
35–49	233	7.9	90	2	3	4	9	18	25	46
50–64	182	9.6	121	2	3	5	12	24	37	>99
65+	69	9.3	103	2	3	5	8	30	36	39
GRAND TOTAL	1,020	7.3	79	2	3	4	8	17	25	45

823.80: CLSD FX TIBIA NOS

Type of Patients	Observed Patients	Avg. Stay	Variance	10th	25th	50th	75th	90th	95th	99th
1. SINGLE DX										
A. Not Operated										
0–19 Years	8	1.1	<1	1	1	1	1	2	2	2
20–34	0									
35–49	0									
50–64	0									
65+	1	1.0	0	1	1	1	1	1	1	1
B. Operated										
0–19 Years	7	1.9	1	1	1	2	3	4	4	4
20–34	14	2.0	<1	1	1	2	3	3	4	4
35–49	11	2.4	2	1	1	2	3	4	6	6
50–64	8	2.4	4	1	1	1	2	6	6	6
65+	0									
2. MULTIPLE DX										
A. Not Operated										
0–19 Years	8	3.3	10	1	1	2	5	10	10	10
20–34	5	2.6	1	1	2	3	3	3	4	4
35–49	7	2.3	2	1	2	2	3	5	5	5
50–64	14	3.9	4	2	2	4	5	7	7	7
65+	28	4.2	12	1	3	3	5	8	13	16
B. Operated										
0–19 Years	8	2.8	4	1	2	2	3	5	6	6
20–34	21	3.8	6	1	2	3	5	7	8	9
35–49	18	4.4	9	1	2	3	7	8	11	11
50–64	21	5.5	30	2	3	4	5	10	16	24
65+	13	5.1	44	1	2	3	6	8	26	26
SUBTOTALS:										
1. SINGLE DX										
A. Not Operated	9	1.1	<1	1	1	1	1	2	2	2
B. Operated	40	2.2	2	1	1	2	3	4	5	6
2. MULTIPLE DX										
A. Not Operated	62	3.7	8	1	2	3	5	7	8	16
B. Operated	81	4.5	19	1	2	3	6	8	10	26
1. SINGLE DX	49	2.0	2	1	1	1	2	4	5	6
2. MULTIPLE DX	143	4.1	14	1	2	3	5	8	10	24
A. NOT OPERATED	71	3.4	8	1	1	3	4	6	8	16
B. OPERATED	121	3.7	14	1	1	3	5	7	9	24
TOTAL										
0–19 Years	31	2.3	4	1	1	1	3	5	6	10
20–34	40	3.0	4	1	2	2	4	7	7	9
35–49	36	3.4	7	1	1	3	4	7	8	11
50–64	43	4.4	18	1	2	3	5	7	10	24
65+	42	4.4	21	1	2	3	5	8	13	26
GRAND TOTAL	192	3.6	12	1	1	3	4	7	9	24

Western Region, October 2006–September 2007 Data, by Diagnosis

823.82: CLSD FX TIB W FIBULA NOS

Type of Patients	Observed Patients	Avg. Stay	Variance	10th	25th	50th	75th	90th	95th	99th
1. SINGLE DX										
A. Not Operated										
0–19 Years	20	1.5	<1	1	1	1	2	2	3	3
20–34	8	2.4	6	1	1	1	2	8	8	8
35–49	4	1.7	2	1	1	1	1	4	4	4
50–64	1	1.0	0	1	1	1	1	1	1	1
65+	0									
B. Operated										
0–19 Years	36	1.9	1	1	1	2	2	4	5	5
20–34	81	2.5	3	1	1	2	3	5	5	9
35–49	60	3.0	9	1	1	2	3	5	12	17
50–64	31	3.0	7	1	2	2	4	4	5	16
65+	2	5.5	4	4	4	4	7	7	7	7
2. MULTIPLE DX										
A. Not Operated										
0–19 Years	13	1.5	<1	1	1	1	2	2	4	4
20–34	9	1.6	<1	1	1	1	2	3	3	3
35–49	21	2.5	2	1	2	2	3	4	5	6
50–64	27	3.7	4	1	2	3	5	7	8	9
65+	44	3.0	3	1	3	3	4	6	6	7
B. Operated										
0–19 Years	32	4.0	11	2	2	3	5	8	12	13
20–34	123	3.9	15	1	2	3	4	6	10	21
35–49	161	4.8	22	1	2	3	5	12	16	20
50–64	169	5.4	39	1	2	3	6	11	14	27
65+	77	4.9	10	2	3	4	6	9	10	20
SUBTOTALS:										
1. SINGLE DX										
A. Not Operated	33	1.7	2	1	1	1	2	3	4	8
B. Operated	210	2.6	5	1	1	2	3	4	5	15
2. MULTIPLE DX										
A. Not Operated	114	2.8	3	1	1	3	4	5	6	8
B. Operated	562	4.7	23	1	2	3	5	10	14	22
1. SINGLE DX	243	2.5	5	1	1	2	3	4	5	15
2. MULTIPLE DX	676	4.4	21	1	2	3	5	9	13	21
A. NOT OPERATED	147	2.5	3	1	1	2	3	5	6	8
B. OPERATED	772	4.2	19	1	2	3	5	9	13	21
TOTAL										
0–19 Years	101	2.4	5	1	1	2	3	4	7	13
20–34	221	3.3	10	1	2	2	4	6	9	20
35–49	246	4.1	17	1	2	3	4	10	14	19
50–64	228	4.8	31	1	2	3	5	9	14	25
65+	123	4.2	8	2	2	4	5	8	9	15
GRAND TOTAL	919	3.9	17	1	2	3	4	8	12	20

823.92: OPEN FX TIBIA W FIB NOS

Type of Patients	Observed Patients	Avg. Stay	Variance	10th	25th	50th	75th	90th	95th	99th
1. SINGLE DX										
A. Not Operated										
0–19 Years	0									
20–34	1	2.0	0	2	2	2	2	2	2	2
35–49	0									
50–64	0									
65+	0									
B. Operated										
0–19 Years	12	3.4	4	2	2	3	4	7	8	8
20–34	14	4.7	21	2	2	3	4	9	19	19
35–49	15	3.3	5	2	2	2	5	6	10	10
50–64	10	3.4	1	2	2	3	4	5	5	5
65+	3	3.3	<1	3	3	3	4	4	4	4
2. MULTIPLE DX										
A. Not Operated										
0–19 Years	0									
20–34	1	3.0	0	3	3	3	3	3	3	3
35–49	1	2.0	0	2	2	2	2	2	2	2
50–64	2	3.5	<1	3	3	4	4	4	4	4
65+	0									
B. Operated										
0–19 Years	23	10.8	186	3	3	5	15	26	28	62
20–34	54	9.1	61	4	4	6	12	22	29	29
35–49	87	7.8	50	2	3	5	11	17	24	40
50–64	54	7.1	42	2	3	5	8	14	24	32
65+	29	7.4	34	3	4	5	9	15	17	29
SUBTOTALS:										
1. SINGLE DX										
A. Not Operated	1	2.0	0	2	2	2	2	2	2	2
B. Operated	54	3.7	8	2	2	3	4	6	9	19
2. MULTIPLE DX										
A. Not Operated	4	3.0	<1	2	3	3	3	4	4	4
B. Operated	247	8.2	61	2	3	5	11	18	25	32
1. SINGLE DX	55	3.7	8	2	2	3	4	6	9	19
2. MULTIPLE DX	251	8.1	61	2	3	5	11	17	25	32
A. NOT OPERATED	5	2.8	<1	2	2	3	3	4	4	4
B. OPERATED	301	7.4	55	2	3	4	9	17	24	29
TOTAL										
0–19 Years	35	8.3	135	2	3	4	8	22	28	62
20–34	70	8.0	54	2	3	5	10	19	27	29
35–49	103	7.1	45	2	3	4	7	16	24	26
50–64	66	6.4	37	2	3	4	7	14	21	25
65+	32	7.0	32	3	3	5	9	12	17	29
GRAND TOTAL	306	7.3	54	2	3	4	9	17	24	29

824: ANKLE FRACTURE

Type of Patients	Observed Patients	Avg. Stay	Variance	10th	25th	50th	75th	90th	95th	99th
1. SINGLE DX										
A. Not Operated										
0–19 Years	97	1.6	1	1	1	1	2	3	4	8
20–34	86	1.5	<1	1	1	1	2	3	4	5
35–49	53	1.7	1	1	1	1	2	3	4	7
50–64	21	1.6	<1	1	1	1	2	3	3	4
65+	6	2.0	2	1	1	2	3	4	4	4
B. Operated										
0–19 Years	413	1.8	2	1	1	2	2	3	4	8
20–34	991	2.3	4	1	1	2	3	4	6	10
35–49	735	2.2	3	1	1	2	3	4	5	10
50–64	508	2.3	3	1	1	2	3	4	5	12
65+	104	2.4	2	1	1	2	3	4	6	8
2. MULTIPLE DX										
A. Not Operated										
0–19 Years	109	1.7	<1	1	1	2	2	3	3	5
20–34	156	2.5	4	1	1	2	3	5	6	12
35–49	237	2.9	9	1	1	2	3	6	9	14
50–64	379	3.5	11	1	2	3	4	7	9	16
65+	814	3.7	8	1	2	3	4	6	8	15
B. Operated										
0–19 Years	507	2.8	12	1	2	2	3	5	8	19
20–34	1,777	3.4	20	1	2	3	4	7	10	22
35–49	2,501	3.6	20	1	2	3	4	7	10	25
50–64	3,624	3.7	17	1	2	3	4	7	9	20
65+	3,239	4.2	12	2	2	3	5	7	10	19
SUBTOTALS:										
1. SINGLE DX										
A. Not Operated	263	1.6	1	1	1	1	2	3	4	5
B. Operated	2,751	2.2	3	1	1	2	3	4	5	10
2. MULTIPLE DX										
A. Not Operated	1,695	3.3	9	1	1	3	4	6	8	15
B. Operated	11,648	3.7	17	1	2	3	5	7	10	20
1. SINGLE DX	3,014	2.1	3	1	1	2	3	4	5	10
2. MULTIPLE DX	13,343	3.7	16	1	2	3	5	7	10	20
A. NOT OPERATED	1,958	3.1	8	1	1	3	4	6	8	14
B. OPERATED	14,399	3.5	14	1	2	3	4	6	9	19
TOTAL										
0–19 Years	1,126	2.3	7	1	1	2	3	4	5	15
20–34	3,010	2.9	14	1	1	2	4	5	8	18
35–49	3,526	3.2	16	1	1	3	4	6	9	19
50–64	4,532	3.5	15	1	2	3	4	7	9	19
65+	4,163	4.1	11	1	2	3	5	7	10	18
GRAND TOTAL	16,357	3.4	14	1	1	3	4	6	9	18

Length of Stay by Diagnosis and Operation, Western Region, 2008

727

Western Region, October 2006–September 2007 Data, by Diagnosis

824.0: CLSD FX MEDIAL MALLEOLUS

Type of Patients	Observed Patients	Avg. Stay	Vari-ance	10th	25th	50th	75th	90th	95th	99th
1. SINGLE DX										
A. *Not Operated*										
0–19 Years	7	2.0	7	1	1	1	1	8	8	8
20–34	10	1.6	2	1	1	1	2	2	5	5
35–49	8	1.5	1	1	1	1	2	4	4	4
50–64	1	3.0	0	3	3	3	3	3	3	3
65+	1	2.0	0	2	2	2	3	2	2	2
B. *Operated*										
0–19 Years	35	1.4	<1	1	1	1	1	2	3	6
20–34	53	2.6	5	1	1	2	3	6	8	9
35–49	32	2.4	5	1	1	2	3	5	6	7
50–64	20	3.1	8	1	1	2	4	7	7	11
65+	1	1.0	0	1	1	1	1	1	1	1
2. MULTIPLE DX										
A. *Not Operated*										
0–19 Years	13	1.5	<1	1	1	2	2	2	2	2
20–34	26	3.2	5	1	1	2	4	7	7	8
35–49	36	2.5	6	1	1	2	3	4	8	14
50–64	35	3.3	11	1	2	3	4	6	8	20
65+	53	3.5	3	2	2	3	4	6	7	10
B. *Operated*										
0–19 Years	53	3.0	12	1	2	2	3	5	13	17
20–34	153	3.6	12	1	2	3	4	7	10	17
35–49	137	3.4	9	1	1	2	4	7	11	15
50–64	149	3.4	7	1	1	3	4	8	10	14
65+	86	4.2	14	1	2	3	5	8	11	22
SUBTOTALS:										
1. SINGLE DX										
A. Not Operated	27	1.7	3	1	1	1	2	4	5	8
B. Operated	141	2.3	5	1	1	1	3	5	7	11
2. MULTIPLE DX										
A. Not Operated	163	3.0	6	1	2	2	4	6	7	14
B. Operated	578	3.5	11	1	1	3	4	8	10	17
1. SINGLE DX	168	2.3	4	1	1	1	2	5	7	11
2. MULTIPLE DX	741	3.4	10	1	1	3	4	7	10	16
A. NOT OPERATED	190	2.8	6	1	1	2	3	6	7	14
B. OPERATED	719	3.3	10	1	1	2	4	7	10	16
TOTAL										
0–19 Years	108	2.2	7	1	1	1	2	4	7	15
20–34	242	3.2	10	1	1	2	4	7	9	16
35–49	213	3.0	8	1	1	2	4	6	9	14
50–64	205	3.3	8	1	2	3	4	7	10	14
65+	141	3.9	10	1	2	3	5	7	8	19
GRAND TOTAL	909	3.2	9	1	1	2	4	7	9	16

824.2: CLSD FX LAT MALLEOLUS

Type of Patients	Observed Patients	Avg. Stay	Vari-ance	10th	25th	50th	75th	90th	95th	99th
1. SINGLE DX										
A. *Not Operated*										
0–19 Years	0									
20–34	5	1.8	<1	1	1	2	2	2	3	3
35–49	2	1.0	0	1	1	1	1	1	1	1
50–64	1	1.0	0	1	1	1	1	1	1	1
65+	0									
B. *Operated*										
0–19 Years	25	1.7	2	1	1	1	2	2	3	8
20–34	89	1.6	1	1	1	1	2	3	3	6
35–49	65	1.9	2	1	1	2	2	3	4	7
50–64	30	1.9	2	1	1	2	3	4	4	6
65+	8	2.0	2	1	1	2	3	5	5	5
2. MULTIPLE DX										
A. *Not Operated*										
0–19 Years	3	1.7	1	1	1	2	3	3	3	3
20–34	20	2.7	4	1	2	2	3	5	9	9
35–49	29	3.2	7	1	2	2	4	7	8	12
50–64	55	3.1	6	1	1	2	4	6	8	13
65+	150	3.8	9	1	2	3	4	6	10	16
B. *Operated*										
0–19 Years	41	2.1	13	1	1	1	2	3	4	24
20–34	144	2.4	7	1	2	2	3	4	6	12
35–49	192	2.5	6	1	1	2	3	4	6	17
50–64	290	2.9	10	1	1	2	3	6	8	14
65+	224	3.5	8	2	2	3	4	6	7	12
SUBTOTALS:										
1. SINGLE DX										
A. Not Operated	8	1.5	<1	1	1	1	2	3	3	3
B. Operated	217	1.8	1	1	1	1	2	3	4	6
2. MULTIPLE DX										
A. Not Operated	257	3.5	7	1	2	3	4	6	8	15
B. Operated	891	2.8	8	1	1	2	3	5	7	15
1. SINGLE DX	225	1.8	1	1	1	1	2	3	4	6
2. MULTIPLE DX	1,148	3.0	8	1	1	2	4	5	7	15
A. NOT OPERATED	265	3.4	7	1	2	3	4	6	8	15
B. OPERATED	1,108	2.6	7	1	1	2	3	5	7	12
TOTAL										
0–19 Years	69	1.9	9	1	1	1	2	4	6	15
20–34	258	2.1	5	1	1	1	3	4	6	10
35–49	288	2.4	5	1	1	2	3	4	6	15
50–64	376	2.8	9	1	1	2	4	5	8	13
65+	382	3.6	8	2	2	3	4	6	7	16
GRAND TOTAL	1,373	2.8	7	1	1	2	3	5	7	13

824.4: CLSD FX BIMALLEOLAR

Type of Patients	Observed Patients	Avg. Stay	Vari-ance	10th	25th	50th	75th	90th	95th	99th
1. SINGLE DX										
A. *Not Operated*										
0–19 Years	5	1.4	<1	1	1	1	1	1	3	3
20–34	15	1.4	1	1	1	1	1	2	5	5
35–49	13	1.4	<1	1	1	1	2	2	3	3
50–64	3	1.7	<1	1	1	2	2	2	2	2
65+	1	3.0	0	3	3	3	3	3	3	3
B. *Operated*										
0–19 Years	92	1.7	<1	1	1	2	2	2	3	4
20–34	226	2.2	5	1	1	2	2	4	5	10
35–49	186	2.1	3	1	1	2	2	4	5	10
50–64	138	2.1	3	1	1	2	3	4	5	12
65+	40	2.1	1	1	1	2	3	3	4	5
2. MULTIPLE DX										
A. *Not Operated*										
0–19 Years	14	1.3	<1	1	1	1	1	2	3	3
20–34	25	2.1	2	1	1	2	2	4	5	7
35–49	38	3.1	13	1	1	2	3	6	14	18
50–64	88	3.9	12	1	1	3	5	8	9	20
65+	211	3.8	6	1	2	3	5	7	8	11
B. *Operated*										
0–19 Years	102	2.5	7	1	1	2	3	4	6	13
20–34	387	2.7	7	1	1	2	3	4	7	13
35–49	612	3.2	13	1	2	2	3	5	8	18
50–64	1,048	3.7	21	1	2	3	4	6	9	23
65+	1,198	4.2	12	1	2	3	5	7	10	19
SUBTOTALS:										
1. SINGLE DX										
A. Not Operated	37	1.5	<1	1	1	1	2	3	3	5
B. Operated	682	2.1	3	1	1	2	2	3	5	10
2. MULTIPLE DX										
A. Not Operated	376	3.6	8	1	2	3	4	7	9	16
B. Operated	3,347	3.6	14	1	2	3	4	6	9	19
1. SINGLE DX	719	2.0	3	1	1	2	2	3	5	10
2. MULTIPLE DX	3,723	3.6	14	1	2	3	4	6	9	19
A. NOT OPERATED	413	3.4	8	1	1	3	4	7	9	15
B. OPERATED	4,029	3.3	13	1	2	2	4	6	8	18
TOTAL										
0–19 Years	213	2.0	4	1	1	2	2	3	4	13
20–34	653	2.5	6	1	1	2	3	5	7	11
35–49	849	2.9	11	1	1	2	3	5	7	16
50–64	1,277	3.5	19	1	2	2	4	6	9	21
65+	1,450	4.1	11	1	2	3	5	7	9	18
GRAND TOTAL	4,442	3.3	12	1	2	3	4	6	8	18

Western Region, October 2006–September 2007 Data, by Diagnosis

824.5: OPEN FX BIMALLEOLAR

Type of Patients	Observed Patients	Avg. Stay	Variance	10th	25th	50th	75th	90th	95th	99th
1. SINGLE DX										
A. Not Operated										
0–19 Years	0									
20–34	1	1.0	0							
35–49	0									
50–64	0									
65+	0									
B. Operated										
0–19 Years	13	1.9	1	1	1	2	3	3	4	4
20–34	23	2.3	4	1	1	2	3	5	6	9
35–49	12	1.9	<1	1	1	2	3	3	3	3
50–64	20	2.7	6	1	1	2	3	4	12	12
65+	4	4.5	10	1	3	6	8	8	8	8
2. MULTIPLE DX										
A. Not Operated										
0–19 Years	1	4.0	0	4	4	4	4	4	4	4
20–34	1	2.0	0	2	2	2	2	2	2	2
35–49	1	2.0	0	2	2	2	2	2	2	2
50–64	1	6.0	0	6	6	6	6	6	6	6
65+	7	4.9	18	2	2	3	6	14	14	14
B. Operated										
0–19 Years	23	3.4	5	2	2	3	4	5	8	11
20–34	70	5.1	26	1	2	3	6	12	15	29
35–49	80	5.3	52	1	2	3	5	10	25	44
50–64	140	5.5	32	1	2	4	7	12	20	40
65+	131	5.4	17	2	3	4	7	11	14	20
SUBTOTALS:										
1. SINGLE DX										
A. Not Operated	1	1.0	0	1	1	1	1	1	1	1
B. Operated	72	2.4	4	1	1	2	3	4	6	12
2. MULTIPLE DX										
A. Not Operated	11	4.4	12	2	2	3	6	6	14	14
B. Operated	444	5.3	29	2	2	4	6	11	14	30
1. SINGLE DX	73	2.4	4	1	1	2	3	4	6	12
2. MULTIPLE DX	455	5.2	29	2	2	4	6	11	14	30
A. NOT OPERATED	12	4.1	12	2	2	3	4	6	14	14
B. OPERATED	516	4.9	26	2	2	3	5	10	14	29
TOTAL										
0–19 Years	37	2.9	4	1	2	2	4	5	8	11
20–34	95	4.3	22	1	2	3	5	11	15	29
35–49	93	4.8	46	2	2	3	4	9	13	44
50–64	161	5.2	30	1	2	3	6	11	14	40
65+	142	5.3	17	2	3	4	6	11	14	20
GRAND TOTAL	528	4.8	26	2	2	3	5	10	14	29

824.6: CLSD FX TRIMALLEOLAR

Type of Patients	Observed Patients	Avg. Stay	Variance	10th	25th	50th	75th	90th	95th	99th
1. SINGLE DX										
A. Not Operated										
0–19 Years	6	2.0	2	1	1	1	3	4	4	4
20–34	20	1.5	1	1	1	1	2	2	5	5
35–49	10	2.3	4	1	1	1	3	3	7	7
50–64	5	1.4	<1	1	1	1	1	3	3	3
65+	3	1.0	0	1	1	1	1	1	1	1
B. Operated										
0–19 Years	42	2.2	4	1	1	2	3	3	6	12
20–34	238	2.5	6	1	1	2	3	5	7	17
35–49	182	2.0	2	1	1	2	3	3	4	7
50–64	175	2.1	2	1	1	2	3	3	4	8
65+	27	2.4	1	1	1	2	3	4	4	6
2. MULTIPLE DX										
A. Not Operated										
0–19 Years	3	1.3	<1	1	1	1	2	2	2	2
20–34	22	1.4	<1	1	1	1	1	3	3	3
35–49	38	3.4	21	1	1	2	3	10	14	25
50–64	62	3.0	21	1	1	2	3	5	6	35
65+	109	3.6	11	1	2	3	4	6	9	18
B. Operated										
0–19 Years	47	2.3	2	1	1	2	3	4	5	7
20–34	326	2.5	5	1	1	2	3	5	6	12
35–49	621	3.1	10	1	2	2	3	5	8	16
50–64	1,104	3.3	7	1	2	3	4	6	8	13
65+	1,035	4.0	11	1	2	3	5	7	9	18
SUBTOTALS:										
1. SINGLE DX										
A. Not Operated	44	1.7	2	1	1	1	2	3	4	7
B. Operated	664	2.2	4	1	1	2	3	4	5	10
2. MULTIPLE DX										
A. Not Operated	234	3.2	14	1	1	2	3	6	9	19
B. Operated	3,133	3.4	9	1	2	3	4	6	8	15
1. SINGLE DX	708	2.2	3	1	1	2	3	4	5	9
2. MULTIPLE DX	3,367	3.4	9	1	2	3	4	6	8	16
A. NOT OPERATED	278	2.9	13	1	1	2	3	5	9	19
B. OPERATED	3,797	3.2	8	1	2	3	4	6	8	15
TOTAL										
0–19 Years	98	2.2	3	1	1	2	3	4	6	12
20–34	606	2.4	5	1	1	2	3	5	6	13
35–49	851	2.9	9	1	1	2	3	5	7	15
50–64	1,346	3.1	7	1	2	2	4	6	8	13
65+	1,174	3.9	11	1	2	3	4	7	9	18
GRAND TOTAL	4,075	3.2	9	1	2	3	4	6	8	15

824.8: CLSD FX ANKLE NOS

Type of Patients	Observed Patients	Avg. Stay	Variance	10th	25th	50th	75th	90th	95th	99th
1. SINGLE DX										
A. Not Operated										
0–19 Years	71	1.5	<1	1	1	1	2	2	3	5
20–34	31	1.5	<1	1	1	1	2	3	3	4
35–49	19	1.7	1	1	1	1	3	3	4	4
50–64	11	1.5	<1	1	1	1	2	2	4	4
65+	1	4.0	0	4	4	4	4	4	4	4
B. Operated										
0–19 Years	176	1.7	1	1	1	1	2	3	4	6
20–34	299	2.1	2	1	1	2	2	4	4	8
35–49	197	2.3	4	1	1	2	3	4	5	13
50–64	89	2.6	7	1	1	2	3	5	9	14
65+	19	2.9	5	1	1	2	4	6	9	9
2. MULTIPLE DX										
A. Not Operated										
0–19 Years	68	1.8	<1	1	1	2	2	3	4	5
20–34	53	2.7	6	1	1	2	3	5	6	14
35–49	91	2.6	8	1	1	2	3	6	7	11
50–64	130	3.6	8	1	1	3	4	8	9	14
65+	280	3.7	10	1	2	3	4	7	8	13
B. Operated										
0–19 Years	154	2.3	4	1	1	2	3	4	6	10
20–34	471	3.3	21	1	1	3	3	6	8	18
35–49	615	3.4	12	1	2	3	4	6	9	18
50–64	609	3.8	18	1	2	3	4	7	10	19
65+	380	4.1	8	1	2	3	5	7	10	15
SUBTOTALS:										
1. SINGLE DX										
A. Not Operated	133	1.6	<1	1	1	1	2	3	3	4
B. Operated	780	2.1	3	1	1	2	2	4	5	11
2. MULTIPLE DX										
A. Not Operated	622	3.2	8	1	1	3	4	6	8	13
B. Operated	2,229	3.5	14	1	2	3	4	7	9	18
1. SINGLE DX	913	2.0	3	1	1	2	2	3	4	10
2. MULTIPLE DX	2,851	3.5	13	1	2	3	4	7	9	17
A. NOT OPERATED	755	2.9	7	1	1	2	4	6	8	12
B. OPERATED	3,009	3.2	12	1	1	2	4	6	8	16
TOTAL										
0–19 Years	469	1.9	2	1	1	2	2	3	4	8
20–34	854	2.8	13	1	1	3	3	5	7	15
35–49	922	3.1	10	1	1	3	3	6	8	17
50–64	839	3.6	15	1	2	3	4	7	9	17
65+	680	3.9	9	1	2	3	5	7	9	14
GRAND TOTAL	3,764	3.1	11	1	1	2	4	6	8	15

Length of Stay by Diagnosis and Operation, Western Region, 2008

Western Region, October 2006–September 2007 Data, by Diagnosis

824.9: OPEN FX ANKLE NOS

Type of Patients	Observed Patients	Avg. Stay	Variance	10th	25th	50th	75th	90th	95th	99th
1. SINGLE DX										
A. Not Operated										
0–19 Years	7	1.6	1	1	1	1	2	4	4	4
20–34	4	2.2	2	1	1	2	2	4	4	4
35–49	1	1.0	0	1	1	1	1	1	1	1
50–64	0									
65+	0									
B. Operated										
0–19 Years	26	3.2	15	1	2	2	3	5	8	21
20–34	38	3.7	9	1	2	3	4	8	13	13
35–49	41	3.1	4	1	2	3	4	5	5	13
50–64	21	2.4	1	1	2	2	3	3	5	5
65+	2	2.5	<1	2	2	2	3	3	3	3
2. MULTIPLE DX										
A. Not Operated										
0–19 Years	6	1.7	<1	1	1	1	2	3	3	3
20–34	7	1.9	<1	1	1	2	3	3	3	3
35–49	4	6.0	6	4	4	4	7	9	9	9
50–64	5	2.0	<1	1	2	2	3	3	3	3
65+	1	8.0	0	8	8	8	8	8	8	8
B. Operated										
0–19 Years	52	4.2	31	1	2	3	3	6	16	31
20–34	133	6.0	33	2	3	4	7	15	20	25
35–49	149	7.4	76	2	3	4	9	18	25	54
50–64	145	5.9	42	2	3	4	6	11	17	39
65+	84	5.7	15	3	3	4	6	10	14	27
SUBTOTALS:										
1. SINGLE DX										
A. Not Operated	12	1.7	1	1	1	1	2	4	4	4
B. Operated	128	3.2	7	1	2	2	4	5	8	13
2. MULTIPLE DX										
A. Not Operated	23	2.8	5	1	2	2	3	7	8	9
B. Operated	563	6.1	44	2	3	4	7	14	18	32
1. SINGLE DX	140	3.1	7	1	2	2	3	5	8	13
2. MULTIPLE DX	586	6.0	43	2	3	4	7	14	18	32
A. NOT OPERATED	35	2.4	4	1	2	2	3	4	8	9
B. OPERATED	691	5.6	39	2	2	4	6	13	18	31
TOTAL										
0–19 Years	91	3.6	23	1	2	2	3	5	14	31
20–34	182	5.3	27	2	2	3	6	13	17	25
35–49	195	6.5	62	2	2	4	7	16	21	54
50–64	171	5.4	37	2	2	4	6	10	16	39
65+	87	5.6	15	3	3	4	7	10	14	27
GRAND TOTAL	726	5.4	38	2	2	3	6	12	17	31

825: FX OF TARSAL/METATARSAL

Type of Patients	Observed Patients	Avg. Stay	Variance	10th	25th	50th	75th	90th	95th	99th
1. SINGLE DX										
A. Not Operated										
0–19 Years	19	1.4	<1	1	1	1	2	2	2	2
20–34	49	2.4	5	1	1	1	2	5	8	11
35–49	35	1.9	1	1	1	2	2	3	4	5
50–64	17	1.7	<1	1	1	1	2	3	3	3
65+	1	2.0	0	2	2	2	2	2	2	2
B. Operated										
0–19 Years	73	2.1	2	1	1	2	3	4	4	8
20–34	203	2.1	2	1	1	2	3	4	4	7
35–49	154	2.1	3	1	1	2	3	3	4	10
50–64	87	2.1	2	1	1	2	2	3	4	7
65+	12	2.3	<1	1	2	2	3	3	4	4
2. MULTIPLE DX										
A. Not Operated										
0–19 Years	40	2.2	2	1	1	2	3	4	6	8
20–34	159	3.0	25	1	1	2	3	6	8	27
35–49	167	2.8	11	1	1	2	3	5	7	25
50–64	187	3.4	15	1	1	2	4	7	9	28
65+	185	3.4	4	1	2	3	4	6	7	11
B. Operated										
0–19 Years	138	3.5	13	1	1	2	4	8	12	17
20–34	585	4.5	29	1	2	3	5	10	14	27
35–49	590	4.2	22	1	2	3	5	9	12	28
50–64	526	4.1	24	1	2	3	4	9	13	22
65+	167	4.3	22	1	2	3	5	8	12	31
SUBTOTALS:										
1. SINGLE DX										
A. Not Operated	121	2.0	3	1	1	1	2	3	5	10
B. Operated	529	2.1	2	1	1	2	3	4	4	7
2. MULTIPLE DX										
A. Not Operated	738	3.1	13	1	1	2	4	6	8	21
B. Operated	2,006	4.2	24	1	2	3	4	9	13	26
1. SINGLE DX	650	2.1	2	1	1	2	3	4	4	8
2. MULTIPLE DX	2,744	3.9	21	1	2	3	4	8	12	26
A. NOT OPERATED	859	3.0	12	1	1	2	3	5	8	16
B. OPERATED	2,535	3.8	20	1	2	2	4	8	12	25
TOTAL										
0–19 Years	270	2.8	8	1	1	2	3	6	8	17
20–34	996	3.7	22	1	2	2	4	7	12	26
35–49	946	3.5	17	1	2	2	4	7	11	26
50–64	817	3.7	19	1	2	2	4	8	11	21
65+	365	3.8	12	1	2	3	4	6	9	18
GRAND TOTAL	3,394	3.6	18	1	2	2	4	7	11	24

825.0: CLSD FRACTURE CALCANEUS

Type of Patients	Observed Patients	Avg. Stay	Variance	10th	25th	50th	75th	90th	95th	99th
1. SINGLE DX										
A. Not Operated										
0–19 Years	5	1.6	<1	1	1	2	2	2	2	2
20–34	28	3.0	8	1	1	2	5	8	10	11
35–49	21	1.7	<1	1	1	1	2	3	3	4
50–64	14	1.8	<1	1	1	2	3	3	3	3
65+	1	2.0	0	2	2	2	2	2	2	2
B. Operated										
0–19 Years	12	2.5	4	1	1	2	3	4	8	8
20–34	88	2.1	1	1	1	2	3	4	4	7
35–49	97	2.3	3	1	1	2	3	4	4	14
50–64	50	1.9	2	1	1	2	2	4	4	7
65+	12	2.3	<1	1	2	2	3	3	4	4
2. MULTIPLE DX										
A. Not Operated										
0–19 Years	10	2.7	<1	1	2	3	3	4	4	4
20–34	72	4.0	42	1	1	2	4	7	9	50
35–49	106	3.0	11	1	2	2	3	5	7	16
50–64	92	3.4	10	1	2	2	4	8	10	21
65+	45	4.0	4	2	3	3	5	6	8	11
B. Operated										
0–19 Years	11	3.3	4	1	2	3	3	6	8	8
20–34	166	4.6	31	1	2	3	4	13	18	27
35–49	257	3.7	14	1	2	3	4	7	12	21
50–64	245	3.7	16	1	2	3	4	8	12	22
65+	75	4.0	13	2	2	3	5	9	12	18
SUBTOTALS:										
1. SINGLE DX										
A. Not Operated	69	2.3	4	1	1	2	3	5	7	11
B. Operated	259	2.2	2	1	1	2	3	4	4	8
2. MULTIPLE DX										
A. Not Operated	325	3.5	17	1	2	2	4	6	9	21
B. Operated	754	3.9	18	1	2	3	4	8	13	23
1. SINGLE DX	328	2.2	2	1	1	2	3	4	4	10
2. MULTIPLE DX	1,079	3.8	18	1	2	3	4	8	12	23
A. NOT OPERATED	394	3.3	15	1	1	2	4	6	9	21
B. OPERATED	1,013	3.5	15	1	2	2	4	7	11	21
TOTAL										
0–19 Years	38	2.7	3	1	1	3	3	4	8	8
20–34	354	3.7	25	1	1	2	3	7	13	26
35–49	481	3.2	11	1	1	2	3	6	9	17
50–64	401	3.4	12	1	2	2	4	7	10	21
65+	133	3.9	9	1	2	3	5	7	11	18
GRAND TOTAL	1,407	3.4	15	1	2	2	4	7	10	21

Western Region, October 2006–September 2007 Data, by Diagnosis

825.21: CLSD FX ASTRAGALUS

Type of Patients	Observed Patients	Avg. Stay	Variance	10th	25th	50th	75th	90th	95th	99th
1. SINGLE DX										
A. Not Operated										
0–19 Years	3	1.3	<1	1	1	1	1	2	2	2
20–34	4	1.8	2	1	1	1	1	4	4	4
35–49	2	1.0	0	1	1	1	1	1	1	1
50–64	1	1.0	0	1	1	1	1	1	1	1
65+	0									
B. Operated										
0–19 Years	11	1.6	1	1	1	1	2	3	4	4
20–34	27	1.9	<1	1	1	2	2	3	4	4
35–49	14	2.4	3	1	1	2	2	4	8	8
50–64	6	2.5	5	1	1	2	2	7	7	7
65+	0									
2. MULTIPLE DX										
A. Not Operated										
0–19 Years	4	2.3	2	1	2	2	4	4	4	4
20–34	22	1.8	2	1	1	1	2	4	5	6
35–49	12	4.4	44	1	1	2	4	5	25	25
50–64	13	2.0	1	1	1	3	3	4	4	4
65+	8	2.9	<1	1	3	3	3	4	4	4
B. Operated										
0–19 Years	24	3.5	11	1	2	3	3	6	9	17
20–34	114	4.1	21	1	2	3	4	8	10	26
35–49	81	3.7	13	1	2	3	4	7	8	27
50–64	32	4.8	13	2	2	3	6	9	13	15
65+	11	3.8	4	2	3	3	5	6	8	8
SUBTOTALS:										
1. SINGLE DX										
A. Not Operated	10	1.4	<1	1	1	1	1	2	2	4
B. Operated	58	2.0	2	1	1	2	2	4	4	8
2. MULTIPLE DX										
A. Not Operated	59	2.6	11	1	1	2	3	4	5	25
B. Operated	262	4.0	16	1	2	3	4	8	10	26
1. SINGLE DX	68	1.9	2	1	1	2	2	4	4	8
2. MULTIPLE DX	321	3.7	15	1	2	3	4	8	9	25
A. NOT OPERATED	69	2.4	9	1	1	2	3	4	5	25
B. OPERATED	320	3.6	14	1	2	3	4	8	9	17
TOTAL										
0–19 Years	42	2.7	7	1	1	2	3	4	6	17
20–34	167	3.4	16	1	1	2	4	7	9	26
35–49	109	3.6	15	1	1	3	4	7	8	25
50–64	52	3.8	11	1	2	3	5	8	12	15
65+	19	3.4	3	1	3	3	4	6	8	8
GRAND TOTAL	389	3.4	13	1	1	2	4	7	9	25

825.25.25: CLSD FX METATARSAL BONE

Type of Patients	Observed Patients	Avg. Stay	Variance	10th	25th	50th	75th	90th	95th	99th
1. SINGLE DX										
A. Not Operated										
0–19 Years	6	1.2	<1	1	1	1	1	2	2	2
20–34	13	1.5	<1	1	1	1	2	2	3	3
35–49	4	2.5	3	1	1	2	2	5	5	5
50–64	2	1.5	<1	1	1	2	2	2	2	2
65+	0									
B. Operated										
0–19 Years	26	1.9	2	1	1	1	3	4	5	6
20–34	41	2.0	2	1	1	2	2	4	4	7
35–49	20	1.4	<1	1	1	1	2	2	5	5
50–64	18	2.1	1	1	1	2	2	4	5	5
65+	0									
2. MULTIPLE DX										
A. Not Operated										
0–19 Years	12	1.5	<1	1	1	2	2	2	2	2
20–34	37	2.8	18	1	1	2	3	4	6	27
35–49	29	1.9	<1	1	1	2	2	3	3	4
50–64	63	4.0	29	1	1	2	4	8	9	32
65+	110	3.3	3	1	2	3	4	6	7	9
B. Operated										
0–19 Years	29	2.9	8	1	1	2	3	6	10	13
20–34	90	2.7	5	1	1	2	4	5	7	14
35–49	110	3.6	16	1	2	2	4	8	12	16
50–64	113	2.9	6	1	1	2	3	7	9	12
65+	47	4.2	30	2	2	3	5	6	8	31
SUBTOTALS:										
1. SINGLE DX										
A. Not Operated	25	1.6	<1	1	1	1	2	2	3	5
B. Operated	105	1.9	2	1	1	2	2	4	5	6
2. MULTIPLE DX										
A. Not Operated	251	3.1	12	1	1	2	4	5	7	27
B. Operated	389	3.2	12	1	1	2	4	6	9	16
1. SINGLE DX	130	1.8	1	1	1	2	2	4	5	6
2. MULTIPLE DX	640	3.2	12	1	1	2	4	6	8	16
A. NOT OPERATED	276	3.0	11	1	1	2	3	5	7	27
B. OPERATED	494	2.9	10	1	1	2	3	6	8	16
TOTAL										
0–19 Years	73	2.1	4	1	1	2	3	4	6	13
20–34	181	2.4	7	1	1	2	3	5	6	14
35–49	163	3.0	12	1	1	2	3	6	11	16
50–64	196	3.2	14	1	1	2	4	7	9	28
65+	157	3.5	11	1	2	3	4	6	7	25
GRAND TOTAL	770	2.9	10	1	1	2	3	6	8	16

826: FRACTURE PHALANGES FOOT

Type of Patients	Observed Patients	Avg. Stay	Variance	10th	25th	50th	75th	90th	95th	99th
1. SINGLE DX										
A. Not Operated										
0–19 Years	2	1.0	0	1	1	1	1	1	1	1
20–34	5	1.2	<1	1	1	1	1	2	2	2
35–49	3	2.0	<1	1	1	2	3	3	3	3
50–64	0									
65+	0									
B. Operated										
0–19 Years	13	1.7	<1	1	1	2	2	3	3	3
20–34	15	1.8	<1	1	1	2	2	3	3	3
35–49	8	2.0	<1	1	1	2	2	3	3	3
50–64	3	1.7	1	1	1	1	3	3	3	3
65+	0									
2. MULTIPLE DX										
A. Not Operated										
0–19 Years	5	1.4	<1	1	1	1	2	2	2	2
20–34	16	1.7	1	1	1	1	2	4	4	4
35–49	16	1.9	1	1	2	2	3	4	4	4
50–64	15	3.1	3	1	2	3	5	5	7	7
65+	42	3.3	3	2	2	3	4	5	7	8
B. Operated										
0–19 Years	23	3.1	7	1	1	3	4	6	7	12
20–34	41	4.3	37	1	1	3	5	9	10	39
35–49	41	4.0	20	2	2	3	4	7	9	23
50–64	38	4.8	30	1	1	3	6	10	19	28
65+	22	3.2	4	1	2	3	4	7	7	7
SUBTOTALS:										
1. SINGLE DX										
A. Not Operated	10	1.4	<1	1	1	1	2	2	2	3
B. Operated	39	1.8	<1	1	1	2	2	3	3	3
2. MULTIPLE DX										
A. Not Operated	94	2.7	3	1	1	2	4	4	6	8
B. Operated	165	4.1	23	1	1	3	4	8	10	28
1. SINGLE DX	49	1.7	<1	1	1	2	2	3	3	3
2. MULTIPLE DX	259	3.6	16	1	1	3	4	7	9	23
A. NOT OPERATED	104	2.5	2	1	1	2	4	4	5	7
B. OPERATED	204	3.6	19	1	1	2	4	7	10	23
TOTAL										
0–19 Years	43	2.4	5	1	1	2	3	4	6	12
20–34	77	3.1	22	1	1	2	4	5	9	39
35–49	68	3.2	13	1	1	3	3	5	8	23
50–64	56	4.2	22	1	2	3	5	10	11	28
65+	64	3.3	3	2	2	3	4	6	7	8
GRAND TOTAL	308	3.3	14	1	1	2	4	6	8	20

Length of Stay by Diagnosis and Operation, Western Region, 2008

Western Region, October 2006–September 2007 Data, by Diagnosis

Type of Patients	826.1: OPEN FX PHALANX FOOT										827: LOWER LIMB FRACTURE NEC										828: FX LEGS W ARM/RIB									
	Observed Patients	Avg. Stay	Vari-ance	10th	25th	50th	75th	90th	95th	99th	Observed Patients	Avg. Stay	Vari-ance	10th	25th	50th	75th	90th	95th	99th	Observed Patients	Avg. Stay	Vari-ance	10th	25th	50th	75th	90th	95th	99th
1. SINGLE DX																														
A. Not Operated																														
0–19 Years	1	1.0	0	1	1	1	1	1	1	1	0										0									
20–34	3	1.3	<1	1	1	1	2	2	2	2	0										0									
35–49	2	1.5	<1	1	1	2	2	2	2	2	0										0									
50–64	0										0											0									
65+	0										0											0									
B. Operated																														
0–19 Years	12	1.8	<1	1	1	1	2	3	3	3	1	2.0	0	2	2	2	2	2	2	2	0									
20–34	11	2.0	<1	1	1	2	3	3	3	3	0										0									
35–49	8	2.0	<1	1	1	2	2	3	3	3	1	2.0	0	2	2	2	2	2	2	2	0									
50–64	3	1.7	1	1	1	1	3	3	3	3	0										0									
65+	0										0											0									
2. MULTIPLE DX																														
A. Not Operated																														
0–19 Years	4	1.5	<1	1	1	2	2	2	2	2	0										0									
20–34	7	1.4	<1	1	1	1	2	2	2	2	0										0									
35–49	5	1.6	<1	1	1	2	2	2	2	2	0										0									
50–64	8	2.8	2	1	2	3	4	5	5	5	2	4.5	<1	4	4	5	5	5	5	5	0									
65+	10	3.0	2	1	2	3	4	4	5	5	1	4.0	0	4	4	4	4	4	4	4	0									
B. Operated																														
0–19 Years	21	3.0	8	1	1	2	4	6	7	12	0										0									
20–34	33	4.1	45	1	1	2	4	7	10	39	0										0									
35–49	35	4.3	23	1	2	3	5	8	20	23	0										0									
50–64	32	4.4	27	1	1	3	5	10	11	28	1	3.0	0	3	3	3	3	3	3	3	1	8.0	0	8	8	8	8	8	8	8
65+	19	3.2	4	1	2	3	4	7	7	7	0										0									
SUBTOTALS:																														
1. SINGLE DX																														
A. Not Operated	6	1.3	<1	1	1	1	2	2	2	2	0										0									
B. Operated	34	1.9	<1	1	1	2	3	3	3	3	2	2.0	0	2	2	2	2	2	2	2	0									
2. MULTIPLE DX																														
A. Not Operated	34	2.2	2	1	1	2	3	4	5	5	3	4.3	<1	4	4	5	5	5	5	5	0									
B. Operated	140	3.9	24	1	1	3	4	7	10	28	1	3.0	0	3	3	3	3	3	3	3	1	8.0	0	8	8	8	8	8	8	8
1. SINGLE DX	40	1.8	<1	1	1	2	2	3	3	3	2	2.0	0	2	2	2	2	2	2	2	0									
2. MULTIPLE DX	174	3.6	20	1	1	2	4	7	10	28	4	4.0	<1	3	4	4	5	5	5	5	1	8.0	0	8	8	8	8	8	8	8
A. NOT OPERATED	40	2.1	2	1	1	2	2	4	4	5	3	4.3	<1	4	4	4	5	5	5	5	0									
B. OPERATED	174	3.5	20	1	1	2	4	7	10	28	3	2.3	<1	2	2	2	3	3	3	3	1	8.0	0	8	8	8	8	8	8	8
TOTAL																														
0–19 Years	38	2.4	5	1	1	2	3	4	7	12	1	2.0	0	2	2	2	2	2	2	2	0									
20–34	54	3.2	29	1	1	2	3	5	9	39	0										0									
35–49	50	3.5	17	1	2	2	4	7	9	23	1	2.0	0	2	2	2	2	2	2	2	0									
50–64	43	3.9	21	1	1	3	4	8	10	28	3	4.0	<1	3	3	4	5	5	5	5	1	8.0	0	8	8	8	8	8	8	8
65+	29	3.1	3	1	2	3	4	7	7	7	1	4.0	0	4	4	4	4	4	4	4	0									
GRAND TOTAL	214	3.3	17	1	1	2	4	6	9	23	6	3.3	1	2	2	4	4	5	5	5	1	8.0	0	8	8	8	8	8	8	8

Length of Stay by Diagnosis and Operation, Western Region, 2008

Western Region, October 2006–September 2007 Data, by Diagnosis

829: FRACTURE NOS

Type of Patients	Observed Patients	Avg. Stay	Variance	10th	25th	50th	75th	90th	95th	99th
1. SINGLE DX										
A. Not Operated										
0–19 Years	0									
20–34	0									
35–49	0									
50–64	0									
65+	0									
B. Operated										
0–19 Years	0									
20–34	0									
35–49	0									
50–64	0									
65+	0									
2. MULTIPLE DX										
A. Not Operated										
0–19 Years	0									
20–34	0									
35–49	0									
50–64	1	1.0	0	1	1	1	1	1	1	1
65+	0									
B. Operated										
0–19 Years	1	4.0	0	4	4	4	4	4	4	4
20–34	0									
35–49	0									
50–64	0									
65+	1	2.0	0	2	2	2	2	2	2	2
SUBTOTALS:										
1. SINGLE DX										
A. Not Operated	0									
B. Operated	0									
2. MULTIPLE DX										
A. Not Operated	1	1.0	0	1	1	1	1	1	1	1
B. Operated	2	3.0	2	2	2	2	4	4	4	4
1. SINGLE DX	0									
2. MULTIPLE DX	3	2.3	2	1	1	2	4	4	4	4
A. NOT OPERATED	1	1.0	0	1	1	1	1	1	1	1
B. OPERATED	2	3.0	2	2	2	2	4	4	4	4
TOTAL										
0–19 Years	1	4.0	0	4	4	4	4	4	4	4
20–34	0									
35–49	0									
50–64	1	1.0	0	1	1	1	1	1	1	1
65+	1	2.0	0	2	2	2	2	2	2	2
GRAND TOTAL	3	2.3	2	1	1	2	4	4	4	4

830: JAW DISLOCATION

Type of Patients	Observed Patients	Avg. Stay	Variance	10th	25th	50th	75th	90th	95th	99th
1. SINGLE DX										
A. Not Operated										
0–19 Years	2	2.5	4	1	1	3	4	4	4	4
20–34	0									
35–49	0									
50–64	0									
65+	0									
B. Operated										
0–19 Years	0									
20–34	0									
35–49	0									
50–64	0									
65+	0									
2. MULTIPLE DX										
A. Not Operated										
0–19 Years	0									
20–34	2	2.0	2	1	1	2	3	3	3	3
35–49	3	1.7	1	1	1	1	3	3	3	3
50–64	3	4.7	6	2	2	5	7	7	7	7
65+	9	4.1	22	1	2	2	5	16	16	16
B. Operated										
0–19 Years	0									
20–34	0									
35–49	1	2.0	0	2	2	2	2	2	2	2
50–64	0									
65+	0									
SUBTOTALS:										
1. SINGLE DX										
A. Not Operated	2	2.5	4	1	1	3	4	4	4	4
B. Operated	0									
2. MULTIPLE DX										
A. Not Operated	17	3.5	13	1	1	2	5	7	16	16
B. Operated	1	2.0	0	2	2	2	2	2	2	2
1. SINGLE DX	2	2.5	4	1	1	3	4	4	4	4
2. MULTIPLE DX	18	3.4	13	1	1	2	5	7	16	16
A. NOT OPERATED	19	3.4	12	1	1	2	5	7	16	16
B. OPERATED	1	2.0	0	2	2	2	2	2	2	2
TOTAL										
0–19 Years	2	2.5	4	1	1	3	4	4	4	4
20–34	2	2.0	2	1	1	2	3	3	3	3
35–49	4	1.8	<1	1	1	2	3	3	3	3
50–64	3	4.7	6	2	2	5	7	7	7	7
65+	9	4.1	22	1	2	2	5	16	16	16
GRAND TOTAL	20	3.3	12	1	1	2	4	5	7	16

831: SHOULDER DISLOCATION

Type of Patients	Observed Patients	Avg. Stay	Variance	10th	25th	50th	75th	90th	95th	99th
1. SINGLE DX										
A. Not Operated										
0–19 Years	5	2.8	16		1	1	1	10	10	10
20–34	9	1.3	<1	1	1	1	1	1	4	4
35–49	4	1.0	0	1	1	1	1	1	1	1
50–64	5	1.4	<1	1	1	1	2	2	2	2
65+	1	1.0	0	1	1	1	1	1	1	1
B. Operated										
0–19 Years	6	1.3	<1		2	1	2	2	2	2
20–34	15	1.3	<1	1	2	1	2	2	3	3
35–49	8	1.1	<1	1	1	1	1	2	2	2
50–64	5	1.2	<1	1	1	1	1	2	2	2
65+	1	3.0	0	3	3	3	3	3	3	3
2. MULTIPLE DX										
A. Not Operated										
0–19 Years	13	1.8	2	1	1	1	3	3	5	5
20–34	47	2.3	5	1	1	1	3	4	7	11
35–49	42	2.4	3	1	1	2	3	6	6	8
50–64	52	2.4	5	1	1	2	3	5	7	15
65+	187	3.0	5	1	1	3	4	6	7	12
B. Operated										
0–19 Years	2	2.0	0	2	2	2	2	2	2	2
20–34	17	3.7	9	1	2	3	4	7	12	12
35–49	23	3.4	11	1	1	2	4	8	10	14
50–64	24	2.2	3	1	2	2	3	4	5	7
65+	20	3.4	4	1	2	3	4	6	7	8
SUBTOTALS:										
1. SINGLE DX										
A. Not Operated	24	1.6	4	1	1	1	1	2	4	10
B. Operated	35	1.3	<1	1	1	1	2	2	3	3
2. MULTIPLE DX										
A. Not Operated	341	2.7	4	1	1	2	3	5	7	11
B. Operated	86	3.1	6	1	2	2	4	7	8	14
1. SINGLE DX	59	1.4	2	1	1	1	1	2	3	10
2. MULTIPLE DX	427	2.8	5	1	1	2	3	6	7	12
A. NOT OPERATED	365	2.6	4	1	1	2	3	5	7	11
B. OPERATED	121	2.6	5	1	1	2	3	5	7	12
TOTAL										
0–19 Years	26	1.9	4	1	1	1	2	3	5	10
20–34	88	2.3	5	1	1	1	3	4	7	12
35–49	77	2.5	6	1	1	2	3	6	8	14
50–64	86	2.2	4	1	1	2	3	4	5	15
65+	209	3.0	4	1	1	3	4	6	7	9
GRAND TOTAL	486	2.6	5	1	1	2	3	5	7	12

Length of Stay by Diagnosis and Operation, Western Region, 2008

Western Region, October 2006–September 2007 Data, by Diagnosis

831.01: CLSD ANT DISLOC HUMERUS

Type of Patients	Observed Patients	Avg. Stay	Vari-ance	10th	25th	50th	75th	90th	95th	99th
1. SINGLE DX										
A. Not Operated										
0–19 Years	0									
20–34	5	1.6	2	1	1	1	1	4	4	4
35–49	1	1.0	0	1	1	1	1	1	1	1
50–64	5	1.4	<1	1	1	1	2	2	2	2
65+	0									
B. Operated										
0–19 Years	0									
20–34	1	1.0	0	1	1	1	1	1	1	1
35–49	0									
50–64	2	1.0	0	1	1	1	1	1	1	1
65+	1	3.0	0	3	3	3	3	3	3	3
2. MULTIPLE DX										
A. Not Operated										
0–19 Years	3	1.7	1	1	1	1	3	3	3	3
20–34	17	2.1	1	1	1	2	3	3	4	4
35–49	18	2.4	3	1	1	2	2	6	6	6
50–64	29	2.6	8	1	1	2	3	5	7	15
65+	108	2.6	4	1	1	2	3	5	6	9
B. Operated										
0–19 Years	0									
20–34	5	2.8	2	1	2	3	4	4	4	4
35–49	7	5.1	18	2	2	4	7	14	14	14
50–64	2	3.5	<1	3	3	4	4	4	4	4
65+	7	3.6	3	2	3	3	4	7	7	7
SUBTOTALS:										
1. SINGLE DX										
A. Not Operated	11	1.5	<1	1	1	1	1	2	2	4
B. Operated	4	1.5	1	1	1	1	1	3	3	3
2. MULTIPLE DX										
A. Not Operated	175	2.5	4	1	1	2	3	5	6	12
B. Operated	21	3.9	7	2	3	3	4	7	7	14
1. SINGLE DX	15	1.5	<1	1	1	1	2	3	4	4
2. MULTIPLE DX	196	2.7	5	1	1	2	3	5	7	14
A. NOT OPERATED	186	2.5	4	1	1	2	3	5	6	12
B. OPERATED	25	3.5	7	1	2	3	4	7	7	14
TOTAL										
0–19 Years	3	1.7	1	1	1	1	3	3	3	3
20–34	28	2.1	2	1	1	2	3	4	4	4
35–49	26	3.1	8	1	1	2	4	6	7	14
50–64	38	2.4	6	1	1	2	3	4	7	15
65+	116	2.7	4	1	1	2	3	5	7	9
GRAND TOTAL	211	2.6	5	1	1	2	3	5	6	12

832: ELBOW DISLOCATION

Type of Patients	Observed Patients	Avg. Stay	Vari-ance	10th	25th	50th	75th	90th	95th	99th
1. SINGLE DX										
A. Not Operated										
0–19 Years	13	1.1	<1	1	1	1	1	1	2	2
20–34	4	1.8	2	1	1	1	1	4	4	4
35–49	5	1.0	0	1	1	1	1	1	1	1
50–64	6	1.5	<1	1	1	1	2	3	3	3
65+	1	1.0	0	1	1	1	1	1	1	1
B. Operated										
0–19 Years	3	1.3	<1	1	1	1	2	2	2	2
20–34	3	1.3	<1	1	1	1	2	2	2	2
35–49	3	1.0	0	1	1	1	1	1	1	1
50–64	2	1.0	0	1	1	1	1	1	1	1
65+	1	1.0	0	1	1	1	1	1	1	1
2. MULTIPLE DX										
A. Not Operated										
0–19 Years	11	1.5	<1	1	1	1	2	3	3	3
20–34	14	1.8	2	1	1	2	2	4	5	5
35–49	12	1.9	<1	1	1	2	2	3	4	4
50–64	21	2.2	3	1	1	2	3	5	6	6
65+	18	2.2	2	1	1	2	3	5	5	5
B. Operated										
0–19 Years	2	1.0	0	1	1	1	1	1	1	1
20–34	12	4.1	17	1	1	3	7	7	15	15
35–49	13	4.1	32	1	2	2	3	14	19	19
50–64	15	5.1	31	1	3	3	6	17	17	17
65+	8	1.5	<1	1	1	2	2	3	3	3
SUBTOTALS:										
1. SINGLE DX										
A. Not Operated	29	1.2	<1	1	1	1	1	2	3	3
B. Operated	12	1.2	<1	1	1	1	1	2	2	2
2. MULTIPLE DX										
A. Not Operated	76	2.0	2	1	1	2	3	4	5	6
B. Operated	50	3.8	22	1	1	2	4	14	17	19
1. SINGLE DX	41	1.2	<1	1	1	1	1	2	2	4
2. MULTIPLE DX	126	2.7	11	1	1	2	3	5	7	17
A. NOT OPERATED	105	1.8	1	1	1	1	2	3	5	6
B. OPERATED	62	3.3	19	1	1	2	3	7	15	19
TOTAL										
0–19 Years	29	1.2	<1	1	1	1	2	2	3	3
20–34	33	2.6	8	1	1	1	3	5	7	15
35–49	33	2.6	14	1	1	2	2	4	14	19
50–64	44	3.0	14	1	1	2	3	6	12	17
65+	28	1.9	1	1	1	2	3	3	5	5
GRAND TOTAL	167	2.3	9	1	1	2	3	4	6	17

833: WRIST DISLOCATION

Type of Patients	Observed Patients	Avg. Stay	Vari-ance	10th	25th	50th	75th	90th	95th	99th
1. SINGLE DX										
A. Not Operated										
0–19 Years	1	1.0	0	1	1	1	1	1	1	1
20–34	3	1.0	0	1	1	1	1	1	1	1
35–49	3	1.3	<1	1	1	1	1	2	2	2
50–64	0									
65+	0									
B. Operated										
0–19 Years	0									
20–34	3	1.7	1	1	1	1	3	3	3	3
35–49	2	3.5	4	2	2	5	5	5	5	5
50–64	2	1.0	0	1	1	1	1	1	1	1
65+	0									
2. MULTIPLE DX										
A. Not Operated										
0–19 Years	1	1.0	0	1	1	1	1	1	1	1
20–34	3	1.0	0	1	1	1	1	1	1	1
35–49	1	2.0	0	2	2	2	2	2	2	2
50–64	2	1.0	0	1	1	1	1	1	1	1
65+	1	1.0	0	1	1	1	1	1	1	1
B. Operated										
0–19 Years	3	1.3	<1	1	1	2	2	2	2	2
20–34	18	2.4	3	1	1	2	3	6	7	7
35–49	10	2.7	2	1	2	2	4	5	5	5
50–64	5	1.8	<1	1	1	1	2	3	3	3
65+	5	2.2	5	1	1	1	2	6	6	6
SUBTOTALS:										
1. SINGLE DX										
A. Not Operated	7	1.1	<1	1	1	1	1	2	2	2
B. Operated	7	2.0	2	1	1	3	3	5	5	5
2. MULTIPLE DX										
A. Not Operated	8	1.1	<1	1	1	1	1	2	2	2
B. Operated	41	2.3	3	1	1	2	3	5	6	7
1. SINGLE DX	14	1.6	1	1	1	1	2	3	5	5
2. MULTIPLE DX	49	2.1	2	1	1	2	3	5	6	7
A. NOT OPERATED	15	1.1	<1	1	1	1	1	2	2	2
B. OPERATED	48	2.3	3	1	2	2	3	5	6	7
TOTAL										
0–19 Years	5	1.2	<1	1	1	1	2	2	2	2
20–34	27	2.0	3	1	1	1	3	4	6	7
35–49	16	2.5	2	1	1	2	4	5	5	5
50–64	9	1.4	<1	1	1	1	2	3	3	3
65+	6	2.0	4	1	1	1	2	6	6	6
GRAND TOTAL	63	2.0	2	1	1	1	2	4	5	7

Length of Stay by Diagnosis and Operation, Western Region, 2008

834: DISLOCATION OF FINGER

Type of Patients	Observed Patients	Avg. Stay	Variance	10th	25th	50th	75th	90th	95th	99th
1. SINGLE DX										
A. Not Operated										
0–19 Years	4	1.3	<1	1	1	1	1	2	2	2
20–34	5	1.6	2	1	1	1	1	4	4	4
35–49	2	1.0	0	1	1	1	1	1	1	1
50–64	3	1.3	<1	1	1	1	2	2	2	2
65+	0									
B. Operated										
0–19 Years	5	1.6	<1	1	1	1	2	3	3	3
20–34	12	1.3	<1	1	1	1	1	2	2	2
35–49	5	1.0	0	1	1	1	1	1	1	1
50–64	1	1.0	0	1	1	1	1	1	1	1
65+	1	3.0	0	3	3	3	3	3	3	3
2. MULTIPLE DX										
A. Not Operated										
0–19 Years	1	1.0	0	1	1	1	1	1	1	1
20–34	9	1.1	<1	1	1	1	1	2	2	2
35–49	8	2.8	6	1	1	2	6	7	7	7
50–64	2	1.0	0	1	1	1	1	1	1	1
65+	6	1.7	1	1	1	1	2	4	4	4
B. Operated										
0–19 Years	9	1.1	<1	1	1	1	1	2	2	2
20–34	17	2.4	3	1	1	2	3	4	7	7
35–49	30	1.7	<1	1	1	1	2	3	4	5
50–64	9	1.5	<1	1	1	1	2	3	3	3
65+	18	1.7	2	1	1	1	2	4	5	5
SUBTOTALS:										
1. SINGLE DX										
A. Not Operated	14	1.4	<1	1	1	1	1	2	4	4
B. Operated	24	1.3	<1	1	1	1	2	2	3	3
2. MULTIPLE DX										
A. Not Operated	26	1.7	2	1	1	1	2	4	6	7
B. Operated	83	1.8	1	1	1	1	2	3	4	7
1. SINGLE DX	38	1.3	<1	1	1	1	1	2	3	4
2. MULTIPLE DX	109	1.8	2	1	1	1	2	4	4	7
A. NOT OPERATED	40	1.6	2	1	1	1	2	2	6	7
B. OPERATED	107	1.7	1	1	1	1	2	3	4	5
TOTAL										
0–19 Years	19	1.3	<1	1	1	1	1	2	3	3
20–34	43	1.7	2	1	1	1	2	4	4	7
35–49	45	1.8	2	1	1	1	2	3	5	7
50–64	15	1.3	<1	1	1	1	2	2	3	3
65+	25	1.8	1	1	1	1	2	4	4	5
GRAND TOTAL	147	1.6	1	1	1	1	2	3	4	7

835: DISLOCATION OF HIP

Type of Patients	Observed Patients	Avg. Stay	Variance	10th	25th	50th	75th	90th	95th	99th
1. SINGLE DX										
A. Not Operated										
0–19 Years	16	1.2	<1	1	1	1	1	2	2	2
20–34	5	2.6	13	1	1	1	1	9	9	9
35–49	2	1.5	<1	1	1	1	2	2	2	2
50–64	3	1.3	<1	1	1	1	2	2	2	2
65+	4	1.8	<1	1	1	2	3	3	3	3
B. Operated										
0–19 Years	3	1.7	<1	1	1	2	2	2	2	2
20–34	1	1.0	0	1	1	1	1	1	1	1
35–49	1	4.0	0	4	4	4	4	4	4	4
50–64	0									
65+	0									
2. MULTIPLE DX										
A. Not Operated										
0–19 Years	34	1.9	1	1	1	2	3	3	4	5
20–34	41	1.9	1	1	1	1	2	4	4	5
35–49	27	2.8	7	1	1	2	3	8	9	10
50–64	22	3.7	10	1	1	3	4	9	10	12
65+	49	3.1	6	1	1	2	5	7	8	9
B. Operated										
0–19 Years	19	4.6	12	1	3	4	6	9	15	15
20–34	16	5.1	14	2	3	3	6	11	16	16
35–49	8	8.4	7	5	6	8	9	13	13	13
50–64	8	6.9	6	4	4	8	9	11	11	11
65+	5	6.0	7	2	5	7	7	9	9	9
SUBTOTALS:										
1. SINGLE DX										
A. Not Operated	30	1.5	2	1	1	1	2	2	3	9
B. Operated	5	2.0	1	1	1	2	2	4	4	4
2. MULTIPLE DX										
A. Not Operated	173	2.6	5	1	1	2	3	6	8	10
B. Operated	56	5.7	12	2	3	5	8	11	13	16
1. SINGLE DX	35	1.6	2	1	1	1	2	2	4	9
2. MULTIPLE DX	229	3.4	8	1	1	2	4	8	9	13
A. NOT OPERATED	203	2.4	5	1	1	2	3	5	8	10
B. OPERATED	61	5.4	12	2	3	5	7	9	11	16
TOTAL										
0–19 Years	72	2.5	5	1	1	2	3	5	6	15
20–34	63	2.7	7	1	1	2	3	5	7	16
35–49	38	3.9	12	1	1	2	6	9	11	13
50–64	33	4.3	11	1	1	4	6	9	11	12
65+	58	3.2	7	1	1	2	5	7	9	9
GRAND TOTAL	264	3.1	8	1	1	2	4	7	9	13

836: DISLOCATION OF KNEE

Type of Patients	Observed Patients	Avg. Stay	Variance	10th	25th	50th	75th	90th	95th	99th
1. SINGLE DX										
A. Not Operated										
0–19 Years	3	1.3	<1	1	1	1	2	2	2	2
20–34	1	1.0	0	1	1	1	1	1	1	1
35–49	3	2.0	0	2	2	2	2	2	2	2
50–64	4	3.3	15	1	1	2	9	9	9	9
65+	1	1.0	0	1	1	1	1	1	1	1
B. Operated										
0–19 Years	10	3.7	34	1	1	1	2	19	19	19
20–34	14	1.6	<1	1	1	1	2	3	4	4
35–49	4	1.8	<1	1	1	1	3	3	3	3
50–64	4	1.5	1	1	1	1	3	3	3	3
65+	1	3.0	0	3	3	3	3	3	3	3
2. MULTIPLE DX										
A. Not Operated										
0–19 Years	7	2.2	3	1	1	2	2	6	6	6
20–34	22	1.7	<1	1	1	2	2	2	3	5
35–49	27	2.5	2	1	1	2	3	5	5	7
50–64	42	3.7	8	1	2	3	4	6	7	17
65+	64	3.8	9	1	2	3	5	6	8	19
B. Operated										
0–19 Years	25	2.2	4	1	1	2	2	4	5	10
20–34	57	4.5	63	1	1	2	4	8	19	49
35–49	67	3.6	17	1	1	2	4	9	10	26
50–64	64	4.5	45	1	1	3	5	9	12	44
65+	45	3.3	6	3	3	3	4	7	8	13
SUBTOTALS:										
1. SINGLE DX										
A. Not Operated	12	2.1	5	1	1	2	2	2	9	9
B. Operated	33	2.3	11	1	1	1	2	3	8	19
2. MULTIPLE DX										
A. Not Operated	162	3.2	7	1	2	2	4	6	7	17
B. Operated	258	3.8	31	1	1	2	4	8	12	30
1. SINGLE DX	45	2.3	9	1	1	1	2	3	8	19
2. MULTIPLE DX	420	3.6	22	1	1	2	4	7	10	26
A. NOT OPERATED	174	3.1	7	1	2	2	4	6	7	17
B. OPERATED	291	3.7	29	1	1	2	4	8	11	30
TOTAL										
0–19 Years	45	2.5	10	1	1	2	2	5	8	19
20–34	94	3.4	40	1	1	2	3	5	11	49
35–49	101	3.2	12	1	1	2	4	7	10	13
50–64	114	4.1	29	1	1	3	5	8	12	29
65+	111	3.6	8	1	2	3	5	6	8	14
GRAND TOTAL	465	3.5	21	1	1	2	4	7	10	26

Length of Stay by Diagnosis and Operation, Western Region, 2008

Western Region, October 2006–September 2007 Data, by Diagnosis

836.0: TEAR MED MENISC KNEE-CUR

Type of Patients	Observed Patients	Avg. Stay	Variance	10th	25th	50th	75th	90th	95th	99th
1. SINGLE DX										
A. Not Operated										
0–19 Years	0									
20–34	0									
35–49	0									
50–64	0									
65+	0									
B. Operated										
0–19 Years	2	1.0	0		1			1	1	1
20–34	3	1.3	<1	1	1	1	2	2	2	2
35–49	3	1.3	<1	1	1	1	2	2	2	2
50–64	1	1.0	0	1	1	1	1	1	1	1
65+	0									
2. MULTIPLE DX										
A. Not Operated										
0–19 Years	1	2.0	0	2	2	2	2	2	2	2
20–34	0									
35–49	5	3.2	6	1	2	2	4	7	7	7
50–64	13	3.0	7	1	2	2	3	5	11	11
65+	30	4.1	15	1	2	3	5	7	14	19
B. Operated										
0–19 Years	5	1.4	<1	1	1	1	2	2	2	2
20–34	20	1.8	3	1	1	1	2	3	3	3
35–49	27	1.9	2	1	1	1	2	4	4	4
50–64	30	2.7	6	1	1	1	4	6	6	12
65+	30	3.1	8	1	1	2	4	7	8	13
SUBTOTALS:										
1. SINGLE DX										
A. Not Operated	0									
B. Operated	9	1.2	<1	1	1	1	1	2	2	2
2. MULTIPLE DX										
A. Not Operated	49	3.7	11	1	2	3	4	7	11	19
B. Operated	112	2.4	5	1	1	1	3	5	7	12
1. SINGLE DX	9	1.2	<1	1	1	1	1	2	2	2
2. MULTIPLE DX	161	2.8	7	1	1	2	3	6	7	14
A. NOT OPERATED	49	3.7	11	1	2	3	4	7	11	19
B. OPERATED	121	2.3	5	1	1	1	3	5	7	12
TOTAL										
0–19 Years	8	1.4	<1	1	1	1	2	2	2	2
20–34	23	1.7	2	1	1	1	2	3	3	3
35–49	35	2.0	3	1	1	1	2	4	7	8
50–64	44	2.8	6	1	1	2	4	5	6	12
65+	60	3.6	11	1	2	3	5	7	13	19
GRAND TOTAL	170	2.7	7	1	1	2	3	6	7	14

837: DISLOCATION OF ANKLE

Type of Patients	Observed Patients	Avg. Stay	Variance	10th	25th	50th	75th	90th	95th	99th
1. SINGLE DX										
A. Not Operated										
0–19 Years	1	1.0	0	1	1	1	1	1	1	1
20–34	6	1.5	<1	1	1	1	2	2	2	2
35–49	2	1.0	0	1	1	1	1	1	1	1
50–64	3	1.3	<1	1	1	1	2	2	2	2
65+	0									
B. Operated										
0–19 Years	1	2.0	0	2	2	2	2	2	2	2
20–34	7	2.3	2	1	2	2	2	5	5	5
35–49	5	2.2	3	1	2	2	2	5	5	5
50–64	2	1.5	<1	1	1	1	2	2	2	2
65+	0									
2. MULTIPLE DX										
A. Not Operated										
0–19 Years	0									
20–34	10	1.3	<1	1	1	1	1	2	3	3
35–49	5	4.0	17	1	1	3	4	11	11	11
50–64	12	2.2	4	1	1	1	4	5	7	7
65+	8	5.6	19	1	3	4	9	13	13	13
B. Operated										
0–19 Years	7	2.4	2	1	2	2	3	5	5	5
20–34	23	2.6	6	1	1	2	3	7	7	10
35–49	12	4.4	30	2	2	2	4	7	21	21
50–64	13	4.3	36	1	1	2	4	8	23	23
65+	3	6.7	12	3	3	7	10	10	10	10
SUBTOTALS:										
1. SINGLE DX										
A. Not Operated	12	1.3	<1	1	1	1	2	2	2	2
B. Operated	15	2.1	2	1	1	2	2	5	5	5
2. MULTIPLE DX										
A. Not Operated	35	3.0	10	1	1	2	4	9	11	13
B. Operated	58	3.5	17	1	1	2	4	7	10	23
1. SINGLE DX	27	1.8	1	1	1	2	2	2	2	2
2. MULTIPLE DX	93	3.3	15	1	2	2	4	7	10	23
A. NOT OPERATED	47	2.6	8	1	1	2	3	7	9	13
B. OPERATED	73	3.3	14	1	1	2	3	7	10	23
TOTAL										
0–19 Years	9	2.2	1	1	2	2	2	5	5	5
20–34	46	2.1	3	1	1	2	2	3	7	10
35–49	24	3.6	19	1	1	2	4	7	11	21
50–64	30	3.0	18	1	1	2	4	7	8	23
65+	11	5.9	16	3	3	5	9	10	13	19
GRAND TOTAL	120	3.0	12	1	1	2	3	7	9	21

838: DISLOCATION OF FOOT

Type of Patients	Observed Patients	Avg. Stay	Variance	10th	25th	50th	75th	90th	95th	99th
1. SINGLE DX										
A. Not Operated										
0–19 Years	1	1.0	0	1	1	1	1	1	1	1
20–34	2	1.0	0	1	1	1	1	1	1	1
35–49	2	1.0	0	1	1	1	1	1	1	1
50–64	0									
65+	0									
B. Operated										
0–19 Years	4	1.5	<1	1	1	2	2	2	2	2
20–34	7	1.0	0	1	1	1	1	1	1	1
35–49	1	2.0	0	2	2	2	2	2	2	2
50–64	0									
65+	2	2.0	2	1	1	3	3	3	3	3
2. MULTIPLE DX										
A. Not Operated										
0–19 Years	0									
20–34	3	1.3	<1	1	1	1	2	2	2	2
35–49	8	2.0	5	1	1	1	3	7	7	7
50–64	2	1.5	<1	1	1	2	2	2	2	2
65+	3	4.0	<1	3	3	4	5	5	5	5
B. Operated										
0–19 Years	0									
20–34	15	2.5	6	1	1	2	3	6	9	9
35–49	11	3.3	3	1	2	3	5	5	5	5
50–64	13	3.5	9	1	2	2	3	9	10	10
65+	10	2.3	2	1	1	2	3	5	5	5
SUBTOTALS:										
1. SINGLE DX										
A. Not Operated	5	1.0	0	1	1	1	1	1	1	1
B. Operated	9	1.6	<1	1	1	1	2	3	3	3
2. MULTIPLE DX										
A. Not Operated	16	2.2	3	1	1	1	3	5	7	7
B. Operated	49	2.9	5	1	1	2	4	6	9	10
1. SINGLE DX	14	1.4	<1	1	1	1	2	2	3	3
2. MULTIPLE DX	65	2.7	5	1	1	2	3	5	7	10
A. NOT OPERATED	21	1.9	3	1	1	2	2	4	5	7
B. OPERATED	58	2.7	5	1	1	2	3	5	9	10
TOTAL										
0–19 Years	5	1.4	<1	1	1	1	2	2	2	2
20–34	22	2.1	4	1	1	1	2	5	6	9
35–49	22	2.5	3	1	1	2	4	5	5	7
50–64	15	3.2	8	1	1	2	4	9	10	10
65+	15	2.6	2	1	1	3	4	5	5	5
GRAND TOTAL	79	2.5	4	1	1	2	3	5	7	10

736

839: DISLOCATION NEC

Type of Patients	Observed Patients	Avg. Stay	Variance	10th	25th	50th	75th	90th	95th	99th
1. SINGLE DX										
A. *Not Operated*										
0–19 Years	4	1.3	<1	1	1	1	1	2	2	2
20–34	9	1.8	2	1	1	1	2	4	4	4
35–49	6	2.7	<1	2	2	3	3	4	4	4
50–64	4	1.0	0	1	1	1	1	1	1	1
65+	0									
B. *Operated*										
0–19 Years	1	1.0	0	1	1	1	1	1	1	1
20–34	14	2.8	4	1	1	3	4	5	8	8
35–49	16	1.5	2	1	1	1	1	5	5	5
50–64	5	2.2	2	1	1	2	3	4	4	4
65+	0									
2. MULTIPLE DX										
A. *Not Operated*										
0–19 Years	22	2.2	2	1	1	2	3	4	4	6
20–34	42	2.7	4	1	1	2	4	5	6	10
35–49	57	3.4	8	1	1	2	4	8	10	12
50–64	39	3.4	4	1	2	3	5	7	7	7
65+	37	4.5	16	1	2	3	5	8	15	19
B. *Operated*										
0–19 Years	17	6.2	37	1	3	4	9	26	>99	>99
20–34	78	4.4	30	1	2	3	5	10	16	31
35–49	125	6.2	80	1	1	3	6	14	24	44
50–64	112	5.5	69	1	1	3	6	11	18	44
65+	39	5.9	20	1	3	5	8	13	16	19
SUBTOTALS:										
1. SINGLE DX										
A. *Not Operated*	23	1.8	1	1	1	1	2	4	4	4
B. *Operated*	36	2.1	3	1	1	1	3	5	5	8
2. MULTIPLE DX										
A. *Not Operated*	197	3.3	8	1	1	2	4	7	9	15
B. *Operated*	371	5.6	58	1	2	3	6	12	19	44
1. SINGLE DX	59	2.0	2	1	1	1	3	4	5	8
2. MULTIPLE DX	568	4.8	41	1	2	3	5	10	15	31
A. NOT OPERATED	220	3.2	7	1	1	2	4	7	8	14
B. OPERATED	407	5.3	54	1	1	3	6	11	18	44
TOTAL										
0–19 Years	44	3.6	19	1	1	2	4	9	12	>99
20–34	143	3.6	19	1	1	3	4	6	10	30
35–49	204	4.9	54	1	1	3	5	10	17	31
50–64	160	4.8	50	1	1	3	6	8	14	44
65+	76	5.2	19	1	2	4	7	12	16	19
GRAND TOTAL	627	4.5	38	1	1	3	5	9	14	31

839.20: CL DISLOC LUMBAR VERT

Type of Patients	Observed Patients	Avg. Stay	Variance	10th	25th	50th	75th	90th	95th	99th
1. SINGLE DX										
A. *Not Operated*										
0–19 Years	0									
20–34	4	2.0	2	1	1	1	2	4	4	4
35–49	3	3.0	<1	2	2	3	4	4	4	4
50–64	2	1.0	0	1	1	1	1	1	1	1
65+	0									
B. *Operated*										
0–19 Years	1	1.0	0	1	1	1	1	1	1	1
20–34	10	2.3	2	1	1	2	3	5	5	5
35–49	14	1.0	0	1	1	1	1	1	1	1
50–64	3	1.3	<1	1	1	1	2	2	2	2
65+	0									
2. MULTIPLE DX										
A. *Not Operated*										
0–19 Years	3	3.7	4	2	2	3	6	6	6	6
20–34	12	3.7	9	2	2	2	4	9	10	10
35–49	23	3.5	10	1	1	2	4	10	10	12
50–64	16	4.4	4	2	3	3	5	7	7	7
65+	10	3.9	8	1	1	5	7	8	8	8
B. *Operated*										
0–19 Years	0									
20–34	43	2.8	3	1	1	2	4	5	5	10
35–49	52	4.0	24	1	1	2	5	9	17	25
50–64	38	2.9	7	1	1	2	4	6	7	14
65+	13	3.6	7	1	1	3	5	7	9	9
SUBTOTALS:										
1. SINGLE DX										
A. *Not Operated*	9	2.1	2	1	1	2	3	4	4	4
B. *Operated*	28	1.5	1	1	1	1	2	3	4	5
2. MULTIPLE DX										
A. *Not Operated*	64	3.8	7	1	2	3	5	7	10	12
B. *Operated*	146	3.3	12	1	1	2	4	6	9	20
1. SINGLE DX	37	1.7	1	1	1	1	2	4	4	5
2. MULTIPLE DX	210	3.5	11	1	1	3	5	7	9	17
A. NOT OPERATED	73	3.6	7	1	2	3	5	7	10	12
B. OPERATED	174	3.0	11	1	1	2	4	6	9	20
TOTAL										
0–19 Years	4	3.0	5	1	1	3	4	6	6	6
20–34	69	2.8	4	1	1	3	4	6	6	10
35–49	92	3.4	17	1	1	2	4	9	10	25
50–64	59	3.1	6	1	1	3	5	7	7	14
65+	23	3.8	7	1	1	3	6	7	8	9
GRAND TOTAL	247	3.2	10	1	1	2	4	7	9	17

840: SHOULDER & ARM SPRAIN

Type of Patients	Observed Patients	Avg. Stay	Variance	10th	25th	50th	75th	90th	95th	99th
1. SINGLE DX										
A. *Not Operated*										
0–19 Years	1	1.0	0	1	1	1	1	1	1	1
20–34	1	1.0	0	1	1	1	1	1	1	1
35–49	1	1.0	0	1	1	1	1	1	1	1
50–64	0									
65+	0									
B. *Operated*										
0–19 Years	2	1.5	<1	1	1	2	2	2	2	2
20–34	11	1.6	2	1	1	1	2	2	6	6
35–49	24	1.3	<1	1	1	1	1	2	2	4
50–64	34	1.4	<1	1	1	1	2	2	3	3
65+	11	1.7	<1	1	2	2	2	2	4	4
2. MULTIPLE DX										
A. *Not Operated*										
0–19 Years	0									
20–34	13	1.4	<1	1	1	1	2	2	3	3
35–49	26	2.1	1	1	1	2	3	4	4	5
50–64	54	2.9	8	1	1	2	4	6	8	17
65+	125	3.7	9	1	2	3	5	7	9	14
B. *Operated*										
0–19 Years	1	1.0	0	1	1	1	1	1	1	1
20–34	33	1.3	<1	1	1	1	2	2	2	3
35–49	140	1.6	1	1	1	1	2	2	4	8
50–64	368	1.7	2	1	1	1	2	3	4	8
65+	475	1.8	2	1	1	1	2	3	4	7
SUBTOTALS:										
1. SINGLE DX										
A. *Not Operated*	3	1.0	0	1	1	1	1	1	1	1
B. *Operated*	82	1.4	<1	1	1	1	2	2	3	6
2. MULTIPLE DX										
A. *Not Operated*	218	3.2	8	1	1	2	4	6	8	14
B. *Operated*	1,017	1.7	2	1	1	1	2	3	4	7
1. SINGLE DX	85	1.4	<1	1	1	1	2	2	3	6
2. MULTIPLE DX	1,235	2.0	3	1	1	1	2	4	5	9
A. NOT OPERATED	221	3.1	8	1	1	2	4	6	8	14
B. OPERATED	1,099	1.7	2	1	1	1	2	3	4	7
TOTAL										
0–19 Years	4	1.3	<1	1	1	1	2	2	2	2
20–34	58	1.4	<1	1	1	1	2	2	3	6
35–49	191	1.6	1	1	1	2	2	3	4	8
50–64	456	1.8	3	1	1	1	2	3	5	8
65+	611	2.2	4	1	1	2	3	4	6	9
GRAND TOTAL	1,320	1.9	3	1	1	1	2	4	5	8

737

Length of Stay by Diagnosis and Operation, Western Region, 2008

Western Region, October 2006–September 2007 Data, by Diagnosis

840.4: ROTATOR CUFF SPRAIN

Type of Patients	Observed Patients	Avg. Stay	Vari-ance	10th	25th	50th	75th	90th	95th	99th
1. SINGLE DX										
A. Not Operated										
0–19 Years	0									
20–34	0									
35–49	0									
50–64	0									
65+	0									
B. Operated										
0–19 Years	1	1.0	0	1	1	1	1	1	1	1
20–34	1	1.0	0	1	1	1	1	1	1	1
35–49	12	1.4	<1	1	1	1	2	2	4	4
50–64	24	1.4	<1	1	1	1	2	2	3	3
65+	11	1.7	<1	1	1	2	2	2	4	4
2. MULTIPLE DX										
A. Not Operated										
0–19 Years	0									
20–34	1	2.0	0	2	2	2	2	2	2	2
35–49	5	2.4	<1	2	2	2	2	4	4	4
50–64	21	3.9	15	1	1	2	5	8	8	17
65+	66	4.5	12	2	2	3	5	9	10	22
B. Operated										
0–19 Years	1	1.0	0	1	1	1	1	1	1	1
20–34	11	1.4	<1	1	1	1	2	2	2	2
35–49	95	1.7	2	1	1	1	2	3	5	9
50–64	300	1.7	1	1	1	1	2	3	4	8
65+	444	1.8	2	1	1	1	2	3	4	6
SUBTOTALS:										
1. SINGLE DX										
A. Not Operated	0									
B. Operated	49	1.5	<1	1	1	1	2	2	3	4
2. MULTIPLE DX										
A. Not Operated	93	4.2	12	1	2	3	5	8	10	22
B. Operated	851	1.7	2	1	1	1	2	3	4	7
1. SINGLE DX	49	1.5	<1	1	1	1	2	2	3	4
2. MULTIPLE DX	944	2.0	3	1	1	1	2	4	5	9
A. NOT OPERATED	93	4.2	12	1	2	3	5	8	10	22
B. OPERATED	900	1.7	2	1	1	1	2	3	4	7
TOTAL										
0–19 Years	2	1.0	0	1	1	1	1	1	1	1
20–34	13	1.4	<1	1	1	1	2	2	2	2
35–49	112	1.7	2	1	1	1	2	3	4	8
50–64	345	1.8	2	1	1	1	2	3	5	8
65+	521	2.1	4	1	1	2	2	4	5	9
GRAND TOTAL	993	2.0	3	1	1	1	2	4	5	9

841: ELBOW & FOREARM SPRAIN

Type of Patients	Observed Patients	Avg. Stay	Vari-ance	10th	25th	50th	75th	90th	95th	99th
1. SINGLE DX										
A. Not Operated										
0–19 Years	0									
20–34	0									
35–49	1	6.0	0	6	6	6	6	6	6	6
50–64	0									
65+	0									
B. Operated										
0–19 Years	0									
20–34	1	1.0	0	1	1	1	1	1	1	1
35–49	2	1.0	0	1	1	1	1	1	1	1
50–64	3	1.0	0	1	1	1	1	1	1	1
65+	0									
2. MULTIPLE DX										
A. Not Operated										
0–19 Years	1	1.0	0	1	1	1	1	1	1	1
20–34	3	5.0	28	1	1	3	11	11	11	11
35–49	2	1.0	0	1	1	1	1	1	1	1
50–64	3	1.3	<1	1	1	1	2	2	2	2
65+	1	11.0	0	11	11	11	11	11	11	11
B. Operated										
0–19 Years	1	1.0	0	1	1	1	1	1	1	1
20–34	2	2.5	4	1	1	1	4	4	4	4
35–49	7	2.3	7	1	1	1	2	8	8	8
50–64	9	1.4	<1	1	1	1	2	3	3	3
65+	2	1.0	0	1	1	1	1	1	1	1
SUBTOTALS:										
1. SINGLE DX										
A. Not Operated	1	6.0	0	6	6	6	6	6	6	6
B. Operated	6	1.0	0	1	1	1	1	1	1	1
2. MULTIPLE DX										
A. Not Operated	10	3.3	17	1	1	1	3	11	11	11
B. Operated	21	1.8	3	1	1	1	2	3	4	8
1. SINGLE DX	7	1.7	4	1	1	1	1	6	6	6
2. MULTIPLE DX	31	2.3	7	1	1	1	2	4	11	11
A. NOT OPERATED	11	3.6	16	1	1	1	6	11	11	11
B. OPERATED	27	1.6	2	1	1	1	2	3	4	8
TOTAL										
0–19 Years	3	1.0	0	1	1	1	1	1	1	1
20–34	5	4.0	17	1	1	3	4	11	11	11
35–49	12	2.2	5	1	1	1	2	6	8	8
50–64	15	1.3	<1	1	1	1	2	2	3	3
65+	3	4.3	33	1	1	11	11	11	11	11
GRAND TOTAL	38	2.2	7	1	1	1	2	6	11	11

842: WRIST & HAND SPRAIN

Type of Patients	Observed Patients	Avg. Stay	Vari-ance	10th	25th	50th	75th	90th	95th	99th
1. SINGLE DX										
A. Not Operated										
0–19 Years	0									
20–34	0									
35–49	0									
50–64	0									
65+	0									
B. Operated										
0–19 Years	3	1.0	0	1	1	1	1	1	1	1
20–34	2	3.5	<1	3	3	4	4	4	4	4
35–49	2	2.0	2	1	1	3	3	3	3	3
50–64	2	1.5	<1	1	1	2	2	2	2	2
65+	1	1.0	0	1	1	1	1	1	1	1
2. MULTIPLE DX										
A. Not Operated										
0–19 Years	2	1.0	0	1	1	1	1	1	1	1
20–34	6	1.2	<1	1	1	1	1	2	2	2
35–49	3	1.0	0	1	1	1	1	1	1	1
50–64	4	1.5	<1	1	1	1	2	2	2	2
65+	15	2.0	1	1	1	2	3	3	4	4
B. Operated										
0–19 Years	2	1.0	0	1	1	1	1	1	1	1
20–34	5	1.4	<1	1	1	1	2	2	2	2
35–49	4	1.8	<1	1	1	2	2	3	3	3
50–64	5	1.4	<1	1	1	1	2	3	3	3
65+	1	1.0	0	1	1	1	1	1	1	1
SUBTOTALS:										
1. SINGLE DX										
A. Not Operated	0									
B. Operated	10	1.8	1	1	1	1	3	4	4	4
2. MULTIPLE DX										
A. Not Operated	30	1.6	<1	1	1	1	2	3	3	4
B. Operated	17	1.4	<1	1	1	1	2	3	3	3
1. SINGLE DX	10	1.8	1	1	1	1	3	4	4	4
2. MULTIPLE DX	47	1.5	<1	1	1	1	2	3	3	4
A. NOT OPERATED	30	1.6	<1	1	1	1	2	3	3	4
B. OPERATED	27	1.6	<1	1	1	1	2	3	3	4
TOTAL										
0–19 Years	7	1.0	0	1	1	1	1	1	1	1
20–34	13	1.6	<1	1	1	1	2	3	4	4
35–49	9	1.6	<1	1	1	1	2	3	3	3
50–64	11	1.5	<1	1	1	1	3	3	3	3
65+	17	1.9	1	1	1	1	3	3	4	4
GRAND TOTAL	57	1.6	<1	1	1	1	2	3	3	4

Western Region, October 2006–September 2007 Data, by Diagnosis

843: HIP & THIGH SPRAIN

Type of Patients	Observed Patients	Avg. Stay	Vari-ance	10th	25th	50th	75th	90th	95th	99th
1. SINGLE DX										
A. Not Operated										
0–19 Years	3	1.7	<1	1	1	1	3	3	3	3
20–34	1	1.0	0	1	1	1	1	1	1	1
35–49	1	2.0	0	2	2	2	2	2	2	2
50–64	1	2.0	0	2	2	2	2	2	2	2
65+	1	3.0	0	3	3	3	3	3	3	3
B. Operated										
0–19 Years	0									
20–34	2	2.0	2	1	1	3	3	3	3	3
35–49	3	1.3	<1	1	1	1	1	2	2	2
50–64	5	1.6	<1	1	1	2	2	2	2	2
65+	0									
2. MULTIPLE DX										
A. Not Operated										
0–19 Years	10	2.8	3	1	1	3	3	7	7	7
20–34	16	1.9	1	1	1	2	2	4	5	5
35–49	26	2.2	1	1	1	2	3	4	4	4
50–64	52	3.7	12	1	2	3	4	5	10	24
65+	252	3.4	5	1	2	3	4	5	7	12
B. Operated										
0–19 Years	1	1.0	0	1	1	1	1	1	1	1
20–34	8	1.6	2	1	1	1	1	5	5	5
35–49	16	2.8	6	1	1	2	3	8	9	9
50–64	26	2.6	3	1	1	2	4	6	6	7
65+	24	3.5	8	2	2	2	4	7	9	12
SUBTOTALS:										
1. SINGLE DX										
A. Not Operated	7	1.9	<1	1	1	2	3	3	3	3
B. Operated	10	1.6	<1	1	1	2	2	3	3	3
2. MULTIPLE DX										
A. Not Operated	356	3.2	6	1	2	3	4	5	7	12
B. Operated	75	2.8	5	1	1	2	3	6	8	12
1. SINGLE DX	17	1.7	<1	1	1	2	2	3	3	3
2. MULTIPLE DX	431	3.2	6	1	2	3	4	5	7	12
A. NOT OPERATED	363	3.2	6	1	2	3	4	5	7	12
B. OPERATED	85	2.7	5	1	1	2	3	6	7	12
TOTAL										
0–19 Years	14	2.4	3	1	1	3	3	4	7	7
20–34	27	1.8	1	1	1	1	1	4	5	5
35–49	46	2.3	3	1	1	3	3	4	4	9
50–64	84	3.2	9	1	2	2	4	5	7	24
65+	277	3.4	5	1	2	3	4	6	7	12
GRAND TOTAL	448	3.1	5	1	2	3	4	5	7	12

843.8: HIP & THIGH SPRAIN NEC

Type of Patients	Observed Patients	Avg. Stay	Vari-ance	10th	25th	50th	75th	90th	95th	99th
1. SINGLE DX										
A. Not Operated										
0–19 Years	2	2.0	2	1	1	3	3	3	3	3
20–34	1	1.0	0	1	1	1	1	1	1	1
35–49	1	2.0	0	2	2	2	2	2	2	2
50–64	1	2.0	0	2	2	2	2	2	2	2
65+	0									
B. Operated										
0–19 Years	0									
20–34	2	2.0	2	1	1	3	3	3	3	3
35–49	2	1.0	0	1	1	1	1	1	1	1
50–64	4	1.5	<1	1	1	2	2	2	2	2
65+	0									
2. MULTIPLE DX										
A. Not Operated										
0–19 Years	8	3.0	4	1	2	3	4	7	7	7
20–34	11	1.8	<1	1	1	2	2	4	4	4
35–49	15	2.1	3	1	1	2	3	4	4	4
50–64	22	3.8	6	1	2	4	4	7	10	10
65+	148	3.4	4	1	2	3	4	5	7	8
B. Operated										
0–19 Years	0									
20–34	6	1.2	<1	1	1	1	1	2	2	2
35–49	15	2.9	6	1	1	2	3	8	9	9
50–64	19	2.8	4	1	1	2	4	6	7	7
65+	20	3.6	9	2	2	2	4	7	12	12
SUBTOTALS:										
1. SINGLE DX										
A. Not Operated	5	1.8	<1	1	1	2	2	3	3	3
B. Operated	8	1.5	<1	1	1	2	2	3	3	3
2. MULTIPLE DX										
A. Not Operated	204	3.3	4	1	2	3	4	5	7	10
B. Operated	60	2.9	6	1	1	2	3	6	8	12
1. SINGLE DX	13	1.6	<1	1	1	1	2	3	3	3
2. MULTIPLE DX	264	3.2	4	1	2	3	4	6	7	10
A. NOT OPERATED	209	3.2	4	1	2	3	4	5	7	10
B. OPERATED	68	2.7	6	1	1	2	3	7	8	12
TOTAL										
0–19 Years	10	2.8	3	1	1	3	3	7	7	7
20–34	20	1.6	<1	1	1	1	2	3	4	4
35–49	33	2.4	4	1	1	2	3	4	8	9
50–64	46	3.1	5	1	2	2	4	6	7	10
65+	168	3.4	4	1	2	3	4	6	7	12
GRAND TOTAL	277	3.1	4	1	2	3	4	5	7	10

844: KNEE & LEG SPRAIN

Type of Patients	Observed Patients	Avg. Stay	Vari-ance	10th	25th	50th	75th	90th	95th	99th
1. SINGLE DX										
A. Not Operated										
0–19 Years	5	1.8	1	1	1	1	3	3	3	3
20–34	3	2.0	3	1	1	1	4	4	4	4
35–49	2	1.5	<1	1	1	2	2	2	2	2
50–64	0									
65+	1	1.0	0	1	1	1	1	1	1	1
B. Operated										
0–19 Years	17	1.6	1	1	1	1	2	3	4	4
20–34	52	1.9	1	1	1	1	3	4	5	6
35–49	49	2.0	2	1	1	2	2	4	5	7
50–64	32	2.3	3	1	1	2	3	5	6	9
65+	7	2.0	4	1	1	1	3	6	6	6
2. MULTIPLE DX										
A. Not Operated										
0–19 Years	10	1.9	2	1	1	1	3	4	4	4
20–34	28	2.8	6	1	1	2	3	6	7	12
35–49	43	2.7	3	1	1	2	4	5	6	8
50–64	70	3.4	7	1	2	3	4	6	9	14
65+	191	3.8	8	1	2	3	5	6	7	20
B. Operated										
0–19 Years	67	1.6	<1	1	1	1	1	3	3	5
20–34	138	2.1	4	1	1	2	3	4	5	12
35–49	199	2.6	13	1	1	2	3	5	7	17
50–64	193	2.8	12	1	1	2	3	5	8	12
65+	212	3.4	7	2	2	3	4	6	8	11
SUBTOTALS:										
1. SINGLE DX										
A. Not Operated	11	1.7	1	1	1	1	3	3	4	4
B. Operated	157	2.0	2	1	1	1	2	4	5	7
2. MULTIPLE DX										
A. Not Operated	342	3.4	7	1	2	3	4	6	7	14
B. Operated	809	2.7	9	1	1	2	3	5	7	12
1. SINGLE DX	168	2.0	2	1	1	1	3	4	5	7
2. MULTIPLE DX	1,151	2.9	8	1	1	3	4	6	7	12
A. NOT OPERATED	353	3.4	7	1	2	3	4	6	7	14
B. OPERATED	966	2.6	8	1	1	2	3	5	7	11
TOTAL										
0–19 Years	99	1.6	<1	1	1	1	2	3	4	4
20–34	221	2.1	4	1	1	1	3	4	5	12
35–49	293	2.5	10	1	1	2	3	5	6	11
50–64	295	2.9	10	1	1	2	3	5	8	13
65+	411	3.5	7	1	2	3	4	6	7	12
GRAND TOTAL	1,319	2.8	8	1	1	2	3	5	7	12

Length of Stay by Diagnosis and Operation, Western Region, 2008

Western Region, October 2006–September 2007 Data, by Diagnosis

844.2: KNEE CRUCIATE LIG SPRAIN

Type of Patients	Observed Patients	Avg. Stay	Vari-ance	10th	25th	50th	75th	90th	95th	99th
1. SINGLE DX										
A. Not Operated										
0–19 Years	0									
20–34	1	1.0	0	1	1	1	1	1	1	1
35–49	1	2.0	0	2	2	2	2	2	2	2
50–64	0									
65+	0									
B. Operated										
0–19 Years	15	1.5	<1	1	1	1	2	3	4	4
20–34	17	1.2	<1	1	1	1	1	2	3	3
35–49	3	1.3	<1	1	1	1	2	2	2	2
50–64	4	2.0	<1	1	2	2	3	3	3	3
65+	0									
2. MULTIPLE DX										
A. Not Operated										
0–19 Years	4	1.3	<1	1	1	1	1	2	2	2
20–34	4	5.5	25	1	1	2	7	12	12	12
35–49	13	2.5	2	1	1	3	3	4	6	6
50–64	7	4.1	10	1	2	3	8	9	9	9
65+	13	4.8	23	2	3	4	4	6	20	20
B. Operated										
0–19 Years	52	1.5	<1	1	1	1	2	3	3	4
20–34	82	1.9	4	1	1	1	2	3	4	14
35–49	84	1.9	3	1	1	1	2	3	5	11
50–64	27	1.6	2	1	1	2	2	3	3	7
65+	6	2.0	<1	1	1	2	3	3	3	3
SUBTOTALS:										
1. SINGLE DX										
A. Not Operated	2	1.5	<1	1	1	1	2	2	2	2
B. Operated	39	1.4	<1	1	1	1	2	3	3	4
2. MULTIPLE DX										
A. Not Operated	41	3.7	13	1	2	3	4	7	9	20
B. Operated	251	1.8	3	1	1	1	2	3	4	11
1. SINGLE DX	41	1.4	<1	1	1	1	2	3	3	4
2. MULTIPLE DX	292	2.0	4	1	1	1	2	4	5	12
A. NOT OPERATED	43	3.6	12	1	1	1	4	7	9	20
B. OPERATED	290	1.7	2	1	1	1	2	3	4	11
TOTAL										
0–19 Years	71	1.5	<1	1	1	1	2	3	3	4
20–34	104	1.9	5	1	1	1	2	3	5	12
35–49	101	2.0	3	1	1	1	2	4	5	7
50–64	38	2.1	4	1	1	2	3	4	8	9
65+	19	3.9	17	2	3	3	4	6	20	20
GRAND TOTAL	333	2.0	2	1	1	1	2	3	5	12

844.8: KNEE & LEG SPRAIN NEC

Type of Patients	Observed Patients	Avg. Stay	Vari-ance	10th	25th	50th	75th	90th	95th	99th
1. SINGLE DX										
A. Not Operated										
0–19 Years	2	1.0	0	1	1	1	1	1	1	1
20–34	1	1.0	0	1	1	1	1	1	1	1
35–49	0									
50–64	0									
65+	1	1.0	0	1	1	1	1	1	1	1
B. Operated										
0–19 Years	2	2.0	2	1	1	2	3	3	3	3
20–34	33	2.2	3	1	1	1	3	5	6	6
35–49	45	2.1	2	1	1	2	2	4	5	7
50–64	26	2.4	4	1	1	2	3	5	6	9
65+	6	2.2	4	1	2	3	3	6	6	6
2. MULTIPLE DX										
A. Not Operated										
0–19 Years	2	2.5	4	1	1	4	4	4	4	4
20–34	9	2.1	2	1	1	2	3	5	5	5
35–49	14	2.6	3	1	1	2	4	4	7	7
50–64	19	2.6	4	1	2	2	4	5	9	9
65+	48	3.8	11	1	2	3	4	7	11	19
B. Operated										
0–19 Years	4	1.3	<1	1	1	1	1	2	2	2
20–34	46	2.4	4	1	1	2	3	5	5	12
35–49	99	2.8	5	1	1	2	3	6	7	17
50–64	149	3.0	14	1	1	2	3	6	8	10
65+	184	3.3	7	1	2	3	4	6	7	11
SUBTOTALS:										
1. SINGLE DX										
A. Not Operated	4	1.0	0	1	1	1	1	1	1	1
B. Operated	112	2.2	3	1	1	2	3	5	6	7
2. MULTIPLE DX										
A. Not Operated	92	3.2	7	1	2	3	4	5	9	19
B. Operated	482	3.0	9	1	1	2	4	6	7	11
1. SINGLE DX	116	2.2	2	1	1	2	3	5	6	7
2. MULTIPLE DX	574	3.0	8	1	1	2	4	6	7	11
A. NOT OPERATED	96	3.1	7	1	1	2	4	5	9	19
B. OPERATED	594	2.9	8	1	1	2	4	5	7	11
TOTAL										
0–19 Years	10	1.6	1	1	1	1	2	4	4	4
20–34	89	2.3	3	1	1	2	3	5	5	12
35–49	158	2.6	4	1	1	2	3	5	6	8
50–64	194	2.9	12	1	1	2	3	5	6	10
65+	239	3.4	8	1	2	3	4	6	8	11
GRAND TOTAL	690	2.9	7	1	1	2	4	5	7	11

844.9: KNEE & LEG SPRAIN NOS

Type of Patients	Observed Patients	Avg. Stay	Vari-ance	10th	25th	50th	75th	90th	95th	99th
1. SINGLE DX										
A. Not Operated										
0–19 Years	3	2.3	1	1	1	3	3	3	3	3
20–34	0									
35–49	0									
50–64	0									
65+	0									
B. Operated										
0–19 Years	0									
20–34	0									
35–49	1	1.0	0	1	1	1	1	1	1	1
50–64	1	2.0	0	2	2	2	2	2	2	2
65+	1	1.0	0	1	1	1	1	1	1	1
2. MULTIPLE DX										
A. Not Operated										
0–19 Years	3	1.7	1	1	1	1	3	3	3	3
20–34	10	2.4	2	1	1	3	3	6	6	6
35–49	10	3.1	5	1	1	3	4	8	8	8
50–64	33	3.6	9	1	2	3	4	6	13	14
65+	113	3.7	6	1	2	3	5	7	7	9
B. Operated										
0–19 Years	0									
20–34	1	1.0	0	1	1	1	1	1	1	1
35–49	3	2.7	<1	2	2	3	3	3	3	3
50–64	10	3.5	10	1	2	2	4	4	12	12
65+	14	3.8	4	1	2	5	5	6	7	7
SUBTOTALS:										
1. SINGLE DX										
A. Not Operated	3	2.3	1	1	1	3	3	3	3	3
B. Operated	3	1.3	<1	1	1	2	2	2	2	2
2. MULTIPLE DX										
A. Not Operated	169	3.6	6	1	2	3	3	6	7	14
B. Operated	28	3.5	6	1	2	3	5	6	7	12
1. SINGLE DX	6	1.8	<1	1	1	2	2	3	3	3
2. MULTIPLE DX	197	3.6	6	1	2	3	5	6	7	14
A. NOT OPERATED	172	3.5	6	1	2	3	4	6	7	14
B. OPERATED	31	3.3	6	1	2	3	5	6	6	12
TOTAL										
0–19 Years	6	2.0	1	1	1	3	3	3	3	3
20–34	11	2.3	2	1	1	2	3	3	6	6
35–49	14	2.9	4	1	1	3	4	5	8	8
50–64	44	3.6	9	1	2	3	5	6	12	14
65+	128	3.7	6	1	2	3	5	7	7	9
GRAND TOTAL	203	3.5	6	2	2	3	4	6	7	13

Length of Stay by Diagnosis and Operation, Western Region, 2008

Western Region, October 2006–September 2007 Data, by Diagnosis

845: ANKLE & FOOT SPRAIN

Type of Patients	Observed Patients	Avg. Stay	Vari-ance	10th	25th	50th	75th	90th	95th	99th
1. SINGLE DX										
A. Not Operated										
0–19 Years	3	1.7	1	1	1	1	1	3	3	3
20–34	5	2.2	5	1	1	1	2	6	6	6
35–49	1	1.0	0	1	1	1	1	1	1	1
50–64	1	3.0	0	3	3	3	3	3	3	3
65+	0									
B. Operated										
0–19 Years	1	1.0	0	1	1	1	1	1	1	1
20–34	29	1.4	1	1	1	1	1	2	2	7
35–49	51	1.2	<1	1	1	1	1	2	3	4
50–64	23	1.2	<1	1	1	1	1	2	2	2
65+	2	1.0	0	1	1	1	1	1	1	1
2. MULTIPLE DX										
A. Not Operated										
0–19 Years	13	2.0	1	1	1	2	3	3	4	4
20–34	17	2.0	1	1	1	2	3	4	4	4
35–49	23	2.1	4	1	1	2	2	3	4	10
50–64	41	3.2	10	1	1	2	3	5	9	16
65+	137	3.3	3	1	2	3	4	5	7	10
B. Operated										
0–19 Years	8	1.5	<1	1	1	1	3	3	3	3
20–34	26	2.0	1	1	1	2	3	4	4	5
35–49	41	1.6	<1	1	1	1	2	2	3	5
50–64	50	2.5	11	1	1	1	3	5	6	22
65+	42	2.5	3	1	2	2	3	4	4	11
SUBTOTALS:										
1. SINGLE DX										
A. Not Operated	10	2.0	3	1	1	1	3	6	6	6
B. Operated	106	1.3	<1	1	1	1	1	2	2	4
2. MULTIPLE DX										
A. Not Operated	231	3.0	5	1	1	3	4	5	7	10
B. Operated	167	2.2	5	1	1	2	3	4	5	11
1. SINGLE DX	116	1.3	<1	1	1	1	1	2	3	6
2. MULTIPLE DX	398	2.6	5	1	1	2	3	5	6	11
A. NOT OPERATED	241	2.9	4	1	1	3	4	5	7	10
B. OPERATED	273	1.8	3	1	1	1	2	3	4	11
TOTAL										
0–19 Years	25	1.8	1	1	1	1	3	3	3	4
20–34	77	1.8	2	1	1	1	2	3	4	7
35–49	116	1.5	1	1	1	1	2	2	3	5
50–64	115	2.5	9	1	1	2	3	5	6	16
65+	181	3.1	3	1	2	3	4	5	7	10
GRAND TOTAL	514	2.3	4	1	1	2	3	4	5	10

845.09: ANKLE SPRAIN NEC

Type of Patients	Observed Patients	Avg. Stay	Vari-ance	10th	25th	50th	75th	90th	95th	99th
1. SINGLE DX										
A. Not Operated										
0–19 Years	1	3.0	0	3	3	3	3	3	3	3
20–34	4	2.5	6	1	1	2	2	6	6	6
35–49	1	1.0	0	1	1	1	1	1	1	1
50–64	0									
65+	0									
B. Operated										
0–19 Years	0									
20–34	29	1.4	1	1	1	1	1	2	2	7
35–49	49	1.2	<1	1	1	1	1	2	3	4
50–64	23	1.2	<1	1	1	1	1	2	2	2
65+	2	1.0	0	1	1	1	1	1	1	1
2. MULTIPLE DX										
A. Not Operated										
0–19 Years	2	1.0	0	1	1	1	1	1	1	1
20–34	6	2.3	1	1	2	2	3	4	4	4
35–49	3	4.3	24	1	1	2	10	10	10	10
50–64	11	2.9	3	1	1	3	4	5	6	6
65+	27	3.6	4	1	2	3	5	6	7	10
B. Operated										
0–19 Years	3	1.7	1	1	1	1	3	3	3	3
20–34	14	1.8	<1	1	1	2	3	3	4	4
35–49	32	1.5	<1	1	1	1	2	2	3	3
50–64	40	2.5	12	1	1	1	3	5	5	22
65+	39	2.5	3	1	2	3	3	4	6	11
SUBTOTALS:										
1. SINGLE DX										
A. Not Operated	6	2.3	4	1	1	2	3	6	6	6
B. Operated	103	1.3	<1	1	1	1	1	2	2	4
2. MULTIPLE DX										
A. Not Operated	49	3.2	4	1	2	3	4	5	7	10
B. Operated	128	2.1	5	1	1	2	3	4	4	11
1. SINGLE DX	109	1.3	<1	1	1	1	1	2	3	6
2. MULTIPLE DX	177	2.4	5	1	1	2	3	4	6	11
A. NOT OPERATED	55	3.1	4	1	2	3	4	5	7	10
B. OPERATED	231	1.8	3	1	1	1	2	3	4	7
TOTAL										
0–19 Years	6	1.7	1	1	1	1	3	3	3	3
20–34	53	1.7	2	1	1	1	2	3	4	7
35–49	85	1.4	1	1	1	1	2	2	3	5
50–64	74	2.1	7	1	1	2	3	5	6	22
65+	68	2.9	4	1	2	3	3	5	6	11
GRAND TOTAL	286	2.0	4	1	1	1	2	4	5	10

846: SACROILIAC REGION SPRAIN

Type of Patients	Observed Patients	Avg. Stay	Vari-ance	10th	25th	50th	75th	90th	95th	99th
1. SINGLE DX										
A. Not Operated										
0–19 Years	0									
20–34	5	1.6	<1	1	1	1	2	3	3	3
35–49	4	1.3	<1	1	1	1	2	2	2	2
50–64	2	1.5	<1	1	1	1	2	2	2	2
65+	0									
B. Operated										
0–19 Years	0									
20–34	0									
35–49	0									
50–64	0									
65+	0									
2. MULTIPLE DX										
A. Not Operated										
0–19 Years	5	2.0	1	1	1	2	2	4	4	4
20–34	17	2.5	<1	2	2	2	3	3	4	4
35–49	51	2.8	3	1	2	2	3	5	5	11
50–64	44	2.5	2	1	1	3	3	5	6	6
65+	97	3.6	6	1	2	3	4	7	10	12
B. Operated										
0–19 Years	0									
20–34	0									
35–49	0									
50–64	1	4.0	0	4	4	4	4	4	4	4
65+	0									
SUBTOTALS:										
1. SINGLE DX										
A. Not Operated	11	1.5	<1	1	1	1	2	2	3	3
B. Operated	0									
2. MULTIPLE DX										
A. Not Operated	214	3.1	4	1	2	3	4	5	7	11
B. Operated	0									
1. SINGLE DX	11	1.5	<1	1	1	1	2	2	3	3
2. MULTIPLE DX	215	3.1	4	1	2	3	4	5	7	11
A. NOT OPERATED	225	3.0	4	1	2	3	4	5	6	11
B. OPERATED	1	4.0	0	4	4	4	4	4	4	4
TOTAL										
0–19 Years	5	2.0	1	1	1	1	2	2	4	4
20–34	22	2.3	<1	1	2	2	3	3	3	4
35–49	55	2.7	3	1	2	3	3	5	5	11
50–64	47	2.5	2	1	1	3	3	5	6	6
65+	97	3.6	6	1	2	3	4	7	10	12
GRAND TOTAL	226	3.0	4	2	2	3	4	5	6	11

(Percentiles)

Length of Stay by Diagnosis and Operation, Western Region, 2008

Western Region, October 2006–September 2007 Data, by Diagnosis

847: BACK SPRAIN NEC & NOS

Type of Patients	Observed Patients	Avg. Stay	Variance	Percentiles						
				10th	25th	50th	75th	90th	95th	99th
1. SINGLE DX										
A. Not Operated										
0–19 Years	19	1.3	<1	1	1	1	1	3	4	4
20–34	28	1.4	<1	1	1	1	2	2	2	5
35–49	26	1.8	1	1	1	2	2	3	3	5
50–64	12	1.1	<1	1	1	1	1	1	2	2
65+	3	2.3	2	1	1	2	4	4	4	4
B. Operated										
0–19 Years	1	1.0	0	1	1	1	1	1	1	1
20–34	0									
35–49	0									
50–64	0									
65+	0									
2. MULTIPLE DX										
A. Not Operated										
0–19 Years	82	1.5	<1	1	1	1	2	3	3	6
20–34	276	2.0	3	1	1	1	2	4	5	9
35–49	331	2.3	3	1	1	2	3	4	5	10
50–64	307	2.6	4	1	1	2	3	5	7	10
65+	487	3.2	5	2	2	3	4	6	7	13
B. Operated										
0–19 Years	4	7.8	15	3	6	11	11	11	11	11
20–34	1	8.0	0	8	8	8	8	8	8	8
35–49	9	4.3	17	1	1	3	6	12	12	12
50–64	5	7.6	26	2	5	5	12	14	14	14
65+	7	4.0	7	1	2	4	5	9	9	9
SUBTOTALS:										
1. SINGLE DX A. Not Operated	88	1.5	<1	1	1	1	2	2	4	5
1. SINGLE DX B. Operated	1	1.0	0	1	1	1	1	1	1	1
2. MULTIPLE DX A. Not Operated	1,483	2.6	4	1	1	2	3	5	6	11
2. MULTIPLE DX B. Operated	26	5.6	16	1	2	5	9	12	14	14
1. SINGLE DX	89	1.5	<1	1	1	1	2	2	4	5
2. MULTIPLE DX	1,509	2.6	5	1	1	2	3	5	6	11
A. NOT OPERATED	1,571	2.5	4	1	1	2	3	5	6	11
B. OPERATED	27	5.4	16	2	2	4	9	12	12	14
TOTAL										
0–19 Years	106	1.7	3	1	1	1	2	3	4	11
20–34	305	2.0	3	1	1	1	2	4	5	8
35–49	366	2.3	4	1	1	2	3	4	5	10
50–64	324	2.6	5	1	1	2	3	5	7	12
65+	497	3.2	5	2	2	3	4	6	7	13
GRAND TOTAL	1,598	2.6	4	1	1	2	3	5	6	11

847.0: NECK SPRAIN

Type of Patients	Observed Patients	Avg. Stay	Variance	Percentiles						
				10th	25th	50th	75th	90th	95th	99th
1. SINGLE DX										
A. Not Operated										
0–19 Years	16	1.2	<1	1	1	1	1	1	4	4
20–34	20	1.4	<1	1	1	1	2	5	5	5
35–49	10	1.6	2	1	1	2	2	5	5	5
50–64	7	1.1	<1	1	1	1	1	2	2	2
65+	1	4.0	0	4	4	4	4	4	4	4
B. Operated										
0–19 Years	1	1.0	0	1	1	1	1	1	1	1
20–34	0									
35–49	0									
50–64	0									
65+	0									
2. MULTIPLE DX										
A. Not Operated										
0–19 Years	68	1.5	<1	1	1	1	2	3	3	6
20–34	168	1.7	1	1	1	1	2	3	4	6
35–49	166	2.1	4	1	1	2	2	4	5	11
50–64	118	2.2	3	1	1	2	3	4	5	10
65+	139	2.9	4	1	1	2	4	5	7	11
B. Operated										
0–19 Years	3	6.7	16	3	3	6	6	11	11	11
20–34	1	8.0	0	8	8	8	8	8	8	8
35–49	6	4.3	17	1	1	3	6	12	12	12
50–64	4	8.2	32	2	2	5	12	14	14	14
65+	5	4.0	10	1	2	3	5	9	9	9
SUBTOTALS:										
1. SINGLE DX A. Not Operated	54	1.4	<1	1	1	1	1	2	4	4
1. SINGLE DX B. Operated	1	1.0	0	1	1	1	1	1	1	1
2. MULTIPLE DX A. Not Operated	659	2.1	3	1	1	2	3	4	5	10
2. MULTIPLE DX B. Operated	19	5.6	18	1	2	5	9	12	14	14
1. SINGLE DX	55	1.4	<1	1	1	1	1	2	4	5
2. MULTIPLE DX	678	2.2	4	1	1	2	3	4	5	11
A. NOT OPERATED	713	2.1	3	1	1	1	3	4	5	11
B. OPERATED	20	5.4	18	2	2	5	9	12	14	14
TOTAL										
0–19 Years	88	1.6	2	1	1	1	2	3	4	11
20–34	189	1.7	2	1	1	1	2	3	4	8
35–49	182	2.2	4	1	2	2	3	4	5	10
50–64	129	2.3	5	1	1	2	3	4	5	12
65+	145	2.9	4	1	1	2	4	5	7	11
GRAND TOTAL	733	2.2	4	1	1	2	3	4	5	11

847.2: LUMBAR REGION SPRAIN

Type of Patients	Observed Patients	Avg. Stay	Variance	Percentiles						
				10th	25th	50th	75th	90th	95th	99th
1. SINGLE DX										
A. Not Operated										
0–19 Years	2	2.5	<1	2	2	3	3	3	3	3
20–34	6	1.3	<1	1	1	1	2	2	2	2
35–49	16	1.9	<1	1	1	2	2	3	4	4
50–64	5	1.0	0	1	1	1	1	1	1	1
65+	2	1.5	<1	1	1	2	2	2	2	2
B. Operated										
0–19 Years	0									
20–34	0									
35–49	0									
50–64	0									
2. MULTIPLE DX										
A. Not Operated										
0–19 Years	9	1.9	1	1	1	2	2	4	4	4
20–34	87	2.8	5	1	1	2	4	5	7	12
35–49	140	2.6	3	1	1	2	3	5	5	10
50–64	158	2.9	5	1	2	3	3	6	8	11
65+	266	3.5	6	1	2	3	4	6	8	15
B. Operated										
0–19 Years	0									
20–34	0									
35–49	3	4.4	24	1	1	2	10	10	10	10
50–64	1	5.0	0	5	5	5	5	5	5	5
65+	1	4.0	0	4	4	4	4	4	4	4
SUBTOTALS:										
1. SINGLE DX A. Not Operated	31	1.7	<1	1	1	2	2	3	3	4
1. SINGLE DX B. Operated	0									
2. MULTIPLE DX A. Not Operated	660	3.0	5	1	1	3	4	6	7	12
2. MULTIPLE DX B. Operated	5	4.4	12	1	2	4	5	10	10	10
1. SINGLE DX	31	1.7	<1	1	1	2	2	3	3	4
2. MULTIPLE DX	665	3.1	5	1	1	3	4	6	7	12
A. NOT OPERATED	691	3.0	5	1	1	2	4	5	7	12
B. OPERATED	5	4.4	12	2	2	4	5	10	10	10
TOTAL										
0–19 Years	11	2.0	1	1	1	2	2	3	4	4
20–34	93	2.7	5	1	1	2	4	5	7	12
35–49	159	2.5	3	1	1	2	3	5	5	10
50–64	164	2.9	5	1	2	3	4	6	8	11
65+	269	3.5	6	1	2	3	4	6	8	15
GRAND TOTAL	696	3.0	5	1	1	3	4	6	7	12

Western Region, October 2006–September 2007 Data, by Diagnosis

848: SPRAIN & STRAIN NEC

Type of Patients	Observed Patients	Avg. Stay	Variance	10th	25th	50th	75th	90th	95th	99th
1. SINGLE DX										
A. Not Operated										
0–19 Years	2	1.5	<1	1	1	2	2	2	2	2
20–34	4	1.5	<1	1	1	1	2	2	2	2
35–49	9	1.1	<1	1	1	1	1	2	2	2
50–64	1	1.0	0	1	1	1	1	1	1	1
65+	0									
B. Operated										
0–19 Years	0									
20–34	3	1.0	0	1	1	1	1	1	1	1
35–49	2	1.0	0	1	1	1	1	1	1	1
50–64	1	1.0	0	1	1	1	1	1	1	1
65+	0									
2. MULTIPLE DX										
A. Not Operated										
0–19 Years	5	1.0	0	1	1	1	1	1	1	1
20–34	31	1.6	<1	1	1	1	2	2	3	5
35–49	43	1.8	2	1	1	1	2	3	4	7
50–64	82	2.0	2	1	1	2	3	4	4	10
65+	114	2.7	6	1	1	2	3	6	9	10
B. Operated										
0–19 Years	1	1.0	0	1	1	1	1	1	1	1
20–34	2	14.0	332	1	1	14	27	27	27	27
35–49	3	1.3	<1	1	1	1	2	2	2	2
50–64	5	2.6	4	1	1	2	3	6	6	6
65+	2	3.5	4	2	2	5	5	5	5	5
SUBTOTALS:										
1. SINGLE DX										
A. Not Operated	16	1.3	<1	1	1	1	1	2	2	2
B. Operated	6	1.0	0	1	1	1	1	1	1	1
2. MULTIPLE DX										
A. Not Operated	275	2.2	3	1	1	2	3	4	6	10
B. Operated	13	4.1	50	1	1	2	3	6	27	27
1. SINGLE DX	22	1.2	<1	1	1	1	1	2	2	2
2. MULTIPLE DX	288	2.3	6	1	1	2	3	4	6	10
A. NOT OPERATED	291	2.1	3	1	1	1	3	4	6	10
B. OPERATED	19	3.1	36	1	1	1	2	6	27	27
TOTAL										
0–19 Years	8	1.1	<1	1	1	1	1	2	2	2
20–34	40	2.2	17	1	1	1	2	3	5	27
35–49	57	1.6	1	1	1	1	2	3	4	7
50–64	89	2.0	2	1	1	2	3	4	4	10
65+	116	2.7	6	1	1	2	3	6	9	10
GRAND TOTAL	310	2.2	5	1	1	1	2	4	6	10

848.8: OTHER SPRAINS & STRAINS

Type of Patients	Observed Patients	Avg. Stay	Variance	10th	25th	50th	75th	90th	95th	99th
1. SINGLE DX										
A. Not Operated										
0–19 Years	1	1.0	0	1	1	1	1	2	2	2
20–34	4	1.5	<1	1	1	1	2	2	2	2
35–49	9	1.1	<1	1	1	1	1	2	2	2
50–64	1	1.0	0	1	1	1	1	1	1	1
65+	0									
B. Operated										
0–19 Years	0									
20–34	3	1.0	0	1	1	1	1	1	1	1
35–49	2	1.0	0	1	1	1	1	1	1	1
50–64	1	1.0	0	1	1	1	1	1	1	1
65+	0									
2. MULTIPLE DX										
A. Not Operated										
0–19 Years	4	1.0	0	1	1	1	1	1	1	1
20–34	24	1.6	<1	1	1	1	2	2	3	5
35–49	28	2.1	2	1	1	2	2	4	6	7
50–64	49	2.1	3	1	1	1	3	4	5	10
65+	73	3.0	7	1	1	2	4	7	9	13
B. Operated										
0–19 Years	1	1.0	0	1	1	1	1	1	1	1
20–34	2	14.0	332	1	1	14	27	27	27	27
35–49	3	1.3	<1	1	1	1	2	2	2	2
50–64	5	2.6	4	1	1	2	3	6	6	6
65+	2	3.5	4	2	2	5	5	5	5	5
SUBTOTALS:										
1. SINGLE DX										
A. Not Operated	15	1.2	<1	1	1	1	1	2	2	2
B. Operated	6	1.0	0	1	1	1	1	1	1	1
2. MULTIPLE DX										
A. Not Operated	178	2.4	4	1	1	2	3	5	7	10
B. Operated	13	4.1	50	1	1	2	3	6	27	27
1. SINGLE DX	21	1.1	<1	1	1	1	1	2	2	2
2. MULTIPLE DX	191	2.5	7	1	1	2	3	5	7	13
A. NOT OPERATED	193	2.3	4	1	1	2	3	4	7	10
B. OPERATED	19	3.1	36	1	1	1	2	6	27	27
TOTAL										
0–19 Years	6	1.0	0	1	1	1	1	2	2	2
20–34	33	2.3	20	1	1	1	2	3	5	27
35–49	42	1.8	2	1	1	1	2	3	4	7
50–64	56	2.1	3	1	1	2	3	4	4	10
65+	75	3.0	7	1	1	2	4	7	9	13
GRAND TOTAL	212	2.4	7	1	1	2	3	5	7	10

850: CONCUSSION

Type of Patients	Observed Patients	Avg. Stay	Variance	10th	25th	50th	75th	90th	95th	99th
1. SINGLE DX										
A. Not Operated										
0–19 Years	255	1.1	<1	1	1	1	1	2	2	2
20–34	83	1.4	<1	1	1	1	1	2	3	7
35–49	42	1.2	<1	1	1	1	1	2	2	3
50–64	25	1.2	<1	1	1	1	1	2	2	2
65+	4	1.5	<1	1	1	2	2	2	2	2
B. Operated										
0–19 Years	0									
20–34	0									
35–49	0									
50–64	0									
65+	0									
2. MULTIPLE DX										
A. Not Operated										
0–19 Years	1,192	1.6	1	1	1	1	2	3	4	7
20–34	1,869	1.7	3	1	1	1	2	3	4	8
35–49	1,242	2.2	6	1	1	1	2	4	6	12
50–64	1,081	2.4	6	1	1	2	3	5	7	13
65+	1,139	3.2	7	1	1	2	4	6	8	13
B. Operated										
0–19 Years	75	4.9	49	1	2	4	6	8	10	60
20–34	134	5.5	28	1	2	4	7	13	17	28
35–49	103	9.8	104	2	3	5	13	26	31	43
50–64	73	11.1	177	2	3	7	11	29	48	60
65+	46	9.0	64	1	4	6	11	20	23	35
SUBTOTALS:										
1. SINGLE DX										
A. Not Operated	409	1.2	<1	1	1	1	1	2	2	3
B. Operated	0									
2. MULTIPLE DX										
A. Not Operated	6,523	2.2	5	1	1	1	3	4	6	11
B. Operated	431	7.7	84	1	2	5	9	17	27	48
1. SINGLE DX	409	1.2	<1	1	1	1	1	2	2	3
2. MULTIPLE DX	6,954	2.5	11	1	1	1	3	5	7	16
A. NOT OPERATED	6,932	2.1	4	1	1	1	2	4	6	11
B. OPERATED	431	7.7	84	1	2	5	9	17	27	48
TOTAL										
0–19 Years	1,522	1.7	4	1	1	2	2	3	4	7
20–34	2,086	2.0	5	1	1	1	3	4	5	12
35–49	1,387	2.7	17	1	1	1	3	4	8	24
50–64	1,179	3.0	21	1	2	3	4	6	9	21
65+	1,189	3.4	10	1	1	3	4	7	9	18
GRAND TOTAL	7,363	2.4	11	1	1	1	3	5	7	15

Length of Stay by Diagnosis and Operation, Western Region, 2008

Western Region, October 2006–September 2007 Data, by Diagnosis

850.0: CONCUSSION W/O LOC

Type of Patients	Observed Patients	Avg. Stay	Vari-ance	Percentiles						
				10th	25th	50th	75th	90th	95th	99th
1. SINGLE DX										
A. Not Operated										
0–19 Years	94	1.1	<1	1	1	1	1	1	2	2
20–34	13	1.1	<1	1	1	1	1	2	2	2
35–49	11	1.5	<1	1	1	1	2	2	3	3
50–64	4	1.3	<1	1	1	1	1	2	2	2
65+	1	2.0	0	2	2	2	2	2	2	2
B. Operated										
0–19 Years	0									
20–34	0									
35–49	0									
50–64	0									
65+	0									
2. MULTIPLE DX										
A. Not Operated										
0–19 Years	257	1.5	<1	1	1	1	2	2	4	7
20–34	272	1.7	2	1	1	1	2	3	4	7
35–49	208	2.2	6	1	1	1	3	4	6	11
50–64	188	2.4	4	1	1	2	3	5	5	12
65+	362	3.2	5	1	2	3	4	6	8	12
B. Operated										
0–19 Years	8	3.6	12	1	1	2	5	11	11	11
20–34	17	4.7	21	1	2	4	6	11	19	19
35–49	14	6.7	39	1	2	4	8	13	24	24
50–64	10	8.8	95	1	3	7	10	35	35	35
65+	12	6.2	22	4	4	4	7	11	19	19
SUBTOTALS:										
1. SINGLE DX										
A. Not Operated	123	1.1	<1	1	1	1	1	2	2	2
B. Operated	0									
2. MULTIPLE DX										
A. Not Operated	1,287	2.3	4	1	1	2	3	4	6	11
B. Operated	61	6.0	37	1	2	4	8	11	19	35
1. SINGLE DX	123	1.1	<1	1	1	1	1	2	2	2
2. MULTIPLE DX	1,348	2.4	6	1	1	2	3	5	7	12
A. NOT OPERATED	1,410	2.2	4	1	1	1	3	4	6	10
B. OPERATED	61	6.0	37	1	2	4	8	11	19	35
TOTAL										
0–19 Years	359	1.4	1	1	1	1	2	2	4	7
20–34	302	1.9	3	1	1	1	2	3	4	11
35–49	233	2.5	9	1	1	1	3	5	8	19
50–64	202	2.7	10	1	2	2	3	5	8	12
65+	375	3.3	6	1	2	3	4	6	8	13
GRAND TOTAL	1,471	2.3	6	1	1	1	3	5	6	12

850.11: CONCUSSION W LOC <31 MIN

Type of Patients	Observed Patients	Avg. Stay	Vari-ance	Percentiles						
				10th	25th	50th	75th	90th	95th	99th
1. SINGLE DX										
A. Not Operated										
0–19 Years	82	1.1	<1	1	1	1	1	1	2	3
20–34	25	1.1	<1	1	1	1	1	1	2	3
35–49	11	1.1	<1	1	1	1	1	1	2	2
50–64	9	1.2	<1	1	1	1	1	2	2	2
65+	3	1.3	<1	1	1	1	2	2	2	2
B. Operated										
0–19 Years	0									
20–34	0									
35–49	0									
50–64	0									
65+	0									
2. MULTIPLE DX										
A. Not Operated										
0–19 Years	423	1.5	<1	1	1	1	2	3	3	6
20–34	618	1.7	1	1	1	1	2	3	4	6
35–49	400	2.2	4	1	1	1	2	4	6	12
50–64	397	2.3	5	1	1	2	3	5	6	11
65+	287	3.1	7	1	1	2	4	6	8	15
B. Operated										
0–19 Years	30	4.5	6	1	2	4	6	8	9	10
20–34	49	5.5	18	1	2	5	7	13	15	17
35–49	40	7.9	59	2	3	5	11	17	27	32
50–64	30	13.1	245	2	3	9	12	40	48	60
65+	18	9.0	52	2	3	6	13	21	23	23
SUBTOTALS:										
1. SINGLE DX										
A. Not Operated	130	1.1	<1	1	1	1	1	2	2	3
B. Operated	0									
2. MULTIPLE DX										
A. Not Operated	2,125	2.0	4	1	1	1	2	4	6	10
B. Operated	167	7.6	77	1	3	5	9	17	23	48
1. SINGLE DX	130	1.1	<1	1	1	1	1	2	2	3
2. MULTIPLE DX	2,292	2.4	11	1	1	1	3	5	7	15
A. NOT OPERATED	2,255	2.0	3	1	1	1	2	4	5	10
B. OPERATED	167	7.6	77	1	3	5	9	17	23	48
TOTAL										
0–19 Years	535	1.6	2	1	1	1	2	3	4	8
20–34	692	1.9	4	1	1	1	2	4	5	11
35–49	451	2.7	12	1	1	2	3	5	8	17
50–64	436	3.0	28	1	1	2	3	6	9	27
65+	308	3.4	12	1	1	2	4	7	11	18
GRAND TOTAL	2,422	2.4	10	1	1	1	2	5	7	15

850.5: CONCUSSION W COMA NOS

Type of Patients	Observed Patients	Avg. Stay	Vari-ance	Percentiles						
				10th	25th	50th	75th	90th	95th	99th
1. SINGLE DX										
A. Not Operated										
0–19 Years	60	1.1	<1	1	1	1	1	2	2	2
20–34	38	1.5	2	1	1	1	1	3	5	7
35–49	18	1.2	<1	1	1	1	1	2	2	2
50–64	11	1.2	<1	1	1	1	1	2	2	2
65+	0									
B. Operated										
0–19 Years	0									
20–34	0									
35–49	0									
50–64	0									
65+	0									
2. MULTIPLE DX										
A. Not Operated										
0–19 Years	426	1.7	2	1	1	1	2	3	4	7
20–34	794	1.7	3	1	1	1	2	3	4	8
35–49	504	2.1	5	1	1	1	2	4	6	11
50–64	385	2.6	7	1	1	2	3	6	8	15
65+	304	3.2	7	1	2	2	4	6	8	11
B. Operated										
0–19 Years	29	3.9	8	1	2	3	5	7	10	13
20–34	49	5.1	27	1	2	3	6	11	14	28
35–49	38	12.5	164	2	3	8	17	38	43	49
50–64	25	8.6	99	1	4	6	10	29	29	47
65+	12	13.0	119	3	4	9	18	32	35	35
SUBTOTALS:										
1. SINGLE DX										
A. Not Operated	127	1.2	<1	1	1	1	1	2	2	5
B. Operated	0									
2. MULTIPLE DX										
A. Not Operated	2,413	2.1	4	1	1	1	2	4	6	11
B. Operated	153	7.9	87	1	2	5	10	18	29	47
1. SINGLE DX	127	1.2	<1	1	1	1	1	2	2	5
2. MULTIPLE DX	2,566	2.5	11	1	1	1	3	5	7	16
A. NOT OPERATED	2,540	2.1	4	1	1	1	2	4	6	10
B. OPERATED	153	7.9	87	1	2	5	10	18	29	47
TOTAL										
0–19 Years	515	1.7	2	1	1	1	2	3	5	7
20–34	881	1.9	5	1	1	1	2	4	5	11
35–49	560	2.8	22	1	1	1	3	5	8	27
50–64	421	2.9	14	1	2	2	3	7	9	15
65+	316	3.5	14	1	3	3	4	7	9	18
GRAND TOTAL	2,693	2.4	11	1	1	1	3	5	7	15

Length of Stay by Diagnosis and Operation, Western Region, 2008

Western Region, October 2006–September 2007 Data, by Diagnosis

850.9: CONCUSSION NOS

Type of Patients	Observed Patients	Avg. Stay	Vari-ance	10th	25th	50th	75th	90th	95th	99th
1. SINGLE DX										
A. Not Operated										
0–19 Years	17	1.1	<1	1	1	1	1	2	2	2
20–34	5	1.4	<1	1	1	1	2	2	2	2
35–49	2	1.0	0	1	1	1	1	1	1	1
50–64	1	1.0	0	1	1	1	1	1	1	1
65+	0									
B. Operated										
0–19 Years	0									
20–34	0									
35–49	0									
50–64	0									
65+	0									
2. MULTIPLE DX										
A. Not Operated										
0–19 Years	74	1.7	2	1	1	1	2	3	4	8
20–34	156	1.9	5	1	1	1	2	3	4	17
35–49	107	2.4	9	1	1	2	2	5	7	14
50–64	97	2.4	8	1	1	1	2	5	6	23
65+	172	3.3	7	1	1	3	4	7	9	12
B. Operated										
0–19 Years	4	5.0	7	2	4	6	6	8	8	8
20–34	12	3.3	5	1	1	3	4	6	8	8
35–49	7	6.4	40	2	3	3	11	19	19	19
50–64	5	7.2	25	3	3	5	11	14	14	14
65+	4	5.7	31	1	1	1	9	12	12	12
SUBTOTALS:										
1. SINGLE DX										
A. Not Operated	25	1.2	<1	1	1	1	1	2	2	2
B. Operated	0									
2. MULTIPLE DX										
A. Not Operated	606	2.4	7	1	1	2	3	5	7	13
B. Operated	32	5.1	19	1	2	3	6	11	14	19
1. SINGLE DX	25	1.2	<1	1	1	1	2	2	2	2
2. MULTIPLE DX	638	2.6	8	1	1	2	3	5	8	14
A. NOT OPERATED	631	2.4	7	1	1	1	3	5	7	13
B. OPERATED	32	5.1	19	1	2	3	6	11	14	19
TOTAL										
0–19 Years	95	1.7	2	1	1	1	2	3	6	8
20–34	173	2.0	5	1	1	1	2	3	6	17
35–49	116	2.7	12	1	1	2	3	5	11	19
50–64	103	2.6	10	1	1	2	3	5	9	14
65+	176	3.4	7	1	1	3	4	7	9	12
GRAND TOTAL	663	2.5	8	1	1	2	3	5	8	14

851: CEREBRAL LAC/CONTUSION

Type of Patients	Observed Patients	Avg. Stay	Vari-ance	10th	25th	50th	75th	90th	95th	99th
1. SINGLE DX										
A. Not Operated										
0–19 Years	60	1.9	5	1	1	1	2	3	4	18
20–34	36	3.2	39	1	1	2	3	5	7	39
35–49	16	2.0	5	1	1	1	2	5	9	9
50–64	15	2.0	2	1	1	2	2	3	7	7
65+	4	2.5	2	2	2	3	3	4	4	4
B. Operated										
0–19 Years	4	3.8	2	2	3	5	5	5	5	5
20–34	3	9.7	132	3	3	5	23	23	23	23
35–49	1	3.0	0	3	3	3	3	3	3	3
50–64	3	5.0	0	5	5	5	5	5	5	5
65+	1	9.0	0	9	9	9	9	9	9	9
2. MULTIPLE DX										
A. Not Operated										
0–19 Years	270	3.8	19	1	1	2	5	7	13	23
20–34	485	4.2	30	1	1	2	5	9	13	28
35–49	398	5.3	46	1	2	3	6	13	19	39
50–64	481	5.3	47	1	2	3	6	11	16	28
65+	915	4.9	22	1	2	4	6	10	13	23
B. Operated										
0–19 Years	69	15.9	144	4	7	12	22	34	38	66
20–34	149	15.9	219	3	6	11	23	39	45	63
35–49	119	19.1	277	4	7	14	27	43	65	80
50–64	100	18.3	242	4	6	14	26	41	48	74
65+	138	12.2	152	3	5	9	15	23	30	76
SUBTOTALS:										
1. SINGLE DX										
A. Not Operated	131	2.3	14	1	1	2	2	4	5	18
B. Operated	12	5.9	32	3	3	5	5	9	23	23
2. MULTIPLE DX										
A. Not Operated	2,549	4.8	32	1	2	3	6	10	15	28
B. Operated	575	16.1	215	3	6	11	22	35	46	77
1. SINGLE DX	143	2.6	16	1	1	2	3	5	6	23
2. MULTIPLE DX	3,124	6.8	85	1	2	4	8	17	25	47
A. NOT OPERATED	2,680	4.6	31	1	2	3	5	10	14	28
B. OPERATED	587	15.9	213	3	6	11	22	35	46	77
TOTAL										
0–19 Years	403	5.6	60	1	2	3	6	16	22	38
20–34	673	6.7	96	1	2	3	7	17	28	49
35–49	534	8.3	130	1	2	4	9	22	33	65
50–64	599	7.4	102	1	2	4	8	18	26	50
65+	1,058	5.8	45	1	2	4	7	12	17	30
GRAND TOTAL	3,267	6.7	83	1	2	4	7	16	25	47

851.80: OTH CEREB LAC/CONTU-NOS

Type of Patients	Observed Patients	Avg. Stay	Vari-ance	10th	25th	50th	75th	90th	95th	99th
1. SINGLE DX										
A. Not Operated										
0–19 Years	7	4.5	37	1	1	3	3	18	18	18
20–34	4	11.4	332	1	1	2	4	39	39	39
35–49	1	1.0	0	1	1	1	1	1	1	1
50–64	0									
65+	0									
B. Operated										
0–19 Years	0									
20–34	0									
35–49	1	3.0	0	3	3	3	3	3	3	3
50–64	2	5.0	0	5	5	5	5	5	5	5
65+	0									
2. MULTIPLE DX										
A. Not Operated										
0–19 Years	19	4.6	21	1	1	2	7	13	15	15
20–34	55	4.4	20	1	1	3	6	10	12	28
35–49	45	5.2	40	1	2	3	6	14	20	>99
50–64	50	6.4	30	2	3	5	7	13	19	26
65+	124	5.8	42	1	2	4	6	11	21	38
B. Operated										
0–19 Years	4	16.1	33	9	15	17	23	23	23	23
20–34	13	21.2	301	5	10	11	33	47	52	52
35–49	9	17.5	78	7	11	18	18	35	35	35
50–64	16	17.9	328	5	6	9	21	41	74	74
65+	25	9.3	40	2	4	8	11	19	22	22
SUBTOTALS:										
1. SINGLE DX										
A. Not Operated	12	6.5	125	1	1	2	3	18	39	39
B. Operated	3	4.3	1	3	3	5	5	5	5	5
2. MULTIPLE DX										
A. Not Operated	293	5.5	34	1	2	4	7	12	18	38
B. Operated	67	15.1	178	4	6	11	18	33	41	74
1. SINGLE DX	15	6.0	99	1	1	3	5	18	39	39
2. MULTIPLE DX	360	7.3	75	1	2	5	8	17	24	47
A. NOT OPERATED	305	5.5	38	1	2	4	7	12	18	38
B. OPERATED	70	14.7	175	4	6	11	18	33	41	74
TOTAL										
0–19 Years	30	6.1	40	1	2	3	9	17	18	23
20–34	72	7.8	122	1	2	4	8	14	39	52
35–49	56	7.0	65	1	2	3	8	18	35	>99
50–64	68	9.1	120	2	4	6	10	15	26	74
65+	149	6.4	43	1	2	4	7	21	22	38
GRAND TOTAL	375	7.2	76	1	2	5	8	18	24	47

Length of Stay by Diagnosis and Operation, Western Region, 2008

Western Region, October 2006–September 2007 Data, by Diagnosis

851.81: OTH C LAC/CONTU W/O LOC

Type of Patients	Observed Patients	Avg. Stay	Variance	10th	25th	50th	75th	90th	95th	99th
1. SINGLE DX										
A. Not Operated										
0–19 Years	9	1.7	1	1	1	1	2	4	4	4
20–34	8	2.8	6	1	1	2	6	7	7	7
35–49	5	1.2	<1	1	1	1	1	2	2	2
50–64	3	2.0	<1	1	1	2	3	3	3	3
65+	0									
B. Operated										
0–19 Years	1	2.0	0	2	2	2	2	2	2	2
20–34	1	3.0	0	3	3	3	3	3	3	3
35–49	0									
50–64	1	5.0	0	5	5	5	5	5	5	5
65+	0									
2. MULTIPLE DX										
A. Not Operated										
0–19 Years	43	2.1	3	1	1	1	3	5	5	9
20–34	67	3.2	10	1	1	2	4	5	10	17
35–49	59	3.9	17	1	1	2	5	9	13	21
50–64	102	4.5	19	1	2	3	6	8	10	26
65+	300	4.4	14	1	2	3	5	9	10	19
B. Operated										
0–19 Years	3	3.7	5	1	1	5	5	5	5	5
20–34	6	12.9	186	1	4	6	16	39	39	39
35–49	14	14.5	239	2	3	6	25	34	55	55
50–64	10	13.5	178	1	4	9	18	20	46	46
65+	37	9.5	54	2	4	7	15	20	25	30
SUBTOTALS:										
1. SINGLE DX										
A. Not Operated	25	2.0	3	1	1	1	2	4	6	7
B. Operated	3	3.3	2	2	2	3	5	5	5	5
2. MULTIPLE DX										
A. Not Operated	571	4.0	14	1	2	3	5	8	10	19
B. Operated	70	11.1	117	2	4	7	17	25	34	55
1. SINGLE DX	28	2.1	3	1	1	1	3	5	6	7
2. MULTIPLE DX	641	4.8	30	1	2	3	6	10	15	28
A. NOT OPERATED	596	4.0	14	1	2	3	5	8	10	19
B. OPERATED	73	10.8	115	2	4	6	16	25	34	55
TOTAL										
0–19 Years	56	2.1	3	1	1	1	3	5	5	9
20–34	82	3.9	27	1	1	2	4	7	12	39
35–49	78	5.6	71	1	1	2	6	14	25	55
50–64	116	5.2	38	1	2	4	7	10	18	28
65+	337	5.0	20	1	2	4	6	10	13	25
GRAND TOTAL	669	4.7	29	1	2	3	6	10	14	28

851.82: OTH CEREB LAC/CONTU-BRF

Type of Patients	Observed Patients	Avg. Stay	Variance	10th	25th	50th	75th	90th	95th	99th
1. SINGLE DX										
A. Not Operated										
0–19 Years	18	1.5	1	1	1	1	2	2	5	5
20–34	6	2.3	<1	2	2	2	3	3	3	3
35–49	3	1.3	<1	1	1	1	2	2	2	2
50–64	3	1.3	<1	1	1	1	2	2	2	2
65+	1	1.0	0	1	1	1	1	1	1	1
B. Operated										
0–19 Years	1	5.0	0	5	5	5	5	5	5	5
20–34	0									
35–49	0									
50–64	0									
65+	0									
2. MULTIPLE DX										
A. Not Operated										
0–19 Years	53	3.4	20	1	1	2	3	5	10	30
20–34	96	2.8	5	1	1	2	4	6	7	15
35–49	65	4.2	17	1	2	3	5	8	13	21
50–64	81	4.2	19	1	2	3	5	9	12	28
65+	129	5.0	20	1	2	4	6	11	12	22
B. Operated										
0–19 Years	4	8.5	39	2	7	8	17	17	17	17
20–34	22	8.4	59	3	3	7	11	14	28	30
35–49	15	13.5	54	5	7	13	20	27	27	27
50–64	11	11.2	31	5	6	11	17	17	23	23
65+	18	10.2	124	2	5	8	10	20	51	51
SUBTOTALS:										
1. SINGLE DX										
A. Not Operated	31	1.6	<1	1	1	1	2	3	3	5
B. Operated	1	5.0	0	5	5	5	5	5	5	5
2. MULTIPLE DX										
A. Not Operated	424	4.0	16	1	2	3	5	8	12	22
B. Operated	70	10.4	69	3	5	9	13	20	27	51
1. SINGLE DX	32	1.7	1	1	1	1	2	3	5	7
2. MULTIPLE DX	494	4.9	29	1	2	3	6	11	14	28
A. NOT OPERATED	455	3.9	16	1	1	2	5	8	12	22
B. OPERATED	71	10.3	69	3	5	8	13	20	27	51
TOTAL										
0–19 Years	76	3.2	18	1	1	2	3	5	5	9
20–34	124	3.7	19	1	1	2	4	7	11	28
35–49	83	5.8	36	1	2	4	6	13	20	27
50–64	95	4.9	25	1	2	3	7	10	14	28
65+	148	5.6	34	1	2	4	7	11	15	25
GRAND TOTAL	526	4.7	28	1	2	3	6	11	14	27

851.86: OTH CEREB LAC/CONTU-NEC

Type of Patients	Observed Patients	Avg. Stay	Variance	10th	25th	50th	75th	90th	95th	99th
1. SINGLE DX										
A. Not Operated										
0–19 Years	7	1.9	<1	1	1	2	2	3	3	3
20–34	8	2.0	1	1	1	2	3	4	4	4
35–49	3	3.7	21	1	1	1	9	9	9	9
50–64	3	1.3	<1	1	1	1	2	2	2	2
65+	2	2.5	<1	2	2	3	3	3	3	3
B. Operated										
0–19 Years	0									
20–34	0									
35–49	0									
50–64	0									
65+	1	9.0	0	9	9	9	9	9	9	9
2. MULTIPLE DX										
A. Not Operated										
0–19 Years	48	4.7	23	1	1	4	6	9	17	23
20–34	95	3.6	17	1	2	3	6	7	12	27
35–49	80	6.5	55	1	2	3	8	17	25	31
50–64	77	5.9	132	1	2	4	6	13	20	96
65+	92	5.3	26	2	2	4	7	10	13	41
B. Operated										
0–19 Years	21	14.9	248	3	5	9	18	34	38	66
20–34	39	15.6	323	3	4	9	20	45	55	93
35–49	24	16.4	269	2	5	11	22	42	50	65
50–64	24	23.7	280	3	12	23	34	42	47	69
65+	17	15.4	136	5	6	12	19	32	45	45
SUBTOTALS:										
1. SINGLE DX										
A. Not Operated	23	2.1	3	1	1	2	2	3	4	9
B. Operated	1	9.0	0	9	9	9	9	9	9	9
2. MULTIPLE DX										
A. Not Operated	392	5.2	51	1	2	3	6	11	17	31
B. Operated	125	17.2	269	3	5	12	25	41	47	69
1. SINGLE DX	24	2.4	5	1	1	2	3	4	9	9
2. MULTIPLE DX	517	8.1	129	1	2	4	9	19	30	55
A. NOT OPERATED	415	5.0	48	1	2	3	6	11	17	28
B. OPERATED	126	17.1	267	3	5	12	25	41	47	69
TOTAL										
0–19 Years	76	7.2	104	1	2	4	7	18	27	66
20–34	142	6.8	128	1	1	3	7	16	25	55
35–49	107	8.6	117	1	2	4	11	22	29	50
50–64	104	9.9	218	2	3	4	11	29	39	69
65+	112	6.8	55	2	3	5	8	13	19	41
GRAND TOTAL	541	7.8	125	1	2	4	8	18	29	55

Length of Stay by Diagnosis and Operation, Western Region, 2008

Western Region, October 2006–September 2007 Data, by Diagnosis

852: TRAUMATIC SAH/SDH/EXDH

Type of Patients	Observed Patients	Avg. Stay	Variance	10th	25th	50th	75th	90th	95th	99th
1. SINGLE DX										
A. *Not Operated*										
0–19 Years	129	2.0	11	1	1	1	2	3	4	7
20–34	67	2.1	2	1	1	2	2	4	4	11
35–49	22	2.3	6	1	1	1	3	4	7	11
50–64	29	1.7	2	1	1	1	2	3	3	9
65+	19	2.3	2	1	1	2	3	5	5	5
B. *Operated*										
0–19 Years	22	3.6	3	2	2	3	4	5	7	9
20–34	12	3.8	8	1	2	3	5	7	11	11
35–49	8	3.5	2	2	3	3	4	6	6	6
50–64	18	3.1	2	1	2	3	4	5	6	6
65+	19	3.7	5	2	2	3	5	7	9	9
2. MULTIPLE DX										
A. *Not Operated*										
0–19 Years	398	3.5	18	1	1	2	4	7	12	25
20–34	668	3.5	24	1	1	2	4	7	9	23
35–49	726	4.4	35	1	1	3	5	9	14	28
50–64	1,099	4.7	39	1	2	3	5	10	15	34
65+	3,435	4.6	19	1	2	3	6	9	12	20
B. *Operated*										
0–19 Years	138	12.9	141	3	4	10	17	31	39	51
20–34	221	17.5	270	3	5	12	25	37	52	93
35–49	295	14.6	262	3	5	9	19	35	55	>99
50–64	531	12.4	167	3	4	8	15	29	40	75
65+	1,539	9.6	53	3	5	7	12	19	24	37
SUBTOTALS:										
1. SINGLE DX										
A. *Not Operated*	266	2.0	7	1	1	2	2	3	4	11
B. *Operated*	79	3.5	4	1	2	3	4	6	7	11
2. MULTIPLE DX										
A. *Not Operated*	6,326	4.4	25	1	2	3	5	9	12	25
B. *Operated*	2,724	11.5	126	3	5	8	14	25	34	63
1. SINGLE DX	345	2.4	6	1	1	2	3	4	5	11
2. MULTIPLE DX	9,050	6.5	66	1	2	4	7	15	21	43
A. NOT OPERATED	6,592	4.3	24	1	2	3	5	9	12	25
B. OPERATED	2,803	11.3	124	3	5	8	14	24	34	62
TOTAL										
0–19 Years	687	5.1	57	1	1	2	5	13	20	39
20–34	968	6.6	113	1	1	3	6	18	29	55
35–49	1,051	7.2	119	2	2	4	8	18	28	72
50–64	1,677	7.1	92	2	2	4	8	17	26	57
65+	5,012	6.1	34	1	2	4	7	13	18	29
GRAND TOTAL	9,395	6.4	64	1	2	4	7	14	21	42

852.00: TRAUMATIC SAH-NOS

Type of Patients	Observed Patients	Avg. Stay	Variance	10th	25th	50th	75th	90th	95th	99th
1. SINGLE DX										
A. *Not Operated*										
0–19 Years	5	1.2	<1	1	1	1	1	2	2	2
20–34	2	2.5	<1	2	2	2	3	3	3	3
35–49	3	4.0	7	2	2	3	7	7	7	7
50–64	2	1.0	0	1	1	1	1	1	1	1
65+	0									
B. *Operated*										
0–19 Years	0									
20–34	0									
35–49	0									
50–64	0									
65+	0									
2. MULTIPLE DX										
A. *Not Operated*										
0–19 Years	28	4.2	28	1	1	2	4	7	11	26
20–34	46	4.1	64	1	1	2	4	7	9	55
35–49	72	6.2	92	1	2	3	6	13	23	72
50–64	87	4.9	25	1	2	3	6	10	13	31
65+	213	5.5	36	1	2	3	6	12	16	38
B. *Operated*										
0–19 Years	9	20.7	303	6	7	11	34	49	49	49
20–34	17	16.4	154	4	5	11	24	36	38	38
35–49	5	27.3	953	5	10	12	29	80	80	80
50–64	11	18.2	263	4	6	14	22	33	58	58
65+	18	10.4	50	3	4	10	14	20	30	30
SUBTOTALS:										
1. SINGLE DX										
A. *Not Operated*	12	2.1	3	1	1	1	2	3	7	7
B. *Operated*	0									
2. MULTIPLE DX										
A. *Not Operated*	446	5.3	45	1	2	3	6	12	15	38
B. *Operated*	60	16.5	232	4	5	11	22	34	45	80
1. SINGLE DX	12	2.1	3	1	1	1	3	3	7	7
2. MULTIPLE DX	506	6.6	80	1	2	4	7	14	23	45
A. NOT OPERATED	458	5.2	44	1	2	3	6	12	15	38
B. OPERATED	60	16.5	232	4	5	11	22	34	45	80
TOTAL										
0–19 Years	42	7.3	128	1	1	3	7	13	19	49
20–34	65	7.2	114	1	2	3	6	18	23	55
35–49	80	7.4	159	1	2	4	8	15	25	80
50–64	100	6.3	66	2	2	4	7	13	22	33
65+	231	5.9	39	1	2	4	7	13	17	38
GRAND TOTAL	518	6.5	79	1	2	4	7	14	23	45

852.01: TRAUMATIC SAH W/O LOC

Type of Patients	Observed Patients	Avg. Stay	Variance	10th	25th	50th	75th	90th	95th	99th
1. SINGLE DX										
A. *Not Operated*										
0–19 Years	37	1.4	<1	1	1	1	2	3	3	4
20–34	10	1.9	1	1	1	2	2	4	4	4
35–49	5	1.2	<1	1	1	1	1	2	2	2
50–64	2	1.5	<1	1	1	2	2	2	2	2
65+	2	4.5	<1	4	4	4	5	5	5	5
B. *Operated*										
0–19 Years	0									
20–34	0									
35–49	0									
50–64	0									
65+	0									
2. MULTIPLE DX										
A. *Not Operated*										
0–19 Years	44	3.1	8	1	1	2	3	6	8	16
20–34	81	2.6	10	1	1	2	2	5	8	24
35–49	97	3.4	12	1	1	2	4	7	9	20
50–64	149	5.1	51	1	2	3	5	13	18	36
65+	473	4.6	23	1	2	3	6	10	13	23
B. *Operated*										
0–19 Years	9	7.5	29	1	4	7	9	19	19	19
20–34	8	16.8	237	3	7	15	20	52	52	52
35–49	10	16.7	859	1	3	6	13	19	99	99
50–64	10	18.7	186	4	12	14	24	34	49	49
65+	41	13.8	81	4	7	12	19	25	29	41
SUBTOTALS:										
1. SINGLE DX										
A. *Not Operated*	56	1.6	1	1	1	1	2	3	4	5
B. *Operated*	0									
2. MULTIPLE DX										
A. *Not Operated*	844	4.3	25	1	1	3	5	9	13	23
B. *Operated*	78	14.4	198	3	6	11	19	27	41	99
1. SINGLE DX	56	1.6	1	1	1	1	2	3	4	5
2. MULTIPLE DX	922	5.2	48	1	2	3	6	12	16	34
A. NOT OPERATED	900	4.1	24	1	2	3	5	9	13	23
B. OPERATED	78	14.4	198	3	6	11	19	27	41	99
TOTAL										
0–19 Years	90	2.8	10	1	1	2	3	6	9	19
20–34	99	3.7	41	1	1	2	3	6	15	52
35–49	112	4.5	95	1	1	2	5	8	13	20
50–64	161	5.9	69	1	2	3	6	15	22	49
65+	516	5.4	34	1	2	3	6	12	16	28
GRAND TOTAL	978	5.0	46	1	1	3	6	12	16	34

Length of Stay by Diagnosis and Operation, Western Region, 2008

Western Region, October 2006–September 2007 Data, by Diagnosis

852.02: TRAUMATIC SAH-BRIEF

Type of Patients	Observed Patients	Avg. Stay	Vari-ance	10th	25th	50th	75th	90th	95th	99th
1. SINGLE DX										
A. Not Operated										
0–19 Years	3	2.7	2	1	1	3	4	4	4	4
20–34	13	1.2	<1	1	1	1	1	2	2	2
35–49	4	1.3	<1	1	1	1	1	2	2	2
50–64	8	1.1	<1	1	1	1	1	2	2	2
65+	4	2.2	4	1	1	1	2	5	5	5
B. Operated										
0–19 Years	0									
20–34	0									
35–49	0									
50–64	0									
65+	0									
2. MULTIPLE DX										
A. Not Operated										
0–19 Years	51	2.6	5	1	1	2	3	5	9	10
20–34	100	2.7	12	1	1	2	3	5	6	21
35–49	83	2.8	9	1	1	2	4	5	6	24
50–64	133	3.3	16	1	1	2	4	7	10	14
65+	196	4.3	16	2	2	3	6	9	14	20
B. Operated										
0–19 Years	3	6.7	14	4	4	5	11	11	11	11
20–34	9	14.1	342	3	4	5	17	61	61	61
35–49	13	11.9	152	3	4	7	11	24	46	46
50–64	17	12.4	102	2	5	10	13	32	36	36
65+	24	10.0	54	3	5	9	15	21	27	28
SUBTOTALS:										
1. SINGLE DX										
A. Not Operated	32	1.5	<1	1	1	1	2	2	4	5
B. Operated	0									
2. MULTIPLE DX										
A. Not Operated	563	3.4	13	1	1	2	4	7	10	20
B. Operated	66	11.4	118	3	4	8	13	24	32	61
1. SINGLE DX	32	1.5	<1	1	1	1	2	2	4	5
2. MULTIPLE DX	629	4.2	30	1	1	3	5	9	14	27
A. NOT OPERATED	595	3.3	13	1	1	2	4	7	10	20
B. OPERATED	66	11.4	118	3	4	8	13	24	32	61
TOTAL										
0–19 Years	57	2.9	6	1	1	2	4	6	9	11
20–34	122	3.4	42	1	1	2	3	5	10	23
35–49	100	3.9	36	1	1	2	4	7	11	46
50–64	158	4.2	32	1	2	2	5	10	12	36
65+	224	4.9	23	2	2	3	6	11	16	22
GRAND TOTAL	661	4.1	29	1	1	2	5	9	13	27

852.06: TRAUMATIC SAH-NEC

Type of Patients	Observed Patients	Avg. Stay	Vari-ance	10th	25th	50th	75th	90th	95th	99th
1. SINGLE DX										
A. Not Operated										
0–19 Years	8	2.1	2	1	1	2	3	3	5	5
20–34	8	2.0	<1	2	2	2	3	3	3	3
35–49	1	1.0	0	1	1	1	1	1	1	1
50–64	5	3.2	11	1	2	2	2	9	9	9
65+	2	3.5	4	2	2	5	5	5	5	5
B. Operated										
0–19 Years	0									
20–34	0									
35–49	0									
50–64	0									
65+	0									
2. MULTIPLE DX										
A. Not Operated										
0–19 Years	43	4.2	26	1	1	2	5	5	13	23
20–34	119	3.9	34	1	1	2	4	7	12	22
35–49	103	4.5	30	1	1	2	5	10	16	25
50–64	128	5.2	40	1	2	3	5	11	18	34
65+	159	5.6	37	1	2	4	7	10	17	36
B. Operated										
0–19 Years	12	22.6	254	10	10	20	32	38	63	63
20–34	42	21.2	280	7	10	17	27	37	44	93
35–49	30	25.2	441	7	10	18	43	64	85	>99
50–64	38	17.5	153	5	7	14	23	36	41	51
65+	23	16.8	161	5	7	16	19	34	49	50
SUBTOTALS:										
1. SINGLE DX										
A. Not Operated	24	2.4	3	1	1	2	3	5	5	9
B. Operated	0									
2. MULTIPLE DX										
A. Not Operated	552	4.8	35	1	2	3	6	10	16	34
B. Operated	145	20.5	262	5	9	16	27	43	54	93
1. SINGLE DX	24	2.4	3	1	2	2	3	5	5	9
2. MULTIPLE DX	697	8.1	122	1	2	4	9	20	32	54
A. NOT OPERATED	576	4.7	34	1	2	3	5	10	15	34
B. OPERATED	145	20.5	262	5	9	16	27	43	54	93
TOTAL										
0–19 Years	63	7.5	118	1	1	3	6	10	23	63
20–34	169	8.1	150	1	2	3	9	25	30	56
35–49	134	9.1	195	1	2	3	10	25	44	85
50–64	171	7.9	90	1	2	4	9	20	32	41
65+	184	7.0	65	1	2	4	9	16	19	49
GRAND TOTAL	721	7.9	119	1	2	4	9	20	30	54

852.20: TRAUMATIC SDH-NOS

Type of Patients	Observed Patients	Avg. Stay	Vari-ance	10th	25th	50th	75th	90th	95th	99th
1. SINGLE DX										
A. Not Operated										
0–19 Years	7	1.4	<1	1	1	1	2	3	3	3
20–34	0									
35–49	4	2.0	0	2	2	2	2	2	2	2
50–64	2	3.0	0	3	3	3	3	3	3	3
65+	2	1.0	0	1	1	1	1	1	1	1
B. Operated										
0–19 Years	0									
20–34	1	4.0	0	4	4	4	4	4	4	4
35–49	3	3.3	<1	3	3	3	4	4	4	4
50–64	7	3.0	2	2	2	2	5	5	5	5
65+	6	3.7	8	1	2	2	4	9	9	9
2. MULTIPLE DX										
A. Not Operated										
0–19 Years	26	3.1	7	1	1	2	5	6	7	12
20–34	44	3.7	9	1	1	3	5	8	9	14
35–49	79	5.5	38	1	2	4	7	12	16	37
50–64	135	6.3	74	1	2	4	6	13	29	43
65+	551	4.8	15	1	2	4	6	9	12	21
B. Operated										
0–19 Years	11	6.5	36	3	3	4	8	16	20	20
20–34	18	18.5	378	4	5	12	30	76	>99	>99
35–49	65	10.2	96	3	5	8	10	21	28	55
50–64	108	8.5	62	3	4	6	11	19	24	58
65+	456	8.4	39	3	4	6	10	17	23	30
SUBTOTALS:										
1. SINGLE DX										
A. Not Operated	12	1.7	<1	1	1	1	2	3	3	3
B. Operated	17	3.4	4	2	2	3	4	5	9	9
2. MULTIPLE DX										
A. Not Operated	835	5.0	26	1	2	4	6	10	13	29
B. Operated	658	8.8	60	3	4	6	10	18	24	52
1. SINGLE DX	29	2.7	3	1	2	2	3	5	5	9
2. MULTIPLE DX	1,493	6.7	45	2	3	5	8	14	20	36
A. NOT OPERATED	847	5.0	26	1	2	4	6	9	13	29
B. OPERATED	675	8.7	60	3	4	6	10	18	24	52
TOTAL										
0–19 Years	44	3.7	16	1	1	2	5	7	12	20
20–34	63	7.9	155	1	3	4	8	24	31	>99
35–49	148	7.5	68	2	3	5	9	15	26	49
50–64	252	7.1	68	2	3	5	7	15	25	55
65+	1,015	6.4	29	2	3	5	8	13	18	27
GRAND TOTAL	1,522	6.6	44	2	3	5	8	14	20	36

Length of Stay by Diagnosis and Operation, Western Region, 2008

Western Region, October 2006–September 2007 Data, by Diagnosis

852.21: TRAUMATIC SDH W/O LOC

Type of Patients	Observed Patients	Avg. Stay	Variance	10th	25th	50th	75th	90th	95th	99th
1. SINGLE DX										
A. *Not Operated*										
0–19 Years	25	1.5	<1	1	1	1	2	2	3	3
20–34	14	2.8	7	1	1	2	3	4	11	11
35–49	1	1.0	0	1	1	1	1	1	1	1
50–64	8	1.5	<1	1	1	1	2	3	3	3
65+	9	1.8	<1	1	1	2	2	3	3	3
B. *Operated*										
0–19 Years	3	6.0	13	2	2	7	9	9	9	9
20–34	3	5.3	2	4	4	5	7	7	7	7
35–49	3	3.7	4	2	2	3	6	6	6	6
50–64	7	3.1	2	1	2	3	4	5	5	5
65+	11	4.1	3	2	2	4	6	6	7	7
2. MULTIPLE DX										
A. *Not Operated*										
0–19 Years	83	3.2	18	1	1	2	3	7	9	32
20–34	83	3.0	8	1	1	2	4	6	8	18
35–49	121	3.8	27	1	1	2	4	8	10	27
50–64	217	4.0	13	1	2	3	5	6	8	19
65+	1,311	4.3	16	1	2	3	5	8	11	19
B. *Operated*										
0–19 Years	23	9.9	63	3	4	8	13	21	27	33
20–34	29	10.8	93	2	4	6	14	24	34	38
35–49	73	9.6	81	3	4	7	10	22	34	43
50–64	201	8.6	68	2	4	6	11	18	25	52
65+	766	9.1	43	3	5	7	11	17	21	36
SUBTOTALS:										
1. SINGLE DX										
A. *Not Operated*	57	1.8	2	1	1	1	2	3	4	11
B. *Operated*	27	4.1	4	2	2	4	6	7	7	9
2. MULTIPLE DX										
A. *Not Operated*	1,815	4.1	16	1	2	3	5	8	11	19
B. *Operated*	1,092	9.1	52	3	4	7	11	18	24	38
1. SINGLE DX	84	2.6	4	1	1	2	3	5	7	11
2. MULTIPLE DX	2,907	6.0	35	1	2	4	7	12	17	30
A. NOT OPERATED	1,872	4.1	16	1	2	3	5	8	11	19
B. OPERATED	1,119	9.0	51	3	4	7	11	18	23	37
TOTAL										
0–19 Years	134	4.1	29	1	1	2	4	10	14	32
20–34	129	4.8	36	1	1	3	5	12	16	34
35–49	198	5.9	54	1	2	3	7	12	22	43
50–64	433	6.1	44	1	2	4	7	13	19	40
65+	2,097	6.1	31	1	3	4	8	12	17	27
GRAND TOTAL	2,991	5.9	35	1	2	4	7	12	17	30

852.22: TRAUMATIC SDH-BRIEF

Type of Patients	Observed Patients	Avg. Stay	Variance	10th	25th	50th	75th	90th	95th	99th
1. SINGLE DX										
A. *Not Operated*										
0–19 Years	14	2.4	3	1	1	2	3	5	7	7
20–34	6	1.8	<1	1	1	2	2	3	3	3
35–49	2	6.0	49	1	1	11	11	11	11	11
50–64	0									
65+	0									
B. *Operated*										
0–19 Years	1	2.0	0	2	2	2	2	2	2	2
20–34	1	3.0	0	3	3	3	3	3	3	3
35–49	1	5.0	0	5	5	5	5	5	5	5
50–64	0									
65+	0									
2. MULTIPLE DX										
A. *Not Operated*										
0–19 Years	46	3.1	18	1	1	2	3	7	8	25
20–34	63	3.1	5	1	1	2	4	6	8	10
35–49	56	3.4	13	1	1	2	4	7	13	20
50–64	110	3.3	12	1	1	3	4	6	8	19
65+	210	3.9	11	2	2	3	5	8	10	15
B. *Operated*										
0–19 Years	10	9.6	29	3	6	7	14	16	19	19
20–34	15	6.8	57	1	2	5	6	19	29	29
35–49	10	7.6	50	3	3	4	13	17	22	22
50–64	28	15.5	243	3	4	10	25	39	45	67
65+	56	12.4	82	3	6	10	18	28	31	38
SUBTOTALS:										
1. SINGLE DX										
A. *Not Operated*	22	2.6	6	1	1	2	3	5	7	11
B. *Operated*	3	3.3	2	2	2	3	5	5	5	5
2. MULTIPLE DX										
A. *Not Operated*	485	3.5	11	1	2	3	4	7	9	19
B. *Operated*	119	11.8	115	3	4	8	15	28	34	45
1. SINGLE DX	25	2.6	5	1	1	2	3	5	7	11
2. MULTIPLE DX	604	5.2	43	1	2	3	6	11	18	31
A. NOT OPERATED	507	3.5	11	1	1	2	4	7	9	19
B. OPERATED	122	11.6	114	3	4	7	15	28	31	45
TOTAL										
0–19 Years	71	3.8	21	1	1	2	4	8	14	25
20–34	85	3.7	16	1	1	3	5	9	16	29
35–49	69	4.1	20	1	1	3	7	11	14	22
50–64	138	5.8	82	1	2	3	5	13	19	45
65+	266	5.7	38	2	2	4	7	12	20	31
GRAND TOTAL	629	5.1	41	1	2	3	6	11	18	31

852.26: TRAUMATIC SDH-NEC

Type of Patients	Observed Patients	Avg. Stay	Variance	10th	25th	50th	75th	90th	95th	99th
1. SINGLE DX										
A. *Not Operated*										
0–19 Years	6	1.7	<1	1	1	2	2	3	3	3
20–34	6	1.7	<1	1	1	1	2	3	3	3
35–49	3	1.7	1	1	1	1	3	3	3	3
50–64	3	1.0	0	1	1	1	1	1	1	1
65+	0									
B. *Operated*										
0–19 Years	1	4.0	0	4	4	4	4	4	4	4
20–34	1	11.0	0	11	11	11	11	11	11	11
35–49	1	2.0	0	2	2	2	2	2	2	2
50–64	4	3.2	4	1	1	3	3	6	6	6
65+	1	2.0	0	2	2	2	2	2	2	2
2. MULTIPLE DX										
A. *Not Operated*										
0–19 Years	39	5.7	52	1	1	3	8	13	25	32
20–34	74	4.5	50	1	1	2	5	9	14	51
35–49	72	4.1	12	1	1	3	6	9	11	17
50–64	106	5.6	78	1	1	3	6	12	23	48
65+	174	4.5	13	1	2	3	6	8	11	20
B. *Operated*										
0–19 Years	20	14.0	109	2	4	13	19	31	39	39
20–34	27	18.5	170	2	5	19	27	39	41	45
35–49	40	15.5	182	3	5	11	29	35	62	>99
50–64	61	19.1	407	3	6	14	23	47	67	>99
65+	93	12.0	74	4	5	10	16	24	27	47
SUBTOTALS:										
1. SINGLE DX										
A. *Not Operated*	16	1.6	<1	1	1	1	2	3	3	3
B. *Operated*	8	4.0	10	1	2	3	4	11	11	11
2. MULTIPLE DX										
A. *Not Operated*	465	4.8	37	1	2	3	6	9	13	31
B. *Operated*	241	15.3	196	3	5	11	21	33	45	>99
1. SINGLE DX	24	2.4	5	1	1	2	3	4	6	11
2. MULTIPLE DX	706	8.4	116	1	2	5	10	22	31	62
A. NOT OPERATED	481	4.7	36	1	2	3	6	9	13	31
B. OPERATED	249	14.9	194	3	5	11	21	32	45	>99
TOTAL										
0–19 Years	66	7.8	80	1	1	3	12	23	30	39
20–34	108	7.9	114	1	2	3	9	24	32	45
35–49	116	8.0	100	1	2	4	9	26	33	>99
50–64	172	10.3	233	1	2	5	12	27	47	92
65+	268	7.1	47	2	3	5	8	16	23	34
GRAND TOTAL	730	8.2	113	1	2	4	9	21	31	62

Length of Stay by Diagnosis and Operation, Western Region, 2008

Western Region, October 2006–September 2007 Data, by Diagnosis

Type of Patients	853: OTHER TRAUMATIC ICH										853.00: OTH TRAUM ICH-NOS										853.01: OTH TRAUM ICH W/O LOC									
	Observed Patients	Avg. Stay	Vari-ance	10th	25th	50th	75th	90th	95th	99th	Observed Patients	Avg. Stay	Vari-ance	10th	25th	50th	75th	90th	95th	99th	Observed Patients	Avg. Stay	Vari-ance	10th	25th	50th	75th	90th	95th	99th
1. SINGLE DX																														
A. Not Operated																														
0–19 Years	36	1.7	1	1	1	1	2	3	5	5	2	1.5	<1	1	1	2	2	2	2	2	21	1.8	2	1	1	1	2	5	5	5
20–34	17	1.9	2	1	1	1	3	4	5	5	0										8	1.6	1	1	1	1	2	4	4	4
35–49	6	2.2	2	1	1	2	3	4	4	4	2	2.0	0	2	2	2	2	2	2	2	0									
50–64	1	1.0	0	1	1	1	1	1	1	1	0										1	1.0	0	1	1	1	1	1	1	1
65+	2	1.5	<1	1	1	2	2	2	2	2	1	1.0	0	1	1	1	1	1	1	1	0									
B. Operated																														
0–19 Years	0										0										0									
20–34	1	8.0	0	8	8	8	8	8	8	8	0										0									
35–49	1	12.0	0	12	12	12	12	12	12	12	0										0									
50–64	0										0										0									
65+	0										0										0									
2. MULTIPLE DX																														
A. Not Operated																														
0–19 Years	91	3.3	18	1	1	2	4	7	10	25	10	1.3	<1	1	1	1	1	3	3	3	24	2.9	21	1	1	2	2	4	8	23
20–34	160	3.5	25	1	1	2	4	7	11	26	26	5.1	81	1	1	2	4	13	14	46	35	2.5	18	1	1	2	2	4	7	26
35–49	152	5.4	38	1	1	3	7	13	22	27	26	7.7	50	2	3	6	10	22	24	28	54	6.1	46	1	1	3	9	14	24	26
50–64	220	5.7	65	1	2	3	6	14	20	38	38	6.1	59	1	2	3	7	14	29	38	94	5.5	52	1	1	3	6	15	21	48
65+	674	4.9	23	1	2	4	6	10	12	21	148	5.4	33	1	2	4	6	11	14	21	378	4.7	17	1	2	3	6	9	12	23
B. Operated																														
0–19 Years	25	17.2	224	2	3	15	24	37	48	50	3	13.3	58	5	5	15	20	20	20	20	0									
20–34	43	18.3	210	4	5	15	26	38	41	65	11	17.0	124	5	6	16	19	33	40	40	5	10.0	11	5	8	12	12	13	13	13
35–49	31	19.3	265	3	5	13	30	39	54	59	8	25.7	293	21	21	28	39	54	54	54	3	4.0	3	2	2	5	5	5	5	5
50–64	40	17.3	139	5	7	15	26	38	40	>99	14	15.7	145	5	7	10	23	38	40	40	6	11.2	25	4	9	10	17	17	17	17
65+	41	10.4	50	3	5	9	13	20	25	32	9	8.5	46	1	4	7	9	20	20	20	18	11.5	34	5	8	11	13	21	25	25
SUBTOTALS:																														
1. SINGLE DX																														
A. Not Operated	62	1.8	1	1	1	1	2	3	5	5	5	1.6	<1	1	1	2	2	2	2	2	30	1.7	2	1	1	1	2	5	5	5
B. Operated	2	10.0	8	8	8	12	12	12	12	12	0										0									
2. MULTIPLE DX																														
A. Not Operated	1,297	4.8	32	1	2	3	6	11	14	26	248	5.5	43	1	2	4	6	12	15	38	585	4.7	26	1	2	3	6	10	14	26
B. Operated	180	16.3	176	3	6	12	23	37	41	65	45	16.2	158	4	6	14	21	38	40	54	32	10.5	29	5	7	10	13	17	21	25
1. SINGLE DX	64	2.0	4	1	1	1	2	4	5	12	5	1.6	<1	1	1	2	2	2	2	2	30	1.7	2	1	1	1	2	5	5	5
2. MULTIPLE DX	1,477	6.2	64	1	2	3	7	14	22	41	293	7.2	75	1	2	4	9	16	27	46	617	5.0	28	1	2	3	6	11	16	26
A. NOT OPERATED	1,359	4.6	31	1	2	3	5	10	14	26	253	5.5	42	1	2	3	6	12	15	38	615	4.6	25	1	2	3	5	10	14	26
B. OPERATED	182	16.2	174	3	6	12	23	37	41	65	45	16.2	158	4	6	14	21	38	40	54	32	10.5	29	5	7	10	13	17	21	25
TOTAL																														
0–19 Years	152	5.2	75	1	2	2	4	15	24	48	15	3.7	33	1	1	2	3	15	20	20	45	2.4	12	1	1	1	2	5	8	23
20–34	221	6.3	93	1	3	3	6	18	26	46	37	8.6	121	1	1	3	13	19	40	46	48	3.1	20	1	1	2	2	8	12	26
35–49	190	7.6	100	1	3	3	9	22	28	54	36	11.4	156	2	2	6	21	28	39	54	57	6.0	44	2	2	4	8	14	24	26
50–64	261	7.4	94	1	2	4	9	20	29	48	52	8.7	99	1	2	4	10	23	38	40	101	5.8	51	1	1	3	7	16	19	48
65+	717	5.2	26	1	2	4	6	11	14	24	158	5.5	34	1	2	4	7	12	15	21	396	5.0	20	1	2	4	6	10	13	24
GRAND TOTAL	1,541	6.0	62	1	2	3	7	14	21	40	298	7.1	74	1	2	4	9	16	27	46	647	4.9	27	1	2	3	6	11	15	26

Length of Stay by Diagnosis and Operation, Western Region, 2008

750

Western Region, October 2006–September 2007 Data, by Diagnosis

853.06: OTH TRAUM ICH-NEC

Type of Patients	Observed Patients	Avg. Stay	Variance	10th	25th	50th	75th	90th	95th	99th
1. SINGLE DX										
A. Not Operated										
0–19 Years	4	1.3	<1	1	1	1	1	2	2	2
20–34	5	2.6	3	1	1	3	3	5	5	5
35–49	0									
50–64	0									
65+	1	2.0	0	2	2	2	2	2	2	2
B. Operated										
0–19 Years	0									
20–34	0									
35–49	1	12.0	0	12	12	12	12	12	12	12
50–64	0									
65+	0									
2. MULTIPLE DX										
A. Not Operated										
0–19 Years	24	4.8	19	1	1	4	7	10	15	16
20–34	46	4.3	20	1	1	3	5	11	11	21
35–49	28	3.9	22	1	1	2	4	13	14	19
50–64	42	4.8	24	1	2	2	6	11	14	20
65+	62	5.4	51	1	2	4	6	11	14	51
B. Operated										
0–19 Years	13	16.3	245	2	3	15	24	36	50	50
20–34	12	16.8	190	3	3	10	26	38	38	38
35–49	14	20.6	306	6	7	10	37	46	59	59
50–64	11	21.9	149	6	10	20	35	38	41	41
65+	5	13.8	114	4	9	11	13	32	32	32
SUBTOTALS:										
1. SINGLE DX										
A. Not Operated	10	2.0	2	1	1	2	3	3	5	5
B. Operated	1	12.0	0	12	12	12	12	12	12	12
2. MULTIPLE DX										
A. Not Operated	202	4.7	30	1	2	3	6	11	14	21
B. Operated	55	18.4	210	3	6	17	30	38	46	59
1. SINGLE DX	11	2.9	11	1	1	2	3	5	5	12
2. MULTIPLE DX	257	7.7	99	1	2	4	9	20	34	50
A. NOT OPERATED	212	4.6	29	1	1	3	5	11	14	21
B. OPERATED	56	18.3	207	3	6	15	26	38	46	59
TOTAL										
0–19 Years	41	8.1	118	1	2	4	9	17	34	50
20–34	63	6.5	73	1	1	3	7	9	26	38
35–49	43	9.5	171	1	2	4	12	24	37	59
50–64	53	8.3	97	1	2	4	11	20	35	41
65+	68	6.0	58	1	2	4	7	12	16	51
GRAND TOTAL	268	7.5	97	1	2	4	9	20	32	50

854: OTHER IC INJURY

Type of Patients	Observed Patients	Avg. Stay	Variance	10th	25th	50th	75th	90th	95th	99th
1. SINGLE DX										
A. Not Operated										
0–19 Years	19	1.5	1	1	1	1	1	3	6	6
20–34	4	1.5	<1	1	1	1	1	3	3	3
35–49	5	2.0	5	1	1	1	1	6	6	6
50–64	2	1.0	0	1	1	1	1	1	1	1
65+	2	1.0	0	1	1	1	1	1	1	1
B. Operated										
0–19 Years	0									
20–34	0									
35–49	1	5.0	0	5	5	5	5	5	5	5
50–64	0									
65+	0									
2. MULTIPLE DX										
A. Not Operated										
0–19 Years	113	3.1	29	1	1	1	3	6	12	27
20–34	167	2.7	33	1	1	1	2	5	7	20
35–49	100	3.6	29	1	1	2	3	8	16	26
50–64	88	4.5	59	1	2	2	4	8	15	45
65+	73	5.5	31	1	2	4	6	13	19	25
B. Operated										
0–19 Years	18	12.6	102	3	5	8	19	29	37	37
20–34	27	18.7	453	2	4	10	24	56	68	78
35–49	20	15.6	398	3	5	8	13	34	47	86
50–64	9	24.1	698	3	5	12	33	75	75	75
65+	5	16.8	94	7	12	13	20	32	32	32
SUBTOTALS:										
1. SINGLE DX										
A. Not Operated	32	1.5	2	1	1	1	2	3	6	6
B. Operated	1	5.0	0	5	5	5	5	5	5	5
2. MULTIPLE DX										
A. Not Operated	541	3.6	36	1	1	2	3	7	13	30
B. Operated	79	17.0	359	3	5	10	22	47	68	86
1. SINGLE DX	33	1.6	2	1	1	1	3	3	6	6
2. MULTIPLE DX	620	5.3	97	1	1	2	5	12	22	56
A. NOT OPERATED	573	3.5	35	1	1	2	3	7	13	30
B. OPERATED	80	16.9	356	3	5	9	22	47	68	86
TOTAL										
0–19 Years	150	4.0	44	1	1	2	4	10	19	37
20–34	198	4.8	118	1	1	2	5	9	20	69
35–49	126	5.4	103	1	1	2	5	13	22	47
50–64	99	6.2	143	1	1	2	5	12	36	75
65+	80	6.1	42	1	2	4	7	15	20	32
GRAND TOTAL	653	5.1	93	1	1	2	5	11	21	56

860: TRAUM PNEUMOHEMOTHORAX

Type of Patients	Observed Patients	Avg. Stay	Variance	10th	25th	50th	75th	90th	95th	99th
1. SINGLE DX										
A. Not Operated										
0–19 Years	54	2.6	2	1	1	2	3	5	5	7
20–34	124	2.6	2	1	2	2	3	5	6	7
35–49	61	2.6	2	1	2	2	3	4	5	6
50–64	25	2.9	3	1	2	2	4	5	6	9
65+	2	3.5	<1	3	3	4	4	4	4	4
B. Operated										
0–19 Years	2	5.0	0	5	5	5	5	5	5	5
20–34	4	7.2	3	5	5	7	8	9	9	9
35–49	3	3.3	<1	3	3	3	4	4	4	4
50–64	1	8.0	0	8	8	8	8	8	8	8
65+	1	4.0	0	4	4	4	4	4	4	4
2. MULTIPLE DX										
A. Not Operated										
0–19 Years	475	3.6	8	1	2	3	5	7	9	14
20–34	1,043	4.2	19	1	2	3	5	8	10	18
35–49	1,087	4.4	13	1	2	4	5	8	11	17
50–64	1,193	5.1	27	1	2	4	6	9	12	28
65+	956	5.7	20	2	3	5	7	11	14	23
B. Operated										
0–19 Years	76	11.8	162	4	5	7	12	26	31	87
20–34	185	9.5	49	3	5	8	12	17	25	38
35–49	156	12.6	152	4	5	10	15	25	32	98
50–64	141	12.4	169	4	5	8	15	22	39	99
65+	77	15.2	255	3	7	10	20	29	59	>99
SUBTOTALS:										
1. SINGLE DX										
A. Not Operated	266	2.6	2	1	2	2	3	5	6	7
B. Operated	11	5.5	4	3	4	5	8	8	9	9
2. MULTIPLE DX										
A. Not Operated	4,754	4.7	19	1	2	4	6	9	11	22
B. Operated	635	11.9	141	4	5	8	14	24	31	87
1. SINGLE DX	277	2.8	3	1	2	2	4	5	6	8
2. MULTIPLE DX	5,389	5.6	39	1	2	4	7	11	15	29
A. NOT OPERATED	5,020	4.6	18	1	2	4	6	9	11	20
B. OPERATED	646	11.7	140	4	5	8	14	23	29	87
TOTAL										
0–19 Years	607	4.6	34	1	2	3	5	8	12	26
20–34	1,356	4.8	25	1	2	3	6	8	13	25
35–49	1,307	5.3	36	1	2	4	6	10	14	27
50–64	1,360	5.8	46	1	2	4	7	11	15	38
65+	1,036	6.4	43	2	3	5	8	12	17	31
GRAND TOTAL	5,666	5.4	37	1	2	4	6	10	14	28

Length of Stay by Diagnosis and Operation, Western Region, 2008

751

Western Region, October 2006–September 2007 Data, by Diagnosis

860.0: TRAUM PNEUMOTHORAX-CLSD

Type of Patients	Observed Patients	Avg. Stay	Variance	10th	25th	50th	75th	90th	95th	99th
1. SINGLE DX										
A. Not Operated										
0–19 Years	19	2.1	<1	1	1	2	2	4	4	4
20–34	42	2.2	1	1	1	2	3	3	4	6
35–49	34	2.5	2	1	2	2	3	3	5	5
50–64	18	2.5	2	1	2	2	4	4	5	5
65+	1	3.0	0	3	3	3	3	3	3	3
B. Operated										
0–19 Years	0									
20–34	0									
35–49	0									
50–64	0									
65+	0									
2. MULTIPLE DX										
A. Not Operated										
0–19 Years	262	3.1	6	1	1	2	4	6	8	11
20–34	460	3.5	9	1	2	3	4	7	9	14
35–49	615	3.8	7	1	2	3	5	7	8	12
50–64	724	4.4	24	1	2	3	5	8	10	23
65+	547	5.1	16	2	3	4	6	9	12	18
B. Operated										
0–19 Years	16	10.9	180	3	6	7	9	26	57	57
20–34	37	10.3	69	3	6	9	11	19	28	45
35–49	31	12.1	121	3	5	7	17	31	39	41
50–64	35	12.1	309	3	5	7	13	17	50	99
65+	15	10.5	67	3	3	8	18	21	29	29
SUBTOTALS:										
1. SINGLE DX										
A. Not Operated	114	2.3	1	1	2	2	3	4	5	6
B. Operated	0									
2. MULTIPLE DX										
A. Not Operated	2,608	4.1	14	1	2	3	5	8	10	16
B. Operated	134	11.3	153	3	5	8	12	26	31	57
1. SINGLE DX	114	2.3	1	1	2	2	3	4	5	6
2. MULTIPLE DX	2,742	4.5	23	1	2	3	5	8	11	22
A. NOT OPERATED	2,722	4.0	14	1	2	3	5	8	10	16
B. OPERATED	134	11.3	153	3	5	8	12	26	31	57
TOTAL										
0–19 Years	297	3.5	18	1	2	2	4	6	8	18
20–34	539	3.9	16	1	2	3	5	8	11	19
35–49	680	4.1	15	1	2	3	5	7	10	21
50–64	777	4.7	39	1	2	3	6	9	11	27
65+	563	5.2	18	2	3	4	6	10	13	21
GRAND TOTAL	2,856	4.4	23	1	2	3	5	8	11	21

860.1: TRAUM PNEUMOTHORAX-OPEN

Type of Patients	Observed Patients	Avg. Stay	Variance	10th	25th	50th	75th	90th	95th	99th
1. SINGLE DX										
A. Not Operated										
0–19 Years	16	2.5	2	1	2	2	3	3	5	5
20–34	35	2.5	2	1	1	2	3	4	5	6
35–49	10	2.7	1	2	2	3	3	5	5	5
50–64	4	3.5	4	2	2	4	6	6	6	6
65+	1	4.0	0	4	4	4	4	4	4	4
B. Operated										
0–19 Years	1	5.0	0	5	5	5	5	5	5	5
20–34	0									
35–49	2	3.5	<1	3	3	4	4	4	4	4
50–64	0									
65+	0									
2. MULTIPLE DX										
A. Not Operated										
0–19 Years	61	3.1	3	1	2	3	4	5	6	8
20–34	139	3.2	3	1	2	3	4	6	7	9
35–49	59	3.1	4	1	2	3	4	5	6	12
50–64	22	3.1	3	1	2	3	4	5	5	8
65+	1	3.0	0	3	3	3	3	3	3	3
B. Operated										
0–19 Years	6	3.8	4	2	2	4	5	7	7	7
20–34	15	6.8	40	1	2	5	8	20	22	22
35–49	9	4.9	5	2	4	4	6	9	9	9
50–64	2	11.5	83	5	5	12	18	18	18	18
65+	1	23.0	0	23	23	23	23	23	23	23
SUBTOTALS:										
1. SINGLE DX										
A. Not Operated	66	2.6	2	1	2	2	3	5	5	6
B. Operated	3	4.0	<1	3	3	4	5	5	5	5
2. MULTIPLE DX										
A. Not Operated	282	3.1	3	1	2	3	4	5	6	9
B. Operated	33	6.5	34	2	3	5	7	18	22	23
1. SINGLE DX	69	2.7	2	1	2	3	3	5	5	6
2. MULTIPLE DX	315	3.5	7	1	2	3	4	6	7	18
A. NOT OPERATED	348	3.0	3	1	2	3	4	5	6	16
B. OPERATED	36	6.3	32	2	3	4	7	18	22	23
TOTAL										
0–19 Years	84	3.1	3	1	2	3	4	5	6	8
20–34	189	3.3	7	1	2	3	4	6	7	20
35–49	80	3.3	4	1	2	3	4	6	7	12
50–64	28	3.8	11	1	2	3	4	6	8	18
65+	3	10.0	126	3	3	4	23	23	23	23
GRAND TOTAL	384	3.3	7	1	2	3	4	6	7	18

860.2: TRAUM HEMOTHORAX-CLOSED

Type of Patients	Observed Patients	Avg. Stay	Variance	10th	25th	50th	75th	90th	95th	99th
1. SINGLE DX										
A. Not Operated										
0–19 Years	0									
20–34	6	3.8	3	2	3	3	5	7	7	7
35–49	3	2.7	2	1	1	3	3	4	4	4
50–64	1	4.0	0	4	4	4	4	4	4	4
65+	0									
B. Operated										
0–19 Years	0									
20–34	0									
35–49	1	3.0	0	3	3	3	3	3	3	3
50–64	0									
65+	1	4.0	0	4	4	4	4	4	4	4
2. MULTIPLE DX										
A. Not Operated										
0–19 Years	7	4.7	10	1	2	5	8	9	9	9
20–34	39	3.8	8	1	2	3	5	8	10	13
35–49	80	5.3	32	2	2	4	6	9	14	46
50–64	111	6.1	56	1	2	4	7	10	17	41
65+	197	6.2	24	2	3	5	8	11	15	31
B. Operated										
0–19 Years	12	6.6	12	3	5	6	6	13	13	13
20–34	12	10.2	29	4	6	9	12	21	23	25
35–49	29	9.4	78	4	5	7	11	20	22	53
50–64	42	9.4	78	4	5	7	11	20	22	53
65+	38	13.1	208	4	7	9	14	29	87	>99
SUBTOTALS:										
1. SINGLE DX										
A. Not Operated	10	3.5	3	2	2	3	3	4	4	7
B. Operated	2	3.5	<1	3	3	4	4	4	4	4
2. MULTIPLE DX										
A. Not Operated	434	5.8	32	2	3	4	7	10	14	36
B. Operated	121	10.4	103	4	5	8	12	20	25	87
1. SINGLE DX	12	3.5	2	2	3	4	4	5	7	7
2. MULTIPLE DX	555	6.8	51	2	3	5	8	12	19	41
A. NOT OPERATED	444	5.7	32	2	3	4	7	10	13	36
B. OPERATED	123	10.3	102	4	5	8	12	20	25	87
TOTAL										
0–19 Years	7	4.7	10	1	2	5	8	9	9	9
20–34	57	4.4	9	2	2	4	6	8	13	13
35–49	113	6.4	35	2	3	5	8	12	14	25
50–64	154	7.0	63	2	3	5	7	12	21	45
65+	236	7.3	60	2	3	5	9	13	19	37
GRAND TOTAL	567	6.7	50	2	3	5	8	12	18	41

Length of Stay by Diagnosis and Operation, Western Region, 2008

Western Region, October 2006–September 2007 Data, by Diagnosis

860.4: TRAUM PNEUMOHEMOTHOR-CL

Type of Patients	Observed Patients	Avg. Stay	Vari-ance	10th	25th	50th	75th	90th	95th	99th
1. SINGLE DX										
A. Not Operated										
0–19 Years	3	3.3	2	2	2	3	5	5	5	5
20–34	3	2.7	4	1	1	2	5	5	5	5
35–49	4	1.8	<1	1	1	1	3	3	3	3
50–64	1	1.0	0	1	1	1	1	1	1	1
65+	0									
B. Operated										
0–19 Years	0									
20–34	1	5.0	0	5	5	5	5	5	5	5
35–49	0									
50–64	1	8.0	0	8	8	8	8	8	8	8
65+	0									
2. MULTIPLE DX										
A. Not Operated										
0–19 Years	52	5.4	13	2	3	5	6	9	14	22
20–34	159	5.6	17	2	3	4	7	10	14	26
35–49	253	6.0	19	2	3	5	7	10	14	23
50–64	306	6.2	19	2	3	5	8	11	15	22
65+	207	7.0	26	2	4	6	9	13	16	24
B. Operated										
0–19 Years	12	13.7	107	6	8	9	26	31	34	34
20–34	36	12.7	51	5	8	12	16	23	25	35
35–49	50	18.3	275	6	10	15	23	27	78	>99
50–64	49	14.2	113	5	7	12	18	24	28	67
65+	21	21.7	453	6	8	17	23	38	59	97
SUBTOTALS:										
1. SINGLE DX										
A. Not Operated	11	2.4	2	1	1	2	3	5	5	5
B. Operated	2	6.5	4	5	5	5	8	8	8	8
2. MULTIPLE DX										
A. Not Operated	977	6.2	20	2	3	5	8	11	15	24
B. Operated	168	16.0	195	5	8	13	20	27	38	98
1. SINGLE DX	13	3.0	5	1	1	2	5	5	8	8
2. MULTIPLE DX	1,145	7.6	58	2	4	6	9	15	21	34
A. NOT OPERATED	988	6.2	20	2	3	5	8	11	14	24
B. OPERATED	170	15.9	194	5	8	13	20	26	38	98
TOTAL										
0–19 Years	67	6.8	39	2	3	5	8	12	22	34
20–34	199	6.9	31	2	3	5	8	15	18	26
35–49	307	7.9	81	2	4	5	10	17	23	39
50–64	357	7.3	40	2	4	6	9	15	18	28
65+	228	8.4	82	2	4	6	10	17	22	38
GRAND TOTAL	1,158	7.6	57	2	4	6	9	15	21	34

860.5: TRAUM PNEUMOHEMOTHOR-OPN

Type of Patients	Observed Patients	Avg. Stay	Vari-ance	10th	25th	50th	75th	90th	95th	99th
1. SINGLE DX										
A. Not Operated										
0–19 Years	12	3.3	4	1	1	3	5	6	7	7
20–34	30	3.0	4	1	2	2	4	7	7	7
35–49	5	3.4	4	1	2	4	4	6	6	6
50–64	0									
65+	0									
B. Operated										
0–19 Years	1	5.0	0	5	5	5	5	5	5	5
20–34	1	8.0	0	8	8	8	8	8	8	8
35–49	0									
50–64	0									
65+	0									
2. MULTIPLE DX										
A. Not Operated										
0–19 Years	81	4.5	8	2	3	4	6	8	11	13
20–34	196	5.4	49	2	3	4	6	10	11	26
35–49	60	5.6	14	2	4	4	6	10	11	23
50–64	28	6.5	45	2	3	5	8	10	11	38
65+	3	8.3	4	6	6	9	10	10	10	10
B. Operated										
0–19 Years	36	13.5	216	4	5	8	17	25	29	87
20–34	71	8.8	46	3	5	7	11	16	25	38
35–49	22	8.4	24	4	5	7	10	14	17	23
50–64	9	13.7	191	5	7	11	16	>99	>99	>99
65+	0									
SUBTOTALS:										
1. SINGLE DX										
A. Not Operated	47	3.1	4	1	1	3	5	6	7	7
B. Operated	2	6.5	4	5	5	8	8	8	8	8
2. MULTIPLE DX										
A. Not Operated	368	5.4	34	2	3	4	6	10	11	23
B. Operated	138	10.3	99	4	5	7	12	21	27	87
1. SINGLE DX	49	3.3	4	1	2	3	5	7	7	8
2. MULTIPLE DX	506	6.7	56	2	3	5	8	12	17	38
A. NOT OPERATED	415	5.1	31	2	3	4	6	9	11	23
B. OPERATED	140	10.2	97	4	5	7	12	20	25	87
TOTAL										
0–19 Years	130	6.9	81	2	3	5	7	13	21	29
20–34	298	6.0	46	2	3	4	7	11	16	35
35–49	87	6.1	18	2	4	5	8	11	14	23
50–64	37	8.3	86	2	4	6	9	16	49	>99
65+	3	8.3	4	6	6	9	10	10	10	10
GRAND TOTAL	555	6.4	52	2	3	5	7	11	17	38

861: HEART & LUNG INJURY

Type of Patients	Observed Patients	Avg. Stay	Vari-ance	10th	25th	50th	75th	90th	95th	99th
1. SINGLE DX										
A. Not Operated										
0–19 Years	13	1.5	<1	1	1	1	2	3	3	3
20–34	12	1.2	<1	1	1	1	2	2	2	2
35–49	6	1.3	<1	1	1	1	2	2	2	2
50–64	1	10.0	0	10	10	10	10	10	10	10
65+	0									
B. Operated										
0–19 Years	1	6.0	0	6	6	6	6	6	6	6
20–34	3	2.0	<1	1	1	2	3	3	3	3
35–49	1	2.0	0	2	2	2	2	2	2	2
50–64	0									
65+	0									
2. MULTIPLE DX										
A. Not Operated										
0–19 Years	188	2.8	6	1	2	2	3	5	8	13
20–34	314	3.1	18	1	2	2	4	6	9	14
35–49	200	3.8	18	1	2	2	4	8	12	25
50–64	167	4.1	21	1	3	3	5	9	13	26
65+	169	5.4	73	1	2	4	6	10	18	24
B. Operated										
0–19 Years	52	10.9	163	3	5	8	11	16	39	83
20–34	144	10.6	72	4	6	8	13	20	27	47
35–49	63	14.0	119	4	7	11	18	30	35	60
50–64	41	14.6	131	5	7	11	18	26	33	52
65+	18	16.4	63	5	9	18	21	32	>99	>99
SUBTOTALS:										
1. SINGLE DX										
A. Not Operated	32	1.6	3	1	1	1	2	2	3	10
B. Operated	5	2.8	4	1	2	2	3	6	6	6
2. MULTIPLE DX										
A. Not Operated	1,038	3.7	26	1	2	2	4	7	11	23
B. Operated	318	12.2	106	4	6	9	15	24	33	52
1. SINGLE DX	37	1.8	3	1	1	1	2	2	6	10
2. MULTIPLE DX	1,356	5.7	57	2	3	3	7	13	19	39
A. NOT OPERATED	1,070	3.6	25	1	2	2	4	7	11	23
B. OPERATED	323	12.0	105	4	6	9	15	24	33	52
TOTAL										
0–19 Years	254	4.4	49	1	2	2	5	9	12	39
20–34	473	5.3	46	1	3	3	6	11	17	37
35–49	270	6.2	60	1	2	3	7	15	23	40
50–64	209	6.2	59	1	2	3	7	14	21	37
65+	187	6.5	83	1	2	4	7	18	21	99
GRAND TOTAL	1,393	5.6	56	1	2	3	7	13	19	39

753

Length of Stay by Diagnosis and Operation, Western Region, 2008

Western Region, October 2006–September 2007 Data, by Diagnosis

861.21: LUNG CONTUSION-CLOSED

Type of Patients	Observed Patients	Avg. Stay	Variance	10th	25th	50th	75th	90th	95th	99th
1. SINGLE DX										
A. Not Operated										
0–19 Years	9	1.5	<1	1	1	1	2	3	3	3
20–34	7	1.3	<1	1	1	1	2	2	2	2
35–49	4	1.3	<1	1	1	1	1	2	2	2
50–64	1	10.0	0	10	10	10	10	10	10	10
65+	0									
B. Operated										
0–19 Years	0									
20–34	0									
35–49	1	2.0	0	2	2	2	2	2	2	2
50–64	0									
65+	0									
2. MULTIPLE DX										
A. Not Operated										
0–19 Years	157	2.7	5	1	1	2	3	5	8	13
20–34	238	2.5	5	1	1	2	3	5	6	10
35–49	159	3.7	17	1	1	2	4	8	12	31
50–64	123	4.3	25	1	1	2	6	9	13	26
65+	106	5.2	22	2	2	4	6	11	16	23
B. Operated										
0–19 Years	9	8.8	30	2	2	11	12	16	16	16
20–34	28	10.2	97	3	4	7	15	21	37	41
35–49	19	16.6	153	1	6	17	24	36	40	40
50–64	14	17.3	176	4	8	15	24	33	52	52
65+	13	13.5	42	5	9	17	19	20	21	21
SUBTOTALS:										
1. SINGLE DX										
A. Not Operated	21	1.8	4	1	1	1	2	2	3	10
B. Operated	1	2.0	0	2	2	2	2	2	2	2
2. MULTIPLE DX										
A. Not Operated	783	3.4	14	1	1	2	4	7	10	23
B. Operated	83	13.2	113	2	5	11	19	26	36	52
1. SINGLE DX	22	1.8	4	1	1	1	2	2	3	10
2. MULTIPLE DX	866	4.4	32	1	1	2	5	10	15	33
A. NOT OPERATED	804	3.4	14	1	1	2	4	7	10	22
B. OPERATED	84	13.1	114	2	5	11	18	26	36	52
TOTAL										
0–19 Years	175	2.9	8	1	1	2	3	6	10	14
20–34	273	3.2	20	1	1	2	4	6	9	23
35–49	183	5.0	46	1	1	2	5	12	21	40
50–64	138	5.7	54	1	2	3	7	13	19	37
65+	119	6.1	31	1	2	4	8	17	19	23
GRAND TOTAL	888	4.3	31	1	1	2	5	10	15	33

862: INTRATHORACIC INJURY NEC

Type of Patients	Observed Patients	Avg. Stay	Variance	10th	25th	50th	75th	90th	95th	99th
1. SINGLE DX										
A. Not Operated										
0–19 Years	3	1.7	<1	1	1	2	2	2	2	2
20–34	4	1.7	2	1	1	1	2	4	4	4
35–49	3	1.3	<1	1	1	1	2	2	2	2
50–64	2	2.0	0	2	2	2	2	2	2	2
65+	1	1.0	0	1	1	1	1	1	1	1
B. Operated										
0–19 Years	1	8.0	0	8	8	8	8	8	8	8
20–34	1	4.0	0	4	4	4	4	4	4	4
35–49	1	1.0	0	1	1	1	1	1	1	1
50–64	0									
65+	0									
2. MULTIPLE DX										
A. Not Operated										
0–19 Years	21	4.6	12	1	2	4	5	8	13	14
20–34	43	3.5	8	1	1	3	5	8	9	10
35–49	27	4.6	21	1	1	3	6	11	12	20
50–64	42	3.4	9	1	1	2	4	7	8	14
65+	52	6.3	45	2	3	4	7	11	21	39
B. Operated										
0–19 Years	54	8.8	37	2	4	7	13	17	19	30
20–34	127	10.6	107	3	5	7	12	26	35	58
35–49	55	10.2	92	3	5	7	12	18	30	61
50–64	42	15.2	187	5	7	11	18	27	38	74
65+	10	11.3	73	4	5	10	14	32	32	32
SUBTOTALS:										
1. SINGLE DX										
A. Not Operated	13	1.6	<1	1	1	2	2	2	4	4
B. Operated	3	4.3	12	1	1	4	8	8	8	8
2. MULTIPLE DX										
A. Not Operated	185	4.6	22	1	2	3	6	9	12	23
B. Operated	288	10.9	104	3	5	8	13	23	31	61
1. SINGLE DX	16	2.1	3	1	1	1	2	4	8	8
2. MULTIPLE DX	473	8.4	81	2	3	6	10	18	26	54
A. NOT OPERATED	198	4.4	21	1	2	3	5	9	12	23
B. OPERATED	291	10.8	103	3	5	8	13	23	31	61
TOTAL										
0–19 Years	79	7.4	33	2	3	6	11	16	19	30
20–34	175	8.6	90	1	3	6	10	20	31	58
35–49	86	8.0	74	1	3	6	11	16	20	61
50–64	86	9.1	130	2	5	5	11	23	27	74
65+	63	7.0	52	2	3	4	8	14	21	39
GRAND TOTAL	489	8.2	80	3	3	5	10	18	26	54

863: GI TRACT INJURY

Type of Patients	Observed Patients	Avg. Stay	Variance	10th	25th	50th	75th	90th	95th	99th
1. SINGLE DX										
A. Not Operated										
0–19 Years	16	3.5	38	1	1	2	3	6	26	26
20–34	5	2.0	2	1	1	2	2	4	4	4
35–49	6	1.8	<1	1	1	2	2	3	3	3
50–64	1	1.0	0	1	1	1	1	1	1	1
65+	0									
B. Operated										
0–19 Years	20	4.9	7	2	3	5	6	9	12	12
20–34	26	4.8	4	3	3	4	6	8	8	10
35–49	15	4.6	5	2	3	4	6	8	9	9
50–64	6	5.4	3	3	5	5	6	8	8	8
65+	1	4.0	0	4	4	4	4	4	4	4
2. MULTIPLE DX										
A. Not Operated										
0–19 Years	34	4.5	19	1	2	2	6	12	16	16
20–34	47	3.2	7	1	2	2	4	6	7	16
35–49	32	3.8	10	1	2	3	4	9	10	14
50–64	31	3.1	5	1	1	3	3	6	7	10
65+	32	4.1	25	2	2	3	4	7	15	27
B. Operated										
0–19 Years	296	10.1	100	4	5	7	11	19	30	57
20–34	748	9.8	97	3	5	7	10	18	28	54
35–49	381	10.3	89	3	5	7	11	22	30	59
50–64	153	11.9	106	5	6	9	15	21	29	62
65+	49	17.1	316	5	7	10	21	42	65	76
SUBTOTALS:										
1. SINGLE DX										
A. Not Operated	28	2.8	22	1	1	2	3	4	6	26
B. Operated	68	4.8	5	2	3	4	6	8	9	12
2. MULTIPLE DX										
A. Not Operated	176	3.7	13	1	2	3	4	7	10	16
B. Operated	1,627	10.4	104	4	5	7	11	20	29	61
1. SINGLE DX	96	4.2	10	1	2	4	5	7	9	26
2. MULTIPLE DX	1,803	9.7	99	3	5	7	11	20	28	57
A. NOT OPERATED	204	3.6	14	1	2	2	4	7	10	16
B. OPERATED	1,695	10.1	102	4	5	7	11	20	29	61
TOTAL										
0–19 Years	366	9.0	90	2	4	6	10	17	26	56
20–34	826	9.2	91	3	5	6	10	17	27	54
35–49	434	9.5	83	3	4	7	10	21	30	51
50–64	191	10.2	97	3	5	7	13	20	25	62
65+	82	11.9	238	2	3	7	14	25	42	76
GRAND TOTAL	1,899	9.4	96	3	4	7	10	19	28	57

Length of Stay by Diagnosis and Operation, Western Region, 2008

864: LIVER INJURY

Type of Patients	Observed Patients	Avg. Stay	Variance	10th	25th	50th	75th	90th	95th	99th
1. SINGLE DX										
A. Not Operated										
0–19 Years	55	2.2	1	1	1	2	3	4	4	5
20–34	28	2.3	2	1	1	2	3	5	5	5
35–49	9	2.0	1	1	1	2	3	4	4	4
50–64	10	1.3	<1	1	1	1	2	2	2	2
65+	0									
B. Operated										
0–19 Years	4	2.0	<1	1	2	2	3	3	3	3
20–34	10	3.0	2	1	2	3	4	5	5	5
35–49	1	2.0	0	2	2	2	2	2	2	2
50–64	0									
65+	0									
2. MULTIPLE DX										
A. Not Operated										
0–19 Years	278	3.5	10	1	2	3	4	7	9	17
20–34	344	3.5	9	1	2	3	4	6	9	16
35–49	176	3.7	11	1	2	3	5	7	9	19
50–64	111	4.5	21	1	2	3	5	8	11	23
65+	62	5.5	17	2	3	4	7	10	13	21
B. Operated										
0–19 Years	125	9.8	76	3	5	7	13	20	25	41
20–34	228	12.6	222	3	4	7	16	30	53	99
35–49	117	13.4	233	3	4	7	15	36	48	72
50–64	46	11.0	80	3	4	8	14	28	28	39
65+	16	14.5	118	5	8	13	20	22	49	49
SUBTOTALS:										
1. SINGLE DX										
A. Not Operated	102	2.1	1	1	1	2	3	4	4	5
B. Operated	15	2.7	2	1	2	3	3	5	5	5
2. MULTIPLE DX										
A. Not Operated	971	3.8	12	1	2	3	5	7	9	21
B. Operated	532	12.0	176	3	4	7	15	28	39	72
1. SINGLE DX	117	2.2	1	1	1	2	3	4	5	5
2. MULTIPLE DX	1,503	6.7	85	1	2	4	7	15	23	53
A. NOT OPERATED	1,073	3.6	11	1	2	3	4	7	9	19
B. OPERATED	547	11.8	173	3	4	7	14	27	39	72
TOTAL										
0–19 Years	462	5.0	35	1	2	3	6	11	16	35
20–34	610	6.8	108	1	2	4	7	16	26	64
35–49	303	7.4	118	1	2	4	7	17	27	53
50–64	167	6.1	45	1	2	4	7	14	23	31
65+	78	7.4	50	2	3	5	8	14	21	49
GRAND TOTAL	1,620	6.4	80	1	2	4	7	14	22	50

864.05: LIVER LAC NOS-CLOSED

Type of Patients	Observed Patients	Avg. Stay	Variance	10th	25th	50th	75th	90th	95th	99th
1. SINGLE DX										
A. Not Operated										
0–19 Years	16	2.3	<1	1	2	2	3	4	4	4
20–34	9	2.7	2	1	2	3	3	5	5	5
35–49	3	1.7	1	1	1	1	3	3	3	3
50–64	2	1.5	<1	1	1	1	2	2	2	2
65+	0									
B. Operated										
0–19 Years	0									
20–34	0									
35–49	0									
50–64	0									
65+	0									
2. MULTIPLE DX										
A. Not Operated										
0–19 Years	71	4.1	16	2	2	3	4	7	11	30
20–34	100	3.6	8	1	2	3	4	6	8	22
35–49	48	3.9	7	1	2	3	5	8	9	12
50–64	30	4.5	30	1	2	3	5	5	19	28
65+	20	5.0	12	2	2	4	7	13	13	13
B. Operated										
0–19 Years	15	10.1	74	4	5	7	9	25	31	31
20–34	21	21.7	850	4	4	7	18	57	95	99
35–49	13	13.1	97	4	5	12	13	27	37	37
50–64	6	11.5	61	6	6	8	17	25	25	25
65+	5	22.2	253	8	13	20	21	49	49	49
SUBTOTALS:										
1. SINGLE DX										
A. Not Operated	30	2.3	1	1	1	2	3	4	4	5
B. Operated	0									
2. MULTIPLE DX										
A. Not Operated	269	4.0	13	1	2	3	5	7	10	22
B. Operated	60	15.9	375	4	5	8	20	37	53	99
1. SINGLE DX	30	2.3	1	1	1	2	3	4	4	5
2. MULTIPLE DX	329	6.2	99	2	2	4	6	12	20	53
A. NOT OPERATED	299	3.8	12	1	2	3	4	7	10	22
B. OPERATED	60	15.9	375	4	5	8	20	37	53	99
TOTAL										
0–19 Years	102	4.7	27	1	2	3	5	8	12	30
20–34	130	6.5	182	1	2	4	7	16	18	95
35–49	64	5.7	38	1	2	4	7	12	13	37
50–64	38	5.5	39	1	2	4	5	17	25	28
65+	25	8.5	101	2	3	5	8	20	21	49
GRAND TOTAL	359	5.8	92	1	2	3	5	11	20	53

865: SPLEEN INJURY

Type of Patients	Observed Patients	Avg. Stay	Variance	10th	25th	50th	75th	90th	95th	99th
1. SINGLE DX										
A. Not Operated										
0–19 Years	147	2.9	2	1	2	3	4	5	5	7
20–34	55	2.7	2	1	2	2	3	4	6	7
35–49	16	2.7	1	2	2	3	3	4	5	5
50–64	4	3.8	<1	3	3	4	5	5	5	5
65+	1	5.0	0	5	5	5	5	5	5	5
B. Operated										
0–19 Years	10	4.2	<1	3	4	4	5	5	6	6
20–34	9	4.2	1	3	3	4	5	6	6	6
35–49	7	5.9	3	3	5	6	7	8	8	8
50–64	1	6.0	0	6	6	6	6	6	6	6
65+	1	5.0	0	5	5	5	5	5	5	5
2. MULTIPLE DX										
A. Not Operated										
0–19 Years	401	3.6	4	1	2	3	5	6	7	11
20–34	364	3.9	13	1	2	3	5	6	8	19
35–49	245	3.9	6	1	2	3	5	7	8	12
50–64	198	4.8	20	2	2	4	6	9	11	29
65+	93	5.4	30	2	3	4	6	9	14	48
B. Operated										
0–19 Years	173	7.8	63	3	4	5	8	15	20	40
20–34	294	9.2	106	3	4	6	10	18	27	70
35–49	223	11.7	185	4	5	7	12	21	37	79
50–64	189	14.2	230	4	5	9	18	36	59	>99
65+	90	13.0	111	5	7	10	15	23	32	72
SUBTOTALS:										
1. SINGLE DX										
A. Not Operated	223	2.8	2	1	2	3	4	5	5	7
B. Operated	28	4.7	2	3	4	5	6	7	7	8
2. MULTIPLE DX										
A. Not Operated	1,301	4.0	12	1	2	3	5	7	9	17
B. Operated	969	10.9	146	4	5	7	12	22	35	79
1. SINGLE DX	251	3.0	2	1	2	3	4	5	6	7
2. MULTIPLE DX	2,270	7.0	80	2	3	5	7	13	21	59
A. NOT OPERATED	1,524	3.9	10	1	2	3	5	6	8	15
B. OPERATED	997	10.7	143	4	5	7	11	22	34	76
TOTAL										
0–19 Years	731	4.5	21	2	2	4	5	7	10	21
20–34	722	6.0	57	2	3	4	6	10	17	35
35–49	491	7.4	102	2	3	5	8	14	20	67
50–64	392	9.3	143	2	3	5	10	23	36	>99
65+	185	9.1	84	3	4	7	11	16	24	48
GRAND TOTAL	2,521	6.6	74	2	3	4	7	12	20	48

Length of Stay by Diagnosis and Operation, Western Region, 2008

Western Region, October 2006–September 2007 Data, by Diagnosis

865.00: SPLEEN INJURY NOS-CLOSED

Type of Patients	Observed Patients	Avg. Stay	Vari-ance	10th	25th	50th	75th	90th	95th	99th
1. SINGLE DX										
A. Not Operated										
0–19 Years	26	2.5	2	1	2	2	3	4	5	6
20–34	14	2.2	1	1	1	2	3	3	4	4
35–49	3	3.0	<1	2	2	3	4	4	4	4
50–64	1	4.0	0	4	4	4	4	4	4	4
65+	0									
B. Operated										
0–19 Years	1	4.0	0	4	4	4	4	4	4	4
20–34	1	3.0	0	3	3	3	3	3	3	3
35–49	1	3.0	0	3	3	3	3	3	3	3
50–64	0									
65+	0									
2. MULTIPLE DX										
A. Not Operated										
0–19 Years	86	3.0	4	1	2	2	4	5	6	12
20–34	81	4.1	33	1	2	3	4	6	7	41
35–49	55	3.2	3	1	2	3	4	6	8	9
50–64	51	4.0	12	2	2	3	5	6	8	24
65+	19	4.4	8	1	2	4	6	8	12	12
B. Operated										
0–19 Years	18	6.8	8	5	5	6	8	10	15	15
20–34	22	15.4	267	3	5	8	18	40	45	67
35–49	23	12.2	257	3	4	6	17	20	25	79
50–64	15	6.9	9	4	6	7	9	13	>99	>99
65+	6	11.8	53	3	5	11	18	22	22	22
SUBTOTALS:										
1. SINGLE DX										
A. Not Operated	44	2.5	1	1	2	2	3	4	4	6
B. Operated	3	3.3	<1	3	3	3	4	4	4	4
2. MULTIPLE DX										
A. Not Operated	292	3.6	13	1	2	3	4	6	7	24
B. Operated	84	10.9	154	3	5	7	12	22	40	>99
1. SINGLE DX	47	2.5	1	1	2	2	3	4	4	6
2. MULTIPLE DX	376	5.3	54	1	2	3	6	9	16	45
A. NOT OPERATED	336	3.5	12	1	2	3	4	6	7	12
B. OPERATED	87	10.7	151	3	5	7	12	22	40	>99
TOTAL										
0–19 Years	131	3.4	6	1	2	3	5	6	7	12
20–34	118	6.0	91	1	2	3	6	10	11	45
35–49	82	5.7	88	1	2	3	5	10	12	79
50–64	67	4.7	12	2	2	4	6	9	12	>99
65+	25	6.2	27	2	3	4	7	12	18	22
GRAND TOTAL	423	4.9	49	1	2	3	5	9	14	41

865.02: SPLEEN CAPS TEAR-CLOSED

Type of Patients	Observed Patients	Avg. Stay	Vari-ance	10th	25th	50th	75th	90th	95th	99th
1. SINGLE DX										
A. Not Operated										
0–19 Years	17	2.7	1	1	2	3	4	4	5	5
20–34	6	2.2	1	1	1	2	3	4	4	4
35–49	2	2.0	0	2	2	2	2	2	2	2
50–64	0									
65+	0									
B. Operated										
0–19 Years	0									
20–34	1	4.0	0	4	4	4	4	4	4	4
35–49	1	5.0	0	5	5	5	5	5	5	5
50–64	0									
65+	0									
2. MULTIPLE DX										
A. Not Operated										
0–19 Years	53	3.5	3	2	2	3	4	5	7	11
20–34	54	3.6	4	1	2	3	4	6	8	11
35–49	20	3.9	7	1	2	3	5	7	12	12
50–64	35	4.4	9	2	2	3	5	9	12	14
65+	12	4.3	7	1	2	4	5	8	9	9
B. Operated										
0–19 Years	10	5.8	19	1	4	5	8	10	16	16
20–34	11	10.8	92	5	5	6	17	20	35	35
35–49	13	11.8	520	3	4	4	12	87	87	87
50–64	17	14.5	90	4	7	12	18	27	36	36
65+	9	17.9	420	6	11	11	13	72	72	72
SUBTOTALS:										
1. SINGLE DX										
A. Not Operated	25	2.5	1	1	2	3	3	4	4	5
B. Operated	2	4.5	<1	4	4	5	5	5	5	5
2. MULTIPLE DX										
A. Not Operated	174	3.8	6	2	2	3	5	7	8	12
B. Operated	60	12.3	220	4	5	7	13	26	36	87
1. SINGLE DX	27	2.7	2	1	2	2	4	4	5	5
2. MULTIPLE DX	234	6.0	73	2	3	4	6	11	16	36
A. NOT OPERATED	199	3.7	5	1	2	3	5	7	8	12
B. OPERATED	62	12.0	215	4	5	6	13	26	35	87
TOTAL										
0–19 Years	80	3.6	6	1	2	3	5	6	7	16
20–34	72	4.6	23	1	2	3	5	8	11	35
35–49	36	6.7	197	2	2	4	6	12	12	87
50–64	52	7.7	57	2	3	4	6	9	16	36
65+	21	10.1	220	4	4	7	11	13	16	72
GRAND TOTAL	261	5.7	67	2	2	4	6	9	14	36

865.03: SPLEEN PARENCHYMA LAC-CL

Type of Patients	Observed Patients	Avg. Stay	Vari-ance	10th	25th	50th	75th	90th	95th	99th
1. SINGLE DX										
A. Not Operated										
0–19 Years	48	3.3	3	1	2	3	4	5	6	8
20–34	9	2.5	<1	2	2	2	3	3	3	3
35–49	5	2.0	<1	1	2	2	2	3	3	3
50–64	1	3.0	0	3	3	3	3	3	3	3
65+	0									
B. Operated										
0–19 Years	3	4.3	<1	4	4	4	5	5	5	5
20–34	3	4.3	2	3	3	4	6	6	6	6
35–49	1	8.0	0	8	8	8	8	8	8	8
50–64	1	6.0	0	6	6	6	6	6	6	6
65+	1	5.0	0	5	5	5	5	5	5	5
2. MULTIPLE DX										
A. Not Operated										
0–19 Years	106	4.1	7	2	3	4	5	6	7	17
20–34	96	4.5	11	2	3	4	6	7	9	26
35–49	64	4.2	9	1	3	4	5	7	9	20
50–64	33	4.9	12	2	3	4	6	11	11	17
65+	23	7.7	92	2	3	5	8	15	17	48
B. Operated										
0–19 Years	34	7.9	52	3	4	5	9	14	22	40
20–34	64	9.1	56	4	6	6	10	22	27	35
35–49	54	16.1	291	5	7	10	17	35	67	82
50–64	28	14.3	186	3	6	10	18	35	38	60
65+	12	12.5	45	5	6	12	15	24	24	24
SUBTOTALS:										
1. SINGLE DX										
A. Not Operated	63	3.1	2	1	2	3	4	5	6	8
B. Operated	9	5.0	2	3	4	5	6	8	8	8
2. MULTIPLE DX										
A. Not Operated	322	4.6	16	2	3	4	5	7	10	19
B. Operated	192	11.8	148	4	5	7	14	24	35	74
1. SINGLE DX	72	3.3	3	1	2	3	4	5	6	8
2. MULTIPLE DX	514	7.3	77	2	3	5	7	15	22	46
A. NOT OPERATED	385	4.3	14	2	2	4	5	7	9	19
B. OPERATED	201	11.5	144	4	5	7	13	24	35	67
TOTAL										
0–19 Years	191	4.6	16	2	3	4	5	7	11	22
20–34	172	6.1	32	2	3	4	6	10	21	29
35–49	124	9.3	166	2	3	5	9	19	29	74
50–64	63	9.0	109	2	3	6	11	18	33	60
65+	36	9.2	78	3	4	6	12	17	24	48
GRAND TOTAL	586	6.8	70	2	3	4	7	14	20	46

865.04: SPLEEN DISRUPTION-CLSD

Type of Patients	Observed Patients	Avg. Stay	Variance	Percentiles 10th	25th	50th	75th	90th	95th	99th
1. SINGLE DX										
A. Not Operated										
0–19 Years	17	3.1	2	1	2	3	4	5	6	6
20–34	4	4.0	3	2	2	3	6	6	6	6
35–49	3	3.3	2	2	2	3	5	5	5	5
50–64	1	3.0	0	3	3	3	3	3	3	3
65+	0									
B. Operated										
0–19 Years	1	3.0	0	3	3	3	3	3	3	3
20–34	1	5.0	0	5	5	5	5	5	5	5
35–49	2	5.5	<1	5	5	6	6	6	6	6
50–64	0									
65+	0									
2. MULTIPLE DX										
A. Not Operated										
0–19 Years	23	3.9	3	2	3	3	5	6	6	9
20–34	19	4.3	5	2	2	4	6	8	8	8
35–49	14	5.1	7	2	3	5	7	8	10	10
50–64	11	5.0	14	1	3	5	6	6	15	15
65+	6	6.8	24	3	3	7	10	15	15	15
B. Operated										
0–19 Years	57	7.2	23	3	4	5	8	15	17	26
20–34	80	7.3	15	4	5	6	9	11	13	28
35–49	66	10.1	102	4	5	7	10	17	35	59
50–64	73	15.9	358	4	6	8	20	42	86	>99
65+	40	12.1	92	4	7	9	14	18	32	46
SUBTOTALS:										
1. SINGLE DX										
A. Not Operated	25	3.3	2	2	2	3	4	5	6	6
B. Operated	4	4.8	2	3	3	5	6	6	6	6
2. MULTIPLE DX										
A. Not Operated	73	4.6	8	2	3	4	6	8	10	15
B. Operated	316	10.4	134	4	5	7	10	20	37	86
1. SINGLE DX	29	3.5	2	2	2	3	5	6	6	6
2. MULTIPLE DX	389	9.3	115	3	4	6	10	17	32	86
A. NOT OPERATED	98	4.3	7	2	3	4	5	7	9	15
B. OPERATED	320	10.4	132	4	5	7	10	19	35	86
TOTAL										
0–19 Years	98	5.7	18	2	3	5	6	13	17	26
20–34	104	6.6	14	3	4	6	8	10	13	19
35–49	85	8.9	85	3	5	6	9	15	31	59
50–64	85	14.3	324	4	5	7	15	39	76	>99
65+	46	11.4	85	3	7	9	14	18	32	46
GRAND TOTAL	418	8.9	109	3	4	6	9	16	31	76

865.09: SPLEEN INJURY NEC-CLOSED

Type of Patients	Observed Patients	Avg. Stay	Variance	Percentiles 10th	25th	50th	75th	90th	95th	99th
1. SINGLE DX										
A. Not Operated										
0–19 Years	26	2.9	1	2	2	3	4	4	5	6
20–34	14	3.1	3	2	2	2	4	6	7	7
35–49	1	3.0	0	3	3	3	3	3	3	3
50–64	1	5.0	0	5	5	5	5	5	5	5
65+	0									
B. Operated										
0–19 Years	2	5.5	<1	5	5	5	5	6	6	6
20–34	0									
35–49	0									
50–64	0									
65+	0									
2. MULTIPLE DX										
A. Not Operated										
0–19 Years	77	3.6	3	2	2	3	4	7	7	9
20–34	63	3.4	5	1	2	3	4	6	8	13
35–49	49	3.8	7	1	2	3	5	8	10	12
50–64	33	5.3	36	1	2	4	6	9	10	35
65+	15	5.1	12	3	3	5	6	10	14	14
B. Operated										
0–19 Years	25	6.4	17	3	4	6	7	10	14	21
20–34	44	7.4	38	2	4	6	8	17	21	30
35–49	27	11.0	172	3	4	8	10	20	40	65
50–64	25	16.1	206	4	7	14	23	57	58	>99
65+	10	13.4	80	3	7	10	19	23	32	32
SUBTOTALS:										
1. SINGLE DX										
A. Not Operated	42	3.0	2	2	2	3	4	5	6	7
B. Operated	2	5.5	<1	5	5	5	6	6	6	6
2. MULTIPLE DX										
A. Not Operated	237	3.9	10	1	2	3	5	7	9	13
B. Operated	131	10.0	107	3	4	7	11	22	30	65
1. SINGLE DX	44	3.1	2	2	2	3	4	5	6	7
2. MULTIPLE DX	368	6.1	53	2	3	4	7	11	20	57
A. NOT OPERATED	279	3.8	9	1	2	3	5	7	8	13
B. OPERATED	133	10.0	105	3	4	7	10	22	30	65
TOTAL										
0–19 Years	130	4.0	7	2	2	3	5	7	8	14
20–34	121	4.8	20	1	2	4	6	8	13	25
35–49	77	6.3	75	1	3	4	7	11	15	65
50–64	59	9.9	134	1	4	6	10	24	57	>99
65+	25	8.4	54	1	4	5	10	19	23	32
GRAND TOTAL	412	5.8	48	2	2	4	7	10	18	40

866: KIDNEY INJURY

Type of Patients	Observed Patients	Avg. Stay	Variance	Percentiles 10th	25th	50th	75th	90th	95th	99th
1. SINGLE DX										
A. Not Operated										
0–19 Years	33	2.2	2	1	1	2	3	4	5	6
20–34	18	1.8	<1	1	1	2	2	3	4	4
35–49	6	1.7	1	1	1	1	3	3	3	3
50–64	4	2.0	<1	1	1	2	2	3	3	3
65+	0									
B. Operated										
0–19 Years	0									
20–34	3	5.0	<1	4	4	5	6	6	6	6
35–49	0									
50–64	0									
65+	0									
2. MULTIPLE DX										
A. Not Operated										
0–19 Years	136	3.1	6	1	1	2	4	6	9	10
20–34	171	2.9	4	1	1	2	4	6	7	9
35–49	86	3.7	14	1	2	3	4	7	9	28
50–64	85	3.3	4	1	2	3	5	6	7	8
65+	62	4.1	6	1	3	4	5	7	8	13
B. Operated										
0–19 Years	44	9.7	63	3	6	8	12	15	25	43
20–34	65	13.1	122	5	6	7	17	31	38	49
35–49	27	11.5	106	5	6	7	11	29	35	43
50–64	14	15.2	333	5	6	12	15	22	75	75
65+	6	15.4	313	4	5	9	15	51	51	51
SUBTOTALS:										
1. SINGLE DX										
A. Not Operated	61	2.0	2	1	1	2	3	3	4	6
B. Operated	3	5.0	<1	4	4	5	6	6	6	6
2. MULTIPLE DX										
A. Not Operated	540	3.3	7	1	2	3	4	6	8	11
B. Operated	156	12.1	127	4	6	8	14	27	38	51
1. SINGLE DX	64	2.1	2	1	1	2	3	4	5	6
2. MULTIPLE DX	696	5.3	47	1	2	3	6	10	15	40
A. NOT OPERATED	601	3.1	6	1	1	3	4	6	8	11
B. OPERATED	159	12.0	126	4	5	7	14	27	38	51
TOTAL										
0–19 Years	213	4.3	25	1	1	3	5	9	13	25
20–34	257	5.4	53	1	2	3	6	11	22	40
35–49	119	5.4	45	1	2	3	6	10	21	35
50–64	103	4.9	63	1	3	3	6	10	13	22
65+	68	5.1	39	1	3	4	5	9	11	51
GRAND TOTAL	760	5.0	44	1	2	3	6	9	15	38

Length of Stay by Diagnosis and Operation, Western Region, 2008

757

Western Region, October 2006–September 2007 Data, by Diagnosis

867: PELVIC ORGAN INJURY

Type of Patients	Observed Patients	Avg. Stay	Vari-ance	10th	25th	50th	75th	90th	95th	99th
1. SINGLE DX										
A. Not Operated										
0–19 Years	1	1.0	0	1	1	1	1	1	1	1
20–34	2	1.5	<1	1	1	2	2	2	2	2
35–49	3	1.7	1	1	1	1	3	3	3	3
50–64	0									
65+	0									
B. Operated										
0–19 Years	4	3.5	25	1	1	1	1	11	11	11
20–34	8	2.9	2	1	2	3	4	5	5	5
35–49	0									
50–64	0									
65+	0									
2. MULTIPLE DX										
A. Not Operated										
0–19 Years	12	2.8	13	1	1	2	2	4	14	14
20–34	33	3.0	14	1	1	2	2	9	12	18
35–49	38	3.4	5	1	2	3	5	6	9	9
50–64	60	3.6	30	1	2	3	4	5	6	43
65+	274	3.9	10	1	2	3	5	8	10	15
B. Operated										
0–19 Years	29	7.6	44	2	4	6	10	13	35	>99
20–34	71	7.6	42	2	3	6	9	15	21	38
35–49	39	8.5	48	2	5	7	9	17	27	37
50–64	19	8.9	77	3	5	6	10	23	38	38
65+	40	6.9	45	2	3	5	9	12	17	40
SUBTOTALS:										
1. SINGLE DX										
A. Not Operated	6	1.5	<1	1	1	1	2	2	3	3
B. Operated	12	3.1	8	1	1	2	4	5	11	11
2. MULTIPLE DX										
A. Not Operated	417	3.7	13	1	2	3	4	8	10	15
B. Operated	198	7.7	47	2	4	6	9	16	23	40
1. SINGLE DX	18	2.6	6	1	1	2	3	5	11	11
2. MULTIPLE DX	615	5.0	27	1	2	4	6	10	14	35
A. NOT OPERATED	423	3.7	13	1	2	3	4	8	10	15
B. OPERATED	210	7.5	45	2	3	6	9	15	21	38
TOTAL										
0–19 Years	46	5.9	38	2	2	4	8	13	20	>99
20–34	114	5.8	35	1	2	4	8	12	18	28
35–49	80	5.8	32	2	2	5	7	10	16	37
50–64	79	4.9	45	2	2	3	5	10	17	43
65+	314	4.3	15	1	2	3	5	9	11	16
GRAND TOTAL	633	5.0	27	1	2	3	6	10	14	35

867.0: BLAD/URETHRA INJURY-CLSD

Type of Patients	Observed Patients	Avg. Stay	Vari-ance	10th	25th	50th	75th	90th	95th	99th
1. SINGLE DX										
A. Not Operated										
0–19 Years	1	1.0	0	1	1	1	1	1	1	1
20–34	1	2.0	0	2	2	2	2	2	2	2
35–49	1	3.0	0	3	3	3	3	3	3	3
50–64	0									
65+	0									
B. Operated										
0–19 Years	2	1.0	0	1	1	1	1	1	1	1
20–34	3	1.7	1	1	1	1	3	3	3	3
35–49	0									
50–64	0									
65+	0									
2. MULTIPLE DX										
A. Not Operated										
0–19 Years	9	3.2	17	1	1	2	2	14	14	14
20–34	23	3.7	19	1	1	2	3	10	12	18
35–49	32	3.7	5	1	2	3	5	6	9	9
50–64	54	3.7	33	1	2	3	4	6	9	43
65+	263	3.8	9	1	2	3	5	8	10	15
B. Operated										
0–19 Years	14	8.3	81	3	3	5	8	20	35	35
20–34	30	8.0	51	3	4	6	9	15	21	38
35–49	27	8.5	53	2	5	6	9	17	20	37
50–64	9	13.3	125	3	5	10	17	38	38	38
65+	38	7.0	47	2	3	5	9	12	17	40
SUBTOTALS:										
1. SINGLE DX										
A. Not Operated	3	2.0	<1	1	1	2	3	3	3	3
B. Operated	5	1.4	<1	1	1	1	1	3	3	3
2. MULTIPLE DX										
A. Not Operated	381	3.8	13	1	2	3	4	8	10	16
B. Operated	118	8.2	59	2	4	6	10	17	23	38
1. SINGLE DX	8	1.6	<1	1	1	1	2	3	3	3
2. MULTIPLE DX	499	4.8	27	1	2	3	6	10	12	35
A. NOT OPERATED	384	3.8	13	1	2	3	4	8	10	16
B. OPERATED	123	7.9	59	2	3	6	10	16	21	38
TOTAL										
0–19 Years	26	5.7	56	1	1	3	6	14	20	35
20–34	57	5.8	39	1	2	3	8	12	18	38
35–49	60	5.8	32	1	2	5	7	10	16	37
50–64	63	5.1	56	1	2	3	5	10	17	43
65+	301	4.2	15	1	2	3	5	9	11	17
GRAND TOTAL	507	4.8	27	1	2	3	6	10	12	35

868: OTH INTRA-ABD INJURY

Type of Patients	Observed Patients	Avg. Stay	Vari-ance	10th	25th	50th	75th	90th	95th	99th
1. SINGLE DX										
A. Not Operated										
0–19 Years	14	1.7	<1	1	1	2	2	3	3	3
20–34	12	1.8	2	1	1	1	3	3	5	5
35–49	4	1.3	<1	1	1	1	1	1	2	2
50–64	4	1.2	<1	1	1	1	1	2	2	2
65+	1	1.0	0	1	1	1	1	1	1	1
B. Operated										
0–19 Years	14	3.4	5	1	2	3	4	5	9	9
20–34	26	2.6	2	1	1	3	4	4	5	5
35–49	9	2.6	2	1	1	3	3	4	4	4
50–64	1	4.0	0	4	4	4	4	4	4	4
65+	0									
2. MULTIPLE DX										
A. Not Operated										
0–19 Years	42	2.1	5	1	1	2	2	3	4	15
20–34	66	3.4	19	1	2	2	4	6	9	32
35–49	53	3.1	8	1	1	3	5	7	8	16
50–64	47	5.0	26	1	2	3	6	10	13	30
65+	69	5.4	17	2	3	4	7	10	12	25
B. Operated										
0–19 Years	66	5.5	47	1	2	4	6	9	15	48
20–34	192	6.0	77	2	3	4	6	11	16	43
35–49	109	6.6	56	2	3	5	7	14	19	53
50–64	59	9.7	170	2	3	6	8	26	40	74
65+	18	9.2	56	3	4	6	15	20	29	29
SUBTOTALS:										
1. SINGLE DX										
A. Not Operated	35	1.6	<1	1	1	1	2	3	3	5
B. Operated	50	2.8	3	1	1	3	4	5	5	9
2. MULTIPLE DX										
A. Not Operated	277	3.9	17	1	2	3	4	8	11	25
B. Operated	444	6.7	80	2	3	4	7	13	20	53
1. SINGLE DX	85	2.3	2	1	1	2	3	4	5	9
2. MULTIPLE DX	721	5.6	57	1	2	4	6	10	17	43
A. NOT OPERATED	312	3.7	16	1	1	2	4	8	11	17
B. OPERATED	494	6.3	73	2	3	4	6	11	19	53
TOTAL										
0–19 Years	136	3.8	27	1	2	2	4	8	9	25
20–34	296	5.0	56	1	2	3	5	8	13	40
35–49	175	5.2	41	1	2	4	6	10	17	53
50–64	111	7.4	107	2	3	5	7	13	30	53
65+	88	6.1	27	2	3	5	8	12	17	29
GRAND TOTAL	806	5.3	53	1	2	4	6	10	16	40

869: INTERNAL INJURY NOS

Type of Patients	Observed Patients	Avg. Stay	Variance	Percentiles						
				10th	25th	50th	75th	90th	95th	99th
1. SINGLE DX										
A. *Not Operated*										
0–19 Years	0									
20–34	1	7.0	0	7	7	7	7	7	7	7
35–49	0									
50–64	0									
65+	0									
B. *Operated*										
0–19 Years	0									
20–34	0									
35–49	0									
50–64	0									
65+	0									
2. MULTIPLE DX										
A. *Not Operated*										
0–19 Years	2	5.0	31	1	1	1	9	9	9	9
20–34	1	2.0	0	2	2	2	2	2	2	2
35–49	1	2.0	0	2	2	2	2	2	2	2
50–64	2	2.5	4	1	1	1	4	4	4	4
65+	1	2.0	0	2	2	2	2	2	2	2
B. *Operated*										
0–19 Years	1	9.0	0	9	9	9	9	9	9	9
20–34	2	20.0	711	1	1	20	39	39	39	39
35–49	0									
50–64	0									
65+	0									
SUBTOTALS:										
1. SINGLE DX										
A. *Not Operated*	1	7.0	0	7	7	7	7	7	7	7
B. *Operated*	0									
2. MULTIPLE DX										
A. *Not Operated*	7	3.0	8	1	1	2	4	9	9	9
B. *Operated*	3	16.3	398	1	1	9	39	39	39	39
1. SINGLE DX	1	7.0	0	7	7	7	7	7	7	7
2. MULTIPLE DX	10	7.0	136	1	1	2	9	9	39	39
A. NOT OPERATED	8	3.5	9	1	1	2	7	9	9	9
B. OPERATED	3	16.3	398	1	1	9	39	39	39	39
TOTAL										
0–19 Years	3	6.3	21	1	1	9	9	9	9	9
20–34	4	12.3	324	1	1	7	39	39	39	39
35–49	1	2.0	0	2	2	2	2	2	2	2
50–64	2	2.5	4	1	1	1	4	4	4	4
65+	1	2.0	0	2	2	2	2	2	2	2
GRAND TOTAL	11	7.0	122	1	1	2	9	39	39	39

870: OCULAR ADNEXA OPEN WOUND

Type of Patients	Observed Patients	Avg. Stay	Variance	Percentiles						
				10th	25th	50th	75th	90th	95th	99th
1. SINGLE DX										
A. *Not Operated*										
0–19 Years	8	1.3	<1	1	1	1	1	2	2	2
20–34	7	1.3	<1	1	1	1	2	2	2	2
35–49	3	2.0	3	1	1	1	4	4	4	4
50–64	2	1.0	0	1	1	1	1	1	1	1
65+	0									
B. *Operated*										
0–19 Years	7	1.1	<1	1	1	1	1	2	2	2
20–34	5	1.2	<1	1	1	1	1	2	2	2
35–49	2	2.0	0	2	2	2	2	2	2	2
50–64	1	1.0	0	1	1	1	1	1	1	1
65+	0									
2. MULTIPLE DX										
A. *Not Operated*										
0–19 Years	29	1.4	<1	1	1	1	2	2	3	3
20–34	40	1.4	<1	1	1	1	2	2	2	3
35–49	26	1.5	<1	1	1	1	2	3	3	5
50–64	16	2.2	3	1	1	2	3	4	7	7
65+	28	2.7	3	1	1	3	4	5	6	8
B. *Operated*										
0–19 Years	29	1.5	<1	1	1	1	2	3	3	3
20–34	43	3.5	37	1	1	1	3	5	20	30
35–49	31	2.4	4	1	1	1	3	5	7	8
50–64	14	2.4	2	1	1	3	3	5	5	5
65+	9	2.5	3	1	1	2	3	6	6	6
SUBTOTALS:										
1. SINGLE DX										
A. *Not Operated*	20	1.4	1	1	1	1	2	2	4	4
B. *Operated*	15	1.3	<1	1	1	1	2	2	2	2
2. MULTIPLE DX										
A. *Not Operated*	139	1.8	2	1	1	1	2	3	4	7
B. *Operated*	126	2.6	14	1	1	1	3	5	6	24
1. SINGLE DX	35	1.3	<1	1	1	1	2	2	2	4
2. MULTIPLE DX	265	2.1	8	1	1	1	2	4	5	20
A. NOT OPERATED	159	1.7	1	1	1	1	2	3	4	7
B. OPERATED	141	2.4	13	1	1	1	3	4	6	24
TOTAL										
0–19 Years	73	1.4	<1	1	1	1	2	2	3	3
20–34	95	2.3	18	1	1	1	2	3	5	30
35–49	62	2.0	3	1	1	1	2	4	5	8
50–64	33	2.2	2	1	1	2	3	4	5	7
65+	37	2.6	3	1	1	2	4	5	6	8
GRAND TOTAL	300	2.1	7	1	1	1	2	4	5	8

871: EYEBALL OPEN WOUND

Type of Patients	Observed Patients	Avg. Stay	Variance	Percentiles						
				10th	25th	50th	75th	90th	95th	99th
1. SINGLE DX										
A. *Not Operated*										
0–19 Years	0									
20–34	0									
35–49	2	2.0	2	1	1	1	3	3	3	3
50–64	0									
65+	0									
B. *Operated*										
0–19 Years	53	1.6	<1	1	1	1	2	2	3	5
20–34	41	1.4	<1	1	1	1	2	2	3	5
35–49	34	1.9	2	1	1	2	2	4	7	7
50–64	18	1.9	1	1	1	2	3	4	5	5
65+	1	4.0	0	4	4	4	4	4	4	4
2. MULTIPLE DX										
A. *Not Operated*										
0–19 Years	3	1.3	<1	1	1	1	2	2	2	2
20–34	2	1.5	<1	1	1	2	2	2	2	2
35–49	1	1.0	0	1	1	1	1	1	1	1
50–64	3	4.0	27	1	1	1	10	10	10	10
65+	3	2.0	3	4	4	4	4	4	4	4
B. *Operated*										
0–19 Years	81	2.1	3	1	1	2	3	3	5	12
20–34	116	2.7	15	1	1	3	3	6	7	23
35–49	102	2.5	7	1	1	3	3	5	6	14
50–64	78	2.5	11	1	1	3	3	4	7	26
65+	125	3.1	16	1	4	4	4	6	8	14
SUBTOTALS:										
1. SINGLE DX										
A. *Not Operated*	2	2.0	2	1	1	1	3	3	3	3
B. *Operated*	147	1.7	1	1	1	1	2	3	3	7
2. MULTIPLE DX										
A. *Not Operated*	12	2.2	7	1	1	2	2	4	10	10
B. *Operated*	502	2.6	11	1	1	2	3	5	7	18
1. SINGLE DX	149	1.7	1	1	1	1	2	3	4	7
2. MULTIPLE DX	514	2.6	11	1	1	2	3	5	7	18
A. NOT OPERATED	14	2.1	6	1	1	1	2	4	10	10
B. OPERATED	649	2.4	9	1	1	2	3	4	6	14
TOTAL										
0–19 Years	137	1.9	2	1	1	1	2	3	5	7
20–34	159	2.4	12	1	1	1	2	4	7	23
35–49	139	2.3	6	1	1	1	3	5	7	14
50–64	99	2.4	10	1	1	1	3	4	7	13
65+	129	3.1	16	1	1	2	4	6	8	14
GRAND TOTAL	663	2.4	9	1	1	2	3	4	6	14

Length of Stay by Diagnosis and Operation, Western Region, 2008

Western Region, October 2006–September 2007 Data, by Diagnosis

871.1: OCULAR LAC W PROLAPSE

Type of Patients	Observed Patients	Avg. Stay	Variance	10th	25th	50th	75th	90th	95th	99th
1. SINGLE DX										
A. Not Operated										
0–19 Years	0									
20–34	0									
35–49	0									
50–64	0									
65+	0									
B. Operated										
0–19 Years	23	1.5	1	1	1	1	2	3	3	5
20–34	18	1.2	<1	1	1	1	1	1	2	2
35–49	14	1.9	3	1	1	1	2	2	7	7
50–64	7	1.6	<1	1	1	1	2	3	3	3
65+	0									
2. MULTIPLE DX										
A. Not Operated										
0–19 Years	0									
20–34	0									
35–49	0									
50–64	1	1.0	0	1	1	1	1	1	1	1
65+	1	1.0	0	1	1	1	1	1	1	1
B. Operated										
0–19 Years	38	2.3	4	1	1	2	3	3	5	12
20–34	51	3.0	23	1	1	2	3	5	10	27
35–49	54	1.9	2	1	1	1	3	3	5	6
50–64	29	2.0	3	1	1	1	2	4	5	10
65+	68	3.2	25	1	1	2	3	6	10	39
SUBTOTALS:										
1. SINGLE DX										
A. Not Operated	0									
B. Operated	62	1.5	1	1	1	1	2	2	3	3
2. MULTIPLE DX										
A. Not Operated	2	1.0	0	1	1	1	1	1	1	1
B. Operated	240	2.6	13	1	1	2	2	3	6	23
1. SINGLE DX	62	1.5	1	1	1	1	2	2	3	3
2. MULTIPLE DX	242	2.6	13	1	1	2	3	5	6	23
A. NOT OPERATED	2	1.0	0	1	1	1	1	1	1	1
B. OPERATED	302	2.4	11	1	1	1	3	4	5	12
TOTAL										
0–19 Years	61	2.0	3	1	1	2	2	3	5	12
20–34	69	2.5	18	1	1	1	2	4	6	27
35–49	68	1.9	2	1	1	1	2	4	5	7
50–64	37	1.9	3	1	1	1	2	3	5	10
65+	69	3.2	24	1	1	2	3	6	10	39
GRAND TOTAL	304	2.3	11	1	1	1	3	4	5	12

872: OPEN WOUND OF EAR

Type of Patients	Observed Patients	Avg. Stay	Variance	10th	25th	50th	75th	90th	95th	99th
1. SINGLE DX										
A. Not Operated										
0–19 Years	2	1.0	0	1	1	1	1	1	1	1
20–34	4	1.5	<1	1	1	1	1	3	3	3
35–49	1	1.0	0	1	1	1	1	1	1	1
50–64	1	3.0	0	3	3	3	3	3	3	3
65+	0									
B. Operated										
0–19 Years	2	1.0	0	1	1	1	1	1	1	1
20–34	2	2.0	2	1	1	3	3	3	3	3
35–49	3	3.3	6	1	1	3	3	6	6	6
50–64	0									
65+	0									
2. MULTIPLE DX										
A. Not Operated										
0–19 Years	23	1.8	1	1	1	2	2	3	4	5
20–34	28	1.4	<1	1	1	1	2	2	3	4
35–49	24	1.8	3	1	1	1	2	3	3	9
50–64	12	1.9	2	1	1	1	2	3	5	5
65+	18	2.1	2	1	1	2	3	5	6	6
B. Operated										
0–19 Years	6	2.5	4	1	1	2	3	3	6	6
20–34	16	2.8	9	1	1	2	3	5	13	13
35–49	14	3.4	9	1	1	2	5	8	8	8
50–64	13	2.9	3	1	2	2	5	6	6	6
65+	4	3.0	5	1	1	2	3	6	6	6
SUBTOTALS:										
1. SINGLE DX										
A. Not Operated	8	1.5	<1	1	1	1	1	3	3	3
B. Operated	7	2.3	4	1	1	1	3	6	6	6
2. MULTIPLE DX										
A. Not Operated	105	1.8	2	1	1	1	2	3	4	6
B. Operated	53	3.0	6	1	2	2	3	6	8	13
1. SINGLE DX	15	1.9	2	1	1	1	2	3	6	6
2. MULTIPLE DX	158	2.2	3	1	1	2	2	5	6	9
A. NOT OPERATED	113	1.8	2	1	1	1	2	3	4	6
B. OPERATED	60	2.9	6	1	1	2	3	6	8	13
TOTAL										
0–19 Years	33	1.9	2	1	1	2	2	3	5	6
20–34	50	1.9	4	1	1	1	2	3	4	13
35–49	42	2.4	6	1	1	1	3	8	8	9
50–64	26	2.5	2	1	1	2	3	5	5	6
65+	22	2.3	2	1	1	2	3	5	6	6
GRAND TOTAL	173	2.1	3	1	1	2	2	5	6	9

873: OTHER OPEN WOUND OF HEAD

Type of Patients	Observed Patients	Avg. Stay	Variance	10th	25th	50th	75th	90th	95th	99th
1. SINGLE DX										
A. Not Operated										
0–19 Years	61	1.1	<1	1	1	1	1	2	2	3
20–34	47	1.2	<1	1	1	1	1	2	2	3
35–49	14	1.1	<1	1	1	1	1	2	2	2
50–64	9	1.1	<1	1	1	1	1	2	2	2
65+	3	3.3	4	1	1	4	5	5	5	5
B. Operated										
0–19 Years	24	1.4	<1	1	1	1	2	2	3	3
20–34	9	1.8	<1	1	1	2	3	3	3	3
35–49	10	1.7	<1	1	1	2	2	3	3	3
50–64	4	2.3	2	1	1	2	4	4	4	4
65+	2	1.0	0	1	1	1	1	1	1	1
2. MULTIPLE DX										
A. Not Operated										
0–19 Years	312	1.5	1	1	1	1	2	3	4	6
20–34	536	1.7	3	1	1	1	2	3	4	7
35–49	397	2.0	3	1	1	1	2	4	5	8
50–64	356	2.4	8	1	1	2	3	4	6	13
65+	731	2.7	7	1	1	2	3	5	7	17
B. Operated										
0–19 Years	125	2.9	58	1	1	2	3	5	5	13
20–34	171	2.9	14	1	1	2	3	5	8	25
35–49	127	3.3	15	1	1	2	4	7	10	18
50–64	91	3.5	13	1	1	2	4	9	13	19
65+	83	4.2	40	1	1	2	4	10	14	45
SUBTOTALS:										
1. SINGLE DX										
A. Not Operated	134	1.2	<1	1	1	1	1	2	2	4
B. Operated	49	1.6	<1	1	1	1	2	3	3	4
2. MULTIPLE DX										
A. Not Operated	2,332	2.1	5	1	1	1	2	4	5	11
B. Operated	597	3.2	27	1	2	2	4	6	10	25
1. SINGLE DX	183	1.3	<1	1	1	1	1	2	3	4
2. MULTIPLE DX	2,929	2.4	10	1	1	1	3	4	6	14
A. NOT OPERATED	2,466	2.1	5	1	1	1	2	4	5	10
B. OPERATED	646	3.1	25	1	2	2	3	6	10	19
TOTAL										
0–19 Years	522	1.8	15	1	1	1	2	3	4	9
20–34	763	1.9	5	1	1	1	2	4	5	10
35–49	548	2.3	6	1	1	1	3	4	6	13
50–64	460	2.6	9	1	1	2	3	5	8	15
65+	819	2.8	11	1	1	2	3	5	7	17
GRAND TOTAL	3,112	2.3	9	1	1	1	3	4	6	14

Length of Stay by Diagnosis and Operation, Western Region, 2008

Western Region, October 2006–September 2007 Data, by Diagnosis

873.0: OPEN WOUND OF SCALP

Type of Patients	Observed Patients	Avg. Stay	Vari-ance	10th	25th	50th	75th	90th	95th	99th
1. SINGLE DX										
A. Not Operated										
0–19 Years	12	1.1	<1	1	1	1	1	1	2	2
20–34	26	1.1	<1	1	1	1	1	1	2	2
35–49	4	1.0	0	1	1	1	1	1	1	1
50–64	5	1.0	0	1	1	1	1	1	1	1
65+	2	2.5	4	1	1	1	4	4	4	4
B. Operated										
0–19 Years	1	1.0	0	1	1	1	1	1	1	1
20–34	2	3.0	0	3	3	3	3	3	3	3
35–49	2	2.5	<1	2	2	3	3	3	3	3
50–64	2	1.5	<1	1	1	1	2	2	2	2
65+	0									
2. MULTIPLE DX										
A. Not Operated										
0–19 Years	80	1.4	<1	1	1	1	2	3	3	6
20–34	191	1.5	2	1	1	1	2	2	3	7
35–49	150	1.8	2	1	1	1	2	3	4	8
50–64	142	2.4	13	1	1	1	2	4	7	14
65+	360	2.5	8	1	1	2	3	5	6	17
B. Operated										
0–19 Years	16	2.1	2	1	1	3	3	5	5	5
20–34	24	4.3	63	1	1	2	3	5	25	34
35–49	20	4.0	12	1	2	3	5	10	15	15
50–64	19	5.8	29	1	2	4	5	16	19	19
65+	16	6.8	48	3	3	4	12	15	27	27
SUBTOTALS:										
1. SINGLE DX										
A. Not Operated	49	1.1	<1	1	1	1	1	1	2	2
B. Operated	7	2.1	<1	1	1	1	1	3	3	3
2. MULTIPLE DX										
A. Not Operated	923	2.1	6	1	1	1	2	4	5	13
B. Operated	95	4.6	34	1	1	3	5	12	16	34
1. SINGLE DX	56	1.3	<1	1	1	1	1	2	3	4
2. MULTIPLE DX	1,018	2.3	9	1	1	1	3	4	6	16
A. NOT OPERATED	972	2.0	6	1	1	1	2	4	5	13
B. OPERATED	102	4.4	32	1	1	3	5	11	15	27
TOTAL										
0–19 Years	109	1.5	<1	1	1	1	1	3	4	5
20–34	243	1.7	8	1	1	1	2	3	4	14
35–49	176	2.1	4	1	1	1	2	4	6	13
50–64	168	2.7	15	1	1	1	3	5	10	19
65+	378	2.7	10	1	1	2	3	5	6	19
GRAND TOTAL	1,074	2.3	9	1	1	1	2	4	5	16

873.42: OPEN WOUND OF FOREHEAD

Type of Patients	Observed Patients	Avg. Stay	Vari-ance	10th	25th	50th	75th	90th	95th	99th
1. SINGLE DX										
A. Not Operated										
0–19 Years	18	1.2	<1	1	1	1	1	2	3	3
20–34	8	1.0	0	1	1	1	1	1	1	1
35–49	4	1.0	0	1	1	1	1	1	1	1
50–64	1	1.0	0	1	1	1	1	1	1	1
65+	1	5.0	0	5	5	5	5	5	5	5
B. Operated										
0–19 Years	2	1.5	<1	1	1	1	2	2	2	2
20–34	2	1.0	0	1	1	1	1	1	1	1
35–49	1	1.0	0	1	1	1	1	1	1	1
50–64	0									
65+	0									
2. MULTIPLE DX										
A. Not Operated										
0–19 Years	59	1.5	<1	1	1	1	2	3	4	5
20–34	117	1.6	1	1	1	1	2	3	4	6
35–49	94	1.8	2	1	1	1	2	4	5	8
50–64	89	2.2	3	1	1	2	3	4	5	12
65+	205	2.8	6	1	1	2	3	5	7	14
B. Operated										
0–19 Years	14	2.2	10	1	1	2	2	5	13	13
20–34	15	2.5	5	1	1	2	4	5	9	9
35–49	22	4.0	26	1	2	2	4	13	17	18
50–64	20	3.3	17	1	1	2	3	13	13	14
65+	14	2.4	4	1	1	2	4	6	6	6
SUBTOTALS:										
1. SINGLE DX										
A. Not Operated	32	1.2	<1	1	1	1	1	1	3	5
B. Operated	5	1.2	<1	1	1	1	2	2	2	2
2. MULTIPLE DX										
A. Not Operated	564	2.1	4	1	1	1	2	4	5	10
B. Operated	85	3.0	14	1	1	3	5	6	13	18
1. SINGLE DX	37	1.2	<1	1	1	1	1	2	3	5
2. MULTIPLE DX	649	2.3	5	1	1	2	3	4	6	13
A. NOT OPERATED	596	2.1	4	1	1	1	3	4	5	10
B. OPERATED	90	2.9	13	1	1	1	3	6	13	18
TOTAL										
0–19 Years	93	1.6	2	1	1	1	2	3	4	13
20–34	142	1.7	2	1	1	1	2	3	4	6
35–49	121	2.2	7	1	1	1	2	4	5	17
50–64	110	2.4	6	1	1	2	3	4	6	13
65+	220	2.7	6	1	1	2	3	5	7	14
GRAND TOTAL	686	2.2	5	1	1	1	3	4	5	13

873.43: OPEN WOUND OF LIP

Type of Patients	Observed Patients	Avg. Stay	Vari-ance	10th	25th	50th	75th	90th	95th	99th
1. SINGLE DX										
A. Not Operated										
0–19 Years	2	1.0	0	1	1	1	1	1	1	1
20–34	3	1.3	<1	1	1	1	2	2	2	2
35–49	2	2.0	0	2	2	2	2	2	2	2
50–64	0									
65+	0									
B. Operated										
0–19 Years	3	1.7	1	1	1	1	3	3	3	3
20–34	1	1.0	0	1	1	1	1	1	1	1
35–49	1	2.0	0	2	2	2	2	2	2	2
50–64	0									
65+	1	1.0	0	1	1	1	1	1	1	1
2. MULTIPLE DX										
A. Not Operated										
0–19 Years	28	1.5	<1	1	1	1	2	3	3	5
20–34	40	1.4	<1	1	1	1	2	2	3	4
35–49	29	2.1	5	1	1	1	2	5	8	10
50–64	26	2.1	2	1	1	1	4	4	5	6
65+	35	2.0	2	1	1	1	3	4	5	6
B. Operated										
0–19 Years	11	1.3	<1	1	1	1	1	2	2	2
20–34	17	1.5	<1	1	1	1	2	3	3	3
35–49	12	1.8	<1	1	1	2	2	3	3	3
50–64	15	2.3	2	1	1	2	3	5	5	5
65+	5	2.8	6	1	1	2	3	7	7	7
SUBTOTALS:										
1. SINGLE DX										
A. Not Operated	7	1.4	<1	1	1	1	1	2	2	2
B. Operated	6	1.5	<1	1	1	1	2	3	3	3
2. MULTIPLE DX										
A. Not Operated	158	1.8	2	1	1	1	2	4	5	8
B. Operated	60	1.8	1	1	1	2	2	3	5	7
1. SINGLE DX	13	1.5	<1	1	1	1	2	2	3	3
2. MULTIPLE DX	218	1.8	2	1	1	1	2	3	5	7
A. NOT OPERATED	165	1.8	2	1	1	1	2	4	4	8
B. OPERATED	66	1.8	1	1	1	1	2	3	3	7
TOTAL										
0–19 Years	44	1.4	<1	1	1	1	2	3	3	5
20–34	61	1.4	<1	1	1	1	2	2	3	4
35–49	44	2.0	3	1	1	2	3	4	5	10
50–64	41	2.2	2	1	1	2	3	4	5	6
65+	41	2.0	2	1	1	2	3	4	5	7
GRAND TOTAL	231	1.8	2	1	1	1	2	3	4	7

Length of Stay by Diagnosis and Operation, Western Region, 2008

Western Region, October 2006–September 2007 Data, by Diagnosis

874: OPEN WOUND OF NECK

Type of Patients	Observed Patients	Avg. Stay	Variance	10th	25th	50th	75th	90th	95th	99th
1. SINGLE DX										
A. Not Operated										
0–19 Years	17	1.5	<1	1	1	1	1	3	4	4
20–34	20	1.1	<1	1	1	1	1	1	1	2
35–49	5	1.4	<1	1	1	1	1	3	3	3
50–64	5	1.0	0	1	1	1	1	1	1	1
65+	1	1.0	0	1	1	1	1	1	1	1
B. Operated										
0–19 Years	9	1.2	<1	1	1	1	1	2	2	2
20–34	9	2.0	3	1	1	1	2	5	5	5
35–49	5	3.4	14	1	1	2	3	10	10	10
50–64	1	1.0	0	1	1	1	1	1	1	1
65+	1	1.0	0	1	1	1	1	1	1	1
2. MULTIPLE DX										
A. Not Operated										
0–19 Years	45	1.9	6	1	1	1	2	4	5	16
20–34	137	2.0	4	1	1	1	2	4	5	13
35–49	76	3.6	33	1	1	2	5	7	10	46
50–64	40	2.8	6	1	1	1	4	7	9	9
65+	19	4.2	10	1	2	3	6	10	10	10
B. Operated										
0–19 Years	23	7.0	67	1	2	4	12	17	18	36
20–34	96	4.9	38	1	2	2	7	7	17	46
35–49	56	5.2	37	1	2	2	6	16	18	29
50–64	30	5.3	32	1	2	3	7	18	21	22
65+	9	10.0	94	1	3	7	11	30	30	30
SUBTOTALS:										
1. SINGLE DX										
A. Not Operated	48	1.2	<1	1	1	1	1	2	3	4
B. Operated	25	1.9	4	1	1	1	2	5	5	10
2. MULTIPLE DX										
A. Not Operated	317	2.6	12	1	1	1	3	6	8	13
B. Operated	214	5.5	43	1	1	3	7	12	19	30
1. SINGLE DX	73	1.5	2	1	1	1	1	3	4	10
2. MULTIPLE DX	531	3.8	27	1	1	2	4	9	12	25
A. NOT OPERATED	365	2.4	11	1	1	1	3	5	7	13
B. OPERATED	239	5.1	40	1	1	2	7	11	18	30
TOTAL										
0–19 Years	94	3.0	24	1	1	1	2	6	14	36
20–34	262	3.0	18	1	1	1	3	7	9	22
35–49	142	4.1	33	1	1	2	5	9	15	29
50–64	76	3.7	18	1	1	2	5	8	9	22
65+	30	5.7	41	1	2	3	8	10	21	30
GRAND TOTAL	604	3.5	24	1	1	2	4	8	11	23

874.8: OPEN WOUND OF NECK NEC

Type of Patients	Observed Patients	Avg. Stay	Variance	10th	25th	50th	75th	90th	95th	99th
1. SINGLE DX										
A. Not Operated										
0–19 Years	13	1.2	<1	1	1	1	1	2	3	3
20–34	13	1.1	<1	1	1	1	1	1	2	2
35–49	5	1.4	<1	1	1	1	1	1	3	3
50–64	3	1.0	0	1	1	1	1	1	1	1
65+	1	1.0	0	1	1	1	1	1	1	1
B. Operated										
0–19 Years	3	1.3	<1	1	1	1	2	2	2	2
20–34	7	1.6	2	1	1	1	2	5	5	5
35–49	2	1.5	<1	1	1	2	2	2	2	2
50–64	0									
65+	1	1.0	0	1	1	1	1	1	1	1
2. MULTIPLE DX										
A. Not Operated										
0–19 Years	28	1.4	<1	1	1	1	2	2	2	5
20–34	103	1.6	1	1	1	1	2	3	4	5
35–49	63	3.4	37	1	1	2	3	7	8	46
50–64	32	2.7	7	1	1	2	4	7	9	9
65+	8	2.5	4	1	1	2	5	6	6	6
B. Operated										
0–19 Years	8	3.6	13	2	2	2	4	12	12	12
20–34	52	2.4	7	1	1	2	4	6	10	11
35–49	29	3.7	16	1	2	2	3	9	16	17
50–64	17	4.2	23	1	2	3	5	9	21	21
65+	3	8.3	14	4	4	10	11	11	11	11
SUBTOTALS:										
1. SINGLE DX										
A. Not Operated	35	1.2	<1	1	1	1	1	2	3	3
B. Operated	13	1.5	1	1	1	1	2	2	5	5
2. MULTIPLE DX										
A. Not Operated	234	2.3	12	1	1	1	2	5	7	10
B. Operated	109	3.3	13	1	2	2	4	9	11	17
1. SINGLE DX	48	1.3	<1	1	1	1	1	2	3	5
2. MULTIPLE DX	343	2.6	13	1	1	1	3	5	8	16
A. NOT OPERATED	269	2.1	11	1	1	1	2	5	6	10
B. OPERATED	122	3.1	12	1	1	2	3	7	11	17
TOTAL										
0–19 Years	52	1.7	3	1	1	1	2	2	4	12
20–34	175	1.8	3	1	1	1	2	4	5	11
35–49	99	3.3	29	1	1	2	3	7	10	46
50–64	52	3.1	12	1	1	2	5	7	9	21
65+	13	3.6	12	1	1	3	5	10	11	11
GRAND TOTAL	391	2.4	11	1	1	1	2	5	8	16

875: OPEN WOUND OF CHEST

Type of Patients	Observed Patients	Avg. Stay	Variance	10th	25th	50th	75th	90th	95th	99th
1. SINGLE DX										
A. Not Operated										
0–19 Years	11	1.0	0	1	1	1	1	1	1	1
20–34	29	1.3	<1	1	1	1	1	2	4	4
35–49	12	1.0	0	1	1	1	1	1	1	1
50–64	3	1.0	0	1	1	1	1	1	1	1
65+	0									
B. Operated										
0–19 Years	1	2.0	0	2	2	2	2	2	2	2
20–34	7	1.3	<1	1	1	1	2	2	2	2
35–49	3	1.7	<1	1	1	2	2	2	2	2
50–64	1	1.0	0	1	1	1	1	1	1	1
65+	1	1.0	0	1	1	1	1	1	1	1
2. MULTIPLE DX										
A. Not Operated										
0–19 Years	65	1.7	2	1	1	1	2	3	3	8
20–34	157	1.9	5	1	1	1	2	3	4	13
35–49	77	1.6	1	1	1	1	2	3	5	6
50–64	27	2.8	6	1	1	2	4	5	9	10
65+	14	5.6	33	1	1	5	9	11	21	21
B. Operated										
0–19 Years	8	7.0	27	1	4	5	6	18	18	18
20–34	50	4.4	47	1	1	2	5	8	17	43
35–49	22	4.5	15	1	1	3	7	10	11	15
50–64	5	5.4	13	2	2	5	8	10	10	10
65+	1	8.0	0	8	8	8	8	8	8	8
SUBTOTALS:										
1. SINGLE DX										
A. Not Operated	55	1.2	<1	1	1	1	1	1	2	4
B. Operated	13	1.4	<1	1	1	1	2	2	2	2
2. MULTIPLE DX										
A. Not Operated	340	2.0	5	1	1	1	2	4	5	11
B. Operated	86	4.8	34	1	3	3	6	10	15	43
1. SINGLE DX	68	1.2	<1	1	1	1	1	2	2	4
2. MULTIPLE DX	426	2.6	12	1	1	1	3	5	8	18
A. NOT OPERATED	395	1.9	5	1	1	1	2	4	5	11
B. OPERATED	99	4.3	31	1	2	2	5	10	15	43
TOTAL										
0–19 Years	85	2.1	6	1	1	1	2	4	6	18
20–34	243	2.3	14	1	1	1	2	4	6	21
35–49	114	2.1	5	1	1	2	4	5	7	11
50–64	36	3.0	7	1	1	2	4	8	10	10
65+	16	5.4	31	1	1	5	9	11	21	21
GRAND TOTAL	494	2.4	11	1	1	1	2	5	8	18

Length of Stay by Diagnosis and Operation, Western Region, 2008

Western Region, October 2006–September 2007 Data, by Diagnosis

875.0: OPEN WOUND CHEST

Type of Patients	Observed Patients	Avg. Stay	Variance	10th	25th	50th	75th	90th	95th	99th
1. SINGLE DX										
A. Not Operated										
0–19 Years	9	1.0	0	1	1	1	1	1	1	1
20–34	24	1.3	<1	1	1	1	1	2	4	4
35–49	10	1.0	0	1	1	1	1	1	1	1
50–64	3	1.0	0	1	1	1	1	1	1	1
65+	0									
B. Operated										
0–19 Years	1	2.0	0	2	2	2	2	2	2	2
20–34	5	1.2	<1	1	1	1	1	2	2	2
35–49	2	2.0	0	2	2	2	2	2	2	2
50–64	1	1.0	0	1	1	1	1	1	1	1
65+	0									
2. MULTIPLE DX										
A. Not Operated										
0–19 Years	58	1.5	1	1	1	1	2	2	3	7
20–34	126	1.6	1	1	1	1	2	3	4	6
35–49	71	1.6	1	1	1	1	2	3	5	6
50–64	23	2.6	5	1	1	2	4	5	5	10
65+	13	5.8	36	1	1	5	9	11	21	21
B. Operated										
0–19 Years	3	3.3	4	1	1	4	5	5	5	5
20–34	31	2.5	4	1	1	1	3	5	8	9
35–49	18	4.2	15	1	1	3	6	10	15	15
50–64	3	3.0	3	2	2	2	5	5	5	5
65+	1	8.0	0	8	8	8	8	8	8	8
SUBTOTALS:										
1. SINGLE DX										
A. Not Operated	46	1.2	<1	1	1	1	1	1	2	4
B. Operated	9	1.4	<1	1	1	1	1	2	2	2
2. MULTIPLE DX										
A. Not Operated	291	1.9	4	1	1	1	2	4	5	11
B. Operated	56	3.3	8	1	1	2	5	8	9	15
1. SINGLE DX	55	1.2	<1	1	1	1	1	2	2	4
2. MULTIPLE DX	347	2.1	5	1	1	1	2	5	6	11
A. NOT OPERATED	337	1.8	3	1	1	1	2	4	5	10
B. OPERATED	65	3.0	7	1	1	2	4	7	8	15
TOTAL										
0–19 Years	71	1.6	1	1	1	1	2	2	4	7
20–34	186	1.7	2	1	1	1	2	3	4	8
35–49	101	2.0	5	1	1	1	2	5	6	10
50–64	30	2.5	4	1	1	2	3	5	5	10
65+	14	5.9	33	1	1	5	9	11	21	21
GRAND TOTAL	402	2.0	4	1	1	1	2	4	5	10

876: OPEN WOUND OF BACK

Type of Patients	Observed Patients	Avg. Stay	Variance	10th	25th	50th	75th	90th	95th	99th
1. SINGLE DX										
A. Not Operated										
0–19 Years	16	1.3	<1	1	1	1	1	3	4	4
20–34	25	1.0	<1	1	1	1	1	1	2	2
35–49	7	1.1	<1	1	1	1	1	2	2	2
50–64	1	1.0	0	1	1	1	1	1	1	1
65+	0									
B. Operated										
0–19 Years	2	1.0	0	1	1	1	1	1	1	1
20–34	2	1.0	0	1	1	1	1	1	1	1
35–49	0									
50–64	0									
65+	0									
2. MULTIPLE DX										
A. Not Operated										
0–19 Years	46	2.0	9	1	1	1	1	2	5	20
20–34	109	1.9	4	1	1	1	2	4	6	12
35–49	30	1.7	3	1	1	1	2	3	7	8
50–64	6	1.8	4	1	1	2	4	6	6	6
65+	2	2.0	2	1	1	3	3	3	3	3
B. Operated										
0–19 Years	7	2.9	5	1	1	2	4	7	7	7
20–34	15	2.3	4	1	1	2	3	4	9	9
35–49	6	3.7	6	1	2	2	6	7	7	7
50–64	4	2.2	4	1	1	1	2	5	5	5
65+	1	7.0	0	7	7	7	7	7	7	7
SUBTOTALS:										
1. SINGLE DX										
A. Not Operated	49	1.1	<1	1	1	1	1	1	2	4
B. Operated	4	1.0	0	1	1	1	1	1	1	1
2. MULTIPLE DX										
A. Not Operated	193	1.9	5	1	1	1	2	4	6	14
B. Operated	33	2.8	5	1	1	2	4	7	7	9
1. SINGLE DX	53	1.1	<1	1	1	1	1	2	2	4
2. MULTIPLE DX	226	2.0	5	1	1	1	2	4	6	12
A. NOT OPERATED	242	1.7	4	1	1	1	1	3	5	12
B. OPERATED	37	2.6	5	1	1	2	4	7	7	9
TOTAL										
0–19 Years	71	1.9	7	1	1	1	2	4	5	20
20–34	151	1.8	4	1	1	1	2	3	6	12
35–49	43	1.9	3	1	1	1	2	5	7	8
50–64	11	1.9	3	1	1	1	2	5	6	10
65+	3	3.7	9	1	1	3	7	11	21	21
GRAND TOTAL	279	1.9	4	1	1	1	2	4	6	12

877: OPEN WOUND OF BUTTOCK

Type of Patients	Observed Patients	Avg. Stay	Variance	10th	25th	50th	75th	90th	95th	99th
1. SINGLE DX										
A. Not Operated										
0–19 Years	14	1.3	<1	1	1	1	1	2	3	3
20–34	10	1.4	<1	1	1	1	1	3	3	3
35–49		1.0	0	1	1	1	1	1	1	1
50–64	2	2.0	0	2	2	2	2	2	2	2
65+	0									
B. Operated										
0–19 Years	0									
20–34	6	3.3	23	1	1	2	2	13	13	13
35–49	0									
50–64	0									
65+	0									
2. MULTIPLE DX										
A. Not Operated										
0–19 Years	27	1.6	1	1	1	1	2	3	3	6
20–34	50	2.6	18	1	1	1	2	4	13	24
35–49	11	1.6	2	1	1	1	2	2	6	6
50–64	4	3.3	4	2	2	2	3	6	6	6
65+	6	5.2	30	1	3	3	5	16	16	16
B. Operated										
0–19 Years	10	4.3	10	1	1	4	4	6	10	10
20–34	19	5.3	18	1	2	4	4	9	11	16
35–49	10	3.5	3	1	2	3	5	6	6	6
50–64	9	5.2	13	1	2	3	9	10	10	10
65+	3	9.7	57	1	1	13	15	15	15	15
SUBTOTALS:										
1. SINGLE DX										
A. Not Operated	27	1.4	<1	1	1	1	2	3	3	3
B. Operated	6	3.3	23	1	1	2	2	13	13	13
2. MULTIPLE DX										
A. Not Operated	98	2.4	12	1	1	1	2	4	6	24
B. Operated	51	5.0	15	1	2	3	8	10	13	16
1. SINGLE DX	33	1.7	5	1	1	1	2	3	3	13
2. MULTIPLE DX	149	3.3	15	1	1	2	4	9	11	17
A. NOT OPERATED	125	2.2	10	1	1	1	2	4	6	17
B. OPERATED	57	4.8	16	1	2	3	7	11	13	16
TOTAL										
0–19 Years	51	2.1	4	1	1	1	3	4	6	10
20–34	85	3.1	17	1	1	1	3	9	13	24
35–49	22	2.5	4	1	1	2	3	6	6	6
50–64	15	4.3	10	2	2	3	8	6	10	16
65+	9	6.7	38	1	3	3	13	16	16	16
GRAND TOTAL	182	3.0	13	1	1	1	3	7	11	17

Length of Stay by Diagnosis and Operation, Western Region, 2008

Western Region, October 2006–September 2007 Data, by Diagnosis

878: OPEN WOUND GENITAL ORGAN

Type of Patients	Observed Patients	Avg. Stay	Vari-ance	10th	25th	50th	75th	90th	95th	99th
1. SINGLE DX										
A. Not Operated										
0–19 Years	7	1.0	0	1	1	1	1	1	1	1
20–34	5	2.6	7	1	1	1	3	7	7	7
35–49	5	1.4	<1	1	1	1	2	2	2	2
50–64	1	1.0	0	1	1	1	1	1	1	1
65+	0									
B. Operated										
0–19 Years	19	1.1	<1	1	1	1	1	1	2	2
20–34	21	1.1	<1	1	1	1	1	1	2	2
35–49	5	2.0	5	1	1	1	1	6	6	6
50–64	3	2.3	<1	2	2	2	3	3	3	3
65+	0									
2. MULTIPLE DX										
A. Not Operated										
0–19 Years	15	2.0	5	1	1	1	2	6	8	8
20–34	23	2.6	12	1	1	1	2	6	10	15
35–49	18	2.0	1	1	1	2	3	3	5	5
50–64	5	2.6	7	1	1	1	3	7	7	7
65+	5	4.6	14	1	1	5	6	10	10	10
B. Operated										
0–19 Years	50	2.5	10	1	1	1	2	5	11	18
20–34	71	3.0	19	1	1	2	3	5	9	32
35–49	36	6.6	282	1	1	5	5	10	29	98
50–64	28	2.9	21	1	1	1	3	7	14	22
65+	3	2.0	3	1	1	2	4	4	4	4
SUBTOTALS:										
1. SINGLE DX										
A. Not Operated	18	1.6	2	1	1	1	1	3	7	7
B. Operated	48	1.3	<1	1	1	1	1	2	2	6
2. MULTIPLE DX										
A. Not Operated	66	2.4	7	1	1	1	3	6	8	15
B. Operated	188	3.5	68	1	1	1	3	6	12	32
1. SINGLE DX	66	1.3	1	1	1	1	1	2	3	7
2. MULTIPLE DX	254	3.3	52	1	1	1	3	6	10	29
A. NOT OPERATED	84	2.3	6	1	1	1	2	6	7	15
B. OPERATED	236	3.1	55	1	1	1	2	5	10	29
TOTAL										
0–19 Years	91	2.0	7	1	1	1	2	4	6	18
20–34	120	2.6	14	1	1	1	2	5	8	15
35–49	64	4.5	163	1	1	1	3	6	10	98
50–64	37	2.8	17	1	1	1	3	7	14	22
65+	8	3.6	11	1	1	4	6	10	10	10
GRAND TOTAL	320	2.9	42	1	1	1	2	5	10	23

879: OPEN WOUND SITE NEC

Type of Patients	Observed Patients	Avg. Stay	Vari-ance	10th	25th	50th	75th	90th	95th	99th
1. SINGLE DX										
A. Not Operated										
0–19 Years	47	1.2	<1	1	1	1	1	2	2	4
20–34	75	1.2	<1	1	1	1	1	2	2	4
35–49	12	1.2	<1	1	1	1	1	1	3	3
50–64	1	2.0	0	2	2	2	2	2	2	2
65+	0									
B. Operated										
0–19 Years	31	1.6	<1	1	1	1	2	3	3	4
20–34	26	2.6	3	1	1	1	4	5	6	7
35–49	9	1.2	<1	1	1	1	1	3	3	3
50–64	2	5.0	2	4	4	5	6	6	6	6
65+	0									
2. MULTIPLE DX										
A. Not Operated										
0–19 Years	87	1.8	2	1	1	1	2	4	4	7
20–34	217	1.6	3	1	1	1	2	3	3	9
35–49	124	2.2	9	1	1	2	2	4	5	14
50–64	53	3.1	21	1	1	1	3	6	9	28
65+	9	3.9	11	1	2	3	5	10	11	11
B. Operated										
0–19 Years	72	3.2	16	1	1	2	4	6	11	25
20–34	157	3.5	19	1	1	2	4	6	11	28
35–49	84	3.3	15	1	1	2	4	6	7	30
50–64	39	5.1	60	1	2	3	5	11	47	>99
65+	11	6.2	21	3	3	5	8	12	17	17
SUBTOTALS:										
1. SINGLE DX										
A. Not Operated	135	1.2	<1	1	1	1	1	2	2	4
B. Operated	68	2.0	2	1	1	1	3	4	5	7
2. MULTIPLE DX										
A. Not Operated	490	2.0	6	1	1	1	2	4	5	14
B. Operated	363	3.7	22	1	1	2	4	7	11	38
1. SINGLE DX	203	1.5	1	1	1	1	1	3	4	6
2. MULTIPLE DX	853	2.7	14	1	1	1	3	5	7	25
A. NOT OPERATED	625	1.8	5	1	1	1	2	3	5	10
B. OPERATED	431	3.4	19	1	1	2	4	6	10	30
TOTAL										
0–19 Years	237	2.1	6	1	1	1	2	4	5	12
20–34	475	2.2	9	1	1	1	2	4	6	15
35–49	229	2.5	11	1	1	1	3	5	6	19
50–64	95	4.0	37	1	1	1	5	9	19	>99
65+	20	5.2	17	2	2	4	7	11	12	17
GRAND TOTAL	1,056	2.5	12	1	1	1	3	5	7	19

879.2: OPN WND ANTERIOR ABDOMEN

Type of Patients	Observed Patients	Avg. Stay	Vari-ance	10th	25th	50th	75th	90th	95th	99th
1. SINGLE DX										
A. Not Operated										
0–19 Years	24	1.3	<1	1	1	1	1	2	2	4
20–34	39	1.1	<1	1	1	1	1	1	2	4
35–49	8	1.3	<1	1	1	1	1	3	3	3
50–64	0									
65+	0									
B. Operated										
0–19 Years	12	1.8	1	1	1	2	3	3	4	4
20–34	19	2.1	2	1	1	1	3	4	5	5
35–49	7	1.3	<1	1	1	1	1	3	3	3
50–64	1	6.0	0	6	6	6	6	6	6	6
65+	0									
2. MULTIPLE DX										
A. Not Operated										
0–19 Years	38	1.4	<1	1	1	1	2	3	3	3
20–34	108	1.3	<1	1	1	1	1	3	3	3
35–49	64	1.9	2	1	1	1	2	4	5	6
50–64	28	1.9	2	1	1	1	3	4	5	7
65+	2	7.0	32	3	3	11	11	11	11	11
B. Operated										
0–19 Years	35	3.3	19	1	1	2	4	6	11	25
20–34	84	3.3	20	1	1	2	4	5	7	38
35–49	56	2.9	8	1	1	2	3	6	7	19
50–64	21	3.2	4	2	2	3	4	5	7	9
65+	7	5.4	12	2	3	4	8	12	12	12
SUBTOTALS:										
1. SINGLE DX										
A. Not Operated	71	1.2	<1	1	1	1	1	2	2	4
B. Operated	39	2.0	2	1	1	1	3	4	5	6
2. MULTIPLE DX										
A. Not Operated	240	1.6	2	1	1	1	2	3	4	6
B. Operated	203	3.2	14	1	2	2	4	6	7	19
1. SINGLE DX	110	1.5	1	1	1	1	1	3	4	5
2. MULTIPLE DX	443	2.4	8	1	1	1	3	5	6	12
A. NOT OPERATED	311	1.5	1	1	1	1	2	3	4	6
B. OPERATED	242	3.0	13	1	2	2	4	5	7	19
TOTAL										
0–19 Years	109	2.0	7	1	1	1	2	4	4	11
20–34	250	2.0	8	1	1	1	2	4	5	11
35–49	135	2.2	5	1	1	1	3	5	6	7
50–64	50	2.6	3	1	1	3	5	7	9	12
65+	9	5.8	13	2	4	6	8	12	12	12
GRAND TOTAL	553	2.2	7	1	1	1	3	4	6	11

Length of Stay by Diagnosis and Operation, Western Region, 2008

Western Region, October 2006–September 2007 Data, by Diagnosis

880: OPN WND SHOULD/UPPER ARM

Type of Patients	Observed Patients	Avg. Stay	Vari- ance	Percentiles						
				10th	25th	50th	75th	90th	95th	99th
1. SINGLE DX										
A. Not Operated										
0–19 Years	15	1.2	<1	1	1	1	1	2	3	3
20–34	17	1.1	<1	1	1	1	1	1	3	3
35–49	6	1.3	<1	1	1	1	2	2	2	2
50–64	1	1.0	0	1	1	1	1	1	1	1
65+	1	2.0	0	2	2	2	2	2	2	2
B. Operated										
0–19 Years	8	1.6	1	1	1	1	2	4	4	4
20–34	7	1.7	<1	1	1	1	2	3	3	3
35–49	3	1.7	1	1	1	2	3	3	3	3
50–64	2	2.5	<1	2	2	3	3	3	3	3
65+	0									
2. MULTIPLE DX										
A. Not Operated										
0–19 Years	57	1.6	1	1	1	1	2	3	4	7
20–34	98	1.8	2	1	1	1	2	4	6	9
35–49	57	3.1	18	1	1	1	3	8	16	19
50–64	26	2.1	3	1	1	1	3	4	6	7
65+	19	2.8	4	1	1	2	4	5	8	8
B. Operated										
0–19 Years	31	4.6	63	1	1	2	4	9	25	40
20–34	64	3.9	32	1	1	2	4	7	12	31
35–49	41	4.6	40	1	2	3	5	8	15	36
50–64	17	4.2	13	1	2	3	6	12	12	12
65+	8	4.3	30	1	1	2	6	17	17	17
SUBTOTALS:										
1. SINGLE DX										
A. Not Operated	40	1.2	<1	1	1	1	1	2	3	3
B. Operated	20	1.8	<1	1	1	1	2	3	4	4
2. MULTIPLE DX										
A. Not Operated	257	2.2	6	1	1	1	2	4	6	16
B. Operated	161	4.3	37	1	1	2	4	8	15	36
1. SINGLE DX	60	1.4	<1	1	1	1	2	3	3	4
2. MULTIPLE DX	418	3.0	19	1	1	1	3	6	9	25
A. NOT OPERATED	297	2.0	5	1	1	1	2	4	6	16
B. OPERATED	181	4.0	34	1	1	2	4	8	12	36
TOTAL										
0–19 Years	111	2.4	20	1	1	1	2	4	5	25
20–34	186	2.4	13	1	1	1	3	5	8	25
35–49	107	3.6	25	1	1	2	3	8	15	20
50–64	46	2.9	7	1	1	2	4	7	8	12
65+	28	3.2	11	1	1	2	4	6	8	17
GRAND TOTAL	478	2.8	17	1	1	1	3	5	8	25

881: OPEN WOUND OF LOWER ARM

Type of Patients	Observed Patients	Avg. Stay	Vari- ance	Percentiles						
				10th	25th	50th	75th	90th	95th	99th
1. SINGLE DX										
A. Not Operated										
0–19 Years	19	1.3	<1	1	1	1	1	2	2	3
20–34	9	1.5	<1	1	1	1	2	3	3	3
35–49	9	1.7	2	1	1	1	2	5	5	5
50–64	5	1.8	1	1	1	1	3	3	3	3
65+	0									
B. Operated										
0–19 Years	28	1.9	4	1	1	2	2	4	7	9
20–34	50	1.8	4	1	1	1	2	3	4	9
35–49	26	1.6	2	1	1	1	2	4	5	9
50–64	10	1.6	2	1	1	1	2	3	5	6
65+	1	1.0	0	1	1	1	1	1	1	1
2. MULTIPLE DX										
A. Not Operated										
0–19 Years	57	1.6	1	1	1	1	2	3	4	5
20–34	136	1.9	3	1	1	1	2	4	5	9
35–49	114	2.5	4	1	1	2	3	5	8	10
50–64	80	2.9	8	1	1	2	3	6	9	16
65+	76	3.3	7	1	2	3	3	6	10	15
B. Operated										
0–19 Years	100	2.6	12	1	1	2	2	4	7	20
20–34	306	3.0	14	1	1	2	3	6	10	20
35–49	191	2.9	10	1	1	2	3	6	9	17
50–64	100	4.0	30	1	1	2	4	9	12	38
65+	56	4.2	14	1	1	3	6	9	10	19
SUBTOTALS:										
1. SINGLE DX										
A. Not Operated	42	1.5	<1	1	1	1	2	3	3	5
B. Operated	115	1.8	2	1	1	1	2	4	5	9
2. MULTIPLE DX										
A. Not Operated	463	2.4	5	1	1	2	3	5	6	12
B. Operated	753	3.2	15	1	1	2	3	6	10	20
1. SINGLE DX	157	1.7	2	1	1	1	2	3	5	9
2. MULTIPLE DX	1,216	2.9	11	1	1	2	3	6	9	17
A. NOT OPERATED	505	2.3	4	1	1	2	3	4	6	12
B. OPERATED	868	3.0	14	1	1	2	3	6	9	20
TOTAL										
0–19 Years	204	2.1	7	1	1	1	2	4	5	17
20–34	501	2.6	10	1	1	2	3	5	8	17
35–49	340	2.6	7	1	1	2	3	5	8	13
50–64	195	3.4	19	1	1	2	3	7	10	27
65+	133	3.6	10	1	2	3	4	8	10	15
GRAND TOTAL	1,373	2.7	10	1	1	2	3	6	9	17

881.00: OPEN WOUND OF FOREARM

Type of Patients	Observed Patients	Avg. Stay	Vari- ance	Percentiles						
				10th	25th	50th	75th	90th	95th	99th
1. SINGLE DX										
A. Not Operated										
0–19 Years	7	1.1	<1	1	1	1	1	2	2	2
20–34	2	1.0	0	1	1	1	1	1	2	2
35–49	2	1.0	0	1	1	1	1	1	1	1
50–64	2	1.0	0	1	1	1	1	1	1	1
65+	0									
B. Operated										
0–19 Years	3	3.0	12	1	1	1	7	7	7	7
20–34	6	2.5	10	1	1	1	2	7	9	9
35–49	6	1.5	1	1	1	1	2	4	4	4
50–64	2	2.0	2	1	1	3	3	3	3	3
65+	0									
2. MULTIPLE DX										
A. Not Operated										
0–19 Years	22	1.4	<1	1	1	1	1	2	3	4
20–34	47	1.5	1	1	1	1	2	3	4	5
35–49	27	1.9	2	1	1	2	3	3	4	6
50–64	17	2.2	3	1	1	2	3	4	7	7
65+	25	3.3	5	2	2	3	4	5	6	12
B. Operated										
0–19 Years	11	2.4	5	1	1	2	4	6	7	7
20–34	24	3.2	7	1	1	2	5	5	8	10
35–49	13	2.4	3	1	1	2	3	5	5	17
50–64	14	3.3	24	1	1	1	3	3	12	17
65+	14	5.0	8	1	3	4	8	8	10	10
SUBTOTALS:										
1. SINGLE DX										
A. Not Operated	13	1.1	<1	1	1	1	1	1	2	2
B. Operated	17	2.2	6	1	1	1	2	7	9	9
2. MULTIPLE DX										
A. Not Operated	138	2.0	2	1	1	1	2	4	5	7
B. Operated	76	3.3	10	1	1	2	4	8	10	17
1. SINGLE DX	30	1.7	3	1	1	1	1	3	7	9
2. MULTIPLE DX	214	2.5	5	1	1	2	3	5	7	12
A. NOT OPERATED	151	1.9	2	1	1	1	2	4	5	7
B. OPERATED	93	3.1	9	1	1	2	4	8	9	17
TOTAL										
0–19 Years	43	1.7	2	1	1	1	2	4	6	7
20–34	79	2.1	4	1	1	1	2	5	8	10
35–49	48	1.9	2	1	1	1	3	4	5	7
50–64	35	2.6	11	1	1	1	3	4	12	17
65+	39	3.9	5	1	2	3	5	8	10	12
GRAND TOTAL	244	2.4	5	1	1	1	3	5	7	12

Length of Stay by Diagnosis and Operation, Western Region, 2008

Western Region, October 2006–September 2007 Data, by Diagnosis

881.10: OPEN WOUND FOREARM-COMP

Type of Patients	Observed Patients	Avg. Stay	Variance	10th	25th	50th	75th	90th	95th	99th
1. SINGLE DX										
A. Not Operated										
0–19 Years	3	1.3	<1	1	1	1	2	2	2	2
20–34	1	2.0	0	2	2	2	2	2	2	2
35–49	3	1.0	0	1	1	1	1	1	1	1
50–64	2	2.0	2	1	1	3	3	3	3	3
65+	0									
B. Operated										
0–19 Years	4	3.5	14	1	1	3	9	9	9	9
20–34	4	1.5	1	1	1	1	3	3	3	3
35–49	4	1.0	0	1	1	1	1	1	1	1
50–64	3	2.3	5	1	1	1	5	5	5	5
65+	0									
2. MULTIPLE DX										
A. Not Operated										
0–19 Years	12	1.9	<1	1	1	2	3	3	3	3
20–34	24	2.0	1	1	1	2	3	3	4	5
35–49	21	3.1	5	1	2	2	4	5	8	10
50–64	21	2.6	6	1	1	2	3	5	5	12
65+	19	3.7	9	2	2	3	4	6	15	15
B. Operated										
0–19 Years	13	2.8	4	1	1	3	4	5	7	7
20–34	41	3.9	16	1	1	2	5	7	12	17
35–49	38	3.3	8	1	2	2	4	7	12	13
50–64	20	8.8	92	2	3	4	9	22	27	38
65+	9	5.8	35	1	2	3	9	19	19	19
SUBTOTALS:										
1. SINGLE DX										
A. Not Operated	9	1.5	<1	1	1	1	2	2	3	3
B. Operated	15	2.1	5	1	1	2	3	3	9	9
2. MULTIPLE DX										
A. Not Operated	97	2.7	5	1	1	2	3	5	6	15
B. Operated	121	4.6	29	1	1	3	5	9	13	27
1. SINGLE DX	24	1.8	3	1	1	1	2	3	5	9
2. MULTIPLE DX	218	3.7	19	1	1	2	4	8	12	22
A. NOT OPERATED	106	2.6	5	1	1	2	3	5	5	12
B. OPERATED	136	4.3	27	1	1	3	5	9	13	27
TOTAL										
0–19 Years	32	2.4	4	1	1	2	3	4	7	9
20–34	70	3.1	10	1	1	2	4	7	11	17
35–49	66	3.0	7	1	1	2	3	7	9	13
50–64	46	5.3	52	1	2	3	5	12	22	38
65+	28	4.4	17	1	2	3	5	9	15	19
GRAND TOTAL	242	3.5	18	1	1	2	4	8	11	22

881.20: OPN WND FOREARM W TENDON

Type of Patients	Observed Patients	Avg. Stay	Variance	10th	25th	50th	75th	90th	95th	99th
1. SINGLE DX										
A. Not Operated										
0–19 Years	1	2.0	0	2	2	2	2	2	2	2
20–34	2	2.0	2	1	1	3	3	3	3	3
35–49	2	2.0	0	2	2	2	2	2	2	2
50–64	0									
65+	0									
B. Operated										
0–19 Years	4	1.8	<1	1	1	2	3	3	3	3
20–34	16	1.7	2	1	1	1	2	3	6	6
35–49	8	1.8	2	1	1	1	1	5	5	5
50–64	4	1.0	0	1	1	1	1	1	1	1
65+	1	1.0	0	1	1	1	1	1	1	1
2. MULTIPLE DX										
A. Not Operated										
0–19 Years	1	1.0	0	1	1	1	1	1	1	1
20–34	6	2.2	<1	1	2	2	3	3	3	3
35–49	3	1.7	1	1	1	1	3	3	3	3
50–64	2	3.0	0	3	3	3	3	3	3	3
65+	0									
B. Operated										
0–19 Years	36	2.1	7	1	1	2	2	3	6	17
20–34	106	2.9	12	1	1	2	3	6	8	18
35–49	66	3.2	15	1	1	2	4	6	9	25
50–64	13	1.9	2	1	1	1	2	3	6	6
65+	10	1.8	0	1	1	1	2	3	4	4
SUBTOTALS:										
1. SINGLE DX										
A. Not Operated	4	2.0	<1	2	2	2	3	3	3	3
B. Operated	33	1.6	1	1	1	1	2	3	5	6
2. MULTIPLE DX										
A. Not Operated	12	2.1	<1	1	1	2	3	3	3	3
B. Operated	231	2.7	11	1	1	2	3	5	8	18
1. SINGLE DX	37	1.7	1	1	1	1	2	3	5	6
2. MULTIPLE DX	243	2.7	11	1	1	2	3	5	7	18
A. NOT OPERATED	16	2.1	<1	1	1	2	3	3	3	3
B. OPERATED	264	2.6	10	1	1	2	3	5	6	18
TOTAL										
0–19 Years	42	2.1	6	1	1	2	3	4	6	17
20–34	130	2.7	10	1	1	2	3	5	6	18
35–49	78	2.9	13	1	1	2	3	6	9	25
50–64	19	1.8	2	1	1	2	3	5	6	6
65+	11	1.7	1	1	1	2	3	4	4	4
GRAND TOTAL	280	2.6	10	1	1	2	3	5	6	18

882: OPEN WOUND OF HAND

Type of Patients	Observed Patients	Avg. Stay	Variance	10th	25th	50th	75th	90th	95th	99th
1. SINGLE DX										
A. Not Operated										
0–19 Years	10	2.0	2	1	2	2	2	5	5	5
20–34	32	2.1	1	1	1	2	3	3	5	5
35–49	17	1.7	<1	1	1	1	2	3	4	4
50–64	7	1.6	<1	1	1	2	2	2	2	2
65+	0									
B. Operated										
0–19 Years	16	2.8	18	1	1	1	3	4	18	18
20–34	31	1.9	2	1	1	1	2	4	6	7
35–49	20	2.1	3	1	1	1	2	4	9	9
50–64	8	2.0	3	1	1	2	3	6	6	6
65+	2	2.0	2	1	1	2	3	3	3	3
2. MULTIPLE DX										
A. Not Operated										
0–19 Years	29	2.0	2	1	1	2	3	4	5	6
20–34	88	2.3	3	1	1	2	3	5	6	12
35–49	55	2.3	4	1	1	2	3	5	7	12
50–64	63	2.3	3	1	1	2	3	4	5	7
65+	60	2.8	3	1	1	3	4	5	6	10
B. Operated										
0–19 Years	63	3.4	16	1	1	2	3	7	13	23
20–34	197	2.7	9	1	1	2	3	5	7	14
35–49	106	4.0	33	1	1	3	4	6	12	21
50–64	86	3.1	8	1	1	3	4	6	8	16
65+	50	3.1	5	1	1	3	4	6	8	10
SUBTOTALS:										
1. SINGLE DX										
A. Not Operated	66	1.9	1	1	1	2	3	3	4	5
B. Operated	77	2.1	6	1	1	1	2	4	6	18
2. MULTIPLE DX										
A. Not Operated	295	2.4	3	1	1	2	3	4	6	10
B. Operated	502	3.2	15	1	1	2	4	6	8	16
1. SINGLE DX	143	2.0	4	1	1	1	2	4	5	9
2. MULTIPLE DX	797	2.9	10	1	1	2	3	5	7	14
A. NOT OPERATED	361	2.3	3	1	1	2	3	4	5	8
B. OPERATED	579	3.0	14	1	1	2	3	6	8	18
TOTAL										
0–19 Years	118	2.9	12	1	1	2	3	6	10	18
20–34	348	2.5	6	1	1	2	3	5	6	12
35–49	198	3.1	20	1	1	2	4	5	9	21
50–64	164	2.7	5	1	1	2	3	5	6	14
65+	112	2.9	4	1	1	3	4	6	7	10
GRAND TOTAL	940	2.7	9	1	1	2	3	5	7	14

Length of Stay by Diagnosis and Operation, Western Region, 2008

Western Region, October 2006–September 2007 Data, by Diagnosis

882.1: OPEN WOUND HAND-COMP

Type of Patients	Observed Patients	Avg. Stay	Variance	10th	25th	50th	75th	90th	95th	99th
1. SINGLE DX										
A. Not Operated										
0–19 Years	6	2.5	2	1	2	2	3	5	5	5
20–34	19	2.4	2	1	1	2	3	5	5	5
35–49	14	1.9	1	1	1	2	3	3	4	4
50–64	5	1.8	<1	1	2	2	2	2	2	2
65+	0									
B. Operated										
0–19 Years	7	3.6	41	1	1	1	2	18	18	18
20–34	16	1.9	<1	1	1	1	2	3	6	6
35–49	8	2.3	<1	2	2	2	3	3	3	3
50–64	4	2.8	6	1	1	3	6	6	6	6
65+	0									
2. MULTIPLE DX										
A. Not Operated										
0–19 Years	14	2.2	2	1	1	2	3	5	6	6
20–34	52	2.6	3	1	1	2	3	5	6	8
35–49	41	2.4	4	1	1	2	3	4	4	12
50–64	44	2.5	2	2	2	2	4	4	5	7
65+	41	3.1	4	1	2	3	4	6	6	10
B. Operated										
0–19 Years	27	4.4	27	1	2	2	4	13	15	23
20–34	79	2.8	4	1	1	2	3	5	7	14
35–49	53	4.8	57	1	2	3	5	7	18	52
50–64	38	3.8	7	1	2	3	5	7	9	14
65+	27	3.5	7	1	1	3	6	8	9	10
SUBTOTALS:										
1. SINGLE DX										
A. Not Operated	44	2.2	1	1	1	2	3	4	5	5
B. Operated	35	2.4	9	1	1	2	2	4	6	18
2. MULTIPLE DX										
A. Not Operated	192	2.6	3	1	1	2	3	5	6	10
B. Operated	224	3.7	21	1	2	3	4	6	9	21
1. SINGLE DX	79	2.3	5	1	1	2	3	4	5	18
2. MULTIPLE DX	416	3.2	13	1	2	2	4	6	8	15
A. NOT OPERATED	236	2.5	3	1	1	2	3	5	6	8
B. OPERATED	259	3.5	19	1	2	2	4	6	9	21
TOTAL										
0–19 Years	54	3.5	20	1	1	2	3	7	15	23
20–34	166	2.6	3	1	1	2	3	5	6	8
35–49	116	3.4	29	1	2	2	4	5	9	21
50–64	91	3.0	4	2	2	2	4	5	7	14
65+	68	3.3	5	2	2	3	4	6	8	10
GRAND TOTAL	495	3.1	12	1	1	2	4	6	7	18

882.2: OPEN WOUND HAND W TENDON

Type of Patients	Observed Patients	Avg. Stay	Variance	10th	25th	50th	75th	90th	95th	99th
1. SINGLE DX										
A. Not Operated										
0–19 Years	0									
20–34	2	1.5	<1	1	1	1	2	2	2	2
35–49	0									
50–64	1	1.0	0	1	1	1	1	1	1	1
65+	0									
B. Operated										
0–19 Years	8	2.3	2	1	1	2	4	4	4	4
20–34	9	1.7	<1	1	1	1	2	3	3	3
35–49	10	2.1	7	1	1	2	1	9	9	9
50–64	4	1.3	<1	1	1	2	2	2	2	2
65+	1	3.0	0	3	3	3	3	3	3	3
2. MULTIPLE DX										
A. Not Operated										
0–19 Years	2	2.5	4	1	1	3	4	4	4	4
20–34	4	2.0	4	1	1	1	1	5	5	5
35–49	5	1.2	<1	1	1	1	1	2	2	2
50–64	2	1.5	<1	1	1	1	2	2	2	2
65+	1	3.0	0	3	3	3	3	3	3	3
B. Operated										
0–19 Years	29	2.6	8	1	1	2	3	7	8	14
20–34	89	2.6	14	1	1	2	3	5	6	32
35–49	43	3.3	11	1	1	2	4	7	12	14
50–64	36	2.8	11	1	1	2	3	6	13	16
65+	13	2.9	3	3	3	3	4	5	7	7
SUBTOTALS:										
1. SINGLE DX										
A. Not Operated	3	1.3	<1	1	1	1	1	2	2	2
B. Operated	32	1.9	3	1	1	1	3	4	6	9
2. MULTIPLE DX										
A. Not Operated	14	1.8	2	1	1	2	3	4	5	5
B. Operated	210	2.8	11	1	1	2	4	6	8	14
1. SINGLE DX	35	1.9	3	1	1	2	3	4	5	9
2. MULTIPLE DX	224	2.7	10	1	1	2	3	5	8	14
A. NOT OPERATED	17	1.7	1	1	1	2	2	4	5	5
B. OPERATED	242	2.7	10	1	1	2	3	5	8	14
TOTAL										
0–19 Years	39	2.5	6	1	1	2	3	4	5	14
20–34	104	2.5	12	1	1	2	3	4	6	12
35–49	58	2.9	9	1	1	2	4	5	7	14
50–64	43	2.5	9	1	1	2	3	5	6	16
65+	15	2.9	3	1	1	3	4	6	8	7
GRAND TOTAL	259	2.6	9	1	1	2	3	5	8	14

883: OPEN WOUND OF FINGER

Type of Patients	Observed Patients	Avg. Stay	Variance	10th	25th	50th	75th	90th	95th	99th
1. SINGLE DX										
A. Not Operated										
0–19 Years	8	1.9	<1	1	1	1	3	3	3	3
20–34	19	1.9	2	1	1	1	2	3	6	6
35–49	19	1.7	<1	1	1	1	2	4	4	4
50–64	7	1.6	<1	1	1	2	2	2	2	2
65+	0									
B. Operated										
0–19 Years	22	1.5	<1	1	1	1	2	2	3	3
20–34	60	2.1	2	1	1	2	3	4	4	7
35–49	35	1.9	2	1	1	1	2	3	5	8
50–64	21	2.0	4	1	1	1	2	4	4	9
65+	2	1.0	0	1	1	1	1	1	1	1
2. MULTIPLE DX										
A. Not Operated										
0–19 Years	11	2.6	2	1	1	2	3	4	6	6
20–34	57	1.9	2	1	1	2	3	3	3	9
35–49	61	2.8	7	1	1	2	3	5	8	15
50–64	45	2.4	4	1	1	2	3	4	4	7
65+	29	2.3	4	1	1	3	3	5	8	9
B. Operated										
0–19 Years	64	2.6	5	1	1	2	3	6	8	11
20–34	252	2.6	5	1	1	2	3	5	6	11
35–49	206	2.9	6	1	1	2	4	6	7	13
50–64	139	3.1	16	1	1	2	3	6	9	28
65+	49	2.9	7	1	1	2	4	6	9	14
SUBTOTALS:										
1. SINGLE DX										
A. Not Operated	53	1.8	1	1	1	1	2	3	4	6
B. Operated	140	1.9	2	1	1	1	2	3	4	8
2. MULTIPLE DX										
A. Not Operated	203	2.4	4	1	1	2	3	4	6	10
B. Operated	710	2.7	8	1	1	2	3	5	7	13
1. SINGLE DX	193	1.9	2	1	1	1	2	3	4	8
2. MULTIPLE DX	913	2.7	7	1	1	2	3	5	7	13
A. NOT OPERATED	256	2.3	3	1	1	2	3	4	5	10
B. OPERATED	850	2.6	7	1	1	2	3	5	7	13
TOTAL										
0–19 Years	105	2.3	3	1	1	2	3	4	6	8
20–34	388	2.3	4	1	1	2	3	4	5	10
35–49	321	2.7	6	1	1	2	3	5	7	13
50–64	212	2.8	11	1	1	2	3	6	7	16
65+	80	2.6	6	1	1	2	3	6	8	14
GRAND TOTAL	1,106	2.5	6	1	1	2	3	5	7	12

Length of Stay by Diagnosis and Operation, Western Region, 2008

Western Region, October 2006–September 2007 Data, by Diagnosis

883.1: OPEN WND FINGER-COMP

Type of Patients	Observed Patients	Avg. Stay	Variance	10th	25th	50th	75th	90th	95th	99th
1. SINGLE DX										
A. Not Operated										
0–19 Years	4	1.5	1	1	1	1	3	3	3	3
20–34	13	1.8	1	1	1	2	3	3	5	5
35–49	14	1.8	1	1	1	2	2	4	4	4
50–64	4	1.8	<1	1	1	2	2	2	2	2
65+	0									
B. Operated										
0–19 Years	4	1.8	<1	1	1	1	3	3	3	3
20–34	17	2.2	<1	1	2	2	3	3	4	4
35–49	18	2.3	3	1	1	2	3	5	8	8
50–64	10	2.7	6	1	1	2	4	4	9	9
65+	0									
2. MULTIPLE DX										
A. Not Operated										
0–19 Years	8	2.6	3	1	1	2	3	6	6	6
20–34	29	2.1	3	1	1	2	3	3	3	9
35–49	48	3.2	8	1	2	3	3	8	10	15
50–64	37	2.5	2	1	1	3	3	4	6	7
65+	14	2.7	4	1	1	3	3	5	8	8
B. Operated										
0–19 Years	20	3.9	6	2	2	3	5	8	11	11
20–34	74	3.3	10	1	2	2	4	6	10	22
35–49	85	3.3	5	1	2	2	4	6	7	14
50–64	49	4.0	20	1	2	3	4	7	11	28
65+	16	2.9	5	1	1	2	4	5	9	9
SUBTOTALS:										
1. SINGLE DX — A. Not Operated	35	1.8	1	1	1	2	2	3	4	5
1. SINGLE DX — B. Operated	49	2.3	3	1	1	2	3	4	5	9
2. MULTIPLE DX — A. Not Operated	136	2.7	4	1	1	2	3	4	8	10
2. MULTIPLE DX — B. Operated	244	3.5	10	1	2	3	4	6	9	16
1. SINGLE DX	84	2.1	2	1	1	2	2	4	4	9
2. MULTIPLE DX	380	3.2	8	1	2	3	4	6	8	15
A. NOT OPERATED	171	2.5	4	1	1	2	3	4	6	10
B. OPERATED	293	3.3	9	1	2	2	4	6	8	16
TOTAL										
0–19 Years	36	3.1	5	1	2	3	4	6	8	11
20–34	133	2.7	7	1	1	2	3	5	7	13
35–49	165	3.0	5	1	2	2	4	6	8	14
50–64	100	3.3	12	1	1	2	4	6	7	28
65+	30	2.8	4	1	1	2	4	6	8	9
GRAND TOTAL	464	3.0	7	1	1	2	4	5	8	14

883.2: OPEN WND FINGER W TENDON

Type of Patients	Observed Patients	Avg. Stay	Variance	10th	25th	50th	75th	90th	95th	99th
1. SINGLE DX										
A. Not Operated										
0–19 Years	0									
20–34	1	6.0	0	6	6	6	6	6	6	6
35–49	0									
50–64	2	1.5	<1	1	1	2	2	2	2	2
65+	0									
B. Operated										
0–19 Years	14	1.4	<1	1	1	1	2	3	3	3
20–34	38	1.9	1	1	1	2	2	3	4	5
35–49	16	1.4	<1	1	1	1	1	3	3	3
50–64	9	1.3	<1	1	1	1	1	3	3	3
65+	1	1.0	0	1	1	1	1	1	1	1
2. MULTIPLE DX										
A. Not Operated										
0–19 Years	0									
20–34	8	1.8	<1	1	1	1	3	3	3	3
35–49	4	2.0	1	1	1	1	3	3	3	3
50–64	0									
65+	2	1.0	0	1	1	1	1	1	1	1
B. Operated										
0–19 Years	39	2.1	3	1	1	1	2	5	8	8
20–34	161	2.1	2	1	1	2	3	4	5	8
35–49	113	2.5	7	1	1	2	3	5	7	13
50–64	78	2.6	14	1	1	2	3	5	7	31
65+	28	2.8	7	1	1	2	3	4	6	14
SUBTOTALS:										
1. SINGLE DX — A. Not Operated	3	3.0	7	1	1	2	2	6	6	6
1. SINGLE DX — B. Operated	78	1.6	<1	1	1	1	2	3	4	5
2. MULTIPLE DX — A. Not Operated	14	1.7	<1	1	1	1	3	3	3	3
2. MULTIPLE DX — B. Operated	419	2.4	6	1	2	2	3	5	6	13
1. SINGLE DX	81	1.7	1	1	1	1	2	3	4	6
2. MULTIPLE DX	433	2.3	6	1	1	2	3	5	6	13
A. NOT OPERATED	17	1.9	2	1	1	1	3	3	6	6
B. OPERATED	497	2.2	5	1	1	2	3	4	6	10
TOTAL										
0–19 Years	53	1.9	3	1	1	1	2	4	6	8
20–34	208	2.1	2	1	1	2	2	4	5	8
35–49	133	2.4	6	1	1	1	3	4	6	13
50–64	89	2.4	12	1	1	2	3	4	7	31
65+	31	2.6	7	1	1	2	3	6	6	14
GRAND TOTAL	514	2.2	5	1	1	2	3	4	6	10

884: MULT/NOS OPEN WOUND ARM

Type of Patients	Observed Patients	Avg. Stay	Variance	10th	25th	50th	75th	90th	95th	99th
1. SINGLE DX										
A. Not Operated										
0–19 Years	1	1.0	0	1	1	1	1	1	1	1
20–34	2	2.0	2	1	1	2	3	3	3	3
35–49	1	1.0	0	1	1	1	1	1	1	1
50–64	0									
65+	0									
B. Operated										
0–19 Years	1	3.0	0	3	3	3	3	3	3	3
20–34	1	1.0	0	1	1	1	1	1	1	1
35–49	0									
50–64	0									
65+	0									
2. MULTIPLE DX										
A. Not Operated										
0–19 Years	3	4.0	27	1	1	1	10	10	10	10
20–34	7	2.7	7	1	2	3	4	8	8	8
35–49	9	4.1	11	2	2	3	10	10	10	10
50–64	5	4.8	23	1	4	4	10	10	10	10
65+	3	4.0	0	4	4	4	4	4	4	4
B. Operated										
0–19 Years	3	6.7	32	2	2	5	13	13	13	13
20–34	12	5.3	44	1	1	3	5	14	22	22
35–49	8	2.3	2	1	1	2	3	5	5	5
50–64	7	3.8	4	1	3	3	6	7	7	7
65+	2	6.0	8	4	4	6	8	8	8	8
SUBTOTALS:										
1. SINGLE DX — A. Not Operated	4	1.5	<1	1	1	1	3	3	3	3
1. SINGLE DX — B. Operated	2	2.0	2	1	1	2	3	3	3	3
2. MULTIPLE DX — A. Not Operated	27	3.8	11	1	1	3	4	10	10	10
2. MULTIPLE DX — B. Operated	32	4.4	21	1	1	3	5	9	14	22
1. SINGLE DX	6	1.7	1	1	1	1	3	3	3	3
2. MULTIPLE DX	59	4.1	17	1	1	3	5	10	13	22
A. NOT OPERATED	31	3.5	10	1	1	2	4	10	10	10
B. OPERATED	34	4.2	21	1	1	3	5	9	14	22
TOTAL										
0–19 Years	8	4.5	21	1	1	3	5	13	13	13
20–34	21	4.1	28	1	1	2	4	9	14	22
35–49	19	3.0	7	1	1	2	3	10	10	10
50–64	12	4.2	11	1	3	3	6	10	10	10
65+	5	4.8	3	4	4	4	4	8	8	8
GRAND TOTAL	65	3.9	16	1	1	3	4	10	10	22

Length of Stay by Diagnosis and Operation, Western Region, 2008

Western Region, October 2006–September 2007 Data, by Diagnosis

885: TRAUM AMPUTATION THUMB

Type of Patients	Observed Patients	Avg. Stay	Variance	10th	25th	50th	75th	90th	95th	99th
1. SINGLE DX										
A. Not Operated										
0–19 Years	1	4.0	0	4	4	4	4	4	4	4
20–34	0									
35–49	0									
50–64	1	1.0	0	1	1	1	1	1	1	1
65+	0									
B. Operated										
0–19 Years	5	1.8	2	1	1	1	2	4	4	4
20–34	13	3.5	3	2	2	3	5	6	7	7
35–49	9	2.2	5	1	1	1	2	6	6	6
50–64	11	2.2	7	1	1	1	2	5	9	9
65+	2	1.5	<1	1	1	2	2	2	2	2
2. MULTIPLE DX										
A. Not Operated										
0–19 Years	0									
20–34	1	3.0	0	3	3	3	3	3	3	3
35–49	1	1.0	0	1	1	1	1	1	1	1
50–64	1	1.0	0	1	1	1	1	1	1	1
65+	1	1.0	0	1	1	1	1	1	1	1
B. Operated										
0–19 Years	9	4.2	11	1	3	3	5	12	12	12
20–34	53	3.2	11	1	1	2	4	7	11	17
35–49	58	3.2	12	1	1	2	5	8	12	13
50–64	52	2.7	5	1	1	2	4	6	7	9
65+	16	3.1	3	1	2	3	4	5	7	7
SUBTOTALS:										
1. SINGLE DX										
A. Not Operated	2	2.5	4	1	1	4	4	4	4	4
B. Operated	40	2.5	4	1	1	2	4	6	6	9
2. MULTIPLE DX										
A. Not Operated	4	1.5	<1	1	1	1	1	1	3	3
B. Operated	188	3.1	9	1	1	2	4	7	9	13
1. SINGLE DX	42	2.5	4	1	1	2	4	6	6	9
2. MULTIPLE DX	192	3.1	9	1	1	2	4	7	9	13
A. NOT OPERATED	6	1.8	2	1	1	1	3	4	4	4
B. OPERATED	228	3.0	8	1	1	2	4	7	9	13
TOTAL										
0–19 Years	15	3.4	8	1	1	3	5	5	12	12
20–34	67	3.2	9	1	1	2	4	7	10	17
35–49	68	3.1	11	1	1	1	4	8	12	13
50–64	65	2.6	5	1	1	2	3	6	7	9
65+	19	2.8	3	1	1	2	4	5	7	7
GRAND TOTAL	234	3.0	8	1	1	2	4	7	9	13

886: TRAUM AMPUTATION FINGER

Type of Patients	Observed Patients	Avg. Stay	Variance	10th	25th	50th	75th	90th	95th	99th
1. SINGLE DX										
A. Not Operated										
0–19 Years	1	1.0	0	1	1	1	1	1	1	1
20–34	2	1.0	0	1	1	1	1	1	1	1
35–49	2	1.5	<1	1	1	2	2	2	2	2
50–64	1	1.0	0	1	1	1	1	1	1	1
65+	0									
B. Operated										
0–19 Years	32	2.3	5	1	1	1	2	6	8	10
20–34	33	1.6	2	1	1	1	2	3	5	6
35–49	26	1.6	1	1	1	1	2	3	4	6
50–64	24	2.3	6	1	1	1	2	8	8	9
65+	3	1.0	0	1	1	1	1	1	1	1
2. MULTIPLE DX										
A. Not Operated										
0–19 Years	1	1.0	0	1	1	1	1	1	1	1
20–34	6	2.7	3	1	1	2	4	5	5	5
35–49	3	2.0	3	1	1	1	1	1	4	4
50–64	3	1.7	<1	1	1	2	2	2	2	2
65+	4	1.3	<1	1	1	1	1	2	2	2
B. Operated										
0–19 Years	53	3.5	13	1	1	2	5	9	10	18
20–34	160	2.6	7	1	1	2	3	6	9	16
35–49	176	2.7	10	1	1	2	3	5	8	20
50–64	129	2.7	8	1	1	2	3	6	9	13
65+	63	2.2	2	1	1	2	3	5	5	8
SUBTOTALS:										
1. SINGLE DX										
A. Not Operated	6	1.2	<1	1	1	1	1	2	2	2
B. Operated	118	1.9	3	1	1	1	2	4	6	9
2. MULTIPLE DX										
A. Not Operated	17	1.9	2	1	1	1	2	4	5	5
B. Operated	581	2.7	8	1	1	2	3	6	8	17
1. SINGLE DX	124	1.9	3	1	1	1	2	4	6	9
2. MULTIPLE DX	598	2.7	8	1	1	2	3	6	8	16
A. NOT OPERATED	23	1.7	1	1	1	1	2	4	4	5
B. OPERATED	699	2.6	8	1	1	2	3	6	8	16
TOTAL										
0–19 Years	87	3.0	10	1	1	2	3	5	9	18
20–34	201	2.4	6	1	1	1	3	5	7	16
35–49	207	2.5	9	1	1	2	3	5	7	18
50–64	157	2.6	8	1	1	2	3	6	9	13
65+	70	2.1	2	1	1	2	2	4	5	7
GRAND TOTAL	722	2.5	8	1	1	2	3	5	8	16

886.0: AMPUTATION FINGER

Type of Patients	Observed Patients	Avg. Stay	Variance	10th	25th	50th	75th	90th	95th	99th
1. SINGLE DX										
A. Not Operated										
0–19 Years	1	1.0	0	1	1	1	1	1	1	1
20–34	2	1.0	0	1	1	1	1	1	1	1
35–49	2	1.5	<1	1	1	2	2	2	2	2
50–64	1	1.0	0	1	1	1	1	1	1	1
65+	0									
B. Operated										
0–19 Years	30	2.2	5	1	1	1	2	5	8	10
20–34	28	1.5	1	1	1	1	2	3	4	6
35–49	22	1.6	1	1	1	1	2	2	4	6
50–64	21	2.0	5	1	1	1	2	3	8	9
65+	3	1.0	0	1	1	1	1	1	1	1
2. MULTIPLE DX										
A. Not Operated										
0–19 Years	1	1.0	0	1	1	1	1	1	1	1
20–34	5	2.2	2	1	1	2	3	4	4	4
35–49	2	2.5	4	1	1	1	2	2	4	4
50–64	3	1.7	<1	1	1	2	2	2	2	2
65+	4	1.3	<1	1	1	1	1	2	2	2
B. Operated										
0–19 Years	42	3.5	15	1	1	2	5	9	10	18
20–34	137	2.4	5	1	1	2	3	6	7	13
35–49	143	2.6	10	1	1	2	3	5	6	20
50–64	108	2.7	9	1	1	2	3	6	9	13
65+	54	2.2	2	1	1	2	3	4	5	6
SUBTOTALS:										
1. SINGLE DX										
A. Not Operated	6	1.2	<1	1	1	1	1	2	2	2
B. Operated	104	1.8	3	1	1	2	2	4	6	9
2. MULTIPLE DX										
A. Not Operated	15	1.8	1	1	1	1	2	4	4	4
B. Operated	484	2.6	8	1	1	2	3	5	8	17
1. SINGLE DX	110	1.8	3	1	1	1	2	3	6	9
2. MULTIPLE DX	499	2.6	8	1	1	2	3	5	8	16
A. NOT OPERATED	21	1.6	<1	1	1	1	2	3	4	4
B. OPERATED	588	2.5	7	1	1	2	3	5	7	16
TOTAL										
0–19 Years	74	2.9	11	1	1	2	3	7	10	18
20–34	172	2.2	5	1	1	1	3	4	6	13
35–49	169	2.5	9	1	1	2	3	5	6	20
50–64	133	2.5	8	1	1	2	2	6	9	13
65+	61	2.0	2	1	1	1	2	4	5	6
GRAND TOTAL	609	2.4	7	1	1	1	3	5	7	14

Length of Stay by Diagnosis and Operation, Western Region, 2008

Western Region, October 2006–September 2007 Data, by Diagnosis

887: TRAUMATIC AMP ARM/HAND

Type of Patients	Observed Patients	Avg. Stay	Vari-ance	Percentiles						
				10th	25th	50th	75th	90th	95th	99th
1. SINGLE DX										
A. Not Operated										
0–19 Years	0									
20–34	0									
35–49	0									
50–64	0									
65+	0									
B. Operated										
0–19 Years	1	3.0	0		3	3	3	3	3	3
20–34	7	4.4	7	3	3	3	8	8	8	8
35–49	0									
50–64	3	7.6	17	3	3	9	11	11	11	11
65+	0									
2. MULTIPLE DX										
A. Not Operated										
0–19 Years	0									
20–34	1	2.0	0	2	2	2	2	2	2	2
35–49	0									
50–64	0									
65+	0									
B. Operated										
0–19 Years	4	11.7	248	1	3	3	8	35	35	35
20–34	25	10.3	72	2	4	7	15	22	24	32
35–49	17	12.0	151	2	3	8	18	30	48	48
50–64	8	15.4	268	3	7	11	20	53	53	53
65+	5	8.6	12	4	6	10	11	12	12	12
SUBTOTALS:										
1. SINGLE DX										
A. Not Operated	0									
B. Operated	11	5.2	10	3	3	3	8	9	11	11
2. MULTIPLE DX										
A. Not Operated	1	2.0	0	2	2	2	2	2	2	2
B. Operated	70	10.4	108	2	3	7	12	22	32	53
1. SINGLE DX	11	5.2	10	3	3	3	8	9	11	11
2. MULTIPLE DX	60	11.2	120	2	4	7	15	22	32	53
A. NOT OPERATED	1	2.0	0	2	2	2	2	2	2	2
B. OPERATED	70	10.4	108	2	3	7	12	22	32	53
TOTAL										
0–19 Years	5	10.0	201	1	3	3	8	35	35	35
20–34	33	8.8	62	2	3	5	11	22	24	32
35–49	17	12.0	151	2	3	8	18	30	48	48
50–64	11	13.3	204	3	4	9	18	20	53	53
65+	5	8.6	12	4	6	10	11	12	12	12
GRAND TOTAL	71	10.3	108	2	3	7	12	22	32	53

890: OPEN WOUND OF HIP/THIGH

Type of Patients	Observed Patients	Avg. Stay	Vari-ance	Percentiles						
				10th	25th	50th	75th	90th	95th	99th
1. SINGLE DX										
A. Not Operated										
0–19 Years	30	1.5	<1	1	1	1	2	2	3	4
20–34	49	1.3	<1	1	1	1	1	2	2	4
35–49	26	1.6	<1	1	1	1	2	3	3	5
50–64	4	1.3	<1	1	1	1	2	2	2	2
65+	0									
B. Operated										
0–19 Years	15	3.1	11	1	1	2	5	10	11	11
20–34	24	1.8	2	1	1	1	3	5	5	5
35–49	13	2.3	6	1	1	1	3	5	9	9
50–64	4	1.5	<1	1	1	2	3	3	3	3
65+	0									
2. MULTIPLE DX										
A. Not Operated										
0–19 Years	53	1.8	2	1	1	1	2	3	5	8
20–34	125	1.7	2	1	1	1	2	3	4	8
35–49	48	2.3	4	1	1	2	2	5	7	9
50–64	30	2.9	5	1	1	2	3	5	8	11
65+	11	3.6	8	1	2	3	4	6	11	11
B. Operated										
0–19 Years	43	5.2	45	1	1	2	6	14	22	29
20–34	83	5.3	49	1	2	3	6	11	14	46
35–49	52	5.5	42	1	2	4	6	16	23	29
50–64	29	8.4	120	1	3	3	13	30	33	42
65+	11	7.2	60	1	2	4	10	18	25	25
SUBTOTALS:										
1. SINGLE DX										
A. Not Operated	109	1.4	<1	1	1	1	2	2	3	4
B. Operated	56	2.3	5	1	1	1	2	5	9	11
2. MULTIPLE DX										
A. Not Operated	267	2.0	3	1	1	1	2	4	5	11
B. Operated	218	5.8	56	1	2	3	6	16	23	38
1. SINGLE DX	165	1.7	2	1	1	1	2	3	5	10
2. MULTIPLE DX	485	3.8	31	1	1	2	4	8	14	30
A. NOT OPERATED	376	1.9	3	1	1	1	2	3	5	9
B. OPERATED	274	5.1	48	1	1	3	5	13	21	38
TOTAL										
0–19 Years	141	2.9	18	1	1	1	3	6	10	23
20–34	281	2.7	18	1	1	1	3	5	8	22
35–49	139	3.4	20	1	1	2	4	6	9	24
50–64	67	5.1	62	1	2	2	5	15	20	42
65+	22	5.4	36	2	2	4	6	11	18	25
GRAND TOTAL	650	3.2	24	1	1	2	3	6	11	29

890.0: OPEN WND HIP/THIGH

Type of Patients	Observed Patients	Avg. Stay	Vari-ance	Percentiles						
				10th	25th	50th	75th	90th	95th	99th
1. SINGLE DX										
A. Not Operated										
0–19 Years	17	1.4	<1	1	1	1	1	1	3	4
20–34	35	1.3	<1	1	1	1	1	2	3	4
35–49	20	1.6	<1	1	1	1	2	2	3	5
50–64	2	1.5	<1	1	2	2	2	2	2	2
65+	0									
B. Operated										
0–19 Years	9	3.3	17	1	1	1	2	11	11	11
20–34	9	2.3	3	1	1	1	4	5	5	5
35–49	5	1.8	1	1	1	1	3	3	3	3
50–64	0									
65+	0									
2. MULTIPLE DX										
A. Not Operated										
0–19 Years	25	1.3	<1	1	1	1	1	2	3	3
20–34	81	1.6	2	1	1	1	2	3	3	12
35–49	28	1.9	3	1	1	1	2	3	5	9
50–64	18	3.1	5	1	2	2	3	5	11	11
65+	8	2.5	2	1	1	2	4	4	4	4
B. Operated										
0–19 Years	17	6.6	67	1	2	2	7	23	29	29
20–34	26	4.7	25	1	2	3	6	13	13	22
35–49	22	3.4	6	1	1	2	5	8	8	9
50–64	4	1.3	<1	1	1	1	2	2	2	2
65+	2	2.5	<1	2	2	3	3	3	3	3
SUBTOTALS:										
1. SINGLE DX										
A. Not Operated	74	1.4	<1	1	1	1	2	2	3	5
B. Operated	23	2.6	8	1	1	1	3	5	10	11
2. MULTIPLE DX										
A. Not Operated	160	1.8	2	1	1	1	2	3	4	11
B. Operated	71	4.5	28	1	2	3	6	9	14	29
1. SINGLE DX	97	1.7	3	1	1	1	2	3	5	11
2. MULTIPLE DX	231	2.6	12	1	1	2	3	5	8	22
A. NOT OPERATED	234	1.7	2	1	1	1	2	3	4	9
B. OPERATED	94	4.0	24	1	1	2	5	9	13	29
TOTAL										
0–19 Years	68	2.9	23	1	1	1	2	7	11	29
20–34	151	2.1	7	1	1	1	2	4	6	13
35–49	75	2.3	4	1	1	2	3	5	8	9
50–64	24	2.7	4	1	2	2	4	5	5	11
65+	10	2.5	1	1	2	2	4	4	4	4
GRAND TOTAL	328	2.4	9	1	1	1	2	4	8	14

890.1: OPEN WND HIP/THIGH-COMP

Type of Patients	Observed Patients	Avg. Stay	Variance	10th	25th	50th	75th	90th	95th	99th
1. SINGLE DX										
A. Not Operated										
0–19 Years	13	1.5	<1	1	1	1	2	2	3	3
20–34	14	1.2	<1	1	1	1	1	2	2	2
35–49	6	1.7	<1	1	1	2	2	3	3	3
50–64	2	1.0	0	1	1	1	1	1	1	1
65+	0									
B. Operated										
0–19 Years	6	2.8	5	1	1	2	5	6	6	6
20–34	12	1.6	2	1	1	1	2	3	5	5
35–49	7	2.7	10	1	1	1	5	9	9	9
50–64	3	1.7	1	1	1	1	3	3	3	3
65+	0									
2. MULTIPLE DX										
A. Not Operated										
0–19 Years	28	2.2	3	1	1	1	3	5	5	8
20–34	44	2.0	5	1	1	1	2	4	5	8
35–49	20	2.8	5	1	1	2	4	6	8	8
50–64	12	2.6	6	1	1	1	3	7	8	8
65+	3	6.7	16	3	3	6	11	11	11	11
B. Operated										
0–19 Years	23	3.7	20	1	1	2	4	7	10	22
20–34	51	5.8	66	1	2	3	6	10	16	46
35–49	27	7.0	65	1	2	4	6	23	24	29
50–64	19	11.0	152	2	2	5	17	33	42	42
65+	5	8.8	33	4	4	8	10	18	18	18
SUBTOTALS:										
1. SINGLE DX										
A. Not Operated	35	1.4	<1	1	1	1	2	2	3	3
B. Operated	28	2.1	4	1	1	1	2	5	6	9
2. MULTIPLE DX										
A. Not Operated	107	2.4	4	1	1	2	3	5	7	8
B. Operated	125	6.6	72	1	2	4	6	18	24	42
1. SINGLE DX	63	1.7	2	1	1	1	2	3	5	9
2. MULTIPLE DX	232	4.7	45	1	1	2	5	9	18	38
A. NOT OPERATED	142	2.1	3	1	1	1	3	5	6	8
B. OPERATED	153	5.8	63	1	1	3	6	15	23	42
TOTAL										
0–19 Years	70	2.6	9	1	1	2	3	5	7	22
20–34	121	3.5	33	1	1	2	4	7	9	38
35–49	60	4.6	37	1	1	2	5	9	21	29
50–64	36	6.8	100	1	1	3	8	20	33	42
65+	8	8.0	25	3	4	6	11	18	18	18
GRAND TOTAL	295	4.0	37	1	1	2	4	8	16	38

891: OPEN WND KNEE/LEG/ANKLE

Type of Patients	Observed Patients	Avg. Stay	Variance	10th	25th	50th	75th	90th	95th	99th
1. SINGLE DX										
A. Not Operated										
0–19 Years	37	1.4	<1	1	1	1	2	2	4	4
20–34	36	1.9	2	1	1	1	2	3	6	9
35–49	10	1.4	<1	1	1	2	2	3	3	3
50–64	5	1.2	<1	1	1	1	1	2	2	2
65+	0									
B. Operated										
0–19 Years	57	2.3	6	1	1	2	3	4	6	17
20–34	87	2.7	8	1	1	2	3	5	11	15
35–49	39	1.7	1	1	1	1	2	3	4	5
50–64	15	2.5	3	1	1	2	3	5	7	7
65+	6	2.7	3	1	1	2	3	6	6	6
2. MULTIPLE DX										
A. Not Operated										
0–19 Years	56	2.2	3	1	1	2	3	5	6	9
20–34	86	2.3	7	1	1	1	2	4	5	21
35–49	51	3.4	28	1	1	2	4	6	7	38
50–64	72	4.5	28	1	2	3	5	9	13	40
65+	152	3.7	7	1	2	3	5	7	10	12
B. Operated										
0–19 Years	90	3.8	36	1	1	2	4	6	13	46
20–34	250	4.2	30	1	1	2	4	10	16	29
35–49	156	5.3	61	1	2	3	6	10	21	48
50–64	130	5.9	31	1	2	4	8	14	19	24
65+	159	5.5	18	2	3	4	7	11	15	22
SUBTOTALS:										
1. SINGLE DX										
A. Not Operated	88	1.6	1	1	1	1	2	3	3	9
B. Operated	204	2.4	6	1	1	2	3	4	6	14
2. MULTIPLE DX										
A. Not Operated	417	3.3	13	1	1	2	4	7	9	14
B. Operated	785	4.9	35	1	2	3	6	11	16	29
1. SINGLE DX	292	2.2	4	1	1	2	3	4	6	14
2. MULTIPLE DX	1,202	4.4	28	1	1	3	5	9	14	28
A. NOT OPERATED	505	3.0	11	1	1	2	4	6	8	13
B. OPERATED	989	4.4	30	1	1	3	5	10	15	28
TOTAL										
0–19 Years	240	2.7	16	1	1	2	3	5	6	21
20–34	459	3.4	20	1	1	2	4	7	12	25
35–49	256	4.2	45	1	1	2	4	7	14	38
50–64	222	5.1	29	1	2	3	6	11	15	24
65+	317	4.6	13	2	3	3	6	9	12	18
GRAND TOTAL	1,494	3.9	24	1	1	2	4	8	12	24

891.0: OPEN WND LOW LEG

Type of Patients	Observed Patients	Avg. Stay	Variance	10th	25th	50th	75th	90th	95th	99th
1. SINGLE DX										
A. Not Operated										
0–19 Years	22	1.3	<1	1	1	1	1	2	2	4
20–34	19	1.9	3	1	1	1	2	3	9	9
35–49	7	1.3	<1	1	1	1	1	3	3	3
50–64	3	1.0	0	1	1	1	1	1	1	1
65+	0									
B. Operated										
0–19 Years	19	2.3	13	1	1	2	2	4	17	17
20–34	19	3.7	11	1	2	3	4	11	14	14
35–49	16	1.4	<1	1	1	1	2	2	3	3
50–64	6	3.3	5	1	2	3	5	7	7	7
65+	1	2.0	0	2	2	2	2	2	2	2
2. MULTIPLE DX										
A. Not Operated										
0–19 Years	29	1.6	<1	1	1	2	2	3	3	4
20–34	51	1.8	3	1	1	1	2	3	5	11
35–49	19	3.5	71	1	1	1	2	5	38	38
50–64	22	3.4	11	1	2	2	4	9	9	13
65+	84	3.3	6	1	2	3	4	5	7	15
B. Operated										
0–19 Years	19	2.1	<1	1	1	2	3	4	4	4
20–34	58	3.7	22	1	1	2	4	10	13	28
35–49	34	4.8	49	1	1	2	5	9	23	33
50–64	33	4.5	19	1	2	3	6	10	11	23
65+	49	5.2	18	1	3	4	6	10	13	22
SUBTOTALS:										
1. SINGLE DX										
A. Not Operated	51	1.5	2	1	1	1	2	2	3	9
B. Operated	61	2.6	9	1	1	2	3	5	7	17
2. MULTIPLE DX										
A. Not Operated	205	2.7	11	1	1	2	3	5	7	13
B. Operated	193	4.2	24	1	2	3	5	9	13	28
1. SINGLE DX	112	2.1	6	1	1	2	3	4	6	14
2. MULTIPLE DX	398	3.5	18	1	1	2	4	7	11	23
A. NOT OPERATED	256	2.5	9	1	1	2	3	5	7	13
B. OPERATED	254	3.9	21	1	2	2	4	9	12	23
TOTAL										
0–19 Years	89	1.8	3	1	1	1	2	3	4	17
20–34	147	2.8	12	1	1	2	3	5	10	19
35–49	76	3.4	41	1	1	3	5	9	21	38
50–64	64	3.8	14	1	1	3	5	9	11	23
65+	134	4.0	11	2	3	3	5	9	11	16
GRAND TOTAL	510	3.2	15	1	2	2	3	6	10	22

771

Length of Stay by Diagnosis and Operation, Western Region, 2008

Western Region, October 2006–September 2007 Data, by Diagnosis

891.1: OPEN WND LOW LEG-COMP

Type of Patients	Observed Patients	Avg. Stay	Vari-ance	10th	25th	50th	75th	90th	95th	99th
1. SINGLE DX										
A. Not Operated										
0–19 Years	15	1.7	<1	1	1	1	2	3	4	4
20–34	15	2.0	2	1	1	1	2	3	6	6
35–49	2	1.5	<1	1	1	2	2	2	2	2
50–64	1	2.0	0	2	2	2	2	2	2	2
65+	0									
B. Operated										
0–19 Years	23	2.3	2	1	1	2	3	4	4	6
20–34	54	2.2	4	1	1	2	2	4	7	12
35–49	12	1.8	2	1	1	1	3	4	5	5
50–64	8	1.9	<1	1	1	2	2	4	4	4
65+	3	3.3	6	1	2	3	6	6	6	6
2. MULTIPLE DX										
A. Not Operated										
0–19 Years	25	3.0	5	1	1	2	2	6	7	9
20–34	33	3.0	14	1	1	2	3	5	9	21
35–49	32	3.4	4	1	2	3	4	7	7	9
50–64	48	5.0	36	1	2	4	6	11	13	40
65+	65	4.1	7	1	2	3	6	8	10	11
B. Operated										
0–19 Years	45	4.5	57	1	1	2	5	10	13	46
20–34	137	4.5	37	1	1	2	5	11	17	35
35–49	84	6.1	86	1	2	3	6	14	24	57
50–64	79	6.7	37	1	2	5	9	15	21	28
65+	88	5.9	20	2	3	5	8	13	15	23
SUBTOTALS:										
1. SINGLE DX										
A. Not Operated	33	1.8	1	1	1	2	2	3	4	6
B. Operated	100	2.2	3	1	1	2	3	4	5	12
2. MULTIPLE DX										
A. Not Operated	203	3.9	15	1	2	3	5	7	9	14
B. Operated	433	5.5	45	1	2	3	7	13	18	35
1. SINGLE DX	133	2.1	3	1	1	2	2	4	5	8
2. MULTIPLE DX	636	5.0	36	1	2	3	6	11	15	34
A. NOT OPERATED	236	3.6	13	1	2	3	5	7	9	14
B. OPERATED	533	4.9	39	1	1	3	6	11	16	34
TOTAL										
0–19 Years	108	3.3	26	1	1	2	3	6	9	24
20–34	239	3.6	25	1	1	2	4	8	13	25
35–49	130	5.0	59	1	1	3	5	16	16	48
50–64	136	5.8	35	1	2	4	7	13	19	28
65+	156	5.1	15	1	3	4	7	10	14	18
GRAND TOTAL	769	4.5	31	1	1	3	5	9	14	28

892: OPEN WOUND OF FOOT

Type of Patients	Observed Patients	Avg. Stay	Vari-ance	10th	25th	50th	75th	90th	95th	99th
1. SINGLE DX										
A. Not Operated										
0–19 Years	19	1.6	1	1	1	1	2	3	5	5
20–34	2	1.0	0	1	1	1	1	1	1	1
35–49	1	8.0	0	8	8	8	8	8	8	8
50–64	2	2.0	2	1	1	2	3	3	3	3
65+	0									
B. Operated										
0–19 Years	19	2.8	10	1	1	1	5	6	13	13
20–34	16	1.7	3	1	1	1	2	2	8	8
35–49	6	1.7	<1	1	1	2	2	3	3	3
50–64	3	1.7	<1	1	1	2	2	2	2	2
65+	0									
2. MULTIPLE DX										
A. Not Operated										
0–19 Years	35	2.7	5	1	1	2	3	5	5	13
20–34	30	2.5	2	1	1	2	3	5	6	6
35–49	40	4.0	11	1	1	3	6	9	10	14
50–64	31	3.8	8	1	2	3	5	6	9	14
65+	23	3.6	5	2	2	3	5	7	8	9
B. Operated										
0–19 Years	44	6.6	38	3	3	4	7	15	21	24
20–34	46	4.5	25	1	2	3	5	13	17	21
35–49	51	4.6	15	1	2	4	6	10	11	19
50–64	39	7.8	180	1	3	4	7	13	43	74
65+	18	8.9	234	2	3	5	6	12	69	69
SUBTOTALS:										
1. SINGLE DX										
A. Not Operated	24	1.8	3	1	1	1	2	3	5	8
B. Operated	44	2.2	6	1	1	1	2	5	6	13
2. MULTIPLE DX										
A. Not Operated	159	3.4	7	1	1	3	4	7	9	14
B. Operated	198	6.0	75	1	2	4	6	13	19	69
1. SINGLE DX	68	2.1	5	1	1	1	2	5	6	13
2. MULTIPLE DX	357	4.8	46	1	2	3	6	10	14	29
A. NOT OPERATED	183	3.2	7	1	1	2	4	6	8	14
B. OPERATED	242	5.3	65	1	1	3	6	11	17	43
TOTAL										
0–19 Years	117	4.0	21	1	1	2	3	6	9	24
20–34	94	3.3	15	1	1	2	4	8	13	25
35–49	98	4.2	13	1	1	3	5	11	11	19
50–64	75	5.7	100	1	2	4	6	9	14	74
65+	41	5.9	109	2	2	4	6	9	10	69
GRAND TOTAL	425	4.4	41	1	1	3	5	9	13	24

892.1: OPEN WOUND FOOT-COMP

Type of Patients	Observed Patients	Avg. Stay	Vari-ance	10th	25th	50th	75th	90th	95th	99th
1. SINGLE DX										
A. Not Operated										
0–19 Years	16	1.4	<1	1	1	1	2	3	3	3
20–34	1	1.0	0	1	1	1	1	1	1	1
35–49	1	8.0	0	8	8	8	8	8	8	8
50–64	2	2.0	2	1	1	2	3	3	3	3
65+	0									
B. Operated										
0–19 Years	8	3.0	5	1	1	4	5	6	6	6
20–34	5	2.4	10	1	1	1	1	8	8	8
35–49	3	1.7	1	1	1	1	3	3	3	3
50–64	0									
65+	0									
2. MULTIPLE DX										
A. Not Operated										
0–19 Years	27	2.8	5	1	2	2	3	4	5	13
20–34	19	2.7	3	1	1	2	3	6	6	6
35–49	29	3.9	7	1	2	3	6	8	9	10
50–64	22	4.1	9	1	2	4	4	6	9	14
65+	18	3.7	6	1	2	3	5	8	9	9
B. Operated										
0–19 Years	23	7.0	43	1	3	4	7	19	21	23
20–34	29	5.6	35	1	2	3	7	17	19	21
35–49	30	5.4	15	2	2	5	6	11	11	19
50–64	27	10.1	243	1	3	6	8	29	43	74
65+	10	6.1	8	4	4	6	6	12	12	12
SUBTOTALS:										
1. SINGLE DX										
A. Not Operated	20	1.8	3	1	1	1	2	3	3	8
B. Operated	16	2.6	5	1	1	1	5	6	8	8
2. MULTIPLE DX										
A. Not Operated	115	3.4	6	1	2	3	4	7	9	13
B. Operated	119	6.9	77	1	2	4	7	14	21	43
1. SINGLE DX	36	2.1	4	1	1	1	3	5	8	8
2. MULTIPLE DX	234	5.2	45	1	2	3	6	10	14	29
A. NOT OPERATED	135	3.2	6	1	1	2	4	6	8	13
B. OPERATED	135	6.4	71	1	2	4	7	13	19	43
TOTAL										
0–19 Years	74	3.8	20	1	1	3	4	7	15	23
20–34	54	4.2	23	1	1	2	5	12	17	21
35–49	63	4.5	11	1	2	4	6	9	10	19
50–64	51	7.2	140	1	2	4	6	9	29	74
65+	28	4.5	8	2	3	4	6	9	10	12
GRAND TOTAL	270	4.8	41	1	2	3	6	9	13	29

Length of Stay by Diagnosis and Operation, Western Region, 2008

Western Region, October 2006–September 2007 Data, by Diagnosis

893: OPEN WOUND OF TOE

Type of Patients	Observed Patients	Avg. Stay	Variance	10th	25th	50th	75th	90th	95th	99th
1. SINGLE DX										
A. Not Operated										
0–19 Years	3	1.7	1	1	1	1	3	3	3	3
20–34	3	1.3	<1	1	1	1	2	2	2	2
35–49	0									
50–64	2	1.5	<1	1	1	2	2	2	2	2
65+	0									
B. Operated										
0–19 Years	1	1.0	0	1	1	1	1	1	1	1
20–34	2	1.5	<1	1	1	2	2	2	2	2
35–49	1	1.0	0	1	1	1	1	1	1	1
50–64	1	1.0	0	1	1	1	1	1	1	1
65+	0									
2. MULTIPLE DX										
A. Not Operated										
0–19 Years	2	2.0	0	2	2	2	2	2	2	2
20–34	4	1.8	<1	1	1	1	2	3	3	3
35–49	6	6.2	9	1	4	8	8	9	9	9
50–64	6	2.2	1	1	1	2	3	4	4	4
65+	6	2.5	<1	2	2	3	3	4	4	4
B. Operated										
0–19 Years	4	3.3	4	1	2	2	5	5	5	5
20–34	7	2.0	<1	1	1	2	3	3	3	3
35–49	13	4.6	14	2	2	4	5	7	15	15
50–64	7	4.6	23	1	1	4	4	15	15	15
65+	7	3.9	7	1	2	4	5	9	9	9
SUBTOTALS:										
1. SINGLE DX										
A. Not Operated	8	1.5	<1	1	1	1	2	3	3	3
B. Operated	5	1.2	<1	1	1	1	1	2	2	2
2. MULTIPLE DX										
A. Not Operated	24	3.2	6	1	2	2	4	8	8	9
B. Operated	38	3.9	11	2	2	3	5	7	15	15
1. SINGLE DX	13	1.4	<1	1	1	1	2	2	3	3
2. MULTIPLE DX	62	3.6	9	1	2	3	4	7	9	15
A. NOT OPERATED	32	2.8	5	1	1	2	3	7	8	9
B. OPERATED	43	3.5	10	1	2	2	5	7	9	15
TOTAL										
0–19 Years	10	2.3	2	1	1	2	3	5	5	5
20–34	16	1.8	<1	1	1	2	2	3	3	3
35–49	20	4.9	12	1	2	5	7	9	15	15
50–64	16	3.1	12	1	1	2	4	4	15	15
65+	13	3.2	4	2	2	2	4	5	9	9
GRAND TOTAL	75	3.2	8	1	1	2	4	7	9	15

894: OPEN WOUND OF LEG NEC

Type of Patients	Observed Patients	Avg. Stay	Variance	10th	25th	50th	75th	90th	95th	99th
1. SINGLE DX										
A. Not Operated										
0–19 Years	0									
20–34	0									
35–49	0									
50–64	0									
65+	1	6.0	0	6	6	6	6	6	6	6
B. Operated										
0–19 Years	2	2.5	<1	2	2	2	3	3	3	3
20–34	2	1.5	<1	1	1	2	2	2	2	2
35–49	0									
50–64	0									
65+	0									
2. MULTIPLE DX										
A. Not Operated										
0–19 Years	0									
20–34	2	3.5	12	1	1	4	6	6	6	6
35–49	1	1.0	0	1	1	1	1	1	1	1
50–64	4	3.8	7	1	2	2	6	6	6	6
65+	2	5.0	18	2	2	8	8	8	8	8
B. Operated										
0–19 Years	2	13.0	96	6	6	13	20	20	20	20
20–34	3	3.0	0	3	3	3	3	3	3	3
35–49	1	3.0	0	3	3	3	3	3	3	3
50–64	0									
65+	1	7.0	0	7	7	7	7	7	7	7
SUBTOTALS:										
1. SINGLE DX										
A. Not Operated	1	6.0	0	6	6	6	6	6	6	6
B. Operated	4	2.0	<1	1	2	2	3	3	3	3
2. MULTIPLE DX										
A. Not Operated	9	3.7	8	3	1	2	6	8	8	8
B. Operated	5	7.8	50	3	3	6	7	20	20	20
1. SINGLE DX	5	2.8	4	1	2	2	3	6	6	6
2. MULTIPLE DX	14	5.2	24	1	2	6	6	8	20	20
A. NOT OPERATED	10	3.9	7	1	1	2	3	7	8	8
B. OPERATED	9	5.2	35	1	2	3	6	8	20	20
TOTAL										
0–19 Years	4	7.7	69	2	3	3	6	20	20	20
20–34	5	2.6	4	1	1	2	3	6	6	6
35–49	2	2.0	2	1	1	1	5	9	15	15
50–64	4	3.8	7	1	2	2	6	6	8	8
65+	4	5.8	7	2	6	7	8	8	8	8
GRAND TOTAL	19	4.5	20	1	2	3	4	7	20	20

895: TRAUMATIC AMPUTATION TOE

Type of Patients	Observed Patients	Avg. Stay	Variance	10th	25th	50th	75th	90th	95th	99th
1. SINGLE DX										
A. Not Operated										
0–19 Years	0									
20–34	0									
35–49	0									
50–64	0									
65+	0									
B. Operated										
0–19 Years	7	2.4	3	1	1	2	4	5	5	5
20–34	4	1.5	<1	1	1	2	2	2	2	2
35–49	1	2.0	0	2	2	2	2	2	2	2
50–64	0									
65+	0									
2. MULTIPLE DX										
A. Not Operated										
0–19 Years	0									
20–34	0									
35–49	0									
50–64	0									
65+	0									
B. Operated										
0–19 Years	12	4.8	21	2	2	3	6	7	18	18
20–34	14	4.2	21	1	2	3	6	8	18	18
35–49	10	3.3	9	1	1	3	4	9	9	9
50–64	12	2.6	3	1	2	2	3	4	7	7
65+	7	4.9	11	2	2	5	5	10	10	10
SUBTOTALS:										
1. SINGLE DX										
A. Not Operated	0									
B. Operated	12	2.1	2	1	1	2	3	4	5	5
2. MULTIPLE DX										
A. Not Operated	0									
B. Operated	55	3.9	13	1	2	2	5	8	10	18
1. SINGLE DX	12	2.1	2	1	1	2	3	4	5	5
2. MULTIPLE DX	55	3.9	13	1	2	2	5	8	10	18
A. NOT OPERATED	0									
B. OPERATED	67	3.6	12	1	2	2	5	7	9	18
TOTAL										
0–19 Years	19	3.9	15	1	2	3	5	7	18	18
20–34	18	3.6	18	1	1	2	4	8	18	18
35–49	11	3.2	8	1	1	2	3	4	9	9
50–64	12	2.6	3	1	2	2	3	4	7	7
65+	7	4.9	11	2	2	5	5	10	10	10
GRAND TOTAL	67	3.6	12	1	2	2	5	7	9	18

773

Length of Stay by Diagnosis and Operation, Western Region, 2008

Western Region, October 2006–September 2007 Data, by Diagnosis

896: TRAUMATIC AMP FOOT

Type of Patients	Observed Patients	Avg. Stay	Vari- ance	10th	25th	50th	75th	90th	95th	99th
1. SINGLE DX										
A. Not Operated										
0–19 Years	0									
20–34	0									
35–49	0									
50–64	0									
65+	0									
B. Operated										
0–19 Years	1	7.0	0	7	7	7	7	7	7	7
20–34	1	3.0	0	3	3	3	3	3	3	3
35–49	0									
50–64	1	6.0	0	6	6	6	6	6	6	6
65+	0									
2. MULTIPLE DX										
A. Not Operated										
0–19 Years	0									
20–34	0									
35–49	0									
50–64	0									
65+	0									
B. Operated										
0–19 Years	3	13.4	263	2	2	6	32	32	32	32
20–34	4	15.0	37	11	11	13	24	24	24	24
35–49	5	12.8	42	5	9	11	19	20	20	20
50–64	8	13.1	51	3	8	13	26	26	26	26
65+	1	31.0	0	31	31	31	31	31	31	31
SUBTOTALS:										
1. SINGLE DX — A. Not Operated	0									
1. SINGLE DX — B. Operated	3	5.4	4	3	3	6	7	7	7	7
2. MULTIPLE DX — A. Not Operated	0									
2. MULTIPLE DX — B. Operated	21	14.3	74	5	8	13	19	26	31	32
1. SINGLE DX	3	5.4	4	3	3	6	7	7	7	7
2. MULTIPLE DX	21	14.3	74	5	8	13	19	26	31	32
A. NOT OPERATED	0									
B. OPERATED	24	13.2	74	3	7	11	19	26	31	32
TOTAL										
0–19 Years	4	11.8	187	2	6	7	32	32	32	32
20–34	5	12.6	56	3	11	12	13	24	24	24
35–49	5	12.8	42	5	9	11	19	20	20	20
50–64	9	12.3	50	3	8	13	14	26	26	26
65+	1	31.0	0	31	31	31	31	31	31	31
GRAND TOTAL	24	13.2	74	3	7	11	19	26	31	32

897: TRAUMATIC LEG AMPUTATION

Type of Patients	Observed Patients	Avg. Stay	Vari- ance	10th	25th	50th	75th	90th	95th	99th
1. SINGLE DX										
A. Not Operated										
0–19 Years	0									
20–34	0									
35–49	0									
50–64	0									
65+	0									
B. Operated										
0–19 Years	0									
20–34	0									
35–49	0									
50–64	0									
65+	0									
2. MULTIPLE DX										
A. Not Operated										
0–19 Years	0									
20–34	0									
35–49	0									
50–64	0									
65+	1	2.0	0	2	2	2	2	2	2	2
B. Operated										
0–19 Years	8	20.1	121	8	10	21	26	40	40	40
20–34	20	15.2	49	4	11	13	22	26	27	27
35–49	14	13.1	79	5	7	11	16	38	>99	>99
50–64	13	18.1	423	5	8	10	20	34	80	80
65+	5	7.0	8	4	5	6	9	11	11	11
SUBTOTALS:										
1. SINGLE DX — A. Not Operated	0									
1. SINGLE DX — B. Operated	0									
2. MULTIPLE DX — A. Not Operated	1	2.0	0	2	2	2	2	2	2	2
2. MULTIPLE DX — B. Operated	60	15.3	146	5	8	13	21	27	38	>99
1. SINGLE DX	0									
2. MULTIPLE DX	61	15.1	146	5	8	13	21	27	38	>99
A. NOT OPERATED	1	2.0	0	2	2	2	2	2	2	2
B. OPERATED	60	15.3	146	5	8	13	21	27	38	>99
TOTAL										
0–19 Years	8	20.1	121	8	10	21	26	40	40	40
20–34	20	15.2	49	4	11	13	22	26	27	27
35–49	14	13.1	79	5	7	11	16	38	>99	>99
50–64	13	18.1	423	5	8	10	20	34	80	80
65+	6	6.2	11	2	4	6	9	11	11	11
GRAND TOTAL	61	15.1	146	5	8	13	21	27	38	>99

900: HEAD/NECK VESSEL INJURY

Type of Patients	Observed Patients	Avg. Stay	Vari- ance	10th	25th	50th	75th	90th	95th	99th
1. SINGLE DX										
A. Not Operated										
0–19 Years	0									
20–34	1	3.0	0	3	3	3	3	3	3	3
35–49	1	6.0	0	6	6	6	6	6	6	6
50–64	0									
65+	0									
B. Operated										
0–19 Years	2	3.5	<1	3	3	3	4	4	4	4
20–34	4	1.8	<1	1	1	2	3	3	3	3
35–49	2	5.0	31	1	1	1	9	9	9	9
50–64	0									
65+	0									
2. MULTIPLE DX										
A. Not Operated										
0–19 Years	3	1.7	1	1	1	1	3	3	3	3
20–34	8	5.6	20	1	1	7	7	14	14	14
35–49	6	4.0	21	1	1	2	5	13	13	13
50–64	10	2.8	8	1	1	1	4	4	10	10
65+	3	1.3	<1	1	1	1	2	2	2	2
B. Operated										
0–19 Years	29	5.8	27	1	2	4	8	15	16	19
20–34	70	6.0	55	1	2	3	7	15	20	45
35–49	47	6.6	132	1	1	3	6	12	22	64
50–64	39	5.7	123	1	1	3	4	12	23	67
65+	18	5.8	65	1	2	3	5	21	32	32
SUBTOTALS:										
1. SINGLE DX — A. Not Operated	2	4.5	4	3	3	5	6	6	6	6
1. SINGLE DX — B. Operated	8	3.0	7	1	1	3	3	9	9	9
2. MULTIPLE DX — A. Not Operated	30	3.5	13	1	1	2	5	14	13	14
2. MULTIPLE DX — B. Operated	203	6.0	81	1	1	3	6	14	20	46
1. SINGLE DX	10	3.3	6	1	1	3	4	6	9	9
2. MULTIPLE DX	233	5.7	73	1	1	3	6	14	19	46
A. NOT OPERATED	32	3.6	13	1	1	2	5	7	13	14
B. OPERATED	211	5.9	79	1	1	3	6	14	20	46
TOTAL										
0–19 Years	34	5.3	24	1	2	3	6	14	16	19
20–34	83	5.7	49	1	1	3	7	14	18	45
35–49	56	6.2	114	1	1	3	6	14	22	64
50–64	49	5.1	100	1	2	2	4	11	15	67
65+	21	5.1	58	1	2	2	5	10	21	32
GRAND TOTAL	243	5.6	71	1	1	3	6	14	18	46

Western Region, October 2006–September 2007 Data, by Diagnosis

901: THOR BLOOD VESSEL INJURY

Type of Patients	Observed Patients	Avg. Stay	Variance	10th	25th	50th	75th	90th	95th	99th
1. SINGLE DX										
A. Not Operated										
0–19 Years	0									
20–34	0									
35–49	1	1.0	0							
50–64	0									
65+	0									
B. Operated										
0–19 Years	1	2.0	0	2	2	2	2	2	2	2
20–34	0									
35–49	0									
50–64	0									
65+	0									
2. MULTIPLE DX										
A. Not Operated										
0–19 Years	1	3.0	0	3	3	3	3	3	3	3
20–34	3	5.0	19	2	2	3	10	10	10	10
35–49	1	16.0	0	16	16	16	16	16	16	16
50–64	2	28.8	>999	3	3	55	55	55	55	55
65+	5	9.8	42	4	5	8	12	20	20	20
B. Operated										
0–19 Years	21	13.2	113	6	6	8	21	29	35	38
20–34	56	11.6	108	3	5	8	13	25	35	52
35–49	29	16.7	353	4	7	11	18	58	58	94
50–64	20	19.5	309	6	6	11	34	55	59	59
65+	7	16.7	160	6	6	12	23	42	42	42
SUBTOTALS:										
1. SINGLE DX										
A. Not Operated	1	1.0	0	1	1	1	1	1	1	1
B. Operated	1	2.0	0	2	2	2	2	2	2	2
2. MULTIPLE DX										
A. Not Operated	12	11.8	219	3	3	8	16	20	55	55
B. Operated	133	14.4	198	4	6	10	18	34	42	59
1. SINGLE DX	2	1.5	<1	1	1	1	2	2	2	2
2. MULTIPLE DX	145	14.2	199	3	6	10	18	34	42	59
A. NOT OPERATED	13	10.9	210	2	3	5	12	20	55	55
B. OPERATED	134	14.3	198	3	6	10	18	34	42	59
TOTAL										
0–19 Years	23	12.3	112	3	6	8	21	29	35	38
20–34	59	11.3	106	2	4	8	13	25	35	52
35–49	31	16.2	337	4	7	11	18	21	58	94
50–64	22	20.3	352	3	6	11	34	55	59	59
65+	12	13.9	116	5	6	11	23	42	42	42
GRAND TOTAL	147	14.0	198	3	6	9	18	34	42	59

902: ABD/PELVIC VESSEL INJURY

Type of Patients	Observed Patients	Avg. Stay	Variance	10th	25th	50th	75th	90th	95th	99th
1. SINGLE DX										
A. Not Operated										
0–19 Years	1	2.0	0	2	2	2	2	2	2	2
20–34	0									
35–49	0									
50–64	0									
65+	0									
B. Operated										
0–19 Years	0									
20–34	1	3.0	0	3	3	3	3	3	3	3
35–49	0									
50–64	0									
65+	0									
2. MULTIPLE DX										
A. Not Operated										
0–19 Years	2	4.5	12	2	2	7	7	7	7	7
20–34	7	5.7	10	1	4	6	9	9	9	9
35–49	5	3.8	1	2	1	4	4	5	5	5
50–64	1	1.0	0	1	1	1	1	1	1	1
65+	3	6.3	57	1	1	3	15	15	15	15
B. Operated										
0–19 Years	16	14.9	228	3	4	9	22	36	55	55
20–34	39	10.5	130	2	4	5	12	26	39	54
35–49	26	6.4	27	2	3	5	8	13	15	24
50–64	17	8.6	39	2	5	6	10	23	23	23
65+	14	9.2	34	4	5	9	13	17	22	22
SUBTOTALS:										
1. SINGLE DX										
A. Not Operated	1	2.0	0	2	2	2	2	2	2	2
B. Operated	1	3.0	0	3	3	3	3	3	3	3
2. MULTIPLE DX										
A. Not Operated	18	4.9	13	1	2	4	7	9	15	15
B. Operated	112	9.7	98	2	4	6	12	22	27	54
1. SINGLE DX	2	2.5	<1	2	2	2	3	3	3	3
2. MULTIPLE DX	130	9.1	89	2	4	5	11	22	26	54
A. NOT OPERATED	19	4.7	13	1	2	4	7	9	15	15
B. OPERATED	113	9.7	97	2	4	6	11	22	27	54
TOTAL										
0–19 Years	19	13.1	208	2	3	5	22	36	55	55
20–34	47	9.6	112	2	4	6	11	21	37	54
35–49	31	6.0	23	2	3	4	7	13	15	24
50–64	18	8.2	40	2	5	6	10	23	23	23
65+	17	8.7	36	2	4	6	13	17	22	22
GRAND TOTAL	132	9.0	88	2	4	5	11	21	26	54

903: ARM BLOOD VESSEL INJURY

Type of Patients	Observed Patients	Avg. Stay	Variance	10th	25th	50th	75th	90th	95th	99th
1. SINGLE DX										
A. Not Operated										
0–19 Years	0									
20–34	2	2.0	2	1	1	3	3	3	3	3
35–49	0									
50–64	1	3.0	0	3	3	3	3	3	3	3
65+	0									
B. Operated										
0–19 Years	4	1.3	<1	1	1	1	1	2	2	2
20–34	15	1.4	<1	1	1	1	2	2	4	4
35–49	9	2.1	5	1	1	1	2	8	8	8
50–64	2	2.5	4	1	1	3	4	4	4	4
65+	1	3.0	0	3	3	3	3	3	3	3
2. MULTIPLE DX										
A. Not Operated										
0–19 Years	1	2.0	0	2	2	2	2	2	2	2
20–34	10	3.2	10	1	1	1	6	6	10	10
35–49	2	1.5	<1	1	1	1	2	2	2	2
50–64	3	3.3	10	1	1	2	7	7	7	7
65+	3	5.0	<1	4	4	5	6	6	6	6
B. Operated										
0–19 Years	51	2.8	10	1	1	2	2	4	5	20
20–34	186	2.7	6	1	1	2	3	5	8	12
35–49	101	3.4	14	1	1	2	4	6	11	21
50–64	50	4.4	34	1	1	2	6	12	14	34
65+	19	2.7	3	1	1	2	4	6	6	6
SUBTOTALS:										
1. SINGLE DX										
A. Not Operated	3	2.3	1	1	1	3	3	3	3	3
B. Operated	31	1.7	2	1	1	1	2	3	4	8
2. MULTIPLE DX										
A. Not Operated	19	3.3	7	1	1	2	4	6	10	10
B. Operated	407	3.1	12	1	1	2	4	6	10	17
1. SINGLE DX	34	1.8	2	1	1	1	2	3	4	8
2. MULTIPLE DX	426	3.1	12	1	1	2	4	6	10	17
A. NOT OPERATED	22	3.1	6	1	1	2	5	6	7	10
B. OPERATED	438	3.0	11	1	1	2	4	6	10	17
TOTAL										
0–19 Years	56	2.7	9	1	1	2	2	5	5	20
20–34	213	2.6	6	1	1	2	2	5	8	11
35–49	112	3.3	13	1	1	2	4	6	11	21
50–64	56	4.2	31	1	1	3	5	12	14	34
65+	23	3.0	3	1	1	3	5	6	6	6
GRAND TOTAL	460	3.0	11	1	1	2	4	6	10	17

Length of Stay by Diagnosis and Operation, Western Region, 2008

Western Region, October 2006–September 2007 Data, by Diagnosis

904: BLOOD VESSEL INJURY NEC

Type of Patients	Observed Patients	Avg. Stay	Variance	10th	25th	50th	75th	90th	95th	99th
1. SINGLE DX										
A. Not Operated										
0–19 Years	1	2.0	0	2	2	2	2	2	2	2
20–34	1	1.0	0	1	1	1	1	1	1	1
35–49	0									
50–64	0									
65+	0									
B. Operated										
0–19 Years	2	2.0	2	1	1	1	3	3	3	3
20–34	2	2.0	2	1	1	2	3	3	3	3
35–49	0									
50–64	0									
65+	0									
2. MULTIPLE DX										
A. Not Operated										
0–19 Years	2	1.0	0	1	1	1	1	1	1	1
20–34	7	2.3	3	1	1	2	4	5	5	5
35–49	12	3.0	4	1	2	2	3	5	8	8
50–64	10	3.8	5	1	2	3	6	7	7	7
65+	12	3.7	4	1	2	4	5	6	6	6
B. Operated										
0–19 Years	45	7.2	59	2	3	5	8	13	16	49
20–34	100	9.0	73	2	3	6	12	19	26	40
35–49	37	9.9	155	2	2	4	11	33	43	49
50–64	20	7.4	78	1	3	6	8	12	42	42
65+	11	8.5	48	1	3	7	14	19	21	21
SUBTOTALS:										
1. SINGLE DX										
A. Not Operated	2	1.5	<1	1	1	2	2	2	2	2
B. Operated	4	2.0	1	1	1	1	3	3	3	3
2. MULTIPLE DX										
A. Not Operated	43	3.2	4	1	1	2	5	6	6	8
B. Operated	213	8.6	83	2	3	5	11	19	27	46
1. SINGLE DX	6	1.8	<1	1	1	2	3	3	3	3
2. MULTIPLE DX	256	7.7	74	1	2	5	9	18	24	46
A. NOT OPERATED	45	3.1	4	1	1	2	5	6	6	8
B. OPERATED	217	8.5	82	2	3	5	11	19	27	46
TOTAL										
0–19 Years	50	6.6	56	1	3	4	8	13	16	49
20–34	110	8.4	70	2	2	5	12	19	26	40
35–49	49	8.2	126	1	2	4	8	24	38	49
50–64	30	6.2	56	2	2	5	7	11	12	42
65+	23	6.0	29	2	2	4	7	14	19	21
GRAND TOTAL	262	7.5	73	1	2	4	9	18	23	46

905: LATE EFFECT MS INJURY

Type of Patients	Observed Patients	Avg. Stay	Variance	10th	25th	50th	75th	90th	95th	99th
1. SINGLE DX										
A. Not Operated										
0–19 Years	0									
20–34	0									
35–49	0									
50–64	0									
65+	0									
B. Operated										
0–19 Years	0									
20–34	1	1.0	0	1	1	1	1	1	1	1
35–49	0									
50–64	1	1.0	0	1	1	1	1	1	1	1
65+	0									
2. MULTIPLE DX										
A. Not Operated										
0–19 Years	0									
20–34	2	1.0	0	1	1	1	1	1	1	1
35–49	3	6.3	56	2	2	2	15	15	15	15
50–64	2	11.9	71	6	6	6	18	18	18	18
65+	4	3.5	2	2	2	4	5	5	5	5
B. Operated										
0–19 Years	5	1.2	<1	1	1	1	1	2	2	2
20–34	6	1.7	<1	1	1	2	2	2	3	3
35–49	7	2.3	<1	1	2	2	3	4	4	4
50–64	11	2.9	8	1	1	2	3	7	10	10
65+	5	6.0	8	3	4	6	7	10	10	10
SUBTOTALS:										
1. SINGLE DX										
A. Not Operated	0									
B. Operated	2	1.0	0	1	1	1	1	1	1	1
2. MULTIPLE DX										
A. Not Operated	11	5.3	33	1	2	3	6	15	18	18
B. Operated	34	2.8	6	1	1	2	3	7	10	10
1. SINGLE DX	2	1.0	0	1	1	1	1	1	1	1
2. MULTIPLE DX	45	3.4	13	1	1	2	4	7	10	10
A. NOT OPERATED	11	5.3	33	1	2	3	6	15	18	18
B. OPERATED	36	2.7	6	1	1	2	3	7	10	10
TOTAL										
0–19 Years	5	1.2	<1	1	1	1	1	2	2	2
20–34	9	1.5	<1	1	1	1	2	3	3	3
35–49	10	3.5	17	1	2	2	3	15	15	15
50–64	14	4.0	23	1	1	2	6	10	18	18
65+	9	4.9	6	2	3	4	6	10	10	10
GRAND TOTAL	47	3.3	13	1	1	2	4	7	10	10

906: LATE EFF SKIN/SUBCU INJ

Type of Patients	Observed Patients	Avg. Stay	Variance	10th	25th	50th	75th	90th	95th	99th
1. SINGLE DX										
A. Not Operated										
0–19 Years	0									
20–34	0									
35–49	0									
50–64	0									
65+	0									
B. Operated										
0–19 Years	0									
20–34	4	2.0	4	1	1	1	5	5	5	5
35–49	0									
50–64	1	1.0	0	1	1	1	1	1	1	1
65+	0									
2. MULTIPLE DX										
A. Not Operated										
0–19 Years	1	2.0	0	2	2	2	2	2	2	2
20–34	0									
35–49	1	2.0	0	2	2	2	2	2	2	2
50–64	4	3.8	3	2	3	4	5	6	6	6
65+	4	2.8	<1	2	2	3	3	4	4	4
B. Operated										
0–19 Years	1	7.0	0	7	7	7	7	7	7	7
20–34	2	7.0	50	2	7	12	12	12	12	12
35–49	2	13.5	<1	13	13	13	14	14	14	14
50–64	4	3.8	9	1	1	3	8	8	8	8
65+	7	4.6	8	1	2	5	8	8	8	8
SUBTOTALS:										
1. SINGLE DX										
A. Not Operated	0									
B. Operated	5	1.8	3	1	1	1	1	5	5	5
2. MULTIPLE DX										
A. Not Operated	10	3.0	2	2	2	3	4	6	6	6
B. Operated	16	5.9	18	1	3	5	8	13	14	14
1. SINGLE DX	5	1.8	3	1	1	1	1	5	5	5
2. MULTIPLE DX	26	4.8	14	2	2	3	7	12	13	14
A. NOT OPERATED	10	3.0	2	2	2	3	4	6	6	6
B. OPERATED	21	5.0	18	1	1	3	8	12	13	14
TOTAL										
0–19 Years	2	4.5	12	2	2	7	7	7	7	7
20–34	6	3.7	19	1	1	2	5	12	12	12
35–49	3	9.7	44	2	2	13	14	14	14	14
50–64	9	3.5	5	2	2	3	4	8	8	8
65+	11	3.9	6	2	2	3	5	8	8	8
GRAND TOTAL	31	4.3	13	1	2	3	6	8	13	14

Length of Stay by Diagnosis and Operation, Western Region, 2008

Western Region, October 2006–September 2007 Data, by Diagnosis

907: LATE EFF NERV SYSTEM INJ

Type of Patients	Observed Patients	Avg. Stay	Vari-ance	Percentiles						
				10th	25th	50th	75th	90th	95th	99th
1. SINGLE DX										
A. *Not Operated*										
0–19 Years	0									
20–34	0									
35–49	0									
50–64	0									
65+	0									
B. *Operated*										
0–19 Years	0									
20–34	0									
35–49	0									
50–64	0									
65+	0									
2. MULTIPLE DX										
A. *Not Operated*										
0–19 Years	0									
20–34	2	9.5	12	7	7	10	12	12	12	12
35–49	8	8.1	61	1	1	3	14	22	22	22
50–64	4	5.5	35	1	2	5	14	>99	>99	>99
65+	5	11.8	59	6	7	9	12	25	25	25
B. *Operated*										
0–19 Years	0									
20–34	0									
35–49	4	3.3	5	1	1	4	4	6	6	6
50–64	3	3.3	10	1	1	2	7	7	7	7
65+	3	3.7	2	2	2	4	5	5	5	5
SUBTOTALS:										
1. SINGLE DX										
A. *Not Operated*	0									
B. *Operated*	0									
2. MULTIPLE DX										
A. *Not Operated*	19	8.7	49	1	2	9	14	25	>99	>99
B. *Operated*	10	3.4	4	1	2	2	5	6	7	7
1. SINGLE DX	0									
2. MULTIPLE DX	29	6.9	39	1	2	6	12	22	25	>99
A. NOT OPERATED	19	8.7	49	1	2	9	14	25	>99	>99
B. OPERATED	10	3.4	4	1	2	2	5	6	7	7
TOTAL										
0–19 Years	0									
20–34	2	9.5	12	7	7	10	12	12	12	12
35–49	12	6.5	46	1	1	3	11	14	22	22
50–64	7	4.6	22	1	2	5	14	>99	>99	>99
65+	8	8.8	53	2	5	7	12	25	25	25
GRAND TOTAL	29	6.9	39	1	2	6	12	22	25	>99

908: LATE EFF INJURY NEC&NOS

Type of Patients	Observed Patients	Avg. Stay	Vari-ance	Percentiles						
				10th	25th	50th	75th	90th	95th	99th
1. SINGLE DX										
A. *Not Operated*										
0–19 Years	0									
20–34	1	4.0	0	4	4	4	4	4	4	4
35–49	0									
50–64	0									
65+	0									
B. *Operated*										
0–19 Years	0									
20–34	0									
35–49	0									
50–64	0									
65+	0									
2. MULTIPLE DX										
A. *Not Operated*										
0–19 Years	0									
20–34	1	8.0	0	8	8	8	8	8	8	8
35–49	1	1.0	0	1	1	1	1	1	1	1
50–64	1	74.0	0	74	74	74	74	74	74	74
65+	1	6.0	0	6	6	6	6	6	6	6
B. *Operated*										
0–19 Years	0									
20–34	2	2.0	0	2	2	2	2	2	2	2
35–49	1	3.0	0	3	3	3	3	3	3	3
50–64	1	1.0	0	1	1	1	1	1	1	1
65+	2	3.5	<1	3	3	4	4	4	4	4
SUBTOTALS:										
1. SINGLE DX										
A. *Not Operated*	1	4.0	0	4	4	4	4	4	4	4
B. *Operated*	0									
2. MULTIPLE DX										
A. *Not Operated*	4	22.3	>999	1	6	8	74	74	74	74
B. *Operated*	6	2.5	1	1	2	3	3	4	4	4
1. SINGLE DX	1	4.0	0	4	4	4	4	4	4	4
2. MULTIPLE DX	10	10.5	506	1	2	3	6	74	74	74
A. NOT OPERATED	5	18.6	962	1	4	6	8	74	74	74
B. OPERATED	6	2.5	1	1	2	3	3	4	4	4
TOTAL										
0–19 Years	0									
20–34	4	4.0	8	2	2	4	4	8	8	8
35–49	2	2.0	2	1	1	1	3	3	3	3
50–64	2	37.8	>999	1	1	74	74	74	74	74
65+	3	4.3	2	3	3	4	6	6	6	6
GRAND TOTAL	11	9.9	459	1	2	3	6	8	74	74

909: LATE EFF OTHER EXT CAUSE

Type of Patients	Observed Patients	Avg. Stay	Vari-ance	Percentiles						
				10th	25th	50th	75th	90th	95th	99th
1. SINGLE DX										
A. *Not Operated*										
0–19 Years	0									
20–34	0									
35–49	0									
50–64	0									
65+	0									
B. *Operated*										
0–19 Years	0									
20–34	0									
35–49	0									
50–64	0									
65+	0									
2. MULTIPLE DX										
A. *Not Operated*										
0–19 Years	1	5.0	0	5	5	5	5	5	5	5
20–34	0									
35–49	1	1.0	0	1	1	1	1	1	1	1
50–64	1	4.0	0	4	4	4	4	4	4	4
65+	2	3.5	13	1	1	4	6	6	6	6
B. *Operated*										
0–19 Years	0									
20–34	2	2.0	2	1	1	1	3	3	3	3
35–49	1	2.0	0	2	2	2	2	2	2	2
50–64	2	5.5	24	2	2	9	9	9	9	9
65+	2	4.5	<1	4	4	5	5	5	5	5
SUBTOTALS:										
1. SINGLE DX										
A. *Not Operated*	0									
B. *Operated*	0									
2. MULTIPLE DX										
A. *Not Operated*	5	3.4	5	1	1	4	5	6	6	6
B. *Operated*	7	3.7	7	1	2	3	5	9	9	9
1. SINGLE DX	0									
2. MULTIPLE DX	12	3.6	6	1	1	4	5	6	9	9
A. NOT OPERATED	5	3.4	5	1	1	4	5	6	6	6
B. OPERATED	7	3.7	7	2	2	3	5	9	9	9
TOTAL										
0–19 Years	1	5.0	0	5	5	5	5	5	5	5
20–34	2	2.0	2	1	1	1	3	3	3	3
35–49	2	1.5	<1	1	1	2	2	2	2	2
50–64	3	5.0	13	2	2	4	9	9	9	9
65+	4	4.0	5	1	4	5	5	6	6	6
GRAND TOTAL	12	3.6	6	1	1	4	5	6	9	9

777

Length of Stay by Diagnosis and Operation, Western Region, 2008

Western Region, October 2006–September 2007 Data, by Diagnosis

910: SUPERFICIAL INJURY HEAD

Type of Patients	Observed Patients	Avg. Stay	Variance	10th	25th	50th	75th	90th	95th	99th
1. SINGLE DX										
A. Not Operated										
0–19 Years	24	1.1	<1	1	1	1	1	1	2	3
20–34	5	1.6	2	1	1	1	1	4	4	4
35–49	2	1.5	<1	1	1	2	2	2	2	2
50–64	1	1.0	0	1	1	1	1	1	1	1
65+	0									
B. Operated										
0–19 Years	0									
20–34	0									
35–49	0									
50–64	0									
65+	0									
2. MULTIPLE DX										
A. Not Operated										
0–19 Years	57	1.2	<1	1	1	1	1	2	2	3
20–34	56	1.6	2	1	1	1	1	3	5	9
35–49	43	1.7	2	1	1	1	2	4	4	6
50–64	47	1.8	2	1	1	1	2	4	4	7
65+	49	2.6	7	1	1	2	3	4	5	17
B. Operated										
0–19 Years	1	1.0	0	1	1	1	1	1	1	1
20–34	0									
35–49	1	44.0	0	44	44	44	44	44	44	44
50–64	1	3.0	0	3	3	3	3	3	3	3
65+	0									
SUBTOTALS:										
1. SINGLE DX										
A. Not Operated	32	1.2	<1	1	1	1	1	2	2	3
B. Operated	0									
2. MULTIPLE DX										
A. Not Operated	252	1.8	3	1	1	1	2	3	4	9
B. Operated	3	16.1	587	1	1	3	44	44	44	44
1. SINGLE DX	32	1.2	<1	1	1	1	1	2	2	3
2. MULTIPLE DX	255	1.9	10	1	1	1	2	3	4	11
A. NOT OPERATED	284	1.7	2	1	1	1	2	3	4	9
B. OPERATED	3	16.1	587	1	1	3	44	44	44	44
TOTAL										
0–19 Years	82	1.2	<1	1	1	1	1	2	2	3
20–34	61	1.6	2	1	1	1	1	3	4	9
35–49	46	2.7	40	1	1	1	2	4	5	44
50–64	49	1.8	2	1	1	1	2	4	4	7
65+	49	2.6	7	1	1	2	3	4	5	17
GRAND TOTAL	287	1.9	9	1	1	1	2	3	4	11

911: SUPERFICIAL INJURY TRUNK

Type of Patients	Observed Patients	Avg. Stay	Variance	10th	25th	50th	75th	90th	95th	99th
1. SINGLE DX										
A. Not Operated										
0–19 Years	10	1.1	<1	1	1	1	1	1	2	2
20–34	4	1.3	<1	1	1	1	1	2	2	2
35–49	3	1.3	<1	1	1	1	2	2	2	2
50–64	1	1.0	0	1	1	1	1	1	1	1
65+	0									
B. Operated										
0–19 Years	0									
20–34	1	2.0	0	2	2	2	2	2	2	2
35–49	0									
50–64	0									
65+	0									
2. MULTIPLE DX										
A. Not Operated										
0–19 Years	19	1.2	<1	1	1	1	1	2	3	3
20–34	51	1.7	5	1	1	2	2	3	4	5
35–49	39	2.5	7	1	1	1	3	5	8	12
50–64	18	2.6	7	1	1	1	4	5	11	11
65+	18	2.7	3	1	1	3	4	4	8	8
B. Operated										
0–19 Years	3	1.7	1	1	1	1	3	3	3	3
20–34	10	3.1	9	1	1	2	6	9	9	9
35–49	7	6.3	11	2	3	6	9	11	11	11
50–64	2	3.0	8	1	1	3	5	5	5	5
65+	2	7.0	0	7	7	7	7	7	7	7
SUBTOTALS:										
1. SINGLE DX										
A. Not Operated	18	1.2	<1	1	1	1	1	2	2	2
B. Operated	1	2.0	0	2	2	2	2	2	2	2
2. MULTIPLE DX										
A. Not Operated	145	2.1	3	1	1	1	3	4	5	11
B. Operated	24	4.2	10	1	1	3	7	9	9	11
1. SINGLE DX	19	1.2	<1	1	1	1	1	2	2	2
2. MULTIPLE DX	169	2.4	5	1	1	1	3	5	8	11
A. NOT OPERATED	163	2.0	3	1	1	1	2	4	4	11
B. OPERATED	25	4.1	10	1	1	3	7	9	9	11
TOTAL										
0–19 Years	32	1.2	<1	1	1	1	1	2	3	3
20–34	66	1.9	2	1	1	1	2	3	4	9
35–49	49	3.0	7	1	1	2	3	8	9	12
50–64	21	2.5	6	1	1	1	4	5	5	11
65+	20	3.2	5	1	1	3	4	7	8	8
GRAND TOTAL	188	2.2	4	1	1	1	3	4	7	11

912: SUPERF INJURY SHLDR/UA

Type of Patients	Observed Patients	Avg. Stay	Variance	10th	25th	50th	75th	90th	95th	99th
1. SINGLE DX										
A. Not Operated										
0–19 Years	0									
20–34	0									
35–49	0									
50–64	0									
65+	0									
B. Operated										
0–19 Years	0									
20–34	0									
35–49	0									
50–64	0									
65+	1	1.0	0	1	1	1	1	1	1	1
2. MULTIPLE DX										
A. Not Operated										
0–19 Years	6	1.8	3	1	1	1	2	5	5	5
20–34	15	1.2	<1	1	1	1	1	2	3	3
35–49	10	2.5	3	1	1	2	4	4	6	6
50–64	0									
65+	0									
B. Operated										
0–19 Years	0									
20–34	4	5.8	15	3	3	8	8	10	10	10
35–49	1	1.0	0	1	1	1	1	1	1	1
50–64	1	8.0	0	8	8	8	8	8	8	8
65+	0									
SUBTOTALS:										
1. SINGLE DX										
A. Not Operated	0									
B. Operated	1	1.0	0	1	1	1	1	1	1	1
2. MULTIPLE DX										
A. Not Operated	31	1.7	2	1	1	1	2	4	5	6
B. Operated	6	5.4	14	2	2	8	8	10	10	10
1. SINGLE DX	1	1.0	0	1	1	1	1	1	1	1
2. MULTIPLE DX	37	2.3	5	1	1	1	3	6	8	10
A. NOT OPERATED	31	1.7	2	1	1	1	2	4	5	6
B. OPERATED	7	4.7	15	1	1	3	8	10	10	10
TOTAL										
0–19 Years	6	1.8	3	1	1	1	2	5	5	5
20–34	19	2.2	6	1	1	1	2	8	10	10
35–49	11	2.4	3	1	1	2	4	4	6	6
50–64	1	8.0	0	8	8	8	8	8	8	8
65+	1	1.0	0	1	1	1	1	1	1	1
GRAND TOTAL	38	2.3	5	1	1	1	3	6	8	10

Length of Stay by Diagnosis and Operation, Western Region, 2008

Western Region, October 2006–September 2007 Data, by Diagnosis

913: SUPERF INJURY FOREARM

Type of Patients	Observed Patients	Avg. Stay	Vari-ance	10th	25th	50th	75th	90th	95th	99th
1. SINGLE DX										
A. *Not Operated*										
0–19 Years	2	1.0	0	1	1	1	1		1	1
20–34	2	2.0	2	1	1	3	3		3	3
35–49	1	1.0	0	1	1	1	1		1	1
50–64	0									
65+	0									
B. *Operated*										
0–19 Years	0									
20–34	0									
35–49	0									
50–64	0									
65+	0									
2. MULTIPLE DX										
A. *Not Operated*										
0–19 Years	17	2.8	8	1	1	2	2	7	12	12
20–34	38	2.6	6	1	1	2	3	6	10	12
35–49	22	2.5	3	1	1	2	4	4	7	7
50–64	13	3.6	13	1	1	2	4	7	14	14
65+	20	2.5	8	1	1	2	3	4	4	14
B. *Operated*										
0–19 Years	0									
20–34	6	7.4	14	5	6	6	6	15	15	15
35–49	1	8.0	0	8	8	8	8	8	8	8
50–64	3	4.3	2	3	3	4	6	6	6	6
65+	0									
SUBTOTALS:										
1. SINGLE DX										
A. *Not Operated*	5	1.4	<1	1	1	1	1		3	3
B. *Operated*	0									
2. MULTIPLE DX										
A. *Not Operated*	110	2.7	7	1	1	2	3	6	7	14
B. *Operated*	10	6.5	11	3	5	6	6	15	15	15
1. SINGLE DX	5	1.4	<1	1	1	1	1	3	3	3
2. MULTIPLE DX	120	3.1	8	1	1	2	4	6	10	14
A. NOT OPERATED	115	2.7	7	1	1	2	3	6	7	14
B. OPERATED	10	6.5	11	3	5	6	6	15	15	15
TOTAL										
0–19 Years	19	2.6	8	1	1	2	2	7	12	12
20–34	46	3.2	9	1	1	2	4	6	10	15
35–49	24	2.7	4	1	1	2	4	7	7	8
50–64	16	3.8	11	1	2	3	6	7	14	14
65+	20	2.5	8	1	1	2	3	4	4	14
GRAND TOTAL	125	3.0	8	1	1	2	3	6	8	14

914: SUPERF INJ HAND X FINGER

Type of Patients	Observed Patients	Avg. Stay	Vari-ance	10th	25th	50th	75th	90th	95th	99th
1. SINGLE DX										
A. *Not Operated*										
0–19 Years	5	2.0	3	1	1	1	2	2	5	5
20–34	2	1.0	0	1	1	1	1	1	1	1
35–49	1	1.0	0	1	1	1	1	1	1	1
50–64	0									
65+	0									
B. *Operated*										
0–19 Years	0									
20–34	0									
35–49	0									
50–64	0									
65+	0									
2. MULTIPLE DX										
A. *Not Operated*										
0–19 Years	7	1.4	<1	1	1	1	2	2	2	2
20–34	12	2.1	8	1	1	2	4	4	5	5
35–49	15	3.1	8	1	1	3	4	6	12	12
50–64	9	3.8	6	1	2	3	5	9	9	9
65+	5	4.4	18	1	1	3	6	11	11	11
B. *Operated*										
0–19 Years	0									
20–34	0									
35–49	0									
50–64	0									
65+	0									
SUBTOTALS:										
1. SINGLE DX										
A. *Not Operated*	8	1.6	2	1	1	1	2	5	5	5
B. *Operated*	0									
2. MULTIPLE DX										
A. *Not Operated*	48	2.9	6	1	1	2	3	6	9	12
B. *Operated*	0									
1. SINGLE DX	8	1.6	2	1	1	1	2	5	5	5
2. MULTIPLE DX	48	2.9	6	1	1	2	3	6	9	12
A. NOT OPERATED	56	2.7	6	1	1	2	3	6	9	12
B. OPERATED	0									
TOTAL										
0–19 Years	12	1.7	1	1	1	1	2	2	2	2
20–34	14	1.9	2	1	1	1	2	4	5	5
35–49	16	3.0	8	1	1	2	3	6	12	12
50–64	9	3.8	6	1	2	3	5	9	9	9
65+	5	4.4	18	1	1	3	6	11	11	11
GRAND TOTAL	56	2.7	6	1	1	2	3	6	9	12

915: SUPERF INJURY FINGER

Type of Patients	Observed Patients	Avg. Stay	Vari-ance	10th	25th	50th	75th	90th	95th	99th
1. SINGLE DX										
A. *Not Operated*										
0–19 Years	1	1.0	0	1	1	1	1	1	1	1
20–34	1	1.0	0	1	1	1	1	1	1	1
35–49	1	1.0	0	1	1	1	1	1	1	1
50–64	2	4.5	<1	4	4	5	5	5	5	5
65+	0									
B. *Operated*										
0–19 Years	1	1.0	0	1	1	1	1	1	1	1
20–34	1	3.0	0	3	3	3	3	3	3	3
35–49	0									
50–64	0									
65+	0									
2. MULTIPLE DX										
A. *Not Operated*										
0–19 Years	7	1.9	1	1	1	2	2	4	4	4
20–34	5	2.2	<1	1	2	2	3	3	3	3
35–49	12	2.7	2	1	2	2	3	5	5	5
50–64	7	1.9	1	1	1	2	2	4	4	4
65+	5	1.8	1	1	1	1	3	3	3	3
B. *Operated*										
0–19 Years	1	2.0	0	2	2	2	2	2	2	2
20–34	3	2.7	4	1	1	2	5	5	5	5
35–49	3	2.7	4	1	1	2	5	5	5	5
50–64	3	6.0	7	3	3	7	8	8	8	8
65+	3	4.3	6	2	2	4	7	7	7	7
SUBTOTALS:										
1. SINGLE DX										
A. *Not Operated*	5	2.4	4	1	1	1	4	5	5	5
B. *Operated*	2	2.0	2	1	1	3	3	3	3	3
2. MULTIPLE DX										
A. *Not Operated*	36	2.2	1	1	1	2	3	4	5	5
B. *Operated*	13	3.8	6	1	2	3	5	7	8	8
1. SINGLE DX	7	2.3	3	1	1	1	4	5	5	5
2. MULTIPLE DX	49	2.6	3	1	1	2	3	5	7	8
A. NOT OPERATED	41	2.2	2	1	1	2	3	4	5	5
B. OPERATED	15	3.5	6	1	2	3	5	7	8	8
TOTAL										
0–19 Years	10	1.7	<1	1	1	2	2	2	4	4
20–34	10	2.3	2	1	1	2	3	3	5	5
35–49	16	2.6	2	1	1	2	3	5	5	5
50–64	12	3.3	5	1	2	3	3	7	8	8
65+	8	2.8	4	1	1	3	3	7	7	7
GRAND TOTAL	56	2.6	3	1	1	2	3	5	7	8

Length of Stay by Diagnosis and Operation, Western Region, 2008

Western Region, October 2006–September 2007 Data, by Diagnosis

916: SUPERF INJURY HIP/LEG

Type of Patients	Observed Patients	Avg. Stay	Variance	10th	25th	50th	75th	90th	95th	99th
1. SINGLE DX										
A. Not Operated										
0–19 Years	3	1.0	0	1	1	1	1	1	1	1
20–34	2	2.0	2	1	1	3	3	3	3	3
35–49	3	1.3	<1	1	1	1	2	2	2	2
50–64	1	1.0	0	1	1	1	1	1	1	1
65+	0									
B. Operated										
0–19 Years	1	1.0	0	1	1	1	1	1	1	1
20–34	1	8.0	0	8	8	8	8	8	8	8
35–49	1	1.0	0	1	1	1	1	1	1	1
50–64	0									
65+	0									
2. MULTIPLE DX										
A. Not Operated										
0–19 Years	35	2.0	3	1	1	1	2	4	6	8
20–34	41	2.4	4	1	1	2	3	6	6	7
35–49	45	2.8	6	1	1	2	3	7	7	13
50–64	39	4.0	9	1	2	3	5	9	10	16
65+	48	3.3	4	1	2	3	4	6	8	11
B. Operated										
0–19 Years	5	8.4	75	4	4	5	5	24	24	24
20–34	3	2.3	1	1	1	3	3	3	3	3
35–49	5	3.8	5	1	2	5	5	6	6	6
50–64	2	12.4	179	3	3	3	22	22	22	22
65+	9	5.5	7	3	3	5	8	9	9	9
SUBTOTALS:										
1. SINGLE DX										
A. Not Operated	9	1.3	<1	1	1	1	1	3	3	3
B. Operated	3	3.4	16	1	1	1	8	8	8	8
2. MULTIPLE DX										
A. Not Operated	208	2.9	6	1	1	2	4	6	7	11
B. Operated	24	5.9	32	2	3	5	6	9	22	24
1. SINGLE DX	12	1.8	4	1	1	1	2	3	8	8
2. MULTIPLE DX	232	3.2	9	1	1	2	4	6	8	16
A. NOT OPERATED	217	2.9	5	1	1	2	4	6	7	11
B. OPERATED	27	5.6	30	1	3	4	6	9	22	24
TOTAL										
0–19 Years	44	2.6	13	1	1	1	3	5	6	24
20–34	47	2.5	4	1	1	2	3	6	7	8
35–49	54	2.8	6	1	1	2	3	6	7	13
50–64	42	4.3	17	1	2	3	5	9	10	22
65+	57	3.7	5	1	2	3	4	8	9	11
GRAND TOTAL	244	3.2	9	1	1	2	4	6	8	16

917: SUPERF INJURY FOOT/TOE

Type of Patients	Observed Patients	Avg. Stay	Variance	10th	25th	50th	75th	90th	95th	99th
1. SINGLE DX										
A. Not Operated										
0–19 Years	7	1.3	<1	1	1	1	1	1	3	3
20–34	1	2.0	0	2	2	2	2	2	2	2
35–49	0									
50–64	0									
65+	0									
B. Operated										
0–19 Years	0									
20–34	1	1.0	0	1	1	1	1	1	1	1
35–49	1	9.0	0	9	9	9	9	9	9	9
50–64	0									
65+	0									
2. MULTIPLE DX										
A. Not Operated										
0–19 Years	8	2.6	5	1	1	2	3	8	8	8
20–34	10	1.9	<1	1	1	2	3	3	3	3
35–49	9	2.9	2	1	1	3	4	5	5	5
50–64	20	2.6	2	1	2	2	3	5	5	5
65+	21	3.5	8	1	2	3	3	6	7	14
B. Operated										
0–19 Years	6	1.7	<1	1	1	2	2	3	3	3
20–34	2	4.5	12	2	2	7	7	7	7	7
35–49	2	5.0	0	5	5	5	5	5	5	5
50–64	5	5.2	4	3	4	5	6	8	8	8
65+	5	6.4	3	4	6	6	8	8	8	14
SUBTOTALS:										
1. SINGLE DX										
A. Not Operated	8	1.4	<1	1	1	1	2	3	3	3
B. Operated	2	4.9	32	1	1	1	9	9	9	9
2. MULTIPLE DX										
A. Not Operated	68	2.8	4	1	2	3	3	5	6	14
B. Operated	20	4.3	6	1	2	4	6	8	8	8
1. SINGLE DX	10	2.1	6	1	1	1	2	3	9	9
2. MULTIPLE DX	88	3.2	5	1	2	3	4	6	8	14
A. NOT OPERATED	76	2.7	4	1	1	2	3	5	6	14
B. OPERATED	22	4.4	7	1	2	4	6	8	8	9
TOTAL										
0–19 Years	22	1.9	2	1	1	1	2	3	3	8
20–34	13	2.3	3	1	1	2	3	3	7	7
35–49	12	3.7	5	2	2	4	5	9	9	9
50–64	25	3.1	3	1	2	3	4	5	6	8
65+	26	4.1	8	1	2	3	6	6	8	14
GRAND TOTAL	98	3.1	5	1	3	3	4	6	8	14

918: SUPERF INJURY EYE/ADNEXA

Type of Patients	Observed Patients	Avg. Stay	Variance	10th	25th	50th	75th	90th	95th	99th
1. SINGLE DX										
A. Not Operated										
0–19 Years	3	1.0	0	1	1	1	1	1	1	1
20–34	0									
35–49	0									
50–64	0									
65+	0									
B. Operated										
0–19 Years	0									
20–34	0									
35–49	0									
50–64	0									
65+	0									
2. MULTIPLE DX										
A. Not Operated										
0–19 Years	13	1.5	<1	1	1	1	2	3	3	3
20–34	8	1.8	2	1	1	1	2	5	5	5
35–49	5	1.6	<1	1	1	1	2	3	3	3
50–64	5	1.8	<1	1	1	2	3	3	3	3
65+	2	1.5	<1	1	1	2	2	2	2	2
B. Operated										
0–19 Years	1	2.0	0	2	2	2	2	2	2	2
20–34	0									
35–49	0									
50–64	1	1.0	0	1	1	1	1	1	1	1
65+	1	1.0	0	1	1	1	1	1	1	1
SUBTOTALS:										
1. SINGLE DX										
A. Not Operated	3	1.0	0	1	1	1	1	1	1	1
B. Operated	0									
2. MULTIPLE DX										
A. Not Operated	33	1.6	<1	1	1	1	2	3	3	5
B. Operated	3	1.3	<1	1	1	1	2	2	2	2
1. SINGLE DX	3	1.0	0	1	1	1	1	1	1	1
2. MULTIPLE DX	36	1.6	<1	1	1	1	2	3	3	5
A. NOT OPERATED	36	1.6	<1	1	1	1	2	3	3	5
B. OPERATED	3	1.3	<1	1	1	1	2	2	2	2
TOTAL										
0–19 Years	17	1.4	<1	1	1	1	2	3	3	3
20–34	8	1.8	2	1	1	1	2	5	5	5
35–49	5	1.6	<1	1	1	1	2	3	3	3
50–64	6	1.7	<1	1	1	2	2	2	2	2
65+	3	1.3	<1	1	1	1	2	2	2	2
GRAND TOTAL	39	1.5	<1	1	1	1	2	3	3	5

Length of Stay by Diagnosis and Operation, Western Region, 2008

919: SUPERF INJURY NEC

Type of Patients	Observed Patients	Avg. Stay	Vari-ance	Percentiles						
				10th	25th	50th	75th	90th	95th	99th
1. SINGLE DX										
A. Not Operated										
0–19 Years	5	1.2	<1	1	1	1	1	2	2	2
20–34	4	1.0	0	1	1	1	1	1	1	1
35–49	1	1.0	0	1	1	1	1	1	1	1
50–64	2	1.0	0	1	1	1	1	1	1	1
65+	1	1.0	0	1	1	1	1	1	1	1
B. Operated										
0–19 Years	0									
20–34	0									
35–49	0									
50–64	0									
65+	0									
2. MULTIPLE DX										
A. Not Operated										
0–19 Years	10	1.6	<1	1	1	1	2	3	3	3
20–34	15	1.3	<1	1	1	1	2	2	3	3
35–49	9	1.3	<1	1	1	1	2	2	2	2
50–64	11	2.8	4	1	1	2	4	6	7	7
65+	7	2.7	3	1	1	2	4	5	5	5
B. Operated										
0–19 Years	0									
20–34	0									
35–49	1	4.0	0	4	4	4	4	4	4	4
50–64	1	1.0	0	1	1	1	1	1	1	1
65+	0									
SUBTOTALS:										
1. SINGLE DX										
A. Not Operated	13	1.1	<1	1	1	1	1	1	2	2
B. Operated	0									
2. MULTIPLE DX										
A. Not Operated	52	1.9	2	1	1	1	2	4	5	7
B. Operated	2	2.5	4	1	1	1	4	4	4	4
1. SINGLE DX	13	1.1	<1	1	1	1	1	1	2	2
2. MULTIPLE DX	54	1.9	2	1	1	1	2	4	5	7
A. NOT OPERATED	65	1.7	2	1	1	1	2	3	4	7
B. OPERATED	2	2.5	4	1	1	1	4	4	4	4
TOTAL										
0–19 Years	15	1.5	<1	1	1	1	2	3	3	3
20–34	19	1.3	<1	1	1	1	1	2	3	3
35–49	11	1.5	<1	1	1	1	2	2	2	4
50–64	14	2.4	4	1	1	2	3	6	7	7
65+	8	2.5	3	1	1	2	4	5	5	5
GRAND TOTAL	67	1.8	2	1	1	1	2	4	4	7

920: CONTUSION HEAD X EYE

Type of Patients	Observed Patients	Avg. Stay	Vari-ance	Percentiles						
				10th	25th	50th	75th	90th	95th	99th
1. SINGLE DX										
A. Not Operated										
0–19 Years	64	1.2	<1	1	1	1	1	2	2	4
20–34	11	1.1	<1	1	1	1	1	1	2	2
35–49	7	1.3	<1	1	1	1	2	2	2	2
50–64	4	2.7	4	1	1	2	5	5	5	5
65+	1	1.0	0	1	1	1	1	1	1	1
B. Operated										
0–19 Years	0									
20–34	0									
35–49	0									
50–64	0									
65+	0									
2. MULTIPLE DX										
A. Not Operated										
0–19 Years	140	1.4	<1	1	1	1	2	3	3	5
20–34	133	1.5	1	1	1	1	2	3	3	6
35–49	120	2.6	13	1	1	1	3	5	7	26
50–64	147	2.6	12	1	1	2	3	6	8	22
65+	548	2.9	5	1	1	2	4	5	7	10
B. Operated										
0–19 Years	2	4.0	2	3	3	5	5	5	5	5
20–34	1	1.0	0	1	1	1	1	1	1	1
35–49	6	4.2	4	1	3	5	6	6	6	6
50–64	1	2.0	0	2	2	2	2	2	2	2
65+	11	3.8	5	2	2	3	5	5	9	9
SUBTOTALS:										
1. SINGLE DX										
A. Not Operated	87	1.3	<1	1	1	1	1	2	2	5
B. Operated	0									
2. MULTIPLE DX										
A. Not Operated	1,088	2.5	6	1	1	2	3	4	5	13
B. Operated	21	3.7	4	2	2	3	5	6	6	9
1. SINGLE DX	87	1.3	<1	1	1	1	1	1	2	5
2. MULTIPLE DX	1,109	2.5	6	1	1	2	3	5	7	13
A. NOT OPERATED	1,175	2.4	6	1	1	1	3	5	6	13
B. OPERATED	21	3.7	4	1	2	3	5	6	6	9
TOTAL										
0–19 Years	206	1.4	<1	1	1	1	2	3	3	5
20–34	145	1.5	<1	1	1	1	2	3	3	6
35–49	133	2.6	12	1	1	1	3	5	6	26
50–64	152	2.6	12	1	1	2	3	6	8	22
65+	560	2.9	5	1	1	2	4	5	7	10
GRAND TOTAL	1,196	2.4	6	1	1	2	3	5	6	13

921: CONTUSION EYE & ADNEXA

Type of Patients	Observed Patients	Avg. Stay	Vari-ance	Percentiles						
				10th	25th	50th	75th	90th	95th	99th
1. SINGLE DX										
A. Not Operated										
0–19 Years	8	2.3	2	1	1	3	4	4	4	4
20–34	2	1.5	<1	1	1	2	2	2	2	2
35–49	1	4.0	0	4	4	4	4	4	4	4
50–64	0									
65+	0									
B. Operated										
0–19 Years	0									
20–34	0									
35–49	0									
50–64	0									
65+	0									
2. MULTIPLE DX										
A. Not Operated										
0–19 Years	37	1.7	1	1	1	1	2	3	3	5
20–34	24	1.5	<1	1	1	1	2	3	3	3
35–49	23	2.3	4	1	1	1	3	4	8	8
50–64	22	2.3	7	1	1	2	3	4	4	13
65+	73	2.5	3	1	2	2	3	5	7	9
B. Operated										
0–19 Years	5	7.4	11	4	6	7	7	13	13	13
20–34	1	6.0	0	6	6	6	6	6	6	6
35–49	2	2.0	2	1	1	3	3	3	3	3
50–64	6	1.8	4	1	1	1	1	6	6	6
65+	3	5.3	2	4	4	5	7	7	7	7
SUBTOTALS:										
1. SINGLE DX										
A. Not Operated	11	2.3	2	1	1	2	4	4	4	4
B. Operated	0									
2. MULTIPLE DX										
A. Not Operated	179	2.2	3	1	1	2	3	4	6	9
B. Operated	17	4.4	11	1	1	4	6	7	13	13
1. SINGLE DX	11	2.3	2	1	1	2	4	4	4	4
2. MULTIPLE DX	196	2.3	4	1	1	2	3	5	7	13
A. NOT OPERATED	190	2.2	3	1	1	2	3	4	5	9
B. OPERATED	17	4.4	11	1	1	4	6	7	13	13
TOTAL										
0–19 Years	50	2.3	5	1	1	1	3	5	7	13
20–34	27	1.7	1	1	1	1	2	3	3	6
35–49	26	2.3	4	1	1	1	3	4	8	8
50–64	28	2.2	6	1	1	1	2	4	6	13
65+	76	2.6	4	1	1	2	3	5	7	9
GRAND TOTAL	207	2.3	4	1	1	2	3	5	7	9

Western Region, October 2006–September 2007 Data, by Diagnosis

922: CONTUSION OF TRUNK

Type of Patients	Observed Patients	Avg. Stay	Variance	10th	25th	50th	75th	90th	95th	99th
1. SINGLE DX										
A. Not Operated										
0–19 Years	40	1.2	<1	1	1	1	1	2	3	3
20–34	31	1.6	1	1	1	1	1	2	5	6
35–49	29	1.4	<1	1	1	1	1	3	3	3
50–64	14	1.3	<1	1	1	1	1	2	3	3
65+	4	1.8	<1	1	1	2	2	3	3	3
B. Operated										
0–19 Years	10	1.6	<1	1	1	1	2	3	3	3
20–34	5	1.4	<1	1	1	1	1	3	3	3
35–49	4	1.8	<1	1	1	2	2	3	3	3
50–64	0									
65+	0									
2. MULTIPLE DX										
A. Not Operated										
0–19 Years	131	1.3	<1	1	1	1	2	2	3	3
20–34	220	1.7	1	1	1	1	2	3	4	6
35–49	248	2.3	7	1	1	2	3	5	6	16
50–64	382	2.6	5	1	1	2	3	5	6	12
65+	953	3.3	7	2	2	3	4	6	8	16
B. Operated										
0–19 Years	6	2.2	3	1	1	1	3	5	5	5
20–34	19	3.8	15	1	1	3	5	7	18	18
35–49	11	3.1	6	1	1	1	4	7	8	8
50–64	15	7.5	60	2	2	5	9	21	29	29
65+	27	6.5	38	1	3	4	7	13	23	27
SUBTOTALS:										
1. SINGLE DX										
A. Not Operated	118	1.4	<1	1	1	1	1	2	3	3
B. Operated	19	1.6	<1	1	1	1	2	3	3	3
2. MULTIPLE DX										
A. Not Operated	1,934	2.7	6	1	1	2	3	5	7	13
B. Operated	78	5.2	32	1	2	4	6	11	21	29
1. SINGLE DX	137	1.4	<1	1	1	1	2	2	3	5
2. MULTIPLE DX	2,012	2.8	8	1	1	2	3	5	7	15
A. NOT OPERATED	2,052	2.7	6	1	1	2	3	5	7	13
B. OPERATED	97	4.5	28	1	1	3	5	9	18	29
TOTAL										
0–19 Years	187	1.4	<1	1	1	1	2	2	3	5
20–34	275	1.8	2	1	1	1	2	3	5	6
35–49	292	2.3	7	1	1	1	3	5	6	16
50–64	411	2.7	8	1	1	2	3	5	8	13
65+	984	3.4	9	1	2	3	4	6	8	17
GRAND TOTAL	2,149	2.7	7	1	1	2	3	5	7	15

922.1: CONTUSION OF CHEST WALL

Type of Patients	Observed Patients	Avg. Stay	Variance	10th	25th	50th	75th	90th	95th	99th
1. SINGLE DX										
A. Not Operated										
0–19 Years	7	1.0	0	1	1	1	1	1	1	1
20–34	8	1.1	<1	1	1	1	1	2	2	2
35–49	10	1.2	<1	1	1	1	1	2	2	2
50–64	7	1.0	0	1	1	1	1	1	1	1
65+	4	1.8	<1	1	1	2	2	3	3	3
B. Operated										
0–19 Years	0									
20–34	0									
35–49	0									
50–64	0									
65+	0									
2. MULTIPLE DX										
A. Not Operated										
0–19 Years	45	1.3	<1	1	1	1	1	2	3	5
20–34	101	1.5	<1	1	1	1	2	3	3	4
35–49	123	2.1	6	1	1	2	3	4	6	16
50–64	200	2.2	3	1	1	2	3	4	6	9
65+	539	3.0	5	1	1	3	4	6	7	12
B. Operated										
0–19 Years	0									
20–34	2	6.5	<1	6	6	7	7	7	7	7
35–49	2	2.0	2	1	1	1	1	3	3	3
50–64	2	25.0	32	21	21	21	29	29	29	29
65+	8	6.9	9	4	4	5	5	9	12	12
SUBTOTALS:										
1. SINGLE DX										
A. Not Operated	36	1.2	<1	1	1	1	1	2	2	3
B. Operated	0									
2. MULTIPLE DX										
A. Not Operated	1,008	2.5	5	1	1	2	3	5	7	12
B. Operated	14	8.7	58	3	4	6	10	21	29	29
1. SINGLE DX	36	1.2	<1	1	1	1	1	2	2	3
2. MULTIPLE DX	1,022	2.6	6	1	1	2	3	5	7	12
A. NOT OPERATED	1,044	2.5	5	1	1	2	3	5	6	12
B. OPERATED	14	8.7	58	3	4	6	10	21	29	29
TOTAL										
0–19 Years	52	1.3	<1	1	1	1	1	2	3	5
20–34	111	1.5	1	1	1	1	2	3	4	6
35–49	135	2.0	6	1	1	1	2	4	6	16
50–64	209	2.4	8	1	1	2	3	5	7	12
65+	551	3.1	5	1	1	3	4	6	7	12
GRAND TOTAL	1,058	2.6	6	1	1	2	3	5	7	12

922.2: CONTUSION ABDOMINAL WALL

Type of Patients	Observed Patients	Avg. Stay	Variance	10th	25th	50th	75th	90th	95th	99th
1. SINGLE DX										
A. Not Operated										
0–19 Years	29	1.3	<1	1	1	1	1	2	3	3
20–34	16	1.6	2	1	1	1	2	3	6	6
35–49	10	1.5	<1	1	1	1	2	3	3	3
50–64	5	1.4	<1	1	1	1	1	3	3	3
65+	0									
B. Operated										
0–19 Years	0									
20–34	0									
35–49	1	3.0	0	3	3	3	3	3	3	3
50–64	0									
65+	0									
2. MULTIPLE DX										
A. Not Operated										
0–19 Years	64	1.3	<1	1	1	1	2	2	3	3
20–34	78	1.8	1	1	1	1	2	3	4	6
35–49	78	2.3	4	1	1	2	3	5	6	13
50–64	95	2.7	8	1	1	3	3	5	7	21
65+	143	3.8	12	2	2	3	4	7	10	19
B. Operated										
0–19 Years	2	1.5	<1	1	1	2	2	2	2	2
20–34	4	2.0	<1	1	2	2	3	3	3	3
35–49	4	3.5	5	1	2	4	4	7	7	7
50–64	6	4.5	5	2	2	5	6	8	8	8
65+	11	8.2	80	2	2	4	13	23	27	27
SUBTOTALS:										
1. SINGLE DX										
A. Not Operated	60	1.4	<1	1	1	1	2	2	3	3
B. Operated	1	3.0	0	3	3	3	3	3	3	3
2. MULTIPLE DX										
A. Not Operated	458	2.6	7	1	1	2	3	5	7	16
B. Operated	27	5.3	40	1	2	4	6	13	23	27
1. SINGLE DX	61	1.4	<1	1	1	1	2	3	3	6
2. MULTIPLE DX	485	2.8	9	1	1	2	3	5	7	19
A. NOT OPERATED	518	2.5	7	1	1	2	3	5	7	15
B. OPERATED	28	5.2	38	1	2	4	6	13	23	27
TOTAL										
0–19 Years	95	1.3	<1	1	1	1	1	2	3	3
20–34	98	1.8	1	1	1	1	2	3	4	6
35–49	93	2.3	4	1	1	2	3	5	6	13
50–64	106	2.8	8	1	2	3	3	5	7	15
65+	154	4.1	18	1	2	3	4	8	13	23
GRAND TOTAL	546	2.6	9	1	1	2	3	5	7	18

Western Region, October 2006–September 2007 Data, by Diagnosis

922.31: CONTUSION OF BACK

Type of Patients	Observed Patients	Avg. Stay	Variance	10th	25th	50th	75th	90th	95th	99th
1. SINGLE DX										
A. Not Operated										
0–19 Years	0									
20–34	3	1.3	<1	1	1	1	2	2	2	2
35–49	2	1.5	<1	1	1	2	2	2	2	2
50–64	0									
65+	0									
*B. Operated**										
0–19 Years	0									
20–34	0									
35–49	0									
50–64	0									
65+	0									
2. MULTIPLE DX										
A. Not Operated										
0–19 Years	13	1.4	<1	1	1	1	2	2	3	3
20–34	22	2.1	2	1	1	2	3	4	5	6
35–49	23	3.7	26	1	1	3	3	6	6	26
50–64	31	2.6	6	1	1	1	3	6	8	11
65+	131	3.8	10	1	2	3	5	6	8	18
B. Operated										
0–19 Years	1	5.0	0	5	5	5	5	5	5	5
20–34	1	18.0	0	18	18	18	18	18	18	18
35–49	0									
50–64	1	11.0	0	11	11	11	11	11	11	11
65+	2	2.5	4	1	1	4	4	4	4	4
SUBTOTALS:										
1. SINGLE DX										
A. Not Operated	5	1.4	<1	1	1	1	2	2	2	2
B. Operated	0									
2. MULTIPLE DX										
A. Not Operated	220	3.3	10	1	1	3	3	6	8	18
B. Operated	5	7.9	46	1	4	5	11	18	18	18
1. SINGLE DX	5	1.4	<1	1	1	1	2	2	2	2
2. MULTIPLE DX	225	3.4	11	1	1	3	4	6	8	18
A. NOT OPERATED	225	3.3	10	1	1	3	4	6	8	18
B. OPERATED	5	7.9	46	1	4	5	11	18	18	18
TOTAL										
0–19 Years	14	1.6	1	1	1	1	2	3	5	5
20–34	26	2.6	12	1	1	2	3	5	6	18
35–49	25	3.5	25	1	1	2	3	6	8	26
50–64	32	2.9	8	1	1	2	3	7	11	11
65+	133	3.8	10	1	2	3	4	6	8	18
GRAND TOTAL	230	3.4	11	1	1	3	4	6	8	18

923: CONTUSION OF UPPER LIMB

Type of Patients	Observed Patients	Avg. Stay	Variance	10th	25th	50th	75th	90th	95th	99th
1. SINGLE DX										
A. Not Operated										
0–19 Years	6	1.8	2	1	1	1	3	4	4	4
20–34	2	1.0	0	1	1	1	1	1	1	1
35–49	0									
50–64	0									
65+	0									
*B. Operated**										
0–19 Years	0									
20–34	0									
35–49	0									
50–64	0									
65+	0									
2. MULTIPLE DX										
A. Not Operated										
0–19 Years	13	1.4	<1	1	1	1	1	3	4	4
20–34	27	1.8	3	1	1	1	2	4	6	7
35–49	31	2.7	13	1	1	2	3	4	8	20
50–64	47	2.8	4	1	1	2	4	6	7	8
65+	168	3.1	6	1	2	3	4	6	7	13
B. Operated										
0–19 Years	1	17.0	0	17	17	17	17	17	17	17
20–34	1	3.0	0	3	3	3	3	3	3	3
35–49	3	3.7	<1	3	3	4	4	4	4	4
50–64	5	4.4	<1	4	4	4	4	6	6	6
65+	5	6.8	83	3	3	3	4	23	23	23
SUBTOTALS:										
1. SINGLE DX										
A. Not Operated	8	1.6	1	1	1	1	3	4	4	4
B. Operated	0									
2. MULTIPLE DX										
A. Not Operated	286	2.8	6	1	1	2	4	6	7	13
B. Operated	15	5.8	35	3	3	4	4	17	23	23
1. SINGLE DX	8	1.6	1	1	1	1	3	4	4	4
2. MULTIPLE DX	301	3.0	8	1	1	2	4	6	7	17
A. NOT OPERATED	294	2.8	6	1	1	2	3	6	7	13
B. OPERATED	15	5.8	35	3	3	4	4	17	23	23
TOTAL										
0–19 Years	20	2.3	13	1	1	1	1	4	4	17
20–34	30	1.8	2	1	1	1	3	4	6	7
35–49	34	2.8	12	1	1	2	3	4	8	20
50–64	52	3.0	4	1	1	2	4	6	7	8
65+	173	3.2	8	1	2	3	4	6	8	18
GRAND TOTAL	309	2.9	8	1	1	2	4	6	7	17

924: CONTUSION LEG & OTH SITE

Type of Patients	Observed Patients	Avg. Stay	Variance	10th	25th	50th	75th	90th	95th	99th
1. SINGLE DX										
A. Not Operated										
0–19 Years	23	1.4	<1	1	1	1	2	2	3	3
20–34	14	1.6	<1	1	1	1	2	3	3	4
35–49	13	2.1	2	1	1	2	2	4	5	5
50–64	3	1.3	<1	1	1	1	2	2	2	2
65+	8	1.9	2	1	1	1	3	4	4	4
*B. Operated**										
0–19 Years	1	1.0	0	1	1	1	1	1	1	1
20–34	3	1.7	1	1	1	1	3	3	3	3
35–49	0									
50–64	1	8.0	0	8	8	8	8	8	8	8
65+	2	2.0	2	1	1	3	3	3	3	3
2. MULTIPLE DX										
A. Not Operated										
0–19 Years	41	1.5	1	1	1	1	2	3	3	6
20–34	97	1.9	2	1	1	1	2	4	6	8
35–49	148	2.7	9	1	1	2	3	5	6	18
50–64	290	3.3	7	1	2	3	4	6	8	13
65+	1,674	3.7	7	1	2	3	5	7	8	15
B. Operated										
0–19 Years	2	1.0	0	1	1	1	1	1	1	1
20–34	8	5.1	33	2	2	3	6	19	19	19
35–49	11	4.6	23	1	1	3	6	9	17	17
50–64	31	7.8	103	1	3	4	9	16	18	56
65+	96	7.7	37	2	3	6	11	17	20	28
SUBTOTALS:										
1. SINGLE DX										
A. Not Operated	61	1.6	1	1	1	1	2	3	4	5
B. Operated	7	2.6	7	1	1	1	3	8	8	8
2. MULTIPLE DX										
A. Not Operated	2,250	3.5	7	1	2	3	4	6	8	15
B. Operated	148	7.3	49	2	3	5	9	17	19	28
1. SINGLE DX	68	1.7	2	1	1	1	2	3	4	8
2. MULTIPLE DX	2,398	3.7	11	1	2	3	4	7	9	18
A. NOT OPERATED	2,311	3.4	7	1	2	3	4	6	8	15
B. OPERATED	155	7.1	48	1	3	5	9	16	19	28
TOTAL										
0–19 Years	67	1.5	<1	1	1	1	2	3	3	6
20–34	122	2.1	5	1	1	1	3	4	6	8
35–49	172	2.8	9	1	1	2	3	5	6	18
50–64	325	3.7	17	1	2	3	4	7	9	17
65+	1,780	3.9	10	1	2	3	5	7	9	18
GRAND TOTAL	2,466	3.7	10	1	2	3	4	7	9	17

Length of Stay by Diagnosis and Operation, Western Region, 2008

Western Region, October 2006–September 2007 Data, by Diagnosis

924.00: CONTUSION OF THIGH

Type of Patients	Observed Patients	Avg. Stay	Variance	10th	25th	50th	75th	90th	95th	99th
1. SINGLE DX										
A. Not Operated										
0–19 Years	9	1.3	<1	1	1	1	1	3	3	3
20–34	3	1.7	<1	1	1	2	2	2	2	2
35–49	6	2.3	3	1	1	2	2	5	5	5
50–64	1	1.0	0	1	1	1	1	1	1	1
65+	2	2.0	2	1	1	3	3	3	3	3
B. Operated										
0–19 Years	2	1.0	0	1	1	1	1	1	1	1
20–34	1	2.0	2	1	1	1	3	3	3	3
35–49	0									
50–64	1	8.0	0	8	8	8	8	8	8	8
65+	1	3.0	0	3	3	3	3	3	3	3
2. MULTIPLE DX										
A. Not Operated										
0–19 Years	6	1.7	1	1	1	1	3	3	3	3
20–34	19	2.2	3	1	1	1	3	4	7	7
35–49	31	3.0	6	1	2	2	4	5	10	11
50–64	58	3.3	7	1	1	2	4	6	9	15
65+	171	4.3	11	1	2	4	5	8	11	16
B. Operated										
0–19 Years	3	1.0	0	1	1	1	1	1	1	1
20–34	3	7.7	96	2	2	5	19	19	19	19
35–49	4	7.3	44	3	3	5	12	17	17	17
50–64	9	12.9	284	3	3	8	14	56	56	56
65+	12	9.2	61	3	4	6	10	19	28	28
SUBTOTALS:										
1. SINGLE DX										
A. Not Operated	21	1.7	1	1	1	1	2	3	4	5
B. Operated	5	3.2	8	1	1	3	3	8	8	8
2. MULTIPLE DX										
A. Not Operated	285	3.7	9	1	2	3	5	7	10	16
B. Operated	29	9.7	124	2	3	6	14	19	28	56
1. SINGLE DX	26	2.0	3	1	1	1	3	4	5	8
2. MULTIPLE DX	314	4.3	22	1	2	3	5	9	12	19
A. NOT OPERATED	306	3.6	9	1	2	3	5	7	10	15
B. OPERATED	34	8.7	112	1	3	4	10	19	28	56
TOTAL										
0–19 Years	17	1.4	<1	1	1	1	1	3	3	3
20–34	27	2.7	13	1	1	2	3	4	7	19
35–49	41	3.3	10	1	2	2	4	6	10	17
50–64	69	4.5	50	1	2	3	5	9	14	56
65+	186	4.6	15	1	2	4	5	12	12	19
GRAND TOTAL	340	4.1	21	1	2	3	5	8	12	19

924.01: CONTUSION OF HIP

Type of Patients	Observed Patients	Avg. Stay	Variance	10th	25th	50th	75th	90th	95th	99th
1. SINGLE DX										
A. Not Operated										
0–19 Years	3	1.3	<1	1	1	1	2	2	2	2
20–34	3	2.7	2	1	1	3	4	4	4	4
35–49	0									
50–64	0									
65+	3	2.0	3	1	1	1	4	4	4	4
B. Operated										
0–19 Years	0									
20–34	0									
35–49	0									
50–64	0									
65+	0									
2. MULTIPLE DX										
A. Not Operated										
0–19 Years	5	1.2	<1	1	1	1	1	2	2	2
20–34	14	2.5	4	1	1	2	3	6	7	7
35–49	35	3.5	21	1	2	2	4	5	12	26
50–64	99	3.4	8	1	2	3	4	6	8	13
65+	948	3.5	5	1	2	3	4	6	7	12
B. Operated										
0–19 Years	0									
20–34	3	4.0	8	2	1	6	6	6	6	6
35–49	3	4.0	19	1	1	2	9	9	9	9
50–64	4	3.0	<1	2	3	3	3	4	4	4
65+	15	8.3	58	2	2	4	13	24	24	24
SUBTOTALS:										
1. SINGLE DX										
A. Not Operated	9	2.0	2	1	1	1	3	4	4	4
B. Operated	0									
2. MULTIPLE DX										
A. Not Operated	1,101	3.5	6	1	2	3	4	6	7	13
B. Operated	24	6.5	43	2	2	4	9	15	24	24
1. SINGLE DX	9	2.0	2	1	1	1	3	4	4	4
2. MULTIPLE DX	1,125	3.6	7	1	2	3	4	6	8	14
A. NOT OPERATED	1,110	3.5	6	1	2	3	4	6	7	12
B. OPERATED	24	6.5	43	2	2	4	9	15	24	24
TOTAL										
0–19 Years	8	1.3	<1	1	1	1	1	2	2	2
20–34	19	2.7	4	1	1	2	4	6	7	7
35–49	38	3.6	20	2	2	2	4	9	12	26
50–64	103	3.4	8	1	2	3	4	6	8	13
65+	966	3.6	6	1	2	3	4	6	8	14
GRAND TOTAL	1,134	3.6	7	2	2	3	4	6	8	14

924.10: CONTUSION OF LOWER LEG

Type of Patients	Observed Patients	Avg. Stay	Variance	10th	25th	50th	75th	90th	95th	99th
1. SINGLE DX										
A. Not Operated										
0–19 Years	3	2.0	1	1	1	2	2	3	3	3
20–34	3	1.3	<1	1	1	1	1	2	2	2
35–49	2	1.5	<1	1	1	2	2	2	2	2
50–64	2	1.5	<1	1	1	2	2	2	2	2
65+	3	1.7	1	1	1	1	3	3	3	3
B. Operated										
0–19 Years	0									
20–34	0									
35–49	0									
50–64	0									
65+	1	1.0	0	1	1	1	1	1	1	1
2. MULTIPLE DX										
A. Not Operated										
0–19 Years	10	1.5	<1	1	1	1	1	2	2	2
20–34	15	2.0	4	1	1	1	2	6	8	8
35–49	30	2.7	10	1	1	2	3	5	5	18
50–64	57	2.9	5	1	1	2	4	6	8	11
65+	170	4.4	13	1	2	3	6	8	12	20
B. Operated										
0–19 Years	0									
20–34	0									
35–49	1	5.0	0	5	5	5	5	5	5	5
50–64	9	7.3	45	1	1	7	11	18	18	18
65+	51	8.0	33	2	3	6	12	17	18	24
SUBTOTALS:										
1. SINGLE DX										
A. Not Operated	13	1.6	<1	1	1	1	2	3	3	3
B. Operated	1	1.0	0	1	1	1	1	1	1	1
2. MULTIPLE DX										
A. Not Operated	282	3.7	11	1	1	3	5	7	10	18
B. Operated	61	7.8	34	1	3	6	11	17	18	24
1. SINGLE DX	14	1.6	<1	1	1	1	2	3	3	3
2. MULTIPLE DX	343	4.4	17	1	2	3	5	9	15	20
A. NOT OPERATED	295	3.6	11	1	1	3	4	7	10	18
B. OPERATED	62	7.7	34	2	3	5	11	17	18	24
TOTAL										
0–19 Years	13	1.6	<1	1	1	1	2	3	4	4
20–34	18	1.9	4	1	1	1	2	6	8	8
35–49	33	2.7	9	1	1	2	3	5	5	18
50–64	68	3.5	12	1	2	2	4	8	11	18
65+	225	5.2	20	1	2	4	6	11	15	20
GRAND TOTAL	357	4.3	17	1	2	3	5	9	15	20

Length of Stay by Diagnosis and Operation, Western Region, 2008

Western Region, October 2006–September 2007 Data, by Diagnosis

924.11: CONTUSION OF KNEE

Type of Patients	Observed Patients	Avg. Stay	Vari-ance	10th	25th	50th	75th	90th	95th	99th
1. SINGLE DX										
A. Not Operated										
0–19 Years	3	1.7	<1	1	1	2	2	2	2	2
20–34	2	1.0	0	1	1	1	1	1	1	1
35–49	2	3.0	2	2	2	4	4	4	4	4
50–64	0									
65+	0									
B. Operated										
0–19 Years	0									
20–34	0									
35–49	0									
50–64	0									
65+	0									
2. MULTIPLE DX										
A. Not Operated										
0–19 Years	5	1.4	<1	1	1	1	2	2	2	2
20–34	10	1.4	<1	1	1	1	2	2	3	3
35–49	21	2.4	2	1	1	2	3	4	5	5
50–64	44	4.3	9	1	3	3	6	8	10	13
65+	250	3.4	6	1	2	3	4	6	7	14
B. Operated										
0–19 Years	1	1.0	0	1	1	1	1	1	1	1
20–34	0									
35–49	2	2.0	2	1	1	2	3	3	3	3
50–64	3	4.0	13	1	1	3	8	8	8	8
65+	12	4.3	8	2	2	3	4	6	11	11
SUBTOTALS:										
1. SINGLE DX										
A. Not Operated	7	1.9	1	1	1	2	2	4	4	4
B. Operated	0									
2. MULTIPLE DX										
A. Not Operated	330	3.4	6	1	2	3	4	6	8	13
B. Operated	18	3.8	8	1	2	3	6	8	11	11
1. SINGLE DX	7	1.9	1	1	1	2	2	4	4	4
2. MULTIPLE DX	348	3.4	6	1	2	3	4	6	8	13
A. NOT OPERATED	337	3.3	6	1	2	3	4	6	8	13
B. OPERATED	18	3.8	8	1	2	3	6	8	11	11
TOTAL										
0–19 Years	9	1.5	<1	1	1	1	2	2	2	2
20–34	12	1.3	<1	1	1	1	1	2	2	3
35–49	25	2.4	2	1	1	2	3	4	5	5
50–64	47	4.3	9	1	3	3	6	8	10	13
65+	262	3.5	6	1	2	3	4	6	7	14
GRAND TOTAL	355	3.4	6	1	2	3	4	6	8	13

925: CRUSH INJ FACE/SCALP/NK

Type of Patients	Observed Patients	Avg. Stay	Vari-ance	10th	25th	50th	75th	90th	95th	99th
1. SINGLE DX										
A. Not Operated										
0–19 Years	0									
20–34	0									
35–49	0									
50–64	0									
65+	0									
B. Operated										
0–19 Years	0									
20–34	0									
35–49	0									
50–64	0									
65+	0									
2. MULTIPLE DX										
A. Not Operated										
0–19 Years	1	3.0	0	3	3	3	3	3	3	3
20–34	3	1.7	<1	1	1	2	2	2	2	2
35–49	1	1.0	0	1	1	1	1	1	1	1
50–64	1	1.0	0	1	1	1	1	1	1	1
65+	0									
B. Operated										
0–19 Years	2	17.4	532	1	1	1	34	34	34	34
20–34	4	4.0		1	3	4	4	8	8	8
35–49	4	17.7	185	6	6	6	28	31	31	31
50–64	1	2.0	0	2	2	2	2	2	2	2
65+	3	9.0	57	2	2	8	17	17	17	17
SUBTOTALS:										
1. SINGLE DX										
A. Not Operated	0									
B. Operated	0									
2. MULTIPLE DX										
A. Not Operated	6	1.7	<1	1	1	2	2	3	3	3
B. Operated	14	10.8	138	1	2	6	17	31	34	34
1. SINGLE DX	0									
2. MULTIPLE DX	20	8.0	113	1	1	3	8	31	34	34
A. NOT OPERATED	6	1.7	<1	1	1	2	2	3	3	3
B. OPERATED	14	10.8	138	1	2	6	17	31	34	34
TOTAL										
0–19 Years	3	12.7	340	1	1	3	34	34	34	34
20–34	7	3.0	6	1	1	2	6	8	8	8
35–49	5	14.3	194	1	6	6	28	31	31	31
50–64	2	1.5	<1	1	1	1	2	2	2	2
65+	3	9.0	57	2	2	8	17	17	17	17
GRAND TOTAL	20	8.0	113	1	1	3	8	31	34	34

926: CRUSH INJURY TRUNK

Type of Patients	Observed Patients	Avg. Stay	Vari-ance	10th	25th	50th	75th	90th	95th	99th
1. SINGLE DX										
A. Not Operated										
0–19 Years	0									
20–34	3	1.3	<1	1	1	1	2	2	2	2
35–49	0									
50–64	0									
65+	0									
B. Operated										
0–19 Years	1	1.0	0	1	1	1	1	1	1	1
20–34	0									
35–49	0									
50–64	1	1.0	0	1	1	1	1	1	1	1
65+	0									
2. MULTIPLE DX										
A. Not Operated										
0–19 Years	7	1.9	<1	1	1	2	3	3	3	3
20–34	20	2.8	5	1	1	2	4	7	7	8
35–49	26	4.7	26	1	2	3	5	8	11	27
50–64	13	3.7	7	2	2	3	5	6	11	11
65+	5	3.2	7	1	1	2	6	6	6	6
B. Operated										
0–19 Years	4	6.5	25	1	1	6	13	13	13	13
20–34	11	13.0	154	2	2	9	22	33	37	37
35–49	8	15.3	311	6	9	9	10	59	59	59
50–64	3	15.3	72	9	9	12	25	25	25	25
65+	2	2.0	2	1	1	1	3	3	3	3
SUBTOTALS:										
1. SINGLE DX										
A. Not Operated	3	1.3	<1	1	1	1	2	2	2	2
B. Operated	2	1.0	0	1	1	1	1	1	1	1
2. MULTIPLE DX										
A. Not Operated	71	3.6	13	1	2	3	4	7	8	27
B. Operated	28	12.2	163	1	6	9	13	33	37	59
1. SINGLE DX	5	1.2	<1	1	1	1	1	2	2	2
2. MULTIPLE DX	99	6.0	69	1	2	3	7	12	22	37
A. NOT OPERATED	74	3.5	13	1	1	3	4	7	8	27
B. OPERATED	30	11.4	160	1	3	9	13	25	37	59
TOTAL										
0–19 Years	12	3.3	13	1	1	2	3	6	13	13
20–34	34	6.0	74	1	1	3	7	14	33	37
35–49	34	7.2	106	1	3	4	8	11	27	59
50–64	17	5.6	36	1	2	3	6	12	25	25
65+	7	2.9	5	1	1	2	6	6	6	6
GRAND TOTAL	104	5.8	67	1	2	3	7	11	22	37

Length of Stay by Diagnosis and Operation, Western Region, 2008

Western Region, October 2006–September 2007 Data, by Diagnosis

927: CRUSH INJURY UPPER LIMB

Type of Patients	Observed Patients	Avg. Stay	Vari-ance	Percentiles						
				10th	25th	50th	75th	90th	95th	99th
1. SINGLE DX										
A. Not Operated										
0–19 Years	1	1.0	0	1	1	1	1	1	1	1
20–34	1	4.0	0	4	4	4	4	4	4	4
35–49	3	1.7	1	1	1	1	3	3	3	3
50–64	0									
65+	0									
B. Operated										
0–19 Years	2	1.5	<1	1	1	2	2	2	2	2
20–34	2	2.5	4	1	1	4	4	4	4	4
35–49	4	1.8	2	1	1	1	4	4	4	4
50–64	0									
65+	0									
2. MULTIPLE DX										
A. Not Operated										
0–19 Years	4	1.5	1	1	1	1	3	3	3	3
20–34	16	2.4	5	1	1	2	2	7	8	8
35–49	16	1.7	<1	1	1	1	2	3	4	4
50–64	6	2.3	<1	1	2	3	3	3	3	3
65+	2	1.5	<1	1	1	1	1	2	2	2
B. Operated										
0–19 Years	34	3.7	32	1	1	4	4	8	21	22
20–34	110	4.1	17	1	1	5	5	11	13	20
35–49	97	3.7	19	1	1	2	4	12	15	21
50–64	80	3.8	24	1	1	2	4	8	13	25
65+	18	5.4	76	1	1	2	5	25	32	32
SUBTOTALS:										
1. SINGLE DX										
A. Not Operated	5	2.0	2	1	1	1	3	4	4	4
B. Operated	8	1.9	2	1	1	2	4	4	4	4
2. MULTIPLE DX										
A. Not Operated	44	2.0	2	1	1	2	3	3	4	8
B. Operated	339	4.0	24	1	1	2	4	10	14	24
1. SINGLE DX	13	1.9	2	1	1	1	3	4	4	4
2. MULTIPLE DX	383	3.7	22	1	1	2	4	9	14	24
A. NOT OPERATED	49	2.0	2	1	1	2	3	3	4	8
B. OPERATED	347	3.9	23	1	1	2	4	10	14	24
TOTAL										
0–19 Years	41	3.3	28	1	1	1	2	8	19	22
20–34	129	3.9	16	1	1	2	5	10	13	20
35–49	120	3.3	16	1	1	2	3	10	14	17
50–64	86	3.7	23	1	1	2	4	8	13	25
65+	20	5.0	69	1	1	2	4	8	25	32
GRAND TOTAL	396	3.7	21	1	1	2	4	9	14	24

928: CRUSH INJURY LOWER LIMB

Type of Patients	Observed Patients	Avg. Stay	Vari-ance	Percentiles						
				10th	25th	50th	75th	90th	95th	99th
1. SINGLE DX										
A. Not Operated										
0–19 Years	6	1.0	0	1	1	1	1	1	1	1
20–34	14	1.7	<1	1	1	1	2	3	4	4
35–49	1	4.0	0	4	4	4	4	4	4	4
50–64	1	1.0	0	1	1	1	1	1	1	1
65+	0									
B. Operated										
0–19 Years	1	2.0	0	2	2	2	2	2	2	2
20–34	1	4.0	0	4	4	4	4	4	4	4
35–49	2	3.5	4	2	2	4	5	5	5	5
50–64	0									
65+	0									
2. MULTIPLE DX										
A. Not Operated										
0–19 Years	15	1.9	<1	1	1	2	2	4	4	4
20–34	33	2.6	3	1	1	3	3	5	6	7
35–49	34	2.7	8	1	1	2	3	5	7	16
50–64	33	2.7	5	1	1	2	4	5	6	11
65+	15	4.0	50	1	1	2	4	5	29	29
B. Operated										
0–19 Years	30	7.3	48	1	3	5	12	20	25	>99
20–34	94	8.0	122	1	2	5	9	21	32	67
35–49	54	9.1	98	2	3	5	11	26	30	43
50–64	53	9.1	124	2	3	5	9	26	41	51
65+	19	10.0	73	2	3	8	14	23	36	36
SUBTOTALS:										
1. SINGLE DX										
A. Not Operated	22	1.6	1	1	1	1	2	3	4	4
B. Operated	4	3.3	2	2	2	2	5	5	5	5
2. MULTIPLE DX										
A. Not Operated	130	2.8	10	1	1	2	3	5	6	16
B. Operated	250	8.6	104	1	3	5	10	22	32	58
1. SINGLE DX	26	1.9	2	1	1	1	2	4	4	5
2. MULTIPLE DX	380	6.6	79	1	2	3	7	17	26	51
A. NOT OPERATED	152	2.6	8	1	1	2	3	5	6	16
B. OPERATED	254	8.5	103	1	2	5	10	22	32	58
TOTAL										
0–19 Years	52	4.9	36	1	1	3	6	17	22	>99
20–34	142	6.1	88	1	2	3	6	15	21	58
35–49	91	6.6	70	1	2	3	7	16	27	43
50–64	87	6.6	87	1	2	4	6	15	32	51
65+	34	7.4	70	1	2	4	10	18	29	36
GRAND TOTAL	406	6.3	75	1	2	3	7	17	25	43

929: MULT CRUSH INJURY & NOS

Type of Patients	Observed Patients	Avg. Stay	Vari-ance	Percentiles						
				10th	25th	50th	75th	90th	95th	99th
1. SINGLE DX										
A. Not Operated										
0–19 Years	0									
20–34	0									
35–49	0									
50–64	0									
65+	0									
B. Operated										
0–19 Years	0									
20–34	0									
35–49	0									
50–64	0									
65+	0									
2. MULTIPLE DX										
A. Not Operated										
0–19 Years	0									
20–34	1	4.0	0	4	4	4	4	4	4	4
35–49	1	2.0	0	2	2	2	2	2	2	2
50–64	0									
65+	0									
B. Operated										
0–19 Years	0									
20–34	0									
35–49	2	19.6	540	3	3	36	36	36	36	36
50–64	0									
65+	1	25.0	0	25	25	25	25	25	25	25
SUBTOTALS:										
1. SINGLE DX										
A. Not Operated	0									
B. Operated	0									
2. MULTIPLE DX										
A. Not Operated	2	3.0	2	2	2	4	4	4	4	4
B. Operated	3	21.5	278	3	3	25	36	36	36	36
1. SINGLE DX	0									
2. MULTIPLE DX	5	14.1	241	2	3	4	25	36	36	36
A. NOT OPERATED	2	3.0	2	2	2	4	4	4	4	4
B. OPERATED	3	21.5	278	3	3	25	36	36	36	36
TOTAL										
0–19 Years	0									
20–34	1	4.0	0	4	4	4	4	4	4	4
35–49	3	13.8	375	2	2	3	36	36	36	36
50–64	0									
65+	1	25.0	0	25	25	25	25	25	25	25
GRAND TOTAL	5	14.1	241	2	3	4	25	36	36	36

Length of Stay by Diagnosis and Operation, Western Region, 2008

Western Region, October 2006–September 2007 Data, by Diagnosis

930: FB IN EYE

Type of Patients	Observed Patients	Avg. Stay	Variance	Percentiles 10th	25th	50th	75th	90th	95th	99th
1. SINGLE DX										
A. Not Operated										
0–19 Years	1	1.0	0	1	1	1	1	1	1	1
20–34	0									
35–49	0									
50–64	1	5.0	0	5	5	5	5	5	5	5
65+	0									
B. Operated										
0–19 Years	0									
20–34	0									
35–49	0									
50–64	0									
65+	0									
2. MULTIPLE DX										
A. Not Operated										
0–19 Years	2	1.5	<1	1	1	1	2	2	2	2
20–34	6	1.5	<1	1	1	1	2	3	3	3
35–49	2	3.5	<1	3	3	4	4	4	4	4
50–64	1	1.0	0	1	1	1	1	1	1	1
65+	0									
B. Operated										
0–19 Years	0									
20–34	0									
35–49	0									
50–64	0									
65+	1	2.0	0	2	2	2	2	2	2	2
SUBTOTALS:										
1. SINGLE DX										
A. Not Operated	2	3.0	8	1	1	5	5	5	5	5
B. Operated	0									
2. MULTIPLE DX										
A. Not Operated	11	1.8	1	1	1	1	3	3	4	4
B. Operated	1	2.0	0	2	2	2	2	2	2	2
1. SINGLE DX	2	3.0	8	1	1	5	5	5	5	5
2. MULTIPLE DX	12	1.8	1	1	1	2	3	3	4	4
A. NOT OPERATED	13	2.0	2	1	1	1	3	4	5	4
B. OPERATED	1	2.0	0	2	2	2	2	2	2	2
TOTAL										
0–19 Years	3	1.3	<1	1	1	1	2	2	2	2
20–34	6	1.5	<1	1	1	1	2	3	3	3
35–49	2	3.5	<1	3	3	4	4	4	4	4
50–64	2	3.0	8	1	1	5	5	5	5	5
65+	1	2.0	0	2	2	2	2	2	2	2
GRAND TOTAL	14	2.0	2	1	1	2	3	4	5	5

931: FB IN EAR

Type of Patients	Observed Patients	Avg. Stay	Variance	Percentiles 10th	25th	50th	75th	90th	95th	99th
1. SINGLE DX										
A. Not Operated										
0–19 Years	3	1.0	0	1	1	1	1	1	1	1
20–34	0									
35–49	1	1.0	0	1	1	1	1	1	1	1
50–64	0									
65+	0									
B. Operated										
0–19 Years	0									
20–34	0									
35–49	0									
50–64	0									
65+	0									
2. MULTIPLE DX										
A. Not Operated										
0–19 Years	3	1.0	0	1	1	1	1	1	1	1
20–34	0									
35–49	1	2.0	0	2	2	2	2	2	2	2
50–64	1	1.0	0	1	1	1	1	1	1	1
65+	0									
B. Operated										
0–19 Years	0									
20–34	0									
35–49	0									
50–64	1	1.0	0	1	1	1	1	1	1	1
65+	0									
SUBTOTALS:										
1. SINGLE DX										
A. Not Operated	4	1.0	0	1	1	1	1	1	1	1
B. Operated	0									
2. MULTIPLE DX										
A. Not Operated	5	1.2	<1	1	1	1	1	2	2	2
B. Operated	1	1.0	0	1	1	1	1	1	1	1
1. SINGLE DX	4	1.0	0	1	1	1	1	1	1	1
2. MULTIPLE DX	6	1.2	<1	1	1	1	1	2	2	2
A. NOT OPERATED	9	1.1	<1	1	1	1	1	1	2	2
B. OPERATED	1	1.0	0	1	1	1	1	1	1	1
TOTAL										
0–19 Years	6	1.0	0	1	1	1	1	1	1	1
20–34	0									
35–49	3	1.3	<1	1	1	1	2	2	2	2
50–64	1	1.0	0	1	1	1	1	1	1	1
65+	0									
GRAND TOTAL	10	1.1	<1	1	1	1	1	1	2	2

932: FB IN NOSE

Type of Patients	Observed Patients	Avg. Stay	Variance	Percentiles 10th	25th	50th	75th	90th	95th	99th
1. SINGLE DX										
A. Not Operated										
0–19 Years	11	1.0	0	1	1	1	1	1	1	1
20–34	0									
35–49	0									
50–64	0									
65+	0									
B. Operated										
0–19 Years	0									
20–34	0									
35–49	0									
50–64	0									
65+	0									
2. MULTIPLE DX										
A. Not Operated										
0–19 Years	7	1.3	<1	1	1	1	2	2	2	2
20–34	0									
35–49	1	1.0	0	1	1	1	1	1	1	1
50–64	0									
65+	0									
B. Operated										
0–19 Years	0									
20–34	0									
35–49	0									
50–64	0									
65+	0									
SUBTOTALS:										
1. SINGLE DX										
A. Not Operated	11	1.0	0	1	1	1	1	1	1	1
B. Operated	0									
2. MULTIPLE DX										
A. Not Operated	8	1.3	<1	1	1	1	1	2	2	2
B. Operated	0									
1. SINGLE DX	11	1.0	0	1	1	1	1	1	1	1
2. MULTIPLE DX	8	1.3	<1	1	1	1	1	2	2	2
A. NOT OPERATED	19	1.1	<1	1	1	1	1	2	2	2
B. OPERATED	0									
TOTAL										
0–19 Years	18	1.1	<1	1	1	1	1	2	2	2
20–34	0									
35–49	1	1.0	0	1	1	1	1	1	1	1
50–64	0									
65+	0									
GRAND TOTAL	19	1.1	<1	1	1	1	1	2	2	2

Length of Stay by Diagnosis and Operation, Western Region, 2008

Western Region, October 2006–September 2007 Data, by Diagnosis

933: FB IN PHARYNX & LARYNX

Type of Patients	Observed Patients	Avg. Stay	Variance	10th	25th	50th	75th	90th	95th	99th
1. SINGLE DX										
A. Not Operated										
0–19 Years	46	1.2	<1	1	1	1	1	2	2	2
20–34	5	1.2	<1	1	1	1	1	2	2	2
35–49	7	1.0	0	1	1	1	1	1	1	1
50–64	2	1.0	0	1	1	1	1	1	1	1
65+	1	2.0		2	2	2	2	2	2	2
B. Operated										
0–19 Years	0									
20–34	0									
35–49	0									
50–64	1	1.0	0	1	1	1	1	1	1	1
65+	0									
2. MULTIPLE DX										
A. Not Operated										
0–19 Years	57	1.7	2	1	1	2	2	3	5	8
20–34	10	2.2	2	1	1	2	4	4	4	4
35–49	24	2.9	14	1	1	2	3	4	13	16
50–64	42	2.5	5	1	1	2	3	5	6	11
65+	172	2.8	5	1	1	2	4	5	7	13
B. Operated										
0–19 Years	1	12.0	0	12	12	12	12	12	12	12
20–34	0									
35–49	1	11.0	0	11	11	11	11	11	11	11
50–64	2	12.5	24	9	9	16	16	16	16	16
65+	3	8.7	97	3	3	3	20	20	20	20
SUBTOTALS:										
1. SINGLE DX										
A. Not Operated	61	1.2	<1	1	1	1	1	2	2	2
B. Operated	1	1.0	0	1	1	1	1	1	1	1
2. MULTIPLE DX										
A. Not Operated	305	2.5	5	1	1	2	3	5	6	13
B. Operated	7	10.6	39	3	3	11	16	20	20	20
1. SINGLE DX	62	1.1	<1	1	1	1	1	2	2	2
2. MULTIPLE DX	312	2.7	7	1	1	2	3	5	8	15
A. NOT OPERATED	366	2.3	5	1	1	1	3	5	6	13
B. OPERATED	8	9.4	45	1	3	11	16	20	20	20
TOTAL										
0–19 Years	104	1.6	2	1	1	1	2	2	3	8
20–34	15	1.9	1	1	1	1	2	4	4	4
35–49	32	2.8	13	1	1	1	3	4	13	16
50–64	47	2.8	10	1	1	2	3	6	10	16
65+	176	2.9	7	1	1	2	4	5	7	15
GRAND TOTAL	374	2.5	6	1	1	1	3	5	7	15

933.1: FB IN LARYNX

Type of Patients	Observed Patients	Avg. Stay	Variance	10th	25th	50th	75th	90th	95th	99th
1. SINGLE DX										
A. Not Operated										
0–19 Years	26	1.2	<1	1	1	1	1	2	2	2
20–34	2	1.5	<1	1	1	2	2	2	2	2
35–49	4	1.0	0	1	1	1	1	1	1	1
50–64	0									
65+	0									
B. Operated										
0–19 Years	0									
20–34	0									
35–49	0									
50–64	0									
65+	0									
2. MULTIPLE DX										
A. Not Operated										
0–19 Years	45	1.7	2	1	1	2	2	3	5	8
20–34	7	1.9	1	1	1	2	2	4	4	4
35–49	11	3.1	12	1	1	2	4	4	13	13
50–64	27	2.7	6	1	1	2	3	4	10	11
65+	138	2.9	5	1	1	2	4	5	7	13
B. Operated										
0–19 Years	1	12.0	0	12	12	12	12	12	12	12
20–34	0									
35–49	1	11.0	0	11	11	11	11	11	11	11
50–64	1	16.0	0	16	16	16	16	16	16	16
65+	2	11.6	143	3	3	20	20	20	20	20
SUBTOTALS:										
1. SINGLE DX										
A. Not Operated	32	1.2	<1	1	1	1	1	2	2	2
B. Operated	0									
2. MULTIPLE DX										
A. Not Operated	228	2.6	5	1	1	2	3	5	7	13
B. Operated	5	12.4	40	11	11	12	16	20	20	20
1. SINGLE DX	32	1.2	<1	1	1	2	2	2	2	2
2. MULTIPLE DX	233	2.8	8	1	1	2	3	5	9	15
A. NOT OPERATED	260	2.5	5	1	1	2	3	5	6	13
B. OPERATED	5	12.4	40	3	11	12	16	20	20	20
TOTAL										
0–19 Years	72	1.7	3	1	1	1	2	3	3	12
20–34	9	1.8	<1	1	1	2	2	4	4	4
35–49	16	3.1	14	1	1	2	4	11	13	13
50–64	28	3.2	13	1	1	2	4	10	11	16
65+	140	3.1	7	1	1	2	4	5	8	15
GRAND TOTAL	265	2.7	7	1	1	2	3	5	8	15

934: FB IN TRACH/BRONCH/LUNG

Type of Patients	Observed Patients	Avg. Stay	Variance	10th	25th	50th	75th	90th	95th	99th
1. SINGLE DX										
A. Not Operated										
0–19 Years	45	1.1	<1	1	1	1	1	2	2	2
20–34	1	1.0	0	1	1	1	1	1	1	1
35–49	1	1.0	0	1	1	1	1	1	1	1
50–64	1	1.0	0	1	1	1	1	1	1	1
65+	0									
B. Operated										
0–19 Years	2	1.0	0	1	1	1	1	1	1	1
20–34	2	5.0	31	1	1	1	9	9	9	9
35–49	0									
50–64	0									
65+	0									
2. MULTIPLE DX										
A. Not Operated										
0–19 Years	63	2.1	3	1	1	2	2	4	5	11
20–34	14	3.3	7	1	1	3	5	7	9	9
35–49	28	3.9	10	1	1	3	5	8	11	13
50–64	61	4.0	20	1	1	3	4	9	14	22
65+	145	3.5	10	1	1	2	4	8	10	14
B. Operated										
0–19 Years	2	9.5	<1	9	9	10	10	10	10	10
20–34	0									
35–49	3	10.7	46	3	3	13	16	16	16	16
50–64	7	10.0	7	5	9	10	12	13	13	13
65+	13	9.2	123	2	3	7	9	13	44	44
SUBTOTALS:										
1. SINGLE DX										
A. Not Operated	48	1.1	<1	1	1	1	1	2	2	2
B. Operated	4	3.0	16	1	1	1	1	9	9	9
2. MULTIPLE DX										
A. Not Operated	311	3.4	11	1	1	2	4	8	11	14
B. Operated	25	9.6	67	2	5	9	12	13	16	44
1. SINGLE DX	52	1.3	1	1	1	1	1	2	2	9
2. MULTIPLE DX	336	3.8	17	1	1	2	5	9	12	17
A. NOT OPERATED	359	3.1	10	1	1	2	4	7	10	14
B. OPERATED	29	8.7	65	1	3	9	11	13	16	44
TOTAL										
0–19 Years	112	1.8	3	1	1	1	2	4	5	10
20–34	17	3.4	8	1	1	3	5	9	9	9
35–49	32	4.5	16	1	1	3	5	11	13	16
50–64	69	4.6	21	1	1	3	5	12	14	22
65+	158	4.0	21	1	1	2	5	9	12	17
GRAND TOTAL	388	3.5	16	1	1	2	4	9	11	17

Length of Stay by Diagnosis and Operation, Western Region, 2008

Western Region, October 2006–September 2007 Data, by Diagnosis

935: FB IN MOUTH/ESOPH/STOM

Type of Patients	Observed Patients	Avg. Stay	Vari-ance	10th	25th	50th	75th	90th	95th	99th
1. SINGLE DX										
A. *Not Operated*										
0–19 Years	259	1.1	<1	1	1	1	1	1	2	4
20–34	22	1.7	4	1	1	1	1	2	7	9
35–49	16	1.4	<1	1	1	1	2	2	3	3
50–64	3	1.0	0	1	1	1	1	1	1	1
65+	8	1.1	<1	1	1	1	1	2	2	2
B. *Operated*										
0–19 Years	2	3.5	4	2	2	5	5	5	5	5
20–34	0									
35–49	0									
50–64	1	1.0	0	1	1	1	1	1	1	1
65+	0									
2. MULTIPLE DX										
A. *Not Operated*										
0–19 Years	158	1.6	2	1	1	1	1	4	5	8
20–34	144	3.4	13	1	1	2	4	8	11	17
35–49	184	2.7	14	1	1	1	3	6	8	20
50–64	193	2.6	13	1	1	1	2	5	8	22
65+	377	2.7	7	1	1	2	3	6	8	15
B. *Operated*										
0–19 Years	14	6.4	5	4	5	6	8	10	11	11
20–34	17	9.2	42	3	5	7	11	18	28	28
35–49	21	9.2	32	3	6	8	11	16	18	26
50–64	14	13.7	94	5	7	10	16	26	40	40
65+	16	7.0	31	2	4	6	8	14	24	24
SUBTOTALS:										
1. SINGLE DX										
A. *Not Operated*	308	1.2	<1	1	1	1	1	1	2	5
B. *Operated*	3	2.7	4	1	1	2	5	5	5	5
2. MULTIPLE DX										
A. *Not Operated*	1,056	2.6	10	1	1	2	3	6	8	16
B. *Operated*	82	9.1	44	3	5	7	11	16	24	40
1. SINGLE DX	311	1.2	<1	1	1	1	1	2	2	5
2. MULTIPLE DX	1,138	3.1	15	1	1	2	3	7	10	18
A. NOT OPERATED	1,364	2.3	8	1	1	1	2	5	7	16
B. OPERATED	85	8.9	44	3	5	7	11	16	24	40
TOTAL										
0–19 Years	433	1.5	2	1	1	1	1	2	5	8
20–34	183	3.7	18	1	1	2	4	10	12	18
35–49	221	3.2	18	1	1	1	3	7	10	20
50–64	211	3.3	25	1	1	1	3	8	16	24
65+	401	2.8	9	1	1	2	3	6	8	15
GRAND TOTAL	1,449	2.7	12	1	1	1	3	6	9	18

935.1: FB IN ESOPHAGUS

Type of Patients	Observed Patients	Avg. Stay	Vari-ance	10th	25th	50th	75th	90th	95th	99th
1. SINGLE DX										
A. *Not Operated*										
0–19 Years	225	1.1	<1	1	1	1	1	1	2	3
20–34	13	1.0	0	1	1	1	1	1	1	1
35–49	16	1.4	<1	1	1	1	2	2	3	3
50–64	3	1.0	0	1	1	1	1	1	1	1
65+	8	1.1	<1	1	1	1	1	2	2	2
B. *Operated*										
0–19 Years	1	2.0	0	2	2	2	2	2	2	2
20–34	0									
35–49	0									
50–64	0									
65+	0									
2. MULTIPLE DX										
A. *Not Operated*										
0–19 Years	117	1.6	2	1	1	1	1	3	5	8
20–34	60	2.0	2	1	1	2	3	4	5	8
35–49	106	1.5	1	1	1	1	2	2	4	6
50–64	166	2.1	6	1	1	2	2	3	5	16
65+	352	2.6	7	1	1	2	3	5	8	15
B. *Operated*										
0–19 Years	3	8.0	9	5	5	8	11	11	11	11
20–34	3	9.3	24	6	6	7	15	15	15	15
35–49	2	11.0	8	9	9	9	13	13	13	13
50–64	3	27.3	144	16	16	26	40	40	40	40
65+	8	6.4	15	2	4	6	10	14	14	14
SUBTOTALS:										
1. SINGLE DX										
A. *Not Operated*	265	1.1	<1	1	1	1	1	1	2	3
B. *Operated*	1	2.0	0	2	2	2	2	2	2	2
2. MULTIPLE DX										
A. *Not Operated*	801	2.1	5	1	1	2	2	4	6	12
B. *Operated*	19	10.9	82	4	5	8	14	26	40	40
1. SINGLE DX	266	1.1	<1	1	1	1	1	1	2	3
2. MULTIPLE DX	820	2.3	8	1	1	1	2	5	7	15
A. NOT OPERATED	1,066	1.9	4	1	1	1	2	4	5	12
B. OPERATED	20	10.5	81	4	5	7	14	16	26	40
TOTAL										
0–19 Years	346	1.3	1	1	1	1	1	2	3	8
20–34	76	2.1	5	1	1	1	2	4	6	15
35–49	124	1.6	3	1	1	1	1	3	5	9
50–64	172	2.5	19	1	1	2	2	4	8	26
65+	368	2.7	7	1	1	2	3	6	8	15
GRAND TOTAL	1,086	2.0	7	1	1	1	2	4	6	14

935.2: FB IN STOMACH

Type of Patients	Observed Patients	Avg. Stay	Vari-ance	10th	25th	50th	75th	90th	95th	99th
1. SINGLE DX										
A. *Not Operated*										
0–19 Years	31	1.1	<1	1	1	1	1	1	2	2
20–34	9	2.7	9	1	1	1	2	9	9	9
35–49	0									
50–64	0									
65+	0									
B. *Operated*										
0–19 Years	1	5.0	0	5	5	5	5	5	5	5
20–34	0									
35–49	0									
50–64	0									
65+	0									
2. MULTIPLE DX										
A. *Not Operated*										
0–19 Years	34	1.9	2	1	1	2	2	4	6	6
20–34	83	4.3	19	1	1	2	7	11	13	17
35–49	74	4.4	27	1	2	3	5	8	11	37
50–64	27	6.0	42	1	2	3	6	18	21	24
65+	25	4.0	14	1	2	3	4	11	14	14
B. *Operated*										
0–19 Years	11	6.0	4	4	4	6	8	8	10	10
20–34	13	9.7	49	4	5	8	11	18	28	28
35–49	18	9.4	34	3	6	7	11	18	26	26
50–64	11	10.0	23	5	6	9	15	16	17	17
65+	8	7.6	50	2	3	4	8	24	24	24
SUBTOTALS:										
1. SINGLE DX										
A. *Not Operated*	40	1.5	2	1	1	1	1	2	2	9
B. *Operated*	1	5.0	0	5	5	5	5	5	5	5
2. MULTIPLE DX										
A. *Not Operated*	243	4.2	22	1	1	2	5	10	14	21
B. *Operated*	61	8.7	32	3	5	7	10	16	18	28
1. SINGLE DX	41	1.5	3	1	1	1	1	2	5	9
2. MULTIPLE DX	304	5.1	27	1	2	3	7	11	16	24
A. NOT OPERATED	283	3.8	20	1	1	2	5	8	12	21
B. OPERATED	62	8.7	32	3	5	7	10	16	18	28
TOTAL										
0–19 Years	77	2.2	4	1	1	2	2	6	7	10
20–34	105	4.9	24	1	1	2	8	11	15	18
35–49	92	5.4	32	1	2	4	7	11	18	37
50–64	38	7.1	39	1	2	5	10	17	21	24
65+	33	4.8	24	1	2	3	5	11	14	24
GRAND TOTAL	345	4.7	25	1	1	3	6	11	16	24

Length of Stay by Diagnosis and Operation, Western Region, 2008

Western Region, October 2006–September 2007 Data, by Diagnosis

936: FB IN INTESTINE & COLON

Type of Patients	Observed Patients	Avg. Stay	Vari-ance	Percentiles						
				10th	25th	50th	75th	90th	95th	99th
1. SINGLE DX										
A. Not Operated										
0–19 Years	12	1.3	<1	1	1	1	1	1	3	3
20–34	1	2.0	0		2	2	2	2	2	2
35–49	0									
50–64	2	1.0	0	1	1	1	1	1	1	1
65+	0									
B. Operated										
0–19 Years	2	6.0	8	4	4	8	8	8	8	8
20–34	1	1.0	0	1	1	1	1	1	1	1
35–49	2	4.5	24	1	1	5	8	8	8	8
50–64	2	4.0	8	2	2	6	6	6	6	6
65+	0									
2. MULTIPLE DX										
A. Not Operated										
0–19 Years	13	2.5	3	1	1	2	3	6	6	6
20–34	36	4.8	27	1	2	4	6	9	13	30
35–49	34	4.0	14	1	1	3	6	9	12	18
50–64	24	3.9	17	1	2	3	5	7	7	21
65+	12	3.2	1	2	2	3	4	4	5	5
B. Operated										
0–19 Years	9	7.8	66	2	4	5	7	29	29	29
20–34	23	7.5	23	3	4	6	12	14	15	21
35–49	31	8.6	57	3	5	6	9	18	19	41
50–64	34	6.7	9	3	4	7	9	10	13	15
65+	32	13.2	266	4	6	8	15	24	28	94
SUBTOTALS:										
1. SINGLE DX										
A. Not Operated	15	1.3	<1	1	1	1	1	1	2	3
B. Operated	7	4.3	10	1	1	2	8	8	8	8
2. MULTIPLE DX										
A. Not Operated	119	4.0	16	1	1	3	5	7	10	21
B. Operated	129	9.0	95	3	5	7	9	18	23	41
1. SINGLE DX	22	2.2	5	1	1	1	2	6	8	8
2. MULTIPLE DX	248	6.6	63	1	3	5	7	13	18	30
A. NOT OPERATED	134	3.7	15	1	1	3	5	7	10	21
B. OPERATED	136	8.7	91	3	4	6	9	15	23	41
TOTAL										
0–19 Years	36	3.6	24	1	1	2	4	7	8	29
20–34	61	5.7	27	1	2	4	6	13	14	30
35–49	67	6.2	39	1	2	5	7	14	18	41
50–64	62	5.4	14	1	3	5	7	9	12	21
65+	44	10.5	213	2	4	7	10	23	28	94
GRAND TOTAL	270	6.2	60	1	2	5	7	12	18	30

937: FB IN ANUS & RECTUM

Type of Patients	Observed Patients	Avg. Stay	Vari-ance	Percentiles						
				10th	25th	50th	75th	90th	95th	99th
1. SINGLE DX										
A. Not Operated										
0–19 Years	9	1.0	0	1	1	1	1	1	1	1
20–34	11	1.1	<1	1	1	1	1	1	2	2
35–49	29	1.1	<1	1	1	1	1	2	2	3
50–64	17	1.1	<1	1	1	1	1	1	2	2
65+	4	1.0	0	1	1	1	1	1	1	1
B. Operated										
0–19 Years	0									
20–34	1	3.0	0	3	3	3	3	3	3	3
35–49	7	3.0	2	1	2	3	5	5	5	5
50–64	1	4.0	0	4	4	4	4	4	4	4
65+	0									
2. MULTIPLE DX										
A. Not Operated										
0–19 Years	7	1.4	<1	1	1	1	2	3	3	3
20–34	23	1.7	1	1	1	1	2	3	4	5
35–49	47	1.3	1	1	1	1	1	2	3	7
50–64	49	1.3	<1	1	1	1	2	2	3	6
65+	6	1.3	<1	1	1	1	2	2	2	2
B. Operated										
0–19 Years	2	6.0	2	5	5	6	7	7	7	7
20–34	6	5.0	8	1	3	6	7	9	9	9
35–49	19	4.7	9	1	2	4	6	10	12	12
50–64	19	5.4	28	1	1	4	6	11	23	23
65+	2	7.5	12	5	5	5	10	10	10	10
SUBTOTALS:										
1. SINGLE DX										
A. Not Operated	70	1.1	<1	1	1	1	1	1	2	3
B. Operated	9	3.1	2	1	2	3	4	5	5	5
2. MULTIPLE DX										
A. Not Operated	132	1.4	<1	1	1	1	1	2	3	6
B. Operated	48	5.2	16	1	3	4	7	10	11	23
1. SINGLE DX	79	1.3	<1	1	1	1	1	2	3	5
2. MULTIPLE DX	180	2.4	8	1	1	1	3	6	8	12
A. NOT OPERATED	202	1.3	<1	1	1	1	1	2	3	5
B. OPERATED	57	4.9	14	1	3	4	6	10	11	23
TOTAL										
0–19 Years	18	1.7	3	1	1	1	2	5	7	7
20–34	41	2.1	3	1	1	1	3	4	6	9
35–49	102	2.0	4	1	1	1	2	5	6	10
50–64	86	2.2	9	1	1	1	2	5	6	23
65+	12	2.3	7	1	1	1	2	5	10	10
GRAND TOTAL	259	2.1	6	1	1	1	2	5	7	11

938: FB IN DIGESTIVE SYST NOS

Type of Patients	Observed Patients	Avg. Stay	Vari-ance	Percentiles						
				10th	25th	50th	75th	90th	95th	99th
1. SINGLE DX										
A. Not Operated										
0–19 Years	12	1.1	<1	1	1	1	1	1	2	2
20–34	6	3.0	4	1	1	4	4	6	6	6
35–49	1	2.0	0	2	2	2	2	2	2	2
50–64	1	1.0	0	1	1	1	1	1	1	1
65+	0									
B. Operated										
0–19 Years	0									
20–34	1	1.0	0	1	1	1	1	1	1	1
35–49	1	5.0	0	5	5	5	5	5	5	5
50–64	0									
65+	0									
2. MULTIPLE DX										
A. Not Operated										
0–19 Years	17	1.7	<1	1	1	2	3	3	3	3
20–34	29	3.5	21	1	1	2	2	6	9	25
35–49	15	3.8	10	1	2	3	6	9	11	11
50–64	10	3.3	3	1	1	3	4	6	6	6
65+	5	1.8	<1	1	1	2	2	3	3	3
B. Operated										
0–19 Years	1	6.0	0	6	6	6	6	6	6	6
20–34	0									
35–49	1	4.0	0	4	4	4	4	4	4	4
50–64	1	4.0	0	4	4	4	4	4	4	4
65+	0									
SUBTOTALS:										
1. SINGLE DX										
A. Not Operated	20	1.7	2	1	1	1	2	4	4	6
B. Operated	2	3.0	8	1	1	3	5	5	5	5
2. MULTIPLE DX										
A. Not Operated	76	3.0	11	1	1	2	3	6	9	25
B. Operated	4	4.5	1	4	4	4	6	6	6	6
1. SINGLE DX	22	1.8	2	1	1	1	2	4	5	6
2. MULTIPLE DX	80	3.1	11	1	1	2	4	6	9	25
A. NOT OPERATED	96	2.7	9	1	1	2	3	6	7	25
B. OPERATED	6	4.0	3	4	4	4	6	6	6	6
TOTAL										
0–19 Years	31	1.6	1	1	1	1	2	3	3	6
20–34	36	3.4	17	1	1	2	4	6	9	25
35–49	18	3.7	8	1	2	3	5	9	11	11
50–64	12	3.2	3	1	2	3	4	6	6	6
65+	5	1.8	<1	1	1	2	2	3	3	3
GRAND TOTAL	102	2.8	9	1	1	2	4	6	6	11

Western Region, October 2006–September 2007 Data, by Diagnosis

939: FB IN GU TRACT

Type of Patients	Observed Patients	Avg. Stay	Variance	Percentiles						
				10th	25th	50th	75th	90th	95th	99th
1. SINGLE DX										
A. Not Operated										
0–19 Years	1	1.0	0	1	1	1	1	1	1	1
20–34	3	1.0	0	1	1	1	1	1	1	1
35–49	3	1.3	<1	1	1	1	2	2	2	2
50–64	1	1.0	0	1	1	1	1	1	1	1
65+	1	1.0	0	1	1	1	1	1	1	1
B. Operated										
0–19 Years	0									
20–34	0									
35–49	5	1.6	<1	1	1	1	2	3	3	3
50–64	0									
65+	0									
2. MULTIPLE DX										
A. Not Operated										
0–19 Years	7	5.7	21	1	1	6	9	13	13	13
20–34	17	1.8	<1	1	1	2	2	3	4	4
35–49	16	1.3	<1	1	1	1	1	2	4	4
50–64	8	1.9	2	1	1	1	3	4	4	4
65+	6	2.7	7	1	1	1	5	7	7	7
B. Operated										
0–19 Years	2	2.0	0	2	2	2	2	2	2	2
20–34	3	3.6	14	1	1	2	8	8	8	8
35–49	10	4.2	15	2	2	2	5	14	14	14
50–64	11	1.6	<1	1	1	1	2	2	3	3
65+	2	1.5	<1	1	1	1	2	2	2	2
SUBTOTALS:										
1. SINGLE DX										
A. Not Operated	9	1.1	<1	1	1	1	1	2	2	2
B. Operated	5	1.6	<1	1	1	1	2	3	3	3
2. MULTIPLE DX										
A. Not Operated	54	2.3	6	1	1	1	2	5	8	13
B. Operated	28	2.7	8	1	1	2	2	7	8	14
1. SINGLE DX	14	1.3	<1	1	1	1	1	2	3	3
2. MULTIPLE DX	82	2.4	6	1	1	2	2	5	8	14
A. NOT OPERATED	63	2.1	5	1	1	1	2	4	7	13
B. OPERATED	33	2.6	7	1	1	2	2	5	8	14
TOTAL										
0–19 Years	10	4.5	18	1	1	2	8	13	13	13
20–34	23	1.9	2	1	1	1	2	3	3	4
35–49	34	2.2	6	1	1	1	2	4	7	14
50–64	20	1.7	<1	1	1	1	2	3	4	4
65+	9	2.2	5	1	1	1	2	7	7	7
GRAND TOTAL	96	2.3	6	1	1	1	2	5	8	14

940: BURN OF EYE & ADNEXA

Type of Patients	Observed Patients	Avg. Stay	Variance	Percentiles						
				10th	25th	50th	75th	90th	95th	99th
1. SINGLE DX										
A. Not Operated										
0–19 Years	1	1.0	0	1	1	1	1	1	1	1
20–34	0									
35–49	0									
50–64	0									
65+	0									
B. Operated										
0–19 Years	0									
20–34	0									
35–49	0									
50–64	0									
65+	0									
2. MULTIPLE DX										
A. Not Operated										
0–19 Years	6	1.2	<1	1	1	1	1	2	2	2
20–34	3	1.0	0	1	1	1	1	1	1	1
35–49	1	1.0	0	1	1	1	1	1	1	1
50–64	1	2.0	0	2	2	2	2	2	2	2
65+	2	1.0	0	1	1	1	1	1	1	1
B. Operated										
0–19 Years	0									
20–34	1	28.0	0	28	28	28	28	28	28	28
35–49	1	22.0	0	22	22	22	22	22	22	22
50–64	1	2.0	0	2	2	2	2	2	2	2
65+	0									
SUBTOTALS:										
1. SINGLE DX										
A. Not Operated	1	1.0	0	1	1	1	1	1	1	1
B. Operated	0									
2. MULTIPLE DX										
A. Not Operated	13	1.2	<1	1	1	1	1	2	2	2
B. Operated	3	17.4	183	2	2	22	28	28	28	28
1. SINGLE DX	1	1.0	0	1	1	1	1	1	1	1
2. MULTIPLE DX	16	4.2	67	1	1	1	2	22	28	28
A. NOT OPERATED	14	1.1	<1	1	1	1	1	2	2	2
B. OPERATED	3	17.4	183	2	2	22	28	28	28	28
TOTAL										
0–19 Years	7	1.1	<1	1	1	1	1	2	2	2
20–34	4	7.7	181	1	1	1	22	28	28	28
35–49	2	11.4	215	1	1	1	22	22	22	22
50–64	2	2.0	0	2	2	2	2	2	2	2
65+	2	1.0	0	1	1	1	1	1	1	1
GRAND TOTAL	17	4.0	64	1	1	1	2	22	28	28

941: BURN OF HEAD/FACE/NECK

Type of Patients	Observed Patients	Avg. Stay	Variance	Percentiles						
				10th	25th	50th	75th	90th	95th	99th
1. SINGLE DX										
A. Not Operated										
0–19 Years	1	1.0	0	1	1	1	1	1	1	1
20–34	0									
35–49	2	1.5	<1	1	1	1	2	2	2	2
50–64	0									
65+	1	1.0	0	1	1	1	1	1	1	1
B. Operated										
0–19 Years	0									
20–34	0									
35–49	0									
50–64	0									
65+	0									
2. MULTIPLE DX										
A. Not Operated										
0–19 Years	174	3.3	11	1	1	2	4	8	10	17
20–34	129	3.4	14	1	1	2	4	9	12	15
35–49	118	4.1	19	1	2	2	7	12	13	16
50–64	123	4.6	28	1	1	2	6	12	15	24
65+	58	6.2	55	1	1	3	8	21	24	31
B. Operated										
0–19 Years	34	18.6	412	2	5	16	19	43	73	93
20–34	34	19.5	283	5	8	14	32	52	70	>99
35–49	37	22.4	334	3	10	15	34	53	57	69
50–64	35	16.3	222	6	9	12	19	31	52	81
65+	13	32.3	390	13	19	28	45	61	64	64
SUBTOTALS:										
1. SINGLE DX										
A. Not Operated	4	1.3	<1	1	1	1	1	2	2	2
B. Operated	0									
2. MULTIPLE DX										
A. Not Operated	602	4.0	21	1	1	2	5	10	13	22
B. Operated	153	20.3	328	3	8	15	28	52	61	93
1. SINGLE DX	4	1.3	<1	1	1	1	1	1	2	2
2. MULTIPLE DX	755	7.3	126	1	1	3	9	18	30	61
A. NOT OPERATED	606	4.0	21	1	1	2	5	10	13	22
B. OPERATED	153	20.3	328	3	8	15	28	52	61	93
TOTAL										
0–19 Years	209	5.8	106	1	1	3	5	15	19	54
20–34	163	6.8	111	1	1	3	8	16	32	70
35–49	157	8.4	152	1	1	3	11	21	37	57
50–64	158	7.2	94	1	2	4	10	23	52	52
65+	72	10.8	214	3	3	14	29	45	64	64
GRAND TOTAL	759	7.3	126	1	1	3	9	18	30	61

Length of Stay by Diagnosis and Operation, Western Region, 2008

Western Region, October 2006–September 2007 Data, by Diagnosis

941.29: 2ND DEG BURN HEAD MULT

Type of Patients	Observed Patients	Avg. Stay	Vari-ance	10th	25th	50th	75th	90th	95th	99th
1. SINGLE DX										
A. Not Operated										
0–19 Years	0									
20–34	0									
35–49	0									
50–64	0									
65+	0									
B. Operated										
0–19 Years	0									
20–34	0									
35–49	0									
50–64	0									
65+	0									
2. MULTIPLE DX										
A. Not Operated										
0–19 Years	62	3.3	9	1	1	2	5	8	8	17
20–34	55	4.9	22	1	1	3	8	12	14	19
35–49	50	5.7	25	1	1	3	9	13	13	20
50–64	36	4.4	23	1	1	3	6	9	15	23
65+	16	5.4	44	1	2	3	3	19	21	21
B. Operated										
0–19 Years	8	26.5	543	4	10	16	39	73	73	73
20–34	10	13.6	112	2	6	8	19	23	36	36
35–49	7	28.5	386	14	15	21	37	69	69	69
50–64	9	28.4	574	8	11	22	32	81	81	81
65+	2	27.5	<1	27	27	28	28	28	28	28
SUBTOTALS:										
1. SINGLE DX										
A. Not Operated	0									
B. Operated	0									
2. MULTIPLE DX										
A. Not Operated	219	4.6	21	1	1	3	7	12	14	20
B. Operated	36	23.8	377	6	11	19	28	52	73	81
1. SINGLE DX	0									
2. MULTIPLE DX	255	7.3	115	1	1	3	9	16	23	69
A. NOT OPERATED	219	4.6	21	1	1	3	7	12	14	20
B. OPERATED	36	23.8	377	6	11	19	28	52	73	81
TOTAL										
0–19 Years	70	6.0	119	1	1	3	6	11	19	73
20–34	65	6.2	44	1	1	3	9	14	19	36
35–49	57	8.5	120	1	1	6	12	16	27	69
50–64	45	9.2	216	1	1	4	9	23	32	81
65+	18	7.9	90	1	2	3	14	27	28	28
GRAND TOTAL	255	7.3	115	1	1	3	9	16	23	69

942: BURN OF TRUNK

Type of Patients	Observed Patients	Avg. Stay	Vari-ance	10th	25th	50th	75th	90th	95th	99th
1. SINGLE DX										
A. Not Operated										
0–19 Years	3	2.3	<1	2	2	2	3	3	3	3
20–34	0									
35–49	0									
50–64	0									
65+	0									
B. Operated										
0–19 Years	1	1.0	0	1	1	1	1	1	1	1
20–34	1	5.0	0	5	5	5	5	5	5	5
35–49	0									
50–64	0									
65+	0									
2. MULTIPLE DX										
A. Not Operated										
0–19 Years	215	3.8	11	1	1	2	5	8	9	14
20–34	70	4.6	14	1	1	4	6	10	12	18
35–49	71	5.4	23	1	2	4	8	12	15	25
50–64	59	4.8	15	1	2	4	6	11	15	17
65+	48	4.8	12	2	2	4	6	12	12	15
B. Operated										
0–19 Years	84	14.4	173	2	5	12	18	31	40	71
20–34	53	16.9	198	5	9	13	23	42	70	>99
35–49	67	18.6	205	6	9	17	24	37	41	89
50–64	73	20.7	199	5	10	17	30	39	42	67
65+	44	18.4	234	4	7	14	22	43	53	65
SUBTOTALS:										
1. SINGLE DX										
A. Not Operated	3	2.3	<1	2	2	2	3	3	3	3
B. Operated	2	3.0	8	1	1	5	5	5	5	5
2. MULTIPLE DX										
A. Not Operated	463	4.4	14	1	2	3	6	10	12	16
B. Operated	321	17.7	201	4	8	14	24	38	45	71
1. SINGLE DX	5	2.6	2	1	2	2	3	5	5	5
2. MULTIPLE DX	784	9.8	133	1	2	6	13	25	34	63
A. NOT OPERATED	466	4.4	14	1	2	3	6	10	12	16
B. OPERATED	323	17.6	201	4	7	14	24	38	45	71
TOTAL										
0–19 Years	303	6.7	79	1	2	3	6	11	15	43
20–34	124	9.9	128	1	3	7	12	24	34	>99
35–49	138	11.8	154	1	3	8	17	27	37	49
50–64	132	13.6	179	2	4	8	20	33	40	60
65+	92	11.3	163	2	3	6	14	27	43	65
GRAND TOTAL	789	9.8	133	1	2	6	13	25	34	63

943: BURN OF ARM

Type of Patients	Observed Patients	Avg. Stay	Vari-ance	10th	25th	50th	75th	90th	95th	99th
1. SINGLE DX										
A. Not Operated										
0–19 Years	0									
20–34	1	1.0	0	1	1	1	1	1	1	1
35–49	0									
50–64	0									
65+	0									
B. Operated										
0–19 Years	0									
20–34	0									
35–49	1	1.0	0	1	1	1	1	1	1	1
50–64	0									
65+	0									
2. MULTIPLE DX										
A. Not Operated										
0–19 Years	87	3.3	10	1	1	2	4	8	10	16
20–34	76	4.4	18	1	1	3	6	8	14	21
35–49	68	5.1	35	1	2	3	7	11	13	44
50–64	44	5.4	36	1	2	4	8	13	15	33
65+	15	4.8	10	1	2	4	7	9	12	12
B. Operated										
0–19 Years	46	15.3	130	6	8	13	21	33	45	>99
20–34	58	12.4	103	4	7	10	15	21	32	71
35–49	72	19.1	296	5	10	15	22	40	50	97
50–64	59	16.8	215	4	8	13	19	52	52	74
65+	25	19.6	179	6	10	18	25	40	42	59
SUBTOTALS:										
1. SINGLE DX										
A. Not Operated	1	1.0	0	1	1	1	1	1	1	1
B. Operated	1	1.0	0	1	1	1	1	1	1	1
2. MULTIPLE DX										
A. Not Operated	290	4.4	22	1	1	3	6	10	13	21
B. Operated	260	16.4	198	5	8	13	20	32	44	81
1. SINGLE DX	2	1.0	0	1	1	1	1	1	1	1
2. MULTIPLE DX	550	10.1	141	1	2	7	13	22	32	71
A. NOT OPERATED	291	4.4	22	1	1	3	6	10	13	21
B. OPERATED	261	16.4	198	5	8	13	20	32	44	81
TOTAL										
0–19 Years	133	7.4	84	1	1	4	10	19	25	57
20–34	135	7.8	70	1	2	6	11	16	21	32
35–49	141	12.2	216	1	3	8	16	25	43	81
50–64	103	11.9	169	1	3	9	16	25	34	72
65+	40	14.0	166	2	5	10	22	33	42	59
GRAND TOTAL	552	10.1	141	1	2	7	13	22	32	71

Length of Stay by Diagnosis and Operation, Western Region, 2008

Western Region, October 2006–September 2007 Data, by Diagnosis

944: BURN OF HAND & WRIST

Type of Patients	Observed Patients	Avg. Stay	Vari-ance	Percentiles 10th	25th	50th	75th	90th	95th	99th
1. SINGLE DX										
A. *Not Operated*										
0–19 Years	3	1.0	0	1	1	1	1	1	1	1
20–34	4	1.0	0	1	1	1	1	1	1	1
35–49	2	1.0	0	1	1	1	1	1	1	1
50–64	1	1.0	0	1	1	1	1	1	1	1
65+	0									
B. *Operated*										
0–19 Years	1	1.0	0	1	1	1	1	1	1	1
20–34	2	1.0	0	1	1	1	1	1	1	1
35–49	3	2.0	1	1	1	2	3	3	3	3
50–64	0									
65+	0									
2. MULTIPLE DX										
A. *Not Operated*										
0–19 Years	142	2.9	8	1	1	2	4	7	8	13
20–34	111	2.7	9	1	1	2	3	5	7	12
35–49	94	3.7	13	1	1	2	5	8	12	18
50–64	87	4.0	25	1	1	2	5	9	13	33
65+	13	4.5	11	1	2	5	7	8	11	11
B. *Operated*										
0–19 Years	52	7.5	43	1	1	6	11	18	21	25
20–34	61	12.3	159	2	4	10	15	22	39	66
35–49	58	12.6	178	2	5	9	15	24	45	71
50–64	49	15.9	139	3	8	13	21	34	40	51
65+	13	13.0	146	1	4	7	17	25	43	43
SUBTOTALS:										
1. SINGLE DX										
A. *Not Operated*	10	1.0	0	1	1	1	1	1	1	1
B. *Operated*	6	1.5	<1	1	1	1	2	3	3	3
2. MULTIPLE DX										
A. *Not Operated*	447	3.3	13	1	1	2	4	7	10	17
B. *Operated*	233	12.1	139	1	4	9	16	23	37	58
1. SINGLE DX	16	1.2	<1	1	1	1	1	2	3	3
2. MULTIPLE DX	680	6.3	73	1	1	3	8	15	22	47
A. NOT OPERATED	457	3.2	12	1	1	2	4	7	10	17
B. OPERATED	239	11.9	138	1	4	9	16	23	37	58
TOTAL										
0–19 Years	198	4.0	21	1	1	2	6	10	14	22
20–34	178	5.9	81	1	1	2	7	15	22	57
35–49	157	6.9	92	1	1	4	9	16	21	58
50–64	137	8.3	98	1	1	4	12	21	33	49
65+	26	8.8	94	1	2	7	11	23	25	43
GRAND TOTAL	696	6.2	72	1	1	3	7	15	21	47

945: BURN OF LEG

Type of Patients	Observed Patients	Avg. Stay	Vari-ance	Percentiles 10th	25th	50th	75th	90th	95th	99th
1. SINGLE DX										
A. *Not Operated*										
0–19 Years	7	2.3	5	1	1	1	3	7	7	7
20–34	0									
35–49	2	3.0	8	1	1	1	5	5	5	5
50–64	1	1.0	0	1	1	1	1	1	1	1
65+	1	2.0	0	2	2	2	2	2	2	2
B. *Operated*										
0–19 Years	7	4.3	40	1	1	1	6	18	18	18
20–34	2	3.5	12	1	1	6	6	6	6	6
35–49	2	2.5	4	1	1	4	4	4	4	4
50–64	0									
65+	0									
2. MULTIPLE DX										
A. *Not Operated*										
0–19 Years	153	3.9	16	1	1	2	5	9	12	20
20–34	80	4.3	14	1	1	3	6	10	11	21
35–49	127	5.5	42	1	2	3	7	12	18	32
50–64	114	4.1	12	1	2	3	5	10	12	14
65+	86	6.5	44	1	3	4	7	13	22	36
B. *Operated*										
0–19 Years	92	12.2	95	2	6	11	16	22	26	60
20–34	97	14.1	170	2	6	10	18	30	46	>99
35–49	150	13.0	130	2	6	10	16	25	32	59
50–64	172	13.2	139	3	5	10	17	29	40	>99
65+	76	16.1	235	3	7	12	21	34	47	96
SUBTOTALS:										
1. SINGLE DX										
A. *Not Operated*	11	2.3	4	1	1	1	3	5	7	7
B. *Operated*	11	3.8	26	1	1	1	6	6	18	18
2. MULTIPLE DX										
A. *Not Operated*	560	4.8	26	1	2	3	6	10	13	27
B. *Operated*	587	13.5	148	3	6	11	17	27	40	81
1. SINGLE DX	22	3.1	15	1	1	1	4	6	7	18
2. MULTIPLE DX	1,147	9.2	107	1	3	6	12	21	29	58
A. NOT OPERATED	571	4.7	25	1	2	3	6	10	13	27
B. OPERATED	598	13.3	147	2	6	11	17	27	38	68
TOTAL										
0–19 Years	259	6.8	60	1	2	4	10	17	20	40
20–34	179	9.6	122	1	3	7	11	21	30	81
35–49	281	9.5	103	1	3	7	12	21	30	44
50–64	287	9.6	108	2	3	6	12	22	30	68
65+	163	10.9	156	2	3	7	13	24	34	58
GRAND TOTAL	1,169	9.1	106	1	2	6	12	21	29	58

946: BURN OF MULTIPLE SITE

Type of Patients	Observed Patients	Avg. Stay	Vari-ance	Percentiles 10th	25th	50th	75th	90th	95th	99th
1. SINGLE DX										
A. *Not Operated*										
0–19 Years	0									
20–34	0									
35–49	0									
50–64	0									
65+	0									
B. *Operated*										
0–19 Years	0									
20–34	0									
35–49	0									
50–64	0									
65+	0									
2. MULTIPLE DX										
A. *Not Operated*										
0–19 Years	1	4.0	0	4	4	4	4	4	4	4
20–34	2	5.0	31	1	1	1	9	9	9	9
35–49	4	5.7	9	3	4	4	6	10	10	10
50–64	2	17.0	49	12	12	22	22	22	22	22
65+	3	4.0	9	1	1	4	7	7	7	7
B. *Operated*										
0–19 Years	0									
20–34	0									
35–49	1	62.0	0	62	62	62	62	62	62	62
50–64	0									
65+	1	45.0	0	45	45	45	45	45	45	45
SUBTOTALS:										
1. SINGLE DX										
A. *Not Operated*	0									
B. *Operated*	0									
2. MULTIPLE DX										
A. *Not Operated*	12	6.9	34	1	4	6	9	12	22	22
B. *Operated*	2	53.5	142	45	45	62	62	62	62	62
1. SINGLE DX	0									
2. MULTIPLE DX	14	13.6	325	1	4	6	12	45	62	62
A. NOT OPERATED	12	6.9	34	1	4	6	9	12	22	22
B. OPERATED	2	53.5	142	45	45	62	62	62	62	62
TOTAL										
0–19 Years	1	4.0	0	4	4	4	4	4	4	4
20–34	2	5.0	31	1	1	1	9	9	9	9
35–49	5	17.0	635	3	4	6	10	62	62	62
50–64	2	17.0	49	12	12	22	22	22	22	22
65+	4	14.2	422	1	4	7	7	45	45	45
GRAND TOTAL	14	13.6	325	1	4	6	12	45	62	62

Length of Stay by Diagnosis and Operation, Western Region, 2008

Western Region, October 2006–September 2007 Data, by Diagnosis

947: BURN OF INTERNAL ORGANS

Type of Patients	Observed Patients	Avg. Stay	Variance	10th	25th	50th	75th	90th	95th	99th
1. SINGLE DX										
A. Not Operated										
0–19 Years	1	6.0	0	6	6	6	6	6	6	6
20–34	1	1.0	0	1	1	1	1	1	1	1
35–49	0									
50–64	0									
65+	0									
B. Operated										
0–19 Years	0									
20–34	0									
35–49	0									
50–64	0									
65+	0									
2. MULTIPLE DX										
A. Not Operated										
0–19 Years	7	2.0	2	1	1	2	2	5	5	5
20–34	14	6.2	27	1	2	4	10	14	15	15
35–49	12	3.9	14	1	1	2	7	11	11	11
50–64	8	4.6	30	1	2	2	8	17	17	17
65+	8	12.4	120	1	4	5	18	34	34	34
B. Operated										
0–19 Years	0									
20–34	0									
35–49	1	29.0	0	29	29	29	29	29	29	29
50–64	3	38.7	562	19	19	32	65	65	65	65
65+	0									
SUBTOTALS:										
1. SINGLE DX										
A. Not Operated	2	3.5	13	1	1	4	6	6	6	6
B. Operated	0									
2. MULTIPLE DX										
A. Not Operated	49	5.8	43	1	2	3	8	16	17	34
B. Operated	4	36.3	398	19	19	29	65	65	65	65
1. SINGLE DX	2	3.5	13	1	1	4	6	6	6	6
2. MULTIPLE DX	53	8.1	130	1	2	3	11	18	32	65
A. NOT OPERATED	51	5.7	42	1	1	3	8	15	17	34
B. OPERATED	4	36.3	398	19	19	29	65	65	65	65
TOTAL										
0–19 Years	8	2.5	4	1	1	2	2	6	6	6
20–34	15	5.9	26	1	1	4	10	14	15	15
35–49	13	5.9	62	1	1	2	7	11	29	29
50–64	11	13.9	387	2	2	3	19	32	65	65
65+	8	12.4	120	1	4	5	18	34	34	34
GRAND TOTAL	55	8.0	126	1	2	3	11	18	32	65

948: BURN BY % BODY SURFACE

Type of Patients	Observed Patients	Avg. Stay	Variance	10th	25th	50th	75th	90th	95th	99th
1. SINGLE DX										
A. Not Operated										
0–19 Years	0									
20–34	0									
35–49	0									
50–64	0									
65+	0									
B. Operated										
0–19 Years	0									
20–34	0									
35–49	0									
50–64	0									
65+	0									
2. MULTIPLE DX										
A. Not Operated										
0–19 Years	0									
20–34	1	6.0	0	6	6	6	6	6	6	6
35–49	1	8.0	0	8	8	8	8	8	8	8
50–64	1	1.0	0	1	1	1	1	1	1	1
65+	0									
B. Operated										
0–19 Years	0									
20–34	0									
35–49	0									
50–64	0									
65+	0									
SUBTOTALS:										
1. SINGLE DX										
A. Not Operated	0									
B. Operated	0									
2. MULTIPLE DX										
A. Not Operated	3	5.0	13	1	1	6	6	8	8	8
B. Operated	0									
1. SINGLE DX	0									
2. MULTIPLE DX	3	5.0	13	1	1	6	6	8	8	8
A. NOT OPERATED	3	5.0	13	1	1	6	6	8	8	8
B. OPERATED	0									
TOTAL										
0–19 Years	0									
20–34	1	6.0	0	6	6	6	6	6	6	6
35–49	1	8.0	0	8	8	8	8	8	8	8
50–64	1	1.0	0	1	1	1	1	1	1	1
65+	0									
GRAND TOTAL	3	5.0	13	1	1	6	6	8	8	8

949: BURN UNSPECIFIED

Type of Patients	Observed Patients	Avg. Stay	Variance	10th	25th	50th	75th	90th	95th	99th
1. SINGLE DX										
A. Not Operated										
0–19 Years	1	3.0	0	3	3	3	3	3	3	3
20–34	0									
35–49	0									
50–64	0									
65+	0									
B. Operated										
0–19 Years	0									
20–34	0									
35–49	0									
50–64	0									
65+	0									
2. MULTIPLE DX										
A. Not Operated										
0–19 Years	0									
20–34	0									
35–49	0									
50–64	0									
65+	0									
B. Operated										
0–19 Years	0									
20–34	0									
35–49	0									
50–64	1	2.0	0	2	2	2	2	2	2	2
65+	0									
SUBTOTALS:										
1. SINGLE DX										
A. Not Operated	1	3.0	0	3	3	3	3	3	3	3
B. Operated	0									
2. MULTIPLE DX										
A. Not Operated	0									
B. Operated	1	2.0	0	2	2	2	2	2	2	2
1. SINGLE DX	1	3.0	0	3	3	3	3	3	3	3
2. MULTIPLE DX	1	2.0	0	2	2	2	2	2	2	2
A. NOT OPERATED	1	3.0	0	3	3	3	3	3	3	3
B. OPERATED	1	2.0	0	2	2	2	2	2	2	2
TOTAL										
0–19 Years	1	3.0	0	3	3	3	3	3	3	3
20–34	0									
35–49	0									
50–64	1	2.0	0	2	2	2	2	2	2	2
65+	0									
GRAND TOTAL	2	2.5	<1	2	2	2	3	3	3	3

Length of Stay by Diagnosis and Operation, Western Region, 2008

Western Region, October 2006–September 2007 Data, by Diagnosis

950: INJ OPTIC NERV/PATHWAYS

Type of Patients	Observed Patients	Avg. Stay	Vari-ance	Percentiles 10th	25th	50th	75th	90th	95th	99th
1. SINGLE DX										
A. Not Operated										
0–19 Years	0									
20–34	0									
35–49	1	2.0	0	2	2	2	2	2	2	2
50–64	0									
65+	1	1.0	0	1	1	1	1	1	1	1
B. Operated										
0–19 Years	0									
20–34	0									
35–49	0									
50–64	0									
65+	0									
2. MULTIPLE DX										
A. Not Operated										
0–19 Years	0									
20–34	2	3.0	8	1	1	3	5	5	5	5
35–49	0									
50–64	0									
65+	1	3.0	0	3	3	3	3	3	3	3
B. Operated										
0–19 Years	1	5.0	0	5	5	5	5	5	5	5
20–34	0									
35–49	0									
50–64	0									
65+	0									
SUBTOTALS:										
1. SINGLE DX										
A. Not Operated	2	1.5	<1	1	1	2	2	2	2	2
B. Operated	0									
2. MULTIPLE DX										
A. Not Operated	3	3.0	4	1	1	3	5	5	5	5
B. Operated	1	5.0	0	5	5	5	5	5	5	5
1. SINGLE DX	2	1.5	<1	1	1	2	2	2	2	2
2. MULTIPLE DX	4	3.5	4	1	2	4	5	5	5	5
A. NOT OPERATED	5	2.4	3	1	1	2	3	5	5	5
B. OPERATED	1	5.0	0	5	5	5	5	5	5	5
TOTAL										
0–19 Years	1	5.0	0	5	5	5	5	5	5	5
20–34	2	3.0	8	1	1	3	5	5	5	5
35–49	1	2.0	0	2	2	2	2	2	2	2
50–64	0									
65+	2	2.0	2	1	1	1	3	3	3	3
GRAND TOTAL	6	2.8	3	1	1	2	5	5	5	5

951: INJURY OTH CRANIAL NERVE

Type of Patients	Observed Patients	Avg. Stay	Vari-ance	Percentiles 10th	25th	50th	75th	90th	95th	99th
1. SINGLE DX										
A. Not Operated										
0–19 Years	0									
20–34	0									
35–49	0									
50–64	0									
65+	0									
B. Operated										
0–19 Years	0									
20–34	0									
35–49	0									
50–64	0									
65+	0									
2. MULTIPLE DX										
A. Not Operated										
0–19 Years	0									
20–34	3	1.0	0	1	1	1	1	1	1	1
35–49	5	1.6	<1	1	1	2	2	3	3	3
50–64	1	3.0	0	3	3	3	3	3	3	3
65+	1	1.0	0	1	1	1	1	1	1	1
B. Operated										
0–19 Years	5	2.2	2	1	1	2	3	4	4	4
20–34	10	4.1	10	2	2	3	5	6	12	12
35–49	3	2.0	<1	1	1	2	3	3	3	3
50–64	2	3.5	5	2	2	4	5	5	5	5
65+	0									
SUBTOTALS:										
1. SINGLE DX										
A. Not Operated	0									
B. Operated	0									
2. MULTIPLE DX										
A. Not Operated	10	1.5	<1	1	1	1	2	3	3	3
B. Operated	20	3.3	6	1	2	2	4	6	12	12
1. SINGLE DX	0									
2. MULTIPLE DX	30	2.7	5	1	1	2	3	5	6	12
A. NOT OPERATED	10	1.5	<1	1	1	1	2	3	3	3
B. OPERATED	20	3.3	6	1	2	2	4	6	12	12
TOTAL										
0–19 Years	5	2.2	2	1	1	2	3	4	4	4
20–34	13	3.4	9	1	1	2	4	6	12	12
35–49	8	1.8	<1	1	1	2	3	3	3	3
50–64	3	3.3	2	1	2	3	5	5	5	5
65+	1	1.0	0	1	1	1	1	1	1	1
GRAND TOTAL	30	2.7	5	1	1	2	3	5	6	12

952: SPINAL CORD INJ W/O FX

Type of Patients	Observed Patients	Avg. Stay	Vari-ance	Percentiles 10th	25th	50th	75th	90th	95th	99th
1. SINGLE DX										
A. Not Operated										
0–19 Years	14	2.4	3	1	1	1	3	5	7	7
20–34	8	2.4	3	1	1	1	3	5	5	5
35–49	7	3.6	6	1	1	4	4	8	8	8
50–64	4	2.0	2	1	1	1	4	4	4	4
65+	0									
B. Operated										
0–19 Years	1	8.0	0	8	8	8	8	8	8	8
20–34	1	3.0	0	3	3	3	3	3	3	3
35–49	1	9.0	0	9	9	9	9	9	9	9
50–64	0									
65+	0									
2. MULTIPLE DX										
A. Not Operated										
0–19 Years	41	2.2	2	1	1	2	3	4	4	6
20–34	59	5.2	127	1	1	2	4	15	21	80
35–49	85	4.0	11	1	2	3	5	8	10	21
50–64	121	4.8	25	1	2	3	6	9	11	26
65+	119	5.2	19	2	3	4	6	10	15	21
B. Operated										
0–19 Years	11	16.2	123	8	9	12	25	31	40	40
20–34	27	9.2	49	2	4	8	12	19	25	30
35–49	61	11.9	138	3	3	7	16	27	35	53
50–64	68	12.6	198	3	5	9	14	25	38	86
65+	66	11.8	88	4	7	9	14	25	27	65
SUBTOTALS:										
1. SINGLE DX										
A. Not Operated	33	2.6	3	1	1	2	4	5	7	8
B. Operated	3	6.7	10	3	3	8	9	9	9	9
2. MULTIPLE DX										
A. Not Operated	425	4.6	33	1	2	3	5	9	11	25
B. Operated	233	12.0	130	3	5	9	14	25	31	65
1. SINGLE DX	36	2.9	5	1	1	2	4	7	8	9
2. MULTIPLE DX	658	7.2	80	1	2	4	9	16	25	47
A. NOT OPERATED	458	4.4	31	1	2	3	5	8	11	25
B. OPERATED	236	11.9	129	3	5	9	14	25	31	65
TOTAL										
0–19 Years	67	4.6	48	1	1	2	4	10	16	40
20–34	95	6.1	97	1	2	3	8	15	21	80
35–49	154	7.1	75	1	2	4	8	17	27	47
50–64	193	7.5	99	2	2	5	9	14	25	65
65+	185	7.6	53	2	3	5	9	16	21	30
GRAND TOTAL	694	7.0	77	2	2	4	8	15	23	47

Length of Stay by Diagnosis and Operation, Western Region, 2008

Western Region, October 2006–September 2007 Data, by Diagnosis

953: INJ NERVE ROOT/SP PLEXUS

Type of Patients	Observed Patients	Avg. Stay	Variance	10th	25th	50th	75th	90th	95th	99th
1. SINGLE DX										
A. Not Operated										
0–19 Years	0									
20–34	3	1.3	<1	1	1	1	2	2	2	2
35–49	0									
50–64	0									
65+	0									
B. Operated										
0–19 Years	0									
20–34	5	1.6	<1	1	1	1	2	3	3	3
35–49	0									
50–64	0									
65+	0									
2. MULTIPLE DX										
A. Not Operated										
0–19 Years	6	4.0	7	1	3	3	4	9	9	9
20–34	15	3.2	5	1	2	2	5	6	8	8
35–49	18	4.2	11	1	2	3	5	8	14	14
50–64	14	2.9	2	1	2	3	4	5	5	5
65+	12	5.6	13	3	3	4	6	11	12	12
B. Operated										
0–19 Years	2	8.0	96	1	1	3	15	15	15	15
20–34	7	6.3	54	1	1	3	13	20	20	20
35–49	5	2.0	2	1	1	1	3	4	4	4
50–64	3	6.7	54	1	1	4	15	15	15	15
65+	1	2.0	0	2	2	2	2	2	2	2
SUBTOTALS:										
1. SINGLE DX										
A. Not Operated	3	1.3	<1	1	1	1	2	2	2	2
B. Operated	5	1.6	<1	1	1	1	2	2	3	3
2. MULTIPLE DX										
A. Not Operated	65	3.9	8	1	2	3	5	8	11	14
B. Operated	18	5.1	37	1	1	2	4	15	20	20
1. SINGLE DX	8	1.5	<1	1	1	1	2	2	3	3
2. MULTIPLE DX	83	4.2	14	1	2	3	5	9	13	20
A. NOT OPERATED	68	3.8	8	1	2	3	5	8	11	14
B. OPERATED	23	4.4	31	1	1	2	4	15	15	20
TOTAL										
0–19 Years	8	5.0	23	1	1	3	4	15	15	15
20–34	27	3.7	18	1	1	2	5	8	13	20
35–49	26	3.5	9	1	1	3	5	7	8	14
50–64	17	3.5	11	1	2	3	4	5	15	15
65+	13	5.3	13	2	3	4	6	11	12	12
GRAND TOTAL	91	3.9	14	1	1	3	5	8	13	20

954: INJURY OTH TRUNK NERVE

Type of Patients	Observed Patients	Avg. Stay	Variance	10th	25th	50th	75th	90th	95th	99th
1. SINGLE DX										
A. Not Operated										
0–19 Years	1	2.0	0	2	2	2	2	2	2	2
20–34	0									
35–49	0									
50–64	0									
65+	0									
B. Operated										
0–19 Years	0									
20–34	0									
35–49	0									
50–64	0									
65+	0									
2. MULTIPLE DX										
A. Not Operated										
0–19 Years	1	3.0	0	3	3	3	3	3	3	3
20–34	1	6.0	0	6	6	6	6	6	6	6
35–49	2	4.5	4	3	3	6	6	6	6	6
50–64	0									
65+	0									
B. Operated										
0–19 Years	0									
20–34	1	5.0	0	5	5	5	5	5	5	5
35–49	0									
50–64	0									
65+	0									
SUBTOTALS:										
1. SINGLE DX										
A. Not Operated	1	2.0	0	2	2	2	2	2	2	2
B. Operated	0									
2. MULTIPLE DX										
A. Not Operated	4	4.5	3	3	3	6	6	6	6	6
B. Operated	1	5.0	0	5	5	5	5	5	5	5
1. SINGLE DX	1	2.0	0	2	2	2	2	2	2	2
2. MULTIPLE DX	5	4.6	2	3	3	5	6	6	6	6
A. NOT OPERATED	5	4.0	3	2	3	3	6	6	6	6
B. OPERATED	1	5.0	0	5	5	5	5	5	5	5
TOTAL										
0–19 Years	2	2.5	<1	2	2	3	3	3	3	3
20–34	2	5.5	<1	5	5	5	6	6	6	6
35–49	2	4.5	4	3	3	6	6	6	6	6
50–64	0									
65+	0									
GRAND TOTAL	6	4.2	3	2	3	5	6	6	6	6

955: INJ PNS SHOULDER/ARM

Type of Patients	Observed Patients	Avg. Stay	Variance	10th	25th	50th	75th	90th	95th	99th
1. SINGLE DX										
A. Not Operated										
0–19 Years	0									
20–34	2	1.5	<1	1	1	2	2	2	2	2
35–49	1	1.0	0	1	1	1	1	1	1	1
50–64	0									
65+	0									
B. Operated										
0–19 Years	1	3.0	0	3	3	3	3	3	3	3
20–34	5	2.6	3	1	1	2	4	5	5	5
35–49	0									
50–64	0									
65+	0									
2. MULTIPLE DX										
A. Not Operated										
0–19 Years	7	1.3	<1	1	1	1	1	3	3	3
20–34	15	2.4	7	1	1	2	2	4	11	11
35–49	10	3.6	15	1	2	2	2	8	13	13
50–64	7	3.1	13	1	1	2	4	11	11	11
65+	10	3.5	6	1	2	3	4	6	9	9
B. Operated										
0–19 Years	34	2.3	3	1	1	2	3	6	6	7
20–34	122	2.8	9	1	1	2	3	5	8	16
35–49	66	3.4	30	1	1	2	4	5	10	39
50–64	36	2.6	3	1	1	2	3	6	6	7
65+	8	2.4	4	1	1	2	2	7	7	7
SUBTOTALS:										
1. SINGLE DX										
A. Not Operated	3	1.3	<1	1	1	1	2	2	2	2
B. Operated	6	2.7	3	1	1	3	4	5	5	5
2. MULTIPLE DX										
A. Not Operated	49	2.8	8	1	1	2	3	8	11	13
B. Operated	266	2.9	12	1	1	2	3	6	7	17
1. SINGLE DX	9	2.2	2	1	1	2	3	5	5	5
2. MULTIPLE DX	315	2.8	12	1	1	2	3	6	8	16
A. NOT OPERATED	52	2.7	8	1	1	2	3	6	11	13
B. OPERATED	272	2.9	12	1	1	2	3	6	7	17
TOTAL										
0–19 Years	42	2.1	3	1	1	1	3	5	6	7
20–34	144	2.7	8	1	1	2	3	5	8	16
35–49	77	3.4	27	1	1	2	4	7	12	39
50–64	43	2.7	5	1	2	2	3	6	6	11
65+	18	3.0	5	1	1	2	4	7	9	9
GRAND TOTAL	324	2.8	11	1	1	2	3	6	8	16

Western Region, October 2006–September 2007 Data, by Diagnosis

956: INJ PERIPH NERV PELV/LEG

Type of Patients	Observed Patients	Avg. Stay	Vari-ance	Percentiles 10th	25th	50th	75th	90th	95th	99th
1. SINGLE DX										
A. Not Operated										
0–19 Years	2	3.0	2	2	2	2	4	4	4	4
20–34	3	5.0	7	2	2	6	7	7	7	7
35–49	0									
50–64	0									
65+	0									
B. Operated										
0–19 Years	0									
20–34	1	1.0	0	1	1	1	1	1	1	1
35–49	0									
50–64	0									
65+	0									
2. MULTIPLE DX										
A. Not Operated										
0–19 Years	4	2.7	6	1	1	3	3	6	6	6
20–34	11	6.6	71	1	1	3	9	23	23	23
35–49	3	2.0	<1	1	1	2	3	3	3	3
50–64	8	4.2	15	1	2	3	4	13	13	13
65+	5	4.6	14	1	2	3	7	10	10	10
B. Operated										
0–19 Years	6	2.2	1	1	1	2	3	4	4	4
20–34	7	1.7	<1	1	1	1	3	3	3	3
35–49	1	3.0	0	3	3	3	3	3	3	3
50–64	7	1.6	<1	1	1	1	2	3	3	3
65+	1	1.0	0	1	1	1	1	1	1	1
SUBTOTALS:										
1. SINGLE DX										
A. Not Operated	5	4.2	5	2	2	4	6	7	7	7
B. Operated	1	1.0	0	1	1	1	1	1	1	1
2. MULTIPLE DX										
A. Not Operated	31	4.7	32	1	1	3	6	10	23	23
B. Operated	22	1.8	<1	1	1	1	3	3	3	4
1. SINGLE DX	6	3.7	6	1	2	4	6	7	7	7
2. MULTIPLE DX	53	3.5	21	1	1	2	3	7	13	23
A. NOT OPERATED	36	4.7	28	1	2	3	6	10	23	23
B. OPERATED	23	1.8	<1	1	1	1	3	3	3	4
TOTAL										
0–19 Years	12	2.5	2	1	1	2	3	4	6	6
20–34	22	4.6	40	1	1	3	5	9	23	23
35–49	4	2.3	<1	1	2	3	3	3	3	3
50–64	15	3.0	10	1	1	2	3	6	13	13
65+	6	4.0	14	1	1	3	7	10	10	10
GRAND TOTAL	59	3.6	19	1	1	2	3	7	13	23

957: INJURY TO NERVE NEC&NOS

Type of Patients	Observed Patients	Avg. Stay	Vari-ance	Percentiles 10th	25th	50th	75th	90th	95th	99th
1. SINGLE DX										
A. Not Operated										
0–19 Years	0									
20–34	1	1.0	0	1	1	1	1	1	1	1
35–49	2	2.5	<1	2	2	3	3	3	3	3
50–64	0									
65+	0									
B. Operated										
0–19 Years	1	1.0	0	1	1	1	1	1	1	1
20–34	1	1.0	0	1	1	1	1	1	1	1
35–49	1	1.0	0	1	1	1	1	1	1	1
50–64	0									
65+	0									
2. MULTIPLE DX										
A. Not Operated										
0–19 Years	1	1.0	0	1	1	1	1	1	1	1
20–34	3	2.0	<1	1	1	2	3	3	3	3
35–49	8	2.5	7	1	1	2	2	9	9	9
50–64	4	2.3	2	1	1	2	3	4	4	4
65+	1	6.0	0	6	6	6	6	6	6	6
B. Operated										
0–19 Years	7	2.7	3	1	1	2	4	6	6	6
20–34	8	1.3	<1	1	1	1	1	2	2	2
35–49	6	2.5	5	1	1	2	2	7	7	7
50–64	8	5.8	83	1	1	2	4	28	28	28
65+	0									
SUBTOTALS:										
1. SINGLE DX										
A. Not Operated	3	2.0	<1	1	1	2	3	3	3	3
B. Operated	3	1.0	0	1	1	1	1	1	1	1
2. MULTIPLE DX										
A. Not Operated	17	2.5	5	1	1	2	3	6	9	9
B. Operated	29	3.1	26	1	1	2	2	7	7	28
1. SINGLE DX	6	1.5	<1	1	1	1	2	3	3	3
2. MULTIPLE DX	46	2.9	18	1	1	2	3	6	7	28
A. NOT OPERATED	20	2.4	4	1	1	2	3	6	9	9
B. OPERATED	32	2.9	23	1	1	2	2	6	7	28
TOTAL										
0–19 Years	9	2.3	3	1	1	2	3	4	6	6
20–34	13	1.4	<1	1	1	1	1	3	3	3
35–49	17	2.4	5	1	1	2	2	7	9	9
50–64	12	4.6	57	1	2	2	4	7	28	28
65+	1	6.0	0	6	6	6	6	6	6	6
GRAND TOTAL	52	2.7	16	1	1	2	3	6	7	28

958: EARLY COMP OF TRAUMA

Type of Patients	Observed Patients	Avg. Stay	Vari-ance	Percentiles 10th	25th	50th	75th	90th	95th	99th
1. SINGLE DX										
A. Not Operated										
0–19 Years	14	1.8	<1	1	1	1	3	3	3	3
20–34	14	2.0	3	1	1	1	2	5	7	7
35–49	6	2.2	4	1	1	1	2	6	6	6
50–64	3	3.0	12	1	1	1	7	7	7	7
65+	0									
B. Operated										
0–19 Years	10	4.1	12	1	2	3	4	11	11	11
20–34	19	3.5	11	1	1	3	4	10	13	13
35–49	12	5.1	24	1	2	3	6	11	18	18
50–64	4	2.3	2	1	1	1	4	4	4	4
65+	0									
2. MULTIPLE DX										
A. Not Operated										
0–19 Years	51	2.8	7	1	1	2	4	6	9	15
20–34	74	3.2	8	1	1	2	4	6	7	15
35–49	61	4.8	16	1	2	4	6	8	12	22
50–64	58	4.5	14	1	2	3	7	9	12	21
65+	90	4.2	6	2	2	4	6	8	9	10
B. Operated										
0–19 Years	69	6.2	32	2	3	5	7	15	18	34
20–34	155	6.9	31	1	3	6	9	14	19	27
35–49	158	6.9	54	1	3	6	8	16	21	41
50–64	121	8.2	62	2	3	6	9	18	28	37
65+	96	6.8	22	2	4	6	9	14	16	24
SUBTOTALS:										
1. SINGLE DX										
A. Not Operated	37	2.0	3	1	1	1	2	5	7	7
B. Operated	45	4.0	14	1	1	3	4	10	11	18
2. MULTIPLE DX										
A. Not Operated	334	3.9	10	1	2	3	5	8	10	16
B. Operated	599	7.1	42	2	3	5	9	15	20	34
1. SINGLE DX	82	3.1	10	1	1	2	4	7	10	18
2. MULTIPLE DX	933	5.9	33	1	2	4	7	13	18	29
A. NOT OPERATED	371	3.7	10	1	2	3	5	8	9	16
B. OPERATED	644	6.8	41	2	3	5	9	15	19	34
TOTAL										
0–19 Years	144	4.4	22	1	2	3	6	9	15	21
20–34	262	5.3	25	1	2	4	7	13	15	26
35–49	237	6.2	42	1	2	4	8	13	19	40
50–64	186	6.8	49	1	3	5	8	16	21	37
65+	186	5.5	16	2	3	4	7	10	14	20
GRAND TOTAL	1,015	5.7	32	1	2	4	7	12	17	29

Length of Stay by Diagnosis and Operation, Western Region, 2008

Western Region, October 2006–September 2007 Data, by Diagnosis

958.3: POSTTRAUM WND INFECT NEC

Type of Patients	Observed Patients	Avg. Stay	Vari-ance	10th	25th	50th	75th	90th	95th	99th
1. SINGLE DX										
A. Not Operated										
0–19 Years	3	3.0	0	3	3	3	3	3	3	3
20–34	4	4.0	6	2	3	4	7	7	7	7
35–49	1	6.0	0	6	6	6	6	6	6	6
50–64	1	7.0	0	7	7	7	7	7	7	7
65+	0									
B. Operated										
0–19 Years	1	1.0	0	1	1	1	1	1	1	1
20–34	1	1.0	0	1	1	1	1	1	1	1
35–49	3	7.0	16	3	3	7	11	11	11	11
50–64	3	1.7	1	1	1	1	3	3	3	3
65+	0									
2. MULTIPLE DX										
A. Not Operated										
0–19 Years	15	2.9	5	1	1	2	4	6	9	9
20–34	19	4.9	19	2	2	3	6	14	15	15
35–49	28	3.9	5	1	2	3	5	7	8	9
50–64	16	3.8	6	1	2	4	7	7	8	8
65+	23	4.5	6	2	2	4	7	8	8	9
B. Operated										
0–19 Years	10	8.7	94	2	3	7	8	15	34	34
20–34	37	7.5	30	2	4	6	9	15	20	23
35–49	39	6.7	41	2	3	6	8	22	22	29
50–64	33	6.9	65	2	3	4	7	17	28	40
65+	30	7.0	21	2	4	5	9	13	15	20
SUBTOTALS:										
1. SINGLE DX										
A. Not Operated	9	4.2	4	2	3	3	6	7	7	7
B. Operated	8	3.5	13	1	1	1	7	11	11	11
2. MULTIPLE DX										
A. Not Operated	101	4.0	8	1	2	4	5	7	9	14
B. Operated	149	7.1	42	2	3	5	8	15	20	34
1. SINGLE DX	17	3.9	8	1	2	3	6	7	11	11
2. MULTIPLE DX	250	5.9	30	2	2	4	7	13	17	29
A. NOT OPERATED	110	4.1	8	1	2	3	5	7	9	14
B. OPERATED	157	7.0	41	2	3	5	8	15	20	34
TOTAL										
0–19 Years	29	4.8	41	1	2	3	6	9	15	34
20–34	61	6.3	26	2	3	5	7	14	15	23
35–49	71	5.6	26	2	2	4	7	10	18	29
50–64	53	5.7	45	2	2	5	7	8	17	40
65+	53	5.9	16	2	3	5	8	12	15	20
GRAND TOTAL	267	5.8	29	2	2	4	7	13	17	29

958.92: TRAUM COMPART SYND-LE

Type of Patients	Observed Patients	Avg. Stay	Vari-ance	10th	25th	50th	75th	90th	95th	99th
1. SINGLE DX										
A. Not Operated										
0–19 Years	0									
20–34	2	1.0	0	1	1	1	1	1	1	1
35–49	1	1.0	0	1	1	1	1	1	1	1
50–64	1	1.0	0	1	1	1	1	1	1	1
65+	0									
B. Operated										
0–19 Years	3	5.7	21	3	3	5	11	11	11	11
20–34	14	3.4	10	1	1	3	4	6	13	13
35–49	5	3.2	4	1	2	3	6	6	6	6
50–64	1	4.0	0	4	4	4	4	4	4	4
65+	0									
2. MULTIPLE DX										
A. Not Operated										
0–19 Years	2	4.0	0	4	4	4	4	4	4	4
20–34	3	3.7	1	3	3	3	5	5	5	5
35–49	1	1.0	0	1	1	1	1	1	1	1
50–64	1	4.0	0	4	4	4	4	4	4	4
65+	3	2.7	2	1	1	3	4	4	4	4
B. Operated										
0–19 Years	37	5.3	14	2	3	5	7	9	15	18
20–34	67	7.1	28	3	3	6	10	13	18	27
35–49	74	7.3	64	2	3	5	8	19	21	44
50–64	42	9.0	49	3	5	7	11	18	21	37
65+	23	7.2	22	2	4	7	9	11	11	24
SUBTOTALS:										
1. SINGLE DX										
A. Not Operated	4	1.0	0	1	1	1	1	1	1	1
B. Operated	23	3.7	9	2	2	3	4	6	11	13
2. MULTIPLE DX										
A. Not Operated	10	3.2	2	1	3	3	4	5	5	5
B. Operated	243	7.2	40	2	3	6	9	15	19	37
1. SINGLE DX	27	3.3	9	1	1	3	4	6	11	13
2. MULTIPLE DX	253	7.1	39	2	3	5	9	13	19	37
A. NOT OPERATED	14	2.6	2	1	1	3	4	4	5	5
B. OPERATED	266	6.9	39	2	3	5	9	13	19	37
TOTAL										
0–19 Years	42	5.3	13	2	3	5	7	9	11	18
20–34	86	6.2	26	1	3	5	8	13	18	27
35–49	81	6.9	60	2	3	4	8	16	21	44
50–64	45	8.6	48	3	5	7	10	18	21	37
65+	26	6.6	22	2	4	6	9	11	11	24
GRAND TOTAL	280	6.7	38	2	3	5	8	13	19	37

959: INJURY NEC & NOS

Type of Patients	Observed Patients	Avg. Stay	Vari-ance	10th	25th	50th	75th	90th	95th	99th
1. SINGLE DX										
A. Not Operated										
0–19 Years	90	1.2	<1	1	1	1	1	2	2	4
20–34	52	1.3	<1	1	1	1	1	3	3	4
35–49	18	1.8	<1	1	1	1	2	3	4	4
50–64	11	1.6	<1	1	1	1	2	2	4	4
65+	7	2.0	1	1	1	2	3	4	4	4
B. Operated										
0–19 Years	4	1.3	<1	1	1	1	2	2	2	2
20–34	17	1.9	5	1	1	1	2	5	10	10
35–49	17	1.5	1	1	1	1	2	3	5	5
50–64	7	1.0	0	1	1	1	1	1	1	1
65+	1	2.0	0	2	2	2	2	2	2	2
2. MULTIPLE DX										
A. Not Operated										
0–19 Years	440	1.5	2	1	1	1	2	2	4	7
20–34	551	1.7	4	1	1	1	2	3	4	10
35–49	451	2.1	4	1	1	2	3	4	6	13
50–64	460	2.5	8	1	1	2	4	5	7	14
65+	943	3.0	8	1	1	2	4	6	7	15
B. Operated										
0–19 Years	21	12.0	597	1	1	3	5	41	70	91
20–34	57	4.1	26	1	2	2	4	15	16	22
35–49	58	6.1	207	1	2	2	4	13	31	96
50–64	41	5.7	96	1	2	2	5	23	30	>99
65+	22	6.4	70	2	3	5	7	10	11	42
SUBTOTALS:										
1. SINGLE DX										
A. Not Operated	178	1.4	<1	1	1	1	1	2	3	4
B. Operated	46	1.6	2	1	1	1	2	2	5	10
2. MULTIPLE DX										
A. Not Operated	2,845	2.3	6	1	1	1	3	5	6	12
B. Operated	199	6.1	159	1	1	2	5	14	27	91
1. SINGLE DX	224	1.4	<1	1	1	1	1	2	3	5
2. MULTIPLE DX	3,044	2.6	17	1	1	1	3	5	7	16
A. NOT OPERATED	3,023	2.3	6	1	1	1	3	4	6	12
B. OPERATED	245	5.3	133	1	1	2	4	11	22	91
TOTAL										
0–19 Years	555	1.8	27	1	1	1	1	3	4	10
20–34	677	1.9	6	1	1	1	2	3	5	15
35–49	544	2.5	27	1	1	2	2	4	6	16
50–64	519	2.7	15	1	1	2	3	3	8	27
65+	973	3.1	9	1	1	2	4	6	7	15
GRAND TOTAL	3,268	2.5	16	1	1	1	3	5	7	15

Length of Stay by Diagnosis and Operation, Western Region, 2008

959.01: HEAD INJURY NOS

Type of Patients	Observed Patients	Avg. Stay	Variance	10th	25th	50th	75th	90th	95th	99th
1. SINGLE DX										
A. Not Operated										
0–19 Years	56	1.2	<1	1	1	1	1	2	2	4
20–34	7	1.4	<1	1	1	1	2	3	3	3
35–49	6	1.5	<1	1	1	1	2	2	2	2
50–64	1	2.0	0	2	2	2	2	2	2	2
65+	1	1.0	0	1	1	1	1	1	1	1
B. Operated										
0–19 Years	0									
20–34	0									
35–49	0									
50–64	0									
65+	0									
2. MULTIPLE DX										
A. Not Operated										
0–19 Years	300	1.5	2	1	1	1	1	2	4	8
20–34	322	1.8	5	1	1	1	2	3	5	12
35–49	249	2.1	5	1	1	1	2	4	6	13
50–64	226	2.4	5	1	1	2	3	5	7	11
65+	482	3.0	10	1	1	2	4	5	7	16
B. Operated										
0–19 Years	6	3.7	15	1	1	1	7	10	10	10
20–34	12	5.2	30	1	1	4	8	15	17	17
35–49	10	13.7	850	1	2	3	9	17	96	96
50–64	9	6.9	51	1	2	5	10	23	23	23
65+	11	4.0	6	1	2	4	6	7	8	8
SUBTOTALS:										
1. SINGLE DX										
A. Not Operated	71	1.2	<1	1	1	1	1	2	2	2
B. Operated	0									
2. MULTIPLE DX										
A. Not Operated	1,579	2.2	6	1	1	1	3	4	6	13
B. Operated	48	6.8	195	1	1	3	7	15	17	96
1. SINGLE DX	71	1.2	<1	1	1	1	1	2	2	4
2. MULTIPLE DX	1,627	2.4	12	1	1	1	3	5	7	14
A. NOT OPERATED	1,650	2.2	6	1	1	1	3	5	6	13
B. OPERATED	48	6.8	195	1	1	3	7	15	17	96
TOTAL										
0–19 Years	362	1.5	2	1	1	1	1	2	3	8
20–34	341	2.0	6	1	1	1	2	3	5	15
35–49	265	2.5	38	1	1	1	2	4	6	16
50–64	236	2.6	7	1	1	1	3	5	8	12
65+	494	3.0	9	1	1	2	4	6	7	16
GRAND TOTAL	1,698	2.3	12	1	1	1	3	4	7	14

959.11: CHEST WALL INJURY NEC

Type of Patients	Observed Patients	Avg. Stay	Variance	10th	25th	50th	75th	90th	95th	99th
1. SINGLE DX										
A. Not Operated										
0–19 Years	0									
20–34	5	1.4	<1	1	1	1	2	2	2	2
35–49	1	2.0	0	2	2	2	2	2	2	2
50–64	5	1.4	<1	1	1	1	2	2	2	2
65+	2	1.0	0	1	1	1	1	1	1	1
B. Operated										
0–19 Years	0									
20–34	0									
35–49	0									
50–64	0									
65+	0									
2. MULTIPLE DX										
A. Not Operated										
0–19 Years	17	1.4	1	1	1	1	1	2	2	5
20–34	49	1.2	<1	1	1	1	1	2	2	3
35–49	37	1.8	2	1	1	1	2	3	7	8
50–64	62	1.8	2	1	1	2	2	3	4	7
65+	112	2.4	4	1	1	2	3	4	7	10
B. Operated										
0–19 Years	0									
20–34	0									
35–49	2	6.5	4	5	5	8	8	8	8	8
50–64	1	48.0	0	48	48	48	48	48	48	48
65+	0									
SUBTOTALS:										
1. SINGLE DX										
A. Not Operated	13	1.4	<1	1	1	1	2	2	2	2
B. Operated	0									
2. MULTIPLE DX										
A. Not Operated	277	1.9	2	1	1	1	2	3	5	9
B. Operated	3	20.3	568	5	5	8	48	48	48	48
1. SINGLE DX	13	1.4	<1	1	1	1	2	2	2	2
2. MULTIPLE DX	280	2.1	10	1	1	1	2	4	5	10
A. NOT OPERATED	290	1.9	2	1	1	1	2	3	5	9
B. OPERATED	3	20.3	568	5	5	8	48	48	48	48
TOTAL										
0–19 Years	17	1.4	1	1	1	1	1	2	2	5
20–34	54	1.2	<1	1	1	1	2	2	2	3
35–49	40	2.1	3	1	1	1	2	4	8	8
50–64	68	2.4	33	1	1	2	3	5	8	48
65+	114	2.4	4	1	1	2	3	4	7	10
GRAND TOTAL	293	2.1	10	1	1	1	2	4	5	10

959.12: ABDOMINAL INJURY NEC

Type of Patients	Observed Patients	Avg. Stay	Variance	10th	25th	50th	75th	90th	95th	99th
1. SINGLE DX										
A. Not Operated										
0–19 Years	20	1.2	<1	1	1	1	1	2	2	2
20–34	18	1.2	<1	1	1	1	1	2	3	3
35–49	2	2.0	2	1	1	1	1	3	3	3
50–64	1	1.0	0	1	1	1	1	1	1	1
65+	1	2.0	0	2	2	2	2	2	2	2
B. Operated										
0–19 Years	0									
20–34	0									
35–49	0									
50–64	0									
65+	0									
2. MULTIPLE DX										
A. Not Operated										
0–19 Years	62	1.5	<1	1	1	1	2	2	3	7
20–34	85	1.3	<1	1	1	1	1	2	2	6
35–49	49	1.7	1	1	1	1	2	3	3	8
50–64	51	2.4	15	1	1	1	2	4	6	28
65+	31	3.4	8	1	1	2	5	8	9	10
B. Operated										
0–19 Years	2	2.0	2	1	1	3	3	3	3	3
20–34	3	3.0	<1	2	2	3	4	4	4	4
35–49	2	8.5	40	4	4	13	13	13	13	13
50–64	4	3.5	19	1	1	1	2	10	10	10
65+	1	5.0	0	5	5	5	5	5	5	5
SUBTOTALS:										
1. SINGLE DX										
A. Not Operated	42	1.2	<1	1	1	1	1	2	2	3
B. Operated	0									
2. MULTIPLE DX										
A. Not Operated	278	1.8	5	1	1	1	2	3	6	9
B. Operated	12	4.1	14	1	1	3	4	10	13	13
1. SINGLE DX	42	1.2	<1	1	1	1	1	2	2	3
2. MULTIPLE DX	290	1.9	5	1	1	1	2	3	6	10
A. NOT OPERATED	320	1.8	4	1	1	1	2	3	4	9
B. OPERATED	12	4.1	14	1	1	3	4	10	13	13
TOTAL										
0–19 Years	84	1.4	<1	1	1	1	1	2	3	7
20–34	106	1.3	<1	1	1	1	1	2	3	4
35–49	53	2.0	4	1	1	1	2	3	4	13
50–64	56	2.4	15	1	1	1	2	5	8	28
65+	33	3.4	7	1	1	2	5	8	9	10
GRAND TOTAL	332	1.8	5	1	1	1	2	3	5	10

Length of Stay by Diagnosis and Operation, Western Region, 2008

Western Region, October 2006–September 2007 Data, by Diagnosis

960: POISONING BY ANTIBIOTICS

Type of Patients	Observed Patients	Avg. Stay	Vari-ance	10th	25th	50th	75th	90th	95th	99th
1. SINGLE DX										
A. Not Operated										
0–19 Years	0									
20–34	0									
35–49	0									
50–64	0									
65+	0									
B. Operated										
0–19 Years	0									
20–34	0									
35–49	0									
50–64	0									
65+	0									
2. MULTIPLE DX										
A. Not Operated										
0–19 Years	10	3.6	20	1	1	1	6	14	14	14
20–34	9	1.9	1	1	1	2	2	2	4	4
35–49	13	2.3	6	1	1	1	2	6	9	9
50–64	7	3.7	6	1	2	2	5	8	8	8
65+	9	3.8	4	1	3	3	5	7	7	7
B. Operated										
0–19 Years	0									
20–34	0									
35–49	0									
50–64	0									
65+	0									
SUBTOTALS:										
1. SINGLE DX										
A. Not Operated	0									
B. Operated	0									
2. MULTIPLE DX										
A. Not Operated	48	3.0	8	1	1	2	5	7	8	8
B. Operated	0									
1. SINGLE DX	0									
2. MULTIPLE DX	48	3.0	8	1	1	2	5	7	8	8
A. NOT OPERATED	48	3.0	8	1	1	2	5	7	8	8
B. OPERATED	0									
TOTAL										
0–19 Years	10	3.6	20	1	1	1	6	14	14	14
20–34	9	1.9	1	1	1	2	2	4	4	4
35–49	13	2.3	6	1	1	1	2	6	9	9
50–64	7	3.7	6	1	2	3	5	8	8	8
65+	9	3.8	4	1	3	3	5	7	7	7
GRAND TOTAL	48	3.0	8	1	1	2	5	7	8	14

961: POISON-ANTI-INFECT NEC

Type of Patients	Observed Patients	Avg. Stay	Vari-ance	10th	25th	50th	75th	90th	95th	99th
1. SINGLE DX										
A. Not Operated										
0–19 Years	1	1.0	0	1	1	1	1	1	1	1
20–34	0									
35–49	0									
50–64	0									
65+	0									
B. Operated										
0–19 Years	0									
20–34	0									
35–49	0									
50–64	0									
65+	0									
2. MULTIPLE DX										
A. Not Operated										
0–19 Years	12	3.6	8	1	1	3	6	8	9	9
20–34	8	1.9	<1	1	1	2	3	3	3	3
35–49	5	3.0	8	1	2	2	2	8	8	8
50–64	12	3.1	3	1	2	3	4	5	7	7
65+	16	4.5	20	1	2	2	8	13	15	15
B. Operated										
0–19 Years	0									
20–34	0									
35–49	0									
50–64	0									
65+	0									
SUBTOTALS:										
1. SINGLE DX										
A. Not Operated	1	1.0	0	1	1	1	1	1	1	1
B. Operated	0									
2. MULTIPLE DX										
A. Not Operated	53	3.4	10	1	1	2	4	8	10	15
B. Operated	0									
1. SINGLE DX	1	1.0	0	1	1	1	1	1	1	1
2. MULTIPLE DX	53	3.4	10	1	1	2	4	8	10	15
A. NOT OPERATED	54	3.4	10	1	1	2	4	8	10	15
B. OPERATED	0									
TOTAL										
0–19 Years	13	3.4	8	1	1	2	6	8	9	9
20–34	8	1.9	<1	1	1	2	3	3	3	3
35–49	5	3.0	8	1	2	2	2	8	8	8
50–64	12	3.1	3	1	2	3	4	5	7	7
65+	16	4.5	20	1	2	2	8	13	15	15
GRAND TOTAL	54	3.4	10	1	1	2	4	8	10	15

962: POISONING BY HORMONES

Type of Patients	Observed Patients	Avg. Stay	Vari-ance	10th	25th	50th	75th	90th	95th	99th
1. SINGLE DX										
A. Not Operated										
0–19 Years	34	1.0	<1	1	1	1	1	1	1	2
20–34	0									
35–49	0									
50–64	1	1.0	0	1	1	1	1	1	1	1
65+	1	1.0	0	1	1	1	1	1	1	1
B. Operated										
0–19 Years	0									
20–34	0									
35–49	0									
50–64	0									
65+	0									
2. MULTIPLE DX										
A. Not Operated										
0–19 Years	87	1.5	2	1	1	1	2	2	3	11
20–34	146	2.4	5	1	1	2	3	5	6	13
35–49	311	2.9	10	1	1	2	3	5	7	17
50–64	318	2.8	15	1	1	2	3	5	9	23
65+	493	2.9	6	1	1	2	4	6	8	13
B. Operated										
0–19 Years	0									
20–34	0									
35–49	3	11.0	31	6	6	10	17	17	17	17
50–64	5	27.6	>999	4	5	7	26	96	96	96
65+	7	8.7	21	1	5	10	12	14	14	14
SUBTOTALS:										
1. SINGLE DX										
A. Not Operated	36	1.0	<1	1	1	1	1	1	1	2
B. Operated	0									
2. MULTIPLE DX										
A. Not Operated	1,355	2.7	9	1	1	2	3	5	8	15
B. Operated	15	15.5	534	4	5	10	14	26	96	96
1. SINGLE DX	36	1.0	<1	1	1	1	1	1	1	2
2. MULTIPLE DX	1,370	2.9	16	1	1	2	3	6	8	15
A. NOT OPERATED	1,391	2.7	8	1	1	2	3	5	8	15
B. OPERATED	15	15.5	534	4	5	10	14	26	96	96
TOTAL										
0–19 Years	121	1.4	1	1	1	1	1	2	3	4
20–34	146	2.4	5	1	1	2	3	5	6	13
35–49	314	3.0	10	1	1	2	3	6	7	17
50–64	324	3.2	43	1	1	2	3	5	10	26
65+	501	3.0	6	1	1	2	4	6	8	13
GRAND TOTAL	1,406	2.8	15	1	1	2	3	6	8	15

Length of Stay by Diagnosis and Operation, Western Region, 2008

Western Region, October 2006–September 2007 Data, by Diagnosis

962.3: POISON-INSULIN/ANTIDIAB

Type of Patients	Observed Patients	Avg. Stay	Vari-ance	10th	25th	50th	75th	90th	95th	99th
1. SINGLE DX										
A. Not Operated										
0–19 Years	33	1.0	<1	1	1	1	1	1	1	2
20–34	0									
35–49	0									
50–64	1	1.0	0					1	1	1
65+	1	1.0	0	1	1	1	1	1	1	1
B. Operated										
0–19 Years	0									
20–34	0									
35–49	0									
50–64	0									
65+	0									
2. MULTIPLE DX										
A. Not Operated										
0–19 Years	79	1.5	2	1	1	1	2	3	3	11
20–34	136	2.4	5	1	1	2	3	5	6	13
35–49	299	2.9	10	1	1	2	3	6	7	17
50–64	297	2.9	16	1	1	2	3	5	9	23
65+	471	2.9	6	1	1	2	4	6	8	13
B. Operated										
0–19 Years	0									
20–34	0									
35–49	3	11.0	31	6	6	10	17	17	17	17
50–64	5	27.6	>999	4	5	7	26	96	96	96
65+	7	8.7	21	1	5	10	12	14	14	14
SUBTOTALS:										
1. SINGLE DX										
A. Not Operated	35	1.0	<1	1	1	1	1	1	1	2
B. Operated	0									
2. MULTIPLE DX										
A. Not Operated	1,282	2.8	9	1	1	2	3	5	6	15
B. Operated	15	15.5	534	4	5	10	14	26	96	96
1. SINGLE DX	35	1.0	<1	1	1	1	1	1	1	2
2. MULTIPLE DX	1,297	2.9	16	1	1	2	3	6	8	15
A. NOT OPERATED	1,317	2.7	9	1	1	2	3	5	8	15
B. OPERATED	15	15.5	534	4	5	10	14	26	96	96
TOTAL										
0–19 Years	112	1.4	1	1	1	1	1	2	3	4
20–34	136	2.4	5	1	1	2	3	5	5	13
35–49	302	3.0	11	1	1	2	4	6	7	17
50–64	303	3.3	46	1	1	2	3	6	10	26
65+	479	3.0	6	1	1	2	4	6	8	13
GRAND TOTAL	1,332	2.9	16	1	1	2	3	6	8	15

963: POISONING-SYSTEMIC AGENT

Type of Patients	Observed Patients	Avg. Stay	Vari-ance	10th	25th	50th	75th	90th	95th	99th
1. SINGLE DX										
A. Not Operated										
0–19 Years	13	1.1	<1	1	1	1	1	1	2	2
20–34	2	1.5	<1	1	1	2	1	2	2	2
35–49	4	1.3	<1	1	1	1	1	2	2	2
50–64	4	1.0	0	1	1	1	1	1	1	1
65+	0									
B. Operated										
0–19 Years	0									
20–34	0									
35–49	0									
50–64	0									
65+	0									
2. MULTIPLE DX										
A. Not Operated										
0–19 Years	170	1.6	3	1	1	1	2	3	3	9
20–34	316	2.0	5	1	1	1	3	3	5	9
35–49	209	2.6	19	1	1	2	3	5	6	13
50–64	98	2.8	6	1	2	2	4	5	7	15
65+	52	4.5	19	2	2	3	5	10	11	26
B. Operated										
0–19 Years	0									
20–34	1	2.0	0	2	2	2	2	2	2	2
35–49	1	24.0	0	24	24	24	24	24	24	24
50–64	1	26.0	0	26	26	26	26	26	26	26
65+	1	6.0	0	2	2	2	2	2	2	6
SUBTOTALS:										
1. SINGLE DX										
A. Not Operated	23	1.1	<1	1	1	1	1	2	2	2
B. Operated	0									
2. MULTIPLE DX										
A. Not Operated	845	2.3	9	1	1	2	3	4	6	15
B. Operated	5	12.0	143	2	2	6	14	26	26	26
1. SINGLE DX	23	1.1	<1	1	1	1	1	2	2	2
2. MULTIPLE DX	850	2.4	11	1	1	2	3	4	6	16
A. NOT OPERATED	868	2.3	9	1	1	2	3	4	6	15
B. OPERATED	5	12.0	143	2	2	6	14	26	26	26
TOTAL										
0–19 Years	184	1.6	3	1	1	1	1	2	3	9
20–34	319	2.0	6	1	1	2	3	5	5	11
35–49	214	2.7	22	1	1	2	3	6	8	23
50–64	103	2.7	6	1	1	2	4	6	7	15
65+	53	4.5	19	1	2	3	5	10	11	26
GRAND TOTAL	873	2.3	10	1	1	1	2	4	6	16

963.0: POIS-ANTIALLRG/ANTIEMET

Type of Patients	Observed Patients	Avg. Stay	Vari-ance	10th	25th	50th	75th	90th	95th	99th
1. SINGLE DX										
A. Not Operated										
0–19 Years	10	1.1	<1	1	1	1	1	1	2	2
20–34	2	1.5	<1	1	1	2	1	2	2	2
35–49	4	1.3	<1	1	1	1	1	2	2	2
50–64	4	1.0	0	1	1	1	1	1	1	1
65+	0									
B. Operated										
0–19 Years	0									
20–34	0									
35–49	0									
50–64	0									
65+	0									
2. MULTIPLE DX										
A. Not Operated										
0–19 Years	163	1.5	<1	1	1	1	2	3	3	4
20–34	306	1.9	3	1	1	1	2	3	5	9
35–49	195	2.6	20	1	1	2	3	4	6	23
50–64	84	2.5	5	1	2	2	3	5	7	15
65+	29	3.4	11	1	2	3	3	6	10	18
B. Operated										
0–19 Years	1	2.0	0	2	2	2	2	2	2	2
20–34	1	24.0	0	24	24	24	24	24	24	24
35–49	1	26.0	0	26	26	26	26	26	26	26
50–64	0									
65+	1	2.0	0	2	2	2	2	2	2	2
SUBTOTALS:										
1. SINGLE DX										
A. Not Operated	20	1.2	<1	1	1	1	1	2	2	2
B. Operated	0									
2. MULTIPLE DX										
A. Not Operated	777	2.1	7	1	1	2	2	4	5	11
B. Operated	4	13.5	176	2	2	2	24	26	26	26
1. SINGLE DX	20	1.2	<1	1	1	1	1	2	2	2
2. MULTIPLE DX	781	2.2	9	1	1	1	2	4	5	13
A. NOT OPERATED	797	2.1	7	1	1	1	2	4	5	11
B. OPERATED	4	13.5	176	2	2	2	24	26	26	26
TOTAL										
0–19 Years	174	1.5	<1	1	1	1	2	3	3	4
20–34	309	1.9	4	1	1	1	2	3	5	9
35–49	200	2.7	23	1	1	2	3	5	6	26
50–64	88	2.4	5	1	2	2	3	5	7	15
65+	30	3.3	11	1	2	3	3	5	10	18
GRAND TOTAL	801	2.1	9	1	1	1	2	4	5	13

Length of Stay by Diagnosis and Operation, Western Region, 2008

Western Region, October 2006–September 2007 Data, by Diagnosis

964: POIS-AGENT AFF BLOOD

Type of Patients	Observed Patients	Avg. Stay	Vari-ance	10th	25th	50th	75th	90th	95th	99th
1. SINGLE DX										
A. Not Operated										
0–19 Years	5	1.4	<1	1	1	1	2	2	2	2
20–34	0									
35–49	0									
50–64	0									
65+	2	4.0	2	3	3	5	5	5	5	5
B. Operated										
0–19 Years	0									
20–34	0									
35–49	0									
50–64	0									
65+	0									
2. MULTIPLE DX										
A. Not Operated										
0–19 Years	16	2.2	6	1	1	2	2	4	11	11
20–34	38	1.9	1	1	1	2	2	4	5	6
35–49	54	3.2	4	1	2	3	4	6	7	9
50–64	97	3.5	8	1	2	3	4	7	11	15
65+	236	3.5	11	1	2	3	4	7	9	15
B. Operated										
0–19 Years	0									
20–34	1	7.0	0	7	7	7	7	7	7	7
35–49	3	13.3	349	2	2	3	35	35	35	35
50–64	3	5.3	5	4	4	4	8	8	8	8
65+	5	5.4	25	1	3	4	5	14	14	14
SUBTOTALS:										
1. SINGLE DX										
A. Not Operated	7	2.1	2	1	1	2	3	5	5	5
B. Operated	0									
2. MULTIPLE DX										
A. Not Operated	441	3.3	8	1	2	2	4	6	8	14
B. Operated	12	7.5	87	2	3	4	7	14	35	35
1. SINGLE DX	7	2.1	2	1	1	2	3	5	5	5
2. MULTIPLE DX	453	3.4	11	1	2	2	4	6	8	15
A. NOT OPERATED	448	3.2	8	1	2	2	4	6	8	14
B. OPERATED	12	7.5	87	2	3	4	7	14	35	35
TOTAL										
0–19 Years	21	2.0	5	1	1	1	2	3	4	11
20–34	39	2.1	2	1	1	2	2	4	6	7
35–49	57	3.7	22	1	2	3	4	6	7	35
50–64	100	3.5	8	1	2	3	4	7	11	14
65+	243	3.5	11	1	2	3	4	7	9	15
GRAND TOTAL	460	3.4	11	1	2	2	4	6	8	15

964.2: POISONING-ANTICOAGULANTS

Type of Patients	Observed Patients	Avg. Stay	Vari-ance	10th	25th	50th	75th	90th	95th	99th
1. SINGLE DX										
A. Not Operated										
0–19 Years	0									
20–34	0									
35–49	0									
50–64	0									
65+	2	4.0	2	3	3	5	5	5	5	5
B. Operated										
0–19 Years	0									
20–34	0									
35–49	0									
50–64	0									
65+	0									
2. MULTIPLE DX										
A. Not Operated										
0–19 Years	3	4.3	33	1	1	2	11	11	11	11
20–34	21	2.3	2	1	1	3	3	4	5	6
35–49	49	3.3	4	1	2	3	5	6	7	9
50–64	97	3.5	8	1	2	3	4	7	11	15
65+	232	3.5	11	1	2	3	4	7	9	15
B. Operated										
0–19 Years	0									
20–34	0									
35–49	3	13.3	349	2	2	3	35	35	35	35
50–64	2	6.0	8	4	4	8	8	8	8	8
65+	5	5.4	25	1	3	4	5	14	14	14
SUBTOTALS:										
1. SINGLE DX										
A. Not Operated	2	4.0	2	3	3	5	5	5	5	5
B. Operated	0									
2. MULTIPLE DX										
A. Not Operated	402	3.4	9	1	2	3	4	6	8	14
B. Operated	10	7.9	105	1	3	4	8	35	35	35
1. SINGLE DX	2	4.0	2	3	3	5	5	5	5	5
2. MULTIPLE DX	412	3.5	11	1	2	3	4	7	9	15
A. NOT OPERATED	404	3.4	9	1	2	3	4	6	8	14
B. OPERATED	10	7.9	105	1	3	4	8	35	35	35
TOTAL										
0–19 Years	3	4.3	33	1	1	2	11	11	11	11
20–34	21	2.3	2	1	1	3	3	4	5	6
35–49	52	3.9	23	1	2	3	5	6	7	35
50–64	99	3.5	8	1	2	3	4	7	11	14
65+	239	3.5	11	1	2	3	4	7	9	15
GRAND TOTAL	414	3.5	11	1	2	3	4	7	9	15

965: POIS-ANALGESIC/ANTIPYR

Type of Patients	Observed Patients	Avg. Stay	Vari-ance	10th	25th	50th	75th	90th	95th	99th
1. SINGLE DX										
A. Not Operated										
0–19 Years	116	1.4	<1	1	1	1	2	2	2	3
20–34	34	1.2	<1	1	1	1	1	2	3	3
35–49	9	1.3	<1	1	1	1	2	2	2	2
50–64	2	2.0	2	1	1	2	3	3	3	3
65+	0									
B. Operated										
0–19 Years	0									
20–34	0									
35–49	0									
50–64	0									
65+	0									
2. MULTIPLE DX										
A. Not Operated										
0–19 Years	1,433	2.1	6	1	1	2	2	4	5	9
20–34	2,864	2.5	8	1	1	2	3	5	6	16
35–49	2,803	3.2	13	1	1	2	4	6	9	19
50–64	2,592	3.7	19	1	1	3	4	7	11	22
65+	1,281	3.9	11	1	2	3	5	8	10	17
B. Operated										
0–19 Years	4	21.9	300	4	15	23	45	45	45	45
20–34	21	11.7	163	3	4	7	14	23	24	59
35–49	30	9.8	57	1	5	9	13	18	26	35
50–64	31	11.8	135	3	4	7	14	28	29	53
65+	25	12.3	99	5	6	11	15	20	21	53
SUBTOTALS:										
1. SINGLE DX										
A. Not Operated	161	1.4	<1	1	1	1	2	2	3	3
B. Operated	0									
2. MULTIPLE DX										
A. Not Operated	10,973	3.1	12	1	1	2	4	6	9	18
B. Operated	111	11.7	116	3	5	8	14	24	29	53
1. SINGLE DX	161	1.4	<1	1	1	1	2	2	3	3
2. MULTIPLE DX	11,084	3.2	14	1	1	2	4	6	9	19
A. NOT OPERATED	11,134	3.0	12	1	1	2	3	6	9	18
B. OPERATED	111	11.7	116	3	5	8	14	24	29	53
TOTAL										
0–19 Years	1,553	2.1	7	1	1	2	2	4	5	10
20–34	2,919	2.5	9	1	1	2	3	5	6	16
35–49	2,842	3.2	14	1	1	2	4	6	10	20
50–64	2,625	3.8	21	1	2	3	4	8	11	23
65+	1,306	4.1	14	1	2	3	5	8	11	17
GRAND TOTAL	11,245	3.1	14	1	1	2	4	6	9	19

965.00: POISONING-OPIUM NOS

Type of Patients	Observed Patients	Avg. Stay	Variance	10th	25th	50th	75th	90th	95th	99th
1. SINGLE DX										
A. Not Operated										
0–19 Years	2	2.0	0	2	2	2	2	2	2	2
20–34	0									
35–49	0									
50–64	0									
65+	0									
B. Operated										
0–19 Years	0									
20–34	0									
35–49	0									
50–64	0									
65+	0									
2. MULTIPLE DX										
A. Not Operated										
0–19 Years	28	3.4	22	1	1	2	3	10	18	19
20–34	114	3.2	14	1	1	2	4	6	13	18
35–49	293	3.6	17	1	1	2	4	8	13	21
50–64	359	4.4	36	1	2	3	5	9	15	34
65+	152	3.5	7	1	2	3	4	6	9	12
B. Operated										
0–19 Years	0									
20–34	3	13.0	109	3	3	12	24	24	24	24
35–49	4	9.0	28	2	8	12	14	14	14	14
50–64	6	20.3	88	7	11	24	28	28	28	28
65+	3	13.6	65	5	5	15	21	21	21	21
SUBTOTALS:										
1. SINGLE DX										
A. Not Operated	2	2.0	0	2	2	2	2	2	2	2
B. Operated	0									
2. MULTIPLE DX										
A. Not Operated	946	3.8	23	1	1	2	4	8	12	23
B. Operated	16	14.9	81	3	8	12	24	28	28	28
1. SINGLE DX	2	2.0	0	2	2	2	2	2	2	2
2. MULTIPLE DX	962	4.0	26	1	1	3	4	9	13	28
A. NOT OPERATED	948	3.8	23	1	1	2	4	8	12	23
B. OPERATED	16	14.9	81	3	8	12	24	28	28	28
TOTAL										
0–19 Years	30	3.3	20	1	1	2	3	5	18	19
20–34	117	3.5	18	1	1	2	4	8	16	18
35–49	297	3.7	18	1	1	2	4	9	13	20
50–64	365	4.7	41	1	2	3	5	10	15	34
65+	155	3.7	10	1	2	3	4	7	10	19
GRAND TOTAL	964	4.0	26	1	1	3	4	9	13	28

965.01: POISONING-HEROIN

Type of Patients	Observed Patients	Avg. Stay	Variance	10th	25th	50th	75th	90th	95th	99th
1. SINGLE DX										
A. Not Operated										
0–19 Years	1	1.0	0	1	1	1	1	1	1	1
20–34	1	1.0	0	1	1	1	1	1	1	1
35–49	0									
50–64	0									
65+	0									
B. Operated										
0–19 Years	0									
20–34	0									
35–49	0									
50–64	0									
65+	0									
2. MULTIPLE DX										
A. Not Operated										
0–19 Years	14	1.8	<1	1	1	1	2	3	4	4
20–34	176	2.8	10	1	1	2	3	6	9	20
35–49	160	4.0	40	1	1	2	4	8	14	42
50–64	113	3.2	11	1	1	2	3	6	12	14
65+	12	5.8	37	2	3	3	4	13	22	22
B. Operated										
0–19 Years	1	45.0	0	45	45	45	45	45	45	45
20–34	3	8.0	13	4	4	9	11	11	11	11
35–49	2	13.5	4	12	12	12	15	15	15	15
50–64	0									
65+	0									
SUBTOTALS:										
1. SINGLE DX										
A. Not Operated	2	1.0	0	1	1	1	1	1	1	1
B. Operated	0									
2. MULTIPLE DX										
A. Not Operated	475	3.3	21	1	1	2	3	6	12	22
B. Operated	6	16.0	216	4	9	11	15	45	45	45
1. SINGLE DX	2	1.0	0	1	1	1	1	1	1	1
2. MULTIPLE DX	481	3.5	25	1	1	2	4	7	12	28
A. NOT OPERATED	477	3.3	21	1	1	2	3	6	12	22
B. OPERATED	6	16.0	216	4	9	11	15	45	45	45
TOTAL										
0–19 Years	16	4.5	119	1	1	1	3	4	45	45
20–34	180	2.8	11	1	1	2	3	6	10	20
35–49	162	4.1	41	1	1	2	4	8	14	42
50–64	113	3.2	11	1	1	2	3	6	12	14
65+	12	5.8	37	2	3	3	4	13	22	22
GRAND TOTAL	483	3.5	25	1	1	2	4	7	12	28

965.02: POISONING-METHADONE

Type of Patients	Observed Patients	Avg. Stay	Variance	10th	25th	50th	75th	90th	95th	99th
1. SINGLE DX										
A. Not Operated										
0–19 Years	1	1.0	0	1	1	1	1	1	1	1
20–34	1	1.0	0	1	1	1	1	1	1	1
35–49	0									
50–64	0									
65+	0									
B. Operated										
0–19 Years	0									
20–34	0									
35–49	0									
50–64	0									
65+	0									
2. MULTIPLE DX										
A. Not Operated										
0–19 Years	60	2.9	25	1	1	1	3	5	7	35
20–34	185	3.4	21	1	1	2	4	6	10	29
35–49	286	3.5	14	1	1	2	4	7	11	23
50–64	320	3.8	26	1	2	3	4	7	10	24
65+	69	3.6	5	1	2	3	5	7	8	9
B. Operated										
0–19 Years	1	23.0	0	23	23	23	23	23	23	23
20–34	4	22.7	674	2	6	23	59	59	59	59
35–49	4	12.5	228	3	3	5	35	35	35	35
50–64	6	6.7	10	3	5	6	8	12	12	12
65+	1	14.0	0	14	14	14	14	14	14	14
SUBTOTALS:										
1. SINGLE DX										
A. Not Operated	2	1.0	0	1	1	1	1	1	1	1
B. Operated	0									
2. MULTIPLE DX										
A. Not Operated	920	3.6	19	1	1	2	4	7	10	23
B. Operated	16	13.6	232	3	5	7	23	35	59	59
1. SINGLE DX	2	1.0	0	1	1	1	1	1	1	1
2. MULTIPLE DX	936	3.7	25	1	1	2	4	7	10	27
A. NOT OPERATED	922	3.6	19	1	1	2	4	7	10	23
B. OPERATED	16	13.6	232	3	5	7	23	35	59	59
TOTAL										
0–19 Years	62	3.2	30	1	1	1	3	5	7	35
20–34	190	3.8	39	1	1	2	4	6	12	39
35–49	290	3.6	17	1	1	2	4	7	11	27
50–64	326	3.9	26	1	2	3	4	8	10	24
65+	70	3.8	7	1	2	3	6	8	8	14
GRAND TOTAL	938	3.7	25	1	1	2	4	7	10	27

Length of Stay by Diagnosis and Operation, Western Region, 2008

803

Western Region, October 2006–September 2007 Data, by Diagnosis

965.09: POISONING-OPIATES NEC

Type of Patients	Observed Patients	Avg. Stay	Variance	10th	25th	50th	75th	90th	95th	99th
1. SINGLE DX										
A. Not Operated										
0–19 Years	7	1.1	<1	1	1	1	1	2	2	2
20–34	0									
35–49	1	1.0	0	1	1	1	1	1	1	1
50–64	0									
65+	0									
B. Operated										
0–19 Years	0									
20–34	0									
35–49	0									
50–64	0									
65+	0									
2. MULTIPLE DX										
A. Not Operated										
0–19 Years	79	2.9	30	1	1	1	2	5	12	33
20–34	313	2.9	14	1	1	2	3	6	9	20
35–49	705	3.3	15	1	1	2	4	6	10	19
50–64	971	3.6	16	1	1	2	4	7	11	18
65+	627	3.9	12	1	2	3	5	8	10	17
B. Operated										
0–19 Years	3	4.0	0	4	4	4	4	4	4	4
20–34	3	15.3	17	12	12	14	20	20	20	20
35–49	14	9.4	49	1	4	8	13	16	26	26
50–64	13	12.6	225	3	4	5	9	29	53	53
65+	11	8.5	16	5	5	7	13	14	15	17
SUBTOTALS:										
1. SINGLE DX										
A. Not Operated	8	1.1	<1	1	1	1	1	2	2	2
B. Operated	0									
2. MULTIPLE DX										
A. Not Operated	2,695	3.5	15	1	1	2	4	7	10	19
B. Operated	42	10.4	92	3	4	8	13	20	27	53
1. SINGLE DX	8	1.1	<1	1	1	1	1	2	2	2
2. MULTIPLE DX	2,737	3.6	17	1	1	2	4	7	11	19
A. NOT OPERATED	2,703	3.5	15	1	1	2	4	7	10	19
B. OPERATED	42	10.4	92	3	4	8	13	20	27	53
TOTAL										
0–19 Years	87	2.7	27	1	1	1	2	4	7	33
20–34	316	3.0	15	1	1	2	3	6	9	20
35–49	720	3.4	16	1	1	2	4	7	11	20
50–64	984	3.8	19	1	1	2	4	8	11	19
65+	638	4.0	12	2	2	3	5	8	11	17
GRAND TOTAL	2,745	3.6	17	1	1	2	4	7	11	19

965.1: POISONING-SALICYLATES

Type of Patients	Observed Patients	Avg. Stay	Variance	10th	25th	50th	75th	90th	95th	99th
1. SINGLE DX										
A. Not Operated										
0–19 Years	23	1.1	<1	1	1	1	1	1	2	2
20–34	8	1.3	<1	1	1	1	2	2	2	2
35–49	1	1.0	0	1	1	1	1	1	1	1
50–64	0									
65+	0									
B. Operated										
0–19 Years	0									
20–34	0									
35–49	0									
50–64	0									
65+	0									
2. MULTIPLE DX										
A. Not Operated										
0–19 Years	243	1.6	<1	1	1	1	2	3	3	5
20–34	311	2.1	9	1	1	2	2	3	5	9
35–49	149	2.6	11	1	1	2	3	4	7	25
50–64	119	3.3	14	1	2	3	4	5	7	25
65+	68	4.0	11	1	2	3	5	8	9	23
B. Operated										
0–19 Years	0									
20–34	1	7.0	0	7	7	7	7	7	7	7
35–49	1	6.0	0	6	6	6	6	6	6	6
50–64	2	7.0	0	7	7	7	7	7	7	7
65+	5	20.3	375	4	7	18	20	53	53	53
SUBTOTALS:										
1. SINGLE DX										
A. Not Operated	32	1.1	<1	1	1	1	1	2	2	2
B. Operated	0									
2. MULTIPLE DX										
A. Not Operated	890	2.4	8	1	1	2	3	4	5	9
B. Operated	9	14.3	239	4	7	7	18	53	53	53
1. SINGLE DX	32	1.1	<1	1	1	1	1	2	2	2
2. MULTIPLE DX	899	2.5	12	1	1	2	3	4	6	16
A. NOT OPERATED	922	2.3	8	1	1	2	3	4	5	9
B. OPERATED	9	14.3	239	4	7	7	18	53	53	53
TOTAL										
0–19 Years	266	1.5	<1	1	1	1	2	3	3	5
20–34	320	2.1	9	1	1	2	2	3	5	9
35–49	151	2.7	11	1	1	2	3	4	7	25
50–64	121	3.4	14	2	2	3	4	5	7	25
65+	73	5.1	48	2	2	3	5	9	18	53
GRAND TOTAL	931	2.4	12	1	1	2	3	4	6	16

965.4: POIS-AROMA ANALGES NEC

Type of Patients	Observed Patients	Avg. Stay	Variance	10th	25th	50th	75th	90th	95th	99th
1. SINGLE DX										
A. Not Operated										
0–19 Years	70	1.5	<1	1	1	1	2	3	3	4
20–34	24	1.3	<1	1	1	1	1	2	3	3
35–49	6	1.5	<1	1	1	1	2	2	2	2
50–64	2	2.0	2	1	2	2	3	3		3
65+	0									
B. Operated										
0–19 Years	0									
20–34	0									
35–49	0									
50–64	0									
65+	0									
2. MULTIPLE DX										
A. Not Operated										
0–19 Years	890	2.1	4	1	1	2	3	4	5	8
20–34	1,546	2.4	5	1	1	3	3	5	6	11
35–49	1,006	2.9	7	1	1	2	3	6	8	14
50–64	498	3.6	16	1	2	2	4	8	10	22
65+	214	4.6	14	1	2	3	6	11	13	16
B. Operated										
0–19 Years	1	15.0	0	15	15	15	15	15	15	15
20–34	7	5.6	17	2	2	5	7	14	14	14
35–49	5	9.0	39	1	6	9	11	18	18	18
50–64	1	3.0	0	3	3	3	3	3	3	3
65+	1	10.0	0	10	10	10	10	10	10	10
SUBTOTALS:										
1. SINGLE DX										
A. Not Operated	102	1.5	<1	1	1	1	2	2	3	3
B. Operated	0									
2. MULTIPLE DX										
A. Not Operated	4,154	2.7	8	1	1	2	3	5	7	14
B. Operated	15	7.5	27	2	3	6	18	15	18	18
1. SINGLE DX	102	1.5	<1	1	1	1	2	2	3	3
2. MULTIPLE DX	4,169	2.7	8	1	1	2	3	5	7	14
A. NOT OPERATED	4,256	2.7	7	1	1	2	3	5	7	14
B. OPERATED	15	7.5	27	2	3	6	11	15	18	18
TOTAL										
0–19 Years	961	2.1	4	1	1	2	2	3	5	8
20–34	1,577	2.4	5	1	1	2	3	5	6	11
35–49	1,017	2.9	8	1	1	2	3	6	8	14
50–64	501	3.6	16	1	2	2	4	8	10	20
65+	215	4.6	14	1	2	3	6	11	13	16
GRAND TOTAL	4,271	2.7	8	1	1	2	3	5	7	14

Length of Stay by Diagnosis and Operation, Western Region, 2008

Western Region, October 2006–September 2007 Data, by Diagnosis

965.61: POISON-PROP ACID DERIV

Type of Patients	Observed Patients	Avg. Stay	Vari-ance	Percentiles						
				10th	25th	50th	75th	90th	95th	99th
1. SINGLE DX										
A. Not Operated										
0–19 Years	8	1.3	<1	1	1	1	1	3	3	3
20–34	0									
35–49	0									
50–64	0									
65+	0									
B. Operated										
0–19 Years	0									
20–34	0									
35–49	0									
50–64	0									
65+	0									
2. MULTIPLE DX										
A. Not Operated										
0–19 Years	106	1.9	2	1	1	1	2	4	6	7
20–34	146	1.9	2	1	1	1	2	3	4	8
35–49	57	2.9	8	1	1	2	3	7	9	13
50–64	30	2.4	2	1	1	2	3	3	5	7
65+	15	2.8	9	1	1	2	3	4	13	13
B. Operated										
0–19 Years	0									
20–34	0									
35–49	0									
50–64	1	6.0	0	6	6	6	6	6	6	6
65+	1	6.0	0	6	6	6	6	6	6	6
SUBTOTALS:										
1. SINGLE DX										
A. Not Operated	8	1.3	<1	1	1	1	1	3	3	3
B. Operated	0									
2. MULTIPLE DX										
A. Not Operated	354	2.1	4	1	1	1	3	4	6	12
B. Operated	2	6.0	0	6	6	6	6	6	6	6
1. SINGLE DX	8	1.3	<1	1	1	1	1	3	3	3
2. MULTIPLE DX	356	2.1	4	1	1	1	3	4	6	12
A. NOT OPERATED	362	2.1	3	1	1	1	2	4	6	12
B. OPERATED	2	6.0	0	6	6	6	6	6	6	6
TOTAL										
0–19 Years	114	1.9	2	1	1	1	2	4	6	7
20–34	146	1.9	2	1	1	1	2	3	4	8
35–49	57	2.9	8	1	1	2	3	7	9	13
50–64	31	2.5	2	1	1	2	3	4	6	7
65+	16	3.0	9	1	1	2	3	6	13	13
GRAND TOTAL	364	2.1	4	1	1	1	3	4	6	12

965.8: POIS-ANALGES/ANTIPYR NEC

Type of Patients	Observed Patients	Avg. Stay	Vari-ance	Percentiles						
				10th	25th	50th	75th	90th	95th	99th
1. SINGLE DX										
A. Not Operated										
0–19 Years	4	1.3	<1	1	1	1	1	2	2	2
20–34	0									
35–49	0									
50–64	0									
65+	0									
B. Operated										
0–19 Years	0									
20–34	0									
35–49	0									
50–64	0									
65+	0									
2. MULTIPLE DX										
A. Not Operated										
0–19 Years	13	1.7	2	1	1	1	2	3	6	6
20–34	55	1.9	2	1	1	1	2	4	6	6
35–49	122	3.1	14	1	1	2	3	6	9	18
50–64	167	3.6	10	1	1	3	4	7	11	17
65+	107	3.3	5	1	2	3	4	6	8	10
B. Operated										
0–19 Years	0									
20–34	0									
35–49	0									
50–64	2	7.9	71	2	2	2	14	14	14	14
65+	3	14.3	16	12	12	12	14	19	19	19
SUBTOTALS:										
1. SINGLE DX										
A. Not Operated	4	1.3	<1	1	1	1	1	2	2	2
B. Operated	0									
2. MULTIPLE DX										
A. Not Operated	464	3.1	9	1	1	2	4	6	9	17
B. Operated	5	11.7	39	2	12	12	14	19	19	19
1. SINGLE DX	4	1.3	<1	1	1	1	1	2	2	2
2. MULTIPLE DX	469	3.2	10	1	1	2	4	6	9	17
A. NOT OPERATED	468	3.1	9	1	1	2	4	6	9	17
B. OPERATED	5	11.7	39	2	12	12	14	19	19	19
TOTAL										
0–19 Years	17	1.6	2	1	1	1	2	3	6	6
20–34	55	1.9	2	1	1	1	2	4	6	6
35–49	122	3.1	14	1	1	2	3	6	9	18
50–64	169	3.6	11	1	1	3	4	7	11	17
65+	110	3.6	8	1	1	3	4	7	10	12
GRAND TOTAL	473	3.2	10	1	1	2	4	6	9	17

966: POISON-ANTICONVULSANTS

Type of Patients	Observed Patients	Avg. Stay	Vari-ance	Percentiles						
				10th	25th	50th	75th	90th	95th	99th
1. SINGLE DX										
A. Not Operated										
0–19 Years	10	1.3	<1	1	1	1	1	3	3	3
20–34	2	1.5	<1	1	1	1	2	2	2	2
35–49	2	2.5	4	1	1	4	4	4	4	4
50–64	0									
65+	0									
B. Operated										
0–19 Years	0									
20–34	0									
35–49	0									
50–64	0									
65+	0									
2. MULTIPLE DX										
A. Not Operated										
0–19 Years	132	2.2	4	1	1	1	2	4	7	10
20–34	350	2.6	8	1	1	2	3	5	7	11
35–49	480	3.0	8	1	1	2	4	6	9	13
50–64	331	3.6	8	1	2	3	4	7	9	14
65+	167	3.9	13	1	2	3	5	8	10	18
B. Operated										
0–19 Years	0									
20–34	4	23.5	997	2	4	11	44	70	70	70
35–49	2	4.0	2	3	3	5	5	5	5	5
50–64	4	4.3	2	3	3	3	5	6	6	6
65+	1	9.0	0	9	9	9	9	9	9	9
SUBTOTALS:										
1. SINGLE DX										
A. Not Operated	14	1.5	<1	1	1	1	2	3	4	4
B. Operated	0									
2. MULTIPLE DX										
A. Not Operated	1,460	3.1	8	1	1	2	4	6	8	15
B. Operated	11	11.7	392	3	3	5	9	17	70	70
1. SINGLE DX	14	1.5	<1	1	1	1	2	3	4	4
2. MULTIPLE DX	1,471	3.1	11	1	1	2	4	6	9	16
A. NOT OPERATED	1,474	3.0	8	1	1	2	4	6	8	15
B. OPERATED	11	11.7	392	3	3	5	9	17	70	70
TOTAL										
0–19 Years	142	2.1	4	1	1	1	2	4	6	10
20–34	356	2.8	21	1	1	2	3	5	7	21
35–49	484	3.0	8	1	1	2	4	6	9	13
50–64	335	3.6	8	1	2	3	4	7	9	14
65+	168	4.0	13	1	2	3	5	8	10	16
GRAND TOTAL	1,485	3.1	11	1	1	2	4	6	9	16

Length of Stay by Diagnosis and Operation, Western Region, 2008

Western Region, October 2006–September 2007 Data, by Diagnosis

966.1: POISON-HYDANTOIN DERIV

Type of Patients	Observed Patients	Avg. Stay	Variance	10th	25th	50th	75th	90th	95th	99th
1. SINGLE DX										
A. Not Operated										
0–19 Years	0									
20–34	1	2.0								
35–49	1	4.0								
50–64	0									
65+	0									
B. Operated										
0–19 Years	0									
20–34	0									
35–49	0									
50–64	0									
65+	0									
2. MULTIPLE DX										
A. Not Operated										
0–19 Years	9	2.8	5	1	1	2	3	7	7	7
20–34	64	3.6	10	1	2	3	4	6	10	21
35–49	134	3.5	6	1	2	3	4	7	9	11
50–64	140	4.2	8	2	2	3	5	7	10	14
65+	94	4.0	8	2	2	3	5	7	9	18
B. Operated										
0–19 Years	0									
20–34	2	9.5	110	2	2	10	17	17	17	17
35–49	0									
50–64	0									
65+	0									
SUBTOTALS:										
1. SINGLE DX										
A. Not Operated	2	3.0	2	2	2	3	4	4	4	4
B. Operated	0									
2. MULTIPLE DX										
A. Not Operated	441	3.8	8	1	2	3	5	7	9	14
B. Operated	2	9.5	110	2	2	10	17	17	17	17
1. SINGLE DX	2	3.0	2	2	2	3	4	4	4	4
2. MULTIPLE DX	443	3.8	8	1	2	3	5	7	9	17
A. NOT OPERATED	443	3.8	8	1	2	3	5	7	9	14
B. OPERATED	2	9.5	110	2	2	10	17	17	17	17
TOTAL										
0–19 Years	9	2.8	5	1	2	2	3	7	7	7
20–34	67	3.7	12	1	2	3	4	7	11	21
35–49	135	3.5	6	1	2	3	4	7	9	11
50–64	140	4.2	8	2	2	3	5	7	10	14
65+	94	4.0	8	2	2	3	5	7	9	18
GRAND TOTAL	445	3.8	8	1	2	3	5	7	9	17

966.3: POIS-ANTICONVULS NEC&NOS

Type of Patients	Observed Patients	Avg. Stay	Variance	10th	25th	50th	75th	90th	95th	99th
1. SINGLE DX										
A. Not Operated										
0–19 Years	9	1.3	<1	1	1	1	1	3	3	3
20–34	1	1.0	0	1	1	1	1	1	1	1
35–49	1	1.0	0	1	1	1	1	1	1	1
50–64	0									
65+	0									
B. Operated										
0–19 Years	0									
20–34	0									
35–49	0									
50–64	0									
65+	0									
2. MULTIPLE DX										
A. Not Operated										
0–19 Years	122	2.1	4	1	1	2	2	4	6	10
20–34	283	2.4	7	1	1	2	3	5	6	11
35–49	338	2.8	9	1	1	2	3	5	8	16
50–64	181	3.1	6	1	2	2	4	6	8	13
65+	53	3.6	12	1	1	2	4	8	12	17
B. Operated										
0–19 Years	0									
20–34	2	37.5	>999	5	5	38	70	70	70	70
35–49	2	4.0	2	3	3	5	5	5	5	5
50–64	2	5.5	<1	5	5	6	6	6	6	6
65+	1	9.0	0	9	9	9	9	9	9	9
SUBTOTALS:										
1. SINGLE DX										
A. Not Operated	11	1.3	<1	1	1	1	1	2	3	3
B. Operated	0									
2. MULTIPLE DX										
A. Not Operated	977	2.7	8	1	1	2	3	5	8	13
B. Operated	7	14.8	598	3	5	5	9	70	70	70
1. SINGLE DX	11	1.3	<1	1	1	1	1	2	3	3
2. MULTIPLE DX	984	2.8	12	1	1	2	3	5	8	15
A. NOT OPERATED	988	2.7	7	1	1	2	3	5	8	13
B. OPERATED	7	14.8	598	3	5	5	9	70	70	70
TOTAL										
0–19 Years	131	2.0	4	1	1	1	2	4	6	10
20–34	286	2.6	23	1	1	2	3	5	7	22
35–49	341	2.8	9	1	1	2	3	5	9	16
50–64	183	3.1	9	1	2	2	4	6	8	13
65+	54	3.7	12	1	2	2	5	9	12	17
GRAND TOTAL	995	2.8	12	1	1	2	3	5	8	15

967: POISON-SEDATIVE/HYPNOTIC

Type of Patients	Observed Patients	Avg. Stay	Variance	10th	25th	50th	75th	90th	95th	99th
1. SINGLE DX										
A. Not Operated										
0–19 Years	3	1.0	0	1	1	1	1	1	1	1
20–34	1	1.0	0	1	1	1	1	1	1	1
35–49	1	4.0	0	4	4	4	4	4	4	4
50–64	0									
65+	0									
B. Operated										
0–19 Years	0									
20–34	0									
35–49	0									
50–64	0									
65+	0									
2. MULTIPLE DX										
A. Not Operated										
0–19 Years	60	1.5	<1	1	1	1	2	2	3	5
20–34	207	2.2	4	1	1	1	2	5	6	11
35–49	427	2.8	24	1	1	2	3	5	8	26
50–64	439	3.1	9	1	1	2	4	6	9	15
65+	339	3.4	9	1	1	3	4	6	8	15
B. Operated										
0–19 Years	1	2.0	0	2	2	2	2	2	2	2
20–34	4	11.5	18	7	7	14	16	16	16	16
35–49	12	18.2	278	2	3	13	30	41	51	51
50–64	13	11.2	45	4	5	11	14	23	24	24
65+	0									
SUBTOTALS:										
1. SINGLE DX										
A. Not Operated	5	1.6	2	1	1	1	1	4	4	4
B. Operated	0									
2. MULTIPLE DX										
A. Not Operated	1,472	2.9	12	1	1	2	3	6	8	15
B. Operated	30	13.7	142	3	4	11	18	30	41	51
1. SINGLE DX	5	1.6	2	1	1	1	1	4	4	4
2. MULTIPLE DX	1,502	3.1	17	1	1	2	4	6	9	21
A. NOT OPERATED	1,477	2.9	12	1	1	2	3	6	8	15
B. OPERATED	30	13.7	142	3	4	11	18	30	41	51
TOTAL										
0–19 Years	64	1.5	<1	1	1	1	2	2	3	5
20–34	208	2.2	4	1	1	1	2	5	6	11
35–49	432	2.9	24	1	1	2	3	6	8	26
50–64	451	3.5	22	1	1	2	4	7	11	25
65+	352	3.7	12	1	2	3	4	7	11	21
GRAND TOTAL	1,507	3.1	17	1	1	2	4	6	9	21

Length of Stay by Diagnosis and Operation, Western Region, 2008

Western Region, October 2006–September 2007 Data, by Diagnosis

967.0: POISONING-BARBITURATES

Type of Patients	Observed Patients	Avg. Stay	Vari- ance	10th	25th	50th	75th	90th	95th	99th
1. SINGLE DX										
A. Not Operated										
0–19 Years	1	1.0	0	1	1	1	1	1	1	1
20–34	0									
35–49	1	4.0	0	4	4	4	4	4	4	4
50–64	0									
65+	0									
B. Operated										
0–19 Years	0									
20–34	0									
35–49	0									
50–64	0									
65+	0									
2. MULTIPLE DX										
A. Not Operated										
0–19 Years	8	1.9	1	1	1	1	2	4	4	4
20–34	37	3.0	4	1	1	2	5	6	7	7
35–49	94	4.7	82	1	1	2	4	8	14	73
50–64	67	4.1	14	1	2	3	6	9	11	22
65+	22	4.3	22	1	2	3	5	8	10	22
B. Operated										
0–19 Years	1	2.0	0	2	2	2	2	2	2	2
20–34	0									
35–49	0									
50–64	1	30.0	0	30	30	30	30	30	30	30
65+	1	23.0	0	23	23	23	23	23	23	23
SUBTOTALS:										
1. SINGLE DX										
A. Not Operated	2	2.5	4	1	1	3	4	4	4	4
B. Operated	0									
2. MULTIPLE DX										
A. Not Operated	228	4.1	41	1	1	3	4	7	11	30
B. Operated	3	18.4	210	2	2	23	30	30	30	30
1. SINGLE DX	2	2.5	4	1	1	3	4	4	4	4
2. MULTIPLE DX	231	4.3	45	1	1	3	4	8	12	30
A. NOT OPERATED	230	4.1	40	1	1	3	4	7	11	30
B. OPERATED	3	18.4	210	2	2	23	30	30	30	30
TOTAL										
0–19 Years	10	1.8	1	1	1	1	2	4	4	4
20–34	37	3.0	4	1	1	2	5	6	7	7
35–49	95	4.7	81	1	1	2	4	8	14	73
50–64	68	4.5	24	1	2	3	6	9	12	30
65+	23	5.1	36	1	2	3	6	10	22	23
GRAND TOTAL	233	4.3	44	1	1	3	4	8	12	30

967.8: POIS-SEDAT/HYPNOTIC NEC

Type of Patients	Observed Patients	Avg. Stay	Vari- ance	10th	25th	50th	75th	90th	95th	99th
1. SINGLE DX										
A. Not Operated										
0–19 Years	2	1.0	0	1	1	1	1	1	1	1
20–34	1	1.0	0	1	1	1	1	1	1	1
35–49	0									
50–64	0									
65+	0									
B. Operated										
0–19 Years	0									
20–34	0									
35–49	0									
50–64	0									
65+	0									
2. MULTIPLE DX										
A. Not Operated										
0–19 Years	43	1.5	<1	1	1	1	2	2	3	5
20–34	144	2.0	5	1	1	1	2	4	5	11
35–49	261	2.3	7	1	1	1	3	4	7	12
50–64	256	2.5	7	1	1	2	3	5	8	15
65+	217	3.1	7	1	1	2	4	6	7	13
B. Operated										
0–19 Years	0									
20–34	0									
35–49	1	16.0	0	16	16	16	16	16	16	16
50–64	4	12.0	370	2	2	3	3	41	41	41
65+	8	9.1	21	4	5	6	13	15	15	15
SUBTOTALS:										
1. SINGLE DX										
A. Not Operated	3	1.0	0	1	1	1	1	1	1	1
B. Operated	0									
2. MULTIPLE DX										
A. Not Operated	921	2.5	6	1	1	2	3	5	7	13
B. Operated	13	10.5	110	2	4	6	14	16	41	41
1. SINGLE DX	3	1.0	0	1	1	1	1	1	1	1
2. MULTIPLE DX	934	2.6	9	1	1	2	3	5	7	15
A. NOT OPERATED	924	2.5	6	1	1	2	3	5	7	13
B. OPERATED	13	10.5	110	2	4	6	14	16	41	41
TOTAL										
0–19 Years	45	1.5	<1	1	1	1	2	2	3	5
20–34	145	2.0	5	1	1	1	2	4	5	11
35–49	262	2.3	8	1	1	1	3	4	7	16
50–64	260	2.7	13	1	1	2	3	5	8	19
65+	225	3.3	9	1	1	2	4	6	8	15
GRAND TOTAL	937	2.6	9	1	1	2	3	5	7	15

967.9: POIS-SEDAT/HYPNOTIC NOS

Type of Patients	Observed Patients	Avg. Stay	Vari- ance	10th	25th	50th	75th	90th	95th	99th
1. SINGLE DX										
A. Not Operated										
0–19 Years	0									
20–34	0									
35–49	0									
50–64	0									
65+	0									
B. Operated										
0–19 Years	0									
20–34	0									
35–49	0									
50–64	0									
65+	0									
2. MULTIPLE DX										
A. Not Operated										
0–19 Years	8	1.4	<1	1	1	1	2	2	2	2
20–34	26	2.2	3	1	1	2	3	5	6	7
35–49	68	2.4	3	1	1	2	3	5	6	9
50–64	112	3.7	10	1	2	3	5	7	11	15
65+	96	4.0	9	1	2	3	5	7	10	21
B. Operated										
0–19 Years	0									
20–34	0									
35–49	3	10.0	13	7	7	9	14	14	14	14
50–64	6	19.0	316	3	4	16	25	51	51	51
65+	4	12.2	70	4	4	10	11	24	24	24
SUBTOTALS:										
1. SINGLE DX										
A. Not Operated	0									
B. Operated	0									
2. MULTIPLE DX										
A. Not Operated	310	3.3	8	1	1	3	4	6	9	15
B. Operated	13	14.8	168	4	7	11	18	25	51	51
1. SINGLE DX	0									
2. MULTIPLE DX	323	3.8	19	1	1	3	4	7	11	21
A. NOT OPERATED	310	3.3	8	1	1	3	4	6	9	15
B. OPERATED	13	14.8	168	4	7	11	18	25	51	51
TOTAL										
0–19 Years	8	1.4	<1	1	1	1	2	2	2	2
20–34	26	2.2	3	1	1	2	3	5	6	7
35–49	71	2.7	6	1	1	2	3	6	8	14
50–64	118	4.4	34	1	2	3	5	9	15	25
65+	100	4.3	14	1	2	3	5	8	12	24
GRAND TOTAL	323	3.8	19	1	1	3	4	7	11	21

Length of Stay by Diagnosis and Operation, Western Region, 2008

Western Region, October 2006–September 2007 Data, by Diagnosis

968: POISONING-CNS DEPRESSANT

Type of Patients	Observed Patients	Avg. Stay	Vari-ance	10th	25th	50th	75th	90th	95th	99th
1. SINGLE DX										
A. Not Operated										
0–19 Years	1	1.0	0	1	1	1	1	1	1	1
20–34	1	1.0	0	1	1	1	1	1	1	1
35–49	0									
50–64	0									
65+	0									
B. Operated										
0–19 Years	0									
20–34	0									
35–49	0									
50–64	0									
65+	0									
2. MULTIPLE DX										
A. Not Operated										
0–19 Years	53	1.9	2	1	1	1	2	4	5	8
20–34	204	2.2	12	1	1	1	2	4	6	8
35–49	319	2.3	4	1	1	2	3	5	6	9
50–64	193	2.8	12	1	1	2	3	5	9	18
65+	29	3.6	11	1	1	3	4	9	9	16
B. Operated										
0–19 Years	0									
20–34	1	10.0	0	10	10	10	10	10	10	10
35–49	3	9.6	72	1	1	10	18	18	18	18
50–64	4	9.5	265	1	1	1	2	34	34	34
65+	0									
SUBTOTALS:										
1. SINGLE DX										
A. Not Operated	2	1.0	0	1	1	1	1	1	1	1
B. Operated	0									
2. MULTIPLE DX										
A. Not Operated	798	2.4	8	1	1	2	3	5	7	14
B. Operated	8	9.6	135	1	1	2	10	34	34	34
1. SINGLE DX	2	1.0	0	1	1	1	1	1	1	1
2. MULTIPLE DX	806	2.5	10	1	1	2	3	5	7	15
A. NOT OPERATED	800	2.4	8	1	1	2	3	5	7	14
B. OPERATED	8	9.6	135	1	1	2	10	34	34	34
TOTAL										
0–19 Years	55	2.0	4	1	1	1	2	4	7	10
20–34	205	2.2	12	1	1	1	2	4	6	8
35–49	322	2.4	5	1	1	2	3	5	6	10
50–64	197	2.9	16	1	1	3	3	5	10	32
65+	29	3.6	11	1	1	3	4	9	9	16
GRAND TOTAL	808	2.5	10	1	1	2	3	5	7	15

968.0: POIS-CNS MUSCLE DEPRESS

Type of Patients	Observed Patients	Avg. Stay	Vari-ance	10th	25th	50th	75th	90th	95th	99th
1. SINGLE DX										
A. Not Operated										
0–19 Years	1	1.0	0	1	1	1	1	1	1	1
20–34	1	1.0	0	1	1	1	1	1	1	1
35–49	0									
50–64	0									
65+	0									
B. Operated										
0–19 Years	0									
20–34	0									
35–49	0									
50–64	0									
65+	0									
2. MULTIPLE DX										
A. Not Operated										
0–19 Years	41	1.8	3	1	1	1	2	4	5	8
20–34	174	2.1	13	1	1	1	3	4	4	15
35–49	277	2.2	3	1	1	2	3	4	6	9
50–64	165	2.4	5	1	1	2	3	5	8	11
65+	22	3.9	13	1	1	3	4	9	9	16
B. Operated										
0–19 Years	1	10.0	0	10	10	10	10	10	10	10
20–34	0									
35–49	2	9.4	143	1	1	1	18	18	18	18
50–64	2	17.5	536	1	1	18	34	34	34	34
65+	0									
SUBTOTALS:										
1. SINGLE DX										
A. Not Operated	2	1.0	0	1	1	1	1	1	1	1
B. Operated	0									
2. MULTIPLE DX										
A. Not Operated	679	2.3	6	1	1	1	3	4	6	10
B. Operated	5	12.8	191	1	1	10	18	34	34	34
1. SINGLE DX	2	1.0	0	1	1	1	1	1	1	1
2. MULTIPLE DX	684	2.3	8	1	1	1	3	4	6	12
A. NOT OPERATED	681	2.3	6	1	1	1	3	4	6	10
B. OPERATED	5	12.8	191	1	1	10	18	34	34	34
TOTAL										
0–19 Years	43	2.0	4	1	1	1	2	4	7	10
20–34	175	2.1	13	1	1	1	2	4	4	15
35–49	279	2.2	4	1	1	2	3	4	6	10
50–64	167	2.6	11	1	1	2	3	5	8	12
65+	22	3.9	13	1	1	3	4	9	9	16
GRAND TOTAL	686	2.3	8	1	1	1	3	4	6	12

968.5: POIS-TOP/INFILTR ANES

Type of Patients	Observed Patients	Avg. Stay	Vari-ance	10th	25th	50th	75th	90th	95th	99th
1. SINGLE DX										
A. Not Operated										
0–19 Years	0									
20–34	0									
35–49	0									
50–64	0									
65+	0									
B. Operated										
0–19 Years	0									
20–34	0									
35–49	0									
50–64	0									
65+	0									
2. MULTIPLE DX										
A. Not Operated										
0–19 Years	3	2.3	1	1	1	3	3	3	3	3
20–34	12	2.2	1	1	1	2	3	3	5	5
35–49	29	2.7	5	1	1	2	3	7	7	9
50–64	18	2.7	5	1	1	1	4	7	8	8
65+	4	1.8	2	1	1	1	4	4	4	4
B. Operated										
0–19 Years	0									
20–34	0									
35–49	1	10.0	0	10	10	10	10	10	10	10
50–64	1	2.0	0	2	2	2	2	2	2	2
65+	0									
SUBTOTALS:										
1. SINGLE DX										
A. Not Operated	0									
B. Operated	0									
2. MULTIPLE DX										
A. Not Operated	66	2.5	4	1	1	2	3	6	7	9
B. Operated	2	6.0	31	2	2	2	10	10	10	10
1. SINGLE DX	0									
2. MULTIPLE DX	68	2.6	5	1	1	2	3	6	7	10
A. NOT OPERATED	66	2.5	4	1	1	2	3	6	7	9
B. OPERATED	2	6.0	31	2	2	2	10	10	10	10
TOTAL										
0–19 Years	3	2.3	1	1	1	3	3	3	3	3
20–34	12	2.2	1	1	1	2	3	3	5	5
35–49	30	2.9	7	1	1	2	4	7	9	10
50–64	19	2.6	5	1	1	1	4	7	8	8
65+	4	1.8	2	1	1	1	4	4	4	4
GRAND TOTAL	68	2.6	5	1	1	2	3	6	7	10

Length of Stay by Diagnosis and Operation, Western Region, 2008

Western Region, October 2006–September 2007 Data, by Diagnosis

969: POIS-PSYCHOTROPIC AGENT

Type of Patients	Observed Patients	Avg. Stay	Vari-ance	Percentiles						
				10th	25th	50th	75th	90th	95th	99th
1. SINGLE DX										
A. *Not Operated*										
0–19 Years	54	1.1	<1	1	1	1	1	1	2	4
20–34	9	1.3	<1	1	1	1	2	2	2	2
35–49	4	1.0	0	1	1	1	1	1	1	1
50–64	4	1.3	<1	1	1	1	1	2	2	2
65+	0									
B. *Operated*										
0–19 Years	0									
20–34	0									
35–49	0									
50–64	0									
65+	0									
2. MULTIPLE DX										
A. *Not Operated*										
0–19 Years	864	2.0	4	1	1	2	2	4	5	12
20–34	2,723	2.4	9	1	1	2	3	4	6	14
35–49	3,877	2.7	9	1	2	2	3	5	7	16
50–64	2,427	3.3	17	1	2	3	4	7	10	19
65+	801	4.0	16	2	3	3	5	8	12	19
B. *Operated*										
0–19 Years	3	3.7	8	2	2	2	7	7	7	7
20–34	16	13.3	209	1	2	8	22	27	57	57
35–49	30	8.2	67	1	2	5	12	17	28	32
50–64	14	11.2	211	2	3	6	12	20	58	58
65+	5	18.5	331	4	5	9	28	46	46	46
SUBTOTALS:										
1. SINGLE DX										
A. *Not Operated*	71	1.1	<1	1	1	1	1	1	2	4
B. *Operated*	0									
2. MULTIPLE DX										
A. *Not Operated*	10,692	2.8	11	1	2	2	3	5	8	17
B. *Operated*	68	10.6	148	1	2	6	13	27	32	58
1. SINGLE DX	71	1.1	<1	1	1	1	1	1	2	4
2. MULTIPLE DX	10,760	2.9	13	1	2	2	3	6	8	17
A. NOT OPERATED	10,763	2.8	11	1	2	2	3	5	8	16
B. OPERATED	68	10.6	148	2	2	6	13	27	32	58
TOTAL										
0–19 Years	921	2.0	4	1	1	1	2	4	5	11
20–34	2,748	2.5	11	1	1	2	3	4	6	16
35–49	3,911	2.7	9	1	1	2	3	5	8	17
50–64	2,445	3.4	19	1	2	2	4	7	10	20
65+	806	4.1	19	2	3	3	5	8	12	19
GRAND TOTAL	10,831	2.8	12	1	1	2	3	6	8	17

969.0: POISONING-ANTIDEPRESSANT

Type of Patients	Observed Patients	Avg. Stay	Vari-ance	Percentiles						
				10th	25th	50th	75th	90th	95th	99th
1. SINGLE DX										
A. *Not Operated*										
0–19 Years	19	1.1	<1	1	1	1	1	2	2	2
20–34	2	1.0	0	1	1	1	1	1	2	1
35–49	1	1.0	0	1	1	1	1	1	1	1
50–64	0									
65+	0									
B. *Operated*										
0–19 Years	0									
20–34	0									
35–49	0									
50–64	0									
65+	0									
2. MULTIPLE DX										
A. *Not Operated*										
0–19 Years	259	1.7	2	1	1	2	2	3	4	6
20–34	683	2.3	5	1	1	2	3	4	6	14
35–49	918	2.7	10	1	1	2	3	5	7	14
50–64	523	3.0	7	1	1	2	4	6	8	13
65+	133	3.8	12	2	2	3	5	7	11	19
B. *Operated*										
0–19 Years	2	2.0	0	2	2	2	2	2	2	2
20–34	0									
35–49	3	10.4	58	2	2	12	17	17	17	17
50–64	0									
65+	0									
SUBTOTALS:										
1. SINGLE DX										
A. *Not Operated*	22	1.1	<1	1	1	1	1	1	2	2
B. *Operated*	0									
2. MULTIPLE DX										
A. *Not Operated*	2,516	2.6	8	1	1	2	3	5	7	14
B. *Operated*	5	7.0	50	2	2	2	12	17	17	17
1. SINGLE DX	22	1.1	<1	1	1	1	1	1	2	2
2. MULTIPLE DX	2,521	2.6	8	1	1	2	3	5	7	14
A. NOT OPERATED	2,538	2.6	8	1	1	2	3	5	7	14
B. OPERATED	5	7.0	50	2	2	2	12	17	17	17
TOTAL										
0–19 Years	280	1.7	2	1	1	1	2	3	4	6
20–34	685	2.2	5	1	1	2	3	4	6	14
35–49	922	2.8	10	1	1	2	3	5	7	16
50–64	523	3.0	7	1	1	2	4	6	8	13
65+	133	3.8	12	2	2	3	5	7	11	19
GRAND TOTAL	2,543	2.6	8	1	1	2	3	5	7	14

969.3: POISON-ANTIPSYCHOTIC NEC

Type of Patients	Observed Patients	Avg. Stay	Vari-ance	Percentiles						
				10th	25th	50th	75th	90th	95th	99th
1. SINGLE DX										
A. *Not Operated*										
0–19 Years	4	1.0	0	1	1	1	1	1	1	1
20–34	0									
35–49	0									
50–64	0									
65+	0									
B. *Operated*										
0–19 Years	0									
20–34	0									
35–49	0									
50–64	0									
65+	0									
2. MULTIPLE DX										
A. *Not Operated*										
0–19 Years	191	2.3	7	1	1	2	2	4	6	19
20–34	561	2.6	10	1	1	2	3	5	7	16
35–49	637	2.9	8	1	1	2	3	6	8	16
50–64	284	3.2	21	1	1	2	4	6	8	19
65+	61	4.1	18	1	2	3	5	8	10	26
B. *Operated*										
0–19 Years	1	7.0	0	7	7	7	7	7	7	7
20–34	1	21.0	0	21	21	21	21	21	21	21
35–49	5	3.6	12	1	1	2	5	9	9	9
50–64	1	1.0	0	1	1	1	1	1	1	1
65+	1	46.0	0	46	46	46	46	46	46	46
SUBTOTALS:										
1. SINGLE DX										
A. *Not Operated*	4	1.0	0	1	1	1	1	1	1	1
B. *Operated*	0									
2. MULTIPLE DX										
A. *Not Operated*	1,734	2.8	11	1	1	2	3	5	8	17
B. *Operated*	9	10.3	220	1	1	5	9	46	46	46
1. SINGLE DX	4	1.0	0	1	1	1	1	1	1	1
2. MULTIPLE DX	1,743	2.9	12	1	1	2	3	5	8	18
A. NOT OPERATED	1,738	2.8	11	1	1	2	3	5	8	17
B. OPERATED	9	10.3	220	1	1	5	9	46	46	46
TOTAL										
0–19 Years	196	2.3	7	1	1	2	2	4	6	19
20–34	562	2.6	11	1	1	2	3	5	7	17
35–49	642	2.9	8	1	1	2	3	5	8	16
50–64	285	3.2	21	1	1	2	4	6	8	19
65+	62	4.8	46	2	3	3	6	8	11	46
GRAND TOTAL	1,747	2.9	12	1	1	2	3	5	8	18

Length of Stay by Diagnosis and Operation, Western Region, 2008

Western Region, October 2006–September 2007 Data, by Diagnosis

969.4: POIS-BENZDIAZ TRANQ

Type of Patients	Observed Patients	Avg. Stay	Vari-ance	10th	25th	50th	75th	90th	95th	99th
1. SINGLE DX										
A. Not Operated										
0–19 Years	16	1.0	0	1	1	1	1	1	1	1
20–34	5	1.4	<1	1	1	1	2	2	2	2
35–49	2	1.0	0	1	1	1	1	1	1	1
50–64	3	1.3	<1	1	1	1	2	2	2	2
65+	0									
B. Operated										
0–19 Years	0									
20–34	0									
35–49	0									
50–64	0									
65+	0									
2. MULTIPLE DX										
A. Not Operated										
0–19 Years	193	2.0	6	1	1	1	2	4	5	19
20–34	894	2.3	13	1	1	2	3	4	5	15
35–49	1,696	2.5	7	1	1	2	3	5	7	14
50–64	1,279	3.1	12	1	1	2	3	6	10	19
65+	532	3.9	16	1	2	3	5	8	12	17
B. Operated										
0–19 Years	0									
20–34	6	19.0	462	2	2	5	27	57	57	57
35–49	11	10.4	142	1	1	4	22	28	32	32
50–64	8	12.9	344	3	3	6	11	58	58	58
65+	4	11.6	126	4	5	9	28	28	28	28
SUBTOTALS:										
1. SINGLE DX										
A. Not Operated	26	1.1	<1	1	1	1	1	2	2	2
B. Operated	0									
2. MULTIPLE DX										
A. Not Operated	4,594	2.8	11	1	1	2	3	5	8	17
B. Operated	29	13.0	244	1	3	5	22	32	57	58
1. SINGLE DX	26	1.1	<1	1	1	1	1	2	2	2
2. MULTIPLE DX	4,623	2.8	13	1	1	2	3	6	8	18
A. NOT OPERATED	4,620	2.8	11	1	1	2	3	5	8	17
B. OPERATED	29	13.0	244	1	3	5	22	32	57	58
TOTAL										
0–19 Years	209	1.9	5	1	1	1	2	4	5	9
20–34	905	2.4	17	1	1	1	3	4	5	19
35–49	1,709	2.5	8	1	1	2	3	5	7	15
50–64	1,290	3.2	14	1	2	3	6	8	10	20
65+	536	4.0	17	1	2	3	5	8	12	19
GRAND TOTAL	4,649	2.8	13	1	1	2	3	6	8	18

969.7: POISON-PSYCHOSTIMULANTS

Type of Patients	Observed Patients	Avg. Stay	Vari-ance	10th	25th	50th	75th	90th	95th	99th
1. SINGLE DX										
A. Not Operated										
0–19 Years	10	1.3	<1	1	1	2	1	4	4	4
20–34	1	2.0	0	2	2	2	2	2	2	2
35–49	0									
50–64	0									
65+	0									
B. Operated										
0–19 Years	0									
20–34	0									
35–49	0									
50–64	0									
65+	0									
2. MULTIPLE DX										
A. Not Operated										
0–19 Years	138	2.2	5	1	1	2	2	4	5	11
20–34	392	2.7	10	1	1	2	3	5	7	19
35–49	405	3.3	13	1	2	2	4	7	10	21
50–64	168	5.0	79	1	2	3	5	9	13	59
65+	15	2.9	3	1	1	3	4	6	6	6
B. Operated										
0–19 Years	0									
20–34	9	8.6	45	1	6	8	11	22	22	22
35–49	7	7.4	15	2	4	9	10	13	13	13
50–64	3	10.3	20	6	6	10	15	15	15	15
65+	0									
SUBTOTALS:										
1. SINGLE DX										
A. Not Operated	11	1.4	<1	1	1	1	1	2	4	4
B. Operated	0									
2. MULTIPLE DX										
A. Not Operated	1,118	3.2	22	1	1	2	3	6	9	22
B. Operated	19	8.5	28	1	5	8	11	15	22	22
1. SINGLE DX	11	1.4	<1	1	1	1	1	2	4	4
2. MULTIPLE DX	1,137	3.3	22	1	1	2	4	6	10	22
A. NOT OPERATED	1,129	3.2	21	1	1	2	3	6	9	22
B. OPERATED	19	8.5	28	1	5	8	11	15	22	22
TOTAL										
0–19 Years	148	2.1	5	1	1	2	2	4	5	11
20–34	402	2.8	12	1	1	2	3	5	8	19
35–49	412	3.3	13	1	1	2	4	7	10	21
50–64	171	5.1	79	1	2	3	5	10	13	59
65+	15	2.9	3	1	1	3	4	6	6	6
GRAND TOTAL	1,148	3.3	22	1	1	2	4	6	9	22

969.8: POISON-PSYCHOTROPIC NEC

Type of Patients	Observed Patients	Avg. Stay	Vari-ance	10th	25th	50th	75th	90th	95th	99th
1. SINGLE DX										
A. Not Operated										
0–19 Years	1	1.0	0	1	1	1	1	1	1	1
20–34	1	1.0	0	1	1	1	1	1	1	1
35–49	1	1.0	0	1	1	1	1	1	1	1
50–64	0									
65+	0									
B. Operated										
0–19 Years	0									
20–34	0									
35–49	0									
50–64	0									
65+	0									
2. MULTIPLE DX										
A. Not Operated										
0–19 Years	34	1.7	1	1	1	2	2	3	5	6
20–34	114	2.1	2	1	1	2	2	4	5	7
35–49	128	3.1	17	1	1	3	3	7	8	17
50–64	120	4.9	22	1	2	3	6	12	13	22
65+	31	7.9	26	2	4	7	12	15	16	19
B. Operated										
0–19 Years	0									
20–34	0									
35–49	4	7.5	24	2	5	10	10	13	13	13
50–64	2	11.0	158	2	2	20	20	20	20	20
65+	0									
SUBTOTALS:										
1. SINGLE DX										
A. Not Operated	3	1.0	0	1	1	1	1	1	1	1
B. Operated	0									
2. MULTIPLE DX										
A. Not Operated	427	3.6	16	1	1	2	4	8	12	17
B. Operated	6	8.7	50	2	2	8	13	20	20	20
1. SINGLE DX	3	1.0	0	1	1	1	1	1	1	1
2. MULTIPLE DX	433	3.7	17	1	1	2	4	8	12	19
A. NOT OPERATED	430	3.6	16	1	1	2	4	8	12	17
B. OPERATED	6	8.7	50	2	2	8	13	20	20	20
TOTAL										
0–19 Years	35	1.7	1	1	1	1	2	3	5	6
20–34	115	2.1	2	1	1	2	2	4	5	7
35–49	133	3.2	17	1	1	2	3	7	10	17
50–64	122	5.0	23	1	2	3	6	12	13	22
65+	31	7.9	26	2	4	7	12	15	16	19
GRAND TOTAL	436	3.6	17	1	1	2	4	8	12	19

Length of Stay by Diagnosis and Operation, Western Region, 2008

Western Region, October 2006–September 2007 Data, by Diagnosis

970: POISONING-CNS STIMULANTS

Type of Patients	Observed Patients	Avg. Stay	Vari-ance	10th	25th	50th	75th	90th	95th	99th
1. SINGLE DX										
A. *Not Operated*										
0–19 Years	1	1.0	0	1	1	1	1	1	1	1
20–34	1	2.0	0	2	2	2	2	2	2	2
35–49	0									
50–64	0									
65+	0									
B. *Operated*										
0–19 Years	0									
20–34	0									
35–49	0									
50–64	0									
65+	0									
2. MULTIPLE DX										
A. *Not Operated*										
0–19 Years	57	2.5	9	1	1	2	3	4	8	21
20–34	273	3.2	17	1	1	2	4	6	8	26
35–49	459	3.3	23	1	1	2	3	6	12	29
50–64	334	3.9	37	1	1	2	4	7	13	64
65+	37	3.9	7	1	2	3	5	6	9	15
B. *Operated*										
0–19 Years	0									
20–34	3	20.0	48	13	13	20	27	27	27	27
35–49	8	13.0	50	4	6	14	18	24	24	24
50–64	7	10.3	53	3	5	7	20	21	21	21
65+	0									
SUBTOTALS:										
1. SINGLE DX										
A. *Not Operated*	2	1.5	<1	1	1	2	2	2	2	2
B. *Operated*	0									
2. MULTIPLE DX										
A. *Not Operated*	1,160	3.4	24	1	1	2	4	7	11	29
B. *Operated*	18	13.1	57	4	6	13	20	24	27	27
1. SINGLE DX	2	1.5	<1	1	1	2	2	2	2	2
2. MULTIPLE DX	1,178	3.6	26	1	1	2	4	7	12	29
A. NOT OPERATED	1,162	3.4	24	1	1	2	4	7	11	29
B. OPERATED	18	13.1	57	4	6	13	20	24	27	27
TOTAL										
0–19 Years	58	2.5	9	1	1	2	3	4	8	21
20–34	277	3.4	20	1	1	2	4	6	12	27
35–49	467	3.5	25	1	1	2	3	7	12	29
50–64	341	4.1	38	1	1	2	4	8	14	64
65+	37	3.9	7	1	2	3	5	6	9	15
GRAND TOTAL	1,180	3.6	26	1	1	2	4	7	12	29

970.8: POIS-CNS STIMULANTS NEC

Type of Patients	Observed Patients	Avg. Stay	Vari-ance	10th	25th	50th	75th	90th	95th	99th
1. SINGLE DX										
A. *Not Operated*										
0–19 Years	0									
20–34	1	2.0	0	2	2	2	2	2	2	2
35–49	0									
50–64	0									
65+	0									
B. *Operated*										
0–19 Years	0									
20–34	0									
35–49	0									
50–64	0									
65+	0									
2. MULTIPLE DX										
A. *Not Operated*										
0–19 Years	54	2.5	9	1	1	2	3	4	8	21
20–34	261	3.2	17	1	1	2	4	6	8	26
35–49	433	3.3	24	1	1	2	3	6	12	29
50–64	309	4.0	39	1	1	2	4	7	14	64
65+	19	3.6	2	1	2	3	5	6	6	6
B. *Operated*										
0–19 Years	0									
20–34	2	16.6	24	13	13	20	20	20	20	20
35–49	7	14.0	49	4	7	14	19	24	24	24
50–64	7	10.3	53	3	5	7	20	21	21	21
65+	0									
SUBTOTALS:										
1. SINGLE DX										
A. *Not Operated*	1	2.0	0	2	2	2	2	2	2	2
B. *Operated*	0									
2. MULTIPLE DX										
A. *Not Operated*	1,076	3.5	26	1	1	2	4	7	12	29
B. *Operated*	16	12.7	48	4	7	13	20	21	24	24
1. SINGLE DX	1	2.0	0	2	2	2	2	2	2	2
2. MULTIPLE DX	1,092	3.6	27	1	1	2	4	7	13	29
A. NOT OPERATED	1,077	3.5	26	1	1	2	4	7	12	29
B. OPERATED	16	12.7	48	4	7	13	20	21	24	24
TOTAL										
0–19 Years	54	2.5	9	1	1	2	3	4	8	21
20–34	264	3.3	19	1	1	2	4	6	12	26
35–49	440	3.5	26	1	1	2	3	7	13	29
50–64	316	4.1	40	1	1	2	4	8	14	64
65+	19	3.6	2	1	2	3	5	6	6	6
GRAND TOTAL	1,093	3.6	27	1	1	2	4	7	13	29

971: POISON-AUTONOMIC AGENT

Type of Patients	Observed Patients	Avg. Stay	Vari-ance	10th	25th	50th	75th	90th	95th	99th
1. SINGLE DX										
A. *Not Operated*										
0–19 Years	4	1.0	0	1	1	1	1	1	1	1
20–34	0									
35–49	0									
50–64	0									
65+	0									
B. *Operated*										
0–19 Years	0									
20–34	0									
35–49	0									
50–64	0									
65+	0									
2. MULTIPLE DX										
A. *Not Operated*										
0–19 Years	38	1.5	1	1	1	1	2	2	4	6
20–34	59	2.3	3	1	1	2	3	4	7	10
35–49	58	2.7	5	1	1	1	4	6	9	9
50–64	46	3.1	6	1	1	2	5	7	8	9
65+	65	2.7	4	1	1	2	4	5	6	9
B. *Operated*										
0–19 Years	0									
20–34	1	7.0	0	7	7	7	7	7	7	7
35–49	0									
50–64	0									
65+	2	3.5	<1	3	3	3	4	4	4	4
SUBTOTALS:										
1. SINGLE DX										
A. *Not Operated*	4	1.0	0	1	1	1	1	1	1	1
B. *Operated*	0									
2. MULTIPLE DX										
A. *Not Operated*	266	2.5	4	1	1	2	3	6	7	9
B. *Operated*	3	4.7	4	3	3	4	7	7	7	7
1. SINGLE DX	4	1.0	0	1	1	1	1	1	1	1
2. MULTIPLE DX	269	2.5	4	1	1	2	4	6	7	9
A. NOT OPERATED	270	2.5	4	1	1	2	3	6	7	9
B. OPERATED	3	4.7	4	3	3	4	7	7	7	7
TOTAL										
0–19 Years	42	1.5	<1	1	1	1	2	2	3	6
20–34	60	2.4	3	1	1	2	3	4	7	10
35–49	58	2.7	5	1	1	1	4	6	9	9
50–64	46	3.1	6	1	1	2	5	7	8	9
65+	67	2.7	3	1	1	2	4	5	6	9
GRAND TOTAL	273	2.5	4	1	1	2	3	6	7	9

Length of Stay by Diagnosis and Operation, Western Region, 2008

Western Region, October 2006–September 2007 Data, by Diagnosis

972: POISON-CV AGENT

Type of Patients	Observed Patients	Avg. Stay	Variance	10th	25th	50th	75th	90th	95th	99th
1. SINGLE DX										
A. Not Operated										
0–19 Years	25	1.1	<1	1	1	1	1	1	2	2
20–34	2	1.0	0	1	1	1	1	1	1	1
35–49	2	1.5	<1	1	1	2	2	2	2	2
50–64	1	1.0	0	1	1	1	1	1	1	1
65+	0									
B. Operated										
0–19 Years	0									
20–34	0									
35–49	0									
50–64	0									
65+	0									
2. MULTIPLE DX										
A. Not Operated										
0–19 Years	116	1.4	<1	1	1	1	2	2	3	5
20–34	110	2.0	2	1	1	2	3	3	4	6
35–49	230	2.5	8	1	1	2	3	5	7	16
50–64	305	3.2	24	1	1	2	4	6	6	17
65+	461	3.0	7	1	1	2	4	6	8	14
B. Operated										
0–19 Years	0									
20–34	2	13.0	280	1	1	13	25	25	25	25
35–49	3	16.3	320	4	4	8	37	37	37	37
50–64	4	9.8	43	4	5	12	18	18	18	18
65+	4	11.7	80	5	5	8	9	25	25	25
SUBTOTALS:										
1. SINGLE DX										
A. Not Operated	30	1.1	<1	1	1	1	1	1	2	2
B. Operated	0									
2. MULTIPLE DX										
A. Not Operated	1,222	2.7	11	1	1	2	3	5	6	16
B. Operated	13	12.4	115	4	5	8	18	25	37	37
1. SINGLE DX	30	1.1	<1	1	1	1	1	1	2	2
2. MULTIPLE DX	1,235	2.8	13	1	1	2	3	5	6	17
A. NOT OPERATED	1,252	2.7	10	1	1	2	3	5	6	16
B. OPERATED	13	12.4	115	4	5	8	18	25	37	37
TOTAL										
0–19 Years	141	1.3	<1	1	1	1	1	2	3	5
20–34	114	2.2	7	1	1	2	3	3	5	12
35–49	235	2.6	13	1	1	2	3	5	7	17
50–64	310	3.3	24	1	1	2	4	6	8	17
65+	465	3.0	8	1	1	2	4	6	8	16
GRAND TOTAL	1,265	2.8	12	1	1	2	3	5	7	17

972.6: POISON-ANTIHTN AGENT

Type of Patients	Observed Patients	Avg. Stay	Variance	10th	25th	50th	75th	90th	95th	99th
1. SINGLE DX										
A. Not Operated										
0–19 Years	14	1.1	<1	1	1	1	1	1	2	2
20–34	1	1.0	0	1	1	1	1	1	1	1
35–49	1	1.0	0	1	1	1	1	1	1	1
50–64	1	1.0	0	1	1	1	1	1	1	1
65+	0									
B. Operated										
0–19 Years	0									
20–34	0									
35–49	0									
50–64	0									
65+	0									
2. MULTIPLE DX										
A. Not Operated										
0–19 Years	70	1.3	<1	1	1	1	2	2	3	5
20–34	53	2.0	3	1	1	2	3	3	4	12
35–49	114	2.4	5	1	1	2	3	5	7	10
50–64	122	2.5	5	1	1	2	3	5	6	10
65+	151	2.7	9	1	1	2	3	5	7	20
B. Operated										
0–19 Years	0									
20–34	0									
35–49	1	4.0	0	4	4	4	4	4	4	4
50–64	0									
65+	0									
SUBTOTALS:										
1. SINGLE DX										
A. Not Operated	17	1.1	<1	1	1	1	1	1	2	2
B. Operated	0									
2. MULTIPLE DX										
A. Not Operated	510	2.3	5	1	1	2	3	4	6	12
B. Operated	1	4.0	0	4	4	4	4	4	4	4
1. SINGLE DX	17	1.1	<1	1	1	1	1	1	2	2
2. MULTIPLE DX	511	2.3	5	1	1	2	3	4	6	12
A. NOT OPERATED	527	2.3	5	1	1	2	3	4	6	12
B. OPERATED	1	4.0	0	4	4	4	4	4	4	4
TOTAL										
0–19 Years	84	1.3	<1	1	1	1	1	2	2	5
20–34	54	2.0	3	1	1	1	2	3	4	12
35–49	116	2.4	5	1	1	2	3	5	7	10
50–64	123	2.5	5	1	1	2	3	5	6	10
65+	151	2.7	9	1	1	2	3	5	7	20
GRAND TOTAL	528	2.3	5	1	1	2	3	4	6	12

972.9: POISON-CV AGENT NEC

Type of Patients	Observed Patients	Avg. Stay	Variance	10th	25th	50th	75th	90th	95th	99th
1. SINGLE DX										
A. Not Operated										
0–19 Years	5	1.2	<1	1	1	1	1	1	2	2
20–34	1	1.0	0	1	1	1	1	1	1	1
35–49	0									
50–64	0									
65+	0									
B. Operated										
0–19 Years	0									
20–34	0									
35–49	0									
50–64	0									
65+	0									
2. MULTIPLE DX										
A. Not Operated										
0–19 Years	22	1.4	1	1	1	1	2	2	3	6
20–34	34	2.0	2	1	1	2	2	4	6	6
35–49	66	2.1	2	1	1	2	2	4	5	7
50–64	104	3.9	54	1	1	2	4	7	13	17
65+	87	3.0	5	1	1	2	4	6	7	10
B. Operated										
0–19 Years	0									
20–34	1	1.0	0	1	1	1	1	1	1	1
35–49	1	37.0	0	37	37	37	37	37	37	37
50–64	0									
65+	0									
SUBTOTALS:										
1. SINGLE DX										
A. Not Operated	6	1.2	<1	1	1	1	1	2	2	2
B. Operated	0									
2. MULTIPLE DX										
A. Not Operated	313	2.9	20	1	1	2	3	5	7	15
B. Operated	2	18.9	633	1	1	1	37	37	37	37
1. SINGLE DX	6	1.2	<1	1	1	1	1	2	2	2
2. MULTIPLE DX	315	3.0	24	1	1	2	3	5	7	16
A. NOT OPERATED	319	2.8	20	1	1	2	3	5	7	15
B. OPERATED	2	18.9	633	1	1	1	37	37	37	37
TOTAL										
0–19 Years	27	1.3	1	1	1	1	2	2	3	6
20–34	36	2.0	2	1	1	2	2	4	6	6
35–49	67	2.6	20	1	1	2	3	4	5	37
50–64	104	3.9	54	1	1	2	4	7	13	17
65+	87	3.0	5	1	1	2	4	6	7	10
GRAND TOTAL	321	2.9	24	1	1	2	3	5	7	16

973: POISONING-GI AGENTS

Type of Patients	Observed Patients	Avg. Stay	Variance	Percentiles						
				10th	25th	50th	75th	90th	95th	99th
1. SINGLE DX										
A. Not Operated										
0–19 Years	8	1.0	0	1	1	1	1	1	1	1
20–34	0									
35–49	0									
50–64	0									
65+	0									
B. Operated										
0–19 Years	0									
20–34	0									
35–49	0									
50–64	0									
65+	0									
2. MULTIPLE DX										
A. Not Operated										
0–19 Years	9	1.4	1	1	1	1	1	4	4	4
20–34	8	2.3	2	1	1	2	4	5	5	5
35–49	13	2.5	2	1	1	3	3	4	5	5
50–64	8	4.8	24	1	2	2	5	16	16	16
65+	23	5.8	43	1	2	4	6	11	12	32
B. Operated										
0–19 Years	0									
20–34	0									
35–49	0									
50–64	0									
65+	0									
SUBTOTALS:										
1. SINGLE DX										
A. Not Operated	8	1.0	0	1	1	1	1	1	1	1
B. Operated	0									
2. MULTIPLE DX										
A. Not Operated	61	3.8	22	1	1	3	4	6	11	32
B. Operated	0									
1. SINGLE DX	8	1.0	0	1	1	1	1	1	1	1
2. MULTIPLE DX	61	3.8	22	1	1	3	4	6	11	32
A. NOT OPERATED	69	3.5	20	1	1	2	4	6	11	32
B. OPERATED	0									
TOTAL										
0–19 Years	17	1.2	<1	1	1	1	1	2	4	4
20–34	8	2.3	2	1	1	2	4	5	5	5
35–49	13	2.5	2	1	1	3	3	4	5	5
50–64	8	4.8	24	1	2	2	5	16	16	16
65+	23	5.8	43	1	2	4	6	11	12	32
GRAND TOTAL	69	3.5	20	1	1	2	4	6	11	32

974: POIS-WATER METAB AGENT

Type of Patients	Observed Patients	Avg. Stay	Variance	Percentiles						
				10th	25th	50th	75th	90th	95th	99th
1. SINGLE DX										
A. Not Operated										
0–19 Years	1	1.0	0	1	1	1	1	1	1	1
20–34	0									
35–49	0									
50–64	0									
65+	0									
B. Operated										
0–19 Years	0									
20–34	0									
35–49	0									
50–64	0									
65+	0									
2. MULTIPLE DX										
A. Not Operated										
0–19 Years	7	1.3	<1	1	1	1	2	2	2	2
20–34	13	3.0	7	1	2	2	3	7	10	10
35–49	32	2.5	6	1	1	2	3	5	7	13
50–64	62	3.5	15	1	1	2	4	7	9	22
65+	101	3.7	10	1	2	3	4	8	9	20
B. Operated										
0–19 Years	0									
20–34	0									
35–49	0									
50–64	0									
65+	1	13.0	0	13	13	13	13	13	13	13
SUBTOTALS:										
1. SINGLE DX										
A. Not Operated	1	1.0	0	1	1	1	1	1	1	1
B. Operated	0									
2. MULTIPLE DX										
A. Not Operated	215	3.3	10	1	1	2	4	7	9	18
B. Operated	1	13.0	0	13	13	13	13	13	13	13
1. SINGLE DX	1	1.0	0	1	1	1	1	1	1	1
2. MULTIPLE DX	216	3.4	11	1	1	2	4	7	9	18
A. NOT OPERATED	216	3.3	10	1	1	2	4	7	9	18
B. OPERATED	1	13.0	0	13	13	13	13	13	13	13
TOTAL										
0–19 Years	8	1.3	<1	1	1	1	2	2	2	2
20–34	13	3.0	7	1	2	2	3	7	10	10
35–49	32	2.5	6	1	1	2	3	5	7	13
50–64	62	3.5	15	1	1	2	4	7	9	22
65+	102	3.8	11	1	2	3	5	8	9	18
GRAND TOTAL	217	3.4	11	1	1	2	4	7	9	18

975: POISONING-MUSCLE AGENT

Type of Patients	Observed Patients	Avg. Stay	Variance	Percentiles						
				10th	25th	50th	75th	90th	95th	99th
1. SINGLE DX										
A. Not Operated										
0–19 Years	6	1.0	0	1	1	1	1	1	1	1
20–34	2	1.0	0	1	1	1	1	1	1	1
35–49	0									
50–64	0									
65+	0									
B. Operated										
0–19 Years	0									
20–34	0									
35–49	0									
50–64	0									
65+	0									
2. MULTIPLE DX										
A. Not Operated										
0–19 Years	86	1.7	3	1	1	1	2	3	3	14
20–34	138	2.0	4	1	1	1	2	3	6	8
35–49	177	2.8	6	1	1	2	4	6	8	11
50–64	101	3.1	7	1	2	2	4	5	8	17
65+	39	4.8	22	1	2	3	6	11	20	20
B. Operated										
0–19 Years	0									
20–34	0									
35–49	1	7.0	0	7	7	7	7	7	7	7
50–64	3	11.0	84	1	1	13	19	19	19	19
65+	0									
SUBTOTALS:										
1. SINGLE DX										
A. Not Operated	8	1.0	0	1	1	1	1	1	1	1
B. Operated	0									
2. MULTIPLE DX										
A. Not Operated	541	2.6	7	1	1	2	3	5	8	14
B. Operated	4	10.0	60	1	7	7	7	19	19	19
1. SINGLE DX	8	1.0	0	1	1	1	1	1	1	1
2. MULTIPLE DX	545	2.7	8	1	1	2	3	5	8	16
A. NOT OPERATED	549	2.6	7	1	1	2	3	5	8	14
B. OPERATED	4	10.0	60	1	7	7	19	19	19	19
TOTAL										
0–19 Years	92	1.7	3	1	1	1	2	3	3	14
20–34	140	1.9	4	1	1	1	2	3	6	8
35–49	178	2.8	6	1	1	2	4	6	8	11
50–64	104	3.3	10	1	1	2	4	6	11	17
65+	39	4.8	22	1	2	3	6	11	20	20
GRAND TOTAL	553	2.6	8	1	1	2	3	5	8	16

Length of Stay by Diagnosis and Operation, Western Region, 2008

Western Region, October 2006–September 2007 Data, by Diagnosis

975.2: POIS-SKEL MUSCLE RELAX

Type of Patients	Observed Patients	Avg. Stay	Vari-ance	10th	25th	50th	75th	90th	95th	99th
1. SINGLE DX										
A. Not Operated										
0–19 Years	2	1.0	0	1	1	1	1	1	1	1
20–34	1	1.0	0	1	1	1	1	1	1	1
35–49	0									
50–64	0									
65+	0									
B. Operated										
0–19 Years	0									
20–34	0									
35–49	0									
50–64	0									
65+	0									
2. MULTIPLE DX										
A. Not Operated										
0–19 Years	38	1.9	2	1	1	1	3	3	3	8
20–34	103	1.9	4	1	1	1	2	3	4	8
35–49	160	2.8	6	1	1	2	4	6	9	11
50–64	85	3.2	8	1	2	2	4	5	10	17
65+	29	5.6	27	2	2	3	7	14	20	20
B. Operated										
0–19 Years	0									
20–34	0									
35–49	1	7.0	0	7	7	7	7	7	7	7
50–64	2	16.0	18	13	13	19	19	19	19	19
65+	0									
SUBTOTALS:										
1. SINGLE DX										
A. Not Operated	3	1.0	0	1	1	1	1	1	1	1
B. Operated	0									
2. MULTIPLE DX										
A. Not Operated	415	2.8	8	1	1	2	3	6	8	16
B. Operated	3	13.0	36	7	7	13	19	19	19	19
1. SINGLE DX	3	1.0	0	1	1	1	1	1	1	1
2. MULTIPLE DX	418	2.8	9	1	1	2	3	6	9	17
A. NOT OPERATED	418	2.7	8	1	1	2	3	6	8	16
B. OPERATED	3	13.0	36	7	7	13	19	19	19	19
TOTAL										
0–19 Years	40	1.9	2	1	1	1	2	3	3	8
20–34	104	1.9	4	1	1	1	2	3	4	8
35–49	161	2.8	6	1	1	2	4	6	8	11
50–64	87	3.5	12	1	2	2	4	7	12	19
65+	29	5.6	27	2	2	3	7	14	20	20
GRAND TOTAL	421	2.8	9	1	1	2	3	6	9	17

976: POIS-SKIN/EENT AGENT

Type of Patients	Observed Patients	Avg. Stay	Vari-ance	10th	25th	50th	75th	90th	95th	99th
1. SINGLE DX										
A. Not Operated										
0–19 Years	3	1.0	0	1	1	1	1	1	1	1
20–34	0									
35–49	0									
50–64	0									
65+	0									
B. Operated										
0–19 Years	0									
20–34	0									
35–49	0									
50–64	0									
65+	0									
2. MULTIPLE DX										
A. Not Operated										
0–19 Years	10	2.2	6	1	1	1	2	3	9	9
20–34	6	1.8	<1	1	1	1	2	3	3	3
35–49	17	2.0	2	1	1	1	2	5	6	6
50–64	13	8.2	442	1	1	2	3	9	78	78
65+	12	2.8	3	1	2	3	4	5	6	6
B. Operated										
0–19 Years	0									
20–34	0									
35–49	1	5.0	0	5	5	5	5	5	5	5
50–64	0									
65+	0									
SUBTOTALS:										
1. SINGLE DX										
A. Not Operated	3	1.0	0	1	1	1	1	1	1	1
B. Operated	0									
2. MULTIPLE DX										
A. Not Operated	58	3.6	102	1	1	2	3	5	9	78
B. Operated	1	5.0	0	5	5	5	5	5	5	5
1. SINGLE DX	3	1.0	0	1	1	1	1	1	1	1
2. MULTIPLE DX	59	3.6	100	1	1	2	3	5	9	78
A. NOT OPERATED	61	3.4	97	1	1	2	3	5	6	78
B. OPERATED	1	5.0	0	5	5	5	5	5	5	5
TOTAL										
0–19 Years	13	1.9	5	1	1	1	2	3	9	9
20–34	6	1.8	<1	1	1	1	2	3	3	3
35–49	17	2.0	2	1	1	2	2	5	6	8
50–64	14	8.0	409	1	2	3	4	9	78	78
65+	12	2.8	3	1	2	3	4	5	6	6
GRAND TOTAL	62	3.5	96	1	1	2	3	5	6	78

977: POISON-MEDICINAL NEC&NOS

Type of Patients	Observed Patients	Avg. Stay	Vari-ance	10th	25th	50th	75th	90th	95th	99th
1. SINGLE DX										
A. Not Operated										
0–19 Years	17	1.2	<1	1	1	1	1	1	2	2
20–34	3	1.0	0	1	1	1	1	1	1	1
35–49	0									
50–64	1	1.0	0	1	1	1	1	1	1	1
65+	0									
B. Operated										
0–19 Years	0									
20–34	0									
35–49	0									
50–64	0									
65+	1	1.0	0	1	1	1	1	1	1	1
2. MULTIPLE DX										
A. Not Operated										
0–19 Years	84	1.7	7	1	1	1	2	3	3	7
20–34	161	2.4	5	1	1	2	3	5	7	11
35–49	276	3.6	23	1	1	2	4	9	12	29
50–64	277	3.3	12	1	1	2	4	7	10	20
65+	154	4.0	24	1	2	2	4	7	16	29
B. Operated										
0–19 Years	0									
20–34	0									
35–49	2	28.4	215	18	18	18	39	39	39	39
50–64	2	6.5	24	3	3	7	10	10	10	10
65+	0									
SUBTOTALS:										
1. SINGLE DX										
A. Not Operated	21	1.2	<1	1	1	1	1	2	2	2
B. Operated	1	1.0	0	1	1	1	1	1	1	1
2. MULTIPLE DX										
A. Not Operated	952	3.2	15	1	1	2	3	6	10	22
B. Operated	4	17.5	241	3	10	18	39	39	39	39
1. SINGLE DX	22	1.2	<1	1	1	1	1	2	2	2
2. MULTIPLE DX	956	3.3	17	1	1	2	3	7	10	22
A. NOT OPERATED	973	3.2	15	1	1	2	3	6	10	22
B. OPERATED	5	14.2	235	3	10	18	39	39	39	39
TOTAL										
0–19 Years	101	1.6	1	1	1	1	2	3	3	6
20–34	164	2.3	5	1	1	2	3	5	7	11
35–49	278	3.8	28	1	1	2	4	9	13	31
50–64	280	3.3	12	1	2	2	4	7	10	20
65+	155	4.0	24	1	2	2	4	7	16	29
GRAND TOTAL	978	3.2	16	1	1	2	3	6	10	22

Western Region, October 2006–September 2007 Data, by Diagnosis

977.8: POISON-MED AGENT NEC

Type of Patients	Observed Patients	Avg. Stay	Vari-ance	Percentiles						
				10th	25th	50th	75th	90th	95th	99th
1. SINGLE DX										
A. *Not Operated*										
0–19 Years	5	1.4	<1	1	1	1	2	2	2	2
20–34	1	1.0	0	1	1	1	1	1	1	1
35–49	0									
50–64	0									
65+	0									
B. *Operated*										
0–19 Years	0									
20–34	0									
35–49	0									
50–64	0									
65+	0									
2. MULTIPLE DX										
A. *Not Operated*										
0–19 Years	40	1.5	<1	1	1	1	2	3	3	4
20–34	87	2.2	4	1	1	2	2	5	7	11
35–49	135	3.5	18	1	1	2	4	8	11	22
50–64	147	3.6	17	1	1	2	4	7	11	24
65+	90	4.1	23	1	2	3	4	7	15	31
B. *Operated*										
0–19 Years	0									
20–34	0									
35–49	0									
50–64	2	6.5	24	3	3	7	10	10	10	10
65+	0									
SUBTOTALS:										
1. SINGLE DX										
A. *Not Operated*	6	1.3	<1	1	1	1	2	2	2	2
B. *Operated*	0									
2. MULTIPLE DX										
A. *Not Operated*	499	3.3	15	1	1	2	4	7	10	22
B. *Operated*	2	6.5	24	3	3	7	10	10	10	10
1. SINGLE DX	6	1.3	<1	1	1	1	2	2	2	2
2. MULTIPLE DX	501	3.3	15	1	1	2	4	7	10	22
A. NOT OPERATED	505	3.2	15	1	1	2	4	7	10	22
B. OPERATED	2	6.5	24	3	3	7	10	10	10	10
TOTAL										
0–19 Years	45	1.5	<1	1	1	1	2	3	3	4
20–34	88	2.2	4	1	1	2	2	5	7	11
35–49	135	3.5	18	1	1	2	4	8	11	22
50–64	149	3.7	17	1	1	2	4	8	11	24
65+	90	4.1	23	1	2	3	4	7	15	31
GRAND TOTAL	507	3.2	15	1	1	2	4	7	10	22

977.9: POISON-MED AGENT NOS

Type of Patients	Observed Patients	Avg. Stay	Vari-ance	Percentiles						
				10th	25th	50th	75th	90th	95th	99th
1. SINGLE DX										
A. *Not Operated*										
0–19 Years	12	1.2	<1	1	1	1	1	1	2	2
20–34	2	1.0	0	1	1	1	1	1	1	1
35–49	0									
50–64	1	1.0	0	1	1	1	1	1	1	1
65+	0									
B. *Operated*										
0–19 Years	0									
20–34	0									
35–49	0									
50–64	0									
65+	0									
2. MULTIPLE DX										
A. *Not Operated*										
0–19 Years	41	1.8	1	1	1	1	2	3	3	7
20–34	68	2.5	6	1	1	2	3	6	6	17
35–49	133	3.8	29	1	1	2	4	10	13	29
50–64	119	3.0	5	1	1	2	4	6	8	11
65+	61	4.0	26	1	2	2	3	8	16	29
B. *Operated*										
0–19 Years	0									
20–34	0									
35–49	2	28.4	215	18	18	18	39	39	39	39
50–64	0									
65+	0									
SUBTOTALS:										
1. SINGLE DX										
A. *Not Operated*	15	1.1	<1	1	1	1	1	2	2	2
B. *Operated*	0									
2. MULTIPLE DX										
A. *Not Operated*	422	3.2	16	1	1	2	3	6	10	19
B. *Operated*	2	28.4	215	18	18	18	39	39	39	39
1. SINGLE DX	15	1.1	<1	1	1	1	1	2	2	2
2. MULTIPLE DX	424	3.3	19	1	1	2	3	7	10	22
A. NOT OPERATED	437	3.1	15	1	1	2	3	6	10	19
B. OPERATED	2	28.4	215	18	18	18	39	39	39	39
TOTAL										
0–19 Years	53	1.6	1	1	1	1	2	3	3	7
20–34	70	2.5	6	1	1	2	3	6	6	17
35–49	135	4.2	39	1	1	2	4	10	15	39
50–64	120	3.0	5	1	1	2	4	6	7	11
65+	61	4.0	26	1	2	2	3	8	16	29
GRAND TOTAL	439	3.3	19	1	1	2	3	7	10	22

978: POISONING-BACT VACCINES

Type of Patients	Observed Patients	Avg. Stay	Vari-ance	Percentiles						
				10th	25th	50th	75th	90th	95th	99th
1. SINGLE DX										
A. *Not Operated*										
0–19 Years	0									
20–34	0									
35–49	0									
50–64	0									
65+	0									
B. *Operated*										
0–19 Years	0									
20–34	0									
35–49	0									
50–64	0									
65+	0									
2. MULTIPLE DX										
A. *Not Operated*										
0–19 Years	0									
20–34	1	1.0	0	1	1	1	1	1	1	1
35–49	0									
50–64	0									
65+	0									
B. *Operated*										
0–19 Years	0									
20–34	0									
35–49	0									
50–64	0									
65+	0									
SUBTOTALS:										
1. SINGLE DX										
A. *Not Operated*	0									
B. *Operated*	0									
2. MULTIPLE DX										
A. *Not Operated*	1	1.0	0	1	1	1	1	1	1	1
B. *Operated*	0									
1. SINGLE DX	0									
2. MULTIPLE DX	1	1.0	0	1	1	1	1	1	1	1
A. NOT OPERATED	1	1.0	0	1	1	1	1	1	1	1
B. OPERATED	0									
TOTAL										
0–19 Years	0									
20–34	1	1.0	0	1	1	1	1	1	1	1
35–49	0									
50–64	0									
65+	0									
GRAND TOTAL	1	1.0	0	1	1	1	1	1	1	1

Length of Stay by Diagnosis and Operation, Western Region, 2008

Western Region, October 2006–September 2007 Data, by Diagnosis

979: POIS-OTH VACC/BIOLOGICAL

Type of Patients	Observed Patients	Avg. Stay	Variance	10th	25th	50th	75th	90th	95th	99th
1. SINGLE DX										
A. *Not Operated*										
0–19 Years	0									
20–34	0									
35–49	0									
50–64	0									
65+	0									
B. *Operated*										
0–19 Years	0									
20–34	0									
35–49	0									
50–64	0									
65+	0									
2. MULTIPLE DX										
A. *Not Operated*										
0–19 Years	0									
20–34	0									
35–49	1	1.0	0	1	1	1	1	1	1	1
50–64	0									
65+	0									
B. *Operated*										
0–19 Years	0									
20–34	0									
35–49	0									
50–64	0									
65+	0									
SUBTOTALS:										
1. SINGLE DX										
A. *Not Operated*	0									
B. *Operated*	0									
2. MULTIPLE DX										
A. *Not Operated*	1	1.0	0	1	1	1	1	1	1	1
B. *Operated*	0									
1. SINGLE DX	0									
2. MULTIPLE DX	1	1.0	0	1	1	1	1	1	1	1
A. NOT OPERATED	1	1.0	0	1	1	1	1	1	1	1
B. OPERATED	0									
TOTAL										
0–19 Years	0									
20–34	0									
35–49	1	1.0	0	1	1	1	1	1	1	1
50–64	0									
65+	0									
GRAND TOTAL	1	1.0	0	1	1	1	1	1	1	1

980: ALCOHOL TOXICITY

Type of Patients	Observed Patients	Avg. Stay	Variance	10th	25th	50th	75th	90th	95th	99th
1. SINGLE DX										
A. *Not Operated*										
0–19 Years	8	1.0	0	1	1	1	1	1	1	1
20–34	1	1.0	0	1	1	1	1	1	1	1
35–49	0									
50–64	0									
65+	0									
B. *Operated*										
0–19 Years	0									
20–34	0									
35–49	0									
50–64	0									
65+	0									
2. MULTIPLE DX										
A. *Not Operated*										
0–19 Years	135	1.4	<1	1	1	1	2	2	3	3
20–34	226	2.3	7	1	1	1	3	4	7	13
35–49	331	3.2	14	1	1	2	4	6	9	17
50–64	185	3.0	6	1	1	2	4	6	8	14
65+	50	3.0	5	1	1	2	4	7	8	10
B. *Operated*										
0–19 Years	0									
20–34	2	9.0	49	4	4	14	14	14	14	14
35–49	1	14.0	0	14	14	14	14	14	14	14
50–64	1	22.0	0	22	22	22	22	22	22	22
65+	0									
SUBTOTALS:										
1. SINGLE DX										
A. *Not Operated*	9	1.0	0	1	1	1	1	1	1	1
B. *Operated*	0									
2. MULTIPLE DX										
A. *Not Operated*	927	2.7	9	1	1	2	3	5	8	14
B. *Operated*	4	13.5	54	4	14	14	14	22	22	22
1. SINGLE DX	9	1.0	0	1	1	1	1	1	1	1
2. MULTIPLE DX	931	2.7	9	1	1	2	3	5	8	15
A. NOT OPERATED	936	2.6	9	1	1	2	3	5	8	14
B. OPERATED	4	13.5	54	4	14	14	14	22	22	22
TOTAL										
0–19 Years	143	1.4	<1	1	1	1	2	2	3	3
20–34	229	2.4	7	1	1	1	3	4	8	14
35–49	332	3.2	14	1	1	2	4	6	10	17
50–64	186	3.1	8	1	1	2	4	6	8	16
65+	50	3.0	5	1	1	2	4	7	8	10
GRAND TOTAL	940	2.7	9	1	1	2	3	5	8	15

980.0: TOXIC EFF ETHYL ALCOHOL

Type of Patients	Observed Patients	Avg. Stay	Variance	10th	25th	50th	75th	90th	95th	99th
1. SINGLE DX										
A. *Not Operated*										
0–19 Years	4	1.0	0	1	1	1	1	1	1	1
20–34	0									
35–49	0									
50–64	0									
65+	0									
B. *Operated*										
0–19 Years	0									
20–34	0									
35–49	0									
50–64	0									
65+	0									
2. MULTIPLE DX										
A. *Not Operated*										
0–19 Years	122	1.4	<1	1	1	1	2	2	3	3
20–34	163	2.1	7	1	1	1	2	4	5	18
35–49	244	3.1	10	1	1	2	4	6	9	17
50–64	141	3.2	7	1	1	3	4	6	9	14
65+	40	2.8	5	1	1	2	4	7	8	10
B. *Operated*										
0–19 Years	0									
20–34	1	14.0	0	14	14	14	14	14	14	14
35–49	0									
50–64	0									
65+	0									
SUBTOTALS:										
1. SINGLE DX										
A. *Not Operated*	4	1.0	0	1	1	1	1	1	1	1
B. *Operated*	0									
2. MULTIPLE DX										
A. *Not Operated*	710	2.6	7	1	1	2	3	5	8	14
B. *Operated*	1	14.0	0	14	14	14	14	14	14	14
1. SINGLE DX	4	1.0	0	1	1	1	1	1	1	1
2. MULTIPLE DX	711	2.6	7	1	1	2	3	5	8	14
A. NOT OPERATED	714	2.6	7	1	1	2	3	5	8	14
B. OPERATED	1	14.0	0	14	14	14	14	14	14	14
TOTAL										
0–19 Years	126	1.4	<1	1	1	1	2	2	3	3
20–34	164	2.2	8	1	1	1	2	4	6	18
35–49	244	3.1	10	1	1	2	4	6	9	17
50–64	141	3.2	7	1	1	3	4	6	9	14
65+	40	2.8	5	1	1	2	4	7	8	10
GRAND TOTAL	715	2.6	7	1	1	2	3	5	8	14

Length of Stay by Diagnosis and Operation, Western Region, 2008

Western Region, October 2006–September 2007 Data, by Diagnosis

981: TOXIC EFF PETROLEUM PROD

Type of Patients	Observed Patients	Avg. Stay	Vari-ance	10th	25th	50th	75th	90th	95th	99th
1. SINGLE DX										
A. *Not Operated*										
0–19 Years	3	1.0	0		1	1	1	1	1	1
20–34	0									
35–49	1	1.0	0	1	1	1	1	1	1	1
50–64	0									
65+	0									
B. *Operated*										
0–19 Years	0									
20–34	0									
35–49	0									
50–64	0									
65+	0									
2. MULTIPLE DX										
A. *Not Operated*										
0–19 Years	10	1.8	1	1	1	1	3	3	3	3
20–34	2	6.5	12	4	4	9	9	9	9	9
35–49	3	2.0	<1	1	1	2	3	3	3	3
50–64	1	2.0	0	2	2	2	2	2	2	2
65+	2	1.0	0	1	1	1	1	1	1	1
B. *Operated*										
0–19 Years	0									
20–34	0									
35–49	0									
50–64	0									
65+	0									
SUBTOTALS:										
1. SINGLE DX										
A. *Not Operated*	4	1.0	0	1	1	1	1	1	1	1
B. *Operated*	0									
2. MULTIPLE DX										
A. *Not Operated*	18	2.3	4	1	1	2	3	4	9	9
B. *Operated*	0									
1. SINGLE DX	4	1.0	0	1	1	1	1	1	1	1
2. MULTIPLE DX	18	2.3	4	1	1	2	3	4	9	9
A. NOT OPERATED	22	2.1	3	1	1	1	3	3	4	9
B. OPERATED	0									
TOTAL										
0–19 Years	13	1.6	<1	1	1	1	3	3	3	3
20–34	2	6.5	12	4	4	9	9	9	9	9
35–49	4	1.8	<1	1	1	2	2	3	3	3
50–64	1	2.0	0	2	2	2	2	2	2	2
65+	2	1.0	0	1	1	1	1	1	1	1
GRAND TOTAL	22	2.1	3	1	1	1	3	3	4	9

982: TOXIC EFFECT SOLVENT NEC

Type of Patients	Observed Patients	Avg. Stay	Vari-ance	10th	25th	50th	75th	90th	95th	99th
1. SINGLE DX										
A. *Not Operated*										
0–19 Years	4	1.0	0	1	1	1	1	1	1	1
20–34	1	1.0	0	1	1	1	1	1	1	1
35–49	0									
50–64	1	2.0	0	2	2	2	2	2	2	2
65+	0									
B. *Operated*										
0–19 Years	0									
20–34	0									
35–49	0									
50–64	0									
65+	0									
2. MULTIPLE DX										
A. *Not Operated*										
0–19 Years	21	2.5	5	1	1	2	3	6	8	9
20–34	33	6.5	45	2	2	3	10	16	21	26
35–49	52	4.7	19	2	2	3	6	12	13	21
50–64	28	5.9	31	2	2	4	7	18	18	19
65+	10	5.7	32	1	1	3	13	14	14	14
B. *Operated*										
0–19 Years	0									
20–34	0									
35–49	1	24.0	0	24	24	24	24	24	24	24
50–64	1	12.0	0	12	12	12	12	12	12	12
65+	2	15.0	0	15	15	15	15	15	15	15
SUBTOTALS:										
1. SINGLE DX										
A. *Not Operated*	6	1.2	<1	1	1	1	1	2	2	2
B. *Operated*	0									
2. MULTIPLE DX										
A. *Not Operated*	144	5.1	27	1	2	3	6	13	16	21
B. *Operated*	4	16.5	27	12	15	15	24	24	24	24
1. SINGLE DX	6	1.2	<1	1	1	1	1	2	2	2
2. MULTIPLE DX	148	5.4	30	1	2	3	7	14	17	24
A. NOT OPERATED	150	4.9	26	1	1	3	6	13	16	21
B. OPERATED	4	16.5	27	12	15	15	24	24	24	24
TOTAL										
0–19 Years	25	2.3	5	1	1	2	3	6	8	9
20–34	34	6.3	44	2	2	3	10	16	21	26
35–49	53	5.1	26	1	2	3	6	13	16	24
50–64	30	5.9	30	2	2	4	8	15	18	19
65+	12	7.2	39	1	1	4	14	15	15	15
GRAND TOTAL	154	5.2	30	1	1	3	6	14	17	24

983: TOXIC EFFECT CAUSTICS

Type of Patients	Observed Patients	Avg. Stay	Vari-ance	10th	25th	50th	75th	90th	95th	99th
1. SINGLE DX										
A. *Not Operated*										
0–19 Years	4	1.0	0	1	1	1	1	1	1	1
20–34	1	1.0	0	1	1	1	1	1	1	1
35–49	0									
50–64	0									
65+	0									
B. *Operated*										
0–19 Years	0									
20–34	0									
35–49	0									
50–64	0									
65+	0									
2. MULTIPLE DX										
A. *Not Operated*										
0–19 Years	20	2.4	4	1	1	2	3	4	5	9
20–34	48	2.6	11	1	1	2	2	5	7	21
35–49	35	3.6	19	1	1	2	4	5	14	24
50–64	33	5.0	25	1	1	3	6	12	16	21
65+	21	5.1	39	1	1	2	7	12	15	26
B. *Operated*										
0–19 Years	0									
20–34	1	51.0	0	51	51	51	51	51	51	51
35–49	1	21.0	0	21	21	21	21	21	21	21
50–64	0									
65+	1	12.0	0	12	12	12	12	12	12	12
SUBTOTALS:										
1. SINGLE DX										
A. *Not Operated*	5	1.0	0	1	1	1	1	1	1	1
B. *Operated*	0									
2. MULTIPLE DX										
A. *Not Operated*	157	3.6	19	1	1	2	4	9	14	24
B. *Operated*	3	27.9	413	12	21	21	51	51	51	51
1. SINGLE DX	5	1.0	0	1	1	1	1	1	1	1
2. MULTIPLE DX	160	4.1	35	1	1	2	4	10	15	26
A. NOT OPERATED	162	3.5	19	1	1	2	4	8	12	24
B. OPERATED	3	27.9	413	12	21	21	51	51	51	51
TOTAL										
0–19 Years	24	2.1	3	1	1	1	2	4	5	9
20–34	50	3.5	57	1	1	2	2	6	10	51
35–49	36	4.1	27	1	1	3	4	10	21	24
50–64	33	5.0	25	1	1	3	6	12	16	21
65+	22	5.4	40	1	1	2	8	12	15	26
GRAND TOTAL	165	4.0	34	1	1	2	4	10	15	26

Length of Stay by Diagnosis and Operation, Western Region, 2008

Western Region, October 2006–September 2007 Data, by Diagnosis

984: TOXIC EFF LEAD/COMPOUND

Type of Patients	Observed Patients	Avg. Stay	Variance	10th	25th	50th	75th	90th	95th	99th
1. SINGLE DX										
A. Not Operated										
0-19 Years	0									
20-34	0									
35-49	0									
50-64	0									
65+	0									
B. Operated										
0-19 Years	0									
20-34	0									
35-49	0									
50-64	0									
65+	0									
2. MULTIPLE DX										
A. Not Operated										
0-19 Years	4	3.7	13	1	1	3	3	9	9	9
20-34	0									
35-49	1	3.0	0	3	3	3	3	3	3	3
50-64	2	3.5	<1	3	3	3	4	4	4	4
65+	1	2.0	0	2	2	2	2	2	2	2
B. Operated										
0-19 Years	0									
20-34	0									
35-49	0									
50-64	0									
65+	0									
SUBTOTALS:										
1. SINGLE DX										
A. Not Operated	0									
B. Operated	0									
2. MULTIPLE DX										
A. Not Operated	8	3.4	6	1	2	3	3	9	9	9
B. Operated	0									
1. SINGLE DX	0									
2. MULTIPLE DX	8	3.4	6	1	2	3	3	9	9	9
A. NOT OPERATED	8	3.4	6	1	2	3	3	9	9	9
B. OPERATED	0									
TOTAL										
0-19 Years	4	3.7	13	1	1	3	3	9	9	9
20-34	0									
35-49	1	3.0	0	3	3	3	3	3	3	3
50-64	2	3.5	<1	3	3	3	4	4	4	4
65+	1	2.0	0	2	2	2	2	2	2	2
GRAND TOTAL	8	3.4	6	1	2	3	3	9	9	9

985: TOXIC EFFECT OTH METALS

Type of Patients	Observed Patients	Avg. Stay	Variance	10th	25th	50th	75th	90th	95th	99th
1. SINGLE DX										
A. Not Operated										
0-19 Years	1	1.0	0	1	1	1	1	1	1	1
20-34	1	1.0	0	1	1	1	1	1	1	1
35-49	0									
50-64	0									
65+	0									
B. Operated										
0-19 Years	0									
20-34	0									
35-49	0									
50-64	0									
65+	0									
2. MULTIPLE DX										
A. Not Operated										
0-19 Years	9	2.7	5	1	1	2	3	8	8	8
20-34	21	2.7	7	1	1	2	3	3	8	12
35-49	31	3.5	22	1	1	2	3	7	13	23
50-64	19	2.9	4	1	1	3	4	5	6	9
65+	5	6.2	15	2	4	5	8	12	12	12
B. Operated										
0-19 Years	0									
20-34	0									
35-49	0									
50-64	1	6.0	0	6	6	6	6	6	6	6
65+	0									
SUBTOTALS:										
1. SINGLE DX										
A. Not Operated	2	1.0	0	1	1	1	1	1	1	1
B. Operated	0									
2. MULTIPLE DX										
A. Not Operated	85	3.3	12	1	1	2	3	8	12	23
B. Operated	1	6.0	0	6	6	6	6	6	6	6
1. SINGLE DX	2	1.0	0	1	1	1	1	1	1	1
2. MULTIPLE DX	86	3.3	12	1	1	2	3	8	12	23
A. NOT OPERATED	87	3.2	12	1	1	2	3	8	12	23
B. OPERATED	1	6.0	0	6	6	6	6	6	6	6
TOTAL										
0-19 Years	10	2.5	4	1	1	2	3	3	8	8
20-34	22	2.6	7	1	1	2	3	3	8	12
35-49	31	3.5	22	1	1	2	3	7	13	23
50-64	20	3.1	4	1	1	3	4	6	6	9
65+	5	6.2	15	2	4	5	8	12	12	12
GRAND TOTAL	88	3.2	12	1	1	2	3	8	12	23

986: TOX EFF CARBON MONOXIDE

Type of Patients	Observed Patients	Avg. Stay	Variance	10th	25th	50th	75th	90th	95th	99th
1. SINGLE DX										
A. Not Operated										
0-19 Years	3	1.0	0	1	1	1	1	1	1	1
20-34	2	1.0	0	1	1	1	1	1	1	1
35-49	1	1.0	0	1	1	1	1	1	1	1
50-64	0									
65+	0									
B. Operated										
0-19 Years	1	1.0	0	1	1	1	1	1	1	1
20-34	0									
35-49	0									
50-64	0									
65+	0									
2. MULTIPLE DX										
A. Not Operated										
0-19 Years	16	3.1	16	1	1	2	5	8	16	16
20-34	33	2.4	8	1	1	2	3	5	7	16
35-49	62	2.8	14	1	1	2	3	7	8	24
50-64	76	3.0	16	1	1	2	3	5	10	27
65+	46	2.9	14	1	1	2	3	6	8	24
B. Operated										
0-19 Years	0									
20-34	2	15.1	161	6	6	24	24	24	24	24
35-49	0									
50-64	3	23.1	297	3	3	33	33	33	33	33
65+	0									
SUBTOTALS:										
1. SINGLE DX										
A. Not Operated	6	1.0	0	1	1	1	1	1	1	1
B. Operated	1	1.0	0	1	1	1	1	1	1	1
2. MULTIPLE DX										
A. Not Operated	233	2.8	14	1	1	2	3	6	8	24
B. Operated	5	19.9	209	3	6	24	33	33	33	33
1. SINGLE DX	7	1.0	0	1	1	1	1	1	1	1
2. MULTIPLE DX	238	3.2	23	1	1	2	3	6	10	27
A. NOT OPERATED	239	2.8	13	1	1	2	3	6	8	24
B. OPERATED	6	16.7	226	1	3	24	33	33	33	33
TOTAL										
0-19 Years	20	2.7	14	1	1	1	2	6	8	16
20-34	37	3.0	20	1	1	2	2	6	16	24
35-49	63	2.8	13	1	1	1	3	7	8	24
50-64	79	3.7	38	1	1	2	4	7	19	33
65+	46	2.9	14	1	1	2	3	6	8	24
GRAND TOTAL	245	3.1	22	1	1	2	3	6	9	27

Length of Stay by Diagnosis and Operation, Western Region, 2008

Western Region, October 2006–September 2007 Data, by Diagnosis

987: TOXIC EFF GAS/VAPOR NEC

Type of Patients	Observed Patients	Avg. Stay	Variance	10th	25th	50th	75th	90th	95th	99th
1. SINGLE DX										
A. Not Operated										
0–19 Years	3	1.0	0	1	1	1	1	1	1	1
20–34	1	1.0	0	1	1	1	1	1	1	1
35–49	3	1.0	0	1	1	1	1	1	1	1
50–64	1	1.0	0	1	1	1	1	1	1	1
65+	0									
B. Operated										
0–19 Years	0									
20–34	0									
35–49	0									
50–64	0									
65+	0									
2. MULTIPLE DX										
A. Not Operated										
0–19 Years	33	2.1	8	1	1	1	2	4	6	17
20–34	33	3.8	46	1	1	2	3	7	17	37
35–49	46	3.5	22	1	1	2	5	8	13	26
50–64	41	4.6	103	1	1	2	3	5	21	58
65+	32	3.2	18	1	1	2	3	7	10	23
B. Operated										
0–19 Years	0									
20–34	1	2.0	0	2	2	2	2	2	2	2
35–49	1	20.0	0	20	20	20	20	20	20	20
50–64	0									
65+	2	6.0	0	6	6	6	6	6	6	6
SUBTOTALS:										
1. SINGLE DX										
A. Not Operated	8	1.0	0	1	1	1	1	1	1	1
B. Operated	0									
2. MULTIPLE DX										
A. Not Operated	185	3.5	41	1	1	2	3	7	13	37
B. Operated	4	8.6	63	2	6	6	20	20	20	20
1. SINGLE DX	8	1.0	0	1	1	1	1	1	1	1
2. MULTIPLE DX	189	3.6	42	1	1	2	3	7	15	37
A. NOT OPERATED	193	3.4	39	1	1	1	3	6	13	37
B. OPERATED	4	8.6	63	2	6	6	20	20	20	20
TOTAL										
0–19 Years	36	2.0	8	1	1	1	2	4	6	17
20–34	35	3.7	43	1	1	1	3	7	17	37
35–49	50	3.7	26	1	1	2	5	8	15	26
50–64	42	4.5	101	1	1	2	3	5	21	58
65+	34	3.4	17	1	1	2	4	7	10	23
GRAND TOTAL	197	3.5	40	1	1	1	3	7	15	37

988: TOXIC EFF NOXIOUS FOOD

Type of Patients	Observed Patients	Avg. Stay	Variance	10th	25th	50th	75th	90th	95th	99th
1. SINGLE DX										
A. Not Operated										
0–19 Years	4	1.5	<1	1	1	2	2	2	2	2
20–34	0									
35–49	0									
50–64	0									
65+	0									
B. Operated										
0–19 Years	0									
20–34	0									
35–49	0									
50–64	0									
65+	0									
2. MULTIPLE DX										
A. Not Operated										
0–19 Years	48	1.8	2	1	1	1	2	3	5	8
20–34	18	2.1	2	1	1	2	3	4	5	5
35–49	10	2.2	3	1	1	2	3	4	6	6
50–64	17	2.4	2	1	2	2	3	4	7	7
65+	17	2.1	2	1	1	2	3	4	5	5
B. Operated										
0–19 Years	0									
20–34	0									
35–49	1	2.0	0	2	2	2	2	2	2	2
50–64	0									
65+	0									
SUBTOTALS:										
1. SINGLE DX										
A. Not Operated	4	1.5	<1	1	1	2	2	2	2	2
B. Operated	0									
2. MULTIPLE DX										
A. Not Operated	110	2.0	2	1	1	2	2	4	5	7
B. Operated	1	2.0	0	2	2	2	2	2	2	2
1. SINGLE DX	4	1.5	<1	1	1	2	2	2	2	2
2. MULTIPLE DX	111	2.0	2	1	1	2	2	4	5	7
A. NOT OPERATED	114	2.0	2	1	1	2	2	4	5	7
B. OPERATED	1	2.0	0	2	2	2	2	2	2	2
TOTAL										
0–19 Years	52	1.8	2	1	1	1	2	3	5	8
20–34	18	2.1	2	1	1	2	3	4	5	5
35–49	11	2.2	3	1	1	2	3	5	6	6
50–64	17	2.4	2	1	2	2	3	4	7	7
65+	17	2.1	2	1	1	2	3	4	5	5
GRAND TOTAL	115	2.0	2	1	1	2	2	4	5	7

989: TOX EFF NONMED SUBSTANCE

Type of Patients	Observed Patients	Avg. Stay	Variance	10th	25th	50th	75th	90th	95th	99th
1. SINGLE DX										
A. Not Operated										
0–19 Years	75	1.5	<1	1	1	1	2	2	3	3
20–34	34	1.6	<1	1	1	1	2	3	4	5
35–49	27	1.3	<1	1	1	1	2	2	3	3
50–64	17	1.6	<1	1	1	1	2	3	3	3
65+	6	1.8	<1	1	1	2	2	3	3	3
B. Operated										
0–19 Years	1	2.0	0	2	2	2	2	2	2	2
20–34	0									
35–49	1	5.0	0	5	5	5	5	5	5	5
50–64	0									
65+	0									
2. MULTIPLE DX										
A. Not Operated										
0–19 Years	153	2.0	4	1	1	1	2	3	5	14
20–34	193	2.7	8	1	1	2	3	5	6	11
35–49	242	2.6	4	1	1	2	3	5	6	10
50–64	201	2.3	4	1	1	2	3	4	6	10
65+	109	2.7	9	1	1	2	3	6	7	16
B. Operated										
0–19 Years	5	5.6	11	2	4	5	6	11	11	11
20–34	10	6.9	83	2	2	5	7	32	32	32
35–49	12	5.5	23	1	2	5	7	19	19	19
50–64	6	5.3	6	3	4	4	8	9	9	9
65+	5	6.4	30	3	3	4	6	16	16	16
SUBTOTALS:										
1. SINGLE DX										
A. Not Operated	159	1.5	<1	1	1	1	2	3	3	4
B. Operated	2	3.5	4	2	2	2	5	5	5	5
2. MULTIPLE DX										
A. Not Operated	898	2.5	5	1	1	2	3	5	6	11
B. Operated	38	6.0	33	2	3	5	7	11	19	32
1. SINGLE DX	161	1.5	<1	1	1	1	2	3	3	5
2. MULTIPLE DX	936	2.6	7	1	1	2	3	5	7	13
A. NOT OPERATED	1,057	2.3	5	1	1	2	3	4	6	11
B. OPERATED	40	5.9	31	2	3	5	7	11	19	32
TOTAL										
0–19 Years	234	1.9	3	1	1	2	2	3	5	11
20–34	237	2.7	11	1	1	2	3	5	6	11
35–49	282	2.6	5	1	1	2	3	5	7	10
50–64	224	2.3	4	1	1	2	3	4	6	10
65+	120	2.8	10	1	2	2	3	6	7	16
GRAND TOTAL	1,097	2.4	6	1	1	2	3	5	6	12

Length of Stay by Diagnosis and Operation, Western Region, 2008

819

Western Region, October 2006–September 2007 Data, by Diagnosis

989.5: TOXIC EFFECT VENOM

Type of Patients	Observed Patients	Avg. Stay	Vari-ance	10th	25th	50th	75th	90th	95th	99th
1. SINGLE DX										
A. Not Operated										
0–19 Years	67	1.5	<1	1	1	1	2	3	3	3
20–34	34	1.6	<1	1	1	1	2	3	4	5
35–49	25	1.4	<1	1	1	1	2	2	3	3
50–64	17	1.6	<1	1	1	1	2	3	3	3
65+	6	1.8	<1	1	1	2	2	3	3	3
B. Operated										
0–19 Years	1	2.0	0	2	2	2	2	2	2	2
20–34	0									
35–49	1	5.0	0	5	5	5	5	5	5	5
50–64	0									
65+	0									
2. MULTIPLE DX										
A. Not Operated										
0–19 Years	113	1.8	2	1	1	1	2	3	5	7
20–34	133	2.3	2	1	1	2	3	4	5	8
35–49	173	2.5	3	1	1	2	3	5	6	9
50–64	159	2.1	3	1	1	2	2	4	5	7
65+	73	2.5	10	1	1	2	2	4	6	20
B. Operated										
0–19 Years	4	5.8	15	2	4	5	11	11	11	11
20–34	8	4.4	6	1	3	5	7	7	8	8
35–49	12	5.5	23	1	2	5	7	7	19	19
50–64	6	5.3	6	3	4	5	8	9	9	9
65+	4	4.0	2	3	3	3	6	6	6	6
SUBTOTALS:										
1. SINGLE DX										
A. Not Operated	149	1.5	<1	1	1	1	2	3	3	4
B. Operated	2	3.5	4	2	2	2	5	5	5	5
2. MULTIPLE DX										
A. Not Operated	651	2.2	3	1	1	2	3	4	5	9
B. Operated	34	5.1	12	2	3	4	7	8	11	19
1. SINGLE DX	151	1.6	<1	1	1	1	2	3	3	5
2. MULTIPLE DX	685	2.4	4	1	1	2	3	5	6	10
A. NOT OPERATED	800	2.1	3	1	1	2	2	4	5	9
B. OPERATED	36	5.0	11	2	3	4	7	8	11	19
TOTAL										
0–19 Years	185	1.8	2	1	1	1	2	3	4	7
20–34	175	2.3	3	1	1	2	3	4	5	8
35–49	211	2.5	5	1	1	2	3	5	7	9
50–64	182	2.1	2	1	1	2	3	4	5	9
65+	83	2.5	9	1	1	2	3	4	6	20
GRAND TOTAL	836	2.2	4	1	1	2	3	4	5	9

990: EFFECTS RADIATION NOS

Type of Patients	Observed Patients	Avg. Stay	Vari-ance	10th	25th	50th	75th	90th	95th	99th
1. SINGLE DX										
A. Not Operated										
0–19 Years	0									
20–34	0									
35–49	0									
50–64	0									
65+	0									
B. Operated										
0–19 Years	0									
20–34	0									
35–49	0									
50–64	0									
65+	0									
2. MULTIPLE DX										
A. Not Operated										
0–19 Years	0									
20–34	0									
35–49	1	10.0	0	10	10	10	10	10	10	10
50–64	2	1.5	<1	1	1	2	2	2	2	2
65+	4	6.3	44	2	2	5	16	16	16	16
B. Operated										
0–19 Years	0									
20–34	0									
35–49	0									
50–64	0									
65+	2	7.0	18	4	4	4	10	10	10	10
SUBTOTALS:										
1. SINGLE DX										
A. Not Operated	0									
B. Operated	0									
2. MULTIPLE DX										
A. Not Operated	7	5.5	31	1	2	2	10	16	16	16
B. Operated	2	7.0	18	4	4	4	10	10	10	10
1. SINGLE DX	0									
2. MULTIPLE DX	9	5.8	26	1	2	4	10	16	16	16
A. NOT OPERATED	7	5.5	31	1	2	2	10	16	16	16
B. OPERATED	2	7.0	18	4	4	4	10	10	10	10
TOTAL										
0–19 Years	0									
20–34	0									
35–49	1	10.0	0	10	10	10	10	10	10	10
50–64	2	1.5	<1	1	1	2	2	2	2	2
65+	6	6.5	30	2	2	5	10	16	16	16
GRAND TOTAL	9	5.8	26	1	2	4	10	16	16	16

991: EFF REDUCED TEMPERATURE

Type of Patients	Observed Patients	Avg. Stay	Vari-ance	10th	25th	50th	75th	90th	95th	99th
1. SINGLE DX										
A. Not Operated										
0–19 Years	0									
20–34	2	5.0	18	2	2	8	8	8	8	8
35–49	0									
50–64	1	1.0	0	1	1	1	1	1	1	1
65+	0									
B. Operated										
0–19 Years	0									
20–34	0									
35–49	0									
50–64	1	9.0	0	9	9	9	9	9	9	9
65+	0									
2. MULTIPLE DX										
A. Not Operated										
0–19 Years	15	2.6	8	1	1	2	2	9	10	10
20–34	23	4.1	37	1	1	2	5	8	9	30
35–49	94	4.5	23	1	2	3	6	11	15	29
50–64	120	5.0	33	1	2	3	6	12	21	25
65+	124	5.0	31	1	2	3	6	10	13	25
B. Operated										
0–19 Years	8	16.0	0	16	16	16	16	16	16	16
20–34	8	10.0	86	2	4	8	9	32	32	32
35–49	12	9.3	58	2	4	7	13	20	27	27
50–64	21	20.4	506	6	8	12	23	42	71	90
65+	10	13.3	30	8	9	13	17	25	25	25
SUBTOTALS:										
1. SINGLE DX										
A. Not Operated	3	3.7	14	1	1	2	8	8	8	8
B. Operated	1	9.0	0	9	9	9	9	9	9	9
2. MULTIPLE DX										
A. Not Operated	376	4.7	29	1	2	3	6	10	15	29
B. Operated	52	14.8	252	4	7	11	16	27	42	90
1. SINGLE DX	4	5.0	17	1	1	8	9	9	9	9
2. MULTIPLE DX	428	5.9	67	1	2	3	7	13	19	36
A. NOT OPERATED	379	4.7	29	1	2	3	6	10	15	29
B. OPERATED	53	14.7	248	4	7	11	15	27	42	90
TOTAL										
0–19 Years	16	3.5	19	1	1	2	3	10	16	16
20–34	33	5.6	52	1	2	3	8	9	30	32
35–49	106	5.0	29	1	1	3	6	12	17	27
50–64	143	7.2	130	1	2	3	8	15	24	71
65+	134	5.6	36	1	2	4	7	13	17	25
GRAND TOTAL	432	5.9	66	1	2	3	7	13	19	36

Western Region, October 2006–September 2007 Data, by Diagnosis

991.6: HYPOTHERMIA

Type of Patients	Observed Patients	Avg. Stay	Variance	10th	25th	50th	75th	90th	95th	99th
1. SINGLE DX										
A. Not Operated										
0–19 Years	0									
20–34	0									
35–49	0									
50–64	1	1.0	0	1	1	1	1	1	1	1
65+	0									
B. Operated										
0–19 Years	0									
20–34	0									
35–49	0									
50–64	0									
65+	0									
2. MULTIPLE DX										
A. Not Operated										
0–19 Years	8	1.6	<1	1	1	1	2	3	3	3
20–34	11	1.8	2	1	1	1	2	3	6	6
35–49	54	3.9	19	1	1	2	5	11	14	18
50–64	101	4.1	20	1	2	2	5	10	13	22
65+	115	5.1	33	1	2	3	6	10	15	25
B. Operated										
0–19 Years	0									
20–34	0									
35–49	0									
50–64	5	31.6	>999	8	12	13	35	90	90	90
65+	8	12.2	17	6	9	13	17	17	17	17
SUBTOTALS:										
1. SINGLE DX										
A. Not Operated	1	1.0	0	1	1	1	1	1	1	1
B. Operated	0									
2. MULTIPLE DX										
A. Not Operated	289	4.3	24	1	1	3	5	10	13	25
B. Operated	13	19.7	501	8	9	13	17	35	90	90
1. SINGLE DX	1	1.0	0	1	1	1	1	1	1	1
2. MULTIPLE DX	302	5.0	53	1	2	3	6	11	15	25
A. NOT OPERATED	290	4.3	24	1	1	3	5	10	13	25
B. OPERATED	13	19.7	501	8	9	13	17	35	90	90
TOTAL										
0–19 Years	8	1.6	<1	1	1	1	2	3	3	3
20–34	11	1.8	2	1	1	1	2	3	6	6
35–49	54	3.9	19	1	1	2	5	11	14	18
50–64	107	5.4	98	1	2	3	5	12	15	35
65+	123	5.5	35	1	2	4	7	13	17	25
GRAND TOTAL	303	5.0	53	1	2	3	6	11	15	25

992: EFFECT OF HEAT/LIGHT

Type of Patients	Observed Patients	Avg. Stay	Variance	10th	25th	50th	75th	90th	95th	99th
1. SINGLE DX										
A. Not Operated										
0–19 Years	3	1.3	<1	1	1	1	1	2	2	2
20–34	0									
35–49	0									
50–64	0									
65+	0									
B. Operated										
0–19 Years	0									
20–34	0									
35–49	0									
50–64	0									
65+	0									
2. MULTIPLE DX										
A. Not Operated										
0–19 Years	23	1.3	<1	1	1	1	1	2	2	3
20–34	67	3.0	12	1	1	2	3	6	8	20
35–49	87	3.4	17	1	1	2	3	7	9	28
50–64	112	2.9	11	1	1	2	3	6	10	17
65+	205	2.8	6	1	1	2	4	5	7	11
B. Operated										
0–19 Years	0									
20–34	1	13.0	0	13	13	13	13	13	13	13
35–49	0									
50–64	2	17.5	12	15	15	18	20	20	20	20
65+	4	32.3	>999	4	4	13	20	94	94	94
SUBTOTALS:										
1. SINGLE DX										
A. Not Operated	3	1.3	<1	1	1	1	2	2	2	2
B. Operated	0									
2. MULTIPLE DX										
A. Not Operated	494	2.9	10	1	1	2	3	6	8	20
B. Operated	7	25.3	918	4	13	15	20	94	94	94
1. SINGLE DX	3	1.3	<1	1	1	1	2	2	2	2
2. MULTIPLE DX	501	3.2	27	1	1	2	3	6	9	20
A. NOT OPERATED	497	2.9	10	1	1	2	3	6	8	20
B. OPERATED	7	25.3	918	4	13	15	20	94	94	94
TOTAL										
0–19 Years	26	1.3	<1	1	1	1	1	2	3	3
20–34	68	3.1	13	1	1	2	3	6	8	20
35–49	87	3.4	17	1	1	2	3	7	9	28
50–64	114	3.2	14	1	1	2	3	7	11	20
65+	209	3.4	47	1	1	2	4	6	8	20
GRAND TOTAL	504	3.2	27	1	1	2	3	6	9	20

992.5: HEAT EXHAUSTION NOS

Type of Patients	Observed Patients	Avg. Stay	Variance	10th	25th	50th	75th	90th	95th	99th
1. SINGLE DX										
A. Not Operated										
0–19 Years	0									
20–34	0									
35–49	0									
50–64	0									
65+	0									
B. Operated										
0–19 Years	0									
20–34	0									
35–49	0									
50–64	0									
65+	0									
2. MULTIPLE DX										
A. Not Operated										
0–19 Years	11	1.3	<1	1	1	1	2	2	2	2
20–34	21	1.8	<1	1	1	1	2	3	4	4
35–49	33	2.2	1	1	1	2	2	4	4	5
50–64	40	2.1	3	1	1	1	3	4	5	10
65+	71	2.6	6	1	1	2	3	5	7	14
B. Operated										
0–19 Years	0									
20–34	0									
35–49	0									
50–64	0									
65+	1	13.0	0	13	13	13	13	13	13	13
SUBTOTALS:										
1. SINGLE DX										
A. Not Operated	0									
B. Operated	0									
2. MULTIPLE DX										
A. Not Operated	176	2.2	3	1	1	2	2	4	5	10
B. Operated	1	13.0	0	13	13	13	13	13	13	13
1. SINGLE DX	0									
2. MULTIPLE DX	177	2.3	4	1	1	2	3	4	7	13
A. NOT OPERATED	176	2.2	3	1	1	2	2	4	5	10
B. OPERATED	1	13.0	0	13	13	13	13	13	13	13
TOTAL										
0–19 Years	11	1.3	<1	1	1	1	2	2	2	2
20–34	21	1.8	<1	1	1	1	2	3	4	4
35–49	33	2.2	1	1	1	2	2	4	4	5
50–64	40	2.1	3	1	1	1	3	4	5	10
65+	72	2.7	7	1	1	2	3	5	8	14
GRAND TOTAL	177	2.3	4	1	1	2	3	4	7	13

Length of Stay by Diagnosis and Operation, Western Region, 2008

Western Region, October 2006–September 2007 Data, by Diagnosis

993: EFFECTS OF AIR PRESSURE

Type of Patients	Observed Patients	Avg. Stay	Vari-ance	10th	25th	50th	75th	90th	95th	99th
1. SINGLE DX										
A. Not Operated										
0–19 Years	0									
20–34	2	1.0	0	1	1	1	1	1	1	1
35–49	2	1.0	0	1	1	1	1	1	1	1
50–64	2	1.0	0	1	1	1	1	1	1	1
65+	0									
B. Operated										
0–19 Years	0									
20–34	0									
35–49	0									
50–64	0									
65+	0									
2. MULTIPLE DX										
A. Not Operated										
0–19 Years	8	1.4	<1	1	1	1	2	2	2	2
20–34	12	1.8	<1	1	1	2	2	2	3	3
35–49	24	2.0	2	1	1	2	3	3	4	6
50–64	25	1.7	2	1	1	1	2	3	6	6
65+	46	1.8	1	1	1	2	2	3	4	5
B. Operated										
0–19 Years	0									
20–34	0									
35–49	2	5.0	0	5	5	5	5	5	5	5
50–64	0									
65+	0									
SUBTOTALS:										
1. SINGLE DX										
A. Not Operated	6	1.0	0	1	1	1	1	1	1	1
B. Operated	0									
2. MULTIPLE DX										
A. Not Operated	115	1.8	1	1	1	2	2	3	4	6
B. Operated	2	5.0	0	5	5	5	5	5	5	5
1. SINGLE DX	6	1.0	0	1	1	1	1	1	1	1
2. MULTIPLE DX	117	1.8	1	1	1	2	2	3	5	6
A. NOT OPERATED	121	1.7	1	1	1	1	2	3	4	6
B. OPERATED	2	5.0	0	5	5	5	5	5	5	5
TOTAL										
0–19 Years	8	1.4	<1	1	1	1	2	2	2	2
20–34	14	1.6	<1	1	1	1	2	2	3	3
35–49	28	2.2	2	1	1	2	3	5	5	6
50–64	27	1.7	2	1	1	1	2	3	6	6
65+	46	1.8	1	1	1	2	2	3	4	5
GRAND TOTAL	123	1.8	1	1	1	1	2	3	4	6

994: EFFECT EXT CAUSE NEC

Type of Patients	Observed Patients	Avg. Stay	Vari-ance	10th	25th	50th	75th	90th	95th	99th
1. SINGLE DX										
A. Not Operated										
0–19 Years	102	1.1	<1	1	1	1	1	1	2	2
20–34	8	1.0	0	1	1	1	1	1	1	1
35–49	5	1.4	<1	1	1	1	2	2	2	2
50–64	2	1.0	0	1	1	1	1	1	1	1
65+	0									
B. Operated										
0–19 Years	0									
20–34	0									
35–49	0									
50–64	0									
65+	0									
2. MULTIPLE DX										
A. Not Operated										
0–19 Years	202	3.5	48	1	1	1	3	5	15	42
20–34	119	3.8	25	1	1	2	5	8	13	19
35–49	78	5.1	118	1	1	2	4	10	23	85
50–64	41	3.7	17	1	1	2	5	8	14	19
65+	41	4.2	24	1	2	3	5	7	14	27
B. Operated										
0–19 Years	7	34.9	314	19	22	27	43	70	70	70
20–34	7	13.1	181	3	5	6	18	41	41	41
35–49	2	14.1	126	6	6	22	22	22	22	22
50–64	2	12.6	24	9	9	16	16	16	16	16
65+	0									
SUBTOTALS:										
1. SINGLE DX										
A. Not Operated	117	1.1	<1	1	1	1	1	2	2	2
B. Operated	0									
2. MULTIPLE DX										
A. Not Operated	481	3.9	49	1	1	2	4	8	14	42
B. Operated	18	21.6	302	5	6	19	27	43	70	70
1. SINGLE DX	117	1.1	<1	1	1	1	1	2	2	2
2. MULTIPLE DX	499	4.6	68	1	1	2	4	9	19	43
A. NOT OPERATED	598	3.4	40	1	1	1	3	6	12	37
B. OPERATED	18	21.6	302	5	6	19	27	43	70	70
TOTAL										
0–19 Years	311	3.4	61	1	1	1	2	4	19	43
20–34	134	4.2	35	1	1	2	5	8	13	41
35–49	85	5.1	113	1	1	2	4	10	22	85
50–64	45	3.9	20	1	1	2	5	9	15	19
65+	41	4.2	24	1	2	3	5	7	14	27
GRAND TOTAL	616	3.9	57	1	1	1	3	8	16	42

994.1: DROWNING/NONFATAL SUBMER

Type of Patients	Observed Patients	Avg. Stay	Vari-ance	10th	25th	50th	75th	90th	95th	99th
1. SINGLE DX										
A. Not Operated										
0–19 Years	95	1.1	<1	1	1	1	1	1	2	3
20–34	2	1.0	0	1	1	1	1	1	1	1
35–49	1	2.0	0	2	2	2	2	2	2	2
50–64	0									
65+	0									
B. Operated										
0–19 Years	0									
20–34	0									
35–49	0									
50–64	0									
65+	0									
2. MULTIPLE DX										
A. Not Operated										
0–19 Years	156	3.3	47	1	1	2	2	5	15	45
20–34	34	4.8	61	1	1	2	5	9	19	43
35–49	14	7.1	110	1	2	3	4	23	38	38
50–64	14	4.6	29	1	2	2	5	14	19	19
65+	21	5.6	32	2	3	4	6	8	14	27
B. Operated										
0–19 Years	7	34.9	314	19	22	27	43	70	70	70
20–34	4	17.6	279	5	6	18	41	41	41	41
35–49	0									
50–64	0									
65+	0									
SUBTOTALS:										
1. SINGLE DX										
A. Not Operated	98	1.1	<1	1	1	1	1	1	2	3
B. Operated	0									
2. MULTIPLE DX										
A. Not Operated	239	4.0	50	1	1	2	3	8	19	43
B. Operated	11	28.5	348	6	18	25	41	43	70	70
1. SINGLE DX	98	1.1	<1	1	1	1	1	1	2	3
2. MULTIPLE DX	250	5.1	88	1	1	2	4	13	25	45
A. NOT OPERATED	337	3.2	37	1	1	1	2	6	13	38
B. OPERATED	11	28.5	348	6	18	25	41	43	70	70
TOTAL										
0–19 Years	258	3.3	64	1	1	1	2	4	19	45
20–34	40	5.9	90	1	1	2	6	18	41	43
35–49	15	6.7	104	1	2	3	4	23	38	38
50–64	14	4.6	29	1	2	2	5	14	19	19
65+	21	5.6	32	2	3	4	6	8	14	27
GRAND TOTAL	348	4.0	66	1	1	1	3	7	19	43

Length of Stay by Diagnosis and Operation, Western Region, 2008

Western Region, October 2006–September 2007 Data, by Diagnosis

995: CERTAIN ADVERSE EFF NEC

Type of Patients	Observed Patients	Avg. Stay	Vari-ance	10th	25th	50th	75th	90th	95th	99th
1. SINGLE DX										
A. Not Operated										
0–19 Years	51	1.3	<1	1	1	1	1	2	3	4
20–34	29	1.5	<1	1	1	1	1	4	4	4
35–49	21	1.1	<1	1	1	1	1	2	2	2
50–64	18	1.1	<1	1	1	1	1	2	2	2
65+	7	1.0	0	1	1	1	1	1	1	1
B. Operated										
0–19 Years	0									
20–34	0									
35–49	0									
50–64	0									
65+	0									
2. MULTIPLE DX										
A. Not Operated										
0–19 Years	369	4.1	34	1	1	2	4	10	15	26
20–34	338	2.5	6	1	1	2	3	5	7	14
35–49	652	2.8	21	1	1	2	3	5	7	15
50–64	936	3.1	19	1	1	2	3	6	9	24
65+	1,357	3.8	26	1	1	2	4	8	12	23
B. Operated										
0–19 Years	22	14.8	124	1	6	14	20	28	35	42
20–34	19	7.6	42	1	3	5	10	22	22	22
35–49	30	12.4	335	1	3	7	13	25	40	97
50–64	56	15.4	231	3	5	11	21	41	61	>99
65+	70	12.2	88	3	5	10	16	24	32	42
SUBTOTALS:										
1. SINGLE DX										
A. Not Operated	126	1.3	<1	1	1	1	1	2	3	4
B. Operated	0									
2. MULTIPLE DX										
A. Not Operated	3,652	3.3	23	1	1	2	4	7	11	22
B. Operated	197	13.0	167	2	4	10	18	29	40	97
1. SINGLE DX	126	1.3	<1	1	1	1	1	2	3	4
2. MULTIPLE DX	3,849	3.8	34	1	1	2	4	8	13	29
A. NOT OPERATED	3,778	3.3	22	1	1	2	4	7	11	22
B. OPERATED	197	13.0	167	2	4	10	18	29	40	97
TOTAL										
0–19 Years	442	4.3	41	1	1	2	4	11	17	34
20–34	386	2.6	8	1	1	2	3	5	8	15
35–49	703	3.1	37	1	1	2	3	6	9	19
50–64	1,010	3.7	38	1	1	2	4	8	14	32
65+	1,434	4.2	32	1	1	2	5	10	14	28
GRAND TOTAL	3,975	3.8	34	1	1	2	4	8	13	28

995.0: OTHER ANAPHYLACTIC SHOCK

Type of Patients	Observed Patients	Avg. Stay	Vari-ance	10th	25th	50th	75th	90th	95th	99th
1. SINGLE DX										
A. Not Operated										
0–19 Years	4	1.3	<1	1	1	1	1	2	2	2
20–34	5	1.6	<1	1	1	1	2	3	3	3
35–49	4	1.5	<1	1	1	2	2	2	2	2
50–64	2	1.5	<1	1	1	2	2	2	2	2
65+	0									
B. Operated										
0–19 Years	0									
20–34	0									
35–49	0									
50–64	0									
65+	0									
2. MULTIPLE DX										
A. Not Operated										
0–19 Years	31	1.9	3	1	1	1	2	3	7	7
20–34	82	2.0	2	1	1	1	2	4	5	8
35–49	130	2.1	3	1	1	1	2	4	6	7
50–64	159	2.5	17	1	1	1	3	4	5	25
65+	149	3.2	16	1	1	2	3	6	9	25
B. Operated										
0–19 Years	1	1.0	0	1	1	1	1	1	1	1
20–34	1	16.0	0	16	16	16	16	16	16	16
35–49	5	2.0	5	1	1	1	1	6	6	6
50–64	4	8.8	68	3	5	6	21	21	21	21
65+	8	5.8	31	1	2	4	8	14	14	14
SUBTOTALS:										
1. SINGLE DX										
A. Not Operated	15	1.5	<1	1	1	1	2	2	3	3
B. Operated	0									
2. MULTIPLE DX										
A. Not Operated	551	2.5	11	1	1	1	3	4	6	17
B. Operated	19	5.7	38	1	1	3	8	16	21	21
1. SINGLE DX	15	1.5	<1	1	1	1	2	2	3	4
2. MULTIPLE DX	570	2.6	12	1	1	2	3	5	7	21
A. NOT OPERATED	566	2.4	10	1	1	1	3	4	6	17
B. OPERATED	19	5.7	38	1	1	3	8	16	21	21
TOTAL										
0–19 Years	36	1.8	2	1	1	1	2	3	7	7
20–34	88	2.1	4	1	1	1	2	4	5	16
35–49	139	2.1	3	1	1	1	2	4	6	7
50–64	165	2.6	19	1	1	1	3	4	6	25
65+	157	3.3	17	1	1	2	4	7	14	25
GRAND TOTAL	585	2.5	12	1	1	2	3	5	7	21

995.1: ANGIONEUROTIC EDEMA

Type of Patients	Observed Patients	Avg. Stay	Vari-ance	10th	25th	50th	75th	90th	95th	99th
1. SINGLE DX										
A. Not Operated										
0–19 Years	9	1.3	<1	1	1	1	2	2	2	2
20–34	17	1.7	1	1	1	1	2	4	4	4
35–49	14	1.1	<1	1	1	1	1	1	1	2
50–64	12	1.0	0	1	1	1	1	1	1	1
65+	7	1.0	0	1	1	1	1	1	1	1
B. Operated										
0–19 Years	0									
20–34	0									
35–49	0									
50–64	0									
2. MULTIPLE DX										
A. Not Operated										
0–19 Years	42	1.8	2	1	1	1	2	4	5	6
20–34	102	2.2	2	1	1	2	3	4	5	6
35–49	262	2.1	3	1	1	1	2	5	6	10
50–64	479	2.1	6	1	1	1	2	4	6	12
65+	631	2.2	6	1	1	1	2	4	5	13
B. Operated										
0–19 Years	0									
20–34	2	1.5	<1	1	1	1	2	2	2	2
35–49	1	9.0	0	9	9	9	9	9	9	9
50–64	9	6.9	31	2	4	5	6	20	20	20
65+	9	7.8	49	1	3	7	10	24	24	24
SUBTOTALS:										
1. SINGLE DX										
A. Not Operated	59	1.3	<1	1	1	1	1	2	4	4
B. Operated	0									
2. MULTIPLE DX										
A. Not Operated	1,516	2.1	5	1	1	1	2	4	6	11
B. Operated	21	6.9	36	2	3	5	9	11	20	24
1. SINGLE DX	59	1.3	<1	1	1	1	1	2	4	4
2. MULTIPLE DX	1,537	2.2	6	1	1	1	2	4	6	12
A. NOT OPERATED	1,575	2.1	5	1	1	1	2	4	5	11
B. OPERATED	21	6.9	36	2	3	5	9	11	20	24
TOTAL										
0–19 Years	51	1.7	2	1	1	1	2	3	5	6
20–34	121	2.1	3	1	1	2	3	4	5	6
35–49	277	2.1	3	1	1	1	2	5	6	10
50–64	500	2.2	6	1	1	1	2	4	6	12
65+	647	2.2	7	1	1	1	2	4	6	13
GRAND TOTAL	1,596	2.2	6	1	1	1	2	4	6	12

Length of Stay by Diagnosis and Operation, Western Region, 2008

Western Region, October 2006–September 2007 Data, by Diagnosis

995.91: SEPSIS

Type of Patients	Observed Patients	Avg. Stay	Variance	Percentiles						
				10th	25th	50th	75th	90th	95th	99th
1. SINGLE DX										
A. Not Operated										
0–19 Years	0									
20–34	0									
35–49	0									
50–64	0									
65+	0									
B. Operated										
0–19 Years	0									
20–34	0									
35–49	0									
50–64	0									
65+	0									
2. MULTIPLE DX										
A. Not Operated										
0–19 Years	14	2.9	1	1	2	3	4	4	5	5
20–34	26	5.5	16	2	3	4	7	14	14	15
35–49	58	5.1	11	2	3	4	6	10	12	19
50–64	78	6.9	31	3	3	5	8	13	19	34
65+	252	6.8	48	2	3	5	8	13	17	33
B. Operated										
0–19 Years	8	10.6	61	3	5	8	14	22	22	22
20–34	11	15.0	107	7	7	11	19	25	40	40
35–49	16	16.3	176	5	9	12	21	57	>99	>99
50–64										
65+	33	13.3	73	5	7	12	16	24	32	42
SUBTOTALS:										
1. SINGLE DX										
A. Not Operated	0									
B. Operated	0									
2. MULTIPLE DX										
A. Not Operated	428	6.4	37	2	3	5	8	12	16	32
B. Operated	68	14.0	100	5	7	12	18	27	40	>99
1. SINGLE DX	0									
2. MULTIPLE DX	496	7.4	52	2	3	5	9	15	20	40
A. NOT OPERATED	428	6.4	37	2	3	5	8	12	16	32
B. OPERATED	68	14.0	100	5	7	12	18	27	40	>99
TOTAL										
0–19 Years	14	2.9	1	1	2	3	4	4	5	5
20–34	34	6.7	30	2	3	5	7	14	22	22
35–49	69	6.7	38	2	3	5	7	13	19	40
50–64	94	8.5	67	3	4	6	10	19	27	>99
65+	285	7.6	55	2	3	5	10	15	18	34
GRAND TOTAL	496	7.4	52	2	3	5	9	15	20	40

996: REPLACEMENT & GRAFT COMP

Type of Patients	Observed Patients	Avg. Stay	Variance	Percentiles						
				10th	25th	50th	75th	90th	95th	99th
1. SINGLE DX										
A. Not Operated										
0–19 Years	32	3.6	13	1	1	2	6	8	10	15
20–34	35	2.3	4	1	1	2	3	6	7	8
35–49	32	2.8	5	1	1	2	4	6	7	11
50–64	50	2.1	2	1	1	1	3	4	5	6
65+	28	1.9	2	1	1	2	2	3	5	7
B. Operated										
0–19 Years	54	2.7	11	1	1	1	3	7	11	18
20–34	148	2.5	7	1	1	1	3	5	8	14
35–49	224	2.5	4	1	1	2	3	4	5	12
50–64	262	2.5	5	1	1	2	3	5	6	10
65+	207	2.2	2	1	1	2	3	4	5	6
2. MULTIPLE DX										
A. Not Operated										
0–19 Years	1,359	6.0	39	1	2	4	8	13	17	27
20–34	2,681	5.4	30	1	2	4	7	11	15	29
35–49	5,391	5.3	31	1	2	4	6	11	14	29
50–64	9,218	5.6	30	1	2	4	7	11	16	27
65+	12,564	5.3	24	1	2	4	7	11	14	24
B. Operated										
0–19 Years	1,116	6.4	81	2	2	3	7	15	24	53
20–34	2,647	5.7	50	1	2	3	7	12	19	36
35–49	6,842	5.2	42	1	2	3	6	11	17	32
50–64	15,428	5.2	40	1	2	3	6	11	16	32
65+	23,371	5.1	28	1	2	4	6	10	15	26
SUBTOTALS:										
1. SINGLE DX										
A. Not Operated	177	2.5	5	1	1	2	3	6	7	11
B. Operated	895	2.5	5	1	1	2	3	4	6	13
2. MULTIPLE DX										
A. Not Operated	31,213	5.4	28	1	2	4	7	11	15	26
B. Operated	49,404	5.2	36	1	2	4	6	11	15	30
1. SINGLE DX	1,072	2.5	5	1	1	2	3	5	6	12
2. MULTIPLE DX	80,617	5.3	33	1	2	4	6	11	15	29
A. NOT OPERATED	31,390	5.4	28	1	2	4	7	11	15	26
B. OPERATED	50,299	5.2	36	1	2	3	6	11	15	30
TOTAL										
0–19 Years	2,561	6.1	57	1	2	4	7	14	20	39
20–34	5,511	5.5	39	1	2	4	7	11	17	33
35–49	12,489	5.2	37	1	2	3	6	11	15	30
50–64	24,958	5.3	36	1	2	4	6	11	16	30
65+	36,170	5.2	27	1	2	4	6	11	15	26
GRAND TOTAL	81,689	5.3	33	1	2	4	6	11	15	28

996.01: MECH COMP CARD PACEMAKER

Type of Patients	Observed Patients	Avg. Stay	Variance	Percentiles						
				10th	25th	50th	75th	90th	95th	99th
1. SINGLE DX										
A. Not Operated										
0–19 Years	0									
20–34	0									
35–49	0									
50–64	0									
65+	1	1.0	0	1	1	1	1	1	1	1
B. Operated										
0–19 Years	0									
20–34	4	1.0	0	1	1	1	1	1	1	1
35–49	4	1.0	0	1	1	1	1	1	1	1
50–64	3	1.0	0	1	1	1	1	1	1	1
65+	34	1.2	<1	1	1	1	1	2	3	3
2. MULTIPLE DX										
A. Not Operated										
0–19 Years	5	3.2	7	1	1	2	2	6	6	6
20–34	1	2.0	0	2	2	2	2	2	2	2
35–49	12	2.7	6	1	1	2	3	4	7	10
50–64	37	2.3	3	1	1	2	3	4	5	8
65+	209	2.8	6	1	2	2	3	5	7	13
B. Operated										
0–19 Years	17	2.6	5	1	1	2	3	6	7	7
20–34	25	2.9	6	1	1	2	4	5	8	10
35–49	67	2.3	4	1	1	1	3	5	7	12
50–64	189	2.2	3	1	1	2	3	5	5	9
65+	1,200	2.6	7	1	2	2	3	6	8	13
SUBTOTALS:										
1. SINGLE DX										
A. Not Operated	1	1.0	0	1	1	1	1	1	1	1
B. Operated	45	1.1	<1	1	1	1	1	1	2	3
2. MULTIPLE DX										
A. Not Operated	264	2.7	6	1	1	2	3	5	7	13
B. Operated	1,498	2.6	6	1	1	2	3	6	7	13
1. SINGLE DX	46	1.1	<1	1	1	1	1	1	2	3
2. MULTIPLE DX	1,762	2.6	6	1	1	2	3	6	7	13
A. NOT OPERATED	265	2.7	6	1	1	2	3	5	7	13
B. OPERATED	1,543	2.5	6	1	1	2	3	5	7	13
TOTAL										
0–19 Years	22	2.8	5	1	1	2	2	6	6	7
20–34	30	2.6	5	1	1	1	1	5	8	10
35–49	83	2.3	4	1	1	2	3	5	7	12
50–64	229	2.2	3	1	1	1	3	5	5	9
65+	1,444	2.6	7	1	2	2	3	6	7	13
GRAND TOTAL	1,808	2.6	6	1	1	2	3	5	7	13

Length of Stay by Diagnosis and Operation, Western Region, 2008

996.02: MALFUNCT PROSTH HRT VALV

Type of Patients	Observed Patients	Avg. Stay	Vari-ance	10th	25th	50th	75th	90th	95th	99th
1. SINGLE DX										
A. Not Operated										
0–19 Years	0									
20–34	0									
35–49	0									
50–64	0									
65+	0									
B. Operated										
0–19 Years	0									
20–34	0									
35–49	0									
50–64	0									
65+	0									
2. MULTIPLE DX										
A. Not Operated										
0–19 Years	1	4.0	0	4	4	4	4	4	4	4
20–34	2	2.5	4	1	1	4	4	4	4	4
35–49	13	5.8	47	1	2	3	7	14	25	25
50–64	10	4.0	11	1	1	3	6	11	11	11
65+	31	5.3	15	2	2	5	8	12	13	14
B. Operated										
0–19 Years	6	20.2	>999	1	2	8	8	98	98	98
20–34	14	6.4	17	4	4	5	7	10	10	19
35–49	23	10.5	63	4	6	8	12	18	19	41
50–64	69	12.5	244	4	7	8	12	23	44	95
65+	102	12.0	68	5	7	9	15	23	27	39
SUBTOTALS:										
1. SINGLE DX										
A. Not Operated	0									
B. Operated	0									
2. MULTIPLE DX										
A. Not Operated	57	5.1	20	1	2	3	6	12	14	25
B. Operated	214	11.9	156	4	6	8	13	22	30	81
1. SINGLE DX	0									
2. MULTIPLE DX	271	10.5	135	3	5	8	12	19	27	81
A. NOT OPERATED	57	5.1	20	1	2	3	6	12	14	25
B. OPERATED	214	11.9	156	4	6	8	13	22	30	81
TOTAL										
0–19 Years	7	17.9	>999	1	2	4	8	98	98	98
20–34	16	6.0	16	3	4	5	7	10	19	19
35–49	36	8.8	61	1	3	8	12	18	25	41
50–64	79	11.4	222	3	5	7	11	21	44	95
65+	133	10.5	64	3	6	9	13	21	26	39
GRAND TOTAL	271	10.5	135	3	5	8	12	19	27	81

996.04: MECH COMP AICD

Type of Patients	Observed Patients	Avg. Stay	Vari-ance	10th	25th	50th	75th	90th	95th	99th
1. SINGLE DX										
A. Not Operated										
0–19 Years	0									
20–34	0									
35–49	0									
50–64	0									
65+	0									
B. Operated										
0–19 Years	0									
20–34	1	1.0	0	1	1	1	1	1	1	1
35–49	0									
50–64	5	2.2	5	1	1	1	2	6	6	6
65+	6	1.2	<1	1	1	1	1	2	2	2
2. MULTIPLE DX										
A. Not Operated										
0–19 Years	2	1.5	<1	1	1	1	2	2	2	2
20–34	14	2.8	6	1	1	1	4	7	8	8
35–49	39	2.8	13	1	1	2	3	4	8	23
50–64	108	2.8	6	1	1	2	3	5	8	14
65+	198	3.1	8	1	1	2	4	7	8	13
B. Operated										
0–19 Years	5	2.2	5	1	1	1	2	6	6	6
20–34	30	3.5	7	2	2	3	5	7	10	10
35–49	78	2.5	7	1	1	2	3	5	7	18
50–64	266	2.4	6	1	1	1	3	5	7	12
65+	469	2.7	8	1	1	2	3	6	8	15
SUBTOTALS:										
1. SINGLE DX										
A. Not Operated	0									
B. Operated	12	1.6	2	1	1	1	2	2	6	6
2. MULTIPLE DX										
A. Not Operated	361	3.0	8	1	1	2	4	6	8	14
B. Operated	848	2.6	7	1	1	2	3	6	8	13
1. SINGLE DX	12	1.6	2	1	1	1	2	2	6	6
2. MULTIPLE DX	1,209	2.7	7	1	1	2	3	6	8	13
A. NOT OPERATED	361	3.0	8	1	1	2	4	6	8	14
B. OPERATED	860	2.6	7	1	1	2	3	6	8	13
TOTAL										
0–19 Years	7	2.0	3	1	1	1	2	6	6	6
20–34	45	3.2	7	1	1	2	4	7	8	10
35–49	117	2.6	9	1	1	2	3	4	7	18
50–64	379	2.5	6	1	1	2	3	5	8	13
65+	673	2.8	8	1	1	2	3	6	8	14
GRAND TOTAL	1,221	2.7	7	1	1	2	3	6	8	13

996.1: MECH COMP OTH VASC DEV

Type of Patients	Observed Patients	Avg. Stay	Vari-ance	10th	25th	50th	75th	90th	95th	99th
1. SINGLE DX										
A. Not Operated										
0–19 Years	0									
20–34	0									
35–49	0									
50–64	0									
65+	3	1.0	0	1	1	1	1	1	1	1
B. Operated										
0–19 Years	0									
20–34	1	9.0	0	9	9	9	9	9	9	9
35–49	2	2.0	2	1	1	1	3	3	3	3
50–64										
65+	5	1.6	<1	1	1	2	2	2	2	2
2. MULTIPLE DX										
A. Not Operated										
0–19 Years	81	3.1	9	1	1	2	4	7	9	18
20–34	54	3.4	11	1	1	2	4	7	12	15
35–49	150	2.8	8	1	1	2	3	6	9	17
50–64	204	3.0	8	1	1	2	4	6	8	16
65+	277	3.4	15	1	1	2	4	7	9	24
B. Operated										
0–19 Years	15	4.9	28	1	1	3	7	7	22	22
20–34	32	4.1	20	1	2	3	5	9	10	24
35–49	106	4.4	26	1	1	3	5	10	15	22
50–64	183	4.6	25	1	1	3	5	10	15	27
65+	401	4.7	34	1	2	3	6	11	17	28
SUBTOTALS:										
1. SINGLE DX										
A. Not Operated	3	1.0	0	1	1	1	1	1	1	1
B. Operated	8	2.6	7	1	1	2	2	9	9	9
2. MULTIPLE DX										
A. Not Operated	766	3.2	11	1	1	2	4	7	9	17
B. Operated	737	4.6	30	1	1	3	6	10	16	28
1. SINGLE DX	11	2.2	6	1	1	1	2	3	9	9
2. MULTIPLE DX	1,503	3.9	21	1	1	2	5	8	12	24
A. NOT OPERATED	769	3.2	11	1	1	2	4	7	9	17
B. OPERATED	745	4.6	29	1	1	3	6	10	16	28
TOTAL										
0–19 Years	96	3.4	12	1	1	2	4	7	10	22
20–34	87	3.7	14	1	1	2	5	9	11	24
35–49	258	3.5	16	1	1	2	4	7	11	19
50–64	387	3.8	17	1	1	2	4	8	12	20
65+	686	4.2	26	1	1	2	5	9	14	28
GRAND TOTAL	1,514	3.9	21	1	1	2	5	8	12	24

Length of Stay by Diagnosis and Operation, Western Region, 2008

Western Region, October 2006–September 2007 Data, by Diagnosis

996.2: MECH COMP NERV SYST DEV

Type of Patients	Observed Patients	Avg. Stay	Variance	10th	25th	50th	75th	90th	95th	99th
1. SINGLE DX										
A. *Not Operated*										
0–19 Years	1	1.0	0	1	1	1	1	1	1	1
20–34	0									
35–49	1	4.0	0	4	4	4	4	4	4	4
50–64	0									
65+	0									
B. *Operated*										
0–19 Years	10	1.7	<1	1	1	2	2	3	3	3
20–34	14	2.8	6	1	1	2	4	7	8	8
35–49	6	2.7	7	1	1	2	2	8	8	8
50–64	4	2.3	6	1	1	1	1	6	6	6
65+	3	1.3	<1	1	1	1	2	2	2	2
2. MULTIPLE DX										
A. *Not Operated*										
0–19 Years	62	3.3	30	1	1	2	3	5	6	33
20–34	56	2.6	6	1	1	2	3	5	8	14
35–49	58	2.9	6	1	1	2	3	7	8	12
50–64	58	3.8	20	1	1	2	4	7	17	26
65+	45	5.5	30	1	1	4	7	13	17	27
B. *Operated*										
0–19 Years	461	4.4	34	1	1	3	5	9	13	38
20–34	456	4.6	28	1	2	3	5	10	14	27
35–49	390	4.6	45	1	1	3	5	10	14	29
50–64	359	5.1	75	1	1	2	5	12	18	50
65+	280	3.9	20	1	1	2	5	10	13	22
SUBTOTALS:										
1. SINGLE DX										
A. *Not Operated*	2	2.5	4	1	1	3	4	4	4	4
B. *Operated*	37	2.3	4	1	1	2	2	6	8	8
2. MULTIPLE DX										
A. *Not Operated*	279	3.5	19	1	1	2	4	7	12	27
B. *Operated*	1,946	4.5	40	1	1	2	5	10	15	29
1. SINGLE DX	39	2.3	4	1	1	2	3	6	8	8
2. MULTIPLE DX	2,225	4.4	38	1	1	2	5	10	14	29
A. NOT OPERATED	281	3.5	19	1	1	2	4	7	11	27
B. OPERATED	1,983	4.5	40	1	1	2	5	10	14	29
TOTAL										
0–19 Years	534	4.2	33	1	1	2	4	9	12	33
20–34	526	4.4	26	1	1	3	5	10	13	26
35–49	455	4.3	40	1	1	2	5	9	14	29
50–64	421	4.9	67	1	1	2	5	11	18	42
65+	328	4.1	21	1	1	2	5	10	14	22
GRAND TOTAL	2,264	4.4	37	1	1	2	5	10	14	29

996.31: MECH COMP URETHRAL CATH

Type of Patients	Observed Patients	Avg. Stay	Variance	10th	25th	50th	75th	90th	95th	99th
1. SINGLE DX										
A. *Not Operated*										
0–19 Years	1	1.0	0	1	1	1	1	1	1	1
20–34	0									
35–49	0									
50–64	1	1.0	0	1	1	1	1	1	1	1
65+	0									
B. *Operated*										
0–19 Years	0									
20–34	0									
35–49	0									
50–64	0									
65+	0									
2. MULTIPLE DX										
A. *Not Operated*										
0–19 Years	3	1.3	<1	1	1	1	2	2	2	2
20–34	11	2.1	2	1	1	2	3	3	5	5
35–49	21	3.2	6	1	1	2	5	7	8	8
50–64	29	3.4	5	1	2	3	4	7	8	12
65+	133	4.0	14	1	2	3	5	8	12	17
B. *Operated*										
0–19 Years	0									
20–34	1	3.0	0	3	3	3	3	3	3	3
35–49	1	5.0	0	5	5	5	5	5	5	5
50–64	6	4.0	4	2	3	3	6	7	7	7
65+	17	3.5	6	1	1	3	4	8	10	10
SUBTOTALS:										
1. SINGLE DX										
A. *Not Operated*	2	1.0	0	1	1	1	1	1	1	1
B. *Operated*	0									
2. MULTIPLE DX										
A. *Not Operated*	197	3.7	11	1	2	3	5	8	10	17
B. *Operated*	25	3.7	5	1	3	3	4	7	8	10
1. SINGLE DX	2	1.0	0	1	1	1	1	1	1	1
2. MULTIPLE DX	222	3.7	10	1	2	3	5	8	10	16
A. NOT OPERATED	199	3.7	11	1	2	3	5	8	10	17
B. OPERATED	25	3.7	5	1	3	3	4	7	8	10
TOTAL										
0–19 Years	4	1.3	<1	1	1	1	2	2	2	2
20–34	12	2.2	1	1	1	2	3	3	5	5
35–49	22	3.3	5	1	1	2	5	7	8	8
50–64	36	3.5	5	1	2	3	4	7	8	12
65+	150	4.0	13	1	2	3	5	8	11	17
GRAND TOTAL	224	3.7	10	1	2	3	4	8	10	16

996.39: MALFUNCT GU DEV/GRFT NEC

Type of Patients	Observed Patients	Avg. Stay	Variance	10th	25th	50th	75th	90th	95th	99th
1. SINGLE DX										
A. *Not Operated*										
0–19 Years	1	1.0	0	1	1	1	1	1	1	1
20–34	3	1.0	0	1	1	1	1	1	1	1
35–49	0									
50–64	1	4.0	0	4	4	4	4	4	4	4
65+	0									
B. *Operated*										
0–19 Years	1	1.0	0	1	1	1	1	1	1	1
20–34	1	1.0	0	1	1	1	1	1	1	1
35–49	2	1.5	<1	1	1	2	2	2	2	2
50–64	5	1.0	0	1	1	1	1	1	1	1
65+	6	1.0	0	1	1	1	1	1	1	1
2. MULTIPLE DX										
A. *Not Operated*										
0–19 Years	6	3.0	5	1	2	2	2	7	7	7
20–34	41	2.3	2	1	1	2	3	4	5	6
35–49	88	3.6	15	1	1	2	5	9	12	21
50–64	102	3.5	12	1	2	3	4	6	8	14
65+	153	4.2	12	1	2	3	6	9	11	17
B. *Operated*										
0–19 Years	2	4.5	24	1	1	8	8	8	8	8
20–34	14	4.3	7	1	2	5	6	8	10	10
35–49	50	3.2	13	1	1	2	4	11	12	15
50–64	97	3.0	15	1	1	3	3	8	13	18
65+	241	2.6	11	1	1	1	3	6	9	17
SUBTOTALS:										
1. SINGLE DX										
A. *Not Operated*	5	1.6	2	1	1	1	1	4	4	4
B. *Operated*	15	1.1	<1	1	1	1	1	1	2	2
2. MULTIPLE DX										
A. *Not Operated*	390	3.7	12	1	1	3	4	8	10	18
B. *Operated*	404	2.9	12	1	1	1	3	7	11	17
1. SINGLE DX	20	1.2	<1	1	1	1	1	2	2	4
2. MULTIPLE DX	794	3.3	12	1	1	2	4	7	10	17
A. NOT OPERATED	395	3.6	12	1	1	3	4	8	10	18
B. OPERATED	419	2.8	12	1	1	1	3	7	11	17
TOTAL										
0–19 Years	10	2.9	7	1	1	2	4	8	8	8
20–34	59	2.7	4	1	1	2	3	6	6	10
35–49	140	3.4	14	1	1	2	4	9	12	18
50–64	205	3.2	13	1	2	2	4	7	9	17
65+	400	3.2	12	1	1	2	4	7	11	17
GRAND TOTAL	814	3.2	12	1	1	2	4	7	10	17

Western Region, October 2006–September 2007 Data, by Diagnosis

996.41: MECH LOOSENING JT PROSTH

Type of Patients	Observed Patients	Avg. Stay	Vari-ance	10th	25th	50th	75th	90th	95th	99th
1. SINGLE DX										
A. *Not Operated*										
0–19 Years	0									
20–34	0									
35–49	0									
50–64	0									
65+	0									
B. *Operated*										
0–19 Years	0									
20–34	0									
35–49	4	2.5	1	1	1	3	3	3	3	3
50–64	15	2.7	<1	1	2	3	3	4	4	4
65+	10	3.1	1	2	2	3	3	5	5	5
2. MULTIPLE DX										
A. *Not Operated*										
0–19 Years	0									
20–34	1	3.0	0	3	3	3	3	3	3	3
35–49	3	2.7	8	1	1	1	6	6	6	6
50–64	12	4.2	14	2	2	3	4	6	15	15
65+	45	3.2	5	1	2	3	4	6	7	10
B. *Operated*										
0–19 Years	0									
20–34	17	7.7	126	1	3	4	6	14	49	49
35–49	158	3.8	4	2	3	3	4	6	7	13
50–64	762	3.6	4	2	3	3	4	5	7	10
65+	1,416	4.2	7	2	3	4	5	7	8	15
SUBTOTALS:										
1. SINGLE DX										
A. *Not Operated*	0									
B. *Operated*	29	2.8	<1	1	2	3	3	4	5	5
2. MULTIPLE DX										
A. *Not Operated*	61	3.4	7	1	2	3	4	6	7	15
B. *Operated*	2,353	4.0	7	2	3	3	5	6	8	14
1. SINGLE DX	29	2.8	<1	1	2	3	4	4	5	5
2. MULTIPLE DX	2,414	4.0	7	2	3	3	5	6	8	14
A. NOT OPERATED	61	3.4	7	1	2	3	4	6	7	15
B. OPERATED	2,382	4.0	7	2	3	4	4	6	8	14
TOTAL										
0–19 Years	0									
20–34	18	7.4	119	1	3	4	6	14	49	49
35–49	165	3.7	4	2	3	3	4	6	7	13
50–64	789	3.6	4	2	3	3	4	5	7	10
65+	1,471	4.2	7	2	3	4	5	7	8	15
GRAND TOTAL	2,443	4.0	7	2	3	3	4	6	8	14

996.42: DISLOCATION JOINT PROSTH

Type of Patients	Observed Patients	Avg. Stay	Vari-ance	10th	25th	50th	75th	90th	95th	99th
1. SINGLE DX										
A. *Not Operated*										
0–19 Years	0									
20–34	0									
35–49	0									
50–64	10	1.0	0	1	1	1	1	1	1	1
65+	9	1.4	<1	1	1	1	2	2	2	2
B. *Operated*										
0–19 Years	0									
20–34	1	2.0	0	2	2	2	2	2	2	2
35–49	7	6.2	27	2	2	4	12	15	15	15
50–64	14	3.4	10	2	2	3	3	4	14	14
65+	13	2.9	1	1	3	3	4	4	4	4
2. MULTIPLE DX										
A. *Not Operated*										
0–19 Years	2	2.0	2	1	1	1	3	3	3	3
20–34	3	2.3	2	1	1	2	4	4	4	4
35–49	87	1.8	2	1	1	1	2	4	5	6
50–64	334	2.3	6	1	1	2	3	5	6	13
65+	989	2.8	9	1	1	2	3	5	7	14
B. *Operated*										
0–19 Years	1	1.0	0	1	1	1	1	1	1	1
20–34	16	4.1	7	1	2	4	5	8	10	10
35–49	149	4.2	17	2	2	3	5	6	8	30
50–64	661	4.4	19	2	3	3	5	7	9	20
65+	1,419	5.0	16	2	3	4	6	9	12	19
SUBTOTALS:										
1. SINGLE DX										
A. *Not Operated*	19	1.2	<1	1	1	1	1	2	2	2
B. *Operated*	35	3.7	11	2	2	3	4	5	14	15
2. MULTIPLE DX										
A. *Not Operated*	1,415	2.6	8	1	1	2	3	5	7	13
B. *Operated*	2,246	4.7	17	2	3	4	5	8	11	20
1. SINGLE DX	54	2.8	8	1	1	2	3	4	12	15
2. MULTIPLE DX	3,661	3.9	14	1	2	3	5	7	9	18
A. NOT OPERATED	1,434	2.6	8	1	1	2	3	5	7	13
B. OPERATED	2,281	4.7	17	2	3	4	5	8	11	20
TOTAL										
0–19 Years	3	1.7	1	1	1	1	1	3	3	3
20–34	20	3.7	7	1	2	3	5	8	10	10
35–49	243	3.4	13	1	1	3	4	6	8	18
50–64	1,019	3.6	16	1	2	3	4	5	8	16
65+	2,430	4.1	14	2	3	4	5	7	10	18
GRAND TOTAL	3,715	3.9	14	2	3	3	5	7	9	18

996.43: PROSTH JOINT FAILURE

Type of Patients	Observed Patients	Avg. Stay	Vari-ance	10th	25th	50th	75th	90th	95th	99th
1. SINGLE DX										
A. *Not Operated*										
0–19 Years	0									
20–34	0									
35–49	0									
50–64	0									
65+	0									
B. *Operated*										
0–19 Years	0									
20–34	0									
35–49	4	3.8	<1	3	4	4	4	4	4	4
50–64	13	2.4	2	1	2	2	3	3	7	7
65+	8	3.3	2	1	3	3	3	5	5	5
2. MULTIPLE DX										
A. *Not Operated*										
0–19 Years	0									
20–34	0									
35–49	0									
50–64	10	3.2	7	1	1	2	4	7	9	9
65+	34	3.3	9	1	1	3	4	5	7	18
B. *Operated*										
0–19 Years	3	5.3	10	3	3	4	9	9	9	9
20–34	24	3.9	10	2	2	3	4	8	12	14
35–49	141	4.5	14	2	3	3	5	8	10	23
50–64	522	3.7	4	2	3	3	4	6	7	11
65+	922	4.1	9	2	3	3	4	6	8	17
SUBTOTALS:										
1. SINGLE DX										
A. *Not Operated*	0									
B. *Operated*	25	2.9	2	1	2	3	3	5	5	7
2. MULTIPLE DX										
A. *Not Operated*	44	3.3	9	1	1	3	4	6	7	18
B. *Operated*	1,612	4.0	8	2	3	3	4	6	8	15
1. SINGLE DX	25	2.9	2	1	2	3	3	5	5	7
2. MULTIPLE DX	1,656	4.0	8	2	3	3	4	6	8	16
A. NOT OPERATED	44	3.3	9	1	1	3	4	6	7	18
B. OPERATED	1,637	4.0	8	2	3	3	4	6	8	15
TOTAL										
0–19 Years	3	5.3	10	3	3	4	9	9	9	9
20–34	24	3.9	10	2	2	3	4	8	12	14
35–49	145	4.5	13	2	3	3	4	5	10	23
50–64	545	3.6	4	2	3	3	4	6	7	11
65+	964	4.1	9	2	3	3	4	6	8	17
GRAND TOTAL	1,681	4.0	8	2	3	3	4	6	8	16

Length of Stay by Diagnosis and Operation, Western Region, 2008

Western Region, October 2006–September 2007 Data, by Diagnosis

996.44: PERI-PROSTHETIC FRACTURE

Type of Patients	Observed Patients	Avg. Stay	Variance	Percentiles 10th	25th	50th	75th	90th	95th	99th
1. SINGLE DX										
A. *Not Operated*										
0–19 Years	0									
20–34	0									
35–49	0									
50–64	0									
65+	1	5.0	0	5	5	5	5	5	5	5
B. *Operated*										
0–19 Years	0									
20–34	0									
35–49	0									
50–64	1	9.0	0	9	9	9	9	9	9	9
65+	1	5.0	0	5	5	5	5	5	5	5
2. MULTIPLE DX										
A. *Not Operated*										
0–19 Years	0									
20–34	0									
35–49	3	4.7	9	2	2	4	8	8	8	8
50–64	28	5.1	13	1	2	5	6	11	13	13
65+	204	4.2	9	2	3	3	5	7	10	14
B. *Operated*										
0–19 Years	3	4.3	1	3	3	5	5	5	5	5
20–34	7	5.3	10	2	3	5	7	11	11	11
35–49	43	5.1	9	2	3	4	6	9	11	17
50–64	203	6.3	55	3	4	5	7	11	13	21
65+	965	6.4	14	3	4	6	8	11	13	21
SUBTOTALS:										
1. SINGLE DX										
A. *Not Operated*	1	5.0	0	5	5	5	5	5	5	5
B. *Operated*	3	6.4	5	5	5	5	9	9	9	9
2. MULTIPLE DX										
A. *Not Operated*	235	4.3	9	2	3	3	5	8	10	14
B. *Operated*	1,221	6.3	21	3	4	5	7	10	13	21
1. SINGLE DX	4	6.0	4	5	5	5	9	9	10	21
2. MULTIPLE DX	1,456	6.0	19	3	4	5	7	10	13	21
A. NOT OPERATED	236	4.3	9	2	3	3	5	8	10	14
B. OPERATED	1,224	6.3	20	3	4	5	7	10	13	21
TOTAL										
0–19 Years	3	4.3	1	3	3	5	5	5	5	5
20–34	8	5.8	10	2	3	6	9	11	11	11
35–49	46	5.1	9	2	3	4	6	9	11	17
50–64	232	6.2	50	3	4	5	7	11	13	21
65+	1,171	6.0	14	3	4	6	8	11	12	21
GRAND TOTAL	1,460	6.0	19	3	4	5	7	10	13	21

996.45: PERI-PROSTH OSTEOLYSIS

Type of Patients	Observed Patients	Avg. Stay	Variance	Percentiles 10th	25th	50th	75th	90th	95th	99th
1. SINGLE DX										
A. *Not Operated*										
0–19 Years	0									
20–34	0									
35–49	0									
50–64	0									
65+	0									
B. *Operated*										
0–19 Years	0									
20–34	0									
35–49	0									
50–64	1	2.0	0	2	2	2	2	2	2	2
65+	2	7.5	<1	7	7	8	8	8	8	8
2. MULTIPLE DX										
A. *Not Operated*										
0–19 Years	0									
20–34	0									
35–49	0									
50–64	0									
65+	7	4.0	8	1	1	4	6	8	8	8
B. *Operated*										
0–19 Years	1	39.0	0	39	39	39	39	39	39	39
20–34	4	3.5	<1	3	3	3	4	5	5	5
35–49	37	3.6	3	2	2	3	4	5	8	10
50–64	125	3.1	1	2	2	3	4	5	5	7
65+	213	4.2	11	2	3	3	4	7	9	11
SUBTOTALS:										
1. SINGLE DX										
A. *Not Operated*	0									
B. *Operated*	3	5.6	10	2	2	7	8	8	8	8
2. MULTIPLE DX										
A. *Not Operated*	7	4.0	8	1	1	4	6	8	8	8
B. *Operated*	380	3.9	10	2	3	3	4	6	8	11
1. SINGLE DX	3	5.6	10	2	2	7	8	8	8	8
2. MULTIPLE DX	387	3.9	10	2	3	3	4	6	8	11
A. NOT OPERATED	7	4.0	8	1	1	4	6	8	8	8
B. OPERATED	383	3.9	10	2	3	3	4	6	8	11
TOTAL										
0–19 Years	1	39.0	0	39	39	39	39	39	39	39
20–34	4	3.5	<1	3	3	3	4	5	5	5
35–49	37	3.6	3	2	2	3	4	5	8	10
50–64	126	3.1	1	2	2	3	4	5	5	7
65+	222	4.2	11	2	3	3	4	7	9	11
GRAND TOTAL	390	3.9	10	2	3	3	4	6	8	11

996.46: JT PROSTH SURFACE WEAR

Type of Patients	Observed Patients	Avg. Stay	Variance	Percentiles 10th	25th	50th	75th	90th	95th	99th
1. SINGLE DX										
A. *Not Operated*										
0–19 Years	0									
20–34	0									
35–49	0									
50–64	0									
65+	0									
B. *Operated*										
0–19 Years	0									
20–34	0									
35–49	0									
50–64	1	3.0	0	3	3	3	3	3	3	3
65+	1	2.0	0	2	2	2	2	2	2	2
2. MULTIPLE DX										
A. *Not Operated*										
0–19 Years	0									
20–34	0									
35–49	2	1.0	0	1	1	1	1	1	1	1
50–64	2	5.0	32	1	1	9	9	9	9	9
65+	3	1.0	0	1	1	1	1	1	1	1
B. *Operated*										
0–19 Years	0									
20–34	10	3.0	2	1	2	3	4	4	6	6
35–49	55	3.5	3	2	2	3	4	6	6	11
50–64	143	3.2	3	2	2	3	4	5	5	8
65+	403	3.5	2	2	3	3	4	5	6	9
SUBTOTALS:										
1. SINGLE DX										
A. *Not Operated*	0									
B. *Operated*	2	2.5	<1	2	2	2	3	3	3	3
2. MULTIPLE DX										
A. *Not Operated*	7	2.2	9	1	1	1	1	9	9	9
B. *Operated*	611	3.4	2	2	3	3	4	5	6	9
1. SINGLE DX	2	2.5	<1	2	2	2	3	3	3	3
2. MULTIPLE DX	618	3.4	2	2	3	3	4	5	6	9
A. NOT OPERATED	7	2.2	9	1	1	1	1	9	9	9
B. OPERATED	613	3.4	2	2	3	3	4	5	6	9
TOTAL										
0–19 Years	0									
20–34	10	3.0	2	1	2	3	4	4	6	6
35–49	57	3.4	3	2	2	3	4	6	6	11
50–64	146	3.2	3	2	2	3	4	5	5	9
65+	407	3.5	2	2	3	3	4	5	6	9
GRAND TOTAL	620	3.4	2	2	3	3	4	5	6	9

Western Region, October 2006–September 2007 Data, by Diagnosis

996.47: MECH COMP JT PROSTH NEC

Type of Patients	Observed Patients	Avg. Stay	Vari-ance	10th	25th	50th	75th	90th	95th	99th
1. SINGLE DX										
A. *Not Operated*										
0–19 Years	0									
20–34	0									
35–49	1	3.0	0		3	3	3	3	3	3
50–64	0									
65+	0									
B. *Operated*										
0–19 Years	0									
20–34	0									
35–49	5	2.4	<1	1	2	3	3	3	3	3
50–64	8	2.8	2	1	2	3	4	5	5	5
65+	8	3.6	2	2	3	3	5	6	6	6
2. MULTIPLE DX										
A. *Not Operated*										
0–19 Years	0									
20–34	0									
35–49	8	1.6	<1	1	1	1	3	3	3	3
50–64	21	1.8	1	1	1	1	2	3	3	5
65+	37	3.0	9	1	1	2	3	5	11	14
B. *Operated*										
0–19 Years	2	4.0	2	3	3	3	5	5	5	5
20–34	12	4.6	13	2	2	3	5	9	13	13
35–49	100	3.6	4	2	2	3	4	6	8	14
50–64	369	3.6	7	2	3	3	4	5	7	17
65+	575	4.0	5	2	3	3	4	6	8	13
SUBTOTALS:										
1. SINGLE DX										
A. *Not Operated*	1	3.0	0	3	3	3	3	3	3	3
B. *Operated*	21	3.0	2	1	2	3	3	5	5	5
2. MULTIPLE DX										
A. *Not Operated*	66	2.4	6	1	1	2	3	4	5	14
B. *Operated*	1,058	3.8	6	2	3	3	4	6	8	14
1. SINGLE DX	22	3.0	2	1	2	3	4	5	5	6
2. MULTIPLE DX	1,124	3.8	6	2	3	3	4	6	8	14
A. NOT OPERATED	67	2.4	6	1	1	2	3	4	5	14
B. OPERATED	1,079	3.8	6	2	3	3	4	6	8	14
TOTAL										
0–19 Years	2	4.0	2	3	3	3	3	5	5	5
20–34	12	4.6	13	2	2	3	5	9	13	13
35–49	114	3.4	4	1	2	3	4	6	7	10
50–64	398	3.5	7	1	2	3	4	5	6	17
65+	620	3.9	5	2	3	3	5	6	8	13
GRAND TOTAL	1,146	3.7	6	2	3	3	4	6	8	14

996.49: MECH COMP INT ORTH NEC

Type of Patients	Observed Patients	Avg. Stay	Vari-ance	10th	25th	50th	75th	90th	95th	99th
1. SINGLE DX										
A. *Not Operated*										
0–19 Years	1	1.0	0	1	1	1	1	1	1	1
20–34	0									
35–49	2	1.5	<1	1	1	1	2	2	2	2
50–64	4	2.3	2	1	1	2	4	4	4	4
65+	2	1.5	<1	1	1	1	2	2	2	2
B. *Operated*										
0–19 Years	7	2.1	1	1	1	2	3	4	4	4
20–34	31	2.4	12	1	1	1	3	3	5	20
35–49	68	2.4	2	1	1	2	3	4	5	6
50–64	64	2.5	2	1	2	2	3	4	5	7
65+	30	2.2	1	1	1	2	3	4	4	5
2. MULTIPLE DX										
A. *Not Operated*										
0–19 Years	3	3.3	16	1	1	1	8	8	8	8
20–34	18	2.6	6	1	1	2	3	4	12	12
35–49	31	3.4	11	1	1	2	4	8	11	13
50–64	66	3.5	11	1	1	2	6	9	11	13
65+	97	3.9	15	1	1	3	5	9	11	22
B. *Operated*										
0–19 Years	94	4.1	51	1	1	3	4	7	10	63
20–34	274	3.8	15	1	1	3	4	8	11	22
35–49	920	3.6	15	1	2	3	4	6	10	18
50–64	1,688	4.0	18	1	2	3	5	7	10	21
65+	1,852	4.5	12	2	3	4	6	8	11	19
SUBTOTALS:										
1. SINGLE DX										
A. *Not Operated*	9	1.8	<1	1	1	2	2	4	4	4
B. *Operated*	200	2.4	3	1	1	2	3	4	5	6
2. MULTIPLE DX										
A. *Not Operated*	215	3.6	12	1	1	2	5	8	11	14
B. *Operated*	4,828	4.1	15	1	2	3	5	7	10	20
1. SINGLE DX	209	2.4	3	1	1	2	3	4	5	6
2. MULTIPLE DX	5,043	4.1	15	1	2	3	5	8	10	20
A. NOT OPERATED	224	3.5	12	1	1	2	4	8	11	14
B. OPERATED	5,028	4.1	15	1	2	3	5	7	10	20
TOTAL										
0–19 Years	105	4.0	46	1	1	3	4	7	9	29
20–34	323	3.6	14	1	1	3	4	7	11	20
35–49	1,021	3.5	14	1	2	3	4	6	9	18
50–64	1,822	4.0	17	1	2	3	4	7	10	20
65+	1,981	4.5	12	2	3	4	5	8	11	19
GRAND TOTAL	5,252	4.0	15	1	2	3	5	7	10	20

996.56: MECH COMP PD CATH

Type of Patients	Observed Patients	Avg. Stay	Vari-ance	10th	25th	50th	75th	90th	95th	99th
1. SINGLE DX										
A. *Not Operated*										
0–19 Years	0									
20–34	0									
35–49	0									
50–64	0									
65+	0									
B. *Operated*										
0–19 Years	0									
20–34	0									
35–49	0									
50–64	0									
65+	0									
2. MULTIPLE DX										
A. *Not Operated*										
0–19 Years	8	4.5	26	1	1	4	6	16	16	16
20–34	14	3.8	7	1	2	4	5	6	9	9
35–49	22	2.9	13	1	1	1	2	9	10	15
50–64	30	3.9	12	1	1	2	6	7	8	17
65+	27	3.9	5	1	2	4	6	7	7	8
B. *Operated*										
0–19 Years	12	4.3	7	2	3	4	5	9	10	10
20–34	20	3.9	6	1	1	3	6	8	9	9
35–49	37	4.6	17	1	2	3	5	11	14	20
50–64	49	5.2	23	1	1	4	8	12	14	22
65+	34	6.5	35	1	2	4	10	17	19	21
SUBTOTALS:										
1. SINGLE DX										
A. *Not Operated*	0									
B. *Operated*	0									
2. MULTIPLE DX										
A. *Not Operated*	101	3.7	10	1	1	3	5	7	9	17
B. *Operated*	152	5.1	21	1	2	4	7	11	16	21
1. SINGLE DX	0									
2. MULTIPLE DX	253	4.6	17	2	2	3	6	9	14	20
A. NOT OPERATED	101	3.7	10	1	1	3	5	7	9	17
B. OPERATED	152	5.1	21	1	2	4	7	11	16	21
TOTAL										
0–19 Years	20	4.4	14	1	1	4	6	10	13	16
20–34	34	3.9	6	1	2	3	5	8	9	9
35–49	59	4.0	16	1	1	2	5	10	14	20
50–64	79	4.7	19	1	2	4	7	12	14	22
65+	61	5.4	23	1	2	4	7	12	17	21
GRAND TOTAL	253	4.6	17	2	3	3	6	9	14	20

Length of Stay by Diagnosis and Operation, Western Region, 2008

Western Region, October 2006–September 2007 Data, by Diagnosis

996.59: MECH COMP DEV/GRAFT NEC

Type of Patients	Observed Patients	Avg. Stay	Variance	10th	25th	50th	75th	90th	95th	99th
1. SINGLE DX										
A. Not Operated										
0–19 Years	0									
20–34	3	3.3	6	1	1	3	6	6	6	6
35–49	1	1.0	0	1	1	1	1	1	1	1
50–64	3	1.3	<1	1	1	1	2	2	2	2
65+	1	2.0	0	2	2	2	2	2	2	2
B. Operated										
0–19 Years	2	1.5	<1	1	1	2	2	2	2	2
20–34	3	1.0	0	1	1	1	1	1	1	1
35–49	2	1.0	0	1	1	1	1	1	1	1
50–64	1	1.0	0	1	1	1	1	1	1	1
65+	1	1.0	0	1	1	1	1	1	1	1
2. MULTIPLE DX										
A. Not Operated										
0–19 Years	27	2.7	6	1	1	1	4	8	8	9
20–34	55	3.4	11	1	1	2	4	6	13	17
35–49	117	3.6	10	1	1	3	4	8	9	12
50–64	259	4.2	13	2	2	3	5	8	10	20
65+	387	4.2	11	2	2	3	5	8	10	17
B. Operated										
0–19 Years	11	4.0	16	1	2	2	5	9	14	14
20–34	55	4.8	53	1	2	2	5	11	18	46
35–49	88	3.9	21	1	2	2	4	8	14	26
50–64	162	4.9	46	1	3	3	6	12	16	30
65+	110	8.0	130	2	2	5	10	19	22	44
SUBTOTALS:										
1. SINGLE DX										
A. Not Operated	8	2.1	3	1	1	2	3	6	6	6
B. Operated	9	1.1	<1	1	1	1	1	2	2	2
2. MULTIPLE DX										
A. Not Operated	845	4.0	12	1	2	3	5	8	10	17
B. Operated	426	5.4	65	1	1	3	6	13	19	30
1. SINGLE DX	17	1.6	2	1	1	1	2	3	6	6
2. MULTIPLE DX	1,271	4.5	30	1	2	3	5	9	13	24
A. NOT OPERATED	853	4.0	12	1	2	3	5	8	10	17
B. OPERATED	435	5.4	64	1	1	3	6	13	19	30
TOTAL										
0–19 Years	40	3.0	9	1	1	2	4	8	9	14
20–34	116	4.0	31	1	1	2	4	10	13	24
35–49	208	3.7	15	1	2	2	4	8	11	22
50–64	425	4.5	26	1	2	3	5	10	13	25
65+	499	5.0	40	1	2	4	6	10	15	27
GRAND TOTAL	1,288	4.5	30	1	2	3	5	9	13	24

996.61: INFECT D/T HEART DEVICE

Type of Patients	Observed Patients	Avg. Stay	Variance	10th	25th	50th	75th	90th	95th	99th
1. SINGLE DX										
A. Not Operated										
0–19 Years	0									
20–34	0									
35–49	0									
50–64	0									
65+	0									
B. Operated										
0–19 Years	0									
20–34	1	3.0	0	3	3	3	3	3	3	3
35–49	1	1.0	0	1	1	1	1	1	1	1
50–64	2	1.5	<1	1	1	2	2	2	2	2
65+	2	2.0	0	2	2	2	2	2	2	2
2. MULTIPLE DX										
A. Not Operated										
0–19 Years	1	7.0	0	7	7	7	7	7	7	7
20–34	11	11.1	43	5	5	10	20	20	22	22
35–49	45	8.8	162	1	3	5	9	19	35	72
50–64	104	8.3	70	2	3	6	10	19	26	39
65+	313	7.9	37	2	4	6	11	16	20	25
B. Operated										
0–19 Years	3	5.7	4	4	4	5	8	8	8	8
20–34	18	12.1	80	4	8	9	15	29	37	37
35–49	59	13.4	146	3	6	10	15	26	41	67
50–64	159	11.6	109	2	5	8	15	24	30	52
65+	483	9.2	66	2	4	7	11	18	24	43
SUBTOTALS:										
1. SINGLE DX										
A. Not Operated	1	7.0	0	7	7	7	7	7	7	7
B. Operated	6	1.8	<1	1	1	2	2	3	3	3
2. MULTIPLE DX										
A. Not Operated	474	8.2	56	2	4	6	10	17	22	39
B. Operated	722	10.2	84	2	4	8	13	21	28	51
1. SINGLE DX	7	2.6	4	1	1	2	3	7	7	7
2. MULTIPLE DX	1,196	9.4	74	2	4	7	11	19	25	51
A. NOT OPERATED	475	8.2	56	2	4	6	10	17	22	39
B. OPERATED	728	10.1	83	2	4	8	13	21	28	51
TOTAL										
0–19 Years	4	6.0	3	4	5	6	7	8	8	8
20–34	31	11.3	63	4	5	9	15	20	29	37
35–49	105	11.3	156	2	4	8	13	24	35	67
50–64	265	10.2	96	2	4	7	13	23	29	52
65+	798	8.7	55	2	4	7	11	17	22	41
GRAND TOTAL	1,203	9.3	73	2	4	7	11	19	25	51

996.62: INFECT D/T VASC DEVICE

Type of Patients	Observed Patients	Avg. Stay	Variance	10th	25th	50th	75th	90th	95th	99th
1. SINGLE DX										
A. Not Operated										
0–19 Years	1	1.0	0	1	1	1	1	1	1	1
20–34	0									
35–49	1	1.0	0	1	1	1	1	1	1	1
50–64	1	1.0	0	1	1	1	1	1	1	1
65+	0									
B. Operated										
0–19 Years	0									
20–34	0									
35–49	0									
50–64	0									
65+	0									
2. MULTIPLE DX										
A. Not Operated										
0–19 Years	555	8.3	41	2	4	7	11	16	20	30
20–34	846	6.9	39	2	3	5	8	14	18	34
35–49	1,827	6.7	39	2	3	5	8	13	17	31
50–64	2,945	7.3	35	2	4	6	9	14	19	30
65+	3,065	7.8	34	2	4	6	10	15	18	29
B. Operated										
0–19 Years	21	16.2	136	6	8	16	28	>99	>99	>99
20–34	127	11.8	158	3	5	9	13	24	40	57
35–49	398	10.5	86	2	5	8	13	22	28	47
50–64	757	11.6	112	3	5	8	15	25	30	55
65+	905	10.9	77	3	5	9	14	21	27	43
SUBTOTALS:										
1. SINGLE DX										
A. Not Operated	3	1.0	0	1	1	1	1	1	1	1
B. Operated	0									
2. MULTIPLE DX										
A. Not Operated	9,238	7.4	37	2	4	6	9	14	18	30
B. Operated	2,208	11.2	96	3	5	9	14	23	29	51
1. SINGLE DX	3	1.0	0	1	1	1	1	1	1	1
2. MULTIPLE DX	11,446	8.1	50	2	4	6	10	16	21	36
A. NOT OPERATED	9,241	7.4	37	2	4	6	9	14	18	30
B. OPERATED	2,208	11.2	96	3	5	9	14	23	29	51
TOTAL										
0–19 Years	577	8.6	47	2	4	7	11	17	21	51
20–34	973	7.6	57	2	3	6	9	15	21	41
35–49	2,226	7.4	50	2	3	5	9	14	19	34
50–64	3,703	8.2	54	2	4	6	10	16	22	39
65+	3,970	8.5	46	3	4	7	11	16	21	34
GRAND TOTAL	11,449	8.1	50	2	4	6	10	16	21	36

Western Region, October 2006–September 2007 Data, by Diagnosis

996.63: INFECT D/T NERV DEVICE

Type of Patients	Observed Patients	Avg. Stay	Variance	10th	25th	50th	75th	90th	95th	99th
1. SINGLE DX										
A. Not Operated										
0–19 Years	0									
20–34	0									
35–49	0									
50–64	0									
65+	0									
B. Operated										
0–19 Years	0									
20–34	0									
35–49	1	5.0	0	5	5	5	5	5	5	5
50–64	2	1.0	0	1	1	1	1	1	1	1
65+	0									
2. MULTIPLE DX										
A. Not Operated										
0–19 Years	16	5.2	25	1	3	4	6	17	18	18
20–34	20	5.6	19	3	3	4	7	11	12	19
35–49	45	5.4	12	2	3	4	8	11	13	14
50–64	62	6.2	23	2	2	5	10	14	17	21
65+	33	5.6	18	2	2	5	8	10	14	20
B. Operated										
0–19 Years	83	17.8	116	7	10	15	23	31	38	58
20–34	97	13.6	96	3	5	12	18	33	33	51
35–49	119	9.7	127	2	4	6	12	23	27	50
50–64	162	9.9	128	2	3	6	13	21	29	57
65+	117	9.4	113	2	3	5	11	22	30	52
SUBTOTALS:										
1. SINGLE DX										
A. Not Operated	0									
B. Operated	3	2.3	5	1	1	1	5	5	5	5
2. MULTIPLE DX										
A. Not Operated	176	5.7	19	2	3	4	8	12	15	20
B. Operated	578	11.5	126	2	4	8	16	24	31	53
1. SINGLE DX	3	2.3	5	1	1	1	5	5	5	5
2. MULTIPLE DX	754	10.2	107	2	3	6	14	23	29	52
A. NOT OPERATED	176	5.7	19	2	3	4	8	12	15	20
B. OPERATED	581	11.5	126	2	4	8	16	24	31	53
TOTAL										
0–19 Years	99	15.8	123	4	7	14	21	31	38	53
20–34	117	12.2	92	2	5	11	18	24	30	46
35–49	165	8.5	98	2	3	5	10	14	22	50
50–64	226	8.8	101	2	3	5	11	19	26	53
65+	150	8.5	95	2	3	5	10	20	24	52
GRAND TOTAL	757	10.1	107	2	3	6	14	23	29	52

996.64: INFECT D/T URETHRAL CATH

Type of Patients	Observed Patients	Avg. Stay	Variance	10th	25th	50th	75th	90th	95th	99th
1. SINGLE DX										
A. Not Operated										
0–19 Years	0									
20–34	0									
35–49	0									
50–64	0									
65+	0									
B. Operated										
0–19 Years	0									
20–34	0									
35–49	0									
50–64	0									
65+	0									
2. MULTIPLE DX										
A. Not Operated										
0–19 Years	12	4.7	15	1	2	3	5	12	13	13
20–34	127	4.5	12	1	2	4	6	9	10	18
35–49	291	6.2	41	2	3	4	7	11	16	42
50–64	569	5.3	17	2	3	4	6	10	14	24
65+	2,110	5.1	16	2	3	4	6	10	12	20
B. Operated										
0–19 Years	0									
20–34	3	5.3	26	1	1	4	11	11	11	11
35–49	22	16.0	174	3	8	13	23	36	37	55
50–64	27	14.6	191	4	6	9	18	31	34	69
65+	83	11.6	93	4	6	9	15	22	25	64
SUBTOTALS:										
1. SINGLE DX										
A. Not Operated	0									
B. Operated	0									
2. MULTIPLE DX										
A. Not Operated	3,109	5.2	18	2	3	4	6	10	13	22
B. Operated	135	12.8	126	4	6	9	16	25	34	64
1. SINGLE DX	0									
2. MULTIPLE DX	3,244	5.5	25	2	3	4	7	10	14	25
A. NOT OPERATED	3,109	5.2	18	2	3	4	6	10	13	22
B. OPERATED	135	12.8	126	4	6	9	16	25	34	64
TOTAL										
0–19 Years	12	4.7	15	1	2	3	5	12	13	13
20–34	130	4.5	12	1	2	4	6	9	10	18
35–49	313	6.9	56	2	3	5	8	14	22	42
50–64	596	5.7	28	2	3	4	7	11	14	30
65+	2,193	5.4	20	2	3	4	6	10	13	22
GRAND TOTAL	3,244	5.5	25	2	3	4	7	10	14	25

996.65: INFECT D/T GU DEVICE NEC

Type of Patients	Observed Patients	Avg. Stay	Variance	10th	25th	50th	75th	90th	95th	99th
1. SINGLE DX										
A. Not Operated										
0–19 Years	0									
20–34	1	3.0	0	3	3	3	3	3	3	3
35–49	0									
50–64	0									
65+	0									
B. Operated										
0–19 Years	0									
20–34	0									
35–49	0									
50–64	0									
65+	1	1.0	0	1	1	1	1	1	1	1
2. MULTIPLE DX										
A. Not Operated										
0–19 Years	9	3.3	7	1	2	2	5	9	9	9
20–34	66	5.2	32	2	2	4	6	9	12	33
35–49	104	5.7	22	2	3	4	7	11	15	20
50–64	122	6.0	29	2	3	4	7	11	17	27
65+	248	5.1	15	2	3	4	6	10	13	18
B. Operated										
0–19 Years	0									
20–34	16	7.9	51	2	4	7	8	20	27	27
35–49	34	5.8	44	1	2	4	6	10	27	33
50–64	58	8.3	104	3	3	5	10	23	36	53
65+	132	5.8	37	1	2	4	7	14	19	29
SUBTOTALS:										
1. SINGLE DX										
A. Not Operated	1	3.0	0	3	3	3	3	3	3	3
B. Operated	1	1.0	0	1	1	1	1	1	1	1
2. MULTIPLE DX										
A. Not Operated	549	5.4	22	2	3	4	6	10	14	27
B. Operated	240	6.5	56	1	2	4	8	15	23	36
1. SINGLE DX	2	2.0	2	1	1	1	3	3	3	3
2. MULTIPLE DX	789	5.7	32	2	2	4	7	11	18	30
A. NOT OPERATED	550	5.4	22	2	3	4	6	10	14	27
B. OPERATED	241	6.5	55	1	2	4	8	15	23	36
TOTAL										
0–19 Years	9	3.3	7	1	2	2	5	9	9	9
20–34	83	5.7	36	2	2	4	7	12	20	33
35–49	138	5.7	27	1	2	4	7	11	17	29
50–64	180	6.7	54	2	3	4	7	14	23	38
65+	381	5.3	23	2	3	4	6	10	16	27
GRAND TOTAL	791	5.7	32	2	2	4	7	11	18	30

Length of Stay by Diagnosis and Operation, Western Region, 2008

Western Region, October 2006–September 2007 Data, by Diagnosis

996.66: INFECT D/T JOINT PROSTH

Type of Patients	Observed Patients	Avg. Stay	Vari-ance	10th	25th	50th	75th	90th	95th	99th
1. SINGLE DX										
A. Not Operated										
0–19 Years	0									
20–34	0									
35–49	1	6.0	0	6	6	6	6	6	6	6
50–64	0									
65+	1	3.0	0	3	3	3	3	3	3	3
B. Operated										
0–19 Years	0									
20–34	1	6.0	0	6	6	6	6	6	6	6
35–49	4	3.3	<1	3	3	3	3	4	4	4
50–64	5	8.0	94	1	3	5	6	25	25	25
65+	4	3.2	2	2	2	2	4	5	5	5
2. MULTIPLE DX										
A. Not Operated										
0–19 Years	0									
20–34	7	6.0	7	3	3	7	8	10	10	10
35–49	39	4.3	7	1	2	4	6	7	9	12
50–64	154	5.3	24	2	2	4	6	11	13	23
65+	274	6.0	28	2	3	5	7	11	16	30
B. Operated										
0–19 Years	6	5.8	4	3	4	6	7	8	8	8
20–34	58	7.8	44	2	4	6	9	16	22	35
35–49	269	7.5	71	3	4	6	8	13	19	45
50–64	1,223	7.0	33	3	4	6	8	13	17	35
65+	2,148	7.4	40	3	4	6	9	13	18	31
SUBTOTALS:										
1. SINGLE DX										
A. Not Operated	2	4.5	4	3	3	6	6	6	6	6
B. Operated	14	5.1	35	2	3	3	5	6	25	25
2. MULTIPLE DX										
A. Not Operated	474	5.6	25	2	3	4	7	11	14	25
B. Operated	3,704	7.3	40	3	4	6	8	13	18	33
1. SINGLE DX	16	5.1	31	2	3	3	5	6	25	25
2. MULTIPLE DX	4,178	7.1	39	3	4	5	8	13	18	33
A. NOT OPERATED	476	5.6	25	2	3	4	7	11	14	25
B. OPERATED	3,718	7.3	40	3	4	5	8	13	18	33
TOTAL										
0–19 Years	6	5.8	4	3	4	6	7	8	8	8
20–34	66	7.5	39	2	4	6	8	13	18	35
35–49	313	7.0	63	2	3	5	8	13	16	43
50–64	1,382	6.8	32	3	4	5	8	13	17	35
65+	2,427	7.2	39	3	4	6	9	13	18	31
GRAND TOTAL	4,194	7.1	38	3	4	5	8	13	18	33

996.67: INFECT D/T ORTH DEV NEC

Type of Patients	Observed Patients	Avg. Stay	Vari-ance	10th	25th	50th	75th	90th	95th	99th
1. SINGLE DX										
A. Not Operated										
0–19 Years	2	2.0	2	1	1	3	3	3	3	3
20–34	7	2.7	6	1	1	2	3	8	8	8
35–49	8	3.3	11	1	1	3	4	11	11	11
50–64	3	3.3	6	1	1	3	6	6	6	6
65+	0									
B. Operated										
0–19 Years	10	5.5	39	1	1	3	11	18	18	18
20–34	18	3.6	12	1	1	3	4	9	14	14
35–49	22	4.3	10	1	2	4	5	8	8	15
50–64	17	3.1	4	1	2	2	5	7	7	7
65+	5	2.4	1	1	2	2	3	4	4	4
2. MULTIPLE DX										
A. Not Operated										
0–19 Years	21	6.1	53	2	2	5	6	8	11	36
20–34	62	4.7	22	2	2	3	5	9	11	28
35–49	80	4.8	13	2	3	4	6	8	13	19
50–64	108	6.1	40	2	3	4	7	13	16	25
65+	96	6.6	19	2	4	5	8	12	14	24
B. Operated										
0–19 Years	73	6.6	76	1	3	4	7	11	24	58
20–34	265	6.7	53	3	3	5	7	13	18	34
35–49	473	7.8	57	2	3	6	10	16	22	42
50–64	678	8.1	79	2	3	6	9	15	24	47
65+	577	7.8	46	3	4	6	9	15	21	36
SUBTOTALS:										
1. SINGLE DX										
A. Not Operated	20	3.0	7	1	1	2	3	6	11	11
B. Operated	72	3.9	12	1	2	3	5	8	13	18
2. MULTIPLE DX										
A. Not Operated	367	5.7	27	2	3	5	7	11	15	25
B. Operated	2,066	7.7	61	2	3	5	9	15	22	42
1. SINGLE DX	92	3.7	11	1	2	3	5	8	11	18
2. MULTIPLE DX	2,433	7.4	57	2	3	5	9	15	21	41
A. NOT OPERATED	387	5.6	26	2	2	4	7	11	15	25
B. OPERATED	2,138	7.6	60	2	3	5	9	15	21	42
TOTAL										
0–19 Years	106	6.3	66	1	2	4	7	11	22	38
20–34	352	6.1	46	1	3	4	7	12	18	32
35–49	583	7.2	50	2	3	5	8	15	20	37
50–64	806	7.7	73	2	3	6	8	15	22	43
65+	678	7.6	42	3	4	6	9	15	19	36
GRAND TOTAL	2,525	7.3	55	2	3	5	8	15	21	40

996.68: INFECT D/T PD CATH

Type of Patients	Observed Patients	Avg. Stay	Vari-ance	10th	25th	50th	75th	90th	95th	99th
1. SINGLE DX										
A. Not Operated										
0–19 Years	0									
20–34	0									
35–49	0									
50–64	0									
65+	0									
B. Operated										
0–19 Years	0									
20–34	0									
35–49	0									
50–64	0									
65+	0									
2. MULTIPLE DX										
A. Not Operated										
0–19 Years	9	3.4	4	1	2	4	5	7	7	7
20–34	76	4.5	9	2	3	4	6	9	10	18
35–49	116	5.1	12	2	3	4	7	10	13	18
50–64	195	5.2	19	2	3	4	6	9	13	29
65+	164	6.1	30	2	3	4	7	13	17	28
B. Operated										
0–19 Years	4	5.2	7	3	4	5	5	9	9	9
20–34	50	11.4	159	3	4	7	13	29	44	49
35–49	96	9.4	71	3	5	7	11	17	25	50
50–64	152	9.6	62	3	5	7	12	19	30	35
65+	115	11.0	123	2	4	9	14	24	38	70
SUBTOTALS:										
1. SINGLE DX										
A. Not Operated	0									
B. Operated	0									
2. MULTIPLE DX										
A. Not Operated	560	5.3	20	2	3	4	6	10	13	24
B. Operated	417	10.1	92	2	4	7	13	22	30	49
1. SINGLE DX	0									
2. MULTIPLE DX	977	7.4	56	2	3	5	9	15	22	42
A. NOT OPERATED	560	5.3	20	2	3	4	6	10	13	24
B. OPERATED	417	10.1	92	2	4	7	13	22	30	49
TOTAL										
0–19 Years	13	4.0	5	1	2	4	5	7	9	9
20–34	126	7.3	79	2	3	5	8	13	28	48
35–49	212	7.1	43	2	3	5	8	13	18	36
50–64	347	7.2	43	2	3	5	9	15	21	34
65+	279	8.1	74	2	3	5	10	19	24	53
GRAND TOTAL	977	7.4	56	2	3	5	9	15	22	42

Length of Stay by Diagnosis and Operation, Western Region, 2008

Western Region, October 2006–September 2007 Data, by Diagnosis

996.69: INFECT DUE TO DEVICE NEC

Type of Patients	Observed Patients	Avg. Stay	Variance	10th	25th	50th	75th	90th	95th	99th
1. SINGLE DX										
A. Not Operated										
0–19 Years	0									
20–34	4	3.2	7	1	1	2	3	7	7	7
35–49	4	4.5	4	2	4	4	5	7	7	7
50–64	3	1.7	1	1	1	1	3	3	3	3
65+	0									
B. Operated										
0–19 Years	1	10.0	0	10	10	10	10	10	10	10
20–34	3	2.7	2	1	1	3	4	4	4	4
35–49	6	2.7	5	1	1	2	3	7	7	7
50–64	4	3.3	10	1	1	2	2	8	8	8
65+	1	6.0	0	6	6	6	6	6	6	6
2. MULTIPLE DX										
A. Not Operated										
0–19 Years	40	6.7	31	2	3	5	10	14	17	28
20–34	70	5.9	36	1	2	4	6	15	18	29
35–49	218	4.8	11	2	3	4	6	9	12	17
50–64	318	6.3	33	2	3	4	8	13	18	31
65+	283	6.4	25	2	3	5	8	12	15	28
B. Operated										
0–19 Years	28	5.2	14	1	2	5	7	10	14	15
20–34	85	5.6	35	1	2	4	6	13	17	38
35–49	348	6.7	77	2	3	4	7	14	20	46
50–64	512	7.1	48	2	3	5	9	14	22	35
65+	366	7.3	45	2	3	5	9	15	19	37
SUBTOTALS:										
1. SINGLE DX										
A. Not Operated	11	3.3	5	1	1	3	5	7	7	7
B. Operated	15	3.5	8	1	1	2	6	8	10	10
2. MULTIPLE DX										
A. Not Operated	929	6.0	26	2	3	4	7	12	16	28
B. Operated	1,339	6.9	54	2	3	5	8	15	20	38
1. SINGLE DX	26	3.4	7	1	1	2	5	7	8	10
2. MULTIPLE DX	2,268	6.5	42	2	3	5	8	13	18	32
A. NOT OPERATED	940	5.9	26	2	3	4	7	12	16	28
B. OPERATED	1,354	6.9	53	2	3	5	8	14	19	38
TOTAL										
0–19 Years	69	6.1	24	1	3	5	8	14	16	28
20–34	162	5.6	34	1	2	4	6	12	17	29
35–49	576	6.0	52	2	3	4	7	12	17	44
50–64	837	6.8	43	2	3	5	8	14	19	34
65+	650	6.9	36	2	3	5	9	14	18	29
GRAND TOTAL	2,294	6.5	42	2	3	5	8	13	18	32

996.71: COMP D/T HRT VALV PROSTH

Type of Patients	Observed Patients	Avg. Stay	Variance	10th	25th	50th	75th	90th	95th	99th
1. SINGLE DX										
A. Not Operated										
0–19 Years	0									
20–34	0									
35–49	0									
50–64	0									
65+	0									
B. Operated										
0–19 Years	0									
20–34	2	4.5	<1	4	4	5	5	5	5	5
35–49	1	5.0	0	5	5	5	5	5	5	5
50–64	0									
65+	0									
2. MULTIPLE DX										
A. Not Operated										
0–19 Years	1	1.0	0	1	1	1	1	1	1	1
20–34	8	4.7	13	1	1	3	7	10	10	10
35–49	9	10.0	136	1	2	5	11	33	33	33
50–64	25	5.3	22	2	3	3	5	14	16	18
65+	55	7.1	49	2	2	5	9	19	24	31
B. Operated										
0–19 Years	14	13.1	187	2	4	8	21	37	44	44
20–34	9	8.8	17	3	4	10	12	14	14	14
35–49	22	12.6	146	4	5	7	18	23	29	55
50–64	44	12.6	126	4	6	8	18	23	31	59
65+	66	12.2	55	6	7	10	16	23	26	40
SUBTOTALS:										
1. SINGLE DX										
A. Not Operated	0									
B. Operated	3	4.7	<1	4	4	5	5	5	5	5
2. MULTIPLE DX										
A. Not Operated	98	6.7	47	1	2	4	8	17	24	33
B. Operated	155	12.3	96	4	6	8	16	23	31	55
1. SINGLE DX	3	4.7	<1	4	4	5	5	5	5	5
2. MULTIPLE DX	253	10.1	84	2	4	7	13	22	28	44
A. NOT OPERATED	98	6.7	47	1	2	4	8	17	24	33
B. OPERATED	158	12.1	95	4	6	8	16	23	31	55
TOTAL										
0–19 Years	15	12.3	184	2	4	6	21	37	44	44
20–34	19	6.6	17	1	3	7	10	12	14	14
35–49	32	11.7	137	2	4	6	14	26	33	55
50–64	69	10.0	100	2	4	6	14	22	28	59
65+	121	9.9	58	2	5	7	12	21	24	33
GRAND TOTAL	256	10.0	84	2	4	7	13	22	28	44

996.72: COMP NEC D/T HRT DEV NEC

Type of Patients	Observed Patients	Avg. Stay	Variance	10th	25th	50th	75th	90th	95th	99th
1. SINGLE DX										
A. Not Operated										
0–19 Years	0									
20–34	0									
35–49	0									
50–64	0									
65+	0									
B. Operated										
0–19 Years	0									
20–34	0									
35–49	3	2.0	3	1	1	1	4	4	4	4
50–64	3	1.0	0	1	1	1	1	1	1	1
65+	7	1.1	<1	1	1	1	1	2	2	2
2. MULTIPLE DX										
A. Not Operated										
0–19 Years	2	1.0	0	1	1	1	1	1	1	1
20–34	13	4.5	23	1	1	2	9	11	15	15
35–49	53	2.6	6	1	1	2	3	5	7	15
50–64	188	2.8	5	1	1	2	4	6	7	10
65+	339	3.2	8	1	1	2	4	7	8	15
B. Operated										
0–19 Years	37	5.4	28	3	3	5	6	10	14	31
20–34	24	6.4	147	1	1	3	6	12	61	>99
35–49	260	2.7	10	1	1	2	3	5	8	19
50–64	986	2.6	10	1	1	1	3	6	8	15
65+	1,498	2.5	11	1	1	1	3	5	8	17
SUBTOTALS:										
1. SINGLE DX										
A. Not Operated	0									
B. Operated	13	1.3	<1	1	1	1	1	2	4	4
2. MULTIPLE DX										
A. Not Operated	595	3.0	7	1	1	2	4	6	8	15
B. Operated	2,805	2.6	12	1	1	1	3	6	8	17
1. SINGLE DX	13	1.3	<1	1	1	1	1	2	4	4
2. MULTIPLE DX	3,400	2.7	11	1	1	1	3	6	8	16
A. NOT OPERATED	595	3.0	7	1	1	2	4	6	8	15
B. OPERATED	2,818	2.6	12	1	1	1	3	6	8	17
TOTAL										
0–19 Years	39	5.2	28	2	3	4	6	10	14	31
20–34	37	5.7	102	1	1	3	8	12	61	>99
35–49	316	2.7	9	1	1	2	3	5	8	17
50–64	1,177	2.6	9	1	1	1	3	6	8	15
65+	1,844	2.6	11	1	1	1	3	6	8	16
GRAND TOTAL	3,413	2.7	11	1	1	1	3	6	8	16

Length of Stay by Diagnosis and Operation, Western Region, 2008

Western Region, October 2006–September 2007 Data, by Diagnosis

996.73: COMP D/T RENAL DIALY DEV

Type of Patients	Observed Patients	Avg. Stay	Vari-ance	Percentiles						
				10th	25th	50th	75th	90th	95th	99th
1. SINGLE DX										
A. Not Operated										
0–19 Years	0									
20–34	0									
35–49	0									
50–64	2	2.5	<1	2	2	2	3	3	3	3
65+	2	4.0	18	1	1	7	7	7	7	7
B. Operated										
0–19 Years	0									
20–34	0									
35–49	0									
50–64	2	1.0	0	1	1	1	1	1	1	1
65+	2	1.5	<1	1	1	2	2	2	2	2
2. MULTIPLE DX										
A. Not Operated										
0–19 Years	11	1.9	<1	1	1	2	3	3	3	3
20–34	148	3.3	8	1	2	2	4	6	9	15
35–49	321	3.4	11	1	1	2	4	4	9	17
50–64	585	3.4	14	1	1	2	4	7	10	20
65+	936	3.6	14	1	1	2	5	7	10	17
B. Operated										
0–19 Years	11	4.9	18	2	2	3	7	10	15	15
20–34	246	4.7	34	1	1	3	6	10	16	30
35–49	712	4.1	19	1	1	3	5	8	12	21
50–64	1,519	4.1	28	1	1	3	5	8	12	22
65+	2,309	3.9	17	1	1	2	5	9	12	20
SUBTOTALS:										
1. SINGLE DX										
A. Not Operated	4	3.3	7	1	2	2	7	7	7	7
B. Operated	4	1.3	<1	1	1	1	2	2	2	2
2. MULTIPLE DX										
A. Not Operated	2,001	3.5	13	1	1	2	4	7	10	18
B. Operated	4,797	4.1	22	1	1	2	5	9	12	21
1. SINGLE DX	8	2.3	4	1	1	2	2	2	7	7
2. MULTIPLE DX	6,798	3.9	19	1	1	2	5	8	12	21
A. NOT OPERATED	2,005	3.5	13	1	1	2	4	7	10	18
B. OPERATED	4,801	4.1	22	1	1	2	5	9	12	21
TOTAL										
0–19 Years	22	3.4	11	1	2	2	3	7	10	15
20–34	394	4.2	25	1	1	2	5	9	14	29
35–49	1,033	3.9	17	1	1	3	5	8	11	20
50–64	2,108	3.9	24	1	1	2	5	8	12	21
65+	3,249	3.8	16	1	1	2	5	8	12	19
GRAND TOTAL	6,806	3.9	19	1	1	2	5	8	12	21

996.74: COMP NEC D/T VASC DEVNEC

Type of Patients	Observed Patients	Avg. Stay	Vari-ance	Percentiles						
				10th	25th	50th	75th	90th	95th	99th
1. SINGLE DX										
A. Not Operated										
0–19 Years	1	3.0	0	3	3	3	3	3	3	3
20–34	1	1.0	0	1	1	1	1	1	1	1
35–49	0									
50–64	2	3.5	12	1	1	6	6	6	6	6
65+	1	2.0	0	2	2	2	2	2	2	2
B. Operated										
0–19 Years	0									
20–34	0									
35–49	1	7.0	0	7	7	7	7	7	7	7
50–64	4	2.3	2	1	1	1	3	4	4	4
65+	8	2.1	2	1	1	1	3	4	4	4
2. MULTIPLE DX										
A. Not Operated										
0–19 Years	46	4.2	17	1	2	3	5	11	13	18
20–34	88	5.7	47	1	2	4	6	11	19	52
35–49	238	4.3	14	1	2	3	6	9	12	17
50–64	396	4.3	15	1	2	3	5	8	11	23
65+	493	4.8	18	1	2	4	6	10	12	24
B. Operated										
0–19 Years	23	10.2	358	1	1	4	8	27	50	81
20–34	57	5.9	34	1	2	4	7	11	20	35
35–49	199	5.3	31	1	2	4	7	12	16	46
50–64	838	5.4	25	1	2	4	7	12	15	24
65+	1,591	5.7	32	1	2	4	8	12	16	26
SUBTOTALS:										
1. SINGLE DX										
A. Not Operated	5	2.6	4	1	1	2	3	6	6	6
B. Operated	13	2.5	3	1	1	2	4	4	7	7
2. MULTIPLE DX										
A. Not Operated	1,261	4.6	18	1	2	3	6	9	12	22
B. Operated	2,708	5.6	33	1	2	4	7	12	16	27
1. SINGLE DX	18	2.6	3	1	1	2	4	6	7	7
2. MULTIPLE DX	3,969	5.3	28	1	2	4	7	11	15	26
A. NOT OPERATED	1,266	4.6	18	1	2	3	6	9	12	22
B. OPERATED	2,721	5.6	33	1	2	4	7	12	15	27
TOTAL										
0–19 Years	70	6.2	133	1	1	3	6	12	18	81
20–34	146	5.7	41	1	2	4	7	11	19	35
35–49	438	4.8	22	1	2	3	6	10	14	28
50–64	1,240	5.0	22	1	2	4	7	10	14	24
65+	2,093	5.5	29	1	2	4	7	11	15	26
GRAND TOTAL	3,987	5.3	28	1	2	4	7	11	15	26

996.75: COMP NEC D/T NERVOUS DEV

Type of Patients	Observed Patients	Avg. Stay	Vari-ance	Percentiles						
				10th	25th	50th	75th	90th	95th	99th
1. SINGLE DX										
A. Not Operated										
0–19 Years	1	1.0	0	1	1	1	1	1	1	1
20–34	0									
35–49	0									
50–64	0									
65+	0									
B. Operated										
0–19 Years	0									
20–34	1	1.0	0	1	1	1	1	1	1	1
35–49	1	1.0	0	1	1	1	1	1	1	1
50–64	2	1.5	<1	1	1	1	2	2	2	2
65+	0									
2. MULTIPLE DX										
A. Not Operated										
0–19 Years	13	2.6	4	1	1	2	3	5	7	7
20–34	8	2.9	4	1	1	3	3	7	7	7
35–49	16	3.4	5	1	1	3	5	6	10	10
50–64	21	3.2	9	1	1	3	5	5	5	14
65+	25	3.8	12	1	2	3	4	7	8	17
B. Operated										
0–19 Years	36	4.4	20	1	2	3	5	10	17	21
20–34	45	3.8	27	1	1	2	5	8	11	33
35–49	54	3.4	24	1	1	2	4	7	12	30
50–64	70	3.8	12	1	1	3	5	9	12	16
65+	61	3.9	23	1	2	3	5	8	12	29
SUBTOTALS:										
1. SINGLE DX										
A. Not Operated	1	1.0	0	1	1	1	1	1	1	1
B. Operated	4	1.3	<1	1	1	1	1	2	2	2
2. MULTIPLE DX										
A. Not Operated	83	3.3	8	1	1	3	4	6	7	17
B. Operated	266	3.8	20	1	1	2	5	8	12	29
1. SINGLE DX	5	1.2	<1	1	1	1	1	2	2	2
2. MULTIPLE DX	349	3.7	17	1	1	2	5	8	11	21
A. NOT OPERATED	84	3.3	8	1	1	3	4	6	7	17
B. OPERATED	270	3.8	20	1	1	2	5	8	12	29
TOTAL										
0–19 Years	50	3.9	16	1	2	2	5	8	10	21
20–34	54	3.6	24	1	1	2	4	7	11	33
35–49	71	3.4	19	1	1	2	4	6	10	30
50–64	93	3.6	11	1	1	3	5	8	12	16
65+	86	3.9	20	1	1	2	5	8	12	29
GRAND TOTAL	354	3.7	17	1	1	2	4	8	11	21

Western Region, October 2006–September 2007 Data, by Diagnosis

996.76: COMP NEC D/T GU DEVICE

Type of Patients	Observed Patients	Avg. Stay	Variance	10th	25th	50th	75th	90th	95th	99th
1. SINGLE DX										
A. Not Operated										
0–19 Years	1	1.0	0	1	1	1	1	1	1	1
20–34	1	1.0	0	1	1	1	1	1	1	1
35–49	1	2.0	0	2	2	2	2	2	2	2
50–64	0									
65+	0									
B. Operated										
0–19 Years	0									
20–34	2	1.0	0	1	1	1	1	1	1	1
35–49	1	2.0	0			2	2			
50–64	2	4.0	18	3	3	4	7	7	7	7
65+	1	3.0	0	3	3	3	3	3	3	3
2. MULTIPLE DX										
A. Not Operated										
0–19 Years	9	2.9	5	1	1	2	3	7	7	7
20–34	43	3.4	9	1	1	3	5	6	9	14
35–49	86	3.3	9	1	1	2	4	7	9	20
50–64	105	3.5	9	1	1	3	4	7	9	16
65+	334	3.6	9	1	1	3	5	7	9	15
B. Operated										
0–19 Years	3	15.0	584	1	1	1	43	43	43	43
20–34	26	2.5	2	1	2	2	3	5	5	5
35–49	31	3.3	21	1	1	2	4	6	15	22
50–64	62	3.8	15	1	1	2	5	10	13	17
65+	117	4.8	32	1	1	2	7	11	13	33
SUBTOTALS:										
1. SINGLE DX										
A. Not Operated	3	1.3	<1	1	1	1	2	2	2	2
B. Operated	6	2.5	6	1	1	1	3	7	7	7
2. MULTIPLE DX										
A. Not Operated	577	3.5	9	1	1	3	5	7	9	15
B. Operated	239	4.2	29	1	1	2	5	10	13	33
1. SINGLE DX	9	2.1	4	1	1	1	2	7	7	7
2. MULTIPLE DX	816	3.7	15	1	1	2	5	8	11	17
A. NOT OPERATED	580	3.5	9	1	1	2	4	7	9	15
B. OPERATED	245	4.2	29	1	1	2	5	10	13	33
TOTAL										
0–19 Years	13	5.6	131	1	1	2	3	7	43	43
20–34	72	3.0	6	1	1	2	4	6	7	14
35–49	119	3.3	12	1	1	2	4	7	10	20
50–64	169	3.6	11	1	1	3	4	8	11	17
65+	452	3.9	15	1	1	3	5	8	11	15
GRAND TOTAL	825	3.7	15	1	1	2	5	8	11	17

996.77: COMP NEC D/T JT PROSTH

Type of Patients	Observed Patients	Avg. Stay	Variance	10th	25th	50th	75th	90th	95th	99th
1. SINGLE DX										
A. Not Operated										
0–19 Years	0									
20–34	0									
35–49	2	1.5	<1	1	1	1	2	2	2	2
50–64	1	1.0	0			1	1		1	1
65+	3	2.3	<1	2	2	2	3	3	3	3
B. Operated										
0–19 Years	1	2.0				2	2	2	2	2
20–34	0									
35–49	7	2.7	1	1	2	3	4	4	4	4
50–64	14	2.9	5	1	1	3	3	4	10	10
65+	14	3.0	2	2	2	3	4	4	6	6
2. MULTIPLE DX										
A. Not Operated										
0–19 Years	0									
20–34	4	2.8	4	1	1	4	5	5	5	5
35–49	39	3.2	8	1	1	3	4	6	10	16
50–64	128	2.9	8	1	1	2	3	6	7	16
65+	166	3.3	7	1	1	3	4	6	8	13
B. Operated										
0–19 Years	4	5.5	59	1	1	1	3	17	17	17
20–34	25	3.0	3	1	2	3	4	5	6	8
35–49	184	3.3	4	2	2	3	4	5	6	14
50–64	666	3.4	6	2	2	3	4	5	7	12
65+	1,010	3.7	4	2	3	3	4	6	7	12
SUBTOTALS:										
1. SINGLE DX										
A. Not Operated	6	1.8	<1	1	1	2	2	3	3	3
B. Operated	36	2.9	3	1	2	3	3	4	6	10
2. MULTIPLE DX										
A. Not Operated	337	3.1	7	1	1	2	4	6	8	16
B. Operated	1,889	3.5	5	2	2	3	4	5	7	13
1. SINGLE DX	42	2.7	3	1	2	3	3	4	4	7
2. MULTIPLE DX	2,226	3.5	5	1	2	3	4	6	7	13
A. NOT OPERATED	343	3.1	7	1	1	2	4	6	7	16
B. OPERATED	1,925	3.5	5	2	2	3	4	5	7	12
TOTAL										
0–19 Years	5	4.8	47	1	1	2	3	17	17	17
20–34	29	3.0	3	1	2	3	4	5	6	8
35–49	232	3.2	4	1	2	3	4	5	7	14
50–64	809	3.3	6	2	2	3	4	5	7	15
65+	1,193	3.6	5	2	3	3	4	6	7	13
GRAND TOTAL	2,268	3.5	5	2	2	3	4	6	7	13

996.78: COMP NEC ORTH DEV NEC

Type of Patients	Observed Patients	Avg. Stay	Variance	10th	25th	50th	75th	90th	95th	99th
1. SINGLE DX										
A. Not Operated										
0–19 Years	1	2.0	0	2	2	2	2	2	2	2
20–34	2	1.5	<1	1	1	1	2	2	2	2
35–49	2	2.0	2	1	1	3	3	3	3	3
50–64	1	2.0	0	2	2	2	2	2	2	2
65+	1	2.0	0	2	2	2	2	2	2	2
B. Operated										
0–19 Years	20	1.3	<1	1	1	1	1	2	4	4
20–34	44	1.8	1	1	1	1	2	3	3	6
35–49	52	1.7	<1	1	1	2	2	3	3	4
50–64	42	2.1	1	1	1	2	2	4	4	5
65+	19	2.5	2	1	2	2	3	5	6	6
2. MULTIPLE DX										
A. Not Operated										
0–19 Years	3	2.4	5	1	1	1	5	5	5	5
20–34	9	2.5	6	1	1	1	3	8	8	8
35–49	23	3.4	12	1	1	2	3	6	10	16
50–64	28	2.5	7	1	1	2	3	4	5	14
65+	42	4.1	10	1	2	3	5	9	12	12
B. Operated										
0–19 Years	61	2.4	8	1	1	1	3	4	6	21
20–34	234	2.3	3	1	1	2	3	4	5	8
35–49	594	2.4	6	1	1	2	3	4	5	15
50–64	844	3.0	10	1	1	2	4	5	7	17
65+	718	3.4	7	2	2	3	4	6	8	15
SUBTOTALS:										
1. SINGLE DX										
A. Not Operated	7	1.9	<1	1	1	2	2	3	3	3
B. Operated	177	1.9	1	1	1	2	3	3	4	6
2. MULTIPLE DX										
A. Not Operated	105	3.3	9	1	1	3	4	6	10	14
B. Operated	2,451	2.9	7	1	2	2	4	5	7	14
1. SINGLE DX	184	1.9	1	1	1	2	3	3	4	6
2. MULTIPLE DX	2,556	2.9	7	1	2	2	4	5	7	14
A. NOT OPERATED	112	3.2	9	1	1	3	4	6	10	14
B. OPERATED	2,628	2.8	7	1	1	2	3	5	7	12
TOTAL										
0–19 Years	85	2.1	6	1	1	1	2	4	6	21
20–34	289	2.2	2	1	1	2	3	4	5	8
35–49	671	2.4	5	1	1	2	3	4	5	15
50–64	915	2.9	9	1	1	2	3	5	7	14
65+	780	3.4	7	2	2	3	4	6	8	15
GRAND TOTAL	2,740	2.8	7	1	1	2	3	5	7	14

Length of Stay by Diagnosis and Operation, Western Region, 2008

Western Region, October 2006–September 2007 Data, by Diagnosis

996.79: COMP NEC D/T DEVICE NEC

Type of Patients	Observed Patients	Avg. Stay	Variance	10th	25th	50th	75th	90th	95th	99th
1. SINGLE DX										
A. Not Operated										
0–19 Years	0									
20–34	4	1.7	<1	1	1	1	2	3	3	3
35–49	2	1.5	<1	1	1	2	2	2	2	2
50–64	1	1.0	0	1	1	1	1	1	1	1
65+	2	2.0	2	1	1	2	3	3	3	3
B. Operated										
0–19 Years	0									
20–34	2	2.0	2	1	1	3	3	3	3	3
35–49	9	2.2	2	1	1	2	3	4	4	4
50–64	5	4.2	10	1	1	5	6	8	8	8
65+	1	1.0	0	1	1	1	1	1	1	1
2. MULTIPLE DX										
A. Not Operated										
0–19 Years	10	3.7	13	1	2	2	5	6	13	13
20–34	23	3.2	11	1	2	2	4	5	5	17
35–49	70	4.0	11	1	2	3	6	9	9	18
50–64	103	3.9	9	1	1	3	5	9	10	12
65+	105	4.2	14	1	2	3	5	10	11	19
B. Operated										
0–19 Years	12	7.7	103	1	1	4	24	24	25	25
20–34	24	4.8	25	1	1	3	9	12	12	21
35–49	121	3.8	12	1	1	3	5	8	10	15
50–64	155	4.6	41	1	2	2	5	9	19	39
65+	98	5.0	26	1	2	3	7	12	16	28
SUBTOTALS:										
1. SINGLE DX										
A. Not Operated	9	1.7	<1	1	1	1	2	3	3	3
B. Operated	17	2.7	4	1	1	2	4	6	8	8
2. MULTIPLE DX										
A. Not Operated	311	3.9	11	1	2	3	5	9	11	17
B. Operated	410	4.6	30	1	1	3	5	10	15	25
1. SINGLE DX	26	2.3	3	1	1	1	3	5	6	8
2. MULTIPLE DX	721	4.3	22	1	1	3	5	9	12	24
A. NOT OPERATED	320	3.9	11	1	2	3	5	9	11	17
B. OPERATED	427	4.5	29	1	1	3	5	10	14	25
TOTAL										
0–19 Years	22	5.9	64	1	1	2	5	24	24	25
20–34	53	3.8	17	1	1	2	4	9	12	21
35–49	202	3.8	11	1	1	3	5	8	9	15
50–64	264	4.3	28	1	1	3	5	9	12	25
65+	206	4.5	20	1	2	3	6	10	13	21
GRAND TOTAL	747	4.2	21	1	1	3	5	9	12	24

996.81: COMP KIDNEY TRANSPLANT

Type of Patients	Observed Patients	Avg. Stay	Variance	10th	25th	50th	75th	90th	95th	99th
1. SINGLE DX										
A. Not Operated										
0–19 Years	10	3.3	12	1	1	1	6	10	10	10
20–34	3	1.3	<1	1	1	1	2	2	2	2
35–49	3	4.0	4	2	2	4	6	6	6	6
50–64	3	3.3	4	1	1	4	5	5	5	5
65+	0									
B. Operated										
0–19 Years	0									
20–34	1	2.0	0	2	2	2	2	2	2	2
35–49	0									
50–64	0									
65+	0									
2. MULTIPLE DX										
A. Not Operated										
0–19 Years	209	4.4	17	1	1	3	6	11	13	18
20–34	446	5.0	19	1	2	4	6	10	12	22
35–49	684	4.6	26	1	2	3	5	9	12	18
50–64	822	5.3	20	1	2	3	7	10	14	21
65+	325	5.7	25	1	2	4	7	12	16	25
B. Operated										
0–19 Years	31	8.6	74	2	4	6	9	13	31	43
20–34	114	7.3	41	2	4	6	8	14	21	35
35–49	183	7.9	64	2	4	6	9	16	21	62
50–64	209	7.2	53	2	4	5	8	13	18	31
65+	69	7.8	51	2	3	6	10	17	20	39
SUBTOTALS:										
1. SINGLE DX										
A. Not Operated	19	3.1	8	1	1	2	5	8	10	10
B. Operated	1	2.0	0	2	2	2	2	2	2	2
2. MULTIPLE DX										
A. Not Operated	2,486	5.0	22	1	2	4	6	10	13	21
B. Operated	606	7.6	55	2	4	6	9	15	21	42
1. SINGLE DX	20	3.1	7	1	1	2	5	8	10	10
2. MULTIPLE DX	3,092	5.5	29	1	2	4	7	11	14	27
A. NOT OPERATED	2,505	5.0	22	1	2	4	6	10	13	21
B. OPERATED	607	7.6	55	2	4	6	9	15	21	42
TOTAL										
0–19 Years	250	4.9	25	1	1	3	7	11	13	23
20–34	564	5.4	24	1	2	4	7	10	13	29
35–49	870	5.3	36	1	2	4	6	11	14	29
50–64	1,034	5.7	27	1	3	4	7	11	14	26
65+	394	6.0	30	1	2	4	8	13	17	28
GRAND TOTAL	3,112	5.5	29	1	2	4	7	11	14	27

996.82: COMP LIVER TRANSPLANT

Type of Patients	Observed Patients	Avg. Stay	Variance	10th	25th	50th	75th	90th	95th	99th
1. SINGLE DX										
A. Not Operated										
0–19 Years	9	6.3	16	1	3	6	7	15	15	15
20–34	1	1.0	0	1	1	1	1	1	1	1
35–49	0									
50–64	13	2.2	2	1	1	2	3	4	4	4
65+	1	1.0	0	1	1	1	1	1	1	1
B. Operated										
0–19 Years	0									
20–34	0									
35–49	0									
50–64	0									
65+	0									
2. MULTIPLE DX										
A. Not Operated										
0–19 Years	65	5.1	31	1	1	3	6	13	18	25
20–34	80	6.5	42	2	2	4	8	15	18	32
35–49	159	5.9	30	1	2	4	8	12	17	30
50–64	462	5.9	33	1	2	4	7	12	18	29
65+	84	5.0	20	1	2	3	7	11	16	20
B. Operated										
0–19 Years	7	11.2	64	2	6	8	16	26	26	26
20–34	3	13.7	16	10	10	13	18	18	18	18
35–49	14	15.2	190	4	6	8	24	30	51	51
50–64	52	13.2	118	2	6	10	18	18	37	52
65+	2	6.0	0	6	6	6	6	6	6	6
SUBTOTALS:										
1. SINGLE DX										
A. Not Operated	24	3.6	11	1	1	3	6	7	8	15
B. Operated	0									
2. MULTIPLE DX										
A. Not Operated	850	5.8	32	1	2	4	7	12	18	29
B. Operated	78	13.2	118	2	6	10	18	26	37	52
1. SINGLE DX	24	3.6	11	1	1	3	6	7	8	15
2. MULTIPLE DX	928	6.4	43	1	2	4	8	14	20	31
A. NOT OPERATED	874	5.8	32	1	2	4	7	12	17	29
B. OPERATED	78	13.2	118	2	6	10	18	26	37	52
TOTAL										
0–19 Years	81	5.7	34	1	1	4	8	14	18	26
20–34	84	6.7	43	2	3	4	8	15	18	32
35–49	173	6.7	49	1	3	5	8	13	17	31
50–64	527	6.5	46	1	2	4	8	14	20	32
65+	87	5.0	19	1	2	3	7	11	16	20
GRAND TOTAL	952	6.4	43	1	2	4	8	14	19	31

Length of Stay by Diagnosis and Operation, Western Region, 2008

996.83: COMP HEART TRANSPLANT

Type of Patients	Observed Patients	Avg. Stay	Vari-ance	10th	25th	50th	75th	90th	95th	99th
1. SINGLE DX										
A. Not Operated										
0–19 Years	0									
20–34	0									
35–49	0									
50–64	0									
65+	0									
B. Operated										
0–19 Years	0									
20–34	0									
35–49	0									
50–64	0									
65+	0									
2. MULTIPLE DX										
A. Not Operated										
0–19 Years	27	4.9	11	1	3	4	7	10	11	14
20–34	45	6.3	20	1	3	5	8	15	16	19
35–49	59	6.7	62	1	2	4	7	17	30	36
50–64	85	6.9	38	1	3	5	9	15	19	37
65+	66	6.3	49	1	2	5	7	15	18	46
B. Operated										
0–19 Years	9	14.5	116	5	7	10	18	38	38	38
20–34	14	7.5	38	1	1	7	13	16	20	20
35–49	6	15.5	62	8	9	14	17	30	30	30
50–64	31	10.8	186	1	1	7	16	25	34	65
65+	6	8.6	106	1	2	4	14	27	27	27
SUBTOTALS:										
1. SINGLE DX										
A. Not Operated	0									
B. Operated	0									
2. MULTIPLE DX										
A. Not Operated	282	6.4	40	1	2	5	8	14	18	36
B. Operated	66	10.8	128	1	1	8	15	25	30	65
1. SINGLE DX	0									
2. MULTIPLE DX	348	7.3	59	1	2	5	9	16	21	37
A. NOT OPERATED	282	6.4	40	1	2	5	8	14	18	36
B. OPERATED	66	10.8	128	1	1	8	15	25	30	65
TOTAL										
0–19 Years	36	7.3	53	2	3	5	9	14	25	38
20–34	59	6.6	24	1	3	5	9	16	16	20
35–49	65	7.5	68	1	3	5	7	17	30	36
50–64	116	7.9	79	1	2	6	11	18	22	37
65+	72	6.5	53	1	2	5	8	15	20	46
GRAND TOTAL	348	7.3	59	1	2	5	9	16	21	37

996.84: COMP LUNG TRANSPLANT

Type of Patients	Observed Patients	Avg. Stay	Vari-ance	10th	25th	50th	75th	90th	95th	99th
1. SINGLE DX										
A. Not Operated										
0–19 Years	0									
20–34	1	2.0	0	2	2	2	2	2	2	2
35–49	0									
50–64	1	5.0	0	5	5	5	5	5	5	5
65+	0									
B. Operated										
0–19 Years	0									
20–34	0									
35–49	0									
50–64	0									
65+	0									
2. MULTIPLE DX										
A. Not Operated										
0–19 Years	5	2.4	<1	2	2	2	3	3	3	3
20–34	73	5.8	20	1	3	5	7	11	17	23
35–49	60	5.1	12	2	3	5	6	8	11	21
50–64	167	7.0	56	2	3	5	8	16	19	42
65+	44	7.7	81	2	4	5	7	17	20	57
B. Operated										
0–19 Years	3	20.0	714	3	3	6	51	51	51	51
20–34	24	8.9	49	2	4	8	11	18	22	30
35–49	27	7.1	28	3	4	5	9	14	21	22
50–64	81	10.2	133	2	4	6	11	28	38	>99
65+	17	8.1	36	3	4	6	9	19	22	22
SUBTOTALS:										
1. SINGLE DX										
A. Not Operated	2	3.5	4	2	2	2	5	5	5	5
B. Operated	0									
2. MULTIPLE DX										
A. Not Operated	349	6.4	44	2	3	5	7	13	18	33
B. Operated	152	9.4	100	2	4	6	11	21	36	58
1. SINGLE DX	2	3.5	4	2	2	2	5	5	5	5
2. MULTIPLE DX	501	7.3	63	2	3	5	8	15	21	51
A. NOT OPERATED	351	6.4	44	2	3	5	7	13	18	33
B. OPERATED	152	9.4	100	2	4	6	11	21	36	58
TOTAL										
0–19 Years	8	9.0	291	2	2	3	6	51	51	51
20–34	98	6.6	28	2	3	5	8	14	18	30
35–49	87	5.7	18	2	3	5	6	11	14	22
50–64	249	8.0	82	2	3	5	9	18	28	58
65+	61	7.8	68	2	4	5	8	17	20	57
GRAND TOTAL	503	7.3	62	2	3	5	8	15	21	51

996.85: COMP MARROW TRANSPLANT

Type of Patients	Observed Patients	Avg. Stay	Vari-ance	10th	25th	50th	75th	90th	95th	99th
1. SINGLE DX										
A. Not Operated										
0–19 Years	0									
20–34	0									
35–49	0									
50–64	0									
65+	0									
B. Operated										
0–19 Years	0									
20–34	0									
35–49	0									
50–64	0									
65+	0									
2. MULTIPLE DX										
A. Not Operated										
0–19 Years	48	7.3	54	1	2	4	10	20	23	30
20–34	70	9.4	126	2	3	5	10	23	40	55
35–49	55	11.5	141	2	4	7	15	33	51	>99
50–64	113	11.9	205	2	3	6	14	25	44	72
65+	26	10.5	79	2	4	6	16	24	25	32
B. Operated										
0–19 Years	2	26.3	607	9	9	44	>99	>99	>99	>99
20–34	1	6.0	0	6	6	6	6	6	6	6
35–49	1	51.0	0	51	51	51	51	51	51	51
50–64	6	17.5	184	3	5	8	31	32	32	32
65+	1	36.0	0	36	36	36	36	36	36	36
SUBTOTALS:										
1. SINGLE DX										
A. Not Operated	0									
B. Operated	0									
2. MULTIPLE DX										
A. Not Operated	312	10.5	143	2	3	6	14	24	39	56
B. Operated	11	22.8	297	5	6	26	36	51	>99	>99
1. SINGLE DX	0									
2. MULTIPLE DX	323	10.9	153	2	3	6	14	27	40	72
A. NOT OPERATED	312	10.5	143	2	3	6	14	24	39	56
B. OPERATED	11	22.8	297	5	6	26	36	51	>99	>99
TOTAL										
0–19 Years	50	8.1	78	1	2	5	12	21	30	>99
20–34	71	9.4	124	2	3	5	10	23	40	55
35–49	56	12.2	166	2	4	7	15	33	51	>99
50–64	119	12.2	204	2	3	6	15	25	44	72
65+	27	11.4	100	2	4	6	21	25	32	36
GRAND TOTAL	323	10.9	153	2	3	6	14	27	40	72

Length of Stay by Diagnosis and Operation, Western Region, 2008

Western Region, October 2006–September 2007 Data, by Diagnosis

997: SURG COMP-BODY SYST NEC

Type of Patients	Observed Patients	Avg. Stay	Vari-ance	10th	25th	50th	75th	90th	95th	99th
1. SINGLE DX										
A. Not Operated										
0–19 Years	10	2.5	2	1	2	2	3	6	6	6
20–34	21	3.8	5	1	2	3	4	7	8	10
35–49	26	3.2	3	1	2	3	5	5	6	6
50–64	16	2.8	6	1	1	2	4	8	9	9
65+	13	5.0	23	1	2	3	7	10	17	17
B. Operated										
0–19 Years	6	2.3	11	1	1	1	1	9	9	9
20–34	24	3.5	7	1	1	5	5	7	7	11
35–49	27	3.2	5	1	1	2	5	7	8	9
50–64	31	3.2	4	1	1	3	4	7	7	8
65+	8	4.0	11	1	2	3	8	10	10	10
2. MULTIPLE DX										
A. Not Operated										
0–19 Years	319	3.9	16	1	1	3	4	8	11	25
20–34	994	3.9	14	1	2	3	5	8	11	22
35–49	2,147	4.1	14	1	2	3	5	8	10	19
50–64	3,117	4.4	16	1	2	3	5	9	11	20
65+	3,546	4.7	18	1	2	4	6	9	12	22
B. Operated										
0–19 Years	181	5.9	45	1	2	4	7	14	19	32
20–34	506	6.7	55	1	2	5	8	14	19	33
35–49	1,328	7.6	69	1	3	5	9	15	22	45
50–64	2,384	7.7	66	1	3	5	10	16	23	45
65+	2,654	7.2	52	1	2	5	9	15	20	35
SUBTOTALS:										
1. SINGLE DX										
A. Not Operated	86	3.5	7	1	2	3	5	7	9	17
B. Operated	96	3.3	6	1	1	3	4	7	8	11
2. MULTIPLE DX										
A. Not Operated	10,123	4.4	16	1	2	3	6	8	12	21
B. Operated	7,053	7.4	60	1	3	5	9	16	21	39
1. SINGLE DX	**182**	**3.4**	**7**	**1**	**2**	**3**	**4**	**7**	**8**	**11**
2. MULTIPLE DX	**17,176**	**5.6**	**36**	**1**	**2**	**4**	**7**	**12**	**16**	**30**
A. NOT OPERATED	**10,209**	**4.4**	**16**	**1**	**2**	**3**	**5**	**8**	**11**	**21**
B. OPERATED	**7,149**	**7.3**	**60**	**1**	**3**	**5**	**9**	**15**	**21**	**39**
TOTAL										
0–19 Years	516	4.6	27	1	2	3	5	10	15	27
20–34	1,545	4.8	29	1	2	3	6	10	14	26
35–49	3,528	5.4	37	1	2	4	6	11	15	32
50–64	5,548	5.8	40	1	2	4	7	12	16	33
65+	6,221	5.8	34	1	2	4	7	12	16	29
GRAND TOTAL	**17,358**	**5.6**	**36**	**1**	**2**	**4**	**7**	**12**	**16**	**30**

997.01: CNS SURG COMP

Type of Patients	Observed Patients	Avg. Stay	Vari-ance	10th	25th	50th	75th	90th	95th	99th
1. SINGLE DX										
A. Not Operated										
0–19 Years	0									
20–34	0									
35–49	0									
50–64	0									
65+	1	10.0	0	10	10	10	10	10	10	10
B. Operated										
0–19 Years	1	1.0	0	1	1	1	1	1	1	1
20–34	2	6.0	49	1	1	11	11	11	11	11
35–49	5	3.4	7	2	2	2	3	5	7	7
50–64	2	4.5	12	2	2	2	7	7	7	7
65+	0									
2. MULTIPLE DX										
A. Not Operated										
0–19 Years	3	5.4	4	3	3	6	6	8	8	8
20–34	11	3.6	8	1	2	3	5	7	7	10
35–49	14	3.2	3	1	2	4	4	5	7	7
50–64	14	4.4	8	1	2	4	5	8	11	11
65+	22	6.9	21	2	4	5	10	14	14	17
B. Operated										
0–19 Years	13	3.5	12	1	2	2	3	8	13	13
20–34	35	10.6	204	4	4	7	11	18	37	78
35–49	64	5.3	25	1	3	4	6	9	13	36
50–64	91	6.7	34	1	3	4	9	14	20	28
65+	48	6.9	41	1	2	5	8	15	23	30
SUBTOTALS:										
1. SINGLE DX										
A. Not Operated	1	10.0	0	10	10	10	10	10	10	10
B. Operated	10	3.9	12	1	2	2	7	11	11	11
2. MULTIPLE DX										
A. Not Operated	64	4.9	13	1	2	4	6	10	14	17
B. Operated	251	6.8	58	1	3	5	8	14	20	36
1. SINGLE DX	**11**	**4.5**	**14**	**1**	**2**	**3**	**8**	**10**	**11**	**11**
2. MULTIPLE DX	**315**	**6.4**	**49**	**1**	**2**	**4**	**7**	**14**	**18**	**33**
A. NOT OPERATED	**65**	**5.0**	**13**	**1**	**2**	**4**	**6**	**10**	**14**	**17**
B. OPERATED	**261**	**6.6**	**56**	**1**	**2**	**5**	**8**	**14**	**19**	**36**
TOTAL										
0–19 Years	17	3.7	10	1	2	3	4	8	13	13
20–34	48	8.8	159	1	2	6	10	17	33	78
35–49	83	4.9	21	1	2	4	6	9	12	36
50–64	107	6.3	31	1	3	4	8	14	19	25
65+	71	7.0	34	2	3	5	9	14	22	30
GRAND TOTAL	**326**	**6.3**	**48**	**1**	**2**	**4**	**7**	**13**	**17**	**33**

997.02: IATROGEN CV INFARCT/HEM

Type of Patients	Observed Patients	Avg. Stay	Vari-ance	10th	25th	50th	75th	90th	95th	99th
1. SINGLE DX										
A. Not Operated										
0–19 Years	0									
20–34	0									
35–49	0									
50–64	0									
65+	1	2.0	0	2	2	2	2	2	2	2
B. Operated										
0–19 Years	0									
20–34	0									
35–49	0									
50–64	1	3.0	0	3	3	3	3	3	3	3
65+	0									
2. MULTIPLE DX										
A. Not Operated										
0–19 Years	2	18.6	141	10	10	27	27	27	27	27
20–34	4	6.3	16	3	3	4	4	12	12	12
35–49	22	7.6	111	1	1	4	9	13	21	49
50–64	29	5.6	16	1	3	5	8	10	12	18
65+	85	5.2	12	2	3	5	6	10	13	18
B. Operated										
0–19 Years	2	4.0	0	4	4	4	4	4	4	4
20–34	6	18.5	462	3	4	9	9	31	57	57
35–49	11	10.3	57	5	6	7	10	25	25	25
50–64	20	8.8	49	2	3	6	16	20	22	22
65+	15	11.9	115	3	3	6	21	26	37	37
SUBTOTALS:										
1. SINGLE DX										
A. Not Operated	1	2.0	0	2	2	2	2	2	2	2
B. Operated	1	3.0	0	3	3	3	3	3	3	3
2. MULTIPLE DX										
A. Not Operated	142	5.9	31	2	3	5	7	11	14	27
B. Operated	53	11.0	114	3	4	6	15	25	31	57
1. SINGLE DX	**2**	**2.5**	**<1**	**2**	**2**	**3**	**3**	**3**	**3**	**3**
2. MULTIPLE DX	**195**	**7.3**	**58**	**2**	**3**	**5**	**8**	**15**	**22**	**49**
A. NOT OPERATED	**143**	**5.9**	**31**	**2**	**3**	**5**	**7**	**11**	**14**	**27**
B. OPERATED	**54**	**10.8**	**113**	**3**	**4**	**6**	**15**	**25**	**31**	**57**
TOTAL										
0–19 Years	3	13.7	141	4	4	10	10	27	27	27
20–34	10	13.6	301	3	4	6	12	31	57	57
35–49	33	8.5	92	1	3	6	10	21	21	49
50–64	50	6.8	31	2	3	6	8	17	20	22
65+	101	6.2	32	2	3	5	7	13	17	26
GRAND TOTAL	**197**	**7.2**	**58**	**2**	**3**	**5**	**8**	**15**	**22**	**49**

Length of Stay by Diagnosis and Operation, Western Region, 2008

Western Region, October 2006–September 2007 Data, by Diagnosis

997.09: NERV SYST SURG COMP NEC

Type of Patients	Observed Patients	Avg. Stay	Vari-ance	Percentiles						
				10th	25th	50th	75th	90th	95th	99th
1. SINGLE DX										
A. *Not Operated*										
0–19 Years	1	2.0	0	2	2	2	2	2	2	2
20–34	3	4.0	3	3	3	3	6	6	6	6
35–49	7	3.7	2	2	3	3	5	5	5	5
50–64	2	3.0	8	1	1	5	5	5	5	5
65+	4	2.5	2	1	1	3	3	4	4	4
B. *Operated*										
0–19 Years	1	9.0	0	9	9	9	9	9	9	9
20–34	12	4.3	3	3	3	4	6	7	7	7
35–49	10	3.0	2	1	2	3	4	5	5	5
50–64	14	3.5	3	1	2	4	4	5	7	7
65+	4	3.5	10	1	1	3	3	8	8	8
2. MULTIPLE DX										
A. *Not Operated*										
0–19 Years	12	3.0	3	1	2	3	4	4	7	7
20–34	40	3.9	13	1	2	3	6	9	15	16
35–49	55	3.8	6	1	2	3	5	7	9	10
50–64	62	5.1	16	2	3	4	6	9	10	27
65+	49	4.9	19	1	2	3	7	13	15	17
B. *Operated*										
0–19 Years	16	5.6	21	1	2	4	7	14	16	16
20–34	76	7.4	42	3	3	6	8	19	22	29
35–49	134	6.3	23	2	3	5	8	13	17	22
50–64	186	6.9	39	2	3	5	9	15	17	32
65+	108	8.2	72	1	4	6	9	16	24	42
SUBTOTALS:										
1. SINGLE DX										
A. *Not Operated*	17	3.3	2	1	2	3	5	5	6	6
B. *Operated*	41	3.7	4	1	2	4	5	7	7	9
2. MULTIPLE DX										
A. *Not Operated*	218	4.4	13	1	2	3	6	9	12	16
B. *Operated*	520	7.0	42	2	3	5	9	15	20	32
1. SINGLE DX	58	3.6	3	1	2	3	5	6	7	9
2. MULTIPLE DX	738	6.2	35	1	3	5	8	14	17	29
A. NOT OPERATED	235	4.3	12	1	2	3	6	8	11	16
B. OPERATED	561	6.8	40	1	3	5	8	15	19	32
TOTAL										
0–19 Years	30	4.6	14	1	2	3	5	9	14	16
20–34	131	6.0	31	1	2	4	7	13	19	26
35–49	206	5.4	18	1	2	4	7	11	15	20
50–64	264	6.2	32	2	3	5	7	13	17	29
65+	165	7.0	56	1	2	5	9	14	19	42
GRAND TOTAL	796	6.1	33	1	3	4	7	13	17	29

997.1: SURG COMP-HEART

Type of Patients	Observed Patients	Avg. Stay	Vari-ance	Percentiles						
				10th	25th	50th	75th	90th	95th	99th
1. SINGLE DX										
A. *Not Operated*										
0–19 Years	0									
20–34	0									
35–49	0									
50–64	0									
65+	0									
B. *Operated*										
0–19 Years	0									
20–34	0									
35–49	0									
50–64	0									
65+	0									
2. MULTIPLE DX										
A. *Not Operated*										
0–19 Years	6	7.3	56	1	1	1	11	19	19	19
20–34	17	2.0	2	1	1	2	2	4	5	5
35–49	47	2.6	3	1	1	2	2	4	6	8
50–64	168	3.4	9	1	1	2	4	8	9	14
65+	383	3.6	10	1	1	3	5	7	10	16
B. *Operated*										
0–19 Years	7	9.7	270	2	2	4	5	47	47	47
20–34	17	2.4	4	1	1	3	3	6	6	6
35–49	38	4.2	17	1	1	3	6	11	14	17
50–64	93	4.4	28	1	1	3	6	8	12	39
65+	254	4.0	19	1	1	3	5	8	12	25
SUBTOTALS:										
1. SINGLE DX										
A. *Not Operated*	0									
B. *Operated*	0									
2. MULTIPLE DX										
A. *Not Operated*	621	3.5	10	1	1	2	4	7	10	16
B. *Operated*	409	4.1	24	1	1	3	5	8	12	25
1. SINGLE DX	0									
2. MULTIPLE DX	1,030	3.7	16	1	1	2	5	8	11	18
A. NOT OPERATED	621	3.5	10	1	1	2	4	7	10	16
B. OPERATED	409	4.1	24	1	1	3	5	8	12	25
TOTAL										
0–19 Years	13	8.6	159	1	2	4	11	19	47	47
20–34	34	2.2	3	1	1	2	3	5	6	6
35–49	85	3.3	9	1	1	3	4	7	10	17
50–64	261	3.7	16	1	1	3	5	8	11	21
65+	637	3.8	14	1	1	3	5	8	11	18
GRAND TOTAL	1,030	3.7	16	1	1	2	5	8	11	18

997.2: SURG COMP-PERIPH VASC

Type of Patients	Observed Patients	Avg. Stay	Vari-ance	Percentiles						
				10th	25th	50th	75th	90th	95th	99th
1. SINGLE DX										
A. *Not Operated*										
0–19 Years	0									
20–34	0									
35–49	1	1.0	0	1	1	1	1	1	1	1
50–64	1	1.0	0	1	1	1	1	1	1	1
65+	0									
B. *Operated*										
0–19 Years	0									
20–34	1	4.0	0	4	4	4	4	4	4	4
35–49	0									
50–64	1	1.0	0	1	1	1	1	1	1	1
65+	0									
2. MULTIPLE DX										
A. *Not Operated*										
0–19 Years	3	2.3	2	1	1	2	4	4	4	4
20–34	58	3.1	4	1	1	3	4	6	8	9
35–49	181	3.3	6	1	2	3	4	6	8	14
50–64	247	3.2	5	1	1	3	4	6	7	11
65+	369	3.4	7	1	2	3	4	7	9	15
B. *Operated*										
0–19 Years	9	7.5	66	1	4	4	5	24	24	24
20–34	15	4.0	9	1	1	3	6	8	11	11
35–49	53	6.2	18	2	3	5	8	11	16	21
50–64	166	4.8	19	1	2	4	6	10	16	21
65+	325	5.4	20	1	2	4	7	11	13	23
SUBTOTALS:										
1. SINGLE DX										
A. *Not Operated*	2	1.0	0	1	1	1	1	1	1	1
B. *Operated*	2	2.5	4	1	1	1	4	4	4	4
2. MULTIPLE DX										
A. *Not Operated*	858	3.3	6	1	2	3	4	6	8	12
B. *Operated*	568	5.3	20	1	1	4	7	11	15	22
1. SINGLE DX	4	1.8	2	1	1	1	1	4	4	4
2. MULTIPLE DX	1,426	4.1	13	1	2	3	5	8	11	18
A. NOT OPERATED	860	3.3	6	1	2	3	4	6	8	12
B. OPERATED	570	5.3	20	1	2	4	7	11	15	22
TOTAL										
0–19 Years	12	6.2	54	1	3	4	4	19	24	24
20–34	74	3.3	5	1	1	3	5	5	8	11
35–49	235	4.0	10	1	2	3	5	8	10	16
50–64	415	3.9	11	1	2	3	5	7	10	19
65+	694	4.4	14	1	2	3	6	9	12	18
GRAND TOTAL	1,430	4.1	12	1	2	3	5	8	11	18

839

Length of Stay by Diagnosis and Operation, Western Region, 2008

Western Region, October 2006–September 2007 Data, by Diagnosis

Type of Patients	997.3: SURG COMP-RESP NEC										997.4: SURG COMP-DIGESTIVE										997.5: SURG COMP-URINARY NEC									
	Observed Patients	Avg. Stay	Variance	10th	25th	50th	75th	90th	95th	99th	Observed Patients	Avg. Stay	Variance	10th	25th	50th	75th	90th	95th	99th	Observed Patients	Avg. Stay	Variance	10th	25th	50th	75th	90th	95th	99th
1. SINGLE DX																														
A. Not Operated																														
0–19 Years	1	1.0	0	1	1	1	1	1	1	1	8	2.8	3	1	2	2	3	6	6	6	0									
20–34	0										17	3.8	6	1	2	3	4	6	10	10	0									
35–49	0										15	3.1	3	1	1	3	5	5	6	6	0									
50–64	0										9	3.6	9	1	2	2	4	9	9	9	1	2.0	0	2	2	2	2	2	2	2
65+	0										4	3.8	8	1	2	4	5	7	7	7	1	17.0	0	17	17	17	17	17	17	17
B. Operated																														
0–19 Years	0										0										0									
20–34	0										1	2.0	0	2	2	2	2	2	2	2	0									
35–49	0										6	3.3	10	1	1	3	5	9	9	9	0									
50–64	0										3	5.0	7	3	3	4	8	8	8	8	1	1.0	0	1	1	1	1	1	1	1
65+	0										0										0									
2. MULTIPLE DX																														
A. Not Operated																														
0–19 Years	55	3.9	22	1	1	3	4	7	17	26	198	4.0	14	1	2	3	5	8	10	25	21	2.6	4	1	1	2	3	7	7	7
20–34	52	3.0	6	1	1	2	4	7	9	10	689	4.1	16	1	2	3	5	8	11	23	62	3.0	11	1	1	2	3	5	8	22
35–49	140	3.1	8	2	2	2	4	7	7	13	1,313	4.3	15	1	2	3	5	8	11	21	131	3.2	7	1	1	3	4	5	7	11
50–64	229	3.7	20	1	1	3	5	7	10	23	1,644	4.8	17	1	2	4	6	9	12	21	280	3.1	6	1	1	2	4	6	8	11
65+	399	4.3	14	2	2	3	6	9	11	14	1,421	5.3	21	2	2	4	6	10	14	24	442	4.0	17	1	2	3	5	8	11	19
B. Operated																														
0–19 Years	17	2.6	11	1	1	1	2	7	14	14	84	7.2	49	2	3	5	8	18	23	32	9	2.8	7	1	1	2	3	6	9	9
20–34	17	3.2	11	1	1	2	4	9	11	11	223	6.9	45	2	3	5	9	14	19	28	30	3.0	3	1	1	2	4	6	7	7
35–49	46	3.8	32	1	1	2	4	8	13	35	500	8.5	88	2	3	6	10	18	25	51	76	5.2	34	1	2	4	6	9	14	37
50–64	92	4.8	35	1	1	2	5	14	17	29	708	9.2	89	2	4	7	11	20	27	69	145	5.0	51	1	1	3	6	9	15	41
65+	129	6.1	62	1	2	4	8	13	17	35	426	10.7	91	2	5	9	14	21	27	54	243	4.6	32	1	1	2	6	10	16	31
SUBTOTALS:																														
1. SINGLE DX																														
A. Not Operated	1	1.0	0	1	1	1	1	1	1	1	53	3.4	5	1	2	3	4	7	8	10	2	9.5	109	2	2	10	17	17	17	17
B. Operated	0										10	3.7	8	1	1	3	5	9	9	9	1	1.0	0	1	1	1	1	1	1	1
2. MULTIPLE DX																														
A. Not Operated	875	3.9	15	1	2	3	5	7	10	19	5,265	4.7	18	1	2	3	6	9	12	23	936	3.5	12	1	2	3	4	7	9	15
B. Operated	301	5.0	44	1	1	2	6	13	15	30	1,941	9.0	84	2	4	6	11	19	26	54	503	4.7	36	1	1	3	6	9	15	32
1. SINGLE DX	1	1.0	0	1	1	1	1	1	1	1	63	3.5	5	1	2	3	5	7	8	10	3	6.7	79	1	1	2	17	17	17	17
2. MULTIPLE DX	1,176	4.1	22	1	2	3	5	9	12	24	7,206	5.8	39	1	2	4	7	12	16	31	1,439	3.9	20	1	1	3	5	8	11	23
A. NOT OPERATED	876	3.9	15	1	2	3	5	7	10	19	5,318	4.6	17	1	2	3	6	9	12	22	938	3.6	12	1	2	3	4	7	9	15
B. OPERATED	301	5.0	44	1	1	2	6	13	15	30	1,951	9.0	84	2	4	6	11	19	26	54	504	4.7	36	1	1	3	6	9	15	32
TOTAL																														
0–19 Years	73	3.6	20	1	1	2	4	7	14	26	290	4.9	26	1	2	3	6	10	15	29	30	2.6	5	1	1	2	3	7	7	9
20–34	69	3.1	7	1	1	2	4	8	9	11	930	4.8	24	1	2	3	6	10	14	24	92	3.0	9	1	1	2	4	6	8	22
35–49	186	3.3	14	1	1	2	4	7	8	23	1,834	5.4	39	1	2	4	7	11	15	30	207	4.0	18	1	2	3	5	7	9	23
50–64	321	4.0	24	1	1	3	5	8	14	25	2,364	6.1	43	2	2	4	8	12	17	34	427	3.8	22	1	1	2	5	7	9	22
65+	528	4.7	26	1	2	3	6	10	12	24	1,851	6.5	42	2	3	5	8	14	18	32	686	4.3	22	1	2	3	5	9	12	26
GRAND TOTAL	1,177	4.1	22	1	2	3	5	9	12	24	7,269	5.8	39	1	2	4	7	12	16	31	1,442	4.0	20	1	1	3	5	8	11	23

Length of Stay by Diagnosis and Operation, Western Region, 2008

Western Region, October 2006–September 2007 Data, by Diagnosis

997.62: INFECT AMPUTATION STUMP

Type of Patients	Observed Patients	Avg. Stay	Vari-ance	10th	25th	50th	75th	90th	95th	99th
1. SINGLE DX										
A. Not Operated										
0–19 Years	0									
20–34	1	2.0	0	2	2	2	2	2	2	2
35–49	3	3.0	7	1	1	2	6	6	6	6
50–64	3	1.3	<1	1	1	1	2	2	2	2
65+	0									
B. Operated										
0–19 Years	1	1.0	0	1	1	1	1	1	1	1
20–34	0									
35–49	0									
50–64	1	2.0	0	2	2	2	2	2	2	2
65+	1	3.0	0	3	3	3	3	3	3	3
2. MULTIPLE DX										
A. Not Operated										
0–19 Years	1	4.0	0	4	4	4	4	4	4	4
20–34	28	6.3	30	2	3	5	7	14	20	25
35–49	160	5.4	16	2	3	5	7	10	13	17
50–64	281	5.5	23	2	2	4	7	11	14	26
65+	220	6.1	25	2	3	5	7	11	14	24
B. Operated										
0–19 Years	3	9.4	21	4	4	12	12	12	12	12
20–34	42	8.5	39	2	4	7	10	14	21	29
35–49	247	10.2	95	3	5	8	12	19	30	55
50–64	538	10.1	81	3	5	8	13	19	29	50
65+	579	9.4	48	3	5	8	12	17	22	34
SUBTOTALS:										
1. SINGLE DX										
A. Not Operated	7	2.1	3	1	1	2	2	6	6	6
B. Operated	3	2.0	<1	1	1	2	3	3	3	3
2. MULTIPLE DX										
A. Not Operated	690	5.7	23	2	3	5	7	11	14	26
B. Operated	1,409	9.8	68	3	5	8	12	18	25	45
1. SINGLE DX	10	2.1	2	1	1	2	2	3	6	6
2. MULTIPLE DX	2,099	8.4	57	2	4	7	10	16	21	40
A. NOT OPERATED	697	5.7	23	2	3	5	7	11	14	26
B. OPERATED	1,412	9.8	68	3	5	8	12	18	25	45
TOTAL										
0–19 Years	5	6.7	26	1	4	4	12	12	12	12
20–34	71	7.6	36	2	3	6	10	14	21	29
35–49	410	8.3	69	2	4	6	10	16	22	45
50–64	823	8.5	66	2	3	6	11	16	23	45
65+	800	8.5	44	3	4	7	11	16	20	33
GRAND TOTAL	2,109	8.4	57	2	4	7	10	16	21	40

997.69: AMP STUMP COMP NEC

Type of Patients	Observed Patients	Avg. Stay	Vari-ance	10th	25th	50th	75th	90th	95th	99th
1. SINGLE DX										
A. Not Operated										
0–19 Years	0									
20–34	0									
35–49	0									
50–64	0									
65+	2	5.5	40	1	1	10	10	10	10	10
B. Operated										
0–19 Years	1	1.0	0	1	1	1	1	1	1	1
20–34	5	2.2	5	1	1	1	2	6	6	6
35–49	4	2.8	8	1	1	2	7	7	7	7
50–64	6	2.7	6	1	1	2	4	7	7	7
65+	3	5.0	21	1	1	4	10	10	10	10
2. MULTIPLE DX										
A. Not Operated										
0–19 Years	0									
20–34	4	2.2	2	1	1	2	2	4	4	4
35–49	27	4.3	10	2	2	4	5	8	9	15
50–64	53	5.3	26	1	2	4	7	9	13	33
65+	54	6.7	37	1	3	5	8	15	19	33
B. Operated										
0–19 Years	12	5.2	39	2	2	3	5	10	23	23
20–34	25	4.6	9	3	3	4	5	9	9	15
35–49	125	6.8	59	1	2	5	8	16	24	36
50–64	278	6.0	31	1	2	4	7	13	18	31
65+	407	6.2	31	2	2	5	8	13	19	27
SUBTOTALS:										
1. SINGLE DX										
A. Not Operated	2	5.5	40	1	1	10	10	10	10	10
B. Operated	19	2.9	7	1	1	1	4	7	10	10
2. MULTIPLE DX										
A. Not Operated	138	5.6	27	1	2	4	7	10	15	33
B. Operated	847	6.2	35	1	2	4	8	13	19	31
1. SINGLE DX	21	3.1	9	1	1	1	4	7	10	10
2. MULTIPLE DX	985	6.1	34	1	2	4	8	13	18	31
A. NOT OPERATED	140	5.5	27	1	2	4	7	10	15	33
B. OPERATED	866	6.1	34	1	2	4	8	13	18	31
TOTAL										
0–19 Years	13	4.9	37	1	2	2	5	10	23	23
20–34	34	3.9	9	1	2	4	5	9	9	15
35–49	156	6.3	50	1	2	4	7	14	22	36
50–64	337	5.8	30	1	2	4	7	12	15	31
65+	466	6.2	32	1	2	5	8	13	19	29
GRAND TOTAL	1,006	6.0	33	1	2	4	7	13	18	31

997.99: SURG COMP OTH SYST NEC

Type of Patients	Observed Patients	Avg. Stay	Vari-ance	10th	25th	50th	75th	90th	95th	99th
1. SINGLE DX										
A. Not Operated										
0–19 Years	0									
20–34	0									
35–49	0									
50–64	0									
65+	0									
B. Operated										
0–19 Years	0									
20–34	0									
35–49	0									
50–64	0									
65+	0									
2. MULTIPLE DX										
A. Not Operated										
0–19 Years	16	2.8	4	1	1	2	4	6	8	8
20–34	19	3.1	8	1	1	2	4	6	13	13
35–49	39	2.9	4	1	2	2	4	5	7	12
50–64	73	3.3	7	1	2	2	4	6	9	13
65+	50	3.7	8	1	2	3	5	7	9	15
B. Operated										
0–19 Years	6	2.7	2	1	2	2	4	5	5	5
20–34	13	4.5	9	1	2	4	6	7	12	12
35–49	19	2.8	7	1	1	2	4	7	11	11
50–64	37	2.7	5	1	1	2	3	6	8	10
65+	66	3.4	14	1	1	2	4	7	12	20
SUBTOTALS:										
1. SINGLE DX										
A. Not Operated	0									
B. Operated	0									
2. MULTIPLE DX										
A. Not Operated	197	3.3	7	1	2	2	4	6	9	13
B. Operated	141	3.2	10	1	1	2	4	7	10	13
1. SINGLE DX	0									
2. MULTIPLE DX	338	3.2	8	1	1	2	4	7	9	13
A. NOT OPERATED	197	3.3	7	1	2	2	4	6	9	13
B. OPERATED	141	3.2	10	1	1	2	4	7	10	13
TOTAL										
0–19 Years	22	2.7	4	1	1	2	4	5	6	8
20–34	32	3.7	9	1	2	3	5	5	12	13
35–49	58	2.9	5	1	2	2	4	5	7	12
50–64	110	3.1	6	1	1	2	4	6	8	12
65+	116	3.5	11	1	2	2	4	7	11	15
GRAND TOTAL	338	3.2	8	1	1	2	4	7	9	13

Length of Stay by Diagnosis and Operation, Western Region, 2008

Western Region, October 2006–September 2007 Data, by Diagnosis

998: OTH SURGICAL COMP NEC

Type of Patients	Observed Patients	Avg. Stay	Variance	10th	25th	50th	75th	90th	95th	99th
1. SINGLE DX										
A. Not Operated										
0–19 Years	150	2.0	3	1	1	1	2	4	5	7
20–34	182	2.5	3	1	1	2	3	5	6	8
35–49	238	2.4	4	1	1	2	3	4	6	12
50–64	166	2.4	4	1	1	2	3	4	6	9
65+	57	2.1	1	1	1	2	3	4	4	5
B. Operated										
0–19 Years	160	1.9	6	1	1	1	2	4	7	14
20–34	188	2.3	11	1	1	2	2	6	8	17
35–49	179	2.6	5	1	1	2	3	6	7	13
50–64	130	2.8	5	1	1	2	4	5	7	11
65+	38	2.1	3	1	1	1	3	5	7	7
2. MULTIPLE DX										
A. Not Operated										
0–19 Years	912	3.9	12	1	2	3	5	8	11	17
20–34	2,107	3.9	13	1	2	3	5	7	10	18
35–49	4,817	4.2	16	1	2	3	5	8	11	20
50–64	6,792	4.5	20	1	2	3	5	9	12	22
65+	7,721	4.8	19	1	2	4	6	9	13	22
B. Operated										
0–19 Years	538	5.4	44	1	2	3	7	13	17	31
20–34	1,442	6.1	50	1	2	3	7	12	17	35
35–49	3,122	6.5	48	1	3	5	8	13	18	35
50–64	4,794	7.2	63	1	3	5	9	15	21	42
65+	5,327	7.6	63	1	3	5	9	16	22	41
SUBTOTALS:										
1. SINGLE DX										
A. Not Operated	793	2.3	3	1	1	2	3	4	6	9
B. Operated	695	2.4	7	1	1	1	3	5	7	13
2. MULTIPLE DX										
A. Not Operated	22,349	4.5	18	1	2	3	5	9	12	21
B. Operated	15,223	7.0	58	1	3	5	8	15	21	40
1. SINGLE DX	1,488	2.4	5	1	1	2	3	5	6	12
2. MULTIPLE DX	37,572	5.5	36	1	2	4	7	11	16	30
A. NOT OPERATED	23,142	4.4	17	1	2	3	5	8	12	21
B. OPERATED	15,918	6.8	57	1	2	5	8	14	20	39
TOTAL										
0–19 Years	1,760	4.0	22	1	1	3	5	9	12	22
20–34	3,919	4.6	28	1	2	3	5	9	13	24
35–49	8,356	5.0	29	1	2	3	6	10	14	27
50–64	11,882	5.5	39	1	2	4	7	11	16	32
65+	13,143	5.9	39	1	2	4	7	12	17	30
GRAND TOTAL	39,060	5.4	35	1	2	4	6	11	15	29

998.11: HEMORRHAGE COMP PX

Type of Patients	Observed Patients	Avg. Stay	Variance	10th	25th	50th	75th	90th	95th	99th
1. SINGLE DX										
A. Not Operated										
0–19 Years	64	1.3	<1	1	1	1	1	2	2	3
20–34	37	1.6	2	1	1	1	2	3	5	8
35–49	41	1.4	<1	1	1	1	2	2	2	4
50–64	30	1.5	<1	1	1	1	2	3	3	3
65+	12	1.9	<1	1	1	2	3	3	4	4
B. Operated										
0–19 Years	122	1.2	<1	1	1	1	1	2	3	3
20–34	113	1.2	<1	1	1	1	1	2	2	6
35–49	47	1.8	4	1	1	1	2	4	6	12
50–64	25	1.6	2	1	1	1	2	3	3	7
65+	7	1.3	<1	1	1	1	2	2	2	2
2. MULTIPLE DX										
A. Not Operated										
0–19 Years	113	1.9	2	1	1	1	2	3	5	7
20–34	200	2.5	6	1	1	2	3	5	6	15
35–49	436	2.7	12	1	1	2	3	5	7	15
50–64	1,133	2.5	4	1	1	2	3	5	6	10
65+	1,789	3.1	7	1	1	2	4	6	8	14
B. Operated										
0–19 Years	159	1.7	2	1	1	2	3	4	4	9
20–34	193	2.4	4	1	1	2	3	5	6	11
35–49	248	2.9	10	1	1	2	3	6	9	16
50–64	318	3.9	21	1	1	2	4	9	12	23
65+	543	5.0	38	2	3	3	6	11	15	26
SUBTOTALS:										
1. SINGLE DX										
A. Not Operated	184	1.5	<1	1	1	1	2	2	3	5
B. Operated	314	1.3	1	1	1	1	1	2	3	6
2. MULTIPLE DX										
A. Not Operated	3,671	2.8	7	1	1	2	3	5	7	14
B. Operated	1,461	3.7	22	1	1	2	4	8	12	22
1. SINGLE DX	498	1.4	<1	1	1	1	1	2	3	6
2. MULTIPLE DX	5,132	3.0	11	1	1	2	3	6	8	16
A. NOT OPERATED	3,855	2.7	7	1	1	2	3	5	7	14
B. OPERATED	1,775	3.3	19	1	1	2	4	7	11	22
TOTAL										
0–19 Years	458	1.6	1	1	1	1	2	3	4	6
20–34	543	2.1	4	1	1	1	2	4	6	11
35–49	772	2.6	10	1	1	2	3	5	7	15
50–64	1,506	2.8	8	1	1	2	3	5	8	14
65+	2,351	3.5	15	1	2	2	4	7	10	18
GRAND TOTAL	5,630	2.9	11	1	1	2	3	6	8	15

998.12: HEMATOMA COMPLICATING PX

Type of Patients	Observed Patients	Avg. Stay	Variance	10th	25th	50th	75th	90th	95th	99th
1. SINGLE DX										
A. Not Operated										
0–19 Years	9	2.0	2	1	1	2	2	5	5	5
20–34	40	2.3	2	1	1	2	3	5	5	6
35–49	52	2.0	2	1	1	2	2	3	5	7
50–64	26	2.3	2	1	1	2	4	4	5	6
65+	11	1.5	<1	1	1	1	2	2	4	4
B. Operated										
0–19 Years	4	1.3	<1	1	1	1	2	2	2	2
20–34	13	1.9	3	1	1	1	3	3	7	7
35–49	21	2.1	3	1	1	2	3	4	4	5
50–64	16	2.4	6	1	1	2	3	3	11	11
65+	6	2.3	6	1	1	1	3	7	7	7
2. MULTIPLE DX										
A. Not Operated										
0–19 Years	30	4.5	18	1	2	3	5	11	14	17
20–34	181	3.1	7	1	1	2	4	6	6	20
35–49	473	3.4	9	1	1	3	4	6	9	14
50–64	631	3.5	11	1	1	3	5	7	9	15
65+	871	3.9	10	1	2	3	5	8	10	15
B. Operated										
0–19 Years	13	6.3	32	1	2	5	7	16	19	19
20–34	121	4.5	11	1	2	4	6	9	11	16
35–49	233	4.5	14	1	2	4	6	9	11	20
50–64	346	5.3	29	1	2	4	6	11	16	28
65+	505	5.4	28	1	2	4	6	10	15	29
SUBTOTALS:										
1. SINGLE DX										
A. Not Operated	138	2.1	2	1	1	2	3	3	5	6
B. Operated	60	2.1	3	1	1	1	3	4	5	11
2. MULTIPLE DX										
A. Not Operated	2,186	3.6	10	1	2	3	5	7	9	15
B. Operated	1,218	5.1	24	1	2	4	6	10	14	25
1. SINGLE DX	198	2.1	2	1	1	2	3	4	5	7
2. MULTIPLE DX	3,404	4.2	16	1	2	3	5	8	11	20
A. NOT OPERATED	2,324	3.6	10	1	2	3	5	7	9	15
B. OPERATED	1,278	5.0	23	1	2	4	6	10	14	25
TOTAL										
0–19 Years	56	4.3	19	1	1	3	5	11	16	19
20–34	355	3.4	8	1	2	3	4	6	9	16
35–49	779	3.6	10	1	2	3	5	7	10	15
50–64	1,019	4.1	18	1	2	3	6	8	12	21
65+	1,393	4.4	17	1	2	3	6	9	11	20
GRAND TOTAL	3,602	4.1	15	1	2	3	5	8	11	19

Length of Stay by Diagnosis and Operation, Western Region, 2008

998.13: SEROMA COMPLICATING PX

Type of Patients	Observed Patients	Avg. Stay	Variance	10th	25th	50th	75th	90th	95th	99th
1. SINGLE DX										
A. *Not Operated*										
0–19 Years	6	1.8	<1	1	1	1	3	3	3	3
20–34	6	1.2	<1	1	1	1	1	2	2	2
35–49	17	1.7	<1	1	1	1	2	3	4	4
50–64	11	2.2	3	1	1	2	3	4	6	6
65+	6	1.8	1	1	1	1	2	4	4	4
B. *Operated*										
0–19 Years	0									
20–34	3	2.0	1	1	1	2	3	3	3	3
35–49	5	3.2	5	1	2	3	3	7	7	7
50–64	5	2.0	0	1	2	2	2	4	4	4
65+	1	2.0	0	2	2	2	2	2	2	2
2. MULTIPLE DX										
A. *Not Operated*										
0–19 Years	10	3.1	2	1	2	3	4	6	6	6
20–34	45	3.1	4	1	2	3	4	6	6	9
35–49	142	3.5	11	1	1	2	4	7	9	20
50–64	187	3.7	8	1	2	3	5	7	10	16
65+	153	4.0	10	1	2	3	5	8	10	17
B. *Operated*										
0–19 Years	1	4.0	0	4	4	4	4	4	4	4
20–34	22	4.6	15	2	2	4	5	6	14	17
35–49	39	4.0	13	1	2	3	5	8	13	18
50–64	109	4.6	17	1	2	3	6	8	12	17
65+	104	4.1	9	2	2	3	5	8	10	13
SUBTOTALS:										
1. SINGLE DX										
A. *Not Operated*	46	1.8	1	1	1	1	2	3	3	4
B. *Operated*	14	2.4	3	1	1	2	3	4	7	7
2. MULTIPLE DX										
A. *Not Operated*	537	3.7	9	1	2	3	5	7	10	16
B. *Operated*	275	4.3	13	1	2	3	6	8	12	17
1. SINGLE DX	60	1.9	2	1	1	1	2	3	4	7
2. MULTIPLE DX	812	3.9	11	1	2	3	5	7	10	17
A. NOT OPERATED	583	3.5	9	1	2	3	4	7	9	16
B. OPERATED	289	4.2	13	1	2	3	5	8	11	17
TOTAL										
0–19 Years	17	2.7	2	1	2	3	3	5	6	6
20–34	76	3.4	7	1	2	3	4	6	9	17
35–49	203	3.4	11	1	1	2	4	7	9	18
50–64	312	3.9	11	1	2	3	5	7	10	16
65+	264	4.0	10	1	2	3	5	8	10	16
GRAND TOTAL	872	3.8	10	1	2	3	5	7	10	17

998.2: ACCIDENTAL OP LACERATION

Type of Patients	Observed Patients	Avg. Stay	Variance	10th	25th	50th	75th	90th	95th	99th
1. SINGLE DX										
A. *Not Operated*										
0–19 Years	1	3.0	0	3	3	3	3	3	3	3
20–34	1	1.0	0	1	1	1	1	1	1	1
35–49	5	1.6	<1	1	1	1	2	3	3	3
50–64	2	2.5	<1	2	2	3	3	3	3	3
65+	1	2.0	0	2	2	2	2	2	2	2
B. *Operated*										
0–19 Years	0									
20–34	4	4.5	16	1	1	2	5	10	10	10
35–49	6	3.8	7	1	1	3	6	7	7	7
50–64	4	4.8	<1	4	4	5	5	5	5	5
65+	0									
2. MULTIPLE DX										
A. *Not Operated*										
0–19 Years	5	2.0	1	1	1	2	3	3	3	3
20–34	23	6.9	90	1	2	3	7	18	20	43
35–49	69	4.0	13	1	2	3	5	8	11	21
50–64	110	4.3	13	1	2	3	5	8	10	15
65+	163	5.5	25	2	2	4	6	11	17	22
B. *Operated*										
0–19 Years	7	6.6	51	2	2	4	7	22	22	22
20–34	71	5.8	17	3	3	4	8	11	14	21
35–49	159	7.1	32	3	3	5	8	14	18	33
50–64	251	7.0	35	4	4	6	9	14	17	32
65+	402	9.3	75	5	5	7	10	18	25	52
SUBTOTALS:										
1. SINGLE DX										
A. *Not Operated*	10	1.9	<1	1	1	2	3	3	3	3
B. *Operated*	14	4.3	6	1	2	5	5	7	10	10
2. MULTIPLE DX										
A. *Not Operated*	370	4.9	23	1	2	3	6	10	14	22
B. *Operated*	890	8.0	53	2	4	6	9	15	20	40
1. SINGLE DX	24	3.3	5	1	1	3	5	6	7	10
2. MULTIPLE DX	1,260	7.1	46	2	3	5	8	14	18	35
A. NOT OPERATED	380	4.8	23	1	2	3	6	9	14	22
B. OPERATED	904	7.9	53	2	4	6	9	15	20	37
TOTAL										
0–19 Years	13	4.6	31	1	2	3	4	7	22	22
20–34	99	5.9	34	1	3	4	8	13	17	21
35–49	239	6.0	28	1	3	5	7	13	16	28
50–64	367	6.2	30	2	3	5	8	12	15	29
65+	566	8.2	64	2	4	6	9	16	21	43
GRAND TOTAL	1,284	7.0	46	2	3	5	8	14	18	35

998.31: DISRUPT INTERNAL OP WND

Type of Patients	Observed Patients	Avg. Stay	Variance	10th	25th	50th	75th	90th	95th	99th
1. SINGLE DX										
A. *Not Operated*										
0–19 Years	1	3.0	0	3	3	3	3	3	3	3
20–34	1	4.0	0	4	4	4	4	4	4	4
35–49	0									
50–64	1	8.0	0	8	8	8	8	8	8	8
65+	0									
B. *Operated*										
0–19 Years	1	7.0	0	7	7	7	7	7	7	7
20–34	4	2.3	<1	1	1	3	3	3	3	3
35–49	7	1.9	<1	1	1	2	3	3	3	3
50–64	8	2.9	5	1	1	2	4	7	7	7
65+	0									
2. MULTIPLE DX										
A. *Not Operated*										
0–19 Years	5	2.4	2	1	2	2	2	5	5	5
20–34	7	4.3	38	1	1	3	3	18	18	18
35–49	20	4.1	14	1	2	2	4	10	12	13
50–64	28	7.1	51	1	3	5	9	18	22	31
65+	27	4.0	11	1	1	4	7	8	11	13
B. *Operated*										
0–19 Years	9	4.4	31	1	1	1	4	16	16	16
20–34	44	3.9	12	1	1	3	5	7	8	17
35–49	108	5.9	36	2	2	4	7	14	21	27
50–64	180	6.4	70	2	2	4	7	12	17	73
65+	209	6.4	34	2	2	4	7	14	18	27
SUBTOTALS:										
1. SINGLE DX										
A. *Not Operated*	3	5.0	7	3	3	4	8	8	8	8
B. *Operated*	20	2.6	3	1	1	2	3	7	7	7
2. MULTIPLE DX										
A. *Not Operated*	87	5.0	28	1	2	3	7	12	17	31
B. *Operated*	550	6.1	44	1	2	4	7	13	17	31
1. SINGLE DX	23	2.9	4	1	1	2	4	4	7	8
2. MULTIPLE DX	637	5.9	42	1	2	4	7	13	17	31
A. NOT OPERATED	90	5.0	27	1	2	3	7	12	17	31
B. OPERATED	570	5.9	43	1	2	4	7	13	17	31
TOTAL										
0–19 Years	16	3.9	19	1	1	2	4	12	16	16
20–34	56	3.8	14	1	2	3	4	7	15	18
35–49	135	5.4	32	1	2	3	7	13	19	27
50–64	217	6.4	65	1	2	4	8	13	21	58
65+	236	6.1	32	2	2	4	7	13	17	27
GRAND TOTAL	660	5.8	41	1	2	4	7	13	17	31

Length of Stay by Diagnosis and Operation, Western Region, 2008

Western Region, October 2006–September 2007 Data, by Diagnosis

998.32: DISRUPT EXTERNAL OP WND

Type of Patients	Observed Patients	Avg. Stay	Variance	10th	25th	50th	75th	90th	95th	99th
1. SINGLE DX										
A. Not Operated										
0–19 Years	5	1.2	<1	1	1	1	1	2	2	2
20–34	8	2.5	4	1	1	2	4	7	7	7
35–49	11	3.5	4	1	2	3	6	6	7	7
50–64	11	2.5	3	1	1	2	4	4	6	6
65+	3	1.7	<1	1	1	2	2	2	2	2
B. Operated										
0–19 Years	4	1.5	<1	1	1	1	3	3	3	3
20–34	9	3.0	5	1	1	3	4	8	8	8
35–49	18	3.0	10	1	1	2	3	6	14	14
50–64	13	3.2	4	2	2	3	4	6	8	8
65+	7	1.9	2	1	1	1	3	5	5	5
2. MULTIPLE DX										
A. Not Operated										
0–19 Years	21	3.1	10	1	1	2	3	5	9	14
20–34	47	3.6	22	1	1	2	4	7	10	30
35–49	128	3.9	11	1	2	3	5	8	10	17
50–64	222	4.8	26	1	2	3	6	9	14	29
65+	243	4.9	20	1	2	4	6	9	12	28
B. Operated										
0–19 Years	22	5.1	21	1	2	3	7	13	14	16
20–34	50	4.3	15	1	2	3	5	8	11	19
35–49	159	5.2	27	1	2	4	7	11	13	>99
50–64	386	6.8	56	1	2	5	8	15	22	46
65+	416	6.9	57	1	3	5	8	14	19	42
SUBTOTALS:										
1. SINGLE DX — A. Not Operated	38	2.5	3	1	1	2	4	6	7	7
1. SINGLE DX — B. Operated	51	2.8	6	1	1	2	3	5	8	14
2. MULTIPLE DX — A. Not Operated	661	4.5	20	1	2	3	6	9	13	28
2. MULTIPLE DX — B. Operated	1,033	6.4	50	1	2	4	8	13	19	42
1. SINGLE DX	89	2.7	5	1	1	2	3	6	7	14
2. MULTIPLE DX	1,694	5.7	39	1	2	4	7	12	16	36
A. NOT OPERATED	699	4.4	20	1	2	3	5	9	12	27
B. OPERATED	1,084	6.2	48	1	2	4	7	13	18	42
TOTAL										
0–19 Years	52	3.6	14	1	1	2	4	9	14	16
20–34	114	3.8	16	1	1	3	4	8	11	19
35–49	316	4.5	19	1	2	3	6	10	13	26
50–64	632	6.0	44	1	2	4	7	13	19	35
65+	669	6.1	44	1	2	4	7	12	17	41
GRAND TOTAL	1,783	5.5	38	1	2	4	7	11	16	35

998.51: INFECTED POSTOP SEROMA

Type of Patients	Observed Patients	Avg. Stay	Variance	10th	25th	50th	75th	90th	95th	99th
1. SINGLE DX										
A. Not Operated										
0–19 Years	2	3.0	2	2	2	2	4	4	4	4
20–34	4	2.2	2	1	1	1	3	4	4	4
35–49	7	2.1	1	1	2	2	3	4	4	4
50–64	3	4.0	7	1	1	5	6	6	6	6
65+	1	4.0	0	4	4	4	4	4	4	4
B. Operated										
0–19 Years	0									
20–34	2	1.5	<1	1	1	2	2	2	2	2
35–49	4	2.3	<1	1	2	3	3	3	3	3
50–64	3	2.0	<1	1	1	2	3	3	3	3
65+	0									
2. MULTIPLE DX										
A. Not Operated										
0–19 Years	7	5.6	32	1	3	4	5	18	18	18
20–34	39	5.6	29	1	3	4	7	15	19	26
35–49	170	4.6	13	1	2	4	6	9	12	19
50–64	201	5.2	16	2	3	4	7	9	13	22
65+	168	5.9	29	2	3	4	7	12	15	29
B. Operated										
0–19 Years	5	8.8	65	1	3	5	7	18	18	18
20–34	24	7.8	26	3	4	6	5	14	16	23
35–49	85	6.1	29	2	2	5	7	12	17	35
50–64	119	6.9	38	2	3	5	8	13	20	42
65+	113	7.5	31	3	4	6	8	13	19	24
SUBTOTALS:										
1. SINGLE DX — A. Not Operated	17	2.7	2	1	1	2	4	5	6	6
1. SINGLE DX — B. Operated	9	2.0	<1	1	1	2	3	3	3	3
2. MULTIPLE DX — A. Not Operated	585	5.3	20	2	2	4	7	10	14	24
2. MULTIPLE DX — B. Operated	346	7.0	33	2	3	6	9	13	18	29
1. SINGLE DX	26	2.5	2	1	1	2	3	4	5	6
2. MULTIPLE DX	931	5.9	26	2	3	4	7	11	15	24
A. NOT OPERATED	602	5.2	20	2	2	4	7	10	14	24
B. OPERATED	355	6.9	33	2	3	6	9	13	18	29
TOTAL										
0–19 Years	14	6.3	39	1	3	4	5	9	14	16
20–34	69	6.0	28	1	3	4	7	14	19	26
35–49	266	5.0	19	1	2	4	6	10	12	20
50–64	326	5.8	24	2	3	5	7	11	14	24
65+	282	6.6	30	2	3	5	8	12	18	41
GRAND TOTAL	957	5.8	25	2	3	4	7	11	15	24

998.59: POSTOP INFECTION NEC

Type of Patients	Observed Patients	Avg. Stay	Variance	10th	25th	50th	75th	90th	95th	99th
1. SINGLE DX										
A. Not Operated										
0–19 Years	56	3.0	4	1	2	2	4	5	6	13
20–34	73	3.3	4	1	2	3	5	6	7	8
35–49	91	3.0	5	1	2	2	4	6	8	12
50–64	74	2.8	4	1	2	2	3	5	7	10
65+	18	2.8	2	1	2	3	4	5	5	5
B. Operated										
0–19 Years	20	5.4	19	2	2	4	8	12	12	19
20–34	27	5.7	41	1	2	4	7	16	17	30
35–49	40	3.2	3	1	1	2	5	7	8	9
50–64	34	2.9	3	1	2	2	4	6	7	8
65+	10	1.7	<1	1	1	1	2	3	3	3
2. MULTIPLE DX										
A. Not Operated										
0–19 Years	598	4.6	13	1	2	4	6	9	11	17
20–34	1,375	4.2	13	1	2	3	5	8	10	18
35–49	2,990	4.6	16	1	2	3	6	9	11	20
50–64	3,744	5.1	20	2	3	4	6	10	13	22
65+	3,792	5.7	22	2	3	4	7	11	14	24
B. Operated										
0–19 Years	259	7.7	63	2	3	5	10	16	21	46
20–34	732	7.3	49	2	3	5	9	14	20	35
35–49	1,646	7.6	58	2	3	5	9	15	21	41
50–64	2,342	8.4	70	2	4	6	10	18	23	44
65+	2,315	9.0	70	2	4	7	11	18	25	44
SUBTOTALS:										
1. SINGLE DX — A. Not Operated	312	3.0	4	1	2	2	4	5	7	11
1. SINGLE DX — B. Operated	131	3.9	15	1	2	2	5	7	9	19
2. MULTIPLE DX — A. Not Operated	12,499	5.0	19	2	3	4	6	10	13	22
2. MULTIPLE DX — B. Operated	7,294	8.3	65	2	4	6	10	17	23	44
1. SINGLE DX	443	3.3	8	1	2	2	4	6	8	13
2. MULTIPLE DX	19,793	6.2	38	2	3	4	7	12	17	31
A. NOT OPERATED	12,811	5.0	18	2	2	4	6	9	13	22
B. OPERATED	7,425	8.2	65	2	3	6	10	17	23	44
TOTAL										
0–19 Years	933	5.4	29	1	2	4	6	11	14	28
20–34	2,207	5.2	27	1	3	4	6	10	14	25
35–49	4,767	5.6	32	2	3	4	7	11	15	29
50–64	6,194	6.3	41	2	3	4	8	12	17	34
65+	6,135	6.9	42	2	3	5	8	14	19	33
GRAND TOTAL	20,236	6.2	38	2	3	4	7	12	17	31

Western Region, October 2006–September 2007 Data, by Diagnosis

998.6: PERSIST POSTOP FISTULA

Type of Patients	Observed Patients	Avg. Stay	Variance	Percentiles						
				10th	25th	50th	75th	90th	95th	99th
1. SINGLE DX										
A. Not Operated										
0–19 Years	2	1.5	<1	1	1	2	2	2	2	2
20–34	4	2.8	6	1	1	2	6	6	6	6
35–49	5	3.8	26	1	1	2	2	13	13	13
50–64	1	2.0	0	2	2	2	2	2	2	2
65+	1	3.0	0	3	3	3	3	3	3	3
B. Operated										
0–19 Years	6	2.3	4	1	1	1	5	5	5	5
20–34	3	1.0	0	1	1	1	1	1	1	1
35–49	10	1.8	1	1	1	1	3	4	4	4
50–64	0									
65+	1	4.0	0	4	4	4	4	4	4	4
2. MULTIPLE DX										
A. Not Operated										
0–19 Years	9	3.5	9	1	2	2	4	9	9	9
20–34	33	5.3	29	1	2	4	6	11	16	28
35–49	66	6.9	82	1	2	4	8	14	19	54
50–64	140	9.4	124	1	3	5	11	24	31	55
65+	132	8.3	71	2	3	6	11	17	25	43
B. Operated										
0–19 Years	26	4.3	34	1	1	1	4	18	18	18
20–34	58	10.8	229	1	2	6	13	27	44	91
35–49	161	7.6	78	1	3	6	9	16	21	81
50–64	256	9.8	170	1	3	6	11	20	30	74
65+	244	11.3	179	1	3	7	15	25	37	83
SUBTOTALS:										
1. SINGLE DX										
A. Not Operated	13	2.9	11	1	1	2	3	6	13	13
B. Operated	20	2.0	2	1	1	1	3	5	5	5
2. MULTIPLE DX										
A. Not Operated	380	8.1	89	1	3	5	10	18	28	48
B. Operated	745	9.7	155	1	3	6	12	21	32	77
1. SINGLE DX	33	2.3	6	1	1	1	3	5	6	13
2. MULTIPLE DX	1,125	9.2	133	1	3	6	11	20	30	72
A. NOT OPERATED	393	7.9	87	1	3	4	9	17	28	48
B. OPERATED	765	9.5	152	1	3	6	11	21	30	77
TOTAL										
0–19 Years	43	3.7	23	1	1	2	4	9	18	18
20–34	98	8.3	154	1	2	4	10	19	33	91
35–49	242	7.1	76	1	2	5	9	15	21	54
50–64	397	9.7	153	1	3	6	11	21	31	72
65+	378	10.2	142	2	3	6	13	22	33	75
GRAND TOTAL	1,158	9.0	131	1	3	5	11	20	29	72

998.83: NON-HEALING SURG WND

Type of Patients	Observed Patients	Avg. Stay	Variance	Percentiles						
				10th	25th	50th	75th	90th	95th	99th
1. SINGLE DX										
A. Not Operated										
0–19 Years	1	1.0	0	1	1	1	1	1	1	1
20–34	3	2.0	<1	1	1	2	3	3	3	3
35–49	2	2.0	2	1	1	1	2	3	3	3
50–64	2	1.5	<1	1	1	1	2	2	2	2
65+	0									
B. Operated										
0–19 Years	3	6.7	44	1	1	5	5	14	14	14
20–34	8	5.9	17	1	2	6	8	12	12	12
35–49	12	4.4	14	1	2	4	4	10	13	13
50–64	15	4.0	9	1	2	4	5	7	12	12
65+	2	4.0	2	3	3	5	5	5	5	5
2. MULTIPLE DX										
A. Not Operated										
0–19 Years	6	3.0	3	1	2	2	4	5	5	5
20–34	13	3.4	22	1	2	3	6	6	19	19
35–49	59	4.8	39	1	1	3	8	11	17	36
50–64	96	5.6	30	1	3	4	7	12	18	34
65+	86	6.0	34	1	2	4	7	13	16	33
B. Operated										
0–19 Years	15	4.9	13	1	2	4	6	12	13	13
20–34	71	7.9	148	1	3	5	8	15	29	91
35–49	142	6.4	73	1	2	5	8	13	17	40
50–64	292	6.0	38	1	2	4	7	12	18	35
65+	279	5.5	29	1	2	4	7	12	15	26
SUBTOTALS:										
1. SINGLE DX										
A. Not Operated	8	1.8	<1	1	1	1	2	3	3	3
B. Operated	40	4.7	13	1	2	4	6	12	12	14
2. MULTIPLE DX										
A. Not Operated	260	5.4	33	1	2	4	6	12	17	33
B. Operated	799	6.0	51	1	2	4	7	13	17	34
1. SINGLE DX	48	4.2	12	1	1	3	5	10	12	14
2. MULTIPLE DX	1,059	5.9	46	1	2	4	7	13	17	34
A. NOT OPERATED	268	5.3	32	1	2	4	6	12	17	33
B. OPERATED	839	6.0	49	1	2	4	7	13	17	34
TOTAL										
0–19 Years	25	4.5	14	1	2	4	5	12	13	14
20–34	95	7.1	116	1	2	4	7	14	19	91
35–49	215	5.8	60	1	2	4	7	11	17	36
50–64	405	5.8	35	1	2	4	7	12	18	34
65+	367	5.6	30	1	2	4	7	12	15	27
GRAND TOTAL	1,107	5.8	45	1	2	4	7	12	17	33

998.89: OTH SPEC POSTOP COMP NEC

Type of Patients	Observed Patients	Avg. Stay	Variance	Percentiles						
				10th	25th	50th	75th	90th	95th	99th
1. SINGLE DX										
A. Not Operated										
0–19 Years	1	1.0	0	1	1	1	1	1	1	1
20–34	5	2.0	<1	1	2	2	2	3	3	3
35–49	4	4.7	11	1	1	4	5	9	9	9
50–64	3	1.7	1	1	1	1	3	3	3	3
65+	4	1.3	<1	1	1	1	1	2	2	2
B. Operated										
0–19 Years	0									
20–34	1	1.0	0	1	1	1	1	1	1	1
35–49	6	1.5	<1	1	1	2	2	2	2	2
50–64	3	4.7	21	2	2	2	10	10	10	10
65+	2	4.5	12	2	2	7	7	7	7	7
2. MULTIPLE DX										
A. Not Operated										
0–19 Years	105	2.3	6	1	1	2	3	4	6	7
20–34	129	2.7	4	1	1	2	3	5	7	12
35–49	243	3.2	11	1	1	2	4	6	8	22
50–64	266	2.9	5	1	1	2	4	6	8	10
65+	260	3.2	11	1	1	2	4	6	9	16
B. Operated										
0–19 Years	21	4.7	31	1	1	2	5	12	16	21
20–34	45	3.2	5	1	2	2	4	6	8	10
35–49	114	3.0	8	1	1	2	4	6	9	15
50–64	162	3.9	19	1	1	2	4	7	14	24
65+	149	3.5	13	1	2	2	4	7	11	18
SUBTOTALS:										
1. SINGLE DX										
A. Not Operated	17	2.4	4	1	1	2	3	5	9	9
B. Operated	12	2.8	8	1	1	2	2	7	10	10
2. MULTIPLE DX										
A. Not Operated	1,003	3.0	8	1	1	2	4	6	8	15
B. Operated	491	3.6	14	1	1	2	4	7	11	21
1. SINGLE DX	29	2.5	6	1	1	2	2	7	9	10
2. MULTIPLE DX	1,494	3.2	10	1	1	2	4	6	9	16
A. NOT OPERATED	1,020	3.0	8	1	1	2	4	6	8	15
B. OPERATED	503	3.5	14	1	1	2	4	7	11	21
TOTAL										
0–19 Years	127	2.7	11	1	1	2	3	5	9	15
20–34	180	2.8	5	1	1	2	3	5	8	12
35–49	367	3.2	10	1	1	2	4	6	8	15
50–64	434	3.3	11	1	1	2	4	6	9	21
65+	415	3.3	12	1	1	2	4	7	10	17
GRAND TOTAL	1,523	3.1	10	1	1	2	4	6	9	16

Length of Stay by Diagnosis and Operation, Western Region, 2008

Western Region, October 2006–September 2007 Data, by Diagnosis

999: COMP MEDICAL CARE NEC

Type of Patients	Observed Patients	Avg. Stay	Variance	\Percentiles 10th	25th	50th	75th	90th	95th	99th
1. SINGLE DX										
A. Not Operated										
0–19 Years	9	1.3	<1	1	1	1	2	2	2	2
20–34	2	2.5	5	1	1	3	4	4	4	4
35–49	1	2.0	0	2	2	2	2	2	2	2
50–64	1	4.0	0	4	4	4	4	4	4	4
65+	0									
B. Operated										
0–19 Years	0									
20–34	0									
35–49	0									
50–64	0									
65+	0									
2. MULTIPLE DX										
A. Not Operated										
0–19 Years	78	3.2	11	1	1	2	3	6	11	17
20–34	134	4.8	35	1	2	3	5	10	14	26
35–49	221	3.5	8	1	2	3	4	6	9	15
50–64	291	4.6	19	1	2	3	5	9	13	19
65+	399	4.6	15	1	2	4	6	9	11	22
B. Operated										
0–19 Years	2	3.0	2	2	2	3	4	4	4	4
20–34	7	10.1	107	2	4	7	10	33	33	33
35–49	29	8.2	35	2	4	6	12	21	21	22
50–64	31	7.3	52	2	3	4	8	17	18	35
65+	37	10.6	76	3	4	8	14	23	30	40
SUBTOTALS:										
1. SINGLE DX										
A. Not Operated	13	1.8	1	1	1	1	2	2	4	4
B. Operated	0									
2. MULTIPLE DX										
A. Not Operated	1,123	4.3	17	1	2	3	5	9	11	18
B. Operated	106	8.8	59	2	4	6	12	19	23	35
1. SINGLE DX	13	1.8	1	1	1	1	2	4	4	4
2. MULTIPLE DX	1,229	4.7	22	1	2	3	6	10	14	22
A. NOT OPERATED	1,136	4.3	17	1	2	3	5	9	11	18
B. OPERATED	106	8.8	59	2	4	6	12	19	23	35
TOTAL										
0–19 Years	89	3.0	10	1	1	2	3	6	11	17
20–34	143	5.1	39	1	2	3	6	10	14	33
35–49	251	4.0	13	1	2	3	5	8	9	21
50–64	323	4.9	23	1	2	4	6	10	15	19
65+	436	5.1	23	1	2	4	6	10	13	23
GRAND TOTAL	1,242	4.7	22	1	2	3	6	9	14	22

999.2: VASC COMP MED CARE NEC

Type of Patients	Observed Patients	Avg. Stay	Variance	\Percentiles 10th	25th	50th	75th	90th	95th	99th
1. SINGLE DX										
A. Not Operated										
0–19 Years	0									
20–34	0									
35–49	0									
50–64	0									
65+	0									
B. Operated										
0–19 Years	0									
20–34	0									
35–49	0									
50–64	0									
65+	0									
2. MULTIPLE DX										
A. Not Operated										
0–19 Years	3	7.3	22	2	2	9	11	11	11	11
20–34	28	3.3	10	1	1	2	4	6	9	16
35–49	50	3.6	10	1	1	3	4	8	10	15
50–64	49	3.6	9	1	2	2	5	7	7	19
65+	57	4.3	8	1	2	4	5	9	11	13
B. Operated										
0–19 Years	0									
20–34	0									
35–49	6	8.7	50	2	4	9	12	21	21	21
50–64	5	8.4	52	1	4	5	14	18	18	18
65+	5	2.4	2	1	1	3	3	4	4	4
SUBTOTALS:										
1. SINGLE DX										
A. Not Operated	0									
B. Operated	0									
2. MULTIPLE DX										
A. Not Operated	187	3.8	9	1	2	3	5	7	10	16
B. Operated	16	6.6	40	1	3	4	12	18	21	21
1. SINGLE DX	0									
2. MULTIPLE DX	203	4.1	12	1	2	3	5	9	11	18
A. NOT OPERATED	187	3.8	9	1	2	3	5	7	10	16
B. OPERATED	16	6.6	40	1	3	4	12	18	21	21
TOTAL										
0–19 Years	3	7.3	22	2	2	9	11	11	11	11
20–34	28	3.3	10	1	1	2	4	6	9	16
35–49	56	4.2	16	1	2	3	6	10	13	21
50–64	54	4.0	14	1	2	3	5	7	14	19
65+	62	4.2	8	1	2	4	5	8	11	13
GRAND TOTAL	203	4.1	12	1	2	3	5	9	11	18

999.3: INFECT COMP MED CARE NEC

Type of Patients	Observed Patients	Avg. Stay	Variance	\Percentiles 10th	25th	50th	75th	90th	95th	99th
1. SINGLE DX										
A. Not Operated										
0–19 Years	1	1.0	0	1	1	1	1	1	1	1
20–34	0									
35–49	0									
50–64	0									
65+	0									
B. Operated										
0–19 Years	0									
20–34	0									
35–49	0									
50–64	0									
65+	0									
2. MULTIPLE DX										
A. Not Operated										
0–19 Years	31	3.4	7	1	1	3	4	6	9	13
20–34	69	4.7	18	1	2	3	5	10	12	26
35–49	114	3.8	6	1	2	3	5	8	8	14
50–64	156	5.0	20	2	3	4	6	9	13	17
65+	166	5.1	13	2	3	4	6	9	11	22
B. Operated										
0–19 Years	6	3.0	2	2	2	3	4	4	4	4
20–34	6	10.8	125	2	5	9	10	33	33	33
35–49	19	8.5	33	3	5	6	13	21	22	22
50–64	20	8.3	62	3	4	6	12	18	35	35
65+	28	11.4	67	4	5	9	15	23	26	40
SUBTOTALS:										
1. SINGLE DX										
A. Not Operated	1	1.0	0	1	1	1	1	1	1	1
B. Operated	0									
2. MULTIPLE DX										
A. Not Operated	536	4.6	14	1	2	4	6	9	11	17
B. Operated	75	9.6	60	3	4	7	13	20	26	40
1. SINGLE DX	1	1.0	0	1	1	1	1	1	1	1
2. MULTIPLE DX	611	5.2	23	2	2	4	6	10	14	23
A. NOT OPERATED	537	4.6	14	1	2	4	6	9	11	17
B. OPERATED	75	9.6	60	3	4	7	13	20	26	40
TOTAL										
0–19 Years	34	3.3	7	1	1	3	4	6	9	13
20–34	75	5.2	28	1	2	3	7	10	15	33
35–49	133	4.4	13	1	2	4	5	8	14	21
50–64	176	5.4	26	2	3	4	6	10	15	35
65+	194	6.0	26	2	3	5	7	11	15	26
GRAND TOTAL	612	5.2	23	1	2	4	6	10	14	23

V01: COMMUNICABLE DIS CONTACT

Type of Patients	Observed Patients	Avg. Stay	Vari-ance	10th	25th	50th	75th	90th	95th	99th
						Percentiles				
1. SINGLE DX										
A. *Not Operated*										
0–19 Years	0									
20–34	0									
35–49	0									
50–64	0									
65+	0									
B. *Operated*										
0–19 Years	0									
20–34	0									
35–49	0									
50–64	0									
65+	0									
2. MULTIPLE DX										
A. *Not Operated*										
0–19 Years	0									
20–34	0									
35–49	0									
50–64	0									
65+	0									
B. *Operated*										
0–19 Years	0									
20–34	0									
35–49	0									
50–64	0									
65+	0									
SUBTOTALS:										
1. SINGLE DX										
A. *Not Operated*	0									
B. *Operated*	0									
2. MULTIPLE DX										
A. *Not Operated*	0									
B. *Operated*	0									
1. SINGLE DX	0									
2. MULTIPLE DX	0									
A. NOT OPERATED	0									
B. OPERATED	0									
TOTAL										
0–19 Years	0									
20–34	0									
35–49	0									
50–64	0									
65+	0									
GRAND TOTAL	0									

V02: INFECTIOUS DIS CARRIER

Type of Patients	Observed Patients	Avg. Stay	Vari-ance	10th	25th	50th	75th	90th	95th	99th
						Percentiles				
1. SINGLE DX										
A. *Not Operated*										
0–19 Years	0									
20–34	0									
35–49	0									
50–64	0									
65+	0									
B. *Operated*										
0–19 Years	0									
20–34	0									
35–49	0									
50–64	0									
65+	0									
2. MULTIPLE DX										
A. *Not Operated*										
0–19 Years	0									
20–34	0									
35–49	0									
50–64	0									
65+	0									
B. *Operated*										
0–19 Years	0									
20–34	0									
35–49	0									
50–64	0									
65+	0									
SUBTOTALS:										
1. SINGLE DX										
A. *Not Operated*	0									
B. *Operated*	0									
2. MULTIPLE DX										
A. *Not Operated*	0									
B. *Operated*	0									
1. SINGLE DX	0									
2. MULTIPLE DX	0									
A. NOT OPERATED	0									
B. OPERATED	0									
TOTAL										
0–19 Years	0									
20–34	0									
35–49	0									
50–64	0									
65+	0									
GRAND TOTAL	0									

V03: BACTERIAL DIS VACCINE

Type of Patients	Observed Patients	Avg. Stay	Vari-ance	10th	25th	50th	75th	90th	95th	99th
						Percentiles				
1. SINGLE DX										
A. *Not Operated*										
0–19 Years	0									
20–34	0									
35–49	0									
50–64	0									
65+	0									
B. *Operated*										
0–19 Years	0									
20–34	0									
35–49	0									
50–64	0									
65+	0									
2. MULTIPLE DX										
A. *Not Operated*										
0–19 Years	0									
20–34	0									
35–49	0									
50–64	0									
65+	0									
B. *Operated*										
0–19 Years	0									
20–34	0									
35–49	0									
50–64	0									
65+	0									
SUBTOTALS:										
1. SINGLE DX										
A. *Not Operated*	0									
B. *Operated*	0									
2. MULTIPLE DX										
A. *Not Operated*	0									
B. *Operated*	0									
1. SINGLE DX	0									
2. MULTIPLE DX	0									
A. NOT OPERATED	0									
B. OPERATED	0									
TOTAL										
0–19 Years	0									
20–34	0									
35–49	0									
50–64	0									
65+	0									
GRAND TOTAL	0									

847

Length of Stay by Diagnosis and Operation, Western Region, 2008

Western Region, October 2006–September 2007 Data, by Diagnosis

V04: VIRAL DISEASE VACCINE   **V05: SNGL DISEASE VACCINE NEC**   **V06: DISEASE COMB VACCINE**

Type of Patients	V04 Observed Patients	V04 Avg. Stay	V04 Vari-ance	V04 10th	V04 25th	V04 50th	V04 75th	V04 90th	V04 95th	V04 99th	V05 Observed Patients	V05 Avg. Stay	V05 Vari-ance	V05 10th	V05 25th	V05 50th	V05 75th	V05 90th	V05 95th	V05 99th	V06 Observed Patients	V06 Avg. Stay	V06 Vari-ance	V06 10th	V06 25th	V06 50th	V06 75th	V06 90th	V06 95th	V06 99th
1. SINGLE DX																														
A. *Not Operated*																														
0–19 Years	0										0										0									
20–34	0										0										0									
35–49	0										0										0									
50–64	0										0										0									
65+																														
B. *Operated*																														
0–19 Years	0										0										0									
20–34	0										0										0									
35–49	0										0										0									
50–64	0										0										0									
65+	0										0																			
2. MULTIPLE DX																														
A. *Not Operated*																														
0–19 Years	0										0										0									
20–34	0										0										0									
35–49	0										0										0									
50–64	0										0										0									
65+	0										0										0									
B. *Operated*																														
0–19 Years	0										0										0									
20–34	0										0										0									
35–49	0										0										0									
50–64	0										0										0									
65+	0										0																			
SUBTOTALS:																														
1. SINGLE DX																														
A. *Not Operated*	0										0										0									
B. *Operated*	0										0										0									
2. MULTIPLE DX																														
A. *Not Operated*	0										0										0									
B. *Operated*	0										0										0									
1. SINGLE DX	0										0										0									
2. MULTIPLE DX	0										0										0									
A. NOT OPERATED	0										0										0									
B. OPERATED	0										0										0									
TOTAL																														
0–19 Years	0										0										0									
20–34	0										0										0									
35–49	0										0										0									
50–64	0										0										0									
65+	0										0																			
GRAND TOTAL	0										0										0									

Length of Stay by Diagnosis and Operation, Western Region, 2008

Western Region, October 2006–September 2007 Data, by Diagnosis

V07: PROPHYLACTIC MEASURES

Type of Patients	Observed Patients	Avg. Stay	Variance	Percentiles 10th	25th	50th	75th	90th	95th	99th
1. SINGLE DX										
A. Not Operated										
0–19 Years	0									
20–34	0									
35–49	0									
50–64	1	1.0	0		1	1	1	1	1	1
65+	0									
B. Operated										
0–19 Years	0									
20–34	0									
35–49	0									
50–64	0									
65+	0									
2. MULTIPLE DX										
A. Not Operated										
0–19 Years	2	2.0	2	1	1	3	3	3	3	3
20–34	1	1.0	0	1	1	1	1	1	1	1
35–49	0									
50–64	2	1.5	<1	1	1	1	2	2	2	2
65+	2	4.0	2	3	3	5	5	5	5	5
B. Operated										
0–19 Years	0									
20–34	2	3.5	4	2	2	2	5	5	5	5
35–49	7	2.0	2	1	1	2	2	5	5	5
50–64	7	2.0	<1	1	1	2	3	3	3	3
65+	1	3.0	0	3	3	3	3	3	3	3
SUBTOTALS:										
1. SINGLE DX										
A. Not Operated	1	1.0	0	1	1	1	1	1	1	1
B. Operated	0									
2. MULTIPLE DX										
A. Not Operated	7	2.3	2	1	1	2	3	5	5	5
B. Operated	17	2.2	2	1	1	2	3	5	5	5
1. SINGLE DX	1	1.0	0	1	1	1	1	1	1	1
2. MULTIPLE DX	24	2.3	2	1	1	2	3	5	5	5
A. NOT OPERATED	8	2.1	2	1	1	1	3	5	5	5
B. OPERATED	17	2.2	2	1	1	2	3	5	5	5
TOTAL										
0–19 Years	2	2.0	2	1	1	3	3	3	3	3
20–34	3	2.7	4	1	1	2	5	5	5	5
35–49	7	2.0	2	1	1	2	2	5	5	5
50–64	10	1.8	<1	1	1	2	2	3	3	3
65+	3	3.7	1	3	3	3	5	5	5	5
GRAND TOTAL	25	2.2	2	1	1	2	3	5	5	5

V08: ASYMPTOMATIC HIV STATUS

Type of Patients	Observed Patients	Avg. Stay	Variance	Percentiles 10th	25th	50th	75th	90th	95th	99th
1. SINGLE DX										
A. Not Operated										
0–19 Years	0									
20–34	0									
35–49	0									
50–64	0									
65+	0									
B. Operated										
0–19 Years	0									
20–34	0									
35–49	0									
50–64	0									
65+	0									
2. MULTIPLE DX										
A. Not Operated										
0–19 Years	0									
20–34	0									
35–49	0									
50–64	0									
65+	0									
B. Operated										
0–19 Years	0									
20–34	0									
35–49	0									
50–64	0									
65+	0									
SUBTOTALS:										
A. Not Operated	0									
B. Operated	0									
A. Not Operated	0									
B. Operated	0									
1. SINGLE DX	0									
2. MULTIPLE DX	0									
A. NOT OPERATED	0									
B. OPERATED	0									
TOTAL										
0–19 Years	0									
20–34	0									
35–49	0									
50–64	0									
65+	0									
GRAND TOTAL	0									

V09: INF W DRUG-RESISTANT ORG

Type of Patients	Observed Patients	Avg. Stay	Variance	Percentiles 10th	25th	50th	75th	90th	95th	99th
1. SINGLE DX										
A. Not Operated										
0–19 Years	0									
20–34	0									
35–49	0									
50–64	0									
65+	0									
B. Operated										
0–19 Years	0									
20–34	0									
35–49	0									
50–64	0									
65+	0									
2. MULTIPLE DX										
A. Not Operated										
0–19 Years	0									
20–34	0									
35–49	0									
50–64	0									
65+	0									
B. Operated										
0–19 Years	0									
20–34	0									
35–49	0									
50–64	0									
65+	0									
SUBTOTALS:										
A. Not Operated	0									
B. Operated	0									
A. Not Operated	0									
B. Operated	0									
1. SINGLE DX	0									
2. MULTIPLE DX	0									
A. NOT OPERATED	0									
B. OPERATED	0									
TOTAL										
0–19 Years	0									
20–34	0									
35–49	0									
50–64	0									
65+	0									
GRAND TOTAL	0									

Length of Stay by Diagnosis and Operation, Western Region, 2008

Western Region, October 2006–September 2007 Data, by Diagnosis

V10: HX OF MALIGNANT NEOPLASM

Type of Patients	Observed Patients	Avg. Stay	Variance	10th	25th	50th	75th	90th	95th	99th
1. SINGLE DX										
A. Not Operated										
0–19 Years	0									
20–34	0									
35–49	0									
50–64	0									
65+	0									
B. Operated										
0–19 Years	0									
20–34	0									
35–49	0									
50–64	0									
65+	0									
2. MULTIPLE DX										
A. Not Operated										
0–19 Years	0									
20–34	0									
35–49	0									
50–64	0									
65+	0									
B. Operated										
0–19 Years	0									
20–34	0									
35–49	0									
50–64	0									
65+	0									
SUBTOTALS:										
1. SINGLE DX										
A. Not Operated	0									
B. Operated	0									
2. MULTIPLE DX										
A. Not Operated	0									
B. Operated	0									
1. SINGLE DX	0									
2. MULTIPLE DX	0									
A. NOT OPERATED	0									
B. OPERATED	0									
TOTAL										
0–19 Years	0									
20–34	0									
35–49	0									
50–64	0									
65+	0									
GRAND TOTAL	0									

V11: HX MENTAL DISORDER

Type of Patients	Observed Patients	Avg. Stay	Variance	10th	25th	50th	75th	90th	95th	99th
1. SINGLE DX										
A. Not Operated										
0–19 Years	0									
20–34	0									
35–49	0									
50–64	0									
65+	0									
B. Operated										
0–19 Years	0									
20–34	0									
35–49	0									
50–64	0									
65+	0									
2. MULTIPLE DX										
A. Not Operated										
0–19 Years	0									
20–34	0									
35–49	0									
50–64	0									
65+	0									
B. Operated										
0–19 Years	0									
20–34	0									
35–49	0									
50–64	0									
65+	0									
SUBTOTALS:										
1. SINGLE DX										
A. Not Operated	0									
B. Operated	0									
2. MULTIPLE DX										
A. Not Operated	0									
B. Operated	0									
1. SINGLE DX	0									
2. MULTIPLE DX	0									
A. NOT OPERATED	0									
B. OPERATED	0									
TOTAL										
0–19 Years	0									
20–34	0									
35–49	0									
50–64	0									
65+	0									
GRAND TOTAL	0									

V12: HX CERTAIN OTHER DISEASE

Type of Patients	Observed Patients	Avg. Stay	Variance	10th	25th	50th	75th	90th	95th	99th
1. SINGLE DX										
A. Not Operated										
0–19 Years	0									
20–34	0									
35–49	0									
50–64	0									
65+	0									
B. Operated										
0–19 Years	0									
20–34	0									
35–49	0									
50–64	0									
65+	0									
2. MULTIPLE DX										
A. Not Operated										
0–19 Years	1	4.0	0	4	4	4	4	4	4	4
20–34	0									
35–49	0									
50–64	0									
65+	0									
B. Operated										
0–19 Years	0									
20–34	0									
35–49	0									
50–64	0									
65+	0									
SUBTOTALS:										
1. SINGLE DX										
A. Not Operated	0									
B. Operated	0									
2. MULTIPLE DX										
A. Not Operated	1	4.0	0	4	4	4	4	4	4	4
B. Operated	0									
1. SINGLE DX	0									
2. MULTIPLE DX	1	4.0	0	4	4	4	4	4	4	4
A. NOT OPERATED	1	4.0	0	4	4	4	4	4	4	4
B. OPERATED	0									
TOTAL										
0–19 Years	1	4.0	0	4	4	4	4	4	4	4
20–34	0									
35–49	0									
50–64	0									
65+	0									
GRAND TOTAL	1	4.0	0	4	4	4	4	4	4	4

Length of Stay by Diagnosis and Operation, Western Region, 2008

Western Region, October 2006–September 2007 Data, by Diagnosis

V13: HX OTHER DISEASE

Type of Patients	Observed Patients	Avg. Stay	Variance	10th	25th	50th	75th	90th	95th	99th
1. SINGLE DX										
A. Not Operated										
0–19 Years	0									
20–34	0									
35–49	0									
50–64	0									
65+	0									
B. Operated										
0–19 Years	0									
20–34	0									
35–49	0									
50–64	0									
65+	0									
2. MULTIPLE DX										
A. Not Operated										
0–19 Years	0									
20–34	0									
35–49	0									
50–64	0									
65+	0									
B. Operated										
0–19 Years	0									
20–34	0									
35–49	0									
50–64	0									
65+	0									
SUBTOTALS:										
1. SINGLE DX										
A. Not Operated	0									
B. Operated	0									
2. MULTIPLE DX										
A. Not Operated	0									
B. Operated	0									
1. SINGLE DX	0									
2. MULTIPLE DX	0									
A. NOT OPERATED	0									
B. OPERATED	0									
TOTAL										
0–19 Years	0									
20–34	0									
35–49	0									
50–64	0									
65+	0									
GRAND TOTAL	0									

V14: HX DRUG ALLERGY

Type of Patients	Observed Patients	Avg. Stay	Variance	10th	25th	50th	75th	90th	95th	99th
1. SINGLE DX										
A. Not Operated										
0–19 Years	0									
20–34	0									
35–49	0									
50–64	0									
65+	0									
B. Operated										
0–19 Years	0									
20–34	0									
35–49	0									
50–64	0									
65+	0									
2. MULTIPLE DX										
A. Not Operated										
0–19 Years	0									
20–34	0									
35–49	0									
50–64	0									
65+	0									
B. Operated										
0–19 Years	0									
20–34	0									
35–49	0									
50–64	0									
65+	0									
SUBTOTALS:										
1. SINGLE DX										
A. Not Operated	0									
B. Operated	0									
2. MULTIPLE DX										
A. Not Operated	0									
B. Operated	0									
1. SINGLE DX	0									
2. MULTIPLE DX	0									
A. NOT OPERATED	0									
B. OPERATED	0									
TOTAL										
0–19 Years	0									
20–34	0									
35–49	0									
50–64	0									
65+	0									
GRAND TOTAL	0									

V15: HX OTHER HEALTH HAZARDS

Type of Patients	Observed Patients	Avg. Stay	Variance	10th	25th	50th	75th	90th	95th	99th
1. SINGLE DX										
A. Not Operated										
0–19 Years	0									
20–34	0									
35–49	0									
50–64	0									
65+	0									
B. Operated										
0–19 Years	0									
20–34	0									
35–49	0									
50–64	0									
65+	0									
2. MULTIPLE DX										
A. Not Operated										
0–19 Years	0									
20–34	0									
35–49	0									
50–64	0									
65+	1	3.0	0	3	3	3	3	3	3	3
B. Operated										
0–19 Years	0									
20–34	0									
35–49	0									
50–64	0									
65+	0									
SUBTOTALS:										
1. SINGLE DX										
A. Not Operated	0									
B. Operated	0									
2. MULTIPLE DX										
A. Not Operated	1	3.0	0	3	3	3	3	3	3	3
B. Operated	0									
1. SINGLE DX	0									
2. MULTIPLE DX	1	3.0	0	3	3	3	3	3	3	3
A. NOT OPERATED	1	3.0	0	3	3	3	3	3	3	3
B. OPERATED	0									
TOTAL										
0–19 Years	0									
20–34	0									
35–49	0									
50–64	0									
65+	1	3.0	0	3	3	3	3	3	3	3
GRAND TOTAL	1	3.0	0	3	3	3	3	3	3	3

851

Length of Stay by Diagnosis and Operation, Western Region, 2008

Western Region, October 2006–September 2007 Data, by Diagnosis

V16: FAMILY HX CA / V17: FAM HX CHR DISABLING DIS / V18: FAMILY HX OTH CONDITION

Type of Patients	V16 Observed Patients	V16 Avg. Stay	V16 Vari-ance	V16 10th	V16 25th	V16 50th	V16 75th	V16 90th	V16 95th	V16 99th	V17 Observed Patients	V17 Avg. Stay	V17 Vari-ance	V17 10th	V17 25th	V17 50th	V17 75th	V17 90th	V17 95th	V17 99th	V18 Observed Patients	V18 Avg. Stay	V18 Vari-ance	V18 10th	V18 25th	V18 50th	V18 75th	V18 90th	V18 95th	V18 99th
1. SINGLE DX																														
A. *Not Operated*																														
0–19 Years	0										0										0									
20–34	0										0										0									
35–49	0										0										0									
50–64	0										0										0									
65+																														
B. *Operated*																														
0–19 Years	0										0										0									
20–34	0										0										0									
35–49	0										0										0									
50–64	0										0										0									
65+	0										0										0									
2. MULTIPLE DX																														
A. *Not Operated*																														
0–19 Years	0										0										0									
20–34	0										0										0									
35–49	0										0										0									
50–64	0										0										0									
65+	0										0										0									
B. *Operated*																														
0–19 Years	0										0										0									
20–34	0										0										0									
35–49	0										0										0									
50–64	0										0										0									
65+	0										0										0									
SUBTOTALS:																														
1. SINGLE DX																														
A. *Not Operated*	0										0										0									
B. *Operated*	0										0										0									
2. MULTIPLE DX																														
A. *Not Operated*	0										0										0									
B. *Operated*	0										0										0									
1. SINGLE DX	0										0										0									
2. MULTIPLE DX	0										0										0									
A. NOT OPERATED	0										0										0									
B. OPERATED	0										0										0									
TOTAL																														
0–19 Years	0										0										0									
20–34	0										0										0									
35–49	0										0										0									
50–64	0										0										0									
65+	0										0										0									
GRAND TOTAL	0										0										0									

Length of Stay by Diagnosis and Operation, Western Region, 2008

Western Region, October 2006–September 2007 Data, by Diagnosis

V19: FAMILY HX CONDITIONS NEC

Type of Patients	Observed Patients	Avg. Stay	Variance	10th	25th	50th	75th	90th	95th	99th
1. SINGLE DX										
A. *Not Operated*										
0–19 Years	0									
20–34	0									
35–49	0									
50–64	0									
65+	0									
B. *Operated*										
0–19 Years	0									
20–34	0									
35–49	0									
50–64	0									
65+	0									
2. MULTIPLE DX										
A. *Not Operated*										
0–19 Years	0									
20–34	0									
35–49	0									
50–64	0									
65+	0									
B. *Operated*										
0–19 Years	0									
20–34	0									
35–49	0									
50–64	0									
65+	0									
SUBTOTALS:										
1. SINGLE DX										
A. *Not Operated*	0									
B. *Operated*	0									
2. MULTIPLE DX										
A. *Not Operated*	0									
B. *Operated*	0									
1. SINGLE DX	0									
2. MULTIPLE DX	0									
A. NOT OPERATED	0									
B. OPERATED	0									
TOTAL										
0–19 Years	0									
20–34	0									
35–49	0									
50–64	0									
65+	0									
GRAND TOTAL	0									

V20: HEALTH SUPERVISION CHILD

Type of Patients	Observed Patients	Avg. Stay	Variance	10th	25th	50th	75th	90th	95th	99th
1. SINGLE DX										
A. *Not Operated*										
0–19 Years	0									
20–34	0									
35–49	0									
50–64	0									
65+	0									
B. *Operated*										
0–19 Years	0									
20–34	0									
35–49	0									
50–64	0									
65+	0									
2. MULTIPLE DX										
A. *Not Operated*										
0–19 Years	2	1.5	<1	1	1	1	2	2	2	2
20–34	0									
35–49	0									
50–64	0									
65+	0									
B. *Operated*										
0–19 Years	0									
20–34	0									
35–49	0									
50–64	0									
65+	0									
SUBTOTALS:										
1. SINGLE DX										
A. *Not Operated*	0									
B. *Operated*	0									
2. MULTIPLE DX										
A. *Not Operated*	2	1.5	<1	1	1	1	2	2	2	2
B. *Operated*	0									
1. SINGLE DX	0									
2. MULTIPLE DX	2	1.5	<1	1	1	1	2	2	2	2
A. NOT OPERATED	2	1.5	<1	1	1	1	2	2	2	2
B. OPERATED	0									
TOTAL										
0–19 Years	2	1.5	<1	1	1	1	2	2	2	2
20–34	0									
35–49	0									
50–64	0									
65+	0									
GRAND TOTAL	2	1.5	<1	1	1	1	2	2	2	2

V21: CONSTIT DEVELOPMENT

Type of Patients	Observed Patients	Avg. Stay	Variance	10th	25th	50th	75th	90th	95th	99th
1. SINGLE DX										
A. *Not Operated*										
0–19 Years	0									
20–34	0									
35–49	0									
50–64	0									
65+	0									
B. *Operated*										
0–19 Years	0									
20–34	0									
35–49	0									
50–64	0									
65+	0									
2. MULTIPLE DX										
A. *Not Operated*										
0–19 Years	0									
20–34	0									
35–49	0									
50–64	0									
65+	0									
B. *Operated*										
0–19 Years	0									
20–34	0									
35–49	0									
50–64	0									
65+	0									
SUBTOTALS:										
1. SINGLE DX										
A. *Not Operated*	0									
B. *Operated*	0									
2. MULTIPLE DX										
A. *Not Operated*	0									
B. *Operated*	0									
1. SINGLE DX	0									
2. MULTIPLE DX	0									
A. NOT OPERATED	0									
B. OPERATED	0									
TOTAL										
0–19 Years	0									
20–34	0									
35–49	0									
50–64	0									
65+	0									
GRAND TOTAL	0									

853

Length of Stay by Diagnosis and Operation, Western Region, 2008

Western Region, October 2006–September 2007 Data, by Diagnosis

V22: NORMAL PREGNANCY   V23: SUPERVIS HIGH-RISK PREG   V24: POSTPARTUM CARE & EXAM

Type of Patients	V22 Obs. Pts	V23 Obs. Pts	V24 Obs. Pts	V24 Avg. Stay	V24 Variance	V24 10th	V24 25th	V24 50th	V24 75th	V24 90th	V24 95th	V24 99th
1. SINGLE DX												
A. Not Operated												
0–19 Years	0	0	48	1.6	<1	1	1	2	2	2	2	3
20–34	0	0	437	1.5	<1	1	1	1	2	2	2	3
35–49	0	0	74	1.6	<1	1	1	2	2	2	3	3
50–64	0	0	4	1.3	<1	1	1	1	1	2	2	2
65+	0	0	0									
B. Operated												
0–19 Years	0	0	2	2.0	2	1	1	2	3	3	3	3
20–34	0	0	13	1.5	<1	1	1	2	2	2	2	2
35–49	0	0	3	1.7	<1	1	1	2	2	2	2	2
50–64	0	0	0									
65+	0	0	0									
2. MULTIPLE DX												
A. Not Operated												
0–19 Years	0	0	18	1.6	<1	1	1	2	2	2	2	2
20–34	0	0	115	1.6	<1	1	1	2	2	2	3	3
35–49	0	0	14	1.6	<1	1	1	2	2	2	2	2
50–64	0	0	0									
65+	0	0	0									
B. Operated												
0–19 Years	0	0	0									
20–34	0	0	20	1.8	<1	1	2	2	2	2	3	3
35–49	0	0	3	2.0	0	2	2	2	2	2	2	2
50–64	0	0	0									
65+	0	0	0									
SUBTOTALS:												
1. SINGLE DX												
A. Not Operated	0	0	563	1.5	<1	1	1	1	2	2	2	3
B. Operated	0	0	18	1.6	<1	1	1	2	2	2	3	3
2. MULTIPLE DX												
A. Not Operated	0	0	147	1.6	<1	1	1	2	2	2	2	3
B. Operated	0	0	23	1.8	<1	1	2	2	2	2	2	3
1. SINGLE DX	0	0	581	1.5	<1	1	1	1	2	2	2	3
2. MULTIPLE DX	0	0	170	1.6	<1	1	1	2	2	2	2	3
A. NOT OPERATED	0	0	710	1.5	<1	1	1	1	2	2	2	3
B. OPERATED	0	0	41	1.7	<1	1	1	2	2	2	2	3
TOTAL												
0–19 Years	0	0	68	1.6	<1	1	1	2	2	2	2	3
20–34	0	0	585	1.5	<1	1	1	1	2	2	2	3
35–49	0	0	94	1.6	<1	1	1	2	2	2	3	3
50–64	0	0	4	1.3	<1	1	1	1	1	2	2	2
65+	0	0	0									
GRAND TOTAL	0	0	751	1.5	<1	1	1	2	2	2	2	3

Western Region, October 2006–September 2007 Data, by Diagnosis

V24.0: PP CARE IMMED AFTER DEL

Type of Patients	Observed Patients	Avg. Stay	Vari-ance	10th	25th	50th	75th	90th	95th	99th
1. SINGLE DX										
A. Not Operated										
0–19 Years	48	1.6	<1	1	1	2	2	2	2	3
20–34	437	1.5	<1	1	1	1	2	2	2	3
35–49	74	1.6	<1	1	1	2	2	2	3	3
50–64	4	1.3	<1	1	1	1	1	2	2	2
65+	0									
B. Operated										
0–19 Years	2	2.0	2	1	1	2	3	3	3	3
20–34	13	1.5	<1	1	1	2	2	2	2	2
35–49	3	1.7	<1	1	1	2	2	2	2	2
50–64	0									
65+	0									
2. MULTIPLE DX										
A. Not Operated										
0–19 Years	18	1.6	<1	1	1	2	2	2	2	2
20–34	115	1.6	<1	1	1	2	2	2	3	3
35–49	14	1.6	<1	1	1	2	2	2	2	2
50–64	0									
65+	0									
B. Operated										
0–19 Years	0									
20–34	20	1.8	<1	1	2	2	2	2	3	3
35–49	3	2.0	0	2	2	2	2	2	2	2
50–64	0									
65+	0									
SUBTOTALS:										
1. SINGLE DX										
A. Not Operated	563	1.5	<1	1	1	1	2	2	2	3
B. Operated	18	1.6	<1	1	1	2	2	3	3	3
2. MULTIPLE DX										
A. Not Operated	147	1.6	<1	1	1	2	2	2	2	3
B. Operated	23	1.8	<1	1	2	2	2	2	3	3
1. SINGLE DX	581	1.5	<1	1	1	2	2	2	2	3
2. MULTIPLE DX	170	1.6	<1	1	1	2	2	2	2	3
A. NOT OPERATED	710	1.5	<1	1	1	1	2	2	2	3
B. OPERATED	41	1.7	<1	1	1	2	2	2	3	3
TOTAL										
0–19 Years	68	1.6	<1	1	1	2	2	2	3	3
20–34	585	1.5	<1	1	1	2	2	2	3	3
35–49	94	1.6	<1	1	1	2	2	2	3	3
50–64	4	1.3	<1	1	1	1	1	2	2	2
65+	0									
GRAND TOTAL	751	1.5	<1	1	1	2	2	2	2	3

V25: CONTRACEPTIVE MANAGEMENT

Type of Patients	Observed Patients	Avg. Stay	Vari-ance	10th	25th	50th	75th	90th	95th	99th
1. SINGLE DX										
A. Not Operated										
0–19 Years	0									
20–34	0									
35–49	0									
50–64	0									
65+	0									
B. Operated										
0–19 Years	0									
20–34	13	1.5	<1	1	1	1	2	2	3	3
35–49	13	1.3	<1	1	1	1	1	2	3	3
50–64	2	1.0	0	1	1	1	1	1	1	1
65+	0									
2. MULTIPLE DX										
A. Not Operated										
0–19 Years	0									
20–34	2	1.0	0	1	1	1	1	1	1	1
35–49	1	1.0	0	1	1	1	1	1	1	1
50–64	0									
65+	0									
B. Operated										
0–19 Years	1	2.0	0	2	2	2	2	2	2	2
20–34	71	2.0	3	1	1	1	2	3	4	14
35–49	50	1.7	6	1	1	1	2	2	3	18
50–64	5	1.4	<1	1	1	1	2	2	2	2
65+	0									
SUBTOTALS:										
1. SINGLE DX										
A. Not Operated	0									
B. Operated	28	1.4	<1	1	1	1	1	2	3	3
2. MULTIPLE DX										
A. Not Operated	3	1.0	0	1	1	1	1	1	1	1
B. Operated	127	1.9	4	1	1	1	2	3	4	14
1. SINGLE DX	28	1.4	<1	1	1	1	2	2	3	3
2. MULTIPLE DX	130	1.8	4	1	1	1	2	3	4	14
A. NOT OPERATED	3	1.0	0	1	1	1	1	1	1	1
B. OPERATED	155	1.8	3	1	1	1	2	3	4	14
TOTAL										
0–19 Years	1	2.0	0	2	2	2	2	2	2	2
20–34	86	1.9	3	1	1	1	2	3	4	14
35–49	64	1.6	5	1	1	1	2	2	3	18
50–64	7	1.3	<1	1	1	1	2	2	2	2
65+	0									
GRAND TOTAL	158	1.8	3	1	1	1	2	3	4	14

V26: PROCREATIVE MANAGEMENT

Type of Patients	Observed Patients	Avg. Stay	Vari-ance	10th	25th	50th	75th	90th	95th	99th
1. SINGLE DX										
A. Not Operated										
0–19 Years	0									
20–34	0									
35–49	0									
50–64	0									
65+	0									
B. Operated										
0–19 Years	0									
20–34	12	1.3	<1	1	1	1	1	2	2	3
35–49	14	1.6	<1	1	1	1	2	3	3	3
50–64	2	1.0	0	1	1	1	1	1	1	1
65+	0									
2. MULTIPLE DX										
A. Not Operated										
0–19 Years	0									
20–34	0									
35–49	0									
50–64	0									
65+	0									
B. Operated										
0–19 Years	0									
20–34	9	1.6	<1	1	1	2	2	2	2	2
35–49	13	2.2	3	1	1	2	2	3	7	7
50–64	0									
65+	0									
SUBTOTALS:										
1. SINGLE DX										
A. Not Operated	0									
B. Operated	28	1.4	<1	1	1	1	2	3	3	3
2. MULTIPLE DX										
A. Not Operated	0									
B. Operated	22	2.0	2	1	1	2	2	3	3	7
1. SINGLE DX	28	1.4	<1	1	1	1	2	3	3	3
2. MULTIPLE DX	22	2.0	2	1	1	2	2	3	3	7
A. NOT OPERATED	0									
B. OPERATED	50	1.7	1	1	1	1	2	3	3	7
TOTAL										
0–19 Years	0									
20–34	21	1.4	<1	1	1	1	2	3	3	3
35–49	27	1.9	2	1	1	2	2	3	3	7
50–64	2	1.0	0	1	1	1	1	1	1	1
65+	0									
GRAND TOTAL	50	1.7	1	1	1	1	2	3	3	7

Length of Stay by Diagnosis and Operation, Western Region, 2008

Western Region, October 2006–September 2007 Data, by Diagnosis

V27: OUTCOME OF DELIVERY

Type of Patients	Observed Patients	Avg. Stay	Variance	Percentiles 10th	25th	50th	75th	90th	95th	99th
1. SINGLE DX										
A. Not Operated										
0–19 Years	0									
20–34	0									
35–49	0									
50–64	0									
65+	0									
B. Operated										
0–19 Years	0									
20–34	0									
35–49	0									
50–64	0									
65+	0									
2. MULTIPLE DX										
A. Not Operated										
0–19 Years	0									
20–34	0									
35–49	0									
50–64	0									
65+	0									
B. Operated										
0–19 Years	0									
20–34	0									
35–49	0									
50–64	0									
65+	0									
SUBTOTALS:										
1. SINGLE DX — A. Not Operated	0									
1. SINGLE DX — B. Operated	0									
2. MULTIPLE DX — A. Not Operated	0									
2. MULTIPLE DX — B. Operated	0									
1. SINGLE DX	0									
2. MULTIPLE DX	0									
A. NOT OPERATED	0									
B. OPERATED	0									
TOTAL										
0–19 Years	0									
20–34	0									
35–49	0									
50–64	0									
65+	0									
GRAND TOTAL	0									

V28: ENCOUNT ANTENATAL SCRN

Type of Patients	Observed Patients	Avg. Stay	Variance	Percentiles 10th	25th	50th	75th	90th	95th	99th
1. SINGLE DX										
A. Not Operated										
0–19 Years	0									
20–34	0									
35–49	0									
50–64	0									
65+	0									
B. Operated										
0–19 Years	0									
20–34	0									
35–49	0									
50–64	0									
65+	0									
2. MULTIPLE DX										
A. Not Operated										
0–19 Years	0									
20–34	0									
35–49	0									
50–64	0									
65+	0									
B. Operated										
0–19 Years	0									
20–34	0									
35–49	0									
50–64	0									
65+	0									
SUBTOTALS:										
1. SINGLE DX — A. Not Operated	0									
1. SINGLE DX — B. Operated	0									
2. MULTIPLE DX — A. Not Operated	0									
2. MULTIPLE DX — B. Operated	0									
1. SINGLE DX	0									
2. MULTIPLE DX	0									
A. NOT OPERATED	0									
B. OPERATED	0									
TOTAL										
0–19 Years	0									
20–34	0									
35–49	0									
50–64	0									
65+	0									
GRAND TOTAL	0									

V29: OBS-INFNT SUSPECTED COND

Type of Patients	Observed Patients	Avg. Stay	Variance	Percentiles 10th	25th	50th	75th	90th	95th	99th
1. SINGLE DX										
A. Not Operated										
0–19 Years	93	2.1	<1	1	1	2	3	3	4	6
20–34	0									
35–49	0									
50–64	0									
65+	0									
B. Operated										
0–19 Years	2	1.5	<1	1	1	1	2	2	2	2
20–34	0									
35–49	0									
50–64	0									
65+	0									
2. MULTIPLE DX										
A. Not Operated										
0–19 Years	239	2.8	7	1	2	2	3	4	6	13
20–34	0									
35–49	0									
50–64	0									
65+	0									
B. Operated										
0–19 Years	5	2.8	5	1	1	2	4	6	6	6
20–34	0									
35–49	0									
50–64	0									
65+	0									
SUBTOTALS:										
1. SINGLE DX — A. Not Operated	93	2.1	<1	1	1	2	3	3	4	6
1. SINGLE DX — B. Operated	2	1.5	<1	1	1	1	2	2	2	2
2. MULTIPLE DX — A. Not Operated	239	2.8	7	1	2	2	3	4	6	13
2. MULTIPLE DX — B. Operated	5	2.8	5	1	2	2	4	6	6	6
1. SINGLE DX	95	2.1	<1	1	1	2	3	3	4	6
2. MULTIPLE DX	244	2.8	7	1	2	2	3	4	6	13
A. NOT OPERATED	332	2.6	5	1	2	2	3	4	5	12
B. OPERATED	7	2.4	4	1	1	2	4	6	6	6
TOTAL										
0–19 Years	339	2.6	5	1	2	2	3	4	5	12
20–34	0									
35–49	0									
50–64	0									
65+	0									
GRAND TOTAL	339	2.6	5	1	2	2	3	4	5	12

Length of Stay by Diagnosis and Operation, Western Region, 2008

Western Region, October 2006–September 2007 Data, by Diagnosis

V30: SINGLE LIVEBORN

Type of Patients	Observed Patients	Avg. Stay	Vari-ance	Percentiles						
				10th	25th	50th	75th	90th	95th	99th
1. SINGLE DX										
A. Not Operated										
1–999 Grams	0									
1000–1499	0									
1500–1749	0									
1750–2499	333	1.9	<1	1	1	2	2	3	4	4
2500+	15,166	1.7	<1	1	1	2	2	3	3	4
B. Operated										
1–999 Grams	0									
1000–1499	0									
1500–1749	0									
1750–2499	102	2.1	<1	1	2	2	2	3	4	4
2500+	7,509	1.8	<1	1	1	2	2	3	3	4
2. MULTIPLE DX										
A. Not Operated										
1–999 Grams	558	70.9	286	50	61	77	94	>99	>99	>99
1000–1499	1,951	41.7	325	20	28	40	54	68	78	99
1500–1749	2,011	24.7	148	11	16	22	31	41	49	67
1750–2499	20,728	8.1	71	2	2	4	12	19	25	39
2500+	43,380	3.1	12	1	2	2	3	6	9	17
B. Operated										
1–999 Grams	183	80.6	231	72	85	>99	>99	>99	>99	>99
1000–1499	287	52.5	379	29	39	54	74	>99	>99	>99
1500–1749	218	32.6	334	14	18	28	44	60	74	91
1750–2499	2,583	10.9	170	2	2	5	16	27	36	79
2500+	15,742	2.9	14	1	2	2	3	4	6	19
SUBTOTALS:										
1. SINGLE DX										
A. Not Operated	255,480	1.8	<1	1	1	2	2	3	3	4
B. Operated	36,935	2.0	<1	1	1	2	2	3	4	4
2. MULTIPLE DX										
A. Not Operated	472,471	3.0	25	1	1	2	3	4	7	25
B. Operated	79,259	3.3	48	1	2	2	3	4	7	52
1. SINGLE DX	292,415	1.8	<1	1	1	2	2	3	3	4
2. MULTIPLE DX	551,730	3.0	28	1	2	2	3	4	7	27
A. NOT OPERATED	727,951	2.6	17	1	1	2	3	4	4	18
B. OPERATED	116,194	2.9	33	1	2	2	3	4	4	32
TOTAL										
1–999 Grams	741	73.3	290	53	68	86	>99	>99	>99	>99
1000–1499	2,238	43.1	344	21	29	42	56	72	83	>99
1500–1749	2,229	25.5	172	12	16	23	31	43	51	73
1750–2499	23,746	8.3	82	2	2	4	12	20	25	42
2500+	81,797	2.7	9	1	2	2	3	4	4	16
GRAND TOTAL	844,145	2.6	19	1	1	2	3	4	4	20

V30.00: SINGLE LB-HOSP W/O CD

Type of Patients	Observed Patients	Avg. Stay	Vari-ance	Percentiles						
				10th	25th	50th	75th	90th	95th	99th
1. SINGLE DX										
A. Not Operated										
1–999 Grams	0									
1000–1499	0									
1500–1749	0									
1750–2499	255	1.6	<1	1	1	2	2	2	2	3
2500+	12,265	1.5	<1	1	1	2	2	2	2	3
B. Operated										
1–999 Grams	0									
1000–1499	0									
1500–1749	0									
1750–2499	72	1.8	<1	1	1	2	2	2	2	4
2500+	5,897	1.6	<1	1	1	2	2	2	2	3
2. MULTIPLE DX										
A. Not Operated										
1–999 Grams	124	76.2	236	60	70	85	94	>99	>99	>99
1000–1499	630	44.9	344	21	30	45	58	69	78	97
1500–1749	802	25.7	155	12	17	24	32	42	49	67
1750–2499	12,370	7.3	64	1	2	3	10	18	23	36
2500+	30,021	2.6	8	1	1	2	3	4	7	16
B. Operated										
1–999 Grams	60	84.5	107	76	86	>99	>99	>99	>99	>99
1000–1499	93	53.8	388	30	42	58	76	>99	>99	>99
1500–1749	87	31.8	261	15	20	26	39	58	61	90
1750–2499	1,529	9.2	134	2	2	3	13	23	32	64
2500+	10,837	2.3	8	1	2	2	3	4	5	14
SUBTOTALS:										
1. SINGLE DX										
A. Not Operated	192,061	1.5	<1	1	1	1	2	2	2	3
B. Operated	26,878	1.6	<1	1	2	2	2	2	2	3
2. MULTIPLE DX										
A. Not Operated	326,470	2.3	15	1	1	2	2	3	5	18
B. Operated	52,481	2.5	28	1	2	2	2	3	4	27
1. SINGLE DX	218,939	1.5	<1	1	1	1	2	2	2	3
2. MULTIPLE DX	378,951	2.4	17	1	1	2	2	3	5	19
A. NOT OPERATED	518,531	2.0	10	1	1	1	2	2	4	13
B. OPERATED	79,359	2.2	19	1	1	2	2	3	4	18
TOTAL										
1–999 Grams	184	78.9	208	65	76	92	>99	>99	>99	>99
1000–1499	723	46.0	358	21	32	46	61	74	86	>99
1500–1749	889	26.3	168	12	17	24	33	43	51	69
1750–2499	14,226	7.3	72	1	2	3	10	18	24	38
2500+	59,020	2.2	6	1	2	2	3	3	5	13
GRAND TOTAL	597,890	2.0	11	1	1	2	2	3	3	13

V30.01: SINGLE LB-HOSPITAL BY CD

Type of Patients	Observed Patients	Avg. Stay	Vari-ance	Percentiles						
				10th	25th	50th	75th	90th	95th	99th
1. SINGLE DX										
A. Not Operated										
1–999 Grams	0									
1000–1499	0									
1500–1749	0									
1750–2499	75	2.8	<1	2	2	3	3	4	4	5
2500+	2,865	2.6	<1	2	2	3	3	3	4	4
B. Operated										
1–999 Grams	0									
1000–1499	0									
1500–1749	0									
1750–2499	30	2.8	<1	2	2	3	3	4	4	4
2500+	1,595	2.7	<1	2	2	3	3	4	4	4
2. MULTIPLE DX										
A. Not Operated										
1–999 Grams	432	69.3	291	48	58	74	91	>99	>99	>99
1000–1499	1,307	40.2	310	20	27	38	51	67	78	99
1500–1749	1,197	24.3	143	11	16	21	30	40	48	68
1750–2499	8,260	9.4	79	3	3	6	13	21	26	44
2500+	13,248	4.3	17	2	3	3	4	8	11	21
B. Operated										
1–999 Grams	120	78.6	288	67	85	>99	>99	>99	>99	>99
1000–1499	194	51.8	376	28	38	53	70	96	>99	>99
1500–1749	128	31.8	382	14	29	46	62	78	78	87
1750–2499	1,048	13.3	206	3	4	8	19	31	40	87
2500+	4,882	4.1	27	3	3	3	4	5	10	28
SUBTOTALS:										
1. SINGLE DX										
A. Not Operated	62,994	2.8	<1	2	2	3	3	4	4	4
B. Operated	10,020	2.9	<1	2	2	3	3	4	4	4
2. MULTIPLE DX										
A. Not Operated	144,816	4.4	46	2	2	3	4	5	11	40
B. Operated	26,697	4.9	82	2	3	3	4	5	15	86
1. SINGLE DX	73,014	2.8	<1	2	2	3	3	4	4	4
2. MULTIPLE DX	171,513	4.4	51	2	2	3	4	5	11	46
A. NOT OPERATED	207,810	3.9	33	2	2	3	3	4	7	31
B. OPERATED	36,717	4.3	60	2	2	3	4	4	8	70
TOTAL										
1–999 Grams	552	71.3	305	51	64	82	>99	>99	>99	>99
1000–1499	1,501	41.7	333	21	28	40	54	71	83	>99
1500–1749	1,325	25.0	173	11	16	22	31	43	50	75
1750–2499	9,413	9.8	94	3	3	6	13	22	28	48
2500+	22,590	3.9	16	2	3	3	4	4	6	21
GRAND TOTAL	244,527	3.9	37	2	2	3	3	4	8	35

Length of Stay by Diagnosis and Operation, Western Region, 2008

Western Region, October 2006–September 2007 Data, by Diagnosis

V30.1: SINGLE LB-BEFORE ADMIT

Type of Patients	Observed Patients	Avg. Stay	Vari-ance	10th	25th	50th	75th	90th	95th	99th
1. SINGLE DX										
A. *Not Operated*										
1–999 Grams	0									
1000–1499	0									
1500–1749	0									
1750–2499	3	1.7	<1	1	1	2	2	2	2	2
2500+	36	1.6	<1	1	1	1	2	2	3	4
B. *Operated*										
1–999 Grams	0									
1000–1499	0									
1500–1749	0									
1750–2499	0									
2500+	17	1.5	<1	1	1	2	2	2	2	2
2. MULTIPLE DX										
A. *Not Operated*										
1–999 Grams	2	81.0	2	80	80	80	82	82	82	82
1000–1499	14	44.0	258	26	34	43	64	70	>99	>99
1500–1749	12	28.5	115	16	23	28	37	47	48	48
1750–2499	98	7.8	42	1	3	6	12	17	22	>99
2500+	111	3.5	21	1	2	2	3	6	11	26
B. *Operated*										
1–999 Grams	3	86.0	19	83	83	84	91	91	91	91
1000–1499	0									
1500–1749	3	25.7	645	11	11	11	55	55	55	55
1750–2499	6	22.0	>999	2	2	2	23	94	94	94
2500+	23	3.1	11	1	2	2	3	8	10	15
SUBTOTALS:										
1. SINGLE DX										
A. *Not Operated*	425	1.6	<1	1	1	1	2	2	3	4
B. *Operated*	37	1.5	<1	1	1	1	2	2	2	2
2. MULTIPLE DX										
A. *Not Operated*	1,185	4.3	62	1	2	2	3	8	15	50
B. *Operated*	81	8.3	381	1	2	2	4	11	55	94
1. SINGLE DX	462	1.6	<1	1	1	1	2	2	3	4
2. MULTIPLE DX	1,266	4.6	83	1	2	2	3	9	15	55
A. NOT OPERATED	1,610	3.6	47	1	1	2	3	7	11	43
B. OPERATED	118	6.2	271	1	1	2	3	10	23	91
TOTAL										
1–999 Grams	5	84.0	17	80	82	83	84	91	91	91
1000–1499	14	44.0	258	26	34	43	64	70	>99	>99
1500–1749	15	27.9	183	11	16	26	37	48	55	55
1750–2499	107	8.4	111	1	2	6	11	19	23	94
2500+	187	2.9	15	1	1	2	2	5	9	26
GRAND TOTAL	1,728	3.8	63	1	1	2	3	7	12	48

V31: TWIN MATE LIVEBORN

Type of Patients	Observed Patients	Avg. Stay	Vari-ance	10th	25th	50th	75th	90th	95th	99th
1. SINGLE DX										
A. *Not Operated*										
1–999 Grams	0									
1000–1499	0									
1500–1749	0									
1750–2499	48	2.7	<1	2	2	3	3	4	4	4
2500+	144	2.8	<1	2	2	3	4	4	4	5
B. *Operated*										
1–999 Grams	0									
1000–1499	0									
1500–1749	0									
1750–2499	18	2.8	<1	2	2	3	3	4	4	4
2500+	90	2.8	<1	2	2	3	3	4	4	4
2. MULTIPLE DX										
A. *Not Operated*										
1–999 Grams	129	70.8	284	48	62	74	89	>99	>99	>99
1000–1499	627	41.3	303	20	28	40	51	66	75	91
1500–1749	841	26.2	173	12	16	24	33	44	52	69
1750–2499	6,574	9.7	73	2	3	4	5	21	26	37
2500+	2,635	5.0	21	2	3	4	5	11	14	24
B. *Operated*										
1–999 Grams	52	83.0	190	73	89	>99	>99	>99	>99	>99
1000–1499	127	51.4	312	27	39	54	66	80	>99	>99
1500–1749	123	30.0	103	13	18	29	39	51	60	86
1750–2499	1,048	10.6	103	2	3	4	7	15	23	54
2500+	724	5.3	39	2	3	4	4	10	15	30
SUBTOTALS:										
1. SINGLE DX										
A. *Not Operated*	2,782	2.9	<1	2	2	3	3	4	4	5
B. *Operated*	534	3.0	<1	2	2	3	4	4	4	4
2. MULTIPLE DX										
A. *Not Operated*	15,957	9.6	163	2	3	4	12	24	36	67
B. *Operated*	3,068	11.0	275	2	3	4	13	36	67	>99
1. SINGLE DX	3,316	2.9	<1	2	2	3	4	4	4	5
2. MULTIPLE DX	19,025	9.9	181	2	3	4	12	25	39	84
A. NOT OPERATED	18,739	8.6	145	2	3	4	9	22	33	65
B. OPERATED	3,602	9.8	242	2	3	4	10	29	60	>99
TOTAL										
1–999 Grams	181	74.3	286	55	67	87	>99	>99	>99	>99
1000–1499	754	43.0	318	21	30	42	54	69	79	>99
1500–1749	964	26.7	181	12	16	24	34	45	53	73
1750–2499	7,688	9.8	77	2	3	6	14	21	27	39
2500+	3,593	4.9	24	2	2	4	5	10	14	24
GRAND TOTAL	22,341	8.8	160	2	3	4	10	23	36	78

V31.00: TWIN MATE LB-HOSP W/O CD

Type of Patients	Observed Patients	Avg. Stay	Vari-ance	10th	25th	50th	75th	90th	95th	99th
1. SINGLE DX										
A. *Not Operated*										
1–999 Grams	0									
1000–1499	0									
1500–1749	0									
1750–2499	18	2.0	<1	1	2	2	2	3	4	4
2500+	43	2.1	<1	1	2	2	2	3	4	5
B. *Operated*										
1–999 Grams	0									
1000–1499	0									
1500–1749	0									
1750–2499	5	2.0	0	2	2	2	2	2	2	2
2500+	36	2.2	<1	2	2	2	2	4	4	4
2. MULTIPLE DX										
A. *Not Operated*										
1–999 Grams	13	75.9	258	57	73	86	97	>99	>99	>99
1000–1499	82	40.5	214	22	31	41	52	60	66	>99
1500–1749	164	24.9	168	10	15	23	33	39	45	72
1750–2499	1,486	8.5	60	2	2	5	13	19	24	31
2500+	599	3.8	14	2	2	2	4	9	13	18
B. *Operated*										
1–999 Grams	6	84.0	170	70	94	>99	>99	>99	>99	>99
1000–1499	18	54.5	345	31	45	57	75	87	>99	>99
1500–1749	24	30.5	264	13	21	26	38	53	64	74
1750–2499	249	9.3	95	2	2	6	13	20	26	45
2500+	169	5.1	83	2	2	4	7	10	15	45
SUBTOTALS:										
1. SINGLE DX										
A. *Not Operated*	718	2.0	<1	1	2	2	2	3	3	5
B. *Operated*	154	2.2	<1	2	2	2	2	3	4	4
2. MULTIPLE DX										
A. *Not Operated*	3,535	7.6	115	2	2	3	10	19	28	56
B. *Operated*	716	8.7	216	2	2	3	9	22	45	>99
1. SINGLE DX	872	2.1	<1	1	2	2	2	3	3	5
2. MULTIPLE DX	4,251	7.8	132	2	2	3	10	20	30	69
A. NOT OPERATED	4,253	6.7	100	2	2	2	7	18	26	54
B. OPERATED	870	7.6	184	2	2	2	7	20	37	>99
TOTAL										
1–999 Grams	19	78.5	234	64	73	93	>99	>99	>99	>99
1000–1499	100	43.1	264	23	33	42	55	67	80	>99
1500–1749	188	25.6	182	10	16	23	34	41	51	74
1750–2499	1,758	8.5	65	2	2	5	13	19	24	32
2500+	847	3.9	27	2	2	2	4	8	13	21
GRAND TOTAL	5,123	6.8	114	2	2	2	7	18	27	61

Length of Stay by Diagnosis and Operation, Western Region, 2008

Western Region, October 2006–September 2007 Data, by Diagnosis

V31.01: TWIN MATE LB-HOSP BY CD

Type of Patients	Observed Patients	Avg. Stay	Variance	Percentiles 10th	25th	50th	75th	90th	95th	99th
1. SINGLE DX										
A. Not Operated										
1–999 Grams	0									
1000–1499	0									
1500–1749	0									
1750–2499	30	3.0	<1	2	2	3	4	4	4	4
2500+	101	3.1	<1	2	3	3	4	4	4	5
B. Operated										
1–999 Grams	0									
1000–1499	0									
1500–1749	0									
1750–2499	13	3.2	<1	3	3	3	3	4	4	4
2500+	54	3.3	<1	3	3	3	4	4	4	4
2. MULTIPLE DX										
A. Not Operated										
1–999 Grams	115	70.3	288	48	60	74	88	97	>99	>99
1000–1499	544	41.4	317	19	28	40	51	66	76	91
1500–1749	677	26.5	175	13	16	24	33	45	53	69
1750–2499	5,081	10.1	76	3	4	7	14	22	27	39
2500+	2,035	5.4	23	3	3	4	5	11	15	25
B. Operated										
1–999 Grams	46	82.9	196	74	89	>99	>99	>99	>99	>99
1000–1499	109	50.8	307	27	39	53	65	79	>99	>99
1500–1749	99	29.8	210	13	18	29	41	50	60	>99
1750–2499	799	11.1	105	3	4	7	15	24	30	57
2500+	555	5.4	25	3	3	4	4	10	15	25
SUBTOTALS:										
1. SINGLE DX										
A. Not Operated	2,063	3.2	<1	2	3	3	4	4	4	5
B. Operated	380	3.4	<1	2	3	3	4	4	4	4
2. MULTIPLE DX										
A. Not Operated	12,407	10.2	175	3	3	4	12	25	38	69
B. Operated	2,351	11.7	290	3	3	4	14	40	74	>99
1. SINGLE DX	2,443	3.2	<1	2	3	3	4	4	4	5
2. MULTIPLE DX	14,758	10.5	193	3	3	4	13	27	42	86
A. NOT OPERATED	14,470	9.2	156	3	3	4	10	23	35	66
B. OPERATED	2,731	10.6	259	3	3	4	11	33	64	>99
TOTAL										
1–999 Grams	161	73.9	293	54	67	87	>99	>99	>99	>99
1000–1499	653	43.0	327	20	29	42	54	69	79	>99
1500–1749	776	26.9	180	13	17	24	34	45	53	73
1750–2499	5,923	10.2	80	3	4	7	15	22	28	41
2500+	2,745	5.2	22	3	3	4	5	11	14	25
GRAND TOTAL	17,201	9.4	173	3	3	4	10	24	38	82

V32: TWIN MATE STILLBORN

Type of Patients	Observed Patients	Avg. Stay	Variance	Percentiles 10th	25th	50th	75th	90th	95th	99th
1. SINGLE DX										
A. Not Operated										
1–999 Grams	0									
1000–1499	0									
1500–1749	0									
1750–2499	0									
2500+	2	2.0	2	1	1	3	3	3	3	3
B. Operated										
1–999 Grams	0									
1000–1499	0									
1500–1749	0									
1750–2499	0									
2500+	1	2.0	0	2	2	2	2	2	2	2
2. MULTIPLE DX										
A. Not Operated										
1–999 Grams	3	85.0	398	62	94	99	>99	>99	>99	>99
1000–1499	13	41.7	205	23	37	38	49	63	66	66
1500–1749	10	28.7	143	15	20	22	34	43	53	53
1750–2499	46	12.8	104	2	4	11	18	26	36	39
2500+	16	3.9	10	1	2	3	4	10	12	12
B. Operated										
1–999 Grams	0									
1000–1499	5	53.7	126	44	45	48	62	69	69	69
1500–1749	0									
1750–2499	6	10.5	92	3	4	6	11	29	29	29
2500+	4	3.5	<1	3	3	3	4	4	4	4
SUBTOTALS:										
1. SINGLE DX										
A. Not Operated	15	2.1	<1	1	1	2	3	3	3	3
B. Operated	1	2.0	0	2	2	2	2	2	2	2
2. MULTIPLE DX										
A. Not Operated	126	14.9	341	2	3	6	21	43	62	>99
B. Operated	21	21.6	749	3	3	10	69	>99	>99	>99
1. SINGLE DX	16	2.1	<1	1	1	2	3	3	3	3
2. MULTIPLE DX	147	15.8	400	2	3	7	25	53	99	>99
A. NOT OPERATED	141	13.5	320	2	3	4	19	38	53	>99
B. OPERATED	22	20.7	730	3	3	10	69	>99	>99	>99
TOTAL										
1–999 Grams	3	85.0	398	62	99	>99	>99	>99	>99	>99
1000–1499	18	45.0	205	23	38	45	51	66	69	69
1500–1749	10	28.7	143	15	20	22	34	43	53	53
1750–2499	52	12.6	101	2	3	10	18	26	36	39
2500+	23	3.6	7	1	2	3	4	6	10	12
GRAND TOTAL	163	14.5	377	2	3	4	22	49	94	>99

V33: TWIN NOS

Type of Patients	Observed Patients	Avg. Stay	Variance	Percentiles 10th	25th	50th	75th	90th	95th	99th
1. SINGLE DX										
A. Not Operated										
1–999 Grams	0									
1000–1499	0									
1500–1749	0									
1750–2499	0									
2500+	0									
B. Operated										
1–999 Grams	0									
1000–1499	0									
1500–1749	0									
1750–2499	0									
2500+	0									
2. MULTIPLE DX										
A. Not Operated										
1–999 Grams	0									
1000–1499	4	31.5	27	27	27	30	30	39	39	39
1500–1749	7	28.4	78	12	25	29	36	39	39	39
1750–2499	33	8.9	53	3	3	5	14	17	25	27
2500+	10	2.9	2	2	2	3	3	4	6	6
B. Operated										
1–999 Grams	0									
1000–1499	0									
1500–1749	0									
1750–2499	0									
2500+	6	3.5	<1	3	3	4	4	4	4	4
SUBTOTALS:										
1. SINGLE DX										
A. Not Operated	13	3.0	<1	2	3	3	3	4	4	4
B. Operated	0									
2. MULTIPLE DX										
A. Not Operated	90	8.7	98	2	3	3	12	27	30	39
B. Operated	16	3.6	8	2	2	3	3	4	14	14
1. SINGLE DX	13	3.0	<1	2	3	3	3	4	4	4
2. MULTIPLE DX	106	7.9	87	2	3	3	10	25	30	39
A. NOT OPERATED	103	8.0	89	2	3	3	10	25	30	39
B. OPERATED	16	3.6	8	2	2	3	3	4	14	14
TOTAL										
1–999 Grams	0									
1000–1499	4	31.5	27	27	27	30	30	39	39	39
1500–1749	7	28.4	78	12	25	29	36	39	39	39
1750–2499	33	8.9	53	3	3	5	14	17	25	27
2500+	16	3.1	1	2	3	3	4	6	6	6
GRAND TOTAL	119	7.4	80	2	3	3	6	25	30	39

Length of Stay by Diagnosis and Operation, Western Region, 2008

Western Region, October 2006–September 2007 Data, by Diagnosis

V34: MULT LIVEBORN NEC

Type of Patients	Observed Patients	Avg. Stay	Variance	10th	25th	50th	75th	90th	95th	99th
1. SINGLE DX										
A. Not Operated										
1–999 Grams	0									
1000–1499	0									
1500–1749	0									
1750–2499	0									
2500+	0									
B. Operated										
1–999 Grams	0									
1000–1499	0									
1500–1749	0									
1750–2499	0									
2500+	0									
2. MULTIPLE DX										
A. Not Operated										
1–999 Grams	12	62.2	297	43	55	72	81	>99	>99	>99
1000–1499	143	41.1	257	22	30	39	51	62	72	79
1500–1749	140	25.6	146	13	18	23	31	41	50	60
1750–2499	343	14.5	121	4	7	12	19	28	35	57
2500+	27	8.5	57	3	3	6	11	15	23	35
B. Operated										
1–999 Grams	5	81.6	30	80	83	>99	>99	>99	>99	>99
1000–1499	25	49.0	355	28	34	45	61	80	90	>99
1500–1749	20	31.2	175	17	20	31	41	44	46	66
1750–2499	82	16.6	105	4	8	16	23	31	34	44
2500+	8	12.5	95	4	7	10	27	28	28	28
SUBTOTALS:										
1. SINGLE DX										
A. Not Operated	5	4.0	0	4	4	4	4	4	4	4
B. Operated	1	4.0	0	4	4	4	4	4	4	4
2. MULTIPLE DX										
A. Not Operated	736	21.8	309	3	9	17	32	48	58	76
B. Operated	147	25.6	425	4	10	22	37	80	>99	>99
1. SINGLE DX	6	4.0	0	4	4	4	4	4	4	4
2. MULTIPLE DX	883	22.4	330	4	9	18	33	51	62	>99
A. NOT OPERATED	741	21.6	309	3	8	17	32	48	58	76
B. OPERATED	148	25.4	425	4	10	22	37	80	>99	>99
TOTAL										
1–999 Grams	17	67.9	295	48	72	83	>99	>99	>99	>99
1000–1499	168	42.3	277	22	30	40	52	67	74	90
1500–1749	160	26.3	152	14	18	23	33	43	50	66
1750–2499	425	14.9	118	4	7	12	20	29	35	56
2500+	35	9.4	66	3	4	7	12	23	28	35
GRAND TOTAL	889	22.3	330	4	9	18	33	51	62	>99

V34.01: MULT LB NEC-HOSP BY CD

Type of Patients	Observed Patients	Avg. Stay	Variance	10th	25th	50th	75th	90th	95th	99th
1. SINGLE DX										
A. Not Operated										
1–999 Grams	0									
1000–1499	0									
1500–1749	0									
1750–2499	0									
2500+	0									
B. Operated										
1–999 Grams	0									
1000–1499	0									
1500–1749	0									
1750–2499	0									
2500+	0									
2. MULTIPLE DX										
A. Not Operated										
1–999 Grams	12	62.2	297	43	55	72	81	>99	>99	>99
1000–1499	139	41.1	263	22	30	39	51	62	73	79
1500–1749	140	25.6	146	13	18	23	31	41	50	60
1750–2499	343	14.5	121	4	7	12	19	28	35	57
2500+	26	8.3	58	3	3	5	11	15	23	35
B. Operated										
1–999 Grams	5	81.6	30	80	83	>99	>99	>99	>99	>99
1000–1499	22	48.1	359	28	34	45	61	80	90	>99
1500–1749	20	31.2	175	17	20	31	41	44	46	66
1750–2499	82	16.6	105	4	8	16	23	31	34	44
2500+	8	12.5	95	4	7	10	27	28	28	28
SUBTOTALS:										
1. SINGLE DX										
A. Not Operated	5	4.0	0	4	4	4	4	4	4	4
B. Operated	1	4.0	0	4	4	4	4	4	4	4
2. MULTIPLE DX										
A. Not Operated	727	21.8	308	3	9	17	32	48	58	76
B. Operated	143	25.1	408	4	10	22	37	80	>99	>99
1. SINGLE DX	6	4.0	0	4	4	4	4	4	4	4
2. MULTIPLE DX	870	22.3	326	4	9	18	33	51	62	>99
A. NOT OPERATED	732	21.7	308	3	9	17	32	48	58	76
B. OPERATED	144	24.9	408	4	10	22	37	80	>99	>99
TOTAL										
1–999 Grams	17	67.9	295	48	72	83	>99	>99	>99	>99
1000–1499	161	42.1	280	22	30	40	52	67	74	90
1500–1749	160	26.3	152	14	18	23	33	43	50	66
1750–2499	425	14.9	118	4	7	12	20	29	35	56
2500+	34	9.3	68	3	4	6	11	23	28	35
GRAND TOTAL	876	22.2	326	4	9	18	33	51	62	>99

V35: MULT NEC MATES STILLBORN

Type of Patients	Observed Patients	Avg. Stay	Variance	10th	25th	50th	75th	90th	95th	99th
1. SINGLE DX										
A. Not Operated										
1–999 Grams	0									
1000–1499	0									
1500–1749	0									
1750–2499	0									
2500+	0									
B. Operated										
1–999 Grams	0									
1000–1499	0									
1500–1749	0									
1750–2499	0									
2500+	0									
2. MULTIPLE DX										
A. Not Operated										
1–999 Grams	0									
1000–1499	0									
1500–1749	0									
1750–2499	0									
B. Operated										
1–999 Grams	0									
1000–1499	0									
1500–1749	0									
1750–2499	0									
SUBTOTALS:										
1. SINGLE DX A. Not Operated	0									
B. Operated	0									
2. MULTIPLE DX A. Not Operated	0									
B. Operated	0									
1. SINGLE DX	0									
2. MULTIPLE DX	0									
A. NOT OPERATED	0									
B. OPERATED	0									
TOTAL										
1–999 Grams	0									
1000–1499	0									
1500–1749	0									
1750–2499	0									
2500+	0									
GRAND TOTAL	0									

Length of Stay by Diagnosis and Operation, Western Region, 2008

Western Region, October 2006–September 2007 Data, by Diagnosis

V36: MULT BIRTH NEC LB&SB

Type of Patients	Observed Patients	Avg. Stay	Variance	10th	25th	50th	75th	90th	95th	99th
1. SINGLE DX										
A. *Not Operated*										
1–999 Grams	0									
1000–1499	0									
1500–1749	0									
1750–2499	0									
2500+	0									
B. *Operated*										
1–999 Grams	0									
1000–1499	0									
1500–1749	0									
1750–2499	0									
2500+	0									
2. MULTIPLE DX										
A. *Not Operated*										
1–999 Grams	1	96.0	0	96	96	>99	>99	>99	>99	>99
1000–1499	1	23.0	0	23	23	23	23	23	23	23
1500–1749	0									
1750–2499	7	9.1	72	3	4	5	20	23	23	23
2500+	1	3.0	0	3	3	3	3	3	3	3
B. *Operated*										
1–999 Grams	0									
1000–1499	1	56.0	0	56	56	56	56	56	56	56
1500–1749	0									
1750–2499	0									
2500+	0									
SUBTOTALS:										
1. SINGLE DX										
A. *Not Operated*	2	3.0	0	3	3	3	3	3	3	3
B. *Operated*	0									
2. MULTIPLE DX										
A. *Not Operated*	11	22.9	938	3	4	20	66	>99	>99	>99
B. *Operated*	1	56.0	0	56	56	84	>99	>99	>99	>99
1. SINGLE DX	2	3.0	0	3	3	3	3	3	3	3
2. MULTIPLE DX	12	25.6	944	3	4	23	96	>99	>99	>99
A. NOT OPERATED	13	19.8	837	3	3	5	66	>99	>99	>99
B. OPERATED	1	56.0	0	56	56	84	>99	>99	>99	>99
TOTAL										
1–999 Grams	1	96.0	0	96	96	>99	>99	>99	>99	>99
1000–1499	2	39.5	545	23	23	40	56	56	56	56
1500–1749	0									
1750–2499	7	9.1	72	3	4	5	20	23	23	23
2500+	1	3.0	0	3	3	3	3	3	3	3
GRAND TOTAL	14	22.4	866	3	4	20	66	>99	>99	>99

V37: MULTIPLE BIRTH NEC&NOS

Type of Patients	Observed Patients	Avg. Stay	Variance	10th	25th	50th	75th	90th	95th	99th
1. SINGLE DX										
A. *Not Operated*										
1–999 Grams	0									
1000–1499	0									
1500–1749	0									
1750–2499	0									
2500+	0									
B. *Operated*										
1–999 Grams	0									
1000–1499	0									
1500–1749	0									
1750–2499	0									
2500+	0									
2. MULTIPLE DX										
A. *Not Operated*										
1–999 Grams	0									
1000–1499	2	36.0	98	29	29	36	43	43	43	43
1500–1749	0									
1750–2499	2	18.6	417	4	4	33	33	33	33	33
2500+	0									
B. *Operated*										
1–999 Grams	0									
1000–1499	0									
1500–1749	0									
1750–2499	1	54.0	0	54	54	54	54	54	54	54
2500+	0									
SUBTOTALS:										
1. SINGLE DX										
A. *Not Operated*	1	4.0	0	4	4	4	4	4	4	4
B. *Operated*	0									
2. MULTIPLE DX										
A. *Not Operated*	4	27.3	274	4	29	33	33	43	43	43
B. *Operated*	1	54.0	0	54	54	54	>99	>99	>99	>99
1. SINGLE DX	1	4.0	0	4	4	4	4	4	4	4
2. MULTIPLE DX	5	32.7	348	4	29	43	54	>99	>99	>99
A. NOT OPERATED	5	22.6	314	4	4	29	33	43	43	43
B. OPERATED	1	54.0	0	54	54	54	>99	>99	>99	>99
TOTAL										
1–999 Grams	0									
1000–1499	2	36.0	98	29	29	43	>99	>99	>99	>99
1500–1749	0									
1750–2499	3	30.5	625	4	4	33	54	54	54	54
2500+	0									
GRAND TOTAL	6	27.9	416	4	4	33	54	>99	>99	>99

V39: LIVEBORN NOS

Type of Patients	Observed Patients	Avg. Stay	Variance	10th	25th	50th	75th	90th	95th	99th
1. SINGLE DX										
A. *Not Operated*										
1–999 Grams	0									
1000–1499	0									
1500–1749	0									
1750–2499	0									
2500+	0									
B. *Operated*										
1–999 Grams	0									
1000–1499	0									
1500–1749	0									
1750–2499	0									
2500+	0									
2. MULTIPLE DX										
A. *Not Operated*										
1–999 Grams	0									
1000–1499	0									
1500–1749	0									
1750–2499	1	2.0	0	2	2	2	2	2	2	2
2500+	0									
B. *Operated*										
1–999 Grams	0									
1000–1499	0									
1500–1749	0									
1750–2499	0									
2500+	0									
SUBTOTALS:										
1. SINGLE DX										
A. *Not Operated*	0									
B. *Operated*	0									
2. MULTIPLE DX										
A. *Not Operated*	1	2.0	0	2	2	2	2	2	2	2
B. *Operated*	0									
1. SINGLE DX	0									
2. MULTIPLE DX	1	2.0	0	2	2	2	2	2	2	2
A. NOT OPERATED	1	2.0	0	2	2	2	2	2	2	2
B. OPERATED	0									
TOTAL										
1–999 Grams	0									
1000–1499	0									
1500–1749	0									
1750–2499	0									
2500+	0									
GRAND TOTAL	1	2.0	0	2	2	2	2	2	2	2

861

Length of Stay by Diagnosis and Operation, Western Region, 2008

862

Western Region, October 2006–September 2007 Data, by Diagnosis

V40: MENTAL/BEHAVIORAL PBX | V41: PBX W SPECIAL FUNCTIONS | V42: ORGAN TRANSPLANT STATUS

Type of Patients	V40 Observed Patients	V40 Avg. Stay	V40 Vari-ance	V40 10th	V40 25th	V40 50th	V40 75th	V40 90th	V40 95th	V40 99th	V41 Observed Patients	V41 Avg. Stay	V41 Vari-ance	V41 10th	V41 25th	V41 50th	V41 75th	V41 90th	V41 95th	V41 99th	V42 Observed Patients	V42 Avg. Stay	V42 Vari-ance	V42 10th	V42 25th	V42 50th	V42 75th	V42 90th	V42 95th	V42 99th
1. SINGLE DX																														
A. Not Operated																														
0–19 Years	0										0										0									
20–34	0										0										0									
35–49	0										0										0									
50–64	0										0										0									
65+																														
B. Operated																														
0–19 Years	0										0										0									
20–34	0										0										0									
35–49	0										0										0									
50–64	0										0										0									
65+																														
2. MULTIPLE DX																														
A. Not Operated																														
0–19 Years	0										0										0									
20–34	0										0										0									
35–49	0										0										0									
50–64	0										0										0									
65+																														
B. Operated																														
0–19 Years	0										0										0									
20–34	0										0										0									
35–49	0										0										0									
50–64	0										0										0									
65+																														
SUBTOTALS:																														
1. SINGLE DX																														
A. Not Operated	0										0										0									
B. Operated	0										0										0									
2. MULTIPLE DX																														
A. Not Operated	0										0										0									
B. Operated	0										0										0									
1. SINGLE DX	0										0										0									
2. MULTIPLE DX	0										0										0									
A. NOT OPERATED	0										0										0									
B. OPERATED	0										0										0									
TOTAL																														
0–19 Years	0										0										0									
20–34	0										0										0									
35–49	0										0										0									
50–64	0										0										0									
65+																														
GRAND TOTAL	0										0										0									

Western Region, October 2006–September 2007 Data, by Diagnosis

V43: ORGAN REPLACEMENT NEC

Type of Patients	Observed Patients	Avg. Stay	Vari-ance	Percentiles						
				10th	25th	50th	75th	90th	95th	99th
1. SINGLE DX										
A. *Not Operated*										
0–19 Years	0									
20–34	0									
35–49	0									
50–64	0									
65+	0									
B. *Operated*										
0–19 Years	0									
20–34	0									
35–49	0									
50–64	0									
65+	0									
2. MULTIPLE DX										
A. *Not Operated*										
0–19 Years	0									
20–34	0									
35–49	0									
50–64	0									
65+	0									
B. *Operated*										
0–19 Years	0									
20–34	0									
35–49	0									
50–64	0									
65+	0									
SUBTOTALS:										
1. SINGLE DX										
A. *Not Operated*	0									
B. *Operated*	0									
2. MULTIPLE DX										
A. *Not Operated*	0									
B. *Operated*	0									
1. SINGLE DX	0									
2. MULTIPLE DX	0									
A. NOT OPERATED	0									
B. OPERATED	0									
TOTAL										
0–19 Years	0									
20–34	0									
35–49	0									
50–64	0									
65+	0									
GRAND TOTAL	0									

V44: ARTIF OPENING STATUS

Type of Patients	Observed Patients	Avg. Stay	Vari-ance	Percentiles						
				10th	25th	50th	75th	90th	95th	99th
1. SINGLE DX										
A. *Not Operated*										
0–19 Years	0									
20–34	0									
35–49	0									
50–64	0									
65+	0									
B. *Operated*										
0–19 Years	0									
20–34	0									
35–49	0									
50–64	0									
65+	0									
2. MULTIPLE DX										
A. *Not Operated*										
0–19 Years	0									
20–34	0									
35–49	0									
50–64	0									
65+	0									
B. *Operated*										
0–19 Years	0									
20–34	0									
35–49	0									
50–64	0									
65+	0									
SUBTOTALS:										
1. SINGLE DX										
A. *Not Operated*	0									
B. *Operated*	0									
2. MULTIPLE DX										
A. *Not Operated*	0									
B. *Operated*	0									
1. SINGLE DX	0									
2. MULTIPLE DX	0									
A. NOT OPERATED	0									
B. OPERATED	0									
TOTAL										
0–19 Years	0									
20–34	0									
35–49	0									
50–64	0									
65+	0									
GRAND TOTAL	0									

V45: OTH POSTPROCEDURE STATES

Type of Patients	Observed Patients	Avg. Stay	Vari-ance	Percentiles						
				10th	25th	50th	75th	90th	95th	99th
1. SINGLE DX										
A. *Not Operated*										
0–19 Years	0									
20–34	0									
35–49	0									
50–64	0									
B. *Operated*										
0–19 Years	0									
20–34	0									
35–49	4	3.0	2	2	2	3	5	5	5	5
50–64	4	2.0	4	1	1	1	5	5	5	5
65+	0									
2. MULTIPLE DX										
A. *Not Operated*										
0–19 Years	0									
20–34	1	1.0	0	1	1	1	1	1	1	1
35–49	2	1.0	0	1	1	1	1	1	1	1
50–64	3	1.7	1	1	1	1	3	3	3	3
65+	0									
B. *Operated*										
0–19 Years	1	1.0	0	1	1	1	1	1	1	1
20–34	30	3.0	3	1	1	3	4	5	5	7
35–49	379	3.2	4	1	2	3	4	6	7	9
50–64	524	3.1	4	1	2	3	4	5	6	10
65+	101	2.8	4	1	1	2	4	5	6	9
SUBTOTALS:										
1. SINGLE DX										
A. *Not Operated*	0									
B. *Operated*	8	2.5	3	1	1	2	5	5	5	5
2. MULTIPLE DX										
A. *Not Operated*	6	1.3	<1	1	1	1	1	3	3	3
B. *Operated*	1,035	3.1	4	1	2	3	4	5	6	9
1. SINGLE DX	8	2.5	3	1	1	2	5	5	5	5
2. MULTIPLE DX	1,041	3.1	4	1	2	3	4	5	6	9
A. NOT OPERATED	6	1.3	<1	1	1	1	1	3	3	3
B. OPERATED	1,043	3.1	4	1	2	3	4	5	6	9
TOTAL										
0–19 Years	1	1.0	0	1	1	1	1	1	1	1
20–34	31	2.9	3	1	1	3	4	5	5	7
35–49	385	3.2	4	1	2	3	4	6	7	9
50–64	531	3.1	4	1	2	3	4	5	6	10
65+	101	2.8	4	1	1	2	4	5	6	9
GRAND TOTAL	1,049	3.1	4	1	2	3	4	5	6	9

Length of Stay by Diagnosis and Operation, Western Region, 2008

Western Region, October 2006–September 2007 Data, by Diagnosis

V45.71: ACQ ABSENCE OF BREAST

Type of Patients	Observed Patients	Avg. Stay	Vari-ance	10th	25th	50th	75th	90th	95th	99th
1. SINGLE DX										
A. *Not Operated*										
0–19 Years	0									
20–34	0									
35–49	0									
50–64	0									
65+	0									
B. *Operated*										
0–19 Years	0									
20–34	0									
35–49	4	3.0	2	2	2	3	5	5	5	5
50–64	4	2.0	4	1	1	1	5	5	5	5
65+	0									
2. MULTIPLE DX										
A. *Not Operated*										
0–19 Years	0									
20–34	1	1.0	0	1	1	1	1	1	1	1
35–49	2	1.0	0	1	1	1	1	1	1	1
50–64	3	1.7	1	1	1	1	3	3	3	3
65+	0									
B. *Operated*										
0–19 Years	1	1.0	0	1	1	1	1	1	1	1
20–34	30	3.0	3	1	1	3	4	5	5	7
35–49	379	3.2	4	1	2	3	4	6	7	9
50–64	524	3.1	4	1	2	3	4	5	6	10
65+	101	2.8	4	1	1	2	4	5	6	9
SUBTOTALS:										
1. SINGLE DX										
A. *Not Operated*	0									
B. *Operated*	8	2.5	3	1	1	2	5	5	5	5
2. MULTIPLE DX										
A. *Not Operated*	6	1.3	<1	1	1	1	1	3	3	3
B. *Operated*	1,035	3.1	4	1	2	3	4	5	6	9
1. SINGLE DX	8	2.5	3	1	1	2	5	5	5	5
2. MULTIPLE DX	1,041	3.1	4	1	2	3	4	5	6	9
A. NOT OPERATED	6	1.3	<1	1	1	1	1	3	3	3
B. OPERATED	1,043	3.1	4	1	2	3	4	5	6	9
TOTAL										
0–19 Years	1	1.0	0	1	1	1	1	1	1	1
20–34	31	2.9	3	1	1	3	4	5	5	7
35–49	385	3.2	3	1	2	3	4	6	7	9
50–64	531	3.1	4	1	2	3	4	5	6	10
65+	101	2.8	4	1	1	2	4	5	6	9
GRAND TOTAL	1,049	3.1	4	1	2	3	4	5	6	9

V46: OTHER MACHINE DEPENDENCE

Type of Patients	Observed Patients	Avg. Stay	Vari-ance	10th	25th	50th	75th	90th	95th	99th
1. SINGLE DX										
A. *Not Operated*										
0–19 Years	0									
20–34	0									
35–49	0									
50–64	0									
65+	0									
B. *Operated*										
0–19 Years	0									
20–34	0									
35–49	0									
50–64	0									
65+	0									
2. MULTIPLE DX										
A. *Not Operated*										
0–19 Years	4	1.0	0	1	1	1	1	1	1	1
20–34	3	2.3	5	1	1	1	5	5	5	5
35–49	1	1.0	0	1	1	1	1	1	1	1
50–64	3	6.0	13	2	2	7	9	9	9	9
65+	5	6.6	130	1	1	2	2	27	27	27
B. *Operated*										
0–19 Years	0									
20–34	0									
35–49	0									
50–64	0									
65+	1	1.0	0	1	1	1	1	1	1	1
SUBTOTALS:										
1. SINGLE DX										
A. *Not Operated*	0									
B. *Operated*	0									
2. MULTIPLE DX										
A. *Not Operated*	16	3.9	44	1	1	1	2	9	27	27
B. *Operated*	1	1.0	0	1	1	1	1	1	1	1
1. SINGLE DX	0									
2. MULTIPLE DX	17	3.8	42	1	1	1	2	9	27	27
A. NOT OPERATED	16	3.9	44	1	1	1	2	9	27	27
B. OPERATED	1	1.0	0	1	1	1	1	1	1	1
TOTAL										
0–19 Years	4	1.0	0	1	1	1	1	1	1	1
20–34	3	2.3	5	1	1	1	5	5	5	5
35–49	1	1.0	0	1	1	1	1	1	1	1
50–64	3	6.0	13	2	2	7	9	9	9	9
65+	6	5.7	109	1	1	2	2	27	27	27
GRAND TOTAL	17	3.8	42	1	1	1	2	9	27	27

V47: OTH PBX W INTERNAL ORGAN

Type of Patients	Observed Patients	Avg. Stay	Vari-ance	10th	25th	50th	75th	90th	95th	99th
1. SINGLE DX										
A. *Not Operated*										
0–19 Years	0									
20–34	0									
35–49	0									
50–64	0									
65+	0									
B. *Operated*										
0–19 Years	0									
20–34	0									
35–49	0									
50–64	0									
65+	0									
2. MULTIPLE DX										
A. *Not Operated*										
0–19 Years	0									
20–34	0									
35–49	0									
50–64	0									
65+	0									
B. *Operated*										
0–19 Years	0									
20–34	0									
35–49	0									
50–64	0									
65+	0									
SUBTOTALS:										
1. SINGLE DX / A. *Not Operated*	0									
B. *Operated*	0									
2. MULTIPLE DX / A. *Not Operated*	0									
B. *Operated*	0									
1. SINGLE DX	0									
2. MULTIPLE DX	0									
A. NOT OPERATED	0									
B. OPERATED	0									
TOTAL										
0–19 Years	0									
20–34	0									
35–49	0									
50–64	0									
65+	0									
GRAND TOTAL	0									

Length of Stay by Diagnosis and Operation, Western Region, 2008

Western Region, October 2006–September 2007 Data, by Diagnosis

V48: HEAD/NECK/TRUNK PROBLEMS

Type of Patients	Observed Patients	Avg. Stay	Vari-ance	10th	25th	50th	75th	90th	95th	99th
1. SINGLE DX										
A. Not Operated										
0–19 Years	0									
20–34	0									
35–49	0									
50–64	0									
65+	0									
B. Operated										
0–19 Years	0									
20–34	0									
35–49	0									
50–64	0									
65+	0									
2. MULTIPLE DX										
A. Not Operated										
0–19 Years	0									
20–34	0									
35–49	0									
50–64	0									
65+	0									
B. Operated										
0–19 Years	0									
20–34	0									
35–49	0									
50–64	0									
65+	0									
SUBTOTALS:										
1. SINGLE DX A. Not Operated	0									
1. SINGLE DX B. Operated	0									
2. MULTIPLE DX A. Not Operated	0									
2. MULTIPLE DX B. Operated	0									
1. SINGLE DX	0									
2. MULTIPLE DX	0									
A. NOT OPERATED	0									
B. OPERATED	0									
TOTAL										
0–19 Years	0									
20–34	0									
35–49	0									
50–64	0									
65+	0									
GRAND TOTAL	0									

V49: OTH COND INFLU HEALTH

Type of Patients	Observed Patients	Avg. Stay	Vari-ance	10th	25th	50th	75th	90th	95th	99th
1. SINGLE DX										
A. Not Operated										
0–19 Years	0									
20–34	0									
35–49	0									
50–64	0									
65+	0									
B. Operated										
0–19 Years	0									
20–34	0									
35–49	0									
50–64	0									
65+	0									
2. MULTIPLE DX										
A. Not Operated										
0–19 Years	0									
20–34	0									
35–49	0									
50–64	0									
65+	0									
B. Operated										
0–19 Years	0									
20–34	0									
35–49	0									
50–64	0									
65+	0									
SUBTOTALS:										
1. SINGLE DX A. Not Operated	0									
1. SINGLE DX B. Operated	0									
2. MULTIPLE DX A. Not Operated	0									
2. MULTIPLE DX B. Operated	0									
1. SINGLE DX	0									
2. MULTIPLE DX	0									
A. NOT OPERATED	0									
B. OPERATED	0									
TOTAL										
0–19 Years	0									
20–34	0									
35–49	0									
50–64	0									
65+	0									
GRAND TOTAL	0									

V50: OTHER ELECTIVE SURGERY

Type of Patients	Observed Patients	Avg. Stay	Vari-ance	10th	25th	50th	75th	90th	95th	99th
1. SINGLE DX										
A. Not Operated										
0–19 Years	0									
20–34	0									
35–49	0									
50–64	1	1.0	0	1	1	1	1	1	1	1
65+	1	1.0	0	1	1	1	1	1	1	1
B. Operated										
0–19 Years	5	1.0	0	1	1	1	1	1	1	1
20–34	16	1.6	<1	1	1	1	2	2	4	4
35–49	16	1.5	<1	1	1	2	2	2	2	2
50–64	35	1.3	<1	1	1	1	1	2	2	2
65+	1	1.0	0	1	1	1	1	1	1	1
2. MULTIPLE DX										
A. Not Operated										
0–19 Years	0									
20–34	2	1.0	0	1	1	1	1	1	1	1
35–49	4	2.8	6	1	1	3	6	6	6	6
50–64	2	1.0	0	1	1	1	1	1	1	1
65+	2	1.0	0	1	1	1	1	1	1	1
B. Operated										
0–19 Years	3	1.3	<1	1	1	1	2	2	2	2
20–34	102	1.9	1	1	1	2	2	3	4	5
35–49	512	1.8	1	1	1	1	2	3	4	6
50–64	639	1.7	2	1	1	1	2	3	4	7
65+	118	1.6	2	1	1	1	2	3	4	7
SUBTOTALS:										
1. SINGLE DX A. Not Operated	2	1.0	0	1	1	1	1	1	1	1
1. SINGLE DX B. Operated	73	1.4	<1	1	1	1	2	2	2	4
2. MULTIPLE DX A. Not Operated	10	1.7	3	1	1	1	2	6	6	6
2. MULTIPLE DX B. Operated	1,374	1.8	2	1	1	1	2	3	4	6
1. SINGLE DX	75	1.4	<1	1	1	1	2	2	2	4
2. MULTIPLE DX	1,384	1.8	2	1	1	1	2	3	4	6
A. NOT OPERATED	12	1.6	2	1	1	1	1	3	6	6
B. OPERATED	1,447	1.7	1	1	1	1	2	3	4	6
TOTAL										
0–19 Years	8	1.1	<1	1	1	1	1	2	2	2
20–34	120	1.9	<1	1	1	1	2	3	4	5
35–49	532	1.8	1	1	1	1	2	3	4	6
50–64	677	1.7	2	1	1	1	2	3	4	7
65+	122	1.6	2	1	1	1	2	3	4	7
GRAND TOTAL	1,459	1.7	1	1	1	1	2	3	4	6

Length of Stay by Diagnosis and Operation, Western Region, 2008

Western Region, October 2006–September 2007 Data, by Diagnosis

V50.1: PLASTIC SURGERY NEC

Type of Patients	Observed Patients	Avg. Stay	Vari-ance	10th	25th	50th	75th	90th	95th	99th
1. SINGLE DX										
A. *Not Operated*										
0–19 Years	0									
20–34	0									
35–49	0									
50–64	1	1.0	0	1	1	1	1	1	1	1
65+	1	1.0	0	1	1	1	1	1	1	1
B. *Operated*										
0–19 Years	0									
20–34	5	1.2	<1	1	1	1	1	2	2	2
35–49	10	1.4	1	1	1	1	2	2	2	2
50–64	29	1.2	<1	1	1	1	1	2	2	2
65+	1	1.0	0	1	1	1	1	1	1	1
2. MULTIPLE DX										
A. *Not Operated*										
0–19 Years	0									
20–34	2	1.0	0	1	1	1	1	1	1	1
35–49	3	3.4	6	1	1	3	6	6	6	6
50–64	1	1.0	0	1	1	1	1	1	1	1
65+	2	1.0	0	1	1	1	1	1	1	1
B. *Operated*										
0–19 Years	0									
20–34	43	1.7	<1	1	1	1	2	3	3	4
35–49	130	1.6	1	1	1	1	2	3	3	5
50–64	307	1.4	<1	1	1	1	1	2	3	5
65+	55	1.3	<1	1	1	1	1	2	2	5
SUBTOTALS:										
1. SINGLE DX										
A. *Not Operated*	2	1.0	0	1	1	1	1	1	1	1
B. *Operated*	45	1.2	<1	1	1	1	1	2	2	2
2. MULTIPLE DX										
A. *Not Operated*	8	1.9	3	1	1	1	3	6	6	6
B. *Operated*	535	1.4	<1	1	1	1	2	2	3	5
1. SINGLE DX	47	1.2	<1	1	1	1	1	2	2	2
2. MULTIPLE DX	543	1.4	<1	1	1	1	2	2	3	5
A. NOT OPERATED	10	1.7	3	1	1	1	1	6	6	6
B. OPERATED	580	1.4	<1	1	1	1	2	2	3	5
TOTAL										
0–19 Years	0									
20–34	50	1.6	<1	1	1	1	2	2	3	4
35–49	143	1.6	1	1	1	1	2	2	3	6
50–64	338	1.4	<1	1	1	1	1	2	3	5
65+	59	1.3	<1	1	1	1	1	2	2	5
GRAND TOTAL	590	1.4	<1	1	1	1	2	2	3	5

V50.41: PROPHYLACTIC BREAST RMVL

Type of Patients	Observed Patients	Avg. Stay	Vari-ance	10th	25th	50th	75th	90th	95th	99th
1. SINGLE DX										
A. *Not Operated*										
0–19 Years	0									
20–34	0									
35–49	0									
50–64	0									
65+	0									
B. *Operated*										
0–19 Years	0									
20–34	0									
35–49	0									
50–64	1	2.0	0	2	2	2	2	2	2	2
65+	0									
2. MULTIPLE DX										
A. *Not Operated*										
0–19 Years	0									
20–34	0									
35–49	0									
50–64	0									
65+	0									
B. *Operated*										
0–19 Years	0									
20–34	32	1.9	<1	1	1	2	2	3	4	4
35–49	159	2.2	3	1	1	2	3	4	5	9
50–64	153	2.2	3	1	1	2	3	4	5	9
65+	39	1.7	2	1	1	1	2	3	5	7
SUBTOTALS:										
1. SINGLE DX										
A. *Not Operated*	0									
B. *Operated*	1	2.0	0	2	2	2	2	2	2	2
2. MULTIPLE DX										
A. *Not Operated*	0									
B. *Operated*	383	2.1	3	1	1	2	2	4	5	9
1. SINGLE DX	1	2.0	0	2	2	2	2	2	2	2
2. MULTIPLE DX	383	2.1	3	1	1	2	2	4	5	9
A. NOT OPERATED	0									
B. OPERATED	384	2.1	3	1	1	2	2	4	5	9
TOTAL										
0–19 Years	0									
20–34	32	1.9	<1	1	1	2	2	3	4	4
35–49	159	2.2	3	1	1	2	3	4	5	9
50–64	154	2.2	3	1	1	2	3	4	5	9
65+	39	1.7	2	1	1	1	2	3	5	7
GRAND TOTAL	384	2.1	3	1	1	2	2	4	5	9

V50.42: PROPHYLACTIC OVARY RMVL

Type of Patients	Observed Patients	Avg. Stay	Vari-ance	10th	25th	50th	75th	90th	95th	99th
1. SINGLE DX										
A. *Not Operated*										
0–19 Years	0									
20–34	0									
35–49	0									
50–64	0									
65+	0									
B. *Operated*										
0–19 Years	0									
20–34	0									
35–49	0									
50–64	0									
65+	0									
2. MULTIPLE DX										
A. *Not Operated*										
0–19 Years	0									
20–34	0									
35–49	1	1.0	0	1	1	1	1	1	1	1
50–64	1	1.0	0	1	1	1	1	1	1	1
65+	0									
B. *Operated*										
0–19 Years	0									
20–34	15	2.3	1	1	1	2	3	4	5	5
35–49	173	1.7	<1	1	1	1	2	3	3	5
50–64	133	1.8	<1	1	1	1	2	3	3	6
65+	20	2.3	4	1	1	2	2	3	4	10
SUBTOTALS:										
1. SINGLE DX										
A. *Not Operated*	0									
B. *Operated*	0									
2. MULTIPLE DX										
A. *Not Operated*	2	1.0	0	1	1	1	1	1	1	1
B. *Operated*	341	1.8	1	1	1	2	2	3	3	6
1. SINGLE DX	0									
2. MULTIPLE DX	343	1.8	1	1	1	2	2	3	3	6
A. NOT OPERATED	2	1.0	0	1	1	1	1	1	1	1
B. OPERATED	341	1.8	1	1	1	2	2	3	3	6
TOTAL										
0–19 Years	0									
20–34	15	2.3	1	1	1	2	3	4	5	5
35–49	174	1.7	<1	1	1	1	2	3	3	5
50–64	134	1.8	<1	1	1	1	2	3	3	6
65+	20	2.3	4	1	1	2	2	3	4	10
GRAND TOTAL	343	1.8	1	1	1	2	2	3	3	6

Length of Stay by Diagnosis and Operation, Western Region, 2008

Western Region, October 2006–September 2007 Data, by Diagnosis

V51: AFTERCARE W PLASTIC SURG

Type of Patients	Observed Patients	Avg. Stay	Variance	Percentiles						
				10th	25th	50th	75th	90th	95th	99th
1. SINGLE DX										
A. Not Operated										
0–19 Years	0									
20–34	0									
35–49	1	1.0	0		1	1	1	1	1	1
50–64	0									
65+	0									
B. Operated										
0–19 Years	1	1.0	0	1	1	1	1	1	1	1
20–34	1	1.0	0	1	1	1	1	1	1	1
35–49	0									
50–64	2	1.0	0	1	1	1	1	1	1	1
65+	0									
2. MULTIPLE DX										
A. Not Operated										
0–19 Years	0									
20–34	0									
35–49	0									
50–64	2	1.0	0	1	1	1	1	1	1	1
65+	0									
B. Operated										
0–19 Years	0									
20–34	7	3.7	6	1	2	3	5	8	8	8
35–49	54	3.3	4	1	2	3	4	6	7	10
50–64	60	3.0	4	1	1	3	4	6	6	11
65+	25	2.8	4	1	1	2	4	5	8	8
SUBTOTALS:										
1. SINGLE DX										
A. Not Operated	1	1.0	0	1	1	1	1	1	1	1
B. Operated	4	1.0	0	1	1	1	1	1	1	1
2. MULTIPLE DX										
A. Not Operated	2	1.0	0	1	1	1	1	1	1	1
B. Operated	146	3.1	4	1	1	3	4	6	7	10
1. SINGLE DX	5	1.0	0	1	1	1	1	1	1	1
2. MULTIPLE DX	148	3.1	4	1	1	3	4	6	7	10
A. NOT OPERATED	3	1.0	0	1	1	1	1	1	1	1
B. OPERATED	150	3.1	4	1	1	3	4	6	7	10
TOTAL										
0–19 Years	1	1.0	0	1	1	1	1	1	1	1
20–34	8	3.4	6	1	2	2	5	8	8	8
35–49	55	3.3	4	1	1	3	4	6	7	10
50–64	64	2.8	4	1	1	2	4	6	6	11
65+	25	2.8	4	1	1	2	4	5	8	8
GRAND TOTAL	153	3.0	4	1	1	3	4	6	7	10

V52: FITTING OF PROSTHESIS

Type of Patients	Observed Patients	Avg. Stay	Variance	Percentiles						
				10th	25th	50th	75th	90th	95th	99th
1. SINGLE DX										
A. Not Operated										
0–19 Years	0									
20–34	0									
35–49	0									
50–64	0									
65+	0									
B. Operated										
0–19 Years	0									
20–34	1	3.0	0	3	3	3	3	3	3	3
35–49	0									
50–64	1	1.0	0	1	1	1	1	1	1	1
65+	0									
2. MULTIPLE DX										
A. Not Operated										
0–19 Years	0									
20–34	1	1.0	0	1	1	1	1	1	1	1
35–49	0									
50–64	0									
65+	1	2.0	0	2	2	2	2	2	2	2
B. Operated										
0–19 Years	1	1.0	0	1	1	1	1	1	1	1
20–34	3	1.7	<1	1	1	2	2	2	2	2
35–49	16	2.1	2	1	1	1	3	4	6	6
50–64	22	1.6	1	1	1	1	2	3	3	5
65+	11	2.4	2	1	1	2	4	4	5	5
SUBTOTALS:										
1. SINGLE DX										
A. Not Operated	0									
B. Operated	2	2.0	2	1	1	1	3	3	3	3
2. MULTIPLE DX										
A. Not Operated	2	1.5	<1	1	1	2	2	2	2	2
B. Operated	53	1.9	2	1	1	1	3	4	5	6
1. SINGLE DX	2	2.0	2	1	1	1	3	3	3	3
2. MULTIPLE DX	55	1.9	2	1	1	1	3	4	5	6
A. NOT OPERATED	2	1.5	<1	1	1	2	2	2	2	2
B. OPERATED	55	1.9	2	1	1	1	3	4	5	6
TOTAL										
0–19 Years	1	1.0	0	1	1	1	1	1	1	1
20–34	5	1.8	<1	1	1	2	2	3	3	3
35–49	16	2.1	2	1	1	1	3	4	6	6
50–64	23	1.6	2	1	1	1	2	3	3	5
65+	12	2.3	2	1	1	2	3	4	5	5
GRAND TOTAL	57	1.9	2	1	1	1	3	4	5	6

V53: ADJUSTMENT OF OTH DEVICE

Type of Patients	Observed Patients	Avg. Stay	Variance	Percentiles						
				10th	25th	50th	75th	90th	95th	99th
1. SINGLE DX										
A. Not Operated										
0–19 Years	0									
20–34	2	1.0	0	1	1	1	1	1	1	1
35–49	0									
50–64	0									
65+	0									
B. Operated										
0–19 Years	3	1.0	0	1	1	1	1	1	1	1
20–34	3	1.7	1	1	1	1	3	3	3	3
35–49	0									
50–64	4	2.0	4	1	1	1	1	5	5	5
65+	36	1.1	<1	1	1	1	1	1	3	3
2. MULTIPLE DX										
A. Not Operated										
0–19 Years	36	1.7	2	1	1	1	2	3	5	7
20–34	14	1.2	<1	1	1	1	1	2	3	3
35–49	20	1.9	2	1	1	1	3	3	5	5
50–64	28	2.0	2	1	1	1	2	4	4	6
65+	59	2.2	5	1	1	2	2	5	6	12
B. Operated										
0–19 Years	46	1.6	3	1	1	1	1	2	5	12
20–34	60	2.1	8	1	1	1	2	3	8	19
35–49	109	1.9	3	1	1	1	2	4	6	8
50–64	348	1.7	2	1	1	1	2	3	5	7
65+	1,433	1.7	3	1	1	1	2	3	5	9
SUBTOTALS:										
1. SINGLE DX										
A. Not Operated	2	1.0	0	1	1	1	1	1	1	1
B. Operated	46	1.2	<1	1	1	1	1	2	3	5
2. MULTIPLE DX										
A. Not Operated	157	1.9	3	1	1	1	2	4	5	10
B. Operated	1,996	1.8	3	1	1	1	2	3	5	9
1. SINGLE DX	48	1.2	<1	1	1	1	1	2	3	5
2. MULTIPLE DX	2,153	1.8	3	1	1	1	2	3	5	9
A. NOT OPERATED	159	1.9	3	1	1	1	2	4	5	10
B. OPERATED	2,042	1.7	3	1	1	1	2	3	5	9
TOTAL										
0–19 Years	85	1.6	2	1	1	1	2	2	5	12
20–34	79	1.9	7	1	1	1	2	3	7	19
35–49	129	1.9	3	1	1	1	2	4	6	8
50–64	380	1.7	3	1	1	1	2	4	5	7
65+	1,528	1.7	3	1	1	1	2	3	5	9
GRAND TOTAL	2,201	1.8	3	1	1	1	2	3	5	9

Length of Stay by Diagnosis and Operation, Western Region, 2008

Western Region, October 2006–September 2007 Data, by Diagnosis

V53.31: ADJUST CARDIAC PACEMAKER

Type of Patients	Observed Patients	Avg. Stay	Variance	10th	25th	50th	75th	90th	95th	99th
1. SINGLE DX										
A. Not Operated										
0–19 Years	0									
20–34	0									
35–49	0									
50–64	0									
65+	0									
B. Operated										
0–19 Years	2	1.0	0	1	1	1	1	1	1	1
20–34	2	1.0	0	1	1	1	1	1	1	1
35–49	0									
50–64	0									
65+	33	1.2	<1	1	1	1	1	1	3	3
2. MULTIPLE DX										
A. Not Operated										
0–19 Years	1	1.0	0	1	1	1	1	1	1	1
20–34	0									
35–49	2	2.0	2	1	1	1	3	3	3	3
50–64	6	1.5	<1	1	1	1	2	3	3	3
65+	26	1.7	2	1	1	1	2	4	6	6
B. Operated										
0–19 Years	23	1.8	6	1	1	2	2	2	5	12
20–34	24	2.0	4	1	1	1	3	4	7	8
35–49	31	2.3	3	1	1	2	3	4	5	9
50–64	144	1.7	2	1	1	1	2	4	5	7
65+	961	1.8	4	1	1	1	2	4	5	9
SUBTOTALS:										
1. SINGLE DX										
A. Not Operated	0									
B. Operated	37	1.1	<1	1	1	1	1	1	3	3
2. MULTIPLE DX										
A. Not Operated	35	1.7	2	1	1	1	2	3	6	6
B. Operated	1,183	1.8	4	1	1	1	2	4	5	9
1. SINGLE DX	37	1.1	<1	1	1	1	1	1	3	3
2. MULTIPLE DX	1,218	1.8	4	1	1	1	2	4	5	9
A. NOT OPERATED	35	1.7	2	1	1	1	2	3	6	6
B. OPERATED	1,220	1.8	3	1	1	1	2	4	5	9
TOTAL										
0–19 Years	26	1.7	5	1	1	1	1	2	5	12
20–34	26	1.9	3	1	1	1	2	4	7	8
35–49	33	2.3	3	1	1	2	3	4	5	9
50–64	150	1.7	2	1	1	1	2	4	5	7
65+	1,020	1.8	4	1	1	1	2	3	5	9
GRAND TOTAL	1,255	1.8	3	1	1	1	2	4	5	9

V53.32: ADJUSTMENT AICD

Type of Patients	Observed Patients	Avg. Stay	Variance	10th	25th	50th	75th	90th	95th	99th
1. SINGLE DX										
A. Not Operated										
0–19 Years	0									
20–34	0									
35–49	0									
50–64	0									
65+	0									
B. Operated										
0–19 Years	0									
20–34	0									
35–49	0									
50–64	0									
65+	3	1.0	0	1	1	1	1	1	1	1
2. MULTIPLE DX										
A. Not Operated										
0–19 Years	1	1.0	0	1	1	1	1	1	1	1
20–34	1	1.0	0	1	1	1	1	1	1	1
35–49	2	1.0	0	1	1	1	1	1	1	1
50–64	8	2.0	2	1	1	1	2	4	4	4
65+	17	2.4	8	1	1	1	2	5	12	12
B. Operated										
0–19 Years	3	1.0	0	1	1	1	1	1	1	1
20–34	12	1.3	<1	1	1	1	1	2	3	3
35–49	34	1.4	2	1	1	1	1	2	5	5
50–64	141	1.7	2	1	1	1	2	3	6	7
65+	405	1.6	2	1	1	1	2	3	5	8
SUBTOTALS:										
1. SINGLE DX										
A. Not Operated	0									
B. Operated	3	1.0	0	1	1	1	1	1	1	1
2. MULTIPLE DX										
A. Not Operated	29	2.1	5	1	1	1	2	4	5	12
B. Operated	595	1.6	2	1	1	1	1	3	5	8
1. SINGLE DX	3	1.0	0	1	1	1	1	1	1	1
2. MULTIPLE DX	624	1.6	2	1	1	1	1	3	5	8
A. NOT OPERATED	29	2.1	5	1	1	1	2	4	5	12
B. OPERATED	598	1.6	2	1	1	1	1	3	5	8
TOTAL										
0–19 Years	4	1.0	0	1	1	1	1	1	1	1
20–34	13	1.2	<1	1	1	1	1	2	3	3
35–49	36	1.4	1	1	1	1	1	2	5	5
50–64	149	1.7	2	1	1	1	2	3	6	7
65+	425	1.6	2	1	1	1	1	3	5	8
GRAND TOTAL	627	1.6	2	1	1	1	1	3	5	8

V54: OTH ORTHOPEDIC AFTERCARE

Type of Patients	Observed Patients	Avg. Stay	Variance	10th	25th	50th	75th	90th	95th	99th
1. SINGLE DX										
A. Not Operated										
0–19 Years	14	3.1	11	1	1	2	4	6	13	13
20–34	9	3.8	19	1	1	3	3	15	15	15
35–49	4	1.8	<1	1	1	2	2	2	3	3
50–64	5	2.4	3	1	1	2	3	5	5	5
65+	1	1.0	0	1	1	1	1	1	1	1
B. Operated										
0–19 Years	57	1.6	2	1	1	1	2	2	3	12
20–34	53	1.9	2	1	1	2	2	4	6	7
35–49	36	2.4	5	1	1	2	3	5	7	12
50–64	19	2.3	6	1	1	2	3	5	11	11
65+	4	1.3	<1	1	1	1	2	2	2	2
2. MULTIPLE DX										
A. Not Operated										
0–19 Years	31	2.2	2	1	1	2	3	4	5	6
20–34	39	4.2	34	1	1	2	5	13	29	>99
35–49	59	5.1	62	1	2	3	4	12	25	49
50–64	94	5.7	47	1	2	3	7	12	18	40
65+	255	8.3	68	2	3	6	11	18	20	48
B. Operated										
0–19 Years	92	2.2	2	1	1	2	3	4	5	8
20–34	203	2.6	6	1	1	2	3	4	7	16
35–49	201	2.5	3	1	1	2	3	5	6	8
50–64	251	3.0	8	1	1	2	3	5	8	16
65+	162	3.6	14	2	2	3	4	7	10	21
SUBTOTALS:										
1. SINGLE DX										
A. Not Operated	33	3.0	10	1	1	2	3	6	13	15
B. Operated	169	1.9	3	1	1	1	2	4	5	12
2. MULTIPLE DX										
A. Not Operated	478	6.7	59	1	2	4	8	15	20	48
B. Operated	909	2.8	7	1	1	2	3	5	7	16
1. SINGLE DX	202	2.1	5	1	1	1	2	4	6	12
2. MULTIPLE DX	1,387	4.1	29	1	1	2	4	9	14	25
A. NOT OPERATED	511	6.4	57	1	2	4	8	15	19	41
B. OPERATED	1,078	2.7	7	1	1	2	3	5	7	16
TOTAL										
0–19 Years	194	2.1	3	1	1	2	2	4	5	12
20–34	304	2.7	10	1	1	2	3	5	7	19
35–49	300	3.0	16	1	1	2	3	5	7	25
50–64	369	3.6	19	1	2	2	4	8	11	22
65+	422	6.4	52	1	2	4	8	15	19	39
GRAND TOTAL	1,589	3.9	26	1	1	2	4	8	13	23

Western Region, October 2006–September 2007 Data, by Diagnosis

V54.01: REMOVAL INT FIXATION DEV

Type of Patients	Observed Patients	Avg. Stay	Variance	10th	25th	50th	75th	90th	95th	99th
1. SINGLE DX										
A. *Not Operated*										
0–19 Years	0									
20–34	0									
35–49	0									
50–64	0									
65+	0									
B. *Operated*										
0–19 Years	32	1.3	<1	1	1	1	1	2	3	4
20–34	19	1.3	<1	1	1	1	2	2	3	3
35–49	14	1.6	1	1	1	1	2	3	4	4
50–64	9	2.0	2	1	1	2	2	5	5	5
65+	4	1.3	<1	1	1	1	2	2	2	2
2. MULTIPLE DX										
A. *Not Operated*										
0–19 Years	2	1.0	0	1	1	1	1	1	1	1
20–34	1	1.0	0	1	1	1	1	1	1	1
35–49	3	1.3	<1	1	1	1	2	2	2	2
50–64	1	2.0	0	2	2	2	2	2	2	2
65+	2	1.0	0	1	1	1	1	1	1	1
B. *Operated*										
0–19 Years	38	1.7	1	1	1	1	2	3	4	5
20–34	36	1.9	3	1	1	1	2	3	7	10
35–49	55	1.7	<1	1	1	1	2	3	3	5
50–64	115	2.1	1	1	1	2	3	4	4	5
65+	57	2.6	5	1	1	2	3	4	8	13
SUBTOTALS:										
1. SINGLE DX										
A. *Not Operated*	0									
B. *Operated*	78	1.5	<1	1	1	1	2	3	3	5
2. MULTIPLE DX										
A. *Not Operated*	9	1.2	<1	1	1	1	1	2	2	2
B. *Operated*	301	2.1	2	1	1	2	3	4	4	8
1. SINGLE DX	78	1.5	<1	1	1	1	2	3	3	5
2. MULTIPLE DX	310	2.0	2	1	1	2	3	4	4	8
A. NOT OPERATED	9	1.2	<1	1	1	1	1	2	2	2
B. OPERATED	379	1.9	2	1	1	2	3	4	4	8
TOTAL										
0–19 Years	72	1.5	<1	1	1	1	2	3	4	5
20–34	56	1.7	2	1	1	1	2	3	5	10
35–49	72	1.7	1	1	1	1	2	3	3	5
50–64	125	2.1	1	1	1	2	3	4	4	5
65+	63	2.5	5	1	1	2	3	4	7	13
GRAND TOTAL	388	1.9	2	1	1	1	2	3	4	8

V54.89: ORTHOPEDIC AFTERCARE NEC

Type of Patients	Observed Patients	Avg. Stay	Variance	10th	25th	50th	75th	90th	95th	99th
1. SINGLE DX										
A. *Not Operated*										
0–19 Years	6	2.8	4	1	1	2	4	6	6	6
20–34	5	2.4	3	1	1	2	3	5	5	5
35–49	2	2.0	2	1	1	1	3	3	3	3
50–64	3	3.0	4	1	1	3	5	5	5	5
65+	0									
B. *Operated*										
0–19 Years	15	2.4	8	1	1	1	2	3	12	12
20–34	18	2.1	3	1	1	1	3	5	7	7
35–49	16	2.6	3	1	1	2	3	5	7	7
50–64	6	3.0	16	1	1	1	2	11	11	11
65+	0									
2. MULTIPLE DX										
A. *Not Operated*										
0–19 Years	21	2.1	2	1	1	2	3	4	4	5
20–34	18	1.7	<1	1	1	2	2	3	>99	>99
35–49	26	4.0	28	1	1	2	4	12	13	25
50–64	27	5.3	60	1	1	2	8	12	13	40
65+	27	6.7	32	3	3	4	10	17	17	22
B. *Operated*										
0–19 Years	41	2.5	3	1	2	2	3	4	6	8
20–34	135	2.9	6	1	2	2	3	5	7	16
35–49	107	2.7	4	1	2	2	3	5	5	8
50–64	82	4.0	13	1	2	3	5	8	11	22
65+	41	4.3	26	2	2	3	4	9	10	27
SUBTOTALS:										
1. SINGLE DX										
A. *Not Operated*	16	2.6	3	1	1	2	4	5	6	6
B. *Operated*	55	2.4	5	1	1	2	3	5	7	12
2. MULTIPLE DX										
A. *Not Operated*	119	4.2	30	1	1	2	4	12	17	40
B. *Operated*	406	3.1	9	1	2	2	3	6	8	16
1. SINGLE DX	71	2.5	5	1	1	2	3	5	7	12
2. MULTIPLE DX	525	3.4	14	1	2	2	4	7	10	22
A. NOT OPERATED	135	4.0	27	1	1	2	4	10	13	40
B. OPERATED	461	3.1	9	1	2	2	3	5	8	16
TOTAL										
0–19 Years	83	2.4	3	1	1	2	3	4	6	12
20–34	176	2.6	5	1	1	2	3	5	7	19
35–49	151	2.9	8	1	1	2	3	5	7	16
50–64	118	4.2	24	1	2	3	5	9	12	22
65+	68	5.2	30	1	2	3	5	13	17	27
GRAND TOTAL	596	3.3	13	1	2	2	4	6	10	22

V55: ATTEN TO ARTIF OPENING

Type of Patients	Observed Patients	Avg. Stay	Variance	10th	25th	50th	75th	90th	95th	99th
1. SINGLE DX										
A. *Not Operated*										
0–19 Years	11	1.1	<1	1	1	1	1	1	2	2
20–34	4	1.0	0	1	1	1	1	1	1	1
35–49	0									
50–64	3	2.3	2	1	1	2	4	4	4	4
65+	1	1.0	0	1	1	1	1	1	1	1
B. *Operated*										
0–19 Years	30	4.1	2	3	3	4	5	5	7	8
20–34	67	4.3	3	2	3	4	5	6	7	12
35–49	104	4.4	4	2	3	4	5	7	8	11
50–64	78	4.3	2	3	3	4	5	7	7	8
65+	25	4.2	1	3	4	4	5	5	6	7
2. MULTIPLE DX										
A. *Not Operated*										
0–19 Years	80	2.7	9	1	1	2	2	6	10	15
20–34	38	3.1	21	1	1	2	3	6	14	26
35–49	67	3.9	17	1	1	3	5	10	11	20
50–64	128	3.0	7	1	1	2	4	7	8	13
65+	281	3.6	26	1	1	2	4	8	11	20
B. *Operated*										
0–19 Years	195	6.3	58	2	3	5	7	10	14	30
20–34	422	5.5	11	3	4	5	7	9	10	15
35–49	1,103	6.4	23	3	4	5	7	10	15	25
50–64	1,975	6.5	25	3	4	5	8	10	14	27
65+	1,770	7.4	31	3	4	6	8	12	16	29
SUBTOTALS:										
1. SINGLE DX										
A. *Not Operated*	19	1.3	<1	1	1	1	1	2	4	4
B. *Operated*	304	4.3	3	2	3	4	5	7	7	10
2. MULTIPLE DX										
A. *Not Operated*	594	3.4	18	1	1	2	4	7	11	19
B. *Operated*	5,465	6.7	27	3	4	6	8	11	15	28
1. SINGLE DX	323	4.1	3	2	3	4	5	6	7	10
2. MULTIPLE DX	6,059	6.4	27	2	4	5	7	11	14	27
A. NOT OPERATED	613	3.3	18	1	1	2	4	7	11	18
B. OPERATED	5,769	6.6	26	3	4	5	8	11	14	27
TOTAL										
0–19 Years	316	5.0	41	2	2	4	6	9	12	25
20–34	531	5.2	11	2	3	5	6	8	10	15
35–49	1,274	6.1	22	3	4	5	7	10	14	25
50–64	2,184	6.2	24	2	4	5	7	10	13	27
65+	2,077	6.9	31	2	4	6	8	12	16	29
GRAND TOTAL	6,382	6.3	26	2	4	5	7	10	14	27

Length of Stay by Diagnosis and Operation, Western Region, 2008

869

Western Region, October 2006–September 2007 Data, by Diagnosis

V55.1: ATTEN TO GASTROSTOMY

Type of Patients	Observed Patients	Avg. Stay	Variance	10th	25th	50th	75th	90th	95th	99th
1. SINGLE DX										
A. Not Operated										
0–19 Years	7	1.0	0	1	1	1		1	1	1
20–34	0									
35–49	0									
50–64	0									
65+	0									
B. Operated										
0–19 Years	0									
20–34	0									
35–49	0									
50–64	0									
65+	0									
2. MULTIPLE DX										
A. Not Operated										
0–19 Years	36	2.8	11	1	1		3	6	13	15
20–34	18	3.2	11	1	1	2	4	8	14	14
35–49	30	3.2	13	1	1	2	4	6	9	19
50–64	51	3.5	8	1	1	2	5	7	9	13
65+	189	3.4	9	1	1	2	4	7	10	16
B. Operated										
0–19 Years	5	3.8	9	2	2	3	3	9	9	9
20–34	2	5.0	0	5	5	5	5	5	5	5
35–49	0									
50–64	5	6.2	7	3	5	5	9	9	9	9
65+	3	3.3	4	1	1	4	5	5	5	5
SUBTOTALS:										
1. SINGLE DX										
A. Not Operated	7	1.0	0	1	1	1		1	1	1
B. Operated	0									
2. MULTIPLE DX										
A. Not Operated	324	3.3	10	1	1	2	4	7	10	15
B. Operated	15	4.7	7	2	3	5	5	9	9	9
1. SINGLE DX	7	1.0	0	1	1	1		1	1	1
2. MULTIPLE DX	339	3.4	10	1	1	2	4	7	10	15
A. NOT OPERATED	331	3.2	10	1	1	2	4	7	10	15
B. OPERATED	15	4.7	7	2	3	5	5	9	9	9
TOTAL										
0–19 Years	48	2.6	10	1	1	1	3	6	10	15
20–34	20	3.4	10	1	1	2	5	8	14	14
35–49	30	3.2	13	1	1	2	4	6	9	19
50–64	56	3.7	8	1	2	3	5	7	9	13
65+	192	3.4	9	1	1	2	4	7	10	16
GRAND TOTAL	346	3.3	10	1	1	2	4	7	10	15

V55.2: ATTEN TO ILEOSTOMY

Type of Patients	Observed Patients	Avg. Stay	Variance	10th	25th	50th	75th	90th	95th	99th
1. SINGLE DX										
A. Not Operated										
0–19 Years	0									
20–34	0									
35–49	0									
50–64	1	4.0	0	4	4	4	4	4	4	4
65+	0									
B. Operated										
0–19 Years	6	3.8	3	2	3	3	4	7	7	7
20–34	30	3.7	4	2	3	4	5	5	6	12
35–49	36	3.3	1	2	3	3	4	5	6	7
50–64	28	3.6	1	2	3	3	4	5	6	6
65+	13	4.3	2	3	4	4	5	6	7	7
2. MULTIPLE DX										
A. Not Operated										
0–19 Years	1	12.0	0	12	12	12	12	12	12	12
20–34	2	14.2	284	2	2	26	26	26	26	26
35–49	1	2.0	0	2	2	2	2	2	2	2
50–64	5	3.8	13	1	1	2	6	9	9	9
65+	1	3.0	0	3	3	3	3	3	3	3
B. Operated										
0–19 Years	67	6.0	22	3	4	5	7	9	12	30
20–34	189	4.7	8	2	3	4	6	8	10	15
35–49	362	6.0	28	2	3	4	6	11	16	34
50–64	728	6.0	38	2	3	4	7	11	14	32
65+	577	6.8	36	3	3	5	8	12	17	34
SUBTOTALS:										
1. SINGLE DX										
A. Not Operated	1	4.0	0	4	4	4	4	4	4	4
B. Operated	113	3.6	2	2	3	3	4	5	6	7
2. MULTIPLE DX										
A. Not Operated	10	6.4	62	1	2	2	9	26	26	26
B. Operated	1,923	6.1	32	2	3	5	7	11	15	30
1. SINGLE DX	114	3.6	2	2	3	3	4	5	6	7
2. MULTIPLE DX	1,933	6.1	32	2	3	5	7	11	15	30
A. NOT OPERATED	11	6.2	56	1	2	3	9	12	26	26
B. OPERATED	2,036	6.0	31	2	3	4	7	11	15	29
TOTAL										
0–19 Years	74	5.9	21	3	3	5	7	9	12	30
20–34	221	4.7	9	2	3	4	5	8	10	15
35–49	399	5.7	26	2	3	4	7	10	15	32
50–64	762	5.9	37	2	3	4	8	11	14	32
65+	591	6.7	36	3	3	5	8	12	17	34
GRAND TOTAL	2,047	6.0	31	2	3	4	7	11	15	29

V55.3: ATTEN TO COLOSTOMY

Type of Patients	Observed Patients	Avg. Stay	Variance	10th	25th	50th	75th	90th	95th	99th
1. SINGLE DX										
A. Not Operated										
0–19 Years	0									
20–34	0									
35–49	0									
50–64	0									
65+	1	1.0	0	1	1	1	1	1	1	1
B. Operated										
0–19 Years	24	4.2	2	3	3	4	5	5	6	8
20–34	37	4.7	2	3	4	5	6	6	8	8
35–49	68	4.9	4	3	4	4	6	8	9	11
50–64	50	4.6	2	3	3	5	6	7	7	8
65+	12	4.0	<1	3	3	4	5	5	5	5
2. MULTIPLE DX										
A. Not Operated										
0–19 Years	1	2.0	0	2	2	2	2	2	2	2
20–34	4	1.8	<1	1	1	1	3	3	3	3
35–49	10	2.2	8	1	1	1	2	2	10	10
50–64	18	2.1	5	1	1	1	2	6	8	8
65+	21	1.5	1	1	1	1	1	2	4	5
B. Operated										
0–19 Years	106	6.9	89	3	4	5	7	10	15	26
20–34	227	6.3	13	3	5	6	7	9	11	20
35–49	727	6.7	21	3	5	6	7	10	14	25
50–64	1,220	6.8	17	4	5	6	8	10	14	26
65+	1,168	7.7	26	4	5	7	8	12	16	28
SUBTOTALS:										
1. SINGLE DX										
A. Not Operated	1	1.0	0	1	1	1	1	1	1	1
B. Operated	191	4.7	3	3	3	4	6	7	8	11
2. MULTIPLE DX										
A. Not Operated	54	1.9	3	1	1	1	2	4	6	10
B. Operated	3,448	7.1	23	4	5	6	8	11	15	27
1. SINGLE DX	192	4.7	3	3	3	4	5	7	8	11
2. MULTIPLE DX	3,502	7.0	23	4	5	6	8	11	15	26
A. NOT OPERATED	55	1.8	3	1	1	1	2	4	6	10
B. OPERATED	3,639	6.9	22	4	5	6	8	11	14	26
TOTAL										
0–19 Years	131	6.4	73	3	4	5	7	9	14	26
20–34	268	6.0	12	3	4	5	7	9	10	20
35–49	805	6.5	20	3	4	6	7	10	13	24
50–64	1,288	6.7	17	3	4	6	8	10	13	26
65+	1,202	7.6	26	4	5	7	8	12	16	28
GRAND TOTAL	3,694	6.9	22	3	4	6	8	11	14	26

Length of Stay by Diagnosis and Operation, Western Region, 2008

Western Region, October 2006–September 2007 Data, by Diagnosis

V56: DIALYSIS & CATH CARE

Type of Patients	Observed Patients	Avg. Stay	Vari-ance	10th	25th	50th	75th	90th	95th	99th
1. SINGLE DX										
A. Not Operated										
0–19 Years	0									
20–34	0									
35–49	2	1.0	0	1	1	1	1	1	1	1
50–64	1	1.0	0	1	1	1	1	1	1	1
65+	0									
B. Operated										
0–19 Years	0									
20–34	0									
35–49	0									
50–64	0									
65+	0									
2. MULTIPLE DX										
A. Not Operated										
0–19 Years	26	1.7	2	1	1	1	2	3	6	6
20–34	134	2.2	11	1	1	1	2	4	6	18
35–49	396	1.8	5	1	1	1	2	3	6	15
50–64	480	2.0	7	1	1	1	2	4	6	15
65+	416	2.5	5	1	1	2	3	5	7	10
B. Operated										
0–19 Years	2	10.4	111	3	3	3	18	18	18	18
20–34	10	4.2	11	1	2	3	5	7	12	12
35–49	29	5.7	58	2	2	4	6	10	28	35
50–64	49	4.6	25	1	1	3	7	10	11	26
65+	59	4.3	25	1	1	2	6	11	15	26
SUBTOTALS:										
1. SINGLE DX										
A. Not Operated	3	1.0	0	1	1	1	1	1	1	1
B. Operated	0									
2. MULTIPLE DX										
A. Not Operated	1,452	2.1	6	1	1	1	2	4	6	14
B. Operated	149	4.8	31	1	1	3	6	10	15	28
1. SINGLE DX	3	1.0	0	1	1	1	1	1	1	1
2. MULTIPLE DX	1,601	2.4	9	1	1	1	2	5	7	16
A. NOT OPERATED	1,455	2.1	6	1	1	1	2	4	6	14
B. OPERATED	149	4.8	31	1	1	3	6	10	15	28
TOTAL										
0–19 Years	28	2.4	11	1	1	1	2	6	6	18
20–34	144	2.3	11	1	1	1	2	4	5	18
35–49	427	2.1	9	1	1	1	2	3	6	16
50–64	530	2.3	8	1	1	1	2	4	7	16
65+	475	2.7	8	1	1	2	3	6	7	15
GRAND TOTAL	1,604	2.4	9	1	1	1	2	5	7	16

V56.0: RENAL DIALYSIS ENCOUNTER

Type of Patients	Observed Patients	Avg. Stay	Vari-ance	10th	25th	50th	75th	90th	95th	99th
1. SINGLE DX										
A. Not Operated										
0–19 Years	0									
20–34	0									
35–49	2	1.0	0	1	1	1	1	1	1	1
50–64	1	1.0	0	1	1	1	1	1	1	1
65+	0									
B. Operated										
0–19 Years	0									
20–34	0									
35–49	0									
50–64	0									
65+	0									
2. MULTIPLE DX										
A. Not Operated										
0–19 Years	23	1.8	2	1	1	1	2	3	6	6
20–34	128	2.1	11	1	1	1	2	4	6	18
35–49	386	1.8	5	1	1	1	2	3	5	15
50–64	462	2.0	6	1	1	1	2	4	6	13
65+	400	2.5	5	1	1	2	3	5	7	10
B. Operated										
0–19 Years	1	3.0	0	3	3	3	3	3	3	3
20–34	9	4.3	12	1	2	3	5	12	12	12
35–49	22	6.7	72	1	2	4	6	10	28	35
50–64	33	5.0	32	1	1	3	7	10	21	26
65+	34	5.8	36	1	2	3	7	14	20	26
SUBTOTALS:										
1. SINGLE DX										
A. Not Operated	3	1.0	0	1	1	1	1	1	1	1
B. Operated	0									
2. MULTIPLE DX										
A. Not Operated	1,399	2.1	6	1	1	1	2	4	6	14
B. Operated	99	5.5	40	1	2	3	7	12	21	35
1. SINGLE DX	3	1.0	0	1	1	1	1	1	1	1
2. MULTIPLE DX	1,498	2.3	9	1	1	1	2	5	7	16
A. NOT OPERATED	1,402	2.1	6	1	1	1	2	4	6	14
B. OPERATED	99	5.5	40	1	2	3	7	12	21	35
TOTAL										
0–19 Years	24	1.8	2	1	1	1	2	3	6	6
20–34	137	2.2	11	1	1	1	2	5	6	18
35–49	410	2.1	9	1	1	1	2	4	6	16
50–64	496	2.2	8	1	1	1	2	4	7	16
65+	434	2.7	9	1	1	2	3	6	7	15
GRAND TOTAL	1,501	2.3	9	1	1	1	2	5	7	16

V57: REHABILITATION PROCEDURE

Type of Patients	Observed Patients	Avg. Stay	Vari-ance	10th	25th	50th	75th	90th	95th	99th
1. SINGLE DX										
A. Not Operated										
0–19 Years	0									
20–34	1	7.0	0	7	7	7	7	7	7	7
35–49	0									
50–64	0									
65+	1	87.0	0	87	87	87	87	87	87	87
B. Operated										
0–19 Years	0									
20–34	0									
35–49	0									
50–64	0									
65+	0									
2. MULTIPLE DX										
A. Not Operated										
0–19 Years	169	18.6	237	4	7	13	27	40	49	80
20–34	594	15.5	173	4	7	11	21	33	42	63
35–49	1,203	14.6	155	4	7	11	18	29	39	72
50–64	3,390	13.5	110	4	7	11	17	26	32	55
65+	10,166	12.5	52	5	8	11	16	21	26	37
B. Operated										
0–19 Years	2	43.5	<1	43	43	44	>99	>99	>99	>99
20–34	22	26.7	402	10	13	21	39	66	88	>99
35–49	43	27.1	247	11	18	24	34	43	56	>99
50–64	57	22.5	219	11	12	19	28	42	74	>99
65+	124	19.0	70	8	13	18	24	31	33	39
SUBTOTALS:										
1. SINGLE DX										
A. Not Operated	2	47.3	>999	7	7	87	87	87	87	87
B. Operated	0									
2. MULTIPLE DX										
A. Not Operated	15,522	13.1	80	5	7	11	16	23	29	49
B. Operated	248	22.1	175	10	13	20	27	39	47	>99
1. SINGLE DX	2	47.3	>999	7	7	87	87	87	87	87
2. MULTIPLE DX	15,770	13.2	83	5	7	11	16	23	29	50
A. NOT OPERATED	15,524	13.1	81	5	7	11	16	23	29	49
B. OPERATED	248	22.1	175	10	13	20	27	39	47	>99
TOTAL										
0–19 Years	171	18.9	241	5	7	14	28	42	50	83
20–34	617	15.9	185	4	7	11	21	35	43	69
35–49	1,246	15.1	163	4	7	12	20	30	41	79
50–64	3,447	13.7	113	4	7	11	17	26	33	55
65+	10,291	12.6	53	5	8	11	16	21	26	38
GRAND TOTAL	15,772	13.2	83	5	7	11	16	23	29	50

Length of Stay by Diagnosis and Operation, Western Region, 2008

Western Region, October 2006–September 2007 Data, by Diagnosis

V57.1: PHYSICAL THERAPY NEC

Type of Patients	Observed Patients	Avg. Stay	Variance	10th	25th	50th	75th	90th	95th	99th
1. SINGLE DX										
A. Not Operated										
0-19 Years	0									
20-34	0									
35-49	0									
50-64	0									
65+	0									
B. Operated										
0-19 Years	0									
20-34	0									
35-49	0									
50-64	0									
65+	0									
2. MULTIPLE DX										
A. Not Operated										
0-19 Years	0									
20-34	10	12.3	214	5	5	6	15	20	51	51
35-49	33	11.5	52	4	6	10	16	26	28	>99
50-64	145	10.3	68	4	6	9	12	19	29	>99
65+	433	11.2	93	4	6	9	13	20	31	98
B. Operated										
0-19 Years	0									
20-34	0									
35-49	1	8.0	0	8	8	8	8	8	8	8
50-64	1	19.0	0	19	19	19	19	19	19	19
65+	6	10.6	13	5	9	10	12	16	16	16
SUBTOTALS:										
1. SINGLE DX										
A. Not Operated	0									
B. Operated	0									
2. MULTIPLE DX										
A. Not Operated	621	11.0	87	4	6	8	13	20	29	>99
B. Operated	8	11.4	20	5	8	10	12	19	19	19
1. SINGLE DX	0									
2. MULTIPLE DX	629	11.0	86	4	6	9	13	20	29	>99
A. NOT OPERATED	621	11.0	87	4	6	8	13	20	29	>99
B. OPERATED	8	11.4	20	5	8	10	12	19	19	19
TOTAL										
0-19 Years	0									
20-34	10	12.3	214	5	5	6	15	20	51	51
35-49	34	11.4	50	4	6	9	16	26	28	>99
50-64	146	10.3	68	4	6	9	12	19	29	>99
65+	439	11.2	92	4	6	9	13	20	29	98
GRAND TOTAL	629	11.0	86	4	6	9	13	20	29	>99

V57.89: REHABILITATION PX NEC

Type of Patients	Observed Patients	Avg. Stay	Variance	10th	25th	50th	75th	90th	95th	99th
1. SINGLE DX										
A. Not Operated										
0-19 Years	0									
20-34	1	7.0	0	7	7	7	7	7	7	7
35-49	0									
50-64	0									
65+	1	87.0	0	87	87	87	87	87	87	87
B. Operated										
0-19 Years	0									
20-34	0									
35-49	0									
50-64	0									
65+	0									
2. MULTIPLE DX										
A. Not Operated										
0-19 Years	168	18.6	238	4	7	13	27	40	49	80
20-34	581	15.5	173	4	7	11	21	33	42	63
35-49	1,166	14.7	158	4	7	11	21	29	40	72
50-64	3,233	13.7	112	4	7	11	17	26	32	54
65+	9,710	12.6	50	5	8	11	16	21	26	36
B. Operated										
0-19 Years	2	43.5	<1	43	43	44	>99	>99	>99	>99
20-34	22	26.7	402	10	13	21	39	66	88	>99
35-49	42	27.5	244	12	19	24	34	43	56	>99
50-64	56	22.5	223	11	12	19	28	42	74	>99
65+	118	19.4	69	13	13	19	25	32	35	39
SUBTOTALS:										
1. SINGLE DX										
A. Not Operated	2	47.3	>999	7	7	87	87	87	87	87
B. Operated	0									
2. MULTIPLE DX										
A. Not Operated	14,858	13.2	80	5	7	11	16	23	29	49
B. Operated	240	22.4	177	10	14	20	28	39	47	>99
1. SINGLE DX	2	47.3	>999	7	7	87	87	87	87	87
2. MULTIPLE DX	15,098	13.3	83	5	7	11	16	23	29	49
A. NOT OPERATED	14,860	13.2	80	5	7	11	16	23	29	49
B. OPERATED	240	22.4	177	10	14	20	28	39	47	>99
TOTAL										
0-19 Years	170	18.9	243	5	7	14	28	42	50	83
20-34	604	15.9	185	4	7	11	21	35	43	69
35-49	1,208	15.2	167	4	7	12	20	30	42	76
50-64	3,289	13.8	115	5	8	11	18	26	33	55
65+	9,829	12.7	51	5	8	11	16	21	26	37
GRAND TOTAL	15,100	13.3	83	5	7	11	16	23	29	49

V58: PX & AFTERCARE NEC & NOS

Type of Patients	Observed Patients	Avg. Stay	Variance	10th	25th	50th	75th	90th	95th	99th
1. SINGLE DX										
A. Not Operated										
0-19 Years	13	2.8	5	1	1	2	5	6	7	7
20-34	22	2.0	2	1	1	1	2	4	5	5
35-49	19	3.1	22	1	1	1	2	13	19	19
50-64	28	1.3	<1	1	1	1	1	2	3	3
65+	9	1.3	4	1	1	1	1	4	4	4
B. Operated										
0-19 Years	8	3.9	12	1	1	1	7	9	9	9
20-34	13	3.0	3	1	2	3	4	5	7	7
35-49	5	2.0	3	1	1	1	2	5	5	5
50-64	7	1.9	2	1	1	1	3	5	5	5
65+	3	3.4	4	1	1	4	5	5	5	5
2. MULTIPLE DX										
A. Not Operated										
0-19 Years	3,349	4.3	22	1	2	3	5	6	9	29
20-34	2,857	5.4	38	2	3	4	5	8	17	30
35-49	4,645	4.9	25	1	2	4	5	7	14	28
50-64	7,638	4.8	36	1	2	4	5	8	17	33
65+	5,199	5.1	40	1	2	3	5	9	19	33
B. Operated										
0-19 Years	64	5.4	56	1	1	2	5	19	25	29
20-34	84	9.4	116	1	2	5	14	23	29	64
35-49	163	7.9	130	1	2	4	7	25	29	52
50-64	257	8.2	118	1	2	4	9	22	30	61
65+	166	6.2	58	1	1	3	7	18	22	32
SUBTOTALS:										
1. SINGLE DX										
A. Not Operated	91	2.0	6	1	1	2	2	4	5	19
B. Operated	36	2.9	5	1	1	4	4	7	8	9
2. MULTIPLE DX										
A. Not Operated	23,688	4.9	33	1	2	4	5	8	16	30
B. Operated	734	7.6	102	2	2	4	8	21	28	47
1. SINGLE DX	127	2.3	6	1	1	1	3	5	7	13
2. MULTIPLE DX	24,422	5.0	36	1	2	4	5	8	17	31
A. NOT OPERATED	23,779	4.9	33	1	2	4	5	8	16	30
B. OPERATED	770	7.4	99	1	2	4	8	20	28	47
TOTAL										
0-19 Years	3,434	4.3	23	1	2	3	5	6	10	29
20-34	2,976	5.5	41	2	3	4	5	9	18	31
35-49	4,832	5.0	29	1	2	4	5	8	15	29
50-64	7,930	4.9	39	1	2	4	5	8	18	34
65+	5,377	5.1	41	1	2	3	5	9	19	33
GRAND TOTAL	24,549	5.0	35	1	2	4	5	8	17	31

Length of Stay by Diagnosis and Operation, Western Region, 2008

Western Region, October 2006–September 2007 Data, by Diagnosis

V58.0: RADIOTHERAPY ENCOUNTER

Type of Patients	Observed Patients	Avg. Stay	Variance	10th	25th	50th	75th	90th	95th	99th
1. SINGLE DX										
A. Not Operated										
0–19 Years	0									
20–34	1	2.0	0	2	2	2	2	2	2	2
35–49	0									
50–64	0									
65+	0									
B. Operated										
0–19 Years	0									
20–34	0									
35–49	0									
50–64	0									
65+	0									
2. MULTIPLE DX										
A. Not Operated										
0–19 Years	13	4.3	7	1	1	5	6	6	10	10
20–34	42	2.7	5	1	2	2	3	4	4	16
35–49	120	2.7	4	1	1	2	3	5	7	17
50–64	178	4.4	22	1	2	3	5	8	17	27
65+	150	6.3	32	2	3	5	7	14	19	29
B. Operated										
0–19 Years	0									
20–34	7	4.7	51	1	2	2	3	21	21	21
35–49	19	2.2	<1	1	2	2	3	3	4	4
50–64	22	2.8	4	1	2	2	3	4	4	11
65+	16	3.3	17	1	1	1	3	12	14	14
SUBTOTALS:										
1. SINGLE DX										
A. Not Operated	1	2.0	0	2	2	2	2	2	2	2
B. Operated	0									
2. MULTIPLE DX										
A. Not Operated	503	4.4	21	1	2	3	5	8	14	25
B. Operated	64	3.0	11	1	1	2	3	4	11	21
1. SINGLE DX	1	2.0	0	2	2	2	2	2	2	2
2. MULTIPLE DX	567	4.2	20	1	2	3	5	8	14	25
A. NOT OPERATED	504	4.4	21	1	2	3	5	8	14	25
B. OPERATED	64	3.0	11	1	1	2	3	4	11	21
TOTAL										
0–19 Years	13	4.3	7	1	1	5	6	6	10	10
20–34	50	2.9	11	1	1	2	3	4	5	21
35–49	139	2.6	4	1	1	2	3	5	6	17
50–64	200	4.2	20	1	2	3	4	7	14	25
65+	166	6.0	31	2	2	4	7	14	18	29
GRAND TOTAL	568	4.2	20	1	2	3	5	8	14	25

V58.11: ANTINEO CHEMO ENCOUNTER

Type of Patients	Observed Patients	Avg. Stay	Variance	10th	25th	50th	75th	90th	95th	99th
1. SINGLE DX										
A. Not Operated										
0–19 Years	3	5.0	4	3	3	5	7	7	7	7
20–34	3	4.7	<1	4	4	5	5	5	5	5
35–49	1	2.0	0	2	2	2	2	2	2	2
50–64	3	1.3	<1	1	1	1	2	2	2	2
65+	1	1.0	0	1	1	1	1	1	1	1
B. Operated										
0–19 Years	0									
20–34	0									
35–49	0									
50–64	0									
65+	0									
2. MULTIPLE DX										
A. Not Operated										
0–19 Years	3,211	4.4	23	1	2	4	5	6	9	29
20–34	2,658	5.5	40	2	3	4	5	8	18	31
35–49	4,092	5.0	26	1	2	4	5	8	15	28
50–64	6,742	4.9	38	1	2	3	5	8	18	34
65+	4,628	5.0	42	1	2	3	5	9	20	34
B. Operated										
0–19 Years	31	8.1	94	1	1	4	15	25	28	29
20–34	29	17.4	179	5	8	14	24	34	42	64
35–49	55	14.0	273	2	2	6	25	31	45	92
50–64	100	14.5	207	2	5	10	18	36	41	87
65+	47	12.6	117	2	4	8	21	28	31	50
SUBTOTALS:										
1. SINGLE DX										
A. Not Operated	11	3.3	4	1	1	3	5	5	7	7
B. Operated	0									
2. MULTIPLE DX										
A. Not Operated	21,331	4.9	35	1	2	4	5	8	17	31
B. Operated	262	13.6	191	2	4	8	20	30	40	87
1. SINGLE DX	11	3.3	4	1	1	3	5	5	7	7
2. MULTIPLE DX	21,593	5.0	37	1	2	4	5	8	18	32
A. NOT OPERATED	21,342	4.9	35	1	2	4	5	8	17	31
B. OPERATED	262	13.6	191	2	4	8	20	30	40	87
TOTAL										
0–19 Years	3,245	4.4	23	1	2	4	5	6	10	29
20–34	2,690	5.7	43	2	3	4	5	9	19	33
35–49	4,148	5.1	30	1	2	4	5	8	16	29
50–64	6,845	5.0	42	1	2	3	5	9	19	36
65+	4,676	5.1	43	1	2	3	5	9	20	34
GRAND TOTAL	21,604	5.0	37	1	2	4	5	8	18	32

V58.12: IMMUNOTX ENCOUNT NEOPL

Type of Patients	Observed Patients	Avg. Stay	Variance	10th	25th	50th	75th	90th	95th	99th
1. SINGLE DX										
A. Not Operated										
0–19 Years	0									
20–34	0									
35–49	0									
50–64	0									
65+	0									
B. Operated										
0–19 Years	0									
20–34	0									
35–49	0									
50–64	0									
65+	0									
2. MULTIPLE DX										
A. Not Operated										
0–19 Years	30	3.6	6	1	2	4	4	6	6	14
20–34	97	4.7	10	2	3	4	5	7	9	23
35–49	307	4.4	8	2	4	4	5	6	7	11
50–64	534	4.7	8	2	3	4	5	6	8	17
65+	196	4.6	22	1	2	4	5	7	10	35
B. Operated										
0–19 Years	0									
20–34	0									
35–49	1	26.0	0	26	26	26	26	26	26	26
50–64	3	12.7	93	2	2	15	21	21	21	21
65+	0									
SUBTOTALS:										
1. SINGLE DX										
A. Not Operated	0									
B. Operated	0									
2. MULTIPLE DX										
A. Not Operated	1,164	4.6	9	2	3	4	5	6	8	17
B. Operated	4	16.0	107	2	15	18	21	26	26	26
1. SINGLE DX	0									
2. MULTIPLE DX	1,168	4.6	10	2	3	4	5	6	8	19
A. NOT OPERATED	1,164	4.6	9	2	3	4	5	6	8	17
B. OPERATED	4	16.0	107	2	15	18	21	26	26	26
TOTAL										
0–19 Years	30	3.6	6	1	2	4	4	6	6	14
20–34	97	4.7	10	2	3	4	5	7	9	23
35–49	308	4.5	6	2	4	4	5	6	7	12
50–64	537	4.7	8	2	3	4	5	6	9	17
65+	196	4.6	22	1	2	4	5	7	10	35
GRAND TOTAL	1,168	4.6	10	2	3	4	5	6	8	19

Length of Stay by Diagnosis and Operation, Western Region, 2008

Western Region, October 2006–September 2007 Data, by Diagnosis

Type of Patients	V58.49 Observed Patients	V58.49 Avg. Stay	V58.49 Variance	V58.49 10th	V58.49 25th	V58.49 50th	V58.49 75th	V58.49 90th	V58.49 95th	V58.49 99th	V58.89 Observed Patients	V58.89 Avg. Stay	V58.89 Variance	V58.89 10th	V58.89 25th	V58.89 50th	V58.89 75th	V58.89 90th	V58.89 95th	V58.89 99th	V59 Observed Patients	V59 Avg. Stay	V59 Variance	V59 10th	V59 25th	V59 50th	V59 75th	V59 90th	V59 95th	V59 99th
1. SINGLE DX																														
A. Not Operated																														
0–19 Years	4	2.0	4	1	1	1	1	5	5	5	1	1.0	0	1	1	1	1	1	1	1	14	1.1	<1	1	1	1	1	1	2	2
20–34	6	1.7	<1	1	1	2	2	2	3	3	4	1.0	0	1	1	1	1	1	1	1	5	1.2	<1	1	1	1	1	2	2	2
35–49	7	1.9	1	1	1	2	2	4	4	4	1	13.0	0	13	13	13	13	13	13	13	11	2.0	6	1	1	1	2	3	9	9
50–64	7	1.6	<1	1	1	1	2	3	3	3	0										3	1.3	<1	1	1	1	2	2	2	2
65+	2	1.0	0	1	1	1	1	1	1	1	0										0									
B. Operated																														
0–19 Years	1	1.0	0	1	1	1	1	1	1	1	2	1.0	0	1	1	1	1	1	1	1	8	2.3	<1	2	2	2	2	3	3	3
20–34	1	3.0	0	3	3	3	3	3	3	3	5	2.8	2	1	2	2	3	5	5	5	157	2.7	1	2	2	3	3	4	5	6
35–49	0										1	1.0	0	1	1	1	1	1	1	1	194	2.8	2	1	2	3	3	4	5	8
50–64	1	1.0	0	1	1	1	1	1	1	1	0										140	2.5	2	1	2	2	3	4	4	6
65+	0										0										4	3.5	<1	3	3	4	4	4	4	4
2. MULTIPLE DX																														
A. Not Operated																														
0–19 Years	11	3.2	7	1	1	2	2	7	7	7	11	4.6	35	1	1	2	5	14	18	18	1	1.0	0	1	1	1	1	1	1	1
20–34	9	4.9	15	1	1	5	7	13	13	13	12	3.8	31	1	1	5	7	7	21	21	2	1.0	0	1	1	1	1	1	1	1
35–49	37	2.7	7	1	1	2	3	5	9	14	18	8.3	49	1	1	7	12	21	25	25	9	1.6	1	1	1	1	2	4	4	4
50–64	51	4.3	27	1	2	3	4	9	19	22	29	10.6	154	1	2	7	11	26	26	59	9	1.3	<1	1	1	1	2	2	2	2
65+	31	5.7	33	1	2	3	8	12	21	23	60	7.4	32	2	3	6	11	15	17	27	0									
B. Operated																														
0–19 Years	10	1.5	<1	1	1	1	2	2	4	4	3	3.3	10	1	1	2	7	7	7	7	3	3.3	5	2	2	2	6	6	6	6
20–34	3	2.0	3	1	1	1	1	4	4	4	11	4.3	24	1	2	3	7	7	18	18	105	3.5	3	2	3	3	4	5	6	8
35–49	12	5.0	61	1	1	3	5	6	29	29	12	7.5	81	1	1	5	11	21	29	29	203	3.2	2	2	2	3	4	5	6	7
50–64	24	3.7	19	1	1	1	5	7	8	21	4	4.3	11	1	3	4	4	9	9	9	188	3.3	13	1	2	3	4	5	6	21
65+	15	2.1	3	1	1	1	5	5	7	7	5	6.0	54	3	3	3	4	19	19	19	19	3.5	13	3	3	4	4	4	18	18
SUBTOTALS:																														
1. SINGLE DX																														
A. Not Operated	26	1.7	1	1	1	1	2	3	4	5	6	3.0	24	1	1	1	1	13	13	13	33	1.4	2	1	1	1	1	2	3	9
B. Operated	3	1.7	1	1	1	1	3	3	3	3	8	2.1	2	1	1	2	3	5	5	5	503	2.7	1	1	2	3	3	4	5	6
2. MULTIPLE DX																														
A. Not Operated	139	4.1	21	1	1	3	5	9	16	22	130	7.7	64	1	2	5	11	17	25	27	21	1.4	<1	1	1	1	2	2	2	4
B. Operated	64	3.1	20	1	1	1	4	6	7	29	35	5.5	44	1	1	3	7	18	21	29	518	3.3	6	2	2	3	4	5	6	14
1. SINGLE DX	29	1.7	1	1	1	1	2	3	4	5	14	2.5	10	1	1	1	2	5	13	13	536	2.6	2	1	2	3	3	4	5	7
2. MULTIPLE DX	203	3.8	21	1	1	2	4	8	14	22	165	7.2	60	1	2	4	10	17	24	29	539	3.2	6	2	2	3	4	5	6	14
A. NOT OPERATED	165	3.8	19	1	1	2	4	8	14	22	136	7.5	63	1	2	5	11	17	25	27	54	1.4	1	1	1	1	1	2	3	9
B. OPERATED	67	3.1	19	1	1	1	4	6	7	29	43	4.9	38	1	1	3	5	11	19	29	1,021	3.0	4	1	2	3	4	4	5	8
TOTAL																														
0–19 Years	26	2.3	4	1	1	1	3	7	7	7	17	3.7	25	1	1	3	4	14	18	18	26	1.7	1	1	1	1	2	3	3	6
20–34	19	3.3	10	1	1	2	5	7	13	13	32	3.5	20	1	1	2	4	5	18	21	269	3.0	2	1	2	3	4	4	5	7
35–49	56	3.1	18	1	1	2	3	5	9	29	32	7.9	58	1	1	6	12	21	25	29	417	2.9	2	1	2	3	4	5	6	8
50–64	83	3.9	22	1	1	2	4	8	17	22	33	9.8	140	2	2	7	11	25	26	59	340	2.9	8	1	2	3	4	4	5	15
65+	48	4.4	25	2	2	2	5	12	16	23	65	7.3	33	3	3	6	11	15	17	27	23	3.5	11	1	3	3	4	4	4	18
GRAND TOTAL	232	3.6	19	1	1	2	4	7	13	22	179	6.8	58	1	2	4	10	17	24	29	1,075	2.9	4	1	2	3	3	4	5	8

Column groups: **V58.49: POSTSURG AFTERCARE NEC**, **V58.89: AFTERCARE NEC**, **V59: DONOR**

Western Region, October 2006–September 2007 Data, by Diagnosis

V59.4: KIDNEY DONOR

Type of Patients	Observed Patients	Avg. Stay	Variance	Percentiles						
				10th	25th	50th	75th	90th	95th	99th
1. SINGLE DX										
A. Not Operated										
0–19 Years	0									
20–34	0									
35–49	1	1.0	0	1	1	1	1	1	1	1
50–64	0									
65+	0									
B. Operated										
0–19 Years	8	2.3	<1	2	2	2	2	3	3	3
20–34	152	2.6	1	1	2	3	3	4	4	5
35–49	187	2.6	1	1	2	3	3	4	4	6
50–64	137	2.4	<1	1	2	2	3	4	4	4
65+	4	3.5	<1	3	3	4	4	4	4	4
2. MULTIPLE DX										
A. Not Operated										
0–19 Years	0									
20–34	1	1.0	0	1	1	1	1	1	1	1
35–49	3	1.0	0	1	1	1	1	1	1	1
50–64	1	1.0	0	1	1	1	1	1	1	1
65+	0									
B. Operated										
0–19 Years	2	2.0	0	2	2	2	2	2	2	2
20–34	96	3.2	1	2	3	3	4	4	5	7
35–49	195	3.1	2	2	2	3	4	5	5	7
50–64	177	2.7	1	1	2	3	3	4	5	6
65+	19	3.5	13	1	2	3	4	4	18	18
SUBTOTALS:										
1. SINGLE DX										
A. Not Operated	1	1.0	0	1	1	1	1	1	1	1
B. Operated	488	2.6	1	1	2	3	3	4	4	5
2. MULTIPLE DX										
A. Not Operated	5	1.0	0	1	1	1	1	1	1	1
B. Operated	489	3.0	2	2	2	3	4	4	5	7
1. SINGLE DX	**489**	**2.6**	**1**	**1**	**2**	**3**	**3**	**4**	**4**	**5**
2. MULTIPLE DX	**494**	**3.0**	**2**	**2**	**2**	**3**	**4**	**4**	**5**	**7**
A. NOT OPERATED	**6**	**1.0**	**0**	**1**	**1**	**1**	**1**	**1**	**1**	**1**
B. OPERATED	**977**	**2.8**	**2**	**1**	**2**	**3**	**4**	**4**	**5**	**6**
TOTAL										
0–19 Years	10	2.2	<1	2	2	2	2	3	3	3
20–34	249	2.8	1	1	2	3	3	4	5	6
35–49	386	2.8	1	1	2	3	3	4	5	6
50–64	315	2.6	1	1	2	3	3	4	4	5
65+	23	3.5	11	1	2	3	4	4	4	18
GRAND TOTAL	**983**	**2.8**	**2**	**1**	**2**	**3**	**3**	**4**	**5**	**6**

V60: HOUSEHOLD CIRCUMSTANCES

Type of Patients	Observed Patients	Avg. Stay	Variance	Percentiles						
				10th	25th	50th	75th	90th	95th	99th
1. SINGLE DX										
B. Operated (0–19)	0									
B. Operated (20–34)	0									
B. Operated (35–49)	0									
B. Operated (50–64)	0									
B. Operated (65+)	0									
2. MULTIPLE DX										
A. Not Operated (20–34)	0									
A. Not Operated (35–49)	0									
A. Not Operated (50–64)	0									
B. Operated (0–19)	0									
B. Operated (20–34)	0									
B. Operated (35–49)	0									
B. Operated (50–64)	0									
B. Operated (65+)	0									
SINGLE DX A. Not Operated	0									
SINGLE DX B. Operated	0									
MULTIPLE DX A. Not Operated	0									
MULTIPLE DX B. Operated	0									
1. SINGLE DX	**0**									
2. MULTIPLE DX	**0**									
A. NOT OPERATED	**0**									
B. OPERATED	**0**									
TOTAL 0–19	0									
TOTAL 20–34	0									
TOTAL 35–49	0									
TOTAL 50–64	0									
TOTAL 65+	0									
GRAND TOTAL	**0**									

V61: OTH FAMILY CIRCUMSTANCES

Type of Patients	Observed Patients	Avg. Stay	Variance	Percentiles						
				10th	25th	50th	75th	90th	95th	99th
1. SINGLE DX										
B. Operated (0–19)	0									
B. Operated (20–34)	0									
B. Operated (35–49)	0									
B. Operated (50–64)	0									
B. Operated (65+)	0									
2. MULTIPLE DX										
A. Not Operated (20–34)	0									
A. Not Operated (35–49)	0									
A. Not Operated (50–64)	0									
B. Operated (0–19)	0									
B. Operated (20–34)	0									
B. Operated (35–49)	0									
B. Operated (50–64)	0									
B. Operated (65+)	0									
SINGLE DX B. Operated	0									
MULTIPLE DX B. Operated	0									
1. SINGLE DX	**0**									
2. MULTIPLE DX	**0**									
A. NOT OPERATED	**0**									
B. OPERATED	**0**									
TOTAL 0–19	0									
TOTAL 20–34	0									
TOTAL 35–49	0									
TOTAL 50–64	0									
GRAND TOTAL	**0**									

Length of Stay by Diagnosis and Operation, Western Region, 2008

Western Region, October 2006–September 2007 Data, by Diagnosis

V62: PSYCHOSOCIAL CIRCUM NEC

Type of Patients	Observed Patients	Avg. Stay	Vari-ance	Percentiles						
				10th	25th	50th	75th	90th	95th	99th
1. SINGLE DX										
A. Not Operated										
0–19 Years	1	1.0	0	1	1	1	1	1	1	1
20–34	0									
35–49	0									
50–64	1	2.0	0	2	2	2	2	2	2	2
65+	0									
B. Operated										
0–19 Years	0									
20–34	0									
35–49	0									
50–64	0									
65+	0									
2. MULTIPLE DX										
A. Not Operated										
0–19 Years	13	1.8	2	1	1	1	2	4	5	5
20–34	8	3.6	5	1	2	3	5	8	8	8
35–49	7	2.2	<1	1	1	2	3	3	3	3
50–64	6	5.0	63	1	1	2	4	21	21	21
65+	1	2.0	0	2	2	2	2	2	2	2
B. Operated										
0–19 Years	0									
20–34	0									
35–49	0									
50–64	1	10.0	0	10	10	10	10	10	10	10
65+	0									
SUBTOTALS:										
1. SINGLE DX										
A. Not Operated	2	1.5	<1	1	1	1	2	2	2	2
B. Operated	0									
2. MULTIPLE DX										
A. Not Operated	35	2.9	13	1	1	2	3	5	8	21
B. Operated	1	10.0	0	10	10	10	10	10	10	10
1. SINGLE DX	2	1.5	<1	1	1	1	2	2	2	2
2. MULTIPLE DX	36	3.1	14	1	1	2	3	5	10	21
A. NOT OPERATED	37	2.8	12	1	1	2	3	5	8	21
B. OPERATED	1	10.0	0	10	10	10	10	10	10	10
TOTAL										
0–19 Years	14	1.8	2	1	1	1	2	4	5	5
20–34	8	3.6	5	1	2	3	5	8	8	8
35–49	7	2.2	<1	1	1	2	3	3	3	3
50–64	8	5.3	50	1	1	2	10	21	21	21
65+	1	2.0	0	2	2	2	2	2	2	2
GRAND TOTAL	38	3.0	13	1	1	2	3	5	10	21

V63: NO MED FACILITY FOR CARE

Type of Patients	Observed Patients	Avg. Stay	Vari-ance	Percentiles						
				10th	25th	50th	75th	90th	95th	99th
1. SINGLE DX										
A. Not Operated										
0–19 Years	0									
20–34	0									
35–49	0									
50–64	0									
65+	0									
B. Operated										
0–19 Years	0									
20–34	0									
35–49	0									
50–64	0									
65+	0									
2. MULTIPLE DX										
A. Not Operated										
0–19 Years	0									
20–34	0									
35–49	0									
50–64	0									
65+	0									
B. Operated										
0–19 Years	0									
20–34	0									
35–49	0									
50–64	0									
65+	0									
SUBTOTALS:										
1. SINGLE DX										
A. Not Operated	0									
B. Operated	0									
2. MULTIPLE DX										
A. Not Operated	0									
B. Operated	0									
1. SINGLE DX	0									
2. MULTIPLE DX	0									
A. NOT OPERATED	0									
B. OPERATED	0									
TOTAL										
0–19 Years	0									
20–34	0									
35–49	0									
50–64	0									
65+	0									
GRAND TOTAL	0									

V64: PROCEDURES NOT DONE

Type of Patients	Observed Patients	Avg. Stay	Vari-ance	Percentiles						
				10th	25th	50th	75th	90th	95th	99th
1. SINGLE DX										
A. Not Operated										
0–19 Years	0									
20–34	0									
35–49	1	1.0	0	1	1	1	1	1	1	1
50–64	0									
65+	0									
B. Operated										
0–19 Years	0									
20–34	0									
35–49	0									
50–64	0									
65+	0									
2. MULTIPLE DX										
A. Not Operated										
0–19 Years	0									
20–34	0									
35–49	0									
50–64	0									
65+	0									
B. Operated										
0–19 Years	0									
20–34	0									
35–49	0									
50–64	0									
65+	0									
SUBTOTALS:										
1. SINGLE DX										
A. Not Operated	1	1.0	0	1	1	1	1	1	1	1
B. Operated	0									
2. MULTIPLE DX										
A. Not Operated	0									
B. Operated	0									
1. SINGLE DX	1	1.0	0	1	1	1	1	1	1	1
2. MULTIPLE DX	0									
A. NOT OPERATED	1	1.0	0	1	1	1	1	1	1	1
B. OPERATED	0									
TOTAL										
0–19 Years	0									
20–34	0									
35–49	1	1.0	0	1	1	1	1	1	1	1
50–64	0									
65+	0									
GRAND TOTAL	1	1.0	0	1	1	1	1	1	1	1

Length of Stay by Diagnosis and Operation, Western Region, 2008

Western Region, October 2006–September 2007 Data, by Diagnosis

V65: OTH PERSON SEEK CONSULT

Type of Patients	Observed Patients	Avg. Stay	Variance	10th	25th	50th	75th	90th	95th	99th
1. SINGLE DX										
A. Not Operated										
0–19 Years	8	1.5	<1	1	1	1	2	3	3	3
20–34	6	3.0	2	1	2	3	4	4	4	4
35–49	1	2.0	0	2	2	2	2	2	2	2
50–64	2	2.0	0	2	2	2	2	2	2	2
65+	1	1.0	0	1	1	1	1	1	1	1
B. Operated										
0–19 Years	0									
20–34	0									
35–49	0									
50–64	0									
65+	0									
2. MULTIPLE DX										
A. Not Operated										
0–19 Years	6	2.7	5	1	1	2	3	7	7	7
20–34	21	3.0	12	1	1	2	4	5	6	16
35–49	28	2.9	4	1	1	2	4	6	6	8
50–64	12	2.4	8	1	1	1	2	3	11	11
65+	2	2.0	0	2	2	2	2	2	2	2
B. Operated										
0–19 Years	0									
20–34	0									
35–49	0									
50–64	0									
65+	0									
SUBTOTALS:										
1. SINGLE DX										
A. Not Operated	18	2.1	1	1	1	2	3	4	4	4
B. Operated	0									
2. MULTIPLE DX										
A. Not Operated	69	2.8	7	1	1	2	4	6	7	16
B. Operated	0									
1. SINGLE DX	18	2.1	1	1	1	2	3	4	4	4
2. MULTIPLE DX	69	2.8	7	1	1	2	4	6	7	16
A. NOT OPERATED	87	2.7	6	1	1	2	4	5	6	16
B. OPERATED	0									
TOTAL										
0–19 Years	14	2.0	3	1	1	2	2	3	7	7
20–34	27	3.0	9	1	1	2	4	4	6	16
35–49	29	2.9	4	1	1	2	4	6	6	8
50–64	14	2.4	7	1	1	2	2	3	11	11
65+	3	1.7	<1	1	2	2	2	2	2	2
GRAND TOTAL	87	2.7	6	1	1	2	4	5	6	16

V66: CONVALESCENCE

Type of Patients	Observed Patients	Avg. Stay	Variance	10th	25th	50th	75th	90th	95th	99th
1. SINGLE DX										
A. Not Operated										
0–19 Years	1	1.0	0	1	1	1	1	1	1	1
20–34	3	26.0	645	1	1	25	52	52	52	52
35–49	3	1.3	<1	1	1	1	1	1	1	1
50–64	4	2.0	<1	1	2	2	2	3	3	3
65+	0									
B. Operated										
0–19 Years	0									
20–34	0									
35–49	0									
50–64	0									
65+	0									
2. MULTIPLE DX										
A. Not Operated										
0–19 Years	3	2.7	4	1	1	2	5	5	5	5
20–34	4	7.1	88	2	2	3	21	21	21	21
35–49	6	10.1	224	2	2	3	9	40	40	40
50–64	5	2.4	<1	1	1	3	3	4	4	4
65+	10	9.1	193	1	1	5	8	14	47	47
B. Operated										
0–19 Years	0									
20–34	0									
35–49	0									
50–64	0									
65+	0									
SUBTOTALS:										
1. SINGLE DX										
A. Not Operated	11	8.3	259	1	1	2	3	25	52	52
B. Operated	0									
2. MULTIPLE DX										
A. Not Operated	28	7.1	126	1	2	3	7	21	40	47
B. Operated	0									
1. SINGLE DX	11	8.3	259	1	1	2	3	25	52	52
2. MULTIPLE DX	28	7.1	126	1	2	3	7	21	40	47
A. NOT OPERATED	39	7.4	158	1	1	2	5	25	47	52
B. OPERATED	0									
TOTAL										
0–19 Years	4	2.3	4	1	1	1	2	3	5	5
20–34	7	15.2	364	1	2	3	25	52	52	52
35–49	9	7.1	159	1	2	2	4	40	40	40
50–64	9	2.2	1	1	1	2	3	4	4	4
65+	10	9.1	193	1	1	5	8	14	47	47
GRAND TOTAL	39	7.4	158	1	1	2	5	25	47	52

V67: FOLLOW-UP EXAMINATION

Type of Patients	Observed Patients	Avg. Stay	Variance	10th	25th	50th	75th	90th	95th	99th
1. SINGLE DX										
A. Not Operated										
0–19 Years	4	3.0	4	2	2	2	6	6	6	6
20–34	1	2.0	0	2	2	2	2	2	2	2
35–49	1	1.0	0	1	1	1	1	1	1	1
50–64	1	3.0	0	3	3	3	3	3	3	3
65+	1	1.0	0	1	1	1	1	1	1	1
B. Operated										
0–19 Years	0									
20–34	0									
35–49	0									
50–64	0									
65+	0									
2. MULTIPLE DX										
A. Not Operated										
0–19 Years	23	1.7	2	1	1	1	2	4	5	6
20–34	6	1.5	<1	1	1	1	2	3	3	3
35–49	8	2.3	13	1	1	2	3	5	5	5
50–64	24	2.9	13	1	1	1	3	7	13	13
65+	15	2.1	2	1	1	2	3	4	5	5
B. Operated										
0–19 Years	0									
20–34	3	4.0	27	1	1	1	10	10	10	10
35–49	7	3.0	4	1	2	3	3	7	7	7
50–64	12	4.0	4	1	2	4	5	6	7	7
65+	6	3.0	5	1	1	3	3	7	7	7
SUBTOTALS:										
1. SINGLE DX										
A. Not Operated	8	2.4	3	1	2	2	3	6	6	6
B. Operated	0									
2. MULTIPLE DX										
A. Not Operated	76	2.2	5	1	1	1	3	5	6	13
B. Operated	28	3.5	6	1	1	3	5	7	7	10
1. SINGLE DX	8	2.4	3	1	2	2	3	6	6	6
2. MULTIPLE DX	104	2.6	6	1	1	1	3	6	7	13
A. NOT OPERATED	84	2.2	5	1	1	1	3	5	6	13
B. OPERATED	28	3.5	6	1	1	3	5	7	7	10
TOTAL										
0–19 Years	27	1.9	2	1	1	1	2	5	6	6
20–34	10	2.3	8	1	1	1	2	10	10	10
35–49	16	2.5	3	1	1	2	3	5	7	7
50–64	37	3.3	10	1	1	1	5	5	13	13
65+	22	2.3	7	1	1	2	3	4	5	7
GRAND TOTAL	112	2.5	6	1	1	1	3	6	7	13

Length of Stay by Diagnosis and Operation, Western Region, 2008

Western Region, October 2006–September 2007 Data, by Diagnosis

V68: ADMINISTRATIVE ENCOUNTER

Type of Patients	Observed Patients	Avg. Stay	Variance	10th	25th	50th	75th	90th	95th	99th
1. SINGLE DX										
A. Not Operated										
0–19 Years	14	1.0	0	1	1	1	1			1
20–34	20	1.3	<1	1	1	1	1	3	3	3
35–49	9	1.6	3	1	1	1	1	6	6	6
50–64	12	1.3	1	1	1	1	1	1	5	5
65+	23	1.5	1	1	1	1	1	3	5	5
B. Operated										
0–19 Years	0									
20–34	0									
35–49	0									
50–64	0									
65+	1	4.0	0	4	4	4	4	4	4	4
2. MULTIPLE DX										
A. Not Operated										
0–19 Years	1	1.0	0	1	1	1	1	1	1	1
20–34	0									
35–49	3	2.7	<1	2	2	3	3	>99	>99	>99
50–64	1	1.0	0	1	1	1	1	1	1	1
65+	3	3.3	4	1	1	4	5	5	5	5
B. Operated										
0–19 Years	0									
20–34	0									
35–49	0									
50–64	0									
65+	0									
SUBTOTALS:										
1. SINGLE DX A. Not Operated	78	1.3	1	1	1	1	1	2	5	6
B. Operated	1	4.0	0	4	4	4	4	4	4	4
2. MULTIPLE DX A. Not Operated	8	2.5	2	1	1	3	4	>99	>99	>99
B. Operated	0									
1. SINGLE DX	79	1.4	1	1	1	1	1	3	5	6
2. MULTIPLE DX	8	2.5	2	1	1	3	4	>99	>99	>99
A. NOT OPERATED	86	1.4	1	1	1	1	1	3	5	>99
B. OPERATED	1	4.0	0	4	4	4	4	4	4	4
TOTAL										
0–19 Years	15	1.0	0	1	1	1	1	1	1	1
20–34	20	1.3	<1	1	1	1	1	3	3	3
35–49	12	1.8	2	1	1	1	3	6	>99	>99
50–64	13	1.3	1	1	1	1	2	5	5	5
65+	27	1.8	2	1	1	1	2	3	5	5
GRAND TOTAL	87	1.5	1	1	1	1	1	3	5	>99

V69: LIFESTYLE PROBLEMS

Type of Patients	Observed Patients	Avg. Stay	Variance	10th	25th	50th	75th	90th	95th	99th
1. SINGLE DX										
A. Not Operated										
0–19 Years	0									
20–34	0									
35–49	0									
50–64	0									
65+	0									
B. Operated										
0–19 Years	0									
20–34	0									
35–49	0									
50–64	0									
65+	0									
2. MULTIPLE DX										
A. Not Operated										
0–19 Years	0									
20–34	0									
35–49	0									
50–64	0									
65+	0									
B. Operated										
0–19 Years	0									
20–34	0									
35–49	0									
50–64	0									
65+	0									
SUBTOTALS:										
1. SINGLE DX A. Not Operated	0									
B. Operated	0									
2. MULTIPLE DX A. Not Operated	0									
B. Operated	0									
1. SINGLE DX	0									
2. MULTIPLE DX	0									
A. NOT OPERATED	0									
B. OPERATED	0									
TOTAL										
0–19 Years	0									
20–34	0									
35–49	0									
50–64	0									
65+	0									
GRAND TOTAL	0									

V70: GENERAL MEDICAL EXAM

Type of Patients	Observed Patients	Avg. Stay	Variance	10th	25th	50th	75th	90th	95th	99th
1. SINGLE DX										
A. Not Operated										
0–19 Years	176	1.3	<1	1	1	1	1	2	2	4
20–34	625	2.8	13	1	1	2	3	5	11	20
35–49	287	2.6	16	1	1	2	2	5	11	20
50–64	280	1.9	10	1	1	1	1	3	5	20
65+	62	2.9	9	1	1	1	5	8	8	8
B. Operated										
0–19 Years	0									
20–34	9	1.0	0	1	1	1	1	1	1	1
35–49	11	1.0	0	1	1	1	1	1	1	1
50–64	0									
65+	0									
2. MULTIPLE DX										
A. Not Operated										
0–19 Years	152	1.4	1	1	1	1	2	2	2	4
20–34	314	6.6	49	1	2	3	11	17	20	27
35–49	270	4.7	52	1	1	2	5	15	20	34
50–64	368	4.1	36	1	1	1	4	14	18	27
65+	135	2.8	13	1	1	1	3	8	8	17
B. Operated										
0–19 Years	0									
20–34	0									
35–49	5	6.4	120	1	1	2	26	>99	>99	>99
50–64	3	31.5	>999	1	1	1	92	92	92	92
65+	0									
SUBTOTALS:										
1. SINGLE DX A. Not Operated	1,430	2.4	11	1	1	1	2	4	8	20
B. Operated	20	1.0	0	1	1	1	1	1	1	1
2. MULTIPLE DX A. Not Operated	1,239	4.4	38	1	1	2	4	14	18	27
B. Operated	8	15.8	>999	1	1	2	26	>99	>99	>99
1. SINGLE DX	1,450	2.4	11	1	1	1	2	4	8	20
2. MULTIPLE DX	1,247	4.5	45	1	1	2	4	14	18	27
A. NOT OPERATED	2,669	3.3	25	1	1	1	3	8	17	27
B. OPERATED	28	5.3	313	1	1	1	1	26	92	>99
TOTAL										
0–19 Years	328	1.3	<1	1	1	1	2	2	2	4
20–34	948	4.0	28	1	1	2	3	12	17	27
35–49	573	3.6	34	1	1	1	3	9	18	28
50–64	651	3.3	38	1	1	1	3	7	17	27
65+	197	2.8	12	1	1	1	3	8	8	17
GRAND TOTAL	2,697	3.3	28	1	1	1	3	8	17	27

Length of Stay by Diagnosis and Operation, Western Region, 2008

Western Region, October 2006–September 2007 Data, by Diagnosis

V70.7: EXAM-CLINICAL TRIAL

Type of Patients	Observed Patients	Avg. Stay	Vari-ance	10th	25th	50th	75th	90th	95th	99th
1. SINGLE DX										
A. Not Operated										
0–19 Years	175	1.3	<1	1	1	1	1	2	2	4
20–34	624	2.8	13	1	1	2	3	5	11	20
35–49	287	2.6	16	1	1	1	2	5	11	20
50–64	279	1.9	10	1	1	1	1	3	5	20
65+	62	2.9	9	1	1	1	5	8	8	8
B. Operated										
0–19 Years	0									
20–34	9	1.0	0	1	1	1	1	1	1	1
35–49	11	1.0	0	1	1	1	1	1	1	1
50–64	0									
65+	0									
2. MULTIPLE DX										
A. Not Operated										
0–19 Years	150	1.4	1	1	1	1	2	2	2	4
20–34	312	6.5	46	1	2	3	11	17	20	27
35–49	264	4.7	52	1	1	2	5	14	20	34
50–64	359	4.0	35	1	1	1	4	14	18	27
65+	131	2.7	13	1	1	1	2	8	8	17
B. Operated										
0–19 Years	0									
20–34	0									
35–49	5	6.4	120	1	1	2	26	>99	>99	>99
50–64	3	31.5	>999	1	1	1	92	92	92	92
65+	0									
SUBTOTALS:										
1. SINGLE DX										
A. Not Operated	1,427	2.4	12	1	1	1	2	4	8	20
B. Operated	20	1.0	0	1	1	1	1	1	1	1
2. MULTIPLE DX										
A. Not Operated	1,216	4.3	38	1	1	2	4	14	18	27
B. Operated	8	15.8	>999	1	1	2	26	>99	>99	>99
1. SINGLE DX	1,447	2.4	11	1	1	1	2	4	8	20
2. MULTIPLE DX	1,224	4.4	44	1	1	2	4	14	18	27
A. NOT OPERATED	2,643	3.3	25	1	1	1	3	8	17	27
B. OPERATED	28	5.3	313	1	1	1	1	26	92	>99
TOTAL										
0–19 Years	325	1.3	<1	1	1	1	2	2	2	4
20–34	945	4.0	27	1	1	2	3	12	17	27
35–49	567	3.6	34	1	1	1	3	9	18	28
50–64	641	3.2	38	1	1	1	3	7	17	27
65+	193	2.8	12	1	1	1	3	8	8	17
GRAND TOTAL	2,671	3.3	27	1	1	1	3	8	17	27

V71: OBSERVATION SUSPECT COND

Type of Patients	Observed Patients	Avg. Stay	Vari-ance	10th	25th	50th	75th	90th	95th	99th
1. SINGLE DX										
A. Not Operated										
0–19 Years	110	1.3	<1	1	1	1	1	2	3	3
20–34	67	1.4	<1	1	1	1	2	2	3	4
35–49	37	2.1	10	1	1	2	2	2	3	20
50–64	20	2.0	3	1	1	1	2	4	5	7
65+	6	1.0	0	1	1	1	1	1	1	1
B. Operated										
0–19 Years	0									
20–34	0									
35–49	0									
50–64	1	3.0	0	3	3	3	3	3	3	3
65+	0									
2. MULTIPLE DX										
A. Not Operated										
0–19 Years	380	1.5	1	1	1	1	1	3	4	7
20–34	629	1.3	<1	1	1	1	1	2	3	4
35–49	378	1.6	1	1	1	1	2	3	3	6
50–64	282	1.9	6	1	1	1	2	4	5	11
65+	307	2.0	3	1	1	1	3	4	5	8
B. Operated										
0–19 Years	9	6.2	32	2	2	5	8	19	19	19
20–34	6	4.7	21	1	1	3	7	13	13	13
35–49	8	2.5	4	1	1	1	3	6	6	6
50–64	10	3.2	3	2	2	3	4	5	7	7
65+	9	4.1	6	1	3	3	7	8	8	8
SUBTOTALS:										
1. SINGLE DX										
A. Not Operated	240	1.5	2	1	1	1	2	2	3	5
B. Operated	1	3.0	0	3	3	3	3	3	3	3
2. MULTIPLE DX										
A. Not Operated	1,976	1.6	2	1	1	1	2	3	4	7
B. Operated	42	4.1	13	1	2	3	6	8	10	19
1. SINGLE DX	241	1.5	2	1	1	1	2	2	3	5
2. MULTIPLE DX	2,018	1.7	2	1	1	1	2	3	4	7
A. NOT OPERATED	2,216	1.6	2	1	1	1	2	3	4	7
B. OPERATED	43	4.1	13	1	2	3	6	8	10	19
TOTAL										
0–19 Years	499	1.5	2	1	1	1	1	3	4	9
20–34	702	1.3	<1	1	1	1	2	3	3	5
35–49	423	1.7	2	1	1	1	2	3	3	6
50–64	313	2.0	5	1	1	1	2	4	5	7
65+	322	2.1	4	1	1	1	3	4	5	8
GRAND TOTAL	2,259	1.6	2	1	1	1	2	3	4	7

V71.4: OBSERVATION ACCIDENT NEC

Type of Patients	Observed Patients	Avg. Stay	Vari-ance	10th	25th	50th	75th	90th	95th	99th
1. SINGLE DX										
A. Not Operated										
0–19 Years	57	1.0	<1	1	1	1	1	1	1	2
20–34	34	1.1	<1	1	1	1	1	1	2	2
35–49	11	1.1	<1	1	1	1	1	2	2	2
50–64	10	1.8	2	1	1	1	2	4	5	5
65+	4	1.0	0	1	1	1	1	1	1	1
B. Operated										
0–19 Years	0									
20–34	0									
35–49	0									
50–64	0									
65+	0									
2. MULTIPLE DX										
A. Not Operated										
0–19 Years	231	1.3	<1	1	1	1	1	2	2	5
20–34	486	1.2	<1	1	1	1	1	2	2	4
35–49	221	1.3	<1	1	1	1	1	2	3	3
50–64	138	1.6	3	1	1	1	2	3	4	11
65+	186	2.1	4	1	1	1	3	3	5	12
B. Operated										
0–19 Years	6	8.5	32	3	5	6	8	19	19	19
20–34	3	3.7	9	1	1	3	7	7	7	7
35–49	3	4.0	7	1	1	5	6	6	6	6
50–64	0									
65+	1	3.0	0	3	3	3	3	3	3	3
SUBTOTALS:										
1. SINGLE DX										
A. Not Operated	116	1.1	<1	1	1	1	1	1	2	4
B. Operated	0									
2. MULTIPLE DX										
A. Not Operated	1,262	1.4	1	1	1	1	2	2	3	5
B. Operated	13	5.9	22	1	3	5	7	10	19	19
1. SINGLE DX	116	1.1	<1	1	1	1	1	1	2	4
2. MULTIPLE DX	1,275	1.5	2	1	1	1	2	2	3	6
A. NOT OPERATED	1,378	1.4	1	1	1	1	2	2	3	5
B. OPERATED	13	5.9	22	1	3	5	7	10	19	19
TOTAL										
0–19 Years	294	1.4	2	1	1	1	1	2	3	10
20–34	523	1.2	<1	1	1	1	1	2	2	4
35–49	235	1.3	<1	1	1	1	1	2	3	4
50–64	148	1.6	4	1	1	1	2	3	4	11
65+	191	2.1	4	1	1	1	3	3	5	12
GRAND TOTAL	1,391	1.4	2	1	1	1	1	2	3	6

Length of Stay by Diagnosis and Operation, Western Region, 2008

Western Region, October 2006–September 2007 Data, by Diagnosis

V71.89: OBS SUSPECT COND NEC | V72: SPECIAL EXAMINATIONS | V73: VIRAL & CHLAMYD SCREEN

Type of Patients	V71.89 Obs. Patients	Avg. Stay	Vari-ance	10th	25th	50th	75th	90th	95th	99th	V72 Obs. Patients	Avg. Stay	Vari-ance	10th	25th	50th	75th	90th	95th	99th	V73 Obs. Patients	Avg. Stay	Vari-ance	10th	25th	50th	75th	90th	95th	99th
1. SINGLE DX																														
A. *Not Operated*																														
0–19 Years	43	1.6	<1	1	1	1	2	3	3	4	0										0									
20–34	11	1.3	<1	1	1	1	2	2	2	2	0										0									
35–49	5	1.4	<1	1	1	1	1	3	3	3	0										0									
50–64	2	1.0	0	1	1	1	1	1	1	1	1	11.0	0	11	11	11	11	11	11	11	0									
65+	0										1	1.0	0	1	1	1	1	1	1	1	0									
B. *Operated*																														
0–19 Years	0										0										0									
20–34	0										0										0									
35–49	0										0										0									
50–64	0										0										0									
65+	0										0										0									
2. MULTIPLE DX																														
A. *Not Operated*																														
0–19 Years	96	1.8	2	1	1	1	2	4	4	9	1	1.0	0	1	1	1	1	1	1	1	0									
20–34	58	1.6	2	1	1	1	2	3	5	6	3	2.7	4	1	1	2	5	5	5	5	0									
35–49	56	2.1	2	1	1	2	3	4	4	6	8	1.5	1	1	1	1	1	4	4	4	0									
50–64	57	2.4	17	1	1	1	2	5	6	32	20	2.3	7	1	1	1	2	6	11	11	0									
65+	75	1.7	1	1	1	1	2	3	4	7	16	1.5	1	1	1	1	2	4	4	4	0									
B. *Operated*																														
0–19 Years	3	1.7	<1	1	1	2	2	2	2	2	0										0									
20–34	1	1.0	0	1	1	1	1	1	1	1	1	1.0	0	1	1	1	1	1	1	1	0									
35–49	1	1.0	0	1	1	1	1	1	1	1	1	3.0	0	3	3	3	3	3	3	3	0									
50–64	7	2.4	<1	1	1	2	3	4	4	4	5	1.0	0	1	1	1	1	1	1	1	0									
65+	3	4.0	13	1	1	3	8	8	8	8	2	14.0	157	5	5	14	23	23	23	23	0									
SUBTOTALS:																														
1. SINGLE DX																														
A. *Not Operated*	61	1.5	<1	1	1	1	2	3	3	4	2	6.0	49	1	1	1	11	11	11	11	0									
B. *Operated*	0										0										0									
2. MULTIPLE DX																														
A. *Not Operated*	342	1.9	4	1	1	1	2	4	4	6	48	1.9	4	1	1	1	2	5	6	11	0									
B. *Operated*	15	2.4	3	1	1	2	3	4	8	8	9	4.1	52	1	1	1	3	23	23	23	0									
1. SINGLE DX	**61**	**1.5**	**<1**	**1**	**1**	**1**	**2**	**3**	**3**	**4**	**2**	**6.0**	**49**	**1**	**1**	**1**	**11**	**11**	**11**	**11**	**0**									
2. MULTIPLE DX	**357**	**1.9**	**4**	**1**	**1**	**1**	**2**	**4**	**5**	**7**	**57**	**2.2**	**11**	**1**	**1**	**1**	**2**	**5**	**6**	**23**	**0**									
A. NOT OPERATED	**403**	**1.8**	**4**	**1**	**1**	**1**	**2**	**3**	**4**	**6**	**50**	**2.0**	**5**	**1**	**1**	**1**	**2**	**5**	**6**	**11**	**0**									
B. OPERATED	**15**	**2.4**	**3**	**1**	**1**	**2**	**3**	**4**	**8**	**8**	**9**	**4.1**	**52**	**1**	**1**	**1**	**3**	**23**	**23**	**23**	**0**									
TOTAL																														
0–19 Years	142	1.8	1	1	1	1	2	3	4	6	1	1.0	0	1	1	1	1	1	1	1	0									
20–34	70	1.5	1	1	1	1	2	3	4	6	4	2.3	4	1	1	1	5	5	5	5	0									
35–49	62	2.0	1	1	1	2	3	4	4	6	9	1.7	1	1	1	2	2	4	4	4	0									
50–64	66	2.4	15	1	1	2	2	4	5	32	26	2.4	9	1	1	1	2	6	11	11	0									
65+	78	1.8	2	1	1	1	2	3	4	8	19	2.8	26	1	1	1	2	5	23	23	0									
GRAND TOTAL	**418**	**1.9**	**4**	**1**	**1**	**1**	**2**	**3**	**4**	**6**	**59**	**2.4**	**12**	**1**	**1**	**1**	**2**	**5**	**11**	**23**	**0**									

Length of Stay by Diagnosis and Operation, Western Region, 2008

Western Region, October 2006–September 2007 Data, by Diagnosis

V74: BACT/SPIRO DIS SCREENING

Type of Patients	Observed Patients	Avg. Stay	Variance	Percentiles						
				10th	25th	50th	75th	90th	95th	99th
1. SINGLE DX										
A. Not Operated										
0–19 Years	0									
20–34	0									
35–49	0									
50–64	0									
65+	0									
B. Operated										
0–19 Years	0									
20–34	0									
35–49	0									
50–64	0									
65+	0									
2. MULTIPLE DX										
A. Not Operated										
0–19 Years	0									
20–34	1	6.0	0	6	6	6	6	6	6	6
35–49	3	1.7	<1	1	1	2	2	2	2	2
50–64	3	3.7	4	2	2	3	6	6	6	6
65+	1	4.0	0	4	4	4	4	4	4	4
B. Operated										
0–19 Years	0									
20–34	0									
35–49	0									
50–64	0									
65+	0									
SUBTOTALS:										
1. SINGLE DX *A. Not Operated*	0									
B. Operated	0									
2. MULTIPLE DX *A. Not Operated*	8	3.3	4	1	2	3	6	6	6	6
B. Operated	0									
1. SINGLE DX	0									
2. MULTIPLE DX	8	3.3	4	1	2	3	6	6	6	6
A. NOT OPERATED	8	3.3	4	1	2	3	6	6	6	6
B. OPERATED	0									
TOTAL										
0–19 Years	0									
20–34	1	6.0	0	6	6	6	6	6	6	6
35–49	3	1.7	<1	1	1	2	2	2	2	2
50–64	3	3.7	4	2	2	3	6	6	6	6
65+	1	4.0	0	4	4	4	4	4	4	4
GRAND TOTAL	8	3.3	4	1	2	3	6	6	6	6

V75: INFECT DIS SCREENING NEC

Type of Patients	Observed Patients	Avg. Stay	Variance	10th	25th	50th	75th	90th	95th	99th
1. SINGLE DX *A. Not Operated* 0–19 Years	0									
20–34	0									
35–49	0									
50–64	0									
65+	0									
B. Operated 0–19 Years	0									
20–34	0									
35–49	0									
50–64	0									
65+	0									
2. MULTIPLE DX *A. Not Operated* 0–19 Years	0									
20–34	0									
35–49	0									
50–64	0									
65+	0									
B. Operated 0–19 Years	0									
20–34	0									
35–49	0									
50–64	0									
65+	0									
SUBTOTALS: 1. SINGLE DX *A. Not Operated*	0									
B. Operated	0									
2. MULTIPLE DX *A. Not Operated*	0									
B. Operated	0									
1. SINGLE DX	0									
2. MULTIPLE DX	0									
A. NOT OPERATED	0									
B. OPERATED	0									
TOTAL 0–19 Years	0									
20–34	0									
35–49	0									
50–64	0									
65+	0									
GRAND TOTAL	0									

V76: CANCER SCREENING

Type of Patients	Observed Patients	Avg. Stay	Variance	Percentiles						
				10th	25th	50th	75th	90th	95th	99th
1. SINGLE DX										
A. Not Operated										
0–19 Years	0									
20–34	0									
35–49	0									
50–64	0									
65+	0									
B. Operated										
0–19 Years	0									
20–34	0									
35–49	0									
50–64	0									
65+	0									
2. MULTIPLE DX										
A. Not Operated										
0–19 Years	0									
20–34	1	1.0	0	1	1	1	1	1	1	1
35–49	1	1.0	0	1	1	1	1	1	1	1
50–64	8	1.5	2	1	1	1	1	5	5	5
65+	0									
B. Operated										
0–19 Years	0									
20–34	0									
35–49	1	1.0	0	1	1	1	1	1	1	1
50–64	2	3.0	2	2	2	2	4	4	4	4
65+	0									
SUBTOTALS:										
1. SINGLE DX *A. Not Operated*	0									
B. Operated	0									
2. MULTIPLE DX *A. Not Operated*	10	1.4	2	1	1	1	1	5	5	5
B. Operated	3	2.3	2	1	1	2	4	4	4	4
1. SINGLE DX	0									
2. MULTIPLE DX	13	1.6	2	1	1	1	1	4	5	5
A. NOT OPERATED	10	1.4	2	1	1	1	1	5	5	5
B. OPERATED	3	2.3	2	1	1	2	4	4	4	4
TOTAL										
0–19 Years	0									
20–34	1	1.0	0	1	1	1	1	1	1	1
35–49	2	1.0	0	1	1	1	1	1	1	1
50–64	10	1.8	2	1	1	1	2	5	5	5
65+	0									
GRAND TOTAL	13	1.6	2	1	1	1	1	4	5	5

Length of Stay by Diagnosis and Operation, Western Region, 2008

Western Region, October 2006–September 2007 Data, by Diagnosis

V77: ENM/IMMUNITY SCREENING

Type of Patients	Observed Patients	Avg. Stay	Vari-ance	Percentiles 10th	25th	50th	75th	90th	95th	99th
1. SINGLE DX										
A. *Not Operated*										
0–19 Years	0									
20–34	0									
35–49	0									
50–64	0									
65+	0									
B. *Operated*										
0–19 Years	0									
20–34	0									
35–49	0									
50–64	0									
65+	0									
2. MULTIPLE DX										
A. *Not Operated*										
0–19 Years	0									
20–34	1	1.0	0	1	1	1	1	1	1	1
35–49	0									
50–64	0									
65+	0									
B. *Operated*										
0–19 Years	0									
20–34	0									
35–49	0									
50–64	0									
65+	0									
SUBTOTALS:										
1. SINGLE DX										
A. *Not Operated*	0									
B. *Operated*	0									
2. MULTIPLE DX										
A. *Not Operated*	1	1.0	0	1	1	1	1	1	1	1
B. *Operated*	0									
1. SINGLE DX	0									
2. MULTIPLE DX	1	1.0	0	1	1	1	1	1	1	1
A. NOT OPERATED	1	1.0	0	1	1	1	1	1	1	1
B. OPERATED	0									
TOTAL										
0–19 Years	0									
20–34	1	1.0	0	1	1	1	1	1	1	1
35–49	0									
50–64	0									
65+	0									
GRAND TOTAL	1	1.0	0	1	1	1	1	1	1	1

V78: BLOOD DISORDER SCREENING

Type of Patients	Observed Patients	Avg. Stay	Vari-ance	Percentiles 10th	25th	50th	75th	90th	95th	99th
1. SINGLE DX										
A. *Not Operated*										
0–19 Years	0									
20–34	0									
35–49	0									
50–64	0									
65+	0									
B. *Operated*										
0–19 Years	0									
20–34	0									
35–49	0									
50–64	0									
65+	0									
2. MULTIPLE DX										
A. *Not Operated*										
0–19 Years	0									
20–34	0									
35–49	0									
50–64	0									
65+	0									
B. *Operated*										
0–19 Years	0									
20–34	0									
35–49	0									
50–64	0									
65+	0									
SUBTOTALS:										
1. SINGLE DX										
A. *Not Operated*	0									
B. *Operated*	0									
2. MULTIPLE DX										
A. *Not Operated*	0									
B. *Operated*	0									
1. SINGLE DX	0									
2. MULTIPLE DX	0									
A. NOT OPERATED	0									
B. OPERATED	0									
TOTAL										
0–19 Years	0									
20–34	0									
35–49	0									
50–64	0									
65+	0									
GRAND TOTAL	0									

V79: MENTAL DISORD SCREENING

Type of Patients	Observed Patients	Avg. Stay	Vari-ance	Percentiles 10th	25th	50th	75th	90th	95th	99th
1. SINGLE DX										
A. *Not Operated*										
0–19 Years	0									
20–34	0									
35–49	0									
50–64	0									
65+	0									
B. *Operated*										
0–19 Years	0									
20–34	0									
35–49	0									
50–64	0									
65+	0									
2. MULTIPLE DX										
A. *Not Operated*										
0–19 Years	0									
20–34	0									
35–49	0									
50–64	0									
65+	0									
B. *Operated*										
0–19 Years	0									
20–34	0									
35–49	0									
50–64	0									
65+	0									
SUBTOTALS:										
1. SINGLE DX										
A. *Not Operated*	0									
B. *Operated*	0									
2. MULTIPLE DX										
A. *Not Operated*	0									
B. *Operated*	0									
1. SINGLE DX	0									
2. MULTIPLE DX	0									
A. NOT OPERATED	0									
B. OPERATED	0									
TOTAL										
0–19 Years	0									
20–34	0									
35–49	0									
50–64	0									
65+	0									
GRAND TOTAL	0									

Length of Stay by Diagnosis and Operation, Western Region, 2008

Western Region, October 2006–September 2007 Data, by Diagnosis

V80: NEURO/EYE/EAR DIS SCREEN

Type of Patients	Observed Patients	Avg. Stay	Vari-ance	Percentiles 10th	25th	50th	75th	90th	95th	99th
1. SINGLE DX										
A. *Not Operated*										
0–19 Years	0	0								
20–34	0	0								
35–49	0	0								
50–64	0	0								
65+	0	0								
B. *Operated*										
0–19 Years	0	0								
20–34	0	0								
35–49	0	0								
50–64	0	0								
65+	0	0								
2. MULTIPLE DX										
A. *Not Operated*										
0–19 Years	0	0								
20–34	0	0								
35–49	0	0								
50–64	0	0								
65+	0	0								
B. *Operated*										
0–19 Years	0	0								
20–34	0	0								
35–49	0	0								
50–64	0	0								
65+	0	0								
SUBTOTALS:										
1. SINGLE DX										
A. *Not Operated*	0	0								
B. *Operated*	0	0								
2. MULTIPLE DX										
A. *Not Operated*	0	0								
B. *Operated*	0	0								
1. SINGLE DX	0	0								
2. MULTIPLE DX	0	0								
A. NOT OPERATED	0	0								
B. OPERATED	0	0								
TOTAL										
0–19 Years	0	0								
20–34	0	0								
35–49	0	0								
50–64	0	0								
65+	0	0								
GRAND TOTAL	0	0								

V81: CV/RESP/GU DIS SCREENING

Type of Patients	Observed Patients	Avg. Stay	Vari-ance	Percentiles 10th	25th	50th	75th	90th	95th	99th
1. SINGLE DX										
A. *Not Operated*										
0–19 Years	0									
20–34	0									
35–49	0									
50–64	0									
B. *Operated*										
0–19 Years	0									
2. MULTIPLE DX										
A. *Not Operated*										
0–19 Years	2	1.5	<1	1	1	2	2	2	2	2
20–34	0									
35–49	0									
50–64	1	2.0	0	2	2	2	2	2	2	2
65+	1	1.0	0	1	1	1	1	1	1	1
B. *Operated*										
0–19 Years	0									
20–34	0									
35–49	0									
50–64	0									
65+	0									
SUBTOTALS:										
1. SINGLE DX										
A. *Not Operated*	0									
B. *Operated*	0									
2. MULTIPLE DX										
A. *Not Operated*	4	1.5	<1	1	1	2	2	2	2	2
B. *Operated*	0									
1. SINGLE DX	0									
2. MULTIPLE DX	4	1.5	<1	1	1	2	2	2	2	2
A. NOT OPERATED	4	1.5	<1	1	1	2	2	2	2	2
B. OPERATED	0									
TOTAL										
0–19 Years	2	1.5	<1	1	1	2	2	2	2	2
20–34	0									
35–49	0									
50–64	1	2.0	0	2	2	2	2	2	2	2
65+	1	1.0	0	1	1	1	1	1	1	1
GRAND TOTAL	4	1.5	<1	1	1	2	2	2	2	2

V82: SCREENING FOR OTHER COND

Type of Patients	Observed Patients	Avg. Stay	Vari-ance	Percentiles 10th	25th	50th	75th	90th	95th	99th
1. SINGLE DX										
A. *Not Operated*										
0–19 Years	0									
20–34	0									
35–49	0									
50–64	0									
B. *Operated*										
0–19 Years	0									
20–34	0									
35–49	0									
2. MULTIPLE DX										
A. *Not Operated*										
0–19 Years	0									
20–34	1	1.0	0	1	1	1	1	1	1	1
35–49	1	1.0	0	1	1	1	1	1	1	1
50–64	0									
B. *Operated*										
0–19 Years	0									
20–34	0									
35–49	0									
50–64	0									
65+	0									
SUBTOTALS:										
1. SINGLE DX										
A. *Not Operated*	0									
B. *Operated*	0									
2. MULTIPLE DX										
A. *Not Operated*	2	1.0	0	1	1	1	1	1	1	1
B. *Operated*	0									
1. SINGLE DX	0									
2. MULTIPLE DX	2	1.0	0	1	1	1	1	1	1	1
A. NOT OPERATED	2	1.0	0	1	1	1	1	1	1	1
B. OPERATED	0									
TOTAL										
0–19 Years	0									
20–34	1	1.0	0	1	1	1	1	1	1	1
35–49	1	1.0	0	1	1	1	1	1	1	1
50–64	0									
65+	0									
GRAND TOTAL	2	1.0	0	1	1	1	1	1	1	1

883

Length of Stay by Diagnosis and Operation, Western Region, 2008

Western Region, October 2006–September 2007 Data, by Diagnosis

V83: GENETIC CARRIER STATUS

Type of Patients	Observed Patients	Avg. Stay	Variance	10th	25th	50th	75th	90th	95th	99th
1. SINGLE DX										
A. *Not Operated*										
0–19 Years	0									
20–34	0									
35–49	0									
50–64	0									
65+	0									
B. *Operated*										
0–19 Years	0									
20–34	0									
35–49	0									
50–64	0									
65+	0									
2. MULTIPLE DX										
A. *Not Operated*										
0–19 Years	0									
20–34	0									
35–49	0									
50–64	0									
65+	0									
B. *Operated*										
0–19 Years	0									
20–34	0									
35–49	0									
50–64	0									
65+	0									
SUBTOTALS:										
1. SINGLE DX A. Not Operated	0									
B. Operated	0									
2. MULTIPLE DX A. Not Operated	0									
B. Operated	0									
1. SINGLE DX	0									
2. MULTIPLE DX	0									
A. NOT OPERATED	0									
B. OPERATED	0									
TOTAL										
0–19 Years	0									
20–34	0									
35–49	0									
50–64	0									
65+	0									
GRAND TOTAL	0									

V84: GENETIC SUSCEPTIBILITY

Type of Patients	Observed Patients	Avg. Stay	Variance	10th	25th	50th	75th	90th	95th	99th
1. SINGLE DX										
A. *Not Operated*										
0–19 Years	0									
20–34	0									
35–49	0									
50–64	0									
65+	0									
B. *Operated*										
0–19 Years	0									
20–34	0									
35–49	0									
50–64	0									
65+	0									
2. MULTIPLE DX										
A. *Not Operated*										
0–19 Years	0									
20–34	0									
35–49	0									
50–64	0									
65+	0									
B. *Operated*										
0–19 Years	0									
20–34	1	1.0	0	1	1	1	1	1	1	1
35–49	2	2.5	5	1	1	3	4	4	4	4
50–64	3	1.3	<1	1	1	1	2	2	2	2
65+	1	4.0	0	4	4	4	4	4	4	4
SUBTOTALS:										
1. SINGLE DX A. Not Operated	0									
B. Operated	0									
2. MULTIPLE DX A. Not Operated	0									
B. Operated	7	2.0	2	1	1	1	1	4	4	4
1. SINGLE DX	0									
2. MULTIPLE DX	7	2.0	2	1	1	1	1	4	4	4
A. NOT OPERATED	0									
B. OPERATED	7	2.0	2	1	1	1	1	4	4	4
TOTAL										
0–19 Years	0									
20–34	1	1.0	0	1	1	1	1	1	1	1
35–49	2	2.5	5	1	1	3	4	4	4	4
50–64	3	1.3	<1	1	1	1	2	2	2	2
65+	1	4.0	0	4	4	4	4	4	4	4
GRAND TOTAL	7	2.0	2	1	1	1	1	4	4	4

V85: BODY MASS INDEX

Type of Patients	Observed Patients	Avg. Stay	Variance	10th	25th	50th	75th	90th	95th	99th
1. SINGLE DX										
A. *Not Operated*										
0–19 Years	0									
20–34	0									
35–49	0									
50–64	0									
65+	0									
B. *Operated*										
0–19 Years	0									
20–34	0									
35–49	0									
50–64	0									
65+	0									
2. MULTIPLE DX										
A. *Not Operated*										
0–19 Years	0									
20–34	0									
35–49	0									
50–64	0									
65+	0									
B. *Operated*										
0–19 Years	0									
20–34	0									
35–49	0									
50–64	1	2.0	0	2	2	2	2	2	2	2
65+	0									
SUBTOTALS:										
1. SINGLE DX A. Not Operated	0									
B. Operated	0									
2. MULTIPLE DX A. Not Operated	0									
B. Operated	1	2.0	0	2	2	2	2	2	2	2
1. SINGLE DX	0									
2. MULTIPLE DX	1	2.0	0	2	2	2	2	2	2	2
A. NOT OPERATED	0									
B. OPERATED	1	2.0	0	2	2	2	2	2	2	2
TOTAL										
0–19 Years	0									
20–34	0									
35–49	0									
50–64	1	2.0	0	2	2	2	2	2	2	2
65+	0									
GRAND TOTAL	1	2.0	0	2	2	2	2	2	2	2

Length of Stay by Diagnosis and Operation, Western Region, 2008

V86: ESTROGEN RECEPTOR STATUS

Type of Patients	Observed Patients	Avg. Stay	Vari-ance	Percentiles						
				10th	25th	50th	75th	90th	95th	99th
1. SINGLE DX										
A. *Not Operated*										
0–19 Years	0									
20–34	0									
35–49	0									
50–64	0									
65+	0									
B. *Operated*										
0–19 Years	0									
20–34	0									
35–49	0									
50–64	0									
65+	0									
2. MULTIPLE DX										
A. *Not Operated*										
0–19 Years	0									
20–34	0									
35–49	0									
50–64	0									
65+	0									
B. *Operated*										
0–19 Years	0									
20–34	0									
35–49	0									
50–64	0									
65+	0									
SUBTOTALS:										
1. SINGLE DX										
A. *Not Operated*	0									
B. *Operated*	0									
2. MULTIPLE DX										
A. *Not Operated*	0									
B. *Operated*	0									
1. SINGLE DX	0									
2. MULTIPLE DX	0									
A. NOT OPERATED	0									
B. OPERATED	0									
TOTAL										
0–19 Years	0									
20–34	0									
35–49	0									
50–64	0									
65+	0									
GRAND TOTAL	0									

APPENDIX A
Hospital Characteristics
Short-Term, General, Nonfederal Hospitals[1]

HOSPITAL CATEGORY	U.S. TOTAL
Bed Size	
6–24 Beds	1,013
25–49	1,575
50–99	1,377
100–199	1,386
200–299	702
300–399	405
400–499	175
500+	254
Unknown	56
Total	**6,943**
Region and Census Division	
Northeast	**967**
New England	305
Middle Atlantic	662
North Central	**1,898**
East North Central	1,040
West North Central	858
South	**2,775**
South Atlantic	1,051
East South Central	566
West South Central	1,158
West	**1,303**
Mountain	521
Pacific	782
Location	
Urban	4,595
Rural	2,349
Teaching Intensity	
High/Medium	423
Low	6,521

---

[1] For a definition of short-term, general, and nonfederal hospitals, see "Description of the Database."

APPENDIX B
States Included in Each Region

Northeast

Connecticut
Maine
Massachusetts
New Hampshire
New Jersey
New York
Pennsylvania
Rhode Island
Vermont

North Central

Illinois
Indiana
Iowa
Kansas
Michigan
Minnesota
Missouri
Nebraska
North Dakota
Ohio
South Dakota
Wisconsin

South

Alabama
Arkansas
Delaware
District of Columbia
Florida
Georgia
Kentucky
Louisiana
Maryland
Mississippi
North Carolina
Oklahoma
South Carolina
Tennessee
Texas
Virginia
West Virginia

West

Alaska
Arizona
California
Colorado
Hawaii
Idaho
Montana
Nevada
New Mexico
Oregon
Utah
Washington
Wyoming

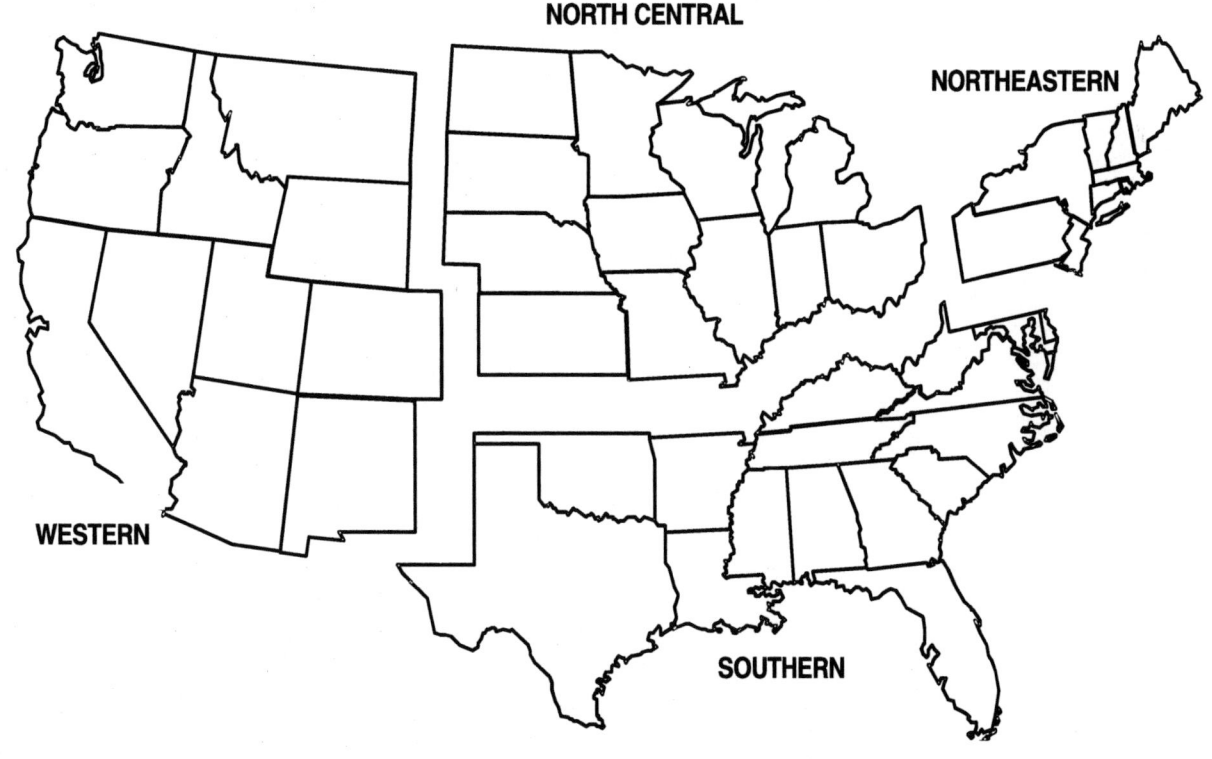

Length of Stay by Diagnosis and Operation, Western Region, 2008   889

GLOSSARY

Average Length of Stay Calculated from the admission and discharge dates by counting the day of admission as the first day; the day of discharge is not included. The average is figured by adding the lengths of stay for each patient and then dividing by the total number of patients. Patients discharged on the day of admission are counted as staying one day in the calculation of average length of stay. Patients with stays over 99 days (>99) are excluded from this calculation.

Distribution Percentiles A length of stay percentile for a stratified group of patients is determined by arranging the individual patient stays from low to high. Counting up from the lowest stay to the point where one-half of the patients have been counted yields the value of the 50th percentile. Counting one-tenth of the total patients gives the 10th percentile, and so on. The 10th, 25th, 50th, 75th, 90th, 95th, and 99th percentiles of stay are displayed in days. If, for example, the 10th percentile for a group of patients is four, then 10 percent of the patients stayed four days or less. The 50th percentile is the median. Any percentile with a value of 100 days or more is listed as >99. Patients who were hospitalized more than 99 days (>99) are not included in the total patients, average stay, and variance categories. The percentiles, however, do include these patients.

Multiple Diagnoses Patients Patients are classified in the multiple diagnoses category if they had at least one valid secondary diagnosis in addition to the principal one. The following codes are not considered valid secondary diagnoses for purposes of this classification

1. Manifestation codes (conditions that evolved from underlying diseases [etiology] and are in italics in ICD-9-CM, Volume 1)

2. Codes V27.0-V27.9 (outcome of delivery)

3. E Codes (external causes of injury and poisoning)

Observed Patients The number of patients in the stratified group as reported in our projected inpatient database. Patients with stays longer than 99 days (>99) are not included. This data element does not use the projection factor.

Operated Patients In the diagnosis tables, operated patients are those who had at least one procedure that is classified by CMS as an operating room procedure. CMS physician panels classify every ICD-9-CM procedure code according to whether the procedure would in most hospitals be performed in the operating room. This classification system differs slightly from that used in Length of Stay publications published previous to 1995, in which patients were categorized as operated if any of their procedures were labeled as Uniform Hospital Discharge Data Set (UHDDS) Class 1. Appendix C contains a list of procedure codes included in this book and their CMS-defined operative status.

Variance A measure of the spread of the data around the average, the variance shows how much individual patient lengths of stay from the average. The smallest variance is zero, indicating that all lengths of stay are equal. In tables in which there is a large variance and the patient group size is relatively small, the average stay may appear high. This sometimes occurs when one or two patients with long hospitalizations fall into the group.

ALPHABETIC INDEX

This index provides an alphabetical listing by descriptive title for all chapter ICD-9-CM diagnoses and procedures codes included in the book. For ease of use, titles are grouped into major classification chapters (i.e., *Diseases of the Circulatory System*). These classification chapters are listed for your reference below.

ICD-9-CM Classification Chapters

Diagnosis Chapters

Infectious and Parasitic Diseases	Codes 001–139
Neoplasms	Codes 140–239
Endocrine, Nutritional and Metabolic Diseases, and Immunity Disorders	Codes 240–279
Diseases of the Blood and Blood-Forming Organs	Codes 280–289
Mental Disorders	Codes 290–319
Diseases of the Nervous System and Sense Organs	Codes 320–389
Diseases of the Circulatory System	Codes 390–459
Diseases of the Respiratory System	Codes 460–519
Diseases of the Digestive System	Codes 520–579
Diseases of the Genitourinary System	Codes 580–629
Complications of Pregnancy, Childbirth, and the Puerperium	Codes 630–677
Diseases of the Skin and Subcutaneous Tissue	Codes 680–709
Diseases of the Musculoskeletal System and Connective Tissue	Codes 710–739
Congenital Anomalies	Codes 740–759
Certain Conditions Originating in the Perinatal Period	Codes 760–779
Symptoms, Signs, and Ill-Defined Conditions	Codes 780–799
Injury and Poisoning	Codes 800–999
Supplementary Classification of Factors Influencing Health Status and Contact with Health Services	Codes V01–V83

Diagnosis Codes

Diagnosis Codes

ENDOCRINE, NUTRITIONAL, AND METABOLIC DISEASES, AND IMMUNITY DISORDERS (240-279)

DISEASES OF THE BLOOD AND BLOOD-FORMING ORGANS (280-289)

MENTAL DISORDERS (290-319)

Diagnosis Codes

Code	Description	Page	Code	Description	Page
303	Alcohol dependence synd	208	346	Migraine	242
300	Anx/dissoc/somat disord	205	355	Mononeuritis leg & NOS	251
312	Conduct disturbance NEC	219	354	Mononeuritis upper limb	251
297	Delusional disorders	203	340	Multiple sclerosis	236
290	Dementias	183	359	Muscular dystrophies	255
311	Depressive disorder NEC	219	358	Myoneural disorders	254
304	Drug dependence	209	381	NOM & ET disorders	264
292	Drug-induced mental dis	187	349	Nerv syst disord NEC&NOS	248
313	Emotional dis child/ADOL	221	353	Nerve root/plexus disord	250
296	Episodic mood disorder	195	327	Organic sleep disorders	227
314	Hyperkinetic syndrome	221	384	Oth disord tympanic memb	266
319	Mental retardation NOS	223	321	Oth organism meningitis	224
317	Mild mental retardation	223	344	Oth paralytic syndromes	238
305	Nondependent drug abuse	212	341	Other CNS demyelination	236
310	Nonpsychotic OBS	218	348	Other brain conditions	245
298	Oth nonorganic psychoses	204	387	Otosclerosis	269
318	Other mental retardation	223	338	Pain NEC	234
294	Persist ment dis D/T CCE	190	332	Parkinson's disease	230
301	Personality disorders	207	325	Phlebitis IC ven sinus	227
299	Pervasive devel disorder	204	361	Retinal detachment	256
316	Psychic factor w DCE	222	362	Retinal disorders NEC	256
306	Psychophysiologic pbx	214	336	Spinal cord disease NEC	233
295	Schizophrenic disorders	190	334	Spinocerebellar disease	232
302	Sex/gender ID disorders	207	378	Strabismus	263
307	Special symptom NEC	215	382	Suppurative/NOS OMed	264
315	Specific develop delays	222	350	Trigem nerve disorder	249
293	Trans mental dis D/T CCE	189	386	Vertiginous syndromes	266
			368	Visual disturbances	258

DISEASES OF THE NERVOUS SYSTEM AND SENSE ORGANS (320-389)

Code	Description	Page
335	Ant horn cell disease	232
337	Autonomic nerve disorder	233
320	Bacterial meningitis	224
369	Blindness & low vision	259
324	CNS abscess	226
347	Cataplexy & narcolepsy	244
366	Cataract	257
330	Cereb degen in child	228
331	Cerebral degeneration	228
363	Choroidal disorders	256
371	Corneal opacity & NEC	259
352	Disorder cran nerve NEC	250
380	Disorder of external ear	263
372	Disorders of conjunctiva	260
388	Disorders of ear NEC	269
374	Disorders of eyelids NEC	261
377	Disorders of optic nerve	262
367	Disorders of refraction	258
360	Disorders of the globe	255
376	Disorders of the orbit	261
323	Encephalomyelitis	225
345	Epil & recur seizures	238
333	Extrapyramid disord NEC	231
379	Eye disorders NEC	263
351	Facial nerve disorders	249
365	Glaucoma	257
389	Hearing loss	269
342	Hemiplegia	237
356	Hered periph neuropat	252
343	Infantile cerebral palsy	237
357	Inflam/toxic neuropathy	253
373	Inflammation of eyelids	260
364	Iris/ciliary body disord	257
370	Keratitis	259
375	Lacrimal system disorder	261
326	Late eff IC abscess	227
383	Mastoiditis et al	265
322	Meningitis cause NOS	225
385	Mid ear/mastoid pbx NEC	266

DISEASES OF THE CIRCULATORY SYSTEM (390-459)

Code	Description	Page
410	AMI	281
421	Ac/subac endocarditis	293
436	Acute ill-defined CVD	314
422	Acute myocarditis	294
420	Acute pericarditis	292
415	Acute pulmonary hrt dis	289
413	Angina pectoris	286
441	Aortic aneurysm	321
444	Arterial embolism	326
445	Atheroembolism	327
440	Atherosclerosis	318
427	Cardiac dysrhythmias	299
425	Cardiomyopathy	296
434	Cerebral artery occlus	311
416	Chr pulmonary heart dis	290
393	Chr rheumatic pericard	271
426	Conduction disorders	297
448	Disease of capillaries	330
395	Diseases of aortic valve	271
394	Diseases of mitral valve	271
397	Endocardial disease NEC	273
401	Essential hypertension	274
404	HTN heart & CKD	278
428	Heart failure	303
455	Hemorrhoids	335
403	Hypertensive CKD	277
402	Hypertensive heart dis	275
458	Hypotension	338
432	ICH NEC & NOS	308
429	Ill-defined heart dis	307
431	Intracerebral hemorrhage	308
438	Late eff cerebrovasc dis	316
454	Leg varicose veins	334
396	Mitral/aortic valve dis	272
457	NonINF lymphatic disord	337
412	Old myocardial infarct	286
411	Oth ac ischemic hrt dis	285
437	Oth cerebrovasc disease	314
414	Oth chr ischemic hrt dis	287

Diagnosis Codes

Code	Description	Page	Code	Description	Page
459	Oth circulatory disorder	340	502	Silica pneumocon NEC	368
424	Oth endocardial disease	295	507	Solid/liq pneumonitis	370
423	Oth pericardial disease	294	480	Viral pneumonia	353
443	Oth periph vasc disease	325			
417	Oth pulmon circ disease	292	**DISEASES OF THE DIGESTIVE SYSTEM (520-579)**		
398	Oth rheumatic heart dis	273	540	Acute appendicitis	407
453	Oth venous thrombosis	332	570	Acute liver necrosis	438
442	Other aneurysm	324	566	Anal & rectal abscess	430
447	Other arterial disease	329	565	Anal fissure & fistula	429
446	Polyarterit nodosa et al	328	541	Appendicitis NOS	408
452	Portal vein thrombosis	332	574	Cholelithiasis	444
433	Precerebral occlusion	309	571	Chr liver dis/cirrhosis	439
391	RhF w heart involvement	270	524	Dentofacial anomalies	384
390	RhF w/o heart involv	270	530	Diseases of esophagus	388
392	Rheumatic chorea	270	577	Diseases of pancreas	454
405	Secondary hypertension	280	562	Diverticula of intestine	426
430	Subarachnoid hemorrhage	308	532	Duodenal ulcer	395
451	Thrombophlebitis	331	564	Funct digestive dis NEC	428
435	Transient cereb ischemia	313	538	GI mucositis	407
456	Varicose veins NEC	336	531	Gastric ulcer	393
			535	Gastritis & duodenitis	398
DISEASE OF THE RESPIRATORY SYSTEM (460-519)			578	Gastrointestinal hemor	456
465	Ac URI mult sites/NOS	344	534	Gastrojejunal ulcer	397
466	Ac bronchitis/bronchiol	345	523	Gingival/periodontal dis	384
464	Ac laryngitis/tracheitis	343	521	Hard tissue dis of teeth	383
460	Acute nasopharyngitis	341	550	Inguinal hernia	410
462	Acute pharyngitis	343	579	Intestinal malabsorption	457
461	Acute sinusitis	341	560	Intestinal obstruction	423
463	Acute tonsillitis	343	526	Jaw diseases	385
477	Allergic rhinitis	351	528	Oral soft tissue disease	386
501	Asbestosis	368	551	Oth abd hernia w gangr	412
493	Asthma	363	552	Oth abd hernia w obstr	412
494	Bronchiectasis	366	543	Oth diseases of appendix	409
490	Bronchitis NOS	360	576	Oth disord biliary tract	452
485	Bronchopneumonia org NOS	358	575	Oth gallbladder disorder	450
474	Chr T & A disease	349	537	Oth gastroduodenal dis	405
476	Chr laryng/laryngotrach	350	569	Oth intestinal disorders	434
472	Chr pharyn/nasopharyng	347	573	Oth liver disorders	443
496	Chronic airway obstr NEC	367	558	Oth nonINF gastroent	422
491	Chronic bronchitis	360	568	Oth peritoneal disorders	432
473	Chronic sinusitis	348	553	Other abdominal hernia	415
500	Coal workers' pneumocon	367	542	Other appendicitis	409
470	Deviated nasal septum	347	525	Other dental disorder	385
504	Dust pneumonopathy NEC	369	533	Peptic ulcer site NOS	396
492	Emphysema	362	567	Periton/retroperit INF	431
510	Empyema	371	522	Pulp & periapical dis	383
495	Extr allergic alveolitis	367	555	Regional enteritis	417
506	Fume/vapor resp diseases	369	527	Salivary gland diseases	386
487	Influenza	359	572	Sequela of chr liver dis	441
503	Inorg dust pneumocon NEC	368	536	Stomach function disord	403
517	Lung involv in DCE	376	529	Tongue disorders	387
513	Lung/mediastinum abscess	374	520	Tooth develop/erupt pbx	382
471	Nasal polyps	347	556	Ulcerative colitis	419
516	Oth alveo pneumonopathy	375	557	Vasc insuff intestine	421
519	Oth resp system diseases	380			
478	Oth up respiratory dis	351	**DISEASES OF THE GENITOURINARY SYSTEM (580-629)**		
482	Other bact pneumonia	354	580	Acute nephritis	458
518	Other lung diseases	377	584	Acute renal failure	459
475	Peritonsillar abscess	350	610	Benign mammary dysplasia	482
511	Pleurisy	371	585	Chronic kidney disease	461
484	Pneum in oth INF dis	358	582	Chronic nephritis	459
481	Pneumococcal pneumonia	354	595	Cystitis	469
505	Pneumoconiosis NOS	369	593	Disord kidney/ureter NEC	466
483	Pneumonia organism NEC	357	626	Disorder of menstruation	502
486	Pneumonia organism NOS	359	607	Disorders of penis	480
512	Pneumothorax	373	621	Disorders of uterus NEC	495
515	Postinflam pulm fibrosis	375	617	Endometriosis	488
514	Pulmonary congestion	375	619	Female genital fistula	493
508	Resp cond D/T ext agent	370	625	Female genital symptoms	500

Diagnosis Codes

Code	Description	Page
628	Female infertility	504
614	Female pelvic inflam dis	483
618	Genital prolapse	489
603	Hydrocele	478
591	Hydronephrosis	465
600	Hyperplasia of prostate	475
588	Impaired renal function	462
590	Kidney infection	463
594	Lower urinary calculus	469
606	Male infertility	480
627	Menopausal disorders	503
583	Nephritis NOS	459
581	Nephrotic syndrome	458
620	Noninfl disord ov/FALL	493
622	Noninfl disorder cervix	498
624	Noninfl disorder vulva	500
623	Noninflam disord vagina	499
604	Orchitis & epididymitis	478
608	Oth disord male genital	481
616	Oth female genit inflam	486
629	Oth female genital dis	504
602	Oth prostatic disorders	477
599	Oth urinary tract disord	474
596	Other bladder disorders	471
611	Other breast disorders	482
601	Prostatic inflammation	476
605	Redun prepuce & phimosis	479
586	Renal failure NOS	462
587	Renal sclerosis NOS	462
592	Renal/ureteral calculus	465
589	Small kidney	463
598	Urethral stricture	473
597	Urethritis/urethral synd	473
615	Uterine inflammatory dis	486

COMPLICATIONS OF PREGNANCY, CHILDBIRTH, AND THE PUERPERIUM (630-677)

Code	Description	Page
641	AP hemor & plac prev	511
654	Abn pelvic organ in preg	541
631	Abnormal POC NEC	505
661	Abnormal forces of labor	557
668	Comp anes in delivery	569
639	Comp following abortion	510
653	Disproportion	540
644	Early/threatened labor	520
633	Ectopic pregnancy	506
643	Excess vomiting in preg	519
638	Failed attempted AB	510
655	Fetal abn affect mother	545
640	Hemorrhage in early preg	511
630	Hydatidiform mole	505
642	Hypertension comp preg	514
636	Illegal induced abortion	509
675	Infect breast in preg	574
647	Infective dis in preg	526
677	Late effect OB comp	575
645	Late pregnancy	522
635	Legally induced abortion	508
662	Long labor	559
670	Maj puerperal infection	571
652	Malposition of fetus	537
632	Missed abortion	505
651	Multiple gestation	536
650	Normal delivery	536
673	OB pulmonary embolism	572
660	Obstructed labor	555
658	Oth amniotic cavity prob	549
676	Oth breast/lact dis preg	574
669	Oth comp labor/delivery	569

Code	Description	Page
649	Oth cond/status in preg	534
648	Oth current cond in preg	528
656	Oth fetal pbx aff mother	546
659	Oth indication care-del	551
646	Other comp of pregnancy	523
665	Other obstetrical trauma	565
664	Perineal trauma w del	563
657	Polyhydramnios	548
666	Postpartum hemorrhage	567
674	Puerperal comp NEC & NOS	573
672	Puerperal pyrexia NOS	572
667	Ret plac/memb w/o hemor	568
634	Spontaneous abortion	507
663	Umbilical cord comp	560
637	Unspecified abortion	509
671	Venous comp in preg & PP	572

DISEASES OF THE SKIN AND SUBCUTANEOUS TISSUE (680-709)

Code	Description	Page
683	Acute lymphadenitis	580
691	Atopic dermatitis	582
694	Bullous dermatoses	583
680	Carbuncle & furuncle	575
682	Cellulitis & abscess NEC	576
707	Chronic ulcer of skin	588
692	Contact dermatitis	582
700	Corns & callosities	585
693	Derm D/T internal agent	583
703	Diseases of nail	587
705	Disorders of sweat gland	587
690	Erythematosquamous derm	581
695	Erythematous conditions	584
681	Finger & toe cellulitis	575
704	Hair & follicle disease	587
684	Impetigo	580
697	Lichen	585
686	Oth local skin infection	581
701	Oth skin hypertr/atrophy	586
702	Other dermatoses	586
709	Other skin disorders	593
685	Pilonidal cyst	580
698	Pruritus & like cond	585
696	Psoriasis/like disorders	584
706	Sebaceous gland disease	588
708	Urticaria	593

DISEASES OF THE MUSCULOSKELETAL SYSTEM AND CONNECTIVE TISSUE (710-739)

Code	Description	Page
735	Acq deformities of toe	636
716	Arthropathies NEC & NOS	603
713	Arthropathy in CCE	597
711	Arthropathy w infection	595
712	Crystal arthropathies	597
737	Curvature of spine	637
710	Dif connective tiss dis	594
729	Disord soft tiss NEC	625
734	Flat foot	636
720	Inflam spondylopathies	610
717	Internal derang knee	606
722	Intervertebral disc dis	612
719	Joint disorder NEC & NOS	607
728	Muscle/LIG/fascia disord	623
739	Nonallopathic lesions	639
731	Osteitis deformans	630
715	Osteoarthrosis et al	598
732	Osteochondropathies	631
730	Osteomyelitis	627
736	Oth acq limb deformities	636
733	Oth bone/cart disorder	631

Diagnosis Codes

Code	Description	Page	Code	Description	Page
727	Oth dis synov/tend/bursa	621	789	Oth abdomen/pelvis Sx	681
738	Other acquired deformity	638	799	Oth ill-def morb/mort	689
723	Other cerv spine disord	615	796	Other abnormal findings	688
718	Other joint derangement	606	786	Resp syst/oth chest Sx	673
724	Other/unspec back disord	617	797	Senility w/o psychosis	688
726	Periph enthesopathies	619	782	Skin & integument NEC Sx	667
725	Polymyalgia rheumatica	619	798	Sudden death cause unkn	689
714	RA & inflam polyarthrop	598	784	Sx involving head/neck	670
721	Spondylosis et al	610	788	Urinary system symptoms	679

CONGENITAL ANOMALIES (740-759)

INJURY AND POISONING (800-999)

Code	Description	Page	Code	Description	Page
740	Anencephalus et al	640	902	Abd/pelvic vessel injury	775
745	Card septal close anomal	642	980	Alcohol toxicity	816
758	Chromosomal anomalies	649	845	Ankle & foot sprain	741
749	Cleft palate & cleft lip	644	824	Ankle fracture	727
754	Cong MS deformities	647	903	Arm blood vessel injury	775
744	Cong anomal ear/face/nk	641	847	Back sprain NEC & NOS	742
759	Cong anomalies NEC & NOS	650	904	Blood vessel injury NEC	776
757	Cong skin anomalies	649	948	Burn by % body surface	794
743	Congenital eye anomaly	641	943	Burn of arm	792
752	Genital organ anomalies	646	940	Burn of eye & adnexa	791
751	Oth anom digestive syst	645	944	Burn of hand & wrist	793
747	Oth cong circ syst anom	643	941	Burn of head/face/neck	791
755	Oth cong limb anomaly	647	947	Burn of internal organs	794
742	Oth nerv syst anomalies	640	945	Burn of leg	793
756	Other MS anomalies	648	946	Burn of multiple site	793
746	Other cong anomaly heart	643	942	Burn of trunk	792
750	Other upper GI anomaly	645	949	Burn unspecified	794
748	Respiratory syst anomaly	644	814	Carpal fracture	714
741	Spina bifida	640	851	Cerebral lac/contusion	745
753	Urinary system anomalies	646	995	Certain adverse eff NEC	823
			810	Clavicle fracture	706

CERTAIN CONDITIONS ORIGINATING IN THE PERINATAL PERIOD (760-779)

Code	Description	Page	Code	Description	Page
			999	Comp medical care NEC	846
			850	Concussion	743
767	Birth trauma	653	921	Contusion eye & adnexa	781
762	Comp plac/cord aff NB	651	920	Contusion head X eye	781
772	Fetal/neonatal hemor	656	924	Contusion leg & oth site	783
776	Hematological dis of NB	659	922	Contusion of trunk	782
778	Integument/temp cond NB	660	923	Contusion of upper limb	783
768	Intrauterine asphyxia	653	925	Crush inj face/scalp/nk	785
766	Long gestation/high BWT	652	928	Crush injury lower limb	786
760	MTL cond aff fetus/NB	650	926	Crush injury trunk	785
761	Maternal comp aff NB	650	927	Crush injury upper limb	786
775	NB endocr/metabol dis	658	839	Dislocation NEC	737
773	NB hemoly dis-isoimmun	656	837	Dislocation of ankle	736
770	Oth NB respiratory cond	654	834	Dislocation of finger	735
763	Oth comp del aff NB	651	838	Dislocation of foot	736
779	Oth perinatal condition	660	835	Dislocation of hip	735
774	Other perinatal jaundice	657	836	Dislocation of knee	735
777	Perinatal GI system dis	659	958	Early comp of trauma	797
771	Perinatal infection	655	991	Eff reduced temperature	820
769	Resp distress syndrome	653	994	Effect ext cause NEC	822
765	Short gestation/low BWT	652	992	Effect of heat/light	821
764	Slow fetal growth/malnut	651	993	Effects of air pressure	822
			990	Effects radiation NOS	820

SYMPTOMS, SIGNS, AND ILL-DEFINED CONDITIONS (780-799)

Code	Description	Page	Code	Description	Page
			841	Elbow & forearm sprain	738
			832	Elbow dislocation	734
			871	Eyeball open wound	759
795	Abn cytolog/hist/DNA	687	939	FB in GU tract	791
793	Abn find-body struct NOS	686	937	FB in anus & rectum	790
792	Abn find-oth body subst	686	938	FB in digestive syst NOS	790
790	Abnormal blood findings	685	931	FB in ear	787
794	Abnormal function study	687	930	FB in eye	787
791	Abnormal urine findings	686	936	FB in intestine & colon	790
785	Cardiovascular syst Sx	672	935	FB in mouth/esoph/stom	789
787	GI system symptoms	677	932	FB in nose	787
780	General symptoms	661	933	FB in pharynx & larynx	788
781	Nervous/MS syst symptoms	665	934	FB in trach/bronch/lung	788
783	Nutrit/metabol/devel Sx	669	829	Fracture NOS	733

Diagnosis Codes

Code	Description	Page	Code	Description	Page
818	Fracture arm mult/NOS	716	979	Pois-oth vacc/biological	816
820	Fracture neck of femur	717	969	Pois-psychotropic agent	809
802	Fracture of face bones	693	976	Pois-skin/EENT agent	814
809	Fracture of trunk bones	705	974	Pois-water metab agent	813
826	Fracture phalanges foot	731	972	Poison-CV agent	812
816	Fracture phalanges hand	715	961	Poison-anti-infect NEC	800
819	Fx arms w rib/sternum	717	966	Poison-anticonvulsants	805
828	Fx legs w arm/rib	732	971	Poison-autonomic agent	811
825	Fx of tarsal/metatarsal	730	977	Poison-medicinal NEC&NOS	814
807	Fx rib/stern/lar/trach	700	967	Poison-sedative/hypnotic	806
863	GI tract injury	754	960	Poisoning by antibiotics	800
900	Head/neck vessel injury	774	962	Poisoning by hormones	800
861	Heart & lung injury	753	968	Poisoning-CNS depressant	808
843	Hip & thigh sprain	739	970	Poisoning-CNS stimulants	811
812	Humerus fracture	707	973	Poisoning-GI agents	813
955	Inj PNS shoulder/arm	796	978	Poisoning-bact vaccines	815
953	Inj nerve root/sp plexus	796	975	Poisoning-muscle agent	813
950	Inj optic nerv/pathways	795	963	Poisoning-systemic agent	801
956	Inj periph nerv pelv/leg	797	813	Radius & ulna fracture	710
959	Injury NEC & NOS	798	996	Replacement & graft comp	824
951	Injury oth cranial nerve	795	846	Sacroiliac region sprain	741
954	Injury oth trunk nerve	796	811	Scapula fracture	707
957	Injury to nerve NEC&NOS	797	840	Shoulder & arm sprain	737
869	Internal injury NOS	759	831	Shoulder dislocation	733
862	Intrathoracic injury NEC	754	801	Skull base fracture	691
830	Jaw dislocation	733	800	Skull vault fracture	690
866	Kidney injury	757	952	Spinal cord inj w/o fx	795
844	Knee & leg sprain	739	865	Spleen injury	755
908	Late eff injury NEC&NOS	777	848	Sprain & strain NEC	743
907	Late eff nerv system inj	777	914	Superf inj hand X finger	779
909	Late eff other ext cause	777	919	Superf injury NEC	781
906	Late eff skin/subcu inj	776	918	Superf injury eye/adnexa	780
905	Late effect MS injury	776	915	Superf injury finger	779
864	Liver injury	755	917	Superf injury foot/toe	780
827	Lower limb fracture NEC	732	913	Superf injury forearm	779
815	Metacarpal fracture	715	916	Superf injury hip/leg	780
929	Mult crush injury & NOS	786	912	Superf injury shldr/UA	778
804	Mult fx skull w oth bone	697	910	Superficial injury head	778
884	Mult/NOS open wound arm	768	911	Superficial injury trunk	778
817	Multiple hand fractures	716	997	Surg comp-body syst NEC	838
870	Ocular adnexa open wound	759	901	Thor blood vessel injury	775
891	Open WND knee/leg/ankle	771	823	Tibia & fibula fracture	724
878	Open wound genital organ	764	986	Tox eff carbon monoxide	818
876	Open wound of back	763	989	Tox eff nonmed substance	819
877	Open wound of buttock	763	987	Toxic eff gas/vapor NEC	819
875	Open wound of chest	762	984	Toxic eff lead/compound	818
872	Open wound of ear	760	988	Toxic eff noxious food	819
883	Open wound of finger	767	981	Toxic eff petroleum prod	817
892	Open wound of foot	772	983	Toxic effect caustics	817
882	Open wound of hand	766	985	Toxic effect oth metals	818
890	Open wound of hip/thigh	770	982	Toxic effect solvent NEC	817
894	Open wound of leg NEC	773	886	Traum amputation finger	769
881	Open wound of lower arm	765	885	Traum amputation thumb	769
874	Open wound of neck	762	860	Traum pneumohemothorax	751
893	Open wound of toe	773	852	Traumatic SAH/SDH/EXDH	747
879	Open wound site NEC	764	887	Traumatic amp arm/hand	770
880	Opn WND should/upper arm	765	896	Traumatic amp foot	774
868	Oth intra-abd injury	758	895	Traumatic amputation toe	773
998	Oth surgical comp NEC	842	897	Traumatic leg amputation	774
854	Other IC injury	751	805	Vert fx w/o cord inj	697
821	Other femoral fracture	720	806	Vertebral fx w cord inj	700
873	Other open wound of head	760	842	Wrist & hand sprain	738
803	Other skull fracture	696	833	Wrist dislocation	734
853	Other traumatic ICH	750			
822	Patella fracture	723			
808	Pelvic fracture	704			
867	Pelvic organ injury	758			
964	Pois-agent aff blood	802			
965	Pois-analgesic/antipyr	802			

SUPPLEMENTARY CLASSIFICATION OF FACTORS INFLUENCING HEALTH STATUS (V01-V83)

Code	Description	Page
V53	Adjustment of oth device	867
V68	Administrative encounter	878
V51	Aftercare w plastic surg	867

Diagnosis Codes